STROKE

STROKE
Pathophysiology, Diagnosis, and Management

Third Edition

HENRY J. M. BARNETT, OC, MD, FRCP(C)
Professor Emeritus, Department of Clinical Neurological Sciences
University of Western Ontario
London, Ontario, Canada

J. P. MOHR, MD
Sciarra Professor, Department of Neurology
Columbia University College of Physicians and Surgeons
Director, Division of Cerebrovascular Research
Department of Neurology
Neurological Institute
Columbia-Presbyterian Medical Center
New York, New York

BENNETT M. STEIN, MD
Professor Emeritus, Department of Neurological Surgery
Columbia University College of Physicians and Surgeons
New York, New York

FRANK M. YATSU, MD
Professor and Emeritus Chairman, Department of Neurology
The University of Texas
Health Science Center at Houston
Houston, Texas

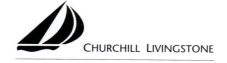

CHURCHILL LIVINGSTONE

A Harcourt Health Sciences Company
New York, Edinburgh, London, Philadelphia

CHURCHILL LIVINGSTONE

A *Harcourt Health Sciences Company*

The Curtis Center
Independence Square West
Philadelphia, Pennsylvania 19106

Library of Congress Cataloging-in-Publication Data

Stroke : pathophysiology, diagnosis, and management / [edited by]
Henry J.M. Barnett . . . [et al.]. — 3rd ed.

    p.   cm.

Includes bibliographical references and index.

ISBN 0–443–07551–4

1. Cerebrovascular disease.   I. Barnett, H. J. M. (Henry J. M.)
[DNLM: 1. Cerebrovascular Disorders.   WL 355 S92134 1998]

RC388.5.S8528   1998   616.8′1—dc21

DNLM/DLC   98–3396

Stroke: Pathophysiology, Diagnosis, and Management   ISBN 0–443–07551–4

Last digit is the print number: 9   8   7   6   5   4

To our wives
Kathleen B, Joan M, Bonita S, and Mich Y
whose forbearance is herewith
acknowledged with gratitude.

Preface to the First Edition

Over the past decade, there has been a rapid explosion of the advancing diagnostic and research technologies on stroke and a burgeoning interest in interventional therapies which have reduced the occurrence and severity of stroke. As we elbow our way past failed treatments and abandon therapeutic nihilism, we in the field are optimistic that the unfolding investigations on stroke pathophysiology and treatment will result in a better outlook for various stroke syndromes.

These exciting advances in treatment and the absence of an encyclopedic work on the subject convinced the editors to put together a comprehensive work on stroke. *Stroke: Pathophysiology, Diagnosis, and Management* is broad in scope and detailed in presentation and is intended to address the needs of the internist, surgeon, neurological practitioner, and students of these disciplines. The book provides current information on stroke pathophysiology, diagnosis, and therapy in a single reference. The reader is not spared technical details but is introduced to these details in understandable terms presented in a readable style. Each of the five major sections—pathophysiology, diagnosis, clinical manifestations, medical therapy, and surgical therapy—is self-contained, although a certain degree of arbitrary separation of topics has been necessary to minimize redundancy.

We have organized the book to provide practical and ready access to the conventional approaches to stroke syndromes but have also examined viable future options in stroke therapy and prevention. More importantly, we hope we have conveyed a sense of the excitement of stroke research, the enthusiasm for which is fueled by the certain knowledge that stroke occurrences can be further curtailed to an irreducible minimum.

HENRY J. M. BARNETT, MD
J. P. MOHR, MD
BENNETT M. STEIN, MD
FRANK M. YATSU, MD

Preface to the Third Edition

Twelve years have elapsed since the writing of the first edition of this book. In the field of stroke, very important changes have occurred in this short period. The components of this revolution involve a number of exciting developments. Our understanding of the biochemical and cellular changes in ischemia has leaped ahead. Our improved ability to image the arteries and to visualize the brain—both anatomically and, most recently, biochemically—has been nothing short of dramatic. Epidemiologists, biostatisticians, methodologists, pharmacologists, biochemists, hematologists, and clinical neurological and surgical scientists have joined forces to devise and evaluate preventive therapy and now, most recently, postischemic treatments.

In developed, as well as developing, countries, academic institutions and many hospitals have been aggressively seeking new staff sophisticated about stroke. This departure from the immediate past is reflective of the fact that treatment, prevention, and the attraction of basic research in this field have matured to the point where the demand for scientists and practitioners with stroke expertise exceeds the supply. More news of progress over a wide range of activity will be coming, extending all the way from genetic studies to the evaluation of endovascular therapy.

It is the hope of the editors that this comprehensive third edition of the book covering all aspects of stroke will help those in the academic and the practicing communities to keep abreast of a rapidly evolving and stimulating branch of neuroscience. Readers will note new sections and will be introduced to additions to our list of authors. In keeping with our traditional approach, we have invited the participation of experts from a number of countries. It is very satisfying to take note of the international enthusiasm that exists to tackle the thorny problems presented by the most common disorders that affect the brain.

HENRY J. M. BARNETT, MD
J. P. MOHR, MD
BENNETT M. STEIN, MD
FRANK M. YATSU, MD

Contributors

Harold P. Adams, Jr., MD
Professor of Neurology
Director of the Division of
    Cerebrovascular Diseases
Department of Neurology
University of Iowa College of Medicine
Attending Neurologist and Director,
    Acute Stroke Care and Monitoring Unit
University of Iowa Hospitals and Clinics
Consultant Neurologist, Iowa City
    Veterans Affairs Hospital
Iowa City, Iowa
    *Medical Management of Aneurysmal
        Subarachnoid Hemorrhage*

Pierre Amarenco, MD
Professor of Neurology
Pierre and Marie Curie University
Department of Neurology
Hôpital Lariboisière
Paris, France
    *Vertebrobasilar Occlusive Disease
    Atherosclerotic Disease of the Aortic Arch*

Robert W. Barnes, MD
Professor and Chair, Department of
    Surgery
Department of Surgery
University of Arkansas for Medical
    Sciences
Attending Surgeon, Surgical Service
University Hospital of Arkansas and Little
    Rock Veterans Affairs Medical Center
Little Rock, Arkansas
    *Atherosclerotic Disease of the Carotid
        Arteries: Surgical Considerations in
        Asymptomatic Disease*

Henry J. M. Barnett, OC, MD, FRCP(C)
Professor Emeritus, Division of Neurology
Department of Clinical Neurological
    Sciences
University of Western Ontario
London, Ontario, Canada
    *Cerebral Venous Thrombosis
    Spinal Cord Ischemia
    Antithrombotic Therapy in Diseases of the
        Cerebral Vasculature
    Cardiogenic Brain Embolism: Incidence,
        Varieties, and Treatment
    Atherosclerotic Disease of the Carotid
        Arteries: Overview: A Medical Perspective*

Jean-Claude Baron, MD
Director, Institut National de la Santé et
    de la Recherche Médicale
Consultant, Department of Neurology
University Hospital "Côte de Nâcre"
Caen, France
    Positron Emission Tomography

Oscar Benavente, MD, FRCP(C)
Assistant Professor, Division of Neurology,
    Department of Medicine
University of Texas Medical School at San
    Antonio
University of Texas Health Science Center
San Antonio, Texas
    Spinal Cord Ischemia

Serge Blecic, MD
Associate Professor in Neurology
Department of Neurology
Free University of Brussels
Department of Neurology
Erasme Hospital
Brussels, Belgium
    Stroke in Young Adults

Julien Bogousslavsky, MD
Professor and Chairman, Department of
    Neurology
Professor of Cerebrovascular Disease
University of Lausanne
Chief, Service de Neurologie
Centre Hospitalier Universitaire Vaudois
Lausanne, Switzerland
    Stroke in Young Adults

Marie-Germaine Bousser, MD
Professor of Neurology
Paris VII Lariboisiere University
Head, Neurology Department
Hôpital Lariboisière
Paris, France
    *Cerebral Venous Thrombosis
    CADASIL (Cerebral Autosomal Dominant
        Arteriopathy with Subcortical Infarcts and
        Leukoencephalopathy)*

Thomas G. Brott, MD
Professor of Neurology
University of Cincinnati, College of
    Medicine
Cincinnati, Ohio
    *Thrombolytic and Defibrinogenating Agents
        for Ischemic and Hemorrhagic Stroke*

John C. M. Brust, MD
Department of Neurology
College of Physicians and Surgeons of
    Columbia University
Harlem Hospital Center
New York, New York
    Anterior Cerebral Artery Disease
    Stroke and Substance Abuse

Louis R. Caplan, MD
Professor and Chair, Department of
    Neurology
Professor of Medicine
Tufts University School of Medicine
Neurologist, New England Medical
    Center
Boston, Massachusetts
    Vertebrobasilar Occlusive Disease
    Intracerebral Hemorrhage

H. Chabriat, MD
Department of Neurology
University of Paris
Consultant, Service de Neurologie
Hôpital Lariboisière
Paris, France
    CADASIL (Cerebral Autosomal Dominant
    Arteriopathy with Subcortical Infarcts and
    Leukoencephalopathy)

David Chiu, MD
Cerebrovascular Disease Fellow
University of Texas Medical
    Center–Houston
University of Texas Health Sciences
    Center
Houston, Texas
    Pharmacologic Modification of Acute
    Cerebral Ischemia

Tanvir F. Choudhri, MD
Instructor, Department of Neurosurgery
Columbia University College of Physicians
    and Surgeons
Post Doctoral Residency Fellow in
    Neurosurgery
Columbia-Presbyterian Medical Center
New York, New York
    Management of Spinal Vascular
    Malformations

G. Patrick Clagett, MD
Professor and Chairman, Division of
    Vascular Surgery
Department of Surgery
University of Texas Southwestern Medical
    Center
Dallas, Texas
    Atherosclerotic Disease of the Carotid
    Arteries: Surgical Considerations in
    Symptomatic Disease

Ariel Cohen, MD
Professor of Cardiology
Department of Cardiology
Pierre and Marie Curie University
Department of Cardiology
Hopital Saint-Antoine
Paris, France
    Atherosclerotic Disease of the Aortic Arch

Bruce M. Coull, MD
Professor and Head, Department of
    Neurology
Arizona Health Sciences Center
University of Arizona
Tucson, Arizona
    Coagulation Abnormalities in Stroke

Robert M. Crowell, MD
Berkshire Associates
Pittsfield, Massachusetts
    Intercerebral Hemorrhage: Surgical
    Considerations

Mark A. Crowther, MD, FRCPC
Hamilton Civic Hospitals Research Centre
McMaster University
Henderson General Hospital
Hamilton, Ontario, Canada
    Principles of Hemostasis and Antithrombotic
    Therapy

Ralph B. D'Agostino, PhD
Professor of Mathematics/
    Statistics and Public Health
Department of Mathematics
Boston University College of Arts and
    Sciences
Boston, Massachusetts
    Epidemiology of Stroke

Stephen M. Davis, MD, FRACP
Associate Professor, Department of
    Neurology
University of Melbourne
Director of Neurology, Department of
    Neurology
Melbourne Neuroscience Centre
Royal Melbourne Hospital
Parkville, Victoria, Australia
    Single-Photon Emission Computed
    Tomography

Thomas J. DeGraba, MD
National Institute of NDS
Bethesda, Maryland
    Medical Complications of Stroke

R. L. DeLaPaz, MD
Professor of Radiology
Columbia University
College of Physicians and Surgeons
Director of Neuroradiology
Columbia-Presbyterian Medical Center
New York, New York
  Magnetic Resonance Scanning

Thomas G. DeLoughery, MD
Assistant Professor of Medicine and
  Pathology
Oregon Health Sciences University School
  of Medicine
Portland, Oregon
  Coagulation Abnormalities in Stroke

**Henry B. Dinsdale, MD, FRCPC, FACP,
FRSA, FRCP**
Professor of Medicine (Neurology)
  Emeritus, Queen's University
President, The National Council on
  Bioethics in Human Research
Immediate Past-President
The Royal College of Physicians and
  Surgeons of Canada
Kingston, Ontario, Canada
  Hypertensive Encephalopathy

Marco R. Di Tullio, MD
Assistant Professor of Clinical Medicine
Division of Cardiology, Department of
  Medicine
Associate Director, Echocardiography
  Laboratories
Columbia-Presbyterian Medical Center
New York, New York
  Patent Foramen Ovale and Ischemic Stroke

Geoffrey Donnan, MD
Department of Neurology
Austin Hospital
Heidelberg/Melbourne, Victoria, Australia
  Overview of Laboratory Studies

Gary Duckwiler, MD
Associate Professor, Radiological Sciences
University of California at Los Angeles
Los Angeles, California
  *Intracranial Aneurysms: Interventional
    Neuroradiological Management*

Hoang Duong, MD
Assistant Professor of Radiology
Columbia University
Interventional Neuroradiologist
Columbia-Presbyterian Medical Center
New York, New York
  Brachiocephalic Angioplasty

J. Donald Easton, MD
Professor and Chairman
Department of Clinical Neurosciences
Brown University School of Medicine
Chairman, Department of Medicine
Rhode Island Hospital
Providence, Rhode Island
  *Dissections and Trauma of Cervicocerebral
    Arteries*

Michael Eliasziw, PhD
Associate Professor, Department of
  Clinical Epidemiology and Biostatistics
University of Western Ontario
Scientist, The John P. Robarts Research
  Institute
London, Ontario, Canada
  *Antithrombotic Therapy in Diseases of the
    Cerebral Vasculature*
  *Atherosclerotic Disease of the Carotid
    Arteries: Overview: A Medical Perspective*

Frank M. Faraci, PhD
Associate Professor, Departments of
  Internal Medicine and Pharmacology
University of Iowa College of Medicine
Iowa City, Iowa
  Vascular Biology of Cerebral Arteries

William M. Feinberg, MD
Professor of Neurology, Arizona Health
  Sciences Center
University of Arizona
Tucson, Arizona
  Coagulation Abnormalities in Stroke

Robert Fern, MD
Department of Neurology
University of Washington School of
  Medicine
Seattle, Washington
  *Molecular Pathophysiology of White Matter
    Anoxic/Ischemic Injury*

Allan J. Fox, MD
Professor, Departments of Diagnostic
  Radiology and Clinical Neurological
  Sciences
University of Western Ontario
Director, Neuroradiology
Department of Radiology
London Health Sciences Centre
London, Ontario, Canada
  *Intracranial Aneurysms: Interventional
    Neuroradiological Management*

Peter T. Fox, MD
Professor and Director, Research Imaging
  Center
University of Texas Health Science Center
San Antonio, Texas
  Functional Magnetic Resonance Imaging

Juergen Froehlich, MD, MFPM
Senior Clinical Scientist, Department of
  Medical Affairs
Genentech, Inc.
South San Francisco, California
  *Basic Science of Fibrinolysis: Coronary and
  Cerebral Thrombolysis*

Anthony J. Furlan, MD
Assistant Clinical Professor, Department
  of Neurology
Case Western Reserve University
School of Medicine
Cleveland, Ohio
Assistant Clinical Professor, Department
  of Neurology
Pennsylvania State University College of
  Medicine
Hershey, Pennsylvania
Head, Section of Adult Neurology
Cleveland Clinic Foundation
Medical Director, Cerebral Vascular
  Center
Department of Neurology
Cleveland Clinic Foundation
Cleveland, Ohio
  *Cardiogenic Brain Embolism: Incidence,
  Varieties, and Treatment*

Jia-Hong Gao, PhD
Assistant Professor, Department of
  Radiology and Research Imaging
  Center
University of Texas Health Science Center
San Antonio, Texas
  Functional Magnetic Resonance Imaging

Julio H. Garcia, MD
Professor of Pathology
Case Western Reserve University
Cleveland, Ohio
Division Head, Department of
  Neuropathology
Henry Ford Hospital
Detroit, Michigan
  Pathology

J.C. Gautier, MD
Professor of Neurology, (Hon)
Faculté Pitié-Salpêtrière
Médecin (Hon) de la Salpêtrière
Membre de l'Académie Nationale de
  Médecin
Paris, France
  Internal Carotid Artery Disease
  Middle Cerebral Artery Disease

Jeffrey Ginsberg, MD, FRCP(C)
Associate Professor, Department of
  Medicine
McMaster University
Director, Thromboembolism Unit
McMaster University Medical Center
Hamilton, Ontario, Canada
  *Principles of Hemostasis and Antithrombotic
  Therapy*

Glen E. Gresham, MD
Professor and Chairman, Department of
  Rehabilitation Medicine
State University of New York at Buffalo
Attending Physician, Erie County Medical
  Center
Buffalo, New York
  Rehabilitation of the Stroke Survivor

Marina Grisoli, MD
Assistant Chief, Department of Diagnostic
  Neuroradiology
Istituto Nazionale Neurologico "Carlo
  Besta"
Milan, Italy
  Computed Tomography Scanning

James C. Grotta, MD
Professor of Neurology
Adjunct Professor of Radiology
University of Texas Medical School–
  Houston
Director of Stroke Program
Hermann Hospital and University of Texas
  Health Medical School–Houston
Houston, Texas
  *Pharmacologic Modification of Acute
  Cerebral Ischemia*

**Vladimir Hachinski, MD, FRCP(C), MSc
(DME), DSc (Med)**
Richard and Beryl Ivey Professor and
  Chair
The University of Western Ontario
Chief, Department of Clinical
  Neurological Sciences
London Health Sciences Centre
London, Ontario, Canada
  Multi-Infarct Dementia

Werner Hacke, MD, PhD
Professor and Chairman, Department of
  Neurology
University of Heidelberg
Heidelberg, Germany
  The Intensive Care of the Stroke Patient
  *Thrombolytic and Defibrinogenating Agents
  for Ischemic and Hemorrhagic Stroke*

Sandra Hanson, MD
Neurology Consultant, Department of
    Neuroscience
Parc Nicollet Clinic
St. Louis Park, Minnesota
    Medical Complications of Stroke

Edward B. Healton, MD
Associate Clinical Professor, Department
    of Neurology
Associate Dean, Columbia University
    College of Physicians and Surgeons
New York, New York
    Cerebrovascular Fibromuscular Dysplasia

Donald D. Heistad, MD
Professor, Departments of Internal
    Medicine and Pharmacology
Director, Cardiovascular Division
University of Iowa College of Medicine
Iowa City, Iowa
    Vascular Biology of Cerebral Arteries

Michael Hennerici, MD
Professor and Chairman, Department of
    Neurology
University of Heidelberg
Mannheim Medical School
Mannheim, Germany
    *Ultrasound Imaging and Doppler
        Sonography*

Daniel B. Hier, MD
Professor and Chairman, Department of
    Neurology
University of Illinois College of Medicine
Chicago, Illinois
    Middle Cerebral Artery Disease

Judith A. Hinchey, MD
Clinical Associate, Cerebrovascular Center
Department of Neurology
Cleveland Clinic Foundation
Cleveland, Ohio
    *Cardiogenic Brain Embolism: Incidence,
        Varieties, and Treatment*

Khang-Loon Ho, MD
Clinical Associate Professor, Pathology
Wayne State University
Senior Staff, Department of
    Neuropathology
Henry Ford Hospital
Detroit, Michigan
    Pathology

Shunichi Homma, MD
Associate Professor of Clinical Medicine
Division of Cardiology, Department of
    Medicine
Director, Echocardiography Laboratories
Columbia-Presbyterian Medical Center
New York, New York
    Patent Foramen Ovale and Ischemic Stroke

Jari Honkaniemi
Department of Neurology
University of California, San Francisco
    School of Medicine
Veterans Adminsitration Medical Center
San Francisco, California
University of Tampere
Tampere, Finland
    Neurochemistry and Molecular Biology

Bernard Infeld, MD
Postgraduate Medical Research Fellow in
    Cerebrovascular Disease
Department of Neurology
University of Melbourne
Neurology
Royal Melbourne Hospital
Parkville, Victoria, Australia
    *Single-Photon Emission Computed
        Tomography*

Steven R. Isaacson, MD, FACS
Associate Professor of Clinical Radiation
    Oncology and Clinical Otolaryngology
College of Physicians and Surgeons of
    Columbia University
Associate Attending, Radiation Oncology
    Service
Columbia-Presbyterian Medical Center
New York, New York
    *Vascular Malformations of the Brain and
        Dura*

A. Joutel, MD, PhD
Institut National de la Santé et de la
    Recherche Médicale
Faculte de Médecine Necker Enfants-
    Malades
Paris, France
    *CADASIL (Cerebral Autosomal Dominant
        Arteriopathy with Subcortical Infarcts and
        Leukoencephalopathy)*

Carlos S. Kase, MD
Professor, Department of Neurology
Boston University School of Medicine
Associate Neurologist, Neurology
Boston Medical Center
Boston, Massachusetts
    *Intracerebral Hemorrhage
    Intracerebral Hemorrhage: Medical
        Considerations*

Bruce A. Keyt, PhD
Senior Scientist, Department of
  Pharmacokinetics and Metabolism
Genentech, Inc.
South San Francisco, California
  *Basic Science of Fibrinolysis: Coronary and
    Cerebral Thrombolysis*

J. Philip Kistler, MD
Professor of Neurology
Department of Neurology
Harvard Medical School
Director, Stroke Service
Massachusetts General Hospital
Boston, Massachusetts
  Intracranial Aneurysms

Kyuya Kogure, MD
Professor of Neurology
Institute of Neuropathology
Kumagay-shi
Saitama, Japan
  Neurochemistry and Molecular Biology

Derk Krieger, MD
Assistant Professor of Neurology
University of Texas
Houston, Texas
  The Intensive Care of the Stroke Patient

R. M. Lazar, MD
Associate Professor of Clinical
  Neuropsychology
Department of Neurology
Columbia University College of Physicians
  and Surgeons
Neurological Institute
Columbia-Presbyterian Medical Center
New York, New York
  Middle Cerebral Artery Disease

Donald H. Lee, MB, BCh
Associate Professor, Departments of
  Diagnostic Radiology and Clinical
  Neurological Sciences
University of Western Ontario
Staff Neuroradiologist, Department of
  Radiology
London Health Sciences Centre
London, Ontario, Canada
  *Cerebral Angiography: Magnetic Resonance
    Angiography*

Betsy B. Love, MD
Assistant Professor, Department of
  Neurology
University of Iowa College of Medicine
Iowa City, Iowa
  *Medical Management of Aneurysmal
    Subarachnoid Hemorrhage*

Stephen P. Lownie, MD, FRCSC
Assistant Professor, Division of
  Neuroradiology and Neurosurgery
Departments of Diagnostic Radiology and
  Clinical Neurological Sciences
University of Western Ontario Faculty of
  Medicine
Consultant Neurosurgeon and
  Interventional Neuroradiologist,
  Departments of Clinical Neurological
  Sciences and Diagnostic Radiology
London Health Sciences Centre
London, Ontario, Canada
  *Cerebral Angiography: Conventional
    Angiography*

R. S. Marshall, MD
Assistant Professor of Neurology
Columbia University College of Physicians
  and Surgeons
Neurological Institute
Columbia-Presbyterian Medical Center
New York, New York
  Middle Cerebral Artery Disease

José-Luis Marti-Vilalta, MD
Fundacio de Gestio Sanitaria de l'Hospital
  de la Santa Creu i Sant Pau
Barcelona, Spain
  Lacunes

Pablo Martinez-Lage MD, PhD
Clinical Fellow, Department of Neurology
University of Western Ontario
London, Ontario, Canada
  Multi-Infarct Dementia

Stephen M. Massa, MD, PhD
Assistant Professor, Department of
  Neurology
University of California, San Francisco,
  School of Medicine
Assistant Professor, Neurology
Veterans Administration Medical Center
San Francisco, California
  Neurochemistry and Molecular Biology

H. Mast, MD
Abteilung fuer Neurologie und
  Krisenintervention
Universitaetsklinikum Benjamin Franklin
Freie Universitaet Berlin
Berlin, Germany
  Binswanger's Disease

Junichi Masuda, MD
Professor, Department of Laboratory
  Medicine
Shimane Medical University
Shimane, Japan
  Moyamoya Disease

Paul C. McCormick, MD
Associate Professor of Neurosurgery
Columbia University College of Physicians
   and Surgeons
Associate Attending Neurosurgeon
Columbia-Presbyterian Medical Center
New York, New York
   Management of Spinal Vascular
     Malformations

Stephen Meairs, MD
Assistant Professor, Department of
   Neurology
University of Heidelberg
Mannheim Medical School
Mannheim, Germany
   Ultrasound Imaging and Doppler
     Sonography

Heather E. Meldrum, BA
The John P. Robarts Research Institute
London, Ontario, Canada
   Antithrombotic Therapy in Diseases of the
     Cerebral Vasculature
   Atherosclerotic Disease of the Carotid
     Arteries: Overview: A Medical Perspective

J. P. Mohr, MD
Sciarra Professor, Department of
   Neurology
Columbia University College of Physicians
   and Surgeons
Director, Division of Cerebrovascular
   Research
Department of Neurology
Neurological Institute
Columbia-Presbyterian Medical Center
New York, New York
   Overview of Laboratory Studies
   Magnetic Resonance Scanning
   Ultrasound Imaging and Doppler
     Sonography
   Classification of Ischemic Stroke
   Internal Carotid Artery Disease
   Middle Cerebral Artery Disease
   Posterior Cerebral Artery Disease
   Choroidal Artery Disease
   Lacunes
   Intracerebral Hemorrhage
   Intracranial Aneurysms
   Arteriovenous Malformations and Other
     Vascular Anomalies
   Stroke in the Setting of Collagen Vascular
     Disease
   Cerebrovascular Fibromuscular Dysplasia
   Migraine and Stroke
   Hypertensive Encephalopathy
   Binswanger's Disease

J. W. Norris, MD, FRCP
Professor, Department of Neurology
University of Toronto
Director, Stroke Research Unit
Sunnybrook Health Science Centre
Toronto, Ontario, Canada
   Atherosclerotic Disease of the Carotid
     Arteries: Medical Considerations

Jun Ogata, MD
Director, Department of Preventive
   Medicine
National Cardiovascular Center
Osaka, Japan
   Moyamoya Disease

Christopher S. Ogilvy, MD
Assistant Professor, Department of
   Surgery
Harvard Medical School
Boston, Massachusetts
   Intercerebral Hemorrhage: Surgical
     Considerations

Robert G. Ojemann, MD
Massachusetts General Hospital
Boston, Massachusetts
   Intercerebral Hemorrhage: Surgical
     Considerations

Leonardo Pantoni, MD
Research Associate, Neurological and
   Psychiatric Sciences
University of Florence
Fellow, Neurological and Psychiatric
   Sciences
University of Florence
Florence, Italy
   Pathology

Michael S. Pessin, MD (deceased)
Professor, Department of Neurology
Tufts University School of Medicine
Senior Neurologist, New England Medical
   Center Hospitals
Boston, Massachusetts
   Internal Carotid Artery Disease
   Posterior Cerebral Artery Disease
   Vertebrobasilar Occlusive Disease

George W. Petty, MD
Associate Professor, Department of
   Neurology
Mayo Medical School
Consultant, Department of Neurology
Mayo Clinic and Mayo Foundation
Rochester, Minnesota
   Stroke in the Setting of Collagen Vascular
     Disease

John Pile-Spellman, MD
Associate Professor of Radiology and
    Neurosurgery
Columbia University College of Physicians
    and Surgeons
Director of Interventional Neuroradiology
Columbia-Presbyterian Medical Center
New York, New York
    *Arteriovenous Malformations and Other
        Vascular Anomalies*
    Brachiocephalic Angioplasty
    *Vascular Malformations of the Brain and
        Dura*

Bruce R. Ransom, MD, PhD
Department of Neurology
University of Washington School of
    Medicine
Seattle, Washington
    Molecular Pathophysiology of White Matter

James T. Robertson, MD
Professor, Department of Neurosurgery
Consultant
University of Tennessee, Memphis
    School of Medicine
Memphis, Tennessee
    *Atherosclerotic Disease of the Carotid
        Arteries: Surgical Considerations in
        Symptomatic Disease*
    *Athersclerotic Disease of the Carotid
        Arteries: Surgical Considerations in
        Asymptomatic Disease*

Ralph L. Sacco, MS, MD
Associate Professor of Neurology and
    Public Health (Epidemiology) in the
    Sergievsky Center
Director
Northern Manhattan Stroke Study
Columbia University College of Physicians
    and Surgeons
Associate Attending, Presbyterian Hospital
    of the City of New York
New York, New York
    Classification of Ischemic Stroke
    Patent Foramen Ovale and Ischemic Stroke

Jeffrey L. Saver, MD
Assistant Professor of Clinical Neurology
University of California, Los Angeles
Neurology Director, UCLA Stroke Center
Los Angeles, California
    *Dissections and Trauma of Cervicocerebral
        Arteries*

Mario Savoiardo, MD
Chief, Department of Diagnostic
    Neuroradiology
Istituto Nazionale Neurologico "Carlo
    Besta"
Milan, Italy
    Computed Tomography Scanning

Frank R. Sharp, MD
Professor, Department of Neurology
University of California, San Francisco
    School of Medicine
Professor, Neurology
Veterans Administration Medical Center
San Francisco, California
    Neurochemistry and Molecular Biology

Christopher G. Sobey, PhD
NHMRC C. J. Martin Fellow
Department of Pharmacology
The University of Melbourne
Parkville, Victoria, Australia
    Vascular Biology of Cerebral Arteries

Robert F. Spetzler, MD
Director, Barrow Neurological Institute
J. N. Harber Chairman of Neurological
    Surgery
Professor, Section of Neurosurgery
University of Arizona
Phoenix, Arizona
    *Intracranial Aneurysms: Surgical
        Management*

William B. Stason, MD
Department of Health Policy and
    Management
Harvard School of Public Health
Boston, Massachusetts
    Rehabilitation of the Stroke Survivor

Bennett M. Stein, MD
Professor Emeritus, Department of
    Neurological Surgery
Columbia University College of Physicians
    and Surgeons
New York, New York
    *Arteriovenous Malformations and Other
        Vascular Anomalies*
    Vascular Malformations of the Brain and Dura
    Management of Spinal Vascular Malformations

Wolfgang Steinke, MD
Associate Clinical Professor
Chief, Department of Neurology
Marienhospital
Düsseldorf, Germany
    *Ultrasound Imaging and Doppler
        Sonography*

Raymond A. Swanson, MD
Associate Professor of Neurology
Department of Neurology
University of California, San Francisco
    School of Medicine
Associate Professor, Neurology
Veterans Administration Medical Center
San Francisco, California
    Neurochemistry and Molecular Biology

T. K. Tatemichi, MD (deceased)
Associate Professor, Department of
    Neurology
Columbia University College of Physicians
    and Surgeons
Neurological Institute
Columbia-Presbyterian Medical Center
New York, New York
    Migraine and Stroke

Philip A. Teal, MD, FRCP(C)
Assistant Professor of Neurology
University of British Columbia
Director, Stroke Prevention Clinic
Vancouver General Hospital
Vancouver, British Columbia, Canada
    *Atherosclerotic Disease of the Carotid
        Arteries: Medical Considerations*

G. Roger Thomas, PhD
Senior Scientist, Department of
    Cardiovascular Research
Genentech, Inc.
South San Francisco, California
    *Basic Science of Fibrinolysis: Coronary and
        Cerebral Thrombolysis*

Serge Timsit, MD
Assistant Neurologist, Department of
    Neurology
Pitié-Salpêtrière
Paris, France
    Choroidal Artery Disease

Danilo Toni, MD
Universitá degli Studi di Roma
    'la Sapienza'
Rome, Italy
    Classification of Ischemic Stroke

E. Tournier-Lasserve, MD
Director of Research
Faculte de Medecine Necker Enfants-
    Malades
Institut National de la Santé et de la
    Recherche Médicale
Paris, France
    *CADASIL (Cerebral Autosomal Dominant
        Arteriopathy with Subcortical Infarcts and
        Leukoencephalopathy)*

K. Vahedi, MD
Department of Neurology
University of Paris
Clinical Assistant, Service de Neurologie
Hôpital Lariboisière
Paris, France
    *CADASIL (Cerebral Autosomal Dominant
        Arteriopathy with Subcortical Infarcts and
        Leukoencephalopathy)*

Carlos Villar-Cordova, MD
Instructor, Department of Neurology
University of Texas Medical School at
    Houston
Houston, Texas
    Atherosclerosis
    Medical Complications of Stroke

Harry V. Vinters, MD, FRCP(C)
Professor of Pathology and Laboratory
    Medicine
Chief, Division of Neuropathology
University of California, Los Angeles
    Medical Center
Los Angeles, California
    Cerebral Amyloid Angiopathy

Fernando Viñuela, MD
Professor, Department of Radiology
University of California, Los Angeles
    School of Medicine
Director, Division of Interventional
    Neuroradiology
Neurovascular Clinic
Los Angeles, California
    *Intracranial Aneurysms: Interventional
        Neuroradiological Management*

Stephen G. Waxman, MD, PhD
Professor and Chairman, Department of
    Neurology
Director, PVA/EPVA Neuroscience and
    Regeneration Research Center
Yale University School of Medicine
New Haven, Connecticut
    *Molecular Pathology of White Matter
        Anoxic/Ischemic Injury*

Babette B. Weksler, MD
Professor of Medicine
Cornell University Medical Center
Attending Physician, Department of
    Medicine
The New York Hospital
New York, New York
    Platelet Function and Antiplatelet Agents

K. M. A. Welch, MD
William T. Gossett Chair, Department of
    Neurology
Henry Ford Hospital
Detroit, Michigan
    Migraine and Stroke

Christine A. C. Wijman, MD
Teaching Fellow of Neurology
Department of Neurology
Boston University School of Medicine
Boston, Massachusetts
*Intracerebral Hemorrhage: Medical
Considerations*

Philip A. Wolf, MD
Professor, Department of Neurology
Research Professor, Department of
Medicine
Neurological Epidemiology and Genetics
Boston University School of Medicine
Senior Visiting Physician in Neurology
Section of Preventive Medicine and
Epidemiology
Department of Clinical Research
Boston Medical Center
Boston, Massachusetts
Epidemiology of Stroke

Takenori Yamaguchi, MD
Cerebrovascular Division
Department of Internal Medicine
Director General of the Hospital
National Cardiovascular Center
Osaka, Japan
Moyamoya Disease

Frank M. Yatsu, MD
Professor and Emeritus Chairman,
Department of Neurology
The University of Texas Health Science
Center at Houston
Houston, Texas
*Atherosclerosis
Medical Complications of Stroke*

Joseph M. Zabramski, MD
Chief, Section of Cerebrovascular Surgery
Barrow Neurology Institute
Mercy Healthcare Arizona
Phoenix, Arizona
*Intracranial Aneurysms: Surgical
Management*

Jianhui Zhong, PhD
Associate Professor, Department of
Diagnostic Radiology
Yale University School of Medicine
New Haven, Connecticut
Functional Magnetic Resonance Imaging

Contents

Color Plates

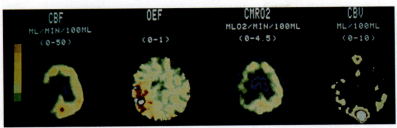

Plate 6.1

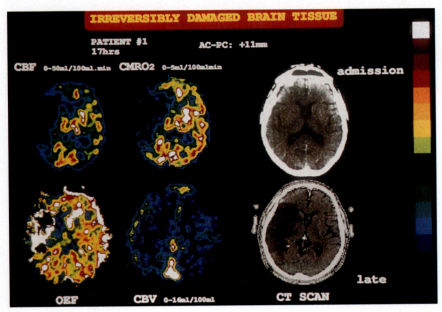

Plate 6.2

Plate 6.1 Quantitative positron emission tomographic (PET) images showing the cerebral blood flow (CBF), oxygen extraction fraction (OEF), cerebral metabolic rate of oxygen (CMRO₂), and cerebral blood volume (CBV) according to a pseudocolor scale ranging from 0 to a maximum pixel vlaue of 50 ml/100 ml/min; unity, 4.5 ml/100 ml/min and 10 ml/100 ml, respectively. The data were obtained using the [15]O continuous inhalation technique at a level 60 mm above and parallel to the orbitomeatal line in a 76-year-old patient 30 hours after the abrupt onset of right hemiparesis and global aphasia due to middle cerebral artery embolism from a cardiac source; at time of PET study, clinical recovery was rapid. On these images, the left side of the brain is to the reader's left, and anterior is at the top. There is a marked reduction of CBF in the left parietorolandic cortex (minimum value, 13 ml/100 ml/min) associated with a markedly increased OEF (maximum value, 1.90 ml/100 ml/min) and a marginally increased CBV. This pattern of critical cerebral ischemia (? ``penumbra'') corresponds to pattern 2 of Marchal et al.[78] In this case, it was still present 30 hours after the onset of stroke and was associated with an excellent clinical outcome and normal corresponding CT scan at follow-up, suggesting potentially viable tissue.

Plate 6.2 Quantitative positron emission tomographic (PET) images of cerebral blood flow (CBF), cerebral metabolic rate of oxygen (CMRO₂), oxygen extraction fraction (OEF), and cerebral blood volume (CBV), obtained at the level of the basal ganglia in a 77-year-old patient, 17 hours after onset of right-sided MCA territory stroke. On the right are shown CT scans of this patient obtained at admission (top) and about 1 month later (bottom, coregistered three-dimensionally with PET). There was near-zero CBF and CMRO₂ in the whole affected MCA territory together with patchy OEF (black pixels represent unmeasurable OEF), representing presumably irreversible damage. The patient made a poor recovery and the initially severely hypometabolic area was infarcted at follow-up CT scan (right). This example would correspond to pattern 1 of Marchal et al.[78]

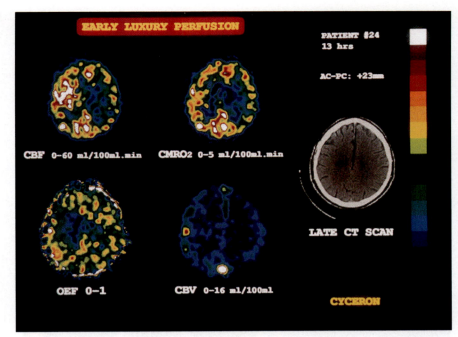

Plate 6.3

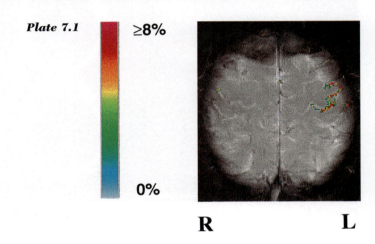

Plate 7.1

R   L

Plate 6.3 Quantitative positron emission tomographic (PET) images of cerebral blood flow (CBF), cerebral metabolic rate of oxygen (CMRO$_2$), oxygen extraction fraction (OEF), and cerebral blood volume (CBV) obtained at the level of the corona radiata in a 61-year-old patient 15 hours after onset of left hemiparesis presumably due to right middle cerebral artery embolism of cardiac origin. The images are shown according to a pseudocolor scale ranging from 0 to a maximum pixel value of 60 ml/100 ml/min; unity, 5 ml/100 ml/min; and 16 ml/100 ml for CBF, CMRO$_2$, OEF, and CBV, respectively; the right side of the brain is on the reader's left side. The data demonstrate an area of increased CBF in the right cortical mantle, associated with an increased CBV and a decreased OEF (luxury perfusion with absolute hyperemia, documenting early reperfusion of previously ischemic tissue). The CMRO$_2$ is preserved or even slightly increased in the hyperperfused regions, which were morphologically intact at follow-up CT scan (obtained at day 62 post stroke). This pattern of changes corresponds to pattern 3 of Marchal et al.[78]

Plate 7.1 Functional MR image of a healthy right-handed male volunteer during the finger-tapping task ($P<0.01$). For the activation state, the volunteer touched each of the fingertips of his right hand to the thumb consecutively. For the resting state, the volunteer was simply instructed to relax. The significantly activated area in motor cortex is superimposed in color onto the anatomic image. The color scale corresponds to the percentage of signal change in the finger-tapping task relative to the rest condition.

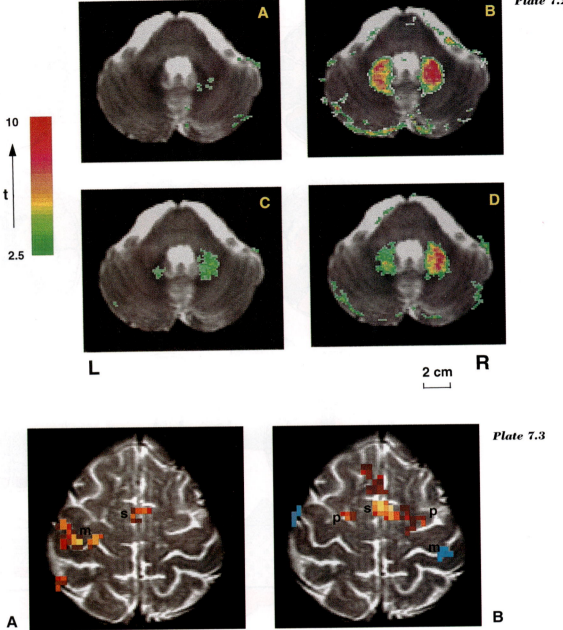

Plate 7.2

Plate 7.3

Plate 7.2 Functional MR images illustrate that the cerebellum is engaged in cognitive tasks. Functional activations (in color) are overlaid on anatomic MR images (in gray) for four behavioral tasks: **(A)** simple finger movement, **(B)** finger movement and sensory discrimination, **(C)** sensory acquisition, and **(D)** sensory discrimination. (A more detailed description can be found in ref. 43.)

Plate 7.3 Functional MRI of a 33-year-old right-handed woman who had a left internal carotid artery dissection and a sustained left striatocapsular infarct 10 days prior to the imaging study. **(A)** Left hand (normal). **(B)** right hand (affected by stroke). The patient had minimal awkwardness in fine movements with the right hand. The color represents pixels with significant t-values ($P<0.05$). (See text for detailed description.)

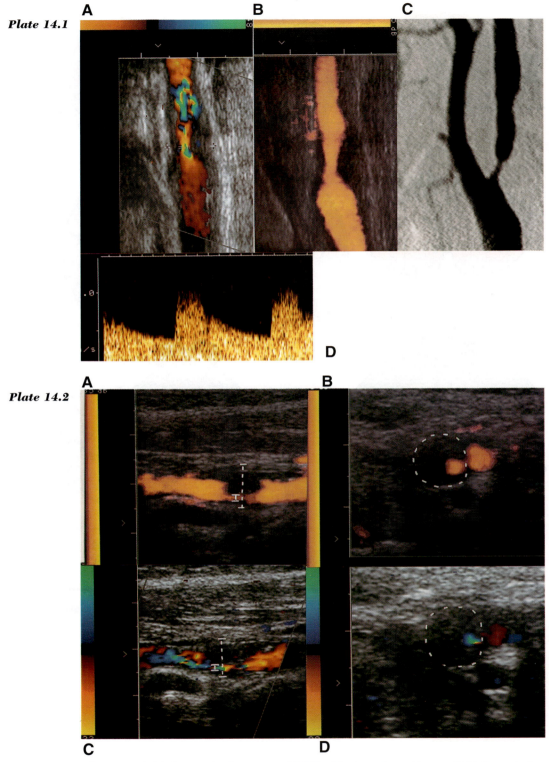

Plate 14.1 (**A**) Color Doppler flow imaging (CDFI) of the internal carotid artery (ICA) demonstrating decreased color saturation, some aliasing, and turbulent poststenotic flow, features characteristic of moderate stenosis. (**B**) Power Doppler imaging (PDI) shows excellent contrast of the plaque surface, extending distally beyond the stenotic area. (**C**) The corresponding angiogram correlates well with the plaque configuration documented with CDFI and PDI. (**D**) Maximum peak velocity of approximately 200 cm/s is consistent with a diagnosis of moderate stenosis of the ICA.

Plate 14.2 Measurement of high-grade stenosis of the internal carotid artery. Calculation of the residual lumen/vessel diameter ratio with either (**A**) power Doppler imaging or (**C**) color Doppler flow imaging results in a good approximation of the degree of stenosis. More accurate results are obtained with (**B** & **D**) residual lumen/cross-sectional area measurements.

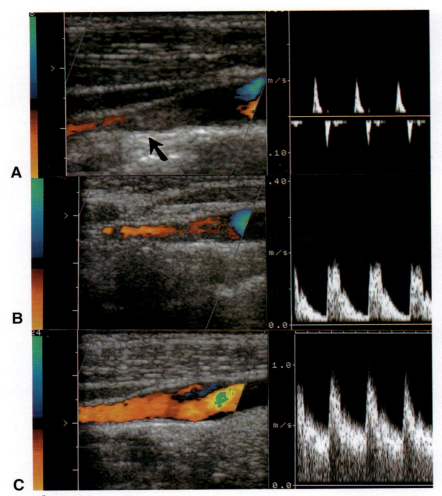

Plate 14.3 Diagnosis and follow-up of internal carotid artery dissection. **(A)** Color Doppler flow imaging (CDFI) depicts inhomogenous floating material attached to the internal carotid wall, presumably representing an intimal flap or thrombus. Slight residual flow is detected distal to the dissection. The corresponding Doppler spectrum on the right shows high-resistance signals with absent diastolic flow and low-flow bidirectional signal components. **(B)** Two weeks later CDFI demonstrates improved flow in the internal carotid artery. The Doppler spectrum shows low peak systolic velocity and reduced diastolic flow. **(C)** Follow-up with CDFI after 6 weeks shows good flow in the internal carotid artery with some residual turbulence. The Doppler spectrum has normalized.

Plate 14.4 **(A)** Subclavian steal with low flow and bidirectional signal components in the vertebral artery during inflation of a blood pressure cuff on the ipsilateral arm. **(B)** Release of the blood pressure cuff (arrow) results in reversed flow. **(C)** In another patient with subclavian steal the vertebral artery shows reversed flow during brachial artery compression, as indicated by the characteristic Doppler spectrum. **(D)** Release of the blood pressure cuff (arrow) results in increased reversed flow, thus verifying the subclavian steal phenomenon.

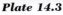

Plate 14.3

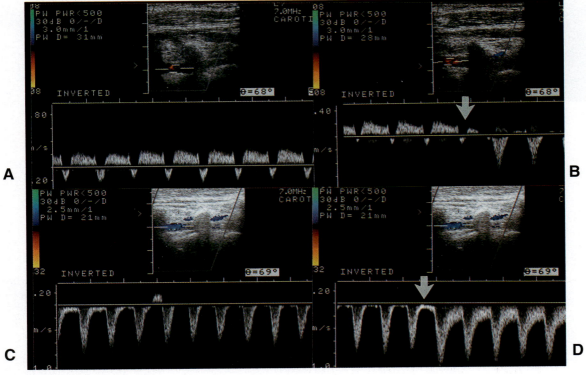

Plate 14.4

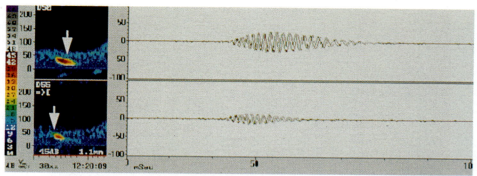

Plate 14.5

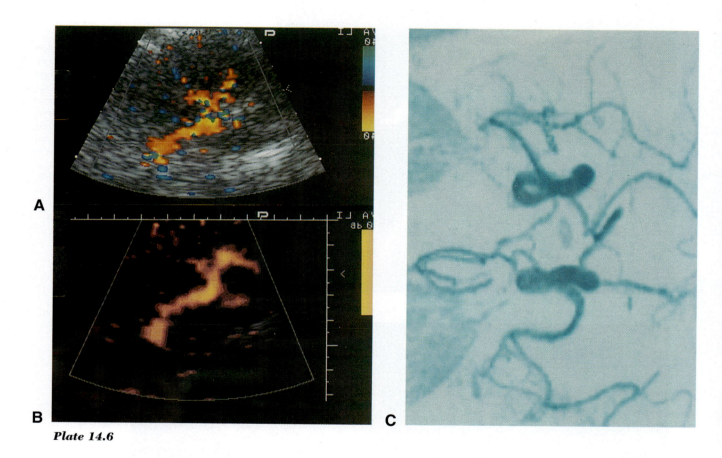

Plate 14.6

Plate 14.5 Detection of high-intensity transient signal (HITS) using a multigate technique. At the first gate (bottom), high-intensity signals of short duration appear in the Doppler spectrum as an oval area of increased color saturation (arrow). The corresponding FFT analysis of the Doppler spectrum identifies the HITS. At the second Doppler gate (top), HITS with a slight temporal delay are detected, thus excluding an artifact as the source of these HITS.

Plate 14.6 Demonstration of normal middle cerebral artery with (**A**) color Doppler flow imaging, (**B**) power Doppler imaging, and (**C**) magnetic resonance angiography (MRA). The configuration of the M1 and initial M2 segments depicted with both Doppler methods correlate well with MRA.

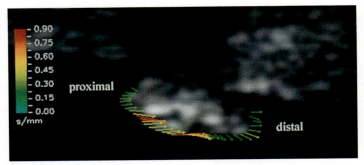

Plate 14.7

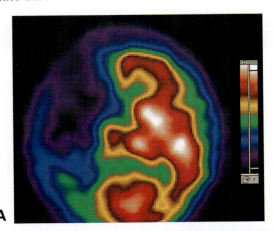

A

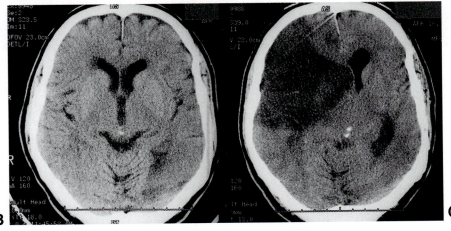

B   C

Plate 15.1

Plate 14.7 Representative motion measurements for the surface of a symptomatic plaque during systole. Motion vectors, achieved through model-based hierarchical motion estimation, are color-coded to vector magnitude (color legend on left indicates corresponding movement in millimeters). Proximal and distal surfaces of the plaque are labeled. Note the disparity of both magnitude and direction of motion vectors demonstrating plaque deformation.

Plate 15.1 Example of a large hypoperfusion deficit, predicting early mortality. **(A)** Single-photon emission computed tomography (SPECT) scan of a patient with severe right middle cerebral artery (MCA) territory infarction within 4 hours of symptom onset. The clinical features were left hemiplegia and gaze palsy with visual and sensory neglect. The SPECT scan demonstrates severe perfusion reduction involving the entire MCA territory. **(B)** CT scan showing minor early infarct changes contrasting with the striking hypoperfusion on SPECT. **(C)** CT scan showing severe infarction, mass effect, and transtentorial herniation. The patient died 3 days later as the result of cerebral edema and transtentorial herniation.

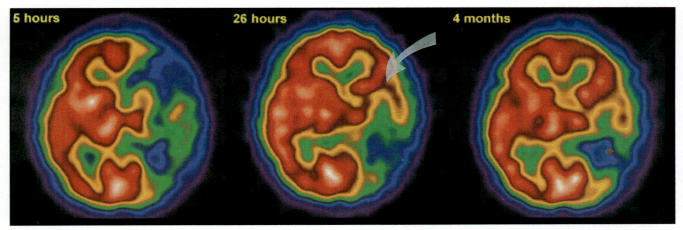

Plate 15.2

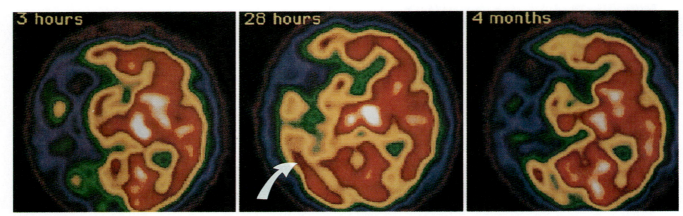

Plate 15.3

Plate 15.2 Example of nutritional reperfusion. Serial SPECT scans of a patient with left middle cerebral artery cortical infarction at 5 hours, 26 hours, and 4 months after stroke onset. There is reperfusion (arrow) between the first two scans, which was accompanied by clinical improvement. This reperfusion is maintained at the chronic stage, and is therefore *nutritional* in nature.

Plate 15.3 Example of non-nutritional reperfusion. Serial SPECT scans of a patient with right middle cerebral artery cortical infarction at 3 hours, 28 hours, and 4 months after stroke onset. Although there is reperfusion between the first two scans (arrow), this was not accompanied by clinical improvement. Furthermore, hypoperfusion increases at the chronic stage and is similar in severity to that on the initial scan. This indicates *non-nutritional reperfusion*.

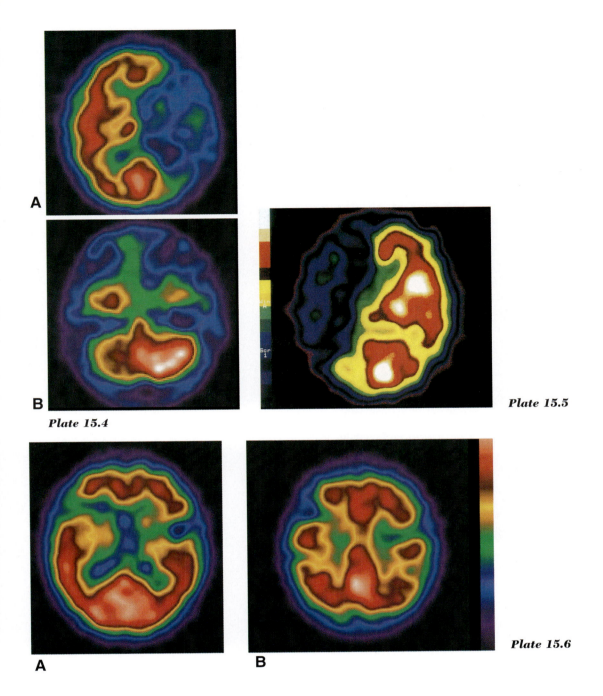

Plate 15.4 Example of crossed cerebellar diaschisis. SPECT scan of a patient with acute left middle cerebral artery cortical infarction. This demonstrates (**A**) left cerebral hypoperfusion associated with (**B**) right cerebellar hypoperfusion. The cerebellum was structurally normal on a correlative CT scan.

Plate 15.5 Right cerebral hypoperfusion due to severe symptomatic cerebral vasospasm following subarachnoid hemorrhage.

Plate 15.6 (**A & B**) Multifocal perfusion defects in a patient with dementia, indicating a multi-infarct etiology.

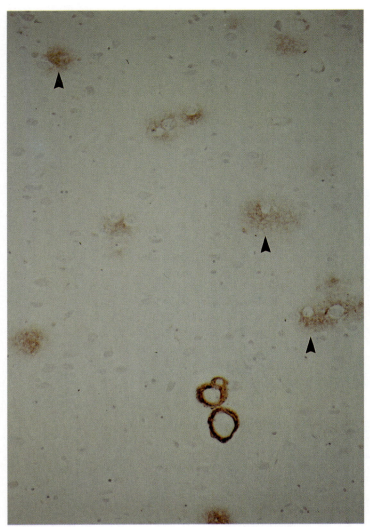

Plate 39.1

Plate 39.1 CAA in a patient with Dutch familial cerebral hemorrhage (HCHWA-D). Brain section immunostained with anti beta/A4 1-42. Note prominent microvascular staining, and small diffuse beta/A4 immunoreactive deposits (arrowheads) within brain parenchyma. (×175) (Material studied courtesy of Dr. Marion Maat and Prof. R.A.C. Roos, Department of Neurology, Leiden University Medical Center, The Netherlands.)

Pathophysiology of Stroke

FRANK M. YATSU

Fueled by the first successful treatment of acute ischemic strokes with the use of the thrombolytic agent, tissue plasminogen activator (tPA), research interests have been further galvanized in detailing the complex pathophysiologic mechanisms of strokes. In addition to greater insights into the mechanisms of thrombosis and molecular tools in developing more effective and safer thrombolytic agents (as reviewed expertly by Bruce Keyt and his colleagues from Genentech), application of modern neuroimaging tools such as positron emission tomography (PET) (reviewed extensively by Jean Claude Baron of the Institut National de la Santé et de la Récherche Médicale in Caen, France) and functional magnetic resonance imaging (rigorously surveyed by Peter Fox and his colleagues at the University of Texas at San Antonio) provide palpable excitement in the investigation of the mechanisms provoking irreversible ischemic brain damage and a means to intervene and analyze "on line" with advanced technologies. The expertise of Julio Garcia and his colleagues at the Henry Ford Hospital in the newer aspects of the neuropathology of various stroke syndromes provides the clinician with an easy grasp of pathologic changes. The explosion of molecular biologic techniques and advances has been translated to the study of brain ischemia, and these important insights, provided by Frank Sharp and his colleagues at the University of California at San Francisco and elsewhere and by Bruce Ransom of the University of Washington, furnish an understanding of the tremendous opportunities to avert irreversible brain damage caused by secondary ischemic changes and opportunities for reperfusion following recanalization with thrombolytic agents. Finally, the relevant field of vascular biology as it relates to potential interventions to prevent or reverse vascular diseases with techniques such as gene therapy is reviewed expertly by Donald Heistad and his colleagues at the University of Iowa, and the primary condition of atherosclerosis as the primary cause of ischemic strokes is summarized by this author and his colleagues at the University of Texas at Houston.

The in-depth and rigorous review of the pathophysiology of strokes in this section should provide the interested clinician with an overview of the exciting state of the art and science of stroke pathophysiology.

CHAPTER 1

Epidemiology of Stroke

PHILIP A. WOLF

RALPH B. D'AGOSTINO

Epidemiology is "the study of the distribution and determinants of disease frequency" in human populations.[64] Any consideration of the epidemiology of stroke, therefore, needs to include both elements, distribution (disease mortality, incidence, prevalence, and secular trends) and determinants (predisposing conditions and risk factors). Since stroke results from a number of pathologic processes, the distribution and determinants of specific stroke subtypes must be considered as well. Recent studies have provided new insights into risk factors for thrombotic and embolic ischemic stroke, as well as for intracerebral hemorrhage (IH) and subarachnoid hemorrhage (SAH).

Although several medical and surgical therapies to reduce the damage from impending or recent onset stroke have recently been shown to be effective in carefully selected patients and must be pursued in the future, it seems likely that prevention will continue to be the most effective strategy to reduce the health and economic consequences of cerebrovascular disease. Prevention is facilitated by an understanding of predisposing host and environmental factors. The relative impact of each of these factors has become clearer, chiefly through prospective epidemiologic study. Controlled clinical trials have demonstrated the effectiveness of risk factor modification in stroke prevention. In this chapter, in addition to including pertinent studies from the literature, we rely on up to 40 years of follow-up data from the Framingham Study. This prospective study of a general population sample is ideal for the examination of the determinants, incidence, and manifestations of stroke. Assessment of risk factors that were measured systematically and prospectively, often many years prior to the overt appearance of disease, provides the least distorted picture of the evolution of these host and environmental factors into stroke.

Stroke Mortality

Stroke is the most common life-threatening neurologic disease and the third leading cause of death in the United States, after heart disease and cancer, accounting for 1 of every 15 deaths. Although stroke is more often disabling than lethal, 158,061 deaths were attributed to stroke in 1995, corresponding to 1 death every 3.4 minutes.[6] In 1997, the American Heart Association estimates there were 500,000 initial strokes and 3,890,000 stroke survivors in the United States, many of whom required chronic care.[6] In the elderly, the segment of the population in which stroke occurs most frequently, it is a major cause of disability requiring long-term institutionalization.

Death rates for stroke are quite heterogeneous around the world and even vary widely within national boundaries, suggesting that powerful environmental factors are operating and indicating that stroke occurrence is not an inevitable consequence of aging or genetic influences.[70] There are wide variations in death rates from stroke from country to country, with the highest rates reported from eastern Europe and Portugal[70] (Fig. 1.1). There is no striking male predominance in stroke mortality. Even within the United States, reported deaths attributed to stroke vary widely. The lowest rates (20 to 24 deaths/100,000 population) occur largely in the Southwest, while the highest 29 to 42/100,000 population[70] occur in the southeastern states, which have been designated the *stroke belt*, (Fig. 1.2). Within the stroke belt, the coastal plains of Georgia, North Carolina, and South Carolina have the highest rates, a remarkable 40% overall excess risk of stroke compared with other regions.[46] This increased stroke mortality occurs in blacks and whites and in men and women.

SECULAR TRENDS

In the United States, stroke mortality has declined approximately 1.5% annually between 1915 and 1968. It is believed that this steady decrease is a result of improvements in the general public health and nutritional status of citizens in the United States (and in other western societies), rather than improvements in medical care. From 1972 to 1990 the slope of the decline steepened, and stroke mortality rates fell approximately 5% a year[70] (Fig. 1.3). Although the mechanism underlying this rapid acceleration of the decline is unclear, it occurred concurrent with a decline in other cardiovascular disease deaths, notably coronary heart disease. Since it began when programs to detect and control hypertension were initiated, some have attributed the decline to these efforts. Others

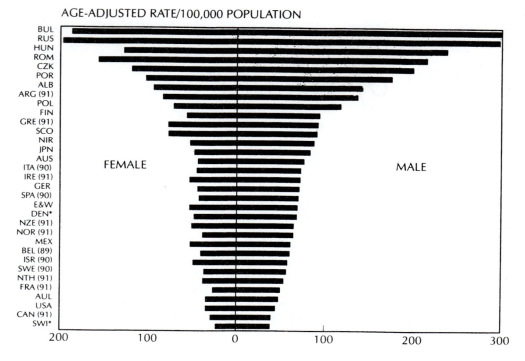

AGE-ADJUSTED RATE/100,000 POPULATION

FEMALE | MALE

* Eighth revision of the ICD.

Figure 1.1 Death rates for a stroke age 35 to 74, by country and sex (1992). Among 33 industrial countries, the United States has one of the lowest death rates for stroke. Eastern European countries and Portugal have markedly higher rates compared with other countries. (From National Institutes of Health,[70] with permission.)

have concluded that the success of programs to manage hypertension was relatively modest and insufficient to account for the magnitude of the observed decline.[15,18] Nevertheless, between 1972 and 1990, stroke mortality *rates* fell a remarkable 60%. This rapid pace of decline more than counterbalanced the aging of the population, so the *number* of persons dying from stroke also declined steadily. However, the decline in both the number and in the age-adjusted death rate for stroke reached a nadir in 1992 and 1993 and is now rising for the first time since 1915[6] (Fig. 1.4).[6]

It is of interest that substantial variability exists in the rates of decline around the world. There has been a long-term

Figure 1.2 Age-adjusted death rates for stroke by state, U.S., 1989 to 1991. Death rates for stroke are the highest in the southeastern states, most of which compose "the stroke belt." (from NIH,[70] with permission.)

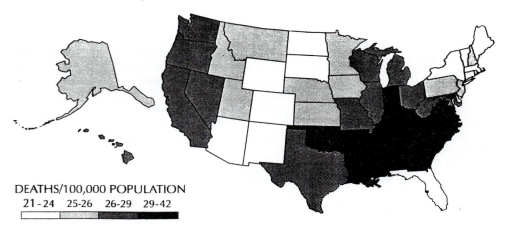

DEATHS/100,000 POPULATION

21 - 24   25-26   26-29   29-42

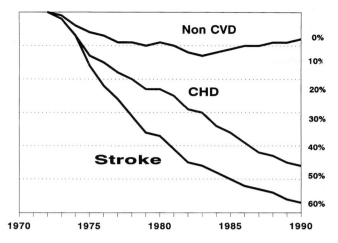

Figure 1.3 Decline in age-adjusted mortality rates for cardio-vascular diseases, United States, 1972 to 1990. (from Wolf,[123] with permission.)

steady steep decline between 1970 and 1985 exceeding 30% in 29 nations, with similar magnitudes in men and women.[110] The pace of decline varied from country to country, with Japan having an extraordinary 75% decrease, at the same time death rates in Eastern Europe actually *increased*. These data serve to confirm the importance of environmental influences including the varied intensity of effort and commitment of resources to implementing preventive measures in different countries.

SECULAR TRENDS IN STROKE SEVERITY

The dramatic decline in mortality from stroke in the past 30 years is real and not an artifact of death certification or coding practices. It has occurred in most industrialized nations, in men and women, and in all age and racial groups.[110] Furthermore, death rates attributable to stroke have declined in the face of falling total death rates. In fact, the diminution in

Figure 1.4 Mortality from stroke in the United States, 1979 to 1995. °, provisional; °°, 9 months (estimated) ending September, 1995. (Data from Vital Statistics of U.S., NCHS.)

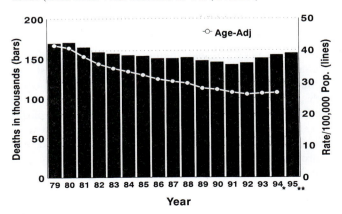

stroke death has been a major contributor to the decline in total cardiovascular diseases, providing further substantiation that the stroke decline is real (Fig. 1.3). The decline in death rates from stroke could come from either decreased incidence of stroke, improved survival of stroke patients, or a combination of these effects. Evidence supporting the role of declining incidence of stroke came from the community-based study of Rochester, Minnesota where stroke incidence was documented to decline between 1945 and 1985.[37] In addition, there was a particularly striking decline in the incidence of intracerebral hemorrhage, a stroke subtype with the highest case-fatality rate.[35] The decline in stroke had initially been noted for intracerebral hemorrhage by clinicians in Göteberg, Sweden.[10] They noted a decreased frequency of hemorrhage and a 10-year "delay" in onset of this disease, both of which they attributed to more effective treatment of severe hypertension.[10] However, studies of secular trends of stroke incidence in other populations have not uniformly disclosed a decline in incidence.[43,130] This suggested that improved stroke survival was playing a role in these populations, since in most reported studies death rates were declining.[67]

Evidence to support improved survival following stroke was found in the National Hospital Discharge Survey, which showed a decreasing case-fatality rate from stroke from 1970 to 1983. Three mechanisms are probably operating to reduce the case-fatality rates for stroke: improved acute stroke care has prolonged survival; stroke events in recent years are less severe and life-threatening than formerly; or, stroke cases that previously went undetected, and were milder in severity, are now routinely diagnosed. Improved medical and supportive care of acute stroke patients may be responsible for some degree of improvement in survival, although few data are available and no new effective treatment modality has emerged in the past 10 to 20 years. However, considerable evidence shows that the severity of strokes has been decreasing. There are fewer lethal stroke types such as IH, and even ischemic strokes seem to be less severe. Hospital case-fatality rates in Allegheny County, Pennsylvania decreased significantly from 19.6% to 11% from 1971 to 1980.[67] This decline in death rates coincided with a reduction in the severity of stroke. Fewer stroke patients were comatose, and this reduction in the prevalence of coma was thought to be responsible for more than 80% of the decline in the case-fatality rate.[67]

It is quite likely that small cerebral infarctions or hemorrhages, with mild or minimal neurologic deficits, which would not have been accurately diagnosed in the past, are now identified as definite strokes through the routine use of computed tomography (CT). The widespread availability of a diagnostic test for stroke, particularly for stroke in the elderly, may be particularly important here. The increase in diagnostic sensitivity afforded by the CT scan, and in the 1990s by magnetic resonance imaging (MRI), may counterbalance the impact of declining mortality and incidence. In Rochester, Minnesota, incidence rates have leveled off and perhaps even started to rise coincident with the availability of the CT scan and stroke severity has fallen dramatically where there was a significant ($P < 0.001$) reduction in 30-day case-fatality rates from 33% during 1945 to 1949 to 17% during 1980 to 1984 (the 1980 to 1984 quinquennium coincided with the availability of head CT scan).[17,36] In Allegheny County, Pennsylvania the advent of CT was accompanied by a twofold increase in survivorship of stroke patients.[5]

Aside from the improved sensitivity permitting diagnosis of smaller strokes with milder deficits, there has, additionally, been evidence of declining stroke severity.[45] In a study of stroke outcome in Allegheny County, Pennsylvania, age-adjusted mortality rates declined significantly from 1971 to 1980 for four sex-race groups while hospital case-fatality rates also fell from 19.6% to 11% between 1971 and 1980. The decline in death rates corresponded to a reduction in the severity of stroke with fewer patients in coma. The authors found that reduced severity of stroke events was responsible for more than 80% of the decline in case-fatality rates.[5]

Survival following stroke also improved from 49% to 62% in a five-county rural area of North Carolina from 1970 to 1973 and 1979 to 1980.[45] The decline in death rates corresponded to U.S. vital statistics and census data reports for the same five-county area, where a 24% decline from 1970 to 1980 had occurred. The decrease in deaths from stroke mortality resulted only slightly from a decrease in incidence and in substantial measure from improved survival following stroke.[47]

In Framingham, although the incidence of atherothrombotic brain infarction (ABI) fell in women age 55 to 64 years between the 1950s and the 1970s, no decline occurred in men. Nevertheless, stroke severity declined, with fewer severe deficits or unconscious stroke victims on admission to the hospital in the latest decade studied.[45]

There are a number of possible mechanisms contributing to the decline in stroke severity. First, increased awareness and recognition of transient ischemic attacks (TIAs) on the part of the general population and physicians must explain some portion of the increase in prevalence of these events. This increased recognition would tend to increase the incidence of total cerebrovascular events while reducing the case-fatality rate. Second, reduction in severity might result from a differential decline in the incidence of specific stroke subtypes with high case-fatality rates such as in IH and SAH. In the Rochester, Minnesota population, a decline in intracerebral hemorrhage incidence occurred over 25 years, 1945 to 1979. It was estimated that 24% of hemorrhages in the years prior to the advent of the CT scan had incorrectly been attributed to cerebral infarction and that these hemorrhages tended to be smaller and less severe.

There has been a clear decline in case-fatality rates for IH in Hisayama, Japan due in part to a decrease in the incidence of massive ganglionic hemorrhages from 1961 to 1983 in the two cohorts studied in that area. In addition, decreased case-fatality rates following SAH have been reported in the period 1975 to 1984 in Rochester, Minnesota and for white men and women in the United States as a whole.[45]

AGING AND PROSPECTS FOR THE FUTURE

As the population ages, the number of persons affected by stroke is likely to increase. It is estimated that by the year 2025 in the United States, the portion of the population age 65 years and older will increase to 18.4% from 12.6% in 1995.[111] For black Americans, who have higher stroke rates, the over-65 population will increase from 8.2% of the United States population in 1995 to 12.3% by 2025.[111] This increase in the size of the elderly population, both white and black,

forecasts an increase in the burden imposed by a number of diseases including stroke. The average remaining years of life in white and black adults after attaining age 65 years, now 17.3 and 15.4 years, respectively, are likely to increase in the future. Since most stroke victims survive the stroke with residual neurologic deficits, disability from stroke is almost certain to increase substantially. Stroke, although ranking 11th among the leading chronic conditions causing limitation of activity, currently disables more than 1.1 million Americans.

COST

Based on mortality and health survey data from the National Center for Health Statistics, health expenditure data from the Health Care Financing Administration, and income data from the U.S. Bureau of the Census, it is estimated that the economic cost of stroke in the United States in 1997 was $40.9 billion.[6] Some $26.2 billion was the direct cost of hospital care, professional care, and drugs, and $14.7 billion represented lost output. These estimates are crude and are derived from multiple indirect sources.[6] Recent attempts to quantify inpatient and poststroke costs by stroke subtype should lead to more precise estimates of the actual costs of these diseases.[6] Hence, successful preventive efforts are likely to yield economic as well as medical and human benefits.

Incidence

Incidence of stroke was determined over 40 years of follow-up of 5,184 men and women, ages 30 to 62, who were free of stroke at entry to the Framingham Study in 1950. The population has been examined every 2 years, and follow-up has been satisfactory, with approximately 85% of subjects participating in each examination. Study subjects suspected of stroke have been evaluated neurologically in the hospital at the time of the stroke since 1968. Since 1982, 91.5% have had at least one CT or MRI scan of the brain and arteries; many have had more than one study. Aside from confirming or ruling out a hemorrhage as the basis for the stroke, the stroke has been confirmed by CT/MRI study in 60.9% of cases. It has been possible, therefore, to distinguish clearly hemorrhage from infarction and to classify the ischemic stroke events into lacunar, large artery, and cardioembolic subtypes with a reasonable degree of assurance utilizing established criteria.[83] Over 40 years, since the study began, the neurologic deficit of the stroke was verified by a Framingham Study neurologist. Since 1981 when surveillance was intensified, the neurologic deficit was confirmed by a Framingham Study neurologist in 56.3% of cases. Follow-up of the population has been satisfactory; approximately 7% have been completely lost to follow-up for death.

Table 1.1 Annual Incidence of Atherothrombotic Brain Infarction (ABI) and Completed Strokes in Men and Women, Ages 35–94 Years

Age (yr)	Men		Women	
	No.	Rate/1,000	No.	Rate/1,000
ABI				
35–44	1	0.13	1	0.11
45–54	14	0.96	14	0.77
55–64	41	2.24	37	1.55
65–74	76	5.25	76	3.61
75–84	58	10.42	87	8.55
85–94	4	—	28	12.17
Total	194	3.78[a]	243	2.80[a]
Completed stroke				
35–44	3	0.40	4	0.44
45–54	26	1.79	18	0.99
55–64	64	3.50	62	2.60
65–74	122	8.43	129	6.12
75–84	90	16.17	137	13.46
85–94	7	—	56	24.34
Total	312	6.03[a]	406	4.53[a]

[a] Age-adjusted, 45–84 years.

(Data from the Framingham Study: 40-year Follow-up.)

After 40 years of follow-up in the Framingham Study, there were 718 cases of initial completed strokes and 113 instances of isolated TIAs. The average annual incidence of stroke events increased with age and doubled in successive decades (Table 1.1). This was true for ABIs, and for *completed* strokes (ischemic stroke and hemorrhages combined) (Table 1.1). There were too few cases in men aged 85 to 94 years to permit computation of rates; in women, stroke incidence continued to rise into this oldest decade of life without reaching a plateau. Overall, the annual age-adjusted (ages 45 to 84 years) total completed stroke rates were 6.03/1,000 in men and 4.53/1,000 in women, approximately 33% higher in men than in women (Table 1.1). The annual age-adjusted (ages 45 to 84 years) incidence of isolated TIAs also increased with age and was 1.05/1,000 in men and 0.69/1,000 in women, a male excess of approximately 52%. A perspective concerning the incidence of symptomatic coronary artery disease (CAD) and stroke may be gained by comparing analogous manifestations, myocardial infarction (MI), and ischemic stroke with no clear cardiac source for emboli, termed ABI (Fig. 1.5). Comparing these two major manifestations of atherosclerotic disease, in men, the age-adjusted average annual incidence rate of MI was three times that of ABI; in women, MI incidence was approximately twice that of ABI. Comparing incidence by gender, overall MI developed 2.8 times more often in men than in women, while ABI was approximately 1.35 times more frequent in men. In both sexes, rates doubled with each advancing decade. The 20-year lag in incidence of MI in women was not seen for ABI: age-specific rates were similar in both men and women.

Frequency of Stroke By Type

The in-hospital assessment of stroke at Framingham by a study neurologist has helped to document the stroke and determine stroke subtype and also to differentiate stroke from other neurologic diseases. Utilizing the in-person neurologic evaluations, and at least one CT scan of the brain obtained on admission to the hospital (and available on most stroke patients since 1978), it was usually possible to determine if the stroke mechanism was hemorrhage or infarction and to distinguish SAH from intraparenchymatous hemorrhage. Diagnosis of lacunar infarction was based on clinical and CT scan findings, while criteria for embolic infarction required a definite cardiac

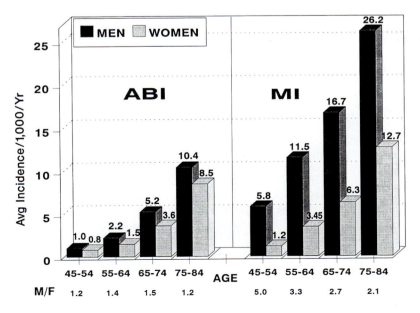

Figure 1.5 Incidence of myocardial and brain infarction in men and women according to age categories: 40-year follow-up. (Data from the Framingham Study.)

source for embolism. Distinguishing cerebral infarction resulting from extracranial versus intracranial arterial disease was made on clinical grounds relying on noninvasive carotid studies and magnetic resonance angiography. Contrast angiography was requested only infrequently by the study subjects' personal physicians, chiefly in cases of extracranial carotid stenosis prior to endarterectomy or with SAH. The occurrence of TIA was revealed by systematic routine questioning on each biennial examination since 1971 and by scrutiny of physician records and hospital notes. This surveillance for TIA has been comprehensive and systematic and extended over more than 25 years. In addition to the 15.1% of ABI preceded by TIA, there were 113 persons whose initial cerebrovascular symptom fulfilled criteria for TIA but who did not sustain a subsequent stroke. These isolated TIAs accounted for 14.8% of total cerebrovascular events in men and 12.7% of events in women.

The relative frequency of completed stroke by type was nearly identical in men and women (Table 1.2). ABI, including infarction secondary to large vessel atherothrombosis, lacunar infarction, and infarct of undetermined cause, occurred most frequently, in 62.2% in men and 59.9% in women. Intracranial hemorrhage accounted for 14.4% of completed strokes in men and 13.8% in women. There were roughly equal numbers of IHs and SAHs in men and women. Since IH is more prevalent at older ages and since more women survived to the oldest age groups, it is not appropriate simply to compare numbers. Age-adjusted rates of intracerebral hemorrhage were 9.01/100 person-years in men and 7.12/100 person-years in women for ages 75 to 94 years. Rates of SAH were roughly equivalent in the two sexes. In men, age-adjusted SAH rates were 2.75/100 person-years for ages 35 to 74 and 4.26/100 person-years for ages 75 to 94. In women, age-adjusted SAH rates were 2.16/100 person-years and 5.22/100 person-years for ages 35 to 74 and 75 to 94 years, respectively. The relative frequency of IH and SAH varies according to the age of population studied, the intensity of the neurologic workup, and other undetermined reasons.

In Framingham, SAH due to a ruptured berry aneurysm was nearly always confirmed by neurologic workup including angiography, surgery, or autopsy, while IH was usually verified by CT scan of the brain (and in the years prior to CT scan by the clinical picture, lumbar puncture, or autopsy). In prior tabulations and publications, when the Framingham cohort was younger in age, SAH incidence exceeded that of IH. This finding differed from that found in other defined populations, notably the population of Rochester, Minnesota, where, between 1945 and 1976, primary IH was five times more frequent than SAH.[35] More recent data from Rochester suggest that the incidence of IH was twice that of SAH.[15] On the other hand, in the National Survey of Stroke, a pre-CT-scan era sample of hospitalized strokes in the United States in 1971 to 1976, rates were more like those in Framingham, with 5.9% of stroke due to SAH and 6.3% attributed to IH.[79]

Risk Factors

Identification of risk factors for stroke as well as an awareness of the relative importance of each and of their interaction should facilitate stroke prevention. Since the pathogenetic

Table 1.2 Frequency of Complete Stroke by Type in Men and Women, Ages 35–94 Years

Completed Stroke	Men	Women	Total	%
Atherothrombotic brain infarction	194	243	437	60.9
Cerebral embolus	69	101	170	23.7
Intracerebral hemorrhage	25	28	53	6.7
Subarachnoid hemorrhage	20	28	48	7.3
Other	4	6	10	1.4
Total	312	406	718	100.0
Isolated transient ischemic attack	54	59	113	

(*Data from the Framingham Study: 40-Year Follow-up.*)

processes underlying the various stroke types differ, it is reasonable to expect that risk factors for infarction differ from risk factors for hemorrhage. Furthermore, precursors of intraparenchymatous bleeding are likely to differ from those for SAH. There is reason to believe that risk factors for stroke from atherosclerosis of the carotid and vertebral arteries may differ in their impact when compared with stroke resulting from lacunar infarction, and precursors of embolic stroke are also likely to be different. Nevertheless, certain predisposing factors, particularly elevated blood pressure, are common to most stroke types.

ATHEROGENIC HOST FACTORS

Assessment of the importance of the major atherogenic risk factors was made utilizing data from Framingham and other prospective epidemiologic studies. These risk factors include elevated blood pressure; blood lipid levels; diabetes; fibrinogen and other clotting factors; obesity; cardiac diseases (coronary heart disease, congestive heart failure, atrial fibrillation, left ventricular hypertrophy, and echocardiographic abnormalities); race; family history; and several recently recognized factors such as homocysteine and indices of inflammation.

Hypertension

Hypertension is the principal risk factor for thrombotic stroke as well as for intracerebral hemorrhage. Hypertension also predisposes to the cardiac conditions promoting cardiogenic cerebral embolism and to a lesser extent to SAH from aneurysm. Thus hypertension serves the unique role of prime risk factor for stroke resulting from the most frequent mechanisms.

Risk of stroke in the presence of *definite* hypertension (a blood pressure level of ≥160 mmHg systolic and/or ≥95 mmHg diastolic), when compared with risk in normotensives, is 3.1 in men and 2.9 in women. Even *borderline* levels (be-

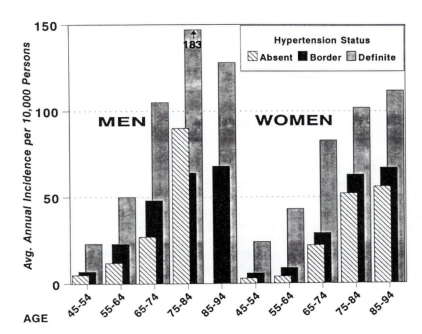

Figure 1.6 Incidence atherothrombotic brain infarction and hypertensive status, 40-year follow-up, the Framingham Study.

tween 140 and 159 mmHg systolic and 90 to 94 mmHg diastolic) carry a 50% increased stroke risk. Although there is evidence of a diminishing impact of hypertension with advancing age, risk of stroke is increased even in hypertensives aged 75 to 84 years. For nonembolic ischemic stroke (ABI), incidence of stroke increases with increasing severity of hypertension in men and women and in all age categories from 45 to 84 years (Fig. 1.6). Categorical designation of increased blood pressure fails to depict the strong and consistent relationship between level of blood pressure and incidence of stroke. From an analysis of 13,000 stroke events occurring in 450,000 persons in 45 prospective cohorts, there is a clear relationship between level of diastolic blood pressure and incidence of stroke in all adult age groups: <45 years, 45 to 64 years, and ≥65 years[77] (Fig. 1.7). With increasing age, as arterial elasticity declines, systolic blood pressure levels increase through the 70s, while diastolic pressures begin to level off in the 50s, and then fall substantially (Fig. 1.8). As a result, after age 65 years, stroke risk is more strongly related to level of systolic blood pressure and increases incrementally with each 10 mmHg increase in systolic level (Fig. 1.9). Although risk of stroke is strongly related to systolic blood pressure level, there are relatively few persons in the general population with pressures above 180 mmHg systolic (Fig. 1.10). Most stroke cases occur in persons whose systolic blood pressure is in the moderately elevated range. In Framingham, after 38 years of follow-up with more than 500 initial strokes, approximately 30% of stroke events occurred at systolic levels between 140 and 159 mmHg. Only 36% of strokes in men and 41% of strokes in women occurred in persons whose systolic pressure was ≥160 mmHg. Thus, approximately 60% of all initial stroke events occurred at systolic blood pressure levels of <160 mmHg. These persons, who would not be categorized as having *definite* hypertension, constitute the majority of stroke victims. Clearly, attention to mild and moderate systolic blood pressure elevations in the elderly will be necessary if stroke is to be prevented by antihypertensive treatment.

A substantial portion of stroke incidence is directly attributable to hypertension, and a portion of stroke in the population would be eliminated if hypertension were effectively treated. This portion, the *population-attributable fraction*, was estimated to be 56.4% of strokes in men and 66.1% in women based on an analysis of 26-year follow-up of Framingham data. The above classification of hypertension clearly fails to characterize adequately the risk of stroke and other cardiovascular disease events. Accordingly, the Fifth Report of the Joint National Committee on Detection, Evaluation, and Treatment

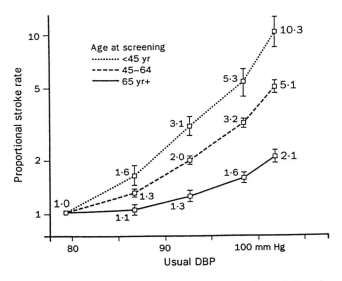

Figure 1.7 Proportional stroke risk, by age and usual diastolic blood pressure. Floating absolute risk, adjusted for study, sex, total cholesterol, history of coronary heart disease, and ethnicity. (From Prospective Studies Collaboration,[77] with permission.)

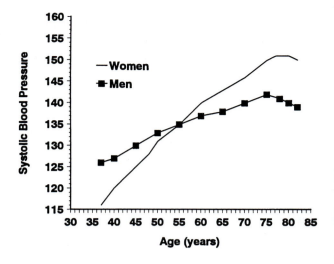

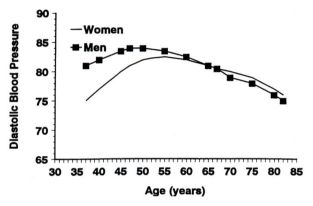

Figure 1.8 Cross-sectional age trends in blood pressure levels (mmHg), the Framingham Study, examinations 3 to 16. (From Wilson and Kannel,[122] with permission.)

of High Blood Pressure has proposed a new nomenclature[50] (Table 1.3).

Systolic Versus Diastolic Pressure Level

As noted, both systolic and diastolic blood pressure levels are strongly related to stroke incidence. Diastolic blood pressure has been thought to be of greater importance than systolic pressure. Clinical trials of antihypertensive treatment have used diastolic blood pressure as the basis for categorization of subjects. However, evidence for the ascendancy of diastolic blood pressure over systolic is lacking.[82] Diastolic blood pressure is more difficult to measure accurately, varies within a narrower range than systolic, and offers little advantage in predicting cardiovascular complications of hypertension. For example, at each level of diastolic blood pressure, incidence of stroke rises as systolic blood pressure rises, in both men and women, and at normal, borderline, and hypertensive systolic blood pressure levels (Table 1.4). In persons with systolic hypertension (systolic blood pressure ≥160 mmHg), stroke risk does not increase with increasing levels of diastolic blood pressure (Fig. 1.11). On the other hand, among persons with diastolic blood pressure ≥95 mmHg (i.e., *diastolic hypertensives*), incidence of stroke rises steadily as systolic blood pressure levels rise, in men and women.

Isolated Systolic Hypertension

As noted above, with increasing age, there is a disproportionate rise in systolic blood pressure, while the diastolic pressure levels off and then declines (Fig. 1.8). Above age 65, this elevation of systolic pressure, isolated systolic hypertension (ISH), defined as a systolic pressure <160 mmHg and diastolic pressure <90 mmHg, becomes increasingly prevalent (Fig. 1.12). ISH is present in approximately 20% of men and 30% of women above age 80.[120] Elevated systolic blood pressure in the presence of normal diastolic levels in the elderly results

Figure 1.9 Incidence of stroke according to systolic blood pressure, 40-year follow-up, men and women, 65 to 84 years of age. (Data from the Framingham Study.)

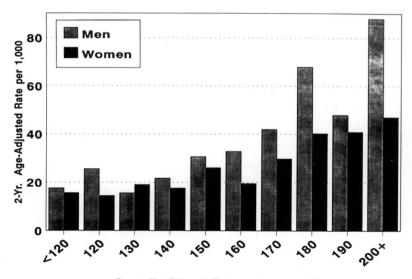

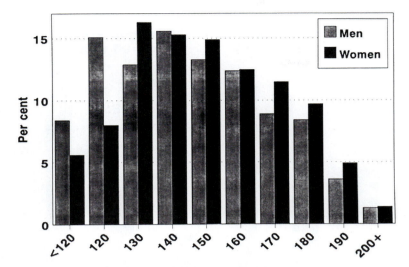

Figure 1.10 Frequency of stroke according to systolic blood pressure, 40-year follow-up, men and women, 65 to 84 years of age. (Data from the Framingham Study.)

from decreased elasticity of the walls of the aorta and other large arteries. As such, these isolated systolic pressure elevations were considered to be a consequence rather than a precursor of cardiovascular disease. However, it has been demonstrated in Framingham and in other epidemiologic studies that stroke and cardiovascular disease incidence were significantly increased in persons with isolated systolic hypertension.[23] Risk was proportionately related to the level of systolic pressure even after diastolic pressure, age, and digital pulse-wave configuration (an index of arterial rigidity) were taken into account.[55] Recently, even *borderline ISH* (systolic blood pressure level of 140 to 159 mmHg and diastolic pressure of >90 mmHg) was found to increase the risk of developing *definite*

hypertension.[88] Furthermore, there was a 42% increase in the incidence of stroke or TIAs in borderline isolated systolic hypertensives, even after other pertinent risk factors were taken into account.[88] The landmark report of a striking beneficial effect of blood pressure reduction in isolated systolic hypertensives gives these data added significance[93] and is discussed below.

Blood Lipids

With increasing levels of total serum cholesterol, there is a steady increase in the incidence of CHD. This relationship holds in both men and women and persists after accounting for other risk factors. The impact declines with advancing age and is no longer significant above age 60, particularly in men. However, when the components of cholesterol (high-, low-, and very low-density lipoprotein) are related to incidence of CHD, even in persons older than age 60, a relationship re-

Table 1.3 Classification of Blood Pressure for Adults Age 18 Years and Older[a]

Category	Blood Pressure (mmHg)	
	Systolic	*Diastolic*
Normal	<130	<85
High normal	130–139	85–89
Hypertension stage[b]		
1 (mild)	140–159	90–99
2 (moderate)	160–179	100–109
3 (severe)	180–209	110–119
4 (very severe)	≥210	≥120

[a] *Not taking antihypertensive drugs and not acutely ill. When systolic (SBP) and diastolic (DBP) pressures fall into different categories, the higher category should be selected to classify the individual's blood pressure status. For instance, 160/92 mmHg should be classified as stage 2, and 180/120 mmHg should be classified as stage 4. Isolated systolic hypertension (ISH) is defined as SBP ≥140 mmHg and DBP <90 mmHg and is staged appropriately (e.g., 170/85 mmHg is defined as stage 2 ISH). (From JHC.[50])*

[b] *Based on the average of two or 'more' readings taken at each of two or more visits following an initial screening.*

Table 1.4 Two-Year Age-Adjusted Rate[a] of Stroke per 1,000[b]

	Systolic Pressure	Diastolic Pressure		
		<90	*90–94*	*95+*
Men	<140	8.0	6.3	6.6
	140–159	12.5	7.8	13.0
	160+	23.8	13.0	13.7
Women	<140	7.5	8.2	12.2
	140–159	9.2	12.4	11.9
	160+	14.5	15.9	17.7

[a] *Direct method using entire (sex-specific) population as standard.*

[b] *By sex and level of systolic and diastolic blood pressure (mmHg), men and women ages 35–94 years.*

(Data from the Framingham Study: 40-Year Follow-up.)

Figure 1.11 Incidence of stroke in systolic and diastolic hypertensive patients according to diastolic and systolic blood pressure levels, men and women, ages 35 to 94 years; 40-year follow-up. (Data from the Framingham Study.)

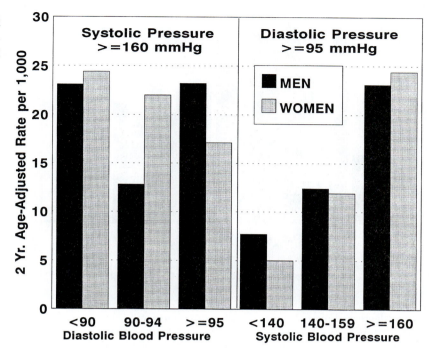

emerges. The level of total cholesterol, and specifically low density lipoprotein cholesterol (LDL), is directly related to incidence of CHD. However, at any level of LDL cholesterol, the incidence of CHD is inversely related to the level of high density lipoprotein (HDL) cholesterol. The relationship of blood cholesterol to CHD incidence is best expressed by the ratio of total serum cholesterol to HDL cholesterol, which demonstrates a significant impact on CHD incidence until age 80. For example, in persons aged 75 to 79 years, the risk ratio for CHD with an elevated total/HDL cholesterol ratio

is 1.6 for men and 1.8 for women. However, for stroke generally and for nonembolic ischemic stroke in particular, there is no clear or consistent relationship to blood lipid levels. For example, in a meta-analysis of 45 prospective epidemiologic studies comprising 450,000 subjects among whom 13,000 strokes occurred, no significant association between total serum cholesterol and total stroke incidence was seen.[77] However, a relationship was found in the Honolulu Heart Study of Hawaiian men of Japanese ancestry and in the Multiple Risk Factor Intervention Trial (MRFIT) screenees.[49] In Hon-

Figure 1.12 Prevalence of isolated systolic hypertension in men and women, ages 35 to 84 years, 36-year follow-up. (Data from the Framingham Study.)

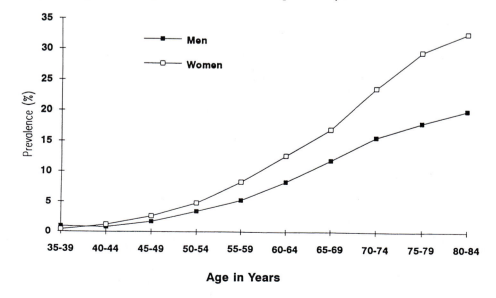

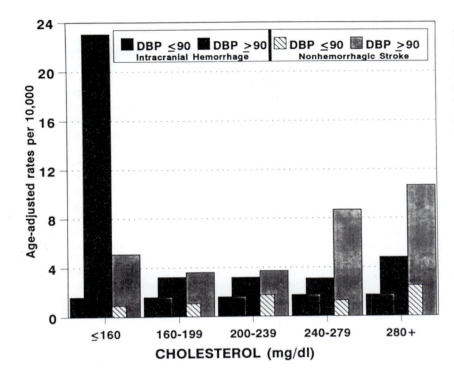

Figure 1.13 Ischemic stroke and intracerebral hemorrhage death rates in men with normal and elevated diastolic blood pressure (DBP) according to screening serum cholesterol level. Multiple Risk Factor Intervention Trial screenees, 6-year follow-up. (Figure adapted from data published in Ito et al,[49] with permission.)

olulu, the level of total cholesterol measured years before was directly related to the incidence of thromboembolism.[12] No such direct relationship, long or short term, between ischemic stroke and total or LDL cholesterol has been found in Framingham, and no protective effect of HDL cholesterol was seen.[127] In MRFIT, the incidence of ischemic stroke, diagnosed on death certificates, was greater in those with the highest levels of serum total cholesterol obtained 6 years before (Fig. 1.13).

Although the relationship between blood lipids and stroke is unclear, serum lipid levels have been directly related to extracranial carotid artery atherosclerosis including increased extracranial carotid artery wall thickness.[31,73,121] HDL cholesterol exerts a protective influence, while LDL cholesterol and total serum cholesterol appear to increase the intimal-medial thickness (IMT) of the carotid artery wall and promote the development of atheromata. Atherosclerosis of the carotid arteries and other arteries of the circle of Willis has been demonstrated in autopsy studies to be directly related to levels of blood lipids. A meta-analysis of the older cholesterol-lowering trials showed a definite benefit in reduction in myocardial infarction rates but no significant benefit in stroke prevention in the treated groups.[8] However, in 1987 a new class of lipid-lowering compounds, the 3-hydroxy-3-methylglutaryl coenzyme A (HMG-CoA) reductase inhibitors, was introduced in the United States. The Asymptomatic Carotid Artery Progression Study (ACAPS) demonstrated that lovastatin (20 to 40 mg/day) was effective in reducing the mean maximum IMT in the extracranial carotid arteries of asymptomatic subjects with early carotid atherosclerosis and moderately elevated LDL cholesterol levels.[34] There was a 28% decline in LDL cholesterol level from 156.6 mg/dl to 113.1 mg/dl at 6 months and a significant regression of the mean maximum IMT by 36 months. The lovastatin group experienced a regression of

plaque thickness of -0.009 ± 0.003 mm/year ($P = 0.001$), while the IMTs of subjects in the other arms of this randomized clinical trial demonstrated progression of $+0.006 \pm 0.003$ mm/year.[34] Of particular note was the striking reduction in cardiovascular events observed in the lovastatin group (from 14 to 5). The 14 events in subjects not receiving lovastatin included four CHD deaths, five strokes, and five nonfatal MIs compared with only five nonfatal MIs (and no strokes) in the lovastatin group. Of the five strokes, four occurred in the groups receiving warfarin.[4] Of these, there were two hemorrhages from berry aneurysms, one had a pontine lacune, and one had a capsular infarction associated with high-grade ICA stenosis. One woman, aged 70, who sustained an IH was in neither the lovastatin nor the warfarin groups.[4]

Several other trials of lipid lowering by these drugs, also known as statins, confirmed this rather dramatic effect.[20] In the 4S study (the Scandinavian Simvastatin Survival Study), 4,444 patients with angina pectoris or prior MI and a total serum cholesterol level of 5.5 to 8.0 mmol/L were randomized to a HMG-CoA inhibitor or placebo.[89] After a median follow-up of 5.4 years, there were substantial reductions in total cholesterol (-28%) and LDL cholesterol (-38%) in the simvastatin group and an increase in HDL cholesterol ($+8\%$). At 1 year, 72% had reached the goal of a total cholesterol of <5.2 mmol/L. As in the ACAPS study, a striking reduction in mortality was seen: 12% in placebo versus 8% in the simvastatin group, relative risk 0.70 (95% confidence interval [CI] 0.58 to 0.85; $P = 0.0003$).[89] A 42% reduction in fatal CHD was responsible for the reduced overall mortality. For cerebrovascular end points, there was no difference in fatal strokes between treatment and placebo groups, with 14 and 12 events, respectively. For nonfatal cerebrovascular events, there were 2.7% versus 4.3% in the treatment and placebo groups, respectively. A post hoc analysis of all cerebrovascular events, fatal and nonfatal, showed a relative risk of 0.70 (95% CI 0.52 to 0.96; $P = 0.024$). Among stroke subtypes the most striking reductions were in the TIA, nonembolic, and intervention-related stroke categories. The reduction in intervention-related and TIA categories seems to correspond to the reduction in total fatal and nonfatal cerebrovascular events to 70 events in the simvastatin and 98 in the placebo group (relative risk 0.70; 95% CI 0.52 to 0.96; $P = 0.024$) in a post hoc analysis.[89]

These findings raised the question of whether statins would exert a similarly beneficial effect in persons with lesser elevations of LDL cholesterol. Two recent reports, again principally studies for the prevention of CHD end points, have provided data to help answer this question.[87,94] In the West of Scotland Coronary Prevention Study Group, 6,595 men, 45 to 64 years of age, with a mean ($\pm$SD) cholesterol level of 272 ± 23 mg/dl were randomly assigned to receive pravastatin (40 mg daily) or placebo. These men had hypercholesterolemia but no history of myocardial infarction and were followed for 4.9 years. A significant reduction occurred in the level of LDL cholesterol in the treated group. This was accompanied by a 31% relative risk reduction in definite coronary events and a 32% decrease in deaths from all cardiovascular causes. There were 46 strokes (6 of which were fatal) in the pravastatin group and 51 (4 fatal) in the placebo group, representing an overall 10% relative risk reduction, which was not significant. In the Cholesterol and Recurrent Events (CARE) Trial, pravastatin and placebo were randomly allocated to 4,159 survivors of a myocardial infarction (3,583 men and 576 women) with *average* cholesterol levels (total cholesterol levels below 240 mg/dl and LDL cholesterol levels of 115 to 174 mg/dl (mean 139 mg/dl).[87] The specified primary end point of death from CHD or nonfatal MI was reduced by 24% (95% CI 9 to 36; $P = 0.003$) in the pravastatin group. Other CHD end points were similarly reduced during the 5 years of follow-up. Stroke occurred in 78 (3.8%) of the placebo group and 54 (2.6%) of the pravastatin group, a relative risk reduction of 31% (95% CI 3 to 52; $P = 0.03$).[87] It was estimated that 25 strokes would be prevented by treating 1,000 such patients ≥60 years of age with pravastatin for 5 years. This compares favorably with the 27 fatal CHD events and 46 nonfatal MIs prevented in this relatively young group for stroke (mean age 59 ± 9 years).[87]

It seems likely that the significant reductions in stroke and MI in the ACAPS trial did not result from the fraction of a hundredth of a millimeter reduction in plaque thickness in the extracranial carotid artery wall. It is similarly unlikely in the 4S and CARE studies that a reduction in plaque thickness was responsible for the striking benefit. Some have suggested the statin drugs acted by altering the lipid composition of the plaque, reducing the tendency to rupture or fissure, as well as by improving the hemorrheologic environment. These important relative risk reductions in stroke incidence, if confirmed in other elderly populations with higher stroke rates, may lead to the use of these agents for either primary or secondary stroke prevention.[112]

LOW CHOLESTEROL AND HEMORRHAGE
Low total serum cholesterol has been consistently related to an increased incidence of IH.[131] This finding was first noted following World War II among rural Japanese, who had very low serum cholesterol levels by Western standards (i.e., <160

mg/dl) and also had a marked increase in incidence of IH.[95] Initially, no cause and effect relationship was seriously considered. However, as nutrient intake of animal fat increased and sodium chloride intake fell, there was a corresponding increase in total serum cholesterol in this population.[95] In men and women ages 40 to 49, the total serum cholesterol levels rose from 155 mg/dl in 1963 to 1966, to 175 mg/dl in 1972 to 1975, and to 181 mg/dl in 1980 to 1983. Total serum protein levels and relative weight rose significantly during these 20 years, while systolic and diastolic blood pressures declined. Accompanying these profound changes in risk factor levels were similar remarkable declines in the incidence of IH, which fell 65% in men (P <0.05) and 94% in women (P <0.001) between 1964 to 1968 and 1979 to 1983.[95] Serum cholesterol levels were quite low, frequently <160 mg/dl. An etiologic link has been suggested by the recent confirmation of this relationship in other Oriental populations, in Hawaiian Japanese, and in Caucasian men in the United States. Of 350,977 men aged 35 to 57 years screened for entry into MRFIT, after 6 years of follow-up, there were 83 deaths from IH and 55 deaths from SAH.[49] In the lowest serum cholesterol category, <160 mg/dl, the risk factor-adjusted relative risk of intracranial hemorrhage was 1.0, and the relative risk at all higher levels of serum cholesterol was approximately 0.32. When deaths from intracranial hemorrhage were examined by entry diastolic blood pressure, the age-adjusted rate of death was significant only in persons with pressures ≥90 mmHg (Fig. 1.13). Death rates per 10,000 were 23.07 in the lowest serum cholesterol category, <160 mg/dl, and ranged from 3.09 to 4.83 in the four higher categories.[49] The mechanism by which an elevated diastolic blood pressure and a very low serum cholesterol promotes IH has been suggested to be an alteration in the cell membranes, which weakens the endothelium of intracerebral arteries.

Still another link is the direct relationship between elevated total serum cholesterol and LDL cholesterol and the inverse relationship of HDL cholesterol and extracranial carotid artery atherosclerosis.[31,72,73,109,121] This finding is obviously related to the diminution of plaque or IMT by lovastatin seen in the ACAPS trial.

Diabetes

Diabetics are known to have an increased susceptibility to coronary, femoral, and cerebral artery atherosclerosis. Surveys of stroke patients and prospective studies have confirmed the increased risk of stroke in diabetics. The Honolulu Heart Program of Japanese men living in Hawaii found that increasing degrees of glucose intolerance conferred an increasing risk of thromboembolic stroke that was independent of other risk factors. There was no relationship to hemorrhage[19] (Fig. 1.14). Evaluation of the impact of diabetes on stroke in a population-based cohort in Rancho Bernardo disclosed a relative risk of stroke that was 1.8 in men and 2.2 in women even after adjusting for the effect of other pertinent risk factors.[11]

In Framingham, peripheral arterial disease with intermittent claudication occurs more than four times as often in diabetics. The coronary and cerebral arteries are also affected, but to a lesser extent.[53] For atherothrombotic brain infarction, the impact of glucose intolerance, (i.e., physician-diagnosed diabetes, glycosuria, or a blood sugar >150 mg/100 ml) is greater in women than men and was significant as an independent contributor to incidence only in older women. However,

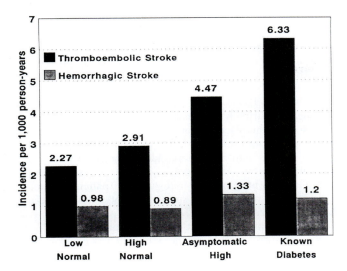

Figure 1.14 Incidence of stroke and glucose intolerance, Honolulu Heart Study, 22-year follow-up. (From Burchfiel) et al,[19] with permission.)

at all ages both men and women with glucose intolerance have approximately double the risk of ABI compared with nondiabetics.

Obesity

Obese persons have higher levels of blood pressure, blood glucose, and atherogenic serum lipids, and on that account alone could be expected to have an increased stroke incidence. Obesity, expressed as a Metropolitan Relative Weight that is >30% above average, is a significant independent contributor to ABI incidence in younger men and elderly women. However, in all age groups and in both sexes, obesity exerts an adverse influence on health status that is probably mediated through elevated blood pressure, impaired glucose tolerance, and other mechanisms. Recent studies have suggested that abdominal obesity, rather than elevated body mass index, is

more strongly related to stroke incidence. In 28,643 male health professionals, the relative risk of stroke was 2.33 in the highest compared with the lowest quintile. Relative risk using body mass index or waist circumference alone were less strongly related to stroke incidence.[114]

Heart Disease and Impaired Cardiac Function

Cardiac diseases and impaired cardiac function are disease states or organ dysfunction that predispose to stroke. Although hypertension is the pre-eminent risk factor for stroke of all types, at each blood pressure level persons with impaired cardiac function have a significantly increased stroke risk.[131] The prevalence of these cardiac contributors to stroke increases with age (Fig. 1.15). Cardiovascular disease is highly prevalent among stroke cases. In Framingham, after 36 years of follow-up 80.8% were hypertensive, 32.7% had prior CHD, 14.5% had cardiac failure, 14.5% had atrial fibrillation, and (AF) only 13.6% had none of these. Cardiac disease is an important precursor of stroke and is dealt with in detail in several other chapters.

CORONARY HEART DISEASE   In Framingham, CHD was ascertained prospectively on biennial examination as well as by monitoring hospitalizations over 36 years of follow-up. CHD predisposes to stroke by a variety of mechanisms: as a source for embolism from the heart; by virtue of shared risk factors; as an untoward effect of medical and surgical treatments for coronary atherosclerotic disease; and, as a consequence of pump failure. In the 2-week period after acute myocardial infarction, stroke occurs most frequently at a rate estimated to be between 0.7% and 4.7%.[62] As expected, older age and ventricular dysfunction (chiefly decreased ejection fraction) following MI increased stroke risk.[62] Treatment with aspirin, and particularly with warfarin anticoagulation, decreased the incidence of stroke in a large group of MI survivors.[62,97] Stroke occurs most frequently following *anterior* wall MI, in 2% to 6% of cases. The mechanism is cerebral embolism principally from left ventricular mural thrombus, which is demonstrable on echocardiographic studies in 40% of cases.

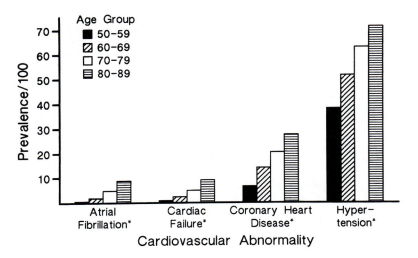

Figure 1.15 Prevalence of cardiovascular abnormality with increasing age, men and women combined: 34-year follow-up.* Significant trend for age ($P < .001$) (Data from the Framingham Study.)

Inferior wall MI is an infrequent basis for mural thrombus or stroke. Often, however, the mechanism of stroke in persons with CHD is less apparent. Persons with uncomplicated angina pectoris, non–Q-wave infarction, and clinically silent MI also have an increased incidence of ischemic stroke. Recent data from Framingham suggest that silent or unrecognized MI survivors had a 10-year incidence of stroke of 17.8% in men and 17.3% in women, an incidence not that much less than the 19.5% and 29.3% in men and women, respectively, that is seen following recognized MI.

ATRIAL FIBRILLATION   In association with rheumatic heart disease and mitral stenosis, AF is acknowledged to predispose to stroke. In recent years, chronic AF without valvular heart disease, previously considered to be innocuous, has been associated with approximately a fivefold increase in stroke incidence. AF is also the most prevalent persistent cardiac arrhythmia in the elderly. In the Framingham Study, AF incidence more than doubled in successive decades and rose from 0.2:1,000 for ages 30 to 39 to 39.0:1,000 for ages 80 to 89 years. AF was particularly important in the elderly since the proportion of total strokes associated with this arrhythmia increased steadily with age, reaching 36.2% for ages 80 to 89 years.[125] Although the prevalence of other cardiac contributors to stroke also increased with age, the increased incidence of stroke in persons with AF was more likely to be a consequence of the AF and not the associated CHD or cardiac failure. This becomes apparent when age trends in risk of stroke are examined (Fig. 1.16). Relative risk of stroke declines with each successive decade for hypertension, congestive heart failure, and CHD, while AF continues to exert a significant impact even into the 80s (Fig. 1.16). In addition, while attributable risk of stroke increased with age for AF, risk of stroke attributable to cardiac failure, CHD, and hypertension declined with age.[125] Notably, in the oldest age group (80 to 89 years), the percent of stroke attributable to AF was 23.5% and approached that of hypertension (33.4%), a far more prevalent disorder. A dispute as to whether AF is an independent risk factor or merely a risk marker for other conditions predisposing to stroke raged for several years.[22,126] This issue would seem to have been settled by the remarkable concordance of a half-dozen randomized clinical trials demonstrating a 68% stroke risk reduction on intention-to-treat analyses and over 80% on efficacy (on-treatment) analyses of warfarin for stroke prevention in AF.[9] The reduction in risk of stroke far outweighs the risk of serious and particularly intracranial bleeding. Aspirin has a far less potent impact and seems to prevent milder noncardioembolic strokes.[69] From a pooled analysis of the five primary prevention trials, four risk factors were shown to increase stroke risk: increasing age; a history of prior stroke or TIAs; diabetes; or hypertension.[9] Warfarin reduced the incidence of stroke in persons with any one of these risk factors and in all three age groups: younger than 65 years, 65 to 75 years and older than age 75 (Fig. 1.17) In all age groups, in the presence or absence of risk factors, the fourfold increased incidence of stroke was reduced to approximately 1% by warfarin anticoagulation. In the youngest age group, persons younger than age 65 who had no risk factors, the incidence without warfarin was 1% and it is only this group for which anticoagulation is not currently indicated. These individuals, denoted as having "lone AF," may be treated with aspirin

alone. This conclusion is based on relatively sparse data and will require more studies to refine further who may safely be followed without warfarin. The relative lack of efficacy of aspirin was clearly demonstrated in a large secondary prevention trial, the European Atrial Fibrillation Trial, in patients with a stroke or TIA within 3 months of enrollment. The annual stroke rate of 12% was not significantly reduced by aspirin 300 mg/day. Virtually identical rates occurred with aspirin as were seen in the placebo group,[29] and no case of intracranial bleeding was seen in the warfarin group, although many were elderly. In this high-risk group, elderly persons with AF and a prior cerebrovascular event, 90 events (mostly strokes) would be prevented in 1 year for every 1,000 patients anticoagulated. These authors have suggested that a target international normalized ratio (INR) of 3.0 would produce the lowest rates of ischemic stroke without an increase in the risk of serious hemorrhage.[30] In another study the risk of stroke rose steeply below an INR of 2.0.[48] At an INR of 1.7, the adjusted odds ratio (OR) for stroke was 2.0 (95% confidence interval, 1.6 to 2.4); at an INR of 1.5, it was 3.3 (95% confidence interval, 2.4 to 4.6).[48] Combinations of subtherapeutic doses of warfarin combined with aspirin provided little protection. There were no lower rates of hemorrhage, and stroke prevention was far less effective than therapeutic levels of warfarin anticoagulation.[107] Nevertheless, physicians and patients are reluctant to use warfarin, particularly in elderly patients, in whom the risk of stroke is highest.[100] Patients 80 years or older were least likely to be given warfarin. In 1992 to 1993, only 19% of eligible octogenarians were treated. On the positive side, overall, warfarin use for stroke prevention in AF has increased from 7% in 1980 to 1981 to 32% in 1992 to 1993.[100]

LEFT VENTRICULAR HYPERTROPHY BY ELECTROCARDIOGRAM   Left ventricular hypertrophy by electrocardiogram, (LVH by ECG), increases in prevalence with age and blood pressure. Risk of ABI increased by more than fourfold in men and sixfold in women with this abnormal ECG pattern. The increased risk persisted even after the influence of age and other atherogenic precursors, including systolic blood pressure, were taken into account.

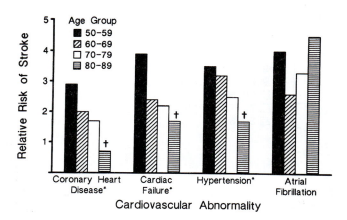

Figure 1.16 Estimated relative risk of stroke with advancing age according to the presence of coronary heart disease, cardiac failure, hypertension, and atrial fibrillation: 34-year follow-up.† No significant excess of strokes; °, significant *inverse* trend for age (*P* <.05) (Data from the Framingham Study.)

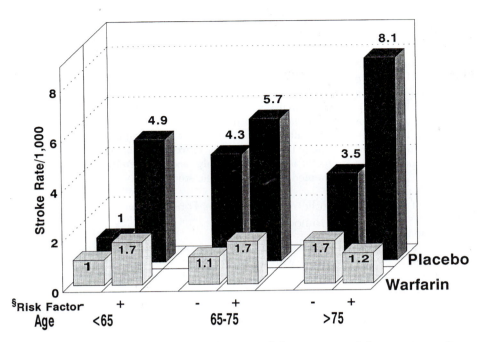

Figure 1.17 Efficacy of warfarin by risk category§ (hypertension, diabetes, prior stroke or TIA), pooled analysis of atrial fibrillation trials.

A more sensitive and precise measure of cardiac muscle hypertrophy, left ventricular mass (LVM-to-height ratio), on echocardiography is now frequently available. LVM as determined on M-mode echocardiography was directly related to incidence of stroke.[13] The hazard ratio for stroke and TIA, comparing the uppermost quartile of LVM-to-height ratio with the lowest, was 2.72 after adjusting for age, gender, and cardiovascular risk factors. There was a graded response with a hazard ratio of 1.45 for each quartile increment of LVM-to-height ratio. Thus, echocardiography provides prognostic information beyond that provided by traditional risk factors.

Fibrinogen

Serum fibrinogen has been implicated in atherogenesis and in arterial thrombus formation. A number of epidemiologic studies have shown a substantial and significant independent impact of fibrinogen on cardiovascular disease incidence including stroke. In a prospective study of 54-year-old Swedish men, fibrinogen in combination with elevated systolic blood pressure was found to be a potent risk factor for stroke.[119] Level of fibrinogen, measured at the 10th biennial examination in Framingham, was also significantly related to incidence of cardiovascular disease including stroke.[54]

However, fibrinogen was also positively associated with most of the major risk factors for stroke including age, hypertensive status, hematocrit level, obesity, and diabetes.[33,54,60] There is considerable optimism that further study of fibrinogen and other clotting factors will yield important clues into the pathogenesis of atherosclerotic cardiovascular disease.

Race

Comparisons of variability in the occurrence of stroke in different races are often confounded by factors other than racial differences. These include socioeconomic, life style, and nutri-tional factors, as well as a variation in risk factor abnormalities in different racial groups. In recent years attempts have been made to determine risk factor differences in different racial groups in a single geographic location[85] and to determine the contribution of these risk factor differences to differences in the frequency of stroke. In addition, differences in the proportion of strokes due to differences in stroke mechanisms between racial groups and the susceptibility of one group to more severe or lethal stroke subtypes are being explored. Much of what is known about racial differences in stroke susceptibility derives from isolated circumstances and studies that have been confounded by unique dietary and socioeconomic factors.

Compared with whites, blacks have higher death rates from stroke. Age-adjusted incidence rates are 1.5 times higher for black men and 2.3 times higher for black women than for whites.[38] In the National Health and Nutrition Examination Survey I Epidemiologic Follow-up Study, age-adjusted mortality for blacks from stroke was 1.98 times that of whites.[74] It is of interest that 31% of excess mortality could be accounted for by six key risk factors for cardiovascular disease. A further 38% of the excess deaths could be accounted for by family income; 31% of the excess black total mortality remained unexplained. When compared with whites, blacks had increased prevalence rates of hypertension and diabetes. They also had more IH and less extracranial and large artery atherosclerotic disease than whites.[38,59] The National Longitudinal Mortality Study estimated that in men, lower socioeconomic status accounted for 14% to 46% of the excess black stroke risk, but no association was present for black women.[74] Epidemiologic studies of Hispanics in the United States are hampered by the different origins and the heterogeneity of the groups; however, stroke death rates were similar in Hispanics and whites younger than age 65 and lower above age 65. This may be changing. In a hospital- and community-based cohort study of all cases of first stroke in northern Manhattan, blacks and Hispanics had an overall age-adjusted 1-year stroke incidence rate of 2.4 and 1.6 times, respectively, that of whites.[84]

Stroke was a leading cause of death among U.S. Native Americans in 1990, but death rates were lower than in whites.[39] In 1988 through 1990, stroke death rates were similar in Native Americans and whites under age 65 and, as for Hispanics, were lower in whites older than age 65. The epidemiology of stroke in blacks and Hispanics is being investigated with increased intensity in a number of multiracial populations in the United States.

Asians have had a low rate of CHD and a high prevalence of stroke. A high incidence and prevalence of stroke in Chinese was found in a survey of six mainland cities with rates that were comparable to those of native Japanese in Japan.[61] The disparity between the stroke and CHD death rates, and presumably a similar disparity in incidence rates, is usually attributed to the high prevalence of hypertension and the low levels of blood lipids in orientals.[78] Hypertension was generally related to high salt intake and perhaps to genetic factors while the low serum lipids were related to the low levels of animal fat and protein in the oriental diet. Cerebrovascular disease was the most frequently certified cause of death in Japan during the three decades following World War II, and the mechanism of stroke was thought to be IH. By 1980, stroke death rates had fallen, and cancer became the leading cause of death. In Japanese men in Hawaii and San Francisco, deaths attributed to stroke also fell relative to those from CHD and cancer. In 1985, heart disease became the second leading cause of death in Japan (114.8:100,000) following cancer (156.4:100,000), and stroke fell to the third position (110.6:100,000).[78]

It is now well established that infarction, not hemorrhage, is the most frequent stroke mechanism and accounts for two-thirds of stroke events in Japanese, be they resident in Japan or Hawaii. However, IH does occur several times more frequently in Japanese than in U.S. whites or blacks. There is also a difference in the site of the atherosclerotic arterial pathology with a predominance of intracranial disease in Japanese in contrast to the pattern in white Americans, in whom the extracranial arteries are the focus of most of the atherosclerotic occlusive disease. In Japan, including rural Japan, substantial changes have occurred in the diet since World War II. These include an increase in animal fat and animal protein and a reduction in the amount of sodium chloride in the diet.[95] This has been associated with a remarkable >75% decline in stroke deaths during the past 2 decades.[95]

Family History of Stroke

Although family history of stroke is perceived to be an important marker of increased stroke risk, confirmation by epidemiologic study has been lacking. In a recent report, maternal history of death from stroke was significantly related to stroke incidence in a cohort of Swedish men born in 1913.[116] Other significant risk factors included hypertension, abdominal pattern of obesity, and fibrinogen level; however, maternal history of fatal stroke was independently related to stroke even after these variables were taken into account.

In a study of familial predisposition to stroke in Framingham, there was no relationship between a history of stroke *death* in parents and documented stroke in subjects. However, definite nonfatal and fatal strokes in these cohort members were related to the occurrence of stroke in their children (members of the Framingham Offspring Study cohort). In these analyses, both maternal and paternal stroke were associated with approximately a 1.5-fold increased risk of stroke even after other risk factors were taken into account.[57] Thus, family history of stroke, so frequently acknowledged as a risk factor for stroke, has only recently been identified and documented by epidemiologic study.

Folic Acid to Reduce Total Plasma Homocysteine Levels

Elevated plasma levels of total homocysteine (tHcy) are associated with a higher incidence of CHD (OR 1.6/5-μmol/L tHcy) and an increased incidence of stroke, OR 1.5 per 5-μmol/L tHcy.[16] When folic acid is supplemented by approximately 200 μg/day in the diet, a reduction in tHcy levels of approximately 4 μmol/L is seen. The level of tHcy is directly related to most of the major components of the cardiovascular risk profile: male sex; increasing age; cigarette smoking; high blood pressure; elevated blood cholesterol level; and lack of exercise.[71] Clearly these risk factors need to be accounted for to estimate the independent impact of elevated tHcy levels on stroke incidence. A recent nested case-control study within the British Regional Heart Study cohort has demonstrated a powerful and independent relationship between nonfasting tHcy level and stroke incidence.[75] There was a graded increase in risk with increasing levels of tHcy (Fig. 1.18). Levels of <10.3 μmol/L (representing the lowest quartile) were the referent group; the risk factor-adjusted OR increased from 1.2 (10.3 to 12.49 μmol/L), to 2.6 (12.5 to 15.39 μmol/L), to 4.7 ($\geq$15.4 μmol/L) in successive quartiles of tHcy (P = 0.03 for trend). The risk in the uppermost quartile was 4.7-fold greater than in the lowest quartile. This was a graded response with no discernible threshold occurring after adjustment for serum creatinine (associated with increased tHcy levels), age, social class, blood pressure, and other pertinent risk factors.[75] However, in other large population studies no statistically significant relationship was found.[105,113] In the Atherosclerosis Risk in Communities study, a strong independent relationship was found between fasting plasma tHcy concentrations and carotid artery intimal-medial wall thickening.[66] Increased levels of fasting plasma Hcy were related to ultrasound-assessed extracranial common carotid artery stenosis $\geq$25% in the Framingham cohort.[90] Furthermore, levels of Hcy are inversely related to levels of dietary and plasma folic acid, as well as vitamins B_{12} and B_6.[90,91] The *fasting* tHcy level may miss persons with impaired Hcy metabolism since approximately 40% of persons with elevated Hcy levels in response to a methionine challenge, who are thought to be at increased cardiovascular risk, have normal fasting levels. Furthermore, the Hcy level is similar to other physiologic measures such as blood pressure or serum cholesterol—as a graded and continuous variable without clear threshold effect. A number of investigators have either called for or begun to mount clinical trials using dietary folic acid, 0.4 mg/day, to prevent MI and stroke recurrence[102,103] Dietary supplementation with folic acid (B_6)

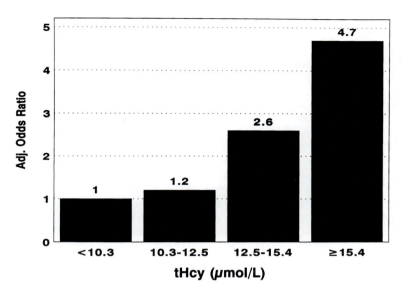

Figure 1.18 Homocysteine level and stroke risk in men; a case-control study. (from Wolf,[124] with permission.)

will reduce Hcy levels to their lowest even in persons with adequate dietary intake and normal plasma vitamin levels.[80,92,104] However, there is little or no risk to dietary supplementation, and the cost of these vitamins is minimal. Adding 1 mg of cyanocobalamin should alleviate concerns about masking pernicious anemia or B_{12} deficiency. It may well be that, in the near future, patients will be expected to know their Hcy levels as they are currently supposed to know their blood pressure and cholesterol levels.

ENVIRONMENTAL FACTORS

Cigarette Smoking

Cigarette smoking, a powerful risk factor for MI and sudden death, has been clearly linked to brain infarction, as well as to IH and SAH.[24,129] A similar relationship between cigarette smoking and stroke has been seen in Hawaiian Japanese men after 10 years of follow-up in the Honolulu Heart Study, with cigarette smoking making a significant independent contribution to cerebral infarction and intracranial hemorrhage risk.[2]

In the late 1970s, several studies of oral contraceptives (OCs) and stroke in young women identified cigarette smoking as an important risk factor. Surprisingly, the association among cigarette smoking, OCS, and stroke was primarily related to SAH. In the Royal College of General Practitioners Study of OC use, the increased risk of SAH occurred principally in women older than age 35, who were current or former OC users, and who smoked cigarettes.[81] In the Nurses' Health Study, a cohort of nearly 120,000 women was followed prospectively for 8 years for the development of stroke. There was an increased risk of SAH as well as thrombotic stroke in cigarette smokers. Relative risk of SAH showed a dose-response relationship from 4-fold in light smokers to 9.8-fold in smokers of 25 or more cigarettes daily.[81] In each smoking category the relative risk of SAH, whether or not other associated risk factors were taken into account, was twice as great as for thromboembolic stroke.

The association between cigarette smoking and SAH from aneurysm was also found in men (as well as women) in Framingham[86] and in New Zealand[14] in case-control analyses. In a case-control study of 114 patients with SAH in a defined region in Finland, cigarette smokers were significantly more prevalent in cases than in controls matched for age, sex, and domicile.[32] Relative risk of SAH in smokers, compared with nonsmokers, was 2.7 in men and 3.0 in women. The authors suggested that smoking promoted a temporary increase in blood pressure, which, acting in concert with the "metastatic emphysema effect," was responsible for SAH from cerebral aneurysm. No more reasonable hypothesis has been promulgated to explain this powerful relationship.

That cigarette smoking increases the risk of thrombotic stroke and SAH is generally accepted; the relationship of cigarette smoking to IH is less well established. Data from the Honolulu Heart Program firmly link cigarette smoking in Hawaiian men of Japanese ancestry to stroke both "thromboembolic and hemorrhagic".[2]

Risk of "hemorrhagic" stroke was significantly greater (relative risk 2.5) in cigarette smokers than in nonsmokers; this excess risk of stroke was independent and persisted at a relative risk of 2.8 even after the other associated risk factors of age, diastolic blood pressure, serum cholesterol, alcohol consumption, hematocrit, and body mass were taken into account.

In a meta-analysis of 32 separate studies, including those cited above, cigarette smoking was a significant independent contributor to stroke incidence in both sexes and at all ages, and was associated with an approximately 50% increased risk overall compared with nonsmokers.[96] The risk of stroke generally, and of ABI specifically, rose as the number of cigarettes smoked a day increased, in both men and women.

Oral Contraceptives

In the 1970s, risk of stroke was estimated to be increased five-fold in women using OCs. This increased risk was most marked in older women (i.e., older than age 35), predominantly in those with other cardiovascular risk factors, particularly hypertension and cigarette smoking.[98] The relative risk of stroke was higher in OC users and former users with risk concentrated in cigarette smokers older than age 35, However, the mechanism of stroke in OC users is unclear. Cerebral infarction is more likely to be due to thrombotic disease than to atherosclerosis; it is known that clotting is enhanced by the OC-induced increased platelet aggregability and by its alteration of clotting factors to favor thrombogenesis. In young women with unexplained ischemic stroke, the use of OCs is presumed to be the "cause" of the infarct; however, the stroke was attributed to OC use in no more than 10% of a series of carefully studied patients.[3] Of particular interest is the interaction among the older preparations of OCs (containing high doses of estrogens), cigarette smoking, and SAH. Prospective observation of over 40,000 women, half of whom were taking OCs, showed an increased risk of fatal SAH (not cerebral infarction) in women taking OCs. The risk was increased fourfold in cigarette smokers older than age 35, with most cases confined to this group.[81]

There was no increase in stroke or other cardiovascular disease in the Nurses' Health Study among former users of OCs.[106] An international ischemic stroke and OC study assessed the risk of stroke in women in Europe and in less developed countries.[118] The risk of stroke was increased, with an OR of 2.99 (95% CI 1.65 to 5.40) and was lowest in younger women, nonsmokers with recently checked and not elevated blood pressure. Women with hypertension had an OR of 10.7 (95% CI 2.04 to 56.6). In Europe, with the current use of low-dose OCs (<50 μg estrogen), the OR was 1.53 (95% CI 0.71 to 3.31).[118] In the United States, a population-based case-control study of OC use in women with stroke, in which the OC preparations contained the current low dose of estrogen, was conducted using the California Kaiser Permanente Medical Care Program.[76] Comparing current with former and never-users of OCs, the OR for ischemic stroke was 1.18 (95% CI 0.54 to 2.59) after adjustment for other risk factors for stroke.[76] Thus risk of ischemic stroke is quite low in women of childbearing age and is not definitely increased in nonsmokers without hypertension.

The OR for hemorrhagic stroke in OC users in the California Kaiser Permanente Program study was also not significantly increased. There was a positive (nonsignificant) interaction for hemorrhage in current users who smoked, with an OR of 3.64 (95% CI 0.95 to 13.87).[76] In the World Health Organization Collaborative Study, the risk of hemorrhagic stroke was not increased in younger women and was only slightly increased in older women.[117] The bulk of these hemorrhages were subarachnoid, 200 of 248 in Europe, and the risk was significantly increased in women aged 35 years or older. The OR for hemorrhage among current OC users aged 35 years or older who were current cigarette smokers was 3.91 (95% CI 1.54 to 9.89).[117]

Postmenopausal Estrogen

Although postmenopausal estrogen therapy, with and without progestin, has been associated with a decreased risk of coronary heart disease, little information is available on the influence on stroke incidence.[42] No convincing benefit has been demonstrated for stroke. On the other hand, there is little clear evidence that combined estrogen-progestin has an adverse influence on stroke risk, and it may be safely used for its cardioprotective and beneficial influence in reducing osteoporosis.

Alcohol Consumption

As in myocardial infarction, the impact of alcohol consumption on stroke risk is related to the amount of alcohol consumed. Heavy alcohol use, either habitual daily heavy alcohol consumption or binge drinking, seems to be related to higher rates of cardiovascular disease. Light or moderate alcohol consumption, on the other hand, is convincingly associated with a reduced incidence of CHD.[101] Light and moderate alcohol use tends to raise the HDL cholesterol and may be associated with a reduction in CHD incidence, while high levels of alcohol intake are linked to hypertension and hypertriglyceridemia and may, in this way, predispose to fatal and nonfatal CHD.

The relationship of alcohol consumption to stroke occurrence is less clearly elucidated. Available evidence suggests the existence of a U-shaped relationship between level of alcohol consumption and ischemic stroke risk. Minimal consumption or total abstinence and heavy alcohol consumption seem to increase ischemic stroke occurrence, while moderate alcohol use is associated with the lowest risk. The risk of stroke due to hemorrhage increases with the amount of alcohol consumed.[27] In the Honolulu Heart Study of men of Japanese ancestry, a powerful dose-response relationship was found between alcohol consumption and incidence of IH and SAH even after taking other pertinent risk factors, particularly blood pressure, into account. Increases in alcohol consumption were related to increasing levels of blood pressure and cigarette smoking and to lower serum cholesterol levels, all risk factors for IH. However, even after taking these factors into account, alcohol consumption was independently related to incidence of intracranial hemorrhage, both subarachnoid and intracerebral; no significant relationship was found between alcohol and thromboembolic stroke. The age-adjusted relative risk of IH for light drinkers (1 to 14 oz/month), compared with nondrinkers, was 2.1, for moderate drinkers (15 to 39 oz/month) it was 2.4, and for heavy drinkers (40+ oz/month) it was 4.0. After adjustment was made for the other associated risk factors, IH was 2.0, 2.0, and 2.4 times as frequent, respectively, in these alcohol consumption categories.[27] However, there was no significant relationship to thromboembolic stroke. Data from the Framingham study also suggest an increased incidence of brain infarction and stroke with increased levels of alcohol use, but only in men.

There are a number of mechanisms by which heavy alcohol consumption may predispose to and moderate alcohol consumption protect from stroke.[21] Cigarette smoking is more frequent in heavy drinkers and contributes to the hemoconcentration accompanying heavy alcohol consumption, which increases hematocrit and viscosity.[44] In addition, rebound thrombocytosis during abstinence has been observed. Cardiac rhythm disturbances, particularly AF, occur with alcohol intoxication, producing what has been termed *holiday heart*.[28] Acute alcohol intoxication has been named as a precipitating factor in stroke in young people, in both thrombotic stroke and SAH.[44,108] Others have found a relationship to acute intoxication; a case-control study failed to find an effect that was independent of other risk factors, particularly cigarette smoking.[41]

Physical Activity

Leisure-time and work-associated vigorous physical activity has been linked to lower CHD incidence. Vigorous exercise may exert a beneficial influence on risk factors for atherosclerotic disease by reducing elevated blood pressure as a result of weight loss and by reducing the pulse rate, raising the HDL and lowering the LDL cholesterol, improving glucose tolerance, and promoting a life style conducive to favorably changing detrimental health habits such as cigarette smoking. However, only recently has physical activity been found to be associated with reduced stroke incidence.[1,40,58,68,115] In Framingham, physical activity in subjects with a mean age of 65 years was associated with a reduced stroke incidence.[58] In men, the relative risk was 0.41 (95% CI 0.24 to 0.69; $P = 0.0007$) after accounting for the effects of potential confounders including systolic blood pressure; serum cholesterol; glucose intolerance; vital capacity; obesity; LVH on the ECG; AF; valvular heart disease; congestive heart failure; coronary heart disease; and occupation. However, there was no evidence of a protective effect of physical activity on risk of stroke in women. As in coronary heart disease, *moderate* physical activity conferred no less benefit than *heavy* activity levels. In a number of other population studies and in a series of case-control studies, low levels of physical activity were associated with increased incidence of stroke. Recently, a beneficial effect was found in women.[68]

A graded response to exercise was seen in 7,735 male British civil servants, aged 40 to 59 years, with the greatest benefit in reduced stroke incidence derived from the most intense level of exercise and an intermediate protective effect from medium levels.[115] In the Honolulu Heart Study of Hawaiian Japanese men, higher levels of physical activity (after adjustment for other risk factors) were associated with lower rates of both ischemic and hemorrhagic stroke.[1] Recent data from the NHANES 1 Epidemiologic Follow-up Study disclosed a consistent association of low levels of physical activity and an increased risk of stroke in women as well as men and in both blacks and whites.[40] Moderate levels of activity tended to provide an intermediate level of protection.[40]

Physical activity exerts a beneficial influence on risk factors for atherosclerotic disease by reducing blood pressure and weight, reducing the pulse rate, raising the HDL cholesterol and lowering the LDL cholesterol, decreasing platelet aggregability, and increasing insulin sensitivity and improving glucose tolerance, and promoting a life style conducive to changing diet and promoting cessation of cigarette smoking. Increased physical activity levels have now been rather convincingly associated with reduced incidence of stroke. Moderate levels of recreational and nonrecreational physical activity provide substantial benefit and may be recommended as a sensible life style modification to reduce the risk of cardiovascular disease including stroke.

Stroke Prevention Through Risk Factor Management

The rapid and remarkable 60% decline in death rates from stroke in the United States, and in most other industrialized nations since 1972, offers strong support to the hypothesis that modifiable environmental influences are operating. Part of the decline results from a reduction in the incidence and severity of stroke, which may be attributed to improved detection and treatment of hypertension over a 20-year span.[15] Based on data from randomized clinical trials and from observational study, we can conclude that stroke may be prevented, and perhaps stroke recurrence risk reduced, by a number of risk factor interventions. These include reducing elevated blood pressure; cessation of cigarette smoking; warfarin anticoagulation in AF; increasing physical activity and promoting weight reduction; and perhaps reducing elevated blood lipids with HMG-CoA reductase inhibitors. It is possible that by lowering plasma Hcy and by achieving better control of blood sugar in diabetics that further reductions may be achieved. It is probable that prevention and treatment of predisposing cardiac diseases (CHD, congestive heart failure, AF, increased left ventricular mass, and valvular heart disease) would also reduce stroke occurrence.

CONTROL OF HYPERTENSION AND STROKE PREVENTION

On the basis of a combined analysis of nine major prospective (observational) studies of 420,000 individuals, a graded relationship between diastolic pressure and stroke and CHD incidence was apparent.[65] There was no threshold level below which risk gradients were flat, implying a steadily increasing risk with increasing diastolic pressure *even in the normal range.* This impact was also seen in another meta-analysis of drug treatment for hypertension.[65] The incidence of stroke increased 46% and CHD increased 29% with a 7.5-mmHg increase in diastolic pressure.

These findings were validated by randomized trials of blood pressure reduction demonstrating that reducing elevated blood pressure prevented stroke.[25,63] The findings of 14 treatment trials in 37,000 hypertensive subjects should finally put to rest the long-standing concern that control of elevated blood pressure in hypertensives precipitates stroke. The average blood pressure reduction of 5.8 mmHg resulted in a reduction in stroke incidence of 42%. This observed reduction in stroke incidence closely approximated that expected on the basis of prospective observational studies.[25,63] In these studies, the duration of blood pressure reduction was brief, from 2 to 5 years. The dramatic impact on stroke incidence within this short period suggests that the treatment interrupted a precipitating factor rather than interfered with atherogenesis. Presumably, more prolonged blood pressure control would have both effects.

In virtually all treatment trials the diastolic pressure has been emphasized, although stroke risk is clearly directly related to systolic pressure levels.[52] In the elderly, in whom isolated elevation of the systolic pressure is common, it was thought that treatment would be ineffective in reducing pressure, hazardous in terms of side effects, and unwarranted on the basis of available epidemiologic data. In the Systolic Hypertension in the Elderly Program (SHEP Trial), 4,736 persons older than 60 years with systolic blood pressure levels >160 mmHg and diastolic pressures <90 mmHg were enrolled.[93] In the treated group, blood pressure reduction was associated with a 36% reduction in stroke and a 27% reduction in MI and coronary death after 4.5 years of follow-up. These findings have enormous importance, since two-thirds of all individuals with hypertension between the ages of 65 and 89 years have isolated systolic hypertension, and most strokes occur in this age group.[120]

It is clear from the SHEP Trial and from the European Working Party on Hypertension in the Elderly study that antihypertensive medication was well tolerated by the elderly.[7,99,120] SHEP demonstrated that reduction of pressure was accomplished with relative ease; approximately half of the patients were controlled with chlorthalidone alone, and reduction was well tolerated, as evidenced by 90% compliance rates in the active treatment group at 5 years. Since increased blood pressure is the most powerful risk factor for stroke, and since the benefits of treatment occur so promptly, control of increased blood pressure, systolic as well as diastolic, is the cornerstone of stroke prevention.

Only a small portion of the benefits derived from the treatment of elevated blood pressure in hypertensives has been achieved to date. An estimated 50 million Americans have elevated blood pressure (systolic blood pressure ≥ 140 mmHg and/or diastolic blood pressure ≥ 90 mmHg) or are taking antihypertensive medication.[50] While 65% of these 50 million are aware their blood pressure is elevated, and 49% are on treatment, in only 21% has blood pressure control been achieved. Thus, using the $\geq 140/\geq 90$ mmHg level, four-fifths of Americans are either unaware, untreated, or uncontrolled. Using the older classification, $\geq 160/\geq 95$ mmHg, the figures are 84% aware, 73% treated, and 55% controlled, which still leaves nearly half of American hypertensives uncontrolled.[50]

CESSATION OF CIGARETTE SMOKING

Based on data from Framingham and the Nurses' Health Study, it is clear that stroke risk in cigarette smokers is reduced by about 60% by smoking cessation.[56,129] This reduction in

risk occurs in a remarkably short time and is similar to the reduction in CHD risk, which decreases by approximately 50% within 1 year of smoking cessation and reaches the level of those who never smoked within 5 years. In Framingham, in both men and women, the risk of stroke in former cigarette smokers did not differ from that of persons who never smoked by the end of 5 years.[129] There was no interaction with age, suggesting that cigarette smoking exerted a precipitating effect on stroke regardless of age or duration of smoking. Similar findings from the Nurses' Health Study show a sizable reduction of risk within 2 years and a reduction to a relative risk of 0.4 (the same as for women who never smoked) from a referent level for current smokers of 1.0[56] (Fig. 1.19) Since smoking confers an increase in stroke risk of 40% in men and 60% in women, after all other pertinent risk factors have been taken into account, cessation may be expected to reduce the risk of stroke significantly.

WARFARIN ANTICOAGULATION IN ATRIAL FIBRILLATION

Prophylactic anticoagulation with warfarin is indicated in all persons with AF, with the possible exception of persons younger than age 65 with no history of hypertension, diabetes, TIA, or stroke, who are free of structural heart disease. Persons in whom anticoagulants are contraindicated may be placed on aspirin 325 mg/day. Based on currently available information, anticoagulation may be safely administered to persons older than age 75 years and should be continued indefinitely at an intensity of INR >2.0, with a target INR of 3.0.[30,48] Since there appears to be no lower risk of stroke in the presence of paroxysmal AF, warfarin is indicated in these patients as well. It is likely that further refinement of treatment guidelines will be forthcoming and high- and low-risk groups better defined.

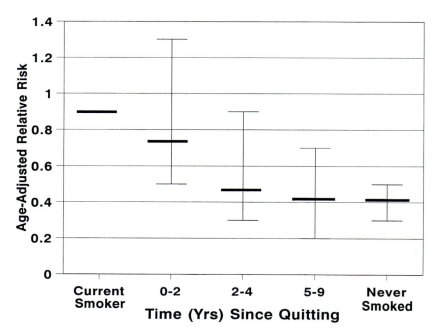

Figure 1.19 Smoking cessation and risk of stroke in women. Age-adjusted relative risks of total stroke in relation to time since stopping smoking. Current smoker was the reference category. Error bars represent 95% confidence intervals. (From Kawachi et al,[56] with permission.)

REDUCTION IN LDL CHOLESTEROL WITH STATINS

The recent evidence (from trials of HMG-CoA reductase inhibitors in men with elevated LDL cholesterol and usually pre-existing CHD) that treatment reduced stroke incidence opens a new area for stroke prevention. Since the influence of cholesterol on stroke appears to be less important than for CHD, some have speculated that other actions of the statins are responsible for the reduction in stroke incidence (which is equivalent to the reduction in CHD incidence in some studies).[112] The influence on hemorrheologic factors, plaque geometry, and plaque thrombogenicity and promotion of plaque regression[112] have been suggested.

PREVENTION AND TREATMENT OF HEART DISEASE INCLUDING ATRIAL FIBRILLATION

Since CHD, congestive heart failure, and AF predispose to stroke, prevention of these cardiovascular contributors can be anticipated to reduce incidence of stroke.[126] On the basis of current knowledge of the epidemiology of congestive heart failure, prevention of obesity and treatment of hypertension may be beneficial. Reduction of CHD risk requires, in addition to hypertension control and smoking cessation, dietary or pharmacologic treatment to reduce elevated total and LDL cholesterol and to increase the HDL cholesterol fraction. Prevention of AF might best be accomplished by preventing the appearance of the major precursor of AF, which is heart disease, particularly CHD.

PHYSICAL ACTIVITY

As with cigarette smoking, recently published data from observational studies strongly suggest an association between increased levels of physical activity and longer life span, and reduced cardiovascular disease including CHD and stroke. Whether benefit accrues from physical fitness and training over and above that achieved from weight reduction, blood pressure reduction, improved glucose tolerance, and other physiologic effects on clotting factors is unknown. There are conflicting data on the benefit of intensive versus moderate exercise. No randomized clinical trial data are likely to appear to bolster these data, but better measures of physical activity (recreational and nonrecreational) and physical fitness may help to clarify these issues. Nevertheless, the beneficial effects on vigor and feeling of well-being, as well as the positive effects on cardiovascular risk factors are compelling. It is clear that regular moderate physical activity should be an integral part of a life style that will help to reduce the risk of stroke and other cardiovascular diseases.

FOLIC ACID TO REDUCE TOTAL PLASMA HOMOCYSTEINE LEVELS

Several clinical trials are underway to determine if reduction of plasma Hcy levels by vitamin supplementation will reduce stroke or MI recurrence. It seems likely that the adverse effects of homocysteine will receive greater attention in the future.

INTENSIVE DIABETES THERAPY

Intensive therapy with insulin at three or more doses a day to achieve tight control of hyperglycemia in recent onset insulin-dependent diabetes mellitus was shown to reduce microvascular complications, nephropathy, and retinopathy as well as peripheral neuropathy.[26] The demonstration that improved glycemic control reduces some complications is the first clear evidence of what was previously thought likely but was unproved prior to the publications by the Diabetes Control and Complications Trial Research Group.[26] Whether improved glycemic control will reduce the risk of stroke and other cardiovascular diseases in diabetics remains to be seen, but such a reduction seems plausible. Reasoning by analogy, improved glycemic control in non–insulin-dependent diabetics, who constitute the majority of adult-onset diabetics, might be associated with decreased stroke occurrence.

IDENTIFICATION OF HIGH-RISK CANDIDATES FOR STROKE PREVENTION

Each physician can identify those patients at increased risk of stroke. Those with severe and moderately severe hypertension will definitely require aggressive pharmacologic treatment to achieve and maintain normotension and help to prevent stroke. However, the bulk of hypertensives are those with borderline elevations of blood pressure, (class 2 hypertension), accounting for 70% of all hypertensives.[50] Treatment of this entire large population with mild and borderline blood pressure elevation using drugs may not be necessary since non-pharmacologic measures may be effective. What is needed is a way of selecting persons at substantially increased risk of stroke and other cardiovascular diseases for intensive preventive intervention including pharmacologic treatment of hypertension. For the remainder, whose risk of stroke is average or only mildly increased, hygienic measures should be prescribed. These include weight loss and attention to diet, with reduction of salt, calories, and fat, and assurance of adequate amounts of fruits, vegetables, and potassium in the diet. In addition, cigarette smoking cessation, weight reduction, and moderate physical activity are all measures that can be advocated for most people.

To help identify persons at increased risk of stroke, a risk profile has been developed (utilizing data from 36 years of follow-up from Framingham) that allows the physician to de-

Figure 1.20 Bar graph of probability of stroke during 10 years in men aged 70 years at two systolic blood pressure levels: impact of other risk factors. Hyp Rx, antihypertensive therapy; DM, diabetes mellitus; Cigs, cigarette smoking; CVD, previously diagnosed coronary heart disease, cardiac failure, or intermittent claudication; AF, atrial fibrillation; LVH-ECG, left ventricular hypertrophy by electrocardiogram. (From Wolf et al,[128] with permission.)

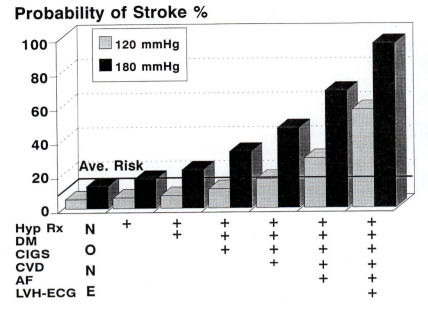

termine a patient's probability of stroke.[128] This can be done based on information collected from a medical history and physical examination, plus an ECG. Using a table that is sex specific, probability is determined by a point system depending on age; systolic blood pressure; antihypertensive therapy use; presence of diabetes; cigarette smoking; history of cardiovascular disease (CHD or congestive heart failure); and ECG abnormalities (LVH or AF). Risk is distributed over a wide range and permits the physician to relate a particular patient's probability of stroke quite quickly to that of an average person of the same age and sex.

The stroke risk profile will help the physician to identify which borderline hypertensives warrant pharmacologic treatment by virtue of an increased probability of stroke usually attributable to the presence of several other risk factor abnormalities (Fig. 1.20). Using the risk profile of a man aged 70 years with two systolic blood pressure levels (120 and 180 mmHg), it can be seen that the probability of stroke in 10 years ranges from less than half the average level to nearly 100% depending on the risk factor burden. In the presence of multiple risk factor abnormalities, the probability of stroke may be higher in the presence of a normal systolic blood pressure of 120 mmHg than in a man with a pressure of 180 mmHg who is free of diabetes and cardiovascular disease and who is a nonsmoker. This risk profile provides a quantitative assessment of the level of risk that is particularly helpful in the presence of multiple borderline risk factor abnormalities. The graphic and percentage display provides the patient (and the physician) with a concrete estimate that the probability of stroke is below, at, or several fold above average. It also provides an illustration of how certain risk factors, treatment of which has been demonstrated to reduce stroke risk, may result in a decrease in stroke probability. A patient can be shown that reduction of the systolic blood pressure from 180 mmHg to ≤140 mmHg by treatment, cessation of cigarette smoking, and administration of warfarin anticoagulation if AF is present may reduce a significantly elevated risk to nearly normal.[128]

The profile may be used to select persons at highest probability of stroke for antihypertensive drug treatment. For example, by restricting drug treatment to persons with a borderline systolic blood pressure level who have two or more other risk factor abnormalities, (not including age and male sex), it is possible to identify a group consisting of 22% of the men and 14% of women at high risk. In this group approximately 40% of strokes will occur within the subsequent 10 years.[128]

A substantially increased risk of stroke also exists in other situations: recent TIA, particularly in the presence of internal carotid artery stenosis ≥70%; recent onset AF; recent MI; during and immediately following cardiac surgery and cerebral angiography; and others dealt with elsewhere in this volume.

Acknowledgements

This study was supported in part by grants 2-RO1-NS-17950-13 (National Institute of Neurological Disorders and Stroke), RO1-HL40423 (National Institute on Aging, National Heart, Lung, and Blood Institute), and contract NIH-NO1-HC-38038 (National Heart, Lung, Blood Institute).

References

1. Abbott RD, Yin Y, Reed DM, Yano K: Risk of stroke in male cigarette smokers. N Engl J Med 315:717–720, 1986
2. Abbott RD, Rodriguez BL, Burchfiel CM, Curb JD: Physical activity in older middle-aged men and reduced

risk of stroke: the Honolulu Heart Program. Am J Epidemiol 139:881–893, 1994

3. Adams HP Jr, Butler MJ, Biller J, Toffol GJ: Nonhemorrhagic cerebral infarction in young adults. Arch Neurol 43:793–796, 1986

4. Adams HP Jr, Byington RP, Hoen H et al: Effect of cholesterol-lowering medications on progression of mild atherosclerotic lesions of the carotid arteries and on the risk of stroke. Cerebrovasc Dis 5:171–177, 1995

5. Ahmed OI, Orchard TJ, Sharma R et al: Declining mortality from stroke in Allegheny County, Pennsylvania. Trends in case fatality and severity of disease, 1971–1980. Stroke 19:181–184, 1988

6. American Heart Association: Heart and Stroke Facts Statistics: 1997 Statistical Supplement. American Heart Association, Dallas, 1997

7. Amery A, Birkenhager W, Brixko P et al: Mortality and morbidity results from the European Working Party on High Blood Pressure in the Elderly trial. Lancet 1:1349–1354, 1985

8. Atkins D, Psaty BM, Koepsell TD et al: Cholesterol reduction and the risk for stroke in men. A meta-analysis of randomized, controlled trials. Ann Intern Med 119:136–145, 1993

9. Atrial Fibrillation Investigators: Risk factors for stroke and efficacy of antithrombotic therapy in atrial fibrillation. Arch Intern Med 154:1449–1457, 1994

10. Aurell M, Hood B: Cerebral hemorrhage in a population after a decade of active antihypertensive treatment. Acta Med Scand 176:377–383, 1964

11. Barrett Connor E, Khaw KT: Diabetes mellitus: an independent risk factor for stroke? Am J Epidemiol 128:116–123, 1988

12. Benfante R, Yano K, Hwang LJ et al: Elevated serum cholesterol is a risk factor for both coronary heart disease and thromboembolic stroke in Hawaiian Japanese men. Implications for shared risk. Stroke 25:814–820, 1994

13. Bikkina M, Levy D, Evans JC et al: Left ventricular mass and risk of stroke in an elderly cohort. JAMA 272:33–36, 1994

14. Bonita R: Cigarette smoking, hypertension and the risk of subarachnoid hemorrhage: a population-based case-control study. Stroke 17:831–835, 1986

15. Bonita R, Beaglehole R: The enigma of the decline in stroke deaths in the United States. The search for an explanation. Stroke 27:370–372, 1996

16. Boushey CJ, Beresford SAA, Omenn GS, Motulsky AG: A quantitative assessment of plasma homocysteine as a risk factor for vascular disease. Probable benefits of increasing folic acid intakes. JAMA 274:1049–1057, 1995

17. Broderick JP, Phillips SJ, Whisnant JP: Incidence rates of stroke in the eighties: the end of the decline in stroke? Stroke 20:577–582, 1989

18. Brown RD, Whisnant JP, Sicks JD et al: Stroke incidence, prevalence, and survival: secular trends in Rochester, Minnesota, through 1989. Stroke 27:373–380, 1996

19. Burchfiel CM, Curb JD, Rodriguez BL et al: Glucose intolerance and 22-year stroke incidence. The Honolulu Heart Program. Stroke 25:951–957, 1994

20. Byington RP, Jukema JW, Salonen JT et al: Reduction in cardiovascular events during pravastatin therapy. Pooled analysis of clinical events of the pravastatin atherosclerosis intervention program. Circulation 92:2419–2425, 1995

21. Camargo CA Jr: Moderate alcohol consumption and stroke. The epidemiologic evidence. Stroke 20:1611–1626, 1989

22. Chesebro JH, Fuster V, Halperin JL: Atrial fibrillation—risk marker for stroke. N Engl J Med 323:1556–1558, 1990

23. Colandrea MA, Friedman GD, Nichaman MZ, Lynd CN: Systolic hypertension in the elderly. An epidemiologic assessment. Circulation 41:239–245, 1970

24. Colditz GA, Bonita R, Stampfer MJ et al: Cigarette smoking and risk of stroke in middle-aged women. N Engl J Med 318:937–941, 1988

25. Collins R, Peto R, MacMahon S et al: Blood pressure, stroke, and coronary heart disease. Part 2, Short-term reductions in blood pressure: overview of randomised drug trials in their epidemiological context. Lancet 335:827–838, 1990

26. Diabetes Control and Complications Trial Research Group: The effect of intensive diabetes therapy on the development and progression of neuropathy. The Diabetes Control and Complications Trial Research Group. Ann Intern Med 122:561–568, 1995

27. Donahue RP, Abbott RD, Reed DM, Yano K: Alcohol and hemorrhagic stroke. The Honolulu Heart Program. JAMA 255:2311–2314, 1986

28. Ettinger PO, Wu CF, De La Cruz C Jr et al: Arrhythmias and the "holiday heart": alcohol-associated cardiac rhythm disorders. Am Heart J 95:555–562, 1978

29. European Atrial Fibrillation Trial Study Group (EAFT): Secondary prevention in non-rheumatic atrial fibrillation after transient ischaemic attack or minor stroke. Lancet 342:1255–1262, 1993

30. European Atrial Fibrillation Trial Study Group: Optimal oral anticoagulant therapy in patients with nonrheumatic atrial fibrillation and recent cerebral ischemia. The European Atrial Fibrillation Trial Study Group. N Engl J Med 333:5–10, 1995

31. Fine-Edelstein JS, Wolf PA, O'Leary DH et al: Precursors of extracranial carotid atherosclerosis in the Framingham Study. Neurology 44:1046–1050, 1994

32. Fogelholm R, Murros K: Cigarette smoking and subarachnoid haemorrhage: a population-based case-control study. J Neurol Neurosurg Psychiatry 50:78–80, 1987

33. Folsom AR, Qamhieh HT, Flack JM et al: Plasma fibrinogen: levels and correlates in young adults. Am J Epidemiol 138:1023–1036, 1993

34. Furberg CD, Adams HP Jr, Applegate WB et al: Effect of lovastatin on early carotid atherosclerosis and cardiovascular events. Asymptomatic Carotid Artery Progression Study (ACAPS) Research Group. Circulation 90:1679–1687, 1994

35. Furlan AJ, Whisnant JP, Elveback LR: The decreasing incidence of primary intracerebral hemorrhage: a population study. Ann Neurol 5:367–373, 1979

36. Garraway WM, Whisnant JP, Drury I: The changing pat-

tern of survival following stroke. Stroke 14:699–703, 1983

37. Garraway WM, Whisnant JP, Furlan AJ et al: The declining incidence of stroke. N Engl J Med 300:449–452, 1979

38. Gillum RF: Stroke in blacks. Stroke 19:1–9, 1988

39. Gillum RF: The epidemiology of stroke in Native Americans. Stroke 26:514–521, 1995

40. Gillum RF, Mussolino ME, Ingram DD: Physical activity and stroke incidence in women and men. The NHANES I Epidemiologic Follow-Up Study. Am J Epidemiol 143:860–869, 1996

41. Gorelick PB: The status of alcohol as a risk factor for stroke. Stroke 20:1607–1610, 1989

42. Grodstein F, Stampfer MJ, Manson JE et al: Postmenopausal estrogen and progestin use and the risk of cardiovascular disease. N Engl J Med 335:453–461, 1996

43. Harmsen P, Tsipogianni A, Wilhelmsen L: Stroke incidence rates were unchanged, while fatality rates declined, during 1971–1987 in Goteborg, Sweden. Stroke 23:1410–1415, 1992

44. Hillbom M, Kaste M, Rasi V: Can ethanol intoxication affect hemocoagulation to increase the risk of brain infarction in young adults? Neurology 33:381–384, 1983

45. Howard G, Craven TE, Sanders L, Evans GW: Relationship of hospitalized stroke rate and in-hospital mortality to the decline in US stroke mortality. Neuroepidemiology 10:251–259, 1991

46. Howard G, Evans GW, Pearce K et al: Is the stroke belt disappearing? An analysis of racial, temporal, and age effects. Stroke 26:1153–1158, 1995

47. Howard G, Toole JF, Becker C et al: Changes in survival following stroke in five North Carolina counties observed during two different periods. Stroke 20:345–350, 1989

48. Hylek EM, Skates SJ, Sheehan MA, Singer DE: An analysis of the lowest effective intensity of prophylactic anticoagulation for patients with nonrheumatic atrial fibrillation. N Engl J Med 335:540–546, 1996

49. Iso H, Jacobs DR Jr, Wentworth D et al: Serum cholesterol levels and six-year mortality from stroke in 350,977 men screened for the multiple risk factor intervention trial. N Engl J Med 320:904–910, 1989

50. JNC: The Fifth Report of the Joint National Committee on Detection, Evaluation, and Treatment of High Blood Pressure. NIH Publication no. 93–1088. NIH, Bethesda, MD, 1993

51. Kannel WB, D'Agostino RB, Belanger AJ: Fibrinogen, cigarette smoking, and risk of cardiovascular disease: insights from the Framingham Study. Am Heart J 113: 1006–1010, 1987

52. Kannel WB, Dawber TR, Sorlie P, Wolf PA: Components of blood pressure and risk of atherothrombotic brain infarction: the Framingham study. Stroke 7: 327–331, 1976

53. Kannel WB, McGee DL: Diabetes and cardiovascular disease, the Framingham Study. JAMA 241:2035–2038, 1979

54. Kannel WB, Wolf PA, Castelli WP, D'Agostino RB: Fibrinogen and risk of cardiovascular disease. The Framingham Study. JAMA 258:1183–1186, 1987

55. Kannel WB, Wolf PA, McGee DL et al: Systolic blood pressure, arterial rigidity, and risk of stroke. The Framingham study. JAMA 245:1225–1229, 1981

56. Kawachi I, Colditz GA, Stampfer MJ et al: Smoking cessation and decreased risk of stroke in women. JAMA 269:232–236, 1993

57. Kiely DK, Wolf PA, Cupples LA et al: Familial aggregation of stroke: the Framingham Study. Stroke 24: 1366–1371, 1993

58. Kiely DK, Wolf PA, Cupples LA et al: Physical Activity and Stroke Risk: The Framingham Study. Am J Epidemiol 140:608–620, 1994

59. Kittner SJ, White LR, Losonczy KG et al: Black-white differences in stroke incidence in a national sample. The contribution of hypertension and diabetes mellitus. JAMA 264:1267–1270, 1990

60. Lee AJ, Lowe GD, Woodward M, Tunstall-Pedoe H: Fibrinogen in relation to personal history of prevalent hypertension, diabetes, stroke, intermittent claudication, coronary heart disease, and family history: the Scottish Heart Health Study. Br Heart J 69:338–342, 1993

61. Li S, Schoenberg BS, Wang C, et al: Cerebrovascular disease in the People's Republic of China: epidemiologic and clinical features. Neurology (Cleve) 35:1708–1713, 1985

62. Loh E, Sutton MSJ, Wun CC et al: Ventricular dysfunction and the risk of stroke after myocardial infarction. N Engl J Med 336:251–257, 1997

63. MacMahon S, Peto R, Cutler J, et al: Blood pressure, stroke, and coronary heart disease. Part 1, Prolonged differences in blood pressure: prospective observational studies corrected for the regression dilution bias. Lancet 335:765–774, 1990

64. MacMahon B, Pugh TF, Ipsen J: Epidemiologic Methods. Little, Brown, Boston, 1960

65. MacMahon S, Rodgers A: The epidemiological association between blood pressure and stroke: implications for primary and secondary prevention. Hypertens Res, Suppl. 17:S23–S32, 1994

66. Malinow MR, Nieto FJ, Szklo M et al: Carotid artery intimal-medical wall thickening and plasma homocysteine in asymptomatic adults. The Atherosclerosis Risk in Communities Study. Circulation 87:1107–1113, 1993

67. Malmgren R, Warlow C, Bamford J, Sandercock P: Geographical and secular trends in stroke incidence. Lancet 2:1196–1200, 1987

68. Manson JE, Stampfer MJ, Willett WC et al: Physical activity and incidence of coronary heart disease and stroke in women. Circulation 91:927, 1995

69. Miller VT, Rothrock JF, Pearce LA et al: Ischemic stroke in patients with atrial fibrillation: effect of aspirin according to stroke mechanism. Neurology 43:32–36, 1993

70. National Institutes of Health: Morbidity and mortality: 1996 Chartbook on Cardiovascular, Lung, and Blood Diseases. NIH, Bethesda, MD, 1996

71. Nygard O, Vollset SE, Refsum H, et al: Total plasma homocysteine and cardiovascular risk profile. The Hordaland Homocysteine Study. JAMA 274:1526–1533, 1995

72. O'Leary DH, Anderson KM, Wolf PA et al: Cholesterol

and carotid atherosclerosis in older persons: the Framingham Study. Ann Epidemiol 2:147–153, 1992

73. O'Leary DH, Polak JF, Kronmal RA et al: Thickening of the carotid wall. A marker for atherosclerosis in the elderly? Stroke 27:224–231, 1996

74. Otten MW Jr, Teutsch SM, Williamson DF, Marks JS: The effect of known risk factors on the excess mortality of black adults in the United States. JAMA 263:845–850, 1990

75. Perry IJ, Refsum H, Morris RW et al: Prospective study of serum total homocysteine concentration and risk of stroke in middle-aged British men. Lancet 346: 1395–1398, 1995

76. Petitti DB, Sidney S, Bernstein A et al: Stroke in users of low-dose oral contraceptives. N Engl J Med 335:8–15, 1996

77. Prospective Studies Collaboration: Cholesterol, diastolic blood pressure and stroke: 13,000 strokes in 450,000 people in 45 prospective cohorts. Lancet 346: 1647–1653, 1995

78. Reed DM: The paradox of high risk of stroke in populations with low risk of coronary heart disease. Am J Epidemiol 131:579–588, 1990

79. Robins M, Baum HM: The National Survey of Stroke. Stroke 75:I–45–I–57, 1981

80. Robinson K, Mayer EL, Miller DP et al: Hyperhomocysteinemia and low pyridoxal phosphate. Common and independent reversible risk factors for coronary artery disease. Circulation 92:2825–2830, 1995

81. Royal College of General Practitioners' Oral Contraception Study: Further analyses of mortality in oral contraceptive users. Lancet 1:541–546, 1981

82. Rutan GH, McDonald RH, Kuller LH: A historical perspective of elevated systolic vs diastolic blood pressure from an epidemiological and clinical trial viewpoint. J Clin Epidemiol 42:663–673, 1989

83. Sacco RL, Ellenberg JH, Mohr JP et al: Infarcts of undetermined cause: the NINCDS Stroke Data Bank. Ann Neurol 25:382–390, 1989

84. Sacco RL, Hauser WA, Mohr JP, Foulkes MA: One-year outcome after cerebral infarction in whites, blacks, and Hispanics. Stroke 22:305–311, 1991

85. Sacco RL, Shi T, Zamanillo MC, Kargman DE: Predictors of mortality and recurrence after hospitalized cerebral infarction in an urban community: the Northern Manhattan Stroke Study. Neurology 44:626–634, 1994

86. Sacco RL, Wolf PA, Bharucha NE et al: Subarachnoid and intracerebral hemorrhage: natural history, prognosis, and precursive factors in the Framingham Study. Neurology 34:847–854, 1984

87. Sacks FM, Pfeffer MA, Moye LA et al: The effect of pravastatin on coronary events after myocardial infarction in patients with average cholesterol levels. Cholesterol and Recurrent Events Trial investigators. N Engl J Med 335:1001–1009, 1996

88. Sagie A, Larson MG, Levy D: The natural history of borderline isolated systolic hypertension. N Engl J Med 329:1912–1917, 1993

89. Scandinavian Simvastatin Survival Study Group: Randomised trial of cholesterol lowering in 4444 patients with coronary heart disease: the Scandinavian Simvastatin Survival Study (4S). Lancet 344:1383–1389, 1994

90. Selhub J, Jacques PF, Bostom AG et al: Association between plasma homocysteine concentrations and extracranial carotid-artery stenosis. N Engl J Med 332: 286–291, 1995

91. Selhub J, Jacques PF, Bostom AG et al: Relationship between plasma homocysteine, vitamin status and extracranial carotid-artery stenosis in the Framingham Study population. J Nutr 126:1258S–1265S, 1996

92. Selhub J, Jacques PF, Wilson PWF et al: Vitamin status and intake as primary determinants of homocysteinemia in an elderly population. JAMA 270:2693–2698, 1993

93. SHEP Cooperative Research Group: Prevention of Stroke by antihypertensive drug treatment in older persons with isolated systolic hypertension. Final results of the Systolic Hypertension in the Elderly Program (SHEP). JAMA 265:3255–3264, 1991

94. Shepherd J, Cobbe SM, Ford I et al: Prevention of coronary heart disease with pravastatin in men with hypercholesterolemia. West of Scotland Coronary Prevention Study Group. N Engl J Med 333:1301–1307, 1995

95. Shimamoto T, Komachi Y, Inada H et al: Trends for coronary heart disease and stroke and their risk factors in Japan. Circulation 79:503–515, 1989

96. Shinton R, Beevers G: Meta-analysis of relation between cigarette smoking and stroke. BMJ 298:789–794, 1989

97. Smith P, Arnesen H, Holme I: The effect of warfarin on mortality and reinfarction after myocardial infarction. N Engl J Med 323:147–152, 1990

98. Stadel BV: Oral contraceptives and cardiovascular disease (second of two parts). N Engl J Med 305:672–677, 1981

99. Staessen J, Amery A, Birkenhager W et al: Syst-Eur—a multicenter trial on the treatment of isolated systolic hypertension in the elderly: first interim report. J Cardiovasc Pharmacol 19:120–125, 1992

100. Stafford RS, Singer DE: National patterns of warfarin use in atrial fibrillation. Arch Intern Med 156: 2537–2541, 1996

101. Stampfer MJ, Colditz GA, Willett WC et al: A prospective study of moderate alcohol consumption and the risk of coronary disease and stroke in women. N Engl J Med 319:267–273, 1988

102. Stampfer MJ, Malinow MR: Can lowering homocysteine levels reduce cardiovascular risk? N Engl J Med 332: 328–329, 1995

103. Stampfer MJ, Rimm EB: Folate and cardiovascular disease. Why we need a trial now. JAMA 275:1929–1930, 1996

104. Stampfer M, Willett W: Homocysteine and marginal vitamin deficiency: the importance of adequate vitamin intake. JAMA 270:2726–2727, 1993

105. Stampfer MJ, Malinow MR, Willett WC et al: A prospective study of plasma homocyst(e)ine and risk of myocardial infarction in US physicians. JAMA 268:877–881, 1992

106. Stampfer MJ, Willett WC, Colditz GA et al: A prospective study of past use of oral contraceptive agents and risk of cardiovascular diseases. N Engl J Med 319: 1313–1317, 1988b

107. Stroke Prevention in Atrial Fibrillation Investigators: Adjusted-dose warfarin versus low-intensity, fixed-dose warfarin plus aspirin for high-risk patients with atrial fibrillation: Stroke Prevention in Atrial Fibrillation III randomized clinical trial. Lancet 348:633–638, 1996
108. Taylor JR, Combs Orme T: Alcohol and strokes in young adults. Am J Psychiatry 142:116–118, 1985
109. Tell GS, Crouse JR, Furberg CD: Relation between blood lipids, lipoproteins, and cerebrovascular atherosclerosis. A review. Stroke 19:423–430, 1988
110. Thom TJ: Stroke mortality trends. An international perspective. Ann Epidemiol 3:509–518, 1993
111. US Bureau of the Census: Statistical Abstract of the United States: 1995. 115th Ed. US Bureau of the Census, Washington, DC, 1995
112. Vaughan CJ, Murphy MB, Buckley BM: Statins do more than just lower cholesterol. Lancet 348:1079–1082, 1996
113. Verhoef P, Hennekens CH, Malinow MR et al: A prospective study of plasma homocyst(e)ine and risk of ischemic stroke. Stroke 25:1924–1930, 1994
114. Walker SP, Rimm EB, Ascherio A et al: Body size and fat distribution as predictors of stroke among US men. Am J Epidemiol 144:1143–1150, 1996
115. Wannamethee G, Shaper AG: Physical activity and stroke in British middle aged men. BMJ 304:597–601, 1992
116. Welin L, Svardsudd K, Wilhelmsen L et al: Analysis of risk factors for stroke in a cohort of men born in 1913. N Engl J Med 317:521–526, 1987
117. WHO Collaborative Study of Cardiovascular Disease and Steroid Hormone Contraception: Haemorrhagic stroke, overall stroke risk, and combined oral contraceptives: results of an international, multicentre, case-control study. Lancet 348:505–510, 1996
118. WHO Collaborative Study of Cardiovascular Disease and Steroid Hormone Contraception: Ischaemic stroke and combined oral contraceptives: results of an international, multicentre, case-control study. Lancet 348:498–505, 1996
119. Wilhelmsen L, Svardsudd K, Korsan Bengtsen K et al: Fibrinogen as a risk factor for stroke and myocardial infarction. N Engl J Med 311:501–505, 1984
120. Wilking SV, Belanger A, Kannel WB et al: Determinants of isolated systolic hypertension. JAMA 260:3451–3455, 1988
121. Wilson PWF, Hoeg JM, Belanger AJ et al: Cholesterol-years, blood pressure-years, pack-years and carotid stenosis. Circulation 92:I–519, 1995
122. Wilson WF, Kannel WB: Hypertension, other risk factors, and the risk of cardiovascular disease. pp. 99–114. In: Laragh JH, Brenner BM (eds): Hypertension: Pathophysiology, Diagnosis, and Management. Raven Press, New York, 1995. Vol. I.
123. Wolf PA: Cereorovascular disease in the elderly. pp. 125–148. In Tresch DD, Aronow WS (eds): Cardiovascular Disease in the Elderly Patient. Marcel Dekker, New York, 1993
124. Wolf PA: Epidemiology and risk factor management. pp. 751–757. In Welch M et al (eds): Primer on Cerebrovascular Disease. Academic Press, San Diego, 1997
125. Wolf PA, Abbott RD, Kannel WB: Atrial fibrillation: a major contributor to stroke in the elderly. The Framingham Study. Arch Intern Med 147:1561–1564, 1987
126. Wolf PA, Abbott RD, Kannel WB: Atrial fibrillation as an independent risk factor for stroke: the Framingham Study. Stroke 22:983–988, 1991
127. Wolf PA, D'Agostino RB, Belanger AJ et al: Are blood lipids risk factors for stroke? Stroke 22:26, 1991
128. Wolf PA, D'Agostino RB, Belanger AJ, Kannel WB: Probability of stroke: a risk profile from the Framingham Study. Stroke 22:312–318, 1991
129. Wolf PA, D'Agostino RB, Kannel WB et al: Cigarette smoking as a risk factor for stroke. The Framingham Study. JAMA 259:1025–1029, 1988
130. Wolf PA, D'Agostino RB, O'Neal MA et al: Secular trends in stroke incidence and mortality. The Framingham Study. Stroke 23:1551–1555, 1992
131. Wolf PA, Kannel WB, McNamara PM, Gordon T: The role of impaired cardiac function in atherothrombotic brain infarction: the Framingham study. Am J Public Health 63:52–58, 1973
132. Yano K, Reed DM, MacLean CJ: Serum cholesterol and hemorrhagic stroke in the Honolulu Heart Program. Stroke 20:1460–1465, 1989

CHAPTER 2

Atherosclerosis

FRANK M. YATSU

CARLOS VILLAR-CORDOVA

Since the review of atherosclerosis in the second edition of *Stroke* in 1992, a tremendous amount of research has defined with greater precision the cellular and molecular defects accounting for the causes of atherosclerosis, the major etiology of strokes.[19] Despite this literal explosion of research worldwide, the exact mechanisms causing atherosclerosis have not yet been defined, although clearly they are multifactorial.[14,19,44,46,66] In this update on atherosclerosis as it relates to strokes or atherothrombotic brain infarction (ABI), emphasis is placed on the current studies without repeating important previous findings, particularly those reviewed in the second edition of *Stroke*.[19] These older studies focused on molecular biologic investigations, such as sequencing of various lipoproteins that carry cholesterol and triglycerides in the bloodstream as well as the various receptors for the lipoproteins, like the low density lipoprotein (LDL) receptor.[1,6,10,19,76]

Since 1992, further insights into the pathophysiology of atherosclerosis have been gained by investigations into the mechanisms regulating smooth muscle cell (SMC) proliferation (an important and integral factor in atherogenesis), the role of lipids in aggravating and indeed provoking atherogenesis, and the now recognized functions played by inflammatory factors.[18,25,35,36,40,48–53] In addition to a review of these aspects, a practical approach toward the treatment of risk factors for atherosclerosis is outlined, to reduce both stroke and myocardial infarction.[37]

Figure 2.1 depicts a static view of the dynamic arterial wall. The major constituents of the artery include (1) the endothelial cell (EC); (2) the basement membrane; (3) the media, made up primarily of SMCs; and (4) the adventitia. The artery exists in a dynamic state with a turnover of its constituents, such as ECs, and a constant change in its reactivity to its environment, such as arterial pressure changes, ischemia, shear stress, and inflammation. In the process of atherogenesis, the major changes occur both intraluminally and within the arterial wall. Although the atheroma is primarily an expression of endothelial overgrowth of SMCs and monocyte-derived macrophages, which become foam cells, each constituent is involved in this pathologic conversion to an atheromatous plaque.[10,15,17,18,20,21,25,29,35,40,48–54,57,58,65,71,72,74,75,77]

Although all ECs are everywhere continuous and nonthrombogenic, like "Teflon," the ECs throughout the body are not identical. ECs in different organs have subtle but distinct differences, reflecting in part the special requirements of the organs or the EC environment.[3] For example, upregulation of surface antigens for the liver or brain would be expected to have differing requirements (as they indeed do) than do those of the adipose tissue.[3] As discussed in the chapter on thrombolysis (Chapter 9), EC surfaces possess both procoagulant and anticoagulant activities with, for example, the surface expression of tissue plasminogen activator and plasminogen activator inhibitor-1. Although these factors may not play a direct role in atherogenesis, their aberration under pathologic states of atherosclerosis may favor thrombosis.[20,24,54]

The atheromatous plaque is characterized histologically by five factors: (1) increase in cholesterol, particularly cholesterol-esters; (2) increase in connective tissue elements, especially elastins and glycosaminoglycans; (3) SMC proliferation, an important hallmark of atherosclerosis; (4) presence of foam cells, the lipid-laden macrophages; and (5) inflammatory cells. Each of these abnormalities has been the focus of research investigations, although abnormalities in cholesterol metabolism and increase in the proliferation of SMCs have received the most attention. This review focuses primarily on studies dealing with these abnormalities as well as those showing an involvement of inflammatory reactions. The theory supporting an abnormality in lipid metabolism is known as the *lipid hypothesis*, and that favoring the abnormal proliferation of SMCs is known as the *injury-healing hypothesis*.[10,38,62,77]

Lipid Hypothesis of Atherogenesis

The oldest and most popular theory of the cause of atherosclerosis is the lipid hypothesis; it has morphologic plus animal and human studies to support its relevance and importance.

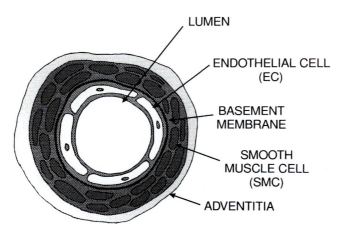

Figure 2.1 Normal arterial histology. Diagrammatic cross section showing the lumen, endothelial cell, basement membrane, and smooth muscle cells of the media and the adventitia. Each constituent of the arterial wall is in dynamic equilibrium and is metabolically active.

Morphologically, the oldest observations of atheromas related to the high lipids content, particularly cholesterol-esters. As a result, earlier studies focused primarily on the obviously important role of cholesterol in atherogenesis, although for a long time this association was not thought to be relevant for cerebrovascular atherosclerosis.[47,69] This notion arose in part from the frequent finding that elderly subjects, who are most likely to suffer from strokes, have reduced levels of plasma cholesterol, unlike coronary artery disease patients. However, since the development of cerebrovascular atherosclerosis typically takes a much longer time than coronary artery disease, the antecedent, as opposed to proximate, history of a subject's lipid profile is more important; the relatively earlier appearance of coronary artery disease is provoked by the mechanical motion to which these arteries are constantly exposed. Even so, recent studies show a relationship between blood lipids and atherosclerosis.[30] For example, studies show a correlation between carotid bifurcation atheroma progression and plasma concentration of LDL as well as abnormal metabolism of both LDL and high density lipoprotein (HDL) in strokes due to atherosclerosis; changes are seen that favor retention of LDL (the bad cholesterol), whereas HDL (the good cholesterol) is catabolized more rapidly.[30,77]

Plasma cholesterol (particularly LDL) has a relationship with ABI; in addition, treatment of subjects with elevated cholesterol using cholesterol-lowering drugs (such as the statins, which inhibit the rate-limiting step in cholesterol synthesis of hydroxy-methyl-glutaryl coenzyme A reductase [HMG-CoA reductase]), has shown that both carotid artery thickness and stroke incidence are reduced.[22,64] For coronary artery disease, the benefits of cholesterol lowering are apparent for both marked and moderately elevated LDL, but no appreciable differences are seen when LDL levels are relatively normal (≤125 mg/dl).[64] Since the arterial tree is continuous everywhere in the body, these findings have implications for the prevention of ABI: prudent approaches to cholesterol levels for coronary artery disease subjects would be similarly applicable to those at risk of ABIs.[4,45]

Advances in atherosclerosis research over the past 4 decades (since the time plasma lipoproteins were first isolated in the mid-1950s by ultracentrifugation) have paralleled the remarkable progress made in research techniques, methodologies, and insights, for example, improved techniques for particle separation of molecular biologic probes. The focus of research progressed from the relatively crude measurement of plasma cholesterol to identifying the precise apoprotein envelope of these lipids with the gene sequence of the apoproteins and their receptors, discussed in the second edition of *Stroke*. At the present time, over 100 potential genes and their abnormalities or dysregulation may contribute to atherogenesis, a clearly multifactorial disease process.[44]

Since lipoprotein metabolism and its understanding will give the clinician insights into rational treatment strategies aimed at reducing atherosclerosis, the metabolism of LDL and HDL is reviewed. Following a discussion of the role of SMC proliferation in atherogenesis (which forms the second most popular theory on atherosclerosis), the two are discussed together, as they are probably synergistic in humans. Historically, the various lipid fractions in isolation were compared with plasma, and the nomenclature that persists today is descriptive without providing pathophysiologic clues. Thus LDL, HDL, and very low density lipoprotein (VLDL), the most abundant apolipoproteins, are named according to their relative densities (relative amounts of protein to lipid). For example, relative to plasma, HDL has a high density because more protein is present relative to lipid, thus making it less buoyant and heavier.[5,19]

LOW DENSITY LIPOPROTEINS

LDL carries about two thirds of the plasma cholesterol and is the conduit for the delivery of cholesterol to cells, including those of the arterial wall. Approximately 1 g of cholesterol is synthesized daily in the liver and is packaged, together with triglyceride, as a VLDL[77] (Fig. 2.2). An increased amount of cholesterol is produced in genetically predisposed individuals, like those with type IIa and IIb hypercholesterolemia. Cholesterol is an essential component of body cells and is needed for the formation of bile by liver and as a backbone for steroid moieties; the daily requirements are relatively small, however. As a result, dietary cholesterol will add on to the plasma concentrations made in the liver. Although the relationship between dietary cholesterol and liver production is complex (with the presence of feedback inhibition), for elevated, primarily LDL plasma cholesterol, dietary cholesterol reduced to under 300 mg daily will substantially decrease plasma LDL. Some subjects are high responders and develop high levels of plasma LDL with elevated dietary cholesterol; conversely, the plasma level drops substantially on a low cholesterol diet.[16]

The LDL molecule is submicroscopic and has a diameter of approximately 200 Å. Each LDL has approximately 500 molecules of cholesterol on its surface and approximately 1,500 cholesterol-esters in its core, and each LDL has but one surface apoprotein, namely, apoprotein B (apo B). The apoproteins, all alphabetized in sequence, make the water-insoluble lipids water soluble; apo B is made in the liver and

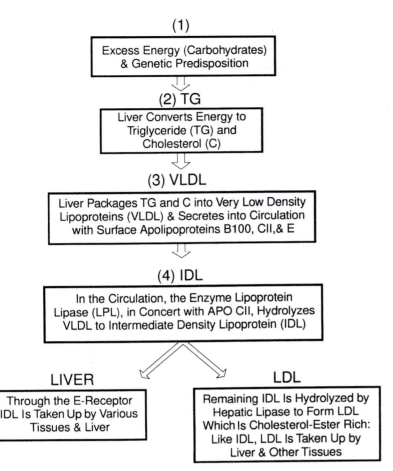

(1)

Excess Energy (Carbohydrates) & Genetic Predisposition

(2) TG

Liver Converts Energy to Triglyceride (TG) and Cholesterol (C)

(3) VLDL

Liver Packages TG and C into Very Low Density Lipoproteins (VLDL) & Secretes into Circulation with Surface Apolipoproteins B100, CII,& E

(4) IDL

In the Circulation, the Enzyme Lipoprotein Lipase (LPL), in Concert with APO CII, Hydrolyzes VLDL to Intermediate Density Lipoprotein (IDL)

LIVER

Through the E-Receptor IDL Is Taken Up by Various Tissues & Liver

LDL

Remaining IDL Is Hydrolyzed by Hepatic Lipase to Form LDL Which Is Cholesterol-Ester Rich: Like IDL, LDL Is Taken Up by Liver & Other Tissues

Figure 2.2 Low density lipoprotein (LDL), the "bad" cholesterol, and its metabolic pathway. As discussed in the text, the metabolism of LDL is complex, and not linear as depicted in the diagram. For simplicity's sake, however, this view makes the pathway more understandable. In general, the higher the quantity of LDL in the plasma, the greater the risk of arterial atherosclerosis.

is called apo B-100. The apo B made in the intestinal tract is called B-48, but it is of lesser quantity. LDL accounts for approximately two-thirds of the plasma cholesterol and has a half-life of about 2.5 days.[76,77]

As shown in Figure 2.2, a more or less linear reaction occurs in the bloodstream after VLDL is secreted by the liver, following the packaging of cholesterol and triglycerides, which are also synthesized in the liver. The amount of cholesterol and triglyceride is determined to a large degree by genetic predisposition, as well as by dietary intake of cholesterol and energy sources, particularly carbohydrates. The major apoproteins that make up the outer shell of VLDL are apo B-100, apo CII, and apo E, among others. The half-life of VLDL in the bloodstream is on the order of several hours, and it will quickly release its triglycerides to muscle and adipose tissue by the action of vessel lipases in those tissues. By the interaction of a number of modifying EC and plasma enzymes, VLDL is converted by lipoprotein lipase, in concert with apo CII, and hydrolyzed to an intermediate density lipoprotein (IDL) (Fig. 2.2). IDL in turn may be directly taken up by the liver and other tissues through the E-receptors. By contrast, IDL may be hydrolyzed by hepatic lipase to form LDL, which is cholesterol-ester rich. As with IDL, LDL is also taken up by the liver and other tissues and is the major source of cholesterol for body tissues (Fig. 2.2). LDL has only apo B-100 left on its shell; by way of B-receptors on liver cells and other

tissue membranes, the LDL, which is rich in cholesterol, is taken up by the process of endocytosis.[10,73] The LDL receptor has been cloned and sequenced and was found on chromosome 19; the gene has 18 exons and 17 introns.[77]

It should be noted that one of the means of reducing cholesterol is to interfere with the enterohepatic cycle. Normally cholesterol is converted to bile in the liver to produce sufficient detergent action of bile to solubilize and thereby take up lipids. The bile formed is largely reabsorbed and thus does not require a continuous large conversion of plasma cholesterol. By binding bile with a resin, such as cholestyramine or colestipol, which will not permit its uptake by the intestinal tract, the requirement for bile will cause an increase in the conversion of cholesterol to bile, thereby reducing plasma cholesterol levels.[4,7,8,13,42,43]

HIGH DENSITY LIPOPROTEINS

As depicted in Figure 2.3, HDL (the "good cholesterol") has a similar more or less linear reaction in the bloodstream as does LDL. The popular term "good cholesterol" comes from observations that elevated levels of HDL are associated with a decreased risk of atherosclerosis, presumably in part by con-

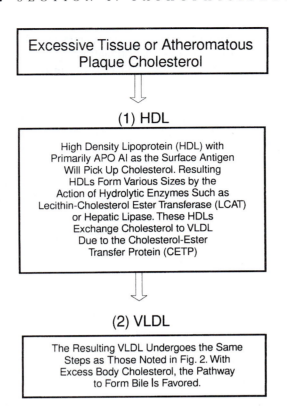

Figure 2.3 flow chart:

Excessive Tissue or Atheromatous Plaque Cholesterol

(1) HDL

High Density Lipoprotein (HDL) with Primarily APO AI as the Surface Antigen Will Pick Up Cholesterol. Resulting HDLs Form Various Sizes by the Action of Hydrolytic Enzymes Such as Lecithin-Cholesterol Ester Transferase (LCAT) or Hepatic Lipase. These HDLs Exchange Cholesterol to VLDL Due to the Cholesterol-Ester Transfer Protein (CETP)

(2) VLDL

The Resulting VLDL Undergoes the Same Steps as Those Noted in Fig. 2. With Excess Body Cholesterol, the Pathway to Form Bile Is Favored.

Figure 2.3 High density lipoprotein (HDL), the "good cholesterol" and its role in reverse cholesterol transport, which conveys excessive tissue cholesterol to the liver for conversion into bile. As with LDL metabolism, HDL metabolism is complex and not simply linear. HDL's action in helping to clear arteries of excess cholesterol and assist in delivering it to the liver for bile formation (hence the reverse direction of LDL, which is atherogenic) is associated with reduced incidences of atherosclerosis. The exact factors regulating the direction in which the intravascular lipids go in favoring their pro- or antiatherogenic effects are not clearly understood. In general, the higher the HDL in plasma, the lower the incidence of atherosclerosis.

veying cholesterol in tissues, such as atheromas, to the liver to convert it into bile. HDL, made in the liver, picks up tissue cholesterol by as yet uncertain mechanisms, although the presence of apo AI is important.[28,77] The resulting HDLs form a variety of HDL particles of differing sizes, resulting from the action of enzymes that rearrange them. These include the hydrolytic enzymes such as lecithin cholesterol-ester transferase, which takes the fatty acid from the phospholipid lecithin and transfers it to cholesterol to make a cholesterol-ester; the action of hepatic lipase is similar. These HDLs, primarily HDL2 and HDL3, will ultimately exchange their cholesterol molecules to VLDL, resulting from the action of cholesterol-ester transfer protein. After the formation of VLDL, the same steps occur: it is converted to IDL and then taken up by the liver, when the dynamics of cholesterol excess favor that pathway.[2,27–29,53]

HDL is about one-third the size of LDL (approximately 100 Å in diameter), and its major apoproteins are AI, CIII,

and AIV, although others are present. As inferred in Figure 2.3, defects in the pathway of reverse cholesterol transport can provoke atherosclerosis. By contrast, elevated HDL, especially the AI-Milano variant, will efficiently rid the body of excess cholesterol.[53] Efforts to rid the body of excess cholesterol using liver transplants with a normal complement of B-receptors or by using plasmapheresis to lower plasma LDL have resulted in marked reduction in the size of atherosclerotic lesions. These techniques have been used in patients with rapidly accelerating atherosclerosis due to familial hypercholesterolemia.[38,53]

Figure 2.4 shows a lateral section of an arterial wall with an expansion of the space between the ECs and the underlying SMCs. The action of HDL in preventing the oxidation of LDL to form modified and minimally modified LDL (mLDL and mmLDL) is noteworthy; mLDL and mmLDL have been shown to be highly atherogenic.[61] Thus, in addition to carrying cholesterol from tissue to liver to form bile, in the process of reverse cholesterol transport, HDL also functions to minimize oxidative reactions and to carry lipid hydroperoxides to the liver for disposal.[57] As shown in Figure 2.4, the metabolic activities of the ECs and SMCs result in the formation of oxidants, which in turn oxidize LDL. The mmLDL will by its toxic action provoke the ECs and SMCs to secrete monocyte chemoattractant protein-1 (MCP-1), which, as the name implies, causes monocytes to enter the subendothelial space and the ECs to produce a variety of cellular adhesion molecules (X-CAMs), which further attracts monocytes. In turn, the monocytes, by engulfing the mmLDL and mLDL, are converted to foam cells, which look foamy in appearance histologically because of the abundant lipid in their cytoplasm. Although foam cells, by scavenging lipids, might have a beneficial effect in taking up mLDL and mmLDL, the evidence appears to favor a destructive role, in part by their ability to induce an inflammatory response (discussed below) but also by releasing a variety of hydrolytic and toxic enzymes, particularly in the atheroma, to which they migrate[50] (Fig. 2.4).

In addition to the action of MCP-1 in causing monocyte migration to the subendothelial area, EC injury results in an inflammatory reaction caused by ischemia with the production of intercellular adhesion molecules, such as ICAM-1 and ICAM-2, vascular cell adhesion molecule-1, selection carbohydrates (such as E- and P-selection), and others, including mucin and CD31. Along with the mechanisms noted above, these adhesion molecules cause the blood monocytes to increase their rolling and adhesive activity along the vessel ECs, preceding migration into the subendothelial space.[24,25,49,50]

ARTERIAL VASODILATATION

Although lipids and the proliferation of SMCs are critical features of atherogenesis, factors influencing arterial wall vasodilatation and constriction (normal functions required for the regulating of blood flow) play a role in provoking SMC proliferation in atherogenesis, as depicted in Figures 2.5 and 2.6. In Figure 2.5, the normal sequence of events in arterial vasodilatation is depicted: the normal activities of blood flow and the factors it carries (such as acetylcholine and thrombin) plus

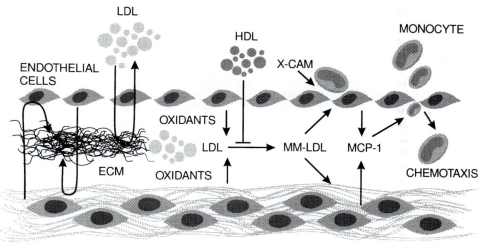

Figure 2.4 Interaction of low density lipoprotein (LDL) and high density lipoprotein (HDL) within the arterial wall. Interaction of LDL and HDL within the arterial wall (subendothelial space) in provoking or hindering atherosclerosis and related events such as the oxidation of LDL to produce minimally modified LDL (mmLDL), monocyte chemoattractant proteins (MCP-1), and a variety of endothelial cell adhesion molecules (X-CAM). In this sequence (from left to right), both endothelial cells (ECs) and smooth muscle cells (SMCs) produce, as a side product, a fibrillar extracellular matrix of (ECM), which can bind LDL. The metabolic products of these cells also produce oxidants that will convert LDL to mmLDL. HDL, as discussed in the text, has an antiatherogenic effect by inhibiting the oxidation of LDL to mmLDL. The production of mmLDL, as oxidized from LDL, causes the production of adhesion molecules. These molecules will cause monocytes to stick to the ECs and eventually enter the subendothelial space to become, ultimately, the foam cells of the atheroma. The mmLDL also causes production of MCP-1 by both EC and SMC, which in turn causes the monocyte to migrate subendothelially. (From Navab et al,[50] with permission.)

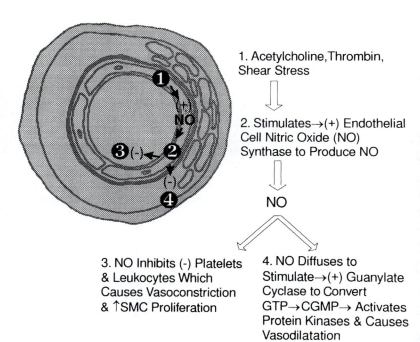

Figure 2.5 Arterial vasodilatations. Although arterial vasodilatation and vasoconstriction are constantly occurring depending on circulating peptides, ions, pH, and arterial pressure changes, the forces of vasodilatation depicted in this diagram tend to be antiatherogenic in minimizing the proliferation of smooth muscle cells (SMCs). GTP, guanosine triphosphate; cGMP, cyclic guanosine monophosphate.

Figure 2.6 Vasoconstriction and smooth muscle cell (SMC) proliferation and atherosclerosis. The intent of this diagram is to show forces opposite to those seen in Fig. 2.5. (i.e., atherogenic). When the arterial wall cannot compensate for the stresses it is exposed to, inhibition of nitric oxide (NO) synthesis occurs. Reduction of NO by endothelial cells (ECs) precedes the atherogenic processes, leading to SMC proliferation provoked by growth factors from platelets and leukocytes, such as platelet-derived growth factors (PDGF). HTN, hypertension; DM, diabetes mellitus; NO, nitric oxide.

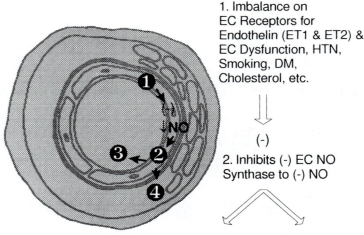

1. Imbalance on EC Receptors for Endothelin (ET1 & ET2) & EC Dysfunction, HTN, Smoking, DM, Cholesterol, etc.

(-)

2. Inhibits (-) EC NO Synthase to (-) NO

3. Lack of (-) of Platelets & Leukocytes, Whose Growth Factors, e.g., PDGF, Stimulates SMC Proliferation

4. Reduced NO, no SMC & Lack of Vasodilator Drive Allow Stimulus for SMC Proliferation

the mild shear stress of the blood pressure stimulate the nitric oxide (NO) synthase of the ECs to produce NO. In turn, NO will affect both the lumen and the SMCs, by its proximate location. By diffusing into the lumen, NO will inhibit platelets and leukocytes, which will release factors that cause vasoconstriction and SMC proliferation, such as platelet-derived growth factor (PDGF). Then, by diffusing from the ECs to the media, NO will stimulate guanylate cyclase to convert guanosine triphosphate to cyclic guanosine monophosphate, which activates a number of cellular protein kinases to phosphorylate proteins and finally results in vasodilatation. Whereas vasodilatation and vasoconstriction are normal and alternating responses to changes in blood pressure and other factors, the heightened vasoconstrictive activity will help to accelerate SMC proliferation and thereby provoke atherosclerosis.[52]

ARTERIAL VASOCONSTRICTION AND SMOOTH MUSCLE CELL PROLIFERATION AND ATHEROSCLEROSIS

As depicted in Figure 2.5, various stress factors (e.g., hypertension, smoking, diabetes mellitus, elevated cholesterol, homocyst(e)ine, and other factors like excessive shear stresses) will negatively impact on the ECs. For example, EC receptors such as endothelin 1 and 2 (ET1 and ET2) affected and cause EC dysfunction. The resulting effect is to negate the differentially affected sequences seen with vasodilatation in Figure 2.4 with inhibition of EC NO synthase and reduced synthesis of NO. In turn, the lack of NO will allow platelets and leukocytes to secrete their growth factors, such as PDGF, and will cause SMC cell proliferation by diffusing to the media.[62,63] A

variety of studies show that the major growth factor of platelets that provokes SMC proliferation is the PDGF-BB chains, not the AA chains.[60] Our laboratory has explored the regulation of SMC proliferation and found that certain protein kinase Cs are involved, specifically protein kinase C-γ, and that calcium channel blockers, such as clentiazem, may be highly effective in blocking PDGF-BB-induced SMC proliferation, as is butyrate.[60] These findings have clinical implications in preventing important aspects of atherogenesis, but they require verification in humans.

The mechanism of excessive shear stress in causing atherosclerosis may relate to increased deposition of lipoproteins by dynamic pressure and to regulation of the ICAM-1 gene at the site of its shear stress response element, resulting in its increased synthesis. The same mechanism may occur with MCP-1.[40,48-51,59]

SEQUENCE OF ENDOTHELIAL CELL INJURY, LIPID UPTAKE, AND SMOOTH MUSCLE CELL PROLIFERATION

Figure 2.7 attempts to unify the major atherogenesis theories into one composite view. As with Figure 2.6 and arterial vasoconstriction, an important etiologic, perhaps parallel, event is the occurrence of EC injury through the action of hypertension, smoking, diabetes mellitus, elevated cholesterol, homocyst(e)ine, and other factors. As a result of injured ECs and the lack of NO, production of SMC growth factors such as PDGF in platelets and leukocytes is not halted.[71] Meanwhile (in parallel), the damaged endothelium, aided by the actions of lipid oxidation (discussed with Figure 2.4), promotes monocyte adhesion to ECs and migration into the subendothelial

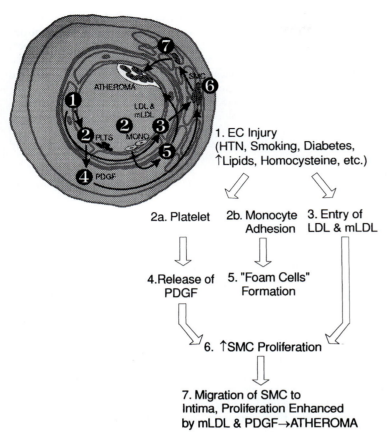

Figure 2.7 Atherosclerosis: sequence of endothelial cell (EC) injury, lipid uptake and smooth muscle cell (SMC) proliferation. Diagram showing an amalgamation of the injury healing theory and the lipid theory of atherogenesis discussed in the text. Although the diagram depicts the simultaneous occurrence of factors in the second stage of affecting platelets, monocytes, and the lipoproteins, this is a prolonged process that is probably partially serial, but with periods of regression and progression. Thus, the sequence of events shown in 1 to 7 probably takes years, if not decades to develop. HTN, hypertension; LDL, low density liprotein; mLDL, modified LDL; PDGF, platelet-derived growth factor.

cell spaces, where the monocytes engulf lipids to become foam cells. At the same time, EC injury allows the entry of LDL and also oxidized or mLDL, the production of which is then taken up by monocytes, which also assist in SMC proliferation. With the robust proliferative activity of SMCs, albeit over a long time course, the monocytes, along with the foam cells, migrate to the intima to constitute the atheroma, which is variably filled with cholesterol-esters, SMCs, inflammatory cells, and foam cells, making up nearly one-half of all the cellular structures in the atheroma.[21,41,55,67,68,75] In addition to these components of the atheroma, up to 15% of the cells may be T lymphocytes.[29] The makeup of the atheroma appears to play a role in causing thrombosis, since those high in free cholesterol-esters and foam cells rupture to expose collagen surfaces that are highly thrombogenic.[9,35,54,70]

Dietary Aspects of Plasma Lipids

Dietary cholesterol and saturated fats will increase plasma levels of cholesterol, although the relationship between dietary lipids and plasma levels is not a simple linear one and is controversial according to some. Nonetheless, studies of Mattson et al[45] show that for every 100 mg of dietary cholesterol per 1,000 calories taken in, the plasma cholesterol will rise approximately 10 mg/dl. Although it is arguable whether dietary lipids add on to plasma levels, the clinical validity of this hypothesis is supported by data showing that reduction of dietary lipids is associated with a significant reduction in plasma lipids.[32] High fat intake (40% of total calories) is associated with increased incidence of symptomatic and early atherosclerotic diseases, including strokes. The American Heart Association and the National Cholesterol Education Program have advocated diets lower in cholesterol (i.e., fat should compose <30% of caloric intake).[26,32,39]

As alluded to above, the initial treatment for increased cholesterol levels should be dietary reduction of both cholesterol and saturated fats. Some patients are high responders, showing dramatic rises in cholesterol with high dietary content and also substantially reduced plasma cholesterol with concomitant decreases in dietary lipids. If dietary lipid reduction is not coupled with medical therapy, the latter is of no practical value. The recommended relative reduction of cholesterol (as LDL) depends to some extent on the symptomatic burden of disease. For example, in subjects with coronary heart disease or two major risk factors such as hypertension and diabetes mellitus, the targeted LDL-cholesterol level should be <130 mg/dl; for those without these risks, it should be <160 mg/dl.[39]

Institution of dietary guidelines will usually require expert input from trained dieticians. As a general guideline, for achieving cholesterol reduction, total dietary fat should be reduced to no more than 30% of the total caloric intake, with saturated fats making up <10%; total dietary cholesterol should be <300 mg/day. As a reminder, one egg has nearly that much cholesterol alone. A simple rule is to cut down or stop eating the four major foods containing cholesterol and saturated fats, namely, red meat, eggs (yolks), butter, and whole milk.[16,34,77]

Whether to lower plasma cholesterol aggressively in subjects at risk of strokes, such as those who have had a mild or moderate stroke due to atherosclerosis, depends on a number of factors, not least of which are the age of the patient and the cost/benefit ratio. Recently, data on the value of reducing plasma cholesterol for preventing strokes have finally surfaced, with studies using the HMG-CoA reductase inhibitor pravastatin.[22,64] Ultimately, the decision to institute a cholesterol-lowering diet requires good clinical judgment that balances the best interests of the patient with practicality.

Therapy for Atherothrombotic Brain Infarctions: Primary and Secondary Prevention

Although the recent data noted above on the benefits of lowering cholesterol for preventing progression of carotid atherosclerosis and averting strokes support this strategy, the best data thus far involve coronary heart disease.[22] The first persuasive study was the Lipid Research Clinics Coronary Primary Prevention Trial in 1984.[42,43] Approximately 4,000 middle-aged men with elevated cholesterol (>260 mg/dl) who were asymptomatic of coronary disease were randomly assigned to either a low fat/low cholesterol diet plus placebo or this diet plus cholestyramine, a bile sequestrant that will lower cholesterol. In the over 7-year follow-up, the cholestyramine-treated group had reductions of total cholesterol and LDL cholesterol of 9% and 12%, respectively, as well as an aggregate decrease in coronary events of 19% compared with controls. These beneficial findings translate to a 2% reduction in coronary artery events for each 1% reduction in plasma cholesterol.

Subsequent to this study, a number of investigations on the use of cholesterol-lowering drugs or techniques were published, all of which bolster their value in preventing primary and secondary coronary events.[4,7–9,11,31–34,36,56] Studies on the value of lowering cholesterol to prevent strokes due to atherosclerosis are limited, but further investigations similar to those for coronary artery disease will be forthcoming. As with coronary disease, it can be predicted that those who will benefit the most from lowering cholesterol will be those at heightened risk of strokes or those who may be genetically predisposed.[79] For example, we studied restriction fragment length polymorphism at two sites with LDL and HDL plus the three alleles of apo E in VLDL and the known polymorphism of angiotensin-converting enzyme, which correlates with coronary artery disease, in over 200 patients with strokes due to atherosclerosis as well as controls. Interestingly, white subjects with strokes, making up two-thirds of this group, had a significant elevation of total cholesterol plus polymorphism of LDL, compared with their white controls. By contrast, black American stroke subjects had significant polymorphisms for HDL and angio-

tensin-converting enzyme plus an increase in expression of the E4 allele (phenotype) in VLDL, compared with their controls. Although we will probably need 800 to 1,000 stroke subjects plus matching controls in each group to make the results statistically significant because of normal random variation in gene mutations, should our preliminary results hold up (as we suspect they will), it would be possible to identify a genetic stroke profile; such a profile could form the basis for interventional therapy as well as education at an earlier age on the relative risk burden the subject carries the effects of cholesterol and hypertension later in life.[79]

Lipid-Lowering Drugs

The various drugs used to lower lipids include bile sequestrants, such as cholestyramine and colestipol; HMG-CoA reductase inhibitors, namely, the statins such as mevinolin and pravastatin; fibric acid compounds, such as gemfibrozil; niacin; and probucol, the antioxidant. Familiarity with each drug will guide choices, but elderly individuals frequently have difficulty with bile sequestrants because of gastrointestinal symptoms such as bloating, eructations, and nausea. Perhaps the most popular drugs among clinicians are the statins, which are effective and have few side effects and drug interactions. When using any of these drugs, the physician should be aware of side effects and complications, whether baseline and follow-up studies are required, and drug interactions.[1,12,16,32,34]

Whether calcium channel blockers are antiatherogenic has been the subject of a long-term debate. Recent in vitro studies suggest that certain calcium channel blockers may be more effective in inhibiting the proliferation of SMC, a necessary process in atherogenesis.[23,60,78] As noted above, for spectacularly elevated cholesterol levels, as seen with familial hypercholesterolemia, normal liver transplants with a high complement of B- and B/E-receptors have promptly lowered elevated cholesterol levels, as has lipoprotein apheresis.[38]

Summary and Conclusions

Stroke due to atherosclerosis remains the most common neurologic disorder, particularly among the elderly population. This chapter has reviewed current theories on pathogenesis, such as the lipid hypothesis and the injury healing hypothesis, as well as the role of inflammation. From clues in treating coronary artery disease due to atherosclerosis, it can now be inferred that successful treatment strategies for coronary disease will be beneficial for stroke prevention. These strategies have been directed primarily toward cholesterol reduction, but in the future other simultaneous therapies are expected, particularly those affecting SMC proliferation and the associated inflammatory responses. The future is bright for better identification of those subjects who will benefit from interventional therapies to prevent stroke occurrence or recurrence; clearly, despite advances in acute ischemic stroke therapies, such as the use of thrombolytic drugs acutely, the best treatment of strokes remains their prevention.

References

1. Alberts AW, Chen J, Kuron G et al: Mevinolin: a highly potent competitive inhibitor of hydroxymethylglutaryl-coenzyme A reductase and a cholesterol-lowering agent. Proc Natl Acad Sci USA 77:3957–3961, 1980
2. Badimon JJ, Badimon L, Fuster V: Regression of atherosclerotic lesions by high density lipoprotein plasma fraction in the cholesterol-fed rabbit. J Clin Invest 85:1234–1241, 1990
3. Bicknell R: Heterogeneity of the endothelial cell. Behring Institute Mitteilungen 92:1–7, 1993
4. Blankenhorn DHG, Nessim SA, Johnson RL et al: Coronary beneficial effects of combined colestipol-niacin therapy on atherosclerosis and coronary venous bypass grafts. JAMA 257:3233, 1987
5. Bonanome A, Grundy SM: Effects of dietary stearic acid on plasma cholesterol and lipoprotein levels. N Engl J Med 318:1244–1248, 1989
6. Bowry VW, Stanley KK, Stocker R: High density lipoprotein is the major carrier of lipid hydroperoxides in human blood plasma from fasting donors. Proc Natl Acad Sci USA 89:10316–10320, 1992
7. Brensike JF, Levy RI, Kelsey SF et al: Effects of therapy with cholestyramine on progression of coronary arteriosclerosis: results of the NHLBI type II Coronary Intervention Study. Circulation 69:313–324, 1984
8. Brown BG: Effect of lovastatin or niacin combined with colestipol and regression of coronary atherosclerosis. Eur Heart J 13:17–20, 1992
9. Brown BG, Albers JJ, Fisher LD et al: Progression of coronary artery disease as a result of intensive lipid-lowering therapy in men with high levels of apolipoprotein B. N Engl J Med 323:1289–1298, 1990
10. Brown MS, Goldstein JL: A receptor-mediated pathway for cholesterol homeostasis. Science 232:34–47, 1986
11. Canner PL, Berge KG, Wenger NK et al: Fifteen year mortality in Coronary Drug Project patients: long-term benefit with niacin. J Am Coll Cardiol 8:1245–1255, 1986
12. Carew TE, Schwenke DC, Steinberg D: Antiatherogenic effect of probucol unrelated to its hypocholesterolemic effect: evidence that antioxidants in vivo can selectively inhibit low density lipoprotein degradation in macrophage-rich fatty streaks and slow the progression of atherosclerosis in the Watanabe heritable hyperlipidemic rabbit. Proc Natl Acad Sci USA 84:7725–7729, 1987
13. Cashin-Hemphill L, Mack WJ, Pogoda J et al: Beneficial effects of colestipol-niacin on coronary atherosclerosis: a 4-year follow-up. JAMA 264:3013–3017, 1990
14. Castelli WP, Wilson PW, Levy D et al: Cardiovascular risk factors in the elderly. Am J Cardiol 63:12H–19H, 1989
15. Charo I: Monocyte-endothelial cell interactions. Curr Opin, Lipidol 3:335–343, 1992
16. Connor WE, Connor SL: The dietary treatment of hyperlipidemia. Rationale, technique and efficacy. Med Clin North Am 66:485–518, 1982
17. Cushing SD, Berliner JA, Valente AJ et al: Minimally modified low-density lipoprotein induces monocyte chemotactic protein-1 in human endothelial cells and smooth muscle cells. Proc Natl Acad Sci USA 87:5134–5138, 1990
18. Cybulsky MI, Gimbrone MA: Endothelial expression of a mononuclear leukocyte adhesion molecule during atherogenesis. Science 251:788–791, 1991
19. DeGraba T, Fisher M, Yatsu FM: Atherogenesis and Strokes. pp. 28–48. In Barnett HJM, Mohr JP, Stein B, Yatsu FM (eds): *Strokes: Pathophysiology, Diagnosis and Management.* 2nd Ed. Churchill Livingstone, New York, 1992
20. Fisher M, Blumenfeld A, Smith TW: The importance of carotid artery plaque disruption and hemorrhage. Arch Neurol 44:1086–1089, 1987
21. Fogelman AM, Schechter I, Seager J et al: Malondialdehyde alteration of low density lipoproteins leads to cholesteryl ester accumulation in human monocyte-macrophages. Proc Natl Acad Sci USA 77:2214–2218, 1980
22. Furberg CD, Adams HP Jr, Applegate WB et al: Effect of lovastatin on early cartoid atherosclerosis and cardiovascular events. Asymptomatic Carotid Artery Progression study (ACAPS) Research Group. Circulation 90:1679–1687, 1994
23. Fronek K: Calcium antagonists and experimental atherosclerosis. Cardiovasc Drug Rev 8:229–237, 1990
24. Galis ZS, Sukhova GK, Lark MW et al: Increased expression of matrix metalloproteinases and matrix degrading activity in vulnerable regions of human atherosclerotic plaques. J Clin Invest 94:2493–2503, 1994
25. Gimbrone MAJ, Bevilacqua MP, Cybulsky MI: Endothelial-dependent mechanisms of leukocyte adhesion in inflammation and atherosclerosis. Ann NY Acad Sci 598:77–85, 1990
26. Ginsberg HN, Barr SL, Gilbert A et al: Reduction of plasma cholesterol levels in normal men on an American Heart Association step-1 diet or a step-1 diet with added monounsaturated fat. N Engl J Med 322:574–579, 1990
27. Glomset JA: The plasma lecithin: cholesterol acyltransferase reaction. J Lipid Res 9:155–167, 1968
28. Gordon T, Castelli WP, Hjortland MC et al: High density lipoprotein as a protective factor against coronary heart disease. The Framingham Study. Am J Med 62:707–714, 1977
29. Gown AM, Tsukada T, Ross R: Human atherosclerosis. II. Immunocytochemical analysis of the cellular composition of human atherosclerotic lesions. Am J Pathol 125:191–207, 1986
30. Grotta JC, Yatsu FM, Pettigrew LC et al: Prediction of carotid stenosis progression by lipid and hematologic measurements. Neurol 39:1325–1331, 1989
31. Grundy SM: Comparison of monounsaturated fatty acid and carbohydrates for lowering plasma cholesterol. N Engl J Med 314:745–748, 1986
32. Grundy SM, Bilheimer D, Blackburn H et al: Rationale of the diet-heart statement of the American Heart Association: report of Nutrition Committee. Circulation 65:839A–854A, 1982

33. Hoeg JM, Brewer HB Jr: 3-Hydroxy-3-methyl-glutaryl-coenzyme A reductase inhibitors in the treatment of hypercholesterolemia. JAMA 258:3532–3536, 1987

34. Illingworth DR: Management of hyperlipidemia: goals for the prevention of atherosclerosis. Clin Invest Med 13: 211–218, 1990

35. Jonasson L, Holm J, Skalli O et al: Regional accumulation of T cells, macrophages, and smooth muscle cells in the human atherosclerotic plaque. Arteriosclerosis 6: 131–138, 1986

36. Kane JP, Malloy MJ, Ports TA et al: Regression of coronary atherosclerosis during treatment of familial hypercholesterolemia with combined drug regimen. JAMA 264: 3007–3012, 1990

37. Kannel WB, Wolf PA, Verter J: Manifestations of coronary disease predisposing to stroke: The Framingham Study. JAMA 250:2942–2946, 1983

38. Kottke BA, Pineda AA, Case MT et al: Hypercholesterolemia and atherosclerosis: present and future therapy including LDL-apheresis. J Clin Apheresis 4:35–46, 1988

39. Lenfant C: A new challenge for America: the National Cholesterol Education Program. Circulation 73:855–856, 1986

40. Li H, Cybulsky MI, Gimbrone MA Jr et al: An atherogenic diet rapidly induces VCAM-1, a cytokine regulatable mononuclear leukocyte adhesion molecule, in rabbit aortic endothelium. Arterioscler Throm 13:197–204, 1993

41. Libby P, Clinton SK: The role of macrophages in atherogenesis. Curr Opin Lipidol 4:355–363, 1993

42. Lipid Research Clinics Program: The Lipid Research Clinics Coronary Primary Prevention Trial results. I. Reduction in incidence of coronary heart disease. JAMA 251: 351–364, 1984

43. Lipid Research Clinics Program: The Lipid Research Clinics Coronary Primary Prevention Trial results. II. The relationship of reduction in incidence of coronary heart disease to cholesterol lowering. JAMA 251:365–374, 1984

44. Lusis AJ: Genetic factors affecting blood lipoproteins: the candidate gene approach. J Lip Res 29:397–429, 1988

45. Mattson FH, Erickson BA, Kligman AM: Effect of dietary cholesterol on serum cholesterol in man. Am J Clin Nutr 25:589–594, 1972

46. McGill HC Jr: Relationship of atherosclerosis in young men to serum lipoprotein cholesterol concentrations and smoking: a preliminary report from the Pathobiological Determinants of Atherosclerosis in Youth (PDAY) Research Group. JAMA 264:3018, 1990

47. Mendez I, Hachinski V, Wolfe B: Serum lipids after stroke. Neurology. 37:507–511, 1987

48. Mitchison MJ, Ball RY: Macrophages and atherogenesis. Lancet 2:146–149, 1987

49. Nagel T, Resnick N, Atkinson WJ et al: Shear stress selectively upregulates intercellular adhesion molecule-1 expression in cultured human vascular endothelial cells. J Clin Invest 94:885–891, 1994

50. Navab M, Berliner JA, Watson AD et al: The Yin and Yang of oxidation in the development of the fatty streak. Arterioscler Thromb Vasc Biol 16:831–842, 1996

51. Nelken N, Coughlin SR, Gordon D et al: Monocyte chemoattractant protein-1 in human atheromatous plaques. J Clin Invest 88:1121–1127, 1991

52. Neren RM, Harris DG, Taylor WR et al: Hemodyanamics and vascular endothelial biology. J Cardiovasc Pharm 21: S6–S10, 1993

53. Norum KR, Berg T, Helgerud P et al: Transport of cholesterol. Physiol Rev 63:1343–1419, 1983

54. Ogata J, Masuda J, Yutani C et al: Rupture of atheromatous plaque as a cause of thrombotic occlusion of stenotic internal carotid artery. Stroke 21:1740, 1990

55. Ohara Y, Petersen TE, Harrison DG: Hypercholesterolemia increases endothelial superoxide anion production. J Clin Invest 91:2546–2551, 1993

56. Ornish D, Brown SE, Scherwitz LW et al: Can lifestyle changes reverse coronary heart disease?—The Lifestyle Heart Trial. Lancet 336:129–133, 1990

57. Parthasarathy S, Barnett J, Fong LG: High-density lipoprotein inhibits the oxidative modification of low-density lipoprotein. Biochim Biophys Acta 1044:275–283, 1990

58. Poston RN, Haskard DO, Coucher JR et al: Expression of intercellular adhesion molecule-1 in atherosclerotic plaques. Am J Pathol 140:665–673, 1992

59. Printseva O, Peclo MM, Gown AM: Various cell types in human atherosclerotic lesions express ICAM-1. Further immunocytochemical and immunochemical studies employing monoclonal antibody 10F3. Am J Pathol 140: 889–896, 1992

60. Ranganna K, Joshi T, Yatsu FM: Sodium butyrate inhibits platelet-derived growth factor-induced proliferation of vascular smooth muscle cells. Arterioscler Thromb Vasc Biol 15:2273–2283, 1995

61. Reaven PD: Mechanisms of atherosclerosis: role of LDL oxidation. Adv Exp Med Biol 366:113–128, 1994

62. Ross R: The pathogenesis of atherosclerosis: a perspective for the 1990s. Nature 362:801–809, 1993

63. Ross R, Raines WE, Bowen-Pope DF: The biology of platelet-derived growth factor. Cell 46:155–169, 1986

64. Sacks FM, Pfeffer MA, Moye LA et al: The effect of pravastatin on coronary events after myocardial infarction in patients with average cholesterol levels. Cholesterol and Recurrent Event Trial Investigators. N Engl J Med 335:1001–1009, 1996

65. Salomon RN, Underwood R, Doyle MV et al: Increased apolipoprotein E and c-fms gene expression without elevated interleukin 1 or 6 mRNA levels indicate selective activation of macrophage functions in advanced human atheroma. Proc Natl Acad Sci USA 89:2814–2818, 1992

66. Scheffler E, Wiest E, Woehrle J et al: Smoking influences the atherogenic potential of low-density lipoprotein. Clin Invest 70:263–268, 1992

67. Serhan CN: Lipoxin biosynthesis and its impact in inflammation and vascular events. Biochim Biophys Acta 212: 1–25, 1994

68. Tanaka H, Sukhova GK, Swanson SJ et al: Sustained activation of vascular cells and leukocytes in the rabbit aorta after balloon injury. Circulation 88:1788–1803, 1993

69. Tell GS, Crouse JR, Furberg CD: Relation between blood lipids, lipoproteins, and cerebrovascular atherosclerosis: a review. Stroke 19:423–430, 1988

70. Van der Wal AC, Becker AE, van der Loos CM et al: Site of intimal rupture or erosion of thrombosed coronary

atherosclerotic plaques is characterized by an inflammatory process irrespective of the dominant plaque morphology. Circulation 89:36–44, 1994

71. Walker LN, Bowen Pope DF, Ross R et al: Production of platelet-derived growth factor-like molecules by culture of arterial smooth muscle cells accompanies proliferation after arterial injury. Proc Natl Acad Sci USA 83: 7311, 1986

72. Wang J, Sica A, Peri G et al: Expression of monocyte chemotactic protein and interleukin-8 by cytokine-activated human vascular smooth muscle cells. Arterioscler Thromb 11:1166–1174, 1991

73. Weisgraber KH, Innerarity TL, Mahley RW: Abnormal lipoprotein receptor-binding activity of the human apoprotein E due to cysteine-arginine interchange at a single site. J Biol Chem 257:2518–2521, 1982

74. Wilson AC, Schaub RG, Goldstein RC et al: Suppression of aortic atherosclerosis in cholesterol-fed rabbits by purified rabbit interferon. Arteriosclerosis 10:208–214, 1990

75. Witznum JL, Steinberg D: Role of oxidized low density lipoprotein in atherogenesis. J Clin Invest 88:1785–1792, 1991

76. Yang CY, Chen SH, Gianturco SH et al: Sequence, structure, receptor-binding domains and internal repeats of human apolipoprotein B-100. Nature 323:738–742, 1986

77. Yatsu FM, Fisher M: Atherosclerosis: current concepts on pathogenesis and interventional therapies. Ann Neurol 26:3–12, 1989

78. Yatsu FM, Alam R, Alam SS: Enhancement of cholesteryl ester metabolism in cultured human monocyte-derived macrophages by verapamil. Biochim Biophys Acta 847: 77–81, 1985

79. Yatsu FM, Kasturi R, Alam R et al: Molecular biology of atherothrombotic strokes. Stroke, suppl. II, 21:131–133, 1990

CHAPTER 3

Vascular Biology of Cerebral Arteries

CHRISTOPHER G. SOBEY

FRANK M. FARACI

DONALD D. HEISTAD

Cerebral perfusion is compromised by several pathophysiologic conditions that are associated with altered vascular responses and increased risk of stroke. Recently significant progress has been made in the understanding of mechanisms that normally regulate cerebral blood flow, and of abnormalities of cerebral vascular function in pathophysiologic states. Disease states may produce cerebral vascular abnormalities by a variety of mechanisms, including endothelial dysfunction, impaired relaxation of vascular muscle, and augmented vasoconstriction.

This chapter summarizes the current understanding of some important mechanisms of cerebral vascular function and dysfunction. Recent development in techniques of gene transfer to cerebral vessels are also described briefly, with speculation on the potential applications of this technology for the study of vascular biology and for therapy. We have not addressed other aspects of vascular biology including mechanisms of vasoconstriction, vascular proliferation, remodeling, and formation of collateral vessels.

Physiologic Dilator Mechanisms in Cerebral Vessels

NITRIC OXIDE AND CYCLIC GMP-MEDIATED MECHANISMS

The endothelium modulates vascular tone by producing and releasing potent vasoactive substances.[14,50] One of these important substances is endothelium-derived relaxing factor (EDRF), which diffuses to vascular muscles and produces relaxation by activation of the soluble form of guanylate cyclase, resulting in an increased intracellular concentration of cyclic guanosine monophosphate (cGMP) and relaxation. The EDRF-guanylate cyclase mechanism represents a major mechanism of cerebral vasodilatation.

EDRF has been identified as nitric oxide (NO), or an NO-containing substance, produced by the endothelial isoform of nitric oxide synthase (NOS), which uses L-arginine as a substrate.[50] NO is a potent dilator of cerebral vessels.[14] Soluble guanylate cyclase, which is cytosolic, can also be activated by pharmacologic agents, including nitroglycerin and sodium nitroprusside.[50,97] NO is produced in cerebral vessels under basal conditions, and activity of NOS can be further stimulated by increases in intracellular calcium that occur in response to receptor-mediated agonists like acetylcholine, or in response to increase in shear stress.[14]

Under normal conditions, NO is released both luminally and abluminally by endothelium. Endothelial release of both NO and prostacyclin, a product of arachidonic acid metabolism, into the vascular lumen contributes to the antithrombogenic properties of endothelium, because both substances inhibit aggregation of platelets and adherence of leukocytes to endothelium.

Particulate guanylate cyclase, the second form of guanylate cyclase in vascular muscle, can be activated by the members of the natriuretic peptide family—atrial natriuretic peptide, brain natriuretic peptide, and C-type natriuretic peptide.[97] Atrial and brain natriuretic peptides produce relaxation of cerebral blood vessels when administered exogenously, but it is not clear whether endogenously produced natriuretic peptides contribute to regulation of cerebral vascular tone.

In addition to the constitutively expressed endothelial and neuronal isoforms of NOS, an inducible (or immunologic) isoform may be expressed in endothelium, vascular muscle, and

41

other cell types in brain.[14] The gene of inducible NOS is probably not expressed in blood vessels under normal conditions but can be expressed in the brain and can produce large amounts of NO during pathophysiologic conditions including ischemia and meningitis.

CYCLIC AMP-MEDIATED MECHANISMS

Activation of adenylate cyclase and production of cyclic adenosine monophosphate (cAMP) in vascular muscle mediates relaxation of blood vessels in response to a variety of endogenous substances, and represents a second major mechanism of vasodilatation in cerebral vessels.[54] Stimuli that activate adenylate cyclase include prostanoids (prostacyclin and prostaglandin E_2), adenosine, calcitonin gene-related peptide (CGRP), vasoactive intestinal peptide, β-adrenergic agonists, pituitary adenylate cyclase activating peptide, and adrenomedullin. A new concept is that increases in intracellular AMP in vascular muscle produces vasodilatation only in part by a direct effect and in part by activation of K^+ channels (see below).

K^+ CHANNELS

A third vasodilator mechanism that has received considerable attention in the last few years involves activation of K^+ channels. Increases in activity of K^+ channels result in membrane hyperpolarization of vascular muscle.[69] Several types of K^+ channels are present in cerebral blood vessels, but adenosine triphosphate (ATP)-sensitive K^+ channels and calcium-dependent K^+ channels have been studied most extensively.

Activity of ATP-sensitive K^+ channels is inhibited by intracellular ATP or an increased ratio of ATP to adenosine diphosphate (ADP). The intracellular concentration of ATP is normally sufficient to inhibit opening of these K^+ channels completely, and in cerebral vascular muscle these channels appear to be closed under normal conditions.[48] Because intracellular ATP levels are tightly regulated, it is likely that ATP-sensitive K^+ channels are rarely activated by reductions in ATP. Reductions in levels of intracellular PO_2 and pH also open these channels and produce vasorelaxation. Thus, activity of ATP-sensitive K^+ channels appears to reflect, in part, the metabolic state of cells.[69]

Several endogenous substances produce hyperpolarization and relaxation of cerebral vascular muscle that is mediated, in part, by activation of ATP-sensitive K^+ channels. These substances include CGRP,[46] norepinephrine, and increased intracellular concentration of cAMP.[44] The concept that ATP-sensitive K^+ channels may be activated by increased concentrations of cAMP is supported by evidence that dilatation of the basilar artery in response to forskolin, a direct activator of adenylate cyclase, can be attenuated with glibenclamide, a selective inhibitor of ATP-sensitive K^+ channels.[44,46] By contrast, vasodilators that increase cGMP in cerebral vessels are usually not inhibited by glibenclamide.[16,48,92]

Systemic hypoxia is a potent dilator stimulus in the cerebral circulation, and relaxation of cerebral vessels during hypoxia appears to involve activation of K^+ channels.[70] Relaxation of both large cerebral arteries and cerebral arterioles during hypoxia is inhibited by glibenclamide. These findings suggest that responses to hypoxia are mediated by activation of ATP-sensitive K^+ channels.[48]

Activity of calcium-dependent K^+ channels is increased in response to elevations in intracellular calcium. Calcium-dependent K^+ channels in blood vessels appear to act as a negative feedback mechanism during increases in intracellular concentrations of calcium, so that opening of these channels occurs more frequently during increases in blood pressure and with membrane depolarization. Tone of cerebral vessels, particularly during elevations of arterial pressure, may potentially be influenced by activity of calcium-dependent K^+ channels (see Hypertension section below).[70] In contrast to ATP-sensitive K^+ channels, calcium-dependent K^+ channels may be active in large cerebral arteries under basal conditions, and selective inhibition of this channel (e.g., with tetraethylammonium or iberiotoxin) leads to constriction of cerebral arteries.[2,6]

Calcium-dependent K^+ channels are responsive to other stimuli in addition to the intracellular concentration of calcium. Activation of calcium-dependent K^+ channels appears to contribute to relaxation of cerebral arterioles in response to activation of adenylate cyclase and accumulation of cAMP.[75,94] Because a variety of endogenous vasoactive stimuli increase the concentration of cAMP in vascular muscle, activation of calcium-dependent K^+ channels by cAMP may play a major role in regulation of cerebral vascular tone. Evidence also shows that increases in cGMP can increase activity of calcium-dependent K^+ channels in some vessels.[75]

Pathophysiologic Alterations in Cerebral Vessel Function

PLATELETS AND LEUKOCYTES

Activated platelets release potent vasoactive substances, including ADP (an endothelium-dependent vasodilator), serotonin (a vasoconstrictor or endothelium-dependent vasodilator, depending on vascular bed and vessel size), and thromboxane A_2 (a vasoconstrictor). In normal vessels, the vasomotor response to platelet products may therefore potentially be dilatation, constriction, or little net effect, depending on the relative influence of individual mediators. Under pathophysiologic conditions in which endothelial function is impaired, release of EDRF in response to ADP will be reduced, and a greater portion of the net vasomotor response to platelet products will be shifted to vasoconstrictor influences.

Polymorphonuclear leukocytes and monocytes also produce a variety of vasoactive agents, but the identities and conditions for release of many of these mediators are still poorly understood. In general, it is uncertain whether vasoconstrictor or vasodilator responses prevail in response to leukocytes.[1] Endothelium appears to mediate dilator responses (or attenuate constrictor responses) to leukocytes (as well as platelets) in some vascular preparations. In contrast to platelets, however, leukocytes produce endothelium-dependent constriction of normal arteries.[1,84] The mechanism of this latter effect appears to be through inactivation or inhibition of basally produced NO. The effect of endothelial dysfunction on vascular responses to leukocytes is therefore difficult to predict, and it will be important to evaluate vasoactive influences of leukocytes on cerebral vessels under specific pathophysiologic conditions.

ATHEROSCLEROSIS

Endothelium-Dependent Relaxation in Atherosclerosis

Both basal and agonist-induced release or activity of EDRF is impaired in extracranial blood vessels by atherosclerosis.[9,19,27,66,85] Superoxide dismutase improves endothelium-dependent relaxation in atherosclerotic arteries, suggesting that the mechanism of impairment involves excess generation of superoxide anion and inactivation of EDRF rather than reduced production of NO by NOS.[66]

The effect of atherosclerosis on endothelium-dependent relaxation of cerebral vessels is less clear. Compared with noncerebral vessels, intracranial vessels appear to develop atherosclerosis more slowly than extracranial vessels.[33] Relaxation of cerebral vessels to endothelium-dependent stimuli can be normal in the same atherosclerotic animals that exhibit marked impairment of endothelium-dependent relaxation in the aorta.[33,43,83] By contrast, some studies suggest that atherosclerosis or hypercholesterolemia produces cerebral endothelial dysfunction. For example, hypercholesterolemia is associated with impaired endothelium-dependent relaxation of the basilar artery.[80] Administration of L-arginine, the substrate for EDRF synthesis, restores dilator responses of the basilar artery to acetylcholine to normal.[80] This confirmed finding is surprising, because it seems unlikely that L-arginine deficiency contributes to impairment of endothelial function in atherosclerosis.

Cerebral Vascular Responses to Platelet and Leukocyte Products in Atherosclerosis

In the carotid and other large arteries supplying the brain, constrictor responses to serotonin and thromboxane A_2 are enhanced in the presence of atherosclerosis.[17,18,31,85,95] Collagen, which activates platelets, increases carotid blood flow normally but produces decreases in blood flow in the presence of atherosclerosis.[85] The normal increase in carotid blood flow produced by collagen is probably due largely to endothelium-dependent vasodilatation mediated by release of EDRF from small cerebral arteries in response to ADP, a major product of platelet activation.[25,96] Because EDRF normally inhibits constrictor responses of large cerebral arteries to serotonin, impairment of release or activity of EDRF may contribute to

augmented vasoconstrictor responses during atherosclerosis.[7,15] However, it appears that endothelial dysfunction alone is not sufficient to account for the marked increases in constrictor responsiveness of large cerebral arteries to serotonin.[31,95]

Analogous results have been obtained concerning effects of leukocytes on cerebral arteries during atherosclerosis.[1] Leukocytes in vitro induce greater contraction of atherosclerotic arteries than of normal vessels.[1] Intravascular activation of leukocytes leads to prolonged contraction of cerebral arteries of the atherosclerotic monkey, whereas in normal animals the constrictor effects of activated leukocytes are trivial.[18] Leukocytes from hypercholesterolemic rabbits release greater amounts of at least one unidentified contracting factor that inhibits NO-dependent vascular relaxation.[28]

Most transient ischemic attacks (TIAs) are thought to be produced by platelet adhesion, aggregation, and embolization from plaques in large extracranial arteries.[3] Release of serotonin during aggregation of platelets, coupled with augmented constrictor responses to serotonin in atherosclerotic arteries, may produce pronounced vasoconstriction and perhaps contribute to cerebral ischemia.[95]

Importantly, vasoactive effects of platelets and leukocytes are likely to be closely interdependent. When leukocytes and platelets are activated together, release of vasoactive products appears to be enhanced, and activation of leukocytes inhibits vasodilatation in response to platelets.[39] Furthermore, the action of platelet- and leukocyte-derived vasoconstrictors on vascular tone is synergistic.[1] Abnormal cerebral vascular responses to activated platelets, and possibly leukocytes, may thus contribute to the pathophysiology of TIAs and cerebral ischemia in the presence of atherosclerosis.[31]

Effects of Therapy to Lower Plasma Cholesterol

Reduction in dietary cholesterol produces regression of atherosclerosis and restores endothelium-dependent relaxation of extracranial arteries toward normal in experimental animals.[19,27,85] Susceptibility to vasoconstriction in response to activation of platelets and leukocytes is reduced or abolished by regression of atherosclerosis.[72]

Augmented constrictor responses of large cerebral arteries to serotonin are also largely restored to normal during regression of atherosclerosis.[31,85] Significant functional improvement appears to precede structural regression and occurs within only a few months of dietary treatment of hypercholesterolemia in cerebral and noncerebral arteries of atherosclerotic monkeys.[4,85] Thus, the benefits of cholesterol-lowering therapy may be relatively fast. Hypercholesterolemia alters platelets, as well as blood vessels, and part of the rapid improvement in vascular responses during treatment of hypercholesterolemia may be related to normalization of platelet function.[38]

Of considerable interest is the finding that in patients with coronary heart disease who received a cholesterol-lowering agent for approximately 5 years, reduction of cholesterol reduced cerebral vascular events by one-third.[81] Improvement of endothelial function during regression of atheroscle-

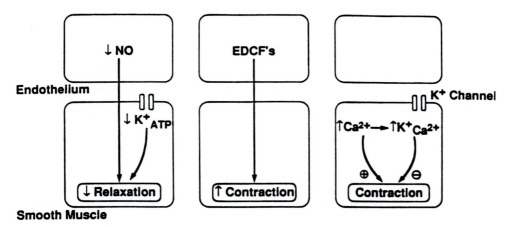

Figure 3.1 Some abnormalities in cerebral vessels during chronic hypertension. Decreased production or activity of nitric oxide (NO) may occur during chronic hypertension. Activity of adenosine triphosphate (ATP)-sensitive potassium channels (K^+_{ATP}) may also be reduced during hypertension. Production of endothelium-derived contracting factors (EDCFs) may occur and may counteract normal vasodilator mechanisms. Activity of calcium-activated K^+ channels (K^+Ca^{2+}) appears to be increased during chronic hypertension, perhaps in response to increased levels of intracellular calcium.

rosis may thus contribute to reduction of cerebral vascular events.

CHRONIC HYPERTENSION

Endothelial Function in Chronic Hypertension

Endothelium-dependent relaxation is impaired in the cerebral circulation during chronic hypertension (Fig. 3.1). Dilatation of cerebral arterioles and the basilar artery in response to endothelium-dependent agonists such as acetylcholine and ADP is impaired in the chronically hypertensive rat.[57,60,63,64,100,101] Cerebral vasodilatation in response to endothelium-independent agonists (which act directly on vascular muscle) such as NO, nitroglycerin, and adenosine is not impaired during chronic hypertension, suggesting that endothelial function is impaired, but vascular muscle relaxation is preserved.[45,57,60,63,64,100,101] Thus, the cAMP and cGMP mechanisms appear to be relatively normal during chronic hypertension.

Mechanisms that account for impaired endothelium-dependent relaxation during chronic hypertension appear to be different in cerebral arterioles and in the basilar artery. In cerebral arterioles, this impairment may be related to release of an endothelium-derived contracting factor (EDCF) that counteracts the normal dilator effects of EDRF/NO[60,64] (Fig. 3.1). This EDCF appears to be a prostanoid (not, for example, endothelin) because indomethacin restores responses to endothelium-dependent agonists to or toward normal.[60,64] In contrast to cerebral arterioles, impaired endothelium-dependent relaxation of the basilar artery does not appear to be due to production of an EDCF and is restored by L-arginine in stroke-prone spontaneously hypertensive rats.[49,57] The abnor-

mality of endothelial function in the basilar artery during chronic hypertension may therefore be related to reduced production or activity of EDRF/NO.

We speculate that altered responses of cerebral arterioles to endothelium-dependent agonists (acetylcholine and serotonin) in chronic hypertension may impair cerebral vasodilatation in response to vasoactive substances released by platelets. It is possible that, when platelets aggregate at plaques in the carotid arteries and release serotonin, impairment of endothelium-dependent responses during chronic hypertension may predispose to cerebral ischemia and stroke. Evidence consistent with that possibility is that serotonin produces greater constriction of large cerebral arteries in spontaneously hypertensive stroke-prone rats than in Wistar-Kyoto rats.[51]

K⁺ Channels in Chronic Hypertension

Dilator responses of cerebral arteries of chronically hypertensive rats are impaired in response to activation of ATP-sensitive K^+ channels[45] (Fig. 3.1). Because ATP-sensitive K^+ channels are important mediators of vasodilator responses to hypoxia and hypotension, one might speculate that cerebral dilator responses to hypoxia and hypotension are impaired in chronic hypertension.[48,92]

Specific inhibitors of calcium-dependent K^+ channels produce greater contraction of cerebral vessels in hypertensive than normotensive animals. Thus, basal activity of calcium-dependent K^+ channels appears to be increased in cerebral arteries during chronic hypertension[76] (Fig. 3.1). Our interpretation of this finding is that increased intracellular concentration of calcium or changes in sensitivity to calcium during chronic hypertension cause increased activation of the calcium-dependent K^+ channel, which may function as a compensatory mechanism to modulate increased constriction of cerebral arteries.

SUBARACHNOID HEMORRHAGE

Function of Endothelium and Soluble Guanylate Cyclase

Subarachnoid hemorrhage produces several abnormalities of vascular function (Fig. 3.2). Cerebral vascular muscle is partially depolarized after subarachnoid hemorrhage,[26] contributing to cerebral vasospasm, which often occurs following subarachnoid hemorrhage.[12] Several mechanisms, including endothelial function, may contribute to vasospasm. Endothelium-dependent relaxation is impaired in large cerebral arteries in experimental models of subarachnoid hemorrhage.[34,40–42,67,73,74] Similar impairment has been observed in the basilar artery from humans following subarachnoid hemorrhage.[29]

Several mechanisms have been proposed to account for impaired endothelium-dependent relaxation following subarachnoid hemorrhage.[12] Both the amount and the activity of endothelial NOS protein are relatively unchanged in large cerebral arteries following subarachnoid hemorrhage.[36,68] These findings are consistent with previous reports that release of EDRF is normal following subarachnoid hemorrhage.[40–42]

Some findings suggest that impaired endothelium-dependent relaxation following subarachnoid hemorrhage is due to reduced protein levels, or activity of soluble guanylate cyclase, or both[8,36,42] (Fig. 3.2). By contrast, other studies report that vasorelaxation in response to nitrovasodilators is unaltered.[34,37]

The presence of hemoglobin in the cerebrospinal fluid may contribute to vasospasm following subarachnoid hemorrhage by inhibition of EDRF. Hemoglobin avidly binds EDRF and thus may prevent diffusion of EDRF from endothelium to smooth muscle. In addition, hemoglobin may destroy EDRF by generation of superoxide anion.[12] Thus, more than one mechanism may contribute to impairment of endothelium-dependent relaxation of cerebral arteries following subarachnoid hemorrhage.

Endothelin

Endothelin is a vasoactive peptide produced by endothelial cells and is thus an EDCF.[99] It is not clear whether endothelin plays a role in physiologic regulation of the cerebral circulation. Because endothelin-mediated constriction is long lasting, it seems unlikely that endothelin contributes to the fine, short-term regulation of cerebral blood flow. Topical application of endothelin receptor antagonists does not alter diameter of cerebral vessels in vivo, suggesting that endothelin does not contribute to basal cerebrovascular tone.[20,47]

Several findings suggest that endothelin may contribute to cerebral vasospasm following subarachnoid hemorrhage[82] (Fig. 3.2). Hemoglobin and thrombin, which are present in cerebrospinal fluid following subarachnoid hemorrhage, can enhance endothelin gene expression and endothelin release[11,35,71,91] (Fig. 3.2). Concentrations of endothelin in the basilar artery and in cerebrospinal fluid are increased following subarachnoid hemorrhage.[32,51,55,90,98] Intracisternal administration of antagonists for endothelin type A

Figure 3.2 Some abnormalities in cerebral vessels following subarachnoid hemorrhage. Thrombin and hemoglobin cause increased gene expression of endothelin—a potent vasoconstrictor. Superoxide anion ($O_2^{\bullet-}$) may be formed from hemoglobin and may inactivate nitric oxide (NO), thus impairing relaxation. Vasodilatation in response to activation of adenosine triphosphate (ATP)-sensitive K^+ channels (K^+_{ATP}) appears to be augmented following subarachnoid hemorrhage. This latter mechanism, in contrast to the first two, has implications for treatment of vasospasm following subarachnoid hemorrhage.

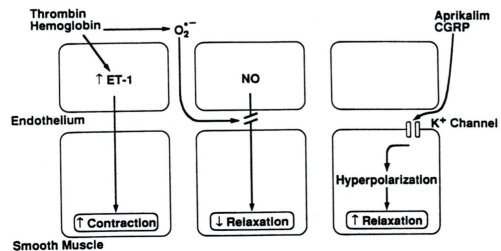

(ET$_A$) receptors reduces vasospasm following subarachnoid hemorrhage.[10,20,32,102,103] By contrast, other studies report no correlation between cerebrospinal fluid endothelin levels and cerebral vasospasm[22] and failure of ET$_A$ antagonists to reverse cerebral vasospasm.[13] However, most evidence is consistent with the concept that endothelin and activation of ET$_A$ receptors contribute to the onset or maintenance of cerebral vasospasm following subarachnoid hemorrhage.

K$^+$ Channel Function after Subarachnoid Hemorrhage

Another mechanism that may contribute to vasospasm following subarachnoid hemorrhage may involve changes in activity of K$^+$ channels in cerebral vessels. Partial depolarization of cerebral vascular muscle after subarachnoid hemorrhage appears to be due to decreased membrane conductance to K$^+$.[26] Depolarization and vasospasm can be inhibited by nicorandil, a vasodilator that activates both potassium channels and soluble guanylate cyclase.[26] These findings suggest that activators of K$^+$ channels in vascular muscle may have beneficial effects during vasospasm following subarachnoid hemorrhage (Fig. 3.2).

Consistent with these findings are recent reports that dilatation of the basilar artery in response to openers of ATP-sensitive K$^+$ channels is enhanced following subarachnoid hemorrhage[86,87] (Fig. 3.2). Interestingly, K$^+$ channel-mediated dilatation of large cerebral vessels may be especially enhanced following subarachnoid hemorrhage during chronic hypertension.[86] Thus, augmented responses to activation of K$^+$ channels despite the presence of hypertension are unusual and potentially useful.

HYPERHOMOCYSTEINEMIA

Moderate elevation of plasma homocysteine appears to be an independent risk factor for stroke and is associated with peripheral vascular disease and myocardial infarction.[5] Like hypercholesterolemia, hyperhomocysteinemia is caused by both genetic and dietary factors and may possibly contribute to vascular disease in a large number of patients.[89] Moderate elevations of plasma homocysteine can be decreased by dietary supplementation with folic acid, which suggests that hyperhomocysteinemia may be a treatable risk factor for stroke and other vascular diseases.

Mechanisms responsible for the association between hyperhomocysteinemia and vascular disease may involve generation of hydrogen peroxide or other reactive oxygen species. High concentrations of homocysteine in vitro impair NO-mediated inhibition of platelet aggregation[88] and inhibit thrombomodulin-dependent activation of protein C, a clinically important anticoagulant.[52,78] Homocysteine also induces cultured endothelial cells to express procoagulant molecules[21,79] and alters binding of tissue plasminogen activator to endothelium.[24] Recent findings in monkeys suggest that diet-induced moderate hyperhomocysteinemia leads to increased platelet-mediated vasoconstriction, impaired endothelium-dependent dilatation of extracranial vessels, and decreased endothelial thrombomodulin-dependent activation of protein C.[53] These effects were reversible by dietary folate treatment. The findings suggest that endothelial dysfunction may be a plausible mechanism for predisposition to cerebral vascular disease and atherosclerosis in hyperhomocysteinemia.

DIABETES MELLITUS

Endothelial dysfunction also occurs in cerebral vessels during diabetes mellitus.[56,59,65,77] Mechanisms that account for impairment appear to be similar in diabetes to those observed during chronic hypertension. Altered responses of cerebral arterioles to endothelium-dependent agonists are probably due to production of an EDCF that activates a prostaglandin H$_2$/thromboxane A$_2$ receptor[65] with activation of protein kinase C.[77] In the basilar artery, impaired responses to endothelium-dependent stimuli are not due to production of a cyclooxygenase-derived EDCF.[59]

As in chronic hypertension, activity of ATP-sensitive K$^+$ channels appears to be altered in diabetes. Dilatation of the basilar artery in response to aprikalim, an activator of ATP-sensitive K$^+$ channels, is reduced in diabetic rats, suggesting that function of the ATP-sensitive K$^+$ channel may be abnormal in diabetes mellitus.[61]

Recent findings suggest that hyperglycemia per se produces impairment of endothelium-dependent dilatation of cerebral arterioles. This impairment during acute elevations of glucose appears to involve activation of protein kinase C.[62]

Gene Transfer to Cerebral Blood Vessels

At present, gene transfer is a promising tool for the study of vascular biology; and despite great obstacles, such therapy for cerebrovascular disease has considerable potential.[30] The goal is to introduce cDNA into a cerebral artery or perivascular tissue and to stimulate production of a protein that favorably modulates vascular growth or function. Theoretically, this could be accomplished using naked DNA, but in reality this approach provides very inefficient gene transfer. Thus, other more efficient vectors have been developed including viral vectors (adenovirus, retrovirus, adeno-associated virus, and herpesvirus), complexes of DNA-cationic lipids, and viral conjugate vectors (liposomes with a viral coat).[30] It is important to note, however, that at present, each of these vectors has limitations, and the development of more efficient and safe vectors is an active area of investigation.

Gene transfer can potentially be "targeted" to appropriate tissues, such as adventitia, endothelium, or specific receptors on the cell surface. Transgene expression may be driven by tissue-specific promoters. In addition, gene transfer can be used to express antisense oligonucleotides that inhibit expression of selected genes. For example, an antisense construct for astrocyte glial fibrillary acidic protein has been used to inhibit gliosis in astrocytes.[23]

We envision several potential applications of gene therapy for intracranial vascular disease. First, gene therapy might be used to prevent vasospasm following subarachnoid hemorrhage by transient transfection of a gene whose product produces (either directly or indirectly) marked vasodilatation. Possible candidates are NOS and CGRP. It is now possible to alter function of intracranial blood vessels in tissue culture using a gene to overexpress endothelial NOS.[8] Second, gene transfer might be used to stimulate growth of collateral vessels in the presence of ischemia. This approach appears feasible in other organs. Third, gene therapy might be used to treat brain tumors by inhibiting vascular proliferation and thus produce ischemia in the tumor.

In extracranial vascular disease, gene therapy might be useful for treatment of disease in the carotid or vertebral artery. Gene transfer approaches have been used to interrupt the cell cycle and thereby inhibit proliferation of vascular muscle. Therefore, a goal of gene therapy might be to transfect an atherosclerotic lesion in an extracranial artery with a gene that inhibits proliferation of the lesion. However, the problems presently related to transient expression of transgenes provide major obstacles for the use of gene therapy to inhibit the chronic proliferation characteristic of atherosclerosis.

Summary

Abnormalities of cerebral vessel function occur in several pathophysiologic conditions. Although the mechanisms are complex and multifactorial, increased understanding of several mechanisms of cerebral vessel dysfunction has been achieved in recent years. Many of these abnormalities are likely to compromise cerebral blood flow and increase the risk of stroke. Therapy for cerebral vascular dysfunction may involve pharmacologic or dietary interventions, or both, and may potentially utilize gene transfer technology.

Acknowledgments

Original studies cited in this review were supported by NIH grants NS 24621, HL 38901, HL 14388, HL 16066, and AG 10269; by Research Funds from the Veterans Administration; and by a Grant-In-Aid from the American Heart Association (95014510). F.M. Faraci is an Established Investigator of the American Heart Association. Dr. Sobey is supported by a C.J. Martin Fellowship from the National Health and Medical Research Council of Australia and is the recipient of a Michael J. Brody Fellowship in Basic Cardiovascular Research from the University of Iowa.

References

1. Akopov S, Sercombe R, Seylaz J: Cerebrovascular reactivity: role of endothelium/platelet/leukocyte interactions. Cerebrovasc Brain Metab Rev 8:11, 1996
2. Asano M, Masuzawa-Ito K, Matsuda T: Charybdotoxin-sensitive K + channels regulate the myogenic tone in the resting state of arteries from spontaneously hypertensive rats. Br J Pharmacol 108:214, 1993
3. Barnett HJM: Progress towards stroke prevention: Robert Wartenberg Lecture. Neurology 30:1212, 1980
4. Benzuly KH, Padgett RC, Kaul S et al: Functional improvement precedes structural regression of atherosclerosis. Circulation 89:1810, 1994
5. Boushey CJ, Beresford SAA, Omenn GS, Motulsky AG: A quantitative assessment of plasma homocysteine as a risk factor for vascular disease: probable benefits of increasing folic acid intakes. JAMA 274:1049, 1995
6. Brayden JE, Nelson MT: Regulation of arterial tone by activation of calcium-activated potassium channels. Science 256:532, 1992
7. Brian JE, Kennedy RH: Modulation of cerebral arterial tone by endothelium-derived relaxing factor. Am J Physiol 264:H1245, 1993
8. Chen AFY, Kinoshita H, Tsutsui M et al: Effect of recombinant endothelial nitric oxide synthase gene expression on reactivity of isolated canine basilar artery, abstracted. FASEB J 10:A303, 1996
9. Chester AH, O'Neil GS, Moncada S et al: Low basal and stimulated release of nitric oxide in atherosclerotic epicardial coronary arteries. Lancet 336:897, 1990
10. Clozel M, Watanabe H: BQ-123, a peptidic endothelin ETA receptor antagonist, prevents the early cerebral vasospasm following subarachnoid hemorrhage after intracisternal but not intravenous injection. Life Sci 52: 825, 1993
11. Cocks TM, Malta E, King SJ et al: Oxyhaemoglobin increases the production of endothelin-1 by endothelial cells in culture. Eur J Pharmacol 196:177, 1991
12. Cook DA: Mechanisms of cerebral vasospasm in subarachnoid hemorrhage. Pharmacol Ther 66:259, 1995
13. Cosentino F, McMahon EG, Carter JS, Katusic ZS: Effect of endothelin A-receptor antagonist BQ-123 and phosphoramidon on cerebral vasospasm. J Cardiovasc Pharmacol, suppl. 8, 22:S332, 1993
14. Faraci FM, Brian JE: Nitric oxide and the cerebral circulation. Stroke 25:692, 1994
15. Faraci FM, Heistad DD: Endothelium-derived relaxing factor inhibits constrictor responses of large cerebral arteries to serotonin. J Cereb Blood Flow Metab 12:500, 1992
16. Faraci FM, Heistad DD: Role of ATP-sensitive potassium channels in the basilar artery. Am J Physiol 264: H8, 1993
17. Faraci FM, Williams JK, Breese KR et al: Atherosclerosis potentiates constrictor responses of cerebral and ocular blood vessels to thromboxane. Stroke 20:242, 1989
18. Faraci FM, Lopez JAG, Breese K et al: Effect of atherosclerosis on cerebral vascular responses to activation of leukocytes and platelets in monkeys. Stroke 22:790, 1991
19. Faraci FM, Orgren K, Heistad DD: Impaired relaxation of the carotid artery during activation of ATP-sensitive potassium channels in atherosclerotic monkeys. Stroke 25:178, 1994
20. Foley PL, Caner HH, Kassell NF, Lee KS: Reversal of subarachnoid hemorrhage-induced vasoconstriction

with an endothelin receptor antagonist. Neurosurgery 34:108, 1994

21. Fryer RH, Wilson BD, Gubler DB et al: Homocysteine, a risk factor for premature vascular disease and thrombosis, induces tissue factor activity in endothelial cells. Arterioscler Thromb Vasc Biol 13:1327, 1993

22. Gaetani P, Rodriguez y Baena R, Grignani G et al: Endothelin and aneurysmal subarachnoid hemorrhage: a study of subarachnoid cisternal cerebrospinal fluid. J Neurol Neurosurg Psychiatry 57:66, 1994

23. Ghirnikar RS, Yu AC, Eng LF: Astrogliosis in culture: III. Effect of recombinant retrovirus expressing antisense glial fibrillary acidic protein RNA. J Neurosci Res 38:376, 1994

24. Hajjar KA: Homocysteine-induced modulation of tissue plasminogen activator binding to its endothelial cell membrane receptor. J Clin Invest 91:2873, 1993

25. Hardebo JE, Kahrstrom J, Owman C: P1-P2-purine receptors in brain circulation. Eur J Pharmacol 144:343, 1987

26. Harder DR, Dernbach P, Waters A: Possible cellular mechanism for cerebral vasospasm after experimental subarachnoid hemorrhage in the dog. J Clin Invest 80:875, 1987

27. Harrison DG, Armstrong ML, Freiman PC, Heistad DD: Restoration of endothelium-dependent relaxation by dietary treatment of atherosclerosis. J Clin Invest 80:1808, 1987

28. Hart JL, Sobey CG, Woodman OL: Cholesterol feeding enhances the vasoconstrictor effects of products from rabbit polymorphonuclear leukocytes. Am J Physiol 269:H1, 1995

29. Hatake K, Wakabayashi I, Kakishita E, Hishida S: Impairment of endothelium-dependent relaxation in human basilar artery after subarachnoid hemorrhage. Stroke 23:1111, 1992

30. Heistad DD, Faraci FM: Gene therapy for cerebral vascular disease. Stroke 27:1688, 1996

31. Heistad DD, Breese K, Armstrong ML: Cerebral vasoconstrictor responses to serotonin after dietary treatment of atherosclerosis: implications for transient ischemic attacks. Stroke 18:1068, 1987

32. Hirose H, Ide K, Sasaki T et al: The role of endothelin and nitric oxide in modulation of normal and spastic cerebral vascular tone in the dog. Eur J Pharmacol 277:77, 1995

33. Kanamura K, Waga S, Tochio H, Nagatani K: The effect of atherosclerosis on endothelium-dependent relaxation in the aorta and intracranial arteries of rabbits. J Neurosurg 70:793, 1989

34. Kanamura K, Weir BKA, Findlay JM et al: Pharmacological studies on relaxation of spastic primate cerebral arteries in subarachnoid hemorrhage. J Neurosurg 71:909, 1989

35. Kasuya H, Weir BKA, White DM, Steffansson K: Mechanisms of oxyhemoglobin-induced release of endothelin-1 from cultured vascular endothelial cells and smooth muscle cells. J Neurosurg 79:892, 1993

36. Kasuya H, Weir BKA, Nakane M et al: Nitric oxide synthase and guanylate cyclase levels in canine basilar artery

after subarachnoid hemorrhage. J Neurosurg 82:250, 1995

37. Katusic ZS, Milde JH, Cosentino F, Mitrovic BS: Subarachnoid hemorrhage and endothelial L-arginine pathway in small brain stem arteries in dogs. Stroke 24:392, 1993

38. Kaul S, Waack BJ, Padgett RC et al: Altered vascular responses to platelets from hypercholesterolemic humans. Circ Res 72:737, 1993

39. Kaul S, Waack BJ, Padgett RC et al: Interaction of platelets and leukocytes in modulation of vascular tone. Am J Physiol 266:H1706, 1994

40. Kim P, Sundt TM, Vanhoutte PM: Alterations in endothelium-dependent responsiveness of the canine basilar artery after subarachnoid hemorrhage. J Neurosurg 69:239, 1988

41. Kim P, Lorenz RR, Sundt TM, Vanhoutte PM: Release of endothelium-derived relaxing factor after subarachnoid hemorrhage. J Neurosurg 70:108, 1989

42. Kim P, Schini VB, Sundt TM, Vanhoutte PM: Reduced production of cGMP underlies the loss of endothelium-dependent relaxations in the canine basilar artery after subarachnoid hemorrhage. Circ Res 70:248, 1992

43. Kitagawa S, Yamaguchi Y, Sameshima E, Kunitomo M: Differences in endothelium-dependent relaxation in various arteries from Watanabe heritable hyperlipidaemic rabbits with increasing age. Clin Exp Pharmacol Physiol 21:963, 1994

44. Kitazono T, Faraci FM, Heistad DD: Effect of norepinephrine on rat basilar artery in vivo. Am J Physiol 264:H178, 1993

45. Kitazono T, Heistad DD, Faraci FM: ATP-sensitive potassium channels in the basilar artery during chronic hypertension. Hypertension 22:677, 1993

46. Kitazono T, Heistad DD, Faraci FM: Role of ATP-sensitive K + channels in CGRP-induced dilatation of basilar artery in vivo. Am J Physiol 265:H581, 1993

47. Kitazono T, Heistad DD, Faraci FM: Enhanced responses of the basilar artery to activation of endothelin B receptors in stroke-prone spontaneously hypertensive rats. Hypertension 25:490, 1995

48. Kitazono T, Faraci FM, Taguchi H, Heistad DD: Role of potassium channels in cerebral blood vessels. Stroke 26:1713, 1995

49. Kitazono T, Faraci FM, Heistad DD: L-arginine restores dilator responses of the basilar artery to acetylcholine during chronic hypertension. Hypertension 27:893, 1996

50. Knowles RG, Moncada S: Nitric oxide synthases in mammals. Biochem J 298:249, 1994

51. Kraus GE, Bucholz RD, Yoon K-W et al: Cerebrospinal fluid endothelin-1 and endothelin-3 levels in normal and neurosurgical patients. A clinical and literature review. Surg Neurol 35:20, 1991

52. Lentz SR, Sadler JE: Inhibition of thrombomodulin surface expression and protein C activation by the thrombogenic agent homocysteine. J Clin Invest 88:1906, 1991

53. Lentz SR, Sobey CG, Piegors DJ et al: Vascular dysfunction in monkeys with diet-induced hyperhomocyst(e)inemia. J Clin Invest 98:24, 1996

54. Lincoln TM, Cornwell TL: Towards an understanding of the mechanism of action of cyclic AMP and cyclic

GMP in smooth muscle relaxation. Blood Vessels 28: 129, 1991

55. Masaoka H, Suzuki R, Hirata Y et al: Raised plasma endothelin in aneurysmal subarachnoid hemorrhage. Lancet Dec 9:1402, 1989

56. Mayhan WG: Impairment of endothelium-dependent dilatation of cerebral arterioles during diabetes mellitus. Am J Physiol 256:H621, 1989

57. Mayhan WG: Impairment of endothelium-dependent responses of basilar artery during chronic hypertension. Am J Physiol 259:H1455, 1990

58. Mayhan WG: Responses of the basilar artery to products released by platelets during chronic hypertension. Brain Res 545:97, 1991

59. Mayhan WG: Impairment of endothelium-dependent dilation of the basilar artery in diabetes mellitus. Brain Res 580:297, 1992

60. Mayhan WG: Role of prostaglandin H2-thromboxane A2 in responses of cerebral arterioles during chronic hypertension. Am J Physiol 262:H539, 1992

61. Mayhan WG: Effect of diabetes mellitus on response of the basilar artery to activation of ATP-sensitive potassium channels. Brain Res 636:35, 1994

62. Mayhan WG, Patel KP: Acute effects of glucose on reactivity of cerebral microcirculation: role of activation of protein kinase C. Am J Physiol 269:H1297, 1995

63. Mayhan WG, Faraci FM, Heistad DD: Impairment of endothelium-dependent responses of cerebral arterioles in chronic hypertension. Am J Physiol 253:H1435, 1987

64. Mayhan WG, Faraci FM, Heistad DD: Impairment of endothelium-dependent responses of cerebral arterioles in chronic hypertension. Hypertension 12:556, 1988

65. Mayhan WG, Simmons LK, Sharpe GM: Mechanism of impaired responses of cerebral arterioles during diabetes mellitus. Am J Physiol 260:H319, 1991

66. Mugge A, Elwell JH, Peterson TE et al: Chronic treatment with polyethylene-glycolated superoxide dismutase partially restores endothelium-dependent vascular relaxations in cholesterol-fed rabbits. Circ Res 69:1293, 1991

67. Nakagomi T, Kassell NF, Sasaki T et al: Impairment of endothelium-dependent vasodilatation induced by acetylcholine and adenosine triphosphate following experimental subarachnoid hemorrhage. Stroke 18:482, 1987

68. Naveri L, Stromberg C, Saavedra JM: Angiotensin IV reverses the acute cerebral blood flow reduction after experimental subarachnoid hemorrhage in the rat. J Cereb Blood Flow Metab 14:1096, 1994

69. Nelson MT, Quayle JM: Physiological roles and properties of potassium channels in arterial smooth muscle. Am J Physiol 268:C799, 1995

70. Nelson MT, Cheng H, Rubart M et al: Relaxation of arterial smooth muscle by calcium sparks. Science 270: 588, 1995

71. Ohlstein EH, Storer BL: Oxyhemoglobin stimulation of endothelin production in cultured endothelial cells. J Neurosurg 77:274, 1992

72. Padgett RC, Heistad DD, Mugge A et al: Vascular responses to activated leukocytes after regression of atherosclerosis. Circ Res 70:423, 1992

73. Pasqualin A, Hongo K, Van Beek O et al: Cerebrovascular effects of substance P after experimental hemorrhage. Acta Neurochir (Wien) 119:139, 1992

74. Pasqualin A, Tsukahara T, Kassell NF, Torner JC: Effect of nicardipine on basilar artery vasoactive responses after subarachnoid hemorrhage. Neurosurgery 31:697, 1992

75. Paterno R, Faraci FM, Heistad DD: Role of Ca^{++}-dependent K$^+$ channels in cerebral vasodilatation induced by increases in cyclic GMP and cyclic AMP. Stroke 27: 1603, 1996

76. Paterno K, Heistad DD, Faraci FM: Functional activity of calcium-dependent potassium channels is increased in the basilar artery in vivo during chronic hypertension. Am J Physiol 272:H1287–H1291, 1997

77. Pelligrino DA, Koenig HM, Wang Q, Albrecht RF: Protein kinase C suppresses receptor-mediated pial arteriolar relaxation in the diabetic rat. Neuroreport 5:417, 1994

78. Rodgers GM, Conn MT: Homocysteine, an atherogenic stimulus, reduces protein C activation by arterial and venous endothelial cells. Blood 75:895, 1990

79. Rodgers GM, Kane WH: Activation of endogenous factor V by a homocysteine-vascular endothelial cell activator. J Clin Invest 77:1909, 1986

80. Rossitch E, Alexander E, Black PMcL, Cooke JP: L-arginine normalizes endothelial function in cerebral vessels from hypercholesterolemic rabbits. J Clin Invest 87: 1295, 1991

81. Scandinavian Simvastatin Survival Study Group: Randomised trial of cholesterol lowering in 4444 patients with coronary heart disease: the Scandinavian Simvastatin Survival Study (4S). Lancet 344:1383, 1994

82. Seifert V, Loffler B-M, Zimmerman M et al: Endothelin concentrations in patients with aneurysmal subarachnoid hemorrhage. J Neurosurg 82:55, 1995

83. Simonsen U, Ehrnrooth E, Gerdes LU et al: Functional properties in vitro of systemic small arteries from rabbits fed a cholesterol-rich diet for 12 weeks. Clin Sci 80:119, 1991

84. Sobey CG, Woodman OL: Myocardial ischaemia: what happens to the coronary arteries? Trends Pharmacol Sci 14:448, 1993

85. Sobey CG, Faraci FM, Piegors DJ, Heistad DD: Effect of short-term regression of atherosclerosis on reactivity of carotid and retinal arteries. Stroke 27:927, 1996

86. Sobey CG, Heistad DD, Faraci FM: Effect of subarachnoid hemorrhage on cerebral vasodilatation in response to activation of ATP-sensitive K+ channels in chronically hypertensive rats. Stroke 27:14, 1996

87. Sobey CG, Heistad DD, Faraci FM: Effect of subarachnoid hemorrhage on dilatation of rat basilar artery in vivo. Am J Physiol 271:H126, 1996

88. Stamler JS, Osborne JA, Jaraki O et al: Adverse vascular effects of homocysteine are modulated by endothelium-derived relaxing factor and related oxides of nitrogen. J Clin Invest 91:308, 1993

89. Stampfer MJ, Malinow MR: Can lowering homocysteine levels reduce cardiovascular risk? N Engl J Med 332: 328, 1995

90. Suzuki H, Sato S, Suzuki Y et al: Increased endothelin contraction in CSF from patients with subarachnoid hemorrhage. Acta Neurol Scand 81:553, 1990

91. Suzuki M, Ogawa A, Sakurai Y et al: Thrombin activity in cerebrospinal fluid after subarachnoid hemorrhage. Stroke 23:1181, 1992

92. Taguchi H, Heistad DD, Kitazono T, Faraci FM: ATP-sensitive potassium channels mediate dilatation of cerebral arterioles during hypoxia. Circ Res 74:1005, 1994

93. Taguchi H, Faraci FM, Kitazono T, Heistad DD: Relaxation of the carotid artery during hypoxia is impaired in Watanabe heritable hyperlipidemic rabbits. Arterioscler Thromb Vasc Biol 15:1641, 1995

94. Taguchi H, Heistad DD, Kitazono T, Faraci FM: Dilatation of cerebral arterioles in response to activation of adenylate cyclase is dependent on activation of Ca + + - dependent K+ channels. Circ Res 76:1057, 1995

95. Tamaki K, Armstrong M, Heistad D: Effects of atherosclerosis on cerebral vessels: hemodynamic and morphometric studies. Stroke 17:1209, 1986

96. Vanhoutte PM, Houston DS: Platelets, endothelium and vasospasm. Circulation 72:728, 1985

97. Wong SKF, Garbers DL: Receptor guanylyl cyclases. J Clin Invest 90:299, 1992

98. Yamaura I, Tani E, Maeda Y et al: Endothelin-1 of canine basilar artery in vasospasm. J Neurosurg 76:99, 1992

99. Yanagisawa M, Kurihara H, Kimura S et al: A novel potent vasoconstrictor peptide produced by vascular endothelial cells. Nature 332:411, 1988

100. Yang SY, Mayhan WG, Faraci FM, Heistad DD: Endothelium-dependent responses of cerebral blood vessels during chronic hypertension. Hypertension 17:612, 1991

101. Yang SY, Mayhan WG, Faraci FM, Heistad DD: Mechanisms of impaired endothelium-dependent cerebral vasodilatation in response to bradykinin during chronic hypertension. Stroke 22:1177, 1991

102. Zuccarello M, Lewis AI, Rapoport RM: Endothelin ETA and ETB receptors in subarachnoid hemorrhage-induced cerebral vasospasm. Eur J Pharmacol 259:R1, 1994

103. Zuccarello M, Romano A, Passalacqua M, Rapoport RM: Decreased endothelium-dependent relaxation in subarachnoid hemorrhage-induced vasospasm: role of ET-1. Am J Physiol 269:H1009, 1995

Neurochemistry and Molecular Biology

FRANK R. SHARP

RAYMOND A. SWANSON

JARI HONKANIEMI

KYUYA KOGURE

STEPHEN M. MASSA

Definitions

The term *stroke* and its synonym *cerebrovascular accident* refer to irreversible brain injury resulting from cerebral ischemia. Cerebral ischemia occurs when blood flow decreases to the point that metabolic substrate delivery fails to meet the metabolic demand of the tissue. The actual flow rate at which this occurs is variable, since brain metabolic demand is variable from region to region and varies during different conditions.[348]

Hypoxia refers to decreases of the partial pressure of oxygen, and anoxia refers to the complete absence of oxygen in either the air or in tissue. The role of oxygen deficits in the production of ischemic injury is complicated by the fact that reduction in the FIO_2 below 6% to 8% produces cardiac dysfunction, which leads secondarily to cerebral ischemia. The confusing term *hypoxia/ischemia* is sometimes used in reference to this complex circumstance. Hypoxia alone, without superimposed ischemia or acidosis, does not appear to cause brain injury. Experimental delivery of cyanide, an inhibitor of the complex IV enzymes in the mitochondrial respiratory chain, to the rat carotid artery produces a flat electroencephalogram (EEG) but only modest reductions in adenosine triphosphate (ATP) and no neuronal death.[245]

Cerebral infarction is defined as either the death of both neuronal and glial cells in a specific region, or the combined death of all cellular elements, including neurons, glia, and endothelial cells, the latter being termed *pan-necrosis*.[104] A second pattern of brain injury, selective neuronal necrosis, is observed after brief periods of cerebral ischemia and at the margins of cerebral infarcts.[107] Pyramidal neurons in the CA1 sector of hippocampus and Purkinje cells of the cerebellum appear to be the neuronal populations most sensitive to global ischemia.[193,310,311] Selective neuronal cell death can also occur following hypoglycemia and status epilepticus.

Ischemia may be classified as either complete or incomplete, temporary or permanent. Occlusion of a cerebral artery results in complete ischemia in regions with no collateral flow, and incomplete ischemia in a surrounding penumbra region with collateral blood supply. This condition is termed *focal ischemia* and may be either temporary or permanent. Cardiac arrest or severe hypotension causes complete ischemia to the entire brain, a condition also referred to as *global ischemia*. A confusion in the experimental literature arises from the fact that the term global ischemia is often used interchangeably with complete ischemia. Animal models of complete (or global) ischemia often use occlusion and reperfusion of multiple vessels, such as the two-vessel gerbil global ischemia model,[167,193] the two-vessel model with combined hypotension,[354] and the four-vessel rodent global ischemia model.[311,312] Since global ischemia of sufficient duration is fatal, all animal models of global or complete ischemia are models of temporary rather than permanent ischemia.

Experimental Models of Focal and Global Ischemia

COMPLETE ISCHEMIA

Models

Most experimental studies of global ischemia use the gerbil model. In the gerbil, which has no collaterals between the anterior and posterior circulation, 2 minutes of bilateral ca-

Figure 4.1 (**A**) ATP loss and (**B**) lactate accumulation in brain after decapitation of anesthetized animals.

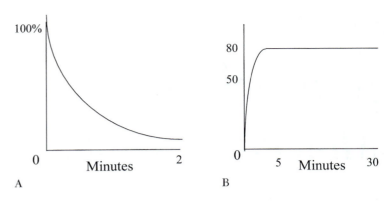

A

B

rotid occlusion produces no cell death. Five-minute occlusions of both carotid arteries produce selective, delayed cell death of most pyramidal neurons in the CA1 sector of the hippocampus without any cell death elsewhere.[194] In the gerbil model there is no ischemia of the brain stem and cerebellum. The two-vessel rat global ischemia model involves bilateral carotid occlusion combined with systemic hypotension.[354] The Pulsinelli rat model includes permanent occlusion of the vertebrals, temporary occlusion of both carotids, and compression of cervical collaterals with a neck suture.[312] Decapitation ischemia is the ultimate global ischemia model, although it has been used relatively little since it is not reversible. The EEG becomes isoelectric approximately 12 seconds after decapitation when ATP is still preserved. ATP falls to about 50% of control by 30 seconds and was approximately 10% of control by 2 minutes following decapitation[365] (Fig. 4.1). Electrical failure occurs before energy failure. Following decapitation ischemia, lactate increases to 50 to 70 nmol/mg protein, values below the 90 nmol/mg protein considered neurotoxic during cerebral ischemia.[274] This may help to explain why infarction does not usually occur in global ischemia in humans and in experimental animals.

Selective Vulnerability of Neurons to Global (Complete) Ischemia

Following brief global (complete) ischemia in the gerbil[167,194] rat,[311] monkey,[409] and human,[356] no immediate changes are evident in the brain. However, evidence of pyknotic, eosinophillic neurons becomes evident in the CA1 pyramidal hippocampal neurons sometime between 1 and 4 days later. This CA1 neuronal death has been described as *delayed* since cells appear to be morphologically normal for as long as a day following the ischemia. This selective vulnerability of CA1 neurons appears to be related to this cell type since the same neurons can be selectively injured in rodents and primates, and since CA1 neurons even in tissue slice preparations are the cells most vulnerable to hypoxia/glucose deprivation.[301]

With more prolonged global ischemia other neurons also die—with a well-defined hierarchy of susceptibility to ischemia. Following 5 minutes of ischemia CA1, hippocampal neurons die. Following 10 and 15 minutes of global ischemia in the gerbil, neurons die in the striatum, inferior colliculus, septum, and pyramidal neurons in layers 3 and 5 of the cortex, CA3 neurons of the hippocampus, and lateral, reticular, and geniculate nuclei of thalamus, and the substantia nigra.[16] In the four-vessel rat global ischemia model a similar pattern of vulnerability is noted, in addition to the finding that cerebellar Purkinje cells are particularly vulnerable.

Various mechanisms of cell death are discussed below and their relation to global and focal ischemic injury pointed out. It is worth stating that the selective, delayed cell death that occurs in the CA1 region and possibly elsewhere in the brain has been the subject of several possibly interrelated theories. These include (1) an *excitotoxic hypothesis*—ischemic cell death is related to glutamate actions at excitatory amino acid receptors, which is mediated by calcium[58,323]; (2) a *mitochondrial hypothesis*—ischemia disrupts axonal transport, which disturbs mitochondrial synthesis, since the subunits of mitochondrial respiratory enzymes are synthesized in the nucleus as well as from mitochondrial DNA in axons and dendrites[4]; (3) an *inflammatory hypothesis*—ischemia-induced changes in cells, perhaps with calcium and free radicals as a central mediator, result in inflammatory attack and cell death from leukocytes and/or microglia[51,72]; and (4) *apoptosis*—ischemia initiates the programmed death of cells with the activation of killer proteins.[153,171,224]

FOCAL ISCHEMIA

Models

Three general approaches have been used to produce focal ischemia. The first utilizes ligatures to tie off one or more arteries. Occlusion of the rat middle cerebral artery (MCA) has been achieved using an intracranial approach with or without carotid artery occlusion in the neck.[157] MCA occlusion has also been accomplished by enlarging the foramen ovale.[344] Intracranial surgery must be performed for these two approaches. A recently developed focal ischemia model utilizes a nylon suture. The suture is threaded into the external carotid artery in the neck and then advanced intracranially to occlude the MCA. This method, called the suture or thread model, has gained popularity because it is easy, does not require intracranial surgery, and can be temporary or permanent.[235] Other models include photocoagulation of vessels with laser light and photosensitive dyes introduced into the vascular system.[75]

Ischemic Core Versus Ischemic Penumbra

The core region of focal ischemia receives insufficient blood supply to maintain energy metabolism.[130] If blood flow is not restored to this region within a critical period—which may

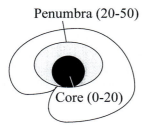

Figure 4.2 Diagram of a human brain showing an area of infarction (black) where blood flow is very low (0 to 20 ml/100 g/min) surrounded by an area called the penumbra (gray area) where blood flow is reduced (20 to 50 ml/100 g/min) below normal.

be as short as 5 minutes or as long as many hours in some brain regions—this region cannot be saved using any known means.

Between the area of dense ischemia and the region of normal perfusion is an intermediate area, called the penumbra (Fig. 4.2), where blood flow is reduced to a level that interrupts neuronal function, but ATP levels are maintained at normal or near-normal levels.[367] The neuronal dysfunction manifests as decreased voltage and eventually a flat EEG and failure to detect sensory evoked potentials. Membrane pumps and ionic gradients are generally maintained. In baboons with occlusion of the MCA, Symon[367] showed that sensory evoked potentials disappeared with blood flows below 18 ml/100 g/min and infarction occurred when flows fell below 12 ml/100 g/min. The penumbra was defined as areas of cerebral blood between 12 and 18 ml/100 g/min in primate brain, and about double this in the rodent brain (Fig. 4.2).

When blood perfusion pressure falls below the value at which vasodilatation can compensate and autoregulation can be maintained (about 60 mmHg), then oxygen extraction increases from a normal resting value of around 30% to 40% up to values between 90% and 100%.[305,306] Thus, even though blood flow decreases, tissue hypoxia does not result because increases in the oxygen extraction fraction (OEF) can maintain normal tissue oxygen concentrations. When blood flow falls below the point to which OEF can compensate, oxygen delivery falls. However, since the amount of glucose in blood normally far exceeds the extractable oxygen in blood, anaerobic metabolism of glucose ensues, with the production of lactic acid.[305] The threshold for production of lactate is about 50% of the normal cerebral blood flow (CBF). The metabolic changes in brain following decreases in CBF are outlined in Figure 4.3.

Based on positron emission tomography studies in patients, it appears that the pH in penumbra is around 6.7 compared with lower levels in infarcts and 7.0 in normal brain. The oxygen metabolic rate is 60 to 80 mmol/100 g/min in the penumbra compared with lower values in infarcts and 130 to 160 mmol/100 g/min in normal brain. The glucose metabolic rate in the penumbra is around 17 mmol/100 g/min compared with 12 mmol/100 g/min and below in infarcts and 25 mmol/100 g/min in normal brain.[130]

The time windows during which the penumbra is no longer viable depend on the degree of blood flow reduction. Selective necrosis of gray matter occurs if the CBF does not

Figure 4.3 As blood flow falls in rat brain, the rates of protein synthesis begin to decrease well before any changes in brain adenosine triphosphate (ATP) occur. CBV, cerebral blood flow; OEF, oxygen extraction fraction; IEGs, immediate early genes; DWI, diffusion-weighted imaging.

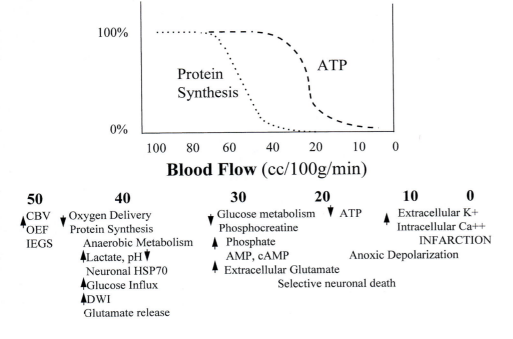

increase above 5 to 15 ml/100 g/min for 1 to 3 hours.[250] With flows of 5 ml/100 g/min neurons appear to be viable for 30 minutes, whereas this period is doubled when blood flow is increased to 10 ml/100 g/min. In cats a direct cortical response (DCR) was attenuated when CBF decreased to 23.7 ml/100 g/min (half normal) and was obliterated when blood flow fell to 8.7 ml/100 g/min.[49] The duration of ischemia after which the DCR was unlikely to recover was 30 minutes for a CBF of 5 ml/100 g/min, 60 minutes for a CBF of 10 ml/100 g/min, 90 minutes for a CBF of 15 ml/100 g/min, and 2 hours for a CBF of 17 ml/100 g/min.[49]

Protein, Glucose, and RNA Metabolism Following Ischemia

Regional protein and glucose metabolism has been well studied following ischemia. Decreases in total protein synthesis are one of the earliest responses to decreased CBF (Fig. 4.3). In rodent brain protein synthesis decreases almost linearly when flow is decreased even slightly below normal values (80 ml/100 g/min), with protein synthesis being decreased by 50% when blood flow fell to about 50 ml/100 g/min.[156,202] Protein synthesis decreased to nearly zero when blood flows reached values between 40 and 20 ml/100 g/min.[260] In regions that infarct and in regions where delayed neuronal death occurs, protein metabolism in those areas goes to near zero within 1 hour and remains at this level until the cells die.[154,374]

The mechanism of decreased protein synthesis is still not clear.[285] Recent studies suggest that an inhibition of the initiation of protein translation follows ischemia. The most likely site of block is in the assembly of the 80S initiation complex of the ribosome (Fig. 4.4). The elongation initiation factor-2 (eIF-2) plays a particularly important role since a 30% phosphorylation of eIF-2 is sufficient to inhibit protein synthesis.[45] The phosphorylation of eIF-2 is modulated by a heme-regulated kinase, also called protein kinase J, and a double-stranded RNA-activated inhibitor and a phosphatase.[215] Although the kinase is regulated by heme, phosphorylated heat shock protein 90, heavy metals/iron, and arachidonic acid, how

hypoxia or ischemia might activate the eIF-2 kinase is unknown.

Regional glucose metabolism also changes following focal ischemia. In areas where blood flow is severely reduced and infarction is rapid, glucose metabolism falls rapidly. Glucose utilization is zero in areas of infarction. In the penumbra [^{14}C] 2-deoxyglucose autoradiography studies have demonstrated increased glucose utilization.[114,277,344] The increased glucose metabolic rate in the ischemic penumbra could be due to (1) increased neuronal activity in the penumbra caused by increased extracellular concentrations of excitatory amino acids and/or potassium; or (2) increased anaerobic metabolism of glucose, with greater glucose uptake occurring because glucose is being metabolized to lactate rather than aerobically in the Krebs cycle.

RNA metabolism has been studied to a lesser degree. Following global ischemia it appears that many mRNAs are made, including those for the heat shock proteins and immediate early genes. However, the protein products of these mRNAs are not synthesized.[283]

Mechanisms of Ischemic Brain Injury

PRIMARY EFFECTS OF ISCHEMIA

The primary effects of ischemia are reduced supply of substrate for energy metabolism (oxygen and glucose) and reduced removal of lactic acid. These derangements cause neuronal and glial death directly in severe ischemia, such as in the ischemic core of focal ischemia. These primary abnormalities can also trigger secondary processes leading to cell death in regions of incomplete ischemia and after reperfusion. Some of these secondary mechanisms of injury are unique to the brain and probably contribute to the extreme vulnerability of brain to ischemic injury.

Figure 4.4 Diagram of roles of elongation initiation factors (eIFs) in protein synthesis. Ischemia probably depresses protein synthesis by phosphorylation of eIF-2 via protein kinase J, which may be activated by hypoxia.

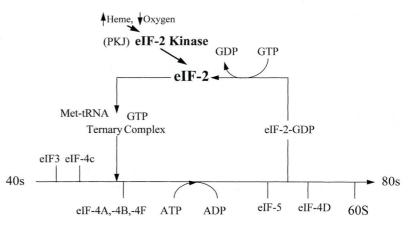

SECONDARY EFFECTS OF ISCHEMIA

Although energy charge clearly decreases following global ischemia, increasing data suggest that the fall in energy-related molecules is not the actual cause of selective or delayed neuronal cell death. The major reason for this supposition is that following restoration of CBF there is rapid normalization of hydrogen, sodium, potassium, and water in cells and a fairly rapid normalization of ATP levels.[348] Moreover, the cells that die following global ischemia may die a slow or delayed death. In addition, similar changes in energy charge appear to occur throughout the hippocampus, even though CA1 neurons generally die whereas dentate granule cell neurons generally survive the ischemia. This finding suggests that transient energy depletion and loss of ionic homeostasis sets in motion a series of secondary cellular events that kill vulnerable neurons. It is clear that the initiator of this injury is energy failure; it is less clear why some cells live and other cells die. Interventions aimed at blocking the secondary effects of ischemia have shown promise as a means of reducing ischemic injury in animal models of stroke.

Secondary effects of ischemia in the brain include release of neurotransmitters, calcium influx into cells, activation of proteases and lipases, production of free radicals and pro-inflammatory molecules, activation of intracellular second messengers, and induction of genes that promote cell death via apoptosis.

Glutamate-Mediated Excitotoxicity

One of the leading theories about mechanisms of secondary injury in the brain relates to glutamate and its receptors. Glutamate normally functions as an excitatory neurotransmitter in the brain, but under pathologic conditions such as ischemia prolonged glutamate receptor activation can lead to neuronal death (excitotoxicity).[58] Glutamate binding to its receptors causes membrane depolarization and increased cytosolic Ca^{2+} levels. Under normal conditions glutamate is quickly cleared from the synaptic cleft by uptake into surrounding astrocytes, allowing neuronal Ca^{2+} levels to normalize (Fig. 4.5). During ischemia, glutamate receptor activation is markedly prolonged due to both excessive glutamate release and impaired glutamate uptake. The resulting sustained elevations in cytosol Ca^{2+} are thought to trigger protease and lipase production as well as other processes that eventually cause neuronal death.

Neurons and astrocytes maintain an extracellular glutamate concentrations in the range of 1 to 5 μmol/L, whereas concentrations in the cytoplasm are 5 to 10 mmol/L. This difference is maintained by using the transmembrane Na^+, K^+, and charge gradients to drive glutamate uptake.[19] These gradients are maintained by membrane Na^+, K^+ ATPase. Compromise in ATP production resulting from ischemia will therefore impair glutamate uptake and lead to increased extracellular concentrations.

Nonsynaptic (or nonvesicular) release of glutamate differs from synaptic, neurotransmitter glutamate release. Synaptic release is an early event during ischemia, triggered by membrane depolarization. This process stops as ATP levels decline because synaptic release is ATP dependent. Nonsynaptic release can occur from both neuronal and glial cytoplasm. The major route of this release appears to be via reversed flow of glutamate across the glutamate uptake transporters when the normal Na^+, K^+, and charge gradients fail to be maintained.[237] The total amount of glutamate in the brain pool that could be released nonsynaptically far exceeds the amount that could be released via synaptic vesicles.[89]

Extracellular glutamate may also increase following spreading depression, which is a slowly moving (2 to 5 mm/s) wave of glial and neuronal depolarization associated with a massive efflux of K^+ and glutamate into the extracellular space.[134] Spreading depression spreads when local elevations in $[K^+]_o$ exceed the ability of astrocytes to buffer or limit these elevations. Repeated waves of spreading depression pass through the ischemic penumbra during focal ischemia and are believed to exacerbate injury by causing increased energy demand and increased levels of extracellular glutamate.[75,155,276]

Potential Mediators of Injury

ROLE OF CALCIUM AND EXCITATORY NEUROTRANSMITTERS/ RECEPTORS

Following ischemia a number of events increase excitability or produce persistent depolarization of cells. This results in abnormal increases in intracellular calcium $[Ca^{2+}]_i$. The increases in $[Ca^{2+}]_i$ produce cellular injury by (1) activating proteases (2) activating lipases, (3) activating endonucleases, and (4) producing release of cytokines and other factors that either directly or indirectly lead to injury and death.

Calcium homeostasis therefore plays a central role in whether ischemia results in selective neuronal cell death or infarction (Fig. 4.5). The resting $[Ca^{2+}]_i$ in neurons is around 100 nM and is maintained in the face of millimolar extracellular calcium concentrations via a number of mechanisms. These include (1) a plasma membrane calcium ATPase that pumps calcium out of cells; (2) a plasma membrane Na^+/Ca^{2+} exchanger that removes calcium from cellular cytoplasm except when the membrane is persistently depolarized, when the exchanger may change directions and pump calcium into cells; (3) a sarcoplasmic endoplasmic reticulum ATPase that pumps calcium into the endoplasmic reticulum and other organelles; and (4) increased expression of calcium binding proteins including calbindin, calmodulin, and others[257,258,349] (Fig. 4.5).

Following ischemia calcium enters cells and increases $[Ca^{2+}]_i$ through a number of different mechanisms. Spreading depression occurs, which can proceed to ischemic depolarization.[21,75,405] Both of these events would result in release of K^+, which would depolarize the membrane of the ischemic cells, resulting in calcium influx into cells through voltage-dependent calcium channels (VDCC). Drugs that are potas-

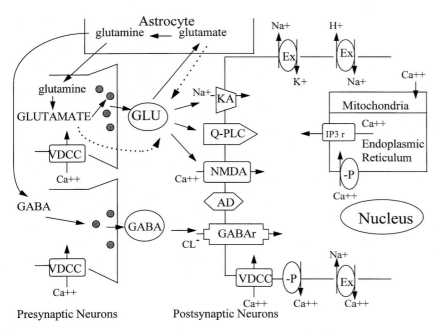

Figure 4.5 Extracellular glutamate increases following ischemia, which can have a number of effects on neurons and eventual cellular injury.

sium channel openers and hence block potassium channels decrease ischemic injury.[142] There are several known types of VDCCs, including n, p, and others, which are located on different types of cells, have different thresholds for calcium entry, and have different capacities for flux of calcium.[111,115] Although drugs acting at VDCCs have not been effective in human stroke—possibly because of their use beyond an appropriate therapeutic window—a wide range of drugs acting at several different VDCCs have decreased ischemic injury in both focal and global ischemia models.[6,32,42,115,168,225,264,290,315,321,391,395,408]

Ischemic depolarization, spreading depression, and calcium entry via VDCCs would be expected to increase the release of glutamate from presynaptic processes of excitatory neurons, which utilize glutamate as neurotransmitters. Glutamate release occurs when CBF falls to about half normal (20 ml/100 g/min in humans; 40 to 50 in rodents). The normal extracellular glutamate concentration is in the 1- to 10-μM range, whereas intracellular glutamate is around 8 to 10 mmol/L. Release of glutamate would be expected to act at several postsynaptic receptors including the (1) N-methyl-D-aspartate (NMDA) receptor; (2) kainic acid/alpha amino-3-hydroxy-5-methyl-4-isoxazole propionic acid (KA/AMPA) receptor; and (3) quisqualate receptor.[36,146,147,261] Glutamate binding to the NMDA receptor results in calcium and some sodium flux through its calcium-associated ion channel, with the calcium flux being modulated by zinc, glycine, hydrogen ion, and redox sites on the NMDA receptor.[147] Competitive NMDA receptor antagonists compete with the glutamate binding site, noncompetitive NMDA receptor antagonists compete within the calcium channel of the NMDA receptor, and glycine and other more novel NMDA antagonists compete at other sites within the calcium channel. Recently, the relative role of zinc has been emphasized since it might modu-late the NMDA receptor, and its prolonged presence within cells might exacerbate calcium-related injury since it acts something like calcium but is not cleared as readily.[57] The potential importance of the NMDA receptors in ischemic injury is emphasized by (1) the prevention of neurotoxicity of ischemia and glucose deprivation in in vitro models; and (2) the improvement of stroke outcome in focal ischemia models in rodents.[100,112,251,289,296] It is notable that NMDA receptor antagonists do not affect cell death in global ischemia models, when brain temperature is controlled for.[40,41,386] Many NMDA antagonists produce hallucinations and psychosis in people and have been shown to produce neuronal damage including cell death and induction of stress proteins in specific populations of neurons in adult rodents.[94,336,337]

Glutamate release also results in the activation of KA/AMPA receptors as well as metabotropic quisqualate receptors. The activation of KA/AMPA receptors is critical in normal fast neurotransmission at glutamate receptors and normally results in sodium entry into the postsynaptic neuron.[36] Sodium entry would depolarize neurons, resulting in calcium influx through VDCCs, and possibly calcium entry via the sodium/calcium exchanger. Some KA/AMPA receptors have also been shown to flux calcium through associated calcium channels.[146] In addition, it has been suggested that ischemia, specifically global ischemia, can result in the upregulation of subunits of the KA/AMPA receptor that are known to flux calcium.[300] This has led to the hypothesis that ischemia may induce the type of KA/AMPA receptor subunit leading to the receptor subtype that fluxes calcium and thus leading to increased calcium entry into ischemic cells and eventual death of cells.[299] KA/AMPA antagonists decrease injury in CA1 neurons following global ischemia and decrease stroke size in focal ischemia models.[43,341] However, even these effects might be due in part to the effects of these drugs on brain temperature.

Glutamate actions at quisqualate receptors would activate G proteins, which would (1) modulate the activity of the NMDA and KA/AMPA receptors; and (2) activate hydrolysis of inositol phospholipids and release of inositol triphosphate, which would bind to IP_3 receptors in the endoplasmic membrane, and lead to release of calcium stores in the endoplasmic membrane and possibly from the mitochondria.[172] Whether the calcium release from the internal cellular stores is sufficient to lead to cellular injury is uncertain. However, the release of these internal cellular stores might contribute to injury.

Energy failure, rather than just effects of transmitters and their receptors, will also increase intracellular calcium.[400] This occurs by failure of the plasma membrane ATPase, failure of the endoplasmic reticulum ATPase, and possibly reversal of the sodium/calcium plasma membrane exchanger. In addition, with energy failure there may be substantial effects on the normal mechanisms of glutamate removal from the extracellular space.[237,362,363] Since glial uptake of glutamate is the major mechanism of glutamate removal from the extracellular space, glial energy failure would contribute to excess glutamate in the extracellular space (Fig. 4.5). In addition, with energy failure the normal sodium/glutamate exchanger might reverse directions, resulting in intracellular sodium flux and efflux of glutamate, which would lead to cellular swelling combined with excess stimulation of cellular glutamate receptors.[237,368] Also, neuronal glutamate transporters almost certainly play important roles in the modulation of extracellular glutamate and determine the balance between neurotoxic and stimulatory concentrations of extracellular amino acids.[176,324] With the recognition of non-NMDA (KA/AMPA) receptors on certain types of glial cells, this might also provide a mechanism by which extracellular glutamate would affect glial calcium homeostasis.[46,261]

Other excitatory neurotransmitters could also increase calcium influx into neurons and thereby exacerbate calcium-mediated injury due to ischemia. Thus, acetylcholine actions on excitatory muscarinic receptors[15] and dopamine actions at excitatory dopamine receptors (including D1 and D5)[44] might tend to increase ischemic injury. Therefore, cholinergic[293] and dopaminergic antagonists[122,165,204] might be predicted to improve ischemic injury. The relative innervation of various cell groups by these excitatory transmitters might dictate which cells groups were more or less vulnerable.

ACIDOSIS

Once oxygen delivery decreases below a threshold where it does not match the delivery of glucose and the tissue metabolic demand, then anaerobic metabolism of glucose occurs. Although glucose is normally metabolized to pyruvate, which enters the Krebs cycle, in the absence of oxygen the pyruvate is metabolized to lactate to yield 2ATP rather than the 36ATP produced by aerobic metabolism.[347] A large body of data shows that tissue lactate and pH fall during cerebral ischemia.[85,99,113,313,346] A threshold for pH appears to occur around 5.9, where lactate infusions sufficient to produce this pH result in tissue infarction—in the absence of ischemia or decreased oxygen delivery.[213] Very low pH produces pannecrosis.[212]

During the course of focal ischemia tissue pH usually falls to a level around 6.4 to 6.6, which occurs when the serum glucose is in the normal range. With plasma hyperglycemia, tissue pH can fall to around 6.0 to 6.1 because of the continued delivery of glucose and production of lactate during glycolysis. With decapitation ischemia, in which blood flow and delivery of glucose are not continuous, tissue pH is in the upper 6.6 to 6.8 range because of the finite amount of glucose and glycogen in brain.[113,365]

This and other data led Plum[304] to suggest that tissue acidosis was the major factor determining whether selective neuronal death or focal infarction occurred following ischemia. Since global ischemia results in the complete cessation of blood flow, tissue pH only falls a relatively small amount. These investigators proposed that as long as pH was above a certain threshold, glial cells could derive sufficient energy and survive entirely via glycolysis. This hypothesis is consistent with studies of cultured astrocytes showing that either chemical or atmospheric hypoxia does not result in glial cell death—unless either glucose deprivation or acidosis also occurs.[360] Plum[304] suggested that in focal ischemia pH fell below the threshold at which glia could survive only via glycolysis and also maintain cellular homeostasis in the face of severe acidosis. The precise mechanism by which acidosis kills cells is not clear, although direct protein denaturation is possible. It is also possible that acidosis results in severe derangements of calcium metabolism with activation of proteases, lipases, and other degradative enzymes. It is unlikely that acidosis per se accounts for differences in vulnerability of neurons and glia to ischemia since neurons and glia in culture die at about the same pH value.[124,274]

It is of note that very mild acidosis may be beneficial. Once hydrogen ion concentrations fall below 6.8, the NMDA receptor no longer fluxes calcium ions. Very mild acidosis has been shown to protect against focal ischemia in experimental focal ischemia models.[353]

These findings have suggested that clinically it is probably better to maintain euglycemia in patients with cerebral infarctions. Hyperglycemia would only be beneficial when complete cessation of blood flow occurs as in global ischemia and in the distributions of end arteries where there are no collaterals.[74,99,164,182,222,273,307,314,378]

SECOND MESSENGER SYSTEMS

Second messengers, such as calcium, cyclic adenosine monophosphate (cAMP), cyclic guanosine monophosphate (cGMP), diacylglycerol (DAG) and inositol triphosphate ($InsP_3$), are effectors that act with other molecules to mediate the extracellular, receptor-transmitted signals to produce the subsequent intracellular changes (Fig. 4.6). As discussed above, ischemia-induced stimulation of the glutamatergic system appears to have a central role in mediating neuronal injury. The increases in the intracellular calcium levels mediated by ionotropic glutamate receptors elicit several profound responses in cellular metabolism. Calcium also activates calmodulin, which activates adenylyl cyclase, nitric oxide synthase (NOS), calmodulin kinase 2 (CaM), and protein kinase C (PKC). Changes in

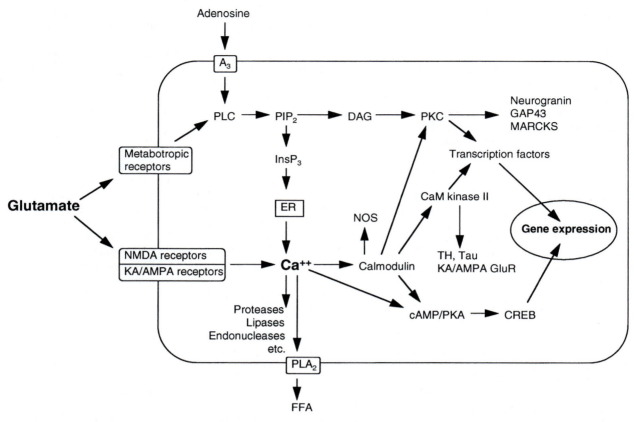

Figure 4.6 Glutamate can produce injury via activation of a number of intracellular messengers.

CaM[144,269,294,335] and PKC[47,76,139] have been noted in ischemia. CaM phosphorylates transcription factors, leading to changes in gene expression. Calcium also affects gene expression by activating transcription through cAMP response element (CRE) binding protein (CREB).[68,265] Stimulation of adenylyl cyclase induces formation of cAMP, which by activating protein kinase A (PKA) phosphorylates CREB in concert with calcium and thereby activates transcription. CREB is a constitutively expressed transcription factor, and the promoter regions of several genes, such as c-*fos*, contain CRE.[265] These calcium-elicited changes in gene expression mediated by CREB and CaM may contribute to ischemic cell death by affecting the expression of a number of genes, including those inducing apoptosis.

Calcium entry into postsynaptic neurons via the ionotropic glutamatergic receptors activates phospholipase A₂ (PLA₂). Activation of PLA₂ activates the formation of platelet activating factor (PAF) and the formation of arachidonic acid (AA, 20:4). As discussed below, AA is metabolized by cyclooxygenase 1 and 2 to produce prostaglandins and leukotrienes. PAF can also be synthesized from phosphorylcholine and alkylacetylglycerol.[25,27] PAF is inactivated by PAF acetylhydrolase. PAF appears to have binding sites within cells as well as on the surface membranes of cells. PAF induces immediate early genes, including c-fos, possibly via the calcium response element (CREB). PAF actions on extracellular receptors may modulate glutamate release and the release of other excitatory

neurotransmitters. PAF may also modulate inducible prostaglandin synthase via actions on the intracellular PAF receptors.[26] The role of PAF in mediating ischemic injury is supported by the findings that PAF antagonists, including BN 52021, restore blood flow and decrease damage in cerebral ischemia.[359] PAF antagonists decrease phospholipid degradation by PLA₂ and protect CA1 pyramidal neurons in the gerbil global ischemia model, and the PAF antagonist 52021 prevents postischemic hypoperfusion and edema formation in a spinal cord ischemic model.[27]

Glutamate activation of metabotropic receptors activates the G protein-coupled phospholipase C (PLC). Furthermore, ischemia induces a rapid and transient increase in PLC transcription. PLC apparently participates in mediating ischemic injury, since the PLC inhibitor phenylmethylsulfonyl fluoride prevents ischemic injury.[377] Furthermore, PLC is also stimulated by A₃ adenosine receptors, and acute administration of A₃ agonists attenuates ischemic cell death after global ischemia.[382] PLC cleaves phosphoinositol 4,5-biphosphate into DAG and InsP₃. DAG and PKC activities increase following ischemia.[4,217,226,403] InsP₃ acts on receptors on the endoplasmic reticulum to release internal calcium stores. Blockade of the endoplasmic reticulum receptors or calcium release from internal stores can influence ischemic injury.[2] Furthermore, the InsP₃-mediated calcium release appears to mediate ischemic injury, since InsP₃ accelerates the cell death of ischemic hippocampal neurons, and this change can be prevented by calcium chelator.[376]

DAG activates PKC, which is also activated by calmodulin (see above). PKC phosphorylates a number of molecules and may be a key regulator of K channels, glutamate transporters, and other molecules in hippocampal and other excitatory neurons, determining the degree and extent of excitotoxic injury. PKC appears to participate in ischemic injury, since inhibition of PKC activity by staurosporine and other kinase inhibitors reduces ischemic cell death in the CA1 neurons following global ischemia.[140] cGMP, microtubule-associated protein (MAP) kinases and many other intracellular second messengers almost certainly have some role in ischemic cell death. The challenge for research in this area is to identify the second messenger systems that are most important in modulating neuronal injury or recovery.

INFLAMMATORY MECHANISMS

The role of leukocytes and inflammatory mediators in the production of ischemic injury has been the subject of recent studies in brain and other organs. Leukocyte recruitment to areas of ischemic injury can occur as early as 30 minutes after cerebral ischemia and reperfusion.[107] The accumulation of these leukocytes, in combination with fibrin and platelets,[72] may contribute to vascular plugging.[86] The finding that depletion of the accumulating leukocytes can attenuate brain damage after focal cerebral ischemia has stimulated interest in the mechanisms of leukocyte adhesion and specific treatments aimed at these mechanisms. The mechanisms by which leukocytes might exacerbate injury are under investigation but could include the production of free radicals.[196,393]

A variety of cell surface adhesion molecules are either activated or induced following ischemia. Although the mechanisms of induction are not entirely clear, many of these molecules play a role in injury. The CD11b/18 molecule is an integrin adhesion molecule constitutively expressed on the surface of activated leukocytes. Administration of antibodies against this molecule or against intercellular adhesion molecule (ICAM) decreases ischemic injury.[38,62,256,404] The CD18 molecule binds to its receptor, ICAM-1. Following activation, ICAM-1 is expressed on the surface of endothelial cells. ICAM-1 can be induced by interferon-α, interleukin-1 (IL-1), and tumor necrosis factor-α (TNF-α). Following ischemia ICAM-1 is upregulated on microvessels,[61,256,384] perhaps because of local release of IL-1 by endothelial cells, brain microglia, or leukocytes themselves.[96,119,,385] Administration of antibodies to ICAM-1 decreases leukocyte accumulation and ischemic injury following transient focal ischemia.[37,62,256,404]

Selectins are a recently identified family of adhesion molecules that regulate early leukocyte adhesion to endothelium. They slow down leukocytes, cause rolling, and promote the firm attachment of leukocytes to ICAM-related molecules.[72,266] L selectin is a constitutive molecule on the surface of specific leukocytes. E-selectin is induced on the surface of endothelial cells by cytokines. P-selectin is transferred to the surface of platelets and endothelial cells after activation.[292] The selectins bind to calcium-dependent lectins that can bind to a variety of carbohydrate ligands found on platelets, leukocytes, and endothelial cells. Treatment with a synthetic oligopeptide that blocks the lectin domain of selectin decreases stroke size.[266] This peptide could act on any of the selectins, since all are expressed following ischemia, P-selectin being expressed within 1 to 2 hours,[292] E-selectin within 12 to 24 hours, and L-selectin being expressed constitutively.[384]

Since IL-1 plays an important role in the activation of adhesion molecules and in activating many proinflammatory response genes, several studies have targeted either this molecule or its receptor. IL-1 and IL-6 receptor antagonists decrease ischemic injury.[28,106,318,394] Overexpression of an IL-1 antagonist in brain endothelial and choroidal cells by an adenoviral vector also protects against focal ischemic injury.[33]

The cytokines and the leukocyte response appear to be most important in ischemic models where there is reperfusion. Antibodies against the adhesion molecules do not appear to work well in permanent MCA occlusion models, suggesting that this approach to ischemia therapy may be limited to reperfusion injury. In addition, the role of the cytokines and leukocytes in selective neuronal cell death following global ischemic injury is being investigated. As noted below, this type of cell death may occur via apoptosis, may not incite a leuckocyte response, and may involve activation of macrophages or microglia in the final death scene.[281] During the process of selective neuronal cell death following either global or focal ischemia, dying neurons release a soluble factor, perhaps a cytokine.[63,358] This signals either microglia or macrophages to engulf the cell, a process that occurs without a great deal of inflammation.[109,221] Following global ischemia, microglial activation occurs about 24 hours later, and microglial and macrophage invasion of the CA1 region is quite prominent by 72 hours.[179]

FREE RADICALS, LIPID PEROXIDATION, AND ARACHIDONIC ACID

The term *oxygen free radical* refers to reactive, partially reduced forms of oxygen: superoxide (O_2^-·), peroxyl radical (RO_2^-·), nitric oxide (NO·), the very reactive hydroxyl radical (OH·), and species such as singlet oxygen.[133] Free radicals can be injurious because they react indiscriminately with other cell constituents. The carbon double bonds of polyunsaturated fatty acids are particularly vulnerable to free radical attack. Ischemia appears to increase free radical production markedly, particularly during reperfusion, as evidenced by lipid peroxidation, protein oxidation, and depletion of the antioxidants glutathione and ascorbate.[50,51] Identified sources of free radical production during ischemia/reperfusion include mitochondria,[82] endothelial xanthine dehydrogenase (which is converted to superoxide-producing xanthine oxidase under ischemic conditions), marginating leukocytes,[255] delocalized iron stores,[317] and NOS.[70]

Free radical stress and excitotoxicity amplify one another.[81] Impairment in brain free radical defenses may also contribute to increased vulnerability to free radical stress during ischemia. Astrocytes appear to have higher concentrations of glutathione and equal or greater activities of catalase, super-

Figure 4.7 Diagram of pathways responsible for the production of oxygen free radicals and other free radicals that produce lipid peroxidation, denature proteins, and damage DNA.

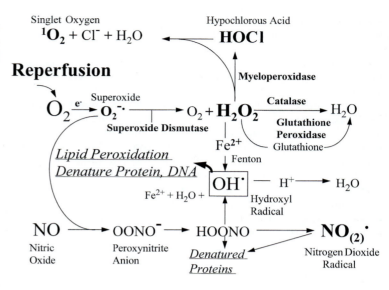

oxide dismutase, glutathione peroxidase, and glutathione reductase than do neurons.[248,401] This arrangement suggests that free radical scavenging mechanisms in glia may serve to support neuronal survival.

Free radicals are produced in cells during the course of normal oxidation reactions. The conversion of oxygen to water and ATP in the electron transport chain results in the formation of (O_2^-), hydrogen peroxide (H_2O_2), and OH.[133] H_2O_2 is not a radical. However, interactions of H_2O_2 and O_2^- with metals, particularly iron, results in the formation of the highly reactive and toxic OH· radical[133] (Fig. 4.7). The oxidation of phospholipids to AA and its metabolites results in free radicals.[39,113] Self-oxidation of flavins, catecholamines, dopamine, and other compounds is also a source of free radicals. Free radicals can attack the unsaturated bonds in fatty acids and cholesterol and produce lipid peroxides, which are free radicals themselves.[117] Hence, free radical production must ordinarily be tightly controlled since free radicals tend to produce more free radicals.[196] A number of proteins are also vulnerable to inactivation by free radicals, the activity of glutamate synthase being used as a sensitive measure of free radical injury.[98] Free radicals can also be produced by the actions of calcium on PLA_2 xanthine oxidase, and NOS (Fig. 4.7). Calcium-activated proteolysis results in formation of xanthine oxidase from xanthine dehydrogenase, which oxidizes hypoxanthine or xanthine to produce uric acid and superoxide radicals. The superoxide radicals can produce injury in part by binding to nitric oxide (NO), with the formation of the highly injurious free radical peroxynitrite (Fig. 4.7). NO, as discussed below, is produced by one of several NOS enzymes.

Lipid peroxidation and the production of free radicals often occurs in association with activation of phospholipases.[24,27] Calcium activation of PLA_2[35] results in the release of arachidonic acid (AA)[4] from phosphoinositol.[2] AA can directly damage vascular cells[209] and inhibit glutamate uptake in glia.[397] AA is metabolized by cyclooxygenase 2 to prostaglandins and thromboxanes, and AA is metabolized via 5-lipoxygenase to leukotrienes, lipoxins, and hepoxilins.[291] An AA epoxygenase has recently been localized to astrocytes in the brain, where the production of epoxyeicosatetraenoic acids

occurs, which are known to dilate cerebral arteries and enhance calcium currents in these cells.[5] Indocin, the prototypic cyclooxygenase inhibitor, has been shown to decrease ischemic injury in some systems.[77,332,410] Leukotrienes, produced by the actions of a specific lipoxygenase, affect permeability of the cerebral vessels and promote edema formation.[54,199]

Normal cells have antioxidant enzymes and free radical scavengers present to protect against endogenous and exogenous sources of free radicals (Fig. 4.7). The enzymes that directly metabolize free radicals include superoxide dismutase (SOD), which catalyzes the superoxide radical to form (H_2O_2). Catalase metabolizes H_2O_2 to H_2O and O_2. Glutathione peroxidase also converts H_2O_2 to H_2O and O_2 but uses glutathione as a cofactor.[248] Free radical scavengers present within cells include ascorbic acid (millimolar concentrations), vitamin E (α-tocopherol), β-carotene, and free glutathione.[132] Ascorbate scavenges free radicals. Vitamin E blocks peroxidation in membranes. β-Carotene quenches excited molecules and binds free radicals. Free glutathione is a reducer that reacts with oxidizing species before they bind to lipids or proteins. The regulation of free radical production is also important for calcium homeostasis since free radicals affect the function of NMDA receptors, VDCCs, calcium ATPases, calcium exchangers, calcium binding proteins, and others.

The precise roles of the above reactions in cerebral ischemia have not been delineated with certainty but are the subjects of many ongoing studies. Several studies suggest that the superoxide radical is important since exogenous administration of SOD can decrease stroke size in experimental models.[50,52,141,163] SOD transgenic mice have decreased stroke volumes following temporary MCA occlusions but not following permanent MCA occlusions, suggesting that SOD is particularly important in ischemic injury where there is reperfusion and production of free radicals.[51]

Inhibition of cyclooxygenase and lipoxygenase with piroxicam and flurbiprofen has been shown to improve neuronal survival in the gerbil global ischemia model,[271] as does the cyclooxygenase inhibitor indocin.[332] Inhibition of free radical and lipid peroxidation with vitamin E improves ischemic neuronal injury.[136] Free radical scavengers such as dimethylthiourea decrease neuronal injury in focal and global ischemia models,[201,239,295,308] as does the compound tirilazad or U74006F[8,20,131,186] and related antioxidants.[137] Spin trapping compounds, including N-tert-butyl-alpha-phenylnitrone, reduced ischemic brain injury and prevented the age-associated increased in brain protein oxidation and decline in memory function in gerbils.[48]

NITRIC OXIDE

NO is a gas that serves as a potent vasodilator and was initially identified as the endothelium-dependent relaxation factor.[70,93,159] All cells in the brain can potentially produce NO, which in turn can have large effects on blood vessels and neighboring cells. NO concentrations increase markedly in ischemic brain. Mounting evidence suggests that modulation of NO production can either decrease or worsen ischemic injury depending on which cells produce the NO.[69,93,159]

NOS metabolizes L-arginine to NO and citrulline (Fig. 4.8). At least three forms of NOS have been identified and cloned from brain: the neuronal (nNOS), the endothelial cell-derived (eNOS), and an inducible NOS (iNOS).[70] iNOS can be induced in a variety of cells including macrophages, astrocytes, and microglia.[406] In the presence of adequate arginine, NOS forms citrulline and NO. In the absence of arginine NOS can generate superoxide and H_2O_2.[93]

Although the role of eNOS is still being examined, it appears that a variety of mediators can activate it, including acetylcholine, substance P, histamine, arginine vasopressin, bradykinin, prostaglandin F, and the endothelin receptor.[406] The activation of eNOS results in the increased production of NO within the endothelial cell. The NO diffuses out of the endothelial cell into the adjacent smooth muscle cell, where the NO activates GMP, which produces relaxation of the muscle, vasodilatation, and increased CBF (Fig. 4.8). The NO released also decreases aggregation and adherence of platelets and leukocytes. Drugs that inhibit eNOS (including L-NMMA, L-NNA, and L-NAME) produce vasconstriction in vitro and in vivo and probably worsen ischemic injury.[102] Mice with knockouts of the eNOS gene have larger strokes than wild-type mice with normal eNOS function.

The role of nNOS has been controversial but is becoming clearer with genetic experiments and more specific drugs. Approximately 2% of the neurons in brain contain nNOS, which often co-localizes with an enzyme reduced nicotinamide adenosine dinucleotide phosphate, diaphorase. These neurons are evenly scattered over the basal ganglia, cortex, and other brain regions. Nonspecific drugs that inhibit one or all forms of NOS have been variably reported as either worsening stroke or improving stroke. Chemical lesioning of the neurons containing nNOS improves ischemic injury.[95] More recently mice with knockouts of the nNOS gene have been shown to have smaller stroke sizes than wild-type animals with normal nNOS function.[158] These data suggest that production of NO by nNOS neurons can contribute to stroke-related injury. How this occurs is still somewhat unclear. Activation of both NMDA and non-NMDA receptors causes neurons to produce NO and release it. In vitro studies suggest that NMDA-mediated neurotoxicity is NO dependent and could relate to NO effects on the NMDA receptor.[231] In addition, NO can interact with the superoxide radical to form peroxynitrite, which is a cytotoxic free radical (Fig. 4.7). Oxidation of NO produces the nitrosonium ion, which can nitrosylate proteins, resulting in their dysfunction. If arginine were limiting during ischemia, then NOS would produce superoxide and H_2O_2, both of which are cytotoxic.[93]

Both eNOS and nNOS would be expected to be present at the time of ischemia. The effects of ischemia on both enzymes would probably be rapid, occurring within seconds to minutes of the initial ischemia. Therefore, the clinical usefulness of manipulating these enzymes might be limited to prophylaxis against ischemic injury. The role of iNOS in cerebral ischemia has been studied the least. During and immediately after ischemia, iNOS levels would be very low. However, iNOS would be induced within hours in microglia, astrocytes, and vessels.[87,103,160,268] The role of this glial NOS could be

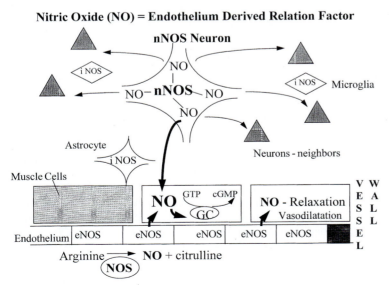

Nitric Oxide (NO) = Endothelium Derived Relation Factor

Figure 4.8 Sites of production of nitric oxide (NO) include neurons (neuronal NOS), endothelial cells (eNOS), and microglia and other cells (inducible NOS). At the moment of ischemia, nNOS and eNOS would be responsible for NO release. iNOS is induced many hours after ischemia and would produce NO for several days following a stroke. NOS, nitric oxide synthase.

harmful in as much as neuronal production of NO also appears to be harmful. Preliminary studies suggest that inhibition of NOS activity several hours after ischemia may improve neuronal survival.[161,142] These results suggest that facilitation of eNOS and inhibition of nNOS and perhaps iNOS, might improve ischemic injury. The development of specific drugs that target each form of NOS will help to answer these questions.

PROTEASES

Calpains are calcium-activated neutral cysteine proteases that have been implicated in dynamic remodeling of the cytoskeleton as part of several physiologic mechanisms, such as mitosis and synaptic plasticity, as well as cytoskeletal disruption in some pathologic states.[333] They comprise two major isoforms distinguished functionally by their calcium requirements: μ- or type I calpain (activated by low calcium concentrations) and m- or type II calpain, which requires higher calcium. μ-Calpain is found associated with cytoskeletal elements in neurons and glia throughout the brain and is particularly prominent in neurons that are susceptible to injury and degenerative processes.[350] Calpain substrates generally contain calmodulin-binding domains near their cleavage site that interact with and modulate the activity of the protease. Among the calpain substrates are numerous critical structural and catalytic molecules including fodrin (nonerythroid spectrin), troponins I and C, tropomyosin, filamin, desmin, talin, vinculin α-actinin, integrins, MAP2, and plasma membrane Ca^{2+}-ATPase. Calpains also undergo autolysis. Sensitive and specific detection of calpain activity in situ has been accomplished through the use of monoclonal antibodies specific for one or the other of the peptide ends generated by calpain cleavage of fodrin.[319]

Calpain activation is an early marker of injury following excitotoxic insults and ischemia. Increases in fodrin breakdown have been demonstrated within 1 to 2 hours in areas of rat cortex destined to infarct following focal ischemia,[23] and in gerbil hippocampus within 15 to 30 minutes following transient global ischemia.[396] In addition, μ-calpain autolysis, another indicator of calpain activation, has been found to occur in the brains of rabbits following cardiac arrest.[278] It is likely that the supraphysiologic levels of cytosolic calcium that occur during excitotoxicity and ischemia are directly responsible for this rapid calpain activation.

Inhibition of calpain proteolysis can reduce the effects of ischemia. Peptide calpain inhibitors have been shown to decrease neuronal loss following global ischemia[316] and in several models of focal ischemia.[23,149] In one study in which the drug was superfused over the cortical surface, up to a 75% reduction in infarct size was observed even when drug administration was begun 3 hours after the initiation of ischemia. These studies suggest that calpain activation is an early and ongoing contributor to cellular damage during and following ischemia and that inhibition of these proteases is a promising avenue for the amelioration of ischemic injury.

Other proteases are involved in neuronal injury. The proteases involved in apoptosis are mentioned in the next section. Matrix metalloproteinases may be involved in opening the blood-brain barrier following ischemia and other types of brain injury.[322] Intravascular proteases could be important in clot formation and propagation but are not discussed here.

PROGRAMMED CELL DEATH

Apoptosis occurs in the nervous system during development. Apoptosis is mediated by DNA cleavage and by other autolytic processes causing nuclear shrinkage, chromatin clumping, cytoplasmic blebbing, and ultimate cell death. Apoptosis may also be induced by ischemia.[171] This may occur by depriving surviving neurons of their normal synaptic connections, by disrupting normal exposure to trophic factors, or by inducing enough cellular injury to trigger a suicide program. Apoptosis in many settings can be prevented by the administration of trophic factors or by intervening at various points in the cell death program. The relative importance of apoptosis to the overall cell death resulting from ischemia remains to be established.

During apoptosis nuclear damage occurs first. The integrity of the plasma and mitochondrial membranes is maintained until late in the process. By contrast, during necrotic cell death the nuclei, organelles, and plasma membrane all swell and lyse, with the early loss of plasmalemmal integrity.[184] During apoptosis cells often require the production of new mRNAs and proteins to complete the suicide program.[334] The activation of calcium-dependent endonucleases that cleave between nucleosomes, producing a DNA ladder on electrophoresis, has been widely used as evidence of apoptosis, as has in situ nick end labeling, although this is less specific.[126]

The molecular biology of apoptosis (Fig. 4.9) has been the subject of intense research, fueled by the findings of bcl-2 inhibition of cell death,[381] cloning of genes involved in C. elegans apoptosis and some of their mammalian analogues like interleukin-converting enzyme (ICE),[399] and the discovery of other cell death-related genes like reaper.[357] Three major classes of genes control apoptosis (Fig. 4.9). These include (1) those that prevent cell death, like bcl-2 and bcl-xL; (2) those that promote death, like bax and bcl-xs and (3) those that promote the engulfment and destruction of cells. Increased production of the protective proteins promotes cell survival, and production of the death proteins produces cell death. One interesting feature of apoptosis is that the cell death does not evoke an inflammatory response with leukocyte invasion. Instead, cells appear to be engulfed quietly, probably by microglia or macrophages without surrounding tissue damage or inflammation.[281]

Once cells are pushed toward the death pathway, specific proteases and endonucleases are activated to carry out the death program. ICE (interleukin-1β converting enzyme) is a cysteine protease first isolated as the processing enzyme for IL-1β but then found to be related to a C. elegans cell death gene.[375] ICE belongs to a growing family of proteases that generally share between 20% and 45% sequence identity, but all have the invariant sequence . . . QACRG . . . containing the active site cysteine. Related proteases include CPP32 and Nedd-2/ICH-1. All the known enzymes have isoforms that can promote apoptosis. Expression of these proteases in a variety of cells can cause apoptosis, which can be prevented

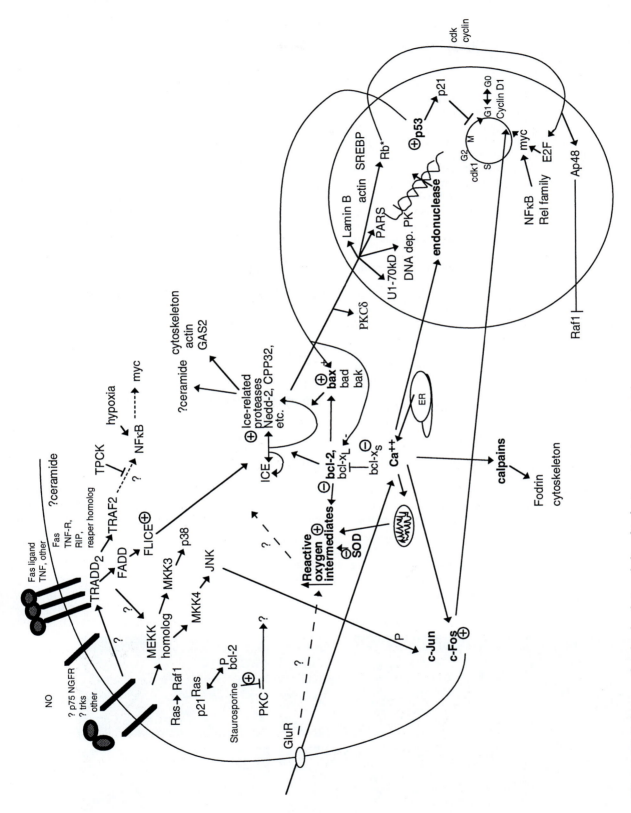

Figure 4.9 Pathways and molecules that are believed to be important in apoptosis/programmed cell death.

by inhibitors of the proteases or introduction of the protective gene, bcl-2.[216]

Many recent studies have suggested that at least some of the cell death observed in ischemic brain may be related to apoptotic mechanisms. Shigeno et al[343] found that treatment with anisomycin, a protein synthesis inhibitor, reduced CA1 cell death following global ischemia in the gerbil. Subsequently, MacManus et al[242–244] showed DNA laddering indicative of apoptosis in the hippocampi of rats following global ischemia, and Linnik et al[230] reported laddering in a model of rat focal ischemia and found that infarct size could be partially reduced by infusion of the protein synthesis inhibitor cycloheximide. Since 1993, many reports, generally using the same basic techniques of evaluation—morphology, nick end labeling, and DNA laddering—have found evidence of cell death resembling apoptosis in a variety of systems including adult rat global and focal ischemia, newborn rat and piglet hypoxia/ischemia, and focal ischemia in mice.[31,80,145,153,166,224,259]

Consideration of other molecules and systems reveals connections between the basic mechanisms of apoptosis and postischemic injury. Reactive oxygen intermediates (e.g. superoxide [·OH]), which are upregulated during excitotoxicity in culture and reperfusion injury in vivo,[65] have been implicated in signaling during the early phases of apoptosis,[127] although the sustained generation of such compounds may kill cells through other mechanisms. c-fos and c-jun are upregulated following ischemia, and in a study by Dragunow et al[79] hyperexpression of c-jun best correlated with injured cells. bcl-2, an antiapoptotic molecule, can modulate the outcome of ischemia. bcl-2- overexpressing transgenic mice have reduced stroke size in response to permanent focal ischemia.[252] Also, delivery of bcl-2 message to the brain in defective herpesvirus vectors prior to focal ischemia was shown to decrease injury at the injection sites.[229] p53 is a tumor suppressor/transcription factor implicated in mediation of apoptosis in response to DNA damage.[129] It is upregulated in regions of neuronal injury following focal ischemia.[223] Moreover, transgenic animals with decreased p53 expression show decreased stroke size in response to MCA occlusion.[67] Finally, it has recently been shown that bax, a bcl-2-associated proapoptotic protein that is a downstream effector of p53, is markedly upregulated in cells that degenerate following ischemia due to transient cardiac arrest.[214]

Specific apoptosis-related genes are induced in cells that will die.[151] Following 5 and 10 minutes of global ischemia, the bcl-2 and bcl-x mRNAs are induced selectively in the CA1 pyramidal neurons of hippocampus 12 to 24 hours later (Fig. 4.10). The bcl-2 induction would likely serve to protect cells, and the bcl-x induction could serve to protect or produce cell death depending on which form of bcl-x predominated. In addition, ICE-like mRNA was induced in the CA1 region at 24 hours with a peak at 72 hours. This induction probably did not occur in CA1 neurons since most of the CA1 neurons are dead by 72 hours following 5 minutes of global ischemia. Although these results do not prove that apoptosis is the mechanism of CA1 neuronal cell death, they are consistent with such a hypothesis. It is possible that ischemia suppression of protein synthesis could prevent the synthesis of bcl-2, bcl-xl, and other protective proteins. In the absence of these protective proteins, activation of ICE-like proteases and calcium activation of endonucleases could occur, with eventual death of the cells. The delayed death of CA1 neurons could be explained by the temporary production of protective proteins, which then fail, followed by activation of death proteins.

Potential Protective Responses to Ischemia

ROLE OF ASTROCYTES

Astrocytes are able to maintain function under hypoxic conditions, at least for limited periods, by glycolytic ATP production alone.[361] Like other cells capable of anaerobic function, astro-

Figure 4.10 In situ hybridization autoradiographs showing the mRNA for several apoptosis-related genes in the hippocampus of gerbils subjected to sham surgery (control) and 24 and 72 hours following global ischemia.

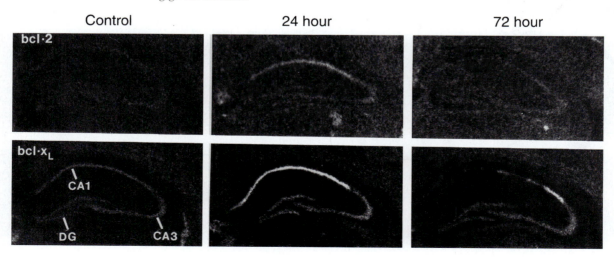

cytes contain glycogen and may produce lactate during periods of high energy demand. The ability of astrocytes to function with only glycolytic ATP production may be important in the ischemic penumbra because the residual blood flow to this region carries far more glucose than extractable oxygen. The capacity of astrocytes to maintain nonoxidative ATP production from glucose is severely compromised, however, as pH falls below 6.6.[360] The failure to maintain ATP is accompanied by irreversible astrocyte injury and tissue infarction.

During complete ischemia, astrocytes are completely deprived of energy substrates. ATP levels quickly fall, and transmembrane ion gradients collapse. Complete ischemia lasting longer than 20 to 30 minutes causes astrocyte death and thus infarction of the involved tissue. Hyperglycemia is found to *promote* infarction in most ischemic models. This effect of hyperglycemia is probably due to increased lactic acidosis in the ischemic territory.[304] The mechanism by which acidosis promotes astrocyte death is via blockade of nonoxidative ATP production.[360] The potential beneficial effect of increased substrate delivery is apparently outweighed by the faster and more extreme production of acidosis during hyperglycemia.

ATP depletion causes both failure of glutamate uptake and a massive efflux of glutamate via reversed operation of the glutamate transporters, resulting in marked elevations in extracellular glutamate concentrations.[58] During incomplete ischemia, continued supply of glucose to the penumbral region could potentially fuel continued ATP production by glycolysis, even in the absence of oxygen. This glycolytic ATP production may suffice to fuel glutamate uptake and prevent cytoplasmic release of glutamate.[236] pH is a significant factor determining the ability of astrocytes to maintain ATP levels in the absence of oxygen delivery, and the ability of astrocytes to maintain glutamate uptake during hypoxia is markedly impaired by acidosis over the range produced by ischemia.[363]

Although elevated extracellular $[K^+]_o$ does not induce reversal of transport in intact astrocytes, elevated $[K^+]_o$ does induce glutamate efflux via volume-sensitive ion channels. Astrocyte swelling is the first morphologic change observed during ischemia and is thought to result from a massive influx of K^+, Cl^-, and water. The efflux of glutamate and other organic osmolytes through volume-sensitive anion channels appears to be a volume-regulatory mechanism. These channels can be blocked by a variety of pharmacologic agents.[187,330]

Astrocytes can actively sequester H^+ by a variety of mechanisms and thereby reduce acidification of the extracellular space. It is not known whether these active mechanisms can function during ischemia or whether they are capable of buffering the massive acidosis caused by ischemia. However, Kraig and Chesler[210] have shown that the internal pH of some astrocytes may fall as much as an order of magnitude below the extracellular pH during terminal ischemia. This occurs in the absence of ATP hydrolysis, possibly as a passive function of astrocyte membranes that allows an inward conductance for H^+ substantially greater than conductance outward. Astrocyte sequestration of H^+ by either active or passive means will lessen acidification of the extracellular space but may have detrimental effects on continued astrocyte function and survival.

Not all astrocyte functions are neuroprotective during ischemia. Astrocytes under hypoxic conditions can continue to produce and release glutamine.[364] This would permit continued formation of neurotransmitter glutamate, release of which could exacerbate neuronal injury. Pharmacologic inhibition of glutamine synthetase reduces brain glutamine levels, reduces K^+-evoked glutamate release, and has been reported to reduce infarct size in a focal ischemia model of stroke.[366]

INHIBITORY NEUROTRANSMITTERS

Following ischemia, a number of transmitters and amino acids are released from cells. Included among these are the inhibitory transmitters γ-aminobutyric acid (GABA) and adenosine.[121,303] GABA is the major inhibitory neurotransmitter found in the brain (Fig. 4.5). It acts at two major classes of receptors, GABAa and GABAb. It seems reasonable that if excitatory neurotransmitters can kill neurons and possibly even initiate infarction, then promoting the functions of inhibitory transmitters might be beneficial.[123] Barbiturates, which act at a specific site on GABAa receptors, do decrease ischemic injury in some models but not others.[17,174,240] Muscimol, which is a specific GABAa agonist acting at the benzodiazepine site, and other GABA agonists also decreases ischemic injury.[241,246,345] GABA uptake inhibitors promote cell survival in cerebral ischemia.[169,302] GABAb agonists, like baclofen, have not proved reliable in decreasing neuronal injury.[13]

Adenosine appears to act as an inhibitory neuromodulator or transmitter in many systems. Adenosine receptors, of which there are three known, are upregulated following ischemia.[18,270] Actions at the A3 receptor activates IP_3 and produces release of intracellular calcium stores. Adenosine agonists have been reported to decrease ischemic injury in several different models.[71,297,382]

IMMEDIATE EARLY GENES AND SPREADING DEPRESSION

Although ischemia initiates a large number of ionic and enzymatic changes that may damage cells, these changes may also initiate new gene expression. Immediate early genes (IEGs), heat shock genes, and other stress genes, as well as many other families of genes are induced during and following cerebral ischemia. The induction of these genes may be very important to the cells since they are being induced in the face of energy deprivation. Many of these genes may be induced to protect cells against further injury and to promote survival, although some inducible genes, like iNOS and pro-apoptotic genes, may mediate injury.

Focal Ischemia

IEGs are induced by a variety of stimuli, including calcium, and are translated into transcription factor proteins, which regulate expression of specific target genes.[265,325,326,339] Following MCA occlusion in rodent models there is induction of the c-fos, junB, NGFI-A,-B, and -C and many other related leucine-zipper and zinc finger IEGs throughout the entire

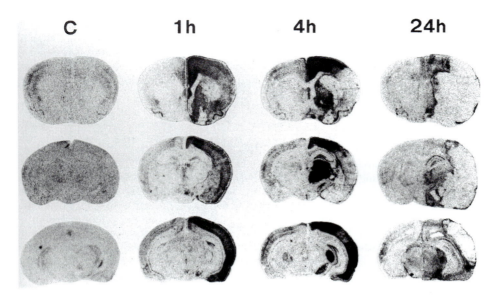

Figure 4.11 In situ hybridization autoradiographs showing c-fos mRNA in the brains of control animals (C) and in rats 1 hour, 4 hours, and 24 hours following middle cerebral artery, (MCA) infarctions. Note induction of c-fos mRNA throughout cortex 1 hour following the MCA occlusion. By 4 hours after the stroke, c-fos mRNA has decreased in the cortex in the area of the infarction but is still induced in the cortex outside the infarction as well as in the ipsilateral thalamus, hippocampus, and substantia nigra.

hemisphere.[7,108,152,153,157,173,188,190,232] This IEG induction occurs within minutes of the MCA ischemia, and occurs inside the MCA territory as well as throughout the anterior (ACA) and posterior cerebral artery (PCA) territories (Fig. 4.11). This IEG induction is maximal around 4 hours after ischemia, decreases in regions of MCA infarction by 24 hours after the MCA inclusion, and can persist for several days in regions outside the infarction.[188]

Although the mechanism for this induction is not clear, we proposed that ischemia-induced spreading depression accounts for IEG induction in the ischemic MCA territory as well as in the nonischemic PCA territory.[190] Following focal ischemia, waves of depolarization spread throughout an ischemic hemisphere and may occur repeatedly depending on the severity and duration of the ischemia.[21,75,275,370] MK801, which is a noncompetitive NMDA receptor antagonist, has been shown to block this spreading depression. Since we showed that MK801 also blocked the cortical induction of IEGs following focal ischemia, the depolarization produced by the spreading depression was proposed to induce the IEGs.[190,340]

Induction of the IEGs following ischemia is important because these genes are transcription factors that regulate the expression of many other target genes. The Fos and Jun family members form dimers, which then bind to sites in the promoters of other genes called AP1 sites. Genes with AP1 sites in their promoters include the glial fibrillary acidic protein-(GFAP) gene; the dopamine-synthesizing tyrosine hydroxylase gene; the growth factors BDNF, FGF, and others; the inducible NOS gene; the heme-catabolizing hemeoxygenase gene; the amyloid preprotein expressed in brains with Alzheimer's disease; and others. It is likely that ischemia-induced

spreading depression leads to induction of Fos, Jun, Zif268, and many other transcription factors, which then act on these target genes to induce them throughout the ischemic hemisphere in rodent models. This would explain induction of GFAP in glia throughout an ischemic hemisphere even though ischemia was restricted to the MCA territory.[211]

Global Ischemia

Spreading depression is not the only mechanism of IEG induction in ischemic brain, since global ischemia also induces virtually every IEG studied in the hippocampus. Global ischemia in gerbil and rat models induces c-fos, c-jun, fosB, junB, NGFI-A, -B, and -C, and many other genes in either all parts or only specific portions of the hippocampus.[34,78,142,185,233,284,355] The expression of these genes has been of interest since only CA1 pyramidal neurons die in these models, whereas most of the genes are induced in CA1, CA3, and dentate granule cell neurons, that is, neurons that will live as well as die following the global ischemia. It appears that ischemia-induced depolarization and calcium entry into almost all hippocampal neurons results in induction of most IEGs in ischemic hippocampus. However, expression of the IEGs occurs both in cells that will die and in cells that will survive the injury. Therefore, the induction appears to be more a feature of the occurrence of ischemia and calcium influx rather than with the outcome of the cells.

A number of important findings have been published about gene regulation in the CA1 cells destined to die. First, the messenger RNA (mRNA) expression of a number of IEGs including c-fos, c-jun, and others remains quite elevated in CA1 neurons that will eventually die.[79,153,287] Although the mRNA for these genes appears to be increased, in many cases the proteins are not expressed.[287] When cells continue to express the mRNA for an IEG, but do not express the protein, at 24 hours following global ischemia this is an indication of a prolonged translational block and in molecular terms may indicate that the cells are dying or dead.

GROWTH AND TROPHIC FACTORS

The interest in growth factors in cerebral ischemia has been focused on the possibility that they might be useful in treatment of ischemic injury.[258] BDNF is a major growth factor expressed in most mature neurons. Its receptor, trkB, is expressed throughout the brain. NGF is essential for the survival of peripheral sympathetic neurons and appears to be important for the normal function of central nervous system cholinergic neurons in the septum and basal forebrain. Its receptor, trkA, is expressed in the basal forebrain, the hippocampus, and to a lesser extent in the cortex. Neurotrophin-3 (NT-3) and its receptor (trkC) are expressed throughout brain. bFGF and IGF-1 and their receptors are distributed throughout the brain.[320] Astrocytes, microglia, and neurons are a source of bFGF, NGF, BDNF, IGF, IL-1, TNF, and other growth factors and cytokines.[109,118,398]

Several growth factors are induced in the brain following ischemia. Some of these may be induced by transcription factors, including leucine zipper (Fos/Jun, AP1) and zinc finger proteins, acting on AP1 sites or other responsive sites in the promoters of the growth factor genes (AP1 site in NGF; BDNF).[325] bFGF is induced at the sites of stab wound injuries and is also in the hippocampus following transient forebrain ischemia.[201] bFGF mRNA is induced throughout an ischemic hemisphere following MCA occlusions, suggesting possible bFGF induction via spreading depression. bFGF is also induced in ischemic cells.[88,201,369] Transient global ischemia in the gerbil and hypoxia in the rat transiently increases NGF expression followed by a fall when cells die.[228] IGF-2 is increased in hypoxic/ischemic neonatal rat brain.[203] Hypoxia increases trkB levels in rat brain following hypoglycemia and hypoxia, and BDNF is induced following brain injury/ischemia.[207,228]

Growth factors have proved effective in decreasing cellular injury in many culture models of ischemia and in decreasing ischemic injury in many animal models.[257] Although a single injection of bFGF into CA1 did not protect against CA1 pyramidal cell damage in rats,[138] bFGF does protect against hypoxia/ischemia and NMDA neurotoxicity in neonatal rats.[288] bFGF also decreases infarct size following MCA occlusions in adult rats.[97,208] Acidic FGF protects CA1 pyramidal neurons in the gerbil global ischemia model.[331] NGF infusions or NGF pellets prevent CA1 neuronal death in rat and gerbil models of global ischemia[342,392] and in a neonatal ischemia model.[148] Insulin, presumably through actions on IGF-like receptors, protects cortical and striatal neurons against ischemia.[20,219] TGF-β protects rabbit cortex against ischemic

injury.[128,308] BDNF also protects ischemic brain,[29,56] as does CNTF.[389]

HEAT SHOCK/STRESS GENES

Heat Shock Proteins

A number of genes have evolved to deal with normal and extraordinary cellular stress.[387] Heat shock proteins (HSPs) are stress proteins induced by heat shock in response to denatured proteins within cells. The denatured proteins activate heat shock factors (HSFs). HSFs form a trimer and bind to the heat shock element of the gene promoter, which then activates transcription of the mRNA. The mRNA is translated into the HSPs, which are then targeted to various cellular compartments where the HSPs serve as chaperones to renature proteins or to keep them from folding abnormally.[66,83,227,254,267,286]

The HSC70 HSP is the 70-kd chaperone normally found in all cells. This protein functions as an ATPase to bind to other proteins. HSC70 binds to all proteins as they are being formed on the ribosome to prevent them from folding abnormally during the synthesis of the mature protein.[30] HSC70 also participates in the regulation of formation of clathrin-coated vesicles and regulates the function of actin.[150] Following heat shock, HSC70 is modestly upregulated in most tissues. Following global ischemia, HSC70 is also upregulated. Very short durations of ischemia (2 minutes) that do not damage cells induce HSC70 mRNA and protein two-to threefold in CA1 pyramidal neurons.[3,9,183] This induction may persist for some time.[383] There is little increase in HSC70 expression with increased durations of ischemia.[11] HSC70 functions as a normal cellular chaperone that can respond to modest degrees of cellular stress.

The inducible HSP70 heat shock gene is found in multiple copies in most cells. Some inducible hsp70 genes are found in low levels in normal cells, whereas others are not expressed at all in normal cells.[254] Following heat shock and a wide variety of injurious stimuli, HSP70 mRNA and protein can be massively induced to become the most abundant proteins within the cell. The induced HSP70 proteins bind to denatured and partially denatured proteins and serve to prevent further denaturation and to renature partially denatured proteins. Following heat shock of the brain, HSP70 protein is induced almost exclusively in glial cells in the gray and white matter.[249]

HSP70 Induction Following Global Ischemia

The inducible HSP70 protein has been examined in several global ischemia models, including the gerbil model and the rat two-vessel model. Following very brief durations of ischemia in the rat, HSP70 protein can be expressed in small groups of CA1 pyramidal neurons (see Fig. 4.12) or all the pyramidal neurons in the CA1 sector.[125] This CA1 induction occurs without induction of HSP70 in any other cell type, supporting the idea that CA1 neurons are the most vulnerable cell to global ischemia in the brain. In the gerbil global is-

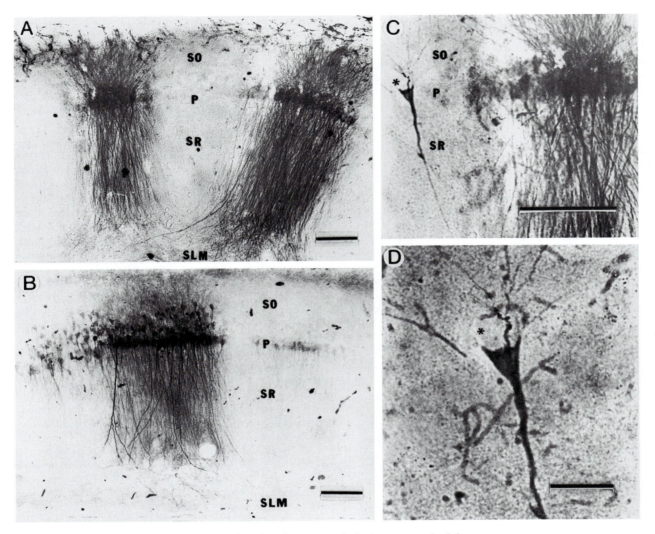

Figure 4.12 (**A–D**) HSP70 protein is induced in hippocampal CA1 neurons of adult gerbils 24 hours following global ischemia. Note HSP70 induction in clumps of neurons (A–C) as well as in isolated, single neurons (C–D).

chemia model, hsp70 mRNA can be selectively induced in CA1 pyramidal neurons without hsp70 stress gene induction in any other brain region.[282,380]

With more prolonged durations of ischemia, HSP70 protein was induced in selected dentate hilar neurons.[125] This induction may well occur in the hilar interneurons that contain somatostatin since these cells are among the most vulnerable to ischemia in the hippocampus.[170] Longer durations of ischemia result in marked HSP70 induction in CA3 pyramidal neurons and variable induction in the dentate granule cell neurons.[180,380] Once HSP70 is induced in CA3 regions of hippocampus, there is significantly less HSP70 induction in CA1 neurons. This appears to occur because longer durations of ischemia produce more and more severe CA1 neuronal damage, which results in the inability of the cells to translate hsp70 mRNA into HSP70 protein. Once severe prolonged ischemia occurs, then the hippocampus is infarcted with failure to synthesize HSP70 protein in either neurons or glial cells. How-

ever, HSP70 protein is synthesized in endothelial cells throughout the infarcted hippocampus. These studies have confirmed the heirarchy of ischemic neurons, dentate granule cells, glial cells, and finally capillary endothelial cells.[125]

Following 5 minutes of ischemia, which results in CA1 neuronal cell death, hsp70 mRNA is expressed throughout all CA1 neurons. This induction occurs within 1 hour of the ischemia and persists for at least 24 hours and probably up until the death of the CA1 neurons (between 2 and 4 days or longer). Although the CA1 neurons express large amounts of hsp70 mRNA, these cells express very little protein.[162,282,380] It appears that these cells have a translation block for formation of HSP70 protein. Since these cells are known to go on to die, cells that make hsp70 mRNA but are unable to synthesize HSP70 protein are destined to die.

Following global ischemia produced using the four-vessel model HSP70 protein is similarly expressed in CA1 neurons first. However, unlike the gerbil model, HSP70 protein appears to be expressed in CA1 neurons that will go on to die.[351] Therefore, a spectrum of injury results in a spectrum of hsp70 stress gene expression. First, hsp70 mRNA and HSP70 protein can be induced with very short durations of ischemia in cells that appear to be histologically normal and that survive the ischemic injury. More prolonged ischemia will result in greater induction of hsp70 mRNA and HSP70 protein. Once the ischemic duration and severity reach a threshold, hsp70 mRNA and HSP70 protein can be induced in cells that go on to die, although this is a zone of ischemia not often seen in the gerbil global ischemia model.[351] With more prolonged ischemia a translation block occurs. hsp70 mRNA (and probably many other stress gene mRNAs) is synthesized, but the cells are so damaged so that they cannot synthesize HSP70 protein. This translation block for stress genes probably indicates a lethal injury. Even more severe ischemia can result in the abrupt failure of hsp70 mRNA as well as HSP70 protein synthesis in cells that probably undergo rapid necrosis following ischemia.

HSP70 Induction Following Focal Ischemia—Molecular Definition of the Penumbra

Following brief MCA occlusions, using the suture model in the rat, it is possible to induce hsp70 mRNA and HSP70 protein throughout the MCA distribution, even without evidence of infarction or overt cell death.[338] MCA occlusions of 30 minutes' duration using this suture model typically result in infarction of the lateral portion of striatum. Following these 30-minute occlusions hsp70 mRNA is induced throughout the MCA distribution including the neocortex and the striatum.[188,191,192,388] The hsp70 mRNA peaks around 4 hours after the ischemia.[192] There is little mRNA induction in the core of the ischemic territory, apparently because of the limited availability of ATP.[206] In the region of striatal infarction HSP70 protein is expressed mainly in capillary endothelial cells. At the margins of the infarctions HSP70 protein is expressed in glial cells, which include astrocytes and microglia. In the cortex, which is not infarcted, HSP70 protein is expressed almost entirely in neurons that can be found in most cortical layers, but especially layers 2 3, and 5.[191] These HSP70, stained cortical neurons are located in the distribution of the ischemic MCA.[188,191,192]

MCA occlusions of 3 hours duration, or permanent MCA occlusions, result in infarction of most of the striatum and cortex in the MCA distribution. Again, HSP70 protein is localized mainly to endothelial cells within the areas of striatal and cortical infarction and also to glial cells, which are mainly located at the margins of the infarctions. HSP70-immunostained neurons are found in a small rim of cortex immediately adjacent to the cortical infarction, in the border zone between the MCA and ACA arteries.[188,191,192]

These data support a number of long-held concepts in experimental cerebral ischemia research. First, there is a hierarchy of cellular damage in both global and focal ischemia: neurons are most vulnerable to ischemia, glia are the next most vulnerable, and endothelial cells are the most resistant. Second, an ischemic penumbra can be described in terms of the hsp70 response. *The ischemic penumbra can be defined as the region outside an infarction where hsp70 mRNA and HSP70 protein are expressed exclusively in neurons.* Following short durations of ischemia (30 minutes), the ischemic penumbra can include all of the cortex in the MCA distribution (see Fig. 4.13). As the duration of ischemia extends (3 hours) the ischemic penumbra progressively decreases in size so that following permanent MCA occlusion the penumbra of HSP70-immunostained neurons is restricted to very small cortical zones immediately adjacent to the cortical infarctions (Fig. 4.13).

Glucose-Regulated Proteins

A class of stress proteins that are less studied but of similar importance to the HSPs includes the glucose-regulated proteins (GRPs). These proteins are induced by low glucose and calcium ionophores in cultured cells, and many are also induced by hypoxia/anoxia.[253,254] The GRPs do not appear to have heat shock elements in their promoters and hence respond poorly to heat shock stress and are not called HSPs. GRP78 is a glucose-regulated protein found in the endoplasmic reticulum that is important for chaperoning proteins through the endoplasmic reticulum and regulating the glycosylation of target proteins.[254,263] GRP78 is modestly upregulated by ischemia and prolonged seizures.[238,383] The glucose transporter 1 (GLUT1), which is found in brain endothelial cells, is also a glucose-regulated protein whose expression is upregulated by low glucose and calcium ionophore in culture[84] and is induced following ischemia.[110,220,379] This finding suggests that decreased delivery of glucose to endothelium and brain cells during focal ischemia is a sufficient stimulus to promote the upregulation of the brain endothelial glucose transporters.

Another glucose-regulated protein, GRP75, a recently cloned glucose-regulated gene, is localized to mitochondria.[253] GRP75 probably plays an important chaperone function in moving proteins across mitochondrial membranes. GRP75 is only modestly induced by heat shock but is markedly induced following ischemia.[253] Following very brief ischemia GRP75 is induced in the distribution of the MCA ischemia similar to glucose transporter induction in the ischemic territory. Following permanent MCA occlusions, GRP75 is expressed in the cortex outside the MCA distribution: cingulate and parietal cortex in the ACA and PCA territories, respectively.[253] The stimulus for this GRP75 induction is still unclear but could be related to prolonged ischemic depolarization produced by the MCA occlusions.

Hemeoxygenase-1

Hemeoxygenase metabolizes heme-containing proteins to biliverdin, carbon monoxide, and iron.[90] The carbon monoxide released by this reaction could have important effects for controlling cerebrovascular responses to changes in neuronal activity. In the brain there are inducible (hemeoxygenase-1 [HO-1]) and constitutive (HO-2) forms of hemeoxygenase. The HO-2 protein is found mainly in neurons and is not inducible.[90] The HO-1 gene is expressed mainly in glial cells following heat shock and is inducible by a variety of stimuli.[90–92,247] The HO-1 gene has multiple responsive elements in its promoter: a heat shock element that makes it responsive

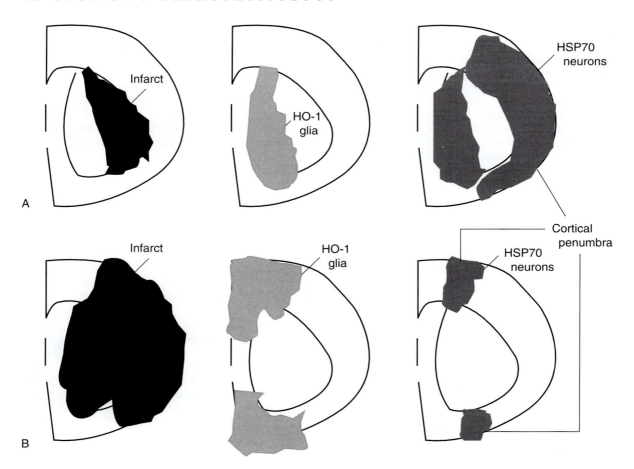

Figure 4.13 Diagrams of infarction (black), HO-1 stress protein induction (light gray), and HSP70 heat shock protein induction (dark gray) following (**A**) 30-minute MCA occlusions and (**B**) 2-hour MCA occlusions. Note that following 30-minute occlusion lateral striatum infarction occurred with HO-1 expression in glia in medial striatum and HSP70 protein expression in medial striatum and cortex in the MCA distribution. Based on this finding and the lower panel, it is suggested that neuronal HSP70 protein expression can be used as a biochemical and anatomical marker of the penumbra shown in Figure 4.2 (gray).

to heat shock; an AP1 element that may render it responsive to certain c-fos and c-jun family members; an NFKB element that may render the gene responsive to hypoxia and oxidative stress; and an element that makes the gene responsive to free heme.

HO-1 is also induced by cerebral ischemia. Following 30-minute MCA occlusions, infarction of the lateral striatum was noted 24 hours later. HO-1 was induced in glial cells, mainly microglia, in the regions around the striatal infarction.[279] HSP70 was also induced in glial cells around the infarction. However, in the cortex HSP70 protein was expressed in neurons throughout the MCA distribution whereas HO-1 protein was not expressed at all (Fig. 4.13). These data are important for showing different ischemic thresholds for the induction of these two stress proteins, with HSP70 being expressed in areas of ischemic injury where no HO-1 induction was detectable.

Following permanent MCA occlusions there was another major difference in the patterns of HO-1 and HSP70 protein expression. Within areas of cortical infarction both HO-1 and

HSP70 were expressed in endothelial cells and in scattered glial cells. At the margins of the infarction both HSP70 and HO-1 proteins were expressed in glial cells and neurons. There was no HSP70 expression in the cingulate or occipital cortex following the MCA occlusions. HO-1 protein, on the other hand, was expressed in glial cells throughout an ischemic hemisphere—in the cingulate cortex as well as in posterior parietal cortex (Fig. 4.13). This HO-1 microglial expression occurred well outside any area of ischemia. This finding suggests that the focal MCA ischemia is affecting stress gene function in glia throughout an ischemic hemisphere. It is possible that ischemia-induced spreading depression or depolarization leads to induction of IEGs. The induction of specific c-fos or c-jun family members within the microglia would lead to activation of AP-1 sites of the HO-1 gene, increased glial transcription, and eventual translation of HO-1 protein.

HO-1 expression has also been examined following global ischemia. With 5 minutes of global ischemia in the gerbil model, there is substantial induction of HO-1 in microglia throughout the hippocampus, particularly around the CA1 neurons that will die.[298,371] This glial HO-1 induction is occurring presumably in the absence of any glial cell death, and in response to damaged and dying CA1 pyramidal neurons. This finding suggests a signal between damaged neurons and a resultant stress response in the surrounding glial cells.

Repeated Focal Ischemia—Increased Vulnerability versus Tolerance

Following hyperthermia, the vulnerability of the brain and cells to ischemia varies with time. Hyperthermia worsens ischemic damage, when the hyperthermia occurs during or shortly after the ischemia.[53,73,218,262,407] Hyperthermia, however, can improve neural injury and decrease ischemic damage when the hyperthermia occurs 24 hours prior to the ischemia.[22,59] Hypothermia can improve ischemic injury in a wide variety of models.[41,64,73,116]

Like hypothermia, the vulnerability of the brain to ischemia after short periods of ischemia (transient ischemic attacks) is a function of the duration of the initial ischemia and also a function of the time between the periods of ischemia. If brief episodes of nonlethal ischemia are paired close in time, brain damage occurs. For example, 2-minute episodes of global ischemia in the gerbil produce no cell death. However, 2-minute episodes of ischemia given 1 hour apart for 3 hours produce neuronal cell death. In addition, the neuronal cell death produced by these three separate 2-minute ischemic episodes is much more severe than a single 6-minute episode of ischemia.[14,178,180]

If the periods of ischemia spread out further in time, however, the phenomenon of *ischemic tolerance* can also be demonstrated in the brain.[197] Following brief periods of ischemia that do not injure the brain, a triphasic response has been described. Following two periods of ischemia of 2 minutes each, the brain is initially more vulnerable to ischemia. However, if enough time elapses between the ischemic preconditioning and the exposure to any otherwise lethal duration of ischemia (times between 1 and 3 days depending upon the model and durations of ischemia), then CA1 pyramidal neurons may be partially or fully protected[55,195,198] or the size of focal ischemic injury will be decreased.[120,352] If more time lapses between the preconditioning and the ischemic injury, then the degree of injury returns to baseline levels (tolerance having been induced) and disappears.

The factors that determine the occurrence of ischemic tolerance are still unclear. Ischemic tolerance in the brain clearly takes a day to many days to develop. It has been suggested that tolerance can be blocked by the simultaneous administration of MK801 when the preconditioning ischemia occurs.[181] This suggests that tolerance relates to some change in the NMDA receptor.[205] Induction of HSPs may induce tolerance.[10] It is possible that ischemic induction of HSP70 and other HSPs, induction of the endothelial glucose transporter and other GRPs, and induction of HO-1 and other oxygen-regulated stress proteins may also play some role in the phenomenon of ischemic tolerance.[175,177,234,272,280]

It has also been suggested that adenosine receptors mediate ischemic tolerance in the brain.[143] Adenosine agonists produce partial protection against CA1 neuronal injury in the gerbil brain. Adenosine antagonists partially block ischemic tolerance. It appears, however, that adenosine does not account for the entire phenomenon of ischemic tolerance in brain because the degree of tolerance produced by ischemia is greater than compounds acting at adenosine receptors. Ischemic tolerance involves, at least in part, a cascade of events including liberation of adenosine, stimulation of A1 adenosine receptors, and opening of sulfonylurea-sensitive ATP-sensitive K+ channels.[143]

Remote Neuronal Cell Injury Following Focal Ischemia

Following MCA occlusions in both rodents and humans there is not only infarction of the cortex and striatum, but slow atrophy of the ipsilateral thalamus[60,135,373,390] and in some cases atrophy of ipsilateral substantia nigra pars reticulata (SNr).[101,372] In rodent models of MCA occlusions there is consistent gene induction in the thalamus and SNr as well as in the hippocampus.[188,189] Rodent studies also demonstrate neuronal cell death in the hippocampus following permanent MCA occlusions.[32] These regions of injury in the thalamus, SNr, and hippocampus are outside the region of MCA ischemia and therefore must be due to remote trans-synaptic effects of the cortical and striatal infarcts on cellular function in these nonischemic, but interconnected brain regions.

Following MCA occlusions the c-fos IEG is induced in the ipsilateral thalamus (Fig. 4.11). This thalamic IEG induction occurs in thalamic nuclei that project to the areas of infarction (e.g., the ventrolateral and ventroposterolateral nuclei). However, the IEG induction also occurs in thalamic nuclei that project to cortical areas that do not infarct, including the lateral geniculate (visual cortex) and anterior thalamic (cingulate cortex, frontal cortex) nuclei. This IEG induction throughout the thalamus has been suggested to be due to spreading depression affecting the entire cortex, depolarizing thalamocortical neurons and inducing IEGs in all thalamic neurons receiving cortical inputs.[188] hsp 70 mRNA, however, is also expressed in thalamus following MCA occlusions. The thalamic hsp 70 induction was restricted to a relatively few thalamic nuclei that were proposed to innervate selectively areas of cortex that sustained ischemic injury.[188] This hsp 70 induction in specific thalamic nuclei suggests that denatured proteins might be present in selected thalamic neurons following ischemic cortical injury.[188] FGF infusions have been reported to prevent thalamic atrophy following MCA occlusions,[390] as have cortical transplants to areas of cortical ablation.[60]

Atrophy of ipsilateral SNr has also been described following large MCA infarctions in humans and rodents.[12,101,372] Infarction or damage to large regions of the striatum is required to produce SNr cellular damage, and the volume of striatal damage correlates with the degree of SNr damage.[327,329] Infusions of GABA agonists may prevent the substantia nigra cell loss.[328]

References

1. Abe K, Aoki M, Kawagoe J et al: Ischemic delayed neuronal death. A mitochondrial hypothesis. Stroke 26:1478, 1995

2. Abe K, Araki T, Kawagoe J et al: Phospholipid metabolism and second messenger system after brain ischemia. Adv Exp Med Biol 318:183, 1992

3. Abe K, Kawagoe J, Aoki M, Kogure K: Dissociation of HSP70 and HSC70 heat shock mRNA inductions as an early biochemical marker of ischemic neuronal death. Neurosci Lett 149:165, 1993

4. Abe K, Kogure K, Yamamoto H et al: Mechanism of arachidonic acid liberation during ischemia in gerbil cerebral cortex. J Neurochem 48:503, 1987

5. Alkayed NJ, Narayanan J, Gebremedhin D et al: Molecular characterization of an arachidonic acid epoxygenase in rat brain astrocytes. Stroke 27:971, 1996

6. Alps BJ, Calder C, Hass WK, Wilson AD: Comparative protective effects of nicardipine, flunarizine, lidoflazine and nimodipine against ischaemic injury in the hippocampus of the Mongolian gerbil. Br J Pharmacol 93:877, 1988

7. An G, Lin TN, Liu JS et al: Expression of c-fos and c-jun family genes after focal cerebral ischemia [see comments]. Ann Neurol 33:457, 1993

8. Andrus PK, Taylor BM, Sun FF, Hall ED: Effects of the lipid peroxidation inhibitor tirilazad mesylate (U-74006F) on gerbil brain eicosanoid levels following ischemia and reperfusion. Brain Res 659:126, 1994

9. Aoki M, Abe K, Kawagoe J et al: Acceleration of HSP70 and HSC70 heat shock gene expression following transient ischemia in the preconditioned gerbil hippocampus. J Cereb Blood Flow Metab 13:781, 1993

10. Aoki M, Abe K, Kawagoe J et al: The preconditioned hippocampus accelerates HSP70 heat shock gene expression following transient ischemia in the gerbil. Neurosci Lett 155:7, 1993

11. Aoki M, Abe K, Kawagoe J et al: Temporal profile of the induction of heat shock protein 70 and heat shock cognate protein 70 mRNAs after transient ischemia in gerbil brain. Brain Res 601:185, 1993

12. Araki T, Kato H, Kogure K: Selective neuronal vulnerability following transient cerebral ischemia in the gerbil: distribution and time course. Acta Neurol Scand 80:548, 1989

13. Araki T, Kato H, Kogure K: Neuronal damage and calcium accumulation following repeated brief cerebral ischemia in the gerbil. Brain Res 528:114, 1990

14. Araki T, Kato H, Kogure K, Inoue T: Regional neuroprotective effects of pentobarbital on ischemia-induced brain damage. Brain Res Bull 25:861, 1990

15. Araki T, Kato H, Kogure K: Comparative protective effects of vinconate, baclofen, and pentobarbital against neuronal damage following repeated brief cerebral ischemia in the gerbil brain. Res Exp Med (Berl) 191:371, 1991

16. Araki T, Kato H, Kogure K, Saito T: Postischemic alteration of muscarinic acetylcholine, adenosine A1 and calcium antagonist binding sites in selectively vulnerable areas: an autoradiographic study of gerbil brain. J Neurol Sci 106:206, 1991

17. Araki T, Kato H, Kogure K: Postischemic alteration of muscarinic acetylcholine and adenosine A1 binding sites in gerbil brain. Protective effects of a novel vinca alkaloid derivative, vinconate, and pentobarbital using an autoradiographic study. Res Exp Med (Berl) 192:79, 1992

18. Araki T, Kato H, Kanai Y, Kogure K: Long-term observations in gerbil brain following transient cerebral ischemia: autoradiographic and histological study. Metab Brain Dis 8:181, 1993

19. Attwell D, Barbour B, Szatkowski M: Nonvesicular release of neurotransmitter. Neuron 11:401, 1993

20. Auer RN: Combination therapy with U74006F (tirilazad mesylate), MK-801, insulin and diazepam in transient forebrain ischaemia. Neurol Res 17:132, 1995

21. Back T, Ginsberg MD, Dietrich WD, Watson BD: Induction of spreading depression in the ischemic hemisphere following experimental middle cerebral artery occlusion: effect on infarct morphology. J Cereb Blood Flow Metab 16:202, 1996

22. Barbe MF, Tytell M, Gower DJ, Welch WJ: Hyperthermia protects against light damage in the rat retina. Science 241:1817, 1988

23. Bartus RT, Hayward NJ, Elliott PJ et al: Calpain inhibitor AK295 protects neurons from focal brain ischemia. Effects of postocclusion intra-arterial administration. Stroke 25:2265, 1994

24. Bazan NG: Second messengers derived from excitable membranes are involved in ischemic and seizure-related brain damage. Patol Fiziol Eksp Ter 11, 1992

25. Bazan NG, Allan G, Rodriguez de Turco EB: Role of phospholipase A2 and membrane-derived lipid second messengers in membrane function and transcriptional activation of genes: implications in cerebral ischemia and neuronal excitability. Prog Brain Res 96:247, 1993

26. Bazan NG, Marcheselli VL, Mukherjee PK: Inducible prostaglandin synthase in cell injury. Adv Prostaglandin Thromboxane Leukotriene Res 23:317, 1995

27. Bazan NG, Rodriguez de Turco EB, Allan G: Mediators of injury in neurotrauma: intracellular signal transduction and gene expression. J Neurotrauma 12:791, 1995

28. Beamer NB, Coull BM, Clark WM et al: Interleukin-6 and interleukin-1 receptor antagonist in acute stroke. Ann Neurol 37:800, 1995

29. Beck T, Lindholm D, Castren E, Wree A: Brain-derived neurotrophic factor protects against ischemic cell damage in rat hippocampus. J Cereb Blood Flow Metab 14:689, 1994

30. Beckmann RP, Mizzen LE, Welch WJ: Interaction of Hsp 70 with newly synthesized proteins: implications for protein folding and assembly. Science 248:850, 1990

31. Beilharz EJ, Williams CE, Dragunow M et al: Mechanisms of delayed cell death following hypoxic-ischemic injury in the immature rat: evidence for apoptosis during

selective neuronal loss. Brain Res Mol Brain Res 29:1, 1995

32. Benyo Z, De Jong GI, Luiten PG: Nimodipine prevents early loss of hippocampal CA1 parvalbumin immuno-reactivity after focal cerebral ischemia in the rat. Brain Res Bull 36:569, 1995

33. Betz AL, Yang GY, Davidson BL: Attenuation of stroke size in rats using an adenoviral vector to induce overexpression of interleukin-1 receptor antagonist in brain. J Cereb Blood Flow Metab 15:547, 1995

34. Blumenfeld KS, Welsh FA, Harris VA, Pesenson MA: Regional expression of c-fos and heat shock protein-70 mRNA following hypoxia-ischemia in immature rat brain. J Cereb Blood Flow Metab 12:987, 1992

35. Bonventre JV, Koroshetz WJ: Phospholipase A_2 (PLA_2) activity in gerbil brain: characterization of cytosolic and membrane-associated forms and effects of ischemia and reperfusion on enzymatic activity. J Lipid Mediat 6:457, 1993

36. Boulter J, Hollmann M, O'Shea-Greenfield A et al: Molecular cloning and functional expression of glutamate receptor subunit genes. Science 249:1033, 1990

37. Bowes MP, Rothlein R, Fagan SC, Zivin JA: Monoclonal antibodies preventing leukocyte activation reduce experimental neurologic injury and enhance efficacy of thrombolytic therapy. Neurology 45:815, 1995

38. Bowes MP, Zivin JA, Rothlein R: Monoclonal antibody to the ICAM-1 adhesion site reduces neurological damage in a rabbit cerebral embolism stroke model. Exp Neurol 119:215, 1993

39. Braughler JM, Hall ED: Involvement of lipid peroxidation in CNS injury. J Neurotrauma suppl 1, 9: S1, 1992

40. Buchan AM, Gertler SZ, Li H et al: A selective N-type Ca(2+)-channel blocker prevents CA1 injury 24 h following severe forebrain ischemia and reduces infarction following focal ischemia. J Cereb Blood Flow Metab 14:903, 1994

41. Buchan AM, Li H, Cho S, Pulsinelli WA: Blockade of the AMPA receptor prevents CA1 hippocampal injury following severe but transient forebrain ischemia in adult rats. Neurosci Lett 132:255, 1991

42. Buchan A, Li H, Pulsinelli WA: The N-methyl-D-aspartate antagonist, MK-801, fails to protect against neuronal damage caused by transient, severe forebrain ischemia in adult rats. J Neurosci 11:1049, 1991

43. Buchan A, Pulsinelli WA: Hypothermia but not the N-methyl-D-aspartate antagonist, MK-801, attenuates neuronal damage in gerbils subjected to transient global ischemia. J Neurosci 10:311, 1990

44. Buisson A, Callebert J, Mathieu E et al: Striatal protection induced by lesioning the substantia nigra of rats subjected to focal ischemia. J Neurochem 59:1153, 1992

45. Burda J, Martin ME, Garcia A et al: Phosphorylation of the alpha subunit of initiation factor 2 correlates with the inhibition of translation following transient cerebral ischaemia in the rat. Biochem J 302:335, 1994

46. Burnashev N, Khodorova A, Jonas P et al: Calcium-permeable AMPA-kainate receptors in fusiform cerebellar glial cells. Science 256:1566, 1992

47. Busto R, Globus MY, Neary JT, Ginsberg MD: Regional alterations of protein kinase C activity following transient cerebral ischemia: effects of intraischemic brain temperature modulation. J Neurochem 63:1095, 1994

48. Carney JM, Floyd RA: Brain antioxidant activity of spin traps in Mongolian gerbils. Methods Enzymol 234: 523, 1994

49. Carter LP, Yamagata S, Erspamer R: Time limits of reversible cortical ischemia. Neurosurgery 12:620, 1983

50. Chan PH: Oxygen radicals in focal cerebral ischemia. Brain Pathol 4:59, 1994

51. Chan PH, Epstein CJ, Li Y et al: Transgenic mice and knockout mutants in the study of oxidative stress in brain injury. J Neurotrauma 12:815, 1995

52. Chan PH, Kinouchi H, Epstein CJ et al: Role of superoxide dismutase in ischemic brain injury: reduction of edema and infarction in transgenic mice following focal cerebral ischemia. Prog Brain Res 96:97, 1993

53. Chen H, Chopp M, Welch KM: Effect of mild hyperthermia on the ischemic infarct volume after middle cerebral artery occlusion in the rat. Neurology 41:1133, 1991

54. Chen ST, Hsu CY, Hogan EL et al: Thromboxane, prostacyclin, and leukotrienes in cerebral ischemia. Neurology 36:466, 1986

55. Chen T, Kato H, Liu XH et al: Ischemic tolerance can be induced repeatedly in the gerbil hippocampal neurons. Neurosci Lett 177:159, 1994

56. Cheng B, Mattson MP: NT-3 and BDNF protect CNS neurons against metabolic/excitotoxic insults. Brain Res 640:56, 1994

57. Choi DW: Calcium-mediated neurotoxicity: relationship to specific channel types and role in ischemic damage. Trends Neurosci 11:465, 1988

58. Choi DW: Glutamate neurotoxicity and diseases of the nervous system. Neuron 1:623, 1988

59. Chopp M, Chen H, Ho KL et al: Transient hyperthermia protects against subsequent forebrain ischemic cell damage in the rat. Neurology 39:1396, 1989

60. Ciricillo SP, Hill MP, Gonzalez MF et al: Whisker stimulation metabolically activates thalamus following cortical transplantation but not following cortical ablation. Neuroscience 59:975, 1994

61. Clark WM, Coull BM, Briley DP et al: Circulating intercellular adhesion molecule-1 levels and neutrophil adhesion in stroke. J Neuroimmunol 44:123, 1993

62. Clark WM, Lauten JD, Lessov N et al: The influence of antiadhesion therapies on leukocyte subset accumulation in central nervous system ischemia in rats. J Mol Neurosci 6:43, 1995

63. Clemens JA, Stephenson DT, Smalstig EB et al: Reactive glia express cytosolic phospholipase A_2 after transient global forebrain ischemia in the rat. Stroke 27:527, 1996

64. Colbourne F, Corbett D: Delayed postischemic hypothermia: a six month survival study using behavioral and histological assessments of neuroprotection. J Neurosci 15:7250, 1995

65. Coyle JT, Puttfarcken P: Oxidative stress, glutamate, and neurodegenerative disorders. Science 262:689, 1993

66. Craig EA, Gambill BD, Nelson RJ: Heat shock proteins: molecular chaperones of protein biogenesis. Microbiol Rev 57:402, 1993

67. Crumrine RC, Thomas AL, Morgan PF: Attenuation of p53 expression protects against focal ischemic damage in transgenic mice. J Cereb Blood Flow Metab 14:887, 1994

68. Curran T, Morgan JI: Fos: an immediate-early transcription factor in neurons. J Neurobiol 26:403, 1995

69. Dalkara T, Moskowitz MA: The complex role of nitric oxide in the pathophysiology of focal cerebral ischemia. Brain Pathol 4:49, 1994

70. Dawson DA: Nitric oxide and focal cerebral ischemia: multiplicity of actions and diverse outcome. Cerebrovasc Brain Metab Rev 6:299, 1994

71. Deckert J, Gleiter CH: Adenosine—an endogenous neuroprotective metabolite and neuromodulator. J Neural Transm Suppl 43:23, 1994

72. del Zoppo GJ: Microvascular changes during cerebral ischemia and reperfusion. Cerebrovasc Brain Metab Rev 6:47, 1994

73. Dietrich WD: The importance of brain temperature in cerebral injury. J Neurotrauma, suppl. 2, 9: S475, 1992

74. Dietrich WD, Alonso O, Busto R: Moderate hyperglycemia worsens acute blood-brain barrier injury after forebrain ischemia in rats. Stroke 24:111, 1993

75. Dietrich WD, Feng ZC, Leistra H et al: Photothrombotic infarction triggers multiple episodes of cortical spreading depression in distant brain regions. J Cereb Blood Flow Metab 14:20, 1994

76. Domanska-Janik K, Zablocka B: Protein kinase C as an early and sensitive marker of ischemia-induced progressive neuronal damage in gerbil hippocampus. Mol Chem Neuropathol 20:111, 1993

77. Dougherty JH, Jr, Levy DE, Rawlinson DG et al: Experimental cerebral ischemia produced by extracranial vascular injury: protection with indomethacin and prostacyclin. Neurology 32:970, 1982

78. Dragunow M, Beilharz E, Sirimanne E et al: Immediate-early gene protein expression in neurons undergoing delayed death, but not necrosis, following hypoxic-ischaemic injury to the young rat brain. Brain Res Mol Brain Res 25:19, 1994

79. Dragunow M, Young D, Hughes P et al: Is c-Jun involved in nerve cell death following status epilepticus and hypoxic-ischaemic brain injury? Brain Res Mol Brain Res 18:347, 1993

80. Du C, Hu R, Csernansky CA et al: Very delayed infarction after mild focal cerebral ischemia: a role for apoptosis? J Cereb Blood Flow Metab 16:195, 1996

81. Dugan LL, Lin TS, He YY et al: Detection of free radicals by microdialysis/spin trapping EPR following focal cerebral ischemia-reperfusion and a cautionary note on the stability of 5,5-dimethyl-1-pyrroline N-oxide (DMPO).Free Radic Res 23:27, 1995

82. Dugan LL, Sensi SL, Canzoniero LM et al: Mitochondrial production of reactive oxygen species in cortical neurons following exposure to N-methyl-D-aspartate. J Neurosci 15:6377, 1995

83. Dwyer BE, Nishimura RN: Heat shock proteins in hypoxic-ischemic brain injury: a perspective. Brain Pathol 2:245, 1992

84. Ebert BL, Firth JD, Ratcliffe PJ: Hypoxia and mitochondrial inhibitors regulate expression of glucose transporter-1 via distinct Cis-acting sequences. J Biol Chem 270:29083, 1995

85. Ekholm A, Katsura K, Siesjo BK: Tissue lactate content and tissue PCO_2 in complete brain ischaemia: implications for compartmentation of H^+. Neurol Res 13:74, 1991

86. Ember JA, del Zoppo GJ, Mori E et al: Polymorphonuclear leukocyte behavior in a nonhuman primate focal ischemia model. J Cereb Blood Flow Metab 14:1046, 1994

87. Endoh M, Maiese K, Wagner J: Expression of the inducible form of nitric oxide synthase by reactive astrocytes after transient global ischemia. Brain Res 651:92, 1994

88. Endoh M, Pulsinelli WA, Wagner JA: Transient global ischemia induces dynamic changes in the expression of bFGF and the FGF receptor. Brain Res Mol Brain Res 22:76, 1994

89. Erecinska M, Silver IA: Metabolism and role of glutamate in mammalian brain. Prog Neurobiol 35:245, 1990

90. Ewing JF, Haber SN, Maines MD: Normal and heat-induced patterns of expression of heme oxygenase-1 (HSP32) in rat brain: hyperthermia causes rapid induction of mRNA and protein. J Neurochem 58:1140, 1992

91. Ewing JF, Maines MD: Glutathione depletion induces heme oxygenase-1 (HSP32) mRNA and protein in rat brain. J Neurochem 60:1512, 1993

92. Ewing JF, Raju VS, Maines MD: Induction of heart heme oxygenase-1 (HSP32) by hyperthermia: possible role in stress-mediated elevation of cyclic 3′:5′-guanosine monophosphate. J Pharmacol Exp Ther 271:408, 1994

93. Faraci FM, Brain JE Jr: Nitric oxide and the cerebral circulation. Stroke 25:692, 1994

94. Farber NB, Price MT, Labruyere J et al: Antipsychotic drugs block phencyclidine receptor-mediated neurotoxicity [see comments]. Biol Psychiatry 34:119, 1993

95. Ferriero DM, Sheldon RA, Black SM, Chuai J: Selective destruction of nitric oxide synthase neurons with quisqualate reduces damage after hypoxia-ischemia in the neonatal rat. Pediatr Res 38:912, 1995

96. Feuerstein GZ, Liu T, Barone FC: Cytokines, inflammation, and brain injury: role of tumor necrosis factor-alpha. Cerebrovasc Brain Metab Rev 6:341, 1994

97. Fisher M, Meadows ME, Do T et al: Delayed treatment with intravenous basic fibroblast growth factor reduces infarct size following permanent focal cerebral ischemia in rats. J Cereb Blood Flow Metab 15:953, 1995

98. Floyd RA, Carney JM: Free radical damage to protein and DNA: mechanisms involved and relevant observations on brain undergoing oxidative stress. Ann Neurol, suppl. 32:S22, 1992

99. Folbergrova J, Memezawa H, Smith ML, Siesjo BK: Focal and perifocal changes in tissue energy state during middle cerebral artery occlusion in normo- and hyperglycemic rats. J Cereb Blood Flow Metab 12:25, 1992

100. Foster AC, Gill R, Woodruff GN: Neuroprotective effects of MK-801 in vivo: selectivity and evidence for delayed degeneration mediated by NMDA receptor activation. J Neurosci 8:4745, 1988

101. Fujioka M, Okuchi K, Sakaki T et al: Specific changes in

human brain following reperfusion after cardiac arrest. Stroke 25:2091, 1994

102. Furfine ES, Harmon MF, Paith JE et al: Potent and selective inhibition of human nitric oxide synthases. Selective inhibition of neuronal nitric oxide synthase by S-methyl-L-thiocitrulline and S-ethyl-L-thiocitrulline. J Biol Chem 269:26677, 1994

103. Galea E, Reis DJ, Xu H, Feinstein DL: Transient expression of calcium-independent nitric oxide synthase in blood vessels during brain development. Faseb J 9:1632, 1995

104. Garcia JH: The evolution of brain infarcts. A review. J Neuropathol Exp Neurol 51:387, 1992

105. Garcia JH, Lasen NA, Weiller C et al: Ischemic stroke and incomplete infarction. Stroke 27:761, 1996

106. Garcia JH, Liu KF, Relton JK: Interleukin-1 receptor antagonist decreases the number of necrotic neurons in rats with middle cerebral artery occlusion. Am J Pathol 147:1477, 1995

107. Garcia JH, Liu KF, Yoshida Y et al: Influx of leukocytes and platelets in an evolving brain infarct (Wistar rat). Am J Pathol 144:188, 1994

108. Gass P, Spranger M, Herdegen T et al: Induction of FOS and JUN proteins after focal ischemia in the rat: differential effect of the N-methyl-D-aspartate receptor antagonist MK-801. Acta Neuropathol (Berl) 84:545, 1992

109. Gehrmann J, Banati RB, Wiessner C et al: Reactive microglia in cerebral ischaemia: an early mediator of tissue damage? Neuropathol Appl Neurobiol 21:277, 1995

110. Gerhart DZ, Leino RL, Taylor WE et al: GLUT1 and GLUT3 gene expression in gerbil brain following brief ischemia: an in situ hybridization study. Brain Res Mol Brain Res 25:313, 1994

111. Giacoia GP: Asphyxial brain damage in the newborn: new insights into pathophysiology and possible pharmacologic interventions. South Med J 86:676, 1993

112. Gill R, Foster AC, Woodruff GN: Systemic administration of MK-801 protects against ischemia-induced hippocampal neurodegeneration in the gerbil. J Neurosci 7:3343, 1987

113. Ginsberg MD: Local metabolic responses to cerebral ischemia. Cerebrovasc Brain Metab Rev 2:58, 1990

114. Ginsberg MD, Graham DI, Busto R: Regional glucose utilization and blood flow following graded forebrain ischemia in the rat: correlation with neuropathology. Ann Neurol 18:470, 1985

115. Ginsberg MD, Lin B, Morikawa E et al: Calcium antagonists in the treatment of experimental cerebral ischemia. Arzneimittelforschung 41:334, 1991

116. Ginsberg MD, Sternau LL, Globus MY et al: Therapeutic modulation of brain temperature: relevance to ischemic brain injury. Cerebrovasc Brain Metab Rev 4:189, 1992

117. Ginsberg MD, Watson BD, Busto R et al: Peroxidative damage to cell membranes following cerebral ischemia. A cause of ischemic brain injury? Neurochem Pathol 9:171, 1988

118. Giulian D: Reactive glia as rivals in regulating neuronal survival. Glia 7:102, 1993

119. Giulian D, Baker TJ, Shih LC, Lachman LB: Interleukin 1 of the central nervous system is produced by ameboid microglia. J Exp Med 164:594, 1986

120. Glazier SS, OR Rourke DM, Graham DI, Welsh FA: Induction of ischemic tolerance following brief focal ischemia in rat brain. J Cereb Blood Flow Metab 14:545, 1994

121. Globus MY, Busto R, Dietrich WD et al: Effect of ischemia on the in vivo release of striatal dopamine, glutamate, and gamma-aminobutyric acid studied by intracerebral microdialysis. J Neurochem 51:1455, 1988

122. Globus MY, Busto R, Dietrich WD et al: Intra-ischemic extracellular release of dopamine and glutamate is associated with striatal vulnerability to ischemia. Neurosci Lett 91:36, 1988

123. Globus MY, Ginsberg MD, Busto R: Excitotoxic index—a biochemical marker of selective vulnerability. Neurosci Lett 127:39, 1991

124. Goldman SA, Pulsinelli WA, Clarke WY et al: The effects of extracellular acidosis on neurons and glia in vitro. J Cereb Blood Flow Metab 9:471, 1989

125. Gonzalez MF, Lowenstein D, Fernyak S et al: Induction of heat shock protein 72-like immunoreactivity in the hippocampal formation following transient global ischemia. Brain Res Bull 26:241, 1991

126. Grasl KB, Ruttkay NB, Koudelka H et al: In situ detection of fragmented DNA (TUNEL assay) fails to discriminate among apoptosis, necrosis, and autolytic cell death: a cautionary note. Hepatology 21:1465, 1995

127. Greenlund LJ, Deckwerth TL, Johnson EJ: Superoxide dismutase delays neuronal apoptosis: a role for reactive oxygen species in programmed neuronal death. Neuron 14:303, 1995

128. Gross CE, Bednar MM, Howard DB, Sporn MB: Transforming growth factor-beta 1 reduces infarct size after experimental cerebral ischemia in a rabbit model. Stroke 24:558, 1993

129. Hainaut P: The tumor suppressor protein p53: a receptor to genotoxic stress that controls cell growth and survival. Curr Opin Oncol 7:76, 1995

130. Hakim AM: The cerebral ischemic penumbra. Can J Neurol Sci 14:557, 1987

131. Hall ED: Neuroprotective actions of glucocorticoid and nonglucocorticoid steroids in acute neuronal injury. Cell Mol Neurobiol 13:415, 1993

132. Hall ED, Braughler JM, McCall JM: Antioxidant effects in brain and spinal cord injury. J Neurotrauma, suppl. 91:S165, 1992

133. Halliwell B: Reactive oxygen species and the central nervous system. J Neurochem 59:1609, 1992

134. Hansen AJ, Quistorff B, Gjedde A: Relationship between local changes in cortical blood flow and extracellular K + during spreading depression. Acta Physiol Scand 109:1, 1980

135. Hara H, Harada K, Sukamoto T: Chronological atrophy after transient middle cerebral artery occlusion in rats. Brain Res 618:251, 1993

136. Hara H, Kato H, Kogure K: Protective effect of alpha-tocopherol on ischemic neuronal damage in the gerbil hippocampus. Brain Res 510:335, 1990

137. Hara H, Kogure K: Prevention of hippocampus neuronal damage in ischemic gerbils by a novel lipid peroxidation

inhibitor (quinazoline derivative). J Pharmacol Exp Ther 255:906, 1990

138. Hara H, Onodera H, Kawagoe J, Kogure K: Failure of basic fibroblast growth factor to prevent postischemic neuronal damage in the rat. Eur J Pharmacol 209:195, 1991

139. Hara H, Onodera H, Kogure K: Protein kinase C activity in the gerbil hippocampus after transient forebrain ischemia: morphological and autoradiographic analysis using [3H]phorbol 12, 13-dibutyrate. Neurosci Lett 120:120, 1990

140. Hara H, Onodera H, Yoshidomi M et al: Staurosporine, a novel protein kinase C inhibitor, prevents postischemic neuronal damage in the gerbil and rat. J Cereb Blood Flow Metab 10:646, 1990

141. He YY, Hsu CY, Ezrin AM, Miller MS: Polyethylene glycol-conjugated superoxide dismutase in focal cerebral ischemia-reperfusion. Am J Physiol 265:H252, 1993

142. Heurteaux C, Bertaina V, Widmann C, Lazdunski M: K+ channel openers prevent global ischemia-induced expression of c-fos, c-jun, heat shock protein, and amyloid beta-protein precursor genes and neuronal death in rat hippocampus. Proc Natl Acad Sci USA 90:9431, 1993

143. Heurteaux C, Lauritzen I, Widmann C, Lazdunski M: Essential role of adenosine, adenosine A1 receptors, and ATP-sensitive K+ channels in cerebral ischemic preconditioning. Proc Natl Acad Sci USA 92:4666, 1995

144. Hiestand DM, Haley BE, Kindy MS: Role of calcium in inactivation of calcium/calmodulin dependent protein kinase II after cerebral ischemia. J Neurol Sci 113:31, 1992

145. Hill IE, MacManus JP, Rasquinha I, Tuor UI: DNA fragmentation indicative of apoptosis following unilateral cerebral hypoxia-ischemia in the neonatal rat. Brain Res 676:398, 1995

146. Hollmann M, Hartley M, Heinemann S: Ca^{2+} permeability of KA-AMPA–gated glutamate receptor channels depends on subunit composition. Science 252:851, 1991

147. Hollmann M, Heinemann S: Cloned glutamate receptors. Annu Rev Neurosci 17:31, 1994

148. Holtzman DM, Sheldon RA, Jaffe W et al: Nerve growth factor protects the neonatal brain against hypoxic-ischemic injury. Ann Neurol 39:114, 1996

149. Hong SC, Lanzino G, Goto Y et al: Calcium-activated proteolysis in rat neocortex induced by transient focal ischemia. Brain Res 661:43, 1994

150. Honing S, Kreimer G, Robenek H, Jockusch BM: Receptor-mediated endocytosis is sensitive to antibodies against the uncoating ATPase (hsc70). J Cell Sci 107:1185, 1994

151. Honkaniemi J, Massa SM, Sharp FR: Global ischemia induces apoptosis associated genes in gerbil hippocampus. Brain Res Mol Brain Res 42:79, 1996

152. Honkaniemi J, Sagar SM, Pyykonen I et al: Focal brain injury induces multiple immediate early genes encoding zinc finger transcription factors. Brain Res Mol Brain Res 28:157, 1995

153. Honkaniemi J, Sharp FR: Global ischemia induces immediate-early genes encoding zinc finger transcription factors. Cereb Blood Flow Metab 16:557, 1996

154. Hossmann KA: Disturbances of cerebral protein synthesis and ischemic cell death. Prog Brain Res 96:161, 1993

155. Hossmann KA: Glutamate-mediated injury in focal cerebral ischemia: the excitotoxin hypothesis revised. Brain Pathol 4:23, 1994

156. Hossmann KA: Viability thresholds and the penumbra of focal ischemia [see comments]. Ann Neurol 36:557, 1994

157. Hsu CY, An G, Liu JS, Xue JJ et al: Expression of immediate early gene and growth factor mRNAs in a focal cerebral ischemia model in the rat. Stroke 24:178, 1993

158. Huang Z, Huang PL, Panahian N et al: Effects of cerebral ischemia in mice deficient in neuronal nitric oxide synthase. Science 265:1883, 1994

159. Iadecola C, Pelligrino DA, Moskowitz MA, Lassen NA: Nitric oxide synthase inhibition and cerebrovascular regulation. J Cereb Blood Flow Metab 14:175, 1994

160. Iadecola C, Zhang F, Xu S et al: Inducible nitric oxide synthase gene expression in brain following cerebral ischemia. J Cereb Blood Flow Metab 15:378, 1995

161. Iadecola C, Zhang F, Xu X: Inhibition of inducible nitric oxide synthase ameliorates cerebral ischemic damage. Am J Physiol 268:R286, 1995

162. Ikeda J, Nakajima T, Osborne OC et al: Coexpression of c-fos and hsp 70 mRNAs in gerbil brain after ischemia: induction threshold, distribution and time course evaluated by in situ hybridization. Brain Res Mol Brain Res 26:249, 1994

163. Imaizumi S, Woolworth V, Fishman RA, Chan PH: Liposome-entrapped superoxide dismutase reduces cerebral infarction in cerebral ischemia in rats. Stroke 21:1312, 1990

164. Inamura K, Olsson Y, Siesjo BK: Substantia nigra damage induced by ischemia in hyperglycemic rats. A light and electron microscopic study. Acta Neuropathol (Berl) 75:131, 1987

165. Ishii H, Stanimirovic DB, Chang CJ et al: Dopamine metabolism and free-radical related mitochondrial injury during transient brain ischemia in gerbils. Neurochem Res 18:1193, 1993

166. Islam N, Aftabuddin M, Moriwaki A, Hori Y: Detection of DNA damage induced by apoptosis in the rat brain following incomplete ischemia. Neurosci Lett 188:159, 1995

167. Ito U, Spatz M, Walker JT Jr, Klatzo I: Experimental cerebral ischemia in mongolian gerbils. I. Light microscopic observations. Acta Neuropathol (Berl) 32:209, 1975

168. Jacewicz M, Brint S, Tanabe J, Pulsinelli WA: Continuous nimodipine treatment attenuates cortical infarction in rats subjected to 24 hours of focal cerebral ischemia. J Cereb Blood Flow Metab 10:89, 1990

169. Johansen FF, Diemer NH: Enhancement of GABA neurotransmission after cerebral ischemia in the rat reduces loss of hippocampal CA1 pyramidal cells. Acta Neurol Scand 84:1, 1991

170. Johanson FF, Zimmer J, Diemer NH: Early loss of somatostatin neurons in dentate hilus after cerebral ischemia in the rat precedes CA-1 pyramidal cell loss. Acta Neuropathol (Berl) 73:110, 1987

171. Johnson EJ, Greenlund LJ, Akins PT, Hsu CY: Neuronal

apoptosis: current understanding of molecular mechanisms and potential role in ischemic brain injury. J Neurotrauma 12:843, 1995

172. Jorgensen MB: The role of signal transduction in the delayed necrosis of the hippocampal CA1 pyramidal cells following transient ischemia. Acta Neurol Scand Suppl 143:1, 1993

173. Kamii H, Kinouchi H, Sharp FR et al: Expression of c-fos mRNA after a mild focal cerebral ischemia in SOD-1 transgenic mice. Brain Res 662:240, 1994

174. Kanai Y, Araki T, Kato H, Kogure K: Effect of pentobarbital on postischemic MK-801, muscimol, and naloxone bindings in the gerbil brain. Brain Res 657:51, 1994

175. Kanemitsu H, Kirino T, Nakagomi T et al: Key of induced tolerance to ischaemia in gerbil hippocampal CA1 is not at transcriptional level of hsp70 gene: in situ hybridization of hsp70 mRNA. Neurol Res 16:209, 1994

176. Kanner BI: Glutamate transporters from brain. A novel neurotransmitter transporter family. FEBS Lett 325:95, 1993

177. Kato H, Araki T, Itoyama Y et al: An immunohistochemical study of heat shock protein-27 in the hippocampus in a gerbil model of cerebral ischemia and ischemic tolerance. Neuroscience 68:65, 1995

178. Kato H, Araki T, Kogure K: Repeated focal cerebral ischemia in gerbils is associated with development of infarction. Brain Res 596:315, 1992

179. Kato H, Kogure K, Araki T, Itoyama Y: Astroglial and microglial reactions in the gerbil hippocampus with induced ischemic tolerance. Brain Res 664:69, 1994

180. Kato H, Liu XH, Nakata N, Kogure K: Immunohistochemical visualization of heat shock protein-70 in the gerbil hippocampus following repeated brief cerebral ischemia. Brain Res 615:240, 1993

181. Kato H, Liu Y, Araki T, Kogure K: MK-801, but not anisomycin, inhibits the induction of tolerance to ischemia in the gerbil hippocampus. Neurosci Lett 139:118, 1992

182. Katsura K, Kristian T, Smith ML, Siesjo BK: Acidosis induced by hypercapnia exaggerates ischemic brain damage. J Cereb Blood Flow Metab 14:243, 1994

183. Kawagoe J, Abe K, Kogure K: Regional difference of HSP70 and HSC70 heat shock mRNA inductions in rat hippocampus after transient global ischemia. Neurosci Lett 153:165, 1993

184. Kerr JF, Wyllie AH, Currie AR: Apoptosis: a basic biological phenomenon with wide-ranging implications in tissue kinetics. Br J Cancer 26:239, 1972

185. Kiessling M, Stumm G, Xie Y et al: Differential transcription and translation of immediate early genes in the gerbil hippocampus after transient global ischemia. J Cereb Blood Flow Metab 13:914, 1993

186. Kim H, Koehler RC, Hurn PD et al: Amelioration of impaired cerebral metabolism after severe acidotic ischemia by tirilazad posttreatment in dogs. Stroke 27:114, 1996

187. Kimelberg HK, Goderie SK, Higman S et al: Swelling-induced release of glutamate, aspartate, and taurine from astrocyte cultures. J Neurosci 10:1583, 1990

188. Kinouchi H, Sharp FR, Chan PH et al: Induction of c-fos, junB, c-jun, and hsp70 mRNA in cortex, thalamus, basal ganglia, and hippocampus following middle cerebral artery occlusion. J Cereb Blood Flow Metab 14:808, 1994

189. Kinouchi H, Sharp FR, Chan PH et al: Induction of NGFI-A mRNA following middle cerebral artery occlusion in rats: in situ hybridization study. Neurosci Lett 171:163, 1994

190. Kinouchi H, Sharp FR, Chan PH et al: MK-801 inhibits the induction of immediate early genes in cerebral cortex, thalamus, and hippocampus, but not in substantia nigra following middle cerebral artery occlusion. Neurosci Lett 179:111, 1994

191. Kinouchi H, Sharp FR, Hill MP et al: Induction of 70-kDa heat shock protein and hsp70 mRNA following transient focal cerebral ischemia in the rat. J Cereb Blood Flow Metab 13:105, 1993

192. Kinouchi H, Sharp FR, Koistinaho J et al: Induction of heat shock hsp70 mRNA and HSP70 kDa protein in neurons in the 'penumbra' following focal cerebral ischemia in the rat. Brain Res 619:334, 1993

193. Kirino T: Delayed neuronal death in the gerbil hippocampus following ischemia. Brain Res 239:57, 1982

194. Kirino T, Sano K: Selective vulnerability in the gerbil hippocampus following transient ischemia. Acta Neuropathol (Berl) 62:201, 1984

195. Kirino T, Tsujita Y, Tamura A: Induced tolerance to ischemia in gerbil hippocampal neurons. J Cereb Blood Flow Metab 11:299, 1991

196. Kirsch JR, Helfaer MA, Lange DG, Traystman RJ: Evidence for free radical mechanisms of brain injury resulting from ischemia/reperfusion-induced events. J Neurotrauma, suppl. 1:S157, 1992

197. Kitagawa K, Matsumoto M, Kuwabara K et al: 'Ischemic tolerance' phenomenon detected in various brain regions. Brain Res 561:203, 1991

198. Kitagawa K, Matsumoto M, Tagaya M et al: 'Ischemic tolerance' phenomenon found in the brain. Brain Res 528:21, 1990

199. Kiwak KJ, Moskowitz MA, Levine L: Leukotriene production in gerbil brain after ischemic insult, subarachnoid hemorrhage, and concussive injury. J Neurosurg 62:865, 1985

200. Kiyota Y, Pahlmark K, Memezawa H et al: Free radicals and brain damage due to transient middle cerebral artery occlusion: the effect of dimethylthiourea. Exp Brain Res 95:388, 1993

201. Kiyota Y, Takami K, Iwane M et al: Increase in basic fibroblast growth factor-like immunoreactivity in rat brain after forebrain ischemia. Brain Res 545:322, 1991

202. Kleihues P, Hossmann KA: Protein synthesis in the cat brain after prolonged cerebral ischemia. Brain Res 35:409, 1971

203. Klempt M, Klempt ND, Gluckman PD: Hypoxia and hypoxia/ischemia affect the expression of insulin-like growth factor binding protein 2 in the developing rat brain. Brain Res Mol Brain Res 17:347, 1993

204. Knollema S, Aukema W, Hom H et al: L-deprenyl reduces brain damage in rats exposed to transient hypoxia-ischemia. Stroke 26:1883, 1995

205. Kobayashi S, Harris VA, Welsh FA: Spreading depres-

sion induces tolerance of cortical neurons to ischemia in rat brain. J Cereb Blood Flow Metab 15:721, 1995

206. Kobayashi S, Welsh FA: Regional alterations of ATP and heat-shock protein-72 mRNA following hypoxia-ischemia in neonatal rat brain. J Cereb Blood Flow Metab 15:1047, 1995

207. Kokaia Z, Metsis M, Kokaia M et al: Brain insults in rats induce increased expression of the BDNF gene through differential use of multiple promoters. Eur J Neurosci 6:587, 1994

208. Koketsu N, Berlove DJ, Moskowitz MA et al: Pretreatment with intraventricular basic fibroblast growth factor decreases infarct size following focal cerebral ischemia in rats. Ann Neurol 35:451, 1994

209. Kontos HA, Wei EP, Povlishock JT et al: Cerebral arteriolar damage by arachidonic acid and prostaglandin G2. Science 209:1242, 1980

210. Kraig RP, Chesler M: Astrocytic acidosis in hyperglycemic and complete ischemia. J Cereb Blood Flow Metab 10:104, 1990

211. Kraig RP, Dong LM, Thisted R, Jaeger CB: Spreading depression increases immunohistochemical staining of glial fibrillary acidic protein. J Neurosci 11:2187, 1991

212. Kraig RP, Petito CK, Plum F, Pulsinelli WA: Hydrogen ions kill brain at concentrations reached in ischemia. J Cereb Blood Flow Metab 7:379, 1987

213. Kraig RP, Pulsinelli WA, Plum F: Hydrogen ion buffering during complete brain ischemia. Brain Res 342:281, 1985

214. Krajewski S, Mai JK, Krajewska M et al: Upregulation of bax protein levels in neurons following cerebral ischemia. J Neurosci 15:6364, 1995

215. Krause GS, Tiffany BR: Suppression of protein synthesis in the reperfused brain. Stroke 24:747, 1993

216. Kumar S: Inhibition of apoptosis by the expression of antisense Nedd2. Febs Lett 368:69, 1995

217. Kunievsky B, Bazan NG, Yavin E: Generation of arachidonic acid and diacylglycerol second messengers from polyphosphoinositides in ischemic fetal brain. J Neurochem 59:1812, 1992

218. Kuroiwa T, Bonnekoh P, Hossmann KA: Prevention of postischemic hyperthermia prevents ischemic injury of CA1 neurons in gerbils. J Cereb Blood Flow Metab 10:550, 1990

219. Lee WH, Bondy C: Insulin-like growth factors and cerebral ischemia. Ann NY Acad Sci 679:418, 1993

220. Lee WH, Bondy CA: Ischemic injury induces brain glucose transporter gene expression. Endocrinology 133:2540, 1993

221. Lees GJ: The possible contribution of microglia and macrophages to delayed neuronal death after ischemia. J Neurol Sci 114:119, 1993

222. Li PA, Shamloo M, Smith ML et al: The influence of plasma glucose concentrations on ischemic brain damage is a threshold function. Neurosci Lett 177:63, 1994

223. Li Y, Chopp M, Zhang ZG et al: p53-immunoreactive protein and p53 mRNA expression after transient middle cerebral artery occlusion in rats. Stroke 25:849, 1994

224. Li Y, Sharov VG, Jiang N et al: Ultrastructural and light microscopic evidence of apoptosis after middle cerebral artery occlusion in the rat. Am J Pathol 146:1045, 1995

225. Lin BW, Dietrich WD, Busto R, Ginsberg MD: (S)-emopamil protects against global ischemic brain injury in rats. Stroke 21:1734, 1990

226. Lin TA, Zhang JP, Sun GY: Metabolism of inositol, 1,4,5-trisphosphate in mouse brain due to decapitation ischemic insult: effects of acute lithium administration and temporal relationship to diacylglycerols, free fatty acids and energy metabolites. Brain Res 606:200, 1993

227. Lindquist S: Heat-shock proteins and stress tolerance in microorganisms. Curr Opin Genet Dev 2:748, 1992

228. Lindvall O, Ernfors P, Bengzon J et al: Differential regulation of mRNAs for nerve growth factor, brain-derived neurotrophic factor, and neurotrophin 3 in the adult rat brain following cerebral ischemia and hypoglycemic coma. Proc Natl Acad Sci USA 89:648, 1992

229. Linnik MD, Zahos P, Geschwind MD, Federoff HJ: Expression of bcl-2 from a defective herpes simplex virus-1 vector limits neuronal death in focal cerebral ischemia Stroke 26:1670, 1995

230. Linnik MD, Zobrist RH, Hatfield MD: Evidence supporting a role for programmed cell death in focal cerebral ischemia in rats. Stroke 24:2002, 1993

231. Lipton SA, Singel DJ, Stamler JS: Nitric oxide in the central nervous system. Prog Brain Res 103:359, 1994

232. Liu HM: Correlation between proto-oncogene, fibroblast growth factor and adaptive response in brain infarct. Prog Brain Res 105:239, 1995

233. Liu HM, Chen HH: c-fos protein expression and ischemic changes in neurons vulnerable to ischemia/hypoxia, correlated with basic fibroblast growth factor immunoreactivity. J Neuropathol Exp Neurol 53:598, 1994

234. Liu Y, Kato H, Nakata N, Kogure K: Temporal profile of heat shock protein 70 synthesis in ischemic tolerance induced by preconditioning ischemia in rat hippocampus. Neuroscience 56:921, 1993

235. Longa EZ, Weinstein PR, Carlson S, Cummins R: Reversible middle cerebral artery occlusion without craniectomy in rats. Stroke 20:84, 1989

236. Longuemare MC, Hill MP, Swanson RA: Glycolysis can prevent non-synaptic excitatory amino acid release during hypoxia. Neuroreport 5:1789, 1994

237. Longuemare MC, Swanson RA: Excitatory amino acid release from astrocytes during energy failure by reversal of sodium-dependent uptake. J Neurosci Res 40:379, 1995

238. Lowenstein DH, Gwinn RP, Seren MS et al: Increased expression of mRNA encoding calbindin-D28K, the glucose-regulated proteins, or the 72 kDa heat-shock protein in three models of acute CNS injury. Brain Res Mol Brain Res 22:299, 1994

239. Lundgren J, Smith ML, Siesjo BK: Effects of dimethylthiourea on ischemic brain damage in hyperglycemic rats. J Neurol Sci 113:187, 1992

240. Lust WD, Assaf HM, Ricci AJ et al: A role for gamma-aminobutyric acid (GABA) in the evolution of delayed neuronal death following ischemia. Metab Brain Dis 3:287, 1988

241. Lyden P, Lonzo L, Nunez S: Combination chemotherapy extends the therapeutic window to 60 minutes after stroke. J Neurotrauma 12:223, 1995

242. MacManus JP, Buchan AM, Hill IE et al: Global is-

chemia can cause DNA fragmentation indicative of apoptosis in rat brain. Neurosci Lett 164:89, 1993

243. MacManus JP, Hill IE, Huang ZG et al: DNA damage consistent with apoptosis in transient focal ischaemic neocortex. Neuroreport 5:493, 1994

244. MacManus JP, Hill IE, Preston E et al: Differences in DNA fragmentation following transient cerebral or decapitation ischemia in rats. J Cereb Blood Flow Metab 15:728, 1995

245. MacMillan VH: Cerebral energy metabolism in cyanide encephalopathy. J Cereb Blood Flow Metab 9:156, 1989

246. Madden KP: Effect of gamma-aminobutyric acid modulation on neuronal ischemia in rabbits. Stroke 25:2271, 1994

247. Maines MD, Eke BC, Weber CM, Ewing JF: Corticosterone has a permissive effect on expression of heme oxygenase-1 in CA1-CA3 neurons of hippocampus in thermal-stressed rats. J Neurochem 64:1769, 1995

248. Makar TK, Nedergaard M, Preuss A et al: Vitamin E, ascorbate, glutathione, glutathione disulfide, and enzymes of glutathione metabolism in cultures of chick astrocytes and neurons: evidence that astrocytes play an important role in antioxidative processes in the brain. J Neurochem 62:45, 1994

249. Manzerra P, Rush SJ, Brown IR: Temporal and spatial distribution of heat shock mRNA and protein (hsp70) in the rabbit cerebellum in response to hyperthermia. J Neurosci Res 36:480, 1993

250. Marcoux FW, Morawetz RB, Crowell RM et al: Differential regional vulnerability in transient focal cerebral ischemia. Stroke 13:339, 1982

251. Margaill I, Parmentier S, Callebert J et al: Short therapeutic window for MK-801 in transient focal cerebral ischemia in normotensive rats. J Cereb Blood Flow Metab 16:107, 1996

252. Martinou JC, Dubois-Dauphin M, Staple JK et al: Overexpression of BCL-2 in transgenic mice protects neurons from naturally occurring cell death and experimental ischemia. Neuron 13:1017, 1994

253. Massa SM, Longo FM, Zuo J et al: Cloning of rat grp75, an hsp70-family member, and its expression in normal and ischemic brain. J Neurosci Res 40:807, 1995

254. Massa SM, Swanson RA, Sharp FR: The stress gene response in brain. Cerebrovasc Brain Metab Rev 8:95, 1996

255. Matsuo Y, Kihara T, Ikeda M et al: Role of neutrophils in radical production during ischemia and reperfusion of the rat brain: effect of neutrophil depletion on extracellular ascorbyl radical formation. J Cereb Blood Flow Metab 15:941, 1995

256. Matsuo Y, Onodera H, Shiga Y et al: Role of cell adhesion molecules in brain injury after transient middle cerebral artery occlusion in the rat. Brain Res 656:344, 1994

257. Mattson MP, Cheng B, Smith-Swintosky VL: Mechanisms of neurotrophic factor protection against calcium- and free radical-mediated excitotoxic injury: implications for treating neurodegenerative disorders. Exp Neurol 124:89, 1993

258. Mattson MP, Scheff SW: Endogenous neuroprotection factors and traumatic brain injury: mechanisms of action and implications for therapy. J Neurotrauma 11:3, 1994

259. Mehmet H, Yue X, Squier MV et al: Increased apoptosis in the cingulate sulcus of newborn piglets following transient hypoxia-ischaemia is related to the degree of high energy phosphate depletion during the insult. Neurosci Lett 181:121, 1994

260. Mies G, Ishimaru S, Xie Y et al: Ischemic thresholds of cerebral protein synthesis and energy state following middle cerebral artery occlusion in rat. J Cereb Blood Flow Metab 11:753, 1991

261. Miller S, Kesslak JP, Romano C, Cotman CW: Roles of metabotropic glutamate receptors in brain plasticity and pathology. Ann NY Acad Sci 757:460, 1995

262. Minamisawa H, Smith ML, Siesjo BK: The effect of mild hyperthermia and hypothermia on brain damage following 5, 10, and 15 minutes of forebrain ischemia. Ann Neurol 28:26, 1990

263. Mizzen LA, Chang C, Garrels JI, Welch WJ: Identification, characterization, and purification of two mammalian stress proteins present in mitochondria, grp 75, a member of the hsp 70 family and hsp 58, a homolog of the bacterial groEL protein. J Biol Chem 264:20664, 1989

264. Moller A, Christophersen P, Drejer J et al: Pharmacological profile and anti-ischemic properties of the Ca(2+)-channel blocker NS-638. Neurol Res 17:353, 1995

265. Morgan JI, Curran T: Immediate-early genes: ten years on. Trends Neurosci 18:66, 1995

266. Morikawa E, Zhang SM, Seko Y et al: Treatment of focal cerebral ischemia with synthetic oligopeptide corresponding to lectin domain of selectin. Stroke 27:951, 1996

267. Morimoto RI: Cells in stress: transcriptional activation of heat shock genes. Science 259:1409, 1993

268. Murphy S, Simmons ML, Agullo L et al: Synthesis of nitric oxide in CNS glial cells [see comments]. Trends Neurosci 16:323, 1993

269. Nagafuji T, Sugiyama M, Matsui T: Temporal profiles of Ca^{2+}/calmodulin-dependent and -independent nitric oxide synthase activity in the rat brain microvessels following cerebral ischemia. Acta Neurochir Suppl (Wien) 60:285, 1994

270. Nagasawa H, Araki T, Kogure K: Alteration of adenosine A1 receptor binding in the post-ischaemic rat brain. Neuroreport 5:1453, 1994

271. Nakagomi T, Sasaki T, Kirino T et al: Effect of cyclooxygenase and lipoxygenase inhibitors on delayed neuronal death in the gerbil hippocampus. Stroke 20:925, 1989

272. Nakata N, Kato H, Kogure K: Inhibition of ischaemic tolerance in the gerbil hippocampus by quercetin and anti-heat shock protein-70 antibody. Neuroreport 4:695, 1993

273. Nedergaard M: Transient focal ischemia in hyperglycemic rats is associated with increased cerebral infarction. Brain Res 408:79, 1987

274. Nedergaard M, Goldman SA, Desai S, Pulsinelli WA: Acid-induced death in neurons and glia. J Neurosci 11:2489, 1991

275. Nedergaard M, Hansen AJ: Characterization of cortical depolarizations evoked in focal cerebral ischemia. J Cereb Blood Flow Metab 13:568, 1993

276. Nedergaard M, Hansen AJ: Spreading depression is not

associated with neuronal injury in the normal brain. Brain Res 449:395, 1988

277. Nedergaard M, Jakobsen J, Diemer NH: Autoradiographic determination of cerebral glucose content, blood flow, and glucose utilization in focal ischemia of the rat brain: influence of the plasma glucose concentration. J Cereb Blood Flow Metab 8:100, 1988

278. Neumar RW, Hagle SM, DeGracia DJ et al: Brain mu-calpain autolysis during global cerebral ischemia. J Neurochem 66:421, 1996

279. Nimura T, Massa SM, Panter S et al: Heme oxygenase-1 (HO-1) protein induction in rat brain following focal ischemia. Brain Res Mol Brain Res 37:201, 1996

280. Nishi S, Taki W, Uemura Y et al: Ischemic tolerance due to the induction of HSP70 in a rat ischemic recirculation model. Brain Res 615:281, 1993

281. Nitatori T, Sato N, Waguri S et al: Delayed neuronal death in the CA1 pyramidal cell layer of the gerbil hippocampus following transient ischemia is apoptosis. J Neurosci 15:1001, 1995

282. Nowak TS Jr: Localization of 70 kDa stress protein mRNA induction in gerbil brain after ischemia. J Cereb Blood Flow Metab 11:432, 1991

283. Nowak TS Jr: Protein synthesis and the heart shock/stress response after ischemia. Cerebrovasc Brain Metab Rev 2:345, 1990

284. Nowak TS Jr: Synthesis of heat shock/stress proteins during cellular injury. Ann NY Acad Sci 679:142, 1993

285. Nowak TS Jr, Fried RL, Lust WD, Passonneau JV: Changes in brain energy metabolism and protein synthesis following transient bilateral ischemia in the gerbil. J Neurochem 44:487, 1985

286. Nowak TS Jr, Jacewicz M: The heat shock/stress response in focal cerebral ischemia. Brain Pathol 4:67, 1994

287. Nowak TS Jr, Osborne OC, Suga S: Stress protein and proto-oncogene expression as indicators of neuronal pathophysiology after ischemia. Prog Brain Res 96:195, 1993

288. Nozaki K, Finklestein SP, Beal MF: Basic fibroblast growth factor protects against hypoxia-ischemia and NMDA neurotoxicity in neonatal rats. J Cereb Blood Flow Metab 13:221, 1993

289. Ohno M, Yamamoto T, Ueki S, Watanabe S: Protection by N-methyl-D-aspartate receptor antagonists against impairment of working memory in rats following transient cerebral ischemia. Neurosci Lett 138:1, 1992

290. Ohta S, Smith ML, Siesjo BK: The effect of a dihydropyridine calcium antagonist (isradipine) on selective neuronal necrosis. J Neurol Sci 103:109, 1991

291. Ohtsuki T, Matsumoto M, Hayashi Y et al: Reperfusion induces 5-lipoxygenase translocation and leukotriene C4 production in ischemic brain. Am J Physiol 268:H1249, 1995

292. Okada Y, Copeland BR, Mori E et al: P-selectin and intercellular adhesion molecule-1 expression after focal brain ischemia and reperfusion. Stroke 25:202, 1994

293. Olney JW: Excitatory transmitter neurotoxicity. Neurobiol Aging 15:259, 1994

294. Onodera H, Yamasaki Y, Kogure K, Miyamoto E: Calcium/calmodulin-dependent protein kinase II and protein phosphatase 2B (calcineurin) immunoreactivity in the rat hippocampus long after ischemia. Brain Res 684:95, 1995

295. Pahlmark K, Folbergrova J, Smith ML, Siesjo BK: Effects of dimethylthiourea on selective neuronal vulnerability in forebrain ischemia in rats. Stroke 24:731, 1993

296. Park CK, Nehls DG, Graham DI et al: The glutamate antagonist MK-801 reduces focal ischemic brain damage in the rat. Ann Neurol 24:543, 1988

297. Parkinson FE, Rudolphi KA, Fredholm BB: Propentofylline: a nucleoside transport inhibitor with neuroprotective effects in cerebral ischemia. Gen Pharmacol 25:1053, 1994

298. Paschen W, Uto A, Djuricic B, Schmitt J: Hemeoxygenase expression after reversible ischemia of rat brain. Neurosci Lett 180:5, 1994

299. Pellegrini-Giampietro DE, Pulsinelli WA, Zukin RS: NMDA and non-NMDA receptor gene expression following global brain ischemia in rats: effect of NMDA and non-NMDA receptor antagonists. J Neurochem 62:1067, 1994

300. Pellegrini-Giampietro DE, Zukin RS, Bennett MV et al: Switch in glutamate receptor subunit gene expression in CA1 subfield of hippocampus following global ischemia in rats [published erratum appears in Proc Natl Acad Sci USA 90:780, 1993]. Proc Natl Acad Sci USA 89:10499, 1992

301. Perez-Pinzon MA, Tao L, Nicholson C: Extracellular potassium, volume fraction, and tortuosity in rat hippocampal CA1, CA3, and cortical slices during ischemia. J Neurophysiol 74:565, 1995

302. Phillis JW: CI-966, a GABA uptake inhibitor, antagonizes ischemia-induced neuronal degeneration in the gerbil. Gen Pharmacol 26:1061, 1995

303. Phillis JW, Smith-Barbour M, Perkins LM, O'Regan MH: Characterization of glutamate, aspartate, and GABA release from ischemic rat cerebral cortex. Brain Res Bull 34:457, 1994

304. Plum F: What causes infarction in ischemic brain?: The Robert Wartenberg Lecture. Neurology 33:222, 1983

305. Powers WJ: Cerebral hemodynamics in ischemic cerebrovascular disease. Ann Neurol 29:231, 1991

306. Powers WJ, Grubb RL Jr, Raichle ME: Physiological responses to focal cerebral ischemia in humans. Ann Neurol 16:546, 1984

307. Prado R, Ginsberg MD, Dietrich WD et al: Hyperglycemia increases infarct size in collaterally perfused but not end-arterial vascular territories. J Cereb Blood Flow Metab 8:186, 1988

308. Prehn JH, Backhauss C, Krieglstein J: Transforming growth factor-beta 1 prevents glutamate neurotoxicity in rat neocortical cultures and protects mouse neocortex from ischemic injury in vivo. J Cereb Blood Flow Metab 13:521, 1993

309. Prehn JH, Karkoutly C, Nuglisch J et al: Dihydrolipoate reduces neuronal injury after cerebral ischemia. J Cereb Blood Flow Metab 12:78, 1992

310. Pulsinelli WA: Selective neuronal vulnerability: morphological and molecular characteristics. Prog Brain Res 63:29, 1985

311. Pulsinelli WA, Brierley JB, Plum F: Temporal profile

of neuronal damage in a model of transient forebrain ischemia. Ann Neurol 11:491, 1982

312. Pulsinelli WA, Buchan AM: The four-vessel occlusion rat model: method for complete occlusion of vertebral arteries and control of collateral circulation. Stroke 19: 913, 1988

313. Pulsinelli WA, Duffy TE: Regional energy balance in rat brain after transient forebrain ischemia. J Neurochem 40:1500, 1983

314. Pulsinelli WA, Waldman S, Rawlinson D, Plum F: Moderate hyperglycemia augments ischemic brain damage: a neuropathologic study in the rat. Neurology 32:1239, 1982

315. Rami A, Krieglstein J: Neuronal protective effects of calcium antagonists in cerebral ischemia. Life Sci 55:2105, 1994

316. Rami A, Krieglstein J: Protective effects of calpain inhibitors against neuronal damage caused by cytotoxic hypoxia in vitro and ischemia in vivo. Brain Res 609:67, 1993

317. Rehncrona S, Hauge HN, Siesjo BK: Enhancement of iron-catalyzed free radical formation by acidosis in brain homogenates: differences in effect by lactic acid and CO_2. J Cereb Blood Flow Metab 9:65, 1989

318. Relton JK, Martin D, Thompson RC, Russell DA: Peripheral administration of interleukin-1 receptor antagonist inhibits brain damage after focal cerebral ischemia in the rat. Exp Neurol 138:206, 1996

319. Roberts-Lewis JM, Savage MJ, Marcy VR et al: Immunolocalization of calpain I-mediated spectrin degradation to vulnerable neurons in the ischemic gerbil brain. J Neurosci 14:3934, 1994

320. Rocamora N, Massieu L, Boddeke HW et al: Neuronal death and neurotrophin gene expression: long-lasting stimulation of neurotrophin-3 messenger RNA in the degenerating CA1 and CA4 pyramidal cell layers. Neuroscience 53:905, 1993

321. Rod MR, Auer RN: Combination therapy with nimodipine and dizocilpine in a rat model of transient forebrain ischemia. Stroke 23:725, 1992

322. Rosenberg GA, Navratil M, Barone F, Feuerstein G: Proteolytic cascade enzymes increase in focal cerebral ischemia in rat. J Cereb Blood Flow Metab 16:360, 1996

323. Rothman SM, Olney JW: Glutamate and the pathophysiology of hypoxicischemic brain damage. Ann Neurol 19: 105, 1986

324. Rothstein JD, Martin L, Levey AI et al: Localization of neuronal and glial glutamate transporters. Neuron 13: 713, 1994

325. Sagar SM, Edwards RH, Sharp FR: Epidermal growth factor and transforming growth factor alpha induce c-fos gene expression in retinal Muller cells in vivo. J Neurosci Res 29:549, 1991

326. Sagar SM, Sharp FR, Curran T: Expression of c-fos protein in brain: metabolic mapping at the cellular level. Science 240:1328, 1988

327. Saji M, Cohen M, Blau AD et al: Transient forebrain ischemia induces delayed injury in the substantia nigra reticulata: degeneration of GABA neurons, compensatory expression of GAD mRNA. Brain Res 643:234, 1994

328. Saji M, Reis DJ: Delayed transneuronal death of substantia nigra neurons prevented by gamma-aminobutyric acid agonist. Science 235:66, 1987

329. Saji M, Volpe BT: Delayed histologic damage and neuron death in the substantia nigra reticulata following transient forebrain ischemia depends on the extent of initial striatal injury. Neurosci Lett 155:47, 1993

330. Sanchez-Olea R, Pena C, Moran J, Pasantes-Morales H: Inhibition of volume regulation and efflux of osmoregulatory amino acids by blockers of C1-transport in cultured astrocytes. Neurosci Lett 156:141, 1993

331. Sasaki K, Oomura Y, Suzuki K et al: Acidic fibroblast growth factor prevents death of hippocampal CA1 pyramidal cells following ischemia. Neurochem Int 21:397, 1992

332. Sasaki T, Nakagomi T, Kirino T et al: Indomethacin ameliorates ischemic neuronal damage in the gerbil hippocampal CA1 sector. Stroke 19:1399, 1988

333. Schollmeyer JE: Calpain II involvement in mitosis [see comments]. Science 240:911, 1988

334. Schwartz LM, Kosz L, Kay BK: Gene activation is required for developmentally programmed cell death. Proc Natl Acad Sci USA 87:6594, 1990

335. Shackelford DA, Yeh RY, Zivin JA: Inactivation and subcellular redistribution of Ca^{2+}/calmodulin-dependent protein kinase II following spinal cord ischemia. J Neurochem 61:738, 1993

336. Sharp FR, Butman M, Wang S et al: Haloperidol prevents induction of the hsp 70 heat shock gene in neurons injured by phencyclidine (PCP), MK801, and ketamine. J Neurosci Res 33:605, 1992

337. Sharp FR, Jasper P, Hall J et al: MK-801 and ketamine induce heat shock protein HSP72 in injured neurons in posterior cingulate and retrosplenial cortex. Ann Neurol 30:801, 1991

338. Sharp FR, Kinouchi H, Koistinaho J et al: HSP70 heat shock gene regulation during ischemia. Stroke 24:172, 1993

339. Sharp FR, Sagar SM, Swanson RA: Metabolic mapping with cellular resolution: c-fos vs. 2-deoxyglucose. Crit Rev Neurobiol 7:205, 1993

340. Sharp JW, Sagar SM, Hisanaga K et al: The NMDA receptor mediates cortical induction of fos and fos-related antigens following cortical injury. Exp Neurol 109: 323, 1990

341. Sheardown MJ, Nielsen EO, Hansen AJ et al: 2,3-Dihydroxy-6-nitro-7-sulfamoyl-benzo (F) quinoxaline: a neuroprotectant for cerebral ischemia. Science 247:571, 1990

342. Shigeno T, Mima T, Takakura K et al: Amelioration of delayed neuronal death in the hippocampus by nerve growth factor. J Neurosci 11:2914, 1991

343. Shigeno T, Yamasaki Y, Kato G et al: Reduction of delayed neuronal death by inhibition of protein synthesis. Neurosci Lett 120:117, 1990

344. Shiraishi K, Sharp FR, Simon RP: Sequential metabolic changes in rat brain following middle cerebral artery occlusion: a 2-deoxyglucose study. J Cereb Blood Flow Metab 9:765, 1989

345. Shuaib A, Mazagri R, Ijaz S: GABA agonist "muscimol" is neuroprotective in repetitive transient forebrain ischemia in gerbils. Exp Neurol 123:284, 1993

346. Siesjo BK: Acidosis and ischemic brain damage. Neurochem Pathol 9:31, 1988

347. Siesjo BK, Ekholm A, Katsura K, Theander S: Acid-base changes during complete brain ischemia. Stroke 21: III194, 1990

348. Siesjo BK, Katsura K, Zhao Q et al: Mechanisms of secondary brain damage in global and focal ischemia: a speculative synthesis. J Neurotrauma 12:943, 1995

349. Siesjo BK, Zhao Q, Pahlmark K et al: Glutamate, calcium, and free radicals as mediators of ischemic brain damage. Ann Thorac Surg 59:1316, 1995

350. Siman R, Gall C, Perlmutter LS et al: Distribution of calpain I, an enzyme associated with degenerative activity, in rat brain. Brain Res 347:399, 1985

351. Simon RP, Cho H, Gwinn R, Lowenstein DH: The temporal profile of 72-kDa heat-shock protein expression following global ischemia. J Neurosci 11:881, 1991

352. Simon RP, Niiro M, Gwinn R: Prior ischemic stress protects against experimental stroke. Neurosci Lett 163: 135, 1993

353. Simon RP, Niro M, Gwinn R: Brain acidosis induced by hypercarbic ventilation attenuates focal ischemic injury. J Pharmacol Exp Ther 267:1428, 1993

354. Smith ML, Auer RN, Siesjo BK: The density and distribution of ischemic brain injury in the rat following 2–10 min of forebrain ischemia. Acta Neuropathol (Berl) 64: 319, 1984

355. Sommer C, Gass P, Kiessling M: Selective c-JUN expression in CA1 neurons of the gerbil hippocampus during and after acquisition of an ischemia-tolerant state. Brain Pathol 5:135, 1995

356. Squire LR: Memory and the hippocampus: a synthesis from findings with rats, monkeys, and humans [published erratum appears in Psychol Rev 99:582, 1992]. Psychol Rev 99:195, 1992

357. Steller H, Abrams JM, Grether ME, White K: Programmed cell death in *Drosophila*. Philos Trans R Soc Lond [Biol] 345:247, 1994

358. Streit WJ: Microglial-neuronal interactions. J Chem Neuroanat 6:261, 1993

359. Sun D, Kintner D, Fitzpatric JH et al: The effect of a free radical scavenger and platelet-activating factor antagonist on FFA accumulation in post-ischemic canine brain. Neurochem Res 19:525, 1994

360. Swanson RA: Acidosis potentiates hypoxic death of astrocytes by blocking glycolysis. Blood Flow Metab 15:S266, 1995

361. Swanson RA: Physiologic coupling of glial glycogen metabolism to neuronal activity in brain. Can J Physiol Pharmacol, suppl. 70:S138, 1992

362. Swanson RA, Chen J, Graham SH: Glucose can fuel glutamate uptake in ischemic brain. J Cereb Blood Flow Metab 14:1, 1994

363. Swanson RA, Farrell K, Simon RP: Acidosis causes failure of astrocyte glutamate uptake during hypoxia. J Cereb Blood Flow Metab 15:417, 1995

364. Swanson RA, Graham SH: Fluorocitrate and fluoroacetate effects on astrocyte metabolism in vitro. Brain Res 664:94, 1994

365. Swanson RA, Sagar SM, Sharp FR: Regional brain glycogen stores and metabolism during complete global ischaemia. Neurol Res 11:24, 1989

366. Swanson RA, Shiraishi K, Morton MT, Sharp FR: Methionine sulfoximine reduces cortical infarct size in rats after middle cerebral artery occlusion. Stroke 21:322, 1990

367. Symon L: The relationship between CBF, evoked potentials and the clinical features in cerebral ischaemia. Acta Neurol Scand Suppl 78:175, 1980

368. Szatkowski M, Barbour B, Attwell D: Non-vesicular release of glutamate from glial cells by reversed electrogenic glutamate uptake. Nature 348:443, 1990

369. Takami K, Iwane M, Kiyota Y et al: Increase of basic fibroblast growth factor immunoreactivity and its mRNA level in rat brain following transient forebrain ischemia. Exp Brain Res 90:1, 1992

370. Takano K, Latour LL, Formato JE et al: The role of spreading depression in focal ischemia evaluated by diffusion mapping. Ann Neurol 39:308, 1996

371. Takeda A, Onodera H, Sugimoto A et al: Increased expression of heme oxygenase mRNA in rat brain following transient forebrain ischemia. Brain Res 666:120, 1994

372. Tamura A, Kirino T, Sano K et al: Atrophy of the ipsilateral substantia nigra following middle cerebral artery occlusion in the rat. Brain Res 510:154, 1990

373. Tamura A, Tahira Y, Nagashima H et al: Thalamic atrophy following cerebral infarction in the territory of the middle cerebral artery. Stroke 22:615, 1991

374. Thilmann R, Xie Y, Kleihues P, Kiessling M: Persistent inhibition of protein synthesis precedes delayed neuronal death in postischemic gerbil hippocampus. Acta Neuropathol (Berl) 71:88, 1986

375. Thornberry NA, Bull HG, Calaycay JR et al: A novel heterodimeric cysteine protease is required for interleukin-1 beta processing in monocytes. Nature 356:768, 1992

376. Tsubokawa H, Oguro K, Robinson HP et al: Abnormal Ca^{2+} homeostasis before cell death revealed by whole cell recording of ischemic CA1 hippocampal neurons. Neuroscience 49:807, 1992

377. Umemura A, Mabe H, Nagai H, Sugino F: Action of phospholipases A2 and C on free fatty acid release during complete ischemia in rat neocortex. Effect of phospholipase C inhibitor and N-methyl-D-aspartate antagonist. J Neurosurg 76:648, 1992

378. Vannucci RC, Mujsce DJ: Effect of glucose on perinatal hypoxic-ischemic brain damage. Biol Neonate 62: 215, 1992

379. Vannucci SJ, Seaman LB, Vannucci RC: Effects of hypoxia-ischemia on GLUT1 and GLUT3 glucose transporters in immature rat brain. J Cereb Blood Flow Metab 16:77, 1996

380. Vass K, Welch WJ, Nowak TS, Jr: Localization of 70-kDa stress protein induction in gerbil brain after ischemia. Acta Neuropathol (Berl) 77:128, 1988

381. Vaux DL, Cory S, Adams JM: Bcl-2 gene promotes haemopoietic cell survival and cooperates with c-myc to immortalize pre-B cells. Nature 335:440, 1988

382. Von Lubitz DK, Lin RC, Popik P et al: Adenosine A3

receptor stimulation and cerebral ischemia. Eur J Pharmacol 263:59, 1994

383. Wang S, Longo FM, Chen J et al: Induction of glucose regulated protein (grp78) and inducible heat shock protein (hsp70) mRNAs in rat brain after kainic acid seizures and focal ischemic. Neurochem Int 23:575, 1993

384. Wang X, Feuerstein GZ: Induced expression of adhesions molecules following focal brain ischemia. J Neurotrauma 12:825, 1995

385. Wang X, Yue TL, Barone FC et al: Concomitant cortical expression of TNF-alpha and IL-1 beta mRNAs follows early response gene expression in transient focal ischemia. Mol Chem Neuropathol 23:103, 1994

386. Warner MA, Nadler JV, Crain BJ: Effects of NMDA receptor antagonists and body temperature in the gerbil carotid occlusion model of transient forebrain ischemia. Prog Clin Biol Res 361:409, 1990

387. Welch WJ: Heat shock proteins functioning as molecular chaperones: their roles in normal and stressed cells. Philos Trans R Soc Lond [Biol] 339:327, 1993

388. Welsh FA: Regional expression of immediate-early genes and heat-shock genes after cerebral ischemia. Ann NY Acad Sci 723:318, 1994

389. Wen TC, Matsuda S, Yoshimura H et al: Ciliary neurotrophic factor prevents ischemia-induced learning disability and neuronal loss in gerbils. Neurosci Lett 191:55, 1995

390. Yamada K, Kinoshita A, Kohmura E et al: Basic fibroblast growth factor prevents thalamic degeneration after cortical infarction. J Cereb Blood Flow Metab 11:472, 1991

391. Yamada K, Teraoka T, Morita S et al: Omega-conotoxin GVIA protects against ischemia-induced neuronal death in the Mongolian gerbil but not against quinolinic acid-induced neurotoxicity in the rat. Neuropharmacology 33:251, 1994

392. Yamamoto S, Yoshimine T, Fujita T et al: Protective effect of NGF atelocollagen mini-pellet on the hippocampal delayed neuronal death in gerbils. Neurosci Lett 141:161, 1992

393. Yamasaki Y, Kogure K: Possible contribution of free radicals and lipid peroxidations on pathogenesis of post-ischemic brain damage. Hum Cell 5:341, 1992

394. Yamasaki Y, Shozuhara H, Onodera H, Kogure K: Blocking of interleukin-1 activity is a beneficial approach to ischemia brain edema formation. Acta Neurochir Suppl (Wien) 60:300, 1994

395. Yamashita A, Ozaki A, Ikegami A, et al: Effects of a new diphenylpiperazine calcium antagonist, KB-2796, on cerebral ischemic neuronal damage in rats. Gen Pharmacol 24:1473, 1993

396. Yokota M, Saido TC, Tani E et al: Three distinct phases of fodrin proteolysis induced in postischemic hippocampus. Involvement of calpain and unidentified protease. Stroke 26:1901, 1995

397. Yu AC, Chan PH, Fishman RA: Arachidonic acid inhibits uptake of glutamate and glutamine but not of GABA in cultured cerebellar granule cells. J Neurosci Res 17:424, 1987

398. Yu AC, Lee YL, Fu WY, Eng LF: Gene expression in astrocytes during and after ischemia. Prog Brain Res 105:245, 1995

399. Yuan J, Shaham S, Ledoux S et al: The C. elegans cell death gene ced-3 encodes a protein similar to mammalian interleukin-1 beta-converting enzyme. Cell 75:641, 1993

400. Yudkoff M, Nissim I, Daikhin Y et al: Brain glutamate metabolism: neuronal-astroglial relationships. Dev Neurosci 15:343, 1993

401. Yudkoff M, Pleasure D, Cregar L et al: Glutathione turnover in cultured astrocytes: studies with [^{15}N] glutamate. J Neurochem 55:137, 1990

402. Zhang F, Casey RM, Ross ME, Iadecola C: Aminoguanidine ameliorates and L-arginine worsens brain damage from intraluminal middle cerebral artery occlusion. Stroke 27:317, 1996

403. Zhang JP, Sun GY: Free fatty acids, neutral glycerides, and phosphoglycerides in transient focal cerebral ischemia. J Neurochem 64:1688, 1995

404. Zhang RL, Chopp M, Jiang N et al: Anti-intercellular adhesion molecule-1 antibody reduces ischemic cell damage after transient but not permanent middle cerebral artery occlusion in the Wistar rat. Stroke 26:1438, 1995

405. Zhang ZG, Chopp M, Maynard KI, Moskowitz MA: Cerebral blood flow changes during cortical spreading depression are not altered by inhibition of nitric oxide synthesis. J Cereb Blood Flow Metab 14:939, 1994

406. Zhang ZG, Chopp M, Zaloga C et al: Cerebral endothelial nitric oxide synthase expression after focal cerebral ischemia in rats. Stroke 24:2016, 1993

407. Zhao Q, Memezawa H, Smith ML, Siesjo BK: Hyperthermia complicates middle cerebral artery occlusion induced by an intraluminal filament. Brain Res 649:253, 1994

408. Zhao Q, Smith ML, Siesjo BK: The omega-conopeptide SNX-111, an N-type calcium channel blocker, dramatically ameliorates brain damage due to transient focal ischaemia. Acta Physiol Scand 150:459, 1994

409. Zola-Morgan S, Squire LR, Rempel NL et al: Enduring memory impairment in monkeys after ischemic damage to the hippocampus. J Neurosci 12:2582, 1992

410. Zuckerman SL, Mirro R, Armstead WM et al: Indomethacin reduces ischemia-induced alteration of blood-brain barrier transport in piglets. Am J Physiol 266:H2198, 1994

CHAPTER 5

Molecular Pathophysiology of White Matter Anoxic/Ischemic Injury

BRUCE R. RANSOM

STEPHEN G. WAXMAN

ROBERT FERN

Ischemia of the mammalian central nervous system (CNS), including the secondary vascular embarrassment that frequently accompanies traumatic brain and spinal cord insults,[89] damages both gray (GM) and white matter (WM). In fact, about 20% of ischemic strokes involve predominantly WM, as a result of occlusion of small penetrating arteries that supply the deep parenchymal areas of the cerebral hemispheres[21] (see Ch. 23, Lacunes). Clinically, damage to WM can result in serious disability, as seen in stroke, spinal cord and traumatic brain injury, and some forms of vascular dementia.[37,40]

The pathophysiology of anoxic injury is likely to be different in WM than in GM, since WM contains no neuronal cell bodies or synapses, but does contain myelinated axons that have a unique, highly specialized structure.[86] Axons respond differently to ischemia than either neurons or glial cells. Because axons can extend for great distances from their cell bodies of origin, they must depend on local production of adenosine triphosphate (ATP) to maintain ion gradients and sustain energy-consuming functions. This metabolic isolation also means that axons suffer energy deprivation in a manner that is independent of neuron cell bodies. The pathophysiology of WM damage can now be effectively studied at a molecular level; what we know about the sequence of cellular events that lead to irreversible CNS axon injury is reviewed here.

Isolated Rat Optic Nerve Model

The WM of the mammalian CNS consists of the afferent and efferent axonal tracts that interconnect neuron cell body-containing areas of the brain and spinal cord. WM consists exclusively of axons and glial cells and is devoid of synapses. Many axons in these tracts are myelinated, lending a white appearance to this tissue.

We have studied the pathophysiology of injury mediated by anoxia in CNS WM using the isolated rat optic nerve.[12,51] The optic nerve is not, in fact, a conventional nerve but a typical WM tract. Optic nerves from Long-Evans rats (50 to 70 days old) are dissected free and placed in a tissue slice chamber.[74] Optic nerves, consisting entirely of astrocytes, oligodendrocytes, and myelinated axons, have mature physiologic properties at this age.[11,23] Experiments are conducted at 37°C, and the nerves are perfused continuously with a physiologic saline containing 3 mM K^+ and 2 mM Ca^{2+}.[74] The tissue is oxygenated in a 95% O_2/5% CO_2 atmosphere, and anoxia is achieved by switching to a 95% N_2/5% CO_2 gas mixture (chamber O_2 tension falls to zero in about 2.5 minutes)[52]; combined zero-glucose/anoxia is produced by switching to a bath solution that contains no glucose at the same time as anoxia is induced.[49]

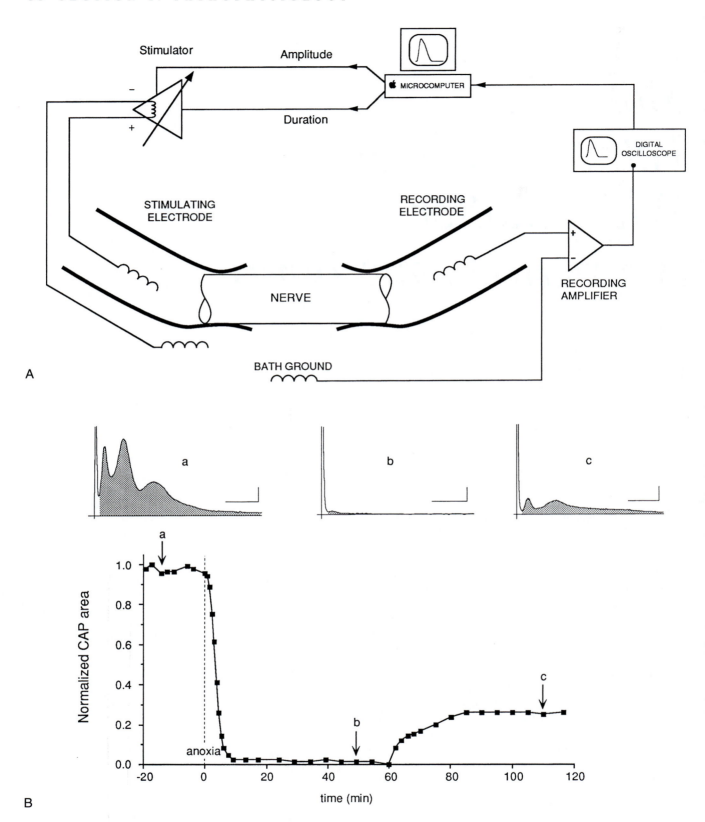

The effects of anoxia on optic nerve function are assessed by measuring the compound action potential (CAP), using quantitative electrophysiologic techniques. Stimulation and recording from optic nerves are accomplished using suction electrodes (Fig. 5.1A). The stimulus strength is set to 25% above the strength that elicits a maximum CAP. Area under the CAP is measured before and after experimental manipulations, using computer-assisted techniques[72] (Fig. 5.1A); CAP area is shown as percent of the control CAP integral. Activities of individual axons within a myelinated nerve bundle sum linearly to form the CAP[6] so that CAP area reflects the number of axons that are capable of conducting action potentials.[72] By monitoring the CAP in the optic nerve at various times before, during, and after anoxia or ischemia (i.e., combined zero glucose/anoxia), function in this WM tract can be quantitatively evaluated.

WM function, monitored as CAP area, is rapidly lost during anoxia (Fig. 5.1B) or ischemia. With anoxia, the CAP begins to decline within 2 to 3 minutes and virtually disappears after 8 to 10 minutes.[74] In most experiments we subjected the optic nerve to a standardized anoxic insult lasting for 60 minutes. During reoxygenation following anoxia, the CAP partially returns to a new stable level within 1 hour[12,74] (Fig. 5.1B). Thus, for quantitative studies we typically assessed the magnitude of CAP recovery at 60 minutes following anoxic exposure. The speed and magnitude of CAP recovery decrease as the duration of anoxia increases.[12] Following the standardized anoxic period of 60 minutes, the mean recovery of optic nerve CAP area is about 30%.[74]

Glucose deprivation in combination with anoxia is used to mimic ischemia. Optic nerve function is more rapidly lost under these conditions than with anoxia alone, and the degree of irreversible injury is greater.[18] The damaging sequence of ionic and molecular events that are set in motion by anoxia in WM[51] (see below) probably also occurs with anoxia plus zero glucose. This has not been explicitly proved, however.

The effects of pure glucose deprivation on optic nerve function and survival are of special interest.[18,49] The optic nerve operates normally for about 40 minutes in the absence of glucose (with oxyen maintained at normal levels[18]). Current evidence strongly suggests that during glucose withdrawal glycogen in optic nerve astrocytes breaks down to lactate, which then is transferred to axons, where it is used as fuel.[49] Astrocytes, therefore, may play a crucial role in protecting CNS axons from the disastrous consequences of energy failure associated with hypoglycemia.

Postnatal White Matter Sensitivity to Anoxia

Sensitivity to anoxia or ischemia develops postnatally in the rat between days 10 and 20.[12,18] The optic nerve is less susceptible to anoxic injury at earlier stages of development. Neonatal optic nerve axons have no myelin.[23,85] These premyelinated axons conduct action potentials, but with much slower conduction velocities than in the adult, as expected.[11,23] Conduction in these premyelinated axons is supported by very low densities ($2/\mu m^2$) of Na^+ channels. The CAP of the neonatal optic nerve, in contrast to the adult, is unchanged during anoxic exposure for periods as long as 90 minutes.[18,85] Susceptibility to anoxia-induced dysfunction and injury are acquired by the optic nerve with a time course similar to the proliferation of oligodendrocytes and development of myelination.[18] Interestingly, Na^+ channels (see below) cluster at nodes of Ranvier in the optic nerve with a similar time course.[82]

In the myelin-deficient (*md*) rat, myelination is absent due to an abnormality of oligodendrocytes.[14] We used this mutant to test the hypothesis that myelination contributes to the development of anoxic susceptibility in developing WM. The *md* optic nerve, like normal premyelinated optic nerve, is relatively insensitive to anoxia.[85] Excitability is lost within a few minutes of onset of anoxia in normals but is not lost entirely in *md* nerves even after 60 minutes. In addition, the *md* optic nerves show significantly greater CAP recovery after

Figure 5.1 Method of measuring rat optic nerve function before and after anoxia. (**A**) Diagram of recording arrangement. The rat optic nerve is stimulated with a supramaximal voltage pulse via one suction electrode. The CAP is recorded from the other end of the nerve with a second suction electrode; signals are amplified, digitized, and transferred to a microcomputer for processing and storage. (**B**) Effects of anoxia on WM function. The function of the optic nerve was monitored as the area under the CAP (a–c); this is shown graphically as percent of the control CAP integral. Anoxia was begun at time zero by switching from a 95% O_2 5% CO_2 to a 95% N_2 5% CO_2 atmosphere. CAP area rapidly declined, becoming virtually zero after 10 minutes of anoxia. (Residual area was mostly stimulus artifact.) A standard 60-minute period of anoxia was used in most experiments. After O_2 was reintroduced, the CAP area gradually recovered to a mean of about 30% of control in perfusate containing 2.0 mM $[Ca^{2+}]_o$. For quantification, postanoxic CAP measurements were routinely made 60 minutes after the end of anoxia since recovery always reached a plateau by this time. Specimen records of the CAP under control (a), anoxic (b), and postanoxic (c) conditions are shown. Calibration marks are 1 ms and 1 mV. (Modified from Stys et al.[74])

60 minutes of anoxia ($71 \pm 25\%$ of control CAP area versus $33 \pm 21\%$ in controls[85]). These findings support the idea that myelination, or changes associated with it, may be important in the development of anoxic susceptibility in WM.

Other changes occur postnatally in the rat brain that may be important for the development of sensitivity to oxygen or glucose deprivation, or both. For example, key enzymes of energy metabolism, such as hexokinase, pyruvate dehydrogenase, lactate dehydrogenase, and citrate synthetase show marked increases in activity 10 to 15 days postnatally,[4] suggesting, perhaps, a shift to greater dependency on aerobic energy production. In addition, antioxidant enzymes such as superoxide dismutase, catalase, glutathione peroxidase, and glutathione reductase show an increase in their activities in the brain during development.[42] Changes in these enzyme systems could logically be involved in the development of susceptibility to anoxic injury in WM.

Anoxia and Rapid Derangement of Transmembrane Ion Gradients

Rapid changes in brain extracellular ion concentrations occur with anoxia.[27] These changes reflect the metabolic state of local brain tissue[66,67] and can have direct effects on neural behavior. Elevated $[K^+]_o$ depolarizes neuronal membranes (reducing and then blocking action potentials), causes uncontrolled transmitter release,[2] reduces electrogenic glial uptake of neurotransmitters including the excitotoxin glutamate,[63] induces cell swelling,[30] and may affect cerebral blood flow.[45] Extracellular acidosis can have direct toxic effects on both neuronal and glial membranes,[25,33,70] may alter ion channel function,[7] and blocks currents generated by activation of *N*-methyl-D-aspartate (NMDA) receptors.[78] In the case of WM, the extracellular ionic changes produced by anoxia predispose to other ionic events that are critical for injury (see below).

In WM, anoxia causes rapid changes in the extracellular concentrations of K^+ and H^+ that are qualitatively similar to those seen in GM, but smaller[27,34,52] (Fig. 5.2A). Within 3 or 4 minutes of the onset of anoxia, $[K^+]_o$ in the optic nerve begins to increase and reaches a final concentration of 14.0 ± 2.9 mM. No spreading depression-like event occurs in WM during anoxia, in contrast to most GM areas,[27,68] and this partially explains why $[K^+]_o$ increases less in WM than in GM.[32,52]

An acid shift in pH_o develops during anoxia with a maximum value of 0.31 ± 0.07 pH unit in standard physiologic solution.[52] After anoxia, pH_o returns slowly to its baseline level and exhibits a secondary acidification phase of unknown significance. The acid shifts in pH_o seen in WM and GM during anoxia are probably the consequence of increased anaerobic metabolism, leading to accumulation of extracellular lactic acid.[31,34,66] Lactic acid can exit cells by diffusion, in its undisso-

ciated form, or by a direct transport mechanism.[81] *In vitro* studies suggest that during anoxia glial cells and neurons contain equivalent amounts of intracellular lactate, but that glial cells transport more lactic acid to the extracellular space (ECS).[81] Mammalian glial cells, but not neurons,[13] exhibit intracellular alkalinization with depolarization,[8,48] and this is also likely to cause extracellular acidification. Glia, therefore, may have an important role in producing the acid shift in pH_o seen with anoxia.[48]

As in GM,[34] the magnitude of the extracellular acid shift increases with higher levels of bath glucose concentration, and this is associated with smaller increases in $[K^+]_o$ and delayed loss of the CAP[52] (Fig. 5.2B). In the presence of 20 mM glucose, compared with 10 mM, there is more substrate for anaerobic metabolism and presumably greater generation of lactic acid and ATP. The higher levels of ATP would act to slow the deterioration of ion gradients during anoxia, accounting for the smaller increases in $[K^+]_o$ (Fig. 5.2B).

Although the rate of oxygen consumption is lower in WM than in GM,[43] in the absence of oxygen neither tissue appears able to meet its energy demands by anaerobic metabolism alone.[38,66] The decline of ATP causes energy-dependent ion pumps to fail, including the Na^+/K^+ and Ca^{2+}-ATPases, and this would affect both axons and glial cells (see below). As a consequence, ions redistribute down their concentration gradients, leading to membrane depolarization that activates voltage-dependent ion channels. Other K^+ channels may be activated and contribute to the increase on $[K^+]_o$, including Ca^{2+}-dependent K^+ channels, ATP-dependent K^+ channels, and Na^+-dependent K^+ channels.[26,27] Anoxia causes the volume of the ECS of the rat optic nerve to decrease by as much as 20%,[52] probably because of glial swelling triggered by increases in $[K^+]_o$.[30,55]

In WM, glial cells have been shown to contribute directly to anoxia-induced changes in extracellular ions, based on studies using optic nerves that (as a result of retinal ablation and resultant loss of axons) contain only glial cells.[50,54] In "glial" nerves, anoxia causes abrupt increases in $[K^+]_o$ and decreases in pH_o that develop and recover with time courses similar to those of the corresponding ionic changes seen in intact rat optic nerves.

GM appears to suffer more damage when anoxia/ischemia occurs in the presence of higher than usual glucose concentrations.[46] WM, on the other hand is functionally protected under these conditions,[52] even though the elevated bath glucose concentration causes a greater acid shift (Fig. 5.2B), which is believed to worsen outcome.[46,47] The protective effect of elevated bath glucose concentration is probably the simple consequence of greater amounts of ATP available for the maintenance of ion gradients (see above). Curiously, *in vitro* studies, in contrast to *in vivo* studies, indicate that GM and WM are both protected from anoxic injury by elevated glucose.[62] The worse outcome noted *in vivo*, after anoxic exposure in the presence of elevated glucose, could depend on vascular factors that have been largely removed in the *in vitro* situation. *In vivo*, a more pronounced acid shift associated with elevated glucose may worsen the functional recovery of the capillary or precapillary systems necessary for reperfusion.

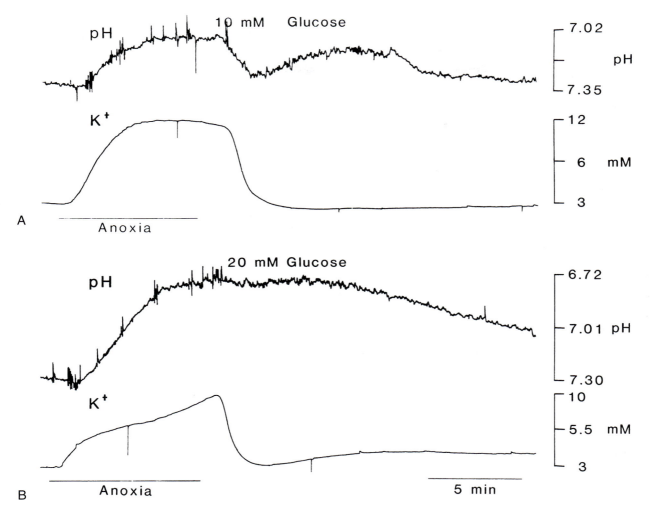

Figure 5.2 The effects of anoxia on pH_o and $[K^+]_o$ in the optic nerve. Separate ion-selective microelectrodes, placed within 100 μm of one another, were used to measure pH_o and $[K^+]_o$ in an adult rat optic nerve. Anoxia duration is indicated by the bar. (**A**) Reponses obtained while bathing the nerve in 10 mM glucose. (**B**) Reponses obtained while bathing in 20 mM glucose. The acid shift was much larger (average maximal acid shift, 0.58 ± 0.08 pH unit) in 20 mM glucose, and the rise in $[K^+]_o$ was slower and less extreme. Note the secondary acid shift that occurred during the recovery period following anoxia. The abrupt vertical deflections in the pH_o recordings are artifacts related to vapor condensation on the electrodes. (From Ransom et al,[52] with permission.)

Extracellular Ca^{2+} and Anoxic White Matter Injury

The calcium hypothesis holds that unregulated increases in intracellular $[Ca^{2+}]$ represent a final common pathway for cellular damage.[60,65] This appears to be true for WM damage due to anoxia.

To study this question we tested the effect of varying perfusate $[Ca^{2+}]$ concentrations on CAP recovery from the standard 60-minute period of anoxia (Fig. 5.3). Test solutions with different concentrations of Ca^{2+} are applied for a period extending from 10 minutes before the onset of anoxia to 10 minutes after the end of anoxia (Fig. 5.3B, inset). As the $[Ca^{2+}]$ of the test solution is decreased from 4 mM to zero, the degree of CAP recovery from anoxia gradually increases (Fig. 5.3B). Even a 50% reduction in $[Ca^{2+}]$ (i.e., from 2 to 1 mM) results in significant enhancement of CAP recovery. The CAP area recovers to 100% of control with zero $[Ca^{2+}]$ perfusate (Fig. 5.3A), indicating that axons are strongly protected from the injury associated with exposure to 60 minutes of anoxia by perfusion with zero $[Ca^{2+}]$. Some axons appeared to conduct more slowly, as evidenced by delays in the CAP peaks[74] (Fig. 5.3A). If the postanoxic nerves are permitted to recover for several more hours, the CAP area remains rela-

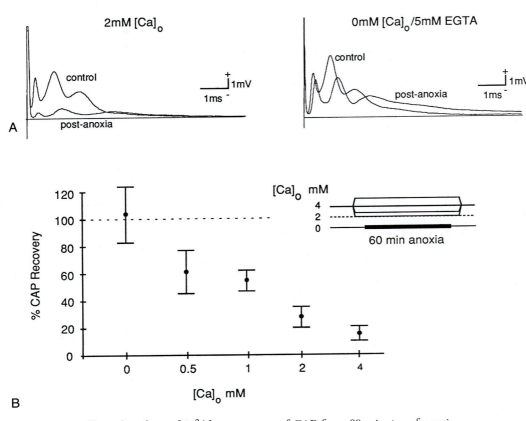

Figure 5.3 Effect of perfusate $[Ca^{2+}]$ on recovery of CAP from 60 minutes of anoxia. (**A**) CAPs before (control) and 60 minutes after anoxia in 2.0 mM $[Ca^{2+}]$ or zero $[Ca^{2+}]/5$ mM EGTA are shown. CAP recovery from anoxia is enhanced in the zero Ca^{2+} solution. (**B**) Graph showing average (± 1 SD) percent CAP recovery after a standard 60-minute period of anoxia as a function of perfusate $[Ca^{2+}]$ during anoxia. Test solutions were begun 10 minutes before anoxia onset and continued until 10 minutes after the end of anoxia (see inset). The percent recovery of the CAP gradually diminished as perfusate $[Ca^{2+}]$ increased from 0 to 4 mM. The mean recovery in 2.0 mM $[Ca^{2+}]_o$ was 28.5 $\pm$ 10.6%, whereas in zero $[Ca^{2+}]/5$ mM EGTA the area under the CAP recovered to 103 $\pm$ 23% of the control value. All points were significantly different from the normal $[Ca^{2+}]$ of 2 mM ($P < 0.005$). (Modified from Stys et al.[74])

tively unchanged, but the peak latencies tend to improve (P.K. Stys, unpublished observations).

These data indicate that the presence of extracellular Ca^{2+} is critical for the development of irreversible anoxic injury in WM and suggest that the degree of injury is related to the transmembrane Ca^{2+} gradient. Extracellular Ca^{2+}, therefore, probably acts as a source for inward Ca^{2+} flux into a cytoplasmic compartment. This ion seems to produce its deleterious effects by moving from the ECS into an intracellular space throughout the 60-minute anoxic interval.[74]

Because it is the axons that become dysfunctional during anoxia, based on the loss of the CAP, a damaging increase in intra-axonal $[Ca^{2+}]$ seems likely. Indeed, 60 minutes of anoxia causes striking pathologic alterations within axons.[84] Large vacuolar spaces appear between axons and their myelin sheaths, axoplasmic mitochondria are swollen and disrupted, and neurofilaments and microtubules disappear from the axoplasm (Fig.

5.4). Similar alterations of the axonal cytoskeleton and intracellular organelles have been reported in peripheral axons exposed to the calcium ionophore A23187,[61] which presumably causes elevated $[Ca^{2+}]_i$. Ultrastructural changes following WM anoxia were most prominent in large axons. Some axons exhibited paranodal myelin retraction from the node, and this may adversely affect saltatory conduction (Fig. 5.4B, arrow). Although some of the ultrastructural changes seen after 60 minutes of anoxia show partial recovery after 60 minutes of reoxygenation, neurofilament and microtubule damage persists. The relationship between paranodal myelin and axon membrane is partially restored in some axons, which might represent the anatomic substrate for partial return of the CAP (Fig. 5.1B). It is clear, however, that the return of the CAP to a new steady level after anoxia is a multifactorial process and must also involve the reestablishment of critical transmembrane ion gradients that are the basis of axonal excitability.[29]

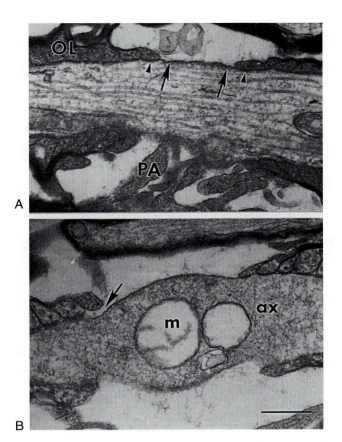

Figure 5.4 Electron micrographs of nodes of Ranvier in the optic nerve under control or anoxic conditions. Note, in control optic nerve (**A**), the close apposition of terminating oligodendroglial loops (OL) to the axon in the paranode (arrowheads) and the dense undercoating of the normal axon membrane (arrows). Perinodal astrocyte processes (PA) approach the node. The axoplasm contains a dense network of microtubules. In the anoxic optic nerve (**B**), there is occasional detachment of terminal myelin loops from the axon (arrow). Mitochondria are swollen with distorted cristae (m). There is destruction of microtubules within the axoplasm (ax). **A, B:** × 40,000. Bar = 0.5 μm. (Modified from Waxman et al.[84])

If the nerve is exposed to anoxia in the absence of bath calcium, the ultrastructural abnormalities described above are not seen.[83] The correlation, therefore, between changes in axonal structure and changes in axonal function (i.e., CAP area) is excellent; in the presence of normal extracellular [Ca^{2+}], anoxia disrupts both axonal structure and function, while in the absence of extracellular [Ca^{2+}], anoxia fails to produce long-term disruption of either. The available evidence is indirect, but all of it points to the conclusion that during anoxia Ca^{2+} rushes into axonal cytoplasm, probably at nodes of Ranvier where the axon membrane is most exposed, leading to the loss of normal architecture and excitability. There are also changes in the surrounding glial cells and myelin, but the way that these changes contribute to the patho-

physiology of disrupted energy metabolism in WM is still to be worked out.

Ca^{2+} Influx During Anoxia

REVERSAL OF Na^+/Ca^{2+} EXCHANGE

The central role of Ca^{2+} influx in mediating anoxic/ischemic damage in neuron cell bodies is well established.[9,10] In GM, where synapses abound, the predominant mechanism for Ca^{2+} entry into neurons is through NMDA-type glutamate receptors. Given the anatomic and physiologic differences between WM and GM, it seemed likely at the outset that the mechanism in WM would be different than in GM. WM has no synapses and is resistant to prolonged application of high concentrations of glutamate,[53] concentrations that would quickly kill neuron cell bodies. Moreover, the NMDA antagonist ketamine, at low concentrations that are relatively specific for blocking this receptor, does not protect against anoxia-induced WM injury. At very high concentrations, ketamine is protective, but this effect is probably related to the drug's anesthetic-like actions on Na^+ channel permeability and not to NMDA receptor blockade.[39,53,87] Studies have now established that during anoxia Ca^{2+} enters axons by two mechanisms: (1) reverse operation of the Na^+/Ca^{2+} exchanger, a ubiquitous (with the exception of red blood cells) membrane protein that normally operates to extrude cytoplasmic Ca^{2+} in exchange for Na^+ influx; and (2) via voltage-gated Ca^{2+} channels.

The Na^+/Ca^{2+} exchanger does not consume ATP and is primarily driven by the transmembrane Na^+ gradient. The exchanger can function equally well in the forward or reverse direction and is a high-capacity, relatively low-affinity transporter of Ca^{2+} ions.[3] The stoichiometry of this process, at least in some instances, is that 3 Na^+ ions exchange for each Ca^{2+} ion; this exchange ratio causes the process to be electrogenic and, in fact, membrane current is generated by its operation.[35,59] For this reason, the exchanger is also influenced by membrane potential[3,35]; membrane depolarization favors reverse exchange (i.e., Na^+ efflux and Ca^{2+} influx). The manner in which [Ca^{2+}]$_i$ can be modulated by changes in the transmembrane Na^+ gradient or membrane potential (or both) is illustrated in Figure 5.5.[76] It is important to note that relatively small changes in intracellular [Na^+] ([Na^+]$_i$) or membrane potential can markedly alter [Ca^{2+}]$_i$. Specifically, increases in [Na^+]$_i$ and membrane depolarization would lead to large increases in [Ca^{2+}]$_i$.

We hypothesized that anoxic/ischemic injury of WM axons involves the following sequence of events. Anoxia/ischemia causes a rapid drop in ATP with an increase in [K^+]$_o$ (see above), resulting in axonal depolarization. Na^+ influx through voltage-dependent Na^+ channels would lead to an increase in [Na^+]$_i$ because the Na^+ pump function would be impaired.[1] Both membrane depolarization and the increase in [Na^+]$_i$ favor reverse operation of the Na^+/Ca^{2+} exchanger,

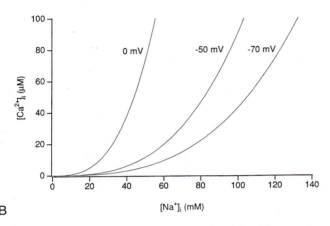

$$E_{NaCa} = \frac{n\,E_{Na} - 2\,E_{Ca}}{n - 2} \qquad \text{eq.1}$$

$$[Ca]_i = [Ca]_o \; Exp\left[\frac{F\,V_m\,(n-2)}{R\,T}\right]\left[\frac{[Na]_i}{[Na]_o}\right]^n \qquad \text{eq.2}$$

A

B

Figure 5.5 Effects of membrane potential and $[Na^+]_i$ on $Na^+/$ Ca^{2+} exchange. (**A**) Equations describing the behavior of the Na^+/Ca^{2+} exchanger.[3,64] E_{NaCa}, E_{Na}, and E_{Ca} are reversal potentials of the exchanger, Na^+ and Ca^{2+} ions, respectively, and n represents the exchanger stoichiometry. The exchanger will operate in the direction required to bring its reversal potential closer to membrane potential, V_m. At thermodynamic equilibrium, $E_{NaCa} = V_m$. Substituting V_m into Eq. [1], expanding the expressions for E_{Na} and E_{Ca}, and rearranging, we obtain an expression (Eq. [2]) for the $[Ca^{2+}]_i$ that would be maintained by the $Na^+/$ Ca^{2+} exchanger. (**B**) Graphical representation of Eq.[2] at three values of membrane potential assuming a stoichiometry of 3 Na^+: 1 Ca^{2+}. With increasing $[Na^+]_i$ and/or membrane depolarization, both of which occur during anoxia, the Na^+/Ca^{2+} exchanger will tend to increase $[Ca^{2+}]_i$. (From Stys et al,[76] with permission.)

which would continue until a higher, steady-state $[Ca^{2+}]_i$ is reached (Fig. 5.5).

If reversal of Na^+/Ca^{2+} exchange mediates Ca^{2+} loading during anoxia in WM, then blocking the exchanger during anoxia should improve outcome, and it does. Inhibitors of this transporter (bepridil and benzamil) markedly improve postanoxic recovery (Fig. 5.6). The degree of postanoxic CAP recovery, seen following treatments that limit operation of the $Na^+/$ Ca^{2+} exchanger, approaches the level of recovery seen when the nerve is bathed in zero Ca^{2+} solution during anoxia. We also carried out experiments in which we manipulated the transmembrane gradient of Na^+ and observed the changes that would be expected from Ca^{2+} flux mediated by the $Na^+/$

Ca^{2+} exchanger.[76,77] These results indicate that reverse operation of the Na^+/Ca^{2+} exchanger is responsible for damaging Ca^{2+} influx into axons during anoxia.

It follows from the above sequence that increases in $[Na^+]_i$ strongly propel reverse Na^+/Ca^{2+} exchange. The probable way that axons would accumulate net amounts of Na^+ during disruption of energy metabolism is activation of voltage-dependent Na^+ channels, and myelinated axons possess extremely high densities ($>10^3/\mu m^2$) of these channels at nodes of Ranvier.[86] Blocking Na^+ channels with tetrodotoxin (TTX) significantly improves CAP recovery following anoxia (Fig. 5.7) and proves that these channels are involved in the pathophysiology of WM anoxic injury. Concentrations of TTX that do not significantly alter optic nerve excitability as measured by the CAP also protect against anoxic injury, but to a lesser extent than higher concentrations, which do block action potential electrogenesis.[76] TTX application during anoxia yields a maximum of about 80% recovery of CAP area, which may underestimate the protective effect of Na^+ channel blockade because the postanoxic CAP may have been partially depressed due to incomplete washout of TTX. In GM, Na^+ influx during anoxia also contributes to acute injury, but the mechanism of this is not clear.[24,57]

In the optic nerve, Na^+ entry during anoxia continues throughout the entire 60-minute period of exposure.[76] Conventional Na^+ channels quickly inactivate with depolarization and would not be available to mediate persistent Na^+ influx. Some Na^+ channels, however, inactivate slowly or not at all.[69,79] Non-inactivating Na^+ channels are present in optic nerve axons[75] and appear to account for the pathologic Na^+ influx that leads to axonal dysfunction in WM.

It is theoretically possible that Na^+ channels contribute to Ca^{2+}-dependent anoxic injury by acting directly as a route of Ca^{2+} entry. The Na^+ channel possesses finite permeability to other ionic species including Ca^{2+}; the Na^+/Ca^{2+} permeability ratio of this channel can be as low as 10:1.[28,41] To test this possibility, the optic nerve was exposed to a solution containing no Na^+ (with equimolar substitution by choline or Li^+) during anoxia.[76] If the damaging influx of Ca^{2+} occurs directly via Na^+ channels, then the removal of Na^+ during anoxia should have no effect on outcome measured by the degree of CAP recovery because Na^+ channels would still be fully available to allow Ca^{2+} entry. In fact, Na^+ removal during anoxia strikingly improves recovery (Fig. 5.7). This result indicates that irreversible anoxic injury in WM does not arise from Ca^{2+} entering through voltage-gated Na^+ channels.

VOLTAGE-GATED Ca^{2+} CHANNELS

Voltage-gated Ca^{2+} channels are known to participate in irreversible dysfunction in some models of anoxic injury.[36] Calcium channel blockers reduce the extent of this injury, presumably by preventing damaging Ca^{2+} influx into neurons that are depolarized due to anoxia.[36,88] Initially it appeared that organic and inorganic Ca^{2+} channel antagonists did not improve the outcome of WM exposed to anoxia.[73] It was later shown, however, that these antagonists have unexpectedly complex actions in WM.[17] Indeed, a more complete study

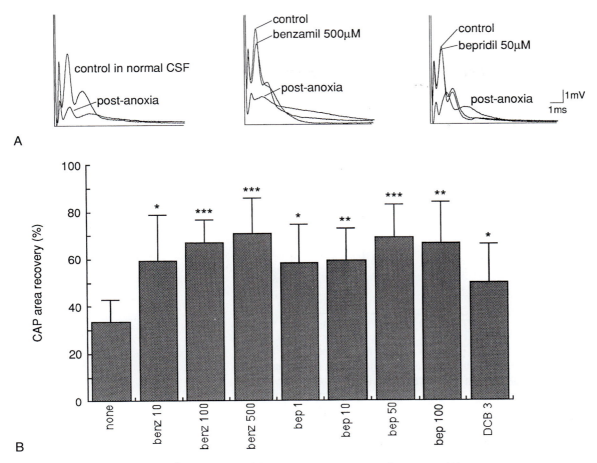

A

B

Figure 5.6 Effects of Na^+/Ca^{2+} exchange inhibitors on CAP recovery after anoxia. (**A**) Benzamil (benz), bepridil (bep), or dichlorobenzamil (DCB) were applied 60 minutes before the start of anoxia and continued until 15 minutes after reoxygenation, when normal solution was resumed. Postanoxic activity was measured 1 hour after reoxygenation. (**B**) Benzamil significantly improves recovery of CAP area in a dose-dependent manner over a concentration range of 10 to 500 μM. Bepridil (1 to 100 μM) and dichlorobenzamil (3 μM) also significantly improve recovery. Benzamil has no effect on the preanoxic response at 10 and 100 μM and reduces CAP area modestly to 61.1 ± 20% of control at 500 μM in a reversible manner. Bepridil and dichlorobenzamil have no effect on preanoxic responses at the concentrations shown. *, $P < 0.01$; **, $P < 0.001$; ***, $P < 0.0001$; N = 7 to 10 for each drug and concentration. (Modified from Stys et al.[76])

clearly establishes that both L-type and N-type Ca^{2+} channels are involved in the development of anoxic injury in CNS white matter.[17] Ca^{2+} channels are expressed in optic nerve axons and glia,[17] although their cellular location and function are not known.

Reverse operation of the Na^+/Ca^{2+} exchanger and activation of Ca^{2+} channels may act in parallel to allow Ca^{2+} entry into axons during anoxia. Alternatively, Ca^{2+} influx may be initiated through Ca^{2+} channels, leading to an increase in $[Ca^{2+}]_i$ that subsequently triggers reverse Na^+/Ca^{2+} exchange. For unclear reasons, higher $[Ca^{2+}]_i$ than normal is a necessary precondition for reversal of Na^+/Ca^{2+} exchange.[15] In this latter view, axonal Ca^{2+} channels act to kick start the phase of Ca^{2+} accumulation mediated by the Na^+/Ca^{2+} exchanger.

A summary diagram of how anoxia leads to Ca^{2+} accumulation in WM is shown in Figure 5.8. In the presence of oxygen and glucose, sufficient energy is generated in the form of ATP to maintain normal Na^+ pump operation. The Na^+ pump maintains a low $[Na^+]_i$ and prevents large increases in $[Na^+]_i$ from occurring when the nerve fires action potentials.[56] It is also responsible for the axon's high negative resting membrane potential. These conditions, normal transmembrane Na^+ gradient and negative membrane potential, dictate that the Na^+/Ca^{2+} exchanger operates in the forward mode, so that it acts as a Ca^{2+} extruder (Fig. 5.8A). In the absence of oxygen, ATP drops to very low levels in 2 to 3 minutes (Fig. 5.8B). The Na^+ pump, which consumes about half of all the energy used in neurons,[1] is no longer able to maintain transmembrane gradients of K^+ and Na^+. Increases in $[Na^+]_i$ secondary to

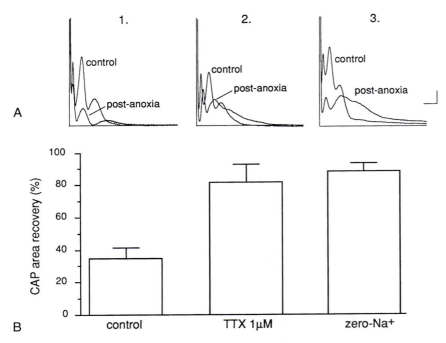

Figure 5.7 Protective effect of TTX and perfusion in zero-[Na$^+$] solution on the anoxic optic nerve. (**A**) Representative CAPs, before and after 60 minutes of anoxia, are shown in normal solution (1), with the addition of 1 μM TTX (2), and with perfusion with zero-[Na$^+$] solution (3). These agents were applied beginning 15 minutes (TTX) or 20 minutes (zero-[Na$^+$] solution) before the onset of anoxia and were continued until 15 minutes after the anoxic period. The TTX-treated optic nerves were perfused for 3 hours in normal solution following reoxygenation to allow TTX to wash out as completely as possible before postanoxic measurements were taken. Recovery of the CAP area is improved with both TTX and zero-[Na$^+$] solution, although peak latencies were delayed. (**B**) Pretreatment with 1 μM TTX or zero-[Na$^+$] significantly improves CAP recovery (81.5 $\pm$ 11%; $P <$ 0.0001 and 88.0 $\pm$ 5%; $P <$ 0.0001, respectively) compared with normal solution (CAP recovery, 36.7 $\pm$ 7%). (Modified from Stys et al.[76])

influx through Na$^+$ channels can no longer be corrected.[56] Myelinated axons may be especially susceptible to this cascade of events because they express very high densities of Na$^+$ channels in the axon at the nodes of Ranvier.[86] In fact, the association of the myelination process and susceptibility to anoxic injury during development (see above) might be explained on this basis. The very high densities of Na$^+$ channels at nodes of Ranvier would predispose to local increases in [Na$^+$]$_i$. Increases in [K$^+$]$_o$ cause membrane depolarization and opening of non-inactivating, voltage-dependent Na$^+$ channels[75] that elevate [Na$^+$]$_i$. Ca^{2+} channels would be open persistently under these conditions, and the resulting Ca^{2+} influx would lead to elevation of [Ca^{2+}]$_i$. The progressive deterioration of membrane potential and transmembrane Na$^+$ gradient, along with an increase in [Ca^{2+}]$_i$, causes reverse operation of the Na$^+$/Ca^{2+} exchanger, which can rapidly cause [Ca^{2+}]$_i$ to rise into the micromolar range[3] (Fig. 5.5). This outline emphasizes the disruption in ionic regulation that leads to an increase of [Ca^{2+}]$_i$ and ultimately to irreversible damage.[60] The downstream events that are the ultimate cause of cell death[22,44,67] have yet to be defined in WM. They are likely to include a set of biochemical reactions mediated by enzymes such as proteases and lipases, and the generation of free radicals.

Autoprotective Events in WM Involving GABA and Adenosine

Nerve fiber tracts in the CNS do not contain synapses, but they do contain the inhibitory neurotransmitter γ-aminobutyric acid (GABA)[80] and GABA receptors.[5] While the normal physiologic function of GABA in WM is not known, GABA appears in the ECS when WM is also made ischemic.[64] Adenosine is also found in WM and, like GABA, is produced when oxygen demand outstrips its supply.[58] Both GABA and adenosine affect the outcome of WM subjected to anoxia; at very low concentrations they both attenuate the severity of injury. Because they are released into the ECS of WM with anoxia, they constitute a unique autoprotective system for this tissue.[19,20]

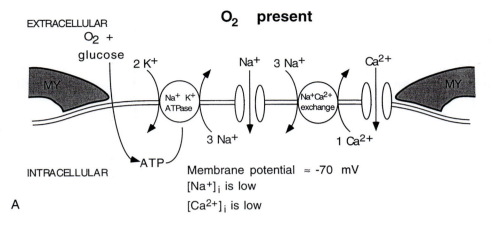

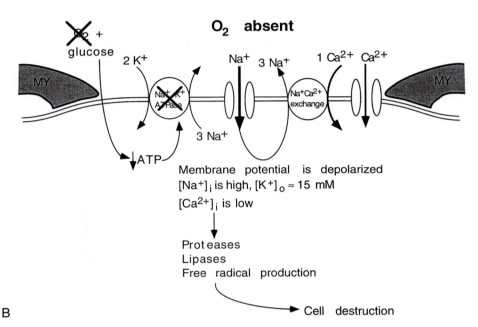

Figure 5.8 Key ionic events that lead to intracellular Ca^{2+} accumulation during anoxia at nodes of Ranvier of CNS axons. (**A**) Under normal conditions there is sufficient oxygen and glucose present to generate enough ATP to operate the necessary ion pumps for maintaining excitability. If $[Na^+]_i$ increases due to action potentials, this increase is easily compensated for by enhanced Na^+ pump activity. The steep Na^+ gradient produced by the Na^+ pump, in conjunction with a high negative membrane potential, drives the high-capacity Na^+/Ca^{2+} exchanger in the forward direction, which helps maintain low $[Ca^{2+}]_i$. There is reason to believe that both the Na^+ pump and the Na^+/Ca^{2+} exchanger might be preferentially located at the nodes because this is where activity-dependent ion fluxes occur in myelinated axons. Voltage-gated Ca^{2+} channels are also present but are not necessary for action potential generation. (**B**) In the absence of oxygen the generation of ATP is seriously reduced because it is now exclusively coming from glycolysis. The shortfall of ATP (the extent of which depends on glucose availability; see text) causes ion gradients to deteriorate, and the speed of deterioration is augmented by voltage-gated Na^+ channels, some of which are non-inactivating, which increases the workload on the Na^+ pump. As the transmembrane Na^+ gradient falls and the membrane depolarizes, the Na^+/Ca^{2+} exchanger is driven to work in reverse and begins loading the axon with Ca^{2+}. Ca^{2+} also enters the axon by way of voltage-gated Ca^{2+} channels. The ultimate destruction of cellular integrity is probably mediated by Ca^{2+}-activated destructive enzmyes, such as proteases and lipases, and the generation of free radicals.

The effect of GABA on the extent of CAP recovery from a standard 60-minute period of anoxia is shown in Figure 5.9. Application of GABA (1 μM) to the optic nerve during anoxia significantly enhances improvement. The beneficial effect of GABA was mediated by GABA-B type receptors; thus, GABA-induced protection was duplicated by the selective GABA-B agonist baclofen and blocked by the GABA-B antagonist phaclofen. High concentrations of GABA or baclofen failed to afford protection probably because of receptor desensitization.[20] That GABA was being released from endogenous stores and was providing a protective effect in the absence of bath application was demonstrated by the fact that the GABA-B receptor blocker phaclofen significantly worsens outcome.[20]

GABA-B receptors are known to act through G-proteins, and the protective effect of GABA against anoxic injury was blocked by G-protein antagonists. The second messenger sequence of GABA's action was followed one step further and was found to involve protein kinase C (PKC). Direct activation of PKC, in the absence of added GABA, mimicked the action of GABA, which is to say it was significantly protective.[20] Blockade of PKC prevented expression of GABA's protection action. The model shown in Figure 5.10 summarizes our current understanding of how GABA acts to protect WM from anoxic injury. Anoxia induces a sequence of ionic disruptions that increase $[K^+]_o$, $[Na^+]_i$, and Ca^{2+} influx via reverse Na^+/Ca^{2+} exchange and activation of voltage-gated Ca^{2+} channels.

(The latter is not shown in this model.) At the same time, anoxia causes release of GABA into the ECS, presumably from endogenous stores. The cellular origin of GABA under these conditions has not been determined, but glial cells contain GABA and have the capacity to release it if the ionic gradients that sustain uptake are degraded, as would be the case during anoxia.[20] Once released, GABA acts at GABA-B receptors and through a G-protein/PKC pathway to protect the optic nerve partially from anoxia-induced injury. The protection is believed to be due to the phosphorylation by PKC of a critical protein within axons, but presently this target is not known. Phosphorylation and downregulation of the Na^+/Ca^{2+} exchanger would be one possibility (as indicated by the arrow with a ? in Fig. 5.10). Curtailing the conductance of non-inactivating Na^+ channels or voltage-gated Ca^{2+} channels is another possibility that could serve to lessen the impact of a period of anoxia.

Adenosine acts at specific receptors within WM to reduce the extent of CAP loss associated with anoxic exposure, and in this way closely mimics the behavior of GABA described above.[20] In fact, GABA and adenosine act synergistically to protect WM via the same G-protein/PKC pathway. Both are believed to be released at nanomolar concentrations during anoxia to recruit the autoprotection mechanism.[20] The extent to which this novel aspect of the pathophysiology of WM damage can be pharmacologically manipulated remains to be investigated.

Figure 5.9 The inhibitory neurotransmitter GABA acted at low concentrations to protect rat optic nerve axons from anoxia-induced damage. Superimposed pre- and postanoxic CAPs taken under control conditions and in the presence of various agents are shown along with a graphic summary of these results. The larger of each CAP pair is the preanoxic recording and the smaller CAP is the postanoxic recovery. (**A**) Under control conditions, the mean postanoxic CAP recovery is 36.5 $\pm$ 2.9%. (**B**) GABA at 1 μM significantly increased recovery to a mean of 55.7 $\pm$ 2.5%. (**C**) The selective GABA-B antagonist phaclofen (500 μM) blocked GABA's protective effect against anoxic injury. (**D**) The selective GABA-B agonist baclofen (1 μM) protected against anoxic injury. (**E**) Summarized results from numerous experiments like those shown in A–D. (Modified from Fern et al.[19])

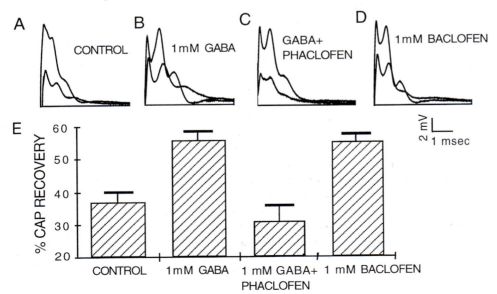

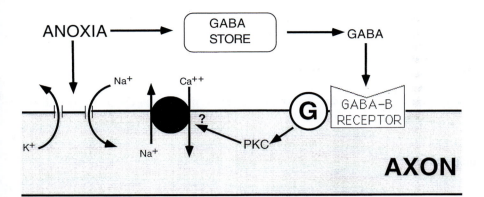

Figure 5.10 A model for the mechanism of GABA's protective effect during anoxia in the rat optic nerve. Anoxia induces GABA release from endogenous stores within the nerve. The resulting increase in extracellular GABA concentration triggers the activation of GABA-B receptors and initiates an intracellular pathway involving a G-protein/protein kinase C (PKC) cascade. The optic nerve axons are rendered more resistant to anoxia-induced injury as a result. The target of PKC phosphorylation is unknown, but it could be the Na^+/Ca^{2+} exchanger (see arrow with ?), or Ca^{2+} channels, phosphorylation and downregulation of which would limit Ca^{2+} influx (see text). (From Fern et al,[19] with permission.)

Strategies for Protecting WM from Anoxic Injury

The complexity of the injury process in WM presents many potential strategies for therapeutic intervention. Experiments with isolated WM have shown that inhibitors of voltage-gated Na^+ channels, voltage-gated Ca^{2+} channels, or the Na^+/Ca^{2+} exchanger are all protective against anoxic injury.[17,51,76] Potentiation of the GABA/adenosine autoprotective system is also protective in isolated WM.[19,20] These pharmacologic manipulations act to occlude events that occur relatively early in the injury cascade. For example, the Na^+/Ca^{2+} exchanger inhibitor bepridil is protective because it prevents Ca^{2+} influx during anoxia, eliminating the downstream events that follow from high intracellular Ca^{2+} such as the activation of destructive enzymes. In one sense this is advantageous, since interrupting the chain of events during the early stages represents the best opportunity for complete arrest of the injury process. The disadvantage of these drugs is that they must be present either before or immediately after the onset of an anoxic/ischemic event, if they are to have a significantly protective effect. This suggests that identification of high-risk patients and chronic treatment with prophylactic concentrations of drugs will represent the most effective way of reducing the impact of WM ischemic injuries such as lacunar infarcts. Such drugs will need to be very well tolerated and have few side effects to justify their use in this preemptive way.

Based on our present understanding, the utility of a therapeutic strategy will therefore be governed both by its efficacy and the degree to which it is tolerated by patients. Bearing this in mind, two types of intervention seem most promising. A number of drugs currently in clinical use for other conditions have been shown to protect WM from anoxic/ischemic injury as a result of blocking Na^+ channels. These include antiarrhythmic drugs such as prajmaline and tocainide,[71] the antiepileptic drugs phenytoin and carbamazepine,[16] and the antidepressant diazepam.[16] Some of these drugs have been shown to protect isolated WM from injury at concentrations below those currently used clinically. For example, phenytoin increases recovery from a 60-minute period of anoxia by about 80% at 1 μM, a concentration below that found in the cerebrospinal fluid of patients taking phenytoin to treat epilepsy.[16]

Drugs that interfere with GABA uptake and degradation represent a second way of interrupting the injury cascade with minimal side effects in patients. These drugs, which include vigabatrin and gabapentin, have been developed recently to treat epilepsy; they act, it appears, by increasing the extracellular concentration of GABA. Raising extracellular GABA is protective against anoxic injury in WM,[19,20] suggesting a secondary use for these drugs in WM ischemia. This kind of drug therapy would have the advantage that it involves potentiation of an existing protective mechanism, a strategy that has proved highly effective in other disease states. The relatively benign therapeutic profile of drugs like vigabatrin and low concentrations of carbamazepine suggest that long-term use in patients at high risk of WM injury may be a beneficial clinical practice.

Acknowledgments

Work in the authors' laboratories has been supported in part by grants from the National Institutes of Health (B.R.R.) and by the Medical Research Service, U.S. Department of Veterans Affairs (S.G.W.).

References

1. Ames A III, Li Y, Heher EC, Kimble CR: Energy metabolism of rabbit retina as related to function: high cost of Na^+ transport. J Neurosci 12:840, 1992

2. Benveniste H, Drejer J, Shousboe A, Diemer NH: Elevation of the extracellular concentrations of glutamate aspartate in rat hippocampus during transient cerebral ischemia monitored by intracerebral microdialysis. J Neurochem 43:1369, 1984

3. Blaustein MP: Calcium transport and buffering in neurons. TINS 11:438, 1988

4. Booth RFG, Patel TB, Clark JB: The development of enzymes of energy metabolism in brain of a precocial (guinea pig) and non-cocial (rat) specimen. J Neurochem 34:17, 1980

5. Bowery NG, Hudson AL, Price GW: GABA-A and GABA-B receptor site distribution in the rat central nervous system. Neuroscience 20:365, 1987

6. Buchthal F, Rosenfalck A: Evoked action potentials and conduction velocity in human sensory nerves. Brain Res 3:1, 1966

7. Chesler M: The regulation and modulation of pH in the nervous system. Prog Neurobiol 34:401, 1990

8. Chesler M, Kraig, RP: Intracellular pH of astrocytes increases rapidly with cortical stimulation. Am J Physiol 253:R666, 1987

9. Choi DW: Calcium-mediated neurotoxicity: relationship to specific channel types and role in ischemic damage. Trends Neurosci 11:465, 1988

10. Choi DW: Glutamate neurotoxicity and diseases of the nervous system. Neuron 1:624, 1988

11. Connors BW, Ransom BR, Kunis DM, Gutnick MJ: Activity-dependent K^+ accumulation in the developing rat optic nerve. Science 216:1341, 1982

12. Davis P, Ransom BR: Anoxia and CNS white matter: *in vitro* studies using the rat optic nerve. Soc Neurosci Abstr 13:1634, 1987

13. Deitmer JW, Szatkowski M: Membrane potential dependence of intracellular pH regulation by identified glial cells in the leech central nervous system. J Physiol (Lond) 421:617, 1990

14. Dentinger MP, Barron KD, Csiza CK: Ultrastructure of the central nervous system in a myelin deficient rat. J Neurocytol 11:671, 1982

15. DiPolo R, Beauge L: Regulation of Na^+-Ca^{2+} exchange. An overview. Ann NY Acad Sci 639:100, 1991

16. Fern R, Ransom BR, Stys PK, Waxman SG: Pharmacological protection of CNS white matter during anoxia. J Pharmacol Exp Ther 266:1549, 1993

17. Fern R, Ransom BR, Waxman SG: Voltage-gated calcium channels in CNS white matter: role in anoxic injury. J Neurophysiol 74:369, 1995

18. Fern R, Davis PK, Waxman SG, Ransom BR: Axon conduction and survival in CNS white matter during energy deprivation: A developmental study. J Neurophysiol 1998, in press

19. Fern R, Waxman SG, Ransom BR: Endogenous GABA attenuates CNS white matter dysfunction following anoxia. J Neurosci 15:699, 1995

20. Fern R, Waxman SG, Ransom BR: Modulation of anoxic injury in CNS white matter by adenosine, and interaction between adenosine and GABA. J Neurophysiol 72:2609, 1994

21. Fisher CM: Capsular infarcts: the underlying vascular lesions. Arch Neurol 36:65, 1979

22. Flamm ES, Demopoulos HB, Seligman ML et al: Free radicals in cerebral ischemia. Stroke 9:445, 1978

23. Foster RE, Connors BW, Waxman SG: Rat optic nerve: electrophysiological, pharmacological and anatomical studies during development. Dev Brain Res 3:371, 1982

24. Goldberg WT, Kadingo RM, Barrett JN: Effects of ischemia-like conditions on cultured neurons: protection by low Na^+, low Ca^{2+} solutions. J Neurosci 6:3144, 1986

25. Goldman SA, Pulsinelli WA, Clarke WY et al: The effects of extracellular acidosis on neurons and glia *in vitro*. J Cereb Blood Flow Metab 9:471, 1989

26. Haimann C, Bernheim L, Bertrand D, Bader CR: Potassium current activated by intracellular sodium in quail trigeminal ganglion neurons. J Gen Physiol 95:961, 1990

27. Hansen AJ: Effect of anoxia on ion distribution in the brain. Physiol Rev 65:101, 1985

28. Hille B: Ionic Channels of Excitable Membranes. Sinauer, Sunderland, MA, 1984

29. Hodgkin AL: The Conduction of the Nervous Impulse. Liverpool University Press, London, 1964

30. Kimelberg HK, Ransom BR: Physiological and pathological aspects of astrocytic swelling. p. 129. In Fedoroff S, Vernadakis A (eds): Astrocytes. Vol. 3. Academic Press, Orlando, 1986

31. Kraig R, Ferreira-Filho CR, Nicholson C: Alkaline and acid transients in cerebellar microenvironment. J Neurophysiol 49:831, 1983

32. Kraig RP, Nicholson C: Extracellular ionic variations during spreading depression. Neuroscience 3:1045, 1978;

33. Kraig RP, Petito CK, Plum F, Pulsinelli WA: Hydrogen ions kill brain at concentrations reached in ischemia. J Cereb Blood Flow Metab 7:379, 1987

34. Kraig RP, Pulsinelli WA, Plum F: Hydrogen ion buffering during complete brain ischemia. Brain Res 342:281, 1985

35. Lagnado L, Cervetto L, Mcnaughton PA: Ion transport by the Na-Ca exchanger in isoated rod outer segments. Procl Natl Acad Sci USA 85:4548, 1988

36. Lipton SA: Calcium channel antagonists in the prevention of neurotoxicity. Adv Pharmacol 22:271, 1991

37. Loizou LA, Kendall BE, Marshall J: Subcortical arteriosclerotic encephalopathy: a clinical and radiological investigation. J Neurol Neurosurg Psychiatry 44:294, 1981

38. Lowry OH, Passonneau JV, Hasselberger FX, Schlutz PW: Effect of ischemia on known substrates and cofactors of the glycolytic pathway in the brain. J Biol Chem 239:18, 1964

39. Marcoux FW, Goodrich JE, Dominick MA: Ketamine prevents ischemic neuronal injury. Brain Res 452:329, 1988

40. McQuinn BA, O'Leary DH: White matter lucencies on computed tomography, subacute arteriosclerotic encephalopathy (Binswanger's disease), and blood pressure. Stroke 18:900, 1987

41. Meves H, Vogel W: Calcium inward currents in internally perfused giant axons. J Physiol (Lond) 235:225, 1973

42. Mishra OP, Deliveria-Papadopoulos M: Anti-oxidant enzymes in fetal guinea pig brain during development and the effect of maternal hypoxia. Dev Brain Res 42:173, 1988

43. Nishizaki T, Yamauchi R, Tanimoto M, Okada Y: Effects of temperature on the oxygen consumption in thin slices from different brain regions. Neurosci Lett 86:301, 1988

44. Orrenius S, McConkey DJ, Jones DP, Nicotera P: Ca^{2+}-activated mechanisms in toxicity and programmed cell death. ISI Atlas of Science: Pharmacology 2:319, 1988

45. Paulson OB, Newman EA: Does the release of potassium from astrocyte endfeet regulate cerebral blood flow? Science 237:896, 1987

46. Plum F: What causes infarction in ischemic brain? Neurology 33:222, 1983

47. Pulsinelli WA, Waldman S, Rawlinson D, Plum F: Moderate hyperglycemia augments ischemic brain damage: a neuropathologic study in the rat. Neurology 32:1239, 1982

48. Ransom BR: Glial modulation of neural excitability mediated by extracellular pH: a hypothesis. p. 37. In Yu A, Sykova E, Hertz L et al (eds): Progress in Brain Research. Vol. 94. Elsevier, Amsterdam, 1992

49. Ransom BR, Fern R: Does astrocytic glycogen benefit axon function and survival in CNS white matter during glucose deprivation? Glia 21:134, 1997

50. Ransom BR, Philbin DM: Anoxia-induced extracellular ionic changes in CNS white matter: the role of glial cells. Can J Physiol Pharmacol 70:181, 1992

51. Ransom BR, Stys PK, Waxman SG: The pathophysiology of anoxic injury in CNS white matter. Stroke, suppl. III, 21:52, 1990

52. Ransom BR, Walz W, Davis PK, Carlini WG: Anoxia-induced changes in extracellular K$^+$ and pH in mammalian central white matter. J Cereb Blood Flow Metab 12:593, 1992

53. Ransom BR, Waxman SG, Davis PK: Anoxic injury of CNS white matter: protective effect of ketamine. Neurology 40:1399, 1990

54. Ransom BR, Yamate CL: The rat optic nerve following enucleation: a pure preparation of mammalian glia. Soc Neurosci Abstr 10:949, 1984

55. Ransom BR, Yamate CL, Connors BW: Activity-dependent shrinkage of extracellular space in rat optic nerve: a developmental study. J Neurosci 5:532, 1985

56. Rose CR, Ransom BR: Regulation of intracellular sodium in cultured rat hippocampal neurones. J Physiol (Lond) 499:573, 1997

57. Rothman SM, Olney JW: Glutamate and the pathophysiology of hypoxic-ischemic brain damage. Ann Neurol 19:105, 1986

58. Rudolphi KA, Schubert P, Parkinson FE, Fredholm BB: Neuroprotective role of adenosine in cerebral ischemia. TIPS 13:439, 1992

59. Russell JM, Blaustein MP: Calcium efflux from barnacle muscle fibers: dependence on external cations. J Gen Physiol 63:144, 1974

60. Schanne FA, Kane AB, Young EE, Farber JL: Calcium-dependence of toxic cell death: a final common pathway. Science 206:700, 1979

61. Schlaepfer WW: Structural alterations of peripheral nerve induced by the calcium ionophore A23817, Brain Res 136:1, 1977

62. Schurr A, West CA, Reid KG et al: Increased glucose improves recovery of neuronal function after cerebral hypoxia in vitro. Brain Res 421:135, 1987

63. Schwartz EA, Tachibana M: Electrophysiology of glutamate and sodium co-transport in a glial cell of the salamander retina. J Physiol (Lond) 426:43, 1990

64. Shimada N, Graf R, Rosner G, Heiss WD: Ischemia-induced accumulation of extracellular amino acids in cerebral cortex, white matter, and cerebrospinal fluid. J Neurochem 60:66, 1993

65. Siesjö BK: Calcium and ischemic brain damage. Eur Neurol 25:45, 1986

66. Siesjö BK: Cell damage in the brain: a speculative synthesis. J Cereb Blood Flow Metab 1:155, 1981

67. Siesjö BK, Wieloch T: Brain injury: neurochemical aspects. p. 513. In Central Nervous System Trauma Status Report. NIH, NINCDS, Bethesda, MD, 1985

68. Somjen GG, Aitken PG, Balestrino M et al: Spreading depression-like depolarization and selective vulnerability of neurons; a brief review. Stroke 21:111–179, 1990

69. Stafstrom CE, Schwindt PC, Chubb MC, Crill WE: Properties of persistent sodium conductance and calcium conductance of layer V neurons from cat sensorimotor cortex. J Neurophysiol 53:153, 1985

70. Staub F, Baethmann A, Peters J et al: Effects of lactacidosis on glial cell volume and viability. J Cereb Blood Flow Metab 10:866, 1990

71. Stys PK: Protective effects of antiarrhythmic agents against anoxic injury in CNS white matter. J Cereb Blood Flow Metab 15:425, 1995

72. Stys PK, Ransom BR, Waxman SG: Compound action potential of nerve recorded by suction electrode: a theoretical and experimental analysis. Brain Res 546:18, 1991

73. Stys PK, Ransom BR, Waxman SG: Effects of polyvalent cations and dihydropyridine calcium channel blockers on recovery of CNS white matter from anoxia. Neurosci Lett 115:293, 1990

74. Stys PK, Ransom BR, Waxman SG, Davis PK: The role of extracellular calcium in anoxic injury of mammalian white matter. Proc Natl Acad Sci USA 87:4212, 1990

75. Stys PK, Sontheimer H, Ransom BR, Waxman SG: Non-inactivating, tetrodotoxin-sensitive Na$^+$ conductance in rat optic nerve axons. Proc Natl Acad Sci USA 90:6976, 1993

76. Stys PK, Waxman SG, Ransom BR: Ionic mechanisms of anoxic injury in mammalian CNS white matter: role of Na$^+$ channels and Na$^+$-Ca^{2+} exchanger. J Neurosci 12:430, 1992

77. Stys PK, Waxman SG, Ransom BR: Na$^+$-Ca^{2+} exchanger mediates Ca^{2+} influx during anoxia in mammalian CNS white matter. Ann Neurol 30:375, 1991

78. Tang CM, Dichter M, Morad M: Modulation of the N-methyl-D-aspartate channel by extracellular H$^+$. Proc Natl Acad Sci USA 87:6445, 1990

79. Taylor CP: Na$^+$ currents that fail to inactivate. TINS 16: 455, 1993

80. Van De Hayden JAM, De Kloet ER, Versteeg DHL: GABA content of discrete brain nuclei and spinal cord of the rat. J Neurochem 33:857, 1979

81. Walz W, Mukerji S: Lactate release from cultured astrocytes and neurons: a comparison. Glia 1:366, 1988

82. Waxman SG, Black JA, Foster RE: Freeze-fracture heterogeneity of the axolemma of premyelinated fibers in the CNS. Neurology 32:418, 1982

83. Waxman SG, Black JA, Ransom BR, Stys PK: Protection of the axonal cytoskeleton in anoxic optic nerve by decreased extracellular calcium. Brain Res 614:137, 1993

84. Waxman SG, Black JA, Stys PK, Ransom BR: Ultrastructural concomitants of anoxic injury and early post-anoxic recovery in rat optic nerve. Brain Res 574:105, 1992

85. Waxman SG, Davis PK, Black JA, Ransom BR: Anoxic injury of mammalian central white matter: decreased susceptibility in myelin-deficient optic nerve. Ann Neurol 28:335, 1990

86. Waxman SG, Ritchie JM: Organization of ion channels in the myelinated nerve fiber. Science 228:1502, 1985

87. Weiss J, Goldberg MP, Choi DW: Ketamine protects cultured neocortical neurons from hypoxic injury. Brain Res 380:186, 1986

88. Weiss JH, Hartley DM, Koh J, Choi DW: The calcium channel blocker nifedipine attenuates slow excitatory amino acid neurotoxicity. Science 247:107, 1990

89. Young W: Blood flow, metabolic and neurophysiological mechanisms in spinal cord injury. p. 463. In Becker D, Povlishock JT (eds): Central Nervous System Trauma Status Report. NIH, NINCDS, Bethesda, MD, 1985

CHAPTER 6

Positron Emission Tomography

JEAN-CLAUDE BARON

By allowing quantitative tomographic maps of cerebral blood flow (CBF), cerebral blood volume (CBV), cerebral metabolic rate of oxygen (CMRO$_2$), brain glucose utilization (CMRGlc), and intracellular pH (pH$_i$) in humans, positron emission tomography (PET) provides better delineation of pathophysiologic mechanisms contributing to ischemic stroke.[109,112] In addition, PET has allowed the development of new functional concepts for the therapy of acute brain ischemia[15] and for mechanisms of functional recovery.[4,24,46,142]

Although several of the above-mentioned physiologic variables are accessible by other investigative methods (e.g., xenon CBF and the Kety-Schmidt N$_2$O techniques), only PET allows the concomitant measurement, in absolute quantitative terms, of several of these variables in the same subject and according to high-resolution images.[12] In addition, access to CBF and CBV allows one to compute the CBV/CBF ratio, which represents the local circulatory mean transit time (t).[38,109] Likewise, the measurement of CBF and CMRO$_2$ allows quantitative mapping of both oxygen extraction fraction (OEF) and the end-capillary partial oxygen tension, which reflects the partial tissue oxygen tension (PtO$_2$); CMRGlc/CMRO$_2$ reflects the stoichiometric relationship between glucose use and oxygen consumption.[12] Finally, using selective plasma and red cell markers, quantitation of local cerebral plasma and erythrocyte volumes (and hence local cerebral hematocrit) can be accomplished.[12]

Table 6.1 shows the main physiologic variables quantifiable with PET, the most accepted and best validated methods allowing their measurement, and the average value measured in regions of interest predominantly containing normal gray matter. The reader is referred to technical articles published elsewhere for further details and methodologic references.[12] A point worthy of mention relates to the quantitation of these variables in absolute terms, which necessitates obtaining arterial blood for radioactivity counting (input function). Although this is achieved safely using fine catheters inserted in the radial artery (with which no complications have been reported thus far), its performance has medical contraindications and is not always possible to perform.

In addition to the nonspecific physiologic variables given above, PET also allows the investigation of specific binding sites/receptors. For example, changes in specific glial and neuronal markers can be assessed with ^{11}C-PK 1195 and ^{11}C-flumazenil, respectively.[118,126] Another potentially interesting variable is essential amino acid uptake in normal and acutely injured brain tissue after stroke, which may provide insights into the phenomena of breakdown and rebound of protein synthesis in relation to ultimate tissue outcome.[54]

The instrumentation characteristics of PET cameras as well as the description and problems related to cyclotron use, radiochemistry, and computer science are outside the scope of this chapter. The interested reader is referred to specialized articles and books. Present-day PET cameras are capable of acquiring up to 64 contiguous brain slices simultaneously, which allows true three-dimensional (3D) imaging with a practical spatial resolution in the order of 4 mm and a temporal resolution of <5 seconds. The complexity of computer PET science has recently advanced rapidly with, for example, development of full 3D volume acquisition, stereotaxic localization/normalization, automatic realignment in 3D with structural magnetic resonance imaging (MRI), and multiparameter, nonlinear, compartmental analysis of dynamic PET data.

The problem of the partial volume effect has considerably diminished with new-generation PET cameras, which have exquisite spatial resolution. However, quantitative values obtained with the newest machines for the physiologic variables listed in Table 6.1 have not yet appeared. Thus, and as a result of the difficulty in analyzing pure tissue compartments, absolute gray matter values for several of the physiologic variables listed in Table 6.1 are on the low side, particularly CBF, CMRO$_2$, and CMRGlc.

Normal Coupling of CBF, CMRO$_2$, CMRGlc, and CBV

With physiologic conditions, there exists in each subject a matching of local values of CBF, CMRO$_2$, and CBV, according to a linearly proportional relationship.[9,125] The CBF-CMRO$_2$

Table 6.1 Physiologic Variables Measured by Positron Emission Tomography

Physiologic Variable	*Abbreviation*	*Normal Values (Gray Matter)*	*Main Radiotracers*	*Method*
Cerebral blood flow	CBF	50 ml/1–100 ml/min	^{15}O–CO_2	Bolus or steady-state
			–^{15}O–H_2O	Bolus or steady-state
			^{11}C or [^{15}O]Butanol	Bolus
			[^{18}F] or [^{11}C]Fluoromethane	Bolus
Cerebral blood volume	CBV	4 ml/100 ml	^{15}O–CO	Bolus or steady-state
			^{11}C–CO	Bolus to equilibrium
Cerebral metabolic rate of oxygen	$CMRO_2$[a]	4 ml/100 ml/min	^{15}O–O_2	Bolus or steady-state
Cerebral metabolic rate of glucose	CMRGlc[a]	8 mg/100 ml/min	[^{18}F]fluoro-2-deoxy-D-glucose	Bolus
			[^{11}C]2-deoxy-D-glucose	Bolus
			[^{11}C]1-D-glucose	Bolus
Tissular pH	pHt	7.04	^{11}C-DMO (intracellular pH)	Bolus
			^{11}C–CO_2	Continuous inhalation
Oxygen extraction fraction	OEF	0.40	^{15}O–CO_2 (or ^{15}O–H_2O) and ^{15}O–O_2	From CBF and $^{15}O_2$ distribution
Mean transit time	t	0.08 min	—	Ratio CBV/CBF (inversely proportional to the cerebral perfusion pressure)
Tissue partial O_2 tension	PtO_2	31.2 mmHg	—	From CBF and $CMRO_2$
Local tissue hematocrit	tHt	0.28	[^{11}C]albumin-^{11}C–CO	Bolus to equilibrium

[a] *The conversion factors to obtain $CMRO_2$ and CMRGlc in micromolar units are 44.6 $\mu mol/ml$ and 5.56 $\mu mol/mg$, respectively.*

matching is such that local CBF values are highest in areas of highest $CMRO_2$ and vice versa; this describes the metabolic regulation of the cerebral circulation and explains why the distribution of CBF, as demonstrated in PET images, is superimposable on that of $CMRO_2$ and why the OEF image is uniform. Thus, in the normal resting human brain, the local CBF reliably reflects the prevailing $CMRO_2$, although this coupling phenomenon may be altered during focal brain activation.

In individual normal subjects, there also exists a coupling between local CBF and CBV, which indicates that the degree of local vasodilatation in brain is strictly proportional to local tissue perfusion.[125] Since CBV, as measured by PET, reflects mainly the resistance (arteriolar) and capacitance (venular) blood volume, PET is able to evaluate the flow-to-resistance relationships. Studies in normal subjects also demonstrate a linear relationship between local CBV and $CMRO_2$ values.[125] Overall, the coupling among CBF, CBV, and $CMRO_2$ observed by PET reflects the metabolic regulation of cerebrovascular resistance and, in turn, of tissue perfusion, which operates at the local level in the normal brain.

Investigations of the relationships between CBF and CMRGlc have shown that in normal subjects the perfusion-metabolism coupling also applies to CMRGlc.[9] Likewise, excellent linear correlations between local $CMRO_2$ and CMRGlc values exist in control subjects, indicating coupling between oxygen consumption and glucose utilization in resting (but perhaps not during activated) human gray matter. The calculated stoichiometric relationship ($CMRO_2$/CMRGlc ratio) is close to the expected value of 6, indicating that glucose metabolism in the brain is almost exclusively oxidative.[9]

Inter-relationships of CBF, CBV, $CMRO_2$, and Brain Glucose Utilization in Ischemic Cerebrovascular Diseases

PET studies in stroke have delineated a variably altered interplay among local CBF, CBV, $CMRO_2$, and CMRGlc values, thereby allowing one to define distinct profiles of changes in physiologic coupling, each underscoring a different pathophysiologic situation. Four main profiles have been described: hemodynamic failure, irreversible damage, luxury perfusion, and primary metabolic depression.

HEMODYNAMIC FAILURE

Hemodynamic failure, defined by a fall in the cerebral perfusion pressure (CPP) below the lower threshold of CBF autoregulation, is characterized by a reduction in CBF unaccompanied by a proportional reduction in $CMRO_2$—a disruption in the physiologic flow-metabolism coupling. Such a state of uncoupling, immediately detectable on the PET images as a focal increase in the OEF, has been termed *misery perfusion*.[7] This increase in the OEF above the normal value of 0.40, up to values approaching the theoretical maximum of 1.00, draws on the wide reserve of oxygen extraction that allows the brain, despite a reduced CBF, to maintain a normal $CMRO_2$—albeit at the expense of reduced PtO_2. This initial phase, in which $CMRO_2$ is fully preserved thanks to tapping the perfusion reserve, is called *oligemia*.[70] Beyond this phase, if CPP drops further, $CMRO_2$ begins to fall precipitously, characterizing the phase of *true ischemia*, in which tissue function is definitely impaired.[70] Thus, misery perfusion goes from simple oligemia to true ischemia, since CBF is reduced and OEF is elevated across the whole continuum of hemodynamic failure (Plate 6.1).

The phenomenon of *autoregulation*, which is based on vasodilatation of resistance vessels to counteract any reduction in CPP, expresses itself in CBV images as clear-cut increases in cortical blood volume during both oligemia and ischemia.[109] This increase in CBV is maximal in the former condition but returns toward normal values in the latter as a result of vascular collapse and metabolic depression.[125] Furthermore, CBV imaging allows one to identify the phase of autoregulation in

which vasodilatation efficiently maintains CBF, also called the *hemodynamic reserve* (see Table 6.2). Measurement of CBV and CBF also allows one to measure the CBV/CBF ratio and its converse, the CBF/CBV ratio. The former has a unit of time and represents the local mean circulatory transit time, t, a physiologic parameter indicative of flow velocity.[109] With PET, t is obtained by dividing, pixel by pixel, the CBV parametric map (in ml/100 ml) by the corresponding CBF map (in ml/100 ml/min). It indicates the coupling between blood flow and velocity in a given block of tissue and therefore increases as soon as CBF autoregulation is tapped. The converse ratio (CBF/CBV) has a unit of minutes^{-1} and is a reliable index of the local CPP under circumstances of unaltered vasomotor tone.[38] The use of this ratio for small brain regions in single patients has allowed demonstration in the living human brain of the successive stages of declining CPP from autoregulation to overt ischemia[125] (Fig. 6.1). These studies have delineated a threshold value of the CBF/CBV ratio of about 7

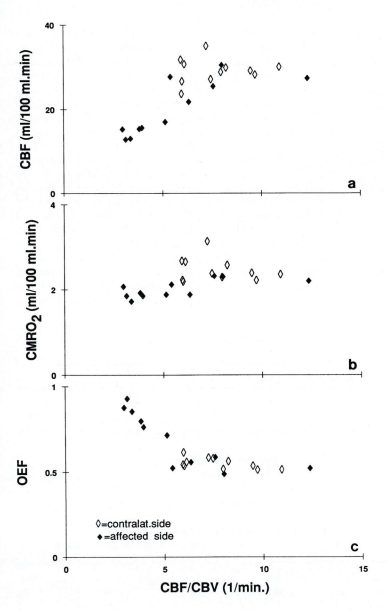

Figure 6.1 Local values of cortical cerebral blood flow (CBF), oxygen extraction fraction (OEF), and cerebral metabolic rate of oxygen ($CMRO_2$) obtained in the patient described in Plate 6.1 from various areas of the hemispheres ipsilateral and contralateral to the left middle cerebral artery blood flow/cerebral blood volume (CBF/CBV) ratios. The data show that the theoretically expected behavior of CBF, $CMRO_2$, and OEF as the local cerebral perfusion pressure (CCP), which is reflected in the CBF/CBV ratio, falls from normal to extremely low values. The data demonstrate efficient CBF autoregulation down to CBF/CBV ratios around 7 minutes^{-1}, followed by a fall in CBF in proportion to that of CPP; at this stage, the OEF rises to values close to 100% and the $CMRO_2$ is well maintained for moderately low CPP (oligemia) but falls at lower CPP (true ischemia). These data demonstrate the capability of positron emission tomography to estimate in vivo the local CPP and to relate the brain hemodynamics and oxygen metabolism to the effects of arterial occlusion in a single patient. (From Sette et al,[125] with permission.)

minutes^{-1} (normal value in controls 10 to 12 minutes^{-1}), below which the CBF falls and the OEF rises, corresponding to the lower limit of autoregulation[38,125]; the OEF value at which the CBV is maximally elevated (lower limit of the vasodilatory reserve) has been recorded at 0.53.[57] The CBF/CBV ratio below which the $CMRO_2$ begins to fall, signaling ischemia, is approximately 4 minutes^{-1}.[125]

Other, more direct, ways to assess the vasodilatory capacity of the brain use agents such as CO_2 (inhalation of 5% CO_2 in air) or acetazolamide.[50,63,76,77] Whereas in the normal brain these agents induce marked increases in CBF, a blunted or even absent response characterizes brain regions with an already vasodilated (autoregulated) vascular bed despite normal perfusion at rest; paradoxical decreases in CBF may even occur in areas with already exhausted reserve (*hemodynamic steal*).

IRREVERSIBLE DAMAGE

Analysis of the relationships between PET parametric values and final tissue outcome (assessed by computed tomography [CT]) has revealed well-defined CBF and $CMRO_2$ thresholds separating structurally intact areas from necrotic areas[10] (Plate 6.2). In the acute stage of stroke, two reports indicate that tissue with $CMRO_2$ below about 1.4 ml/100 g/min is eventually always infarcted.[2,112] Above this threshold, tissue outcome is uncertain, which is consistent with the concept of reversible ischemia (i.e., "penumbra")[117]; however, as these studies were performed with low-resolution machines, concerned mainly gray matter, and did not rely on co-registered CT scans for infarct mapping, this value may be overestimated. Corresponding thresholds for CBF, if any, have not yet been defined with enough reliability.

LUXURY PERFUSION

In 1966, luxury perfusion was recognized by Lassen[69] as the cause of both the red vein syndrome seen by neurosurgeons and the early angiographic blush of recanalized brain infarc-

tion. Characterized by an oxygen supply in excess of demand, its hallmark with PET is a focal reduction of the OEF.[6] This situation, the converse of misery perfusion, indicates re-establishment of perfusion, and hence of CPP, in a previously ischemic tissue. However, luxury perfusion can have diverse appearances as well as mechanisms. Thus, CBF may be increased (hyperperfusion) (Plate 6.3), normal, or even decreased (relative luxury perfusion), although by definition it is in excess of prevailing $CMRO_2$. The latter may itself be either close to normal, as in the reactive hyperemia that immediately sets in a reperfused ischemic but non-necrotic tissue, or reduced—to an extent that depends on the severity of damage incurred during ischemia. Reports indicate that CBV is increased (true hyperemia) in hyperperfused areas, documenting abnormal vasodilatation with *vasoparalysis*.[82]

PRIMARY METABOLIC DEPRESSION

Primary metabolic depression is defined as a matched decrease in CBF, CBV, and $CMRO_2$, without alteration in the OEF, indicating that the normal perfusion-metabolism coupling is preserved.[5,6] The available data also suggest a matched reduction in CMRGlc, indicating a physiologic oxidative use of glucose.[9] Thus, primary metabolic depression reflects a global reduction in synaptic activity/density in an otherwise normally regulated tissue. Following stroke, primary metabolic depression is prone to affect widely both cortical and subcortical structures as a result of disconnection (see the section Remote Metabolic Effects and Their Clinical Correlates below). In the chronic stage and in the peri-infarcted tissue, it may also reflect partial ischemic necrosis or selective neuronal loss.[141]

The various profiles of altered physiologic variables encountered in stroke are summarized in Table 6.2. PET allows not only delineation of widely different pathophysiologic situations but also differentiation of the three conditions with reduced CBF (misery perfusion, primary metabolic depression, and relative luxury perfusion). In addition, PET reveals abnormal hemodynamic changes despite normal CBF (i.e., during

Table 6.2 Patterns of Multiparameter Relationships as Revealed by Positron Emission Tomography in Acute Stroke

Pattern	CBF	CBV	OEF	CMRO₂	Mechanism
Autoregulatory range	N	+	N	N	Vasodilatation (hemodynamic) reserve
Misery perfusion					
Oligemia	−	+ +	+ to + +	N	Oxygen extraction reserve (perfusion reserve)
Ischemia	− −	+	+ +	−	Metabolic impairment (neuronal shutdown)
Irreversible damage	Variable	Variable	Variable	− −	Ischemic pan-necrosis
Luxury perfusion					
Relative	− − or N	+	−	− −	Reperfused necrotic tissue
Absolute	+	+	− −	Variable	Reactive hyperemia or reperfused necrosis
Primary metabolic depression	−	−	N	−	Decreased synaptic activity/density (neuronal death, diaschisis)

Abbreviations and symbols: N, normal; +, increased; + +, extremely increased; −, reduced; − −, extremely reduced; CBF, cerebral blood flow; CBV, cerebral blood volume; OEF, oxygen extraction fraction; $CMRO_2$, cerebral metabolic rate of oxygen.

autoregulatory challenge and luxury perfusion), which emphasizes how misleading isolated CBF measurements may be.

CMRO₂ AND CMRGlc UNCOUPLING IN CEREBROVASCULAR DISEASE

Because of the logistics involved in performing both ^{15}O and ^{18}fluorodeoxyglucose (^{18}FDG) studies in the same setting, only a few reports have appeared on the relationship of CMRO₂ and CMRGlc in stroke. In addition, problems exists with the use of the ^{18}FDG model to evaluate CMRGlc in acutely ischemic tissue.[12] Hence, both the ^{18}FDG rate constant and the lumped constant can be grossly altered in this model, potentially resulting in spurious calculated CMRGlc. Studies that have attempted to overcome these problems have demonstrated clear-cut CMRO₂-CMRGlc uncoupling.[9,12] In acutely ischemic or necrotic tissue, CMRGlc is better preserved than CMRO₂, indicating anaerobic shift of glycolysis.[9,43,144] The reverse uncoupling has also been observed, mainly in tissues surrounding the actual infarct, suggesting the oxidative use of substrates other than glucose.[9]

Acute Ischemic Stroke

HEMODYNAMIC AND METABOLIC PARAMETERS IN THE ISCHEMIC AREAS

Despite the logistics involved, a few studies focusing on the acute stage of stroke (defined as <24 hours from onset) have appeared concerning middle cerebral artery (MCA) territory ischemic stroke (i.e., the most frequent and most typical stroke subtype).[2,45,78–82,111,112] PET studies on acute stroke are not only difficult for logistical reasons; they also have limitations (which they share with all other brain imaging techniques, however). The main limitation is to allow only one or two "snapshot" evaluations despite the highly dynamic and complex nature of the ischemic process. Additional limitations relate to the lack of premorbid assessment to serve as an internal reference to assess the changes observed and to the lack of systematic postmortem mapping of damage. Because all these limitations vanish with animal models, the MCA occlusion model has been implemented for PET applications in the dog,[26] the cat,[48] and the baboon.[102,126,134,152] An additional bonus with such models is that many of the factors that underlie the heterogeneity of clinical stroke, such as site and duration of the occlusion, age, and premorbid associated conditions (e.g., arterial hypertension, diabetes, anemia), can be strictly controlled. One drawback, however, is the need to perform these studies under general anesthesia, which may interfere with the natural history of the disease. In the text that follows, the results from these animal studies are incorporated together with, and for further illumination of, the clinical results.

Both animal and the human studies show three main patterns of changes in the affected areas: irreversible damage, hyperperfusion, and misery perfusion.

Irreversibly Damaged Tissue

TOPOGRAPHY. In a large proportion of patients, irreversible damage (as revealed by profoundly reduced CMRO₂; see above) affects the deep MCA territory very early and is associated in most instances with cortical misery perfusion.[78,146] Presumably because of its poor collaterals, and at variance with the cerebral cortex, the lenticulostriate territory constitutes the core of ischemia and rapidly suffers irreversible damage. This is supported by findings in baboons subjected to MCA occlusion: reduced CMRO₂ and falling OEF is seen in this area as early as 1 to 2 hours postocclusion,[102,152] although the subsequent expansion of this deep-seated hypometabolic area suggests it is not immediately destroyed in its entirety.[134]

In a patient subset, however, the irreversibly damaged area also affects wide parts of the cortical territory very early[78] presumably as a result of inadequate pial collaterals (Plate 6.2).

ASSOCIATED CBF CHANGES. In most instances, the CBF is also profoundly reduced in irreversibly damaged tissues[78] (Plate 6.2), but partial reperfusion with variably reduced or even essentially normal CBF is occasionally encountered, especially in deep infarcts.[82]

IMPLICATIONS FOR TISSUE OUTCOME. Marchal et al[79] have shown that the volume of profoundly hypometabolic tissue, as assessed with PET 5 to 18 hours after onset of stroke, is highly linearly correlated to final infarct volume, as measured by CT scan about 1 month later; the former, however, generally underestimated the latter, because of subsequent metabolic deterioration of the surrounding penumbra (see below). Thus, mapping the profoundly hypometabolic tissue in the acute stage of stroke may provide an early assessment of already established damage and may predict a minimum volume of final infarction.

Early Hyperperfusion

Early hyperperfusion (Plate 6.3), which indicates recanalization of the occluded artery, has been observed in up to one third of cases studied between the 5th and the 18th hour after stroke onset.[80] In most of the cases, it was not associated with reduced metabolism, but instead with a significantly increased CMRO₂, suggesting postischemic rebound of cellular energy-dependent processes.[82] However, the OEF was significantly reduced, indicating that perfusion was indeed overabundant relative to the metabolic needs (i.e., luxury perfusion). In this sample, the hyperperfused areas consistently exhibited intact morphology at chronic-stage CT.[82] Thus, at variance with the idea that sudden tissue reoxygenation might exacerbate ischemic damage, but consistent with the animal literature showing reduction of infarct size by early recanalization, these findings suggest that in humans *early* reperfusion is harmless, and even, presumably, beneficial.

Misery Perfusion

PENUMBRAL TISSUE. One major finding from PET studies has been the demonstration, hours into the episode, of still critically ischemic tissue (Plate 6.1). Wide zones of cerebral cortex with reduced CBF (often below the penumbral threshold of 20 ml/100 g/min),[117] massively increased OEF (often >0.80), and mildly to moderately reduced $CMRO_2$ (i.e., above the generally accepted threshold for irreversibility) have been reported in 50%, 37%, and 25% of the patients studied within 9, 18, and 24 hours, respectively,[2,80,143] and occasionally as late as 30 or 48 hours[11,45] after onset of stroke. These alterations would be consistent with at-risk but still recuperable (i.e., penumbral) tissue.

Transition of such "penumbral" areas toward infarction has been documented within hours of stroke onset and entails a decline in $CMRO_2$ despite stable CBF.[8,44,45,143] Marchal et al[81] have documented the presence within the finally infarcted tissue of still metabolically active but severely ischemic tissue up to 16 hours after onset, with subsequent metabolic deterioration. This process is also strikingly illustrated by the associated dramatic fall in the OEF, from very high to very low values, which signals exhaustion of the tissue's oxygen needs. Occasionally, however, such a deleterious course does not take place, which is consistent with the potential for reversibility that characterizes the penumbra.[11,111] Experiments in baboons with MCA occlusion have strikingly illustrated this process of metabolic deterioration. Following permanent MCA occlusion, both Pappata et al[102] and Touzani et al[134] in the baboon, as well as Heiss et al[48] in the cat, have documented a progressive expansion of the volume of profoundly hypometabolic tissue for up to 24 hours and possibly beyond,[134] indicating a prolonged window of therapeutic opportunity. This was demonstrated by subsequent experiments by the same group documenting that tissue reperfusion by MCA reopening 6 hours after occlusion significantly reversed the previously observed volume expansion of severe hypometabolism.[133]

In a systematic PET-CT correlative data analysis, Furlan et al[37] documented that the final outcome (infarction or preserved integrity) of the penumbral tissue was indeed variable from subject to subject and, more importantly, from one region to the next in the same subject. The interpretation provided was that some favorable event (e.g., partial reperfusion) occurred after the PET study to save part or all of the penumbra.

OLIGEMIC TISSUE. Wide areas of oligemic tissue (i.e., with moderately reduced CBF, increased OEF, and normal $CMRO_2$) are occasionally seen surrounding the core of ischemia and the penumbral tissue.[11] Although acutely hypoxic, these areas are generally characterized by favorable tissue outcome.[37]

CLINICAL CORRELATES OF PET FINDINGS

Marchal et al[78,80] conducted a study that systematically and prospectively assessed the relationships between acute-stage PET findings and clinical outcome. They studied 30 patients and compared the changes in CBF and $CMRO_2$ observed 5 to 18 hours after onset of stroke against the subsequent spontaneous neurologic course. They identified three distinct patterns of PET changes into which each patient could be classified as follows: (1) *pattern 1* (Plate 6.2) was characterized by a large subcorticocortical area of already extensive necrosis (see above); (2) *pattern 2* (Plate 6.1) was consistent with cortical penumbra and absent or only deep-seated established necrosis; and (3) *pattern 3* (Plate 6.3) was characterized by hyperperfusion with either essentially normal $CMRO_2$, or only a very limited area of profound hypometabolism. There was a statistically highly significant relationship between PET patterns and neurologic recovery. Thus, all patients classified as pattern 1 did poorly (death from massive infarct, or poor outcome with recovery index <25%), and all patients classified as pattern 3 did well (recovery index >75%); patients classified as pattern 2 had a highly variable course, ranging from death to full recovery. This predictive value of PET patterns 1 and 3 remained statistically significant even when initial neurologic scores were taken into account in the model such that PET better predicted outcome than neurologic scores, especially so for intermediate severity scores.

These findings are important because they demonstrated for the first time that the long-documented clinical variability in stroke prognosis is subtended by comparable heterogeneity at the pathophysiologic level, and that it is possible with PET performed in the acute stage to predict the individual clinical outcome accurately for two of three CBF-$CMRO_2$ patterns. Another conclusion from that study was that early spontaneous reperfusion appears to be beneficial, whereas the unpredictable outcome associated with pattern 2 suggested that the ischemic tissue progressed to necrosis to some variable extent subsequent to the PET study. Furthermore, the volume of the eventually noninfarcted penumbral tissue was found to influence subsequent neurologic recovery strongly, documenting that survival of the penumbra is indeed a key determinant of neurologic recovery after stroke[37] (see the section Mechanisms of Recovery below).

IMPLICATIONS FOR CLINICAL MANAGEMENT AND CLINICAL TRIALS

Demonstration of misery perfusion (high OEF) in the setting of acute stroke implies that the autoregulation of CBF has been over-ridden in the affected territory. This finding is especially important in view of the frequent occurrence of reactive arterial hypertension in this clinical setting. Thus, any lowering of the systemic arterial pressure (SAP) is likely to reduce the CPP further and, in turn, the CBF, in the affected tissue, effects that can be potentially damaging if the tissue was already penumbral. This may explain why reductions of SAP in acute stroke are associated with poorer outcome.[56] Accordingly, pharmacologic increases of SAP in instances of marked misery perfusion were associated in at least one patient with increased CBF in the penumbra together with an improvement in oxygen metabolism; clinical outcome was excellent in this case.[2] In another patient, studied at day 4 after stroke, the increase in SAP resulted in a marked elevation of CBF in the affected area but was associated with an inverse change in OEF of the same magnitude, without improvement either in $CMRO_2$ or the clinical deficit.[143] However, the $CMRO_2$ in this case was already well below the above-mentioned infarction threshold, and the tissue outcome at day 4 was presumably already settled.

If *low OEF with hyperfusion* (absolute luxury perfusion) is found, management of arterial hypertension may be warranted, particularly if early edema is demonstrated by CT or MRI. Experimental studies suggest that hyperperfusion in necrotic tissue may promote the development of malignant brain swelling. However, this remains to be documented in humans.

Regarding patient screening for clinical trials, the available data suggest the following tentative guidelines[15]: (1) the finding of *hyperfusion* earlier than 18 hours after onset suggests that spontaneous recanalization has already occurred and almost invariably predicts good outcome; thus, these patients need not be entered into therapeutic trials, although whether antioxidants may further reduce tissue damage is a remote possibility; (2) the finding of *a large volume of irreversibly damaged tissue*, when observed <6 hours after onset, suggests poor outcome with a great risk of massive brain swelling and early death. Patients with this profile should similarly be excluded a priori from therapeutic trials. However, because vasogenic edema in itself could cause further tissue damage in the penumbra, this category of patients might benefit from early preventive antiedema therapy with or without surgical brain decompression; and (3) the finding of *high OEF, low CBF but relatively preserved CMRO$_2$* suggests that penumbral tissue is still present. As patients with this pattern have an unpredictable spontaneous outcome, and their potential for recovery depends on the extent of penumbra, they would be the best candidates for trials of neuroprotective agents; furthermore, that this pattern has been observed up to 18 hours after stroke onset suggests that the concept of a rigid (e.g., <6 hours) therapeutic window may have to be reconsidered.[15] However, patients with misery perfusion should be spared any untoward reduction of the SAP as a side effect of the agent being investigated (see above).

Time Course of Changes in CBF and Oxygen Metabolism in Subacute Cerebral Infarction

One almost invariable finding is that of luxury perfusion in the necrotic tissue, starting as early as the 2nd or 3rd day and lasting for several weeks.[16,43,74] During this phase, the CBF increases progressively and often reaches normal or above-normal values around the 8th to 12th day, with a resulting loss of sensitivity. The focal OEF varies in a mirror fashion, falling to very low values around the 10th day. This rise in CBF takes place without any significant increase, and in most cases with a further decline, in CMRO$_2$, indicating useless reperfusion in an irreversibly damaged tissue and presumably reflecting neovascularization with abnormal flow-metabolism regulation. In established infarction, a positive linear correlation exists between local CBF and the magnitude of CT contrast enhancement, indicating leakage of proteins through a damaged blood-brain barrier.[8]

In areas surrounding the infarct, mild physiologic changes are seen in the subacute phase in over 75% of the cases.[11] Thus, luxury perfusion may persist for several days in the areas surrounding the final infarct associated with either normal or only mildly decreased CMRO$_2$.[11] Misery perfusion may be seen in ultimately viable areas as late as the 12th day.[11,116] In a number of instances, CMRO$_2$ was reduced despite a mildly increased OEF, suggesting the superimposition of mild oligemia on a background of synaptic depression, presumably reflecting selective neuronal loss or deafferentation (see the section Remote Metabolic Effects and Their Clinical Correlates below).

Following this subacute phase, the infarcted area progressively takes its final appearance: that of close to zero CBF and CMRO$_2$. This process of cavitation lasts about 2 months, during which the CBF slowly falls while the OEF returns to baseline. The surrounding tissue often exhibits normal CBF and CMRO$_2$, but in many cases a matched decrease in CBF and CMRO$_2$ affects widely remote areas (see the section Remote Metabolic Effects and Their Clinical Correlates below). Finally, in patients with minor stroke and persistent carotid or MCA stenosis/occlusion, protracted hemodynamic impairment is occasionally encountered (see the section Carotid Artery Obstructive Disease below).

The Coupling Among CBF, CMRO$_2$, and Brain Glucose Utilization

Using ^{13}NH$_3$ as a perfusion tracer and ^{18}FDG to measure CMRGlc, Kuhl et al[62] found two opposite patterns of uncoupling among these two variables in early infarcts. Initially, ^{13}N uptake was low but ^{18}FDG uptake was relatively preserved, suggesting persistent ischemia with enhanced anaerobic glycolysis; later the data suggested reperfusion within the hypometabolic tissue. However, firm conclusions cannot be drawn from such data because of uncertainties with applying the ^{18}FDG model in recent infarcts. In three studies, both CMRO$_2$ and CMRGlc were measured.[9,43,144] Preservation of CMRGlc relative to CMRO$_2$ was observed within the core of the infarct, implying enhanced anaerobic glycolysis; as luxury perfusion was constant, anaerobic glycolysis occurred in the face of tissue hyperoxia, inferring that mechanisms other than hypoxia were at play. By contrast, Hakim et al[43] observed preserved CMRGlc/CMRO$_2$ coupling in acutely ischemic tissue, despite local acidosis. Finally, zones of depressed CMRGlc but preserved CMRO$_2$ immediately surrounding the area of tissue damage have been reported, suggesting that substrates other than blood-borne glucose were oxidized for energy production in this tissue.[9] The evidence for a disruption of the CMRGlc/CMRO$_2$ coupling suggests that the measurement of glucose utilization does not reliably reflect the tissue's synaptic activity in recent stroke. These findings presumably explain, in part, the weak correlations reported between neurologic outcome and ipsilateral hemisphere CMRGlc.[66]

Studies of Tissue pH

Using ^{11}C-DMO, Syrota et al[130] found markedly increased intracellular pH in subacute carotid artery infarcts. Since combined ^{15}O studies revealed prominent luxury perfusion in the affected brain area in these four patients, the results exclude tissue acidosis as the causal factor of luxury perfusion. Because the degree of alkalosis was correlated with the decrease in local OEF, the hypothesis was advanced that perfusion in excess of local metabolic demand could have triggered tissular tissue alkalosis by removing the metabolically produced CO_2 and, in turn, decreasing the local H^+ content. The intracellular alkalosis observed within the necrotic area could be due to the infiltration of phagocytic cells, using glycolysis to synthesize hydrogen peroxide. Hakim et al[43] reported a normal pH in the core of reperfused infarction, but this result may have reflected the more acutely studied nature of the patients, or that the ^{11}C-DMO method used provided only whole-tissue pH. In patients with hypoperfusion, Hakim et al[43] reported a reduced pH, indicating tissue acidosis unrelated to enhanced anaerobic glycolysis, which was ruled out by a normal CMRGlc/CMRO$_2$ ratio. Using the ^{11}CO$_2$-whole-tissue pH method, Senda et al[122] also observed tissue acidosis in hypoperfused, acutely ischemic tissue; in less acute conditions, and in the setting of hyperperfusion and lowered OEF, these authors found an increased pH, in agreement with earlier findings.

PET Studies of Other Markers of Neuronal Death and Glial Proliferation

Sette et al[126] conducted a series of studies in baboons with temporary MCA occlusion to assess the relative sensitivity of the two BZ radioligands ^{11}C-flumazenil and ^{11}C-PK 11195 as markers of neuronal membranes and microglial/macrophagic proliferation, respectively. They found that, in the areas destined to infarction as assessed by chronic stage CT, significant reductions in ^{11}C-flumazenil–specific binding were already observed as early as 24 hours after the insult, with sensibility maintained thereafter, whereas increased ^{11}C-PK 11195–specific binding only developed after 1 week and was only a transient phenomenon (as also reported in a case study by Ramsey et al[118]). This study indicated that ^{11}C-flumazenil could be a useful indicator of early neuronal damage after stroke.[129] One further argument supporting this view was that of specificity, as ^{11}C-flumazenil uptake was not significantly altered in hypometabolic areas remote from the site of infarction (i.e., diaschitic but undamaged). One limitation of the approach, however, is its poor sensitivity to subcortical damage, due to the very low density of central BZ receptors outside the cortical mantle. Also, it is unknown how early after stroke this method is able to document neuronal damage.

Remote Metabolic Effects and Their Clinical Correlates

Remote metabolic effects are widely explained as depressed synaptic activity at sites distant from, but neurally connected with (either directly or transneurally), the damaged area.[14,33,95] As such, they allow one to map the disruption in distributed networks as a result of focal infarction. Although they are often referred to collectively as *diaschisis*,[33] behind this term is concealed a variety of cellular derangements, from reversible hypofunction to evolving degeneration, which all have the same PET expression.[4] Because some of these effects may represent purely functional (i.e., potentially recoverable) trans-synaptic derangement, and thus may participate in both the acute clinical expression of and the subsequent recovery from stroke, they have attracted considerable interest over the last 15 years.

CROSSED CEREBELLAR DIASCHISIS

Description and Mechanisms

Crossed cerebellar diaschisis (CCD), a striking phenomenon, affects the cerebellar hemisphere contralateral to supratentorial stroke[5] (Fig. 6.2). It occurs in about 50% of patients with either cortical or subcortical stroke but is more frequent and severe the larger the frontoparietal infarcts and with subcortical lesions affecting the internal capsule, including posterior limb lacunes.[55,65,74,83,89,92,97,101,123] These and other topographic correlations suggest that CCD results from damage to the corticopontocerebellar system (CPCS), inducing transneuronal functional depression.[5,36] Although CCD is correlated with both the presence and severity of hemiparesis, this association is not systematic, indicating that damage to the pyramidal system is neither necessary nor sufficient to induce CCD and presumably simply reflects the proximity of the pyramidal and the corticopontine fibers.[5,97] Furthermore, CCD has been reported after unilateral damage to the CPCS at the level of the crus cerebri or basis pontis.[32,119,135]

Time Course

In the vast majority of patients, CCD exhibits no tendency for recovery, and this chronicity suggests CCD might evolve into transneuronal degeneration in the long run.[74,92,97] However, that CCD may develop within the first hours of stroke and subsequently disappear within a few days indicates that it can be one acute manifestation of deafferentation and may not unavoidably precede degeneration.[5,67,92,124] This view is further documented by the fact that CCD can manifest transiently during transient ischemic attacks,[105] unilateral carotid infusion of barbiturates in epileptic patients,[64] or balloon occlusion of the internal carotid artery.[20] Finally, even in cases with chronic CCD, crossed cerebellar atrophy is not demonstrated by MRI,[100] even though ipsilateral atrophy of the cerebral peduncle is occasionally seen, which further documents CPCS damage.[107]

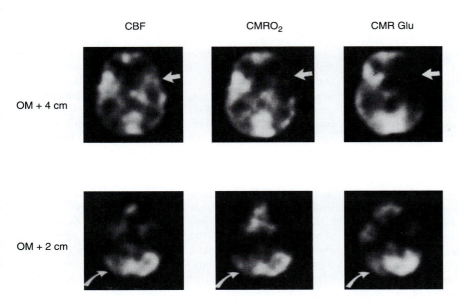

CBF CMRO₂ CMR Glu

OM + 4 cm

OM + 2 cm

Figure 6.2 Quantitative images of cerebral blood flow (CBF), cerebral metabolic rate of oxygen (CMRO₂), and cerebral metabolic rate of glucose (CMRGlc) obtained at two brain levels in a 37-year-old patient 6 days after massive right MCA infarction due to cardiac embolism. On these images, the right side of the brain is on the reader's right. The data show on level OM + 4 cm a profoundly reduced CMRO₂ and CMRGlc in the infarcted area associated with a heterogeneous CBF showing combined areas of markedly reduced, moderately reduced, and increased flow (luxury perfusion, straight arrows); on level OM + 2 cm, a proportional reduction in flow, oxygen consumption, and glucose utilization in the entire left cerebellar hemisphere (crossed cerebellar diaschisis, curved arrows), demonstrating primary metabolic depression, is seen. This is a remote transneuronal effect of right MCA infarction, which damages the crossed corticoponto-cerebellar pathway. (Adapted from Baron et al,[9] with permission.)

Clinical Correlates

Although a relationship between CCD and ipsilateral ataxia has been anecdotally reported,[16,42,119] other reports suggest a lack of both sensitivity and specificity of CCD for ataxia.[101] It appears that a strong link between CCD and ataxia holds only when a retrograde mechanism for CCD is likely, such as in lateral thalamic infarction.[132] Apart from ataxia, a significant relationship has been reported between CCD and ipsilateral flaccidity,[98] but again this was not a one-to-one association; the observed relationship appeared to be in fact indirect, reflecting striatal damage.[99] In the acute stage of MCA territory stroke, CCD is not a reliable predictor of outcome.[123,124] However, on an individual basis, all patients without significant CCD made an excellent recovery, suggesting that the lack of CCD in the acute stage may help predict good outcome.[123,124]

CONTRALATERAL CEREBRAL HYPOMETABOLISM

Widely hypothesized as transcallosal in nature, the classic phenomenon of contralateral cerebral hypometabolism has attracted great interest as it may underlie some "diffuse" symp-toms of acute supratentorial stroke such as agitation, confusion, and coma; it may also exacerbate the initial focal deficit.[3,33] However, it has proved difficult to document in either humans or the animals in the acute stage.[3] Quite unexpectedly, metabolism in the contralateral hemisphere appears to reach its lowest level several days after stroke onset.[52,74,103] Early PET studies of this effect in heterogeneous samples of carotid territory stroke patients were inconsistent,[74,145] presumably because confounding factors such as subject's age, lesion topography, and underlying large vessel occlusion were not considered, while comparison with controls not matched for prestroke cerebrovascular risk factors is now considered inappropriate.[145] Furthermore, studies that used CBF to evaluate this phenomenon in acutely ill patients were limited by the dependence of this parameter on extracerebral physiologic variables, such as PaCO₂ or hematocrit.[30] In patients with unilateral thalamic stroke, however, a significant reduction in contralateral cortical glucose utilization has been repeatedly shown[10,68,131]; furthermore, this effect was found to develop following VL-Vim nucleus thalamotomy, compared with preoperative status[13] and to recover monoexponentially in parallel with the clinical improvement.[14] A study in anterior circulation ischemic stroke that controlled for most of the above-mentioned confounding factors also revealed a significantly reduced contralateral CBF in the subacute stage, but this effect did not correlate with the subject's lethargy score.[30]

Previously, Lenzi et al[74] had reported a significant contralateral hemispheric hypometabolism in MCA stroke patients with impairment of consciousness occurring a few days after onset, possibly in relation to brain swelling. Likewise, Heiss et al[47] reported reduced contralateral hemisphere CMRGlc in the subacute stage of MCA stroke, which to some extent predicted poor subsequent recovery. Recently, however, Iglesias et al[52] reported no correlation between the degree and time course of contralateral cerebral CMRO$_2$ and either initial neurologic deficit or recovery therefrom, suggesting that the level of contralateral metabolism plays little or no part in the clinical expression of acute stroke. Overall, therefore, the presently available data suggest that contralateral cerebral hypometabolism does not develop acutely after MCA territory stroke (as also documented in baboon models of MCA occlusion) but may slowly creep in within the first week and recover partly thereafter, an effect presumably related to transcallosal fiber degeneration that lacks clear clinical implications thus far.[102,134,152] Conversely, the contralateral cerebral effect after unilateral thalamic stroke, which is fairly well established, may be involved in functional recovery (see the section Mechanisms of Recovery below).

SUBCORTICAL EFFECTS

Subcortical Aphasia

Metter et al[85,86] described four patients with subcortical stroke and the association of aphasia and hypometabolism of the left cortical mantle and suggested that some aspects of the language impairment could be related to this remote effect. In patients with verbal memory impairment and left thalamic or thalamocapsular stroke, Baron et al[10] similarly reported significant ipsilateral neocortical hypometabolism (Fig. 6.3). Metter et al[90] subsequently reported that although the subcortical lesion itself did have a direct relationship with some of the aphasic measures, left frontal and temporal hypometabolism indirectly played a role in verbal fluency and comprehension tasks, respectively. Likewise, positive correlations between impairment in several aphasic items (oral and written comprehension, naming, and repetition) and left parietotemporal hypometabolism have been documented.[58] In the special case of insular cortex hypometabolism overlying large striatocapsular infarcts, direct ischemic neuronal damage of the insula may, however, occasionally partly sustain language impairment.[141]

Recovery from subcortical aphasia or pure alexia is generally associated with a return toward normality of cortical hypometabolism,[10,13,128] although discrepancies at the individual level do occur.[13] Patients with lesser defects in resting CMRGlc around Wernicke's and Broca's areas in the subacute stage of stroke have better outcomes in terms of language comprehension and verbal fluency, respectively[59]; likewise, performing the PET study during a language activation task may allow an improved prediction of subsequent recovery from aphasia.[46]

Subcortical Neglect

In right-sided subcortical infarcts with left hemineglect, a marked ipsilateral cortical hypometabolism has been consistently reported.[10,34,104] Predominance of these effects over the frontal and parietal cortices, especially in the case of motor neglect, with relative sparing of the primary motor circuit (striatum, cerebellum, and motor strip) and a relative impairment of a supramotor circuit (premotor, prefrontal, and cingulate and parietal cortices), suggests involvement of Mesulam's subcorticocortical network of directed attention, which involves parieto-frontal interactions.[34,41]

Hemianopia

Damage to the optic radiations as a result of MCA territory stroke induces a significant reduction in glucose utilization in the disconnected part of the ipsilateral primary visual cor-

Figure 6.3 (**A**) Computed tomography scan and (**B & C**) positron emission tomography (PET) images obtained in a 57-year-old woman 2 months following a left paramedian thalamic infarct associated with persisting impairment in verbal fluency and memory. The PET images of cerebral glucose utilization, obtained at the levels of the corona radiata (**B**) and of the basal ganglia (**C**) show significant metabolic depression affecting the entire cortical mantle on the side of the thalamic infarct. (The left side of the images corresponds to the left side of the brain.)

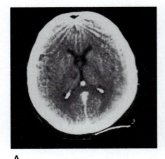
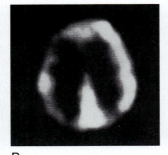
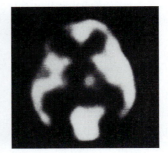

A   B   C

tex,[17,22,62,108] sometimes spreading to the visual association areas[108] and even to the contralateral visual cortex.[60]

Thalamocortical Diaschisis

PET studies have demonstrated that even small unilateral infarcts in the anterior, medial, or lateral thalamus often induce a metabolic depression of the entire ipsilateral cortical mantle[10,13,19,68,100,131] (Fig. 6.3). Accentuation of this diffuse effect in the projection area corresponding to the apparent nuclear topography of the thalamic infarct suggests involvement of the excitatory thalamocortical fibers.[10] In addition to the ipsilateral cortex, the metabolic depression also affects—albeit to a lesser degree—the contralateral cortical ribbon.[10,13,68,131] As the magnitude of ipsilateral neocortical hypometabolism significantly correlates with the severity of global cognitive impairment,[13] and cognitively intact patients with posterolateral thalamic infarcts exhibit no significant cortical metabolic impairment,[23] a link between cognitive impairment and cortical hypometabolism after thalamic stroke has been suggested. In addition to the above-noted relationships between the pattern of cortical hypometabolism and the aphasia or hemineglect profile, more specific cognitive-metabolic patterns also emerge. For instance, a syndrome of verbal amnesia and anhedonia after left anteropolar thalamic infarct has been related to preferential hypometabolism of the amygdala and posterior cingulate cortex.[25] However, dissociations between cognitive status and cortical metabolic asymmetry after unilateral thalamic stroke are not exceptional, presumably because asymmetries do not reflect actual bilateral metabolic depression.[13]

Both the bilateral metabolic depression and the cortical asymmetry that follow unilateral thalamic stroke tend to recover monoexponentially over the ensuing months[13,14] in parallel with recovery from cognitive impairment, which is consistent with findings after nonthalamic subcortical stroke.[136] Thus, recovery of cortical metabolism presumably partly underlies functional recovery after subcortical infarction and is one expression of network reorganization after thalamocortical system damage. However, such a capacity appears to be severely limited in the event of bilateral thalamic infarction, which induces long-lasting cortical hypometabolism[75] (see below).

White Matter Infarcts, Leukoaraiosis, Multiple Strategic Infarcts, and Subcortical Dementia

Lacunes of the posterior limb of the internal capsule without neuropsychological sequelae as a rule do not significantly alter cortical metabolism.[71,101] Conversely, in a patient with multiple lacunes and cognitive impairment of the frontal type, Metter et al[88] found left frontal hypometabolism, which they attributed to a lacune in the anterior limb of the left internal capsule, probably interrupting the thalamocortical fibers from the mediodorsal nucleus. Large corona radiata infarcts are also prone to induce hypoperfusion of the overlying cerebral cortex, presumably as a result of disconnection.[49]

In patients with leukoaraiosis, Delpla et al[27] reported a significant, predominantly frontal hypometabolism that was associated with a mild but preferentially frontal-type cognitive impairment. Conversely, cognitively intact subjects (despite extensive white matter T_2 hypersignals at MRI scans) exhibit only a mild and nonsignificant depression of cortical oxygen consumption.[84] Other studies on leukoaraiosis have presented the idea that cortical hypometabolism is prominent only when cognitive impairment is significant.[28] In agreement with this view, there exists in Binswanger's dementia a profound cortical hypometabolism that tends to predominate in the frontal lobe.[35,150] In the bilateral paramedian thalamic infarction syndrome, which includes severe amnesia and apathy, marked neocortical hypometabolism (occasionally with frontal predominance) has similarly been reported consistent with the idea that thalamocortical deafferentation underlies the clinical presentation of thalamic dementia.[75,131]

OTHER REMOTE EFFECTS

PET studies have clearly demonstrated the frequent occurrence of a significant hypometabolism affecting the striatum and the thalamus ipsilateral to subcortical stroke.[6,22,33,62,91,95,100] Striatal hypometabolism resulted preferentially from prerolandic cortical lesions, whereas thalamic hypometabolism sets in only a few days after stroke.[93] Published data suggest that deep nuclei hypometabolism is associated with specific measures of cognitive and language performance,[87,90] whereas left caudal and thalamic hypometabolism are significantly associated with Broca's aphasia, as compared with Wernicke's or conduction aphasia.[91] The cellular basis of striatal and thalamic hypometabolism after superficial infarction is probably different, with the former presumably reflecting loss of glutamatergic input from the cortex and the latter a process of active retrograde degeneration of the damaged thalamocortical neurons.[4]

Mechanisms of Recovery: Insights from PET

Several distinct although presumably synergistic mechanisms are thought to underlie recovery from neurologic impairment after ischemic stroke. Each of these mechanisms seems to have its own time course and to be operational within a distinct time window after stroke. Clinically, neurologic recovery can start as early as hours after onset and be spectacular and rapid; in other cases it can be slow or delayed, or both, occasionally spanning several years. In most instances, however, it has an exponential-like shape, usually reaching close to final values within 4 to 6 months. Although across subjects final outcome is well correlated to early neurologic score, the relationship is unreliable at the individual level—except if the initial deficit is either very mild or very severe. This is not the place to review all the putative mechanisms of recovery, and the reader is referred to dedicated overviews.[33,55] Here I address three mechanisms that have been more specifically assessed using the PET technology. Two of them, alleviation of penumbra and alleviation of remote metabolic effects, have already been alluded to above. The last mechanism, which concerns the

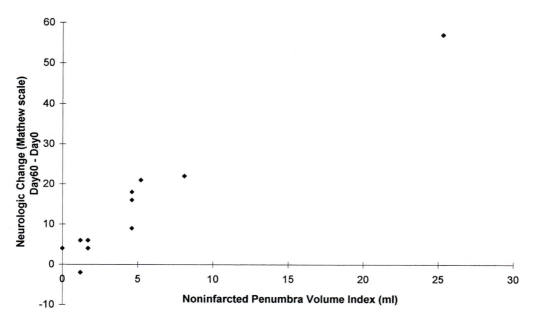

Figure 6.4 Graph showing the relationship between neurologic recovery (expressed in absolute changes in Mathew scale scores between day 0 and day 60) and the volume of ultimately noninfarcted penumbra, as determined in a sample of 11 survivors from acute ischemic stroke in the middle cerebral artery all studied by PET within 18 hours of stroke onset and in whom a CT scan was performed 1 to 2 months later to determine the boundaries of the final infarct. This relationship is highly significant by nonparametric rank correlation ($P = 0.00003$) and documents that the fate of the ischemic penumbra is a major determinant of early neurologic recovery after ischemic stroke. (From Furlan et al,[37] with permission.)

reorganization of cortical maps, is described below in some detail.

ALLEVIATION OF PENUMBRA

Alleviation of penumbra (Fig. 6.4) has long been hypothesized as one major mechanism underlying early recovery from ischemic stroke.[33,55,96] The subsequent finding that early hyperperfusion is invariably associated with good outcome was interpreted as further evidence for this hypothesis.[78,80,82] However, this mechanism was only recently documented quantitatively in a prospective and longitudinal fashion by Furlan et al.[37] In 11 patients with MCA territory stroke evaluated by PET within 18 hours of onset, these authors found that the extent of subsequent neurologic recovery was highly linearly correlated to the individual volume of acute stage penumbral tissue that ultimately escaped infarction, as assessed with chronic stage CT. Somewhat unexpectedly, the best correlations were observed with 2-month recovery scores, which suggests that survival of the penumbra influences not only early, but also late, recovery. One hypothesis put forward by the authors to explain this finding was that survival of the penumbra not only allowed for early return of function in the peri-infarct tissue, but also provided an important opportunity for subsequent neural reorganization processes, in a synergistic rather than simply cumulative way.[37] Thus, survival of the

penumbra would appear to be the most important early mechanism for subsequent functional recovery.

ALLEVIATION OF REMOTE METABOLIC DEPRESSION

As described above, the only remote metabolic effect that regularly exhibits either full or partial reversal with time is neocortical hypometabolism after unilateral subcortical stroke. Several studies have documented that, across subjects, this return toward more symmetric neocortical metabolism parallels the remarkable recovery from neurologic or cognitive impairment that often follows subcortical infarcts, although quantitative correlations between these two variables have yet to be reported.[7,13,14,18,106,136] This parallel improvement has been particularly well documented after unilateral thalamic or juxtathalamic stroke inducing verbal or visual spatial impairment,[7,13,14,106,136] but it has also been seen in variously located subcortical lesions, such as in patients with reversible lateral homonymous hemianopia (including one patient with reversible pure alexia) due to white matter infarction.[18,128] Recovery of neocortical hypometabolism implies a mechanism of synaptic plasticity at the level of deafferented neocortical fields, in relation to, for example, sprouting of undamaged, excitatory thalamocortical neurons (reactivating the postsynaptic neuron) or reorganization of postsynaptic circuits, or both.[33] This considerable capacity for thalamocortical system plasticity in the adult human brain may be probed by evaluating the response of the neocortex ipsilateral to and surrounding the infarct to behavioral activation. Thus, Heiss et al[46] found that the extent of increase in CMRGlc in the peri-infarcted tissue in patients with subchronic aphasia performing a verbal comprehension and expression task was well correlated with subsequent language recovery. More generally, the more severe the metabolic defect in the subacute stage of stroke, the poorer the neurologic outcome[46]; specifically, severe resting hypometabolism around Wernicke's and Broca's areas was associated with poor outcome in terms of language comprehension and verbal fluency, respectively.[59]

At variance with the ipsilateral neocortical hypometabolism, neither the contralateral cerebellar nor the contralateral cerebral metabolic effects have been shown to abate in parallel with early neurologic recovery.[52,123,124] This finding suggests that both are epiphenomena that only reflect the severity of damage in the affected hemisphere. However, long-term increments in contralateral cerebral metabolism have been reported, although the implications of this finding in long-term recovery remain unclear.[14,103,106]

REORGANIZATION OF CORTICAL MAPS

As described above, studying *resting* brain metabolism after stroke provides maps of integrated synaptic disruption spatially distant from the actual focus of damage and reflecting deafferentation/de-efferentation-induced neuronal death, selective synapse loss, synaptic dysfunction, and/or neurotransmitter imbalance. As such, mapping the changes over time in these metabolic effects may provide insight into the pre- and postsynaptic neurobiologic adaptive mechanisms that influence functional recovery, such as with the above-described metabolic increments in the neocortex ipsilateral to subcortical lesions occurring in parallel with neuropsychological improvement. However, studies in the resting state do not provide information on the changes in selective neural networks specifically underlying a given behavioral process during the course of recovery.

This can now be investigated according to the so-called PET activation paradigm, which allows one to isolate the brain regions involved in a specific neural process by subtracting the cerebral perfusion images obtained during a given behavioral task from those obtained either during rest or during a lower-level task. Although this paradigm is in its principles extremely attractive in that it allows one to investigate reorganization of large-scale neural networks in relation to recovery, it has proved extremely difficult to implement for the investigation of the recovery process. This is so because until recently it was applicable only to groups of subjects, implying that it was impossible to control adequately for several potentially confounding factors that may affect the individual recovery process (e.g., topography and age of infarct, subject's age and gender, premorbid brain organization and hemispheric dominance, personal behavioral strategy). Indeed, to assemble a sample of patients identical in each one of these clinical aspects would be almost impossible. Although until recently this limitation has greatly impeded research, the recent implementation of individual activation mapping should resolve this issue. However, other problems arise with the statistical analysis, such as what should constitute the control group is not always clear.

Two other issues complicate the application of the activation paradigm to the study of recovery processes, either with the group or with the individual type of analysis. One relates to the fact that unless one studies only fully recovered subjects the task performance during scanning is by definition impaired, and thus the comparison to normally performing controls may not be appropriate. Although the group of controls may be asked to perform equally poorly, this may not constitute an appropriate behavioral match. The second issue relates to the very nature of mechanistic studies of recovery, which ideally require one to compare in a longitudinal fashion the *changes* in brain activation maps with the concomitant *changes* in behavioral performance, according to a prospective, quantitative design; unless this is done, interpretation of findings from transversal studies are of uncertain significance in terms of recovery mechanisms. At the time of writing this chapter, no PET study fulfilling all these requirements has appeared in peer-reviewed journals. In what follows, I summarize the main findings from the available PET literature on activation studies in relation to recovery.

Motor Recovery

In a group of patients with complete to near-complete recovery from hemiparesis (either left- or right-sided) studied <2 months after stroke, Chollet et al[24] reported that sequential finger-to-thumb opposition of the recovered hand induced *bilateral* activation of the sensorimotor cortex and the cerebellum, whereas movement of the unaffected hand induced essentially contralateral activation; in addition, motion of the recovered hand also activated bilaterally the insula, inferior parietal, and premotor cortices. In a subsequent similar study on 10 patients recovering from striatocapsular hemiparesis, this time comparing the results with control subjects, Weiller et al[139] confirmed the finding of abnormal activation of the ipsilateral motor, insular, parietal, prefrontal, and cingulate cortices. Some of these changes may represent recruitment of both the contralateral motor system—possibly responsible for the contralateral synkinesias observed in these patients—and a left-sided attentional motor system, as in this sample most strokes were in the nondominant hemisphere. Such a bilateral activation of the motor cortex has also been reported in five patients by Weder et al,[138] although the use of a heavily sensory-weighted paradigm and the lack of control data in this work made interpretation of the findings somewhat uncertain.

Subsequent studies, also carried out in capsular stroke patients with complete motor recovery but this time according to the individual paradigm, documented that this activation of the motor pathways ipsilateral to the recovered hand was in fact inconsistent from patient to patient, and that its presence was related to the occurrence of synkinesias.[140] In contrast to these inconsistent activations in the inappropriate hemisphere, one feature common to half the patients in this sample was a ventral extension into the face area of the hand field of the contralateal (i.e., appropriate) sensory-motor cortex, together with an excessive activation of the supplementary motor, insular, frontal opercular, and parietal cortices on the same side.[140] Activation of the face field during hand motion in recovered hemiparetics suggests a considerable reorganization of cortical maps within the motor strip following deafferentation from capsular damage, implying the unmasking of pre-existing but physiologically silent hand muscle-specific connections.[140]

Cognitive Impairment

Weiller et al[142] reported on a group study of six unusual patients who had recovered from Wernicke's aphasia caused by a left posterior temporal infarct. Compared with control subjects, increased activation of right hemisphere language zones, as well as increased activation of the left prefrontal cortex, was observed in the patients during pseudoword repetition and verb generation tasks. All these areas, except a right prefrontal area, were already activated, although to a lesser extent, in control subjects, suggesting that in the patients there was a redistribution of activity within the framework of a pre-existing, parallel processing, and bilateral network. However, altered performance in the verb generation task somewhat complicated the interpretation of the findings. Also, because this was a group study that only analyzed those cortical gyri that physically still existed in all the subjects studied, a role for the peri-infarct borders in the recovery process could not be assessed. Likewise, because in that study the controls were much younger than the patients, changes in the activation pattern due to aging per se could not be completely excluded. In one rare patient with partial recovery from auditory agnosia due to bilateral perisylvian strokes, Engelien et al[31] reported individual changes in the brain activation pattern during categorization of environmental sounds (compared with passive listening) of the same nature as Weiller et al's[142] findings just described (i.e., bilateral activation with recruitment of areas homologous to those in the left hemisphere known to be responsible for normal function); in addition, these authors were able to document an abnormal engagement of peri-infarct regions in the left hemisphere, suggesting plasticity.

The above findings in relation to both motor and cognitive paradigms concur in suggesting that following unilateral brain infarction regions in the hemisphere contralateral to the lesion are abnormally recruited during performance of the recovered functions; however, as this effect seemingly represents an exaggeration of the normal response, it may only reflect a differential distribution of activation in a pre-existing bilateral network rather than truly plasticity changes. It has not been shown to be quantitatively related to recovery according to a longitudinal design. However, these changes in the contralateral hemisphere fit well with the long-suspected role of this hemisphere in recovery from hemiparesis or aphasia, which was based until now on clinical observations only. Over and above these effects in the contralateral hemisphere, changes in the affected hemisphere also occur, involving not only parts of the networks distant from the damaged or deafferented area, but seemingly also the tissue immediately surrounding the infarcted cortex, which may represent the initially penumbral but ultimately noninfarcted tissue (see the section Alleviation of Penumbra). However, the same comments as to the lack of a longitudinal, prospective study also apply here. Finally, the presumably tight topographic and temporal relationships between patterns of abnormal activations and depressed

metabolism in the resting state have scarcely been addressed thus far.

Carotid Artery Obstructive Disease

Since the first report in 1981 of misery perfusion in a patient with carotid artery occlusion and continuing reversible ischemic attacks,[7] PET studies have repeatedly documented that internal carotid artery disease may have hemodynamic consequences on the distal cerebral vascular bed.[38,54,73,110,113,120,146] Overall, these investigations have shown that the severity of such effects is related both to the degree of obstruction (i.e., only >50% stenosis or occlusion may have measurable effects) and to the compensation afforded by the circle of Willis (with the most marked effects seen when compensation is essentially or exclusively from the ipsilateral ophthalmic artery). Similar effects have been reported in patients with long-standing MCA stem stenosis or occlusion.[109] The hemodynamic effects observed, which reflect the extent to which the CPP is reduced, range from simple autoregulation (i.e., tapping the *hemodynamic reserve*, with normal resting CBF but increased CBV, reduced CBF/CBV ratio, and reduced vasodilatory capacity to CO_2 or acetazolamide stress) to true oligemia (i.e., tapping the *perfusion reserve*, with reduced resting CBF, increased OEF, increased CBV, markedly reduced CBF/CBV ratio, and abolished vasodilatory capacity with occasional hemodynamic steal).[76,77] Whatever their severity, these changes, as expected, are pressure dependent[121] and in many cases predominate in watershed territories[6,72,120,147]; for controversial findings, see ref. 21. Furthermore, focal chronic misery perfusion has been documented to forerun the development of watershed infarction in occasional patients with tight carotid artery stenosis or occlusion.[53,148]

Although the clinical correlates of these hemodynamic changes can be straightforward, as in the rare instances of orthostatic transient ischemic attacks, in many instances they are difficult to ascertain.[7] Furthermore, hemodynamic abnormalities can be found in asymptomatic subjects or in the asymptomatic hemisphere of symptomatic subjects. Although in the early 1980s the documentation of a clear-cut compromise of brain circulation was considered the only rational basis for extra-intracranial arterial bypass (EIAB), this surgical procedure has now been largely abandoned due to lack of demonstrated clinical benefit.[7,39,72,109,120] Consistent with this, the retrospective nonrandomized studies of Powers et al[114,115] suggested that the finding of hemodynamic compromise accurately predicted neither poor outcome if medical therapy was elected, nor good outcome if EIAB was performed. However, several recent studies now suggest that, if cerebrovascular reactivity is severely impaired, there is an increased risk of ipsilateral stroke despite best medical treatment.[29,61,63,137,149,151]

It has been repeatedly shown that successful cerebral revascularization by means of either carotid endarterectomy or EIAB at least partially reverses the preoperatively observed hemodynamic compromise, documenting that the latter truly results from carotid artery obstruction and not from distal bed disease such as watershed microembolic angiopathy.[7,39,40,51,73,94,109,120] However, it has also been suggested that patients with the most compromised cerebrovascular physiology may also be those most at risk of perioperative complications such as low-pressure breakthrough of autoregulation (presumably as a result of long-term dysregulation of the cerebral circulation).[29] Thus, the results from PET, transcranial Doppler, and angiographic data of each candidate for revascularization surgery need to be weighed carefully to assess the risk/benefit ratio, as well as to tailor the surgical procedure to each case.

Apart from the issue of surgical management, impaired brain hemodynamics in a patient with carotid artery disease should be considered in planning the best medical management. For instance, systemic hypotension (as a result of drug therapy or any surgical procedure, especially cardiac) should be carefully avoided in such cases. Conversely, because embolic events may have more serious tissue consequences in a dysregulated vascular bed than they would in the normal brain, medical measures to prevent embolism should also be considered.

References

1. Ackerman RH, Correia JA, Alpert NM et al: Positron imaging in ischemic stroke disease using compounds labelled with oxygen-15. Arch Neurol 38:537–543, 1981

2. Ackerman RH, Lev MH, Mackay BC et al: PET studies in acute stroke: findings and relevance to therapy. J Cereb Blood Flow Metab, suppl. 1, 9:S359, 1989

3. Andrews RJ: Transhemispheric diaschisis, a review and comment. Stroke 22:943–949, 1991

4. Baron JC: Testing cerebral function: will it help the understanding or diagnosis of CNS disease. CIBA Found Symp 163:250–264, 1991

5. Baron JC, Bousser MG, Comar D, Castaigne P: "Crossed cerebellar diaschisis" in human supratentorial brain infarction. Trans Am Neurol Assoc 105:459–461, 1980

6. Baron JC, Bousser MG, Comar D et al: Noninvasive tomographic study of cerebral blood flow and oxygen metabolism in vivo: potentials, limitations and clinical applications in cerebral ischemic disorders. Eur Neurol 20:273–284, 1981

7. Baron JC, Bousser MG, Rey A et al: Reversal of focal "misery-perfusion syndrome" by extra-intracranial arterial bypass in hemodynamic cerebral ischemia: a case study with [15]O positron tomography. Stroke 12:454–459, 1981

8. Baron JC, Delattre JY, Chiras J et al: Comparison study of CT and positron emission tomographic data in recent cerebral infarction. AJNR 4:536–540, 1983

9. Baron JC, Rougemont D, Soussaline F et al: Local interrelationships of cerebral oxygen consumption and glucose utilization in normal subjects and in ischemic stroke patients: a positron tomography study. J Cereb Blood Flow Metab 4:140–149, 1984

10. Baron JC, D'Antona R, Pantano P et al: Effects of thalamic stroke on energy metabolism of the cerebral cortex. Brain 109:1243–1259, 1986

11. Baron JC, Samson Y, Pantano P et al: Interrelationships of local CBF, OEF and $CMRO_2$ in ischemic areas with variable outcome: further PET studies in humans. J Cereb Blood Flow Metab, suppl. 1, 7:41, 1987

12. Baron JC, Frackowiak RSJ, Herholz K et al: Use of positron emission tomography in the investigation of cerebral hemodynamics and energy metabolism in cerebrovascular disease. J Cereb Blood Flow Metab 9:723–742, 1989

13. Baron JC, Levasseur M, Mazoyer B et al: Thalamo-cortical diaschisis: PET study in humans. J Neurol Neurosurg Psychiatry, 55:935–942, 1992

14. Baron JC, Levasseur M, Mazoyer B et al: Cortical hypometabolism and neuropsychological impairment in unilateral thalamic lesions. p. 437. In Vallar G et al (ed): Neuropsychological Disorders and Subcortical Lesions. Oxford University Press, New York, 1992

15. Baron JC, Von Kummer R, Del Zoppo GJ: Treatment of acute ischemic stroke. Challenging the concept of a rigid and universal time window. Stroke 26:2219–2221, 1995

16. Bogousslavsky J, Regli F, Delaloye B et al: Hemiataxie et déficit sensitif ipsilateral: infarctus du territoire de l'artère choroïdienne antérieure, diaschisis cérébelleux croisé. Rev Neurol 142:671–676, 1986

17. Bosley T, Rosenquist AC, Kushner M et al: Ischemic lesions of the occipital cortex and optic radiations: positron emission tomography. Neurology 35:470–484, 1985

18. Bosley TM, Dann R, Silver FL et al: Recovery of vision after ischemic lesions: positron emission tomography. Ann Neurol 21:444–450, 1987

19. Boysen G, Hogh P, Pedersen H et al: Thalamic infarcts: effects on cerebral blood flow, metabolism, and neuropsychological function. J Stroke Cerebrovasc Dis 3:81–89, 1993

20. Brunberg JA, Frey KA, Horton JA et al: [15]O]H2O positron emission tomography determination of cerebral blood flow during balloon test occlusion of the internal carotid artery. AJNR 15:725–732, 1994

21. Carpenter DA, Grubb RL, Powers WJ: Border zone hemodynamics in cerebrovascular disease. Neurology 40:1587–1592, 1990

22. Celesia GG, Polcyn RE, Holden JE et al: Determination of regional cerebral blood flow in patients with cerebral infarction—use of fluoromethane labeled with fluorine 18 and positron emission tomography. Arch Neurol 41:262–267, 1984

23. Chabriat H, Levasseur M, Pappata S et al: Cortical energy metabolism in posterolateral thalamic stroke. Acta Neurol Scand 86:285–290, 1992

24. Chollet F, Di Piero V, Wise RJS et al: The functional anatomy of motor recovery after stroke in humans: a study with positron emission tomography. Ann Neurol 29:63–71, 1991

25. Clarke S, Assal G, Bogousslavsky J et al: Pure amnesia after unilateral left polar thalamic infarct: topographic and sequential neuropsychological and metabolic (PET)

correlations. J Neurol Neurosurg Psychiatry 57:27–34, 1994

26. De Ley G, Weyne J, Demeester G et al: Experimental thromboembolic stroke studied by positron emission tomography: immediate versus delayed reperfusion by fibrinolysis. J Cereb Blood Flow Metab 8:539–545, 1988

27. Delpla PA, Zatorre R, Meyer E et al: Leucoaraïose et dysfonctionnement frontal précoce chez le sujet âgé non dément: approche neuropsychologique et par la caméra à positons. p. 123. In Bes A, Géraud G (eds): Cerveau et Hypertension Artérielle. J. Libbey, Paris, 1990

28. De Reuck J, Van Aken J, Decoo D et al: Cerebral blood flow and oxygen metabolism in leuko-araiosis. Cerebrovasc Dis 1:25–30, 1991

29. Derlon JM, Bouvard G, Viader F et al: Impaired cerebral hemodynamics in internal carotid occlusion. Cerebrovas Dis 2:72–81, 1992

30. Dobkin JA, Levine RL, Lagoze HL et al: Evidence for transhemispheric diaschisis in unilateral stroke. Arch Neurol 46:1333–1336, 1989

31. Engelien A, Silbersweig D, Stern E et al: The functional anatomy of recovery from auditory agnosia. A PET study of sound categorization in a neurological patient and normal controls. Brain 118:1395–1409, 1995

32. Fazekas F, Payer F, Valetitsch H et al: Brain stem infarction and diaschisis. A SPECT cerebral perfusion study. Stroke 24:1162–1166, 1993

33. Feeney D, Baron JC: Diaschisis. Stroke 17:817–830, 1986

34. Fiorelli M, Blin J, Bakchine S, Laplane D, Baron JC: PET studies of cortical diaschisis in patients with motor hemi-neglect. J Neurol Sci 104:136–142, 1991

35. Fukuyama H, Doi T, Yamaguchi S et al: Cerebral circulation and metabolism in progressive subcortical arteriosclerotic encephalopathy (Binswanger type) examined by PET. J Cereb Blood Flow Metab, suppl 2.11, S796, 1991

36. Fulham MJ, Brooks RA, Hallett M, Di Chiro G: Cerebellar diaschisis revisited: pontine hypometabolism and dentate sparing. Neurology 42:2267–2273, 1992

37. Furlan M, Marchal G, Viader F et al: Spontaneous neurological recovery after stroke and the fate of the ischemic penumbra. Ann Neurol 40:216–226, 1996

38. Gibbs JM, Wise RJS, Leenders KL, Jones T: Evaluation of cerebral perfusion reserve in patients with carotid-artery occlusion. Lancet 8372:310–314, 1984

39. Gibbs JM, Wise RJS, Mansfield AO et al: Regional cerebral blood flow and blood volume before and after EC-IC bypass surgery and carotid endarterectomy in patients with occlusive carotid disease. J Cereb Blood Flow Metab, suppl. 1, 5:S19–S20, 1985

40. Gibbs JM, Wise RJS, Thomas DJ et al: Cerebral haemodynamic changes after extracranial-intracranial bypass surgery. J Neurol Neurosurg Psychiatry 50:140–150, 1987

41. Giesen HJ von, Schlaug G, Steinmetz H et al: Cerebral network underlying unilateral motor neglect: evidence from positron emission tomography. J Neurol Sci 125:29–38, 1994

42. Giroud M, Creisson E, Fayolle H et al: Homolateral ataxia and crural paresis: a crossed cerebral-cerebellar diaschisis. J Neurol Neurosurg Psychiatry 57:221–222, 1994

43. Hakim AM, Pokrupa RP, Villaneuva J et al: The effects of spontaneous reperfusion on metabolic function in early human cerebral infarcts. Ann Neurol 21:279–289, 1987

44. Hakim AM, Evans AC, Berger L et al: The effect of nimodipine on the evolution of human cerebral infarction studied by PET. J Cereb Blood Flow Metab 9:523–534, 1989

45. Heiss WD, Huber M, Fink GR et al: Progressive derangement of periinfarct viable tissue in ischemic stroke. J Cereb Blood Flow Metab 12:193–203, 1992

46. Heiss WD, Kessler J, Karbe H et al: Cerebral glucose metabolism as a predictor of recovery from aphasia in ischemic stroke. Arch Neurol 50:958–964, 1993

47. Heiss WD, Emunds HG, Herholz K: Cerebral glucose metabolism as a predictor of rehabilitation after ischemic stroke. Stroke 24:1784–1788, 1993

48. Heiss WD, Graf R, Wienhard K et al: Dynamic penumbra demonstrated by sequential multitracer PET after middle cerebral artery occlusion in cats. J Cereb Blood Flow Metab 14:892–902, 1994

49. Herholz K, Heindel W, Racki A et al: Regional cerebral blood flow in patients with leuko-araiosis and atherosclerotic carotid artery disease. Arch Neurol 47:392–396, 1990

50. Herold S, Brown M, Frackowiak RSJ et al: Assessment of cerebral haemodynamic reserve: correlation between PET parameters and CO_2 reactivity measured by the intravenous[133] xenon injection technique. J Neurol Neurosurg Psychiatry 51:1045–1050, 1988

51. Hino A, Tenjin H, Ohmori Y et al: Hemodynamic and metabolic insufficiency in patients with high degree carotid artery stenosis. J Cereb Blood Flow Metab, suppl. 1, 13:S344, 1993

52. Iglesias S, Marchal G, Rioux P et al: Do changes in oxygen metabolism in the unaffected cerebral hemisphere underlie early neurological recovery after stroke?: a PET study. Stroke 27:1192–1199, 1996

53. Itoh M, Hatazawa J, Pozzilli C et al: Positron CT imaging of an impending stroke. Neuroradiology 30:276–279, 1988

54. Jacobs A: Amino acid uptake in ischemically compromised brain tissue. Stroke 26:1859–1866, 1995

55. Johansson BB, Grabowski M: Functional recovery after brain infarction: plasticity and neural transplantation. Brain Pathol 4:85–95, 1994

56. Jorgensen H, Nakayama H, Raaschou HO, Olsen TJ: Effect of blood pressure and diabetes on stroke in progression. Lancet 344:156–159, 1994

57. Kanno I, Uemura K, Higano S et al: I. Oxygen extraction fraction at maximally vasodilated tissue in the ischemic brain estimated from the regional CO_2 responsiveness measured by positron emission tomography. J Cereb Blood Flow Metab 8:227–235, 1988

58. Karbe H, Szelies B, Herholz K, Heiss WD: Impairment of language is related to left parieto-temporal glucose metabolism in aphasic stroke patients. J Neurol 237:19–23, 1990

59. Karbe H, Kessler J, Herholz K et al: Long-term prog-

nosis of poststroke aphasia studied with positron emission tomography. Arch Neurol 52:186–190, 1995

60. Kiyosawa M, Bosley TM, Kushner M et al: Middle cerebral artery strokes causing homonymous hemianopia: positron emission tomography. Ann Neurol 28:180–183, 1990

61. Kleiser B, Widder B: Course of carotid artery occlusions with impaired cerebrovascular reactivity. Stroke 23:171–174, 1992

62. Kuhl DE, Phelps ME, Kowell AP et al: Effects of stroke on local cerebral metabolism and perfusion. Mapping by emission computed tomography of ^{18}FDG and ^{13}NH3. Ann Neurol 8:47–60, 1980

63. Kuroda S, Kamiyama H, Abe H et al: Acetazolamide test in detecting reduced cerebral perfusion reserve and predicting long-term prognosis in patients with internal carotid artery occlusion. Neurosurgery 32:912–919, 1993

64. Kurthen M, Reichman K, Linke DB et al: Crossed cerebellar diaschisis in intracarotid sodium amytal procedures: a SPECT study. Acta Neurol Scand 81:416–422, 1990

65. Kushner M, Alair A, Reivich M et al: Contralateral cerebellar hypometabolism following cerebral insult: a positron emission tomographic study. Ann Neurol 15:425–434, 1984

66. Kushner M, Reivich M, Fieschi C et al: Metabolic and clinical correlates of acute ischemic infarction. Neurology 37:1103–1110, 1987

67. Kushner M, Kassik AE, Nencini P et al: Contralateral cerebellar hypometabolism following cerebral infarction: an acute and follow-up study. Neurology, suppl. 1, 38:147, 1988

68. Kuwert T, Hennerici M, Langen KL et al: Regional cerebral glucose consumption measured by positron emission tomography in patients with unilateral thalamic infarction. Cerebrovasc Dis 1:327–336, 1991

69. Lassen NA: The luxury perfusion syndrome and its possible relation to acute metabolic acidosis localized within the brain. Lancet 2:1113–1115, 1966

70. Lassen NA: Pathophysiology of brain ischemia as it relates to the therapy of acute ischemic stroke. Clin Neuropharmacol 13:S1–S85, 1990

71. Laterre EC, De Volder AG, Goffinet AM: Brain glucose metabolism in thalamic syndrome. J Neurol Neurosurg Psychiatry 51:427–428, 1988

72. Leblanc R, Tyler JL, Mohr G et al: Hemodynamic and metabolic effects of cerebral revascularization. J Neurosurg 66:529–535, 1987

73. Leblanc R, Yamamoto YL, Tyler JL, Hakim A: Hemodynamic and metabolic effects of extracranial carotid disease. Can J Neurol Sci 16:51–57, 1989

74. Lenzi GL, Frackowiak RSJ, Jones T: Cerebral oxygen metabolism and blood flow in human cerebral ischemic infarction. J Cereb Blood Flow Metab 2:231–235, 1982

75. Levasseur M, Baron JC, Sette G et al: Brain energy metabolism in bilateral paramedian thalamic infarcts: a positron emission tomography study. Brain 115:795–807, 1992

76. Levine RL, Sunderland JJ, Lagreze HL et al: Cerebral perfusion reserve indexes determined by fluoromethane positron emission scanning. Stroke 19:19–27, 1988

77. Levine RL, Dobkin JA, Rozental JM et al: Blood flow reactivity to hypercapnia in strictly unilateral carotid disease: preliminary results. J Neurol Neurosurg Psychiatry 54:204–209, 1991

78. Marchal G, Serrati C, Rioux P et al: PET imaging of cerebral perfusion and oxygen consumption in acute ischaemic stroke: relation to outcome. Lancet 341:925–927, 1993

79. Marchal G, Rioux P, Beaudoin V et al: Severe hypoperfusion/hypometabolism in acute stroke: an index of the minimum extent of irreversible damage. Cerebrovasc Dis 5:230, 1995

80. Marchal G, Rioux P, Serrati C et al: Value of acute-stage PET in predicting neurological outcome after ischemic stroke: further assessment. Stroke 26:524–525, 1995

81. Marchal G, Beaudouin V, Rioux P et al: Prolonged persistance of substantial volumes of potentially viable brain tissue after stroke: a correlate PET-CT study with voxel-based data analysis. Stroke 27:599–606, 1996

82. Marchal G, Furlan M, Beaudoin V et al: Early spontaneous hyperperfusion after stroke: a marker of favorable tissue outcome? Brain 119:409–419, 1996

83. Martin WR, Raichle ME: Cerebellar blood flow and metabolism in cerebral hemisphere infarction. Ann Neurol 14:168–176, 1983

84. Meguro K, Hatazawa J, Yamaguchi T et al: Cerebral circulation and oxygen metabolism associated with subclinical periventricular hyperintensity as shown by magnetic resonance imaging. Ann Neurol 28:378–383, 1990

85. Metter EJ, Wasterlain CG, Kuhl DE et al: ^{18}FDG positron emission tomography in a study of aphasia. Ann Neurol 10:173–183, 1981

86. Metter EJ, Riege WH, Hanson WR et al: Comparison of metabolic rates, language and memory in subcortical aphasia. Brain Language 19:33–47, 1983

87. Metter EJ, Riege WH, Hanson WR et al: Correlations of glucose metabolism and structural damage to language function in aphasia. Brain Language 21:187–207, 1984

88. Metter EJ, Mazziotta JC, Itabaschi HA et al: Comparison of glucose metabolism, X-ray CT and postmortem data in a patient with multiple cerebral infarcts. Neurology 35:1695–1701, 1985

89. Metter EJ, Kempler D, Jackson CA et al: Cerebellar glucose metabolism in chronic aphasia. Neurology 37:1599–1606, 1987

90. Metter EJ, Riege WH, Hanson WR et al: Subcortical structures in aphasia. Arch Neurol 45:1229–1234, 1988

91. Metter EJ, Kempler D, Jackson C et al: Cerebral glucose metabolism in Wernicke's, Broca's, and conduction aphasia. Arch Neurol 46:27–34, 1989

92. Miura H, Nagata K, Hirata Y et al: Evolution of crossed cerebellar diaschisis in middle cerebral artery infarction. J Neuroimag 4:91–96, 1994

93. Miyashita K, Naritomi H, Yamamoto H et al: Progressive metabolic reduction in the thalamus following ipsilateral embolic cortical infarction found by positron emission tomography. J Cereb Blood Flow Metab 15(suppl 1):676, 1995

94. Muraishi K, Kameyama M, Sato K et al: Cerebral circulatory and metabolic changes following EC/IC bypass surgery in cerebral occlusive diseases. Neurol Res 15: 97–103, 1993

95. Nagasawa H, Kogure K, Fujiwara T, Itoh T: Metabolic disturbances in exo-focal brain areas after cortical stroke studied by positron emission tomography. J Neurol Sci 123:147–153, 1994

96. Olsen TS, Bruhn P, Öberg GE: Cortical hypoperfusion as a possible cause of subcortical aphasia. Brain 109: 393–410, 1986

97. Pantano P, Baron JC, Samson Y et al: Crossed cerebellar diaschisis: further studies. Brain 109:677–694, 1986

98. Pantano P, Ricci M, Formisano R et al: Crossed cerebellar diaschisis and prolonged muscular flaccidity after stroke. Cerebrovasc Dis 2:206, 1992

99. Pantano P, Formisano R, Ricci M et al: Prolonged muscular flaccidity after stroke. Morphological and functional brain alterations. Brain 118:1329–1338, 1995

100. Pappata S, Tran Dinh S, Samson Y et al: Remote metabolic effects of cerebrovascular lesions: magnetic resonance and positron tomography imaging. Neuroradiology 29:1–6, 1987

101. Pappata S, Mazoyer B, Tran-Dinh S et al: Cortical and cerebellar hypometabolic effects of capsular, thalamocapsular, and thalamic stroke: a positron tomography study. Stroke 21:519–524, 1990

102. Pappata S, Fiorelli M, Rommel T et al: PET study of changes in local brain hemodynamics and oxygen metabolism after unilateral middle cerebral artery occlusion in baboons. J Cereb Blood Flow Metab 13:416–424, 1993

103. Pawlik G, Herholz K, Beil C et al: Remote effects of focal lesions on cerebral blood flow and metabolism. pp. 59–83. In Heiss WD (ed): Functional Mapping of the Brain in Vascular Disorders. Springer-Verlag, Berlin, 1985

104. Perani D, Vallar G, Cappa S et al: Aphasia and neglect after subcortical stroke. A clinical cerebral perfusion correlation study, Brain 110:1211–1229, 1987

105. Perani D, Di Piero V, Lucignani G et al: Remote effects of cerebrovascular lesions: a SPECT cerebral perfusion study. J Cereb Blood Flow Metab 8:560–567, 1988

106. Perani D, Vallar G, Paulesu E et al: Left and right hemisphere contribution to recovery from neglect after right hemisphere damage—an [^{18}F]FDG PET study of two cases. Neuropsychologia 31:115–125, 1993

107. Perlman S, Blood K, Sackett J et al: Anatomic and functional changes associated with crossed cerebellar diaschisis in chronic brain injured subjects. J Neurol Rehab 4:219–227, 1991

108. Phelps ME, Mazziotta JC, Kuhl DE et al: Tomographic mapping of human cerebral metabolism: visual stimulation and deprivation. Neurology 31:517–529, 1981

109. Powers WJ: Cerebral hemodynamics in ischemic cerebrovascular disease. Ann Neurol 29:231–240, 1991

110. Powers WJ, Martin WRW, Herscovitch P et al: Extracranial-intracranial bypass surgery: hemodynamic and metabolic effects. Neurology 34:1168–1174, 1984

111. Powers WJ, Grubb RL, Baker RP et al: Regional cerebral blood flow and metabolism in reversible ischemia due to vasospasm. J Neurosurg 62:539–546, 1985

112. Powers WJ, Grubb RL Jr, Darriet D, Raichle ME: Cerebral blood flow and cerebral metabolic rate of oxygen requirements for cerebral function and viability in humans. J Cereb Blood Flow Metab 5:600–608, 1985

113. Powers WJ, Press GA, Grubb RL et al: The effect of hemodynamically significant carotid artery disease on the hemodynamic status of the cerebral circulation. Ann Intern Med 106:27–35, 1987

114. Powers WJ, Grubb RL, Raichle M: Clinical results of extracranial-intracranial bypass surgery in patients with hemodynamic cerebrovascular disease. J Neurosurg 70: 61–67, 1989

115. Powers WJ, Tempel LW, Grubb RL: Influence of cerebral hemodynamics on stroke risk: one-year follow-up of 30 medically treated patients. Ann Neurol 25:325–330, 1989

116. Pozzilli C, Itoh M, Matsuzawa T et al: Positron emission tomography in minor ischemic stroke using oxygen-15 steady-state technique. J Cereb Blood Flow Metab 7: 137–142, 1987

117. Pulsinelli W: Pathophysiology of acute ischaemic stroke. Lancet 339:16–19, 1992

118. Ramsay SC, Weiller C, Myers R et al: Monitoring by PET of macrophage accumulation in brain after ischaemic stroke. Lancet 239:1054–1055, 1992

119. Sakai F, Aoki S, Kan S et al: Ataxic hemiparesis with reduction of ipsilateral cerebellar blood flow. Stroke 17: 1016–1018, 1986

120. Samson Y, Baron JC, Bousser MG et al: Effects of extra-intracranial arterial bypass on cerebral blood flow and oxygen metabolism in humans. Stroke 16:609–616, 1985

121. Samson Y, Baron JC, Pappata S et al: Angiotensin II infusion improves perfusion and oxygen consumption in both cerebral hemispheres in patients with bilateral carotid artery obstruction. J Cereb Blood Flow Metab 7(suppl. 1):177, 1987

122. Senda M, Alpert NM, Mackay BC et al: Evaluation of the $^{11}CO_2$ positron emission tomographic method for measuring brain pH. II. Quantitative pH mapping in patients with ischemic cerebrovascular diseases. J Cereb Blood Flow Metab 9:859–873, 1989

123. Serrati C, Marchal G, Furlan M et al: Predictive value of crossed cerebellar hypoperfusion (CCHP) in acute ischemic stroke (AIS): a PET study. Cerebrovasc Dis 4: 255, 1994

124. Serrati C, Marchal G, Rioux P et al: JC Contralateral cerebellar hypometabolism: a predictor for stroke outcome. J Neurol Neurosurg Psychiatry 57:174–179, 1994

125. Sette G, Baron JC, Mazoyer B et al: Local brain hemodynamics and oxygen metabolism in cerebro-vascular disease: positron emission tomography. Brain 112:931–951, 1989

126. Sette G, Sette G, Baron JC et al: In vivo mapping of brain benzodiazepine receptor changes by positron emission tomography following focal ischemia in the anesthetized baboon. Stroke 24:2046–2058, 1993

127. Sgouropoulos P, Baron JC, Samson Y et al: Sténoses et occlusions persistantes de l'artère cérébrale moyenne; conséquences hémodynamiques et métaboliques étudiées par tomographie á positions. Rev Neurol (Paris) 141:698–705, 1985

128. Silver FL, Chawluk JB, Bosley TM et al: Resolving metabolic abnormalities in a case of pure alexia; Neurology 38:730–735, 1988

129. Spelle S, Delforge J, Rancurel G et al: Chronic cortical hypoperfusion in partial middle cerebral artery stroke: deactivation or partial neuronal loss? A ^{11}C-flumazenil PET study of benzodiazepine receptors. Neurology, suppl. 1, 46:A195, 1996

130. Syrota A, Samson Y, Boullais C et al: Tomographic mapping of brain intracellular pH and extracellular water space in stroke patients. J Cereb Blood Flow Metab 5: 358, 1985

131. Szelies B, Herholz K, Pawlik G et al: Widespread functional effects of discrete thalamic infarction. Arch Neurol 48:178–182, 1991

132. Tanaka M, Kondo S, Hirai S et al: Crossed cerebellar diaschisis accompanied by hemiataxia: a PET study. J Neurol Neurosurg Psychiatry 55:121–125, 1992

133. Touzani O, Young AR, Derlon JM et al: Evolution of severely hypometabolic tissue: temporary versus permanent middle cerebral artery occlusion (MCAO) in the baboon. J Cereb Blood Flow Metab, 15(suppl 1):S327, 1995

134. Touzani O, Young AR, Derlon JM et al: Sequential studies of severely hypometabolic tissue volumes after permanent middle cerebral artery occlusion: a positron emission tomographic investigation in anaesthetized baboons. Stroke 26:2112–2119, 1995

135. Tsuda Y, Ayada Y, Izumi Y et al: Cerebellar diaschisis in pontine infarctions: a report of five cases. Eur J Nucl Med 22:413–418, 1995

136. Vallar G, Perani D, Cappa S et al: Recovery from aphasia and neglect after subcortical stroke: neuropsychological and cerebral perfusion study; J Neurol Neurosurg Psychiatry 51:1269–1276, 1988

137. Webster MW, Makaroun MS, Steed DL et al: Compromised cerebral blood flow reactivity is a predictor of stroke in patients with symptomatic carotid artery occlusive disease. J Vasc Surg 21:338–345, 1995

138. Weder B, Knorr U, Herzog H et al: Tactile exploration of shape after subcortical ischaemic infarction studied with PET. Brain 117:593–605, 1994

139. Weiller C, Chollet F, Friston KJ et al: Functional reorganization of the recovery from striatocapsular infarction in man. Ann Neurol 31:463–472, 1992

140. Weiller C, Ramsay SC, Wise RJS et al: Individual patterns of functional reorganization in the human cerebral cortex after capsular infarction. Ann Neurol 33:181–189, 1993

141. Weiller C, Willmes K, Reiche W et al: The case of aphasia or neglect after striatocapsular infarction. Brain 116: 1509–1525, 1993

142. Weiller C, Isensee C, Rijntjes M et al: Recovery from Wernicke's aphasia: a positron emission study tomographic study. Ann Neurol 37:723–732, 1995

143. Wise RJS, Bernardi S, Frackowiak RSJ et al: Serial observations on the pathophysiology of acute stroke. The transition from ischaemia to infarction as reflected in regional oxygen extraction. Brain 106:197–222, 1983

144. Wise RJS, Rhodes CG, Gibbs JM et al: Disturbances of oxidative metabolism of glucose in recent human cerebral infarcts. Ann Neurol 14:627–637, 1983

145. Wise RJS, Gibbs J, Frackowiak RSJ et al: No evidence for transhemispheric diaschisis after human cerebral infarction. Stroke 17:853–860, 1986

146. Yamauchi H, Fukuyama H, Kimura J et al: Hemodynamics in internal carotid artery occlusion examined by positron emission tomography. Stroke 21:1400–1406, 1990

147. Yamauchi H, Fukuyama H, Yamaguchi S et al: High-intensity area in the deep white matter indicating hemodynamic compromise in internal carotid artery occlusive disorders. Arch Neurol 48:1067–1071, 1991

148. Yamauchi H, Fukuyama H, Fujimoto N et al: Significance of low perfusion with increased oxygen extraction fraction in a case of internal carotid artery stenosis. Stroke 23:431–432, 1992

149. Yamauchi H, Fukuyama H, Nagahama Y et al: PET evidence of misery perfusion and risk for recurrent stroke in major cerebral arterial occlusive disease. J Neurol Neurosurg Psychiatry 61:18–25, 1996

150. Yao H, Sadoshima S, Kuwabara Y et al: Cerebral blood flow and oxygen metabolism in patients with vascular dementia of the Binswanger type. Stroke 21:1694–1699, 1990

151. Yonas H, Smith HA, Durham SR et al: Increased stroke risk predicted by compromised cerebral blood flow reactivity. J Neurosurg 79:483–489, 1993

152. Young AR, Sette G, Touzani O et al: Relationships between high oxygen extraction fraction in the acute stage and final infarction in reversible middle cerebral artery occlusion. An investigation in anaesthetized baboons with positron emission tomography. J Cereb Blood Flow Metab 16:1176–1188, 1996

CHAPTER 7

Functional Magnetic Resonance Imaging

JIA-HONG GAO

JIANHUI ZHONG

PETER T. FOX

Conventional magnetic resonance imaging (MRI) based on proton-density, T_1, or T_2 contrast provides images of human anatomy with high spatial resolution and excellent soft tissue contrast. MRI has been used extensively in the past decade or so to distinguish adequately hemorrhagic lesions from infarction and to depict ischemic stroke 12 to 24 hours after onset. As treatment regimens for ischemic stroke proliferate, however, early, accurate diagnosis of ischemic infarction has become increasingly important. The overall goal of acute stroke imaging is to diagnose precisely the type of stroke, allowing prompt implementation of appropriate management. The possibility of identifying the ischemic penumbra—regions with low blood flow in the range of about 15 to 20 ml/100 g/min outside of structural ischemic damage—and of delaying the extension of ultimate lesion size is the primary target of active treatment of stroke patients in the hospital.

Functional magnetic resonance imaging (fMRI) has already shown its superiority over conventional MRI or computed tomography (CT) in verifying stroke within minutes (or within the first few hours) of onset. Presently, several fMRI techniques are being developed or used in the early diagnosis of stroke and follow-up stroke treatment; they include magnetic resonance angiography (MRA), diffusion/perfusion imaging, and brain activation MRI.

MRA provides an accurate means to evalute the patency of cerebral arteries and veins. It gives functional information about the cerebrovascular system, such as differentiation of arteries and veins, determination of flow direction, source of vascular supply, and identification of collateral flow patterns. MRA can be used to visualize pathologies such as stenoses of vessels, occlusions, displacements, elongations, aneurysms, and ateriovenous malformations.

Diffusion/perfusion MRI are new techniques that monitor water transport in the microenvironment at cellular or capillary levels. They provide information about the temporal evolution of the destruction of brain tissue secondary to vascular disease and will potentially enhance our ability to evaluate ischemic stroke shortly after onset (within the first few hours).

Brain activation MRI depicts the regions of the brain that are responsible for specific actions. In the MRI literature, brain activation MRI has been termed fMRI, even though all these methods (MRA, diffusion/perfusion, and brain activation MRI) can technically provide images of brain function. fMRI has the ability to provide information regarding functional recovery and reorganization following cerebral infarction. An increased understanding of brain plasticity may be useful for improving stroke rehabilitation.

Fundamental aspects of brain function can be investigated using the interrelationship among cerebral activity, metabolism, and regional hemodynamics. fMRI techniques, such as MRA, diffusion/perfusion, and brain activation MRI, are of relevance to neurologic and vascular diseases not only because they can provide direct information about cerebrovascular disease (i.e., ischemia), but because they are positively correlated to tissue function. Therefore, in many disease states, altered diffusion/perfusion and vascular structures are coupled to altered cerebral function. For example, in the field of ischemic stroke, diffusion-weighted MR images can depict the location and extent of the ischemic lesion as soon as a stroke patient is available for examination. Perfusion measurements of blood flow within the brain's microvasculature can reveal regions of perfusion deficits corresponding to major vascular territories. Combined diffusion and perfusion measurements potentially correlate to the ischemic penumbra and are likely to have a central role in the evaluation of new therapies and in guiding early clinical management of patients. With the implementation of more and more whole-body MRI scanners equipped with fast scanning capability, such as echo planar imaging

(EPI), in clinical settings, it is becoming practical to perform diffusion, perfusion, MRA, and fMRI for a single stroke patient using the same machine. The prospect of acquiring such a wide range of highly valuable structural and functional information on individual patients by a single visit to a single site provides strong motivation for developing the necessary capabilities.

To understand the role of fMRI in the assessment and treatment of stroke, it is appropriate to review the basic physical principles and the methods for implementation of MRA, diffusion/perfusion MRI, and fMRI.

Magnetic Resonance Angiography

MRA, which uses blood flow as an intrinsic contrast agent, has attracted a great deal of attention since the mid-1980s when it was first proposed. MRA techniques include many variations of sequences that exploit basic contrast mechanisms, such as phase and inflow enhancement.[25,45,63,83,85,96] Although numerous variations exist in principle, all MRA methods belong to one of two classes. The first is time-of-flight (TOF) angiography, which is based on the principle of signal enhancement due to the inflow of fresh blood with nonsaturated magnetization into the imaging region. The other is phase contrast (PC) angiography, which is based on the principle that flow along a magnetic field gradient induces a phase shift that is proportional to velocity. TOF MRA requires the acquisition of only one image data set. By contrast, PC MRA requires the acquisition of two imaging data sets, which are substracted from one another. The subtraction eliminates background stationary signals and leaves only vascular structures with high signal intensity. Although PC MRA requires the collection of more data and requires more post-processing time than TOF MRA, its unique ability to assess flow velocity accurately and its superior suppression of background stationary tissues still motivates researchers to improve this technique. Generally, PC MRA methods use the shortest possible repetition time (TR) (e.g., 16 ms), whereas TOF MRA methods require a longer TR (e.g., 40 to 50 ms) to maximize blood vessel contrast. This results in comparable total imaging times for PC (multiple data sets) and TOF MRA (single data set).

A three-dimensional (3D) MRA image is commonly displayed using the maximum intensity projection (MIP) algorithm.[80] An MIP image is computed from the volume image by selecting the highest voxel value intercepted along a ray path defined by a pixel position in the projection plane (Fig. 7.1). MIP has found widespread use because it reliably and automatically produces useful results with a high contrast/noise ratio between flowing blood and stationary tissues. Figure 7.2 shows several MIP projections sequentially at a variety of view angles on a display monitor, which greatly enhances the illusion of the 3D vascular structure. This simple multiple-view display procedure provides accurate locations of each blood vessel, information that is lost if the image is viewed only from a single angle.

Compared with the gold standard, x-ray angiography, MRA has significant advantages. These include noninva-

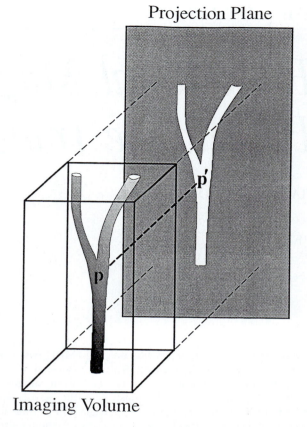

Figure 7.1 Illustration of the maximum intensity projection (MIP) algorithm. In this procedure, parallel rays are cast along the projection direction across the 3D imaging volume. A 2D projection image is created by reducing the data encountered by each ray to a single value of highest intensity hit by the ray on its path through the imaging volume.

siveness, the ability to image a target organ and its blood supply and vessels in a broad range of sites, the ability to obtain retrospective projections, and the possibility of obtaining flow and velocity information directly.

MRA image quality is closely related to the degree to which background stationary tissue can be suppressed. A PC MRA image does not have a problem in this respect because it is obtained by subtracting two imaging data sets that completely cancel out the stationary tissues, provided the MRI system has a high degree of stability and the patient does not move. However, the stationary tissue suppression in TOF MRA is based on saturation of the magnetization of stationary spins that have been excited by multiple radiofrequency (rf) pulses. In some situations, the steady-state nuclear magnetic resonance (NMR) signal of the stationary spins in 3D TOF MRA pulse sequences may not necessarily be very small compared with the signal from the blood. Slowly moving blood, which is likely to be excited by multiple rf pulses in the imaging volume, is easily saturated and quickly becomes invisible in the angiogram. Although this is less of a problem in two-dimensional (2D) TOF MRA, 2D TOF MRA has poorer spatial resolution in the slice dimension than 3D TOF MRA. A mul-

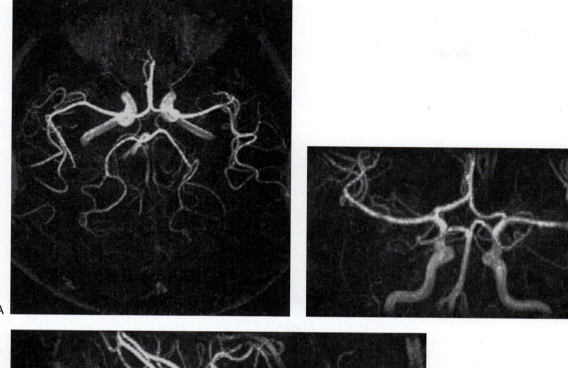

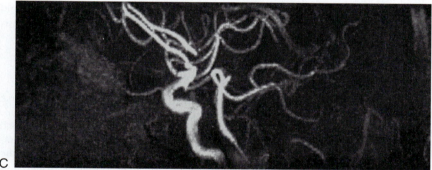

Figure 7.2 3D time-of-flight (TOF) MRA depicting the circle of Willis, obtained from 64 1.0-mm 3D partitions (TR, 57 ms, TE, 8 ms, flip angles, 30 degrees), (**A–C**) MIP images from three different views. It shows that the MIP image has a clear illusion of vascular structure.

tislab 3D data acquisition strategy has recently been proposed to combine the 2D and 3D advantages to solve slowly moving blood saturation problems.[74] In addition, during the past several years major progress has been made in significantly improving background suppression in 3D TOF MRA. The currently used techniques are summarized below.

TECHNIQUES TO SUPPRESS BACKGROUND

Imaging Parameters Optimization

By properly selecting sequence TR and the excitation pulse angle, the contrast between stationary and flowing blood may be maximized. Typical parameters used in neurovascular applications of 3D TOF MRA include

TR = 40 to 50 ms

TE = minimum

Flip angle = 30 degrees

Field-of-view (FOV) = as small as practical

Slice thickness = 0.7 to 1.5 mm

Magnetization Transfer Contrast Technique

Magnetization transfer contrast (MTC) is an efficient way to improve the contrast between blood vessels and surrounding tissues in MRA images.[75] The exchange of magnetization between protons in water and those in macromolecules contributes significantly to the observed relaxation rate of water in biologic tissues. It has been experimentally determined that cerebral white matter, gray matter, and skeletal muscle all show significant magnetization transfer, resulting in an observed signal attenuation of more than 40%. However, blood has a signal loss of <17%. In other words, the background tissues have more signal loss than blood, further increasing the signal difference between blood vessels and surrounding tissues.

Tilted, Optimized, Nonsaturating Excitation Technique

In 3D TOF MRA, the tilted, optimized, nonsaturating excitation technique (TONE) improves blood uniformity and contrast significantly when the blood flow is predominantly unidirectional.[89] 3D TOF MRA can produce excellent angiographic images of the vessels in relatively thin slabs of tissue. As blood traverses the slab, its signal is weakened by saturation, setting a practical limit to the slab thickness. A balanced signal distribution can be obtained from blood flowing roughly perpendicular to the slab by using small tip angles for the unsaturated blood entering from one side of the slab, and increasingly large tip angles for the partially saturated blood traversing the slab. This can be accomplished with an rf pulse having a tilted slice profile. Incorporating the TONE pulse into existing 3D MRA clinical sequences results in an improvement of the quality of renal, carotid, and intracranial angiograms. A combination of MTC and TONE techniques will result in a further increase in intracranial vessel contrast.

Contrast Agent Technique

Intravenous injections of relaxation agents, such as gadolinium diethylene-triamine-penta-acetic acid (Gd-DTPA), are widely used to alter the T_1 of selected tissues. Contrast agents can shorten the T_1 of blood, thereby making the blood more difficult to saturate and thus increasing the penetration of relaxed blood into the imaged volume. Slowly moving blood, such as that found in many veins, becomes more readily detected. Unfortunately, tissues such as mucous membranes, neoplasms, and regions of hemorrhage are also highlighted and become more readily visible, reducing the efficiency of the contrast agent's usefulness. In addition, the use of contrast agents in 3D TOF MRA studies significantly increases the examination cost.

TECHNIQUES TO REDUCE TURBULENCE-RELATED EFFECTS

Besides the background tissue problem encountered in the TOF MRA, as discussed above, the nature of the time-dependent blood flow also potentially generates MRA imaging artifacts. Turbulence and complex blood flow may produce false-positive results from turbulence-induced spin dephasing and the concomitant signal loss. Currently, turbulence-related effects can be reduced in two ways: short echo time (TE) strategy and black blood strategy.

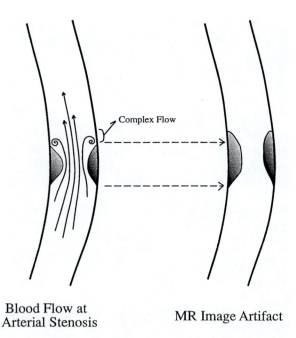

Blood Flow at Arterial Stenosis   MR Image Artifact

***Figure* 7.3** Demonstration of the turbulent or complex flow appearing around a stenosis, which will result in a signal void and make the NMR image appear to have a larger area of stenosis than it truly does.

Short TE Strategy

Turbulence and complex flow can cause serious transverse magnetization phase dispersion, resulting in signal loss. This signal loss is often seen in areas of bifurcation and in blood vessels with stenosis. Signal voids due to turbulent and complex flow can cause clinicians to diagnose stenosis in some cases when it does not exist or to diagnose stenosis to a greater degree than truly exists (Fig. 7.3). The tendency to overestimate the degree of stenosis may seriously affect the diagnostic reliability of MRA. In general, phase dispersion depends on TE, magnetic field gradient strength, and the nature of the flow. Smaller TE and weaker magnetic field gradient strengths will introduce a smaller phase dispersion. However, TE and magnetic field gradient strength usually have an inverse relationship in the imaging process; if one reduces TE, the gradient strength should increase accordingly. Experimental data and detailed theoretical calculations show that phase dispersion, while proportional to gradient strength, has a second-order dependence on TE. Therefore, reducing TE, at the cost of increasing the magnetic field gradient, is a more efficient way to reduce phase dispersion. Half-k space sampling techniques are also recommended for use in MRA because they can reduce data acquisition time up to 50%, resulting in a significant reduction in TE. Flow compensation can be applied as well to compensate for the coherent part of turbulent and complex flow.[39] Higher spatial resolution also helps to reduce signal loss resulting from turbulence and complex flow, because it minimizes intravoxel dephasing.

Black Blood Strategy

Black blood techniques, which aim to provide a more reliable depiction of the arterial lumen in regions of complex flow, use saturation or dephasing mechanisms to suppress rather than preserve flow signal. These accomplishments may have advantages in regions in which signal loss plagues bright blood techniques. This approach is subject to effects associated with nonvascular anatomy, which also produces low signal intensity.

APPLICATIONS IN STROKE

The major extracranial and intracranial cerebral vessels and their main branches can be seen on TOF or PC MRAs. The pathologies that can be visualized include stenoses of vessels, occlusions, displacements and elongations, aneurysms, and arteriovenous malformations. A comprehensive review of the role of MRA in the diagnosis of stroke has recently been published by Mattle and co-workers.[58] MRA has clearly demonstrated its clinical role in accurate diagnosis of stroke. Figure 7.4 shows an example of MRA and MRI images of a patient with cerebral infarction. This stroke patient is a 37-year-old man. MRI and MRA of the patient were acquired 40 hours after stroke onset. MIP images show occlusion of the right middle cerebral artery (Fig. 7.4A). The MRA finding was further confirmed by the T_2-weighted MR image (Fig. 7.4B) which shows that the right temporal lobe, insula and basal ganglia are hyperintense. Conventional T_1-weighted MR images of this patient (Fig. 7.4C) do not show apparent abnormalities.

Although MRA is extremely valuable in the diagnosis of stroke in its early stage, it cannot provide quantitative information about the extent of the effects of the abnormalities on the surrounding tissues, as it provides information only for blood flow in relatively large blood vessels. Diffusion/perfusion MRI can address these problems.

Diffusion/Perfusion MRI

PHYSICAL PRINCIPLES OF DIFFUSION MEASUREMENTS

Comprehensive reviews of diffusion measurements in clinical studies have been given in the past few years.[32,33,47,55,56,68] Only concepts that are directly relevant to in vivo stroke studies are discussed in this section.

Diffusion is a fundamental physical process that occurs in variety of physical systems. Subject to the perpetually changing interaction with their surroundings, the individual water molecules are induced to carry out an irregular motion—diffusion or random brownian motion, in which molecules constantly change their direction of motion with respect to each other. Einstein first showed that a diffusion coefficient can be defined to characterize the linear relationship between the mean square displacement a molecule travels and the time it needs to travel that distance. In the brain, the cellular structures and the cerebral vasculature affect the motion of water, which is the main constituent of the brain tissue. In a cerebrovascular accident, such as a stroke event, profound alterations

in the microenvironment occur. Monitoring the water molecule displacements due to diffusion in the tissues in vivo thus has enormous potential to aid in understanding of the pathophysiology of ischemia and the emergency management of stroke patients. In fact, MRI is the only noninvasive means available today that allows molecular movement to be studied at the cellular or microvascular level in vivo.

Diffusion in Heterogeneous Biologic Systems

Diffusion-weighted imaging (DWI) uses MRI pulse sequences sensitive to the thermally driven random motion of water molecules. Stejskal and Tanner[84] first used pulsed magnetic field gradients to determine the diffusion coefficient. The molecular diffusion process in the presence of gradients results in a random distribution of phase shifts, which reduce signal amplitude. Although diffusion effects are always present in samples, the contribution to signal loss is minimal in usual NMR measurements. Only when strong field gradients of the proper arrangement are added to the sequences does the attenuation due to diffusion of the observed signal become directly related to the gradients (Fig. 7.5).

In a typical pulsed gradient spin-echo sequence, the diffusion sensitization is achieved by adding two strong, rapidly switched gradient pulses around the 180-degree pulse[54,84] (Fig. 7.6). With diffusion in isotropic free space, the molecules undergo free brownian motion and the resulting signal intensity (SI) is given by:

$$SI(b) = SI(0)e^{-(\gamma \delta G)^2 (\Delta - \delta/3)D} = SI(0)e^{-bD} \quad [1]$$

where γ is the gyromagnetic ratio, D is the diffusion coefficient, δ and G are the duration and amplitude of the applied pulsed gradient, respectively, and Δ is the time interval between the two gradient pulses as indicated in Figure 7.6. Equation [1] predicts a linear dependence of one ln [SI(b)] on the amplitude of the squared external gradient strength G and a linear dependence on the so-called gradient factor b = $(\gamma \delta G)^2 (\Delta - \delta/3)$. In the above expression SI(0) is the signal intensity without the diffusion-sensitizing gradients.

In biologic tissues and other heterogeneous media, complex microstructure, such as cell membranes, compartments of cellular structure, flow in microvasculature, and inhomogeneous distribution of macromolecules in different cellular compartments, may affect the water diffusion process (Fig. 7.7). The diffusing water molecules may also experience effects due to variations in magnetic susceptibility on a microscopic scale and internal field gradients (e.g., gradients aroused from placement of the sample into an NMR spectrometer). Diffusion of nuclei through these gradients causes attenuation of the amplitude of the spin-echo.[104] In this kind of situation, Eq. [1] is no longer valid. However, an apparent diffusion coefficient ADC can still be defined according to

$$ADC = -\frac{\ln \left[\frac{SI(b)}{SI(0)} \right]}{b} \quad [2]$$

where b is the gradient factor defined above. The ADC now

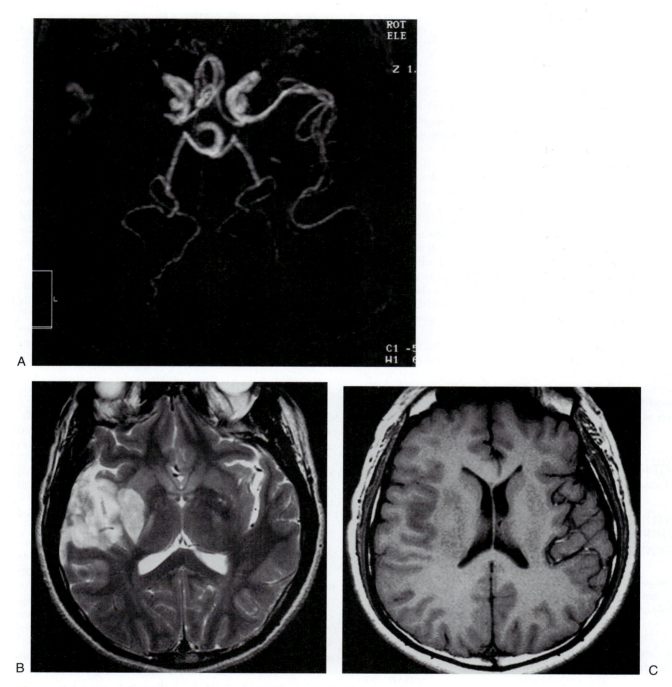

Figure 7.4 MRA and MRI images of a patient with cerebral infarction. (**A**) Maximum intensity projection (MIP) images show an occlusion of the right middle cerebral artery. The right temporal lobe, insula, and basal ganglia are (**B**) hyperintense on T_2-weighted MR images, and (**C**) isointense on T_1-weighted images.

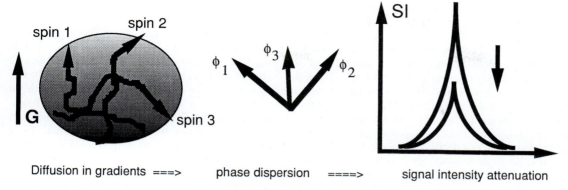

Figure 7.5 Signal reduction due to random motion. The molecular diffusion process in the presence of gradients results in a random distribution of phases of the individual spins, which reduces the signal amplitude.

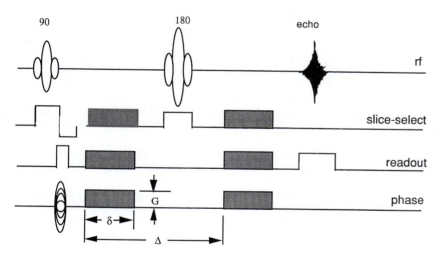

Figure 7.6 Pulsed gradient spin-echo imaging sequence diagram for diffusion measurements. Shaded magnetic field gradient pulses are diffusion-sensitizing pulses.

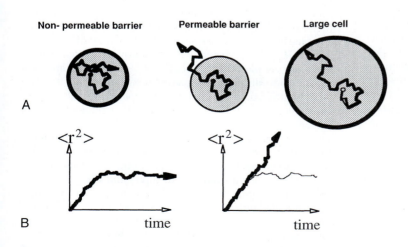

Figure 7.7 (**A**) Effects of compartment sizes and permeability of diffusion barriers on water diffusion. (**B**) Restriction of diffusion and deviations of mean squared displacement from linear dependence on time in small, nonpermeable compartments.

becomes dependent on the choice of experimental parameters, and its value reflects the microscopic environment that the diffusing spins experience.

The mean distance traveled by molecules in a time, t, is proportional to $\sqrt{Dt}$ and is typically 20 μm in 80 ms for water at body temperature. Thus, on the time scale of a typical T_2-weighted spin-echo sequence, molecules diffuse a mean distance that is comparable to cellular dimensions. DWI experiments are therefore capable of probing molecular displacements in vivo in the range well below the spatial resolution of conventional MRI experiments. In the case of whole-body imaging systems, it is by about 3 orders of magnitude. DWI thus offers a unique opportunity for obtaining information from morphologies otherwise inaccessible to other MRI methods. Another example of the impact of the tissue structure on the apparent diffusion of water is an apparent anisotropy of diffusion in both white matter and muscle. The measured apparent diffusion coefficient of water depends on the angle between the fiber-tract axis and the applied magnetic field gradient. This effect may be exploited to identify tissue structures, as we shall see later.

Diffusion-Weighted Imaging and ADC Measurements in the Clinical Setting

Different terminology is often used in the literature, leading to confusion. A diffusion-weighted image is generated by applying a pair of diffusion-sensitizing gradients in imaging sequences so that the signal intensity in each image pixel reflects the effects of diffusion in that pixel, in addition to the usual effects of spin density (SD) and longitudinal or transverse relaxation times (T_1 and T_2). Since the diffusion of water molecules in applied external gradients causes dephasing of the spin population and therefore reduction of observed signal, in a diffusion-weighted image, regions of low SI correspond to fast diffusion spins (such as in cerebrospinal fluid), and regions of higher SI correspond to spins that diffuse more slowly (such as in the brain parenchyma). However, simultaneously existing SD, T_1, and T_2 effects can obscure diffusion effects, and the image contrast will depend on the strength of the diffusion weighting in comparison with the imaging parameters that determine the magnitudes of these other contrast mechanisms.

A qualitative diffusion image is often obtained by subtracting an image from a standard spin-echo sequence performed with normal gradient pulses and diffusion-sensitizing gradients from an image generated by a pulse sequence that differs from the first only by the lack of diffusion-sensitizing gradient pulses. Thus, the effects of SD, T_1, and T_2 are removed and the SI of the calculated image qualitatively reflects difference in diffusion only.

For a more quantitative analysis of diffusion effects, a parametric map of diffusion coefficients in individual pixels may be required. This kind of analysis may be important if the diffusion measurements are used to identify regions of different levels of damage after ischemia. When the signal attenuation due to diffusion weighting gradients follows a monoexponential decay function, as suggested by Eq. [1], in principle only two images of different diffusion sensitivities are needed to calculate diffusion coefficients. In that case, the natural logarithmic of the ratio of the signal intensity in the two images can be taken and the apparent diffusion coefficient will be given by ADC = $- \ln [\text{SI}(b_2)/\text{SI}(b_1)]/(b_2 - b_1)$. It can be shown that measurements with two b-fact chosen so that $(b_2 - b_1) = 1/D$, and with the ratio of the number of measurements using these values ($b_1 < b_2$) at 1:3, provide an optimum measurement of the diffusion coefficient D (measurements result in the smallest standard deviation).[12] In brain imaging, in which deviations from single exponential decay usually exist due to the mixing of different types of tissue (i.e., partial volume effects in gray matter with cerebrospinal fluid mixing), a quantitative diffusion coefficient parametric map is usually created by fitting the SI in the images acquired with different sensitivities to diffusion on a pixel-by-pixel basis according to Eq. [1]. With more images, a better signal/noise ratio can be achieved in the calculated ADC map, and contamination due to cerebrospinal fluid mixing can be readily corrected.[21] Frequently, a series of six to eight images is acquired with a fixed set of δ and Δ values, and then G is incremented to achieve different sensitivities to diffusion.

It should be noted that in MRI sequences, magnetic field gradients are also used for spatial encoding. Unless the diffusion-sensitizing gradients are much larger than these other gradients, their effects should also be taken into consideration when calculating the diffusion-sensitizing gradient factor, b.

A major challenge for in vivo imaging of diffusion arises from irregular motion of the object. Although DWI of subacute and chronic infarcts was demonstrated several years ago, methodologic limitations prevented DWI from being practical for use in acute stroke patients until recently with the advance of fast-imaging techniques such as EPI.[19,54] The diffusion measurement sequences used are deliberately sensitized to motion by the addition of large gradients, and hence gross motions may lead to widely dispersed and potentially misleading artifacts. With conventional spin-warp MRI techniques, artifacts arise from discontinuities when successive cycles of the 2D Fourier transformation sequence are separated by a time interval, TR, that is close to the motion period. The requirement of voluntarily maintaining the head in a completely immobile position for the 10 minutes or more required to perform DWI with conventional MRI strategies is not practical for many patients with acute stroke. With EPI, the entire set of echoes needed to form an image is collected in a single acquisition period (single shot) of 25 to 100 ms. Therefore, problems with motion artifacts in DWI are minimized. In echo-planar DWI pulse sequences, a series of gradient echoes (usually 64 or 128, created with a train of fast switching gradients) are sampled to form a complete image. In comparison with the conventional DW spin-echo sequences, such as the one in Figure 7.6, the readout part is replaced with a series of gradient echoes, but the diffusion-sensitizing gradients remain the same.

Another issue commonly encountered in diffusion measurements in the brain is the anisotropic characteristic of diffusion in tissues such as the white matter tract. In a homogeneous medium, the diffusion is isotropic, and the same ADC is obtained in spite of the orientation of applied diffusion-sensitizing gradients. In brain tissues, however, the diffusional motion of water is influenced by the presence of the cell membranes and myelin fibers, and the ADC values become dependent on spatial orientation. If the plane of the applied gradient pulses is perpendicular to (or across) myelin fibers, the ADC values are lower than when the gradients are applied along the length of the fibers.[18,66,81] This anisotropy may be caused by a different restriction size in the respective directions; as axons of the cells in the brain tissue are mostly cylindrically shaped, the diffusion in two perpendicular directions is much lower than in the diffusion along the axon axis.

This important observation has prompted studies to determine nerve fiber tract orientations in white matter with diffusion measurements by applying diffusion-sensitizing gradients of different orientations.[24,70,71] In recent years, more quantitative approaches have been sought to relate diffusion measurements with structural anisotropy (e.g., brain white matter) based on tensor analysis.[9,10] Water diffusive motion in anisotropic systems is described by a tensor, with its three orthotropic axes given by the eigenvectors, and the effective diffusivities along these axes given by the eigenvalues of the tensor. This kind of analysis may lead to methods for determining fiber orientation in vivo and to the ability to infer the microscopic displacements of protons and other moieties in vivo. The scalar invariants of the diffusion tensor (the trace of the diffusion tensor being one of them), which are independent of orientation of the tissue in the laboratory frame of reference, reveal useful information about molecular mobility reflective of local microstructure and anatomy. Technically, however, this kind of analysis requires the acquisition of multiple images with high signal/noise ratios, and its usefulness in clinical settings still needs to be explored. As seen below, to define the extent of the pathologic attacks in ischemic injury with DWI better, it is important to separate the effects of changes in ADC due to pathophysiologic alterations from the dependence of ADC values on the orientations of the sensitizing gradients.

PHYSICAL PRINCIPLES OF PERFUSION MEASUREMENTS

In the broadest sense, the term *brain perfusion* has been used for various aspects of cerebrovascular circulation, although with the more classical definition, blood perfusion refers to the delivery of oxygen and nutrients to cells through capillaries, measured in units of ml blood/100 g tissue/min. The different techniques of MR perfusion imaging typically deal with blood volume, transit times, and blood flow. The two perfusion strategies that have found clinical and scientific applicability are based either on induced changes in intravascular magnetic susceptibility or on tagging inflowing arterial spins.

The susceptibility-based techniques utilize either injected paramagnetic contrast agents (such as chelated Gd-DTPA) or endogenous changes in the concentration of the intrinsic paramagnetic molecule deoxyhemoglobin to induce susceptibility changes related to brain perfusion. The latter technique is referred to as blood oxygenation level dependent (BOLD) and is the basis for most of the somatosensory or cognitive functional MRI studies in stroke discussed in this chapter.

Because magnetic susceptibility contrast is one of the most powerful means of affecting tissue signal intensity, dynamic MRI techniques based on tracking of paramagnetic contrast agents have shown considerable promise in providing the ability to generate maps of hemodynamic parameters. The susceptibility differences induced by paramagnetic agents set up local magnetic field gradients in the tissue, causing a loss of phase coherence and thus a decrease in signal intensity in the tissue surrounding the vessels. Following intravenous injection, these agents produce significant signal changes during first-pass cerebral transit. Dramatic loss of signal is seen ($\leq 50\%$) when sequences sensitive to susceptibility effects, such as gradient echo, are used with a normal clinical dose of contrast agent (0.1 to 0.3 mmol/kg). Typically, a short bolus of Gd-DTPA is injected intravenously and MR images are sequentially obtained at short time intervals. The transit of the contrast agent is monitored for 1 minute or less.[46,79] Tracer kinetic theory is then applied to the resulting series of images. Calculation of fractional cerebral blood volume (rCBV) is straightforward if the flow is assumed to be in steady-state, and the integrated arterial concentration of the contrast agent has the same value for all tissues in the brain. The rCBV is then simple integration of the concentration vs. time curves[2]:

$$rCBV \propto \int_0^\infty C_t(t)dt \propto \int_0^\infty \Delta R^\circ_2(t)dt \qquad [3]$$

where $C_t(t)$ is the contrast agent concentration in tissue, and ΔR°_2 is the change in the transverse relaxation rates measured with a susceptibility-sensitive pulse sequence. In the MRI contrast agent bolus tracking experiments, a linear relationship is assumed between the observed change in the transverse relaxation rate and the concentration of contrast agents. Calculation of regional cerebral blood flow (rCBF) or perfusion requires knowledge of the arterial input function of the contrast agent.[79,97] The measurement of absolute tissue perfusion is currently an active area of research, but it is not yet routinely performed in stroke studies. Because cerebral transit times are on the order of seconds, a rapid imaging technique is needed to resolve the passage of the intravascular agent through the capillary bed. In most successful applications in human studies, the EPI technique is usually used. Figure 7.8 is an example of a SI-versus-time curve and an rCBV map generated with bolus tracking.

Another group of MR perfusion methods uses blood water as a contrast agent. In a method first suggested by Detre and co-workers,[22,23,100–103] the proton spins in the arterial blood at the neck are prepared, using rapidly repeated slice-selective saturation or inversion pulses. Continuous proximal (with respect to blood flow) magnetic labeling of arterial water proton spins is applied to generate a steady-state change in distal tissue water magnetization, and difference MR images with or without this arterial blood labeling are calculated to produce quantitative perfusion imaging. This type of measurement yields a tissue-specific perfusion rate (f) (i.e., blood flow per gram of tissue per unit time):

$$f = \left(1 - \frac{M}{M_0}\right)\frac{1}{T_1} \qquad [4]$$

where M/M_0 is the ratio of the tissue signal in the presence

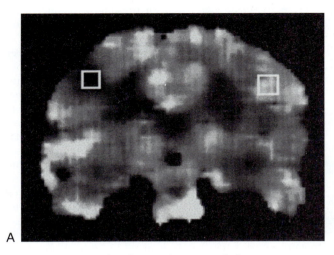

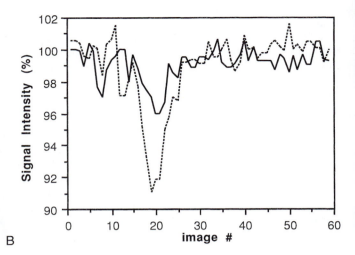

Figure 7.8 Example of a signal intensity (SI)-versus-time curve and fractional cerebral blood volume (rCBV) map generated with bolus tracking. A spin-echo echo planar imaging (EPI) sequence with TR = 1,200 ms and TE = 100 ms was used to acquire 60 images/slice in 5 slices. **(A)** rCBV map in a seizure patient that depicts the location of the hypoperfusion lesion very well. **(B)** Plot of the change in image signal intensity from a region of interest (ROI) inside the lesion and on the contralateral side.

or absence of the blood labeling, and T_1 is the spin-lattice relaxation time in tissue measured with blood labeling pulses.

Arterial blood labeling can also be achieved via dynamic approaches.[28,52,53,99] In pulsed arterial spin labeling techniques, a slab of arterial blood is magnetically tagged, and the inflow of this tagged blood into an imaging slice is measured. Images are acquired both with and without application of the tag, and the difference signal in each pixel is proportional to the amount of tagged blood that has entered that voxel. Images of these difference signals can be considered qualitative maps of the volume of blood delivered to capillary beds in a given volume of tissue per unit time. Arterial labeling techniques are rooted in the same principles that underlie positron emission tomography (PET) tracer methods and potentially provide noninvasive, accurate quantitation of perfusion.[16] Currently, a number of confounding theoretical and technical effects are being actively investigated in different research groups, and the role of this promising technique in stroke studies is just starting to emerge.

APPLICATIONS OF DIFFUSION/PERFUSION MEASUREMENTS IN STROKE

Early Detection of Ischemia with Diffusion-Weighted Imaging

A major application of diffusion/perfusion MRI within the field of cerebrovascular disease involves the study of cerebral ischemia. The progress of DWI in the study of stroke arises from the long-standing concern that conventional MRI has been largely unable to characterize changes quickly and accu-

rately following acute ischemia. Since the detection of ischemic stroke by diffusion-weighted MRI within minutes after vascular occlusion was first demonstrated by Moseley and co-workers[66,67] in a cat model, it has been predicted that this technique might become an important tool for both the identification of very early ischemic injury in patients and the quantitative assessment of severity and volume of ischemic injury (Fig. 7.9).

In animals of different species it has been found that within minutes after the onset of ischemia, the ADC of water molecules in brain tissues is reduced by as much as 50%.[15,50,59–62,67] In one of the first clinical studies of human stroke, Chien et al[19] performed DWI in 15 patients with cerebral infarction. These patients had mostly chronic stroke, with infarcts up to 4 years in age. Warach and co-workers[92–94] studied patients as early as 3 hours after onset of signs and symptoms of cerebral ischemia. They found that the ADC was reduced in acute infarction and was confirmed on T_2-weighted MR and CT images acquired days later. In all cases, studies 24 hours or more postocclusion showed lesion sizes that were similar in T_2-weighted and DW images. More importantly, as T_2-weighted hyperintensity increased, the ADC value remained reduced and only reached control values at 5 to 10 days. Chronic infarcts displayed elevated ADC values. These studies suggest that the relative ADC progress with time in stroke patients makes the distinction of acute lesions adjacent to chronic infarcts readily apparent. Recently, with the development of more robust imaging techniques—one of the important developments being the correction of motion artifacts using either navigator pulses or single-shot EPI sequences—more clinical studies of acute stroke are being performed.[21,95]

It is now established that DWI can detect lesions within minutes after the onset of stroke in comparison with the days

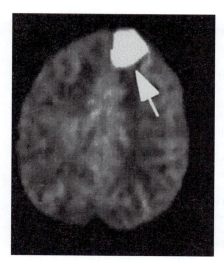
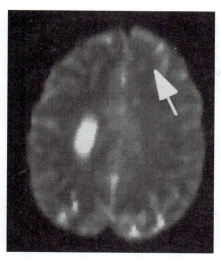

Figure 7.9 Detection of acute ischemia with DWI; embolization in an arteriovenous malformation (AVM) patient causes acute cerebral ischemia, which can be easily detected in (**A**) a diffusion-weighted image, but not in (**B**) a T_2-weighted image.

required with other imaging techniques, while at the same time maintaining all the advantages of MRI that have made MRI the choice of diagnosis in most neurologic examinations. The full potential of the technique, however, can only be realized with a better understanding of the underlying mechanisms that account for the changes in the ADC. Specifically, the correlation between the appearance of image changes and the underlying pathologic damage, and subsequent treatment planning, will require a deeper understanding of what causes the changes in the images under different conditions. Many of the basic properties that affect DWI in tissues are now qualitatively well understood[87]: the ADCs of water are greatly affected by the cellular architecture of a tissue, mainly because cellular membranes are relatively impermeable to water. For long diffusion times Δ, and small signal attenuation, the ADC is relatively insensitive to how it is measured. For given measuring conditions, the ADC depends on intra- and extracellular diffusion coefficients, membrane permeabilities, cell sizes, and the cellular volume fraction. Studies of water diffusion in a tissue model with analytical analysis and numerical Monte Carlo simulations suggest that the reduction in ADC in ischemia is a result of the combined effects of changes in cellular volume fraction and extracellular and intracellular diffusion.[87]

Since an image pixel contains many segments of cellular structure that can lead to anisotropic diffusion, the effective anisotropy in imaging is an average of the range of orientations within a voxel. The contrast in a diffusion image will therefore be due to a combination of the anisotropy, the orientation of the applied diffusion gradient relative to the cell axis, and the true local differences in diffusion. In a study of a rat occlusion model, van Gelderen et al[91] suggested using the trace of the diffusion tensor to quantify the reduction in ADC in ischemia. The trace of the diffusion tensor is calculated as the sum of the ADC values measured at three orthogonal orientations when the effects of the spatial encoding imaging gradients on diffusion can be ignored. The absence of any anisotropy and

orientation effects in the trace images made the differences in healthy and affected tissue unambiguous in the animals studied. The trace images showed a slight contrast between white and gray matter. The diffusion coefficient in white matter is decreased in acute stroke to approximately the same extent as in gray matter. Images representing the trace of the diffusion tensor provide a much more accurate delineation of the affected area than images representing the diffusion in one direction only.

Identification of the Ischemic Penumbra

Noninvasive measurements of the hemodynamic variables, such as rCBV and the mean transit time of the bolus, have been shown to have significant impact on the diagnosis and management of patients with ischemia. With ischemic disease, this kind of functional data offers the potential both to detect hypoperfusion well before conventional MRI studies and to quantify the degree of hypoperfusion within the central lesion and the surrounding ischemic penumbra. Dynamic first-pass bolus tracking of susceptibility contrast agents has been used to demonstrate the reduction in perfusion in focal ischemia in animal models and stroke patients.[20,27,92,93,98] In a preliminary study by Warach et al,[92,93] dynamic contrast agent tracking and MRA were used to evaluate rCBV and the intracranial arterial system in 34 patients within 48 hours of cerebral ischemia. There was good correlation between the lesions on MRA images and the regions of decreased blood volume in acute infarcts, and both techniques demonstrated lesions early in the clinical course.

Perfusion and diffusion imaging techniques are able to delineate, respectively, areas of hypoperfusion and ischemic neuronal injury within minutes after the induction of cerebral ischemia in animal models.[4,15,60,64,65] Since diffusion and perfusion MRI can identify very early ischemic lesions, it is reasonable to hypothesize that these techniques could distinguish regions destined for infarction from those that will not progress to infarction. Combined perfusion and DWI were used in a rat model of reversible middle carotid artery occlusion.[69] Hyperintensity in DWI was found to reverse after 45 minutes but not after 120 minutes of middle carotid artery occlusion. Analysis of the signal-reduction and time-delay parametric maps from these measurements demonstrated regions of different perfusion changes in the ischemic hemisphere. In a recent study by Warach et al,[95] in a small group of patients with severe clinical deficits, it was found that perfusion and diffusion MRI were highly accurate in distinguishing those who would improve from those who would not. The authors suggest possible future roles of diffusion/perfusion measurements in the initial screening, selection, and evaluation of patients with stroke for acute pharmacologic interventions.

Sorensen and co-workers[86] performed EPI DWI using three or more directions to calculate tensor trace maps of 17 to 20 slices, and perfusion imaging using dynamic EPI during bolus injection of 0.2 mmol/kg of standard gadolinium-based contrast agent. The signal reduction caused by the contrast agent bolus was converted into relative rCBV maps using a numerical integration technique. Volumes of lesions on hyperacute cases (<6 hours from onset of deficit) from diffusion/perfusion measurements were presented. In the nine patients with both diffusion and perfusion abnormalities, the initial DWI abnormality volume was 58% of the follow-up infarct volume, whereas the perfusion abnormality volume was 138% of the final infarct volume. The authors hypothesized that DWI may represent, in humans, tissue that is damaged and unlikely to recover without intervention, whereas perfusion-deficit volume represents total affected tissue. The difference between these two may represent tissue at risk, or alternatively, imaging correlates of the ischemic penumbra.

Arterial spin tagging techniques and DWI were used in a thromboembolic stroke model of rats in a recent study.[1,14] The combination of perfusion and diffusion MRI was shown to give direct insight into the consequences of perfusion deficits with high temporal resolution. A good correlation between the regions of perfusion deficit and ADC reduction were observed. Quantitative assessment of both perfusion and ADC changes in ischemic regions revealed a gradual worsening of the tissue impairment in regions of severe perfusion deficits. Thus, the relationship between perfusion deficit and degree of tissue damage emphasizes the importance of including perfusion measurements to investigate the pathophysiologic processes.

Time Course in Human Complete and Progressing Stroke

In a study by Ebisu and co-workers,[26] the ADC was measured with a single-shot DW spin-echo EPI sequence in symptomatic stroke patients. Relative ADC (rADC, the ratio of lesion to contralateral control) was used to compensate for the global differences in each MR parameter that is independent of focal ischemia. The DWI hyperintensity and reduced ADC were observed in all acute stroke patients. The initially reduced rADC in completed stroke cases began to increase 1 day after onset, returning to the normal range in 15 to 24 days. By contrast, the rADC in a progressive stroke case continued to decrease even after 28 days. These findings suggest that the observation of ADC changes in complete stroke may be a greater indicator of asymptomatic infarction age than conventional T_2-weighted MR signal changes. Furthermore, ADC changes could discriminate between complete and progressive stroke.

Warach and co-workers[95] studied 19 patients with severely disabling clinical deficits attributable to ischemia in at least an entire division of the middle cerebral artery. Their findings demonstrated that initial perfusion and diffusion MRI were more accurate than conventional MRI in predicting no, partial, or complete improvement. Seventeen of 19 cases were accurately predicted by perfusion/diffusion MRI versus 10 of 19 cases, which were accurately predicted by conventional MRI. In a subset of patients studied within 6 hours of onset, diffusion/perfusion MRI was an even better predictor of improvement than conventional MRI—11 of 12 versus 4 of 12, respectively. They have begun to screen the entire brain in stroke patients, and lesions as small as 4 mm are being detected. Echo-planar DWI of the entire brain takes only 3 seconds, and perfusion imaging of the entire brain can be complete in less than 1 minute; thus their use as screening tests would not unduly delay urgent therapies.

These studies suggest that the progression of the relative ADC with time in stroke patients allows the distinction of acute lesions adjacent to chronic infarcts to be readily apparent. In addition, the use of rapid diffusion and perfusion techniques in the evaluation of stroke promises to allow more accurate localization and better prognosis than are possible with conventional imaging methods alone.

Brain Activation MRI

PRINCIPLES

Brain activation MRI (known as fMRI) has become a powerful tool for studying functional organization within the living human brain in recent years. Although fMRI initially followed leads set by PET and single-photon emission CT, fMRI has leapt beyond its nuclear forebears. fMRI is establishing its role in the assessment of brain disorders such as stroke, tumors, epilepsy, and dementia.

The first fMRI brain activation study was reported by Belliveau and co-workers[11] at Massachusetts General Hospital in 1991. They administered an intravascular paramagnetic contrast agent (Gd-DTPA) as a rapidly injected bolus. The paramagnetic contrast agents produce a heterogeneous magnetic field in and around vessels, thereby decreasing the MRI signal from the tissue surrounding the vessels in the brain. The MRI signal loss is approximately proportional to the concentration of the contrast agents in the blood. By integrating over the first passage of the contrast agents through the brain, a map of relative blood volume can be generated. The rCBV change during functional brain activation relative to the control state can then be determined.

In 1992, Kwong et al[51] and others[73] first mapped human brain activity using fMRI techniques without any administration of tracer (contrast agent). Their technique relied solely on endogenous contrast resulting from physiologic changes in the brain during activation. Task-associated changes in brain neural activity are associated with local changes in blood flow,[34,35,38] blood volume,[11,36] blood oxygenation,[36,37,72] and carbohydrate metabolism.[36,37] These physiologic changes have been used to map the location of neural activity with a variety of techniques, including PET, single-photon emission CT, and infrared reflectance imaging. MRI is sensitive to blood flow, blood volume, and the blood oxygenation state of hemoglobin, all of which can be used to generate noninvasive images of human brain activity. Several factors contribute to the brain activation MRI signal and are related to the physiologic changes of the brain during activation. The two major contributions are described below.

Blood Oxygenation Level-Dependent Effects

Previous PET experiments have shown a large increase in rCBF and a small increase in oxygen consumption during brain activation.[34,36,37] This results in a reduced concentration of deoxyhemoglobin in capillaries and veins. The magnetic state of hemoglobin in red cells is strongly dependent on oxygen saturation, and the deoxyhemoglobin is more paramagnetic (higher magnetic susceptibility) than oxygenated blood. Thus, the paramagnetic deoxyhemoglobin creates a local magnetic field gradient in the surrounding diamagnetic brain tissue. This magnetic field heterogeneity within an imaging voxel results in an MRI signal loss on T°_2-weighted images.[72] As the concentration of deoxyhemoglobin in the capillaries and veins decreases during activation, the resulting decrease in the tissue-blood magnetic susceptibility difference leads to less intravoxel dephasing of the MRI signal and therefore to an increased MRI signal on T°_2-weighted images. Consequently, a T°_2-weighted gradient echo pulse sequence is a good candidate for mapping the neural activity of the brain.

Blood Flow Effects

It is well known that changes in the blood flow (either in large vessels or in the capillary bed) will significantly change the magnitude of the MRI signal.[3,23,40–42,44] The signal changes from moving blood are dependent on the nature of the flow, the parameters of the MRI protocol, and the history of the rf pulses. In general, the washin of fresh blood with full magnetization into the image slice will enhance the MRI signal, whereas blood washout of an image slice without experiencing the refocusing 180 degrees for spin-echo-type pulse sequences will decrease the MRI signal. For large vessels, Gao and co-workers[42] evaluated the contribution of inflow effects to the fMRI signal. They concluded that for T°_2-weighted gradient-echo EPI sequences, the blood oxygenation level-dependent (BOLD) signal will dominate the fMR image. However, for the conventional (non-EPI) gradient-echo sequences, the inflow effects may suppress the BOLD contribution to fMRI signal. In functional brain mapping, signals coming from large vessels cause poor localization of the true function area. It is apparent that EPI imaging sequences, compared with non-EPI imaging sequences, will have advantages in identifying the exact location of the brain functional area.

In the capillary bed, blood flow (perfusion) changes can

result in a change in the apparent longitudinal relaxation time T_1. The relationship between T_1 and regional blood flow has been modeled by the following equation[23,51]:

$$\frac{1}{T_{1a}} = \frac{1}{T_1} + \frac{f}{\lambda} \qquad [5]$$

where T_{1a} is the apparent longitudinal relaxation time with flow effects included, T_1 is the true tissue longitudinal relaxation time in the absence of flow, f is the flow in milliliters per gram per unit time, and λ is the brain-blood partition coefficient of water; $\lambda = 0.95$ ml/g.[77] Assuming the true tissue longitudinal relaxation time T_1 remains constant between activation and control states, a change in blood flow, Δf, will lead to a change in the apparent T_{1a}:

$$\Delta\left(\frac{1}{T_{1a}}\right) = \frac{\Delta f}{\lambda} \qquad [6]$$

Thus, a T_1-weighted pulse sequence can be used to detect the blood flow changes between activation and control states.

fMRI techniques have been widely used for neuroscience research and are presently being developed for clinical applications. Of particular relevance to stroke applications is the study of the brain function of normal volunteers when they perform motor tasks. Activation in the primary motor cortex has been clearly demonstrated (Plate 7.1) during the execution of simple tasks such as finger tapping.[5,6,51] The intensity of the fMRI signal change increased with the tapping rate.[8] Later studies with these simple paradigms also showed hemispheric asymmetry in the functional activation of the motor cortex during contralateral and ipsilateral movements.[48] The right motor cortex was activated mostly during left finger movements, and the left motor cortex was activated substantially during both right and left finger movements. The premotor and supplementary motor areas were activated by complex finger movements and mental rehearsal of the finger movements.[7,8,31,88,90] Challenging the classical view of separable motor representations, overlapped representations in the primary motor cortex, M1, for different finger movements were revealed by Sanes et al.[82] In addition, task-related activations for finger and wrist movements have been observed in the cerebellum, demonstrating the involvement of the cerebellum in voluntary movements.[29] It was also found (Plate 7.2) that the dentate nucleus of the cerebellum activated more intensely during cognitive processing[49] and sensory-perceptual acquisition[43] even if no voluntary movement was involved relative to contributions of simple movements. These fMRI findings not only improve our understanding in human brain function, but also will help in the assessment of neurologic diseases such as stroke.

fMRI APPLICATION IN STROKE

Studying functional recovery of the human brain is an important clinical issue. Motor recovery following cerebral infarction from hemiparesis due to stroke was demonstrated by fMRI using a finger-tapping task.[13,30,57] Early motor recovery was reported to be characterized by increased activation in ipsilateral sensory and contralateral motor areas. The reorganization of the hand sensorimotor area after unilateral brain injury in the prenatal period was reported by Cao et al.[17] Unlike normal subjects, who exhibit cortical activation primarily contralateral to voluntary finger movements, the hemiparetic patients' intact hemispheres were equally activated by contralateral and ipsilateral finger movements.

Plate 7.3 shows a brain activation MR image from a study of a stroke patient. This patient is a 33-year-old right-handed woman who had a left internal carotid artery dissection and a sustained left striatocapsular infarct 10 days prior to the imaging study. The patient had minimal awkwardness in fine movements with the right hand. In brain activation studies, the patient performed an index finger-tapping task at a rate of 1 tap/s, cued verbally. To standardize the task performance, the arm was strapped to a wooden tapping device with levers of fixed resistance for the tapping finger. Each task at a different resistance was performed two or three times. Sixty sets of images per task performance (20 at rest, 20 during task performance, and 20 at rest) were acquired. To identify significantly activated pixels, t-tests were used. With index finger tapping by the normal left hand, there is activation of the right primary motor cortex (m). There is also an area of activation that includes supplementary motor cortex (s) bilaterally. Small areas of activation were occasionally seen in this area in normal subjects. With index finger tapping by the right hand, which was affected by the stroke, there is bilateral activation of premotor cortex (p) and also an area of activation medially that includes supplementary motor cortex and is larger and stronger than the activation seen in this region with tapping by the normal left hand. There is also an area of signal decrease that includes part of the left primary motor cortex.

Using functional imaging techniques to study plasticity has aroused great interest. Even before fMRI techniques were developed, Powers and co-workers[76] used PET brain activation methods to evaluate patients with transient ischemic attacks but with no residual neurologic deficit. In 16 patients with severe carotid artery disease, brain activations were able to detect functional abnormalities despite normal resting-state PET scans and normal brain CT scans. This indicates that the brain activation measures, both PET and fMRI, can assess cerebral perfusion reserve.

Given that several limitations exist with PET techniques, we anticipate that fMRI, especially as it is further developed, will play a major role in the study of recovery and plasticity and in stroke management. fMRI techniques, including MRA, diffusion/perfusion, and brain activation MRI, have already shown great promise in the diagnosis of early stage stroke and will hopefully also have a great impact on assessment of new stroke pharmaceuticals.

References

1. Allegrini PR, Busch E, Hoehn-Berlage M et al: A new approach to follow ADC in relation to perfusion changes assessed by ultrafast arterial spin tagging in a thrombo-embolic stroke model. p. 488. In: Proceedings of ISMRM, New York, 1996

2. Axel L: Cerebral blood flow determination by rapid-sequence computed tomography. Radiology 137:679, 1980

3. Axel L: Blood flow effects in magnetic resonance imaging. AJR 143:1157, 1984

4. Back T, Berlage M, Hoehn M et al: Diffusion nuclear magnetic resonance imaging in experimental stroke. Correlation with cerebral metabolites. Stroke 25:494, 1994

5. Bandettini PA, Wong EC, Hinks RS et al: Time course EPI of human brain function during task activation. Magn Reson Med 25:390, 1992

6. Bandettini PA, Jesmanowicz A, Wong EC, Hyde JS: Processing strategies for time-course data sets in functional MRI of the human brain. Magn Reson Med 30:161, 1993

7. Bandettini PA, Rao SM, Binder JR et al: Magnetic resonance functional neuroimaging of the entire brain activation during rehearsal of complex finger tasks. Proc Soc Magn Reson Med 1396, 1993

8. Bandettini PA, Wong EC, DeYoe EA et al: The functional dynamics of blood oxygen level dependent contrast in the motor cortex. Proc Soc Magn Reson Med 1382, 1993

9. Basser PJ, Mattiello J, LeBihan D: Estimation of the effective self-diffusion tensor from the NMR spin echo. J Magn Reson [B] 103:247, 1994

10. Basser PJ, Mattiello J, LeBihan D: MR diffusion tensor spectroscopy and imaging. Biophys J 66:259, 1994

11. Belliveau JW, Kennedy DN, McKinstry RC et al: Functional mapping of the human visual cortex by magnetic resonance imaging. Science 254:716, 1991

12. Bito Y, Hiratada S, Yamamoto E: Optimum gradient factors for apparent diffusion coefficient measurements. p. 913. In: Proceeding of SMR/ESMRMB, Nice, France, 1996

13. Bookheimer SY, Cohen MS, Dobkin B, Mazziotta JC: Functional MRI during motor activation following stroke. Hum Brain Map S1:429, 1995

14. Busch E, Krüger K, Allegrini PR et al: rt-PA treatment of thromboembolic stroke in rat: assessment by repeated ultrafast arterial spin tagging perfusion and diffusion MRI. p. 320. In: Proceedings of ISMRM, New York, 1996

15. Busza AL, Allen KL, King MD et al: Diffusion-weighted imaging studies of cerebral ischemia in gerbils: potential relevance to energy failure. Stroke 23:1602, 1992

16. Buxton RB: Quantitative perfusion imaging. p. 2. In: Proceedings of ISMRM, New York, 1996

17. Cao Y, Vikingstad EM, Huttenlocher PR et al: Functional magnetic resonance studies of the reorganization of the human hand sensorimotor area after unilateral brain injury in the prenatal period. Proc Natl Acad Sci USA 91:9612, 1994

18. Chenevert TL, Brunberg JA, Pipe JG: Anisotropic diffusion in human white matter: demonstration with MR techniques in vivo [see comments]. Radiology 177:401, 1990

19. Chien D, Kwong KK, Gress DR et al: MR diffusion imaging of cerebral infarction in humans. AJNR Am J Neuroradiol 13:1097, 1992

20. de Crespigny AJ, Tsuura M, Mosley ME, Kucharczyky J: Perfusion and diffusion MR imaging of thromboembolic stroke. J Magn Reson Imaging 3:746, 1993

21. de Crespigny AJ, Marks MP, Enzmann DR, Moseley ME: Navigated diffusion imaging of normal and ischemic human brain. Magn Reson Med 33:720, 1995

22. Detre JA, Eskey CJ, Koretsky AP: Measurement of cerebral blood flow in rat brain by 19F-NMR detection of trifluoromethane washout [published erratum appears in Magn Reson Med 16:179, 1990]. Magn Reson Med 15:45, 1990

23. Detre JA, Leigh JS, Williams SS, Koretsky AP: Perfusion imaging. Magn Reson Med 23:37, 1992

24. Douek P, Turner R, Pekar J et al: MR color mapping of myelin fiber orientation. JCAT 15:923, 1991

25. Dumoulin CL, Hart HR: Magnetic resonance angiography. Radiology 161:717, 1986

26. Ebisu T, Tanaka C, Umeda M et al: Time course in human completed and progressing stroke studied by diffusion-weighted echo-planar imaging. p. 573. In: Proceedings of ISMRM, New York, 1996

27. Edelman RR, Mattle HP, Atkinson DJ et al: Cerebral blood flow: assessment with dynamic contrast-enhanced T_2^*-weighted MR imaging at 1.5T. Radiology 176:211, 1990

28. Edelman RR, Siever B, Wielopolski P et al: Noninvasive mapping of cerebral perfusion by using EPISTAR angiography. J Magn Reson Imaging 4(P):68, 1994

29. Ellermann JM, Flament D, Kim SG et al: Spatial patterns of functional activation of the cerebellum investigation using high field (4T) MRI. Nuclear Magn Reson Biomed 7:63, 1994

30. Faiss JH, Rijntjes M, Weiller CS et al: Motor recovery following cerebral infarction visualized by functional MRI. Proc Soc Magn Reson Med 333, 1994

31. Fieldman JB, Cohen LG, Jezzard P et al: Functional neuroimaging with echo-planar imaging in humans during execution and mental rehearsal of a simple motor task. Proc Soc Magn Reson Med 1416, 1993

32. Fisher M, Sotak CH, Minematsu K, Li L: New magnetic resonance techniques for evaluating cerebrovascular disease. Ann Neurol 32:115, 1992

33. Fisher M, Prichard JW, Warach S: New magnetic resonance techniques for acute ischemic stroke. JAMA 274:908, 1995

34. Fox PT, Raichle ME: Stimulus rate dependence of regional cerebral blood flow in human striate cortex, demonstrated by positron emission tomography. J Neurophysiol 51:1109, 1984

35. Fox PT, Raichle ME: Stimulus rate determines regional blood flow in striate cortex. Ann Neurol 17:303, 1985

36. Fox PT, Raichle ME: Focal physiological uncoupling of cerebral blood flow and oxidative metabolism during somatosensory stimulation in human subjects. Proc Natl Acad Sci USA 83:1140, 1996

37. Fox PT, Raichle ME, Mintun MA, Dence C: Nonoxidative glucose consumption during focal physiological neural activity. Science 241:462, 1988

38. Fox PT, Mintun MA, Raichle ME et al: Mapping human visual cortex with positron emission tomography. Nature 323:806, 1996

39. Gao JH, Gore JC: Turbulent flow effects on NMR imaging: measurement of turbulent intensity. Med Phys 18:1045, 1991

40. Gao JH, Gore JC: NMR signal from flowing nuclei in fast gradient-echo pulse sequences with refocusing. Phys Med Biol 39:2305, 1994

41. Gao JH, Holland SK, Gore JC: Nuclear magnetic resonance signal from flowing nuclei in rapid imaging using gradient echoes. Med Phys 15:809, 1988

42. Gao JH, Miller I, Lai S et al: Quantitative assessment of blood inflow effects in functional MRI signals. Magn Reson Med 36:314, 1996

43. Gao JH, Parsons LM, Bower JM et al: Cerebellum implicated in sensory acquisition and discrimination rather than motor control. Science 272:545, 1996

44. Gullberg GT, Simons MA, Wehrli FW: A mathematical model for signal from spins flowing during the application of spin echo pulse sequences. Magn Reson Imaging 6:437, 1988

45. Hahn EL: Detection of sea-water motion by nuclear precession. J Geophys Res 65:776, 1960

46. Hamberg LM, Macfarlane R, Tasdemiroglu E et al: Measurement of cerebrovascular changes in cats after transient ischemia using dynamic magnetic resonance imaging. Stroke 24:444, 1993

47. Hazlewood CF, Rorschach HE, Lin C: Diffusion of water in tissues and MRI. Magn Reson Med 19:214, 1991

48. Kim SG, Ashe J, Hendrich K et al: Functional magnetic resonance imaging of motor cortex: hemispheric asymmetry and handiness. Science 261:613, 1993

49. Kim SG, Ugurbil K, Strick PL: Activation of a cerebellar output nucleus during cognitive processing. Science 256:949, 1994

50. Knight RA, Ordidge RJ, Helpern JA et al: Temporal evolution of ischemic damage in rat brain measured by proton nuclear magnetic resonance imaging. Stroke 22:802, 1991

51. Kwong KK, Belliveau JW, Chesler DA et al: Dynamic magnetic resonance imaging of human brain activity during primary sensory stimulation. Proc Natl Acad Sci USA 89:5675, 1992

52. Kwong KK, Rosen BR et al: Real time imaging of perfusion change and blood oxygenation change with EPI. p. 301. In: SMRM, Berlin, 1992

53. Kwong KK, Chesler DA, Weisskoff RM et al: MR perfusion studies with T_1-weighted echo planar imaging. Magn Reson Med 34:878, 1995

54. Le Bihan D, Breton E, Lallemand D et al: MR imaging of intravoxel incoherent motions: application to diffusion and perfusion in neurologic disorders. Radiology 161:401, 1986

55. Le Bihan D, Turner R, Moonen CTW, Pekar J: Imaging of diffusion and microcirculation with gradient sentization: design, strategy, and significance. J Magn Reson Imaging 1:7, 1991

56. Le Bihan D, Douek P, Argyropoulou M et al: Diffusion and perfusion magnetic resonance imaging in brain tumors. Top Mag Reson Imaging 5:25, 1993

57. Leifer D, Zhong J, Graham GD et al: Functional mag-

netic resonance imaging of motor activity during recovery from stroke. Neurology A339:46, 1996

58. Mattle HP, Wentz KU, Tuncdogan E, Vock P: Intracranial manifestation of thrombosis and vascular occlusion. p. 432. In Potchen EJ, Haacke EM, Siebert JE, Gottschalk A (eds): Magnetic Resonance Angiography. 1st Ed. Mosby-Year Book, St. Louis, 1993

59. Minematsu K, Li L, Fisher M et al: Diffusion-weighted magnetic resonance imaging: rapid and quantitative detection of focal brain ischemia. Neurology 42:235, 1992

60. Minematsu K, Li L, Sotak CH et al: Reversible focal ischemic injury demonstrated by diffusion-weighted magnetic resonance imaging in rats. Stroke 23:1304, 1992

61. Mintorovitch J, Baker LL, Yang GY: Diffusion weighted hyperintensity in early cerebral ischemia: correlation with brain water content and ATPase activity. p. 329. In the Tenth Annual Meeting of the Society for Magnetic Resonance in Medicine, 1991

62. Mintorovitch J, Moseley ME, Chileutt L et al: Comparison of diffusion- and T_2-weighted MRI for the early detection of cerebral ischemia and reperfusion in rats. Magn Reson Med 18:39, 1991

63. Moran PR: A flow velocity zeugmatographic interlace for NMR imaging in humans. Magn Reson Imaging 1:197, 1982

64. Moseley ME, Cohen Y, Kucharczyk J et al: Diffusion-weighted MR imaging of anisotropic water diffusion in cat central nervous system. Radiology 176:439, 1990

65. Moseley ME, Cohen Y, Mintorovitch J et al: Early detection of regional cerebral ischemia in cats: comparison of diffusion- and T_2-weighted MRI and spectroscopy. Magn Reson Med 14:330, 1990

66. Moseley ME, Kucharczyk J, Asgari HS, Morman D: Anisotropy in diffusion-weighted MRI. Magn Reson Med 19:321, 1991

67. Moseley ME, Mintorovitch J, Asgari H et al: Diffusion/perfusion MR characterization of hyperacute cerebral ischemia. p. 330. In The Tenth Annual Meeting of the Society for Magnetic Resonance in Medicine, 1991

68. Moseley ME, Wendland MF, Kucharczyk J: Magnetic resonance imaging of diffusion and perfusion. Top Magn Reson Imaging 3:50, 1991

69. Muller TB, Haraldseth O, Jones RA: Combined perfusion and diffusion-weighted magnetic resonance imaging in a rat model of reversible middle cerebral artery occlusion. Stroke 26:451, 1995

70. Nakada T, Matsuzawa H: Three-dimensional anisotropy contrast magnetic resonance imaging of the rat nervous system: MR axonography. Neurosci Res 22:389, 1995

71. Nakada T, Matsuzawa H, Kwee IL: Magnetic resonance axonography of the rat spine cord. Neuroreport 5:2053, 1994

72. Ogawa S, Lee TM, Kay AR, Tank DW: Brain magnetic resonance imaging with contrast dependent on blood oxygenation. Proc Natl Acad Sci USA 87:9868, 1990

73. Ogawa S, Tank DW, Menon R et al: Intrinsic signal changes accompanying sensory stimulation: functional brain mapping with magnetic resonance imaging. Proc Natl Acad Sci USA 89:5951, 1992

74. Parker DL, Yuan C, Blatter DD: MR angiography by multiple thin slab acquisition. Magn Reson Med 17:434, 1991

75. Pike GB, Hu BS, Glove GH, Enzmann DR: Magnetization transfer time-of-flight magnetic resonance angiography. Magn Reson Med 25:372, 1992

76. Powers WJ, Fox PT, Raichle ME: The effect of carotid artery disease on the cerebrovascular response to physiogic stimulation. Neurology 38:1475, 1988

77. Raichle ME, Eichling JO, Straatmann MG et al: Blood-brain barrier permeability of ^{11}C-labeled alcohols and ^{15}O-labeled water. Am J Physiol 230:543, 1976

78. Rao SM, Binder JR, Bandettini PA et al: Functional magnetic resonance imaging of complex human movements. Neurology 43:2311, 1993

79. Rosen BR, Belliveau JW, Vevea JM, Brady TJ: Perfusion imaging with NMR contrast agents. Magn Reson Med 14:249, 1990

80. Rossnick S, Laub G, Braeckle R et al: Three dimensional display of blood vessels in MRI. pp. 193–196. In: *Proceedings of the IEEE Computers in Cardiology Conference*, New York, 1986

81. Sakuma H, Nomura Y, Takeda K et al: Adult and neonatal human brain: diffusional anisotropy and myelination with diffusion-weighted MR imaging. Radiology 180:229, 1991

82. Sanes JN, Donoghue JP, Thangaraj V et al: Shared neural substrates controlling hand movements in human motor cortex. Science 268:1775, 1995

83. Singer JR: Blood flow rates by nuclear magnetic resonance measurements. Science 130:1652, 1959

84. Stejskal EO, Tanner JE: Spin diffusion measurements: spin echoes in the presence of a time-dependent field gradient. J Chem Phys 52:288, 1965

85. Suryan G: Nuclear resonance in flowing liquids. Proc Indian Acad Sci 33:107, 1951

86. Sorensen AG, Koroshetz WJ, Buonanno FS et al: Diffusion/perfusion mismatch in MRI of acute human stroke. p. 91. In: Proceedings of ISMRM, New York, 1996

87. Szafer A, Zhong J, Gore J: Theoretical model for water diffusion in tissue. Magn Reson Med 22:697, 1995

88. Takahashi T, Takiguchi K, Itagaki H et al: Real time imaging of brain activation during imagination of finger tasks. Proc Soc Magn Reson Med 1415, 1993

89. Tkach JA, Masaryk TJ, Ruggieri PK et al: Use of tilted optimised nonsaturating excitation (TONE) rf pulses and MTC to improve the quality of MR angiograms of the carotid bifurcations. p. 3905. In: *Book of Abstracts*. The 11th Annual Meeting of the SMRM, Berlin, 1992

90. Tyszka JM, Grafton ST, Chew W et al: Parcellation of mesial frontal motor areas during ideation and movement using functional magnetic resonance imaging at 1.5 tesla. Ann Neurol 35:746, 1994

91. van Gelderen P, Vleeschouwer MHM, DesPres D et al: Water diffusion and acute stroke. Magn Reson Med 31:154, 1994

92. Warach S, Chien D, Li W et al: Fast magnetic resonance diffusion-weighted imaging of acute human stroke. Neurology 42:1717, 1992

93. Warach S, Li W, Ronthal M, Edelman RR: Acute cerebral ischemia: evaluation with dynamic contrast-en-

hanced MR imaging and MR angiography. Radiology 182:41, 1992

94. Warach S, Gaa J, Siewert B et al: Acute human stroke studied by whole brain echo planar diffusion-weighted magnetic resonance imaging. Ann Neurol 37:231, 1995

95. Warach S, Dashe JF, Edelman RR: Clinical outcome in ischemic stroke predicted by early diffusion-weighted and perfusion magnetic resonance imaging: a preliminary analysis. J Cereb Blood Flow Metab 16:53, 1996

96. Wedeen VJ, Meuli RA, Edelman RR et al: Projective imaging of pulsatile flow with magnetic resonance. Science 230:946, 1985

97. Weisskoff RM, Chesler D, Boxerman JL, Rosen BR: Pitfalls in MR measurement of tissue blood flow with intravascular tracers: which mean transit time? Magn Reson Med 29:553, 1993

98. Wendland MF, White DL, Aicher KP et al: Detection with echo-planar MR imaging of transit of susceptibility contrast medium in a rat model of regional brain ischemia. J Magn Reson Imaging 1:285, 1991

99. Wong EC, Buxton RB, Frank LR: Quantitative perfusion imaging using EPISTAR and FAIR. p. 10. In: Proceedings of ISMRM, New York, 1996

100. Williams DS, Detre JA, Leigh JS, Koretsky AP: Magnetic resonance imaging of perfusion using spin inversion of arterial water. Proc Natl Acad Sci USA 89:212, 1992

101. Williams DS, Grandis DJ, Zhang W, Koretsky AP: Magnetic resonance imaging of perfusion in the isolated rat heart using spin inversion of arterial water. Magn Reson Med 30:361, 1993

102. Zhang W, Williams DS, Detre JA, Koretsky AP: Measurement of brain perfusion by volume-localized NMR spectroscopy using inversion of arterial water spins: accounting for transit time and cross-relaxation. Magn Reson Med 25:362, 1992

103. Zhang W, Williams DS, Koretsky AP: Measurement of rat brain perfusion by NMR using spin labeling of arterial water: in vivo determination of the degree of spin labeling. Magn Reson Med 29:416, 1993

104. Zhong J, Gore JC: Studies of restricted diffusion in heterogeneous media containing variations in susceptibility. Magn Reson Med 19:276, 1991

CHAPTER 8

Pathology

JULIO H. GARCIA

KHANG-LOON HO

LEONARDO PANTONI

The abrupt development of a focal neurologic deficit is called a *stroke* if the deficit is thought to be the consequence of a local disturbance in the cerebral circulation. In most instances, these sudden changes in brain function result from either the obstruction of an intracranial artery or the rupture of a vessel supplying the brain or spinal cord. This chapter describes selected vascular diseases and structural deformities affecting the brain parenchyma as a consequence of either ischemic or hemorrhagic events. Angiopathies discussed in individual chapters of this book, such as aneurysms, are not included in this chapter. Intracerebral hemorrhage is covered in depth elsewhere; only the histologic responses to intraparenchymal bleeding are included here.

Vascular Diseases

ATHEROSCLEROSIS

Atherosclerosis in the intracranial arteries usually involves the terminal portion of the internal carotid artery, the basilar artery, and, to a lesser extent, the middle cerebral artery, the anterior and pericallosal arteries, and the posterior cerebral arteries.[15] Carotid atherosclerotic plaques frequently develop at the origin of the common carotid as it arises from the aortic arch, at the origin of the internal carotid artery, and, intracranially, in the internal carotid artery siphon.[101]

The atheromatous plaque is characterized by focal subendothelial deposits of lipid derived from the blood plasma accompanied by smooth muscle proliferation, influx of T lymphocytes and monocytes, and collagen deposition.[33,76] Both smooth muscle cells and circulating monocytes play significant roles in lipid deposition.[134] Certain factors, both genetic and acquired, increase the risk of carotid atherosclerosis. Four of them have been well characterized: hyperlipidemia, arterial hypertension, cigarette smoking, and diabetes mellitus.

Early atheromatous lesions localize in the carotid bulb along the outer and posterior walls of the artery in a region characterized by low wall shear stress, flow separation, flow stasis, increased particle residence time, and shear stress oscillation.[135] Most carotid atheromatous plaques are smooth, nonstenotic, covered by a well-formed fibrous cap, and asymptomatic.

Plaques become symptomatic when they cause marked stenosis (>70% narrowing), are accompanied by thrombotic occlusion of the lumen, or become the source of embolism.[123] Complicated or symptomatic plaques develop at the same location where fibrous plaques form; they are more complex than the fibrous plaques and are characterized by intimal cellular proliferation, lipid accumulation, calcification, hemorrhage, ulceration, and thrombosis.[113] The mechanisms underlying the progression of carotid atherosclerosis and the appearance of symptoms are poorly understood. Ulceration and intraplaque hemorrhage are prominent features of symptomatic carotid plaques and may be responsible for the development of ischemic symptoms, but the issue remains controversial.[36] Rupture of the fibrous cap could be one of the factors promoting thrombotic occlusion of the internal carotid artery.[92] Ulceration or breakdown of the fibrous cap covering the atheroma may be the result of hemodynamic alterations secondary to marked stenosis; this is because blood flow velocity and shear stress increase as the lumen narrows.[116] A high level of shear stress may promote erosion of the endothelial cell lining and exposure to the circulation of the debris normally covered by the fibrous cap. Debris may be released into the cerebral circulation, and these particles may occlude distal arteries and become the cause of either transient ischemic attacks or cerebral infarcts.[116] The term *atheroembolism* is generically used to indicate microembolism by either cholesterol crystals or atherothrombotic material.

Intraplaque hemorrhage may result from the entry of blood into the plaque through an erosion of the fibrous cap; this may produce an intramural dissection or an intraplaque hemorrhage. Such an event may also result from the disruption of vasa vasorum;[6] advanced or complicated atherosclerotic lesions contain abundant vasa vasorum that presumably originate from vessels normally present in the tunica adventitia of the extradural arteries.[9] Intraplaque hemorrhage is a feature of both symptomatic and asymptomatic carotid atherosclerosis with marked stenosis.[36] The relationship between intraplaque hemorrhage and the development of symptoms of cerebral ischemia remains unclear. The factors that promote intraplaque hemorrhage are unknown. Some authors suggest that both chronic and transient hypertension might result in intraplaque hemorrhage.[6]

ARTERIOLOSCLEROSIS

Cerebral arteriolosclerosis (small blood vessel disease; microangiopathy) describes structural changes affecting perforating arterial vessels ($\leq$500 μm in average diameter) such as the lenticulostriate branches of the anterior and middle cerebral arteries, as well as the thalamopenetrating branches of the basilar artery.[104] Two types of arterial vessels penetrate the brain: (1) those endowed with an internal elastic lamina and a tunica media composed of three to four layers of smooth muscle cells are arteries with internal diameters ranging between 100 and 400 μm; and (2) those devoid of continuous elastic lamina and having a tunica media composed of one to two layers of smooth muscle cells are called arterioles; most arterioles measure $\leq$100 μm in average diameter. Both penetrating arteries and arterioles arise directly from large parent arteries located in the subarachnoid space; this exposes these vessels to intraluminal pressures that scarcely reach arteries or arterioles of similar caliber outside the brain.[56] The best known causes of cerebral arteriolosclerosis are arterial hypertension, diabetes mellitus, and aging. The following are some of the elements of arteriolosclerosis.

Microatheroma

Chronic arterial hypertension promotes atherosclerosis of the large arteries and may also be accompanied by the formation of atheromatous plaques (microatheroma) at the orifice or initial segment of penetrating arteries with a diameter of 300 to 700 μm.[14] Microatheroma is characterized by subintimal proliferation of fibroblasts and lipid-laden macrophages as well as deposits of cholesterol; this process probably contributes to the occlusion of small arteries.

Lipohyalinosis

This lesion is not unique to the brain and, in about one half of the cases, lipohyalinosis is related to the effects of hypertension as seen elsewhere in the body. Lipohyalinosis has features of both arterial (lipidoses, atheroma) and arteriolar (hyalinization) disease.[34] The combination of these lesions in a single vessel reflects the fact that the progression of both processes (hyalinization and atheromatous lipid deposit) is influenced by a common factor (i.e., arterial hypertension). The caudate nucleus, putamen, thalamus, internal capsule, pons, and cerebellum are the sites where lipohyalinosis is most common; these are the same sites where hypertensive hemorrhages and lacunes are frequent.

Fibrinoid Necrosis

The term *fibrinoid necrosis* describes a bright, eosinophilic, finely granular material that is deposited in the tunica media of intraparenchymal arteries and arterioles. The material represents a combination of necrotic smooth muscle cells and extravasated plasma proteins. Fibrinoid necrosis occurs predominantly in acute, malignant hypertension and is the most characteristic vascular change observed in hypertensive encephalopathy.

Microaneurysms

Originally described by Charcot and Bouchard in 1868, microaneurysms were classified by Fisher[34] into four types: (1) miliary saccular aneurysms (300 to 1,100 μm) are symmetric outpouchings with a wall devoid of endothelial lining; (2) lipohyalinotic aneurysms (0.5 to 1.5 mm) are common in the cerebral cortex and are often associated with small hemorrhages; (3) fusiform dilatations or pseudoaneurysms (700 to 800 μm) are seldom associated with hypertensive intracerebral hemorrhages; and (4) bleeding globes or pseudoaneurysms (0.3 mm to 1 cm in diameter) consist of masses of red blood cells and platelets wrapped in concentric layers of fibrin and reticulin fibers. The prevalence of microaneurysms of the Charcot-Bouchard type has been questioned recently; using a combined histochemical stain for alkaline phosphatase and microradiographic methods, Challa et al[18] have suggested that many intracerebral vessels with coils, twists, and overlapping loops have been misinterpreted as being microaneurysms. These newer interpretations based on the application of combined methods are probably correct.

CEREBRAL AMYLOID ANGIOPATHY

Cerebral amyloid angiopathy (CAA), also known as congophilic angiopathy, selectively affects the cerebral vessels, often in the absence of systemic amyloidosis.[23] CAA is characterized by the deposition of proteinaceous, intensively eosinophilic material that thickens the vessel walls. Amyloid stains with periodic acid-Schiff and toluidine blue; amyloid is apple-green birefringent under polarized light when stained with Congo red; and it fluoresces under ultraviolet light when stained with thioflavin S or T.[106] Amyloid infiltrates the tunicae media and adventitia of arteries and veins of medium or small caliber; most amyloid-containing vessels are located either in the cerebral cortex or in the subarachnoid space. In the cerebral hemispheres, all lobes may be involved by CAA, although the parietal and occipital lobes are more frequently affected.[126] The injured vessels, particularly those located in the leptomeninges, may show segmental dilatation, microaneurysm formation, a double-barrel lumen, fibrinoid necrosis, or luminal occlusion.[80] The amyloid of CAA consists of randomly arranged, nonbranching, nonparallel filaments 7 to 9 nm in diameter. The β-amyloid protein of CAA shares its antigenicity with the amyloid β-protein of Alzheimer's disease plaques, and identical amino acid sequences have been identified in the β-amyloid protein of both conditions.[103] The origin of amyloid and the mechanism by which amyloid is deposited in the vessel wall remain unknown.[37,103] CAA is associated with several entities: intracerebral hemorrhage, Alzheimer's disease, Down syndrome, dementia pugilistica, cerebral microinfarcts, vasculitis, periventricular leukoencephalopathy, late postirradiation encephalopathy, spongiform encephalopathy (especially the

Gerstmann-Strässler-Scheinker syndrome), and cerebral vascular malformations.[127] Deposits of tumor-like amyloid (amyloidoma) in the brain have been reported in a few cases.[20]

CAA is frequently associated with intracerebral hemorrhage in persons with or without Alzheimer's disease.[129] CAA-related intracerebral hemorrhage (sporadic type) is a disease of the elderly (mean age, 72 years). Thirty percent of these patients have mixed microangiopathy (with both arteriolosclerosis and CAA changes). Over 40% of patients with CAA-related intracerebral hemorrhage are demented, and a similar percentage show neuropathologic changes of Alzheimer's disease. Intracerebral hemorrhages in CAA patients are usually lobar, often involving the frontal and parietal lobes, and rarely involving deep ganglionic structures or the cerebellum. Multiple, old, microscopic hemorrhages and microscopic infarcts are common in CAA, but subarachnoid and subdural hemorrhages are rare.

Two important hereditary syndromes have been recognized among patients with CAA. Hereditary cerebral hemorrhage with amyloidosis-Dutch type (HCHWA-D) is an autosomal dominant disease caused by deposition of β-amyloid on the leptomeningeal arteries and cortical arterioles as well as amyloid plaques in the brain parenchyma.[10] β-Amyloid deposition in arteries and arterioles seemingly starts at the junction of the media and adventitia and proceeds to spread to the tunica media, eventually replacing the smooth muscle cells. HCHWA-D is characterized by recurrent strokes and dementia, which can occur after the first stroke but also may precede it. Neuroimaging studies in these patients reveal focal lesions (hemorrhages and hemorrhagic and nonhemorrhagic infarcts) and diffuse white matter damage. The relationship of the β-amyloid angiopathy to the hemorrhages and to other brain lesions remains to be elucidated. The genetic defect in HCHWA-D has been traced to a point mutation at codon 693 of the amyloid precursor protein gene at chromosome 21.

Hereditary cystatin C amyloid angiopathy (HCCAA), also called hereditary cerebral hemorrhage with amyloidosis-Icelandic type (HCHWA-I), is an autosomal dominant trait causing fatal cerebral hemorrhages in young adults (20 to 40 years of age).[96] Recurrent cerebral hemorrhages accompanied by increasing motor disability and gradual loss of mental functions are common. HCCAA is now classified as a systemic amyloidosis with amyloid depositions in the brain and various tissues as well. Amyloid deposits in HCCAA are present in the cerebral arteries as well as in interstitial tissues of the brain, vessels of the optic nerve, lymphoid tissue, skin, and other organs. A mutation in the gene encoding the cysteine proteinase inhibitor cystatin C has been demonstrated in several patients with HCCAA. Most patients with HCCAA have decreased concentration of cystatin C in the cerebrospinal fluid (CSF).[81]

SYSTEMIC LUPUS ERYTHEMATOSUS

A multisystem disease of autoimmune origin, systemic lupus erythematosus (SLE) is a chronic, remitting and relapsing illness characterized by injury to the vessels of the skin, joints, kidney, and serosal membranes. SLE predominates among women, who usually become symptomatic in the second or third decade of life, and appears to be a heterogeneous disorder resulting from complex interactions among genetic, hormonal, and environmental factors. The morphologic changes in SLE are extremely protean, reflecting the variability of the clinical manifestations in individual patients. The arterial lesion includes deposits of immunoglobulins, DNA, and C3 protein, as demonstrated in selected patients; these observations support the theory that the vascular changes may be mediated by immune complexes. Most manifestations of cerebral lupus may have a vascular etiology, and the neuropsychiatric symptoms could be induced by various mechanisms, including vasculopathy, hemorrhage, embolism, and damage by either antineuronal antibodies[8] or demyelinating factors.[12] An autopsy study based on the examination of 50-plus cases revealed that most cerebral lesions were brain infarcts of probable embolic origin.[25] Approximately 40% of lupus patients have detectable antiphospholipid antibodies, and as many as 15% of SLE patients exhibit features of the antiphospholipid syndrome, which includes repeated episodes of arterial or venous thrombosis, recurrent spontaneous abortions, and thrombocytopenia.[1] Patients with antiphospholipid syndrome, either primary or associated with SLE, may develop chronic cerebral vasculopathy and repeated cerebral infarcts or hemorrhages.[21] In these patients, the leptomeningeal arteries show widespread luminal obstructions by a proliferation of intimal fibrous tissue or myointimal cells and superimposed fibrin thrombi.[1] The involved vessels do not exhibit inflammatory infiltrates or immune complex deposits.

THROMBOTIC THROMBOCYTOPENIC PURPURA

The primary process of thrombotic thrombocytopenic purpura (TTP) involves intravascular platelet aggregation with fibrin deposition in arterioles and capillaries but not in venules. Cellular inflammation is not seen in the involved vessels. Thrombi may be covered by endothelial cells and thus become intramural components. Neurologic manifestations are recorded in 74% to 90% of the patients and include headache, confusion, seizures, paresis, and coma.[2] These findings may change rapidly and be transient, reflecting the fleeting nature of the microvascular lesions. Microscopic confirmation of the diagnosis may be based on blood smears to demonstrate schistocytes, as well as gingival biopsy, which may reveal thrombotic microangiopathy.[16]

SNEDDON SYNDROME

As originally described in 1965, patients with Sneddon syndrome have repeated, multifocal ischemic strokes accompanied by cutaneous livedo reticularis.[118] The lesions in both the brain and the skin are attributed to alterations involving small and medium-sized arteries. The angiopathic changes, as described by Zegler et al,[136] have a distinctive time sequence in which the initial phase consists of a loosening and detachment of the endothelial cells, accompanied by surface adhesion of inflammatory cells interspersed with fibrin. Affected vessels then undergo subendothelial proliferation of smooth

Figure 8.1 Sneddon syndrome. (**A**) Sub-arachnoid artery with subendothelial proliferation of smooth muscle cells. (**B**) Nearly complete obliteration of the lumen is visible in another brain artery of the same patient. (H&E, original magnification × 36.) (Courtesy of Dr. W. Roggendorf, Würzburg, Germany.)

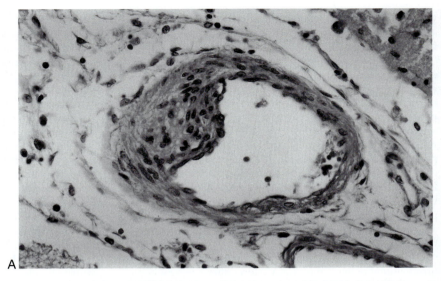

A

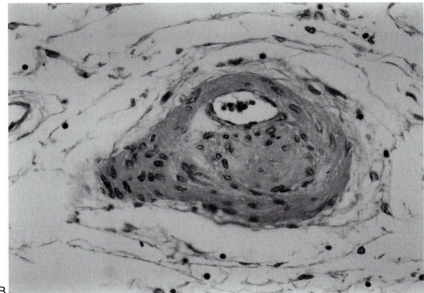

B

muscle cells and eventual partial or complete obliteration of the vessel lumen[40] (Fig. 8.1). An undetermined percentage of patients with Sneddon syndrome have detectable serum antiphospholipid antibodies, but the relationship of this finding to the vascular changes is undefined.[50]

Hereditary Disorders Associated with CNS Angiopathy

Genetic disorders associated with angiopathies of the central nervous system (CNS) may be divided into metabolic and nonmetabolic diseases. Table 8.1 lists a selected number of genetic syndromes associated with CNS angiopathy.

HOMOCYSTINURIA AND HOMOCYSTEINEMIA

Patients with homocystinuria have extremely high levels of total plasma homocysteine. They also have a high incidence of cardiovascular and cerebrovascular disease in early adolescence and childhood. Homocystinuria results from several enzymatic defects in homocysteine metabolism; the most common defect is an autosomal recessive deficiency of cystathionine-β-synthase. Premature vascular disease develops irrespective of the site of metabolic deletion, however, suggesting that homocysteine is responsible for most of the vascular damage.[83] Plasma homocysteine refers to the sum of protein-bound, free-oxidized, and reduced species of homocysteine; this sum usually measures 5 to 15 μmol/L in healthy subjects. Moderate hyperhomocysteinemia (15 to 30 μmol/L) is related to genetic or acquired factors. In young adults,

Table 8.1 Hereditary Angiopathies of the Central Nervous System

Metabolic disorders
    Homocystinuria and homocysteinemia[82,114]
        Autosomal recessive
        Premature atherosclerotic occlusion of carotid artery and large
            cerebral arteries
    MELAS[58] (mitochondrial myopathy, encephalopathy, lactic acidosis,
        and stroke-like episodes)
        Transmitted maternally
        Proliferated mitochondria in smooth muscle cells of cerebral
            vessels (mitochondrial microangiopathy)
    Fabry disease (angiokeratoma corporis diffusum)[53]
        X-linked recessive
        Glycosphingolipid deposit in endothelial cells, cerebral aneu-
            rysms
Nonmetabolic disorders
    Sturge-Weber syndrome (encephalofacial angiomatosis)[128]
        Possibly autosomal dominant
        Leptomeningeal venous angioma, AVM, venous and dural sinus
            abnormalities
    von Hippel-Lindau syndrome[88]
        Autosomal dominant
        Cerebellar, brain stem, and spinal cord hemangioblastoma
    Tuberous sclerosis (Bourneville disease)[51]
        Autosomal dominant
        Intracranial aneurysm, moyamoya syndrome
    Rendu-Osler-Weber syndrome (hereditary hemorrhagic telangiec-
        tasia)[54]
        Autosomal dominant
        AVM, aneurysm, meningeal telangiectasia, venous angioma
    Angiodysgenetic myelomalacia of Foix-Alajounine[22]
        Spinal AVM
    Wyburn-Mason syndrome[133]
        Cerebral AVM (usually brain stem)

Ehlers-Danlos (type IV) syndrome[102]
    Genetically heterogeneous
    Saccular aneurysm, carotid-cavernous fistulas, artery dissection
Pseudoxanthoma elasticum[62]
    Genetically heterogeneous
    Premature atherosclerosis, saccular and microaneurysms, ca-
        rotid-cavernous fistulas
Menkes syndrome (kinky hair disease)[132]
    X-linked recessive
    Tortuosity, elongation, and occlusion of cerebral arteries
Marfan syndrome[105]
    Autosomal dominant
    Aortic dissection; intracranial aneurysm
Klippel-Trénaunay-Weber Syndrome[26]
    Spinal cord vascular malformation
Bannayan-Zonana syndrome[84]
    Hemangioma (usually cerebellum)
Moyamoya syndrome[75]
    Noninflammatory occlusive intracranial vasculopathy (may be
        associated with other hereditary disorders such as neurofibro-
        matosis, tuberous sclerosis, Sturge-Weber syndrome, fibro-
        muscular dysplasia, Marfan syndrome)
Fibromuscular dysplasia[111]
    May be autosomal dominant
    Arterial stenosis, arterial dissection; carotid-cavernous fistulae
Hereditary cerebral amyloid angiopathy[96]
    Autosomal dominant
    HCHWA-Dutch type (β-amyloid)
    HCHWA-Iceland type (cystatin C)
CADASIL[107]
    Autosomal dominant
    Nonatherosclerotic, nonamyloidotic angiopathy of leptomenin-
        geal and small penetrating arteries

Abbreviations: AVM, arteriovenous malformation; HCHWA, hereditary cerebral hemorrhage with amyloidosis; CADASIL, cerebral autosomal dominant arteriopathy with subcortical infarcts and leukoencephalopathy.

moderate hyperhomocysteinemia and cerebrovascular disease may be genetically linked, whereas in elderly patients homocysteinemia is more likely to be acquired. Studies conducted on more than 3,300 patients have established a significant relationship between moderate homocysteinemia and premature vascular disease in the coronary, cerebral, and peripheral arteries.[3] Increased plasma homocysteine is an independent risk factor for atherosclerosis, but an association between homocysteine levels and other cardiovascular risk factors such as high serum cholesterol level, high blood pressure, and cigarette smoking has also been demonstrated.[90] Brain infarction in patients with homocysteinemia is caused by the atheromatous occlusion of the large intracranial vessels. Large arteries in homocystinuria patients demonstrate features typical of atherosclerosis such as fibrous plaques, medial fibrosis, and disruption of the internal elastic membranes. The mechanism by which homocysteinemia promotes atherosclerosis may involve a biochemical pathway through which the sulfur atom of homocysteine thiolactone is oxidized and converted to phosphoadenosine phosphosulfate, the coenzyme that forms the sulfated glycosaminoglycans of atherosclerotic plaques.[82]

MELAS

The term *mitochondrial disease* encompasses a heterogenous group of disorders in which a primary mitochondrial dysfunction is either suspected or proved by morphologic, genetic, or biochemical means.[87] Mitochondrial disease (or mitochondrial DNA-related syndromes) can be divided into two groups: mitochondrial *encephalomyopathies*, characterized by the presence in muscle biopsies of ragged-red fibers as the morphologic hallmark, or pure *encephalopathies* without muscle abnormalities.[137] The first group (encephalomyopathies) includes myoclonic epilepsy with ragged-red fibers, mitochondrial encephalomyopathy with lactic acidosis and strokelike episodes (MELAS), Kearns-Sayre syndrome, chronic progressive external ophthalmoplegia, and a newly described entity, maternally inherited myopathy and cardiomyopathy.

The second group (encephalopathies) includes Leber's hereditary optic neuroretinopathy and the newly recognized ataxia-retinitis pigmentosa-dementia complex.[137]

The stroke-like episodes observed in patients with MELAS are often preceded by prolonged migrainous headaches accompanied by nausea and vomiting occurring in clusters over a few days.[86] Neuropathologic studies of tissues from MELAS patients describe multiple either solitary or confluent foci of necrosis in cerebral cortex and white matter. The distribution of the lesions does not correspond to the territory of a single large artery. Evidence of thromboembolism, vascular inflammation, or arteriosclerotic changes are not visible in the cerebral vessels of patients with MELAS. A marked increase in the number of mitochondria in the small muscle cells of cerebral vessels has been described by one group.[94] Such a change appears to be especially prominent in the walls of leptomeningeal and penetrating arteries with a diameter of up to 250 μm. The basic mechanism of the stroke-like episodes in MELAS may be a mitochondrial dysfunction of the smooth muscle cells of cerebral vessels, a 'mitochondrial microangiopathy.'

Among six patients with a diagnosis of MELAS, the walls of almost all arteries of the biopsied skeletal muscle exhibited large granular deposits with high succinate dehydrogenase activity, and the smooth muscle cells of the sites with strong succinate dehydrogenase activity contained large numbers of mitochondria.[58]

CADASIL

The acronym CADASIL stands for cerebral autosomal dominant arteriopathy with subcortical infarcts and leukoencephalopathy[124] and designates the syndrome previously called "hereditary multi-infarct dementia."[120] CADASIL patients have recurrent subcortical ischemic strokes starting in adulthood, sometimes leading to pseudobulbar palsy and dementia. Other disturbances include migraine and psychiatric symptoms.[17] Magnetic resonance imaging (MRI) of the brain shows small, cavitary lesions (lacunes) in the basal ganglia, as well as diffuse leukoencephalopathy with ventricular dilation. Genetic linkage analysis in two unrelated French families assigned the disease locus to chromosome 19q12.[124]

Marked white matter atrophy, pallor of subcortical myelin with sparing of U-fibers, and multiple lacunes involving the central gray matter, white matter, and pons are the major features of CADASIL. The underlying vascular lesion is a nonatherosclerotic, nonamyloidotic angiopathy of the leptomeningeal and small penetrating arteries of the subcortical white matter and basal ganglia.[5] The arterial walls are thickened by deposits of unidentified material in the tunica media; duplication or fragmentation of the elastic lamina are additional features. The tunica media is thickened by electrondense, osmiophilic granules of unknown origin (Fig. 8.2). Similar changes may be seen in vessels of the sural nerve, skeletal muscle, and skin, suggesting that CADASIL is a systemic disorder.[107]

Ischemic Lesions

Ischemia, or decreased blood flow below the levels of autoregulatory compensation (60 mmHg mean arterial blood pressure) can be the consequence of (1) hypotensive or hemody-

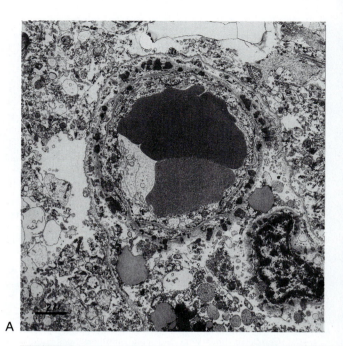

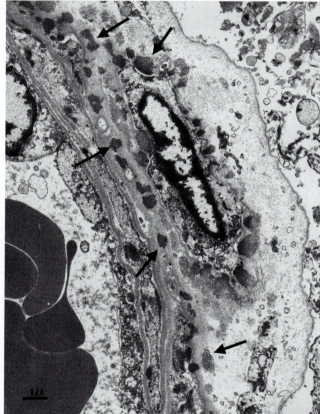

Figure 8.2 CADASIL (**A**) osmiophilic granular deposits in an arteriole of the cerebellar cortex. (**B**) Detail of the osmiophilic granular deposits (arrows) in an arteriole of the cerebral cortex; a few erythrocytes occupy the lumen of the vessel. (Courtesy of Dr. M.M. Ruchoux, Lille, France.)

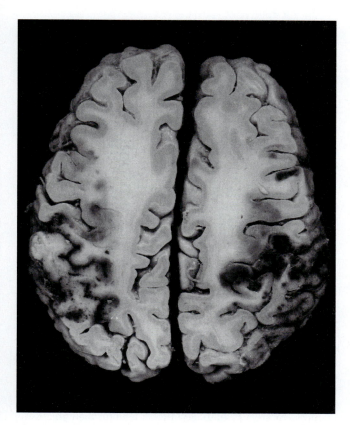

Figure 8.3 Effects of transient global ischemia on the brain. Bilateral areas of hemorrhagic ischemic injury (especially prominent in the arterial boundary zones) in a patient who survived an episode of cardiac arrest for 5 days.

namic crises and (2) occlusive vascular disease involving the arterial vessels of the CNS. A diagnosis of ischemic stroke implies the development of a focal neurologic deficit in a patient who is presumed to have suffered a focal injury secondary to the occlusion of an intracranial artery or arteriole.

LESIONS OF HYPOTENSIVE (OR HEMODYNAMIC) ORIGIN

Ischemic lesions of the CNS having a hemodynamic origin are the consequence of episodic cardiac arrest, abrupt drops in systemic blood pressure, shock, peripheral vascular collapse, and, less frequently, cardiac dysrhythmias. The resulting parenchymal lesions are of a highly diverse nature and may involve one or more of the following sites: cerebral cortical mantle, basal ganglia, cerebellar cortex, cerebral white matter, brain stem, spinal cord, and various combinations of these CNS sites.[40]

Selective Vulnerability

Brain injuries secondary to an episode of cardiac arrest, as an example, selectively involve specific sites of the CNS such as the arterial border (or boundary) zones of the cerebral hemispheres (Fig. 8.3), the cerebellum, and the spinal cord. This

selective involvement is attributed to the precarious nature of the arterial blood supply at sites identified as the *distal end* of an arterial territory. *Selective vulnerability* also applies to the involvement of specific cell types following a systemic injury; thus the pyramidal neurons in the CA-1 sector of the hippocampus and the Purkinje cell layer of the cerebellum are two neuronal groups that are most susceptible to necrosis following a global ischemic crisis. In the cerebral cortex, layers III to V (more than the rest of the cortical layers) are likely to be injured by systemic ischemia. Likewise, in the basal ganglia, the globus pallidus is more susceptible to the ischemic injury than the striatum, and after an episode of systemic hypotension or transient cardiac arrest, small striatal neurons become necrotic before large neurons show morphologic changes of necrosis.[40]

After an episode of cardiac arrest or a hypotensive crisis, the extent of the resultant brain injury is influenced by both the duration of the event and the severity (measured by the blood pressure level on recovery) of the ischemic episode; additional factors influencing the outcome of an injury caused by hypotensive ischemic crises include age of the patient (the younger the individual the longer the tolerance for ischemia); body temperature (hypothermia protects neurons from the ischemic injury, whereas hyperthermia may have the opposite effect), and serum glucose content (hypoglycemia at the time of the ischemic event is said to protect the ischemic brain by limiting the rate of production of lactic acid). Length of survival after the cardiac arrest, or duration of reperfusion, may be an additional factor that determines the extent of the injury to the hippocampus.[100]

The ischemic brain lesions attributed to the effects of hypotensive crises are almost always bilateral and relatively symmetric regardless of their location in the CNS. Some ischemic lesions of hypotensive origin may have a hemorrhagic component (Fig. 8.3) consisting of numerous petechiae scattered throughout the gray matter structures. This hemorrhagic quality is attributed to the effects of reperfusion on a previously ischemic territory; alternatively, the nonocclusive nature of the ischemic event may be such that during the hypotensive crisis a trickle of blood flow is retained into the injured area.[40]

Subcortical Leukoencephalopathy

Systemic hypoperfusion of the brain may be one of the mechanisms that induce diffuse injury to the periventricular white matter of the cerebral hemispheres; this morphologic alteration, as seen on neuroimaging studies, is descriptively known as *leukoaraiosis* or white matter rarefaction. Leukoaraiosis, or areas of hypodensity on computed tomography (CT) scans or hyperintensity on MRI, is a common finding among persons older than 60 years. The clinical significance of this abnormality is a subject of much controversy; analyses of several epidemiological studies suggest that (1) the condition is more common after the age of 60 years; (2) leukoaraiosis is more prevalent among persons with a history of cardiac disease and stroke than in appropriately matched controls; and (3) although leukoaraiosis exists in psychologically intact persons, the more severe degrees of white matter rarefaction are encountered in persons with subtle cognitive deficits and decreased velocity in mental processing.[97] Among premature newborns, the condition of periventricular leukomalacia is at-

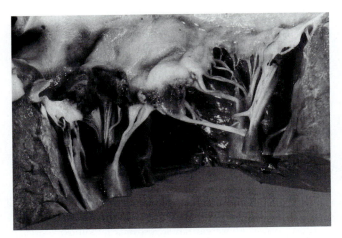

Figure 8.4 Nonbacterial thrombotic vegetations on the anterior leaflet of the mitral valve. Rheumatic thickening of the cordae tendinae and leaflets is also apparent.

tributed to the effects of hypoxemia (caused by pulmonary immaturity) and ischemia (caused by combined systemic hypotension and cardiac failure).[40]

ISCHEMIC LESIONS OF OCCLUSIVE ORIGIN

Brain infarcts may be the consequence of either arterial embolism or thrombosis. Some of the thrombotic events are intuitively attributed to local vascular disease; however, in a significant percentage of cases, the causes of the intracranial vascular occlusions accompanying a brain infarct remain undetected.[108] Some of the patients with intracranial vascular occlusions of unknown etiology may have hematologic abnormalities that promote intravascular coagulation, such as antiphospholipid antibodies[21] or deficiency of proteins C or S.[70,71,109]

Brain Infarcts of Embolic Origin

Two common sources of embolism to the brain are the left-sided cardiac valves, the left-sided chambers of the heart (especially among patients who have had a transmural myocardial infarct), and the origin of the internal carotid artery (ICA). Vegetations, made of fibrin platelets, may form at the mitral and aortic valves in patients who have hypercoagulable states; the classic example of this condition is represented by a patient with adenocarcinoma of the pancreas who develops multiple thrombi in several veins as well as in the cardiac valves. Valvular vegetations in these patients are sometimes called "marantic endocarditis"; this designation is inappropriate because marasmus is not essential for the formation of vegetations and because no inflammatory component is present. The preferred designation is *nonbacterial thrombotic vegetations* (Fig. 8.4), which among patients with SLE are called Libman-Sacks vegetations. Congenital valvular defects and systemic infections are two of many factors that promote the formation of

infected vegetations; this results in the condition of bacterial endocarditis (subacute or acute depending on the microorganism responsible for the infection). The origin of cerebral emboli among patients with atrial fibrillation is disputed; this is because postmortem studies in these patients seldom show mural thrombi in the atrial appendages of the heart. Nevertheless, patients with nonvalvular atrial fibrillation (NAF) have a 33% increased risk of developing brain infarcts that are presumed to be of embolic origin. Repeated CT evaluation of the brain in NAF patients has disclosed increasing numbers of asymptomatic brain lesions (mostly of the lacunar type) currently known as silent infarcts.[29]

Artery-to-artery embolism frequently results from the detachment of mural thrombi from the origin of the ICA, at the site of an ulcerated atheromatous plaque. In such cases, the material occluding small branches of either the retinal artery or the middle cerebral arteries (MCAs) is composed primarily of platelets and fibrin. Ophthalmoscopic examination of the retina, shortly after an embolic event (manifested in amaurosis fugax), sometimes allows visualization of the embolic material, which is identifiable by the bright yellow color of the cholesterol crystals and the lipid components. Most brain emboli are distributed in the territory of the MCA, which is the main and most direct branch of the ICA. Emboli to the cerebral hemispheres commonly lodge at the junction between the cortex and white matter and preferentially involve the bottom of the sulcus rather than the crest of the gyrus. Many brain infarcts of cardioembolic origin are hemorrhagic; additional features common to embolic infarcts include their relatively small size (usually <2 cm in average diameter) and their multiplicity within a single arterial territory. The inflammatory response by polymorphonuclear leukocytes at the site of an embolic infarct is usually more pronounced than it is at sites of thrombotic infarcts; this is reflected in a high increase in the neutrophil count of the CSF, which, in addition, may also contain numerous erythrocytes.[40]

Thrombotic Arterial Infarcts: Early Events

Examples of brain infarcts, secondary to the thrombotic occlusion of an artery, are frequently seen in hypertensive, diabetic patients with advanced atherosclerosis of the basilar artery or other intracranial arteries; at the site where the vascular lumen is maximally narrowed, a thrombus that completely occludes the arterial lumen may develop either abruptly or over a period of several days. As studied serially in experimental models of ischemic stroke, occlusion of an intracranial artery results in a concomitant decrease of the local cerebral blood flow (CBF) and loss of function of the tissues supplied by the occluded vessel. During the initial 45 to 90 minutes, the tissue changes induced by an experimental arterial occlusion are detectable by diffusion-weighted MRI. In rats with intraluminal occlusion of the MCA (of ≤ 90 minutes' duration), the degree of change in apparent diffusion coefficient (ADC) correlates well with each of the following factors: degree of astrocyte/endothelial cell swelling, number of microvessels with impaired patency, and number of neuronal perikarya with acute ischemic changes.[77] The reversibility of some of these changes, induced by brief periods (<45 minutes) of arterial occlusion, has been demonstrated in humans who suffer tran-

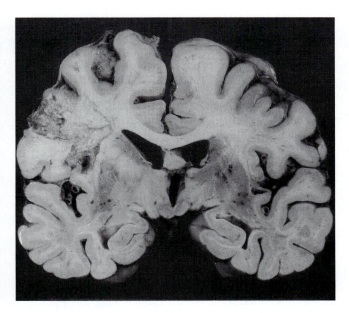

Figure 8.5 Subacute brain infarct (about 2 to 3 weeks old by clinical history) in the territory of a middle cerebral artery branch.

sient neurologic deficits as a result of either carotid endarterectomy or carotid angioplasty.[30]

ANEMIC BRAIN INFARCTS

The word infarct, used by most authors interchangably with infarction, describes an area of coagulation necrosis (or pannecrosis) that in most instances is secondary to an arterial occlusion.[27] The clinical manifestations produced by an intracranial artery occlusion are called ischemic strokes, which in most patients are expressed in focal neurologic deficits. In contrast to the effects of an arterial occlusion, most intracranial venous occlusions do not result in focal neurologic deficits and induce brain edema and hemorrhages rather than tissue necrosis.[39] Based on their grossly visible features, brain infarcts associated with arterial occlusions are divided into *white* (or bland, anemic) infarcts and *red* (or hemorrhagic) infarcts. The main difference between the two resides on the number of grossly visible petechiae; these hemorrhages are very abundant in red infarcts and are either very scant or absent in white infarcts. Sequential CT evaluations of patients with ischemic strokes demonstrate that a significant percentage of initially anemic infarcts undergo spontaneous hemorrhagic transformation, which can take one of two expressions: multiple petechiae that usually remain confined to the gray matter structures (cortex and basal ganglia), or massive hemorrhage that entirely replaces the originally ischemic tissues.[11]

Traditional descriptions of the morbid gross anatomy of arterial brain infarcts divide the evolution of these lesions into four stages: (1) acute ischemia occurs 0 hours to 2 days after the beginning of symptoms; the brain lesion is invisible to the naked eye until 3 to 4 days after the stroke; (2) maximal swelling (days 4 to 5) becomes appreciable by the significant softening of the injured tissues and the displacement of neighboring

structures (this effect is called by some authors mass effect); (3) a subacute stage begins between days 5 and 10 and is characterized by the disappearance of the swelling and the sharp demarcation of the previously blurred boundary of the ischemic or infarcted tissue (Fig. 8.5); and (4) the chronic or healed stage (appearing weeks or months later) corresponds to the time when reabsorption of the necrotic debris takes place; the completion of this stage leaves behind a fluid-filled cavity.[95,99] In contrast to what happens in the heart, kidney, and other viscera, necrotic tissues in the brain are not replaced by collagenous scar; instead, the cavity left by the activity of macrophages (Fig. 8.6) is filled with fluid with a protein content similar to that of the CSF. Possibly because the tissue is replaced by liquid, some authors refer to this process as liquefaction necrosis. The precise timing of these events is extremely difficult to ascertain in human specimens because, as demonstrated in experimental models of ischemic stroke, the duration of the arterial occlusion significantly alters the tissue responses, and in most instances of human ischemic stroke it is extremely difficult to determine the duration of the arterial occlusion.[49]

The previously described sequence of events raises several questions: how long must an intracranial artery be occluded before coagulation necrosis appears? If the duration of the

Figure 8.6 Cavitary stage of brain infarction involving the territory supplied by a middle cerebral artery branch on the left hemisphere. The clinical history indicated that the patient had had a stroke several years before death.

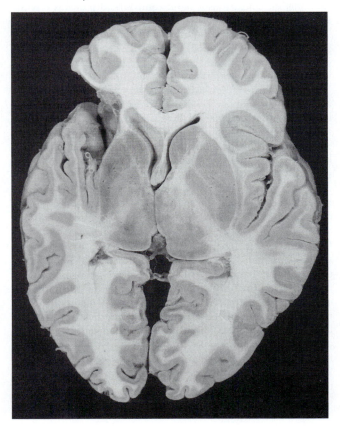

arterial occlusion influences the extent of the necrosis, what are the tissue responses that develop after a short, transient arterial occlusion? Finally, are there differences in terms of topographic location about the time when various neuronal groups die following an arterial occlusion?

The answers to these questions and related ones cannot be sought in human brains and for this reason it has become necessary to study the chronologic evolution of ischemic strokes in animal models in which the arterial occlusion can be reproducibly induced without opening the skull; the resulting brain lesion has features similar or identical to those induced in humans by arterial occlusions (see below).

HEMORRHAGIC (RED) BRAIN INFARCTS

A hemorrhagic brain lesion is generally attributed to an arterial occlusion, and most red infarcts are believed to evolve from an initially white or bland infarct. The mechanisms responsible for the hemorrhagic transformation of ischemic brain lesions are remarkably complex, and a single cause does not apply to every situation. In autopsy studies, $\leq 42\%$ of brain infarcts were classified as hemorrhagic, and $> 70\%$ of all brain infarcts thought to have an embolic origin had hemorrhagic components. By contrast, only 22% of the brain infarcts with a presumed thrombotic etiology were hemorrhagic.[57] The lack of reliable, objective criteria that may tell the difference between an embolus and a thrombus on microscopic examination constitutes a significant difficulty in this type of study.

Based on autopsy observations, Fisher and Adams[35] suggested that the hemorrhagic transformation of a white infarct could be the result of a thromboembolus fragmentation and the subsequent reperfusion of the ischemic territory. Support for that hypothesis exists in the results of experiments conducted in cats that had transient (6-hour) MCA occlusion followed by a 24-hour period of reperfusion; in those animals multiple petechiae appeared in the gray matter of the ischemic tissues according to a pattern similar to that observed in human ischemic strokes that undergo hemorrhagic transformation.[66]

The beneficial effects of early ($\leq$1-hour) reperfusion in the treatment of an experimental ischemic stroke have been demonstrated in rats that had the right MCA occluded with a nylon filament and were allowed to survive for 1 week after the arterial occlusion.[49] Untimely reperfusion carries with it several potential hazards, however, including (1) increased generation of oxygen free radicals, (2) hemorrhagic transformation of the brain lesion, and (3) aggravation of the postischemic brain edema.[24] The optimal time when reperfusion may be helpful probably varies for each individual, and the limit of reversibility may be primarily influenced by the adequacy of the collateral anastomoses that exist among arteries located in the subarachnoid space. Brain microvessels are known to dilate and rupture in increasing numbers as a function of the duration of the arterial occlusion in primates with transient MCA occlusion of 3-hour duration followed by a 24-hour period of reperfusion.[46]

Hemorrhagic Transformation of Brain Infarcts

The hemorrhagic transformation of white infarcts has become the focus of great interest because this is the most frequent and serious complication of thrombolytic therapy.[55,89] The percentage of ischemic (white) brain infarcts undergoing hemorrhagic transformation increases as a function of the frequency with which neuroimaging studies are carried out in patients with ischemic strokes.[11] Hemorrhagic transformation detected by CT occurred in 43% of brain infarcts involving tissues in the territory of the carotid artery.[122]

The biologic factor(s) responsible for the hemorrhagic transformation of brain infarcts has not been identified, and reopening the occluded artery does not appear to be indispensable for bleeding to occur in an evolving white infarct.[61] Late ($\leq$6-hour) reperfusion in rats with MCA occlusion increases the incidence of hemorrhagic transformation and the volume of the hemorrhages,[32] but hemorrhagic transformation also occurs in 48% of animals in which the MCA remains occluded for 72 hours.[98] Ogata et al[93] reported a series of 14 patients with persistent embolic arterial occlusions studied at autopsy. In seven of these brain specimens the infarcts were hemorrhagic; in the other seven there were no grossly visible petechiae. The authors suggested that higher blood pressure readings in the group with hemorrhagic brain lesions may have accounted for the hemorrhagic transformation that occurred in the absence of arterial reopening.[93] Support for this hypothesis was derived from observations made on cats with surgical clipping of the MCA; induced hypertension correlated with hemorrhagic transformation in one-half of these animals.[110] Among humans the incidence of hemorrhagic transformation in brain infarcts correlates with the volume of the brain lesion[79] and with the administration of anticoagulants.[13]

CELLULAR EVENTS IN AN EXPERIMENTAL MODEL OF ISCHEMIC STROKE

A detailed, chronologic analysis of the cellular events initiated by the occlusion of an intracranial artery cannot be conducted in humans. Significant advances have been made through observations conducted on a reproducible experimental model of MCA occlusion in the rat. The laboratory method to occlude the orifice of a MCA in adult rats is based on the intracarotid insertion of a nylon monofilament that does not require opening the skull, is compatible with the reperfusion of the ischemic tissues, and is minimally invasive. The difficulty in interpreting the widely variable results, a consequence of individual variations in the responses to this type of insult, is partially overcome by averaging the results of observations made in groups of 5 to 10 animals, each submitted to identical experimental conditions.

Leukocytes, Microvessels, and Astrocytes

Permanent MCA occlusion of ≤ 7 days, duration evaluated at short, hourly intervals reveals a progressive growth of the brain lesion (i.e., area of pallor) that peaks 3 to 4 days after

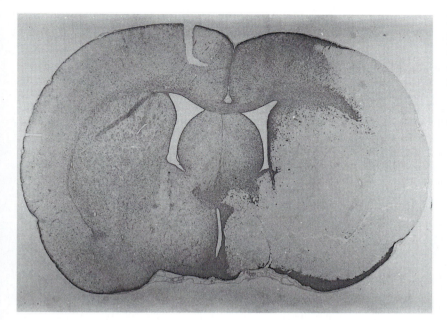

Figure 8.7 Brain infarct (Wistar rat). The right middle cerebral artery was permanently occluded 7 days before death. (Glial fibrillary acidic protein immunoreaction, original magnification × 2.5.)

the arterial occlusion. A progressive spread or growth of the lesion from the basal ganglia-preoptic area to the cerebral cortex has been noted both in histologic preparations[48] and in vivo, as studied by positron emission tomography in cats with MCA occlusion.[59,60] The appearance of areas of pale staining and coagulation necrosis in this experimental model is delayed by several days[48] (Fig. 8.7) and follows a chronology similar to the CT changes in density observed in humans with MCA occlusions.[73] In addition to the progressive spread of the lesion, reflected in the growth of an area of decreased stainability, there is a time-dependent increase in the number of necrotic neurons that peaks at about 24 hours in the caudo-putamen and several hours later in the cerebral cortex.[43] The progressive worsening of the brain lesion at a time when no additional injury has been induced suggests that some biologic events, initiated by the arterial occlusion, are time dependent and that some of these may account for the eventual appearance of neuronal necrosis.

MCA occlusion in rats elicits brain upregulation of interleukin-1α (IL-1α) and tumor necrosis factor.[44] Since both these cytokines have potent proinflammatory effects that include the activation of circulating polymorphonuclear leukocytes (PMN), IL-1α upregulation may be responsible for the continuous influx of leukocytes into the ischemic territory. Leukocyte influx in rats with permanent MCA occlusion starts within 1 hour after the arterial occlusion and peaks about 24 hours later when the numbers of PMN visible in the ischemic parenchyma begin to decrease.[45] The presence of PMN leukocytes in the lumen of microvessels ($\leq$15 μm in average diameter) may impair the circulation of erythrocytes and thus may aggravate the conditions of the microcirculation. In addition, PMN leukocytes may contribute to the necrosis of endothelial and neuronal cells through the release of oxygen free radicals.[112] The hypothesis that the influx of PMN leukocytes may contribute to the neuronal injury was tested in experiments in which the

effects of the proinflammatory cytokine IL-1 were blocked by injecting rats with human recombinant IL-1 receptor antagonist (IL-1ra), a polypeptide that specifically binds to the receptor sites for IL-1 on endothelial cells. The mechanism of action for IL-1ra may involve the inhibition of IL-1 and the prevention of endothelial cells from secreting IL-8, a cytokine necessary for the transendothelial migration of PMN leukocytes.[67] Injecting human recombinant IL-1ra into rats with permanent MCA occlusion significantly decreased the number of necrotic neurons at 24 hours and 7 days and also resulted in significant improvement of the animals' sensorimotor functions as well as in a decreased number of PMN leukocytes entering the ischemic brain.[44]

Additional support for the hypothesis that microvascular alterations, occurring shortly after the arterial occlusion, may contribute to the subsequent neuronal injury has been obtained in experiments based on arterial occlusions of short duration. In these experiments, the brain lesion induced by MCA occlusion lasting 45 to 90 minutes was mapped by diffusion-weighted MRI; this method revealed multiple, scattered foci of the ischemic hemisphere in which the apparent diffusion coefficient (ADC) changed either moderately or severely. A close correlation was established between the severity of change in the ADC and each of the following morphometric parameters: numbers of microvessels with narrowed or occluded lumen, degree of swelling of astrocytes, and numbers of neurons with shrunken perikarya.[77] These and other observations suggest that the sequence of biologic events initiated by an arterial occlusion involve, during the early stages of the lesion, structural and functional changes in microvessels ($\leq$15 μm in diameter) and astrocytes. The second stage of the ischemic lesion, beginning about 6 hours after the arterial occlusion, would be characterized by the beginning of the death of selected neurons (i.e., those located in the striatum). Therefore, considerable interest exists in exploring mechanisms of neuronal death under conditions of ischemia.

Neuronal Injury: Necrosis and Apoptosis

Neuronal function disappears as soon as the artery is occluded, as demonstrated by the loss of spontaneous and evoked action potentials.[47] However, this functional loss is reversible, and the period of tolerance is directly related to the severity of the ischemia: moderate ischemia (15 to 20 ml/100 g/min) may be reversible after hours, while severe ischemia (≤10 ml/100 g/min) may lead to neuronal death within a few minutes.[60]

The occlusion of a large intracranial artery in both humans[74] and laboratory animals[4] creates at least two areas where the degree of ischemia is significantly different. The center (or core) is characterized by very low CBF values, whereas the marginal (or penumbral) zone maintains CBF at levels higher than in the core. This heterogeneity in blood flow changes and the *selective vulnerability* of isolated neuronal groups may explain why necrosis appears at predictable sites at different times after the arterial occlusion.[43] Additional factors that contribute to the heterogeneous and multicentric distribution of the necrotic neurons may be related to the diverse mechanisms by which neurons die after an ischemic event: necrosis, apoptosis, or other.

Necrosis

The traditional concept of irreversible cell injury after focal ischemia is based on observations showing that energy failure and hypoxemia result in the shutdown of the plasma membrane protein (adenosine triphosphatase) responsible for maintaining the normal ion distribution across cell membranes. This results in a prompt efflux of K^+ into the extracellular space. In the CNS, the resultant depolarization promotes massive release of glutamate,[7] which leads to an indiscriminate opening of the glutamate-gated channels, many of which are permeant to Ca^{2+}. The intracellular entry of Ca^{2+} is further aggravated by the fact that depolarization opens voltage-gated Ca^{2+} channels as well. Excessive cytosolic Ca^{2+} exerts several deleterious effects: (1) it enhances lipolysis, (2) it promotes disaggregation of tubulin and polyribosomes, and (3) it damages plasma membranes, thus promoting additional influx of Ca^{2+} into the ischemic cell.[115] At the structural level, cells undergoing necrosis initially display pyknosis followed by breakdown of nuclear and plasma membranes and eventual phagocytosis and removal of all cellular fragments. This type of cell death, traditionally known as necrosis, is attributed to the effects of physical, chemical, or osmotic damage to the plasma membrane.[72]

Apoptosis

The term *apoptosis*, originally coined by Kerr et al,[68] refers to the process whereby deciduous trees shed their leaves during the fall; some authors use the word interchangeably with the term *programmed cell death* (PCD). Apoptosis may be part of the normal organogenic process during which excessive numbers of cells are eliminated; this is supported by the observation that failure to undergo apoptosis during organogenesis causes malformations in insects and mammals.[125]

In contrast to the phenomena occurring after necrosis, cells undergoing PCD exhibit intact plasma membranes until the late phases of the metabolic suicide, allowing adjacent cells to engulf the entire dying cell and to eliminate it before its content is released.[72] The *induction* stage of PCD probably occurs in response to hypoxemia. Cytoplasmic structures, including mitochondria, participate in the *effector* stage, with the nuclear abnormalities occurring in the *late* stage. A decrease in mitochondrial transmembrane potential followed by uncoupling and generation of reactive oxygen species precedes the nuclear alterations.[72]

The progression of myocyte death after focal ischemia was studied in rats with coronary artery ligation of up to 7 days' duration. The authors concluded that in these experiments most myocytes die, in a progressive manner, through *apoptotic* mechanisms beginning at 2 hours. By contrast, *necrosis* (as indicated by plasma membrane injury) began in earnest 6 hours after the arterial occlusion.[65]

Two aspects of these experiments deserve special attention: first, as in the case of the MCA occlusion, the ischemic injury killed cells over a period of several hours (2 to 48 hours); second, not all cells died by the same mechanism. The possibility that apoptotic and necrotic injuries occur in the brain after an arterial occlusion remains unproved. In addition to anoxia, apoptosis may be inducible by neurotransmitters such as glutamate.[91] Both apoptosis and the effects of glutamate on the N-methyl-D-aspartate receptors can be counteracted in ways that in the opinion of some authors could become the basis of future therapeutic interventions in human ischemic stroke.[91]

INCOMPLETE BRAIN INFARCTION

Arterial occlusions in both humans[74] and experimental animals,[4,47] produce heterogeneous changes in local CBF that in cases of permanent arterial occlusion probably become homogeneous after several hours and lead to a widespread area of coagulation necrosis that appears 3 to 4 days later.[48] This suggests that the process leading to necrosis may be interrupted at least in some portions of the ischemic territory by interventions based on the administration of neuroprotective agents reopening the artery, or a combination of both. A sequential angiographic study demonstrated that thrombolytic mechanisms in humans are fairly efficient in that, in the absence of any therapy, most occluded arteries reopen within 24 to 48 hours.[119] The effects of this form of delayed reperfusion are not known; it is possible that in many cases the arterial reopening occurs at a time when the effects of reperfusion on the ischemic brain are insignificant.

Among rats with intrinsic MCA occlusion, reopening the artery as much as 60 minutes later resulted in significant improvement of sensory motor functions. More importantly, early reperfusion modified the brain lesion so that after 7 days cavitation was either absent or present only in very small isolated foci of the ischemic territory. The bulk of the brain lesion induced in these animals by short-term arterial occlusion was characterized by partial (or selective) loss of neurons accompanied by reactive astrogliosis with preservation of the brain tissue architecture and tissue density[49] (Figs. 8.8 and

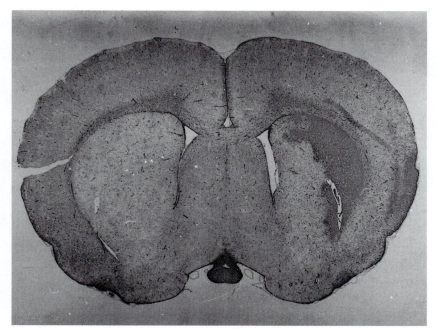

Figure 8.8 Incomplete infarct (Wistar rat). The right middle cerebral artery was occluded for 30 minutes; the subject was allowed to survive for 21 days. The darker areas on the right hemisphere correspond to sites of selective neuronal injury and activation of microglia. (ED-1 immuno-reaction, original magnification × 2.5.)

8.9). A hyperintense area in the territory of the occluded MCA, detected by diffusion-weighted MRI as early as 30 minutes after the arterial occlusion, disappeared in the cortex but not in the caudoputamen as a result of reopening the artery.[85]

These two experimental observations offer strong support to the concept that *moderate* ischemia of the type produced by an arterial occlusion of short duration (less than 60 minutes) results in ischemic injury to the brain that cannot be classified as an infarct because it is at least partially reversible. The histopathology of the brain lesion produced by moderate tran-

sient ischemia include selective neuronal death and astrogliosis; because this lesion does not lead to cavitation of the type visible in the chronic stage after permanent arterial occlusion, we suggest that the injury induced in the brain by moderate ischemia be called *incomplete infarct*.[42] Lesions that correspond to the current designation of incomplete infarctions were observed by Spatz in 1939 and Scholz in 1957 among human autopsy specimens of MCA occlusion.[42] Lassen et al[74] have described brain lesions in which neuronal destruction was partial in two patients, each of whom had (1) angiographic

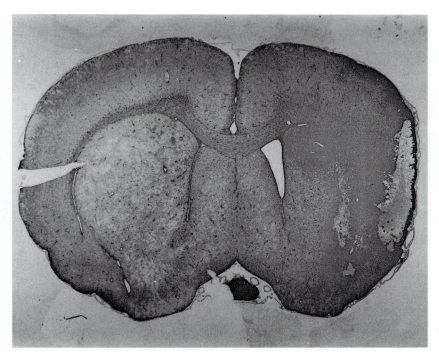

Figure 8.9 Incomplete infarct and small areas of infarction (Wistar rat). The right middle cerebral artery was occluded for 30 minutes (day 1), 15 minutes (day 2), and 15 minutes (day 3); the experiment was terminated on day 21. On the right hemisphere the lateral ventricle is enlarged, and the architecture of the basal ganglia and cortex are blurred by the increased astrogliosis. Localized sites of pan-necrosis appear white on the photograph. (Glial fibrillary acidic protein immunoreaction, original magnification × 2.5.)

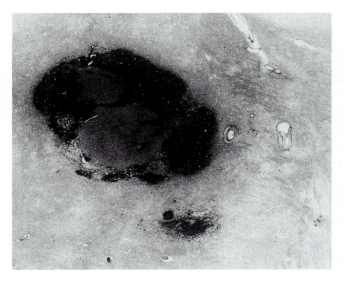

Figure 8.10 Intracerebral hemorrhage (basal ganglia) of recent age. Hyalinization is visible in two arteries at the periphery of the hemorrhage. (H&E, original magnification × 2.5.)

evidence of arterial occlusion, (2) evidence of heterogeneous changes in the CBF secondary to the arterial occlusion, and (3) autopsy confirmation of partial neuronal destruction with astrogliosis in areas where the local CBF values had been only moderately lowered. Incorporating the concept of incomplete infarction is significant because, although conventional neuroimaging methods cannot detect this type of lesion, functional neuroimaging with radioligands can identify areas of the brain where the ischemic injury may be at least partially reversed or ameliorated either by reperfusion or by other therapeutic interventions.[42]

Intracerebral Hemorrhage

MORPHOLOGY

The sequential changes affecting the brain parenchyma after a spontaneous intracerebral hemorrhage (ICH) have interested pathologists for over a century. The histologic changes occurring in ICH were outlined by Neumann and Spatz and include three stages as defined in autopsy specimens. During the first 4 days, there is deformation, edema, and necrosis of the surrounding brain tissues; the second stage, absorption of the hematoma, lasts for 5 to 15 days; and conversion of the hematoma into either a fibroglial scar or a cavity occurs in the final stage.[41]

In the acute stages, the ICH consists of a liquid or semiliquid mass of erythrocytes (Fig. 8.10) that may contain small fragments of necrotic brain tissue. The edema that develops around the hemorrhage is particularly prominent in ICH located in the white matter. Petechiae visible within the rim of brain tissue surrounding the ICH are called Stäemller mar-

ginal hemorrhages. After a few days, the hematoma increases in consistency and adopts a brownish color, while the peripheral edema begins to recede. The formation of hemoglobin-derived pigments in macrophages confers a golden green tinge to the edge of the tissue around the ICH. After several months or years, depending on the size of the hematoma, the erythrocytes are replaced by a cavity lined by cells containing brownish pigment; this is sometimes called an *apoplectic cyst*. There are significant differences of opinion concerning the evolution of an ICH. Some authors state that an ICH becomes a solid clot a few hours after the original bleeding and that partial liquefaction begins 12 to 15 hours later, while others opine that clotting in ICH occurs only after the first day.[78] Most authors maintain that an ICH becomes at least partially liquefied by the end of the first week, but nonliquefied clots are known to remain unchanged for several weeks.[78,131]

In contrast to the cavities left at sites where reabsorption of the hematoma is complete, some ICH become encapsulated by a fibroglial membrane that is established 5 to 6 weeks after the original bleeding. The earliest tissue reactions include edema of adjacent tissues and neutrophilic infiltrates; macrophages begin a slow process of digestion. The resulting cavity becomes encapsulated after a period of several weeks and is finally surrounded by collagen fibers.[63] In the early stages, the extravasated erythrocytes preserve their shape and color, and the interphase with the adjacent brain is well defined. The edge of the hematoma contacts partly edematous parenchyma, and cellular inflammatory infiltrates are not visible. After several hours or days, depending on the size and site of the hemorrhage, extracellular brain edema may become evident in the parenchyma adjacent to the hematoma. The hemispheric white matter expands and displays pale-staining and swollen, vacuolated myelin sheaths. After approximately 4 to 10 days, depending on the size of the ICH, the red blood cells membranes begin to break up. Individual erythrocytes are difficult to identify as their shape becomes blurred or swollen and eventually their plasma membranes rupture; at this time, the bright red erythrocytes are replaced by amorphous masses of methemoglobin. Once the metabolic reserves are depleted, deoxygenated hemoglobin and methemoglobin (oxidized deoxyhemoglobin) become abundant at the site of ICH.[41]

Cellular infiltrates appear at the periphery of the hemorrhage within a few days. One of the earliest events is the influx of PMNs and activated microglial cells. Studies detailing the chronology of the arrival of PMNs in human brain hemorrhages are not available, but experimental observations suggest that PMNs begin to infiltrate the margin of the ICH after 2 days and that their numbers peak at 4 days.[64] The appearance of macrophages is better documented in human hematomas than is the appearance of PMNs. Macrophages display a round shape, few cytoplasmic processes, foamy or granular cytoplasm, and round nuclei located close to the plasma membrane; macrophages have strong acid phosphatase activity and can be immunostained by antibodies to macrophages such as KP-1 or Mac 387 and also with biotinylated lectins, such as *Ricinus comunis* agglutinin.[28]

The time-dependent appearance of hemoglobin-derived products in the ICH is of interest, especially because the interpretation of neuroimaging studies is based on the presence of these products of blood breakdown. The two major hemoglobin-derived pigments identifiable in tissue sections are hemosiderin and hematoidin. Hemosiderin represents aggregates of ferritin micelles within phagosomes (lysosomes of phagocytic cells); hemosiderin is a coarse, golden brown, granular intracytoplasmic pigment. The ferritin micelles contain ferric ions, which makes hemosiderin demonstrable with histochemical methods. Hematoidin, by contrast, is chemically identical to bilirubin, a pigment that forms locally as a result of hemoglobin breakdown; this process is favored by reduced oxygen tension.[41] Hematoidin has a golden yellow color, appears as more coarse and globular deposits than hemosiderin, and is frequently extracellular. The main difference between the two pigments is that hematoidin does not contain iron and for this reason is Prussian blue negative. In human ICH, hemosiderin appears first at 6 days and remains visible for a long time; hematoidin becomes visible 10 days after the hemorrhage, and its appearance is always more delayed than that of hemosiderin.[41]

One of the final events in the microscopic changes of cerebral hematomas involves the astrocytes. These cells proliferate at the periphery of the hemorrhage in a manner similar to that observed after other types of focal cerebral injury. The precise sequence of astrocyte reactions after ICH is not known, but experimental studies suggest that the increased glial fibrillary acidic protein reactivity of these cells may take place as early as 2 to 3 days after the hemorrhage.[64]

ICHs in newborn, premature infants evolve in a manner similar to that observed in adults; however, a major difference is that the hemosiderin is completely cleared from the premature brains, while in the adult brain the pigment remains for years. This may be related to the transfer of hemosiderin from macrophages to astrocytes, an event that rarely happens in infants but is common in the adult. Cavitation after an ICH is much more rapid in the premature infant, but the biologic reasons for this difference are not known.[52]

Few studies of experimental ICH detail the sequence of pathologic changes. Most experiments are based on either the intracerebral injection of coagulated venous blood or the insertion of intracerebral balloons; neither of these experimental conditions reproduce the arterial bleeding of human ICH. Enzmann et al[31] and Takasugi et al[121] report good correlation between their observations on canine hemorrhages and the stages described in human ICH by Spatz.[52] Experimental ICH in the rat has been induced by injecting at arterial pressure an aliquot of liquid blood; the sequence of histologic changes observed in that model agrees with the timetable suggested by Spatz.[64] The extent of brain edema in these rats was greater than the original size of the ICH, suggesting that, in rats, brain edema may be more harmful than the initial bleeding. PMNs appeared around the ICH at 48 hours, and their numbers peaked at 4 days. Hemosiderin-laden macrophages appeared between 4 and 14 days, and astroglial proliferation was well established by 14 days. This latter event resulted in the formation of a membrane (glia limitans) that separates the residual hematoma from the adjacent neuropil.[64] Observations made on an animal model of ICH, recently developed, emphasize the early leakage of macromolecules and the concomitant perihematoma edema as significant determinants of the clinical outcome.[130] The evolution of cellular changes elicited by the presence of blood within the brain has been studied in rabbits by Koeppen et al.[69] In these animals,

conversion of hemoglobin to hemosiderin began 5 days after the injection of either whole blood or erythrocytes. Astrocytes that did not succumb to the initial ICH re-entered the margins of the hematoma and intermingled with microglia and macrophages. This interaction among glial cells may have reversed the uncoupling of ferritin biosynthesis and may have initiated iron storage and formation of hemosiderin.[69]

ICH, especially in subcortical locations, is a known complication of fibrinolytic therapy for coronary artery occlusion. Analysis of a large epidemiologic study suggests that among these patients, ICH may be associated with additional risk factors such as cerebral amyloid angiopathy, acute or persistent arterial hypertension, severe ventricular arrhythmias, and hypofibrinogenemia.[117]

ICH has long been considered a one-time event in which the postictal worsening of the patient's condition has been attributed to the development of brain edema around the hematoma, progressive increases in intracranial pressure, and miscellaneous systemic factors. However, repeated CT evaluations reveal frequent spontaneous expansion of the ICH that may contribute to the worsening of the symptoms observed 2 to 3 days after the stroke.[19,38] One of the factors that may contribute to the continuous or repeated bleeding at the site of an ICH may be a persistently raised mean arterial blood pressure.[19] Patients with ICH who have associated liver dysfunction, hematomas of large volume (as seen on the initial CT scan), or nonspherical ICH are at increased risk of having repeated intracerebral bleeding.[38]

References

1. Alarcón-Segovia D, Deleze M et al: Antiphospholipid antibodies and the antiphospholipid syndrome in systemic lupus erythematosus. A prospective analysis of 500 consecutive patients. Medicine 68:353, 1989

2. Amorosi EL, Ultmann JE: Thrombotic thrombocytopenic purpura: a report of 16 cases and review of the literature. Medicine 45:139, 1966

3. Arnesen E, Refsum H, Bonaa KH et al: Serum total homocysteine and coronary heart disease. Int J Epidemiol 24:704–709, 1995

4. Astrup J, Symon L, Siesjö BK: Thresholds in cerebral ischemia: the ischemic penumbra. Stroke 12:723–725, 1981

5. Baudrimont M, Dubas F, Joutel A et al: Autosomal dominant leukoencephalopathy and subcortical ischemic stroke: a clinicopathological study. Stroke 24:122–125, 1993

6. Beach KW, Hatsukami T, Detmer PR et al: Carotid artery intraplaque hemorrhage and stenotic velocity. Stroke 24:314–319, 1993

7. Benveniste H, Drejer J, Schousboe A, Diemer H: Elevation of the extracellular concentrations of glutamate and aspartate in rat hippocampus during transient cerebral ischemia monitored by microdialysis. J Neurochem 43:1369–1374, 1984

8. Bluestein HG, Zvaifler NT: Antibodies reactive with

central nervous system antigens. Hum Pathol 14: 424–428, 1983

9. Bo WJ, McKinney WM, Bowden RL: The origin and distribution of vasa vasorum at the bifurcation of the common carotid artery with atherosclerosis. Stroke 20: 1484–1487, 1989

10. Bornebroek M, Haan J, Maat-Schieman MLC et al: Hereditary cerebral hemorrhage with amyloidosis—Dutch type (HCHWA-D): I. A review of clinical, radiologic and genetic aspects. Brain Pathol 6:111–114, 1996

11. Bogousslavsky J, Regli F, Uské A et al. Early spontaneous hematoma in cerebral infarct: is primary cerebral hemorrhage overdiagnosed? Neurology (NY) 41:837, 1991

12. Brown MM, Swash M: Polyarteritis nodosa and other systemic vasculitides. pp. 353–368. In Toole JF (ed): Handbook of Clinical Neurology. Vol. 11. Vascular Diseases. Part III. Elsevier, Amsterdam 1989

13. Calandre L, Ortega JF, Bermejo F: Anticoagulation and hemorrhagic infarction in cerebral embolism secondary to rheumatic heart disease. Arch Neurol 41:1152–1154, 1984

14. Caplan LR: Intracranial branch atheromatous disease: a neglected, understudied, and underused concept. Neurology 39:1246–1250, 1989

15. Capron L: Extra and intracranial atherosclerosis. pp. 91–106. In Toole JF (ed): Handbook of Clinical Neurology. Vol. 9. Vascular Diseases. Part I. Elsevier, Amsterdam 1988

16. Case Records of the Massachusetts General Hospital (Case 30, 1991). N Engl J Med 325:265, 1991

17. Chabriat H, Vahedi K, Iba-Zizen MT et al: Clinical spectrum of CADASIL: a study of seven families. Lancet 346:934–939, 1995

18. Challa VR, Moody DM, Bell MA: The Charcot-Bouchard aneurysm controversy: impact of a new histologic technique. J Neuropath Exp Neuropathol 51:264–271, 1992

19. Chen ST, Chen SD, Hsu CY, Hogan EL: Progression of hypertensive intracerebral hemorrhage. Neurology 39: 1509–1514, 1989

20. Cohen M, Lanska D, Roessmann U et al: Amyloidoma of the CNS. I. Clinical and pathologic study. Neurology 42:2019–2023, 1992

21. Coull BM, Levine SR, Brey RL: The role of antiphospholipid antibodies in stroke. Neurol Clin 10:125, 1992

22. Criscuolo GR, Oldfield EH, Doppman JL: Reversible acute and subacute myelopathy in patients with dural arteriovenous fistulae: Foix-Alajouanine syndrome reconsidered. J Neurosurg 70:354–359, 1989

23. Crooks DA: Cerebral amyloid angiopathy. J Neurol Neurosurg Psychiatry 57:1457, 1994

24. de Graba TJ: Editorial comment on the effects of reperfusion. Stroke 24:463–464, 1993

25. Devinsky O, Petito CK, Alonso DR: Clinical and neuropathological findings in systemic lupus erythematosus. The role of vasculitis, heart emboli, and thrombotic thrombocytopenic purpura. Ann Neurol 23:380, 1988

26. Djindjian M, Djindjian R, Hurth M et al: Spinal cord arteriovenous malformations and the Klippel-Trenaunay-Weber syndrome. Surg Neurol 8:229–237, 1977

27. Dorland's Illustrated Medical Dictionary. 28th Ed. p. 837. WB Saunders, Philadelphia, 1994

28. Duchen LW: General pathology of neurons and neuroglia. pp. 1–68. In Adams JH, Duchen LW (eds): Greenfield's Neuropathology. 5th Ed. Oxford University Press, New York, 1992

29. EAFT Study Group: Silent brain infarction in nonrheumatic atrial fibrillation. Neurology 46:159–165, 1996

30. Eckert B, Zanella FB, Thie A et al: Angioplasty of the internal carotid artery: results, complications, and follow-up in 61 cases. Cerebrovasc Dis 6:97–105, 1996

31. Enzmann DR, Britt RH, Lyons BE: Natural history of experimental intracranial haemorrhage: sonography, computed tomography and neuropathology. AJNR 2: 517–526, 1981

32. Fagan SC, Garcia JH: Reperfusion hemorrhage after middle cerebral artery occlusion in the rat. Neurology 46:A195, 1996

33. Feeley TM, Leen EJ, Cogan MP et al: Histologic characteristics of carotid artery plaque. J Vasc Surg 13: 719–724, 1991

34. Fisher CM: Cerebral miliary aneurysms in hypertension. Am J Pathol 66:313–330, 1971

35. Fisher CM, Adams RD: Observations on brain embolism with special reference to the mechanism of hemorrhagic infarction. J Neuropathol Exp Neurol 10:92–94, 1951

36. Fisher M, Martin A, Cosgrove M et al: Carotid artery plaques in the NASCET and ACAS projects. Neurology, suppl. 3, 42:204, 1992

37. Frackowiak J, Zoltowska A, Wisniewski HM: Nonfibrillar beta-amyloid protein is associated with smooth muscle cells of vessel walls in Alzheimers disease. J Neuropathol Exp Neurol 53:637–645, 1994

38. Fuji Y, Tanaka R, Takeuchi S et al: Hematoma enlargement in spontaneous intracerebral hemorrhage. J Neurosurg 80:51–57, 1994

39. Garcia JH: Thrombosis of cranial veins and sinuses: brain parenchymal effects. pp. 27–35. In Einhäupl K, Kempski O, Baethmann A (eds): Cerebral Sinus Thrombosis. Plenum Press, New York, 1990

40. Garcia JH, Anderson ML: Circulatory disorders and their effects on the brain. pp. 715–822. In Davis RL, Robertson DM (eds): Textbook of Neuropathology. 3rd Ed. Williams & Wilkins, Baltimore, 1997

41. Garcia JH, Ho K-L, Caccamo D: Intracerebral hemorrhage: pathology of selected topics. pp. 45–72. In Kase CS, Caplan LR (eds): Intracerebral Hemorrhage. Butterworths, Boston, 1994

42. Garcia JH, Lassen NA, Weiller C et al: Ischemic stroke and incomplete infarction. Stroke 27:161–165, 1996

43. Garcia JH, Liu K-F, Ho K-L: Neuronal necrosis after middle cerebral artery occlusion in Wistar rats progresses at different time intervals in the caudoputamen and the cortex. Stroke 26:636–643, 1995

44. Garcia JH, Liu K-F, Relton JK: Interleukin-1 receptor antagonist decreases the number of necrotic neurons in rats with middle cerebral artery occlusion. Am J Pathol 147:1477–1486, 1995

45. Garcia JH, Liu K-F, Yoshida Y et al: Influx of leukocytes and platelets in an evolving brain infarct (Wistar rat). Am J Pathol 144:188–199, 1994

46. Garcia JH, Lowry SL, Briggs L et al: Brain capillaries expand and rupture in areas of ischemia and reperfusion. pp. 169–179. In Revich M, Hurtig HI (eds): Cerebrovascular Diseases. Thirteenth Conference. Lippincott-Raven, Philadelphia, 1983

47. Garcia JH, Mitchem HL, Briggs L et al: Transient focal ischemia in subhuman primates: neuronal injury as a function of local cerebral blood flow. J Neuropathol Exp Neurol 42:44–60, 1983

48. Garcia JH, Yoshida Y, Chen H et al: Progression from ischemic injury to infarct following middle cerebral artery occlusion in the rat. Am J Pathol 142:623–635, 1993

49. Garcia JH, Wagner S, Liu K-F, Hu X-J: Neurological deficit and the extent of neuronal necrosis attributable to middle cerebral artery occlusion: Statistical validation. Stroke 26:627–635, 1995

50. Geschwind DH, FitzPatrick M, Mischel PS, Cummings JL: Sneddon's syndrome is a thrombotic vasculopathy, neuropathologic and neuroradiologic evidence. Neurology 45:557–560, 1995

51. Gomez MR. Phenotypes of the tuberous sclerosis complex with a revision of diagnostic criteria. Ann NY Acad Sci 615:1, 1991

52. Gomori JM, Grossman RI, Hackney DB et al. Variable appearance of subacute intracranial hematomas on high-field spin-echo MR. AJNR 8:1019–1026, 1987

53. Grewal RP, Barton NW. Fabry's disease presenting with stroke. Clin Neurol Neurosurg 94:177–179, 1992

54. Guttmacher AE, Marchuk DA, White RI Jr: Hereditary hemorrhagic telangiectasia. N Engl J Med 333:918–924, 1995

55. Hacke W, Kaste M, Fieschi C et al: Intravenous thrombolysis with recombinant tissue plasminogen activator for acute hemispheric stroke: The European Cooperative Acute Stroke Study (ECASS). JAMA 274:1017–1025, 1995

56. Harper SL, Bohlen HG: Microvascular adaptation in cerebral cortex of adult spontaneously hypertensive rats. Hypertension 6:408–419, 1984

57. Hart RG, Easton JH: Hemorrhagic infarcts. Stroke 17:586–589, 1986

58. Hasegawa H, Matsuoka T, Goto Y, Nonaka I: Strongly succinate dehydrogenase—reactive blood vessels in muscles from patients with mitochondrial myopathy, encephalopathy, lactic acidosis and stroke-like episodes. Ann Neurol 29:601–605, 1991

59. Heiss WD, Graf R, Wienhard K et al: Dynamic penumbra demonstrated by sequential multitracer PET after middle cerebral artery occlusion in cats. J Cereb Blood Flow Metab 14:892–902, 1994

60. Heiss WD, Rosner G: Functional recovery of cortical neurons as related to degree and duration of ischemia. Ann Neurol 14:294–301, 1983

61. Hornig CR, Dorndorf W, Agnoli AL: Hemorrhagic cerebral infarction—a prospective study. Stroke 17:179–185, 1986

62. Iqbal A, Alter M, Lee SH: Pseudoxanthoma elasticum: a review of neurological complications. Ann Neurol 4:18–20, 1978

63. Jellinger K: Pathology and aetiology of ICH. pp. 131–135. In Pia HW, Langmaid C, Zierski J (eds): Spontaneous Intracerebral Hematomas. Advances in Diagnosis and Therapy. Springer-Verlag, Berlin, 1980

64. Jenkins A, Maxwell W, Graham D: Experimental intracerebral hematoma in the rat: sequential light microscopic changes. Neuropathol Appl Neurobiol 15:477–486, 1989

65. Kajstura J, Cheng W, Reiss K et al: Apoptotic and necrotic myocyte cell deaths are independent contributing variables of infarct size in rats. Lab Invest 74:86–107, 1996

66. Kamijyo Y, Garcia JH, Cooper J: Temporary middle cerebral artery occlusion: a model of hemorrhagic and subcortical infarction. J Neuropathol Exp Neurol 36:338–350, 1977

67. Kaplanski G, Farnarier C, Kaplanski S et al: Interleukin-1 induces interleukin-8 secretion from endothelial cells by a juxtacrine mechanism. Blood 84:4242–4248, 1994

68. Kerr JFR, Wyllie AH, Currie AR: Apoptosis: a basic biological phenomenon with wide ranging implications in tissue kinetics. Br J Cancer 26:239–257, 1972

69. Koeppen AH, Dickson AC, McEvoy JA: The cellular reactions to experimental intracerebral hemorrhage. J Neurol Sci, suppl. 134:102–112, 1995

70. Kohler J, Kasper J, Witt I, von Reuthern GM: Ischemic stroke due to protein C deficiency. Stroke 21:107–108, 1990

71. Koster T, Rosendaal FR, de Ronde H et al: Venous thrombosis due to poor anticoagulant response to activated protein C: Leiden thrombophilia study. Lancet 342:1503–1506, 1993

72. Kroemer G, Pepit P, Zamzami N et al: The biochemistry of programmed cell death. FASEB J 9:1277–1287, 1995

73. von Kummer R, Holle R, Rosin L et al: Does arterial recanalization improve outcome in carotid territory stroke? Stroke 26:581–587, 1995

74. Lassen NA, Losen TS, Højggard K, Skriver E: Incomplete infarction: a CT-negative irreversible ischemic brain lesion. J Cereb Blood Flow Metab, suppl. B:S602–S603, 1983

75. Li B, Wang CC, Zhao ZZ et al: A histological, ultrastructural and immunohistochemical study of superficial temporal arteries in moyamoya disease. Acta Pathol Jpn 41:521–530, 1991

76. Libby P, Hansson GK: Involvement of the immune system in human atherogenesis: current knowledge and unanswered questions. Lab Invest 64:5–15, 1991

77. Liu K-F, Garcia JH, Tatlisumak T et al: Focal brain ischemia: endothelial/astrocyte swelling precedes neuronal necrosis, abstracted. J Neuropathol Exper Neurol 55:621, 1996.

78. Luyendjik W: Intracerebral haematoma. Vascular diseases of the nervous system, Part I. pp. 660–719. In Vinken PJ, Bruyn GW (eds): Handbook of Clinical Neurology. North-Holland, Amsterdam, 1972

79. Lyden PD, Zivin JA: Hemorrhagic transformation after cerebral ischemia: mechanisms and incidence. Cerebrovasc Brain Metab Rev 5:1–16, 1993

80. Mandybur TI: Cerebral amyloid angiopathy: the vascular pathology and complications. J Neuropathol Exp Neurol 45:79–83, 1986

81. Maruyama K, Ikeda S, Ishihara T et al: Immuno-histo-

chemical characterization of cerebrovascular amyloid in 46 autopsied cases using antibodies to beta protein and cystatin C. Stroke 21:397–403, 1990

82. McCully KS: Homocysteine and vascular disease. Nature Med 2:386–389, 1996

83. McCully KS, Wilson RB: Homocysteine theory of arteriosclerosis. Atherosclerosis 22:215–227, 1975

84. Miles JH, Zonana J, MacFarlane JP et al: Macrocephaly with hamartomas: Bannayan-Zonana syndrome. Am J Genet 19:225–234, 1984

85. Minematsu K, Li L, Sotak CH et al: Reversible focal ischemic injury demonstrated by diffusion-weighted magnetic resonance imaging in rats. Stroke 23: 1304–1311, 1992

86. Montagna P, Gallassi R, Medori R et al: MELAS syndrome: characteristic migrainous and epileptic features and maternal transmission. Neurology 38:751, 1988

87. Moraes CT, Schon EA, DiMauro S: Mitochondrial disease: toward a rational classification. pp. 83–120. In Appel SH (ed): Current Neurology. Mosby–Year Book, St. Louis, 1991

88. Neumann HPH, Eggert HR, Scheremet R et al: Central nervous system lesions in von Hippel-Lindau syndrome. J Neurol Neurosurg Psychiatry 55:898–901, 1992

89. NINDS rt-PA Stroke Study Group: Tissue plasminogen activator for acute ischemic stroke. N Engl J Med 333: 1581–1587, 1995

90. Nygard O, Vollset SE, Refsum H et al: Total plasma homocysteine and cardiovascular risk profile. The Hordaland Homocysteine Study. JAMA 274:1526–1533, 1995

91. Obrenovitch TP, Richards DA: Extracellular neurotransmitter changes in cerebral ischaemia. Cerebrovasc Brain Metab Rev 7:1–54, 1995

92. Ogata J, Masuda J, Yutani C et al: Rupture of atheromatous plaque as a cause of thrombotic occlusion of stenotic internal carotid artery. Stroke 21:1740–1745, 1990

93. Ogata J, Yutani C, Imakita M et al: Hemorrhagic infarct of the brain without a reopening of the occluded arteries in cardioembolic stroke. Stroke 20:76–83, 1989

94. Ohama E, Ohara S, Ikuta F et al: Mitochondrial angiopathy in cerebral blood vessels of mitochondrial encephalomyopathy. Acta Neuropathy 74:226, 1987

95. Okazaki H: Fundamentals of Neuropathology. pp. 25–81. Igaku-Shoin, New York, 1983

96. Ólafsson E, Thorsteinsson L, Jensson O: The molecular pathology of hereditary cystatin C amyloid angiopathy causing brain hemorrhage. Brain Pathol 6:121–126, 1996

97. Pantoni L, Garcia JH: The significance of cerebral white matter abnormalities 100 years after Binswanger's report: a review. Stroke 26:1293–1301, 1995

98. Pantoni L, Hagiwara M, Gutierrez JA, Garcia JH: Hemorrhagic transformation of cerebral infarcts in a rat model, abstracted. Cerebrovasc Dis 6:187, 1996

99. Petito CK: Cerebrovascular diseases. pp. 436–458. In Nelson JS, Parisi JE, Schochet SS (eds): Principles and Practice of Neuropathology. Mosby–Year Book, St. Louis, 1993

100. Petito CK, Feldmann E, Pulsinelli WA et al: Delayed hippocampal damage in humans following cardiorespiratory arrest. Neurology (NY) 37:1281, 1987

101. Prati P, Vanuzzo D, Casaroli M et al: Prevalence and determinants for carotid atherosclerosis in a general population. Stroke 23:1705–1711, 1992

102. Pretorius ME, Butler IJ: Neurologic manifestations of Ehlers-Danlos syndrome. Neurology 33:1087–1089, 1983

103. Price DL, Sisodia SS, Gandy SE: Amyloid beta amyloidosis in Alzheimer's disease. Curr Opin Neurol 8: 268–274, 1995

104. Pullicino PM: The course and territories of cerebral small arteries. pp. 11–39. In Pullicino PM, Caplan LT, Hommel M (eds): Advances in Neurology: Cerebral Small Artery Disease. Vol. 62. Lippincott-Raven, Philadelphia, 1993

105. Pyeritz RE, McKusick VA: Basic defects in the Marfan syndrome. N Engl J Med 305:1011–1012, 1981

106. Richardson EP Jr: Amyloid in the human brain. West J Med 143:518, 1985

107. Ruchoux MM, Gueronaou D, Vanderhaute B et al: Systemic vascular smooth muscle cell impairment in cerebral autosomal dominant arteriopathy with subcortical infarcts and leukoencephalopathy. Acta Neuropathol 89: 500–512, 1995

108. Sacco RL, Ellenberg JH, Mohr JP et al: Infarcts of undetermined cause: the NINCDS Stroke Data Bank. Ann Neurol 25:382, 1989

109. Sacco RL, Owen J, Mohr JP et al: Free protein S deficiency: a possible association with cerebrovascular occlusion. Stroke 20:1657–1661, 1989

110. Saku Y, Choki J, Waki R et al: Hemorrhagic infarct induced by arterial hypertension in cat brain following middle cerebral artery occlusion. Stroke 21:589–595, 1990

111. Sandok BA: Fibromuscular dysplasia of the cephalic arterial system. pp. 283–292. In Toole JF (ed): Handbook of Clinical Neurology. Vol. II. Vascular Diseases. Part III. Elsevier, Amsterdam 1989

112. Schmid-Schönbein GW: Capillary plugging by granulocytes and the no-reflow phenomenon in the microcirculation. FASEB J 46:2397–2401, 1987

113. Seeger JM, Barratt E, Lawson GA, Hingman N: The relationship between carotid plaque composition, plaque morphology, and neurologic symptoms. J Surg Res 58:330–336, 1995

114. Selhub J, Jacques PF, Bostom AG et al: Association between plasma homocysteine concentrations and extracranial carotid-artery stenosis. N Engl J Med 332: 286–291, 1995

115. Siesjö BK: Cell damage in the brain: a speculative synthesis. J Cereb Blood Flow Metab 1:155–185, 1981

116. Sitzer M, Müller W, Siebler M et al: Plaque ulceration and lumen thrombus are the main sources of cerebral microemboli in high-grade internal carotid artery stenosis. Stroke 26:1231–1233, 1995

117. Sloan MA: Stroke associated with thrombolytic therapy for acute myocardial infarction. Heart Dis Stroke 1: 287–294, 1992

118. Sneddon JB: Cerebral vascular lesions and livedo reticularis. Br J Dermatol 77:180–185, 1965

119. Solis OJ, Roberson GR, Taveras JM et al: Cerebral angiography in acute cerebral infarction. Rev Interam Radiol 2:19–25, 1977

120. Sourander P, Walinder J: Hereditary multi-infarct dementia. Acta Neuropathol 39:247–254, 1977

121. Takasugi S, Ueda S, Matsumoto K: Chronological changes in spontaneous intracerebral hematoma: an experimental and clinical study. Stroke 16:651–658, 1985

122. Toni D, Fiorelli M, Bastianello S et al: Hemorrhagic transformation of brain infarct: predictability in the first 5 hours from stroke onset and influence on clinical outcome. Neurology 46:341–345, 1996

123. Torvik A, Svindland A, Lindboe DV: Pathogenesis of carotid thrombosis. Stroke 20:1477, 1989

124. Tournier-Lasserne E, Joutel A, Melki J et al: Cerebral autosomal dominant arteriopathy with subcortical infarcts and leukoencephalopathy maps on chromosome 19q12. Nature Genet 3:256–259, 1993

125. Vaux DL, Haecker C, Strasser A: An evolutionary perspective on apoptosis. Cell 76:777–781, 1994

126. Vinters HV, Gilbert JJ: Cerebral amyloid angiopathy: incidence and complications in the aging brain. II. The distribution of amyloid vascular changes. Stroke 14:924–928, 1983

127. Vinters HV, Wang ZZ, Secor DL: Brain parenchymal and microvascular amyloid in Alzheimer's disease. Brain Pathol 6:179–195, 1996

128. Vogl TJ, Semonler J, Bergman C et al: MR and MR angiography of Sturge-Weber syndrome. AJNR 14:417–425, 1993

129. Vonsattel JPG, Myers RH, Hedley-Whyte ET et al: Cerebral amyloid angiopathy without and with cerebral hemorrhages: a comparative histological study. Ann Neurol 30:637–649, 1991

130. Wagner KH, Xi G, Hua Y et al: Lobar intracerebral hemorrhage model in the pig. Rapid edema development in perihematomal white matter. Stroke 27:490–497, 1996

131. Weller RO: Spontaneous intracranial hemorrhage. pp. 269–301. In Adams J, Duchen L (eds): Greenfield's Neuropathology. Oxford University Press, New York, 1992

132. Williams RS, Marshall PC, Lott IT et al: The cellular pathology of Menke's steely hair syndrome. Neurology 28:575–583, 1978

133. Willinsky RA, Làsjauniàs P, Terbrugge K, Burrows P: Multiple cerebral arteriovenous malformations (AVMs): review of our experience from 203 patients with cerebral vascular lesions. Neuroradiology 32:207, 1990

134. Yatsu FM, Fisher M: Atherosclerosis: current concepts on pathogenesis and interventional therapies. Ann Neurol 20:3–12, 1989

135. Zarins CK, Zatina MA, Giddens DP et al: Shear stress regulation of artery lumen diameter in experimental atherogenesis. J Vasc Surg 5:413, 1987

136. Zegler B, Sepp N, Schmid KW et al: Life history of cutaneous vascular lesions in Sneddon's syndrome. Hum Pathol 23:668–675, 1992

137. Zeviani M, Antozzi C: Defects of mitochondrial DNA. Brain Pathol 2:121–132, 1992

CHAPTER 9

Basic Science of Fibrinolysis: Coronary and Cerebral Thrombolysis

BRUCE A. KEYT

JUERGEN FROEHLICH

G. ROGER THOMAS

Stroke is the third most common cause of death and hospitalization, and the most common cause of disability in the United States. Nearly 500,000 Americans suffer strokes each year. The mortality rate from this disease is approximately 30%. Clinical data indicate that most strokes are ischemic, whereas hemorrhagic strokes occur less frequently. Cerebral angiography performed shortly after the onset of symptoms reveals arterial occlusion in 75% of acute cerebral infarctions.[194] Animal models of acute ischemic stroke show that thrombolytic therapy reduces brain injury if reperfusion of the occluded artery can be achieved before the infarction process has been completed.[159,220,229]

A landmark randomized, placebo-controlled trial has recently been completed. It demonstrated consistent and significant improvement in long-term clinical benefit for acute ischemic stroke patients treated with alteplase tissue plasminogen activator (tPA) within 3 hours of symptom onset.[167] On the basis of this study and other clinical trials of thrombolytic therapy, the Food and Drug Administration approved the use of tissue plasminogen activator for the treatment of acute ischemic stroke. This is the first step in what may lead to a major change in the way stroke patients are managed in acute care.[1]

The utility of fibrinolytic agents in the treatment of cerebral ischemic stroke has been examined since the late 1950s.[230] Optimally, the goal of thrombolytic therapy for the treatment of stroke is to achieve rapid lysis of the ischemic occlusion and restore cerebral perfusion in the area affected by the thrombus/embolus and its periphery or the so-called penumbra. If the occlusion remains, the loss of tissue perfusion leads to infarction and necrosis of the affected area. In contrast to the infarcted area, the ischemic penumbra is not irreversibly damaged. Timely reperfusion to at least a part of the ischemic penumbra may allow a reduction in total infarction size, a decrease of functional deficit, and possibly restoration of normal neuronal function.

Three different types of fibrinolytic agents have been clinically evaluated during the last 30 years: streptokinase, urokinase-type plasminogen activator (uPA) and recombinant tPA. These fibrinolytic agents differ by mechanism of action and represent various degrees of fibrin specificity; from non-fibrin specific (streptokinase) to increasingly fibrin selective (uPA and tPA). Understanding the biochemical mechanism of fibrin-specific plasminogen activation stimulated the development of more specific thrombolytic agents in the hope of achieving greater efficacy. Both intravenous and intra-arterial routes of administration have been tested with thrombolytic agents; however, optimal dosages and routes of administration for these agents have not been fully established for treatment of stroke. In this chapter, we discuss the process of clot dissolution and the biochemical processes involved in plasminogen activation by the different thrombolytic agents. The current status of preclinical testing in animal models of embolic stroke is also presented and summarized in view of clinical trials with thrombolytic treatment of acute myocardial infarction and ischemic stroke. Finally, we present recent results with a variant of tPA that exhibits inhibitor resistance, increased fibrin specificity, and increased plasma half-life.

Thrombus Formation

Thrombosis is a multifactorial process that includes components of circulating plasma proteins, platelets, and the vascular endothelium. The pathogenesis of thrombosis varies considerably depending on the vascular location. Clot formation differs among arterial, venous, cardiac, or microvascular thromboses, in part due to the effects of flow, to platelet activation, and to cell surface proteins of the endothelium. The initial event in thrombosis (especially in the arterial system, where the flow rate is high and vascular lesions are more common) is often the adhesion of platelets and formation of a platelet clump, usually observed at the origin of such thrombi. Arterial and venous thrombi are morphologically different (red versus white thrombus), but the distinction is more quantitative rather than qualitative. Activation of the coagulation system, by stimulated platelets exposure of plasma to extravascular tissue factor (or by both mechanisms), triggers a cascade of molecular events whereby circulating pro-enzymes are converted to coagulation proteases, resulting in the formation of thrombin (Fig. 9.1). The result of thrombin formation is positive feedback acceleration, by which factors V and VIII are activated, creating more thrombin. Thrombin is a potent stimulator of platelets, which can lead to rapid and extensive platelet aggregation. Platelets are prominent components of the thrombotic process. Activated platelets aid coagulation and also inhibit fibrinolysis by releasing inhibitors. The major sub-

strate of thrombin generated during coagulation is fibrinogen, which is proteolytically cleaved to form a fibrin clot (Fig. 9.1).

It may be instructive to describe the steps in the clotting process. Fibrinogen, the soluble precursor of fibrin, circulates in plasma at concentrations of approximately 3 mg/ml. Fibrinogen is a symmetric glycoprotein with a molecular weight of 340 kd.[72,73,103] It is composed of six polypeptide chains: two Aα-, two Bβ-, and two γ-chains with molecular weights of 67 kd, 57 kd, and 47 kd, respectively (Fig. 9.2A). The six chains of fibrinogen are cross-linked by disulfides. Fibrinogen appears as a trinodal structure by electron microscopy, with one central relatively small nodule connected by thin filamentous structures to two larger outer nodules (Fig. 9.2B). From numerous biochemical studies, the amino termini of all six polypeptide chains are located in the central region, with the carboxy termini in the polypeptides in the outer nodules. Fibrinogen is converted to fibrin by a proteolytic cleavage catalyzed by thrombin. The activation of the coagulation system leads to the generation of thrombin, which is a serine protease that catalyzes fibrin formation by cleaving fibrinopeptides A and B from the amino termini of fibrinogen. The newly formed amino termini of the α-chains interact with sites on other molecules of fibrinogen or fibrin, which leads to the formation of aggregates and polymerization of fibrin (Fig. 9.2C). The polymeric form of fibrin can then be cross-linked by factor XIII in the presence of calcium to stabilize the fibrin clot. Platelets indirectly stimulate factor XIII and increase fibrin cross-linking by activating blood coagulation and elaborating thrombin.

Conversely, fibrin is degraded by plasmin (Fig. 9.2D). This proteolytic enzyme splits insoluble fibrin and releases soluble fibrin degradation products (FDPs). As a result of this degradation of fibrin, thrombi lose their mechanical stability

Figure 9.1 Schematic diagram of the fibrinolytic system. The proenzyme plasminogen is activated to the enzyme, plasmin, by tissue-type plasminogen activator (tPA) or urinary-type plasminogen activator (u-PA). The activation of plasminogen by tPA is stimulated in the presence of fibrin. Plasmin can also convert one-chain tPA to the two-chain species, resulting in feedback activation. Inactivation of tPA (either one-chain or two-chain species) and u-PA occurs by reaction with plasminogen activator inhibitor-type 1 (PAI-1). Fibrin is formed by the action of thrombin on fibrinogen. A fibrin clot is dissolved by active plasmin, which is capable of degrading fibrin to low molecular weight fibrin degradation products. Active plasmin may be inactivated by α_2-antiplasmin (as indicated by the dashed line).

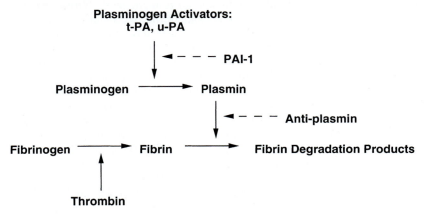

A

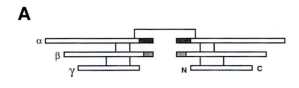

B

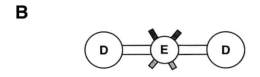

C

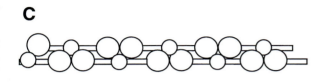

D

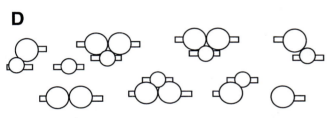

Figure 9.2 Structure of fibrinogen, and schematic representation of fibrin polymerization and fibrinolysis. (**A**) Primary structure model of human fibrinogen with α-, β-, and γ-chains indicated. The chains have been aligned according to homology, with the N termini pointing towards the middle. The connecting lines represent disulfide bridges, and the black and shaded bars indicate A- and B-peptides that contain cleavage sites for thrombin. (**B**) Diagram depicting the fibrinogen molecule as a model of three globular domains, one central E-domain and two distal D-domains, connected by linear coils of α-, β-, and γ-chains. Fibrinopeptides A and B (at the amino termini of α- and β-chains, respectively) are shown as dark and light shaded bars. (**C**) After thrombin has cleaved the A- and B-fibrinopeptides, fibrin monomers assemble into fibrin polymers by end to end and side to side noncovalent associations. These fibrin polymers are insoluble in plasma. In the presence of calcium and factor XIIIa, the fibrin polymers are covalently cross-linked for increased stability. (**D**) Fibrin is degraded by plasmin, a proteolytic enzyme that splits the insoluble polymer into soluble fibrin degradation products (FDPs). FDPs are a heterogeneous mix of fragments, termed X, Y, D, and E, with molecular weights of 240, 150, 80, and 53 kd, respectively.

and disintegrate. Fibrin and FDPs inhibit the polymerization of fibrin monomers during the conversion of fibrinogen into fibrin clots. Elevated FDPs (fragments X and Y) are particularly effective inhibitors and may be responsible for reduced rates of coagulation.

Main Components of the Fibrinolytic System

Fibrinolysis is the dissolution of fibrin via a proteolytic process catalyzed by plasmin. tPA and urokinase (or uPA) are plasma proteins that convert plasminogen (an inactive zymogen) to its active form, plasmin (Fig. 9.1). tPA and plasminogen bind to the fibrin clot, and the rate of plasminogen activation is greater in the presence of fibrin. Hence, fibrin acts as a cofactor or template in forming the complex of tPA and plasminogen. tPA is fibrin specific in that plasminogen activation by tPA is stimulated by fibrin much more than by fibrinogen. Activities of tPA and plasmin are regulated by *ser*ine *p*rotease *in*hibitors (serpins) present in plasma, such as plasminogen activator inhibitor type I (PAI-1) and α_2-antiplasmin, respectively. These inhibitors serve to localize the action of tPA and plasmin to the site of a fibrin clot by rapidly inhibiting the enzymes in circulation, whereas tPA bound to fibrin is not as rapidly inhibited by PAI-1.[246] In addition to the interactions of tPA with its substrate (plasminogen), cofactor (fibrin or fibrinogen), and inhibitor (PAI-1), there is evidence for multiple receptors that rapidly remove tPA from plasma in vivo.[35,174]

PLASMINOGEN AND PLASMIN

Plasminogen, the pro-enzyme of plasmin, is a single-chain glycoprotein of 92 kd (consisting of 791 amino acids) and is present in most extravascular fluid as well as in blood (Fig. 9.3). It is synthesized as the inactive pro-enzyme, secreted from the liver, and circulates in plasma at a concentration of approximately 2 μM. In its predominant form, the amino-terminal residue is glutamic acid. As such, Glu-plasminogen is activated by the cleavage of a single peptide bond at Arg561-Val562, yielding the active enzyme plasmin.[204] Plasmin is composed of two polypeptide chains connected by a disulfide bond; the A-chain (60 kd) and B-chain (25 kd) contain the amino-terminal and carboxy-terminal regions of plasmin, respectively. The A-chain is composed of an amino-terminal domain (77 amino acids) plus five homologous kringle domains (about 90 amino acids each) and confers the specific properties of plasmin, such as binding to fibrin, α_2-antiplasmin, and other proteins. The kringles of plasminogen (and plasmin) have lysine binding sites and amino-hexyl binding sites that target the pro-enzyme (and the enzyme) to exposed lysines of fibrin (or fibrinogen), α_2-antiplasmin, and/or cell surface proteins.[51,190,236] The B-chain of plasmin is a serine protease with homology to trypsin and contains a catalytic triad including residues His603,

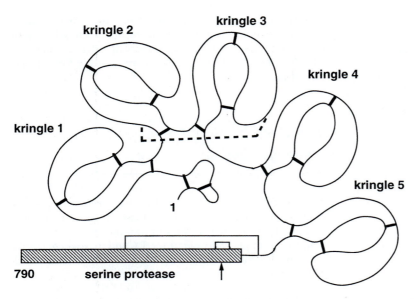

Figure 9.3 Structure of plasminogen. The amino and carboxy termini are indicated by the numbers 1 and 790. Plasminogen has an amino-terminal domain followed by five kringle modules, some of which have binding specificity for internal and carboxy-terminal lysines as presented by intact and partially degraded fibrinogen, respectively. The disulfides are indicated as solid black lines that connect intradomain cysteines, with the exception of the dashed line, which bridges cysteines in kringle 2 to kringle 3. The cross-hatched bar represents the serine protease region, which is homologous to trypsin.

Asp646, and Ser741. Plasmin is specific for cleavage of Arg- and Lys-containing sequences, particularly those between the D- and E-domains of fibrin. The structural characterization of plasminogen has been previously reviewed.[247]

Plasmin is a relatively unspecific protease and can cleave molecules other than fibrin. In certain circumstances, plasmin degrades fibrinogen and the clotting factors V, XII, and XIII. This process, known as fibrinogenolysis, can lead to a transient hemorrhagic or lytic state due to the lack of clotting factors. Under normal physiologic conditions, plasminogen activation proceeds slowly except in the case of formation of ternary complexes of plasminogen with tPA on fibrin or cell surfaces.[90,109,158,218,226] In addition to its role in intravascular thrombolysis, the proteolytic activity of plasmin contributes to a variety of normal and pathologic conditions including cell migration, inflammation, and tissue remodeling.[60,207] These cellular processes require specific mechanisms for the localization of plasminogen and plasmin on cell surfaces.

Over the past decade, the existence of cell surface receptors for plasminogen and plasmin has been demonstrated. Plasminogen receptors have been identified on virtually all cell types tested, and occupancy has been observed in various biologic situations. These receptors are characterized by their relatively low affinity and remarkably high density on many cells. Plasminogen receptors recognize the lysine binding domains (i.e., the kringle structures) of plasminogen and plasmin. These receptors include proteins with carboxy-terminal lysines, such as α-enolase. Plasminogen binding to cells enhances plasmin activity by increasing plasminogen activation, increasing plasmin activity, and protecting plasmin from inhibitors such as α_2-antiplasmin.[198]

Lipoprotein(a) [Lp(a)] is an atherogenic lipoprotein; increased plasma levels of Lp(a) are highly correlated with heart disease. However, the mechanisms by which Lp(a) promotes the atherosclerotic process are not known. The apolipoprotein(a) [apo(a)] portion of Lp(a) shares remarkable homology with plasminogen, including multiple, tandem repeating domains similar to the kringle 4 of plasminogen, a single kringle 5, and an inactive protease domain.[74,156] The homology of apo(a) and plasminogen has stimulated much investigation on competitive inhibition of fibrinolysis by Lp(a).[97] Lp(a) binds to fibrin, and the affinity between fibrin surfaces and Lp(a) appears related to the degree of oxidation in the lipoprotein particle. Recent findings suggest that, depending on the oxidative conditions, Lp(a) can either promote or inhibit in vitro plasmin formation.[144,145] Studies with recombinant apo(a) have demonstrated that the inhibition of fibrinolysis by apo(a) is due to decreased tPA-mediated activation of Glu-plasminogen, but not that of Lys-plasminogen.[210] Apo(a) did not inhibit the conversion of plasminogen by urokinase. Lp(a) also inhibits endothelial cell surface-dependent plasmin generation.[91]

PLASMIN INHIBITORS

The activity of plasmin is regulated by the formation of irreversible enzyme-inhibitor complexes with a fast-acting inhibitor, α_2-antiplasmin, and a slower-acting inhibitor, α_2-macroglobulin. α_2-Antiplasmin is a 67-kd glycoprotein of the serpin superfamily. This inhibitor circulates in plasma at a concentration of approximately 1 μM, approximately half that of plasminogen.[162] Activated platelets inhibit fibrinolysis by releasing α_2-antiplasmin from platelet α-granules, which contributes to the inhibition of plasminogen conversion. α_2-Antiplasmin reacts very rapidly with plasmin, initially forming a reversible, inactive 1:1 complex that slowly converts to an irreversible complex. The active site (or bait region) of α_2-antiplasmin is the Arg364-Met365 peptide bond. The carboxy-terminal extension of α_2-antiplasmin contains a secondary binding site that interacts with the lysine binding sites of kringles 1 to 3 of plasminogen or plasmin, or both. The amino-terminal Gln 14 of α_2-antiplasmin can cross-link to the A-chain of fibrin, in a calcium-dependent reaction catalyzed by the coagulation factor XIII.[122] This inhibitor functions such that circulating plasmin is rapidly inactivated (half-life of approximately 0.1 seconds), whereas fibrin-bound plasmin remains active for a longer period (half-life of 10 to 100 seconds).[253] Therefore, the fibrinolytic process is initiated by fibrin and kinetically localized to the clot surface.

Plasminogen Activators

Plasminogen is activated by a set of proteins known as plasminogen activators. The physiologic activators of plasminogen are tPA and uPA. There are also plasminogen activators of bacterial origin, SK and staphylokinase. In fact, the modern era of fibrinolysis began more than 60 years ago with the observation that streptococci release a substance that dissolved blood clots.[237] This streptococcal factor, called streptokinase, activated plasminogen to plasmin, and this discovery led to a rapid growth in the field of fibrinolysis.[47] Shortly thereafter, a fibrinolytic activity of tissues in culture was observed as a tissue-specific plasminogen activator,[4] followed by the demonstration of a fibrinolytic activity in urine, which is now called urokinase.[251]

BACTERIAL ACTIVATOR: STREPTOKINASE

Streptokinase is a secreted product of group C β-hemolytic streptococci; in the purified form, it has been widely used as a therapeutic agent for thrombolysis. Streptokinase is a single-chain protein of 47 kd that exhibits no intrinsic enzymatic activity. In circulation, exogenous streptokinase can form a 1:1 stoichiometric, noncovalent complex with plasminogen, which results in a conformational change in plasminogen and exposes an active site in the plasminogen moiety. This bimolecular complex (streptokinase/plasminogen) exhibits proteolytic activity and can convert other molecules of plasminogen to plasmin.[29] Thus, streptokinase is capable of activating plasminogen; as such, it functions as a potent plasminogen activator. Significant clinical experience has accumulated for the therapeutic use of streptokinase in treating acute myocardial infarction.[51,152,217]

Plasminogen activators have been classified as 'fibrin specific' or 'non-fibrin specific'.[53] Streptokinase is an example of a non-fibrin-specific fibrinolytic agent since it activates both circulating and fibrin-bound plasminogen. In a sufficient dose, streptokinase activates plasminogen within a thrombus, resulting in thrombolysis. However, plasma plasminogen is also activated, creating a transient state of hyperplasminemia. Extensive systemic activation of plasminogen (normal plasma concentration 1.5 to 2 μM) to plasmin will result in the depletion of the physiologic inhibitor α_2-antiplasmin followed by the release of unregulated plasmin. Excess plasmin can degrade several plasma proteins including fibrinogen, factor V, and factor VIII and can induce a lytic state defined as a 50% reduction in plasma fibrinogen from pretreatment levels. As a result of the transient phase of hyperplasminemia, a partial degradation of fibrinogen and factors V and VIII occurs. This lytic state is characterized by hemostatic failure, which is partly due to the coagulation defect and partly to fibrinogen degradation products, which exert an antithrombotic action and inhibit fibrin polymerization. Degradation of platelet-bound fibrinogen also interferes with platelet aggregation. By contrast, fibrin-specific plasminogen activators such as pro-urokinase and tPA preferentially activate plasminogen at the fibrin surface.

Staphylokinase is another bacterial profibrinolytic agent that forms a 1:1 stoichiometric complex with plasminogen; like streptokinase, it leads to the activation of other plasminogen molecules to plasmin. Unlike streptokinase, staphylokinase is remarkably fibrin specific due to the inability of α_2-antiplasmin to inhibit fibrin-bound complexes of staphylokinase/plasmin, whereas in circulation, the unbound complexes of staphylokinase/plasmin and staphylokinase/plasminogen are readily inhibited by α_2-antiplasmin.[54] Thus, staphylokinase is highly fibrin specific, causing little breakdown of fibrinogen, plasminogen, and α_2-antiplasmin. Recently, staphylokinase was demonstrated to be a potent and fibrin-specific thrombolytic agent in patients with acute myocardial infarction.[58] However, the administration of staphylokinase is associated with the induction of high levels of neutralizing antibodies.[211]

URINARY-TYPE PLASMINOGEN ACTIVATORS: UROKINASE AND PRO-UROKINASE

Urokinase (uPA) is a trypsin-like serine protease that directly activates plasminogen to plasmin. The first isolation of uPA was from human urine and cultured human embryonic kidney cells as a two-chain molecule with polypeptide chains of 20 and 34 kd.[21] More recently, uPA has been isolated from urine, plasma, and cultured cells as the inactive precursor, single-chain uPA or pro-uPA.[75,112,254] Pro-uPA is synthesized and secreted as a single-chain glycoprotein of 54 kd that has very little activity toward low molecular weight substrates in vitro, but does have intrinsic plasminogen-activating potential.[106] The catalytic efficiency of pro-uPA is approximately 100-fold less than that of uPA.[2] Limited proteolysis by plasmin or kallekrein cleaves pro-uPA at the Lys 158-Ile 159 peptide bond (Fig. 9.4). This yields the two-chain form comprised of a light chain (158 amino acids) linked to the heavy chain (253 amino acids) by a disulfide bond. The amino-terminal light chain is composed of an epidermal growth factor (EGF)-like domain and one kringle domain. The EGF domain mediates the binding of uPA and pro-uPA to its receptor, which is present on a variety of cells, such as migrating macrophages and vascular endothelial cells.[6,15,205] The carboxy-terminal heavy chain (33 kd) of two-chain uPA consists of the serine protease domain. The catalytic triad is composed of Asp255, His204, and Ser356. An additional plasmin-catalyzed cleavage of two-chain uPA at the peptide bond between Lys 135 and Lys 136 generates low molecular weight uPA, which consists of only the protease domain and has a molecular weight of 32 kd.[228]

Urokinase has no fibrin specificity and as such it activates fibrin-bound and circulating plasminogen equally and relatively indiscriminately. Extensive plasminogen activation and depletion of α_2-antiplasmin may occur during uPA treatment of patients with thromboembolic disorders. Degradation of fibrinogen and factors V and VIII is often associated with loss of α_2-antiplasmin. By contrast, pro-uPA exhibits significant fibrin specificity, albeit with lower levels of plasmin generation. Recent studies indicate that this clot selectivity may be mediated by the preferential conversion of pro-uPA to uPA at the fibrin surface by the following mechanism.[64,143] Pro-uPA preferentially activates plasminogen that is bound to the fibrin surface. The resulting plasmin converts pro-uPA to uPA, which is significantly more active with respect to plasminogen activation. This positive feedback activation appears to function in in vitro and in vivo model systems.[56] The molecular mechanisms that regulate the fibrin-specific activity of pro-uPA are not fully understood.

Urokinase receptor (uPAR) is a specific cell surface receptor for uPA. It is a glycosylated protein of approximately 55 kd initially synthesized as a 313-amino acid length polypeptide. Following a post-translational cleavage near the carboxy terminus, the 283-amino acid receptor is anchored to the plasma membrane by a glycosyl phosphatidylinositol moiety.[189] uPAR is expressed on a wide variety of cells, and it binds to all forms of uPA that contain the EGF-like domain (Fig. 9.4) with a high affinity characterized by binding constants of 0.1 to 1 nM for most cell types.[14] The receptor is composed of three distantly related domains that appear structurally homologous; the first one mediates binding to the EGF region of uPA.[13] The expression of uPAR and localization of uPA activity to the surface of certain cell types is thought to play a major role in migration of cells during development and wound healing as well as the metastatic processes of invasive tumor cells.[125,151] Recently, studies of homozygous deletion of the uPA gene in mice have shown a remarkably normal phenotype with little effect on endogenous vascular fibrinolytic processes given the complete lack of uPA.[38]

TISSUE-TYPE PLASMINOGEN ACTIVATOR: ALTEPLASE tPA

tPA is a plasma serine protease with a molecular weight of approximately 65 kd. Native single-chain tPA is converted by plasmin to a two-chain form by limited proteolysis of the Arg275-Ile276 peptide bond (Fig. 9.5). Endogenous tPA is synthesized by endothelial cells, and it circulates in normal human plasma at a low concentration (0.1 to 0.2 nM).[203] tPA (activase tPA) for clinical use (alteplase tPA) is predominantly in the single-chain form (approximately 70%). The two-chain form of tPA consists of an amino-terminal A-chain (residues 1 to 275) linked by a disulfide bond (Cys264 to Cys395) to the carboxy-terminal B-chain (residues 276 to 527). The cloning and cDNA sequencing indicated that tPA is organized in five distinct modules.[187] The A-chain is composed of the finger (F), growth factor (G), and two kringle regions (K1, K2); the B-chain is a serine protease domain (P). All the tPA domains are homologous with modules found in numerous other

Figure 9.4 Structure of urinary-type plasminogen activator (uPA) or urokinase. High molecular weight single-chain urokinase consists of a growth factor domain, one kringle structure, and a serine protease (indicated by a cross-hatched bar). Amino and carboxy termini are shown as amino acids 1 and 411. Intradomain disulfide bonds are indicated as solid black lines connecting cysteines. The single-chain form of urokinase is an inactive zymogen, which is activated by cleavage at Lys158, generating the enzyme two-chain urokinase. Cleavage at Lys135 releases low molecular weight urokinase.

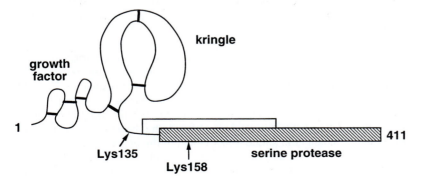

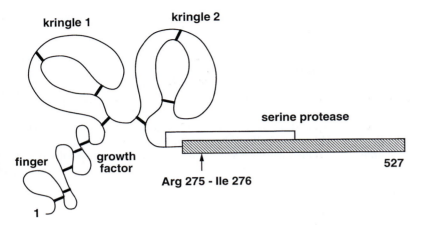

Figure 9.5 Structure of tissue-type plasminogen activator (tPA). Amino and carboxy termini are shown by the residue numbers 1 and 527, respectively. tPA is composed of fibronectin-like finger and epidermal growth factor-like domains, two kringle structures, and a serine protease. Intra-domain disulfide bonds are indicated as solid black lines connecting cysteines. The single-chain form of tPA is an active zymogen, but is converted to the more active two-chain enzyme by the action of plasmin, which cleaves the Arg275-Ile276 peptide bond.

plasma proteins.[5] The protease domain of tPA is homologous with trypsin and contains a catalytic site composed of His322, Asp371, and Ser478. tPA has 35 cysteines that form 17 disulfide bonds, with one unpaired cysteine.[213] Most of the disulfides are intradomain linkages, which have been assigned on the basis of homology with other proteins, such as fibronectin, EGF, and plasminogen.[5,187] Identification of the intron/exon splice junctions in the gene led to the suggestion that the mosaic tPA gene was the result of evolutionary exon shuffling.[170,186] Accordingly, the domain structures of tPA may be correlated with individual functions such as the F- and K2-domains mediating fibrin binding and the GF-domain interacting with cell receptors that mediate plasma clearance.[241] However, more recent data have demonstrated that it is difficult to assign specific functions of tPA to individual modules.[19]

Fibrin Binding and Localization of tPA Activity to the Site of a Clot

tPA displays high affinity for fibrin, which targets the enzymatic activity of tPA to the clot. The domain structures on tPA that mediate fibrin binding are located predominantly within the A-chain of tPA. Isolation of A- and B-chains after mild reduction of two-chain tPA[201] provided evidence for the targeting function of the A-chain domain, separate from the enzymatic activity of the protease domain.[107] These studies indicated that the isolated A-chain bound fibrin, whereas the protease domain did not. Studies with domain deletion variants of tPA demonstrated that the F- and K2-domains of tPA were involved in fibrin binding.[242] Verheijen et al[243] also demonstrated the requirement of the F-domain for high-affinity fibrin binding. If either F- or G-domains (or both) were deleted, the fibrin affinity of the variant tPA decreased by 10-fold.[135] Of the tPA variants with individual domain deletions, the des-K1 tPA was the least defective with respect to fibrin binding.[65]

Charged-to-alanine scanning mutagenesis was used to identify the fibrin binding determinants on tPA.[19] Alanine variants of tPA were labeled at the active site and tested for fibrin binding.[119] Mutations in all domains had some effects on high-affinity fibrin binding, especially mutations located in the K1-domain. Interestingly, mutations in the K2-domain had minimal effect on fibrin binding. A novel fibrin binding site localized in tPA protease was observed.[19] Fibrin binding-deficient variants involving charged residues at positions 403, 432, 434, 460, and 462 co-localized in a patch on a three-dimensional model of the tPA protease. In contrast to the earlier view of autonomous functions for individual domains,[241] results with the alanine scan variants indicate that all domains of tPA are involved in fibrin binding.[19] Many site-directed variants of tPA, constructed with a variety of protein engineering strategies, have resulted in decreased fibrin binding. However, high-affinity fibrin binding is a sensitive indicator of overall intact tPA structure. This is in contrast to lysine binding, which is affected by a limited set of mutations localized in one domain.[19] Furthermore, little correlation appears to exist between lysine binding function (mediated by the K2-domain) and binding to nondegraded, intact fibrin (mediated by multiple domain interactions).

Plasminogen Activation and Fibrin Stimulation

Tissue plasminogen activator and plasminogen bind to the fibrin clot, and the rate of plasminogen activation is greater in the presence of fibrin. tPA is a poor activator in the absence of fibrin, but it binds specifically to fibrin and activates plasminogen at the fibrin surface several hundred-fold more efficiently than in circulation. tPA both binds to and is stimulated by fibrin. Unlike some of the other plasminogen activators, such as uPA or streptokinase, tPA is fibrin-specific in that its activity is stimulated by fibrin much more than by fibrinogen.[109,195,202] Fibrin stimulation of tPA activity has been shown to be the result of a large increase in the affinity of the enzyme (tPA) for the substrate (plasminogen) induced by the cofactor (fibrin). In the absence of fibrin, the Michaelis-Menten constant (K_m) of tPA for Glu-plasminogen is 65 μM. The value for K_m decreases to 0.16 μM in the presence of fibrin, which represents a 400-fold increase in affinity of tPA for plasminogen on fibrin.[109] This increased affinity appears to be the result of a surface assembly of tPA and plasminogen on the fibrin clot. Since the circulating concentration of plasminogen is 2 μM in vivo,[193] the activity of tPA on plasminogen is predominantly localized to the site of the clot. This property of tPA is important as it restricts the production of plasmin to sites of fibrin deposition and limits systemic activation of plasminogen, which can lead to a loss of circulating fibrinogen and an increased risk of hemorrhage. The fibrin-specific nature of tPA is considered a significant advantage compared with other fibrinolytic agents for the treatment of thrombotic disorders.

Inhibition by PAI-1: Regulation of tPA Activity

The activity of tPA is regulated by the serine protease inhibitor in plasma (PAI-1). This serpin localizes the action of tPA to the site of a fibrin clot by rapidly inhibiting the enzyme in circulation, whereas tPA bound to fibrin is not as rapidly inhibited by PAI-1.[246] The activity of exogenous tPA is thought to be primarily localized at the surface of a clot by the fibrin-specific activity of tPA as well as the affinity of both tPA and plasminogen for fibrin. The activity of tPA is further regulated and localized by the action of plasma serine protease inhibitors. The most rapid and specific inhibitor of tPA is PAI-1, which is a fast-acting inhibitor of tPA (and uPA) occurring at very low concentration in the blood. The plasma concentrations of tPA and PAI-1 are approximately 0.1 to 0.2 nM and 0.4 nM, respectively, indicating that this inhibitor plays a central role in regulation of tPA activity.[25,203] Furthermore, the concentration of PAI-1 may be significantly increased in several disease states, including venous thromboembolism and ischemic heart disease.[212] PAI-1 rapidly inactivates tPA by forming a stable and specific 1:1 complex, with a second-order rate constant of approximately 10^7/M/s.[46,101]

PAI-1 is synthesized by vascular endothelial cells and released into plasma as a 45-kd molecular weight protein.[63] In addition to plasma PAI-1, platelet α-granules also contain high concentrations of PAI-1 (as well as α_2-antiplasmin); however, >90% of platelet PAI-1 is thought to be inactive.[24] Although most PAI-1 in platelets is the latent form, the concentration of PAI-1 in platelet-rich clots is orders of magnitude greater than that found in platelet-poor plasma. Thus, the contribution of active PAI-1 from platelets can represent a significant inhibitory activity when localized at the site of a clot. The release of PAI-1 from activated platelets during thrombus formation has led many investigators to suggest that PAI-1 may play a role in stabilizing platelet-rich arterial thrombi, which are known to be resistant to thrombolysis.[139,192] A PAI-1-resistant variant of tPA may therefore display increased potency as a fibrinolytic agent, especially toward platelet-rich thrombi.[132]

Intracranial bleeding is the most catastrophic potential complication of thrombolytic therapy for treatment of both stroke and acute myocardial infarction. Interestingly, recent evidence suggests that plasminogen activators may be associated with decreased synthesis and release of PAI-1 from brain endothelium. In vitro, human cerebral microvascular cells showed decreased secretion of PAI-1 protein in the culture medium and exhibited decreased levels of PAI-1 mRNA in response to tPA, uPA, or streptokinase/plasminogen.[215] These results indicate that brain endothelial cells exposed to tPA exhibit decreased elaboration of PAI-1, which may allow for proteolytic degradation of cerebral vasculature and may predispose some patients to subsequent intracranial hemorrhage.

Binding to Hepatic Receptors Mediates the Plasma Clearance of tPA

In vivo, tPA interacts with plasminogen, fibrin or fibrinogen, PAI-1, and multiple receptors that rapidly remove it from plasma.[35,131,174] tPA receptors serve two major functions, clearance and cell surface localization. Clearance of tPA is quite rapid, as indicated by the short initial half-life of tPA in the circulation, which is 4 to 6 minutes in humans.[82] Rapid clearance of human tPA occurs in mice, rats, rabbits, dogs, and rhesus monkeys.[12,20,76] The pharmacokinetic profile is characterized by a fast α-phase that removes most of the circulating tPA, followed by a slower β-phase of elimination. Early pharmacokinetic studies of tPA in rabbits indicated that the liver is the major organ of clearance.[129] Hepatic parenchymal, endothelial, and Kupffer cells are all capable of tPA uptake. Clearance receptors on these cells are heterogenous and include those that recognize carbohydrate side chains and others that bind and internalize t-PA/PAI-1 complexes. These and other observations provide evidence for different types of hepatic receptors that bind, internalize, and degrade tPA. In vitro and in vivo evidence implicates at least two types of receptor-mediated clearance, carbohydrate-dependent and carbohydrate-independent clearance pathways.

Glycosylation represents the major source of heterogeneity in recombinant tPA. There are three sites of N-linked carbohydrate in t-PA: a high-mannose carbohydrate site located at Asn117 and complex carbohydrate sites at Asn184 and Asn448.[191,224] Glycosylation at Asn184 occurs in approximately 50% of tPA molecules, hence the presence or absence of carbohydrate at position 184 differentiates tPA isozymes known as type I and type II, respectively.[18,196] In addition to the three N-linked glycosylation sites, there is an unusual O-linked glycosylation site that was identified in the growth factor module of tPA. More than 95% of Thr-61 is modified with a single fucose.[98] The presence of O-linked fucose has also been established in other proteins of fibrinolysis and coagulation (i.e., uPA, factor VII, and factor XII).[22,99,118]

The clearance of tPA has been shown to be mediated, in part, by its glycosylation. In vitro studies have confirmed the binding of wild-type tPA to the hepatic mannose receptor.[174] Competition binding studies with labeled tPA incubated with isolated rat hepatocytes in the presence of excess mannosylated ovalbumin showed that much of the tPA uptake in vitro was mannose dependent.[134] Furthermore, antibodies to the mannose receptor decreased the binding and uptake of tPA to rat hepatocytes.[134] These studies indicate that the high-mannose carbohydrate at Asn117 contributes to carbohydrate-mediated tPA clearance via the mannose receptor.[174] Additionally, the presence of exposed terminal galactose residues has also been implicated in tPA clearance. Lack of complete sialylation of the complex carbohydrate on tPA leads to accelerated clearance[50] via the hepatic asialoglycoprotein receptor.[3]

The recent discovery of fucose on Thr61 has been considered as another mechanism for hepatic binding of tPA. Hajjar and Reynolds[94] reported on the binding and uptake of tPA by the hepatic cell line HepG2. In these studies, tPA binding was inhibited by the monosaccharides fucose and galactose, as well as by fucosylated albumin. Fucosidase was used to remove the O-linked sugar at Thr61 of tPA. Hep-G2 cells exhibited 60% reduced binding and uptake of the fucosidase-treated tPA. These results indicate that O-linked α-fucose may mediate tPA binding and degradation by Hep-G2 cells and suggest a potential mechanism for carbohydrate-mediated clearance of tPA.[94]

An additional carbohydrate-independent mechanism for tPA clearance has been demonstrated by a number of investigators.[35,163] These studies suggest that the low density lipoprotein receptor related protein (LRP)[104] can bind and internalize both tPA and the complex of tPA with PAI-1.[33,173] LRP, also identified as the α_2-macroglobulin receptor,[84,133,227] is a complex of 515 kd and 85 kd proteins present on hepatic parenchymal cells.[34,248] LRP can bind and mediate endocytosis of a number of unrelated ligands including tPA,[173] t-PA/PAI-1 complex,[173] uPA/PAI-1 complex,[171] activated α_2-macroglobulin,[227] lipoprotein lipase,[16] lactoferrin,[252] and apolipoprotein E-bound very low density lipoprotein.[130] This receptor may constitute the carbohydrate-independent mechanism for hepatic clearance of tPA.

Cell Surface Proteins that Localize t-PA Activity

In addition to clearance receptors, there are cell surface proteins that bind, localize, and augment the activity of tPA and plasminogen. The endothelium contributes to fibrinolysis by binding plasminogen, plasminogen activators, and plasminogen activator inhibitors on the cell surface. Vascular endothelium also maintains high fluidity of blood flow by constitutively synthesizing and secreting both tPA and uPA.[26,140] In recent years, several types of cell surface receptors for fibrinolytic proteins have been isolated and identified. Hajjar and co-workers[42,93] have demonstrated that the phospholipid binding protein annexin II, which is highly expressed on human endothelial cells, induces a profibrinolytic effect by colocalizing plasminogen and tPA on vascular surfaces. Annexin II has an accessible carboxy-terminal lysine that binds the kringle structure of plasminogen and also contains a distinct binding motif that mediates the interaction with tPA. Furthermore, a phospholipid binding domain (KGLGT) contained within the second endonexin repeat module interacts with and mediates endothelial plasma membrane binding.[92]

Cells of neural origin are capable of binding tPA with high affinity. Plasminogen activators are associated with the surface of several types of neuronal cells, where they are considered to mediate localized degradation of extracellular matrix to facilitate cell motility. Also, tPA mRNA expression in granule neurons is coincident with the neuronal migration in the developing cerebellum.[81] Amphoterin is a 30-kd heparin binding protein that is developmentally regulated in the brain and is functionally involved in neurite outgrowth. Interestingly, amphoterin contains a high mobility group 1 sequence. Amphoterin strongly enhanced plasminogen activation by tPA or uPA, which led to the generation of surface bound plasmin. These results, plus the extracellular localization of amphoterin, suggest a role for amphoterin as a neuronal receptor for tPA in various migrating or invasive cells.[184]

Deposition of amyloid β-protein fibrils in the brain or in neuritic plaques, or associated with the vessel surface, is typical of such disorders as Alzheimer's disease, hereditary cerebral hemorrhage with Dutch-type amyloidosis, and cerebral amyloid angiopathy. Cerebral amyloid angiopathy is an important cause of intracerebral hemorrhage in the elderly. Amyloid β-protein deposits also occur in normal aging. Amyloid β-peptide analogs were found to have a marked stimulatory effect on plasminogen activation by tPA.[123] This stimulatory activity increased when the β-peptides formed aggregated fibrillar structures similar to amyloid deposits. These investigators suggest that the interaction of tPA with amyloid β-protein deposits may contribute to the intracerebral hemorrhage that occurs with low incidence (<1%) in patients receiving thrombolytic therapy with tPA for treatment of myocardial infarction.[88]

DOMAIN DELETION VARIANTS OF tPA WITH LONGER CIRCULATING HALF-LIFE

Considerable effort has been exerted to reducing the rate of tPA clearance to create a more convenient therapeutic agent that can be effectively administered by a single bolus injection. Since tPA is rapidly cleared from circulation, thrombolytic therapy in the coronary setting requires a 100-mg dose of tPA administered as a continuous intravenous infusion for 1.5 to 3 hours to maintain adequate lytic concentrations in plasma. Many variants of tPA that clear more slowly have been constructed, using the techniques of molecular biology, to allow the therapeutic use of bolus intravenous administration. Selected examples are summarized in the following sections.

Several groups have made domain deletion variants, although the amino acid sequence and expression systems have varied.[83,241,243] Variants were constructed by mutagenesis: single or multiple domains were excised from the gene sequence, and the resulting proteins were evaluated in pharmacokinetic studies. Most of the domain deletion variants exhibited increased in vivo half-life in animals. Des-finger tPA (lacking residues 6 to 50) had a 10-fold increased area under the curve (AUC) in rats, which correlated with 10-fold decreased clearance rate compared with that of full-length tPA.[136] Similar results were observed with the des-growth factor tPA (des 51-87) in a variety of species.[31,115,136] Deletion of finger and growth factor domains (des 6-86 tPA) resulted in 6-fold longer initial half-life in rabbits, and the clearance was reduced 10-fold compared with wild-type tPA.[55,57,136] Des-kringle 1 tPA displayed reduced clearance similar to that of des-G tPA, whereas des-kringle 2 tPA was cleared more rapidly than full-length tPA.[32] These studies indicate that the major clearance determinants of tPA are located in the F-, G-, and K1-domains. A mutant of plasminogen activator was constructed that lacked the finger and growth factor domains and deleted the glycosylation site in kringle 1, substituting Asn 117 by Gln (N117Q).[137] This mutant, termed Δ-FE 1X plasminogen activator (ΔFE1X), has been developed for phase III clinical testing in Japan as the thrombolytic agent SUN 9216 (Suntory, Japan). In the United States, phase II clinical trials have been completed for ΔFE1X, or NPA, which is currently being investigated by Bristol Myers Squibb as the thrombolytic agent lanoteplase (BMS-200980).[172]

Although many domain deletion variants have substantially reduced clearance, the thrombolytic activity of these variants has usually been compromised. Specific in vivo thrombolytic potency is a measure of the amount of clot lysis in an animal model for a given plasma concentration of lytic agent.[55] For example, the in vivo thrombolytic potency of des-FG tPA was similar to that of tPA despite a 10-fold increase in plasma concentration.[55,57] Thus, the specific in vivo thrombolytic activity of des-FG tPA was markedly reduced compared with tPA. Numerous domain deletion, insertion, and chimeric variants of tPA have been constructed with reduced plasma clearance; however, all exhibited reduced in vivo specific thrombolytic activity.[55]

The strategy of domain deletion has been employed in the construction of another variant of tPA that lacks the finger, growth factor, and kringle 1 domains. These modifications result in a molecule with decreased fibrin affinity and fibrin specificity but with increased circulating half-life.[153,221] This molecule, termed reteplase, consists of the kringle 2 and protease domains of tPA and has recently been approved by the Food and Drug Administration for therapeutic use in treatment of acute myocardial infarction (manufactured by Boehringer Mannheim and DuPont-Merck). Reteplase is produced by recombinant DNA technology in an unglycosylated form by expression in *Escherichia coli*, is then denatured in guanidine, and refolded during purification.[126,127] This process results in a 355-amino acid single-chain protein that can be converted to the two-chain form during fibrinolysis (Fig. 9.6). Deletion of the three amino-terminal domains and the absence of glycosylation present in native tPA alter the pharmacokinetic properties such that reteplase has a plasma half-life of 13 to 16 minutes compared with the 3- to 6-minute half-life observed for the α-phase of alteplase tPA.[154,155,231] The longer half-life of reteplase permits a double bolus intravenous dosing, with the second dose given 30 minutes after the first. Reteplase and streptokinase were evaluated as equivalent in a large (n = 6,010 patients), randomized, double-blind clinical trial comparing double-bolus administration of reteplase with streptokinase in acute myocardial infarction.[113]

TNK-tPA: LONGER HALF-LIFE, MORE FIBRIN-SPECIFIC FORM OF tPA

The use of tPA for coronary or cerebral thrombolysis has been demonstrated as an effective means of resolving the acute ischemic event.[88,167] The fibrin specificity of tPA compared with that of streptokinase or uPA results in decreased degradation of fibrinogen, factor V, and factor VIII, which reduces the potential for hemorrhage. Despite the theoretic advantage of tPA, intracranial hemorrhage was reported in trials of coronary thrombolysis.[37,185] The development of new plasminogen activators with enhanced biochemical and pharmacologic properties such as prolonged half-life and increased fibrin specificity, in conjunction with preclinical studies,[183] may allow adjustments to thrombolytic therapies that may potentially decrease intracranial bleeding.

Many investigators have produced longer half-life versions of tPA that could be administered as a bolus.[105,141] However, virtually all the tPA variants with reduced clearance yielded significantly decreased fibrinolytic activities.[55] In a series of comprehensive mutagenesis and screening efforts, the most effective, long-half-life tPA identified was a variant with an extraglycosylation site in kringle 1 created by the substitution of Asn for Thr at 103 (T103N, henceforth called T).[182] In another variant, the high mannose structure at position 117 was removed by a deglycosylation substitution, N117Q (abbreviated N). This variant exhibited a modest reduction in clearance in rabbits with minimal perturbation of fibrinolytic activity.[108,223] A combination variant (TN-tPA) was created with extraglycosylation and deglycosylation at positions 103 and 117, respectively, which effectively moved the glycosylation site on kringle 1 from position 117 to position 103.

Alanine scanning mutagenesis was used to identify KHRR(296–299)AAAA, a mutation that confers both fibrin specificity and PAI-1 resistance.[19,149] This variant (abbreviated as 'K') has improved fibrin specificity, because it has eight-fold less activity in the absence of fibrin while retaining full activity in the presence of fibrin. The K variant of tPA was shown to be approximately 90-fold more resistant to PAI-1 as determined by the second-order inhibition rate constants of variant and wild-type t-PA.[182] To create a variant of tPA with reduced clearance, enhanced fibrin specificity, and PAI-1 resistance, the mutations at three loci [T103N, N117Q, KHRR(296–299)AAAA][121] were combined as the TNK variant of tPA (Fig. 9.7).

TNK-tPA has been engineered to be more fibrin specific than tPA. This property is the result of the KHRR (296–299)AAAA mutation (K of TNK-tPA). To determine the effect of increased fibrin specificity on fibrinogen degradation, various concentrations of tPA or TNK-tPA were incubated in human citrated plasma (for 1 hour at 37°C) and subsequently assayed for residual fibrinogen by the Clauss method.[49] The concentration of activator at which 50% of the initial fibrinogen concentration was depleted (EC_{50}) was determined from a four-parameter fit of the fibrinogen versus activator concentration data. These data, shown in Figure 9.8, indicate that the K mutation allows TNK-tPA to be present at approximately 12-fold higher concentrations before significant fibrinogen depletion is observed in human plasma.[199]

TNK-tPA was constructed to have a longer circulating plasma half-life compared with that of tPA. The elimination of tPA from systemic circulation has been demonstrated to be due primarily to binding, uptake, and degradation in liver parenchymal cells.[174] Freshly isolated rat hepatocytes were used to evaluate the binding and uptake of TNK-tPA and variants that contained one or more of the mutations T, N, or K (Fig. 9.9). These data show that any variant of tPA con-

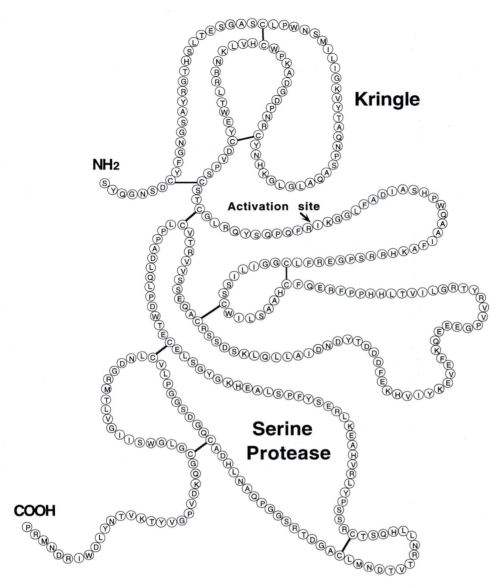

Figure 9.6 Schematic representation of the primary structure of kringle 2-protease as exemplified by Reteplase. Reteplase is a 354 amino acid, nonglycosylated recombinant molecule, composed of the kringle 2 and serine protease domains of t-PA. The first three amino acids, Ser-Tyr-Gln, correspond to the amino-terminal sequence of tPA, followed by residues 176 to 527 of tPA. Plasmin cleaves the activation site of K2-P at the Arg-Ile peptide bond similar to conversion of one-chain to two-chain tPA. Disulfide bonds are indicated by solid black lines between appropriate cysteines.

taining the T103N mutation does not exhibit a high degree of specific binding to hepatocytes in vitro.[120] The N117Q- and KHRR(296–299)AAAA-containing variants exhibit binding similar to that observed with tPA, such that these mutations do not contribute to the reduced hepatocyte binding characteristic of TNK-tPA.

The binding of tPA or TNK-tPA to liver cells mediates the rate of plasma clearance in vivo and therefore determines the requirement for an infusion or bolus administration to achieve effective thrombolysis. Although tPA can restore

blood flow to occluded coronary or cerebral arteries, it may also provoke brain damage by causing cerebral hemorrhage. To determine the relevance of tPA activity and brain hemorrhage, Yatsu and co-workers evaluated the relative binding kinetics of tPA and TNK-tPA on brain endothelial cells.[256] The binding of radiolabeled tPA to cultured rat brain endothelial cells was specific and saturable. Labeled tPA was competitively displaced in the presence of unlabeled excess tPA, but less effectively by excess unlabeled TNK-tPA, suggesting that TNK-tPA binds to some but not all the tPA binding sites on

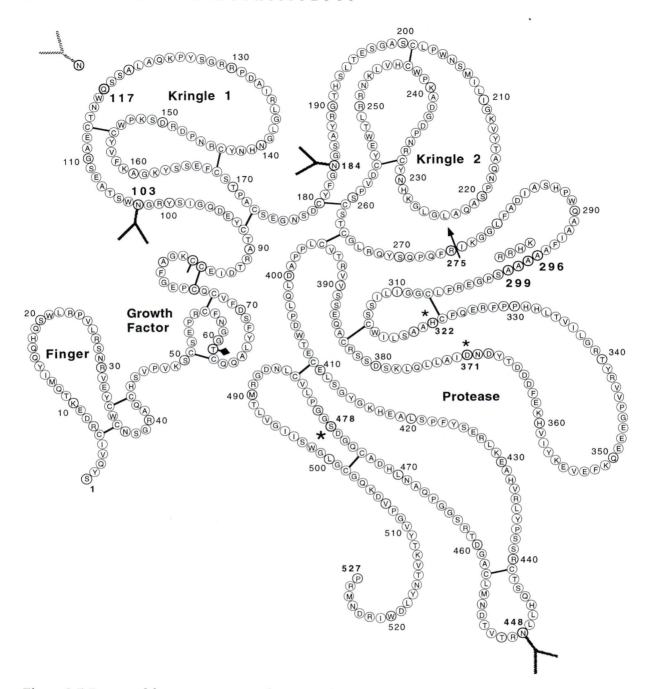

Figure 9.7 Diagram of the primary structure of TNK-tPA showing domains, disulfides, and glycosylation sites. Domain structures or modules are indicated as finger, growth factor, kringle 1, kringle 2, and protease. Proposed disulfides are represented as black lines between cysteines. The cysteine at position 83 is an unpaired sulfhydryl. O-linked fucosylated threonine is represented by a black diamond at position 61. N-linked glycosylation sites are indicated by Y-shaped black bars at Asn103, Asn184, and Asn448. The deglycosylation of the 117 site in native tPA is indicated by the detached Y-shaped shaded bar. The plasmin-catalyzed conversion of one-chain tPA to two-chain tPA occurs with cleavage of the Arg275-Ile276 peptide bond (arrow). Tetra-alanine substitutions for Lys296, His297, Arg298, and Arg299 are shown by bold circles. Active site residues His322, Asp371, and Ser478 are marked by asterisks.

In Vitro Fibrinogenolysis in Human Plasma

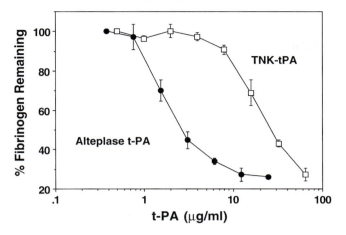

Figure 9.8 Effect of alteplase t-PA and the TNK-tPA variant on fibrinogen consumption in human plasma. The samples of tPA were incubated at various concentrations in human plasma at 37°C for 1 hour as indicated. The percent residual fibrinogen was then determined using the Clauss clotting time method.[49] Approximately 12-fold higher concentrations of TNK-tPA were required for the process of in vitro fibrinogenolysis to result in 50% decreased fibrinogen compared with alteplase t-PA.

Figure 9.9 Binding of tPA or variants of TNK-tPA to freshly isolated rat hepatocytes in vitro. tPA and variants of TNK-tPA were radiolabeled using the YPACK technique.[119] Rat hepatocytes were prepared from male Sprague-Dawley rats by collagenase perfusion. The binding of ^{125}I-tPA (0.1 μC at 15 ng/ml) to 10^6 cells was evaluated in vitro at 37°C for 0.5 hour with intermittant shaking. The hepatocytes were centrifuged and washed with incubation buffer (Krebs-Henseleit buffer containing 2% BSA); bound tPA was then determined by counting the radioactivity associated with the cell pellet. Nonspecific binding was evaluated in the presence of 1,000-fold excess unlabeled tPA. Specific binding of the TNK variants was normalized to that observed with tPA.

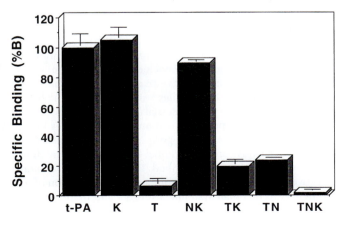

the brain endothelium. Radioligand blotting of brain endothelial cell membranes indicated that a protein of approximately 40 kd bound tPA, which is consistent with the studies by Hajjar et al[93] identifying annexin II as the tPA binding protein of human umbilical vein endothelium. Further work is necessary to evaluate more fully the role of tPA binding to brain endothelium and its potential relevance in the mechanism of intracerebral hemorrhage.

Pharmacokinetics and Pharmacodynamics of TNK-tPA in Rabbits

The clearance of TNK-tPA and tPA was compared in rabbits following bolus intravenous injections. The AUC was 8.4-fold greater than for wild-type tPA, which yielded clearance values of 1.9 versus 16.1 ml/min/kg for TNK-tPA and tPA, respectively.[121] Pharmacokinetic analysis of TNK-tPA indicated α- and β-phase half-lives of approximately 9 and 31 minutes, compared with tPA, which exhibited α-, β-, and γ-phases with half-lives of 1.3, 6, and 33 minutes, respectively. The thrombolytic potency of TNK-tPA (by bolus) was compared with that of tPA (by infusion) in a rabbit arteriovenous shunt model of clot lysis.[200] Clots were made from fresh rabbit whole blood or citrate collected plasma spiked with rabbit platelet-enriched plasma to a platelet concentration of approximately 10^9 platelets/ml. Extent of lysis after 2 hours was evaluated with doses ranging from 7 to 180 μg/kg for TNK-tPA, and 20 to 540 μg/kg for tPA. Relative potency of TNK-tPA was determined from the ED$_{50}$ of a fit of the dose-response curves. From this analysis, TNK-tPA was found to be 7.5 and 13.5 times more potent than tPA in lysing rabbit whole blood and platelet enriched clots, respectively.[121] These experimental data, although useful, do not measure the dissolution of a clot within a blood vessel. The next step in evaluation of tPA, TNK-tPA, and other thrombolytic agents is to show efficacy in more relevant preclinical models of thromboembolic vascular occlusion. The use of TNK-tPA and its comparison with tPA in rabbit models of occlusive cerebral and carotid artery thrombolysis have been described previously.[17,232] The progress of TNK-tPA in phase I trials for treatment of acute myocardial infarction is described later in this chapter.

Preclinical Studies of Cerebral Thrombolysis: Animal Models

Numerous reports have described the effects of thrombolytic agents in embolic stroke models. This work was initiated in response to the difficulties that arose from early clinical trials with streptokinase or uPA, plus the lack of predictable animal models to optimize the use of thrombolytic therapy for treatment acute ischemic stroke. Since then the primary focus of these studies has been to test the efficacy of various thrombolytic agents and regimens as well as to investigate the interactions between thrombolytic therapy and other pharmacologic approaches.

PHARMACOLOGIC EFFICACY AND SAFETY

Most of the preclinical studies have been conducted in the rabbit, in which two types of models have evolved. In the fragmented clot model the animal is injected with 2,000 to 4,000 clots, each <100 μm in diameter, and totaling 15 to 150 mg in weight. Although this is not an exact model of the clinical situation, it does have great relevance since its primary readout is neurologic status.[260] In the second and more commonly employed model, a single preformed clot is instilled into the cerebral circulation. In most cases this will lodge in the middle cerebral artery (MCA), resulting in focal ischemia of the MCA territory.[148] Variations of this model have been developed using small clots that selectively block the MCA or larger emboli to occlude larger portions of the circle of Willis. In addition, various labeling techniques have been used for monitoring clot lysis.

These range from tin granules[10,44,124] for roentgenographic evaluation and ^{125}I-labeled microspheres for clot localization[261] to ^{99m}Tc-labeled sulfur colloids for sequential γ-scintigraphy.[235]

The use of other animal models has been somewhat limited by the species-specificity of human tPA.[128] Nevertheless, a number of significant studies have been conducted in the rat with two basic modes reported. The first is similar to the fragmented clot model in the rabbit: a suspension of emboli is prepared from whole blood and injected into the cerebral circulation. End-point measurements include not only cerebral blood flow (^{133}Xe clearance) and angiography but also infarct size.[176] The alternative to introducing preformed emboli is to make the thrombus in situ. This is the basis of the photochemical model, whereby damage to the endothelium is induced by photoillumination with green light (540-nm wave length) of an exposed segment of the MCA. Concomitant injection of rose bengal dye causes the formation of reactive oxygen species that damage the endothelial cells in the illuminated area to yield a highly thrombogenic surface and subsequent thrombus formation.[240]

The baboon has also played an important role in the study of thrombolysis within the central nervous system. The model most often described involves the surgical implantation of a Silastic balloon cuff assembly around the MCA. Inflation of the balloon occludes the MCA, and reperfusion of the artery is controlled by deflation of the cuff.[225] Not only does the model have a period of regional ischemia due to the MCA occlusion but also subsequent perfusion deficits due to the formation of microthrombi. This model has yielded some important insights into the effects of thrombolytics (and their interactions with other therapies) on infarction, hemorrhage, and neurologic outcome in a non-human primate following a period of cerebral ischemia.[66–68] For a comprehensive list of the various models and the readout from each model see Overgaard's review of "Thrombolytic Therapy in Experimental Embolic Stroke."[175]

Hemorrhage

Of paramount concern in the clinical use of thrombolytics is the balance between safety and efficacy, especially considering the risk of cerebral hemorrhage. In some of the earliest animal experiments it was shown that there was no significant increase in the risk of hemorrhage if the thrombolytics were administered early[44,147,219] or even if delayed to 24 hours after embolization.[147] In a non-human primate model, neither intracarotid uPA nor intravenous tPA caused an increase in the incidence or severity of hemorrhage despite increases in fibrinogenolysis and incidence of peripheral bleeding.[66,68]

Indications that there may have been differences in the hemorrhagic rates between streptokinase and tPA were noticed as early as 1990.[146] In a series of experiments it was shown that, although both drugs were effective at producing thrombolysis, streptokinase caused significantly more hemorrhages than the saline-treated controls whereas tPA did not. Since then it was shown that streptokinase is very fibrinogen conserving in the rabbit and does not cause the systemic effects reported in humans.[142] In a recent study, using a rabbit model of embolic stroke, equipotent doses of streptokinase and tPA caused cerebral hemorrhage with equal regularity and increased template bleeding time to the same degree. However, circulating plasminogen amounts remaining after streptokinase (88%) and tPA (49%) administration were markedly different. This would suggest that the mechanisms responsible for bleeding events associated with the two molecules are probably different.[234]

Apart from the enzymatic actions of the thrombolytic agents, the physiologic hypertensive response to cerebral ischemia[28] or manipulations that increase blood pressure[85,138,208] may also play a significant role in the pathogenesis of hemorrhagic transformations. These studies would certainly argue that careful blood pressure management is probably required to decrease the incidence of hemorrhage when using thrombolytic therapy for acute ischemic stroke.

DOSE AND ROUTE OF ADMINISTRATION FOR TREATMENT OF STROKE

One of the confounding issues in preclinical studies is the inconsistency in the route of administration and dose of tPA used by the various investigators. In 1992 Russell et al[206] showed that front loading of tPA to yield a short, square wave infusion was preferable to a constant infusion of the drug. This was confirmed in a rat model of thromboembolic stroke.[180] The best route of administration is, however, controversial. Two similar studies were conducted to compare intra-arterial and intravenous administration. The first study concluded that when a low dose (3 mg/kg) was given intra-arterially it was superior to intravenous administration.[206] Conversely, the second study concludes that intravenous administration is the more effective treatment.[10] The main difference between the two studies was the site at which the clots were instilled; proximal internal carotid in the first versus middle cerebral and posterior communicating arteries in the second study. These represent peripheral and intracranial arteries, respectively, and differential effects of tPA in these blood vessels have been described. tPA appears to be more effective in the treatment of thromboembolic occlusion of intracranial arteries than systemic arteries[43] and therefore may be more susceptible to overdose. Additionally, the susceptibility of tPA-induced bleeding to tranexamic acid was shown to be greater in the cerebral vasculature than in cutaneous vascular beds.[61] Del Zoppo et al[66] had also noted a disparity between the incidence of peripheral hemorrhages and the absence of significant ischemia-related hemorrhagic transformations in his baboon model. These observations, taken together, suggest that a real difference may exist between cerebral and peripheral vascular responses to tPA in particular and perhaps to other thrombolytic agents.

Although the route of administration was being addressed, the exact dose response to tPA was still not adequately resolved. In 1993, we reported the results of a study in rabbits showing that either short (30-minute) or longer (2-hour) square wave infusions of tPA were comparable in their ability to lyse cerebral embolic clots as long as the doses were adjusted accordingly to yield similar plasma concentrations.[235] Moreover, we observed a bell-shaped dose-response curve for tPA. The optimal doses given either as short or long infusions correlated with consumption of about 50% of the available plasminogen, fibrinogen, and α_2-antiplasmin. The decreased activity at the higher doses, which caused significantly more systemic plasminogen activation, was probably attributable to the plasminogen steal effect previously described by Sobel et al.[222] From this study, it was predicted that the optimal dose in humans would be 1.3 mg/kg over 2 hours or 0.7 mg/kg over 30 minutes and that overdosing of the drug would lead to decreased thrombolytic activity.[235]

It is also clear that the type of thromboembolic obstruction is important. Fibrin-rich clots appear to be much more susceptible to tPA lysis than the platelet-rich white clots. In a series of reports describing the results of autopsy examinations, Jörgensen and Torvic[116,117] conclude that the composition of emboli and thrombi vary considerably and that no single clot type is predominant. However, the optimal substrate for thrombolytic therapy would be fresh thrombi consisting of fibrin and blood cells, since, as described previously, all thrombolytic agents ultimately work via the activation of plasminogen and the enzymatic action of plasmin. It is also probable that this is the least likely type of clot to be found in autopsy studies since they are the most likely to be degraded by endogenous tPA.

NEUROLOGIC OUTCOME

Although cerebral hemorrhage is of considerable importance to the clinician, overall neurologic status is the principal measure of any successful outcome. Few investigators have attempted to measure this in animal models using thrombolytic therapy. One of the earliest observations was the work of Zivin et al,[260] who demonstrated that tPA was beneficial in their fragmented clot model. This was confirmed in subsequent studies in 1988 and 1995.[27,261] Del Zoppo et al also showed that intracarotid administration of uPA[68] but not intravenous tPA[66] improved neurologic outcome in the baboon. In a series of observations it was also shown that in a rat model tPA, in a dose-dependent manner, induced recanalization (by angiography), reduced infarct volume (by histology), decreased mortality,[177–179] and improved neurologic function.[209]

COMBINATION WITH OTHER AGENTS

The need to use thrombolytics as part of a comprehensive multifaceted treatment for thromboembolic stroke was investigated in many of the preclinical studies. Early observations[148] showed that anticoagulation with heparin, even when administered to excess (partial thromboplastin time greater than three-fold over control), did not affect intracranial hemorrhage after experimental embolic stroke. However, in a follow-up study using the same single-clot model in the rabbit the authors found that while tPA alone or the combination of tPA and heparin carried no greater risk of hemorrhage than saline treatment, intravenous aspirin either alone or in combination with tPA significantly increased the chance of hemorrhagic conversion in this model.[48] This result was later re-examined using an optimal dose of tPA. This time the propensity for cerebral bleeding after thrombolytic therapy with tPA was not influenced by intravenous aspirin. However, it was demonstrated that intravenous aspirin (5 to 20 mg/kg) markedly attenuated the thrombolytic action of tPA. There seems to be no clear-cut reason for this effect. Moreover, the attenuation of tPA clot lysis was fully reversed by coadministration of a prostacyclin analog (Iloprost), suggesting that aspirin treatment may affect cerebral blood flow, especially under ischemic conditions.[233] This hypothesis is not supported by the work of Copeland et al,[59] who show that much higher doses of intravenous aspirin (90 mg/kg) are required to inhibit cyclo-oxygenase activity in cerebral microvessels. It should be stressed that these experiments were done using intravenous aspirin, and it has been shown that the route of aspirin administration can dramatically affect its interaction with the cardiovascular system.[41] Nevertheless, at very high doses of aspirin even oral administration has been shown to have a thrombogenic effect.[259] The overriding conclusion from these experiments is that at least in rabbit models of stroke, aspirin did not improve the outcome of tPA treatment. This was also confirmed in a rat model of embolic stroke.[180] Conversely, combined therapy with tPA and ticlopidine showed no such paradoxic results.[11]

The potential use of excitatory amino acid receptor antagonists for the treatment of stroke prompted their study in combination with thrombolytics. Rat studies were carried out by selective inhibition of the α-amino-3-hydroxy-5-methylisoxazol-4-propionic acid (AMPA) subtype of the glutamate receptor using the antagonist 2,3-dihydro-6-nitro-7-sulphamoyl-benzo(f)quinoxaline (NBQX) in combination with tPA. The results from these studies were encouraging and showed that neuroprotection afforded by NBQX augmented the benefit from thrombolysis in this model.[157,181] Similar effects were seen with the N-methyl-D-aspartic acid (NMDA) antagonist MK-801 (dizocilpine).[214] The additive effect of these two therapeutic approaches (glutamate receptor blockade plus thrombolysis) is probably due to improved accessibility of the receptor antagonists to the ischemic area after recanalization of the vessels by tPA.

It has long been thought that reopening of an occluded vessel will bring its own problems of reperfusion injury. Thus, antineutrophil agents have also been tested in combination with tPA in the setting of thromboembolic stroke. The combination of these two therapeutic approaches was tested in the rabbit fragmented clot model.[27] The study showed that by blocking the intercellular cell adhesion molecule ICAM-1 (using anti-ICAM-1 antibodies) on endothelial cells or the MAC-1 integrin on neutrophils (using anti-CD-18 antibodies), the window of opportunity for successful treatment with tPA could be extended. This is an important finding and corresponds well with the observation that anti-adhesion molecules alone are effective at reducing infarct volumes[258] and abrogating the no-reflow phenomenon due to microvascular plugging.[160] However, early clinical experience with a murine full-length antibody to human ICAM as sole therapy for stroke has not proved to be as promising as the preclinical data would have suggested. It is also noteworthy that although tPA modulates ex vivo platelet aggregation, it has no effect on ex vivo neutrophil activation.[9]

VARIANTS OF tPA

Genetic variants of tPA have recently become available, and some of these have been tested in animal models of ischemic stroke. Probably the first molecule of this type to be tested in a rabbit model of stroke was Fb-Fb-CF. This molecule is composed of the catalytic fragment of tPA (CF) and a dimer of fragment B (Fb) from staphylococcal protein A. This chimeric molecule displayed a prolonged plasma half-life (90 minutes), presumably due to interaction of the protein A domains with circulating immunoglobulin. Fb-Fb-CF exhibited fibrin specificity, as indicated by conservation of fibrinogen in vivo. When administered as a bolus 15 or 90 minutes after embolization, Fb-Fb-CF resulted in rapid reperfusion and consumed less than 20% of the circulating fibrinogen.[188] Another variant of tPA, SUN9216, has been evaluated in animal models of embolic stroke. This molecule was constructed by deleting the growth factor and finger domains of tPA with the inclusion of a single substitution made in the first kringle domain, which eliminates an N-linked glycosylation site (Asn117 to Gln117). The resultant molecule exhibits a 20-fold slower clearance in rats compared with that observed with native tPA. A single bolus dose of SUN9216 (1 mg/kg) given to a rat model of photochemically induced acute cerebral thrombosis resulted in reperfusion in 6 of 19 animals within 38 ± 6 minutes. Interestingly, the coinfusion of vapiprost (a thromboxane receptor antagonist) given to combat the postischemic hypoperfusion had no significant effect on the number of vessels recannulated but significantly reduced the time to opening (i.e., 21 ± 3 minutes) as well as the area of cerebral infarction.[240] The SUN9216 molecule, also known as nPA or lanoteplase, is currently in clinical testing for treatment of acute myocardial infarction under development by Bristol Myers Squibb.[172]

TNK-tPA is another thrombolytic agent that contains a substitution at amino acid residue 117, which is part of the strategy used to construct longer half-life molecules. As described previously, this variant exhibited increased fibrin specificity, reduced plasma clearance, and resistance to PAI-1.[121] This molecule was very potent in a rabbit single-clot model of embolic stroke, giving equivalent rates of lysis after a single bolus dose of 0.6 mg/kg compared with a 2-hour infusion of tPA (3 mg/kg/h). There was significantly less systemic plasmin-

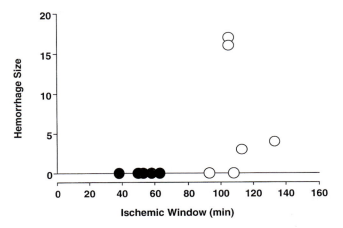

Figure 9.10 A relationship between ischemic period and hemorrhage conversion is shown by plotting the hemorrhage size measured 24 hours after treatment against the time to achieve 50% clot lysis in a rabbit model of embolic acute ischemic stroke treated with TNK-tPA. The treatment was given as a bolus administration at either 20 minutes (●) or 75 minutes (○) after embolization. The data show that early treatment with a very fibrin-specific thrombolytic agent does not cause hemorrhagic transformations. However, delayed treatment, even with fibrinogen-conserving agents such as TNK-tPA, is more likely to cause cerebral bleeding.

ogen activation, as indicated by reduced fibrinogenolysis, and less depletion of α_2-antiplasmin and factor VIII.[232,234] What was surprising in these studies using TNK-tPA, and another highly fibrin-specific variant of tPA having only the tetra-alanine substitutions at 296,297,298, and 299 (K-variant of tPA), was that the frequency of hemorrhagic conversions (measured as any form of hemorrhage seen at 24 hours after treatment and not limited to hematoma) was decreased dramatically from the 50% frequency rate observed in the animals in the buffer and tPA-treated groups.[234] However, as seen in Figure 9.10, when thrombolytic treatment is delayed and the time to reperfusion increased from 55 to 110 minutes, the number of hemorrhages increased. Although thrombolysis carries an inherent risk of cerebral hemorrhage, strong evidence shows that this risk can be offset by increasing the fibrin specificity of the thrombolytic agent. Also, the time to treatment is an important factor and can influence to a large extent the outcome of thrombolytic therapy of acute ischemic stroke.

In conclusion, the data available from the preclinical studies suggest that tPA is effective and (if given early and at an appropriate dose) relatively safe. As with all thrombolytics, tPA carries an inherent risk of cerebral hemorrhage, but by increasing the fibrin specificity this risk may be reduced. On balance, the evidence would suggest that potent anticoagulant or antiplatelet drugs do not enhance the therapeutic benefit seen after thrombolytic therapy. However, other therapeutic approaches such as antineutrophil agents or excitatory amino acid receptor antagonists may have additive or even synergistic effects with thrombolysis. These combinations of diverse therapeutic approaches may form the basis of a comprehensive approach to future stroke management.

Clinical Approaches in Thrombolysis

THROMBOLYSIS IN THE TREATMENT OF ACUTE MYOCARDIAL INFARCTION

Currently, alteplase tPA and streptokinase are used most often for the intravenous treatment of acute myocardial infarction (AMI). Intra-arterial administration does not play a major role in the treatment of AMI. Different types of clinical studies have been performed in AMI to investigate thrombolytic efficacy, function of the heart muscle, or clinical outcome. Angiographic studies were designed either to document an occlusive thrombus before treatment and subsequent recanalization on repeat angiography after administration of thrombolytics or to assess patency with angiography performed only after initiation of treatment. Other trials used functional end points, such as persistent regional myocardial wall motion abnormalities and impaired global left ventricular function, to define indirectly restoration of perfusion to infarct-related myocardial territories. Lastly, high-profile large trials have used mortality as the primary indication of clinical outcome.

Large Clinical Studies with Alteplase and Streptokinase

The Thrombolysis in Myocardial Infarction (TIMI 1) study in AMI patients demonstrated significantly higher recanalization rates 90 minutes after administration of alteplase (80 mg) given over a period of 3 hours compared with the standard streptokinase regimen (1.5 million units) given over 90 minutes (62% versus 31%).[45] Heparin was administered concomitantly with either fibrinolytic agent. A dose regimen for administering 100 mg of alteplase over 3 hours (10 mg bolus, 50 mg in the first hour and 20 mg in each of the second and third hours) yielded patency rates of 70% to 77%.[39,244] Front-loading of alteplase with 50% of a 100-mg dose given in the first 30 minutes demonstrated improved 90-minute patency rates of 81% to 91% compared with the conventional regimen.[39,87,168,169] Other clinical studies for early treatment of AMI have demonstrated improvement in ventricular function,[150,216,250] which reflected salvage of myocardium.

The Gruppo Italiano per lo Studio della Streptochinasi nell'Infarto Miocardico I (GISSI-1)[86] and the Second International Study of Infarct Survival (ISIS-2) trials,[114] both utilizing 1.5 million units of streptokinase administered over 60 minutes, were the first major clinical studies to establish the clinical efficacy of coronary thrombolysis in reducing early mortality by as much as 50% when initiated within the first 6 hours after symptom onset. The clinical results of the large GUSTO study with 41,000 AMI patients treated within 6 hours of symptom onset demonstrated reduced mortality associated with higher patency rates for the front-loaded alteplase dosing regimen and concomitant intravenous heparin compared with 1.5 million units of streptokinase with either subcutaneous or intravenous heparin.[87,88] There were also significant differ-

ences in allergic reactions (1.6% versus 5.7% and 5.8%) and anaphylaxis (0.2% versus 0.7% and 0.6%) between the front-loaded alteplase tPA treatment arm compared with those observed with both the subcutaneous and intravenous heparin/streptokinase arms. These results confirm the low immunogenic potential of alteplase tPA, as expected for a recombinant human protein. The frequency of hemorrhagic stroke with alteplase tPA (0.72%) was not significantly different compared with that seen with the streptokinase groups (0.49% and 0.54% for subcutaneous and intravenous heparin, respectively). The incidence of other bleeding events tended to be less frequent in patients treated with alteplase tPA.

Effects of Alteplase and Streptokinase on the Pathways of Coagulation and Fibrinolysis

In a clinical trial in AMI patients receiving different doses of alteplase tPA and streptokinase, cross-linked fibrin degradation products (XL-FDP) and fibrinopeptides were measured at several time points as an indication of fibrinolysis. Patients given alteplase tPA exhibited higher elevations of XL-FDP than those given streptokinase.[78] This difference was particularly striking 7 hours or more after thrombolysis. The levels of fibrinopeptides were significantly higher after alteplase tPA beginning 3 hours after treatment. These results are consistent with a greater fibrinolytic response to alteplase tPA and prolonged fibrinolytic activity compared with that of streptokinase. In several other studies the decrease in fibrinogen after initiation of fibrinolysis with alteplase tPA was significantly less pronounced compared with streptokinase.[52,150,197] Similar changes were observed for plasminogen and α_2-antiplasmin levels.

ANTITHROMBOTIC/ ANTICOAGULANT THERAPY ADJUNCTIVE TO THROMBOLYSIS IN AMI

Plasminogen activators have either no (i.e., alteplase tPA) or only weak (i.e., streptokinase) intrinsic anticoagulant properties, mainly induced by fibrinogen breakdown and the subsequent release of fibrin and fibrinogen degradation products.[77,100,249] Effective clot lysis by plasminogen activators removes the occluding thrombus but does not affect the underlying vascular lesion that is usually the cause of clot formation. Coronary atherosclerotic plaques, which are the usual underlying culprit of the occlusion in AMI, have a highly thrombogenic surface. Pharmacologic thrombolysis itself, predominantly by inducing thrombin release, represents an additional procoagulant component.[100,249]

Intravenous heparin has been extensively used in AMI to counteract these procoagulant activities and to prevent recurrent coronary thrombosis after thrombolysis. Multiple studies have demonstrated that the short-acting, relatively fibrin-specific plasminogen activators (alteplase tPA and single-chain uPA) should be used with adequately administered intravenous heparin to achieve and sustain therapeutic prolongations of the partial thromboplastin time. Concomitant intravenous heparin administration does not affect the patency rates at 90 minutes after alteplase tPA administration,[238] but it reduced coronary reocclusion rates after initially successful thrombolysis.[23,62,110,166] By contrast, a 5,000-IU regimen of subcutaneous heparin every 12 hours does not result in effective anticoagulation in most patients.[111,239] Even with higher subcutaneous heparin doses, there was a delay of up to 1.5 days from the beginning of the treatment before adequate partial thromboplastin time prolongation was reached.[239]

Aspirin has a direct inhibitory effect on platelet aggregation by inhibiting thromboxane synthesis. Platelets also play a role in reocclusion or reinfarction following successful coronary artery reperfusion. The landmark placebo-controlled ISIS-2 study in 12,000 patients demonstrated the usefulness of aspirin in AMI patients, either alone or in combination with streptokinase.[114] Aspirin (160 mg) reduced mortality by more than 20%. Given concomitantly, aspirin and streptokinase further reduced mortality from 13.2% to 8%. In ISIS-2, the highest rate of reinfarction was seen in the group receiving streptokinase without concomitant aspirin.[114]

INTRAVENOUS THROMBOLYSIS IN ACUTE ISCHEMIC STROKE: LARGE PLACEBO-CONTROLLED TRIALS

Tissue Plasminogen Activator

Two different molecular preparations of rtPA have been investigated in clinical studies of acute stroke: alteplase and duteplase (an investigational, predominantly double-chain rtPA molecule with a substitution of methionine at 245 for valine). Duteplase was investigated in the United States in a pilot dose escalating recanalization study,[70] as well as in a few small clinical trials in Japan.[161,255] In Europe, a clinical efficacy study of alteplase tPA was performed by the European Cooperative Acute Stroke Study (ECASS) investigators.[70] In the United States, alteplase tPA was subjected to a carefully designed and executed sequence of three clinical studies including a dose escalation pilot study[30,95,96] and two long-term clinical efficacy studies sponsored by the National Institute of Neurological Disorders and Strokes (NINDS)[167] These two latter studies described the results of 624 patients with moderate to severe neurologic deficit who were randomized within 3 hours of symptom onset to 0.9 mg/kg activase alteplase tPA or placebo. This is approximately two-thirds of the commonly used AMI dose of 100 mg given within 90 to 180 minutes. By intent-to-treat analysis of both studies, alteplase tPA-treated patients were at least 30% more likely to have minimal or no disability compared with those receiving placebo. Symptomatic intracranial hemorrhage during the first 36 hours occurred more commonly in activase alteplase tPA-treated patients (6.4% versus 0.6%), while the 90-day mortality rate was not statistically different with alteplase tPA (17% versus 21% with placebo). As a result of this comprehensive investigational program, alteplase tPA became the first approved treatment for acute ischemic stroke in the United States.

Many small pilot studies have been performed in Europe with alteplase tPA from a different manufacturer utilizing doses ranging from 70 to 100 mg. Two of the larger clinical trials were recanalization studies following angiographic demonstration of intracerebral arterial occlusion[102,245] within 2 to 18 hours of onset of symptoms. Recently, the results of a clinical efficacy study were reported by the ECASS Investigators.[89] A total of 620 acute hemispheric stroke patients with moderate to severe neurologic deficit were randomized to receive 1.1 mg/kg alteplase tPA or placebo within 6 hours of symptom onset. In the intent-to-treat analysis, there was no difference in functional outcome as measured by the median Barthel Index or the median Modified Rankin Scale at 90 days after treatment. In a prospectively defined target population consisting mainly of patients without major early infarct signs on the baseline computed tomography and lacking some other major exclusion criteria, the Modified Rankin Scale indicated a significant benefit at 90 days for alteplase tPA-treated patients, as was observed using the Scandinavian Stroke Scale for neurologic recovery. For the alteplase tPA group, the frequencies for mortality and intracranial hemorrhages were higher compared with placebo. For a more comprehensive and detailed discussion of clinical experience with alteplase tPA for treatment of stroke, see Chapter 51.

Streptokinase

Three large placebo-controlled multicenter studies have been performed with streptokinase in acute ischemic stroke. The Australian Streptokinase Trial[71] treated patients within 0 to 4 hours of symptom onset, while the Multicenter Acute Stroke Trial (MAST)-Italy[165] and the MAST-Europe[164] used a 0- to 6-hour time window. In contrast to alteplase tPA, no pilot dose finding studies were performed to select a benefit and risk balancing dose. Instead, all three studies utilized a streptokinase dose of 1.5 million units infused over 60 minutes, which is commonly used for AMI treatment. Although previous studies in AMI patients indicated that concomitant administration of heparin and streptokinase resulted in an increased risk of bleeding, there were no protocol-specified provisions to prohibit heparin or aspirin in the first 24 hours after symptom onset or initiation of thrombolysis. In fact, the MAST-Italy study utilized a factorial design of streptokinase, streptokinase plus aspirin, aspirin, and placebo.[165]

All three studies were prematurely terminated due to the observed increase in mortality, ranging from 29% to 45%. These rates were significantly higher compared with the placebo groups, with mortality ranging from 20.5% to 34.4%. Also, the frequency of symptomatic intracranial hemorrhage in the streptokinase groups varied from 6% to 21.2%, which was significantly higher compared to that observed with placebo.

INTRA-ARTERIAL THROMBOLYSIS IN ACUTE ISCHEMIC STROKE

Intra-arterial administration of alteplase tPA, streptokinase, urokinase, or single-chain uPA for the treatment of acute ischemic stroke has been evaluated in small-scale feasibility or dose finding studies.[7,8,40,69,79,80] One recently completed study combined initial intravenous alteplase tPA therapy with intra-arterial administration of alteplase tPA after angiographic demonstration of persistent cerebrovascular occlusion.[79] In these studies the observed recanalization rates were lower than the highest rates observed after either intravenous or intra-arterial thrombolysis in AMI. Observed rates for intracranial hemorrhage were dependent on dose and time to treatment. Follow-up data on outcomes indicated the potential for clinical benefit in patients. Phase III studies focusing on clinical efficacy are currently being performed or considered.

ANTICOAGULANT/ ANTIPLATELET THERAPY IN ACUTE ISCHEMIC STROKE

To date the available data from clinical studies do not support the immediate use of heparin or aspirin with cerebral thrombolysis. The large placebo-controlled studies with alteplase tPA elected not to administer intravenous heparin or aspirin during the first 24 hours after the onset of symptoms or after initiation of thrombolysis to minimize the anticipated risk of intracranial hemorrhage. In the NINDS study,[167] which also did not allow either heparin or aspirin in the first 24 hours after symptom onset, the recurrent stroke rate at 3 months was not different in either the placebo or the alteplase tPA group (5.4% versus 5.8%). In angiographic studies, intravenous heparin was used but was restricted before and during the angiography.

Surprisingly, and disregarding the well-documented effects of streptokinase administration on the coagulation system, no precautions disallowing or restricting the use of aspirin were considered in the three large clinical trials with streptokinase. The MAST-Italy study randomized patients in a four-arm factorial design to treatment with streptokinase, aspirin, combined streptokinase and aspirin, or placebo. In this study, the use of heparin was not restricted during the first 24 hours. All studies using streptokinase for treatment of stroke were prematurely terminated due to higher frequencies of intracranial hemorrhage and mortality in streptokinase or streptokinase plus aspirin-treated patients. In the Italian MAST study, the study group receiving the combination of streptokinase with aspirin exhibited increased event rates for symptomatic cerebral hemorrhage during the hospital stay (10% versus 6% for streptokinase and aspirin versus streptokinase only, respectively) as well as increased mortality at 6 months (44% versus 28%, respectively).[164,165]

CLINICAL EXPERIENCE WITH TNK-tPA

TNK-tPA has undergone initial clinical evaluation in the treatment of AMI in a phase I trial (TIMI 10A). TIMI 10A was an open-label, dose-ranging, pilot trial of single-bolus, intravenous TNK-tPA in patients with AMI. Eligible patients were older than 70 years with symptom onset of <12 hours duration and electrocardiographic evidence of AMI or new left bundle branch block without contraindications to thrombolytic therapy. All patients received oral aspirin and intravenous heparin therapy titrated to an activated partial thromboplastin time of 55 to 85 seconds. End points included pharmacokinetic analysis, effect on hemostatic parameters, angiographic assessment by TIMI flow grade and TIMI frame count, and safety evaluation. Doses ranging from 5 to 50 mg were studied in a total of 113 patients.[36] At the 30-, 40-, and 50-mg doses, TIMI grade 3 patency rates achieved at 90 minutes with TNK-tPA were 57% to 64%, which is at least as good if not superior to patency rates achieved with accelerated alteplase tPA in the GUSTO I trial. Pharmacokinetic data from the TIMI 10A trial showed TNK-tPA to have a plasma clearance of 151 ± 55 ml/min, which is approximately fourfold less than that of alteplase tPA (572 ± 132 ml/min). The plasma half-lives for TNK-tPA and alteplase tPA were 17 ± 7 and 3.5 ± 1.4 minutes, respectively. Little effect was observed on coagulation parameters, and negligible fibrinogen or plasminogen consumption was noted (3% and 13%, respectively). No intracranial bleeding, anaphylaxis, or immunogenicity was observed. Adverse events reported in the TIMI 10A trial, which included escalating bolus doses of TNK-tPA, resulted in a safety profile comparable to that observed in other thrombolytic trials.[36] To define the efficacy and safety profile of TNK-tPA more completely additional larger phase II clinical trials (TIMI 10B and ASSENT) with >3,000 patients have recently been completed.

Summary

In conclusion, fibrin-specific thrombolytic agents exhibit distinctly different biologic and pharmacologic characteristics in comparison with less fibrin-specific molecules. Animal models of acute ischemic stroke indicate that fibrin-specific thrombolysis results in improved reperfusion and less bleeding. Clinical studies of thrombolysis in acute myocardial infarction suggested that improved reperfusion results in reduced mortality as demonstrated by an accelerated regimen of alteplase tPA compared with the less fibrin-specific molecule streptokinase. In treatment of AMI, co-administration of heparin and aspirin sustains reperfusion, leading to reduced rates of reocclusion. Clinical studies in acute ischemic stroke indicate the critical importance of careful dose selection. Lower doses in acute ischemic stroke compared with AMI seem to provide a balance between clinical benefit versus the risk of intracranial hemorrhage and associated mortality. As indicated by animal models, the coadministration of aspirin and heparin with thrombolytic therapy may result in increased frequencies of intracranial hemorrhage and mortality, particularly when streptokinase is administered at doses used for treatment of AMI. As we look to potential improvements in the treatment of acute ischemic stroke, we can anticipate that the ideal thrombolytic would be easy and rapid to administer, be fibrin specific (thus not inducing a systemic lytic state), not be inhibited by endogenous inhibitors (e.g., PAI-1), and have a more favorable safety profile than alteplase tPA. The future of stroke therapy will most probably involve thrombolysis. However, the full potential of early and rapid recanalization of cerebral vessels will only be realized when thrombolytic agents are used in conjunction with other therapeutic approaches.

References

1. Adams HP, Brott TG, Furlan AJ et al: Guidelines for Thrombolytic Therapy for Acute Stroke: A Supplement to the Guidelines for the Management of Patients with Acute Ischemic Stroke. Circulation 94:1167–1174, 1996, also Stroke 27:1711–1718

2. Almeda S, Vovis G: Thrombolytic properties of Lys-158 mutants of recombinant single chain urokinase-type plasminogen activator (scu-PA) in rabbits with jugular vein thrombosis. J Vasc Med Biol 1:46–49, 1989

3. Ashwell G, Harford J: Carbohydrate specific receptors of the liver. Annu Rev Biochem 51:531–554, 1982

4. Astrup T, Permin PM: Fibrinolysis in the animal organism. Nature 159:681–682, 1947

5. Banyai L, Varadi A, Patthy L: Common evolutionary origin of the fibrin-binding structures of fibronectin and tissue-type plasminogen activator. FEBS Lett 163: 37–41, 1983

6. Barnathan ES, Kuo A, Kariko K et al: Characterization of human endothelial cell urokinase-type plasminogen activator receptor protein and messenger RNA. Blood 76:1795–1806, 1990

7. Barr JD, Horowitz MB, Mathis JM et al: Intra-operative urokinase infusion for embolic stroke during carotid endarterectomy. Neurosurgery 36:606–1611, 1995

8. Barr JD, Mathis JM, Wildenhain SL et al: Acute stroke intervention with intra-arterial urokinase infusion. J Vasc Interv Radiol 5:705–713, 1994

9. Bednar MM, Dooley RH, Zanani M et al: Neutrophil and platelet activity and quantification following delayed tPA therapy in a rabbit model of thromboembolic stroke. J Thromb Thrombol 1:179, 1995

10. Bednar MM, Raymond SJ, Gross CE: Tissue plasminogen activator: comparison of dose and route of administration in a rabbit model of thromboembolic stroke. Neurol Res 15:405–408, 1993

11. Bednar MM, Raymond-Russell SJ, Booth CL, Gross CE: Combination tissue plasminogen activator and ticlopidine therapy in a rabbit model of acute thromboembolic stroke. Neurol Res 18:45–48, 1996

12. Beebe DP, Aronson DL: Turnover of tissue-type plasminogen activator (t-PA) in rabbits. Thromb Res 43: 663–674, 1986

13. Behrendt N, Ploug M, Patthy L et al: The ligand-binding domain of the cell surface receptor for the urokinase-type plasminogen activator. J Biol Chem 266: 7842–7847, 1991

14. Behrendt N, Ronne E, Danø K: The structure and function of the urokinase receptor, a membrane protein governing plasminogen activation on the cell surface. Biol Chem Hoppe-Seyler 376:269–279, 1995

15. Behrendt N, Ronne E, Ploug M et al: The human receptor for urokinase plasminogen activator. J Biol Chem 265:6453–6460, 1990

16. Beiseigel U, Weber W, Ihrke G et al: The LDL receptor-related protein, LRP, is an apolipoprotein E-binding protein. Nature 341:162–164, 1989

17. Benedict CR, Refino CJ, Keyt BA et al: New variant of human tissue plasminogen activator (tPA) with enhanced efficacy and lower incidence of bleeding compared with recombinant human tPA. Circulation 92: 3032–3040, 1995

18. Bennett WF: Two forms of tissue-type plasminogen activator (t-PA) differ at a single glycosylation site. Thromb Haemost 50:106, 1983

19. Bennett WF, Paoni NF, Keyt, BA et al: High resolution analysis of functional determinants on human tissue-type plasminogen activator. J Biol Chem 266:5191–5201, 1991

20. Berleau LT, Refino CJ, Modi N et al: Interspecies scaling of wildtype t-PA and TNK-tPA: prediction of TNK-tPA clearance in humans. Fibrinolysis suppl. 1,8:26, 1994

21. Bernik MB, Oller EP: Increased plasminogen activator (urokinase) in tissue culture after fibrin deposition. J Clin Invest 53:823–834, 1973

22. Bjoern S, Foster DC, Thim L et al: Human plasma and recombinant factor VII: characterization of O-glycosylation at serine residues 52 and 60 and effects of site-directed mutagenesis of serine 52 to alanine. J Biol Chem 266:11051–11057, 1991

23. Bleich SD, Nichols TC, Schumacher RR et al: Effect of heparin on coronary arterial patency after thrombolysis with tissue plasminogen activator in acute myocardial infarction. Am J Cardiol 66:1412, 1990

24. Booth NA, Robbie LA, Croll AM, Bennett B: Lysis of platelet-rich thrombi: the role of PAI-1. Ann NY Acad Sci 667:70–80, 1992

25. Booth NA, Simpson AJ, Croll A et al: Plasminogen activator inhibitor (PAI-1) in plasma and platelets. Br J Haematol 70:327–333, 1988

26. Booyse FM, Osikowicz G, Feder S, Scheinbucks J: Isolation and characterization of a urokinase-type plasminogen activator (Mr = 54000) from cultured human endothelial cell indistinguishable from urinary urokinase. J Biol Chem 259:7198–7204, 1984

27. Bowes MP, Rothlein R, Fagan SC, Zivin JA: Monoclonal antibodies preventing leukocyte activation reduce experimental neurologic injury and enhance efficacy of thrombolytic therapy. Neurology 45:815–819, 1995

28. Bowes MP, Zivin JA, Thomas GR et al: Acute hypertension, but not thrombolysis, increases the incidence and severity of hemorrhagic transformation following experimental stroke in rabbits. Exp Neurol 141:40, 1996

29. Brogden RN, Speight TM, Avery GS: Streptokinase: a review of its clinical pharmacology, mechanism of action and therapeutic uses. Drugs 5:357–445, 1973

30. Brott TG, Haley EC, Levy DE et al: Urgent therapy for stroke. Part I. Pilot study of tissue plasminogen activator administered within 90 minutes. Stroke 23:632–640, 1992

31. Browne MJ, Carey JE, Chapman CG et al: A tissue-type plasminogen activator mutant with prolonged clearance *in vivo*. J Biol Chem 263:1599–1602, 1988

32. Browne MJ, Chapman CG, Dodd I et al: The role of

tissue-type plasminogen activator A-chain domains in plasma clearance. Fibrinolysis 3:207–214, 1989

33. Bu G, Williams S, Strickland DK et al: Low density lipoprotein receptor/α_2-macroglobulin receptor is an hepatic receptor for tissue-type plasminogen activator. Proc Natl Acad Sci USA 89:7427–7431, 1992

34. Bu G, Maksymovitch EA, Schwartz AL: Receptor-mediated endocytosis of tissue-type plasminogen activator by low density lipoprotein receptor-related protein on human hepatoma HEP G2 cells. J Biol Chem 268: 13002–13009, 1993

35. Bu G, Warshawsky I, Schwartz AL: Cellular receptors for the plasminogen activators. Blood 83:3427–3436, 1994

36. Cannon CP, McCabe CH, Gibson M et al: TNK-tissue plasminogen activator in acute myocardial infarction, results of thrombolysis in myocardial infarction (TIMI) 10A dose-ranging trial. Circulation 95:351–356, 1997

37. Carlson SE, Aldrich MS, Greenberg HS, Topol EJ: Intra-cerebral hemorrhage complicating intravenous tissue plasminogen activator treatment. Arch Neurol 45: 1070–1073, 1988

38. Carmeliet P, Schoonjans L, Kieckens L et al: Physiological consequences of loss of plasminogen activator gene function in mice. Nature 368:419–424, 1994

39. Carney RJ, Murphy GA, Brandt TR et al: Randomized angiographic trial of recombinant tissue-type plasminogen activator (alteplase) in myocardial infarction. J Am Coll Cardiol 20:17–23, 1992

40. Casto L, Moschini L, Camerlingo M et al: Local intra-arterial thrombolysis for acute stroke in the carotid artery territories. Acta Neurol Scand 86:308–311, 1992

41. Cerletti C, Gambino MC, Garattini S, de Gaetano G: Biochemical selectivity of oral versus intravenous aspirin in rats. J Clin Invest 78:323–326, 1986

42. Cesarman GN, Guevara CA, Hajjar KA: An endothelial cell receptor for plasminogen/tissue plasminogen activator: II. Annexin II-mediated enhancement of t-PA-dependent plasminogen activation. J Biol Chem 269: 21198–21203, 1994

43. Chehrazi BB, Seibert JA, Hein L, Brock J, Kissel P: Differential effect of recombinant tissue plasminogen activator-induced thrombolysis in the central nervous system and systemic arteries. Neurosurgery 28:364–369, 1991

44. Chehrazi BB, Seibert JA, Kissel P et al: Evaluation of recombinant tissue plasminogen activator in embolic stroke. Neurosurg 24:355–360, 1989

45. Chesebro JH, Knatterud G, Roberts R et al: Thrombolysis in myocardial infarction (TIMI) trial. Phase I: a comparison between intravenous tissue plasminogen activator and intravenous streptokinase. Circulation 76:142, 1987

46. Chmielewska J, Ranby M, Wiman B: Kinetics of the inhibition of plasminogen activators by the plasminogen-activator inhibitor. Biochem J 251:327–332, 1988

47. Christensen RL, MacLeod CM: A proteolytic enzyme of serum: characterization, activation and reaction with inhibitors. J Gen Physiol 28:559–583, 1945

48. Clark WM, Madden KP, Lyden PD, Zivin JA: Cerebral hemorrhagic risk of aspirin or heparin therapy with thrombolytic treatment in rabbits Stroke 22:872–876, 1991

49. Clauss A: Gerinnungsphysiologische Schnellmethode zur Bestimmung des Fibrinogens. Acta Haematol (Basel) 17:237–240, 1957

50. Cole ES, Nichols EH, Poisson L et al: In vivo clearance of tissue plasminogen activator: the complex role of sites of glycosylation and level of sialylation. Fibrinolysis 7: 15–22, 1993

51. Collen D: On the regulation and control of fibrinolysis. Thromb Haemost 43:77–89, 1980

52. Collen D, Bounameaux H, De Cock F et al: Analysis of coagulation and fibrinolysis during intravenous infusion of recombinant human tissue-type plasminogen activator in patients with acute myocardial infarction. Circulation 73:511, 1986

53. Collen D, Lijnen HR: Basic and clinical aspects of fibrinolysis and thrombolysis. Blood 78:3114–3124, 1991

54. Collen D, Lijnen HR: Staphylokinase, a fibrin-specific plasminogen activator with therapeutic potential? Blood 84:680–686, 1994

55. Collen D, Lijnen HR, Vanlinthout I et al: Thrombolytic and pharmacokinetic properties of human tissue-type plasminogen activator variants, obtained by deletion and/or duplication of structural/functional domains, in a hamster pulmonary embolism model. Thromb Haemost 65:174–180, 1991

56. Collen D, Mao J, Stassen JM et al: Thrombolytic properties of Lys-158 mutants of recombinant single chain urokinase-type plasminogen activator (scu-PA) in rabbits with jugular vein thrombosis. J Vasc Med Biol 1:46–49, 1989

57. Collen D, Stassen JM, Larsen G: Pharmacokinetics and thrombolytic properties of deletion mutants of human tissue-type plasminogen activator in rabbits. Blood 71: 216–219, 1988

58. Collen D, Van de Werf F: Coronary thrombolysis with recombinant staphylokinase in patients with evolving myocardial infarction. Circulation 87:18503, 1993

59. Copeland JR, Willoughby KA, Tynan TM et al: Endothelial and non-endothelial cyclo-oxygenase mediate rabbit pial arteriole dilation by bradykinin. Am J Physiol 268: H458–H466, 1995

60. Dano K, Andreasen PA, Grondahl-Hansen J et al: Plasminogen activators, tissue degradation, and cancer. Adv Cancer Res 44:139–266, 1985

61. de Bono DP, Pringle S, Underwood I: Differential effects of aprotinin and tranexamic acid on cerebral bleeding and cutaneous bleeding time during rt-PA infusion. Thromb Res 61:159–163, 1991

62. de Bono DP, Simoons ML, Tijssen J et al: Effect of early intravenous heparin on coronary patency, infarct size, and bleeding complications after alteplase thrombolysis: results of a randomised double blind. European Cooperative Study Group Trial. Br Heart J 67:122, 1992

63. DeClerck PJ, Alessi MC, Verstreken M et al: Measurement of plasminogen activator inhibitor 1 in biologic fluids with a murine monoclonal antibody-based enzyme-linked immunosorbant assay. Blood 71:220–225, 1988

64. DeClerck PJ, Lijnen HR, Verstreken M et al: A mono-

clonal antibody specific for two chain urokinase-type plasminogen activator. Application to the study of the mechanism of clot lysis with single-chain urokinase-type plasminogen activator in plasma. Blood 75:1794–1800, 1990

65. de Vries C, Veerman, H, Pannekoek H: Identification of the domains of tissue-type plasminogen activator involved in the augmented binding to fibrin after limited digestion with plasmin. J Biol Chem 264:12604–12610, 1989

66. del Zoppo GJ, Copeland BR, Anderchek K et al: Hemorrhagic transformation following tissue plasminogen activator in experimental cerebral infarction. Stroke 21: 596–601, 1990

67. del Zoppo GJ, Copeland BR, Harker LA et al: Experimental acute thrombotic stroke in baboons. Stroke 17: 1254, 1986

68. del Zoppo GJ, Copeland BR, Waltz TA et al: The beneficial effect of intracarotid urokinase on acute stroke in a baboon model. Stroke 17:638–643, 1986

69. del Zoppo GJ, Higashida R, Furlan A et al: The prolyse in acute cerebral thromboembolism trial (PROACT): results of 6 mg dose tier. Cerebrovasc Dis 6:184, 1996

70. del Zoppo GJ, Poeck K, Pessin MS et al: Recombinant tissue plasminogen activator in acute thrombotic and embolic stroke. Ann Neurol 32:78–86, 1992

71. Donnan GA, Davis SM, Chambers BR et al: Trials of streptokinase in severe acute ischaemic stroke. Lancet 345:578–579, 1995

72. Doolittle RF: Fibrinogen and fibrin. Sci Am 245:92–101, 1981

73. Doolittle RF: Structural aspects of the fibrinogen to fibrin conversion. Adv Protein Chem 27:1–109, 1973

74. Eaton DL, Fless GM, Kohr WJ et al: Partial amino acid sequence of apolipoprotein(a) shows that it is homologous to plasminogen. Proc Natl Acad Sci USA 84: 3224–3228, 1987

75. Eaton DL, Scott RW, Baker JB: Purification of human fibroblast urokinase proenzyme and analysis of its regulation by proteases and protease nexin. J Biol Chem 259: 6241–6247, 1984

76. Einarsson M, Smedrød B, Pertoft H: Uptake and degradation of tissue-type plasminogen activator in rat liver. Thromb Haemost 59:474–479, 1988

77. Eisenberg PR, Sherman L, Rich M et al: Importance of continued activation of thrombin reflected by fibrinopeptide A to the efficacy of thrombolysis. J Am Coll Cardiol 7:1255–1262, 1986

78. Eisenberg PR, Sherman LA, Tiefenbrunn AJ et al: Sustained fibrinolysis after administration of t-PA despite its short half life in the circulation. Thromb Haemost 57:35–40, 1987

79. EMS Bridging Trial Investigators: Combined intravenous and intra-arterial thrombolysis versus intra-arterial thrombolysis alone: preliminary safety and clot lysis. Cerebrovasc Dis 6:184, 1996

80. Fitt GJ, Farrar J, Baird AE et al: Intra-arterial streptokinase in acute ischaemic stroke. A pilot study. Vic Med J Aust 159:331–334, 1993

81. Friedman GC, Seeds NW: Tissue plasminogen activator mRNA expression in granule neurons coincides with their migration in the developing cerebellum. J Comp Neurol 360:658–670, 1995

82. Garabedian HD, Gold HK, Leinbach RC et al: Comparative properties of two clinical preparations of recombinant human tissue-type plasminogen activator in patients with acute myocardial infarction. J Am Coll Cardiol 9:599–607, 1987

83. Gething MJ, Adler B, Boose JA et al: Variants of human tissue-type plasminogen activator that lack specific structural domains of the heavy chain. EMBO J 7:2731–2740, 1988

84. Gliemann J, Davidsen O: Characterization of receptors for α_2-macroglobulin-trypsin complex in rat hepatocytes. Biochim Biophys Acta 885:49–57, 1986

85. Globus JH, Epstein JA: Massive cerebral hemorrhage: spontaneous and experimentally induced. J Neuropathol Exp Neurol 12:107, 1953

86. Gruppo Italiano per lo Studio della Streptochinasi nell'Infarto Miocardico (GISSI): Effectiveness of intravenous thrombolytic treatment in acute myocardial infarction. Lancet 1:397–402, 1986

87. GUSTO Angiographic Investigators: An angiographic study within the global randomized trial of aggressive versus standard thrombolytic strategies in patients with acute myocardial infarction. N Engl J Med 329:1615, 1993

88. GUSTO Investigators: An intenational randomized trial comparing four thrombolytic strategies for acute myocardial infarction. N Engl J Med 329:673–682, 1993

89. Hacke W, Kaste M, Fieschi C et al: Intravenous thrombolysis with recombinant tissue plasminogen activator for acute hemispheric stroke. The European Cooperative Acute Stroke Study (ECASS). JAMA 274: 1017–1025, 1995

90. Hajjar KA: The endothelial cell tissue plasminogen activator receptor: specific interaction with plasminogen. J Biol Chem 266:21962–21970, 1991

91. Hajjar KA, Gavish D, Breslow JL, Nachmann RL: Lipoprotein (a) modulation of endothelial cell surface fibrinolysis and its potential role in atherosclerosis. Nature 339:303–305, 1989

92. Hajjar KA, Guevara CA, Lev E et al: Interaction of the fibrinolytic receptor, annexin II, with the endothelial cell surface: essential role of endonexin repeat 2. J Biol Chem 271:21652–21659, 1996

93. Hajjar KA, Jacovina AT, Chacko J: An endothelial cell receptor for plasminogen and tissue plasminogen activator: I. Identity with annexin II. J Biol Chem 269: 21191–21197, 1994

94. Hajjar KA, Reynolds CM: Alpha-fucose-mediated binding and degradation of tissue-type plasminogen activator by HepG2 cells. J Clin Invest 93:703–710, 1994

95. Haley EC, Brott TG, Sheppard GL et al: Pilot randomized trial of tissue plasminogen activator in acute ischemic stroke. Stroke 24:1000–1004, 1993

96. Haley EC, Levy DE, Brott TG et al: Urgent therapy for stroke, part II pilot study of tissue plasminogen activator administered 91–180 minutes from onset. Stroke 23: 641–645, 1992

97. Harpel PC, Hermann A, Zhang X et al: Lipoprotein(a),

plasmin modulation and atherogenesis. Thromb Haemost 74:382–386, 1995

98. Harris RJ, Leonard CK, Guzzetta AW, Spellman MW: Tissue plasminogen activator has O-linked fucose attached to threonine-61 in the epidermal growth factor domain. Biochem 30:2311–2314, 1991

99. Harris RJ, Ling VT, Spellman, MW: O-linked fucose is present in the first epidermal growth factor domain of factor XII but not protein C. J Biol Chem 267: 5102–5107, 1992

100. Haskel EJ, Prager NA, Adams SP et al: The relative efficacy of antithrombin compared with antiplatelet agents in accelerating coronary thrombolysis and preventing early reocclusion. Circulation 83:1048–1056, 1991

101. Hekman C, Loskutoff DJ: Kinetic analysis of the interactions between plasminogen activator inhibitor 1 and both urokinase and tissue plasminogen activator. Arch Biochem Biophys 262:199–210, 1988

102. Hennerici M, Hacke W, von Kummer R et al: Intravenous tissue plasminogen activator for the treatment of acute thromboembolic ischemia. Cerebrovasc Dis 1: 124–128, 1991

103. Henschen A: Fibrinogen-Blutgerinnungfaktor I. Biochemische Aspekte. Haemostaseologie 1:49–61, 1981

104. Herz J: Surface location and high affinity for calcium of a 500 kd liver membrane protein closely related to the LDL-receptor suggest a physiological role as a lipoprotein receptor. EMBO J 7:4119–4127, 1988

105. Higgins DH, Bennett WF: Tissue plasminogen activator: the biochemistry and pharmacology of variants produced by mutagenesis. Annu Rev Pharmacol Toxicol 30: 91–121, 1990

106. Holmes WE, Pennica D, Blaber M et al: Cloning and expression of the gene for pro-urokinase in *Escherichia coli*. Biotechnology 3:923–929, 1985

107. Holvoet P, Lijnen HR, Collen D: Characterization of functional domains in human tissue-type plasminogen activator with the use of monoclonal antibodies. Eur J Biochem 158:173–177, 1986

108. Hotchkiss A, Refino CJ, Leonard CK et al: The influence of carbohydrate structures on the clearance of recombinant tissue-type plasminogen activator. Thromb Haemost 60:255–261, 1990

109. Hoylaerts M, Rijken DC, Lijnen HR, Collen D: Kinetics of the activation of plasminogen by tissue-type plasminogen activator. J Biol Chem 257:2912–2919, 1982

110. Hsia J, Hamilton WP, Kleiman N et al: A comparison between heparin and low-dose aspirin as adjunctive therapy with tissue plasminogen activator for acute myocardial infarction. N Engl J Med 323:143–147, 1990

111. Hull RD, Raskob GE, Rosenbloom D: Heparin for 5 days as compared with 10 days in the initial treatment of proximal venous thrombosis. N Engl J Med 322:260, 1990

112. Husain SS, Gurewich V, Lipinski B: Purification and partial characterization of a single-chain high-molecular-weight form of urokinase (pro-urokinase) and urokinase from human urine. Arch Biochem Biophys 220:31–38, 1983

113. International Joint Efficacy Comparison of Thrombo-

lytics: Randomized, double-blind comparison of reteplase double-bolus administration with streptokinase in acute myocadial infarction (INJECT), a trial to investigate equivalence. Lancet 346:329–336, 1995

114. ISIS-2 (Second International Study of Infarct Survival) Collaborative Group: Randomised trial of intravenous streptokinase, oral aspirin, both, or neither among 17,187 cases of suspected acute myocardial infarction: ISIS-2. Lancet 2:349–360, 1988

115. Johannessen M, Diness V, Pingel K et al: Fibrin affinity and clearance of t-PA deletion and substitution analogues. Thromb Haemost 6:54–59, 1990

116. Jörgensen L, Torvik A: Ischemic cerebrovascular diseases in a autopsy series. Part 1. Prevalence, location and predisposing factors in verified thrombo-embolic occlusions, and their significance in the pathogenesis of cerebral infarction. J Neurol Sci 3:490, 1966

117. Jörgensen L, Torvik A: Ischemic cerebrovascular diseases in a autopsy series. Part 2. Prevalence, location, pathogenesis, and clinical course of cerebral infarcts. J Neurol Sci 3:490, 1966

118. Kentzer EJ, Buko A, Menon G, Sarin VK: Carbohydrate composition and presence of a fucose-protein linkage in recombinant human pro-urokinase. Biochem Biophys Res Commun 171:410–406, 1990

119. Keyt BA, Berleau LT, Nguyen H, Bennett WF: Radioiodination of the active site of tissue plasminogen activator: a method for radiolabeling serine proteases with tyrosylprolylarginyl chloromethyl ketone. Anal Biochem 206: 73–83, 1992

120. Keyt BA, Berleau LT, Nguyen HV et al: Subtle alterations of tissue plasminogen activator yield reduced plasma clearance with fibrinolytic activity: a novel fibrin specific tPA variant with six-fold increased potency. Thromb Haemost 69:992, 1993

121. Keyt BA, Paoni NF, Refino CJ et al: A faster-acting and more potent form of tissue plasminogen activator. Proc Natl Acad Sci USA 91:3670–3674, 1994

122. Kimura S, Aoki N: Cross-linking site in fibrinogen for α_2-antiplasmin. J Biol Chem 261:15591–15595, 1986

123. Kingston IB, Castro MJ, Anderson S: In vitro stimulation of tissue-type plasminogen activator by Alzheimer amyloid beta-peptide analogues. Nature Medicine 1: 138–142, 1995

124. Kissel P, Chehrazi B, Seibert JA, Wagner FC: Digital angiographic quantification of blood flow dynamics in embolic stroke treated with tissue-type plasminogen activator. J Neurosurg 67:399–405, 1987

125. Kohga S, Harvey SR, Weaver RM, Markus G: Localization of plasminogen activators in human colon cancer by immunoperoxidase staining. Cancer Res 45:1787–1796, 1985

126. Kohnert U, Rudolph R, Prinz H et al: Production of a recombinant human tissue plasminogen activator variant (BM 06.022) from *Escherichia coli* using a novel renaturation technology (abstract). Fibrinolysis, suppl. 3, 4:44, 1990

127. Kohnert U, Rudolph R, Verheijen JH et al: Biochemical properties of the kringle 2 and protease domains are maintained in the refolded t-PA deletion variant BM 06.022. Protein Eng 5:93–100, 1992

128. Korninger C, Collen D: Studies on the specific fibrinolytic effect of human extrinsic (tissue-type) plasminogen activator in human blood and in various animal species in vitro. Thromb Haemost 46:561–565, 1981

129. Korninger C, Stassen JM, Collen D: Turnover of human extrinsic (tissue-type) plasminogen activator in rabbits. Thromb Haemost 46:658–661, 1981

130. Kowal RC, Herz J, Goldstein JL et al: Low density lipoprotein receptor-related protein mediates uptake of cholesteryl esters derived from apoprotein E-enriched lipoproteins. Proc Natl Acad Sci USA 86:5810–5814, 1989

131. Krause J: Catabolism of tissue-type plasminogen activator (t-PA), its variants, mutants and hybrids. Fibrinolysis 2:133–142, 1988

132. Krishnamurti C, Keyt B, Maglasang P, Alving BM: PAI-1 resistant t-PA: low doses prevent fibrin deposition in rabbits with increased PAI-1 activity. Blood 87:14–19, 1996

133. Kristensen T, Moestrup SK, Gliemann J et al: Evidence that the newly cloned low density lipoprotein receptor-related protein (LRP) is the α_2-macroglobulin receptor. FEBS Lett 276:151–155, 1990

134. Kuiper J, Otter M, Rijken DC et al: Characterization of the interaction in vivo of tissue-type plasminogen activator with liver cells. J Biol Chem 263:18220–18224, 1988

135. Larsen GR, Hensen K, Blue Y: Variants of human tissue-type plasminogen activator. J Biol Chem 263:1023–1029, 1988

136. Larsen GR, Metzger M, Hensen K et al: Pharmacokinetic and distribution analysis of variant forms of tissue-type plasminogen activator with prolonged clearance in rat. Blood 73:1842–1850, 1989

137. Larsen GR, Timony GA, Horgan PG et al: Protein engineering of novel plasminogen activators with increased thrombolytic potency in rabbits relative to Activase. J Biol Chem 266:8156–8161, 1991

138. Laurent JP, Molinari GF, Oakley JC: Primate model of cerebral hematoma. J Neuropathol Exp Neurol 35:560, 1976

139. Levi M, Biemond BJ, van Zonneveld AJ et al: Inhibition of plasminogen activator inhibitor-1 activity results in promotion of endogenous thrombolysis and inhibition of thrombus extension in models of experimental thrombosis. Circulation 85:305–312, 1992

140. Levin EG, Loskutoff DJ: Cultured bovine endothelial cells produce both urokinase and tissue-type plasminogen activators. J Cell Biol 94:631–636, 1982

141. Lijnen HR, Collen D: Strategies for the improvement of thrombolytic agents. Thromb Haemost 66:88–110, 1991

142. Lijnen HR, Stassen JM, Vanlinthout I et al: Comparative fibrinolytic properties of staphylokinase and streptokinase in animal models of venous thrombosis. Thromb Haemost 66:468–473, 1991

143. Lijnen HR, Van Hoef B, De Cock F, Collen D: The mechanism of plasminogen activation and fibrin dissolution by single chain urokinase-type plasminogen activator in a plasma milieu in vitro. Blood 73:1864–1872, 1989

144. Liu J, Harpel PC, Gurewich V: Fibrin-bound lipoprotein(a) promotes plasminogen binding but inhibits fibrin

145. Liu J, Harpel PC, Pannell R, Gurewich V: Lipoprotein(a), a kinetic study of its influence on fibrin-dependent plasminogen activation by prourokinase or tissue plasminogen activator. Biochemistry 32:9694–9700, 1993

146. Lyden PD, Madden KP, Clark WM et al: Incidence of cerebral hemorrhage after anti-fibrinolytic treatment for embolic stroke in rabbits. Stroke 21:1589–1593, 1990

147. Lyden PD, Zivin JA, Clark WA et al: Tissue plasminogen activator-mediated thrombolysis of cerebral emboli and its effect on hemorrhagic infarction in rabbits. Neurology 39:703–708, 1989

148. Lyden PD, Zivin JA, Soll M et al: Intracerebral hemorrhage after experimental embolic infarction. Anticoagulation Arch Neurol 44:848–850, 1987

149. Madison EL, Goldsmith EJ, Gerard RD et al: Serpin-resistant mutants of human tissue-type plasminogen activator. Nature 339:721–724, 1989

150. Magnani B, for the PAIMS Investigators: Plasminogen Activator Italian Multicenter Study (PAIMS): comparison of intravenous recombinant single-chain human tissue-type plasminogen activator (rt-PA) with intravenous streptokinase in acute myocardial infarction. J Am Coll Cardiol 13:19–26, 1989

151. Markus G, Camiolo SM, Kohga S et al: Plasminogen activator secretion of human tumors in short term organ culture, including a comparison of primary and metastatic colon tumors. Cancer Res 43:5517–5525, 1983

152. Marsh N: pp. 1–254. In: Fibrinolysis. John Wiley & Sons, New York, 1981

153. Martin U, Bader R, Bohm E et al: BM 06.022. A novel recombinant plasminogen activator. Cardiovasc Drug Rev 11:299–311, 1993

154. Martin U, van Mollendorf E, Akpan W et al: Dose-ranging study of the novel recombinant plasminogen activator BM 06.022 in healthy volunteers. Clin Pharmacol Ther 50:429–436, 1991

155. Martin U, van Mollendorf E, Akpan W et al: Pharmacokinetic and hemostatic properties of the recombinant plasminogen activator BM 06.022 in healthy volunteers. Thrombo Haemost 66:569–574, 1991

156. McLean JW, Tomlinson JE, Kuang WJ et al: cDNA sequence of human apolipoprotein is homologous to plasminogen. Nature 330:132–137, 1987

157. Meden P, Overgaard K, Sereghy T, Boysen G: Enhancing the efficacy of thrombolysis by AMPA receptor blockade with NBQX in a rat embolic stroke model. J Neurol Sci 119:209–216, 1993

158. Miles LA, Plow EF: Binding and activation of plasminogen on the platelet surface. J Biol Chem 260:4303–4311, 1985

159. Molinari GF: Clinical relevance of experimental stroke models. pp. 19–33. In Price TR, Nelson E (eds): Cerebrovascular Disease: Eleventh Princeton Conference. Lippincott-Raven, Philadelphia, 1979

160. Mori E, del Zoppo GJ, Chambers JD et al: Inhibition of polymorphonuclear leukocyte adherence suppresses no-reflow after focal cerebral ischemia in baboons. Stroke 23:712–718, 1992

161. Mori E, Yoneda Y, Tabuchi M et al: Intravenous recombinant tissue plasminogen activator in acute carotid artery territory stroke. Neurology 42:976–982, 1992

162. Moroi M, Aoki N: Isolation and characterization of alpha-2-plasmin inhibitor from human plasma. A novel proteinase inhibitor which inhibits activator-induced clot lysis. J Biol Chem 251:5956–5965, 1976

163. Morton PA, Owensby DA, Sobel BE et al: Catabolism of tissue-type plasminogen activator by the human hepatoma cell line HepG2. J Biol Chem 264:7228–7235, 1989

164. Multicenter Acute Stroke Trial—Europe Study Group: Thrombolytic therapy with streptokinase in acute ischemic stroke. N Engl J Med 335:145–150, 1996

165. Multicenter Acute Stroke Trial—Italy (MAST-I) Group: Randomised controlled trial of streptokinase, aspirin, and combination of both in treatment of acute ischaemic stroke. Lancet 346:1509–1514, 1995

166. National Heart Foundation of Australia Coronary Thrombolysis Group: A randomized comparison of oral aspirin/dipyridamole versus intravenous heparin after rTPA for acute myocardial infarction. Circulation suppl. II, 80:11–114, 1989

167. National Institute of Neurological Disorders and Stroke, rt-PA Stroke Study Group: Tissue plasminogen activator for acute ischemic stroke. N Engl J Med 333:1582–1587, 1995

168. Neuhaus KL, Feurer W, Jeep-Tebbe S et al: Improved thrombolysis with a modified dose regimen of recombinant tissue-type plasminogen activator. J Am Coll Cardiol 14:1566–1569, 1989

169. Neuhaus KL, Von Essen R, Tebbe U et al: Improved thrombolysis in acute myocardial infarction with front-loaded administration of alteplase: results of the rt-PA-APSAC patency study (TAPS). J Am Coll Cardiol 19:885–891, 1992

170. Ny T, Elgh F, Lund B: The structure of the human tissue-type plasminogen activator gene: correlation of intron and exon structures to functional and structural domains. Proc Natl Acad Sci USA 81:5355–5359, 1984

171. Nykaer A, Petersen CM, Møller B et al: Purified α_2-macroglobulin receptor/LDL receptor-related protein binds urokinase: plasminogen activator inhibitor type-1 complex. J Biol Chem 267:14542–14546, 1992

172. Ogata N, Ogata Y, Hokamaki J et al: Serial changes of plasminogen activator inhibitor activity in thrombolytic therapy for acute myocardial infarction: comparison between thrombolytic therapies with mutant TPA (lanoteplase-BMS-) and recombinant TPA (alteplase). Circulation, suppl. 8, 94:I89, 1996

173. Orth K, Madison EL, Gething M-J et al: Complexes of tissue-type plasminogen activator and its serpin inhibitor plasminogen activator inhibitor type I are internalized by means of the low density lipoprotein receptor-related protein/α_2-macroglobulin receptor. Proc Natl Acad Sci USA 89:7422–7426, 1992

174. Otter M, Barrett-Bergshoeff MM, Rijken DC: Binding of tissue-type plasminogen activator by the mannose receptor. J Biol Chem 266:13931–13935, 1991

175. Overgaard K: Thrombolytic therapy in experimental embolic stroke. Cerebrovasc Brain Metab Rev 6:257, 1994

176. Overgaard K, Sereghy T, Boysen G et al: A rat model of reproducible cerebral infarction using thrombotic blood clot emboli. J Cereb Blood Flow Metab 12:484–490, 1992

177. Overgaard K, Sereghy T, Boysen G et al: Reduction of infarct volume and mortality by thrombolysis in a rat embolic stroke model. Stroke 23:1167–1174, 1992

178. Overgaard K, Sereghy T, Boysen G et al: Reduction of infarct volume by thrombolysis with rt-PA in an embolic rat stroke model. Scand J Clin Lab Invest 53:383–393, 1993

179. Overgaard K, Sereghy T, Frellsen M et al: Comparison of emboli influences the efficacy of thrombolysis with rt-PA in a rat stroke model. Fibrinolysis 7:141–148, 1993

180. Overgaard K, Sereghy T, Pedersen H, Boysen G: Dose-response of rt-PA and its combination with aspirin in a rat embolus stroke model. Neuroreport 3:925–928, 1992

181. Overgaard K, Sereghy T, Pedersen H, Boysen G: Neuroprotection with NBQX and thrombolysis with rt-PA in rat embolic stroke. Neurol Res 15:344–349, 1993

182. Paoni NF, Keyt BA, Refino CJ et al: A slow clearing, fibrin-specific, PAI-1 resistant variant of t-PA (T103N, KHRR296–299AAAA). Thromb Haemost 70:307–312, 1993

183. Paoni NF, Steinmetz HG, Gillett N et al: An experimental model of intracranial hemorrhage during thrombolytic therapy with t-PA. Thromb Haemost 75:820–826, 1996

184. Parkkinen J, Raulo E, Merenmies J et al: Amphoterin, the 30 kDa protein in a family of HMF1-type polypeptides, enhanced expression in transformed cells, leading edge localization, and interactions with plasminogen activation. J Biol Chem 268:19726–19738, 1993

185. Passamani E, Hodges M, Herman M: The thrombolysis in myocardial infarction (TIMI) phase II pilot study: tissue plasminogen activator followed by percutaneous transluminal coronary angioplasty. J Am Coll Cardiol 10:51B–64B, 1987

186. Patthy L: Evolution of the proteases of blood coagulation and fibrinolysis by assembly from modules. Cell 41:657–663, 1985

187. Pennica D, Holmes WE, Kohr WJ et al: Cloning and expression of human tissue-type plasminogen activator cDNA in *E. coli*. Nature 301:214–221, 1983

188. Phillips DA, Fisher M, Smith TW et al: The effects of a new tissue plasminogen activator analogue, Fb-Fb-CF, on cerebral reperfusion in a rabbit embolic stroke model. Ann Neurol 25:281–285, 1989

189. Ploug M, Ronne, Behrendt N, Jensen AL et al: Cellular receptor for urokinase plasminogen activator. Carboxyl-terminal processing and membrane anchoring by glycosyl-phosphatidylinositol. J Biol Chem 266:1926–1933, 1991

190. Plow EF, Fele J, Miles LA: Cellular regulation of fibrinolysis. Thromb Haemost 66:32–36, 1991

191. Pohl G, Kenne L, Nilsson B, Einarsson M: Isolation and characterization of three different carbohydrate chains from melanoma tissue plasminogen activator. Eur J Biochem 170:69–75, 1987

192. Potter van Loon BJ, Rijken DC, Brommer EJP, van der Maas APC: The amount of plasminogen, t-PA and PAI-

1 in human thrombi and the relation to ex-vivo lysibility. Thromb Haemost 67:101–105, 1992

193. Rabiner SF, Goldfine JD, Hart A et al: Radioimmunoassay of human plasminogen and plasmin. J Lab Clin Med 74:265–274, 1969

194. Raichle MM: The pathophysiology of brain ischemia. Ann Neurol 13:2–10, 1993

195. Rånby M: Studies on the kinetics of plasminogen activation by tissue plasminogen activator. Biochim Biophys Acta 704:461–469, 1982

196. Rånby M, Bergsdorf N, Pohl G, Wallen P: Isolation of two variants of native one-chain tissue plasminogen activator. FEBS Lett 146:289–292, 1984

197. Rao KA, Pratt C, Berke A et al: Thrombolysis in myocardial infarction trial (TIMI)-phase I: hemorrhagic manifestations, complications, and changes in plasma fibrinogen and the fibrinolytic system in patients treated with recombinant tissue plasminogen activator and streptokinase. J Am Coll Cardiol 11:1, 1988

198. Redlitz A, Plow EF: Receptors for plasminogen and t-PA, an update. Baillieres Clin Haematol 8:313–327, 1995

199. Refino CJ, Keyt BA, Paoni NF et al: A variant of tissue plasminogen activator (T103N, N117Q, KHRR296-299AAAA) with a decreased plasma clearance rate is substantially more potent than Activase rt-PA in a rabbit thrombolysis model. Thromb Haemost 69:841, 1993

200. Refino CJ, Paoni NF, Keyt BA et al: A variant of tPA (T103N, KHRR296-299AAAA) that, by bolus, has increased potency and decreased systemic activation of plasminogen. Thromb Haemost 70:313–319, 1993

201. Rijken DC, Groenveld E: Isolation and functional characterization of the heavy and light chains of human tissue-type plasminogen activator. J Biol Chem 261:3098–3102, 1986

202. Rijken DC, Hoylaerts M, Collen D: Fibrinolytic properties of one-chain and two-chain human extrinsic (tissue-type) plasminogen activator. J Biol Chem 257:2920–2925, 1982

203. Rijken DC, Juhan-Vague I, De Cock F, Collen D: Measurement of human tissue-type plasminogen activator by a two-site immunoradiometric assay. J Lab Clin Med 101:274–284, 1983

204. Robbins KC, Bernabe LA, Summaria L: The primary structure of human plasminogen. The NH-terminal sequence of human plasminogen and the S-carboxymethyl heavy (A) chain and light (B) chain derivates of plasmin. J Biol Chem 247:6757–6762, 1967

205. Roldan AL, Cubellis MV, Masucci MT et al: Cloning and expression of the receptor for human urokinase plasminogen activator, a central molecule in cell surface, plasmin dependent proteolysis. EMBO J 9:467–474, 1990

206. Russell D, Madden KP, Clark WM, Zivin JA: Tissue plasminogen activator cerebrovascular thrombolysis in rabbits is dependent on the rate and route of administration. Stroke 23:388–393, 1992

207. Saksela O, Rijken DB: Cell-associated plasminogen activation: regulation and physiological functions. Annu Rev Cell Biol 4:93–126, 1988

208. Saku Y, Choki J, Waki et al: Hemorrhagic infarct induced by arterial hypertension in cat brain following middle cerebral artery occlusion. Stroke 21:589, 1990

209. Sakurama T, Kitamura R, Kaneko M: Tissue-type plasminogen activator improves neurological functions in a rat model of thromboembolic stroke. Stroke 25:451–456, 1994

210. Sangrar W, Bajzar L, Nesheim ME, Koschinsky ML: Anti-fibrinolytic effect of recombinant apolipoprotein(a) in vitro is primarily due to attenuation of tPA-mediated glu-plasminogen activation. Biochemistry 34:5151–5157, 1995

211. Schlott B, Harmann M, Gührs KH et al: High yield production and purification of recombinant staphylokinase for thrombolytic therapy. Biotechnology 12:185–189, 1994

212. Schneiderman J, Loskutoff DJ: Plasminogen activator inhibitors. Trends Cardiovasc Med 1:99–102, 1991

213. Sehl LC, Nguyen HV, Berleau LT et al: Locating the unpaired cysteine of tissue-type plasminogen activator. Protein Eng 9:283–290, 1996

214. Sereghy T, Overgaard K, Boysen G: Neuroprotection by excitatory amino acid antagonist augments the benefit of thrombolysis in embolic stroke in rats. Stroke 24:1702–1708, 1993

215. Shatos MA, Doherty JM, Penar PL, Sobel BE: Suppression of plasminogen activator inhibitor-1 release from human cerebral endothelium by plasminogen activators, a factor potentially predisposing to intracranial bleeding. Circulation 94:636–642, 1996

216. Sheenan FH, Braunwald E, Canner P et al: The effect of intravenous thrombolytic therapy on left ventricular function: a report on tissue-type plasminogen activator and streptokinase from the Thrombolysis in Myocardial Infarction (TIMI Phase I) trial. Circulation 75:817–829, 1987

217. Sherry S: Streptokinase pharmacology and its application to acute myocardial infarction. Vasc Med 1:64–76, 1983

218. Silverstein RL, Nachman RL, Leung LLK, Harpel PC: Activation of immobilized plasminogen by tissue activator. J Biol Chem 260:10346–10352, 1985

219. Slivka A, Pulsinelli W: Hemorrhagic complications of thrombolytic therapy in experimental stroke. Stroke 18:1148–1156, 1987

220. Sloan MA, Brott TG, del Zoppo GJ: Thrombolysis and stroke. pp. 361–380. In Julian DG, Kubler W, Norris RM et al (eds): Thrombolysis in Cardiovascular Disease. Marcel Dekker, New York, 1989

221. Smalling RW, Bode C, Kalbfleisch J et al: More rapid, complete and stable coronary thrombolysis with bolus administration of Reteplase compared with Alteplase infusion in acute myocardial infarction. Circulation 91:2725–2732, 1995

222. Sobel BE, Nachowiak DA, Fry ETA et al: Paradoxical attenuation of fibrinolysis attributable to "plasminogen steal" and its implications for coronary thrombolysis. Coron Artery Dis 1:111–119, 1990

223. Sobel BE, Sarnoff SJ, Nachowiak BA: Augmented and sustained plasma concentrations after intramuscular injections of molecular variants and deglycosylated forms of tissue-type plasminogen activator. Circulation 81:1362–1373, 1990

224. Spellman MW, Basa LJ, Leonard CK et al: Carbohydrate structures of human tissue plasminogen activator expressed in Chinese hamster ovary cells. J Biol Chem 264:14100–14111, 1989

225. Spetzler RF, Selman WR, Weinstein P et al: Chronic reversible cerebral ischemia: evaluation of a new baboon model. Neurosurg 7:257–261, 1980

226. Stack S, Gonzalez-Gronow M, Pizzo SV: Regulation of plasminogen activation by components of the extracellular matrix. Biochemistry 29:4966–4970, 1990

227. Strickland DK, Ashcom JD, Williams S et al: Sequence identity between the α_2-macroglobulin receptor and low density lipoprotein receptor-related protein suggests that this molecule is a multi-functional receptor. J Biol Chem 265:17401–17404, 1990

228. Stump DC, Lijnen HR, Collen D: Purification and characterization of a novel low molecular weight form of single-chain urokinase-type plasminogen activator. J Biol Chem 261:17120–17126, 1986

229. Sundt TM Jr, Grant WC, Garcia JH: Restoration of middle cerebral artery flow in experimental infarction. J Neurosurg 31:311–321, 1969

230. Sussman BJ, Fitch T: Thrombolysis with fibrinolysin in cerebral arterial occlusion. JAMA 167:1705–1709, 1958

231. Tanswell P, Seifried E, Su PCAF et al: Pharmacokinetics and systemic effects of tissue-type plasminogen activator in normal subjects. Clin Pharmacol Ther 46:155–162, 1989

232. Thomas GR, Thibodeaux H, Errett CJ et al: A long-half-life and fibrin-specific form of tissue plasminogen activator in rabbit models of embolic stroke and peripheral bleeding. Stroke 25:2072–2079, 1994

233. Thomas GR, Thibodeaux H, Errett CJ et al: Intravenous aspirin causes a paradoxical attenuation of cerebrovascular thrombolysis. Stroke 26:1039–1046, 1995

234. Thomas GR, Thibodeaux H, Errett CJ et al: Limiting systemic plasminogenolysis reduces the bleeding potential for tissue-type plasminogen activators but not for streptokinase. Thromb Haemost 75:915–920, 1996

235. Thomas GR, Thibodeaux H, Bennett WF et al: Optimized thrombolysis of cerebral clots with tissue-type plasminogen activator in a rabbit model of embolic stroke. J Pharmacol Exp Ther 264:67–73, 1993

236. Thorsen S: The mechanism of plasminogen activation and the variability of the fibrin effector during tissue-type plasminogen activator-mediated fibrinolysis. Ann NY Acad Sci 667:52–63, 1992

237. Tillet WS, Garner RL: The fibrinolytic activity of hemolytic streptococci. J Exp Med 58:485–502, 1933

238. Topol EJ, George BS, Kereiakes DJ et al: A randomized controlled trial of intravenous tissue plasminogen activator and early intravenous heparin in acute myocardial infarction. Circulation 79:281–286, 1989

239. Turpie AGG, Robinson JG, Doyle DJ et al: Comparison of high-dose with low-dose subcutaneous heparin to prevent left ventricular mural thrombosis in patients with acute transmural anterior myocardial infarction. N Engl J Med 320:352, 1989

240. Umemura K, Wada K, Uematsu T, Nakashima M: Evaluation of the combination of a tissue-type plasminogen activator, SUN9216, and a thromboxane A_2 receptor an-tagonist, vapiprost, in a rat middle cerebral artery thrombus model. Stroke 24:1077–1082, 1993

241. van Zonneveld AJ, Veerman H, Pannekoek HJ: Autonomous functions of structural domains on human tissue-type plasminogen activator. Proc Natl Acad Sci USA 83:4670–4674, 1986

242. van Zonneveld AJ, Veerman H, Pannekoek H: On the interaction of the finger and the kringle-2 domain of tissue-type plasminogen activator with fibrin. J Biol Chem 261:14214–14218, 1986

243. Verheijen JH, Caspers MPM, Chang GTG et al: Involvement of finger domain and kringle 2 domain of tissue-type plasminogen activator in fibrin binding and stimulation of activity of fibrin. EMBO J, 5:3525–3530, 1986

244. Verstraete M, Bernard R, Bory M et al: Randomised trial of intravenous recombinant tissue-type plasminogen activator versus intravenous streptokinase in acute myocardial infarction. Lancet 1:842, 1985

245. von Kummer R, Hacke W: Safety and efficacy of intravenous tissue plasminogen activator and heparin in acute middle cerebral artery stroke. Stroke 23:646–652, 1992

246. Wagner OF, de Vries C, Hohmann C et al: Interaction between plasminogen activator inhibitor 1 (PAI-1) bound to fibrin and either tissue-type plasminogen (t-PA) or urokinase-type plasminogen activator (u-PA). J Clin Invest 84:647–655, 1989

247. Wallen P: Biochemistry of plasminogen. pp. 1–24. In Kline DL, Reddy KNN (eds): Fibrinolysis. CRC Press, Boca Raton, 1981

248. Warshawsky I, Bu G, Schwartz AL: 39 kD protein inhibits tissue-type plasminogen activator clearance in vivo. J Clin Invest 92:937–944, 1993

249. Webster MWI, Chesebro JH, Mruk JS: Antithrombotic therapy during and after thrombolysis for acute myocardial infarction. Coron Artery Dis 1:190–198, 1990

250. White HD, Rivers JT, Norris RM et al: Is rt-PA or streptokinase superior for preservation of left ventricular function after myocardial infarction? (abstract). Circulation, suppl. II, 78:II–303, 1988

251. Williams JRB: The fibrinolytic activity of urine. Br J Exp Pathol 32:530–536, 1951

252. Willnow TE, Goldstein JL, Orth K et al: Low density receptor-related protein and gp330 bind similar ligands, including plasminogen activator-inhibitor complexes and lactoferrin, an inhibitor of chylomicron remnant clearance. J Biol Chem 267:26172–26180, 1992

253. Wiman B, Collen D: Molecular mechanism of physiological fibrinolysis. Nature 272:549–550, 1978

254. Wun TC, Schleuning WD, Reich E: Isolation and characterization of urokinase from human plasma. J Biol Chem 257:3276–3283, 1982

255. Yamaguchi T, Hayakawa T, Kiuchi H, the Japanese Thrombolysis in Stroke Group: Intravenous tissue plasminogen activator ameliorates the outcome of hyperacute embolic stroke. Cerebrovasc Dis 3:269, 1993

256. Yatsu FM, Alam R, Alam S, Bui G: Recombinant tissue plasminogen activator and mutant rt-PA binding kinetics and cytotoxicity on brain endothelial cell—relevance to brain hemorrhage. pp. 315–322. In Yamaguchi T, Mori E, Minematsu K, del Zoppo GJ (eds): Thrombolytic

Therapy in Acute Ischemic Stroke. Vol. 3. Springer-Verlag, Tokyo, 1995

257. Zeumer H, Freitag HJ, Zanella F et al: Local intra-arterial fibrinolytic therapy in patients with stroke: urokinase versus recombinant tissue plasminogen activator (rt-PA). Neuroradiology 35:159–162, 1993

258. Zhang ZG, Chopp M, Tang WX et al: Post-ischemic treatment (2–4 h) with anti-CD11b and anti-CD-18 monoclonal antibodies are neuroprotective after transient (2h) focal cerebral ischemia in the rat. Brain Res 698:79–85, 1995

259. Zimmerman R, Thiessen M, Mörl H, Weckesser G: The paradoxical thrombogenic effects of aspirin in experimental thrombosis. Thromb Res 16:843–846, 1979

260. Zivin JA, Fisher M, DeGirolami U et al: Tissue plasminogen activator reduces neurological damage after cerebral embolism. Science 230:1289–1292, 1985

261. Zivin JA, Lyden PD, DeGirolami U et al: Tissue plasminogen activator reduction of neurological damage after experimental embolic stroke. Arch Neurol 45:387–391, 1988

SECTION II:

Diagnostic Studies for Stroke

J. P. MOHR

The chapters in this section cover those tests in common use for the detection of stroke, with the added attempt to assess the severity and predict the outcome. An overview of their use is presented, including some techniques currently less commonly used. Recent advances in the application of diagnosis algorithms are reflected in the first chapter.

The authors of the individual chapters have attempted to provide succinct descriptions of the individual technologies, not as instruction manuals but to provide insight into their scope and the basis for their selection in clinical management. As in prior editions, the main emphasis is on the findings in acute stroke. Illustrations of brain images in acute stroke are also found throughout the book, which is one reason this section is not more crowded with images.

Further changes in content from prior editions reflect the impact of rapidly developing technologies. Digital venous angiography has all but vanished from the scene, and magnetic resonance angiography and computed tomographic angiography are dominating the field. Magnetic resonance imaging, with its constantly expanding scope and reduction in imaging times, has pushed ahead of computed tomography as a preferred technology, although the most modern devices are not available everywhere. Position emission tomography and single-photon tomography continue to hold their place in centers so equipped. Doppler ultrasonography is now a major technique in the most modern centers, not just for its physiologic measurements, which supplement imaging, but also as a technique that can easily be brought to the bedside.

CHAPTER 10

Overview of Laboratory Studies

J. P. MOHR

GEOFFREY DONNAN

Acute Stroke

Faced with an acute stroke, the physician must determine the cause, estimate the severity, consider the possibility of progression or recurrence, and seek ways of stabilizing or reversing it. Investigations should be designed to assist clinicians in subcategorizing patients at three specific levels: (1) separating strokes from nonstrokes such as cerebral tumors and subdural hematoma; (2) distinguishing hemorrhage from infarction; and (3) identifying specific pathophysiological subtypes of cerebral infarction.[14] Because the possibility of worsening or recurrence is paramount, speedy efforts should be made to arrive at a diagnosis of stroke mechanism using this approach. The ideal test should be inexpensive, noninvasive, accessible, accurate, and informative. If investigations are used in a logical sequence and are related to the clinical syndrome, unnecessary tests can be avoided and more cost-effective approaches adopted. An example of a suggested sequence of investigations, with these points taken into consideration, is given in Table 10-1.[14]

BRAIN IMAGING

In most hospitals the first testing step is an attempt to image the injured site by computed tomography (CT) or magnetic resonance imaging (MRI).[29,41] If neither is available, estimates of risk factor analysis and clinical assessments of the syndrome help greatly but cannot substitute for brain imaging. Rapidly acquired images with spiral CT (seconds only) is now available in many centers.

The initial scan should separate hemorrhage from ischemia or infarction. For the CT scan, high-density signal attenuation (about 80 HU) points to hemorrhage and low density to ischemia; the reverse is the case for MRI scanning, using the most frequent method, long T_2 sequence. In CT scanning,

the high-density abnormality from parenchymatous hemorrhage is usually rather circumscribed in the acute stage and gradually loses its density over 1 week in the smaller hemorrhages, persisting as long as months for the larger or more intense hemorrhage. Infarction followed by hemorrhagic transformation is more easily recognized when it is confined to the cerebral surface,[4] but it may mimic the findings of hematoma, making a certain differential diagnosis difficult.[28] One exception, a finding that seems specific for hemorrhage, is the pooling of blood found in some lobar hemorrhages.[69] Although hemorrhagic infarction is uncommon in the first hours after stroke, no certain rule can be claimed. Hemorrhagic infarction can be inferred when the lesion lies in the territory of a single surface branch or is limited to the cortex in ribbon-like fashion, but even these findings have been mimicked in lobar hemorrhage. MR scanning shows the same uniform density as does CT for hematomas but suffers the same problem as CT in failing to separate dense hemorrhagic infarction from hematoma in all cases. MRI is even more sensitive than CT in showing minor examples of hemorrhagic infarction. In some instances, autopsy-documented hemorrhagic infarction has appeared isodense or even hypodense on CT scan and has been seen as scattered flecks of very low signal peppered through the infarct site.

On CT scan, infarction appearing as a low-density focus occurs as early as 3 hours, but more often does not make an appearance before 6 hours.[24] After 12 hours, almost one-half the cases are positive,[45] and certainly after 48 hours,[62] reaching a plateau within 3 days in more than 60% of cases. Recently completed studies suggest that both CT and MRI are comparable for detecting the lesion in the earliest hours, and neither have much success before about 3 to 4 hours from onset.[45] On CT, the low-density abnormality is seen early more often with embolic infarction, when the infarcts have more complete tissue necrosis and edema, and is seen later with perfusion failure from thrombosis of large arteries, when the necrosis may be more patchy and edema less obvious.[56]

In the cerebrum, the topography of the CT or MRI abnor-

Table 10.1 Investigation of TIA and Stroke

| Investigation Sequence | Clinical Presentation | | | | Reason for Investigation |
| | TIA or Minor Stroke | | | Severe Stroke | |
	Lacunar	Hemispheric	Brain Stem		
CT at presentation (not enhanced)[a]	Yes	Yes	Yes	Yes	Distinguish hemorrhage from infarction, tumor, subdural hematoma
Ultrasound scan of carotid arteries, MRI/A, or both	No[b]	Yes if good recovery	No[b]	No	Assess patency of carotid vessels
Echocardiography	No	Yes if carotid ultrasound/MRA normal	Yes if clinical evidence of cardiac disease	No	Cardiac source of embolism
Intra-arterial digital subtraction angiography	No	Yes if ultrasound/MRA shows significant stenosis[d]	Usually no[c]	No	More precise evaluation of extracranial and intracranial vessels
Repeat CT at day 7–10 (not enhanced) or MRI even earlier	Yes if early CT normal	Yes if early CT normal	Yes if early CT normal	Yes if early CT normal	Topography for infarct mechanism and prognosis

Abbreviations: CT, computed tomography; MRI, magnetic resonance imaging; MRA, magnetic resonance angiography; TIA, transient ischemic attack.

[a] *Standard investigations may also be arranged at this time (see text).*

[b] *May do as risk factor assessment or MRA to detect basilar stenosis in brain stem ischemia.*

[c] *Sometimes if patient is under 55 years or events are repeated.*

[d] *Definition may vary from center to center, but usually >50% stenosis or evidence of ulceration, or both.*

(Modified from Donnan,[14] with permission.)

mality may assist in differentiating distal infarction due to larger artery thrombosis from infarction attributed to embolism: the former is higher over the convexity and usually spares the sylvian region, whereas the latter conforms more to the territory supplied by one or more cerebral surface branches. Small surface infarcts are not always easily visualized on CT scan, since they may be hidden in the gyral pattern of the convexity; MRI is a better tool. In late CT scanning, some low-density lesions are the late effect of parenchymatous hematoma, a diagnosis more easily made by MRI, in which the residual methemoglobin leaves a permanent signal change. A high-density mass in the stem of the middle cerebral artery strongly suggests embolism, but this occurs infrequently.[55,68]

MR scanning offers a clear advantage over CT for imaging flowing blood, which appears black on the MR image, allowing a diagnosis with a high degree of accuracy.[49] This physiologic effect allows the diagnosis of arteriovenous malformation in ways difficult for CT scan, which relies on hemorrhage, calcification, or contrast enhancement to suggest the diagnosis even though it is positive in up to 80% of cases.[33] MRI has also become the tool of choice for the demonstration of cavernous angiomas, which have a low-signal center and a high-signal rim, commonly called a tiger eye. These small angiographically occult lesions may cause brain hemorrhage. MRI may also demonstrate the thrombosed dome of a recently ruptured aneurysm, a difficult imaging feat rarely achieved by CT scan.

Both CT and MRI can document deep infarcts,[58] with MRI showing smaller lesions than those seen by CT, especially in the basal ganglia and thalamus.[43] MRI is preferred over CT for the smaller infarcts deep in the brain and for those in the brain stem.[55] However, the mere imaging of these smaller lesions does not elucidate the mechanism—thrombotic or embolic.[44] When a core of very low signal is seen on MRI, the uncommon deep lesions from old hemorrhage can be differentiated from those of infarction. Coexisting surface infarcts often confound attempts to attribute aphasiologic abnormalities to deep infarcts seen on CT scan.[8,54,64,66] Many of the larger deep infarcts are not due to microatheroma in the lenticulostriates but have had an associated cerebral surface component that reflects their embolic origin. No findings on CT or MRI reliably separate a deep lesion due to thrombosis of a small feeding artery from one occluded by embolism.

DUPLEX AND TRANSCRANIAL DOPPLER

In experienced hands, the duplex and transcranial Doppler methods may provide useful information within minutes, adding to the assessment of acute stroke.[10,63] In a setting of occlusion, in the early hours after stroke, before brain imaging can demonstrate the changes of infarction, duplex Doppler may disclose high-grade stenosis of a carotid or vertebral artery. Transcranial Doppler may infer extracranial carotid occlusion[27] or high-grade stenosis by a collateral across the circle of Willis to the affected side, inferred by reversal of flow in the ipsilateral anterior cerebral, or by blunted wave forms in the cerebral vessels ipsilateral to a hemodynamically significant lesion.[61]

Intracranial disease may also be documented by stenosis of the basilar or a major cerebral artery. When the middle cerebral velocity signal is missing ipsilateral to symptomatic hemispheral dysfunction, a good correlation has been found for angiographic evidence of occlusion.[31] Proof of occlusion of a major cerebral artery is difficult to demonstrate directly, but increased velocity in an adjacent cerebral artery may indicate an augmentation flow-bearing collateral.[5] Recanalization has been demonstrated.[47] When the Doppler waveforms indicate greatly reduced resistance to flow, an arteriovenous shunt may be suspected, helping to suggest arteriovenous malformation in some instances of brain hemorrhage. Although vasospasm after acute aneurysm rupture is not usually found in the first day or so, transcranial Doppler has proved to be a useful tool for the early detection of vasospasm and a means of following its course.[35]

More recently, transcranial Doppler has been shown to be of potential benefit in detecting embolic (high-intensity) signals in the middle cerebral and carotid arteries, but the practical uses of this information are still being determined. Specifically, it remains to be shown whether these signals translate into increased stroke risk in various clinical settings such as symptomatic or asymptomatic carotid stenosis.[57] If this does prove to be the case, the technique will be an extremely useful one.

ECHOCARDIOGRAPHY

Transesophageal echocardiography has recently been used increasingly to identify cardiac or aortic arch sources of embolism not previously realized and is superior to transthoracic echocardiography in this ability.[13] While the procedure is modestly invasive in that it usually requires the patient to be sedated during the passage of the probe down the esophagus, the information provided may help to stratify subsequent stroke risk and possibly aid in therapy. A major issue is now the finding that aortic arch atheroma may be a more common cause of ischemic stroke than previously realized, although which form of therapy is most effective is as yet unclear.[1] Using this technique, cardiac causes of emboli have also been detected that were not able to be visualized using transthoracic echocardiography. Of these, left atrial spontaneous echocontrast, a swirling pattern generated by stasis within the atrium, is the most notable and is usually present in association with atrial fibrillation.

LUMBAR PUNCTURE

Long the mainstay of diagnosis, lumbar puncture has been relegated to a minor role when high-quality brain imaging is available. Widespread subarachnoid hemorrhage or local subarachnoid collections can usually be detected by CT scan, and MRI can image most of the larger aneurysms and all the arteriovenous malformations and cavernous angiomas, obviat-

ing the purpose of lumbar puncture, which simply proves the existence of subarachnoid hemorrhage but not the cause. When imaging is not available, lumbar puncture is distinctive for subarachnoid hemorrhage; it usually shows blood and high-protein and xanthochromic fluid in the major syndrome caused by parenchymatous brain hemorrhage but may appear normal in small brain hemorrhage. In this last setting a diagnosis of hemorrhage versus infarction is important; whether or not to treat with anticoagulants must be decided. Therefore in this case, lumbar puncture alone is not sufficient to rule out hemorrhage when the spinal fluid is clear. In the rare instance of arteritis, lumbar puncture may show elevated white cell counts and elevated protein, findings also encountered in large infarcts.

ANGIOGRAPHY

Angiography remains the preferred tool for demonstrating aneurysms and vasospasm, for easily diagnosing arteriovenous malformation, and for separating embolism from large artery thrombosis.[37] Recent evidence suggests that many embolic occlusions are quite transient; forcing a plan for prompt angiography is a diagnosis of occlusion due to embolism is to be confirmed.[11,25] Thrombosis is expected to persist. The search for a source of embolism is a separate issue from documenting the occurrence of brain embolism. In the case of the former, conventional monitoring of arrhythmias, blood cultures, echocardiography, and the like usually takes days. If delayed until the results of these tests are complete, angiography could yield a negative study. *Digital subtraction angiography*, a technique that underwent rapid development in the last decade,[38] is fast being eclipsed in some centers by *magnetic resonance angiography (MRA)*, which has almost matched conventional angiography in estimation of disease at the carotid bifurcation[40] and is rapidly developing the potential to estimate blood flow and other time-based changes.[60] However, MRA tends to overestimate the degree of stenosis when compared with conventional angiography, which may have the effect of falsely including cases recommended for carotid endarterectomy given the current trial evidence for symptomatic disease (70% stenosis or greater).[36] In both digital angiography and MRA, the circle of Willis and the basilar artery, their main branches, and many of the large surface vessels can be imaged well enough to determine if some are occluded.[9] CT angiography is sometimes used to complement other studies, but the extra computer time required to reconstruct the images can be a disadvantage.[17]

Both digital angiography and MRA demonstrate arteriovenous malformations, but neither method is as yet the equal of *cut-film angiography* in demonstrating vasospasm and the widespread stenoses found in arteritis.

STUDIES OF BLOOD FLOW AND METABOLISM

Xenon Computed Tomography and Single-Photon Emission Computed Tomography

Xenon CT blood flow imaging is occasionally used[32] and has now been supplemented by single photon emission CT (SPECT).[22] Both methods demonstrate both local and distant functional effects after stroke, and some authors have shown effects on resting flows remote from the site of infarction. Applied quickly after infarction, the deficit in local flow may be evident before the tissue signal changes appear on CT or MRI, and reasonable sensitivities and specificities for subsequent infarction have been shown.[6] Neither technique separates hemorrhage from infarction. It remains uncertain whether these methods will predict the potential for clinical recovery.[12] A combination of transcranial Doppler and cerebral blood flow has been helpful in tracking the course of vasospasm in subarachnoid hemorrhage.[26]

Positron Emission Tomography

Positron emission tomography scanning has demonstrated its power in documenting the functional metabolic response of the brain to focal infarction, but its availability remains limited.[16] It remains the best method for demonstrating viable tissue in cerebral ischemia,[53,67] the time window for which may be longer than previously realized.[39] It has been able to demonstrate the remote effects of infarctions, some spread over wide areas[30] and some explained as trans-synaptic depression or diaschisis.[2] Tissue cubes, about 10 to 15 mm to a side, are being resolved.[52]

Magnetic Resonance Techniques

More recently, the techniques of diffusion and perfusion-weighted imaging with MRI have been introduced and may provide further insights into the clinical circumstances during which perfusion changes occur in ischemic stroke.[65] (See Chapter 7.)

TRANSIENT ISCHEMIC ATTACKS

Only after the symptoms have faded is a diagnosis of transient ischemic attack (TIA) justified. In the acute symptomatic phase, the approach is that of an acute stroke. Symptoms may fade or entirely disappear, yet brain imaging demonstrates recent ischemic lesions. The old definition of TIA as any neurologic deficit resolving in 24 hours is now out of date. The actual duration of a brief ischemic event is typically measured in minutes, not hours. When symptoms have lasted longer than 1 hour, a higher frequency of brain lesions has been found than when the symptoms have lasted for minutes.

After it is certain that all symptoms have disappeared, investigation of a TIA is directed at underlying disease, which may predict the risk of recurrence in the same or different vascular territory.

By habit and because of a surgical option for therapy, TIAs are often equated with the surgically correctable disease in the neck at the carotid bifurcation. However, TIAs may occur in territories remote from this site. For those affecting the carotid territory, duplex and transcranial Doppler should suffice to demonstrate whether high-grade stenosis or occlusion exists and any indication of the development of some vascular collateral is present. Embolism may account for many transient ischemic attacks, yet some may be explained by distal

insufficiency in the far fields of the middle cerebral artery or in the border zone between the middle and anterior cerebral arteries.[51] This suprasylvian location would be expected to produce a clinical deficit involving the forearm and hand. A high frequency of stereotypic neurologic deficits has been reported in a patient suffering repeated TIAs.[50] Even in single attacks, distal brachial sensorimotor syndromes lead all others in frequency. *Positron emission tomography* and *single-photon emission CT* can determine whether the brain supplied through the stenosis or by collaterals around the stenosis or occlusion suffers from inadequate flow[2] (i.e., *misery perfusion syndrome*),[3] which has been shown to be surgically reversible in some instances. In the even more severe state of distal intracranial internal carotid artery stenosis with abundant collaterals associated with moyamoya disorder, hyperventilation has been shown to precipitate focal symptoms.[59] The demonstration of such an extreme degree of sensitivity of cerebral flow to alterations in PCO_2 suggests that cerebral claudication may even occur.[43]

Angiography, digital subtraction angiography,[18] *CT angiography*,[17] and MRA have all become popular for demonstrating stenosis or occlusion of the carotid. Venous bolus angiography has become less popular because of poor resolution and the high dose of intravenous contrast required.[15] In experienced centers, the combination of Doppler to demonstrate high-grade stenosis and the degree of collateral, and MRA for anatomy may replace all invasive angiography in the evaluation of extracranial occlusive disease. Even though the risks are small, angiographic complications in direct injection studies remain a risk to be avoided when possible.[21] However, conventional angiography is still the tool of choice to show ulceration, a component of carotid disease that may still explain many forms of stroke. When Doppler or MRA fails to indicate high-grade stenosis, digital angiography may not be fully justified.

Asymptomatic Disease

Asymptomatic disease manifests usually by a bruit discovered on routine office evaluation or stenosis on a Doppler done as a screening test.[42] The bruits of carotid stenosis and from radiated heart murmurs are difficult to distinguish clinically. The improvement in Doppler technology has been so great that a bruit is no longer considered a sign of stenosis of the carotid artery but only as an indication for a Doppler study.[19]

Doppler studies of the flow velocities through arteries have been available for years.[70] Some of the devices using Doppler signals display the different velocities encountered along an artery in different colors according to velocity, allowing the clinician to see the stenosis in one color and the normal flow in another. Like spectral analysis, Doppler studies can be useful to follow the course of a stenosis.[48] Although impressive, the information from conventional continuous-wave Doppler analysis adds little to that available from other methods and has its own sources of error.[70] Pulsed-wave, range-gated Doppler techniques have been developed that can scan the lumen from wall to wall in tiny steps.[18] Newer devices that allow color-coded displays permit better characterization of the flow patterns. Despite such improved characterizations, it has not yet become evident that the extra information obtained relates to stroke risk.[23] To date, the rate of progression of the extracranial carotid stenosis, not the specific characteristics of the velocity profiles, has predicted subsequent symptoms. Virtually nothing is known of the prognosis for asymptomatic stenosis of the intracranial vessels.

Brain imaging may demonstrate prior stroke. In roughly 20% of patients with high-grade carotid stenosis, and in a similar number of patients seen for their first symptomatic stroke, CT scan shows evidence of prior brain infarction. Most of the lesions are small and are in brain regions not likely to cause major symptoms, but a small percentage have been as large as a portion of a cerebral lobe, a finding not easily dismissed, although not in any way explained.

Asymptomatic aneurysms, arteriovenous malformations, cavernous angiomas, and dural fistulas have also been reported by brain imaging. Little is known of the prognostic significance of such findings, except for aneurysms: a few studies have indicated a higher risk of hemorrhage from those 8 to 15 mm in size.

References

1. Amarenco P, Cohen A, Tzourio C et al: Atherosclerotic disease of the aortic arch and the risk of ischemic stroke. N Engl J Med 331:1474, 1994
2. Baron JC, Bousser MG, Comar D, Castaigne P: "Crossed cerebellar diaschesis": a remote functional depression secondary to supratentorial infarction of man. J Cereb Blood Flow Metab, suppl. 1, 1:500, 1981
3. Baron JC, Bousser MG, Rey A et al: Reversal of focal "misery-perfusion syndrome" by extra-intracranial arterial bypass in haemodynamic cerebral ischaemia. Stroke 12:454, 1981
4. Brahme FJ: CT diagnosis of cerebrovascular disorders: a review. Comput Tomogr 2:173, 1978
5. Brass LM, Duterte DL, Mohr JP: Anterior cerebral artery velocity changes in disease of the middle cerebral artery stem. Stroke 20:1737, 1989
6. Brass LM, Walovitch RC, Joseph JL et al: The role of single photon emission computed tomography brain imaging with ^{99m}Tc-bicisate in the localization and definition of mechanism of ischemic stroke. J Cereb Blood Flow Metab, suppl. 1, 14:S91–S98, 1994
7. Buonanno FS, Kistler JP, Dewitt LD et al: Proton (^{1}H) nuclear magnetic resonance (NMR) imaging in stroke syndromes. Neurol Clin North Am 1:243, 1983
8. Castaigne P, Lhermitte F, Buge A et al: Paramedian thalamic and midbrain infarcts: clinical and neuropathological study. Ann Neurol 10:127, 1981
9. Cline HE, Lorensen WE, Souza SP et al: 3D surface rendered MR images of the brain and its vasculature. J Comput Assist Tomogr 15:344, 1991
10. Comerota AJ, Cranley JJ, Cook SE: Real-time B-mode carotid imaging in diagnosis of cerebrovascular disease. Surgery 6:718, 1981
11. Delal PM, Shah PM, Aiyar RR: Arteriographic study of cerebral embolism. Lancet 2:358, 1961
12. Demeurisse M, Verhas M, Capon A, Paternot J: Lack of evolution of the cerebral blood flow during clinical recovery of a stroke. Stroke 14:77, 1983
13. Donaldson RM, Emanuel RW, Earl CJ: The role of two-dimensional echocardiography in the detection of potentially embolic intracardiac masses in patients with cerebral ischaemia. J Neurol Neurosurg Psychiatry 44:803, 1981
14. Donnan GA: Investigation of patients with stroke and transient ischaemic attacks. Lancet 339:473, 1992
15. Ducos de Lahitte M, Marc-Vergnes JP, Rascol A et al: Intravenous angiography of the external cerebral arteries. Radiology 137:705, 1980
16. Frackowiak RSJ, Wise RJS: Positron tomography in ischaemic cerebrovascular disease. Neurol Clin North Am 1:183, 1983
17. Frisen L, Kjällman L, Lindberg B, Svendsen P: Detection of extracranial carotid stenosis by computed tomography. Lancet 1:1319, 1979
18. Furlan AJ, Weinstein MA, Little JR, Modic MT: Digital substraction angiography in the evaluation of cerebrovascular disease. Neurol Clin North Am 1:55, 1983
19. Gautier JC, Rosa A, Lhermitte F: Auscultation carotidienne: correlations chez 200 patients avec 332 angiographies. Rev Neurol 131:175, 1975
20. Gross CR, Kase CS, Mohr JP et al: Stroke in South Alabama: incidence and diagnostic features: a population-based study. Stroke 15:249, 1984
21. Hankey GJ, Warlow CP, Sellar RJ: Cerebral angiographic risk in mild cerebrovascular disease. Stroke 21:209, 1990
22. Hanyu H, Arai H, Kobayashi Y et al: Remote effects in cerebral infarction—1231-IMP SPECT study. Kaku Igaku 27:629, 1990
23. Hennerici M, Steinke W, Rautenberg W, Mohr JP: Symptomatic and asymptomatic high-grade carotid stenosis in Doppler color flow imaging. Neurology (NY) 42:131, 1992
24. Inoue Y, Takemoto K, Miyamoto T et al: Sequential computed tomography scans in acute cerebral infarction. Radiology 135:655, 1980
25. Irino T, Tandea M, Minami T: Angiographic manifestations in postrecanalized cerebral infarction. Neurology 27:471, 1977
26. Jakobsen M, Enevoldsen E, Dalager T: Spasms index in subarachnoid haemorrhage: consequences of vasospasm upon cerebral blood flow and oxygen extraction. Acta Neurol Scand 82:311, 1990
27. Kaps M, Damian MS, Teschendorf U, Dorndorf W: Transcranial Doppler ultrasound findings in middle cerebral artery occlusion. Stroke 21:532, 1990
28. Kase CS, Williams JP, Mohr JP: Lobar intracerebral haematomas. Neurology (NY) 32:1146, 1982
29. Kistler JP, Buonanno FS, Dewitt LD et al: Vertebral basilar posterior cerebral territory stroke delineation by proton nuclear magnetic resonance imaging. Stroke 15:417, 1984
30. Kiyosawa M, Bosley TM, Kushner M et al: Middle cerebral artery strokes causing homonymous hemianopia: positron emission tomography. Ann Neurol 28:180, 1990
31. Kushner MJ, Zanette EM, Bastianello S et al: Transcranial Doppler in acute hemispheric brain infarction. Neurology (NY) 41:109, 1990
32. Lassen N, Ingvar DH, Skinhoj E: Brain function and

blood flow: changes in the amount of blood flowing in areas of the human cerebral cortex, reflecting changes in the activity of those areas, are graphically revealed with the aid of radioactive isotope. Sci Am 239:62, 1978

33. Leblanc R, Ethier R, Little JR: Computerized tomography findings in arteriovenous malformations of the brain. J Neurosurg 51:765, 1979

34. Lees RS, Lees AM, Strauss WH: External imaging of human atherosclerosis. J Nucl Med 24:154, 1983

35. Lennihan L, Petty GW, Mohr JP et al: Transcranial Doppler detection of anterior cerebral artery vasospasm. Stroke 20:151, 1989

36. Levi CR, Donnan GA, Fitt G: Magnetic resonance angiography. Cerebrovasc Dis (in press)

37. Liliequist B, Lindqvist M, Valdimarsson E: Computed tomography and subarachnoid haemorrhage. Neuroradiology 14:21, 1977

38. Ludwig JW, Verhoeven LHJ, Engels PHC: Digital video subtraction angiography (DVSA) equipment: angiographic technique in comparison with conventional angiography in different vascular areas. Br J Radiol 55:54, 1982

39. Marchal G, Beaudouin V, Rioux P et al: Prolonged persistence of substantial volumes of potentially viable brain tissue after stroke: a correlative PET-CT study with voxel-based data analysis. Stroke 27:599, 1996

40. Mattle HP, Kent KC, Edelman RR et al: Evaluation of the extracranial carotid arteries: correlation of magnetic resonance angiography, duplex ultrasonography, and conventional angiography. J Vasc Surg 13:838, 1991

41. McCullough EC, Baker HL Jr: Nuclear magnetic resonance. Radiol Clin North Am 20:3, 1982

42. Mohr JP: Asymptomatic carotid artery disease. Stroke 13:431, 1982

43. Mohr JP: Discussion. In Reivich M (ed): Cerebrovascular Disease. Proceedings of the Thirteenth Princeton Conference in Cerebrovascular Disease. Lippincott-Raven, Philadelphia, 1983

44. Mohr JP: Lacunes. Neurol Clin North Am 1:201, 1983

45. Mohr JP, Biller J, Hilal SK et al: MR vs CT imaging in acute stroke: Stroke 26:807, 1995

46. Mohr JP, Caplan LR, Melski JW et al: The Harvard Cooperative Stroke Registry: a prospective registry of cases hospitalized with stroke. Neurology (NY) 28:754, 1978

47. Mohr JP, Duterte DI, Oliveira VR et al: Recanalization of acute middle cerebral artery occlusion. Neurology (NY) 38:215, 1988

48. Norrving B, Nilsson B, Olsson J: Progression of carotid disease after endarterectomy: a Doppler ultrasound study. Ann Neurol 12:548, 1982

49. Nussel F, Wegmuller H, Huber P: Comparison of magnetic resonance angiography, magnetic resonance imaging and conventional angiography in cerebral arteriovenous malformation. Neuroradiology 33:56, 1991

50. Pessin MS, Duncan GW, Mohr JP, Poskanzer DC: Carotid artery territory transient ischaemic attacks. N Engl J Med 296:358, 1977

51. Pessin MS, Hinton RC, Davis KR et al: Mechanisms of acute carotid stroke: a clinicoangiographic study. Ann Neurol 6:245, 1979

52. Phelps ME, Mazziotta JC, Kuhl DE et al: Tomographic mapping of human cerebral metabolism: visual stimulation and deprivation. Neurology (NY) 31:517, 1981

53. Powers WJ, Martin ERW, Herscovitch P et al: Extracranial-intracranial bypass surgery: hemodynamic and metabolic effects. Neurology (NY) 34:1168, 1984

54. Rascol A, Clanet M, Manelfe: Pure motor hemiplegia: CT study of 30 cases. Stroke 13:11, 1982

55. Savoiardo M, Bracchi M, Passerini A, Visciani A: The vascular territories in the cerebellum and brainstem: CT and MR study. AJNR 8:199, 1987

56. Schuknecht B, Ratzka M, Hofmann E: The "dense artery sign"—major cerebral artery thromboembolism demonstrated by computed tomography. Neuroradiology 32:98, 1990

57. Siebler M, Kleinschmidt A, Sitzer M et al: Cerebral microembolism in symptomatic and asymptomatic high-grade internal carotid artery stenosis. Neurology, 44:615, 1994

58. Sipponen JT, Kaste M, Sepponen RE et al: Nuclear magnetic resonance imaging in reversible cerebral ischaemia. Lancet 1:294, 1983

59. Suzuki J, Kodama N. Moyamoya disease—a review. Stroke 14:104, 1983

60. Tarnawski M, Padayachee S, Graves MJ et al: Measurement of time-averaged flow in the middle cerebral artery by magnetic resonance imaging. Br J Radiol 64:178, 1991

61. Tatemichi TK, Chamorro A, Petty GW et al: Hemodynamic role of ophthalmic artery collateral in internal carotid artery occlusion. Neurology (NY) 40:461, 1990

62. Tatemichi TK, Mohr JP, Rubinstein LV et al: CT findings and clinical course in acute stroke: the NINCDS stroke data bank. Presented at the Tenth International Joint Conference on Stroke and Cerebral Circulation, New Orleans, LA, February 22, 1985

63. Tatemichi TK, Oropeza LA, Saco RL et al: Doppler diagnosis of vertebral artery occlusion: role of runoff into the posterior inferior cerebellar artery. Ann Neurol 26:1;58, 1989

64. Wallesch CW, Kornhuber HH, Kunz T, Brunner RJ: Neuropsychological deficits associated with small unilateral thalamic lesions. Brain 106:141, 1983

65. Warach S, Dashe JR, Edelman RR: Clinical outcome in ischemic stroke predicted by early diffusion-weighted and perfusion magnetic resonance imaging: preliminary analysis. J Cereb Blood Flow Metab 16:53, 1996

66. Weaver RG Jr, Howard G, McKinney WM et al: Comparison of Doppler ultrasonography with arteriography of the carotid bifurcation. Stroke 4:402, 1980

67. Yamauchi H, Fukuyama H, Kimura J et al: Hemodynamics in internal carotid artery occlusion examined by positron emission tomography. Stroke 21:1400, 1990

68. Yock DH Jr: CT demonstration of cerebral emboli. J Comput Assist Tomogr 5:190, 1981

69. Zilkha A: Intraparenchymal fluid-blood level: a CT sign of recent intracerebral haemorrhage. J Comput Assist Tomogr 7:301, 1983

70. Zwiebel WJ, Crummy AB: Sources of error in Doppler diagnosis of carotid occlusive disease. AJNR 2:231, 1982

Computed Tomography Scanning

MARIO SAVOIARDO

MARINA GRISOLI

In the first clinical paper devoted to computed tomography (CT) published in 1973 by Ambrose,[3] the author concludes that "in the overall investigation of cerebrovascular disease, computerized transverse axial scanning will, without doubt, come to be an invaluable means of distinguishing between hemorrhage and infarction." The following year, Paxton and Ambrose[115] reported positive CT studies in 66 of 66 intracranial hemorrhages and in 27 of 55 patients with occlusive cerebrovascular disease and observed density changes in the evolution of the infarction.

In the following years, numerous papers dealing with different aspects of cerebrovascular disease clarified most of the CT features that can be encountered in patients with transient ischemic attack (TIA), ischemic or hemorrhagic infarction, and intracranial hemorrhage.[24] About 15 years ago, magnetic resonance imaging (MRI) appeared; it has since integrated with and often substituted for CT in neuroimaging. CT, however, still retains an important role in the diagnosis of cerebrovascular disease. The sum of the knowledge about CT scanning for different aspects of cerebrovascular disease is outlined in this chapter.

Transient Ischemic Attacks

Before CT was available, TIAs were not usually considered to be associated with permanent focal lesions of the brain. However, CT demonstrated that small infarcts may sometimes manifest clinically as TIAs, and pathologic reports also support this view.[9] Even small hematomas or other lesions such as vascular malformations or tumors may rarely be found (Fig. 11.1). If the occasional unexpected pathologic change is excluded, there is much disagreement about the interpretation of findings in TIAs.

In a few instances of TIA, a normal plain CT with postcontrast cortical enhancement, corresponding to capillary blush and early filling veins on angiography, is observed.[20,22,80] This finding is clearly correlated with the preceding TIA; however, postcontrast enhancement may represent a transient phenomenon, but it may also be associated with a small cortical infarct, even if this is hardly demonstrable by CT (Fig. 11.2). Permanent tiny cortical changes may be more easily demonstrated with MRI.

Small infarcts and atrophy are also a fairly frequent observation; in some series, however, they were considered unrelated to the presenting TIA[21]; however, other authors pointed out that, being on the appropriate side, they were related to the TIAs. Perrone et al[117] reported small infarcts, mainly in the basal ganglia, in 34% of their patients with TIAs; they also pointed out that lateralized atrophy, which is a fairly common finding in patients with occlusion or severe stenosis of the homolateral internal carotid artery, was probably due to insufficient vascular supply to that hemisphere.

The importance of a small infarction in determining permanent or transient neurologic symptoms and signs depends on its strategic location. A small infarction far away from crucial areas may even be completely asymptomatic.[4] Therefore when, in a patient with recent TIAs, CT detects a small recent infarct in the appropriate area, the correlation is obvious. Nevertheless, in most of the cases, a clear correlation between age of the infarct and previous TIAs is not possible, and a small infarct in the basal ganglia has to be regarded as a coincidental finding, an expression, however, of the same cerebrovascular disease that also causes TIAs.

In TIAs occurring in the vertebrobasilar system, CT findings are almost always normal[79,117]; only when the TIA presents as transient global amnesia are a significant number of infarcts found in the territory of the left posterior cerebral artery.[85]

In summary, in patients with TIAs, CT demonstrates a significant number of small infarctions only in the carotid system or in the territory of the posterior cerebral arteries, but never, or very rarely, in the posterior fossa. TIAs without infarction certainly exist but should be differentiated from the

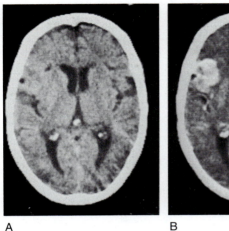 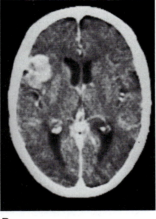

A   B

Figure 11.1 Metastases from unknown primary tumor presenting as TIAs. Patient had repeated, transient episodes of expressive aphasia and/or right hemiparesis for 20 days. (**A**) Plain computed tomography scan only shows minimal compression of left sylvian fissure. (**B**) Postcontrast computed tomography scan shows an enhancing nodule in frontal operculum. A second nodule, not shown, was present in the left motor cortex (left side is on reader's left).

new category suggested by Waxman and Toole[167] of cerebral infarction with transient neurologic signs. CT and other diagnostic tools demonstrate that such cases occur more frequently than previously thought.

In our opinion, it must be borne in mind that TIA is a clinical concept that is perhaps becoming outdated,[31] and that the main role of CT in patients with TIAs is to rule out an unexpected pathologic change. Whether a normal scan or a small infarct is found, this result does not change the investigative approach, which is based on other laboratory and neuroradiologic studies.

Infarction

GENERAL ASPECTS

The possibility of recognizing ischemic cerebral infarction has greatly increased since the early CT studies because of both the higher resolution of currently available CT machines and the knowledge of the density changes of the infarctions in their stages of evolution. Apart from clinical criteria, several CT aspects have to be considered to ascertain that a certain lesion is an infarction: location and distribution of the lesion, density changes and their evolution in serial scans, and modifications of the lesion after intravenous contrast administration.

Location

The infarction within a vascular territory may involve all or part of the territory. One or more territories of the major arteries may be involved; or, on the contrary, the border zones between different vascular territories may be affected. The location of the lesion is, therefore, an important diagnostic element: a lesion straddling different vascular territories is not likely to be an infarction.

The different vascular territories as seen on CT have been studied and have also been correlated with functional areas[14,35,61,133,149,150] (Plate 11.1). In posterior fossa, the vascular territories have also been defined with the help of MRI, which, particularly in the lower part of posterior fossa, is much more useful than CT because of greater contrast sensitivity and lack of bony artifacts[133] (Plate 11.2).

The frequency of infarctions in the areas of the major arterial territories is similar in the series observed in our clinic (the Besta Neurologic Institute) and in various reported series.[17,33,121,132] The middle cerebral artery territory is the most frequently involved (62% in our early series of about 500

Figure 11.2 Small infarcts in a patient with TIA manifested by proximal right arm and leg weakness. (**A**) Plain computed tomography scan, 10 days after TIA, is normal except for cortical atrophy. (**B**) Postcontrast computed tomography scan shows enhancement in the watershed area between left anterior cerebral artery and middle cerebral artery territories. (**C**) Repeat computed tomography scan, 10 months later, shows small cortical infarcts corresponding to the areas of previous enhancement (*arrowheads*). (Left side is on reader's left.)

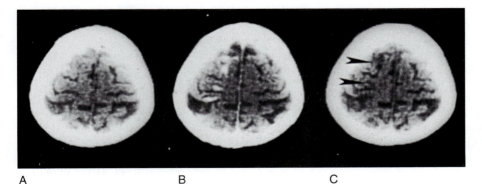

A   B   C

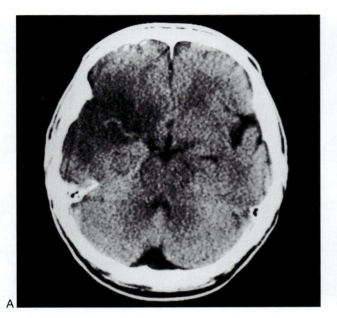 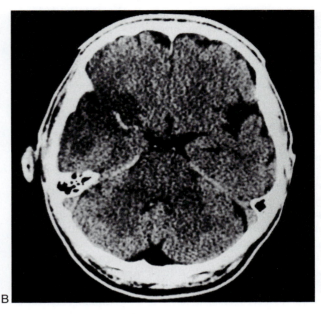

A   B

Figure 11.3 Two-day infarction in right middle cerebral artery distribution. The occluded initial segment of the middle cerebral artery is hyperdense. **(A)** The hyperdense acute thrombus is visible on the 10-mm-thick section. **(B)** The thrombus is better demonstrated in the thin, 3-mm-thick section.

cases), followed by the posterior cerebral artery (14%), and the anterior cerebral artery (5%). Infarcts in the posterior fossa were observed in 5% of our cases, while multiple territories or watershed areas accounted for the remaining 14%.

Localization of an infarct in a certain territory has only a modest value in indicating the occluded or stenotic artery; for this purpose, other studies (ultrasonography, angiography, MR angiography) are necessary. However, occasionally the occluded intracranial vessel can be visualized (see the following section, Density Changes) (Fig. 11.3), and direct or reformatted CT images of the extracranial carotid arteries may be demonstrative[66,69,159] (Fig. 11.4).

Density Changes

The infarcted area appears as a hypodense lesion generally 24 to 48 hours after the stroke, but occasional positive CT scans are observed even 3 hours after onset.[71] The hypodensity is initially mild and poorly defined; in middle cerebral artery infarct, the insular cortex may lose its gray matter density.[161] In proximal occlusion of this artery, slight hypodensity of the lentiform nucleus and loss of definition of its margins may also be visible on CT scans performed within 4 hours after stroke.[19,156] These have been reported as early, subtle signs of middle cerebral artery infarction (Fig. 11.5).

A few large studies have recently been reported. One study comparing CT with MR scanning provided one of the few prospective opportunities to document the evolution of ischemic infarction. Sixty-eight patients were imaged within 4 hours and an additional 12 patients within 24 hours from stroke.[105] Seventy-five cases were due to infarction, 5 to hemorrhage. The median time to first scan was 132 minutes. Although some of the 75 cases with infarction were detected

Figure 11.4 Postcontrast computed tomography scan in a patient with extracranial left internal carotid artery dissection. The patent lumen is hyperdense (*white arrow*), while the subacute intramural hematoma (*black arrows*) is hypodense. The dissection was confirmed by magnetic resonance imaging and angiography.

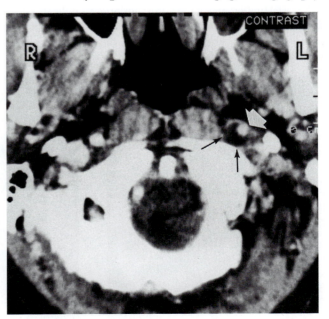

within 1 hour, the fraction of positive first scans approached an asymptote at 2 to 3 hours. Overall, using conventional non-contrast-enhanced CT and the T_1- and T_2-weighted MR techniques available in 1991, neither was superior in the very early detection of infarction. There was a marginally significant correlation between early positive brain imaging and the severity of the stroke. Some patients had initially positive CT or MR scans (or both), but their neurologic examination had returned to normal by 24 hours. After 24 hours, both CT and MR more conspicuously defined the lesion limits than they did at baseline.

Toni et al[157] reported on a consecutive series of 152 patients with first-ever ischemic stroke affecting the cerebral hemispheres who reached the hospital within 5 hours of onset and underwent a first CT scan within 1 hour of arrival. An absence of early hypodensity at first CT proved to be among the independent predictors of early improvement. Patients who showed clinical improvement during the acute course had the highest frequency of small infarcts.

From as early a trial as the American Nimodipine Study[153] to more recent studies of tissue plasminogen activator thrombolysis therapy,[160] a pretreatment scan showing changes consistent with infarction carried a poorer prognosis for response to therapy than did those treated whose scan had not yet become positive.

Within 2 or 3 days the attenuation values become lower, the margins of the lesion become better defined, and the lesion clearly appears to involve both gray and white matter. The best evidence of the lesion in this early phase is, therefore, on the third and fourth days after the stroke. In addition, in this period of edema and necrosis, there is often evidence of mass effect.

Occasionally, the segment of the artery occluded by an embolus or a thrombus may appear hyperdense in early studies.[51,120,174] This sign has been reported particularly in the main trunk of the middle cerebral artery, where it has been observed in up to 50% of the patients with recent infarction in this vessel territory[8,138,154] (Fig. 11.3).

Tomsick et al[155] found a lower initial National Institutes of Health score and a worse 3-month outcome for the 18 patients among 55 studied in a hyperacute trial of intravenous alteplase thrombolytic therapy.

The edema and mass effect of the infarction gradually subside, and the hypodensity becomes less evident in the following days. The hypodensity may almost completely disappear and the infarcted area may become nearly indistinguishable from the normal surrounding brain.

This phenomenon occurs in the second or third week and corresponds to the period in which invasion of macrophages and proliferation of capillaries are observed on pathologic specimens. The rate of this occurrence varies in different series. On scans performed 10 days after stroke, Skriver and Olsen[143] found disappearance of hypodensity in 54% of their 50 cases. Becker et al[11] named this phenomenon the "fogging effect," observing it at some time in all the cases of their smaller series examined with six consecutive CT scans within 42 days after stroke. However, with the high-resolution CT scans now available, some mottling of the infarcted area is usually recognizable.

In large infarcts, the fogging effect is usually partial and

Figure 11.5 Infarction in right middle cerebral artery distribution in a 2-year-old girl. **(A)** The first computed tomography scan, performed 5 hours after stroke, shows slight hypodensity and loss of definition of right lentiform nucleus and head of caudate nucleus. **(B)** The computed tomography scan performed on the 4th day shows more evident hypodensity, also involving the insular cortex and the frontal operculum. **(C)** On the final computed tomography scan 4 months later, the infarction is markedly hypodense, and the frontal horn has enlarged.

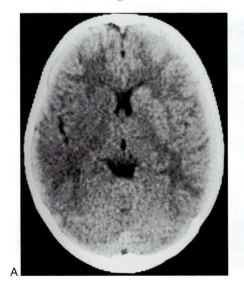

A

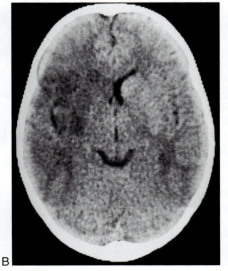

B

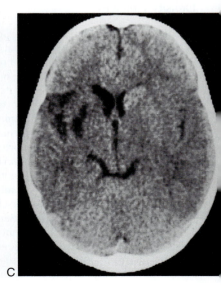

C

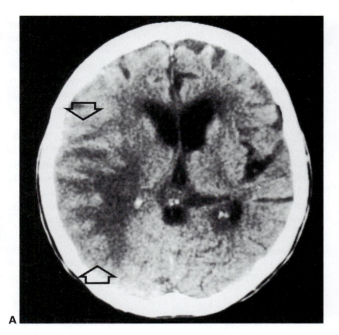
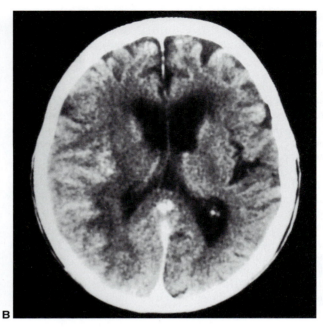

Figure 11.6 Right middle cerebral artery infarction 6 days after stroke. **(A)** On plain computed tomography scan, the "fogging effect" brings the attenuation values of the involved posterior sylvian cortex to normal levels (*arrows*). The underlying white matter remains hypodense. **(B)** On postcontrast computed tomography scan, the infarcted cortical mantle presents slight enhancement.

appears as isodense superficial curvilinear bands; they correspond to the gray matter of the cortical mantle (Fig. 11.6), where the cellular reaction is more marked than in the white matter and where petechial hemorrhages may occur[71,172] (see Fig. 11.16B). This phenomenon has to be kept in mind when one is judging the size of the infarct: a scan performed in the second or third week after stroke may lead one to underestimate the size of the infarct or even to fail to recognize the infarct itself. As the process of tissue breakdown and phagocytosis continues, the infarcted area gradually becomes replaced by cystic spaces filled with fluid; on CT scan, therefore, the hypodensity again becomes more evident, with attenuation values now in the range of cerebrospinal fluid (CSF). The margins of the infarct also become sharply demarcated. Dilatation of the homolateral ventricle and of the adjacent cisterns and even retraction of the midline structures may become evident.

Edema and Mass Effect

In ischemic infarcts, the edema seen in the early stage involves both gray and white matter and is present only in the area affected by ischemia; swelling of the infarcted gray and white matter is actually the first sign visible with the naked eye on the pathologic specimens.[172] This is an important element for the differential diagnosis from tumors; in tumors, the vasogenic edema is confined to the white matter and tends to track along white matter pathways, such as the internal and external capsule; involvement of the subcortical regions gives the characteristic digitate pattern (Fig. 11.7). There are very few exceptions to this general rule: Monajati and Heggeness[107] found that only 4 of their 339 patients with infarct presented edema in the white matter pathways, while only 2 of 155 supra-

tentorial tumors showed edema not only in the white matter but also in the overlying gray matter.

In the fogging phase, the gray matter tends to become isodense, while the white matter may remain hypodense; the plain CT features of infarcts and tumors may be similar, but decrease of mass effect in infarcts and patterns of enhancement help in the differentiation[95] (Fig. 11.6).

Obviously, the extent of mass effect in the early phase of the edema is proportional to the size of the infarct.[71] Mass effect may therefore be life threatening in large infarcts involving the whole territory of the middle cerebral artery or in the posterior fossa. In the posterior fossa, large cerebellar infarcts may compress the brain stem and occlude the fourth ventricle, causing acute triventricular hydrocephalus; in these cases, suboccipital decompression may be a life-saving procedure.[140,152]

Some reports suggested that there is a relationship between hyperglycemia in acute stroke and extent of edema, size of the infarct as documented by CT, and clinical outcome.[12,30,41] This association would require careful measures to control serum glucose levels in early stroke to limit edema and infarct size and improve outcome. However, other series did not confirm the correlation between hyperglycemia and size of the infarct at final CT, even if clinical recovery was significantly poorer.[84]

Contrast Enhancement

Another major aspect to consider in CT scans of infarcts is the pattern observed after intravenous contrast administration.

Variable responses of the infarcted area to administration

of contrast medium in different stages have been noted since early CT studies.[40,170] In the first 5 or 6 days after stroke, intravenous contrast administration usually does not modify the attenuation values of the infarcted area or modifies them very little.

After the first week, contrast enhancement of the infarcted area is prominent in the great majority of cases; contrast enhancement is particularly evident in the second and third week after stroke and may last up to a month or even longer.[11,29,71,121,170] Contrast enhancement coincides with radioisotope uptake.[38,170]

After this stage, contrast enhancement diminishes and on late CT scans the attenuation values of the infarcted area remain unmodified after administration of contrast medium.

The contrast enhancement may appear in different patterns, from small, patchy, scattered areas or long curvilinear bands to large compact areas of intense elevation of attenuation values. The distribution is mostly in the gray matter, either of the cortical mantle or of the basal ganglia[127] (Figs. 11.8, 11.9 and 11.10). However, delayed CT scans demonstrate a diffuse spreading of the enhancement, also involving the white matter in the infarcted area.[71]

A coincidence both in distribution and time between enhancement and the fogging effect has been noted by Skriver and Olsen.[144] This coincidence is an important element for understanding the pathophysiologic mechanism of contrast enhancement in infarcts.

Dysautoregulation with hyperemia and alteration of the blood-brain barrier, vascular necrosis, and vascular proliferation of capillaries with abnormally permeable endothelium have been considered as explanations for contrast enhancement.[29,71,170] It is likely that all these factors may play a role in the contrast enhancement of infarcts[127]; however, dysautoregulation or luxury perfusion, which may explain a more transient, early, and peripheral gray matter enhancement,[80] usu-

ally disappears in a few days.[71] Vascular necrosis involving hemorrhages might explain only a minority of the cases, since hemorrhagic infarctions represent probably about 20% of cerebral infarcts,[34,38,47] while contrast enhancement is a much more frequent phenomenon. Nevertheless, it is not necessary for vascular necrosis to occur to explain extravascular passage of contrast medium; this simply requires an abnormality of the blood-brain barrier.

Therefore, both the progressive accumulation of iodine in extravascular spaces demonstrated by CT scans[128] and the peak of this phenomenon in the second to third week after stroke (a period coinciding with the peak of new capillary growth) demonstrate that contrast enhancement in infarcts mostly depends on leakage of contrast medium through the abnormally permeable endothelium of new capillaries[29,64,71] (Fig. 11.11).

Frequency of contrast enhancement in the appropriate stage of evolution in the infarct is different in various series, ranging from about 50% to almost 100% of the cases.[11,29,71,88,121,144]

Contrast enhancement generally parallels the fogging effect and, similarly to it, is transient, and therefore may not be visible on a single CT study performed in the "appropriate" period. This fact, together with the time interval between injection and CT scan and the improved resolution of CT machines, explains the different frequencies reported. On serial scans repeated at short intervals, contrast enhancement is constantly observed at some time during the evolution of the infarct, particularly if a hyperosmolar medium is injected.[11,29] Contrast enhancement of the infarcted area improves the possibility of recognizing the infarct when the fogging effect is present. However, the elevation of attenuation values by contrast medium in a hypodense area may bring them up to the normal range. The infarct may not be visible and may be overlooked if only postcontrast study is performed. This event,

Figure 11.7 **(A)** Edema and mass effect in infarct in the territory of the middle cerebral artery, 3 days after stroke. The hypodensity also involves the gray matter. **(B)** In tumor, the vasogenic edema tracks along white matter pathways and does not involve gray matter.

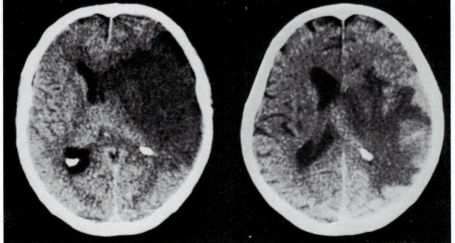

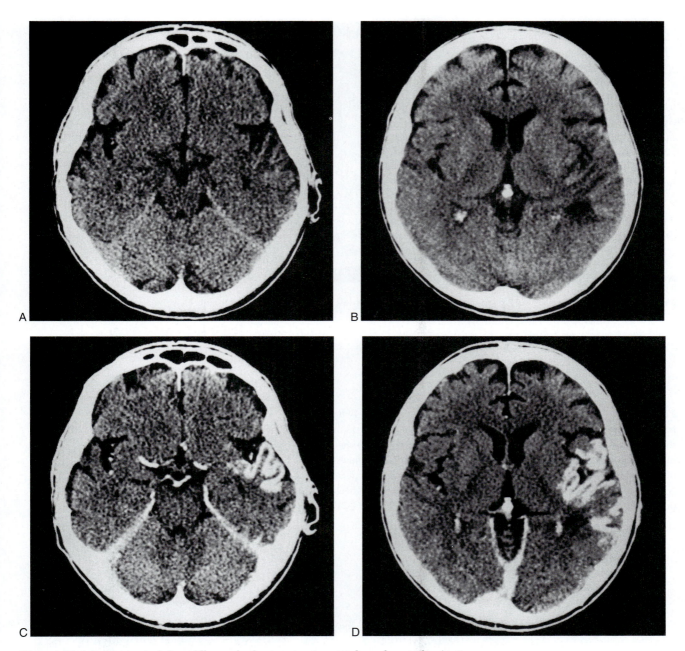

Figure 11.8 Infarction in left middle cerebral artery territory 13 days after stroke. (**A &
B**) In the "fogging" phase the plain computed tomography scans only show minimal white
matter hypodensity. (**C & D**) Postcontrast computed tomography scans show marked cortical enhancement.

which may be called a masking effect, was observed in 5 percent of the cases in the series reported by Wing et al.[170]

Another point, stressed by Skriver and Olsen,[144] is that
the infarct demonstrated by contrast enhancement is usually
smaller than that demonstrated by late plain scans; the best
correlation with the late scan is seen on the plain CT on the
third or fourth day after stroke.

In conclusion, the visibility of an infarct on CT scan fluctuates in the different phases, being good in the phase of

edema, sometimes poor in the phase of proliferation of capillaries and invasion of macrophages, and excellent in the stage
of glial scar and cyst formation. Contrast enhancement may
be helpful in the second phase, when it can obviate the fogging
effect (Fig. 11.12).

The need for contrast medium administration in infarcts
has been questioned. Serial scans may resolve the doubtful
cases, and, moreover, warnings about risks of contrast medium
administration have been expressed.[29,76,121]

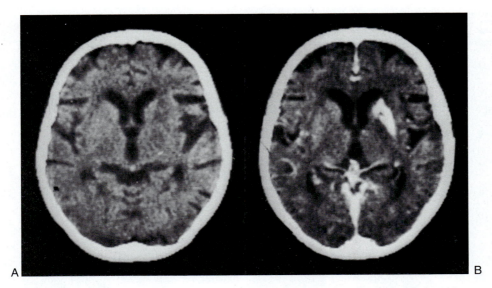

Figure 11.9 **(A)** Barely visible hypodensity in anterior limb of left internal capsule and putamen, 14 days after stroke. **(B)** Intense, homogeneous enhancement is seen on postcontrast scan.

Figure 11.10 Infarction in the territory of the left superior cerebellar artery. **(A)** Postcontrast computed tomography scan 8 days after stroke shows cortical enhancement; observe the pattern of orientation of the cerebellar folia, separated by edematous underlying white matter. **(B)** Plain computed tomography scan 6 months later shows marked hypodensity of the infarct in the territory of central and lateral hemispheric branches of the superior cerebellar artery. Minimal hypodensity (*arrowhead*) probably indicates incomplete infarction in the territory of the superior vermian branch (see Plate 11-2D).

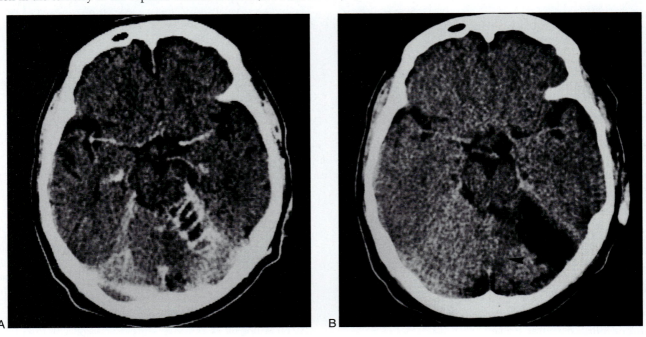

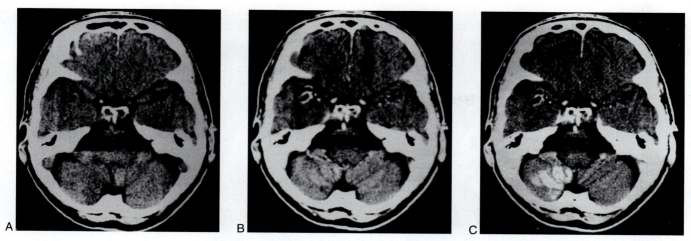

Figure 11.11 Contrast enhancement is due to the abnormal blood-brain barrier in the phase of capillary proliferation. Infarct in the right posterior inferior cerebellar artery distribution, 10 days after stroke. (**A**) Plain computed tomography scan shows only slight hypodensity. (**B**) The hypodensity is masked by minimal enhancement on postcontrast computed tomography scan. (**C**) Delayed computed tomography scan 15 minutes later allows demonstration of progressive accumulation of contrast medium in the extravascular space, thus delineating the infarct. Particularly in infarcts of the posterior fossa (which is scanned first), postcontrast studies starting immediately after injection may be insufficient to demonstrate the abnormality of the blood-brain barrier.

Figure 11.12 (**A**) Schematic representation of density changes of infarcted area on plain computed tomography scan; in the 2nd and 3rd week the density may return to normal level. (**B**) In this period contrast enhancement is most evident. (**C**) Combination of plain computed tomography and contrast-enhanced computed tomography scans improves the possibility of detecting infarcts, but contrast enhancement may mask a hypodense area.

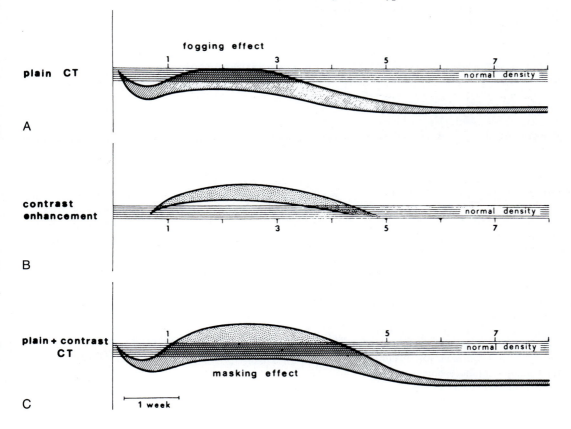

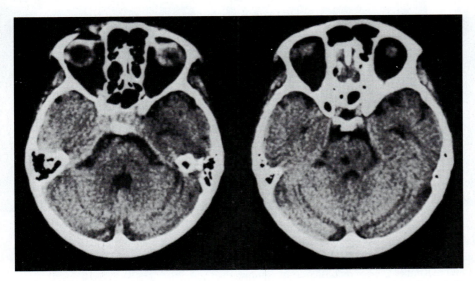

Figure 11.13 (**A & B**) Bilateral infarcts in central and upper pons in a patient with emboli of cardiac origin. The distribution is in the territory of paramedian penetrating arteries.

In particular, Kendall and Pullicino[76] found that the prognosis of patients with infarct who had received contrast medium was poorer than that of the patients who had not received contrast. The difference was not statistically significant; however, it is conceivable that the neurotoxicity of the contrast agents, which extravasate through the abnormal blood-brain barrier, may adversely affect borderline viable neurons, thus influencing negatively the outcome of these patients.[128] The nonionic contrast media currently used are probably less hazardous for the patients than the ionic ones used a few years ago; still, the use of contrast medium in patients with stroke has progressively declined.

An important observation has been made by Hayman et al.[62] In a group of patients examined within 28 hours after stroke with delayed CT and high-dosage contrast medium, seven cases were found to present massive extravasation of contrast medium indicating severe vasogenic edema. Of these seven patients, four subsequently developed large hemorrhagic infarctions. The massive enhancement was regarded as an indicator of patients who are prone to develop hemorrhagic infarction. However, in view of the possible hazard of contrast medium in infarcts, administration of high dosages is hardly recommendable.

Limitations to Recognizability:
Artifacts and Size

Other limitations to the visibility of an infarct, besides its own density changes, are related to its location and size. Infarcts near the skull base, such as in the middle and posterior fossa, may escape detection because of bone-related artifacts. In the posterior fossa, only cerebellar infarctions are easily recognized, particularly in the territory of the superior cerebellar arteries (Fig. 11.10); brain stem infarcts, however, are less easily visible. Even when they are clinically devastating because of their strategic location, brain stem infarcts are relatively small. Therefore, CT demonstration of infarcts in the lower pons and medulla is exceptional because of the combination of small size and artifacts, while, at the level of upper pons and midbrain, infarcts can be more frequently recognized[67,79,147,162] (Fig. 11.13). In the case of lacunar infarcts, the difficulty in recognizing them is directly related to their size.

In suspected posterior fossa infarct, MRI becomes a mandatory examination; it can demonstrate even the small lateral medullary infarction, almost never demonstrated by CT.[133]

LACUNAR INFARCTS

Lacunar infarcts usually occur in the distribution of the penetrating small branches of the middle cerebral, posterior cerebral, anterior choroidal, and basilar arteries and may result in a large number of characteristic syndromes.[46,104] There is a high incidence of hypertension in these patients.[46,102,106]

The lacunes of very few millimeters in diameter may escape detection not only in the brain stem; larger lacunes measuring 0.5 to 1.5 cm in diameter are recognized (Fig. 11.14), and their location has helped in reassessing the anatomic basis for the clinical syndromes for which they are responsible.[44,72,94,116,124,129,146,147,158]

Although the occlusion of the penetrating arteries is most often the result of lipohyalinosis, fibrinoid necrosis, or microatheroma,[46,104] occlusion of small arteries may be caused by emboli of cardiac or carotid origin.[122,124] In patients presenting clinically with a lacunar syndrome, large infarcts can be found at CT in a significant number of cases.[110,165]

It can be concluded, therefore, that CT is essential in establishing that a clinical lacunar syndrome is really due to a lacunar infarct; even in that case, however, CT should not be the final study; in selected cases, further investigation is needed to search for possible sources of emboli.[110,122]

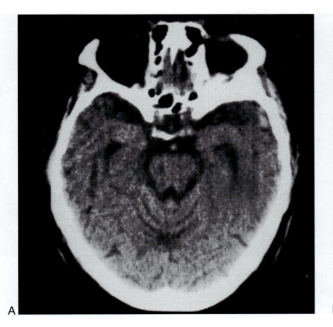 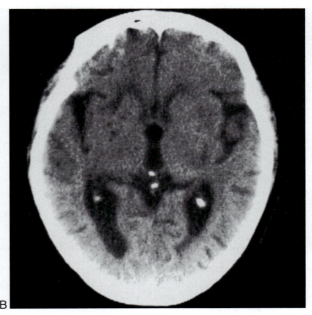

Figure 11.14 Computed tomography scans in a hypertensive patient. **(A)** Lacunar infarct in right upper pons. **(B)** Lacunar infarcts in both thalami and both lentiform nuclei.

SUBCORTICAL ARTERIOSCLEROTIC ENCEPHALOPATHY (BINSWANGER'S DISEASE)

Subcortical arteriosclerotic encephalopathy was first described by Binswanger in 1894, and the subject was reviewed by Olszewski[114] in 1962. In the past few years, the availability of CT studies, and then of MRI, has revived interest in this disease.

The disease affects elderly, usually hypertensive persons, causing progressive dementia and transient, recurrent neurologic deficits that may lead to a pseudobulbar paralysis. Arteriosclerotic changes in the basal arteries and thickening and hyalinosis of the long medullary arteries are prominent. These changes result in lacunar infarcts in the basal ganglia and mostly in extensive demyelination of the periventricular white matter and of the centrum semiovale with relative sparing of the subcortical arcuate fibers. The density of the white matter is therefore the point of interest on CT studies of patients with Binswanger's disease.

Mild changes of white matter density occurring with age have been documented.[5,177] However, in old, hypertensive patients, with the clinical picture of subcortical arteriosclerotic encephalopathy, striking changes of the white matter with low density, either diffuse to the whole centrum semiovale or limited to the periventricular region, mostly around the frontal horns, are often observed. The ventricles are dilated, with ragged margins; cortical sulci may be dilated. Lacunar infarcts are also part of the CT picture (Fig. 11.15). Pathologic correlation has been obtained in a number of cases and strict correspondence between CT and pathologic findings has been observed.[55,91,178]

Similar clinical pictures may be observed in patients with pseudobulbar palsy, corresponding to the *état lacunaire*, and in multi-infarct dementia. A more steady progression of neurologic deficits and the presence on CT scan of the white matter hypodensities without cortical infarcts favor the diagnosis of subcortical arteriosclerotic encephalopathy.

Loizou et al[91] pointed out that the location of the white matter changes corresponds to the deep paraventricular watershed area between the deep, perforating branches and the cortical medullary arteries.[171] Therefore, the anatomic picture of the disease can be considered the result of chronic ischemia in this watershed area, secondary to arteriosclerotic, hypertensive vasculopathy with a peculiar distribution.

Other conditions, such as amyloid angiopathy,[56] leukodystrophies, demyelinating diseases, and cerebral syphilis may cause white matter hypodensity.[52,65] Even excluding these other disorders, white matter hypodensity in elderly patients is much more common than the clinical diagnosis of Binswanger's disease. In these patients, MRI often demonstrates even more dramatically the white matter changes. Dementia and other neurologic disturbances are often absent; therefore, the significance of these changes has been questioned. Hachinski et al[58] proposed a new, neutral, and general term, leukoaraiosis (white matter rarefaction), to label these white matter changes.

Recent positron emission tomography studies and local cerebral blood flow measurements obtained by the stable xenon CT method demonstrated that diffuse cerebral hypoperfusion, particularly in combination with the poor collateral circulation of the periventricular white matter, is responsible for leukoaraiosis.[82,98] We also observed cases of asymmetric white matter changes on MRI in which the side more affected corresponded to the side of the more severely stenotic carotid artery.

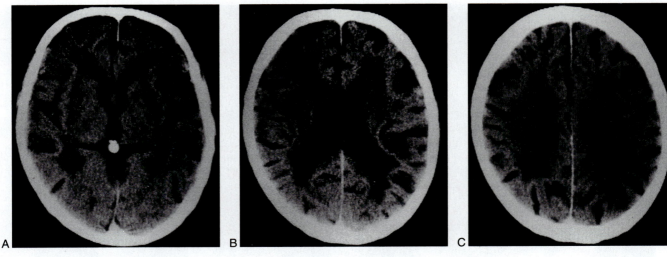

Figure 11.15 Computed tomography scans showing subcortical arteriosclerotic encephalopathy in a 70-year-old hypertensive patient. (**A**) Lacunar infarcts in the basal ganglia. (**B & C**) Hypodensity of periventricular and subcortical white matter; dilated ventricles and sulci.

In conclusion, there is probably a spectrum of white matter changes in elderly people, generally caused by hypoperfusion, that can be called leukoaraiosis. CT and MRI may detect these abnormalities even when they do not cause symptoms and signs. Only when the changes are severe enough and are accompanied by the appropriate neurologic symptomatology are we justified in using the term Binswanger's disease or subcortical arteriosclerotic encephalopathy.

HEMORRHAGIC INFARCTS

Cerebral ischemic infarcts become hemorrhagic when the blood re-enters the capillary bed either through the collateral circulation or after fragmentation of the original embolus. Anticoagulant therapy may also convert an ischemic infarction to a hemorrhagic one.[45] In hemorrhagic infarcts of arterial origin, hemorrhages occur only in the gray matter and are almost constant, provided that the ischemia has lasted long enough to damage the capillary walls and that the systemic blood pressure has remained above 60 mmHg.[172]

The infarcted gray matter may become entirely hemorrhagic, but in large infarcts only the periphery may be affected while the center remains pale.[172] Small and rare petechial hemorrhages are, therefore, an extremely frequent microscopic finding in all infarcts; however, diapedesis of red blood cells significant enough to make an infarct red or hemorrhagic is observed in about 20 percent of cases.[23,38,47,62]

In spite of this reported frequency, CT observations of hemorrhagic infarcts are rare.[17] The reason for this is twofold: small petechiae are not detected because of volume averaging,[2] and the time of increased density due to the extravasated blood (see the section on intracerebral hemorrhages later in this chapter) may be so short as to escape detection if serial scans are not performed. Tiny petechiae contribute to the fogging effect of ischemic infarcts. MRI demonstrates hemorrhagic infarction better than CT, and for a longer time. On CT scan, observation of a single area of high density within an infarction several days after stroke leaves the possibility either of hemorrhagic infarction or of a resolving hematoma within the area of infarction. A peripheral location and a patchy distribution suggest hemorrhagic infarction.[23] Early spontaneous hematoma within a cerebral infarct may occur even in the first 24 hours and may be mistaken for a primary cerebral hemorrhage if a previous CT scan had not been performed. Rapid clinical worsening usually accompanies the intervening hematoma.[16]

The usual CT appearance of hemorrhagic infarction is that of mixed hypodense and hyperdense areas in the cortical or deep gray matter. In cases with large confluent petechiae, the hyperdensity may involve the whole infarcted area (Figs 11.16 and 11.17). Contrast enhancement may be minimal, barely detectable, or massive.[38,71,166,176] When massive bleeding occurs, the enhancement may assume a ring shape as in primary intracerebral hematomas (see the sections on hemorrhages later in this chapter) (Fig. 11.17).

Hemorrhagic infarcts or even hematomas may also result from dural sinus thrombosis; in venous pathologic conditions they more frequently involve the subcortical white matter.[166]

It has not proved easy to develop a method that reliably differentiates nonhemorrhagic from hemorrhagic stroke on clinical grounds alone, independently from imaging. Besson et al[15] suggested a system based on 26 clinical variables, using CT scanning as the gold standard. However, they were able to identify correctly only 40% of the 305 patients studied with a nonhemorrhagic infarct. Furthermore, they found no threshold values that allowed a diagnosis of cerebral hemorrhage entirely on clinical grounds with a high positive predictive value, leaving even this important differentiation unsettled unless brain imaging was undertaken.

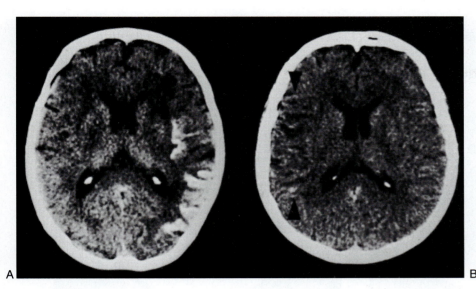

Figure 11.16 Hemorrhagic infarcts in middle cerebral artery distribution: two different cases. **(A)** Marked cortical hyperdensity on plain computed tomography scan 15 days after a stroke indicates diffuse petechial hemorrhages. **(B)** In the second case, the findings are subtle, consistent with rare and smaller petechiae (*arrowheads*).

DURAL SINUS THROMBOSIS

In dural sinus thrombosis, the clinical presentation may be consistent with a stroke, but more often epileptic seizures, lethargy, and signs of increased intracranial pressure are present.[123] In fact, focal, lateralized CT signs are less frequently observed than are small ventricles and direct signs of thrombosed sinus.[49,123] The ventricles may subsequently enlarge.[78]

The focal signs in the brain tissue include hemorrhagic infarctions, hematomas, low-density areas of edema or infarctions, and areas of gyral enhancement. The hemorrhagic infarctions may be single or multiple, unilateral or bilateral; when they occur on both sides in the supraventricular regions, mostly in the parasagittal areas, in a nontraumatized patient, they should suggest superior sagittal sinus thrombosis.[26]

The direct sign of recent sinus thrombosis consists of a small hyperdensity within the sinus representing the clot (Fig. 11.18); more frequently, however, the thrombus, particularly the old thrombus, is only recognized as a nonenhancing area within the sinus on postcontrast CT scan. The empty triangle has been called the delta sign[28,49,123] (Fig. 11.19).

The cord sign, which is a hyperdense streak converging on the superior sagittal sinus seen on plain scan, represents an extension of the thrombosis to a cortical vein and, although rare, is considered a pathognomonic sign.[28,123]

Recognizing the delta sign is often difficult; it is usually not visible with the standard window setting but requires a higher window level and more extended window width. In addition, a subtle line of apparent filling defect at the base of the triangle of the superior sagittal sinus is usually a bone-related artifact,[141] and a delta sign with short extension may be caused by splitting or duplication of the sinus.[28,123] One must, therefore, be very cautious about diagnosing sinus thrombosis based on subtle CT signs; the use of angiography is fully justified to investigate such cases further. MRI may also solve, noninvasively, the diagnostic problem and should be the first examination in a case of suspected dural sinus thrombosis.

STROKE IN CHILDREN

Stroke in children has a widespread range of causes.[180] The problems of perinatal pathologic changes and of intracerebral bleeding or ischemic infarcts occurring as a complication of known underlying diseases such as leukemia, intracranial infections, or trauma will not be analyzed here. Stroke in children, usually manifesting with acute hemiplegia, differs from that of adults in several respects: it is a single event, TIA does not exist (except in moyamoya), and heart disease is the most frequent predisposing condition, but usually no predisposing factors are found.[136] The high frequency of nasopharyngeal and tonsillar infections reported in other series[60] was not observed in our cases.[132]

While the abnormalities observed on angiography are often peculiar, and different from those observed in adults, there are no unusual features in CT findings except for extreme rarity of localization in the vertebrobasilar territory, absence of lacunar infarcts, and discrepancy between frequent extensive parenchymal damage and good functional recovery.

One disease, however, has more distinctive although nonspecific features: moyamoya.

MOYAMOYA

Moyamoya is by no means limited to children but is the cause of stroke in 10% to 15% of children with cerebrovascular disease and is almost the only cause of bilateral disease in children.[60]

Diagnosis of moyamoya is made by angiography, but CT findings are highly suggestive when bilateral infarcts are demonstrated in a child or young adult. Other angiodysplasias or

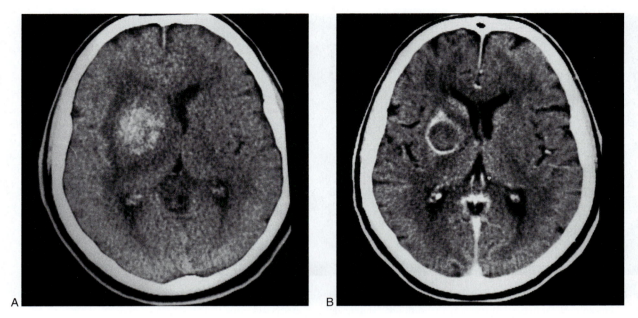

Figure 11.17 **(A)** Plain computed tomography scan 6 days after stroke shows massive bleeding in infarction in the territory of the right lenticulostriate arteries. **(B)** Postcontrast computed tomography scan 6 weeks later shows ring-shaped enhancement.

arteritides may cause the same CT picture; however, they are less frequent than moyamoya, or, as in cases of postmeningitic vasculitis, they are easily diagnosed on the basis of clinical history.

In moyamoya, infarcts in different phases of their evolution, but usually old, cortical, and preferably in distal or watershed areas, are the most common finding, followed in frequency by atrophy with ventricular dilatation[59,151] (Fig. 11.20). Occasionally, intracerebral or subarachnoid bleeding may be observed. However, we found this only in one young adult who also presented with a basilar artery aneurysm.

Since in old infarcts there is no rupture of the blood-

Figure 11.18 **(A & B)** Acute thrombosis of the right transverse sinus (*arrowheads*) in a 5-year-old girl. The recent clot is hyperdense on the plain computed tomography scan.

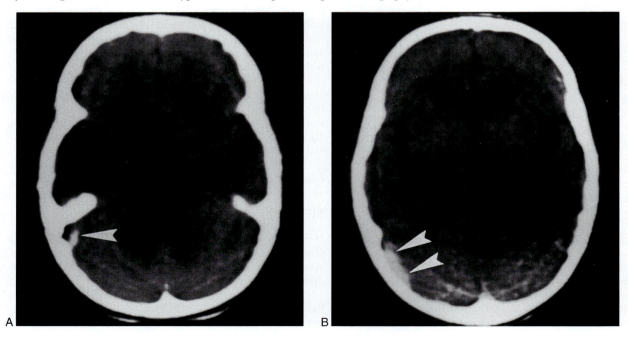

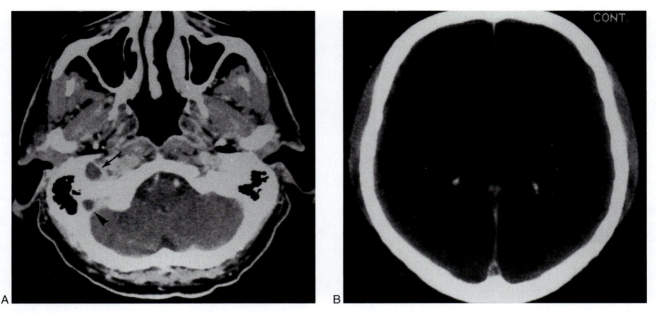

Figure 11.19 Dural sinus thrombosis of more than a month duration in two different cases; postcontrast computed tomography studies. **(A)** The hypodense thrombus of the right sigmoid sinus is delineated by the enhancing dura (*arrowhead*). Thrombosis extends to the internal jugular vein (*arrow*). **(B)** Demonstration of the "delta sign" in a thrombosed superior sagittal sinus may require appropriate window setting.

brain barrier, it is not surprising that postcontrast examination is negative and that demonstration of the tiny vessels that form the typical basal network is obtained only in a minority of cases, sometimes only with high-dosage bolus injection.[151] Scanning on a modified coronal plane, parallel to the long axis

of the supraclinoid segment of the carotid siphons and of the vessels forming the basal network, has been advocated. All five patients examined with this technique showed a nebula-like hyperdensity, corresponding perfectly to the angiographic picture.[6]

Figure 11.20 **(A & B)** Advanced moyamoya disease with bilateral temporoparieto-occipital (middle cerebral arteries and posterior cerebral arteries), right frontal (middle cerebral artery), and left frontoparietal parasagittal (anterior cerebral artery and watershed anterior cerebral artery-middle cerebral artery) infarcts. Irregularities of bone on both sides indicate the site of previous external-internal carotid artery bypasses. (Left side is on reader's left.)

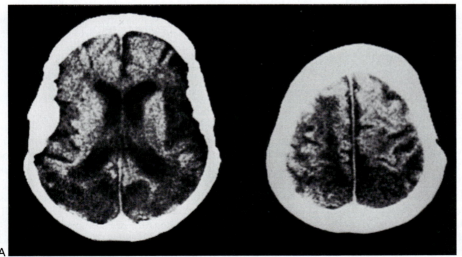

Lack of CT demonstration of the basal network may be related to its actual disappearance during the evolution of the disease[148]; however, monitoring the progression of the disease with repeated angiograms is unjustified.

ASYMPTOMATIC INFARCTION

A growing literature is documenting a range of lesions seen on CT (and on MRI) that are completely or largely asymptomatic. Loeb et al,[90] in the most recent report, studied 383 consecutive stroke patients whose CT was positive and found that fully 34% of the lesions had been asymptomatic. Of these, 88% were small (<2 mm), many considered to be lacunes, while others were in the deep central white matter. However, in 21% larger lesions were seen, also asymptomatic, most of them accompanied by other infarcts, making a differentiation difficult as to whether the syndrome reflected combined lesions. Similarly, Boon et al[18] reviewed 755 consecutive cases of first-ever supratentorial ischemic stroke and found 27% with one or more silent infarcts on CT scan. As in Loeb et al, most (82%) were deep, small infarcts consistent with lacunes, but some were convex. No independent association was found for a cardioembolic source (including atrial fibrillation) or for carotid stenosis with a diameter reduction of >50%. Of especial importance was the demonstration that so-called silent infarcts had no effect on the severity of the initial handicap, or on the 30-day case fatality, or even on the 1-year mortality.

Intracerebral Hemorrhages

CT has brilliantly solved the problem of recognizing intracerebral hematomas: in the first study by Paxton and Ambrose,[115] hemorrhages were recognized in 100% of the cases.

Prior to the availability of CT, intracerebral hematomas were diagnosed on the basis of clinical presentation, evidence of avascular lesion with mass effect on angiography, and occasional ring uptake of radioisotope around the hematoma. Presence of blood in the CSF at lumbar puncture was diagnostic, but it only occurred when the hematoma had ruptured into the ventricles or toward the subarachnoid spaces; in deepseated hematomas, however, this evidence was lacking.

GENERAL ASPECTS

CT studies demonstrate that the intracerebral hematoma appears as a high-density lesion that is immediately recognizable when the bleeding occurs. The circulating blood is also hyperdense with respect to the brain tissue, as is demonstrated by the higher attenuation values observed in large pools of blood such as in giant nonthrombosed aneurysms and arteriovenous malformations (AVMs) (see Fig. 11.31A).

In vitro studies demonstrated that the whole blood with normal hematocrit and normal hemoglobin level has an atten-

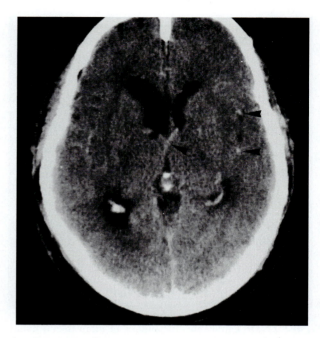

Figure 11.21 Plain computed tomography scan of a patient with secondary polycythemia and hematocrit of 70 percent; high attenuation values in arteries and veins (*arrowheads*) simulate a postcontrast study.

uation value of 55 to 60 Hounsfield units (HU); the freshly extravasated blood is, therefore, immediately demonstrable. Packed red cells at a hematocrit of 90%, representative of clotted blood, and actual retracted clot measure about 80 to 85 HU. The attenuation values depend on the hemoglobin content, while iron has a low influence and the contribution of calcium is negligible.[111,112]

That the attenuation values of circulating blood depend on the hematocrit is also demonstrated by CT scans of patients with polycythemia, which mimics postcontrast examinations because of the high density of all arterial and venous vessels (Fig. 11.21).

At very low hemoglobin levels, therefore, a hematoma may appear with attenuation values similar or even inferior to those of the normal brain tissue (24 to 46 HU). In fact, decreased absorption values were described in a cerebellar hematoma occurring in a severely anemic patient.[73]

Density Changes and Evolution

In clinical situations, it is extremely rare to observe a hematoma in the first minutes; however, cases of continuing intracerebral hemorrhage have been observed and a density of 54 HU, which corresponds exactly to the expected data, was reported.[92,96]

In a very short period of time (about 3 hours), the process of clot formation and clot retraction takes place. The first CT scan, therefore, usually demonstrates a homogeneous, well-defined area of high density, with attenuation values around 80 HU. The spontaneous intracerebral hematoma presents a rounded or oval or, sometimes, a more irregular shape depending on its size and location; spontaneous intracerebral hemorrhages tend to dissect along the fiber tracts with less disruption of the brain tissue than occurs with post-traumatic lacerations.[42,172]

The evolution of intracerebral hematomas has been reviewed by several authors.[13,42,43,57,77,100,109] The hematoma exerts a mass effect that is proportional to its size: extensive surrounding edema is not seen, but a faint, thin rim of low density appears early at the periphery of the hematoma. This peripheral rim may be attributable to a combination of serum separation in clot retraction with edema and ischemic necrosis of the surrounding compressed brain.[33,43,77] The peripheral low-density rim of the serum expressed by the retracted clot was clearly demonstrated in phantom studies by Bergström et al[13] and Kendall and Radue.[77]

Growth of a hematoma has been reported in some detail in a prospective study carried out within 3 hours of stroke onset. Brott et al[27] found evidence of continuing increase in hematoma size in 26% of their 103 cases when comparing the baseline and 1-hour CT scans. A further 12% of hematomas were enlarged in the scans comparing a 1- and 20-hour interval. The enlarging hematomas were correlated with a declining clinical status of the cases under study. One discouraging finding in this study was the failure to identify any clinical or CT features in the baseline evaluation that predicted the continued enlargement.

Intracerebral fluid-blood level is rarely seen in recent hemorrhages; a fluid-blood level observed in a few cases at CT by Zilkha[179] was not found to be associated with bleeding in a cyst, but, at operation or postmortem examination, only layering of clotted and unclotted blood was demonstrated. Since the smaller, nondependent part of the fluid-blood interface was of low density and no cyst cavity was found, separation of serum with subsequent resorption is likely.[179] This phenomenon is transient, as it was observed only in very recent hemorrhages; one should be aware of this to avoid making a hasty judgment of bleeding in a pre-existing tumoral cyst.

After reaching the plateau of about 80 HU in a few hours, the hematoma appears as a well-defined, homogeneous, hyperdense mass lesion with negligible or absent postural changes,[77] even though a mixture of clotted and unclotted blood is found at surgery in virtually all cases. The density of the hematoma then begins to decline because of the breakdown of hemoglobin, progressing concentrically, with consequent enlargement of the peripheral zone of hypodensity. The central area of hyperdensity also fades progressively, but it remains the last to change to normal and then to low-attenuation values.

Dolinskas et al[42] calculated the rate of the density changes in terms of both attenuation values and size: they found an average decrease in density of 1.4 HU/day and of 0.65 mm/day. It follows, therefore, that the central hyperdensity reaches values similar to the normal brain in 3 to 4 weeks and then becomes totally hypodense. Disappearance of the hyperdensity is obviously more rapid in small than in large hematomas (Fig. 11.22). The mass effect, however, remains present because the hematoma has simply changed its density values[100] (Fig. 11.23); the process of resorption with reduction of mass effect and reduction of the hematoma to a slit cavity containing a yellowish fluid takes much longer. After months, therefore, the CT scan may demonstrate only a narrow streak of hypodensity with attenuation values similar to those of CSF, and an enlarged homolateral ventricle. In small hematomas, the residual cavity may even become unrecognizable.

This is a considerable difference between intracerebral hematomas and infarctions. In infarctions, the size of the involved area changes very little with time because there is destruction of the brain tissue, while in spontaneous intracerebral hematomas the reduction in size of the cavity is sometimes surprising because the brain tissue was mainly dissected without much destruction (Figs. 11.24 and 11.25). Therefore, the observation on late scans of a narrow streak of hypodensity in an appropriate site, such as in the external capsule or in the lobar white matter in a patient with previous stroke, indicates previous hematoma rather than infarction. Confirmation may be exquisitely obtained by MRI through demonstration of the rim of decreased signal intensity in T_2-weighted images due to hemosiderin.

Contrast Enhancement

Administration of intravenous contrast medium is usually unnecessary in cases of intracerebral hemorrhages, at least in the early stages. However, when the plain CT scan demonstrates

Figure 11.22 Schematic representation of density changes in intracerebral hematoma. Ring enhancement is present from approximately the 10th day to the 7th week.

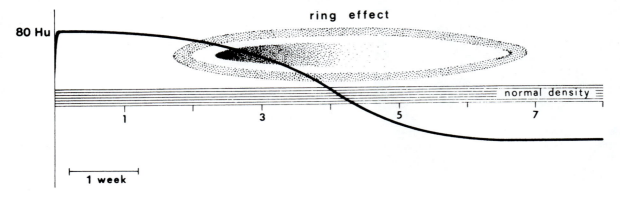

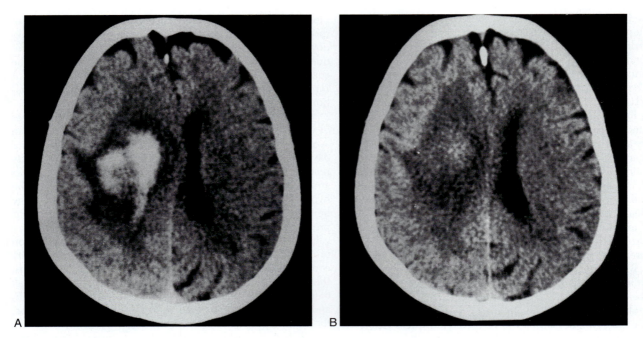

Figure 11.23 **(A)** Hematoma 6 days after stroke. **(B)** Same hematoma 30 days after stroke. Despite the density changes, the size of the hematoma and its mass effect are unchanged.

Figure 11.24 Acute hematoma of the right external capsule. The hematoma dissects the brain tissue along the white matter of the capsule, displacing the insular cortex outward and the lentiform nucleus inward, and tracks around the posterior end of the sylvian fissure.

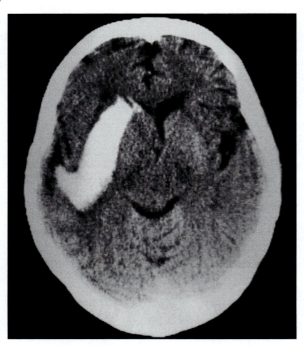

white matter edema around the acute hematoma or abnormal densities adjacent to, or surrounding, the hematoma, postcontrast examination is required because of possible bleeding in a tumor or in a vascular malformation (Fig. 11.26).

In any case, in the first few days after hypertensive spontaneous hemorrhage, no significant changes are observed after contrast enhancement. After 1 week or 10 days, a ring enhancement is observed around the hematoma, at the periphery of the enlarging low-density area. This ring enhancement surrounds the central hyperdensity, which has begun to reduce in size and intensity, forming a target-like image (Fig. 11.27).

The ring of enhancement corresponds to the area of granulation tissue with neovascularity, phagocytosis, and gliosis that surrounds the hematoma. In this zone, the newly formed capillaries have an abnormal blood-brain barrier that allows extravasation of contrast medium or of radioisotopes. The phenomenon is very similar to that observed in infarcts, and it is visible on serial scans for up to 6 to 8 weeks.[43,77,181] If the clinical history is unknown, this pattern of enhancement may be misleading, since it is also seen in abscesses and tumors; follow-up CT scans or MRI studies may be necessary in doubtful cases (Fig. 11.26). On the other hand, a bleeding tumor or vascular malformation may be completely masked by the hyperdensity of the hematoma and its surrounding, enhancing ring. Particularly in cases of lobar hematomas, even if angiography does not show a vascular malformation, in young, nonhypertensive patients, we recommend late CT scans, because of the possibility of detecting the nodule of a cryptic vascular malformation[135] (Fig. 11.28). Also in these cases, early MRI may demonstrate the vascular malformation undetected by CT.

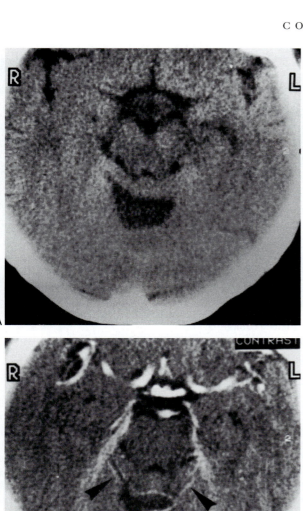

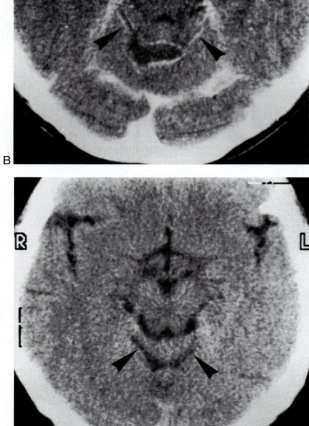

Figure 11.25 **(A)** Subacute, hypodense cerebellar hematoma in the superior vermis 2 weeks after stroke. **(B)** Postcontrast computed tomography scan with thin marginal enhancement 2 weeks later. **(C)** Plain computed tomography 4 months after stroke. Figures B and C demonstrate the pattern of dissection, along the white matter underlying the folia of the cerebellar hemispheres (*arrowheads*). The resolving hematoma becomes a progressively thinner fissure.

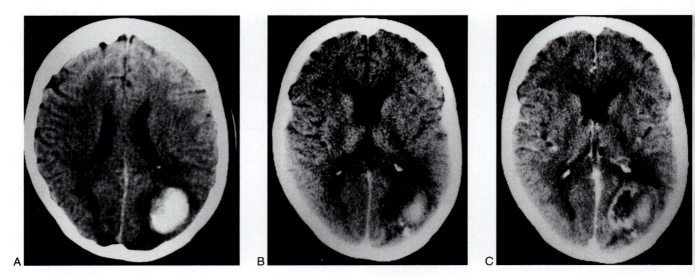

Figure 11.26 **(A)** Acute lobar hematoma in a 64-year-old woman. **(B)** On plain computed tomography scan 16 days later, decrease in density allows easy recognition of calcifications. **(C)** Postcontrast computed tomography demonstrates irregular marginal enhancement. Magnetic resonance imaging confirmed hematoma in tumor, glioblastoma multiforme at histologic examination.

Location

The well-established concept that spontaneous intracerebral bleeding occurs overwhelmingly in the basal ganglia region has come into question. Prognosis is poorer and mortality is higher in deep-seated hematomas, particularly if they are large and rupture into the ventricles.[77] It is obvious, therefore, that autopsy series counted more basal ganglia than lobar hematomas. With the in vivo diagnosis offered by CT, frequency of basal ganglia hemorrhages has been found lower than that of more peripheral bleedings.[33,77,108] Our early series of 150 spontaneous hematomas also supports this view: spontaneous

Figure 11.27 Posterior temporal hematoma, 10 days after stroke. **(A)** Plain computed tomography scan. **(B)** Postcontrast computed tomography scan. The ring enhancement delineates exactly the hematoma, hypodense at the periphery.

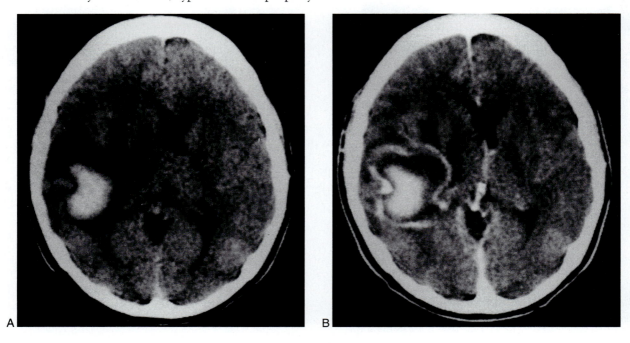

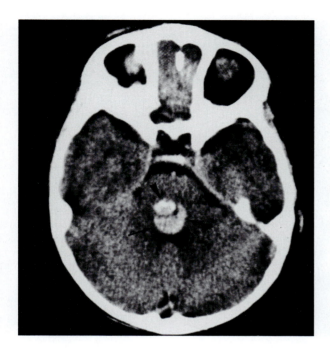

Figure 11.28 Hematoma from cavernous hemangioma of the pons. Eight days after the bleeding, the decrease in density of the hematoma (*arrows*) allows recognition of the nodule of the hemangioma (*arrowhead*). The diagnosis was confirmed by magnetic resonance imaging and proved by operation.

hematomas occurred in the cerebral lobes in 52% of the cases, in the basal ganglia in 37%, and in the posterior fossa in 11%.[132] However, a different selection of patients can play an important role in determining discrepancies.

Cerebellar hematomas occur more frequently in elderly patients, while in the general population frequency of cerebellar hematomas is about 10%, Moseley and Olney[108] reported a frequency of 18% in a series of patients over 70 years of age.

It remains true that hypertension is more frequent in persons with basal ganglia and pontine lesions than lobar hematomas, although hypertension is frequently also observed in persons with the latter.[77]

Rupture into the ventricular system is obviously an aggravating factor; however, CT studies demonstrate that intraventricular rupture, which occurred in 32% of the hematomas reviewed by Kendall and Radue,[77] is not an ominous sign, as previously thought.[32] Communication of the hematomas with the ventricles may lead to a porencephalic cyst.

In conclusion, CT studies in intracerebral hemorrhages are always diagnostic when performed in the early stage. When clinical presentation or plain CT raises the possibility of bleeding in a tumor or from a vascular malformation, postcontrast examination or MRI and angiography are necessary. Postcontrast examination on late CT scan or MRI may demonstrate the nodule of an angiographically occult vascular malformation. Late CT scans are also helpful in monitoring possible late complications of intraventricular or subarachnoid rupture, such as hydrocephalus or expanding porencephalic cysts.

Subarachnoid Hemorrhage: Aneurysms

The blood that extravasates into the subarachnoid spaces from a ruptured aneurysm elevates the attenuation values of these spaces above those of the brain tissue. Therefore, blood in the subarachnoid space is usually easily demonstrated by CT, provided that the examination is performed in the first few days after the hemorrhage (Fig. 11.29). When CT is obtained within 4 or 5 days, a positive scan is found in about 90% of cases.[1,70,139] The high density rapidly declines, and blood may usually be demonstrated for no more than 8 to 10 days. Obviously, the amount of blood in the cerebral cisterns is the key factor determining its recognizability; however, there is no correlation between the amount of blood detected by CT and by lumbar puncture.[37] Moreover, with unquestionable bleeding verified by lumbar puncture, an occasional negative CT scan may be obtained even 1 day after the hemorrhage. Therefore, CT cannot be a complete substitute for lumbar puncture, and an early negative CT scan cannot rule out a subarachnoid hemorrhage (SAH). However, much more information can be obtained by CT in patients with SAH.

First, CT can exclude the possibility that the SAH is due to the rupture into the subarachnoid spaces of an intracerebral hematoma or to bleeding from a silent tumor, which would orient differently both the angiographic study and the management of the patient.[25,119] Second, CT can localize the aneurysm that has bled. Localization can be based either on an uneven distribution of blood in the cisterns or on the presence of a localized hematoma around the aneurysm, which may also rupture into the brain tissue (Fig. 11.30). The most easily predictable aneurysm is that of the anterior communicating artery, which shows a greater amount of blood in the frontal interhemispheric fissure and may cause either a midline hematoma, which extends through the lamina terminalis into the septum, or a lateralized frontal lobe hematoma. In both cases the blood may rupture into the ventricles.

The second most predictable aneurysm is that of the middle cerebral artery, which shows more blood in the homolateral sylvian fissure and may form a hematoma extending all along the fissure, with rare rupture into the opercula.

In aneurysm of the carotid bifurcation or at the origin of the posterior communicating artery, there is usually a more even distribution of blood in the cisterns. Aneurysms of the carotid bifurcation may cause frontal hematomas similar to those of the anterior communicating artery. Prevalence of blood in the posterior fossa points to aneurysms of the vertebrobasilar system.

Finally, a confusing picture may be offered by the rare cases of subdural hematoma caused by aneurysms bleeding into the subdural space through a breached arachnoid and arachnoidal adhesions.[50]

There is, in conclusion, a fairly frequent overlapping of the CT patterns, so that a prediction of the site of the aneurysm is made with a high degree of confidence only if there is a localized hematoma or a well-defined difference in the distribution of the cisternal blood. Only in aneurysm of the anterior communicating artery is the accuracy of localization high,[70,139] in spite of the presence of a typical septal hematoma

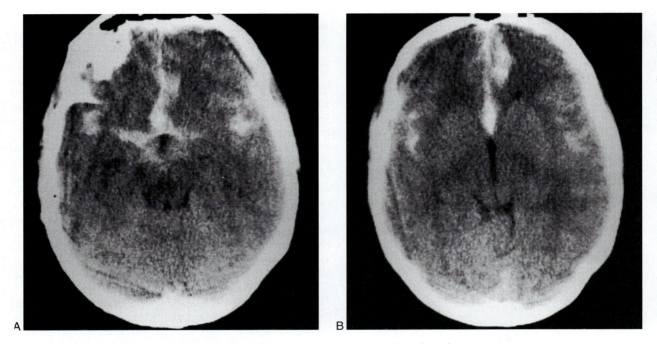

Figure 11.29 (**A & B**) Computed tomography scan performed a few hours after subarachnoid hemorrhage; the distribution of blood in the cisterns suggests bleeding from anterior communicating artery aneurysm that was confirmed by angiography and surgery.

Figure 11.30 Bleeding aneurysms with subarachnoid and intraventricular hemorrhages and intracerebral hematomas. Two different cases. (**A**) Aneurysm of the right middle cerebral artery bifurcation. (**B**) Aneurysm of the anterior communicating artery. The blood filling the 4th ventricle causes acute hydrocephalus.

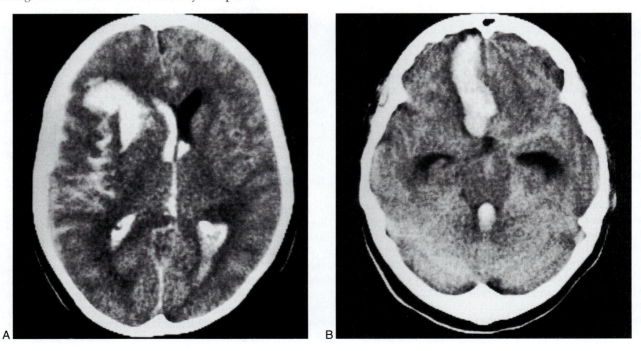

in the minority of cases.[175] However, the much rarer pericallosal aneurysm causes a very similar blood distribution; angiography is always necessary to define the aneurysm.[89]

CT localization of the bleeding aneurysm would seem futile, since angiography demonstrates the aneurysm; in these cases, CT is able, at most, to guide the angiographic study. Localization becomes important when multiple aneurysms are found, which happens in about 15% of the cases. Kendall et al,[75] however, contend that CT localization of the bleeding aneurysm is always essential and that the angiographic study should be limited to the region of bleeding. In their series of multiple aneurysms, there is no evidence that incidental aneurysms carry a significant risk; therefore, they should be ignored. However, this view is not shared by all the neurosurgeons and, when elective surgery for incidental aneurysms is considered, precise CT localization is important only for determining the priority of treatment.

CT without intravenous contrast administration is able to detect giant aneurysms because of their high density and is particularly useful in partially thrombosed, calcified aneurysms. Depending on their location, such aneurysms sometimes must be differentiated from craniopharyngiomas, pituitary adenomas, meningiomas, or other lesions that may calcify. Calcifications and thrombosis, however, are not the rule in giant aneurysms and all the patterns may be encountered, from nonthrombosed to completely thrombosed aneurysms (Figs. 11.31 and 11.32). MRI, of course, is usually very demonstrative.

The thrombosed parts of the aneurysm may have variable densities, sometimes lower than the part where blood is circulating. Comparison of plain with postcontrast CT scan or with angiography demonstrates the relationship of the two parts. Contrast enhancement may also be observed in the thick fibrous layer at the periphery of the thrombus,[118] which may rarely be the source of emboli and thus the cause of distal infarction. The partially thrombosed aneurysm therefore presents a fairly characteristic pattern with a central or eccentric enhancing area (i.e., the patent lumen), a peripheral isodense or slightly hyperdense area (i.e., the thrombus), and a surrounding, hyperdense, enhancing rim. This target sign, in appropriate situations, is highly specific for giant, partially thrombosed aneurysms[118,137] (Fig. 11.32).

Contrast administration is always necessary to demonstrate the smaller-sized aneurysms; MRI or MR angiography, however, may become the examination of choice. On CT scan, the possibility of detection after enhancement is good for anterior communicating and middle cerebral artery aneurysms, while it is poorer for those of the internal carotid and posterior communicating arteries.[53] However, it is our policy to avoid injection of contrast medium in patients with SAH, who are going to be subjected, in any case, to angiography. Only if angiography is negative might one expect to demonstrate on postcontrast CT a lesion that was unsuspected on plain CT and missed by angiography. This is only a theoretical possibility, while more emphasis should be placed on the possibility of a bleeding lesion in the spinal canal, mimicking a ruptured intracranial aneurysm. In patients with SAH, we never found a positive postcontrast CT scan with both normal plain CT and angiography, while we have found two neurinomas of the cauda equina and a spinal cord AVM presenting only with

Figure 11.31 Giant, fusiform basilar artery aneurysm, with compression of the brain stem. **(A)** The circulating blood is normally hyperdense. Tiny calcifications are visible in the aneurysmal wall. **(B)** Postcontrast computed tomography scan with uniform, complete enhancement confirms absence of thrombosis.

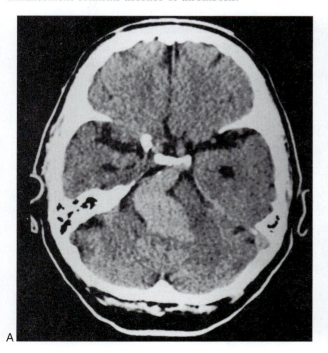
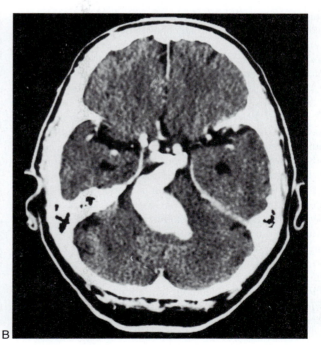

A   B

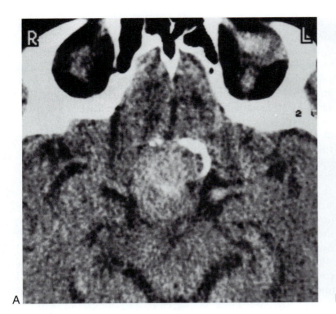 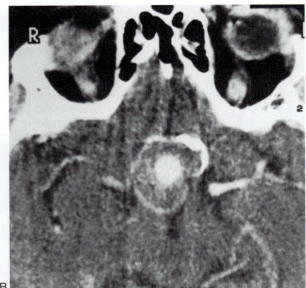

Figure 11.32 Giant, partially thrombosed aneurysm of the anterior communicating artery. **(A)** Plain computed tomography scan. **(B)** Postcontrast computed tomography scan. Comparison of plain with postcontrast study allows recognition of thrombosed peripheral part and of central patent lumen.

SAH, which were diagnosed by myelography after negative results on a four-vessel study. MRI may now demonstrate noninvasively the spinal pathology responsible for bleeding.

Intravenous contrast administration has been found to cause diffuse enhancement in the subarachnoid spaces in a considerable number of patients with SAH, particularly when it was performed in the first few days.[36,68,70,175] The enhancement is usually found in all the basal cisterns and may extend over the convexity. It does not help, therefore, in localizing the aneurysm but seems valuable for predicting vasospasm and cerebral infarcts.[68] The mechanism of subarachnoid enhancement in SAH has not been clearly established; the hypothesis that subarachnoid enhancement is related to thickening of the leptomeninges is unlikely, since this is a local, late reactive change. The most likely explanation is leakage of contrast medium from the vessels whose blood-CSF interface has been altered by the irritating effect of the surrounding blood.[70,145] If this is so, one has to consider the potential risk of adding a neurotoxic contrast agent in the CSF to the blood already present. In patients in poor equilibrium, even if nonionic, less neurotoxic contrast media are now used, it seems safer to rely upon the demonstration of blood in the cisterns for predicting vasospasm. Retrospective and prospective studies have demonstrated that development of symptomatic cerebral vasospasm is predicted with good accuracy on the basis of the presence of clots or thick layers of blood in the cisterns in the first few days after SAH.[36,48,81]

If clinical deterioration occurs, CT easily demonstrates whether it is due to rebleeding, infarction, or development of hydrocephalus. Frequency of hydrocephalus is variable in different series; ventricular dilatation is approximately present in one-third of the cases with SAH.[1,39,99,142] Many cases show spontaneous regression after 1 or 2 weeks.[99] The main factor determining the development of hydrocephalus is the amount of blood present in the cisterns and mostly in the ventricles (Fig. 11.30): all patients with intraventricular hemorrhage have some degree of ventricular dilatation and carry a poor prognosis.[103,142] Periventricular hypodensity, which indicates transependymal passage of CSF, also points to progression of hydrocephalus.[142]

Hydrocephalus is also associated with reduced cerebral blood flow and clinical deterioration.[103] Therefore, many factors, interfering with each other, are involved in determining the clinical evolution of patients with SAH. CT is the main tool for monitoring these patients, and serial CT studies are often needed in the pre- and postoperative period.

Intracranial Hemorrhages: Vascular Malformations

Cerebral vascular malformations may cause hemorrhages in the brain with rupture into the subarachnoid space or the ventricles. However, they may present with seizure disorder or, more rarely, with focal neurologic signs. Different types of vascular malformations have different tendencies to bleed and have different appearances on CT.

Cerebral vascular malformations are classified as (1) AVMs, (2) venous angiomas, (3) cavernous hemangiomas, and (4) capillary angiomas or telangiectases.[126] Some authors also add varices as a separate entity.

AVMs had long been considered the most frequent cerebral vascular malformation[97]; however, a prospective autopsy series of >4,000 consecutive brains challenges previous reported frequences of cerebral vascular malformations. In this series of 177 vascular malformations in 165 brains, the most frequently encountered malformation was the venous angioma (59%), followed by telangiectasis (16%), AVM (14%), cavernous hemangioma (9%), and varix (2%).[130] These findings simply mean that small venous angiomas and telangiectases, which are most often not relevant from the clinical point of view, have also been overlooked in autopsy series.

The relative frequency with which cerebral vascular malformations are observed at CT or MRI has yet to be established.

ARTERIOVENOUS MALFORMATIONS

AVMs are probably the most commonly diagnosed type of cerebral vascular malformation and have the greatest tendency to bleed. Frequency of bleeding is quite variable both in neurosurgical series and in necropsy studies[169]; one-third to one-half of patients with AVM present at CT scan with intracranial hemorrhage.[74,87,168]

CT findings in nonbleeding AVMs are often diagnostic: AVMs usually appear as slightly hyperdense, well-defined lesions with sometimes irregular or multilobular but sharp margins; occasional thin hypodense areas at the periphery or within the lesion are seen; the lesions rarely exhibit mass effect, but are associated instead with dilatation of the homolateral ventricle and of the adjacent sulci. Calcifications are rarely seen, but microcalcifications may contribute to the high density of the lesion.

The low-density areas are sometimes the result of previous hematomas or infarctions or may represent surrounding atrophy or demyelination. Plain CT abnormalities, often suggestive of AVM, are seen in about 80% of the cases.[63,87] However, contrast medium administration is usually crucial for a specific diagnosis: the lesion strongly enhances, and tortuous vascular channels, representing the feeding arteries, but mostly the larger draining veins, are often demonstrated (Fig. 11.33).

Sometimes the features of the lesion are not so typical; MRI usually answers the question.

CT features are less evident when bleeding occurs: the hematoma may mask part of the lesion, and presence of mass effect and edema may lead one to include bleeding tumor in the differential diagnosis, but again MRI and angiography are usually diagnostic.

AVMs are more frequently lobar rather than deep; therefore, a spontaneous lobar hematoma in a young or middle-aged, nonhypertensive person should make one suspect vascular malformation. If angiography gives negative results, CT (or MRI) should, in any case, be repeated after resolution of the hematoma because of the possibility of detecting the nodule of the vascular malformation on late postcontrast CT scan. AVMs may, in fact, be occult on angiography either transiently when the bleeding occurs or permanently if they are thrombosed. CT (like MRI) is able to detect these lesions, which accounted for 11% of the cases reported by Leblanc et al.[87] However, in these cases, definite correct diagnosis is sometimes obtained only at histologic examination, and glioma or other tumors are a possible misdiagnosis.[10,83,86]

Figure 11.33 Arteriovenous malformation. **(A)** Plain computed tomography scan. **(B)** Postcontrast computed tomography scan. Postcontrast study also demonstrates feeding arteries (*arrowheads*).

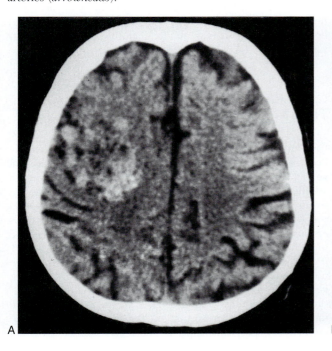
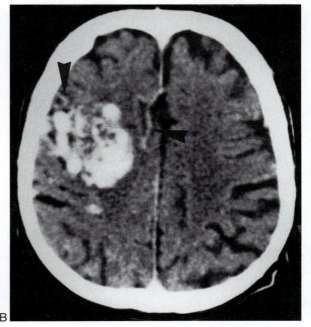

VENOUS ANGIOMAS

Of all cerebral vascular malformations, venous angiomas probably have the lowest tendency to bleed. We observed only two hematomas associated with venous angiomas, while demonstration of venous angiomas at angiography or CT or MRI is an incidental, not rare, occurrence in studies performed for unrelated reasons. The venous angioma is composed of a tuft of venous channels converging on a larger venous collector, interspersed in normal brain tissue. For this reason and because of reduced tendency to bleed, preventive surgery is not indicated and therefore pathologic demonstration is often lacking. The diagnosis, however, must be considered sufficiently proved when angiography demonstrates a group of veins in a medusa or umbrella-like pattern in normal venous phase, and when CT demonstrates that the venous channels cross the brain to reach a subependymal or a superficial vein without any nodule or other abnormalities of the surrounding brain tissue[164] (Fig. 11.34). The umbrella-like pattern reflects the embryologic development of these venous anomalies[163]; unfortunately, it is difficult to demonstrate with either CT or MRI.

A few cases with a small nodular component seen on postcontrast CT scan have been reported.[93,101] It is likely that the nodular component represents the point of convergence of the venous channels combined with tortuosity of the large draining vein. Otherwise, a nodular component on CT scan associated with a large draining vein points more to a cavernous hemangioma; MRI is helpful in defining these cases.

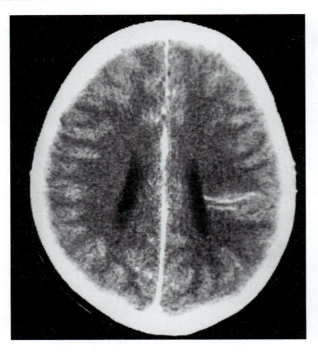

Figure 11.34 Venous angioma. Only postcontrast computed tomography scan shows the anomalous venous channels crossing normal brain tissue.

Mixed angiomas, arteriovenous and venous, telangiectatic and cavernous, are also sometimes observed on histologic examination.

CAVERNOUS HEMANGIOMAS

Cavernous hemangiomas are peculiar vascular malformations because they have no intervening brain tissue among the thin-walled sinusoidal spaces of which they are composed. Even if they do not have a true capsule, cavernous hemangiomas are well circumscribed and are therefore easily removed at surgery.[54] Cavernous hemangiomas are the second most relevant cerebral vascular malformation after AVMs, and MRI demonstrates them with increased frequency. Their frequency of bleeding is uncertain: before CT became available, it seemed high, because cavernous hemangiomas were diagnosed mostly when they had bled. After CT, cavernous hemangiomas presenting only with focal epilepsy were more frequently recognized.[134] However, even in these cases MRI demonstrates that microhemorrhages not detectable by CT are almost the rule.

The most frequent CT pattern consists of a well-defined, slightly inhomogeneous hyperdense area without mass effect (Fig. 11.35). Hypodense areas at the periphery or in the center of the nodule are rarely seen, while calcifications are most frequently observed. In four cases we observed, the cavernous hemangioma was isodense, recognizable only after contrast enhancement. Contrast enhancement is a constant feature.[135]

In our experience, cavernous hemangiomas were the most common angiographically occult vascular malformation. Pathologic circulation or early draining veins were found in only a minority of cases. Therefore, in the appropriate clinical setting, a combination of an avascular area in the capillary phase of the angiogram, with an enhancing nodule without mass effect on CT scan, suggests the possibility of cavernous hemangioma.[7,135] MRI demonstrates cavernous hemangiomas better than CT and may eliminate the necessity of angiography.

CAPILLARY ANGIOMAS OR TELANGIECTASES

Capillary angiomas seem to be the second most frequently occurring cerebral vascular malformation.[130] However, like venous angiomas, they are usually not clinically relevant. In addition, telangiectases are not demonstrated by angiography: to our knowledge, the only case in which pathologic circulation was reported was a mixed angioma, with telangiectases, cavernous angioma, and dilated venous channels.[125] Since the most frequent location of telangiectases is in the pons,[97,126] it is reasonable to suppose that spontaneous hematomas in nonhypertensive patients occurring in the pons are due, at least in part, to ruptured telangiectases. CT easily detects pontine hematomas; less frequently, it is able to demonstrate the underlying vascular malformation. However, in patients without hemorrhage, with symptoms and signs referable to a brain

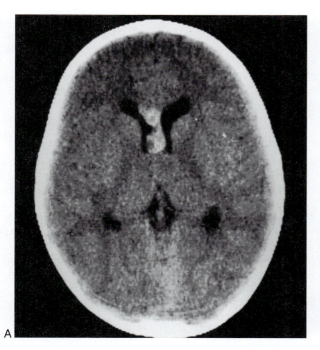
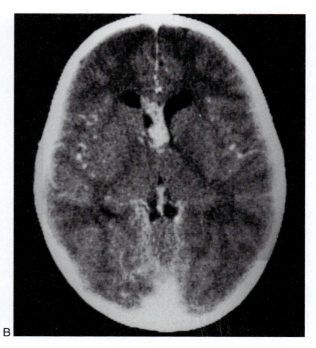

Figure 11.35 Cavernous hemangioma, surgically verified, in unusual, septal location. **(A)** Plain computed tomography scan shows well-defined, hyperdense lesion. **(B)** Lesion slightly enhances on postcontrast study. Magnetic resonance imaging yielded higher diagnostic specificity.

stem lesion, CT may occasionally demonstrate a hyperdense, sometimes calcified, enhancing lesion, without significant mass effect and without growth, consistent with a cryptic vascular malformation. Results of angiography are usually negative.[173] MRI in a few cases may suggest a cavernous hemangioma, but sometimes only a chronic hematoma is recognizable. Pathologic proof is almost always lacking; even in hemorrhagic cases, at evacuation of the hematoma, histologic diagnosis is usually not obtained.[113]

Summary

CT is by no means the only neuroradiologic examination that has to be performed in patients with cerebrovascular disease, and has largely been substituted for or complemented by MRI; but it is safe, noninvasive, and, in some instances, can conclude the neuroradiologic workup. CT studies may also be complemented with dynamic CT and with xenon enhancement to monitor the pathophysiologic changes that occur in cerebrovascular occlusive disease. However, these studies are not routinely performed and have not been included in this chapter.

CT, performed without contrast medium and sometimes with contrast enhancement (using iodine), is usually the first examination in patients with cerebrovascular disease, whether ischemic or hemorrhagic, and is extremely valuable in orienting the subsequent diagnostic and therapeutic approach. In suspected posterior fossa lesions, however, MRI should be the examination of choice. In patients with TIAs and infarcts, CT scan excludes the presence of unexpected lesions and the presence of bleeding, but other investigations are necessary if the site of the stenotic or occluded artery has to be determined. In patients with intracerebral bleeding, CT may be the only examination, but, if a vascular malformation is suspected, angiography becomes necessary. Angiography is always needed in SAH, provided that the patient's condition does not contraindicate the examination. In general, one should always consider the patient's condition and the medical or surgical therapeutic implications expected from the various studies to avoid unnecessary or risky procedures.

Acknowledgments

We would like to thank Dr. Carla Carollo and Dr. Luciano De Lorenzi for their collaboration in selecting CT scans, Ms. Luciana Caposio, x-ray technician, and Mr. Paolo Tinelli for photographic assistance.

References

1. Adams HP, Jr, Kassel NF, Torner JC, Sahs AL: CT and clinical correlations in recent aneurysmal subarachnoid hemorrhage: a preliminary report of the Cooperative Aneurysm Study. Neurology (NY) 33:981, 1983

2. Alcalà H, Gado M, Torack RM: The effect of size, histologic elements, and water content on the visualization of cerebral infarcts: a computerized cranial tomographic study. Arch Neurol 35:1, 1978

3. Ambrose J: Computerized transverse axial scanning (tomography). 2. Clinical application. Br J Radiol 46:1023, 1973

4. Araki G, Mihara H, Shizuka M et al: CT and arteriographic comparison of patients with transient ischemic attacks: correlation with small infarction of basal ganglia. Stroke 14:276, 1983

5. Arimitsu T, Di Chiro G, Brooks RA, Smith PB: White-grey matter differentiation in computed tomography. J Comput Assist Tomogr 1:437, 1977

6. Asari S, Satoh T, Sakurai M et al: The advantage of coronal scanning in cerebral computed angiotomography for diagnosis of moyamoya disease. Radiology 145:709, 1982

7. Bartlett JE, Kishore PRS: Intracranial cavernous angioma. AJR 128:653, 1977

8. Bastianello S, Pierallini A, Colonnese C et al: Hyperdense middle cerebral artery CT sign: comparison with angiography in the acute phase of ischemic supratentorial infarction. Neuroradiology 33:207, 1991

9. Beal MF, Williams RS, Richardson EP Jr, Fisher CM: Cholesterol embolism as a cause of transient ischemic attacks and cerebral infarction. Neurology (NY) 31:860, 1981

10. Becker DH, Townsend JJ, Kramer RA, Newton TH: Occult cerebrovascular malformations: a series of 18 histologically verified cases with negative angiography. Brain 102:249, 1979

11. Becker H, Desch H, Hacker H, Pencz A: CT fogging effect with ischemic cerebral infarcts. Neuroradiology 18:185, 1979

12. Berger L, Hakim AM: The association of hyperglycemia with cerebral edema in stroke. Stroke 17:865, 1986

13. Bergström M, Ericson K, Levander B et al: Variation with time of the attenuation values of intracranial hematomas. J Comput Assist Tomogr 1:57, 1977

14. Berman SA, Hayman LA, Hinck VC: Correlation of CT cerebral vascular territories with function. I. Anterior cerebral artery. AJR 135:253, 1980

15. Besson G, Robert C, Hommel M, Perret J: Is it clinically possible to distinguish nonhemorrhagic infarct from hemorrhagic stroke? Stroke 26:1205, 1995

16. Bogousslavsky J, Regli F, Uské A, Maeder P: Early spontaneous hematoma in cerebral infarct: is primary cerebral hemorrhage overdiagnosed? Neurology (NY) 41:837, 1991

17. Bogousslavsky J, Van Melle G, Regli F: The Lausanne Stroke Registry: analysis of 1,000 consecutive patients with first stroke. Stroke 19:1083, 1988

18. Boon A, Lodder J, Heuts-van Raak L, Kessels F: Silent brain infarcts in 755 consecutive patients with a first-ever supratentorial ischemic stroke. Relationship with index-stroke subtype, vascular risk factors, and mortality. Stroke 25:2384, 1994

19. Bozzao L, Bastianello S, Fantozzi LM et al: Correlation of angiographic and sequential CT findings in patients with evolving cerebral infarction. AJNR 10:1215, 1989

20. Bradac GB: CT and angiography in the diagnosis of cerebrovascular occlusive diseases, p. 199. In Cecchini A, Nappi G, Arrigo A (eds): Cerebral Pathology in Old Age. Neuroradiological and Neurophysiological Correlations. Emiras, Pavia, 1982

21. Bradac GB, Oberson R: CT and angiography in cases with occlusive disease of supratentorial cerebral vessels. Neuroradiology 19:193, 1980

22. Bradac GB, Oberson R: Angiography and Computed Tomography in Cerebro-Arterial Occlusive Disease. 2nd Ed. Springer-Verlag, New York, 1983

23. Brahme FJ: CT diagnosis of cerebrovascular disorders: a review. Comput Tomogr 2:173, 1978

24. Brandt T, Grau AJ, Hacke W: Severe stroke. Baillieres Clin Neurol 5:515, 1996

25. Brismar J: Computed tomography as the primary radiologic procedure in acute subarachnoid hemorrhage. Acta Radiol [Diagn] (Stockh) 20:849, 1979

26. Brismar J: Computed tomography in superior sagittal sinus thrombosis. Acta Radiol [Diagn] (Stockh) 21:321, 1980

27. Brott T, Broderick J, Kothari R et al: Early hemorrhage growth in patients with intracerebral hemorrhage. Stroke 28:1, 1997

28. Buonanno FS, Moody DM, Ball MR, Laster DW. Computed cranial tomographic findings in cerebral sinovenous occlusion. J Comput Assist Tomogr 2:281, 1978

29. Caillé JM, Guibert F, Bidabé AM et al: Enhancement of cerebral infarcts with CT. Comput Tomogr 4:73, 1980

30. Candelise L, Landi G, Orazio EN, Boccardi E: Prognostic significance of hyperglycemia in acute stroke. Arch Neurol 42:661, 1985

31. Caplan LR: Are terms such as completed stroke or RIND of continued usefulness? Stroke 14:431, 1983

32. Caplan LR, Mohr JP: Intracerebral hemorrhage: an update. Geriatrics 33:42, 1978

33. Cecchini A, Cosi V: TC: indicazioni diagnostiche, risultati e limiti nelle malattie cerebro-vascolari. Ital J Neurol Sci, suppl. 1:37, 1979

34. Constant P, Renou AM, Caillé JM et al: Aspects tomodensitométriques des accidents ischémiques cérébraux. J Neuroradiol 4:291, 1977

35. Damasio H: A computed tomographic guide to the identification of cerebral vascular territories. Arch Neurol 40:138, 1983

36. Davis JM, Davis KR, Crowell RM: Subarachnoid hemorrhage secondary to ruptured intracranial aneurysm: prognostic significance of cranial CT. AJNR 1:17, 1980

37. Davis JM, Ploetz J, Davis KR et al: Cranial computed tomography in subarachnoid hemorrhage: relationship between blood detected by CT and lumbar puncture. J Comput Assist Tomogr 4:794, 1980

38. Davis KR, Ackerman RH, Kistler JP, Mohr JP: Computed tomography of cerebral infarction: hemorrhagic, contrast enhancement, and time of appearance. Comput Tomogr 1:71, 1977

39. Davis KR, New PFJ, Ojemann RG et al: Computed tomographic evaluation of hemorrhage secondary to intracranial aneurysm. AJR 127:143, 1976

40. Davis KR, Taveras JM, New PFJ et al: Cerebral infarction diagnosis by computerized tomography: analysis and evaluation of findings. AJR 124:643, 1975

41. de Falco FA, Sepe Visconti O, Fucci G, Caruso G: Correlation between hyperglycemia and cerebral infarct size in patients with stroke. A clinical and X-ray computed tomography study in 104 patients. Schweiz Arch Neurol Psychiatr 144:233, 1993

42. Dolinskas CA, Bilaniuk LT, Zimmerman RA, Kuhl DE: Computed tomography of intracerebral hematomas. I. Transmission CT observations on hematoma resolution. AJR 129:681, 1977

43. Dolinskas CA, Bilaniuk LT, Zimmerman RA et al: Computed tomography of intracerebral hematomas. II. Radionuclide and transmission CT studies of the perihematoma region. AJR 129:689, 1977

44. Donnan GA, Tress BM, Bladin PF: A prospective study of lacunar infarction using computerized tomography. Neurology (NY) 32:49, 1982

45. Drake ME Jr, Shin C: Conversion of ischemic to hemorrhagic infarction by anticoagulant administration: report of two cases with evidence from serial computed tomographic brain scans. Arch Neurol 40:44, 1983

46. Fisher CM: Lacunar strokes and infarcts: a review. Neurology (NY) 32:871, 1982

47. Fisher CM, Adams RD: Observations on brain embolism with special reference to the mechanism of hemorrhagic infarction. J Neuropathol Exp Neurol 10:92, 1951

48. Fisher CM, Kistler JP, Davis JM: Relation of cerebral vasospasm to subarachnoid hemorrhage visualized by computerized tomographic scanning. Neurosurgery 6:1, 1980

49. Ford K, Sarwar M: Computed tomography of dural sinus thrombosis. AJNR 2:539, 1981

50. Friedman MB, Brant-Zawadzki M: Interhemispheric subdural hematoma from ruptured aneurysm. Comput Radiol 7:129, 1983

51. Gács G, Fox AJ, Barnett HJM, Viñuela F: CT visualization of intracranial arterial thromboembolism. Stroke 14:756, 1983

52. Ganti SR, Cohen M, Sane P, Hilal SK: Computed tomography of cerebral syphilis. J Comput Assist Tomogr 5:345, 1981

53. Ghoshhajra K, Scotti L, Marasco J, Baghai-Naiini P: CT detection of intracranial aneurysms in subarachnoid hemorrhage. AJR 132:613, 1979

54. Giombini S, Morello G: Cavernous angiomas of the brain: account of fourteen personal cases and review of the literature. Acta Neurochir (Wien) 40:61, 1978

55. Goto K, Ishii N, Fukasawa H: Diffuse white-matter disease in the geriatric population: a clinical, neuropathological, and CT study. Radiology 141:687, 1981

56. Gray F, Dubas F, Roullet E, Escourolle R: Leukoencephalopathy in diffuse hemorrhagic cerebral amyloid angiopathy. Ann Neurol 18:54, 1985

57. Grumme T, Lanksch W, Wende S: Diagnosis of spontaneous intracerebral hemorrhage by computerized tomography. p. 284. In Lanksch W, Kazner E (eds): Cranial Computerized Tomography. Springer-Verlag, Berlin, 1976

58. Hachinski VC, Potter P, Merskey H: Leukoaraiosis. Arch Neurol 44:21, 1987

59. Handa J, Nakano Y, Okuno T et al: Computerized tomography in moyamoya syndrome. Surg Neurol 7:315, 1977

60. Harwood-Nash DC, Fitz CR: Neuroradiology in Infants and Children. CV Mosby, St Louis, 1976

61. Hayman LA, Berman SA, Hinck VC: Correlation of CT cerebral vascular territories with function. II. Posterior cerebral artery. AJNR 2:219, 1981

62. Hayman LA, Evans RA, Bastion FO, Hinck VC: Delayed high dose contrast CT: identifying patients at risk of massive hemorrhagic infarction. AJNR 2:139, 1981

63. Hayman LA, Fox AJ, Evans RA: Effectiveness of contrast regimens in CT detection of vascular malformations of the brain. AJNR 2:421, 1981

64. Hayman LA, Sakai F, Meyer JS et al: Iodine-enhanced CT patterns after cerebral arterial embolization in baboons. AJNR 1:233, 1980

65. Heinz ER, Drayer BP, Haenggeli CA et al: Computed tomography in white-matter disease. Radiology 130:371, 1979

66. Heinz ER, Pizer SM, Fuchs H et al: Examination of the extracranial carotid bifurcation by thin-section dynamic CT: direct visualization of intimal atheroma in man (Part 1). AJNR 5:355, 1984

67. Hinshaw DB Jr, Thompson JR, Hasso AN, Casselman ES: Infarctions of the brainstem and cerebellum: a correlation of computed tomography and angiography. Radiology 137:105, 1980

68. Hirata Y, Matsukado Y, Fukumura A: Subarachnoid enhancement secondary to subarachnoid hemorrhage with special reference to the clinical significance and pathogenesis. Neurosurgery 11:367, 1982

69. Hodge CJ, Leeson M, Cacayorin E et al: Computed tomographic evaluation of extracranial carotid artery disease. Neurosurgery 21:167, 1987

70. Inoue Y, Saiwai S, Miyamoto T et al: Postcontrast computed tomography in subarachnoid hemorrhage from ruptured aneurysms. J Comput Assist Tomogr 5:341, 1981

71. Inoue Y, Takemoto K, Miyamoto T et al: Sequential computed tomography scans in acute cerebral infarction. Radiology 135:655, 1980

72. Iragui VJ, McCutchen CB: Capsular ataxic hemiparesis. Arch Neurol 39:528, 1982

73. Kasdon DL, Scott RM, Adelman LS, Wolpert SM: Cerebellar hemorrhage with decreased absorption values on computed tomography: a case report. Neuroradiology 13:265, 1977

74. Kendall BE, Claveria LE: The use of computed axial tomography (CAT) for the diagnosis and management of intracranial angiomas. Neuroradiology 12:141, 1976

75. Kendall BE, Lee BCP, Claveria E: Computerized tomography and angiography in subarachnoid hemorrhage. Br J Radiol 49:483, 1976

76. Kendall BE, Pullicino P: Intravascular contrast injection in ischaemic lesions. II. Effect on prognosis. Neuroradiology 19:241, 1980

77. Kendall BE, Radue EW: Computed tomography in spontaneous intracerebral haematoma. Br J Radiol 51:563, 1978

78. Kingsley DPE, Kendall BE, Moseley IF: Superior sagittal sinus thrombosis: an evaluation of the changes dem-

onstrated on computed tomography. J Neurol Neurosurg Psychiatry 41:1065, 1978

79. Kingsley DPE, Radue EW, Du Boulay EPGH: Evaluation of computed tomography in vascular lesions of the vertebrobasilar territory. J Neurol Neurosurg Psychiatry 43:193, 1980

80. Kinkel WR, Jacobs L, Kinkel PR: Gray matter enhancement: a computerized tomographic sign of cerebral hypoxia. Neurology (NY) 30:810, 1980

81. Kistler JP, Crowell RM, Davis KR et al: The relation of cerebral vasospasm to the extent and location of subarachnoid blood visualized by CT scan: a prospective study. Neurology (NY) 33:424, 1983

82. Kobari M, Meyer JS, Ichijo M, Oravez WT: Leukoaraiosis: correlation of MR and CT findings with blood flow, atrophy, and cognition. AJNR 11:273, 1990

83. Kramer RA, Wing SD: Computed tomography of angiographically occult cerebral vascular malformations. Radiology 123:649, 1977

84. Kushner M, Nencini P, Reivich M et al: Relation of hyperglycemia early in ischemic brain infarction to cerebral anatomy, metabolism, and clinical outcome. Ann Neurol 28:129, 1990

85. Ladurner G, Skvarc A, Sager WD: Computer tomography in transient global amnesia. Eur Neurol 21:34, 1982

86. Leblanc R, Ethier R: The computerized tomographic appearance of angiographically occult arteriovenous malformations of the brain. Can J Neurol Sci 8:7, 1981

87. Leblanc R, Ethier R, Little JR: Computerized tomography findings in arteriovenous malformations of the brain. J Neurosurg 51:765, 1979

88. Lee KF, Chambers RA, Diamond C et al: Evaluation of cerebral infarctions by computed tomography with special emphasis on microinfarction. Neuroradiology 16:156, 1978

89. Liliequist B, Lindqvist M, Valdimarsson E: Computed tomography and subarachnoid hemorrhage. Neuroradiology 14:21, 1977

90. Loeb C, Gandolfo C, Del Sette M et al: Asymptomatic cerebral infarctions in patients with ischemic stroke. Eur Neurol 36:343, 1996

91. Loizou LA, Kendall BE, Marshall J: Subcortical arteriosclerotic encephalopathy: a clinical and radiological investigation. J Neurol Neurosurg Psychiatry 44:294, 1981

92. Longo M, Fiumara F, Pandolfo I, D'Avella N: CT observation of an ongoing intracerebral hemorrhage. J Comput Assist Tomogr 7:362, 1983

93. Maehara T, Tasaka A: Cerebral venous angioma: computerized tomography and angiographic diagnosis. Neuroradiology 16:296, 1978

94. Manelfe C, Clanet M, Gigaud M et al: Internal capsule: normal anatomy and ischemic changes demonstrated by computed tomography. AJNR 2:149, 1981

95. Masdeu JC: Enhancing mass on CT: neoplasm or recent infarction? Neurology (NY) 33:836, 1983

96. Mason WG Jr, Latchaw RE, Yock DH, Jr: Spontaneous hemorrhage during cranial computed tomography. AJR 135:181, 1980

97. McCormick WF, Hardman JM, Boulter TR: Vascular malformations ("angiomas") of the brain, with special reference to those occurring in the posterior fossa. J Neurosurg 28:241, 1968

98. Meguro K, Hatazawa J, Yamaguchi T et al: Cerebral circulation and oxygen metabolism associated with subclinical periventricular hyperintensity as shown by magnetic resonance imaging. Ann Neurol 28:378, 1990

99. Menon D, Weir B, Overton T: Ventricular size and cerebral blood flow following subarachnoid hemorrhage. J Comput Assist Tomogr 5:328, 1981

100. Messina AV, Chernik NL: Computed tomography: the "resolving" intracerebral hemorrhage. Radiology 118:609, 1975

101. Michels LG, Bentson JR, Winter J: Computed tomography of cerebral venous angiomas. J Comput Assist Tomogr 1:149, 1977

102. Miller VT: Lacunar stroke: a reassessment. Arch Neurol 40:129, 1983

103. Mohr G, Ferguson G, Khan M et al: Intraventricular hemorrhage from ruptured aneurysm: retrospective analysis of 91 cases. J Neurosurg 58:482, 1983

104. Mohr JP: Lacunes. Stroke 13:3, 1982

105. Mohr JP, Biller J, Hilal SK et al: MR vs CT imaging in acute stroke. Stroke 26:807, 1995

106. Mohr JP, Caplan LR, Melski JW et al: The Harvard Cooperative Stroke Registry: a prospective registry. Neurology (NY) 28:754, 1978

107. Monajati A, Heggeness L: Patterns of edema in tumors vs. infarcts: visualization of white matter pathways. AJNR 3:251, 1982

108. Moseley IF, Olney J: Intracranial hemorrhage in the elderly: neuroradiology. p. 215. In Cecchini A, Nappi G, Arrigo A (eds): Cerebral Pathology in Old Age. Neuroradiological and Neurophysiological Correlations. Emiras, Pavia, 1982

109. Müller HR, Wiggli U: Cerebral, cerebellar and pontine hemorrhages. p. 249. In Du Boulay GH, Moseley IF (eds): CAT in Clinical Practice. Springer-Verlag, Berlin, 1977

110. Nelson RF, Pullicino P, Kendall BE, Marshall J: Computed tomography in patients presenting with lacunar syndromes. Stroke 11:256, 1980

111. New PFJ, Aronow S: Attenuation measurements of whole blood and blood fractions in computed tomography. Radiology 121:635, 1976

112. Norman D, Price D, Boyd D et al: Quantitative aspects of computed tomography of the blood and cerebrospinal fluid. Radiology 123:335, 1977

113. O'Laoire SA, Crockard A, Thomas DGT, Gordon DS: Brain-stem hematoma: a report of six surgically treated cases. J Neurosurg 56:222, 1982

114. Olszewski J: Subcortical arteriosclerotic encephalopathy: review of the literature on the so called Binswanger's disease and presentation of two cases. World Neurol 3:359, 1962

115. Paxton R, Ambrose J: The EMI scanner: a brief review of the first 650 patients. Br J Radiol 47:530, 1974

116. Perman GP, Racy A: Homolateral ataxia and crural paresis: case report. Neurology (NY) 30:1013, 1980

117. Perrone P, Candelise L, Scotti G et al: CT evaluation in patients with transient ischemic attack. Correlation

between clinical and angiographic findings. Eur Neurol 18:217, 1979

118. Pinto RS, Kricheff II, Butler AR, Murali R: Correlation of computed tomographic, angiographic and neuropathological changes in giant cerebral aneurysms. Radiology 132:85, 1979

119. Pluchino F, Lodrini S, Savoiardo M: Subarachnoid hemorrhage and meningioma: report of two cases. Acta Neurochir (Wien) 68:45, 1983

120. Pressman BD, Tourje EJ, Thomson JR: Early CT sign of ischemic infarction: increased density in a cerebral artery. AJNR 8:645, 1987

121. Pullicino P, Kendall BE: Contrast enhancement in ischemic lesions. I. Relationship to prognosis. Neuroradiology 19:235, 1980

122. Pullicino P, Nelson RF, Kendall BE, Marshall J: Small deep infarcts diagnosed on computed tomography. Neurology (NY) 30:1090, 1980

123. Rao KCVG, Knipp HC, Wagner EJ: Computed tomographic findings in cerebral sinus and venous thrombosis. Radiology 140:391, 1981

124. Rascol A, Clanet M, Manelfe C et al: Pure motor hemiplegia: CT study of 30 cases. Stroke 13:11, 1982

125. Roberson GH, Kase CS, Wolpow ER: Telangiectases and cavernous angiomas of the brain stem: "cryptic" vascular malformations: report of a case. Neuroradiology 8:83, 1974

126. Russell DS, Rubinstein LJ: Pathology of Tumours of the Nervous System. 3rd Ed. Edward Arnold, London, 1971

127. Sage MR: Blood-brain barrier: phenomenon of increasing importance to the imaging clinician. AJNR 3:127, 1982

128. Sage MR: Kinetics of water-soluble contrast media in the central nervous system. AJNR 4:897, 1983

129. Saris S: Chorea caused by caudate infarction. Arch Neurol 40:590, 1983

130. Sarwar M, McCormick WF: Intracerebral venous angioma: case report and review. Arch Neurol 35:323, 1978

131. Savoiardo M: The vascular territories of the carotid and vertebrobasilar system. Diagrams based on CT studies. Ital J Neurol Sci 7:405, 1986

132. Savoiardo M, Bracchi M: Neuroradiology of stroke. p. 94. In Callaghan N, Galvin R (eds): Recent Research in Neurology. Pitman, London, 1984

133. Savoiardo M, Bracchi M, Passerini A, Visciani A: The vascular territories in the cerebellum and brainstem: CT and MR study. AJNR 8:199, 1987

134. Savoiardo M, Passerini A: CT, angiography, and RN scans in intracranial cavernous hemangiomas. Neuroradiology 16:256, 1978

135. Savoiardo M, Strada L, Passerini A: Intracranial cavernous hemangiomas: neuroradiologic review of 36 operated cases. AJNR 4:945, 1983

136. Schoenberg BS, Mellinger JF, Schoenberg DG: Cerebrovascular disease in infants and children: a study of incidence, clinical features, and survival. Neurology (NY) 28:763, 1978

137. Schubiger O, Valavanis A, Hayek J: Computed tomography in cerebral aneurysms with special emphasis on giant intracranial aneurysms. J Comput Assist Tomogr 4:24, 1980

138. Schuknecht B, Ratzka M, Hofmann E: The "dense artery sign"—major cerebral artery thromboembolism demonstrated by computed tomography. Neuroradiology 32:98, 1990

139. Scotti G, Ethier R, Melançon D: Computed tomography in the evaluation of intracranial aneurysms and subarachnoid hemorrhage. Radiology 123:85, 1977

140. Scotti G, Spinnler H, Sterzi R, Vallar G: Cerebellar softening. Ann Neurol 8:133, 1980

141. Segall HD, Ahmadi J, McComb JG et al: Computed tomographic observations pertinent to intracranial venous thrombotic and occlusive disease in childhood: state of the art, some new data, and hypotheses. Radiology 143:441, 1982

142. Silver AJ, Pederson ME Jr, Ganti SR et al: CT of subarachnoid hemorrhage due to ruptured aneurysms. AJNR 2:13, 1981

143. Skriver EB, Olsen TS: Transient disappearance of cerebral infarcts on CT scan, the so-called fogging effect. Neuroradiology 22:61, 1981

144. Skriver EB, Olsen TS: Contrast enhancement of cerebral infarcts: incidence and clinical value in different states of cerebral infarction. Neuroradiology 23:259, 1982

145. Sobel DF, Li FC, Norman D, Newton TH: Cisternal enhancement following subarachnoid hemorrhage, abstracted. AJNR 1:374, 1980

146. Soisson T, Cabanis EA, Iba-Zizen MT et al: Pure motor hemiplegia and computed tomography: 19 cases. J Neuroradiol 9:304, 1982

147. Stiller J, Shanzer S, Yang W: Brainstem lesions with pure motor hemiparesis: computed tomographic demonstration. Arch Neurol 39:660, 1982

148. Suzuki J, Takaku A: Cerebrovascular "moyamoya" disease; disease showing abnormal netlike vessels in the base of the brain. Arch Neurol 20:288, 1969

149. Takahashi S, Goto K, Fukasawa H et al: Computed tomography of cerebral infarction along the distribution of the basal perforating arteries. I. Striate arterial group. Radiology 155:107, 1985

150. Takahashi S, Goto K, Fukasawa H et al: Computed tomography of cerebral infarction along the distribution of the basal perforating arteries. II. Thalamic arterial group. Radiology 155:119, 1985

151. Takeuchi S, Kobayashi K, Tsuchida T et al: Computed tomography in moyamoya disease. J Comput Assist Tomogr 6:24, 1982

152. Taneda M, Ozaki K, Wakayama A et al: Cerebellar infarction with obstructive hydrocephalus. J Neurosurg 57:83, 1982

153. The Nimodipine Study Group. American nimodipine trial in acute stroke. Stroke 23:1, 1992

154. Tomsick TA, Brott TG, Chambers AA et al: Hyperdense middle cerebral artery sign on CT: efficacy in detecting middle cerebral artery thrombosis. AJNR 11:473, 1990

155. Tomsick T, Brott T, Barsan W et al: Prognostic value of the hyperdense middle cerebral artery sign and stroke scale score before ultraearly thrombolytic therapy. AJNR 17:79, 1996

156. Tomura N, Uemura K, Inugami A et al: Early CT finding in cerebral infarction: obscuration of the lentiform nucleus. Radiology 168:463, 1988

157. Toni D, Fiorelli M, Bastianello S et al: Acute ischemic strokes improving during the first 48 hours of onset: predictability, outcome, and possible mechanisms. A comparison with early deteriorating strokes. Stroke 28:10, 1997

158. Tredici G, Pizzini G, Bogliun G, Tagliabue M: The site of motor corticospinal fibres in the internal capsule of man: a computerized tomographic study of restricted lesions. J Anat 134:199, 1982

159. Tress BM, Davis S, Lavain J et al: Incremental dynamic computed tomography: practical method of imaging the carotid bifurcation. AJNR 7:49, 1986

160. Trouillas P, Nighoghossian N, Getenet JC et al: Open trial of intravenous tissue plasminogen activator in acute carotid territory stroke. Correlations of outcome with clinical and radiological data. Stroke 27:882, 1996

161. Truwit C, Barkovich AJ, Gean-Marton A et al: Loss of the insular ribbon: another early CT sign of acute middle cerebral artery infarction. Radiology 176:801, 1990

162. Tsai FY, Teal JS, Heishima GB et al: Computed tomography in acute posterior fossa infarcts. AJNR 3:149, 1982

163. Valavanis A, Schefer S, Wichmann W: Cavernomas and venous angiomas of the brain. Riv Neuroradiol, suppl 2, 3:89, 1990

164. Valavanis A, Wellauer J, Yasargil MG: The radiological diagnosis of cerebral venous angioma: cerebral angiography and computed tomography. Neuroradiology 24:193, 1983

165. Van Gijn J, Kraaijeveld CL: Blood pressure does not predict lacunar infarction. J Neurol Neurosurg Psychiatry 45:147, 1982

166. Vonofakos D, Artmann H: CT findings in hemorrhagic cerebral infarct. Comput Radiol 7:75, 1983

167. Waxman SG, Toole JF: Temporal profile resembling TIA in the setting of cerebral infarction. Stroke 14:433, 1983

168. Weisberg LA: Computed tomography in the diagnosis of intracranial vascular malformations. Comput Tomogr 3:125, 1979

169. Weisberg LA, Nice C, Katz M: Cerebral Computed Tomography. A Text-Atlas. WB Saunders, Philadelphia, 1978

170. Wing SD, Norman D, Pollock JA, Newton TH: Contrast enhancement of cerebral infarcts in computed tomography. Radiology 121:89, 1976

171. Wodarz R: Watershed infarctions and computed tomography: a topographical study in cases with stenosis or occlusion of the carotid artery. Neuroradiology 19:245, 1980

172. Yates PO: Vascular disease of the central nervous system. p. 86. In Blackwood W, Corsellis JAN (eds): Greenfield's Neuropathology. 3rd Ed. Edward Arnold, London, 1976

173. Yeates A, Enzmann D: Cryptic vascular malformations involving the brainstem. Radiology 146:71, 1983

174. Yock DH Jr: CT demonstration of cerebral emboli. J Comput Assist Tomogr 5:190, 1981

175. Yock DH Jr, Larson DA: Computed tomography of hemorrhage from anterior communicating artery aneurysms, with angiographic correlation. Radiology 134:399, 1980

176. Yock DH Jr, Marshall WH Jr: Recent ischemic brain infarcts at computed tomography: appearances pre- and postcontrast infusion. Radiology 117:599, 1975

177. Zatz LM, Jernigan TL, Ahumada AJ Jr: White matter changes in cerebral computed tomography related to aging. J Comput Assist Tomogr 6:19, 1982

178. Zeumer H, Schonsky B, Sturm KW: Predominant white matter involvement in subcortical arteriosclerotic encephalopathy (Binswanger disease). J Comput Assist Tomogr 4:14, 1980

179. Zilkha A: Intraparenchymal fluid-blood level: a CT sign of recent intracerebral hemorrhage. J Comput Assist Tomogr 7:301, 1983

180. Zimmerman RA, Bilaniuk LT, Packer RJ et al: Computed tomographic-arteriographic correlates in acute basal ganglionic infarction of childhood. Neuroradiology 24:241, 1983

181. Zimmerman RD, Leeds NE, Naidich TP: Ring blush associated with intracerebral hematoma. Radiology 122:707, 1977

CHAPTER 12

Magnetic Resonance Scanning

R. L. DeLaPaz

J. P. MOHR

Magnetic resonance imaging (MRI) has become the preferred technique of brain imaging because of the wealth of information it offers. It has been limited in the past by long imaging times, compared with computed tomography (CT) scanning, but recent developments such as echo-planar imaging have greatly reduced this problem. The diminished sensitivity for the detection of acute hemorrhage, especially subarachnoid hemorrhage, has been another limiting factor of MRI, but a better understanding of early hemorrhage and recent experience with fluid attenuated inversion recovery (FLAIR) promises sensitivity rivaling CT scanning. The traditional advantages of CT, wider availability and lower cost, are becoming less valuable as MRI availability increases and costs come down. The manufacturers of MRI equipment have also made major strides in standardizing the instrumentation and making its operation within the grasp of most technologists with reasonable training. In addition, recent technical developments have produced capabilities beyond those of CT, including noninvasive imaging of cerebral vascular anatomy, tissue perfusion, and tissue water diffusion. Early experience with these methods suggests a potentially significant role in the identification of the vascular lesions associated with a cerebral ischemia and identification of the salvageable penumbra zone of incomplete ischemic injury. The role of MR spectroscopy continues to be evaluated, but long acquisition times, low spatial resolution, and the uncertain prognostic or therapeutic significance of the observed biochemical changes have limited enthusiasm for its use in the clinical management of cerebral ischemia.

Basic Principles

MRI is based on the interaction between radio waves and certain nuclei of the body tissues, in the presence of a powerful magnetic field. Hydrogen nuclei (protons) are the most common MR-observable nuclei within the human body. They enter into the composition of water, fats, and almost every other organic molecule normally present in tissue. Water protons and fat protons are the most extensively imaged clinically. The nuclei that are visible to MR have specific internal rotation properties, called spin, and are often referred to as "spins." Besides hydrogen, other nuclei such as sodium, phosphorus, carbon, and fluorine are being investigated with MRI and MR spectroscopy at magnetic field strength ranging from 1.5 to 4 Tesla (T). These nuclei are much less abundant than hydrogen and are less sensitive to MR methods, thus producing weaker signals and therefore images of much lower spatial resolution and spectra of lower signal-to-noise ratio than is possible with protons.

When the human body is positioned in a strong magnetic field its MR-observable nuclei become susceptible to excitation by intermittent radiofrequency (rf) pulses. The energy from the rf pulses is absorbed and then released from the tissue at the same frequency as the spins return toward baseline magnetic equilibrium, a process called relaxation. This process can be visualized as an aggregate magnetic vector produced by the population of nuclear spins that is flipped out of alignment with the magnetic field and then returns to alignment. For most clinical imaging, two rf pulses are applied, the first producing a 90° flip and the second a 180° flip of the magnetic vector. This sequence produces a return signal called a spin echo. The energy released from the excited spins as they realign governs the intensity of this echo and is characterized by two relaxation time constants known as T_1 and T_2. MRI methods sample these constants through the timing of the rf pulses applied to the tissue and the timing of the signals that return from the tissue. The most important of the rf timing parameters are the repetition time (TR) of the applied radiofrequency pulse sequence and the time after these pulses that a spin echo returns (TE). The signal elicited from different tissues by these pulse sequences can be predicted by the relative length of the TR and TE times. A short TR is typically in the range of 300 to 600 ms and a long TR in the range of 2,000 to 3,000 ms. A short TE is typically 10 to 30 ms and a long TE 80 to 120 ms. The contrast in a given MR image will depend on the interaction of these timing parameters and the relaxation time constants within each tissue according to the following general rules: (1) in short TR–short TE images, called T_1-weighted images, contrast depends mostly on T_1 differences between tissues (in brain this results in low signal from the cerebrospinal fluid (CSF) relative to the brain while fat has a high signal intensity); (2) in long TR–long TE images, called T_2-weighted images, contrast depends mostly on T_2 differences between tissues (in brain this results in high signal from the CSF relative to brain while fat has a low signal); and (3) in long TR–short TE images, often (incorrectly) called "spin density" or "proton density" images, contrast is the result of a balance between T_1 and T_2 differences in tissues (in brain this results in a similar signal between the CSF and brain). These images are more correctly referred to as "balanced" images. They are not true proton density images (i.e., images in which the signal is dependent only on the abundance of protons in the tissue and independent of T_1 and T_2 relaxation effects). True proton density images would require impractically long TR and short TE times. Although technically erroneous, reference to these balanced images as proton density images has become common practice and is the accepted shorthand term for long TR–short TE images obtained in clinical practice.

Another type of pulse sequence produces T_2°-weighted images. T_2° is a relaxation constant similar to but shorter than T_2 and more directly sensitive to tissue magnetic field inhomogeneities or areas of magnetic susceptibility difference. This sensitivity to variations in tissue magnetic susceptibility is enhanced by the use of long TE times and a gradient shift rather than a second of pulse to produce the signal echo, generating so-called "gradient-echo" or "field-echo" images. Gradient-echo images are also usually obtained with a partial flip angle for the initial rf pulse. A partial flip angle rf pulse produces a $<90°$ flip of the nuclear magnetic vector, typically in the range of 10° to 30°. Use of gradient echoes and partial flip angles allows rapid acquisition of images with T_2 and T_2° sensitivity. T_2° sensitivity is also enhanced by imaging at higher magnetic fields, such as 1.5 or 4 T gradient-echo images which emphasize that the T_2° effect of paramagnetic blood products are often used for the study of patients with stroke to evaluate the presence of hemorrhage.

Finally, the use of flow-sensitive imaging techniques has permitted the depiction of the extracranial and intracranial blood vessels in a totally noninvasive fashion. Arteries and veins can be imaged separately. Images depicting cerebral perfusion and diffusion of water molecules have also been improving in quality and precision and are rapidly becoming important tools in the evaluation of cerebral ischemia.

Techniques

A standard protocol for the study of a patient with stroke includes images with T_1-weighted, T_2-weighted and balanced or proton density images (long TR–short TE images). The T_1-weighted images (TR 300 to 600 ms and TE 20 to 30 ms) provide good anatomic definition and are most useful for the detection

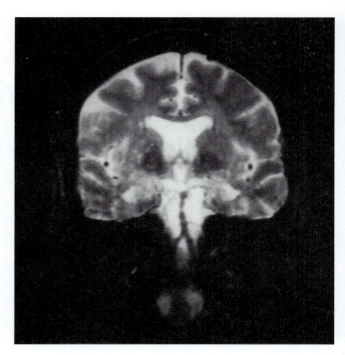

Figure 12.1 Coronal T_2-weighted MR image showing basilar stenosis shown independently by angiogram and insonated by transcranial Doppler.

of subacute or chronic hemorrhage or vascular thrombosis. Gyral swelling can often be appreciated on T_1-weighted images. T_2-weighted images (TR ≳ 2,500 ms and TE 80 to 120 ms) are best suited for the demonstration of cerebral parenchymal damage and the associated increase in tissue water encountered in brain edema and infarction. This pulse sequence is also helpful in depicting the normal signal void from arteries and veins. Occluded or stenotic vessels can often be demonstrated on these images (Fig. 12.1). T_2-weighted images have become the preferred pulse sequence for the demonstration of the site and extent of increased tissue water accompanying subacute edema or chronic infarction. Many lesions well below the size detected on CT are found by MR. A balanced or proton density image (TR 2,500 ms, TE 30 ms) helps in depicting infarctions close to the ventricle or sulci, which may be obscured by high signal from CSF on T_2-weighted images. The recently developed FLAIR imaging sequence appears to carry this advantage further by completely suppressing signal from the CSF and enhancing sensitivity to tissue T_1 and T_2 prolongation. Gradient-echo images with a partial flip angle and a long TE are recommended for the detection of small amounts of acute or chronic hemorrhage.

The greatest strides in very early, hyperacute, stroke detection have come from new methods of imaging the regional perfusion of the brain, with and without paramagnetic contrast agent injection, and imaging of the focal restriction of water (proton) diffusion that occurs with ischemic cytotoxicity. Paramagnetic contrast agents, such as gadolinium-diethylenetri-aminepentaacetic acid (Gd-DTPA), have also been used to enhance arterial signal on T_1-weighted images in the acute stages of major vascular territory infarction.[119] Early arterial enhancement is felt to indicate either proximal occlusion or severe stenosis of enhancing arteries. The use of paramagnetic contrast agents also helps to define areas of blood-brain barrier breakdown. This occurs later than identifiable perfusion defects or arterial enhancement, usually at 3 to 7 days after onset, a period approximately coincident with the parenchymal contrast enhancement seen on CT scans.

The appearance of hemorrhage on T_1- and T_2-weighted images is complex; it varies from hypo- to hyperintense over the first hours and days and evolves differently in different locations, such as parenchymal and subdural spaces. The paramagnetic effect of the naturally occurring methemoglobin and hemosiderin permits dating of hematomas and helps separate hematomas from hemorrhagic infarction.[21] Flowing blood helps diagnose arteriovenous malformations, and the characteristic appearance of hemorrhages of different ages permits a diagnosis of angiographically negative cavernous angioma as never before. MRI is the most sensitive imaging modality for the detection of cavernous angiomas because of the paramagnetic effect of old blood. Subdural and epidural hemorrhages are easily demonstrated, especially in the subacute phase when they appear as high signal on T_1-weighted images, often when asymptomatic because of their age or small size. Also, small chronic subdural hematomas and epidural hematomas often missed on CT can be readily detected by MRI.

MR angiography (MRA) is rapidly gaining acceptance for the diagnosis of intracranial and extracranial vascular disease. Each of the carotid vessels or the vertebral arteries can be depicted individually in multiple projections, providing an accurate assessment of the profile of the vessel that is quite comparable to angiography. Moderate carotid stenosis and vessel occlusion are diagnosed by MRA with almost the same sensitivity and specificity as conventional angiography. At present, the limitation lies in the inability of MRA to image highly stenotic vessels with a minute residual open lumen. Inaccuracy arises from the loss of signal in a stenotic segment caused either by high flow rates through moderate to severe stenoses, which produce loss of signal (dephasing) and apparent discontinuity in the vessel, or by very slow flow in a nearly occluded lumen that is not seen because the lumen signal is obscured by noise or lack of time-of-flight effect. Intracranial aneurysms and arteriovenous malformations can be detected by a variety of imaging techniques including conventional T_2-weighted images and MRA pulse sequences.

Diffusion and Perfusion Imaging of Hyperacute Ischemia

Although early MR experimental studies of cerebral ischemia in animal models suggested that increased signal, due to increased tissue free water, may be seen on T_2-weighted images as early as 30 minutes,[10] it has not been a consistent finding in hyperacute ischemia (<6 hours), and human clinical studies have shown a more prolonged latency of 6 to 12 hours. Recent work indicates that functional MRI imaging of cerebral blood perfusion and tissue water diffusion provide more sensitive and specific measures of tissue metabolic status in hyperacute ischemia, within the therapeutic window for acute stroke treatment.

Perfusion MRI, also referred to as hemodynamically weighted MRI, may be performed using either the first pass contrast bolus method or spin tagging of endogenous protons in blood water.

Both methods measure the definitive physiologic changes in ischemia: reduced cerebral blood flow (CBF) and blood volume (CBV), as well as increased mean transit time (MTT) of blood through the tissue. Although accurate quantitative tissue blood flow and blood volume measures can be obtained with these methods experimentally, the applications currently used in clinical practice generate relative or regional values (rCBF and rCBV) because of the difficulty in deriving accurate arterial input functions and capillary transit times of the contrast agent or tagged spins. The first-pass bolus method, also called bolus tracking or susceptibility-based perfusion imaging, uses an intravenous injection of paramagnetic contrast material, such as Gd-DTPA, which creates local magnetic field gradients around blood vessels as the highly concentrated initial bolus of contrast material passes through the cerebral vessels and capillaries. These local gradients are produced by the difference between the high magnetic susceptibility of the paramagnetic contrast agent and the lower susceptibility of the surrounding tissue. The gradients create microscopic magnetic field inhomogenieties that cause acceleration of T_2 and $T_2°$ relaxation rates, which results in signal loss on T_2- and $T_2°$-weighted MR images. The degree of signal loss over the duration of the bolus passage is proportional to tissue blood volume. The MTT can also be derived from these time-intensity curves, and estimates of CBF can be derived according to the central volume principle (CBF = CBV/MTT). The spin tagging methods, sometimes called time-of-flight methods, do not use an exogenous contrast agent. They are performed by magnetically labeling endogenous water protons in arterial blood and then detecting the difference in magnetization as these protons flow into cerebral tissue. The magnetic labeling is done with MR coils over the neck vessels, and images of the brain are obtained after a short interval. The perfusion images obtained with these methods more directly reflect CBF, rather than CBV, as with susceptibility methods.

Diffusion MRI measures the microscopic motion of water protons in tissue noninvasively and has been quantified using the apparent diffusion coefficient (ADC), which lumps the effects of random and restricted water motion in tissue.[55] A slowed diffusion rate (reduced ADC) appears to be a sensitive marker of the failure of cellular energy metabolism in ischemic cerebral tissue. In experimental studies diffusion-weighted images (DWIs) consistently show increased signal, indicating reduced diffusion rates, as early as 2 to 3 minutes after severe ischemia onset.[13] Other animal experiments suggest that the mechanism for this change in diffusion is the shift of extracellular water into the intracellular space, where the bound fraction of water is higher and water molecule motion is more restricted.[77] This is supported by evidence that electrical impedance of ischemic brain tissue is reduced, which indicates a decrease in the extracellular space.[67] Peri-ischemic depolarization, known to contribute to the evolution of cerebral infarction, evokes disturbances that can be detected by DWI signal increases (reduced diffusion rates).[39] The metabolic correlate of reduced diffusion in cerebral ischemia appears to be the collapse of cellular energy metabolism and failure of the cell membrane Na-K adenosine triphosphate (ATP).[5,13] Diffusion rates have been shown to decrease with experimental inhibition of the Na-K-ATPase pump using ouabain, and diffusion rate decreases coincide with ATP depletion and acidosis in cerebral ischemic lesions.[3,5,76] Severe ADC reductions have also been shown to match closely histopathologic evidence of ischemic injury.[3,59,72,90] Diffusion reductions in acute ischemia are closely related to measures of cerebral perfusion. Absolute tissue perfusion under 15 to 20 ml/100 g/min appears to be the threshold for reduced diffusion and also corresponds to the threshold for dysfunction of Na-K-ATPase activity in cerebral tissue.[13,95] Mild or moderate reductions in CBF may produce no change in ADC or reductions that are reversible with reperfusion in <1 hour or with administration of neuroprotective agents within 15 minutes (e.g., Na^+-Ca^{2+} ion channel modulators such as N-methyl-D-aspartate antagonists).[41,54,59,71]

As sensitive as diffusion imaging appears to be for early cytotoxic changes, diffusion abnormalities alone do not fully define ischemic lesions. Correlation with measures of cerebral perfusion are necessary. Early experience with combined diffusion and perfusion imaging in human ischemic stroke indicates a complex relationship between these parameters.[14,98] The presence of matched diffusion and perfusion abnormalities (reductions in both ADC and CBV) is 90% to 100% predictive of a nonrecoverable clinical deficit.[61,99,114] Mismatches between diffusion and perfusion abnormalities are more difficult to interpret and appear to have variable predictive values for final lesion outcome. Diffusion abnormalities larger than perfusion abnormalities, rare in human studies, may be the counterpart to the reversible diffusion seen in animal studies.[98] The outer zone of normal perfusion and reduced diffusion may represent recovering tissue if reperfusion is sufficiently early or dying tissue if reperfusion is too late. More experience with human stroke is needed to understand this rare mismatch fully. Mismatches between a smaller, central diffusion abnormality and a larger, overlapping perfusion defect appear to identify a partially ischemic penumbra zone of potentially salvageable tissue, sometime called the zone of "misery" perfusion. Early indications also suggest that accurate quantitation of these parameters is important in that there appear to be threshold levels of abnormal diffusion and perfusion above which recovery may occur with reperfusion and/or neuroprotective therapy.[118]

The complexity of applying these imaging methods to clinical lesions is illustrated by recent reports outlining their predictive value. Early experience at one center suggests that CBV may be the best predictor of final lesion size, while another group has found a measure of perfusion delay, the time to peak (TTP), to be the best predictor.[14,102] The first report suggests that the best predictor of final lesion size may be the region of reduced CBV. This appears to be the best match with the chronic lesion seen on T_2-weighted images in followup. The early changes on DWI appear to be smaller, and the CBF abnormality appears to be larger than the final lesion. MTT (derived from the ratio of CBV/CBF) is a sensitive indicator of ischemia but may overestimate the final lesion size in areas where partial ischemia is reversed before permanent tissue damage occurs. In rapidly evolving acute ischemic lesions there may be an initial increase of CBV in response to

reduced CBF, producing an increased MTT, which persists in the periphery of the lesion, while the low CBV in the central lesion represents cerebrovascular collapse and the zone of true infarction.[14] The second report illustrates integration of diffusion and perfusion imaging into clinical evaluation of acute stroke in 38 patients within the first 5 hours.[102] Rapid MRI access (<40 minutes from emergency room presentation) with a short imaging protocol (20 minutes) and quick image processing (5 minutes) of DWI and Gd-DTPA bolustracking perfusion maps allowed incorporation of these studies into acute therapeutic decision making. T_2-weighted and (FLAIR; see below) images were negative in these patients. Both CBV and TTP maps were generated and correlated with the DWI images to assess the potential volume of tissue that was likely to respond to therapy, the penumbra zone. This early experience suggested that the DWI image abnormalities seen after 1 to 2 hours identify the tissue that has already undergone irreversible energy failure and infarction. The TTP maps identified underperfused tissue outside this zone that remained at risk and were the best predictors of final lesion size on follow-up T_2-weighted images. Other centers have seen a more variable predictive value of acute TTP maps with as much as a two times overestimate of the lesion size, probably caused by delayed but effective collateral flow at the borderzones of the perfusion abnormality.[62] Similar experience is accumulating using a related measure of delayed tissue perfusion, the MTT.[14] This field is rapidly evolving, and a consensus on the predictive value of diffusion and perfusion measures in clinical practice is likely to be reached in the near future. Monitoring of reperfusion and neuroprotective experimental therapy with these methods has also begun. These methods are likely to become the best way to assess improved perfusion and/or reduced expansion of the central infarct zone during neuroprotective therapy of hyperacute cerebral ischemia in the clinical setting.

As cerebral infarcts age there is a gradual prolongation of the short ADCs in the central ischemic zone. Histologic examination in animal studies has shown early neuronal injury followed by intense gliotic activity and protein leakage associated with infarction and edema on day 2, as well as cavitation in severely infarcted areas on day 6.[65] These lesions show initial ADC reductions followed by ADC increases on day 2, which may be associated with vasogenic edema and cell lysis. Later elevations in ADC are probably related to cavitation of infarcted tissue. In some cases this ADC prolongation may result in a pseudonormalization of the DWI scans as diffusion rates become similar to normal tissue on the way to prolonged values in the chronic lesion. This normalization may result in disappearance of the lesion on the DWI studies and typically occurs at 5 to 10 days after an infarct but may be delayed to 60 days in some cases.[32,113,114] Typically, after about 10 days the ADC becomes elevated above normal brain and may reach high levels in regions of high signal on T_2-weighted images in which cystic encephalomalacia is the histopathogic end point of the ischemic injury (Fig. 12.2).

TRANSIENT ISCHEMIC ATTACKS

Two of the studies that address early human stroke evaluation with diffusion and perfusion imaging have described absent or reversible changes in these measures with transient symptomatology. In five patients, transient ischemic stroke symptoms lasting for 1 to 48 hours were associated with normal conventional MRI as well as DWI and perfusion images.[63,98] In one patient, early abnormal findings on DWI (low calculated ADC) resolved at 36 hours along with resolution of symptoms.[63] Experimental studies support the insensitivity or reversibility of these measures if cellular injury thresholds are not reached. It appears that DWI images do not change until CBF drops below 15 to 20 ml/100 g/min and usually remain normal until near total occlusion of arterial blood supply occurs (without sufficient collateral flow).[13,95] Reductions in cerebral perfusion (CBV or CBF) may be able to identify the site of transient ischemia, but the current semiquantitative nature of these measures with MRI and the wide variability of normal values make it difficult to rely on these measures alone. The combination of perfusion measures to assess relative ischemia and DWI as a monitor of cellular injury appears to be the best way to use MRI to evaluate the severity of transient or resolving symptoms and to predict the eventual degree of cerebral injury.[98]

The perfusion and diffusion techniques described above require specialized hardware and software upgrades to be used on clinical MRI systems, although many 1.5 T commercial units now in production include these options. The key modification is the ability to acquire multislice imaging data very rapidly, preferably over the whole head. The optimal hardware modification is the addition of echoplanar imaging (EPI), which allows acquisition of a complete image with a single rf echo, in as little as 20 to 100 ms. EPI imaging maximizes the temporal sampling frequency for perfusion studies and virtually eliminates macroscopic tissue motion in diffusion studies.[19] On systems with conventional hardware, software modifications can be used to program fast gradient-echo pulse sequences or spiral techniques, which can provide adequate temporal resolution for perfusion and diffusion studies.[55]

Conventional Imaging of Acute and Subacute Ischemia

Although perfusion and diffusion methods are becoming available on many MRI systems, their use requires hardware and software modifications. The bulk of routine clinical imaging in cerebral ischemia is still done using conventional T_1- and T_2-weighted MRI. The earliest changes observed with these methods in ischemic stroke have been those relating to abnormal vascular dynamics and to morphologic changes resulting from brain swelling (Fig. 12.2). T_2-weighted parenchymal signal increases in some patients with nonhemorrhagic strokes have been seen as early as 45 minutes,[74] but the latency is greater than 6 to 8 hours in 85% to 90% of cases. Newer methods, such as FLAIR, may improve the sensitivity to early ischemia but are unlikely to provide the immediate identification and characterization of lesions that are available from diffusion and perfusion methods. The early changes on conventional MRI in acute stroke can be categorized as follows.

ABNORMAL IMAGES OF THE CEREBRAL VESSELS

The absence of the normal flow void may be an early sign of arterial occlusion. A report by Uchino et al[108] described ten angiographically proven examples of middle cerebral artery stem occlusion with stroke that were identified by the absence of flow void on MR, demonstrated as an isodense or hypodense structure on T_2-weighted images. Absence of the expected flow void on T_2-weighted images was also found in the sylvian fissure in eight cases. Another vascular sign is arterial contrast enhancement, which is observed on the T_1-weighted images and consists of a conspicuous high intensity of the major arteries, commonly in the sylvian fissure and sometimes in cortical sulci. It is seen in the arteries supplying the region of infarctions, where there is substantial slowing of the circulation and vasodilatation. The enhancement may be associated with partial occlusion of the artery or complete occlusion with contrast enhancement supplied by retrograde collateral filling (Fig. 12.3).[15,119] This finding is often the earliest sign of cerebral ischemia available when only conventional T_1-weighted and T_2-weighted images are acquired. It is seen in more than half the patients studied with contrast-enhanced MRI in the first 24 hours after onset of symptoms and in 75% of cases within the first 3 days.[15,25,96,119] These statistics refer to patients who will eventually develop an MR-observable infarction in the area of the clinical stroke. Transient ischemic attacks are excluded from these statistics. Occlusion of the vessel from thrombosis or embolism will also, at some stage, appear as a high-signal vessel, analogous to the hyperdense vessel sign on CT scans. Wall hemorrhage can also been seen in an artery suffering dissection (Fig. 12.4).

LOCAL BRAIN SWELLING

Local brain swelling refers to the observation of swollen gyri or mass effects without alteration of the signal in the brain. This finding is more pronounced in cases of cortical infarction and is seen in the first 24 hours in two-thirds of the patients who will eventually develop an infarction observable on MR. It can precede the T_2 signal changes by several hours.

CHANGES IN THE PARENCHYMAL SIGNAL INTENSITY ON T_1- AND T_2-WEIGHTED AND PROTON DENSITY IMAGES

It is uncommon to see changes on T_2-weighted MR in the first few hours after stroke, at most in 15% of cases within the first 8 hours.[74] At 24 hours almost 90% of patients who eventually develop an MR-observable infarction will show signal change on T_2-weighted sequences.[11,119] This is compared with 50% sensitivity on T_1-weighted images (Fig. 12.5). The lower sensitivity of the T_1-weighted images is due to the opposing effects of T_1 prolongation (which produces lower signal) and T_2 prolongation (which produces higher signal) in areas of increased tissue water content. T_2-weighted images and proton density images

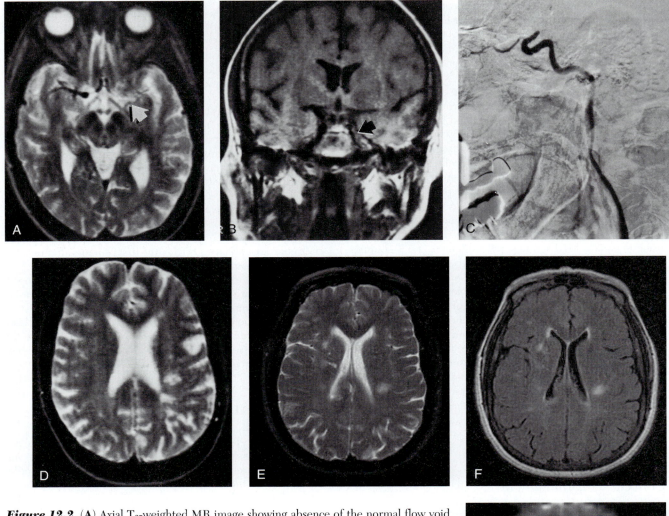

Figure 12.2 (**A**) Axial T$_2$-weighted MR image showing absence of the normal flow void in the middle cerebral artery and no signal changes in the brain. (**B**) Coronal T$_1$-weighted MR image showing the signal void in the middle cerebral artery and early hemispheral edema. (**C**) Angiogram demonstrating the occluded middle cerebral artery. (**D**) Axial T$_2$-weighted MR image showing the high-convexity, centrum semiovale "distal field" infarction. In a different patient (**E**) T$_2$-weighted and (**F**) FLAIR images show nonspecific bilateral periventricular high-signal lesions indicating acute, subacute, or chronic white matter ischemia. (**G**) The DWI shows high signal only in the left-sided lesion, indicating an acute to subacute white matter infarct. The low diffusion rate in this lesion produces DWI high signal, whereas higher diffusion rates in the chronic lesions make them isointense with the surrounding brain.

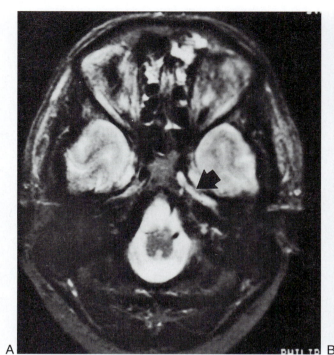

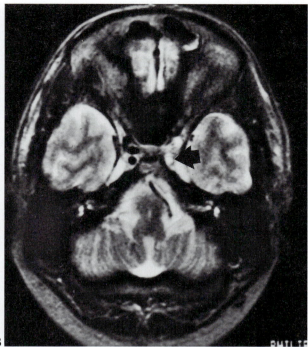

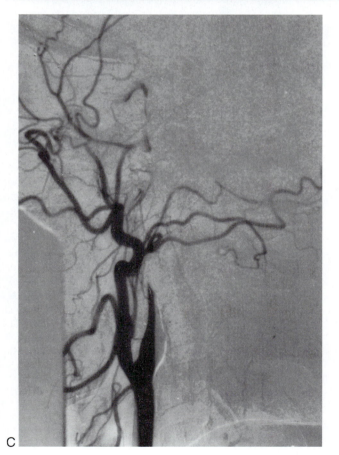

Figure 12.3 (**A**) MR image showing lack of signal void due to occlusion of the carotid (arrows). (**B**) Patent intracranial vertebral (arrow) in the same case. (**C**) Angiogram showing the extracranial carotid dissection in the same angiogram.

Illustration continued on following page

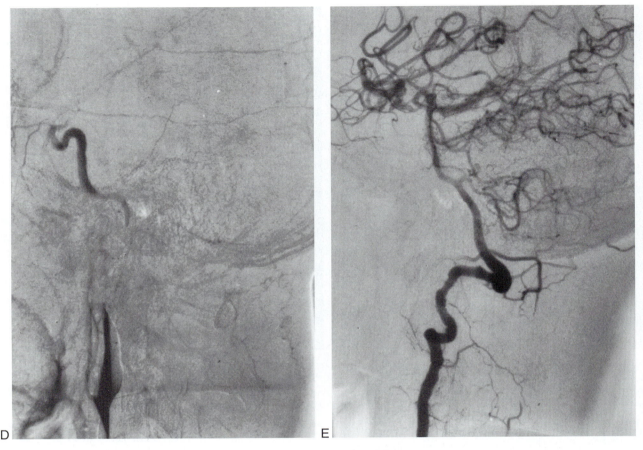

Figure 12.3 *(Continued)* (**D**) Angiogram showing the vertebral dissection. (**E**) Angiogram showing the vertebral dissection in the same angiogram.

are probably equally sensitive to tissue water changes, but proton density images often show lesions more conspicuously in the early phase, especially those that lie close to the ventricles and subarachnoid spaces where the high signal of the CSF can mask them on T_2-weighted images.

The time course of the parenchymal signal changes on T_2-weighted sequences follows the morphologic evidence of brain swelling by several hours. The appearance of the high signal on the T_2-weighted image coincides with the appearance and course of vasogenic edema that results from the blood-brain barrier damage. The initial brain swelling is presumed to coincide with the cytotoxic edema phase, in which a small amount of water (about 3% of tissue volume) is believed to enter the intracellular space as a consequence of the failure of the Na-K-ATP pump. Such a small change of tissue water appears to be insufficient to change the T_2 characteristic of brain tissue. Also, in the early stage of infarction tissue water, particularly intracellular water of cytotoxic edema, may be bound and less available for MR observation.

Signal changes more than 24 hours after the onset of ischemic stroke are seen in most cases (Fig. 12.6). Furthermore, 30% of patients with an infarction visualized in the first 24 hours show an increase in size on the follow-up scan.[11] The size of abnormal T_2 findings gradually reaches a maximum by 5 to 7 days, after which it gradually subsides to a stable

size after about 2 months.[31] In some studies, a "fogging" effect has been seen in the subacute period, analogous to that seen on CT, and has been explained as developing hemorrhagic infarction: the low signal produced by petechial hemorrhage balances the high signal of the ischemic lesion.

The shrinkage of tissue after infarction is a well-known effect. Less well known is the distant effect on pathways and target organs as the degenerating fiber pathways cause tissue shrinkage. Uchino et al[109] studied presumed wallerian degeneration of the corticospinal tract through the brain in 25 patients who had suffered supratentorial infarction. Within 3 months some signal hyperintensities were seen on T_2-weighted images ipsilaterally in the brain stem, and at 6 months the ipsilateral brain stem had become smaller ipsilaterally.

CHANGES IN THE PARENCHYMAL SIGNAL INTENSITY ON FLAIR IMAGES

FLAIR, recently developed conventional pulse sequence, appears to offer improved sensitivity to early ischemic changes over T_1-weighted and T_2-weighted spin-echo or fast spin-echo

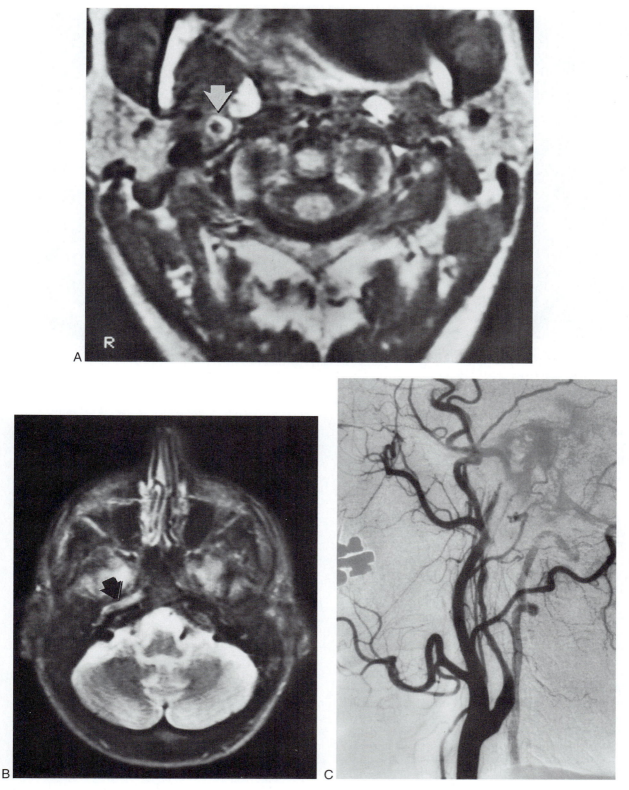

Figure 12.4 (**A**) T₂-weighted MR image showing carotid dissection with hematoma in the extracranial carotid vessel wall (arrow). (**B**) T₂-weighted MR image showing high signal from slowed arterial flow in the petrous portion of the internal carotid. (**C**) The angiogram shows the dissection in the extracranial portion of the internal carotid.

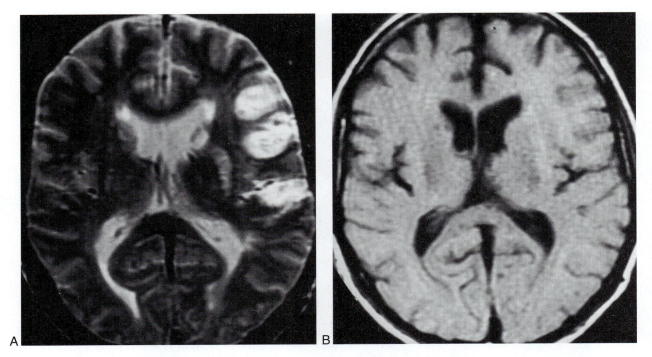

Figure 12.5 (**A**) T$_2$-weighted MR image 27 hours after stroke showing acute hemispheral convexity infarction. (**B**) T$_1$-weighted MR image at 27 hours showing faint changes over the same site that showed prominent changes on T$_2$.

images. FLAIR images are acquired with an inversion rf pulse that is delivered at a time TI before the 90 degree rf imaging pulse. The TI time is approximately equal to the T$_1$ relaxation time of CSF, about 2 seconds at 1.5 T. This results in a nulling of the signal from free water, making the CSF in the basal cisterns, sulci, and ventricles appear black and giving high contrast against the normal signal of the brain parenchyma. In addition, the pulse sequence uses a TR as long as 10 seconds and a TE as long as 160 ms to produce heavy T$_2$-weighting and high signal in most brain lesions, which stand out conspicuously against normal brain parenchyma. Recent comparisons of FLAIR with T$_2$-weighted and proton density spin-echo and fast spin-echo images have indicated an advantage for FLAIR in acute periventricular and cortical ischemic lesions.[9,104] However, these same studies indicate that some brain stem lesions may not be as apparent or may be missed on FLAIR images. This is especially true in subacute lesions in which high water content and/or cystic changes result in a lesion with substantial free water and long T$_1$ relaxation whose signal may be suppressed by the inversion pulse and balanced against the high signal effects of prolonged T$_2$ relaxation. Isointensity may also occur when the inversion time does not closely match the T$_1$ of the free fluid, resulting in only partial signal suppression. One recent study[58] comparing FLAIR with fast spin-echo T$_2$-weighted images and DWI in acute ischemia indicates that FLAIR images show early ischemic lesions less conspicuously than DWI but more clearly than fast spin-echo T$_2$-weighted images. While the general experience with FLAIR in acute cerebral ischemia is limited at this time, it appears that it will become a useful clinical tool for early detection of lesions when DWI is not available. In clinical practice, FLAIR

does not discriminate well between acute and subacute (1 to 2 weeks) lesions, as both are equally bright. DWI appears to be useful for this discrimination, showing acute lesions as high signal and older lesions as isointense. FLAIR may be more helpful in the discrimination between subacute and chronic lesions by showing lower signal or isointensity in microcystic or macrocystic chronic lesions, which often appear similar to subacute lesions on T$_2$-weighted images.

Comparison of Magnetic Resonance and Computed Tomographic Images

Since the early days of MRI it has been clear that elevated signal on T$_2$-weighted images is more sensitive for the detection of early cerebral infarction than CT scanning.[97,100] Direct comparisons within the first 24 hours have demonstrated overall detection rates of 90% for MRI and 58% for CT.[11] Deep lesions and brain stem lesions were seen on 60% of MRI and 39% of CT scans within the first 24 hours. These higher detection rates for MRI are due to its greater sensitivity to abnormal tissue water (edema) for the most part.[44,112] Above the tentorium, MRI lesions are more clearly defined while CT findings are often difficult to identify, leading to a tentative diagnosis. In the posterior fossa a significant advantage for MRI is the absence of the beam-hardening interpetrous artifact that obscures lesions on CT.[48] The multiplanar capability

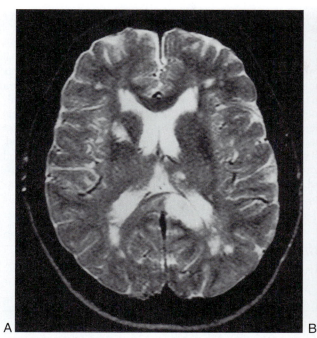

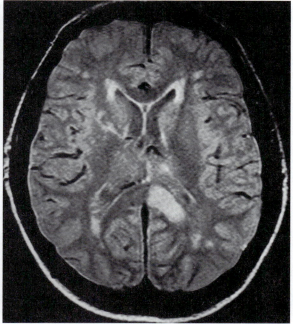

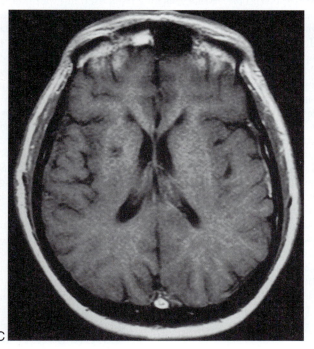

Figure 12.6 (**A**) T$_2$-weighted MR image 3 weeks after acute stroke showing the clinically recent occipital and callosal infarction, and the old contralateral capsular infarction. (**B**) Balanced MR image at the same time. (**C**) T$_1$-weighted MR image at the same time showing only faint signs of the recent infarction and the well-established signs of old infarction.

of MRI also provides multiple views of a lesion in axial, coronal, and sagittal planes, which increases detection rates and confidence in the diagnosis.

Contrast Enhancement

Early hopes that paramagnetic substances as blood-brain barrier markers could separate ischemia from infarction have not been realized.[69] Opening of the blood-brain barrier to a de-

gree detectible on contrast-enhanced T$_1$-weighted MR images does not typically occur until several (3 to 7) days after infarction occurs, approximately the same time course as contrast enhancement seen on CT scans. Several recent studies on the use of MRI contrast agents have revealed interesting insights into the mechanism of enhancement in cerebral infarctions.[15,48,49,73,78,111] Gd-DTPA was the first clinically approved contrast medium for MRI and is currently still the most widely used agent. It is a paramagnetic substance that shortens the T$_1$ relaxation of hydrogen nuclei in unbound water molecules. In most infarcts (more than 80% of cases) the typical sequence of parenchymal enhancement is similar to that seen with contrast-enhanced CT scans and proceeds as follows.[45]

1. Contrast enhancement is not seen before 6 days.

2. It is most visible in the subacute phase (7 to 30 days; peak incidence 14 to 21 days).

3. It slowly fades away in the chronic phase (>30 days).

4. It may persist for as long as 6 weeks.

In one review, Crain et al[15] observed this sequence of parenchymal enhancement in 67 of 82 lesions studied. They called it the "progressive enhancement pattern." In this group the enhancement is seen later than the T_2 signal changes observed 24 hours after the onset of stroke. Furthermore, the enhanced area is smaller than that depicted on the T_2-weighted images. In the remaining 15% there was a pattern of early and/or intense enhancement in the first 7 days after the onset of the stroke. In these cases the gadolinium enhancement appeared at the same time as the T_2 changes and covered the same area. Also, clinically, this second group of patients with early enhancement had a better neurologic outcome. Crain et al.[15] attributed the two types of enhancement pattern to a difference in the underlying pathologic processes. In the progressive enhancement group it is believed that the arterial occlusion is complete and that there is insufficient acute collateral circulation to transport enough contrast agent to the site of infarction. In the early and/or intense enhancement group it is believed that the occlusion is either incomplete or that there is sufficient collateral circulation to transport the contrast agent to the infarction. It is hypothesized that this early enhancement is an indicator of partial ischemia, which would also explain the more favorable clinical outcome in these cases.

Early infarct contrast enhancement, within the first 24 hours, may also be associated with a higher frequency of hemorrhagic transformation, usually occurring in the 24- to 48-hour time period. This is a well-known phenomenon with CT scanning and also appears to be true for MRI.[42,47,53] The basic mechanism for the early contrast enhancement and hemorrhagic transformation is probably the same, early reperfusion of ischemic tissue with damaged capillary endothelial cells.

The use of contrast enhancement in the second week after infarction may help to avoid two critical diagnostic pitfalls. The first is the so-called fogging effect that may occur on T_2-weighted images in this period. As a cortical infarction evolves, the T_2 may become shortened sufficiently to produce isointensity with normal brain, giving the false impression of resolution or disappearance of the lesion. This is analogous to the phenomenon of the same name observed in this period on CT scans and is probably due to the combination of decreasing free water content and increasing cellular protein and membrane debris. Because cortical parenchymal enhancement is seen in 90% to 100% of patients at this time, obtaining a T_1-weighted postgadolinium scan will avoid this misdiagnosis in almost all cases. The other pitfall to avoid is the misdiagnosis of neoplasm in cases of subacute infarction, especially when the clinical history is vague or unavailable. This may be difficult when the enhancement pattern is ill defined, but usually the peripheral, cortical location and areas of gyriform enhancement can be identified to favor the diagnosis of subacute infarct over neoplasm.

As mentioned above, another type of contrast enhancement in stroke patients is the enhancement of arteries. Arterial enhancement is seen in approximately 75% of cortical infarcts in the first 3 days. Meningeal enhancement may also be seen in the first week with peripheral cortical infarction, in approximately 35% of cases, and is thought to be due to meningeal irritation.[25] Arterial, meningeal, and cortical enhancement may be seen together in 35% of cases late in the first week (4 to 7 days) after infarction and has been referred to as mixed compartment or transitional stage enhancement.[25] The cortical enhancement is of the late onset, progressive type, indicating complete ischemia.[15]

Magnetic Resonance Spectroscopy and Cerebral Ischemia

MR spectroscopy (MRS) has long been used in experimental settings to assess metabolite concentrations in vivo but has only recently been available for clinical use. Many commercial 1.5-T scanners are being upgraded to perform MRS, and it appears that clinical applications will increase in the future. Most of the work in cerebral ischemia has been focused on proton (^{1}H) and phosphorus (^{31}P) nuclei. Proton MRS is the most widely available in the clinical setting and generates spectra and spectroscopic images (metabolite maps) with voxels as small as 1 cm^3 at 1.5 T.[40] This translates to an image with 15-mm slice thickness and in-plane resolution of 8 × 8 mm, considerably lower resolution than anatomic proton MRI but still useful for demonstration of metabolite distributions. Acquisition of MRS data is also slower than proton imaging, typically 10 to 15 minutes for single multivoxel images. It is likely that proton MRS imaging will improve to much higher resolutions and faster acquisitions in the future as studies are performed on 3-T and 4-T systems now being developed. The major metabolites identifiable on ^{1}H MRS in brain are N-acetyl aspartate (NAA, a neuronal marker of uncertain metabolic function), choline (Ch, typically a membrane component), and total creatine (Cr, including phosphocreatine (PCr), a cellular energy metabolite).

Lactate may also be observed on proton MRS in pathologic conditions such as ischemia or neoplasm.[29] In animal studies, lactate accumulation, presumably from anaerobic glucose metabolism, has been seen within minutes of onset in experimental cerebral ischemia,[25,89] and it has been suggested that brain infarction may be associated with lactate concentrations 17 mmol/g.[91] It is not clear whether this lactate accumulation is part of the mechanism of ischemic cellular injury or a secondary metabolic effect, or whether these increases are primarily from neuronal or glial metabolism. It is also unclear whether lactate accumulation is directly related to decreases in intracellular pH, as these parameters may change independently in cerebral ischemic lesions.[60,80] The early accumulation of lactate does appear to be correlated with CBF below a threshold of 20 ml/100 g/min, which is similar to that for failure of cellular energy metabolism and appearance of abnormal diffusion on MRI.[16] In subacute and chronic infarctions, brain macrophages may also contribute to increases in lactate concentration.[87] Clinical studies of cerebral infarction in humans have shown similar changes in lactate with elevations in the early hours, peak concentrations at 2 to 3 days, and declining concentration over the next several days.[37] Lactate concentrations were highest in the center of the lesions, where signs of neuronal injury and decreased NAA were most pronounced.[4] Beyond the subacute stage, lactate tends to decline to undetectable levels over 2 to 4 weeks, but some chronic infarcts show persistent elevated levels.[23,26,28]

The other major metabolite studied with proton MRS in cerebral ischemia has been NAA. Because NAA is considered a marker of neuronal viability, reductions in acute and chronic infarction have been interpreted as evidence of neuronal cell loss.[28,37] Evidence for a gradient of neuronal injury in infarctions is the observation that NAA levels are lowest at the center of lesions with gradual increases to normal level at the periphery.[34] NAA levels also appear to decline over the first 2 weeks of an infarction.[37]

Changes in Ch and Cr are not as clearly correlated with ischemia as are lactate and NAA. While one study has found that Ch may remain normal while NAA and Cr decrease, suggesting a pattern specific for neuronal injury,[6] others have seen decreases in Ch as well as NAA and Cr in chronic infarctions.[23]

Phosphorus (^{31}P) MR is the other spectroscopic method that has been used extensively to study cerebral ischemia. Phosphorus MRS has been used to assess the tissue concentrations of the cellular high-energy metabolites ATP, PCr, and inorganic phosphate (Pi), as well as various phosphomonoesters and phosphodiesters. Phosphorus MRS can also be used to determine tissue pH by measuring the chemical shift of the Pi peak.[88] Experimental animal studies have demonstrated rapid depletion of high-energy phosphates, reduced PCr/Pi ratios, and decreases in intracellular pH within minutes of ischemia onset.[46] In recent clinical studies, reductions in ATP, increases in Pi, and reductions in pH have been demonstrated in the first 48 hours. A transition from early acidosis to alkalosis over the first 3 weeks has also been shown.[57] However, the significance of these pH changes is unclear as the clinical neurologic status does not appear to correlate with them.[57] The clinical application of phosphorus MRS to stroke management is currently limited by the low spatial resolution of the method, compared with proton MRS. The typical voxel volume for ^{31}P MRS at 1.5 T is approximately 9 cm^3 (e.g., 30-mm slice with in-plane resolution of 17 × 17 mm). Although this resolution can be improved at higher magnetic fields, phosphorus MRS will always have considerably lower spatial resolution and longer acquisition times than comparable proton MRS because of the severalfold lower NMR sensitivity and lower concentration of phosphorus in tissue.

Other MRS and imaging techniques currently under development may make direct measurement of critical physiologic variables available in the future. These include oxidative metabolism using blood oxygen level dependent techniques,[17] glucose metabolism using ^{13}C MRS,[38] and sodium concentrations using ^{23}Na imaging.[24]

Distribution of Cerebral Infarction

A distinctive diagnostic aspect of infarctions is their location and distribution, which depends on the vascular territory involved. The conformity of an infarction to a vascular territory is an important element in the diagnosis that helps in distinguishing these lesions from brain tumors, inflammation, and trauma. Besides conforming to a known vascular territory, infarctions tend to have less mass effect for their size than neoplasms, particularly rapidly growing neoplasms. Cortical enhancement and cortical hemorrhage also favor the diagnosis of infarction. A brief discussion of the various vascular territories is helpful as a background to the diagnosis of cerebral infarctions.

SUPRATENTORIAL VASCULAR TERRITORIES

Lesions due to vascular occlusions of the anterior, middle, or posterior cerebral arteries or their branches in their course in the subarachnoid space usually result in the characteristic distribution of the infarction.

The *anterior cerebral artery* gives a few perforators (usually including one large one referred to as the recurrent artery of Heubner) that enter the anterior perforated substance supplying the anterior portion of the caudate nucleus and the anterior limb of the internal capsule. These perforators arise from the initial segment of the anterior cerebral artery. More distally, the anterior cerebral artery supplies the orbital surface of the frontal lobe and the frontal pole, the medial aspect of the frontal lobe, a small strip on the convexity aspect of the frontal and parietal lobes, the genu and the anterior two-thirds of the corpus callosum, the fornix, and the septum pellucidum.

The *middle cerebral artery* provides perforating (lenticulostriate) branches through the anterior perforated substance that supply the anterior two-thirds of the internal capsule, most of the globus pallidus, and nearly all the putamen. Distally, the middle cerebral artery supplies the insula, almost 80% of the convexity surface of the frontal and parietal lobes, the entire lateral aspect of the temporal lobe, the tip of the temporal lobe, and a small strip on the inferior surface of the temporal lobe. It receives collaterals via a borderzone network of small anastomosing arteries from the anterior cerebral and posterior cerebral arteries along a strip on the convexity surface of the brain only a few centimeters lateral to the superior sagittal sinus.

The *posterior cerebral artery* supplies the posterior thalamus and midbrain through its perforating thalamic and thalamogeniculate branches. Its peripheral branches supply the medial aspect of the entire occipital and parietal lobes and extend over the convexity aspect of these two lobes to anastomose with middle cerebral branches. The posterior cerebral

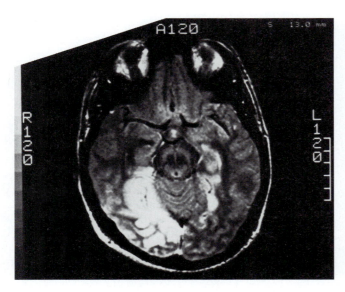

Figure 12.7 Axial T_2-weighted MR image showing bilateral posterior cerebral artery territory infarction.

also supplies the tentorial surface of the occipital lobe and the posterior two-thirds of the temporal lobe (Fig. 12.7).

The *anterior choroidal artery* supplies the optic tract anteriorly, the choroid plexus of the lateral ventricle, the hippocampal formation, the lateral geniculate body, the lateral thalamic nuclei and pulvinar, and the lowest levels of the posterior limb of the internal capsule (Fig. 12.8).

POSTERIOR FOSSA VASCULAR TERRITORIES

Infarctions of the brain stem and cerebral hemispheres are notoriously difficult to appreciate on CT because of the bone artifacts from the skull base. MRI is by far the preferred modality for imaging these lesions. The practical problem, however, is that patients with brain stem lesions are often uncooperative and unable to hold still during the MR examination. This problem with motion artifact is decreasing because of the availability of the fast imaging sequence (fast spin-echo, gradient-echo, and echo-planar techniques), which remarkably reduce examination time and are better tolerated by the sick patient.

Ischemic lesions in the pons are usually due to occlusion of the *basilar artery* or its perforating vessels. Characteristically, they involve one side of the pons and seem to stop abruptly at the midline. This appearance is due to the highly characteristic distribution of the median perforating branches.

The cerebellum is supplied by three artery territories. The *posterior inferior cerebellar artery* territory covers the posterior lateral part of the medulla, the cerebellar tonsils, the inferior lateral aspects of the cerebellar hemispheres, and the inferior vermis. Occlusions of various segments of this vessel will produce a characteristic infarction in the territory described above. The territory of the *anterior inferior cerebellar artery* (AICA) will produce infarctions in the brachium

pontis and the anterior inferior aspect of the cerebellar hemisphere. A small segment of the posterior medulla is also supplied by the AICA. The superior cerebellar artery territory includes the mesencephalon, the quadrigeminal plate, the superior cerebellar peduncle, the superior medullary velum, the superior vermis, and the posterior part of the cerebellar hemispheres. While the collateral anastomoses over the cerebellar hemispheres are generous between the superior cerebellar, the anterior inferior cerebellar, and the posterior inferior cerebellar arteries, the brain stem vascular supply is primarily from end arteries with no significant collateral channels, making it more vulnerable to occlusive vascular disease than the cerebellar hemispheres.

White Matter Lesions

The great sensitivity of MR to changes in water content has created images that may represent more subtle tissue injury than frank infarction with tissue loss. Other possibilities include edema, enlarged vascular spaces, transudation of spinal fluid across incompetent ventricular walls, and even white matter demyelination and thinning of tissue from atrophy and trans-synaptic fiber degeneration.[92] The most common partial ischemic lesions are the patchy white matter high-signal changes on T_2-weighted images that are a sign of arteriolosclerosis. Van Swieten et al[110] found periventricular images of increased signal on T_2-weighted images in 10% of subjects in their sixties, and in 50% of those in their eighties among their 40 subjects. Whole brain sections in 19 subjects showed a correlation with the histologic severity of demyelination and astrocytic gliosis. They noted that demyelination was related to an increased wall thickness of the arterioles up to 150 μm in size. Axonal loss was present to varying degrees in the white matter showing demyelination. They concluded that arteriolosclerosis was the primary factor in the pathogenesis of diffuse white matter lesions in the elderly, setting in train demyelination and axonal loss. Brains showing microvascular ischemic demyelination have shown poor blood flow in the white matter as tested by single-photon emission computed tomography.[18]

Widening of perivascular spaces is a common finding, especially in the elderly, and should not be confused with infarctions or lacunar disease. The perivascular spaces that are seen most frequently are those in the basal ganglia in the area of the anterior perforated substance near the anterior commissure, occasionally in the midbrain, and frequently in the subcortical white matter in the high-convexity centrum semiovale.

Dural Sinus Thrombosis

MRI is the preferred modality for the diagnosis of venous sinus thrombosis clinically. The collateral venous channels on the surface of the brain are quite abundant and have enough capacity to compensate for a slow sinus occlusion. In these

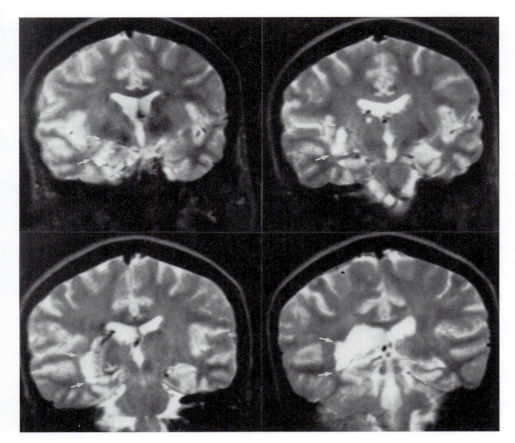

Figure 12.8 Four coronal views of the brain on a T$_2$-weighted MR image showing infarction in the territory of the anterior choroidal artery territory. (From Mohr et al.,[74] with permission.)

cases no clinical symptoms may be observed. If the sinus occlusion is rapid and/or involves a large sinus such as the superior sagittal sinus or the lateral transverse sinus, the process may cause hemorrhagic venous infarction in the affected territory. The presence of brain parenchymal changes appears to be directly correlated with increasing venous sinus pressure and can be classified into five stages: (stage I) no parenchymal changes; (stage II) brain swelling, sulcal effacement, and mass effect without signal changes to indicate edema; (stage III) attenuation and signal intensity changes compatible with mild to moderate edema; (stage IV) severe edema with or without small hemorrhage; and (stage V) massive edema or hemorrhage.[107]

In the case of superior sagittal sinus thrombosis, one sees parasagittal hemorrhagic infarctions, commonly bilateral. The infarctions are characteristically confined to the local cortical vein drainage zone and tend to involve the gray-white matter junction. Hemorrhagic transformation within these infarctions is seen as a high signal on the T$_1$-weighted image or low signal on the T$_2$-weighted images, depending on the age of the hemorrhagic changes. Besides hemorrhagic infarction there is absence of the normal flowing blood signal void in the superior sagittal sinus. This is the most reliable sign of thrombosis and is best observed in imaging planes oriented perpendicular to the normal sinus flow, that is, coronal images for the anterior

superior sagittal sinus, axial images for the posterior descending portion, and sagittal images for the transverse sinuses. Early thrombus (1 to 2 days) may show absence of the signal void and a signal isointense with brain on T$_1$-weighted images, before methemoglobin changes occur. The most common and reliable finding is absence of the signal void with hyperintensity on T$_1$-weighted images, due to thrombus in the methemoglobin phase. The T$_2$-weighted images may show what appears to be signal void in the sinus, which is due to the paramagnetic effect of the blood product such as the intracellular deoxyhemoglobin or methemoglobin phases. The MR image might be confusing in some cases when there is a partial thrombosis of the sinus or recanalization of the previously occluded sinus. In such cases only a fraction of the cross section of the sinus may be blocked by the clot, and the associated infarction may not be hemorrhagic.

Nonocclusive Infarction

Cerebral infarctions result from a variety of mechanisms not requiring a vascular occlusion. Examples are hypotension, anemia, hypoxemia (open heart surgery) hypoglycemia, or metabolic enzymatic deficiencies such as mitochondral encephalopathies. In most cases in children, the gray matter, particularly that of the basal ganglia, seems to be more affected than other parts of the brain. The hippocampus is also highly sensitive to global ischemia. In cases of severe hypotension there may be involvement of the border zones and adjacent distal arterial territories of the major cerebral arteries. This state is also observed in occlusions of the cervical carotid artery with diminished perfusion to the cerebral hemisphere. Other lesions include the changes brought about by occlusive disease of small vessels such as in Binswanger's disease with diffuse increased signal intensity in the subcortical white matter.

Another condition that deserves mention is the transient hyperintensity of white matter in patients with hypertensive encephalopathy or pre-eclampsia and eclampsia. In these cases there is a reversible increase in the white matter signal in the periatrial regions and often also in the cerebellar white matter.

Hemorrhagic Infarction

Hemorrhagic transformation of ischemic brain infarction was found at autopsy to occur more often in embolic strokes than in thrombotic strokes. The rate of hemorrhagic infarctions varies from 54%[27] to 78%.[51] It is believed that the hemorrhagic transformation of a pale infarction results from a two-step process: (1) an ischemic insult that causes damage to the endothelial vascular wall, and (2) restoration of blood flow to the injured vascular territory. The reperfusion may be due either to a recanalization of the occluded vessel or to the establishment of collateral blood supply to the infarction, or both. In recent studies by CT scans and angiography, Bozzao et al[8] found that hemorrhagic infarction developed in 18 of 36 stroke patients with middle cerebral artery occlusion within 7 days after onset, while no hemorrhagic infarction was present on the initial CT scan obtained at 4 hours. Pessin et al[86] comment that "hemorrhagic infarction is a natural and common tissue accompaniment of cerebral embolic infarction. Its clinical significance may have been exaggerated as a consequence of its association with the neurologic effects of the infarct itself." Hemorrhagic transformation is more common in cortical infarction. It was observed in all patients (10 of 10) with a cortical hypotensity seen on CT reported by Bozzao et al,[8] while they found hemorrhagic changes in only 11 of 24 patients with basal ganglia infarctions. The preponderance of hemorrhagic changes in cortical lesions is due to the robust collateral blood supply in the cortex. Mechanisms of hemorrhage in deep strokes depend only on the recanalization of the middle cerebral artery stem and its perforating branches, since there is no potential for establishing a collateral circulation to the deep infarction.

It is important to distinguish between hemorrhagic infarction and parenchymatous hematoma in the assessment of intracranial bleeding, and both should not be casually grouped together. There are undoubtedly some parenchymatous hematomas that arise from severe multicentric bleeding after reperfusion of capillaries injured by ischemia. These cases cannot be distinguished from the rupture of one or more small arterioles without the ischemic insult. Parenchymatous hematomas are known to be associated with clinical worsening, unlike hemorrhagic infarctions. Parenchymatous hematomas on CT generally show a more homogeneous high density, a well-demarcated region with a prominent mass effect, and frequently intraventricular bleeding. Hemorrhagic infarctions, on the other hand, are more inhomogeneous, patchy, and gyriform in distribution.

On MRI, hemorrhagic infarctions are typically recognized after the first 1 to 2 days by a high signal intensity on T_1-weighted images and patchy low signal in the midst of the high signal lesion on T_2-weighted images (Fig. 12.9). The appearance of the high signal on T_1-weighted images, due to methemoglobin, occurs early in ischemic lesions, at 1 to 2 days, compared with the typical 3 to 4 days needed for this evolution in larger hematomas.[36] Cortical hemorrhagic infarctions often show a thin, serpiginous high signal line along the effected gyri. Reliable statistics on hyperacute hemorrhagic transformation identified with MRI are not yet available because of the current reliance on CT and the complex early evolution of acute hemorrhage on MRI. Within the first few hours, tissue hemorrhage is isointense with normal brain on T_1- and T_2-weighted images. The earliest changes of hemorrhagic infarction are low signal areas within the lesion zone on T_1- and T_2-weighted images. $T_2°W$ gradient-echo images are especially sensitive and the most specific MRI method for the detection of early acute hemorrhage in infarcts. These images are maximally sensitive to the local magnetic susceptibility inhomogenieties created by the paramagnetic components in the hemorrhage. It has been suggested in one recent study that $T_2°$-weighted images may allow MRI to substitute for CT as part of the comprehensive prethrombolysis evaluation of stroke symptoms in the hyperacute period.[84] This study found parenchymal hemorrhage in five cases at 2.5 to 5 hours after symptom onset. Hemorrhages appeared as conspicuous low signal on susceptibility sensitive ($T_2°$-weighted) gradient-echo and echo-planar images and were isointense with normal brain on T_1- and T_2-weighted images. They concluded that "MR may be an adequate screen for primary intraparenchymal hemorrhage". More reliance may be placed on MRI in the future as early hemorrhage evolution is better understood and as MRI is more widely used in the evaluation of hyperacute cerebral ischemia.

Cerebral Hematoma

Since the early days of MRI, CT has been deemed more sensitive than MR for the detection of acute cerebral hemorrhage.[52] CT is directly sensitive to the high electron density of hemoglobin in clotted blood while MRI detection depends on multiple factors, including water content, T_1 and T_2 relaxation times, and the oxygenation state of the hemoglobin. Early studies outlined the basics of parenchymal hematoma evolution, from early low signal on T_2W images to high signal on T_1- and T_2-weighted images in subacute and chronic phases.[20] At the time, the limited understanding of MR characteristics of blood and the relatively low mag-

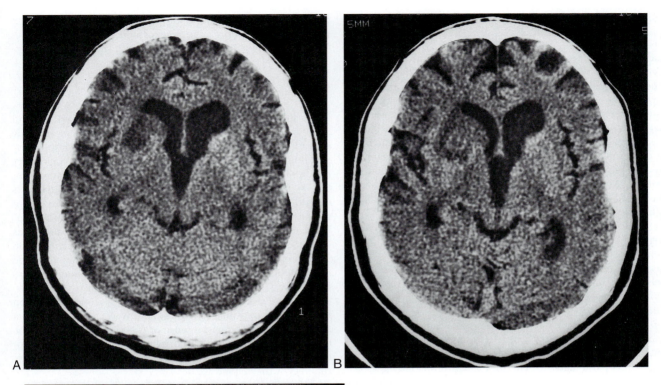

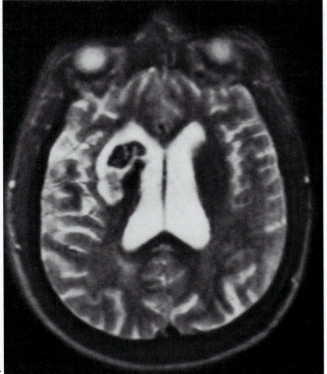

Figure 12.9 (**A**) CT scan showing acute infarction before start of anticoagulant therapy. (**B**) CT scan 10 days later, after institution of anticoagulant therapy. (**C**) Axial T_2-weighted MR image done the same day as the CT scan in Fig. B showing high and low signal changes consistent with hemorrhagic infarction not seen as readily on CT scan.

netic field (0.15 T) used for imaging did not permit the detection of the full spectrum of signal changes and magnetic susceptibility effects of blood and blood breakdown products. It was the work of Gomori and his collaborators[34,35,36] that laid down the foundation of our understanding of the MR characteristics of cerebral hematomas at different fields, especially the higher clinical fields such as 1.5 T. For descriptive purposes the MRI appearances of cerebral hematoma can be classified into four stages: hyperacute, acute, subacute, and chronic.

HYPERACUTE HEMATOMA

Traditionally, it has been unusual that a cerebral hematoma is imaged with MRI in the hyperacute stage in the clinical setting. This stage lasts for only a few hours but with increasing emphasis on early stroke imaging as part of thrombolytic and neuroprotective therapy, it is becoming more common to image this early stage hemorrhage. Hyperacute hematomas consist mostly of freshly extravasated red blood cells containing oxyhemoglobin. Oxyhemoglobin is diamagnetic, meaning it has no paramagnetic properties because it has no unpaired electrons. MRI signal characteristics of oxyhemoglobin collections are similar to those of any other brain lesions, being slightly hypointense on T_1-weighted images and bright on T_2-weighted images because of the higher water content with increased spin density and prolonged relaxation times. The hematoma may be very sharply demarcated with a hypointense rim on T_1-weighted images, representing a serum pocket surrounding the retracted clot. On T_2-weighted images this rim is bright and is surrounded by a zone of high-signal brain edema.

Within the first few minutes to hours after intracerebral clot formation, the hemoglobin begins to evolve from oxyhemoglobin to deoxyhemoglobin, which has four unpaired electrons and is paramagnetic. The iron atom in this molecule is shielded by the surrounding globin protein from the close approach of water molecules. Consequently, deoxyhemoglobin cannot affect the relaxivity of water protons by dipole–dipole interaction precluding a shortening of the T_1 of water. Therefore no bright signal should be expected on the T_1-weighted images from deoxyhemoglobin. The packaging of the paramagnetic deoxyhemoglobin in the red cells, on the other hand, will cause a focal distortion of the magnetic field leading to a significant T_2° effect that reduces the signal on the T_2°- and T_2-weighted images. The changes may occur at varying rates throughout the hematoma but typically begin at the periphery, where the earliest MR signal changes are noted.

T_2°-weighted gradient-echo image hypointensity is more sensitive to hyperacute hemorrhage than T_1- or T_2W-weighted spin-echo images. T_2°W images are maximally sensitive to the local magnetic susceptibility inhomogeneities created by the paramagnetic components in the hemorrhage, and this sensitivity increases at high magnetic fields. The effect of spatial inhomogeneity of clot evolution probably also enhances the paramagnetic changes in hemoglobin.[43] T_2°-weighted image hypointensity is consistent in descriptions of hyperacute hematomas at different magnetic field strengths. Weingarten et al[115,116] studied experimental animals and a series of 50 patients within 72 hours of ictus and showed that neither T_1- nor T_2-weighted sequences can reliably detect small hematomas in the hyperacute stage but that hypointense signals could often be obtained on T_2°-weighted gradient-echo images at 0.6 T. Zyed et al[121] documented a hypointense signal rim on gradient-echo images in 45 of 46 hyperacute to chronic stage lesions studied at 0.5 and 1.0 T. At 1.5 T, Gomori et al[34] compared the appearance of hemorrhage in the first week with later evolution of the hemorrhage and found that the initial central hypointensity and its later disappearance helped to establish the time of onset of hemorrhage retrospectively. As noted above, T_2°-weighted images are also the most sensi-

tive and specific MR method for detecting the hypointensity of hyperacute hemorrhagic transformation of infarctions.[84]

ACUTE HEMATOMA

Acute hematoma signal characteristics usually appear around 24 hours from the bleed, and they consist primarily of a slightly hypointense signal on T1-weighted images and markedly hypointense signal on T2-weighted images. The hypointensity on the T_1 is probably due to the pronounced shortening of the T_2 relaxation. The low signal on T_2-weighted images is caused by the progression of oxyhemoglobin to deoxyhemoglobin evolution throughout the hematoma and is better appreciated on higher field magnet and with longer echo times (TE$\geq$80 ms) (Fig. 12.10). Using a very high field magnet (2.35 T), Zuerrer et al[120] studied the time course of signal change in hematomas in 28 pediatric patients. Hematomas <3 days old showed an isointense to mildly hypointense appearance on T_1-weighted images and were strikingly hypointense on long T_2-weighted images. After about a week the hematoma signal also became hyperintense on T_1-weighted images. The changes were evident in the periphery first, spreading centripetally. The hematomas became uniformly hyperintense by the end of the second week.

SUBACUTE HEMATOMA

At 2 to 7 days after the bleeding, subacute hematoma occurs, marked by conversion of oxyhemoglobin or deoxyhemoglobin (or both) to paramagnetic methemoglobin. At the beginning of the subacute stage the methemoglobin is contained within intact red blood cells and, like deoxyhemoglobin, this produces local magnetic field inhomogeneities whose predominant effect is signal loss from shortening of T_2 and T_2° relaxation times. Toward the end of this stage the red blood cells lyse, freeing methemoglobin, which diffuses throughout the hematoma. At this stage the hematoma is a proteinaceous water solution, and the paramagnetic properties of methemoglobin act directly on water protons through a dipole-dipole interaction, causing a marked shortening of T_1 relaxation, resulting in high signal on T_1-weighted images.[34–36] These changes occur first at the periphery of the hematoma and gradually spread toward the center of the clot (Fig. 12.11).

The evolution of signal changes in subacute hematomas on T_2- and T_2°-weighted images is more complex. These changes depend on (1) the presence of methemoglobin, (2) whether the methemoglobin is still packaged in the red blood cells, and (3) the extent of the phagocytic activities in the periphery of the hematoma. In the early subacute phase, there is low signal at the site of the hematoma as long as there are intact red blood cells containing the methemoglobin. At the same time there is an inflammatory repair response in the tissue surrounding the hematoma with phagocytes and macrophages infiltrating the boundary of the hematoma. This process results in accumulation of iron products such as hemosiderin within these cells at the periphery of the hematoma. These intracellular hemoglobin breakdown products create

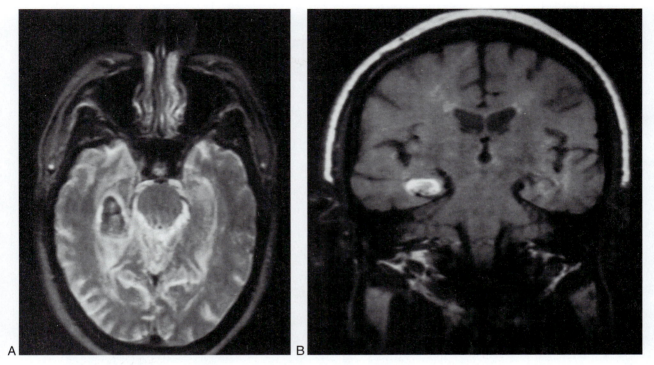

Figure 12.10 (**A**) Axial T_2-weighted MR image showing early changes after parenchymatous hemorrhage. (**B**) Coronal T_1-weighted MR image at the same time showing predominantly bright signal from the recent hemorrhage.

microscopic magnetic field inhomogeneities and produce a dark signal rim on T_2- and T_2°-weighted images.

In the late subacute, or intermediate phase, after the first week, the hematoma is bright on both T_1 and T_2. The high signal on T_1 is due to the shortening of the T_1 of water by dipole-dipole interaction with methemoglobin, and the bright signal on T_2 is due to the increased water spin density in the

proteinaceous watery solution of the hematoma. Again, at this stage, there is a black rim surrounding the hematoma due to ferrous iron stored in hemosiderin (Fig. 12.12).

CHRONIC HEMORRHAGIC CHANGES

In the late stages, beyond 1 month, the T_2-weighted and especially the T_2°-weighted images become even more hypointense.[34] These changes reflect the conversion of methemoglobin to hemosiderin, most of which is found in macrophages. The location of macrophages throughout the hematoma and peripheral zone of the lesion makes the hypointensity diffuse. The low signal margins of the lesion become increasingly indistinct as the hematoma ages. Thulborn et al[105] studied changes in rat hemorrhage and found both ferritin and hemosiderin, two iron-storage substances, in chronic hematomas. These changes have been summarized by Williams et al.[117]

These signs of chronic hemorrhage are not seen on CT scans, which makes MRI the only available method for their detection and investigation. The existence of chronic changes on T_2- and T_2°-weighted images in the rim of the lesion was used by Nakajima et al[81] to document the frequency of hemorrhages in a group of clinically asymptomatic patients. The authors reported (in Japanese) their detection of 17 patients with asymptomatic hemorrhages among 2,757 who had brain MR using a 1.0-T unit. These 17 patients represented a 1.5% frequency among patients with stroke and 9.5% among those with hemorrhage.

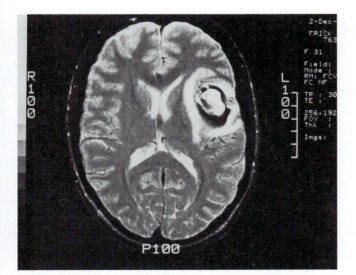

Figure 12.11 Axial T_2-weighted MR, image showing rim of edema, external ring of low signal, and central high signal.

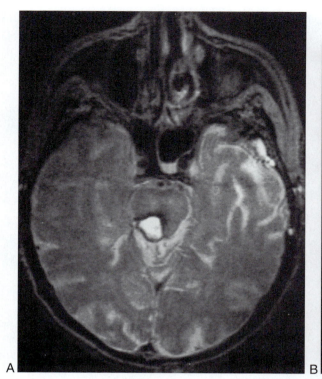

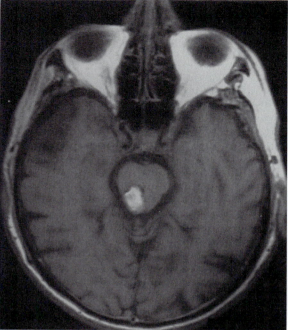

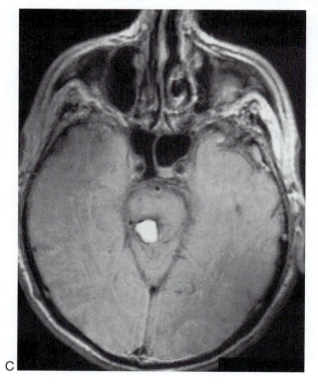

Figure 12.12 (**A**) Axial T$_2$-weighted MR image showing changes several weeks after parenchymatous hemorrhage. (**B**) Axial balanced MR image at the same time showing similar changes. (**C**) Axial T$_1$-weighted MR image at the same time showing similar changes.

SUBARACHNOID HEMORRHAGE

CT has long been accepted as the imaging method of choice for detection of acute subarachnoid hemorrhage. This remains generally true in clinical practice when CT is compared with conventional T$_1$- and T$_2$-weighted MRI studies, despite some studies suggesting otherwise.[66] Acute blood, mixed with CSF in the basal cisterns and sulci, may be isointense with brain, may be indistinguishable from the normal signal of CSF on T$_1$- and T$_2$-weighted images, or may be confused with high

Text continued on page 250

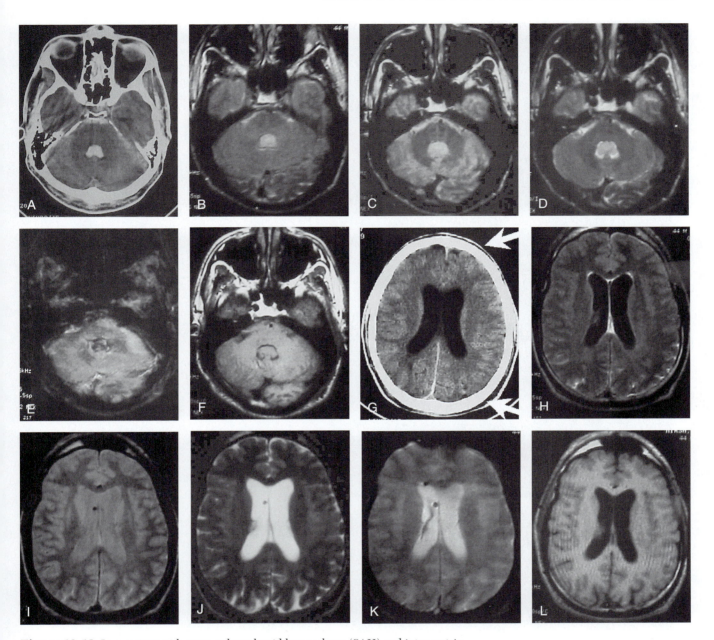

Figure 12.13 In a patient with acute subarachnoid hemorrhage (SAH) and intraventricular hemorrhage (IVH) (**A**), CT scan shows dense prepontine SAH and fourth ventricular IVH. (**B**) FLAIR image shows this hemorrhage as abnormal high signal (vs. normal black CSF as seen in the lateral ventricles in H) (**C**) Balanced and (**D**) T_2-weighted images show intermediate to high signal indistinguishable from normal CSF and motion artifact. (**E**) Gradient echo image shows low signal caused by hemorrhage-induced magnetic susceptibility gradients. (**F**) T_1-weighted image shows this acute hemorrhage as iso-intense with the brain stem and cerebellum. In the same patient (**G**) CT scan shows apparent SAH as extra-axial high density in left parietal and frontal regions (arrows). (**H**) FLAIR image shows more extensive abnormal high signal in parietal sulci bilaterally, probably representing SAH and hemorrhage breakdown products in sulcal CSF. The left frontal hemorrhage is also more specifically shown as a thin subdural collection (SDH). (**I**) Balanced, (**J**) T_2-weighted, and (**K**) gradient echo images show nonspecific high signal similar to CSF in these areas of hemorrhage. (**L**) T_1-weighted image shows normal-appearing low signal CSF in these same areas.

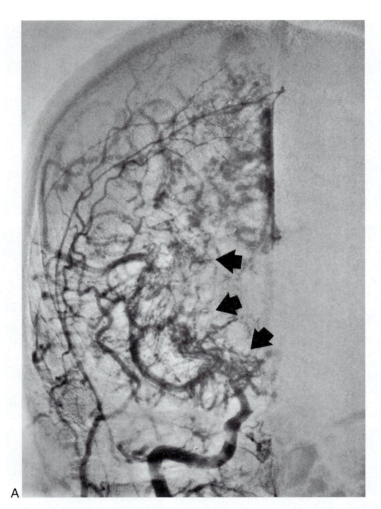

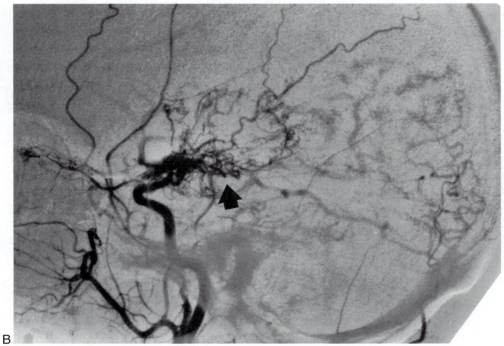

Figure 12.14 (**A&B**) Angiograms showing both moyamoya changes and an arteriovenous malformation, (AVM) the resistance to flow from the carotid stenosis, and associated moyamoya preventing adequate visualization of AVM.

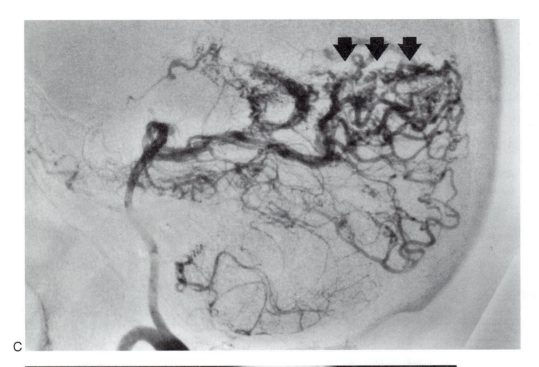

C

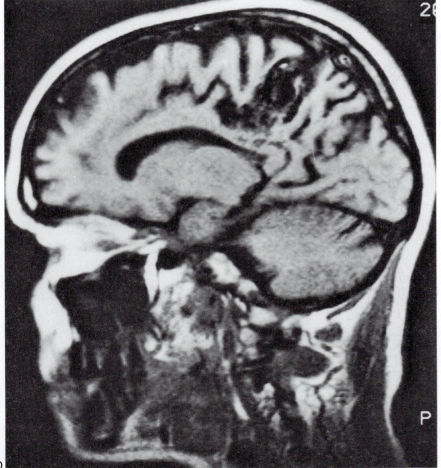

D

Figure 12.14 (*Continued*) (**C D**) T$_1$-weighted sagittal MR image and gradient-recalled echo imaging sequence MR image showing the presence and extent of an arteriovenous malformation better than that that seen by angiogram.
Illustration continued on following page

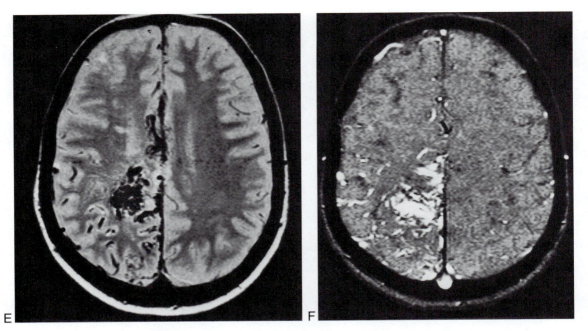

Figure 12.14 (*Continued*) (**E**) Axial T$_2$-weighted MR image and gradient-recalled echo imaging sequence MR image (**F**) showing the presence and extent of an arteriovenous malformation better than that seen by angiogram.

or low signal flow artifacts.[101] Subacute or chronic organized clot in the subarachnoid space may be seen as high signal on T$_1$-weighted images and low signal on T$_2$-weighted images, usually well after the hemorrhage is therapeutically relevant. Recent experience with FLAIR imaging has prompted some to suggest that this MRI method may be comparable to CT for detection of acute subarachnoid hemorrhage (Fig. 12.13). Laboratory studies indicate that a mixture of fresh unclotted blood and CSF is high signal and conspicuous against brain and signal-suppressed CSF on FLAIR images, but that clotted blood tends to be isointense with brain and relatively inconspicuous.[12] Animal studies show that FLAIR is positive in 80% of acute (6 hour) subarachnoid hemorrhage seen on CT. Parenchymal hematomas, within the first 6 hours, are also conspicuous as high signal on FLAIR but are nonspecific in appearance, and the low signal on conventional T$_2$- and T$_2$°-weighted images is needed to establish the diagnosis of hemorrhage.[106] In two clinical series of 57 total patients with acute subarachnoid hemorrhage, 2 hours to 2 days old, FLAIR was equal in sensitivity to CT, showing 100% of subarachnoid and intraventricular hemorrhages. FLAIR was also felt to be of some advantage in the posterior fossa, where beam hardening artifact from bone partially obscured lesions on CT.[70,82]

Arteriovenous Malformations

MR images show rapidly flowing blood as absence of signal, or signal void. The very low intensity signal characteristic of blood flowing through vessels through an area of hemorrhage helps to demonstrate arteriovenous malformations (AVMs) as

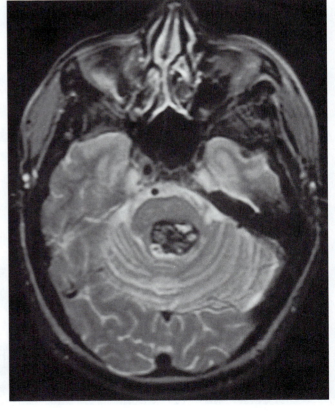

Figure 12.15 Axial T$_2$-weighted MR image of a large cavernous angioma of the brainstem, later removed surgically.

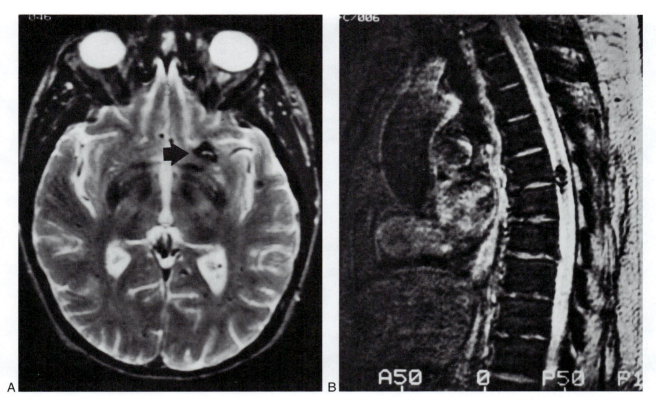

Figure 12.16 (**A & B**) T_2-weighted MR images showing a cavernous angioma in the temporal lobe (**A**) and the spinal cord (**B**) in the same patient.

the underlying cause. These low signal areas can be distinguished from hematoma regions by the presence of low signal on both T_1- and T_2-weighted images and characteristic flow artifacts (phase 'ghosts') that are usually present. As opposed to angiogram, which reveals nothing of the brain parenchyma, MRI shows the relationship between vessels and surrounding brain and is especially useful in defining the local anatomic changes at the AVM nidus[83] and the margins of the lesion.[49] Evidence of prior hemorrhage and its source,[68] the size of the nidus, the source of flow to the lesion, the course of draining veins, and the relation of the malformation to normal brain structures are now regularly shown. The nidus of the AVM may be better seen by MR compared with CT or angiogram,[83] and MRI has become an essential part of the evaluation of AVMs[56] (Fig. 12.14). However, MRI and MR angiography have not yet progressed to the stage where they can replace catheter angiography for the fine details needed by the surgeon.

Cavernous Malformations

Cavernous malformations, small angiomas, can be readily identified by MR. The flow through these lesions is minimal and therefore they are rarely seen on angiograms. This diagnosis is favored when the central focus of high signal is surrounded by or mixed with hypointensity on MRI, creating a 'cat's eye' or 'popcorn' appearance. Although distinctive, this appearance of cavernous angiomas may also be found in AVM[93] and even in tumor.[103] Even so, the distinctive finding has been used by several authors to explain small hematomas found in unusual locations such as in the brain stem[30] (Fig. 12.15). The margins of the cavernous angiomas are often smoother than those found in AVMs.[49]

MRI has allowed study of family members, which in a small series of cases has suggested a hereditary basis for some instances of multiple cavernous malformations.[94] Through this method multiple foci have been seen in the same patient, one quite remote from the other (Fig. 12.16).

Aneurysm

MR angiography is now being used to screen for cerebral aneurysms and is discussed in detail elsewhere. MRI is frequently used to determine vascular causes of large compressive intracranial lesions, including cavernous aneurysms, dolichoectatic basilar arteries (Fig. 12.17), and large basilar aneurysms.[7,64] A few striking examples have been described in which the dome or base of the aneurysm has been visualized by MR when it was not found by angiography.[86] Nagata et al[79] reported (in Japanese) on 12 giant aneurysms studied by

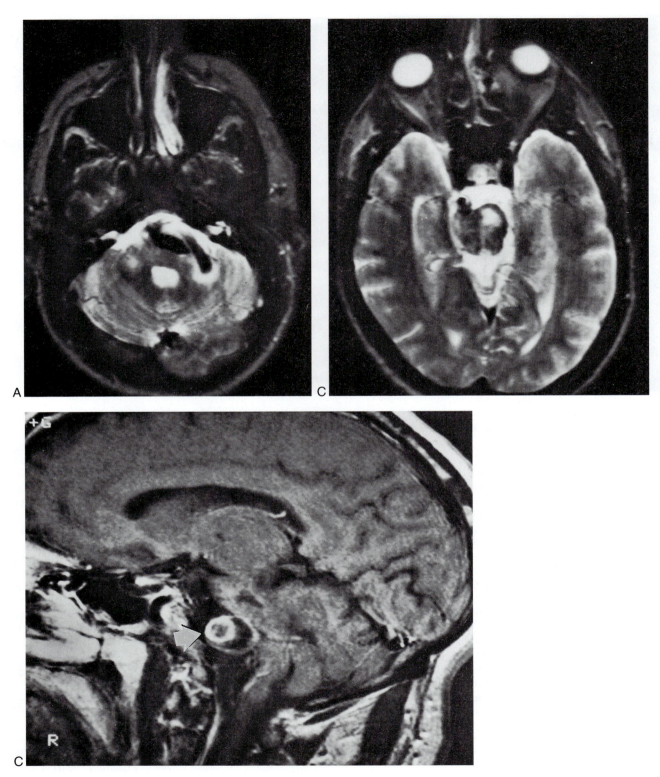

Figure 12.17 (**A & B**) Axial artery T$_2$-weighted (**A**) and sagittal T$_1$-weighted (**B**) MR image showing the thickened basilar artery in a case of dolicho-ectasia with pontine infarction (**C**) in a plane above those showing the dolicho-ectasia.

MR in which intraluminal thrombosis was found in 9. They noted that thrombosis was more frequent in the large aneurysms. The finding that thrombi were more prevalent posteriorly and inferiorly near the neck prompted the suggestion that stagnation of blood flow might be the explanation. The use of ferromagnetic clips initially made MR imaging a risk for postoperative evaluations, but these risks have subsided considerably with the introduction of nonferromagnetic materials. The main current problems are the major changes induced in the MR signal by the presence of the magnetic artifact.[22]

References

1. Alexander JA, Sheppard S, Davis PC, Salverda P: Adult cerebrovascular disease: role of modified rapid fluid-attenuated inversion-recovery sequences. AJNR 17:1507–1513, 1996

2. Awad I, Modic M, Litte JR et al: Focal parenchymal lesions in transient ischemic attacks: correlation of computed tomography and magnetic resonance imaging. Stroke 17:399–404, 1986

3. Back T, Hoehn-Berlage M, Kohno K, Hossmann KA: Diffusion nuclear magnetic resonance imaging in experimental stroke. Correlation with cerebral metabolities. Stroke 25:494–500, 1994

4. Barker PB, Gillard JH, van Zijl PCM et al: Acute stroke: evaluation with serial proton MR spectroscopic imaging. Radiology 192:723–732, 1994

5. Bienveniste H, Hedlund LW, Johnson GA: Mechanism of detection of acute cerebral ischemia in rats by diffusion-weighted magnetic resonance microscopy. Stroke 23:746–754, 1992

6. Birken D, Olendorf WH: N-acetyl aspartic acid: a literature review of a compound prominent in ^{1}H-NMR spectroscopic studies of the brain. Neurosci Biobehav Rev 13:23–31, 1989

7. Bollensen E, Buzanoski JH, Prange HW: Brainstem compression by basilar artery anomalies as visualized by MRI. J Neurol 238:49, 1991

8. Bozzoa L, Angeloni U, Bastianello S et al: Early angiographic and CT findings in patients with hemorrhagic infarction in the distribution of the middle cerebral artery. AJNR 12:1115, 1991

9. Brant-Zawadzki M, Atkinson D, Detrick M et al: Fluid-attenuated inversion recovery (FLAIR) for assessment of cerebral infarction: initial clinical experience in 50 patients, Stroke 27:7 1187–1191, 1996

10. Brant-Zawadski M, Pereira B, Weinstein P et al: MR imaging of acute experimental ischemia in cats. AJNR 7:7, 1986

11. Bryan RN, Levy LM, Whitlow WD et al: Diagnosis of acute cerebral infarction: comparison of CT and MR imaging. AJNR 12:611, 1991

12. Busch E, Beaulieu C, de Crespigny A, Moseley ME: Are subarachnoid blood clots visible on FLAIR MRI? Proc Int Soc Magn Reson Med 5:625, 1997

13. Busza AL, Allen KL, King MD et al: Diffusion-weighted imaging studies of cerebral ischemia in gerbils: potential relevance to energy failure. Stroke 23:1602–1612, 1992

14. Copen WA, Koroshetz WJ, Ostergaard I, et al: Prediction of ischemic injury in acute human stroke with diffusion- and perfusion- weighted MRI. Proc Int. Soc. Magn Reson. Med 5:272, 1997

15. Crain MR, Yuh WTC, Greene GM et al: Cerebral ischemia: evaluation with contrast-enhanced MR imaging. AJNR 12:631, 1991

16. Crockard HA, Gadian DG, Frackowiak et al: Acute cerebral ischaemia: concurrent changes in CBF, energy metabolites, pH and lactate measured with hydrogen clearance and ^{31}P and ^{1}H nuclear magnetic resonance spectroscopy. II. Changes during ischemia. J Cereb Blood Flow Metab 7:394–402, 1987

17. Davis TL, Kwong KK, Bandettini PA et al: Mapping the dynamics of oxidative metabolism by functional MRI. Proce Int Soc Magn Reson Med 5:151, 1997

18. De Cristofaro MT, Mascalchi M, Pupi A et al: Subcortical arteriosclerotic encephalopathy: single photon emission computed tomography magnetic resonance imaging correlation. Am J Physiol Imaging 5:68, 1990

19. DeLaPaz RL: Echo planar imaging. Radiographics 14:1045–1058, 1994

20. DeLaPaz RL, New PFJ, Buonanno: NMR imaging of intracranial hemorrhage. J Comput Assist Tomogr 8:599–607, 1984

21. Demaerel P, Van Hecke P, Marchal G et al: MRI of intraparenchymal hematoma: responsible mechanisms. J Belge Radiol 73:279, 1990

22. Doyon D, David P, Halimi P: Les clips vasculaires cerebraux en IRM. Contre indication absolue ou relative. J Radiol 70:123, 1989

23. Duijn JH, Matson GB, Maudsley AA et al: Human brain infarction: proton MR spectroscopy. Radiology 183:711–718, 1992

24. Duong TQ, Song S-K, Neil JJ et al: Cerebral sodium accumulation in transient focal ischemia in rat: a ^{23}Na MRI study. Proc Int Soc Magn Reson Med 5:502, 1997

25. Elster AD, Moody DM: Early cerebral infarction: gadopentetate dimeglumine enhancement. Radiology 177:627, 1990

26. Fenstermacher MJ, Narayana PA: Serial proton magnetic resonance spectroscopy of ischemic brain injury in humans. Invest Radiol 25:1034–1039, 1990

27. Fisher CM, Adams RD: Observations on brain embolism with special reference to the mechanism of hemorrhagic infarction. J Neuropathol Exp Neurol 10:92, 1951

28. Ford CC, Griffey RH, Matwiyoff NA, Rosenberg GA: Multivoxel^{1}H-MRS of stroke. Neurology 42:1408–1412, 1992

29. Frahm J, Michaelis T, Merboldt K-D et al: On the N-acetylmethyl resonance in localized ^{1}H NMR spectra of the hyman brain. In Vivo NMR Biomed 4:201–204, 1991

30. Froment JC, Bascoulergue Y, Crouzet G et al: Apparently isolated, spontaneous haematomas of the brain stem. Seven cases explored by CT and MRI. J Neuroradiol 16:38, 1989

31. Fukuda O, Sato S, Suzuki T et al: MRI of acute cerebral infarction. No Shinkei Geka 17:31, 1989

32. Gass A, Gaa J, Sommer A et al: Echo planar diffusion

weighted magnetic resonance imaging improves pattern recognition in patients with cerebral ischemia. Proc Int Soc Magn Reson Med 5:270, 1997

33. Gideon P, Henrickson O, Sperling B et al: Early time course of N-acetyl aspartate, creatine, and phosphocreatine, and compounds containing choline in the brain after acute stroke. A proton magnetic resonance spectroscopy study. Stroke 23:1566–1572, 1992

34. Gomori JM, Grossman RI, Goldberg HI et al: Intracranial hematomas: imaging by high-field MR. Radiology 157:87, 1985

35. Gomori JM, Grossman RI, Hackney DB et al: Variable appearances of subacute intracranial hematomas on high field spin echo MR. AJR 150:171, 1988

36. Gomori JM, Grossman RI, Yu IC, Asakura T: NMR relaxation times of blood: dependence on field strength, oxidation state, and cell integrity. J Comput Assist Tomogr. 11:684, 1987

37. Graham GD, Blamire AM, Rothman DL et al: Early temporal variation of cerebral metabolism after human stroke. A proton magnetic resonance spectroscopy study. Stroke 24:1891–1896, 1993

38. Gruetter R, Seaquist ER, Adriany G et al: Localized ^{13}C MRS of the human visual cortex. Proc Int Soc Magn Reson Med 5:1216, 1997

39. Gyngell ML, Back T, Hoehn-Berlage M et al: Transient cell depolarization after permanent middle cerebral artery occlusion: an observation by diffusion-weighted MRI and localized 1H-MRS. Magn Reson Med 31: 337–341, 1994

40. Hanstock CC, Rothman, Prichard JW et al: Spatially localized ^{1}H NMR spectra of metabolites in the human brain. Proc Natl Acad Sci USA 85:1821–1825, 1988

41. Hasegawa Y, Fisher M, Latour I et al: MRI diffusion mapping of reversible and irreversible ischemic injury in focal brain ischemia. Neurology 44:1484–1490, 1994

42. Hayman LA, Evans RA, Bastion FU et al: Delayed high dose contrast CT: identifying patients at risk for massive hemorrhagic infarction. AJR 136:1151–1159, 1981

43. Hayman LA, Taber KH, Ford JJ et al: Mechanisms of MR signal alteration by acute intracerebral blood: old concepts and new theories. AJNR 12:899, 1991

44. Heiss W-D, Herholz K, Boecher-Schwarz HG et al: PET, CT, and MR imaging in cerebrovascular disease. J Comput Tomogr 10:903, 1986

45. Hesselink JR, Press GA: MR contrast enhancement of intracranial lesions with Gd DTPA. Radiol Clin North Am. 26:873, 1988

46. Hope PL, Cady EB, Chu A et al: Brain metabolism and intracellular pH during ischemia and hypoxia: an in vivo ^{31}P and ^{1}H nuclear magnetic resonance study in the lamb. J Neurochem 49:75–82, 1987

47. Hornig CR, Dorndorf W, Agnoli AL: Hemorrhagic cerebral infarction—a prospective study. Stroke 17: 179–185, 1986

48. Imakita S, Nishimura T, Yamada N et al: Magnetic resonance imaging of cerebral infarction: time course of Gd DTPA enhancement and CT comparison. Neuroradiology 30:372, 1988

49. Imakita S, Nishimura T, Yamada N et al: Cerebral vascular malformations: applications of magnetic resonance imaging to differential diagnosis. Neuroradiology 31: 320, 1989

50. Imakita S, Yamada N, Nishimura T et al: Magnetic resonance imaging of cerebrovascular disorders; cerebral infarction. Rinsho-Hoshasen 34:657, 1989

51. Jorgensen L, Rorvik A: Ischemic cerebrovascular disease in an autopsy series. I. Prevalence, location and predisposing factors in verified thromboembolic occlusions, and their significance in the pathogenesis of cerebral infarction. J Neurol Sci 3:490, 1966

52. Kertesz A, Black SE, Nicholson L, Carr T: The sensitivity and specificity of MRI in stroke. Neurology 37:1580, 1987

53. Knight RA, Barker PB, Fagan SC et al: MRI and histopathology of evolving hemorrhagic conversion in ischemic stroke. Proc Int Soc Magn Reson Med 5:501, 1997

54. Kucharczyk J, Mintorovitch J, Moseley ME et al: Ischemic brain damage: reduction by sodium-calcium ion channel modulator RS-87476. Radiology 179:221–227, 1991

55. Le Bihan D (ed): Diffusion and Perfusion Magnetic Resonance Imaging. Lippincott-Raven, Philadelphia, 1995

56. Leblanc R, Levesque M, Comair Y, Ethier R: Magnetic resonance imaging of cerebral arteriovenous malformations. Neurosurgery 21:15, 1987

57. Levine SR, Helpern JA, Welch KMA et al: Human focal cerebral ischemia: evaluation of brain pH and energy metabolism with ^{31}P NMR spectroscopy. Radiology 185: 537–544, 1992

58. Liu Y, Breger R, Blechinger J et al: Stroke evaluation: FLAIR/diffusion-weighted EPI and analysis of EPI perfusion imaging. Proc Int Soc Magn Reson Med 5:566, 1997

59. Lo EH, Matsumoto K, Pierce AR et al: Pharmacologic reversal of acute changes in diffusion-weighted magnetic resonance imaging in focal cerebral ischemia. J Cereb Blood Flow Metab 14:597–603, 1994

60. Lotito S, Blondet P, Francois A et al: Correlation between intracellular pH and lactate levels in the rat brain during potassium cyanide induced metabolism blockade: a combined^{31}P and ^{1}H in vivo nuclear magnetic spectroscopic study. Neurosci Lett 97:91–96, 1989

61. Lutsep H, Albers G, de Crespigny A, Moseley M: Diffusion imaging of human stroke. Proc Int Soc Magn Med 4:89, 1996

62. Maeda M, Crosby DL, Magnotta VA et al: Cerebral hemodynamics in patients with major cerebral artery occlusion or severe stenosis: evaluation with perfusion MR imaging. Proc Int Soc Magn Reson Med 5:594, 1996

63. Marks MP, de Crespigny A, Lentz D et al: acute and chronic stroke: navigated spin-echo diffusion-weighted MR imaging. Radiology 199:403–408, 1996

64. Maruyama K, Tanaka M, Ikeda S et al: A case report of quadriparesis due to compression of the medulla oblongata by the elongated left vertebral artery. Rinsho Shinkeigaku 29:108, 1989

65. Matsumoto K, Lo EH, Pierce AR et al: Diffusion-weighted imaging: comparison with multiparameter MR and immunohistochemistry AJNR 16:1107–1115, 1995

66. Matsumura K, Matsuda M, Handa J, Todo G: Magnetic resonance imaging with aneurysmal subarachnoid hem-

orrhage: comparison with computed tomography scan. Surg Neurol 34:71–87, 1990

67. Matsuoka Y, Hossmann KA: Cortical impedance and extracellular volume changes following middle cerebral artery occlusion in cats. J Cereb Blood Flow Metab 2: 466–474, 1982

68. Mawad ME, Hilal SK, Silver AJ, Sane P: High resolution, high field MR imaging of cerebral arteriovenous malformations. Radiology 153:143, 1984

69. McNamara MT, Brant-Zawadski M, Berry I et al: Acute experimental cerebral ischemia: MR enhancement using Gd-DTPA. Radiology 158:701, 1986

70. Mikami T, Saito K, Oluyama T et al: FLAIR images of subarachnoid hemorrhage (in Japanese). No Shinkei Geka, 24:1087–1092, 1996

71. Minematsu K, Fisher M, Li L, Sotak CH: Diffusion and perfusion magnetic resonance imaging studies to evaluate a noncompetitive N-methyl-D-aspartate antagonist and reperfusion in experimental stroke in rats. Stroke 24:2074–2081, 1993

72. Minematsu K, Li L, Sotak CH et al: Reversible focal ischemic injury demonstrated by diffusion-weighted magnetic imaging in rats. Stroke 23:1304–1311, 1992

73. Miyashita K, Naritomi H, Sawada T, et al: Identification of recent lacunar lesions in cases of multiple small infarctions by magnetic resonance imaging. Stroke 19:834, 1988

74. Mohr JP, Biller J, Hilal SK et al: MR vs CT imaging in acute stroke. Presented at 17th International Conference on Stroke and the Cerebral Circulation, Phoenix A2, 1992

75. Monsein LH, Mathews VP, Barker PB et al: Irreversible regional cerebral ischemia: serial MRI and proton MR spectroscopy in a non-human primate model, AJNR 14: 963–970, 1993

76. Moseley ME, Cohen Y, Mintorovich J: Early detection of cerebral ischemia in cats: comparison of diffusion-and T_2-weighted MRI and spectroscopy. Magn Reson Med 14:330–346, 1990

77. Moseley ME, Kucharczyk J, Mintorovitch J et al: Diffusion-weighted MR imaging of acute stroke: correlation with T_2-weighted and magnetic susceptibility-enhanced MR imaging in cats. AJNR 11:423–429, 1990

78. Muller W, Kramer G, Roder RG, Kuhnert A: Balance of T_1 weighted images before and after application of a paramagnetic substance (Gd DTPA). Neurosurg Rev 10: 117, 1987

79. Nagata I, Kikuchi H, Yamagata S et al: Intraluminal thrombosis and growth mechanism of giant intracranial aneurysms. No Shinkei Geka 18:1115, 1990

80. Nakada T, Houkin D, Hida K, Kwee IL: Rebound alkalosis and persistent lactate: multinuclear (^{1}H, ^{13}C, ^{31}P) NMR spectroscopic studies in rats. Magn Reson Med 18:9–14, 1991

81. Nakajima Y, Ohsuga H, Yamamoto M, Shinohara Y: Asymptomatic cerebral hemorrhage detected by MRI. Rinsho Shinkeigaku 31:270, 1991

82. Noguchi K, Ogawa T, Inugami A et al: Acute subarachnoid hemorrhage: MR imaging with fluid-attenuated inversion recovery pulse sequences, Radiology 196: 773–777, 1995

83. Nussel F, Wegmuller H, Huber P: Comparison of magnetic resonance angiography, magnetic resonance imaging and conventional angiography in cerebral arteriovenous malformation. Neuroradiology 33:56, 1991

84. Patel MR, Edelman RR, Warach S: Detection of hyperacute primary intraparenchymal hemorrhage by magnetic resonance imaging. Stroke 27:2321–2324, 1996

85. Pertuiset B, Haisa T, Bordi L et al: Detection of a ruptured aneurysmal sac by MRI in a case of negative angiogram. Successful clipping of an anterior communicating artery aneurysm. Case report. Acta Neurochir (Wien) 100:84, 1989

86. Pessin MS, Teal PA, Caplan LR: Hemorrhagic infarction: guilt by association. AJNR 12:1123, 1991

87. Petroff OAC, Graham GD, Blamire AM et al: Spectroscopic imaging of stroke in humans: histopathology correlates of spectral changes. Neurology 42:1349–1354, 1992

88. Petroff OAC, Prichard JW, Alger J et al: Cerebral intracellular pH by ^{31}P nuclear magnetic resonance spectroscopy. Neurology 35:781–788, 1985

89. Petroff OAC, Prichard JW, Ogino T, Shulman RG: Proton magnetic resonance spectroscopic studies of agonal carbohydrate metabolism in rabbit brain. Neurology 38: 1569–1574, 1988

90. Pierpoaoli C, Righini A, Linfante I et al: Histopathologic correlations of abnormal water diffusion in cerebral ischemia: diffusion-weighted MR imaging and light and electron microscopy study. Radiology 189:439–449, 1993

91. Plum F: What causes infarction in ischemic brain? Neurology 33:222–233, 1993

92. Prencipe M, Marini C: Leuko-araiosis: definition and clinical correlates—an overview. Eur Neurol 29:27, 1989

93. Rapacki TF, Brantley MJ, Furlow TW Jr et al: Heterogeneity of cerebral cavernous hemangiomas diagnosed by MR imaging. J Comput Assist Tomogr 14:18, 1990

94. Rigamonti D et al: Cerebral cavernous malformations: incidence and familial occurrence. N Engl J Med 319: 343, 1988

95. Roberts TPL, Vexler Z, Derugin N et al: High-speed MR imaging of ischemic brain injury following stenosis of the middle cerebral artery. J Cereb Blood Flow Metab 13:940–946, 1993

96. Sato A, Takahashi S, Soma Y Cerebral infarction: early detection by means of contrast-enhanced cerebral arteries at MR imaging. Radiology 178:433, 1991

97. Sipponen JT, Kaste M, Ketonen L: Serial nuclear magnetic resonance (NMR) imaging in patients with cerebral infarction. J Comput Assist Tomogr 7:585–589, 1993

98. Sorensen AG, Buonanno FS, Gonzalez RG, et al: Hyperacute Stroke: Evaluation with combined multisection diffusion-weighted and hemodynamically weighted echo-planar MR imaging. Radiology 199:391–401, 1996.

99. Sorensen AG, Koroshetz WJ, Buonanno FS et al: Diffusion/perfusion mismatch in MRI of acute human stroke. Proc Int Soc Magn Reson Med 4:91, 1996

100. Spetzler RF, Zabramski JM, Kaufman B, Yeung HN:

Acute NMR changes during MCA occlusions: a preliminary study in primates. Stroke 14:185–191, 1983

101. Spickler E, Lufkin R, Teresi L et al: MR imaging of acute subarachnoid hemorrhage. Comput Med Imaging Graph 14:67, 1990

102. Sunshine JL, Lewin JS, Tarr RW et al: Emergent perfusion/diffusion imaging of the brain in the management of acute stroke. Proc Int Soc Magn Reson Med 5:269, 1997

103. Sze G, Harper PS, Galicich JH et al: Hemorrhagic neoplasms: MR mimics of occult vascular malformations. Am Soc Neuroradiol May 10–15: 125, 1987

104. Taoka T, Iwasaki S, Nakagawa H Fast fluid-attenuated inversion recovery (FAST-FLAIR) of ischemic lesions in the brain: comparison with T2-weighted turbo SE. Radiat Med 14:127–131, 1996

105. Thulborn KR, Sorensen AG, Kowall NW et al: The role of ferritin and hemosiderin in the MR appearance of cerebral hemorrhage: a histopathologic biochemical study in rats. AJNR 11:291, 1990

106. Tkach JA, Perl J, Ding X: Detection of hyperacute parenchymal hematomas and subarachnoid hemorrhage: dog model. Proc Int Soc Magn Reson Med 5:623, 1997

107. Tsai FY, Wang A-M, Matovich VB et al: MR staging of acute dural sinus thrombosis: correlation with venous pressure measurements and implications for treatment and prognosis. AJNR Am J Neuroradiol 16:1021–1029, 1995

108. Uchino A, Ohnari N, Ohno M: MRI of middle cerebral artery occlusion. Nippon Igaku Hoshasen Gakkai Zasshi 49:1355, 1989

109. Uchino A, Onomura K, Ohno M: Wallerian degeneration of the corticospinal tract in the brain stem: MR imaging. Radiat Med 7:74, 1989

110. van Swieten JC, van den Hout JH, van Ketel BA et al: Periventricular lesions in the white matter on magnetic resonance imaging in the elderly. A morphometric correlation with arteriolosclerosis and dilated perivascular spaces. Brain 114:761, 1991

111. Virapongse C, Mancuso A, Quisling R: Human brain infarcts: Gd-DTPA-enhanced MR imaging. Radiology 161:785, 1986

112. Wall SD, Brant-Zawadzki M, Jeffrey RB, Barnes B: High frequency CT findings within 24 hours after cerebral infarction. AJR 138:307–311, 1982

113. Warach S, Chien D, Li D et al: Fast magnetic resonance diffusion-weighted imaging of acute human stroke [published erratum appears in Neurology 42:2192, 1992] Neurology 42:1717–1723, 1992

114. Warach S, Gaa J, Siewert B et al: Acute human stroke studied by whole brain echo planar imaging. Ann Neurol 37:231–241, 1995

115. Weingarten K, Zimmerman RD, Deo-Narine V et al: MR imaging of acute intracranial hemorrhage: findings on sequential spin-echo and gradient-echo images in a dog model. AJNR 12:457, 1991

116. Weingarten K, Filippi C, Zimmerman RD, Deck MD: Detection of hemorrhage in acute cerebral infarction. Evaluation with spin-echo and gradient-echo MRI. Clin Imaging 18:43–55, 1994

117. Williams KD, Drayer BP, Bird CR: Magnetic resonance imaging in the diagnosis of intracerebral hematoma. BNI Q 5:16, 1989

118. Wu O, Weisskoff RM, Copen WA et al: Comparison of scalar metrics of anisotropy in ischemic human brain using diffusion weighted magnetic resonance imaging. Proc Int Soc. Magn Reson Med 5:227, 1997

119. Yuh WT, Crain MR, Loes DJ et al: MR imaging of cerebral ischemia: findings in the first 24 hours. AJNR 12: 62, 1991

120. Zuerrer M, Martin E, Boltshauser E: MR imaging of intracranial hemorrhage in neonates and infants at 2.35 Tesla. Neuroradiology 33:223, 1991

121. Zyed A, Hayman LA, Bryan RN: MR imaging of intracerebral blood: diversity in the temporal pattern at 0.5 and 1.0 T. AJNR 12:469, 1991

Cerebral Angiography

Conventional Angiography

STEPHEN P. LOWNIE

Of the diagnostic measures available to evaluate the blood vessels of the brain, cerebral angiography is the most precise and the most comprehensive. In the 70 years since the neurologist Moniz performed the first such test on a human,[96] it has come to be regarded as the standard for the investigation of cerebral ischemia and hemorrhage.

That designation has been changing. For the patient, cerebral angiography is uncomfortable, and there is a small risk of disabling stroke. For the referring physician, the procedure is not always readily available[56]: the personnel are specialized and the equipment and liquid contrast agent are expensive. In recent years, competing noninvasive technologies have been developed, including Doppler ultrasound, magnetic resonance angiography (MRA), and computed tomographic (CT) angiography (Fig. 13.1). Coupled with standard CT and MR imaging (MRI) they are gradually supplanting angiography in the diagnosis of many, but not all, cerebrovascular disorders.

Indications

ISCHEMIA

Cerebral and ocular ischemia due to atherosclerosis are common indications for angiography, primarily to confirm and quantitate precisely the degree of stenosis at the carotid bifurcation (Table 13.1). Two major clinical trials, the North American Symptomatic Carotid Endarterectomy Trial (NASCET) and the European Carotid Surgery Trial (ECST), have confirmed the benefit of carotid endarterectomy for severe symptomatic carotid stenosis, relying on cerebral angiography to determine whether the stenosis was 70%.[43,103,104]

Currently cerebral angiography is being used not to obtain the diagnosis of carotid bifurcation disease but to define the need for further treatment. In the workup prior to angiography, Doppler ultrasound is used as a reliable screening tool to diagnose carotid bifurcation disease and to exclude patients from angiography with only mild degrees of stenosis or with

sonographically complete occlusion of the internal carotid artery. The latter requires a particularly high level of accuracy using color Doppler if angiography is not undertaken, to ensure that near occlusion is not mistaken for occlusion.[83]

The comprehensive examination obtained with angiography sometimes leads to unexpected findings, which can influence treatment decisions. In the NASCET study of 659 patients, 4 had severe intracranial stenosis and 3 had a cerebral aneurysm, thus a total of 1% was considered technically ineligible for carotid endarterectomy based on angiography.[103] Another 25 (3.8%) had an intraluminal thrombus beyond the stenosis. In the 2,885 patients in NASCET with symptoms due to moderate or severe stenosis, 52 (1.8%) had an intraluminal thrombus (NASCET, unpublished data). In the Veterans Affairs study of asymptomatic carotid stenosis, data from 714 angiograms in 1,935 patients led to exclusion of 23 patients from the study due to severe intracranial stenosis (2.7% of angiograms) or an intraluminal thrombus (0.6% of angiograms).[70] In the Asymptomatic Carotid Atherosclerosis Study (ACAS), in which 415 patients had a postrandomization angiogram prior to surgery, 4 were excluded from surgery due to intracranial abnormalities (aneurysm, arteriovenous malformation [AVM], or severe carotid siphon stenosis in 1%).[44,153] Thus it appears that at least 1% of individuals affected by carotid bifurcation disease will harbor an intracranial vascular lesion of clinical significance and as many as 2% will have thrombus in the arterial lumen. At present, angiography is the best method to detect such lesions prior to carotid surgery.

In the setting of acute ischemic stroke, cerebral angiography is not generally required as part of the diagnostic workup. Cerebral embolism, if detected prior to the development of infarction on CT, may warrant immediate cerebral angiography if the option of intra-arterial thrombolytic therapy exists within the protocol of a clinical investigation.

Extracranial carotid and vertebral artery dissection is often diagnosed on clinical, MRI, and MRA investigations; cerebral angiography may serve as an adjunct to confirm the diagnosis. Fibromuscular dysplasia, which may be present with dissection, is more often detected incidentally during cerebral angiography. In suspected cerebral vasculitis, angiography is considered part of the diagnostic workup along with

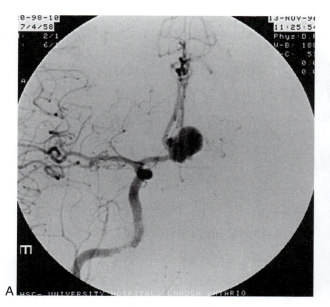
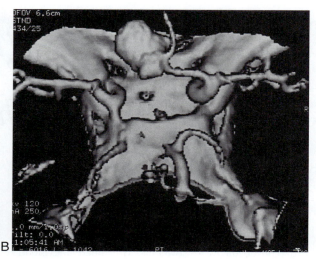

Figure 13.1 (**A**) Right carotid angiogram, anteroposterior projection. Large anterior communicating artery aneurysm. (**B**) CT angiogram, same patient.

MRI and brain biopsy. In moyamoya disease angiography remains critical to the diagnosis and treatment planning. Venous disease and dolichoectasia are now largely diagnosed with CT, MRI, and MRA.

HEMORRHAGE

Nontraumatic intracranial hemorrhage may be intracerebral, subarachnoid, intraventricular, or subdural in location, alone or in combination. Intracerebral hemorrhage, which accounts for 10% of all strokes, is most commonly due to hypertension (about one-half of cases).[46] These hemorrhages are deeply located in the basal ganglia, thalamus, cerebellum, and pons. Angiography is not usually helpful. In the absence of hypertension, clinical evidence of anticoagulant use or the abuse of crack cocaine or alcohol should be sought; these account for another 10% to 20% of cases.[46] Angiography should be considered in most other situations. CT or MRI may provide clues to the presence of underlying glioma or metastasis by the presence of excess edema, contrast enhancement, and multiple or unusual locations of hemorrhage. Intracerebral hemorrhage due to aneurysm or AVM will often be associated with subarachnoid hemorrhage.

Hemorrhage that is purely subarachnoid and/or intraventricular in location warrants an urgent cerebral angiogram. Cerebral aneurysm and cerebral AVM are the most frequent diagnoses, about 75% and 5% of cases respectively (Figs. 13.2 and 13.3). Angiography is negative after subarachnoid hemorrhage in 15% of cases. Consideration should be given to performing a second angiogram 1 week later (Fig. 13.4). The subject of aneurysms is covered extensively in Chapter 26.

Table 13.1 Indications and Nonindications for Cerebral Angiography

Condition	Indication	Relative Indication or Not Indicated
	Quantitation of carotid bifurcation stenosis	Diagnosis of carotid atherosclerosis
	Preoperative assessment of intracranial circulation prior to carotid endarterectomy	Acute stroke
		Cerebral embolism
		Extracranial carotid/vertebral artery dissection
	Suspected intracranial atherosclerosis or dissection	Venous disease
		Dolichoectasia
	Clinically suspected vasculitis with consistent MRI	
Ischemia	Suspected moyamoya disease	
		Hypertensive hemorrhage
	Suspected aneurysm	Anticoagulant/illicit drug use
	Suspected AVM	
	Suspected vasculitis	Neoplasm
Hemorrhage	Suspected moyamoya	Amyloid angiopathy

Abbreviation: AVM, arteriovenous malformation.

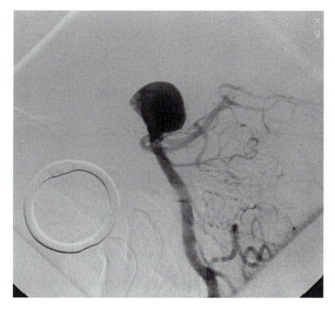

Figure 13.2 Left vertebral angiogram, lateral projection, in a 63-year-old woman with acute subarachnoid hemorrhage. Giant basilar bifurcation aneurysm.

OTHER INDICATIONS

Cerebral angiography is frequently undertaken prior to planned therapeutic procedures. It is important to delineate the vascular anatomy of a cerebral AVM, dural fistula, aneurysm, or tumor prior to surgery or embolization. Angiography is also useful to evaluate vessel narrowing due to vasospasm or atherosclerosis prior to angioplasty. Angiographic evaluation of the collateral circulation with manual compression of the carotid artery is valuable prior to planned surgical or detachable balloon occlusion for the treatment of aneurysm or tumor. In epilepsy, internal carotid artery sodium amytal injection is used to lateralize speech and memory function in the angiography suite.

Safety

From the time of its introduction in 1927[96] until the 1950s and 1960s, virtually all cerebral angiography was performed by direct needle puncture of the carotid and vertebral arteries. As early as 1941 the femoral artery was cannulated using an open approach, passing a catheter up to the abdominal aorta to perform angiography.[45] Ten years later a catheter technique was used to perform carotid angiography in two cancer chemotherapy patients.[14] In 1953 the era of percutaneous angiography was ushered in by Seldinger.[128] He used a needle with a stylet to puncture the artery, through which a flexible metal guidewire was inserted, whereupon the needle was removed, and a polyethylene catheter with the same diameter as the needle was advanced over the wire. He and his colleagues performed 35 aortograms without complications.

In 1963 Lang[81] conducted a survey of 204 physicians who were using the Seldinger technique. There were 89 serious or fatal complications in 11,402 procedures. Local arterial thrombosis accounted for 53% of these, arterial embolism 10%, and remote arterial thrombosis 10%. Thus, thromboembolic phenomena were the cause of three-fourths of all of the serious or fatal complications.

Two potential solutions to the problem of catheter-related thrombosis were considered.[39,50] One was to heparinize the patient systemically. It was found that a small systemic dose of heparin (30 U/kg) was sufficient to eliminate 95% of the surface clot on indwelling catheters in dogs.[100] Clinical trials comparing systemic heparinization with controls (in which heparin was used in the catheter flushing solution only) showed a significantly lower incidence of thromboembolic complications and catheter thrombus.[8,145] However, heparinized patients showed a higher incidence of local hematoma and had longer arterial compression times. The second potential solution was to embed catheters with heparin to make them less thrombogenic.[50] In a controlled study in which heparinized catheters were used, Eldh and Jacobsson[39] detected no catheter thrombus in 26 patients, compared with an 80% detection rate in controls.

At the present time, most centers do not systemically heparinize patients for routine diagnostic cerebral angiography. Many radiologists either intermittently flush the catheter with heparinized saline or run heparinized infusion into the catheter between contrast injections. As a result, a delayed mild systemic anticoagulation usually occurs.[146] It is not known whether routine systemic anticoagulation[29] results in decreased risk of stroke during (or after) the procedure. The risk may be similar whether systemic heparin is used or not.

Besides using either local or systemic heparin, structural factors associated with the formation of catheter thrombus have been identified. Mani[91] found the most significant factor to be the ratio of the diameter of the catheter to the diameter of the artery. In a prospective study of 176 femoral catheterizations using either 5 French (1.6-mm) or 7 French (2.4-mm) diameter catheters, the 9 cases of catheter thrombus all occurred with the use of the larger catheter. Formerly, large-bore catheters were required to allow adequate injection rates of contrast agent to perform arch aortograms. Improvements in catheter material strength have allowed 6 French[38] and more recently 5 French[68] catheters to be used for arch studies instead.

The use of heparin-impregnated catheters (with or without systemic heparinization), the practice of catheter flushing or catheter infusion with heparinized saline, the progressive reductions in catheter diameter, and the heparin coating of guidewires have all contributed to angiography that is safer for the patient.

Factors related to the patient's clinical condition must also be considered in planning safe angiography. Blood pressure should be under good control if the patient is hypertensive. Factors such as advanced age, cerebrovascular disease, elevated creatinine, and diabetes mellitus cannot be modified but should enter into the primary decision to perform cerebral angiography in a particular patient.

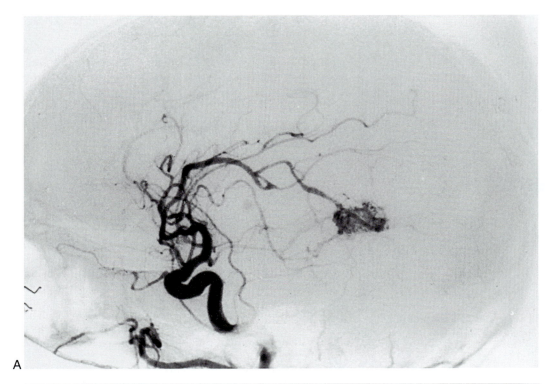

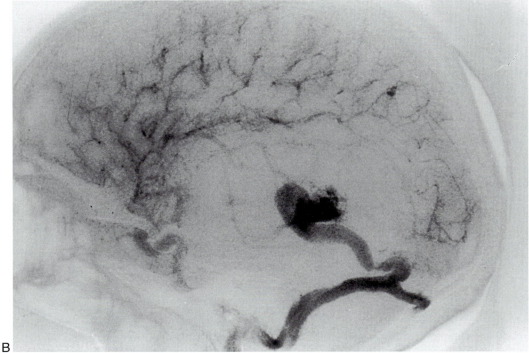

Figure 13.3 (**A**) Left carotid angiogram, lateral projection, in a middle-aged woman with acute headache and aphasia and a large left posterior temporal lobe intracerebral hematoma on CT scan. Early arterial phase shows a small temporal lobe arteriovenous malformation (AVM). Marked elevation of the Sylvian vessels also noted due to mass effect from hematoma. (**B**) Venous phase of same angiogram shows AVM venous drainage into an enlarged vein of Labbe and then into the transverse sinus. Note the stenosis of the draining vein and surrounding loss of the capillary blush due to mass effect from the hematoma.

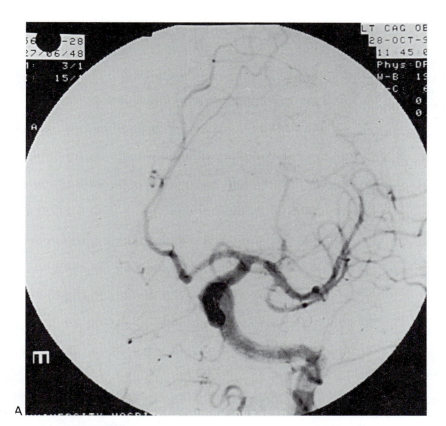

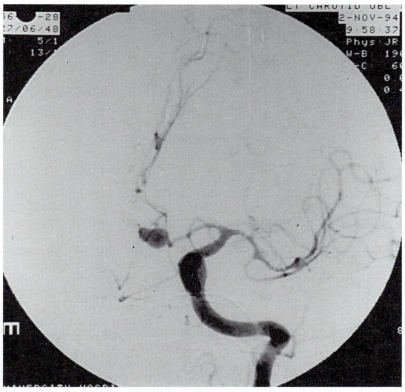

Figure 13.4 (**A**) Left carotid angiogram, oblique view, performed early following subarachnoid hemorrhage. No evidence of aneurysm. (**B**) Same injection, 5 days later. Angiographic appearance of anterior communicating aneurysm in the interim. Also note moderate vasospasm affecting anterior and middle cerebral arteries.

Risk

There is a small but significant risk of major stroke or death during or soon after cerebral angiography. Early prospective studies identified the risk to be <0.5% and to be associated with advanced age (older than 70 years), elevated serum creatinine (>120), hypertension, a lengthy procedure time (> 60 minutes), and the use of several angiographic catheters.[31,32]

Table 13.2 summarizes eight recent studies examining the risk of transient ischemic attack (TIA), stroke, or death following cerebral angiography.[31,32,58,62,66,70,147,153] In most instances, events occurring during or within 24 hours of the angiogram were considered direct complications of angiography. In the study of Dion et al,[31] an additional 0.3% of patients suffered a permanent stroke between 24 and 72 hours. It is uncertain whether such events should be attributed to angiography. The study of Hankey et al[62] included events up to 72 hours after the procedure, with an overall major stroke rate of 1.3%, the highest risk reported. That study involved patients referred to a single neurologist from 1977, of whom one-third underwent direct carotid puncture rather than the transfemoral approach in general use today.

As in studies of carotid endarterectomy for asymptomatic carotid stenosis, neurologic events such as transient cerebral ischemia and minor stroke have in some studies been combined with major stroke, resulting in an inflated assessment of risk. In the Veterans Affairs study, one of the three strokes related to angiography resulted in hemiparesis (0.1%), with the remaining two patients having minimal neurologic deficits.[70] In the ACAS, an angiographic stroke risk of 1.2% was indicated in the first report, although in a subsequent paper two or possibly three disabling strokes were stated to have occurred in 415 patients (0.5% to 0.7%).[44,153]

Except for the study of Hankey et al,[62] the average risk of major stroke or death within 24 hours of angiography from these studies is 0.3% and that of TIA or minor stroke is 1.0%.

Table 13.2 Neurologic Complications of Cerebral Angiography in Recent Major Studies

Author	Year	No. of Patients	Major Stroke or Death within 24 h (%)	TIA or Minor Stroke (%)
Earnest et al[32]	1983	1,387	0.4	1.2
Dion et al[31]	1987	724	0.1	1.2
Hankey et al[62,a]	1990	382	1.3	1.3
Grzyska et al[58]	1990	1,095	0.1	0.5
Waugh and Sacharias[147]	1992	922	0.3	0.6
Veterans Affairs[70]	1993	714	0.1	0.3
Heiserman et al[66]	1994	688	0.7	0.7
ACAS[44,153]	1996	415	0.5	1.0

Abbreviations: TIA, transient ischemic attack; ACAS, Asymptomatic Carotid Atherosclerosis Study.

[a] Events up to 72 hours included in this study.

Technical Aspects

Most angiographers recognize that selective cannulation of the great vessels is mandatory for adequate intracranial angiography. Modified catheters and guidewires have been developed to aid in the negotiation of tortuous atherosclerotic vessels. During retrograde passage up the aorta, the J-shaped guidewire is used to prevent inadvertent vessel injury.[99] Certain catheter configurations, either preshaped by the manufacturer or shaped by the angiographer, facilitate selective cannulation of the origins of the innominate, left common carotid, and left subclavian arteries.[69,142]

In the evaluation of cerebrovascular disease, the angiographer determines from the clinical history and neurologic examination the major arterial territory (i.e., carotid or vertebral, right or left) suspected to be causing the patient's symptoms. That territory is studied first. Extracranial (cervical) and intracranial views in the anteroposterior (AP) and lateral projections are obtained. Arterial, capillary, and venous phases are visualized intracranially. If the major vessel is occluded or flow is compromised, the contralateral artery is studied to evaluate the collateral circulation. In addition, any potential extracranial source of vessel reconstitution is also studied (e.g., the carotid artery in the case of vertebral artery occlusion, since muscular collaterals from the carotid system may reconstitute a proximally occluded vertebral, or vice versa). With symptoms in one carotid territory, both carotid arteries are usually studied: contralateral internal carotid artery occlusion or siphon stenosis is of clinical significance.[153] For carotid disease selective vertebral injections are probably not required unless the intracranial collateral circulation needs to be seen. In vertebrobasilar disease however, the carotids are usually injected in addition to the vertebrals.

The arch aortogram, performed in the right posterior oblique projection to open up the arch of the aorta, provides a survey of the great vessel origins, including the vertebral arteries. Often a routine part of the study of atherosclerotic patients in many centers, its diagnostic yield is low (Fig. 13.5). In one series of 1,000 patients who had arch aortograms, only 18 had significant intrathoracic pathology.[3] Some angiographers only perform an arch aortogram if symptoms remain unexplained after selective carotid and subclavian and/or vertebral injections, about 10% of patients ultimately requiring it.[75]

The advent of digital computer technology has allowed immediate subtraction images to be obtained by digitizing the radiologic image into a matrix before and after the injection of radiographic contrast.[28,35,134] The spatial resolution of this method depends on the size of the matrix, which is 512 to 1,024 for most systems currently in use. Such spatial resolution is less than that obtained with conventional film screen methods, but contrast sensitivity is superior with digital techniques.[28] The advantages of intra-arterial digital subtraction angiography (DSA) include the ability to use smaller doses of contrast agent and smaller catheters. Because images are computerized immediately and can be replayed, there is no time lost in developing, checking, or changing film as there is with conventional methods. The overall procedure time is shortened, decreasing patient discomfort. These advantages

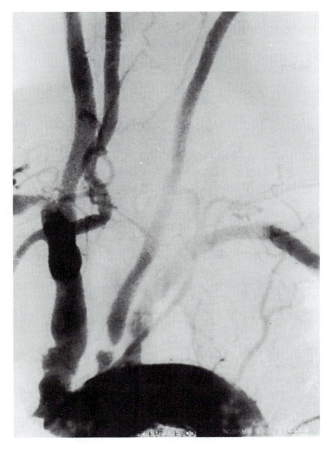

Figure 13.5 Arch aortogram, right posterior oblique projection. Severe stenosis near the origin of the left common carotid artery.

have led to a gradual adoption of intra-arterial DSA by most centers.

Angiographic Indicators of Pathology in Cerebral Ischemia

ANGIOGRAPHY OF ACUTE STROKE

CT and MRI have largely replaced cerebral angiography in the diagnosis of early or completed stroke. The angiographic findings continue to be of importance in acute stroke therapies such as intra-arterial thrombolysis.

Arterial branch occlusion is the most frequent angiographic finding.[82,140] In descending order, the middle, posterior, and anterior cerebral arteries and their branches are affected.[82] A local region of avascularity may be seen during the capillary phase of the angiogram. As a result of the obstruction, regional arteries may take longer to empty themselves

of contrast, and they may still be seen during the capillary or venous phases of the angiogram.[140] Another phenomenon is late filling of the occluded vessel in a retrograde manner from distal collateral branches. Leptomeningeal collateral may be associated with hemorrhagic transformation after ischemic stroke.[21]

When contrast passes rapidly into local cerebral veins, the terms arteriovenous shunting or early venous filling are used.[48] The cause may be either local vasodilatation or a bypass of the occluded capillary bed. The finding is common in the first 2 weeks following infarction. Associated capillary blush in the infarcted region may also occur.[117]

Ultimately, recanalization of occluded cerebral vessels usually takes place. Almost half recanalize within 1 week.[73] Some residual vessel narrowing or local stenosis is common. Distal cerebral branches may occlude in the interim. The only remaining signs of infarction in the subacute stage may be the evidence of mass effect or capillary blush.

COLLATERAL CIRCULATION

Collateral blood flow is most frequently invoked in the preservation of blood flow to an area that would otherwise be rendered ischemic. In addition, collateral circulation is seen in situations not necessarily preserving blood flow. AVMs are an example of this situation. Finally, inappropriate collateral has been postulated to actually cause ischemia by diverting blood away from the brain (the so-called steal effect), as in the subclavian steal phenomenon.

Collateral pathways are divided into intracranial and extracranial types.[86,93,98,129,149] Intracranial collateral includes circle of Willis and leptomeningeal sources. The most physiologically important is the circle of Willis. Leptomeningeal collateral, the connections between superficial cortical branches of the major arterial territories, is much less effective than the circle of Willis in maintaining flow (Fig. 13.6). Extracranial pathways include extracranial-to-intracranial and extracranial-to-extracranial connections. The former comprise numerous branches of the external carotid artery (ECA), which by various routes connect with either the petrous, cavernous, or supraclinoid (ophthalmic) segments of the internal carotid artery (ICA) (Fig. 13.7). Also in this group are the unusual transdural anastomoses (rete mirabile) between dural arteries and superficial cortical vessels.[84,148] The extracranial-to-extracranial group includes reconstitution of the carotid system by the vertebral artery (or vice versa) through muscular collaterals, in the event of more proximal occlusion of the artery (Fig. 13.7). Anatomic variations may also permit such collateral to arise.[111]

In a review of 573 angiograms done for all disorders on the author's unit in 1990, collateral circulation was observed in 24% of patients; half of these patients had atherosclerotic disease (unpublished data). Among these, the circle of Willis collateral was seen in 86% and was the exclusive form of collateral in 44%. Circle of Willis plus ECA-to-ICA collateral accounted for a further 25% of observed collateral. In the atherosclerotic carotid occlusions, the ophthalmic artery was the most frequent (74%) and inferred to be the most hemodynamically significant form of ECA-to-ICA collateral.

A potential consequence of the excellent preservation of cerebral blood flow by the circle of Willis is that stroke may be less common in people with well-developed circles. There is pathologic evidence to substantiate this. "Normal" circles are considered to have all of their constituent vessels at least 1 mm in diameter. In a series comparing 194 infarcted brains with 350 normal ones, the normals had 52% normal circles, while the infarcts had only 33%.[6] Tiny posterior communicating and tiny proximal anterior cerebral arteries were more frequent in the infarcted brains. Another study, comparing 49 infarcted brains with 88 controls, substantiated these findings.[12] More recent investigations undertaken during carotid endarterectomy with electroencephalographic monitoring or using MRA have reached similar conclusions.[89,126]

Collateral blood flow to the brain may present a devious route for cerebral emboli. This could occur if atheromatous disease affected the collateral artery itself. Also, the "stump" of an occluded ICA may act as the source of emboli passing through ECA collateral.[11]

Inappropriate collateral, as in the subclavian steal phenomenon, may be overrated as a cause of neurologic symptoms. In a Doppler study of 324 patients with reversed verte-bral artery flow, 64% had no neurologic symptoms at all, while 31 patients had hemispheric events due to concomitant carotid stenosis.[67] The 5% who clinically had brain stem events all had bilateral flow reversal in the vertebral arteries. Thus, although the condition is angiographically striking (Fig. 13.8), careful clinical and ultrasound evaluation is warranted, as most such patients do not have true brain stem ischemia.

STENOSIS

In a rigid system, as the diameter of a tube decreases, the rate of fluid flowing through it also declines. The relationship is not linear. In fact, the flow decreases as a function of the fourth power of the radius, a very steep rate of decline.

In living systems the relationship is different. In two canine studies arterial blood flow did not decrease until the cross-sectional area was reduced by 80%.[92,94] This corresponds to a reduction in arterial diameter of 50% to 60%. Studies in humans have yielded comparable results. In two studies in which patients underwent application of an external carotid clamp, there was no significant change in pressure or flow until the cross-sectional area was reduced by 70% to

Figure 13.6 (**A**) Left common carotid angiogram, Towne projection, early arterial phase. Tapered occlusion of the proximal middle cerebral artery (arrow). (**B**) Later phase. Lepto-meningeal collateral (arrows) from the distal anterior cerebral to distal middle cerebral territory.

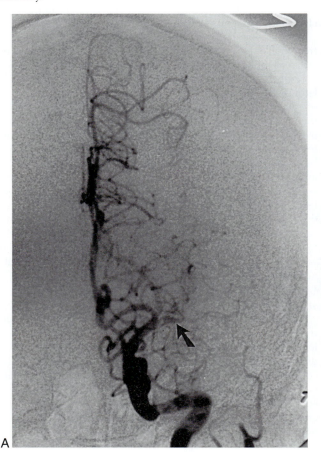

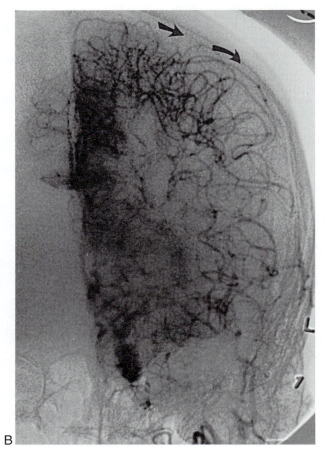

A

B

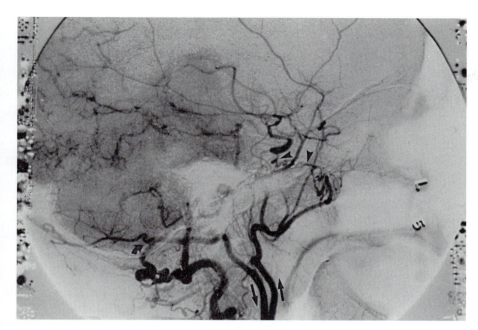

Figure 13.7 Left vertebral angiogram, lateral projection. Case of left common carotid artery occlusion. Muscular branch of vertebral artery (curved arrow) fills the external carotid artery retrogradely via the occipital artery (arrow downward). This fills the internal maxillary artery (arrow upward), which reconstitutes the supraclinoid carotid artery via various branches including the artery of the foramen rotundum (arrowheads).

90%.[22,141] Another study of 61 patients with atherosclerotic narrowing showed that a reduction of luminal diameter by 63% uniformly resulted in a significant distal pressure drop.[30] Stenosis of 48% to 62% had variable effects. Thus in living systems, when the diameter of an artery is decreased by up to 50% there is little or no measurable effect on flow. Above this, flow declines rapidly in proportion to the decrease in the diameter of the vessel.

The degree of a stenosis is more important than its length. Doubling the length of a 1.5-cm stenosis reduces flow by only 5% to 8%.[144] With tandem stenosis, the combined effect is not additive but corresponds approximately to the effect of the more severe stenosis alone.[144]

Although flow is more closely related to luminal area than luminal diameter, conventional angiographic measurements of stenosis are based on the latter. It is important to measure the degree of stenosis objectively on an angiogram rather than use an eyeball approach.[110] In the Joint Study of Extracranial Arterial Occlusion (1969), the segment of arterial stenosis was compared with the lumen of normal-appearing artery at and above the carotid bulb.[17] Others have used the width proximal to the stenosis as the denominator.[7] In the NASCET study, the percentage of luminal narrowing was calculated using the internal carotid diameter distal to the bulb and any post-stenotic dilatation as the denominator[104] (Fig. 13.9). The ECST study used an estimate of the original carotid bulb diameter as the denominator.[43] These different methods can lead to major differences in the estimate of stenosis.[122,123] The NASCET method utilizes a smaller denominator than the ECST method. When the ECST method measures a narrowing at 82%, the corresponding reading in NASCET is 70%.

Fewer patients are designated as "severe" by the NASCET measurement. While controversy persists, most clinicians in North America who do measure stenosis are usually using the NASCET method.[40]

ANGIOGRAPHIC DIFFERENTIAL DIAGNOSIS OF SPECIFIC DISEASES

Generally, the findings seen at cerebral angiography allow for a straightforward radiologic diagnosis. In the case of arterial stenosis, the location is one helpful point of differentiation. Atherosclerosis characteristically involves the proximal ICA, while dissection and fibromuscular dysplasia usually occur in the upper cervical part of the vessel.

The string sign of the ICA is most often due to atheromatous disease, usually near occlusion[95] (Fig. 13.10). The other causes are dissection, intimal fibroplasia, radiation-induced fibrosis, or a congenital small ICA.

Angiographic Findings in Specific Pathologies

ATHEROSCLEROSIS

There have been numerous angiographic studies of the topography of atherosclerotic plaques causing cerebrovascular disease. Comparison is difficult because of differences in the patient demographics and differences in disease severity (stroke versus transient ischemia versus no symptoms). Large angiographic studies from the 1960s allow for certain generalizations in populations of predominantly white male North Americans.[13,65,101] The common carotid bifurcation/proximal ICA is the commonest site of involvement, being affected in 50% to 80%. At this location, stenosis is about two to three times more common than complete arterial occlusion in symptomatic individuals. The next most frequent site of involvement is the vertebral artery, most commonly its origin. Here, stenosis and occlusion are about equal in occurrence. The proximal subclavian arteries are the third most frequently affected, the left side two to three times more often than the right. Intracranially, stenosis or occlusion is less common. Individually, the basilar (Fig. 13.11), intracranial carotid siphon, and proximal circle of Willis arteries are each involved in 1% to 4% of patients.

More recent studies have examined race and sex differences in the topography of atherosclerosis. White race is a strong predictor of extracranial carotid artery disease; blacks, Hispanics, and Asians have a predilection for intracranial disease.[150] Male sex appears to be associated with intracranial stenosis.[13,150] Intracranial disease may be more common than was observed in earlier studies.[13,65,101,150]

Figure 13.8 Right vertebral angiogram, straight anteroposterior projection. Retrograde flow down the left vertebral artery (large arrow), which reconstitutes the left subclavian artery (small arrow). Case of proximal left subclavian occlusion.

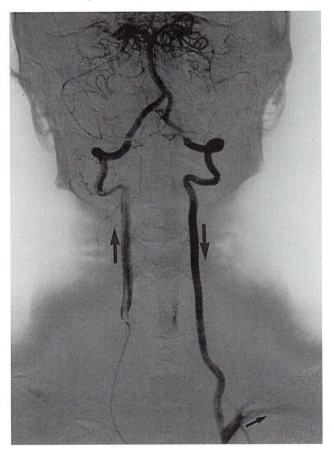

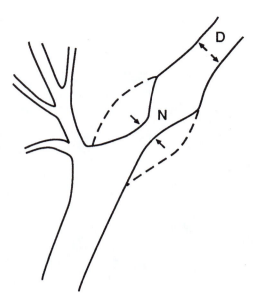

Figure 13.9 N = width in millimeters of lumen at greatest region of stenosis. D = width of the artery distal to the carotid bulb or any poststenotic dilatation. Percentage of stenosis calculated as: $(D-N)/D \times 100$ (NASCET method).

The pathologic features of atherosclerosis include stenosis, ulceration, hemorrhage into a plaque, intraluminal thrombus formation, and occlusion.[132] Stenotic changes at the common carotid bifurcation are most prominent along the posterior wall of the common and internal carotid arteries. The lateral angiographic projection often best depicts this. Stenosis is classified as severe (70% to 99%; Fig. 13.12), moderate (30% to 69%; Fig. 13.13), or mild (< 30%). Markedly severe stenosis causes slowing of internal carotid blood flow, resulting in delayed filling of intracranial branches as compared with extracranial ones (Fig. 13.14).

Atheromatous ulceration was first recognized surgically during carotid endarterectomy, platelet thrombi being seen within the base of the ulcer craters.[74] Ulcer-related debris was invoked as a cause of embolic stroke, even in the absence of hemodynamically significant stenosis.[97] Angiographically, ulcers are often best seen in the lateral projection, although oblique views may be superior.[90] The ICA is the commonest site of ulceration, while external carotid ulceration occurs rarely.[151] Virtually all ulcers are within 2.5 cm of the bifurcation. The best radiographic criterion of ulceration is the so-called penetrating niche, the crater of contrast material seen below overhanging edges of atheroma (Figs. 13.12 and 13.13). The ulcer cavity is contained within the atheroma, not extending beyond the projected line of normal artery wall. Irregularity of the vessel wall is a less reliable criterion of ulceration, since tandem plaque formation may cause such an appearance.[18] If the ulcer is partly or completely superimposed on the artery, a circumscribed double density may be seen, which is another criterion for ulceration[151] (Fig. 13.12).

Reports of the angiographic detection of ulceration, as correlated with the findings at surgery, vary from 50% to 86%.[18,37] The largest multicenter study showed little agreement between biplane angiography and surgical observations.[135] Very severe or very mild degrees of stenosis tend to reduce the accuracy of detection. False-positive interpretations are due to vessel wall irregularities, plaque hemorrhage, and flow phenomena.[34,90] Until recently, the relative inaccuracy of angiography in ulcer detection has hampered studies of the significance of ulceration.[104] Analysis of 659 patients from the NASCET study has shown that angiographic plaque ulceration more than doubles the risk of stroke at higher degrees of stenosis.[41]

Hemorrhage into an atherosclerotic plaque may be un-

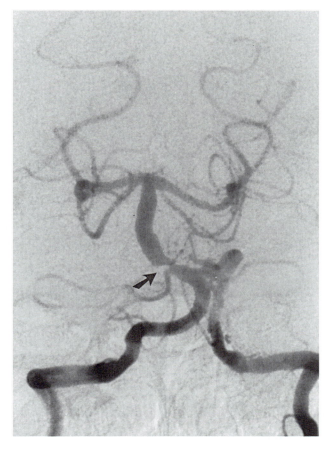

Figure 13.11 Left vertebral angiogram, Towne projection. Stenosis of midbasilar artery distal to the origin of the anterior inferior cerebellar artery (arrow).

Figure 13.10 Left common carotid angiogram, lateral view. Near occlusion of the internal carotid artery due to atherosclerosis with angiographic string sign.

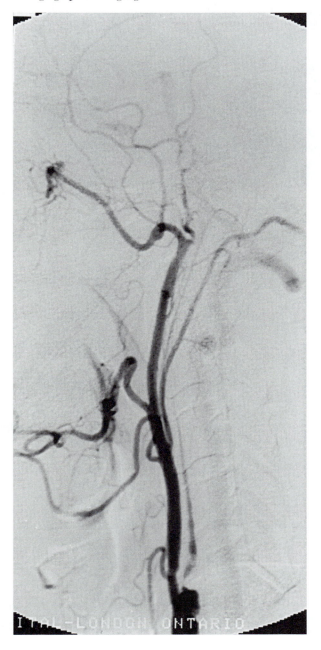

derrated in importance. A study of 50 carotid endarterectomies revealed 12 subintimal hematomas and 20 ulcerated plaques.[33] The distinguishing feature at angiography was a more spheroid shape than the smooth atheromatous plaque, with sharper angles with the adjacent vessel wall. Plaque hemorrhage and its subsequent resolution have been postulated to explain spontaneous disappearance of carotid stenosis at follow-up angiography.[76]

Another local complication of carotid atherosclerosis, frequently associated with ulceration or irregular atheroma, is the formation of intraluminal thrombus. A luminal filling defect, separated from the vessel wall by contrast material on two or more projections, is considered the best angiographic criterion[121] (Fig. 13.15). Multiple views of the carotid bifurcation may be necessary. The thrombus is typically smooth but may be of variable shape, including elongated, tubular, or ball-like.[109] Radiologic differential diagnosis includes a smooth protruding plaque, dissection, and laminar flow caused by severe stenosis.

Internal carotid occlusion may occur in the setting of an acute stroke,[114] or silently, depending on the intracranial collateral circulation and whether distal embolization occurred. The degree to which the collateral pathways can support the intracranial circulation is remarkable; reports exist of occlusion of all four extracranial vessels with minimal neurologic

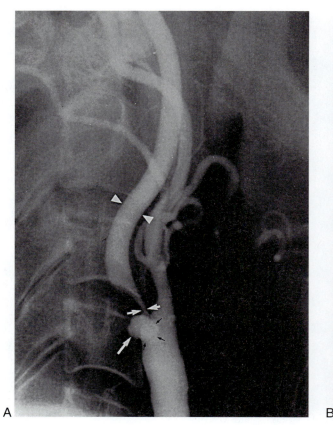
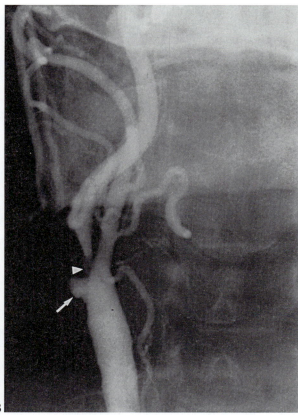

Figure 13.12 (**A**) Right common carotid angiogram, lateral view. Severe stenosis of proximal internal carotid artery: 80% based on width at small white arrows and white arrowheads. Also note the area of ulcer formation (large white arrow), partially superimposed on the carotid bifurcation as a double density (black arrows). (**B**) Anteroposterior view. Laterally pointing ulcer is at large arrow and stenosis at small arrow.

symptoms.[143] It is most important to establish that complete occlusion truly exists. Near-complete occlusion may only be detected with a prolonged imaging run showing very slow antegrade flow.[127] The distal ICA may exhibit collapse down to a tiny string of contrast.[52]

EMBOLISM

Most intracranial arterial occlusions are embolic. Embolic material, derived either from the heart or from the carotid bifurcation atheroma,[59] may lodge virtually anywhere in the cerebrovascular tree, from the high cervical ICA to the peripheral cerebral arterioles.

The middle cerebral artery (MCA) is the most commonly affected vessel.[87] Emboli typically arrest where the artery tapers beyond its first major branch, the anterior temporal artery[5,16] (Fig. 13.16). Larger emboli may lodge more proximally in the MCA trunk, at the level of the internal carotid bifurcation, or where the ICA narrows in the upper cervical region. The posterior cerebral artery, upper basilar artery and its branches, and anterior cerebral artery are less common sites.[24,53]

Radiologically, cerebral embolism was first recognized when follow-up angiography revealed early recanalization of an occluded vessel.[54] Investigators performing serial angiography, beginning in the acute stage, demonstrated actual migration of embolic fragments.[25] Migration occurs within hours to days of the onset of symptoms; the migration itself takes only seconds to minutes.

Without the benefit of repeat angiography showing a patent artery, or the fortuitous observation of clot migration, the angiographic diagnosis of embolism cannot be categorical. Intracranial atheromatous disease (i.e., stenosis with superimposed thrombosis) must also be considered. The classic appearance of an abrupt arrest of contrast is strongly suggestive of an embolus[27] (Fig. 13.16). A convex proximal edge indicates an intraluminal filling defect. Uncommonly, the clot may be only partially occlusive, and the obstructed artery may fill distally (Fig. 13.17).

DISSECTION

Dissections of the craniocervical arteries are traditionally separated according to whether they are extracranial or intracranial and spontaneous or traumatic. Most ICA dissections are extracranial and spontaneous.[36,49,106] Underlying fibromuscular dysplasia (FMD) has been proved in 10% to 20% of these cases.[36,106] Angiographically, the most frequent finding is that of irregular, often eccentric vessel narrowing. The narrowing typically begins distal to the carotid bulb and extends to the level of the skull base, where the vessel resumes its normal caliber (Fig. 13.18). Severe narrowing in such cases has been termed the angiographic string sign.[106]

Dissection of the vertebral artery is most often extracranial. The narrowing begins near the level of the second cervical vertebra and extends a variable distance (Fig. 13.19).

Intracranial dissection is rare and affects the middle cerebral, internal carotid, and vertebral arteries most frequently.[105] Involvement of the zone between the intima and media results in marked stenosis or occlusion, with subsequent infarction.

Dissections involving the media with extension through the vessel wall may result in aneurysm formation and rare but catastrophic subarachnoid hemorrhage. Angiographic stenosis preceded by luminal outpouching has been described as the pearl and string appearance. Vessel encroachment proximal

Figure 13.13 Right common carotid angiogram, lateral view. Moderate stenosis of 40% based on narrowest point (large arrows) compared with normal artery (white arrowheads). There is also a small ulcer (small arrow).

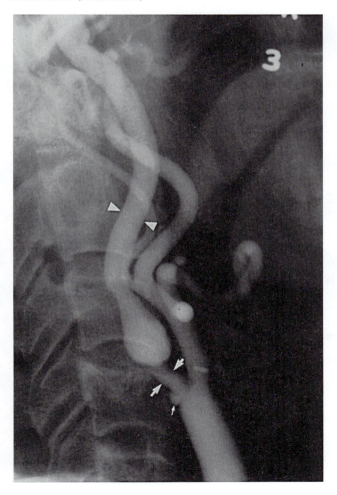

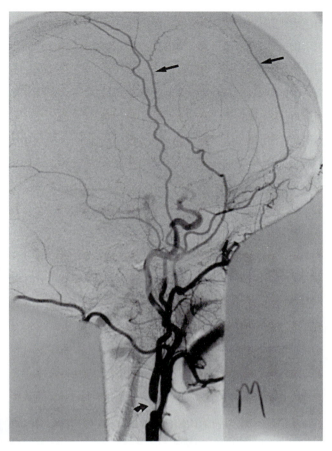

Figure 13.14 Right common carotid angiogram, lateral view. Near occlusion of the proximal internal carotid artery (curved arrow). Delayed internal carotid filling as seen by earlier visualization of external carotid branches (straight arrows).

to an aneurysm, particularly an aneurysm not related to an arterial bifurcation, favors a diagnosis of dissecting aneurysm[88] (Fig. 13.20). Dissecting aneurysms typically arise in the distal vertebral artery. Other sites include the basilar artery and rarely the anterior and middle cerebral arteries.[60,116,118,152]

Definitive angiographic diagnosis requires the visualization of the true and false lumina.[55] Seen in profile, the presence of an intimal flap (Fig. 13.21) is diagnostic. If the two lumina are *en face*, then two strips of contrast of different densities may be seen[80] (Fig. 13.22).

Improved diagnostic accuracy may be obtained with MRI which can demonstrate eccentric high signal intensity blood within the vessel wall (Fig.13.23).

FIBROMUSCULAR DYSPLASIA

Pathologically, arterial FMD most commonly involves the media of the arterial wall. Originally identified in the renal arteries, since 1964 it has also been known to involve extrarenal vessels, including the ICA.[108] Most affected individuals are women.[124]

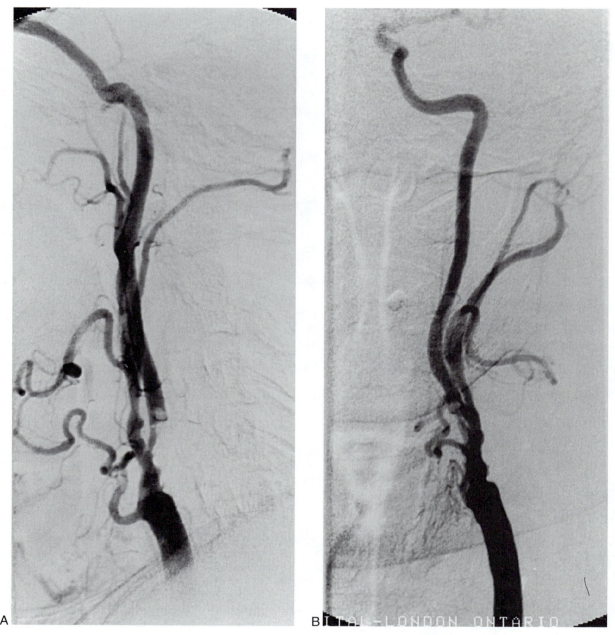

Figure 13.15 (**A**) Left common carotid angiogram, lateral view. Irregular stenosis of the proximal internal carotid artery, with a ball-like intraluminal thrombus. (**B**) Anteroposterior view. Thrombus seen faintly.

In large angiographic series, the incidence of detection of FMD ranges from 0.3% to 0.7%.[71,72] Detection is frequently incidental. In one series of 52 patients, over half were not having symptoms attributable to the disease, and < 20% had cerebral ischemia.[72] Complications of FMD include carotid dissection and carotid-cavernous fistula.[124]

The ICA is affected in 70% to 90% of cases, the vertebral arteries less often.[72,107] Bilateral involvement occurs in more than half. The epicenter of the ICA disease is at the level of the C2 vertebra. The proximal 2.5 cm of the ICA is almost never involved, although a septum or web of fibrous tissue may be seen at the carotid bifurcation.[107,124]

The angiographic hallmark of FMD is the string of beads, contiguous alternating areas of constriction and dilatation, seen in 80% of cases.[107] The areas of dilatation widen the vessel to more than its normal caliber, in contrast to atherosclerosis.[72] Less frequent is the appearance of single or multiple areas of tubular stenosis, without intervening dilatation. Unusually, multiple aneurysmal dilatations of the affected vessel may be seen.[107]

Rarely, FMD may involve the intracranial circulation, in-

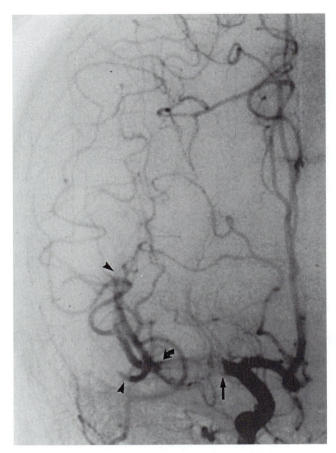

Figure 13.17 Right common carotid angiogram, Towne projection. Embolus of middle cerebral artery just beyond the bifurcation (straight arrow). The artery fills beyond the embolus (curved arrow). Two other distal emboli are noted (arrowheads).

cluding the ICA, MCA, and vertebrobasilar system.[120] It may not be possible to differentiate the arterial beading or tubular stenosis from changes due to cerebral vasculitis if the extracranial vessels are unaffected.

When fibroplasia involves the intima rather than the media, segments of smooth stenosis are seen angiographically.[136] Short segments may resemble atherosclerosis. Long areas of severe stenosis may cause a string sign similar to arterial dissection, particularly since the proximal internal carotid tends to be spared in both conditions.[136] The string sign usually resolves on follow-up angiography in dissection, but not with intimal fibroplasia.

CEREBRAL VASCULITIS/ VASCULOPATHY

The myriad conditions causing cerebral *vasculitis* have in common an inflammatory process that affects the blood vessel wall. Vasculitis may arise as a primary angiitis restricted to the central nervous system or as a secondary angiitis due to other systemic or CNS diseases.[63,64] Systemic vasculitis causing ce-

Figure 13.16 Left common carotid angiogram, Towne projection. Occlusion of the middle cerebral artery just distal to the anterior temporal branch (arrow). The anterior temporal artery also has an embolus within it (arrowhead).

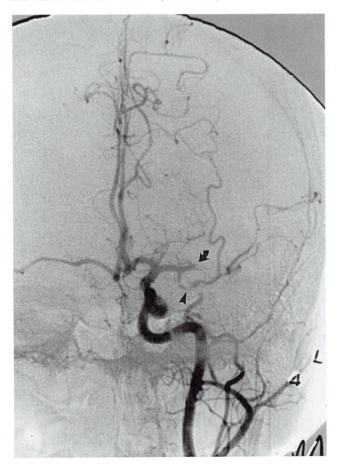

Figure 13.18 (**A**) Right common carotid angiogram, lateral view, cervical level. Irregular narrowing of the internal carotid artery beginning at about the C2 level (arrow). (**B**) Lateral view at level of skull base. The narrowing (curved arrow) continues to the level of the carotid canal where the lumen resumes a normal appearance (straight arrow).

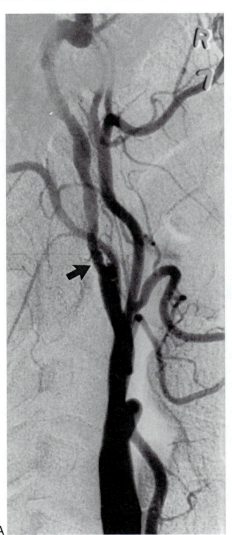

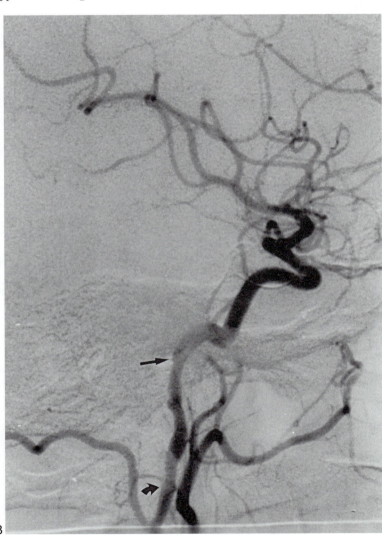

A

B

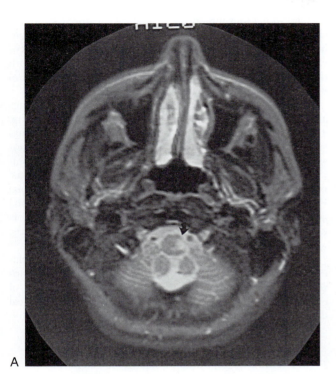

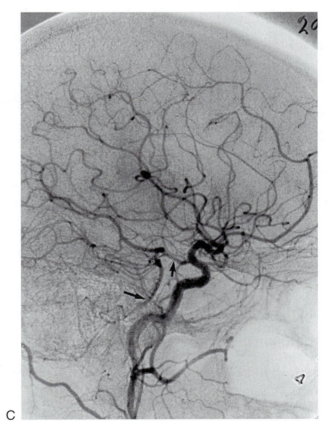

Figure 13.19 (**A**) Axial T$_2$-weighted MR scan showing small infarction in left lateral medulla (arrow). (**B**) Left vertebral angiogram, lateral projection. Irregular narrowing of artery starting at the C1 level (straight arrows). Only a wisp of contrast reaches the basilar artery (curved arrow). (**C**) Right common carotid angiogram, lateral projection. Collateral filling of the basilar artery (large arrow) via the posterior communicating artery (small arrow).

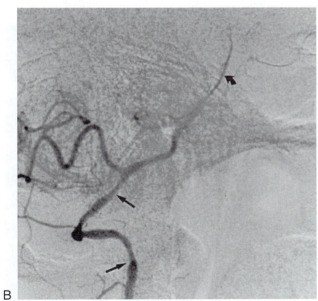

A

B

C

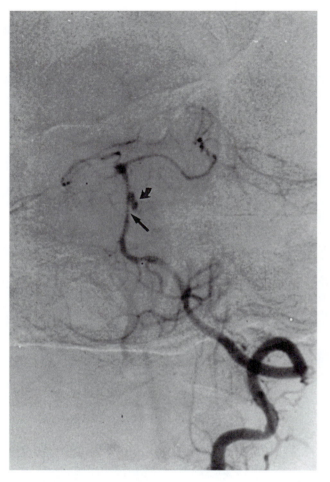

Figure 13.20 Left vertebral angiogram, left anterior oblique Caldwell projection. Aneurysm of the basilar artery (curved arrow). Narrowing of the artery immediately proximal to the aneurysm (straight arrow).

rebral vasculitis is often diagnosed on the basis of systemic involvement rather than neurologic presentation. Polyarteritis nodosa leads to hypertension and multiple organ involvement usually prior to CNS complications.[119] Temporal arteritis presents with headache and elevated sedimentation rate, and temporal artery biopsy is the usual method of diagnosis.[64] Takayasu's arteritis, with its characteristic involvement of the aortic arch and its branches, often requires arch aortography for diagnosis. Ultrasonography is useful to follow the disease progression.[137]

Systemic diseases involving the connective tissue may uncommonly present with an immune-mediated intracranial vasculitis. In systemic lupus erythematosus, neurologic symptoms are usually due to embolic stroke or infection rather than CNS vasculitis.[64] In scleroderma, CNS vasculitis is extremely rare, but four-vessel angiography is felt to be required for diagnosis. Sjögren syndrome, rheumatoid arthritis, and Lyme disease are among others that have been reported to cause CNS vasculitis.

Primary CNS infection often spreads to involve cerebral vessels. Rarely, stroke may even be the first manifestation of meningitis.[112] In bacterial meningitis, angiographically dem-

onstrated vasculitis has been shown to be the most frequent intracranial complication (37%).[115] Meningovascular syphilis can cause an arteritis affecting large and medium-sized cerebral arteries[64] (Fig. 13.24).

Vasculopathy denotes the conditions affecting the blood vessel wall without inflammatory features. These diseases include intracranial atherosclerosis, intracranial FMD, radiation-induced vasculopathy, drug-induced vasculopathy (e.g., cocaine[51]), and moyamoya disease. Diseases associated with thrombosis such as sickle cell disease, protein S deficiency, and Sneddon syndrome may cause an arterial vasculopathy.[2,9,19]

In vasculitis and vasculopathy, the angiographic findings are not specific. The most frequent finding is vessel narrowing. This affects long segments and is circumferential, whereas atherosclerosis tends to cause short segment eccentric stenosis.[47] Irregular narrowing or a shaggy appearance is more common with infectious forms of vasculitis (bacterial, tuberculous, mycotic).[85] Beading is seen but also occurs in intracranial FMD and atherosclerosis rarely.[77] Involvement of extracranial arteries helps to distinguish atherosclerosis, FMD, polyarteritis nodosa, and Takayasu's disease from primary angiitis, which is purely intracranial.

A retrospective study has attempted to evaluate the relative contributions of MRI, CT, and angiography to the diagnosis of vasculitis.[63] Eleven patients out of 92 met criteria of either positive brain biopsy, positive angiography, or typical clinical course and response to therapy. MRI or CT showed

Figure 13.21 Right vertebral angiogram, lateral projection. Widening of the upper basilar artery, with an intimal flap (arrow).

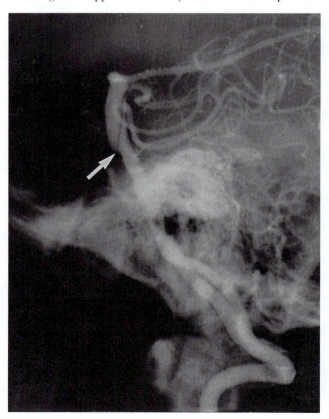

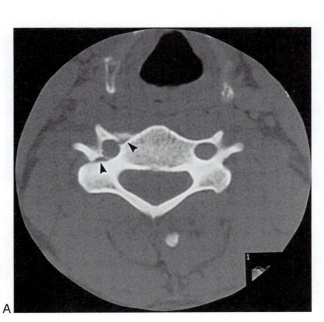

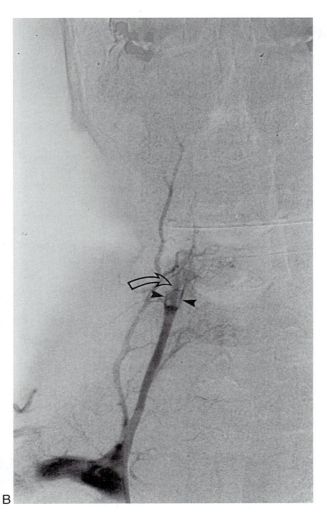

Figure 13.22 (**A**) Axial CT scan of the cervical spine shows fracture line across foramen transversarium (arrowheads). (**B**) Right vertebral angiogram, straight anteroposterior projection. The artery widens (between arrowheads), and bands of contrast are seen peripherally (arrowheads) and centrally (clear arrow), in the true and false lumina.

abnormalities in every patient with vasculitis; a normal MRI excluded the diagnosis. It was suggested that angiography should not be necessary if the screening MRI shows no evidence of infarction or hemorrhage. However, other investigators have observed normal MRI in the presence of primary angiitis proved by angiography or biopsy, or both.[4]

In the same study, angiography showed classic changes of vasculitis in 8 of the 11 cases (72%), a sensitivity level similar to that of other studies.[63] If the involved vessels are of a size below the resolution of angiography, then the test will be falsely negative (20% to 30%). With a clinical suspicion of vasculitis and an abnormal MRI, angiography that is normal should lead the clinician to consider brain biopsy.

MOYAMOYA DISEASE

Kudo[79] described a progressive condition manifested by spontaneous occlusion of the intracranial segments of the ICAs. Associated involvement of other circle of Willis vessels was also observed. The development of exuberant collateral through the small perforating branches of the basal arteries was commonly seen. It was described as *moyamoya*, which is Japanese for hazy, like a puff of smoke.[139]

The moyamoya phenomenon has been observed at angiography in diseases known to cause progressive cerebral arterial occlusion. These include radiation therapy, atherosclerosis, FMD, and neurofibromatosis.[15] These rare cases have been termed either secondary moyamoya or moyamoya syndrome.

Moyamoya disease usually presents with cerebral ischemia in childhood cases and intracranial hemorrhage in adult cases.[138] The disease has been angiographically staged according to the degree of stenosis or occlusion of the ICA and its branches and the amount of moyamoya.[139] Stenosis is initially restricted to the distal supraclinoid ICA. The moyamoya then develops and later intensifies as the anterior and middle cerebral arteries occlude. It diminishes as the disease spreads proximally to the anterior choroidal and posterior communicating arteries, since the basal perforators mainly

Figure 13.23 Axial T1-weighted MR scan shows high signal in or adjacent to the basilar artery (arrow). Same case as in Figure 13.21.

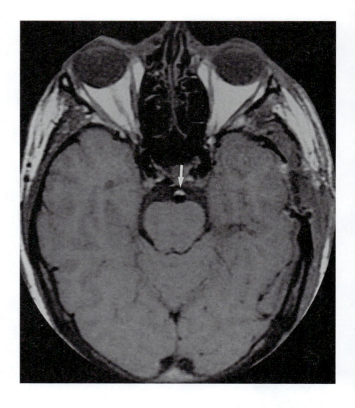

arise from these vessels. Ultimately the brain is supplied only by external carotid collateral vessels as the moyamoya disappears.[84,139,148]

Intracranial hemorrhage is usually subarachnoid or intraventricular in location. Angiography will sometimes reveal an intracranial aneurysm, often on a distal choroidal artery branch (Fig. 13.25) or at the basilar bifurcation.[1,61,78]

VENOUS DISEASE

Cortical venous and dural sinus thrombosis should be considered when the topography of cerebral infarction does not correspond to either an arterial branch or arterial watershed territory.[20,42] Cerebral infarction with patchy areas of hemorrhage can also suggest a venous cause (Fig. 13.26A). MRI is the method of choice for evaluation. However, cerebral angiography may be performed during the course of investigation for presumed arterial disease. Films obtained during the venous phase occasionally lead to the detection of an unsuspected venous thrombosis.

Partial or complete lack of opacification of one or more of the dural sinuses is the angiographic hallmark[20] (Fig. 13.26B). Usually other signs are also present, including lack of cortical venous filling, delayed emptying, or abnormal collateral venous drainage.

DOLICHOECTASIA AND FUSIFORM ANEURYSMS

Apart from presenting clinically with mass effect[26] or hemorrhage,[130] fusiform aneurysms may produce ischemia by one of three mechanisms: thrombosis of the aneurysm itself, small perforating artery occlusion, or distal embolization. Thrombosis of vertebrobasilar fusiform aneurysms with massive brain stem infarction is usually fatal.[102,155] Occlusion of a pontine perforator may cause only unilateral pontine infarction.[113] Embolization into the posterior cerebral or middle cerebral territory distal to fusiform aneurysms has been observed.[133]

Diagnosis can usually be made with MRI and MRA. In a large fusiform sac, thrombus invariably lines the wall, and there is characteristically sluggish blood flow within it (Fig. 13.27). During or after conventional angiography, there is a risk of

Figure 13.24 (A) Left common carotid angiogram, lateral view. Long areas of segmental narrowing affecting the anterior cerebral and middle cerebral arteries. (B) Left vertebral injection, AP Towne projection, same case. Segmental narrowing of the right anterior inferior cerebellar, left posterior inferior cerebellar, both superior cerebellar and both posterior cerebral arteries. Case of meningovascular syphilis.

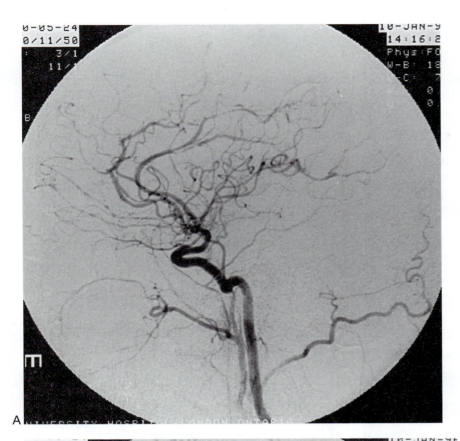

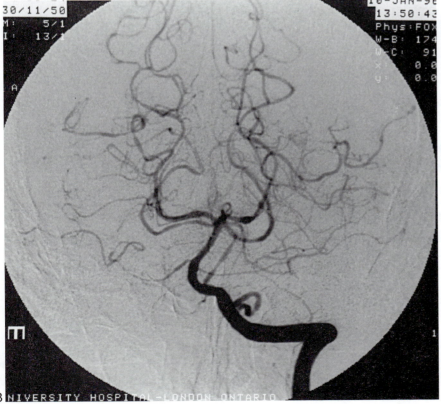

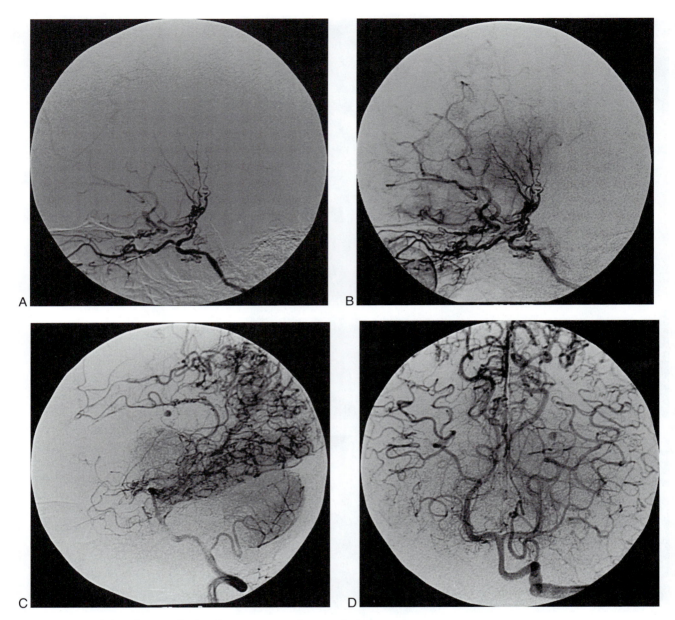

Figure 13.25 (**A**) Left internal carotid angiogram, early arterial phase, in a young man presenting with intraventricular hemorrhage. Marked narrowing of the supraclinoid and cavernous internal carotid artery with poor filling of the middle and anterior cerebral arteries. (**B**) Same injection, later phase. Faint filling of the anterior and middle cerebral territories and marked moyamoya phenomenon. (**C**) Left vertebral angiogram, lateral projection. Collateralization of the distal anterior cerebral territory from cortical and pericallosal branches of the posterior cerebral artery. Note the small aneurysm. (**D**) Same injection, AP Towne projection. Aneurysm seen in the distribution of the lateral posterior choroidal artery.

Figure 13.27 (**A**) Right vertebral angiogram, anteroposterior projection. Large fusiform aneurysm of the basilar artery. (**B**) Same injection, lateral view. Marked thrombus formation along the anterior wall of the aneurysm (arrows).

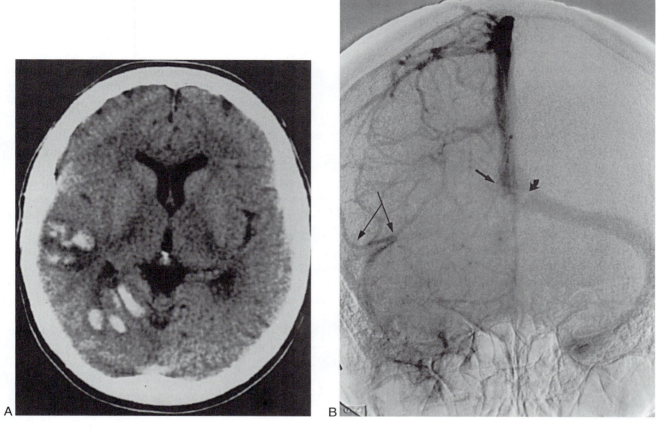

Figure 13.26 (**A**) Axial noncontrast CT scan showing patchy zones of hemorrhage in the right temporal and occipital lobes. (**B**) Right common carotid angiogram, Towne projection, venous phase. Occlusion of the right transverse sinus (between arrows).

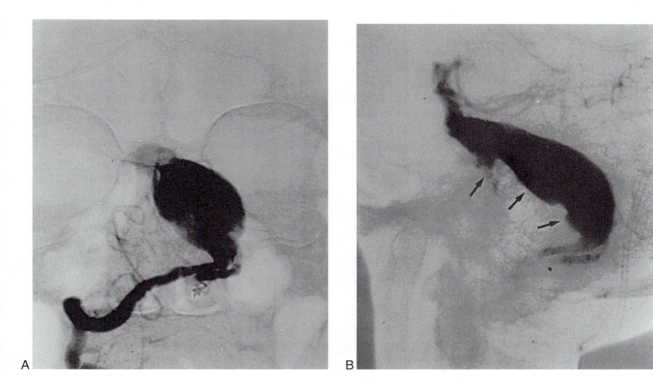

thromboembolism. In one case on the author's unit, complete thrombosis of a fusiform basilar artery and death occurred 3 days after cerebral angiography, probably related to alterations in the dose of anticoagulants. Others encountering such complications postulate that contrast material in stasis interferes with local blood flow.[131] Such untoward events should be considered when diagnostic angiography is contemplated, since CT and MRI will secure the diagnosis in most patients.

References

1. Adams HP, Kassell NF, Wisoff HS, Drake CG: Intracranial saccular aneurysm and moyamoya disease. Stroke 10:174, 1979

2. Adams RJ, Nichols FT, Figueroa R et al: Transcranial Doppler correlation with cerebral angiography in sickle cell disease. Stroke 23:1073, 1992

3. Akers DL, Markowitz IA, Kerstein MD: The value of aortic arch study in the evaluation of cerebrovascular insufficiency. Am J Surg 154:230, 1987

4. Alhalabi M, Moore PM: Serial angiography in isolated angiitis of the central nervous system. Neurology 44:1221, 1994

5. Allcock JM: Occlusion of the middle cerebral artery: serial angiography as a guide to conservative therapy. J Neurosurg 27:353, 1967

6. Alpers BJ, Berry RG: Circle of Willis in cerebral vascular disorders. Arch Neurol 8:398, 1963

7. Alter M, Kieffer S, Resch J, Ansari K: Cerebral infarction: clinical and angiographic correlations. Neurology (NY) 22:590, 1972

8. Antunovic R, Rosch J, Dotter CT: The value of systemic arterial heparinization in transfemoral angiography: a prospective study. AJR 127:223, 1976

9. Barinagarrementeria F, Brito CC, Izaguirre R, de la Pena A: Progressive intracranial occlusive disease associated with deficiency of protein S. Stroke 24:1752, 1993

10. Barnett HJM, Haines SJ: Carotid endarterectomy for asymptomatic carotid stenosis (editorial). N Engl J Med 328:276, 1993

11. Barnett HJM, Peerless SJ, Kaufmann JCE: "Stump" of internal carotid artery—a source for further cerebral embolic ischemia. Stroke 9:448, 1978

12. Battacharji SK, Hutchinson EC, McCall AJ: The circle of Willis—the incidence of developmental abnormalities in normal and infarcted brains. Brain 90:747, 1967

13. Bauer RB, Sheehan S, Wechsler N, Meyer JS: Arteriographic study of sites, incidence and treatment of arteriosclerotic cerebrovascular lesions. Neurology (NY) 12:698, 1962

14. Bierman HR, Miller ER, Byron RL et al: Intra-arterial catheterization of viscera in man. AJR 66:555, 1951

15. Bitzer M, Topka H: Progressive cerebral occlusive disease after radiation therapy. Stroke 26:131, 1995

16. Bladin PF: A radiologic and pathologic study of embolism of the internal carotid-middle cerebral arterial axis. Radiology 82:615, 1964

17. Blaisdell FW, Claus RH, Galbraith JG et al: Joint study of extracranial arterial occlusion. IV. A review of surgical considerations. JAMA 209:1889, 1969

18. Blaisdell FW, Glickman M, Trunkey DD: Ulcerated atheroma of the carotid artery. Arch Surg 108:491, 1974

19. Boortz-Marx RL, Clark HB, Taylor S et al: Sneddon's syndrome with granulomatous leptomeningeal infiltration. Stroke 26:492, 1995

20. Bousser M-G, Chiras J, Bories J, Castaigne P: Cerebral venous thrombosis—a review of 38 cases. Stroke 16:199, 1985

21. Bozzao L, Angeloni U, Bastianello S et al: Early angiographic and CT findings in patients with hemorrhagic infarction in the distribution of the middle cerebral artery. AJNR 12:1115, 1991

22. Brice JG, Dowsett DJ, Lowe RD: Haemodynamic effects of carotid artery stenosis. BMJ 2:1363, 1964

23. Burger PC, Burch JG, Vogel FS: Granulomatous angiitis. An unusual etiology of stroke. Stroke 8:29, 1977

24. Caplan LR: "Top of the basilar" syndrome. Neurology (NY) 30:72, 1980

25. Dalal PM, Shah PM, Sheth SC, Deshpande CK: Cerebral embolism: angiographic observations on spontaneous clot lysis. Lancet 1:61, 1965

26. Dandy WE: Intracranial Arterial Aneurysms. Hafner, New York, 1969

27. Davis DO, Rumbaugh CL, Gilson JM: Angiographic diagnosis of small vessel cerebral emboli. Acta Radiol Diagn 9:264, 1969

28. Davis PC, Hoffman JC: Work in progress: intra-arterial digital subtraction angiography: evaluation in 150 patients. Radiology 148:9, 1983

29. Debrun GM, Viñuela FV, Fox AJ: Aspirin and systemic heparinization in diagnostic and interventional neuroradiology. AJNR 3:337, 1982

30. Deweese JA, May AG, Lipchik EO, Rob CG: Anatomic and hemodynamic correlations in carotid artery stenosis. Stroke 1:149, 1970

31. Dion JE, Gates PC, Fox AJ et al: Clinical events following neuroangiography: a prospective study. Stroke 18:997, 1987

32. Earnest F, Forbes G, Sandok BA et al: Complications of cerebral angiography: prospective assessment of risk. AJNR 4:1191, 1983

33. Edwards JH, Kricheff II, Gorstein F et al: Atherosclerotic subintimal hematoma of the carotid artery. Radiology 133:123, 1979

34. Edwards JH, Kricheff II, Riles T, Imparato A: Angiographically undetected ulceration of the carotid bifurcation as a cause of embolic stroke. Radiology 132:369, 1979

35. Eggers FM, Price AC, Allen JH, James AE: Neuroradiologic applications of intraarterial digital subtraction angiography. AJNR 4:854, 1983

36. Ehrenfeld WK, Wylie EJ: Spontaneous dissection of the internal carotid artery. Arch Surg 111:1294, 1976

37. Eikelboom BC, Riles TR, Mintzer R et al: Inaccuracy of angiography in the diagnosis of carotid ulceration. Stroke 14:882, 1983

38. Eisenberg RL, Mani RL: The six French catheter in arch aortography. Radiology 125:822, 1977

39. Eldh P, Jacobsson B: Heparinized vascular catheters: a clinical trial. Radiology 111:289, 1974

40. Eliasziw M, Smith RF, Singh N et al: Further comments on the measurement of carotid stenosis from angiograms. Stroke 25:2445, 1994

41. Eliasziw M, Streifler JY, Fox AJ et al: Significance of plaque ulceration in symptomatic patients with high-grade carotid stenosis. Stroke 25:304, 1994

42. Enevoldson TP, Ross Russell RW: Cerebral venous thrombosis: new causes for an old syndrome? Q J Med 77:1255, 1990

43. European Carotid Surgery Trialists' Collaborative Group: MRC European Carotid Surgery Trial: interim results for symptomatic patients with severe (70–99%) or with mild (0–29%) carotid stenosis. Lancet 337:1235, 1991

44. Executive Committee for the Asymptomatic Carotid Atherosclerosis Study: Endarterectomy for asymptomatic carotid artery stenosis. JAMA 273:1421, 1995

45. Farinas PL: New technique for arteriographic examination of abdominal aorta and its branches. AJR 46:641, 1941

46. Feldmann E: Intracerebral hemorrhage. Stroke 22:684, 1991

47. Ferris EJ, Levine HL: Cerebral arteritis: classification. Radiology 109:327, 1973

48. Ferris EJ, Shapiro JH, Simeone FA: Arteriovenous shunting in cerebrovascular occlusive disease. AJR 98:631, 1966

49. Fisher CM, Ojemann RG, Roberson GH: Spontaneous dissection of the cervico-cerebral arteries. Can J Neurol Sci 5:9, 1978

50. Formanek G, Frech RS, Amplatz K: Arterial thrombus formation during clinical percutaneous catheterization. Circulation 41:833, 1970

51. Fredericks RK, Lefkowitz DS, Challa VR, Troost BT: Cerebral vasculitis associated with cocaine abuse. Stroke 22:1437, 1991

52. Gabrielson TO, Seeger JF, Knake JE et al: The nearly occluded carotid artery: a diagnostic trap. Radiology 138:611, 1981

53. Gacs G, Fox AJ, Barnett HJM, Viñuela F: Occurrence and mechanisms of occlusion of the anterior cerebral artery. Stroke 14:952, 1983

54. Gannon WE, Chait A: Occlusion of the middle cerebral artery with recanalization. AJR 88:24, 1962

55. Giedke H, Kriebel J, Sindermann F: Dissecting aneurysm of the petrous portion of the internal carotid artery: case report and review of previous cases. Neuroradiology 10:121, 1975

56. Goldstein LB, Bonito AJ, Matchov DB et al: US national survey of physician practices for the secondary and tertiary prevention of ischemic stroke. Stroke 27:801, 1996

57. Greenan TJ, Grossman RI, Goldberg HI: Cerebral vasculitis: MR imaging and angiographic correlation. Radiology 182:65, 1992

58. Grzyska U, Freitag J, Zeumer H: Selective cerebral in-traarterial DSA: complication rate and control of risk factors. Neuroradiology 32:296, 1990

59. Gunning AJ, Pickering GW, Robb-Smith AHT, Ross Russell R: Mural thrombosis of the internal carotid artery and subsequent embolism. Q J Med 33:155, 1964

60. Guridi J, Gallego J, Monzon F, Aguilera F: Intracerebral hemorrhage caused by transmural dissection of the anterior cerebral artery. Stroke 24:1400, 1993

61. Hamada J-I, Hashimoto N, Tsukahara T: Moyamoya disease with repeated intraventricular hemorrhage due to aneurysm rupture. J Neurosurg 80:328, 1994

62. Hankey GJ, Warlow CP, Molyneux AJ: Complications of cerebral angiography for patients with mild carotid territory ischemia being considered for carotid endarterectomy. J Neurol Neurosurg Psychiatry 53:542, 1990

63. Harris KG, Tran DD, Sickels WJ et al: Diagnosing intracranial vasculitis: the role of MR and angiography. AJNR 15:317, 1994

64. Harris KG, Yuh WTC: Intracranial vasculitis. Neuroimaging Clin North Am 4:773, 1994

65. Hass WK, Fields WS, North RR et al: Joint study of extracranial arterial occlusion. II. Arteriography, techniques, sites and complications. JAMA 203:159, 1968

66. Heiserman JE, Dean BL, Hodak JA et al: Neurologic complications of cerebral angiography. AJNR 15:1401, 1994

67. Hennerici M, Klemm C, Rautenberg W: The subclavian steal phenomenon: a common vascular disorder with rare neurological deficits. Neurology (NY) 38:669, 1988

68. Hinck VC: Single catheter for aortic arch and selective cerebral angiography. AJNR 7:159, 1986

69. Hinck VC, Judkins MP, Paxton HD: Simplified selective femorocerebral angiography. Radiology 89:1048, 1967

70. Hobson RW, Weiss DG, Fields WS et al: Efficacy of carotid endarterectomy for asymptomatic carotid stenosis. N Engl J Med 328:221, 1993

71. Houser OW, Baker HL: Fibromuscular dysplasia and other uncommon diseases of the cervical carotid artery: angiographic aspects. AJR 104:201, 1968

72. Houser OW, Baker HL, Sandok BA, Holley KE: Cephalic arterial fibromuscular dysplasia. Radiology 101:605, 1971

73. Irino T, Taneda M, Minami T: Angiographic manifestations in postrecanalized cerebral infarction. Neurology (NY) 27:471, 1977

74. Julian OC, Dye WS, Javid H, Hunter JA: Ulcerative lesions of the carotid artery bifurcation. Arch Surg 86:803, 1963

75. Kerber CW, Cromwell LD, Drayer BP, Bank WO: Cerebral ischemia. I. Current angiographic techniques, complications and safety. AJR 130:1097, 1978

76. Kishore PRS, Dick AR: Spontaneous disappearance of carotid stenosis. Radiology 129:721, 1978

77. Knopman DS, Anderson DC, Mastri A, Larson D: Leptomeningeal artery atherosclerosis visualized by angiography: clinical correlates. Stroke 9:262, 1978

78. Kodama N, Suzuki J: Moyamoya disease associated with aneurysm. J Neurosurg 48:565, 1978

79. Kudo T: Spontaneous occlusion of the circle of Willis:

a disease apparently confined to Japanese. Neurology (NY) 18:485, 1968

80. Kunze S, Schiefer W: Angiographic demonstration of a dissecting aneurysm of the middle cerebral artery. Neuroradiology 2:201, 1971

81. Lang EK: A survey of the complications of percutaneous retrograde arteriography: Seldinger technic. Radiology 81:257, 1963

82. Lanner LO, Rosengren K: Angiographic diagnosis of intracerebral vascular occlusions. Acta Radiol Diagn 2:129, 1964

83. Lee DH, Gao F-Q, Rankin RN et al: Duplex and color Doppler flow sonography of occlusion and near occlusion of the carotid artery. AJNR 17:1267, 1996

84. Leeds NE, Abbott KH: Collateral circulation in cerebrovascular disease in childhood via rete mirabile and perforating branches of anterior choroidal and posterior cerebral arteries. Radiology 85:628, 1965

85. Leeds NE, Goldberg HI: Angiographic manifestations in cerebral inflammatory disease. Radiology 98:595, 1971

86. Lehrer GM: Arteriographic demonstration of collateral circulation in cerebrovascular disease. Neurology (NY) 8:27, 1958

87. Lhermitte F, Gautier JC, Derouesne C: Nature of occlusions of the middle cerebral artery. Neurology (NY) 20:82, 1970

88. Liliequist B: The roentgenologic appearance of spontaneous dissecting aneurysm of the cervical internal carotid artery. Vasc Surg 2:223, 1968

89. Lopez-Bresnahan MV, Kearse LA, Yanez P, Young TI: Anterior communicating artery collateral flow protection against ischemic change during carotid endarterectomy. J Neurosurg 79:379, 1993

90. Maddison FE, Moore WS: Ulcerated atheroma of the carotid artery: arteriographic appearance. AJR 107:530, 1969

91. Mani RL: Computer analysis of factors associated with thrombus formation observed on pullout angiograms. Invest Radiol 10:378, 1975

92. Mann FC, Herrick JF, Essex HE, Baldes EJ: The effect on the blood flow of decreasing the lumen of a blood vessel. Surgery 4:249, 1938

93. Margolis MT, Newton TH: Collateral pathways between the cavernous portion of the internal carotid and external carotid arteries. Radiology 93:834, 1969

94. May AG, Deweese JA, Rob CG: Hemodynamic effects of arterial stenosis. Surgery 53:513, 1963

95. Mehigan JT, Olcott C: The carotid "string" sign: differential diagnosis and management. Am J Surg 140:137, 1980

96. Moniz E: L'encéphalographie artérielle, son importance dans la localisation des tumeurs cérébrales. Rev Neurol 2:72, 1927

97. Moore WS, Hall AD: Ulcerated atheroma of the carotid artery: a cause of transient cerebral ischemia. Am J Surg 116:237, 1968

98. Mount LA, Taveras JM: Arteriography demonstration of the collateral circulation of the cerebral hemispheres. Arch Neurol Psychiatry 78:235, 1957

99. Nebesar RA, Pollard JJ: A curved-tip guide wire for thoracic and abdominal angiography. AJR 97:508, 1966

100. Nejad MS, Klaper MA, Steggerda FR, Gianturco C: Clotting on the outer surface of vascular catheters. Radiology 91:248, 1968

101. Newton TH, Adams JE, Wylie EJ: Arteriography of cerebrovascular occlusive disease. N Engl J Med 270:14, 1964

102. Nishizaki T, Tamaki N, Takeda N et al: Dolichoectatic basilar artery: a review of 23 cases. Stroke 17:1277, 1986

103. North American Symptomatic Carotid Endarterectomy Trial Collaborators: Beneficial effect of carotid endarterectomy in symptomatic patients with high-grade carotid stenosis. N Engl J Med 325:445, 1991

104. North American Symptomatic Carotid Endarterectomy Trial (NASCET) Steering Committee: North American Symptomatic Carotid Endarterectomy Trial: methods, patient characteristics and progress. Stroke 22:711, 1991

105. O'Connell BK, Towfighi J, Brennan RW et al: Dissecting aneurysms of head and neck. Neurology 35:993, 1985

106. Ojemann RG, Fisher CM, Rich JC: Spontaneous dissecting aneurysm of the internal carotid artery. Stroke 3:434, 1972

107. Osborn AG, Anderson RE: Angiographic spectrum of cervical and intracranial fibromuscular dysplasia. Stroke 8:617, 1977

108. Palubinskas AJ, Ripley HR: Fibromuscular hyperplasia in extrarenal arteries. Radiology 82:451, 1964

109. Pelz DM, Buchan A, Fox AJ et al: Intraluminal thrombus of the internal carotid arteries: angiographic demonstration of resolution with anticoagulant therapy alone. Radiology 160:369, 1986

110. Pelz DM, Fox AJ, Eliasziw M, Barnett HJM: Stenosis of the carotid bifurcation: subjective assessment compared with strict measurement guidelines. Can Assoc Radiol J 44:247, 1993

111. Pelz DM, Fox AJ, Viñuela F et al: The ascending pharyngeal artery: a collateral pathway in complete occlusion of the internal carotid artery. AJNR 8:177, 1987

112. Perry JR, Bilbao JM, Gray T: Fatal basilar vasculopathy complicating bacterial meningitis. Stroke 23:1175, 1992

113. Pessin MS, Chimowitz MI, Levine SR et al: Stroke in patients with fusiform vertebrobasilar aneurysms. Neurology (NY) 39:16, 1989

114. Pessin MS, Duncan GW, Davis KR et al: Angiographic appearance of carotid occlusion in acute stroke. Stroke 11:485, 1980

115. Pfister H-W, Borasio GD, Dirnagl U et al: Cerebrovascular complications of bacterial meningitis in adults. Neurology 42:1497, 1992

116. Piepgras DG, McGrail KM, Tazelaar HD: Intracranial dissection of the distal middle cerebral artery as an uncommon cause of distal cerebral artery aneurysm. J Neurosurg 80:909, 1994

117. Pitts FW, Haskin ME, Riggs HE, Groff RA: "Tumorstain" in cerebrovascular disease. J Neurosurg 21:298, 1964

118. Pozzati E, Andreoli A, Padovani R, Nuzzo G: Dissecting

aneurysms of the basilar artery. Neurosurgery 36:254, 1995

119. Provenzale JM, Allen NB: Neuroradiologic findings in polyarteritis nodosa. AJNR 17:1119, 1996

120. Rinaldi I, Harris WO, Kopp JE, Legier J: Intracranial fibromuscular dysplasia: report of two cases, one with autopsy verification. Stroke 7:511, 1976

121. Roberson GH, Scott WR, Rosenbaum AE: Thrombi at the site of carotid stenosis: radiographic diagnosis. Radiology 109:353, 1973

122. Rothwell PM, Gibson RJ, Slattery J et al: Equivalence of measurements of carotid stenosis. Stroke 25:2435, 1994

123. Rothwell PM, Gibson RJ, Slattery J et al: Prognostic value and reproducibility of measurements of carotid stenosis. Stroke 25:2440, 1994

124. Sandok BA: Fibromuscular dysplasia of the cephalic arterial system. p. 283. In Toole JF (ed): Handbook of Clinical Neurology. Vol. 2. Elsevier, New York, 1989

125. Schmalbrock P, Yuan C, Chakeres DW et al: Volume MR angiography: methods to achieve very short echo times. Radiology 175:861, 1990

126. Schomer DF, Marks MP, Steinberg GK et al: The anatomy of the posterior communicating artery as a risk factor for ischemic cerebral infarction. N Engl J Med 330: 1565, 1994

127. Sekhar LN, Heros RC, Lotz PR, Rosenbaum AE: Atheromatous pseudo-occlusion of the internal carotid artery. J Neurosurg 52:782, 1980

128. Seldinger SI: Catheter replacement of the needle in percutaneous arteriography: a new technique. Acta Radiol 39:368, 1953

129. Shapiro R: Thrombosis of the internal carotid artery. Radiology 58:94, 1952

130. Shokunbi MT, Vinters HV, Kaufmann JCE: Fusiform intracranial aneurysms: clinicopathologic features. Surg Neurol 29:263, 1988

131. Smoker WRK, Corbett JJ, Gentry LR et al: High-resolution computed tomography of the basilar artery. 2. Vertebrobasilar dolichoectasia: clinico-pathologic correlation and review. AJNR 7:61, 1986

132. Special report from the National Institute of Neurological Disorders and Stroke: Classification of cerebrovascular diseases. III. Stroke 21:637, 1990

133. Steel JG, Thomas HA, Strollo PJ: Fusiform basilar aneurysm as a cause of embolic stroke. Stroke 13:712, 1982

134. Stevens JM, Barter S, Kerslake R et al: Relative safety of intravenous digital subtraction angiography over other methods of carotid angiography and impact on clinical management of cerebrovascular disease. Br J Radiol 62: 813, 1989

135. Streifler JY, Eliasziw M, Fox AJ et al: Angiographic detection of carotid plaque ulceration. Stroke 25:1130, 1994

136. Sukoff MH, Dorsey TJ, Johnson DA et al: Intimal fibroplasia of the internal carotid arteries. Stroke 2:483, 1971

137. Sun Y, Yip P-K, Jeng J-S et al: Ultrasonographic study and long-term follow-up of Takayasu's arteritis. Stroke 27:2178, 1996

138. Suzuki J, Kodama N: Moyamoya disease—a review. Stroke 14:104, 1983

139. Suzuki J, Takaku A: Cerebrovascular "moyamoya" disease. Arch Neurol 20:288, 1969

140. Taveras JM, Gilson JM, Davis DO et al: Angiography in cerebral infarction. Radiology 93:549, 1969

141. Tindall GT, Odom GL, Cupp HB, Dillon ML: Studies on carotid artery flow and pressure: observations in 18 patients during graded occlusion of proximal carotid artery. J Neurosurg 19:917, 1962

142. Vitek JJ: Femoro-cerebral angiography: analysis of 2,000 consecutive examinations, special emphasis on carotid arteries catheterization in older patients. AJR 118:633, 1973

143. Vitek JJ, Halsey JH, McDowell HA: Occlusion of all four extracranial vessels with minimal clinical symptomatology: case report. Stroke 3:462, 1972

144. VonRuden WJ, Blaisdell FW, Hall AD, Thomas AN: Multiple arterial stenoses: effect on blood flow. Arch Surg 89:307, 1964

145. Walker WJ, Mundall SL, Broderick HG et al: Systemic heparinization for femoral percutaneous coronary arteriography. N Engl J Med 288:826, 1973

146. Wallace S, Medellin H, DeJongh D, Gianturco C: Systemic heparinization for angiography. AJR 116:204, 1972

147. Waugh JR, Sacharias N: Arteriographic complications in the DSA era. Radiology 182:243, 1992

148. Weidner W, Hanafee W, Markham CH: Intracranial collateral circulation via leptomeningeal and rete mirabile anastomoses. Neurology (NY) 15:39, 1965

149. Wilson M: Angiography in cerebrovascular occlusive disease. Am J Med Sci 250:554, 1965

150. Wityk RJ, Lehman D, Klag M et al: Race and sex differences in the distribution of cerebral atherosclerosis. Stroke 27:1974, 1996

151. Wood EH, Correll JW: Atheromatous ulceration in major neck vessels as a cause of cerebral embolism. Acta Radiol Diagn 9:520, 1969

152. Yano H, Sawada M, Shinodi J, Funakoshi T: Ruptured dissecting aneurysm of the peripheral anterior cerebral artery. Neurol Med Chir (Tokyo) 35:450, 1995

153. Young B, Moore WS, Robertson JT et al: An analysis of perioperative surgical mortality and morbidity in the asymptomatic carotid atherosclerosis study. Stroke 27: 2216, 1996

154. Younger DS, Brust JCM, Hays A, Rowland LP: Granulomatous angiitis of the central nervous system: a nonspecific reaction of diverse etiology, abstracted. Ann Neurol 20:157, 1986

155. Yu YL, Moseley IF, Pullicino P, McDonald WI: The clinical picture of ectasia of the intracerebral arteries. J Neurol Neurosurg Psychiatry 45:29, 1982

Magnetic Resonance Angiography

DONALD H. LEE

Magnetic resonance angiography (MRA) is the natural product of the flow-sensitive nature of MR imaging (MRI). The early nuclear (N)MR literature, as well as early MRI literature, using spin echo image acquisition, was replete with discussions of different types of flow effects seen, and the use of MR to produce flow measurement. MRI flow effects described include through-plane flow producing flow void, in-plane flow and even-echo rephasing, diastolic pseudogating, pulsatile cerebrospinal fluid (CSF) flow producing CSF signal loss, and entry slice phenomena, all of which generated variable signals in the intracranial or extracranial vessels or CSF spaces. The addition of flow-compensating gradients removed several of these flow phenomena, while others persisted. Gradient echo imaging added another dimension to MRI of flow; because of the rapid acquisition possible, MRA became reality. Rather than giving an exhaustive description of the physical components of MRA, this chapter briefly outlines the modalities used for MRA, the advantages and disadvantages of each, and the current clinical applications of MRA. Readers wanting more complete physical reviews of MRA techniques and specific scan parameters are advised to read the articles, chapters, and books referenced.[1,12,26,53,63] Techniques of MRA continue to be refined, both because of hardware developments such as gradient coils and faster computers and because of advanced software. Thus, there will likely be continual improvements in MRA that will reflect these ongoing developments. Currently, MRA allows a sensitive noninvasive evaluation of both the intra- and extracranial circulation and can be combined with other MR sequences to allow a comprehensive evaluation of the patient with stroke, all in a clinically relevant total scan time. Like all MRI, however, the techniques are not applicable to all patients; they are currently limited by known contraindications to MRI and by patient motion.

Techniques

MRA techniques (TOF) can be divided into one of two types: (1) time-of-flight (TOF) imaging and (2) phase contrast (PC) imaging.

TIME-OF-FLIGHT IMAGING

TOF MRA techniques[1,26,53] can be subdivided into bright blood and black blood techniques.[1,13] Bright blood techniques utilize the fact that fully magnetized (unsaturated) spins flowing into a slice produce high signal; the slice is saturated—it has received some form of radiofrequency (rf) pulse as part of its acquisition (Fig. 13.28). In black blood techniques, flow is of lower signal than the surrounding tissue; this is because it does not stay long enough in the slice to either receive the rf pulse(s) received by that tissue or to generate a signal back to the coil; thus a slice-selective signal is not formed, which produces the typical flow void seen in vessels on conventional spin echo images.

Both types of TOF MRA techniques can be acquired using two-dimensional (2D), or three-dimensional (3D) scanning. 2D scanning acquires each slice individually, producing a complete slice, before the scan sequence is repeated to produce the next slice. 3D scanning excites a block (or volume) of tissue, which is then subsequently partitioned into individual slices (also termed partitions).

In general, 2D TOF techniques are quicker, and, because each slice is individually acquired, more sensitive to slow flow. They are, however, limited by gradient constraints, so relatively thick slices (1.5- to 2-mm-thick) are produced. They also have lower signal-to-noise ratios. The 3D TOF techniques are capable of very thin slice partitions (potentially 0.5 mm or less, although typically partition thicknesses between 0.7 and 1 mm are chosen to allow coverage of a specific region) and have higher signal-to-noise ratios. Because flow in the slab is subjected to multiple rf pulses during the acquisition sequence, there may be more saturation (signal suppression) of flow through the slice, especially if thicker volumes are used, if the flow through the volume is slow, or if the flip angle of the rf pulse used is large. To show arterial or venous flow selectively when the aortic arch and neck vessels are imaged, additional rf pulses are applied in the plane above, or below the slice or volume imaged. This suppresses signal from blood that will flow into the slice (e.g., for arterial images, an rf pulse is applied superior to the slice to suppress venous flow). More recent innovations in 3D TOF include magnetization transfer (to suppress background signal—used for intracranial MRA),[74] multiple overlapping thin slab angiography (MOTSA),[63] and contrast-enhanced MRA.[7,25,33,37,38,43,57] MOTSA uses small volumes, with multiple volumes acquired over the area needing to be imaged. This modification allows higher resolution imaging (because of the 3D acquisition), but, because of the thinner volumes, there is less saturation of the high signal of the flow as it traverses the volume compared with standard 3D TOF MRA, with improved vessel visualization. Contrast-enhanced MRA started initially as a

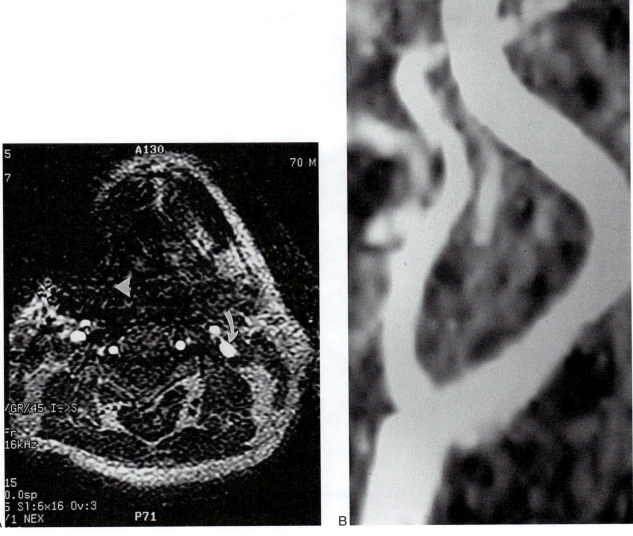

Figure 13.28 (**A**) Individual slice from 3D dataset—high signal in vascular lumen (arrow). Multiple images like this are summed together and the brightest points reprocessed to produce a flow-sensitive rendition of the vessel lumen. Note absence of venous flow, due to application of RF pulse superior to the imaging volume. Note also dephasing producing low signal due to dental work in the right side of the mandible (arrowhead). (**B**) The summed data showing a normal bifurcation.

means of showing smaller intracranial vessels[7,25,38,43] or removing artifact from slower flow in vessels, although with some potentially artifactual enhancement in local tissue such as the cavernous sinus. It has now evolved to pump-assisted contrast injections, with rapidly acquired 3D datasets.[37,57] Recently, images from different vascular phases from arterial to venous during the sequence have been produced; these are termed 3D time-resolved imaging of contrast kinetics (TRICKS)[33] (Fig. 13.29). While still awaiting extensive clinical experience, this technique could revolutionize the depic-

tion of the larger extra- and intracranial arteries, as well as allowing something not yet done to any degree in MRA—temporal sequencing of vascular anatomy and pathology. Obviously, compared with conventional MRA, which relies on intrinsic contrast between the inflowing blood and surrounding tissue, these contrast-enhanced techniques mean that MRA becomes a more invasive study. It is, however, only minimally invasive, as the contrast is given intravenously, with little chance of serious side effects using current MR contrast agents.

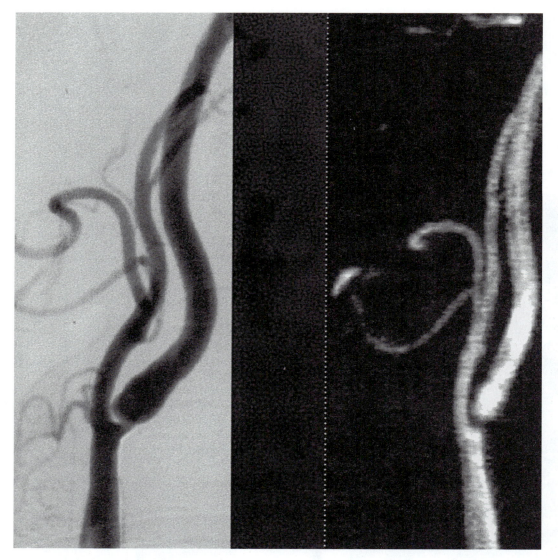

Figure 13.29 Internal carotid origin stenosis demonstrated with TRICKS: the contrast-enhanced MRA of the carotid bifurcation is on the right. The conventional angiogram is shown on the left. (Courtesy of the Vascular Imaging Group, University of Wisconsin-Madison, Wisconsin.)

PHASE CONTRAST IMAGING

In PC MRA,[1,12] a baseline image is first acquired, and then additional gradients are applied in a user-selectable fashion, with the same sequence repeated. The additional gradients produce phase shifts in nonstatic tissue (flow/motion). Then the baseline image is subtracted from the flow-sensitive image or images (those with gradients applied) to produce an image or images in which only flow is shown. This technique allows better background suppression, because of subtraction of static tissue. The potential also exists for both directional information about flow because the applied gradients in the flow-sensitive sequence can be user defined for one of the three main axes of flow—superoinferior, anteroposterior, or side to side) and rate of flow (from slow to fast depending on the strength of the applied gradient in the flow-sensitive image—faster flow is imaged with lower gradient strengths, and slower flow with higher strengths). Again, images can be acquired using either 2D or 3D scanning techniques.

Computerized image processing can yield either magnitude images (showing the background with superimposed flow), speed images (which show flow as high signal), or directional images (where flow in one direction is bright, and in the other direction dark. The speed images are used for MRA image production (Fig. 13.30). Obviously, except by reviewing the directional images, one is not able to suppress arterial or venous flow selectively with this technique. However, because

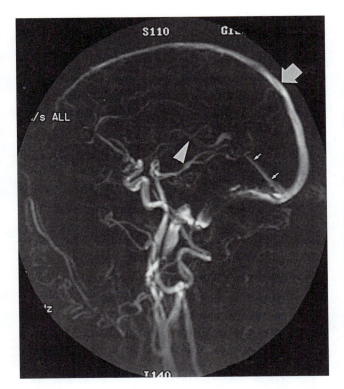

Figure 13.30 Sagittal projection, phase contrast MRA. There is absence of any identifiable signal from brain or soft tissue. Note excellent demarcation of sagittal sinus (thick arrow), straight sinus (arrowhead), and internal cerebral veins (thin arrow). Note also the superimposed carotid and basilar circulations. Imaging time, 1 minute, 36 seconds.

the potential exists to obtain directional information, arteries can be separated from veins on the basis of flow direction, especially in the large arteries of the neck and brain. Some work has documented better vessel depiction with contrast usage in PC MRA, but most centers using PC MRA do not employ contrast enhancement.

Final image processing on the dataset (either 2D or 3D TOF/PC MRA) is done using a workstation. All the images are loaded into the computer, and projection ray tracing software scans through the data volume, extracting either very high signal, or very low signal data (MIP: maximum intensity pixel or minimum intensity pixel reprojection, respectively). Thus an angiogram-like image is produced (Figs. 13.31 and 13.32). This is then displayed in some rotational fashion. Individual arteries/veins can be selected from the full image volume and displayed using the workstation—this is termed targeted MIP (Figs. 13.32 and 13.33). Obviously one is not able to obtain selective images of a specific artery, as is done in conventional angiography with standard TOF MRA. However, using TRICKS, it is possible to image selectively the temporal sequence of the carotids using targeted MIP, as shown in Figure 13.29.

LIMITATIONS

Lower Resolution

MRA provides lower resolution compared with conventional angiography (by at least one-half to one-third). This becomes progressively worse as the luminal size decreases.

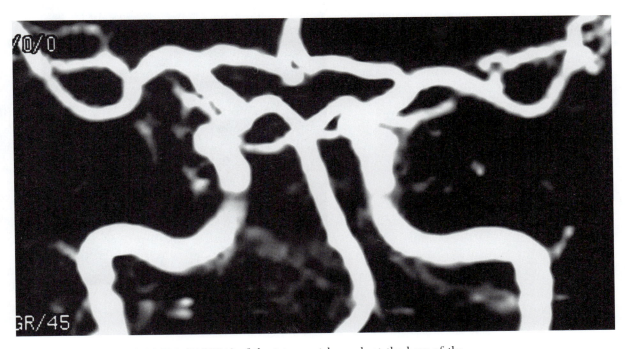

Figure 13.31 3D TOF MRA (MOTSA) of the intracranial vessels at the base of the brain (AP view). Normal appearance of vessels.

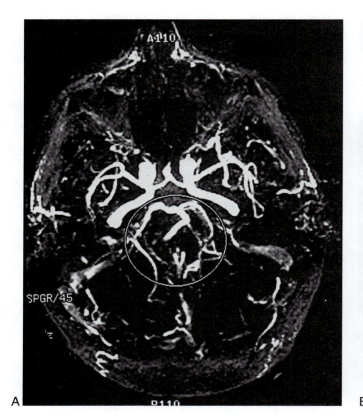

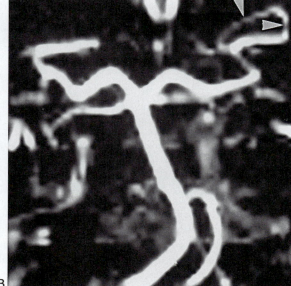

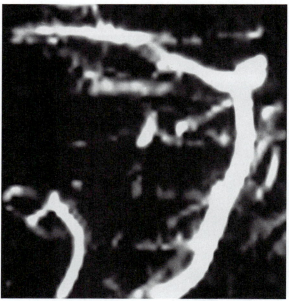

Figure 13.32 (**A**) Axial (collapse) view of the intracranial vasculature; the circle demarcates the basilar artery and its branches. (**B**) The targeted MIP image (AP view) of the vertebrobasilar system. Note artifactual stenosis of the left P2 segment due to saturation effects (arrowheads). (**C**) The same targeted MIP, rotated through 90 degrees.

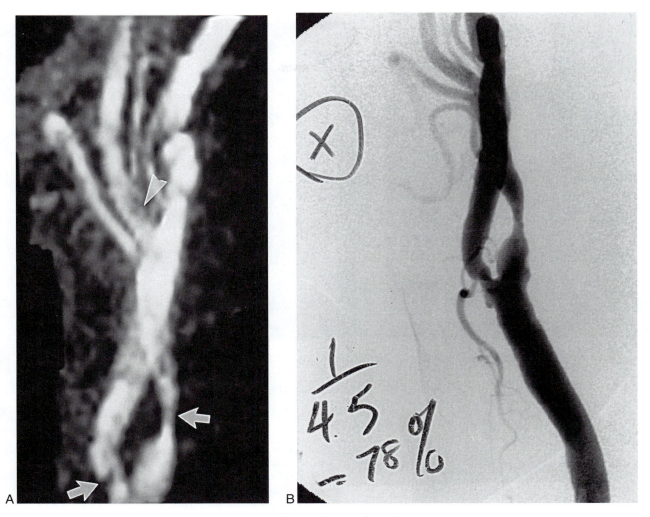

Figure 13.33 (**A**) 3D TOF MRA (MOTSA). Targeted MIP showing the right common carotid bifurcation. Note stenosis of the right internal and external carotid arteries (arrows). There is irregular signal in distal internal carotid artery due to saturation effects (arrowhead). (**B**) The conventional angiogram only shows stenosis of the internal and external carotid arteries.

Artifacts

Slow flow, turbulent flow, and in-plane flow may all show loss of signal with subsequent overestimation of stenosis, or nonvisualization of a vessel or vascular abnormality such as aneurysm (Fig. 13.34). Postprocessing artifacts may show non-vascular structures such as the posterior pituitary, or give the impression of flow, such as in thrombosed aneurysms, because these structures may be as bright as vascular structures on the images produced in the MRA sequence. Black blood MRA suffers from potential overestimation of luminal size when adjacent structures are low signal (e.g., the intracavernous carotid and the local sphenoid sinus), which are summed together during the minimum pixel ray tracing. Metal artifacts (e.g., aneurysm clips, VP shunts, dental appliances, or large amounts of metal in the neck or teeth) may render vessels invisible due to local susceptibility changes with loss of signal.

Limited Area of Coverage

Most studies include either the carotid bifurcation or the intracranial vascular structures of the circle of Willis. Larger coverage is possible with combination coils, but with the trade off of longer imaging times and potential patient motion.

Patient Motion

High-resolution sequences take 5 to 10 minutes to produce. Motion produces minor to major degradations of image quality, and longer imaging times lead to more potential for patient motion.

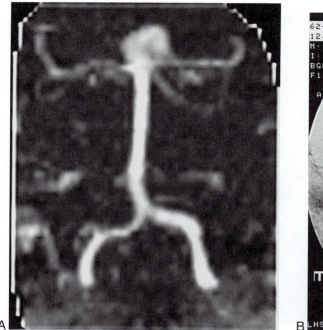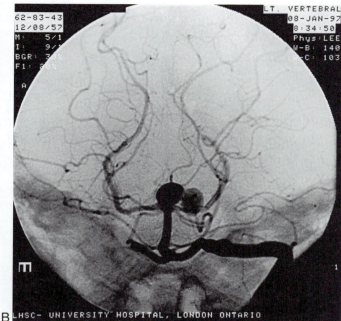

Figure 13.34 (**A**) 3D TOF MRA of bilobed basilar bifurcation aneurysm. The second lobule, shown on the angiogram, is poorly seen due to slower, more turbulent flow in the lobule, which is well seen on the corresponding conventional angiogram (Fig. B). (**B**) Bilobed basilar bifurcation aneurysm—selective left vertebral injection.

Clinical Applications

VASCULAR STENOSIS

Extracranial Stenosis

Numerous papers[2,3,10,11,15,18,20,22,27,28,35,40,42,47–49,50,52,54,56,66,67,71,73] have documented the ability to demonstrate stenosis in the extracranial carotid using MRA. The most commonly used sequences have been 2D or 3D TOF techniques.

With these techniques, sensitivities and specificities for detection of stenosis are similar to those of duplex sonography. However, all these studies have shown overestimation of degree of stenosis by MRA, with high sensitivity (>85%) but lower specificity (74% to 95%, lower with 2D techniques than with 3D techniques). This is well summarized by Rosokovsky and Litt.[59] Because of the relatively small number of studies of patients with carotid stenosis who have been assessed by MRA, it is difficult to know exactly how accurate MRA is for estimation of stenosis according to NASCET measurements. When MRA has been compared with angiographic stenosis measured by NASCET techniques,[20,54] there is a high rate of sensitivity (around 90% to 94%), and a reasonably high rate of specificity (around 88%) for 3D MRA, (about 10% lower for 2D MRA) with false positives on the basis of either kinking or overestimation of stenosis, and false negatives on the basis of nonimaging of stenosis or artifact. It should be noted that the flow gap seen is not absolutely reliable for a high-grade stenosis, being seen in stenosis grades of 40% to 60%, although much more commonly in stenoses of >60%, and invariably in stenoses of >70% with 2D TOF MRA.[18] In all the reported series, there were variable numbers (around 5%) of patients who had nondiagnostic MRA examinations. It has been suggested by some authors that the combination of duplex ultrasound and MRA is the most cost-effective method of determining potential candidates for carotid endarterectomy.[15,27] Others have suggested that ultrasound followed by confirmatory angiography remains a cost-effective way of imaging patients with carotid stenosis.[68] It should be noted that MRA has poor capability to show ulcers in plaques; reported accuracy is around 22%.

Intracranial Stenosis

For the demonstration of intracranial vascular stenosis, 3D techniques have been used, although quick screening can be obtained in the acute stroke setting in <2 minutes using PC MRA (Fig. 13.35). When compared with conventional angiography for showing stenoses of the arteries at the base of the brain, MRA has accuracies of 80% to 90%, with sensitivities and specificities in the 70% to 100% range.[9,16,19,32,41,55,61,69,75,76] It should be noted, however, that some of the literature referenced does not have angiographic correlation.[41,61,69,75] MRA appears to have better interobserver reliability than CT angiography of the intracranial vessels, based on small numbers of cases.[75] It has been suggested that 5 to 10 ml of gadolinium-based MR contrast agent may improve vessel detection in intracranial MRA.[25] This is not, however, common clinical practice. For detection of vasculitis, MRA is probably of little

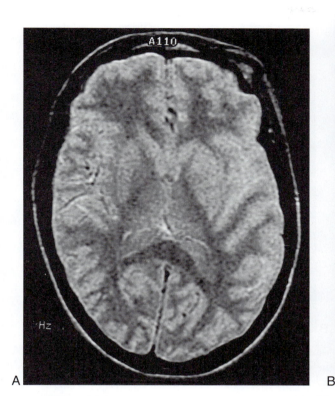

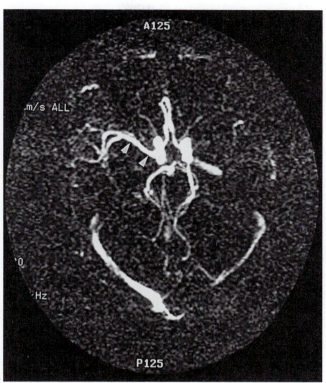

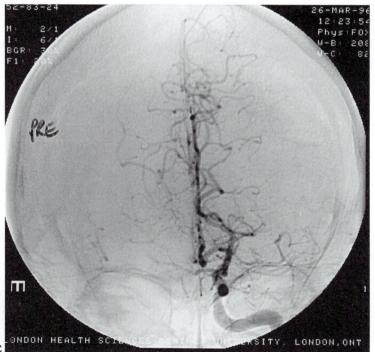

Figure 13.35 (**A**) Patient with acute stroke. Spin echo image (TR/TE 3,000/30 msec). Mild hyperintensity of left cerebral cortex, with absence of flow voids in left middle cerebral artery branches (compared with normal right side). (**B**) 2D phase contrast MRA: absence of flow in left middle cerebral artery compared with right MCA (arrowheads). (**C**) The angiogram prior to thrombolysis confirms occlusion of the left MCA distal to lenticulostriate branches.

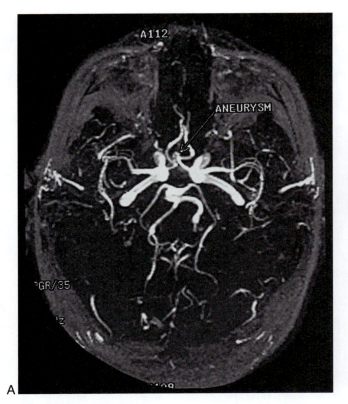

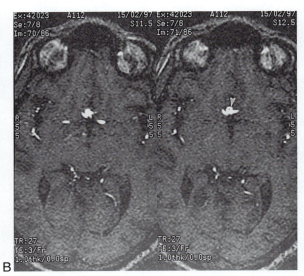

Figure 13.36 (A) Small anterior communicating artery aneurysm—axial collapse view. (B) Source data: two adjacent slices. Note dephasing in the center of the aneurysm (arrowhead), which measures approximately 5 mm.

value, as the resolution needed to show the subtle vessel changes is beyond what is currently achievable with MRA. It can, however, potentially demonstrate stenosis in the basal vessels.

VENOUS OCCLUSION

MR and MRA are highly sensitive for detection of venous sinus thrombosis. Various MRA techniques have been used—2/3D TOF, and 2D PC.[58,65,70] The quickest technique is 2D PC, which allows rapid screening of the venous sinuses in <4 minutes. These techniques also allow an easy method of following the venous sinuses after anticoagulant therapy. All demonstrate absence of normal flow in the venous sinus(es). Thrombus can also be seen on conventional MRI, as high signal in the veins; however, with gradient echo sequences, there may be high signal in the veins that can potentially be confused with thrombus.

ANEURYSMS

After initial demonstration of intracranial aneurysms by MRI and subsequently MRA, much interest arose in the potential use of MRA to demonstrate aneurysms noninvasively (Figs.

13.34 and 13.36). The first papers using 3D MRA showed high degrees of sensitivity (up to 86%) for reliably excluding aneurysms using MRA.[17,24,60,62,64] Unfortunately, this has proved to be premature. Size is important: several studies have shown that for aneurysms >5 mm the sensitivity for detection is up to 90%.[4,23,31,72] For smaller aneurysms, however, the sensitivity drops to <55%. It should be noted that MRA does offer a way of noninvasively following aneurysms of 3 to 5 mm, since, in at least one study, the aneurysms could be seen retrospectively.[23] As in other areas, it is important to evaluate the individual slice images, as well as the reprojected images.[30]

Two studies have evaluated the use of MRA in acute subarachnoid hemorrhage. In the one study, MRA could only be performed in 49% of patients. When it could be done, it was positive in 90% of patients.[4] In the other study, sensitivity for aneurysm detection was 81%, with 100% specificity.[30]

While newer techniques have provided an improvement in the quality of MRA images (for both individual slices and the reprojection images), the limitations of MRA still apply. Probably the most important are limited field of coverage (important in mycotic aneurysms, or more distally located aneurysms) and subacute hemorrhage (methemoglobin) mimicking aneurysm lumen (because it is high signal on T_1-weighted sequences). Also important for aneurysm detection is the fact that current nonferromagnetic clips still produce significant metallic artifact, which precludes assessment of the postoperative aneurysm, neck remnants, or even other local aneurysms. Obviously, ferromagnetic clips cannot be imaged, and there is at least one report of a fatal outcome because of MRI of a ferromagnetic clip.[29] New nonferromagnetic clip materials such as pure titanium have been shown to create significantly less artifact,[34] although these still need to be assessed in general clinical usage. Thus, while MRA may be good for screening patients at higher risk of aneurysms, it may still miss aneurysms and should be used with caution, as at least one author has recommended.[39]

At least one case report exists of an aneurysm that was seen on MRA but not on angiography. MRA is less affected by intra-aneurysm coils[44] and may prove to be better for noninvasive follow-up of patients than CT angiography. Conventional invasive angiography, however, remains the only effective mechanism for evaluating the postcoiling appearance of the aneurysm lumen.

Relatively little is found in the MRA literature about the evaluation of vasospasm after aneurysm rupture; one report documents narrowing of vessels in six of eight arteries showing vasospasm, in three patients with vasospasm.[21] It is currently probably more practical to use Transcranial Doppler to monitor vasospasm, rather than MRA.

ARTERIOVENOUS MALFORMATIONS

Intracranial

MRI can show moderate to large intracranial AVMs well; MRA can do the same.[1,6,14,51,62] While MRA can provide some information about the AVM. (i.e., large local feeders and draining veins and some estimation of nidus size), based on anatomic information, this information is not temporal, and only provides superficial structural information. It should be noted that it may be difficult by MRA to differentiate angiomatous transformation of normal vessels from true feeding vessels/nidus of the AVM. Again, size is an issue—very small AVMs and especially dural AVMs can be missed on MRA and can require angiographic demonstration.[51] The use of intravenous contrast may help in delineating slower venous flow or varices in the AVM. Because it can be programmed to show different velocities, PC MRA may be more useful than conventional 3D TOF MRA; slower velocity sensitivity is good for showing the nidus and slowly draining veins. The higher velocity sensitivity images are good for showing the arterial feeders. When stereotactic radiosurgery has been used, PC MRA may be useful in documenting decrease in flow through the AVM. PC MRA may also show dural sinus occlusion, which has been documented to accompany a large proportion of dural AVMs.

Spinal

Both PC and TOF MRA are good screening tools for showing the large veins of the AVM.[5,6,45,46,50] Resolution is again a problem; usually only the draining vein and nidus are shown, not the feeder, although at least one group believes that, in some cases, the feeding artery can be shown with PC MRA.[46]

It is more likely that the vessel seen with spinal dural AV fistulas is the draining radicular vein.

MISCELLANEOUS

Several papers have been published on carotid dissection, detailing the imaging findings; the most characteristic is the eccentric subintimal hematoma seen in patients with dissection.[36] However, to make the diagnosis of dissection, conventional angiography is still important. Fibromuscular dysplasia is difficult to diagnose with MRA—as for dissection, angiography is necessary.

In summary, MRA is a noninvasive or minimally invasive technique (when contrast material is used) and shows relatively good concordance with angiography or other noninvasive modalities like ultrasound or CT angiography. While it will not replace conventional angiography until time resolution and high resolution are present in the images, it still offers potentially helpful low-resolution imaging of the extra- and intracranial vasculature.

References

1. Anderson CM, Edelman RR, Turski PA: Clinical Magnetic Resonance Angiography. Lippincott-Raven, Philadelphia, 1993
2. Anderson CM, Lee RH, Levin DL et al: Measurement of internal carotid artery stenosis from source MR angiograms. Radiology 193:219–226, 1994
3. Anderson CM, Saloner D, Lee RE et al: Assessment of carotid artery stenosis by MR angiography: comparison with x-ray angiography and color-coded Doppler ultrasound. AJNR 13:989–1003, 1992
4. Anzalone N, Triulzi F, Scotti G: Acute subarachnoid haemorrhage: 3D time-of-flight MR angiography versus intra-arterial digital angiography. Neuroradiology 37:257–261, 1995
5. Bowen BC, DePrima S, Pattany PM et al: MR angiography of normal intradural vessels of the thoracolumbar spine. AJNR 17:483–494, 1996
6. Bowen BC, Kochan JP, Margosina P et al: Time of flight MR angiography of spinal vascular abnormalities. Radiology 185(P):122, 1992
7. Creasy JL, Price RR, Presbey T et al: Gadolinium-enhanced MR angiography. Radiology 175:280–283, 1990
8. Curnes JT, Shogry ME, Clark DC et al: MR angiographic demonstration of an intracranial aneurysm not seen on conventional angiography. AJNR 14:971–973, 1993
9. Dagirmanjian A, Ross JS, Obuchowski N et al: High resolution magnetization transfer saturation variable flip angle, time-of-flight MRA in the detection of intracranial vascular stenoses. J Comput Assist Tomogr 19:700–706, 1995
10. De Marco JK, Nesbit GM, Wesbey CE et al: Prospective evaluation of extracranial carotid stenosis. MR angiography with maximum-intensity projections and multiplanar

reformation compared with conventional angiography. AJR 163:1205–1212, 1994

11. Ding X, Tkach JA, Ruggieri PR et al: Sequential three-dimensional time-of-flight MR angiography of the carotid arteries: value of variable excitation and post-processing in reducing venetian blind artifact. AJR 18:683–688, 1994

12. Dumoulin CL: Phase-contrast magnetic resonance angiography. Neuroimaging Clin North Am 2:657–677, 1992

13. Edelman RR, Mattle HP, Wallner B et al: Extracranial carotid arteries: evaluation with "black blood" MR angiography. Radiology 177:45–50, 1990

14. Edelman RR, Wentz KU, Mattle HP et al: Intracerebral arteriovenous malformations: evaluation with selective MR angiography and venography. Radiology 173: 831–837, 1989

15. Erdoes LS, Marek JM, Mills JL et al. The relative contributions of carotid duplex scanning, magnetic resonance angiography, and cerebral arteriography to clinical decision making: a prospective study in patients with carotid occlusive disease. J Vasc Surg 23:950–956, 1996

16. Furst G, Hofer M, Steinmetz H et al: Intracranial steno-occlusive disease: MR angiography with magnetization transfer and variable flip angle. AJNR 17:1749–1757, 1996

17. Gouliamos A, Gotsis E, Vlahos L et al: Magnetic resonance angiography compared to digital subtraction arteriography in patients with subarachnoid hemorrhage. Neuroradiology 35:46–49, 1992

18. Heiserman JE, Drayer BP, Fram EK et al: Carotid artery stenosis: clinical efficacy of two-dimensional time-of-flight MR angiography. Radiology 182:761–768, 1992

19. Heiserman JE, Drayer BP, Keller PJ, Fram EK: Intracranial vascular stenosis and occlusion: evaluation with three-dimensional time-of-flight MR angiography. Radiology 185:667–673, 1992

20. Heiserman JE, Zabramski JM, Drayer BP, Keller PJ: Clinical significance of the flow gap in carotid magnetic resonance angiography. J Neurosurg 85:384–387, 1996

21. Horikoshi T, Fukamachi A, Nishi H et al: Observation of vasospasm after subarachnoid hemorrhage by magnetic resonance angiography. A preliminary study. Neurol Med Chir (Tokyo) 35:298–304, 1993

22. Huston J III, Lewis BD, Wiebers DO et al: Carotid artery: prospective blinded comparison of two-dimensional time-of-flight MR angiography with conventional angiography and duplex US. Radiology 186:339–344, 1993

23. Huston J III, Nichols DA, Luetmer PH et al: Blinded prospective evaluation of sensitivity of MR angiography to know intracranial aneurysms: importance of aneurysm size. AJNR 15:1607–1614, 1994

24. Huston J III, Rufenacht DA, Ehman D, Wiebers DO: Intracranial aneurysms and vascular malformations: comparison of time-of-flight and phase-contrast MR angiography. Radiology 181:721–730, 1991

25. Jung HW, Chang KH, Choi DS et al: Contrast-enhanced MR angiography for the diagnosis of intracranial vascular disease. AJR 165:1251–1255, 1995

26. Keller PJ: Time-of-flight magnetic resonance angiography. Neuroimaging Clin North Am 2:639–656, 1992

27. Kent KC, Kuntz KM, Patel MR et al: Perioperative imaging strategies for carotid endarterectomy. JAMA 274: 888–893, 1995

28. Kido DK, Barsotti JB, Rice LZ et al: Evaluation of the carotid artery bifurcation: comparison of magnetic resonance angiography and digital subtraction arch aortography. Neuroradiology 33:48–51, 1991

29. Klucznik RP, Carrier DA, Pyka R, Haid RW: Placement of a ferromagnetic intracerebral aneurysm clip in a magnetic field with a fatal outcome. Radiology 187:855–856, 1993

30. Korogi Y, Takahashi M, Mabuchi N et al. Intracranial aneurysms: diagnostic accuracy of MR angiography with evaluation of maximum intensity projection and source images. Radiology 199:199–207, 1996

31. Korogi Y, Takahashi M, Mabuchi N et al: Intracranial aneurysms: diagnostic accuracy of three-dimensional, Fourier transform time-of-flight MR angiography. Radiology 193:181–186, 1994

32. Korogi Y, Takahashi M, Mabuchi N et al: Intracranial vascular stenosis and occlusion: diagnostic accuracy of three-dimensional Fourier transform, time-of-flight MR angiography. Radiology 193:187–193, 1994

33. Korosec FR, Frayne R, Grist TM, Mistretta CA: Time-resolved contrast-enhanced 3D MR angiography. MRM 36:345–351, 1996

34. Lawton MT, Heiserman JE, Prendergast VC et al: Titanium aneurysm clips: part III—clinical application in 16 patients with subarachnoid hemorrhage. Neurosurgery 38:1170–1175, 1996

35. Lassiter RE Jr, Acker JD, Halford HH II, Nauert TC: Assessment of MR angiography versus arteriography for evaluation of cervical carotid bifurcation disease. AJNR 14:681–688, 1993

36. Levy C, Laissy JP, Raveau V et al: Carotid and vertebral artery dissections: three-dimensional time-of-flight MR angiography and MR imaging versus conventional angiography. Radiology 190:97–103, 1994

37. Levy RA, Prince MR: Arterial-phase three-dimensional contrast-enhanced MR angiography of the carotid arteries. AJR 167:211–215, 1996

38. Lin WW, Haacke EM, Smith AS, Clampitt ME: Gadolinium-enhanced high resolution MR angiography with adaptive vessel tracking: preliminary results in the intracranial circulation. J Magn Reson Imaging 2:277–284, 1992

39. Litt AW: MR angiography of intracranial aneurysms. Proceed, but with caution. AJNR 15:1615–1616, 1994

40. Litt AW, Eidelman EM, Pinto RS et al: Diagnosis of carotid artery stenosis: comparison of 2DFT time-of-flight MR angiography with contrast angiography in 50 patients. AJNR 12:149–154, 1991

41. Liu H-M, Tu Y-K, Yip PK, Su C-T: Evaluation of intracranial and extracranial carotid steno-occlusive diseases in Taiwan Chinese patients with MR angiography. Stroke 27:650–653, 1996

42. Lustgarten JH, Solomon RA, Quest DO et al: Carotid endarterectomy after noninvasive evaluation by duplex ultrasonography and magnetic resonance angiography. Neurosurgery 34:612–618, 1994

43. Marchal G, Michiels J, Bosmans H, Van Hecke P: Con-

trast-enhanced MRA of the brain. J Comput Assist Tomogr 16:25–29, 1992

44. Marshall MW, Teitelbaum GP, Kim HS et al: Ferromagnetism and magnetic resonance artefacts of platinum embolization microcoils. Cardiovasc Interv Radiol 14: 163–166, 1991

45. Masalchi M, Bianchi MC, Quilici N et al: MR angiography of spinal vascular malformations. AJNR 16:289–297, 1995

46. Masalchi M, Quilici N, Ferrito G et al: Identification of the feeding arteries of spinal vascular lesions via phase-contrast MR angiography with three-dimensional acquisition and phase display. AJNR 18:351–358, 1997

47. Masaryk AM, Ross JS, DiCello MC et al: 3DFt MR angiography of the carotid bifurcation: potential and limitations as a screening examination. Radiology 179:797–804, 1991

48. Mattle HP, Kent KC, Edelman RR et al: Evaluation of the extracranial carotid arteries: correlation of magnetic resonance angiography, duplex ultrasonography, and conventional angiography. J Vasc Surg 13:838–845, 1991

49. Mittl RLJ, Broderick MD, Carpenter JP et al: Blinded reader comparison of magnetic resonance angiography and duplex ultrasound for carotid bifurcation stenosis. Stroke 25:4–10, 1994

50. Mourier KL, Gelbert F, Reizine D et al: Phase-contrast magnetic resonance of the spinal cord arteriovenous malformations. Acta Neurochir 123:57–63, 1993

51. Mukherji SK, Quisling RG, Kubilis PS et al: Intracranial arteriovenous malformations: quantitative analysis of magnitude contrast MR angiography versus gradient echo MR imaging versus conventional angiography. Radiology 196:187–193, 1995

52. Pan XM, Saloner D, Reilly LM et al: Assessment of carotid artery stenosis by ultrasonography, conventional angiography, and magnetic resonance angiography: correlation with ex vivo measurement of plaque stenosis. J Vasc Surg 21:82–89, 1995

53. Parker DL, Blatter DD: Multiple thin slab magnetic resonance angiography. Neuroimaging Clin North Am 2: 677–692, 1992

54. Patel MR, Kuntz KM, Klufas RA et al: Preoperative assessment of the carotid bifurcation: can magnetic resonance angiography and duplex ultrasonography replace contrast arteriography? Stroke 26:1753–1758, 1995

55. Patrux B, Laissy JP, Jouini S et al: Magnetic resonance angiography of the circle of Willis: a prospective comparison with conventional angiography in 54 subjects. Neuroradiology 36:193–197, 1994

56. Polak JF, Bajakian RL, O'Leary DH et al: Detection of internal carotid artery stenosis: comparison of MR angiography, color Doppler sonography, and arteriography. Radiology 182:35–40, 1992

57. Prince MR, Yucel EK, Kaufmann JA et al: Dynamic gadolinium-enhanced three-dimensional abdominal MR arteriography. J Magn Reson Imaging 3:877–881, 1993

58. Rippe DJ, Boyko OB, Spitzer CE et al: Demonstration of dural sinus occlusion by the use of MR angiography. AJNR 11:199–201, 1990

59. Rosokovsky MA, Litt AW: MR angiography of the extracranial carotid arteries. MRI Clin North Am 3:439–454, 1995

60. Ross JS, Masaryk TJ, Modic MT et al: Intracranial aneurysms: evaluation by MR angiography. AJNR 11:449–456, 1990

61. Seynaeve A, Hasso AN, Thompson JR, Hinshaw DB: Basilar and distal vertebral artery occlusive disease: correlation of MR imaging and MR angiography. JBR-BTR 79: 61–67, 1996

62. Sevick RJ, Tsuruda JS, Schmalbrock P: Three-dimensional time-of-flight MR angiography in the evaluation of cerebral aneurysms. J Comput Assist Tomogr 14: 874–881, 1990

63. Sheppard S: Basic concepts in magnetic resonance angiography. Radiol Clin North Am 33:91–113, 1995

64. Shuierer G, Huk WJ, Laub G: Magnetic resonance angiography of intracranial aneurysms: comparison with intra-arterial subtraction angiography. Neuroradiology 35: 50–54, 1992

65. Tsai FY, Wang A-M, Matovich VB et al: MR staging of acute dural sinus thrombosis: correlation with venous pressure measurements and implications for treatment and prognosis. AJNR 16:1021–1029, 1995

66. Turnipseed WD, Kennel TW, Turski PA et al: Combined use of duplex imaging and magnetic resonance angiography for evaluation of patients with symptomatic ipsilateral high-grade stenosis. J Vasc Surg 17:832–840, 1993

67. Turnipseed WD, Kennel TW, Turski PA et al: Magnetic resonance angiography and duplex imaging. Noninvasive tests for selecting symptomatic carotid endarterectomy candidates. Surgery 114:643–649, 1993

68. Vanninen R, Manninen H, Soimakallio S: Imaging of carotid artery stenosis: clinical efficacy and cost-effectiveness. AJNR 16:1875–1883, 1995

69. Warach S, Li W, Ronthal M, Edelman RR: Acute cerebral ischemia: evaluation with dynamic contrast enhanced MR imaging and MR angiography. Radiology 182:41–47, 1992

70. Wasenko JJ, Holsapple JW, Winfield JA: Cerebral venous thrombosis: demonstration with magnetic resonance angiography. Clin Imaging 19:153–161, 1995

71. White JE, Russell WL, Greer MS et al: Efficacy of screening MR angiography and Doppler ultrasonography in the evaluation of carotid stenosis. Am Surg 60:340–348, 1993

72. Wilcock D, Jaspan T, Holland I et al: Comparison of magnetic resonance angiography with conventional angiography in the detection of intracranial aneurysms in patients presenting with subarachnoid hemorrhage. Clin Radiol 51:330–334, 1996

73. Wilkerson DK, Keller I, Mezrich K et al: The comparative evaluation of three-dimensional magnetic resonance angiography for carotid artery disease. J Vasc Surg 14: 803–811, 1991

74. Wolff SD, Eng J, Balaban RS: Magnetization transfer contrast: method for improving contrast in gradient recalled echo images. Radiology 179:133–137, 1991

75. Wong KS, Lam WWM, Liang E et al: Variability of magnetic resonance angiography and computed tomography angiography in grading middle cerebral artery stenosis. Stroke 27:1084–1087, 1996

76. Yamada I, Suzuki S, Matsushima Y: Moyamoya disease: comparison of assessment with MR angiography and MR imaging versus conventional angiography. Radiology 196: 211–218, 1995

CHAPTER 14

Ultrasound Imaging and Doppler Sonography

STEPHEN MEAIRS

WOLFGANG STEINKE

J. P. MOHR

MICHAEL HENNERICI

The continuous development of noninvasive ultrasound techniques has resulted in an array of clinical applications for assessment of both extracranial and intracranial arterial diseases. More than 2 decades ago continuous-wave (CW) ultrasound became the first method for evaluation of cerebrovascular hemodynamics. Some years later real-time B-mode sonography was introduced; this method images tissue and vessel structures in a two-dimensional gray-scale display. Combined B-mode and pulsed-wave (PW) Doppler-mode technologies in duplex systems allow imaging of tissue and registration of Doppler spectrums simultaneously. More recently, color-coded Doppler flow imaging was developed, displaying real-time visualization of blood flow patterns.[69,101,157,223] These ultrasound techniques provide complementary information for the diagnosis and staging of various cerebrovascular diseases. In particular, their noninvasive nature and high diagnostic accuracy have prompted diversified use in a number of clinical settings.

New approaches for improvement of blood vessel delineation include power Doppler imaging, application of contrast agents, and harmonic imaging. Three-dimensional (3D) ultrasound imaging is a rapidly expanding field with new applications for plaque reconstruction and volume quantification, as well as for 3D extra- and intracranial power Doppler angiography. Four-dimensional analyses of carotid plaques and arterial wall motion are new frontiers in diagnostic ultrasound.[155]

This chapter discusses the clinical merits and limitations of ultrasound imaging and Doppler techniques for assessment of extra- and intracranial cerebrovascular disease and addresses the potential utility of emerging developments in neurosonology.

Extracranial Doppler Sonography

Both CW and PW Doppler are used for examining the intra- and extracranial arteries supplying the brain. Interpretation of Doppler signals is based on analysis of the audio signals and of the frequency spectrum. The Doppler effect, bearing the name of Christian Andreas Doppler, for his 1842 description of the effect of moving objects on the change in frequency of emitted light, is familiar to anyone who has stood in one place and listened to a source of sound passing by: the rising pitch of the passing movement of sound rushes toward the listener and drops away as the source leaves him behind. For modern vascular insonations, the Doppler frequency shift, which is the difference between emitted and received ultrasound frequency, is within the audible range (200 to 20 Hz) and is proportional to the velocity of moving blood cells.

CW Doppler systems use two transducers, one of which emits while the other receives ultrasound continuously (Fig. 14.1A). This system is very useful for the detection of a broad range of flow velocity alterations, including very high blood flow velocities such as those that occur in severe stenosis, but it provides only limited information about the topographic origin of the ultrasound-reflecting source. By contrast, PW Doppler systems, in which ultrasound is both emitted and received subsequently from a single piezocrystal in the transducer (Fig. 14.1B), has the advantage of providing an estimate of depth from the probe to the site being insonated; thus PW Doppler sonography can also be used transcranially for the

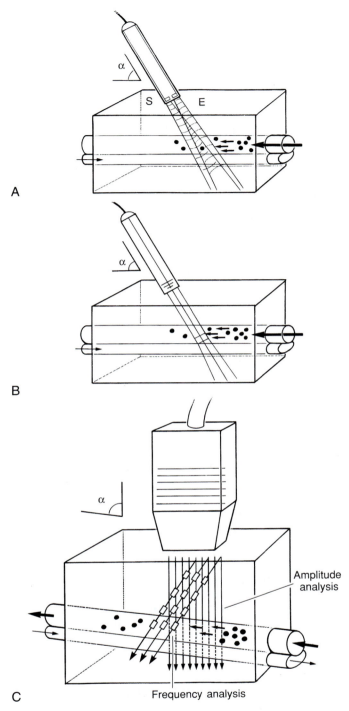

Figure 14.1 Schematic drawing demonstrating different ultrasound methods. **(A)** Continuous-wave Doppler sonography uses a single piezo crystal for both transmitting and receiving ultrasound signals. **(B)** Pulsed-wave Doppler uses separate piezo crystals, one emitting (E) and one receiving (S) ultrasound waves. This allows location of the sample volume. **(C)** Color-coded duplex sonography combines B-mode echo tomography and flow velocity signals for structural and hemodynamic analysis. (From Hennerici et al,[108] with permission.)

evaluation of intracranial cerebral arteries when the examiner takes into account the tissue depth from which the signal is derived.

Freely hand-held Doppler methods are simple, inexpensive, and noninvasive. In experienced hands they provide reliable data about hemodynamically significant lumen narrowing in the carotid system. Small lesions, however, cannot be reliably detected by extracranial Doppler sonography alone, and information on plaque morphology is not available with this method. CW and PW Doppler are good screening procedures for detection of stenoses and occlusions in the extracranial arteries; however, their use for differentiation of pathologic findings is more limited in the vertebral arteries. The diagnostic accuracy of PW Doppler is considerably increased when used in duplex systems.

CAROTID ARTERY

Indirect tests such as insonation of the ophthalmic artery ushered in the initial period of ultrasonography in the study of cerebrovascular disease.[139,149,156,166] This periorbital technique still provides useful and rapidly available information regarding the existence of collateral pathways. In the presence of severe stenosis or occlusion of the internal carotid artery, retrograde blood supply from the external carotid artery via the ophthalmic anastomosis can be easily detected with CW Doppler. With sufficient collateralization from the contralateral carotid or the vertebrobasilar systems, orthograde perfusion of the ophthalmic artery may occur. Accordingly, this indirect test fails to detect even hemodynamically significant ipsilateral carotid obstruction in ≤20% of patients. Thus, whereas detection of retrograde perfusion in the ophthalmic artery is a strong indicator of severe pathology within the ipsilateral extracranial carotid system, findings of normal perfusion of the ophthalmic branches cannot exclude even severe carotid stenosis or occlusion.

Direct Doppler sonography of the extracranial carotid system is used to detect various degrees of obstruction. According to the distribution of abnormal blood flow patterns within, proximal to, or distal to a narrowed arterial segment, this method provides information on the extent, site, and degree of lesions of >40% lumen narrowing. In such lesions the sensitivity (92% to 100%) and specificity (93% to 100%) of various Doppler techniques have been shown to be similar to those of arteriography in large series studied.[41,105] The reliablility of the diagnosis of carotid artery plaques producing <40% stenosis is considerably smaller; such plaques usually remain undetectable for CW and PW Doppler sonography. However, sometimes the audio signal in such cases is altered due to local turbulences, and spectral broadening may be demonstrated in spectrum analysis. For the detection of these small plaques, either simultaneous or complementary use of high-resolution B-mode imaging is necessary.

Low-frequency PW Doppler devices, which were developed for transcranial insonation, can be used to assess distal extracranial lesions of the internal carotid artery (e.g., carotid dissections, fibromuscular dysplasia, or atypically located atherosclerosis). Adequate positioning of the probe in the sub-

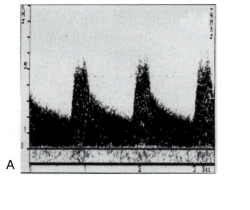
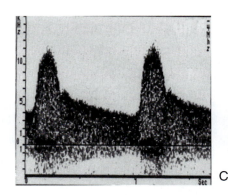
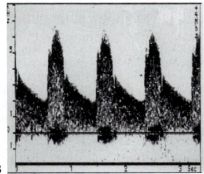
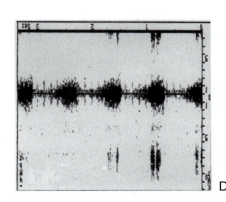

Figure 14.2 Different types of carotid artery stenoses (continuous-wave Doppler). **(A)** Mild stenosis. **(B)** Moderate stenosis. **(C)** Severe stenosis. **(D)** Pseudo-occlusion.

mandibular region allows recording of flow velocity in the internal carotid artery (ICA) up to the base of the skull with a recording depth of 50 to 80 mm.

Several stages of carotid obstruction can be defined with Doppler sonography (Fig. 14.2):

1. *Mild stenosis* (40% to 60%) is characterized by a local increase of peak and mean flow velocities. Systolic peak velocities range above 120 cm/s (4-MHz probe).

2. *Moderate stenosis* (60% to 80%) shows a distortion of normal pulsatile flow in addition to a local increase of peak and mean frequencies. Typically, systolic flow decelerations are found in the poststenotic segment. The systolic peak velocity ranges form 120 to 240 cm/s.

3. *Severe stenosis* (>80%) produces markedly increased peak flow velocities exceeding 240 cm/s and occasionally reaching 500 cm/s. In addition, pre- and poststenotic blood flow velocity is significantly reduced compared with the contralateral unaffected carotid artery. Retrograde flow of the ophthalmic artery may occur.

4. *Subtotal stenosis* (>95%) is characterized by a signal of variable, usually low frequency, which decreases once a stenosis reaches such severity that it becomes pseudo-occlusive. This condition is difficult to separate from complete occlusion and may be misdiagnosed.

5. *ICA occlusion* is characterized by the absence of any signal along the cervical course of the ICA; in some cases a low-velocity Doppler signal with a predominant reversed signal component and absent diastolic can be recorded at the presumed origin of the ICA (stump flow). Blood flow velocity in the common carotid artery (CCA) is reduced, and frequently retrograde perfusion of the ophthalmic artery occurs.

6. *Severe intracranial obstructions* within the carotid siphon or the middle cerebral artery (MCA) may lead to dampened spectra in the ipsilateral extracranial carotid artery. In addition, alterations of flow direction and signal frequency may occur in the ophthalmic artery depending on the site and degree of the lesion. Intracranial arteriovenous malformations (AVMS) and shunts may lead to increased flow velocities in the ipsilateral proximal vessel segments. Such findings on extracranial Doppler examinations should therefore prompt an appropriate workup for suspected intracranial AVM.

VERTEBRAL ARTERY

Stenosis in the vertebral artery can be assessed directly by Doppler sonography if it is located at the origin or at the atlas loop (Fig. 14.3). The criteria for classifying the degree of the lesion are the same as those in the carotid system. Severe lesions in distal or intracranial segments of the vertebral and in the basilar artery may lead to reduced flow velocities at locations where the Doppler signals can be recorded. Without additional information from B-mode imaging it is not possible to separate obstructive lesions from anatomic variations such

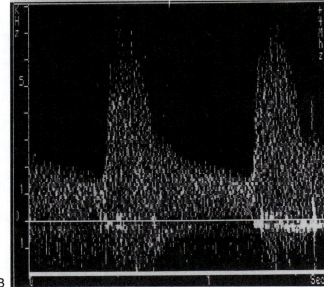

Figure 14.3 Tight stenosis at the origin of the vertebral artery. **(A)** Angiogram **(B)** Doppler spectra.

producing >50% lumen narrowing are lower than those for similar processes in the carotid system.[105] The combination of CW Doppler techniques with high-resolution B-mode imaging and color Doppler flow imaging of the extracranial vertebral arteries, together with transcranial Doppler sonography for the intracranial segments of the vertebral arteries and for the basilar artery, considerably increases diagnostic accuracy in the vertebrobasilar circulation.[59,74]

SUBCLAVIAN AND INNOMINATE ARTERIES

In patients with severe lesions of the proximal subclavian arteries, Doppler methods are excellent noninvasive tools for the detection of associated hemodynamic alterations such as retrograde or alternating blood flow in the ipsilateral vertebral artery[102,240] (Fig. 14.4). A transient increase of retrograde blood flow in the vertebral artery due to postischemic hyperemia following compression maneuver of the ipsilateral arm is another characteristic feature of the subclavian steal phenomenon. Severe obstructions of the innominate artery lead to complex hemodynamic alterations within the ipsilateral carotid and vertebral arteries including reversed flow signals.[185]

Sonographic Vascular Imaging

Sonographic imaging techniques such as conventional duplex scanning and color Doppler flow imaging (CDFI) have been established as routine methods for the evaluation of carotid and vertebral arterial disease. In some neurovascular laboratories, duplex scanning and CDFI are performed in selected patients after CW Doppler sonography, whereas in other centers duplex sonography with Doppler spectrum analysis is used directly for the assessment of extracranial obstructive lesions. Recently, power Doppler imaging (PDI) was introduced as another imaging technique for vascular applications; it provides an angiographic-like visualization of the arterial lumen. Accordingly, several different sonographic techniques are available for evaluation of the extracranial arteries; they all provide complementary information.

All sonographic imaging techniques use high-resolution *B-mode scanning* for display of the morphologic features of normal and pathologic vascular structures[82,109,110,243]; however, today gray-scale B-mode echotomograms are commonly combined with at least one other technique. Since the extracranial carotid and vertebral arteries lie close to the skin surface, linear array transducers are commonly used at an ultrasound frequency of 7.0 to 10.0 MHz.

Until a few years ago, *conventional duplex sonography,* which combines integrated PW Doppler spectrum analysis and B-mode sonography, was the second standard method for examination of the extracranial arteries besides CW Doppler sonography. In duplex sonography the B-mode echotomogram provides information about the presence and echomorphology of arterial lesions; in addition, it serves as a road map for the placement of the PW Doppler sample volume. Distinct

as hypoplasia and deep cervical collateral pathways. The same is true for the differentiation between occlusion and aplasia. Since the vertebral artery can regularly be recorded only at two sites with the hand-held Doppler technique, the sensitivity and specificity for detecting vertebral artery obstructions

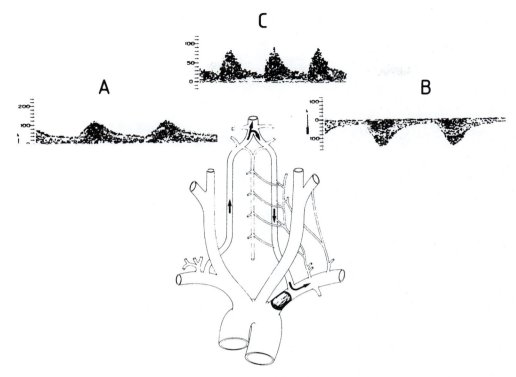

Figure 14.4 Subclavian steal phenomenon. Schematic drawing and Doppler spectra of **(A)** right vertebral artery (orthograde flow direction); **(B)** left vertebral artery (retrograde flow direction), and **(C)** basilar artery (orthograde flow).

criteria of the Doppler spectrum analysis are then used to evaluate hemodynamics and to categorize carotid artery stenoses (Table 14.1). Since the CCA, ICA, and external carotid artery (ECA) are usually characterized by a relatively distinct Doppler frequency spectrum, sample volume placement of the integrated PW Doppler system in these arteries confirms vessel identification (Fig. 14.5). The emission frequency of the integrated PW Doppler system ranges between 4 and 7 MHz.

Color Doppler flow imaging (CDFI) preserves the advantages of conventional duplex sonography and additionally visualizes color-coded blood flow patterns superimposed on the gray-scale B-mode echotomogram.[157,158,224] Using a defined color scale, the direction and the average mean velocity of moving blood cells within the sample volume at a given point in time is endcoded. Generation of color signals is based on the detection of frequency and phase shifts using a special multigate transducer (Fig. 14.1C). To obtain a quasi-real-time visualization of color-coded hemodynamics, additional technical principles such as autocorrelation are implemented. Table 14.2 summarizes the advantages and limitations of CDFI compared with conventional duplex sonography.

In contrast to CDFI, *power Doppler imaging (PDI)* relies on echo amplitudes depending on the density of red cells within the sample volume, the attenuation of the intervening tissue, and the size of the vessel in relation to the sample volume size.[203] Special filter systems further improve blood/tissue discrimination and intravascular surface definition. Since flowing blood undergoes less change in amplitude than in frequency, frame to frame averaging can be used to boost the signal noise ratio. An important feature of PDI is the ability to detect flow orthogonal to the ultrasound beam, thus permitting imaging of tortuous vessels without dropout. Clinical evaluation of power Doppler imaging is currently under way. First reports have demonstrated a diagnostic edge of power Doppler imaging over color Doppler flow imaging in the assessment of carotid stenosis.[86,225] Technical differences between CDFI and PDI are summarized in Table 14.3.

EXAMINATION PROCEDURE

The examination should be performed systematically with the patient in a supine position and the neck slightly hyperextended and rotated away from the transducer, which is

Table 14.1 Criteria for the Classification of Internal Carotid Artery Stenosis by Pulsed-Wave Doppler Sonography

Diameter Stenosis (%)	Peak Systolic Frequency (kHz)	Peak Systolic Velocity (cm/s)	End Diastolic Frequency (kHz)	End Diastolic Velocity (cm/s)
40–60	>4.0	>120	<1.3	<40
61–80	>4.0	>120	>1.3	>40
81–90	>8.0	>240	>3.3	>100

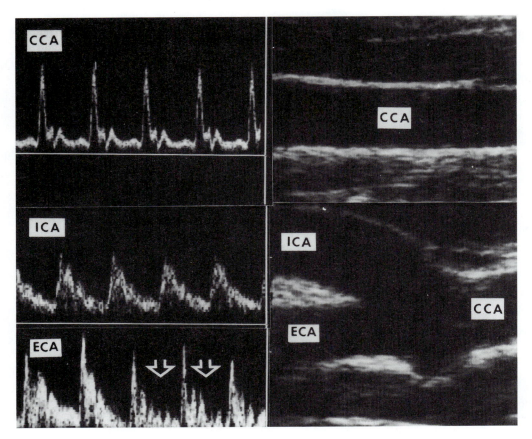

Figure 14.5 Duplex system analysis of a normal carotid artery. Doppler frequency spectra (left) and B-mode echotomograms of the common carotid artery (CCA) and the bifurcation with internal carotid artery (ICA) and external carotid artery (ECA). High systolic and low diastolic flow and transmitted oscillation (open arrows) from tapping the superficial temporal artery in the ECA. Flow in the ICA is higher in diastole, reflecting a low-resistance pattern. The Doppler waveform in the CCA reflects the two vascular beds it supplies, but it is dominated by the low-resistant flow to the brain.

Table 14.2 Advantages and Limitations of Color Doppler Flow Imaging Compared with Conventional Duplex Sonography

Advantages
    Simultaneous real-time image of blood flow and vessel anatomy
    Ease of vessel identification
    Faster data acquisition and shorter examination time
    Improved characterization of plaque surface structure
    Improved measurement of diameter and area stenosis
    Facilitated localization of the point of maximal intrastenotic flow velocity
    High intra- and interobserver reproducibility
    More reliable differential diagnosis of neck masses
Disadvantages
    Variable interpretation of blue-coded signals as reversed blood flow, turbulence, or aliasing phenomenon or due to angle of insonation
    Difficult detection of very slow flow velocity
    Limited temporal resolution of color-coded patterns
    Shadowing of color signals due to calcified plaque

positioned along the longitudinal axis of the carotid artery. Alternatively, posterior-lateral insonation, behind the sterno-cleidomastoid muscle, may provide good visualization of the vessel, in particular of the anterior arterial wall.

Sequential longitudinal and cross-sectional gray-scale scans are displayed from the most proximal segment of the CCA to the bifurcation and along the ICA to the submandibular region. Since both branches of the bifurcation cannot be visualized simultaneously in most cases, the CCA is displayed together with either the ICA or the ECA in longitudinal sections. Structural vascular abnormalities are characterized according to their echomorphologic features.

If color flow imaging is available, color-coded Doppler signals are then superimposed for analysis of the (1) temporal and spatial extent of physiologic flow separation zones in the normal carotid bifurcation; (2) location and pattern of secondary vortices and turbulences adjacent to nonstenotic plaques (3) characterization of pre-, intra-, and poststenotic blood flow patterns; (4) improved visualization of the plaque surface structure and geometric configuration of vascular lesions; and (5) measurement of the relative diameter and area reduction on longitudinal and transverse views of carotid stenosis. In

Table 14.3 Technical Differences Between Color Doppler Flow Imaging (CDFI) and Power Doppler Imaging (PDI)

	CDFI	**PDI**
Physical principle	Frequency and phase shift	Echo amplitude
Color-coded information	Mean velocity and direction	Density of blood cells
Hemodynamic information	Display in real time	None
Angle dependence of color display	Present	Absent
Aliasing phenomenon	Above Nyqist limit	Absent
Intravascular color contrast	Good definition of plaque surface	Improved display of high-grade stenoses Improved visualization in calcified plaques
Motion artifacts	Rare	Frequent

some cases in which complicated partially calcified stenoses cannot be adequately displayed by CDFI, additional use of PDI may better delineate the intravascular surface and the stenotic vessel segments, thus allowing measurements of diameter and area stenosis.

When the examination of the carotid artery is completed, the probe is shifted laterally from the CCA while maintaining a longitudinal position until the cervical vertebrae are displayed to visualize the intertransverse segments of the vertebral artery. Additional adjustment of the insonation angle is often necessary for adequate display of the vessel lumen and intravascular color-coded flow signals. The Doppler sample volume is positioned in the intertransverse segment to record the Doppler frequency spectrum. The vertebral artery is then followed in a proximal direction, and the pretransverse section below the sixth cervical vertebrum is traced to its ostium in the subclavian artery, where another PW Doppler spectrum is recorded. Finally, the atlas loop of the vertebral artery is displayed with the probe positioned below the mastoid process and the insonation beam directed toward the contralateral orbit.

NORMAL CAROTID ARTERY BIFURCATION

Since atherosclerosis in the carotid system is located predominantly at the bifurcation and the origin of the ICA, local hemodynamic patterns have been analyzed in experimental models and in ultrasound studies using conventional duplex scanning and color Doppler flow imaging to identify patterns of hemodynamic and structural interactions relevant in atherogenesis.[126,129,140,159,163,178,223,245,247] The complexity of physiologic flow separation, which is present in 94% to 99% of normal carotid bifurcations, cannot be assessed satisfactorily by means of PW Doppler sonography; however, CDFI displays the distribution of separation zones and their changes during the cardiac cycle in real time. CDFI has confirmed results from in vitro studies showing that secondary flow occurs at the outer wall of the carotid sinus. However, the temporal and spatial in vivo distribution of flow separation visualized by blue-coded Doppler signals is highly variable.[159,223] It frequently occurs at the origin of the ECA as well, and in some cases secondary flow extends from the ICA into the ECA around the flow

divider. Flow separation may be absent if smooth plaques fill the carotid sinus, or if there is no common or internal carotid bulb; by contrast, secondary flow does not exclude small plaques in the carotid bifurcation. However, since the assessment of blood flow direction is still limited by CDFI, complex 3D hemodynamics cannot be analyzed adequately in detail.

INTIMAL-MEDIAL THICKNESS IN ATHEROSCLEROSIS

B-mode ultrasonography has been used to assess the presence and extent of minimal to mild atherosclerosis in the carotid artery by measurement of the intimal-medial thickness (IMT)[70,180,196] (Fig. 14.6). While the severity of IMT reflects the extent of local disease, sequential assessments performed over time may provide documentation on the course of atherosclerosis.[204] In a large number of epidemiologic studies IMT was correlated with all common vascular risk factors and may also predict the degree of coronary artery disease.[51,79] Furthermore, management of risk factors appeared to have an impact on IMT.[7,114,142,175,202] However, methodologic controversies on where, when, and what to measure have yet to be resolved.[112,169,179,241]

CHARACTERIZATION OF ATHEROSCLEROTIC PLAQUES

Small atherosclerotic plaques (luminal narrowing <40%) may be suspected by Doppler sonography if spectral broadening is present, indicating abnormal blood flow components. However, since physiologic flow separation and a variety of other hemodynamic variables may confound the interpretation of spectral broadening, ultrasonic imaging techniques are required to detect atherosclerotic lesions and assess plaque morphology. High-resolution B-mode scanning allows characterization of distinct echomorphologic features of carotid plaques that correlate with different stages of the disease according to histopathologic criteria.[50,82,84,109] By contrasting the intra-

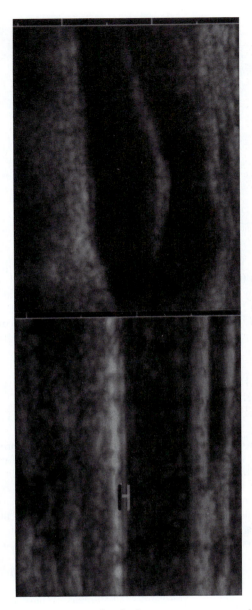

Figure 14.6 Intima media thickness measurements shown in typical B-mode imaging below the carotid bifurcation. (From Hennerici et al,[108] with permission.)

vascular lumen, color signals on CDFI and PDI further improve evaluation of the plaque surface and configuration.[46,158,215,222,223]

Plaque Echogenicity

Plaques with homogeneous echogenicity consist mainly of fibrotic tissue.[82,109] Ulceration is rare in homogeneous plaques, perhaps accounting for the lack of significant correlation with the occurrence of focal cerebral ischemia. Heterogeneous plaques represent matrix deposition, cholesterol accumulation, necrosis, calcification, and intraplaque hemor-

rhage[82,109,243] (Fig. 14.7). Preoperative duplex images have correlated well with plaque histology of endarterectomy specimens except in some cases of recent plaque hemorrhage.[28] Although echolucent areas within the plaque may represent thrombotic material or hemorrhage, it has been recognized that lipid accumulation may produce similar echogenicity.[32] Plaque calcification produces acoustic shadowing in B-mode echotomograms. Depending on plaque location and extent of calcification, this artifact can be a major obstacle for adequate visualization of the vasculature as well as of the plaque itself.

Many studies have reported an association between heterogeneous plaques and the occurrence of cerebrovascular events.[10,30,131,170,229] These conclusions have been based on evaluation of endarterectomy specimens that suggested a correlation of intraplaque hemorrhage and transient ischemic attacks and stroke.[73,116,117,141] More recent studies have not confirmed this hypothesis.[20,133,134]

Plaque Surface Structure

Attempts to characterize plaque surface structure with B-mode echotomography have been disappointing. Although a relatively good differentiation among smooth, irregular, and ulcerative plaque surfaces has been obtained for postmortem carotid artery specimens,[109] the in vivo accuracy compared with findings at carotid endarterectomy has been considerably poorer.[50,199,242] Both B-mode imaging and arteriography failed to provide a satisfactory diagnostic yield for ulcerative plaques, the sensitivities being 47% and 53% respectively.[50] Diagnostic sensitivity for detection of plaque ulceration, however, is affected by the degree of carotid stenosis and increases to 77% in plaques associated with ≤50%, stenosis.[50] Other authors have been unable to distinguish between the presence or absence of intimal ulcerations with B-mode scans and conclude that differentiation between smooth and irregular plaque surface structure does not allow for identification of patients at risk of ulceration.[31] Color signals on both CDFI and PDI contrast the intravascular surface, thus improving the detection of plaque ulceration. Large echolucent components of the plaque can also be assessed more reliably using CDFI and PDI.

Whether plaque surface irregularities or ulcerations are useful parameters for defining patients at risk of carotid embolism is a matter of ongoing debate. Advocates of a pathophysiologic relationship maintain that ulcerations represent fertile ground for potential thrombosis and consequent embolic events. Indeed, a recent report contends that the presence of an angiographically defined ulceration is associated with an increased risk of stroke in medically treated symptomatic patients.[68] Moreover, high-intensity transient signals monitored in the MCAs of patients with carotid stenosis, assumed to represent asymptomatic microembolic events, were found to correlate with the appearance of ipsilateral plaque ulceration on angiography.[239] Pathologic studies, however, have pointed out that in asymptomatic carotid plaques with stenosis exceeding 60% there is an increased frequency of plaque hemorrhages, ulcerations, and mural thrombi, as well as an increase in numerous healed ulcerations and organized thrombi.[231] Likewise, comparisons of symptomatic with asymptomatic large and stenotic carotid endarterectomy plaques have re-

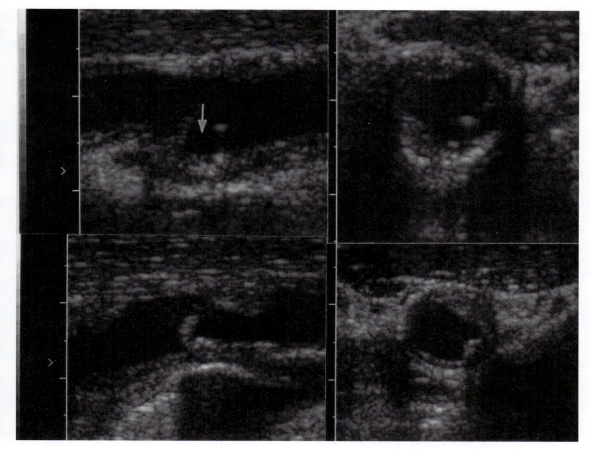

Figure 14.7 Longitudinal and transverse B-mode scans of plaques of the internal carotid artery. (**A**) Plaque with well-defined, echolucent surface defect (arrow), presumably representing an ulceration. (**B**) Corresponding transverse view of Fig. A demonstrating the plaque's circular form and heterogeneous echo pattern. (**C**) Longitudinal scan of a plaque with a hook-like configuration. (**D**) In the transverse plane, this plaque shows an irregular, half-moon shape.

vealed a high incidence of complex plaque structure and complications in each.[20,81] There appears, therefore, to be little difference between plaque specimens from symptomatic and asymptomatic patients.

Quantification of Plaque Size and Volume

The quantitative assessment of plaque size by B-mode imaging alone has important limitations,[49,249] including a low interobserver reproducibility.[191] To overcome these deficits, first attempts at volume quantification of carotid plaques were undertaken several years ago and involved tedious manual tracing of sequential B-mode slices.[220] Since then rapid developments in computer hardware and software have made this task feasible in the routine clinical setting. The use of an advanced imaging system for acquisition and offline analysis of electrocardiogram-gated, equidistant axial

B-mode scans has recently been reported to allow reliable quantification of moderately sized carotid plaques.[60]

QUANTIFICATION AND GRADING OF CAROTID ARTERY STENOSIS

The combination of B-mode echotomography and PW Doppler sonography in duplex instruments has considerably improved the accuracy of the noninvasive diagnosis and grading of carotid stenosis. The degree of stenosis can be estimated from distinct parameters of the Doppler frequency spectrum (Table 14.1). Instead of Doppler shift frequencies, equivalent flow velocity values can be used after correction of the Doppler insonation angle according to the flow direction in the vessel segment. In CDFI three sources of information are available for the classification of carotid stenosis: the Doppler frequency spectrum, measurement of the residual vessel lumen, and characteristic color flow patterns.

Doppler Frequency Spectrum

The time-consuming search for optimal placement of the PW Doppler sample volume is facilitated in CDFI instruments, and reproducibility for the classification of carotid stenosis is significantly improved.[230] Assessment of the Doppler spectrum is particularly important since it can be recorded frequently even when plaque calcification obscures adequate visualization of color flow patterns and the residual vessel lumen. Using distinct parameters from the Doppler spectrum such as the peak systolic frequency/velocity[199,232,250] (Table 14.1), a significantly higher agreement of angiography can be obtained with CDFI (plate 14.1) than with standard duplex sonography (86.6% versus 79.6%, P 0.034). Comparison between color-assisted duplex sonography and planimetry of carotid endarterectomy specimens for the assessment of cross-sectional area reduction revealed a high correlation.[11]

Measurement of Residual Vessel Lumen

The methodologic limitations of measurements of residual vessel lumen with B-mode echotomograms are well documented.[49,191,249] Using sequential longitudinal and transverse sections, both CDFI and PDI allow more reliable assessment of plaque configuration and relative obstruction by contrasting the intravascular surface.[46,69,159,215,222,223] Assuming a concentric stenosis, the percentage area reduction in cross sections is higher than the relative diameter reduction.[11] Although first reports on the use of CDFI for evaluation of the degree of stenosis from the relative reduction in the color flow lumen found a relatively poor agreement with angiography on longitudinal (74%) and transverse (65%) measurements,[69] recent studies have reported a good correlation between transverse lumen reduction on CDFI and diameter reduction on corresponding angiograms of carotid stenosis.[213,222] (Plate 14.2). Measurement of local diameter and area reduction in carotid stenosis can be performed more frequently by PDI than by CDFI due to improved visualization of the residual stenotic lumen.[86,225] In addition, it was recently reported that PDI correlated significantly better than CDFI with angiographic stenosis evaluated according to the European Carotid Surgery Trial method.[71]

Color Doppler Flow Patterns

Color Doppler flow patterns can provide complementary information for establishing the degree of carotid artery stenosis. Low-grade stenosis (40% to 60%) is associated with a relatively long segment of decreased color saturation with absent or minimal poststenotic turbulence.[224] In moderate obstructions (61% to 80%), the decreased color saturation is more circumscribed, while flow velocity remains high during diastole. Poststenotic flow is turbulent, and flow reversal occurs frequently (Plate 14.1). High-grade stenosis is characterized by a mosaic pattern indicating high flow velocity and mixed turbulence.[90] A short segment of maximal color fading or aliasing with severe poststenotic turbulence and flow reversal provides further evidence for high-grade stenosis.[224]

Although good agreement between angiographic findings and color Doppler flow patterns for low-, middle-, and high-grade stenosis can be obtained, several factors can lead to misinterpretation of a semiquantitative analysis of color Doppler results.[224] Color-coded hemodynamic patterns are variable due to different plaque configuration and vessel geometry. Interpretation of blue-coded Doppler signals as turbulence, reversed flow, or aliasing phenomenon may be difficult in some cases. In addition, peak velocities cannot be directly determined from the color signals since each color pixel on CDFI represents the approximate mean velocity, which is particularly lower than the peak velocity if turbulence is present. Other potential color Doppler artifacts include shadowing, reverberation, color bleed, and color noise. In ultrasound systems implementing induced signal amplitude for color suppression, setting the Doppler gain too high or the Doppler reject too low can result in random variations in echo measurements causing hypoechoic regions (e.g., thrombosed vessels) to fill with color. It is therefore essential that color Doppler findings be complemented by spectral analysis.

Recently an international consensus meeting was held to determine criteria for the quantification of ICA stenosis.[56] Recommendations were made for interpretation of maximum Doppler shift velocities, systolic velocity ratios, and residual area. Magnetic resonance angiography (MRA) was considered an efficient complement to ultrasound—when both methods indicate severe carotid stenosis with unaffected intracranial arteries, angiography can be avoided in surgical candidates.

OCCLUSION OF THE CAROTID ARTERY

The diagnosis of carotid occlusion by B-mode echotomography alone without Doppler sonography is not reliable since the residual vascular lumen frequently cannot be visualized adequately in complicated heterogeneous, partially calcified high-grade obstructions. In acute thrombotic occlusion, echolucent material fills the vascular lumen, which can hardly be differentiated on the gray scale from blood flow in a patent ICA. CW Doppler and duplex sonography had a significantly higher accuracy for the diagnosis of ICA occlusion; however, the differentiation from a subtotal stenosis remained difficult. The PW Doppler spectrum and color signals in ICA occlusion typically demonstrate a marked reduction of the systolic and diastolic blood flow velocity in the CCA and an internalized ECA with high diastolic flow velocity, indicating collateral supply via the ophthalmic artery. Color-coded intravascular Doppler signals are absent in the occluded ICA; however, blue-coded flow reversal in the residual stump at the bifurcation (stump flow) may occur. The capacity of modern CDFI and PDI instruments to detect very slow blood flow velocities has markedly improved the sensitivity for the diagnosis of a subtotal ICA stenosis and pseudo-occlusion, which may represent candidates for vascular surgery.

CCA occlusion is a relatively rare condition that can be reliably diagnosed by conventional duplex sonography and color Doppler flow imaging.[136,246] However, it is more difficult to assess the patency of the ICA distal to the CCA occlusion, the precondition for surgical intervention, and collateral flow of the ECA.[26,54,195,228] Typically, CDFI displays blue-coded signals in the ECA due to reversed flow direction and orthograde filling of the ICA in the absence of Doppler signals in the CCA.

CAROTID ARTERY DISSECTION

Several recent studies have demonstrated the usefulness of ultrasound for diagnosis of carotid artery dissection, a cause of transient or permanent neurologic deficits particularly in young patients. ICA dissection usually occurs spontaneously and results in a typical syndrome of focal cerebral deficits, headache, neck pain, and ipsilateral Horner syndrome.

The diagnosis can be suspected when CW Doppler studies detect a high-resistance Doppler signal with bidirectional signal components over the course of the ICA. B-mode scans can demonstrate a tapered lumen and occasionally a floating intimal flap, although the results of this investigation are often unremarkable. CDFI, however, is an important diagnostic tool in this setting and shows marked flow reversal at the origin of the ICA in systole and absent or minimal blood flow in diastole corresponding to the high-resistance bidirectional Doppler signal. Follow-up examinations demonstrate gradual normalization of the Doppler spectrum, indicating recanalization of the ICA within a few weeks to months in more than two-thirds of patients[111,219,226,227] (Plate 14.3).

VERTEBRAL ARTERY

Examination of the vertebral artery with CW, Doppler, PW Doppler, and duplex scanning is limited to its origin from the subclavian artery, the proximal pretransverse segment, short intertransverse segments between the third and sixth cervical vertebrae, and the atlas loop. Although PW Doppler criteria for vertebral artery stenosis are similar to those used for diagnosis of carotid artery stenosis and have been defined by several duplex studies, classification and detection of vertebral artery stenosis or occlusion is more difficult than in the carotid arteries.[5,29,55] One reason for this difficulty is that variations in arterial caliber are frequent in vertebral arteries. Numerous collateral pathways of the vertebral system can permit orthograde flow to the basilar artery even in the face of vertebral occlusion. These features make examination of the vertebral artery at several locations mandatory. Intravascular color Doppler allows noninvasive quantification of flow in the vertebral artery system in greater than 95% of all patients[27] and facilitates identification of the proximal segment and ostium, the predominant location of extracranial vertebral stenosis, as well as of the atlas loop.[15,237]

Correct interpretation of Doppler results from the vertebral artery requires knowledge of Doppler parameters from both the contralateral vertebral artery and from the carotid system. For example, an increase in the systolic or diastolic velocity profile of the proximal vertebral artery, although suggestive of stenosis, can also occur as a compensatory response to a variety of conditions of the contralateral vertebral artery such as hypoplasia, aplasia, stenosis, or occlusion, as well as to severe obstruction of the carotid system.

Normal Findings

The PW Doppler spectrum from an intertransverse segment of a normal vertebral artery shows a high diastolic flow velocity and low pulsatility, indicating low vascular resistance in the territory of supply (Fig. 14.8). In a study of 42 healthy subjects with color-coded duplex imaging, the mean systolic peak velocity was 56 cm/s (range, 19 to 98 cm/s), the mean diastolic flow velocity 17 cm/s (range, 6 to 30 cm/s), and the resistance index between 0.62 and 0.75.[236] Slightly lower values of aver-

Figure 14.8 (**A**) Normal vertebral artery at its origin from the subclavian artery on longitudinal B-mode scan with corresponding Doppler spectrum indicating low vascular resistance. (**B**) An intertransverse segment of the vetebral artery between the cervical vertebrae is well visualized.

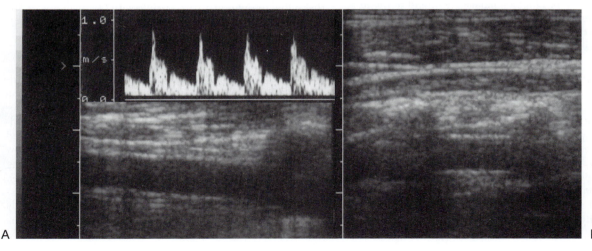

A   B

age maximal systolic velocity (43.0 ± 8.9 cm/s on the right and 43.3 ± cm/s on the left) were obtained in a study of 108 normal vertebral arteries investigated with duplex sonography. Here the average diameter of this vessel in the pretransverse and intertransverse segment C5-C6 was reported as 3.8 ± 0.46 mm on the right and 3.88 ± 0.47 mm on the left.[18] Detection of the origin of the vertebral artery with color-coded duplex is superior to conventional duplex sonography and more accessible on the right (88%) than on the left (73%) side.[15]

Vertebral Hypoplasia

Vertebral hypoplasia has been defined in pathoanatomic studies as a decrease in vascular lumen diameter below 2 mm.[72] A recent study using CDFI has confirmed this definition by showing a reduction in systolic and diastolic flow velocities in vertebral arteries with diameters <2 mm.[59] Through measurement of the vessel lumen, vertebral hypoplasia can be distinguished from proximal or distal obstructive disease, which may also produce abnormal reduction of flow velocity or an intermediate Doppler spectrum characterized by flow reversal in early systole.

Stenosis and Occlusion of the Vertebral Artery

The predominant site of extracranial vertebral artery stenosis is the ostium of the subcalvian artery. The atlas loop and intracranial V4 segment are involved less frequently, and stenoses in the intertransverse segments are rare. A peak systolic frequency exceeding 4 kHz assessed by means of the integrated PW Doppler system indicates a relevant vertebral stenosis. Features of color-coded Doppler signals correspond to those of carotid stenosis. With increasing degree of luminal narrowing decreased color saturation becomes more circumscribed, and turbulence as well as poststenotic flow reversal are more severe. Hemodynamically significant obstruction of the intracranial vertebral artery produces a high-resistance Doppler waveform with a resistivity index exceeding 0.80.[237] However, the Doppler spectrum may be normal if flow to the ipsilateral posterior inferior cerebellar artery is preserved. In acute proximal vertebral artery occlusion PW Doppler spectra cannot be recorded, and color Doppler signals are absent in the pre- and intertransverse segments. However, demonstration of a vascular lumen differentiates this condition from vertebral hypoplasia.

Vertebral Artery Dissection

Vertebral artery dissection is one of the most important causes of brain stem strokes in young patients.[45,94] It presents with neck pain, occipital headache, and signs and symptoms of brain stem or cerebellar ischemia in about 90% of patients and commonly leaves a permanent deficit.[85,125,162] Findings on cerebral angiography are not always diagnostic of vertebral artery dissection. Specific radiographic findings such as pseudoaneurysm or intraluminal clot are infrequent,[1] and more often less specific features such as irregular stenoses or occlusions are found, frequently indistinguishable from those of

atherosclerotic or partially recanalized embolic occlusions of the vertebral artery.[113] Magnetic resonance imaging (MRI) is emerging as the imaging modality of choice for diagnosis of vertebral artery dissection.[183] One primary advantage of this technique is its ability to detect characteristic intramural hematoma as hyperintense signals within the wall of the vertebral artery on T_1-weighted imaging.[42] Although larger studies evaluating the role of MRI and MRA in vertebral artery dissection are not yet available, it is likely that its usefulness in this setting will be similar to that in carotid dissection.[42]

The role of ultrasound in the diagnosis of vertebral artery dissection, however, remains uncertain. In contradistinction to carotid artery dissection, there is no pathognomonic ultrasound finding for vertebral artery dissection if the lesion affects the V2 to V4 segments. Examination of the atlas loop can show absent, low bidirectional or low poststenotic flow signals.[230] In hitherto less frequently considered dissections of the V1 segment, the stenotic segment can be identified directly; absent flow in the intertransverse segments should similarly raise the question of vertebral dissection. Further findings can include a localized increase in the diameter of the artery with hemodynamic signs of stenosis or occlusion at the same level, decreased pulsatility, and the presence of intravascular echoes in the enlarged segment.[17,235] Transcranial Doppler can be helpful in determining the length of dissection.[57] The combined use of extracranial and transcranial Doppler and duplex sonography has been reported to increase the diagnostic yield to detect vertebral artery dissection; consideration of any abnormal sonographic finding resulted in a yield of 86%, whereas reliance on definite abnormal findings (absent flow signal, severely reduced flow velocities, absent diastolic flow, bidirectional flow, or stenosis signal) reduced the diagnostic yield to only 64%.[230] Similar results were obtained in another study in which ultrasound abnormalities (high-resistance signal, occlusion, and bilateral retrograde flow) were found in 8 of 10 vertebral artery dissections.[113]

The relatively good likelihood of detecting abnormal flow characteristics in the vertebral artery suggests a role for ultrasound in guidance of both further diagnostic imaging procedures and therapeutic measures. However, since unremarkable ultrasound findings in the setting of suspected vertebral dissection do not exclude the diagnosis, further workup in these cases is mandatory. Recanalization, occurring in most cases, can be monitored by Doppler sonography, provided that initial findings were compatible with the diagnosis of dissection.

Subclavian Steal Phenomenon

Severe obstruction of the proximal subclavian artery or brachiocephalic trunk often leads to a permanent subclavian steal phenomenon in which the subclavian artery distal to the stenosis is supplied by the ipsilateral vertebral artery. Classical findings include retrograde flow in the vertebral artery associated with abnormal Doppler spectra, reversed color-coded flow patterns, and a transient increase in retrograde flow following postischemic hyperemia of the upper extremities (Plate 14.4). An intermediate flow pattern similar to that seen in hypoplastic vertebral arteries may also be seen in hemodynamically relevant obstruction of the subclavian artery. In cases of marginal steal phenomenon with orthograde flow in the vertebral

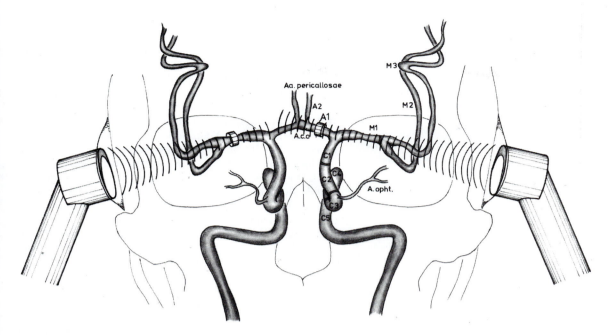

Figure 14.9 Schematic illustration of the position of the sample volume inside the skull, using the transtemporal approach. Aa.pericallosae, pericallosal arteries; A.opht., ophthalmic artery; A.c.a., anterior communicating artery.

artery, a compression test shows a subtle increase in flow velocities directly after inflation of a blood pressure cuff on the ipsilateral arm.

A number of studies have documented the benign nature of the subclavian steal syndrome. In 324 patients with reversed vertebral artery blood flow neither the presence nor the type of vertebral artery steal (permanent [n = 204] or intermediate [n = 120]) determined neurologic symptoms; most patients were asymptomatic, and symptoms that occurred were related to coincidental carotid obstructions or abnormal flow velocity patterns in the basilar artery.[102] Likewise, in a prospective study of 39 patients with subclavian steal syndrome, only 15% of initially asymptomatic patients experienced vertebrobasilar transient ischemic attacks, and spontaneous remission of these attacks occurred in approximately 50%.[4] Surgical treatment is therefore discouraged for most patients with this benign flow abnormality.

Transcranial Doppler

Noninvasive assessment of intracranial arteries and veins can be achieved with transcranial Doppler (TCD). This technique uses high-energy bidirectional pulsed Doppler, typically at a low frequency of 2 MHz, for intracranial vascular examination via transtemporal, transorbital, and transnuchal bone windows (Fig. 14.9). Applications for TCD include detection of intracranial stenosis and occlusion, evaluation of intracranial collateral circulations, detection of vasospasm in subarachnoid hemorrhage, assessment of cerebral autoregulation, and documentation of progressive obstruction of the cerebral circulation as seen in conditions leading to brain death. A rapidly increasing number of TCD monitoring techniques are available for surveillance of intracranial hemodynamics during carotid endarterectomy, for detection of high intensity transient signals suggestive of microembolism, for diagnosis of patent foramen ovale, for assessment of orthostatic dysregulation, and for functional investigations of neuronal coupling. The introduction of color TCD flow imaging has led to greater accuracy in vessel identification, and first reports on the merits of this imaging procedure for detection of cerebral aneurysms, evaluation of AVMs, and characterization of vessel morphology are now available. Recent technologic advances that promise to bring new capabilities to TCD ultrasonography include transcranial power Doppler imaging, insonation after administration of contrast media, harmonic imaging, and 3D transcranial power Doppler angiography.

With conventional TCD, intracranial basal arteries are identified by flow direction, depth of the Doppler sample volume, and probe position (Table 14.4). Since flow velocities of intracranial vessels are known to vary with age and sex,[6] hematocrit,[37] and end-tidal CO_2 partial pressure, a standardized TCD examination procedure is mandatory.[83] Normal values of flow velocities of the basal cerebral arteries are presented in Table 14.5.[3,13,40,41,92,107,138] Optimal performance and correct interpretation of TCD studies require knowledge of the clinical setting and results from extracranial ultrasound examinations.

Compression of the CCA is occasionally useful for the elucidation of complex intracranial hemodynamics. This test may be used with simultaneous measurement of velocity changes in the MCA to predict tolerance to carotid artery occlusion

Table 14.4 Transcranial Doppler Criteria for the Identification of Basal Intracranial Vessels Using the Transtemporal, Transorbital, and Nuchal Approaches

Vessel	Probe	Depth (mm)	Flow Direction
Transtemporal approach			
MCA	Medial	30–65	Toward probe
ACA	Medial	55–80	Away from probe
ICA	Caudal	55–75	Toward probe
PCA, P1	Posterior	55–80	Toward probe
PCA, P2	Posterior	55–75	Away from probe
Transorbital approach			
Ophthalmic artery	30–60	Toward probe	
ICA, C4, C5	60–80	Toward probe	
ICA, C2, C3	60–80	Away from probe	
Nuchal approach			
VA	50–100	Away from probe	
BA	75–120	Away from probe	

Abbreviations: MCA, middle cerebral artery; ACA, anterior cerebral artery; ICA, internal carotid artery; PCA, posterior cerebral artery; VA, vertebral artery; BA, basilar artery.

(e.g., prior to treatment of certain aneurysms when surgical sacrifice of the carotid artery is anticipated[80] or in the preoperative assessment of the effect of clamping during carotid endarterectomy). Since there is evidence that compression of the CCA can provoke embolic strokes on rare occasions, this procedure should be performed only after exclusion of atherosclerotic disease in the CCA and ICA and should be limited to a few seconds in the proximal CCA, avoiding the carotid bulb.[127]

INTRACRANIAL STENOSIS AND OCCLUSION

Significant narrowing of intracranial arteries results in localized increases in mean and peak flow velocities, turbulence and reversed flow phenomena, and reduction of pre- or poststenotic flow velocities.[106,137,218] Stenosis of >50% lumen narrowing can be reliably detected in arterial segments with anatomically favorable insonation angles (Fig. 14.10) such as the M1 segment of the MCA and the P1 segment of the posterior cerebral artery (PCA). In segments approaching perpendicular insonation angles such as those of the distal MCA branches, stenosis is more difficult to evaluate. Assessment of the degree of stenosis is facilitated by using complementary information from TCD and MRA. This dual regimen appears to be superior to conventional angiography for the demonstration and quantification of intracranial stenosis, provided standardized parameters are used for validation of obstructive lesions.[12,200] The difficulty of establishing new criteria for evaluation of intracranial stenosis, in which pathoanatomic correlation is seldom possible, remains a challenge for future studies.

A reliable diagnosis of occlusion in the M1 segment can

only be made when unequivocal evidence of blood flow in the ipsilateral anterior cerebral artery (ACA) or PCA can be obtained, thus differentiating this condition from high ultrasound attenuation and poor echo window insonation. Further findings supporting MCA occlusion are dampened spectra in segments proximal to the occlusion, reversed flow direction in distal MCA branches, and abnormally elevated ipsilateral ACA flow velocities.[151] In a series of 467 patients, the sensitivity for the detection of MCA occlusion by TCD was 79% with a specificity of 100%.[189] Continuous monitoring of the MCA can document early recanalization of an acute occlusion.[161]

TCD examinations of the vertebrobasilar arteries are less reliable than those of the anterior circulation. The junction of the basilar artery is difficult to define by TCD criteria alone, and investigation of the entire course of the basilar artery, usually limited by excessive insonation depth with poor signal/noise ratio, can be achieved in only 30% of patients.[164] As in the anterior circulation, partial obstructions are easier to detect than total occlusions. Using intraarterial digital subtraction angiography as a standard reference, TCD has demonstrated sensitivities of 74% to 87% and specificities of 80% to 86% for detection of large vessel occlusive disease of the intracranial vertebrobasilar system.[47,233] Best results, however, are obtained when TCD is used in combination with cerebral angiography[164] or MRA.[201] Unfortunately, detection of basilar artery occlusion is poor, with a sensitivity of only

Table 14.5 Normal Values of Transcranial Doppler Examination

Vessel	Systolic Peak Velocity (cm/s)	Mean Velocity (cm/s)	Diastolic Velocity (cm/s)	Age Group (yr)
MCA	94.5 ± 13.6	58.4 ± 8.4	45.6 ± 6.6	<40
(50 mm)	91.0 ± 16.9^a	57.7 ± 11.5^a	44.3 ± 9.5^a	40–60
	78.1 ± 15.0^a	44.7 ± 11.1^a	31.9 ± 9.1^a	>60
ACA	76.4 ± 16.9	47.3 ± 13.6	36.0 ± 9.0	<40
(70 mm)	86.4 ± 20.1	53.1 ± 10.5	41.1 ± 7.4^b	40–60
	73.3 ± 20.3	45.3 ± 13.5	34.2 ± 8.8^b	>60
PCA	53.2 ± 11.3	34.2 ± 7.8	25.9 ± 6.5	<40
(60 mm)	60.1 ± 20.6	36.6 ± 9.8	28.7 ± 7.5^b	40–60
	51.0 ± 11.9	29.9 ± 9.3	22.0 ± 6.9^b	>60
VA/BA	56.3 ± 7.8	34.9 ± 7.8	27.0 ± 5.3	<40
(75 mm)	59.5 ± 17.0	36.4 ± 11.7	29.2 ± 8.4^b	40–60
	50.9 ± 18.7	30.5 ± 12.4	21.2 ± 9.2^b	>60
Pulsatility Index (All Age Groups)			
MCA	0.92 ± 0.25		
ACA	0.8 ± 0.16		
PCA	0.88 ± 0.21		

Abbreviations: MCA, middle cerebral artery; ACA, anterior cerebral artery; PCA, posterior cerebral artery; VA, vertebral artery; BA, basilar artery.

$^a P < 0.02.$

$^b P < 0.05.$

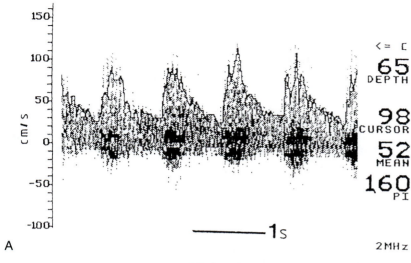

A

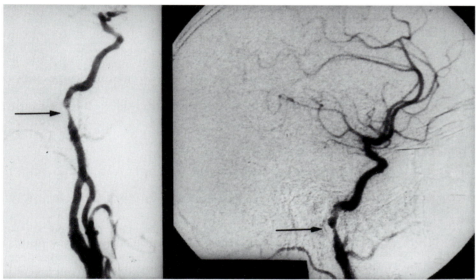

B

Figure 14.10 (**A**) Doppler spectra (recording depth: 65 mm, increased peak velocities, low-frequency signals). (**B**) Angiogram of a patient with an extracranial distal lesion of the internal carotid artery (arrows).

36%.[104] This is of major clinical importance in evaluation of patients suspected of suffering from acute basilar artery thrombosis.

TCD may be valuable in assessment of vertebrobasilar insufficiency due to bilateral extracranial vertebral artery compression resulting from head and neck movements. Provocative maneuvers evoke an immediate and precipitous drop in flow velocity associated with concomitant symptoms of vertebrobasilar insufficiency.[38]

INTRACRANIAL COLLATERALIZATION

The presence of intracranial collateralization in patients with stenosis or occlusion of the extracranial carotid arteries can be investigated with conventional TCD. Findings compatible with collateral flow over the anterior communicating artery

include retrograde flow in the ipsilateral ACA, increased peak and mean velocities in both ACAs, increased velocities and low-frequency signals in the midline indicating functional stenosis of the anterior communicating artery, and decreased MCA velocity during contralateral CCA compression. Collateralization from the posterior circulation is suggested by increased velocities in the ipsilateral P1 segment of the PCA or in the basilar artery as well as by low-frequency signals in the vicinity of the posterior communicating artery. Leptomeningeal anastomosis, although more difficult to assess, may be associated with increased velocities in proximal and distal segments of the PCA and with retrograde flow signals in distal MCA branches. TCD can also detect retrograde flow in the ophthalmic artery, another avenue for collateralization.

Flow velocities in the MCA distal to significant stenosis and occlusion vary with regard to the efficacy of intracranial collateralization. Whereas reduced MCA velocities and pulsatility indexes have been found ipsilateral to symptomatic carotid occlusion,[207,208] normal peak and mean velocities indicating adequate collateralization have been reported for asymptomatic patients.[186]

VASOSPASM IN SUBARACHNOID HEMORRHAGE

TCD has become a standard examination procedure for detection, quantification, and follow-up of vasospasms after subarachnoid hemorrhage (SAH).[2,92,210] Vasospasms generally occur at the 4th day after SAH, while peak flow velocities can be observed between the 11th and 18th days. Normalization of flow velocities occurs within the third or fourth week after SAH. Rapid increase of velocities 4 to 8 days following SAH is associated with an increased risk of ischemic stroke.

Although early reports claimed that TCD results mirror the degree of obstruction commonly demonstrated in angiograms of stroke-prone patients after SAH, recent observations have questioned a simple focal narrowing of the arterial lumen, analogous to that in atherosclerotic disease, as the cause of altered Doppler flow patterns following SAH. The pathophysiology of subarachnoid vasospasm is complex. Elevated intracranial pressure may lead to an increase in vasomotor resistance of capillary and arteriolar vessels with consequent dampening of the Doppler flow velocity in major proximal arteries. This may result in false-negative Doppler results despite angiographically demonstrable vasospasm. Moreover, local flow turbulences may be found despite a normal appearance of the angiogram if peripheral vasomotor dysregulation and large vessel vasoconstriction occur subsequent to SAH. Importantly, TCD findings in patients with SAH are greatly influenced by changing therapeutic concepts. Only 28% of patients treated with calcium channel blockers have a significant increase in flow velocities prior to the onset of delayed ischemic stroke, suggesting that vasospasm may occur in more distal arterial segments inaccessible to TCD insonation.[132] TCD is further limited in patients with SAH by its relatively poor diagnostic accuracy in the ACA territory, a frequent site of aneurysms.[135]

ARTERIOVENOUS MALFORMATIONS

High-flow angiomas are characterized by a low peripheral resistance resulting in high peak and mean velocities with a low pulsatility index in the proximal segments of feeding vessels. Transcranial duplex color flow imaging allows identification of the major afferent feeding vessels, the venous drainage, and the vascular convolution of accessible AVMs.[25] In some AVMs even selective recordings of small secondary feeding vessels may be possible.

Identification of AVM feeding vessels as well as estimation of the relative magnitude of the flow provided to the malformation may be facilitated by evaluation of CO_2 reactivity.[58] Relatively normal vasomotor reactivity in arteries ipsilateral to an AVM have been reported to indicate a high-pressure AVM with an increased risk of hemorrhage, whereas pathologic vasomotor reactivity in arteries both ipsilateral and con-

tralateral to an AVM indicates a low-pressure AVM with a greater prevalence of focal neurologic signs.[63] A linear relationship between mean velocity, diameter of the feeder, and volume of AVM has been reported,[96] and mean flow velocity, pulsatility index, vessel diameter, and flow volume have been found to be significantly different among AVM feeders, nonfeeders, and control arteries.[143] Assessment of hemodynamic changes occurring after surgical resection or embolization of AVMs can be performed with TCD.[93,176]

In a large prospective study of 114 consecutive AVM patients, the sensitivity of TCD for diagnosis of large and medium-sized AVMs was high (>80%), whereas 62% of small AVMs were missed.[150] The results demonstrated no relationship between flow velocity profiles and spontaneous hemorrhage. Moreover, the finding of a poor correlation between flow velocities and focal neurologic deficit unrelated to hemorrhage in this study calls into question the concept of hemodynamic steal in AVMs.

CAROTID SINUS FISTULAS

In patients with carotid-cavernous sinus fistulas both TCD and transcranial color Doppler flow imaging can detect abnormal flow patterns with high velocities and low frequency signals in the region of the shunt.[128,216] TCD is also a useful follow-up technique after therapy for carotid-cavernous sinus fistulas.[165]

DOLICHOECTATIC ARTERIES AND INTRACRANIAL VASCULOPATHIES

Noninvasive diagnosis of intracranial dolichoectatic arteries,[209] a cause of transient ischemic attacks or stroke,[184] can be achieved with TCD in combination with computed tomography or MRI (Fig. 14.11). The dramatic reduction in peak and mean flow velocities often observed in these patients suggests a thromboembolic mechanism of ischemia in slow flow territories. TCD is also sensitive and specific for the detection of arterial vasculopathy in sickle cell disease[8,9] and has been used for assessment of reversible multisegmental narrowing of cerebral arteries in postpartum cerebral angiopathy.[35]

CARBON DIOXIDE REACTIVITY

CO_2 reactivity has been proposed as a parameter for characterization of the hemodynamic reserve capacities within the circle of Willis in patients with significant extracranial arterial disease.[160,190,197,198,238] This test addresses vasomotor regulation by measuring the reactivity of the peripheral cerebral arterioles to changing PCO_2 levels. Hypercapnea, induced by administration of CO_2 in air, leads to vasodilatation and reduced vasomotor resistance in the peripheral arteriolar bed with subsequently increased blood flow velocities in the proximal large arteries of the affected vascular territories. Assuming that the diameter of the proximal large vessels remains relatively constant or is less affected than that of smaller arteries

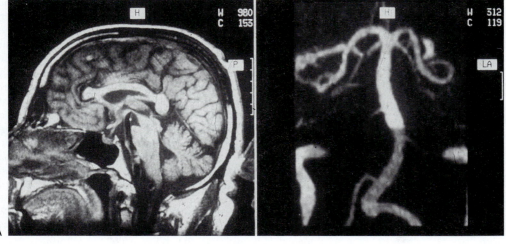

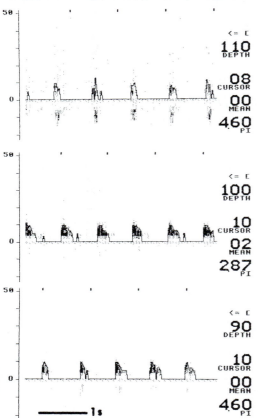

Figure 14.11 (**A**) Dolichoectasia of the basilar artery is well demonstrated by MRI in the sagittal plane. (**B**) Maximal intensity projection of Fig. A resulting in MR angiogram. (**C**) Transcranial Doppler shows reduced velocities in the basilar artery, consistent with dolichoectasia.

by changes in PCO_2, the relative changes in blood flow velocities measured by TCD may mirror cerebral tissue perfusion.[115] Major limitations of the CO_2 reactivity test derive from the adaptation of vessel caliber changes to alternating PCO_2 levels and from the large variability of compensatory networks and perfusion territories by overlapping microcirculatory systems.[74] Moreover, the efficacy of major collateral pathways outside the area of examination (e.g., leptomeningeal anastomosis) may be important. At present, the individual prognostic value of the CO_2 reactivity test for assessment of intracranial reserve capacity in patients with extracranial arterial disease remains unclear.

INTRACRANIAL PRESSURE

Simultaneous recordings of Doppler signals of the basal cerebral arteries, systemic blood pressure, and intracranial pressure (ICP) with epidural devices have shown that a progressive reduction in diastolic and systolic velocities can occur with increasing ICP. Moreover, various patterns of flow alterations have been demonstrated in different regions of the brain, indicating the existence of varying pressure gradients inside the skull.[97] When the ICP rises above that of the diastolic blood pressure, Doppler signals of the basal cerebral arteries are

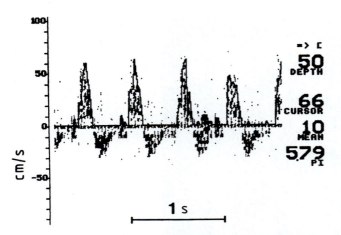

Figure 14.12 Alternating flow profile in the middle cerebral artery in a patient with brain death.

severely altered. Mild or moderate increases in ICP, however, can be compensated for by an increase in the systemic blood pressure, thus resulting in normal TCD findings. Despite these limitations, TCD may prove useful in evaluating strategies to improve cerebral autoregulation as well as in the optimal management of ICP control.[14]

BRAIN DEATH

TCD has been shown to be a reliable tool for confirmation of brain death,[33,99,168,181,248] with a sensitivity of 91.3% and a specificity of 100%.[177] TCD spectra recorded in brain-dead patients consist of short, sharp systolic peaks followed by retrograde flow during diastole, systolic peaks with absent flow in either direction,[248] or zero flow[98] (Fig. 14.12). It is essential that signals suggestive of brain death be detectable in more than one vessel. Zero flow may be misleading if sequential examinations are not available. Early changes in patients progressing to brain death include decreased flow velocity and increased pulse pressures. Later changes consist of a persistent increase in pulse pressure with the appearance of retrograde flow velocities during diastole. In the end stage, complete diastolic retrograde flow gives rise to a characteristic reverberating pattern. One study has emphasized the importance of determination of net flow velocity in conjunction with a reverberating waveform pattern; although an associated net flow velocity of <10 cm/s was found in all cases of brain death, functional recovery was documented in one patient with a net flow velocity of >20 cm/s.[181]

INTRAOPERATIVE MONITORING DURING CAROTID ENDARTERECTOMY

TCD has been used in carotid endarterectomy to monitor MCA velocity during ipsilateral ICA clamping.[99,124,152] Application of carotid clamps causes a significant fall in MCA veloc-

ity[124,167,208] with a linear relationship between MCA velocity and ICA stump pressure.[167,208] Results on the clinical utility of intraoperative TCD monitoring during carotid endarterectomy have been controversial. Proponents argue that continuous surveillance of cerebral hemodynamics with TCD allows immediate ensurance of postoperative ICA patency as well as identification of high-velocity states associated with hyperperfusion syndromes.[182] Moreover, it is argued that intraoperative TCD monitoring may be useful for identification of patients at risk of intracerebral hemorrhage.[121] In one large retrospective study, however, severe reduction in MCA velocity during carotid clamping was found in only 7.2% of patients.[91] Another investigation concluded that TCD was not useful for routine intraoperative monitoring during carotid endarterectomy, especially since monitoring results were normal in the only patient who sustained an operative stroke.[19] Since only a few patients present with postoperative neurologic deficits and since the ability of TCD monitoring of MCA velocity to predict an unfavorable outcome is unclear, TCD results should be interpreted with caution.[91,99,122,205,207,208] On a selective basis, TCD monitoring may be advantageous for decisions regarding shunting during carotid surgery.

HIGH-INTENSITY TRANSIENT SIGNALS

High-intensity transient signals (HITS) suggestive of microembolism (Plate 14.5) have been detected by TCD monitoring during interventions such as angiography,[148,188] carotid angioplasty,[146] open heart surgery,[43,192] and carotid endarterectomy.[76,120,174,217] TCD monitoring has also been used to detect spontaneous HITS in patients with transient ischemic attacks or stroke,[77,88,211,212] asymptomatic carotid stenosis,[147] heart valve prosthesis,[78,87] and intracranial arterial disease.[64] Results on the frequency of HITS suggestive of microemboli from the heart or from the proximal arteries of the intracranial circulation have been variable.[118,187] In patients with heart valve prosthesis, thousands of clinically silent events can be recorded, whereas in patients with symptomatic carotid stenoses, HITS are relatively rare events. It appears that emboli of cardiac and carotid origin may have different ultrasonic characteristics, which are likely to be based on composition and size.[89] The clinical relevance of these features, however, is unclear.

Significant work has been performed in attempts to differentiate between artifact and embolic material in HITS. In animal models this has been accomplished with high sensitivity and specificity.[144] Audio band-pass filters for isolation of frequencies associated with air emboli, implicated in the development of cognitive and neurologic deficits following bypass surgery, have also been implemented.[43] Recently, a multigate Doppler technique has been introduced to improve identification of artifacts (Plate 14.5). Further developments are likely to add better differentiation for different pathologic cerebral embolic materials.[145]

Some evidence shows that HITS detected during the dissection phase of carotid endarterectomy may correlate with clinically silent infarctions demonstrated with MRI.[120] Moreover, in a few cases a relationship between persistent particulate embolization in the immediate postoperative period and both incipient carotid artery thrombosis and the development of major neurologic deficits have been observed.[76] In carotid angioplasty, embolization at the time of intervention is very common but usually asymptomatic. Late embolization, occurring in a minority of patients, may account for the small but significant risk of delayed stroke.[146]

New studies indicate that TCD-detected microemboli in stroke patients may be associated with an increased prevalence of prior cerebrovascular ischemia,[234] thus suggesting a role of HITS as a risk factor for cerebrovascular ischemia. Prospective studies will be necessary to confirm these preliminary findings. In most cases in which HITS are detected, however, it is still unclear whether these phenomena are associated with an increased risk of functional or morphologic brain damage.[101]

Recently, it has been shown that HITS occur predominantly in patients with large vessel territory stroke patterns and persisting deficits, most likely due to artery-to-artery or cardiogenic embolism.[53] By contrast, patients with small vessel disease and rapid recovery only occasionally present with HITS. Thus, the detection of HITS may support the classification of the individual pathogenesis of cerebral ischemia, in particular when multiple risk constellations for stroke coexist.

DETECTION OF RIGHT-TO-LEFT SHUNTS

An increasingly recognized cause of embolic strokes and transient ischemic attacks in patients with stroke of uncertain etiology is paradoxical embolism. TCD monitoring of the basal intracranial vessels during intravenous injection of contrast media can be used for the detection of right-to-left shunts e.g., patent foramen ovale, by documentation of microbubbles reaching the brain.[48,62,119] TCD results correlate well with those of transesophageal echocardiography (sensitivity, 0.93; specificity, 1.0) when a standardized procedure including the Valsalva maneuver is used.[123]

ORTHOSTATIC DYSREGULATION

In patients with autonomic neuropathy, autonomic failure, or pandysautonomia, TCD monitoring is useful for detection of abnormal decreases in flow velocities within basal cerebral arteries during orthostatic stress[52,244] (Fig. 14.13). This technique also allows objective assessment of drug therapy in such patients. Routine measurements of intracranial flow velocities during orthostatic stress may be of value in patients with syncope and orthostatic dysregulation.[39,130]

FUNCTIONAL INVESTIGATIONS

Studies with TCD monitoring have shown that neuronal activation through mental activity or light exposure can be reflected by alterations in blood flow velocity[1,65] (Fig. 14.14). These findings indicate that TCD can detect changes in blood flow during activation of distinct brain areas. Recent studies

Figure 14.13 Topographic registrations of cerebral blood flow velocity, heart beat, and blood pressure during orthostasis. **(A)** Normal response of cerebral blood flow value to orthostasis. Normal intervals are shaded in gray. **(B)** Distal cerebral blood flow value in the middle cerebral artery without pathologic changes of blood pressure and heart rate in a patient with syncope. (From Hennerici et al,[108] with permission.)

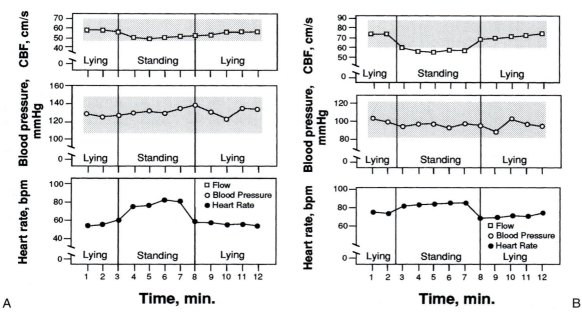

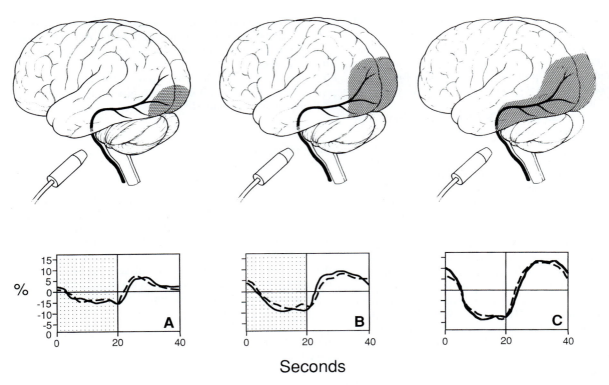

Figure 14.14 Functional analysis of vascular and metabolic coupling. Baseline signal velocity shown in the left sides of the graphs. **(A)** Increase in signal velocity caused by exposure to white light (right side of graph). **(B)** Changes in exposure to checkerboard pattern. **(C)** Changes in exposure to color film. The portions of brain regions activated by a given procedure are indicated by the hatched areas shown in each brain figure (top). (From Hennerici et al,[108] with permission.)

have shown that bilateral simultaneous MCA blood flow velocity monitoring and averaging during cognitive tasks may help to identify hemispheric dominance for cognitive tasks.[194] Moreover, TCD monitoring during nonverbal visuospatial tasks may be useful in neuropsychological research of functional specialization.[95] In patients with migraine with or without aura, blood flow alterations, induced by neuronal coupling with variable visual stimuli, have been found to be significantly higher than in controls. This finding suggests a further role of functional TCD monitoring as a diagnostic tool for assessment of migraine.

TRANSCRANIAL COLOR DOPPLER FLOW IMAGING

Transcranial color Doppler flow imaging (TCDFI) facilitates identification of basal cerebral arteries. While conventional TCD sonography assumes a 0-degree Doppler angle for the calculation of flow velocities, TCDFI allows determination of and correction for the Doppler insonation angle. The magnitude of the angle of insonation and the effect on flow velocity estimates in intracranial vessels have been determined through visually controlled measurements of the Doppler angle of insonation made by color flow imaging: angle-corrected peak systolic flow velocities were 3% to 30% higher compared with uncorrected velocity readings by conventional Doppler sonography.[16] Similar findings were reported in another study: in 14.5% the angle-corrected velocity was 25% to 50% higher and in 10.8% it was more than 50% higher compared with the uncorrected velocity.[66] Further studies are required to elucidate the clinical significance of these differences.

Color-coded representation of blood flow allows unequivocal identification of the circle of Willis within the anatomic B-mode image of the brain parenchyma.[34] Results on criteria and sensitivity of TCDFI for detection of intracranial aneurysms have recently been presented.[22] Aneurysms appear as a round or oval mass divided by a separation zone into red and blue areas and are characterized by lack of both turbulence and spontaneous fluctuations. Using these criteria, 85% of nonthrombosed aneurysms with a diameter of 6 to 25 mm were identified. Since small or thrombosed aneurysms may be missed, it is unlikely that TCDFI will have a role in the acute diagnosis of subarachnoid hemorrhage. These findings suggest, however, that transcranial color Doppler flow imaging may be suited for incidental detection of cerebral aneurysms.

For the morphologic evaluation of intracranial cerebrovascular disease, duplex imaging has been reported to contribute to the etiologic evaluation of MCA stenosis or occlusion. Hyperechogenic stenotic vascular segments may indicate an atherosclerotic vascular lesion with calcium deposits, and normal echogenicity may suggest the presence of a thrombotic or embolic lesion.[24] Further pathoanatomic studies will be necessary to confirm this contention.

Although TCDFI is considered by some as the ultrasonic method of choice in evaluation of the intracranial circulation, no data are available on the failure rate of TCDFI in a large group of patients. Thus the question of whether the diagnostic accuracy of TCDFI for detection of occlusive intracranial arterial disease is superior to that of conventional TCD remains unanswered.

TRANSCRANIAL POWER DOPPLER IMAGING

Recent reports on the diagnostic edge of power Doppler imaging over color Doppler flow imaging in the assessment of carotid stenosis suggest that PDI may be a promising technique for transcranial applications[86,225] (Plate 14.6). Our own first comparisons of transcranial PDI with MR4 have shown good correlation for display of the anterior and posterior communicating arteries. This feature may be useful in a variety of clinical conditions. For example, detection of collateral supply to both posterior arteries via the posterior communicating arteries without evidence of flow from the basilar artery provides additional support for a diagnosis of acute basilar artery thrombosis in the appropriate clinical setting. PDI may also be useful for identification of low flow after intracranial stenoses and occlusions, particularly in patients with suboptimal bone windows.[23]

New Developments in Cerebrovascular Ultrasound

ECHO-ENHANCING AGENTS

The ability of intravenous contrast media to increase the echogenicity of flowing blood has been known for some time.[172] Only recently, however, has there been an increasing demand for use of echo-enhancing agents in assessment of cerebrovascular disease (e.g., transcranial ultrasound studies in patients with severe hyperostosis of the skull, quantification of internal carotid stenosis, and diagnosis of internal carotid occlusion versus pseudo-occlusion).[214] Currently known industrial ultrasound contrast enhancers fall into three physical categories: suspensions of free gas bubbles in a pure liquid vehicle, gas-filled microspheres, and microparticle suspensions. The latter of these categories has received particular attention in the past several years and involves the use of water-soluble microparticles as origin and carrier of air microbubbles with transpulmonary stability (<5 μm diameter) and the ability to reflect transmitted ultrasound at discrete harmonic frequencies.[193] Such features are useful for investigation of slow flow in large vessels and of microvessel flow characteristics where low signal amplitudes are normally obscured by high-intensity border zone reflections (e.g., pseudo-occlusion

of large vessels, abnormal small vessels), in poorly visualized regions (e.g., transcranial vasculature), and in unresolved examinations.[206] Recently, a phase II clinical trial reported an increase in the diagnostic utility of transcranial ultrasound in 77% of the patients studied.[173] Moreover, evidence shows that contrast-enhanced TCDFI may be useful for evaluation of AVMs, aneurysms, and cerebral venous thrombosis.[21] More interesting are further studies on the possible application of contrast agents for differentiation of ischemic versus normal brain tissue and in measurement of cerebral venous flow. Other opportunities, such as using the contrast agent as an indicator for bolus dilution estimates of flow and transit time, remain to be exploited.

HARMONIC IMAGING

Harmonic imaging is a new technique that utilizes resonating gas bubbles that emanate harmonics at exactly twice the frequency of fundamental echoes.[44] By transmitting echoes at one frequency (4 MHz) and receiving at double the frequency (8 MHz), it is possible to generate sonoangiograms. This is because the higher frequency echoes are emitted only from contrast agent bubbles and not from surrounding tissue. Harmonic imaging may allow considerable reduction of color Doppler filter settings for exclusion of shifts from moving tissues, thus improving clutter rejection and allowing Doppler detection of smaller vessels than previously possible. Clinical studies using this method have yet to be performed.

THREE-DIMENSIONAL POWER DOPPLER ANGIOGRAPHY

The superior ability of power Doppler imaging to delineate blood vessels has recently been exploited for 3D applications. For the carotid system, 3D image acquisition can be achieved by mounting a linear transducer onto a computerized motor, which delivers equidistant, electrocardiogram-gated ultrasound slices. Rendering of the 3D volume data sets with maximum intensity projections results in high-quality power Doppler angiograms. A similar method can be implemented to obtain transcranial power Doppler angiograms. By attaching a sector transducer to a computerized fan motor, which tilts the transducer at specified angle increments, a series of images can be acquired that are consequently reconstructed into a 3D volume data set (Fig. 14.15). New technology for image acquisition utilizes 6 degrees of freedom electromagnetic tracking devices to allow free-hand scanning.[61,75,171] Although potentially more robust than motorized systems, further work will be necessary to complement this method with intelligent image acquistion techniques that guarantee adequate scanning for 3D reconstructions. Rapid progress in this field suggests that 3D power Doppler angiography may evolve as a leading diagnostic innovation in cerebrovascular imaging.

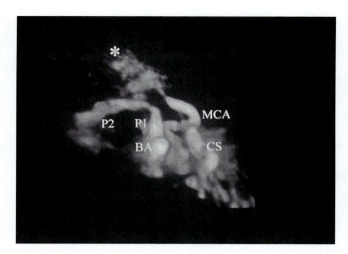

Figure 14.15 Three-dimensional transcranial power Doppler angiography. Ray tracing of 80 transverse sector scans achieved with electrocardiographic-gated fan motor positioned at the transtemporal window (°). Angle displacement was 0.5 degree. The 3D view is from caudal, looking up into the transcranial arteries. CS, carotid siphon; MCA middle cerebral artery; and P1, P2, and BA, segments of the posterior cerebral artery and basilar artery.

FOUR-DIMENSIONAL CEREBROVASCULAR ULTRASOUND

Through application of computer vision and optical flow techniques, ultrasound may be useful for assessment of temporal, four-dimensional (4D) qualitites of pulsatile flow dynamics, plaque geometry, and vessel wall segments.[155] First investigations with noninvasive 4D ultrasound of atherosclerotic plaque motion in the ICA using a hierarchic motion estimator have shown relatively uniform plaque displacement in asymptomatic patients as opposed to complex motion and focal movement disparities in symptomatic plaques (Plate 14.7), thus suggesting a role for motion analysis of atherosclerotic plaques in identification of patients at risk of carotid embolism.[153] Four-dimensional ultrasound may also be useful for investigation of focal alterations in wall motion, possibly reflecting local, endothelial dysfunction at early stages of atherosclerosis.[103] Recently, the feasibility of incorporating 4D ultrasound data into models for computer simulation of complex pathophysiologic interactions among pulsatile flow, plaque and vessel geometry, and wall elasticity has been demonstrated.[154]

Summary

Cerebrovascular ultrasonography has experienced an almost exponential growth over the past 25 years. Today routine ultrasound techniques are available for noninvasive examination of the extracranial arteries for detection and quantification of stenosis, characterization of atherosclerotic plaques, diagnosis and follow-up of dissections, and assessment of relatively rare cerebrovascular disorders such as fibromuscular dysplasia, Takayasu's disease[36] and carotid body tumors.[221] Although ultrasound investigations were previously regarded as screening tools, color flow and power Doppler imaging have claimed their new position as gold standards for quantification of carotid artery stenosis, thus making arteriography an almost obsolete technique for evaluation of this condition.

TCD has assumed a firm role in the detection of intracranial stenosis and has become a valuable tool for evaluation of intracranial collateral circulations, vasculopathies, and progressive obstruction of the cerebral circulation in brain death. TCD monitoring, through its ability to diagnose right-to-left shunts in suspected paradoxical embolism, its capacity to detect HITS as additional evidence for embolism as the pathophysiologic mechanism of stroke, and its ability to offer insights into orthostatic dysregulation and neuronal coupling, has become standard practice in many institutions. The introduction of color Doppler flow imaging in transcranial applications has led to greater confidence in vessel identification and has added new dimensions to assessment of AVMs.

Promising new techniques such as power Doppler imaging and harmonic imaging are being added to the arsenal of cerebrovascular ultrasound. Three-dimensional ultrasound imaging is rapidly evolving, with new applications for plaque reconstruction, plaque volume quantification, and 3D Doppler angiography. Four-dimensional ultrasound, a new tool for elucidation of cerebrovascular pathophysiology, may be useful for assessment of plaque motion patterns associated with symptomatic carotid artery disease, for evaluation of focal wall motion alterations in early stages of atherosclerosis, and as a clinical framework for computer simulation studies.

References

1. Aaslid R: Visually evoked dynamic blood flow response of the human cerebral circulation. Stroke 17:771, 1987
2. Aaslid R, Huber P, Nornes H: Evaluation of cerebrovascular spasm with transcranial Doppler ultrasound. J Neurosurg 60:37, 1984
3. Aaslid R, Markwalder TM, Nornes H: Noninvasive transcranial Doppler ultrasound recording of flow velocity in basal arteries. J Neurosurg 57:769, 1982
4. Ackermann H, Diener HC, Seboldt H, Huth C: Ultrasonographic follow-up of subclavian stenosis and occlusion: natural history and surgical treatment. Stroke 19:431, 1988
5. Ackerstaff RG, Hoeneveld H, Slowikowski JM et al: Ultrasonic duplex scanning in atherosclerotic disease of the innominate, subclavian and vertebral arteries. A comparative study with angiography. Ultrasound Med Biol 10:409, 1984
6. Ackerstaff RG, Keunen RW, van Pelt W et al: Influence of biological factors on changes in mean cerebral blood flow velocity in normal aging: a transcranial Doppler study. Neurol Res 12:187, 1990
7. Adams HP, Byington R, Hoen H et al: Effect of cholesterol-lowering medications on progression of mild ath-

erosclerotic lesions of the carotid arteries and on the risk of stroke. Cerebrovasc Dis 5:171, 1995

8. Adams RJ, Nichols FT III, Aaslid R et al: Cerebral vessel stenosis in sickle cell disease: criteria for detection by transcranial Doppler. Am J Pediatr Hematol Oncol 12:277, 1990

9. Adams RJ, Nichols FT, Figueroa R et al: Transcranial Doppler correlation with cerebral angiography in sickle cell disease. Stroke 23:1073, 1992

10. Aldoori MI, Baird R: Duplex scanning and plaque histology in cerebral ischaemia. Eur J Vasc Surg 1:159, 1987

11. Alexandrov AV, Bladin CF, Magissano R, Norris JW: Measuring carotid stenosis. Stroke 24:1292, 1993

12. Anzola GP, Gasparotti R, Magoni M, Prandini F: Transcranial Doppler sonography and magnetic resonance angiography in the assessment of collateral hemispheric flow in patients with carotid artery disease. Stroke 26:214, 1995

13. Arnolds BJ, von Reutern GM: Transcranial Doppler sonography. Examination technique and normal reference values. Ultraschall Med 12:115, 1987

14. Babikian V, Wechsler L: Recent developments in transcranial Doppler sonography. J Neuroimaging 4:159, 1994

15. Bartels E: [Color coded Doppler sonography of the vertebral arteries. Comparison with conventional duplex sonography] Farbkodierte Dopplersonographie der Vertebralarterien. Vergleich mit der konventionellen Duplexsonographie. Ultraschall Med 13:59, 1992

16. Bartels E, Flugel KA: Quantitative measurements of blood flow velocity in basal cerebral arteries with transcranial duplex color-flow imaging. A comparative study with conventional transcranial Doppler sonography. J Neuroimaging 4:77, 1994

17. Bartels E, Flügel KA: Evaluation of extracranial vertebral artery dissection with duplex color-flow imaging. Stroke 27:290, 1996

18. Bartels E, Fuchs HH, Flugel KA: Duplex ultrasonography of vertebral arteries: examination, technique, normal values, and clinical applications. Angiology 43:169, 1992

19. Bass A, Krupski WC, Schneider PA et al: Intraoperative transcranial Doppler: limitations of the method. J Vasc Surg 10:549, 1989

20. Bassiouny HS, Davis H, Massawa N et al: Critical carotid stenoses: morphologic and chemical similarity between symptomatic and asymptomatic plaques. J Vasc Surg 9:202, 1989

21. Bauer A, Becker G, Krone A et al: Transcranial duplex sonography using ultrasound contrast enhancers. Clin Radiol 51:19, 1996

22. Baumgartner RW, Mattle HP, Kothbauer K, Schroth G: Transcranial color-coded duplex sonography in cerebral aneurysms. Stroke 25:2429, 1994

23. Baumgartner RW, Schmid C, Baumgartner I: Comparative study of power-based versus mean frequency-based transcranial color-coded duplex sonography in normal adults. Stroke 27:101, 1996

24. Becker G, Lindner A, Hofmann E, Bogdahn U: Contribution of transcranial color-coded real-time sonography to the etiopathogenetic classification of middle cerebral artery stenosis. J Clin Ultrasound 22:471, 1994

25. Becker GM, Winkler J, Hoffmann E, Bogdahn U: Imaging of cerebral arterio-venous malformations by transcranial colour-coded real-time sonography. Neuroradiology 32:280, 1990

26. Belkin M, Mackey WC, Pessin MS et al: Common carotid artery occlusion with patent internal and external carotid arteries: diagnosis and surgical management. J Vasc Surg 17:1019, 1993

27. Bendick PJ, Glover JL: Hemodynamic evaluation of vertebral arteries by duplex ultrasound. Surg Clin North Am 70:235, 1990

28. Bendick PJ, Glover JL, Hankin R et al: Carotid plaque morphology: correlation of duplex sonography with histology. Ann Vasc Surg 2:6, 1988

29. Bendick PJ, Jackson VP: Evaluation of the vertebral arteries with duplex sonography. J Vasc Surg 3:523, 1986

30. Bluth EI, Kay D, Merritt CRB et al: Sonographic characterization of carotid plaque: detection of hemorrhage. AJR 11061, 1986

31. Bluth EI, McVay LV III, Merritt CR, Sullivan MA: The identification of ulcerative plaque with high resolution duplex carotid scanning. J Ultrasound Med 7:73, 1988

32. Bock RW, Lusby RJ: Carotid plaque morphology and interpretation of the echolucent lesion. p. 225. In Labs KH, Jäger KA, Fitzgerald DE et al (eds): Diagnostic Vascular Imaging. Arnold, London, 1992

33. Bode H, Sauer M, Pringsheim W: Diagnosis of brain death by transcranial Doppler sonography. Arch Dis Child 63:1474, 1988

34. Bogdahn U, Becker G, Winkler J et al: Transcranial color-coded real-time sonography in adults. Stroke 21:1680, 1990

35. Bogousslavsky J, Despland PA, Regli F, Dubuis PY: Postpartum cerebral angiopathy: reversible vasoconstriction assessed by transcranial Doppler ultrasound. Eur Neurol 29:102, 1989

36. Bond JR, Charboneau JW, Stanson AW: Takayasu's arteritis. Carotid duplex sonographic appearance, including color Doppler imaging. J Ultrasound Med 9:625, 1990

37. Brass LM, Pavlakis SG, DeVivo D et al: Transcranial Doppler measurements of the middle cerebral artery. Effect of hematocrit. Stroke 19:1466, 1988

38. Brautaset NJ: Provokable bilateral vertebral artery compression diagnosed with transcranial Doppler. Stroke 23:288, 1992

39. Briebach T, Fischer PA: [Circulation studies and transcranial Doppler sonography in orthostatic regulation disorders] Kreislaufphysiologische Untersuchungen und transkranielle Dopplersonographie bei orthostatischen Regulationsstorungen. Ultraschall Med 9:223, 1988

40. Büdingen HJ, Staudacher T: Die Identifizierung der Arteria basilaris mit der transkraniellen Dopplersonographie. Ultraschall 8:95, 1987

41. Büdingen HJ, von Reutern GM: Ultraschalldiagnostik der hirnversorgenden Arterien. Thieme, Stuttgart, 1994

42. Bui LN, Brant-Zawadzki M, Verghese P, Gillan G: Magnetic resonance angiography of cervicocranial dissection. Stroke 24:126, 1993

43. Bunegin L, Wahl D, Albin MS: Detection and volume estimation of embolic air in the middle cerebral artery

using transcranial Doppler sonography. Stroke 25:593, 1994

44. Burns PN: Harmonic imaging with ultrasound contrast agents. Clin Radiol 51:50, 1996

45. Caplan LR, Zarins CK, Hemmatti M: Spontaneous dissection of the extrancranial vertebral arteries. Stroke 16:1030, 1985

46. Chan KH, Dearden NM, Miller JD: Transcranial Doppler sonography in severe head injury. Acta Neurochir [Suppl] (Wien) 59:81, 1993

47. Cher LM, Chambers BR, Smidt V: Comparison of transcranial Doppler with DSA in vertebrobasilar ischaemia. Clin Exp Neurol 29:143, 1992

48. Chimowitz MI, Nemec JJ, Marwick TH et al: Transcranial Doppler ultrasound identifies patients with right-to-left cardiac or pulmonary shunts. Neurology 41:1902, 1991

49. Comerota AJ, Cranley A, Cook S: Real-time B-mode imaging in diagnosis of cerebrovascular disease. Surgery 718, 1981

50. Comerota AJ, Katz ML, White JV, Grosh JD: The preoperative diagnosis of the ulcerated carotid atheroma. J Vasc Surg 11:505, 1990

51. Craven TE, Ryu JE, Espeland MA et al: Evaluation of the associations between carotid artery atherosclerosis and coronary artery stenosis. A case-control study. Circulation 82:1230, 1990

52. Daffertshofer M, Diehl RR, Ziems GU, Hennerici M: Orthostatic changes of cerebral blood flow velocity in patients with autonomic dysfunction. J Neurol Sci 104:32, 1991

53. Daffertshofer M, Ries S, Schminke U, Hennerici M: High intensity transient signals in patients with cerebral ischemia. Stroke 27:1844, 1996

54. Dashefsky SM, Cooperberg PL, Harrison PB et al: Total occlusion of the common carotid artery with patient internal carotid artery. Identification with color flow Doppler imaging. J Ultrasound Med 10:417, 1991

55. Davis PC, Nilsen B, Braun IF, Hoffmann JCJ: A prospective comparison of duplex sonography vs angiography of the vertebral arteries. AJNR 7:1059, 1986

56. De Bray JM, Glatt B: Quantification of atheromatous stenosis in the extracranial internal carotid artery. Cerebrovasc Dis 5:414, 1995

57. De Bray JM, Missoum A, Dubas F et al: [Doppler transcranial ultrasonography in carotid and vertebral dissections: 36 cases involving angiography] Le Doppler transcranien dans les dissections carotidiennes et vertébrales: étude de 36 cas arteriographies. J Mal Vasc 19:35, 1994

58. De Salles AA, Manchola I: CO_2 reactivity in arteriovenous malformations of the brain: a transcranial Doppler ultrasound study. J Neurosurg 80:624, 1994

59. Delcker A, Diener HC: Die verschiedenen Ultraschallmethoden zur Untersuchung der Arteria vertebralis—eine vergleichende Wertung. Ultraschall Med 13:213, 1992

60. Delcker A, Diener HC: Quantification of atherosclerotic plaques in carotid arteries by three-dimensional ultrasound. Br J Radiol 67:672, 1994

61. Detmer PR, Baschein G, Hodges TC et al: 3D ultrasonic image feature localization based on magnetic scanhead tracking: in vitro calibration and validation. Ultrasound Med Biol 20:923, 1994

62. Di Tullio M, Sacco RL, Venketasubramanian N et al: Comparison of diagnostic techniques for the detection of a patent foramen ovale in stroke patients. Stroke 1020, 1993

63. Diehl RR, Henkes H, Nahser HC et al: Blood flow velocity and vasomotor reactivity in patients with arteriovenous malformations. A transcranial Doppler study. Stroke 25:1574, 1994

64. Diehl RR, Sliwka U, Rautenberg W, Schwartz A: Evidence for embolization from a posterior cerebral artery thrombus by transcranial Doppler monitoring. Stroke 24:606, 1993

65. Droste DW, Harders AG, Rastogi E: A transcranial Doppler study of blood flow velocity in the middle cerebral arteries performed at rest and during mental activities. Stroke 20:1005, 1989

66. Eicke BM, Tegeler CH, Dalley G, Myers LG: Angle correction in transcranial Doppler sonography. J Neuroimaging 4:29, 1994

67. Eicke BM, von Lorentz J, Paulus W: Embolus detection in different degrees of carotid disease. Neurol Res 17:181, 1995

68. Eliasziw M, Strifler JY, Fox AJ et al: Significance of plaque ulceration in symptomatic patients with high-grade carotid stenosis. Stroke 25:304, 1994

69. Erickson SJ, Mewissen MW, Foley WD et al: Stenosis of the internal carotid artery: assessment using color Doppler imaging compared with angiography. AJR 152:1299, 1989

70. Espeland MA, Hoen H, Byington R et al: Spatial distribution of carotid intimal-medial thickness as measured by B-mode ultrasonography. Stroke 25:1812, 1994

71. European Carotid Surgery Trialists' Collaborative Group: MRC European Surgery Trial: interim results for symptomatic patients with severe (70–99%) or mild (0–29%) carotid stenosis. Lancet 19:45, 1991

72. Fisher CM, Gore I, Okabe N, White PD: Atherosclerosis of the carotid and vertebral arteries—extracranial and intracranial. Neuropathol Exp Neurol 455, 1965

73. Fisher M, Blumenfeld AM, Smith TW: The importance of carotid artery plaque disruption and hemorrhage. Arch Neurol 44:1086, 1987

74. Fujii K, Heistad D, Faraci FM: Flow medicated dilation of the basilar artery in vivo. Circ Res 697, 1991

75. Ganapathy U, Kaufman A: 3D acquisition and visualization of ultrasound data. p. 535. In: Proc SPIE Visualization in Biomedical Computing, 1992

76. Gaunt ME, Martin PJ, Smith JL et al: Clinical relevance of intraoperative embolization detected by transcranial Doppler ultrasonography during carotid endarterectomy: a prospective study of 100 patients. Br J Surg 81:1435, 1994

77. Georgiadis D, Grosset DG, Quin RO et al: Detection of intracranial emboli in patients with carotid disease. Eur J Vasc Surg 8:309, 1994

78. Georgiadis D, Mallinson A, Grosset DG, Lees KR: Coagulation activity and emboli counts in patients with prosthetic cardiac valves. Stroke 25:1211, 1994

79. Geroulaks G, O'Gorman D, Nicolaides A et al: Carotid

intima-media thickness. Correlation with the British Regional Heart Study risk score. J Intern Med 235:431, 1994

80. Giller CA, Mathews D, Walker B et al: Prediction of tolerance to carotid artery occlusion using transcranial Doppler ultrasound. J Neurosurg 81:15, 1994

81. Glagov S, Bassiouny HS, Giddens DP, Zarins CK: Intimal thickening: morphogenesis, functional significance and detection. J Vasc Invest 1:1, 1995

82. Goes E, Janssens W, Maillet B et al: Tissue characterization of atheromatous plaques: correlation between ultrasound image and histological findings. J Clin Ultrasound 18:611, 1990

83. Gomez CR, Brass LM, Tegeler CH et al: The transcranial Doppler standardization project. J Neuroimaging 3: 190, 1993

84. Gray Weale AC, Graham JC, Burnett JR et al: Carotid artery atheroma: comparison of preoperative B-mode ultrasound appearance with carotid endarterectomy specimen pathology. J Cardiovasc Surg Torino 29:676, 1988

85. Greselle JF, Zenteno M, Kien P et al: Spontaneous dissection of the vertebro-basilar system. A study of 18 cases (15 patients). J Neuroradiol 14:115, 1987

86. Griewing B, Morgenstern C, Driesner F et al: Cerebrovascular disease assessed by color-flow and power Doppler ultrasonography: comparison with digital subtraction angiography in internal carotid artery stenosis. Stroke 27:95, 1996

87. Grosset DG, Cowburn P, Georgiadis D et al: Ultrasound detection of cerebral emboli in patients with prosthetic heart valves. J Heart Valve Dis 3:128, 1994

88. Grosset DG, Georgiadis D, Abdullah I et al: Doppler emboli signals vary according to stroke subtype. Stroke 25:382, 1994

89. Grosset DG, Georgiadis D, Kelman AW, Lees KR: Quantification of ultrasound emboli signals in patients with cardiac and carotid disease. Stroke 24:1922, 1993

90. Hallam MJ, Reid JM, Cooperberg PL: Color-flow Doppler and conventional duplex scanning of the carotid bifurcation: prospective, double-blind, correlative study. AJR 152:1101, 1989

91. Halsey JH: Risks and benefits of shunting in carotid endarterectomy. Stroke 23:1583, 1993

92. Harders A: Neurosurgical Applications of Transcranial Doppler Sonography. Springer, New York, 1986

93. Harders A, Bien S, Eggert HR et al: Haemodynamic changes in arteriovenous malformations induced by superselective embolization: transcranial Doppler evaluation. Neurol Res 10:239, 1988

94. Hart RG: Vertebral artery dissection. Neurology 38:987, 1988

95. Hartje W, Ringelstein EB, Kistinger B et al: Transcranial Doppler ultrasonic assessment of middle cerebral artery blood flow velocity changes during verbal and visuospatial cognitive tasks. Neuropsychologia 32:1443, 1994

96. Hassler W: Hemodynamic Aspects of Cerebral Angiomas. Springer, New York, 1986

97. Hassler W, Steinmetz H, Gawlowski J: Transcranial Doppler ultrasonography in raised intracranial pressure and in intracranial circulatory arrest. J Neurosurg 68: 745, 1988

98. Hassler W, Steinmetz H, Pirschel J: Transcranial Doppler study of intracranial circulatory arrest. J Neurosurg 71:195, 1989

99. Hennerici M: Can carotid endarterectomy be improved by neurovascular monitoring? Stroke 24:637, 1993

100. Hennerici M: High intensity transcranial signals (HITS): a questionable "jackpot" for the prediction of stroke risk. J Heart Valve Dis 3:124, 1994

101. Hennerici M, Freund HJ: Efficacy of CW-Doppler and duplex-system examinations for the evaluation of extracranial carotid disease. J Clin Ultrasound 12:155, 1984

102. Hennerici M, Klemm C, Rautenberg W: The subclavian steal phenomenon: a common vascular disorder with rare neurologic deficits. Neurology 38:669, 1988

103. Hennerici M, Meairs S, Daffertshofer M et al: Investigation of wall motion, local hemodynamics and atherosclerotic plaque geometry in carotid arteries using 4-D ultrasound and high resolution magnetic resonance angiography. p. 123. In Moskowitz M, Caplan L (eds): Cerebrovascular Diseases. Butterworth-Heinemann. Boston, 1995

104. Hennerici M, Mohr JP, Rautenberg W, Steinke W: Ultrasound imaging and Doppler sonography in the diagnosis of cerebrovascular diseases. p. 241. In Barnett HJM, Mohr JP, Stein BM, Yatsu F (eds): Stroke: Pathophysiology, Diagnosis, and Management 2nd Ed. Churchill Livingstone, New York, 1992

105. Hennerici M, Neuerburg-Heusler D: Gefässdiagnostik mit Ultraschall. Thieme, Stuttgart, 1994

106. Hennerici M, Rautenberg W, Schwartz A: Transcranial Doppler ultrasound for the assessment of intracranial arterial flow velocity—Part 2. Evaluation of intracranial arterial disease. Surg Neurol 27:523, 1987

107. Hennerici M, Rautenberg W, Sitzer G, Schwartz A: Transcranial Doppler ultrasound for the assessment of intracranial arterial flow velocity—Part 1. Examination technique and normal values. Surg Neurol 27:439, 1987

108. Hennerici M, Rautenberg W, Steinke W: Ultrasonography. p. 185. In Mohr JP, Gautier J-C (eds): Guide to Clinical Neurology. Churchill Livingstone.

109. Hennerici M, Reifschneider G, Trockel U, Aulich A: Detection of early atherosclerotic lesions by duplex scanning of the carotid artery. J Clin Ultrasound 12:455, 1984

110. Hennerici M, Steinke W: Carotid plaque developments: aspects of hemodynamic and vessel wall-platelet interaction. Cerebrovasc Dis 1:142, 1991

111. Hennerici M, Steinke W, Rautenberg W: High-resistance Doppler flow pattern in extracranial carotid dissection. Arch Neurol 46:670, 1989

112. Hodges TC, Detmer PR, Dawson DL et al: Ultrasound determination of total arterial wall thickness. J Vasc Surg 19:745, 1994

113. Hoffmann M, Sacco RL, Chan S, Mohr JP: Noninvasive detection of vertebral artery dissection. Stroke 24:815, 1993

114. Howard G, Burke GL, Evans GW et al: Relations of intimal-medial thickness among sites within the carotid artery as evaluated by B-mode ultrasound. ARIC Investigators. Atherosclerosis Risk in Communities. Stroke 25: 1581, 1994

115. Huber P, Handa J: Effect of contrast material, hypercap-

nea, hyperventilation, hypotonic glucose and papaverine on the diameter of cerebral arteries. Invest Radiol 2:17, 1967

116. Imparato AM, Riles TS, Gostein F: The carotid bifurcation plaque: pathologic findings associated with cerebral ischemia. Stroke 10:238, 1979

117. Imparato AM, Riles TS, Mintzer R, Baumann FG: The importance of hemorrhage in the relationship between gross morphologic characteristics and cerebral symptoms in 376 carotid artery plaques. Ann Surg 197:195, 1983

118. International Workshop on Cerebral Embolism. Cerebrovasc Dis 5:67, 1995

119. Itoh T, Matsumoto M, Handa N et al: Paradoxical embolism as a cause of ischemic stroke of uncertain etiology. A transcranial Doppler sonographic study. Stroke 25:771, 1994

120. Jansen C, Ramos LM, van Heesewijk JP et al: Impact of microembolism and hemodynamic changes in the brain during carotid endarterectomy. Stroke 25:992, 1994

121. Jansen C, Sprengers AM, Moll FL et al: Prediction of intracerebral haemorrhage after carotid endarterectomy by clinical criteria and intraoperative transcranial Doppler monitoring: results of 233 operations. Eur J Vasc Surg 8:220, 1994

122. Jansen C, Vriens EM, Eikelboom BC et al: Carotid endarterectomy with transcranial Doppler and electroencephalographic monitoring: a prospective study in 130 operations. Stroke 24:665, 1993

123. Jauss M, Kaps M, Keberle M et al: A comparison of transesophageal echocardiography and transcranial Doppler sonography with contrast medium for detection of patent foramen ovale. Stroke 25:1265, 1994

124. Jorgensen LG, Schroeder TV: Transcranial Doppler for detection of cerebral ischaemia during carotid endarterectomy. Eur J Vasc Surg 6:142, 1992

125. Josien E: Extracranial vertebral artery dissection: nine cases. J Neurol 239:327, 1992

126. Kerber CW, Heilman CB: Flow dynamics in the human carotid artery: I. Preliminary observations using a transparent elastic model. AJNR 13:173, 1992

127. Khaffaf N, Karnik R, Winkler WB et al: Embolic stroke by compression maneuver during transcranial Doppler sonography. Stroke 25:1056, 1994

128. Kotval PS, Weitzner I Jr, Tenner MS: Diagnosis of carotid-cavernous fistula by periorbital color Doppler imaging and pulsed Doppler volume flow analysis. J Ultrasound Med 9:101, 1990

129. Ku DN, Giddens DP, Phillips DJ, Strandness DEJ: Hemodynamics of the normal carotid bifurcation: in vitro and in vivo studies. Ultrasound Med Biol 11:13, 1985

130. Lagi A, Bacalli S, Cencetti S et al: Cerebral autoregulation in orthostatic hypotension. A transcranial Doppler study. Stroke 25:1771, 1994

131. Langsfeld M, Gray Weale AC, Lusby RJ: The role of plaque morphology and diameter reduction in the development of new symptoms in asymptomatic carotid arteries. J Vasc Surg 9:548, 1989

132. Laumer R, Steinmeier R, Gönner R et al: Cerebral hemodynamics in subarachnoid hemorrhage evaluated by transcranial Doppler sonography. Neurosurgery 31:1, 1993

133. Leen EJ, Feeley TM, Colgan MP et al: "Haemorrhagic" carotid plaque does not contain haemorrhage. Eur J Vasc Surg 4:123, 1990

134. Lennihan L, Kupsky WJ, Mohr JP et al: Lack of association between carotid plaque hematoma and ischemic cerebral symptoms. Stroke 18:879, 1987

135. Lennihan L, Petty GW, Fink E et al: Transcranial Doppler detection of anterior cerebral vasospasm. J Neurol Neurosurg Psychiatry 56:906, 1993

136. Levine SR, Welch KM: Common carotid artery occlusion. Neurology 39:178, 1989

137. Lindegaard KF, Bakke SJ, Aaslid R, Nornes H: Doppler diagnosis of intracranial arterial occlusive disorders. J Neurol Neurosurg Psychiatry 49:510, 1986

138. Lindegaard KF, Bakke SJ, Grolimund P et al: Assessment of intracranial hemodynamics in carotid artery disease by transcranial Doppler ultrasound. J Neurosurg 63:890, 1985

139. LoGerfo FW, Mason GR: Directional Doppler studies of supraorbital artery flow in internal carotid stenosis and occlusion. Surgery 76:723, 1974

140. LoGerfo FW, Nowak MD, Quist WC: Structural details of boundary layer separation in an model human carotid bifurcation under steady and pulsatile flow conditions. J Vasc Surg 2:263, 1985

141. Lusby RJ, Ferrell LD, Ehrenfeld WK et al: Carotid plaque hemorrhage. Its role in production of cerebral ischemia. Arch Surg 117:1479, 1982

142. Mack WJ, Selzer RH, Hodis HN et al: One-year reduction and longitudinal analysis of carotid intima-media thickness associated with colestipol/niacin therapy. Stroke 24:1779, 1993

143. Manchola IF, De Salles AA, Foo TK et al: Arteriovenous malformation hemodynamics: a transcranial Doppler study. Neurosurgery 33:556, 1993

144. Markus H, Loh A, Brown MM: Computerized detection of cerebral emboli and discrimination from artifact using Doppler ultrasound. Stroke 24:1667, 1993

145. Markus HS, Brown MM: Differentiation between different pathological cerebral embolic materials using transcranial Doppler in an in vitro model. Stroke 24:1, 1993

146. Markus HS, Clifton A, Buckenham T, Brown MM: Carotid angioplasty. Detection of embolic signals during and after the procedure. Stroke 25:2403, 1994

147. Markus HS, Droste DW, Brown MM: Detection of asymptomatic cerebral embolic signals with Doppler ultrasound. Lancet 343:1011, 1994

148. Markus HS, Loh A, Isrrael D et al: Microscopic air embolism during cerebral angiography and strategies for avoidance. Lancet 341:784, 1993

149. Maroon JC, Pieroni DW, Campbell RL: Ophthalmosonometry: an ultrasonic method for assessing carotid blood flow. J Neurosurg 30:238, 1969

150. Mast H, Mohr JP, Thompson JL et al: Transcranial Doppler ultrasonography in cerebral arteriovenous malformations. Diagnostic sensitivity and association of flow velocity with spontaneous hemorrhage and focal neurological deficit. Stroke 26:1024, 1995

151. Mattle H, Grolimund P, Huber P et al: Transcranial

Doppler sonographic findings in middle cerebral artery disease. Arch Neurol 45:289, 1988

152. McDowell HA, Jr Gross GM, Halsey JH: Carotid endarterectomy monitored with transcranial Doppler. Ann Surg 215:514, 1992

153. Meairs S, Daffertshofer M, Steinke W, Hennerici M: Altered carotid plaque motion as an indicator of embolic potential. Cerebrovasc Dis 5:227, 1995

154. Meairs S, Hennerici M: Evaluation of wall and atherosclerotic plaque motion in carotid arteries using 4D ultrasound. p. 357. In Liepsch D (ed): Biofluid Mechanics. VDI-Verlag, Düsseldorf, 1994

155. Meairs S, Röther J, Neff W, Hennerici M: New and future developments in cerebrovascular ultrasound, magnetic resonance angiography and related techniques. J Clin Ultrasound 23:139, 1995

156. Melis-Kisman E, Mol JMF: L'application de l'effect Doppler à l'exploration cérébrovasculaire—rapport préliminaire. Rev Neurol (Paris) 122:470, 1970

157. Merritt CR: Doppler color flow imaging. J Clin Ultrasound 15:591, 1987

158. Middleton WD, Foley WD, Lawson TL: Color-flow Doppler imaging of carotid artery abnormalities. AJR 150:419, 1988

159. Middleton WD, Foley WD, Lawson TL: Flow reversal in the normal carotid bifurcation: color Doppler flow imaging analysis. Radiology 167:207, 1988

160. Miller JD, Smith RR, Holaday HR: Carbon dioxide reactivity in the evaluation of cerebral ischemia. Neurosurgery 30:518, 1992

161. Mohr JP, Duterte DI, Oliveira VR et al: Recanalization of acute middle cerebral artery occlusion. Neurology 38:215, 1988

162. Mokri B, Houser OW, Sandok BA, Piepgras DG: Spontaneous dissections of the vertebral arteries. Neurology 38:880, 1988

163. Motomiya M, Karino T: Flow patterns in the human carotid artery bifurcation. Stroke 15:50, 1984

164. Mull M, Aulich A, Hennerici M: Transcranial Doppler ultrasonography versus arteriography for assessment of the vertebrobasilar circulation. J Clin Ultrasound 18:539, 1990

165. Munk PL, Downey D, Pelz D et al: Colour-flow Doppler imaging of a carotid-cavernous fistula. Can Assoc Radiol J 43:227, 1992

166. Müller HR: Direktionelle Dopplersonographie der A. frontalis medialis. EEG EMG 2:816, 1971

167. Naylor AR, Wildsmith JA, McClure J et al: Transcranial Doppler monitoring during carotid endarterectomy. Br J Surg 78:1264, 1991

168. Newell DW, Grady MS, Sirotta P, Winn HR: Evaluation of brain death using transcranial Doppler. Neurosurgery 24:509, 1989

169. Nolsoe CP, Engel U, Karstrup S et al: The aortic wall: an in vitro study of the double-line pattern in high-resolution US. Radiology 175:387, 1990

170. O'Donnell TF, Erdoes L, Mackay WC et al: Correlation of B-mode ultrasound imaging and arteriography with pathologic findings at carotid endarterectomy. Arch Surg 120:443, 1985

171. Ohbuchi R, Chen D, Fuchs H: Incremental volume re-construction and rendering for 3D ultrasound imaging. p. 312. In Proc SPIE Visualization in Biomedical Computing, 1992

172. Ophir J, Parker KJ: Contrast agents in diagnostic ultrasound. Ultrasound Med Biol 15:319, 1989

173. Otis S, Rush M, Boyajian R: Contrast-enhanced transcranial imaging. Results of an American phase-two study. Stroke 26:203, 1995

174. Padayachee TS, Gosling RG, Bishop CCR et al: Monitoring MCA blood velocity during carotid endarterectomy. Br J Surg 73:98, 1986

175. Persson J, Formgren J, Israelsson B, Berglund G: Ultrasound-determined intima-media thickness and atherosclerosis. Direct and indirect validation. Arterioscler Thromb 14:261, 1994

176. Petty GW, Massaro AR, Tatemichi TK et al: Transcranial Doppler ultrasonographic changes after treatment for arteriovenous malformations. Stroke 21:260, 1990

177. Petty GW, Mohr JP, Pedley TA et al: The role of transcranial Doppler in confirming brain death: sensitivity, specificity, and suggestions for performance and interpretation. Neurology 40:300, 1990

178. Phillips DJ, Greene FM, Langlois YJ et al: Flow velocity patterns in the carotid bifurcations of young, presumed normal subjects. Ultrasound Med Biol 9:39, 1983

179. Picano E, Landini L, Lattanzi F et al: Time domain echo pattern evaluations from normal and atherosclerotic arterial walls: a study in vitro. Circulation 77:654, 1988

180. Pignoli P, Tremoli E, Poli A et al: Intimal plus medial thickness of the arterial wall: a direct measurement with ultrasound imaging. Circulation 74:1399, 1986

181. Powers AD, Graeber MC, Smith RR: Transcranial Doppler ultrasonography in the determination of brain death. Neurosurgery 24:884, 1989

182. Powers AD, Smith RR, Graeber MC: Transcranial Doppler monitoring of cerebral flow velocities during surgical occlusion of the carotid artery. Neurosurgery 25:383, 1989

183. Quint DJ, Spickler EM: Magnetic resonance demonstration of vertebral artery dissection. J Neurosurg 72:961, 1990

184. Rautenberg W, Aulich A, Röther J et al: Stroke and dolichoectatic intracranial arteries. Neurol Res 14:201, 1992

185. Rautenberg W, Hennerici M: Pulsed Doppler assessment of innominate artery obstructive disease. Stroke 19:1514, 1988

186. Rautenberg W, Hennerici M: Intracranial hemodynamic measurements in patients with severe asymptomatic extracranial carotid disease. Cerebrovasc Dis 1:216, 1991

187. Rautenberg W, Ries S, Bäzner H, Hennerici M: Emboli detection by TCD monitoring. Can J Neurol Sci 20:138, 1993

188. Rautenberg W, Schwartz A, Hennerici M: Transkranielle Dopplersonographie während der zerebralen Angiographie. p. 144. In Widder B (ed): Transkranielle Dopplersonographie bei zerebrovaskulären Erkrankungen. Springer, New York, 1987

189. Rautenberg W, Schwartz A, Mull M et al: Noninvasive detection of intracranial stenoses and occlusions. Stroke 21:149, 1990

190. Reith W, Pfadenhauer K, Loeprecht H: Significance of

transcranial Doppler CO_2. Reactivity measurements for the diagnosis of hemodynamically relevant carotid obstructions. Ann Vasc Surg 4:359, 1990

191. Ricotta JJ, Bryan FA, Bond MG et al: Multicenter validation study of real-time (B-mode) ultrasound, arteriography, and pathologic examination. J Vasc Surg 6:512, 1987

192. Ries F, Eicke M: Auswirkungen der extrakorporalen Zirkulation auf die intrazerebrale Hämodynamik—Erklärung postoperativer neuropsychiatrischer Komplikationen. p. 100. In Wider B (ed): Transkranielle Doppler-Sonographie bei zerebrovaskulären Erkrankungen. Springer, New York, 1987

193. Ries F, Honisch C, Lambertz M, Schlief R: A transpulmonary contrast medium enhances the transcranial Doppler signal in humans. Stroke 24:1903, 1993

194. Rihs F, Gutbrod K, Gutbrod B et al: Determination of cognitive hemispheric dominance by "stereo" transcranial Doppler sonography. Stroke 26:70, 1995

195. Riles TS, Imparato AM, Posner MP, Eikelboom BC: Common carotid occlusion. Ann Surg 199:363, 1984

196. Riley WA, Barnes RW, Applegate WB et al: Reproducibility of noninvasive ultrasonic measurement of carotid atherosclerosis. The Asymptomatic Carotid Artery Plaque Study. Stroke 23:1062, 1992

197. Ringelstein EB, Sievers C, Ecker S et al: Noninvasive assessment of CO_2-induced cerebral vasomotor response in normal individuals and patients with internal carotid artery occlusions. Stroke 19:963, 1988

198. Ringelstein EB, Van Eyck S, Mertens I: Evaluation of cerebral vasomotor reactivity by various vasodilating stimuli: comparison of CO_2 to acetazolamide. J Cereb Blood Flow Metab 12:162, 1992

199. Robinson ML, Sacks D, Perlmutter GS, Marinelli DL: Diagnostic criteria for carotid duplex sonography. AJR 151:1045, 1988

200. Röther J, Schwartz A, Rautenberg W et al: Middle cerebral artery assessment by magnetic resonance angiography and transcranial Doppler. Neurology 45:414, 1993

201. Röther J, Wentz KU, Rautenberg W et al: Magnetic resonance angiography in vertebrobasilar ischemia. Stroke 24:1310, 1993

202. Rubba P, Mercuri M, Faccenda F et al: Premature carotid atherosclerosis: does it occur in both familial hypercholesterolemia and homocystinuria? Ultrasound assessment of arterial intima-media thickness and blood flow velocity. Stroke 25:943, 1994

203. Rubin JM, Bude RO, Carson PL et al: Power Doppler US: a potentially useful alternative to mean frequency-based color Doppler US. Radiology 190:853, 1994

204. Salonen R, Salonen JT: Progression of carotid atherosclerosis and its determinants: a population-based ultrasonography study. Atherosclerosis 33, 1990

205. Sandmann W, Kolvenbach R, Willeke F: Risks and benefits of shunting in carotid endarterectomy. Stroke 24:1098, 1993

206. Schlief R: Developments in echo-enhancing agents. Clin Radiol 51:5, 1996

207. Schneider PA, Rossman ME, Bernstein EF et al: Effect of internal carotid artery occlusion on intracranial hemodynamics. Transcranial Doppler evaluation and clinical correlation. Stroke 19:589, 1988

208. Schneider PA, Rossman ME, Torem S et al: Transcranial Doppler in the management of extracranial cerebrovascular disease: implications in diagnosis and monitoring. J Vasc Surg 7:223, 1988

209. Schwartz A, Rautenberg W, Hennerici M: Dolichoectatic intracranial arteries: review of selected aspects. Cerebrovasc Dis 3:273, 1993

210. Seiler RW, Grolimund P, Aaslid R et al: Cerebral vasospasm evaluated by transcranial ultrasound correlated with clinical grade and CT-visualized subarachnoid hemorrhage. J Neurosurg 64:594, 1986

211. Siebler M, Sitzer M, Rose G et al: Silent cerebral embolism caused by neurologically symptomatic high-grade carotid stenosis. Event rates before and after carotid endarterectomy. Brain 116:1005, 1993

212. Siebler M, Sitzer M, Steinmetz H: Detection of intracranial emboli in patients with symptomatic extracranial carotid artery disease. Stroke 1992:1652, 1993

213. Sitzer M, Furst G, Fischer H et al: Between-method correlations in quantifying internal carotid stenosis. Stroke 24:1513, 1993

214. Sitzer M, Furst G, Siebler M, Steinmetz H: Usefulness of an intravenous contrast medium in the characterization of high-grade internal carotid stenosis with color Doppler-assisted duplex imaging. Stroke 25:385, 1994

215. Sliwka U, Rother J, Steinke W, Hennerici M: [The value of duplex sonography in cerebral ischemia] Die Bedeutung der Duplexsonographie bei zerebralen Ischamien. Bildgebung 58:182, 1991

216. Sommer C, Mullges W, Ringelstein EB: Noninvasive assessment of intracranial fistulas and other small arteriovenous malformations. Neurosurgery 30:522, 1992

217. Spencer MP, Thomas GI, Nicholls SC, Sauvage LR: Detection of middle cerebral artery emboli during carotid endarterectomy using transcranial Doppler ultrasonography. Stroke 21:415, 1990

218. Spencer MP, Whisler D: Transorbital Doppler diagnosis of intracranial arterial stenosis. Stroke 17:916, 1986

219. Steinke W, Aulich A, Hennerici M: Diagnose und Verlauf von Carotisdissektionen. DMW 114:1869, 1989

220. Steinke W, Hennerici M: Three-dimensional ultrasound imaging of carotid artery plaques. J Cardiovasc Technol 8:15, 1989

221. Steinke W, Hennerici M, Aulich A: Doppler color flow imaging of carotid body tumors. Stroke 20:1574, 1989

222. Steinke W, Hennerici M, Rautenberg W, Mohr JP: Symptomatic and asymptomatic high-grade carotid stenoses in Doppler color-flow imaging. Neurology 42:131, 1992

223. Steinke W, Kloetzsch C, Hennerici M: Variability of flow patterns in the normal carotid bifurcation. Atherosclerosis 84:121, 1990

224. Steinke W, Kloetzsch C, Hennerici M: Carotid artery disease assessed by color Doppler flow imaging: correlation with standard Doppler sonography and angiography. AJNR 11:259, 1990

225. Steinke W, Meairs S, Ries S, Hennerici M: Sonographic assessment of carotid artery stenosis: comparison of power imaging and color Doppler flow imaging. Stroke 27:91, 1996

226. Steinke W, Rautenberg W, Schwartz A, Hennerici M:

Noninvasive monitoring of internal carotid artery dissection. Stroke 25:998, 1994

227. Steinke W, Rautenberg W, Schwartz A et al: Ultrasonographic diagnosis and monitoring of cervicocephalic arterial dissection. Cerebrovasc Dis 2:195, 1992

228. Steinke W, Rautenberg W, Sliwka U, Hennerici M: Common carotid artery occlusion: clinical significance of a patent internal carotid artery. Neurol Sci 20:140, 1993

229. Sterpetti AV, Schultz RD, Feldhaus RJ et al: Ultrasonographic features of carotid plaque and the risk of subsequent neurologic deficits. Surgery 104:652, 1988

230. Sturzenegger M, Mattle HP, Rivoir A et al: Ultrasound findings in spontaneous extracranial vertebral artery dissection. Stroke 24:1910, 1993

231. Svindland A, Torvik A: Atherosclerotic carotid disease in asymptomatic individuals: an histological study of 53 cases. Acta Neurol Scand 78:506, 1988

232. Taylor DC, Strandness DE Jr: Carotid artery duplex scanning. J Clin Ultrasound 15:635, 1987

233. Tettenborn B, Estol C, DeWitt LD et al: Accuracy of transcranial Doppler in the vertebrobasilar circulation. J Neurol 237:159, 1990

234. Tong DC, Albers GW: Transcranial Doppler-detected microemboli in patients with acute stroke. Stroke 26:1588, 1995

235. Touboul PJ, Mas JL, Bousser MG, Laplane D: Duplex scanning in extracranial vertebral artery dissection. Stroke 19:116, 1988

236. Trattnig S, Hubsch P, Schuster H, Polzleitner D: Color-coded Doppler imaging of normal vertebral arteries. Stroke 21:1222, 1990

237. Trattnig S, Schwaighofer B, Hubsch P et al: Color-coded Doppler sonography of vertebral arteries. J Ultrasound Med 10:221, 1991

238. Tuteur P, Reivich M, Goldberg HI et al: Transient responses of cerebral blood flow and ventilation to changes in $PaCO_2$ in normal subjects and patients with cerebrovascular disease. Stroke 7:584, 1976

239. Valton L, Larrue V, Arrué P et al: Asymptomatic cerebral embolic signals in patients with carotid stenosis: correlation with appearance of plaque ulceration on angiography. Stroke 26:813, 1995

240. von Reutern GM, Pourcelot L: Cardiac-cycle dependent alternating flow in vertebral arteries with subclavian artery stenosis. Stroke 9:229, 1978

241. Wendelhag I, Gustavsson T, Suurküla MJ et al: Ultrasound measurement of wall thickness in the carotid artery: fundamental principles and description of a computerized analysing system. Clin Physiol 11:565, 1991

242. Widder B, Paulat K, Hackspacher J et al: Morphological characterization of carotid artery stenoses by ultrasound duplex scanning. Ultrasound Med Biol 16:349, 1990

243. Wolverson MK, Bashiti HM, Peterson GJ: Ultrasonic tissue characterisation of atheromatous plaques using high resolution real time scanner. Ultrasound Med Biol 9:599, 1983

244. Yonehara T, Ando Y, Kimura K et al: Detection of reverse flow by duplex ultrasonography in orthostatic hypotension. Stroke 25:2407, 1994

245. Zarins CK, Giddens DP, Bharadvaj BK et al: Carotid bifurcation atherosclerosis: quantitative correlation of plaque localization with flow velocity profiles and wall shear stress. Circ Res 53:502, 1983

246. Zbornikova V, Lassvik C: Common carotid artery occlusion: haemodynamic features. Cerebrovasc Dis 1:136, 1991

247. Zierler RE, Philips DJ, Beach KW et al: Noninvasive assessment of normal carotid bifurcation hemodynamics with color-flow ultrasound imaging. Ultrasound Med Biol 13:471, 1987

248. Zurynski Y, Dorsch N, Pearson I, Choong R: Transcranial Doppler ultrasound in brain death: experience in 140 patients. Neurol Res 13:248, 1991

249. Zwiebel WJ, Austin CW, Sackett JF, Strother CM: Correlation of high-resolution, B-mode and continuous-wave Doppler sonography with arteriography in the diagnosis of carotid stenosis. Radiology 149:523, 1983

250. Zwiebel WJ, Knighton R: Duplex examination of the carotid arteries. Semin Ultrasound CT MRI 11:97, 1990

CHAPTER 15

Single-Photo Emission Computed Tomography

STEPHEN M. DAVIS

BERNARD INFELD

Single-photon emission computed tomography (SPECT) has become a widely available functional neuroimaging technique, with an expanding role in the investigation and management of a wide range of neurologic disorders. This functional neuroimaging modality complements conventional computed tomographic (CT) and magnetic resonance imaging (MRI) techniques, which image brain structure. Because regional hypoperfusion initiates the pathogenesis of cerebral ischemia, SPECT has found particular application in the study of cerebrovascular disease. Both cortical and subcortical structures are well delineated by modern SPECT systems, but spatial resolution is less than can be achieved by CT, MRI, or positron emission tomography (PET). Using SPECT technology, three-dimensional images representing certain aspects of cerebral function can be generated, mainly perfusion and, to a lesser degree, neuroreceptor distribution. In most nuclear medicine departments, SPECT systems are now available with rotating γ-cameras and commercially marketed radionuclides.

In the assessment of cerebral perfusion, SPECT imaging has largely replaced the earlier planar ^{133}Xe technique, in which the radiotracer was administered via the intravenous, inhalational, or intra-arterial routes, with extracranial detecting probes placed over each hemisphere. It is logistically far simpler and less expensive than PET. Unlike PET, however, regional metabolism cannot be imaged. In normal brain, regional cerebral blood flow (rCBF) and metabolism are matched, and it can generally be assumed that the rCBF information obtained with SPECT corresponds to brain function. However, these parameters may be discordant in various pathologic states, particularly in acute ischemia. Perfusion SPECT has the advantage over the nonradioactive xenon CT technique, also used to image rCBF with excellent spatial resolution, in that the mildly anesthetic effects of the xenon gas are avoided. Echoplanar MR scanning techniques to measure CBF are still in their infancy and are not yet a challenge to SPECT, but they hold great promise.[115,116]

Single-photon, γ-emitting radionuclides are used in SPECT imaging, contrasting with the positron emitters used in PET scanning that generate two photons in coincidence following the annihilation reaction between the positron and tissue electron. Rotating γ-camera or fixed ring detector systems are used to measure these cerebral emissions in SPECT, regional counts correlating with functional activity in different brain regions. Like PET, counts are normally much higher in the gray matter of the cortex, basal ganglia, and cerebellum than in the white matter of the centrum semiovale. Radionuclide SPECT technology can be categorized into perfusion SPECT and neuroreceptor SPECT methods. Virtually all studies in cerebrovascular disease have involved perfusion SPECT. Four principal techniques have been developed. These, described below, include the xenon-133 (^{133}Xe) clearance method and three techniques whereby brain retention of a radioligand generates cerebral images representing regional perfusion.

Perfusion SPECT Techniques

XENON-133 CLEARANCE METHOD

The ^{133}Xe clearance technique was a development of the earlier, nontomographic (planar) ^{133}Xe method, relating the cerebral clearance of ^{133}Xe to rCBF. The method has the advantage of providing quantification of rCBF in ml/100 g/min.

Table 15.1 Perfusion SPECT Techniques

	^{133}Xe	^{123}IMP	^{99m}Tc-HMPAO	^{99m}Tc-ECD
Advantages	Quantification of rCBF Multiple studies can be performed on the same day	Validated rCBF technique	Steady state for several hours Good spatial resolution Readily available radioligand Extensive published experience	Superior to ^{99m}Tc-HMPAO in subacute stroke Good spatial resolution Greater stability in vitro than ^{99m}Tc-HMPAO
Disadvantages	Inferior spatial resolution Requires specialized detection instruments	Inferior imaging quality to technetium-based methods Cerebral imaging has to be performed <1 hour after injection May underestimate rCBF in cerebral acidosis	Quantification of rCBF extremely difficult Hyperfixation artifact in subacute stroke	May not detect luxury perfusion

Abbreviations: ^{133}Xe, xenon-133; ^{123}IMP, iodine-123-*N*-isopropyl-*p*-iodoamphetamine; ^{99m}Tc-HMPAO, technetium-99m-hexamethylpropylene amine oxime; ^{99m}Tc-ECD, technetium-99m-ethyl cysteinate dimer; rCBF, regional cerebral blood flow.

Furthermore, as ^{133}Xe is rapidly cleared, multiple studies can be performed on the same day. However, image quality is inferior to the more recently introduced retention SPECT techniques; the poorer spatial resolution is explained by both the low photon energy of the ^{133}Xe radiotracer and its rapid cerebral clearance (Table 15.1). In addition, this method requires specialized instrumentation.[50] For these reasons, the ^{133}Xe SPECT method is rarely used in clinical practice.

BRAIN RADIOPHARMACEUTICAL PERFUSION (RETENTION) TECHNIQUES

Developments in perfusion SPECT over the past decade have utilized radiotracers that cross the blood-brain barrier, distribute in the brain in proportion to perfusion, and remain fixed for a sufficient time to allow extracranial tomographic imaging of the γ-emission. Three techniques have now come into clinical practice.[111]

^{123}I-IMP Spect

Iodine-123 (^{123}I) requires cyclotron generation and therefore the availability of the ^{123}I-*N*-isopropyl-*p*-iodoamphetamine (IMP) technique is more limited than the technetium-based methods. It has been validated as a reliable rCBF technique.[85,95] Redistribution is fairly rapid, hence cerebral imaging has to be performed within 1 hour of injection. Due to lower dosimetry and lower photon flux, imaging quality is somewhat inferior to the technetium-based methods.[111] The ^{123}I-IMP technique may underestimate rCBF in acidotic brain, which is pertinent in acute cerebral ischemia, and is one potential disadvantage of this technique.[50,67]

^{99m}Tc-HMPAO Spect

The technetium-99m-hexamethylpropylene amine oxime (^{99m}Tc-HMPAO) SPECT technique was developed in the mid-1980s.[52,88,96] It has been the most commonly used method in SPECT research in cerebrovascular disease. It utilizes a technetium-labeled lipophilic agent, which has a high first-pass brain extraction fraction and is fixed intracerebrally in proportion to perfusion. Steady-state conditions within the brain are reached approximately 2 to 3 minutes after injection and remain constant for a few hours.[96] This persistence allows delayed imaging in a nuclear medicine department to be performed several hours after initial injection of the radiopharmaceutical, a longer and more practical interval than allowed by the IMP technique. The retention of ^{99m}Tc-HMPAO appears to be critically dependent on an intracellular reaction with glutathione, and is due to conversion to a hydrophilic form.[87,88]

Precise quantification of CBF cannot be performed using this method, as the biodistribution and kinetics of the radionuclide are unclear.[6,96] However, using arterial sampling, estimates of rCBF can be generated that correlate with other CBF methods.[56,57,97] The lower costs and the ready availability of this ^{99m}Tc labeled perfusion tracer led to its widespread application in the study of various cerebral disorders in the late 1980s.[9]

Other than visual image analysis, a number of several semiquantitative techniques used to measure abnormalities in perfusion have been described. These include the analysis of side-to-side differences in activity distributions in homologous cerebral regions, or normalization with respect to a reference site in an unaffected brain region, such as the cerebellum.[109] Techniques for volumetric analysis of hypoperfusion have also been described.[83] To measure regional infarct hypoperfusion, we have developed a technique involving integrated volumetric analysis (in cubic centimeters), incorporating a measure of both the severity and extent of regional hypoperfusion.[25,53] Quantitative volumetric measurement is useful for statistical comparisons with clinical parameters in cerebrovascular research, but qualitative image analysis is generally used in clinical practice.

Using ^{99m}Tc-HMPAO SPECT, focal hyperfixation of the radionuclide in subacute stroke can give spuriously high, artifactual estimates of rCBF in some patients, with poor clinical correlations at these times between regional perfusion changes and neurologic parameters.[107]

^{99m}Tc-ECD

A newer technetium ligand has high cerebral uptake with slow clearance and optimal characteristics for SPECT imaging.[51] An additional advantage is the stability of the *technetium-99m-ethyl cysteinate dimer* (^{99m}Tc-ECD) ligand in vitro for about 6 hours.[50,111] The intracerebral distribution of ^{99m}Tc-ECD SPECT has been shown to be similar to rCBF measured by ^{133}Xe imaging.[31,38] The ^{99m}Tc-ECD technique appears to be preferable in the assessment of rCBF in subacute stroke, due to lack of the hyperfixation artifact seen in ^{99m}Tc-HMPAO SPECT.[18]

CEREBROVASCULAR RESERVE

Using any of these perfusion SPECT techniques, perfusion reserve can be calculated using a vasodilatory challenge with either 1 g intravenously injected acetazolamide or 5% CO_2 administered by inhalation.[74,113] These vasodilatory agents increase rCBF in normal brain. In ischemic brain regions, which may appear to be normal using structural brain techniques, cerebral arterioles are already vasodilated to optimize microvascular perfusion (rCBF). Following the vasodilatory challenge, an area with impaired perfusion reserve is reflected by lower regional perfusion, compared with the degree of increased rCBF in surrounding normal brain.[72,84] These regions of relative vasoparalysis are identified by comparison of the baseline and postchallenge scans. These focal changes in vasoreactivity can be correlated with other parameters indicating hemodynamic compromise, including occlusive lesions on angiography, arterial flow changes shown by transcranial Doppler, and border zone infarction on CT scans.[65]

Neuroreceptor SPECT

Various neuroreceptor ligands have been developed for muscarinic and cholinergic receptors, dopamine D_2 receptors, and the serotonin-2 and benzodiazepine receptors.[34,50,105] Few studies have been performed in cerebrovascular disease, and these ligands are not used in routine clinical practice.[111]

Imaging Systems

Instrumentation for SPECT imaging relies on the use of rotating γ-cameras or ring-type dedicated imaging systems. The tomographic γ-camera systems can be used for body as well as dedicated head scanning.[50] A spatial resolution of 7 to 10 mm is achieved for full-width half-maximum (FWHM) three and four-head γ-camera systems, reaching 7 to 8 mm FWHM for dedicated ring-type imaging systems.

SPECT in Cerebrovascular Disease

In the 1980s, SPECT was shown to demonstrate regional hypoperfusion in acute stroke and to demonstrate brain ischemia more sensitively than early CT scans, the hypoperfusion deficits being correlated with clinical measures of neurologic severity[35] (Table 15.2). A wide range of SPECT studies in various cerebrovascular conditions over subsequent years have been developed. These include the analysis of serial perfusion changes in acute and evolving stroke through to brain recovery, the use of perfusion SPECT in stroke prognosis, measurement of perfusion abnormalities in patients with clinically transient cerebral ischemia, evaluation of perfusion changes following pharmacologic interventions in acute stroke, analysis of functional perfusion reserve in patients with carotid occlusive disease, and measurement of perfusion abnormalities in patients with subarachnoid hemorrhage and arteriovenous malformations. Other related SPECT studies have focused on the diagnosis of vascular dementia and focal epileptic disorders. Recent interest has focused on the role of SPECT in the selection of patients to be treated with new, interventional stroke therapies such as thrombolysis.

ACUTE ISCHEMIC STROKE: DIAGNOSIS AND CLINICAL CORRELATIONS

Many studies have demonstrated the superior diagnostic sensitivity of perfusion SPECT in acute ischemic stroke, compared with CT or conventional MRI (Plate 15.1). Thi sensitivity is due to the hypoperfusion that is the hallmark of acute ischemia, whereas structural changes shown on CT or conventional T_2-weighted MRI evolve over hours to days.[16,27,30,36,96,98] Other studies emphasized the discrepancy between the larger areas of regional cortical hypoperfusion in acute stroke, compared with the extent of early structural changes.[50] Acute cerebral hypoperfusion has been found to correlate well with both the site and severity of neurologic deficits in ischemic stroke, particularly cortical infarcts. By contrast, false-negative studies in subcortical lacunar strokes are a well-recognized problem using SPECT, due to its reduced spatial resolution compared with CT or MRI.[18,30] Brass et al,[18] using ECD SPECT, showed nonetheless that a normal image or small subcortical hypoperfusion defect was highly predictive of lacunar infarction, while the method was both highly sensitive and specific in the diagnosis and localization of cortical infarction. The technique is also useful in the pathogenetic differentiation between embolic and border zone infarcts.[9] This diagnostic sensitivity of SPECT in acute stroke

Table 15.2 SPECT Abnormalities in Cerebrovascular Disease

Disease Category	SPECT Abnormalities	Clinical Usefulness
Acute stroke		
Early diagnosis	Regional hypoperfusion	Accurate diagnosis of acute cerebral ischemia
Stroke Prognosis	Regional acute hypoperfusion predicts functional outcome	Adds little to clinical prognostic determinants
Diagnosis stroke subtype	Regional hypoperfusion useful in predicting cortical, border zone, lacunar infarcts	Limited
Interventional therapy	Reperfusion correlated with clinical benefits; conflicting results from studies	Potentially useful in selection of patients for reperfusion therapies
Diaschisis	Crossed cerebellar diaschisis correlates with acute stroke severity; may give insight into metabolism at infarct site	Not evaluated
Transient ischemic attacks	Regional hypoperfusion in patients with clinical recovery; impaired perfusion reserve in some patients	May predict high-risk subset of patients
Subarachnoid hemorrhage	Regional hypoperfusion correlates with site of vasospasm producing tissue ischemia; correlates with delayed neurologic deficits	Role in monitoring tissue ischemia due to vasospasm Template for therapy such as angioplasty
Arteriovenous malformations	Pre- and postoperative hypoperfusion linked to clinical deficits and prognosis	Limited
Stroke-related epilepsy	Interictal hypoperfusion; ictal hyperperfusion	Very useful in temporal lobe epilepsy; not specifically evaluated in poststroke epilepsy
Vascular dementia	Multifocal hypoperfusion deficits; distinctly different pattern from Alzheimer's disease	Useful in distinction between multi-infarct and Alzheimer's-type dementia

progressively declines over the first 72 hours, due to the phenomenon of luxury perfusion, marked by the rCBF becoming inappropriately elevated relative to the metabolic needs of the tissue.

STROKE PROGNOSIS

Given the early diagnostic sensitivity of SPECT in acute ischemic stroke, investigators focused on the prognostic potential of the functional imaging technique. Early published reports even suggested a poor correlation between acute hypoperfusion deficits and stroke outcome.[28,29,48,73] However, a number of these studies were flawed by the analysis of patients at substantial time intervals after stroke onset. It became clear that measurements of perfusion in the subacute stage after stroke (i.e., days to weeks after onset) had a poor correlation with neurologic parameters and outcome due to the presence of luxury perfusion shown to be prevalent on SPECT scans at these times.[22]

Other investigators analyzed cerebral hypoperfusion in the acute phase of stroke and established a good correlation with clinical outcome.[28,40,69,75,76] Giubilei et al[40] found that the severity of CBF asymmetry using ^{99m}Tc-HMPAO SPECT within 6 hours of stroke onset predicted stroke outcome. Similar conclusions were reached by Shimosegawa et al,[106] who used this method to distinguish potentially viable brain within 6 hours of the onset of cerebral ischemia. Other studies correlated large regions of hypoperfusion within 24 hours with a high risk of early death from transtentorial herniation.[76] Our group showed that acute hypoperfusion on ^{99m}Tc-HMPAO SPECT strongly predicted both neurologic impairment and

functional disability after 3 months.[25] Large acute hypoperfusion deficits were typically seen in patients at high risk of death or poor functional outcome (Plate 15.1).

To determine whether perfusion SPECT would be useful in routine clinical practice in estimating stroke prognosis, we compared the predictive value of acute hypoperfusion deficits with two clinical prognostic scores, the Canadian Neurological Score[23] and a multifunction clinical prognostic score[5] analyzing survival and functional disability with the Barthel Index at least 3 months after stroke (Fig. 15.1). We concluded that acute hypoperfusion measurements independently added little to the estimation of functional outcome generated by the clinical predictors. However, acute hypoperfusion measurements could be a useful template for the investigation of acute interventional stroke strategies, particularly those aimed at increasing brain perfusion.

Other studies confirmed these findings[17,45,69] Laloux et al[69] found an excellent correlation between acute hypoperfusion and 1-month functional outcome using the Rankin Scale, but also found that the size of the hypoperfusion deficit was not a better predictor of outcome than the Canadian Neurological Score. Another recent study found that the Canadian Neurological Scale was actually a better prognostic indicator than acute hypoperfusion on SPECT.[17] Hanson et al[45] found that acute hypoperfusion within 6 hours of stroke onset, corresponding with the likely time window for the use of acute interventional therapies, correlated with the severity of the acute neurologic deficit measured by the NIH Stroke Scale and long-term functional outcome measured by the Barthel Index. Alexandrov et al[3] suggested that a perfusion index, incorporating both SPECT and transcranial Doppler parameters, could be used as a rapid noninvasive outcome predictor.

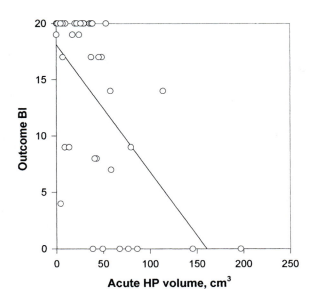

Figure 15.1 Graph showing linear regression of Outcome Barthel Index (BI) as a function of acute hypoperfusion (HP) volume measured by SPECT (B = −0.11 ± 0.02, R = 0.59, n = 4 P < 0.001).

SERIAL PERFUSION CHANGES USING SPECT IN ACUTE STROKE AND BRAIN RECOVERY: THE CONFOUNDING PROBLEM OF LUXURY PERFUSION

An understanding of the evolving infarct stages imaged by SPECT is important in the interpretation of reperfusion changes after acute stroke (Plates 15.2 and 15.3). In the evolution of perfusion changes measured by SPECT, three discrete changes can be recognized. The *acute stage*, lasting between hours and 3 days, is characterized by regional hypoperfusion at the site of the infarct, correlating with the severity of acute neurologic deficits and predicting late functional outcome. This early hypoperfusion typically exceeds the focal deficit demonstrated by acute CT or MRI. In the *subacute stage* however, days to weeks after stroke onset, perfusion SPECT can show reduced, normal, or even increased blood flow (hyperemia).[22,40,77,82,98,101,114] The common finding of hyperemia using ^{99m}Tc-HMPAO SPECT at this stage might in part reflect a hyperfixation artifact, in addition to the presence of luxury perfusion.[107] This artifact was demonstrated in a number of patients with subacute hyperemial in whom discordance between the ^{99m}Tc-HMPAO and the ^{133}Xe perfusion results were shown.[107]

Luxury perfusion was first described by Lassen in 1966[70] and related to tissue acidosis in acute ischemia. Later PET studies showed that the hallmark of luxury perfusion is a mismatch between acute rCBF and metabolism, whereby rCBF is inappropriately elevated in proportion to metabolic needs, and hence is non-nutritional (non-nutritional flow). With stroke recovery, this component of luxury perfusion subsides, and a perfusion vacuum typically develops at the infarct site.[12]

The ^{99m}Tc-ECD SPECT technique may be more useful than ^{99m}Tc-HMPAO SPECT in identifying subacute infarction, showing larger differences between normal and ischemic brain.[82] However, the method may fail to demonstrate luxury perfusion.[71] In a study comparing perfusion data obtained by ^{99m}Tc-ECD and ^{133}Xe SPECT, good agreement was found except in subacute stroke patients, in whom the ^{133}Xe SPECT technique showed normal or elevated flow consistent with reperfusion or luxury perfusion, while the ^{99m}Tc-ECD technique showed low count rates in the infarct region.[71]

In the *chronic stage* of cerebral infarction, weeks to months after onset, regional hypoperfusion is again typically found at the infarct site. In chronic infarction, a region of depressed perfusion around the anatomic area of tissue loss has been identified by some investigators, so that the hypoperfusion region may exceed the area of the infarct size on correlative CT imaging.[100,113] This depressed rCBF in apparently histologically normal tissue may reflect functionally depressed cerebral activity, termed diaschisis, and is consequent on neuronal deafferentation or de-efferentation. In our laboratory, however, we have found that the volume of chronic infarcts on ^{99m}Tc-HMPAO SPECT appears to be quite closely matched to the volume of tissue loss measured on correlative CT scans.

These serial changes in imaged rCBF explain the paradoxical increase in hypoperfusion found by us between studies performed within 3 days of stroke onset and repeated at 3 months, caused by early luxury perfusion imaged on the acute SPECT scans.[25,54,55] Vorstrup et al[114] had earlier documented similar changes, using the ^{133}Xe technique. In assessing reperfusion after stroke, outcome SPECT studies need to be performed to discriminate in retrospect between that proportion of flow that is retained at 3 months, and is hence nutritional, from that proportion of early flow that is not apparent at 3 months, and hence was not supplying viable tissue in the acute stage of stroke. One SPECT study indicated that postinfarction hyperemia could occur with some infarcts as early as 6 hours after onset.[106]

SPECT AND INTERVENTIONAL THERAPY

A number of SPECT studies have addressed the relationship between acute perfusion changes and clinical gains following intravenous thrombolytic therapy.[10,45,49,54,91] These studies chiefly used the ^{99m}Tc-HMPAO SPECT technique, imaging perfusion before and after treatment. The ^{99m}Tc-HMPAO SPECT technique is ideal for this purpose, as the radionuclide can be injected prior to therapy and is fixed in the brain in proportion to regional perfusion. Imaging can be delayed for ≤4 hours, providing an estimate of pretherapy rCBF, and then repeated 24 hours later to measure acute reperfusion. Overgaard et al[91] correlated reperfusion at 24 hours with angiographic recanalization and neurologic benefits. Baird et al[10] linked reperfusion with lower mortality and less functional morbidity. Although they were not evaluating acute therapy, Jorgensen et al[61] studied a large number of cerebral infarcts at various times within the first month after stroke and also concluded that neurologic gains correlated with reperfusion.

By contrast, Herderscheê et al[49] and Hanson et al[45] found essentially no relationship between acute reperfusion and either changes in acute clinical parameters over 24 hours[45] or outcome.[49] Other investigators evaluated longer term neurologic recovery with serial rCBF changes; some reported neurologic improvements with reperfusion over a longer period,[61,77,112] whereas others[17,25,29,98,114] could not confirm this association. As confirmed by our serial studies,[25,53] Bowler et al[17] recently showed a lack of association between reperfusion over the first week after stroke and clinical outcome.

It is likely that the disparity between these reports reflects the variable contributions of nutritional and non-nutritional flow in the reperfusion phase after acute stroke. Although it is possible to analyze the degree of luxury perfusion prospectively using PET scanning, which is marked by depression of the oxygen extraction fraction, outcome SPECT studies are required to differentiate in retrospect between the components of reperfusion that are nutritional or non-nutritional.[2,12]

We studied 24 patients in the Australian Streptokinase Trial with ^{99m}Tc-HMPAO SPECT and found no difference in acute reperfusion between those receiving intravenous streptokinase or placebo therapy.[54] However, streptokinase was associated with a significantly larger amount of non-nutritional reperfusion than placebo. This luxury perfusion was associated with a poor functional outcome. This study also found an association between non-nutritional flow and hemorrhagic transformation, suggesting that luxury perfusion may be an important determinant of reperfusion injury. Luxury perfusion was more prominent in the patients with larger acute hypoperfusion regions, correlating with recent trial results suggesting that established or large infarcts have a worse outcome after thrombolysis.[44] Finally, nutritional reperfusion was more likely with earlier treatment; therapeutic efficacy is critically related to the timing of thrombolysis.[32,110]

ROLE OF SPECT IN ACUTE ISCHEMIC STROKE

Other investigations using SPECT have provided insights into ischemic mechanisms and stroke management. One study demonstrated that pharmacologic reduction of blood pressure after ischemic stroke was associated with impaired CBF, emphasizing the risks of aggressive treatment of hypertension in the acute stroke setting.[78] In addition to acute diagnosis and prognosis, SPECT is useful in the delineation of stroke subtype. Patients with acute hemispheric stroke and normal SPECT imaging are likely to have lacunar infarcts.[18]

The results of the recent intravenous thrombolytic trials using intravenous tissue plasminogen activator (tPA) have led to optimism that a group of patients with acute ischemic stroke will benefit from acute interventional therapy.[44,110] The European Cooperative Acute Stroke Study trial showed benefits using intravenous tPA within 6 hours of stroke onset, but only in those patients in whom CT scans did not show signs of major early ischemia and who were therefore not subject to a high risk of hemorrhagic transformation.[44] The National Institutes of Health Trial showed overall benefits for observed patients treated within 3 hours of stroke onset, a time frame when acute CT changes are not commonly observed.[110] Even in this trial, however, the rate of symptomatic hemorrhagic transformation was at least 10 times greater with tPA than in the placebo-treated patients.[110]

It has therefore been suggested that noninvasive brain perfusion imaging with SPECT, giving evidence about the intensity and extent of ischemia and the degree of collateral flow, may be useful in the selection of patients for thrombolytic therapy.[4,37,80] Patients with small areas of acute hypoperfusion could be expected to have a favorable outcome and probably would not be candidates for thrombolytic therapy.[4] Alternatively, extensive absence of flow might suggest poor collateral flow and little chance of benefit from acute treatment. Patients with moderate perfusion deficits might be ideal candidates for thrombolytic reperfusion. To test these hypotheses and evaluate the role of brain SPECT in acute ischemic stroke and interventional therapy, a clinical trial is now being planned.[4]

DIASCHISIS IN ACUTE STROKE AND BRAIN RECOVERY

Diaschisis, defined as functional depression remote from the infarct site, has been explored in a number of SPECT investigations. These have mainly evaluated crossed cerebellar diaschisis (CCD)[55,81,92,94] (Plate 15.4). This is a matched functional depression of rCBF and metabolism in the cerebellar hemisphere contralateral to supratentorial infarction, originally described using PET scanning.[11] It is considered that CCD is a functional phenomenon without direct neurologic manifestations, secondary to interruption of the cerebropontocerebellar pathway, due to destruction of the supratentorial portion of the cerebropontine connections.[11,55]

In our laboratory, we studied a cohort of patients who had acute middle cerebral cortical infarction with ^{99m}Tc-HMPAO SPECT within 72 hours of onset, followed up after 3 months.[53] CCD was present in most patients, correlating strongly with the size of the infarct hypoperfusion deficit. The degree of CCD could be correlated with the severity of the acute neurologic deficit and was also prognostic of functional outcome and tissue loss at 3 months, although it was not independently predictive after considering the prognostic value of the volume of the acute hypoperfusion deficit. Other workers concluded that CCD had no predictive value.[69] Because CCD in the acute stage is not affected by luxury perfusion, it might reflect the degree of metabolic derangement at the infarct site. It has therefore been suggested that the degree of CCD might indicate the degree of uncoupling of rCBF and metabolism at the infarct site.[55,117] For example, relatively preserved rCBF at the infarct site associated with marked CCD might suggest a significant degree of luxury perfusion.

Other manifestations of diaschisis have been studied using SPECT. Inferior parietal hypoperfusion has been shown in patients with the subcortical ataxic-hemiparesis syndrome.[7] Poststroke depression in patients with subcortical infarction has been correlated with temporal lobe hypoperfusion, suggesting dysfunction in the limbic system.[42]

TRANSIENT ISCHEMIC ATTACKS

Using various SPECT techniques, prolonged disturbances in regional cerebral hemodynamics have been found in patients with clinically transient cerebral ischemic attacks (TIAs). Hartmann[46] reported rCBF abnormalities in 60% of patients on the day of the TIA, falling to 40% the following day. Bogousslavsky et al[14] found that persistent perfusion abnormalities identified a high-risk group of patients, who were predisposed to early infarction. Laloux and colleagues[68] found that SPECT sensitivity was higher than that of CT in TIA patients, although it did not necessarily provide additional clinical information concerning etiology. One group, assessing both baseline rCBF and vasoreactivity following acetazolamide challenge after TIAs, found abnormalities in virtually all patients.[21] In patients with severe carotid disease, marked focal rCBF asymmetry was noted, which was enhanced after injection of the vasodilator acetazolamide. This finding suggested impaired perfusion reserve in patients with symptomatic major carotid disease.

Other investigators have evaluated the intracranial hemodynamic effects of extracranial carotid stenosis. Lord's group[79] found that a significant proportion of patients demonstrated reduced vascular reserve following acetazolamide, the functional abnormality being abolished by carotid endarterectomy. Burt et al[20] reported similar results, concluding that SPECT could provide an objective evaluation of the hemodynamic effects of carotid surgery.

SUBARACHNOID HEMORRHAGE

The most important cause of morbidity after subarachnoid hemorrhage (SAH) is cerebral ischemia due to vasospasm (Plate 15.5), producing delayed neurologic deterioration in approximately 30% of patients. We reported that in patients with aneurysmal SAH, regional hypoperfusion on ^{99m}Tc-HMPAO SPECT could be correlated with the presence and severity of delayed neurologic deficits, providing more information than CT scans.[26] Regional hypoperfusion deficits correlated with clinical evidence of focal neurologic abnormalities and were most severe in the patients who died. By contrast, asymptomatic patients usually had normal rCBF.[26] Similar findings were reported by other groups.[47,64,86] One study correlated hypoperfusion on SPECT with the site of ruptured aneurysms.[99] Localized hypoperfusion has also been shown following aneurysm clipping without clinical deterioration, possibly reflecting local edema.[102]

Because of the established value of transcranial Doppler ultrasonography (TCD) in the diagnosis of large-vessel vasospasm,[1] we compared serial middle cerebral artery (MCA) velocities using TCD and rCBF changes using[99m]Tc-HMPAO SPECT after SAH, correlating the hemodynamic data with clinical evidence of delayed ischemia.[24] In patients who did not exhibit clinical signs of delayed neurologic deterioration, 50% had vasospasm using TCD criteria, but regional hypoperfusion on SPECT was rare. Concordant MCA vasospasm and regional cortical hypoperfusion were typically present in pa-

tients with delayed ischemia and a lateralizing neurologic deficit, such as hemiplegia, dysphasia, and neglect. We concluded that regional hypoperfusion was a more specific indicator of cerebral ischemia after SAH than the demonstration of vasospasm using TCD. Grosset et al[43] also used ^{99m}Tc-HMPAO SPECT to study rCBF changes in patients exhibiting rapid increases in arterial velocities after SAH. They found that correlative focal hypoperfusion occurred in most patients before the onset of any focal neurologic deficit.

These studies highlight the complementary nature of the information provided by these two hemodynamic techniques and show that SPECT is more specific to tissue ischemia. Based on these focal abnormalities in SAH, SPECT imaging has been used to select the type and intensity of therapy for vasospasm. For example, Lewis et al[75] used ^{99m}Tc-HMPAO SPECT to select patients for angioplasty.

ARTERIOVENOUS MALFORMATIONS

The SPECT technique has also been used to study patients with arteriovenous malformations. Cerebrovascular steal in such patients can be evaluated with SPECT. Abnormally enhanced reactivity was linked to postoperative hyperemia and poor outcomes.[13] Postoperative hypoperfusion on SPECT has been correlated with cognitive and behavioral abnormalities.[41] Awad et al[8] correlated intractable postoperative intracranial hypertension in lesions 6 cm or greater with preoperative hypoperfusion.

EPILEPTIC SEIZURES IN ACUTE AND CHRONIC STROKE

Epileptic seizures are a well-recognized complication of acute ischemic stroke. Our group reported a 4.4% incidence of seizures in 1,000 consecutive patients with stroke and TIAs, only occurring in those with cortical ischemia or lobar hemorrhage.[63] In addition, seizures as a late manifestation of cerebral infarction occur in about 10% of patients.[62] The use of SPECT has found increasing application in the investigation and management of patients with intractable seizure disorders, particularly those with complex partial seizures of temporal lobe origin. In this disorder, interictal SPECT demonstrates regional hypoperfusion with a sensitivity of 50% to 90%.[33,59,93] At the time of an epileptic discharge, there is a marked focal increase in rCBF. A number of studies have shown that perfusion SPECT is very valuable in the localization of a seizure focus at the time of the ictus or in the immediate postictal phase.[89,103,104] Although poststroke epilepsy is rarely an intractable problem, the successful application of SPECT in comprehensive epilepsy programs incorporating surgery for selected patients with refractory temporal lobe epilepsy may in the future assist in the management of other medically refractory seizure disorders. In patients with vascular malformations and epilepsy, SPECT has been used to evaluate focal perfusion abnormalities.[66]

MULTI-INFARCT DEMENTIA

Functional neuroimaging with SPECT is useful in the evaluation of dementia, as there are specific differences in the pattern between multi-infarct dementia (Plate 15.6) and the more common Alzheimer's disease. In Alzheimer's disease, SPECT characteristically shows diffuse hypoperfusion in the temporal and parietal lobes, correlating with the clinical manifestations and severity of the dementia.[50,58,60,90] By contrast, the characteristic pattern on SPECT in multi-infarct dementia consists of multiple asymmetric perfusion deficits involving both the cortex and deep structures.[19,39] In addition, unlike Alzheimer's disease, patients with multi-infarct dementia typically show frontal lobe perfusion abnormalities on SPECT.[108] The use of the vasodilator acetazolamide, when vasoparalysis or impaired perfusion reserve is seen in patients with focal regions of brain ischemia, can also be useful in the distinction between a multi-infarct state and Alzheimer's disease.[15]

Conclusions

A variety of SPECT techniques have been available for a decade, but the use of this technology in cerebrovascular disease is still chiefly confined to centers with a special interest in brain perfusion, rather than widespread application in routine clinical practice. This is likely to change if knowledge of cerebral perfusion changes is proved to be relevant to clinical decision making in cerebrovascular disease. Its most important role may well be to facilitate selection of interventional therapies in acute ischemic stroke, particularly thrombolysis, for which a rapid analysis of regional hypoperfusion may be valuable for the predication of responders to a potentially dangerous therapy.[4] The clinical application of SPECT in cerebrovascular disease, which is often dependent on the interpretation of complex imaging data, should involve a close collaboration between neurologists and nuclear medicine physicians.[111]

References

1. Aaslid R, Huber P, Nornes H: Evaluation of cerebrovascular spasm with transcranial Doppler ultrasound. J Neurosurg 60:37–41, 1984
2. Ackerman RH, Alpert NM, Correia JA et al: Positron imaging in ischemic stroke disease. Ann Neurol, suppl. 15:S126–S130, 1984
3. Alexandrov AV, Bladin CF, Ehrlich LE, Norris JW: Noninvasive assessment of intracranial perfusion in acute cerebral ischemia. J Neuroimaging 5:76–82, 1995
4. Alexandrov AV, Grotta JC, Davis SM, Lassen NA: Brain SPECT and thrombolysis in acute ischemic stroke: time for a clinical trial. J Nucl Med 37:1259–1262, 1996
5. Allen CM: Predicting the outcome of acute stroke: a prognostic score. J Neurol Neurosurg Psychiatry 47:475–480, 1984
6. Andersen AR. ^{99m}Tc-D, L-hexamethylenepropyleneamine oxime (^{99m}Tc-HMPAO): basic kinetic studies of a tracer of cerebral blood flow. Cerebrovasc Brain Metab Rev 1:288–318, 1989
7. Attig E: Parieto-cerebellar loop impairment in ataxic hemiparesis: proposed pathophysiology based on an analysis of cerebral blood flow. Can J Neurol Sci 21:15–23, 1994
8. Awad IA, Magdinec M, Schubert A: Intracranial hypertension after resection of cerebral arteriovenous malformations. Predisposing factors and management strategy. Stroke 25:611–620, 1994
9. Baird AE, Donnan GA, Austin M et al: Preliminary experience with 99m Tc-HMPAO SPECT in cerebral ischaemia. Clin Exp Neurol 28:43–49, 1991
10. Baird AE, Donnan GA, Austin MC et al: Reperfusion after thrombolytic therapy in ischemic stroke measured by single-photon emission computed tomography. Stroke 25:79–85, 1994
11. Baron JC, Bousser MG, Comar D, Castaigne P: "Crossed cerebellar diaschisis" in human supratentorial brain infarction. Trans Am Neurol Assoc 105:459–461, 1980
12. Baron JC, Bousser MG, Comar D et al: Noninvasive tomographic study of cerebral blood flow and oxygen metabolism in vivo. Potentials, limitations, and clinical applications in cerebral ischemic disorders. Eur Neurol 20:273–284, 1981
13. Batjer HH, Devous MD Sr: The use of acetazolamide-enhanced regional cerebral blood flow measurement to predict risk of arteriovenous malformation patients. Neurosurgery 31:213–217, 1992
14. Bogousslavsky J, Delaloye-Bischof A, Regli F, Delaloye B: Prolonged hypoperfusion and early stroke after transient ischemic attack. Stroke 21:40–46, 1990
15. Bonte FJ, Devous MD Sr, Reisch JS et al: The effect of acetazolamide on regional cerebral blood flow in patients with Alzheimer's disease or stroke as measured by single-photon emission computed tomography. Invest Radiol 24:99–103, 1989
16. Bose A, Pacia SB, Fayad P et al: Cerebral blood flow imaging compared to CT during the initial 24 hours of cerebral infarction. Neurology 40:190, 1990
17. Bowler JV, Wade JPH, Jones BE et al: Single-photon emission computed tomography using hexamethylpropyleneamine oxime in the prognosis of acute cerebral infarction. Stroke 27:82–86, 1996
18. Brass LM, Walovitch RC, Joseph JL et al: The role of single photon emission computed tomography brain imaging with ^{99m}Tc-bicisate in the localization and definition of mechanism of ischemic stroke. J Cereb Blood Flow Metab, Suppl. 1, 14:S91–S98, 1994
19. Buell U, Costa DC, Kirsch G et al: The investigation of dementia with single photon emission computed tomography. Nucl Med Commun 11:823–841, 1990
20. Burt RW, Witt RM, Cikrit DF, Reddy RV: Carotid artery disease: evaluation with acetazolamide-enhanced Tc-99m HMPAO SPECT. Radiology 182:461–466, 1992
21. Chollet F, Celsis P, Clanet M et al: SPECT study of cerebral blood flow reactivity after acetzolamide in pa-

tients with transient ischemic attacks. Stroke 20: 458–464, 1989

22. Cordes M, Henkes H, Roll D et al: Subacute and chronic cerebral infarctions: SPECT and gadolinium-DTPA enhanced MR imaging. J Comput Assist Tomogr 13: 567–571, 1989

23. Cote R, Battista RN, Wolfson C et al: The Canadian Neurological Scale: validation and reliability assessment. Neurology 39:638–643, 1989

24. Davis SM, Andrews JT, Lichtenstein M et al: Correlations between cerebral arterial velocities, blood flow, and delayed ischemia after subarachnoid hemorrhage. Stroke 23:492–497, 1992

25. Davis SM, Chua MG, Lichtenstein M et al: Cerebral hypoperfusion in stroke prognosis and brain recovery. Stroke 24:1691–1696, 1993

26. Davis S, Andrews J, Lichtenstein M et al: A single-photon emission computed tomography study of hypoperfusion after subarachnoid hemorrhage. Stroke 21: 252–259, 1990

27. De Bruine JF, Limburg M, van Royen EA et al: SPET brain imaging with 201 diethyldithiocarbamate in acute ischaemic stroke. Eur J Nucl Med 17:248–251, 1990

28. Defer G, Moretti JL, Cesaro P et al: Early and delayed SPECT using N-isopropyl p-iodoamphetamine iodine 123 in cerebral ischemia. A prognostic index for clinical recovery. Arch Neurol 44:715–718, 1987

29. Demeurisse G, Verhas M, Capon A, Paternot J: Lack of evolution of the cerebral blood flow during clinical recovery of a stroke. Stroke 14:77–81, 1983

30. De Roo M, Mortelmans L, Devos P et al: Clinical experience with Tc-99m HM-PAO high resolution SPECT of the brain in patients with cerebrovascular accidents. Eur J Nucl Med 15:9–15, 1989

31. Devous MD Sr, Payne JK, Lowe JL, Leroy RF: Comparison of technetium-99m-ECD to Xenon-133 SPECT in normal controls and in patients with mild to moderate regional cerebral blood flow abnormalities. J Nucl Med 34:754–761, 1993

32. Donnan GA, Davis SM, Chambers BR et al: Streptokinase in acute ischaemic stroke: does time of therapy administration affect outcome? JAMA 1996 (in press)

33. Duncan R, Patterson J, Hadley DM et al: CT, MR and SPECT imaging in temporal lobe epilepsy. J Neurol Neurosurg Psychiatry 53:11–15, 1990

34. Eckelman WC, Reba RC, Rzeszotarski WJ et al: External imaging of cerebral muscarinic acetylcholine receptors. Science 223:291–293, 1984

35. Fayad PB, Brass LM: Single photon emission computed tomography in cerebrovascular disease. Curr Concepts Cerebrovasc Dis Stroke 26:7–12, 1991

36. Fieschi C, Argentino C, Lenzi GL et al: Clinical and instrumental evaluation of patients with ischemic stroke within the first six hours. J Neurol Sci 91:311–321, 1989

37. Fisher M, Pessin MS, Furlan AJ: ECASS: lessons for future thrombolytic stroke trials. JAMA 274:1058–1059, 1995

38. Garret K, Villanueva J, Kuperus J et al: A comparison of regional cerebral blood flow with Xe133 to SPECT Tc99mECD. J Nucl Med 29:913, 1988

39. Gemmell HG, Sharp PF, Besson JA et al: Differential

40. Giubilei F, Lenzi GL, Di Piero V et al: Predictive value of brain perfusion single-photon emission computed tomography in acute ischemic stroke. Stroke 21:895–900, 1990

41. Gomez-Tortosa E, Sychra JJ, Martin EM et al: Postoperative cognitive and single photon emission computed tomography assessment of patients with resection of perioperative high-risk arteriovenous malformations. neurosurgery 36:447–457, 1995

42. Grasso MG, Pantano P, Ricci M et al: Mesial temporal cortex hypoperfusion is associated with depression in subcortical stroke. Stroke 25:980–985, 1994

43. Grosset DG, Straiton J, du Trevou M, Bullock R: Prediction of symptomatic vasospasm after subarachnoid hemorrhage by rapidly increasing transcranial Doppler velocity and cerebral blood flow changes. Stroke 23: 674–679, 1992

44. Hacke W, Kaste M, Fieschi C et al: Intravenous thrombolysis with recombinant tissue plasminogen activator for acute hemispheric stroke. The European Cooperative Acute Stroke Study (ECASS). JAMA 274: 1017–1025, 1995

45. Hanson SK, Grotta JC, Rhoades H et al: Value of single-photon emission-computed tomography in acute stroke therapeutic trials. Stroke 24:1322–1329, 1993

46. Hartmann A: Prolonged disturbances of regional cerebral blood flow in transient ischemic attacks. Stroke 16: 932–939, 1985

47. Hasan D, van Peski J, Loeve I et al: Single photon emission computed tomography in patients with acute hydrocephalus or with cerebral ischaemia after subarachnoid haemorrhage. J Neurol Neurosurg Psychiatry 54: 490–493, 1991

48. Hayman LA, Taber KH, Jhingran SG et al: Cerebral infarction: diagnosis and assessment of prognosis by using [123]IMP-SPECT and CT. AJNR 10:557–562, 1989

49. Herderscheê D, Limburg M, van Royen EA et al: Thrombolysis with recombinant tissue plasminogen activator in acute ischemic stroke: evaluation with rCBF-SPECT. Acta Neurol Scand 83:317–322, 1991

50. Holman BL, Devous MD Sr: Functional brain SPECT: the emergence of a powerful clinical method. J Nucl Med 33:1888–1904, 1992

51. Holman BL, Hellman RS, Goldsmith SJ et al: Biodistribution, dosimetry, and clinical evaluation of technetium-99m ethyl cysteinate dimer in normal subjects and in patients with chronic cerebral infarction. J Nucl Med 30:1018–1024, 1989

52. Holmes RA, Chaplin SB, Royston KG et al: cerebral uptake and retention of [99m]Tcm hexamethylpropyleneamine oxime ([99]Tcm-HM-PAO). Nucl Med Commun 6: 443–447, 1985

53. Infeld B, Binns D, Lichtenstein M et al: Volumetric quantitation of cerebral hypoperfusion on SPECT: validation and reliability. (submitted)

54. Infeld B, Davis SM, Donnan GA et al: Streptokinase increases luxury perfusion after stroke. Stroke 27: 1524–1529, 1996

diagnosis in dementia using the cerebral blood flow agent ^{99m}Tc HM-PAO: a SPECT study. J Comput Assist Tomogr 11:398–402, 1987

55. Infeld B, Davis SM, Lichtenstein M et al: Crossed cerebellar diaschisis and brain recovery after stroke. Stroke 26:90–95, 1995

56. Inugami A, Kanno I, Uemura K et al: Linearization correction of ^{99m}Tc-labeled hexamethyl-propylene amine oxime (HM-PAO) image in terms of regional CBF distribution: comparison to $C^{15}O_2$ inhalation steady-state method measured by positron emission tomography. J Cereb Blood Flow Metab 8:S52–S60, 1988

57. Isaka Y, Iloi Y, Imaizumi M et al: Quantification of rCBF by ^{99m}Tc-hexamethylpropyleneamine oxime single photon emission computed tomography combined with ^{133}Xe CBF. J Cereb Blood Flow Metab 14:353–357, 1994

58. Jagust WJ, Budinger TF, Reed BR: The diagnosis of dementia with single photon emission computed tomography. Arch Neurol 44:258–262, 1987

59. Jibiki I, Kubota T, Fujimoto K et al: Regional relationships between focal hyperfixation images in 123I-IMP single photon emission computed tomography and epileptic EEG foci in interictal periods in patients with partial epilepsy. Eur Neurol 31:360–365, 1991

60. Jobst KA, Smith AD, Barker CS et al: Association of atrophy of the medial temporal lobe with reduced blood flow in the posterior parietotemporal cortex in patients with a clinical and pathological diagnosis of Alzheimer's disease. J Neurol Neurosurg Psychiatry 55:190–194, 1992

61. Jørgensen HS, Sperling B, Nakayama H et al: Spontaneous reperfusion of cerebral infarcts in patients with acute stroke. Incidence, time course, and clinical outcome in the Copenhagen Stroke Study. Arch Neurol 51:865–873, 1994

62. Kilpatrick CJ, Davis SM, Hopper JL, Rossiter SC: Early seizures after acute stroke: risk of later seizures. Arch Neurol 49:509–511, 1992

63. Kilpatrick CJ, Davis SM, Tress BM et al: Epileptic seizures in acute stroke. Arch Neurol 47:157–160, 1990

64. Kimura T, Shinoda J, Funakoshi T: Prediction of cerebral infarction due to vasospasm following aneurysmal subarachnoid haemorrhage using acetazolamide-activated 123I-IMP SPECT. Acta Neurochir 123:125–128, 1993

65. Knop J, Thie A, Fuchs C et al: ^{99m}Tc-HMPAO-SPECT with azetazolamide challenge to detect hemodynamic compromise in occlusive cerebrovascular disease. Stroke 23:1733–1742, 1992

66. Kraemer DL, Awad IA: Vascular malformations and epilepsy: clinical considerations and basic mechanisms. Epilepsia 35:S30–43, 1994

67. Kuhl DE, Barrio JR, Huang SC et al: Quantifying local cerebral blood flow by N-isopropyl-p-[^{123}I]iodoamphetamine (IMP) tomography. J Nucl Med 23:196–203, 1982

68. Laloux P, Jamart J, Meurisse H et al: Persisting perfusion defect in transient ischemic attacks. A new clinically useful subgroup? Stroke 27:425–430. 1996

69. Laloux P, Richelle F, Jamart J et al: Comparative correlations of HMPAO SPECT indices, neurological score, and stroke subtypes with clinical outcome in acute carotid infarcts. Stroke 26:816–821, 1995

70. Lassen NA: The luxury-perfusion syndrome and its possible relations to acute metabolic acidosis localised within the brain. Lancet 2:1113–1115, 1966

71. Lassen NA, Sperling B: 99mTc-bicisate reliably images CBF in chronic brain diseases but fails to show reflow hyperemia in subacute stroke: report of a multicenter trial of 105 cases comparing 133Xe and 99mTc-bicisate (ECD, neurolite) measured by SPECT on same day. J Cereb Blood Flow Metab 14:S44–S48, 1994

72. Launes J, Nikkinen P, Lindroth L et al: Brain perfusion defect size in SPECT predicts outcome in cerebral infarction. Nucl Med Commun 10:891–900, 1989

73. Lee RG, Hill TC, Holman BL et al: Predictive value of perfusion defect size using N-isoproyl-(I-123)-p-iodoamphetamine emission tomography in acute stroke. J Neursurg 61:449–452, 1984

74. Leinsinger G, Piepgras A, Einhaupl K et al: Normal values of cerebrovascular reserve capacity after stimulation with acetazolamide measured by xenon 133 single-photon emission CT. AJNR 15:1327–1332, 1994

75. Lewis DH, Eskridge JM, Newell DW et al: Brain SPECT and the effect of cerebral angioplasty in delayed ischemia due to vasospasm. J Nucl Med 33:1789–1796, 1992

76. Limburg M, van Royen EA, Hijdra A et al: Single-photon emission computed tomography and early death in acute ischemic stroke. Stroke 21:1150–1155, 1990

77. Limburg M, van Royen EA, Hijdra A, Verbeeten B Jr: rCBF-SPECT in brain infarction: when does it predict outcome? J Nucl Med 32:382–387, 1991

78. Lisk DR, Grotta JC, Lamki LM et al: Should hypertension be treated after acute stroke? A randomized controlled trial using single photon emission computed tomography. Arch Neurol 50:855–862, 1993

79. Lord RS, Yeates M, Fernandes V et al: Cerebral perfusion defects, dysautoregulation and carotid stenosis. J Cardiovasc Surg 29:670–675, 1988

80. Masdeu JC, Brass LM, Holman BL, Kushner MJ: Brain single-photon emission computed tomography. Neurology 44:1970–1977, 1994

81. Meneghetti G, Vorstrup S, Mickey B et al: Crossed cerebellar diaschisis in ischemic stroke: a study of regional cerebral blood flow by ^{133}Xe inhalation and single photon emission computerized tomography. J Cereb Blood Flow Metab 4:235–240, 1984

82. Moretti JL, Defer G, Cinotti L et al: "Luxury perfusion" with ^{99m}Tc-HMPAO and ^{123}I-IMP SPECT imaging during the subacute phase of stroke. Eur J Nucl Med 16:17–22, 1990

83. Mountz JM: A method of analysis of SPECT blood flow image data for comparison with computed tomography. Clin Nucl Med 14:192–196, 1989

84. Mountz JM, Deutsch G, Khan SH: Regional cerebral blood flow changes in stroke image by Tc-99m HMPAO SPECT with corresponding anatomic image comparison. Clin Nucl Med 18:1067–1082, 1993

85. Nakano S, Kinoshita K, Jinnouchi S et al: Comparative study of regional cerebral blood flow images by SPECT using xenon-133, iodine-123 IMP, and technetium-99m HM-PAO. J Nucl Med 30:157–164, 1989

86. Naderi S, Ozguven MA, Bayham H et al: Evaluation of cerebral vasospasm in patients with subarachnoid hem-

orrhage using single photon emission computed tomography. Neurosurg Rev 17:261–265, 1994

87. Neirinckx RD, Burke JF, Harrison RC et al: The retention mechanism of technetium-99m-HM-PAO: intracellular reaction with glutathione. J Cereb Blood Flow Metab 8:S4–S12, 1988

88. Neirinckx RD, Canning LR, Piper IM et al: Technetium-99m d, 1-HM-PAO: new radiopharmaceutical for SPECT imaging of regional cerebral blood perfusion. J Nucl Med 28:191–202, 1987

89. Newton MR, Berkovic SF, Austin MC et al: Dystonia, clinical lateralization, and regional blood flow changes in temporal lobe seizures. Neurology 42:371–377, 1992

90. O'Brien JT, Eagger S, Syed GM et al: A study of regional cerebral blood flow and cognitive performance in Alzheimer's disease. J Neurol Neurosurg Psychiatry 55: 1182–1187, 1992

91. Overgaard K, Sperling B, Boysen G et al: Thrombolytic therapy in acute ischemic stroke. A Danish pilot study. Stroke 24:1439–1446, 1993

92. Pantano P, Lenzi GL, Guidetti B et al: Crossed cerebellar diaschisis in patients with cerebral ischemia assessed by SPECT and 123I-HIPDM. Eur Neurol 27:142–148, 1987

93. Pantano P, Matteucci C, di Piero V et al: Quantitative assessment of cerebral blood flow in partial epilepsy using Xe-133 inhalation and SPECT. Clin Nucl Med 16: 898:903, 1991

94. Perani D, Di Piero V, Lucignani G et al: Remote effects of subcortical cerebrovascular lesions: a SPECT cerebral perfusion study. J Cereb Blood Flow Metab 8:560–567, 1988

95. Podreka I, Baumgartner C, Suess E et al: Quantification of regional cerebral blood flow with IMP-SPECT. Reproducibility and clinical relevance of flow values. Stroke 20:183–191, 1989

96. Podreka I, Suess E, Goldenberg G et al: Initial experience with technetium-99m HM-PAO Brain SPECT. J Nucl Med 28:1657–1666, 1987

97. Pupi A, De Cristofaro MT, Bacciottini L et al: An analysis of the arterial input curve for technetium-99m-HMPAO: quantification of rCBF using single-photon emission computed tomography. J Nucl Med 32: 1501–1506, 1991

98. Rango M, Candelise L, Perani D et al: Cortical pathophysiology and clinical neurologic abnormalities in acute cerebral ischemia. A serial study with single photon emission computed tomography. Arch Neurol 46: 1318–1322, 1989

99. Rawluk D, Smith FW, Deans HE et al: Technetium 99m HMPAO scanning in patients with subarachnoid haemorrhage: a preliminary study. Br J Radiol 61:26–29, 1988

100. Raynaud C, Rancurel G, Samson Y et al: Pathophysiologic study of chronic infarcts with I-123 isopropyl iodoamphetamine (IMP): the importance of periinfarct area. Stroke 18:21–29, 1987

101. Raynaud C, Rancurel G, Tzourio N et al: SPECT analysis of recent cerebral infarction. Stroke 20:192–204, 1989

102. Rosen JM, Butala AV, Oropello JM et al: Postoperative changes on brain SPECT imaging after aneurysmal subarachnoid hemorrhage. A potential pitfall in the evaluation of vasospasm. Clin Nucl Med 19:595–597, 1994

103. Rowe CC, Berkovic SF, Austin M et al: Postictal SPECT in epilepsy. Lancet 1:389–390, 1989

104. Rowe CC, Berkovic SF, Austin MC et al: Patterns of postictal cerebral blood flow in temporal lobe epilepsy: qualitative and quantitative analysis. Neurology 41: 1096–1103, 1991

105. Savic I, Persson A, Roland P et al: In-vivo demonstration of reduced benzodiazepine receptor binding in human epileptic foci. Lancet 2:863–866, 1988

106. Shimosegawa E, Hatazawa J, Inugami A et al: Cerebral infarction within six hours of onset: prediction of completed infarction with technetium-99m-HMPAO SPECT. J Nucl Med 35:1097–1103, 1994

107. Sperling B, Lassen NA: Hyperfixation of HMPAO in subacute ischemic stroke leading to spuriously high estimates of cerebral blood flow by SPECT. Stroke 24: 193–194, 1993

108. Starkstein SE, Sabe L, Vázquez S et al: Neuropsychological, psychiatric, and cerebral blood flow findings in vascular dementia and Alzheimer's disease. Stroke 27: 408–414, 1996

109. Syed GMS, Eagger S, Toone BK et al: Quantification of regional cerebral blood flow (rCBF) using ^{99m}Tc-HMPAO and SPECT: choice of the reference region. Nucl Med Commun 13:811–816, 1992

110. The National Institute of Neurological Disorders and stroke rt-PA Stroke Study Group: tissue plasminogen activator for acute ischemic stroke. N Engl J Med 333: 1581–1587, 1995

111. Therapeutics and Technology Assessment Subcommittee of the American Academy of neurology: Assessment of brain SPECT. Neurology 46:278–285, 1996

112. Vallar G, Perani D, Cappa SF et al: Recovery from aphasia and neglect after subcortical stroke: neuropsychological and cerebral perfusion study. J Neurol Neurosurg Psychiatry 51:1269–1276, 1988

113. Vorstrup S: Tomographic cerebral blood flow measurements in patients with ischemic cerebrovascular disease and evaluation of the vasodilatory capacity by the acetazolamide test. Acta Neurol Scand, suppl. 114, 77:1–48, 1988

114. Vorstrup S, Paulson OB, Lassen NA: Cerebral blood flow in acute and chronic ischemic stroke using xenon-133 inhalation tomography. Acta Neurol Scand 74: 439–451, 1986

115. Warach S, Dashe JF, Edelman RR: Clinical outcome in ischemic stroke predicted by early diffusion-weighted and perfusion magnetic resonance imaging: a preliminary analysis. J Cereb Blood Flow Metab 16:53–59, 1996

116. Warach S, Li W, Ronthal M, Edelman RR: Acute cerebral ischemia: evaluation with dynamic contrast-enhanced MR imaging and MR angiography. Radiology 182:41–47, 1992

117. Yamauchi H, Fukuyama H, Kimura J et al: Crossed cerebellar hypoperfusion indicates the degree of uncoupling between blood flow and metabolism in major cerebral arterial occlusion. Stroke 25:1945–1951, 1994

SECTION III

Clinical Manifestations of Stroke

J. P. MOHR

This section covers the major stroke syndromes. Emphasis in the overview remains on the issues involved in rapid and accurate differential diagnosis, in keeping with the new developments in therapy. Aids to diagnosis from laboratory techniques are included but the details of the techniques are deferred to the section on diagnostic studies.

In hopes of having in one place many of the clinical points in differential diagnosis, syndromes are described in considerable detail, with reference to many of the original contributors. Notation is made where issues of pathophysiology beyond the scope of earlier investigators have been solved or improved on by current techniques.

Parenchymatous hemorrhage remains one chapter. Malformations now include cavernous angiomas in addition to arteriovenous malformations.

CHAPTER 16

Classification of Ischemic Stroke

RALPH L. SACCO

DANILO TONI

J. P. MOHR

Over the last decade advances in imaging technologies for the brain and blood vessels have improved the diagnostic accuracy of the classification of ischemic stroke. Infarct subtype used to be determined chiefly on clinical grounds, with a heavy reliance on the clinical syndrome, neurologic examination, and coexisting risk factors. In the unfortunate patient who died, autopsy confirmation was often the basis of the classification. With the widespread application of computed tomography (CT), magnetic resonance imaging (MRI), duplex Doppler and transcranial Doppler (TCD), single-photon emission computed tomography, and other diagnostic studies, clinical impressions have been refined and supported by laboratory confirmation of the infarct subtype. Moreover, the evolution of acute stroke therapies aimed at saving brain tissue provided the opportunity to differentiate stroke subtypes in the early hours after stroke onset since the treatment time window was narrow.[115] The need for early differentiation of ischemic subtypes for specific therapies is exemplified by the demonstration of the delicate balance between striking improvement and potentially disastrous hemorrhagic side effects with thrombolysis.[67,141] Excluding patients who have a high likelihood of spontaneous good functional recovery (like those with lacunar infarcts[99,100,147] or those who may be considered less responsive to thrombolysis such as patients with large artery thrombosis[37,150] and selecting those with embolic occlusions of intracranial arteries have become important tasks for the practicing physician.

Forms of Infarction: Bland and Hemorrhagic

When perfusion pressure falls to critical levels, ischemia develops, progressing to infarction if the effect persists long enough. Ischemic infarction is pathologically divided into bland or hemorrhagic infarction. When the cause is thrombus, the usual occlusion persists, preventing reperfusion of the infarcted region and resulting in pale, anemic, or bland infarction.[5] In regions exposed to circulating blood, such as the edge of a bland infarct, widespread leukocyte infiltration occurs within days. For periods of up to several weeks, macrophages invade the infarct and are active for some months until all the products of infarction are carried off. Only scattered red cells are found.

Hemorrhagic infarction, in contrast to the bland form, occurs when varying amounts of red blood cells are found among the necrotic tissues.[13,63] In some cases, the concentration of red blood cells is enough to make a high-density appearance consistent with blood on CT or MRI scan while at autopsy the specimen shows hemorrhagic foci ranging from a few petechiae scattered through the infarct to a mass of confluent petechial foci having almost the appearance of frank hematoma. The timing of hemorrhagic infarction varies widely, as early as a few hours to as late as 2 weeks or more after an arterial occlusion.

The explanation for hemorrhagic infarction has long been thought to result from reperfusion of the vascular bed of the infarct following relief of the occlusion, such as would occur after fragmentation and distal migration of an embolus[57] or after early reopening of a large vessel occlusion in the setting of an established large infarction.[36,133] Presumably, the renewed pressure of arterial blood into capillaries results in a diapedesis of red blood cells through their hypoxic walls. The more intense the reperfusion and the more severely damaged the capillary walls, the more confluent the hemorrhagic infarction. Assuming that hemorrhagic infarction reflects restored lumen patency, it should be a consequence of spontaneous or thrombolytic recanalization of an embolic occlusion, since the occlusion from thrombus would be more difficult to relieve. This hypothesis is supported by the greater frequency of hemorrhagic infarction found among cardioembolic infarcts.[13,15]

More recently, the simple explanation for hemorrhagic infarction given above has been challenged by observations from third-generation CT devices[75,146] and MRI.[74] These studies have demonstrated that hemorrhagic infarction may frequently develop distal to the site of a persisting occlusion in the arterial bed exposed at best only to retrograde collaterals.[103,108] The severity of the hemorrhagic focus may differ from the more or less extended hematoma observed as a consequence of large artery recanalization. In these former cases, the occurrence of petechial, scattered hemorrhagic infarction may be related to surges in arterial blood pressure and the suddenness, severity, and size of the infarction.[13,108,146] It is presumed that edema initially surrounds the large infarct and compresses pial vessels. As edema subsides, retrograde reperfusion through pial collaterals ensues and leads to petechial hemorrhagic infarction.[75,146]

Problems in the Diagnosis of Infarction

Before modern neuroimaging was routinely available, it was the persistent conviction of many physicians that a definite diagnosis as to stroke mechanism was merely a technical problem awaiting the proper laboratory procedures. In most circumstances the clinical features and CT scan suffice to differentiate acute intracerebral hemorrhage from infarction within the first hours after stroke onset. Clinical scores that have been developed to help differentiate infarct from hemorrhage rely on decreased consciousness, headache, and nausea and vomiting as predictors of hemorrhage.[95,109,130,134,149] The present utility of such scales would be to improve diagnoses in studies with no access to CT or to help with early mobilization of stroke teams who are alerted by emergency room personnel of a potential high-probability infarction case. Since small, deep, or lobar hematomas can present with circumscribed focal deficits and can easily lead those relying on the clinical syndrome alone to diagnose infarction mistakenly, these scores can never be relied on for a definitive diagnosis. The advent of CT has led to the correction of these potential misdiagnoses, resulting in a greater proportion of hemorrhages in stroke series[49] and eliminating the inadvertent use of anticoagulation in the case of a masquerading hemorrhage.[42]

For ischemic stroke, the use of CT scan, MRI, noninvasive vascular imaging, and angiography has greatly improved the ability to diagnose stroke, but has still left large issues unresolved. Classification of the ischemic stroke into subtype can now be done well enough to justify the management decisions, but it is far from precise. Clinical grounds alone, using age, risk factors, and so forth, have been the time-honored means of determining the subtype of infarction, such as separating embolism from thrombosis. However, it is often difficult to classify patients by different mechanism of cerebral infarction on clinical criteria alone. A thorough diagnostic workup is required, as the presenting clinical syndromes are usually not distinctive enough to infer the cause. This is even more apparent in the acute setting, when the frequent cognitive impairment, agitation, and poor cooperation of patients may hinder a thorough assessment of neurologic functions.

Even when strenuous efforts are made toward establishing the exact mechanism of infarction, the problem remains difficult. The duplex Doppler, MR angiogram (MRA), or conventional angiogram often fail to show either the expected arterial stenosis or occlusion; also, when a significant carotid stenosis is found, judging whether the clinical syndrome arose from an embolic or hemodynamic mechanism is often difficult.[113] The acute findings on brain imaging may suggest an occlusion of the middle cerebral artery based on the detection of a high attenuation spot along the course of the artery, which has been found in 30% to 50% of cases with angiographically proven arterial occlusion; such findings do not always settle the problem of the underlying mechanism. The identification of early signs of parenchymal damage and brain edema, proved to be useful as a prognostic index,[67,142,148,152] is not that helpful in the differentiation of ischemic pathogenetic mechanisms.

Few studies have collected detailed information on the clinical and radiologic characteristics of large homogeneous subsets of patients with acute cerebral infarction. The Stroke Data Bank provided a large collection of prospectively collected information on patients with different subtypes of infarction.[61] A deliberate attempt was made to classify patients into distinct categories and create new subsets based on the presumed mechanism of infarction. This effort resulted in some changes in the large categories of stroke due to infarction. In particular, the atherothrombosis category was divided into two subgroups: large artery thrombosis with no evidence of embolic infarction and a form of artery-to-artery embolism arising from an atherosclerotic source. A separate category, infarct of undetermined cause, was created to help ensure the homogeneity of the Stroke Data Bank diagnostic groups (Fig. 16.1).

Efforts to establish the diagnosis for the subtype of infarction proved remarkably difficult in a disappointingly high percentage of cases.[126] Despite efforts to arrive at the diagnosis by CT scan or angiogram, it was apparent that the basis for the diagnosis in many of the cases was still a best clinical guess. When laboratory data were available, the results indicated that large artery atherosclerotic occlusive disease was a less frequent cause of stroke; that small vessel or lacunar and cardioembolic infarction were relatively frequent; and that the cause for most cases of infarction could not be classified into these traditional diagnostic categories. The large frequency of surface infarcts in the setting of a normal or distal branch arterial occlusion led most authors to consider these unexplained cerebral infarcts as examples of embolism with an undetected thrombotic source.[47] In the Stroke Data Bank, a separate diagnostic category was created for cases with unproven mechanisms of infarction: infarct of undetermined cause or cryptogenic infarction. Apart from a few common features, infarctions in this category are still poorly understood and have not yet been successfully characterized as a clinical group (Fig. 16.2).

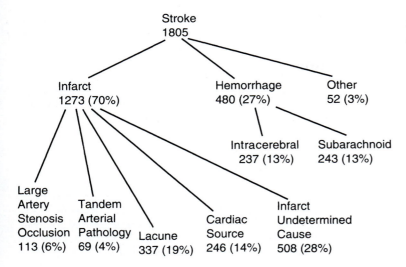

Figure 16.1 Classification of stroke based on data from the NINDS Stroke Data Bank (1983–1986).

Figure 16.2 Stroke diagnostic algorithm. DD, duplex and transcranial Doppler; MRA, magnetic resonance angiography; AG, cerebral angiogram; CT, computed tomography; MRI, magnetic resonance imaging; lac syndrome, currently described classic lacunar syndromes, possibly including other syndromes from focal-deep infarction (e.g., cognitive changes from thalamic or caudate infarcts); AF, atrial fibrillation: AMI, acute myocardial infarction; VHD, valvular heart disease; LV, left ventricular.

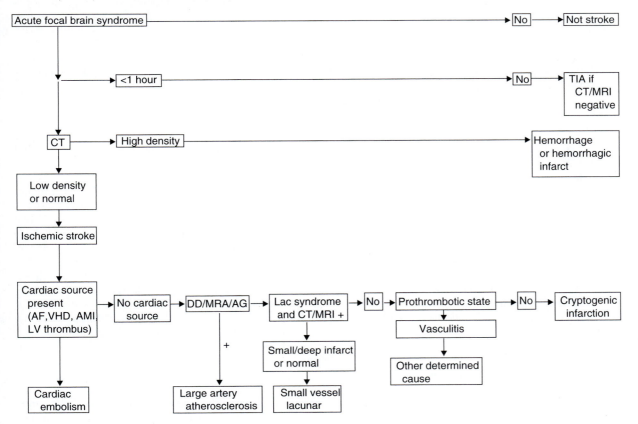

Subtypes of Ischemic Stroke

INFARCT WITH LARGE ARTERY THROMBOSIS

The classification of a stroke patient with an infarction due to large artery thrombosis was sometimes a diagnosis of exclusion in the days of less sophisticated laboratory investigations. Strokes were classified into one of three major diagnostic categories, as follows: hemorrhage if the spinal fluid was bloody, embolism if atrial fibrillation or rheumatic heart disease were present, and thrombosis if the foregoing were not present. Syndromes previously attributed to large artery atherosclerosis, when more closely evaluated with current technology, have been reclassified. The gradual decline in large artery thrombosis as a leading diagnosis has resulted from several factors. Leading among them are the more frequent use of duplex and TCD in the pursuit of stroke diagnosis; the recognition of several clinical subtypes of thrombosis, especially lacunes[8,30,99,145]; documentation proving that some ischemic strokes associated with large artery atherothrombosis are produced by artery-to-artery embolism (local embolism)[45,47,59,77,96]; and discontinuation of the casual classification of a stroke as atherothrombotic in favor of the additional category "undetermined."[17,66,85,102,126]

Many of the descriptions leading to the definition of this subtype stem from pathologic studies of the past.[6] Atherosclerotic lesions were found at bifurcations and curves of the larger vessels, the more proximal the location in the vascular tree the more severe the atherosclerotic lesions.[58,129] Primary occlusion of the arteries distally located over the cerebral surface was rare.[53,101] Atherosclerotic plaque usually led to progressive stenosis with the final large artery occlusion due to thrombosis of the narrowed lumen. Intraplaque hemorrhage sometimes led to accelerated occlusion,[107] although the frequency of this condition is more often a matter of speculation, rather than confirmed in pathologic specimens.[88]

Infarct Mechanism: Perfusion Failure

Stroke in atherothrombus was initially attributed to perfusion failure distal to the site of severe stenosis or occlusion of the major vessel.[16,76,101] In some instances, the major vessel occlusion was rather proximal in the arterial tree, and some degree of collateral flow was interposed between the occlusion and the cerebral territory at risk of infarction.[112] Some cases with interposed collateral were spared infarction of any kind, whereas in others the infarct was located mainly along the most distal brain regions originally supplied by the occluded vessel.[76,101,119,123,139] In the carotid territory, these regions were the suprasylvian frontal, central, and parietal portions of the hemisphere, and in the vertebrobasilar territory, they were the bilateral occipital poles. Internal border zone regions have also been postulated as existing in the white matter of the corona radiata supplied by both superficial middle cerebral artery pial penetrators and lenticulostriate arteries.

The usually accepted mechanism of perfusion failure is more readily accepted in occlusive disease but becomes more difficult to define when, instead, the extracranial vessel is patient but highly stenotic. Some positron emission tomography-based studies have not found supportive evidence for selective hemodynamic impairment among transient ischemic attack (TIA) patients with severe carotid stenosis.[24,113] The development of border zone ischemia is probably dependent on multiple factors, not just the degree of stenosis.[36,114,139]

Infarct Mechanism: Artery-to-Artery Embolism

In addition to vascular occlusion at the site of atherosclerosis, infarcts are also produced by emboli arising from atheromatous lesions situated proximally to otherwise healthy branches located more distal in the arterial tree.[59] Embolic fragments may arise from extracranial arteries affected by stenosis or ulcer[12,33,150]; stenosis of any major cerebral artery stem[2,96] or the basilar artery[27]; the stump of the occluded internal carotid artery[9]; and even from the intracranial tail of the anterograde thrombus atop an occluded carotid.[124] Nowadays embolism from a carotid source has become recognized as another, perhaps more common, cause of stroke in a setting of arterial stenosis and even occlusion.[45,47,77] In the Stroke Data Bank, this mechanism of infarction was labeled tandem arterial pathology. In more recent stroke series, border zone infarcts appear to be less frequent than previously thought, leading to the presumption that embolism was the actual mechanism even in the presence of internal carotid artery tight stenoses or occlusions. To add to the difficulty in distinguishing between these two mechanisms of infarction, cases of perfusion failure due to embolism have been demonstrated. Internal border zone infarcts have been demonstrated after embolic occlusion of MCA pial branches.[4] This may represent an example of an embolic stroke with a possible local hemodynamic effect as the final mechanism of the infarct.

Clinical Features

Focal cortical syndromes are usually found in this group, but syndromes often attributed to lacunar disease such as pure motor or sensorimotor stroke can easily represent the first sign of impending flow failure.[148] Discriminating between infarct subtypes on clinical grounds alone is difficult. To determine some of these distinguishing clinical features in the Stroke Data Bank, demographic, stroke risk, clinical, and radiologic features were compared between the 246 cardioembolic and the 113 large vessel atherosclerotic cerebral infarcts.[143] The Stroke Data Bank definitions ensured more TIAs in atherosclerotic infarcts and more cardiac disease in cardioembolic infarcts, but the diagnosis was distinguished further. Cases with fractional arm weakness (shoulder different from the hand), hypertension, diabetes, and male gender occurred more frequently in atherosclerotic than cardioembolic infarcts. Patients with atherosclerotic infarcts were more likely to have a fractional arm weakness regardless of infarct size.

Distinguishing between the infarct mechanisms (hemodynamic versus embolism) among patients with large artery disease is quite difficult even for the most astute clinician. The sudden mode of onset may suggest, but does not confirm, a diagnosis of embolism.[51] Other clinical features may be indistinguishable. Moreover, it is even more difficult to discriminate between embolisms from a cardiac source and those from an arterial source. Comparisons in the NINDS Stroke Data Bank between the 246 cardioembolic and 66 arterial embolic patients with cerebral infarction demonstrated some differences.[142] Even after controlling for differences in the frequency of cardiac disease, TIAs, and carotid bruits, the probability of an artery-to-artery embolism was increased by the finding of a superficial infarct alone or by a higher hematocrit. The probability of cardiac embolism was greater with an initial decreased consciousness or with an abnormal first CT. These findings suggested that these two embolic infarct subtypes differed in location and extent of the cortical infarction. Smaller and more distal infarction in embolism from an arterial source compared with cardiogenic embolism suggested a smaller embolic particle size. Clinical features observed at stroke onset can help distinguish cerebral infarction subtypes but are not reliable enough to lead to a definite determination of infarct subtype without confirmatory laboratory data.

Results of Diagnostic Tests

BRAIN IMAGING. The only abnormalities on MRI or CT scan directly attributable to cerebral infarction from carotid artery thrombosis are those that can be interpreted to reflect the distal field effect along the border zone between middle and anterior cerebral territories, especially on the middle cerebral side.[16,101,122] This topographic pattern involves the suprasylvian frontal and central regions, shading toward normal in the parieto-occipital region, sparing the region of the sylvian fissure (operculum, insula) and the penetrating territories of the lenticulostriates. The centripetal spread in more severe cases may involve so much of the hemisphere that a differentiation from embolism to the middle cerebral artery stem is impossible.

CT and MRI scans are of help in supporting a diagnosis of embolism when an infarct in the territories of large cerebral arteries or their branches is detected[121] or when a hyperdense spot along the course of the middle cerebral artery is seen,[119] but not in inferring embolism source from the neck. When occlusions involve the territories of the anterior, middle, or posterior cerebral artery, or the basilar artery territory, brain imaging cannot distinguish between thrombosis and embolism if the scan shows low density only in the proximal fields of the arterial territory.

VASCULAR IMAGING. In the clinical setting, for a diagnosis of large artery atherosclerotic occlusive disease, angiography and Doppler scanning remain the most important laboratory tests. On conventional cerebral angiogram, the occlusion of the internal carotid at its origin or in the siphon has the appearance of a pencil point, blunt end, smooth end, or shoulder, with the intracranial portion of the internal carotid or major cerebral artery stems and branches open.[111] Spiral occlusions of the extracranial portion of the internal carotid beyond 2 cm of its origin (a finding consistent with dissection)[116] helps to indicate that the carotid lesion may be the source of the stroke, but not by means of atherosclerosis. Because of the risks of cerebral angiography,[40,68,89] there has been increased reliance on duplex Doppler and TCD to show no or highly resistant flow in the extracranial carotid with dampened pulsatility in the ipsilateral middle cerebral artery.[22,39,65,68,137,154,157] MRA and CT angiography are quickly becoming reliable diagnostic tools for the detection of extracranial and intracranial large artery stenosis and have led to less reliance on conventional angiography.[96]

No satisfactory criteria have yet been developed to certify that a stroke is caused by extracranial arterial disease through the mechanism of embolism. The mechanism is inferred when the clinical syndrome suggests a cortical branch territory; when no obvious cardioembolic source is present and the degree of stenosis is <80% (which would not explain the stroke on the grounds of hemodynamic insufficiency); or when ulcerative plaque is imaged by noninvasive duplex Doppler, MRA or cerebral angiogram.

On the other hand, although angiographic evidence of intracranial occlusion above a carotid stenosis or ulcer is not proof of the source; when present it serves to classify this type of stroke into the present category.[112] The frequency of occurrence of embolism of particles large enough to cause stroke and the variety or severity of carotid lesions giving rise to such embolization remain poorly understood. In a continuous series of patients angiogrammed within the first 6 hours of stroke onset,[47] middle cerebral artery stem or branch occlusion accounted for 60% of the cases. Possible embolic sources included carotid plaque (19%), an occlusion of the ipsilateral internal carotid artery (14%), and a potential source of emboli both arterial and cardiac (27%). Conversely, 58% of patients with internal carotid artery occlusion had a tandem middle cerebral artery occlusion. Despite a normal intracranial arterial tree, the remainder had a territorial infarct on CT, which implied that an artery-to-artery embolism occurred with embolus fragmentation preceding angiography.

Intracranial atherosclerotic artery stem stenoses or occlusions may be due to arteriosclerotic thrombosis but are often difficult to distinguish from embolisms of any extracerebral source.[26,28,140] If one or more appropriate TIAs occurred within the past 30 days, the diagnosis of thrombus may be correct, but the matter can only be settled if a widely patent lumen is subsequently found by serial transcranial Doppler or repeat angiogram.[35] The latter is diagnostic of embolism, while persistence of the occlusion leaves the mechanism unsettled.

Basilar occlusion on angiogram is usually considered the mechanism for brain stem stroke even though in many such cases the clinical syndrome fits the criteria for lacune,[20,21,25,27] since the territory of infarction, however small, is in the field of supply of a vessel thrombosed by the major basilar atheroma.[52] Similar to the case of the carotid, the finding of stenosis of the basilar prevents a definite diagnosis as to the mechanism of infarction, since infarcts more distal in the vertebrobasilar territory might well be the result of distal embolization.[26] Atheromatous disease of the basilar often affects the vessel at sites where local branches directly supply brain tissue.[19,52] In the case of the carotid, the atheroma involves the vessel proximal to the point where its branches supply the brain.[129] When the clinical syndrome of basilar stroke can be localized to the point of the stenosis, infarction may be caused by mural atheroma that only slightly stenoses the basilar but totally occludes a small penetrator departing from the basilar at that point.

This point, established in a few instances by autopsy, can only be inferred in cases studied by angiogram; CT scanning is usually not of technically high enough quality to detect the small brain stem infarcts. However, MRI scanning has defined the lesion and permitted better delineation of such cases.

Blood flow techniques have also helped to confirm the perfusion failure mechanism in cases with atherosclerotic stenosis or occlusive disease through single-photon emission CT,[70] xenon CT,[79] regional cerebral blood flow,[108] MRI,[43] and positron emission tomography.[10,113,132] The more widespread use of these techniques should allow for more accurate distinction between embolism and perfusion failure in the clinical setting.

EMBOLISM ATTRIBUTED TO CARDIAC SOURCES

Embolism from any source probably accounts for between 15% and 70% of all ischemic stroke cases,[17,47,61,85,102] many of which occur from embolism into the territory of the middle cerebral artery. Although the subject of embolism seems clear enough, in that a particle is swept through the blood stream until it jams in an artery too small to allow it to pass, the many complexities of the embolic process make it anything but easy to account for on a case by case basis.

The biggest clinical problem in arriving at a diagnosis of embolism is identifying the source. Embolism was diagnosed in earlier studies mainly when a cardiac source (atrial fibrillation with valvular disease) was obvious.[6] The results of more recent studies have shown that emboli, diagnosed angiographically by isolated branch occlusions, may occur despite all efforts to identify the source.[23,47,102,125] Given the many possibilities and given the traditional use of the term *embolism* to refer to a cardiac source,[29,71,91,131] the following discussion is limited to that subject.

Properties of Emboli

The instability of the embolic material is a point of prime importance in clinical and angiographic analysis of cases of embolism. Mural thrombi and platelet aggregates are the most frequent materials embolized to the brain. This material is remarkably evanescent, as has been repeatedly inferred by findings on angiogram. Embolic fragments are found in >75% of cases angiogrammed within 8 hours of onset of the stroke,[18,47] whereas embolism is demonstrated in 40% of clinically identical cases when angiogram is delayed for up to 72 hours from clinical onset of the stroke[48] and falls to only 15% after 72 hours. These decreasing proportions imply that embolic occlusions are liable to spontaneous recanalization in a sizable number of cases. Serial studies with TCD demonstrated a recanalization of middle cerebral artery mainstem or branch occlusions in up to 52% of cases within the first 48 hours of stroke.[82,155] Repeat angiography, performed in subsets of patients with arterial occlusion at an earlier angiogram, showed recanalization in approximately 30% to 60% of cases.[35,47]

No reliable means have been developed thus far to predict which embolic occlusions will persist and which will disappear, although it is inferred that the more friable materials will disperse more rapidly. In one of the TCD studies mentioned, patients with an arterial source of emboli recanalized less frequently than those with a cardiac source, suggesting a different composition or size of emboli.[155] The size of the emboli is also probably responsible, at least in part, for the highest frequency of both spontaneous[155] and pharmacologic[37,104,120,151] recanalization in cases of distal middle cerebral artery occlusion.

This evanescent quality of embolic material may explain the wide variation in the frequency with which embolism is diagnosed in retrospective or prospective studies of stroke. The size of the material embolized determines the site it initially arrests in the circulation, but it does not determine its final point of arrest. Embolic material arrests where the lumen diameter is too small to permit the material to pass. Bifurcations or foci of atheroma at curves in the artery are the two sites where emboli arrest. Fibrin-platelet complexes and those also laden with bacteria vary considerably in size; some are so huge that they have obstructed the stem of the middle cerebral artery[62] and others have been so small they have lodged asymptomatically in a sensitive region like the Rolandic artery. Calcific plaques have only rarely been described as producing large embolic strokes[33,156]; more often, they seem to produce TIAs, but not persisting cerebral deficits.[12] For noncompressible objects such as shotgun pellets, the site of embolus can easily be predicted by its size.[82] For the more common fibrin-platelet complexes, however, other factors are involved, especially the poorly understood compressibility of the mass and the time required to transit a certain point of narrowing in the arterial tree. The few cases that document the passage of fibrin-platelet emboli through the arterial tree[92] show considerable alteration in the length and width of the material at different points, indicating it possesses a remarkable elasticity and friability. What is sufficient lumen reduction to arrest the material may not be enough to keep it from changing shape or fragmenting within minutes to hours, leaving the site of the original embolic occlusion widely patent.

Embolic obstruction of an arterial lumen is cleared most commonly by recanalization with fibrinolysis. A column of blood develops between the embolus and the arterial wall, enlarges, and erodes the embolus until the lumen is finally cleared. The exact sequence of events is not fully understood in human material, but cases documented at different stages during the process make it clear that it is accomplished within periods as short as hours to days.[92,120,156] The timetable for this process is also poorly understood. In some instances, the erosion takes enough time that noninvasive studies may document stenoses that create turbulence identical to those seen with atheroma. From the angiographic appearance, the gradually eroding embolus is indistinguishable from that found in atherostenosis. During this process, the lumen may appear stenotic.[78,93]

At the site of occlusion, opportunity exists for thrombus to develop anterogradely throughout the length of the vessel, but this event seems to occur only rarely. Lack of anterograde thrombus implies either that an active flow is present proximal to the occlusion or that the occlusion was too short-lived to permit the development of the anterograde thrombus. At autopsy it is common to find the vessel distended by the embolus, yet the histologic appearance of the wall at that point usually shows no significant abnormalities. The frequent finding that the vessel wall itself is not significantly injured by the embolus argues against a role for endothelial injury, vasospasm, or necrotizing effects in the pathogenesis of the infarction from embolism.

Clinical Features

It was once taught that the sudden onset of a clinical deficit was typical of embolism and that a non-sudden onset would be more typical of thrombosis. Numerous case examples have now amply demonstrated that a sudden onset may occur in either condition. Non-sudden or fluctuating onset occurs in 5% to 6% of documented embolic strokes, the syndrome often requiring 36 hours or so to evolve.[60,101] A clinical diagnosis of multiple TIAs is often entertained. The re-establishment of flow, presumed further migration of embolic material, and subsequent repeat of these events are thought to be the mechanisms involved. Embolic material has even been documented to go to the same site on repeated occasions,[153] the opposite of traditional predictions.

In the past, many syndromes were considered almost specific for embolism. In each of these syndromes, it was assumed the infarct was so focal and so far distal in the arterial tree that local atheroma was not a serious possibility. Hemianopia without hemiparesis or hemisensory disturbances, Wernicke's aphasia, ideomotor apraxia, and involvement of specific territories (the posterior division of the middle cerebral artery, the anterior cerebral artery, the cerebellum, multiple territories) were more frequently associated with the presence of a potential cardiac source of embolism in the Lausanne Stroke Registry.[15] CT and MRI scanning have shown that any of these syndromes may arise from hematoma, and modern neurologists have become wary of anticoagulation therapy based on clinical syndrome analysis alone.

One syndrome seems to have held its own as a sign of embolism, although it is met only rarely. A spectacular shrinking deficit can occur when the embolus is introduced into the internal carotid, causing a profound full hemisphere syndrome, after which it passes up the internal carotid to its final resting place in, say, the angular branch of the middle cerebral artery, leaving only a mild aphasia after a few days or a week.[98] Especially characteristic of the middle cerebral artery migratory embolism is the syndrome of fading hemiparesis with Wernicke's aphasia: the embolus lodges initially at the stem of the middle cerebral artery, occluding the penetrating lenticulostriate branches long enough to produce scattered foci of infarction through the basal ganglia and internal capsule, the involvement of the latter producing the hemiparesis. Distal migration of the embolus then occurs, finally occluding the lower division of the middle cerebral artery at the superior temporal plane and beyond. This infarct yields Wernicke's aphasia. Two separate foci of infarction occur, but both result from the same embolic event.

The cardiac history of the patient often provides important clues about a potential embolic source. In the Stroke Data Bank, besides a greater frequency of cardiac disease, patients with cardioembolic infarction more often presented with reduced consciousness.[142,143] Cardioembolic infarcts were more likely to have nonfractional arm weakness, except for those with infarctions of <20 ml, in which fractional weak-

ness was more frequent. In a separate Stroke Data Bank analysis, a history of systemic embolism and an abrupt onset were historical features significantly associated with cardiac sources of embolism.[83] Clinical features observed at stroke onset help to distinguish the cardioembolic group from other subtypes, but the diagnosis largely depends on confirmatory laboratory findings suggesting a definite cardiac source of embolism.[117]

Results of Diagnostic Tests

The role of CT and MRI scans in the diagnosis of embolism is limited. Only when the infarction is confined to the cerebral surface territory of a single branch can embolism be inferred. Infarcts involving branches of different divisions of major cerebral arteries strongly suggest that embolism explains at least some of the clinical strokes that have occurred. A diagnosis of embolism is suggested by a large zone of low density that encompasses what amounts to the entire territory of a major cerebral artery or its main divisions and is larger than one lobe in size. Embolism is also the leading diagnosis when hemorrhagic infarction is seen on brain imaging.[13,15] However, while this assumption is plausible in the presence of a more or less extended hematoma, as already mentioned it may not be true for other cases displaying petechial, scattered high density along the margins or in the infarct zone.[75,146] In some 30% to 50% of cases, the CT (or MRI) may show the occlusion itself, by the presence of this hyperdense middle cerebral artery sign.

Angiography was once considered sufficient to diagnose embolism from any source if the angiogram showed branch occlusion in the absence of other occlusive disease elsewhere.[14,34,35,119] This rule still holds for practical purposes, but isolated branch occlusions may occur in arteritis, and increasing evidence is showing that intracranial atherosclerosis is common enough in some races, especially blacks, that middle cerebral artery stem occlusions may be atheromatous as well as embolic. Recanalizing embolus may mimic all the angiographic features of atherosclerosis.[78] Only when the angiogram is repeated within days of the one demonstrating occlusion, and the initial occlusion is gone, can a diagnosis of embolism be made with confidence. Measures this extreme are impractical for the management of most patients.

In the presence of a cardiac source, the diagnosis is certain for all practical purposes. Establishing the cardiac source is not always a simple task. The most common sources of cardiac embolism include valvular heart disease (mitral stenosis, mitral regurgitation, rheumatic heart disease); intracardiac thrombus particularly along the left ventricular wall (mural thrombus) after anterior myocardial infarction or in the left atrial appendage in patients with atrial fibrillation; ventricular or septal aneurysm; and cardiomyopathies leading to stagnation of blood flow and an increased propensity for the formation of intracardiac thrombus. A paradoxical embolus occurs when a thrombus crosses from the venous circulation to the left side of the heart, most often through a patent foramen ovale. Other possible causes of cardiac embolism are atrial myxoma, atrial septal aneurysm, spontaneous echo contrast, marantic endocarditis, and prolapse of the mitral valve.

The cardiac diagnostic evaluation starts with an electrocardiogram to look for atrial fibrillation, acute myocardial infarction, or other arrhythmias. Holter monitoring for 24 hours is sometimes necessary to detect paroxysmal atrial fibrillation. Identification of the cardiac source is most dependent on transthoracic and transesophageal echocardiography, which has become more sensitive and greatly improved the detection of sources of embolism. Bubble contrast is needed to diagnose a patent foramen ovale. Unfortunately, the size of the embolic material sufficient to produce a focal stroke is so small that it may escape detection by echocardiography and all too often eludes all efforts at diagnosis. Future advances in cardiac imaging may help to increase our sensitivity for detecting cardiac sources of embolism.

LACUNAR INFARCTION

Cases of lacunar infarction represent a special group that warrants description because they often occur as a common set of clinical syndromes, the angiogram is usually negative, and the zone of ischemia is confined to the territory of a single vessel, usually quite small. They are understood to reflect arterial disease of the vessels penetrating the brain to supply the capsule, basal ganglia, thalamus, and paramedian regions of the brain stem.[55] Only a handful have been studied by autopsy, and an even smaller number have been subjected to serial section.[56] The most frequent lesion is a tiny focus of microatheroma or lipohyalinosis stenosing one of the deep penetrating arteries. Less frequent causes include stenosis of the middle cerebral artery stem[5,72] or microembolization to penetrant arterial territories.[56]

More recently, investigators have used the term *lacunar hypothesis* to refer to the clinicopathophysiologic correlation of the condition. The hypothesis consists of two parts: (1) symptomatic lacunes are usually present with a small number of distinct lacunar syndromes, and (2) lacunes are caused by a characteristic disease of the penetrating artery.[8] After satisfying both parts of the hypothesis, then the stroke can be classified as lacunar infarction. Lacunes were slow to gain clinical acceptance, but they are now considered to account for between 15% and 20% of all cases of stroke.[17,61,66,85,99,127,145]

Clinical Features

The diagnosis of lacunar strokes has long been based on clinical characteristics alone, a practice that has contributed little to their popularity among clinical researchers in the field. The term *lacunar syndrome* refers to the constellation of clinical features that may indicate, although not invariably, a lacune. The characteristic features of all these syndromes are their relative purity and their failure to involve higher cerebral functions such as language, praxis, behavior controlled by the nondominant hemisphere, memory, and vision.[105] The classic lacunar syndromes include pure motor, pure sensory, sensorimotor, ataxic hemiparesis, clumsy hand dysarthria, and hemichorea/hemiballism. However, other combinations of findings may be attributed to small, deep infarcts due to a lacunar mechanism. Efforts to expand the diagnosis into new formulae that account for the presence of cognitive changes have shaken the earlier purity and confounded the appealing simplicity of the initial syndromes,[54] leading some to question the separate nosologic identity of lacunar infarcts.[86,97] Some skeptics have suggested the abolition of terms like lacunar syndrome, la-

cune, and lacunar infarction because of confusion. However, most of the investigations that have included analyses of clinical syndromes, results of diagnostic imaging, etiopathophysiologic correlations, and treatment implications justify the continued use of the term lacune.

The correspondence between lacunar syndrome and lacunar infarction is dependent on the timing of presentation and examination. The concordance is greatest among patients examined up to 96 hours after stroke onset[7,8] and is much less when patients are tested in the first few hours of stroke onset.[17,31,45] There are clearly examples of thrombotic or embolic infarcts presenting as pure motor hemiparesis or sensorimotor stroke, and, conversely, large lacunar infarcts in the caudate nucleus or thalamus that may initially present with impairment of higher cerebral functions. The latter syndromes are probably due to a reversible functional disconnection between the subcortical infarcted areas and their cortical projections.[110,136] In the acute setting, therefore, the reliance on clinical grounds alone for the identification of lacunar infarcts can be misleading for both prognostic estimates and therapeutic choices.[147]

Using data from the Northern Manhattan Stroke Study, we were able to evaluate the value of lacunar syndromes in predicting radiologic lacunes, as well as the value of clinicoradiologic lacunes in predicting lacunar infarction as a final stroke mechanism.[64] Lacunar syndromes were found in 225 of 591 patients and the proportions of lacunar infarction in blacks and Hispanics were nearly twice that in whites. The positive predictive value for finding a small, deep infarct on brain imaging after a presenting lacunar syndrome was 87% and was best for pure sensory syndrome (100%) and ataxic hemiparesis (95%), intermediate for sensorimotor syndrome (87%), and least for pure motor hemiparesis (79%). Among the 195 patients who presented with a lacunar syndrome and who were confirmed radiologically to have a small deep infarct, 147 were classified with a final diagnosis of lacunar infarct mechanism (positive predictive value 75%). Extracranial or intracranial atherosclerosis accounted for 16 (8%), cardioembolism for 10 (5%), cryptogenic causes for 19 (10%), and other causes for 3 (2%). It was concluded that lacunar syndromes, especially pure sensory syndrome and ataxic hemiparesis, were highly predictive of small deep infarcts; however, about one in four patients presenting with lacunar syndromes confirmed radiologically may ultimately be proved to have a nonlacunar infarct mechanism. A complete diagnostic evaluation of large vessels and potential cardiogenic sources of embolism is warranted in these patients.

Results of Diagnostic Tests

CT scanning is positive only for roughly half of even the most common form of lacune, pure motor stroke.[30,99,118] Visualizing lacunes depends on their location, and MRI is clearly superior to CT in evaluating lesions, especially in the posterior fossa. Overall, MRI has increased the yield of finding a strategically placed small, deep infarct.[73] In the Northern Manhattan Stroke Study, using either CT or MRI, we were able to detect radiologically small deep infarcts in appropriate locations in 84% of our cases of lacunar syndromes. The radiologic equivalent of a lacune was defined as a small deep lesion on brain imaging usually <1 cm in diameter with a density or signal consistent with an infarct located in the appropriate area of the brain to explain the syndrome, or the absence of a responsible lesion despite a repeat scan. The latter definition is based on the fact that some lacunes are too small to be seen on CT or MRI despite a repeat scan.

Large deep infarcts, some of which have been called super lacunes or giant lacunes, may be seen by CT or MRI scan as a focal, deep site of infarction without involvement of the cerebral surface.[118] A problem arises in the interpretation of these deep lesions, since an embolus may initially be arrested in the stem of the middle cerebral artery, causing a large swath of infarction scattered through the lenticulostriate territories. When accompanied by a separate cerebral surface low density, such large deep infarcts are easily reclassified as examples of embolism, nonthrombotic infarction, or infarction of other cause. Therefore, most of these large, deep infarcts are really not lacunes.

In cases with pure motor hemiparesis, lacunes can be most frequently found in the internal capsule and corona radiata, but they have also been imaged in the basal ganglia, pons, and thalamus. Positive scans in the capsule, adjacent corona radiata, thalamus, or pons have been reported on occasion for the ataxic-hemiparesis, dysarthria-clumsy hand syndrome and hemiballism.[30,135] Pure sensory strokes have been reported from small thalamic infarcts, some so small as to cause selective proprioceptive loss without pain or temperature deficits.[125] Reports of pure sensory stroke from low densities in the centrum semiovale are probably lacunar, although rarely surface infarction has been demonstrated.[38]

Because the vascular lesion lies in vessels some 200 to 400 μm in diameter, it is perhaps no surprise that conventional cerebral angiogram and MRA are normal. Incidental large vessel disease may be found in some series, but whether it is etiologically related to the site of infarction is often unclear.[30] A normal angiogram could also be expected if microembolism was the cause of the deep infarction. Whether the outlook for stenosis of the middle cerebral artery stem or the basilar artery differs if the syndrome is lacunar or not remains unsettled. Because some of the cases of pure motor stroke have been associated with middle cerebral artery stenosis, the mere presence of a such a syndrome has not been an indicator of the status of the major artery in question. TCD of the middle cerebral artery stem or basilar artery has helped to establish the patency of these large vessels. MRA or conventional angiography may be required to settle the matter in some cases, and it remains our technique when the TCD is technically unsatisfactory and the CT or MRI scan shows a large band of low density, one spanning several sections, and one whose abnormality is seen down to the base of the affected basal ganglia.[118] Such a large infarct is not easily accounted for by primary disease in the penetrating artery itself, justifying angiography to seek stenosis of the middle cerebral artery stem. The prognosis for later hemispheral symptoms in cases with stem stenosis presenting as a lacunar infarct is unknown.

CRYPTOGENIC INFARCTION OR INFARCT OF UNDETERMINED CAUSE

Despite efforts to arrive at a diagnosis, the cause of the infarction may remain undetermined. A number of explanations can be offered. The first of the three major reasons for the failure is easily understood: no appropriate laboratory studies are performed. Advanced age, coexisting severe disease with a poor prognosis, and patient or physician unwillingness are only a few of the many reasons for deferring a workup. One reason no longer valid for this approach is that the mechanism of stroke has been diagnosed satisfactorily on clinical grounds alone. Among the syndromes attributed to ischemia, only the Wallenberg syndrome has yet to be reported from hematoma, and causes other than stroke have been so often reported with most of the classical focal brain syndromes that the point need not be labored.

A second common cause for failure to arrive at a diagnosis is improper timing of the appropriate laboratory studies. Angiograms for embolism performed >48 hours after the ictus have a yield as low as 15% for evidence of the responsible occlusion.[18] Brain scans performed once only within a few hours of the onset of an ischemic stroke have a similarly low yield. Brain scans performed no matter how often may remain negative in some cases of small lacunar infarction, when the lesion is below the limits of resolution of the scan technique.

As many as 40% of the cases of ischemic stroke of undetermined cause fall into the third category, in which normal or ambiguous findings are reached despite appropriate laboratory studies performed at the appropriate time. This last group of cases poses special problems for research in stroke diagnosis. It would be comforting should most of these cases fall among those with the milder deficits, perhaps accounting for the negative laboratory studies by virtue of the relative insensitivity of such tests to smaller lesions. However, the scanty data on the subject indicate they are not: they are roughly as severe as ischemic strokes for which a cause is found.

In the Stroke Data Bank, a rigorous diagnostic scheme resulted in a high frequency of infarcts that were difficult to classify into the traditional subtypes. Despite considerable effort at workup, there remained a large percentage, fully 40%, for whom the infarct mechanism escaped explanation and that were classified as infarcts of undetermined cause.[61,126] Not all patients in the Stroke Data Bank were angiogrammed and when it was done it was rarely in the first 48 to 72 hours after stroke. In other series in which patients were angiogrammed within 6 hours of stroke onset,[47] the application of the same diagnostic scheme as that of the Stroke Data Bank has led to a reduction in the number of cases labeled as strokes of undetermined cause to only 15%.

Clinical Features

Cases categorized as ischemic stroke of undetermined cause show no bruit or TIA ipsilateral to the hemisphere affected by stroke and have no obvious source of embolism; in short, they do not have the risk factors or prior history that help to suggest a cardiac embolus or large artery thrombosis.[85,126] In the Stroke Data Bank, the mean age at stroke for infarcts of undetermined cause studied by CT and angiogram was 58 years.[126] Hemispheral syndromes predominated in 66%; basilar syndromes occurred in 15%. Very few have lacunar syndromes. Twenty-seven percent worsened in the hospital, and 41% had a moderate to severe weakness score.

Results of Diagnostic Tests

The CT or MRI scan performed within 7 days may be normal, may show an infarct limited to a surface branch territory, or may show a large zone of infarction affecting regions larger than that accounted for by a single penetrant arterial territory. In the Stroke Data Bank, among those cryptogenic infarcts fully evaluated, CT demonstrated clinically relevant infarcts in 57%; surface infarction was found in 40%.[126] Noninvasive vascular imaging fails to demonstrate an underlying large vessel occlusion or stenosis. No definite cardiac source of embolism is uncovered by echocardiography, electrocardiography, or Holter monitor.

If an angiogram is performed, the study may be normal, or may show a distal branch occlusion or occlusion of a major cerebral artery stem or the top of the basilar. Because middle cerebral artery stem or branch occlusions can be from thrombotic or embolic causes, their demonstration does not settle the mechanism in all cases, particularly among blacks, Asians, and Hispanics, in whom intracranial atheroma has been more frequently detected.[127] In white patients, on the other hand, pathologic examination of middle cerebral artery occlusion rarely demonstrated an organized thrombus,[80,91] so the angiographic identification of an intracranial occlusion may usually be considered typical for embolism despite the absence of a source.[47] In the most extreme case, in which angiography is repeated and the original occlusion is no longer found, a definitive diagnosis of embolism can be made.

Potential Explanations of Cryptogenic Stroke

Some examples of the forms of stroke attributed to meningitis, migraine, lupus anticoagulant, arteritis, dissection, hypercoaguable states, and the like may be represented in the cryptogenic subgroup. Efforts should be made in each case to establish the existence of these unusual causes, and all such instances should be identified and classified as cerebral infarction from *Other determined cause*. Adding together all the estimated frequencies with which such unusual causes present without accompanying evidence of the underlying disease cannot remotely approach the high frequency of the cryptogenic subgroup of stroke documented in the Stroke Data Bank.

Emerging technologies have led to the suggestions that some of the cryptogenic infarct cases may be explained by hematologic disorders causing hypercoaguable states from protein C, free protein S, lupus anticoagulant, or anticardiolipin antibody abnormalities. Others have implicated paradoxical emboli through a patent faramen ovale[41,46,87] or emboli from the ascending tract of the aortic arch,[3] which have both been better identified with the more widespread use of transesophageal echocardiography. The number of cases of cryptogenic infarction attributed to the lack of appropriate diagnostic examinations mentioned above should diminish as newer and more sensitive diagnostic techniques are introduced.

One approach to dealing with this cohort of cases is their forced reclassification into the traditional categories of atherothrombosis, embolism, or lacune. The presentation of a hemispheral syndrome, a surface infarction shown by CT, and a corresponding branch occlusion documented by angiography or normal angiogram has long been considered suggestive of embolism. Nonthrombotic ischemia has been used to describe those cases with normal angiograms. Such findings could be inferred to represent emboli, even though no cardiac source for embolism is documented by clinical or laboratory criteria. Ample evidence exists of many occult sources of emboli, the difficulty in proving their existence, and their role in the first or succeeding ischemic strokes. Reclassification of such cases (and others with limited cerebral infarction seen on CT scan) as embolism with inobvious source would add most of the cryptogenic infarct patients to the embolism category, making embolism from all sources the largest subtype of stroke.[47,126] Alternatively, maintaining a separate category of cryptogenic strokes is useful to determine if this group of cases differs in some way from those in which the mechanism of stroke is better defined and to encourage the continued search for causes of brain infarction and precipitants of thromboembolism.

References

1. Adams RD, Fisher CM: Pathology of Cerebral Arterial Occlusion. In Fields WS (ed): Houston Symposium on Pathogenesis and Treatment of Cerebrovascular Disease. Charles C Thomas, Springfield, IL, 1961
2. Adams HP, Gross CE: Embolism distal to stenosis of the middle cerebral artery. Stroke 12:228, 1981
3. Amarenco P, Duyckaerts C, Tzourioc et al: The prevalence of ulcerated plaques in the aortic arch in patients with stroke. N Engl J Med 326:221–225, 1992
4. Angeloni U, Bozzao L, Fantozzi L et al: Fieschi C. Internal border zone infarction following acute middle cerebral artery occlusion. Neurology 40:1196–1198, 1990
5. Araki G: Small infarctions of the basal ganglia with special reference to transient ischemic attacks. Recent Adv Gerontol 469:161, 1978
6. Aring CD, Merritt HH: Differential diagnosis between cerebral hemorrhage and cerebral thrombosis. Arch Intern Med 56:435, 1935
7. Bamford J, Sandercock P, Dennis M et al: Classification and natural history of clinically identifiable subtypes of cerebral infarction. Lancet 337:1521–1526, 1991
8. Bamford JM, Warlow CP: Evolution and testing of the lacunar hypothesis. Stroke 19:1074–1082, 1988
9. Barnett HJM, Peerless SJ, Kaufmann JCE: "Stump" of internal carotid artery—a source for further cerebral embolic ischemia. Stroke 9:448, 1978
10. Baron JC, Frackowiak RS, Herholz K et al: Use of PET methods for measurement of cerebral energy metabolism and hemodynamics in cerebrovascular disease. J Cereb Blood Flow Metab 9:723–742, 1989
11. Bastianello S, Pierallini A, Colonnese C et al: Hyperdense middle cerebral artery CT sign. Comparison with angiography in the acute phase of ischemic supratentorial infarction. Neuroradiology 33:207–211, 1991
12. Beal MF, Williams RS, Richardson EP, Fisher CM: Cerebral embolism as a cause of transient ischemic attacks and cerebral infarction. Neurology (NY) 31:860, 1981

13. Beghi E, Bogliun G, Cavaletti G et al: Hemorrhagic infarction: risk factors, clinical and tomographic features, and outcome. A case-control study. Acta Neurol Scand 80:226–231, 1989

14. Bladin PF: A radiologic and pathologic study of embolism of the internal carotid-middle cerebral arterial axis. Radiology 82:614, 1964

15. Bogousslavsky J, Cachin C, Regli F et al: Cardiac sources of embolism and cerebral infarction—clinical consequences and vascular concomitants: the Lausanne Stroke Registry. Neurology 41:855–859, 1991

16. Bogousslavsky J, Regli F: Borderzone infarctions distal to internal carotid artery occlusion: prognostic implications. Ann Neurol 20:346–350, 1986

17. Bogousslavsky J, Van Melle G, Regli F: The Lausanne Stroke Registry: Analysis of 1000 consecutive patients with first stroke. Stroke 19:1083–1092, 1988

18. Bozzao L, Fantozzi LM, Bastianello S et al: Ischaemic supratentorial stroke: angiographic findings in patients examined in the very early phase. J Neurol 236:340–342, 1989

19. Caplan LR: Intracranial branch atheromatous disease: a neglected, understudied, and underused concept. Neurology 39:1246–1250, 1989

20. Caplan LR: Occlusion of the vertebral or basilar artery. Follow up analysis of some patients with benign outcome. Stroke 10:277, 1979

21. Caplan LR: "Top of the basilar" syndrome. Neurology 30:72, 1980

22. Caplan LR, Brass LM, DeWitt LD et al: Transcranial Doppler ultrasound: present status. Neurology 40:696–700, 1990

23. Caplan LR, Hier DB, D'Cruz I: Cerebral embolism in the Michael Reese Stroke Registry. Stroke 14:30, 1983

24. Carpenter DA, Grubb RL Jr, Powers WJ: Borderzone hemodynamics in cerebrovascular disease. Neurology 40:1587–1592, 1990

25. Castaigne P, Lhermitte F, Buge A et al: Paramedian thalamic and midbrain infarcts: clinical and neuropathological study. Ann Neurol 10:127, 1981

26. Castaigne P, Lhermitte F, Gautier J-C: Role des lésions artérielles dans les accidents ischemiques cérébraux de l'athérosclerose. Rev Neurol (Paris) 113:1, 1965

27. Castaigne P, Lhermitte F, Gautier J-C et al: Arterial occlusions in the vertebro-basilar system—a study of forty-four patients with post-mortem data. Brain 96:133, 1973

28. Castaigne P, Lhermitte F, Gautier J-C et al: Internal carotid artery occlusion: a study of 61 instances in 50 patients with post-mortem data. Brain 93:231, 1970

29. Cerebral Embolism Task Force second report. Cardiogenic brain embolism. Arch Neurol 46:727–743, 1989

30. Chamorro AM, Sacco RL, Mohr JP et al: Lacunar infarction: clinical-CT correlations in the Stroke Data Bank. Stroke 22:175–181, 1991

31. Chimowitz MI, Furlan AJ, Sila CA et al: Etiology of motor or sensory stroke: a prospective study of the predictive value of clinical and radiological features. Ann Neurol 30:519–525, 1991

32. Cujec B, Polasek P, Voll C, Shuaib A: Transesophageal echocardiography in the detection of potential cardiac source of embolism in stroke patients. Stroke 22:727–733, 1991

33. David NJ, Gordon KK, Friedberg SJ et al: Fatal atheromatous cerebral embolism associated with bright plaques in the retinal arterioles. Neurology 13:708, 1963

34. David DO, Rumbaugh CL, Gilson JM: Angiographic diagnosis of small-vessel cerebral emboli. Acta Radiol (Stockh) 9:264, 1969

35. Dalal PM, Shah PM, Aiyar RR: Arteriographic study of cerebral embolism. Lancet 2:358, 1965

36. De Ley G, Weyne J, Demeester G et al: Experimental thromboembolic stroke studied by positron emission tomography: immediate versus delayed reperfusion by fibrinolysis. J Cereb Blood Flow Metab 8:539–545, 1988

37. del Zoppo GJ, Poeck K, Pessin MS et al: Recombinant tissue plasminogen activator in acute thrombotic and embolic stroke. Ann Neurol 32:78–86, 1992

38. Derouesne C, Mas JL, Bolgert AF, Castaigne P: Pure sensory stroke caused by a small cortical infarct in the middle cerebral artery territory. Stroke 15:660, 1984

39. DeWitt LD, Wechsler LR. Transcranial Doppler. Stroke 19:915–921, 1988

40. Dion JE, Gates PC, Fox AJ et al: Clinical events following neuroangiography: a prospective study. Stroke 18:997–1004, 1987

41. Di Tullio MR, Gopal AS, Sacco RL et al: Prevalence of patent foramen ovale in older cryptogenic stroke patients assessed by contrast echocardiography. J Am Soc Echocardiograph 4:294, 1991

42. Drurys I, Whisnant JP, Garraway WM: Primary intracerebral hemorrhage: impact of CT on incidence. Neurology 34:653–657, 1984

43. Edelman RR, Mattle HP, Atkinson DJ et al: Cerebral blood flow: assessment with dynamic contrast enhanced T2° weighted MR imaging at 1.5 T. Radiology 176:211–220, 1990

44. Edelman RR, Mattle HP, Atkinson DJ, Hoogewoud HM: MR angiography. AJR 154:937–946, 1990

45. Edwards JH, Kricheff II, Riles T, Imparato A: Angiographically undetected ulceration of the carotid bifurcation as a cause of embolic stroke. Radiology 132:369, 1979

46. Falk RH: PFO or UFO? The role of a patent foramen ovale in cryptogenic stroke (editorial). Am Heart J 121:1264–1266, 1991

47. Fieschi C, Argentino C, Lenzi GL et al: Clinical and instrumental evaluation of patients with ischemic stroke within the first six hours. J Neurol Sci 91:311–321, 1989

48. Fieschi C, Bozzao L: Transient embolic occlusion of the middle cerebral and internal carotid arteries in cerebral apoplexy. J Neurol Neurosurg Psychiatry 32:236–240, 1969

49. Fieschi C, Carolei A, Fiorelli M et al: Changing prognosis of primary intracerebral hemorrhage: result of a clinical and computed tomographic study of 104 patients. Stroke 19:192–195, 1988

50. Fieschi C, Rasura M, Anzini A et al: A diagnostic approach to ischemic stroke in young and middle-aged adults. Eur J Neurol 3:324–330, 1996

51. Fieschi C, Sette G, Fiorelli M et al: Clinical presentation and frequency of potential sources of embolism in acute

ischemic stroke patients: the experience of the Rome Acute Stroke Registry. Cerebrovasc Dis 5:75–78, 1995

52. Fisher CM: Bilateral occlusion of basilar artery branches. J Neurol Neurosurg Psychiatry 40:1182, 1977

53. Fisher CM: Cerebral thromboangiitis obliterans. Medicine (Baltimore) 36:169, 1957

54. Fisher CM: Lacunar strokes and infarcts: a review. Neurology (NY) 32:871, 1982

55. Fisher CM: Lacunes: Small deep cerebral infarcts. Neurology (Minneap) 15:774, 1965

56. Fisher CM: The arterial lesions underlying lacunes. Acta Neuropathol (Berl) 12:1, 1969

57. Fisher CM, Adams RD: Observations on brain embolism with special reference to the mechanism of hemorrhagic infarction. J Neuropathol Exp Neurol 10:92, 1951

58. Fisher CM, Gore I, Okabe N, White PD: Atherosclerosis of the carotid and vertebral arteries—extracranial and intracranial. J Neuropathol Exp Neurol 24:455, 1965

59. Fisher CM, Karnes WE: Local embolism. J Neuropathol Exp Neurol 24:174, 1965

60. Fisher CM, Pearlman A: The non-sudden onset of cerebral embolism. Neurology (Minneap) 17:1025, 1967

61. Foulkes MA, Wolf PA, Price TR et al: The Stroke Data Bank: design, methods, and baseline characteristics. Stroke 19:547–554, 1988

62. Friedlich AL, Castleman B, Mohr JP: Case records of the Massachusetts General Hospital. N Engl J Med 278:1109, 1968

63. Gacs G, Fox AJ, Barnett HJM, Vinuela F: CT visualization of intracranial arterial thromboembolism. Stroke 14:756, 1983

64. Gan R, Sacco RL, Kargman DE et al: Testing the validity of the lacunar hypothesis: the Northern Manhattan Stroke Study experience. Neurology 1997 (in press)

65. Grolimund P, Seiler RW, Aaslid R et al: Evaluation of cerebrovascular disease by combined extracranial and transcranial Doppler sonography. Experience in 1,039 patients. Stroke 18:1018–1024, 1987

66. Gross CR, Kase CS, Mohr JP, Cunningham SC: Stroke in south Alabama: incidence and diagnostic features. Stroke 15:249, 1984

67. Hacke W, Kaste M, Fieschi C et al: Safety and efficacy of intravenous thrombolysis with a recombinant tissue plasminogen activator in the treatment of acute hemispheric stroke. JAMA 27:1017–1025, 1995

68. Hankey GJ, Warlow CP, Sellar RJ: Cerebral angiographic risk in mild cerebrovascular disease. Stroke 21:209–222, 1990

69. Hart RG, Kanter MC: Hematologic disorders and ischemic stroke. A selective review. Stroke 21:1111–1112, 1990

70. Heiss WD, Herholz K, Podreka I et al: Comparison of ^{99m}Tc HMPAO SPECT with ^{18}F fluoromethane PET in cerebrovascular disease. J Cereb Blood Flow Metab 10:687–697, 1990

71. Hinton RC, Kistler JP, Fallon JT et al: Influence of etiology of atrial fibrillation on incidence of systemic embolism. Am J Cardiol 40:509, 1977

72. Hinton RC, Mohr JP, Ackerman RA et al: Symptomatic middle cerebral artery stem stenosis. Ann Neurol 5:152, 1979

73. Hommel M, Besson G, Le Bas JF et al: Prospective study of lacunar infarction using magnetic resonance imaging. Stroke 21:546–554, 1990

74. Hornig CR, Bauer T, Simon C et al: Hemorrhagic transformation in cardioembolic cerebral infarction. Stroke 24:465–468, 1993

75. Hornig CR, Dorndorf W, Agnoli AL: Hemorrhagic cerebral infarction—a prospective study. Stroke 17:179–185, 1986

76. Hulqvist GT: Ueber Thrombose und Embolie der Arteria carotis und herbei vorkommende nderungen. Eine pathologisch-anatomische Studie. Gustav Fischer Verlag, Stockholm, 1942

77. Imparato AM, Riles TS, Gorstein F: The carotid bifurcation plaque: pathologic findings associated with cerebral ischemia. Stroke 10:238, 1979

78. Irino T, Tandea M, Minami T: Angiographic manifestations in postrecanalized cerebral infarction. Neurology 27:471, 1977

79. Johnson DW, Stringer WA, Marks MP et al: Stable xenon CT cerebral blood flow imaging: rationale for and role in clinical decision making. AJNR 12:201–213, 1991

80. Jorgensen L, Torvik A: Ischaemic cerebrovascular diseases in an autopsy series. Part I. Prevalence, location and predisposing factors in verified thromboembolic occlusions, and their significance in the pathogenesis of cerebral infarction. J Neurol Sci 3:490–495, 1966

81. Kaps M, Damian MBS, Teschendorf U, Dorndorf W: Transcranial Doppler ultrasound findings in middle cerebral artery occlusion. Stroke 21:532–537, 1990

82. Kase CS, White L, Vinson L, Eichelberger P: Shotgun pellet embolus to the middle cerebral artery. Neurology 31:458, 1981

83. Kittner SJ, Sharkness CM, Price TR et al: Infarcts with a cardiac source of embolism in the NINCDS Stroke Data Bank: historical features. Neurology 40:281–284, 1990

84. Krayenbuehl HA, Yasargil MG: Cerebral Angiography. 2nd Ed. Butterworths, London, 1968

85. Kunitz S, Gross CR, Heyman A et al: The pilot stroke data bank: definition, design, data. Stroke 15:740, 1984

86. Landau WM: Clinical neuromythology VI. Au clair de lacune: holy wholly, holey logic. Neurology 39:725–730, 1989

87. Lechat P, Mas JL, Lascault G et al: Prevalence of patent foramen ovale in patients with stroke. N Engl J Med 318:1148–1152, 1988

88. Lennihan L, Kupsky WJ, Mohr JP et al: Lack of association between carotid plaque hematoma and ipsilateral cerebral symptoms. Stroke 18:879–881, 1987

89. Leow K, Murie JA: Cerebral angiography for cerebrovascular disease: the risks. Br J Surg 75:428–430, 1988

90. Levine SR, Kim S, Deegan MJ, Welch KMA: Ischemic stroke associated with anti-cardiolipin antibodies. Stroke 18:1101–1106, 1987

91. Lhermitte F, Gautier JC, Derouesne C, Guiraud B: Ischemic accidents in the middle cerebral artery territory (a study of the causes in 122 cases). Arch Neurol 19:248, 1968

92. Liebeskind A, Chinichian A, Schechter MM: The mov-

ing embolus seen during serial cerebral angiography. Stroke 2:440, 1971

93. Little JR, Shawhan B, Weinstein M: Pseudo-tandem stenosis of the internal carotid artery. Neurosurgery 7:574, 1980

94. Masaryk TJ, Modic MT, Ross JS et al: Intracranial circulation: preliminary clinical results with three dimensional (volume) MR angiography. Radiology 171: 793–799, 1989

95. Massaro AR, Sacco RL, Timsit SG et al: Early clinical discriminators between cerebral infarction and hemorrhagic stroke. Ann Neurol 30:246–247, 1991

96. Masuda J, Ogata J, Yutani C et al: Artery to artery embolism from a thrombus formed in stenotic middle cerebral artery. Report of an autopsy case. Stroke 18:680–684, 1987

97. Millikan C, Futrell N: The fallacy of the lacunar hypothesis. Stroke 21:1251–1257, 1990

98. Minematsu K, Yamaguchi T, Omae T: Spectacular shrinking deficit: rapid recovery from a full hemispheral syndrome by migration of an embolus. Neurology, suppl. 41:329, 1991

99. Mohr JP: Lacunar infarctions. p. 201. In Barnett HJM (ed): Neurological Clinics of North America. WB Saunders, Philadelphia, 1983

100. Mohr JP: Lacunes. pp. 475–496. In Barnett HJM, Stein BH, Yatsu FM (eds): Stroke: Pathophysiology, Diagnosis and Management. Churchill Livingstone, NY 1986

101. Mohr JP: Neurologic complications of cardiac valvular disease and cardiac surgery. p. 143. In Vinken PJ, Bruyn GW (eds): Handbook of Clinical Neurology. Vol. 34. Medical Conditions. North Holland, Amsterdam, 1979

102. Mohr JP, Caplan LR, Melski JW et al: The Harvard cooperative stroke registry: a prospective registry of cases hospitalized with stroke. Neurology 28:754, 1978

103. Mohr JP, Duterte DI, Oliveira VR et al: Recanalization of acute middle cerebral artery occlusion. Neurology, suppl. 38:215, 1988

104. Mori E, Yoneda Y, Tabuchi M et al: Intravenous recombinant tissue plasminogen activator in acute carotid artery territory stroke. Neurology 42:976–982, 1992

105. Nelson RF, Pullicino P, Kendall BE, Marshall J: Computed tomography on patients presenting with lacunar syndromes. Stroke 11:256, 1980

106. Norrving B, Nilsson B, Risberg J: RCBF in patients with carotid occlusion: resting and hypercapneic flow related to collateral pattern. Stroke 13:155–162, 1982

107. Ogata J, Masuda J, Yutani C, Yamaguchi T: Rupture of atheromatous plaque as a cause of thrombotic occlusion of stenotic internal carotid artery. Stroke 21:1740–1745, 1990

108. Ogata J, Yutani C, Imakita M et al: Hemorrhagic infarct of the brain without a reopening of the occluded arteries in cardioembolic stroke. Stroke 20:876–883, 1989

109. Panzer RJ, Feibel JH, Barker WH, Griner PF: Predicting the likelihood of hemorrhage in patients with stroke. Arch Intern Med 145:1800–1803, 1985

110. Perani D, Vallar G, Cappa S et al: Aphasia and neglect after subcortical stroke: a clinical/cerebral perfusion study. Brain 110:1211–1229, 1987

111. Pessin MS, Duncan GW, Davis KR et al: Angiographic appearance of carotid occlusion in acute stroke. Stroke 11:485, 1980

112. Pessin MS, Hinton RC, Davis KR et al: Mechanisms of acute carotid stroke: a clinicoangiographic study. Ann Neurol 6:245, 1979

113. Powers WJ: Cerebral hemodynamics in ischemic cerebrovascular disease. Ann Neurol 29:231–240, 1991

114. Powers WJ, Tempel LW, Grubb RL Jr: Influence of cerebral hemodynamics on stroke risk: one year follow up of 30 medically treated patients. Ann Neurol 25: 325–330, 1989

115. Pulsinelli W: Pathophysiology of acute ischaemic stroke. Lancet 339:533–536, 1992

116. Quisling RG, Friedman WA, Rhoton AL: High cervical dissection: spontaneous resolution. AJNR 1:463, 1980

117. Ramirez Lassepas M, Cipolle RJ, Bjok RJ et al: Can embolic stroke be diagnosed on the basis of neurologic clinical criteria? Arch Neurol 44:87–89, 1987

118. Rascol A, Clanet M, Manelfe C: Pure motor hemiplegia: CT study of 30 cases. Stroke 13:11, 1982

119. Ring BA: Diagnosis of embolic occlusions of smaller branches of the intracerebral arteries. AJR Radium Ther Nucl Med 97:575, 1966

120. Ringelstein EB, Biniek R, Weiller C et al: Type and extent of hemispheric brain infarctions and clinical outcome in early and delayed middle cerebral artery recanalization. Neurology 42:289–298, 1992

121. Ringelstein EB, Koschorke S, Holling A et al: Computed tomographic patterns of proven embolic brain infarctions. Ann Neurol 26:759–765, 1989

122. Ringelstein EB, Zeumer H, Angelou D: The pathogenesis of strokes from internal carotid artery occlusion. Diagnostic and therapeutic implications. Stroke 14:867, 1983

123. Romanul FCA, Abramowicz A: Changes in brain and pial vessels in arterial borderzones. Arch Neurol (Chic) 11:40, 1964

124. Ross Russell RW: Atheromatous retinal embolism. Lancet 2:1354, 1963

125. Sacco RL, Bello JA, Traub RD, Brust JCM: Selective proprioceptive sensory loss from a thalamic lacunar stroke. Stroke 18:1160–1163, 1987

126. Sacco RL, Ellenberg JA, Mohr JP et al: Infarction of undetermined cause: the NINCDS Stroke Data Bank. Ann Neurol 25:382–390, 1989

127. Sacco RL, Kargman DE, Gu Q, Zamanillo MC: Race-ethnicity and determinants of intracranial atherosclerotic cerebral infarction: the Northern Manhattan Stroke Study. Stroke 26:14–20, 1995

128. Sacco RL, Owen J, Mohr JP, Tatemichi TK: Free protein S deficiency: a possible association with intracranial vascular occlusion. Stroke 20:1657–1661, 1989

129. Samuel KC: Atherosclerosis and occlusion of the internal carotid artery. J Pathol Bacteriol 71:391, 1956

130. Sandercock PAG, Allen CMC, Corston RN et al: Clinical diagnosis of intracranial haemorrhage using Guy's Hospital Score. BMJ 291:1675–1677, 1985

131. Santamaria J, Graus F, Rubio F et al: Cerebraic brain infarctions. sal ganglia due to embolism from the heart. Stroke 14:911, 1983

132. Sette G, Baron JC, Mazoyer B et al: Local brain haemo-

dynamics and oxygen metabolism in cerebrovascular disease. Positron emission tomography. Brain 112:931–951, 1989

133. Sloan MA: Thrombolysis and stroke. Past and future. Arch Neurol 44:748–768, 1987

134. Spitzer K, Thie A, Caplan LR, Kunze K: The MICRO-STROKE expert system for stroke type diagnosis. Stroke 20:1353–1356, 1989

135. Sunohara N, Mukoyama M, Mano Y, Satoyoshi E: Action-induced rhythmic dystonia: an autopsy case. Neurology (Cleveland) 34:321, 1984

136. Takano T, Kimura K, Nakamura M et al: Effect of small deep hemispheric infarction on the ipsilateral cortical blood flow in man. Stroke 16:64–69, 1985

137. Tatemichi TK, Chamorro A, Petty GW et al: Hemodynamic role of ophthalmic artery collateral in internal carotid artery occlusion. Neurology 40:461–464, 1990

138. Tomsick TA, Brott TC, Olinger CP et al: Hyperdense middle cerebral artery: incidence and quantitative significance. Neuroradiology 31:312–315, 1989

139. Torvick A: The pathogenesis of watershed infarcts in the brain. Stroke 15:221–223, 1984

140. Torvik A, Jorgensen L: Thrombotic and embolic occlusions of the carotid arteries in an autopsy material. Part 2. Cerebral lesions and clinical course. J Neurol Sci 3:410, 1966

141. The National Institute of Neurological Disorders and Stroke rt-PA Stroke Study Group: tissue plasminogen activator for acute ischemic stroke. N Engl J Med 333:1581–1587, 1995

142. Timsit S, Sacco RL, Mohr JP et al: Brain infarction severity differs according to cardiac or arterial embolic source: the NINDS Stroke Data Bank. Neurology, suppl. 40:417, 1990

143. Timsit S, Sacco RL, Mohr JP et al: Early clinical differentiation of atherosclerotic and cardioembolic infarction: Stroke Data Bank. J Neurol 237:140, 1990

144. Tohgi H, Kawashima M, Tamura K, Suzuki H: Coagulation fibrinolysis abnormalities in acute and chronic phases of cerebral thrombosis and embolism. Stroke 21:1663–1667, 1990

145. Toni D, Del Duca R, Fiorelli M et al: Pure motor hemiplegia and sensorimotor stroke: accuracy of the very early clinical diagnosis of lacunar stroke. Stroke 25:92–96, 1994

146. Toni D, Fiorelli M, Bastianello S et al: Hemorrhagic transformation of brain infarct: predictability in the first five hours from stroke onset and influence on clinical outcome. Neurology 46:341–345, 1996

147. Toni D, Fiorelli M, De Michele M et al: Clinical and prognostic correlates of stroke subtype misdiagnosis within 12 hours from onset. Stroke 26:1837–1840, 1995

148. Toni D, Fiorelli M, Gentile M et al: Progressing neurological deficit secondary to acute ischemic stroke—study on predictability, pathogenesis and prognosis. Arch Neurol 52:670–675, 1995

149. Von Arbin M, Britton M, de Faire U et al: Accuracy of bedside diagnosis in stroke. Stroke 12:288–293, 1981

150. Von Kummer R, Forsting M, Sartor K, Hacke W: Intravenous recombinant tissue plasminogen activator in acute stroke. pp. 161–167. In Hacke W, del Zoppo GJ, Hirschberg M (eds): Thrombolytic Therapy in Acute Ischemic Stroke. Springer-Verlag, Berlin, 1991

151. Von Kummer R, Hacke W: Safety and efficacy of intravenous tissue plasminogen activator and heparin in acute middle cerebral artery stroke. Stroke 23:646–652, 1992

152. von Kummer R, Meyding-Lamadi U, Forsting M et al: Sensitivity and prognostic value of early CT in occlusion of the middle cerebral artery trunk. AJNR 15:9–15, 1994

153. Whisnant JP: Multiple particles injected may all go to the same cerebral artery branch. Stroke 13:720, 1982

154. Zanette EM, Fieschi C, Bozzao L et al: Comparison of cerebral angiography and transcranial Doppler sonography in acute stroke. Stroke 20:899–903, 1989

155. Zanette EM, Roberti C, Mancini G et al: Spontaneous middle cerebral artery reperfusion in ischemic stroke. A follow-up study with transcranial Doppler. Stroke 26:430–433, 1995

156. Zatz LM, Iannone AM, Eckman PB, Hecker SP: Observations concerning intracerebral vascular occlusion. Neurology 15:390–401, 1965

157. Zierler RE, Kohler TR, Strandness DE Jr: Duplex scanning of normal or minimally diseased carotid arteries: correlation with arteriography and clinical outcome. J Vasc Surg 12:447–454, 1990

Internal Carotid Artery Disease

J. P. MOHR

JEAN-CLAUDE GAUTIER

MICHAEL S. PESSIN (deceased)

The bifurcation of the common carotid artery and the origin of the internal carotid artery (ICA) have been the focus of neurologic attention for many years. They are by far the most common site of significant, atherosclerotic ICA lesions; the extracranial ICA, is, as a rule, devoid of atherosclerosis beyond its origin to its entry into the skull. The extracranial ICA can be examined clinically and by ultrasound and is easy to approach surgically; even some of its less usual disorders such as dissecting aneurysms are to some extent amenable to conventional surgery. The intracranial ICA lends itself poorly to clinical and ultrasound examination, and even angiograms are often difficult to evaluate precisely. Only lately has Doppler ultrasonography been applied to the siphon.[217]

Anatomy

The cervical segment of the ICA extends from the common carotid bifurcation to the skull base. Intracranially, the ICA is divided into the petrosal, cavernous, and supraclinoid portions.

COMMON CAROTID ARTERY

The right common carotid artery usually arises from the innominate and the left directly from the arch. However, the left common carotid often arises from the innominate.[222] The innominate and left common carotid may appear as a fork from the arch of the aorta, or the left common carotid may arise as high as a few centimeters from the origin of the innominate. Instances of agenesis of a common carotid have been reported although rarely,[41,364] as has failure of the carotid to show a bifurcation.[265] The external and internal carotid are

the principal branches of the common carotid artery. The common carotid only very rarely gives rise to the branches usually formed from the external carotid.

Bifurcation

The bifurcation of the common carotid artery is most often found at the level of the thyroid cartilage. However, anatomic variations are great enough that the bifurcation may be found anywhere within 5 cm of this site.[398] The origin of the ICA is usually somewhat dilated (the carotid sinus), extending up to 2 cm from the origin before it assumes a uniform diameter. Although the bifurcation geometry usually places the internal carotid posterior to the external, many variants exist, some in which the internal wraps around the external to a degree that the positions almost appear reversed.

Measurements made on the diameter and angulation of the bifurcation serve to show their modest variations. In their study of 102 normals, Harrison and Marshall[162] found that the common carotid artery was 7.6 mm (± 1.64 mm) in diameter as it entered the bifurcation, the bulb enlarging to 8.3 mm (± 1.95 mm), while the internal carotid beyond the bulb narrowed beyond to 5.1 mm (± 1.1 mm). At the bifurcation, the angle formed between the external and internal was 36.4 degrees (± 18.2 degrees).

The bifurcation area is notable for the presence of the carotid body and the nerve of the carotid sinus. Both receive their blood supply from the external carotid artery. The chemoreceptor function of the carotid body responds to a *decrease* in arterial PO_2, carotid blood flow, or arterial pH and to an *increase* in arterial PCO_2 or blood temperature, in descending order of sensitivity.[71] Its output is mediated by the glossopharyngeal nerve and plays, on the nucleus of the tractus solitarius, nucleus ambiguus, paramedian reticular formation, and lateral reticular nucleus. The carotid body has an important regulatory effect on respiration, being the only mediator of hypoxic ventilatory drive, and has additional effects on blood pressure and heart rate. Stimulation of the carotid body produces increased rate and depth of respiration, increased peripheral vascular resistance, and secondary elevation in blood pressure and bradycardia, among other effects. Unilateral carotid endarterectomy can produce an increase in the PCO_2 and failure of response to hypoxia.[367] The potential sensitivity of the carotid body to manipulation is well demonstrated by the occasional successful conversion of tachyarrhythmia to normal sinus rhythm following carotid body compression (e.g., massage), and here a note of warning is appropriate to recommend against injudicious unilateral or bilateral carotid body compression, which may be followed by severe bradycardia.

Increase in the stretch of the wall of the sinus produces activity of the carotid sinus nerve, which produces reflex hypotension by activation of the sympathoinhibitory effect of the nucleus of the tractus solitarius, and by activating parasympathetic pathways reaching neurons in the dorsal motor nucleus of the vagus that slow the heart rate. Hypofunction caused by reduction in distension of the carotid sinus or by sectioning of the nerve may produce the opposite effect. Such changes rarely persist beyond 48 hours.[71] Bilateral carotid stenosis could be a cause of sustained hypertension.

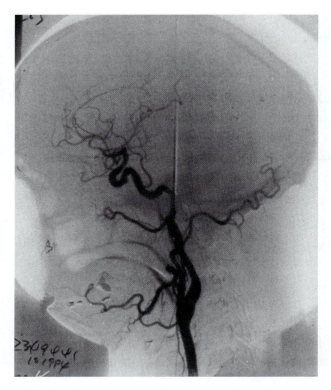

Figure 17.1 Anatomy of the extracranial carotid artery.

EXTERNAL CAROTID ARTERY AND OTHER ASCENDING ARTERIES OF INTEREST

The external carotid artery gives rise to the ascending pharyngeal, superior thyroid, lingual, occipital, facial, posterior auricular, internal maxillary, and superficial temporal branches, in that order. These branches only very rarely arise from the ICA.[276] The superior laryngeal nerve passes posteriorly near its origin, and the hypoglossal nerve courses laterally over the artery. Either of these nerves may be injured in operations on the region of the bifurcation, damage to the latter causing ipsilateral atrophy of the tongue, a distinctive clinical finding.

Occlusion of the ICA at its origin often permits visualization of the ascending pharyngeal artery, which is otherwise often obscured by the contrast in the opacified ICA. The ascending pharyngeal may anastomose with the middle meningeal or occipital arteries or both.[210]

The occipital artery is an important source of collateral blood flow to the extracranial portion of the vertebral artery, by means of a small collateral vessel, the proatlantal artery. In cases of occlusion of the common carotid artery below the bifurcation, collateral flow may arise from the vertebral, pass through the proatlantal, and via retrograde flow through the occipital and to the external carotid reach the bifurcation to supply the ICA in the usual anterograde manner. Likewise, occlusion of the vertebral artery in the neck may allow flow to the distal extracranial segment of the vertebral through the proatlantal from the occipital arteries.

EXTRACRANIAL INTERNAL CAROTID ARTERY

The extracranial ICA extends from the bifurcation to its entry into the carotid canal of the temporal bone without branches or notable change in size[83] (Fig. 17.1). Anomalies are rare.[276] There is considerable variation in the length of the vessel and its degree of tortuosity. In as many as 35% of all cases, some form of tortuosity may be encountered[68] as undulation, coiling, or kinking of the vessel.[374]

Throughout its course, the ICA is intimately associated with ascending sympathetic fibers. Near its origin, it is crossed laterally by the hypoglossal nerve. The superior cervical ganglion and the vagus nerve lie immediately behind. Near its entry into the skull, the artery is separated from the jugular vein by the glossopharyngeal, vagus, spinal accessory, and lingual nerves. It lies just in front of the lateral process of the atlas.

INTRACRANIAL INTERNAL CAROTID ARTERY

The intracranial ICA supplies part of the tympanic cavity and the artery of the pterygoid canal (vidian artery), which may form an anastomosis with the internal maxillary artery.[316]

Cavernous Portion

The cavernous part, approximately 4 to 5 cm in length,[427] enters the cavernous sinus through the foramen lacerum just beneath the gasserian ganglion. It runs rostrally close to the lateral aspect of the sella turcica. This segment of the vessel becomes progressively more tortuous from infancy to old age, ultimately resulting in the S-shaped carotid siphon characteristic of adult humans.[146] The siphon lies within the venous plexus and bears relationships to the third, fourth, fifth, and sixth cranial nerves that run in the lateral wall of the sinus. A detailed study of the relationships of the ICA in the cavernous sinus has been made by Parkinson.[278]

The siphon gives off a few small branches: the meningeal-hypophyseal trunk, the artery of the inferior cavernous sinus (84% of cases), and, less often (28% of cases),[160] McConnell's capsular arteries. Rarely (some 6% to 8% of cases), the ophthalmic and dorsal meningeal arteries arise from the cavernous portion.[160]

The meningeal-hypophyseal trunk is approximately the same size as the ophthalmic artery.[160] It has three tiny branches[222,279]: the artery of the tentorium (the artery of Bernasconi and Cassinari),[24] which courses backward to supply the surface of the tentorium; the dorsal meningeal artery, which supplies the wall of the cavernous sinus, the dura of the clivus, and the sixth cranial nerve and crosses the midline to anastomose with its counterpart; and the inferior hypophyseal artery, which supplies the posterior pituitary gland, resolving into capillaries that enter the pituitary portal system.[357]

The artery of the inferior cavernous sinus supplies the dura of its inferior and lateral wall and in some cases anastomoses with the middle meningeal artery at the foramen spinosum.[160] McConnell's capsular arteries supply the anterior wall of the sella and the anterior lobe of the pituitary, anastomosing with the inferior hypophyseal artery. At this level there are several anastomotic channels between internal and external carotid circulations.

Supraclinoid Portion

The supraclinoid part pierces the dura mater medial to the anterior clinoid process. This short stretch, usually less than 1 cm in length,[402] winds upward and slightly laterally,[200] passing over the oculomotor nerve and below the optic nerve. However short it is, the supraclinoid part of the ICA gives off several important branches and therefore is of great importance for collateral circulation.

The first major branch is the *ophthalmic artery*, which enters the orbit via the optic foramen. The main branches of the ophthalmic artery are the lacrimal, supraorbital, ethmoidal, and palpebral. The artery of the falx arises from the ethmoidal branch. The ophthalmic gives rise to the central retinal artery, which is not usually seen angiographically; a capillary blush from the choroid and retina may be visible, however, in the late arterial phase of the angiogram. The many branches of the ophthalmic artery provide rich anastomotic connections with external carotid artery branches and serve as an important collateral channel between the two circulations, offering some protection in the event of ICA occlusion.

The *posterior communicating artery* is next, arising from the dorsal aspect of the vessel to run caudally and medially and join the posterior cerebral artery. A slight dilatation referred to as *junctional dilatation*[334] or infundibulum may be present. The artery proceeds caudally and medially, where it joins the posterior cerebral artery. The posterior communicating artery supplies the anterior and medial parts of the thalamus and walls of the third ventricle by means of several small branches. When fully developed, keeping in the adult the embryonic disposition, it may serve as an important connection between the carotid and vertebrobasilar circulations. When the posterior cerebral arises from the ICA, occlusion of the ICA can cause particularly devastating infarcts. One to three small perforating arteries may arise just distal to the posterior communicating artery and before the origin of the anterior choroidal artery. These vessels supply the anterior perforating substance. With major intracranial occlusive disease affecting the circle of Willis, these small branches may be visualized angiographically as prominent collateral pathways.

The *anterior choroidal artery* usually arises from the ICA and enters the brain via the choroidal fissure. It is a small branch of the ICA arising just distal to the origin of the posterior communicating artery and supplying the choroid plexus of the temporal horn, hippocampus, basal ganglia, and lower half of the posterior limb of the internal capsule. Although it has been said to raise sometimes from the middle cerebral artery, studies of the anatomy by microdissection show that it almost always arises from the ICA.[145]

The ICA then bifurcates into the anterior and middle cerebral arteries. The latter is the biggest and usually the direct continuation of the ICA. Both the initial segment of the anterior cerebral and the posterior communicating arteries are subject to fairly frequent variations of size that are part of the variations of the circle of Willis.

Anatomic Anomalies

The main anatomic anomaly of the intracranial ICA is the persistence in the adult of the trigeminal artery. This vessel arises from the artery as it enters the cavernous sinus and runs caudally either through the sella turcica or the extradural space under the petroclinoid ligament to join the basilar artery, generally between the origins of the superior cerebellar and anterior inferior cerebellar arteries. A full description of this variation and its embryologic, angiographic, and pathologic significance has been given by Lie[222] and Parkinson and Shields.[279] The other important, if uncommon, variant is that the ophthalmic artery may arise from the middle meningeal artery,[65] with no connection to the intracranial ICA.

Collateral Branches

Apart from the ophthalmic artery, there are few branches of the intracranial ICA (apart from the circle of Willis) that permit collateral with other vessels and are at most very small twigs. They may enlarge and be of great significance under unusual circumstances such as arteriovenous malformations in the dura mater, but ordinarily they remain too small to play a useful role in ameliorating the effects of thrombotic or embolic intracranial ICA occlusions.

Relevant Histology

Extracranial cerebral arteries have the usual structure of elastic or muscular arteries. Intracranial arteries have no external elastic lamina. However, while not visible with routine histologic techniques, the elastic lamina may still be stained with special techniques. Generally, arterial cushions that are often considered precursors of atherosclerotic lesions lie at the curvatures and branchings of the arteries.[18] Intracranial arteries are devoid of vasa vasorum.[16]

The extracranial ICA shares most of the *histology* of other limb and trunk vessels of the same size. The intracranial ICA has some unique anatomy. In its initial stretch it lies in a bony encasement and then, in the cavernous sinus, lies within venous blood, two peculiar situations for an artery. It becomes intracranial in the strict sense only in its short supraclinoid segment. The authors do not know of any histologic study specifically devoted to the intracranial ICA and therefore do not know to what extent the general histologic features of intracranial arteries and their peculiarities affect the histologic structure of the intracranial ICA.

Pathology

ATHEROSCLEROSIS

Atherosclerosis and its complications far exceed all other forms of disease primarily affecting the extracranial and intracranial carotid artery. Because some important differences exist between the lesions in these two sites, they are described separately.

Extracranial Arteriosclerosis

The carotid in the neck has proved to be among the favored sites for development of atherosclerosis. The pathologic process in the carotid seems similar to that found in other vessels. The fibrous plaques that are considered the hallmark of advancing atherosclerosis occur in the carotid arteries as early as age 25 and 40 years but appear in the vertebral and intracranial arteries later, between ages 40 and 50 years.[248]

A recurrent injury to the intima is considered to be the important step in initiation of the atherosclerotic lesion.[268,368] The effects of the injury are influenced by factors such as turbulent flow,[147,267,328,341] hypertension-induced large shearing and vibration forces,[246] chronic hypercholesterolemia,[307] and other less common problems. Platelets adhere to the injured, exposed endothelium[268] and circulating plasma lipids enter the lesion, especially the low-density lipoproteins.[303] Smooth muscle cells migrate from the media to the intima, where they proliferate.[192,391] Views differ as to whether this proliferation occurs from a single cell line[22,291] or as a result of deregulation of proliferation factors from senescence.[240] Whatever the mechanisms involved, the end result is the characteristic histology of the atheroma.[308]

DISTRIBUTION OF EXTRACRANIAL LESIONS
Perhaps the functional importance of the eye and brain and their sensitivity to ischemia have brought about so many studies on atherosclerosis in its various stages of development in the carotid. The disease usually affects the carotid in a uni- or multifocal fashion, not diffusely. The intramural lesions occur

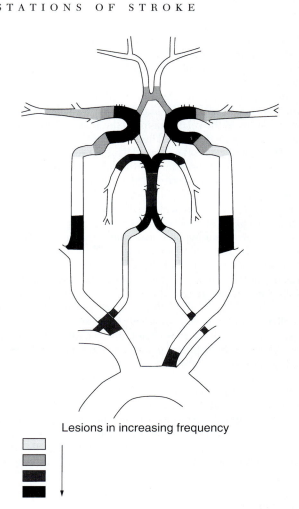

Lesions in increasing frequency

Figure 17.2 Distribution of lesions in the carotid territory.

most frequently at bifurcations and curves[59,127,184,316] (Fig. 17.2). Most lesions are found in the first 2 cm from the origin of the ICA.[59,127,184,316] Fewer lesions occur in the intracranial portion in the siphon and intracraninally at the stems of the anterior and middle cerebral arteries.[59,127] The occurrence and severity of disease in the siphon appears to be unrelated to that in the sinus, and the results of surgical therapy for sinus disease do not appear to be related to disease in the siphon.[304]

CAROTID BIFURCATION ANATOMY AND LESION DEVELOPMENT
Attempts have been made to implicate both vessel size and vascular geometry in the development of atheroma at the bifurcation. For the ICA severely affected by atherosclerosis on one side only, Caplan and Baker[53] found that the smaller vessel was more frequently involved. Flow separation appears to be another factor. LoGerfo et al[231,232] used plastic tubing to demonstrate a flow separation effect that occurs at a fork in a tube and argued that the extent of the flow separation might play a role in the occurrence and positioning of an atheroma at the carotid bifurcation. Wood et al[395] separately demonstrated such boundary separation in human carotid artery bifurcations by painstaking ultrasonic studies. Atheroma opposite the site of the boundary separation was also shown in an autopsy study.[408] Taken together, these findings suggest that the focus of athero-

sclerosis is determined to some degree by the local flow characteristics, for which the carotid bifurcation seems especially suited. This thesis is becoming more widely accepted, although the findings have been challenged by measurements made of a series of cases studied by angiograms, which showed no significant difference between either the size or the angles at the bifurcation in normal or diseased vessels.[162]

HEMODYNAMICALLY SIGNIFICANT STENOSIS

The main variables involved in making a stenosis hemodynamically significant are the reduced cross-sectional area,[26,43,328] the length of the stenosis,[26] the velocity of the blood flow,[405] and the blood viscosity.[49] Of these variables, cross-sectional area is the most important. Brice et al[43] were among the first to define the characteristics of a hemodynamically significant stenosis in vitro. Hemodynamically significant stenosis (i.e., reduced flow) occurred in excised human ICAs when the lumen was constricted along a length of 3 mm to a cross-sectional area of 4 to 5 mm^2 (Fig. 17.3). They extended these studies to humans undergoing clamping of the common carotid artery for intracranial aneurysms. The point of sudden fall in pressure distal to the stenosis occurred when the lumen reached a diameter < 2 mm at its narrowest point. Little detectable change in flow or pressure developed distal to the stenosis until the critical point was reached, after which any further change produced an even more dramatic fall in pressure and flow. The length of the stenosis was far less significant a factor than was the total cross-sectional area at the narrowest point: over a distance of 4 cm, the resistance increased less than twofold. Lesions in tandem produced cumulative effects only if separated by > 3 cm (the usual condition that applies in carotid territory stenoses in tandem). The effects of unilateral carotid stenosis were thought not to be influenced by stenoses elsewhere in the system, although the authors did not document this point in their work.[43] From this study the principle arose that the carotid stenosis must be 2 mm or tighter to be considered hemodynamically significant. Others have used the method of percent reduction in vascular lumen, claiming hemodynamic significance when the diameter is reduced by 50%, a figure corresponding to a cross-section reduction of 75% to 80%.[26,245]

Archie and Feldtman[9] restudied the original observations by Brice in patients with primary arterial disease using electromagnetic blood flow measurements in 47 patients before and after carotid endarterectomy. Normal blood flow was still present up

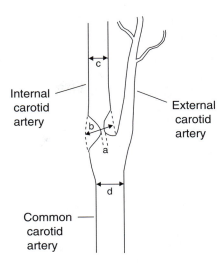

Figure 17.4 Position of measurements for stenosis. a, site of maximum stenosis (whether or not in the carotid bulb); b, original internal carotid lumen; c, internal carotid distal to the stenosis; d, common carotid lumen. (From Young et al,[406] with permission.)

to 60% diameter stenosis and 90% area stenosis. A 40% reduction in blood flow was documented at a 75% diameter and 94% area stenosis, and a 64% reduction of blood flow occurred with 84% diameter stenosis and 96% area stenosis. These data clearly indicate that the stenosis must be rather severe both in diameter and especially in cross-sectional area before significant reductions in blood flow occur. The findings suggested that hemodynamically significant stenosis may not be present until the lumen is more restricted even than the 2 mm lumen diameter suggested by the data of Brice et al.[43]

How the degree of stenosis is established by analysis of angiograms has been the subject of dispute. The methods used have calculated the percent by the formula (1 − minimum residual lumen/normal distal cervical internal carotid artery diameter) × 100 used by the North American Symptomatic Carotid Endarterectomy Trial (NASCET) and the Asymptomatic Carotid Atherosclerosis Study (ACAS). The method for selection of the sites in the vessel is shown in Figure 17.4.[406] Concern has been expressed about whether this method will apply in clinical practice, but the effort by Gagne et al[138] indicated that the technique translates well. The percent stenosis from 219 consecutive angiograms was assessed by two vascular surgeons and two radiologists (blinded as to the results of the other group), who classified stenoses into < or >60% (the break point used in the ACAS) and <30%, 30% to 60%, and ≥70% (as was used in the NASCET). High kappa values (0.825 to 0.903) were found for ACAS criteria; these values were 0.729 to 0.793 for NASCET criteria. By comparison, interobserver agreement on measurements for digital subtraction angiograms and magnetic resonance angiograms has not been high.[431] Practices also differ between continents: in the United States a method of measuring the angiogram may yield a diagnosis of 60% stenosis, whereas the method used in Europe may produce a stenosis of 75% from basically the same angiographic images.[39]

Recent changes in practice are calling into question whether conventional angiography is still the standard of practice. Kuntz

Figure 17.3 Effect of cross-sectional area on pressure and flow.

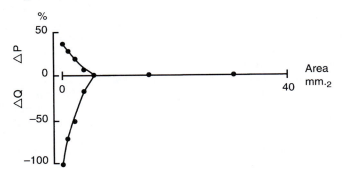

et al[206] undertook a morbidity study drawing on data from the ACAS. Based on the published sensitivity and specificity of the test method (Doppler ultrasound [0.96 and 0.66, respectively] magnetic resonance angiography [1.00 and 0.76, respectively] and Doppler and magnetic resonance angiogram combined [1.00 and 0.86, respectively], they estimated a 5-year reduction in stroke risk of 6.17% for magnetic resonance angiography, 6.35% for Doppler, 6.34% for the combined studies, and 7.12% for conventional angiography. They concluded that noninvasive tests offered an advantage even if the morbidity of conventional angiography could be reduced to 0.4%, a figure that many doubt is obtainable. Many clinics have already largely replaced conventional angiography with noninvasive testing, further reducing the expected overall morbidity in a surgical solution for carotid artery disease, even when symptomatic.[235]

The steady decline in conventional angiography as the primary measure of stenosis and its replacement by Doppler technology (see below) may eventually render moot the issue of measuring stenosis on conventional angiograms.

IN VITRO STUDIES   The hemodynamic effects of stenosis for in vitro models have been hampered by a considerable difference in the dynamics of a static versus compliant stenosis. Santamore et al[318] found that the static stenosis created in a glass rod was little influenced by changes in perfusion pressure or peripheral resistance. However, the hemodynamics of a stenosis created by a balloon catheter in the dog carotid artery proved somewhat different. The stenotic resistance, computed as the pressure gradient across the stenosis divided by the flow, was sensitive to changes in either perfusion pressure or peripheral resistance. When either was decreased, an increase in the stenotic resistance resulted. The loss of compliance may render a given high-degree stenosis its hemodynamic properties. This point is under investigation.

TEMPO OF LESION DEVELOPMENT   Much of the little that is known about the tempo of lesion development is drawn from experience with extracranial ICA disease, as studied by Doppler technology. Judging from studies using conventional angiography, digital subtraction methods, or noninvasive techniques, atheromatous stenoses may develop swiftly over months, slowly over years, or even remain static despite being hemodynamically significant.[189] Only a few studies have addressed the fate of asymptomatic lesions. The early angiogram-based study by Javid et al,[190] whose group reangiogrammed 93 patients whose carotid lesions were asymptomatic at the time of the initial angiogram, found that 35 of 93 arteries showed no change in the severity or configuration of the atheroma over 1 to 9 years: in 19 atheroma size increased by <25% a year, whereas in atheroma size 32 changed >25% a year; 7 developed recurrent stenosis or thrombosis. Bauer et al[20] undertook a similar study in 49 patients using repeat angiography with a mean interval of 25 months. Some degree of progression of the lesions was found in 17 of the 63 unoperated carotid arteries.

The ease of use of Doppler methods for following the course of ICA disease has led to the appearance of reports in increasing numbers. These studies indicate that progression of presymptomatic stenosis may be more common than suspected on clinical grounds alone. Hennerici and Rautenberg[170] documented progression in 85% of 122 prospectively studied asymptomatic patients with extracranial carotid disease followed by continuous-wave Doppler followed for up to 36 months. Norrving et al[270] followed the course of 64 cases of carotid disease over a period of from 1 to 13 years and found a 27% rate of progression on the nonoperated, previously asymptomatic side. About 30% of the cases with progressing disease became symptomatic with transient ischemic attacks (TIAs) or strokes. By contrast, only 5.5% of the vessels showing no progression of the disease process had symptoms, a highly significant difference (P <0.001).

At the time it appeared, the study by Roederer et al[305] of 167 asymptomatic cases was the largest reported cohort to use the duplex Doppler technique. Follow-up at 6 month intervals was attempted and was successful for 103 cases at 6 months, for 95 at 12 months, for 64 at 24 months, and for 17 at 36 months. Some degree of progression was documented in 60% of cases. Overall, symptoms occurred in 10 cases (TIAs in 6 and stroke in 4) and were accompanied by disease progression in 8. Within 6 months, 1 of 5 arteries with 80% to 90% stenosis had occluded; 7 of 46 increased from 50% to 79% to 80% to 99% stenosis; and 4 of 67 increased from 16% to 49% to 50% to 79%. At 24 months, of 33 arteries that were initially 50% to 79%, 2 occluded and 2 increased to 80% to 99% stenosis; of 38 that were initially 16% to 49%, 1 occluded, 1 became 80% to 99% stenosed and 7 increased to 50% to 79% stenosis. At 3 years, of 11 arteries initially 50% to 79% stenosed, 1 occluded and 2 advanced to 80% to 99% stenosis.

PLAQUE MORPHOLOGY   In 1986, Fisher and Ojemann,[130] studying the largest collection of operative specimens up to that time, did not find histologic observations sufficient to support unequivocally the notion of an embolic source from the plaques or ulcerations great enough to settle the matter. Nonetheless, in 1989, Glagov and Zarins[148] still offered the suggestion that such differences could be found and that one or more of them could predict the risk of embolism. In 1997, Hatsukami et al[166] dashed these hopes in their published serial section study of 43 plaques removed at endarterectomy. Fibrous intimal tissue, intraplaque hemorrhage, lipid core, necrotic plaque core, and calcification were studied; no differences were found between the symptomatic and asymptomatic patients, bringing the authors to the conclusion that, "from an imaging perspective, it is unlikely that identification of these plaque features will distinguish severe carotid stenoses that are at higher risk for developing ischemic neurological symptoms."

Hope has been held out for years first that Doppler sonography (and more recently color-coded) Doppler could distinguish features predictive of stroke from those found in patients remaining asymptomatic. That plaques pursue different courses over time is well known. Arbeille et al[8] studied 86 plaques over a period of 24 months, observing increase in volume in 14, decrease in 25, and a stable course in 29. Plaques that increased in volume became more heterogeneous, and those that decreased became more homogeneous. One major observation was the failure of the Doppler velocity profile to parallel the changes in plaque volume, but the exact status of the patients was unclear. Whether ultrasonographic features predicting stroke can be found is less clear. Hennerici et al[171] failed in an attempt that drew on patients from two institutions (Mannheim and the New York Neurological Institute). The Consensus Conference for Carotid Plaque Morphology and Risk (Consensus sur la Morphologie et le Risque des Plaques Carotidiennes)[209] held in December of 1996 in Paris could only conclude that, to date, degree of stenosis is associated with stroke risk, but the ultrasonographic features of the plaque carrying a risk are not settled.

COURSE FOR SEVERE STENOSIS

Little information exists concerning the evolution of lesions already hemodynamically significant when discovered. At times, a dramatic worsening in the degree of stenosis is observed over periods of weeks to months. Other cases, even with pinpoint stenosis, may remain static for years.[190] Five of the 183 cases studied by Roederer et al[305] had 80% to 99% stenosis initially. One artery occluded without symptoms. One of the remaining four patients developed TIAs during the first 6 months and underwent endarterectomy. The fate of the others was unreported, but presumably they also underwent surgery as they were not accounted for in the report at 12 months.

RAPID INCREASE IN STENOSIS

That a minor plaque of atherosclerosis could lead to sudden and dramatic increase of the stenosis was explained in some cases by subintimal hemorrhage.[234] The frequency of such sudden change is not well understood, although estimates ranging up to >85% have been given.[234] Evidence on this point has been the most difficult to develop. Mural thrombus incorporated into the arterial wall may be a cause. Some of the cases may represent arterial dissection, a frequent, if often misdiagnosed, cause of these dramatic sudden lesions. (The subject of dissection is discussed in more detail below.) In the few cases followed, little evidence has shown that sudden worsening occurs. Roederer et al[305] documented only three instances of disease progression from <50% stenosis to occlusion between two successive studies. In all three, the planned 6-month interval examinations did not occur, for various reasons. For two of them, the interval between examinations was 12 months and for two fully 24 months, in all instances too long a period to determine the rate at which the progression occurred. In all the cases studied at regular intervals, no instances of dramatic progression were encountered. In the study of 68 plaques by Arbeille et al,[8] progression occurred in 14, 25 decreased in size, and 29 remained stable.

Intracranial Internal Carotid Artery Atherosclerosis

It is well known that most of the significant atherosclerotic lesions of the ICA develop at the origin (sinus) of the ICA or at the bifurcation of the common carotid artery, or at both sites, yet the incidence of such lesions in the intracranial ICA is not negligible. Hulqvist,[182] in a pioneer work, found that primary ICA occlusion occurred in a third of the cases near the origin of the ophthalmic artery. Torvik and Jörgensen[359–362] found that 14 of 29 recent thrombotic occlusions of the ICA were located in the extracranial compared with 15 in the intracranial part of the vessel. Castaigne et al[58] found that 6 of 27 (22.2%) of atherosclerotic thrombotic occlusions of the ICA had started in the distal ICA.

Although atherosclerotic lesions have been documented in several pathologic studies, further consideration here is given only to those reports in which the ICA was examined throughout its length. Evaluation of the degree of stenosis of the siphon at autopsy is fraught with difficulties resulting from the marked tendency of this part of the artery to calcification, which often results in fracture when it is cut, making detailed studies difficult. Samuel[316] reported on 85 patients over the age of 45 years in whom all ICA lesions were atherosclerotic. Atherosclerosis affected the petrous portion in 27 instances, especially in the regions of its two curvatures. The involvement was less extensive than that of the sinus, cavernous, and supraclinoid segments. In one case an occlusion was present only in the petrous portion. The cavernous part was second after the sinus in order of frequency of atherosclerosis and was involved in 59 instances, twice very severely. Lesions were mostly situated on the inner curves of the artery.

Such a predilection of lesions for inner curvatures has also been reported by others.[253] However, Fisher et al[127] found that the outer curve and other parts (of the siphon) were by no means spared, and Zülch[412] depicted lesions on both the outer and inner curvatures of the siphon.

Yates and Hutchinson[402] reported 100 cases in which the clinical picture had suggested ischemia and from which obvious cases of cerebral embolism in young adults with mitral stenosis had been excluded. Lesions of vessels ≥ 0.5 mm in diameter were either atheromas or occlusions by thrombus. Stenoses that reduced the lumen by about half the cross-sectional area (grade 2) or complete occlusion or severe stenosis in which the lumen was <1 mm in diameter (grade 3) were called significant. Stenoses of the cavernous and supraclinoid (intradural) parts were found in 3 instances compared with 67 instances of such lesions in the sinus. In another three cases the primary occlusion by thrombus was found in the petrous portion.

Torvik and Jörgensen[359–362] studied a consecutive series of 994 autopsies and found 15 recent thrombotic occlusions in the intracranial ICA, "the great majority" of which were superimposed on atherosclerotic stenoses. Other occlusions were either embolic (see below), unclassified, or old. Stenoses found were "roughly averaged" as follows: grade 1, reduction of the lumen by less than one-fourth of the square area; grade 2, reduction by one-fourth to one-half; and grade 3, reduction by more than one-half. Twenty-nine patients with carotid occlusion had grade 2 or 3 atherosclerotic stenoses, but six of them had embolic and eight unclassified occlusions. Ten of 25 patients (40%) with extracranial carotid occlusion had grade 3 stenoses of the intracranial ICA. Among the 25 extracranial occlusions 1 was embolic, 5 unclassified, and 6 old.

Mitchell and Schwartz[253] selected 93 cases on the criterion of age over 35 years. They distinguished the *petrous carotid* and the *terminal carotid*. Stenoses were graded as follows: no stenosis, no reduction in the diameter of the arterial lumen; moderate stenosis, more than one-half the diameter of the original lumen remained; severe stenosis, less than one-half the diameter of the original lumen remained. A low prevalence of severe stenosis was found in the petrous part. A slightly higher prevalence, about 5%, was noted in the terminal carotid. When moderate and severe stenoses were added, figures were of course higher. Among 186 ICAs (93 patients), there were 17 stenoses (9%) on the petrous part and 50 (26%) on the terminal part.

Fisher et al[127] studied atherosclerosis of the carotid and vertebral arteries in 178 unselected autopsies. Although they acknowledged that their series was not entirely random, they deemed that cases of brain diseases probably had a higher incidence than a completely random series would have had. Grades of stenoses were based visually on the cross-sectional area obliterated: 0, 0% to 24%; grade 1, 25% to 49%; grade 2, 50% to 75%; grade 3, >75% but not occluded: and grade 4, total occlusion. There were 15 occlusions in the neck at the sinus. No occlusions were found higher up. All grade 3 stenoses were at the carotid sinus. The second striking site of predilection for atherosclerosis was the region of the siphon. However, in this study stenoses of the intracranial ICA were not graded. Instead Fisher et al[128] stressed the difficulties of assessing correctly the degree of stenosis of the calcified siphon, citing the same reasons mentioned earlier.

Lhermitte et al[219] reported 75 cases from a neurologic ward. Atherosclerotic stenoses were graded on the cross-sectional area obliterated: 0, none or insignificant; 1, <75%; 2, >75%; and 3, occlusion. The intracranial ICA was divided into petrous, and terminal (i.e., cavernous plus supraclinoid) areas. There were 9 stenoses (all grade 1) in the petrous stretch and 20 stenoses (grade 1, 18; grade 2, 2) in the terminal part. For comparison, there were 41 stenoses (grade 1, 28; grade 2, 13) in the sinuses. Occlusion was present in 18 instances, always thrombotic. Thrombosis had started 11 times in the sinus and twice in the siphon; in 5 cases the starting point remained undetermined.

The addition of angiographic evidence sheds further light on the relative prevalence of lesions in the different parts of the intracranial ICA. Marzewski et al[241] reported on 66 patients who had 85 >50% stenoses of the intracranial ICA: 14 stenoses were petrous, 65 cavernous, and 6 supraclinoid. Nineteen patients (28%) had bilateral intracranial ICA stenoses. Craig et al[72] reported on 58 patients with 58 intracranial ICA stenoses that reduced the lumen by at least a third of its diameter: 9 were petrous, 42 cavernous, and 7 supraclinoid. Four patients had lesions in two contiguous segments (e.g., petrous and cavernous). Thirteen patients (22%) had bilateral intracranial ICA stenosis. These data confirm that the cavernous stretch of the artery is the part most often stenosed and show that bilateral intracranial ICA stenoses are by no means rare.

Despite painstaking studies, the problem of the significance of atherosclerotic lesions of the intracranial ICA is still largely unsettled. Discrepancies between studies in which more occlusions occurred in the intracranial ICA than in the extracranial ICA and those in which no occlusion occurred in the intracranial ICA are obvious. Useful comparison between some of the series is difficult if not impossible since grading was different and occlusions were not always separated from stenoses. These studies appeared from 1956 to 1966 when the hemodynamic significance of stenoses may not have been clear to all pathologists. Today terms such as significant or severe would probably not be applied to stenoses that reduce the lumen by about half. However, two main facts stand out: the intracranial ICA, especially the cavernous part, is the second site of predilection of atherosclerosis, but the extent and severity of the lesions are far behind those of the sinus; and a number (unspecified) of atherosclerotic primary occlusive thromboses occur in the intracranial ICA.

Histopathology of Carotid Atheroma

EXTRACRANIAL STENOSIS OR OCCLUSION

In the setting of hemodynamically significant atherostenosis, platelet material, possibly mixed with fibrin complexes, has been shown to be superimposed on the atheroma, perhaps forming the usual means by which stenosis is converted to thrombotic occlusion of the lumen.[19,123] In Samuel's[316] study, the sinus was found to have up to five successive strata of atherosclerosis, which he attributed to the process of layering of mural thrombi.

The carotid lesion found at operation does not always take the form of a thick mound indenting the wall of the artery. In a few instances[227] a thin band of stenosis has been found obstructing cranial or extracranial vessels. The narrow band is thin enough to be invisible on digital substraction studies and was easily overlooked on the conventional angiogram. Presumably, turbulent flow apparent on Doppler analysis should allow a diagnosis when an angiogram fails to demonstrate the appropriate lesion.

Hemorrhage into the wall of the atheroma appears to be a common finding in specimens removed at the time of endarterectomy.[124,185,234,264] Fisher and Ojemann[130] found intraplaque hemorrhages in 34 (38%) of 90 carotid endarterectomy specimens, but their small size was not sufficient to compromise the arterial lumen significantly (Fig. 17.5). However, the hemorrhage in most instances appears to contribute little to the overall mass effect of the stenosis,[264,273] with a few dramatic exceptions.[234] Standard computed tomography (CT)[176] and magnetic resonance imaging (MRI)[149] at the level of arterial injury has documented intramural carotid hemorrhage, thus providing another method of diagnosis. However, in autopsy series, the subject of intramural hemorrhage has rarely been mentioned.[316] Lennihan et al[213] found only 2% of endarterectomy specimens with wall hemorrhages sufficiently large to explain the stenosis.

INTRACRANIAL ATHEROSCLEROSIS

Atherosclerosis in the intracranial ICA has the same general features as elsewhere in the body.[316] However, one peculiar characteristic is that lesions of the cavernous part very often show a high degree of calcification. Such calcifications account for the dense images seen on radiographs and CT scans; moreover, calcification of the siphon by no means indicates significant stenosis of the lumen. Mitchell and Schwartz[253] noted that medial calcification is seen with particular frequency in the petrous and cavernous parts of the artery. Fisher et al[128] studied calcification of the siphon in detail. They found that calcification increased with age and in the older age groups was more pronounced in women. Data on ulceration of plaques are scanty. Mitchell and Schwartz[253] found no ulceration above the sinus, and Fisher et al[128] noted that the intima was not ulcerated.

Occlusion due to pure atherosclerosis is uncommon, although pinpoint atherosclerotic stenoses are frequently encountered. Occlusion usually results from superimposed thrombus. Whether a relationship exists between thrombosis and degree of stenosis is obviously relevant in evaluating the risk of a given stenosis but there are few data on intracranial ICA stenoses. Castaigne et al[59] reported on 19 unilateral atherosclerotic ICA occlusions, 3 of which had started in the siphon, and 12 bilateral atherosclerotic ICA occlusions; 3 of the latter had started in both siphons in one patient, and 1 started in the siphon and contralateral sinus in the other patient. Data suggested differences between unilateral and bilateral occlusions since among the six primary siphon occlusions two were related to more than 75% stenoses, three to 75% to 50% stenoses, and one to a stenosis of <50%. Thus 4 of 6 cases of primary occlusive thromboses of the siphon were related to moderate stenoses, compared with only 2 of 21 primary occlusive thromboses of the sinus, the remaining 19 being related

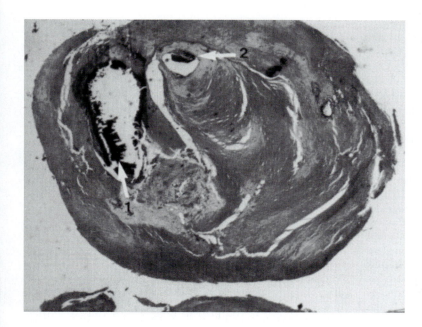

Figure 17.5 Histology of severe stenosis, showing intraplaque hematoma and fibrin-platelet thrombus in lumen. (Courtesy of W. Kupsky, MD.)

to stenoses of >75%. It may be noted that Yates and Hutchinson[402] noted two cases of intracranial ICA primary thrombotic occlusion (case 58: unilateral occlusion of LICA; case 93: bilateral ICA occlusion starting in the petrous-cavernous part on the left) in which thrombosis appeared to have been precipitated by a recent hemorrhage into the plaque. A similar case (case 8) was reported by Castaigne et al.[58] It may be that the calcified siphon is brittle and more liable to intramural hemorrhage with subsequent thrombosis.

TANDEM STENOSES   Stenoses of both the siphon and sinus are another special feature of ICA atherosclerosis. Craig et al[72] found only 6 patients (10%) with ipsilateral 33% to 70% stenoses of siphon and sinus, but Marzewski et al,[241] among their 66 patients with an intracranial ICA stenosis of >50% found 36 (54%) who had 53 extracranial stenoses (24> 50%; 29 <50%). In the series of Castaigne et al[59] only 2 of 6 patients with bilateral ICA occlusion had tandem stenoses of >75%; there were 27 patients with >75% stenosis, and in every case stenoses of <50% were present elsewhere on the ICA; for instance, in 16 unilateral ICA occlusions in which thrombosis had started in the sinus, there were siphon stenoses in every case: 60%, 1 case; 50%, 4 cases; and <50%, 11 cases. The number of reported tandem stenoses of course depends on the degree of stenosis required for admission in a given series, but concomitant lesions of sinus and siphon are at least fairly frequent. This makes it all the more difficult and sometimes impossible to decide which of the two lesions was responsible for a cerebral ischemic event.

Does a siphon stenosis increase the risk of occlusive thrombosis of a sinus stenosis and vice versa? Castaigne et al[59] did not find positive evidence of this. In the series from Craig et al,[72] at the end of follow-up (mean, 30 months) cerebral events had occurred in 25 of the 58 patients (43%), and none of these events were in the 6 patients with tandem stenoses. Marzewski et al[241] followed their 66 patients for a mean of 3.9 years. Eight had isolated TIAs during this period, and seven of the eight had ipsilateral stenoses in their reference angiograms. Among these

seven, five had tandem stenoses. In the same series 10 strokes in all distributions occurred: 2 were in 30 patients (7%) without tandem stenoses on their reference angiograms and 8 were among 36 patients (22%) with tandem stenoses ($P = 0.08$). In five of the eight stroke patients with tandem stenoses the extracranial stenosis was <50%. They concluded that patients with extracranial and intracranial ICA disease appear to have the greater stroke risk, which probably reflects more advanced atherosclerotic disease.

It has been stated that tandem stenoses increase the risk of the carotid endarterectomy, and this is probably a widely held opinion in many neurologic and surgical circles. However, firm evidence is not available. In a report with a particularly disquieting rate of mortality after carotid endarterectomy, a useful comparison between angiographic findings and operative results could not be made.[95] In one,[322] the outcome from carotid bifurcation endarterectomy was compared in 79 cases with 91 stenoses: the 47 stenoses displaying bifurcation disease only were compared with the 44 stenoses showing the tandem lesion of siphon stenosis. No statistically significant differences were encountered among the strokes occurring in the intraoperative (none versus two), perioperative (none versus three), or late postoperative (four versus two) periods, although the crude figures might seem to suggest otherwise.

In some instances, the intracranial stenosis seems to have been an impermanent finding. Little et al[229] found two such instances: the "stenosis" had vanished on the angiogram after endarterectomy. The authors raised the possibility that the finding was an artifact of "pseudo-occlusion." Day et al[78] reported two cases of resolving supraclinoid stenosis following endarterectomy of the ICA origin. It was unclear whether the intracranial ICA narrowing was due to atherosclerosis or atherosclerosis plus mural thrombus or embolism. Such data deserve attention for it may be that unknown relationships exist between tandem stenoses, the understanding of which could shed light on fundamental and therapeutic aspects of atherosclerosis.

Anterograde and retrograde secondary thrombosis of the intracranial ICA is a subject for which only a scanty literature exists. Primary thrombotic occlusion of the sinus is in most cases followed by extensive stagnation thrombosis. However, occlusions occasionally remain segmental. Pathologically well-studied instances of intracranial ICA thrombotic occlusion are rare. In Yates and Hutchinson's[402] cases 58, 72, 78, and 93, the intracranial ICA was occluded by thrombus, but data are lacking about anterograde and retrograde thrombus. In cases 58 and 93 (the latter being a bilateral ICA occlusion), the rostral part of the plug remained proximal to the posterior communicating artery and there was no pericerebral occlusion. In both cases an ipsilateral hemispheral infarct was present. In case 72 there was no cerebral infarct; the occluding material was old. In Torvik and Jörgensen's[359–362] 28 intracranial ICA occlusions, 5 showed anterograde, 6 retrograde, 1 both antero- and retrograde thrombus, and 16 showed none. However, these "primary" occlusions were thrombo-embolic, and the part played by atherosclerotic lesions cannot be estimated. Nevertheless, Torvik and Jörgensen noted that all occlusions more than a month and a half old were longer than 2 cm and that in three of seven cases with retrograde propagation, the thrombus extended down to the extracranial division of the artery. In the study by Castaigne et al[59] of six primary occlusions of the siphon, two had no retrograde thrombosis (one of them was a very short occlusion between the origins of the ophthalmic and posterior communicating arteries), in one a retrograde thrombus extended to the cervical part of the artery, and in three it extended down to the ICA origin. Luessenhop[233] found that when angiography was performed during the first month following the onset of symptoms 31% of the occlusions were in the region of the siphon but that with the passage of time this percentage decreased and became close to zero by 30 months. He thought that this was undoubtedly a consequence of propagation of the thrombi proximally. Most probably, in this series not all occlusions were of atherosclerotic origin. Based on this literature, it seems reasonable to assume that retrograde thrombi developing down to the ICA origin are not rare. Thus arrest of contrast medium at the sinus on angiograms does not allow firm conclusions as to where the primary occlusion started, inasmuch as the angiographic appearance of the proximal end of carotid occlusion is not of predictive value about the age of the occlusion, at least within the first 6 days from stroke onset.[283]

Discontinuous occlusions (i.e., the presence of a patent segment of the ICA between the extracranial occluded ICA and the intracranial ICA) may be found at autopsy, and it may be difficult or impossible to decide whether the distal plug is thrombotic or embolic.[19,59,359–362] This pathologic situation should be kept in mind as a source of technical difficulties in surgical endarterectomies to remove occlusions of the ICA.

Associated Atheromatous Lesions and Conditions

Concomitant stenoses or occlusions of the contralateral ICA sinus and of the intracranial arteries are not rare. In Mitchell and Schwartz's[253] series a strong correlation existed between the degree of carotid and iliac stenosis and the severity of coronary stenosis. The coronary-carotid relationship was present in all age groups in men and in the older age group in women. In men with cardiac infarcts and a high prevalence of severe coronary stenosis, the relationship was even more striking. A positive correlation also existed between compli-

cated (i.e, ulcerated, calcified, or thrombosed) aortic atherosclerosis and carotid stenoses in men. However, in this series the correlations were not specifically studied for the intracranial ICA. In the two recent clinical-angiographic studies of intracranial ICA atherosclerosis already mentioned, coronary artery disease was present in 57.6% and 48% of the patients, peripheral vascular disease in 15.2%, hypertension in 39.4% and 68%, and diabetes mellitus in 50% and 39%, respectively.[72,241] In the 58 patients reported on by Craig et al,[72] most had at least two of the above conditions. Thus atherosclerotic disease of the intracranial ICA is part of a widespread atherosclerosis with a high prevalence of the two main risk factors. This accounts, in part at least, for its poor prognosis.

CARDIAC EMBOLISM

The large series of postmortem cases were often biased toward atherosclerosis. For instance, Fisher et al[127] did not include embolism to the ICA bifurcation, and, as already mentioned, Yates and Hutchinson[402] excluded cases of embolism from mitral stenosis in young patients. Torvik and Jörgensen[359–362] found that less than one-fifth of all cerebral emboli were located in the carotid arteries as emboli tend to lodge in more distal parts of the vessels. Nevertheless, among 43 recent ICA occlusions, 8 were embolic compared with 27 that were thrombotic and 8 unclassified. Blackwood et al[31] found in 105 patients with infarcts in the ICA territory that cardiac embolism was responsible in 48 (45.7%). Among 61 instances of ICA occlusion, Castaigne et al[59] found 13 cases (21.3%) that were due to cardiac embolism.

The true prevalence of ICA embolic occlusion is probably underestimated for three main reasons: first, emboli found at the time of postmortem examination in the pericerebral arteries may well have lodged initially in the ICA and subsequently dislodged and drifted downstream; second, in cases with patent arteries, circumstantial evidence is often suggestive of embolism and at the time of infarction the embolus may well have been lodged in the ICA for some time.[218] Finally, a tendency has always existed to perform fewer angiographies in cases of clinically obvious embolism than in cases presumed to result from atherosclerosis; a recent cooperative study on cerebral embolism did not include angiography in the protocol.[23] This being so, Torvik and Jörgensen[359–362] found seven emboli impacted in the intracranial ICA, at autopsy compared with one in the sinus. Blackwood et al[31] reported that common sites for lodgement of emboli were at the middle cerebral artery trifurcation (commonly referred to as the bifurcation of the stem of the artery) and in the distal ICA, in accordance with the findings of Bladin.[32] Castaigne et al[59] found 8 instances of block of the intracranial ICA among 13 embolic ICA occlusions (one from a thrombus of the aortic arch). The emboli were often several centimeters long, and patterns of occlusion were complex: one had separate embolic occlusion of the external carotid artery/ICA and intracranial ICA, three had occlusions of the intracranial ICA, two had an embolus astride the ICA and the middle cerebral artery, and two were astride the ICA, middle cerebral artery, and anterior cerebral artery.

Anterograde thrombus after intracranial ICA embolic occlusion is probably fairly common.[25,59,359-362] Retrograde thrombus may also develop,[359-362] and it has been reported that a tailing off appearance of the column of contrast material in the more proximal artery is suggestive of retrograde thrombus extension from occlusion of the supraclinoid ICA when angiography is performed in the first 1 or 2 days.[94] However, a significant retrograde thrombus was not found in any of the cases of Castaigne et al's[59] embolic intracranial ICA occlusions; postmortem examinations were performed from 18 hours to 3½ months after the stroke. Probably in some of these cases the ophthalmic and perhaps posterior communicating artery remained patent.

The site of impaction of an embolus in a given artery depends on its size and of the configuration of the vessel, branchings being likely sites of arrest of the traveling plug. In some cardiac diseases emboli of a size such as to block the femoral or iliac arteries are not rare. Therefore, embolic ICA occlusion is not unexpected. The bifurcation of the common carotid artery is the first likely site of arrest, then the tortuous intracranial ICA, and then the bifurcation of its supraclinoid part.

The causes of cardiac embolism have changed during the last decades.[218] Today nonrheumatic atrial fibrillation is likely to be the first responsible condition, followed by postinfarction mural thrombus, although no definite data appear to be available. Conditions like mitral valve prolapse are likely to result in small emboli, which should lodge in pericerebral arteries. In a study of 24 cases of brain events (21 cerebral infarcts or TIAs, one retinal branch occlusion, and two seizures) in patients with mitral valve prolapse (angiography having been performed in 22 patients), no occlusion of the intracranial ICA was reported.[170] The frequency of patent cardiac foramen ovale is now well enough known, occurring in at least 15% of the population, that transcardiac emboli are no longer such rare events (see Ch. 43) as was formerly believed. However, the authors do not know of an example involving occlusion of the carotid itself. Permanent intracranial ICA occlusion from such causes is probably not frequent.

Aortic Arch Atheroma and Embolism

The subject of aortic arch atheroma and embolism has developed so rapidly since the last edition that it now warrants a chapter of its own (see Ch. 36).

OTHER CAUSES OF EXTRACRANIAL CAROTID DISEASE

Apart from atherosclerosis, other causes of carotid artery occlusion include dissection and even embolism from the heart or great vessels. Some causes approach the status of medical curiosities.[122]

Arterial Dissection

In recent years, ICA dissection, either spontaneous or traumatic, has become an important recognized cause of TIAs and stroke within hours or weeks of known trauma, warranting its complete presentation in a separate chapter (see Ch. 29).[46,131,237,260,271,273,296,344]

The pathogenesis of dissection involves the development of a hematoma in the arterial wall either at a subintimal or subadventitial position; the former may lead to narrowing of the true arterial lumen over a long segment, allowing for stagnation thrombus to form a complete occlusion or serve as an embolic source for distal branch occlusion. Hematoma development in the subadventitial portion may not compromise the true arterial lumen, but an aneurysmal dilatation or pouch may collect thrombus and serve as an embolic source into the distal circulation. The arterial disruption seen with dissection is known to heal with time, as documented by serial angiography. Whether this arteriopathy occurs spontaneously because of an underlying arterial defect and/or in response to trivial trauma such as coughing, sneezing, head-turning and other normal activities must be determined on a case-by-case basis.

Hart and Easton[165] have reviewed the major presenting complaints in patients with proven carotid dissection and found that cerebral infarction occurred in 33% (23% minor and 10% major or fatal), TIAs in 45%, head and neck pain in 16%, pulsatile tinnitus in 4%, and asymptomatic bruits in only 2%. Sometimes dissection can be suggested by the clinical presentation if unilateral face or head pain in association with a Horner syndrome and TIAs or if stroke is present in a young, otherwise healthy patient. However, the diagnosis usually rests on angiographic features that include the string sign,[131] which characterizes a tiny, long segment of contrast in the true lumen of the artery, aneurysmal pouch formation, and the distal location of the arteriopathy compared with atheromatous disease, which tends to accumulate at the bifurcation area. Standard CT[176] and MR[149] at the level of arterial injury has documented intramural carotid hemorrhage, thus providing another method of diagnosis.

The natural history and treatment outcome of carotid dissection has not been studied in a controlled fashion, but the weight of case reports strongly suggests that the outcome is benign in over 90% of patients.[165] Surgical treatment either in the form of extracranial carotid thrombectomy or extracranial/intracranial bypass grafting appears unnecessary in the overwhelming majority of patients. The role of anticoagulation and antiplatelet agents is unsettled. A controlled, randomized study will be necessary to establish the efficacy of treatment in those patients with an unstable condition, but such a study would be difficult to mount given the low frequency of the disorder.

Fibromuscular Dysplasia

A rare condition, fibromuscular dysplasia is encountered in <0.6% of cases of ICA disease.[73] It may account for kinks (see below). Intracranial aneurysm occurs in almost 25% of cases (see below). Its clinical importance is unclear, but it has been often enough the subject of publication that it is discussed in a separate chapter (see Ch. 32).

Arterial Kinks

Kinking of the ICA may achieve the same hemodynamic effects as atheromatous stenosis. Kinking of the carotid artery is an acquired condition and is not identical with coiling of the carotid, which is believed to be congenital and of no significance clinically.[63,68] Kinking is thought to be caused by atherosclerosis or to occur as a complication of fibromuscular dysplasia.

Its significance arises when positional head changes produce transient cerebral ischemia, a situation in which dramatic reductions in cerebral blood flow have been documented in some cases during intraoperative studies[338]; as yet, the degree of stenosis observed angiographically has not proved an adequate basis to determine the need for corrective surgery without the additional studies of the effect of head position change.

Kinking caused by alteration in artery position appears to be a rare cause of TIAs. Handa et al described a case of recurrent TIAs following extracranial-intracranial bypass precipitated by yawning.[157] The stretching and kinking of the donor artery by the mouth opening during the yawning was the alleged mechanism.

Extracranial Carotid Aneurysm

Usually the sequelae of a dissecting aneurysm, extracranial carotid aneurysms are highly unusual.[68] Only 34 were reported among 8,500 peripheral vascular aneurysms in one large center over a 12-year period.[247] They usually present as a pulsatile mass in the neck. The neurologic symptoms may include cerebral embolization in addition to the expected syndrome of rupture.[377] Because they are usually very high in the neck, the surgical approach is quite difficult. No clear rules for their medical management have been developed (e.g., whether to treat with warfarin or with aspirin and for how long).

Complications of Head and Neck Cancer

Primary tumors of the vascular structures are uncommon, usually arising from mesoblastic and neural elements such as chemodectomas or paragangliomas.[249] Only 5% are bilateral. The mass grows slowly, presenting as dysphagia and hoarseness, although dyspnea, Horner syndrome, and facial pain may also occur.[159] They produce metastases only in some 2% of cases. Local recurrence is uncommon and is usually delayed for many years.

Involvement of the extracranial carotid by direct extension of local tumor is distinctly uncommon.[153] However, in hospitals with a large oncology case load, this complication occurs often enough to warrant consideration. Direct tumor invasion of the arterial wall was described in 37 of 64 of carotid arteries taken from patients with head or neck cancer in a study at Memorial Hospital in New York.[185] Three examples of such involvement in the siphon from parasellar tumors were reported by Spallone.[335] Two were meningiomas, and the third was a pituitary adenoma. This complication appears to be extremely rare, having been encountered by that author in only 3 cases among more than 10,000 examined angiographically in his institution over a period of approximately 25 years.

Surgical approaches to tumor resection that involve taking the carotid along with the tumor carry considerable risk. Experience at Iowa showed a stroke rate of 25%.[243] Snyderman and D'Amico[333] reviewed the literature to 1991 for all cases of squamous cell carcinoma treated by carotid resection: neurologic complications occurred in 17% of patients but seemed unrelated to the method of attempted carotid reconstruction. Such methods include interposition grafting[274]; the greater saphenous vein graft is preferred, the non-reversed having better patency than the reversed.[397]

Radiation may induce or accelerate atherosclerosis, through means still unclear,[290] but arterial stenosis of the carotid is a recognized complication of radiation to the head and neck. Huvos et al[185] found this form of atherosclerosis in 15 of their 64 cases of head and neck tumor with carotid complication. Supervoltage therapy had been given to 24 of the patients, and 45 had had preoperative radiation therapy to the neck. Levinson et al[216] described three patients with atypical presumably atherosclerotic lesions that developed more than 25 years after external cervical irradiation. The syndromes presented from a variety of inferred mechanisms including cerebral embolization, impaired retinal perfusion, and decreased total cerebral perfusion.

Coexisting Intracranial Arterial Aneurysms

Intracranial aneurysms distal to a symptomatic carotid stenosis are uncommonly encountered.[82,109,293,329] The occurrence appears to be entirely coincidental and not causally related. The main issue is whether surgical management of the carotid disease will influence the course of the aneurysm and encourage its rupture or enlargement. In the handful of cases reported, the aneurysm(s) showed no change in size on follow-up angiography after carotid endarterectomy using intervals of 1 week,[82] 7 months,[329] and 1 year.[109] The difficulty in predicting the course of an asymptomatic aneurysm is well known,[29,403] and some[293] have recommended prophylactic repair. The scanty data that exist seem to indicate the carotid lesion can be attacked with no concerns for acute aneurysmal rupture.

Immediate Postoperative Stenosis or Occlusion

It was long assumed that immediate postoperative stenosis or occlusion was uncommon and that conventional angiography to check on the postoperative status in otherwise asymptomatic patients was counterindicated—because of the risk of complications. A check on the status of the carotid was usually undertaken only in instances of the many and varied focal neurologic deficits apparent postoperatively.[221] Few studies using intraoperative angiography have been reported. Scott et al[324] found 56 defects, 18 requiring surgical revision, among their series of 137 endarterectomies. This worrisome finding is difficult to interpret, as the authors experienced rates of perioperative stroke (6.8%) and death (4.8%) a bit above the lower rates hoped for in a surgical series. However, the point seemed well taken that intraoperative angiography might help to identify the immediate technical problems.

With the introduction of noninvasive scanning and digital subtraction angiography (DSA), the possibilities of morbidity from investigation alone have been reduced to negligible levels. With that reduction has come better documentation of a disappointingly higher incidence of postoperative stenosis and occlusion than was earlier anticipated. As in all clinical series, the incidence of such complications appeared to be inversely proportional to surgical success, which varies considerably. Among 262 carotid reconstructions studied by DSA, Hertzer et al[172] documented five internal carotid occlusions (1.9%), two of which had neurologic complications; stenosis was more than 30% in two. Permanent occult carotid occlusion was not the only cause for stroke: the angiogram was normal in four others with neurologic complications.

Duplex scanning and spectral analysis have shown a higher incidence of postoperative stenosis than is usually appreciated on clinical grounds alone. Ziegler et al[410] found an overall incidence of persistent high-grade stenosis in fully 19% of the cases studied by these methods. Recurrent neurologic symptoms occurred in eight of these cases. The authors believe that the transient nature of some early postoperative stenoses is consistent with proliferation and regression of myointimal lesions in response to arterial injury.

Recurrence of Stenosis or Occlusion after Endarterectomy

For years, recurrent stenosis after successful endarterectomy was thought to be uncommon. Endarterectomy was considered in most cases to be the definitive treatment. In early studies based on recurrent symptoms that lead to reangiogram, the incidence of recurrent stenosis varied from 0.6% to 9.8%.[50] Newer methods of following the course of the postoperative carotid have indicated that recurrence and even residual stenosis may be more common than suspected on clinical grounds alone. The 64 cases followed from 1 to 13 years after endarterectomy by Norrving et al[270] disclosed occlusion or recurrent stenosis (defined as more than 50%) in fully 36% of operated cases, a figure that seemed equivalent to the 27% rate of progression on the nonoperated, previously asymptomatic side. About 30% of the cases with progressing disease became symptomatic with TIAs or strokes. By contrast, only 5.5% of the vessels showing no progression of the disease process had symptoms, a highly significant difference ($P<0.001$).

Two types of recurrence are most frequently recognized. In the first, restenosis develops within a few months up to 2 years. Frequently the finding is that of a fibrous hyperplasia reaction.[50] Stenoses occurring beyond 2 years are frequently conventional atheromatous lesions and are sometimes associated with persistent hypertriglyceridemia or hyperlipidemia. The factors contributing to early restenosis include difficulties with surgical technique and hyperlipidemia that encourages severe atherosclerotic formation.

MISCELLANEOUS PATHOLOGIC DISORDERS OF THE INTRACRANIAL ICA

In this brief review it is convenient to consider the three anatomic parts of the intracranial ICA separately.

Petrous Part

The petrous part is separated from the inner ear by bone that is very thin in the infant and child. In addition, the distal part of the cervical ICA is close to the throat, tonsillar fossa, and lymph nodes. Cases with occlusion or stenosis of the intracranial ICA (and in some of the pericerebral branches) have been reported by Shillito[327] and Bickerstaff[28] in children with infection of the ears, throat, nose, or paranasal sinuses or after tonsillectomy. In some cases of Shillito's and in a comparable case of Banker's,[14] pathologic evidence of acute arteritis was present. When the ICA erodes the bone, it may appear as a red mass in the middle ear when viewed through the tympanic membrane; biopsy in pursuit of a diagnosis can have disastrous consequences.[7] Fractures of the petrous bone can conceivably result in ICA trauma and thus lead to thrombus or embolism, or both, but no positive report of such fracture appears to be available.

Cavernous Part

Stenoses and occlusions of the cavernous segment of the ICA in cavernous sinus infections has been reported in children[28,242,376] and in adults.[32] The intracavernous ICA may also be stenosed by the nonspecific granulomatous arteritis reported by Tolosa.[355] The petrous and cavernous portion can be involved in cranial giant cell arteritis.[383] Meningiomas developed in the sinus can stenose the siphon. Stenosis of the cavernous portion has been described in cluster headache, and it has been speculated that the sympathetic fiber involvement could explain the oculosympathetic paralysis.[103]

Supraclinoid Part

The supraclinoid part of the artery lies in the spinal fluid space. It may thus be involved by the process of endarteritis obliterans in chronic or subacute meningitides due to syphilis (meningovascular syphilis; Heubner's arteritis), tuberculosis, or pyogenic bacteria (e.g., pneumococcus). Stenosis or occlusion results from hyperplasia of subendothelial tissue.[13] Direct invasions of the ICA by hyphae in mucormycosis with infection of the sinus, orbit, and meningitis has been reported in a 3-year-old boy.[314] Dissecting aneurysm may involve intracranial arteries, and in 13 of 58 cases the terminal ICA and its branches were affected.[30] Stenosis and occlusion of the intracranial ICA has been reported in drug addicts.[334,396] Thus the supraclinoid siphon is involved in vasospasm, probably due to acute hypertension.[141]

Moyamoya is a Japanese word meaning "something hazy like a puff of cigarette smoke drifting in the air"[345]; it is also used as a term to denote uncertainty. This disorder is the subject of a separate chapter. Here we make only brief mention of those cases involving the intracranial ICA. The condition refers to an angiographic appearance resulting from the enlargement of numerous small collateral channels associated with stenosis or occlusion of the supraclinoid ICA on both sides. It is rare for the stenosis to extend below the level of the third cervical vertebra.[289] Postmortem examinations have been few, and the characteristics of the obstructing arterial process are poorly known but are attributed to subintimal proliferation. An unusual case without intracranial ICA stenoses has been reported.[64] Data supporting congenital and acquired forms have been recorded. Suzuki and Kodama[345] noted the high prevalence of past inflammations in the head or neck. A stenosis of the siphon with occlusion of the supraclinoid portion and moyamoya have been reported 6 years after irradiation of a pituitary tumor.[23]

Collateral Blood Flow for the Internal Carotid Artery

When the ICA is unable to supply its usual territory distally, five major sources of collateral flow may develop, in a number of variations.[48,204,365] The most readily recognized extracranial source is anastomosis with the external carotid through the orbit. Blood flows anterograde up the external carotid to the orbit, where anastomoses occur with the ophthalmic branch of the intracranial ICA. The anastomoses mainly occur between the maxillary branch of the external carotid and the ophthalmic artery in the floor of the orbit (Fig. 17.6). Smaller anastomoses occur over the roof of the orbit between the facial and frontal branches of the external carotid and the supratrochlear and supraorbital branches of the ophthalmic artery. Blood flows from these anastomoses retrograde in the ophthalmic artery to reach the intracranial portion of the ICA at the siphon. From there the flow continues distally toward the circle of Willis in the usual anterograde fashion. This collateral flow is often demonstrated angiographically. Minor variations exist in the anastomosis pattern in the orbit. Collateral flow to the ophthalmic artery may come from meningeal branches of the external carotid. Rarely, the ophthalmic artery

Figure 17.6 Sources of collateral flow to the internal carotid territory (1, arrow), ophthalmic artery.

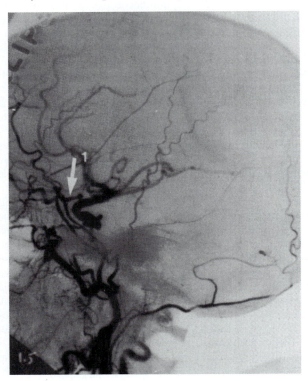

is not a branch of the ICA, receiving instead its entire flow from the meningeal artery, a linkage that offers little intracranial supply to the circle of Willis.

The most important source of collateral for a hemisphere comes from the contralateral ICA via the circle of Willis. In this case, blood flows anterograde up the opposite ICA, and thence across the circle of Willis at the anterior communicating artery, from which it passes on the one hand anterograde along the cortical branches of the anterior cerebral artery and on the other hand retrograde along the stem of the anterior cerebral artery to the middle cerebral stem, and thence distally into the territory of the middle cerebral artery in the usual anterograde fashion. This form of collateral depends on an intact anterior half of the circle of Willis. Many minor variations in the circle of Willis conspire to prevent this collateral flow from developing, among them an azygous anterior cerebral artery, in which the supply to the anterior cerebral artery arises from a common trunk, with no anterior cerebral stem on one side to complete the circle of Willis. In such cases, the two anterior cerebral artery territories may be involved with infarction or spared together, depending on the vascular anatomy.

The vertebrobasilar system may supply the middle and anterior cerebral artery territory by means of collateral flow through the ipsilateral posterior communicating artery. This collateral flow is the posterior equivalent of the collateral flow via the anterior half of the circle of Willis. It depends on patent posterior communicating artery, which occurs far less commonly than does a patent anterior communicating artery. Rarely, the flow into the ICA territory from the basilar artery is by way of a persisting trigeminal artery, which usually reaches the ICA near the base of the skull (Fig. 17.7).

Flow retrograde from cerebral arteries through the border zones over the brain surface may spare some or all of the cortical surface branches of the endangered arterial territories. In this setting, the anatomy of the circle of Willis plays a vital role: should the posterior communicating artery be too small to carry much collateral, the distal ends of the cortical branches of the posterior cerebral artery may supply collateral to the anterior or middle cerebral artery territories through the border zone anastomoses over the hemipshere surface; should the stem of the anterior cerebral artery ipsilateral to the occluded ICA likewise be too small, the anterior cerebral artery may collateralize some or all of the middle cerebral surface branches through the border zone. In such instances, the flow retrograde into the endangered territories varies from full collateral flow all the way to the stem of the recipient vessel to little more than feeble flow into the distal cortical surface branches.

Other paths of collateral may develop under special circumstances. Cerebral surface vessels may anastomose with an extracranial arterial source through a craniotomy site. When the stenosis lies distally, in the intracranial portion of the ICA, preventing collateral flow via the circle of Willis, not only may cerebral surface collaterals develop through the border zones, but the penetrating arteries (the lenticulostriates) may enlarge within the depths of the brain as well. This condition, met commonly in moyamoya disease, has also been encountered in cases of arteriovenous malformations subjected to surgical ligation of the main feeding arteries.[244] Although such anastomoses are rare, they indicate the enormous siphoning effect

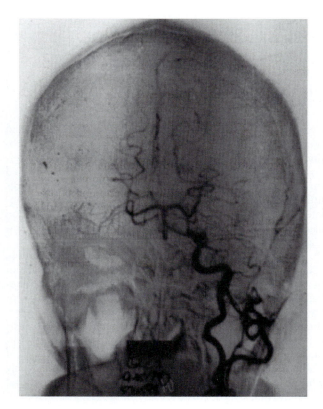

Figure 17.7 Example of a persistent trigeminal artery.

that may exist in underperfused territories. Their occurrence is also important because they demonstrate the occurrence of fusion of arteries in an adult.

CLINICAL SETTINGS FOR DEVELOPMENT OF COLLATERAL BLOOD FLOW

In all arterial territories, low perfusion pressure distal to occlusion, or, in exceptional cases (documented by transcranial Doppler insonation) with severe stenosis, leads to the development of collateral blood flow in the hypoperfused territory. The finding seems to be so familiar to clinicians that few papers on the subject are easily found. Castaigne et al[59] noted collateral flow via the ophthalmic artery in every case of ICA occlusion studied in which the carotid occlusion lay below the ophthalmic artery. The rate at which such collateral flow develops is poorly documented. Opinions vary between days to weeks. From personal experience, it seems certain that retrograde flow through the orbit can develop rather quickly. However, the speed of development almost always seems insufficient to avoid brain ischemia.

In some instances, when carotid artery stenosis has reached the point of hemodynamic significance, collateral flow, whose development can be documented by transcranial Doppler sonography, may develop in response to the flow failure sufficient to cause major symptoms. Cases of asymptomatic carotid occlusion in several autopsy series have shown

a patent circle of Willis, implying that collateral flow has developed to arteries distal to the site of occlusion: five of the internal carotid cases of Fisher et al[127] and three of Hutchinson and Yates[184] were spared infarction. An explanation for the continued risk of stroke involves discussion of the mechanism of stroke in carotid artery occlusion.

The role of the development of collateral flows in protecting the hemisphere against ischemic events is obviously of great importance. It has long been obvious that the mere demonstration of collateral, flow angiographically bears little relationship to its physiologic effect. Accordingly, investigations using regional cerebral blood flow measurements have been undertaken to clarify the role of collateral flow evident angiographically. The results have been somewhat disappointing. Awad et al[10] studied 18 patients with unilateral internal collateral occlusion by both DSA and xenon-133 inhalation measurements. They attempted to correlate distribution of the opacification seen on DSA with regional cerebral blood flow determinations by the xenon-133 inhalation method. The nine patients who showed symmetric filling of the cortical surface branches on DSA showed no significant interhemispheric difference in regional cerebral blood flow. The other nine showed a delayed pattern of cortical filling and varying degrees of asymmetry in the regional cerebral blood flow between the two hemispheres. The authors demonstrated that symmetric filling of the cerebral vessels on DSA correlated with essentially identical regional cerebral blood flow in the two hemispheres. However, they warned that the finding only indicates negligible interhemispheric differences in regional cerebral blood flow but did not refer to normal regional cerebral blood flow. Likewise, since only the larger cortical vessels are seen by DSA and since the regional cerebral blood flow measurements present total flow in both the larger vessels visualized by DSA and the smaller ones are not visualized, the delay in DSA opacification on one side of the brain did not necessarily represent a decrease in regional cerebral blood flow. DSA has not yet reached the point at which it can be used as a predictor of regional cerebral blood flow differences bearing on the risk of subsequent stroke.

Other methods have not been helpful predictors. Using positron emission tomography (PET) measurements (cerebral blood flow, blood volume, oxygen extraction fraction), Powers et al[294] found that neither the percent stenosis nor the residual lumen diameter of the extracranial ICA was a reliable predictor of the hemodynamic state of the cerebral circulation in 19 patients with >66% extracranial carotid lumen diameter reduction. Hemodynamic insufficiency of the hemisphere correlated best with angiographic patterns of meningeal and ophthalmic arterial collaterals. These two angiographic collateral patterns, however, were signs of circulatory inadequacy via the usual carotid and circle of Willis routes, observations further corroborated by Tatemichi et al[346] using transcranial Doppler sonography. These studies indicated that ophthalmic collateral flow is an insufficient source of supply to the brain and, when present, indicates that the more common sources of collateral flow are unavailable or incompetent. Prominent ophthalmic collateral flow is probably a poor, not a favorable, prognostic sign, a finding independently corroborated by Schneider et al[321]

SPONTANEOUS RESOLUTION OF EXTRACRANIAL DISEASE

Spontaneous resolution of occlusive lesions on the carotid artery may be more common than has been appreciated.[195] Resolving lesions include those due to arterial dissection, fibromuscular dysplasia, and even atheromatous lesions. Arbeille et al[8] found that 25 of 86 carotid plaques assessed by Doppler for plaque size underwent reduction in size when re-examined at 6-month intervals over a period of 24 months. The plaques became more homogeneous in the process. How such regression occurred and on what therapy was not detailed in the report; the clinical cohort was described simply as ". . . patients symptomatiques."

Pathophysiology of Carotid Ischemia

GENERAL PRINCIPLES

From disease involving the carotid artery itself, the clinical syndromes that occur result from two basic mechanisms: first, from intracranial arterial occlusion, whether from embolism or from anterograde extension of thrombus across the circle of Willis into the stems of the major cerebral arteries; and second, from perfusion failure due to inadequate collateral distal to hemodynamically significant stenosis or occlusion. Both mechanisms may even be operative in the same patient.[37,286]

The problem in diagnosis and management of carotid artery disease lies mainly in clarifying which one of these principles is at work in a given case, determining the source of an embolus, determining the severity of the perfusion failure, and predicting future events. The problem is compounded by the need to take into account instances of ischemia in the carotid territory from problems unrelated to disease of the carotid itself, especially embolism of cardiac origin and lacunar disease. Although the carotid artery is commonly the site of atherosclosis, severe disease of the carotid is an uncommon finding in autopsy series: Fisher et al[127] found arterial thrombosis with infarction in only 18% of 57 autopsy-studied cases of stroke among 178 collected cases in 1960 to 1961 at the Massachusetts General Hospital. More recent surveys in a multihospital setting in Italy, using Doppler ultrasonography to study 115 men aged 15 to 44 years who presented with TIA or stroke in the carotid artery territory, found a prevalence of 15.8% for carotid stenosis or occlusion.[54]

Most cases of carotid territory ischemia are broadly attributed to atherosclerosis, but a variety of mechanisms of infarction seem to be involved. For TIAs, these mechanisms would entail a temporary cessation of flow either in a distal branch artery from embolus, or over the distal territories of the underperfused carotid while the carotid itself was temporarily blocked. With restoration of blood flow, the ischemic region of the brain quickly recovers and the clinical deficit (TIA) would vanish. For infarction, the processes would presumably be the same, but the effects of the occlusion would persist.

EMBOLISM

From pathologic studies it has been determined that carotid occlusion results when an atheromatous plaque already producing high-grade reduction in the arterial lumen first develops superimposed platelet-fibrin thrombus and later red thrombus, completing the process.[4,19,59,124,127,129] It requires little imagination to envision that as the thrombus accumulates, loose material may be swept into the distal circulation causing permanent or temporary occlusion of small intracranial arteries, leading to TIAs.

Millikan et al[252] were the first to report their success using anticoagulants to treat patients with TIAs, a program quickly copied.[275] The rationale for this therapy was their suggestion that fragments of an enlarging thrombus may be swept away by the blood and temporarily occlude cerebral arteries, producing a TIA. This embolic theory of TIA pathogenesis has received support over the years from several studies. Gunning et al[156] and Castaigne et al[58] found a loose network of fibrin and platelets in patients at the time of endarterectomy who were recently symptomatic with retinal or hemispheral TIAs. By contrast, patients without recent symptoms have relatively clean atheroma at the time of endarterectomy. Fisher[117] and Ross Russell[309,310] observed material passing through the retinal circulation during attacks of transient monocular blindness, documenting that migrating particles could be associated with transient symptoms. Evidence has also been presented for clinically inevident cerebral embolization in patients suffering symptomatic transient monocular blindness.[163] However, Fisher and Ojemann's[130] findings in a study of 90 carotid endarterectomy specimens have challenged the embolic theory of TIAs. They found that three clinical categories—hemispheric TIAs, transient monocular blindness, and asymptomatic, severe carotid obstruction producing subocclusion—led to hemodynamic insufficiency as the cause for the transient symptoms. Mural thrombus, present in many of the specimens, contributed to the overall obstructive process but had little independent serious consequences beyond this effect.

Proof of the embolic mechanism might be difficult to find, since angiographic[77,80,224,301,348,409] and pathologic studies[126] have shown how promptly cerebral emboli fragments disappear, leaving a patent vessel supplying the clinically affected region.

Nature of the Embolic Material

Most of the embolic material has been assumed to be platelet aggregates and red cells enmeshed in fibrin.[2,156,246] Other material has had much less documentation. Beal et al[21] described a syndrome of multiple foci of cerebral infarction due to cholesterol embolization. The patient was a 69-year-old man who experienced several spells over a period of 3 years consistent with hemispheral transient cerebral ischemic attacks (numbness and weakness of one or the other hand with a duration of 5 to 8 minutes). Previously, it had been the opinion of many[44] that such crystals were too small to produce focal signs.

Carotid Artery Sources of the Embolic Material

In a setting of carotid occlusion, embolic material may be swept into the brain from the intracranial portion of the thrombus.[310] One patient described by Countee et al[71] experienced TIAs 3½ years after an ipsilateral carotid endarterectomy.[75] The apparent source was the occluded stump of the ICA, which was found to be filled with atheromatous debris the excision of which was associated with cessation of the TIAs (Fig. 17.8). Unusual rare variations in arterial anatomy may set the stage for an unusual course for the presumed embolic fragments to follow when they leave the ulcerative or stenotic carotid lesion. Waller et al[370] described two cases of TIAs involving the brain stem attributed to microembolization from the carotid via a persistent trigeminal artery.

The usual source for the emboli is assumed to be the carotid stenosis or ulcerated plaque itself. From the stenosis, loose aggregates of platelet-fibrin complexes presumably might be dislodged.[156] Similar fragments could also occur from associated ulcers (Fig. 17.9). The issue of particle size is obviously of great importance. The size of embolic material sufficient to cause retinal ischemia may be too small to affect or block any but the tiny pial surface branches in the hemisphere and are unlikely to cause symptoms. This point alone

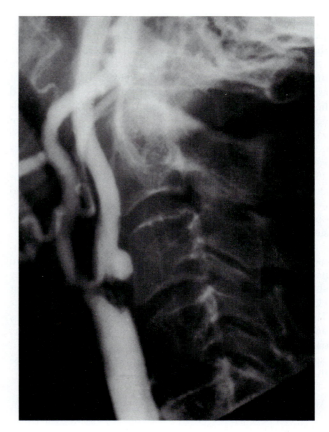

Figure 17.9 Internal carotid artery with combined stenosis and large ulceration.

Figure 17.8 Occluded internal carotid artery with a large stump.

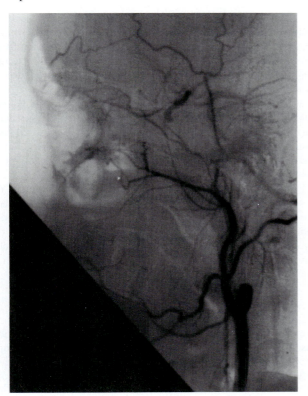

may explain the usually asymptomatic state of cases with cholesterol emboli found in retinal vessels. However, once carotid territory embolism has occurred, no matter how small the particle size, no studies to date permit the inference of continued small particle embolism; subsequent emboli may be quite a bit larger. A few discouraging cases have been reported. In the patient (case 5) reported by Zatz et al[409] a devastating stroke occurred 17 hours after an angiogram. This study was performed for patients with TIAs and documented an irregular nonobstructing plaque at the origin of the ICA. On repeat angiogram 3 hours after the stroke, the plaque was no longer present. Only a minimal irregularity of the wall was seen, and a major occlusion was found in the previously patent stem of the middle cerebral artery above. The authors concluded that the TIAs and the major stroke, respectively, were related to embolism from, and then of, this atheromatous plaque. In this case, it may be argued that the angiogram itself caused or destabilized the lesion, as may have been the case in another dramatic stroke following angiography.[76]

The possibility of a major stroke in a setting of presumably minor carotid disease is the dreaded complication that has dictated many a management decision. The mural hemorrhage thesis of Lusby et al[234] raised this worry. These authors inferred that the presence of a small ulcer or modest atheroma may suffice to allow a subintimal dissection to develop, usually caused by subintimal hemorrhage. The resultant hemorrhage could thus suddenly convert a modest lesion to a severe stenosis. Worse, the unstable intima atop the subintimal hemorrhage would presumably break down, discharging into the arterial lumen as embolic material. The speculation was made that the whole process might be aggravated by the use of aspirin, which might even mask the occurrence of TIAs[56] and help to bring about intramural hemorrhages.[234] If such developments were the result of aspirin therapy, more enthusiasm would be created for elective operative repair of these lesions even in the asymptomatic state. Little evidence has been developed to support these claims. Lennihan et al[213] found only 2% with wall hemorrhages large enough to have caused stenosis. They are often induced by the trauma of the surgery and included as part of the specimen. However, those present preoperatively are only rarely large enough to play a role in the stenosis.[123,213,264]

It should be mentioned in passing that the foregoing arguments assume the source of the embolic material is the carotid itself.[349] However, it is well recognized that the heart may also be the source.[42,79] Furthermore, it is also possible that platelet coagula develop in the circulating blood itself.[81,86,371] Thus far, it has not proved possible to separate the sources on a case-by-case basis. Until a more reliable method of differentiation becomes available, these unsettling possibilities of carotid territory stroke must remain qualitative and not quantitative issues.

Aortic Arch Source of TIA

See Chapter 36.

Embolic TIAs

The embolic theory can account for different types of carotid territory TIAs on the basis of separate embolic material occluding different intracranial branches, and probably many TIAs occur as a result of this short-lived embolic mechanism.

The clinical and angiographic details in many of these cases suggest they are a variant, but not the usual type of TIA. Duration of the TIA deficit is different in embolic cases: Pessin et al[284] postulated emboli as the explanation for at least some of the TIAs encountered in their prospective study of 95 consecutively angiogrammed cases of carotid TIA, but in these cases the deficit tended to last far longer than the usual 5 to 7 minutes that characterize most cases of TIA associated with severe stenosis of the ICA. Their findings echoed the earlier work of Acheson and Hutchinson,[1] who suggested that many of these cases could be interpreted as examples of clinically short-lived strokes arising from a variety of embolic sources, including cardiac, rather than examples of carotid artery stenosis alone. These cases also showed a high incidence of widely patent carotid arteries. This relatively benign form of embolism has been described as acceptable minor embolism by Fisher and Ojemann.[130]

Stereotypic TIAs are a major problem for the embolic theory. In at least one study, however, artificial emboli injected in the carotid circulation gathered in the same vessel.[379] It might be argued that few instances of TIA are truly stereotypic. Exactly repetitive attacks seem rather uncommon.[284] It may be that what seem to be stereotypic attacks are merely attacks with many prominent features commonly occurring in

most cases of embolism to branches of the middle cerebral artery. In the published experience with aberrant embolization from silastic ball therapy for arteriovenous malformations, several cases have been reported in which a similar syndrome occurred from embolism to a variety of different middle cerebral branches: the complaints included focal weakness of the arm[392] persisting for only a few minutes and transient dysesthesia of the contralateral hand,[209] both common symptoms of TIA. Sadly, such details are often lost on physicians from other specialties, as shown by recent studies indicating that many events neurologists label as TIAs are not those of minor stroke, while minor stroke is often included among the conditions labeled as TIA by non-neurologists.[107]

INTRACRANIAL EMBOLISM

Early autopsy studies documented intracranial embolism rising from extracranial carotid occlusive disease as a cause of hemisphere infarction. The outlook is usually serious and often occurs with little warning. Any part of the intracranial carotid circulation may be affected, but frequently the embolus impacts the middle cerebral artery stem or major branches, and a sizable infarct results, causing a serious deficit. The source of the embolus may be fragmentation and distal migration of a thrombus fragment at the time of, or shortly after, acute carotid occlusion, or in the setting of severe stenosis. Alternatively, antegrade propagation of thrombus into the circle of Willis, without fragmentation, may also account for intracranial obstruction.

Embolism arising from extracranial carotid disease may be a frequent cause of stroke. In a series reported by Pessin et al,[283] two-thirds of 64 patients had definite or suggestive angiographic evidence of intracranial embolism. Twenty-five of the 64 patients had definite angiographic evidence of intracranial middle cerebral artery stem or branch cerebral artery occlusion; another 17 had angiographic findings consistent or suggestive of embolism. The clinical picture of these 42 patients contrasted sharply with the 22 patients with no angiographic evidence of embolism. Significantly fewer (40%) of the 42 patients with an embolic (or suspected embolic) mechanism had preceding TIAs, compared with 73% of the 22 patients with a nonembolic mechanism. Stroke deficits were more severe in the embolic compared with the nonembolic group.

This form of embolic infarction has proved difficult, if not impossible, to differentiate from embolism of cardiac sources.[373,391] At our present state of knowledge, there appears to be no essential difference between the type and severity of the syndromes caused by carotid or cardiac embolic sources. These syndromes are discussed more fully in the chapter on the middle cerebral artery (see Ch. 19).

Noninvasive Detection of Emboli

Support for embolism as a cause of TIAs or stroke in carotid diseases seemed clear when reports first began to appear using transcranial Doppler monitoring. These studies found high-intensity transient signals (HITS) appearing in the anterior circle of Willis and its major cerebral artery branches while insonations were being done for evidence of reduction in intracranial velocity profiles distal to high-grade carotid stenosis.[133] Most of this literature has appeared since 1992 as the subject of editorials,[169,353] and the subject was recently surveyed by Gorce and Elias.[151] Considerable variation between study groups exists in the computed hourly rate of HITS and in some of the criteria for reporting them. No disagreement exists on the correlation with stenosis, as HITS are infrequent for other forms of stroke (e.g., lacunes, cardiogenic emboli),[203] but their relationship to ulceration and plaque ultrasonographic characteristics is less certain.

ANTEROGRADE PROPAGATION OF CAROTID THROMBOSIS

Anterograde propagation of carotid thrombosis has been documented in pathologic studies, with extension to and beyond the circle of Willis, involving the stems of the anterior and middle cerebral arteries. The result is usually devastating cerebral infarction.[77,170,284] One result is the rare telodiencephalic syndrome,[412] consisting of contralateral brachiofacial hemiparesis, occasionally accompanied by homonymous hemianopia and aphasia, but associated with ipsilateral hemihypohidrosis, and an ipsilateral Horner syndrome. The authors consider it to be caused by an ischemic lesion of crossed pathways descending from the cerebrum and the uncrossed hypothalamic-spinal sympathetic pathways. The syndrome was attributed to occlusion of the ICA and occasionally the middle cerebral artery.

PERFUSION FAILURE WITH DISTAL INSUFFICIENCY

Distal insufficiency is the other major mechanism that may account for cerebral ischemia. This theory has proved attractive because the topography of cerebral infarcts in many cases of carotid occlusion closely mimics that found in obvious settings of hypotension such as cardiac arrest, and because the most reliable correlation with TIAs is severe stenosis.

The distal insufficiency concept for ischemia or infarction implies decreased vascular perfusion on those areas of the brain parenchyma located at the greatest distance from the site of stenosis or occlusion.[257] As a consequence, stagnation thrombus may develop from local circulatory failure at these distant sites,[115] and infarction follows. The areas at risk include the most distal segments of the cortical branches of the middle cerebral artery, in particular the superior parietal and posterior temporal-occipital area.[36,257]

Distal Field Infarct (Watershed or Border Zone) Topography in Autopsy Studies

Infarction found along the superior frontal, superior parietal, and lateral occipital regions has a long history in the pathology literature (Fig. 17.10).[112,114,225,281,286,302,306,336,358,361,387,388]

The topography of the infarction has been better documented than has the mechanism. Several famous cases have been described. Spatz's[336] case showed infarction affecting the left cerebral hemisphere from the frontal through posterior parietal regions. All the foci of infarction were suprasylvian, that is, sparing the region of the operculum and the insula. A similar suprasylvian topography was described later by Lindenberg and Spatz[225] as the expected topography in cerebral Buerger's disease.

Interest in the subject became more keen after Schneider[320] proposed the thesis of infarction by the process of distal insufficiency, and many of the autopsy-documented cases with such infarct topography were found to be associated with a thrombus or severe stenosis of the carotid artery, a condition known before then as infarction at a distance.[59,112,114,115,127,220,306]

Distal Field Infarct Topography in Radiologic Studies

Studies based on cerebral angiography have attempted to corroborate these findings but have had only modest success. In a clinical-angiographic study of acute cerebral infarction from ICA occlusion or tight stenosis, Pessin et al[286] found a possible mechanism of low flow as the explanation for the infarcts in less than one-third of their cases. Angiography revealed a slowing of circulation throughout the entire middle cerebral artery distribution in those cases, as opposed to direct or indirect evidence of intracranial branch occlusion in those diagnosed as embolic.

CT scanning has commonly been used in settings of carotid territory infarction, but correlations with autopsy findings have only been documented in a few published studies.[388] Ringelstein et al[302] studied 107 cases of internal carotid occlusion documented by Doppler sonograms, angiograms, and CT criteria and attributed 44 of 111 infarcts to a hemodynamic cause, 8 presenting as watershed infarction and 44 as terminal supply area infarction. Harrison and Marshall[161] also carried out similar studies, this time with CT scan and angiograms, and found that the high-convexity lesions on CT scan correlated well with those patients who showed poor collateral flow.

Inhalation studies such as xenon and PET scanning have documented the topography of carotid ischemia. Vorstrup et al[366] showed impaired xenon uptake in suprasylvian areas in a few patients who had suffered TIAs. Single-photon emission tomogram measurements have found documented increased cerebral blood volume, a sign of dilated collaterals, only in those patients with high-grade carotid stenosis.[363] PET has uncovered numerous examples of the distal insufficiency perfusion.[297,399] Known also as the misery perfusion syndrome,[18] it has been explained by reduced cerebral metabolism and has proved to be surgically reversible. Low reactivity of middle cerebral blood vessels in a setting of hypercapnia, a sign of fully dilatated collaterals, was found by Levine et al[215] to have a significant relationship ($P = 0.04$) to high-grade carotid stenosis. Leblanc et al[211] used PET scanning to document the selective vulnerability of the anterior border zone region, with significant reduction in cerebral blood flow and hemodynamic reserve capacity in seven patients (five with TIAs and two asymptomatic) with at least 80% ICA stenosis. Yamauchi et al[399] demonstrated diminished regional cerebral blood flow,

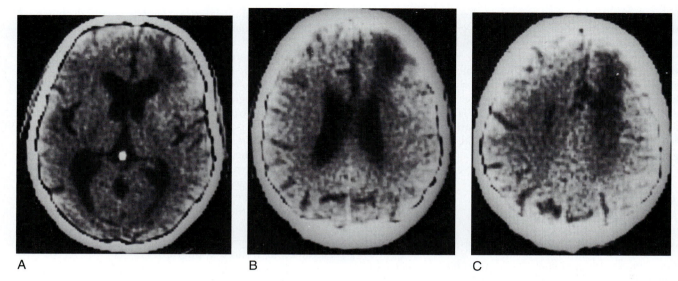

A   B   C

Figure 17.10 CT scan of distal field or border zone infarction.

increased oxygen extraction, and a decrease in the ratio of cerebral blood flow to volume consistent with stagnation thrombus occurring in the border zone areas. All these studies point to a state of hemodynamic insufficiency. Yanagihara et al[401] documented the disappearance of symptoms after endarterectomy but not in patients with disease at the carotid siphon, where surgery was not possible. Carpenter et al,[55] in a study of 32 patients, were unable to document selective border zone hemodynamic impairment in their cohort of patients with varying degrees of carotid stenosis, the notable exception to the general findings of others.

In the even more severe state of distal intracranial ICA artery stenosis with abundant collaterals associated with the moyamoya disorder, hyperventilation has been shown to precipitate focal symptoms.[345] The demonstration of such an extreme degree of sensitivity of cerebral flow to alterations in pCO_2 may help resurrect interest in notions of cerebral claudication,[260] which have been ignored in recent times. The frequency of the misery perfusion syndrome as an explanation for TIAs is unknown. The great expense and effort involved in testing even single patients are certain to discourage studies of large groups. However, the demonstration alone is important since it bears on pathophysiology.

Perfusion Failure TIAs

The principle of distal insufficiency is strongly associated with the high frequency of severe stenosis or occlusion of the carotid[123,273] and with the tendency of TIAs to have the same characteristics from attack to attack.[114,257] The syndromes might vary somewhat from case to case, depending on the collateral arterial pattern for each individual.

The problems of stereotypic TIAs (i.e., repetitive in severity and in clinical details) is not easily accounted for by the embolic theory.[125] The data derived from the pathologic study of carotid endarterectomy specimens by Fisher and Ojemann[130] were viewed by the authors as support for the hemodynamic mechanism of TIAs. Severe stenosis (residual lumen

<1 mm) was present in 33 (98%) of 34 cases with hemispheric TIAs and 19 (90%) of 21 (no information on 2) cases of transient monocular blindness, but in only 5 (15%) of 33 asymptomatic patients. Mural thrombus was present on the atheromatous plaque in 26 (77%) of 34 cases of hemispheric TIAs, 22 (96%) of 23 cases of transient monocular blindness, and 7 (21%) of 33 asymptomatic patients. The absence of mural thrombus, however, in eight TIA patients as well as the tiny amounts (<1 mm) found in an additional five together with the absence of TIAs in seven asymptomatic patients with thrombus, makes the stenosis the most important factor underlying TIAs.

In support of the embolic theory, Whisnant[379] showed the original picture of several embolic pellets that had gone to the same cortical branch by laminar flow. Evidence supporting a hemodynamic insufficiency explanation for repeated stereotyped TIAs has not been forthcoming, and it is also arguable whether hemispheral TIAs are ever truly stereotypic.[284]

INFARCTION MANIFESTING AS TIA

The increase in the use of CT and MRI evaluation[332] in patients with a clinical picture suggesting TIA has demonstrated that a surprisingly large number of such cases already have a focal hypodense area consisting of cerebral infarction in a region clinically related to the symptoms of the TIA. Perrone et al[282] found that 34% of their 35 patients with TIA showed a positive CT scan consisting of small hypodense areas. These lesions were angiographically correlated with arteriosclerotic abnormalities in the ipsilateral carotid. Other investigators have corroborated this observation in a significant number of patients undergoing CT or MRI evaluation, although the duration of TIA is often not specified or, if noted, is generally longer (by hours) than the usual brief (minutes) time frame of more typical carotid TIAs.[11,35,300,372]

ASYMPTOMATIC CAROTID ARTERY DISEASE

Considering the frightening prospects of stroke in a setting of atheromatous lesions of the carotid artery, it is remarkable that asymptomatic disease of the carotid exists at all, let alone seems to be encountered frequently. Perhaps it is the fear of stroke from carotid disease that prompts the efforts to detect the disease in its occult state. Whatever the reasons, when the lesion is discovered, the artery is either occluded or stenotic, or the possibility of carotid disease is raised by the discovery of a bruit in the neck. The risk of stroke differs in each setting.

Asymptomatic Carotid Occlusion

The documentation of carotid occlusion by a noninvasive study or angiogram is fairly common. Dyken et al[91] found a 3% incidence of apparent occult severe stenosis or occlusion of the carotid artery in a hospitalized group of patients older than 50 years. The lesion was documented by reversed flow in the ophthalmic artery, as determined by directional Doppler ultrasound.

Several studies have addressed the issue of stroke in a setting of common carotid artery or ICA occlusion, but few have broken down the data for the strokes that occurred in the territory of the occlusion. The available data show widely scattered results. Furlan and Whisnant[136] documented 6 cases of stroke ipsilateral to a carotid occlusion among their series of 138 angiogrammed cases studied retrospectively, and another 11 that occurred in other vascular territories. The annual stroke rate in their study was 2% a year. Grillo and Paterson[152a] reviewed the angiographic findings of all patients undergoing aortography or cerebral angiography at their hospital over a 5-year period. Forty-four patients with occlusion of the ICA were identified, ranging in age from 45 to 84 years. The incidence of occlusion was essentially the same on both sides. In three, no symptoms attributable to the carotid occlusion were identified. Fully 23 had had a completed stroke before their angiography. An additional three patients had had their stroke at the time of the angiogram. The three otherwise asymptomatic patients had only the nonspecific symptoms of headache and blurred vision. These three experienced no neurologic deficits during the 3 years of the follow-up. Bogousslavsky et al[37] found no strokes among 23 cases of carotid occlusion followed for a mean period of 27 months. Sacquegna et al[315] studied the clinical course of 100 consecutive patients with angiographically proven ICA occlusion. Ninety-three patients presented with stroke, seven with TIAs. Sixty-eight patients were followed from 17 to 69 months; seven patients developed new stroke, but only three were in the territory of the occluded carotid. Four patients had TIAs during follow-up. The observed stroke rate was 4.7% at 1 year, 12.2% at 3 years, and 17.1% at 5 years. In a prospective study of patients with asymptomatic bruits, using noninvasive carotid Doppler evaluation, Bernstein and Norris[27] identified 40 patients with unilateral carotid occlusion. Nineteen were occluded at the study onset. Twenty-one progressed from stenosis to occlusion. More ischemic events occurred in the group that progressed to occlusion than in those already occluded. There were three strokes and nine TIAs in the former group during a mean 30-month follow-up and no strokes and four TIAs in the latter group, which was followed for a mean of 48 months. The annual stroke rate was 3.8% indicating the benign course in asymptomatic patients with carotid occlusion. Cote et al,[70] utilizing the data from the Canadian Cooperative Study, found 47 cases with ICA occlusion who presented either with ipsilateral TIA attack (22 cases), ipsilateral minor infarct (15 cases), or no ipsilateral symptoms (10 cases). The disease affected the origin of the ICA in 87% of cases. Stroke occurred in 11 cases and TIAs in 24 during the follow-up period. The ipsilateral stroke rate was 5% a year.

Data culled from the extracranial/intracranial bypass study provided a large cohort of patients with angiographically proven bilateral ICA occlusion.[368] Seventy-four patients were initially identified of whom 34 were randomized to nonsurgical treatment and followed for a mean of 42 months. Symptoms at initial study entry included nondisabling stroke in 80% or TIAs in 80% or both. Eighteen patients had subsequent ischemic events (11 with stroke, 7 with TIAs) with an annual stroke rate of 13%/patient year. The survival rate was 71% (24 patients); 50% of the survivors were symptom free or had minor disability. The outcome was better than expected considering the seriousness of the vascular disease.

It has not yet been established whether a critical period of vulnerability for stroke exists, what role the presence or absence of certain types of collateral flow plays in the stroke risk, and what risk exists for each of the stroke subtypes—embolism from the stump, the tail, and other sources, distal insufficiency, and so forth. However, these concerns may be excessive, given the low risk of stroke suggested by these studies, even in a setting of occlusion of the ICA.

Asymptomatic Carotid Stenosis

The risk of stroke in a setting of asymptomatic carotid stenosis, once considered unsettled,[108,214,254,292] has been evaluated by the ACAS.[106] This trial, which ended prior to its planned time because of a positive result favoring surgery, randomized all eligible patients with asymptomatic carotid stenosis of ≥60% lumen reduction to 325 mg of aspirin daily or to carotid endarterectomy. All patients received appropriate counseling and treatment for risk factor reduction. The endpoints of TIA or stroke in the distribution of the randomized arteries were used to assess the two treatments.

By the criterion that brain imaging evidence of infarction should mean patients are not symptomatic, the ACAS has already yielded evidence that some patients have lesions on imaging even though they are and have always been clinically asymptomatic. Brott et al[45] reviewed 1,132 patients in ACAS and discovered 126 (15%) with what was characterized as silent infarct. For fully 72%, these were small, deep lesions often considered asymptomatic, but the remainder had convexity infarctions, some as large as half a lobe.

Some earlier studies had suggested an enormous risk for stroke unheralded by TIAs in asymptomatic patients with high-grade carotid stenosis[292]; other studies saw very little risk, and a few addressed the issues of whether the stroke occurs in the territory at risk and by what mechanism. At one end of the spectrum is the recently reported 10-year case-control study of 470 men aged 68 years, selected from among the Malmo population of 230,000.[272] Fifty suffered stroke, 18 with carotid stenosis (21.6 events/1,000 person years), and 43 with normal carotid arteries also had a stroke (14.8 events/1,000 person years), a finding indicating that those with carotid stenosis were not at increased risk of stroke.

In an early study based on Doppler imaging, Hennerici and Rautenberg[170] documented the natural history of 122 prospectively selected neurologically asymptomatic patients with extracranial carotid disease. Only 3 deaths from stroke occurred among 23 deaths during the follow-up period, from 11 to 36 months. Eight of the living patients experienced TIAs, one had a stroke, and the others remained asymptomatic. The cumulative stroke rate was 7%, which the authors estimated to be the same as the average risk of death in a normal population. Eighty-five percent of the patients experienced progression in extracranial arterial disease as documented by repeat examination using continuous-wave Doppler methods. These studies demonstrated development of lesions in previously normal arteries either alone (25 instances) or in combination with a deterioration of the original stenosis (in 14 cases). Deterioration of the original stenosis alone was seen in 9 cases. However, only the occurrence of a combined carotid and vertebral lesion significantly increased the cerebral vascular risk. Under those conditions, the stroke risk was increased sixfold over that for unilateral or bilateral carotid lesions.

Durward et al[90] studied the course of 73 patients with asymptomatic, presumably atheromatous, plaque found in the common carotid bifurcation. Stenosis of more than 50% was found in 50 cases and was accompanied by ulceration in an additional 17. Ulceration was found alone in six cases. The observation period averaged up to 4 years (as little as 6 months to as long as 10 years). Surgical intervention was undertaken only if TIA or minor stroke developed. There was no standard use of antiplatelet or anticoagulant drugs. Twenty-two of the patients developed ischemic symptoms in the follow-up period. In 12, the symptoms occurred in the territory of the previously asymptomatic carotid artery. Among these 12 patients, 2 experienced stroke with no prior TIA. Repeat angiogram in the 6 patients who developed an ischemic event in the previously asymptomatic territory showed that the lesion had progressed significantly in every case, but none had reached complete occlusion. All patients underwent uneventful endarterectomy. Although symptoms occurred in roughly equal frequency in cases with ulceration alone, stenosis alone, or a combination of stenosis and ulceration, the only instances of infarction occurred in a group with stenosis of >50%. Ulceration was not associated with infarction.

A similar experience was documented by Roederer et al[305] who found a 4% annual rate of symptoms in their prospective study of 167 cases referred with bruit. At the extreme benign end of the spectrum was another nonrandomized, noncontrolled study[228] in which 147 cases involving 535 carotid arteries underwent surgery only on the symptomatic side, while the asymptomatic side was left to follow its natural course. No strokes were observed in these patients in a 20-year follow-up period.

The recently reported results of the ACAS have provided data from a clinical trial, adding to the heretofore unclear risk of stroke in this setting. After a median follow-up of 2.7 years, the risk of ipsilateral stroke over 5 years, or any perioperative stroke or death, was 5.1% for surgical patients and 11.0% for medically treated patients. The favorable outcome of surgical patients was predicated on a remarkably low perioperative risk of stroke or death of 2.3%. The 5-year reduction in stroke risk was different for men (67%) and women (17%), in part explained by a higher perioperative complication rate in women. The arteriography-related stroke rate was 1.2% for the 414 patients who underwent arteriography prior to endarterectomy. Despite strong clinical opinions to the contrary, the degree of increasing stenosis (60% to 69%, 70% to 79%, and 80% to 99%) was not statistically related to reduction of the 5-year risk of the primary event. These data provide the first scientifically derived information on the stroke risk and benefits of carotid endarterectomy for asymptomatic carotid disease and are now the new benchmark for this condition.[106]

Despite the outcome of the ACAS, many clinicians have yet to change their former practices: some advise prophylactic endarterectomy; others advise platelet inhibitors; and a few maintain the extreme position of advising no treatment at all. However, none states publicly any doubt that successful surgery removes a major source of risk for stroke.

For a surgical option to apply, the risk of endarterectomy[95,350,351] should be lower than the natural history of the disease if the treatment is to have any place as an alternative. It is this varying risk, study by study, center by center, and even country by country, that continues to provide a basis for controversy. A survey of all published studies from 1980 to 1995, spanning some 51 studies, symptomatic and asymptomatic, found an overall mortality of 1.62% (95% confidence interval 1.3 to 1.9) with a risk of stroke and/or death of 5.64% (95% confidence interval 4.4 to 6.9).[335] Despite the large series thus reviewed, it has proved difficult to tease out the event rates by group subtype. Thus renewed interest has arisen in the ACAS, recent reports from which showed a low rate of stroke attributable to surgery (1.5%), a rate found in the same study to be approximately the same as that for stroke from the arteriogram still being performed in some centers prior to operation.[404] These figures of ≤3% morbidity closely approximate those estimated by Mohr[256] from the experience at the Massachusetts General Hospital, and those calculated by Karis[196] when he recomputed the Jonas and Hass[191] observations to show that a combined morbidity and mortality rate of over 1.4% for arteriography, endarterectomy, and the postoperative period for a surgical approach to carotid territory TIAs would exceed that of the total morbidity and mortality compared with the medical therapy. Current mortality and morbidity data indicate that endarterectomy is being carried out with these acceptably low complications in many centers, certainly for asymptomatic patients, and possibly also for those with TIA. It has been proposed by the ACAS group[106] that these figures be used for future hospital audits of surgical practice. The literature already documents that such efforts are under way (shorter length of stay, sharp decline in the use of angiography over a 4-year period, and no changes in the low [1.9%] incidence of stroke from the procedure as noninvasive preoperative testing replaced conventional angiography).[175]

Asymptomatic Ulcerative Disease

Very few studies have been done on the stroke risk for ulcerative disease alone.[254] Dixon et al[84] followed 153 nonstenotic asymptomatic ulcerative lesions in 141 patients. Over a period of up to 10 years hemispheric strokes without antecedent TIAs occurred in 19% of those with deep complicated ulcers, in 21% with the deep ulcers, and in 3% with small shallow ulcers. Because the calculated annual stroke rate for the more complex ulcers was between 4.5% and 7.6%, the authors considered that this rate was comparable to that of the 6% annual stroke rate in patients with TIAs and recommended prophylactic operation for these cases. Fisher and Ojemann[130] showed that many ulcers are smooth and thick (i.e., they contain no thrombus). The concept of ulcer is mainly based on angiography; the significance of ulcers independent of stenosis may be questioned.

The recently completed NASCET studies produced sobering data on the detection of ulceration when comparing angiographic with surgical specimens. Irrespective of the degree of stenosis, a sensitivity of 45.9% and a specificity of 74.1% were found for the first 500 specimens, yielding a somewhat disappointing positive predictive value of 71.8%.[343] With these data in hand, and with the declining use of conventional angiography, no answer for the risk of stroke in the asymptomatic patients with ulcer disease can confidently be expected, unless data from the ACAS is sufficient to settle the matter.

Asymptomatic Bruit

With widespread availability of Doppler studies, much of the earlier anxieties about bruits have been relieved. A bruit in the neck is commonly encountered in routine clinical examinations. It occurs in 4% to 5% of the population aged 45 to 80 years.[174,390] Except when Doppler technology is not available, the explanation for most bruits can be left to Doppler studies to decide. A local cervical bruit can be detected in approximately 70% to 89% of patients with a tight (75% stenosis, or ≥2 mm residual lumen) stenosis of the ICA.[142,287] The site of maximal intensity of the bruit usually corresponds to the carotid bifurcation area, in front of the upper portion of the thyroid cartilage. It can radiate into the ocular region, and its intensity usually decreases with the Valsalva maneuver. The latter point should be useful in differentiating them from bruits originating from the external carotid artery, which should not change with this maneuver, but the finding is disappointingly unreliable.[212] A bruit may also be absent in some patients with tight stenosis because of a slow-flow state through the patent but severely stenotic artery.[287]

Auscultation of the orbits may also be useful in the clinical diagnosis of extracranial carotid occlusive disease. Fisher[119] noted that an eye bruit may be present on the side contralateral to a carotid occlusion, presumably related to augmentation flow through the open carotid system. Others have corroborated this observation.[40,287] Pessin[287] even found this sign to be present with carotid occlusion more often than an associated cervical bruit. Ocular bruits have a strong relationship to ipsilateral intracranial carotid siphon stenosis.[180]

Bruits with Intracranial Internal Carotid Artery Disease

Auscultation of the eyeball is usually done to detect bruits indicative of intracranial ICA stenoses. However, it has been reported that ocular bruits in relationship with such stenoses are rare.[127,219] In 100 patients with a unilateral ICA stenosis, 4 had a siphon stenosis and in 1 an ocular bruit was heard. In the same report there were 50 patients with a unilateral ICA occlusion and a contralateral angiographically normal ICA. Among the 50 occlusions, the contrast medium stopped in the siphon in 11 (cardiac embolism in 5; atherosclerotic thrombus or embolism in 2; undetermined cause in 4). No ocular bruit but an ipsilateral cervical bruit in one patient and a bilateral cervical bruit in another were heard at the level of the common carotid bifurcation.[50] In 50 patients with tight stenoses or occlusions of the extracranial ICA, a unilateral ocular bruit contralateral to the side of the ICA occlusion occurred in 9 of 10 patients, more often than an associated cervical bruit and was interpreted as a sign of augmentation flow.[287] Twenty-five ocular bruits have been reported in 18 patients with atherothrombotic ischemic cerebrovascular disease. Only 2 patients had a stenosis of the intracranial ICA as the main lesion.[40]

Some large surveys for arterial bruits in relation to cerebral ischemic accidents apparently did not include ocular auscultation, but it seems safe to conclude that the absence of an ocular bruit by no means rules out intracranial ICA lesions and its presence by no means indicates intracranial ICA disease inasmuch as various pathologic conditions may give rise to ocular bruits.[209]

Clinical Syndromes

The basic clinical features of extracranial carotid disease were described many years ago.[60,112–114,182,331] The characteristic clinical syndrome of ICA occlusion has long been taken known to include "premonitory fleeting symptoms including paresthesias, paralysis, monocular blindness and aphasia."[119] Especially remarkable were the episodes of transient monocular blindness (TMB) described by patients with proven ICA occlusion. Interest in TMB later stimulated by actual observations[117,310] of the retinal circulation during an attack led to important ideas concerning the role of embolism in the production of TIAs and stroke. As more clinical detail accumulated about TIAs, it became important to differentiate these spells from others of nonvascular origin. Even today, efforts continue in the difficult task of distinguishing among various types of spells that may have different pathogenesis and prognosis for stroke.

It was the prospect of therapy that prompted so much interest in carotid disease. Fisher[112–114] was mainly responsible for renewed interest in the clinical importance of carotid disease. In his early clinicopathologic studies, he described the prodromal transient neurologic events frequently preceding stroke, discussed possible stroke mechanisms, and even predicted the surgical treatment. Eastcott et al[93] were the first to reconstruct an extracranial internal carotid lesion successfully. Thus began the modern era in diagnosis and management of extracranial carotid artery disease.

TRANSIENT CEREBRAL ISCHEMIC ATTACKS

TIAs have been defined as a temporary, focal neurologic deficit presumably related to ischemia, lasting less than 24 hours.[144,173] The history of this time frame for a TIA seems to have arisen not so much from the documented time course of a typical attack, but more from uncertainty as to its cause. Because it has long been agreed that a focal deficit lasting longer than 24 hours would be expected to have a focus of ischemic infarction found at autopsy, the definition of a TIA as any spell lasting less than this time can be seen as a negative definition.

When the subject has been studied using actual case material, the usual 24-hour criteria has been recognized to be excessive.[284] The typical carotid territory TIAs are brief, typically lasting only some 7 to 10 minutes.[284] The brief spells have a better correlation with angiographic evidence of tight carotid stenosis.[284] However, the prognosis for subsequent stroke appears to be the same whether the spell is brief or long in duration.[230,299]

Natural History

The importance of carotid TIAs is highlighted when viewed from the perspective of carotid stroke. Patients who suffer carotid stroke from extracranial carotid occlusion disease have a known prior TIA incidence of 50% to 75%.[258,286,314]

This contrasts sharply with the low incidence of TIAs (approximately 10%) in association with all types of stroke and reinforces the strong relationship between these transient events and underlying atherothrombotic occlusive disease. The available data, both prospective and retrospective, indicate that the TIAs may be impressive warnings of stroke in some patients, and their recognition provides the opportunity for therapeutic intervention.

Despite the large numbers of studies on TIAs, so many differences exist in definitions and methodology that all too many of them are disappointingly unhelpful. Some studies emphasize incidence, and others describe prevalence. The TIAs have been documented by various methods, some by personal periodic examinations and others by search of clinical records; questionnaires have been tried.[42,197,277,381,384,389] Few have focused on carotid territory TIAs alone, and even fewer have separated transient TMBs from transient hemispheral attacks. The available data show a wide spread of prevalence and incidence. The prevalence varies from 1.1 to 77/1,000 persons and the incidence rate from 2.2 to 8/1,000 persons.[42,381,384] The stroke risk associated with TIAs is significant although no well-designed, controlled, randomized study has provided unequivocal information on the natural history of TIAs, nor is such a study likely to be done today. Past studies have assessed the stroke risk to be between 2% and 50%, results so discrepant as to be useless in any individual case.[12,13,116,134,135,226,238,275,280,330,411] These studies suffer from several limitations including ambiguity of TIA definition, lumping together carotid and vertebral basilar TIAs, and, most importantly, no angiographic verification of underlying vascular disease. Despite the limitations of these early studies, the view emerged that a considerable stroke risk attends TIAs,

namely, in the range of 35% over 5 years, or 5% to 6% a year.[381]

Many of the important questions relating TIAs to specific carotid lesion configurations such as irregular plaque, ulcer, severe stenosis, or occlusion remain unanswered despite all the effort that has gone into the subject thus far.[67] At the least, the available evidence indicates that a serious stroke may follow TIA in a discouraging number of patients, but the factors contributing to the risks for individuals have remained elusive.

In view of the wide variation in reported stroke risk, it may be useful to describe some of the details in the studies representing the extreme ends of the risk spectrum. Acheson and Hutchinson[1] reported the highest incidence of stroke following TIAs. Their 82 cases were confined to TIAs of <1 hour in duration. After an average follow-up of 40 months, 42 (51%) developed a stroke. Twelve died, four were totally disabled, and seven were left with a moderate disability. An important aspect of this study is that the authors defined a stroke as "a clinical episode lasting more than 1 hour." Although they did not indicate how many patients had had such a stroke, 19 patients made a complete recovery. This complete recovery in almost half their cases suggests that many have had only a short-lived deficit. If so, the importance of this study as a predictor of major stroke following TIA may be exaggerated.

At the other end of the prognostic spectrum are three reports, the first one[280] with a very low incidence of stroke: among 61 patients followed for an average of 45 months, only one (2%) suffered a completed stroke. In this study, the inclusion of a large number of patients with vertigo and vertebrobasilar TIAs, whose clinical outlook is thought to be more benign, may have accounted for the difference. Muuronen and Kaste[269] also documented similarly low stroke rate (3.5%) in 228 untreated cases among 314 patients suffering carotid territory TIA. The follow-up period in this study was a mean of 7.8 years. This group contained patients younger than usual for TIA studies. In the other report,[139] treatment with some form of anticoagulant or platelet inhibitor prevented the collection of natural history data. However, the course over an average of 20 months was followed for 241 cases with carotid TIAs, treated with either warfarin or aspirin. During this time only eight cases experienced cerebral infarction. This stroke rate of 3.1% is remarkably lower than any reported on any form of therapy. Of the eight cases of stroke, four occurred in each treatment group, and of the eight, two in each group had the stroke within a few weeks of the onset of treatment. Although both of these studies are important, given their low incidence of stroke in cases with carotid territory TIAs, it may be equally important to note that these cases did not have stenosis or occlusion of the symptomatic carotid, as well as one can judge from the available data. Similar data were reported by Ogren et al[272] (see above).

Much of the variation in outcome data has been set aside by the results of the NASCET. The argument of whether the outlook for TIA cases was too benign for endarterectomy to influence outcome favorably [90,194,269,305,325] has been settled by the dramatic results of the studies for symptomatic patients: both the NASCET and the European Cooperative Study showed a clear advantage of surgery over medical (aspirin) therapy (see Ch. 53 on endarterectomy for further details). Neither trial tested surgery against anticoagulation, and the positive findings were in those patients whose stenosis exceeded 70%. For NASCET, over a period of 18 months, of those symptomatic with TIA and found to have stenosis of 70% to 90%, 7% of the 300 who underwent surgery suffered stroke or death, mostly in the perioperative period, while 24% of the 295 on aspirin therapy had a stroke or died. This difference favoring surgery was highly significant ($P < 0.001$). The outcome and best management plan for those whose stenosis is in the 30% to 70% range remains unsettled, but enrollment has been completed as of December 1996 for this cohort, so a result can be expected by 1998. Judging from the data in the European trial, those whose stenosis is below 30% seem better managed with medical therapy. For patients with TIAs found to have stenosis over 70%, the effect of aspirin therapy alone was unimpressive.

TIAs with Intracranial Internal Carotid Artery Disease

TIAs can be expected to occur in atherosclerosis of the intracranial ICA, as in extracranial ICA disease. However, precise data are lacking. One reason is that most studies of TIAs have not isolated those specifically due to intracranial ICA lesions, and the few that did so have not dealt with symptoms, only with duration or prevalence. The common association is the occurrence of TIAs with lesions elsewhere, and the common occurence of tandem lesions makes it difficult to sort out those TIAs that could specifically result from intracranial ICA disease.

Harrison et al[164] noted seven patients with stenosis ("any narrowing of the lumen") of the siphon in whom TIAs had lasted for <1 hour; none of their 109 other patients had siphon stenosis. Among Marzewski et al's[241] 66 patients, 24 presented with TIAs (17 ICA territory [25.7%]). The onset of attacks before angiography ranged from 3 years to 15 days, with a median interval of 5 months. During follow-up, 8 patients (12.1%) had isolated TIAs (all ICA territory), and 6 of the 10 patients with stroke also experienced TIAs, all in the same territory as the stroke. Seven of the eight patients with isolated TIAs had ipsilateral intracranial ICA stenoses on their reference angiogram, but five had tandem stenoses. For this and other reasons, in only one of the eight patients was the intracranial ICA stenosis the only apparent cause of the ischemic episode. In Craig et al's[72] 58 patients, 16 (28%) presented with TIAs. During follow-up, eight patients suffered TIAs; 25% of these were appropriate to the lesion under study.

Since the ophthalmic artery arises from the intracranial ICA, it might be imagined that amaurosis fugax bears a special relationship to atherosclerosis of that stretch of the vessel. However, in reports of large series of cases, the current authors found no specific data on intracranial ICA atherosclerosis.[3,79,140,239,265,284] Mungas and Baker[266] mentioned that among 107 patients 3 had an isolated intracranial stenosis of the carotid siphon and that a stenosis of the siphon was thought to be the source of an embolus in 5 of 36 patients studied by selective carotid angiography. Wilson et al[385] reported that only the siphon was abnormal in 1 of 44 patients with branch retinal artery occlusion and in none of 18 with central retinal artery occlusion.

Very few specific cases have been recorded. Gerstenfeld[145] reported on a 30-year-old man who suffered many attacks of amaurosis fugax of the right eye. White streaks were seen in the retinal arterioles. Angiography disclosed an ICA occlusion above the level of the ophthalmic artery. In addition, the ophthalmic artery had an unusually early origin from the ICA since it arose from the infraclinoid part. It should be noted that a severe right frontal headache was mentioned, a very uncommon feature of amaurosis fugax, and in that young patient atherosclerosis would appear unlikely. Dyll et al[92] reported on a patient with four attacks of amaurosis fugax and roughening and narrowing of the uncoiled carotid siphon proximal to the origin of the ophthalmic artery. David[75] also reported on a case of amaurosis fugax with siphon lesions and a possible embolic mechanism.

Intracranial ICA atherosclerosis may of course be asymptomatic, and angiography may be performed for reasons not directly or definitely related. In 20 patients (30%) of Marzewski et al,[241] angiography had been performed for asymptomatic carotid bruit in 13, encephalopathy in 2, dizziness in 2, seizures in 2, and cranial nerve palsies in 1. Eleven (19%) of the patients of Craig et al[72] had had an angiography for asymptomatic bruit (four cases), for stroke in other vascular territories (four cases), for confusional state due to metabolic encephalography (two cases), and for investigation prior to major vascular surgery (one case).

Transient Monocular Blindness

TMB, also known as amaurosis fugax, has been recognized as an important manifestation of carotid artery disease since early reports.[105] TMB may be considered a brief monocular visual obscuration described by patients as a fog, blur, cloud, mist, and so forth. A shade or curtain effect occurs in only a minority of cases, approximately 15% to 20%, and is no more predictive of carotid artery disease than other variations of monocular visual loss.[284] Several reports on TMB have corroborated the brief duration of visual impairment, usually <15 minutes, rarely exceeding 30 minutes, with most patients affected for only 1 to 5 minutes.[3,113,266,284,310,369] Flashing lights, scintillations, colors, and fortification spectra rarely occur as TIA manifestations and usually signify a migrainous event.[369] However, the presence of positive visual phenomena during TMB, in patients with ≥75% stenosis, has been recorded by Goodwin et al,[150] making differentiation from retinal migraine difficult, in some cases, on clinical grounds alone.

The number of TMB attacks that occur before a patient seeks medical attention varies greatly. Patients may experience a few or as many as 100 attacks of TMB over a span of several days to a year or more.[284] Vision is usually fully restored following an attack, although in long-term follow-up studies of such patients,[239] a small number may sustain permanent visual loss from retinal infarction. TMB rarely occurs simultaneously with other neurologic deficits, and headache is not part of the disturbance. Hemisphere stroke is an infrequent sequela of TMB alone,[101,178,239] although careful studies of such cases occasionally reveal evidence of clinically inevident cerebral embolism.[163] In most instances, clinically obvious stroke is preceded by one or more transient hemispheral attacks. TMB tends to precede the first transient hemispheral attack if a careful history can be documented.

OPHTHALMOSCOPIC CORRELATIONS.

TMB poses endless diagnostic interpretation difficulties. The failure of the retinal arteries to show any abnormality during a period of TMB has been often described. It has been speculated that the normal appearance of the retinal arteries may be a sign that the inferred embolic material or low flow state applies to the choroidal circulation, which would not be visualized by the ophthalmoscope. However, experimental occlusion of the central retinal artery for up to 98 minutes was not revealed by ophthalmoscopic change, and no significant permanent neurologic damage was observed.[167] Occlusion for 105 minutes or longer, however, produced irreversible damage, but even then no permanent injury was obvious in the retinal vascular bed. Only a transient leakage of fluorescein was observed 2.5 to 3 hours after the occlusion. These findings show that vessels that look normal by ophthalmoscope may be present even in a setting of complete retinal artery occlusion.[140]

INTRAVASCULAR MATERIAL.

It is perhaps only whimsical speculation that Gowers[152] may have found intravascular material over a century ago in his report on embolic material in the vessels supplying the eye. In modern times, Hollenhorst,[177] an ophthalmologist at the Mayo Clinic, is credited with the first description of cholesterol crystals (Hollenhorst plaques) in the retinal circulation. His patients had all types of cerebrovascular symptoms, but he emphasized the association of the retinal material with systemic atherosclerosis and significant cardiovascular mortality, although he was uncertain about concomitant visual symptoms related to this particulate material.[177,295] In fact, in identifying a separate group of patients with TMB who did not have cholesterol plaques in their retinal circulation, he first documented that this embolic material was not necessarily associated with TMB. Clinical experience has corroborated Hollenhorst's observation that patients with TMB do not usually have cholesterol emboli in their retinal circulation during or between TMB attacks. Because of the flat shape and small size of cholesterol emboli, many of them cause no interruption in blood flow.

Reports prompted by the rare opportunity to observe a patient during an attack of TMB have described white or grayish material passing through the retinal circulation, presumably platelet complexes, perhaps mixed with fibrin.[117,310] This material is believed by many to be what is visualized by the ophthalmoscope in the rare instances of TMB studied during an attack. Although he has been credited with the first description of such material observed during an attack, Fisher[117] was careful not to make too great a claim for how the material reached the vascular tree and left open the possibility that it may have been embolic or generated by local events such as sludging from inadequate perfusion. Gerstenfeld[145] found similar white bodies, but the disease was confined to the ICA above the origin of the ophthalmic artery. In other case reports only pallor of the disc was found, even given a source for embolic material in the proximal ICA.[92] McBrien et al[246] succeeded in demonstrating a platelet origin for some of the embolic material seen in the retina in a 37-year-old man who suffered two episodes of blindness, the last one leaving him with a permanent nasal field defect. Platelet material was found in a superior nasal branch (apparently serving a portion of the visual field clinically unaffected). In the rare instances of calcium emboli to the retinal artery, an opportunity was provided to document the visual loss associated with focal branch occlusions. Brockmeier et al[44] described four patients whose accompanying visual loss corresponded to the location of the retinal embolus. Transient visual loss of the type attributed to retinal branch occlusion with platelet aggregates was not encountered. The author suggested that the small size of the calcific emboli was sufficient to plug retinal arteries but insufficient to precipitate clinical symptoms in the cerebrum. However, Beal et al[21] documented several sites of cerebral infarction in a 69-year-old man who experienced numerous brief spells of numbness and weakness consistent with hemispheral transient cerebral ischemic attacks, indicating that some such particles can be large enough to precipitate symptoms. Cattle trucking, a sign described in agonal settings, has also been seen in the vessels during some attacks.[140]

A rare case of transient vertical monocular hemianopsia was described,[393] the attacks being attributed to an anomalous arteriolar pattern in that both the superior and inferior nasal quadrants were supplied by the same arterial branch. Microembolization to this common arteriolar trunk may have accounted for the six episodes of monocular vertical hemianopsia in a 3-day period.

Another interesting cause of TMB was described by Winterkorn et al[386] in nine patients with a variety of medical conditions unrelated to emboli or carotid hypoprofusion. This benign form was attributed to vasoconstriction of the retinal arterioles observed during funduscopic examination in several of their patients. The symptoms were responsive to calcium channel blockers. The clinical features show some variation from TMB associated with carotid disease. Almost one-half of the patients were >50 years old and had had multiple attacks, some as many as 40 and often several a day over a brief period. Retro-orbital ache was noted in four of nine patients. Several of the younger patients had a history of migraine or autoimmune conditions, but these were not present in the older patients. Two older patients had negative temporal artery biopsies. This mechanism may partly explain the well-known clinical recognition of a benign form of TMB in younger patients.

Yet another variant of TMB has been reported by Furlan et al[137] in which exposure to bright light (often sunlight) precipitated transient unilateral visual loss in five patients with high-grade ICA stenosis or occlusion. All the patients also had typical, unprovoked TMB and reduced retinal artery pressure in the affected eye; three also had hemispheric TIAs. Hemodynamic insufficiency of the retinal circulation was the probable mechanism leading to reduced photochemical resynthesis of visual pigments by the retinals, rods and cones. Donnan et al[85] recorded impaired visual evoked responses in four patients with similar symptoms. Wiebers et al[382] extended these observations to include four patients with episodic bilateral visual blurring or dimming in response to bright light; all the patients had severe bilateral carotid occlusive disease. Apart from TMB, persisting visual deficit from ocular infarction may also occur (see below).

Transient Hemispheral Attacks

Symptoms reflecting a transient cerebral disturbance are common in carotid artery disease and have been called transient hemispheral attacks (THAs). Weakness or numbness (or both) of part or all of the contralateral body with or without a speech disturbance, depending on whether the dominant hemisphere is affected, are the general manifestations. It is an inherent problem in studying THAs that an accurate history may be difficult to obtain because the episodes are brief and frightening to the patient, not usually observed by another person, and may involve the right hemisphere, making the patient's report unreliable. Nevertheless, the usual features of THAs have been characterized in several studies.[16,118,238,251,284]

The most common constellation of symptoms involves motor and sensory dysfunction of the contralateral limbs, followed by pure motor dysfunction, pure sensory dysfunction, and lastly, isolated dysphasia.[284] The contralateral distal arm and hand is the body part that most consistently suffers in the attack and may be the only manifestation. The deficit presumably reflects ischemia to a portion of the motor cortex in the distal field of the carotid circulation, by means of either embolism or perfusion failure.

THAs are typically brief in duration (<15 minutes), with most lasting for 1 to 10 minutes. In one study,[284] patients with THAs lasting for 1 hour or more tended to have wide open carotid arteries with evidence of intracranial branch occlusion, suggesting that the THAs reflected a short-lived cerebral embolus.

Patients may have one or many THAs before coming to medical attention; a few have 20 or more.[284] Most patients have THAs over several weeks to a few months, while some patients may have a history spanning months to a year, but rarely longer.

An uncommon form of THA involves limb shaking, a manifestation identified in reports on carotid TIAs.[15,111, 118,311,346,347,400] Patients with major ICA occlusive disease (severe stenosis or occlusion) may experience recurrent, involuntary, irregular, wavering movements of the contralateral arm or leg. The movements are described as shaking, trembling, twitching, flap, or wavering. Other more typical carotid TIAs are usually part of the overall picture, but limb shaking may be an initial manifestation, making distinction from focal epilepsy an important differential point. In the limited number of patients reported to date, it appears that endarterectomy may be beneficial. The mechanism underlying the shaking TIAs is presumed to be hemodynamic insufficiency, well documented in a single case reported by Tatemichi et al.[347] Using xenon-133 regional cerebral blood flow and transcranial ultrasonography with additional challenges of hypercapnia and hypotension, they showed perfusion insufficiency in the distal field of their patient with high-grade carotid stenosis and limb-shaking TIAs. Following endarterectomy, cerebral blood flow and blood velocities improved, and the TIAs ceased.

Nonsimultaneous Transient Monocular Blindness and Transient Hemispheral Attacks

Patients with carotid territory TIAs, depending on when they come to medical attention, may have had TMB, THA, or both types of TIA, although rarely simultaneously. There may be a stronger correlation with severe extracranial carotid artery disease in patients with a history of separate episodes of eye and hemisphere TIAs, compared with either type of spell alone.[284]

Stroke Risk Associated with Transient Monocular Blindness and Transient Hemispheral Attacks

The NASCET[343] provides important information on the stroke risk associated with first-ever retinal versus hemispheral TIAs and high-grade (>70%) carotid stenosis. In the 129 medically treated patients, 59 had retinal TIAs, compared with 70 patients who had hemisphere TIAs. Kaplan-Meier estimates of the risk of ipsilateral stroke at 2 years were 16.6% ± 5.6% for patients with retinal TIAs, and 43.5% ± 6.7% for patients with hemisphere TIAs ($P = 0.002$). Patients with hemispheral TIAs were older and had a higher prevalence of most risk factors for stroke. Patients with TMB had a longer time of delay before seeking medical treatment. The authors speculated that patients with TMB may reflect an earlier stage in the development of carotid atherosclerosis, at which small thromboemboli may have a greater impact on sensitive retinal tissue, but little consequence (because of size) on cortical tissue. An important feature not presented in this report that bears on the conclusions is whether patients with TMB who had stroke had antecedent episodes of THAs.[342]

Angiographic Correlations with TIAs

SEVERE STENOSIS OR OCCLUSION. A strong relationship exists between carotid territory TIAs (either TMB or THA) and extracranial carotid artery disease. Several prospective studies have found an occurrence of significant carotid occlusive disease in 30% to 50% of patients with carotid artery territory TIAs.[102,179,188,284,298,356] One prospective study[284] of patients with carotid artery territory TIAs found a bimodal distribution of angiographically documented extracranial carotid artery disease, either severe stenosis or occlusion, or a widely patent, nonobstructed artery, supporting the view that symptoms do not occur with any degree of stenosis. This severe a stenosis is by no means a chance occurrence. It is prevalent in only 7% of an autopsy population asymptomatic for carotid disease,[127] and in <10% of patients with stroke due to another mechanism such as hemorrhage.[258]

Apart from the degree of stenosis, no distinctive angiographic[312] or ultrasonographic[171] appearances have been found that separate the symptomatic from asymptomatic patients who have the same degree of stenosis. These frustrating observations thus far preclude easy identification of those still asymptomatic who are destined to become symptomatic from stenosis.

Lesser degrees of stenosis do not have the same high correlation with TIA. However, misestimation of the stenosis is common when the imaging is based on conventional angiography. A severe stenosis found at surgery may be misread on angiogram as a lesser degree of stenosis due to minor variations in lumen display or in the judgment of individuals[61,73] (Fig. 17.11). Oblique filming of the carotid bifurcation, in addition to the standard anterior-posterior and lateral views, will disclose irregular or ulcerative lesions not appreciated on the standard views.

ANGIOGRAPHIC COLLATERAL FLOW THROUGH THE OPHTHALMIC ARTERY SYSTEM. Considering the frequency with which angiography has documented the status of ophthalmic collateral flow, it may be somewhat surprising that so little information on its clinical significance is known. For years many authors assumed it was a favorable sign that collateral flow was available. However, Tatemichi et al[346] demonstrated by transcranial Doppler that reversed flow in the ophthalmic artery ipsilateral to high-grade stenosis or occlusion of the ICA correlated with poor or absent ana-

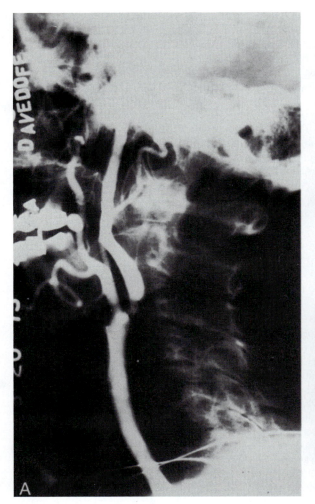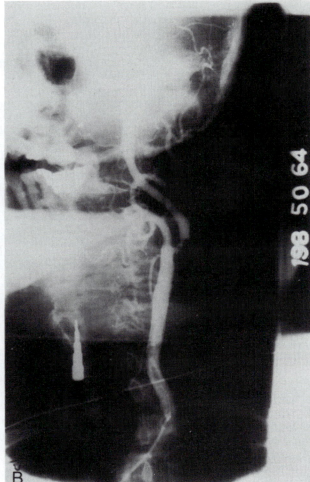

Figure 17.11 (**A & B**) Two views of the same stenosis.

tomic collateral pathways across the circle of Willis. This observation made it possible that ophthalmic flow reversal was a poor, not favorable, prognostic sign.

Recently, a large study of the course followed by patients with severe ($\geq 75\%$) ICA stenosis or occlusion has been reported by Hu et al.[181] The direction of flow of the ophthalmic artery was known. The clinical cohort included 130 patients followed at intervals of from 3 to 6 months for periods of up to 40 months ($\pm$ 16 months). The prevalence of reversal of ophthalmic artery flow was significantly higher ($P <0.001$) in those with stroke or TIA ipsilateral to the carotid lesion (85 patients) compared with those who had symptoms in the contralateral carotid or vertebrobasilar territory (15 patients), or those who were asymptomatic (30 patients). The subgroup with reversed ophthalmic flow also had a higher frequency of neurologic events during follow-up ($P <0.001$).

TIA TYPE AND SEVERE STENOSIS OR OC-
CLUSION. The correlation between TIA and severe stenosis in approximately 50% of patients applies equally as well when the TIA is TMB or THA.

TMB poses a special problem in angiographic correlation. In a few studies, the correlations among the attacks, the funduscopic findings, and angiography have been somewhat disappointing. Sandok et al[317] found 43 patients with TMB among 1,080 patients undergoing carotid angiography. In other studies there has been a poor correlation between the funduscopic and angiographic findings. Ninety-three of 212 patients with TIA had amaurosis fugax. Sixty-six percent had abnormal angiograms with operable atherosclerotic lesions found. The 7-year stroke rate was less in this group than in those with hemisphere attacks.[183]

In a handful of patients TMB was shown by angiogram to be associated with local stenosis of the ophthalmic artery, independent of any disease in the carotid. Angiographic documentation of stenosis of the ophthalmic artery itself is extremely difficult to demonstrate. Weinberger et al[375] documented a 50% stenosis near the origin of the ophthalmic artery in a patient with two episodes of TMB. The details of the visual loss were not described. Their report was the first to correlate TMB with ophthalmic artery stenosis. Gross et al[155] had previously described local stenosis of the ophthalmic artery as a cause of a false-positive pulse delay measured by oculoplethysmography, but they did not describe the visual symptoms in the 2 patients among the 287 studied angiographically.

TIAs AND NONSTENOSING CAROTID LE-SIONS. If TIAs are symptoms and not a unified diseased state, then the clinician's task is to correlate these transient deficits with appropriate carotid lesions. A migrainous event, dizziness, syncope, or seizure in a patient with a carotid lesion should not lead to the erroneous conclusion that the vascular lesion is the cause. That this important effort in clinical vascular correlation is not regularly pursued probably accounts for some of the carotid endarterectomies performed each year in the United States.[380]

The problem arises from the idea that any form of carotid atheromatous plaque can harbor thrombus and serve as an embolic source causing TIAs. Plaque formation, either smooth, irregular, or even with ulceration seen on the angiogram, has been implicated as a significant lesion although no obstruction to flow is present. The natural history of severe carotid stenosis in terms of its stroke risk has never been adequately settled, and even fewer data are available on these other types of lesions. The significance of the presence of intraluminal thrombus removed at endarterectomy and not appreciated at angiography remains unsettled.[261,264] Less has been heard recently of the once-popular argument that intraplaque hemorrhage is the substrate for intraluminal thrombus when endothelialization has not occurred and therefore even minor plaque formation should be removed if the patient has symptoms.[234] Also, if the minor lesions are important, then the difficulty in detecting them by angiography could pose a major treatment dilemma.[100] Many of the concerns have been obviated by the results of the NASCET, but even these results do not settle lingering concerns about the pathophysiology reflected in the attacks.

Plaques and ulcerations have been recognized as potential sources of TIA and stroke since the early years of this century.[60] Early studies seemed to suggest that TIAs could be attributable to any degree of stenosis,[179,263,356] by means of microembolization. Evidence in support of this view arose from individual case reports, to which were later added whole series of cases.[33,76,98,193,201,250,262,394,409] However, compared with stenosis and occlusion, ulcerations are not the common finding in cases with TIAs. In the authors' study of 95 consecutively angiogrammed cases with unilateral carotid territory TIAs,[284] no correlation was found with ulcerations of the carotid artery: ulcerations were present in approximately 6% of cases and occurred with equal frequency ipsilateral and contralateral to the symptomatic side. In other studies as well, although some degree of ulceration was found in 47% of patients suffering amaurosis fugax (TMB) and 49% of cases with THA, fully 50% showed the expected ipsilateral tight stenosis or occlusion.[101,102] In some studies, no information is given as to the frequency of ulcers or stenosis in the nonsymptomatic artery. With Doppler studies, it has been difficult to predict reliably the mechanism of stroke (perfusion failure or embolism) from the ultrasonographic appearance of the plaque in cases of coexisting carotid stenosis. Kessler et al[199] studied 82 patients in a prospective manner and concluded that each type of mechanism can occur, that embolic stroke was slightly more frequent in the cases with heterogeneous plaque, but that smooth plaques are also associated with an embolic mechanism of stroke.

Despite the announced results of the NASCET and European Cooperative Study, debate continues on whether ulcers are important in stroke. They are often found in surgical specimens.[33,98,186,201] The smaller ulcers are difficult to demonstrate angiographically, and considerable interobserver variation exists in the diagnosis of ulceration.[106] As many as 40% are missed on routine angiogram, and many ulcers are found at operation in ". . . smooth, benign-appearing plaques . . ."[98] Ulceration may be an erroneous angiographic diagnosis for a lesion actually due to subintimal hemorrhage into a shallow plaque,[98] a finding that may even resolve spontaneously.[202]

Fisher and Ojemann's[130] pathologic study of carotid endarterectomy plaques found no important clinical correlation with ulcerations or cul-de-sacs (defined as rounded pouches of diverticuli protruding from the lumen into the plaque) in 90 patients who had hemispheric TIAs or TMB or who were asymptomatic, or in a separate group of 51 patients with a persistent neurologic deficit. Of 30 cases of ulceration and 7 cul-de-sacs in the TIA patients, no definite examples of clinical embolic events had occurred. This point is underscored by the observation that nine ulcerations and five cul-de-sacs were found in 33 asymptomatic patients. Similarly, in 51 patients with a persistent neurologic deficit signifying infarction, only 10 had ulcerations or cul-de-sacs, and 6 of these were in association with a severe stenosis (residual lumen <1 mm). The remaining four patients, with widely patent lumens, had minor neurologic signs.

Opinions on the importance of ulceration per se are changing over time. A retrospective study reporting 79 cases with 91 asymptomatic shallow ulcers or ulcerated plaques, followed over a mean of 3 years, showed only a 9% incidence of TIAs and no strokes during that period.[205] The published discussion that followed the paper was conducted by Moore, Machleder, Levin, Javid, and Eastcott, whose combined opinions supported the notion of a benign prognosis for asymptomatic patients with shallow ulcers and ulcerated plaques. This opinion has been repeated in recent years, resulting in a lessening of enthusiasm for surgery for minor ulcerations without coexisting severe stenosis. Although the TIA and stroke risk for complex, deep ulcers is still a subject of dispute,[205,263] the undeniable correlation with high-grade stenosis makes it difficult to perform a separate study of one of the two coexisting elements.

Differential Diagnosis of TIAs

Many types of spells similar or even partly identical to TIAs have different pathogeneses and stroke prognoses.[89,118] The concept of TIA is based on an atherothrombotic mechanism, and this factor alone distinguishes TIAs from other types of spells.

Seizures, migraine accompaniments, syncope, isolated dizziness, and transient memory disturbance are common disturbances that may be confused with TIAs. These spells, however, have no proven atheromatous basis, and their treatments and outcomes differ significantly from TIAs. Even spells considered to meet the definition of TIAs may have an underlying vascular mechanism other than large artery atherothrombotic disease. TIAs may be related to small, penetrating arterial disease that causes lacunar infarction.[258,284] They may occur as a flurry in the hours before stroke, or as isolated events without stroke. The clinical features of lacunar TIAs may be indistinguishable from large artery TIAs, yet diagnostic evaluation, treatment, and stroke risk are probably different. Also, rapidly fading cerebral embolism may give rise to a short-lived neurologic deficit consistent with the time criterion of TIA, but no atherothrombotic mechanism may exist. In one study,[284] such TIAs of a presumed embolic mechanism tended to be of longer duration, ≥ 1 hour, than TIAs from a carotid atheromatous cause.

All these variations should alert the clinician to the heterogeneous nature of TIAs. They are best viewed as symptoms, much like seizure and headache, and not as a homogeneous, pathogenic state. Further clarification of the underlying cerebrovascular mechanisms may lead to more rational therapy and reliable prognostication.

REVERSIBLE ISCHEMIC NEUROLOGIC DEFICIT

The usefulness of the older concept of reversible ischemic neurologic deficit has recently been questioned on the grounds that it has no prognostic value.[51,230] In fact, a clinical deficit that clears off slowly but requires >24 hours to do so probably reflects infarction, as has been corroborated many times by CT scan.[372]

Some carotid-related strokes begin and progress such that accumulation of neurologic deficit occurs over hours to a day or more, giving rise to the term progressive or evolving stroke. Clearly the brain has suffered infarction in this situation, but the patient may have only a submaximal neurologic deficit for the arterial territory affected. For example, if a patient has only mild to moderate right arm and hand weakness but face, leg, speech, and visual field function are spared, then this will be considered a submaximal deficit for the territory involved, although infarction may be present even on CT scan. The mechanism responsible for this deficit might recur, leading to further disability, unless treatment is offered. This approach, which stresses submaximal deficit rather than whether or not the brain has suffered infarction, allows for the opportunity of treatment (surgical or medical) in the hopes of preventing further disability.

ISCHEMIC STROKE FROM CAROTID DISEASE

Ocular Infarction

The ipsilateral eye and brain are the usual sites of clinical symptoms in stroke affecting a given ICA territory. Although both the eye and the brain are susceptible, it is remarkable how infrequently the eye is affected by permanent deficit compared with the brain. Even rarer is the simultaneous occurrence of eye and brain infarction from hemodynamic carotid disease, called optico-cerebral syndrome by Bogousslavsky et al,[38] who found this phenomenon in 3 (0.5%) of 612 consecutive patients with carotid territory stroke. In our experience this syndrome is rare and gives too much emphasis to the notion that the eye and brain are involved at the same time in TIAs, a view that should be de-emphasized, not resurrected.[284]

The relationship between retinal infarction (eye stroke) and extracranial carotid artery disease is complicated. Since Marshall and Meadows's[239] study of the natural history of TMB, it has been known that associated retinal infarction may occur in a small percent of patients followed over the long term. The presumed mechanism is embolic occlusion of either a retinal branch or the central retinal artery. Considerable controversy, however, has centered on the relationship between the embolic material and associated carotid artery disease as a potential source (see above). Cholesterol crystals discovered in the retinal circulation, a marker for systemic atherosclerosis known from Hollenhorst's original reports,[163,281] are often incidentally noted on routine ophthalmologic examination in asymptomatic patients.[47,285,323] Hollenhorst first documented that TMB was not usually associated with cholesterol emboli, an observation corroborated in clinical practice.

Even the role of cholesterol emboli in causing other types of permanent monocular visual loss is unclear. Some studies suggest a relationship to retinal branch occlusion with the carotid artery as the embolic source.[310,385] Other studies, however, identify a strong correlation between retinal infarct from branch occlusion and carotid occlusive disease, but the embolic material is usually platelet debris and not cholesterol. When permanent visual loss related to central retinal artery occlusion is included, a condition in which the embolic obstruction may not be visualized, cardiac embolic sources, albeit occult, as well as the carotid artery, may be the underlying embolic mechanism. The simple and unitary idea that TMB and retinal stroke are all manifestations of one entity with extracranial carotid artery disease giving rise to cholesterol emboli as the offending material is probably incorrect. However, the possibility that moderate to severe carotid disease is similarly associated with different retinal embolic events has been raised by one of the present authors' (M.S.P.) finding that in 39 patients with 42 instances of retinal cholesterol plaques, branch retinal artery occlusion, and central retinal artery occlusion the incidence of carotid disease (56% to 60%) was not different for the three groups.[285]

CENTRAL RETINAL ARTERY OCCLUSION. Several large series of patients with central retinal artery occlusion who had cerebral angiography have documented ipsilateral carotid disease (ulcerative nonstenotic, stenotic without ulceration or irregularity, or occlusive) consistent with an embolic source in 50% to 70% of cases.[87,285,326] Carotid territory TIAs including TMB occurred in many patients before central retinal artery occlusion.

ISCHEMIC OPTIC NEUROPATHY. A host of ocular pathologies included in the term ischemic optic neuropathy may attend chronic orbital ischemia as a result of extracranial carotid occlusive disease. Remarkably, it is an uncommon complication of carotid occlusive disease estimated to affect approximately 5% of patients in one of the early series.[198] Embolism may be the cause in some cases.[236] The ocular abnormalities include pupillary dilatation with poor light reaction; neovascularization of the iris (rubeosis iridis); elevated intraocular pressure with secondary glaucoma; and proliferative retinopathy (Figs. 17.12 and 17.13) with microaneurysms, scattered flame-shaped hemorrhages, and prominent venous stasis.[120,168,198,236,407] Significant visual loss sometimes ending in blindness with optic atrophy makes this a serious condition. The presumed pathogenesis of reduced orbital blood flow has led to claims that the chronic

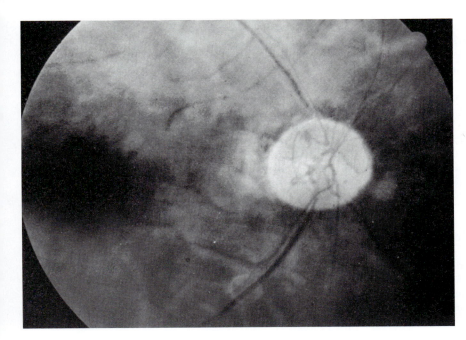

Figure 17.12 Attenuated retinal vessels.

ocular ischemia changes may be reversible with extracranial-intracranial arterial grafting,[99] but others have not found this beneficial.[407]

UNUSUAL SYNDROMES. A small series of cases have been described with symptoms and signs referable to the orbit in cases of carotid disease. For some, a variant of migraine, Raeder syndrome, and the like have been described. Gelmers[143] described two cases with facial pain and ipsilateral oculosympathetic paresis, which he labeled the pericarotid syndrome. The author attributed the ocular disturbance to disease affecting the cervical portion of the ICA, as demonstrated angiographically.

Cerebral Infarction

The number of instances of cerebral infarction in the territory of the ICA far exceeds the instances in which the mechanism of the stroke is determined.[154] Difficulties in determining whether the ICA is occluded, severely stenosed, slightly stenosed, ulcerated, or merely the conduit for the embolic mate-

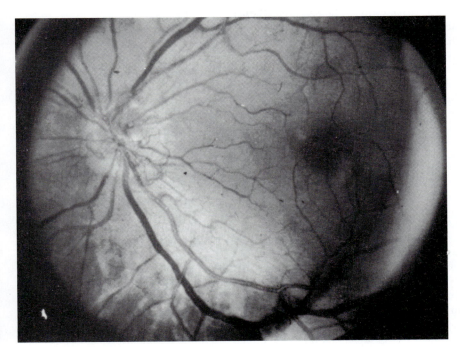

Figure 17.13 Neovascular proliferation affecting the disc.

rial remain a major obstacle to progress in the analysis of cases of stroke in the carotid territory. However, this difficulty is brushed aside when the clinical syndromes of carotid artery disease are discussed in detail, as is apparent in the material that follows.

Following a variable number of TIAs, the completed stroke that results from severe stenosis or occlusion of the ICA reflects infarction from either distal flow failure[112] or embolization.[59,61] The latter mechanism is probably the most common, as it accounts for virtually two-thirds of strokes with ICA occlusion.[286] Distal insufficiency appears to account for the other third. Simultaneous infarction of the eye and brain[152] is rare.[36,284]

INFARCTION WITH DISTAL INSUFFI-CIENCY. The pathophysiologic basis of distal insufficiency has already been covered in detail (see above). The clinical syndromes from cerebral infarction in this distribution should be characterized by a prominent visual field defect, aphasia or hemi-inattention features (from dominant or nondominant hemisphere involvement, respectively), and variable degrees of contralateral sensorimotor deficit. Based on now somewhat outmoded classical clinicopathologic correlations of the homunculus,[259] the latter should affect the proximal more than the distal segments of the upper limb reflecting the location of the infarct along the upper portions of the frontal-parietal convexity.[257] Although the above constellation of symptoms is commonly found (bilaterally) in cases of cardiac arrest and hypotension with resulting bilateral distal field infarction, its unilateral occurrence from ICA atherothrombosis has only recently been documented by CT scan.[35]

In the study of symptoms with carotid occlusion by Pessin et al[286] the clinical differences between the two groups of patients were a higher frequency of preceding TIAs and less severe clinical deficits with infarctions of nonembolic mechanism. These authors could not separate two groups of patients with clinically well-defined neurologic findings to assist in delineating a different topography of the infarcts.

From these considerations, it is apparent that a distal insufficiency mechanism of reduced cerebral flow, although a possible explanation for recurrent stereotypic TIAs,[89] has proved hard to document as the source of cerebral infarction from ICA disease, a situation in which distal embolism appears to account for the great majority of events. As a result, the neurologic examination findings in themselves have no distinctive elements to suggest extracranial ICA atherothrombosis as the cause of the stroke.

Numerous autopsy-documented studies have detailed the clinical picture in suprasylvian unilateral cerebral infarcts, even when the exact cause (e.g., thrombosis with perfusion failure or embolism) of the infarction has been unclear.[59,112,115,120,127,220,257,306,320] Many of these patients developed the infarct in relation to carotid occlusion, under which circumstances the main bulk of the endangered territory lay between the anterior and middle cerebral arteries, which caused the softening in the upper frontal lobe.

The most frequently reported effects have been *unilateral infarction.* The symptoms to be expected in such cases have been described by a number of authors.[112,120,223,225,281,286,302,306,336] Common symptoms have included weakness, paralysis, dyspraxia, numbness and tingling, and stereodysnomia in one or more fingers, or the hand, wrist, or arm and leg. Grasp reflex has been observed. Transient impaired ocular motility is often reported;

when not reported, the meaning of the omission is unclear. Disturbances in higher cerebral function have included episodes of speechlessness and of change in personality,[114,413] as well as dysgraphia of both the paretic and dyspraxic types.

A few well-known examples from the older literature indicate the long-standing recognition of the syndrome. Elder[104] described a 69-year-old messenger who developed stepwise attacks of right arm and leg paresis with slight dysarthria. Sensation was said to be normal, and he had no hemianopia. The left eye was frequently painful. A right grasp was noted. The progressing hemiplegia spared the face. His speech was intact, as was auditory comprehension and repetition. Writing was clumsy, large, and confined to his own name and a few letters; copying was difficult. He named objects presented at sight easily. He was unable to read aloud and could manage only a few letters with frequent repetitions. At autopsy white vessel and extensive infarction was observed extending from the upper frontal region to involve almost the entire lateral parietal and occipital region.

Spatz's[336] famous case was a 43-year-old man whose problems began with attacks of headache and shimmering in the left eye. He later developed a weak right arm and disturbance of speech in which he often failed to find a word. A right homonymous hemianopia was observed. No tests of reading are reported. At autopsy, the suprasylvian territory of the left cerebral hemisphere from the frontal through posterior parietal regions was involved with "granular atrophy."

Attempts to clarify the clinical picture in a setting of carotid occlusion documented in life have been less striking, perhaps because such case material includes a mixture of examples of distal insufficiency, cerebral embolism, and anterograde extension of thrombus into the stem of the middle cerebral artery. In one of the first attempts at such a clinical study, 64 consecutively encountered cases of ICA occlusion among 5,000 angiograms performed over a 3-year period were reported by Pessin et al.[286] They found 22 cases whose clinical picture and radiologic findings suggested that the stroke occurred through the mechanism of distal insufficiency.[286] No angiographic evidence of arterial branch occlusion was found. In this group of 22 cases, 16 had one or more prior TIAs, and the 13 who suffered a stroke had only a modest deficit, mostly confined to weakness in the upper limb. Clinically, the cases attributed to a hemodynamic cause conformed to the formula found by Pessin et al,[286] with a milder deficit and better clinical outlook in such cases compared with those attributed to embolism.

Clinical syndromes of pure dementia have often been alluded to in the literature but have proved difficult to document. Claims of improvement in mental function after carotid endarterectomy have appeared from time to time. One report[187] is of interest for its attempt to focus on those cases presumed to be suffering from the low flow state. Using a battery of tests of memory and mental agility, the authors found a more dramatic change postoperatively in their 12 cases thought to have low flow state preoperatively than they did in the matched controls having no hemodynamically significant lesions.

BILATERAL INFARCTION. Less attention has been paid to bilateral infarcts. Perhaps because of the dramatic clinical picture, some of the literature of symptomatic bilateral cerebral infarction from bilateral carotid occlusion has emphasized the devastating nature of the clinical deficits. Cases of bilateral traumatic thrombosis of the carotid artery, although somewhat unusual, have been particularly striking: Petrov et al[288] described a 30-year-old woman who developed bilateral traumatic carotid occlusions after an automobile accident; she presented in a coma, which deepened over a period of 24 hours. Autopsy appeared to show involvement of virtually the entire territories of both ICAs including not only the proximal and distal fields but also the hypophysis. Castaigne et al[57] reported on the case of a 51-year-old man with bilateral ICA occlusion, the distal end of the occlusion being below the ophthalmic artery on both sides. The patient survived for 2 years and died from cancer of the colon. Neuropathologic examination showed bilateral watershed lesions, more marked on the left hemisphere. On the left side the posterior cerebral artery as well as the anterior and middle cerebral arteries arose from the ICA. Microscopically, the pial arteries were patent, thin-walled, and stained pale pink with eosin. Clinically, the deep reflexes were brisk on both sides; there was a bilateral Babinski sign and *marche à petits pas*. The appearance and demeanor of the patient were quite remarkable. He had a mask-like face with an impressive absence of mimicry. Day after day he lay for hours in his bed, motionless, head and eyes turned toward the left. At long intervals he winked and sighed or made a few clumsy movements with both hands. However, when encouraged he appeared well oriented in time and space. He could name objects and colors and recognized faces. He clumsily and slowly but correctly carried out spoken commands. There was no severe ideomotor apraxia. In Pierre Marie's three-paper test, two of three of the orders were correctly performed. However, as soon as the examination ended the patient reverted to his motionless state.

A few of the cases of bilateral infarction have presented less dramatic clinical syndromes. Romanul and Abramowicz[306] (case 1) described a man with left arm weakness, hyperreflexia, and impaired pin appreciation whose ability to understand newsprint, to draw, and to calculate were impaired. The patient showed bilateral carotid occlusion and bilateral lesions.

HIGH CONVEXITY INFARCTION SYNDROME.

The predominance of high convexity infarction in carotid syndromes of distal insufficiency have yielded some distinctive syndromes. In a study of clinical features separating embolic from carotid thrombotic syndrome, Timsit et al[354] found that the carotid syndrome contained examples of fractional (different degrees of) weakness in the shoulder versus the hand, which was thought to reflect the upper convexity infarction from distal insufficiency. Examples of embolism more often showed comparable degrees of weakness of the hand and shoulder, consistent with the larger and lower convexity infarction. The probability of carotid artery disease increased over embolism when fractional arm weakness (shoulder different from hand) was present (odds ratio, 5.3 95%; confidence interval, 3.1 to 9.0). An example from the records of the Salpêtrière illustrates these points. A 56-year-old right-handed man awoke with a weakness of the right upper and lower limbs without any other symptoms. On neurologic examination 60 hours after onset, he was alert with a slight uneasiness for right finger movements without any other weakness. There was right-sided hypesthesia for warm, cold, pinprick, touch, and joint position sense in the right shoulder extending to the upper third of the arm. Neurologic examination was otherwise unremarkable. CT scan showed an infarct in the upper prero-

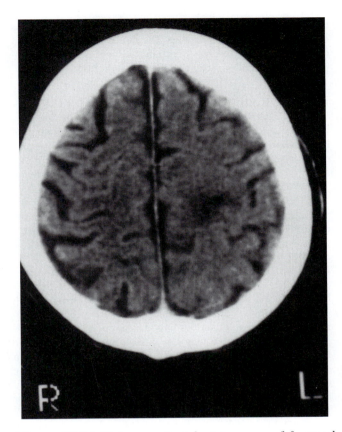

Figure 17.14 High convexity infarct in a case of fractional weakness (see text).

landic region on the left side (Fig. 17.14) and an angiogram showed 75% stenosis of the left ICA. Within several weeks the distal weakness had almost disappeared, but the sensory findings remained unchanged. Carotid endarterectomy was performed without complication.

Another unusual clinical variation of distal insufficiency in carotid occlusive disease has been ipsilateral leg weakness, described in two separate reports.[62,401] Yanagihara et al[401] reported on 19 patients with episodic or progressive lower extremity weakness, contralateral to severe extracranial ICA occlusive disease (16 patients) or carotid siphon stenosis (3 patients). Cerebral blood measurements, using xenon-133 in some of the patients, corroborated reduced hemispheric flow on the appropriate side localized to the border zone in the frontal parietal to parietal areas corresponding to motor function of the lower extremity. Chimowitz et al[62] described a 52-year-old man with separate transient episodes of left eye TMB, right hemiparesis and aphasia, and left leg weakness. The latter occurred on one occasion with simultaneous right arm weakness. When he developed a fixed deficit, his examination showed a right hemiparesis and expressive aphasia, left leg weakness, bilateral hyper-reflexia, and Babinski signs. CT showed bilateral distal field infarcts involving the right frontoparietal, left frontal, and left parietal areas. Angiography showed an 80% stenosis of the left ICA and a 60% stenosis of the right ICA. Both anterior cerebral arteries filled from the left carotid circulation due to a presumably atretic right A1 segment, and the distal right anterior cerebral artery filled incompletely. Following left carotid endarterectomy he improved, and no further TIAs occurred in a 4-month follow-up. The case strongly suggests that distal insufficiency, bilaterally manifested because of an incomplete circle of Willis, accounted for the clinical signs.

INTRACRANIAL INTERNAL CAROTID ARTERY EMBOLISM. Intracranial embolism has also been frequently found in autopsy studies.[62,134,196,234] Embolism has also been the proposed mechanism in prior studies for some of the strokes that are delayed in onset following carotid occlusion.[17,59,74,127,132,220] This type of outlook is far more serious and seems to occur with far less warning.

The embolus may arise from several sources. Anterograde propagation of the thrombosis intracranially may result in a tail of thrombus that lies at the top of the ICA, the tail being available to be swept distally via retrograde flow through the ophthalmic and into the middle and anterior cerebral arteries above.[110,310] Lethal hemispheric stroke has been encountered in one patient 3 days after angiographically documented occlusion of the ipsilateral cerebral ICA. The autopsy evidence was consistent with embolism from the distal intracranial tail of the propagated carotid thrombus. An infarct this large has not previously been reported.[110] Embolization may also arise from the stump of the ICA that remains emanating from the bifurcation of the common carotid after ICA occlusion; the Venturi effect of blood passing up the common to the external carotid artery may sweep material from the stump distally to reach the intracranial arteries.[17] Other sources have not yet been defined.

Embolism may be a frequent cause of stroke associated with carotid thrombosis. In the series reported by Pessin et al,[286] fully 25 of the 64 angiogrammed cases showed angiographic evidence of intracranial main stem or branch middle cerebral artery occlusion, and another 17 had angiographic findings consistent with or suggestive of earlier embolization. The clinical picture in these 43 cases contrasted sharply with the 22 with no signs of embolism: less than half of the patients (17 of 43) had experienced prior TIA, and 12 suffered severe strokes, seven that were moderately severe, and only six that were mild. This difference in TIA frequency and stroke severity was the reverse pattern of the group whose symptoms were attributed to distal insufficiency.

This form of infarction has proved difficult to distinguish on clinical or radiographic grounds from embolism from cardiac source. In the present state of knowledge, there appears to be no essential difference between the type and severity of the syndromes caused by carotid or cardiac sources.[286,302] The subject of such syndromes is discussed in more detail in the middle cerebral artery chapter (see Ch. 19).

ANTEROGRADE EXTENSION OF THROMBUS. Pathologic studies of ICA thrombosis have documented anterograde extension of thrombus intracranially for varying distances. In a number of cases, extension occurred across the circle of Willis into the stems of the anterior and middle cerebral artery, yielding devastating cerebral infarction.[59,112,114,127,220] One result of this form of extension may be the rare telodiencephalic syndrome[341] cited above. The syndrome consists of contralateral brachiofacial hemiparesis occasionally accompanied by hemianopia and aphasia but mainly accompanied by ipsilateral hemihypohidrosis with an ipsilateral Horner syndrome. The authors consider it to be caused by an ischemic lesion of the crossed pathways descending from the cerebrum and the uncrossed hypothalamic-spinal sympathetic pathways. The syndrome was attributed to occlusion of the ICA and occasionally the middle cerebral artery.

Prognosis for Intracranial Internal Carotid Artery Disease

Two reports are available. In Marzewski et al's[241] 66 patients, the mean age at the time of angiography was 61.5 years and follow-up averaged 3.9 years. Ten (15.2%) had a stroke (eight ICA territory), and the observed stroke rate for patients 35 years and older was 13 times the expected infarction rate for a normal population with a similar age and sex distribution. However, due to associated cerebral arterial lesions, the intracranial ICA stenosis was the only apparent cause for only 2 of the 10 strokes. Half of the patients died during follow-up. Eighteen deaths (54.6% of all deaths) were known to be cardiac related. There were no known stroke deaths. The risk of stroke and death appeared to be increased compared with that of ICA occlusion.[241] Craig et al[72] followed for a mean of 30 months (2 to 78 months) 58 patients whose mean age was 62.4 years. At the end of follow-up only 33% were alive and free from subsequent cerebral vascular events, and only 47% were functioning well. Seventeen (29%) had suffered a stroke, and 11 (65%) of these were appropriate to the intracranial ICA stenosis. There were nine fatal strokes, five appropriate to the intracranial ICA stenosis. Twenty-five of the patients (43%) died during follow-up: 44% of the deaths were cardiac related and 36% stroke related. The asymptomatic patients had as poor a prognosis as the symptomatic ones, but women fared better than men, although the number of deaths was similar.[72]

Extracranial Vascular Examination

AUSCULTATION AND PALPATION

Clinical evaluation of cases of carotid territory stroke involves not only the neurologic examination but also assessment of the extracranial vascular tree. The most reliable of these signs are a locally generated bruit and abnormalities in the pattern of facial pulses.

The bruit heard in roughly 70% to 87% of cases with severe stenosis is most often found in front of the upper portion of the thyroid cartilage, which corresponds to the usual location of the carotid bifurcation.[142,281,287] Radiation of the bruit into the ocular region is usually a sign that the carotid below is patent. Because intracranial vascular volume changes dramatically with intrathoracic pressure, great diminution in the bruit intensity with the Valsalva maneuver should be a sign of ICA stenosis. However, this sign has not proved very reliable.[212]

Palpation of the facial pulses is another bedside test that should be of considerable value in the diagnosis of carotid

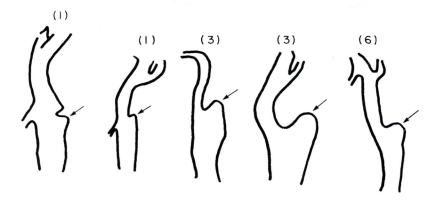

A   Carotid Occlusion, Rounded Stump

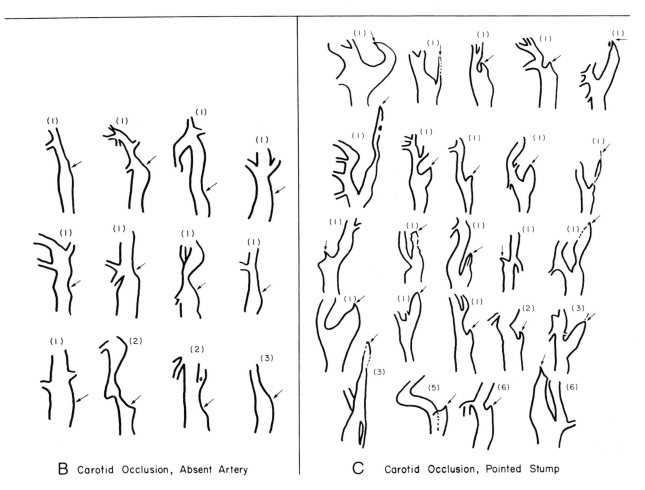

B   Carotid Occlusion, Absent Artery

C   Carotid Occlusion, Pointed Stump

Figure 17.15 Angiographic appearance of different types of internal carotid artery occlusion. Numbers in parentheses indicate days between stroke onset and angiography.

stenosis or occlusion. The collateral flow that develops in a setting of severe stenosis or occlusion of the ICA from branches of the external carotid through anastomoses in the orbit includes the distal orbital branches of the ophthalmic artery.[52] By palpation of these brow arteries, it is common to find an increase in the amplitude of the pulse in external carotid branches (facial, preauricular, temporal arteries) on the side of the ICA disease, resulting from increased collateral flow.[121] A more sensitive sign is the demonstration, by facial palpation, of reversal of flow in the frontal or supratrochlear arteries,[52] which is a fairly reliable indicator of hemodynamically significant stenosis or occlusion of the ICA. However, the pulse is often feeble, and the direction of flow is difficult to demonstrate by palpation alone. Any concern about precipitating a stroke by this maneuver is unwarranted: the flow through these collateral channels is trivial compared with the greater volume carried by the maxillary artery through the floor of the orbit, regions unaccessible to the examiner. This pattern of abnormal collateral flow can be determined more precisely by the use of directional Doppler testing. The demonstration of reversal of flow in frontal or supratrochlear arteries is strong evidence of ipsilateral ICA disease, ranging from residual lumens of 1.5 mm to complete occlusion.[7]

Palpation of the common carotid artery or the bifurcation is unreliable for inference of occlusion and can be dangerous, as it carries an unpredictable risk of dislodgment of thrombi.

DOPPLER EXAMINATION

Doppler technology for carotid artery disease has developed to a degree that it is the subject of a special chapter (see Ch. 14). Meta-analysis of duplex Doppler technology indicates that its current level of sensitivity and specificity rivals that of conventional angiography.[34,340] Suffice it to say that early disappointments with its use in clinical trials[337] have largely faded with its greatly improved sensitivity and specificity for extracranial stenosis, especially at the more severe ends of the spectrum.

Less current enthusiasm exists for the utility of plaque ultrasonographic analysis of plaque echomorphology (by B-mode) and surface characteristics (by color-coded Doppler). Baud et al[19] studied 53 plaques of 0.40% to 80% stenosis, spanning the range from echodense to echolucent, that were analyzed by observers in four centers. Kappa indices of agreement were at best modest: 0.47 for anechoic plaques and 0.52 for luminal surface regularity. Further work is in progress.

ANGIOGRAPHY

Cerebral angiography (see Ch. 13) was for decades the definitive evaluation for assessment of stenosis or occlusion of the extracranial ICA and detailed visualization of the intracranial circulation. Its role as the gold standard has come into question. Digitized angiography[101,126,223] remains popular in many institutions despite its slightly lower image quality compared with conventional angiography. Modern MRI has developed a high level of sensitivity and specificity in depicting severe stenosis or occlusion,[197] even though it overestimates the de-

gree of stenosis in many cases. Modern duplex Doppler has improved to such an extent that it approximates the degree of stenosis seen by angiogram and provides measures of flow patterns and turbulence beyond the scope of the conventional angiogram.[5,6,66,187,362,400] It is also safe. Current information suggests that the hazard of conventional angiography approaches that of carotid endarterectomy itself.[404] Even the status of the collateral circulation at the circle of Willis, once the purview of conventional angiography, has become readily assessable by transcranial Doppler technology. However, conventional angiography still reigns supreme for demonstrating the mechanism of stroke (embolic versus nonembolic) and for imaging the surface branches or the smaller vessels that penetrate the parenchyma (e.g., lenticulostriate branches of the middle cerebral artery).

MR angiography has matured as the noninvasive competitor and even replacement for conventional angiography for initial screening at least.[96,208,228] Combined with duplex Doppler it provides most of the information needed for decisions for endarterectomy.[235]

Symptomatic stenoses leading to either TIAs or infarction are usually tight, with residual lumens of ≤2 mm, a level of stenosis shown to be associated with hemodynamic changes.[9,43] Occluded cervical ICAs can have a number of angiographic patterns, some of which indicate a pathogenetic mechanism for the occlusion: a sharp pointed tapering stenosis of the ICA, distal to which there is a thread-like luminal filling that may open distally into a normal size lumen—the so-called string sign—is a picture commonly seen in carotid dissection.[131] In the atherosclerotic variety of ICA occlusion, on the other hand, several angiographic patterns have been recognized (Fig. 17.15): sharp, pointed stump; amputation of the artery at its origin; and rounded, blunt stump.[283] The old notion that the first pattern indicates recent occlusion and that the other two are found in the chronic stage has not been justified, as all three patterns were seen when arteriograms were performed within 6 days from stroke onset.[283]

OTHER IMAGING METHODS

Quantitative phonoangiography,[77,192,193] which had a short period of limited popularity, has fallen into disuse. Radionuclide imaging of the carotid lesion itself[198] was expected to detect active platelet deposition but has failed to do so in a clinical trial.

References

1. Acheson J, Hutchinson EC: Observations on the natural history of transient cerebral ischemia. Lancet 2:871, 1964
2. Adams HP, Gross CE: Embolism distal to stenosis of the middle cerebral artery. Stroke 12:228, 1981
3. Adams HP Jr, Putnam SF, Corbett JJ et al: Amaurosis fugax. The results of arteriography in 59 patients. Stroke 14:742, 1983

4. Adams RD, Fisher CM: Pathology of cerebral arterial occlusion. In Fields WS (ed): Houston Symposium on Pathogenesis and Treatment of Cerebrovascular Disease. Charles C Thomas, Springfield, IL, 1961.

5. Adiga KR, Fresso SJ, Nayden J: Noninvasive methods in the diagnosis of extracranial carotid artery disease: a correlation with carotid arteriography in eighty patients. Angiology 35:331, 1984

6. Anderson DC, Loewenson R, Yock D et al: B-mode, real-time carotid ultrasonic imaging. Correlation with angiography. Arch Neurol 40:484, 1983

7. Anderson JM, Stevens JC, Sundt TM et al: Ectopic internal carotid artery seen initially as middle ear tumor. JAMA 249:2228, 1983

8. Arbeille P, Bounin-Pineau MH, Philippot M et al: Suivi des paramètres morphologiques des plaques d'athérome sur 24 mois. J Echograph Med Ultrason 17:337, 1996

9. Archie JP, Feldtman RW: Critical stenosis of the internal carotid artery. Surgery 89:67, 1981

10. Awad I, Little JR, Modic MT et al: Intravenous digital subtraction angiography: an index of collateral cerebral blood flow in internal carotid artery occlusion. Stroke 13:469, 1982

11. Awad I, Modic M, Little JR et al: Focal parenchymal lesions in transient ischemic attacks: correlation of computed tomography and magnetic resonance imaging. Stroke 17:399, 1986

12. Baker RN, Broward JA, Fang HC et al: Anticoagulant therapy in cerebral infarction. Neurology 12:823, 1962

13. Baker RN, Ramseyer JG, Schwartz WS: Prognosis in patients with cerebral ischemic attacks. Neurology 18:1157, 1968

14. Banker BQ: Cerebral vascular disease in infancy and childhood. I. Occlusive vascular diseases. J Neuropathol Exp Neurol 20:127, 1961

15. Baquis GD, Pessin MS, Scott RM: Limb shaking—a carotid TIA. Stroke 16:444, 1985

16. Barnett HJM: Delayed cerebral ischemic episodes distal to occlusion of major cerebral arteries. Neurology 28:769, 1978

17. Barnett HJM, Peerless SJ, Kaufmann JCE: The "stump" of internal carotid artery—a source for further cerebral embolic ischemia. Stroke 9:448, 1978

18. Baron JC, Bousser MG, Rey A et al: Reversal of focal "misery-perfusion syndrome" by extra-intracranial arterial bypass in hemodynamic cerebral ischemia. Stroke 12:454, 1981

19. Baud JM, De Bray JM, Delanoy P et al: Reproductibilité ultrasonore dans la caractérisation des plaques carotidiennes. J Echograph Med Ultrason 17:377, 1996

20. Bauer RB, Boulos RS, Myer JS: Natural history and surgical treatment of occlusive cerebral vascular disease evaluated by serial angiography. AJR Radium Ther Nucl Med 104:1, 1968

21. Beal MF, Williams RS, Richardson EP, Fisher CM: Cerebral embolism as a cause of transient ischemic attacks and cerebral infarction. Neurology (NY) 31:860, 1981

22. Benditt EP, Benditt JM: Evidence for a monoclonal origin of atherosclerotic plaques. Proc Natl Acad Sci USA 70:1753, 1973

23. Benoit P, Destée A, Verier A et al: Sténose post-radiothérapeutique de l'artère carotide interne supraclinoï-

dienne. Réseau de moya moya. Rev Neurol 141:666, 1985

24. Bernasconi V, Cassinari V: Caratteristische angiografische bei meningioma del tentorio. Radiol Med 43:1015, 1957

25. Berry RG, Alpers BJ: Occlusion of the carotid circulation. Pathologic considerations. Neurology (Minneapolis) 7:223, 1957

26. Berguer R, Hwang NHC: Critical arterial stenosis: a theoretical and experimental solution. Ann Surg 180:39, 1974

27. Bernstein NM, Norris JW: Benign outcome of carotid occlusion. Neurology 39:6, 1989

28. Bickerstaff ER: Aetiology of acute hemiplegia in childhood. BMJ 2:82, 1964

29. Björkesten G, Troupp H: Changes in the size of intracranial arterial aneurysms. J Neurosurg 19:583, 1962

30. Blackwood W: Pathological aspects of cerebral and spinal vascular disease. In Ross Russell RW (ed): Vascular Disease of the Central Nervous System. 2nd Ed. Churchill Livingstone, Edinburgh, 1983

31. Blackwood W, Hallpike JF, Kocen RS, Mair WGP: Atheromatous disease of the carotid arterial system and embolism from the heart in cerebral infarction: a morbid anatomical study. Brain 92:897, 1969

32. Bladin PF: A radiologic and pathologic study of embolism of the internal-middle cerebral arterial axis. Radiology 82:615, 1964

33. Blaisdell FW, Glickman M, Trunkey DD: Ulcerated atheroma of the carotid artery. Arch Surg 108:491, 1974

34. Blakeley DD, Oddone EZ, Hasselblad V et al: Noninvasive carotid artery testing. A meta-analytic review. Ann Intern Med 122:360, 1995

35. Bogousslavsky J, Regli F: Borderzone infarctions distal to internal carotid artery occlusion: prognostic implications. Ann Neurol 20:346, 1986

36. Bogousslavsky J, Regli F: Cerebral infarction with transient signs (CITS): do TIAs correspond to small deep infarcts in internal carotid artery occlusion? Stroke 15:536, 1984

37. Bogousslavsky J, Regli F, Hungerbühler J-P, Chrzanowski R: Transient ischemic attacks and external carotid artery occlusion. A retrospective study of 23 patients with an occlusion of the internal carotid artery. Stroke 12:627, 1981

38. Bogousslavsky J, Regli F, Zografos L, Uske A: Opticocerebral syndrome: simultaneous hemodynamic infarction of optic nerve and brain. Neurology 37:263, 1987

39. Bousser MG: Faut-il opérer les sténoses carotidiennes asymptomatiques? Rev Neurol 151:363, 1995

40. Bousser MG, Touboul P, Cabanis E et al: The significance of ocular bruits in ischemic cerebro-vascular disease. Neuro-Ophthalmology 1:211, 1981

41. Boyd JD: Absence of the right common carotid artery. J Anat 68:551, 1934

42. Boysen G, Jensen G, Schnor P: Frequency of focal cerebral transient ischemic attacks during a 12 month period. Stroke 10:533, 1979

43. Brice JG, Dowsett DJ, Lowe RD: Haemodynamic effects of carotid artery stenosis. BMJ 2:1363, 1964

44. Brockmeier LB, Adolph RJ, Gustin BW et al: Calcium

emboli to the retinal artery in calcific aortic stenosis. Am Heart J 101:32, 1981

45. Brott T, Tomsick T, Feinberg W et al: Baseline silent cerebral infarction in the Asymptomatic Carotid Atherosclerosis Study. Stroke 25:1122, 1994

46. Brown MF, Graham JM, Feliciano DV et al: Carotid artery injuries. Am J Surg 144:748, 1982

47. Bunt TJ: The clinical significance of the asymptomatic Hollenhorst plaque. J Vasc Surg 4:559, 1986

48. Burnbaum MD, Selhorst JB, Harbison JW, Brush JJ: Amaurosis fugax from disease of the external carotid artery. Arch Neurol 34:532, 1977

49. Byar D, Fiddian RV, Quereau M et al: The fallacy of applying the Poisseulle equation to segmental arterial stenosis. Am Heart J 70:216, 1965

50. Callow AD: Recurrent stenosis after carotid endarterectomy. Arch Surg 117:1082, 1982

51. Caplan LR: Are terms such as completed stroke or RIND of continued usefulness? Stroke 14:431, 1983

52. Caplan LR: The frontal artery sign—a bedside indicator of internal carotid occlusive disease. N Engl J Med 288:1008, 1973

53. Caplan LR, Baker R: Extracranial occlusive vascular disease: does size matter? Stroke 11:63, 1980

54. Carolei A, Marini C, Nencini P et al: Prevalence and outcome of symptomatic carotid lesions in young adults. National Research Council Study Group BMJ May 27:1363, 1995

55. Carpenter DA, Grubb RL Jr, Powers WJ: Borderzone hemodynamics in cerebrovascular disease. Neurology 40:1587, 1990

56. Carson SN, Demling RH, Esquivel CO: Aspirin failure in symptomatic atherosclerotic carotid artery disease. Surgery 90:1084, 1981

57. Castaigne P, Lhermitte F, Gautier JC: Obstruction bilateral des carotids internes. Press Med 71:757, 1963

58. Castaigne P, Lhermitte F, Gautier JC: Role des lesions arterielles dans les accidents ischemiques cerebraux de l'athérosclerose. Rev Neurol (Paris) 113:1, 1965

59. Castaigne P, Lhermitte F, Gautier JC et al: Internal carotid artery occlusion. A study of 61 instances in 50 patients with post-mortem data. Brain 93:321, 1970

60. Chiari H: Ueber das Verhalten der Teilungswinkels der Carotid communis bei der Endarteritis chronica deformans. Verh Dtsch Ges Pathol 9:326, 1905

61. Chikos PM, Fisher LD, Hirsch JH et al: Observer variability in evaluating extracranial cerotid artery stenosis. Stroke 14:885, 1983

62. Chimowitz MI, Lafranchise EF, Furlan AJ, Awad IA: Ipsilateral leg weakness associated with carotid stenosis. Stroke 21:1362, 1990

63. Cioffi FA, Meduri M, Tomasello F et al: Kinking and coiling of the internal carotid artery. J Neurosurg Sci 19:15, 1975

64. Coakham HB, Duchen LW, Scaravilli F: Moyamoya disease: clinical and pathological report of a case with associated myopathy. J Neurol Neurosurg Psychiatry 42:289, 1979

65. Cogan DG: Neurology of the Visual System. Charles C Thomas, Springfield, IL, 1996

66. Comerota AJ, Cranley JJ, Cook SE: Real-time B-mode carotid imaging in diagnosis of cerebrovascular disease. Surgery 6:718, 1981

67. Consensus sur la morphologie et la risque des plaques carotidiennes. J Echograph Med Ultrason 17:300, 1996

68. Correll JW, Quest DO, Carpenter DB: Nonatheromatous lesions of the extracranial cerebral arteries. p. 321. In Smith RR (ed): Stroke and the Extracranial Vessels. Lippincott-Raven, Philadelphia, 1984

69. Corrin LS, Sandok BA, Houser OW: Subsequent cerebral ischemic events in patients with carotid artery fibromuscular hyperplasia, abstracted. Stroke 12:120, 1981

70. Cote R, Barnett HJM, Taylor DW: Internal carotid occlusion: a prospective study. Stroke 14:898, 1983

71. Countee RW, Sapru HN, Vijayanathan T, Wu SZ: "Other syndromes" of the carotid bifurcation. p. 345. In Smith RR (ed): Stroke and the Extracranial Vessels. Lippincott-Raven, Philadelphia, 1984

72. Craig DR, Meguro K, Watridge C et al: Intracranial internal carotid artery stenosis. Stroke 13:825, 1982

73. Croft RJ, Ellam LD, Harrison MJG: Accuracy of carotid angiography in the assessment of atheroma of the internal carotid artery. Lancet 1:997, 1980

74. Dandy WE: Results following ligation of the internal carotid artery. Arch Surg 45:521, 1942

75. David NJ: Amaurosis fugax and after. In Glaser JS (ed): Neuroophthalmology. Vol. IX. CV Mosby, St. Louis, 1979

76. David NJ, Gordon KK, Friedberg SJ et al: Fatal atheromatous cerebral embolism associated with bright plaques in the retinal arterioles. Neurology 13:708, 1963

77. David DO, Rumbaugh CL, Gilson JM: Angiographic diagnosis of small-vessel cerebral emboli. Acta Radiol (Stockh) 9:264, 1969

78. Day AL, Rhoton AL, Quisling RG: Resolving siphon stenosis following endarterectomy. Stroke 11:278, 1980

79. DeBono DP, Warlow CP: Potential sources of emboli in patients with presumed transient cerebral or retinal ischemia. Lancet 1:343, 1981

80. Delal PM, Shah PM, Aiyar RR: Arteriographic study of cerebral embolism. Lancet 2:358, 1965

81. DeMarinis M, Fieschi C, Prencipe M et al: Circulating platelet aggregates: a chronic platelet activation in patients with transient ischaemic attacks. Ital J Neurol Sci 3:163, 1980

82. Denton IC, Gutmann L: Surgical treatment of symptomatic carotid stenosis and asymptomatic ipsilateral intracranial aneurysm. J Neurosurg 38:662, 1973

83. Dilenge D, Heon M: The internal carotid artery. p. 1202. In Newton TH, Potts DG (eds): Radiology of the Skull and Brain. Angiography. Vol. 2. Book 2. CV Mosby, St. Louis, 1974

84. Dixon S, Pais SO, Raviola C et al: Natural history of non stenotic, symptomatic ulcerative lesions of the carotid artery. A further analysis. Arch Surg 117:1493, 1982

85. Donnan GA, Sharbrough FW, Whisnant JP: Carotid occlusive disease. Effect of bright light on visual evoked responses. Arch Neurol 39:687, 1982

86. Doughtery JR Jr, Levy DE, Weksler BB: Platelet activation in acute cerebral ischaemia. Lancet 1:821, 1977

87. Douglas DJ, Schuler JJ, Buchbinder D et al: The association of central retinal artery occlusion and extracranial carotid artery disease. Ann Surg 208:85, 1988

88. Duncan GW, Gruber JO, Dewey CF et al: Evaluation of carotid stenosis by phonoangiography. N Engl J Med 293:1121, 1975

89. Duncan GW, Pessin MS, Mohr JP, Adams RD: Transient cerebral ischemic attacks. p. 1. In Stollerman GH (ed): Advances in Internal Medicine. Vol. 21. Year Book Medical Publishing, Chicago, 1976

90. Durward QJ, Ferguson GG, Barr HWK: The natural history of asymptomatic carotid bifurcation plaques. Stroke 13:459, 1982

91. Dyken ML, Doepker JF, Kiovsky R et al: Asymptomatic occlusion of an internal carotid artery in a hospital population: determined by directional Doppler ophthalmosonometry. Stroke 5:714, 1974

92. Dyll LM, Margolis M, David NJ: Amaurosis fugax. Funduscopic and photographic observations during an attack. Neurology (Minneap) 16:135, 1966

93. Eastcott HG, Pickering GW, Rob CG: Reconstruction of internal carotid artery in a patient with intermittent attacks of hemiplegia. Lancet 2:994, 1954

94. Easton JD, Sherman DG: Management of cerebral embolism of cardiac origin. Stroke 11:433, 1980

95. Easton JD, Sherman DG: Stroke and mortality rate in carotid endarterectomy: 228 consecutive operations. Stroke 8:566, 1977

96. Edelman RR, Mantle HP, Atkinson DJ, Hoogewoud HM: MR angiography. AJR 154:937, 1990

97. Edelman RR, Mantle HP, Wallner B et al: Extracranial carotid arteries: evaluation with "black blood" MR angiography. Radiology 177:45, 1990

98. Edwards JH, Kricheff II, Riles T, Imparato A: Angiographically undetected ulceration of the carotid bifurcation as a cause of embolic stroke. Radiology 132:369, 1979

99. Edwards MS, Chater NL, Stanley JA: Reversal of chronic ocular ischemia by extracranial-intracranial arterial bypass: case report. Neurosurgery 7:480, 1980

100. Eikelboom B, Riles TR, Mintzer F et al: Inaccuracy of angiography of the diagnosis of carotid ulceration. Stroke 14:882, 1983

101. Eisenberg RL, Mani RL: Clinical and arteriographic comparison of amaurosis fugax with hemispheric transient ischemic attacks. Stroke 9:254, 1978

102. Eisenberg RL, Nemzek WR, Moore WS, Mani RL: Relationship of transient ischemic attacks and angiographically demonstrable lesions of carotid artery. Stroke 8:483, 1977

103. Ekbom K, Greitz T: Carotid angiography in cluster headache. Acta Radiol (Diagn) 10:177, 1970

104. Elder W: The clinical varieties of visual aphasia (case 1). Edinb Med J 49:433, 1900

105. Elschnig A: Ueber den Einfluss des Verschlusses der Arteria ophthalmica und der Carotis auf das Sehorgan. Albrecht von Graefes Arch Klin Exp Ophthalmol 39:151, 1893

106. Executive Committee for the Asymptomatic Carotid Atherosclerosis Study: Endarterectomy for asymptomatic carotid artery stenosis. JAMA 273:1421–28, 1995

107. Ferro JM, Falcao I, Rodrigues G et al: Diagnosis of transient ischemic attack by a nonneurologist. Stroke 27:2225, 1996

108. Fields WS: The asymptomatic carotid bruit—operate or not. Stroke 9:269, 1978

109. Fields WS, Weibel J: Coincidental internal carotid stenosis and intra-cranial saccular aneurysm. Trans Am Neurol Assoc 95:237, 1970

110. Finklestein S, Kleinman GM, Cuneo R, Baringer JR: Delayed stroke following carotid occlusion. Neurology (Minneapolis) 30:84, 1980

111. Fisch BJ, Tatemichi TK, Prohovnik I et al: Transient ischemic attacks resembling simple partial motor seizures, abstracted. Neurology, suppl. 1, 38:264, 1988

112. Fisher CM: Occlusion of the internal carotid artery. AMA Arch Neurol Psychiatry 69:346, 1951

113. Fisher CM: Transient monocular blindness associated with hemiplegia. AMA Arch Ophthalmol 47:167, 1952

114. Fisher CM: Occlusion of the carotid arteries. Further experiences. AMA Arch Neurol Psychiatry 72:187, 1954

115. Fisher CM: Cerebral thromboangiitis obliterans. Medicine (Baltimore) 36:169, 1957

116. Fisher CM: The use of anticoagulants in cerebral thrombosis. Neurology 8:311, 1958

117. Fisher CM: Observations of the fundus oculi in transient monocular blindness. Neurology 9:337, 1959

118. Fisher CM: Concerning recurrent transient cerebral ischemic attacks. Can Med Assoc J 86:1091, 1962

119. Fisher CM: Cranial bruit associated with occlusion of the internal carotid artery. Neurology 7:299, 1962

120. Fisher CM: Some neuro-opthalmological observations. J Neurol Neurosurg Psychiatry 30:383, 1967

121. Fisher CM: Facial pulses in internal carotid artery occlusion. Neurology 20:476, 1970

122. Fisher CM: Cerebral ischemia—less familiar types. Clin Neurosurg 18:267, 1971

123. Fisher CM: Clinical syndromes of cerebral thrombosis, hypertensive hemorrhage, and ruptured saccular aneurysm. Clin Neurosurg 22:117, 1975

124. Fisher CM: The natural history of carotid occlusion. p. 194. In Austin GM (ed): Microneurosurgical Anastomoses for Cerebral Ischemia. Charles C Thomas, Springfield, IL, 1976

125. Fisher CM: Discussion at Princeton Conference 1980. In Moosy J, Reinmuth OM (eds): Cerebrovascular Diseases, XIIth Research (Princeton) Conference. Lippincott-Raven, Philadelphia, 1981

126. Fisher CM, Adams RD: Observations on brain embolism with special reference to the mechanism of hemorrhagic infarction. J Neuropathol Exp Neurol 10:92, 1951

127. Fisher CM, Gore I, Okabe N, White PD: Atherosclerosis of the carotid and vertebral arteries—extracranial and intracranial. J Neuropathol Exp Neurol 24:455, 1965

128. Fisher CM, Gore I, Okabe N, White PD: Calcification of the carotid siphon. Circulation 32:538, 1965

129. Fisher CM, Karnes WE: Local embolism. J Neuropathol Exp Neurol 24:174, 1965

130. Fisher CM, Ojemann RG: A clinico-pathologic study of carotid endarterectomy plaques. Rev Neurol (Paris) 142:573, 1986

131. Fisher CM, Ojemann RG, Roberson GH: Spontaneous dissection of cervico-cerebral arteries. Can J Neurol Sci 5:9, 1978

132. Fleming JFR, Petrie D: Traumatic thrombosis of the

internal carotid artery with delayed hemiplegia. Can J Surg 11:166, 1968

133. Forteza AM, Babikian VL, Hyde C et al: Effect of time and cerebrovascular symptoms of the prevalence of microembolic signals in patients with cervical carotid stenosis. Stroke 27:687, 1996

134. Frank G: Comparison of anticoagulation and surgical treatments of TIA. A review and consolidation of recent natural history and treatment studies. Stroke 2:369, 1971

135. Friedman GD, Wilson WS, Mosier JM et al: Transient ischemic attacks in a community. JAMA 210:1428, 1969

136. Furlan AJ, Whisnant JP: Long-term prognosis after carotid artery occlusion. Neurology (Minneapolis) 30:986, 1980

137. Furlan AJ, Whisnant JP, Kearns TP: Unilateral visual loss in bright light. An unusual symptom of carotid artery occlusive disease. Arch Neurol 36:675, 1979

138. Gagne PJ, Matchett J, MacFarland D et al: Can the NASCET technique for measuring carotid stenosis be reliably applied outside the trial?. J Vasc Surg 24:449, 1996

139. Gärde A, Samuelson K, Fahlgren H et al: Treatment after transient ischemic attacks: a comparison between anticoagulant drug and inhibition of platelet aggregation. Stroke 14:677, 1983

140. Gautier JC: Clinical presentation and differential diagnosis of amaurosis fugax. In Bernstein EF (ed): Amaurosis Fugax. Springer-Verlag, New York, 1990

141. Gautier JC: L'angiopathie cérébrale moniliforme des toxicomanes. Signification physiopathologique. Role possible due spasme. Bull Acad Natl Med 172:87, 1988

142. Gautier JC, Rosa A, L'hermitte F: Auscultation carotidienne. Correlations chez 200 patients avec 332 angiographies. Rev Neurol (Paris) 131:175, 1975

143. Gelmers HJ: The pericarotid syndrome. Acta Neurochir (Wien) 57:37, 1981

144. Genton E, Barnett HJM, Fields WS et al: XIV. Cerebral ischemia: the role of thrombosis and of antithrombotic therapy. Joint Committee for Stroke Resources. Stroke 8:147, 1977

145. Gerstenfeld J: The fundus oculi in amaurosis fugax. Am J Ophthalmol 58:198, 1964

146. Gillilan LA: Anatomy of the blood supply to the brain and spinal cord. In: Cerebro-Vascular Survey Report for Joint Council Subcommittee on Cerebrovascular Disease. NINCDS and NHLI, Office of Scientific and Health Reports, Bethesda, MD, 1980

147. Glagov S: Mechanical stresses on vessels and the non-uniform distribution of atherosclerosis. Med Clin North Am 57:63, 1973

148. Glagov S, Zarins CB: What are the determinants of plaque instability and its consequences? J Vasc Surg 9:389, 1989

149. Goldberg HI, Grossman RI, Gomori JM et al: Cervical internal carotid artery dissecting hemorrhage: diagnosis using MR. Radiology 158:157, 1986

150. Goodwin JA, Gorelick PB, Helgason CM: Symptoms of amaurosis fugax in atherosclerotic carotid artery disease. Neurology 37:829, 1987

151. Gorce P, Elias Z: Les microemboli cérébraux (HITS) dans les sténoses carotidiennes cervicales: relation avec la morphologie de la plaque et le risque embolique. J Echograph Med Ultrason 17:364, 1996

152. Gowers WR: On a case of simultaneous embolism of central retinal and middle cerebral arteries. Lancet 2:794, 1875

152a.Grillo P, Paterson RH: Occlusion of the carotid artery: prognosis (natural history) and the possibilities of surgical revascularization. Stroke 6:17, 1975

153. Grobe T: Diagnostik und Behandlungsmöglichkeiten extrakranieller Verschlussprozesse der Arteria carotis. Fortschr Neurol Psychiatr 49:335, 1981

154. Gross CR, Kase CS, Mohr JP et al: Stroke in south Alabama: incidence and diagnostic features. A population-based study. Stroke 15:249, 1984

155. Gross W, Verta MJ, VanBellen B et al: Comparison of non-invasive diagnostic techniques in carotid artery occlusive disease. Surgery 82:271, 1977

156. Gunning AJ, Pickering GW, Robb-Smith AHT et al: Mural thrombosis of the internal carotid artery and subsequent embolism. O J Med 33:155, 1964

157. Handa J, Nakasu Y, Kidooka M: Transient cerebral ischemia evoked by yawning: an experience after superficial temporal artery–middle cerebral artery bypass operation. Surg Neurol 19:46, 1983

158. Hanson MR, Conomy JP, Hodgman JR: Brain events associated with mitral valve prolapse. Stroke 11:499, 1980

159. Harrington HJ, Mayman CI: Carotid body tumor associated with partial Horner's syndrome and facial pain ('Raeder's syndrome'). Arch Neurol 40:564, 1983

160. Harris FS, Rhoton AL: Anatomy of the cavernous sinus. J Neurosurg 45:169, 1976

161. Harrison MJ, Marshall J: The variable clinical and CT findings after carotid occlusion: the role of collateral blood supply. J Neurol Neurosurg Psychiatry 51:269, 1988

162. Harrison MJG, Marshall J: Does the geometry of the carotid bifurcation affect its predisposition to atheroma? Stroke 14:117, 1983

163. Harrison MJG, Marshall J: Evidence of silent cerebral embolism in patients with amaurosis fugax. J Neurol Neurosurg Psychiatry 40:651, 1977

164. Harrison MJG, Marshall J, Thomas DJ: Relevance of duration of transient ischemic attacks in carotid territory. BMJ 2:1578, 1978

165. Hart RG, Easton DF: Dissections of cervical and cerebral arteries. Neurol Clin North Am 1:155, 1983

166. Hatsukami TS, Ferguson MA, Beach KW et al: Carotid plaque morphology and clinical events. Stroke 28:95, 1997

167. Hayreh SS, Weingeist TA: Experimental occlusion of the central artery of the retina. I. Ophthalmoscopic and fluorescein fundus angiographic studies. Br J Ophthalmol 64:896, 1980

168. Hedges TR: Ophthalmoscopic findings in internal carotid artery occlusions. Bull Johns Hopkins Hosp 111:89, 1962

169. Hennerici MG: High intensity transcranial signals (HITS): a questionable 'jackpot' for the prediction of stroke risk. J Heart Valve Dis 3:124, 1994

170. Hennerici M, Rautenberg W: Stroke risk from symp-

tomless extra cranial arterial disease. Lancet 2:1180, 1982

171. Hennerici M, Steinke W, Rautenberg W, Mohr JP: Symptomatic and asymptomatic high-grade carotid stenosis in Doppler color flow imaging. Neurology 42:131, 1992

172. Hertzer NR, Beven EG, Modic MT et al: Early patency of the carotid artery after endarterectomy: digital substraction angiography after 200 operations. Surgery 92:1049, 1982

173. Heyman A, Leviton A, Nefzger D et al: XI. Transient focal cerebral ischemia: epidemiological and clinical aspects. Stroke 5:277, 1974

174. Heyman A, Wilkinson WE, Heyden S et al: Risk of stroke in asymptomatic persons with cervical arterial bruits. N Engl J Med 302:838, 1980

175. Hirko MK, Morasch MD, Burke K et al: The changing face of carotid endarterectomy. J Vasc Surg 23:622, 1996

176. Hodge CJ Jr, Leeson M, Cacayorin E et al: Computed tomographic evaluation of extracranial carotid artery disease. Neurosurgery 21:167, 1987

177. Hollenhorst RW: Significance of bright plaques in the retinal arterioles. JAMA 178:23, 1961

178. Hooshmand H, Vines FS, Lee HM, Grindal A: Amaurosis fugax: diagnostic and therapeutic aspects. Stroke 5:643, 1974

179. Horenstein S, Hambrook G, Roat GW et al: Arteriographic correlates of transient ischemic attacks. Trans Am Neurol Assoc 97:132, 1972

180. Hu HH, Liao KK, Wong WJ et al: Ocular bruits in ischemic cerebrovascular disease. Stroke 19:1229, 1988

181. Hu HH, Wang S, Chern CM et al: Clinical significance of the ophthalmic artery in carotid artery disease. Acta Neurol Scand 92:242, 1995

182. Hulqvist GT: Ueber Thrombose und Embolie der Arteria carotis und herbei vorkommende Gehirnveränderungen. Eine pathologische-anatomische Studie. Gustav Fischer Verlag, Stockholm, 1942

183. Hurwitz BJ, Heyman A, Wilkinson WE, Haynes CS, Utley CM: Comparison of amaurosis fugax and transient cerebral ischemia: a prospective clinical and arteriographic study. Ann Neurol 18:698, 1985

184. Hutchinson EC, Yates PO: Carotico-vertebral stenosis. Lancet 1:2, 1957

185. Huvos AG, Leaming RH, Moore OS: Clinicopathologic study of the resected carotid artery. Am J Surg 126:570, 1973

186. Imparato AM, Riles TS, Gorstein F: The carotid bifurcation plaque: pathologic findings associated with cerebral ischemia. Stroke 10:238, 1979

187. Jacobs LA, Ganji S, Shirley JG et al: Cognitive improvement after extracranial reconstruction for the low flow–endangered brain. Surgery 93:683, 1983

188. Janeway R, Toole JF: Vascular anatomic status of patients with transient ischemic attacks. Trans Am Neurol Assoc 97:137, 1971

189. Javid H, Ostermiller WE, Hengesh JW et al: Carotid endarterectomy for asymptomatic patients. Arch Surg 102:389, 1971

190. Javid H, Ostermiller WE Jr, Hengesh JW et al: Natural history of carotid bifurcation atheroma. Surgery 67:80, 1970

191. Jonas S, Hass WK: An approach to the maximum acceptable stroke complication rate after surgery for transient cerebral ischemia (TIA), abstracted. Stroke 10:104, 1979

192. Jörgensen L, Packham MA, Rowsell HC, Mustard JF: Deposition of formed elements of blood on the intima and signs of intimal injury in the aorta of rabbit, pig, and man. Lab Invest 27:341, 1972

193. Julian OC, Dye WS, Javid H: Ulcerative lesions of the carotid artery bifurcation. Arch Surg 86:803, 1963

194. Kagan A, Popper J, Rhoads GG et al: Epidemiologic studies on coronary artery disease and stroke in Japanese men living in Japan, Hawii, and California: prevalence of stroke. p. 267. In Scheinberg P (ed): Cerebrovascular Diseases. Lippincott-Raven, Philadelphia, 1976

195. Kapp JP, Smith RR: Spontaneous resolution of occlusive lesions on the carotid artery. J Neurosurg 56:73, 1982

196. Karis R: Asymptomatic carotid artery disease (letters to the editors). Stroke 14:443, 1983

197. Karp HR, Heyman A, Heyden S et al: Transient cerebral ischemia. Prevalence and prognosis in a biracial community. JAMA 225:125, 1973

198. Kearns TP, Hollenhorst RW: Venous-stasis retinopathy of occlusive disease of the carotid artery. Staff Meet Mayo Clin 38:304, 1963

199. Kessler C, von Maravic M, Bruckmann H, Kompf D: Ultrasound for the assessment of the embolic risk of carotid plaques. Acta Neurol Scand 92:231, 1995

200. Kirgis MD, Llewellyn RG, Peebles EMcG: Functional trifurcations of the internal carotid artery and its potential clinical significance. J Neurosurg 17:1062, 1960

201. Kishore PRS, Chase NE, Kricheff II: Carotid stenosis and intracranial emboli. Radiology 100:351, 1971

202. Kishore PRS, Dick AR: Spontaneous disappearance of carotid stenosis. Radiology 129:721, 1978

203. Koennecke HC, Mast H, Trocio S, Ma W, Sacco RL, Mohr JP, Thompson JLP: Association of high-intensity transient signals with carotid disease. J Neuroimaging 5:66, 1995

204. Krayenbühl H, Yasargil MG: Die zerebrale Angiographie. George Thieme Verlag, Stuttgart, 1965

205. Kroener JM, Dorn PL, Shoor PM et al: Prognosis of asymptomatic ulcerating carotid lesions. Arch Surg 115:1387, 1980

206. Kuntz KM, Skillman JJ, Whittemore AD, Kent KC: Carotid endarterectomy in asymptomatic patients—is contrast angiography necessary? A morbidity analysis. J Vasc Surg 22:706, 1995

207. Kusske JA, Kelly WA: Embolization and reduction of the "steal" syndrome in cerebral AVMs. J Neurosurg 40:313, 1974

208. Lamparello PJ, Riles TS: MR angiography in carotid stenosis. A clinical prospective. Magn Reson Imaging Clin North Am 3:455, 1995

209. Lancer SR, Guttierrez LF, Pillay VKG: Orbital bruits in patients on maintenance hemodialysis. BMJ 1:481, 1975

210. Lasjaunias P, Moret J: The ascending pharyngeal artery: normal and pathological radioanatomy. Neuroradiology 11:77, 1976

211. Leblanc R, Yamamoto YL, Tyler JL et al: Borderzone ischemia. Ann Neurol 22:707, 1987

212. Lees RS, Kistler JP: Carotid phonoangiography. p. 187.

In Bernstein E (ed): Noninvasive Diagnostic Techniques in Vascular Disease. CV Mosby, St. Louis, 1978

213. Lennihan L, Kupsky WJ, Mohr JP et al: TK: lack of association between carotid plaque hematoma and ipsilateral cerebral symptoms. Stroke 18:879, 1987

214. Levin SM, Sondheimer FK, Levin JM: The contralateral diseased but asymptomatic carotid artery: to operate or not? An update. Am J Surg 140:203, 1980

215. Levine RL, Dobkin JA, Rozental JM et al: Blood flow reactivity to hypercapnia in strictly unilateral carotid disease: preliminary results. J Neurol Neurosurg Psychiatry 54:204, 1991

216. Levinson SA, Close MB, Ehrenfeld WK et al: Carotid artery of occlusive disease following external cervical irradiation. Arch Surg 107:395, 1973

217. Ley-Pozo J, Ringelstein EB: Noninvasive detection of occlusive disease of the carotid siphon and middle cerebral artery. Ann Neurol 28:640, 1990

218. Lhermitte F, Gautier JC: Sites of cerebral arterial occlusions. In Williams D (ed): Modern Trends in Neurology 6. Butterworths, London, 1975

219. Lhermitte F, Gautier JC, Derouesne C: Anatomie et physiopathologie des sténoses carotidiennes. Rev Neurol (Paris) 115:641, 1966

220. Lhermitte F, Gautier JC, Derouesne C: Nature of occlusions of the middle cerebral artery. Neurology (Minneapolis) 20:82, 1970

221. Liapis CD, Satiani B, Florance CL et al: Motor speech malfunction following carotid endarterectomy. Surgery 89:56, 1981

222. Lie TA: Congenital Anomalies of the Carotid Arteries. Exerpta Medica Foundation, Amsterdam, 1968

223. Liebers M: Alzheimerische Krankheit bei schwerer Gehirnarteriosklose. Z Ges Neurol Psychiatr 124:639, 1932

224. Liebeskind A, Chinichian A, Schechter MM: The moving embolus seen during serial cerebral angiography. Stroke 2:440, 1971

225. Lindenberg R, Spatz F: Ueber die Thromboendarteritis obliterans der Hirngefässe. Virchows Arch [A] 305:531, 1940

226. Link H, Lebram G, Johansson I, Radberg C: Prognosis in patients with infarction and TIA in carotid territory during and after anticoagulant therapy. Stroke 10:529, 1979

227. Lipchik EO, DeWeese JA, Schenk EA et al: Diaphragm-like obstructions of the human arterial tree. Radiology 113:43, 1974

228. Litt AW, Eidelman EM, Pinto RS et al: Diagnosis of carotid artery stenosis: comparison of 2DFT time-of-flight MR angiography with contrast angiography in 50 patients. Am J Radiol 156:149, 1991

229. Little JR, Shawhan B, Weinstein M: Pseudo-tandem stenosis of the internal carotid artery. Neurosurgery 7:574, 1980

230. Loeb C, Priano A, Albano C: Clinical features and long-term follow-up of patients with reversible ischemia attacks (RIA). Acta Neurol Scand 57:471, 1978

231. LoGerfo FW, Crawshaw HN, Nowak M et al: Effect of flow split on separation and stagnation in a model vascular bifurcation. Stroke 12:660, 1981

232. LoGerfo FW, Nowak MD, Quist WC et al: Flow studies in a model of carotid bifurcation. Arteriosclerosis 1:235, 1981

233. Luessenhop AJ: Occlusive disease of carotid artery. Observations on the prognosis and surgical treatement. J Neurosurg 16:705, 1959

234. Lusby RJ, Ferrell LD, Ehrenfeld WK et al: Carotid plaque hemorrhage. Its role in production of cerebral ischemia. Arch Surg 117:1479, 1982

235. Lustgarten J, Solomon RA, Quest DW, Mohr JP: Endarterectomy based on Doppler and magnetic resonance angiogram without conventional angiogram. Neurosurgery 34:612, 1994

236. Magargal LE, Sanborn GE, Zimmerman A: Venous stasis retinopathy associated with embolic obstruction of the central retinal artery. J Clin Neuroophthalmol 2:113, 1982

237. Maitland CE, Black JL, Smith WA: Abducens nerve palsy due to spontaneous dissection of the internal carotid artery. Arch Neurol 40:448, 1983

238. Marshall J: The natural history of transient ischemic cerebrovascular attacks. O J Med 33:309, 1964

239. Marshall J, Meadows S: The natural history of amaurosis fugax. Brain 91:419, 1968

240. Martin GM, Sprague CA: Symposium on in vitro studies related to atherogenesis: life histories of hyperplastoid cell lines from aorta and skin. Exp Mol Pathol 18:125, 1973

241. Marzewski DJ, Furlan AJ, St. Louis P et al: Intracranial internal carotid artery stenosis: long term prognosis. Stroke 13:821, 1982

242. Mathew NT, Abraham J, Taori GM et al: Internal carotid artery occlusion in cavernous sinus thrombosis. Arch Neurol 24:11, 1971

243. Maves MD, Bruns MD, Keenan MJ: Carotid artery resection for head and neck cancer. Ann Otol Rhinol Laryngol 101:778, 1992

244. Mawad ME, Hilal SK, Michelsen WJ et al: Occlusive vascular disease associated with cerebral arteriovenous malformations. Radiology 153:401, 1984

245. May AG, DeWeese JA, Rob CG: Hemodynamic effects of arterial stenosis. Surgery 53:513, 1963

246. McBrien DJ, Bradley RD, Ashton N: The nature of retinal emboli in stenosis of the internal carotid artery. Lancet 1:697, 1963

247. McCollum CH, Wheeler WG, Noon GP, DeBakey ME: Aneurysms of the extracranial artery. Am J Surg 137:196, 1979

248. McGill HG Jr, Strong JP: Natural history of human atherosclerotic lesions. p. 39. In Sandler M, Bourne GH (eds): Atherosclerosis and Its Origin. Academic Press, New York, 1963

249. Merino MJ, Livolsi V: Malignant carotid body tumors. Cancer 47:1403, 1981

250. Meyer WW: Cholesterinkrystall embolic kleiner Organarterien und ihre Folgen. Virchows Arch [A] 314:616, 1947

251. Millikan CH: The pathogenesis of transient focal cerebral ischemia. Circulation 32:438, 1965

252. Millikan CH, Siekert RG, Shick RM: Studies in cerebrovascular diseases. V. The use of anticoagulant drugs in the treatment of intermittent insufficiency of the internal carotid arterial system. Mayo Clin Proc 30:578, 1955

253. Mitchell JRA, Schwartz CJ: Arterial Disease. Blackwell Scientific Publications, Oxford, 1965

254. Mohr JP: Asymptomatic carotid artery disease. Stroke 13:431, 1982

255. Mohr JP: Discussion. In Reivich M, Hurtig H (eds): Cerebrovascular Diseases, XIIIth Research (Princeton) Conference. Lippincott-Raven, Philadelphia, 1983

256. Mohr JP: Editorial: transient ischemic attacks and the prevention of strokes. N Engl J Med 1978;299:93, 1978

257. Mohr JP: Neurological complications of cardiac valvular disease and cardiac surgery including systemic hypotension. p. 143. In Klawans HL (ed): Neurological Manifestations of Systemic Diseases. Vol 38. In Vinken PJ, Bruyn GW (eds): Handbook of Clinical Neurology. North-Holland, Amsterdam, 1979

258. Mohr JP, Caplan LR, Melski JW et al: The Harvard cooperative stroke registry: a prospective registry. Neurology 28:754, 1978

259. Mohr JP, Foulkes MA, Polis AB et al: Infarct topography and hemiparesis profiles with cerebral convexity infarction. The Stroke Data Bank. J Neurol Neurosurg Psychiatry 56:344, 1993

260. Mokri B, Sundt TM, Houser OW: Spontaneous internal carotid artery dissection, hemicrania and Horner's syndrome. Arch Neurol 36:677, 1979

261. Moore WS, Boren C, Malone JM et al: Natural history of non-stenotic asymptomatic ulcerative lesions of the carotid artery. Arch Surg 113:1352, 1978

262. Moore WS, Hall AD: Importance of emboli from carotid bifurcation in pathogenesis of cerebral ischemic attacks. Arch Surg 101:708, 1970

263. Moore WS, Hall AD: Ulcerated atheroma of the carotid artery: a major cause of transient cerebral ischemia. Am J Surg 116:237, 1968

264. Moossy J: Cervical and cranial arteries: thrombosis, embolic and infarction. Stroke 14:120, 1983

265. Morax PV, Aron-Rosa D, Gautier JC: Symptomes et signes ophtalmologiques des sténoses et occlusions carotidiennes. Bull Soc Ophtalmol N special, 1970

265a.Morimoto T, Nitta K, Kazekawa K, Hashizume K: The anomaly of a non-bifurcating cervical carotid artery. Case report. J Neurosurg 72:130, 1990

266. Mungas JE, Baker WH: Amaurosis fugax. Stroke 8:232, 1977

267. Murphy EA, Rowsell HC, Downie HG et al: Encrustation and atherosclerosis: the analogy between early in vivo lesions and deposits which occur in extracorporeal circulations. Can Med Assoc J 87:259, 1962

268. Mustard JF, Packham MA: Factors influencing platelet function: adhesion, release, and aggregation. Pharmacol Rev 22:97, 1970

269. Muuronen A, Kaste M: Outcome of 314 patients with transient ischemic attacks. Stroke 13:24, 1982

270. Norrving B, Nilsson B, Olsson J-E: Progression of carotid disease after endarterectomy: a Doppler ultrasound study. Ann Neurol 12:548, 1982

271. O'Dwyer JA, Moscow N, Trevor R et al: Spontaneous dissection of the carotid artery. Radiology 137:379, 1980

272. Ogren M, Hedblad B, Isacsson SO et al: Ten year cerebrovascular morbidity and mortality in 68 year old men with asymptomatic carotid stenosis. BMJ 310:1294, 1995

273. Ojemann RG, Crowell RC, Roberson GH, Fisher CM: Surgical treatment of the extracranial carotid occlusive disease. Clin Neurosurg 22:214, 1975

274. Okamoto Y, Inugami A, Matsuzaki Z et al: Carotid artery resection for head and neck cancer. Surgery 120:54, 1996

275. Olsson JE, Muller R, Berneli S: Long term anticoagulant therapy for TIAs and minor strokes with minimum residuum. Stroke 7:444, 1976

276. Orr AE: A rare anomaly of the carotid arteries (internal and external). J Anat Physiol 41:51, 1906

277. Ostfeld AM, Shekelle RB, Klawans HL: Transient ischemic attacks and risk of stroke in an elderly poor population. Stroke 4:980, 1973

278. Parkinson D: A surgical approach to the cavernous portion of the carotid artery: anatomical studies and case report. J Neurosurg 23:474, 1965

279. Parkinson D, Shields CB: Persistent trigeminal artery: its relationship to the normal branches of the cavernous carotid. J Neurosurg 39:244, 1974

280. Pearce JMS, Gubbay SS, Walton JN: Longterm anticoagulant therapy in transient cerebral ischemic attacks. Lancet 1:6, 1965

281. Pentschew A: Die granuläre Atrophie der Grosshirnrinde. Arch Psychiatr Nervenkr 101:80, 1934

282. Perrone P, Candelise L, Scotti G et al: CT evaluation in patients with transient ischemic attack. Correlation between clinical and angiographic findings. Eur Neurol 18:217, 1979

283. Pessin MS, Duncan GW, Davis KR et al: Angiographic appearance of carotid occlusion in acute stroke. Stroke 11:485, 1982

284. Pessin MS, Duncan GW, Mohr JP, Poskanzer DC: Clinical and angiographic features of carotid transient ischemic attacks. N Engl J Med 296:358, 1977

285. Pessin MS, Estol CJ, DeWitt LD et al: Retinal emboli and carotid disease, abstracted. Neurology suppl. 1, 40: 249, 1990

286. Pessin MS, Hinton RC, Davis KR et al: Mechanisms of acute carotid stroke. Ann Neurol 6:245, 1979

287. Pessin MS, Panis W, Prager RJ et al: Auscultation of cervical and ocular bruits in extracranial carotid occlusive disease: a clinical and angiographic study. Stroke 14:246, 1983

288. Petrov V, Waltregny A, Reznik M et al: Thrombose carotidienne bilaterale post-traumatique. Acta Neurol Belg 73:110, 1973

289. Picard L, Andre JM, Roland J et al: Moyamoya syndrome of the adult. Transient forms. J Neuroradiol 1:69, 1974

290. Piedbois P, Becquemin JP, Pierquin B et al: Les sténoses artérielles après radiothérapie. Bull Cancer Radiother 77:3, 1990

291. Pode JCF: The monoclonal theory of atherosclerosis. Br J Clin Pract 32:219, 1978

292. Podore PC, DeWeese JA, May AG, Rob CG: Asymptomatic contralateral carotid artery stenosis: a five-year follow-up study following carotid endarterectomy. Surgery 88:748, 1980

293. Portnoy HD, Avellanosa A: Carotid aneurysm and contralateral carotid stenosis with successful surgical treatment of both lesions. J Neurosurg 32:476, 1970

294. Powers WJ, Press GA, Grubb RL et al: The effect of hemodynamically significant carotid artery disease on

the hemodynamic status of the cerebral circulation. Ann Intern Med 106:27, 1987

295. Praffenbach DD, Hollenhorst RW: Morbidity and survivorship of patients with embolic cholesterol crystals in the ocular fundus. Am J Ophthalmol 75:66, 1973

296. Quisling RG, Friedman WA, Rhoton AL: High cervical dissection: spontaneous resolution. AJNR 1:463, 1980

297. Raichle M: Discussion. In Reivich M, Hurtig H (eds): Cerebrovascular Disorders. XIIIth Research (Princeton) Conference. Lippincott-Raven, Philadelphia, 1983

298. Ramirez-Lassepas M, Sandok BA, Burton RC: Clinical indicators of extracranial carotid artery disease in patients with transient symptoms. Stroke 4:537, 1973

299. Regli F: Die flüchtigen ischämischen zerebralen Attacken. Deutch Med Wochenschr 96:526, 1971

300. Ricotta JJ, Ouriel K, Green RM, DeWeese JA: Use of computerized cerebral tomography in selection of patients for elective and urgent carotid endarterectomy. Ann Surg 202:783, 1985

301. Ring BA: Diagnosis of embolic occlusions of smaller branches of the intracerebral arteries. Am J Roentgenol Radium Ther Nucl Med 97:575, 1966

302. Ringelstein EB, Zeumer H, Angelou D: The pathogenesis of strokes from internal carotid artery occlusion. Stroke 14:867, 1983

303. Roberts AB, Strauss HW, Lees RS et al: Low density lipoproteins concentrate in damaged arterial wall, abstracted. Circulation, suppl. III, 62:97, 1980

304. Roederer GO, Langlois YE, Chan AT et al: Is siphon disease important in predicting the outcome of carotid endarterectomy?, abstracted. Stroke 14:8, 1983

305. Roederer GO, Langlois YE, Jager KA et al: The natural history of carotid arterial disease in asymptomatic patients with cervical bruits. Stroke 15:605, 1984

306. Romanul FCA, Abramowicz A: Changes in brain and pial vessels in arterial borderzones. Arch Neurol (Chicago) 11:40, 1964

307. Ross R, Glomset JA: Atherosclerosis and the arterial smooth muscle cell. Science 180:1332, 1973

308. Ross R, Glomset J, Kariya B, Harker L: A platelet-dependent serum factor that stimulates the proliferation of arterial smooth muscle cells in vitro. Proc Natl Acad Sci USA 71:1207, 1974

309. Ross Russell RW: Atheromatous retinal embolism. Lancet 2:1354, 1963

310. Ross Russell RW: Observations on the retinal blood vessels in monocular blindness. Lancet 2:1422, 1961

311. Ross Russell RW, Page NGR: Critical perfusion of brain and retina. Brain 106:419, 1983

312. Rothwell PM, Salinas R, Ferrando LA et al: Does the angiographic appearance of a carotid stenosis predict the risk of stroke independently of the degree of stenosis? Clin Radiol 50:830, 1955

313. Rothwell PM, Slattery J, Warlow CP: A systematic comparison of the risks of stroke and death due to carotid endarterectomy for symptomatic and asymptomatic stenosis. Stroke 27:266, 1996

314. Russo LS: Carotid system transient ischemic attacks: clinical, racial, and angiographic correlations. Stroke 12:470, 1981

315. Sacquegna T, DeCarolis P, Pazzaglia P et al: The clinical course and prognosis of carotid artery occlusion. J Neurol Neurosurg Psychiatry 45:1037, 1982

316. Samuel KC: Atherosclerosis and occlusion of the internal carotid artery. J Pathol Bacteriol 71:391, 1956

317. Sandok BA, Tratmann JC, Ramirez-Lassepas M et al: Clinical angiographic correlations in amaurosis fugax. Am J Ophthalmol 78:137, 1974

318. Santamore WP, Bove AA, Carey RA: Hemodynamics of a stenosis in a complaint [sic] artery. Cardiology 69:1, 1982

319. Schiffter R, Reinhart K: The telodiencephalic ischemic syndrome. J Neurol 222:265, 1980

320. Schneider M: Durchblutung und Sauerstoffversorgung des Gehirns. Verh Dtsch Ges Kreislauf forsch 19:3, 1953

321. Schneider PA, Rossman ME, Bernstein EF et al: Noninvasive assessment of cerebral collateral blood supply through the ophthalmic artery. Stroke 22:31, 1991

322. Schuler JJ, Falnigan DP, Lim LT et al: The effect of carotid siphon stenosis on stroke rate, death, and relief of symptoms following elective carotid endarterectomy. Surgery 92:1058, 1982

323. Schwarcz TH, Eton D, Ellenby MI et al: Hollenhorst plaques: Retinal manifestations and the role of carotid endarterectomy. J Vasc Surg 11:635, 1990

324. Scott SN, Sethi GK, Bridgman AH: Perioperative stroke during carotid endarterectomy: the value of intra-operative angiography. J Cardiovasc Surg (Torino) 23:353, 1982

325. Shah AB, Coull BM, Howieson J et al: Does natural history of transient ischemic attacks (TIAs) justify surgery? (Letter to Editor) Stroke 14:828, 1983

326. Sheng FC, Quinones-Baldrich W, Machleder HI et al: Relationship of extracranial carotid occlusive disease and central retinal artery occlusion. Am J Surg 152:175, 1986

327. Shillito J Jr: Carotid arteritis: a cause of hemiplegia in childhood. J Neurosurg 31:540, 1964

328. Shipley RE, Gregg DE: The effect of external constriction of a blood vessel on blood flow. Am J Physiol 141:389, 1944

329. Shoumaker RD, Avant WS, Cohen GH: Coincidental multiple asymptomatic intra-cranial aneurysms and symptomatic carotid stenosis. Stroke 7:504, 1976

330. Siekert RG, Whisnant JP, Millikan CH: Surgical and anticoagulant therapy of occlusive cerebrovascular disease. Ann Intern Med 58:637, 1963

331. Sindermann F: Krankheitsbild und Kollateralkreislauf bei einseitigem und doppleseitigem Carotisverschluss. J Neurol Sci 5:9, 1967

332. Sipponen JT, Kaste M, Sepponen RE et al: Nuclear magnetic resonance imaging in reversible cerebral ischaemia. Lancet 1:294, 1983

333. Snyderman CH, D'Amico F: Outcome of carotid artery resection for neoplastic disease: a meta-analysis. Am J Otolaryngol 13:373, 1992

334. Sobel J, Espinas OE, Friedman SA: Carotid artery obstructions following LSD capsule ingestion. Arch Intern Med 127:290, 1971

335. Spallone A: Occlusion of the internal carotid artery by intracranial tumors. Surg Neurol 15:51, 1981

336. Spatz A: Uber die Beteiligung des Gehirns bei v. Winiwarter-Buergerische Krankheit. Dtsch Z Nervenheilk 136:86, 1935

337. Srinivasan J, Mayberg MR, Weiss DG, Eskridge J: Duplex accuracy compared with angiography in the Veterans Affairs Cooperative Studies Trial for Symptomatic Carotid Stenosis. Neurosurgery 36:648, 1995

338. Stanton PE, McClusky DA, Lamis PA: Hemodynamic assessment and surgical correction of kinking of the internal carotid artery. Surgery 84:793, 1978

339. Stehbens WE: The role of lipid in the pathogenesis of atherosclerosis. Lancet 1:724, 1975

340. Steinke W, Meairs S, Ries S, Hennerici M: Sonographic assessment of carotid artery stenosis. Comparison of power Doppler imaging and color Doppler flow imaging. Stroke 27:91, 1996

341. Stemerman MB: Haemostasis, thrombosis and atherogenesis. Atherosclerotic Rev 6:105, 1979

342. Streifler JY, Eliasziw M, Bonavente OR et al: The risk of stroke in patients with first-ever retinal vs. hemispheric transient ischemic attacks and high-grade carotid stenosis. Arch Neurol 52:246, 1995

343. Streifler JY, Eliasizw M, Fox AJ et al: Angiographic detection of carotid plaque ulceration. Comparison with surgical observations in a multicenter study. North American Symptomatic Carotid Endarterectomy Trial. Stroke 25:1130, 1994

344. Stringer WL, Kelly DL: Traumatic dissection of the extracranial internal carotid artery. Neurosurgery 6:123, 1980

345. Suzuki J, Kodama N: Moyamoya disease—a review. Stroke 14:104, 1983

346. Tatemichi TK, Chamorro A, Petty GW et al: Hemodynamic role of ophthalmic artery collateral in internal carotid artery occlusion. Neurology 40:461, 1990

347. Tatemichi TK, Young WL, Prohovnik I et al: Perfusion insufficiency in limb shaking transient ischemic attacks. Stroke 21:341, 1990

348. Taveras JM, Wood EH: Diagnostic Neuroradiology. 2nd Ed. Vol. 2. Sect. 4. Vascular Diseases. p. 850. Williams & Wilkins, Baltimore, 1976

349. Thiele BL, Young JV, Chikos PM et al: Correlation of arteriographic findings and symptoms in cerebrovascular disease. Neurology 30:1041, 1980

350. Thompson JE: Operative mortality following carotid endarterectomy (letter to the editor). Stroke 14:115, 1983

351. Thompson JE, Patman RD, Persson AV: Management of asymptomatic carotid bruits. Am Surg 42:77, 1977

352. Thompson JE, Patman RD, Talkington CM: Asymptomatic carotid bruit: long-term outcome of patients having endarterectomy compared with unoperated controls. Ann Surg 188:308, 1978

353. Timsit S: HITS (Editorial). Rev Neurol 152:497, 1996

354. Timsit SG, Sacco RL, Mohr JP et al: Early clinical differentiation of atherosclerotic and cardioembolic infarction: the Stroke Data Bank (SDB). In: 1st European Stroke Conference, Duesseldorf, May 10–11, 1990

355. Tolosa E: Periarteritic lesions of the carotid siphon with the clinical features of a carotid infraclinoidal aneurysm. J Neurol Neurosurg Psychiatry 17:300, 1954

356. Toole JF, Janeway R, Choi K et al: Transient ischemic attacks due to atherosclerosis: a prospective study of 160 patients. Arch Neurol 32:5, 1975

357. Toole JF, Patel AN: Cerebrovascular Disorders. 2nd Ed. McGraw-Hill, New York, 1964

358. Torvik A: The pathogenesis of watershed infarcts in the brain. Stroke 15:221, 1984

359. Torvik A, Jörgensen L: Ischemic cerebrovascular disease in an autopsy series. Part 1: Prevalence, location and predisposing factors in verified thrombo-embolic occlusion and their significance in the pathogenesis of cerebral infarction. J Neurol Sci 3:490, 1966

360. Torvik A, Jörgensen L: Ischemic cerebrovascular disease in an autopsy series. Part 2. Prevalence, location, pathogenesis and clinical course of cerebral infarcts. J Neurol Sci 9:285, 1969

361. Torvik A, Jörgensen L: Thrombotic and embolic occlusion of the carotid arteries in an autopsy series: Part 1. Prevalence, location and associated diseases. J Neurol Sci 1:24, 1964

362. Torvik A, Jörgensen L: Thrombotic and embolic occlusion of the carotid arteries in an autopsy series. Part 2. Cerebral lesions and clinical course. J Neurol Sci 3:410, 1966

363. Toyama H, Takeshita G, Takeuchi A et al: SPECT measurement of cerebral hemodynamics in transient ischemic attack patients: evaluation of pathogenesis and detection of misery perfusion. Kaku Igaku 26:1487, 1989

364. Turnbill I: Agenesis of the internal carotid artery. Neurology 12:588, 1962

365. Van der Eecken HM: Anastomoses Between the Leptomeningeal Arteries of the Brain. Charles C Thomas, Springfield IL, 1959

366. Vorstrup S, Hemmingsen R, Henriksen L et al: Regional cerebral blood flow in patients with transient ischemic attacks studied by xenon-133 inhalation and emission tomography. Stroke 14:903, 1983

367. Wade JG, Larson CP, Hickey RR et al: Effect of carotid endarterectomy on carotid chemoreceptor and baroreceptor functions in man. N Engl J Med 282:823, 1970

368. Wade JPH, Wong W, Barnett HJM, Vandervoort P: Bilateral occlusion of the internal carotid arteries. Presenting symptoms in 74 patients and a prospective study of 34 medically treated patients. Brain 110:667, 1987

369. Wagener HP: Amaurosis fugax: a specific type of transient loss of vision. IMJ January: 21, 1957

370. Waller FT, Simons RL, Kerber C et al: Trigeminal artery and micro-emboli to the brain stem. Report of two cases. J Neurosurg 46:104, 1977

371. Walsh PN, Pareti FI, Corbett JJ: Platelet coagulant activation and serum lipids in transient cerebral ischemia. N Engl J Med 295:854, 1976

372. Waxman SG, Toole JF: Temporal profile resembling TIA in the setting of cerebral infarction. Stroke 14:433, 1983

373. Weaver RG Jr, Howard G, McKinney WM et al: Comparison of Doppler ultrasonography with arteriography of the carotid bifurcation. Stroke 4:402, 1980

374. Weibel J, Fields WS: Tortuosity, coiling, and kinking of the internal carotid artery: etiology and radiographic anatomy. Neurology 15:7, 1965

375. Weinberger J, Bender AN, Yang WC: Amaurosis fugax associated with ophthalmic artery stenosis: clinical simulation of carotid artery disease. Stroke 11:290, 1980

376. Weisman AD: Cavernous sinus thrombophlebitis. Re-

port of a case with multiple cerebral infarcts and necrosis of the pituitary body. N Engl J Med 231:118, 1944

377. Welling RE, Taha A, Goel T et al: Extracranial carotid artery aneurysms. Surgery 93:319, 1983

378. Wesolowski SA, Fries CC, Sabini AM, Sawyer PN: The significance of turbulence in hemic systems and in the distribution of the atherosclerotic lesions. Surgery 57: 155, 1965

379. Whisnant JP: Multiple particles injected may all go to the same cerebral artery branch. Stroke 13:720, 1982

380. Whisnant JP: The role of the neurologist in the decline of stroke. Ann Neurol 14:1, 1983

381. Whisnant JP, Matsumoto N, Elveback LR: The effect of anticoagulant therapy on the prognosis of patients with transient cerebral ischemic attacks in a community: Rochester, Minnesota, 1955 through 1969. Mayo Clin Proc 48:844, 1973

382. Wiebers DO, Swanson JW, Cascino TL, Whisnant JP: Bilateral loss of vision in bright light. Stroke 20:554, 1989

383. Wilkinson IMS, Ross Russell RW: Arteries of the head and neck in giant cell arteritis. Arch Neurol 27:378, 1972

384. Wilkinson WE, Heyman A, Burch JG et al: Use of a self-administered questionnaire for detection of transient cerebral ischemic attacks. Survey of elderly persons living in retirement facilities. Ann Neurol 6:40, 1979

385. Wilson LA, Warlow CP, Ross Russell RW: Cardiovascular disease in patients with retinal arterial occlusion. Lancet 1:292, 1979

386. Winterkorn JMS, Kupersmith MJ, Wirtschafter JD, Forman S: Brief Report: treatment of vasospastic amaurosis fugax with calcium-channel blockers. N Engl J Med 329:396, 1993

387. Wodarz R: Watershed infarctions and computed tomography. A topographical study in cases with stenosis or occlusion of the carotid artery. Neuroradiology 19:245, 1980

388. Wodarz R, Ratzka M, Grosse D: Der Grenzzoneninfarkt als besondere Infarktkonstellation bei Karotisinsuffizienz. Fortschr Rontgenstr 134:128, 1981

389. Wolf PA, Dawber TR, Colton T et al: Transient cerebral ischemic attacks and risk of stroke: the Framingham study. CVD Epidemiol Newslett 22:52, 1977

390. Wolf PA, Kannel WB, Sorlie P, McNamara P: Asymptomatic carotid bruit and the risk of stroke. JAMA 245: 1442, 1981

391. Wolinsky H: Mesenchymal response of the blood vessel wall: a potential avenue for understanding and treating atherosclerosis. Circ Res 32:543, 1973

392. Wolpert SM, Stein BM: Catheter embolization of arteriovenous malformations as an aid to surgical excision. Neuroradiology 10:73, 1975

393. Wolpow ER, Lupton RG: Transient vertical monocular hemianopsia with anomalous retinal artery branching. Stroke 12:691, 1981

394. Wood EH, Correll JW: Atheromatous ulceration in major neck vessels as a cause of cerebral embolism. Acta Radiol [Diagn] 9:520, 1969

395. Wood CPL, Smith BR, McKinney CL, Toole JF: Non-invasive detection of boundary layer separation in the normal carotid artery bifurcation. Stroke 13:120, 1982

396. Woods BT, Strewler GJ: Hemiparesis occurring six hours after intravenous heroin injection. Neurology 22:863, 1972

397. Wright JG, Nicholson R, Schuller DE, Smead WL TI: Resection of the internal carotid artery and replacement with greater saphenous vein: a safe procedure for en bloc cancer resections with carotid involvement. J Vasc Surg 23:775, 1996

398. Wylie EJ, Ehrenfeld WK: Extracranial Occlusive Cerebral Vascular Disease—Diagnosis and Management. WB Saunders, Philadelphia, 1970

399. Yamauchi H, Fukuyama H, Kimura J et al: Hemodynamics in internal carotid artery occlusion examined by positron emission tomography. Stroke 21:1400, 1990

400. Yanagihara T, Klass DW: Rhythmic involuntary movement as a manifestation of transient ischemic attacks. Trans Am Neurol Assoc 106:46, 1981

401. Yanagihara T, Sundt TM Jr, Piepgras DG: Weakness of the lower extremity in carotid occlusive disease. Arch Neurol 45:297, 1988

402. Yates PO, Hutchinson EC: Cerebral Infarction: The Role of the Extracranial Cerebral Arteries. Special report series N 300. HM Stationery Office, London, 1961

403. Young B, Meacham WF, Allen JH: Documented enlargement and rupture of a small arterial sacculation. J Neurosurg 34:814, 1971

404. Young B, Moore WS, Robertson JT et al: An analysis of perioperative mortality and morbidity in the asymptomatic carotid atherosclerosis study. Stroke 27:2216, 1996

405. Young DF, Cholvin NR, Kirkeeide RL, Roth AC: Hemodynamics of arterial stenoses at elevated flow rates. Circ Res 41:99, 1977

406. Young GR, Humphrey PR, Nixon TE, Smith ET: Variability in measurement of extracranial internal carotid artery stenosis as displayed by both digital subtraction and magnetic resonance angiography: an assessment of three caliper techniques and visual impression of stenosis. Stroke 27:467, 1996

407. Young LHY, Appen RE: Ischemic oculopathy. A manifestation of carotid artery disease. Arch Neurol 38:358, 1981

408. Zarins CK, Giddens DP, Balasubramanian K et al: Carotid plaques localized in regions of low flow velocity and shear stress. Circulation 64:44, 1981

409. Zatz LM, Iannone AM, Eckman PB, Hecker SP: Observations concerning intracerebral vascular occlusion. Neurology 15:390, 1965

410. Ziegler RE, Bandyk DF, Thiele BL, Strandness DE: Carotid artery stenosis following endarterectomy. Arch Surg 117:1408, 1982

411. Ziegler DK, Hassanein RS: Prognosis in patients with transient ischemic attacks. Stroke 4:666, 1973

412. Zülch KJ: Predilection of cerebral atherosclerotic stenosis: a morphologic and radiologic demonstration. In Zülch KJ, Kaufmann W, Hossmann FA, Hossmann V (eds): Brain and Heart Infarct II. Springer-Verlag, Berlin, 1979

413. Zülch KJ, Kleihues P: Neuropathology of Cerebral Infarction. Thule International Symposium. p. 57. Nordiska Bokhandlung Forlag, Stockholm, 1957

CHAPTER 18

Anterior Cerebral Artery Disease

JOHN C. M. BRUST

Etiology

Infarction in the territory of one or both anterior cerebral arteries (ACAs) is frequently secondary to vasospasm following rupture of saccular aneurysms of the ACA or the anterior communicating artery (ACoA). When such patients are excluded, ACA infarcts have been reported to represent 0.6% to 3% of acute ischemic strokes.[31,114,177] As with middle cerebral artery territory infarcts, those involving the ACA are more often associated with internal carotid artery (ICA) atherosclerosis than with primary stenosis or thrombosis of the ACA itself.[297] In a clinical series of 27 patients, 17 (63%) had probable emboli from the ICA or the heart; other causes were isolated proximal ACA occlusion, paraneoplastic disseminated intravascular coagulation, ICA dissection with embolic occlusion of the opposite ACA, acute ethanol intoxication, and hypertensive occlusion of a small penetrating ACA branch. Six patients with no obvious cause were older than 50 years of age and five of these had risk factors for atherosclerotic stroke.[31] In an autopsy series of 55 patients with ACA infarcts, 10 had probable cardiac emboli and only 5 had atherosclerosis primarily involving the ACA itself.[60] ACA territory infarction has resulted from vessel compression during transfalcial herniation.[302]

Dissecting aneurysms of the ACA have affected either proximal or distal segments, have produced both infarction and subarachnoid hemorrhage, and have occurred either spontaneously or following head trauma.[8,12,161,181,417] Intracranial carotid artery dissection is nearly always associated with ACA occlusion.[392]

A patient with transient ischemic attacks had fibromuscular dysplasia of both pericallosal arteries.[327] In another report, bilateral ACA infarction occurred in a patient with sickle cell trait during acute ethanol intoxication and withdrawal.[349] Bilateral ACA infarction has also followed intracranial extension of Wegener's granulomatosis.[310] ACA occlusion has resulted from arteritis secondary to subarachnoid neurocysticercosis[208] and from radiation vasculitis 19 years after cranial irradiation for acute lymphoblastic leukemia.[108]

Symptoms and signs including weakness, sensory loss, and behavioral disturbance vary widely among patients with ACA infarcts. To understand this variety one must be familiar with the relevant anatomy.

Anatomy

The ACA can be divided into a proximal or A1 segment, from its origin as the medial component of the internal carotid bifurcation to its junction with the ACoA, and a distal or postcommunicating artery segment[74,189,279,280,342] (Fig. 18.1). The distal segment has been variably subdivided by different authors,[19,21,69,103,189,200,213,231,246,247,279,294,309,336,342,393] for example, into an A2 segment beginning at the ACoA and passing in front of the lamina terminalis as far as the junction of the rostrom and genu of the corpus callosum, an A3 segment passing around the genu of the corpus callosum, an A4 segment above the corpus callosum to just beyond the coronal suture, and an A5 segment to the artery's termination.[103] The A2 and A3 segments have together been referred to as the ascending segment, and the A4 and A5 segments as the horizontal segment.[280]

The A1 segment passes over the optic chiasm (in 70% of cases) or optic nerve (30%), varying in length from 7.2 to 18 mm (average 12.7 mm).[279] Its diameter ranges from 0.9 to 4.0 mm (average 2.6 mm) and is >1.5 mm in 90% of brains. In 74% both A1 segments are larger than the ACoA, the diameter of which ranges from 0.2 to 3.4 mm (average 1.5 mm).[279]

The ACAs pass over the corpus callosum side by side in only a minority of cases, and so the ACoA is most often directed obliquely or even anteroposteriorly; thus it is often best seen angiographically on oblique projections.[279]

The recurrent artery of Heubner[154] arises either at the level of the ACoA or just proximal or distal to it[305]; in different series it arose most often from the A1 segment,[264] from the A2 segment,[279] or at the level of the ACoA.[16,92,137,138] Usually the largest branch of the A1 or proximal A2 segments, Heub-

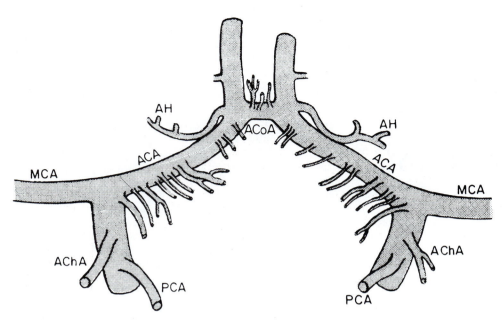

Figure 18.1 Diagram of the dorsal surface of the anterior circle of Willis, showing branches from the A1 segment of the anterior cerebral artery and from the anterior communicating artery. PCA, posterior communicating artery; AChA, anterior choroidal artery; MCA, middle cerebral artery; ACA, anterior cerebral artery; AH, Heubner's artery; ACoA, anterior communicating artery. (From Dunker and Harris,[92] with permission.)

ner's artery doubles back on the ACA for a variable distance and then, either as a single trunk or with as many as 12 branches, penetrates the anterior perforated substance above the ICA bifurcation or lateral to it in the sylvian fissure; some branches enter the olfactory sulcus, the gyrus rectus, or more lateral inferior frontal areas.[2,279] Heubner's artery, of obvious importance to the neurosurgeon,[98,131,151] most consistently supplies the head of the caudate, the anterior inferior part of the internal capsule's anterior limb, the anterior globus pallidus, and parts of the uncinate fasciculus, olfactory regions, and anterior putamen and hypothalamus.[2,5,69,92,130,264,279,305,400]

In addition to Heubner's artery the A1 and A2 segments give off smaller basal perforating branches, ≤15 from each A1[92,279] and ≤10 from each A2.[128,279,280,342] One of these, called the *short central artery*, is considered more consistent than others, in some people supplying part of the caudate nucleus and anterior limb of the internal capsule.[53,22] Other proximal branches penetrate the anterior perforated substance and the optic tract and supply, variably, paraolfactory structures, the medial anterior commissure, globus pallidus, caudate, and putamen, and the anterior limb of the internal capsule; these vessels also frequently supply the genu and contiguous posterior limb of the internal capsule, part of the anterior nucleus of the thalamus, and most of the anterior hypothalamus.[92] More distal A1 penetrating branches are smaller and supply the optic nerve, chiasm, and tract,[82,92] gyrus rectus and inferior frontal lobe, anterior perforated substance, and suprachiasmatic area.[279] Additional supply to the anterior inferior striatum and anterior hypothalamus comes from A2 segment branches, which can arise either separately or from a larger common trunk (the precallosal artery).[280] Similar penetrating branches from the ACoA,[70,92] ≤13 in number,[70,92] supply the suprachiasmatic and paraolfactory

areas, dorsal optic chiasm, anterior perforated substance, inferior frontal lobe, septum pellucidum, columns of the fornix, corpus callosum, septal region, and anterior hypothalamus and cingulum.[70,82,92,279]

Vascular anastomoses are less functional in the diencephalon and basal ganglia than elsewhere in the cerebral hemispheres, and the territories supplied by these ACA penetrating end-zone arteries are no exception. Capillary anastomoses, which are difficult to demonstrate by standard perfusion techniques, exceed arterial.[1,4,21,68,92,326,379]

The distal ACAs, deep in the interhemispheric fissure, are the only example of major cerebral arteries running side by side, although, as noted, one (usually the left) is often posterior to the other, and crossover of branches to the opposite hemisphere means that occlusion of either artery can cause contralateral or bilateral infarction.[280] Beyond the lamina terminalis the main trunk of the ACA, the pericallosal artery, runs above the corpus callosum in the pericallosal cistern (or, less often, over the cingulate gyrus or in the cingulate sulcus[19]), passes around the splenium of the corpus callosum, and terminates in the choroid plexus of the third ventricle; its posterior extent depends on the anterior extent of the posterior cerebral artery (PCA).[214,280] Except most posteriorly, the pericallosal artery lies below the free edge of the falx cerebri and can therefore shift across the midline.

The pericallosal artery has been variably defined as beginning at the ACoA[336,342] or at the point where the ACA gives off the callosomarginal artery; however, the latter is absent in 18% to 60% of brains.[247,280,294] The callosomarginal artery has been defined as that branch of the ACA traveling in or near the cingulate sulcus and giving off at least two major cortical branches.[247] It originates from just beyond the ACoA to the genu of the corpus callosum, most often from the A3 segment,[280] and can be of the same diameter, larger, or smaller than the pericallosal artery.[189,280] Any or all of the callosomarginal's usual branches can arise from the pericallosal artery [280]; these branches supply the inferior frontal lobe (including the gyrus rectus, the orbital part of the superior frontal gyrus, the medial part of the orbital gyri, and the olfactory bulb and tract), the medial surface of the hemisphere (including the cingulate gyrus, the superior frontal gyrus, the paracentral lobule, and the precuneus), and the superior 2 cm of the lateral convexity (including the superior frontal, precentral, central, and postcentral gyri), anastomosing there with branches of the middle cerebral artery (MCA).[19] (These border zones of shared arterial territory are of clinical importance: in a radionuclide study of 365 consecutive stroke patients, infarction in the "watershed" between the ACA and the MCA occurred in 5% of patients, compared with 28% in the MCA territory and 1% in the ACA territory.[34,394,397]) The band of lateral convexity supplied by the ACA is wider anteriorly than posteriorly and may extend into the middle frontal gyrus.

Although variable in number and in whether they arise directly from the pericallosal artery or from its callosomarginal branch, eight major cortical branches of the distal ACA can usually be defined.[280] The orbitofrontal artery arises from the A2 segment except, infrequently, when it shares a common trunk with the frontopolar artery[280] or arises just proximal to the ACoA.[279] Running forward in the floor of the anterior fossa as far as the planum sphenoidale, it supplies the gyrus rectus, olfactory bulb and tract, and orbital surface of the frontal lobe. The frontopolar artery arises from the A2 segment (or, infrequently, from the callosomarginal artery), passes to the frontal pole along the medial hemispheric surface, and supplies parts of the medial and lateral surfaces of the frontal pole.

The anterior, middle, and posterior frontal arteries arise separately from the A2, A3, or A4 segments of the pericallosal artery or from the callosomarginal artery; infrequently they arise from a common stem.[280,294] They supply the anterior, middle, and posterior parts of the superior frontal gyrus and the cingulate gyrus. The paracentral artery, arising from A4 or the callosomarginal artery, supplies premotor, motor, and sensory areas of the paracentral lobule.

The superior parietal artery, arising anterior to the splenium of the corpus callosum from A4, A5, or the callosomarginal artery, passes through the marginal limb of the cingulate sulcus and supplies the superior part of the precuneus. The inferior parietal artery, subdivided by some into the precuneal and parietoccipital arteries,[19,69] is the most frequently absent cortical branch of the ACA (36% of brains in one series[280]); it arises from the A5 segment (or rarely from the callosomarginal artery) just above the splenium of the corpus callosum and supplies the posterior inferior part of the precuneus and portions of the cuneus.

The rostrum, genu, body, and splenium of the corpus callosum are supplied by short callosal arteries, pericallosal artery branches that pass through the callosum to supply, additionally, the septum pellucidum, anterior pillars of the fornix, and anterior commissure.[19,280] Posteriorly the pericallosal artery extends around the splenium of the corpus callosum (the posterior pericallosal artery[342]) and then passes forward, ending on the inferior surface of the splenium[197] or extending all the way to the foramen of Monro.[342]

Of obvious importance in interpreting symptoms and signs is the normal variability of the boundaries (or border zones) between the anterior, middle, and posterior cerebral arteries. Figure 18.2, which is based on injection studies of 25 normal postmortem brains, illustrates the range of cortical distribu-

Figure 18.2 Cortical distribution of the anterior cerebral artery. (**A**) Area of variation on the cerebral convexity. (**B**) Area of variation on the cerebral medial surface. Horizontal or vertical lines represent a composite of maximal extent. Cross-hatched lines represent a composite of minimal extent. SFS, superior frontal sulcus; IFS, inferior frontal sulcus; CS, central sulcus, POS, parieto-occipital sulcus; PCS, precentral sulcus. (From Van der Zwan et al.[383] with permission.)

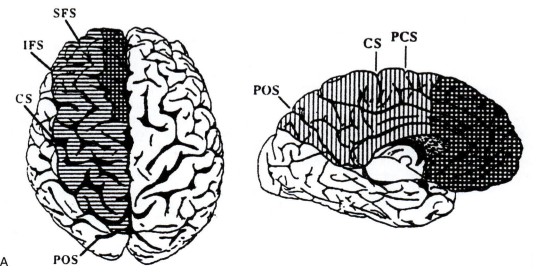

A   B

tion of the ACA.[383] In those with the most extensive ACA distribution, the primary motor and sensory cortices were supplied by the ACA not only medially but also over the convexity as far as the inferior frontal sulcus. In those with the least extensive ACA distribution, the ACA supplied little or none of the primary motor cortex, even medially.

Anomalies and Species Differences

The anatomy of the anterior circle of Willis is so varied among otherwise normal people that it is sometimes difficult to define when a variation should be called an anomaly. Especially common are hypoplastic A1 segments, from mildly narrow to nonfunctionally thread-like, with both distal ACAs filling from the larger A1.[7,98,285,365,405] In one study 7% of brains had a string-like A1 segment and 6% had a hypoplastic ACoA.[293] In another study 22% of brains had A1-segment hypoplasia, severe in 8% and in 82% associated with additional anomalies of the ACA or the posterior cerebral, posterior communicating, or basilar arteries.[230] Such anomalies are associated with an increased frequency of saccular aneurysms, and ACA occlusion secondary to cardiac embolism is often accompanied by hypoplasia of the proximal ACA contralaterally.[185,341,380,405]

A smaller ACA often occurs on the same side as a smaller internal carotid artery,[204] and a hypoplastic A1 segment tends to be associated with an ACoA of larger than usual diameter.[279,366] Small A1 segments are several times more common among patients with symptomatic cerebrovascular disease than in the general population.[400] A young man with episodic vertigo, loss of consciousness, and left leg weakness had, on cerebral angiography, absent ACAs with the MCAs and one intracavernous carotid providing collaterals to the medial cerebral hemispheres.[190]

In 50 adult autopsy specimens, 60% had one ACoA, 30% had two, and 10% three[279]; other investigators have also found doubling and tripling, and some have found absence of the ACoA.[69,406] A1 segment duplication also occurs,[279] as well as a third or median ACA arising from ACoA (arteria termatica), which sometimes is as large as the two other ACAs and may be the major supplier to the posterior medial hemispheres.[25,69,92,342]

The recurrent artery of Heubner rarely arises from the internal carotid at its bifurcation, from the MCA, or from the ACoA itself.[279] Absence or doubling has occurred.[2] Embryologically, the artery of Heubner is a remnant of the primitive olfactory artery, and so when the primitive olfactory artery persists, there is no artery of Heubner.[375]

Another well-recognized anomaly is a supernumerary vessel arising from the internal carotid artery at the level of the ophthalmic artery, coursing below the optic nerve, ascending in front of the optic chiasm, and terminating on the ipsilateral ACA near the ACoA. The A1 segment may be normal, hypoplastic, or absent[44,160,240,257,296]; in one instance both ACAs were absent.[324] Such an anomaly, which may be bilateral,[23] is frequently associated with ACA saccular aneurysm[160,257,265,324,305] and with other anomalies, such as dupli-

cated MCA,[242] median corpus callosum artery, distal moya-moya, aortic coarctation,[203] facial congenital defects, cerebral lipoma[44] and absent internal carotid artery (with the remaining carotid artery giving off a branch that passes beneath the optic nerve and divides into two ACAs, the opposite MCA arising from the PCA).[376] The anomalous vessel itself can cause visual symptoms from compression of the optic nerve or chiasm.[36]

The infraoptic ACA has been considered a remnant of the embryonic primitive maxillary artery, present in 3- to 4-mm embryos as an internal carotid artery branch, and normally becoming a cavernous carotid branch, the inferior hypophyseal artery. (The ACA normally arises from the primitive olfactory artery, eventually becoming the dominant vessel.[36,44,160,266])

Other reported anomalies include, in an autopsied infant, unilaterally absent proximal MCA, ACA, and anterior choroidal artery with much of the ipsilateral inferior frontal lobe supplied by branches from the opposite ACA and secondary porencephaly of the orbital frontal lobe.[343] Autopsy on a neurologically normal man revealed a plexiform anterior communicating system connected to the left internal carotid artery by an anomalous vessel arising from the internal carotid artery near the ophthalmic artery, a single distal ACA, marked right A1 segment hypoplasia, and right plexiform vessels in the area of Heubner's artery, plus other anomalies of the posterior circulation.[236] Such anomalies, rare in combination, are not unusual individually. For example, in a series of 1,250 consecutive autopsies, a plexiform anterior communicating system was found in 15%, hypoplastic ACAs in 4%, and fused distal ACAs in 4%; a plexiform Heubner's artery was much less common.[236] An ophthalmic artery arising from the ACA has also been reported,[147,162,197] as has an accessory MCA arising from the ACA A2 segment.[351]

In a study of 381 brains distal ACA anomalies were present in 25%,[19] including pericallosal artery triplication, absence of ACA pairing, branches from one ACA to the opposite hemisphere, and bihemispheric branches[7,25,69,245,280,381,406] (Fig. 18.3). Triplicate ACAs with a variably developed midline accessory artery arising from the ACoA and supplying little, much, or most of either or both hemispheres have been observed in ≤22% of autopsies.[19,25,89,100,187,201,382,406] Also, long callosal artery (medial artery of the corpus callosum, anterior MCA) can arise from the pericallosal artery and pass parallel to it, giving off callosal perforating branches.[280,342] These anomalies, like a hypoplastic A1 segment, produce at angiography apparent bilateral ACA filling after unilateral carotid injection.[19,72,246,304,307] Bihemispheric ACAs, with either ACA taking over the supply of part or all of the opposite hemisphere, have been reported in up to 64% of brains.[19,245,280,382] (The high figure refers to a study in which any contralateral supply, however small, was included; brains in which most of both hemispheres are supplied by one of two ACAs are less common.[245,280])

In the fetus there is gradual embryonic transition from one to two ACAs.[89,206] An unpaired or azygous ACA, arising by proximal union of the ACAs without an ACoA, occurs in ≤5% of adult brains.[19,25,89,100,187,201,205,350,406] Sometimes the ACAs fuse for ≤3.9 cm with an absent ACoA.[190] Azygous ACAs are associated with a variety of other anomalies, including hydranencephaly, septum pellucidum defects, meningomye-

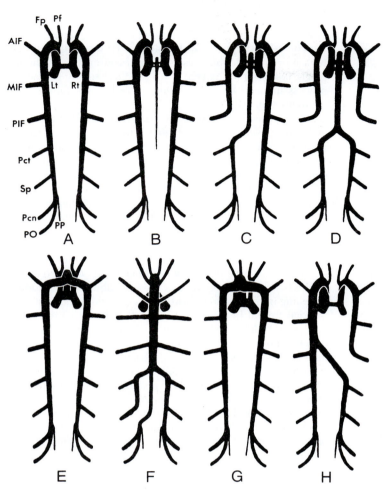

Figure 18.3 Variations in the distal anterior cerebral artery including patterns without (A) and with (B) a medial artery of the corpus callosum, and variously developed accessory (C–E), unpaired (F), and bihemispheric lateral arteries (G & H). Pf, prefrontal (orbitofrontal); Fp, frontopolar; AIF, anterior internal frontal; MIF, middle internal frontal; PIF, posterior internal frontal; Pct, paracentral; Sp, superior parietal; Pcn, precuneal; PO, parieto-occipital; pp, posterior pericallosal. (From Baptista,[19] with permission.)

locele, hydroencephalodysplasia, and vascular malformations[255] and, like other ACA anomalies, with an increased frequency of saccular aneurysm.[112,176] In holoprosencephaly (fusion of the frontal neocortex and absence of the interhemispheric fissure) an azygous ACA courses just beneath the inner table of the skull.[203]

As noted, ACA anomalies are associated with an increased frequency of saccular aneurysms, especially at the ACoA, but also on distal or anomalous branches.[2,111,145,186,243,260,261,308,312,348,369,375] Embryonic prominence of the interhemispheric arterial plexus that develops into the ACoA is the most frequent site for the development of intracranial aneurysms.[374] Of 206 patients with ACoA aneurysms 44 (21.4%) had ACA anomalies, especially a median artery of the corpus callosum and duplication of the ACoA.[261] Ruptured fusiform aneurysm of the ACA A1 segment has been reported.[258] Giant aneurysms have been found on azygous ACAs.[146,328] Following subarachnoid hemorrhage a congenitally narrow A1 segment may be mistaken for vasospasm. Furthermore, proximal ACA ligation in patients with surgically unclippable ACoA aneurysms is not a valid option if one A1 segment fills both distal ACAs or if, in the absence of cross-compression, the aneurysms fill well from either side.[64,71,94,256,285,305]

A common anomaly, ACA fenestration has no clinical significance except when it is mistaken for an aneurysm angiographically.[163] Vestibulocochlear symptoms developed in a 22-year-old patient with fenestration and ectasia of the left ACA and persistence of the right trigeminal artery.[370]

Species differences in the anatomy of the ACA (and other cerebral vessels) must be kept in mind in interpreting animal studies of cerebral ischemia and stroke. For example, birds, amphibians, and anteaters have paired arteries without an ACoA or other left-right anastomoses.[69] In most mammals both ACAs join to form a single pericallosal (azygous) artery, which may or may not bifurcate distally. There is no ACoA.[69] In subhuman primates several recurrent medial striate arteries (the equivalent of Heubner's artery in humans) supplying the anterior caudate, putamen, and globus pallidus have rich preparenchymal anastomoses with lateral lenticulostriate arteries from the MCA; the orbitofrontal artery, supplying most of the orbital surface of the frontal lobe, arises from the MCA and anastomoses with branches of the ACA, and extensive anastomoses exist between the ACA and the proximal MCA in the sylvian fissure.[52,130,174,244,395] In cats the presence of an ACoA has been both claimed[148,149] and denied.[173] The feline ACA supplies the medial hemisphere cortex containing hindlimb motor representation, but cerebral arterial occlusion tends to cause smaller and deeper infarcts than in higher primates.[362] In rats the rostral caudatoputamen is supplied by penetrating ACA branches and a vessel running alongside the lateral olfactory tract, and this area accounts for 25% of strokes in stroke-prone spontaneously hypertensive rats.[292,416]

Symptoms and Signs

WEAKNESS AND SENSORY LOSS

ACA occlusion causes infarction of the paracentral lobule and, as a result, weakness and sensory loss in the contralateral leg[27,46,47,83,290,364] (Fig. 18.4). The deficit is usually greatest distally, in part because the proximal leg is represented on the primary sensorimotor cortex either superiorly on the medial hemisphere or on the high convexity with, therefore, richer collaterals from the MCA, and, in part, because proximal muscles have substantial representation in the ipsilateral hemisphere.[273] If infarction extends to the upper convexity, there may be proximal arm weakness, or, as is usual with cortical lesions, clumsiness or slowness out of proportion to actual loss of strength. Muscle tone is initially most often flaccid, becoming spastic over days or weeks; tendon reflexes at the outset may be decreased, normal, or increased. (This frequent early dissociation between tone and tendon reflexes has been attributed to loss of supraspinal influence upon different kinds of muscle spindle afferents, for example, phasic versus tonic.[45]) Babinski's sign may be present.

The sensory modalities most often affected are discriminative (two-point discrimination, localization, stereognosis) and proprioceptive (position sense). Pain and temperature sensation and gross touch are usually only mildly decreased; the patient can tell sharp from dull, but the pinprick does not feel as sharp or as "normal" as on the unaffected side. Vibratory loss is variable. Depending on the posterior extent of the ACA and collaterals from the PCA, sensory loss may be mild or even absent in the presence of marked crural hemiparesis.[69] Sensation may be similarly spared when occlusion is not of the ACA or the pericallosal artery but of the paracentral branch.[69,220,221,404,407]

Acutely the head and eyes may be deviated toward the side of the lesion.[17,69,107] Forced grasping and groping of the contralateral hand, whether or not it is weak, follows damage to the posterior superior frontal gyrus.[69,212,317,325] Such forced grasping has been considered "a type of limb-kinetic apraxia," and "only one aspect of a total change in behavior, toward a compulsive exploration of the environment"[84]; foot grasping[193] can cause the lower limb to seem "glued to the floor"[84] on attempted walking. Such patients also display sucking and biting,[84] "ansaugen" (a movement of lips and tongue toward stimulation of the skin near the lower lip),[317] bradykinesia (or an "absence of movement intention"[69,135,136]), catalepsy,[33]and "tonic innervation" ("amorphous movements of a pseudo-spontaneous character"[69]) on attempted voluntary action of the affected arm or leg.[135,136,193] During the first few days following ACA territory infarction two patients displayed "hyperkinetic motor behaviors" (including head and eye movements, grimacing, chewing, rubbing body parts, rhythmically moving the fingers, and flexing and extending the thigh) on the contralateral nonparalyzed side.[129] It was suggested that such movements (which also occurred contralateral to hemiplegia following MCA territory infarction) signify "an active process induced by disinhibition, in order to establish new compensatory pathways."

Pronounced weakness of the arm and face in the presence of ACA occlusions has been attributed to involvement of Heubner's artery and its supply to the anterior limb and genu of the internal capsule[69,290] (Fig. 18.5). If the circle of Willis is complete, such proximal thrombosis must extend as far as the ACoA to produce complete hemiplegia, or the contralateral ACA will take over the supply of both medial hemispheres and weakness will be limited to the face and arm. Paralysis of the right arm, paresis of the right face, and only slight weakness of the right leg occurred in a man who at autopsy had infarction of the left putamen, caudate, and anterior limb of the internal capsule, plus a "shrunken and occluded artery of Heubner."[69] (The leg weakness was attributed to additional softening in the territories of the ACA's middle and posterior internal frontal branches.) On the other hand, more recent anatomic studies have shown that Heubner's artery supplies only the most anterior striatum and anterior limb of the internal capsule and is, therefore, probably infrequently the responsible vessel when brachial or facial palsy accompanies ACA occlusion. The more likely possibility in such a situation is involvement of penetrating branches arising from the most proximal ACA and the internal carotid bifurcation that supply, in addition to the hypothalamus and the rostral thalamus, not only the genu but also the anterior part of the internal capsule's posterior limb.[92] Moreover, caudate infarction can cause contralateral limb bradykinesia, clumsiness, and loss of associated movements mistakenly interpreted as weakness.[53] Dysarthria has followed unilateral infarction of either the left or right anterior limb of the internal capsule, and in one report dysarthria followed infarction apparently confined to the caudate nucleus.[53] Five patients with unilateral capsular genu infarction had contralateral facial and lingual weakness with dysarthria; three also had unilateral mastication-palatal-pharyngeal weakness, and one had unilateral vocal cord paresis; the only limb involvement was mild hand weakness in three.[30]

As noted above, in some individuals the ACA territory includes a considerable portion of the upper cerebral convexity, in such a situation infarction would include arm and hand representations on the primary motor (and sensory) cortex.[383] Conversely, in subjects with a smaller than usual ACA territory, leg weakness can be a consequence of MCA or PCA territory infarction. Of 63 patients with acute stroke and "leg-predominant weakness," 12 had infarction in the ACA territory, 9 in the MCA territory, 2 in both territories (not "watershed"), 18 in the internal capsule, 10 in the brain stem, and 2 in the thalamus.[313] Leg weakness was more lasting when infarction involved the motor cortex than when it involved the premotor cortex or supplementary area and spared the motor cortex.

Of 100 patients with "ataxic hemiparesis" after a first stroke, 4 had infarction of the contralateral ACA territory.[248] Pyramidal weakness was greatest in the leg, with ataxia of cerebellar type in the ipsilateral arm. Such ataxia has been attributed to involvement of frontopontocerebellar projec-

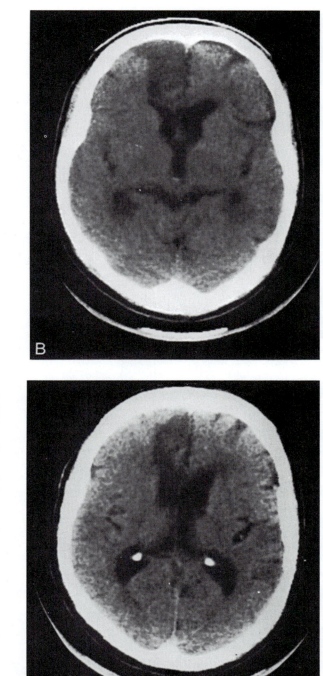

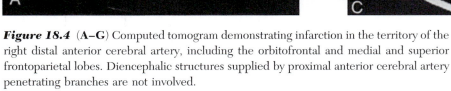

Figure 18.4 (**A–G**) Computed tomogram demonstrating infarction in the territory of the right distal anterior cerebral artery, including the orbitofrontal and medial and superior frontoparietal lobes. Diencephalic structures supplied by proximal anterior cerebral artery penetrating branches are not involved.

tions as well as, on the basis of single-photon emission computed tomographic studies, to transynaptic dysfunction of the contralateral cerebellum (diaschisis).[28,132] A problem with the ataxic hemiparesis syndrome—regardless of the lesion's location—is that upper motor neuron lesions as a rule produce

clumsiness out of proportion to weakness, and so it can be difficult to determine whether the "ataxia" is qualitatively or quantitatively sufficient to label it "cerebellar."

Infarction in the territories of both ACAs causes paraparesis, with or without sensory loss.[345] It occurs most often as a

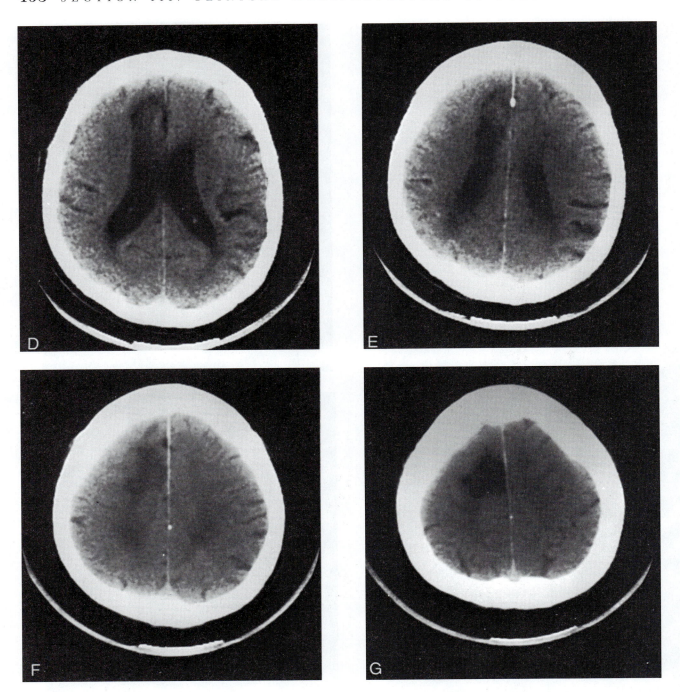

Figure 18.4 (continued)

consequence of bilateral ACA vasospasm following ACA/ACoA aneurysm rupture.[141] In thrombotic or embolic infarction it is especially likely when there is a vascular anomaly, such as a hypoplastic A1 segment or an azygous distal ACA.[17,35,63,69,112,315,316] Particularly when symptoms are stutteringly progressive, spinal cord disease may be erroneously suspected.[19,229,280,378] Even if weakness is mild or absent there may be severe gait disturbance, with inability to initiate the first step with either foot, to lift either foot off the ground, or to turn to either side[241,377] ("slipping clutch syndrome"[86]).

Grasp reflexes of the feet (or hands) are not present in all such patients, and although some can move their legs freely in the air (e.g., bicycling motions),[86] others cannot.[241] When severe, such medial prefrontal damage can produce a pronounced immobility of all four limbs, from bradykinesia to catatonic (perseverative) posturing with gegenhalten, sucking, and biting.[86] In one such report there was unexplained vertical gaze palsy (upward and downward), suggesting midbrain localization.[102]

The gait disability bears obvious resemblance to that found

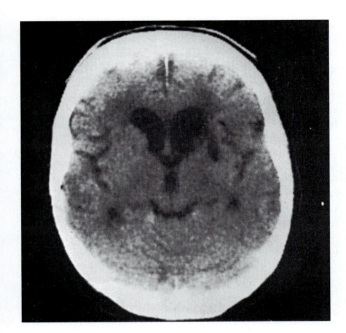

Figure 18.5 Computed tomogram showing infarction in the territory of either the left artery of Heubner or another penetrating branch of the proximal anterior cerebral artery. Brain supplied by the distal anterior cerebral artery was radiographically normal, and at autopsy infarction was limited to the head of the caudate, the anterior part of the internal capsule's anterior limb, and the anterior putamen.

with hydrocephalus and with the paraplegia in flexion of degenerative disease that mainly affects the frontal lobes[40]; in these conditions the pathophysiology is not understood, and the possible roles of descending frontal and prefrontal fibers[104,412] or the globus pallidus[413] are uncertain. Pulsatile flow in the ACAs is decreased in infantile hydrocephalus,[155] and it has been suggested that secondary ACA ischemia may be the cause of lower extremity spasticity in hydrocephalic infants, as well as contributing to the gait disturbance of adult normal pressure hydrocephalus.[235]

CALLOSAL DISCONNECTION SIGNS

In addition to either right or left leg weakness, ACA occlusion can cause left apraxia, agraphia, and tactile anomia.[7,135,207,213,226,317,385,414] Early cases are difficult to interpret, however.[127,150] For example, the patient of Liepmann and Maas[213] had right hemiplegia, including his arm, and so it is uncertain if his agraphia and apraxia were truly unilateral. The patient of Goldstein[135] had left-sided weakness, greatest in the leg, with a pronounced left hand grasp reflex, adding another possible reason for left-sided motor difficulty.[39,86] Agraphia, apraxia, and tactile anomia have occurred, however, in otherwise normal left limbs of patients with ACA occlusion, right leg weakness, and normal right arms.[126,226,314,385] Following surgical occlusion of the left ACA, a patient of

Geschwind and Kaplan[127] had right hemiparesis worse in the leg, a marked grasp reflex in the right hand, and mild right proprioceptive loss. He also had left-handed agraphia, writing incorrectly and paragraphically both spontaneously and to dictation, and could not do written calculations with his left hand. He could not name objects, letters, or numbers placed in his left hand out of vision, but he could identify them afterward with his left hand by pointing to them or demonstrating their use. Using either hand he could not correctly select from a group of objects placed out of sight in the other hand. Finally, he had difficulty performing verbal commands with his left hand (e.g., draw a square, point to the examiner, show how to brush teeth). Despite the grasp reflex his right hand could write normally, and his left hand could slavishly copy writing. Either hand could imitate the examiner's movements or manipulate objects. Following the lead of earlier authors,[213] Geschwind and Kaplan[127] attributed their patient's findings to anterior callosal destruction, with disconnection of the right hemisphere from the left, or, more specifically, of the right sensorimotor cortex from the left language areas. (Earlier writers who claimed that callosal lesions could cause left astereognosis[125,135] were undoubtedly observing tactile anomia rather than true agnosia, although a patient who could identify objects but not letters placed in the left hand is less easily explained.[372]) Preservation of the posterior corpus callosum was manifested by Geschwind and Kaplan's[127] patient's ability to read words presented to either visual field. Retained ability to perform tasks requiring both hands, such as threading a needle, suggested that the two hemispheres could cooperate like two individuals on such visually guided activities.

A left-handed patient had a stroke with weakness of the right leg but not the right arm, plus loss of ability to write with his right but not his left hand; if he is presumed to have had right cerebral language dominance, callosal disconnection might explain his agraphic right hand.[253] Another patient, considered to have pure agraphia, may represent a similar example of ACA occlusion.[283]

Some patients with presumed ACA occlusion and anterior callosal damage have had difficulty not only in performing verbal commands with the left hand but also in imitating the examiner and using actual objects.[33,125,212,225] Inaccessibility of verbal information to the right sensorimotor cortex would not explain this type of apraxia, and it has been suggested that in right-handers engrams for skilled movements (space-time or visuokinesthetic engrams[399]) reside in the left hemisphere and that callosal apraxia with impaired imitation and object use is the result of disconnection between these motor engrams and the right hemisphere.[133,399] In support of such a view is the observation, in a left-hander, that dominance for language and dominance for skilled motor acts appeared to be in different hemispheres.[150] That some patients with ACA occlusion have impaired imitation and object use and some do not has been explained by the hypothesis that verbal motor programs may be transmitted to the right hemisphere across the genu of the corpus callosum, whereas visuokinesthetic engrams may be transmitted across the body.[399]

Not all patients with ACA occlusion and left-sided apraxia perform well on bimanual tasks,[125,133,399] and sometimes the hands actually seem to be fighting one another (the alien hand sign[101,115,133,134,373]). It has been claimed[133] and denied[399] that extracallosal medial hemispheric damage is responsible for this phenomenon. The alien hand phenomenon is possibly related to other bizarre signs associated with callosal (or medial frontal) damage, including diagonistic apraxia (as one hand attempts to perform a voluntary action, the other performs the opposite—e.g., the patient puts on his glasses with his right hand, but his left hand then takes them off)[356,392] and utilization behavior (the patient cannot refrain from picking up and using an object—such as a toothbrush—placed in front of him).[113,210]

A patient with left ACA territory infarction had difficulty naming her left fingers and moving her named left fingers; she also had difficulty pointing to her own body parts with her left hand.[252] It was suggested that this patient's "body schema" was principally organized in her left cerebral hemisphere and was therefore, as a consequence of callosal infarction, disconnected from her right hemisphere.

Occlusion of an ACA that extends around the splenium of the corpus callosum can produce pure alexia in the left visual field or other visual anomic or agnostic problems.[280,399]

A problem in interpreting these patients is the degree to which they differ from those who have undergone surgical callosectomy. Left-sided apraxia to verbal commands occurs acutely following complete section of the corpus callosum and anterior commissure, usually with preserved ability to carry out the act in imitation of the examiner.[116,118] Right-sided movements, when governed by the right hemisphere (e.g., drawing an object seen only in the left visual field), are also impaired.[26] Such deficits tend to improve over days, however,[118] unless severe extracallosal brain damage is present.[116] Lasting deficit after callosal and commissural section is most likely to affect homolateral control of fingers (e.g., moving the left fingers to identify areas corresponding to regions stimulated on the right fingers, or mimicking with the left hand postures shown pictorially to the right visual field). When there is left hemispheric damage early in life, the minor hemisphere can comprehend spoken or written names of familiar objects,[117,122,338,339] but except in the setting of prolonged stimulus exposure[420] or in rare instances of unusual plasticity in speech organization[123,330] it usually cannot comprehend verbs or action nouns.[120–122] Such lack of comprehension accounts for the callosectomized patient's inability to follow verbal commands with either hand when the information is given to the minor hemisphere. Recovery of all but the most distal and subtle apraxia when commands are given to the language hemisphere is explained by each hemisphere's control over homolateral as well as contralateral limbs.

A patient with anterior callosal hemorrhage and bilateral ACA vasospasm had alexia in the left hemifield, anomia for objects held in the left hand, and left-handed agraphia and apraxia (including imitation and object use). She also had bilateral pseudoneglect: visual or tactile line bisection produced left hemineglect with the right hand in the left hemispace and right hemineglect with the left hand in the right hemispace. The explanation offered was disconnection of "the hemisphere important for directing attention-intention into the contralateral hemispace" from "the hemisphere important for controlling sensory motor processing of the limb."[152] By contrast, left hemispatial neglect "confined to right-hand and verbal responses" occurred in a patient with infarction of the posterior genu and whole trunk of the corpus callosum plus the left medial frontal and temporo-occipital lobes.[175] These findings were considered consistent with the hypothesis that "the left hemisphere is only concerned with attending to the contralateral hemispace," whereas "the right hemisphere is specialized for attending to both sides of space." It was further observed, consistent with previous reports, that hemineglect does not seem to occur with lesions restricted to the corpus callosum but requires additional destruction (e.g., medial frontal lobe) that blocks transmission through extracallosal commissures.[134,331]

In a right-handed callosectomized patient with unusually rich right hemispheric verbal comprehension, there was no left-sided apraxia to verbal information presented to the right hemisphere.[121] This finding argues against the notion of motor engrams residing solely in one hemisphere, language-dominant or not.[125,153,182–184,306,388,390] In other callosectomized patients visual nonverbal stimulation has also produced normally coordinated contralateral motor acts.[390]

Consistent with the view that extracallosal damage is probably crucial to the appearance of anterior callosal disconnection syndrome following ACA occlusion is the finding that left tactile anomia, apraxia for verbal commands, and agraphia did not occur in two patients who underwent section of the anterior commissure and only the anterior two-thirds of the corpus callosum.[118] These patients, moreover, performed a variety of nonverbal cross-integration tasks, matching visual or tactile stimuli directed separately to each hemisphere.[139] Conversely, selective sectioning of the splenium, sparing the genu and body, did produce verbal deficits for left visual field and tactile stimuli,[234,372] as well as for tactile-motor tasks requiring interhemispheric integration.[388,390] It appears that "the anterior commissure and the rostral callosum do not transfer either lateralized visual images that elicit motor activity or the specific motor program needed to carry out the appropriate movement."[390] An isolated 3-cm midcallosal section impairs interhemispheric transfer of tactile data but not of information obtained visually.[167] Section of the most posterior 1.5 cm of the callosum disrupts naming of visual stimuli in the left visual field,[119,164,234,346] and an additional 1.5 cm section further impairs sensorimotor integration and tactile naming.[75,390] What information gets transferred across the rostral callosum, that part most often damaged following ACA occlusion is unclear; it has been suggested that the anterior callosum transfers information after processing it into higher order abstraction.[329,390] (Following posterior callosal section, interhemispheric transfer of sensory information from the right hemisphere is lost, but transfer of semantic information is still possible; after complete section, neither sensory nor semantic information can be transferred.[329])

AKINETIC MUTISM (ABULIA)

Coma probably can follow bilateral proximal ACA occlusion, but when aneurysm surgery[269] or vasospasm after subarachnoid hemorrhage[353] is the cause, interpretation is difficult. Dandy[79] believed that left ACA occlusion (i.e., surgical ligation) caused permanent coma and this view was promulgated by Poppen,[286] who, however, considered hypotension during surgery to be a critical factor. Subsequent authors have perpetuated the idea that coma can follow unilateral ACA occlusion.[19,62] However, Dandy's [79] attribution of coma to striatal damage was soon discredited,[251,303] and it is now recognized that coma requires either bihemispheric or ascending reticular activating system lesions.[284] Probably those patients in whom coma seemed to follow ACA occlusion either had, as a result of one of the several vascular anomalies described above, brain damage not restricted to one hemisphere, or were akinetic, mute, and more alert than they seemed.

Akinetic mutism is "a state of limited responsiveness to the environment in the absence of gross alteration of sensory-motor mechanisms operating at a more peripheral level."[320] Neither paralysis nor coma accounts for the symptoms. Patients may open their eyes and seem alert, and brief movement, speech, or even agitation may follow powerful stimuli, but patients are otherwise "indifferent, detached, frozen, and apathetic."[320] The term *akinetic mutism* was used by Cairns et al.[50] to describe such a state in association with a tumor of the third ventricle. With such lesions there is often ophthalmoparesis and fluctuating or continuous somnolence.[41,57,58,97,110,202,209]

Akinetic mutism also occurs with lesions of the anteromedial frontal lobes, including infarction.[49,109,142,269] Ophthalmoparesis (except for early gaze preference) is then not present, and the patient, whose open eyes may follow objects, is more obviously alert than with mesencephalic or thalamic lesions; there may be brief, monosyllabic, but appropriate responses to questions. Striking dissociation occurs between spontaneous verbal communication, which is often totally absent, and solicited communication, which is often retained although restricted.[49] The term *abulia* refers to a continuum of such abnormalities, from mild to severe, having in common decreased spontaneous movement and speech, latency in responding to verbal and other stimuli, and impersistence in responses and tasks.[105,203] While verbal responses are "late, terse, incomplete, and emotionally flat," patients sufficiently prodded sometimes reveal a cognitive capacity much more normal than expected.[53] When the patient is literally akinetic and mute, however, the condition must be differentiated from true stupor or coma, the locked-in state, extrapyramidal akinesia, catatonia, hysteria, and persistent vegetative state. The two structures most often implicated in the production of abulia are the cingulate gyrus and the supplementary motor area (SMA).

Abulia has followed bilateral cingulate gyrus lesions. A woman developed a sudden headache and then "lay staring at the ceiling, not asking for water or food, and never speaking spontaneously." She was incontinent of urine, ate and drank when food or water was brought, comprehended spoken speech, answered questions monosyllabically, and did not display any emotional reaction. Right-sided hyperreflexia and bilateral Babinski signs were present. At autopsy embolic hemorrhagic infarction of the cingulate gyri bilaterally and the corpus callosum was seen.[254] A clinically and pathologically similar patient showed Babinski signs but no hypertonus, and there were "no visible reactions to pain."[20] Inability to walk despite normal strength has been specifically mentioned in other reports.[9] On the other hand, unilateral cingulate infarction in two patients was followed by seizures in one and personality change in another, with no reduction in motor activity.[9] Akinetic mutism occurred in one patient with presumed unilateral cingulate (and pontine) damage, but autopsy findings were incomplete.[332] A patient with hemorrhage into his

right medial frontal lobe had marked bradykinesia of his left limbs, improving when they were placed in his right hemispace. The disturbance was considered motor neglect ("a failure of the intentional systems that lead to preparation and activation of movement"), possibly secondary to SMA damage.[238] It is not unusual for patients with unilateral ACA territory infarction (or medial frontal lobe surgical ablation) to have several days of abulia followed by return of verbal and ipsilateral motor responses, persistence of weakness in the contralateral leg, and a disinclination to move the contralateral arm. Motor neglect thus might be viewed as unilateral abulia.[51,59,69,107,267,311]

With further improvement, signs can become increasingly subtle, for example difficulty with sequential movements involving different joints or coordinating the movements of both arms.[90,311] In one report there was inability to reproduce rhythms from memory,[144] and in another, involving bilateral SMA lesions, there was inability to perceive as separate two successive tactile stimuli applied to the body.[192] Observations such as these have led to the hypotheses that the SMA (and perhaps other premotor structures) are responsible for generating "sequences from memory that fit into a precise timing plan."[144]

Patients with abulia or motor neglect often display relative preservation of reflexic movements, in contrast to anticipated or willed movements. (A comparable dissociation is seen in parkinsonism.) Disinhibition of unanticipated complex motor movements as a result of SMA damage has been invoked to explain such phenomena as alien hand, diagonistic apraxia, and utilization behavior.[270]

Cingulectomy in monkeys caused reduction of motor activity and "loss of social conscience"; the animals treated their fellows as inanimate objects not to be feared.[395] Monkeys in which the medial temporal lobes were removed and with Klüver-Bucy syndrome (quietness, no fear, and increased curiosity with compulsive nosing and smelling of all objects) had gradual clearing of symptoms, which, however, returned following bilateral cingulectomy.[179] In cingulectomized cats, motor signs suggested catatonia.[179] Human surgical cingulate ablation for psychiatric disturbance is difficult to interpret, since the amount of cingulate removed is usually small,[308,401] and the importance of cingulothalamic disconnection in frontal lobotomy has never been defined.[9,85]

The full syndrome of akinetic mutism or abulia has thus not been produced in animals by experimental cingulectomy or in humans by surgical cingulectomy, and even bilateral ACA ligation in humans has on occasion failed to cause the syndrome.[109,286] In an autopsy report of eight patients with akinetic mutism and bilateral cingulate destruction, no difference was seen in the clinical picture whether or not additional lesions existed in the medial orbital cortex or septal region.[9] Most reports, however, have emphasized additional lesions or diffuse compressive cerebral injury,[49,109,284] and electroencephalograms usually show bilateral cerebral slowing.[109,284] An angiographic study of patients with subarachnoid hemorrhage showed correlation of unilateral or bilateral ACA vasospasm with akinetic mutism, but it was unclear if brain damage was limited to one hemisphere in the patients with unilateral vasospasm.[106]

Abulia has also followed unilateral or bilateral caudate infarction (most likely from occlusion of the recurrent artery of Heubner). In one series of unilateral caudate infarctions, it was the most prominent feature in 10 of 17 patients (6 left, 4 right).[53] In four patients the lesions (by computed tomography) were restricted to the caudate; in others the anterior limb of the internal capsule was involved. Three abulic patients had alternating restlessness and hyperactivity, and in four others hyperactivity was present without abulia. In another report it was proposed that abulia resulted from damage to the dorsolateral caudate (which connects to the dorsolateral frontal lobe) and disinhibition from damage to the ventromedial caudate (which connects to orbitofrontal areas).[239]

Following surgical partial section of the anterior corpus callosum, acute akinetic mutism is often seen that tends to recover over days.[337,347] Positron emission tomography studies in baboons have shown that the procedure causes transient depression of cortical metabolism in widespread areas of both frontal lobes (diaschisis).[415]

LANGUAGE DISTURBANCE

Unilateral ACA occlusion can produce language disturbance, but whether it is aphasic is uncertain.[124,168] Details are often lacking in case reports.[305] In some patients "reduction of spontaneous verbal expression"[51] or muteness, often in association with more global psychomotor bradykinesia,[51,78] seems to be a manifestation of abulia; in such patients comprehension of spoken speech may be untestable.[188] Some reports have described truly impaired speech comprehension,[233] word-finding difficulty, alexia,[213] and phonemic or verbal paraphasias on spontaneous speech, reading aloud, or writing.[233,384] Others, however, have emphasized the absence of paraphasias[6,78,211,303] or considered the difficulty "partly defects of an aphasic order and partly those of a dysarthria."[69] A number of reports have described impaired spontaneous speech with normal repetition and sometimes echolalia (transcortical aphasia),[6,15,77,180,188,303,384] and in one instance echolalia and palilalia occurred without other evidence of aphasia.[17] A man with transcortical motor aphasia, although lacking echolalia or echopraxia, could not refrain from completing the sentences of others.[303] Some patients have had transcortical aphasia (or, as Luria calls it, *dynamic aphasia*[223,224]) with a strikingly greater impairment of list naming than naming to confrontation,[6] or particularly impaired speech initiative, as in attempts to narrate stories or describe complex pictures.[303]

In one report a patient with transcortical mixed aphasia had infarction of both the medial frontal and the medial parietal lobes, whereas two other patients with transcortical motor aphasia had infarction of only the medial frontal lobe.[301] One patient following a large left ACA infarct had transcortical motor aphasia and mirror writing.[27] Another, right-handed, had left-handed mirror writing following infarction of the right medial frontal cortex sparing the corpus callosum, leading the authors to conjecture that the SMA is "responsible for nonmirror transformation of motor programs originating in the left hemisphere prior to execution by the primary motor area in the right hemisphere."[55] A woman with aphasia that included impaired comprehension, repetition, reading, and writing had medial frontal infarction plus an old infarct over the rolandic convexity.[288] In some patients speech disturbance was transient, whereas paucity of other movements, including writing, persisted.[233]

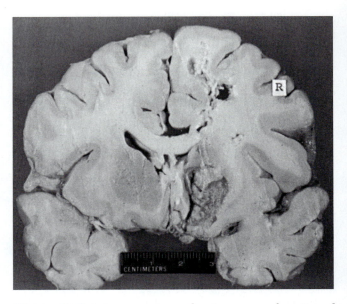

Figure 18.6 Autopsy specimen showing a coronal section of the anterior frontal and temporal lobes. There is infarction in the territories of both the proximal and distal right anterior cerebral artery. Affected areas include the caudate; putamen, internal capsule's anterior limb, cingulate gyrus, and supplementary motor area. (From Brust et al.,[48] with permission.)

Reports of severely impaired language after pathologically documented ACA occlusion have involved left-sided lesions[27] with one exception,[48] a right-handed woman with left hemiparesis, diffuse bradykinesia, speech limited to short replies to questions, and a tendency to echolalia; naming and comprehension of spoken or written language seemed impaired, but were difficult to test. At autopsy there was infarction in the territory of the right ACA, including the head of the caudate, the anterior limb of the internal capsule, the anterior putamen, the anterior cingulate and superior frontal gyri, and the entire SMA (Fig. 18.6). Several reports exist of language disturbance after bilateral ACA occlusion,[156,188,232] and one, with neither postmortem examination nor disclosure of the patient's handedness, of occlusion of the right ACA.[51]

Most investigators, whether or not they consider these abnormalities to be truly aphasic, attribute them to damage to the SMA on the medial surface of the frontal lobe, anterior to the paracentral lobule, and between the cingulate and superior frontal gyri (i.e., the medial hemispheric part of Brodmann's area 6).[124,159,277,278,402] Of 10 right-handed patients with left ACA territory infarcts, four had transcortical motor aphasia, and in each the SMA was involved. Three other patients with sparing of the SMA but involvement of the cingulate had only "alterations of verbal memory."[29] In monkeys, stimulation of this area causes arm and leg movements and head turning,[249] and there seems to be rostral caudal forelimb-hindlimb somatotopy.[43,227,333,358,359,408,411] Unilateral ablation of the SMA in monkeys produces a deficit in tasks of bimanual coordination.[42] In humans SMA stimulation induces bodily postures (e.g., turning of head and eyes toward a contralaterally uplifted arm) or repetitive movements (e.g., stepping or hand-waving).[278] Such responses are often bilateral and can occur after ablation of area 4 (the primary motor cortex). SMA stimulation can also cause speech and movement arrest or vocalization.

Whereas stimulation of the face region of area 4 causes vocalization of continuous vowel sounds,[271,274] SMA stimulation on either hemisphere[273] produces intermittently repeated words, syllables, or meaningless combinations of syllables[278] (saccadic vocalization[402]). The repeated word might be a palilalia of what was being said at the onset of stimulation. Rhythmic mouth and jaw movements sometimes accompany the vocalization. Speech arrest, hesitation, or slowing also occurs, sometimes with mouth movements suggesting attempted speech or with arrest of other voluntary movement. Speech comprehension is usually preserved, but anomia and paraphasias have occurred.[273]

Such symptoms, with or without other motor, sensory, or autonomic phenomena, may be the manifestation of seizures caused by structural lesions affecting the SMA, especially meningiomas.[14,38,55,56,96,143,105,281,354,402] Although experimental stimulation of either the right or left SMA can cause speech arrest or repetition, seizures causing altered speech have only rarely occurred in dextrals with lesions of the right SMA.[37,54] Both stimulation and seizure phenomena raise the questions of whether true aphasia is occurring and which brain structures are in fact responsible.

Destructive lesions, including infarction, are similarly problematic. Medial hemispheric structural lesions such as neoplasm,[66,73,77,95,96,143,228,306] vascular malformation,[225,281] subdural empyema,[199] surgical ablation,[143,194,276,318] and trauma[224] not only can directly affect more regions than the SMA, but can also produce distant effects from edema or brain distortion. SMA excision for the treatment of epilepsy has led to language disturbance, but interpretation of such cases has varied. One group found that excision of the language hemisphere's SMA back to area 4 caused muteness, whereas excision of the language hemisphere's anterior SMA or the nonlanguage hemisphere's entire SMA produced "no specific deficit."[275] Others found, after excision of either SMA, more lasting speech disturbances, which, however, seemed nonaphasic and secondary to bradykinesia.[194] Transcortical motor aphasia followed excision of the left SMA.[318] Bilateral ideomotor apraxia without aphasia affected two patients with ACA infarction involving both the left SMA and the corpus callosum.[398]

The SMA receives afferents from the ipsilateral primary and secondary somatosensory cortex and has reciprocal connections with the ipsilateral area 4, posterior parietal cortex, upper convexity premotor cortex (area 6), several thalamic nuclei, and, across the corpus callosum, the contralateral SMA and convexity area 6.[169–171,402] It has been suggested, therefore, that the SMA is "an area of sensory convergence."[43] Efferents project bilaterally to the cingulate gyrus and striatum,[78,88,167,191] ipsilaterally to the red nucleus, pontine nuclei, and dorsal column nuclei,[43] and contralaterally to area 4 and the midconvexity premotor region (area 8).[78] There are also SMA neurons that project to the spinal cord.[24,227,250] Regional cerebral blood flow (rCBF) increases in the SMA during automatic speech and during repetitive finger movement but not during isometric hand muscle contraction.[57,158,195,198,305] CBF also increases in the SMA during planning of sequential movements.[262,298,299] (By contrast, area 4's CBF increases only during execution of such movements.[298]) In monkeys, medullary pyramidal section did not affect movements produced by SMA stimulation,[410] increased discharge of SMA neurons preceded stereotyped learned motor tasks of either the ipsilateral or contralateral extremities, and SMA neurons fired in response to sensory signals "only when the signal called for a motor response."[359] Neurons in the SMA are, however, less responsive to peripheral stimuli than those in area 4,[43,408] suggesting that part of the SMA's function may be "to 'gate' or suppress the afferent influences on area 4"[407] (perhaps accounting for the transient contralateral grasp reflex frequently seen after SMA ablation[6,273,278,291,334,371,408]). Such suppression would convert area 4's activity from a closed loop to an open loop mode,[403,408] consistent with the further notion that the SMA develops "a preparatory state" for impending movement[359,360] or that it elaborates "programs for motor subroutines necessary in skilled voluntary motion,"[300] including, with its "sequences of fast isolated muscular contraction," human speech.[298] ACA occlusion and SMA damage may therefore affect "an elementary part of language, very primitive, and lacking . . . symbols and intellectual features"[281]; the resulting disturbances would not be, strictly speaking, aphasic.

The oft-cited case of Bonhoeffer[33] may represent ACA occlusion causing language disturbance by a different mechanism. This patient developed right hemiplegia, with the leg weaker than the arm, plus reduction of speech to one or two words, relatively preserved comprehension of spoken speech, alexia, agraphia, and apraxia (difficulty following commands, imitating, and handling objects), that was greater on the left than right. Abnormalities at autopsy included infarction of the posterior left middle and superior frontal gyri, the anterior four-fifths of the corpus callosum, the anterior limb of the left internal capsule, and a small part of the left posterior inferior parietal lobule. Bonhoeffer[33] (and Geschwind,[125] reviewing the case) explained the left apraxia as resulting from the callosal lesion and the aphasia from the combined callosal and capsular lesions, which in effect isolated Broca's area; the posterior parietal lesion probably contributed to the alexia, agraphia, and right apraxia. Neither author discussed the possible contribution of SMA destruction to the language disturbance, which, theoretically, could have occurred without it.

OTHER MENTAL ABNORMALITIES

Besides abulia, apraxia, and language impairment, patients with ACA occlusion can have a variety of other emotional or intellectual disturbances, usually attributed to involvement of structures supplied by branches of the proximal ACA (A1 segment or ACoA).[38,151,323] Anxiety, fear, insomnia, talkativeness, or agitation has occurred with or without weakness, bradykinesia, or grasp and suck reflexes.[9,17,38,69] A young woman, awakening from coma after ACoA aneurysm rupture, had severe withdrawal with unprovoked agitation and screaming; at autopsy there was bilateral infarction of the orbital gyri, gyri recti, septal nuclei, cingulate gyri, hippocampal formations, and right amygdala.[99] Damage to hypothalamic or other limbic structures has also been considered responsible for these symptoms,[92] which, when they predominate, can suggest non-structural neurotic or psychotic illness.[19,62] In any event, the notion that apathy and poor motivation predictably follow dorsolateral frontal lesions, whereas orbitofrontal damage causes disinhibited behavior, appears to be an oversimplification.[140,345]

Confusion, disorientation, and memory loss, sometimes severe, also occur.[81,91,156,173,196,218,219,269,280,289,319,365] Retrograde and anterograde amnesia following ACoA aneurysm rupture may be subtle or severe,[166,268,344,386] with variable denial or confabulation.[84,224,355,389,419] In one report a patient with bilateral infarction of both medial frontal lobes as well as the right inferior temporal lobe and pole had severely impaired recognition of previously presented words or pictures yet could spontaneously recall them.[83] In another report five patients with lesions restricted to basal forebrain structures (sparing the hippocampi and temporal lobes) were able to recall particular stimuli (e.g., someone's name or face) but could not bring such differently learned components together as an integrated memory.[76] Structures implicated in these amnestic syndromes have included the hypothalamus, medial forebrain bundle, septum, nucleus of Meynert, nucleus accumbens, and fornix, with possible secondary dysfunction of medial temporal regions.[76,282,409]

Of 251 patients examined 3 months after an acute ischemic stroke, 66 were demented. Infarction in the territory of the left ACA was more predictive of dementia than infarction in the MCA or PCA territories.[361]

Visuospatial disturbance with difficulty dressing, drawing, or copying or with left hemineglect has followed infarction of the caudate and anterior limb of the internal capsule. Primary dyscalculia followed infarction in the territory of the left ACA.[222] Depression has been associated with left caudate lesions.[340]

INCONTINENCE AND OTHER AUTONOMIC CHANGES

Urinary (and less often fecal) incontinence can occur with either unilateral or bilateral ACA occlusion.[19,54,69,400] Involvement of the paracentral lobule (presuming homuncular representation of motor and sensory components of micturition) has been offered as an explanation,[22,65,280] even though paracentral stimulation produced only contralateral sensation in the penis without motor response.[272] Damage to the superiormedial frontal lobe, especially the midportion of the superior frontal gyrus, the cingulate, and the white matter in between, is a more likely cause, since such damage (e.g., from frontal leukotomy) causes transient or permanent disturbance of urination and defecation, including urgency and incontinence.[10,11,40,295]

Cardiorespiratory alterations are frequent following stroke, whether or not limbic structures are specifically damaged.[217,387] Such changes following ACA occlusion are therefore open to interpretation, but it is not unreasonable to incriminate damage to the hypothalamus, cingulate gyrus, or other limbic areas. Fever not always related to infection, tachycardia, and unexpected death have followed human cingulate infarction.[9,20,269] Human and animal cingulate stimulation can produce altered respirations, bradycardia, temporary respiratory or cardiac arrest, hyper- or hypotension, pupillary dilatation, and piloerection.[20,93,172,321,335,396] Diabetes insipidus, perhaps from anterior hypothalamic infarction, has occurred after surgical occlusion of a proximal ACA for ACoA aneurysm.[69,151] Gastrointestinal bleeding following ACoA aneurysm rupture has also been blamed on hypothalamic damage.[357]

PERIVENTRICULAR LEUKOMALACIA OF INFANCY

Brains of infants dying within hours or months of birth may have necrotic foci along the lateral ventricles, considered by some to be infarcts at border zones between the territories of the ACA, MCA, and PCA.[18,216,391] Others have stressed that the periventricular areas are more properly called end zones and are not in anastomatic areas but rather within a few millimeters of the ventricular wall "between the terminal distributions of ventriculopetal and ventriculofugal branches of small arteries that penetrate deeply into the brain,"[87] including those from the ACA passing through the cingulate gyrus.[352] Such lesions usually spare the cerebral cortex, for the fetus has rich meningeal anastomoses between plial vessels, and the newborn has a relatively higher metabolic rate in white matter.[80,87] Hypotensive newborn dogs develop decreased white matter blood flow and lesions resembling periventricular leukomalacia.[418] Infants with periventricular leukomalacia and no apparent perinatal asphyxia have shown poorly developed ventriculofugal branches at autopsy.[13,352] Affected infants display lethargy, hypotonia, difficulty feeding, and seizures; survivors are usually mentally retarded, with spastic quadriparesis.

Because cerebral autoregulation is impaired in neonates with asphyxia, periventricular hemorrhage in the newborn may be the result of capillary dilatation and rupture in these same deep end zones.[391]

References

1. Abbie AA: The morphology of the fore-brain arteries, with especial reference to the evolution of the basal ganglia. J Anat 68:433, 1934
2. Ahmed DS, Ahmed RH: The recurrent branch of the anterior cerebral artery. Anat Rec 157:699, 1967
3. Alajouanine T, Castaigne P, Sabouraud O, Contamin F: Palilalie paroxystique et vocalisations itératives au cours de crises épileptiques par lesion intéressant l'aire motrice supplémentaire. Rev Neurol 101:685, 1959
4. Alexander L: The vascular supply of the striopallidum. Res Publ Assoc Res Nerv Ment Dis 21:77, 1942
5. Alexander MP, Freedman M: Amnesia after anterior communicating artery aneurysm rupture. Neurology (NY), suppl. 2, 33:104, 1983
6. Alexander MP, Schmitt MA: The aphasia syndrome of stroke in the left anterior cerebral artery territory. Arch Neurol 37:97, 1980

7. Alpers BJ, Berry RG, Paddison RM: Anatomical studies of the circle of Willis in normal brain. Arch Neurol Psychiatry 81:409, 1959

8. Amagasa M, Sato S, Otabe K: Posttraumatic dissecting aneurysm of the anterior cerebral artery: case report. Neurosurgery 23:221, 1988

9. Amyes EW, Nielsen JM: Clinicopathologic study of vascular lesions of the anterior cingulate region. Bull Los Angeles Neurol Soc 20:112, 1955

10. Andrew J, Nathan PW: Lesions of the anterior frontal lobes and disturbances of micturition and defecation. Brain 87:233, 1964

11. Andrew J, Nathan PW: The cerebral control of micturition. Proc R Soc Med 58:553, 1965

12. Araki T, Ouchi M, Ikeda Y: A case of anterior cerebral artery dissecting aneurysm. No Shinkei Geka Neurol Surg 24:87, 1996

13. Armstrong D, Norman MG: Periventricular leukomalacia in neonates: complications and sequelae. Arch Dis Child 49:367, 1974

14. Arseni C, Botez MI: Speech disturbances caused by tumours of the supplementary motor area. Acta Psychiatr Scand 36:279, 1961

15. Atkinson MS: Transcortical motor aphasia associated with left frontal lobe infarction. Trans Am Neurol Assoc 96:136, 1971

16. Aydin IH, Onder A, Takei E et al: Heubner's artery variations in anterior communicating artery aneurysms. Acta Neurochir 127:17, 1994

17. Baldy R: Les Syndromes de l'Artère Cérébrale Antérieure. Jouve, Paris, 1927

18. Banker BQ, Larroche JC: Periventricular leukomalacia of infancy: a form of neonatal anoxic encephalopathy. Arch Neurol 7:386, 1962

19. Baptista AG: Studies on the arteries of the brain. II. The anterior cerebral artery: some anatomic features and their clinical implications. Neurology (NY) 13:825, 1963

20. Barris RW, Schuman HR: Bilateral anterior cingulate gyrus lesions. Syndrome of the anterior cingulate gyri. Neurology (NY) 3:44, 1953

21. Beevor CE: The cerebral arterial supply. Brain 30:403, 1907

22. Berman SA, Hayman LA, Hinck VC: Correlation of CT cerebral vascular territories with function. 1. Anterior cerebral artery. AJR 135:253, 1980

23. Besson G, Leguyader J, Mimassi N et al: Anomalie rare du polygone de Willis: trajet sous-optique des deux artères cérébrales antérieures: aneurysme associé de la bifurcation due tronc basilaire. Neurochirurgie 26:71, 1980

24. Biber MP, Kneisley LW, LaVail JH: Cortical neurons projecting to the cervical and lumbar enlargements of the spinal cord in young and adult rhesus monkeys. Exp Neurol 59:492, 1978

25. Blackburn IW: Anomalies of the encephalic arteries among the insane. J Comp Neurol Psychol 17:493, 1907

26. Bogen JE, Gazzaniga MS: Cerebral commissurotomy in man: minor hemisphere dominance for certain visuospacial functions. J Neurosurg 23:394, 1965

27. Bogousslavsky J, Assal G, Regli F: Infarctus du territoire de l'artère cérébrale antérieure gauche. 2. Troubles du langage. Rev Neurol 143:121, 1987

28. Bogousslavsky J, Martin R, Moulin T: Homolateral ataxia and crural paresis: a syndrome of anterior cerebral artery territory infarction. J Neurol Neurosurg Psychiatry 55:1146, 1992

29. Bogousslavsky J, Regli F: Infarctus du territoire de l'artère cérébrale antérieure gauche. 1. Correlations clinicotomodensitometriques. Rev Neurol 143:21, 1987

30. Bogousslavsky J, Regli F: Capsular genu syndrome. Neurology (NY) 40:1499, 1990

31. Bogousslavsky J, Regli F: Anterior cerebral artery territory infarction in the Lausanne Stroke Registry: clinical and etiological patterns. Arch Neurol 47:144, 1990

32. Bollar A, Martinez R, Gelabert M, Garcia A: Anomalous origin of anterior cerebral artery associated with aneurysm—embryological considerations. Neuroradiology 30:86, 1988

33. Bonhoeffer K: Klischer u. anatomischer Befund zur Lehre von der Apraxie und der motorischen Sprachbahn. Monatsschr Psychiatr Neurol 35:113, 1914

34. Booker J, Morris N, Huang C-Y: Cerebral radionuclide scintigraphy in the stroke syndrome. Med J Aust 1:625, 1978

35. Borggreve F, DeDeyn PP, Marien P et al: Bilateral infarction in the anterior cerebral artery vascular territory due to an unusual anomaly of the circle of Willis. Stroke 25:1279, 1994

36. Bosma NJ: Infra-optic course of anterior cerebral artery and low bifurcation of internal carotid artery. Acta Neurochir 38:305, 1977

37. Botez MI, Wertheim N: Expressive aphasia and amusia following right frontal lesions in a righthanded man. Brain 82:186, 1959

38. Boudouresques J, Bonnal J: Les troubles psychiques des tumeurs frontales. Rev Prat 7:1375, 1957

39. Bouman L, Grunbaum AA: Über motorische Momente der Agraphie. Monatsschr Psychiatr Neurol 77:223, 1930

40. Bradley WE, Timm GW, Scott FB: Innervation of the detrusor muscle and urethra. p. 3. In Lapides J (ed): Symposium on Neurogenic Bladder, The Urologic Clinics of North America. WB Saunders, Philadelphia, 1974

41. Brage D, Morea R, Copello AR: Syndrome nécrotique tegmento-thalamic avec mutisme akinétique. Rev Neurol 104:126, 1961

42. Brinkman C: Lesions in supplementary motor area interfere with a monkey's performance of a bimanual coordination task. Neurosci Lett 27:267, 1981

43. Brinkman C, Porter R: Supplementary motor area in the monkey: activity of neurons during performance of a learned motor task. J Neurophysiol 42:681, 1979

44. Brismar J, Ackerman R, Roberson G: Anomaly of anterior cerebral artery: a case report and embryologic considerations. Acta Radiol [Diagn] (Stockh) 18:154, 1977

45. Brodal A: Neurological Anatomy in Relation to Clinical Medicine. 3rd Ed. Oxford University Press, New York, 1981

46. Brust JCM: Stroke: diagnostic, anatomical, and physiological considerations. p. 667. In Kandel ER, Schwartz JH (ed): Principles of Neural Science. Elsevier/North-Holland, New York, 1981

47. Brust JCM: Cerebral infarction. p. 162. In Rowland LP (ed): Merritt's Textbook of Neurology. 7th Ed. Lea & Febiger, Philadelphia, 1984

48. Brust JCM, Plank C, Burke A et al: Language disorder in a right-hander after occlusion of the right anterior cerebral artery. Neurology (NY) 32:492, 1982

49. Buge A, Escourelle R, Rancurel G: "Mutisme akinétique" et ramollissement bilinguaire: trois observations anatomo-clinique. Rev Neurol 131:121, 1975

50. Cairns H, Oldfield RC, Pennybacker JB: Akinetic mutism with an epidermoid cyst of III ventricle. Brain 64:273, 1941

51. Cambier J, Dehen H: Les syndromes de l'artère cérébrale antérieure. Rev Med Toulouse, suppl.:277, 1973

52. Campbell JB, Forster FM: The anterior cerebral artery in the macaque monkey (Macaca mulatta). J Nerv Ment Dis 99:229, 1944

53. Caplan LR, Schmahmann JD, Kase CS et al: Caudate infarcts. Arch Neurol 47:133, 1990

54. Caplan LR, Zervas NT: Speech arrest in a dextral with a right mesial frontal astrocytoma. Arch Neurol 35:252, 1978

55. Carrieri G: Sindrome da sofferenza dell'area supplementaria motoria sinistra nel corso di un meningioma parasaggitale. Riv Patol Nerv Ment 84:29, 1963

56. Castaigne P: Vocalisations itératives et crises palilaliques dans les lésions prérolandiques de la face interne du lobe frontal. Neurologia 9:39, 1964

57. Castaigne P, Buge A, Cambier J et al: Démence thalamique d'origine vasculaire par ramollissement bilateral, limité au territoire du pedicule retromammilaire. Rev Neurol 114:89, 1966

58. Castaigne P, Buge A, Escourelle R, Masson M: Ramollissement pedonculaire median, tegmento-thalamique avec ophthalmoplegie et hypersomnie. (Étude anatomo-clinique.) Rev Neurol 106:357, 1962

59. Castaigne P, LaPlane D, Degos JD: Trois cas de negligence motrice par lesion frontal prerolandique. Rev Neurol 126:5, 1972

60. Castaigne P, Lhermitte F, Escourelle R et al: Étude anatomopathologique de 74 infarcts de l'artère cérébrale antérieure (55 observations). Rev Med Toulouse, suppl. 339, 1975

61. Chan J-L, Ross ED: Left-handed mirror writing following right anterior cerebral artery infarction: evidence for non-mirror transformation of motor programs by right supplementary motor area. Neurology (NY) 38:59, 1988

62. Chavany JA, Messimy R, Pertuiset B, Hagenmuller D: Les fonctions du territoire cortical de l'artère cérébrale antérieure: parentés séméiologiques des syndromes vasculaires traumatiques et tumoraux. Nouv Presse Med 63:512, 1955

63. Chimowitz MI, Lafranchise EF, Furlan AJ, Awad IA: Ipsilateral leg weakness with carotid stenosis. Stroke 9:1362, 1990

64. Choudhury AR: Proximal occlusion of the dominant anterior cerebral artery for anterior communicating aneurysms. J Neurosurg 45:484, 1976

65. Chusid JG: Correlative Neuroanatomy and Functional Neurology. 16th Ed. Lange Medical, Los Altos, CA, 1976

66. Chusid JG, de Gutiérrez-Mahoney CG, Margules-Lavergne MP: Speech disturbances in association with parasagittal frontal lesions. J Neurosurg 11:193, 1954

67. Claude H, Loyez M: Etude anatomique d'un cas d'apraxie avec hémiplégie droite et cécité verbale. Encephale 8:289, 1913

68. Cobb S: The cerebral circulation. 13. The question of "end-arteries" of the brain and the mechanism of infarction. Arch Neurol Psychiatry 25:273, 1931

69. Critchley M: The anterior cerebral artery and its syndromes. Brain 53:120, 1930

70. Crowell RM, Morawetz RB: The anterior communicating artery has significant branches. Stroke 8:272, 1977

71. Cuatico W: The phenomenon of ipsilateral innervation: one case report. J Neurosurg Sci 23:81, 1979

72. Curry RW, Culbreth GC: The normal cerebral angiogram. AJR 65:345, 1951

73. Cushing H, Eisenhardt L: Meningiomas: Their Classification, Regional Behavior, Life History, and Surgical End Results. Charles C Thomas, Springfield, IL, 1938

74. Czochra M, Kozniewska H, Muszynski A, Trojanowski T: Surgical treatment of aneurysms of the anterior communicating artery using Yasargil's approach. Neurol Neurochir Pol 13:71, 1979

75. Damasio AR, Chui HC, Corbett J, Kassel N: Posterior callosal section in a non-epileptic patient. J Neurol Neurosurg Psychiatry 43:351, 1980

76. Damasio AR, Graff-Radford NR, Eslinger PJ et al: Amnesia following basal forebrain lesions. Arch Neurol 42:263, 1985

77. Damasio AR, Kassel NF: Transcortical motor aphasia in relation to lesions of the supplementary motor area. Neurology (NY) 28:396, 1978

78. Damasio AR, Van Hoesen GW: Structure and function of the supplementary motor area. Neurology (NY) 30:359, 1980

79. Dandy WE: Surgery of the brain. p. 51. In Lewis D (ed): Practice of Surgery. Vol. 12. WF Prior, Hagerstown, MD, 1932

80. Davison AN, Dobbing J: Applied Neurochemistry. FA Davis, Philadelphia, 1968

81. Davison C, Goodhart SP, Needles W: Cerebral localization in cerebrovascular disease. Res Publ Assoc Res Nerv Ment Dis 13:435, 1934

82. Dawson BH: The blood vessels of the human optic chiasma and their relation to those of the hypophysis and thalamus. Brain 81:207, 1958

83. Delbecq-Derouesné J, Beauvois MF, Shallice T: Preserved recall versus impaired recognition: a case study. Brain 113:1045, 1990

84. DeLuca J, Cicerone KD: Cognitive impairments following anterior communicating artery aneurysm. J Clin Exp Neuropsychol 11:47, 1989

85. Denny-Brown D: The frontal lobes and their function. p. 13. In Feiling A (ed): Modern Trends in Neurology. Hoeber, New York, 1951

86. Denny-Brown D: The nature of apraxia. J Nerv Ment Dis 126:9, 1958

87. De Reuck J, Chatta AS, Richardson EP: Pathogenesis and evolution of periventricular leukomalacia in infancy. Arch Neurol 27:229, 1972

88. De Vito JL, Smith OA: Projections from the mesial frontal cortex (supplementary motor area) to the cerebral hemispheres and brain stem of the *Macaca mulatta*. J Comp Neurol 11:261, 1959

89. De Vriese B: Sur la signification morphologique des artères cérébrales. Arch Biol 21:357, 1904/05

90. Dick JPR, Benecke R, Rothwell JC et al: Simple and complex movements in a patient with infarction of the right supplementary area. Mov Disord 1:255, 1986

91. Dimitri V, Victoria M: Sindrome de la arteria cerebral anterior. Rev Neurol Buenos Aires 1:81, 1936

92. Dunker RO, Harris AB: Surgical anatomy of the proximal anterior cerebral artery. J Neurosurg 44:359, 1976

93. Dunsmore RH, Lennox MA: Stimulation and strychninization of supracallosal anterior cingulate gyrus. J Neurophysiol 13:207, 1950

94. Durity F, Logue V: The effect of proximal anterior cerebral occlusion on anterior communicating artery aneurysms. Post-operative radiological survey of 43 cases. J Neurosurg 35:16, 1971

95. Elsberg CA: The parasagittal meningeal fibroblastomas. Bull Neurol Inst NY 1:389, 1931

96. Erickson TC, Woolsey CN: Observations on the supplementary motor area of man. Trans Am Neurol Assoc 76:50, 1951

97. Facon E, Steriade M, Werthein N: Hypersomnie prolongée engendrée par des lesions bilaterales du système activateur médial: le syndrome thrombotique de la bifurcation du tronc basilaire. Rev Neurol 98:117, 1958

98. Falconer MA: The surgical treatment of bleeding intracranial aneurysms. J Neurol Neurosurg Psychiatry 14:153, 1951

99. Faris AA: Limbic system infarction. J Neuropathol Exp Neurol 26:174, 1967

100. Fawcett E, Blachford JV: The circle of Willis: an examination of 700 specimens. J Anat Physiol 40:63a, 1905/06

101. Feinberg TE, Schindler RJ, Flanagan NG, Haber LD: Two alien hand syndromes. Neurology 42:19, 1992

102. Ferbert A, Thron A: Bilateral anterior cerebral artery territory infarction in the differential diagnosis of basilar artery occlusion. J Neurol 239:162, 1992

103. Fischer E: Die Lageabweichungen der vorderen Hirnarterie im Gefässbild. Zentralbl Neurochir 3:300, 1938

104. Fisher CM: Hydrocephalus as a cause of disturbances of gait in the elderly. Neurology (NY) 32:1358, 1982

105. Fisher CM: Abulia minor versus agitated behavior. Clin Neurosurg 31:9, 1983

106. Fisher CM, Kistler JP, David JM: Relation of cerebral vasospasm to subarachnoid hemorrhage by computerized tomographic scanning. Neurosurgery 6:1, 1980

107. Foix C, Hillemand P: Les syndromes de l'artère cérébrale antérieure. Encephale 20:209, 1925

108. Foreman NK, Laitt RD, Chambers EJ et al: Intracranial large vessel vasculopathy and anaplastic meningioma 19 years after cranial irradiation for acute lymphoblastic leukaemia. Med Pediatr Oncol 24:265, 1995

109. Freeman FR: Akinetic mutism and bilateral anterior cerebral artery occlusion. J Neurol Neurosurg Psychiatry 34:693, 1971

110. French JD: Brain lesions associated with prolonged unconsciousness. Arch Neurol Psychiatry 68:727, 1952

111. Friedlander RM, Oglivy CS: Aneurysmal subarachnoid hemorrhage in a patient with bilateral A1 fenestrations associated with an azygous anterior cerebral artery. Case report and literature review. J Neurosurg 84:681, 1996

112. Fujimoto K, Waga S, Kojima T, Shimosaka S: Aneurysm of distal anterior cerebral artery associated with azygous anterior cerebral artery. Acta Neurochir 59:79, 1981

113. Fukui T, Hasegawa Y, Sugita K, Tsukagoshi H: Utilization behavior and concomitant motor neglect by bilateral frontal lobe damage. Eur Neurol 33:325, 1993

114. Gacs G, Fox AJ, Barnett HJM, Vinuela F: Occurrence and mechanism of occlusion of the anterior cerebral artery. Stroke 14:952, 1983

115. Gasquoine PG: Alien hand sign. J Clin Exp Neuropsychol 15:653, 1993

116. Gazzaniga MS, Bogen JE, Sperry RW: Some functional effects of sectioning the cerebral commissures in man. Proc Natl Acad Sci USA 48:1765, 1962

117. Gazzaniga MS, Bogen JE, Sperry RW: Observations on visual perception after disconnection of the cerebral hemispheres in man. Brain 88:221, 1965

118. Gazzaniga MS, Bogen JE, Sperry RW: Dyspraxia following division of the cerebral commissures. Arch Neurol 16:606, 1967

119. Gazzaniga MS, Freedman H: Observations on visual processes after posterior callosal section. Neurology (NY) 23:1126, 1973

120. Gazzaniga MS, Hillyard SA: Language and speech capacity of the right hemisphere. Neuropsychologia 9:273, 1971

121. Gazzaniga MS, LeDoux JE, Wilson DH: Language, praxis, and the right hemisphere: clues to some mechanisms of consciousness. Neurology (NY) 27:1144, 1977

122. Gazzaniga MS, Sperry RW: Language after section of the cerebral commissures. Brain 90:131, 1967

123. Gazzaniga MS, Volpe BT, Smylie CS et al: Plasticity in speech organization following commissurotomy. Brain 102:805, 1979

124. Gelmers HJ: Non-paralytic motor disturbances and speech disorders: the role of the supplementary motor area. J Neurol Neurosurg Psychiatry. 46:1052, 1983

125. Geschwind N: Disconnection syndromes in animals and man. Brain 88:237, 1965

126. Geschwind N: The apraxias: neural mechanisms of disorders of learned movement. Am Sci 63:188, 1975

127. Geschwind N, Kaplan E: A human cerebral disconnection syndrome: a preliminary report. Neurology (NY) 12:675, 1962

128. Ghika JA, Bogousslavsky J, Regli F: Deep perforators from the carotid system: template of the vascular territories. Arch Neurol 47:1097, 1990

129. Ghika J, Bogousslavsky J, van Melle, Regli F: Hyperkinetic motor behaviors contralateral to hemiplegia in acute stroke. Eur Neurol 35:27, 1995

130. Gillilan LA: The arterial and venous blood supplies to the forebrain (including the internal capsule) of primates. Neurology (NY) 18:653, 1968

131. Gillingham FJ: The management of ruptured intracranial aneurysms. Ann R Coll Surg Engl 23:89, 1958

132. Giroud M, Creisson E, Fayolle H et al: Homolateral ataxia and crural paresis: a crossed cerebral-cerebellar diaschisis. J Neurol Neurosurg Psychiatry 57:221, 1994

133. Goldberg G, Mayer NH, Toglia JU: Medial frontal cortex infarction and the alien hand sign. Arch Neurol 38:683, 1981

134. Goldenberg G: Neglect in a patient with partial callosal disconnection. Neuropsychologia 24:397, 1986

135. Goldstein K: Zur Lehre von der motorischen Apraxie. J Psychol Neurol 11:169, 270, 1908

136. Goldstein K: Der makroskopiesche Befund in meinem Fall v. Linksseiter motorischen Apraxie. Zentralbl Neurol 28:898, 1909

137. Gomes F, Dujouny M, Umansky F et al: Microsurgical anatomy of the recurrent artery of Heubner. J Neurosurg 60:130, 1984

138. Gorczyca W, Mohr G: Microvascular anatomy of Heubner's recurrent artery. Neurol Res 9:254, 1987

139. Gordon HW, Bogen JE, Sperry RW: Absence of deconnection syndrome in two patients with partial section of the neocommissures. Brain 94:327, 1971

140. Grafman J, Vance SC, Weingartner H et al: The effects of lateralized frontal lesions on mood regulation. Brain 109:1127, 1986

141. Greene KA, Marciano FF, Dickman CA et al: Anterior communicating artery aneurysm paraparesis syndrome: clinical manifestations and pathologic correlates. Neurology 45:45, 1995

142. Gugliotta MA, Silvestri R, DeDomenico P, Galatioto S: Spontaneous bilateral anterior cerebral artery occlusion resulting in akinetic mutism: a case report. Acta Neurol (Napoli) 11:252, 1989

143. Guidetti B: Désordres de la parole associés à des lésions de la surface interhémisphérique frontale postérieure. Rev Neurol 97:121, 1957

144. Halsband U, Ito N, Tanji J, Freund H-J: The role of premotor cortex and the supplementary motor area in the temporal control of movement in man. Brain 116:243, 1993

145. Hanakita J, Nagayasu S, Nishi S, Suzuki T: An aneurysm of the distal anterior cerebral artery with a remarkably anomalous configuration. No Shinkei Geka 16:781, 1988

146. Hashizume K, Nukui H, Horikoshi T et al: Giant aneurysm of the azygous anterior cerebral artery associated with acute subdural hematoma—case report. Neurol Med Chir (Tokyo) 32:693, 1992

147. Hassler W, Zentner J, Voigt K: Abnormal origin of the ophthalmic artery from the anterior cerebral artery: neuroradiological and intraoperative findings. Neuroradiology 31:85, 1989

148. Hayakawa T, Waltz AG: Immediate effects of cerebral ischemia. Evolution and resolution of neurological deficits after experimental occlusion of one middle cerebral artery in conscious cats. Stroke 6:321, 1975

149. Hayakawa T, Waltz AG: On the importance of the anterior cerebral artery. Stroke 7:523, 1976

150. Hecaen H, Gimeno-Alava A: L'apraxie idéomotrice unilatérale gauche. Rev Neurol 102:648, 1960

151. Hegenholtz H, Morley TP: The results of proximal anterior cerebral artery occlusion for anterior communicating aneurysms. J Neurosurg 37:65, 1972

152. Heilman KM, Bowers D, Watson RT: Pseudoneglect in a patient with partial callosal disconnection. Brain 107:519, 1984

153. Heliman KM, Coyle JM, Gonyea EF, Geschwind N: Apraxia and agraphia in a left-hander. Brain 96:21, 1973

154. Heubner O: Zur Topographie der Ernährungsgebiete der einzelnen Hirnarterien. Zentralbl Med Wissenschaften 10:817, 1872

155. Hill A, Volpe J: Decrease in pulsatile flow in the anterior cerebral arteries in infantile hydrocephalus. Pediatrics 69:4, 1982

156. Hyland HH: Thrombosis of intracranial arteries: report of three cases involving, respectively the anterior cerebral, basilar and internal carotid arteries. Arch Neurol Psychiatry 30:342, 1933

157. Ingvar DH, Philipson L, Torlof P, Ardo A: The average rCBF pattern of resting consciousness studied with a new colour display system. Acta Neurol Scand, suppl. 64, 56:252, 1977

158. Ingvar DH, Schwartz MS: Blood flow patterns induced in the dominant hemisphere by speech and reading. Brain 97:273, 1974

159. Iragui VJ: Ataxic hemiparesis associated with transcortical motor aphasia. Eur Neurol 30:162, 1990

160. Isherwood I, Dutton J: Unusual anomaly of anterior cerebral artery. Acta Radiol [Diagn] (Stockh) 9:345, 1969

161. Ishibashi A, Kubota Y, Yokokura Y et al: Traumatic occlusion of the anterior cerebral artery—case report. Neurol Med Chir (Tokyo) 35:882, 1995

162. Islak C, Ogut G, Numan F et al: Persistent nonmigrated ventral primitive ophthalmic artery. J Neuroradiol 21:46, 1994

163. Ito J, Washiyama K, Kim CH, Ibuchi Y: Fenestration of the anterior cerebral artery. Neuroradiology 21:277, 1981

164. Iwata M, Sugishita M, Toyokura Y et al: Étude sur le syndrome de disconnection visuo-lingual après le transéction du splenium du corps calleux. J Neurol Sci 23:421, 1974

165. Jackson JH: Localized convulsions from tumour of the brain. Brain 5:364, 1882

166. Janowsky JS, Shimamura AP, Kritchevsky M, Squire LR: Cognitive impairment following frontal lobe damage and its relevance to human amnesia. Behav Neurosci 103:548, 1989

167. Jeeves MA, Simpson DA, Geffen G: Functional consequences of the transcollosal removal of intraventricular tumours. J Neurol Neurosurg Psychiatry 42:134, 1979

168. Jonas S: The supplementary motor region and speech emission. J Commun Disord 14:349, 1981

169. Jones EG, Coulter JD, Burton H, Porter R: Cells of origin and terminal distribution of corticostriatal fibers arising in the sensory-motor cortex of monkeys. J Comp Neurol 173:53, 1977

170. Jones EG, Coulter JD, Hendry SHC: Intracortical connectivity of architectonic fields in the somatic sensory, motor, and parietal cortex of monkeys. J Comp Neurol 181:291, 1978

171. Jones EG, Powell TPS: Connections of the somatic sensory cortex of the rhesus monkey. I. Ipsilateral cortical connections. Brain 92:477, 1969

172. Kaada BR, Pribram K, Epstein JA: Respiratory and vascular responses in monkeys from temporal pole, insular, orbital surface, and cingulate gyrus. J Neurophysiol 12: 347, 1949

173. Kamijyo Y, Garcia JH: Carotid arterial supply of the feline brain: applications to the study of regional cerebral ischemia. Stroke 6:361, 1975

174. Kaplan HA: Vascular supply of the base of the brain. p. 138. In Fields WS (ed): Pathogenesis and Treatment of Parkinsonism. Charles C Thomas, Springfield, IL, 1958

175. Kashiwagi A, Kashiwagi T, Nishikawa T et al: Hemispacial neglect in a patient with callosal infarction. Brain 113:1005, 1990

176. Katz RS, Horoupian DS, Zingesser L: Aneurysm of azygous anterior cerebral artery: a case report. J Neurosurg 48:804, 1978

177. Kazui S, Sawada T, Kuriyama Y et al: A clinical study of patients with cerebral infarction localized in the territory of anterior cerebral artery. Jpn J Stroke 9:317, 1987

178. Kazui S, Sawada T, Naritomi H: Angiographic evaluation of brain infarction limited to the anterior cerebral artery territory. Stroke 24:549, 1993

179. Kennard M: The cingulate gyrus in relation to consciousness. J Nerv Ment Dis 121:34, 1955

180. Kertesz A, Lesk D, McCabe P: Isotope localization of infarcts in aphasia. Arch Neurol 34:590, 1977

181. Kidooka M, Okada T, Sonabe M et al: Dissecting aneurysm of the anterior cerebral artery: report of two cases. Surg Neurol 39:53, 1993

182. Kimura D: Neuromotor mechanisms in the evolution of human communication. p. 197. In Steklin HD, Raleigh MJ (eds): Neurobiology of Social Communication in Primates. Academic Press, San Diego, CA, 1979

183. Kimura D, Archibald Y: Motor functions of the left hemisphere. Brain 97:337, 1974

184. Kimura D, Archibald Y: Acquisition of a motor skill after left hemisphere damage. Brain 100:527, 1977

185. Kirgis HD, Fisher WL, Llewellyn RC, Peebles EM: Aneurysms of the anterior communicating artery and gross anomalies of the circle of Willis. J Neurosurg 25:73, 1966

186. Klein SI, Gahbauer H, Goodrich I: Bilateral anomalous anterior cerebral artery and infraoptic aneurysm. AJNR 8:1142, 1987

187. Kleiss E: Die verschiedenen Formen des circulus arteriosus cerebralis Willisi. Anat Anz 92:216, 1942

188. Kornyey E: Aphasie transcorticale et écholalie: le problème de l'initiative de la parole. Rev Neurol 131:347, 1975

189. Krayenbuhl HA, Yasargil MS: Cerebral Angiography. 2nd Ed. Lippincott-Raven, Philadelphia, 1968

190. Kruyt RC: Aplasia of the anterior cerebral arteries: angiographic study of a case. Neurochirurgia 14:172, 1971

191. Kunzle H: Bilateral projections from precentral motor cortex to the putamen and other parts of the basal ganglia: an autoradiographic study in *Macaca fascicularis*. Brain Res 88:195, 1975

192. Lacruz F, Artieda J, Pastor MA, Obeso JA: The anatomical basis of somaesthetic temporal discrimination in humans. J Neurol Neurosurg Psychiatry 54:1077, 1991

193. Landau WM, Clare MH: Pathophysiology of the tonic innervation phenomenon of the foot. Arch Neurol 15: 252, 1966

194. Laplane D, Talairach J, Meininger J et al: Clinical consequences of corticectomies involving the supplementary motor area in man. J Neurol Sci 34:301, 1977

195. Larson B, Skinhoj E, Larsen NA: Variations in regional cortical blood flow in the right and left hemispheres during automatic speech. Brain 101:193, 1978

196. Larsson C, Forssell A, Ronnberg J et al: Subarachnoid blood on CT and memory dysfunction in aneurysmal subarachnoid hemorrhage. Acta Neurol Scand 90:331, 1994

197. Lasjaunias P, Vignaud J, Clay C: Radioanatomie de la vascularisation artérielle de l'orbite, à l'éxception du tronc de l'artère ophtalmique. Ann Radiol 18:181, 1975

198. Lassen NA, Roland PE, Larsen B et al: Mapping of human cerebral functions: a study of the regional cerebral blood flow pattern during rest, its reproducibility and the activation seen during basic sensory and motor functions. Acta Neurol Scand, suppl 64, 56:262, 1977

199. Lazorthes G, Anduze-Acher H, Coll J: Empyème sousdural intérhémisphérique (considérations sur les centres inhibiteurs de la face interne des hémisphères). Rev Otoneuroophtalmol 26:149, 1954

200. Lazorthes G, Bastide G, Gomes FA: Les variations du trajet de la carotide interne d'après une étude artériographe. Arch Anat Pathol 9:129, 1961

201. Lazorthes G, Gaubert J, Poulhes J: La distribution centrale et corticale de l'artère cérébrale antérieure: étude anatomique et incidences neuro-chirurgicales. Neurochirurgie 2:237, 1956

202. Lechi A, Marchi G: Nécrose méso-diencephalique au cours d'une méningo-encephalite subaiguë: observation anatomoclinique. Acta Neurol Belg 67:475, 1967

203. Lehmann G, Vincentelli F, Ebagosti A: Anomalies rares du polygone de Willis: le trajet infraoptique des artères cérébrales antérieures. Neurochirurgie 26:243, 1980

204. Lehrer HZ: Relative calibre of the cervical internal carotid artery. Normal variation with the circle of Willis. Brain 91:339, 1968

205. LeMay M, Gooding CA: The clinical significance of the azygous anterior cerebral artery (ACA). AJR 98:602, 1966

206. Lesem WW: The comparative anatomy of the anterior cerebral artery. Postgrad Med 20:445, 1905

207. Levin HS, Goldstein FC, Ghostine SY et al: Hemispheric disconnection syndrome persisting after anterior cerebral artery aneurysm rupture. Neurosurgery 21:831, 1987

208. Levy AS, Lillehei KO, Rubinstein D, Stears JC: Subarachnoid neurocysticercosis with occlusion of the major intracranial arteries: case report. Neurosurgery 36:183, 1995

209. Lhermitte F, Gautier JC, Marteau R, Chain F: Troubles de la conscience et mutisme akinetique: étude anatomoclinique d'un ramollissement paramedian bilateral du pedoncule cérébral et du thalamus. Rev Neurol 109:115, 1963

210. Lhermitte F, Pillon B, Serdaru M: Human anatomy and the frontal lobes. Part I. Imitation and utilization behav-

ior: a neuropsychological study of 75 patients. Ann Neurol 19:326, 1986

211. Lhermitte J, Schiff P: Le phénomène de la préhension forcée, expression d'un ramollissement complet de la première circonvolution frontale. Rev Neurol 35:175, 1928

212. Lhermitte J, Schiff P, Curtois A: Le phénomène de la préhension forcée, expression d'un ramollissement complet de la première convolution frontale. Rev Neurol 15:1218, 1907

213. Liepmann H, Maas O: Fall von linksseitiger Agraphie und Apraxie bei rechtsseitiger Lähmung. J Psychol Neurol 10:214, 1907

214. Zeal AA, Rhoton AL: Microsurgical anatomy of the posterior cerebral artery. J Neurosurg 48:534, 1978

215. Lin J, Kirsheff I: Normal anterior cerebral artery complex, p. 1319. In Newton TH, Potts DG (eds): Radiology of the Skull and Brain. Vol. 2, Book 2. CV Mosby, St. Louis, 1974

216. Lindenberg R: Patterns of CNS vulnerability in acute hypoxemia including anesthesia accidents. p. 189. In Shade JP, McMenemey WH (eds): Selective Vulnerability of the Brain in Hypoxemia. FA Davis, Philadelphia, 1963

217. Lloyd T Jr: Effect of stroke on lung function and the pulmonary circulation. p. 371. In Price TR, Nelson E (eds): Cerebrovascular Diseases. Proceedings of the Eleventh Research Conference.

218. Löhr W: Erkrankungen des Hirngefässe in arteriographischer Darstellung. Arch Klin Chir 186:298, 1936

219. Löhr W, Jacobi W: Gefässkrankheiten des Gehirns in arteriographischer Darstellung. Arch Klin Chir 177:510, 1933

220. Long E: Contributions à l'étude des fonctions de la zone motrice du cerveau. Rev Neurol 15:1218, 1907

221. Long E: Monoplegia crurale, par lésion du lobule paracentrale. Nouv Icon Salpetr 21:37, 1908

222. Lucchelli F, DeRenzi E: Primary dyscalculia after a medial frontal lesion of the left hemisphere. J Neurol Neurosurg Psychiatry 56:304, 1993

223. Luria AR: Traumatic Aphasia. Mouton, The Hague, 1970

224. Luria AR: Disturbances of memory and consciousness after rupture of an aneurysm of the anterior communicating artery. p. 255. In Luria AR (ed): The Neuropsychology of Memory. Wiley, New York, 1976

225. Luria AR, Tsvetkova LS: Towards the mechanism of "dynamic aphasia." Acta Neurol Belg 67:1045, 1967

226. Maas O: Ein Fall von linksseitiger Apraxie und Agraphie. Zentralbel Neurol 26:789, 1907

227. Macpherson JM, Marangoz C, Miles TS, Wiesendanger M: Microstimulation of the supplementary motor area (SMA) in the awake monkey. Exp Brain Res 45:410, 1982

228. Magnan. On simple aphasia, and aphasia with incoherence. Brain 2:112, 1879/1880

229. Marie P, Foix C: Paraplégie en flexion d'origine cérébrale par nécrose sous épendymaire progressive. Rev Neurol 27:1, 1920

230. Marinkovic S, Kovacevic M, Milisavljevic M: Hypoplasia of the proximal segment of the anterior cerebral artery. Anat Anz 168:145, 1989

231. Marino R: The anterior cerebral artery. I. Anatomo-radiological study of its cortical territories. Surg Neurol 5:81, 1976

232. Masdeu JC: Language disturbance after mesial frontal infarction. Neurology (NY), suppl. 2, 33:243, 1983

233. Masdeu JC, Schoene WC, Funkenstein H: Aphasia following infarction of the left supplementary motor area: a clinical pathological study. Neurology (NY) 28:1220, 1978

234. Maspes PE: Le syndrome expérimental chez l'homme de la section du splenium du corps calleus. Alexie visuelle pure hémianopique. Rev Neurol 80:100, 1948

235. Mathew NT, Hartmann A, Meyer JS et al: The importance of "CSF pressure-regulated cerebral blood flow dysregulation" in the pathogenesis of normal pressure hydrocephalus. p. 145. In Lundberg N, Panton V, Brock M (eds): Intracranial Pressure Two: Proceedings. Springer-Verlag, New York, 1975

236. McCormick WF: A unique anomaly of the intracranial arteries of man. Neurology (NY) 10:77, 1969

237. McNabb AW, Carroll WM, Mastaglia FL: "Alien hand" and loss of bimanual coordination after dominant anterior cerebral artery territory infarction. J Neurol Neurosurg Psychiatry 51:218, 1988

238. Meador KJ, Watson RT, Bowers D, Heilman KM: Hypometria with hemispacial and limb motor neglect. Brain 109:293, 1986

239. Mendez MF, Adams NL, Lewandowski KS: Neurobehavioral changes associated with caudate lesions. Neurology (NY) 39:349, 1989

240. Mercier P, Velvt S, Fournier D et al: A rare embryologic variation: carotid-anterior cerebral artery anastomosis or infraoptic course of the anterior cerebral artery. Surg Radiol Anat 11:73, 1989

241. Meyer JS, Barron DW: Apraxia of gait: a clinicophysiological study. Brain 83:261, 1960

242. Milenkovic Z: Anastomosis between internal carotid artery and anterior cerebral artery with other anomalies of the circle of Willis in a fetal brain. J Neurosurg 55:701, 1981

243. Mishima H, Kim YK, Shiomi K et al: Ruptured anterior communicating artery aneurysm associated with interoptic course of anterior cerebral artery; report of a case and review of the literature. No Shinkei Geka Neurol Surg 22:495, 1994

244. Molinari GF, Moseley JI, Laurent JP: Segmental middle cerebral artery occlusion in primates: an experimental method requiring minimal surgery and anesthesia. Stroke 5:334, 1974

245. Moniz E: Die Cerebral Arteriographie und Phlebographie. Springer-Verlag, Berlin, 1940

246. Morris AA, Peck CM: Roentgenographic study of variation in normal anterior cerebral artery. One hundred cases studied in the lateral plane. AJR 74:818, 1955

247. Moscow N, Michotey P, Salamon G: Anatomy of the cortical branches of the anterior cerebral artery, p. 1411. In Newton TH, Potts DG (eds): Radiology of the Skull and Brain. Vol. 2, Book 2. CV Mosby, St. Louis, 1974

248. Moulin T, Bogousslavsky J, Chopard JL et al: Vascular

ataxic hemiparesis: a reevaluation. J Neurol Neurosurg Psychiatry 58:422, 1995

249. Munk H: Über die Functionen der Grosshirnrinde: Gesammelte Mitteilungen aus den Jahren 1877–80, mit Einleitung und Anmerkungen. Hirschwald, Berlin, 1881

250. Murray EA, Coulter JD: Organization of corticospinal neurons in the monkey. J Comp Neurol 195:339, 1981

251. Myers R: Dandy's striatal theory of "the center of consciousness." Surgical evidence and logical analysis indicating its improbability. Arch Neurol Psychiatry 65:659, 1951

252. Nagumo T, Yamadori A: Callosal disconnection syndrome and knowledge of the body: a case of left hand isolation from the body schema with names. J Neurol Neurosurg Psychiatry 59:548, 1995

253. Nielsen JM: Agnosia, Apraxia, Aphasia. 2nd Ed. Hoeber, New York, 1946

254. Nielsen JM, Jacobs LL: Bilateral lesions of the anterior cingulate gyri. Bull Los Angeles Neurol Soc 16:231, 1951

255. Niizuma H, Kwak R, Uchida K, Susuki J: Aneurysms of the azygous anterior cerebral artery. Surg Neurol 15:225, 1980

256. Nornes H, Wikeby P: Cerebral arterial blood flow and aneurysm surgery. 1. Local arterial flow dynamics. J Neurosurg 47:810, 1977

257. Nutic S, Dilence D: Carotid-anterior cerebral artery anastomosis: case report. J Neurosurg 44:378, 1976

258. Oba M, Suzuki M, Onuma T: Two cases of ruptured fusiform aneurysm of the proximal anterior cerebral artery (A1 segment). No Shinkei Geka 17:365, 1989

259. Odake G: Carotid-anterior cerebral artery anastomosis with aneurysm: case report and review of the literature. Neurosurgery (NY) 23:654, 1988

260. Ogasawara H, Inagawa T, Yamamoto M, Kamiya K: Aneurysm in a fenestrated anterior cerebral artery—case report. Neurol Med Chir 28:575, 1988

261. Ogawa A, Suzuki M, Sakurai Y, Yashimoto T: Vascular anomalies associated with aneurysms of the anterior communicating artery: microsurgical observations. J Neurosurg 72:706, 1990

262. Orgogozo JM, Larsen B: Activation of the supplementary motor area during voluntary movement in man suggests it works as a supramotor area. Science 206:847, 1979

263. Osaka K, Matsumoto S: Holoprosencephaly in neurosurgical practice. J Neurosurg 48:787, 1978

264. Ostrowski AZ, Webster JE, Gurdjian ES: The proximal anterior cerebral artery: an anatomic study. Arch Neurol 3:661, 1960

265. Padget DH: The circle of Willis. Its embryology and anatomy. p. 67. In Dandy WE (ed): Intracranial Arterial Aneurysms. Comstock, Ithaca, NY, 1945

266. Padget DH: The development of the cranial arteries in the human embryo. Contrib Embryol 32:205, 1948

267. Paillard J: À propos de la négligence motrice: issues et perspectives. Rev Neurol 146:600, 1990

268. Parkin AJ, Leng NRC, Stanhope N, Smith AP: Memory impairment following ruptured aneurysm of the anterior communicating artery. Brain Cogn 7:231, 1988

269. Patricolo A, Chiappetta F, Esposito S, Gazzeri G: Complicanze ipotalamiche nel trattamento chirurgio degli aneurismi della communicante anteriore. Minerva Neurochir 15:146, 1971

270. Paus T, Kalina M, Patockova L et al: Medial vs lateral frontal lobe lesions and differential impairment of central-gaze fixation in man. Brain 114:2051, 1991

271. Penfield W: The cerebral cortex in man. I. The cerebral cortex and consciousness. Arch Neurol Psychiatry 40:417, 1938

272. Penfield W, Boldrey E: Somatic motor and sensory representation in cerebral cortex of man as studied by electrical stimulation. Brain 60:384, 1937

273. Penfield W, Jasper H: Epilepsy and the Functional Anatomy of the Human Brain. Little, Brown, Boston, 1954

274. Penfield W, Rasmussen T: Vocalization and arrest of speech. Arch Neurol Psychiatry 61:21, 1949

275. Penfield W, Rasmussen T: The Cerebral Cortex of Man: A Clinical Study of Localization of Function. Macmillan, New York, 1950

276. Penfield W, Roberts L: Speech and Brain Mechanisms. Princeton University Press, Princeton, NJ, 1969

277. Penfield W, Welch K: The supplementary motor area, in the cerebral cortex of man. Trans Am Neurol Assoc 74:179, 1949.

278. Penfield W, Welch K: The supplementary motor area of the cerebral cortex: a clinical and experimental study. Arch Neurol Psychiatry 66:289, 1951

279. Perlmutter D, Rhoton AL: Microsurgical anatomy of the anterior cerebral–anterior communicating–recurrent artery complex. J Neurosurg 45:259, 1976

280. Perlmutter D, Rhoton AL: Microsurgical anatomy of the distal anterior cerebral artery. J Neurosurg 49:204, 1978

281. Petit-Dutaillis D, Guiot G, Messimy R, Bourdillon C: À propos d'une aphémie par atteinte de la zone motrice supplémentaire de Penfield, au cours de l'évolution d'un aneurisme artérioveineux: guérison de l'aphémie par l'ablation de la lesion. Rev Neurol 90:95, 1954

282. Phillips S, Sangalang V, Sterns G: Basal forebrain infarction: a clinicopathologic correlation. Arch Neurol 44:1134, 1987

283. Pitres A: Considerations sur l'agraphie. Rev Med 4:855, 1884

284. Plum P, Posner J: The Diagnosis of Stupor and Coma. 3rd Ed. FA Davis, Philadelphia, 1980

285. Pool JL: Aneurysms of the anterior communicating artery. Bifrontal craniotomy and routine use of temporary clips. J Neurosurg 18:98, 1961

286. Poppen JL: Ligation of the left anterior cerebral artery: its hazards and means of avoidance of its complications. Arch Neurol Psychiatry 41:495, 1939

287. Pozzati E, Galassi E, Godano U, Cordella L: Regressing intracranial carotid occlusions in childhood. Pediatr Neurosurg 21:243, 1994

288. Racy A, Jannotta FS, Lehner LH: Aphasia resulting from occlusion of the left anterior cerebral artery: report of a case with an old infarct in the left rolandic region. Arch Neurol 36:221, 1979

289. Reichert T: Die Arteriographie der Hirngefässe. JF Lehmann, Berlin, 1943

290. Reivich M: Embryology, anatomy, and pathophysiology of the cerebral circulation. p. 749. In Goldensohn ES,

Appel SH (eds): Scientific Approaches to Clinical Neurology. Lea & Febiger, Philadelphia, 1977

291. Richter CP, Hines M: Experimental production of the grasp reflex in adult monkeys by lesions of the frontal lobes. Am J Physiol 101:87, 1932

292. Rieke GK, Bowers DE, Penn P: Vascular supply pattern to rat caudatoputamen and globus pallidus: scanning electronmicroscopic study of vascular endocasts of stroke-prone vessels. Stroke 12:840, 1981

293. Riggs HE, Rupp C: Variation in form of circle of Willis. Arch Neurol 8:8, 1963

294. Ring BA, Waddington MM: Roentgenographic anatomy of the pericallosal arteries. AJR 104:109, 1968

295. Risso M, Poeck K, Creutzfeld O, Pilleri G: Katamnestische Untersuchungen nach frontaler Leukotomie. I. Klinische Beobachtungen. II. Anatomischklinische Korrelationen. Bibl Psychiatr Neurol 116:1, 1962

296. Robinson LR: An unusual human anterior cerebral artery. J Anat 93:131, 1959

297. Rodda RA: The arterial patterns associated with internal carotid disease and cerebral infarcts. Stroke 17:69, 1986

298. Roland PE, Larsen B, Lassen NA, Skinhoj E: Supplementary motor areas in organization of voluntary movements in man. J Neurophysiol 43:118, 1980

299. Roland PE, Meyer E, Shibasaki T et al: Regional cerebral blood flow changes in cortex and basal ganglia during voluntary movements in normal human volunteers. J Neurophysiol 48:467, 1982

300. Roland PE, Skinhoj E, Lassen NA, Larsen B: Different cortical areas in man in organization of voluntary movements in extrapersonal space. J Neurophysiol 43:137, 1980

301. Ross ED: Left medial parietal lobe and receptive language functions: mixed transcortical aphasia after left anterior cerebral artery infarction. Neurology (NY) 30:144, 1980

302. Rothfus WE, Goldberg AL, Tabas JH, Deeb ZL: Callosomarginal infarction secondary to transfalcial herniation. AJNR 8:1073, 1987

303. Rubens AB: Aphasia with infarction in the territory of the anterior cerebral artery. Cortex 11:239, 1975

304. Ruggiero G: Factors influencing the filling of the anterior cerebral artery in angiography. Acta Radiol 37:87, 1952

305. Ryding E, Bradvik B, Ingvar DH: Changes of regional cerebral blood flow measured simultaneously in the right and left hemisphere during automatic speech and humming. Brain 110:1345, 1987

306. Sabouraud O, Pecker J: Suspension de langage non aphasique après intervention sur la region interhémisphérique. Rev Otoneuroophtalmol 1:42, 1960

307. Saita I, Shigeno T, Aritake K et al: Vasospasm assessed by angiography and computerized tomography. J Neurosurg 51:466, 1979

308. Sakai K, Asari S, Fujisawa M, Katagi R: Ruptured aneurysm arising from the anomalous anterior cerebral artery—case report. Neurol Med Chir (Tokyo) 32:846, 1992

309. Salamon G, Huang YP: Radiologic Anatomy of the Brain. Springer-Verlag, Berlin, 1976

310. Satoh J, Miyasaka N, Yamada T et al: Extensive cerebral

infarction due to involvement of both anterior cerebral arteries by Wegener's granulomatosis. Ann Rheum Dis 47:606, 1988

311. Schell G, Hodge CJ, Cacayorin E: Transient neurological deficit after therapeutic embolization of the arteries supplying the medial wall of the hemisphere, including the supplementary motor area. Neurosurgery 18:353, 1986

312. Schick RM, Rumbaugh CL: Saccular aneurysm of the azygous anterior cerebral artery. AJNR, suppl. 10:S73, 1989

313. Schneider R, Gautier J-C: Leg weakness due to stroke. Site of lesions, weakness patterns and causes. Brain 117:347, 1994

314. Schott B, Michel F, Michel D, Dumas R: Apraxie idéomotrice unilatérale gauche avec main gauche anomique: syndrome de déconnection calleuse? Rev Neurol 120:359, 1969

315. Schuster P: Zwangsgreifen u. Nachgreifen, zweiposthemisplegische Bewegungsstörungen. Z Ges Neurol Psychiatr 83:586, 1923

316. Schuster P: Autoptische Befunde bei Zwangsgreifen u. Nachgreifen. Z Ges Neurol Psychiatr 108:751, 1927

317. Schuster P, Pinéas M: Weitere Beobachtungen über Zwangsgreifen u. Nachgreifen u. deren Bezeihungen zu ahnlichen Bewegungsstorungen. Dtsch Z Nervenheilkd 91:16, 1926

318. Schwab O: Über vorübergehende aphasische Störungen nach Rindenexzision aus dem linken Stirnhirn bei Epileptikern. Dtsch Z Nervenheilkd 94:177, 1926

319. Scott M: Ligation of an anterior cerebral artery for aneurysms of the anterior communicating artery complex. J Neurosurg 38:481, 1973

320. Segarra JM: Cerebral vascular disease and behavior. I. The syndrome of the mesencephalic artery (basilar artery bifurcation). Arch Neurol 22:408, 1970

321. Segundo JP, Naquet R, Buser P: Cortical stimulation in monkeys. J Neurophysiol 18:236, 1955

322. Selman J, Dujovny M, Vasquez M et al: Microanatomical basis for lenticulostriate surgery. In: Microsurgery for Cerebral Ischemia. Proceedings of the Ninth International Symposium. Springer-Verlag, Vienna, 1990

323. Sengupta RP: Direct surgery of anterior communicating aneurysms and its effect on intellect and personality. J Neurol Neurosurg Psychiatry 38:406, 1975

324. Senter HJ, Miller DJ: Interoptic course of the anterior cerebral artery associated with anterior cerebral artery aneurysm: case report. J Neurosurg 56:302, 1982

325. Seyffarth H, Denny-Brown D: The grasp reflex and the instinctive grasp reaction. Brain 71:9, 1948

326. Shellshear JC: The basal arteries of the forebrain and their functional significance. J Anat 55:27, 1920

327. Shimauchi M, Kaji Y, Goya T, Kinoshita K: A case report of fibromuscular dysplasia presenting symptoms like moyamoya disease: "string of beads" appearance of the pericallosal artery. No Shinkei Geta 17:981, 1989

328. Shiokawa K, Tanikawa T, Satoh K et al: Two cases of giant aneurysms arising from the distal segment of the anterior cerebral circulation. No Shinkei Geka Neurol Surg 21:467, 1993

329. Sidtsi JJ, Volpe BT, Holtzman JD et al: Cognitive inter-

action after staged callosal section: evidence for transfer of semantic activation. Science 212:344, 1981

330. Sidtis JJ, Volpe BT, Wilson DH et al: Variability in right hemisphere language function after callosal section: evidence for a continuum of generative capacity. J Neurosci 1:323, 1981

331. Sine RD, Soufi A, Shah M: Callosal syndrome: implications for understanding the neuropsychology of stroke. Arch Phys Med Rehab 65:606, 1984

332. Skultety FM: Clinical and experimental aspects of akinetic mutism: report of a case. Arch Neurol 19:1, 1968

333. Smith AM: The activity of supplementary motor area neurons during a maintained precision grip. Brain Res 172:315, 1979

334. Smith AM, Bourbonnais D, Blanchette G: Interaction between forced grasping and learned precision grip after ablation of the supplementary motor area. Brain Res 222:395, 1981

335. Smith WK: The functional significance of the rostral cingular cortex as revealed by its responses to electrical excitation. J Neurophysiol 8:241, 1945

336. Snyckers FD, Drake CG: Aneurysms of the distal anterior cerebral artery: a report on 24 verified cases. S Afr Med J 47:1787, 1973

337. Spencer SS: Corpus callosum section and other disconnection procedures for medically intractable epilepsy. Epilepsia, suppl. 2, 29:S85, 1988

338. Sperry RW, Gazzaniga MS: Language following surgical disconnection of the hemispheres. In Millikan CH (ed): Brain Mechanisms Underlying Speech and Language. Grune & Stratton, New York, 1966

339. Sperry RW, Gazzaniga MS, Bogen JE: Interhemispheric relationships: the neocortical commissures; syndromes of hemispheric disconnection. p. 273. In Vinken PJ, Bruyn GW (eds): Holland Publishing, Amsterdam, 1966

340. Starkstein SE, Robinson RG, Berthier ML et al: Differential mood changes following basal ganglia vs thalamic lesions. Arch Neurol 45:725, 1988

341. Stebbens WE: Aneurysms and anatomic variation of cerebral arteries. Arch Pathol 75:45, 1963

342. Stephens RB, Stilwell DL: Arteries and Veins of the Human Brain. Charles C Thomas, Springfield, IL, 1969

343. Stewart RM, Williams RS, Luhl P, Schoenen J: Ventral porencephaly: a cerebral defect associated with multiple congenital anomalies. Acta Neuropathol 42:231, 1978

344. Stuss DT, Alexander MP, Lieberman A, Levine H: An extraordinary form of confabulation. Neurology (NY) 28:1166, 1978

345. Stuss DT, Benson DF: Neuropsychological studies of the frontal lobes. Psychol Bull 95:3, 1984

346. Sugishita M, Iwata M, Toyokura Y et al: Reading ideograms and phonograms in Japanese patients after partial commissurotomy. Neuropsychologia 16:417, 1978

347. Sussman NM, Gur RC, Gur RE, O'Connor MJ: Mutism as a consequence of callosectomy. J Neurosurg 59:514, 1983

348. Suzuki M, Onuma T, Sakurai Y, et al: Aneurysms arising from the proximal (A1) segment of the anterior cerebral artery. A study of 38 cases. J Neurosurg 76:55, 1992

349. Swanson TH, Zinkel JL, Peterson PL: Bilateral anterior cerebral artery occlusion in an alcohol abuser with sickle cell trait. Henry Ford Hosp Med J 35:67, 1987

350. Szdzuy D, Lehmann R, Nickel B: Common trunk of the anterior cerebral arteries. Neuroradiology 4:51, 1972

351. Tacconi L, Johnston FG, Symon L: Accessory middle cerebral artery. Case report. J Neurosurg 83:916, 1995

352. Takashima S, Tanaka K: Development of cerebrovascular architecture and its relationship to periventricular leukomalacia. Arch Neurol 35:11, 1978

353. Takeuchi K, Hara M, Yokata H et al: Factors influencing the development of moyamoya phenomenon. Acta Neurochir 59:79, 1981

354. Talairach J, Bancaud J: The supplementary motor area in man. Int J Neurol 5:330, 1966

355. Talland GA, Sweet WH, Ballantine HT: Amnestic syndrome with anterior communicating artery aneurysm. J Nerv Ment Dis 145:179, 1967

356. Tanaka Y, Iwasa H, Yoshida M: Diagonistic dyspraxia. Case report and movement-related potentials. Neurology 40:657, 1990

357. Tanaka S, Mori T, Ohara H et al: Gastrointestinal bleeding in cases of ruptured cerebral aneurysms. Acta Neurochir 48:223, 1979

358. Tanji J, Kurata K: Neuronal activity in the cortical supplementary motor area related with distal and proximal forelimb movements. Neurosci Lett 12:201, 1979

359. Tanji J, Kurata K: Comparison of movement-related activity in two cortical motor areas of primates. J Neurophysiol 48:633, 1982

360. Tanji J, Taniguchi K, Saga T: Supplementary motor area: neuronal responses to motor instructions. J Neurophysiol 43:60, 1980

361. Tatemichi TK, Desmond DW, Patik M et al: Clinical determinants of dementia related to stroke. Ann Neurol 33:568, 1993

362. Thompson FJ, Campbell ML: Arterial supply of the feline motor cortex. Stroke 12:233, 1981

363. Thompson GN: Cerebral area essential to consciousness. Bull Los Angeles Neurol Soc 16:311, 1951

364. Tichy F: The syndromes of the cerebral arteries. Arch Pathol 48:475, 1949

365. Tindall GT: The treatment of anterior communicating aneurysms by proximal anterior cerebral artery ligation. Clin Neurosurg 21:134, 1974

366. Tindall GT, Kapp J, Odom GL, Robinson SC: A combined technique for treating certain aneurysms of the anterior communicating artery. J Neurosurg 33:41, 1970

367. Tonnis W, Brandt P, Walter W: The roentgenological diagnosis of tumors of the corpus callosum: with a contribution to the normal roentgenological anatomy of the anterior cerebral artery. J Neurosurg 17:183, 1966

368. Tow PM, Whitty CWM: Personality changes after operations on the cingulate gyrus in man. J Neurol Neurosurg Psychiatry 16:189, 1953

369. Tracy PT: Unusual intracarotid anastomosis associated with anterior communicating artery aneurysm: case report. J Neurosurg 67:765, 1987

370. Tran-Dinh HD, Dorsch NW, Soo YS: Ectasia and fenestration of the anterior cerebral artery associated with persistent trigeminal artery: case report. Neurosurgery 31:125, 1992

371. Travis AM: Neurological deficiencies following supplementary motor area lesions in *Macaca mulatta*. Brain 78:155, 1955

372. Trescher JH, Ford FR: Colloid cyst of the third ventricle. Arch Neurol Psychiatry 37:959, 1937

373. Trojano L, Crisci C, Lanzillo B et al: How many alien hand syndromes? Follow-up of a case. Neurology 43:2710, 1993

374. Truwit CL: Embryology of the cerebral vasculature. Neuroimaging Clin North America 4:663, 1994

375. Tsuji T, Abe M, Tabuchi K: Aneurysm of a persistent primitive olfactory artery. J Neurosurg 83:138, 1995

376. Turnbull I: Agenesis of the internal carotid artery. Neurology (NY) 12:588, 1962

377. Ueno E: Clinical and physiological study of apraxia of gait and frozen gait. Rinsho Shinkeigaku 29:275, 1989

378. Van Bogaert L, Ley R: Contribution à la connaissance de la paraplegie en flexion, type Babinski, d'origine cérébrale. J Neurol Psychiatry 26:547, 1926

379. Van den Bergh R, Vander Eecken H: Anatomy and embryology of cerebral circulation. Prog Brain Res 30:1, 1968

380. VanderArk GD, Kempe LC: Classification of anterior communicating aneurysms as a basis for surgical approach. J Neurosurg 32:300, 1970

381. Van der Eecken HM: Anastomosis Between the Leptomeningeal Arteries of the Brain. Their Morphological, Pathological and Clinical Significance. Charles C Thomas, Springfield, IL, 1959

382. Vander Eecken H: Discussion of "collateral circulation of the brain." Neurology (NY) 11:16, 1961

383. Van der Zwan, Hillen B, Tulleken CAF et al: Variability of the territories of the major cerebral arteries. J Neurosurg 77:927, 1992

384. Van Stockert TR: Aphasia sine aphasia. Brain Lang 1:277, 1974

385. Van Vleuten CF: Linksseitige motorische Apraxie. Z Psychiatr 64:203, 1907

386. Vilkki J: Amnestic syndromes after surgery of anterior communicating artery aneurysms. Cortex 21:431, 1985

387. Vincent GM: Cardiac electrophysiologic abnormalities in the stroke syndrome. p. 365. In Price TR, Nelson E (eds): Cerebrovascular Diseases. Proceedings of the Eleventh Research Conference. Lippincott-Raven, Philadelphia, 1979

388. Volpe BT: Observation of motor control in patients with partial and complete callosal section: implications for current theories of apraxia. In Reeves A (ed): Epilepsy and the Corpus Callosum. Plenum Press, New York, 1983

389. Volpe BT, Hirst W: Amnesia following rupture and repair of an anterior communicating artery aneurysm. J Neurol Neurosurg Psychiatry 46:704, 1983

390. Volpe BT, Sidtis JJ, Holzman JD et al: Cortical mechanisms involved in praxis; observations following partial and complete section of the corpus callosum in man. Neurology (NY) 32:645, 1982

391. Volpe JJ: Cerebral blood flow in the newborn infant: relations to hypoxic-ischemic brain injury and periventricular hemorrhage. J Pediatr 94:170, 1979

392. Wada M, Kajikawa H, Fujii S et al: Ruptured distal ante-rior cerebral artery aneurysm and diagionistic dyspraxia: a case report. No Shinkei Geka Neurol Surg 23:355, 1995

393. Waddington MM: Atlas of Cerebral Angiography with Anatomic Correlations. Little, Brown, Boston, 1974

394. Waltz AG, Sundt TM: The microvascular and microcirculation of the cerebral cortex after arterial occlusion. Brain 90:681, 1967

395. Ward AA: The anterior cingular gyrus and personality. Res Publ Assoc Nerv Ment Dis 27:438, 1948

396. Ward AA: The cingular gyrus: area 24. J Neurophysiol 11:13, 1948

397. Watanabe O, Bremer AM, West CR: Experimental regional cerebral ischemia in the middle cerebral artery territory in primates. 1. Angioanatomy and description of an experimental model with selective embolization of the internal carotid artery bifurcation. Stroke 8:61, 1977

398. Watson RT, Fleet S, Gonzolez-Rothi L, Heilman KM: Apraxia and the supplementary motor area. Arch Neurol 43:787, 1986

399. Watson RT, Heilman KM: Callosal apraxia. Brain 106:391, 1983

400. Webster JE, Gurdjian ES, Lindner DW, Hardy WG: Proximal occlusion of the anterior cerebral artery. Arch Neurol 2:19, 1960

401. Whitty CWM, Duffield JE, Tow PM, Cairns H: Anterior cingulectomy in the treatment of mental disease. Lancet 1:475, 1952

402. Wiesendanger M: Organization of secondary motor areas of cerebral cortex. p. 1121. In Brookhart JM, Mountcastle VB, Brooks VB, Geiger SR (eds): Handbook of Physiology, Section 1: The Nervous System, Volume II: Motor Control, Part 2. American Physiological Society, Bethesda, MD, 1981

403. Wiesendanger M, Ruegg DG, Lucier GE: Why transcortical reflexes? Can J Neurol Sci 2:295, 1975

404. Wilson G. Crucal monoplegia. Arch Neurol Psychiatr 10:699, 1923

405. Wilson G, Riggs HE, Rupp C: The pathologic anatomy of ruptured cerebral aneurysms. J Neurosurg 11:128, 1954

406. Windle BCA: On the arteries forming the circle of Willis. J Anat Physiol 22:289, 1888

407. Winkelman NW: Two brains showing the lesions producing cerebral monoplegia. Arch Neurol Psychiatr 12:241, 1924

408. Wise SP, Tanji J: Supplementary and pre-central motor cortex: contrast in responsiveness to peripheral input in the hindlimb area of the unanesthetized monkey. J Comp Neurol 195:433, 1981

409. Wolfe N, Linn R, Babikian VL et al: Frontal systems impairment following multiple lacunar infarcts. Arch Neurol 47:129, 1990

410. Woolsey CN: Cortical motor map of *Macaca mulatta* after chronic section of the medullary pyramid. p. 19. In Zulch KJ, Creutzfeldt O, Galbraith GC (eds): Springer-Verlag, Berlin, 1975

411. Woolsey CN, Settlage PH, Meyer DR et al: Patterns of localization in precentral and "supplementary" motor

areas. Res Publ Assoc Res Nerv Ment Dis 30:238, 1952

412. Yakovlov PI: Paraplegias of hydrocephalics (clinical note and interpretation). Am J Ment Defic 51:561, 1947

413. Yakovlev PI: Paraplegia in flexion of cerebral origin. J Neuropathol Exp Neurol 13:267, 1954

414. Yamadori A, Osumi Y, Ikeda H, Kanazawa Y: Left unilateral agraphia and tactile anomia: disturbances after occlusion of the anterior cerebral artery. Arch Neurol 37:88, 1980

415. Yamaguchi T, Kunimoto M, Pappata S et al: Effects of anterior corpus callosum section on cortical glucose utilization in baboons: a sequential positron emission tomography study. Brain 113:937, 1990

416. Yamori Y, Horie R, Akiguchi I et al: Pathogenic mechanisms and prevention of stroke in stroke-prone spontaneously hypertensive rats. Prog Brain Res 47:219, 1977

417. Yano H, Sawada M, Shinoda J, Funakoshi T: Ruptured dissecting aneurysm of the peripheral anterior cerebral artery—case report. Neurol Med Chir (Tokyo) 35:450, 1995

418. Young RSK, Hernandez MJ, Yagel SK: Selective reduction of blood flow to white matter during hypotension in newborn dogs: a possible mechanism of periventricular leukomalacia. Ann Neurol 12:445, 1982

419. Youngjohn JR, Altman IM, Van Doren J: Amnesia following anterior communicating aneurysm surgery. J Clin Exp Neuropsychol 11:61, 1989

420. Zaidel E: Unilateral auditory language comprehension on the Token Test following cerebral commissurotomy and hemispherectomy. Neuropsychologia 15:1, 1977

CHAPTER 19

Middle Cerebral Artery Disease

J.P. MOHR

R.M. LAZAR

R.S. MARSHALL

J.C. GAUTIER

DANIEL B. HIER

Anatomy

The middle cerebral artery (MCA) is the artery most commonly affected in stroke syndromes. It is the largest of the major branches of the internal carotid artery and is frequently as much as twice as large as the anterior cerebral artery. Studies of the anatomy of the MCA have been reported over the past century,[1,2,38,141,157,368] some of the more recent utilizing angiography as well as dissections,[175,258] and others using the dissecting microscope to pursue the fine details of vascular anatomy of the MCA stem.[185]

The MCA supplies most of the convex surface of the brain.[312] Only the frontal pole and the superior and extreme posterior rim of the convex surface are supplied by other cerebral arteries. Within the brain, it supplies almost all of the basal ganglia and capsules, including the extreme capsule, claustrum, putamen, the upper parts of the globus pallidus, parts of the substantia innominata of Reichert, the posterior portion of the head and all of the body of the caudate nucleus, and all but the very lowest portions of the anterior and posterior limbs of the internal capsule. The thalamus is supplied almost entirely by the posterior cerebral artery, but a few cases have been reported in which an infarct arising in the thalamus produced slight ischemia in the adjacent internal capsule.[306]

The internal capsule has a complex arterial supply[14]: the inferior part of the anterior limb is supplied by the branch of the anterior cerebral artery known as Heubner's artery, although the MCA supplies even this territory in one-third of cases; the corona radiata and most of the anterior and posterior limbs are fed by the MCA; and the lowest portion of the posterior limb is supplied by the anterior choroidal artery, which usually arises from the internal carotid artery.

CLASSIFICATION

The anatomy of the MCA tree has been classified by two major criteria, one based on the branching of the artery itself and the other based on the relationship between the vessel and the anatomic landmarks of the cerebral surface.

Stem, Divisions, and Branches

The traditional terminology analogizes the vessel as a tree with a trunk and branches (Fig. 19.1). This scheme has proved useful in pathology since emboli tend to arrest at bifurcations, whereas atheromatous lesions occur most often at bifurcations and curves. Because this classification is still commonly used clinically, it will be used throughout this chapter.

The MCA regularly begins as a single trunk or stem. The length of the stem varies from 18 to 26 mm. Its diameter at the site of origin is roughly 3 mm. Actual measurements range from 2.5 to 4.9 mm, averaging 3 mm.[176,185] The *stem* is generally considered to give rise to the lenticulostriate branches, those small arteries given their name because they penetrate the brain to supply the lentiform nucleus (putamen and pallidum) and caudate of the basal ganglia and also supply the internal capsule.[176] (The claustrum and extreme capsule are supplied by vessels from the surface penetrating through the insula.[284]) Between 5 and 17 lenticulostriates arise from a given MCA.[398] A few of the smaller lenticulostriates may arise from the distal internal carotid, but the larger penetrating vessels do not.[185] No clear correlations exist between the

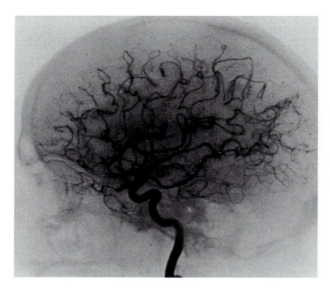

Figure 19.1 Lateral view of the middle cerebral artery anatomy.

length of the MCA stem and the pattern or number of the lenticulostriates, nor does the pattern on one side predict that on the other.[185] Usually, the lenticulostriates arising more medially on the MCA stem are the smaller vessels while the larger are more lateral. Three patterns of origin of the lenticulostriates from the MCA have been described.[185] In the most common variant (49%), one or more of the larger lenticulostriates arise just beyond the major bifurcation. In the next most common permutation (39%), all the larger lenticulostriates arise from the stem just proximal to its bifurcation. In the least commonly encountered pattern, some of the larger penetrators arise from the medial portion of the stem. One important anatomic feature they all share is their lack of anastomoses between themselves and only rare anastomotic links to the cerebral surface vessels (see Ch. 31, Moyamoya Disease). They are, with rare exceptions, end arteries.

The cerebral surface, claustrum, extreme capsule, and the hemispheral cortex and white matter are supplied by those MCA branches that form beyond the lenticulostriates, usually 12 in number. They arise from the MCA stem in a variety of patterns, by far the most common one (78%)[176] being two large divisions whose composition varies considerably. Less often (12%),[176] the 12 branches arise from three major trunks (trifurcation pattern). The least differentiated and least common (10% of cases)[176] is the continuation of the stem with no major divisions, each of the surface branches arising in turn from the common trunk until the primary vessel has given off 11 of the usual 12 branches, after which it terminates as the angular artery.[359]

In the bifurcation patterns, the superior division always contains the orbitofrontal and prefrontal branches; the inferior division always contains the temporal polar, anterior temporal, and middle temporal branches. The distribution of the remaining branches in a given division varies widely. The central (rolandic) branch is almost always in the upper division, while the posterior temporal branch is almost always in the lower division. In like manner, the anterior parietal branch is usually

in the upper while the temporo-occipital branch is usually in the lower division. The posterior parietal and angular branches, which arise in the middle of this fan-like array of vessels, have an almost equal chance of being in either division.

In the trifurcation pattern, the orbitofrontal, prefrontal, and precentral branches supplying the frontal lobe are regularly represented in the upper division. The middle division is made up of the central (rolandic), the anterior parietal, and the angular branches. Less often, the precentral branch is a member of this trunk on the frontal side while in a few other instances the temporo-occipital and superior temporal branches are added on the inferior side. The inferior division regularly contains the temporal polar, anterior, and middle temporal branches, to which the posterior temporal and temporo-occipital branches are less often added.

Although the frequency with which a given branch occurs in a given division may vary, the branches provide a fairly reliable supply to certain brain regions and do not appear to cross one another. No branch arising from the upper division irrigates the brain, which would be expected to be supplied from a branch of the lower division or vice versa. Within their band or wedge of the convexity, remarkable variations have been found in the exact position over gyri and sulci by individual branches.

The brain regions differ in the number and size of the vessels ramifying over their surface. The smallest and the shortest branches supply the frontal lobe.[16,94] Only 27% of the orbital frontal branches are as large as 1 mm.[176] The largest artery is usually the artery of the central (rolandic) sulcus. The more posterior regions of the brain are supplied by fewer arteries, which are larger in size, give off fewer major branches, and have the longest course from the circle of Willis to their termination in a border zone (Fig. 19.2). The temporo-occipital artery is 1 mm in size in 90% of cases and >1.5 mm in size in up to 63% of cases. This large size and ease with which it can be followed on the surface for long distances made this branch preferred by surgeons when the extracra-

Figure 19.2 Anatomy of the border zone anastomoses (individual anastomoses shown by arrows).

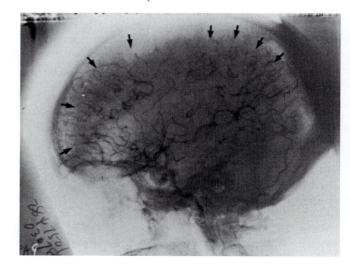

nial-intracranial anastomosis operation was in its heyday. The three vessels with the longest course on the cortical surface are the angular, postparietal, and temporo-occipital arteries.[94,176] Intraluminal diameters >1 mm have been encountered in up to 86% of angular arteries, 68% of temporo-occipital arteries, and 52% of posterior parietal arteries, but only 14% of central sulcus arteries.[401]

Arterial Segments in Relation to Anatomic Landmarks

Another method of classifying the branches of the MCA is based on the relationship of the artery to the major landmarks on the brain, especially the sylvian fissure, the operculum, and the convex surface. This scheme has found its greatest use in angiographic descriptions of the MCA and its branches.[146,246] The MCA is divided into four major segments (Fig. 19.3). The first, or M1, segment occupies the space from the origin of the MCA to the limen insulae. The second, or M2, segment encompasses the portions of the MCA that overlie the insula. The M3 segments are those portions that curve along the surface of the operculum, and the fourth, or M4, segments describe those portions of the branches of the MCA over the convex surface of the brain.

Gibo et al[176] found that the *M1 or sphenoidal* segment was composed of two components. The first was the undivided MCA stem from which the lenticulostriate branches arose; it occupied most of the length of this segment. The second consisted of the short segments from the bifurcation of the MCA into its major divisions to their entry into the sylvian fissure.

Figure 19.3 Classification of the middle cerebral artery by segments.

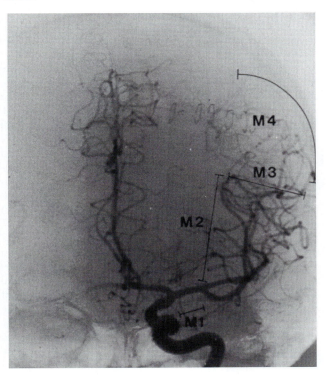

The *M2 or insular* segment gives rise to most of the cerebral surface branches. Most of them develop over the anterior portion of the insula.[176] Branches supplying the frontal and central regions of the convexity ascend sharply upward over the course of the insula, and those supplying the posterior temporal and parietal regions course more or less parallel to the long axis of the insula.

The MCA branches that constitute the *M3 or opercular* segment follow the curve of the operculum back over the surface of the insula. Some of these branches reverse course over as much as 180 degrees,[258] especially those ascending over the frontal and central operculum to gain access to the frontal half of the cerebral convexity. Those passing over the parietal and temporal operculum make less striking reversals of direction, some turning only a few degrees before reaching the convex surface of the temporal and parietal regions.

The *M4 or cortical* segments are those portions of the branches of the MCA after they emerge from the sylvian fissure beyond the operculum and course along the sulci and gyri of the cerebral convexity. Considerable variation in their path is found from brain to brain. Some of them follow a path mainly along the depths of a given sulcus, whereas others pass long distances over the surface of a gyrus.

ANOMALIES

A few anomalies have been described, but all types together appear to occur in no more than 3% of cases.[176,223,383,392] Some dispute even the occurrence of the anomalies.[185] Duplication of the MCA is the more common of the anomalies. The duplicated vessel usually arises from the internal carotid and supplies the same regions that would otherwise have been supplied by the original MCA. In the few cases reported, the regions supplied have mainly been the temporal pole and anterior and middle temporal areas. An accessory MCA has also been described.[223] It arises from the anterior cerebral, usually supplying frontal polar areas.

BORDER ZONE ANASTOMOSES

For each cerebral surface branch of the major cerebral arteries, the terminal twigs end in a narrow network of vessels that form the border zone (Fig. 19.2) between the major arterial territories.[9,77,348] Within the border zone, anastomoses form end to end, end to side, and side to side in remarkable permutations. Although such channels exist, the actual size of the anastomosis at any given point is usually quite small, on the order of 300 to 400 μm.[304] More often, the available anastomotic vessels are 200 to 400 μm, too small to provide adequate collateral to an endangered arterial territory. Only occasionally are the border zone anastomoses >500 μm. There are wide individual variations in the anastomotic artery-to-artery network. Direct, end-to-end anastomoses as large as 1 mm are rare. While these tiny vessels scarcely seem of the size that could sustain collateral flow, it has proved remarkable how useful, but unpredictable, a role they play in limiting the size of a given infarct. The dynamics of their dilation in response to occlusions of proximal arteries are still poorly understood.

Anastomoses between contiguous branches of the MCA are either scanty or quite small and play little or no useful role in collateralizing occlusion of adjacent branches, when compared with the value of end-to-end anastomoses via the border zones.[38,394,395]

HISTOLOGY

The MCA contains the same intima, media, and adventitia as other arteries, but the relative thicknesses of these component parts differ from peripheral arteries of comparable size.[381] The differences begin even within the intracranial internal carotid artery, which changes the histologic character of the MCA in such a way that the two blend in a smooth continuum. Compared with extracranial vessels of comparable size, the MCA has a narrower adventitia with little elastic tissue and little perivascular supporting structures; the media is also thinner, with some 20 circular muscle layers.[26,374] The internal elastic lamina is thicker[423] and finely fenestrated. The intima, although somewhat thin, seems essentially the same as that of comparably sized vessels elsewhere.[374] No evidence of vasa vasorum has been demonstrated to date.[96,374,423]

The implications for pathology of these differences from extracranial vessels is still unclear. The thinner adventitia of intracranial vessels may be a sign of the lower exposure to stretch and trauma compared with the environment in which the extracranial vessels live.[289] As for the elastic tissue, its concentration in the internal elastic lamina, instead of being scattered through the vessel, may make intracranial arteries more prone to dampen pulse waves.[423] Whatever their differences from extracranial arteries, intracranial vessels are susceptible to the same embolization, inflammation, and other diseases as are extracranial vessels. Whether their less frequent involvement by atherosclerosis is for reasons of histology alone is unsettled, as is whether the comparative rigidity of the MCA makes it less compliant in cases of embolization.

Pathology

EMBOLISM

Although atherosclerosis is a major cause of disease of the extracranial carotid and intracranial basilar arteries, embolism is by far the more common cause of occlusion for the major cerebral arteries beyond the circle of Willis. As a cause of stroke, it accounts for between 15% and 30% of cases,[187,247,271] most of which occur in the territory of the MCA.

Particle Size and Composition

To arrest in the stem of the MCA, the embolic mass must be at least a few millimeters in diameter. Rigid materials such as shotgun pellets[229] (first described by Leceve and Lhermitte in 1920), catheter tips, and the like may be this large. Some materials seem too small to be regular candidates, especially calcific plaques.[376] Calcific plaques large enough to occlude the stem occur in unusual circumstances such as direct-puncture carotid arteriography[114] and perhaps from carotid atheroma itself.[376] Rare causes include one case of fibrocartilaginous material.[387] Most of the embolic material is elements of thrombus. These complexes, alone or mixed with bacteria, are a frequent cause of embolism of the middle cerebral stem,[159] the largest diameter vessels in the MCA system. This material seems quite compressible[273] and may alter its length and width remarkably as it passes through the system. The important issue of how large an embolic particle may arise from angiographically inobvious carotid ulceration or from thrombus of the aortic arch remains unresolved.[142,221]

Distribution

Although emboli have access to the entire cerebral arterial tree, their distributions are decidedly nonrandom. The two sides of the brain are equally affected, but the MCA is the most commonly embolized.[162,271] Beyond the stem, flow seems equally directed to the two divisions. In the upper division, the four posterior branches are arranged in series, providing an orderly set of opportunities for emboli to lodge.[59,162,271,285] The orbital frontal branch is rarely embolized, possibly because it is acutely angulated away from the main direction of flow. The lower division passes unbranched across the insula until it reaches the superior temporal plane, where it gives off its three main branches within the space of ≤1 cm. As a result, embolization into lower division often results in the simultaneous occlusion of more than one, or even all, of the branches of the division.

Persistence

It is common to find autopsy evidence of infarction with no occlusion at the site. In the 17 cases attributed to embolism in the series reported by Fisher et al,[153] an embolus at the site of the infarct was not always found. However, in these cases, a source was available in the heart, and no evidence was found for atheromatous stenosis of the branch involved. In other studies of acute ischemic stroke clinically diagnosed as embolism, branch occlusions were found in the first 24 hours in >75% of cases. When the angiogram was delayed >48 hours in cases with the same clinical features, the intracranial branches were widely patent.[123,335] Although it is inferred that the more friable materials will disperse rapidly, no reliable means have been developed thus far to predict which embolic occlusions will persist and which will disappear.[145] Transcranial Doppler studies have documented a few instances in which the occlusion has become recanalized within 40 minutes,[309] but it remains unknown with what frequency and how quickly emboli are dissipated past their point of initial lodgement.[216] From the scant data available, persistence of embolic occlusion seems to be the exception rather than the rule, yet some branches originally affected may be found occluded well beyond 48 hours, and in others the occlusion has disappeared.[430] Persistence of the occlusion seems to carry a worse functional prognosis.[271] When persistent, the material has proved difficult to differentiate from in situ thrombus at autopsy.

Collateral Flow

Unless adequate collateral is present, embolic occlusion of the MCA stem yields a gigantic infarct affecting both the superficial and deep territory of supply. Where collateral is readily available, the resultant infarct may be remarkably circumscribed, sometimes confined to little more than those branches of the lenticulostriates caught by the occluding embolus.[301] Little knowledge is available on what allows collateral flow to be so generous and readily available in some cases and so trivial in others, depending on the variations in the congenitally determined vascular pattern.

Etiology

For this discussion, it is worthwhile separating embolism to the stem from that to the branches of the MCA. It has been known since the time of Chiari[93] that embolic occlusion affecting the distal intracranial internal carotid may also affect the MCA *stem* across the circle of Willis, but particles large enough to lodge in the MCA stem alone are less easily documented. A literature survey was undertaken in an effort to document examples of the variety of settings in which an embolus occluded the MCA stem. Examples for each of the following was found (documented by autopsy or angiogram): "paradoxical" embolus from a leg vein source,[159,177] atrial fibrillation,[143,422] mitral valve prolapse,[31,61] marantic embo-

lus,[245,324] fragmented thrombus complexes from a nonobstructing internal carotid artery plaque,[114,426] shotgun pellet,[229] metal fragment from a penetrating neck wound,[232] traumatic dissection of the internal carotid artery,[217] internal carotid occlusion of various causes,[336] and automobile accident with angiographically normal ipsilateral internal carotid.[217,271]

Embolism to the *surface branches* involves additional considerations. Although it is a commonplace observation that occlusion of one or more branches of the MCA may occur from almost any source of embolism, it is not easy to find autopsy or angiographic evidence in support of such claims.[89,115] In a similar literature survey, the following etiologies were uncovered with an appropriate angiographic finding or autopsy proof: calcific material from the ipsilateral internal carotid[93]; spontaneous dissection of the internal carotid artery from fibromuscular hyperplasia[347]; traumatic internal carotid dissection[380]; mucin and emulsified fat from breast metastasis[118]; endocarditis due to candida[178]; mitral valve prolapse[32]; cardiac myxoma[429]; arterial wall fragments after resuscitation[189]; giant fusiform MCA aneurysm[23,97]; marantic embolus[245]; and internal carotid occlusion from various causes.[30,32,92,304] Recent work has also made clear the importance of transcardiac emboli via a patent cardiac foramen ovale (see Ch. 43).

Clinical Syndromes

The disastrous effects of poorly or uncollateralized occlusion of the MCA are so familiar that only those with limited infarction warrant mention (Fig. 19.4). Collateralization this effective seems to be rare.[1]

Figure 19.4 (A & B) CT scans of a deep infarct, which was the only effect of an occlusion of the stem of the middle cerebral artery. Angiogram showed full collateralization of the surface branches from the adjacent anterior and posterior cerebral arteries.

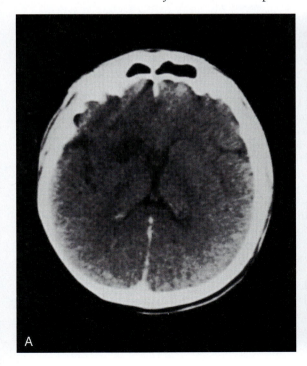 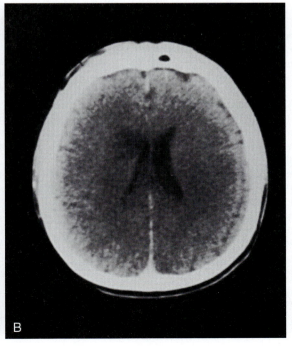

A variety of temporal profiles occur in embolism to *branches* of the MCA. In some instances, the deficits are only transient, even with angiographic evidence of persisting occlusion or brain image evidence of focal infarction that confounds traditional clinical definitions of transient ischemic attack (TIA).[37,336] Aberrant embolism in the days of Silastic pellet therapy for arteriovenous malformations was a well-recognized risk,[425] usually occurring near the end of the embolization procedure when conditions initially favoring the entry of the pellets directly into the AVM vessels changed as the fistula became clogged with pellets.[248,425] In Kusske and Kelly's[248] series of 10 cases, 2 showed focal ischemia, 1 involving the ipsilateral retina and lasting for 5 days, and another involving the contralateral MCA with transient dysesthesia of the left hand. Wolpert and Stein[425] described six patients in whom aberrant embolization occurred. One patient had two beads into an angular branch of the MCA and experienced 15 minutes of contralateral arm numbness—a complaint not entirely predicted by classical clinicopathologic correlation—and also showed immediate distal retrograde collateralization. The pellet remained in place. Single beads occluded parietal branches of the MCA in two others and an ascending frontal in a third, none of whom experienced any deficits; in all patients, immediate collaterals occurred retrograde into the embolized branch.

Emboli initially occluding the MCA stem and then later migrating to the convexity branches may leave lesions in the deep and superficial territories as *discontinuous multifocal infarction*. The lack of collaterals to the lenticulostriates make this territory esecially vulnerable to ischemia. The distally placed embolic fragment in a cortical branch is usually considerably smaller than the mass of which it was a part that initially blocked the MCA stem. The clinical picture may be predominantly that of the deep infarction affecting the penetrating vessels of the MCA stem. A spectacular shrinking deficit (given the initials SSS by Minematsu et al[301]) can occur when the embolus occludes the internal carotid, causing a profound full hemisphere syndrome, after which it passes up the internal carotid to its final resting place in, say, the angular branch of the MCA, leaving only a mild aphasia after a few days or a week. Especially characteristic of this type of migratory embolism is a syndrome of fading hemiparesis with persisting Wernicke's aphasia: the embolus presumably lodges initially at the stem of the MCA, occluding the penetrating lenticulostriate branches long enough to produce scattered foci of infarction through the basal ganglia and internal capsule, the involvement of the latter producing the hemiparesis. Distal migration of the embolus then occurs, usually finally occluding the lower division of the MCA at the superior temporal plane and beyond, yielding Wernicke's aphasia. Two separate foci of infarction occur, but both result from the same embolic event (Fig. 19.5).

Nonsudden or fluctuating onset occurs in 5% to 6% of documented embolic strokes, the syndrome often requiring 36 hours or so to evolve.[154,271] A clinical diagnosis of multiple TIAs is often entertained.

ATHEROSCLEROSIS

Primary atherosclerotic occlusive thrombosis is currently considered a decidedly uncommon cause of symptomatic disease of the MCA,[21] yet for years, most instances of MCA ischemia

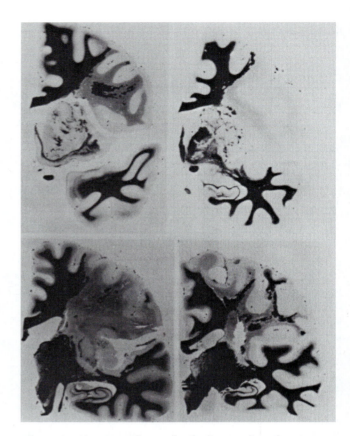

Figure 19.5 Deep and superficial infarction from the same embolic occlusion (myelin stain of celloidin section). (From Friedlich et al,[159] with permission.)

were casually attributed to thrombosis of the MCA.[71,72] As long ago as 1951, Fisher[147] noted that "in case after case neuropathological examination failed to confirm the clinical impression of disease of the middle cerebral artery." In the past 40 years, studies have repeatedly demonstrated that this impression was correct. None of the 178 autopsied cases collected by Fisher and Pearlman[154] to determine the distribution of atherosclerosis in the carotid or vertebrobasilar system showed thrombotic occlusion of an intracranial cerebral artery in the carotid system, including the MCA. Blackwood et al[58] searched back through the records at the National Hospital and found great difficulty uncovering many convincing examples of thrombosis of the MCA, attesting to its rarity. Likewise, in a clinical and autopsy study of 122 cases of infarction in the territory of the MCA, Lhermitte et al[271] diagnosed atherosclerosis in 8 of 94 cases on clinical and angiographic grounds, while in a companion series studied by autopsy, only two (one occlusion, one stenosis) were attributed to atherosclerosis. Resurveying the scene almost 20 years after his initial observation, Fisher[149] diagnosed atherosclerotic thrombosis in only 7% of 68 cases of MCA occlusion by clinical, angiographic, or pathologic criteria.

These findings lend support to the diagnosis of embolism for angiographically documented occlusions of the MCA and its branches, unless shown to be otherwise at autopsy. Angiographically demonstrated middle cerebral stenosis found above a normal internal carotid suggests recanalizing embolism. Except for rare instances, the angiographic appearance of occlusion of the MCA or its branches does not permit a reliable separation between embolism and primary thrombosis. Admittedly, when lysis and disappearance of the initial occlusion occur, the usual cause is embolism,[123,214,222] but the hazards of angiography discourage repeat studies. In those cases with persisting occlusion, the diagnostic problem remains unsettled, defeating the diagnostic efforts of even the best clinicians.[88]

Thrombotic Occlusion

Autopsy studies indicate that thrombotic occlusion accounts for only 2% of cases of ischemic events in the MCA territory.[271] In life, thrombotic occlusion of the MCA is indistinguishable from that caused by embolism. When repeat angiography shows that the lesion has resolved, a diagnosis of embolism can be inferred, but persisting occlusion does nothing to clarify the etiology.

Although the distinction between thrombus and embolus on clinical grounds is difficult, the syndrome of occlusion is worthy of mention in its own right. Asymptomatic occlusion of the MCA stem must be rare, if it occurs at all.[150,254] Lascelles and Burrows[254] found that 18 of their 22 patients had major neurologic deficits, and only 4 experienced satisfactory clinical improvement. Fisher[150] found no such cases among the 40 with occlusion of the MCA stem from his experience at the Massachusetts General Hospital. Almost all the patients had a syndrome featuring hemiplegia or hemiparesis. He uncovered 23 cases; in only 5 of these did the stroke begin with no prodrome. In three the stroke developed in a stepwise fashion, requiring several days to reach the peak. Fully 15 had had previous TIAs, in many instances multiple and over periods as long as a year.

Stenosis

Stenosis, that familiar problem in the extracranial carotid, is uncommon anywhere in the MCA, and when found is almost always in the stem (Fig. 19.6). Thus far, no reliable means have been developed to determine what the lesion represents when seen the first time. Atheroma not fully developed, recent embolus undergoing recanalization, the stenosis of moyamoya disease, dissection, postradiation effects, and other etiologies including infection are all possibilities. Examples of atherosclerosis limited to the MCA stem are difficult to find, the information is somewhat scanty, and the clinical course has been surprisingly mild. Five of the nine cases reported by Lascelles and Burrows[254] made an almost complete recovery. Kawase et al[231] described only examples of TIA. Hinton et al[214] reported on 17 patients, only 3 of whom were left with focal neurologic deficits, although all were treated with warfarin (Coumadin). Minor deficit characterized 8 of the 13 described by Feldmeyer et al.[144] A progressive course was described in five, evolving over ≥12 hours. The leisurely mode of onset even led to a clinical diagnosis of tumor in three instances. Day[117] mentioned TIAs alone or with mild stroke in 12 of the 18 cases of stenosis. The experience of Corston et al[100] was less fortunate: 14 of their 21 patients presented

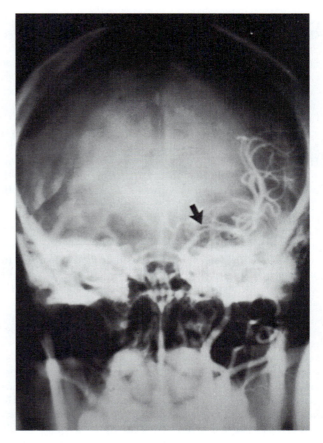

Figure 19.6 Angiogram showing middle cerebral artery stem stenosis.

with stroke, yet even in this series only 3 had a severe disability, and 7 patients presented with TIA alone.

Remarkably enough, the literature is scanty regarding the *clinical syndromes* of stenosis. Judging from the handful of studies available, stenosis can cause lenticulostriate or hemispheral syndromes by at least three mechanisms. Local lacunar-type syndromes affecting the lenticulostriate branches may occur if they become trapped in the atheroma affecting the MCA itself. Ischemic events in the hemisphere distal to the stenosis may occur because of hemodynamic insufficiency[214] or by embolism.[4] Kawase et al[231] found four examples of capsular low density on computed tomography (CT) scans ipsilateral to angiographically documented stenosis of the M1 segment of the MCA in 52 Japanese patients with TIAs affecting the carotid territory. They attributed the clinical syndrome and CT abnormality to the MCA stem stenosis. However, in one, the stenosis was so far distal in the stem that it was beyond the usual point of departure of even the lateral lenticulostriates; in two of the others the stenosis lay at the origin of the stem, and the last lay in its midportion.

Several of the patients (cases 2, 3, and 4) reported by Hinton et al[214] had similar syndromes, limited to pure motor weakness. In each instance, however, there was a considerable shift of the border zone seen angiographically, with anterior cerebral branches collateralizing the MCA. The pure motor character of the attacks and the obvious border zone shift posed a problem in interpretation of the mechanism involved. Corston et al[100] may have had similar experiences, as three of their cases were described with severe hemiplegia, but details on the remainder of the clinical syndrome in these cases were not provided. A shift of the border zone was encountered in some of these cases. Other examples of lacunar syndromes in a setting of MCA stem stenosis may be found scattered through the literature.[18,306]

Hemispheral hemodynamic insufficiency was suggested by the clinical syndromes of 13 of the 16 cases reported by Hinton et al.[214] Their TIAs or minor permanent deficits were accompanied by mutism, dysarthria, or numbness. In each case, an obvious shift had occurred in the borderzone, with striking collateral into the MCA territory. Even given the occurrence of ischemic stroke, the syndromes were quite mild. Less encouraging results were reported by Corston et al,[100] who described nine patients with some disturbance in higher cerebral function, one with no accompanying hemiparesis. In only one was shift of the border zone described. These cases leave no doubt that some patients are left with a severe disability.

Some reports suggest untoward effects may be attributed to surgical intervention. Extracranial-intracranial (EC/IC) bypass surgery, a procedure that at first sight could appear to be a rational step in therapy, has been reported in a few disheartening instances followed by symptomatic occlusion. Furlan et al[160] described a symptomatic patient (case 2) with angiographically documented advancing MCA stem stenosis. He had developed aphasia and right hemiparesis, which cleared within a few days, leaving only mild right hemiparesis. Six days postoperatively, an angiogram demonstrated occlusion of the supraclinoid portion of the left internal carotid artery with good filling of the MCA territory through the anastomosis. Immediately after the angiogram, he developed ". . . fluent dysphasia with jargon speech and numerous paraphasia errors. There was increased right arm weakness." A CT scan showed no evidence of recent infarction. He returned to his postoperative state and was discharged uneventfully. Gumerlock et al[190] found that two of the seven patients with MCA stem stenosis had progressed to occlusion within days of successful EC/IC bypass. One patient presented with a 10-minute episode of aphasia; his postoperative course was described as "stormy," and within 4 days he had ". . . increased speech deficit and generalized weakness, which improved slowly. . . ." The other patient had two episodes of right-sided weakness with dysphasia. Postoperatively, she ". . . demonstrated intermittent right hemiparesis, hyper-reflexia, and Babinski signs." The deficits are not easily explained in any of these three, but some of the features seem reminiscent of the pre-EC/IC bypass deficit. Perhaps the collateral through the bypass was sufficient to permit stagnation at the MCA stem yet insufficient to keep the hemisphere continually perfused. In any case, none of these three had a syndrome obviously of the lenticulostriate or lacunar type, suggesting that the occlusion did not trigger a large deep infarct.

Turning back to the issue faced by the angiographic demonstration of MCA stem stenosis, it is disappointing that no distinctive angiographic criteria permit the separation of recanalizing embolus from stenosis due to atherosclerosis on the basis of a single angiogram.[222] This difficulty nags at every study of the course of angiographic stenosis, since each group

of cases contains an unknown subset of emboli.[100] The angiographic abnormality has been found at various points along the course of the stem, from its origin all the way to the bifurcation.[214]

DISSECTION

Dissection in the MCA is quite rare. It is described here since it seems to pursue a course somewhat different from that of dissection affecting other vessels. Over three dozen cases have been reported. A host of settings for dissection are recognized: trauma,[220] strenuous physical exertion,[424] surgery,[49] fibromuscular hyperplasia,[215] atherosclerosis,[18] mucoid degeneration of the media,[220] moyamoya disease,[427] split or frayed internal elastic lamina,[138] congenital defect of the media,[428] syphilis,[391] and even migraine.[371] The disorder has been most often reported in younger patients, many of them children. The usual site affected is a short section of the stem, although the disorder may spread into adjacent branches[226]; one remarkable case showed a continuous dissection involving the distal intracranial carotid, middle, and anterior cerebral arteries.

When a precipitating factor, such as trauma, has been documented, symptoms developed at that time or were delayed for minutes,[226] hours,[428] or up to 4 days.[139] Once the clinical syndrome was set in motion, events proceeded rapidly, but in a few cases the decline was over a day or more. Since the dissections occur most often in the stem of the MCA, severe clinical deficits usually occur.

As the literature consists of the autopsied cases, the expected fate of patients diagnosed in life is poorly understood. Distinguishing dissection from other causes of stenosis or occlusion of the MCA stem has proved too difficult a diagnosis to be made with confidence.

OTHER DISEASES

The MCA, like other vessels, may fall victim to arteritis, fibromuscular hyperplasia, altered coagulation states, delayed effects of radiation,[230] and the like. From the available literature, not enough features of such involvement in the MCA appear to be present to warrant separate consideration. The reader is referred to the chapters in this book that deal with these topics individually.

Clinical Syndromes of Middle Cerebral Artery Territory Infarction

The major syndromes of MCA disease described by Foix and Levy[157] in their classical article have been repeated over and over in textbooks.[6] In such accounts, the description of the syndrome from each trunk and branch is usually based on the assumption that the entire territory at risk is involved and that a description of the deficit at its maximum will suffice.

However, it has been recognized for some time that the effects of an arterial occlusion are determined by the collateral flow via borderzone vessels shared with the anterior or posterior cerebral arteries. Effective collateralization may rescue the endangered territory, resulting in the striking reduction in symptoms and signs.[350,357] Recent work with CT, positron emission transverse tomography, and now nuclear magnetic resonance (NMR) scanning is demonstrating a wide spectrum of deficits, both acute and chronic, that are occasioned by a given arterial occlusion.

STANDARD SYNDROMES

The main principles of clinical correlation found in textbook accounts[307,312,349] are briefly reviewed here as a backdrop for some of the details that follow. Uncollateralized occlusion of the *main trunk* of the MCA artery causes softening of the basal ganglia and internal capsule within the substance of the hemisphere, as well as a large portion of the cerebral surface and subcortical white matter. The large infarct produces contralateral hemiplegia, deviation of the head and eyes toward the side of the infarct, hemianesthesia, and hemianopia. Major disturbances also occur in behavior: global aphasia occurs when the hemisphere dominant for speech and language is involved, while impaired awareness of the stroke is expected when the nondominant hemisphere is affected. When the infarct is large, the hemianopia may be due to involvement of the visual radiations deep in the brain. More often, the hemianopia is part of a syndrome of hemineglect for the opposite side of the space and is accompanied by failure to turn toward the side of the hemiplegia in response to sounds from that side, a problem separate from the head and eye deviation toward the side of the infarct.

A variant of the syndrome of MCA stem occlusion, colorfully named the malignant infarction (recently described by Hacke et al[191]) referred to those cases experiencing subsequent herniation. Only 12 of the 55 patients studied survived. The mean Scandinavian Stroke Scale score on admission was 20. The time course to severe decline was brief, between 2 and 5 days. The rapid development of a space-occupying mass effect on brain imaging was a particularly predictive sign of poor outcome. Fully 43 patients suffered herniation as the terminating event (see Ch. 44 on tissue plasminogen activator therapy).

When the occlusion is restricted to the *upper division*, the initial deficit mimics that from occlusion of the main trunk: contralateral hemiparesis and hemisensory syndromes are the rule, accompanied by hemineglect for the opposite side of the space, aphasia when the dominant hemisphere is involved, or impaired awareness of the deficit when the opposite hemisphere is affected. However, the hemiparesis usually affects the face and arm more than the leg, a picture opposite from that in anterior cerebral artery disease. Because the occlusions usually affect the anterior branches of the upper division, the aphasia from dominant hemisphere infarction is usually of the motor (Broca) type, while the disturbance in behavior from nondominant hemisphere infarction may be mild.

In the *lower division* syndromes, hemiparesis does not usually occur, head and eye deviation are rarely encountered, and even disorders of sensation are infrequent. When the infarct affects the dominant hemisphere, pure aphasia (Wernicke type) is the rule, while in nondominant hemisphere infarction, the behavior disturbances may appear in relative isolation. Hemianopia may be a prominent sign.

When the involvement is limited to the territory of a small *penetrating artery* branch of the main stem, a small, deep infarct (lacune) occurs, affecting part or all of the internal capsule and producing a syndrome of pure hemiparesis, unaccompanied by sensory, visual, language, or behavior disturbances (see Ch. 23, Lacunes).

Enough exceptions occur that the foregoing can only be accepted as a guide, subject to modification from individual case experience. Analysis of individual cases has also yielded enough data to indicate that the cerebral response to infarction expressed in the clinical picture is more than the effects of ischemia, edema, and collateral blood flow.

In the formulations presented throughout this chapter, efforts have been made to confine the presentation to the case material representing the effects of ischemia in the MCA territory. Those studied by autopsy are given the closest consideration, followed by those documented by CT scan, angiogram, and NMR. Although sorely tempted, the authors have made every effort to avoid analysis based only on textbook descriptions, clinical essays, or case material drawn from other etiologies. In pursuit of this policy, some cases of interest from other etiologies have necessarily been neglected, but in the end it is hoped that the findings reflect the syndromes of ischemia as opposed to other etiologies. Not the least of the points made is the thin support for many of the classical tenets of clinical correlation in neurology.

Clinical Syndromes from Infarction of Either Hemisphere

LOSS OF CONSCIOUSNESS

Transient loss of consciousness seems uncommon in all forms of ischemic stroke. It occurs only rarely in cases of MCA territory infarction. As an initial sign, it occurs in only 8.4% of carotid ischemic strokes,[73] a frequency slightly higher than the 5.7% in vertebrobasilar territory strokes. In half of the cases, the loss is attributable to seizure. The mechanism is unclear in the others. Diaschisis[399] might be considered a possible explanation,[73] assuming it to be secondary to sudden embolization of the stem of the carotid artery with temporary global ischemia.

Delayed loss of consciousness is more common. Following hemispheral infarcts ranging in size from the entire MCA territory to that limited to the frontotemporal region, delays from 36 hours to 4 and 5 days may occur in cases with loss of consciousness.[346] The decline in consciousness is usually part of a larger clinical picture of impending cerebral herniation, and not from an injury to a specific brain region in the MCA territory controlling consciousness (Fig. 19.7).

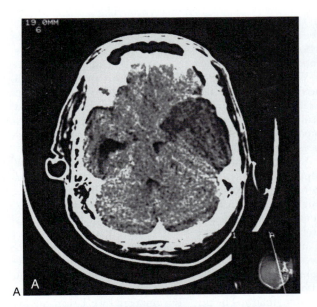

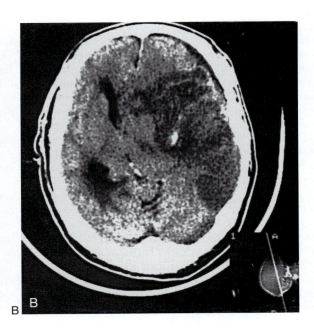

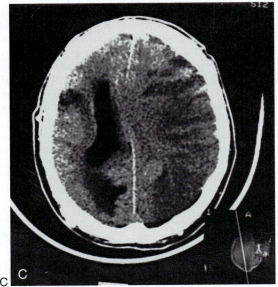

Figure 19.7 Axial CT scans showing infarction of the entire middle cerebral territory. **(A)** From the level of the temporal pole. **(B)** Through the basal ganglia. **(C)** To the upper convexity, with coma and fatal midline shift.

HEMIPLEGIA AND HEMIPARESIS

The terms hemiplegia and hemiparesis have been used too loosely to permit a clear correlation between the formula and severity of weakness and a given site of infarction. Weakness of some degree and type has been encountered most often in infarcts of the branches of the upper division, but it is not regularly reported in infarcts affecting the territory of the lower division.

A disappointingly small number of cases correlate the hemiparesis formula and autopsy findings. Many authors have reviewed large numbers of cases, but not usually in pursuit of the types of hemiparesis. Henschen's[209] review of the published autopsy literature on higher cerebral function was typical of most authors: the occurrence of hemiparesis on a case-by-case basis was mentioned only in passing, and details of the syndrome were rarely given. The literature contains many surprising instances of apparent amelioration of motor deficit following infarction affecting the MCA territory on either side. Since the improvement of the motor deficit was not the main focus of most of the studies, it is difficult to know how seriously to take the findings. A discouraging point is that some of the earlier publications devoted to the clinical correlations of MCA occlusions lack credibility. For example, the effort by Davison et al[116] contains several actual case descriptions, one of which is a photograph of a hemorrhage in a case described as an infarct. Also, among the recent larger series of cases, the basis for the diagnosis of MCA territory infarction varies considerably. For example, branch occlusions documented angiographically were the most common finding in 9 of the 38 cases reported by Barnett et al.[30]

After several attempts, the present author abandoned efforts to assemble the expected syndromes from large review articles and concentrated, instead, on detailed individual case reports found among the huge mass of published material on MCA territory infarcts. The result has been a necessarily haphazard collection of material that may prove little better than the rough collections attempted by his many predecessors, but that is all that appears to be available, as reflected in the following material.

MCA stem occlusions affecting either side of the brain presumably produce the same basic motor deficit and can be described under the same heading. The pilot phase of the NINCDS Stroke Data Bank project,[310] involving some 488 cases of stroke confined to a cerebral hemisphere, showed no difference in the occurrence or the type of the weakness from stroke of comparable source or size affecting either side of the cerebrum. More work is needed on this point since some components of the motor deficit may differ according to the side of the stroke: DeRenzi et al[128] found that the occurrence of conjugate eye deviation from right hemisphere stroke greatly exceeded that of deviation from left hemisphere stroke.

Hemiplegia

The most reliable occurrence of hemiplegia follows complete occlusion of the MCA at its stem. The effect of the occlusion may produce infarction involving both the deep and superficial territory of the MCA, the deep only, or the superficial only. The syndrome of hemiplegia is essentially similar in all three settings but varies enough to warrant separate description.

Foix and Levy[157] described in some detail the *hemiplegia from deep and superficial infarction*. The typical picture includes dense contralateral hemiplegia, hemianesthesia, homonymous hemianopia, and conjugate gaze deviation to the contralateral side. The severity of the syndrome increases when the occlusion approaches the MCA stem.[28,157,254,349] Huge infarctions affecting the territory of the MCA have been documented with a variety of autopsy studies,[5,47,325,346] but the syndrome descriptions echo the same findings as Foix and Levy, with a few embellishments. Among the patients who die within days, contralateral hemiplegia is the rule, usually accompanied by hemianesthesia and hemianopia.[168] Kooiker et al[245] described an example of sudden complete hemiplegia with decerebration associated with angiographic occlusion of the MCA and delayed emptying. Hemorrhagic softening affecting the entire right cerebral hemisphere was found on autopsy 3 days later.

Cases of MCA territory infarction with brain swelling massive enough to promote hemicraniectomy serve to indicate the expected course of hemiplegia in the most extensive strokes. Deterioration with massive brain edema may occur in these cases within periods as early as 36 hours, but often it is more evident by the fourth day. After reversal of the incipient herniation, the persistent neurologic deficit is usually severe hemiplegia. The syndrome among survivors without hemicraniectomy seems similar. For example, complete hemiplegia occurred in the five cases of MCA stem occlusion reported by Irino et al,[222] all of whom were said to survive with severe neurologic deficits. The author's experience includes

an example of occlusion of the MCA stem from foreign body embolism documented by angiogram and CT scan.[229] This previously healthy man suffered a shotgun wound to the chest without neurologic complications but experienced a pellet embolus during resuscitation for cardiac arrest a few days later. His postarrest neurologic deficit featured a complete hemiplegia, with tonic eye deviation, hemihypesthesia, hemianopia, and stupor. An angiogram showed that the pellet had lodged proximal to the lenticulostriate territories. The CT scan showed complete infarction of both the deep and superficial territories of the MCA.

The deficit after hemispherectomy in cases of chronic infarction gives a separate insight into motor functions mediated by the contralateral hemisphere and brain stem. Obrador[330] reported hemispherectomy on 10 patients ranging in age from 3 to 29 years and noted in particular that 3 patients showed only slight facial paresis. Another seven had only moderate lower facial paresis, and four were able to move facial muscles on each side easily. This degree of control of the lower face contrasted with the pattern of weakness of the limbs, which approximated that predicted by the principles attributed to Broadbent.[78] The distal functions of the limbs were very much impaired. Complete paralysis of hand and finger movements was seen in six, and the foot was completely paralyzed in nine. By contrast, the upper limbs moved well at the shoulder and elbow in seven cases, and motility of the muscles of the hip and knee was fairly well preserved, enough for walking in all cases.

Several different syndromes occur when *hemiplegia with deep infarction* occurs. Foix and Levy[157] described two varieties of hemiplegia in the condition they characterize as deep infarction of the sylvian artery. The motor deficit was the same in right and left hemisphere infarcts. In the first type massive hemiplegia occurred that had the same appearances they found when the infarct involved both the superficial and the deep territories. Initial hemiplegia gave way to marked contracture. The authors observed no instances of involuntary movements, choreoathetosis, parkinsonism, or disturbances in balance. A second type was described with a more marked hemiplegia in the leg than in the arm, rendering the patient unable to walk. Contracture in this syndrome was more frequent in the leg and was often associated with a permanent flaccid hemiplegia. The prognosis for recovery was poor, but the outlook for life appeared to be good.

Few cases are to be found in the literature. Some focused on a different problem, and the description of the motor abnormalities was limited to terms such as hemiparesis or hemiplegia. Two described the deficits in some detail. One of the cases described by Fisher and Curry[152] as "pure motor hemiplegia" seems to have been a large, deep infarct, presumably of an embolic mechanism. Hanaway et al[192] encountered an elderly woman with complete hemiplegia and some degree of movement of the face; her autopsy within 2 days of onset showed a larger hemorrhagic infarct affecting the entire lenticulostriate territory of the right MCA. Some of the hemorrhagic component may have been due to therapy with urokinase. Healton et al[195] described an autopsy-documented case with a large, deep, hemorrhagic infarct affecting the head of the caudate nucleus, putamen, and anterior limb, genu, and superior aspect of the posterior limit of the internal capsule and extreme capsule. Contralateral supranuclear facial weakness, deviation of the tongue, paralysis of the arm and leg, hyper-reflexia, and extensor plantar reflex were described. Death occurred 10 days after onset.

Several reports in which lesion topography was documented by CT scan have appeared. Using the term "giant lacunes," Rascol et al[345] have described a small series of cases with capsulo-putamino-caudate infarction. These infarcts spread over both the anterior and posterior limb of the capsule and involved the adjacent striatum. Their large size far exceeded that typical of lacunes, which prompts their inclusion in this discussion. The clinical presentation featured a profound hemiplegia, but, remarkably enough, incomplete syndromes of hemiparesis were also encountered. In a few instances, the course of the hemiparesis was surprisingly mild. Adams et al[3] described two patients with large deep infarcts seen on CT scan associated with arterial occlusion of the first segment of the MCA with no visualization of the lenticulostriate branches. Retrograde filling collateralized the hemisphere surface branches. Severe hemiparesis was present, including the face. In the first patient, no accompanying disturbances were documented in sensation, vision, or language, from an infarct that involved the head of the caudate nucleus, the anterior limit of the internal capsule, and the putamen. In the second patient, flaccid hemiplegia involving the face was associated with mild hypesthesia and normal visual fields and a mild language disturbance. In this instance the CT scan revealed low density involving the head of the caudate nucleus and the anterior limit of the internal capsule and putamen. The clinical course was not further described.

Santamaria et al[360] reported on eight patients with large, deep infarcts seen on CT that they attributed to cerebral embolism. Five suffered complete hemiplegia, but in only one was it a pure syndrome. Complete recovery from the hemiplegia occurred in two and was slight in two; no improvement occurred in the last two. The only adult described by Demierre and Rondot[127] suffered sudden hemiplegia contralateral to a stroke with a CT appearance of hypodensity and central hyperdensity affecting the right lenticulo-capsulo-caudate region. Partial regression of the hemiplegia occurred over 4 days. By 4 weeks, dystonic disorders had developed. Grimes et al[186] described three patients studied by CT scan who showed initial hemiparesis or hemiplegia from infarcts affecting the head of the caudate and the putamen, presumably also affecting the capsule to some degree. In all three, the initial deficit regressed to mild weakness within 3 months.

The senior author's collection includes an elderly woman with a deep infarct whose CT scan showed a high-density lesion outlining the striatum and capsule, interpreted as a hemorrhagic infarct in the lenticulostriate territories (Fig. 19.8). Her clinical presentation featured a complete hemiplegia affecting the face and limbs, involving both the proximal and distal portions of the upper and lower extremity to an equal degree. The deficit improved slightly over the following month only in the hip and foot; the face, shoulder, and hand remained completely paralyzed for the 6-week period she was under clinical observation.

More recent reports describing the syndromes of striatocapsular infarction have emphasized the difficulty of separating the syndrome of large, deep infarction from superficial cortical infarction on clinical grounds alone, and have cited

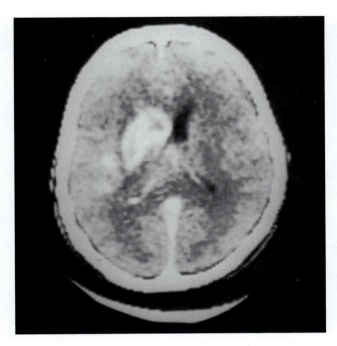

Figure 19.8 Large deep infarction of the middle cerebral artery lenticulostriate territories shown by CT scan.

numerous instances of dysphasia, dyspraxia, and hemineglect among the prominent clinical features.[137,410]

Other case reports have focused on the disturbances in language, and little detailed description of the hemiparesis is available. The subcortical, nonhemorrhagic lesions affected the basal ganglia and capsule and were large enough to be beyond the usual size expected in lacunes.[29,110]

Finally, there are the syndromes of *hemiplegia from surface infarction*. The syndrome of hemiplegia from infarction of the entire surface territory of the MCA is essentially identical to that found when the deep territory is also affected. Few reports are to be found in the literature, and the clinical deficits in those few are described only in part. A case of surface infarction among those in the senior author's collection was a 35-year-old man who suffered a subarachnoid hemorrhage without focal deficit and underwent surgical repair of an aneurysm located at the bifurcation of the MCA. Aneurysmal rupture during the operation necessitated the placement of a clip across the MCA stem just distal to the territory of the lenticulostriate. From the time he awoke postoperatively, he was affected by a dense aphasia, contralateral hemiplegia, and hemisensory syndrome. Re-examination 2 years later showed complete lower facial plegia and deviation of the tongue; his fingers and hand lacked any voluntary movements, and the arm hung by his side with slight flexion at the elbow. The leg supported the body for walking, but the immobile toes and ankle required support by a brace. A few months later he committed suicide. At autopsy the entire MCA surface territory was found to be infarcted, with complete sparing of the territory supplied by the lenticulostriates (Fig. 91.9).

Some examples of surface infarcts confined to the cortical surface of the insula and operculum have been described.[83] The cases have infarcts confined to the region of the insula

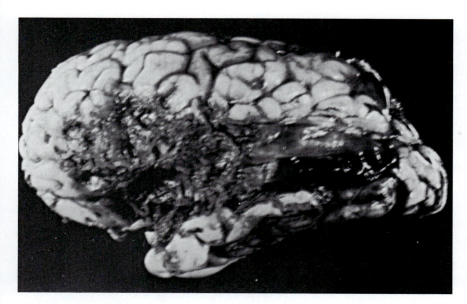

Figure 19.9 Complete infarction of the surface territory of the middle cerebral artery following occlusion of the stem by an aneurysm clip.

and upper and lower banks of the operculum. The syndrome was described as a hemiplegia with faciobrachial predominance that soon fades to a facioplegia with mild predominantly distal paresis of the arm.

Hemiplegia seems rather uncommon from individual branch occlusions.[157] In most cases, hemiparesis occurs, or the syndrome of paralysis is incomplete, confined to one or more body part(s). The most reliable deficit is encountered among those suffering occlusion of the ascending frontal branch. Glew[178] described an example from embolic occlusion of the back branches of the upper division: the patient suffered sudden onset of complete hemiplegia, lethargy, and mumbling of unintelligible sounds. Except for slight movement of the right ankle, the right side was immobile and flaccid, with paralysis of the face and no movement of the tongue. The CT scan showed a large low density in the back branches of the upper division. At autopsy, evidence was found of embolic infarction in the rolandic and ascending parietal regions of the MCA territory.

The clinical course of an initial hemiplegia has been described in disappointingly few cases. A survey of this case material is of interest to indicate that some remarkable improvement may occur, but usually only in cases with branch occlusion. Barnett et al[30] described a patient with sylvian branch occlusion and contralateral hemiplegia who recovered substantially in 1 week. Two years later, only minimal right-sided weakness was found on examination. A second case[30] had total hemiplegia with aphasia, which remitted within 1 week.

Syndromes of Partial Hemiparesis

The most commonly encountered pattern of hemiparesis seems to be one with equivalent weakness of the hand, shoulder, foot, and hip. This type occurred in 71.2% of the 488 unilateral hemisphere strokes studied during the pilot phase of the NINCDS Stroke Data Bank project.[310] A few other types of hemiparesis are also well known. Among them are the classical syndromes of distal predominance to the hemiparesis (Broadbent[78] principle), faciobrachial paresis, and monoplegia.

Few studies of large size have directed attention to the variation in syndromes from convexity infarction. The main phase of the NINDS Stroke Data Bank study provided data for 183 of 1,276 patients with convexity infarction in the middle cerebral artery territory, the largest cohort reported to date. The size of the infarct did not differ between the two sides, but the location of the main site of the infarct differed: on the left side, it was centered in the inferior parietal region, and it was midfrontal on the right. There was a good correlation between infarct size and weakness severity estimated by overall motor function either on one side, or arm, or hand alone. There was a poor correlation, however, for lesion location (lower third, middle third, or upper third on either side of the rolandic fissure) and any of the specific syndromes of focal weakness, no two cases sharing the same lesion for the same syndrome and several cases sharing the same lesion with a different syndrome. The findings indicated a difference in weakness syndromes between the two hemispheres and great individual variation of the acute syndrome caused by a given site of focal infarction along the rolandic convexity. These findings provide a framework for the smaller case studies of incomplete hemiparesis discussed below.

The pattern of hemiparesis with *distal predominance*, attributed to Broadbent,[78] has been widely accepted as typical of MCA territory infarction. The weakness affects the lower face, fingers and the forearm, and toes and lower leg, with relative sparing of the forehead, shoulder and upper arm, hip and thigh, neck, and trunk. This lower facial and distal predominance of hemiparesis has been taken to represent the density of the homuncular representation over the hemispheral surface.[338,339] Although its occurrence is said to typify ischemic stroke involving the MCA territory, it seems a rather uncommon sign. Among the 488 cases with unilateral weakness affecting the cerebrum studied in the pilot phase of the NINCDS Stroke Data Bank project, this pattern was encountered in only 23.5% of cases.[310] Furthermore, it occurred with approximately the same frequency whether the infarct was confined to a single lobe or was as large as several lobes, and whether the area involved was frontal, parietal, temporal, or opercular. As expected, hemiparesis of any kind did not occur in infarcts of the occipital region.

Almost as common is the syndrome of *faciobrachial paresis*. In an angiographic study of MCA occlusion done in the days before CT scanning and with no autopsy data, Lascelles and Burrows[254] found that the lower face was affected in 51 of 59 MCA infarcts; among those who could be assessed, the deficit was greater in the upper than in the lower limb. In cases with involvement of the insula and operculum,[10,83] the weakness of the face and oropharynx may be profound: in addition to the expected lower facial plegia, the upper face may fail to wrinkle for some days or weeks. Obvious weaknesses are present in the muscles of the jaw. Movements of the tongue and oropharynx show impaired swallowing and occasionally impaired vocalization. These lower face and oral pharyngeal disturbances may persist long after the forehead movement has been restored. The initial appearance is sometimes similar to that of a Bell's palsy, but the upper deviation of the eyes characteristic of peripheral facial palsy (Bell phenomenon) is typically not present even in the earliest stages. The involvement of the upper extremity is usually more obvious in the impaired movement of the fingers and hand.

One such autopsied case was studied in life by the author (Fig. 19.10). On the day of the stroke, the patient showed a dense right supranuclear facioplegia, flaccid paralysis of the arm and hand, and moderate paresis of the leg with rare small spontaneous movements of the foot. By the third day the arm could be elevated from the bed, but no movement of the fingers or forearm was found. By the next day she was able to produce a slight pressure on attempted handshake, but the face remained plegic. At 2 weeks the hand was able to produce a moderate grip, the arm could be elevated easily, and the leg supported the patient for standing in a few short steps. Other facial paralysis had improved to the point of moderate paresis and moderate weakness. By the end of the third week, although she showed an obvious extensor plantar response, the weakness of the shoulder and hip were further improved, and a moderate grip with movements of the fingers was observed. The central facial weakness was present at rest and during voluntary movements, but smiling was actually symmetrical, the gag was intact, and the tongue moved freely. At 2 months the deep tendon reflexes had become roughly symmetrical. No further improvements were noted in the limbs, and the face showed a moderate paresis, which was more obvious than the weakness in the arm and leg. By the end of the second month the patient had reached a static condition with regard to hemiparesis; she made no further improvements until her death 14 months later. The autopsy revealed an infarct that had destroyed the insula and adjacent banks of the operculum but spared the internal capsule, centrum semiovale, and cerebral surface above the operculum.

A faciobrachial predominance to the hemiparesis may occur in cases of small surface infarcts of the anterior rolandic

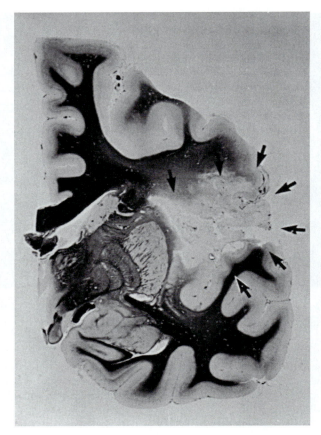

Figure 19.10 Coronal view of insular and upper opercular infarction from embolism to the upper division of the middle cerebral artery. (Myelin stain of celloidin section.)

and opercular area. One of the senior author's autopsied cases[302] with inferior frontal infarction had severe right central facial weakness with only moderate right hemiparesis (Fig. 19.11, case 1). Within a week the face and hand remained plegic, the arm strength improved to the point that the patient could lift the arm off the bed, the leg had full power, and the eyes moved freely. Within 1 month the face and hand remained unchanged, but the arm moved freely, and the patient walked easily. At 5 months the face and fingers remained unchanged, but the wrist was now capable of making moderate movements and the leg remained essentially free of trouble.

Another case (Fig. 19.11, case 2), this one with more extensive spread of the infarct up the rolandic cortex, had a severe right facial and distal arm paralysis (including the hand) that persisted unchanged for 90 days before death. A patient whose focal inferior frontal infarct was documented by angiogram and CT scan was struck mute while talking but did not lose balance. Examination within an hour revealed dense right lower facial plegia during attempts to talk, grimace, or smile, preserved wrinkling of the forehead, deviation of the tongue to the right, slight weakness of the grip, and barely detectable weakness of the shoulder but full movement of the trunk and leg. The right plantar response was extensor. Within 3 weeks the tongue moved freely and the face showed only slight weakness, but the weakness of the hand persisted. By 3 months,

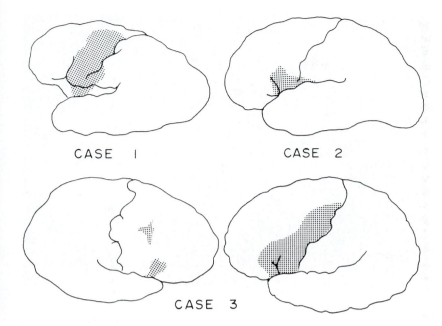

CASE 1   CASE 2

CASE 3

Figure 19.11 Three examples of embolic infarction of the Broca area and surrounding cerebrum. (From Mohr,[302] with permission.)

the facial asymmetry was barely detectable under any conditions and the grip was improved but still noticably weak.

Another similar case indicates that the deficit may follow a similar course when the infarct affects the right hemisphere. Over a 2-hour period, in stuttering fashion, this 54-year-old man developed dysarthria and left facial plegia, with mild weakness of grip, but retained full movement of the shoulder, trunk, and leg. Angiogram revealed occlusion of the MCA at the origin of the upper division, with collateral flow retrograde from the anterior cerebral territory to the point of the occlusion and a normal CT scan. The focal deficit persisted for over a week unchanged and then faded steadily within weeks to a barely detectable lower facial weakness on forced grimace.

Faciobrachial paresis may even occur as an isolated sign. One of the senior author's patients had a mild faciobrachial paresis of sudden onset unaccompanied by other findings, which was correlated with a contrast-enhancing CT scan and branch occlusion on angiogram. Even the possibility of facial weakness as an isolated sign has also been mentioned.[121]

Monoplegias

Monoplegia, a circumscribed disturbance, is described in standard texts on the subject, but is not easily found in the literature. Von Monakow[399] made reference to the possibility of an isolated brachial plegia arising from a lesion confined to the middle of the second frontal gyrus, provided that the lesion is acute and does not extend too deep into the white matter ("... wenn sie akut einsetzt und nicht zu tief in das subcorticale Mark übergrieft . . .").[399] Dejerine and Regnard[122] found a case with weakness limited to the muscles of the thenar, hypothenar, and interosseous muscles; no confirmation of the presumed vascular nature of the lesion was mentioned. Garcin[165] described a monoparesis with weakness predominating in the flexor movements mimicking a median nerve palsy; the locus of the lesion was inferred in the absence of autopsy data.

The only case of focal upper rolandic infarction encoun-

tered by the author with autopsy documentation (Fig. 19.12) was an elderly woman whose examination within hours of onset revealed normal power in the upper extremity including the hands and fingers, sparing the limb entirely. The only clinical signs were slight right facial weakness with initial mutism. She was followed for months, during which time the initial deficit improved, but no disturbance of limb power occurred at any time.

Isolated brachial monoplegia has often been described as a clinical sign in carotid territory TIAs. It has also been encountered as a transient syndrome in aberrant emboli during pellet embolization in treatment of arteriovenous malformations, regardless of the middle cerebral branch embolized. These findings are of great interest but must be interpreted with caution, since the setting (an angiogram suite with the patient under a drape) does not lend itself to detailed evaluation of the leg and axial structures during the frantic period when the physicians are striving to reverse the acute deficit.

Schneider and Gautier,[364] in an extensive review of 1,575 patients with acute stroke and weakness found that only 63 had predominance of the leg. Although 41 patients had hemispheric convexity lesions, in only 1 was the MCA territory affected.

Data from the pilot phase of the NINCDS Stroke Data Bank project contained a mere 31 cases of monoplegia involving the arm among the 488 with cerebral stroke,[310] yet even this small number showed a significant correlation with a single lobe infarct rather than with one involving multiple lobes ($P < 0.002$). Although monoplegia seems to be uncommon, it has some value as a sign of circumscribed infarction. Monoplegia was encountered in infarcts involving the frontal, temporal, or parietal lobes.

Infarcts Without Hemiparesis

Infarction confined to the *lower division* of the MCA is not expected to produce hemiparesis in any form, since the site of the infarct lies so far posterior to the rolandic sulcus. This

Figure 19.12 Small upper rolandic infarction. The pia-arachnoid has been stripped away to show the infarct. (Courtesy of J.M.C. Pearce.)

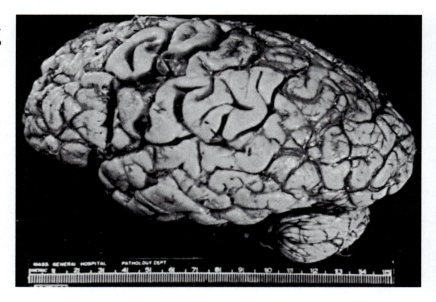

point also seems to apply to the *postrolandic branches of the upper division.* Occlusion of the ascending parietal branch is uncommonly reported, but the few cases documented have been remarkably free of focal motor deficit.[135] The pilot phase of the NINCDS Stroke Data Bank[310] documented a handful of instances of hemiparesis following *opercular infarction.* Several notable cases exist with autopsy correlation in which weakness did not occur in either the face or the limbs at any time during an acute infarct affecting the inferior frontal region, the anterior operculum.[76] Reports of infarction confined to the *orbital frontal branch* of the upper division are exceedingly rare. Waddington and Ring[400] described a 62-year-old man with a grasp reflex, inappropriate laughing *witzelsucht,* inappropriate advances toward his employees, and poor business judgment. His only motor deficit was the grasp reflex and contralateral extensive planar response. The case was studied by angiogram only. Rare reports of occlusion may be a result of the low frequency of embolism into this particular branch.

CONTRAVERSIVE EYE AND HEAD DEVIATION

Deviation of the head and eyes following unilateral lesion was first described clinically by Prevost[343] in 1868. The basic clinicopathologic correlations seem to have been so well accepted that reference to actual clinical cases in review articles has become rather uncommon.[55,332,334] Remarkably little recent documentation has been made of the lesions responsible for the deviation, and even less of the setting in which the deviation either persists or is transient.[384] Most of the authorities writing on the subject seem to infer that the deviation of the eyes represents disruption of the frontal eye fields in and around area 8 alpha, located in the premotor region of the superior frontal lobe.[55,56,113,218,306,332] Given this long-standing assertion, it is remarkable how many cases with deviation of the head or eyes have lesions more centrally located in the

MCA territory, near the operculum or insula, and how few had actually been reported with eye deviation from a superior frontal central infarction.[41,309,362]

Types of Deviation

DeRenzi et al[128] encountered three types of deviations in their 120 patients with occular motility disorders. In the first group the head and eyes were in the midline and moved spontaneously to either side in response to stimulus, but eye movements were less complete to the side of the space served by the damaged hemisphere. In a certain group the head and eyes were found completely to one side with absent spontaneous movements to the contralateral side and only fleeting voluntary deviation of the eyes into the side of the space served by the damaged hemisphere. In the most severely affected group the head or eyes, or both, were completely deviated away from the side of the space served by the damaged hemisphere and failed to turn in response to verbal or sensory stimuli, with no spontaneous or voluntary movements observed to the midline or beyond. In the study by DeRenzi et al,[128] hemi-inattention or neglect of the contralateral side of the space usually accompanied those with head and eye deviation.

Eye Deviation and Infarct Topography

Eye deviation is the expected finding after massive infarction of the *entire* MCA territory. Lascelles and Burrows[254] noted conjugate deviation in a few of their patients with angiographically documented occlusion of the MCA, all of whom died. It seems to have been taken as a sign of major cerebral infarction. In the *upper division* syndromes encountered in studies of Broca's aphasia, the senior author[303] uncovered 10 autopsy cases from the Massachusetts General files; all these patients had experienced head and eye deviation to the site of the lesion persisting for days and clearing within a week. There is less evidence bearing on the occurrence of eye deviation in opercular infarcts. One of the senior author's personal cases showed head and eye deviation as part of the acute clinical syndrome occasioned by a left insula and opercular infarction. The infarct spared the suprasylvian hemispheral surface, centrum semiovale, and capsular and basal ganglia structures. The deviation was reversed by passive head rotation. By the fifth day, ocular motility was normal.

Ocular deviation in cases with *deep infarction* has attracted special interest. Two cases have been described. Hanaway et al[192] found that their elderly woman with a large hemorrhagic infarct involving the entire territory of the lenticulostriates on the right side had deviation of the eyes to the right. The eyes could not be fully moved to the left. She died within 2 days. Healton et al[195] studied a 75-year-old woman whose autopsy showed a large hemorrhagic infarct involving the striatum. The infarct was smeared across the anterior limb, genu, and superior aspect of the posterior limb of the internal capsule. The patient's head and even the trunk remained deviated to the side of the infarct through the 10 days of life after the stroke, despite an alert state and interaction with the examiner sufficient to test language and praxis. In the most recent review, Tijssen[384] studied 133 consecutive patients with "acute supratentorial lesions" of whom 5 showed ipsilateral eye deviation. Four were from hemorrhage (thalamus, frontal or frontotemporal location) and in one it was a subdural hematoma; none were from infarction.

DeRenzi et al[128] found a higher frequency of ocular motor deviation in *right* hemisphere infarcts compared with left. Nearly half of the patients with sensory motor stroke and presumably larger lesions suffered ocular deviation, with less difference between the right and left hemisphere group than in the patients with posterior lesions: 61% of those with right hemisphere lesion experienced deviation compared with 13% of those with left hemisphere lesion. The frequency of ocular deviation in frontal lesions was much lower on both sides, about 5% to 6%. The authors point out the variance of these findings with the traditionally accepted areas for eye movement disturbances. Experience in the NINCDS Stroke Data Bank may bear on this point.[314] Eighty-six cases (16%) of supratentorial type conjugate ocular deviation occurred among the 531 cases of hemispheral stroke diagnosed by clinical or radiologic criteria. The occurrence of ocular deviation was significantly correlated with the larger infarcts, but among the infarcts confined to single lobes, those involving the right side were more frequently associated with ocular deviation. A frontal predominance over parietal infarcts was not found, and a parietal location was not the explanation for the effect of the right-sided stroke. The prevalence of frontal or parietal lobe location did not differ significantly among single lobe infarcts. Ocular deviation occurred from infarction as low on the surface as the operculum. Gaze deviation of <5 days' duration did not correlate with lesion side, size, site, cause, or positive initial CT scan. However, the larger lesions predominated among the nine cases whose ocular deviation persisted beyond 20 days.

Duration of the Deviation and Severity of Infarct

In the study of DeRenzi et al,[128] the severity of the initial ocular motility deficit seemed greater in right hemisphere cases than in left for the first 6 to 9 days, but at the end of 2

and 3 weeks most of the patients showed only mild or no disturbance. Contralateral hemineglect often outlasted the disturbance in ocular motility in these cases. Patients with infarct affecting the *operculum and insula* showed what has been labeled pseudo-ophthalmoplegia for the first few days of the stroke.[83] Conjugate deviation of the head and eyes lasts for several days and then disappears. The lesion causing this condition is far away from area 8 alpha and is considered a reliable feature of infarcts of the insula and operculum.

The duration of ocular deviation following *branch occlusion* in the upper division is less well documented. One of the senior authors' patients[302] had head and eyes deviated to the left for a period of several weeks. The branch occlusion affected the anterior ascending branch of the MCA as high as the border zone with the anterior cerebral artery.

Infarction with No Eye Movement Disturbances

One patient of De Renzi et al[128] who was completely free of any gaze disturbance had a cortical subcortical lesion (a frontal hematoma) on the left involving the areas of the rolandic fissure. The few cases with focal infarction confined to the superior frontal region, near area 8 alpha, have not confirmed the thesis that this region is vital for ocular motility.

SENSORY DISTURBANCES

Because the most attention has been paid to the more obvious deficits in language and motor function, surprisingly few data have described sensory disturbances, outside the usual claims in the textbooks. The presence of a disturbance in sensation carries an important indication of a large lesion when it accompanies hemiparesis: in the pilot data from the NINCDS Stroke Data Bank project, this correlation was highly significant for infarcts greater than a single lobe in size ($P < 0.001$).[310]

Hemispherectomies

Because the sensory disturbance from hemispheral disease may improve with time, it is worth emphasizing that the anatomic substrate may not be the surviving portion of the damaged hemisphere. The data from hemispherectomy cases[330] permit assessment of the sensory disturbance expected under extreme conditions of tissue removal. Studies have shown relative preservation of sensory function in the face. Blunted sensation to several modalities was found the more distally the test were performed in the arm. Complete astereognosia was common in Obrador's[330] patients. Vibration and position sense were heavily affected. No patients showed definite alteration of the body scheme.

Pure Sensory Deficits

Focal sensory deficits have been described in detail in only a handful of cases with autopsy correlation, most of whom were noted because they seemed to show an unusual variant of the expected deficit. One syndrome described has shown a pseudoradicular pattern of sensory loss[121] with impaired joint position sense, stereognosis, graphesthesia, and two-point discrimination. In the few cases studied, the hand is the most severely affected, but two have been described with both hand and foot disturbance. Hemianesthesia has also been described in a few other cases.[156,270,400] The persistence of the deficit outlasts the complaints of sensory disturbances.

Hemisensory Deficits and Lesion Topography

Foix et al[156] are credited with the demonstration that an infarct affecting the anterior parietal region may produce a profound hemisensory loss (pseudothalamic syndrome) with little or no accompanying hemiparesis. Their patient had a large anterior parietal infarct that was so deep it created almost a cleft in the hemisphere to the ventricular wall. Lhermitte et al[270] had a similar patient, studied by CT scan. Few other cases have been described. Derouesne et al[135] reported on a 50-year-old man with sudden numbness of the left thumb and index and middle fingers, which felt frozen or asleep. Normal power was found on examination, but the patient dropped small objects held in the hand. The next day he experienced numbness in the distal foot and clumsiness putting on his slipper. On examination, fine movements of the fingers and toes were inaccurately detected, and severe impairments were noted in graphesthesia, two-point discrimination, and stereognosis although light touch, heat and cold, vibration, and pin prick were normally appreciated. No other disturbances were noted. A hypodense cortical and subcortical lesion was found on CT scan 17 days after the onset consistent with an infarction affecting the parietal region. The symptoms disappeared in 3 weeks, but the sensory deficit persisted unchanged on re-examination 2 months later.

Paillard et al[331] described a case of left MCA lower division occlusion with a large infarct including the posterior parietal region and part of the superior parietal lobule. Very little motor deficit was noted, and deep tendon reflexes were symmetrical. However, a right hemianesthesia persisted for several years. The disturbance affected the right cheek and gums manifested by frequent failure of the patient to notice that food had gone to the right side of the mouth. The hand was so anesthetic that she experienced cuts and burns without noticing them. The foot was anesthetic enough that several times the patient stumbled when climbing stairs. Specific testing of the hand disclosed no joint position sense to point discrimination or ability to report pressure. However, touch could be discriminated both as to direction and general speed (whether fast or slow), and the patient proved capable of discriminating the gross size of an object (large or small) and was also capable of rough location of points of touch along the surface of the limb.

Correlations with Motor Deficits

The correlation of the sensory disturbance with motor disturbance is infrequently reported. A few unusual cases exist suggesting that a sensory disturbance may affect an area far smaller than that of the accompanying motor disturbance. Gacs et al[161] described a 50-year-old woman with a large low-density area in the right frontal region whose clinical deficit

included a dense left hemiplegia including the face with left hemianopia. The sensory disturbance was described only as diminution and pin pricking vibration in the left arm.

VISUAL FIELD DISTURBANCES

Hemianopia

Standard textbook accounts of MCA territory infarction regularly refer to hemianopia accompanying hemiparesis, hemisensory disturbance, and alterations in behavior,[307,312] but little clarification is provided for the value of this sign as an index of infarct site and size, and even less to the pathoanatomic correlate. There is little doubt that hemianopia accompanies the huge infarcts.[157] Traditionally, the hemianopia was ascribed to involvement of the visual radiation, even though the MCA supplies only the upper half of the radiation.[300]

For less global infarcts, hemianopia has been described with infarcts involving the frontal region, some as low as the sylvian fissure.[302] However, hemianopia has been absent in some instances of focal infarction even when impaired opticokinetic nystagmus (OKN) was found. It is difficult to sustain the notion that edema involving the radiations explains hemianopia when the infarct is far away from these structures. Instead, it seems more likely that the hemianopia as described is actually a disturbance in hemispatial response that is part of a hemineglect syndrome.[411] In such cases, other faulty responses to spatial stimuli are noted, such as the patient who is suffering a left hemispheral infarction turning toward the left in response to a voice from the right, and also showing failure to blink to threat stimulus from the right side. The subject requires further investigation.

Quadrantanopia

Parietal infarction deep enough to affect the fibers of the upper half of the visual radiation is presumably responsible for the infrequently described inferior quadrantanopia of MCA territory infarction (Fig. 19.13). Bounds et al[70] described a 45-year-old woman who experienced left inferior quadrantanopia attributed to embolism of the MCA 8 days after aortocoronary bypass surgery. Clinical worsening occurred 5 days later with hemiplegia, coma, and death from herniation. The autopsy report showed softening of most of the right hemisphere, and a specific focus of infarction correlating the earlier quadrantanopia was not described. Remarkably enough, it is difficult to find the clinical setting in which lower quadrantanopia is found; it is even more difficult to determine whether the quadrantanopia indicates a deep cleft of infarction reaching the visual radiation or whether it may occur in a more superficial infarct.

Impaired Opticokinetic Nystagmus

A test for OKN is assumed to detect disorders of the gaze mechanism mild enough that conjugate ocular gaze is not present at rest. Considering the number of patients tested for OKN, it is remarkable that there is still considerable contro-

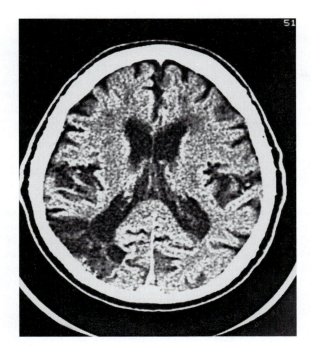

Figure 19.13 Axial CT scan showing a left parietal infarct in a patient with right inferior quadrantanopia.

versy over the usual locus of the lesion, the pathways injured, and even the nature of the disturbance. The early view[167,373] was that OKN was a reflex activity of the cerebral cortex, that the slow component initiated from the occipital region and the fast corrective phase from the frontal region, and that the OKN response was blunted by lesions at any point in the pathway. However, the higher prevalence of abnormal OKN in parietal lesions supported another view,[103,378] namely that the slow component from the occipital region passed directly to the brain stem through a pathway adjacent to the visual radiations, organized in ipsilateral pathways. Still another line of work[167] argued that the pathway runs deep through the parietal region to the frontal lobe, crosses the posterior limb of the corpus callosum, and controls fast phase components generated in the opposite frontal lobe. More recently, arguments have been put forward for separate mechanisms controlling foveal and full-field pursuit.[27] These studies showed the main disturbance to be in the slow component when targets were moved into vision from the side of space served by the damaged hemisphere.

The actual documented sites vary considerably (not all in the parietal lobe), and hemianopia need not occur. Impaired OKN has been encountered in a patient with a small high rolandic infarct whose visual fields were intact (Fig. 19.12). An autopsied patient of the senior author's[302] with superficial infarction confined to the inferior frontal region showed a brisk response by blinking from visual threat to the right side but had absent OKN for targets moving from right to left on initial examination (Fig. 19.10). The patient reported by Baloh et al[27] had a large infarct apparently involving the posterior cerebral artery territory, accompanied by right hemianopia and alexia but no language disturbance. To date, the author has encountered large numbers of cases with abnormal OKN testing when the resting eye position has been normal, but thus far no cases whose OKN testing has been normal in the face of tonic conjugate deviation of the eyes from a hemispheral infarct.

NEGLECT

The term neglect is taken to indicate disturbances shown by patients in responding to stimuli from the right side of space including OKN, turning to the left in response to auditory stimuli from the right, or faulty reading aloud or naming of objects in the right side of space.[12,54]

Neglect from Frontal Lesion

It has long been appreciated that a parietal lesion (from infarct or hemorrhage, or even other etiologies) may be associated with impaired response to stimuli from the opposite side of space, whether from a visual, auditory, or even somatosensory source.[52,99] These deficits are thought to reflect impaired input from sensory to motor regions. However, a similar disturbance occurs from frontal lesions as well,[109,205,206] whether cortical or subcortical.[375] Using positron emission transverse tomography scanning, Deuel and Collins[136] found widespread metabolic suppression in the basal ganglia and thalamus after a unilateral frontal lesion with little evidence of cortical hypometabolism beyond the immediate confines of the lesion. Their findings suggested that part of the syndrome may result from impaired activation of subcortical structures involved in planning motor movements. In the human, the signs of neglect from frontal lesions are remarkably transient, usually fading within a week in all but the largest infarcts.[87] This subject is treated more fully in the section on right hemisphere disease; the discussion below applies mainly to left hemisphere cases.

Motor Neglect

Motor neglect, said to be characterized by underutilization of one side without defects in strength reflex or sensibility, has been described by LaPlane and Degos.[253] Of the 20 cases reported, one of an ischemic type (located only by radionuclide scan in a prerolandic area) manifested by abnormal placement, lack of withdrawal of pain, reduced amplitude of movements, and visual hemineglect of the opposite side of space. This condition has a long history in clinical neurology. Under most circumstances of clinical examination the patient with this syndrome appears to have a hemiparesis, yet with special efforts on examination normal strength and dexterity can be demonstrated. The usual features include a lack of spontaneous placing reaction such as failure to place the hand in the lap or on the arm of a chair when sitting, letting it instead drag down beside the body; delayed or insufficient assumption of correct postures, resulting in heavy falls to the affected side with no attempts to minimize the effect of the fall by reaching out or correcting the balance; impaired automatic withdrawal reaction to pain; and excursions of the limb necessary to achieve a movement such as touching the nose, the patient instead leaning the head forward to compensate for failure to bring the finger far enough up. This disturbance may occur in the absence of a sensory disturbance or demonstrable hemiparesis. A similar autopsy case was described by Hartmann[193] secondary to an infarct affecting the second frontal gyrus of the right frontal lobe. Animal studies in the monkey have demonstrated a similar transitory disturbance observed after selective research high over the prefrontal region.[409]

Neglect for Verbal Material

Leicester et al[262] described a form of visual neglect in which the occurrence and frequency of errors were determined by the verbal content of the test materials. When the patient was required to select from an array of choices displayed directly in front, errors were seen with those materials that the patient found the most difficult to name or write; in such instances, responses were made less frequently to choices on the right-hand side of the display. When the test materials were easily named, little or no evidence of neglect for the right side of space was noted. This form of neglect, which is commonly encountered in testing patients with aphasia, was shown not to be obligatory but highly dependent on the verbal material in the test itself. It was not explained by defective spatial responding nor by defective sensory function, and occurred from left-sided lesions, not right.

MOVEMENT DISORDERS

Temporary or permanent movement disorders including hemichorea, atheosis, or dystonias are uncommon sequelae of MCA territory infarcts. In a few cases the infarct has affected the lenticulostriate territories. The most common cause appears to be lacunes (see Ch. 23), but a few have been associated with relatively large, deep infarcts consistent with occlusion of the MCA stem or embolism into many branches of the lenticulostriate territories.

Despite a large literature on the subject in children, few reports have appeared on adults.[186] Only one has been described with chorea: a 68-year-old woman reported by Austregesilo and Borges-Forte[24] developed immediate torsion spasms with choreiform movements from what was presumed to have been a stroke affecting the head of the caudate nucleus, putamen, and pallidum.

Dystonia has been the subject of the other reports. The one adult described in the series reported by Demierre and Rondot[127] was a 17-year-old with left hemiplegia that improved slightly within 4 weeks, by which time signs of dystonia had appeared. The fingers, wrist, and left elbow extended on walking, the left arm showed retropulsion-abduction with elevation of the shoulders, and the lower limb was held in external rotation. No specific involuntary movements were observed. A large hypodensity affecting the putamen, anterior capsule, and caudate was seen on CT scan. Grimes et al[186] encountered two patients with stroke in adulthood documented by CT scan. The first, a 32-year-old woman, suffered dense hemiplegia and "cortical" sensory loss from a large deep infarct affecting the caudate and putamen that regressed considerably by 5 months. A month later, she began to experience involuntary abduction and extension of the affected fingers with ulnar deviation of the wrist; the arm flexed behind the

back as she walked; and she had coarse tremor of the outstretched hand. The deficit progressed for 2 months and then stabilized. Medical therapy was ineffective. The second patient, a 50-year-old man, pursued a similar course, with the addition of orofacial dyskinesia and dystonia that developed in the fingers and arm, with flexion of the limb behind the back during walking. The syndrome worsened for 3 months before stabilizing and was unaffected by medical therapy.

AUTONOMIC DISTURBANCES

Excess of sweating contralateral to an MCA territory infarction is encountered only rarely. In the small series of cases reported, all patients had major syndromes of hemiparesis, hemisensory problems, hemianopia, and altered behavior states, indicating a large lesion affecting both the superficial and deep territories of the MCA.[249] Sweating in these few cases affected the face, neck, axilla, and upper trunk contralateral to the infarct and faded to normal within days.

Appenzeller[17] published an autopsy case described clinically as showing hyperhidrosis on the contralateral side of the body. No further details were mentioned including none regarding the extent of the other clinical deficits. The published photographs show a site of small hemorrhagic infarction in the upper bank of the insula and adjacent orbital surface of the operculum.

Contralateral rubbery edema of the affected hands and feet may occur from large MCA territory infarction (Fig. 19.14). The syndrome usually becomes evident within a few hours and persists for up to 2 weeks. The exact anatomic correlates are unknown.

Syndromes Referrable to Left Hemisphere Infarction

APHASIA

The cerebrum irrigated by the left MCA is of prime importance in language function. The latter can be defined operationally for clinical purposes as a symbolic system in which the relations between meaningful elements (sounds, print, gestural signs, and so forth) are purely arbitrary. Aphasia (or its more commonly less severe variant known as dysphasia) is thus regarded as a disorder caused by acquired brain injury that results in dysfunctional use of rule-governed, symbolic behavior.[255,413] The sylvian fissure of the hemisphere dominant for speech and language is the region most likely to show symptoms of dysphasia following a focal brain lesion. Over 95% of right-handed people and even most left-handed people have dominance for speech and language in the left hemisphere. Right hemisphere dominance for speech and language in a right-handed person is distinctly uncommon.

Many of the traditional clinicopathologic correlations of brain and language function[74,80] have undergone revisions in recent years. Among them has been that smaller, focal brain

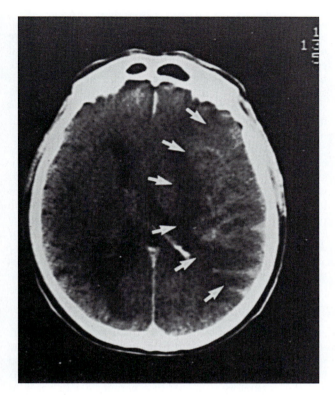

Figure 19.14 Noncontrast-enhanced CT scan showing hemorrhagic infarction of the entire middle cerebral artery territory. Hemihyperhidrosis and distal arm edema were part of the clinical picture.

lesions once thought to produce the major syndromes of aphasia are now known to cause only transient or minor abnormalities in production or comprehension of speech sounds and shapes. Much larger lesions are necessary to produce major disruptions in language function. Recent work has also made it apparent that vital speech and language roles are played by the deeper structures, especially the thalamus.

Global or Total Aphasia

Few studies have indicated the different types of aphasia expected in a setting of acute stroke. Brust et al[82] studied 850 patients admitted to Harlem Hospital, noting that 177 (21%) had acute aphasia. In 57 (32%) the speech disturbance was characterized by fluent aphasia, while in 120 (68%) it was of the nonfluent type (see below for definitions). A significant correlation ($P < 0.01$) was found between the occurrence of nonfluency and a poor prognosis for mortality. For fluent and nonfluent aphasics a greater mortality was associated with hemiparesis or a visual field disturbance. Presumably, the occurrence of the nonfluent type of aphasia was a reflection of larger lesions. CT scanning was not performed in this series of cases. A similar poor outlook for aphasia with acute stroke was noted by Marquardson[285] in his study of 769 acute stroke patients. Aphasia occurred in the acute state in 133 (33%) of these cases. The author noted that hemiplegia was less likely to improve if accompanied by aphasia and that aphasia had a better outlook when unaccompanied by hemiplegia.

CLINICAL FEATURES. Occlusion of the trunk of the MCA or its upper division produces a global disruption of language function. Its effect puts out of action virtually all the brain regions responsible for language. The initial disturbance is so profound that it goes by the term total aphasia. After the acute period, clinicians and family sometimes observe some improved capacity to understand context-related information (e.g., "Are you feeling better?") and to participate in the give and take of simple communication. Within weeks or months, comprehension improves, especially for nongrammatical forms, and the patient shows more disturbances in speaking and writing than in listening and reading.[315] This emphasis on dysphasia more in speaking and writing is known as Broca's aphasia or major motor aphasia.

LESION SIZE. With the advent of CT scanning, a volumetric measure of the lesion became possible, permitting inquiry into the issue not only of the usual lesion size associated with the syndrome, but also of the minimal and maximal dimensions. MR imaging has further improved this capacity. Large lesions have been documented in several CT scan studies.[233,290] Naeser and Hayward[323] documented the lesion volume in two groups of cases, those labeled *mixed* aphasia, a term that broadly encompasses the clinical picture of total aphasia, and those labeled *global* aphasia. The site of the lesion in seven cases of mixed aphasia has proved heterogeneous, usually reflecting a large infarct affecting the sylvian region and beyond, but in a few instances Broca's or Wernicke's areas proper were not mapped in the scanned lesion. The lesion size in these cases was approximately 3.9 by 3.9 cm, and such a lesion was usually seen on five slices. The lesion volume in five cases of global aphasia was considerably larger, on the order of 5.8 by 5.8 cm. Like the mixed aphasia cases, the site of the minimal lesion lay in the sylvian region, and the major contribution to the larger volume was its centrifugal spread into the adjacent frontal, parietal, and temporal regions.

A clinical example should serve to indicate the main features of these cases:

> A 35-year-old man who underwent ligation of the MCA stem just distal to the lenticulostriate branches remained globally aphasic for the remaining 3 years of life. Examined at 2 years, he interacted with the examiner and responded properly on tests that did not obviously require the use of language. Examples representing his consistent failure included his inability to select a picture of a cow on hearing the sound "moo" when presented with eight animal pictures; his inability to point to a picture of a dog when shown a picture of another dog; his inability to point to pots boiling on the stove in the background in a picture showing an elderly lady telling stories to children; and his inability to point to his home state when shown a map of the United States. Other tests of this type were carried out for many trials, demonstrating his ability to see, hear, point, and respond accurately to these stimulus elements when no spoken or written commands were involved from the examiner. However, he obeyed no spoken or printed command, even such single words as the printed word smile. He vocalized only poorly understandable

syllables and did not repeat aloud. He made only crude marks on a page, using his left hand to guide a pen. He was easily dismayed by failure, flushing and bursting into tears when the examiner shook his head after a faulty response. Autopsy over a year later showed complete infarction of the entire hemispheral territory of the MCA, sparing only the basal ganglia and capsule supplied by the lenticulostriate territories (Fig. 19.9).

Motor Aphasia

For almost 100 years a syndrome has been recognized in which the ability to communicate by speaking or writing seems far more impaired than the comprehension of words heard or words seen.[79] Although Boulliaud[69] deserves credit for popularizing the notion that a lesion of both frontal lobes disrupts the power of spoken speech, the surgeon Paul Broca, the friend of Boulliaud's son-in-law, has received most of the credit for the documentation that a left-sided sylvian infarct more reliably causes the syndrome. Broca described two patients who appeared to him to have lost their memory on how to speak. Considerable controversy has persisted concerning whether this characterization is suitable for the findings, the locus of the minimal lesion to precipitate the major syndrome, and whether the effects are the same when the lesion is confined to the third frontal convolution, which Broca took to be the site causing the syndrome that bears his name.

MAJOR MOTOR APHASIA. In its usual form, major motor aphasia develops as a late sign in the course of the major cerebral infarct. The responsible infarct encompasses at least the insula and usually the adjacent frontoparietal operculum, roughly approximating the large sylvian infarct encountered in Broca's original description (Fig. 19.15). In such patients, there is a sharp contrast between the hesitant, agrammatical speech and the relatively better comprehension evident in conversational tests, as long as the examiner keeps the sentences and questions simple.

In the initial period following the acute infarct, attempts at distinction between speech and language production and comprehension are all but impossible given the severe nature of the disturbances encountered. The clinical features of what can be described later as Broca's aphasia cannot be detected, buried as it is in a deficit so profound that the syndrome has long terms like total aphasia or global aphasia.[13,121,197,244,302,303,416] With the passage of a few months, and some improvements in testability, the syndrome of Broca's aphasia begins to appear.

Whether the motor aphasia that emerges is a disturbance confined to speaking and writing or contains a global disturbance in the brain's capacity to deal with grammatical functions has remained the subject of dispute. The difficulties authors have had over the years in settling this point is reflected in the variety of terms used to substitute for Broca's aphasia: expressive dysphasia,[421] efferent motor dysphasia,[280] motor dysphasia,[180] and verbal dysphasia,[194] to name but some. Most authors echo the impression of Liepmann[276] that in such cases the symptoms of motor aphasia predominate; the limited capacity for spoken expression conceals the deeper language disturbances that persist but are less obvious.

The *speech disturbance* is evident to a similar degree whether the utterances are produced in spontaneous conversation or during efforts to repeat aloud or read aloud. The spoken responses are hesitant, demonstrating impaired skilled interaction (dyspraxia) between the settings of the oropharynx and the respiratory elements that permit smooth vocalization.[11] In the production of individual words, the transitions from sound to sound are accomplished with difficulty,[280] an effect of the speech dyspraxia that conveys an impression of stuttering. The effect is especially obvious when polysyllabic words are spoken. The disturbance also impairs the usual clustering of words to form phrases and interferes with the normal melodic intonation that serves to indicate differences among exclamations, questions, and declarative statements. There is a high correlation between the degree of buccolingual dyspraxia and speech loss in patients with Broca's aphasia.[133] Apart from these signs of *speech dyspraxia*, the structure of the spoken phrases may be grammatically simplified, consisting largely of single words that function as predicative elements; these responses strike the listener as having the laconic style of a

Figure 19.15 One of Broca's original cases.

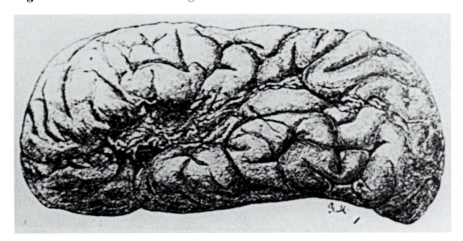

telegram. In more severe cases, the responses consist of single nouns or verbs. These are so condensed that the disorder is not merely one of simplified speaking, but indicates impaired use of grammatical skills. These grossly condensed utterances are labeled *agrammatism*. In some, the utterances have been limited to a single word or phrase[42,327] characterized as verbal stereotypes, a clinical sign carrying a discouraging prognosis for improvement.

Because of its common usage, mention must be made of nonfluency,[244] a term widely used to capture the essence of the complex disturbance in spoken speech and language in these cases. The inherent ambiguities in the term has limited its value, since it is not clear if the user means the hesitancy, the dysmelodic flow of sounds, the condensed grammar, or the groping for words that is part of the disorder of oral naming common to aphasic syndromes of either antero- or retrorolandic origin. Each of the elements alone may thus reflect lesions other than those responsible for motor aphasia. However, the term as defined recently apparently now encompasses all the elements together: ". . . effortful, dysmelodic speech, often with impaired articulation and impoverishment of grammatical form."[244] As often defined, the persistence of nonfluency correlates well with lesion size. Among the group of infarcts studied by Knopman et al,[244] 10 of the 17 patients with persisting nonfluency had lesions whose CT size measured >100 cm^3, six were >25 cm^3, and only one was smaller. Among the cases with smaller lesions, the surface component lay in the inferior rolandic region with a sizable subcortical component, presumably a combination of cortical surface and deep infarction.

Other features of the language deficit are important elements of the syndrome. Numerous authors have commented on the difficulties such patients have in responding to spoken or written material that features small grammatical words such as "the," "are," "then," and so forth or involves spelling.[257] Poorest performance occurs when the meaning is highly dependent on grammatical features, especially when subject-object relations are based less on simple nouns (e.g., "John saw Jane") than on pronouns (e.g., "He saw it"), or when the passive voice is used (e.g., "He was seen by her"). The

disturbances observed extend beyond the acts of speaking or writing into comprehension of the material itself. Silent reading comprehension, which requires no overt vocalization, is usually only a little disturbed unless the material to be read contains a particularly high density of such grammatical words. When it does, the comprehension may be strikingly abnormal. This condition has been termed deep dyslexia and has been described as a third form of dyslexia.[42] Similar disturbances can be documented in tests requiring the patient to point to visual displays containing single letters or grammatical words in response to hearing the names of the letters. Some have even shown faulty selection of a single letter among a visually presented display of letters when the test stimulus was a printed word whose pronounced sound (homophone) is identical to that of a given letter (i.e., "eye" to "i").[315] These examples are indicative of the global disturbances in language that occur and persist in patients with the major syndrome of Broca's aphasia.

The *clinicopathologic correlation* has been better understood in recent years. Major motor or Broca's aphasia is not a syndrome expected from infarction restricted to Broca's area. It usually reflects a major infarction involving most of the territory of supply of the upper division of the left MCA, as was actually shown in Broca's original cases. Accompanying disturbances in motor, sensory, and visual function usually make the diagnosis easy. The usually large size of the sylvian infarct sets the stage for contralateral hemiplegia.[219] At times, however, the main weight of the lesion may fall on the sylvian region alone, which may produce a surprisingly slight hemiparesis considering the major effect on language function[328] (Fig. 19.16). In these cases, the hemiparesis may be limited to the face and hand. Ideomotor dyspraxia of the unaffected left upper extremity is the rule, as is bilateral buccofacial dyspraxia, which has been reported in 90% of patients.[133,171,173] Contralateral hemineglect is the rule in the acute stage.

Autopsy documentation of the major syndrome of Broca's aphasia comes largely from the older literature. In the senior author's[303] review of the 19 autopsy cases found with a syndrome described as Broca's aphasia beyond a period of 10 months, all were examples of major sylvian lesions or insular

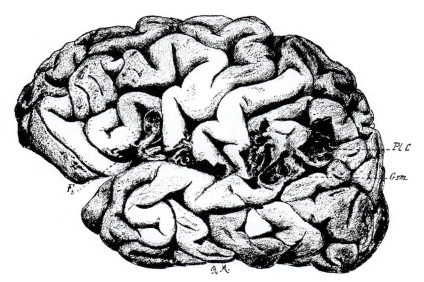

Figure 19.16 Lithograph of an example of infarction limited to the sylvian lip. (From Moutier,[318] with permission.)

opercular lesions at the least. The two notable exceptions were the two original cases reported by Broca himself, in which the author mistakenly considered the responsible lesions to be limited to the third frontal convolution, even though he described the large sylvian opercular infarct that was actually found at autopsy (Fig. 19.15). Fifteen of 39 cases uncovered during a search of the records at the Massachusetts General Hospital for a 10-year period similarly documented large sylvian infarcts.[302] Two cases based on CT scans reported by the same author showed enormous lesions affecting the sylvian region and adjacent operculum and frontoparietal regions of the left hemisphere. In all these cases, hemiplegia was present at onset, no patients were able to stand for a week after onset, and all walked in the chronic state with a circumducted gait carrying a spastic arm and a densely paretic lower face. Head and eye deviation was present for several days after onset, and hemianopia was documented initially and persisted for several days.

Large aphasic populations have been studied using CT scan.[28,237,313,321] In view of the work done with CT scanning, it is perhaps no surprise that a similar large cohort has not been reported by MR, but individual cases continue to appear in the literature. The CT scan lesions with persistent Broca's aphasia have largely been opercular and insular. In Naeser's[321] four cases studied by CT scan, the location was frontosylvian, sparing the temporal lobe, with lesions on the order of 3.1 by 3.1 cm in CT slices where the lesion was present. One such study,[244] focusing on the issue of nonfluency, showed that the larger sylvian lesions were associated with persistent nonfluency. Among the cases with the smaller lesions, destruction of the region taken to represent Broca's area was not necessary for persistent nonfluency but was associated with transient deficits. No details of the remainder of the neurologic deficits were presented in this study. Although rare, a large lesion of the right hemisphere may precipitate the syndrome in a right-handed person.[213]

With regard to the evolution of Broca's syndrome, a 1-year follow-up study by Kertesz[235] showed 15 of 17 patients evolving toward a dysphasia characterized mainly by difficulty in word finding out of proportion to other language disturbances but with a persistent dyspraxia of speech.

A few notable exceptions to the usual clinical picture accompanying Broca's aphasia may occur when the lesion is confined to the insula and adjacent operculum. Moutier's[318] patient Chissadon acutely suffered a hemiplegia but in the chronic state had only the slightest motor deficit. A remarkably circumscribed infarct was found along the lip of the upper bank of the sylvian fissure, which may have sufficed to interfere with language function and not with sensory motor function. A few cases of this type have been described under Benson's term, the sylvian lip syndrome. One of Broca's cases was also described as having no detectable motor disturbance but was examined several years after the onset of his original deficit.

The issue of the smallest lesion that is sufficient to produce the persisting syndrome of Broca's aphasia remains unresolved. To date no known case of an infarct confined to the Broca area alone has produced a lasting severe Broca's aphasia.[269]

MINOR MOTOR APHASIA. Focal infarcts affecting the operculum produce a very different form of disturbance. Infarcts confined to Broca's area are not the expected cause of the syndrome of Broca's aphasia. The syndrome has been described repeatedly in recent years.[250,268,290,302,303] In the acute stages complete mutism with ideomotor and buccofacial dyspraxia is commonly encountered. Auditory and visual comprehension for language is virtually intact, and some individuals are capable of writing properly with the unaffected left hand. Improvement from the initial mutism begins within hours or at the least days and rarely weeks later. Any language deficit evident in speaking and writing is extremely transitory and often disappears before it can be tested in full detail. The accompanying bucco-linguo-facial and ideomotor limb dyspraxia likewise disappears quickly. The dyspraxia appears to contribute to most of the disturbances in speaking. The oral cavity positions closely approximate those desired to generate given sounds, but the slight inaccuracies strike the listener's ears as mispronunciations. Also, the dyspractic disturbance in respiration interferes with the smooth flow of sounds and transition from syllable to syllable in running speech; this has variously been called aphemia, oral-verbal apraxia, or apraxia of speech.[112] The disorder is not a result of weakness of the muscle serving articulation.

The initial mutism is usually accompanied by contralateral hemiparesis, but limitation of the weakness to the lower face and hand is not uncommon. Head and eye deviation have been documented but not often.[302] A few cases of Broca's infarction have presented with no hint of motor paresis.[76] One such patient[288] became mute over a period of 20 minutes after initially experiencing both 5 minutes of numbness affecting the right side of his face and arm and difficulty repeating aloud. The neurologic examination revealed a mild orofacial dyspraxia but no weakness, and sensation and visual fields were normal. The disturbance in speaking faded to normal within 9 days. The CT scan at day 14 showed a low density with abnormal enhancement over the foot of the inferior frontal gyrus and inferior aspect of the second frontal gyrus. The operculum and insula were not involved.

In the six autopsied cases studied by the senior author, three of whom were reported[302] (Fig. 19.11), the initial right-sided motor deficit and ideomotor dyspraxia with initial mutism and language deficit gave way to emerging spoken speech that showed scant evidence of agrammatism. A larger series based on CT scan[313] showed similar findings; only one patient showed any evidence of grammatical condensation and simplified sentence structure at any time. When the speech and language production has been described as nonfluency,[244] a similarly transient disturbance has been seen in the smaller lesions found by CT scan.

The rate and extent of improvement vary considerably. Some patients appear normal within days in all but the most complex language tasks.[313,385] Others become fluent after a few months and appear abnormal only to those most familiar with their daily routines (Fig. 19.17).

The clinicopathologic correlation has proved remarkably reproducible in the reported cases. There appear to be few exceptions to the rule that a Broca's area infarction does not precipitate either the acute or the chronic forms of Broca's aphasia.[95,98,266,303,313] The exceptions to this rule appear infrequent enough to warrant special comment. Van Gehuchten[396] described a 60-year-old man with sudden total loss of speech accompanied by paresis of the right upper limb and a small

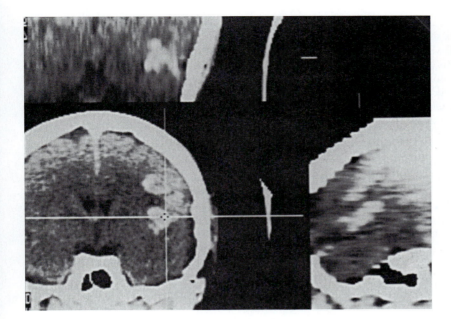

Figure 19.17 CT scan showing three views of an inferior frontal infarct, presenting as minor motor aphasia.

amount of facial involvement. The paresis diminished progressively, but the speech disturbance persisted unchanged until death 1 year later. Van Gehuchten described the clinical picture as " . . . pure motor aphasia with agraphia with no word blindness or deafness." The patient was incapable of speaking. He uttered only a few sounds and sometimes a word or two. However, he could express himself adequately by gestures and wrote some letters or ordinary words from dictation, but was unable to write spontaneously or from dictation under more demanding circumstances. Autopsy revealed an infarct affecting the inferior half of the middle frontal gyrus from the top to the bottom of what was described as Broca's area. The accompanying photograph disclosed the infarct but did not indicate the involvement or sparing of the insula, nor whether the lesion extended deep into the brain. Kleist[243] considered that the rare instances of a persistent and severe deficit associated with a Broca's area infarction could be explained by an extension of the infarct deep into the hemisphere, disrupting the white matter fibers that serve as projection and association pathways for Broca's area. Foix[155] made a similar inference earlier by referring to infarcts effecting the deeper branches of the MCA. Goldstein[180] made similar suggestions but failed to specify the vascular territory involved in these larger lesions.

SPEECH DISTURBANCES WITH LOWER ROLANDIC INFARCTION. The role of the lower rolandic cortex in the motor aphasias has not received wide attention. Few cases have been reported since the days of Moutier,[308] whose studies suggested that infarcts in this region did not cause motor aphasia. Niessl von Mayendorf[328] described a case of infarction involving the rolandic operculum that spread to the supramarginal and angular gyri including the first, second, and third temporal gyri, but that spared Broca's area. The patient was unable to write spontaneously or from dictation. A similar disturbance was suggested by Kleist,[243] using the term aphasic dysarthria. Three autopsied cases have appeared in the literature. Tonkonogy and Good-

glass[385] described a 63-year-old man with moderate right central facial paresis, deviation of the tongue to the right, and slight right hemiparesis predominantly in the right arm with normal sensory function and visual fields. The speech was slow and dysprosadic, involving both stuttering and poor control of pitch. Articulations were deformed to the point of approximating literal paraphasias. A very slight disturbance in word finding was present. Dysprosody and articulatory disturbances remained, and moderate brachial facial dyspraxia was present. Comprehension for reading and writing was practically intact. By 3 weeks the speech function had recovered fully or almost entirely with just mild dysprosody; the right hand had only slight weakness. Autopsy showed an infarct affecting the lower cortex of the rolandic sulcus of superficial size approximately 1.0 by 1.5 cm linked to an infarct in the anterior limb of the internal capsule. LaCours and Lhermitte[250] described a patient whose infarct was limited to the rolandic operculum lacking any disturbance in language but suffering a syndrome of "phonetic disintegration." Levine and Sweet[269] added a third case of rolandic infarction involving most of the precentral gyrus. The patient was only able to vocalize grunting or moaning sounds for the 10 days she was testable before death. Autopsy disclosed a highly focal hemorrhage involving the midportion of the precentral gyrus and sparing the frontal region in Broca's area.

The overlap of this syndrome with cases producing predominantly literal paraphasias has been noted by Luria[282] under the term afferent motor aphasia, attributed to faulty sensory feedback from a postrolandic lesion leading to inaccurate anatomic settings of the oropharynx, with resultant mispronunciations.

The concern over settling the role of the lower rolandic region is not merely an exercise in trivia. Levine and Sweet[268] have updated the long overlooked thesis of the role of the precentral gyrus lesion in the major syndrome of Broca's aphasia. As early as 1926, Niessl von Mayendorf[328] noted the invariable association of precentral gyrus lesions in the larger infarcts that set the stage for motor aphasia. Trojanowski et al[389] encountered a case of persisting Broca's aphasia with infarction limited to the cortex and subcortical white matter of the precentral gyrus sparing the deeper structures and largely sparing the adjacent third frontal convolution. For the present, initial mutism must be considered an expected sign in lower rolandic infarcts, and its occurrence can be taken as a sign predicting against an alternative diagnosis of a deep, lacunar type infarct in a patient presenting with isolated hemiparesis. Should more cases of inferior frontal infarction with persisting Broca's aphasia be described, the current clinical point that such cases mean a larger lesion would lose much of its force.

SPEECH DISTURBANCES FROM DEEP INFARCTS. Two forms of deep infarct speech disorder have occurred. In the first form, infarcts affecting the motor outflow of both sides have produced mutism as part of a syndrome of paralysis of both sides of the face, oropharynx, and tongue. In the second, and more interesting, form, a single deep infarct occurs that has produced enough disturbance in speech and language to be described as an aphasic disorder by the observer. Bonhoeffer's[67] classic patient, unable to speak anything more than a few poorly formed vowels, had a large, deep infarct of the type described as a "giant lacune."[345] However, given its large size and the second infarct in the cortical surface territory of the anterior cerebral, it seems more likely that the cause of the deep infarct was embolism to the MCA stem: the infarct spread from the corner of the lateral ventricle through the caudate and internal capsule, even reaching the external capsule. The speech deficit was formulated as a double disconnection from Broca's area: the giant lacune prevented innervation of the bulbar apparatus from ipsilateral pathways, while the anterior cerebral territory infarct cut off transcallosal projections.

Severe dysarthria and rare paraphasias with little disturbance in comprehension resulting from a single large deep infarct were also reported by Kleist[243] in the patient Bühlmeir. As best as the current authors can make out from the combination of text and pictures, the infarct involved both limbs of the internal capsule, the putamen and caudate, and much of the corona radiata and centrum semiovale; the size was that usually associated with occlusion of the MCA stem. No mention was made of the vascular pathology. The syndrome was formulated as a disruption of both efferent pathways from Broca's area from the single large lesion: one pathway to the bulbar apparatus ipsilaterally was destroyed by the capsular component of the lesion; the other transcallosal pathway through the centrum semiovale was destroyed by another part of the lesion.

Fisher[150] described a case of "modified PMH [pure motor hemiplegia] with 'motor aphasia'" due to a large infarct involving the genu and anterior limb of the internal capsule and adjacent white matter of the corona radiata. Speech was initially dysarthric, progressed later to mispronunciation of words and then to utterance of single-syllable unintelligible sounds, and ended as mutism. Comprehension was reportedly intact. The last of Santamaria et al's[360] series of eight patients had "expressive dysphasia." The language disorder was characterized by ". . . nonfluent conversational speech, naming and reading difficulties, dysgraphia and normal auditory comprehension." The disorder disappeared a year later. Marie[283]

also presented a patient with "anarthria" but no aphasic symptoms, due to a putaminal hemorrhage.

Other cases of mutism with more circumscribed lacunes have been due to bilateral capsular infarction. One of Fisher's cases was documented by microscopic vascular pathology.[149] His patient became mute with the second infarct, which involved the left internal capsule. The left capsular lacune was 4 by 4 by 5 mm and lay at the genu. A case in the senior author's experience at the University of South Alabama was similar, with an earlier infarct in the posterior limb of the right internal capsule and a more recent infarct affecting the left internal capsule at the genu.[306] This last infarct was so small as to be barely visible on CT scan, yet it yielded virtual anarthria, severe dysphonia, and dysphagia but only a mild right arm weakness. None of the purely lacunar cases appear to qualify for the term aphasia, if the term is taken to imply a disturbance in language function independent of impaired articulation.

Imprecise definitions prevent any comparison of these terms with the classic syndrome of subcortical motor aphasia. Unusual syndromes of dysphasia have been described from deep infarcts, but, to date, the neuropathologic nature of the lesions remains unclarified. The six cases reported by Damasio et al[110] were diagnosed by CT scan (with no angiographic or autopsy data), as were the seven cases of ischemic mechanism reported by Naeser et al,[322] at least three of which had accompanying surface infarcts. These uncertainties aside, the CT abnormalities encountered in the wholly deep lesion cases were predominantly in the anterior limb of the internal capsule, putamen, and caudate, and all were among the larger size consistent with the type 1 "giant lacunes" of Rascol et al.[345] Clinically, remarkable dysprosody was seen, at times accompanied by dysarthria, little or no dyspraxia of limbs on either side, and a mixture of deficits in syntactic and semantic functions not typical for any of the classical syndromes of dysphasia.[110,323,410] Other studies showing impaired frontal reactivity in studies of cerebral blood flow suggest that the disorder may be explained by damage to thalamofrontal pathways, the diminished verbal behavior forming part of a syndrome of abulia.[104,251]

Sensory Aphasia

The vast majority of cases labeled Wernicke's aphasia are associated with occlusion of the lower division and its branches. The cause of the occlusion is usually embolism. Because the lower division gives off its branches over an extremely short distance, occlusion at its origin may give rise to several distinct variants in the size and topography of the infarction. Although little effort has been made to pursue the point in the literature on aphasia, there is a rough degree of correlation between the extent of the language deficit and its intensity as a function of the lesion size, which is reflected in the text that follows.

MAJOR SENSORY APHASIA. When the embolus blocks all the branches with no retrograde collateral from the posterior cerebral, a large infarct occurs that encompasses the whole posterior temporal, inferior parietal, and lateral temporo-occipital regions (Fig. 19.18). Infarcts of such huge size generate a profound deficit in language function, often described as *Wernicke's aphasia*.

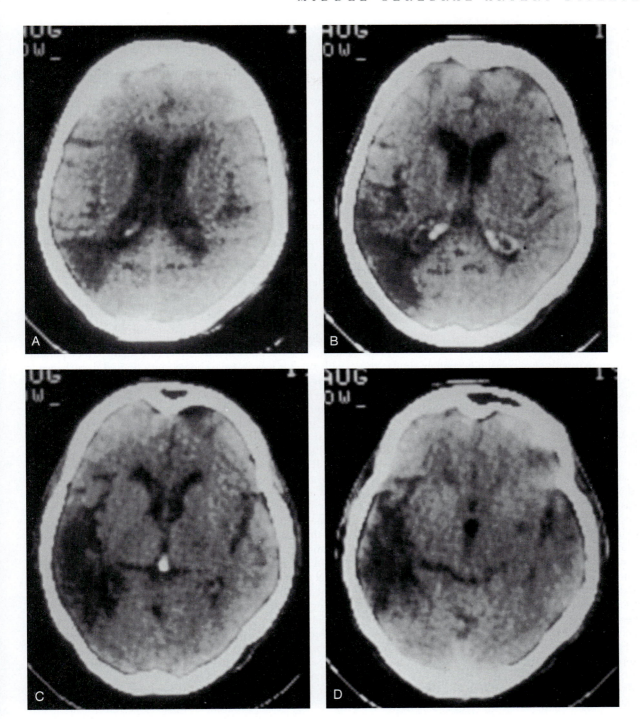

Figure 19.18 (**A–D**) CT evidence of large infarct involving the lower division of the middle cerebral artery in a right-handed woman; no aphasia.

In contrast to motor aphasia, patients with sensory aphasia show little or no disturbance in the ability to vocalize, make smooth transitions between syllables, assemble utterances in the form of phrases, and achieve an intonation of their utterances that sounds like questions, replies, and declarative statements, regardless of the severity of the language disturbance reflected in the content of their speech.[13]

In the acute stage of the major infarcts, the disturbance in language content presents as such gross paraphasias in spontaneous speech that the utterances often contain no understandable words, a condition known as *jargon paraphasia*. The specific words expected to be uttered—the target words—are often distorted (but recognizable) in their phonetic structure (literal paraphasia) both in vowels and consonants, or other words in the same class are substituted (verbal paraphasias); these are occasionally distorted by the addition of unwanted suffixes (less often prefixes) or at times even omitted, and often contaminated by the recurrence (perseverations) of previously uttered words or word fragments. The effects on language behavior are almost the reverse of the insular-opercular syndromes: speech is filled with small grammatical words but is missing the key words (the predicative elements) that contain the essence of the message. The extent of the language disturbance is often revealed only in prolonged conversation. The casual or hurried examiner may find that the patient speaks easily, engages in simple conversational exchanges, and even appears to be making an effort at communication. Because the utterances often flow in a manner suggesting attempts at declarative statements, questions, or explanations, and are accompanied by gestures of the face and limbs, the patients seem to be making efforts to communicate. However, attempts to engage the patient in testing often fail to yield much evidence that the patient has understood the task and is attempting to respond. When the patient does not respond properly, the examiner is faced with the difficulty of deciding whether the fault lies in comprehension, praxis, or failure of the examiner to make clear to the patient what is required.[263]

The writing is usually disturbed in a manner similar to spoken speech. The cursive script is usually legible, since there is no hemiparesis, but the content varies considerably. Instances have been reported with writing far superior to oral naming.[210,311] Because quantitative comparison between written and spoken responses is not the rule for most analyses of cases of Wernicke's aphasia, it remains uncertain whether these observations are exceptions or common.

The disturbance in comprehension of language in the spoken and written forms has been long assumed to be of the same type as that observed in the spoken and written speech, a sign of an essentially unitary nature of the disorder.[181] Although the brain lesion interferes with auditory comprehension, it has been difficult to demonstrate any such disturbance in phonemic processing.[385] Instead of a disturbance in elemental phonemic processing,[166] the problem seems to lie at the level of determining the linguistic significance of the adequately discriminated auditory stimuli.[60] It has likewise proved difficult to determine the extent to which disturbances in reading comprehension parallel those of auditory comprehension. A few patients with rather larger lesions have shown a relative superiority in reading for comprehension compared with auditory comprehension.[210]

The *clinicopathologic correlation* has, like Broca's aphasia, been with a rather large lesion. The cerebral infarction responsible for the major syndrome affects much of the lower division of the MCA.[305] Characteristically, the cause is embolism, the embolic material arresting at the first bifurcation of the lower division. That the lower division gives off many of its branches at this site favors the forward end of the Wernicke area lesion originating in the posterior sylvian region, at the superior temporal plane adjacent to Heschl's transverse gyrus. Uncollateralized occlusion of one or more branches of the lower division can produce an infarct so deep that it creates a schizencephalic cleft, reaching from the surface all the way through the white matter to the ventricular wall. Collateral retrograde into the lower division from the posterior cerebral artery territory may reduce the perimeter of the infarct, in some cases to a fairly small zone just beyond the point of the occlusion.

In most of the recent literature, the full syndrome of Wernicke's aphasia has been correlated mainly with the larger posterior hemispheral extent of the lesions.[323,388] In the four cases clinically diagnosed as Wernicke's aphasia in Naeser's[323] study, the lesions were relatively large, on the order of 2.5 to 3.1 by 3.1 cm on the slices showing low-density lesions, and the findings were seen on three slices around the level of Wernicke's area.

Although the lesion seems to be large in cases labeled clinically as Wernicke's aphasia, little is known about the exact correlation of the lesion site and size and the features of the syndrome. The authors have encountered over 50 such cases of large infarction over the past 10 years. In this group of cases with large lesions, some degree of correlation seems to exist between lesion size and performance in special language studies comparing the spoken and written response to auditory and visual presentation of words, pictures, and sounds: patients suffering the large lesions were no better at language response to words, sounds, or pictures of the same items (i.e., the disturbance was just as severe for words heard as words seen, or for sounds heard as pictures seen). Other patients with smaller lesions have shown more limited disturbance in either auditory or visual comprehension, but not both to the same degree.[210] The authors believe that patients with protracted and exaggerated spontaneous speaking (logorrhea) have been those with the larger infarcts, and that those with the smaller infarcts rarely show this sign, a point that could be studied in more detail.

It has recently been recognized that some of the patients with a fairly large lesion across the lower division may not show a clinical picture of Wernicke's aphasia at all but, instead, show one suggestive of the conduction aphasia syndrome.[5,107,356] In these cases comprehension is so satisfactory that the main finding is difficulty in repeating aloud. The implications are discussed in detail below.

A few cases have been reported in which no detectable initial deficit in language occurred or at the most it was only slight and transient[66,242,291] despite an infarct affecting the posterior superior temporal region large enough to have been expected to produce Wernicke's aphasia. The senior author has had a similar case, an elderly right-handed woman whose cerebral embolus occurred while walking in her garden in the company of her internist son. She was immediately tested: she could read aloud and write correctly and could repeat and converse normally, but she experienced signs of a right hemianopia. Examination by the senior author within days also failed to disclose language disturbance (Fig. 19.18). Cases of this sort serve to indicate the limitations of our present understanding of language organization in the brain.

MINOR SENSORY APHASIA AND VARIANTS. When the embolus occluding at the origin of the lower division is collateralized retrogradely from the branches of the posterior cerebral artery, some reduction in total infarct size occurs, the infarction zone shrinking backward toward the site of occlusion. How often such cases occur is only recently being appreciated with the widespread use of CT or MR scanning. Prior to these techniques, the mere angiographic demonstration of an occluded lower division at its origin left the physician unable to be certain how large an infarction was present distal to the occlusion. However, these cases provide an opportunity to determine how small a lesion is sufficient to precipitate the full syndrome of Wernicke's aphasia. Little is known about the spectrum of syndromes that occur as a function of differences in lesion size.

At issue is the vital question of the precise location and size of Wernicke's area. The thorough review by Bogen and Bogen[63] amply demonstrated that scarcely anyone agrees. Over the decades, the region attributed to Wernicke's area seems to have shrunk steadily from Wernicke's original notion that it was the posterior end of the sylvian fissure and adjacent parieto-temporo-occipital region. From an initially large zone suggested by 19th century authors, actually encompassing much of the arterial supply of the lower division, the area critical for the syndrome is considered by more recent authorities to be smaller and smaller, the most shrunken being the small size of the posterior superior temporal plane in Geschwind's[171] diagrams. As suggested above, the tendency to focus attention on this smaller zone may arise in part from the currently popular means of mapping a lesion by CT or MR scan for several cases in the same cohort, seeking the site where the lesions overlap.[234] The approach has the advantage of targeting the focal lesion site common to all the cases. Since the site common to all cases is the posterior superior temporal plane, it would be easy to assume that this site represents the critical zone. However, this site may simply be an artifact of the diagrammatic method, since it is along the posterior superior temporal plane that the lower division bifurcates, and where most of the embolic infarcts begin. If so, this location may merely be the essential focus of the infarct, not the site of the lesion producing Wernicke's aphasia. The precise relationship needs to be established by patients whose lesions are confined to this small site.

Cases of Wernicke's aphasia with a lesion confined to the superior temporal plane appear to be remarkably rare. A 20-year effort at three large hospital-based populations reviewed by the authors and colleagues has failed to reveal any examples. No less an authority than Charles Foix,[155] writing on vascular causes of Wernicke's aphasia in 1928, admitted he had seen none. In 1939, Nielsen[327] found 12 patients with Wernicke's aphasia in the literature whose deficit included reading disturbances with lesions that spared the angular gyrus. These were the same cases Benson and Geschwind[44] later used to support their claim that severe alexia (part of the full Wernicke's aphasia syndrome) can arise from a lesion confined to the superior temporal plane. However, of these 12 cases, 3 had been reported by the original authors (and also so noted previously by Henschen[209] in his long review) to have had no alexia. Six others had large posterior sylvian lesions of which the superior temporal plane portion was rarely a part. According to the detailed description, two appear to have been old residual subcortical hematomas, a lesion arguably much larger when initially symptomatic than later at autopsy.

Luria[280,281] considered the superior temporal plane to be Wernicke's area, but his cases were of traumatic origin from World War II, a notoriously inadequate source material for precise localization. Kertesz and Benson[236] reported on four autopsied cases with lesions involving the superior temporal plane, but here the lesions in these cases also spread into the insula and supramarginal gyri, even into the angular gyri. Naeser[321] described lesions larger than the superior temporal plane in a study of four cases documented by CT scan.

In our personal literature search, only three superior temporal plane lesions have been found with Wernicke's aphasia among 89 published cases with autopsy correlation. Two are subject to criticisms that minimize their utility, while the third is described too briefly to permit much analysis. The first, Gilbert Ballet's case,[209] was actually reported as an example of pure word deafness, a more restricted syndrome. Examined in March 1900 shortly after the stroke, the patient had pure word deafness, paraphasic speech both spontaneously and on repeating aloud, word blindness, and agraphia. The autopsy description in October 1901, 19 months later, fits that of a residue of an old subcortical (so-called slit) hemorrhage, which one can presume was larger at the time of the evaluation of the original clinical deficit (Fig. 25 in Henschen[209]). In any case, it is certainly not an isolated lesion of the superior temporal plane.

The second, Souques' case,[209] was followed for 14 years clinically. The deficit faded from an initial picture of Wernicke's aphasia to almost normal within 2 years. Unfortunately, the patient was illiterate, so reading and writing were not tested. At autopsy, he appeared to have had an old hematoma, a lesion presumably large enough in the acute stage to have caused the full syndrome of Wernicke's aphasia.

The third case was Kleist's[243] case Papp, who was said to have sensory aphasia for 2 months until another stroke altered the clinical picture. No details of reading tests were described. The lesion was, however, confined to the temporal plane.

Henschen,[209] in a review of the literature up to the mid-1920s, concluded that a superior temporal plane lesion does not cause the full picture of Wernicke's aphasia (i.e., both "pure word deafness" and "alexia"). He based this opinion on a review of 35 cases with temporal lobe lesions, 20 of whom had "pure word deafness." In none was alexia present. Earlier, Bastian[35] had found alexia and sensory (Wernicke's) aphasia in only 5 of 16 temporal lobe cases, and in most of these the lesion was large. Studies based on imaging add no qualitatively new cases: the study of Naeser et al[322] contained cases with medium to large lesions, while that of Mazzocchi and Vignolo[290] reported only one case with a smallish lesion, which the authors described as an exception to the other cases in that "anomias were in the foreground."

These data provide little support for the view that a superior temporal plane lesion alone constitutes the full syndrome of Wernicke's aphasia. The infarction needed to precipitate the full syndrome in the reported cases has been much larger, well beyond the confines of the superior temporal plane. A unique case from our clinical experience further demonstrates this point.

> A 20-year old right-handed man with only a very mild defect in spontaneous word retrieval underwent deliberate embolization of his left angular artery for treatment of a fusiform aneurysm/dysplastic segment. He was asymptomatic for about 4 hours, after which he began to demonstrate mild defects in auditory comprehension. Otherwise reading aloud, reading comprehension, and oral naming of pictures were

normal. An MR scan demonstrated an infarct restricted to the territory of the angular artery, presumably Wernicke's area. His language returned to baseline within a week.

There is no lack of superior temporal plane cases, but simply a lack of such cases showing the full syndrome of Wernicke's aphasia. Many of the cases with an infarct limited to less than the whole lower division territory lesion appear to have been labeled conduction aphasia, pure word deafness, or alexia with agraphia.

Pure word deafness. Over 40 cases with CT or autopsy correlation are reported. According to the classical formulations, the only deficit should be auditory; spontaneous speech should be normal, as should reading comprehension and writing.[279] Eight well-known cases exist with a unilateral lesion confined to the superior temporal plane in the dominant hemisphere. In seven, paraphasic speaking was prominent, a clinical picture not permitted in the formulation of pure word deafness, which, by definition, should be free of a disturbance in speaking. In many, the elements of paraphasic speech later cleared.

Shuster and Taterka's[365] case has been repeatedly cited but is a disappointment: in the acute phase, in addition to the word deafness, the patient had paraphasia for well over a month. More disappointing, at 7-month examination no tests of reading were performed. Finally, autopsy revealed the residue of an old slit hemorrhage, scarcely the stuff of precise correlation. Although this case is famous, the early phase of the illness makes it difficult to maintain the "purity" of a syndrome of pure word deafness. In Nielsen's[326,327] case Sult, a left superior temporal plane lesion was demonstrated, said to be associated with pure word deafness, but there are few satisfying details in the clinical text.

Many of the cases with bilateral lesions also experienced paraphasic speaking with poor comprehension during the acute phase of the stroke.[101,107] In the famous case reported by Pick,[340] bilateral lesions including a large left temporal plane lesion left the patient paraphasic for 4 years. The deficit was only slight when she was examined by the author 10 years later. The most recent case described as pure word deafness[107] had only a few paraphasic errors in spoken speech and in tests indicating comprehension of printed words. He suffered bilateral temporal lobe infarction, documented by CT scan, which the authors inferred had affected the primary auditory cortex. The largest lesion was on the right side.

From the foregoing, it must be concluded that examples of the pure word deafness syndrome occur only rarely. There is not even much current evidence that unilateral infarcts of the left temporal lobe create a state of impaired auditory discrimination.[13] Instead, temporal lobe infarcts of small size or parenchyma residue of an old slit hemorrhage (see Hemorrhage chapter) usually seem to set the stage for a transient form of Wernicke's aphasia whose major clinical feature is a disturbance in auditory comprehension, such as our aneurysm case described above. The spontaneous speech contains many paraphasic errors, especially in the acute stages, enough that the listener may make a preliminary diagnosis of Wernicke's aphasia. Also, when taxed in reading aloud or comprehension tasks, patients make enough errors that the notion of a pure disorder in auditory comprehension is not easily maintained.

Cortical deafness. The issue of cortical deafness is another matter. At least one autopsied patient exists who was well studied clinically and found to have deafness occasioned by an infarct confined to Heschel's transverse gyrus.[261] This case supports Henschen's[209] claim that such an event can occur. Examples are rare enough that the unilateral lesion is difficult to predict on clinical grounds alone. Bilateral infarcts affecting the temporal plane are a well-recognized cause of deafness, although only a few reports have appeared. The 24-year-old man reported by Khurana et al[240] was a typical example: after the second cerebral embolus, he became completely deaf to all sounds, speech and nonspeech in character, and could not be startled by loud noise. The brain stem auditory evoked studies showed normal waveforms through wave V. The patient's spontaneous speech contained the expected paraphasias, which were of the phonetic type; communication was achieved by writing, and occasional paragraphic errors were observed. The bilateral superior temporal plane infarcts were rather circumscribed.

Alexia with agraphia. Alexia with agraphia has proved remarkably difficult to find in case descriptions in the literature. Henschen[209] found five "pure" cases among the more than 250 patients who had dyslexia and dysgraphia as part of a larger clinical syndrome, noting that paraphasia in speaking was a frequent accompaniment of the syndrome.

Its general characteristics have been repeatedly described by a number of authorities[44] as a disturbance in reading comprehension and in the morphology and language content of writing that far exceeds the disturbance in auditory comprehension or in spontaneous speech. The original case of Dejerine's[119,120] suffered a lateral parietal infarct that penetrated as far as the ventricular wall. The disturbance in writing and reading was all out of proportion to the modest dysphasia in conversation, but Dejerine did not see the patient in the acute phase. Touche[388] described a similar case, whose remarkably focal cerebral infarct involved the right posterolateral parietal region in a left-handed man; his case also showed mild paraphasia in spoken speech, but not to the same degree as the disturbance in reading and writing.

Among the many accounts, mention is usually made[44] that ". . . almost all patients suffering alexia with agraphia have some degree of aphasia which ranges from a minimal degree of word-finding difficulty to a more marked sensory aphasia with paraphasia and comprehension disturbance." This observation raises the possibility that the syndrome may be another variant of Wernicke's aphasia. DeMassary[124] suggested that Dejerine himself considered this type of alexia a form of the sensory aphasia syndrome, which is more evident when the patient is seen in the early phase of the stroke. The senior author and colleagues studied such a patient for many years; autopsy eventually showed a large lesion affecting much of the posterior left hemisphere (Fig. 19.19). His deficit began as sensory aphasia, affecting all forms of language and all conditions of testing.[369,370] As time passed, the spoken response to auditory language stimuli improved, but that of written response to any tests and response to printed words remained

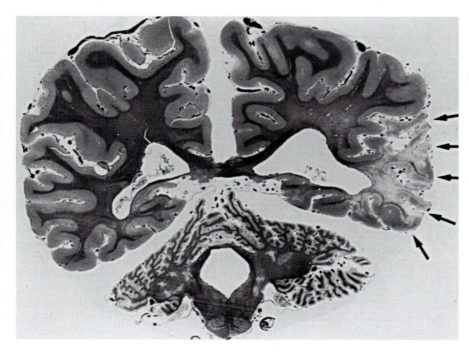

Figure 19.19 Coronal section from posterior half of brain in a patient with Wernicke's aphasia that evolved over years toward a syndrome of dyslexia with dysgraphia.

impaired, a disturbance that could be classified grossly as dyslexia with dysgraphia.

The clinical problem posed by the syndrome is not whether it exists but whether it is only a transient acute disorder, or occurs mainly in the chronic state of an initially more severe Wernicke's aphasia. The anatomy of the lesion requires a circumscribed infarction beyond the superior temporal plane. Embolism is the only reliable source of such an infarct, apart from focal form of vasculitis. In the unusual case in which the posterior cerebral artery takes its origin from the carotid, the main weight of the distal infarction could fall on the parieto-occipital lobe, as happened in our case,[370] but such an event would be most unusual. The available clinical data do not permit the determination of how acutely this syndrome can occur. The cases in the literature suggest it is a late development from an earlier syndrome of more extensive deficits. The few cases of the syndrome from nonvascular causes do not bear on this problem and are beyond the scope of this book.

Conduction Aphasia

This syndrome occupies a special position in aphasiology, mainly because of its theoretical prediction rather than its isolated occurrence as a clinical entity. Wernicke,[414] who first defined the syndrome, offered the opinion that it represented the interruption of fiber pathways connecting the sensory language zone of the posterior half of the brain with the motor language zone in the frontal lobe. For Goldstein,[180] the disorder represented disruption of a brain region located between the major sensory and motor centers, mediating the interaction of both functions simultaneously. As has been well docu-

mented by Levine and Calvanio,[265] its clinical features are not accounted for by either of the two major theories.

The name has become accepted in clinical circles to characterize those patients with poor repetition, especially for unfamiliar material, and far better auditory and visual comprehension of language than that evident in their spontaneous spoken and written efforts. That spontaneous speech is often contaminated by paraphasic utterances is not emphasized. Although auditory and visual language comprehension is relatively preserved, neither is normal at any stage of the disorder.[13] The ease with which disturbances in comprehension and the language content of speech are demonstrated has proved to be a major stumbling block to the satisfactory application of the label conduction aphasia, when the physician is faced with such a patient at the bedside. The disturbance in repeating aloud, on which great stress has been laid,[45,170] is not as useful a distinguishing point in the acute stage of the syndrome, since it is shared with cases of Wernicke's aphasia. In assessing the deficits in conversation, Burns and Canter[85] found a greater incidence of unwanted phonemes and intrusion of semantically related words among those cases classified as Wernicke's aphasia than among those with conduction aphasia, but careful testing was required to make this distinction. Patients with conduction aphasia are also said to have a greater tendency to attempt self-correction than do those with Wernicke's aphasia;[44] in the authors' own experience, this point has applied only to those cases of Wernicke's aphasia with the major syndrome. For ordinary clinical purposes, the distinction between the error patterns in speaking in the two types is not an easy one, except that semantic word substitutions are rare in conduction aphasia.[19,377]

Because the site of the infarct lies behind the rolandic

region, there is usually no contralateral hemiparesis. Disturbances in eye movements and visual fields are also minor or not present. Bucco-linguo-facial dyspraxia is a common accompaniment,[44] as is bimanual ideomotor dyspraxia. The dyspraxia of the latter state is different in the two limbs, the limb served by the infarcted hemisphere taking the form of a deafferentation,[135] while the other conforms more to the picture expected in ideomotor dyspraxia.[172]

The syndrome often proves surprisingly evanescent when seen in an acute setting. More often, the initial syndrome is a Wernicke-type aphasia, evolving later into the picture of conduction aphasia.[356] The syndrome in its late stages may prove difficult to demonstrate. Testing with difficult words that the patient is to repeat aloud is often required.

The clinicopathologic correlation is also at odds with the theory. The most popular current thesis envisions interruption of the arcuate fasciculus as the mechanism for the errors.[45,170,171] The interruption presumably prevents adequate control by the auditory system over the speech apparatus. Because this thesis hinges on a lesion interrupting the arcuate fasciculus, the findings expected on brain imaging or autopsy would be mainly subcortical. However, autopsy evidence in support of this thesis is surprisingly slight. The documented lesions[42] have all been superficial infarcts, whose penetration into the subcortical white matter has varied considerably. In some instances, the infarction was completely superficial; in only a few has it been profound enough to produce a cleft deep enough to injure the arcuate fasciculus. Damasio and Damasio[106,107] offered the suggestion that two projecting systems may exist and may follow pathways susceptible to injury even by superficial lesions. The cases used for their analysis were not "pure," however, since some degree of disturbance in auditory and reading comprehension was present, although no more than in the usual cases classified as conduction aphasia. Over 20 cases with CT, MR, or autopsy correlation are reported with this syndrome, and many show the lesion located in the same area usually attributed to Wernicke's aphasia. Naeser[323] found no difference in the lesion size per slice in cases with conduction or Wernicke's aphasia, but the mean percentage of left hemispheral tissue damage was larger in the Wernicke cases than in those with conduction aphasia ($P < 0.01$).

Another major thesis of the conduction aphasia theory considers the deficit to represent a disturbance in kinesthetic feedback. Luria[280] coined the term *afferent motor aphasia* to characterize the behavior. He assumed that the lesion lay in the sylvian operculum posterior to the rolandic fissure, yielding a disturbance in pronunciation resulting from faulty anatomic oropharyngeal positionings. The words pronounced would contain sounds different from those intended. These errors, analogous to the typing errors of a novice typist, require considerable listener training for their detection, rather like the recognition of typing errors by those familiar with the typewriter keyboard. The novice listener may easily mistake them for language errors (paraphasias) and may assume the speaker has a language disorder. Such an interpretation may be inaccurate, but it remains common medical practice to refer to errors of this type as literal paraphasias. The doubting examiner may well wonder how the patient's language comprehension can be so intact when his speech utterances are so distorted, in some cases to the point of meaningless jargon.

This thesis assumes a surface lesion, such as would be expected from the embolic infarction that is almost invariably the responsible lesion. It matches with studies suggesting that the major difficulty experienced by these patients in repeating aloud can be considered to represent a disturbance in encoding accompanied by a disturbance in short-term memory.[367] A patient with this syndrome showed CT scan evidence of an anterior parietal infarct.

The question of whether the impairment in conduction aphasia represents mere phonologic mistargeting or is truly language based was brought forward again in a recent case of the authors in which a patient with a dilated cardiomyopathy developed a syndrome of fluent conversational speech, normal auditory and reading comprehension, and repetition that was halting and effortful.[287] Nearly all of this patient's paraphasic errors—on naming, on repetition, on reading aloud, and on writing—were semantic substitutions. For example, "The quarterback threw the football down the field on Saturday" became "The quarterback through the baseball into the field." High-resolution MR imaging identified an infarct restricted to the posterior left insular cortex and intrasylvian parietal operculum.

As a result of the more modern studies using brain imaging, it has been recognized for some time that the syndrome may result from a lower division infarct, a point that should further trouble the thesis that Wernicke's aphasia results from superior temporal plane disease. Kleist[243] suggested that some form of mixed hemisphere dominance accounted for the patients with conduction aphasia instead of Wernicke's aphasia from an infarction of the superior temporal plane. For others, including the present authors, the disturbance has been considered merely a mild form of sensory aphasia.[278,379] Many such cases show some degree of decreased auditory comprehension when tested, but their ability to read aloud and for comprehension is so much superior that they do not easily qualify for the full syndrome of Wernicke's aphasia as traditionally defined. However, they would easily be described as examples of the mild form of Wernicke's aphasia.

Transcortical Aphasia

The observation of an aphasic syndrome with relatively intact ability to repeat dictated material aloud is attributed to Wernicke,[414,415] but Goldstein[179,180] has been recognized for his attempt to establish a separate entity characterized by an "isolation of the speech area." The traditional inference has been that the sylvian region is preserved, as demonstrated by intact repetition skills, and that the responsible lesion for the aphasic disorder is elsewhere. The exact anatomic basis is less well established than the term transcortical suggests, but three syndrome subsets have been described—motor, sensory, and mixed—corresponding to the major motor, major sensory, and global aphasias, respectively, except for the presence of otherwise preserved repetition.[48,188]

Transcortical motor aphasia (TCMA) resembles major motor aphasia (limited spontaneous speech, good comprehension) with relatively intact repetition,[158] although significant variations have made any single underlying explanation of the behavioral and anatomic mechanisms problematic. The language of some patients matches the classical behavioral description, but lesions have been found in the white matter anterolateral to the left frontal horn. They have been caused by infarction or hemorrhage in the upper division of the MCA. They demonstrated that the expected lesion location for TCMA produces varying degrees of impaired articulation, mild deficits in auditory comprehension, and stuttering. TCMA has also been described as a phase during the evolution of Broca's syndrome. It has also been observed that motor language syndromes with good repetition occur during the recovery process following infarction in the territory of the anterior cerebral artery, usually involving the supplementary motor area in the paramedian region of the frontal lobe.

Transcortical sensory aphasia (TSCA) resembles a major sensory syndrome with fluent speech, impaired comprehension, alexia with agraphia, and paraphasic errors, but relatively preserved repetition ability.[15] Patients often display compulsive repetition (echolalia), suggesting more linguistic competence than is actually the case. The responsible lesion is usually large, occurring in the territory of the posterior cerebral artery and involving the temporo-parieto-occipital junction;[239] occasionally an isolated thalamic infarct is present. The broad range of cognitive deficits often seen in conjunction with TSCA, including amnestic and attentional disturbances,[183] has clouded its status as a separable aphasic disorder.

Mixed transcortical aphasia is the entity to which Goldstein[179] made reference in 1917 as "isolation of the speech." These are patients with a global aphasia, except for retention of good repetition. There is virtually no other capacity for receptive or expressive propositional language. This is a very unusual syndrome. Only a small number of cases have been reported, mostly in stroke patients, with the study of patients during the evolution of global aphasia or instances of recurrent stroke.[174] In the setting of acute stroke with no prior language disturbance, mixed transcortical aphasia has been said to occur from occlusion of the left internal carotid artery, resulting in simultaneous embolism in the anterior pial territory and perfusion failure in the terminal branches of the middle and posterior cerebral arteries.[65]

Functional Imaging in Aphasia

Following infarction, regional changes in cerebral blood flow and metabolism can be identified by single-photon emission tomography (SPECT), positron emission tomography (PET), or ultrafast MR imaging. Hypoperfusion and hypometabolism may extend into the peri-infarct area or may be seen at a site distant from the lesion itself.[344,382] With the ability to evaluate physiologic effects of structural lesions in regions adjacent to or remote from the territory of infarction has come a re-examination of some clinicopathologic correlations.

Patients with moderate to severe aphasia often show regions of hypometabolism encompassing large frontoparietal or temporoparietal areas, even in the presence of modest cortical or subcortical structural lesions.[47,228,298,333] Larger metabolic defects in the acute phase of hemispheral stroke that extend beyond the borders of infarction correlate with worse initial clinical state and appear to predict poorer recovery from aphasia.[86,299] Reversal of cortical hypometabolism may correlate with clinical improvement when lesions are deep,[393] although in some cases of subcortical stroke cortical hypometab-

olism may persist for at least 3 months despite good clinical recovery.[125]

A recent study by Metter et al[298] suggests that different aphasias may share common regions of hypometabolism regardless of lesion site. Forty-four aphasic patients were studied with (F-18) fluorodeoxyglucose PET. Nineteen patients had "anomic," 10 had "Broca's," 8 had "conduction," 5 had "Wernicke's," 1 had "global," and 1 had "transcortical" aphasia. The authors found that 97% of patients had metabolic decreases in the left angular gyrus, 87% had decreases in the left supramarginal gyrus, and 85% had decreases in the left posterior superior temporal gyrus. Taken all together, 100% had PET abnormalities in the left parietotemporal region. A greater degree of hypometabolism in the prefrontal region was the only imaging feature that distinguished Broca aphasics from Wernicke aphasics. In functional imaging studies of normal controls performing language tasks, hyperperfusion or hypermetabolism has been demonstrated in certain brain regions. The superior temporal gyrus has been implicated both in the early acoustic processing of words and nonwords[51,292,337,421] and in the word-retrieval process required in generating verbs from noun stimuli.[421] The prefrontal region and supplementary motor area may also play a role in word selection and output.[337,421]

Functional imaging has also been used to explore the pathophysiology of atypical aphasias. Cappa et al[91] showed that in two right-handed aphasics with right-sided lesions (periventricular corona radiata and lentiform nucleus), not only was there widespread hypometabolism in right cortical and subcortical structures, but there was decreased metabolism in the left frontal and parietal cortex as well, suggesting that the left hemisphere played a role in the aphasia even though the structural lesion was restricted to the right. Contralateral hemispheral contributions have also been evoked in cases of transcortical aphasias. When structural damage has unexpectedly included the left perisylvian region, SPECT and ^{133}Xe regional cerebral blood flow studies in these instances revealed extensive hypoperfusion throughout the left hemisphere, but showed increased blood flow in the contralateral right temporal lobe.[47] Finally, in a patient with a conduction aphasia in which the paraphasic errors were nearly all semantic substitutions, MRI showed an infarct restricted to the posterior left insular cortex and intrasylvian parietal operculum, but SPECT revealed hypometabolism in the inferomedial and lateral left temporal lobe, suggesting a physiologic—but nonischemic—role for these regions in the syndrome.[286]

Important functional information can also be obtained by imaging aphasic patients while they are actively engaged in a language task. Whereas the pattern of cortical hypoperfusion in one study of 43 patients with subcortical stroke could not differentiate aphasics from nonaphasics,[125] when similar patients were scanned during an object naming task, unique regions of hypoperfusion were identified in the left premotor, frontotemporal, and parieto-temporo-occipital junction.[126] The authors further demonstrated that the contralateral (right) frontal and temporal areas showed increased perfusion during the naming task in a subgroup of patients with less severe aphasia. They hypothesized that in the less affected subgroup a contrahemispheral shift in language function had occurred, to allow partial recovery from the aphasia. The complex question of how the brain recovers from injury remains under intense study. In cases of surface infarction, cortical areas contributing to functional recovery have not been clearly defined. Although some have reported that contrahemispheral mirror locations correlate with the recovery process in mildly affected aphasics, others claim that peri-infarct and other ipsilateral regions are crucial for recovery and that activation in the contralateral hemisphere may correlate with persistence of aphasia.[39] Ipsihemispheral translocation of language function has also been demonstrated in patients with arteriovenous malformations in the posterior, dominant hemisphere.[256] Whatever the mechanism, it seems clear that the brain is capable of reorganization. The pathophysiology of this process remains to be elucidated.

APRAXIA

Apraxias are acquired disorders of execution. They represent an inability to perform a previously learned skilled act that is unexplained by weakness, visual loss, incoordination, dementia, sensory loss, or aphasia. Liepmann[274,275] described apraxia as the "incapacity for purposive movement despite retained mobility." Apraxic patients are unable to perform skilled acts because the motor engrams (programs) that guide skilled acts have either been lost or cannot be accessed. Since these deficits in skilled movement are rarely complete, the term dyspraxia is often used. Apraxic deficits may affect movements of the body, face, or limbs. Liepmann proposed that the left hemisphere possessed the motor engrams necessary for skilled movements just as it possessed the linguistic engrams necessary for speech. Left hemisphere dominance for skilled motor activity has been postulated by Kimura and Archibald[241] as well. The overwhelming proportion of dextrals with motor apraxia have left hemisphere lesions.[201] Ajuriaguerra et al[8] noted 47 cases of ideomotor apraxia and 11 cases of ideational apraxia among 206 left retrorolandic cases and 55 bilateral hemisphere cases. Motor apraxia was absent in their 151 right retrorolandic cases.

Ideomotor Apraxia

The most common type of motor apraxia is ideomotor apraxia. Liepmann believed that a dissociation occurred between the brain areas that contained the "ideas" for movements and the "motor" areas responsible for execution. As a result, skilled movements involving the limbs are not executed accurately. Ideomotor apraxia may be elicited by asking patients to show how they would salute, wave good-bye, hammer a nail, saw wood, and so forth. In the most severe cases, the action cannot be performed at all. In moderately severe cases the actions are vague and confused. In milder cases the actions are clumsy and lack precision. In general, the worst performance is elicited on verbal command. Performance may improve on imitation but still remains abnormal.[196] The best performance is elicited on actual use of the object.[202] Ideomotor apraxia can take two forms: a bilateral ideomotor apraxia in which both extremities are affected and sympathetic apraxia (callosal apraxia) in which the apraxia is limited to the nondominant left arm. Although the left hemisphere is dominant in most dextrals for both language and skilled motor activity, apraxia

does not depend on the presence of dysphasia. Furthermore, although aphasia commonly accompanies ideomotor apraxia, there is no close relationship between either the severity or the type of aphasia.[33,132,260] Geschwind[171] has suggested cerebral disconnection between the language area and the premotor area in the frontal lobe as an explanation for ideomotor apraxia. Lesions in the vicinity of the left supramarginal gyrus with deep extension into the subjacent white matter could interrupt impulses originating in Wernicke's area that were directed toward the premotor area.

Heilman[202] suggests an alternative explanation. He believes that the motor programs for skilled motor movements are stored in the left superior parietal lobe. Skilled motor activity depends on the transmission of these programs to the premotor area in the left frontal lobe. Ideomotor apraxia may then arise from two different mechanisms: direct destruction of motor programs in the left superior parietal lobe or destruction of the pathways from the left superior parietal lobe to the premotor area of the left frontal lobe (i.e., disconnection).[203] Typically, bilateral ideomotor apraxia is associated with retrorolandic lesions in the vicinity of the parietal lobe.[200,202] These lesions are usually superficial cortical infarcts in the distribution of the posterior division of the left MCA. Although ideomotor apraxia is more common with superficial as opposed to deep lesions, larger deep lesions may produce ideomotor apraxia.[7] Ideomotor apraxia does not occur with smaller lacunar-type infarctions. Little is known about recovery from ideomotor apraxia.[202] However, recovery may be surprisingly rapid in certain cases. Anterior lesions have a better prognosis for recovery than posterior cases.[34]

Ideational Apraxia

Ideational apraxia bears an uncertain relation to ideomotor apraxia. Ideational apraxia is a disorder of the sequencing and planning of complex motor acts.[134] It can be elicited by asking the patient to demonstrate complex motor tasks such as lighting a cigarette or mailing a letter. Hecaen and Gimeno[200] reported 8 cases of ideational apraxia among 47 cases of ideomotor apraxia. Sittig[372] believed that ideational apraxia was only a severe form of ideomotor apraxia. Others believe that ideational apraxia is a distinct entity different from ideomotor apraxia.[20,259]

Ideational apraxia is generally observed after dominant hemisphere parietal lobe lesions. Associated findings may include a fluent aphasia (anomic, semantic, or Wernicke's), constructional apraxia,[57] and elements of Gerstmann's syndrome. Dementia and confusion are noted in some cases. The localization is the same as might be expected to produce ideomotor apraxia. Bilateral parietal lesions are present in some cases,[8,131] but isolated right parietal lesions seem to produce ideational apraxia only in individuals with anomalous cerebral dominance.[342] Little is known about recovery from ideational apraxia.

Limb-Kinetic Apraxia

Limb-kinetic (also innervatory or melokinetic) apraxia manifests as a lack of rapidity, skill, and delicacy in the performance of learned motor movements.[201] Liepmann held that in limb-kinetic apraxia "the virtuosity which practice lends to movement is lost. Therefore the movements are . . . clumsy, without precision" (quoted by Kerstesz[233]). The patient is clumsy in the execution of common motor acts such as the manipulation of objects (eating utensils, combs, brushes, saws, hammers, playing cards, and so forth.) Limb-kinetic apraxia is unilateral and affects the limb contralateral to the cerebral lesion. It may be difficult to distinguish between limb-kinetic apraxia and paresis in some cases.[199] Commonly associated neurologic signs include ataxia, choreoathetosis, grasping, spasticity, weakness, and dystonic posturing. However, the clumsiness in using objects is out of proportion to these other deficits. The perseverative and conceptual disturbances that characterize ideational apraxia are not prominent. Patients with limb-kinetic apraxia perform poorly to command or imitation. Performance may improve slightly with use of the object, but patients often act as if they were somewhat unfamiliar with its use.

Limb-kinetic apraxia may occur after injury to either the right or left premotor cortex or subjacent white matter.[327] Slight weakness is usually present, suggesting that injury to the pyramidal pathways is an essential feature of limb-kinetic apraxia. However, injury limited solely to the pyramidal pathways does not produce limb-kinetic apraxia. Patients with pure motor hemiplegia due to lacunar infarction in the internal capsule do not manifest limb-kinetic apraxia. Thus the elicitation of this sign is a useful indicator that surface cortex or subjacent white matter has been injured. The diagnosis of limb-kinetic apraxia is rarely made, reflecting the doubts of some as to its validity as an apraxic entity discrete from either pyramidal weakness or ideomotor apraxia.[199,233]

Callosal Apraxia

Callosal apraxia (sympathetic apraxia) represents a restricted form of ideomotor apraxia in which the apraxia is limited to the nondominant arm. Liepmann and Maas[277] first described a patient with a right hemiplegia who was unable to perform skilled movements with his nonparetic left arm. Similar patients have been described by Geschwind and Kaplan[173] and by Watson and Heilman.[406] Critical to the syndrome is disruption of the anterior portions of the corpus callosum. Infarction of the medial or anterior left frontal lobe with Broca's aphasia and right hemiplegia is often present, but these elements are not critical to the genesis of the apraxia.

The apraxia is unilateral and limited to the nondominant arm. If the right arm is not paretic it can be demonstrated to be free of apraxia. The apraxia of the left arm is similar to the bilateral apraxia that characterizes ideomotor apraxia. Two somewhat similar hypotheses have been offered to explain callosal apraxia. Geschwind[171] has suggested that callosal apraxia is due to a disconnection of the right premotor region from the speech area in the left temporal lobe. Verbal instructions are unable to traverse the anterior corpus callosum and reach the right premotor cortex. Hence, the left arm is deprived of verbal instructions to guide its motor activity. The patient of Geschwind and Kaplan was able to perform skilled movements with his left arm on imitation but not on verbal command. However, this has not been the general experience.[197] Thus, this hypothesis does not explain why patients with callosal apraxia continue to be apraxic upon use of an object or on imitation of the examiner. Heilman[202] suggests that the left arm is apraxic because it is disconnected from the motor engram centers in the left hemisphere.

The lesion producing callosal apraxia may be a rare isolated lesion of the corpus callosum. More commonly the crossing callosal fibers are disrupted in the mesial left hemisphere by either a left anterior cerebral artery territory infarction or an infarction in the distribution of the anterior division of the left MCA. These anterior division left MCA territory infarctions are associated with right hemiplegia and Broca's aphasia. Injury to the corpus callosum rather than injury to the left supplementary motor cortex is critical to the syndrome.[184]

Oral-Buccal-Lingual Apraxia

Orofacial or oral-buccal-lingual apraxia is the inability to perform skilled movements with the oral and facial musculature on command. John Hughlings-Jackson[219] had noted that some patients are unable to protrude their tongue on command. In addition, these patients may be unable to pucker their lips, cough, lick their lips, puff up their cheeks, or whistle on verbal command. These same acts may be performed well spontaneously. DeRenzi et al[133] found oral apraxia in 90% of Broca's aphasics and 33% of conduction aphasics. Oral apraxia is unusual in cases of anomic or Wernicke's aphasia. Although oral apraxia is common in global aphasia, testing for oral apraxia may be difficult due to comprehension disturbances. Hecaen and Albert[197] have emphasized that oral-buccal-lingual apraxia is not synonymous with Broca's aphasia, as some Broca's aphasics will not be dyspraxic and some subjects with oral-buccal-lingual apraxia will not be aphasic.

Oral-buccal-lingual apraxia generally results from an inferior frontal lesion in the premotor cortex adjacent to the face area on the motor strip. Most lesions are cortical and superficial.[386] Occasionally, oral-buccal-lingual apraxia may occur after larger deep lesions.[7]

Syndromes of Right Hemispheral Infarction

A wide variety of behavior abnormalities may follow stroke in the right MCA territory. These deficits are governed in general by several unifying observations:

1. Despite some rudimentary capacity to comprehend language, language plays no important role in the activities subserved by the right hemisphere.

2. The commitment of the cerebral cortex to a specific higher cortical function within the right hemisphere is less precise than in the left hemisphere. While higher cortical functions in the left hemisphere appear to be governed by identifiable "centers" of function, higher cortical functions of the right hemisphere appear to be governed by far-flung "networks."

3. The right hemisphere is dominant for certain aspects of attention[296] including directed attention, focused attention, and vigilance. This specialization for attention may be reflected in a variety of right hemisphere deficits such as neglect, extinction, and impersistence.

4. Many spatial and quasispatial operations are performed by

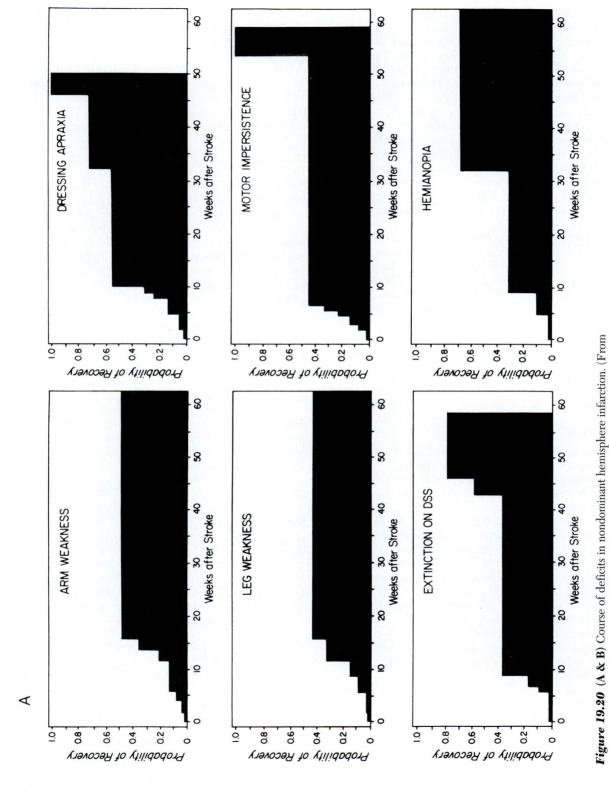

Figure 19.20 (**A & B**) Course of deficits in nondominant hemisphere infarction. (From Hier et al,[212] with permission.) (*Figure continues.*)

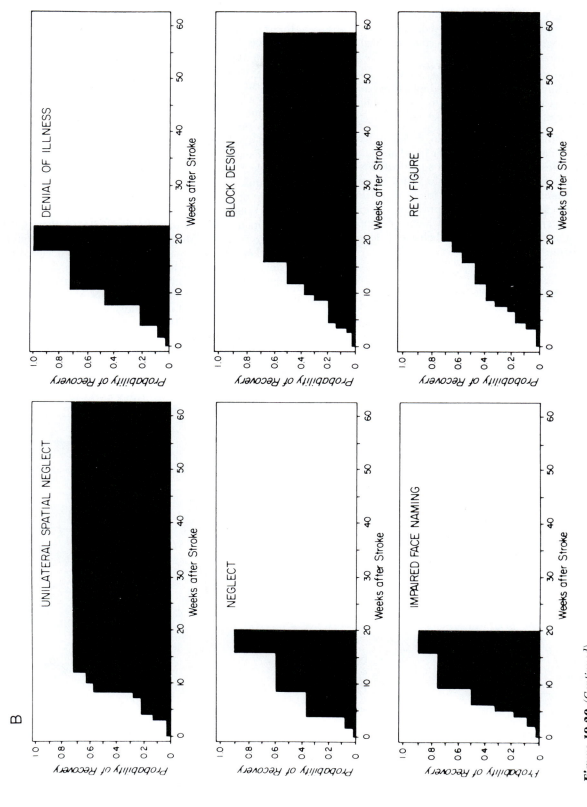

Figure 19.20 (*Continued*)

the right hemisphere. This specialization for spatial operations may be reflected in such right hemisphere deficits as prosopagnosia,[62] topographic disorientation, constructional apraxia, and dressing apraxia.

5. Confabulatory behaviors are more common after right hemisphere injury than left.[170] Both reduplicative paramnesia and anosognosia may be considered forms of confabulation occurring after right hemisphere stroke.

Patients without the many neurologic deficits from right hemispheral infarction do much better in rehabilitation than patients with these deficits. Although some patients show a steady recovery from these deficits (Fig. 19.20), others are left with persistent and disabling behavioral abnormalities that include constructional and dressing apraxia, left neglect, and motor impersistence. The size of the lesion, rather than its exact location, is a better predictor of behavioral deficits after right hemisphere damage (Fig. 19.21).

NEGLECT AND EXTINCTION

Extinction and neglect are two forms of hemi-inattention that may occur after right hemisphere stroke. Extinction implies that a "stimulus is not perceived only when a second stimulus is presented simultaneously—usually but not necessarily on the opposite side of the body."[366] Unilateral spatial neglect (USN) is a restricted syndrome in which patients fail to copy one side (usually the left) of a figure, fail to read one side of words or sentences, and bisect lines far to the right of center. The term neglect implies a more flagrant syndrome characterized by a failure of the patient to attend to new stimuli coming from one side (usually the left).

Neglect is often trimodal (auditory, visual, and tactile). In left-sided neglect, the patient may fail to explore the left side of space; the eyes and body may be turned tonically to the right.[102] Neglect is characterized by "a lack of responsivity to stimuli on one side of the body, in the absence of any sensory or motor deficit severe enough to account for the imperception."[366] Battersby et al[36] found USN in 29% of their right-brain-damaged patients and 12% of their left-brain-damaged patients. Most subjects with USN had lesions involving either the parieto-occipital or temporo-occipital regions. Using a line-bisection test, Schenkenberg et al[361] found USN to be more common after right than left brain damage.

The mechanism underlying USN is uncertain. Neither hemianopia, oculomotor disorders, nor dementia can account for the phenomenon. Heilman and Valenstein[206] suggest that hemispatial hypokinesia due to hypoarousal explains USN on drawing tasks. Related to the syndrome of USN is more gross

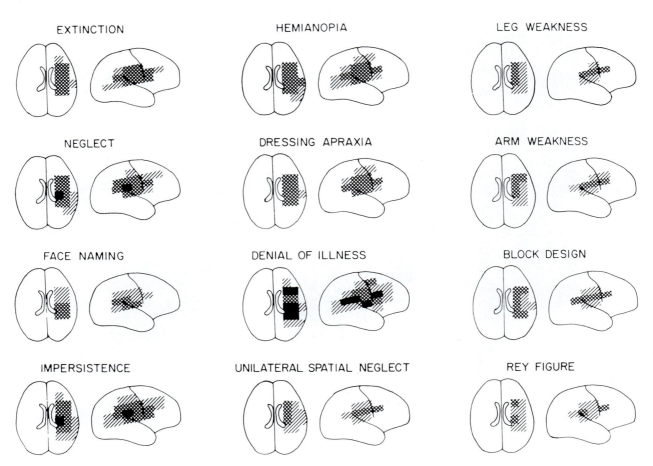

Figure 19.21 Topography of infarction documented by CT scan for cases with nondominant hemisphere deficits. (From Hier et al,[212] with permission.)

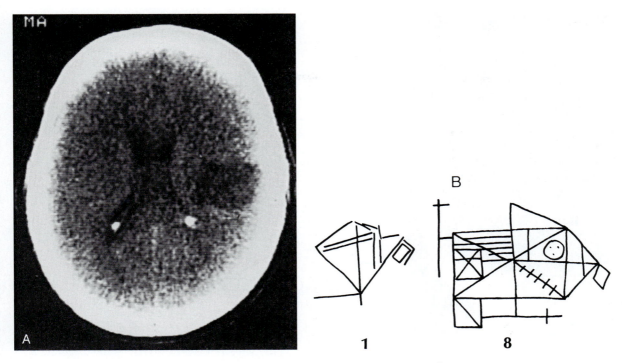

Figure 19.22 **(A)** CT scan of small right middle cerebral artery territory infarct. **(B)** Drawings done at 1 and 8 weeks after stroke.

ignorance of the neglect. These patients behave as if they have completely lost the left side of space and the left side of the body. They may ignore visitors on the left side or fail to attend to sounds coming from the left. Marked left neglect tends to occur in conjunction with other markers of severe right hemisphere damage including anosognosia (i.e., implicit unawareness of illness and its clinical manifestations)[411] and motor impersistence. By contrast, USN may occur with smaller right hemisphere strokes, which usually have a good prognosis (Fig. 19.22).

Neglect has been traditionally attributed to injury in the vicinity of the right parietal lobe. However, neglect may follow injury to the right frontal lobe,[108] right cingulum,[407] right lenticular nucleus, or right thalamus.[64,405,408] Since injury to a variety of cortical and subcortical structures produces left neglect,[105] a cortical network in the right hemisphere underlying directed attention has been proposed.[208,296,402] Mesulam[296] posited a network model for attention that includes a reticular element (providing arousal and vigilance), a parietal element (providing sensory and spatial mapping), a frontal element (providing the motor programs for exploration), and a limbic element prosopagnosia, constructional apraxia, and left-sided neglect. Data from our own series of 34 patients support this notion that the nature of the neglect syndrome may vary depending on whether the lesion lies in the upper or lower division of the right MCA.[50] In a sensory-motor dichotomy analogous to that found with aphasia syndromes, 11 patients with infarction in the lower division of the right MCA demonstrated rightward deviation on line bisection with otherwise minimal or no defect on letter cancellation, suggesting abnormality in perceptual function. By contrast, 10 patients with lesions in the upper division showed neglect on letter cancella-

tion but performed normally on line bisection, suggesting a defect in motor search behavior.

ANOSOGNOSIA

Anosognosia (i.e., unawareness of illness or its clinical manifestations)[411] is more likely to be associated with severe as opposed to mild hemiparesis.[211] Willanger et al[419,420] also noted an association between anosognosia and severity of hemiparesis. Nonetheless, Bisiach et al[53] have shown that anosognosia for either hemianopia or hemiparesis can be dissociated from elementary neurologic deficits or neglect. Babinski[25] noted that the anosognosia often resolves quickly. Hier et al[211,212] found that in 15 cases of acute right hemisphere stroke followed longitudinally, all recovered from anosognosia within 22 weeks.

The lesion producing anosognosia is usually large. Hier et al[211] found that the responsible lesion is often extended beyond the parietal lobe to the frontal and temporal lobes (Fig. 19.23). Extension of the lesion to the deep white matter and basal ganglia was frequent. It is probably incorrect to call anosognosia a "right parietal" phenomenon, since many of the lesions are massive and involve much of the right MCA territory (both deep and superficial structures). Involvement of the occipital lobe does not appear to be essential to development of anosognosia. On occasion smaller deep lesions (often basal ganglionic hemorrhages) may produce anosognosia, presumably by undercutting and isolating the cortex of the right hemisphere.

Neither sensory loss, confusion, nor dementia can ade-

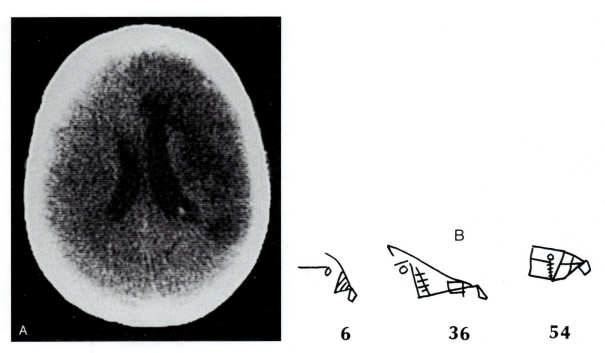

Figure 19.23 (A) CT scan of large right middle cerebral artery territory infarct. (B) Drawings done at 6, 36, and 54 weeks after stroke.

quately account for anosognosia. Gerstmann[169] has viewed anosognosia as a disorder of a hypothetical "body image." Although he believed that this body image was "mapped" in the left parietal lobe, input from the right parietal lobe was essential in updating the left parietal lobe as to the condition of the left side of the body. Injury to the right parietal lobe, or to connecting pathways between right and left parietal lobes could lead to anosognosia. Geschwind[172] suggested that anosognosia may be due to a disconnection syndrome that prevents sensory impressions from reaching the central language zone in the left hemisphere. Another explanation for anosognosia is that structures essential for the recognition of hemiplegia or other body defects are localized to the right hemisphere. Injury to the right hemisphere could produce an agnosia for illness by disrupting structures essential for the recognition of illness. Finally, anosognosia may be viewed as a variation of "neglect" or "inattention" in that the patient with anosognosia fails to "attend" to his hemiplegia.

IMPERSISTENCE

In 1956, Fisher[148] described 10 patients with left hemiplegia who were unable to persist at a variety of willed acts including eye closure, breath holding, conjugate gaze deviation, tongue protrusion, and hand gripping. Fisher introduced the "new term impersistence" to describe "this failure to persist in a motor act." He noted that "mental impairment of some degree was always present" and that impersistence was "encountered almost exclusively in association with left hemiplegia . . . ." Many of the patients had accompanying left neglect, constructional apraxia, and anosognosia.

Joynt et al[227] tested for impersistence in 48 left hemisphere-damaged patients and 34 right hemisphere-damaged patients. Impersistence was found in 26% of the patients with right hemisphere damage and 19% of the patients with left hemisphere damage. Joynt et al[227] found impersistence to be more common in patients with mental impairment, especially visuospatial deficits. However, Levin[264] could not demonstrate an increased incidence of impersistence after right compared with left hemisphere damage. Ben-Yishay et al[40] found a correlation between impersistence and visuomotor and visuospatial deficits. In addition, impersistence proved to bode poorly for rehabilitation efforts. More recent studies confirm a right hemisphere localization for motor impersistence.[238] Hier et al[211] found impersistence in 46% of 41 subjects with acute right hemisphere strokes.

Impersistence correlated with a variety of other deficits including severity of hemiparesis, prosopagnosia, dressing apraxia, constructional apraxia, left neglect, and anosognosia. Motor impersistence occurred only after the largest lesions. Injury generally extended to the frontal, parietal, temporal, and deep structures. No specific locus of injury for "impersistence" was found within the right hemisphere. Rather, impersistence reflected diffuse and widespread dysfunction. Hier et al[211] found recovery from motor impersistence to be quite indolent.

The mechanism underlying impersistence is unknown. Motor impersistence may reflect a depletion of vigilance or sustained attention following widespread injury to the right hemisphere. The anatomic locus of those structures involved in sustained attention and vigilance is unknown. Widespread networks in the right hemisphere may underlie focused attention.

DRESSING APRAXIA

"Apraxia for dressing" was described in 1941 by Brain.[75] Dressing apraxia refers to confusions in the orientation of clothing during dressing. As McFie et al[293] commented, these "difficulties appeared to be due to confusions regarding top and bottom, back and front, and right and left with reference to the garments." Roth[355] noted the close association between constructional apraxia and dressing apraxia. Dressing apraxia occurs almost exclusively with lesions of the right hemisphere.

Although constructional apraxia occurs with either right or left hemisphere lesions, the constructional apraxia that occurs with left hemisphere lesions is rarely associated with dressing apraxia. After right hemisphere damage, strokes large enough to produce both dressing apraxia and constructional apraxia are larger than those strokes producing only constructional apraxia. Unilateral spatial neglect contributes to difficulties in dressing as well. Dressing apraxia should not be diagnosed in the presence of disabling hemiplegia that interferes with dressing.

LOSS OF TOPOGRAPHIC MEMORY AND DISORIENTATION FOR PLACE

Loss of topographic memory is the inability of some patients to find their way in familiar surroundings, to recognize familiar surroundings, and to learn new routes in unfamiliar surroundings. Loss of topographic memory is somewhat different from disorientation to place, which refers to patients who are confused as to their current location.[151] Critchley[103] described several patients who were constantly getting lost in familiar surroundings.

Many of his subjects had biparietal injury. A few had lesions limited to the posterior right hemisphere. Critchley[103] described one patient with a right MCA territory infarction who "will often pass his home without knowing that it is his, and will wander around for many minutes trying to decide where he does live . . . ." In milder cases, patients recognize surroundings as familiar; in more severe cases even very familiar surroundings may seem strange. Critchley described another patient with a right MCA occlusion who could not recognize "the countryside he should have known so well. His home and surroundings are no longer familiar. . . ." Loss of topographic memory is uncommon. Hecaen and Angelergues[198] reported 40 cases of loss of topographic memory, 29 with right hemisphere lesions and 3 with bilateral lesions. Many patients have bilateral parietal lesions, although some have unilateral right parietal lesions. Landis et al[252] described 16 patients with loss of topographic familiarity; all had right medial temporoparietal lesions.

The mechanism underlying loss of topographic memory is uncertain. The failure to recognize familiar surroundings suggests an agnostic defect similar to that underlying prosopagnosia.[403] The inability to follow familiar routes and the inability to orient oneself in space suggest a failure to create an internal spatial representation of the external world. Ross[351] has suggested that visual-modality-specific memory defects may underlie both loss of topographic memory deficits and prosopagnosia.

DISORDERS OF SPATIAL LOCALIZATION

The right hemisphere plays a special role in the spatial localization of stimuli. This effect has been demonstrated for both visual and auditory stimuli. With regard to determination of spatial orientation of objects in space, the severest deficits have been noted after posterior right hemisphere damage.[130,294] Short-term spatial memory (a skill analogous to the auditory short-term memory task of digit span) is a dominant function of the posterior right hemisphere.[129] Auditory localization of sounds in space also depends on an intact posterior right hemisphere.[53]

CONFUSION AND DELIRIUM

Acute confusion and delirium are states characterized by impaired orientation, diminished attention, and aberrant perception. Alertness is usually well maintained, clarity and speed of thinking are diminished, and memories are poorly formed. Inattentiveness, poor concentration, and alerting to irrelevant stimuli are present. There is overlap between confusional and delirious states with delirium considered by some to be a subset of a confusion. Delirium is characterized by disturbed perception with terrifying hallucinations, vivid dreams, fantasies, insomnia, and overactivity.

Acute confusional states have been reported after right MCA infarctions.[363,397] Mesulam and colleagues[297] reported three cases of sudden onset of acute confusion accompanied by retropulsion, unsteady gait, incontinence, difficulty in using common objects, and lack of concern for the illness. Mental agitation evolved into a state of irritable sluggishness, inattention, and memory disorder. Mullaley et al[319,320] reported acute confusion in 13 patients with right parietal lobe lesions and four with right temporal lobe lesions. Levine and Finklestein[267] added eight patients with a behavioral disorder characterized by hallucinations, delusions, agitation, and confusion remotely related (1 month to 11 years) to right temporoparietal stroke or trauma. Dunne et al[140] found that 3% (19) of 661 stroke patients presented with delirium, confusion, dementia, or psychosis. Nearly all had right hemisphere lesions. Elementary neurologic findings were either absent or subtle. In 41 patients with right MCA territory infarctions, Mori and Yamadori[317] found acute confusion in 25 and acute delirium in 6. Caplan et al[90] found that posterior right temporal lesions were more likely to produce acute confusion than posterior right parietal lesions. The propensity of temporal lesions to produce confusional states may be explained by the proximity of these lesions to the underlying limbic system. Confusional states that follow brain infarction may result from one of two processes: disrupted modulation of affective responses in the limbic system or disruption of right hemisphere networks subserving attention.

CONFABULATION AND REDUPLICATIVE PARAMNESIA

Confabulation is the unintentional production of inappropriate and fabricated information. Confabulation is often associated with a failure to inhibit incorrect responses, poor error awareness, and poor self-correction abilities. Impaired memory, poor motivation, and anosognosia are often present. Since many of these associated behaviors are characteristics of frontal lobe pathology, confabulation is often linked to frontal lobe damage. Although impaired memory is often associated with confabulation, the two behaviors vary independently in severity.[43,295] Reduplication is a special form of confabulation. It appears to reflect an attempt of the brain-injured patient to fuse experiences from two disparate periods in his life. In instances of reduplication for place, the patient holds an inaccurate belief that two versions of a geographic location exist. The patient wrongly believes that he is residing in a second version of a familiar setting. The hospitalized patient may persist in a belief that he is at home or at another hospital despite repeated attempts to orient him to his current location. Luria[282] (p. 168) describes several patients with right hemisphere lesions and reduplication for place. He says he "shall never forget a group of patients with deep lesions . . . of the right hemisphere. . . . They firmly believed that at one and the same time they were in Moscow and also in another town. They suggested that they had left Moscow and gone to the other town. They suggested that they were still in Moscow where an operation had been performed on their brain. Yet they found nothing contradictory about these conclusions."

Environmental reduplication occurs most commonly after right frontoparietal lobe injury. Reduplication of person (a false belief that two versions of an individual exist) may also occur after right hemisphere injury. Like reduplication of place, reduplication of person is a restricted form of confabulation.[43]

CONSTRUCTIONAL APRAXIA

In 1934, Kleist[243] described constructional apraxia as "a disturbance which appears in formative activities (arranging, building, drawing) and in which a spatial part of the task is missed, although there is no apraxia of single movements." Kleist's definition includes the key aspects of constructional apraxia: patients fail at tasks that require the manipulation of objects in space. A variety of tests have been utilized to identify constructional apraxia including the copying of block designs, the copying of simple and complex figures, puzzle constructions, mental rotations, and three-dimensional model building. Constructional apraxia is synonymous with other terms including apractognosia, constructional disability, and visual-spatial agnosia.

Constructional apraxia occurs after injury to either cerebral hemisphere. Among 67 patients with constructional apraxia, Piercy et al[341] reported 42 with right-sided lesions and 25 with left-sided lesions. Arrigoni and De Renzi[22] found constructional apraxia to be more prevalent in right-brain-damaged than left-brain-damaged subjects. Most lesions are in the vicinity of the parietal lobe.[358] The nature of constructional apraxia differs according to the hemisphere injured. Patients with left-sided lesions improve their drawings when aided by visual cues, whereas patients with right-sided lesions do not. Warrington et al[404] suggested that the constructional apraxia that follows right hemisphere damage is a visuospatial disorder, whereas the constructional apraxia that follows left hemisphere damage is an executive disorder. The drawings of patients with left hemisphere damage are oversimplified, with reduced detail, whereas left unilateral neglect characterizes the drawings of patients with right hemisphere damage. However, Gainotti et al[163,164] were not able to distinguish right-sided from left-sided constructional apraxia.

Critchley[103] sees constructional apraxia as "an executive defect within a visuospatial domain." Constructional apraxia may also be viewed as a spatial agnosia, that is, a defect in the comprehension of spatial relationships.[352] Similarly, Whitty and Newcombe[418] argued that "the nature of the visual spatial difficulty appears to be of an agnostic rather than simple perceptual type. The term constructional apraxia is not entirely satisfactory." Data from 37 patients in the Neurological Institute Cerebral Localization Laboratory suggest further that abnormal drawing may arise from different behavioral abnormalities correlating with different lesion sites.[286] Those patients with marked drawing hemineglect had infarcts in the dorsal posterior parietal region. Those patients with unrecognizable drawings who performed poorly on line bisection had lesions in the temporo-parieto-occipital junction. Unrecognizable drawings by patients who had normal line bisection were produced by lesions in the anterior, subcortical locations. Similarly, we reported the case of a 66-year-old woman with CT-verified infarction in the region of the right caudate nucleus and putamen who was given traditional clinical measures of perception, attention, and constructional apraxia, followed by the presentation of matching-to-sample procedures.[257] The clinical measures first showed severe constructional apraxia without hemineglect; the matching procedures then provided demonstrable evidence that she could not copy Greek letter forms that she could otherwise match with perfect accuracy, thereby eliminating perceptual dysfunction as a cause of her deficit.

ALLESTHESIA

Allesthesia (also allochiria) is the referral of a sensory stimulus (visual, tactile, or auditory) from one side of the body to the other.[224,225] Allesthesia is most often seen in the setting of right hemisphere damage with left-sided neglect. When the left side is touched, the sensation may be reported by the patient to occur on the right side. Allesthesia may also occur in the setting of spinal cord injury or conversion hysteria.

AMUSIA

Amusia (loss of musical ability secondary to brain disease) has been an elusive deficit to study.[46,68,417] Brust[81] concluded that no simple relationship exists between the location of a lesion and extent of musical disability. Case reports of expressive amusia after right hemisphere lesions are numerous. These patients are unable to sing or whistle but have preserved language function and melody recognition. Receptive amusia may also occur with right hemisphere lesions. Because of its complexity, the neural basis of music remains obscure.[182] Amusia is an isolated phenomenon that may occur after right hemisphere lesions of varying location, size, and etiology.

APROSODY AND AFFECTIVE AGNOSIA

Monrad-Krohn[316] defined prosody as the musical quality of speech produced by "variations in pitch, rhythm, and stress of pronunciation. . . ." After right hemisphere damage, some patients are unable to intone affect into their speech.[84] This deficit is known as aprosody. Based on this work and the work of Heilman et al,[204] Ross and Mesulam[354] proposed that the right hemisphere was dominant for the modulation of affective language and that this modulation was organized in a fashion analogous to left hemisphere organization for propositional language. In a subsequent study, Ross[352] provided additional confirmatory evidence of the functional-anatomic organization of the affective components of language in the right hemisphere. By utilizing a bedside examination strategy, analogous to a routine aphasia examination, combined with CT scan mappings, he observed that the organization of affective language in the right hemisphere mirrored that of propositional language in the left hemisphere. The resulting disturbances of affective modulation were coined the aprosodias. In analogy with the aphasias, Ross[352,353] proposed the existence of motor, sensory, global, conduction, and transcortical aprosodias. In motor aprosody, the patient is unable to utilize prosody to inject affect into speech, nor is the patient able to repeat the affect-laden prosody of others.[412] However, the patient can comprehend the affect conveyed by the prosody of other speakers. The patient with sensory aprosody shows poor comprehension of affective prosody and cannot repeat affective prosody, but has normal spontaneous affective prosody in speech. Global aprosody is reflected in apraxics according to drawing errors. Hecaen and Albert[197] suggest that "constructional apraxia may result from a breakdown in different underlying neuropsychological mechanisms, depending on the hemisphere damaged." Darby[111] reviewed four patients whose syndrome featured impaired response to emotional gestures, evident difficulty in assessing the affective portion of speech heard, and a reduced emotional range of intonations in spontaneous speech and gesture. In all cases studied the syndrome was present in the acute phase of the stroke. In three the lesions were large: two in the inferior divisional area, one affecting a larger region, and one affecting the left side, not the right. The author noted that this finding was not present in healthy controls nor in patients with lacunar infarction.

Heilman and colleagues[207] noted that right temporoparietal lesions caused defects in the comprehension of affective speech and termed this disorder affective agnosia. Tucker and colleagues[390] observed that right temporoparietal lesions caused both affective comprehension deficits and deficits in evoking emotional intonation on a speech repetition task.

References

1. Abbie AA: The morphology of the forebrain arteries with especial reference to the evolution of the basal ganglia. J Anat 68:432, 1934
2. Abbie AA: The vascular supply of the internal capsule. Med J Aust 1934
3. Adams HP, Demasio HC, Putman SF, Demasio AR: Middle cerebral artery occlusion as a cause of isolated subcortical infarction. Stroke 14:948, 1983
4. Adams HP, Gross CE: Embolism distal to stenosis of the middle cerebral artery. Stroke 12:228, 1981
5. Adams JH, Graham DI: Twelve cases of fatal cerebral infarction due to arterial occlusion in the absence of atheromatous stenosis or embolism. J Neurol Surg Psychiatry 30:4379, 1957
6. Adams RD, Victor M: Principles of Neurology. McGraw-Hill, New York, 1984
7. Agostini E, Coletti A, Orlando G, Tredici G: Apraxia in deep cerebral lesions. J Neurol Neurosurg Psychiatry 46:804, 1983
8. Ajuriaguerra J, Hecaen H, Angelergues R: Les apraxies: varietés cliniques et latéralisation lésionelle. Rev Neurol (Paris) 102:494, 1960
9. Akelatis AJ: Symmetrical bilateral granular atrophy of the cerebral cortex of vascular origin. A clinico-pathologic study. Am J Psychiatry 99:447, 1942
10. Alajouanine T, Boudin G, Pertuiset B, Pepin B: Le syndrome operculaire unilatéral avec atteinte contralatérale du territoire des V, VII, IX, XI, XIIème nerfs craniens. Rev Neurol (Paris) 101:167, 1959
11. Alajouanine T, Ombredane A, Durand M: Le Syndrome de Désintégration Phonétique dans l'Aphasie. Masson, Paris, 1939
12. Albert ML: A simple test for neglect. Neurology 23:658, 1973
13. Albert ML, Goodglass H, Helm NA et al: Clinical Aspects of Dysphasia. Springer-Verlag, New York, 1981
14. Alexander L: The vascular supply of the striato-pallidum. Res Publ Assoc Nerv Ment Dis 21:77, 1941
15. Alexander MP, Hiltbrunner B, Fischer RS: Distributed anatomy of transcortical sensory aphasia. Arch Neurol 46:885, 1989
16. Amyes EW, Nielsen JM: Clinicopathologic study of vascular lesions of the anterior cingulate region. Bull Los Angeles Neurol Soc 20:112, 1955
17. Appenzeller O: The Autonomic Nervous System. North Holland Publishing, Amsterdam 1970
18. Araki G: Small infarctions of the basal ganglia with special reference to transient ischemic attacks. Recent Adv Gerontol 469:161, 1978
19. Ardila A, Rosselli M: Language deviations in aphasia: a frequency analysis. Brain Lang 44:165, 1993
20. Arena R, Gainotti G: Constructional apraxia and visuoperceptive disabilities in relation to laterality of cerebral lesions. Cortex 14:463, 1978
21. Aring CD, Merritt HH: Differential diagnosis between cerebral hemorrhage and cerebral thrombosis. Arch Intern Med 56:435, 1935

22. Arrigoni G, DeRenzi E: Constructional apraxia and hemispheric locus of lesion. Cortex 1:170, 1964

23. Auld AW, Shafey S: Transient ischemic attacks not produced by extracranial vascular disease: a plea for early and complete angiographic evaluation. South Med J 69: 722, 1976

24. Austregesilo A, Borges-Forte A: Sur un cas de hemischorée avec lésion du noyau caude. Rev Neurol (Paris) 67:477, 1937

25. Babinski J: Anosognosie. Rev Neurol (Paris) 31:365, 1918

26. Baker AB: Structure of the small cerebral arteries and their changes with age. Am J Pathol 13:453, 1937

27. Baloh RW, Yee RD, Honrubia V: Optokinetic nystagmus and parietal lobe lesions. Ann Neurol 7:269, 1980

28. Barat M, Constant P, Mazaux JM, Caille JM, Arne L: Corrélations anatomo-cliniques dans l'aphasie. Apport de la tomodensitomatrie. Rev Neurol (Paris) 134:611, 1978

29. Barat M, Mazaux JM, Bioulac B et al: Troubles de langage de type aphasique et lésions putamino-caudées. Rev Neurol (Paris) 137:343, 1981

30. Barnett HJM, Boughner DR, Taylor DW et al: Further evidence relating mitral value prolapse to cerebral ischemic events. N Engl J Med 302:139, 1980

31. Barnett HJM, Jones MW, Boughner DR, Kostuk WJ: Cerebral ischemic events associated with prolapsing mitral valve. Arch Neurol 33:777, 1976

32. Barnett HJM, Peerless SJ, Kaufmann JCE: "Stump" of internal carotid artery—a source for further cerebral embolic ischemia. Stroke 9:448, 1978

33. Basso A, Capitani E, Luzzatti C, Spinnler H: Intelligence and left hemisphere disease: the role of aphasia, apraxia and size of lesion. Brain 104:721, 1981

34. Basso A, Luzzatti C, Spinnler H: Is ideomotor apraxia the outcome of damage to well-defined regions of the left hemisphere? J Neurol Neurosurg Psychiatry 43:118, 1980

35. Bastian HC: Some problems in connection with aphasia and other speech defects. Lancet 1:933, 1005, 1131, 1187, 1897

36. Battersby WS, Bender MB, Pollack M: Unilateral spatial agnosia (inattention) in patients with cerebral lesions. Brain 79:68, 1956

37. Beal MF, Williams RS, Richardson EP, Fisher CM: Cerebral embolism as a cause of transient ischemic attacks and cerebral infarction. Neurology (NY) 31:860, 1981

38. Beevor CE: On the distribution of the different arteries supplying the human brain. Philos Trans R Soc [Biol] 1908

39. Belin P, Van Eeckhout P, Zilbovicius M et al: Recovery from nonfluent aphasia after melodic intonation therapy: a PET study. Neurology 47:1504, 1996

40. Ben-Yishay Y, Diller L, Gerstman L et al: The relationship between impersistence, intellectual function and outcome of rehabilitation in patients with left hemiplegia. Neurology 18:852, 1968

41. Bender MB: Brain control of conjugate horizontal and vertical eye movements. A survey of the structural and functional correlates. Brain 103:23, 1980

42. Benson DF: Aphasia, Alexia and Agraphia. Churchill Livingstone, New York, 1979

43. Benson DF, Gardner H, Meadows JC: Reduplicative amnesia. Neurology 26:147, 1976

44. Benson DF, Geschwind N: The aphasias and related disorder. In Baker AB, Baker LH (eds): Clinical Neurology. Vol. 1. Harper & Row, Hagerstown, 1976

45. Benson DF, Sheremata WA, Bouchard R et al: Conduction aphasia. Arch Neurol 28:339, 1973

46. Benton AL: The amusias. In Critchley M, Henson RA (eds): Music and the Brain. Heinemann Medical Books, London, 1977

47. Berry RG, Alpers GJ: Occlusion of the carotid circulation: pathological consideration. Neurology 7:233, 1957

48. Berthier ML, Starkstein SE, Leiguarda R et al: Transcortical aphasia. Brain 114:1409, 1991

49. Bigelow NH: Intracranial dissecting aneurysms. An analysis of their significance. Arch Pathol 60:271, 1955

50. Binder JR, Marshall RS, Lazar RM et al: Distinct syndromes of hemineglect. Arch Neurol 49:1187, 1992

51. Binder JR, Rao SM, Hammeke TA et al: Lateralized human brain language systems demonstrated by task subtraction functional magnetic resonance imaging. Arch Neurol 52:593, 1995

52. Birch HG, Belmont I, Karp E: Delayed information processing and extinction following cerebral damage. Brain 90:113, 1967

53. Bisiach E, Cornacchia L, Sterzi R, Vallar G: Disorder of perceived auditory lateralization after lesions of the hemisphere. Brain 107:37, 1984

54. Bisiach E, Luzzatti C: Unilateral neglect of representational space. Cortex 14:129, 1978

55. Bizzi E: Discharge of frontal eye field neurons during eye movements in unanesthetized monkeys. Science 157:1588, 1967

56. Bizzi E: Discharge of frontal eye field neurons during saccadic and following eye movements in unanesthetized monkeys. Exp Brain Res 6:69, 1968

57. Black FW, Strub RL: Constructional apraxia in patients with discrete missile wounds of the brain. Cortex 12: 212, 1976

58. Blackwood W, Bratty P, Mair WGP: p. 146. In Jakob H (ed): Observations on Occlusive Vascular Disease of the Brain. Vol. 3. Thieme Verlag, Stuttgart, 1963

59. Bladin PF: A radiologic and pathologic study of embolism of the internal carotid-middle cerebral arterial axis. Radiology 82:614, 1964

60. Blumstein SE, Baker E, Goodglass H: Phonological factors in auditory comprehension in aphasia. Neuropsychologia 15:19, 1977

61. Bluschke V, Hennerici M, Scharf RE et al: Mitralklappenprolaps-Syndrom und Thrombozytenaktivität bei jungen Patienten mit zerebralen Ischämien. Dtsch Med Wochenschr 107:410, 1982

62. Bodamer J: Die Prosop-Agnosie. Arch Psychiatr Nervenkr 179:6, 1947

63. Bogen JE, Bogen GM: Wernicke's region—where is it? Ann NY Acad Sci 280:834, 1976

64. Bogousslavsky J, Miklossy J, Regli F et al: Subcortical neglect: neuropsychological, and neuropathological cor-

relations with anterior choroid artery territory infarction. Ann Neurol 23:448, 1988

65. Bogousslavsky J, Regli F, Assal G: Acute transcortical mixed aphasia: a carotid occlusion syndrome with pial and watershed infarcts. Brain 111:631, 1988

66. Boller F: Destruction of Wernicke's area without language disturbance. A fresh look at crossed aphasia. Neuropsychologia 11:243, 1973

67. Bonhoeffer K: Klinischer und anatomischer Befund zur Lehre von der Apraxie und der "Motorischen Sprachbahn." Monatsschr Psychiatr Neurol 35:113, 1914

68. Botez MI, Wertheim N: Expressive aphasia and amusia following right frontal lesion in a right-handed man. Brain 82:186, 1959

69. Boulliaud J: Recherches cliniques propres à demonstrer que la perte de la parole correspond à la lésion des lobules antérieurs du cerveau, et à confirmer l'opinion de M. Gall sur le siège de l'organe du langage articule. Arch Gen Med VIII:25, 1825

70. Bounds JV, Sandok BA, Barnhorst DA: Fatal cerebral embolism following aorto-coronary bypass graft surgery. Stroke 7:611, 1976

71. Bourneville: Athérome généralisé: oblitérations multiples (aphasie; sphàcele du pied, etc.). Prog Med 2:278, 1874

72. Bourneville: Athérome généralisé: oblitérations multiples (aphasie; sphàcele du pied, etc.). Prog Med 2:296, 1874

73. Bousser MG, Dubois B, Castaigne P: Pertes de connaissance brèves au cours des accidents ischemiques cérébraux. Ann Med Interne 132:300, 1981

74. Brain WR: Speech Disorders. Butterworths, London, 1962

75. Brain WR: Visual disorientation with special reference to the lesions of the right hemisphere. Brain 64:244, 1941

76. Bramwell B: A remarkable case of aphasia. Brain 21:343, 1898

77. Brierley JB, Adams JH, Connor RCR, Triep CS: The effects of systemic hypotension upon the human brain. Brain 89:235, 1966

78. Broadbent WH: On the cerebral mechanism of speech and thought. Trans R Med Chiur Soc (Lond) 55:145, 1872

79. Broca P: Remarques sur le siège de la faculté du langage articule, suivies d'une observation d'aphémie (perte de la parole). Bull Soc Anat Paris 6:330, 1861

80. Brown JW: Aphasia, Apraxia, and Agnosia. Charles C Thomas, Springfield, IL, 1972

81. Brust JCM: Music and language. Brain 103:367, 1980

82. Brust JCM, Shafer SQ, Richter RW, Bruun B: Aphasia in acute stroke. Stroke 7:167, 1976

83. Bruyn GW, Gathier JC: The operculum syndrome. p. 776. In Vinken PJ, Bruyn GW (eds): Handbook of Clinical Neurology. Vol. 2. North Holland Publishing, Amsterdam, 1976

84. Buck R, Duffy RJ: Nonverbal communication of affect in brain-damaged patients. Cortex 16:331, 1980

85. Burns MS, Canter GJ: Phonemic behavior of aphasic patients with posterior cerebral languages. Brain Lang 4:492, 1977

86. Bushnell DL, Gupta S, Mlcoch AG, Barnes WE: Prediction of language and neurologic recovery after cerebral infarction with SPECT imaging using N-isopropyl-p-(I 123) iodoamphetamine. Arch Neurol 46:665, 1989

87. Campbell DC, Oxbury JM: Recovery from unilateral visuo-spatial neglect. Cortex 12:303, 1976

88. Caplan LR: A 62 year-old Haitian woman with strokes, renal disease and abdominal pain. N Engl J Med 315:567, 1986

89. Caplan LR, Hier DB, D'Cruz I: Cerebral embolism in the Michael Reese Stroke Registry. Stroke 14:30, 1983

90. Caplan LR, Kelly M, Kase CS et al: Infarcts of the inferior division of the right middle cerebral artery: mirror image of Wernicke's aphasia. Neurology 36:1015, 1986

91. Cappa SF, Perani D, Bressi S et al: Crossed aphasia: a PET follow up study of two cases. J Neurol Neurosurg Psychiatry 56:665, 1993

92. Castaigne P, Lhermitte F, Gautier J-C et al: Internal carotid artery occlusion: a study of 61 instances in 50 patients with post-mortem data. Brain 93:231, 1970

93. Chiari H: Ueber das Verhalten des Teilungswinkels der Carotis communis bei der Endarteritis chronic deformans. Verh Dtsch Ges Pathol 9:326, 1905

94. Chater N, Spetzler R, Tonnemachar K et al: Microvascular bypass surgery. Part I: Anatomical studies. J Neurosurg 44:712, 1976

95. Chouppe: Ramollissement superficiel du cerveau intéressant surtout la troisième circonvolution frontale gauche, sans aphasie. Bull Soc Anat Paris 45:365, 1870

96. Clower BR, Sullivan DM, Smith RR: Intracranial vessels lack vasa vasorum. J Neurosurg 61:44, 1984

97. Cohen MM, Hemalatha CP, D'Addario RT, Goldman HW: Embolism from a fusiform middle cerebral artery aneurysm. Stroke 11:58, 1980

98. Cole MF, Cole M: Comte A: Des paralysies pseudobulbaires (thesis). 8, No. 436, Paris, Steinheil, 1900. In: Pierre Marie's Papers on Speech Disorders. Hafner, New York, 1971

99. Cords R: Optisch-motorisches Feld und optisch-motorishe Bahn. Albrecht von Graefes Arch Ophthalmol 117:58, 1926

100. Corston RN, Kendall BE, Marshall J: Prognosis in middle cerebral artery stenosis. Stroke 15:237, 1984

101. Coslett HB, Brashear HR, Heilman KM: Pure word deafness after bilateral primary auditory cortex infarcts. Neurology (Cleve) 34:347, 1984

102. Costa LD, Vaughan G Jr, Horwitz M, et al: Patterns of behavioral deficit associated with visual spatial neglect. Cortex 5:242, 1969

103. Critchley M: The Parietal Lobes. Hafner, New York, 1953

104. Croisile B, Henry E, Trillet M, Aimard G: Loss of motivation for speaking with bilateral lacunes in the anterior limb of the internal capsule. Clin Neurol Neurosurg 91:3257, 1989

105. Daffner KR, Ahern GL, Weintraub S, Mesulam MM: Dissociated neglect behavior following sequential strokes in the hemisphere. Ann Neurol 28:97, 1990

106. Damasio H, Damasio AR: The anatomic basis of conduction aphasia. Brain 103:337, 1980

107. Damasio H, Damasio AR: Localization of lesions in con-

duction aphasia. p. 231. In Kertesz A (ed): Localization in Neuropsychology. Academic Press, New York, 1983

108. Damasio A, Damasio H, Chang Chi H: Neglect following damage to frontal lobe or basal ganglia. Neuropsychologia 18:123, 1980

109. Damasio H, Damasio AR, Hamsher K, Varney N: CT scan correlates of aphasia and allied disorders. Neurology (Minneap) 29:572, 1979

110. Damasio AR, Damasio H, Rizzo M et al: Aphasia with non-hemorrhagic lesions of the basal ganglia and the internal capsule. Arch Neurol 39:15, 1982

111. Darby DG: Sensory aprosodia: a clinical clue to lesions of the inferior division of the right middle cerebral artery? Neurology 43:567, 1993

112. Darley FL, Aaronson A, Brown J: Motor Speech Disorders. WB Saunders, Philadelphia, 1975

113. Daroff RB, Hoyt WF: Supranuclear disorders of ocular control system in man: clinical, anatomical and physiological correlates. p. 175. In Bach-Y-Rita P, Collins CC et al (eds): The Control of Eye Movements. Academic Press, New York, 1971

114. David NJ, Gordon KK, Friedberg SJ et al: Fatal atheromatous cerebral embolism associated with bright plaques in the retinal arterioles. Neurology 13:708, 1963

115. Davis DO, Rumbaugh CL, Gilson JM: Angiographic diagnosis of small-vessel cerebral emboli. Acta Radiol (Stockh) 9:264, 1969

116. Davison C, Goodhart SP, Needles W: Cerebral localization and cerebral vascular disease. Arch Neurol Psychiatry (Chicago) 30:749, 1933

117. Day AL: Anatomy of the extracranial vessels. p. 9. In Smith RR (ed): Stroke and the Extracranial Vessels. Raven Press, New York, 1984

118. Deck JHN, Lee MA: Mucin embolism to cerebral arteritis: a fatal complication of carcinoma of the breast. J Can Sci Neurol 5:327, 1978

119. Dejerine J: Sur un cas de cecite verbale avec agraphie, suivi d'autopsie. Mem Soc Biol 3:197, 1891

120. Dejerine J: Des différentes variétés de cecite verbale. Mem Soc Biol 1:30, 1892

121. Dejerine J: Séméiologie des Affections du Système Nerveux. Masson, Paris, 1914

122. Dejerine J, Regnard M: Monoplegie brachiale gauche limitée aux muscles des eminences thenar, hypothenar et aux interosseux. Astereognosie, épilepsie jacksonienne. Rev Neurol 1:285, 1912

123. Delal PM, Shah PM, Aiyar RR: Arteriographic study of cerebral embolism. Lancet 2:358, 1965

124. DeMassary J: L'alexie. Encephale 27:134, 1934

125. Demeurisse G, Capon A, Verhas M, Attig E: Pathogenesis of aphasia in deep-seated lesions: likely role of cortical diaschisis. Eur Neurol 30:67, 1990

126. Demeurisse G, Verhas M, Capon A: Remote cortical dysfunction in aphasic stroke patients. Stroke 22:1015, 1991

127. Demierre B, Rondot P: Dystonia caused by putamino-capsulo-caudate vascular lesions. J Neurol Neurosurg Psychiatry 46:404, 1983

128. DeRenzi E, Colombo A, Faglioni P, Gilbertoni N: Conjugate gaze paresis in stroke patients with unilateral damage. Arch Neurol 39:42, 1982

129. DeRenzi E, Faglioni P, Previdi P: Spatial memory and hemispheric locus of lesion. Cortex 13:424, 1977

130. DeRenzi E, Faglioni P, Scotti G: Judgement of spatial orientation in patients with focal brain damage. J Neurol Neurosurg Psychiatry 34:489, 1971

131. DeRenzi E, Lucchelli F: Ideational apraxia. Brain 198:1173, 1988

132. DeRenzi E, Motti F, Nichelli P: Imitating gestures: a quantitative approach to ideomotor apraxia. Arch Neurol 37:6, 1980

133. DeRenzi E, Pieczuro A, Vignola L: Oral apraxia and aphasia. Cortex 2:50, 1966

134. DeRenzi E, Pieczuro A, Vignolo L: Ideational apraxia: a quantitative study. Neuropsychologia 6:41, 1968

135. Derouesne C, Mas JL, Bolgert AF, Castaigne P: Pure sensory stroke caused by a small cortical infarct in the middle cerebral artery territory. Stroke 15:660, 1984

136. Deuel RK, Collins RC: The functional anatomy of frontal lobe neglect in the monkey: behavioral and quantitative 2-deoxyglucose studies. Ann Neurol 15:521, 1984

137. Donnan GA, Bladin PF, Berkovic SF et al: The stroke syndrome of striatocapsular infarction. Brain 114:51, 1991

138. Dratz HM, Woodhall B: Traumatic dissecting aneurysm of left internal carotid, anterior cerebral and middle cerebral arteries. J Neuropathol Exp Neurol 6:286, 1947

139. Duman S, Stephans JW: Post-traumatic middle cerebral artery occlusion. Neurology 13:613, 1963

140. Dunne JW, Leedman PJ, Edis RH: Inobvious stroke: a cause of delirium and dementia. Aust NZ J Med 16:771, 1986

141. Duret H: Recherches anatomiques sur la circulation de l'encéphale. Arch Physiol Norm Pathol 1:919, 1874

142. Edwards JH, Kricheff II, Riles T, Imparato A: Angiographically undetected ulceration of the carotid bifurcation as a cause of embolic stroke. Radiology 132:369, 1979

143. Fairfax AJ, Lambert CD, Leatham A: Systemic embolism in chronic sinoatrial disorder. N Engl J Med 275:190, 1976

144. Feldmeyer JJ, Merendaz C, Regli F: Sténoses symptomatiques de l'artère cérébrale moyenne. Rev Neurol (Paris) 139:725, 1983

145. Fieschi C, Argentino C, Lenzi GL et al: Clinical and instrumental evaluation of patients with ischemic stroke within the first six hours. J Neurol Sci 91:311, 1989

146. Fischer E: Die Lageabweichungen der vorden Hirnarterie im Gefaessbild Zentralbl Neurochir 3:300, 1938

147. Fisher CM: Occlusion of the internal carotid artery. AMA Arch Neurol Psychiatry 69:346, 1951

148. Fisher CM: Left hemiplegia and motor impersistence. J Nerv Ment Dis 123:201, 1956

149. Fisher CM: Cerebral ischemia—less familar types. Clin Neurosurg 18:267, 1971

150. Fisher CM: Capsular infarcts. Arch Neurol 36:65, 1979

151. Fisher CM: Topographic disorientation. Arch Neurol 19:33, 1982

152. Fisher CM, Curry HB: Pure motor hemiplegia of vascular origin. Arch Neurol 13:30, 1965

153. Fisher CM, Gore I, Okabe N, White PD: Atherosclerosis

of the carotid and vertebral arteries—extracranial and intracranial. J Neuropathol Exp Neurol 24:455, 1965

154. Fisher CM, Pearlman A: The non-sudden onset of cerebral embolism. Neurology (Minneap) 17:1025, 1967

155. Foix C: Aphasies. p. 135. In Roger GH, Widal F, Teissier PJ (eds): Nouveau Traité de Medecine. Vol. 18. Masson, Paris, 1928

156. Foix C, Chavany J-A, Levy M: Syndrome pseudo-thalamique d'origine pariétale. Lésion de l'artère du sillon interpariétal (Pa P1 P2 antérieurs, petit territoire insulo-capsulaire). Rev Neurol (Paris) 35:68, 1927

157. Foix C, Levy M: Les ramollissements sylviens. Rev Neurol (Paris) 11:51, 1927

158. Freeman MF, Alexander MP, Naeser MA: Anatomic basis of transcortical motor aphasia. Neurology 34:40, 1984

159. Friedlich AL, Castleman B, Mohr JP: Case records of the Massachusetts General Hospital. N Engl J Med 278:1109, 1968

160. Furlan AJ, Little JR, Dohn DF: Arterial occlusion following anastomoses of the superficial temporal artery to middle cerebral artery. Stroke 11:91, 1980

161. Gacs G, Fox AJ, Barnett HJM, Vinuela F: CT visualization of intracranial arterial thrombo embolism. Stroke 14:756, 1983

162. Gacs G, Merei F, Bodosi M: Balloon catheter as a model of cerebral emboli in humans. Stroke 13:39, 1982

163. Gainotti G, Messerli G, Tissot R: Qualitative analysis of unilateral spatial neglect in relation to laterality of cerebral lesion. J Neurol Neurosurg Psychiatry 35:545, 1972

164. Gainotti G, Tiacci C: The relationships between disorders of visual perception and unilateral spatial neglect. Neuropsychologia 9:451, 1971

165. Garcin R: Paralysie dissociée du median d'origine corticale (sur le caractère durement familial de certains accidents vasculaires cérébraux). Medecine 137, 1932

166. Gardner H, Albert ML, Weintraub S: Comprehending a word: the influence of speed and redundancy on auditory comprehension in aphasia. Cortex 11:155, 1975

167. Gay AJ, Newman NM, Keltner JL: Eye Movement Disorders. CV Mosby, St. Louis, 1974

168. Gazengel JGL: Etude de 276 emboles cérébrales d'origine cardiaque. p. 123. Thèse Faculté de Médécine de Paris. Editions AGEMP, Paris, 1966

169. Gerstmann J: Problem of imperception of disease and of impaired body territories with organic lesions. Arch Neurol Psychiatry 48:890, 1942

170. Geschwind N: Disconnection syndromes in animals and man. Brain 88:237, 1965

171. Geschwind N: Problems in the anatomical understanding of the aphasias. In Benton AL (ed): Contributions to Clinical Neuropsychology. Aldin, Chicago, 1969

172. Geschwind N: The apraxias: neural mechanisms of disorders of learned movement. Am Sci 63:188, 1975

173. Geschwind N, Kaplan E: A human disconnection syndrome. Neurology 12:675, 1962

174. Geschwind N, Quadfasel F, Segarra J: Isolation of the speech area. Neuropsychologia 6:327, 1968

175. Ghika JA, Bogousslavsky J, Regli F: Deep perforators from the carotid system. Template of the vascular territories. Arch Neurol 47:1097, 1990

176. Gibo H, Carver CP, Rhoton AL et al: Microsurgical anatomy of the middle cerebral artery. J Neurosurg 54:151, 1981

177. Gleysteen JJ, Silver D: Paradoxical arterial embolism: collective review. Am Surg 36:47, 1970

178. Glew RH: Case records of the Massachusetts General Hospital. N Engl J Med 301:36, 1979

179. Goldstein K: Die Transkortikal Aphasien. G Fischer, Jena, 1917

180. Goldstein K: Language and Language Disturbances. Grune & Stratton: New York, 1948

181. Goodglass H, Kaplan E: The Assessment of Aphasia and Related Disorders. Lee & Febiger, Philadelphia, 1972

182. Gordon HW, Bogen JE: Hemispheric lateralization of singing after intracarotid sodium amylobarbitone. J Neurol Neurosurg Psychiatry 37:727, 1974

183. Graff-Radford NR, Damasio AR: Disturbances of speech and language associated with thalamic dysfunction. Semin Neurol 4:162, 1984

184. Graff-Radford NR, Welsh K, Godersky J: Callosal apraxia. Neurology 37:100, 1987

185. Grand W: Microsurgical anatomy of the proximal middle cerebral artery and the internal carotid artery bifurcation. Neurosurgery 7:151, 1980

186. Grimes JD, Hassan MN, Quarrington AM, d'Alton J: Delayed-onset post hemiplegic dystonia: CT demonstration of basal ganglia pathology. Neurology (NY) 32:1033, 1982

187. Gross CR, Kase CS, Mohr JP et al: Stroke in south Alabama: incidence and diagnostic features—a population based study. Stroke 15:249, 1984

188. Grossi D, Trohano L, Chiacchio L et al: Mixed transcortical aphasia: clinical features and neuroanatomical correlates: a possible role of the right hemisphere. Eur Neurol 31:204, 1991

189. Gulkin TA, Asbury AK: Fragment of great-vessel wall causing cerebral embolism. N Engl J Med 277:751, 1967

190. Gumerlock MK, Ono H, Neuwelt EA: Can a patent extracranial-intracranial bypass provoke the conversion of an intracranial arterial stenosis to a symptomatic occlusion? Neurosurgery 12:391, 1983

191. Hacke W, Schwab S, Horn M et al: 'Malignant' middle cerebral artery territory infarction: clinical course and prognostic signs. Arch Neurol 53:309, 1996

192. Hanaway J, Torack R, Fletcher AP, Landau WM: Intracranial bleeding associated with urokinase therapy for acute ischemic hemispheral stroke. Stroke 7:143, 1976

193. Hartmann F: Beitrage zur Apraxielehre. Monatsschr Psychiatr Neurol 21:97, 1907

194. Head H: Aphasia and Kindred Disorders of Speech. Cambridge University Press, London, 1926

195. Healton EB, Navarro C, Bressman S, Brust JCM: Subcortical neglect. Neurol (NY) 32:776, 1982

196. Hecaen H: Clinical symptomatology in right and left hemisphere lesions. p. 215. In Mountcastle V (ed): Interhemispheric Relations and Cerebral Dominance. Johns Hopkins University Press, Baltimore, 1962

197. Hecaen H, Albert ML: Human Neuropsychology. John Wiley, New York, 1978

198. Hecaen H, Angelergues R: Etude anatomoclinique de

280 lésions retrorolandiques unilatérales des hémisphères cérébraux. Encephale 6:533, 1961

199. Hecaen H, Angelergues R: Localization of symptoms in aphasia. pp. 223–245. In Dereuck AVS, O'Connor M (eds): Disorders of Language. Little, Brown, Boston, 1978

200. Hecaen H, Gimeno A: L'apraxie idéomotrice unilatérale. Rev Neurol 102:648, 1960

201. Heilbronner K: Die aphasischen, apraktischen und agnostichen Störungen. p. 982. In Lewandowsky M (ed): Handbuch der Neurologie. Vol. 1. Springer-Verlag, Berlin, 1910

202. Heilman KM: Apraxia. In Heilman K, Valenstein E (eds): Clinical Neuropsychology. Oxford University Press, New York, 1979

203. Heilman KM, Rothi LJ, Valenstein E: Two forms of ideomotor apraxia. Neurology (NY) 32:342, 1982

204. Heilman KM, Scholes R, Watson RT: Auditory affective agnosia: disturbed comprehension of affective speech. J Neurol Neurosurg Psychiatry 38:69, 1975

205. Heilman K, Valenstein E: Frontal lobe neglect in man. Neurology (Minneap) 22:660, 1972

206. Heilman KM, Valenstein E: Mechanisms underlying hemispatial neglect. Ann Neurol 5:166, 1979

207. Heilman KM, Van Den Abell T: Right hemispheric dominance for mediating cerebral activation. Neuropsychologia 17:315, 1979

208. Heilman KM, Van Den Abell T: Right hemisphere dominance for attention: the mechanism underlying hemispheric asymmetries of inattention (neglect). Neurology (NY) 30:327, 1980

209. Henschen SE: Klinische und Anatomische Beitrage zur Pathologie des Gehirns. Nordiska Bokhandeln, Stockholm, 1920

210. Hier DB, Mohr JP: Incongruous oral and written naming. Evidence for a subdivision of the syndrome of Wernicke's aphasia. Brain Lang 4:115, 1977

211. Hier DB, Mondlock J, Caplan LR: Behavioral abnormalities after right hemisphere stroke. Neurology (NY) 33:337, 1983

212. Hier DB, Mondlock J, Caplan LR: Recovery of behavioral abnormalities after right hemisphere stroke. Neurology (NY) 33:345, 1983

213. Hindson DA, Westmoreland DE, Carroll WA, Bodmer BA: Persistent Broca's aphasia after right cerebral infarction in a right-hander. Neurology (Cleve) 34:387, 1984

214. Hinton RC, Mohr JP, Ackerman RA, et al: Symptomatic middle cerebral artery stenosis. Ann Neurol 5:152, 1979

215. Hirsch CS, Roessmann U: Arterial dysplasia with ruptured basilar artery aneurysm: report of a case. Hum Pathol 6:749, 1975

216. Hollin SA, Silverstein A: Transient occlusion of the middle cerebral artery. JAMA 194:243, 1965

217. Hollin SA, Sukoff MH, Silverstein A, Gross SW: Posttraumatic middle cerebral artery occlusion. J Neurosurg 25:526, 1966

218. Holmes G: The cerebral integration of the ocular movements. BMJ 2:108, 1938

219. Hughlings-Jackson J: On affections of speech from diseases of the brain. Brain 38:106, 1915

220. Hyland HH: Thrombosis of intracranial arteries. Arch Neurol Psychiatry 30:342, 1933

221. Imparato AM, Riles TS, Gorstein F: The carotid bifurcation plaque: pathologic findings associated with cerebral ischemia. Stroke 10:238, 1979

222. Irino T, Tandea M, Minami T: Angiographic manifestations in postrecanalized cerebral infarction. Neurology 27:471, 1977

223. Jacobs L: Visual allesthesia. Neurology 30:105, 1980

224. Jain KK: Some observations on the anatomy of the middle cerebral artery. Can J Surg 7:134, 1964

225. Joanette Y, Brouchon M: Visual allesthesia in manual pointing: some evidence for a sensorimotor cerebral organization. Brain Cogn 3:152, 1984

226. Johnson AC, Graves VB, Pfaff JP Jr: Dissecting aneurysm of intracranial arteries. Surg Neurol 7:49, 1977

227. Joynt RL, Benton AL, Fogel ML: Behavioral and pathological correlates of motor impersistence. Neurology (NY) 12:876, 1964

228. Karbe H, Szelies B, Herholz K, Heiss WD: Impairment of language is related to left parieto-temporal glucose metabolism in aphasic stroke patients. J Neurol 237:19, 1990

229. Kase CS, White L, Vinson L, Eichelberger P: Shotgun pellet embolus to the middle cerebral artery. Neurology 31:458, 1981

230. Katoh M, Kamiyama H, Abe H et al: Complete occlusion of right middle cerebral artery by radiation therapy after removal of pituitary adenoma: case report. No Shinkei Geka 18:855, 1990

231. Kawase T, Mizukami M, Tazawa T, Araki G: The significance of lenticulostriate arteries in transient ischemic attack—neuroradiological and regional cerebral blood flow studies. Brain Nerve 31:1033, 1979

232. Kerbler S, Schober PH, Steiner H: Traumatische Embolisierung der Arteria cerebri media. Z Kinderchir 45:301, 1990

233. Kertesz A: Aphasia and Associated Disorders: Taxonomy, Localization and Recovery. Grune & Stratton, New York, 1979

234. Kertesz A: Localization of lesions in Wernicke's aphasia. p. 209. In Kertesz A (ed): Localization in Neuropsychology. Academic Press, New York, 1983

235. Kertesz A: Recovery from aphasia. p. 23. In Rose FC (ed): Advances in Neurology. Vol. 42. Progress in Aphasiology. Lippincott-Raven, Philadelphia, 1984

236. Kertesz A, Benson DF: Neologistic jargon: a clinical pathological study. Cortex 6:362, 1970

237. Kertesz A, Harlock W, Coates R: Computer tomographic localization, lesion size and prognosis in aphasia and nonverbal impairment. Brain Lang 8:34, 1979

238. Kertesz A, Nicholson I, Cancelliere A, Kassa K: Motor impersistence: a right-hemisphere syndrome. Neurology 35:662, 1985

239. Kertesz A, Sheppard A, MacKenzie R: Localization in transcortical sensory aphasia. Arch Neurol 39:475, 1982

240. Khurana RK, O'Donnell PP, Suter CM, Inayatullah M: Bilateral deafness of vascular origin. Stroke 12:521, 1981

241. Kimura D, Archibald Y: Motor functions of the left hemisphere. Brain 97:337, 1974

242. Kleist K: Gehirnpathologische und Lokalisatorische Er-

gebnisse uber Horstorungen. Gerauschtaubheiten und Amusie. Monatsschr Psychiatr Neurol 66:853, 1928

243. Kleist K: Gehirnpathologie. Barth, Leipsig, 1934

244. Knopman DS, Selnes OA, Niccum N et al: A longitudinal study of speech fluency in aphasia: CT correlates of recovery and persistent nonfluency. Neurology (Cleve) 33:1170, 1983

245. Kooiker JC, MacLean JM, Sumi SM: Cerebral embolism, marantic endocarditis, and cancer. Arch Neurol 33:260, 1976

246. Krayenbuehl HA, Yasargil MG: Cerebral Angiography. 2nd Ed. Butterworths, London, 1968

247. Kunitz S, Gross CR, Heyman A et al: The pilot stroke data bank: definition, design, data. Stroke 15:740, 1984

248. Kusske JA, Kelly WA: Embolization and reduction of the "steal" syndrome in cerebral AVMs. J Neurosurg 40:313, 1974

249. Labar DR, Mohr JP, Nichols FT, Tatemichi TK: Unilateral hyperhidrosis after cerebral infarction. Neurology 38:1679, 1988

250. LaCours AR, Lhermitte F: The "pure form" of the phonetic disintegration syndrome (pure anathria); anatomical-clinical report of a historical case. Brain Lang 3:88, 1976

251. Laitinen LV: Loss of motivation for speaking with bilateral lacunes in the anterior limb of the internal capsule. Clin Neurol Neurosurg 92:1778, 1990

252. Landis T, Cummings JL, Benson DF, Palmer EP: Loss of topographic familiarity: an environmental agnosia. Arch Neurol 43:132, 1986

253. LaPlane D, Degos JD: Motor neglect. J Neurol Neurosurg Psychiatry 46:152, 1983

254. Lascelles RG, Burrows EH: Occlusion of the middle cerebral artery. Brain 88:85, 1966

255. Lazar RM, Marshall RS, Mohr JP: Aphasia and stroke. p. 118. In Bogousslavsky J, Caplan L (eds): Stroke Syndromes. Cambridge University Press, New York, 1995

256. Lazar RM, Marshall RS, Pile-Spellman J et al: Anterior translocation of language in patients with left cerebral AVMs. Neurology 47:1997 (in press)

257. Lazar RM, Weiner M, Wald HS, Kula RW: Visuoconstructive deficit following infarction in the right basal ganglia: a case report and some experimental data. Arch Clin Neuropsychol 10:543, 1995

258. Lazorthes G, Gouaze A, Salomon G: Vascularisation et Circulation de l'Encéphale. Masson, Paris, 1976

259. Lehmkuhl G, Poeck K: A disturbance in the conceptual organization of actions in patients with ideational apraxia. Cortex 17:153, 1981

260. Lehmkuhl G, Poeck K, Willmes K: Ideomotor apraxia and aphasia: an examination of types and manifestations of apraxic symptoms. Neuropsychologia 21:199, 1983

261. Leicester J: Central deafness and subcortical motor aphasia. Brain Lang 10:224, 1980

262. Leicester J, Sidman M, Stoddard LT, Mohr JP: Some determinants of visual neglect. J Neurol Neurosurg Psychiatry 32:580, 1969

263. Leicester J, Sidman M, Stoddard LT, Mohr JP: The nature of aphasic responses. Neuropsychologia 9:141, 1971

264. Levin HS: Motor impersistence and proprioceptive feedback in patients with unilateral cerebral disease. Neurology (NY) 23:833, 1973

265. Levine DN, Calvanio R: Conduction aphasia. p. 79. In Kirshner HS, Freemon FR (eds): The Neurology of Aphasia. Swets & Zeitlinger, Lisse, 1982

266. Levine DN, Mohr JP: Language after bilateral cerebral infarctions: role of the minor hemisphere and speech. Neurology 29:927, 1979

267. Levine DN, Finkelstein S: Delayed psychosis after right temporoparietal stroke or trauma: relation to epilepsy. Neurology (NY) 32:267, 1982

268. Levine DN, Sweet E: The neuropathologic basis of Broca's aphasia and its implications for the cerebral control of speech. In Arbib M, Kaplan D, Marshall J (eds): Neural Models of Language Processes. Academic Press, New York, 1982

269. Levine DN, Sweet E: Localization in lesions in Broca's motor aphasia. p. 185. In Kertesz A (ed): Localization in Neuropsychology. Academic Press, New York, 1983

270. Lhermitte F, Desi M, Signoret JL, Deloche G: Aphasie kinesthetique associée à un syndrome pseudothalamique. Rev Neurol (Paris) 136:675, 1980

271. Lhermitte F, Gautier JC, Derouesne C: Nature of occlusions of the middle cerebral artery. Neurology (Minneap) 20:82, 1970

272. Lhermitte F, Gautier JC, Derouesne C, Guiraud B: Ischemic accidents in the middle cerebral artery territory (a study of the causes in 122 cases). Arch Neurol 19:248, 1968

273. Liebeskind A, Chinichian A, Schechter MM: The moving embolus seen during serial cerebral angiography. Stroke 2:440, 1971

274. Liepmann H: The syndrome of apraxia (motor asymboly) based on a case of unilateral apraxia. (Translated by Bohne WHO, Liepmann K, Rottenberg DA from Monatsschr Psychiatr Neurol 8:15, 1900.) In Rottenberg DA, Hochberg FH (eds): Neurological Classics in Modern Translation. Hafner, New York, 1977

275. Liepmann H: Aufsätze aus den Apraxiegebeit. S Kargei, Berlin, 1908

276. Liepmann H: Diseases of the brain. p. 467. In Barr CW (ed): Curschmann's Textbook of Nervous Diseases. Vol. 1. Blakiston, Philadelphia, 1915

277. Liepmann H, Maas O: Fall von linksseitiger Agraphie und Apraxie bei rechtsseitiger Lähmung. Z Psychol Neurol 10:214, 1907

278. Liepmann H, Papenheim M: Uber einen Fall von sogenannter Leitungsaphasie mit anatomischen Befund. Z Gesamte Neurol Psychiatry 27:1, 1914

279. Liepmann H, Storch E: Ein Fall Von Reiner Sprachtaubheit. Psychiatr Abhandlung von Wernicke. Hft 7/8, 1898

280. Luria AR: Higher Cortical Functions in Man. Basic Books, New York, 1966

281. Luria AR: Human Brain and Psychological Processes. Harper, New York, 1966

282. Luria AR: The Working Brain. Basic Books, New York, 1976

283. Marie P: Révision de la question de l'aphasie: la troisième circonvolution frontale gauche ne joue aucun role

spécial dans la fonction du langage. Semin Med 26:241, 1906

284. Marinkovic R, Markovic L: The role of the middle cerebral artery in the vascularization of the claustrum. Med Pregl 43:361, 1990

285. Marquardson J: The natural history of acute cerebral vascular disease: a retrospective study of 769 patients. Acta Neurol Scand, suppl. 38, 45, 1969

286. Marshall RS, Lazar RM, Binder JR et al: Intrahemispheric localization of drawing dysfunction. Neuropsychologia 32:493, 1994

287. Marshall RS, Lazar RM, Mohr JP et al: "Semantic" conduction aphasia from a posterior insular cortex infarction. J Neuroimag 6:189, 1996

288. Masdeu JC, O'Hara RJ: Motor aphasia unaccompanied by faciobrachial weakness. Neurology (Cleve) 33:519, 1983

289. Maksimow AA, Bloom W: A Textbook of Histology. 4th Ed. WB Saunders, Philadelphia, 1942

290. Mazzocchi F, Vignolo LA: Localization of lesions in aphasia: clinical-CT scan correlations in stroke patients. Cortex 15:627, 1979

291. Mazzuchi A, Marchini C, Budai R et al: A case of receptive amusia with prominent timbre perception defect. J Neurol Neurosurg Psychiatry 445:644, 1982

292. McClelland JL, Rumelhart DE: An interactive activation model of context effects in letter perception: part 1. An account of basic findings. Psychol Rev 88:375, 1981

293. McFie J, Piercy MF, Zangwill OL: Visual spatial agnosia associated with lesions of the right cerebral hemisphere. Brain 73:167, 1950

294. Meerwaldt JD, Van Harskamp F: Spatial orientation in right-hemisphere infarction. J Neurol Neurosurg Psychiatry 45:586, 1982

295. Mercer B, Wapner W, Gardner H, Benson DF: A study of confabulation. Arch Neurol 34:429, 1977

296. Mesulam M-M: A cortical network for directed attention and unilateral neglect. Ann Neurol 10:309, 1981

297. Mesulam M-M, Waxman SG, Geschwind N et al: Acute confusional states with right middle cerebral artery infarctions. J Neurol Neurosurg Psychiatry 39:84, 1976

298. Metter EJ, Hanson WR, Hackson CA et al: Temporoparietal cortex in aphasia: evidence from positron emission tomography. Arch Neurol 47:1235, 1990

299. Metter EJ, Kempler D, Jackson CA et al: Are remote glucose metabolic effects clinically important? J Cereb Blood Flow Metab, suppl. 1, 7:S196, 1987

300. Miller NR: Walsh and Hoyt's Clinical Neuro-Ophthalmology. 4th Ed. Williams & Wilkins, Baltimore, 1983

301. Minematsu K, Yamaguchi T, Omae T: Spectacular shrinking deficit: rapid recovery from a full hemispheral syndrome by migration of an embolus. Neurology, suppl. 41:329, 1991

302. Mohr JP: Rapid amelioration of motor aphasia. Arch Neurol 28:77, 1973

303. Mohr JP: Broca's area and Broca's aphasia. p. 201. In Whitaker H (ed): Studies in Neurolinguistics. Academic Press, New York, 1976

304. Mohr JP: Neurological complications of cardiac valvular disease and cardiac surgery including systemic hypotension. p. 143. In Klawans HL (ed): Neurological Manifestations of Systemic Diseases. Vol. 38. Vinken PJ, Bruyn GW (eds): Handbook of Clinical Neurology. North-Holland, New York, 1979

305. Mohr JP: The vascular basis of Wernicke aphasia. Trans Am Neurol Assoc 105:133, 1980

306. Mohr JP: Lacunar infarctions. p. 201. In Barnett HJM (ed): Neurological Clinics of North America. WB Saunders, Philadelphia, 1983

307. Mohr JP: Differential diagnosis of stroke. In Rowland LP (ed): Merritt's Textbook of Neurology. 7th Ed. Lea & Febiger, New York, 1984

308. Mohr JP, Caplan LR, Melski JW et al: The Harvard Cooperative Stroke Registry: a prospective registry. Neurology 28:754, 1978

309. Mohr JP, Duterte DI, Oliveira VR et al: Recanalization of acute middle cerebral artery occlusion. Neurology 38:215, 1988

310. Mohr JP, Foulkes MA, Polis AT et al: Infarct topography and hemiparesis profiles with cerebral convexity infarction: the Stroke Data Bank. J Neurol Neurosurg Psychiatry 56:344, 1993

311. Mohr JP, Hier DB, Krishner HS: Modality bias in Wernicke's aphasia. Neurology (NY) 4:395, 1978

312. Mohr JP, Kase CS, Adams RD: Cerebral vascular disorders. In Petersdorf RG et al (eds): Harrison's Principles of Internal Medicine. 10th Ed. McGraw-Hill, New York, 1983

313. Mohr JP, Pessin MS, Finkelstein S et al: Broca aphasia: pathologic and clinical aspects. Neurology 28:311, 1978

314. Mohr JP, Rubinstein LV, Kase CS et al: Gaze palsy in hemispheral stroke: the NINCDS Stroke Data Bank. Presented at the annual meeting of the American Academy of Neurology, Boston, April 12, 1984

315. Mohr JP, Sidman M, Stoddard LT et al: Evolution of the deficit in total aphasia. Neurology 23:1302, 1973

316. Monrad-Krohn GH: The prosodic quality of speech and its disorders. Acta Psychiatr Neurol Scand 22:255, 1947

317. Mori E, Yamadori A: Acute confusional state and acute agitated delirium: occurrence after infarction in the middle cerebral artery territory. Arch Neurol 4:1139, 1987

318. Moutier F: L'Aphasie de Broca. Thèse Médicine, Paris, 1908

319. Mullally W, Huff K, Ronthal M et al: Frequency of acute confusional states with lesions of the right hemisphere. Ann Neurol 12:113, 1982

320. Mullally W, Huff K, Ronthal M et al: Chronic confusional state with right middle cerebral artery occlusion. Neurology (NY) 32:96, 1982

321. Naeser MA: CT scan lesion size and lesion locus in cortical and subcortical aphasias. p. 63. In Kertesz A (ed): Localization in Neuropsychology. Academic Press, New York, 1983

322. Naeser MA, Alexander MP, Helm-Estabrooks N et al: Aphasia with predominantly subcortical lesion sites. Arch Neurol 39:2, 1982

323. Naeser MA, Hayward RW: Lesion localization in aphasia with cranial computerized tomography and The Boston Diagnostic Aphasia Examination. Neurology 28:545, 1978

324. Neufield HN, Cadman NL, Miller AW, Edwards JE:

Embolism from marantic endocarditis as a manifestation of occult carcinoma. Proc Mayo Clin 35:292, 1960

325. Ng LKY, Nimmannitya J: Massive cerebral infarction with severe brain swelling: A clinical pathologic study. Stroke 1:158, 1970

326. Nielsen JM: The unsolved problems in aphasia. Bull Los Angeles Neurol Soc 162, 1939

327. Nielsen JM: Agnosia, Apraxia, Aphasia. Hoeber, New York, 1946

328. Niessl von Mayendorf E: Ueber Die Sognannter Brocasche Windung und ihre Angebliche Bedeutung fur den Motorischen Sprachkt. Monatsschr Psychiatr Neurol 61:129, 1926

329. Niessl von Mayendorf E: Vom lokalisation Problem der articulierte Sprache. Barth, Leipsig, 1930

330. Obrador S: Nervous integration after hemispherectomy in man. p. 133. In Schaltenbrand G, Woolsey CN (eds): Cerebral Localization and Organization. The University of Wisconsin Press, Madison, 1964

331. Paillard J, Michel F, Stelmach G: Localization without content: a tactile analogue of "blind sight." Arch Neurol 40:548, 1983

332. Pederson RA, Troost BT: Abnormalities of gaze in cerebrovascular disease. Stroke 12:251, 1981

333. Perani D, Vallar G, Cappa S et al: Aphasia and neglect after subcortical stroke. Brain 110:1211, 1987

334. Pierrot-Deseilligny C: Saccade and smooth-pursuit impairment after cerebral hemispheric lesions. Eur Neurol 34:121, 1994

335. Pessin MS, Duncan GW, Mohr JP, Poskanzer DC: Clinical and angiographic features of carotid transient ischemic attacks. N Engl J Med 296:358, 1977

336. Pessin MS, Hinton RC, Davis KR et al: Mechanisms of acute carotid stroke. Ann Neurol 6:245, 1979

337. Petersen SE, Fox PT, Posner MI, Mintun M, Raichle ME: Positron emission tomographic studies of the cortical anatomy of single-word processing. Nature 331:585, 1988

338. Phillips CG: Some thoughts on the organization of the motor cortex. In Eccles JC (ed): The Brain and Conscious Experience. Springer-Verlag, New York, 1966

339. Phillips CG: Changing concepts of the precentral motor area. In Eccles JC (ed): Brain and Conscious Experience. Springer-Verlag, New York, 1966

340. Pick A: Studien uber Motorische Apraxie und ihre Mahestehende Erscheinungen. Deuticke, Liepzig, 1905

341. Piercy M, Hecaen H, de Ajuriaguerra J: Constructional apraxia associated with unilateral cerebral lesions: left and right cases compared. Brain 83:225, 1960

342. Poeck P, Lehmkuhl G: Ideatory apraxia in a left-handed patient with right-sided brain lesion. Cortex 16:273, 1980

343. Prevost JL: De la Déviation Conjuguée des Yeux et de la Rotation de la Tête. Thèse, Paris, 1896

344. Rango R, Candelise L, Perani D et al: Cortical pathophysiology and clinical neurologic abnormalities in acute cerebral ischemia. Arch Neurol 46:1318, 1989

345. Rascol A, Clanet M, Manelfe C: Pure motor hemiplegia: CT study of 30 cases. Stroke 13:11, 1982

346. Rengachary SS, Batnitzky S, Morantz RA et al: Hemicra-

niectomy for acute mass of cerebral infarction. Neurosurgery 8:321, 1981

347. Ringel SP, Harrison SH, Norenberg MD, Austin JH: Fibromuscular dysplasia: multiple "spontaneous" dissecting aneurysms of the major cervical arteries. Ann Neurol 1:301, 1977

348. Romanul FCA, Abramowicz A: Changes in brain and pial vessels in arterial borderzones. Arch Neurol 11:40, 1964

349. Rondot P: Syndromes of central motor disorder. p. 169. In Vinken PJ, Bruyn GW (eds): Handbook of Clinical Neurology. Vol 1. Disturbances of Nervous Function. North-Holland, Amsterdam, 1969

350. Rosegay H, Welch KJ: Peripheral collateral circulation between cerebral arteries. J Neurosurg 11:363, 1954

351. Ross ED: Sensory-specific and fractional disorders of recent memory in man: isolated loss of visual recent memory. Arch Neurol 37:193, 1980

352. Ross ED: The aprosodias. Arch Neurol 38:561, 1981

353. Ross ED: Right hemisphere's role in language, affective behavior and emotion. Trends Neurosci 7:342, 1984

354. Ross ED, Mesulam M-M: Dominant language functions of the right hemisphere. Arch Neurol 36:144, 1979

355. Roth M: Disorders of body image caused by lesions of the right parietal lobe. Brain 72:89, 1949

356. Rothi LJ, McFarling D, Heilman KM: Conduction aphasia, syntaxic alexia, and the anatomy of syntactic comprehension. Arch Neurol 39:272, 1982

357. Rovira M, Jacas R, Lay A: The collateral circulation in thrombosis of the internal carotid and its branches. Acta Radiol Stockh 50:101, 1958

358. Ruessman K, Sondag HD, Beneicke U: On the cerebral localization of constructional apraxia. Int J Neurosci 42:59, 1988

359. Salamon G, Huang YP: Radiologic Anatomy of the Brain. Springer-Verlag, New York, 1976

360. Santamaria J, Graus F, Rubio F et al: Cerebral infarction of the basal ganglia due to embolism from the heart. Stroke 14:911, 1983

361. Schenkenberg T, Bradford DC, Ajax ET: Line bisection and unilateral visual neglect in patients with neurological impairment. Neurology (NY) 30:509, 1980

362. Schiller PH, True SD, Conway JL: Effects of frontal eye field and superior colliculus ablations on eye movements. Science 206:590, 1979

363. Schmidley JW, Messing RO: Agitated confusional states: patients with right hemisphere infarctions. Stroke 19:883, 1984

364. Schneider R, Gautier JC: Leg weakness due to stroke. Site of lesions, weakness patterns and causes. Brain 117:347, 1994

365. Schuster P, Taterka H: Beitrag zur Anatomie und Klinik der Reinen Wourttaubheit. Z Neurol Psychiatr 105:494, 1926

366. Schwartz AS, Marchok PL, Kreinick CJ et al: The asymmetric lateralization of tactile extinction in patients with unilateral cerebral dysfunction. Brain 102:669, 1979

367. Shallice T, Warrington EK: The possible role of selective attention in acquired dyslexia. Neuropsychologia 15:31, 1977

368. Shellshear JC: A contribution to our knowledge of the

arterial supply of the cerebral cortex in man. Brain 50: 236, 1927

369. Sidman M: The behavioral analysis of aphasia. J Psychiatr Res 8:413, 1971

370. Sidman M, Stoddard LT, Mohr JP, Leicester J: Behavioral studies of aphasia: methods of investigations and analysis. Neuropsychologia 9:119, 1971

371. Sinclair W Jr: Dissecting aneurysm of the middle cerebral artery associated with migraine syndrome. Am J Pathol 29:1083, 1953

372. Sittig O: Ueber Apraxie. Karger, Berlin, 1931

373. Smith JL: Optokinetic Nystagmus. Charles C Thomas, Springfield, IL, 1963

374. Stehbens WE: Focal intimal proliferation in the cerebral arteries. Am J Pathol 36:289, 1960

375. Stein S, Volpe B: Classical "parietal" neglect syndrome after subcortical right frontal lobe infarction. Neurology (Cleve) 33:797, 1983

376. Steiner TJ, Rail DL, Rose FC: Cholesterol crystal embolization in rat brain—a model for atherosclerotic cerebral infarction. Stroke 11:184, 1980

377. Stengel E, Lodge Patch IC: Central aphasia associated with parietal symptoms. Brain 78:401, 1955

378. Stenvers HW: Ueber die klinische Bedeutung des optischen Nystagmus für die zerebrale Diagnostik. Schweiz Arch Neurol Psychiatr 14:279, 1925

379. Starr A: The pathology of sensory aphasia. Brain 12:82, 1889

380. Stringer WL, Kelly DL: Traumatic dissection of the extracranial internal carotid artery. Neurosurgery 6:123, 1980

381. Strong KC: A study of the structure of the media of the distributing arteries by the method of microdissection. Anat Rec 72:151, 1938

382. Sunderland A, Wade DT, Langton Hewer R: The natural history of visual neglect after stroke: indications from two of assessment. Int Disab Stud 9:55, 1987

383. Teal JS, Rumbaugh CL, Bergeron RT et al: Anomalies of the middle cerebral artery: accessory artery, duplication, and early bifurcation. AJR Radium Ther Nucl Med 118: 567, 1973

384. Tijssen CC: Contralateral conjugate eye deviation in acute supratentorial lesions. Stroke 25:1516, 1994

385. Tonkonogy J, Goodglass H: Language function, foot of the third frontal gyrus, and rolandic operculum. Arch Neurol 38:486, 1981

386. Tognola G, Vignola LA: Brain lesions associated with oral apraxia in stroke patients: a clinico-neuroradiological investigation with the CT scan. Neuropsychologia 18:257, 1980

387. Toro-Gonzalez G, Navarro-Roman L, Roman GC et al: Acute ischemic stroke from fibrocartilaginous embolism to the middle cerebral artery. Stroke 24:738, 1993

388. Touche: Contribution a l'étude anatomo-clinique des aphasies. Arch Gen Med 6:326, 1901

389. Trojanowski JQ, Green RC, Levine DN: Crossed aphasia in a dextral: a clinical pathological study. Neurology 30: 709, 1980

390. Tucker DM, Watson RT, Heilman KM: Discrimination and evocation of affectively intoned speech in patients with right parietal disease. Neurology (NY) 27:947, 1977

391. Turnbull HM: Alterations in arterial structures, and their relation to syphilis. Q J Med 8:201, 1915

392. Umansky F, Dujovny M, Ausman JI et al: Anomalies and variations of the middle cerebral artery: a microanatomical study. Neurosurgery 22:1023, 1988

393. Vallar G, Perani D, Cappa SF et al: Recovery from aphasia and neglect after subcortical stroke: neuropsychological and cerebral perfusion study. J Neurol Neurosurg Psychiatry 51:1269, 1988

394. van der Eecken HM: Anastomoses between the Leptomeningeal Arteries of the Brain. Charles C Thomas, Springfield, IL, 1959

395. van der Eeken HM, Adams RD: The anatomy and functional significance of the meningeal arterial anastomoses of the human brain. J Neuropathol Exp Neurol 12:132, 1953

396. Van Gehuchten P: The Scientific Work of Arthur Van Gehuchten. p. 60. Francqui Fondation, Louvain, 1974

397. Vighetto A, Aimard G, Confavreux C et al: Une observation anatomo-clinique de fabulation (ou delire) topographique. Cortex 16:501, 1980

398. Vincentelli F, Caruso G, Andriamamonji C et al: Modalities of origin of the middle cerebral artery. Incidence on the arrangement of the perforating branches. J Neurosurg Sci 34:7, 1990

399. von Monakow K: Die Lokalisation im Grosshirn und der Abbau der Funktion durch Kortikale Herde. JF Begman, Wiesbaden, 1914

400. Waddington M, Ring BA: Syndromes of occlusion of middle cerebral artery branches, angiographic and clinical correlation. Brain 91:685, 1968

401. Waddington MM: Intraluminal diameter of middle cerebral branches for microanastomosis. Neurol Res 1:65, 1979

402. Walsh KW: Neuropsychology. p. 1197. Churchill Livingstone, Edinburgh, 1978

403. Warrington EK, James M: An experimental investigation of facial recognition in patients with unilateral cerebral lesions. Cortex 3:317, 1967

404. Warrington EK, James M, Kinsbourne M: Drawing disability in relation to laterality of cerebral lesion. Brain 89: 53, 1966

405. Watson RT, Heilman KM: Thalamic neglect. Neurology (NY) 29:690, 1979

406. Watson RT, Heilman KM: Callosal apraxia. Brain 106: 391, 1983

407. Watson RT, Heilman KM, King FA: Neglect after cingulectomy. Neurology (NY) 23:1003, 1973

408. Watson RT, Valenstein E, Heilman KM: Thalamic neglect: possible role of the medial thalamus and nucleus reticularis in behavior. Arch Neurol 38:501, 1981

409. Welch K, Stuteville P: Experimental production of unilateral neglect in monkeys. Brain 81:341, 1958

410. Weiller C, Ringelstein EB, Reiche W et al: The large striatocapsular infarct. A clinical and pathophysiological entity. Arch Neurol 47:1085, 1990

411. Weinstein EA, Kahn RL: The syndrome of anosognosia. Arch Neurol Psychiatry 64:772, 1950

412. Weintraub S, Mesulam M-M, Kramer L: Disturbances in prosody. Arch Neurol 38:742, 1981

413. Weisenberg T, McBride K: Aphasia: A Clinical and Psychological Study. Hafner, New York, 1935

414. Wernicke C: Der Aphasische Symptomencomplex. Breslau, 1874. Reprinted in Gesammelte Aufsatze. Fisher, Berlin, 1893

415. Wernicke C: Lehrbuch der Gehirnkranheiten. Theodore Fischer, Kassel, 1881

416. Wernicke C: The symptom-complex of aphasia. In Church A (ed): Modern Clinical Medical Disease of the Nervous System. Appleton, New York, 1908

417. Wertheim N: The amusias. p. 195. In Vinken PJ, Bruyn GW (eds): Handbook of Clinical Neurology. Vol. 4. North-Holland, Amsterdam, 1969

418. Whitty CWM, Newcombe F: Disabilities associated with lesions in the posterior parietal region of the non-dominant hemisphere. Neuropsychologia 3:175, 1965

419. Willanger R, Danielsen VT, Ankerhus J: Denial and neglect of hemiparesis in right-sided apoplectic lesions. Acta Neurol Scand 64:310, 1981

420. Willanger R, Danielsen UT, Ankerhus J: Visual neglect right-sided apoplectic lesions. Acta Neurol Scand 64: 327, 1981

421. Wise R, Chollet F, Hadar U et al: Distribution of cortical neural networks involved in word comprehension and word retrieval. Brain 114:1803, 1991

422. Wolf PA, Dawber TR, Thomas HE, Kannel WB: Epidemiologic assessment of chronic atrial fibrillation and risk of stroke: the Framingham Study. Neurology (Minneap) 28:973, 1978

423. Wolff HG: The cerebral blood vessels—anatomical principles. In: The Circulation of the Brain and Spinal Cord. Assoc Res Nerv Ment Dis 18:39, 1938

424. Wolman L: Cerebral dissecting aneurysms. Brain 82: 276, 1959

425. Wolpert SM, Stein BM: Catheter embolization of intracranial arteriovenous malformations as an aid to surgical excision. Neuroradiology 10:73, 1975

426. Wood EH, Correll JW: Atheromatous ulceration in major neck vessels as a cause of cerebral embolism. Acta Radiol Diag 9:520, 1969

427. Yamashita M, Tanaka K, Matsuo T et al: Cerebral dissecting aneurysms in patients with moyamoya disease. J Neurosurg 58:120, 1983

428. Yonas H, Agamanolis D, Takaoka Y et al: Dissecting intracranial aneurysms. Surg Neurol 8:407, 1977

429. Yufe R, Karpati G, Carpenter S: Cardiac myxoma: a diagnostic challenge for the neurologist. Neurology 26:1060, 1976

430. Zatz LM, Iannone AM, Eckman PB, Hecker SP: Observations concerning intracerebral vascular occlusion. Neurology 15:390, 1965

Posterior Cerebral Artery Disease

J. P. MOHR

MICHAEL S. PESSIN (deceased)

Anatomy

The posterior cerebral artery usually arises from a terminal bifurcation of the basilar artery. In its initial course across and around the peduncle it gives off the small thalamoperforant branches, which penetrate and supply the midbrain and then supply the thalamus and adjacent lateral geniculate body. During this course it gives rise to the medial and lateral posterior choroidal arteries, which supply the posterior portion of the thalamus and the choroid plexus. It courses downward and backward around the brain stem in the ambient cistern immediately below the tentorium cerebelli just above and slightly lateral to the superior cerebellar artery. Beyond the brain stem, it curves upward and medially in the quadrigeminal cistern. By crossing the free medial edge of the tentorium, it reaches the medial surface of the occipital lobe near the anterosuperior border of the lingual gyrus just below the splenium of the corpus callosum. As it reaches the surface, it usually divides into two major divisions. The anterior division gives rise to the two inferior temporal arteries, the anterior and the posterior. The posterior division yields three major branches in sequence: the first bifurcation gives rise to the occipitotemporal artery and the calcarine artery; the latter gives rise to the occipitoparietal artery. The anterior and posterior inferior temporal arteries and the occipitotemporal artery supply the orbital surface of the temporal and orbital lobes. Their terminal branches anastomose with the middle cerebral artery via a border zone network that runs roughly along the margin of the hemisphere where the orbital surfaces become convex. The calcarine supplies the calcarine cortex and medial surfaces of the occipital lobe as far distally as the occipital pole, anastomosing with terminal branches of the middle cerebral artery. The branches of the occipitoparietal artery supply the precuneus, and along a border zone network the terminal vessels anastomose with branches of the anterior cerebral artery.

In approximately 70% of cases, both the posterior cerebral arteries arise from the basilar artery. In the remainder, one or, rarely, both arise from the internal carotid, fed by a large posterior communicating artery.

BRAIN STEM AND THALAMIC TERRITORY

The posterior cerebral artery branches that supply the midbrain and adjacent thalamus are considered[89] to follow the general plan of the arteries of the brain stem, in which the vessels are divided into three major groups: paramedian penetrating, short circumferential, and long circumferential arteries.[1] The *thalamoperforant* arteries are the midbrain equivalent of the paramedian penetrating branches encountered lower in the brain stem and of the lenticulostriate arteries of the anterior circle of Willis. The thalamoperforants, measuring between 200 and 400 μm in size, arise from the posterior communicating artery and the proximal portions of the posterior cerebral artery, the most constant being those arising from the posterior cerebral.[143] They are divided into three groups: the first two, the premamillary and the postmammillary, follow an upward curvilinear course into the anterior nuclei of the thalamus, and a third group, which pursues a horizontal course, supplies the cerebral peduncle.[143]

The arteries making up the midbrain-thalamic equivalent of the short circumferential group arise from the posterior cerebral artery as it winds around the stem. Measuring from 320 to 800 μm in diameter and numbering between 8 and 10 branches, these *thalamogeniculate, posterior thalamic,* and *pulvinarian* branches curve upward into the posterior portions of the thalamus, supplying the posterolateral nuclei and the pulvinar. One to three thalamogeniculate branches have been found in individual brains.[113]

The medial and lateral posterior choroidal arteries[59] are the equivalent of the lower brain stem long circumferential group. Both arise from the posterior cerebral artery in the circum-mesencephalic course. The *posterolateral choroidal artery* arises first. It follows the curve of the pulvinar, which

Figure 20.1 Arterial supply to the lateral geniculate body showing the course of the arteries. (From Frisen et al,[57] with permission. From BMJ Publishing Group.)

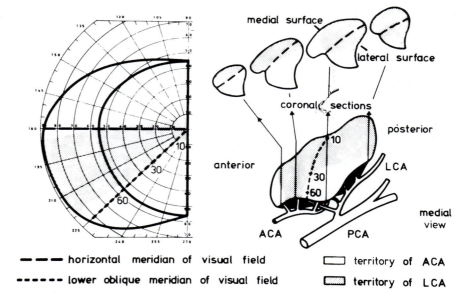

it supplies only superficially, irrigates the optic tract and the lateral geniculate body, and then enters the choroidal fissure to supply the choroid plexus of the lateral ventricle.[119] In the terminal branches, it anastomoses with the anterior choroidal artery. The *posteromedial choroidal artery* arises a few millimeters behind the posterolateral, passing first over the medial and lateral geniculate bodies (Fig. 20.1). This double-humped course gives the vessel the appearance of the number 3 on the angiogram.[143] After entering the choroidal fissure, it supplies the choroid plexus of the third ventricle, and its terminal branches supply the anterior nucleus of the thalamus. The last branch of the arteries supplying the deep territory is the posterior pericallosal or splenial artery.[143] The thalamotuberal artery may rarely take its origin from the middle cerebral artery instead of its more common origination from the posterior communicating artery.[64]

CORTICAL TERRITORY

Although the cortical branches of the posterior cerebral artery are well known, there has been considerable disagreement as to their names. Salamon and Huang[143] label the three major orbital temporal branches the inferior temporal and occipitotemporal arteries, while the vessel supplying the calcarine region is known as the calcarine artery. Kaul et al[81] refer to the former group as the anterior, middle, and posterior temporal arteries. The term parieto-occipital artery describes the branches that supply the calcarine cortex, cuneus, and precuneus (Fig. 20.2).

Whatever their names, three vessels usually supply the entire orbital surface of the temporal and occipital lobes.[101] The anterior inferior temporal and the posterior inferior temporal may arise from a single trunk, separate from the occipitotemporal, or the three may arise from a common trunk. The two anterior arteries supply the entire undersurface (orbital) of the temporal lobe. The undersurface of the occipital lobe,

including the posterior portion of the fusiform and lingual gyri, are supplied by the occipitotemporal branch.

The calcarine artery may be single or double.[81] Although it has been claimed to be the exclusive supply to the visual cortex in the calcarine fissure,[130] the striate area may at times be supplied in part by the occipitotemporal or occipitoparietal arteries.[156] The termination of the supply of the calcarine ar-

Figure 20.2 Anteroposterior view of the posterior cerebral artery territory showing the cerebral surface branches supplying the inferior surface branches, which supply the inferior surface of the temporal lobe and the medial occipital region.

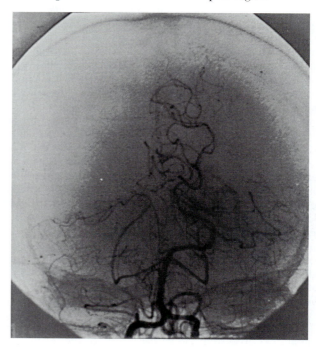

tery and its branches is far posterior along the occipital pole.[102] The supply commonly passes around the edge of the occipital pole and as far forward as 1 cm on the convex surface of the hemisphere, where anastomoses are formed with terminal branches of the middle cerebral artery.

COLLATERALS

The posterior cerebral artery has abundant collaterals with the middle and anterior cerebral arteries.[11] The collaterals occur in the border zone, a narrow (usually 1 mm) strip separating two major arterial territories. Within this zone, anastomoses between end arteries occur freely in a variety of forms, end to end, side to side, and end to side. The actual size of the anastomosing vessels varies considerably, but most are on the order of 300 to 600 μm, only rarely as large as 1 cm. As a result, although a potential collateral exists at any point along a border zone, it is all but impossible to anticipate that a given terminal branch will receive the immediate flow through the border zone it may need to prevent infarction when its territory is suddenly compromised.

The anastomoses with the anterior cerebral usually take place along a narrow border zone of vessels between the precuneus and the parieto-occipital fissure, from the isthmus of the gyrus fornicati inferiorly to the margin of the central sulcus superiorly. Some three to four branches enter the border zone.

With the middle cerebral artery, anastomoses occur from the orbital surface of the anterior tip of the temporal lobe inferolaterally along the margin of the hemisphere as far back as the occipital pole.[148] Between five and eight such branches can be traced into the border zones in most hemispheres.

Pathogenesis

FREQUENCY OF OCCLUSION

Occlusions affecting the posterior cerebral artery or its branches are uncommon compared with involvement of the middle cerebral artery. Reports of frequencies compared with the middle cerebral territory are roughly constant over the decades. Castaigne et al[29] found 22 posterior cerebral arteries occluded in their series of 44 autopsied cases of vertebrobasilar territory occlusions; in only 8 was the posterior cerebral artery occlusion unaccompanied by occlusions in the more proximal vessels. Among 329 cases of infarction reported by Kleihues and Hizawa,[84] the posterior cerebral artery was affected in 35 cases (10.6%). Milandre et al[112] found 82 cases (13.7%) of posterior cerebral artery territory infarction among a nonselected series of 598 cases of cerebral infarction in a stroke registry. Bilateral involvement is rather common, occurring in 13% of the series from Milandre et al,[112] but in 25% of the cases reported by Kleihues and Hizawa.[84]

Table 20.1 Regional Distribution of Infarcts

Infarction	No.
PCA	6
CA	7
PTA	7
ATA	1
POA	2
PTA + ATA	7
CA + POA	6
CA + PTA	10
CA + PTA + ATA	11
CA + PTA + POA	1
CA + PTA + POA + PPA	2

Abbreviations: PCA, posterior cerebral artery; CA, calcarine artery; PTA, posterior temporal artery; ATA, anterior temporal artery; POA, parieto-occipital artery; PPA, posterior pericallosal artery.

(Adapted from Kinkel et al.[83])

TOPOGRAPHY OF INFARCTS

Infarction of the entire deep and superficial territory of the posterior cerebral artery bilaterally must be quite rare. In their 7-year study of infarction documented by computed tomography (CT) scan, Kinkel et al[83] found 6 examples, only one of which was bilateral (Table 20.1). However, posterior cerebral artery territory infarction was an uncommon diagnosis. Only 54 occurred among the 1,050 infarcts (5%). The 6 cases, among only 54 eligible, were fully 11% of the total posterior cerebral artery territory infarcts. Pessin et al[132] found several varieties of infarcts in their series of 35 cases, depending on the mechanism, embolism being the most common (10 cases). Infarction of individual branches, alone or in combination, is the more common. Among the surface branches, the calcarine artery is the most commonly affected.[83] The least commonly affected is the anterior temporal artery, and clinical details in such cases are lacking.

Reports vary as to the frequency of cortical and deep infarction. Six of 38 were diagnosed by Goto et al,[67] but only 2 of 56 by Kinkel and colleagues.[83]

OCCLUSION FROM EMBOLIZATION

Embolism leads all other causes for posterior cerebral artery territory infarction in all series studies.[21,112,120,123,132]

Embolic material may reach the posterior cerebral artery via the vertebral or basilar arteries or internal carotid artery. Uncommonly, the initial presentation of extracranial carotid occlusive disease may be a hemianopia from embolism to the posterior cerebral artery through a fetal origin of the posterior cerebral artery from the internal carotid artery.[133] Compared with other territories, autopsy studies seem to show that a cardiac source for embolism is rare compared with embolic

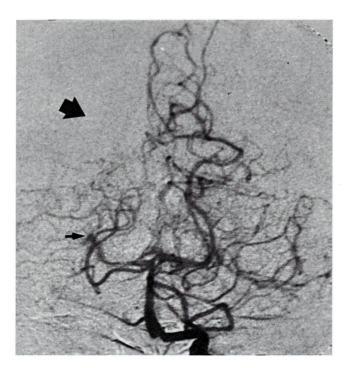

Figure 20.3 Anteroposterior view of a selective left vertebral angiogram. There is occlusion of the ambient segment of the right posterior cerebral artery (*small arrow*). There is no opacification of the terminal branches of this artery (*large arrow*).

material arising from plaques in the vertebrals or the basilar itself: Castaigne et al[29] found 10 atherosclerotic emboli and only 1 from a cardiac cause in their autopsy series.

Emboli up the posterior circulation are often arrested at the top of the basilar,[25] where they may produce bilateral posterior cerebral occlusions, fragment into branches bilaterally, or arrest in one posterior cerebral at any point along its course (Fig. 20.3). Common sites of arrest are the stem of the posterior cerebral where it winds around the brain stem, at the origin of the cortical surface branches, or along the course of the branches serving the occipital lobe. Although embolic occlusions confined to the anterior cortical branches serving the undersurface of the temporal lobe are theoretically possible, no cases were found by the present authors when searching the literature in preparation of this chapter.

Embolic occlusions often produce incomplete infarction of the territory distal to the occluded site. Subcortical infarction, often not obvious on gross inspection of the brain, seems a common finding in many of the case reports.[14,43,92,119,136,174] Complete infarction affecting the gray matter and subcortical white matter to the depths of the ventricular wall is a rather uncommon finding.[22] Patchy infarction is often encountered.[136]

OCCLUSION FROM THROMBOSIS

Atheromatous thrombosis of the posterior cerebral seems rather uncommon.[21,112,123,132] Occlusion in a setting of pre-existing atheromatous stenosis was encountered in only 2 of

22 cases studied by Castaigne et al.[29] In this series, the occlusion was almost always embolic, although the source of the embolus was usually an atherosclerotic lesion more proximally situated in the basilar or vertebral arteries. Posterior cerebral artery stenosis is unusual enough to warrant individual case reports even in current times, given the unusual syndromes such as Benedikt's oculomotor palsy,[51] or reasons to undertake percutaneous transluminal angioplasty.[164]

The atheroma usually affects the posterior cerebral as it winds around the brain stem,[131] at approximately the same sites where embolic material arrest (Fig. 20.4). Thrombus atop pre-existing stenosis is rare.[29] No clinical features specifically distinguish thrombosis from embolic syndromes in which the occlusion is in the proximal posterior cerebral artery stem.

Occlusion may also occur from anterograde extension of thrombus from an occlusion of the upper basilar artery or even from the internal carotid if the posterior communicating artery is patent.[29,86] This mechanism may account for as many

Figure 20.4 Anteroposterior view of a selective left vertebral angiogram with simultaneous compression of the left carotid artery. There is a high-grade stenosis (*arrow*) in the proximal left posterior cerebral artery just distal to its junction with the left posterior communicating artery. Compression of the left carotid artery eliminated the possibility of flow artifact created by nonopacified blood from the anterior circulation. (From Pessin,[131] with permission.)

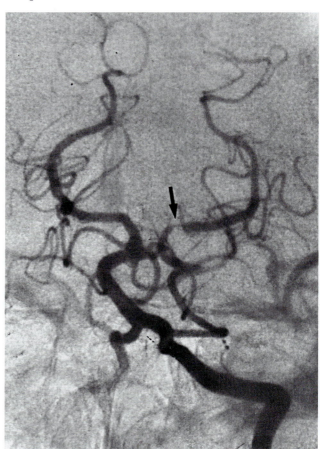

as half the instances of bilateral posterior cerebral artery occlusion.

Reference is often made to the possibility that the occipital lobes may suffer ischemia as a distal field effect from occlusion of the vertebral arteries bilaterally or the basilar itself.[23,108,140,162] Evidence to support this notion is improving, but most of the autopsy material suggests that embolism is the cause.[29]

Few studies have been made of stenosis of the posterior cerebral stem.[21,51,123,131] Duncan and Weidling's[51] patient had diplopia, ipsilateral ptosis, and contralateral hemiataxia, the syndrome reported as a mixture of Benedikt syndrome with pupil-sparing oculomotor palsy. Pessin et al[131] found six examples in a 7-year period. From this slender data base they found that five had had transient ischemic attacks (TIAs) as the major presenting complaint, and two had homonymous visual field defects. The TIAs were predominantly visual disturbances in the contralateral half field, or sensory complaints in the form of paresthesias involving the arm and hand, or occasionally the face and leg. Three patients had visual and sensory spells together. During a period of follow-up ranging from 4 months to 4 years, no patient had a new stroke in the posterior cerebral artery territory, and only one continued to have TIAs.

Syndromes of Infarction

INFARCTION AFFECTING THE BRAIN STEM AND THALAMUS

Brain stem infarction attributable to occlusion of the posterior cerebral arises incidental to a large occlusion affecting the top of the basilar, from local stenosis or thrombus confined to the stem of the posterior cerebral, or from an isolated occlusion of the many penetrating branches of the posterior cerebral itself.

Bilateral Infarcts Affecting the Midbrain and Thalamus

Occlusions affecting the top of the basilar artery are discussed in detail in Chapter 18. In this section, the discussion is confined to those syndromes in which the posterior cerebral is affected as part of the basilar occlusion.

Among the 28 cases of paramedian midbrain and thalamic infarction, Castaigne et al[30] described 4 from pathologically proven occlusion of the posterior cerebral artery: 2 of these had an extension of an occlusion of the upper portion of the basilar or the portion of the posterior cerebral artery between the basilar and the junction with the posterior communicating artery. Atherosclerotic thrombus explained 1 and cardiac embolism 2, but no satisfactory explanation was found for the other. In all 4 the infarct affected the red nucleus and the intralamellary, parafascicular, central, and median nuclei of the thalamus. The clinical picture was dominated by profound deficits in all 4 cases: obtundation, stupor or coma, disturbance

in memory, hemiplegia, varying degrees of hemihypesthesia, and isolated instances of hemianopia or partial third nerve paresis.

Sieben et al[153] described two patients with unilateral thalamopeduncular infarction from occlusion of the posterior cerebral stem between the basilar and the junction of the posterior communicating artery. Hemiparesis occurred in both; somnolence, Horner syndrome, and hemianopia in one; and third nerve paresis with dysarthria in the other.

The literature is also scanty for cases documented only by angiogram or CT scan.[171] Gacs et al[58] described a 60-year-old man with atrial fibrillation who presented with a right third nerve palsy, left hemiparesis, left-sided loss of pain sensation, and left upper quadrant field defect. The CT scan showed a low-density area affecting the posterior cerebral artery territory with enhancement in the right occipital lobe, medial temporal lobe, and thalamus corresponding to the distribution of the right posterior cerebral artery. The motor function improved, but the partial third nerve paresis, diminished pain sensation, and upper quadrant field defect did not change. CT scan showed a high-density area on noncontrast that was considered to reflect occlusion of the posterior cerebral artery stem.

From the limited literature available, it is apparent that occlusion of the posterior cerebral stem between the basilar and the junction with the posterior communicating artery is sufficient to precipitate a hemiparesis from peduncular infarct, ocular motility disorder from deeper infarction of the midbrain, and complex disturbances in consciousness, memory, and even language for those whose infarct penetrates deeper into medial thalamic structures. In some cases, hypersexuality and changes in appetite occur as well.

Unilateral Occlusion of the Posterior Cerebral Stem

Reference has been made above to syndromes from stenosis. For occlusion, a few instances have been reported of unilateral occlusion of the posterior cerebral artery stem, which caused syndromes mimicking those of middle cerebral artery territory infarction (Fig. 20.5). Involvement of both the deep and superficial territory of the posterior cerebral artery (right side) has produced not only contralateral plegia, hemisensory syndrome, hemianopia, and behavioral effects, but also a Horner syndrome and contralateral hyperhydrosis; these last two are explained by involvement of the thalamus and hypothalamus.[9] Brandt et al,[21] Caplan et al,[26] Chambers et al,[33] and Hommel et al[78] have described small case series with occlusion of the proximal posterior cerebral artery. The clinical syndromes affecting the midbrain and cortical territories combined have mimicked many of the elements of middle cerebral artery occlusion, including contralateral hemiparesis, homonymous hemianopia, hemispatial neglect, and sensory loss or sensory inattention. For many patients whose infarction involved the dominant hemisphere, aphasia has been present as well. Brain imaging (CT or magnetic resonance imaging [MRI]) has been needed for accurate diagnosis, suggesting that the specific clinical features do not distinguish the syndromes clearly. Similar frustrations have been recently reported from attempts

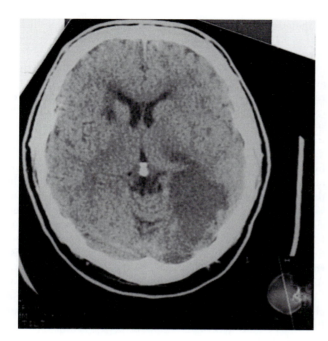

Figure 20.5 Deep thalamic and occipital infarction from occlusion of the posterior cerebral artery in a patient with severe sensory loss and dense hemianopia.

to characterize patients clinically in the hyperacute stage of ischemic stroke.[7]

SENSORY SYNDROMES

Hypesthesia

Hypesthesia or anesthesia might be an expected consequence of posterior cerebral artery occlusion near the stem, since the vascular supply to the ventral tier nuclei of the thalamus is in the territory of its penetrating branches.[153] Most of the literature on this subject is discussed in more detail in the chapter on lacunes in the section on pure sensory stroke (see Ch. 23). The subject of sensory loss has received only passing mention in most of the reviews but has been described in detail in a few case reports. Remarks such as sensorimotor deficit, hypesthesia, and even "considerable anesthesia"[174] are commonly encountered, but not given further elaboration. Rarely, the syndrome may be mentioned as having begun in one part or having been confined to one body part. One of Wyllie's[174] patients with a large autopsy-documented dominant hemisphere occipital infarction but no lesions described in the thalamus (by gross inspection) complained that ". . . the whole right side of the body [felt] cold and heavy . . . the difference of sensation in the two sides being so marked he felt as if a plumb line down the middle of the head and trunk had divided him into two halves."

Among the individual posterior cerebral artery territory branches, the supply to the ventral tier nuclei of the thalamus comes most regularly from the thalamogeniculate branch of the posteromedial choroidal artery (Fig. 20.6). On its course to the thalamus, it passes through the lateral geniculate nucleus. Cases of occlusion of this artery seem uncommon. Frisen et al[57] speculated that its occlusion could produce not only a hemianopia from involvement of the lateral geniculate body, but hemiparesis and hemihypesthesia from involvement of the ventral tier nuclei of the thalamus, although they did not report such a syndrome in their two patients. The only case studied by the present senior author had normal motor function and no abnormality of sensation.[119]

Dejerine-Roussy Syndrome

Despite these negative cases, occlusion of the thalamogeniculate branch of the posteromedial choroidal artery was the source of the thalamic pain syndrome of Dejerine and Roussy,[44] who reviewed the literature up to 1906 showing that its occlusion produced a syndrome of rapidly improving hemiparesis with choreic movements and ataxia, persisting hypesthesia, and severe paroxysmal pain in the hypesthetic side. Their pathologic correlation has been reconfirmed by others over the years[68] and (rarely) by CT scan. The most recent case uncovered by the current authors was reported by Hayman et al[72]; clinical details were limited to the remark that the "patient had Dejerine-Roussy (thalamic) syndrome of altered sensation." Two of the patients reported by Ghika et al[63] with dystonic hands were said to have presented with the Dejerine-Roussy syndrome.

The sensory disturbance in these cases has many features.[100] There is usually some degree of hypesthesia, although rarely sensation may eventually be normal. Dysesthesia, feeling of excessive heaviness, and a disagreeable sensation of coldness are common. Either at the onset or after a period of up to several months, the unusual pain syndrome may appear. This hyperpathia may be spontaneous or precipitated by stimuli, constant or paroxysmal, temporary or permanent. The pain varies from tingling and aching to intense unbearable discomfort. The site stimulated often feels normal at first, but after a brief delay the pain begins and spreads over larger areas, at times increasing steadily in intensity, usually far outlasting the duration of the original stimulus. Once established, such cases may become permanent.

More often, the disorders occur in partial form. Complaints of dysesthesia such as tingling receive frequent mention.[43] The patient described by Caplan and Hedley-Whyte[27] had totally anesthetic right limbs but when pinched firmly experienced a "weak tingling sensation." Geschwind and Fusillo[62] detailed the clinical features of a patient with right hemianopia, alexia, color anomia, and transient memory disturbance due to a large left posterior cerebral territory infarction. He experienced ". . . vague pains over the right side of the body, especially the thorax, which were diffuse and difficult to characterize. They were increased by repetitive sensory stimulation. [They] were repeatedly complained of, [but they] never became agonizing." The serial section autopsy study showed an infarct in the ventral posterolateral nucleus of the thalamus.

No treatment has been devised. Amitriptyline or L-dopamine has been recommended.

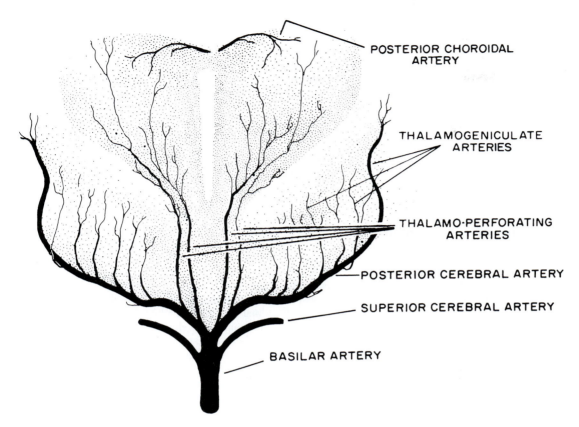

Figure 20.6 Thalamus with the usual arterial distribution. Note the multiple thalamogeniculate arteries.

MOTOR SYNDROMES

Although not expected from classical descriptions, hemiparesis, even hemiplegia, is increasingly recognized as a part of the posterior cerebral artery syndrome.[7,20,21] The clinical features seem identical to those from capsular or middle cerebral artery territory infarction. Instances have been described of a motor syndrome involving abnormal tone and coordination, described as a "jerky dystonic unsteady hand" (three cases attributed to occlusion of the posterior choroidal arteries)[63] or "hyperkinesie volitionnelle."[53] Delayed dystonia has also been described (see also Ch. 23, on lacunes).[90]

Most of the reports have been described as part of the syndrome expected from occlusion of the posterior cerebral stem, affecting the upper brain stem.[123] Some authors have speculated that the posterior portion of the internal capsule could be made ischemic from vessels supplying the medial edges of the thalamus bordering on the capsule.[21,118,124]

VISUAL FIELDS

The lower portions of the visual radiations, throughout their entire course, lie in the territory of the posterior cerebral artery. Most of the upper portion is supplied by branches of the middle cerebral artery, especially the angular and posterior temporal branches. Disruption of the pathway may occur from infarction involving the lateral geniculate body, the radiations along their course in the temporal lobe, or at the calcarine cortex itself.

Bilateral Infarction

The best described bilateral infarctions are the visual field disturbances from infarctions involving the calcarine cortex in one or both territories of the posterior cerebral artery.

COMPLETE INFARCTION. Complete destruction of the entire territory of supply of the cerebral branches of the posterior cerebral artery bilaterally has been reported infrequently and only occasionally have the clinical effects been reviewed in detail.[55,65,84,157,162]

The remarkable patient studied by Brindley and Janota[22] typifies the striking syndrome in massive infarction. Virtually complete infarction of the territories of both posterior cerebral arteries was found at autopsy. Severe stenosis (described as pinhole) was present in both posterior cerebral stems. The infarcts extended bilaterally along the entire undersurface of the temporal and occipital lobes. In the inferior temporal region, the hippocampus, parahippocampal gyrus, and inferior temporal gyrus were destroyed. The medial surface of the occipital lobes was affected including both fusiform gyri, lingual gyrus and cunei, and banks of each calcarine cortex; the infarction affected the posterior portions of the corpus callosum and the pillars of the fornix, and extended as high as the parieto-occipital fissure. Both occipital poles were spared. Throughout the remainder of her life after the stroke, the patient remained blind. She had no response to opticokinetic nystagmus and no visual evoked potentials. She was unable to distinguish steady darkness from steady light, nor could she detect a light moving in front of her. However, she consistently distinguished sudden darkening of a lighted room and sudden lighting of a darkened room.

Electrophysiologic studies of a similar case[32] revealed preservation of visual evoked potentials to pattern stimulation despite a complete lack of vision on testing by clinical methods: the patient was unable to detect a strong light flashed either directly at her face or moved in a vertical, horizontal, or diagonal direction. She vigorously denied visual loss and claimed an ability to see well. In contrast to the patient described above, this patient could not distinguish sudden darkening from sudden lightening in a room. CT scan showed a huge bilateral posterior cerebral territory infarction. More often, the visual evoked responses have been attenuated or absent.

The patient of Goldenberg[65] imaged by MRI showing all but complete bilateral destruction of the calcarine regions denied blindness but was able to describe by recall the shapes of letters and colors typical of certain objects named by the examiners. This last case addresses the issue of whether preservation of the primary visual cortex is necessary to generate conversationally tested recall of images.

Examples in the literature[16] and personal experience suggest that these huge infarcts can be expected to be associated with severe amnestic states, amnestic aphasia, amnestic color dysnomia, topographic disorientation, and implicit unawareness of the extent of the deficit and perhaps even its existence. This last point suggests that the preservation or loss of awareness of the visual loss is of little value in differentiating middle from posterior cerebral territory infarction.[25]

INCOMPLETE BILATERAL INFARCTION. Incomplete bilateral posterior cerebral artery territory infarction produces a remarkable variety of syndromes.[21,112] Such cases have been the basis for the understanding of the projections of the visual fields on the calcarine cortex, the upper radiations in the upper banks, the lower in the lower banks, and the macula at the pole end. Some have begun as complete blindness only to evolve within hours or days to less striking deficits.[108] During the time of complete blindness, the victim commonly volunteers no complaints and is unaware of the deficit.[65] Descriptions of a few of the autopsy cases suffice to indicate an extremely strong correlation between the visual fields and the surviving calcarine cortex. In a series of 25 patients,[18] detection of movement of objects in visual space was present sufficient for localization, but no discrimination of size or shape was noted. Tests were done in the blind areas that possibly proved some extracalcarine vision.

Superficial infarction may involve almost the whole of the calcarine cortex, but if it spares the occipital pole and the subcortical visual radiations, visual function for complex activities such as reading may be spared even if only a tiny portion of the central field remains.[55,110,140,162] Holmes[77] described a case with a narrow wedge of preserved vision extending from the fixation points upward on either side of the vertical meridian, with its apex at the fixation point and its base at the periphery. Serial sections of the autopsy specimen showed total cal-

carine infarction except for a small region, nearly symmetric bilaterally, extending along the inferior lip of the striate cortex from the anterior end to the pole.

Bilateral altitudinal hemianopia is an expected consequence of incomplete occipital infarction but has been reported in detail in only a few cases. The loss of vision is presumed to be from infarction but whether from embolism or otherwise has not been established. The onset in several cases has been preceded by hallucinations of lights, prismatic or geometric forms, and other phenomena suggestive of migrainous scintillations. After the hemianopias have developed, associated visual disturbances have included color dysnomias, difficulties with visual form discrimination, spatial disorientation, and disordered visual search behavior of the type encountered in Balint syndrome. However, others have had little such disturbance,[136] and one of the present author's personal cases, a construction foreman, was annoyed most by his inferior altitudinal hemianopia because it prevented his easy scanning of blueprints and his difficulty in reaching for the floor-mounted gear shift in his pickup truck while driving. Only a handful of autopsy-documented cases have been published, all suffering inferior altitudinal hemianopia.[76,136,162] In each case, however, the superior quadrants were slightly affected as well. Autopsy studies showed foci of infarction scattered through the calcarine cortex with varying degrees of subcortical involvement. The visual field disturbances seemed more homogeneous than was indicated by the discontinuous foci of infarction. Two remarkably homogeneous cases of altitudinal hemianopia were documented by CT scan,[127] one with superior and the other with inferior visual field defects. Neither patient showed a visual field defect that crossed the horizontal meridian as did those documented by autopsy. No angiographic data were provided.

For most of the cases with cortical blindness with bilateral infarction, the deficits are described as persisting and unchanging.[22] However, scattered reports and personal experience indicate that some cases of bilateral cortical blindness may undergo considerable remission of the deficit. Presumably, the infarction is incomplete and the acute syndrome is misleading in its failure to predict the subsequent improvement. Although Bergman[16] addressed the issue of remission in 12 examples of cortical blindness, in only 1 of the 5 due to infarction was any improvement noted. Vision recurred within a month but was confined to the macular region, suggesting sparing of the radiations and the occipital pole. The description of the autopsy specimen does not settle this point.

Clinical events that herald cortical blindness are not often reported. A scattering of cases began with a unilateral hemianopia that was followed by cortical blindness. Bogousslavsky et al[19] followed 58 patients with unilateral infarction in the superficial area supplied by the posterior cerebral artery for a period of up to 39 months. Thirteen of these cases experienced cortical blindness associated with a delayed contralateral occipital infarction. The authors noted that the lack of visual field improvement most accurately predicated a high risk of cortical blindness.

Unilateral Infarction

TEMPORAL CRESCENT SPARING. Preservation of the temporal crescent has been described in a few instances of unilateral infarction with sparing of the anterior end of the inferior lip of the calcarine cortex.[15] More cases need to be reported to understand better the topography of these peripheries of the visual fields.

MACULAR SPARING. Macular sparing is frequently encountered in unilateral (and also in bilateral) infarction of the posterior cerebral artery territory. The most common explanation is that the collateral flow available from the middle cerebral artery territory spares the pole. For macular vision to remain, the infarct must remain superficial enough to spare the visual radiations; when they are involved, anatomic integrity of the occipital pole does not suffice to preserve central vision.[22] Infarcts limited to the middle fields of supply of the posterior cerebral artery involve the anterior portions of the calcarine cortex and lingual gyrus.[11,81,84] The most frequent finding in such instances is a homonymous hemianopia with the most consistent deficit in the area adjacent to the horizontal meridian.[81] What remains unclear is how stable the persisting visual field deficit is. The regions covered by the infarct may have an extremely sharp correlation with the visual field in the chronic state: the autopsy of a well-known pathologist, whose visual field defect showed a small upper quadrantanopia occupying 10 degrees of the vertical and 20 degrees of the horizontal meridians, showed an extremely circumscribed infarct involving the inferior lip of the calcarine fissure almost at the occipital pole; the infarct spread anterolaterally in a broader band, undercutting the lingual gyrus but sparing the radiation[136] (Fig. 20.7). This case is of great interest because of the long period he was under observation and his claims that his vision "cleared up" (see below).

INFARCTION IN THE VISUAL RADIATIONS. Infarctions confined to the visual radiations have been reported rarely. In contrast to middle cerebral artery territory disease, infarctions of the posterior cerebral artery territory have often been reported in which the subcortical component was more evident than was the infarction involving the cortical surface.[14,119,162] However, in most instances, the damage found subcortically affected the white matter of the lingual or fusiform gyrus, often sparing the visual radiations, which pass deeper and are adjacent to the ventricular wall. Infarcts in this deep territory are rare unless they are the result of a full-thickness infarct, one that forms a schizencephalic cleft extending from the pial surface of the cortex all the way to the ependyma of the ventricle.

AWARENESS OF THE VISUAL FIELD DEFICIT. Despite the frequent assumption that implicit unawareness of the visual field deficit should be a property of extensive bilateral infarction, unilateral infarcts have also been reported with such deficits; in the small case series available, no distinct difference in frequency has been found for the right versus the left hemisphere.[112]

LATERAL GENICULATE INFARCTS. Reports of lateral geniculate infarcts make up but a small fraction of the literature[57,98,114,119] (Fig. 20.1). The anterior choroidal artery supplies the anterior hilum and the anterior and lateral aspects of the nucleus. The posterior choroidal artery supplies the remainder, including the crown. The two sources of supply do not anastomose before or in the nucleus and appear to be end arteries with no collaterals. The visual field is represented in three parts in the nucleus: the anteromedial, which subserves inferior quadrant vision; the crown, serving macular vision; and the lateral, which serves upper quadrantic vision. The only pathologically documented infarcts produced a congruous, complete upper quadrantanopsia involving the mac-

ula, with a few degrees of involvement of the upper portion of the lower quadrant.[99,119] From brain imaging, cases of inferred infarcts of the lateral geniculate have shown wedge-shaped homonymous hemianopia, congruent upper quadrantanopia, and a quadruple sector anopia (one case).[98] Upper and lower homonymous sector anopias have also been reported following ligation of the anterior choroidal artery but was documented only by CT scanning.[56,57]

Although such attention to detail might seem excessive, the occlusion of the posterior choroidal artery yields a rather unusual syndrome: the artery supplies the lateral geniculate body, the fornix, the dorsomedial nucleus, and the posterior pulvinar. Infarction of these structures in one autopsied case studied by serial sections caused hemianopia, hemidysesthesia, and disturbance of memory[119]; in some cases reported by brain imaging, such infarction caused homonymous quadrantanopia, with or without sensory disturbances, and a variety of behavioral disturbances characterized as memory disturbance and "transcortical aphasia."[121] That so complex a syndrome can arise from an occlusion very difficult to visualize by angiography and almost as difficult to document by the best CT and MRI scanners keeps this diagnosis at the forefront of clinical concerns.

INFARCTION IN INDIVIDUAL POSTERIOR CEREBRAL ARTERY BRANCHES. Infarction in the territory of individual branches of the posterior cerebral artery other than the calcarine artery has not been found to display a reliable correlation between the severity and type of visual field deficit.[81] CT correlations, by contrast, have been more reliable.[104]

CLINICAL COURSE OF VISUAL FIELD ABNORMALITIES. The clinical course of unilateral partial or complete hemianopia has received little attention. It has been assumed that, like bilateral large infarctions, visual field deficit from unilateral infarctions should also be permanent. However, a few remarkable cases raise the possibility that the initial visual field deficit may undergo gradual shrinkage and that the size of the infarct at autopsy may exceed that predicted by the final, shrunken visual field deficit.[136] The famous pathologist referred to above initially experienced a large visual field defect that later "cleared up."[136] The clinical course was not better characterized historically. As late as 1 year after the onset, he was examined by an ophthalmologist who described a large hemianopic scotoma in the left upper fields "too far from the macula to cause him any disturbances in microscopic work." Twenty-four years later his formal visual fields were plotted by a tangent screen and showed only a dense but highly circumscribed upper quadrantanopsia confined to the macular region some 20 degrees in the horizontal and 10 degrees in the vertical plane (Fig. 20.7). No comments were made on the disparity between the patient's comment that his vision had cleared up and the persisting visual field deficit. At autopsy, years later, the only site of infarction affecting the calcarine cortex was a small wedge of the lower bank near the pole. However, a larger area of infarction had undermined much of the lingual gyrus and adjacent inferior bank of the calcarine cortex, within which the cellular elements were much reduced in number (Fig. 20.6). The findings were interpreted by Polyak[136] as indicating that the surviving cells sufficed to permit the initial visual field defect to undergo functional resolution, a speculation that appears not to have been challenged in his (Polyak's) lifetime.

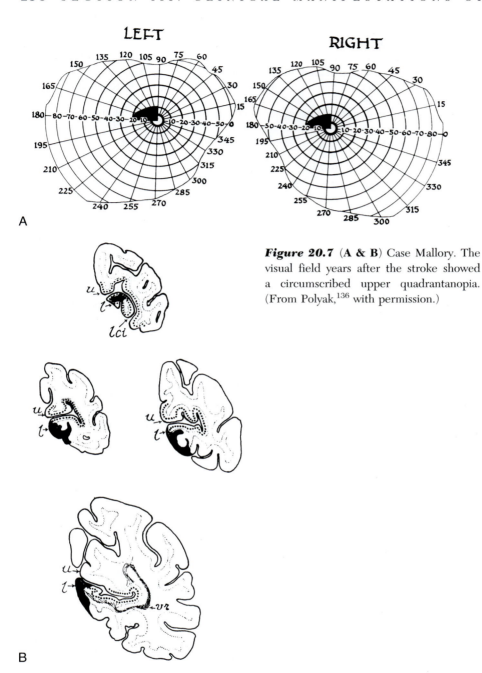

Figure 20.7 (**A & B**) Case Mallory. The visual field years after the stroke showed a circumscribed upper quadrantanopia. (From Polyak,[136] with permission.)

KLÜVER-BUCY SYNDROME

Klüver-Bucy syndrome is described here since its cause is usually bilateral lesions. In the tiny number of cases reported from infarction, some not using this eponym,[160] the lesions have been very large, affecting most of the undersurface of the temporal lobes,[36,79,94,96,106,150] including the fusiform and lingual gyri, hippocampal gyri, and the medial hippocampal structures. In addition to the fearless exploration of environment, the syndromes precipitated by these infarctions frequently include a prominent state of exaggerated motor activity; restlessness, agitation, delirium, crying out, and unwonted excessive reaction to visual, auditory, or cutaneous stimuli may be the most striking features noted in the acute phase.[107] Within hours to days, these states usually subside.

VISUAL AGNOSIA

Extensive bilateral occipital infarction is the usual cause of visual agnosia, a rare disorder. Most of the few cases described occurred in a setting of cardiac arrest. Few have been described from bilateral posterior cerebral artery territory infarction.

A great deal of effort has been expended in asserting[97,142] or denying[10,13,73] that such syndromes exist. Those opposed to the notion argue that the deficits are a combination of a "primary" visual field defect, a secondary perceptual disorder, and some degree of dementia. Those in support of the notion[4,14,108,142] admit that few cases have been fully described but that in those the strict criteria have been met: intact primary visual function and no language disturbance. Two forms are said to exist: an apperceptive, caused by ". . . interference with the processing of primary visual sensory data"[142]; and an associative, ". . . caused by disorders affecting associative cortex where visual percepts were matched with previously processed sensory data for recognition."[142] There are important but seemingly minor differences in the formulae of the deficits.[3] Because no standard method of examining these rare cases has yet been developed, it remains uncertain how many of the differences reflect variations in the syndrome caused by minor differences in lesion site and size, and how many represent nothing more than differences in the approach to testing the individual patients. Included in this notion is whether an "agnosia," or what has labeled an optic aphasia, can be said to exist.[103] The small number of cases from vascular cause show essentially the same syndrome.

Bilateral Posterior Cerebral Artery Territory Infarction

The case reported by Rubens and Benson[142] was later the subject of an autopsy report.[14] The visual agnosia was accompanied by right hemianopia, dyslexia with preserved ability to write, color "agnosia," "impaired verbal learning," and prosopagnosia. The visual agnosia was demonstrated by the patient's ability to produce approximate drawn copies of the picture stimuli he was unable to name or point to after hearing the item named by the examiner. By comparison, he was able to name the same object immediately by palpation or when its characteristic sound was heard. At autopsy, the left posterior cerebral was found to be firmly occluded from its junction with the posterior communicating artery to its first temporal branch. On cut section, a predominantly subcortical infarct was found that undermined the left parahippocampal gyrus, undermined the entire lingual gyrus, and reached the surface at its distal end. A smaller subcortical infarct undermined most of the right lingual gyrus. The authors speculated that the combination of lesions prevented visual stimuli discriminated by the right hemisphere from arousing associations in the left, analogous to the dyslexia and color associative defect also found.

A similar case of the associative type was reported by Albert et al,[4] with later autopsy[5]; this patient's deficit was somewhat more circumscribed. Although able to read aloud, describe pictures, copy by drawing, and match words heard to pictures seen, he had difficulty naming pictures shown to him. He was initially blind but regained some sight within 2 days. By day 8, he showed a right upper quadrantal field defect. The lesion was documented by radionuclide scan with increased uptake in both occipital regions. In a later publication, the results of gross cut sections were reported.[5] On the right side, an infarct was found over the entire parahippocampal and lingual gyrus; on the left, a similar infarct affected the parahippocampal gyrus and another affected part of the lingual and fusiform gyrus. A small infarct was found in the left pulvinar.

One patient reported by Cambier et al[24] had bilateral infarctions, quite large on the right, but the infarct affecting the left side was confined to the fusiform gyrus. Hemianopia was confined to the left side. He had alexia without agraphia, but no ". . . agnosia for colors."

Another variant of the bidirectional disconnection was described in a case studied only by CT scan.[8] Although objects could be matched at sight with one another, naming was deficient and so was the praxic gesture characteristically associated with the use of the object. The authors added the term visual apraxia to the list.

Unilateral Left Posterior Cerebral Artery Territory Infarction

No autopsy cases have been uncovered by the authors, but two cases documented by CT scan have been reported. In the first, a large hemorrhagic infarction was shown by CT scan. The syndrome featured a right homonymous hemianopia, right visual spatial hemineglect, difficulty naming visual stimuli, and alexia with spared writing.[134] The patient was able to copy by drawing; when presented with a picture of an object, he could select the exact picture among six choices or even another pictured item having some functional relationship to the original picture (i.e., another view of the same object). However, he had great difficulty showing the use of an object pictured and also grouping objects together by their functional class. The authors noted that the deficits were not explainable as a bidirectional disconnection but indicated a disorder in the appreciation of the significance or functional value of the stimulus, as might be implied by the original use of the term visual agnosia. They expressed the opinion that these disturbances would not be encountered in right hemispheral infarcts.

The second patient, a 60-year-old right-handed man, had a large left posterior cerebral artery infarct with right homonymous hemianopia said to spare the macula; he had difficulty reading, naming colors, and naming "common objects," with no prosopagnosia (see below) and no aphasia. The basis for the diagnosis of associative visual agnosia seems to have been his difficulty in pointing to visually displayed choices from dictated command.

PROSOPAGNOSIA

This intriguing syndrome may be but a component of the larger problem currently labeled visual agnosia. Prosopagnosia is said to be present when the sufferer fails to name other individuals at sight. In the published literature on the subject, reviewed by Damasio et al,[41] this special deficit has always been associated with unilateral or bilateral visual field defects; dyslexia or color dysnomia is usually also present, and in a few instances, more striking disturbances of visual neglect or the Balint syndrome are present. The patient reported on by Cambier et al[24] (with a large right occipital infarct and a small one on the left limited to the fusiform gyrus) had no trouble with colors. These authors argued for a bilateral mesial occipital lesion in such cases, affecting the inferior visual radiations, and not necessarily caused by large infarcts. They marshaled evidence against the traditional claims that prosopagnosia was a sign of right hemisphere dysfunction.[14,173] Their findings also indicated that the larger of the bilateral lesions could be on the left, not the right, side.

The patient of Landis et al[87] was of importance because she died in the acute phase (after 10 days) and was found to have a large unilateral right occipitotemporal infarct, indicating that unilateral involvement is sufficient for the syndrome to occur. Enough cases have been reported with unilateral right-sided lesion[28,163] to raise the question of whether this syndrome is a feature of the nondominant hemisphere syndrome. The condition does not appear to be confined to difficulty with faces, as many other classes of visual stimuli may be similarly affected. Yet, the syndrome may occur without obvious disturbance in naming other classes of visual stimuli.

PALINOPSIA

Like prosopagnosia, palinopsia has been regarded as a bit of a curiosity, and is not commonly a result of vascular disease.[111] The syndrome is usually encountered when the patient has an impaired visual field but is not entirely blind.[12] Many authors have grouped together the two variants and their frequently associated experiences.[105] In one form, there is a persistence of some or all of a visual image immediately after it has disappeared from the environment. In the other, the image reappears only some time later and persists for varying periods. This last group is quite striking, as the delay between the disappearance of the original stimulus and its reappearance may be hours or days, and the image may persist into the following day. A peculiar feature of the palinopic images is their tendency to be incorporated in the appropriate position into visual stimuli in the present environment, such as a cigar and beard appearing on the faces of the all the people at a party. Frank hallucinations and illusions of visual movement are common accompaniments of both types.[38]

A few reports have appeared on cases of vascular cause, however. Meadows and Munro[105] described three patients with palinopsia, one of whom was autopsied. This patient experienced a severe headache lasting only a few hours and then suffered palinopic images beginning the next day and recurring for the remaining 7 days of her life unaccompanied by any other obvious complaints. A congruous, left upper quadrantanopsia was documented. The autopsy showed a predominantly subcortical infarct undermining the right lingual and fusiform gyri, which seemed to be at least several months old. Michel and Troost,[111] using CT scan only, studied three patients whose palinopic images also occurred in the affected visual field following presumed unilateral occipital infarction, two affecting the right side and one the left. The lesions were all large.

Whether the palinopic effect represents a form of seizure remains unknown, although it remains common practice to treat such patients with anticonvulsants.

MICROPSIA

Micropsia, an unusual complaint in which objects appear smaller than expected, is infrequently reported and rarely described with posterior cerebral artery territory infarction. The example from Yamada et al[175] was a 63-year-old man whose complaint occurred suddenly and was associated with an acute amnestic state (as expected from large posterior cerebral artery territory infarction), but his visual field disturbance was limited to a right upper quadrantanopsia. CT scan and MRI showed an infarct in the left occipital lobe and hippocampus. All the clinical features improved within a month, save for the persistence of the quadrantanopsia. A patient with a migraine history and postmortem right cerebral infarction has also been reported.[35] The infarct was found in the inferolateral occipital region near the inferred border zone shared by the middle and posterior cerebral arteries. The syndrome started as left homonymous hemianopia with prominent prosopagnosia. As these complaints faded over a week's time, he noted that objects seemed somewhat shrunken and compressed in the left visual field, making the plotting of visual fields difficult and producing an awareness that pictures seemed asymmetric. He drew the left-hand side of a pattern larger than the right so it would seem symmetric to him. Autopsy was performed 27 months later with no intervening clinical information.

TOPOGRAPHIC DISORIENTATION

An infrequently described syndrome features a striking inability of patients to find their way around.[71] In most instances, there has been infarction in the right hemisphere and left hemianopia, occasionally a disorder in recognition of faces, and other signs of involvement of the nondominant hemisphere. Topographic syndrome may occur in isolation: in one case studied by the senior author, no other disturbance was discovered despite intense testing. Although suffering a spatial disorientation so severe that he could not find the bathroom in the apartment he had lived in for more than 40 years, he successfully conducted a high-level law practice, with no errors in language, memory, or judgment noted by any of his many colleagues.

DISORDERS OF READING

Ischemic lesions in the territory of the posterior cerebral artery produce a variety of disorders labeled alexia or dyslexia. These syndromes have proved of interest for the opportunity they provide to test mechanisms of cerebral function as well as for the different forms of disturbance encountered. Several distinctive disorders have been encountered. At the present time, all of them are casually classified as alexia or dyslexia, yet the nature of the disorder and the extent of the underlying lesions differ enough that they each deserve a different descriptive term. Unfortunately, no such terms have yet come into common use.

Pure Alexia

Major infarction in the posterior cerebral artery territory of the hemisphere dominant for speech and language may precipitate the striking disorder of pure or absolute alexia, usually the left hemisphere, but reported in the right in some instances.[135] The lexical stimuli are treated as though they are the text of an unfamiliar language. The patient usually rejects truly novel lexical stimuli such as the alphabet of a foreign language sharing no characters in common (like Arabic compared with English), but does not distinguish between languages sharing the same characters as his own (i.e., English and Italian). It makes little difference whether the letters and words are presented in typed, printed, or handwritten form; even the patient's own handwriting is not read successfully. Some words ordinarily presented in a distinctive form (e.g., the script form in which the word Coca-Cola appears in advertisements) may be read aloud easily, but the meaning of the words is derived from the unique shape of the stimuli, not from the letters themselves. This point may be demonstrated by presenting other letters in the same general configuration. When tested, some patients show that the letters can be named when the hand is passively traced over the shapes, which indicates the patient's problem is with the visual forms. Spelling aloud and naming words heard in spelled form are usually spared. In some of the cases, single letters may be read aloud and for comprehension. Characteristically, when presented with lexical stimuli, the patient names them with little hesitation and often displays little awareness his responses are well off the mark. For example, Wyllie's[174] patient III (Fig. 20.8) named the word "Dugald" as a series of single letters "k-a-n-i-o-i," similarly responded to the digit set "123456" as "i-r-e-i-u-e," and even named the mathematical symbols "+ × =" as "n-e-a." Musical notes and digits are classifiable separate from letters, but the items themselves do not convey meaning. The best known example of this effect was described by Dejerine and Vialet[45] in their report of the first patient with absolute alexia; the patient was an accomplished musician, but after his stroke he lost the power to read musical scores, although he retained the ability to play and sing from memory.

This clinical picture has been described in several striking cases and is often accompanied by many other disorders.[47] In some, the alexia has been accompanied by a dense right homonymous hemianopia and also by color dysnomia, amnestic aphasia, and memory disturbance indicative of a major left posterior cerebral artery territory infarction.[27,40,62] In other cases, the deficits accompanying the alexia have been less spectacular.[40] Color dysnomia, in particular, occurs with the larger lesions[40,80,119] and may be absent in some cases.[169] (Fig. 20.9).

The *neuropathology* of this condition has been subject to many interpretations.[40,54,62,69,119,167] In Dejerine's[43] frequently discussed case, the lesion, an old infarct, had damaged the inferior edge of the posterior portion of the corpus callosum, as well as the cortex of the cuneus and adjacent calcarine region, and had completely penetrated the underlying white matter to the wall of the ventricle. Although Dejerine's[43] patient is commonly considered to have had hemianopia, the right visual field function was intact enough that Landolt's[88] original examination demonstrated only a hemiachromatopsia (see section on color); the patient had full, if dim vision in the right visual field to white targets. Dejerine emphasized that the subcortical component of the infarct served to disrupt the projections to the angular gyrus (which he considered to be the site where the lexical information gained access to the language zone) from both the ipsilateral calcarine cortex and the opposite side, this latter pathway via the corpus callosum. Dejerine made little mention of the callosal lesion, nor did Vialet[167] in a thorough review of the case. In both instances, emphasis was placed on the deep paraventricular lesion. Damasio and Damasio[40] resurrected these observations, drew attention to the likelihood that the inferior fibers of the forceps major, which cross in the inferior portion of the corpus callosum and terminate in the inferior visual association cortices, were the fibers of relevance for the conveyance of lexical information from the right to the left hemisphere. The anatomic course of these fibers places them in the position to be caught in a deep infarct that penetrates to the wall of the ventricle.

In his original publication, Dejerine did not specify whether he believed this information was conveyed from the right hemisphere via transcallosal pathways directly to the language zone without interruption, or by an indirect route through the left calcarine region. The lesion shown in his often reproduced diagram can be interpreted either way but is placed laterally enough to emphasize his original point that it served to interrupt the pathway from both calcarine regions. The point is not trivial: should the indirect path be the route, the occurrence of absolute alexia would necessitate a hemianopia; should the the direct route apply, hemianopia from calcarine infarction could occur without alexia if the fibers crossing the callosum are spared (Fig. 20.10).

The widely quoted modern cases[27,39,62] do not bear on this point since the infarcts were so extensive that the entire left calcarine pathway was destroyed. Both of Wyllie's[174] cases showed a major infarction in the proximal calcarine and lingual gyrus region, which spread deep enough to destroy the entire visual radiations, functionally nullifying the intact calcarine cortex farther back toward the occipital pole.

Incomplete right hemianopia, with macular sparing, is commonly encountered without disorders of reading, but such cases should come as no surprise, as the pathway is still intact through the macular zone of the calcarine cortex. Vialet[167] demonstrated that *complete right hemianopia* from a calcarine lesion could occur without alexia provided the deep paraventricular regions are spared. Foix and Hillemand[54] called attention to a role for the posterior portion of the corpus callosum by documenting a similar case. Stommel and col-

Figure 20.8 Case III from Wyllie showing the mesial left occipital infarction that produced absolute alexia. (From Wyllie,[174] with permission.)

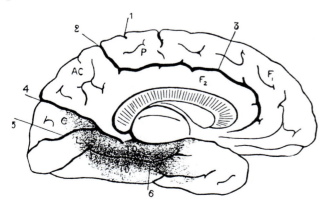

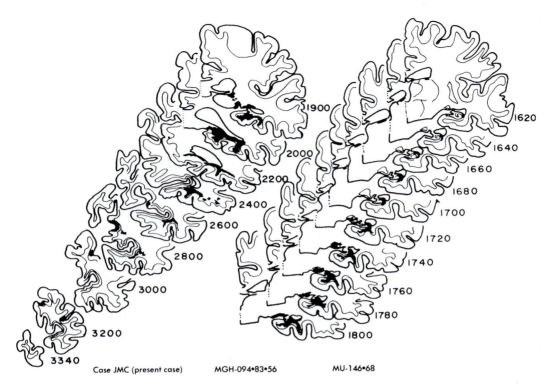

Figure 20.9 Traced serial sections of a posterior cerebral artery territory infarct with involvement of the lateral geniculate body, hippocampus, and subcortical portions of the calcarine region. (From Mohr et al.,[119] with permission.)

leagues[159] described a case of alexia without agraphia with splenogeniculate infarction. In some of the cases with incomplete hemianopia, the disorder of reading has taken the form of slowed and incomplete responses to the stimuli, with particular difficulties in discriminating the right-hand portions of the words (see below).[93]

Orgogozo et al[126] and Damasio and Damasio[40] have described instances of alexia in the presence of a *right upper quadrantanopsia*. The locus of the infarction was documented by CT scan. The authors argued for the original notion of Dejerine and Vialet that the lesion interrupted the deep paraventricular pathways. The patient described by Orgogozo et al[126] was able to read small and large letters without hesitation, but reading words was described as laborious and slow, proceeding from letter to letter to arrive at the syllables and finally the word, but with numerous errors. The reading of long words was impossible. Certain common words such as "good morning" were read as a whole ("globalment"). This patient's deficit seems to strain the notions of pure alexia, arguing instead for some degree of disordered visual discrimination. Patient 3 of Damasio and Damasio[40] was described as having "pure alexia"; no clinical details were given.

Binder and Mohr[17] had different findings in their 17 patients with dominant posterior cerebral artery territory infarction. Patients with dominant posterior cerebral artery infarction in whom reading was unaffected served as an anatomic control group. Normal readers had lesions in the medial and ventral occipital lobe, sparing dorsal white matter pathways and the ventral temporal lobe. Global and permanent alexia

occurred only with additional injury to the splenium, forceps major, or white matter above the occipital horn of the lateral ventricle. These data are different from the more inferomesial location favored by the Damasios and suggest that lesion size large enough to include the forceps major may be needed to create the syndrome of absolute alexia.

A small amount of literature documents that alexia may occur in the *absence* of any evidence of right hemianopia. The first description of the syndrome was made without autopsy data: a 20-year-old woman, walking in the street, suddenly noticed she could not read the letters on a sign or the names of the subway stations.[130] Her alexia was described as complete for all varieties of reading tasks, including musical notes. The handful of autopsied cases, the first of which was described by Greenblatt,[68,70] have been from tumors, arteriovenous malformations, and the like, but not from infarction.

Hemidyslexia

Hemidyslexia, which was described by Wilbrand[172] as a macular hemianopic disturbance of reading (makulär-hemianopische Lesestörung), has received little attention in the literature.[93] In the present authors' experience, it is a frequent accompaniment of a homonymous hemianopia contralateral to infarction affecting the posterior cerebral artery territory of the hemisphere dominant for speech and language. In some instances, the hemianopia is limited to to the macular region, as demonstrated by Polyak's[136] case of Harry Kraft. It may even occur without hemianopia.[31]

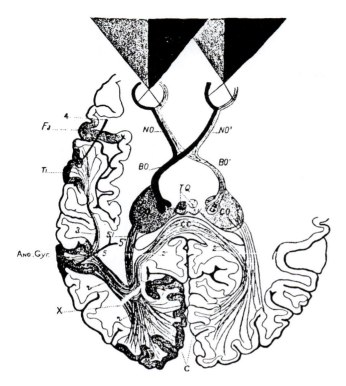

Figure 20.10 Diagram of the possible site (X) of interruption of the visual pathways linking the calcarine cortices (C) with the angular gyrus (Ang. Gyr.). (Adapted from Dejerine and Vialet,[45] with permission.)

For most patients so afflicted, the syndrome occurs from left-sided infarction and presents as misreading of the right-hand end of longer words. The errors occur whether the task is reading aloud or for comprehension, whether the words are printed or written, large or small, and isolated or embedded in text, as long as the words are lengthy, on the order of four letters or more. They occur less often when the right-hand end of the word is easily predicted by the left-hand end (e.g., words such as "eight"). The errors are present more often when the right-hand end has many possibilities not predicted by the left-hand end (e.g., "predator"). The term hemidyslexia is not quite accurate, as the errors do not occur beginning at the midpoint of the stimulus but instead only at some point beyond the midline of the word.

The hemianopia that accompanies hemidyslexia is usually incomplete. Most often it takes the form of upper quadrantanopsia with or without macular sparing, a sign that the lower bank of the calcarine cortex has suffered infarction. At times, colors seem dimmer in the affected field.

The quadrantanopsia with sparing of the other quadrant or the macula indicates that the infarct was not large enough to destroy the underlying visual radiations. The limited infarction appears to spare the pathways involved in conveying the lexical information decoded by the right calcarine cortex; it is inferred that this information concerning the left-hand side of the lexical stimulus does not pass through the left calcarine surface gray matter on its way to whatever brain regions derive the language value of the stimulus.

Hemidyslexia is often part of a complex syndrome of impaired response to complex visual stimuli, which has been explored in detail only rarely, the most elegantly by Levine and Calvanio.[93]

Hemidyslexia for stimuli from the left side of space occurs following sectioning of the corpus callosum but has not been reported in ischemic vascular disease thus far. A small branch of the posterior cerebral artery supplies the posterior corpus callosum. Its occlusion could possibly precipitate such a syndrome.

COLOR DYSNOMIA AND DYSCHROMATOPSIA

Dyschromatopsia

Some degree of faulty color discrimination may occur with dysfunction at any level along the visual pathway.[68,149,166] The lateral geniculate body is considered to play a role in color discrimination,[91] but deficits in color discrimination would be expected to occur only when the lesion is bilateral. However, when infarction is the cause of dyschromatopsia, it usually lies in the occipital lobe inferior to the calcarine cortex in the lingual gyrus.

This type of disturbance has been described in numerous instances of unilateral lingual gyrus involvement, either with full-thickness infarction or with subcortical infarction that undermined the gyrus.[39,43,45,88,109,176] The lesion may be unilateral on either side[88,136,138] or bilateral.[92,129] This correlation has also been established by CT scan studies.[42,85]

Color blindness from cerebral disease shows impaired performance on tests of color discrimination (e.g., Ishihara plates). In typical cases, the colors in the affected field(s) are described as gray, pale, or washed-out. At times, a given color is misnamed for another having a similar hue or brightness. This last finding is of little clinical value since it also occurs in patients whose performance on the Ishihara plates is intact (see below). Recall is normal for the color name characteristically associated with a given object (e.g., green with grass). A degree of improvement over time has been reported, even though an upper quadrantanopsia might remain.[4,85] Prosopagnosia and spatial and topographic disorientation have been reported as associated findings in a few cases with right posterior cerebral artery territory infarction.[34] Dyslexia often accompanies right hemidyschromatopsia.

One[61] among these cases[43,45,88] was explained by subsequent reviewers as a disconnection syndrome. Unfortunately, few of the reports described the exact means of testing for color, often omitting such details as whether the testing was done unilaterally or bilaterally, whether the patient was asked to name the color or simply point to it when named, or whether the patient simply had the visual fields tested with different color stimuli. As a result, the literature remains rather disappointing concerning the clinical points that differentiate between hemidyschromatopsia for the field contralateral to an infarct and a "disconnection" between two sides of the brain.

Color and Color-Name Disconnection

Color and color-name disconnection was named to describe a bidirectional impairment in relating a color to its name in the absence of deficits in color discrimination. The term *color agnosia* has also been used. The absence of deficits in color discrimination is revealed by normal performance on tests such as the Ishihara color plates. The bidirectional impairment in relating a color to its name is shown by errors in naming colors at sight and in matching color names heard or color names seen to color choices, or vice versa.

Geschwind and Fusillo[62] applied the term disconnection syndrome to this type of case to stress the point that the lesion may have separated the adequately discriminated visual input in the right hemisphere from access to the language region of the left hemisphere. As a result, visual stimuli would presumably be unable to be associated with their names, causing alexia (letters and words), defective naming of colors, and defective matching of color names to colors. In support of the disconnection notion, Geschwind and Fusillo[62] stressed that their patient ". . . would answer at random" when shown an object and asked whether it was a certain color. This random quality of color naming has not been a feature of other reported cases, however, even in some other cases with a bidirectional failure in relating colors to their names.

The infarct in the best known case[62] was in the distribution of the left posterior cerebral artery, destroying most of the gray and deep white matter of the medial occipital lobe, including the visual radiation, the inferior longitudinal fasciculus, and the crossing fibers through the splenium of the corpus callosum in the tapetum. A subsequent case[142] showed more circumscribed subcortical infarction underlying the left lingual gyrus. Another case used by these authors in support of their thesis[43,45,97] appears to have had right hemidyschromatopsia; it is not clear from the details of the clinical case report that a disturbance as thoroughly documented as that by Geschwind and Fusillo[62] was present.

Unfortunately, for most of the other reported cases whose deficits might represent the bidirectional disconnection, precise documentation of a disconnection state was lacking.[74,128,139,144,154,155,158] In only a few was complete testing done for color discrimination, impaired color naming, and impaired matching of colors with color names.[62,95,97] Clinically, these cases also showed a right homonymous hemianopia and dyslexia.

Color Dysnomia

Often considered synonymous with the bidirectional disconnection syndromes, color dysnomia appears to be the more common of the acquired cerebral disturbances involving response to color stimuli. Its existence provides another indication that the senior author has had experience with some unusual examples of color dysnomia.[119]

In the initial days after onset, the author's patient (Fig. 20.9) showed errors both in naming colors and in selecting the correct color from among an array of color choices when a color name was dictated aloud to him. However, within several days, he became able to select a color from among several choices when its name was shown to him or dictated to him. He also was easily able to recall the name of color commonly associated with given items and items commonly associated with given a color, yet he persisted in having difficulties in naming a color shown to him and in selecting its name from among several choices. His naming errors were not random or of the confabulatory type. He often named a given color using the name of another color close to it on the spectrum of hue or brightness, such as green for blue, or yellow for orange. The errors were mild enough to be overlooked on casual testing and might have been attributed to dim light in less rigorous test settings. Casual explanations such as these probably account for the infrequency with which the dysnomia is reported in cases with an infarct in a similar locale. When sought in such cases, the deficit is often easily demonstrated. The infarct is often quite modest and may be confined to the subcortical structures of the lingual gyrus.

The syndrome of color dysnomia is also of interest since it may be present without a dyslexia (i.e., with preserved reading). Although the two deficits frequently coexist, color dysnomia and alexia do not reflect a common mechanism for their occurrence, rather they show that spatially proximate regions of the cerebrum serving different functions are susceptible to simultaneous involvement by the same lesion if it is large enough.[137] It usually persists for many months and may be permanent.

Amnestic Color Dysnomia

A syndrome so rare that it is almost nonexistent, termed amnestic color dysnomia, refers to a disturbance in the recall of the names of the colors that are characteristic of a given object (e.g., green for grass) and vice versa. Tests of color discrimination and cross-matching of color with color names are said to be performed well.[66] No definite neuropathologic basis for this disorder has been established.

Unusual Variants

Other types of disturbance in response to colors occur in cerebral disease.[37] However, none of them have as yet been related to a focal lesion. The delineation of most of them requires the examiner to depend on the patient's subjective description of the altered appearance of color and of its relationship to the environment. The syndromes include illusory spread of color.

TRANSCORTICAL SENSORY APHASIA

In unusual disturbance in language function, transcortical sensory aphasia, autopsy correlation is lacking and also disagreements exist concerning its clinical features. Whether to place this syndrome among the consequences of posterior cerebral artery territory infarction is subject to argument, but it is discussed here because of the high frequency of accompanying hemianopia, visual object agnosia, and medial occipital low density seen on CT scan.

That aphasia may occur with posterior cerebral artery territory lesions is well documented, although infrequently.[146]

Kertesz et al[82] worked out a description of these cases. Using CT scanning and the results of the Western Aphasia Battery tests, 15 patients were collected for study. In 12, the lesion was diagnosed by isotope brain scan and in only 6 by CT scan. This manner of documentation probably reflects the very low incidence of the disorder, as well as the long span of time over which the 15 cases were accumulated. A contralateral hemianopia occurred in 12, 1 of whom had only an inferior quadrantanopsia. Eleven had some form of sensory loss. Only 5 had any degree of weakness, in 4 of whom it was described as "slight." In another 5 the disturbed higher cerebral function was accompanied by "visual agnosia." An unusual disturbance in speech and language was described by the authors as fluent and circumlocutory speech, with the content mainly semantic jargon.[82]

The lesion locations were equally unusual, as practically all the cases seem to show massive involvement of the posterior half of the brain, spreading from the occipital pole forward on both the medial and lateral surfaces, and in many the abnormality reached far forward along the mesial occipital lobe, well within the territory of the posterior cerebral artery. The authors suggested that the sites of infarction were ". . . in the posterior cerebral artery territory or in watershed area . . . between posterior cerebral and middle cerebral arteries. . . ."[82]

The mechanism of the infarctions is unclear. It is possible that this syndrome may be the result of an internal carotid occlusion with distal field infarction affecting the parieto-occipital region in the unusual instances in which the posterior cerebral artery is a branch of the internal carotid. For embolism to achieve this result would require some remarkable anatomy. At least one of their cases was an arteriovenous malformation—a lesion suitable for such an unusual location, crossing as it does between two major arterial territories. Little more is currently known of this interesting syndrome, and it awaits further study.

AMNESTIC APHASIA

Amnestic aphasia is characterized by a failure to recall the names of people as well as many other individual nouns when the stimuli are presented in visual or auditory form. Commonly, the expected response fails to occur, with the patient often falling silent or hesitating as if the name is about to be produced momentarily (tip of the tongue phenomenon). When the name fails to appear, it is rare for a neologism or other substitutive error to be produced. Instead, attributes of the item are described, indicating the patient's familiarity with the item in question. The failures in naming are often associated with circumlocutions, lame excuses for failure, and a general acceptance of the correct name when offered.[66]

Although classically considered a sign of deep temporal lobe involvement,[66] amnestic aphasia has occasionally been reported, often incidentally, in cases showing infarction in the territory of the dominant posterior cerebral artery.[74,174] The exact pathologic correlation for such deficits remains unclear, as does the issue of whether memory deficit and amnestic aphasia are functionally related or simply result from a lesion simultaneously involving physically proximate regions of the cerebrum serving separate functions.

MEMORY DEFICITS

Posterior cerebral artery territory infarction may have a profound effect on memory function, as has been fully reviewed.[122,147] Both embolism and thrombus have been found responsible.[162] The occlusions have usually been found proximally in the posterior cerebral artery in the stem and precortical portion. Amnestic disorders have also been reported from occlusion of thalamoperforants, but in these cases the possibility of simultaneous infarction of structures supplied by larger posterior cerebral artery branches is not ruled out. Based on the available literature, the occurrence of an amnestic state is no guide to whether the infarct is of thrombotic or embolic origin.

Bilateral Infarction

The literature contains numerous examples of bilateral posterior cerebral artery territory infarction of varying size described at autopsy[165] or by CT scan.[134,147] In these bilateral cases, the infarcts frequently are found spread along most of the undersurface of the cerebrum, involving the hippocampus and lingual and fusiform gyri, some as far posteriorly as the cuneus[22]; others have been extensive enough to include the fornices and fimbria of the hippocampus.[168] The hippocampus seems to be the most commonly affected of these various structures in amnestic cases. A single case report with infarction confined to the region of the hippocampus lacked most of the essential clinical details needed to determine the clinical features of isolated hippocampal infarction.[46] In case reports where it is described, the memory disorder itself seems to have the characteristics found in surgical removals of the hippocampus bilaterally.

A large literature has accumulated indicating bilateral hippocampal involvement as a necessary condition for amnesia to occur and to persist.[115] A single surgical case suggests that a bilateral disruption of the fornix may achieve the same effect,[161] but no long-term follow-up was reported on this patient. In another similar case,[116] later examination revealed improvement in the memory deficit. Other cases showed that no such effects occur.[2,44,50] The exact role of fornix sectioning in the occurrence and persistence of recent memory deficits has been difficult to determine since instances of isolated bilateral fornix interruption are rare.[75] Cases of isolated infarction have not been found by the present author in a literature search.

The rare case with bilateral posterior cerebral artery territory infarction with unilateral hippocampal or limbic infarction exists to confound efforts to settle the role of the bilateral lesion in memory disorder. Benson et al[14] described a 47-year-old physician with right hemianopia, alexia, visual agnosia, color agnosia, prosopagnosia, and ". . . impaired verbal learning. . . ." This disturbance was manifested by an ". . . inability to learn the names of ward personnel, considerable difficulty in learning the Babcock sentence, and ability to remember only one or two of four unrelated words after five minutes. . . ." He was noted to have made some improvements in the first few months after onset but remained disabled. Although bilateral fusiform gyrus and posterior callosal infarcts were found, the hippocampal infarct was confined to the left side. The autopsy findings were described only on cut section.

Unilateral Infarcts

Few cases have been reported of memory loss with a unilateral nonvascular lesion[49,60,125,147,161] and only a handful from autopsy-documented infarction. Geschwind and Fusillo's[62] case was a man with thrombosis of the left posterior cerebral artery whose infarct was detailed in serial sections. On admission, he was able to recall his name, yet stated his age incorrectly and was unable to recall his address. He failed to recall any of four objects after 1 minute. In addition, prominent deficits were encountered in reading aloud and in naming colors and simple objects. Severe disturbances in topographic orientation and topography were also noted. No further description was given concerning his memory disorder, but when he was seen 7 weeks after onset the recent memory deficits were said to have "... cleared completely." The topographic disorientation "... cleared to normal in the next few weeks." He died 15 months after the stroke occurred. On serial sections, the left hippocampus was infarcted and the left fornix had undergone complete degeneration.

The present senior author's own case[119] showed a severe memory disorder from onset, which persisted unchanged until his death on day 82. On initial examination within 12 hours of onset, this patient also stated his name, failed to recall his exact age, and was unable to state his address or where he had been the evening of his stroke. He repeatedly asked many questions, such as "Where is my wife?"; he accepted the examiner's answer and within seconds asked the question again. When his wife arrived hours after onset and mentioned her brother by name, he asked "Ed who?" He repeatedly attempted to learn the examiner's name, often wrote it on a pad, and when the examiner reappeared, failed to recall the name and failed to consult his notepad. Weeks after discharge, when returning to the laboratory for re-examination, he regularly introduced himself to the staff whom he had met on every previous occasion, and only rarely walked spontaneously in the correct direction toward the examining room. He showed a retrograde and anterograde amnesia for the events surrounding his admission, faulty retention of verbal material, impaired retention of a form discrimination test, and an amnestic dysnomia. Whether his deficit would have persisted over a longer period remains an open question. The pathologic findings indicated only unilateral infarction of the left hippocampus, with secondary degeneration of the left fornix and the precommissural bed nuclei of the septum.

Escourolle and Gray[52] reported an important autopsied case with memory disturbance whose infarct affected the left occipital and temporal lobe with atrophy of the fimbria of the hippocampus, the fornix, and the anterior nucleus of the thalamus. Similar cases have recently been described.[147] The description of an amnestic state from occlusion of the left anterior choroidal artery by Amarenco et al[6] is the first such report.

Clinical Features

When details were provided, the cases reported have shown profound disturbances in memory, especially for recent events when tested by conversational methods. The characteristics of the memory impairments and the performance on special laboratory tests are essentially identical to those reported[151]

from bilateral medial temporal regions that include the hippocampus[145] and from unilateral temporal lobe removals.[49,117,141,170] An acute confusional state in left posterior cerebral artery territory infarction has also been described.[48]

Associated Symptoms and Signs

An isolated amnestic state has yet to be reported from infarction in the posterior cerebral artery territory. To date, such cases have produced other deficits accompanying the amnestic state.

References

1. Abbie AA: The blood supply of the visual pathways. Med J Aust 2:199, 1938
2. Akelaitis AJ: Study of language functions unilaterally following section of the corpus callosum. J Neuropathol Exp Neurol 2:226, 1943
3. Albert NL, Reches A, Silverberg R: Associative visual agnosia with alexia. Neurology 25:322, 1975
4. Albert NL, Reches A, Silverberg R: Hemianopic colour blindness. J Neurol Neurosurg Psychiatry 38:546, 1975
5. Albert NL, Soffer D, Silverberg R, Raches A: The anatomic basis of visual agnosia. Neurology 29:876, 1979
6. Amarenco P, Cohen P, Roullet E et al: Syndrome amnesique lors d'un infarctus du territoire de l'artère choroidienne antérieure gauche. Rev Neurol (Paris) 144:36, 1988
7. Argentino C, De Michele M, Fiorelli M et al: Posterior circulation infarcts simulating anterior circulation stroke. Perspective of the acute phase. Stroke 27:1306, 1996
8. Assal G, Regli F: Syndrome de disconnexion visuo-verbale et visuo-gestuelle. Rev Neurol (Paris) 136:365, 1980
9. Bassetti C, Staikov IN: Hemiplegia vegetativa alterna (ipsilateral Horner's syndrome and contralateral hemihyperhidrosis) following proximal posterior cerebral artery occlusion. Stroke 26:702, 1995
10. Bay E: Agnose und Funktionswandel: Eine Hirnpathologische Studie. Springer-Verlag, Berlin, 1950
11. Beevor CE: On the distribution of the different arteries supplying the human brain. Philos Trans R Soc [Biol] 200:1, 1909
12. Bender MB, Feldman M: The so-called visual agnosias. Brain 95:173, 1972
13. Bender MB, Feldman M, Sobin AJ: Palinopsia. Brain 91:321, 1968
14. Benson DF, Segarra J, Albert ML: Visual agnosia—prosopagnosia. Arch Neurol 30:307, 1974
15. Benton S, Levy I, Swash M: Vision in the temporal crescent in occipital infarction. Brain 103:83, 1980
16. Bergman PS: Cerebral blindness. Arch Psychiatr Neurol 78:568, 1957
17. Binder JR, Mohr JP: The topography of callosal reading pathways. A case-control analysis. Brain 115:1807, 1992
18. Blythe IM, Kennard C, Ruddock KH: Residual vision

in patients with retrogeniculate lesions of the visual pathways. Brain 110:887, 1987

19. Bogousslavsky J, Regli F, van Melle G: Unilateral occipital infarction: evaluating the risks of developing bilateral loss of vision. J Neurol Neurosurg Psychiatry 46:78, 1983

20. Bogousslavsky J, Maeder P, Regli F, Meuli R: Pure midbrain infarction: clinical syndromes, MRI, and etiologic patterns. Neurology 44:2032, 1994

21. Brandt T, Thie A, Caplan LR, Hacke W: Infarkte im Versorgungsgebiet der A. cerebri posterior. Klinik, Pathogenese und Prognose. Nervenarzt 66:267, 1995

22. Brindley GS, Janota I: Observations on cortical blindness and on vascular lesions that cause loss of recent memory. J Neurol Neurosurg Psychiatry 38:459, 1975

23. Bohdiewicz P, Juni JE: Watershed ischemia demonstrated with acetazolamide enhanced Tc-99m HMPAO SPECT. Clin Nucl Med 19:452, 1994

24. Cambier J, Masson M, Elghozi D, Henin D, Viader F: Agnosie visuelle sans hemianopsie droite chez un sujet droitier Rev Neurol (Paris) 136:727 1980

25. Caplan LR: "Top of the basilar" syndrome. Neurology 30:72, 1980

26. Caplan LR, DeWitt LD, Pessin MS et al: Lateral thalamic infarcts. Arch Neurol 45:959, 1988

27. Caplan LR, Hedley-Whyte T: Cuing and memory dysfunction in alexia without agraphia—a case report. Brain 97:251, 1974

28. Carlesimo GA, Caltagirone C: Components in the visual processing of known and unknown faces. J Clin Exp Neuropsychol 17:691, 1995

29. Castaigne P, Lhermitte F, Buge A et al: Paramedian thalamic and midbrain infarcts: clinical and neuropathological study. Ann Neurol 10:127, 1981

30. Castaigne P, Lhermitte F, Gautier JC et al: Arterial occlusions in the vertebro-basilar system—a study of forty-four patients with post-mortem data. Brain 96:133, 1973

31. Castro-Caldas A, Salgado V: Right hemifield alexia without hemianopsia. Arch Neurol 41:84, 1984

32. Celesia GG, Archer CR, Kuriowa Y: Visual function of the extrageniculo-calcarine system in man. Arch Neurol 37:704, 1980

33. Chambers BR, Brooder RJ, Donnan GA: Proximal posterior cerebral artery occlusion simulating middle cerebral artery occlusion. Neurology 41:385, 1991

34. Cogan DG: Visuospatial dysgnosia. Am J Ophthalmol 88:361, 1979

35. Cohen L, Gray F, Meyrignac C et al: Selective deficit of visual size perception: two cases of hemimicropsia. J Neurol Neurosurg Psychiatry 57:73, 1994

36. Conomy JP, Laureno R, Massarweh W: Transient behavioral syndrome associated with reversible vascular lesions of the fusiform-calcarine region in humans, abstracted. Ann Neurol 12:83, 1982

37. Critchley M: Acquired disturbances of color perception of central origin. Brain 88:711, 1965

38. Critchley M: Types of visual perseveration: 'palinopsia' and 'illusory visual spread.' Brain 74:267, 1951

39. Cumming WJK, Hurwitz LJ, Perl NT: A study of a patient who had alexia without agraphia. J Neurol Neurosurg Psychiatry 33:34, 1970

40. Damasio AR, Damasio H: The anatomic basis of pure alexia. Neurology (Cleveland) 33:1573, 1983

41. Damasio A, Damasio H, Van Hoesen GW: Prosopagnosia: anatomic basis and behavioral mechanisms. Neurology (NY) 323:331, 1982

42. Damasio A, Yamada T, Damasio H: Central achromatopsia: behavioral and anatomic and physiologic aspects. Neurology 30:1064, 1980

43. Dejerine J: Différentes variétés de cécite verbale. CR Soc Biol (Paris) 4:61, 1892

44. Dejerine J, Roussy G: La syndrome thalamique. Rev Neurol (Paris) 14:521, 1906

45. Dejerine J, Vialet N: La localisation anatomique de la cécite verbale pure. CR Soc Biol (Paris) 5:790, 1893

46. DeJong RN, Itabashi HH, Olson JR: Memory loss due to hippocampal lesions. Arch Neurol (Chicago) 20:339, 1969

47. De Renzi E, Zambolin A, Crisi G: The pattern of neuropsychological impairment associated with left posterior cerebral artery infarcts. Brain 110:1099, 1987

48. Devinsky O, Bear D, Volpe BT: Confusional states following posterior cerebral artery infarction. Arch Neurol 45:160, 1988

49. Dimsdale H, Logue V, Piercy M: A case of persisting impairment of recent memory following right temporal lobectomy. Neuropsychologia 1:287, 1964

50. Dott NM: The Hypothalamus. Oliver, Boyd, London, 1938

51. Duncan GW, Weidling SM: Posterior cerebral artery stenosis with midbrain infarction. Stroke 26:900, 1995

52. Escourolle R, Gray F: Les accidents vasculaires du système limbique. p. 195. In: Proceedings of the VIIth International Congress of Neuropathology. Excerpta Medica, Amsterdam, 1975

53. Ferroir JP, Feve A, Khalil A et al: Hyperkinesie volitionnelle et d'attitude d'un membre supérieur. Manifestation d'un accident ischemique dans le territoire de l'artère cérébrale postérieure. Presse Med 21:2104, 1992

54. Foix C, Hillemand P: Contribution a l'étude des ramollissements protuberantiels. Rev Neurol (Paris) 43:287, 1925

55. Förster O: Ueber Rindenblindheit. Graefes Arch Ophthalmol 36:94, 1890

56. Frisen L: Quadruple sector anopia and sectorial optic atrophy: a syndrome of the distal anterior choroidal artery. J Neurol Neurosurg Psychiatry 42:590, 1979

57. Frisen L, Holmegaard L, Rosencrantz M: Sectorial optic atrophy and homonymous horizontal sector anopia: a lateral choroidal artery syndrome? J Neurol Neurosurg Psychiatry 41:374, 1978

58. Gacs G, Fox AJ, Barnett HJM, Vinuela F: CT visualization of intracranial arterial thromboembolism. Stroke 14:756, 1983

59. Galloway JR, Greitz T: The medial and lateral choroidal arteries. An anatomic and roentgenographic study. Acta Radiol (Stockh) 53:353, 1960

60. Garcia-Bengochea F, De La Torre O, Esquivel O et al: The section of the fornix in the surgical treatment of certain epilepsies. Trans Am Neurol Assoc 176:1954, 1959

61. Geschwind N: Disconnexion syndromes in animals and man. Brain 88:237, 1965

62. Geschwind N, Fusillo M: Color-naming defects in association with alexia. Arch Neurol (Chicago) 15:137, 1966

63. Ghika J, Bogousslavsky J, Henderson J et al: The "jerky dystonic unsteady hand": a delayed motor syndrome in posterior thalamic infarctions. J Neurol 241:537, 1994

64. Ghika JA, Bogousslavsky J, Regli F: Deep perforators from the carotid system. Template of the vascular territories. Arch Neurol 47:1097, 1990

65. Goldenberg G: Loss of visual imagery and loss of visual knowledge—a case study. Neuropsychologia 30:1081, 1992

66. Goldstein K: Language and Language Disturbances. Grune & Stratton, New York, 1948

67. Goto K, Takagawa K, Uemura K et al: Posterior cerebral artery occlusion: clinical computed tomographic and angiographic correlation. Radiology 132:357, 1979

68. Green GJ, Lessell S: Acquired cerebral dyschromatopsia. Arch Ophthalmol 95:121, 1977

69. Greenblatt SH: Alexia without agraphia or hemianopsia. Brain 96:307, 1973

70. Greenblatt SH: Subangular alexia without agraphia or hemianopia. Brain Lang 3:229, 1976

71. Habib M, Sirigu A: Pure topographical disorientation: a definition and anatomical basis. Cortex 23:73, 1987

72. Hayman LA, Berman SA, Hinck VC: Correlation of CT cerebral vascular territories with function: II. Posterior cerebral artery. Am J Neuroradiol 2:219, 1981

73. Head H: Aphasia: an historical review. Brain 43:340, 1920

74. Heidenhain A: Beitrag zur Kenntnis der Seelenblindheit. Monatsschr Psychiatr Neurol 66:61, 1927

75. Heilman KN, Sypert GW: Korsakoff's syndrome resulting from bilateral fornix lesions. Neurology 27:490, 1977

76. Heller-Bettinger I, Kepes JJ, Preskorn SH et al: Bilateral altitudinal anopia caused by infarction of the calcarine cortex. Neurology 26:1176, 1976

77. Holmes G: Selected Papers of Sir Gordon Holmes. p. 195. London, 1956

78. Hommel M, Besson G, Pollak P et al. Hemiplegia in posterior cerebral artery occlusion. Neurology 40:1496, 1990

79. Horenstein S, Chamberlin W, Conomy J: Infarction of the fusiform and calcarine regions: agitated delirium and hemianopia. Trans Am Neurol Assoc 92:85, 1967

80. Johansson T, Fahlgren H: Alexia without agraphia: lateral and medial infarction of the occipital lobe. Neurology 29:390, 1979

81. Kaul SN, DuBoulay GH, Kendall BE, Ross Russell RW: Relationship between visual field defects and arterial occlusion in the posterior cerebral circulation. J Neurol Neurosurg Psychiatry 37:1033, 1974

82. Kertesz A, Sheppard A, MacKenzie R: Localization in transcortical sensory aphasia. Arch Neurol 39:475, 1982

83. Kinkel WR, Newman RP, Jacobs L: Posterior cerebral artery branch occlusions: CT and anatomic considerations. p. 117. In Berguer R, Bauer RB (eds): Vertebrobasilar Arterial Occlusive Disease: Medical and Surgical Management. Lippincott-Raven, Philadelphia, 1984

84. Kleihues P, Hizawa K: Die Infarkte der A Cerebri posterior. Arch Psychiatr Z Ges Neurol 208:263, 1966

85. Kolmel HW: Pure homonymous hemiachromatopsia. Findings with neuro-ophthalmologic examination and imaging procedures. Eur Arch Psychiatry Neurol Sci 237:237, 1988

86. Kubik CS, Adams RD: Occlusion of the basilar artery: a clinical and pathological study. Brain 69:73, 1946

87. Landis T, Regard M, Bliestle A, Kleihues P: Prosopagnosia and agnosia for noncanonical views. An autopsied case. Brain 111:1287, 1988

88. Landolt E: De la cécite verbale. pp. 418–433. In: Nederlansch Tijdschrift voor geneeskunde Feestbundel oan Franciscus Corneilius Donders. op den 27 Mei 1888. F Van Rossen, Amsterdam, 1888

89. Lazorthes G, Salamon G: Étude anatomique et radioanatomique de la vascularisation arterielle du thalamus. Ann Radiol 14:905, 1971

90. Lazzarino LG, Nicolai A: Late onset unilateral asterixis secondary to posterior cerebral artery infarction. Ital J Neurol Sci 13:361, 1992

91. LeGros Clark WE: The laminar pattern of the lateral geniculate nucleus considered in relation to color vision Doc Ophthalmol 3:57, 1949

92. Lenz G: Zwei Sektionsfalle doppelseitigen zentralen Farbenhemianopsie. Z Ges Neurol Psychiatr 71:135, 1921

93. Levine DN, Calvanio R: A study of the visual defect in verbal alexia—simultanagnosia. Brain 101:65, 1978

94. Levine DN, Finklestein S: Delayed psychosis after right temporoparietal stroke or trauma: relation to epilepsy. Neurology 32:267, 1982

95. Lewandowsky M: Ueber Abspaltung des Farbensinnes. Monatsschr Psychiatr Neurol 23:488, 1908

96. Lilly R, Cummings JL, Benson DF, Frankel M: The human Klüver-Bucy syndrome. Neurology (Cleveland) 33:1141, 1983

97. Lissauer H: Ein Fall von Seelenblindheit nebst einem Beitrage zur Theorie derselben. Arch Psychiatr Nervenkr 21:222, 1890

98. Luco C, Hoppe A, Schweitzer M et al: Visual field defects in vascular lesions of the lateral geniculate body. J Neurol Neurosurg Psychiatry 55:12, 1992

99. Mackenzie I, Meighan S, Pollock EN: On the projection of the retinal quadrants on the lateral geniculate bodies and the relationship of the quadrants to the optic radiations. Trans Ophthalmol Soc UK 53:142, 1933

100. Manfredi M, Curccu G: Thalamic pain revisited. p. 73. In Loeb C (ed): Studies in Cerebrovascular-Disease. Masson Italia Editori, Milan, 1981

101. Margolis MT, Newton TH, Hoyt WF: Cortical branches of the posterior cerebral artery anatomic—radiologic correlation. Neuroradiology 2:127, 1971

102. Margolis MT, Smith CG, Richardson WF: The course and distribution of the arteries supplying the visual (striate) cortex. Am J Ophthalmol 61:1391, 1966

103. Matsuda M, Nakamura K, Fujimoto N et al: Visual agnosia evolving to optic aphasia—a case study. Clin Neurol 32:1179, 1992

104. McAuley DL, Ross Russell RW: Correlation of CAT scan and visual field defects in vascular lesions of the posterior

visual pathways. J Neurol Neurosurg Psychiatry 42:298, 1979

105. Meadows JC, Munro SS: Palinopsia. J Neurol Neurosurg Psychiatry 40:5, 1977

106. Medina JL, Chokroverty S, Rubino FA: Syndrome of agitated delirium and visual impairment: a manifestation of medial temporooccipital infarction. J Neurol Neurosurg Psychiatry 40:861, 1977

107. Medina JL, Rubino FA, Ross E: Agitated delirium caused by infarctions of the hippocampal formation and fusiform and lingual gyri: a case report. Neurology 24: 1181, 1974

108. Melamed E, Abraham FA, Lavy S: Cortical blindness as a manifestation of basilar artery occlusion. Eur Neurol 11:22, 1974

109. Merle P: Aphasie et hemiachromatopsie. Rev Neurol (Paris) 21:1129, 1908

110. Meyer O: Ein- und doppleseitige homonyme Hemianopsia mit Orientirungsstörungen. Monatsschr Psychiatr Neurol 8:440, 1900

111. Michel EM, Troost BT: Palinopsia: cerebral localization with computed tomography. Neurology 30:887, 1980

112. Milandre L, Brosset C, Botti G, Khalil R: Étude de 82 infarctus du territoire des artères cérébrales postérieures. Rev Neurol 150:133, 1994

113. Milisavljevic MM, Marinkovic SV, Gibo H, Puskas LF: The thalamogeniculate perforators of the posterior cerebral artery: the microsurgical anatomy. Neurosurgery 28: 523, 1991

114. Miller NR: Walsh and Hoyt's Clinical Neuro-Ophthalmology. 4th Ed. Vol. 1. Williams & Wilkins, Baltimore, 1982

115. Milner B: Amnesia following operations on the temporal lobes. p. 109. In Whitty CMW, Zangwill OL (eds): Amnesia. Butterworth, London, 1966

116. Milner B: Discussion of Sweet WH et al: Loss of recent memory following section of fornix. Trans Am Neurol Assoc 84:78, 1959

117. Milner B: Laterality effects in audition. p. 177. In VB Mountcastle (ed): Interhemispheric Relations and Cerebral Dominance. Johns Hopkins Press, Baltimore, 1962

118. Mohr JP, Case CS, Meckler RJ, Fisher CM: Sensorimotor stroke due to thalamocapsular ischemia. Arch Neurol 34:739, 1977

119. Mohr JP, Leicester J, Stoddard LT, Sidman M: Right hemianopia with memory and color defects in circumscribed left posterior cerebral artery territory infarction. Neurology 21:1104, 1971

120. Moriyasu H, Yasaka M, Minematsu K et al:. The pathogenesis of brain infarction in the posterior cerebral artery territory. Clin Neurol 35:344, 1995

121. Neau JP, Bogousslavsky J: The syndrome of posterior choroidal artery territory infarction. Ann Neurol 39:779, 1996

122. Nicolai A, Lazzarino LG: Acute confusional states secondary to infarctions in the territory of the posterior cerebral artery in elderly patients. Ital J Neurol Sci 15: 91, 1994

123. North K, Kan A, de Silva M, Ouvrier R: Hemiplegia due to posterior cerebral artery occlusion. Stroke 24:1757, 1993

124. Ortiz N, Barraquer Bordas L, Dourado M et al: La hemiplejia en los infartos de la arteria cerebral posterior. Un analisis de los diversos mecanismos responsables. Neurologia 8:188, 1993

125. Ojemann GA, Blick KI, Ward AA: Improvement and disturbance of short-term verbal memory during human ventrolateral thalamic stimulation. Trans Am Neurol Assoc 94:72, 1969

126. Orgogozo JM, Pere JJ, Strube E: Alexie sans agraphie "agnose" des couleurs et atteinte de l'hémichamp visuel droite: un syndrome de l'artère cérébrale postérieure. Semin Hopit 55:1389, 1979

127. Newman RP, Kinkel WR, Jacobs L: Altitudinal hemianopia caused by occipital infarctions. Arch Neurol 41: 413, 1984

128. Pallis CA: Impaired identification of faces and places with agnosia for colors. J Neurol Neurosurg Psychiatry 18:218, 1955

129. Pearlman AL, Birch J, Meadows JC: Cerebral color blindness: an acquired defect in hue discrimination. Ann Neurol 5:253, 1979

130. Peron N, Goutner V: Alexie pure sans hémianopsie. Rev Neurol (Paris) 76:81, 1944

131. Pessin MS, Kwan ES, DeWitt LD et al: Posterior cerebral artery stenosis. Ann Neurol 21:85, 1987

132. Pessin MS, Kwan ES, Scott RM, Hedges TR: Occipital infarction with hemianopsia from carotid occlusive disease. Stroke 20:409, 1989

133. Pessin MS, Lathi ES, Cohen MB et al: Clinical features and mechanism of occipital infarction. Ann Neurol 21: 290, 1987

134. Pillon B, Bakchine S, Lhermitte F: Alexia without agraphia in a left handed patient with a right occipital lesion. Arch Neurol 44:1257, 1987

135. Pillon B, Signoret J-L, Lhermitte F: Agnosie visuelle associative. Rôle de l'hémisphere gauche dans la perception visuelle. Rev Neurol (Paris) 137:831, 1981

136. Polyak S: The Vertebrate Visual System. University of Chicago Press, Chicago, 1957

137. Pötzl O: Die zweite Gruppe der optischen Agnosien. p. 80. In Aschaffenburg G (ed): Handbuch der Psychiatrie die Aphasielehre: I. Optische-agnostischen Storungen. Franz Deuticke, Wien, 1928

138. Pötzl O: Ueber einige zentrale Probleme des Farbensehens. Wien Klin Wochenschr 61:706, 1949

139. Reinhard C: Zur Frage der Hirnlocalisation mit besonderen Berucksichtigung der cerebralen Sehstorungen. Arch Psychiat Nervenkr 18:240, 1887

140. Riley HA, Yaskin JC, Riggs ME, Torney AS: Bilateral blindness due to lesions in both occipital lobes. NY J Med 43:1619, 1943

141. Ross ED: Sensory-specific and fractional disorders of recent memory in man. I. Isolated loss of visual recent memory. Arch Neurol 37:193, 1980

142. Rubens AB, Benson DF: Associative visual agnosia. Arch Neurol 24:305, 1971

143. Salamon G, Huang YP: Radiologic Anatomy of the Brain. Springer-Verlag, Berlin, 1976

144. Schober H: Erworbene Farbenblindheit nach Schadeltrauma. Graefes Arch Ophthalmol 148:93, 1948

145. Scoville W, Milner B: Loss of recent memory after bilat-

eral hippocampal lesions. J Neurol Neurosurg Psychiatry 20:11, 1957

146. Servan J, Verstichel P, Catala M et al: Aphasia and infarction of the posterior cerebral artery territory. J Neurol 242:87, 1995

147. Servan J, Verstichel P, Catala M, Rancurel G: Syndromes amnesiques et fabulations au cours d'infarctus du territoire de l'artère cérébrale postérieure. Rev Neurol 150: 201, 1994

148. Shellshear JL: A contribution to our knowledge of the arterial supply of the cerebral cortex in man. Brain 50: 236, 1927

149. Sheppard JJ: Human Color Perception. p. 98. Elsevier, New York, 1968

150. Shraberg D, Weisberg L: The Klüver-Bucy syndrome in man. J Nerv Ment Dis 166:130, 1978

151. Sidman M, Stoddard LT, Mohr JP: Some additional quantitative observations of immediate memory in a patient with bilateral hippocampal lesions. Neuropsychologia 6:245, 1968

152. Sidman M, Stoddard LT, Mohr JP, Leicester J: Behavioral studies of aphasia: methods of investigation and analysis. Neuropsychologia 9:119, 1971

153. Sieben G, De Reuck J, Eecken HV: Thrombosis of the mesencephalic artery: a clinico-pathological study of two cases and its correlation with the arterial vascularization. Acta Neurol Belg 77:151, 1977

154. Siemerling: Ein Fall sogenannter Seelenblindheit nebst anderweitigen cerebralen Symptomen. Arch Psychiatr Nervenkr 21:284, 1889

155. Sittig O: Stoerungen in Verhalten gegenuber Farben bei Aphasischen. Monatsschr Psychiatr Neurol 49:63, 1921

156. Smith CG, Richardson WFG: The course and distribution of the arteries supplying the visual striate cortex. Am J Ophthalmol 61:1391, 1966

157. Spector RH, Glaser JS, David NJ, Vining DQ: Occipital lobe infarctions: perimetry and computed tomography. Neurology (NY) 31:1198, 1981

158. Stengel E: The syndrome of visual alexia with color agnosia. Br J Psychiatry 94:46, 1948

159. Stommel EW, Friedman RJ, Reeves AG: Alexia without agraphia associated with spleniogeniculate infarction. Neurology 41:587, 1991

160. Suzuki T, Iwakuma A, Tanaka Y et al: Changes in personality and emotion following bilateral infarction of the posterior cerebral arteries. Jpn J Psychiatr Neurol 46: 897, 1992

161. Sweet WH, Talland GA, Ervin FR: Loss of recent memory following section of fornix. Trans Am Neurol Assoc 84:76, 1959

162. Symonds C, Mackenzie I: Bilateral loss of vision from cerebral infarction. Brain 80:415, 1957

163. Tohgi H, Watanabe K, Takahashi H et al: Prosopagnosia without topographagnosia and object agnosia associated with a lesion confined to the right occipitotemporal region. J Neurol 241:470, 1994

164. Touho H, Takaoka M, Ohnishi H et al: Percutaneous transluminal angioplasty for severe stenosis of the posterior cerebral artery: case report. Surg Neurol 43:42, 1995

165. Trillet M, Fischer C, Serclerat D, Schott B: Le syndrome amnesique des ischemies cérébrales postérieures. Cortex 16:421, 1980

166. Urechia CI, Cremene V, Popescu P: Hémianopsie avec chromoagnosie. Rev Neurol (Paris) 80:70, 1948

167. Vialet N: Les Centres Cérébraux de la Vision et l'Appareil Nerveux Visuel Intra-Cérébral. Faculté de Medecine de Paris, Paris, 1893

168. Victor M, Angevine JB, Mancall EL: Memory loss with lesions of the hippocampal formation. Arch Neurol (Chicago) 5:244, 1961

169. Vincent FM, Sadowsky CH, Saunders RL, Reeves AG: Alexia without agraphia hemianopia or color-naming defect: a disconnection syndrome. Neurology 27:689, 1977

170. Walker AE: Recent memory impairment in unilateral temporal lesions. Arch Neurol Psychiatry (Chicago) 78: 543, 1957

171. Waterston JA, Stark RJ, Gilligan BS: Paramedian thalamic and midbrain infarction: the 'mesencephalothalamic syndrome.' Clin Exp Neurol 24:45, 1987

172. Wilbrand H: Ueber die makulär-hemianopische Lesestörung und die v Monakowsche Projektion der Makula auf die Sehspäre. Klin Monatsbl Augenheilkd 45:1, 1907

173. Whiteley AM, Warrington EK: Prosopagnosia: a clinical psychological and anatomical study of three patients. J Neurol Neurosurg Psychiatry 40:395, 1977

174. Wyllie J: The Disorders of Speech. p. 340. Oliver, Boyd, Edinburgh, 1894

175. Yamada A, Miki H, Nishioka M: A case of posterior cerebral artery territory infarction with micropsia as the chief complaint. Rinsho-Shinkeigaku 30:894, 1990

176. Ziehl-Lübeck: Ueber einem Fall von Alexia and Farbenhemiagnosie. Verh Ges Dtsch Natur Aertze 67:184, 1895

CHAPTER 21

Choroidal Artery Disease

J. P. MOHR
SERGE TIMSIT

Until quite recent times, little attention was paid to the choroidal arteries. Small, not easily seen (even on angiogram), and thought not to be the source of unique supply to structures serving important functions, they often went unmentioned among the vascular clinical syndromes in standard textbooks. Even their territories of supply were not clearly outlined save in the most detailed texts of anatomy, and the maps have been subject to dispute to the present day. With the advent of high-image scanning, magnification angiography, interventional neuroradiology for arteriovenous malformations, and interest in syndromes of small, deep infarction, considerable information has developed concerning the anterior and posterior choroidal arteries, enough to justify a chapter for this third edition. As will be seen, the extent of the anastomosis between the anterior and posterior choroidal arteries, rarely settled in life,[69] has prevented any but generalities to be made concerning what elements of syndromes attributed to each artery are unique to the artery in question or shared by both. Such strokes still seem rare, accounting for only 2% of cases in some series.[61]

Anatomy

ANTERIOR CHOROIDAL ARTERY

The anterior choroidal artery (AChA) usually arises as a small branch of the internal carotid artery (ICA), just distal to the origin of the posterior communicating artery. Rarely, it may arise just proximal to the posterior communicating artery.[36,58] Although it is said to arise sometimes from the middle cerebral artery,[33] studies of the anatomy by microdissection show that it almost always arises from the ICA. The artery is usually divided in many branches soon after it leaves the ICA to course dorsally between the temporal lobe and the cerebral peduncle.

Its course has many variants.[30,47,68,75] The AChA enters the brain via the choroidal fissure as a trunk before dividing into its small branches,[25] passes along the choroid plexus of the temporal horn, and anastomoses with the posterior choroidal artery, the anastomosed vessel then passing around and behind the thalamus to supply the choroid plexus in the third and lateral ventricle.

Early works by anatomists, using autopsy with injection techniques, found the supply to the brain parenchyma roughly paralleling the course of the artery, most of the tissues supplied being stained only to shallow depths, possibly an indication of how lightly the artery is tethered to the ventricular wall throughout its course. The regions supplied include the pyriform cortex, part of the amygdala and the uncus, part of the hippocampus with the fimbria, the medial part of the globus pallidus, the lateral part of the geniculate body, the initial segment of the optic radiations, the subthalamic region, the inferior half of the posterior limb of the internal capsule, part of the cerebral peduncle, the posterior wall of the pulvinar of the thalamus, and, as suggested by the name of the artery, the choroid plexus.[1,3,45] The arterial supply to the uncus may be from quite large arteries.[52]

Despite the classical studies, some controversy remains concerning the supply to the brain parenchyma along the course followed by the AChA, and its overlap with the territory of the posterior cerebral artery (PCA) and the posterior choroidal artery (PChA). For the *amygdala* and *hippocampus*, supply from the PCA, either via its trunk or from the branches of the PChA, was found to predominate over supply from the AChA in a comparative study involving humans and animals.[34] In humans, the 30 hemispheres dissected by Erdem et al[25] showed that the supply to the hippocampus was from several sources in 57% of cases, but in only 3% was the hippocampal supply almost entirely from the AChA. For the remainder, the AChA played no important role, indicating that the PCA is the principal source in most cases. The main site of anastomosis between the AChA and the PCA was at the uncal sulcus.

Figure 21.1 Arterial supply to the lateral geniculate body. (From Frisen et al,[29] with permission. From BMJ Publishing Group.)

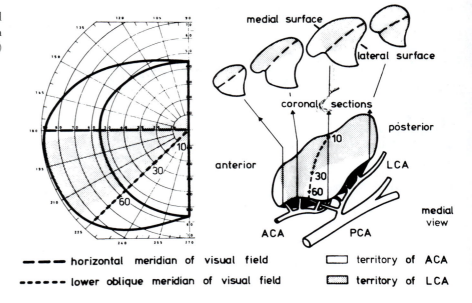

——— horizontal meridian of visual field

------ lower oblique meridian of visual field

☐ territory of ACA

▨ territory of LCA

Supply to the *lateral geniculate body* is of considerable interest (Fig. 21.1). A point of importance is the classical view that both the AChA and the PChA supply the lateral geniculate and do not anastomose before or in the nucleus, but appear to be end arteries with no collaterals,[1] even though the arteries form anastomoses distal to the lateral geniculate. This point has been contradicted by recent studies of Grkovic et al[35]; their work, which we have read only in summary since it was published in Serbo-Croatian, indicated that anastomoses could be found between the AChA and PCA branches supplying the lateral geniculate body. The AChA supplies the anterior hilum and the anterior and lateral aspects of the nucleus. The PChA supplies the remainder, including the crown. These two sites of supply have important clinical implications (see below).

At the extremes of its distal supply, less agreement exists concerning the irrigation of the depth of the brain adjacent to the frontocentral horns of the lateral ventricle, the *periventricular corona radiata*. The early maps did not settle how far up along the lateral wall of the ventricle and how deeply into the adjacent brain (corona radiata) the territory of supply of the AChA extended. The initial templates of vascular territories assembled by Damasio[12] for use in plotting computed tomographic (CT) images were drawn from the diverse information available at the time they were created. As communicated personally from H. Damasio, the maps were intended to show the dominant patterns of vascularization, and the author noted that some areas were especially problematic, the choroidal artery territories among them. The authors did not consider the templates to indicate an extension of the AChA territory into the centrum semiovale, but into the region of transition between the internal capsule and centrum. The matter of the exact areas of supply was not settled.

We mapped the inferred territory in 11 personal patients suffering infarction shown on magnetic resonance imaging (MRI) or CT, and attributed to occlusion of the AChA by angiogram or selective injection of the AChA during CT scanning[57] (Fig. 21.2). The territory involved included the medial temporal lobe, the lowest level of the internal capsule, and the posterior thalamus, but not the brain adjacent to the lateral ventricular wall or corona radiata. Comparison of CT or MR images of 33 other personal consecutive patients whose deep infarction involved the corona radiata at the ventricular wall showed either isolated infarction or extension of the lesion into the adjacent internal capsule. None of the lesions in such cases involved the posterior thalamus or medial temporal lobe. Based on these studies, it was proposed that clinical correlates of AChA territory infarction should not include cases showing involvement of the upper corona radiata or adjacent lateral ventricular wall.

Others have disagreed with this formulation. Hupperts et al[44] undertook a study of 77 patients whose lesion site was based on CT scan, not MRI, the findings arguing for inclusion of the paraventricular posterior corona radiata in the AChA territory, making this artery one of the territories capable of producing small, deep infarcts. More research on this subject is in order.

POSTERIOR CHOROIDAL ARTERY

Often arising as a single trunk from the PCA just distal to its course around the midbrain peduncle, the PChA gives rise to the lateral and medial PChAs (Fig. 21.3).

The poste*rolateral* choroidal artery arises from the PCA just before the posteromedial choroidal artery.[31] It follows the course of the PCA around the midbrain and thereafter passes over the curve of the pulvinar, which it supplies—whether alone or in combination as an anastomosis with the AChA. It also supplies the optic tract and the posterior portion of the lateral geniculate body, thereafter entering the choroidal fis-

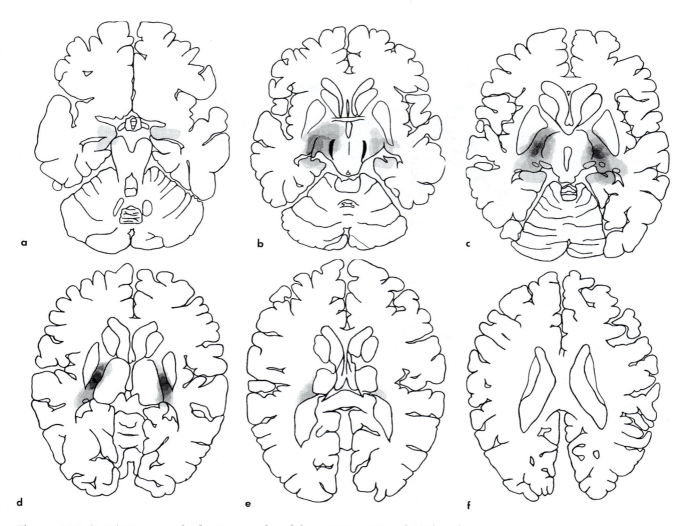

Figure 21.2 (**A–F**) Mapping of infarction as inferred from MRI or CT and attributed to occlusion of the AChA by angiography or selective injection of the AChA during CT.

sure to supply the choroid plexus of the lateral ventricle.[64] In its terminal branches, it anastomoses with the AChA.

The postero*medial* choroidal artery, arising a few millimeters behind the posterolateral choroidal artery, courses over the medial and lateral geniculate bodies, which contributes to its double-humped (number 3) appearance on angiograms.[24] After entering the choroidal fissure, it supplies the habenula, the anterior pulvinar, part of the centromedian nucleus of the thalamus, the paramedian nuclei, and the choroid plexus of the third ventricle; terminal branches may supply the anterior nucleus of the thalamus.[24,62]

Supply to the ventral tier nuclei of the thalamus is the most common from the thalamogeniculate branch of the posteromedial choroidal artery. Milisavljevic et al[54] studied the thalamogeniculate arteries of 30 hemispheres. They arose from several sites along the PCA, 80% from its crural (P2) segment and most from the rest from the quadrigeminal (P3) segment; a few arose from the distal segment of the PCA. A small number supplied the lateral geniculate body.

The posterior pericallosal or splenial artery is a branch of the choroidal system as well.

Etiology of Occlusion

Because of the small size of the AChA and PChA and the deep territories they feed, the infarcts associated with their occlusion could be grouped under small vessel disease in some classifications.[5,46] However, autopsy and clinical studies suggest that small vessel disease is decidedly uncommon. In their series of 35 cases studied at autopsy, Levy et al[47] found that cardioembolism (in 54%) was the most common cause of AChA territory infarction. Artery-to-artery embolism accounted for 17%, and small-artery disease accounted for only 6%. Leys et al[49] reported on 16 patients, including 8 men who underwent extensive evaluation in pursuit of a cause of AChA infarction. Cardioembolism explained four, large vessel atherosclerosis two, and dissection of the ICA two: only one had a diagnosis of "small vessel occlusion." In seven others no cause was found.[49] Tei et al,[72] reporting on 72 cases of presumed capsular infarction, found a source of embolism in only 7% of cases with AChA territory infarction.

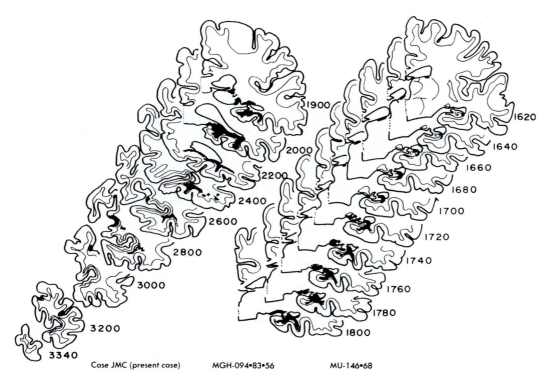

Figure 21.3 Traced serial sections of a PCA territory infarction with involvement of the lateral geniculate body, hippocampus, and subcortical portions of the calcarine body. (From Mohr et al,[56] with permission.)

With an increasing awareness of the clinical features of the syndrome (see below), its occurrence in a setting of surgery for the ICA and aneurysms at the circle of Willis has become increasingly appreciated. Among the mechanisms cited have been vasospasm after subarachnoid hemorrhage, mechanical obstruction, thromboembolism, and distortion of the aneurysm clip.[67]

Embolization for arteriovenous malformations may include the AChA. All the major groups who perform such work regularly have come to have considerable wariness of the hazards of occlusion of this vessel.[23,42]

Clinicopathologic Correlations

ANTERIOR CHOROIDAL ARTERY

Autopsy Material

We have found only 9 single autopsied case reports in the literature and another 35 reported as a group. The information as it exists is summarized in the order in which the cases were reported.

Kolisko[45] reported two cases. His first featured right hemiplegia and hemianesthesia. (No reference was made to visual field disturbances or other signs.) The second also had right hemiplegia and hemianesthesia but no hemianopia.

Foix et al[27] described one case in less than two pages. The patient had right hemiplegia, hemianopia, and hemianesthesia but no aphasia. The postmortem findings on the left side showed infarction in the posterior three-fourths of the internal capsule. The authors were careful to note that this lesion was visible quite high in the internal capsule and also in the superior part of the mesencephalon (pied pes pedunculi). There was also involvement of the optic tract and the optic radiation. The lesion was explained by "obliteration" of the AChA.

Poppi's[63] single case was somewhat complex, because two stroke episodes had occurred. One was related to an infarction in the vertebrobasilar territory and the other to an occlusion in the AChA territory. The patient was a 62-year-old woman with a medical history of chronic cardiopathy whose illness began as coma lasting for 48 hours. On awakening she had a behavior disturbance with disorientation; left hemiplegia with Babinski sign and hyperreflexia; mild dysarthria; right eye ptosis; and vasomotor disturbances (not further defined) but no sensory disturbance and no mention of visual field abnormalities. (It seems likely this was not the choroidal territory infarction.) Six months later, she had a new stroke, this one featuring left-sided dense hemiplegia involving the arm and leg to the same degree; left hemianesthesia involving all sensory modalities, accompanied by what might now be described as a thalamic syndrome: spontaneous pain and contracture of the left hand; worsening of the vasomotor impairment, which consisted of edema and temperature differences between left and right; and worsening of the ptosis but no mention of hemianopia.

Postmortem findings included infarction in numerous structures, some of them anatomically contiguous: the anterior part of the pes pedunculi and the oculomotor nerve complex; the laterodorsal, lateroventral, and centromedian nucleus of the thalamus; the posterior part of the internal capsule; the internal part of the globus pallidus; the ventral part of the subthalamic nucleus; the external part of the tuber cinereum and mamillary body; the anterior and posterior pillar of the trigone; and the right lateral part of the trigone. The optic tract was almost totally spared, as was the lateral geniculate body. The lesions were explained by two infarctions, one in the peduncular artery (branch of the retromamillary pedicle) and the other in the anterior choroidal artery.

Ley[48] detailed the case of a 79-year-old woman with right hemiplegia and contracture in flexion of the arm, brisk reflexes but no Babinski sign, and right hemianopia. All sensory modalities were intact. She had dysarthria but no aphasia. Opticokinetic nystagmus was abolished to the left.

Postmortem findings featured infarction in the internal part of the globus pallidus, posterior part of the internal capsule, pes pedunculi (pied du pedoncule cérébrale), and optic tract and along the lateral ventricle but not in the tail of the caudate nucleus. A large atheromatous plaque was found in the carotid trunk extending into the lumen of the AChA.

Abbie's case (findings communicated by Mackenzie et al[51]) featured a dense right hemiplegia affecting the arm and leg to the same degree, hemianesthesia involving all sensory modalities, and a visual field deficit whose unusual features included an incongruous superior quadrantic hemianopia, with macular sparing and loss of the inferior right nasal field, the first description of what was to become a sectoranopia (see below). The postmortem showed obliteration of both AChAs but infarction limited to the left side involving the pes pedunculi and the internal capsule.

In their collection of cases described as pure motor stroke, Fisher and Curry[26] described a case that postmortem examination related to AChA territory. Clinically, the patient suffered paralysis, which for the most part cleared within a month of the stroke. The lesion measured 7 to 10 mm in diameter, was located at the midlevel of the vertical extent of the capsule in its posterior limb, and extended to the medial part of the globus pallidus. The authors speculated that this lesion "possibly lay in the territory of a penetrating branch of the anterior choroidal artery." In none of the capsular cases was an occluded vessel found, nor was a significant degree of stenosis observed in the vessels. They noted that ". . . occlusion of the anterior choroidal artery or one of its branches may cause an infarct involving only the motor system of the internal capsule."

Buge et al[8] treated a hypertensive, diabetic smoker who presented with an acute pseudobulbar syndrome: dysarthria, right facial weakness, and linguo-pharyngo-laryngeal palsy. In addition, there was no upward gaze and limitation of downward gaze. No weakness was found in the limbs. Postmortem showed a patent foramen ovale, no clot in the stem of the AChA, an old lacunar infarct in the right thalamus, and old hemorrhagic split in the cingulate gyrus. Two recent bilateral infarcts were found, which explained the clinical picture. On the left side, one was in the posterior limb of the internal

capsule (5 mm behind the genu), also involving the nucleus reticularis of the thalamus (affected only superficially in its half inferior part) and the globus pallidus. The lateral geniculate body was spared. On the right side the findings were the same, but the lesion was older. The mechanism of the infarcts was not identified.

Bogousslavsky et al[5] studied an 85-year-old with atrial fibrillation whose stroke featured severe left spastic hemiparesis involving the face, arm, and leg, with left hypesthesia (involving all sensory modalities), left homonymous hemianopia, and left spatial hemineglect. This was the first documentation by CT and single-photon emission CT (SPECT) of infarction in the posterior part of the posterior limb of the internal capsule. The SPECT showed hypoperfusion in the right internal capsule with an associated perfusion decrease in the overlying parietal lobe (35%) and to a lesser extent the right prefrontal region (25%). A 30% cerebellar hypoperfusion was present on the left.

Postmortem showed atheromatous plaques in the basilar and posterior cerebral arteries. The AChA was not examined. An infarct was found in a small part of the pallidus at the level of the pulvinar. The lesion extended from the inferior part of the body of the caudate nucleus to the inferior horn of the lateral ventricle adjacent to the choroidal fissure. Also involved were the lateral half of the retroventricular part of the internal capsule, optic radiation, and right amygdala.

Levy et al[47] reported their retrospective study of 35 patients with cerebral infarcts affecting at least the territory of the AChA. In only two was the AChA alone involved. None of the cases had been diagnosed as AChA territory infarction in life. None of them had the hemiplegia, hemianesthesia, and hemianopia thought typical of AChA territory infarction (see below). The spectrum of findings was thought to reflect to co-involvement of other territories commonly affected along with the AChA including the middle or posterior cerebral artery, which was attributable to concomitant involvement of the ICA (found in 74%).[47]

Efforts to formulate a syndrome from the autopsy material date back to the summaries of Foix and Hillemand.[28] The expansion of their efforts by modern imaging has redefined many of the elements (see below).

Surgery

Knowledge of the anatomic zones of supply of the AChA encouraged surgical occlusion of the artery, in attempts to affect the course of parkinsonism and the dystonias. The effort was led for much of his career by the New York surgeon Irving S. Cooper.[11] The AChA was visualized prior to surgery in 92% of the arteriograms. His technique involved coagulation or silver clip occlusion (total or partial, retrograde collateral unknown). Some 40 operations were performed in 34 patients (bilaterally in 6) with parkinsonism. He coagulated the artery close to its origin and repeated the occlusion more distally.

Some of the occlusions had the desired effect. Tremor was reported to be abolished in 70% of the cases without compromise of motor power. Rigidity was said to be lessened. Some improvement occurred in gait and speech. A 10% mortality was reported. Several patients were somnolent and febrile after operation. Hemiplegia occurred in the contralateral extremities after operation in only 2 patients. Three had slight weakness and fully 29 had no loss of power. Only six patients were followed for more than 1 year.

It may be that Cooper's experience prompted many clinicians to disregard occlusion of the AChA as a source of concern.

Imaging Studies

The bulk of the remaining literature comes from patients studied in a setting of infarction, inferred from angiographically documented occlusion of the AChA or from brain imaging (CT or MRI). A series of cases has been presented, often as single case reports, but some in a series (Fig. 21.4). The predominant finding has been a sensorimotor stroke. In some, the details have been extensive, but in many the summary terms hemiparesis, hemiplegia, and hemianesthesia have been used, often alone, sometimes with hemianopia, and less often with mention of behavior disturbances.

Much of the imaging literature reflected the early publications of several French groups[13,14,43,53,74] and the Chicago group.[40] Apart from documenting the classical syndromes described by Foix and Hillemand, Decroix et al[13] early noted the existence of "incomplete forms of the syndrome" and the association with neuropsychological disorders. Helgason,[38]

heading the Chicago group, is to be credited with rearousing interest in the AChA syndromes in America, adding several variants to the classical grouping including hemiataxia, acute pseudobulbar mutism, pure motor syndrome, pure sensory syndrome, and disorders of higher cortical function. This expanded list prompted considerable effort from others in confirmation or objection to her additions. She also offered the opinion that the most common source of the occlusion was "small-vessel occlusive disease, predominantly found in hypertensive and diabetic patients" but acknowledged that cardioembolism was also a possible cause.[38]

Distinctive Clinical Features

COMBINED MOTOR, SENSORY, AND VISUAL FIELD DEFICITS. Combined deficits have been described by many authors. The setting has been quite striking in some cases. In one, a 27-year-old man with atrial fibrillation who presented with moderate hemiparesis, hemihypesthesia, hemianopia, and dysarthria, the acute syndrome improved with fibrinolysis.[23] Takahashi et al[70] reported 12 cases confirmed by angiogram and imaged by CT or MRI. The extent of the lesion varied from case to case, mirrored by the clinical syndrome.

Figure 21.4 (**A–D**) A series of cases of sensorimotor stroke inferred from angiographically documented occlusion of the AChA, brain imaging, CT, or MRI.

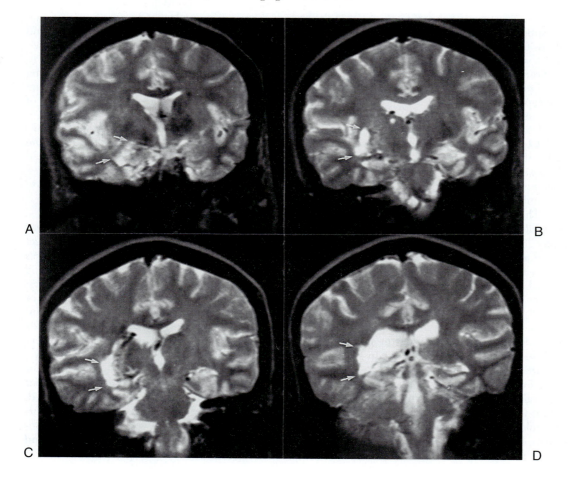

VARIANTS OF THE MOTOR AND SENSORY SYNDROMES.

The variants were the first to attract clinical attention. Helgason and Wilbur[40] noted the possibility that a syndrome of hypesthesia and ataxic hemiparesis could arise from AChA territory infarction. Among 23 cases of hypesthetic ataxic hemiparesis studied by CT or MRI, 15 showed extension of the infarct well outside the boundaries of the capsule into the paraventricular region, while also including the lateral thalamus. These larger infarcts were hypothesized to be in the territory of the AChA. Bogousslavsky et al[6] reported on a single case. The diagnosis was based on CT imaging. The ataxia was said to be of the "cerebellar type," and the sensory disturbance affected all modalities but had a prominent pain component.

It was the severity and duration of the hemiparesis—in some cases hemiplegia—with no infarct found on the crude images of the early CT scans that began to arouse interest in the AChA as a cause. In a survey of pure motor stroke from lacunar infarction, a correlation between syndrome severity and infarct volume was found by Chamorro et al,[10] save for the cases of AChA territory infarction, in which a lesion small enough to cause only partial paresis in other sites in the motor pathway caused hemiplegia. The contralateral hemiplegia (usually severe and affecting the face, arm, and leg equally) portion of the AChA syndrome appears explainable from involvement of the lowest portion of the internal capsule, where the fibers are the most compact.

SENSORY DEFICITS.

Whether sensory disturbance attributed to AChA occlusion and territorial infarction is different from that shared with the PChA is unknown. The only citations referable to this point are the four cases with pure sensory stroke said by Decroix et al[15] to be explained by posterior capsular infarction, possibly from AChA territory infarction, and one case attributed to AChA territory infarction by CT scan.[21]

DISTURBANCES IN BEHAVIOR.

In a few cases, the combined motor, sensory, and visual field deficit has been associated with disturbances in behavior. Delreux et al[19] were among the first to cite the possibility of a nondominant hemisphere syndrome arising in a setting of AChA territory infarction. The extensively studied case of de la Sayette et al[18] was a 72-year-old right-handed woman whose infarct affected the right AChA territory. The accompanying behavior disturbance was characterized as "complete non-determinant hemisphere syndrome that combined disorientation for place and time, anosognosia, hemiasomatognosia, left spatial neglect, constructional apraxia and spatial confabulation concerning both the present time and the weeks that preceded the vascular event. Language and verbal memory were normal." A large lesion was seen on MRI involving the posterior limb of the internal capsule (including the genu), globus pallidus, cerebral peduncle, and amygdala but sparing the thalamus and the corona radiata. This case was unusual in that positron emission tomography (PET) scanning was performed, showing widespread hypometabolism of the right hemisphere, which the authors took as a sign of interruption of deep-to-cortical projection systems from the infarct. Little improvement was seen over time.[18]

MEMORY DISTURBANCES.

We have been able to find only one case of memory disturbance.[17] The details were sketchy at best, reported only in retrospect from chart review. The amnestic state was not fully characterized, and little can be inferred about the syndrome from the case description. The inference that the AChA was the site of occlusion was from the investigators, no actual imaging having been done in life.

The case reported by Amarenco et al[2] had imaging consistent with a left AChA infarct. The patient himself, age 76, was a right-handed smoker and moderate alcohol drinker whose main presenting complaint was a right-sided motor deficit. The weakness started with a right-hand palsy, which then extended to the whole superior limb. Two days later the patient also had bilateral Babinski signs, a mild right-sided sensory deficit, an "intense" right hemianopsia, a right lateral gaze palsy, slight problems with swallowing, and a nasal voice. Language was normal. He was attentive, had a digit span of seven, made an approximation of the day of the week and the date, month, and year, and had a good recall of prior information (retrograde memory) but a dense anterograde amnesia with confabulations: he was unable to recall three words for 1 minute, and on one occasion he said he was minister of different governments (Third Republic, cited Pompidou as president of the Republic). His score on the Wechsler Memory Scale was 34 (normal, 50). Ten days after the deficit began, he was still in a severe anterograde amnestic state, and motor and visual field abnormalities persisted.

VISUAL DISTURBANCES FROM LATERAL GENICULATE INFARCTS.

Visual disturbances make up but a small fraction of the literature on visual field deficits.[29,50,55,56] As noted above, the AChA supplies the anterior hilum and the anterior and lateral aspects of the nucleus. The PChA supplies the remainder, including the crown. The classical view that the two sources of supply do not anastomose before or in the nucleus allows the search for distinctive visual field deficits attributable to involvement of one or the other artery.

The visual field is represented in three parts in the nucleus: the anteromedial, which subserves inferior quadrant vision; the crown, serving macular vision; and the lateral, which serves upper quadrantic vision. In the only autopsy-documented infarcts, there was a congruous, complete upper quadrantanopsia involving the macula, with a few degrees of involvement of the upper portion of the lower quadrant. The source of the infarct was an occlusion of the PCA that involved the PChAs, not the AChA.[76]

POSTERIOR CHOROIDAL ARTERY

Cases of occlusion of the PChA seem uncommon. A handful have had autopsy correlation.[20,22,76] Most of the remainder come from imaging or insightful clinical analysis.[4,9,50,59,65]

The elements of the syndrome inferred from the territories known to be supplied by the PChA (sensory loss [posterior tier nuclei of thalamus], visual field disturbances [lateral geniculate body], possible language disturbance [pulvinar of thalamus], and amnestic states [fimbria of hippocampus]) are only infrequently reported, and rarely in combination.

Autopsy Material

The earliest autopsied case known by the authors is that reported by Mohr et al.[56] At autopsy, an embolus was found occluding the left PCA just at the origin of the PChAs. The brain was embedded for serial section (Fig. 21.3). The lesion included unilateral infarction of the fimbria of the left hippocampus, with secondary degeneration of the left fornix and the precommissural bed nuclei of the septum, as well as sharply circumscribed infarction of the lateral geniculate body.

Other necropsy cases include a 52-year-old man who became confused and aphasic and had an infarct in the thalamus in the distribution of the PChAs at postmortem examination and a 67-year-old woman who had abnormalities of vertical eye movements including retractory nystagmus and who later developed a hemiparesis (see Ch. 22 for details).

Imaging Studies

Frisen et al,[29] drawing on patients whose lesion was imaged or inferred by clinical examination, speculated that infarction in the PChA territory could produce not only a hemianopia from involvement of the lateral geniculate body, but hemiparesis and hemihypesthesia from involvement of the ventral tier nuclei of the thalamus. However, they did not report such a syndrome in their two patients. (Fig. 21.1).

Hayman et al[37] reported a case whose clinical details were limited to the remark that the "patient had Dejerine-Roussy (thalamic) syndrome of altered sensation."

Ortiz et al[60] had two cases, one whose MRI showed infarction in ". . . the posterior arm of the internal capsule . . ." while the other affected the cerebral peduncle. Several different sites for occlusion were suggested, including the PChA.

Luco et al[50] described five patients with "ischaemic lesions of the lateral geniculate body . . ." In two, a homonymous hemianopia was found having wedge-shaped features. In another two, congruent superior homonymous quadrantanopia was found, and one showed a quadruple sector defect. The variations in visual field abnormalities were explained by reference to the dual blood supply of the lateral geniculate body.

Ghika et al[32] described three cases of thalamic infarction attributed to the territory of the PChA. Sensory disturbances were present in all of them, and two had features typical of the Dejerine-Roussy syndrome. They also developed delayed movement disorders, which the authors considered a new syndrome, referred to as the jerky dystonic unsteady hand. Whether these findings were identical to those described by Sunohara et al[66] is unclear. No autopsy data were provided; all cases showing CT or MRI abnormalities in the pulvinar of the thalamus were inferred to be from PChA occlusion.

The Lausanne group added seven more cases to their series. Neau et al[59] selected from 2,925 stroke cases, drew on another 10 published cases, and assembled a syndrome of lateral PChA territory infarction. Theirs featured homonymous quadrantanopsia, with or without hemisensory loss and neuropsychological dysfunction (transcortical aphasia, memory disturbances). They considered a homonymous horizontal sectoranopsia unusual but especially distinctive for the syndrome when present. Attempts to describe a medial PChA territory infarction were less successful, in part due to limited case material. Eye movement disorders were more common, and delayed dystonias and pain were infrequent.

Distinctive Clinical Features

PAIN. Occlusion of the thalamogeniculate branch of the PCA (usually considered separate from the posteromedial choroidal artery but sometimes included with it) was the source of the thalamic pain syndrome of Dejerine and Roussy,[16] who reviewed the literature up to 1906 showing that occlusion into this region of the thalamus can produce a syndrome of rapidly improving hemiparesis with choreic movements and ataxia, persisting hypesthesia, and severe paroxysmal pain in the hypesthetic side. Visual field abnormalities were not reported, and whether these cases belong to the syndrome of either AChA or PChA territory infarction is still open to argument.

Ghika et al[32] reported on a patient with an infarct in the left posterior thalamus involving the internal medullary lamina and the pulvinar in the territory of the left lateral PChA. This patient, who was severely hypertensive, had burning paresthesia in his right hand and foot at the onset of the stroke but later developed restlessness, akathisia, and an irrepressible urge to move the right limbs, symptoms that improved after clonazepam administration. Lateral PChA territory infarcts can involve fibers synapsing in the thalamic sensory nuclei, and hemisensory syndromes can result.

VISUAL FIELD DISTURBANCES. The characteristic visual field defect in patients with PChA territory infarcts is a sectoranopia involving a wedge defect on each side of the horizontal meridian.[32,57] Patients with PChA territory infarcts can also have either an upper or lower quadrantanopia. The only autopsied patient studied by the present senior author (J.P.M.) had normal motor function and no abnormality of sensation.[57] The visual field disturbance was particularly striking (see Fig. 17.6).

MEMORY DEFICITS. The present senior author's (J.P.M.) own case[56] (as described in Ch. 20) showed a severe anterograde memory disorder from onset, which persisted unchanged until his death on day 82. In the early days after onset, there were also signs of retrograde amnestic deficit including failure to recall his own address and names of his family, retrograde and anterograde amnesia for the events surrounding his admission, faulty retention of verbal material, impaired retention of a form discrimination test, and an amnestic dysnomia. There is a rich literature on unilateral infarcts in the PCA territory but little of this documents whether such infarcts affected only the PChA territory (see Ch. 20 for details).

MOTOR AND VISUAL DISTURBANCES WITHOUT SENSORY ABNORMALITIES. Cases of motor and visual disturbances without sensory abnormalities appear to be uncommon. The case described by Tekeuchi et al[71] was in Japanese and not available to the authors in translation; it was said to involve left homonymous hemianopsia and left hemiparesis, but no mention was made of sensory disturbances. MRI was used as the basis for the diagnosis.

OTHER CLINICAL DEFICITS. Some other clinical deficits are less well established. Pulvinar ischemia can cause aphasia, visual hallucinations, and abnormal limb movements and postures. The anterior nucleus of the thalamus with its frontal lobe projections can also be involved. In the Stroke Data Bank series of patients with thalamic infarcts, the most common restricted focal infarcts were in the territory of the PChAs. Two of the patients with PChA territory infarcts had prominent contralateral neglect. Little is known about infarcts limited to the pulvinar or the anterior nucleus of the thalamus.

References

1. Abbie AA: The blood supply of the lateral geniculate body, with a note of the morphology of the choroidal arteries. J Anat 67:491, 1933
2. Amarenco P, Cohen P, Roullet E et al: Syndrome amnésique lors d'un infarctus du territoire de l'artère choroïdienne antérieure gauche. Rev Neurol 144:36, 1988
3. Beevor CE: On the distribution of the different arteries supplying the human brain. Philos Trans R Soc [Biol] 200:1, 1909
4. Besson G, Bogousslavsky J, Regli F: Posterior choroidal artery infarct with homonymous horizontal sectoranopia. Cerebrovasc Dis 1:117, 1991
5. Bogousslavsky J, Misklossy J, Regli F et al: Subcortical neglect: neuropsychological, SPECT, and neuropathological correlations with anterior choroidal artery territory infarction. Ann Neurol 23:448, 1988
6. Bogousslavsky J, Regli F, Delaloye B et al: Hémiataxie et deficit sensitif ipsilatéral. Infarctus du territoire de l'artère choroidienne antérieure. Diaschisis cérébelleux croise. Rev Neurol 142:671, 1986
7. Boiten J, Lodder J: Discrete lesions in the sensorimotor control system. A clinical-topographical study of lacunar infarcts. J Neurol Sci 105:150, 1991
8. Buge A, Escourolle R, Hauw JJ et al: Syndrome pseudobulbaire aigu par infarctus bilatéral limite du territoire des artères choroidiennes antérieures. Rev Neurol 135:313, 1979
9. Caplan LR (ed): Posterior Circulation Disease. Blackwell Science Publications, Cambridge, 1996
10. Chamorro AM, Sacco RL, Mohr JP et al: Lacunar infarction. Clinical-CT correlations in the Stroke Data Bank. Stroke 22:175, 1991
11. Cooper IS: Surgical alleviation of parkinsonism: effects of occlusion of the anterior choroidal artery. J Am Geriatr Soc 2:691, 1954
12. Damasio H: A computed tomographic guide to the identification of cerebral vascular territories. Arch Neurol 43:681, 1983
13. Decroix JP, Cambier J, Masson M: Le syndrome de l'artère choroidienne antérieure. Presse Med 14:1085, 1985
14. Decroix JP, Graveleau P, Masson M, Cambier J: Infarction in the territory of the anterior choroidal artery. A clinical and computerized tomographic study of 16 cases. Brain 109:1071, 1986
15. Decroix JP, Graveleau P, Masson M, Cambier J: Infarctus cérébraux et deficit sensitif pur. Rev Neurol 145:111, 1989
16. Dejerine J, Roussy G: La syndrome thalamique. Rev Neurol 14:521, 1906
17. DeJong RN, Itabashi HH, Olson JR: Memory loss due to hippocampal lesions. Arch Neurol (Chicago) 20:339, 1969
18. de la Sayette V, Petit-Taboue MC, Bouvier F et al: Infarctus dans le territoire de l'artère choroidienne antérieure droite et syndrome de l'hémisphere mineur: étude clinique et metabolique par tomographie à emission de positons. Rev Neurol 151:24, 1995
19. Delreux V, Delreux-Ghilain S, Rectem D et al: Syndrome de l'artère choroidienne antérieure avec troubles neuropsychologiques et oculomoteurs. Acta Neurol Belg 87:5, 1987
20. Denny-Brown D: Basilar artery syndromes. Bull N Engl Med Cent 15:53, 1953
21. Derouesne C, Yelnik A, Castaigne P: Deficit sensitif isolé par infarctus dans le territoire de l'artère choroidienne antérieure. Rev Neurol 141:311, 1985
22. Devic M, Michel F, Lenglet JP: Nystagmus retractorius, paralysie de la verticalité, areflexie pupillaire et anomalie de la posture du regard par ramollissement dans le territoire de la choroidienne postérieure. Rev Neurol 10:399, 1964
23. Dowd CF, Halbach VV, Barnwell SL et al: Particulate embolization of the anterior choroidal artery in the treatment of cerebral arteriovenous malformations. AJNR 12:1055, 1991
24. Duret H: Recherches anatomiques sur la circulation de l'encéphale. Arch Physiol Norm Pathol 60:316, 664, 919, 1874
25. Erdem A, Yasargil G, Roth P: Microsurgical anatomy of the hippocampal arteries. J Neurosurg 79:256, 1993
26. Fisher CM, Curry HP: Pure motor hemiplegia of vascular origin. Arch Neurol 13:30, 1965
27. Foix C, Chavany JA, Hillemand P, Schiff-Wertheimer S: Obliteration de l'artère choroidienne antérieure: ramollissement cérébral, hémiplegie, hémianesthésie et hémianopsie. Bull Soc Ophthalmol Paris 37:221, 1925
28. Foix C, Hillemand P: Contribution à l'étude des ramollissements protuberantiels. Rev Neurol 43:287, 1925
29. Frisen L, Holmegaard L, Rosencrantz M: Sectorial optic atrophy and homonymous horizontal sectoranopia: a lateral choroidal artery syndrome? J Neurol Neurosurg Psychiatry 41:374, 1978
30. Furlani J: The anterior choroidal artery and its blood supply to the internal capsule. Acta Anat 85:108, 1973
31. Galloway JR, Greitz T: The medial and lateral choroidal arteries. An anatomic and roentgenographic study. Acta Radiol (Stockh) 53:353, 1960
32. Ghika J, Bogousslavsky J, Henderson J et al: The "jerky dystonic unsteady hand": a delayed motor syndrome in posterior thalamic infarctions. J Neurol 241:537, 1994
33. Ghika JA, Bogousslavsky J, Regli F: Deep perforators from the carotid system. Template of the vascular territories. Arch Neurol 47:1097, 1990
34. Goetzen B, Sztamska E: Comparative anatomy of the arterial vascularization of the hippocampus in man and in experimental animals (cat, rabbit and sheep). Neuropathol Pol 30:173, 1992
35. Grkovic D, Mihic N, Polzovic A, Draganic V: Characteristics of the human lateral geniculate nucleus vascular network. Karakteristike vaskularne mreze humanog lateralnog genikulatnog jedra. Med Pregl 46:96, 1993

36. Hara N, Koike T, Akiyama K, Toyama M: Anomalous origin of anterior choroidal artery. Neuroradiology 31:88, 1989

37. Hayman LA, Berman SA, Hinck VC: Correlation of CT cerebral vascular territories with function: II. Posterior cerebral artery. AJNR 2:219, 1981

38. Helgason CM: A new view of anterior choroidal artery territory infarction. J Neurol 235:387, 1988

39. Helgason C, Caplan LR, Goodwin J, Hedges T 3d: Anterior choroidal artery-territory infarction. Report of cases and review. Arch Neurol 43:681, 1986

40. Helgason CM, Wilbur AC: Capsular hypesthetic ataxic hemiparesis. Stroke 21:24, 1990

41. Herman LH, Fernando OU, Gurdjian ES: The anterior choroidal artery: an anatomical study of its area of distribution. Anat Rec 154:95, 1966

42. Hodes JE, Aymard A, Casasco A et al: Embolization of arteriovenous malformations of the temporal lobe via the anterior choroidal artery. AJNR 12:775, 1991

43. Hommel M, Dubois F, Pollak P et al: Syndrome de l'artère choroidienne antérieure gauche avec troubles du langage et apraxie constructive. Rev Neurol 141:137, 1985

44. Hupperts RMM, Lodder J, Heuts-van Raak EPM, Kessels F: Infarcts in the anterior choroidal artery territory. Anatomical distribution, clinical syndromes, presumed pathogenesis and early outcome. Brain 117:825, 1994

45. Kolisko A: Ueber die beziehung der Arteria choroidea anterior zum hinteren Schenckel der inneren Kapsel des Gehirns. Holder, Vienna, 1891

46. Lazzarino LG, Nicolai A, Valassi F: L'infarto nel territorio di irrorazione dell'arteria coriodea anteriore. Studio clinico e tomodensitometrico di 11 casi. Minerva Med 82: 821, 1991

47. Levy R, Duyckaerts C, Hauw JJ: Massive infarcts involving the territory of the anterior choroidal artery and cardioembolism. Stroke 26:609, 1995

48. Ley J: Contribution à l'étude du ramollissement cérébral. J Neurol Psychiatr 32:785, 895, 1932

49. Leys D, Mounier-Vehier F, Lavenu I et al: Anterior choroidal artery territory infarcts. Study of presumed mechanisms. Stroke 25:1884, 1994

50. Luco C, Hoppe A, Schweitzer M et al: Visual field defects in vascular lesions of the lateral geniculate body. J Neurol Neurosurg Psychiatry 55:12, 1992

51. Mackenzie I, Meighan S, Pollock EN: On the projection of the retinal quadrants on the lateral geniculate bodies and the relationship of the quadrants to the optic radiations. Trans Ophthalmol Soc UK 53:142, 1933

52. Marinkovic S, Gibo H, Erdem A: Huge uncal branch of the anterior choroidal artery. Neurol Med Chir 34:423, 1994

53. Masson M, Decroix JP, Henin D et al: Syndrome de l'artère choroidienne antérieure. Étude clinique et tomodensitometrique de 4 cas. Rev Neurol 139:547, 1983

54. Milisavljevic M, Marinkovic S, Marinkovic Z, Malobabic S: Anatomic basis for surgical approach to the distal segment of the posterior cerebral artery. Surg Radiol Anat 10:259, 1988

55. Miller NR: Walsh and Hoyt's Clinical Neuro-Ophthalmology. 4th Ed. Vol. 1. Williams & Wilkins, Baltimore, 1982

56. Mohr JP, Leicester J, Stoddard LT, Sidman M: Right hemianopia with memory and colors defects in circumscribed left posterior cerebral artery territory infarction. Neurology 21:1104, 1971

57. Mohr JP, Steinke W, Timsit SG, et al: The anterior choroidal artery does not supply the corona radiata and lateral ventricular wall. Stroke 22:1502–1507, 1991

58. Moyer DJ, Flamm ES: Anomalous arrangement of the origins of the anterior choroidal and posterior communicating arteries. Case report. J Neurosurg 76:1017, 1992

59. Neau J-P, Bogousslavsky J: The syndrome of posterior choroidal artery territory infarction. Ann Neurol 39:779, 1996

60. Ortiz N, Barraquer Bordas L, Dourado M: La hemiplejia en los infartos de la arteria cerebral posterior. Un analisis de los diversos mecanismos responsables. Neurologia 8: 188, 1993

61. Paroni Sterbini GL, Agatiello LM, Stocchi A, Solivetti FM: CT of ischemic infarctions in the territory of the anterior choroidal artery: a review of 28 cases. AJNR 8: 229, 1987

62. Percheron G: Les artères du thalamus humain. Rev Neurol 132:297, 309, 1976

63. Poppi U: Sindrome talamo-capsulare per rammolimento nel territorio dell'arteria coroidea anteriore. Riv Patol Nerv 33:505, 1928

64. Salamon G, Huang YP. Radiologic Anatomy of the Brain. Springer-Verlag, Berlin, 1976

65. Serra Catafan J, Rubio F, Peres Serra J: Peduncular hallucinosis associated with posterior thalamic infarction. J Neurol 239:89, 1992

66. Sunohara N, Mukoyama M, Mano Y, Satoyoshi E: Action induced rhythmic dystonia: an autopsy case. Neurology 34:321, 1984

67. Suzuki H, Fujita K, Ehara K, Tamaki N: Anterior choroidal artery syndrome after surgery for internal carotid artery aneurysms. Neurosurgery 31:132, 1992

68. Takahashi S, Suga T, Kawata Y, Sakamoto K: Anterior choroidal artery: angiographic analysis of variations and anomalies. AJNR 11:719, 1990

69. Takahashi S, Tobita M, Takahashi A, Sakamoto K: Retrograde filling of the anterior choroidal artery: vertebral angiographic sign of obstruction in the carotid system. Neuroradiology 34:504, 1992

70. Takahashi S, Ishii K, Matsumoto K et al: The anterior choroidal artery syndrome. II. CT and/or MR in angiographically verified cases. Neuroradiology 36:340, 1994

71. Takeuchi I, Takagi M, Yamagata S et al: A case of posterior choroidal artery infarction. Clin Neurol 32:1125, 1992

72. Tei H, Uchiyama S, Maruyama S: Capsular infarcts: location, size and etiology of pure motor hemiparesis, sensorimotor stroke and ataxic hemiparesis. Acta Neurol Scand 88:264, 1993

73. Touho H, Karasawa J, Ohnishi H et al: Successful intraarterial fibrinolysis of the anterior choroidal artery in the acute stage of internal carotid artery occlusion: case report. Surg Neurol 41:450, 1994

74. Viader F, Masson M, Marion MH, Cambier J: Infarctus cérébral dans le territoire de l'artère choroidienne antérieure avec trouble oculomoteur. Rev Neurol 140:668, 1984

75. Wackenheim A, Ludwiczak R, Capesius P: The course of the anterior choroidal artery. Neuroradiology 31:73, 1976

76. Waither H: Über einen Dammerzustand mit Triebhafter erregung nach thalamusschadigung. Monatsschr Psychiatr Neurol 111:1, 1945–6

Vertebrobasilar Occlusive Disease

PIERRE AMARENCO

LOUIS R. CAPLAN

MICHAEL S. PESSIN (deceased)

Clinicians of the 19th century described in detail the clinical and pathologic findings in patients with softening or hemorrhage limited to portions of the brain stem. Interest lay primarily in defining the anatomy and function of the various brain stem nuclei and tracts. The nature and location of the responsible vascular lesion and the mechanism of the parenchymatous damage were given little attention because they were at that time of no practical concern.

In the late 19th century and in the early years of the 20th century, attention turned to the pathology and anatomy of the intracranial vessels. Interest in the anatomy of the intracranial vessels started with the landmark descriptions by Henri Duret in 1873 and 1874.[206,207] Although isolated cases[334,443] of basilar artery occlusion, usually attributed to syphilitic endarteritis, had been described in the later 19th century, in 1911 Marburg[464] first reviewed the topic of brain stem infarction and described clinical examples of basilar territory syndromes. In 1932 Pines and Gilinsky[567] published a detailed report that included serial sections of the brain stem in a patient with thrombosis of the rostral basilar artery. Meanwhile Stopford[662,663] in England and Foix and colleagues[122,276,279] in France had defined the anatomy of branches of basilar artery and described syndromes caused by paramedian and lateral ischemia. By 1934, Lhermitte and Trelles,[446] in their review of basilar artery arteriosclerosis and its clinicoanatomic consequences showed that pathologists at that time knew that arteriosclerosis (as well as syphilis) affected the intracranial arteries and led to softening and that the basilar artery and its branches were especially vulnerable to atheroma formation.

In 1946 Kubik and Adams[424] published a meticulous analysis of 18 cases studied clinically and at postmortem of patients with occlusion of the basilar artery. They emphasized the severity of the disorder and believed it was diagnosable during life. In their series, the onset was usually abrupt, and death invariably ensued from extensive brain stem infarction. The possibility of patients occasionally surviving was also enter-tained, and clinical details of four living patients suspected of having basilar artery occlusion were included. This landmark report brought the subject of basilar artery occlusion to the full attention of the neurologic community. With the advent of arteriography, and careful pathologic studies of the entire vascular tree, the 1950s saw awakening of interest in the extracranial vessels. Fisher[254] showed that severe atherosclerotic occlusive vascular disease within the internal carotid artery in the neck was a common cause of hemispheral softening. Hutchinson and Yates[372] carefully dissected the cervical vertebral arteries and demonstrated that severe occlusive disease also occurs frequently in these vessels. Meyer and colleagues[491] corroborated arteriographically the frequency of occlusive disease in the basilar and nuchal vertebral arteries during life. In his seminal article on carotid artery disease, Fisher[254] emphasized that warning spells (transient ischemic attacks) frequently occurred prior to cerebral hemisphere infarctions. Others called these attacks "carotid insufficiency."

As the clinical findings associated with posterior circulation infarction became more widely recognized, Williams and Wilson,[752,753] Denny-Brown,[187] Fang and Palmer,[224] Millikan and Siekert,[496] and others called attention to transient episodes of dysfunction within the posterior circulation territory.[757] The term *vertebrobasilar insufficiency* was born, and interest in the 1960s shifted away from the pathology and clinical symptoms to an attempt to understand the pathophysiology of these vascular lesions. Microembolization, intermittent obstruction of the vertebral arteries by bony osteophytes, and clotting and viscosity factors within the blood were identified as important factors. Intense physiologic studies of Denny-Brown[188] added emphasis to the nature and capability of the collateral circulation with its dependence on systemic factors such as blood pressure, blood volume, cardiac output, body position and activity, and pharmacologic agents.

During the 1970s and 1980s, emphasis had shifted from diagnosis to treatment. As a result of a number of uncontrolled observations, enthusiasm for the use of warfarin anticoagulation grew in the 1960s.[497,498] In a review in 1969 Browne and Poskanzer[102] stated, "If anticoagulation has value, it may be more useful in the patient with vertebrobasilar disease, with its high morbidity, than in other forms of cerebral vascular thrombosis." More recently, aspirin and other agents that affect platelet agglutination, such as dipyridamole, sulfinpyrazone, and ticlopidine, have been used in an attempt to modify coagulation factors in patients with posterior circulation disease. Surgically created shunts from occipital artery to long circumferential cerebellar artery branches of the vertebral and basilar arteries and to the posterior cerebellar artery have been devised to increase circulation to the brain stem and posterior hemispheral regions.[42,405,669] Vertebral[375] and carotid endarterectomy[480] and bypass and transluminal dilatation of the basilar artery[668] involve more direct surgical correction of occlusive disease in the posterior circulation.

Advances in interventional neuroradiology now make it possible to introduce catheters and therapeutic agents into the vertebral artery (VA) and the larger intracranial arteries within the posterior circulation. Intravenous and intra-arterial thrombolytic agents such as streptokinase, urokinase, and recombinant tissue plasminogen activator have been infused to lyse thrombi in patients with VA and basilar artery occlusions.[315,560,770,771]

During the 1980s there were also dramatic improvements in diagnostic technology. Brain imaging became possible in the 1970s after the introduction of computed tomography (CT). CT proved useful for posterior circulation hemorrhages but was less helpful in occlusive disease, since the brain stem was difficult to image. Magnetic resonance imaging (MRI), introduced in the 1980s, permitted far superior imaging of brain stem and cerebellar infarcts.[72,414,645] Axial, sagittal, and coronal sections allow localization of brain stem lesions in rostrocaudal, tegmentobasal, and medial-lateral directions. Flow voids on MRI give information about aneurysm and occlusions in the plane of the section. Technology for study of the posterior circulation arteries has also improved greatly. Duplex scanning, color-coded Doppler imaging, and continuous-wave Doppler sonography allow detection of lesions in the extracranial vertebral arteries,[3,75,215,341,448,704,727] and transcranial Doppler ultrasound has improved detection of intracranial lesions.[134,342,691,727] Magnetic resonance angiography (MRA) has promise in allowing safe imaging of the vertebrobasilar vessels without risk to patients.[204,211,212] Transesophageal echocardiography, cardiac imaging, and sophisticated rhythm monitoring now also allow detection of cardiac sources of embolism to the posterior circulation.[140] Angiography using standard arterial catheterization and dye opacification has also become safer with improvements in catheters, dyes, and filming, and with more experienced personnel. Clearly, physicians practicing in the 1990s have much greater capabilities for defining the brain and vascular lesions in patients with vertebrobasilar arterial occlusive disease than was possible a decade ago. The physicians in the 19th and early 20th centuries had virtually no therapy that could influence the course of serious cerebrovascular disease. In the 1990s, we have a variety of potent treatments. Even more important, we have sophisticated technology. Despite the advances, many basic questions remain. How does disease within the vessels produce transient ischemic attacks[6] or stroke, and why in some cases with severe

occlusive disease do many regions escape damage? Why do clinical signs fluctuate? Which patients do we treat? When? With what? For how long?

Posterior circulation disease is not a homogeneous entity. Many patients are severely disabled or die, whereas others suffer only transient or minor disability. The prognosis varies and is dependent on multiple factors, including (1) the nature, locus, and severity of the vascular lesions; (2) the presence of coexisting vascular lesions elsewhere; (3) hemodynamic, circulatory, and coagulation factors; and (4) the congenital constitution of the individual vascular bed. Somehow the studies of the preceding generations have not provided enough specific details regarding the pathophysiology and diagnosis of posterior circulation disease to allow the present-day clinician to be eclectic and precise in choosing optimal treatment for the individual patient. We need to know more about the less frequent causes of posterior circulation vascular disease such as fibromuscular dysplasia, temporal arteritis, and arterial dissection. Within the large entity of vertebrobasilar occlusive disease, we need to delineate recognizable subdivisions that share a common clinical course and prognosis. Treatment could then be studied within somewhat homogeneous subdivisions, rather than being used indiscriminately against an amalgam of heterogeneous lesions that we list under the loose classification of vertebrobasilar disease.

This chapter begins by summarizing the important anatomic relations within the posterior circulation. The pathology of the diseases that affect the extracranial and intracranial vasculature of the posterior circulation is then reviewed, emphasizing the frequency and locale of lesions. Pathophysiologic mechanisms are discussed briefly, since our knowledge of the relative importance of individual mechanisms is scanty. Clinical findings are then subdivided into groups of patients with known documented vascular lesions in the various vessels within the posterior circulation. Finally, diagnostic techniques and treatments are reviewed briefly, even though the value of individual treatment for each problem is almost entirely speculative at present.

Anatomy

The vertebrobasilar arterial system has several unique features. For a period in the embryologic life of the fetus, most of the blood to the hindbrain structures comes from the carotid circulation. Because of its paired systems and the many changes that it undergoes during fetal development, the vertebrobasilar system has a high incidence of variations, anomalies, and persistent fetal vessels. It is one of the only regions in the body where two large arteries merge into a single larger trunk. The posterior circulation also supplies the anterior spinal artery, which usually forms from smaller arterial branches of each vertebral artery. In addition, because the VAs course through and around many bony structures and ligaments and are fixed in a part of their course, they are especially vulnerable to traumatic injury.

Traditionally, the VA is divided into segments[420,658,680] (Fig. 22.1). In the first segment, the artery courses directly cephalad from its origin as the first branch of the subclavian

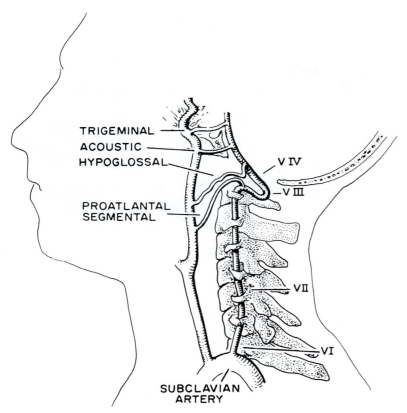

Figure 22.1 Vertebral artery segments and persisting primitive anastomotic connections with the carotid arterial tree (VI to VIV denote vertebral artery segments 1 to 4).

artery to enter the costotransverse foramen of C6 or C5. The second segment is entirely within the transverse foramina from C6 to C2. The third segment is highly tortuous: the VA emerges from the transverse foramen of C2 and courses posteriorly and laterally toward the costotransverse foramen of the atlas. It circles the posterior arch of C1 and passes between the atlas and occiput within the suboccipital triangle. During its course, the third segment of the VA is covered by muscles and nerves and is pressed against bone while being covered by the atlanto-occipital membrane. The fourth segment of the VA is its intracranial portion after the vessel pierces the dura mater to enter the foramen magnum. As the VA pierces the dura, its adventitial and medial coats are less thick, and there is a gross reduction in elastic lamina.[750] Usually at the level of the pontomedullary junction, the two VAs merge to form the basilar artery. The junction is sometimes higher, in which case the VA supplies the mid- and lower pons; occasionally there is a low origin of the basilar artery. The basilar artery becomes somewhat smaller as it travels distally, and frequently it curves slightly in the direction away from the larger VA. It divides near the pontomesencephalic junction to form the two posterior cerebral arteries (PCAs).

Variations are relatively common. In approximately 8% of humans, the left VA originates directly from the aortic arch and not from the subclavian artery (in which case the left VA would not fill from a left brachial injection). Rarely, the right VA arises as a separate branch from the innominate artery and not from the subclavian artery. The VAs are frequently asymmetric (in 45% of people the left is larger, in 21% the right is larger, and in 24% the arteries are of equal size).

The posterior inferior cerebellar artery (PICA) is usually the largest branch of the VA and arises from its intradural segment approximately 1.5 cm from the origin of the basilar artery. The PICA usually arises from the VA an average of 8.6 mm above the foramen magnum but occasionally may originate from the VA as low as 24 mm below the foramen magnum.[279,451] Occasionally, the PICA arises extracranially and courses cephalad within the spinal canal,[225] or originates from the ascending pharyngeal artery.[430] The VA may terminate in the PICA, in which case the distal segment (which usually communicates with the basilar artery) is hypoplastic or nonexistent, and the VA is small compared with the contralateral side.[314] The medial branch of the PICA may also arise directly from the VA, with the lateral branch arising from the basilar artery or more commonly from the anterior inferior cerebellar artery (AICA).[207] One PICA is entirely lacking in 15% of individuals and is hypoplastic in 5%.[465] The posterior spinal arteries may arise from the PICA rather than from their usual VA origin.[293] The PICA and AICA are often reciprocally related in size; for example, a large PICA may supply most of the inferior surface of the cerebellum, whereas the AICA on the same side is quite small and has little cerebellar supply. In the case of a large AICA, the PICA is frequently small. The lateral medulla is rarely fed primarily from the PICA, but in most cases the major blood supply is from direct lateral medullary branches of the VA.[208,271,333] The only part of the medulla that the PICA constantly supplies is the dorsal tegmental area, and this it supplies together with the posterior spinal arteries.[207,208,279] This region is supplied by rami from the medial PICA.[304]

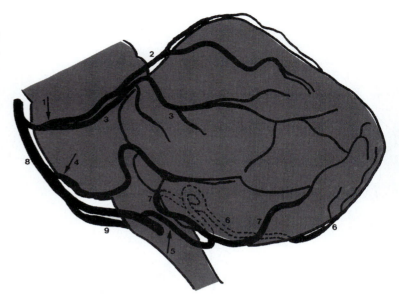

Figure 22.2 Lateral view of cerebellar arteries. 1, Superior cerebellar artery (SCA); 2, medial branch of the SCA; 3, lateral branch of the SCA; 4, anterior inferior cerebellar artery; 5, posterior inferior cerebellar artery (PICA); 6, medial branch of the PICA; 7, lateral branch of the PICA; 8, basilar artery; 9, vertebral artery.

The cerebellum is supplied by the long circumferential vessels[279] (Fig. 22.2); the PICA encircles the medulla and supplies the suboccipital surface in the caudal part of the cerebellum, whereas the AICA encircles the lower pons and relates to a usually small ventral surface in the anteromedial part of the cerebellum, while the superior cerebellar artery (SCA) supplies the tentorial surface (the rostral part of the cerebellum) after encircling the upper pons. When a large AICA is present on one side, the ipsilateral PICA is often hypoplastic, and the AICA territory encompasses the whole anterior inferior aspect of the cerebellum.

The PICA has a sinuous course with several loops (Fig. 22.2). It travels dorsally, lateral to the medulla, below the roots of the 9th and 10th cranial nerves. From there, it goes inferiorly, at a variable level makes the first (caudal) loop, and goes up onto the posterior surface of the medulla in the sulcus separating the medulla and the tonsil. At the top of the tonsil, the PICA makes a second (cranial) loop around the tonsil and then goes downward to the inferior part of the vermis. Sometimes the second loop occurs at the midpoint of the tonsil. Thus, the PICA has lateral medullary, dorsal medullary (ventral tonsillar), superior tonsillar, and dorsal tonsillar segments. The PICA divides into two main branches: the medial (mPICA) and lateral (lPICA) branches.[688] The mPICA climbs along the inferior and dorsal surface of the vermis and the internal part of the hemispheres, making a third loop. The lPICA most often arises from the upper part of the dorsal medullary segment of the parent trunk, between the first and second loops, and then gives rise to several terminal branches to the caudal hemisphere.[310] Sometimes it arises from the first loop. The caudal loop is usually found at the level of the foramen magnum. It can be found below this level, but rami from the lPICA that supply the tonsil are always above the foramen magnum except for instances of tonsillar herniation.[688] Rami from the cranial loop supply the choroid plexus of the fourth ventricle. Two main areas of supply can be distinguished within the PICA territory.[23] The dorsomedial area is supplied by the mPICA, whose territory includes the dorsolat-

eral portion of the medulla. The anterolateral area is supplied by the lPICA, which never supplies the medulla (Fig. 22.3).

The AICA arises from the caudal third of the basilar artery in 75%, sometimes from the middle third, occasionally from its inferior limit, and is lacking in only 4% of individuals.[431,663] However, it can arise from the vertebral or the basilar artery by a common trunk together with the PICA. Rarely, several small vessels arising directly from the basilar artery or from the internal auditory artery replace the AICA. Because of its usual small size, the AICA supplies a small area of the anterior and medial cerebellum (i.e., the middle cerebellar peduncle and the flocculus).[431] Proximal branches of the AICA usually supply the lateral portion of the pons, including the facial, trigeminal, vestibular, and cochlear nuclei, the root of the seventh and eighth cranial nerves, and the spinothalamic tract[24,208] (Fig. 22.3).

The SCA arises from the rostral basilar artery, just before its bifurcation into the posterior cerebral arteries. Each SCA has a short trunk that divides into two main branches: a medial (mSCA) branch and a lateral (lSCA) branch. These two branches sometimes arise separately from the basilar artery, follow the pontomesencephalic sulcus, and pass around the superior cerebellar peduncle to ramify onto the rostral cerebellum (Fig. 22.2). The SCA courses along the anterosuperior margin of the cerebellum. The mSCA starts with a course parallel to that of the lSCA but soon turns medially to reach the lateral surface of the mesencephalon and the inferior colliculus, and from there makes a rostral loop along the superior margin of the colliculus and then courses over the superior vermis (Fig. 22.2). The SCA supplies the rostral half of the cerebellar hemispheres as well as the dentate nucleus.[20] Along its course branches of the SCA supply the laterotegmental portion of the rostral pons (Fig. 22.3).

These three major arteries (the PICA, AICA, and SCA) and their branches are connected by numerous free anastomoses, which limit infarct size in patients who have cerebellar, vertebral, or basilar artery occlusions. Drawings of the territory of each cerebellar artery and their branches conform to the CT and MRI horizontal axial sections (Fig. 22.4).

The major branches of the basilar artery are generally uniform, the most common variation being that the internal auditory artery, usually an AICA branch, may arise directly from the basilar artery. The SCAs are occasionally duplicated or arise from the PCA. Even more uniform are the smaller penetrating branches of the vertebral and basilar arteries.[146,208,271,277,299] There are three groups of arterial penetrators (Fig. 22.5): (1) median arteries, which usually take a slightly caudal course and then penetrate the brain stem and supply the paramedian basal and tegmental regions; (2) short lateral circumferential arteries, which give rise to branches that penetrate the brain stem and supply the intermediate tegmental and basal regions; and (3) long lateral circumferential arteries, which course around the brain stem and supply the lateral basal and tegmental regions. Stephens and Stilwell,[658] using elegant injection techniques, have shown that many lateral circumferential vessels arise from the vertebral and basilar arteries directly, as well as from the long cerebellar vessels. In the medulla and midbrain there are also posterior branches, which arise from the long lateral circumferential cerebellar vessels (the SCA, PICA, and AICA), course in a horizontal and dorsoventral direction, and supply the lateral

Figure 22.3 Anatomic drawings of the territory of cerebellar arteries and their branches at autopsy. (**A**) SCA territory (superior, dorsal view; inferior, lateral view). (**B**) SCA territory (sections from the rostral to the caudal cerebellum). (**C**) lSCA territory. (**D**) Brain stem territory of SCA. (**E**) AICA territory (dorsal and lateral views). (**F**) AICA territory. (**G**) Brain stem territory of AICA. (**H**) PICA territory (dorsal and lateral views). (**I**) PICA territory. (**J**) mPICA territory. (**K**) lPICA territory. 1, flocculus; 2, middle cerebellar peduncle; 3, inferior cerebellar peduncle; 4, superior cerebellar peduncle; 5, dentate nucleus; 6, vestibular nuclei; 7, spinothalamic tract; 8, central tegmental tract; 9, medial lemniscus; 10, nodulus; 11, lateral lemniscus; 12, decussation of trochlear nerve; 13, mesencephalic trigeminal tract; 14, locus ceruleus; 15, medial longitudinal fasciculus. (Data from Amarenco and Hauw[23,24] and Amarenco et al.[31])

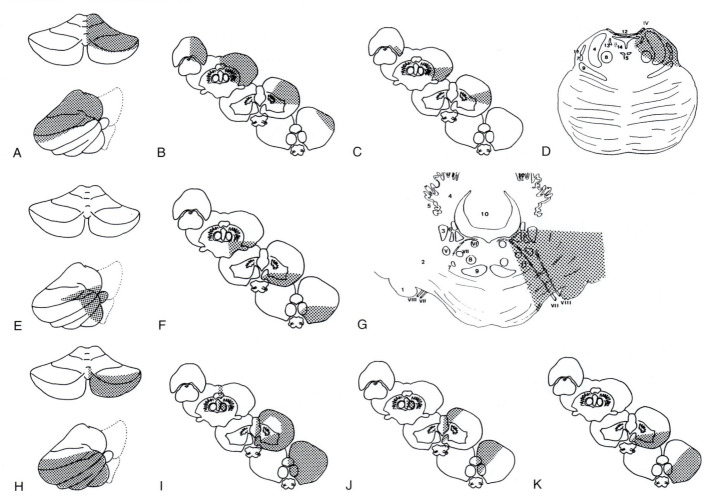

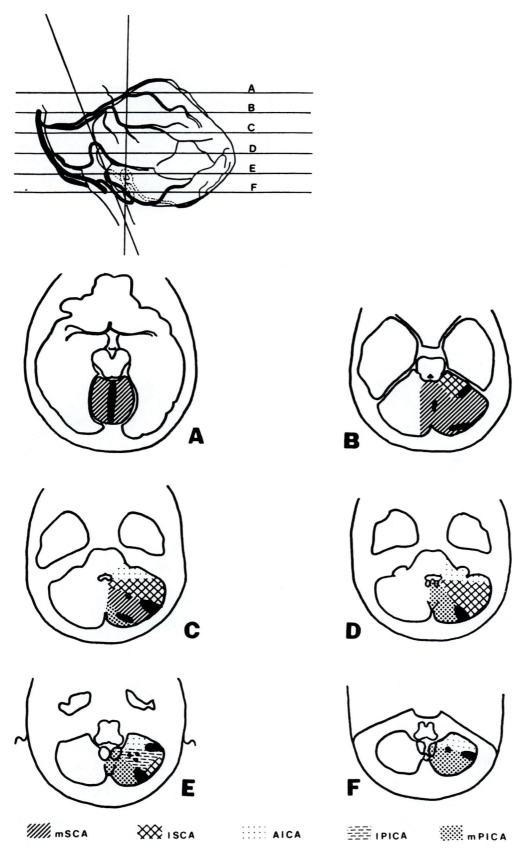

Figure 22.4 Anatomic drawings (**A–F**) of the territory of branches of the cerebellar arteries as they appear on CT and MRI. (Data from Amarenco et al.[27])

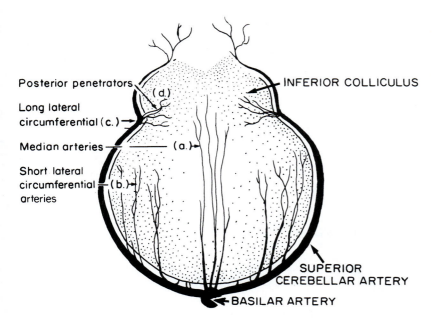

Figure 22.5 Rostral pons with the usual arterial distribution. (**a**) Median penetrating arteries. (**b**) Short lateral circumferential arteries. (**c**) Long lateral circumferential artery. (**d**) Posterior penetrating arteries.

Posterior penetrators

Long lateral circumferential (c.)

Median arteries — (a.)

Short lateral circumferential (b.) arteries

INFERIOR COLLICULUS

SUPERIOR CEREBELLAR ARTERY

BASILAR ARTERY

tegmentum (Fig. 22.5). Penetrating vessels are usually <100 μm in diameter, their size being roughly proportional to their length.[298] The medial penetrating vessels arise from the anterior spinal, vertebral, and basilar arteries as well as from the AICA and PCA; lateral penetrators frequently enter the brain stem along the laterally emerging nerve roots and arise from the vertebral, PICA, AICA, basilar, SCA, and posterior choroidal arteries. The medial tegmental region has a prominent rich collateral supply, making it more resistant to ischemia than the base or lateral tegmentum.

The distal basilar segments are also the source of occasional variations. During early fetal life, the internal carotid artery (ICA) supplies the posterior hemispheres and brain stem via posterior communicating arteries. In one-third of humans, this primitive vascular pattern persists, and the connecting segment from the basilar artery to the PCA (variously called the basilar communicating artery or mesencephalic artery or P1 segment of the PCA) remains vestigial.[298,299,677] In these patients, the PCA may fill from carotid injection, and not after VA opacification. In 2% of humans, this primitive circulatory pattern is bilateral; even more rarely, the basilar artery may be hypoplastic in its distal segment and end in the SCAs.[677] Penetrating branches from the distal basilar communicating artery, SCA, and proximal PCA pass through the posterior perforating substance and supply the paramedian midbrain and diencephalon.

The paramedian mesencephalic arteries arise from the proximal portion of the basilar communicating artery to supply the cerebral peduncle and red nucleus.[208,279,299,359] The lateral midbrain is supplied by peduncular perforating branches arising from the proximal portion of the PCA and from its earliest main branches, the posterior choroidal arteries.[208,359] There are usually two separate paramedian thalamoperforating arteries[131,307,364,553,680,725]: (1) the polar artery (also called tuberothalamic artery) and the preliminary pedicles[145,279,307]; and (2) the thalamic-subthalamic arteries (also called the paramedian thalamic,[552] deep interpeduncular profunda,[307] and the thala-

moperforating pedicle[145,276]). The polar artery arises from the posterior communicating artery and supplies the anterolateral thalamus, including the mamillothalamic tract, the paraventricular region, and a part of the reticular nucleus.[83,131,307] Occasionally the right and left thalamoperforating arteries arise from a common single trunk that originates from the P1 segment of the PCA on one side (Percheron's artery).[552] The lateral portions of the thalamus are supplied by a series of thalamogeniculate arteries, often called the thalamogeniculate pedicle, and not a large vessel, as was formerly believed[148,206,279,658] (Fig. 22.6). The thalamogeniculate pedicle arises from the ambient segment of the PCAs and penetrates the thalamus between the geniculate bodies.[135] These arteries supply the posterolateral and posteromedial ventral somatosensory nuclei, part of the ventralis lateralis, part of the centromedian nucleus, and the rostrolateral portion of the pulvinar. The posterior choroidal arteries arise from the PCAs more laterally and supply portions of the medial nuclei, the habenular nucleus, and the rostromedial pulvinar.

Occasionally, primitive connections from the ICA to the posterior circulation vessels persist into adult life.[446,658,680] The most common persisting channel is the trigeminal artery, which remains in 0.1% to 0.2% of adults.[447] The trigeminal artery arises from the ICA, as it enters the cavernous sinus proximal to the carotid siphon, and penetrates the sella turcica or the dura near the clivus to join the basilar artery between the AICA and SCA branches. The VAs and proximal basilar artery are frequently small or hypoplastic, as is true in many patients with other persistent anastomoses. Persistence of the hypoglossal artery is the next most common variant.[412,447,568] This vessel originates from the ICA in the neck, usually between C1 and C3, and courses posteriorly to enter the hypoglossal canal, from which it joins the basilar artery.[568] A persistent otic artery is a rarer anomaly; this vessel leaves the ICA within the petrous bone and enters the posterior fossa with the seventh and eighth cranial nerves at the internal acoustic meatus, later to join the midbasilar artery. The rarest fetal

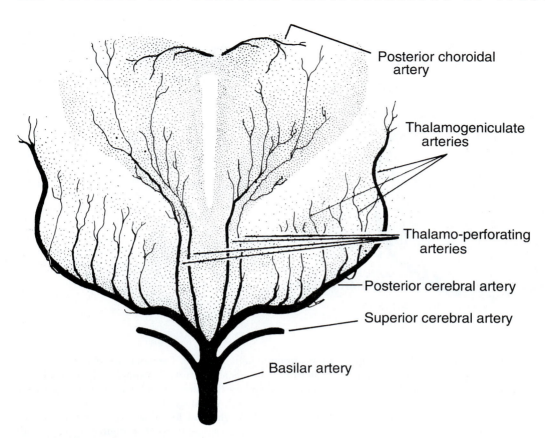

Figure 22.6 Diagram of the thalamic arteries.

communicating channels are the persistent proatlantal intersegmental arteries, which originate from the nuchal internal or external carotid artery at C2 and C3 and join the horizontal (third) segment of the VA suboccipitally.[536] Isolated reports have documented communications between the common or proximal ICA and the lower VAs.[541]

Pathology

ATHEROSCLEROSIS

Atherosclerosis is by far the most common vascular condition responsible for posterior circulation ischemia. Fatty streaks, fibrous plaques, calcified lesions, and complicated lesions (fibrous plaques on which hemorrhage, ulceration, or thrombosis has developed) have all been frequently identified within the larger vessels of the vertebrobasilar system and do not differ qualitatively from atherosclerosis of other vessels.[36,99,124,164,210,230,624] Ulceration in plaques is less frequent in the posterior circulation.[273,624] However, when ulceration occurs, it usually involves the subclavian artery at the origin of the VA or in the most proximal portion of the VA in the neck.[551,624] As in the anterior circulation, thrombosis may

occur in the absence of severe pre-existing atherosclerosis of the vessel wall.[585]

Ulcerated atherosclerotic plaques in the aortic arch have been found in association with posterior circulation ischemia at necropsy.[19,21,218] However, the most common site of atherosclerotic stenosis is at the origin of the VAs.[146,242,372,512,624,745] Plaque forms and may assume a ring-like extension from the subclavian artery to encircle the VA orifice.[242] The left and right VAs are approximately equally affected by atherosclerosis, but there is some indication that when the two vessels are unequal in diameter, the smaller vessel is more frequently occluded.[114,624] The intracranial VA, after it pierces the dura, is another frequent site of occlusive disease.[146,242,512] Aside from these sites, fibrous plaques and fatty streaks are distributed along the VA without any single site of predilection.[146,242,372,512] Often in the second segment of the VA, during its course through the transverse foramina, a ladder-like arrangement of fibrous plaques, seemingly related to the anatomy of the adjacent cervical spine structures, is found.[512] When thrombosis occurs within the extracranial vertebral artery (ECVA), the clot usually develops at a site of atherosclerotic stenosis and seldom forms a long anterograde or retrograde extension.[146,241] By contrast, a thrombus within the extracranial ICA often extends the length of the vessel up to the first branch, the ophthalmic artery. The limited length of the VA thrombus may be related to this vessel's more extensive branching and the possibility that extensive collateral channels keep blood circulating above and below the clot.[237] Thrombus formed within the intracranial VA, however, frequently extends into the proximal basilar artery.[146]

Within the basilar artery, fatty sudanophilic plaques are more prevalent on the ventral surface, and stenosis or occlusion are frequent in the proximal 2 cm of the vessel.[164] In the series of Castaigne et al[144,146] there were six occlusions of the lower third of the basilar artery, five in the middle third, and three in the distal third. In a review of reported cases of basilar artery occlusion, the middle segment of the artery was most often involved, followed in frequency by involvement of the proximal and then the distal third of the artery.[560] In 14% of cases the entire length of the artery was occluded.[560] Atherostenosis of the distal portion of the basilar artery may be common in blacks.[137] Clots within the basilar artery also tend to have limited propagation[145]; frequently they extend only to the orifice of the next long circumferential cerebellar artery (the AICA or SCA). The proximal PCAs are also sites of atherosclerotic lesions, but lesions occur less frequently there than in the middle cerebral artery.[146,512] In Kubik and Adams's[424] pathologic series of 18 patients with basilar artery occlusions, 8 involved the upper third or half basilar artery, 7 the lower half or third basilar artery, and 3 the whole vessel. Embolic material is most often found within the distal basilar tributaries, especially the PCA branches; less often, an embolus lodges in the more proximal vertebral or basilar arteries, especially at sites of luminal encroachment by pre-existing atherosclerotic lesions.[140,146,424] In a series of 30 pathologically verified PCA occlusions studied by Castaigne et al,[146] 15 were artery-to-artery emboli arising as atheromatous debris or clot originating in the more proximal vertebral or basilar artery. One PCA was occluded by an embolus of cardiac origin, and eight occlusions represented extensions of clot from the basilar artery into a PCA. Only three patients had in situ development of thrombosis of the PCA.[146]

Atherosclerotic stenosis of the extracranial ICA occurs approximately twice as often as stenosis of the ECVA,[242,273,512,624] but often both vessels are severely compromised.[371] However, the location and severity of occlusive disease in these two vessels are extremely variable and unpredictable; for example, 60% of the patients studied by Castaigne et al[146] who had occlusions within the vertebrobasilar system had no serious occlusive disease within the anterior circulation. Angiographic studies[60,491,656,719] have corroborated that the origin of the VA, the intradural VA,[699] the basilar artery,[491] and the subclavian artery proximal to the VA origin are the most common sites of occlusive disease. Atherothrombosis in the aortic arch causing artery-to-artery embolism in the posterior circulation has probably been neglected until now because of the lack of clinical diagnostic tools. Its frequency deserves to be investigated now that transesophageal echocardiography is widely available.[716]

The frequency of atherosclerotic lesions in the subclavian and proximal VAs is different in men and women and in persons of different racial backgrounds.[137,231,306] Patients with atheromatous lesions at the origins of the VAs share epidemiologic and demographic features with those who have lesions at the carotid artery bifurcation in the neck.[126,372] There is a strong association of vertebral and carotid artery lesions with coronary and peripheral vascular occlusive disease, smoking, hypertension, and hypercholesterolemia.[126] Men predominate over women.[126] Whites have a relatively higher incidence

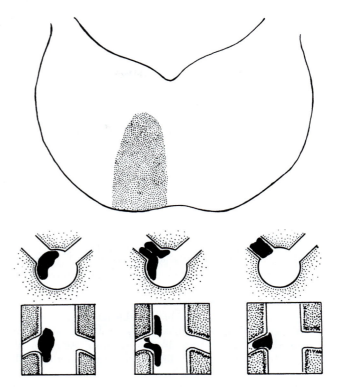

Figure 22.7 Diagrammatic representation of types of branch occlusion. Left to right: Luminal plaque blocking the orifice of a branch, junctional plaque spreading into a branch, and clot in the proximal part of a branch.

of severe extracranial occlusive disease, whereas blacks and persons of Japanese and Chinese ancestry have a preponderance of intracranial occlusive disease, especially of medium-sized branches (the PICA, AICA, SCA, and PCA).[137,231,306,407,582] Blacks, Japanese, Chinese, and women with predominantly intracranial branch disease have a high incidence of hypertension, but a relatively low frequency of coronary and peripheral vascular occlusive disease and hypercholesterolemia. Occlusive lesions of the intracranial vertebral and basilar arteries have less clear sex and racial preponderance.[306]

Atherosclerosis may also compromise the branches of the vertebral and basilar arteries.[123] Whereas AICA occlusions are atherothrombotic in most cases,[21,24,29] either due to basilar artery or in situ occlusions, occlusions of the PICA are equally divided between in situ atherothrombosis and cardioembolism; SCA occlusions are seldom due to atherothrombosis and are most frequently cardioembolic.[21,26,28] Most infarctions in the vascular territories of these vessels are due to narrowing or occlusion of the parent vessel that blocks or diminishes blood flow into these major tributaries.[15,21] The smaller penetrating branches (approximately 0.5 mm in diameter) are vulnerable to occlusive disease. Fisher and Caplan[269] found four such small basilar branch occlusions in a serial section (Fig. 22.7). Two branches were blocked as they traversed the intramural portion of the parent basilar artery, one by a foamy macrophage plaque causing blockage of the orifice of the branch. In the other two vessels, a junctional plaque extended from the parent basilar artery into the proximal branch and occluded the branch lumen. Microatheromata, usually consisting of foamy, fatty macrophage plaques, are frequently seen within the proximal portions of small branches in hypertensive patients. In diabetic patients without documented hypertension, infarction in regions of the pons and diencephalon supplied by paramedian penetrating branches are found three or four times more commonly than in nondiabetics.[554] The morphology of the presumed branch disease in these patients has not been studied but could represent similar microatheromata.[123] Figure 22.7 depicts mechanisms of branch occlusion.

LIPOHYALINOSIS

The pathology of smaller penetrating arteries (<200 μm) within the brain stem parenchyma is qualitatively quite different from atherosclerosis of larger vessels.[124,246,248,263,266] The smaller vessels become occluded by a distinctive process that Fisher[263,266] has called *lipohyalinosis*, which can lead to disorganization and disruption of the lumen of the vessel. In this process, a hyaline material, which readily takes up stains used for fat, accumulates subintimally. The wall of the vessel is weakened, and aneurysmal dilatations occur. At times red blood cells are extravasated through the disintegrating wall.

Lipohyalinosis leads to functional occlusion of the vessel by a subintimal process that obliterates the lumen and leads to ischemia distal to the lesion. Because the ischemic lesions are generally small and somewhat round, the term lacune (hole) has been applied. In addition, the same vascular process can lead to a break in the vessel wall and parenchymatous hemorrhage.[258] Most patients with lipohyalinosis and lacunar

infarctions are or have been hypertensive, although lipohyalinosis is not limited to patients with hypertension. The incidence of lipohyalinosis increases with the age of the patient. Aging itself is associated with adventitial and medial fibrosis in smaller blood vessels but is not correlated with atheroma of larger vessels.

ANEURYSMS

Saccular aneurysms are usually discovered during evaluation of subarachnoid hemorrhage. Occasionally these aneurysms block the orifice of tributary vessels, or a clot within the aneurysm embolizes distally; either mechanism leads to an ischemic stroke.[52] Saccular aneurysms are not common in the posterior circulation but did account for 3.6% (64 of 1,769) of the aneurysms analyzed in the large series of Bull.[104] The most common site within the posterior circulation for saccular aneurysms is the basilar apex (60%); the vertebral-PICA junction (20%) and the basilar-SCA junction (11%) are also common sites, and occasionally aneurysms involve the junction of the vertebral and basilar arteries (3%).[104,543,680] Other sites are quite rare. Aneurysms of the basilar apex may grow quite large, splaying the cerebral peduncle[38] (Fig. 22.8); when these apex aneurysms leak, blood in the interpeduncular fossa may lead to spasm and infarction in the territory of vessels within the posterior perforated substance, producing a complex clinical picture of rostral brain stem ischemia.

Despite their frequency, it is unusual for basilar apex aneurysms to present as an isolated third nerve palsy. Barnes and Ferrario[49] studied 30 patients with posterior circulation aneurysms: all had the clinical features of subarachnoid hemor-

Figure 22.8 Basilar apex aneurysm. (**A**) Anteroposterior view. (**B**) Lateral view.

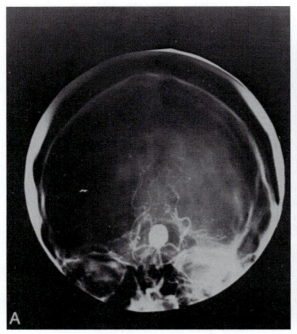
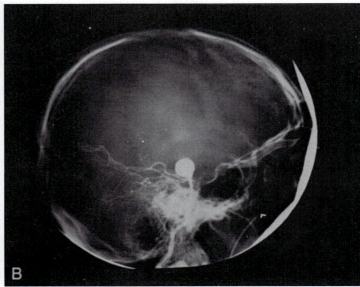

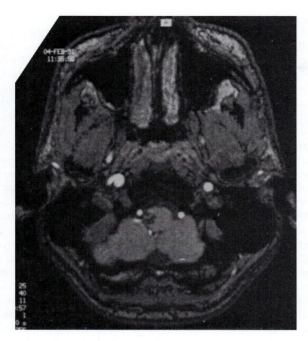

Figure 22.9 T_1-weighted MRI showing lateral medullary infarct sparing the cerebellum.

rhage, and none had a third nerve palsy. Only 4% of aneurysms causing a third nerve palsy arise from the vertebrobasilar system.[49] A single patient with a large aneurysm at the junction of the basilar and left PCAs had paroxysmal hypertension closely simulating a pheochromocytoma[216]; blood pressure normalized after clipping of the aneurysm. Partially thrombosed giant basilar aneurysms are seen on CT scan as calcified, partially enhancing lesions, often near the cerebellopontine angle[524] (Fig. 22.9). However, MRI, MRA, and CT angiography undoubtedly improve their detection.[5,623]

Fusiform (dolichoectatic) aneurysms are tortuous, elongated, ectatic variations of the normal arterial anatomy[768] (Fig. 22.9). Once viewed as uncommon, fusiform aneurysms are now increasingly identified by CT scanning or MRI and MRA, where they appear as dilated enhancing channels crossing the cerebellopontine angle. Fusiform aneurysms of the vertebrobasilar vessels produce symptoms by either compression and traction on posterior fossa structures[516,557] or by ischemia[352] from obstruction of blood flow related to atherostenosis of the vertebrobasilar arteries, local embolism from in situ thrombus within the aneurysm, and compromise of the orifice of tributary vessels.[179,189,214] Headache, located in the occipital-nuchal area, is a common accompaniment. Cranial nerve compression and traction may result in neuropathies, usually affecting the seventh and eighth cranial nerves, resulting in hemifacial spasm, tinnitus, deafness, and occasionally vertigo.[402,530,543,547] Glossopharyngeal and trigeminal-like pain, hiccoughs, and hypoglossal paralysis also result from cranial nerve traction by the aneurysm.[402] Large basilar artery aneurysms may also compress the basis points or cerebral peduncle (leading to spastic paraparesis[493]), may cause hydrocephalus,[214] or may present as cerebellopontine angle masses.[571,579]

VA aneurysms may compress the medulla[469] or upper brain stem.[214]

The pathogenesis of these aneurysms involves congenital and degenerative factors, and occasionally genetic influences. Several reports have documented underlying structural arterial defects, including connective tissue replacement and deficient elastin,[546] fibrous dysplasia and degeneration of internal elastic lamina,[351] and fibrous and collagen replacement of the media. In adults, atherosclerotic changes in the vessels may interact with congenital structural defects to result in fusiform aneurysm formation. Recently, a genetic deficiency in α-glucosidase was found in three adolescent brothers with fusiform basilar aneurysms, two of whom had ruptures of the aneurysms; the third had cerebellar infarction.[461] In some patients with structural defects, the arterial abnormalities are widespread, affecting other vessels.[452,530] An association with aneurysms of the abdominal aorta occurs in up to 45% of patients with dolichoectatic basilar arteries.[291] Fusiform aneurysms therefore appear to represent a heterogeneous mixture of vascular etiologies. Atherosclerosis may be a prominent factor in many adult patients, and other cardiopathies play a role in some patients, especially children.

Dolichoectatic vertebral and basilar artery aneurysms are also readily imaged by MRI and MRA. The heterogeneity of echo densities and morphology of flow voids usually allows detection of thrombus within the aneurysm. MRA accurately detects the vast majority of sizable saccular and fusiform aneurysms.[210–212] Angiography or metrizamide CT cisternography can confirm the diagnosis but are not usually needed if high-quality plain and contrast-enhanced CT or MRI scans have been performed with special attention to the posterior fossa, or if MRA is available.[183]

SPONDYLOSIS

In 1960 Sheehan et al[636] popularized the idea that compression of the VA by osteophytes was a common cause of vertebrobasilar insufficiency. Spondylitic osteophytes project from the vertebral joints adjacent to the transverse foramina through which the VAs course. In cadavers, extreme neck turning can cut off VA flow. When Tatlow and Bammer[686] injected dye into cadavers, turning of the neck revealed minor compression of the VA in the region of C5 to C6 osteophytes. In 26 patients studied clinically and by brachial angiography, the VAs were highly tortuous, with many sigmoid curves, and frequently the lateral concavities of the curves were opposite an intervertebral space.[636] Stenosis was frequent but occlusion rare at the point of maximal concavity.[636] The most frequent loci of disease were the C5 to C6 and C4 to C5 interspaces. However, only two patients developed symptoms on neck turning (dizziness, blurred vision, and confusion), and in only two other patients (not the symptomatic patients) was angiographically measured stenosis worsened by turning. In 6 of the 26 patients, the only symptom was drop attacks, dubiously attributable to vascular disease. Several cogent arguments militate against the argument that spondylosis is a frequent cause of symptomatic vascular compression:

1. In postmortem studies, although slight ridging or streaks are frequently seen in the midcervical area,[512] this region is infrequently a site of severe stenosis or occlusion[146,242,624]; in large radiographic series, severe lateral displacement by osteophytes is rare (2 of 203 cases of Radner[576]).

2. Most reported patients with intermittent posterior circulation ischemia and spondylosis have coexistent atherosclerosis, and some degree of spondylosis is ubiquitous in patients over the age of 40.[323,636]

3. In some patients, spondylosis itself may cause transient rostral spinal cord signs, for example, drop spells.

In other supposed examples of spondylosis-vascular disease, the only symptom is vertigo on neck motion, a common phenomenon in the elderly and one frequently produced by labyrinthine and other nonvascular mechanisms.[268] Blood normally flows in the VAs under arterial pressure; neither cadaver studies nor dye injection in patients accurately depicts the real pressure relationship in each vertebral artery in life.

However, ECVAs can occasionally be intermittently occluded by spondylitic spurs, although this is not common.[153,572,600] In many such patients, the ECVA contralateral to the compressed VA is hypoplastic or previously occluded, or the intracranial vertebral artery (ICVA) ends in PICA. Thus the compressed ECVA is the major supply to the posterior circulation. Chin[153] reported a well-documented example of a patient who developed a left PICA cerebellar and right PCA territory infarct in relation to a high-grade stenosis of the left ECVA at the V4 level. A large vertebral osteophyte projected into the narrowed transverse foramen at this level. My colleagues and I reported a similar case of a patient with intermittent vertigo and downbeat nystagmus provoked by head turning.[600] His ECVA was compressed by a large osteophyte, and symptoms disappeared after removal of the osteophytic obstruction.[600] Similarly, fibrous tissue bands and muscles have occasionally been found to compress the ECVAs, usually in the distal portion of the V1 portions of the ECVAs before they enter the intravertebral foramina.[171,292,324,463] Symptoms are often intermittent and may be precipitated by turning or rotation of the neck during which the ECVA can become occluded. These cases are scarce. Although turning or sudden motion may further compromise kinks or smaller atherosclerotic vessels and can lead to vascular occlusion or dissection, the mechanism only rarely involves spondylosis. Until a clearer relationship between spondylosis and vascular disease can be demonstrated, surgery on spondylitic lesions should not be performed for the sole purpose of treating vertebrobasilar insufficiency.

NECK ROTATION OR TRAUMA

Although earlier reports have described individual case histories of posterior circulation infarction that occurred after neck manipulation, only recently has the mechanism been further elucidated. In 1947 Pratt-Thomas and Berger[574] provided an account of two previously healthy individuals, a 32-year-old man and a 35-year-old woman, who became unconscious during chiropractic manipulation and died in less than 24 hours without regaining consciousness. Occlusion of basilar artery, left AICA, and right PICA with brain stem and bilateral cerebellar hemisphere softenings were found in one patient, and occlusion of the right vertebral and basilar arteries and left PICA in the other. Since this original report, over 50 additional patients have been described in whom posterior circulation stroke followed neck rotation or injury.[281,322,345,422,442,522,592,594,638,762,765] Most cases occur after chiropractic manipulation, but manipulation of the neck by a patient's wife,[281] neck turning while driving a car, wrestling,[594] and practicing archery and yoga[322] have also been implicated. Most of the patients have been young (average age, 37 years)[638] and have had no evidence of pre-existing vascular disease, cervical fractures, or dislocations.

In most patients the syndrome is unilateral, and ischemia is limited to the lateral medulla or pons and the ipsilateral cerebellum.[209,322,442,522,594,638] Arteriography in the patients with predominantly unilateral findings has documented narrowing or occlusion of the VA in its third segment, usually in the region of C2 or C1 before the vessel penetrates the dura. In one patient the occlusive process was in the intracranial vertebral artery;[209] in a single patient with neck trauma and paraplegia the VA was occluded at C6.[658] Only one patient had a lesion at the level of the VA origin, but this patient, who suffered an acute traumatic injury, was studied 7 weeks after the initial injury, a period that would allow retrograde extension of clot.[442] Pseudoaneurysm formation has been seen in five patients, also at the C2 to C1 region. Unilateral lesions tend to develop at the time of neck rotation and often (14 of 21 cases) do not progress.[422] Only 1 of these 21 patients died of the unilateral stroke. Cerebellar softening with subsequent edema and increased posterior fossa pressure may occur and may require surgical decompression.[549]

When initial findings indicate bilateral brain stem lesions, the course is often progressive (9 of 13 cases) and fatal (6 of 13 cases). In approximately one-third of patients, symptoms appear at the time of neck rotation or injury, in one-third symptoms develop minutes or days later, and in one-third symptoms progress after the onset.[638] Autopsy usually confirms extensive brain stem and cerebellar infarctions and thrombosis in the basilar or vertebral arteries. In one patient, the right VA was perforated, with disruption of the media and internal elastic membrane, and hemorrhage surrounded the VA and vein;[638] in one other patient (an 8-year-old boy who fell from a tree), a true traumatic aneurysm of the right VA ruptured, leading to death from subarachnoid hemorrhage.[549] In some patients, the radiographic appearance of pseudoaneurysm suggests dissection of the VA, but this has not often been verified by postmortem examination. Mas et al[472] reported the case of a 35-year-old woman with 3 weeks of cervical pain who developed ischemia in the basilar artery territory following cervical manipulation and died <24 hours later. At postmortem examination, a dissecting aneurysm was found within the third segment of the right VA. Pathologic changes in the lower and upper part of the dissecting aneurysm were different, indicating recurrent bleeding. The hypothesis was that spontaneous dissection had led to the original neck pain, which prompted neck manipulation, which in turn precipitated the stroke by inducing bleeding within the dissecting aneurysm.[472]

Especially susceptible to injury during neck rotation is the third segment of the VA, which lies in relation to the atlas, axis, and atlanto-occipital membrane. Injury to the intima activates clotting mechanisms and leads to the formation of thrombus in the VA, usually at the C2 to C1 region. Thrombus may propagate distally or may embolize to more rostral portions of the basilar arterial tree. Filling defects in the distal vascular bed are occasionally verified angiographically.[119,638] In unusual instances the VA may be perforated, or a dissection may be initiated at the injured segment. Anticoagulation has been occasionally used in an attempt to stop clot propagation and embolization.[638] The variability of the natural course and the scarcity of treated patients make it impossible at present to estimate the utility of anticoagulation in this group of patients.

DISSECTION

Dissection of the vertebral and basilar arteries has been increasingly recognized in recent years following the clinical and angiographic descriptions of ICA dissection.[274] In the posterior circulation, the artery most involved in dissection is the ECVA, usually well above the origin from the subclavian, and below the intradural intracranial penetration of the vessel. The initial reports of dissection of the ECVA were in patients who had had chiropractic or other neck manipulations, but spontaneous dissection or dissection related to trivial trauma has also been recognized.[209,281,289,302,367,422] Minor trauma such as riding on a roller-coaster may cause a VA dissection.[73] VA dissections have been found associated with various pathologic conditions such as Marfan syndrome, Ehlers-Danlos syndrome, pseudoxanthoma elasticum, lentiginosis, systemic lupus erythematosus, fibromuscular dysplasia, and congenital bicuspid aortic valves.[33,616,619,766] Arterial redundancy may predispose to dissections.[48,61] In a series of 51 patients with extracranial artery dissection, 51% had loops, kinks, or coils compared with 16% in 61 controls.[61] Simultaneous dissection of carotid and vertebral arteries are a frequent angiographic finding; however, the occurrence of simultaneous dissection of both cervical and renal arteries in patients with fibromuscular dysplasia suggests that sometimes an underlying morbid systemic process exists.[33] Genetic factors may also predispose to dissection. Whereas the risk of recurrent dissection is 1% a year, it is as high as 50% in patients with a familial history of dissection.[617,618] Recently, several studies of patients with ECVA dissection have been described.[12,119,154,471,509,641] The most common symptom is pain in the head or neck. Usually the pain is in the posterior neck with radiation to the occiput, and sometimes to the shoulder.[641] In some patients, headache and neck pain may be the only complaints. Ischemic symptoms and signs may develop at the same time as the pain or after a delay of hours to a few days. The brain stem regions most susceptible to ischemia from ECVA dissection are the lateral medulla and cerebellum.[154,471,509] The clinical features usually correspond to a partial lateral medullary syndrome. Vertigo and isolated face dysesthesia are common symptoms. Visual blurring, diplopia, and oscillopsia also occur. Ipsilateral cerebellar dysfunction and gait ataxia occur frequently. A Horner syndrome is usually present. If isolated cerebellar infarction occurs, then dizziness and ataxia predominate. Unilateral symptomatic VA dissection may be associated with asymptomatic dissection of the other VA or even the ICA.

ICVA dissection is less common compared with ECVA dissection. Two major clinical presentations have been described: subarachnoid hemorrhage (SAH) and brain stem infarction.[133] Less commonly, the dissection may act as a mass lesion compressing posterior fossa structures.[133] SAH as a complication of ICVA dissection reflects, in part, the differences in vessel morphology of intracranial and extracranial arteries. The intracranial arteries have a thinner media and adventitial layers, and only an internal elastic lamina; extracranial arteries have a thicker media and adventitia and an external as well as an internal elastic lamina. If an intracranial dissection involves the media and spreads to the outer layers, then rupture and SAH may occur. When the dissection occurs in the media and subintimal layers, then obstruction to blood flow from a narrowing of the lumen or local embolism may lead to brain stem infarction. When SAH is present, it is not different from SAH due to saccular aneurysm rupture. Headache, often chronic, is common in all presentations of ICVA dissection. Acute headaches associated with prodromal leaks have been suspected. As with SAH from saccular aneurysms, the outcome is poor. When brain stem infarction occurs, it is usually severe and often fatal. Initial unilateral signs frequently become bilateral with coma and quadriparesis. Deficits limited to the lateral medulla, as in ECVA dissection, are unusual when the dissection involves the ICVA. Dissecting aneurysms of the ICVA may present as mass lesions without SAH or stroke. Headache, neck pain, and progressive lower cranial nerve compressive signs have been the hallmark.[11,116,180]

Dissection of the basilar artery and its major branches is very uncommon compared with VA dissection. Most descriptions are isolated case reports diagnosed at postmortem.[8,217,274,589,740] The commonest clinical presentation is sudden coma with no history of preceding events. Major brain stem infarction correlates with the clinical findings. SAH as the initial presentation of basilar dissection has also been documented. At least one report described dissection beginning in the right ICVA and extending into the basilar artery.[216] Watson[740] described a 32-year-old man who developed headache, confusion, blindness, and pontine dysfunction. The spinal fluid contained no blood. At postmortem examination there was a dissection of the basilar artery between the media and internal elastic lamina, which had narrowed the basilar lumen to a small slit. Unusual loose connective tissue was identified in the media and may have contributed to the dissection. Wolman[758] described a similar case: a 33-year-old man suddenly became comatose and died of brain stem and cerebellar infarction. The basilar artery dissection had begun at the distal end and spread into the PCA and SCA. The lumen of the basilar artery may have predisposed this patient to the dissection. Alexander et al[8] also reported two patients with basilar dissection. One had a month-long chronic course characterized by altered mental state and paraparesis; the basilar dissection had enlarged the vessel, producing considerable mass effect. The other patient, with long-standing migraine, developed sudden brain stem infarction secondary to dissection of the basilar artery. Premonitory symptoms were not noted in any of these cases of basilar dissection. However, Escourolle and colleagues[217] described a patient with a positive serologic test for syphilis who developed severe headache and episodes of left hemiplegia prior to a fixed quadriplegic deficit. Postmortem examination revealed a dissection beginning in the right ICVA extending up the basilar artery to the SCA.

The principal features thought to distinguish carotid artery dissection from atherosclerotic occlusion are (1) local neck or jaw pain, (2) migrainous spells of scintillation, (3) relatively rapid onset with multiple spells (carotid allegro), and (4) Horner syndrome.[274] We have seen several patients in whom VA occlusion was heralded by severe headache, local posterior occipital and nuchal discomfort, and caudal brain stem dysfunction. In some of these cases, angiography has shown a VA occlusion, but the extent of the vascular lesion could not be clarified angiographically, and so the presence of dissection could not be verified. Migraine has been found to be significantly associated with dissection.[172] Some authors have proposed that migraine may predispose to dissection by producing edema of the media of vessels.[740,764] Are we failing to diagnose most examples of VA dissection? Is dissection a more common cause of posterior circulation stroke than is presently appreciated?

VA dissections can be imaged at the C2 and C3 level using high-quality ultrasound with color flow imaging.[705] MRA is also a useful screening test, but the sensitivity and specificity of this method is not yet as good as for carotid artery dissections.[441,603] Standard angiography combined with MRI axial sections of the arteries is still the best way to diagnose VA dissections at present.

FIBROMUSCULAR DYSPLASIA

Fibromuscular dysplasia (FMD) is characterized by hyperplasia of the intima and media of arteries with adventitial sclerosis and breakdown of normal elastic tissue. Thickened septa and ridges protrude into the lumen. At postmortem, basilar occlusion with brain stem infarction has been documented; the basilar artery was severely ectatic and atherosclerotic with focal variations in wall thickness and aneurysm formation. Frens et al[287] and Osborn and Anderson[539] reported patients with homonymous hemianopia and PCA FMD. Cephalic FMD is strongly associated with accompanying intracranial aneurysm.[287,321,488] Six patients in Osborne and Anderson's[539] report presented with SAH from aneurysm rupture. In the Mayo Clinic series reported by Corrin et al[165] 10 of 79 patients had FMD and aneurysm, some with SAH. In a collection of 109 patients with cervical FMD there were 23 intracranial aneurysms. So et al[652] reported 7 patients with Berry aneurysms in their series of 32 patients with FMD and 5 patients with SAH. A relationship between cephalic FMD and dissection has also been noted. In a dramatic example, Ringel et al[589] reported dissecting aneurysms in all four major extracranial arteries in one patient with FMD. The angiographic changes of pseudoaneurysm formation seen in FMD are also commonly described in dissection of cervical vessels.[274] The abnormalities of the media and elastic lamina in patients with FMD may predispose to dissection more often than is presently recognized. The mechanisms of ischemia distal to lesions of FMD are unclear, as are the need for and types of treatment.

TEMPORAL ARTERITIS

Headache and visual loss, the most common clinical manifestations of temporal arteritis, are caused by giant cell granulomatous disease of the ophthalmic branches to the optic nerve and central retinal arteries and the superficial temporal and occipital branches of the external carotid artery. Larger vessels are frequently involved and occasionally lead to symptoms that dominate the clinical picture. Hamrin[320] examined the major branches of the aortic arch in patients with temporal arteritis and found that 10 of 10 had segmental involvement of the subclavian arteries. Klein et al[415] described symptoms related to ischemic involvement of the upper extremities (subclavian artery and its branches) in 20 of 248 patients with temporal arteritis. The subclavian steal syndrome has also been reported as a result of subclavian artery occlusion in temporal arteritis.[571] VA involvement has also been documented in temporal arteritis.[305] The changes invariably affect the VA before it pierces the dura mater, and usually there is an abrupt transition to normal, 5 mm within the dura. Just inside the dura, the normal VA undergoes a decrease in its medial and adventitial coats and thereafter has fewer elastic fibers in the media and external elastic lamina.[751] Similarly, the ICA is affected in its petrous and intracavernous portions just before the artery becomes intradural. VA arteritis can produce brain stem infarction.[751] The most frequently described intracranial vessel pathology in temporal arteritis is thrombus formation without local arteritis; this is probably due to embolization from the extracranial arteritic occlusive disease.[305] Rarely, smaller intracranial vessels, including posterior circulation branches, may demonstrate granulomatous arteritis.[305] The related clinical findings are headache, cerebrospinal fluid pleocytosis, and multifocal cranial nerve and parenchymatous dysfunction, usually without a clear history of strokes.[305]

OTHER PATHOLOGY

Less common diseases affecting vascular structures of the posterior fossa are mentioned only briefly because of their rarity and the lack of data on their special features within the posterior circulation.

Aspergillosis seems to have a special tropism for the posterior circulation vessels.[736] It involves the brain by infarction due to occlusion of distal branches in the cerebellum or occipital lobes. Infarctions are frequently small and hemorrhagic. Later, abscesses may develop at the border zone of the infarcted area. Aspergillosis is a usually nosocomial fungal infection that disseminates via blood route and that develops in the presence of oxygen, which explains why the border zone area of infarcted tissue is the best site for development of an abscess. It rarely occurs together with meningitis, contrary to cryptococcosis, another fungal infection.[767] Mechanisms of arterial occlusion are (1) thromboangiitis with presence of aspergillosis in the arterial wall and in the thrombus, and (2) embolic occlusion from an endocarditis due to *Aspergillus*.[736] Endocarditis is most difficult to diagnose even with transesophageal echocardiography but is found as frequently as in 50% of patients at autopsy.[737] Diagnosis of aspergillosis infection in the presence of brain infarctions is usually very difficult and is based on repeated serology, biopsy, and culture of an associated arthritis or spondylitis infection,[678] culture of a catheter of perfusion, or presence of pneumonia due to *Aspergillus*, especially in severely ill patients in intensive care units, those chronically polyinfected, or drug users.[142,767]

Other fungal and tuberculous meningitis commonly produces changes within vessels, most often in branches of the middle cerebral artery and in arteries that traverse the interpeduncular fossa to penetrate the rostral brain stem. The exudate somehow produces a reaction in the media of these vessels usually referred to as Huebner's arteritis. Sudden stupor may be due to infarctions of the brain stem, often with third cranial nerve palsies and bilateral pyramidal tract dysfunction. Headache, fever, cranial nerve palsies, and confusion dominate the clinical picture, and examination of the cerebrospinal fluid usually confirms the diagnosis.

Fibrous bands crossing the proximal VA before it enters the transverse foramina may constrict the vessel when the neck is turned.[463]

Sickle cell disease is associated with occlusion of small and larger vessels[759]; the larger vessels frequently show extensive intimal proliferation of fibrodysplasia, possibly related to abnormal flow mechanisms.[486] Stroke often occurs during a sickle cell crisis and is heralded by seizures. Few data are available concerning the findings related to posterior circulation occlusion in this group of patients; pseudobulbar signs are more common than bulbar paralysis.

Young women on oral contraceptives may suffer occlusion of the ECVA, and for unclear reasons basilar artery occlusion occasionally occurs in the first 2 decades of life.

Syphilis can also produce an arteritis and can be associated with brain stem infarcts, usually in branch distribution.

Systemic lupus erythematosus and granulomatous angiitis do affect cerebral blood vessels, but a stroke-like picture is rarely found. CT scan or MRI shows very small infarcts often in border zone areas of the cerebellum or occipital lobes.[27]

Homocystinuria, Marfan syndrome, Ehlers-Danlos syndrome, pseudoxanthoma elasticum, polyarteritis nodosa, Kohlmeyer-Degos disease, and *Fabry's disease* are associated with ischemic strokes, but little is known of the incidence and site of involvement in the vertebrobasilar system in these diseases.

Takayasu's pulseless disease often involves the subclavian artery and VA orifices as well as the aorta.[377,459] Occasionally, the intracranial arteries also show intensive inflammation typical of Takayasu's arteritis.[510] Brain stem lesions are especially common in Behçet syndrome.[479]

Behçet's disease was described by a Turk and is common in the Middle East and mediterranean countries. Clinical findings include aphthous stomatitis and genital ulcers, uveitis, cells in the spinal fluid, and multifocal neurologic signs.[346,630] The neurologic symptoms often relate to the brain stem and develop quickly or gradually. CT usually shows a low-density abnormality and T_2-weighted MRI an area of hypersignal in the brain stem, cerebellum, or cerebral white matter that enhances acutely.[346] Mass effect may be seen. With time, enhancement is lost, and the patient stabilizes or improves. Angiography usually does not show arterial occlusions, but dural sinus occlusions are common. At necropsy inflammatory lesions are seen with perivascular lymphocytic cuffing around capillaries and ventricles, especially in the brain stem.[346]

Table 22.1 Pathophysiology of Tenuous Equilibrium after Occlusion of an Artery

Factors Promoting Deficit	Factors Defending Against Deficit
Blood flow to lesion diminished by stenosis of occlusion	Collateral circulation and autoregulation
Embolization from plaque or clot	Passing of emboli
Activation of clotting factors	Thrombolysis (?)

Pathophysiology

LUMINAL OBSTRUCTION

Many factors determine whether or not an ischemic tissue becomes infarcted. Blockage of the lumina of blood vessels by atheroma, clot, or swollen vessel wall, embolization of intraluminal material distally, and activation of clotting factors with propagation of clot all act to increase luminal obstruction and diminish blood flow to a given region. However, concomitantly, reduction of flow to a region leads to accumulation of metabolites, especially lactate, and an increase in collateral circulation. Fibrinolysis and other enzymatic processes act to lyse and solidify the local clot. Embolic fragments pass through the vascular bed, allowing resumption of flow. In addition, systemic factors such as blood pressure, cardiac output, blood viscosity, red blood cell count, and pulmonary function all affect the rheology and oxygen-carrying capacity of the blood reaching a given ischemic region. The sum of these factors determines the survival of a given ischemic zone. The process can be viewed schematically (Table 22.1) as the summation of vectors, those tending to increase ischemia, and those promoting additional blood flow to reduce the ischemic deficit.

Within the posterior circulation, there are multiple collateral channels for augmenting flow. Reduction of flow through a VA can often be compensated for by collaterals from the opposite VA, the thyrocervical trunk, and occipital artery branches of the external carotid artery, which direct flow toward the nuchal vertebral artery. Intracranially, the long circumferential cerebellar arteries (the AICA, PICA, and SCA) form an active collateral system. For example, in a lesion blocking flow in the proximal basilar artery, blood can course from the VA to the PICA, and into hemispheral branches of the AICA and SCA, and back to the basilar artery beyond the region of blockage. Similarly, blood may pass from the SCA to AICA or PICA branches. The ICA may serve as a major source of collateral circulation, with blood flowing via the posterior communicating artery to the PCA and down the basilar artery and SCAs, the latter supplying collaterals to the lower brain stem through the cerebellar hemispheral branches. Collateral circulation is especially rich in the brain stem tegmentum, making this region more resistant to ischemia. The time course of development and progression of symptoms is well correlated with prognosis and gives information about the sum of pathophysiologic factors operative in the individual patient.

Symptoms develop in one of the following temporal patterns: (1) transient ischemic attacks (TIAs), either as an isolated finding or preceding a stroke; (2) sudden-onset deficits that are maximal at onset; (3) fluctuating clinical deficits punctuated by improvements and deteriorations; and (4) gradually progressive stroke. In a series of personally observed cases of vertebral or basilar occlusion, the temporal course was analyzed.[110,138] Most patients had TIAs. These often were multiple and variegated and increased in frequency as the stroke approached. In these patients, the stroke often was noticed on arising. Symptoms and signs of brain stem, cerebellar, and posterior cerebral territory ischemia then fluctuated for a period of 2 to 3 weeks and stabilized thereafter. During this 2- to 3-week period, clinical fluctuations were quite sensitive to blood pressure and postural changes.[110,118] Simply sitting up or raising the head of the bed to eat could cause temporary aggravation of a deficit, which was quickly relieved by lowering the head. The presence of preceding TIAs indicates some chronicity to the occlusive process, allowing more time for collateral circulation to develop. Improvement in function indicates that collateral circulation has developed or the occlusive process is less operant (e.g., lysis of embolic clot). Perhaps for these reasons patients with TIAs and a fluctuating course have a better prognosis. Other patients had sudden-onset deficits sometimes heralded by TIAs or progressive accumulation of deficit without significant temporary improvement in function. Sudden-onset deficits are usually embolic. Prognosis depends on the length of time the embolus blocks the vessel and clot lysis or passage. Steady progression of symptoms without stabilization or improvement indicates poor formation of collaterals and has a bad prognosis.

Few reports have considered the temporal course. Jones et al[384] analyzed the course of 37 patients with vertebrobasilar territory infarction; 12 had had at least one preceding TIA, and in 30 patients the onset of stroke was precipitous. Fluctuations commonly occurred during the first week but were unusual thereafter. Progressive deterioration in function was common (16 of 37 cases), usually reached its maximum within the first 4 days, and had a bad prognosis. Similarly, Patrick et al[545] reviewed 39 patients with vertebrobasilar territory infarction and commented on the instability of the early clinical course but rarity of late (over 3 weeks) progression. In neither series was there frequent corroboration of the nature and locus of the vascular lesion during life.

TIAs are caused by either diminished blood flow (with temporarily insufficient collateral circulation) or embolization of clot or plaque material. In our experience, frequently recurring brief TIAs (machine-gun-like flurries) usually indicate a severe proximal stenosis or occlusion, whereas occasional but longer lasting spells are more likely embolic. The fixed deficit is often noticed in the morning, having accumulated at night during a time of more sluggish flow. Once the vertebral or basilar artery is occluded, propagation of clot, embolization, and diminished blood flow may result. The critical period for development of neurologic deficit is at the time of occlusion and during the next few weeks. During this time collateral circulation is developing, and the clot becomes adherent to the vascular wall and is thereafter more resistant to embolization. Denny-Brown[187] emphasized a contributory role of systemic factors in compounding the clinical deficit and called these fluctuations *reversible hemodynamic crises*. These factors seem most operant in the first 2 weeks after vascular occlusion

and were less clinically important thereafter. Sundt and Piepgras[671] also emphasized the effect of postural changes on flow during the early critical period. Naritomi et al[525] showed that reduction in regional blood flow to the posterior circulation, as measured by xenon inhalation, rarely persisted 3 weeks after transient ischemic symptoms, but that defective autoregulation (i.e., change in flow after induced postural hypotension) was more widespread and long lasting after vertebrobasilar insufficiency than after carotid attacks. Careful scrutiny of blood pressure, maintenance of blood volume and optimal oxygenation, and careful surveillance of patients when they assume sitting or upright postures is very important during the first few weeks after a vertebrobasilar territory stroke, because collateral circulation is still developing. This is especially true in occlusive disease of larger vessels (vertebral or basilar artery), but extension of deficit after reduced blood pressure may also occur in basilar branch occlusion.[264]

INTRA-ARTERIAL EMBOLISM

Embolic occlusion is considered by some to be unusual in patients with vertebrobasilar infarction; this assumption is mostly based on autopsy observations, which included only patients with proven VA, basilar artery, or branch occlusion, ignoring cases coming to autopsy with no more occlusion in the vertebrobasilar system, which is the rule for embolic occlusion after physiologic thrombolysis[146]; however, Castaigne et al[146] have documented the frequency of emboli within the PCAs, and syndromes related to the rostral basilar artery are likely to be more frequently embolic.[112] Other frequent recipient sites for embolism are the SCA, PICA, and distal VAs.[15,19,21]

Artery-to-artery embolisms do occur within the posterior circulation, but their frequency has not been documented. Emboli probably account for the sudden-onset deficits. The most important donor sites for intra-arterial emboli are the aortic arch, subclavian artery, VA origin, and distal VA.[121] The most frequent donor sites are the VA origin (either recent thrombosis[132] or ulcerated plaques[551]) and the ICVA. Among a series of 67 patients with brain stem and cerebellar ischemia, 9 (13%) had intra-arterial embolism as the mechanism of stroke.[140] Among these 9 patients, the donor site was the proximal ECVA in 5, distal ECVA dissection in 3, and a thrombus within the ICVA in 1. Emboli went to the ICVA-PICA in 3, the basilar artery in 3, and the basilar artery-SCA region in another 3.[140] Embolism from VA origin occlusive disease has been recognized in a series of 10 patients with distal intra-arterial embolism. The VA lesions were complete occlusion in 7 patients and severe atherostenosis in 3. Recipient sites were the intracranial VA-PICA in 8 cases and the distal basilar artery and its SCA and PCA branches in 7 patients.[132] Cardiac cavities are other important donor sites of embolism and probably the most prevalent in posterior circulation infarction, especially cerebellar and occipital lobe infarctions.[21,28,150,151]

WORSENING

Generally, progressive neurologic deficits usually imply propagation of clot or failure of collateral circulation to compensate for reduced flow. If a larger vessel is involved, this usually implies a poor prognosis.[110,396] Another cause of worsening of symptoms within the posterior circulation is infarction of the cerebellum with progressive swelling and pressure on the brain stem and ventricular pathways.[435] This problem has high mortality, but it is amenable to surgical decompression. Progression of deficit can also occur within the territory of a basilar branch, but this usually occurs over a shorter period of hours to 1 week, and the deficit is limited to the territory supplied by the single branch or its previously occluded neighboring branches.[247]

Worsening can also be caused by alterations in cardiovascular and respiratory function resulting from ischemic brain stem dysfunction. Lability of blood pressure and blood flow can result from lesions of the medulla and pons.[406] Reis et al[580] have also documented the importance of the fastigial nucleus of the cerebellum in altering vertebral blood flow. Stimulation of regions within the brain stem tegmentum can alter heart rate and rhythm.[50,450] Khurana[406] described persistent tachycardia, orthostatic hypotension without cardiac acceleration, episodic bradycardia, and even cardiorespiratory arrest in four patients with bilateral pontomedullary lesions. Even unilateral lesions can be accompanied by tachycardia and lability of blood pressure. Bogousslavsky et al[80] reported two patients studied clinically and at necropsy with severe hypoventilation related to lateral tegmental pontomedullary infarcts. Intermittent apnea, especially during sleep, and failure to respond during CO_2 retention were prominent features, and each patient died of the complications of respiratory failure.

Activation of clotting factors, polycythemia, or thrombocytosis can exaggerate occlusive disease and in some situations may alone be responsible for sluggish posterior circulation flow and clinical attacks. One patient with an elevated hemoglobin and platelet count and increased platelet agglutination developed frequent spells of vertebrobasilar ischemia and claudication of the legs; no lesion could be seen angiographically, and the spells disappeared after aspirin therapy. This experience prompts the suggestion that a hematologic survey be part of the evaluation of all patients with transient or persisting ischemic symptoms. In the individual patient, the anatomic location of the lesion producing the neurologic signs and the time course development of the deficit help the physician predict the affected vessel, the nature of the pathologic process in the vessel, and the adequacy of collateral circulation. Laboratory investigations, especially angiography, confirm the location of the responsible vascular lesion, give additional information concerning previous pathology or maldevelopment in other extracranial and intracranial vessels, and help define the source and adequacy of collateral circulation.

Clinical Findings in Patients with Vascular Lesions at Various Locations

SUBCLAVIAN AND INNOMINATE ARTERY OCCLUSIVE DISEASE AND SUBCLAVIAN STEAL

In 1961 Reivich and colleagues[581] reported their observations of two patients with TIAs referable to the posterior circulation. Each patient had diminished pulse and blood pressure in the left arm. Attacks were precipitated by exercise in one patient and by change of head posture in the other. Angiography in each case revealed stenosis of the subclavian artery proximal to the origin of the left VA. In one case the left ICA was also occluded. Blood flowed from the normal right VA into the cranium and then down the left VA in a retrograde fashion and filled the distal left subclavian artery. In the laboratory, these investigators occluded the left subclavian artery of dogs and measured blood flow in the other great vessels. In this artificially induced situation they documented a compensatory increase in flow through the right VA. Fisher,[244] in an accompanying editorial in the same edition of the *New England Journal of Medicine*, unsigned, as was the custom at the time, coined the term *subclavian steal*, referring to the siphoning of blood away from its proper cranial destination toward the ischemic arm.

Within the next few years angiography in similar groups of patients documented reversal of flow in the VA due to subclavian artery occlusive disease and showed that the phenomenon was not rare.[174,239,348,534,544,639] The reaction to these reports was immediate and widespread. Coming at a time of rapid growth in the use of angiography and surgical interest in cerebrovascular disease, lesions of the subclavian artery were avidly sought and surgically repaired. More importantly, the concept of blood flowing from one vessel to rescue a more distant circulation gave rise to the concept that the cerebrovascular bed was an open net in which decreased input at any point of entry could conceivably lead to decreased flow in any distant site. To determine ischemia at a distance, clinicians would fully opacify the entire vascular bed, including the aortic arch and the four major extracranial vessels. Any obstructive lesion, even if it did not directly supply the ischemic region, would then be surgically repaired.

In the two decades since the original report, a clearer definition of the clinical findings and further reflections on the place of surgery in the treatment of subclavian steal has been worked out. Patients with subsequently verified subclavian steal may present with one of several types of symptoms: (1) headache, (2) intermittent episodes of cerebral ischemia, or (3) claudication or pain in the ischemic arm. However, many patients have no symptoms referable to the subclavian lesion. They are discovered only when angiographic or noninvasive evaluation of pulse or blood pressure changes in the arm, peripheral vascular disease in the legs, or abnormalities in the carotid circulation reveal the subclavian lesion. In a study of 324 patients with subclavian steal detected by noninvasive techniques, Hennerici and colleagues[340] found that 116 of the 155 patients (74%) who had unilateral isolated subclavian steal and no severe carotid artery disease had no neurologic symptoms.

Headache is common and is usually located in the mastoid, occiput, or neck. The major symptom of the first patient of Reivich et al[581] was recurrent throbbing pain in the left mastoid area, which radiated to the left parietal and occipital regions. The headache may be more generalized and may be isolated or accompany symptoms of cerebral ischemia. The headache may be precipitated by exercise. Surprisingly, symptoms of severe ischemia in the involved arm are rare. Patients may complain of fatigue, claudication on exercise, paresthesia, sensitivity to cold, and sensations of heaviness or coolness in the arm. These are often exercise related. The usual slow development of the occlusion and the richness of collateral supply tend to make upper extremity ischemia a relatively minor problem unless the patient exercises the arm frequently, as would be the case in a golfer or baseball pitcher.

Athletes, especially baseball pitchers, seem to have an increased incidence of subclavian artery occlusive disease, or at least the sufferers are brought more frequently to public attention.[238,240,665] Sudden downward arm motions can cause angulation of the artery over the first rib or a cervical rib where the subclavian artery courses over the flat surface of the first rib on its way out of the thorax. Pitchers and cricket bowlers may subject the subclavian arteries of their throwing arms to chance trauma with subsequent thrombosis. Fatigue, arm pain, loss of pitching velocity and accuracy, and lack of stamina in the throwing arm results. In the large series of Hennerici et al,[340] one-third of patients reported pain, numbness, or fatigue in the arm, but only 15 of 324 patients (4.8%) had objective signs of severe brachial ischemia or embolism.

Cerebral symptoms are common but usually transient, lasting seconds to minutes but often recurring over a period of months or even years.[534,639] In many patients, subclavian stenosis is caused by severe atherosclerotic disease; coexistent significant atherosclerotic lesions in the carotid artery and other extracranial and intracranial vessels are quite common and might even be considered the rule rather than the exception. This fact often makes the origin of transient ischemic cerebral symptoms difficult to discover. For example, the second patient of Reivich et al[581] had a transient episode of aphasia and right-hand paresis. Evaluation revealed complete occlusion of the left ICA, which at surgery contained fresh clot, as well as subclavian steal. Of the nine patients with subclavian steal reported by North et al,[534] only three had permanent deficits; each patient with a lasting deficit had hemiparesis, and all had significant ICA occlusive disease (two bilateral and one unilateral). In all other series, the incidence of associated vascular lesion was high.[340] In the series of Hennerici et al,[340] lateralized hemispheric symptoms of cerebral ischemia were about twice as frequent in patients with unilateral subclavian steal and associated carotid disease as in those without carotid lesions. Hemispheric brain symptoms occurred more often (29 patients, 66%) in patients with severe carotid artery stenosis than in those with less severe obstruction (18 patients, 32%). The arm may show more cyanosis when held above heart level. A bruit may be heard in the supraclavicular region and may radiate into the axilla or along posterior neck to the mastoid region. Sometimes one can distinguish the subclavian or vertebral origin of a bruit by pumping the blood pressure cuff above systolic pressure. This maneuver decreases distal subclavian flow but may increase cephalad flow in the VA, because blood goes into the proximal branches rather than the arm. In disease of the proximal subclavian artery, the bruit usually decreases because of less flow through the stenotic segment and less retrograde vertebral flow; in stenosis of the vertebral artery, the bruit is usually augmented. Focal neurologic deficits caused by subclavian-vertebral siphonage are rare and are usually explained by coexistent carotid artery disease, which should be sought on examination.

The most common etiology of subclavian occlusive disease is atherosclerosis, although congenital lesions such as preductal coarctation of the aorta with patent ductus arteriosus,[180] atresia of the left subclavian artery,[295] and a pseudocoarctation

of the aorta with kinked left subclavian artery[453] occasionally produce the syndrome. Sometimes subclavian steal follows surgical manipulation of the subclavian artery, as in the Blalock-Taussig procedure for tetralogy of Fallot, in which the subclavian artery is anastomosed to the pulmonary artery. Traumatic injury, embolism, and arteritis (temporal arteritis and Takayasu's arteritis) may also cause subclavian steal. In the large series of North et al,[534] the left subclavian artery was affected alone in 33 instances, whereas the right subclavian or innominate artery was affected in 13 cases, and 13 cases were bilateral.

The frequency with which the arteries are affected varies. The left subclavian artery is involved approximately three times more frequently than the right innominate or subclavian arteries. Among 155 patients with a unilateral subclavian steal in one series, 71% were left-sided, and 29% had Raynaud's phenomenon. In the subclavian artery, occlusive disease does not always cause retrograde vertebral flow. Of 20 cases of subclavian artery stenosis evaluated by Berguer et al,[65] only one-half had evidence of reversed VA flow. There are many other possible collateral channels to augment distal subclavian flow, including the inferior and external thyroid, internal mammary, intercostal, and ascending cervical arteries.[47] At times, the VA ipsilateral to the subclavian artery stenosis originates from the aortic arch, ends distally in the PICA, or is tiny or occluded, and so is unavailable as a source of collateral supply.[225]

The anatomy of the right side of the aortic arch differs from that of the left. The innominate artery is larger and usually rises higher in the supraclavicular fossa than its left counterpart. The right subclavian artery has a more intimate relationship with the right common carotid artery. Clot in the right axillary or subclavian artery may propagate into the innominate artery and extend or embolize to the carotid system. Although this phenomenon is rare, most of the patients have been young and have presented a striking clinical picture. Symonds[675] described two patients with diminished arterial pulsation in the right arm, probably due to a cervical rib in which sudden left hemiplegia developed. Yates and Guest[765] reported a patient with progressive pain and weakness in the right arm who had an ununited fracture of the right clavicle. This patient suddenly experienced visual loss, went into a coma, had left hemiplegia, and subsequently died. The right subclavian artery at postmortem was displaced by the fractured bone and occluded. Clot extended into the innominate artery and had embolized to the basilar artery bifurcation. Hoobler[361] reported a similar patient with a cervical rib, weak right arm pulses, and sudden left hemiparesis. Damage to the subclavian artery may be caused by cervical ribs, trauma, or the use of crutches. Clot or aneurysm forms at the site of compression and leads to symptoms of ischemia or Raynaud's phenomenon in the arm; the clot will embolize on the right, into the distal carotid or vertebral arterial tree. Although a similar lesion could occur on the left, it would only involve the left VA and might be difficult to recognize.

Stenosis or occlusion of the innominate artery is less common than is subclavian artery disease. Brewster and colleagues[96] collected 71 patients operated on in one hospital for innominate artery lesions during a 20-year period. In this series, 36 patients had atherosclerotic occlusive disease involving the origin of the innominate artery from the aortic arch or the heart.

Diagnosis of subclavian steal in the early series was usually confirmed by angiography, which is best done by selective transfemoral or transaxillary catheterization of the normal VA with delayed films to show retrograde flow down the contralateral VA. Furthermore, the internal carotid and intracranial circulation can also be visualized during the procedure. Arch angiography provides suboptimal detail of the involved vessels. In addition, more dye is required for arch angiography, and complications are more frequent. Digital subtraction angiography, using intravenous dye instillation, has also been used to show the subclavian-vertebral artery anatomy in the neck.[427,741] However, the complication rate is relatively high, and often opacification and imaging is suboptimal and not diagnostic. Arterial injection using computerized subtraction technology is much more effective and is relatively safe. MRA currently may allow accurate imaging without the need for invasive dye injection.[204,211,212]

Now noninvasive testing accurately documents severe innominate and subclavian artery occlusive disease with a high degree of reliability.[341,342,727] Ekestrom and colleagues[215] used serial measurements to test subclavian flow and detect reversed VA flow; these techniques included forearm blood flow measurement by oscillography, venous occlusive plethysmography of the arm, Doppler ultrasound with the patient in a sitting position, and directional flow recorded in the VA below the transverse process of the atlas. Liljequist et al[448] demonstrated that directional Doppler ultrasound analysis of flow in the VA located just below the transverse process of the atlas reliably detected the presence of retrograde VA blood flow in angiographically verified patients with subclavian steal. Berguer and colleagues[65] measured the relative velocity of pulsed-wave propagation in the two arms and concluded that a delay in propagation was well correlated with angiographically verified reversal of VA flow in the innominate and subclavian arteries. All 21 patients with Doppler-detected innominate stenosis and all 66 patients with subclavian steal had angiography that agreed with the noninvasive findings. Combining the patients with subclavian and vertebral artery extracranial disease, 92% of those that had lesions by Doppler had angiographic agreement. However, provocative tests such as decreasing peripheral resistance in the upper arm could cause temporary basilar artery flow reversal. Transcranial Doppler (TCD) also documents flow changes in the intracranial VA.[134,725] A variety of surgical procedures have been devised to treat subclavian artery occlusive disease.

Endarterectomy of the subclavian lesion usually requires a thoracotomy. Cervical or thoracic prosthetic or venous bypass grafts or ligation of the ipsilateral vertebral artery are other techniques that have been used.[47] Vertebral ligation can cause thrombosis of the VA with later propagation of clot into the cranium or distal embolization.[286,364] The question is not whether surgery can be done to remedy VA siphonage, but whether it should be done in a particular patient. In deciding this question, three points should kept in mind: (1) Subclavian steal is a relatively benign phenomenon. Although transient spells are common, brain stem infarction is rare. Cerebellar infarction has been observed, but only after hypotension. In other words, there is usually more smoke than fire. (2) Coexistent serious extracranial and intracranial vascular disease is

the rule. It is easy to be seduced by the intriguing collateral pathways and the clearly demonstrable physical signs of subclavian disease and miss the more important, more relevant vascular lesion in the individual patient. (3) Subclavian or innominate surgery is somewhat more complex and is associated with more morbidity than other extracranial vascular surgery if a thoracotomy is needed. Patients who could tolerate a local neck procedure such as carotid endarterectomy or venous bypass grafting may not be able to survive a thoracotomy satisfactorily. Unfortunately, the open net theory of cerebral circulation has given license for surgical repair of an angiographic stenosis whether or not it is directly related to the symptomatology.

MOBILE THROMBUS IN THE AORTIC ARCH

Atherosclerotic disease in the aortic arch is frequently ulcerated, and several recent studies have established a statistically significant link between its presence and brain infarction, especially brain infarction of unknown cause.[15,17,19,175,383] This association is even stronger with atherosclerotic plaques ≥4 mm as measured with transesophageal echocardiography. However, plaques ≥4 mm in the aortic arch are also good markers for generalized atherosclerosis and other causes of stroke and carry a high risk of recurrence.[693,717] By contrast, mobile thrombus in the aortic arch that develops on an ulcerated plaque is more likely to be a source for brain and peripheral embolism, and many convincing examples have now been published, including patients with posterior circulation strokes.[391,715,716] Although surgical repair of the aortic arch is feasible, the benefits and risks of such procedures should be evaluated, since patients with aortic thrombi are on average 79 years old.

EXTRACRANIAL VERTEBRAL ARTERY OCCLUSIVE DISEASE

The ECVA is a frequent site of atheromatous disease and also exhibits an unusually high incidence of congenital variability (asymmetry, small size, residual embryologic anastomosis, and termination in the PICA).[242,374,512,624] Atherostenosis at the VA origin is more common in men than in women[137,306] and is often associated with carotid artery occlusive disease.[372] Whites have a higher frequency of vertebral origin disease than blacks or persons of Chinese or Japanese ancestry.[137,306] At times, the proximal VA lesions represent extension of plaque material from the parent subclavian artery.

Despite the high incidence of disease, serious brain stem or posterior circulation strokes have only rarely been caused by occlusive disease limited to an ECVA. During the 19th century Alexander[7] treated epilepsy with apparent impunity by placing a ligature on the VA; he ligated one or both VAs low in the neck in 21 young epileptics, at times tying both vessels at one operation. Surgeons have ligated the VA as a treatment of subclavian steal, eliminating the siphonage through this vessel. Fisher[255] reported in detail five patients in whom bilateral occlusions of the proximal vertebral system could be demonstrated angiographically. All patients had transient ischemic episodes, but in only one was there a persisting neurologic deficit, and that patient also had an occlusion of the ICA at the siphon on the appropriate side to explain the findings. Extensive collateral circulation may develop, especially if the VA occlusion occurs gradually. The occipital branch of the external carotid artery is a prominent source of collateral supply, often filling the deep muscular branches of the VA near the atlas.[255,586] The ascending cervical and transverse cervical branches of the thyrocervical trunk originating from the subclavian artery may also fill the VA in its midcervical course. Compensatory flow from the contralateral VA and retrograde flow down the basilar artery from the carotid-posterior communicating system is also frequently visualized. The most common transient symptoms are dizziness, faint feeling, blurred vision, and imbalance. Fisher[255] has argued that occlusion of the proximal VA, like subclavian steal, is usually a benign syndrome rarely accompanied by serious brain stem infarction.

In the past, proximal VA lesions were said not to ulcerate.[512] However, a report by Pelouze[551] documents the finding of an ulcerated VA plaque as a source of intra-arterial embolism to the intracranial posterior circulation. The patient was a 79-year-old man who had many attacks during a period of months characterized by vertigo, falling, and diplopia. Angiography showed an irregular stenotic lesion at the origin of the left VA, and a B-mode scan of the region suggested the presence of an ulcerated plaque. Two other cases document that embolism may occasionally arise from a previously occluded ECVA.[138] A 58-year-old man had two isolated episodes of brain stem dysfunction, separated by a month, one probably pontine and the other thalamic. Angiography revealed opacification of the left VA only through muscular branches of the thyrocervical trunk. The right VA and intracranial vessels were normal. Spells ceased after anticoagulant therapy. A 39-year-old man suddenly developed headache and quadriparesis some days after a stormy airplane ride.[110] Angiography revealed nonfilling of the right nuchal VA and a midbasilar artery occlusion. After anticoagulation therapy there were no further episodes during the next 3 years. A 34-year-old man had persistent left posterior neck pain and headache for 4 days and then developed a right pontine infarct.[558] Angiography showed a left VA occlusion at the C2 level and an intraluminal filling defect (embolus) in the distal basilar artery and proximal SCA. He was anticoagulated for 6 months. Repeat angiography showed an unchanged left VA occlusion, but the distal basilar artery was now normal. George and Laurian[293] described two patients with VA occlusive disease and suspected basilar embolism. Koroshetz and Ropper[418] studied local embolism of the posterior circulation and found the suspected embolic source in either the extracranial (5 patients), intracranial (3 patients), or both VA segments (3 patients), in 11 patients undergoing angiography. Castaigne et al[146] observed three cases in which emboli had arisen from a tight stenosis of the proximal VA. The frequency of embolism arising in VA occlusive disease or plaques is not known. If a comparable situation in the carotid artery is examined, emboli arising from a fresh occlusion usually occur soon after the occlusion and are rare later. We have reported 10 cases of intra-arterial emboli

distally in the posterior circulation from proximal VA occlusive disease (see above).[132] Our conclusions were that atherosclerotic disease of the VA origin has features in common with disease of the ICA origin, that both have similar risk factors and demography, and both cause strokes by intracranial intra-arterial embolism.[132]

Traumatic occlusions within the nuchal VA are clearly not as benign (see previous section on pathology). Chiropractic and other manipulation and closed head and neck trauma often cause damage to the third segment of the VA just before it pierces the dura. Tears, dissection, and thrombosis develop acutely and may give rise to extension of the clot intracranially or to distal clot embolization. The sudden occurrence of the pathology hampers development of adequate collateral circulation. Furthermore, rapidly developing thrombi are usually less adherent to the vertebral wall and are closer to the intradural VA than in the situation of slowly developing atherosclerotic occlusion of the proximal VAs. In most examples of traumatic injury, the peril of brain stem infarction occurs at the time or soon after the injury. Late occurrences are rarely seen, if ever.

Occasionally, VA aneurysms in the neck can serve as a donor site for intra-arterial emboli. Maruyama et al[470] reported the case of a 40-year-old man who had numerous attacks of double vision, sensory abnormalities, and alternating hemiparesis. Angiography performed after he had developed a fixed quadrantanopia showed a large (nearly 3 by 3 cm) aneurysm near the origin of the left VA. Platelet scintigraphy, using radionuclide-labeled platelets, showed a well-defined focus of activity within the aneurysm. After aspirin, repeat scintigraphy showed no activity in the lesion, but spells persisted. At surgery, a brown thrombus was found firmly attached to the wall of the aneurysm. We recently consulted on an adolescent boy who had been rendered quadriplegic due to a traumatic neck injury and a cervical vertebral fracture with displacement. During the first week, he suddenly went blind and became agitated and later somnolent. Investigation showed that one VA was occluded at the site of the injury, and an intra-arterial embolus had traveled to the rostral basilar artery. We are aware of no prospectively collected series of patients with serious cervical spine injuries who have had systematic studies of the frequency of important accompanying injury to the infraspinous segment of the VAs. In a series of 24 patients with pontine infarcts and a locked-in state, 5 of the 10 patients had neck injuries and delayed onset of brain stem signs. Four patients had cervical fractures, two of whom had documented occlusions of the VA in the neck.[399] Noninvasive ultrasound testing of the VAs should be capable of determining patency of the arteries above the site of bony trauma.

There are few systematic studies of the incidence of symptoms and signs and prognosis in untreated patients with occlusive disease of the proximal VAs. Labauge et al[425] reported 100 personally collected cases of VA occlusion but included lesions at various sites along the ECVA and ICVA. Headache and "cerebellovestibular" symptoms were common. Many patients presented because they were already symptomatic. Moufarrij and colleagues[519,520] performed a prospective study on patients with angiographically detected VA stenosis. Most lesions (93%) were located at the VA origin, and brain stem strokes were rare at presentation or during the follow-up. They followed 89 patients with 75% stenosis of at least one

VA origin for an average of 4.6 years. None developed definite vertebrobasilar TIAs; 19 had nonlocalizing spells, among whom 9 had a stroke. Only two patients had brain stem infarcts, and each also had basilar artery stenosis. Hennerici and colleagues[338] studied a large group of patients who had no neurovascular symptoms but had severe atherosclerosis of the large peripheral arteries, the aorta, or the coronary arteries. In 426 patients, both continuous-wave Doppler insonation and angiograms of the VAs were available; 183 patients (43%) had significant disease of the vertebral or subclavian arteries, indicating that asymptomatic VA disease is quite common. Doppler insonation of the VA origin is quite accurate when performed by sonographers experienced in detecting reduced anterograde flow.[338,727] Insonation at the distal ECVA can detect distal alteration in flow.[117,341,727] In the study of Hennerici et al,[338] the accuracy of continuous-wave Doppler in detecting angiographically confirmed VA lesions was excellent. Among the 183 patients with lesions, the Doppler results did not agree with angiography in only 8%. Considering the total series, 183 patients with lesions and 234 controls without lesions, the accuracy was 90.1%. More recently, duplex scanning has been used to image the proximal VA region.[3,75,704] The technique that combines B-mode ultrasound with Doppler has been shown to detect accurately severe disease from the VA origin to the C3 to C4 level.[468] Color-coded Doppler imaging of the nuchal artery is also quite accurate and useful diagnostically.[709] Kimura and colleagues[411] reported their results using Duplex color-coded ultrasound studies with insonation of the VAs between the C6 and C3 vertebral segments. All 12 patients with unilateral subclavian artery occlusion had retrograde VA flow. In the 11 patients with unilateral VA origin occlusions, no flow signal was detected on the involved side. Even in the 20 patients with ICVA disease, the VA mean and end-diastolic flow velocities in the neck were abnormal and lower than on the side of the normal VA.[411] Insonation of the VA in the neck was only normal in controls with no occlusive disease and in those patients who had basilar artery and PCA occlusions.

TCD is also an essential part of the investigation in patients with posterior circulation occlusive disease whether or not the suspected lesions are thought to be extracranial or intracranial. As in the anterior circulation, the extracranial and intracranial arteries should always be studied together. TCD through the suboccipital window is very accurate in detecting ICVA occlusive disease.[159,160,162] Flow velocities are often reduced on the side of significant extracranial occlusive lesions such as thrombi, atherosclerotic stenosis, and dissections. TCD gives some measure of the functional impact of the extracranial occlusive lesions on intracranial flow. TCD can also be used to assess whether changes in neck position and neck turning cause decreased flow in one or both ICVAs. However, maintenance of optimal consistency of insonation during movement is difficult. When velocities are decreased or lost during motion, it is often hard to be certain if the cause is reduced flow or simply a technical problem due to a change in the insonation angle.

Intravenous digital subtraction angiography can also be helpful. Among 111 patients who had venous digital subtraction angiography in one study, 90% had VA images considered to be of diagnostic quality.[347] MRA may become the diagnostic method of choice because of its capability of noninvasively providing longitudinal images of the arteries, but to date the accuracy of detecting proximal VA lesions is unknown.[204,211,212] In MRA evaluation of proximal extracranial artery disease, often the films of the aortic arch and its branches are suboptimal. In some studies, overlapping of arteries is a problem, and selective views and filming techniques are often needed to obtain images of the regions; these should be performed under the close supervision of an experienced neuroradiologist. The VA origins are particularly difficult to image. The adequacy of films of the VA origins depends on the type of surface coil and the angle of filming. A scarf type coil usually provides the best images.

By contrast, MRA pictures of the V2 and V3 portions of the ECVAs are usually quite good, and hypoplasia or VA occlusion is usually evident on the films. The experience to date with spiral CT angiography is still too little to comment on its relative effectiveness for studying the extracranial VAs. In some patients the ultrasound and MRA results will be concordant and will allow accurate diagnosis of stenosis or occlusion of the proximal arteries, or, on the other hand, the normality of these studies will render the likelihood of significant proximal disease remote. When the noninvasive studies are discordant or technically suboptimal and the presence or absence of proximal VA and subclavian disease is clinically important, standard catheter angiography will be needed to define the vascular lesions better. The data from the noninvasive studies can be used to allow the angiographer to focus on areas of suspicion and may reduce unnecessary injections and opacification of arteries shown to be normal by noninvasive testing.[143] At times cross-section CT or MRI of the neck can be very helpful in the diagnosis of extracranial arterial dissection. MRA and angiography result in images of the residual arterial lumina but do not show the vessel walls. Intramural hematomas and bulging of the arterial wall as seen on cross-section films can document the process as a dissection.

Surgical reconstruction of proximal VA occlusive lesions is most often performed by bypassing the occlusive disease.[64,213,373–375,434,583,601,654] Connections are most often created with the carotid arterial system The operations can be performed safely by surgeons experienced with the procedure, with very low morbidity and mortality. At times, the bypass procedure is performed at the time of carotid endarterectomy.[434] Endarterectomy can also be performed but has been sparingly reported.[551,696] More recently, interventional radiologists have begun to perform angioplasty using catheter techniques. Higashida and colleagues[349] recently reported their experience with angioplasty in 42 vertebrobasilar occlusive lesions, 34 of which involved the proximal VA. They reported two strokes and one vessel rupture as major complications. Four other patients had transient complications consisting of arterial spasm and transient ischemia.[349] Others have reported individual cases or small series of angioplasties.[382,621] Fear of distal intracranial embolization after plaque dilatation has made most neurologists and neurosurgeons wary of the technique until technology is available to trap distally moving emboli at the time of angioplasty. The indications for surgery or angioplasty or both are not clear, since collateral circulation is usually restored naturally, and the risk of severe brain stem infarction without treatment is low.[519,520]

Theoretically, agents that affect platelet function could prevent fibrin-platelet nidi from forming on plaques and nonstenotic lesions. Heparin given during the first week after a recent VA occlusion might prevent propagation and embolization of clot while the thrombus organizes and becomes adherent to the vascular wall. Coumadin could theoretically prevent occlusion or embolization in patients with preocclusive stenosis of the proximal VA. Unfortunately, none of the treatments in use has been systematically studied in trials. Trials would be difficult to perform because the low incidence of adverse events of the lesions would necessitate a very large number of study patients.

INTRACRANIAL VERTEBRAL ARTERY OCCLUSIVE DISEASE

Occlusive disease of the intracranial portion of the VA is much more serious than extracranial disease and is commonly associated with infarction of posterior circulation structures. When the one VA that is responsible for supplying the lion's share of the blood flow (the contralateral VA being tiny, previously occluded, severely narrowed, or ending in the PICA) is occluded, the resulting syndrome is indistinguishable from occlusion of the basilar artery. In fact, Fisher[249] has used the term basilarization of the VA to describe the situation of dependence on one VA for maintenance of the posterior circulation. In addition, clot formed within the distal VA may propagate into the proximal basilar artery, again producing a syndrome indistinguishable from basilar occlusion.

In the more usual situation of bilaterally competent VAs, occlusion of a single VA is usually associated with one of several clinical pictures: (1) lateral medullary infarction, (2) posterior inferior cerebellar infarction due to obstruction of the ostium of the PICA by an occlusive thrombus in the intracranial VA, (3) ischemia of the ipsilateral hemimedulla by obstruction of the ostia of the anterior spinal artery arising from the intracranial portion of the VA, (4) embolic occlusion in vessels of the distal basilar arterial tree, the embolus originating from the VA clot, or (5) transient spells without infarction. Because these syndromes are common, quite distinct, and clinically important, they are considered separately in detail.

Lateral Medullary Infarction

In the comprehensive anatomic description of the brain supply by Duret in 1873,[207] the PICA supplied the lateral region of the medulla. Then Dumenil[203] in 1875 in a clinical and pathologic report realized that unilateral palsy of the palate can be attributed to lateral medullary infarction and PICA occlusion. In 1895 Wallenberg[734] reasoned from the clinical findings in a single case and what he knew of brain stem anatomy and physiology that the responsible lesion should be in the lateral medulla.[749] Furthermore, Wallenberg injected the vessels of seven other autopsied human brains to define the arterial supply to the medulla and concluded that the PICA should be occluded in patients with infarcts in the lateral medulla. In fact, postmortem examination of the single case studied clinically did verify infarction of the cerebellum and medulla and occlusion of the PICA. However, when Fisher et al[271] examined the pattern of vascular occlusion in 17 of

their own cases of lateral medullary infarction, in only 2 cases was the occlusive lesion solely within the PICA. In 13 cases the vertebral artery was occluded, and in 1 case severely stenosed. In 20 earlier reports in which the responsible vascular lesion had been documented, 15 had VA occlusion; only 4 had occlusion within the PICA itself. In about half the cases the thrombus in the VA extended to block the PICA orifice.

Among the patients studied at necropsy, 14 were thought to have atherostenotic thrombotic occlusions, and 3 were thought to represent embolic occlusions. Two patients with embolism had cardiac sources in the form of congenital heart disease and bacterial endocarditis; the other patient with presumed embolism had multiple scattered brain infarcts and no occlusion of the VA or PICA at necropsy, suggesting an embolism that fragmented and passed. Fisher and colleagues[271] also reviewed prior reports of embolism causing lateral medullary infarcts. The first reported case was described by Hallopeau and was a patient, studied at necropsy by Charcot, who was thought to have a distal VA embolus that arose from ulcerated atheromatous plaques in the aorta. A patient of Breuer and Marburg had a cardiac mural thrombus and nonadherent gray embolic thrombus in the ICVA leading to a lateral medullary infarct.[140,271] A patient studied by Richter[586] had a PICA embolus from a bicuspid aortic valve, and Wintler's patient with lateral medullary syndrome had rheumatic heart disease and an atrial thrombus but patent arteries (presumably indicating a migrant clot) leading to the medullary infarct. Escourolle and colleagues[218] found 14 VA occlusions and 3 occlusions of the PICA among 23 examples of lateral medullary infarction. When the infarctions were located in the dorsal medulla the occlusion was more likely to be in the stem of the PICA (four of five patients). Foix and colleagues[280] found in an autopsy case that the lateral medulla was supplied by one single lateral medullary artery that arose from the very proximal portion of the basilar artery and postulated that the syndrome was caused by occlusion of "the artery of the lateral sulcus of the medulla." However, since then, Goodhart and Davison[304] found such an artery only once and Escourolle and colleagues twice.

Fisher and colleagues[271] and Escourolle and colleagues[218] demonstrated that not one (Foix's artery or the PICA as stated by Wallenberg) but several small arteries from the VA usually supply the lateral medullary area. Foix and colleagues probably described an infrequent arterial anomaly, and Wallenberg an unusual lateral medullary supply since the PICA participates in the supply of the lateral medulla in less than one-third of cases. However, the mPICA always participates in the supply of the dorsal medulla along with branches from the posterior spinal arteries.[208] If indeed the intrinsic arterial distribution is usually fixed and divided into medial, lateral, and dorsal areas, the extrinsic arterial supply is extremely variable from one individual to the next.[279] The Lund series[532] was the first study to report the vascular lesions as determined in vivo by either angiography or ultrasound in 43 patients with lateral medullary infarcts. The commonest vascular lesions involved the VAS.[532] Among the 12 angiographically documented VA occlusions, 9 patients had no proximal VA opacification: one VA filled for 4 to 5 cm, and two occlusions involved the distal ECVA. The mechanism by which the ECVA occlusive lesions caused the medullary infarcts was not commented on, but either propagation or embolism of clot into the ICVA must have occurred. Two patients with distal

ECVA stenosis and one patient with PICA stenosis had dissections as the cause of the vascular narrowing. Disease in the contralateral subclavian-VAs was rare. An angiogram of one patient showed contralateral subclavian artery stenosis, and one patient had contralateral VA stenosis at necropsy. Five patients had coexisting carotid artery disease with >50% stenosis in the neck.[532] In the series of Sacco et al[609] 33 patients had vascular studies, and the ipsilateral VA was abnormal in 24 (73%). In 18 patients, VA duplex Doppler showed either high resistance flow or no flow in an imaged artery. Fifteen patients had angiography, which showed that five had VA stenoses, three had VA occlusions, and five had VA dissections. In two patients with VA dissection or stenosis the PICA was also occluded, but no patient had PICA disease as the only finding. In two patients angiography was normal.[609] In another clinical MRI study, ICVA disease was the commonest etiology.[731] Among patients with large dorsolateral infarcts, 75% had severe stenosis or occlusion of the ICVA. Dissections of the VAs and cardioembolism were thought to each account for one-seventh of the cases.[731]

The infarct usually involves a wedge of the medulla extending from the lateral edge (Fig. 22.9). It usually involves a portion of the olive ventrally and in some cases extends dorsally to involve the restiform body. Currier et al[169] divided the pattern of infarction into ventral, superficial, and dorsal lesions, indicating that the extent of infarction was quite variable. When the dorsal medulla is infarcted, the lesion is almost always accompanied by cerebellar infarction.[333] Since the lesion extends dorsally to the olive, the older terminology referred to the lesion as the "retro-olivary" syndrome.[635] The zone of infarction usually extends 7 to 10 mm in a rostrocaudal dimension, occurring most commonly in the middle part of the olive but frequently extending into its upper or lower third.[271] In 9 of 24 lateral medullary infarcts studied by Hauw and colleagues,[333] the lesion extended to the pontomedullary junction. Vuilleumier et al[731] published data from the Lausanne registry on MRI-clinical correlations in 28 patients with medullary infarcts.[731] They showed that the distribution of infarcts suggested earlier by Currier and colleagues[169] could be confirmed by MRI. The commonest locations of medullary infarcts in the Lausanne series were small midlateral, dorsolateral, inferolateral, and inferodorsolateral. Dorsal infarcts were always accompanied by medial PICA territory cerebellar infarcts.[731] In the Sacco series from Columbia University, the selection of cases was predominantly clinical—all patients with a lateral medullary syndrome were included.[609] Although all 33 patients had CT scans (none showed a brain stem infarct but 3 showed cerebellar infarcts), MRI was performed in only 22 (66%); a typical lateral medullary infarct was present in only 12 patients (37% of total patients), and 8 had other brain stem infarcts with or without lateral medullary infarction.[609] In the Korean series of Kim et al,[410] all 33 patients were selected because their MRIs showed unilateral lesions involving mainly the dorsolateral medulla.[410] The infarcts involved the rostral medulla in 8 patients, the middle medulla in 8, and the caudal medulla in 9; among the remaining 8 patients, 4 had rostral and middle infarcts, and 4 had middle and caudal involvement.[410] Accompanying cerebellar infarction was uncommon on neuroimaging scans, occurring in 3 patients (9%) in the New York series,[609] in 7 patients (21%) in the Korean series[410] and in 6 of 30 (20%) patients in the Lund study.[532] As with thrombosis elsewhere, transient attacks frequently precede the stroke by days or weeks, more rarely months, and are noted in about half the patients with lateral medullary infarction.

SYMPTOMS. The symptoms are explained by the distinctive anatomy of the lesion (Fig. 22.10).

Vertigo. The most common symptom is dizziness or vertigo, often accompanied by staggering and double vision. Difficulty in focusing and numbness of the face are other common components of the transient attacks. Headache, especially in the occipital region, may accompany other symptoms or may occur alone. The deficit may develop suddenly, but more commonly it progresses gradually or stepwise over 24 to 48 hours. Fluctuations or stepwise deterioration frequently characterize the first week after the stroke onset, but are less common thereafter and distinctly unusual after 2 weeks.

Headache. Moderate or severe headache is common in lateral medullary infarction and is related to involvement of the descending spinal tract of the fifth cranial nerve and its nucleus, or to vascular distension produced by the occlusive process within the vertebral artery. In 1836 Bright[98] called attention to posterior headache in vascular disease. He described a "gentleman past the meridian of life" who had apoplectic attacks and complained, "I feel completely knocked up and have much pain in the back of the head, like a rheumatic pain, generally at the same spot the right side of the back part of the head." Bright commented, "This pain would itself chiefly direct our suspicions to disease of the vertebral arteries." Steady or, less commonly, pulsatile headache is located most often in the occipital region and is unilateral in about half of cases.[249] Aching headache is usually centered just below the external occipital protuberance and extends into the suboccipital and nuchal regions, usually nearer the midline than the ear. Frequently it extends into the frontal region, and occasionally the headache may be dull and only frontal in location.

Facial pain. Facial pain is more diagnostic and is a cardinal feature of the syndrome. Of 39 patients studied in one large series, 27 had persisting (18 patients) or transient face pain ipsilateral to the lesion.[169] Sharp, single stabs or jolts of pain are felt in the eye or face. Occasionally, these may occur in flurries like a machine gun. Sticking, burning, stinging, tingling, or numbness are other commonly used descriptive terms. The eye is the most commonly affected region, but the pain may be limited to the ear or isolated spots on the forehead or cheeks. Pain frequently affects the entire face, including the lips and inside the mouth but is rarely if ever limited to the mandibular division of the trigeminal nerve. Unpleasant facial sensations, when present, usually appear at the very onset of the stroke and are often the first symptom perceived by the patient. The coexistent contralateral hemianalgesia of the body is seldom mentioned but is usually evident to the patient only after pain or temperature testing. The striking contrast between the spontaneous sudden facial pain due to involvement, presumably, of the nucleus of the descending tract of the fifth cranial nerve and the lack of perception of the hemianalgesia related to ischemia of the spinothalamic

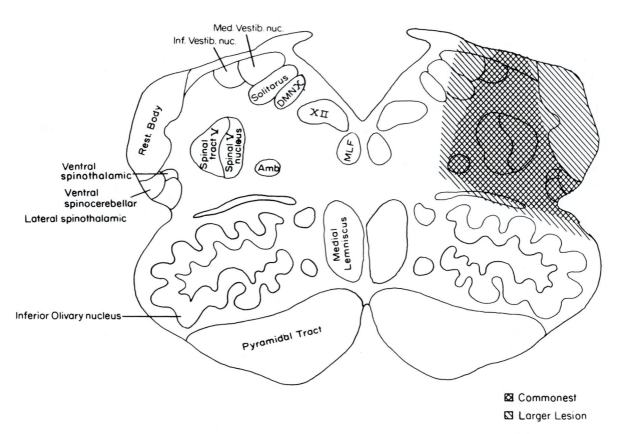

Figure 22.10 Lateral medullary infarction. The most common involvement and largest extent of the lesion are designated by checkerboard markings, as described in the key. (Based on the figure in Currier et al,[169] with permission.)

tract led Fisher[250] to postulate that dysfunction of sensory neurons (either within the dorsal root ganglia or buried within the central nervous system, as in the nucleus of the tract of the fifth cranial nerve or in its main sensory nucleus) produces spontaneous pain, but lesions of white matter or nerves do not generally evoke pain as an early finding. Occasionally burning facial pain, likened by one patient to having salt and pepper thrown on the face, may be seen transiently in tegmental ischemia other than in a lateral medullary location.[117] The presence of facial pain or dysesthetic feelings may not be mentioned spontaneously by the patient because of their bizarre or unusual nature. Since these are so diagnostic of brain stem involvement, their presence should be diligently sought when the patient is questioned.

Feelings of disequilibrium. Vertigo or other feelings of disequilibrium are nearly always present. Although frank whirling or rotational turning may be described, feelings of swaying or falling, feeling seasick, or being off balance are the most common terms used. These perceptions are probably due to involvement of the vestibular nuclei or their connections. Alteration of vision is another frequent complaint and may even be described as diplopia (18 of 39 cases) or, less commonly, as the illusion of objects oscillating or moving.[169] The visual deficit is not monocular, and decreased visual acuity, visual field defects, or extraocular muscle palsies are not found to explain the visual symptoms. In the patient complaining of altered vision, the most common neuro-ophthalmologic finding is nystagmus; the visual complaints are probably due to sudden alteration in the vestibulo-ocular system, sometimes resulting in skew deviation or even in conjugate ipsilateral horizontal gaze palsy. Occasionally patients with lateral medullary infarction complain of tilting of the visual world with a 90- to 180-degree inversion of the visual images.[218] Even with persisting nystagmus, the patient's visual symptoms are usually transient, indicating the nervous system's compensatory ability to adapt to chronic nystagmus and vestibular dysfunction.

Nausea and vomiting. Nausea and vomiting are also common symptoms (18 of 35 patients in the series of Peterman and Siekert[562] and 27 of 39 patients in the series of Currier et al[169]) and are due to vestibular dysfunction or to involvement of the dorsal tegmentum—the *vomiting centers* of Borison and Wang[91] in the floor of the fourth ventricle. Since the nucleus ambiguus is near the vomiting centers, some authors have argued that because signs of 9th and 10th cranial nerve dysfunction frequently occur in patients with vomiting, the floor of the fourth ventricle is incriminated as the site of origin of the vomiting.[169] We have not seen a patient with nausea and vomiting without accompanying dizziness or nystagmus, and we wonder if vomiting is simply a reflection of disease of the vestibular nuclei and their connections.

Ataxia. Ataxia is the rule rather than the exception. Virtually no patient with documented lateral medullary infarction walks normally, and all patients complain of altered gait. Walking is usually characterized by veering to the side, leaning, or stumbling. The patient is also aware of the ipsilateral cerebellar dysfunction and describes the arm as clumsy, unreliable, or weak.

Hiccups. Hiccups (19 of 74 patients in the series of Currier et al[169]) are a frequent complaint, usually developing some time after the onset. In most patients with hiccups, the lateral medullary infarct is typically complete and is usually not ventral or superficial. The origin of the hiccups is uncertain but could relate to dysfunction of "respiratory centers" or to involvement of 10th cranial nerve fibers.[169,455] Difficulty in swallowing is common (55 of 74 patients in the series of Currier et al[169] and Peterman and Siekert[562]). Food or secretions may have unusually free influx into the air passages, a phenomenon unusual in patients with peripheral 9th and 10th cranial nerve involvement at the jugular foramen. Disturbances of the coordination of epiglottic closure and palatal and pharyngeal function may be more likely with a central lesion of the nucleus ambiguus. Food gets stuck in the piriform recess of the pharynx adjacent to the larynx; patients attempt to extricate the material by an unusual cough-like maneuver. This crowing-like cough is characteristic, and its presence in a stroke patient is virtually diagnostic of lateral medullary infarction. Hoarseness is also frequent but may be absent in the ventral or more superficial lesions. Some patients with involvement of the spinothalamic tract mention numbness, burning, or perverted sensations in the contralateral limbs or trunk, but these most commonly occur later in the course, sometimes weeks or months after the stroke.[653] Ipsilateral stuffy nose, altered taste, and dysarthria are less common.

S I G N S . The signs accompanying lateral medullary infarction have been extensively reviewed by others.[169,271,455,487,562,653] A review of the seven main signs follows.

Diminished sensation in the ipsilateral face. Involvement of the descending tract of the fifth cranial nerve and its nucleus usually produces decreased pain and temperature sensation of the ipsilateral face. Almost invariably, the corneal reflex is lost or severely reduced. The forehead and rest of the ophthalmic division are more analgesic than the lower face. Pain and cold sensitivity are generally affected equally. At times, although single pinpricks feel less sharp and less discrete, there may be a dysesthetic quality, with spread and persistence of the perceived stimulus. When the ipsilateral face is severely analgesic, the lower border does not usually conform to the limits of the peripheral mandibular division of the fifth cranial nerve but can be portrayed as a gentle curve sloping downward and medially from the tragus to the mandible where the facial artery lies.[562] Touch may also be diminished in the analgesic face.[653] The facial sensory defect usually clears more quickly than that on the contralateral body, although usually the loss of corneal reflex persists.[653]

Diminished pain and temperature sensation on the contralateral body. Ischemia of the lateral spinothalamic tract is responsible for diminished pain and temperature sensation on the contralateral body. As previously noted, patients infrequently report the contralateral hemianalgesia, but some described a numbness or cold feeling. The sensory loss may affect the entire hemicorpus, but often the cervical region is spared. At onset, a level of pain and temperature sensation

may be delimited either near the nipple line or on the trunk or abdomen, in which case the arm frequently has normal sensibility. Pain and temperature should always be checked in the lower extremity; some examiners will retire their pin to abbreviate the examination when pain has been perceived normally in the arm. The fibers within the spinothalamic tract are laminated, with the sacral fibers most lateral and the arm more medial. The arm and upper neck and trunk are spared in more superficial lesions. When the lesion extends far medially, it may even involve the quintothalamic fibers, which have already crossed to join the medial border of the spinothalamic tract, producing a complete contralateral hemianalgesia including the contralateral face. In patients with bilateral facial analgesia, the pin feels different on the two sides of the face, the loss being more severe ipsilaterally. Without very careful testing, the contralateral face could be passed as normal unless the pin sensibility here is compared with the normal ipsilateral arm or trunk. With time, the hemianalgesia frequently improves, and a level may become apparent over the trunk.[473] Less often the analgesia clears both rostrally and caudally, leaving a band of altered sensibility on the trunk.[455] Although at onset the loss of pain and temperature sensibility tends to be homogeneous over affected areas, greater degrees of sensibility appear later, leaving patches of perverted sensation. The analgesia usually extends to the midline at onset, but the paramedian region of the body often clears more in the front than in the back.[653]

At times, the loss of pain and temperature can be entirely crossed, occurring in the face, arm, trunk, and leg contralateral to the infarct. The lesions that cause this unilateral pattern of sensory loss are located more medially and involve the crossing fibers in the ventral trigeminal thalamic tract and the fibers in the crossed lateral spinothalamic tract. At times, the discomfort is severe and is comparable to thalamic pain, with which it probably shares a common mechanism. Rubbing of the involved part, the pressure of tight clothing, or excessive heat or cold may aggravate the discomfort. When pain makes a delayed appearance in the contralateral body, it generally persists and is relatively resistant to pharmacologic treatments.[653]

Horner syndrome. Sympathetic nervous system fibers course through the lateral reticular substance and are involved in most cases of lateral medullary infarction (25 of 35 patients in the series of Hauw et al[333]), resulting in the Horner syndrome ipsilaterally. Usually the Horner syndrome is incomplete; ptosis is the most common element and leads to drooping of the upper eyelid and some elevation of the lower lid, narrowing the palpebral fissure. Miosis is also very common, the pupil usually retaining its reactivity to light. Anhydrosis is the least common element of the Horner syndrome in lateral medullary infarction.

Ataxia. Gait and limb ataxia are very important signs of lateral stem infarction and are due to ischemia of the restiform body, or to associated infarction of the inferior cerebellum in the territory of the PICA. The gait ataxia seen in the lateral medullary syndrome is different from that seen with the vermal degeneration of alcoholism. Leaning, veering, falling, or toppling to the side when the patient is placed in an erect or sitting position is characteristic of medullary infarction and can be contrasted to wide-based gait with truncal titubation of vermal lesions. The ipsilateral limbs are often called weak by the patient, but on examination striking rebound and finger to nose ataxia are found. The most sensitive test to elicit the cerebellar limb abnormality is to have the patient quickly lift or drop the arms and brake them suddenly: the affected limb will overshoot. When the cerebellum is infarcted, a posterior fossa pressure cone can develop and may lead to a fatal outcome unless medical or surgical decompression is instituted. The presence of cerebellar infarction thus alters the management and prognosis. How can one clinically distinguish involvement of the cerebellum from involvement of the inferior cerebellar components? No study has definitely settled this point. Head tilt, decreased alertness, prominent occipital headache, and a tendency to hold the head stiffly, resisting passive or active movement, probably indicate involvement of the cerebellum itself. In these patients MRI examinations usually show hypersignal on T_2-weighted axial sections of the lower ipsilateral cerebellar hemisphere due to an associated cerebellar infarct in the PICA territory along with lateral medullary infarct. The ataxia of the usual patient with lateral medullary infarction has a tendency to clear remarkably, leaving only minor clumsiness. It is usually safe to reassure the patients that they will be back on their feet within 3 to 6 months.

Nystagmus. The vestibular nuclei and their connections are affected in the lateral tegmentum and very frequently lead to nystagmus. The nystagmus is horizontal and frequently rotatory[169,271]; the quick component of the rotation usually moves the upper border of the iris toward the side of the lesion.[169] Vertical nystagmus is seldom if ever seen with ischemic lesions in the lateral medulla.[271] The eyes frequently drift away from the side of the lesion; small-amplitude, quick nystagmus is present on voluntary gaze to contralateral side, and coarser, larger amplitude, but slower nystagmus is present on ipsilateral gaze. In some cases, this pattern is reversed, with coarser horizontal nystagmus to the opposite side. The directional preponderance of nystagmus probably depends on the rostrocaudal location of the lesion.[514] The nystagmus may be torsional, as it was in three patients reported by Morrow and Sharpe.[514] These patients had skew deviation with hypotropia on the side of the infarct. The torsional nystagmus bears away from the lesion side in all patients, but in one the nystagmus changed direction as the eyes drifted about a neutral position of torsion: most often lateral gaze is characterized by hypermetric saccades to the side of the lesion and hypometric saccades to the opposite side.[220] At times the eyes are forcibly deviated to the side of the lesion, so-called lateropulsion.[74,417,492] Reflex and voluntary eye movements are full, but at rest the eyes may be deviated far to the side, closely mimicking conjugate eye deviation from a hemispheric lesion.[417] Skewing and slight dysconjugacy (the abducting eye lagging on gaze to the ipsilateral side) may explain the patient's complaints of diplopia. Diplopia is relieved in some patients by tilting the head to the side of the lesion.[220] Morrow and Sharpe,[514] Keane,[400] and Brandt and Dieterich[94,198,199] all emphasized torsional changes and skew deviation as common findings in patients with lateral medullary infarcts. Ocular tilt reactions, cyclorotation, and tilt of the subjective determination of the visual vertical axis were often found when tested for in patients with lateral medullary infarcts.

Paralysis of the ipsilateral vocal cord and weakness of the ipsilateral palate. Involvement of the nucleus ambiguus is responsible for paralysis of the ipsilateral vocal cord and weakness of the ipsilateral palate. These signs are frequently absent in more superficial lesions that do not extend far medially. The patient's ability to swallow usually improves despite persistent documentation of pharyngeal and palatal weakness. Unexplained tachycardia has accompanied lateral medullary infarction and could be due to involvement of vagal fibers arising from the dorsal motor nucleus of the vagus.

Slight weakness of the ipsilateral face. Although it is a common occurrence, a slight weakness of the ipsilateral face is difficult to explain, since the lesion is below the facial nucleus. Dejerine and Roussy[181] commented on an aberrant corticobulbar tract that coursed dorsal to the other corticospinal and corticobulbar fibers and looped a bit caudally before traveling rostrally toward the facial nucleus. Involvement of this bundle or, more likely, affection of descending extrapyramidal fibers might explain the facial weakness, which is generally transient and minor in degree.

In a large series of 33 patients with lateral medullary infarcts shown by MRI, aiming to correlate the region and extent of infarction with the clinical findings, Kim et al[410] found a prominent contrast between rostral and caudal lateral medullary infarcts. In this Korean series, patients with rostral lateral medullary infarcts invariably had dysphagia and hoarseness, and although vertigo and ataxia were common, nystagmus was not prominent.[410] By contrast, patients with caudal lateral medullary infarcts had severe vertigo and gait ataxia but did not have dysphagia or hoarseness. Rostral medullary lesions tended to extend more deeply and involve the nucleus ambiguus, whereas caudal medullary lesions were more superficial.[410]

PROGNOSIS. Contralateral hemiparesis or a Babinski sign are not components of the lateral medullary syndrome; their presence indicates a wider zone of ischemia and possibly a more serious prognosis. In the patient with a pure lateral medullary syndrome, the prognosis is usually quite good.[170] However, death may ensue from cerebellar infarction with development of a posterior fossa pressure cone. Some patients with lateral medullary infarction do die unexpectedly without an obvious explanation, that is, either cerebellar infarct or a more extensive occlusion or ischemia.[271]

In 1991, Norrving and Cronqvist[532] reported a study of the prognosis among 43 patients with lateral medullary infarcts collected as part of a population-based stroke registry in Lund, Sweden. During a 6-year period, there were 43 patients with lateral medullary infarcts, representing 1.9% of all admissions for acute stroke during that period. Four patients died during the acute stroke, two from nocturnal apnea, one from an acute myocardial infarct, and one from myocardial infarction, pulmonary embolism, and aspiration pneumonia. Three other patients also had aspiration pneumonia. In two patients new medullary infarcts occurred during the 2 weeks after the lateral medullary infarct, one a medial medullary infarct during hypotension (this patient died 3 weeks later) and one an ipsilateral hemiparesis possibly from caudal spread of the lateral medullary infarct. During follow-up, one patient with a VA occlusion developed a medial medullary infarct, and one patient with severe bilateral VA occlusive disease with extension of thrombus into the basilar artery developed a fatal progressive brain stem infarct. Five patients, four with known VA occlusions and one not studied, had posterior circulation TIAs during follow-up.

Two patients died of myocardial infarcts. The prognosis depended heavily on the nature of the underlying vascular lesions and the coexistence of coronary artery disease.[532]

Levin and Margolis[437] described a single patient with failure of automatic respiration (Ondine's curse) from a unilateral lateral medullary infarct. Others[192] have described altered automatic respiration in bilateral lateral medullary lesions, and one of us (L.R.C.)[109] has examined two stroke patients with failure to initiate respiration: one had postmortem confirmation of a bilateral lateral medullary lesion, and the other patient had a lateral pontine infarct on one side and a lateral medullary infarct on the other. Khurana[406] described a patient with a fatal unilateral lateral medullary infarct with well-documented central hypoventilation, episodic hypotension and hypertension, and profound bradycardia. Bogousslavsky et al[80] described in detail the clinical and autopsy findings in two patients with severe respiratory failure and unilateral lateral medullary infarcts that extended into the lower pons. The patient had a very severe central hypoventilation syndrome with loss of respiratory drive despite high $PaCO_2$. Despite being fully conscious, no ventilatory response could be obtained at 62 mmHg $PaCO_2$ during a CO_2 retention procedure similar to that used for assessment of brain death. Their second patient had periods of apnea during sleep consistent with Ondine's curse. Bogousslavsky and colleagues[80] posited that the hypoventilation was caused by involvement of the nucleus of the solitary tract, nucleus ambiguus, nucleus retroambiguus, nucleus reticularis parvocellularis, and nucleus reticularis gigantocellularis. Evidence that these structures are related to respiratory control and drive is cited. Might apneic periods, arrhythmia, and autonomic abnormalities be more common than is usually recognized in patients with lateral medullary infarcts?[438]

Patients with lateral medullary infarcts may worsen owing to extension of ischemia. Embolization of thrombus from the VA distally to the top of the basilar artery was observable on postmortem examination in 3 of 16 patients examined by Fisher et al.[271] Thrombus may also extend from the VA into the basilar artery, leading to more widespread ischemia. Embolization or thrombus extension occur early in the course (< 7 days) and are very rare after 2 weeks. Prior compromise of the contralateral VA does affect the ultimate prognosis, but in patients with prior contralateral disease the early syndrome, in our experience, is usually not limited to the lateral medulla alone. Insufficient data are available to clarify the risk/benefit ratio of short-term heparin therapy (1 to 3 weeks) in preventing early thrombus extension or embolization. Surely long-term warfarin therapy is not indicated in patients with lateral medullary infarctions.

MRI often defines the location of lateral medullary infarcts on transcranial images of the brain stem and is far superior to CT in sensitivity for detection of these lesions.[410,602,609,731]

Posterior Inferior Cerebellar Infarctions

Posterior inferior cerebellar infarcts are due to PICA occlusion. Occlusion involves the ICVA facing the PICA ostium or (directly) the main stem of the PICA. However, both sites of occlusion share the same causes.[22] Symptoms of cerebellar infarction are nonspecific including vertigo, headache, vomiting, dysarthria, and gait unsteadiness. The major signs include gait and trunk ataxia or ipsilateral axial lateropulsion, or both,

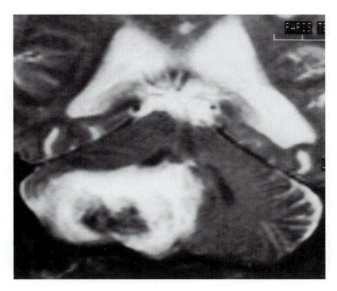

Figure 22.11 Posterior inferior cerebellar artery territory infarction (T_2-weighted MRI).

which usually prevent standing in upright position. Patients able to walk or stand in tandem position normally are unlikely to have important cerebellar infarction.[14] Other signs include nystagmus, ipsilateral limb dysmetria and dysarthria. Impairment of consciousness, ranging from drowsiness to deep coma, occurs in half the patients either at onset or later. In over half the patients, there are signs of associated brain stem infarction (facial palsy, trigeminal involvement, ocular motor abnormalities, motor weakness, and sensory loss) or occipitotemporal infarction (visual field defects, cortical blindness, memory loss). The clinical presentation is similar to that of cerebellar hemorrhage, but unenhanced CT allows distinction between the two conditions.[344,540] In cerebellar infarcts, CT usually shows focal hypodensity in the cerebellum, mass effect on the fourth ventricle, or compression of adjacent posterior fossa cisterns. However, it can be normal or difficult to interpret because of bone artifacts. MRI, now the gold standard for the early and accurate visualization of cerebellar infarctions, shows an area of increased signal on T_2-weighted axial, coronal, and sagittal sections (Fig. 22.11). Outcome of cerebellar infarctions is usually benign, with relatively good recovery, but at times cerebellar infarctions can take a pseudotumoral form due to edema, cerebellar swelling, brain stem compression, obstruction of the fourth ventricle, and hydrocephalus (see below). In that case life-saving surgery is needed when deterioration of consciousness appears.

PICA infarcts were formerly the most studied and presumed to be the most common of all cerebellar infarctions. Most often the pseudotumoral form and the form associated with the Wallenberg syndrome have been emphasized. MRI has shown that these forms are not frequent. Both presentations are very important to know since the former may need life-saving surgical treatment and the latter may require gastrostomy. Other more common presentations have a benign course. Clinicopathologic and clinicoradiologic series show that PICA infarcts are actually about as frequent as SCA infarcts.[22,28,56,150,350,395] In 64 autopsy cases with cerebellar infarctions, 10 of which involved both PICA and SCA territories, there were 28 PICA versus 33 SCA infarcts.[22] In 66 isolated unilateral cerebellar infarcts there were 36 PICA versus 30 SCA infarcts.[395] Macdonell et al[460] found 7 PICA infarcts among 19 autopsy cases of cerebellar infarcts, and Hinshaw et al[350] found that 29% of 42 radiologically demonstrated instances of cerebellar infarction were PICA infarcts. In the Kase et al[395] series, PICA infarcts account for half of the cerebellar infarctions and in a large consecutive series of 115 patients with cerebellar infarctions 35 had PICA infarcts, 30 had SCA infarcts, 9 had AICA infarcts, and 36 had small nonterritorial infarcts not localizable to a given arterial territory.[28]

PICA infarcts were historically, but partly erroneously, closely associated with lateral medullary infarctions (i.e., Wallenberg syndrome). After the anatomic descriptions of Duret (1873)[207] in which only the PICA was posited to supply the lateral region of the medulla, and Wallenberg's description[734,735] of a case of lateral medullary infarction due to PICA occlusion, every lateral medullary infarction was assumed to be due to a PICA occlusion[200,316,370,655,697,754] even when no occlusion could be found.[316,327,370,655,754] In fact, Wallenberg's original patient at necropsy also had an ipsilateral ICVA occlusive lesion. Subsequently the lateral medullary syndrome was confused with the PICA syndrome. Further studies revealed that the lateral region of the medulla is primarily supplied by three or four small branches arising from the distal ICVA between the PICA ostium and the origin of the basilar artery and less frequently by small branches arising from the PICA.[95,218,271,280,577] Krayenbüll and Yasargil[421] estimated that the PICA participated in the supply to this region in ≤22% of individuals. Consequently, PICA infarctions sparing the lateral medullary territory are the most common and, paradoxically, syndromes featuring occlusion of the PICA have been described only during the last 15 years since Duncan et al[205] emphasized the frequency of vertigo as the prominent presenting symptom. In summary, the PICA (1) sometimes participates in the supply of the lateral medullary area usually together with branches from the VA and alone in 22% of individuals and (2) usually participates in the supply of the dorsal medullary area together with the posterior spinal arteries.[421]

CLINICAL ASPECTS.

Involved territories. Two different clinical situations occur depending on whether or not the medulla is involved. In the autopsy series of Amarenco, Hauw, and their colleagues[22] from the Salpêtrière Hospital, the medulla was involved in its dorsolateral aspects in one-third of the patients. No lateral medullary infarction was seen without associated infarction in the dorsal medullary territory. PICA infarctions were much less frequently associated with other vertebrobasilar (pontine, mesencephalic, thalamic, or occipitotemporal) infarctions than AICA or SCA infarctions. The full PICA territory was involved in isolation in only 7% of autopsy cases and was more routinely associated with SCA or AICA infarctions, or both (46%). These combined infarctions were frequently edematous and produced brain stem compression. Partial PICA territory infarctions were very common among autopsy cases (46%). They usually involved the dorsomedial area of the caudal cerebellum, that is, the territory of the mPICA (32%), and less frequently the lateral area, the territory of the lPICA (18%).[22] They represent 75% of PICA infarctions in one clinical series[395] and two-thirds in another series.[28] These partial territory infarctions are never edematous. Thus, when re-

stricted to branch PICA territory, they are often small in size and benign in prognosis.[395] In the Kase et al[395] clinical series, 9 of 36 patients had signs of brain stem compression, and all 9 had full PICA territory infarction. Seven had obstructive hydrocephalus, and four died from cerebellar swelling. No clinically significant differences exist between full PICA and mPICA territory lesions.[32]

Clinical pictures. Several clinical syndromes can be distinguished. The *dorsal lateral medullary syndrome*[203,271,304,734,735] occurred in 25% of autopsy cases of PICA territory infarcts[16] and in one-third of 36 patients in a clinical series of 36 PICA infarctions.[395] Conversely, since dorsal medullary infarctions are almost constantly associated with PICA infarctions and 13% of cases of lateral medullary infarctions occur together with dorsal medullary infarctions,[333] a PICA territory cerebellar infarction is estimated to exist in 13% of cases of lateromedullary infarction.[22] Wallenberg syndrome can be complete or partial, with vertigo, nystagmus, loss of pain and temperature on the ipsilateral face, ninth and tenth cranial nerve palsies, ipsilateral Horner syndrome, appendicular ataxia, and contralateral temperature and pain sensory loss.

When *PICA territory infarctions spare the medulla*, patients mainly present with vertigo, headache, gait ataxia, limb ataxia, and horizontal nystagmus.[355,395,612,613,702] Headache is cervical or occipital, or both, occasionally with periauricular or hemifacial-ocular radiation. Unilateral headaches are ipsilateral to the cerebellar infarction.[395] Nystagmus is the most frequent sign (75%), being either horizontal (ipsilateral in 47% of patients, contralateral in 5%, bilateral in 11%) or vertical (11% of patients).[395] In addition to vertigo, one of the most striking findings in patients with PICA infarctions is ipsilateral axial lateropulsion, a phenomenon suggestive of a lateral displacement of the central representation of the center of gravity.[14] This sign is distinct from lateral deviation of the limbs (i.e., pastpointing) and gait veering. Kase et al also frequently noted that attempts at standing or walking led to falling toward the side of the cerebellar infarction. In one of four patients with this type of PICA infarction, there are signs of brain stem compression such as drowsiness and lateral gaze palsy, followed by progressive coma.[395]

The *isolated acute vertigo* form of PICA infarction, mimicking labyrinthitis, was first described clinicopathologically by Duncan et al[205] in a patient who died of acute myocardial infarction 3 weeks after the onset of vertigo. The autopsy showed a recent medial and caudal cerebellar infarction with no other brain lesions. Subsequently, several convincing clinical cases were reported.[229,312,368,606] We and others have reported a second typical case with necropsy confirmation of an old dorsomedial infarction of the right caudal cerebellum in the territory of mPICA with normal brain stem[20,22] (Fig. 22.12). It was due to an embolic occlusion of the ipsilateral VA involving the V2, V3, and V4 portions due to atrial fibrillation. MRI will probably reveal the actual frequency of PICA infarctions causing isolated vertigo. PICA infarctions should be looked for whenever vascular risk factors exist in vertiginous patients older than 50 years, and in circumstances supporting a vascular mechanism in the young. Normal caloric responses and direction-changing nystagmus on gaze to each side, or after changing head posture or lying down, are additional signs suggesting a pure vestibular syndrome with a PICA territory infarction.[205,613] Vertigo is explained by involvement of the uvulonodular complex of the vermis, which is part of

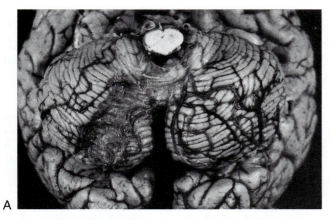

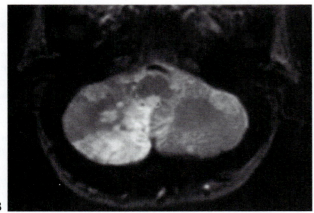

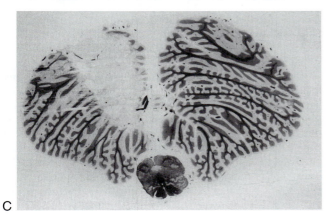

Figure 22.12 Infarctions in the territory of the medial branch of the posterior inferior cerebellar artery (mPICA) (**A**) at autopsy, (**B**) on T$_2$-weighted MRI, and (**C**) on a cartoon.

the vestibular portion of the cerebellum. Since the nodulus is supplied by the PICA and the flocculus by the AICA, these infarctions should not be called "flocculonodular infarctions."

PICA territory cerebellar infarcts are undoubtedly under-recognized and underdiagnosed. Recently Norrving and colleagues[533] studied 24 patients aged 50 to 75 years who came to the hospital in Lund, Sweden, with isolated severe vertigo. Six of the patients had PICA territory cerebellar infarcts (two mPICA, two adjacent parts of mPICA and lPICA, and two full PICA). Among the six patients with cerebellar infarcts,

three had cardiac-origin embolism, and three had VA occlusions. Norrving and colleagues[533] estimated that perhaps one-fourth of elderly patients presenting with severe vertigo and nystagmus might have PICA territory cerebellar infarcts.

PICA territory infarctions associated with AICA or SCA infarctions are much more severe in clinical presentation than isolated PICA territory infarctions.[22] They often present with a pseudotumoral pattern or with deep coma and tetraplegia. *Syndromes of the mPICA* are now frequent MRI findings.[14,28,32,56,136] The first documentation of the territory of the mPICA was reported in 1989[22] (Fig. 22.12). Consistent with its appearance on pathologic sections of the cerebellum at necropsy, Amarenco et al[32] then described the typical territory of mPICA infarctions on T$_2$-weighted MRI axial sections as areas of increased signal in a triangular zone, dorsomedially directed with the dorsal base and the ventral point directed toward the fourth ventricle (Fig. 22.12). Infarctions with occlusion of the medial branch may be clinically silent[22,32] or may present with three principal patterns:[32] (1) isolated vertigo, often misdiagnosed as labyrinthitis; (2) vertigo together with ipsilateral axial lateropulsion of the trunk and gaze,[565] and dysmetria or unsteadiness; and (3) Wallenberg syndrome, when the medulla is also involved. By contrast with PICA, only the mPICA gives rise to rami to the dorsolateral aspect of the medulla.

Clinical manifestations of infarcts of the *lateral branch of the PICA* have been reported as chance autopsy findings with no available clinical information.[22,304] Recently we reported one patient who presented with isolated dysmetria[20] (Fig. 22.13). Then Barth et al[57] reported on a series of 10 patients with cerebellar infarction in the territory of the lateral branch of the PICA. All patients presented with cerebellar dysmetria ipsilateral to the infarct without dysarthria, nystagmus, and rotatory vertigo.

PROGNOSIS. Recent clinical series showed that PICA infarctions have a much more benign outcome than is usually

Figure 22.13 Infarction in the territory of the lateral branch of the PICA (lPICA) (T$_2$-weighted MRI).

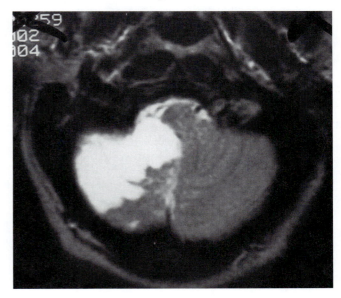

thought.[395] Sypert and Alvord's[676] autopsy series emphasized the high incidence of brain stem compression and tonsillar herniation in acute PICA infarctions, but most acute cases were detected only at necropsy, thus biasing the series to fatal cases with large infarcts. Cerebellar swelling should always be the major concern of clinicians taking care of patients with large cerebellar infarcts (see below). However, Sypert and Alvord[676] excluded from their analysis 46% of their patients with cerebellar infarction not seen acutely and only diagnosed at their autopsy study. Kase et al[395] found signs of brain stem compression in one-fourth of their 36 patients (all of whom had full PICA territory infarcts) and acute hydrocephalus in 7 patients; only 4 patients died from cerebellar swelling. Most full and partial PICA territory infarctions have a relatively benign course.[28,32,395]

CAUSE. The arterial occlusion primarily involves the intracranial portion of the VA facing the PICA ostium and the origin of the PICA. The mechanisms of occlusion are equally divided into cardioembolic and atherosclerotic causes.[22,395] Other mechanisms are VA dissection,[28,395] ulcerated plaques in the aortic arch,[21] and occlusion of the mPICA by tonsillar herniation due to raised posterior fossa pressure.[25]

Hemimedullary Infarction
(Elements of Medial and Lateral Ischemia)

The lateral medulla and inferior cerebellum are the most frequent sites of infarction in patients with occlusion of a single VA intracranially. The ischemia may extend more rostrally to affect the inferolateral pons[202,271] (pyramidal tract; fifth, sixth, and seventh cranial nerves; and motor dysfunction of the fifth cranial nerve) in the territory of the inferolateral pontine artery, which at times may arise from the very proximal basilar artery, but usually is a branch of the AICA.[24,208] Also, the infarction may extend to the medial medulla as well as the lateral tegmentum[202,271,333]; this presumably was the mechanism of hemiparesis or Babinski sign in the Babinski-Nageotte syndrome,[45,46,466] which includes elements of the lateral medullary syndrome with a crossed hemiparesis of Babinski sign. Paramedian arteries supplying the medial medullary territory arise from the anterior spinal arteries, which are branches of the V4 segment of the VAs.[208,333,466] Transient hemiparesis occurring in VA occlusion are presumably due to decreased flow in the medial medullary branches or rostral brain stem ischemia.

The hemiparesis is usually crossed, that is, contralateral to the infarct and on the same side as the body and limb pain and temperature loss. The anatomic basis for the hemiparesis is infarction of the medullary pyramid, a region supplied by the anterior spinal artery.[466,548] Occasionally, the hemiparesis is ipsilateral to the infarct and on the side of the cerebellar signs and contralateral to pain loss.[196] The anatomic explanation is infarction of the pyramid more caudally in the lower medulla and rostral spinal cord after the pyramidal decussation. This results from ischemia in anterior spinal artery supply more distally. Theoretically, a cruciate hemiplegia (one arm and opposite leg) could occur, but we know of no such documented cases.

Medial Medullary Infarction

Each VA usually gives rise to one or several small paramedian anterior spinal branches, which join to form the anterior spinal artery. This disposition usually prevents spinal cord or medial medullary infarction in cases of unilateral VA occlusion.[208,333] However, occasionally, unilateral occlusion of one anterior spinal branch can give rise to a paramedian medullary infarction involving the pyramid, medial lemniscus, and at times the hypoglossal nerve or nucleus.[333] Although the supply of anterior spinal branches is well known, and lesions are frequently postulated, documented occlusion of these vessels is extremely rare. Davison[176] reported one patient with infarction of the right pyramid and medial lemniscus who had severe paralysis of the left arm and leg, with tingling in those limbs. Dementia prevented careful sensory observations. Thrombosis of an anterior spinal artery branch and partial occlusion of the right VA were found at postmortem. Another patient had bilateral but asymmetric signs of damage to the medullary pyramid and medial lemniscus, with bilateral vibration and position sense loss and a unilateral brachiocrural hemiplegia with hyperreflexia and Babinski sign on the other side. Occlusion of the anterior spinal artery after its fusion was verified. Ropper et al[598] described a medullary infarct in the distribution of the anterior spinal artery that had been associated with paralysis of the arm and leg and subjective tingling. Unfortunately, the responsible occlusive lesion could not be identified. Ho and Meyer[354] reviewed the clinical findings in 15 reported cases of medial medullary syndrome. Hypertension was common. Necropsy usually revealed small infarctions involving the pyramid and medial lemniscus; the responsible vascular lesions were usually not identified. In a postmortem analysis of medullary infarcts, 7 of 10 medial infarcts were due to occlusion of the distal intracranial VA blocking the anterior spinal artery branch.[218,333]

Embolic occlusion of the anterior spinal artery territory may be more common than is presently recognized. Reports have now documented unilateral medial medullary infarction[615] and bilateral medial medullary infarcts[416,767] shown during life by MRI. Kase et al[394] described a 23-year-old woman with sudden onset of fibrocartilaginous disc material embolization to the anterior spinal artery branches of the VAs, causing bilateral medial medullary and rostral cord infarction. It is of interest that even though the most rostral level of infarction was below the pontomedullary junction, the patient had bilateral facial weakness, vertical nystagmus, and ocular bobbing, in addition to a flaccid quadriplegia. Flaccid or spastic quadriparesis and impaired control of respiration have been the most consistent clinical findings in patients with bilateral medial medullary infarcts.[176,380,394,416,494,502,707] Tongue weakness, facial weakness, and loss of deep sensations in the limbs have been variable. Mizutani and colleagues[502] also described foreign body emboli in each anterior spinal branch of the VAs; their patient had introduced foreign material into the circulation by intravenous injection of drugs designed for oral use. Nearly one-half of all reported examples of medial medullary infarction are bilateral[354]; usually the lesions occur simultaneously but may rarely develop on separate occasions.[252,711] Emboli reaching a single anterior spinal artery may flow into the point of junction of both anterior spinal branches, or emboli reaching the VA junction might preferentially pass into the anterior spinal artery orifices nearby.

Embolization of Clot from a Region of Vertebral Occlusion

Fisher and colleagues[271] documented distal embolization in three of their patients with vertebral occlusion and the lateral medullary syndrome. In one patient, embolic material blocked both superior cerebellar arteries, and in the other two patients branches of the PCAs were blocked. In cases of PICA infarctions due to VA occlusion, similar observations have been made at autopsy.[22] McCusker and colleagues[475] described a patient with a locked-in syndrome likely due to an embolus to the basilar artery arising from a previously occluded VA. Fisher and Karnes[272] noted 18 examples of local artery-to-artery embolism within the posterior circulation, 5 in relation to a unilateral VA occlusion. Castaigne et al[146] also described examples of artery-to-artery emboli within the posterior circulation, and Caplan[110] reported a patient (case 5) with spells of transient dizziness who developed a stroke when embolic material originating in a unilateral vertebral occlusion embolized to the SCA. George and Laurian[293] described two patients with unilateral VA stenosis and subsequent angiographically verified occlusion, who suffered embolism arising from the diseased VAs. George and Laurian[293] found that 80% of patients with a lateral medullary or cerebellar infarct and 65% of patients with basilar trunk territory infarcts had greater than 50% stenosis of a VA, leading the authors to suspect that the stenotic VA was a common source of embolism.

Koroshetz and Ropper[418] systematically studied patients with PCA territory strokes who also had brain stem symptoms. Six patients had occlusive lesions of the ICVA (combined with extracranial lesions in three patients); the authors considered that these lesions had served as donor sites for intra-arterial emboli to the PCA. Pessin et al[558] reported on a patient with a major basilar artery territory infarct in whom angiography showed occlusion of one intracranial VA and an intraluminal filling defect embolus in the distal basilar artery. Among a series of 85 patients with recent basilar artery thrombi who underwent acute thrombolytic treatment, 16 had stenotic or occlusive lesions of the ICVAs that likely served as a source of artery-to-artery emboli to the basilar artery. Figure 22.14 depicts an example of VA intracranial occlusion with an embolus to the distal basilar artery. In patients with distal basilar artery territory infarction, scant data are available concerning the incidence of coincidentally discovered vertebral occlusion that might have provided an embolic source. Within the anterior circulation, occlusion of the ICA is frequently heralded by a distal embolus.

Transient Ischemic Attacks or No Deficit

As in the case of occlusive disease of other major vessels, some patients suffer an ICVA occlusion without permanent deficit. On some occasions, the occlusion may be totally silent or produce only occipital headache. The most common transient symptom is dizziness or vertigo. In a review of patients who

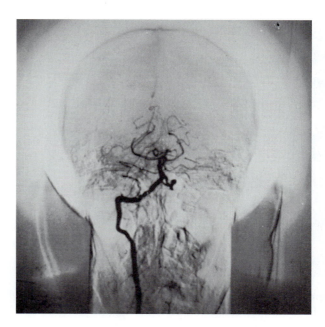

Figure 22.14 Vertebral angiogram showing right vertebral artery intracranial occlusion. The top of the basilar artery and posterior cerebral arteries are not opacified, probably owing to embolus from the vertebral artery clot.

subsequently developed a lateral medullary syndrome, dizziness accompanied other symptoms in 17 of 36 cases and was an unaccompanied symptom in 7 cases.

However, when vertigo was unaccompanied, if an infarct was to develop, it usually did so within 3 weeks. Chronic recurrent unaccompanied spells of vertigo (lasting longer than 6 weeks) are seldom if ever attributable to VA occlusion or other known vascular disease. Similarly, drop attacks (the patient although awake, falls precipitously to the ground, but then arises without a deficit) are considered by some to be typical of vertebrobasilar occlusion. It is often forgotten that similar dropping may occur for a variety of heterogeneous nonvascular reasons; isolated drop spells in the absence of other symptoms of brain stem ischemia have seldom, in our experience, been due to VA occlusion.

Occlusion of the VA can be verified angiographically, although attention must be paid to the specific radiologic features; the VA may be small, originate in an aberrant fashion, or end blindly in the PICA, producing a physiologic occlusion or, more simply, poor opacification.[685,691] Tatsumi and Shenkin[687] consider an irregular or mouse-bitten VA termination and collateral filling of the basilar artery as reliable signs of pathologic occlusion. A smooth vertebral termination and faint basilar opacification are more consistent with physiologic nonfilling. Figure 22.15 depicts occlusion of the VA after the PICA branch, with filling of the SCA from PICA branches.

TCD can now give accurate indications of stenotic and occlusive lesions in the intracranial VAs using insonation through a suboccipital foramen magnum window.[685,691] A study of TCD-angiographic correlation revealed excellent TCD results in patients with intracranial VA disease.[691] MRA may also allow accurate detection of these lesions, although

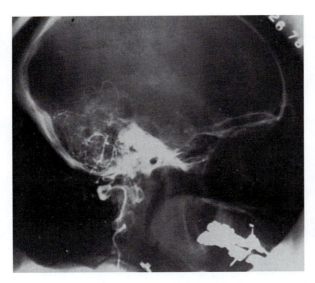

Figure 22.15 Vertebral angiogram. The vertebral artery does not fill past the posterior inferior cerebellar artery branch, and superior cerebellar artery branches fill from the posterior inferior cerebellar artery.

looping of the VA may present technical problems for imaging. Surgeons are now beginning to operate on patients with lesions of the ICVA. Direct endarterectomy in this segment has been performed.[10,40,374] More often bypass procedures are constructed to supply the distal system, especially when there are bilateral occlusive ICVA lesions.[374] Angioplasty using modern endovascular techniques is feasible, but as yet series of treated patients have not been reported.[349]

BILATERAL VERTEBRAL ARTERY OCCLUSION

Occlusion of the origins of the VAs, even when bilateral, can be surprisingly well tolerated because of the potential plethora of available collateral vessels that may supply the more rostral cervical VAs and ICVAs. Intracranial occlusion of both VAs, by contrast, is generally poorly tolerated by the patient and usually leads to severe cerebellar and brain stem infarction. Caplan[109] reviewed his experience with nine patients who had bilateral distal VA occlusion. Most patients had known severe systemic vascular disease as well as diabetes mellitus. The neurologic deficit usually developed gradually. Four patients had discrete TIAs and vague prodromal symptoms that included dizziness, blurred vision, ataxia, and headache; these warning symptoms did not have a discrete onset or end and so could not be easily classified as TIAs. The prodromal period was long and varied from 12 to 60 days (average, 17.3 days) before the stroke. Only one of the nine patients developed a stroke without warnings. The fixed neurologic deficit usually began on awakening or while resting. All patients had prominent cerebellar dysfunction in the form of limb and gait ataxia. Limb weakness was severe in eight patients, six of whom became quadriplegic. Nystagmus, facial weakness, and bilateral

miotic pupils were also common signs. Two patients had an associated PCA hemispheral deficit, and both had a homonymous hemianopia accompanied by an amnestic defect in one. Fluctuation of the neurologic deficits was common early in the course, and some patients became suddenly worse when they sat or stood or when their blood pressure was lowered. All patients died. Only one patient survived for an extended period, and he was the only one in whom a successful surgical posterior circulation shunt had been created. He died 5 months after the surgery but was quadriplegic and locked-in and resided in a nursing home prior to his septic death. Anticoagulation was of no obvious benefit. In the six patients studied postmortem, infarction decimated the medulla, pons, and cerebellar hemispheres, but tended to spare the upper pons and midbrain. Two patients had additional PCA territory infarcts.

Few examples of bilateral ICVA occlusion have been reported in clinical detail. Roski et al[601] reviewed patients treated with occipital artery to PICA bypass including six patients with bilateral ICVA occlusion. Three of these patients had only TIAs, one had a stroke, and two had both TIAs and stroke. Cerebellar, limb, and gait abnormalities were present in four patients, one had nystagmus, and one had a normal neurologic examination. After the shunt, two patients were considered normal or asymptomatic, three were improved, and one was unchanged. None worsened later. These authors also treated five other patients with unilateral ICVA occlusion and contralateral severe VA stenosis with occipital artery to PICA shunts and patients with ICVA occlusion who had many spells, often positional, of vertigo and alternating hemiparesis not responsive to heparin. An external carotid artery to PCA shunt was successful.

By contrast, Bogousslavsky et al[79] followed 10 patients with bilateral ICVA occlusions and reported a more benign prognosis: 4 presented with TIAs only, 4 had nondevastating strokes, and only 2 had severe brain stem infarcts. During follow-up, no severe brain stem strokes occurred, and only one patient died of brain stem infarction. The onset of symptoms was more abrupt than in the series of Caplan.[109]

In patients with basilar artery occlusion the most severely damaged regions are pontine bases bilaterally[426]; the lateral basis pontis, the tegmentum, and the cerebellum are relatively spared. The likely explanation for this distribution is found from analyzing the pattern of collateral circulation that develops when the basilar artery is occluded (Fig. 22.16). When the VA is patent, blood courses from the VA to the PICA and then to the cerebellar hemispheral AICA and SCA branches, ultimately nourishing the lateral brain stem and cerebellum. The pontine and midbrain tegmentum are supplied through the SCA.[70] In patients with bilateral VA occlusion, the PICA supply is usually compromised, leading to cerebellar infarction and poor collateral supply to the lower brain stem. In a clinical pathologic series of 64 patients with cerebellar infarction, five had bilateral ICVA occlusion[22,24,26]: one had devastating cerebellar infarctions involving the SCA territory on the left side and the PICA territory on the right side with intracranial occlusion of the left VA above the PICA ostium and of the right VA just below the PICA ostium; a second patient had SCA and PICA infarcts with bilateral distal occlusion of the VAs below the PICA ostium with an artery-to-artery embolism to the PICA on one side and to the PCA on the other side (this

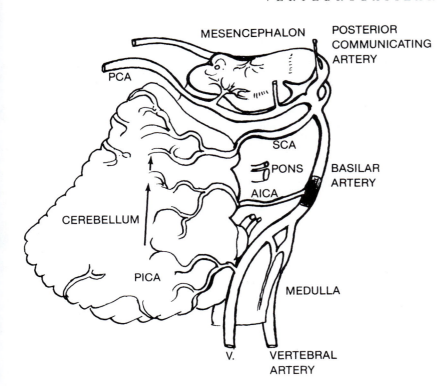

Figure 22.16 Diagrammatic representation of oblique view of the base of the brain. The pattern of collaterals can be seen (*arrows*) when the basilar artery is segmentally occluded.

patient also had severe ulcerated plaques in the aortic arch); one patient had bilateral AICA infarction with bilateral ICVA occlusion above the PICA ostium; another patient had a unilateral AICA infarct with bilateral occlusion of the distal VA above the PICA ostium; finally, the fifth patient had bilateral SCA territory infarction with one occlusion facing the PICA ostium (without PICA or medullary infarction) and the other below the PICA ostium. These observations showed that bilateral VA occlusions above the PICA ostium resulted in limited posterior ischemia whereas occlusions below the PICA ostium were poorly tolerated because of no possible retrograde revascularization of the basilar artery in this case by AICAs and SCAs via anastomoses with the PICAs.

Bilateral distal VA occlusion is usually considered rare (only 1 patient among 115 consecutive patients with cerebellar infarction[28]). The full neurologic deficit in this condition develops over a longer period compared with patients with basilar artery occlusion, branch disease, lacunes, or embolic infarction. The principal pathogenesis of posterior circulation ischemia in this condition is chronically reduced vertebrobasilar perfusion. Desmet and Brucher[191] described a patient with bilateral lateral medullary infarcts and reviewed the clinical and necropsy features of five other cases. Abnormal control of respiratory function may have led to death in these patients. All were considered asymptomatic or normal after surgical treatment. It is of interest that 8 of these 12 patients had orthostatic cerebral ischemia, that is, postural sensitivity of their neurologic signs. Hopkins et al[364] also studied a single patient with recurrent rostral brain stem ischemia, often positional, who had bilateral ICVA occlusion. A superficial temporal artery to PCA shunt seemed to stop his ischemic attacks. Ausman and colleagues[41] described a single patient with bilateral VA occlusion treated with a VA to PICA shunt using an interposed radial artery graft. This patient had intermittent left facial numbness, dysarthria, diplopia, limb and gait ataxia, and a lucent lesion on CT in the left brain stem and cerebellum. Aspirin and warfarin had not stopped the spells. After the surgical shunt, the patient had slight residual gait ataxia. Postural sensitivity was also a feature in this patient. Ausman et al[39] described another patient with unilateral ICVA occlusion and contralateral VA stenosis, who had spells of diplopia, vertigo, and blindness nearly daily, which were not stopped by aspirin, dipyridamole, or heparin. An occipital artery to AICA anastomosis was performed with good results. Sundt et al[669] described 14 patients treated with occipital to PICA bypass: 7 had bilateral VA occlusion, 3 had bilateral VA stenosis, and 3 had unilateral VA occlusion with contralateral stenosis. Cerebellar signs were prominent. In the patients with bilateral VA occlusion, four had an excellent result, two had good results, and one was improved. Sundt et al[669] also emphasized that orthostatic ischemia was present in six of seven patients with bilateral VA occlusion. Sundt and colleagues[667] later also described a single patient with bilateral occlusion, and the success of surgically constructed artificial conduits to bring more blood flow to the posterior circulation provides strong evidence for a low-flow state.[39,41,601,667] As in unilateral VA occlusion, bilateral lateral medullary infarction can lead to sudden death, perhaps due to autonomic, cardiovascular, or respiratory mechanisms.

However, in the New England Medical Center Posterior Circulation Stroke Registry an unexpected very high percentage of patients with ICVA occlusive disease (35%) had bilateral lesions.[126]

The prognosis of bilateral ICVA occlusion is variable. Some patients develop adequate collateral circulation and survive without major subsequent infarction.[79] In others, progressive ischemia develops, and the prognosis is grave.

BASILAR BRANCH DISEASE

A heterogeneous group includes all occlusive disease arising in small or larger branches of the basilar arteries. Convenient subdivisions are (1) intraparenchymatous occlusions resulting in lacunar infarctions due to hypertensive arteriolopathy, usually within the tiny penetrating parenchymatous vessels; (2) extraparenchymatous occlusion of small branches, such as median pontine or thalamogeniculate arteries, usually by miniature atherosclerotic plaques or junctional lesions involving the basilar artery wall[247,269]; and (3) stenosis or occlusion of larger circumferential branches, such as the AICA and SCA.

Lacunar Infarctions

Lacunes are the single most common lesion found in the brain stem at postmortem examination. These small deep infarcts are caused by disruption of vessels <200 μm in diameter by lipohyalinosis or, less commonly, by blockage of arteries 0.1 to 1 mm in diameter by miniature atherosclerotic plaques.[263] Precise clinicopathologic correlation has been infrequent, since the prognosis for recovery from the individual strokes is good, leaving less opportunity for pathologic confirmation. At postmortem, lacunes tend to be multiple, providing a dilemma as to which lacunes were responsible for which symptoms or signs. A lacunar infarct can vary from a tiny pinpoint hole to a larger cavitated lesion 1.5 cm in diameter. They are most common in the pons and thalamus, but do occur in the medulla and midbrain. In the medulla, pons, and midbrain they usually occupy the basal portion, especially medially, seldom extend far into the tegmentum, and are never limited solely to the tegmentum. Fisher's[252] intent in describing specific lacunar syndromes was to call attention to combinations of clinical findings that had an extremely high probability of being caused by lacunar infarctions; many lacunes, however, present a slight deficit impossible to distinguish from an incomplete stroke due to large vessel disease or embolism. Several syndromes known to be caused by brain stem lacunes are reviewed in the following sections.

SYNDROMES. *Pure motor hemiplegia.* Weakness of the face, arm, and leg is not accompanied by visual or sensory signs or deficits of higher cortical function in pure motor hemiplegia. Of the nine original cases studied by Fisher,[259] three had lesions in the basis pontis. One of these patients also had a conjugate gaze paresis to the ipsilateral side, identifying the pontine locus of the stroke. Transient tegmental symptoms or signs (diplopia, dizziness, nystagmus, or internuclear ophthalmoplegia), prominent dysarthria, an ataxic quality to the movements of the hemiparetic side, and bilateral extensor plantar reflexes sometimes give a clue to the brain stem origin. To date, CT has not been effective in predictably verifying these lesions, although we have seen one patient with a past pure motor hemiparesis in whom months after the stroke the definite pontine lacune was seen on CT. MRI is the best imaging technique to show lacunar in-

farcts.[58,358] A lacune in the medial medullary pyramid[354,548,598] or cerebral peduncle[353] can also produce a pure motor hemiparesis, usually with sparing of the face in medullary lesions.

Dysarthria-clumsy hand syndrome. The cardinal features of dysarthria-clumsy hand syndrome are moderate to severe dysarthria, corticobulbar weakness of the lower face and tongue, and slowness of fine movements of one hand. At times there is slight ataxia, hyperreflexia, or a Babinski sign on the side of the clumsy hand. The lesion is a small infarct in the dorsal basis pontis just below the medial lemniscus, which disrupts the corticobulbar fibers in this location.[243] The limb findings are due to dysfunction of extrapyramidal or pyramidal fibers within the basis pontis.

Ataxic hemiparesis. A syndrome in which motor hemiparesis (usually of slight degree) occurs with incoordination of the cerebellar type is termed ataxic hemiparesis.[246] Occasionally the pyramidal and cerebellar dysfunction is limited to the lower extremity; this variant is then called *homolateral ataxia and crural hemiparesis.*[270] The lesion responsible for ataxic hemiparesis is usually in the more rostral pons, interrupting crossing fibers as well as the pyramidal fibers in the pontine base. We have also seen a patient with this syndrome whose postmortem lesion involved the brachium conjunctivum and cerebral peduncle at the midbrain level. Slight ataxia of the contralateral (normal) leg has been a clue to the pontine location of this syndrome. At times, horizontal or vertical nystagmus and dysarthria accompany the limb ataxia and hemiparesis.[246]

Pure sensory stroke. A lacune in the somatosensory nuclei of the thalamus and ventral posterolateral and ventral posteromedial nuclei produces sensory symptoms on the opposite side of the body and face without motor, cerebellar, or higher cortical function abnormalities.[252,260,261,408] Paresthesias are usually characterized as tingling, prickling, or a sleepy, cold, hard, numb, or dead feeling. Usually at least two parts, face and arm or arm and leg, are involved.[260] The limbs are involved more than the face, but often the whole hemicorpus is affected, including the abdomen, chest, and face (including the eye, ear, and inside of the mouth). Cortical representation in the postcentral gyrus for the ear, eye, and trunk is quite small. Involvement of these structures usually means a lesion in a tract or a thalamic nucleus rather than a parietal cortical lesion. When the hand is affected, usually all digits are affected. The symptoms of sensory dysfunction usually far exceed the objective signs; in fact, objective parameters of sensory function may be completely normal. In one reported patient with a right lateral thalamic lacune, the sensory loss consisted only of proprioceptive loss with intact pain and temperature sensation.[608]

Helgason and Wilbur[336] described 10 patients with pontine infarcts identified by MRI in whom sensory symptoms and signs were the most prominent clinical finding. Four of these patients had infarcts that were localized to the lateral pontine tegmentum at various levels.

Sensorimotor stroke. A lacune may involve both the thalamic sensory nuclei and the adjacent posterior limb of the internal capsule. This leads to a combination of hemiparesis, pyramidal signs, and hemisensory loss all on the contralateral side, unaccompanied by visual or intellectual dysfunction.[508]

This syndrome is nearly impossible to differentiate from larger vessel ischemic disease or deep hemorrhage except by CT and angiography.

The tempo of lacunar infarctions in the posterior circulation has been similar to that of infarctions in a supratentorial location.[507] TIAs occur, but are less common than with larger vessel disease. The neurologic deficit usually develops over a period of hours to a few days and rarely evolves over more than 7 days. There is no accompanying headache. The patients generally remain alert. Hypertension, either in the past or present, is the nearly invariable requirement for the development of lacunes; the diagnosis should not be made in its absence. Other syndromes also occur, including pure dysarthria and toppling to the side whenever the erect position is attained, but an absence of symptoms and signs when the patient is examined supine or seated, and pure sensory stroke of just half the face and head. The pathologic basis for these lesions is unknown, but the ecology, tempo of onset, clinical course, and negative radiologic findings do suggest lacunar infarction as the most probable etiology.

Occlusion of Penetrating Branch Arteries in Their Extraparenchymatous Course

Occlusion of medium-sized penetrating vessels is probably quite common, but the pathology within these vessels has only been verified in detail in three cases.[247,269] All these patients were hypertensive and, in addition, two had known diabetes. Atherosclerotic branch disease is probably more common than is presently realized.[123] Diagnosis rests on a clinical syndrome limited to dysfunction in a unilateral branch[276,299,446,663] and findings on CT or MRI[58,684] of infarction in the territory of a single branch. The infarct may extend to the pontine basal surface, confirming that the occlusive process must have involved the branch before penetration of the parenchyma (Fig. 22.17). MRA or standard arterial opacification through catheters shows the patency of the parent basilar artery.

BASILAR BRANCH OCCLUSION WITH PONTINE INFARCTS. The two patients with unilateral basilar branch occlusion had transient tegmental signs: ipsilateral small pupil in one patient, and lateral gaze palsy, internuclear ophthalmoplegia, and horizontal and vertical nystagmus in the other.[269] One patient with bilateral branch occlusion was a hypertensive diabetic man who, 2 months previously, had had a minor stroke characterized by right hemiparesis, dysarthria, and transient diplopia.[123] This lesion was later traced to a bead of atheroma blocking a left pontine paramedian branch. He then developed dysarthria and a severe left hemiparesis. After his blood pressure was lowered precipitously and heparin was given, he became quadriplegic and lost all lateral gaze. Those caring for the patient (including the second author) thought he had an occlusion of the main basilar artery with extensive pontine infarction. To everyone's surprise, the basilar artery was widely patent at postmortem and the vascular lesions were limited to two adjacent paramedian branches. There was an old infarct in the left pons and fresh infarctions superimposed in both the left and right paramedian zones of the pontine base. In this case, prior branch occlusion and rapid reduction in blood pressure led to a large zone of ischemia much wider than would be expected in dis-

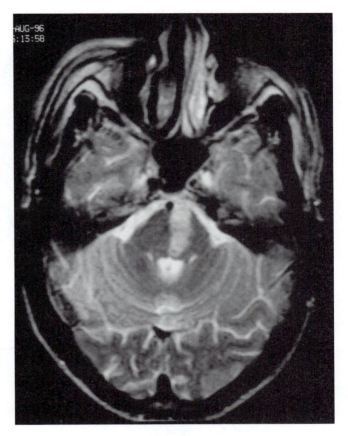

Figure 22.17 Paramedian infarct in the pons (T$_2$-weighted MRI). Note that the basilar artery is patent.

ease of a single branch. The pathology of the branch lesions has been described in the section of this chapter dealing with pathology.

The distribution and size of pontine infarcts depends heavily on the anatomy of the penetrating artery branches. Figure 22.18 shows the distribution within the pons of the arterial territories. These figures were constructed after Foix and Hilemand,[279] Gillilan,[299] and Duvernoy.[208] There are four major arterial territories: anteromedial, anterolateral, lateral tegmental, and posterior.[208] Foix and Hillemand in 1926[276] and then Lhermitte and Trelles in 1934[446] first focused attention on small unilateral pontine infarcts, either paramedian infarcts or small lacunes as infarcts *en chapelet* (Fig. 22.19). In these reports the authors summarized their experience without describing their case material in detail. They realized that these ventral pontine infarcts may have a different clinical presentation than pontine tumors or hemorrhages in which tegmental signs (i.e., cranial nerve involvement) are frequent, giving rise to complex syndromes (Millard-Gübler, Foville, and other alternating syndromes). They called attention to a few patients presenting with clinical symptoms and signs of these paramedian pontine infarcts described as pure motor hemiparesis, hemiparesis with crural predominance at times associated with some ataxia of cerebellar type (forme fruste of cerebellar signs), or some clumsiness of a limb.[276] Bilateral infarcts in the ventromedial area of the pons were responsible for pseu-

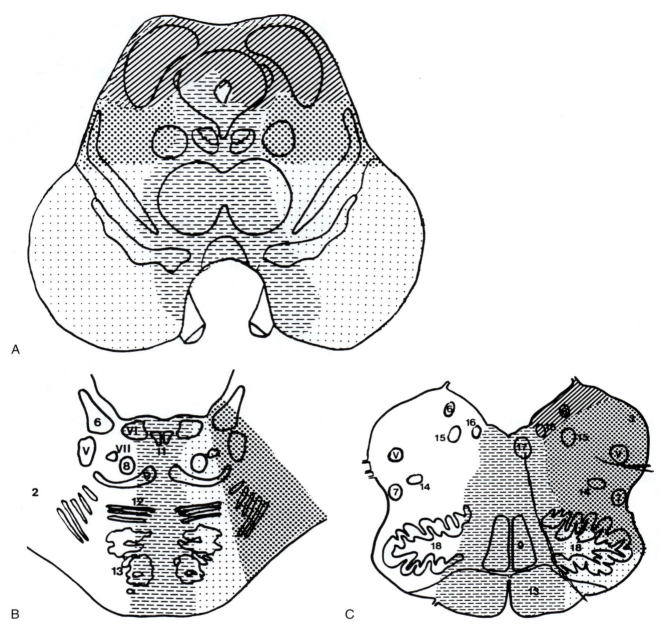

Figure 22.18 Cartoon of the arterial territories in the (**A**) medulla, (**B**) pons, and (**C**) mesencephalon.

dobulbar signs due to bilateral lacunes[276] and for pontine paraplegia in case of larger infarcts.[446]

Foix and Hillemand[276] in their initial description noted that these pontine infarcts are due to involvement of one of the paramedian pontine arteries (i.e., penetrator branches) and that larger paramedian infarcts were due to basilar artery disease that blocks the origin of one or several paramedian arteries.[27] Lhermitte and Trelles[446] established a parallel between small paramedian and short circumferential arteries and lenticulostriate arteries because they arise at right angles from a very large parent artery (the basilar artery for the former and the middle cerebral artery for the latter) and because their ostia may frequently be blocked by atherosclerotic plaques within the basilar artery.[45] Landmark demon-

stration of basilar artery branch occlusions was brought forth in 1971 by Fisher and Caplan,[269] as reported above.[23] Foix and Hillemand[276] also reported on pontine infarcts in the lateral territory of the short circumferential arteries with isolated ipsilateral cerebellar signs involving the arm and leg described as cerebellar hemiplegia.

Infarcts in these territories have been recently re-evaluated with MRI.[58,409,684,708] The most common site of infarction is medial along the base in the territory of the large anteromedial penetrating arteries. Bassetti et al[58] reported the MRI lesions in their patients with infarcts in the pons in anteromedial territory. Of their 36 patients with isolated pontine infarcts, 12 (33%) had lesions in this distribution. Anterolateral infarcts are probably the next most common distribution. These in-

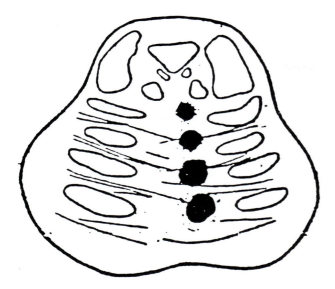

Figure 22.19 Infarcts *en chapelet* by Foix and Hillemand. (From Foix and Hillemand,[276] with permission.)

farcts are located in the basis pontis but more lateral than the medial basal infarcts. Infarcts in this anterolateral distribution tend to be smaller than medial lesions probably because the penetrating arteries are smaller. Hematomas in this location are also smaller than medial pontine hemorrhages. Anterolateral infarcts were found in 9 of the 36 patients (25%) in the series of Bassetti and colleagues.[58] The lateral territory of the caudal pons including the lateral tegmental area is usually supplied by branches arising from the AICA. The lateral portion of the tegmentum in the rostral portion of the pons is fed by penetrating artery branches of the long circumferential arteries (usually the SCAs). Lateral tegmental infarcts are less common than basis pontis infarcts. The posterior (dorsomedial) territories are supplied by a variety of circumferential arteries and are not known to be supplied by penetrating artery branches. Infarcts in the distribution of these circumferential vessels are usually accompanied by cerebellar infarcts or more widespread brain stem infarction due to basilar artery occlusion. The most difficult infarcts to classify by territory are those lesions that are purely tegmental but are not in the midline. This region is probably fed by anteromedial, anterolateral, and lateral tegmental branches varying in individual patients.

BASILAR BRANCH OCCLUSION WITH MIDBRAIN INFARCTS. Lipohyalinosis and atheromatous branch occlusions also occur frequently in arterial penetrating branches of the basilar artery apex and the adjacent basilar communicating, posterior communicating, and proximal posterior cerebral arteries. MRI is now able to identify infarcts limited to the territory of individual penetrating branches.[81,684] However, the only pathologic studies of lesions in penetrating arteries have been Fisher's[260–262] studies of patients with pure sensory stroke due to lateral thalamic infarction.

Paramedian arteries originate from the proximal basilar communicating artery (also called the P1 segment of the PCA by some) and supply the cerebral peduncles, medial portions of the substantia nigra, fascicles of the third cranial nerve, and the red nuclei.[359,769] Peduncular perforating arteries originate

from the distal end of the basilar communicating arteries and the proximal portions (P2a) of the PCAs as they course around the peduncles.[208,279,299,359] These arteries supply the more lateral portions of the ventral midbrain, including the lateral portions of the cerebral peduncles and substantia nigra.

Infarctions in the territory of the paramedian penetrating mesencephalic arteries are probably responsible for some examples of Weber syndrome (ipsilateral third cranial nerve palsy and contralateral hemiplegia), Claude syndrome (ipsilateral third cranial nerve palsy and contralateral limb dysmetria due to involvement of the lower part of the red nucleus), and Benedikt syndrome (ipsilateral third cranial nerve palsy and contralateral movement disorders due to involvement of the upper part of the red nucleus). Some diabetic third cranial nerve palsies probably involve the parenchymatous portions of the third cranial nerve before the fascicle exit from the midbrain.[362] Unilateral nuclear involvement of the third nerve by a small infarct results in vertical gaze paresis[360] and bilateral ptosis.[126] Pure motor hemiplegia could also result from infarction limited to the cerebral peduncle. In the case of peduncular hallucinosis related to bilateral infarcts in the substantia nigra pars reticulata cited earlier, infarction was probably due to bilateral small paramedian artery disease.[476] An organized occlusion with recanalization was identified in one small penetrating artery within the substantia nigra. Some patients with caudal midbrain infarcts have predominant sensory abnormalities.[81]

In the series of Bogousslavsky et al,[81] 12 patients, all with infarcts in the middle midbrain group, had third nerve dysfunction. Five patients with paramedian tegmental infarcts had evidence of involvement of the third nerve nucleus, usually causing bilateral ptosis and bilateral superior rectus weakness. Some also had bilateral mydriasis. Two of these patients also had contralateral limb motor weakness or ataxia. The 7 patients with infarcts that were more ventral and lateral had peripheral-type unilateral third nerve paralysis without other major signs. In one of these patients, the palsy was only partial involving just elevation and adduction of the ipsilateral eye. The other six had weakness of all third nerve innervated muscles, severe ptosis, and mydriasis.[81] In the series of Tatemichi et al,[684] two patients had nuclear third nerve palsies with a complete third nerve palsy on one side and ptosis and elevation palsy on the opposite side. Contralateral weakness or ataxia was often associated.

BASILAR BRANCH OCCLUSION WITH THALAMIC INFARCTS. Four main groups of arteries penetrate the thalamus, arising from the region of the basilar artery bifurcation: two groups of thalamoperforating arteries, the polar (tuberothalamic) arteries and the thalamic-subthalamic (thalamoperforating) arteries, and the thalamogeniculate and the posterior choroidal arteries.

Polar artery. The polar artery (also called the anterior internal optic artery by Duret,[206] the premammillary pedicle by Foix and Hillemand,[279,552,553] and the tuberothalamic artery[131,307]) usually arises from the middle portion of the posterior communicating artery to supply the anterolateral portion of the thalamus. In about a third of cases this artery is absent, and the thalamic-subthalamic artery also supplies this territory. The polar artery supply includes the lateral portion of the anterior thalamic pole, but not the anterior nucleus. Portions of the ventral lateral, dorsomedial, and reticular nuclei are supplied as well as part of mammillothalamic tract.[83,131,307]

Supply is said to be always unilateral by single branches. Infarcts can result from penetrating branch disease or clipping of ICA or posterior communicating artery aneurysm.

Unilateral infarcts cause minor or negligible contralateral motor signs, for example, slight often transient hemiparesis, asymmetric facial expression, slight asymmetry of arm swing, and spontaneous or automatic use of the contralateral limbs. Sensory and oculomotor findings are generally absent.[83,131,307] Cognitive and behavioral abnormalities predominate. Initially, patients may appear confused and disoriented. Later, the predominant findings are lack of initiation and spontaneity, long latency in responding, and inability to persevere with protracted tasks. These deficits have been called abulia by Fisher.[245] They are identical to dysfunction found in patients with disease of the frontal lobes and caudate nuclei[139] and probably indicate loss of function of corticostriatothalamic projections from the anterior thalamic nuclei.[145]

Patients with left anterolateral thalamic infarcts may also have slight aphasic abnormalities with paraphasic errors and verbal perseverations but retain the ability to repeat spoken language.[131] With right anterolateral thalamic infarction, constructional praxis and visual-spatial abnormalities may also be found.[83,131] Verbal memory is affected in left-sided lesions and visual memory in right-sided infarcts.[109,307] The abulia and cognitive and behavioral abnormalities are often transient and usually regress and substantially recover during the 3 to 6 months after the stroke. Kotila and colleagues,[419] using seven patients with left polar artery territory infarcts, studied cognitive functions during the acute phase and after 1 year. The most severe impairments in these patients were in memory functions. The memory performance of all the patients was far below average and five fulfilled criteria for having amnesic syndromes. The most severe deficits were in memorizing verbal material. Intellectual performances generally improved to normal including orientation and visual memory. Verbal memory also improved, but difficulties remained in the learning and recall of verbal material and for names of individuals.[419] The memory deficits prevented three of the four patients who attempted to return to work from succeeding in retaining their previous jobs. The abulia and apathy often improve dramatically in patients with unilateral lesions. Occasional patients have been reported with bilateral, nearly symmetric polar artery territory infarcts.[389] One patient suddenly became abulic and unconcerned after cardiac catheterization and has remained abnormal—very apathetic and unmotivated in the years since. Memory loss and abulia are more severe and more persistent in patients with bilateral lesions. The occurrence of bilateral isolated polar artery territory infarcts suggests that, in some patients, the polar artery, like the thalamic-subthalamic arteries, may emerge from a single artery or an arcade of vessels.[389,553] Polar territory infarcts are responsible for what has been referred to as acute thalamic dementia.

Thalamic-subthalamic arteries. The thalamic-subthalamic arteries (also called interpeduncular profunda arteries, the paramedian thalamic arteries by Percheron,[552,553] the posterior internal optic arteries by Duret,[206] and the thalamoperforating pedicle by Foix and Hillemand[279]) arise from the basilar communicating artery segment of the PCA. The arterial pattern is quite homogeneous. Single arteries to each side can arise, or bilateral branches may arise from a unilateral single artery, or arteries to both sides may arise from a pedicle.[131,145,484,552] These arteries may also supply territory usu-

ally supplied by the polar arteries. Medial thalamic infarcts in the territories of the thalamic-subthalamic arteries usually involve the subthalamus, the rostral interstitial nucleus of the medial longitudinal fasciculus, the nucleus parafascicularis, and the medial part of the centromedian nucleus.[131,145,307,681] Ischemia in the territory of these arteries can be caused by atheromatous branch disease, emboli to the basilar apex, or aneurysms at the basilar bifurcation.

Reported patients with unilateral paramedian left thalamic infarcts all have had upgaze pulses and loss of convergent eye movement.[82,145,307,513,733] Temporary downgaze paresis may also be present. The vertical gaze abnormality affects voluntary saccades, smooth pursuit, and vestibulo-ocular reflex motions.[131] Disorientation and severe amnesic deficits have also been noted.[82,145,307,513] Some patients have also had aphasic abnormalities characterized by occasional paraphasic errors and loss of naming abilities. A minor right hemiparesis characterized by decreased spontaneous and associated movements of the right limbs may be present.[82,145,307] One patient had decreased pain and touch sensation in the right face.[82,131] Insufficient examples of unilateral right-sided paramedian infarction limited to the territory of the thalamic-subthalamic artery are reported that might permit clinicopathologic correlation. Bilateral paramedian infarcts cause hypersomnolence, vertical gaze palsies predominantly of upgaze, loss of ocular convergence, and amnesic syndrome.[131,144,145,484,674,725] Elements of third cranial nerve palsies may also be present. The deficits in patients with bilateral lesions have been qualitatively similar but more severe and more persistent than those found in patients with unilateral posteromedial infarcts. Patients with bilateral paramedian thalamic infarcts usually have persistent severe amnesia and vertical gaze palsies.[462] Malamut and colleagues[462] found that explicit memory (i.e., ability of patients to repeat on confrontation after a delay items that were previously told to them) was very defective but that implicit memory (i.e., unconscious learning as shown from action) was relatively preserved. A permanent Korsakoff-like syndrome often develops in patients with bilateral posteromedial infarcts.

Apathy, disinterest, flattening of emotions, lack of insight, and indifference to people and the environment may be severe. Affective responses to the environment are usually reduced, and patients appear changed in their interpersonal relations: they are described as less warm and caring and more stoical and introverted. Bogousslavsky and colleagues[84] used the term coined by Laplane, "lack of psychic self-activation," to describe aspects of this behavior.[83] One of their patients would "sit at the table to eat only when asked by nurses or family and would stop eating after a few seconds unless repeatedly stimulated. During the day, he would stay in bed or in an armchair unless asked to go for a walk. He did not react to unusual stimuli in the room such as grand mal seizures in another patient. He did not read newspapers and did not watch television.[84] In this patient and some others single-photon emission computed tomography or positron emission tomography have shown medial frontal lobe hypometabolism.[68,84] So-called utilization behavior, in which patients automatically and inappropriately handle and use objects placed before them even though told not to use them, has also been described in patients with posteromedial bilateral thalamic infarcts.[219] This phenomenon, described and named by Lhermitte,[444] has usually been described in patients with frontal lobe disease. Another patient with a large right thalamic infarct that probably included some of the territory of both the polar and thalamic-subthalamic arteries was also noted to have utilization behavior in that she could not inhibit and diffuse decrease in uptake on single-photon emission computed tomography scans in the entire right hemisphere, especially frontally.[329] Hypersomnolence may be more prolonged and severe in patients with bilateral disease. One patient had a compulsive tendency to lie in a sleeping position with her eyes closed throughout the day.[147] She was also apathetic, disinterested, and inactive. It is of great interest that administration of bromocriptine in large doses (≤120 mg/day) resulted in an increase in spontaneous activities and lessening of the sleep-like behavior.[147]

Thalamogeniculate arteries. The thalamogeniculate arteries arise as a pedicle or group of arteries from the ambient segment of the PCA. The pedicle usually consists of six to eight arteries that vary widely in diameter and penetrate the ventral lateral thalamus between the geniculate bodies.[135,279,680] These arteries supply the somatosensory nuclei, the ventral posterolateral and posteromedial nuclei, the inferior and posterior portions of the ventral lateral nucleus, the lateral portion of the centromedial nucleus, and the rostrolateral portion of the pulvinar.[135] In most cases the thalamogeniculate arteries probably also supply a portion of the posterior limb of the internal capsule, as can be seen from the lesions in the original cases of Dejerine and Roussy.[135,181]

Three somewhat distinct syndromes result from infarction in the territory supply of the thalamogeniculate arteries and their branches. These vessels are the posterior circulation counterpart of the lenticulostriate branches of the middle cerebral arteries. Lesions of small branches can produce infarction restricted to the somatosensory nuclei causing the clinical syndromes of pure sensory stroke or sensory loss limited to the face.[260,262] Occlusion of branches supplying the lateral thalamus and posterior limb of the internal capsule can give rise to a sensorimotor stroke in which the deficits are restricted to paresis, decreased pin and touch perception, and pyramidal signs without cognitive or behavioral abnormalities.[135,508] Larger lateral thalamic infarcts cause a syndrome originally described by Dejerine and Roussy,[181] which included hemiataxia, hemichorea, transient hemiparesis, and hemisensory symptoms and signs.[135]

Choroidal arteries. The anterior choroidal artery is also known to supply a small portion of the thalamus,[206] although this is still debated.[279,552,553] However, infarction restricted to the thalamus after occlusion of this artery has not been documented.[335]

Lateral geniculate body infarction can occur secondary to occlusive lesions of either the anterior or posterior choroidal arteries and produce characteristic visual field deficits. Infarcts in the territory of the medial and lateral posterior choroidal arteries are the least well known and most rarely reported of all thalamic infarcts.[77,89] The lateral arteries supply mostly the pulvinar, a portion of the lateral geniculate body, and the anterior nucleus. The medial arteries supply the habenula, anterior pulvinar part of the center median nucleus, and the paramedial nuclei.[279] There have been very few clinicopathologic[76,193,732] and clinicoradiographic reports of patients with posterior choroidal territory infarcts.[67,126,456,527,632] This syndrome is summarized in the series reported by Neau and Bogousslavsky.[527]

The first reported necropsy case was a 52-year-old man who became confused and aphasic and had an infarct in the thalamus in the distribution of the posterior choroidal arteries at postmortem examination.[76,732] The second case involved a 67-year-old woman who had abnormalities of vertical eye movements including retractory nystagmus, and later developed a hemiparesis.[76,193] Although a number of different phenomena may occur in patients with posterior choroidal territory infarction, the most specific abnormality relates to the visual fields. The posterior choroidal arteries and their lateral choroidal artery branches supply a portion of the lateral geniculate body reciprocal to that supplied by the anterior choroidal arteries. The characteristic visual field defect in patients with posterior choroidal artery territory infarcts is a sectoranopia involving a wedge defect on each side of the horizontal meridian.[288,527] By contrast, the visual field defect in patients with anterior choroidal artery territory infarcts can include loss of the upper and lower quadrants with sparing of vision in a line along the median horizontal meridian. Patients with posterior choroidal territory infarcts can also have either an upper or lower quadrantanopia.

Other clinical deficits are less well established. Pulvinar ischemia can cause aphasia, visual hallucinations, and abnormal limb movements and postures. The anterior nucleus of the thalamus with its frontal lobe projections can also be involved. In the Stroke Data Bank series of patients with thalamic infarcts, the most common restricted focal infarcts were in the territory of the posterior choroidal arteries.[657] Two of the patients with posterior choroidal territory infarcts had prominent contralateral neglect. Little is known about infarcts limited to the pulvinar or the anterior nucleus of the thalamus. Ghika et al[296] reported on a patient with an infarct in the left posterior thalamus involving the internal medullary lamina and the pulvinar in the territory of the left lateral posterior choroidal artery. This patient, who was severely hypertensive, had burning paresthesia in his right hand and foot at the onset of the stroke but later developed restlessness, akathisia, and an irrepressible urge to move the right limbs, symptoms that improved after he was given clonazepam.[296] Lateral posterior choroidal territory infarcts can involve fibers synapsing in the thalamic sensory nuclei, and hemisensory syndromes can result.[126]

Occlusion of Long Circumferential Branches: Anterior Inferior and Superior Cerebellar Arteries

The most common mechanism of occlusion of the AICA and SCA is by atheroma or thrombus in the parent basilar artery blocking the orifice of these branches. However, in some cases, atheroma or thrombosis is confined to these branches without major disease of the parent vessel.

ANTERIOR INFERIOR CEREBELLAR ARTERY OCCLUSIONS. AICA infarctions are exceedingly rare, but many probably go undiagnosed.[24] MRI reveals a higher incidence of such strokes than was previously suspected[29] (Fig. 22.4). This type of pontocerebellar infarction differs strikingly from SCA and PICA infarctions in terms of brain stem signs associated with the clinical presentation.

The cerebellar territory of the AICA (Fig. 22.3) varies as a function of its caliber. This is usually not the same from one side to the other. Nearly always the artery supplies the flocculus, the only territory of the cerebellum usually vascularized solely by the AICA.[431] The flocculus is supplied by the PICA rather than the AICA in only 3% to 5% of individuals. In 40% of subjects, the AICA ends on the flocculus.[431] In others, it follows the sulcus separating the anterior lobule and the semilunar lobule and gives rise to terminal branches that supply the neighboring lobules: anterior, simplex, superior semilunar, inferior semilunar, gracilis, and lobulus biventer in 18% to 50% of individuals.[37,431] The AICA can replace a hypoplastic PICA, taking over the supply to most of the inferior surface of the cerebellum, including the anterolateral part of the tonsil but not the vermis. According to Stopford,[663] Foix and Hillemand,[279] Atkinson,[37] Takahashi et al,[681] and Perneczky et al,[556] a balance in size exists between the AICA and the PICA, the artery giving rise to the lateral branch of the PICA being able to arise from AICA. The terminal branches of the AICA anastomose with the ipsilateral SCA and the PICA at the border zone areas of these arteries.

The pontine distribution of the AICA (Fig. 22.3) has been precisely described by Duvernoy.[208] The AICA supplies the middle cerebellar peduncle in every instance, the lower third of the lateral pontine territory in most cases, its middle third frequently, and in a few individuals the superior part of the lateral region of the medulla.

Few reports on AICA infarctions have been published to date, and only recently have series of patients studied pathologically[24] and with MRI been published.[29] The first full report of the AICA syndrome was by Raymond Adams[4] in 1983 in a clinicopathologic study of one patient. Goodhart and Davison[304] had briefly described a patient 7 years before who had an infarct limited to the AICA territory of the cerebellum and whose only symptom was vertigo. The most extensive clinical necropsy study of 20 patients with AICA territory infarcts was by Amarenco and Hauw in 1990.[24] With the advent of MRI, precise localization of brain on nine stem and cerebellar infarcts became possible during life. In 1993, we reported on nine patients with AICA territory infarcts identified by CT and MRI.[29] Matsushita and colleagues[474] also reported on five patients whose AICA territory infarcts were diagnosed by MRI. Fisher[251] reported on one patient diagnosed with MRI.

Clinical aspects. Most AICA infarcts involve a small territory restricted to the lateral region of the caudal pons and, in the cerebellum, to the middle cerebellar peduncle (100% of cases) and flocculus (69% of cases). Involvement of this region accounts for most of the clinical signs described with AICA occlusions.[24] Infarctions often also affect other cerebellar lobules (75% of cases) but usually remain limited in size.

Infarcts commonly involve a small part of the cerebellum comprising the central white matter, the flocculus, and a thin rim of cerebellar cortex located at the junction of the territories of the three major cerebellar arteries, as illustrated in Figure 22.3, but this involvement does not modify the clinical presentation. When the AICA is large (and the PICA is hypoplastic), the AICA territory encompasses the whole anterior inferior cerebellum. There is no significant clinical difference between the signs and symptoms initially observed after infarctions arising with relatively limited AICA involvement and those observed after infarctions arising in vascular systems that have both the AICA and the PICA arising from a common trunk from the vertebral or basilar arteries.[24]

In most AICA infarctions, the inferolateral pontine territory is involved, the infarction sometimes extending up to the middle third of the lateral pons and down to the superior part of the lateral medulla. It involves neither the upper third of the lateral pons, which is supplied by the superior lateral pontine artery, a branch of the basilar artery or of the medial branch of the SCA, nor the ventral aspect of the pons. AICA territory infarctions are associated with PICA and SCA infarcts in 35% of autopsy cases, and this frequently occurs with ventromedian pontine infarction and tonsillar herniation.[24] Other partial AICA infarctions involve at least the middle cerebellar peduncle, the core of the AICA territory.

Four distinct clinical pictures can be distinguished in patients with AICA occlusions (Table 22.2).

The classic syndrome of the AICA, first described by Adams[4] in one patient, is the most common clinical picture described with AICA occlusions.[24] Symptoms include vertigo, vomiting, tinnitus, and dysarthria. Signs include ipsilateral facial palsy, hearing loss, trigeminal sensory loss, Horner syndrome, appendicular dysmetria, and contralateral temperature and pain sensory loss over the limbs and trunk.[4,24] The AICA syndrome may also include ipsilateral conjugate lateral gaze palsy due to involvement of the flocculus rather than damage to the abducens nucleus, dysphagia due to extension of the infarction to the superior part of the lateral medulla, and ipsilateral limb weakness due to contralateral involvement of the corticospinal tract in the pons or mesencephalon.[24] Because some signs are crossed and otherwise some are similar to signs arising with Wallenberg syndrome, an AICA occlusion is often misdiagnosed as lateral medullary infarction. However, signs unusual in Wallenberg syndrome, such as severe facial palsy, deafness, tinnitus, and multimodal sensory impairment over the face, allow accurate clinicotopographic diagnosis.[24]

A complete AICA syndrome was observed in 30% of autopsy cases in individuals with AICA occlusion, an almost complete syndrome in 35%, and an incomplete syndrome in 10%.[24] Limb weakness was found in half these patients.

Coma with tetraplegia from onset occurred in 20% of cases of AICA that came to autopsy.[24] It was due to massive ventromedial involvement of the basis pontis together with cerebellar infarction in the territory of all three cerebellar arteries.

Isolated vertigo, mimicking labyrinthitis, occurs in partial AICA territory infarcts. This was suspected for a long time,[4,304] initially posited in case 1 of Rubenstein et al[606] in which the CT findings were not convincing, and finally demonstrated with MRI by Amarenco et al.[18,20,30] Oas and Baloh[535] reported on two patients who had unilateral AICA territory infarcts in whom attacks of vertigo preceded the strokes by 12 and 3 months, respectively. Each patient also had unilateral hearing loss. However, due to the extent of the territory usually supplied by the AICA, isolated vertigo as the sole clinical presentation is likely to be exceptional. In the case with vertigo as the sole clinical presentation without cranial nerve involvement mimicking a labyrinthitis that we reported,[20,30] only the vestibular nuclei, middle cerebellar peduncle, and flocculus areas were involved on MRI. Surprisingly, the angiogram showed two AICAs on the same side. The one of large caliber arose from the midbasilar artery; the other was hypoplastic and arose from the proximal part of the basilar artery, then reached the flocculus area, where it ended and ramified.[30] This small AICA corresponded to the lower supplementary cerebellar artery described by Jacob.[381] No occlusion was seen on angiography, but this small AICA was thought to be likely responsible for the lesion. Only this very unusual arterial disposition in this patient made possible the small extent of the AICA infarction and its unique clinical pre-

Table 22.2 Cerebellar Stroke Syndromes

Location of Cerebellar Infarct	*Associated Infarcts*	*Clinical Syndrome*
Rostral (SCA)	Mesencephalon, subthalamic area, thalamus, occipitotemporal lobes	Rostral basilar artery syndrome or coma from onset ± tetraplegia
	Laterotegmental area of the upper pons	Dysmetria and Horner syndrome (ipsilateral), temperature and pain sensory loss, and nerve IV palsy (contralateral)
	0	Dysarthria, headache, dizziness, vomiting, ataxia, and delayed coma (pseudotumoral form)
Dorsomedial (mSCA)	0	Dysarthria
		Ataxia
Ventrolateral (lSCA)	0	Dysmetria, axial lateropulsion (ipsilateral) ataxia, and dysarthria
Medial (AICA)	Lateral area of the lower pons	Nerves V, VII, and VIII, Horner syndrome, dysmetria (ipsilateral), temperature and pain sensory loss (contralateral)
	0	Pure vestibular syndrome
Caudal (PICA)	0	Vertigo, headache, vomiting, ataxia, and delayed coma (pseudotumoral form)
Dorsomedial (mPICA)	Dorsolateromedullary area	Wallenberg syndrome
	0	Isolated vertigo or vertigo with dysmetria and axial lateropulsion (ipsilateral) and ataxia
Ventrolateral (lPICA)	0	Vertigo, ipsilateral limb dysmetria
Caudal and medial	Lateral area of the lower pons or lateromedullary area, or both	AICA syndrome ± delayed coma (pseudotumoral form)
Rostrocaudal	0	Vertigo, vomiting, headache, ataxia, dysarthria, and delayed coma (pseudotumoral form)
	Brain stem, thalamus, occipitotemporal lobes	Coma from onset ± tetraplegia

Abbreviations: SCA, superior cerebellar artery; mSCA, medial branch of the SCA; lSCA, lateral branch of the SCA; AICA, anterior inferior cerebellar artery; PICA, posterior inferior cerebellar artery; mPICA, medial branch of the PICA; lPICA, lateral branch of the PICA.

sentation. Another explanation for isolated vertigo in patients with AICA occlusion is occlusion of the internal auditory artery, which supplies the labyrinth and cochlea and arises from the AICA in 80% of individuals. However, good clinical pathologic reports of such cases are lacking. AICA territory infarctions can also cause *isolated cerebellar signs* as demonstrated in a clinical MRI report in a child.[563]

Prognosis. Although most cases reported in the literature have been based on autopsies, AICA infarctions may have a better outcome than would be predicted from these published reports. Most of the reported cases died from remote complications, such as pulmonary embolism and infections. Clinical MRI reports that have been published depict patients with benign outcomes and minimal neurologic residua.[29,30,251] Our clinical report[30] and those of Oas and Baloh[535] of banal, isolated vertigo with benign outcome suggest that partial AICA territory infarctions may be more frequent than has been recognized. Alternatively, AICA occlusion may be a very rare cause of isolated vertigo, as in our patient with an unusual supplementary AICA.

In some cases, AICA territory infarctions may herald massive basilar artery thrombosis, as we have reported.[20,29]

Cause. The arterial occlusion usually seen postmortem involves the lower basilar artery and less frequently the end of the VA above the PICA ostium at postmortem examination.[24] In many cases, there have been associated anomalies of the vertebrobasilar

system, such as a hypoplastic VA, dolichoectatic basilar artery, or patent trigeminal artery. The mechanism was mostly atherosclerotic occlusion.[24] In this study one patient with an isolated AICA territory infarction and one with AICA-SCA-PICA infarctions had no arterial occlusion at necropsy, but each had high-risk cardiac sources of emboli: mitral stenosis with atrial fibrillation and an acute myocardial infarction with a mural thrombus.[21,24] These two cases provide additional evidence that cardiac origin emboli can occasionally cause a unilateral AICA territory infarct. In a series of nine patients with AICA infarction studied during life who were diagnosed with MRI and contrast angiography, we could clearly separate two groups of patients.[29] Four diabetic patients had isolated unilateral AICA infarction, patent basilar artery, and probably basilar branch occlusion due to basilar artery plaques that extended into the AICA or microatheroma that blocked the AICA origin. The other five patients had AICA infarction together with other pontine, midbrain, occipital, PICA, or SCA infarction. They all had basilar artery occlusion including the AICA level and reconstitution of the distal basilar artery by collaterals through hemispheric anastomoses from the PICAs and posterior communicating arteries.[29] Among 79 consecutive patients with territorial cerebellar infarcts, Amarenco et al[28] included 9 patients with AICA territory infarcts. Seven of these nine likely had occlusive branch disease, and the others had ICVA or basilar artery occlusion, or both. Intracranial giant cell arteritis has been shown to cause an occlusion of AICA in one patient studied at necropsy.[478] Cases associated with migraine were also reported.[125]

Figure 22.20 Superior cerebellar artery branches (three-quarter view). The lateral branch of the SCA and medial branch of the SCA and its vermal branches, paravermal branches, and hemispheric branches.

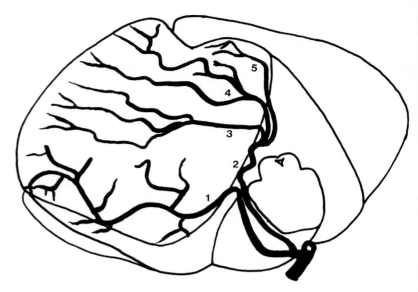

SUPERIOR CEREBELLAR ARTERY OCCLU-SIONS. SCA infarctions are among the most frequent of the cerebellar stroke syndromes. Fifty percent to 65% of all cerebellar infarctions appear in the distribution of this artery.[26,28,56,150,350,395] SCA territory infarctions are characterized by the rarity of clinical involvement of the brain stem territory of the SCA and do not frequently present with the classic SCA syndrome.[26,28,151,395,396] They typically have partial cerebellar involvement, a cardioembolic origin, and a relatively benign prognosis.[28,31,56,150,395,460,664] The SCA supplies the rostral surface of the cerebellum down to the great horizontal sulcus (Fig. 22.3), including the lobulus centralis, culmen, clivus, folium, and tuber of the vermis; the anterior, simplex, and superior semilunar lobules of the cerebellar hemispheres; and, rarely, the upper part of the inferior semilunar lobules.[23] Hemispheric branches can be classified as *medial, intermediate* (both arising from mSCA), and *lateral* (arising from lSCA) groups.[432] The *medial group* supplies the vermis and gives rise to two branches. A paramedian branch on the vermal surface anastomoses with the contralateral mSCA; the other branch runs parallel to the first paramedian branch but more laterally on the medial surface of the hemisphere (Fig. 22.20). Sometimes it is replaced by an artery from the intermediate group.

The *intermediate group* has one to four arteries running obliquely, dorsally, and laterally, giving rise to numerous rami, some of which anastomose with branches from the PICA. One of the arteries from the intermediate group often runs directly down, giving few rami to the rostral cortex and anastomosing directly with one of the PICA branches. The *lateral group*, arising from the lSCA, runs anteriorly on the anterosuperior margin dividing the superior and anterior aspects of the cerebellum (Fig. 22.20). The territory of the lSCA includes the anterior rostral cerebellar cortex and adjacent white matter (the anterior part of the anterior simplex, and superior semilunar lobules) and the ventral aspect of the dentate nucleus.[31] The lSCA probably never supplies the flocculus. Anastomoses exist between the lateral group of the lSCA and branches of the AICA.

The boundary zone between SCA and PICA territories usually lies just above the great horizontal sulcus. The SCA rarely supplies the upper part of the inferior semilunar lobule and never the cerebellar tonsil.[432] As far as the vermis is concerned, the SCA and PICA territories usually overlap on the tuber or the clivus.

The deep territory of the SCA is larger than that of the other two cerebellar arteries. It supplies the dentate, intermediate (the embolus and globulus), and fastigial nuclei and most of the cerebellar white matter.[177,432] The white matter is supplied by branches arising from the cortex that penetrate the cortex perpendicularly and extend toward the dentate nucleus. These branches anastomose in the dentate nucleus with early branches of the parent trunk that follow the superior cerebellar peduncle, giving rise to an internal anastomotic network between deep and superficial branches of the SCA.[432]

In the brain stem, the SCA supplies the dorsolaterotegmental area of the upper pons (Fig. 22.3), which includes the superior cerebellar peduncle, lateral lemniscus, spinothalamic tract, corticotegmental tract, descending sympathetic tracts, mesencephalic trigeminal tract, locus ceruleus, and, more dorsally, the root of the contralateral fourth cranial nerve.[177,208,279,299–301] The SCA participates in the supply of the inferior colliculus[9,279,299] and at times the supply of the superior colliculus as well.[177,279,299] The SCA also supplies the choroid plexus of the fourth ventricle.[177]

The largest early report concerned seven patients with SCA territory infarcts studied by Davison et al in 1935.[177] Then Thompson[698] reported five cases of SCA infarction emphasizing cardioembolic causes. Many of these patients had infarction in the brain stem and cerebellar territory of the SCA. During the first half of the 20th century neurologists and neuroanatomists became very interested in clinicoanatomic correlations and would posit likely symptoms that might result from lesions at various sites. The so-called classic syndrome of the SCA was mostly a product of hypotheses since actual patients with this syndrome are extremely rare. The classic SCA syndrome is said to consist of ipsilateral limb ataxia; ipsilateral Horner syndrome; contralateral loss of pain and temperature sensibility of the face, arm, leg, and trunk; and contralateral fourth nerve palsy.[26] Abnormal ipsilateral spontaneous involuntary movements were also known to occur.[26,313,396]

In 1985, Kase and his colleagues[396] reported on three patients with infarcts that included the SCA. Their patients all had partial infarcts, each identified by CT scan. In 1987 Savoiardo et al[614] published templates of the territories of PICA, AICA, and SCA on axial, coronal, and sagittal sections of CT. On the basis of the complete necropsy analysis of 64 cases of cerebellar infarctions, the territories of the cerebellar arteries and their main branches (mSCA, lSCA, mPICA, and lPICA) have been identified both on pathologic axial sections of the cerebellum and brain stem[23] (Fig. 22.3) and on axial sections of CT and MRI[14,20] (Fig. 22.4). Amarenco and Hauw,[26] 5 years after the article of Kase et al,[396] reported the largest single clinicopathologic analysis of SCA territory infarcts. They reported on findings in 33 patients who had 41 cerebellar infarcts in the territory of the SCA and its main medial and lateral branches; these patients were selected from among all neuropathology specimens studied at the Salpêtrière hospital during a 20-year period.[26] Then the territory and the clinical syndrome of infarction of the lateral branch of the SCA were identified at necropsy and at CT and MRI by the same group.[31] Several large series, including the landmark study of Kase and colleagues[395] and those of Chaves et al[150] and the experience of others,[16,28,56,460,664,701] noted the frequency and locations of cerebellar infarcts identified by CT and/or MRI; these series have often tabulated the underlying vascular lesions, stroke mechanisms, and clinical findings.

Clinical aspects. Infarctions in the full territory of the SCA are usually accompanied by other infarctions in the rostral territory of the basilar artery. In 73% of autopsy cases the involved territory includes the occipitotemporal lobes unilaterally or bilaterally, the thalamic and subthalamic areas, and the mesencephalon.[26] Some infarctions involve the ventral aspect of the pons or occur together with PICA and AICA infarcts (one-third of autopsy cases).[26] Infarctions of the SCA are frequently edematous with brain stem compression and tonsillar herniation sometimes occurring.[25,26] Some SCA infarctions occur together with embolic occlusion of the middle cerebral artery.

Although partial territory SCA infarctions may be associated with rostral basilar artery infarctions,[26] they more frequently involve the rostral cerebellum alone.[28,31,150,395,664] The brain stem territory of the SCA supplied by branches arising early from the parent trunk is usually unaffected in patients with partial territory SCA infarctions. Partial territory infarctions are the most common type of SCA infarctions[28,56,150,395] and differ from infarctions of the full territory in their routinely benign outcome.[28,31,395]

Six distinct clinical patterns arise with SCA occlusion (Table 22.2). The *classic SCA syndrome*, first described by Mills[499,500] and Guillain et al,[313] is rarely seen[26,395,396] and is found in only 3% of patients with SCA occlusions who are examined at autopsy.[26] This syndrome develops with involvement of the brain stem territory of the SCA (Fig. 23.3). Signs characteristic of the syndrome include ipsilateral limb dysmetria, ipsilateral Horner syndrome,[285] contralateral pain and temperature sensory loss,[177,285,301,313,499,607,763] and contralateral fourth nerve palsy.[301] Other signs less frequently reported include ipsilateral loss of emotional expression in the face,[50] unilateral or bilateral hearing loss (possibly due to involvement of the lateral lemniscus), and sleep disorders (due to locus ceruleus damage).[500] Ipsilateral abnormal limb movements

are a more unusual occurrence.[166,177,301,313,396,763] Movement disorders occurring with this syndrome are described as choreiform[396] or athetotic[166,177,301] and consist of slow, undulatory movements[313,763] of large amplitude.[166,301,396] These appear with effort or emotion,[763] at rest, on assuming certain postures, or continuously. Guillain et al[313] noted some unsteadiness of the head in their patient with SCA occlusion and the classic syndrome. Some patients have coarse tremors.[177,285] Movement disorders are presumed to arise from involvement of the dentate nucleus or damage to the superior cerebellar peduncle. A few weeks after ischemic injury, palatal myoclonus and contralateral hypertrophy of the inferior olivary nucleus may occur with dentate nucleus damage.[285] Palatal myoclonus is occasionally accompanied by synchronous myoclonic movements of the jaw, face,[285] tongue, and ipsilateral vocal cord, producing voice disorders.[166] Davison et al[177] described a patient with SCA infarction without palatal myoclonus who had myoclonus of the jaw and a coarse tremor of the hand.

The *rostral basilar artery syndrome* is one of the most striking clinical presentations of SCA occlusion in the autopsy series of Amarenco and Hauw.[26] This syndrome occurs in 25% of patients with SCA territory infarction.[26] The presenting signs include visual field defects, vomiting, dizziness, diplopia, paresthesia, clumsiness of limbs, weakness, and drowsiness. These signs and symptoms suggest occipitotemporal lobe damage. Some patients clearly have cortical blindness or hemianopia, memory loss or confusion, or paralysis of visual fixation (Balint syndrome).

Thalamomesencephalic involvement is manifest in others by multimodal sensory loss, contralateral Horner syndrome, ipsilateral hemianopia, appendicular ataxia or pendular reflexes, behavioral changes, abulia, unilateral spatial neglect, memory loss, transcortical motor aphasia, and vertical gaze palsy. Subthalamic damage may produce hemiballism. Mesencephalic damage is usually manifest as one of several syndromes including Benedikt syndrome of third nerve palsy with contralateral limb movement disorders, Claude syndrome with third nerve palsy and contralateral limb dysmetria, Weber syndrome with contralateral limb weakness, and Parinaud syndrome with vertical gaze paresis. Some individuals with mesencephalic damage also had a pseudo-sixth nerve palsy, tonic deviation of gaze, palpebral retraction, pupillary disturbances, drowsiness, hallucinosis, and confusion.[26,112,481] Additional signs include ipsilateral Horner syndrome, limb dysmetria, hemiplegia, contralateral pain and temperature sensory loss, and internuclear ophthalmoplegia. Usually only two or three of these signs of rostral basilar artery occlusion are present. In these circumstances the SCA involvement is frequently difficult to recognize or is unexpectedly discovered on CT.[26,440]

Coma from onset, together with tetraplegia and oculomotor palsy, is another frequent clinical finding in patients with SCA occlusions seen at autopsy. Patients with this presentation represent about 33% of cases of SCA infarctions that come to autopsy. These clinical findings arise with embolic obstruction of the rostral end of the basilar artery.[26]

SCA occlusion may be *clinically inapparent* if simultaneous embolic infarction exists in the distribution of the ICA with a resultant brachiofacial sensorimotor deficit and aphasia. This occurred in 9% of patients with SCA occlusion who came to autopsy, and it was associated with a cardiac source of embolism.[26] Occasionally this also occurs along with occlusion of the innominate artery with intra-arterial embolism to the right middle cerebral artery and embolism through the VA to the SCA.

Cerebellar and vestibular signs are the prominent presenting features in many clinical series.[28,31,56,151,395,664] This is due to partial SCA territory involvement (Fig. 22.4). Symptoms include headache and gait abnormalities and, in about 35% of patients, dizziness and vomiting.[28,150,395,664] In a series of 30 patients with unilateral, isolated infarctions of the SCA territory as documented by CT,[35] patients most often presented with appendicular (73%) and gait ataxia (67%), nystagmus (50%), and brain stem signs (30%).[395] Nystagmus was horizontal and ipsilateral in 20% of patients, horizontal and contralateral in 3%, horizontal and bilateral in 20%, and vertical in 7%.[395] In an unselected CT series of 17 SCA infarctions, 15 patients had limb ataxia and 12 had truncal ataxia and dysarthria.[664] Dysarthria is one of the main symptoms in SCA infarction and seems to be the counterpart of the vertigo that typically develops with PICA infarctions.[31] Hemiparesis occurs in nearly one-fourth of patients.[664]

The *lSCA syndrome* has been described by Amarenco et al.[31] Occlusions of the lateral branch of the SCA involve the anterior rostral cerebellum (Fig. 23.4). The typical territory of these infarctions has only recently been described by Amarenco and colleagues[26] in one pathologic case and in nine additional patients examined with CT and MRI.[31] Since then, large series of cerebellar infarctions from prospective registries have shown that infarction in the lSCA territory is the most frequent among SCA infarctions, representing about half the cases of SCA infarctions.[28,126] The lSCA syndrome includes dysmetria of the ipsilateral limbs, ipsilateral axial lateropulsion, dysarthria, and gait unsteadiness.[31] The findings can mimic the dysarthria-clumsy hand lacunar syndrome,[706] present with isolated axial lateropulsion,[86] and may be associated with prominent dysmetria, nystagmus, or contrapulsion of saccades.[396,578] Occasionally lSCA infarctions may present with transient symptoms (transient blurring of vision, unsteadiness of gait, and tinnitus lasting a few seconds) and no clinical signs at neurologic examination.[20]

Clinical syndromes due to *dorsomedial infarction* of the rostral cerebellum in the territory of the mSCA have not been fully characterized although some individual patients have been reported.[16,396,591] In large registries of cerebellar infarctions, mSCA infarcts represent 10% to 20% of all SCA infarctions,[26] but no specific clinical syndrome has been reported.[28,126] Among the individual patients that have been reported on, when the most medial branches were involved, isolated unsteadiness of gait was found.[396] When the anterior cerebellar lobe (i.e., the lingula, central, culmen lobules of the vermis, and the anterior lobule of the hemisphere) was involved, some appendicular ataxia and spontaneous posturing of the neck, trunk, and limbs occurred.[591] When more lateral branches were involved in the paravermal territory, isolated dysarthria was found.[16] Lechtenberg and Gilman[433] showed that the paravermal zone of the lateral rostral cerebellum was the most frequently damaged in 31 cases with cerebellar dysarthria and nondegenerative cerebellar disease. However, no patient with pure dysarthria and cerebellar infarction was found. The report of an isolated infarction of this paravermal area demonstrates that this zone is involved in the control of

the voice and that dysarthria should be considered one of the main features of mSCA infarctions.[16]

Prognosis. Superior cerebellar artery territory infarctions can have a pseudotumoral presentation, a characteristic observed in 21% of autopsy cases.[26] However, the course and outcome of SCA infarctions are best evaluated in CT and MRI series of patients.[28,56,150,395,701] When the CT-imaged lesion is limited to the SCA territory, 93% of patients have partial SCA involvement. They have a benign outcome and are left minimally disabled or neurologically intact (93% of the cases).[395] Only 7% of patients have a pseudotumoral pattern leading to coma and occasionally death.[395] This relatively benign course is seen with both lSCA and mSCA infarctions.

Causes. Arterial occlusions leading to strokes in the SCA distribution usually involve the distal tip of the basilar artery, the ICVA, the ECVA at its origin, and less frequently the SCA itself.[21,26,150,395,396,664] However, in most patients with SCA strokes, no arterial occlusion is found. Presumably the thromboembolus has moved on or lysed by the time of angiography or postmortem examination. Thus the frequency of SCA occlusion is probably underestimated.

Every autopsy and clinical series concerned with SCA infarctions emphasizes cardiogenic embolism as the most common cause of SCA territory infarction, whatever the extent of the stroke.[21,26,28,31,150,395,664,698] Cardiac sources of emboli are observed in 35,[664] 40,[28] 61,[395] or 70% of cases.[26] Sometimes the responsible stroke mechanism is artery-to-artery embolism from atherosclerotic occlusion of the VA artery or from ulcerated plaques in the aortic arch,[15,21,26,28,395,664] or VA dissection.[28,133,395,439,664] Atherosclerotic occlusion occurs in 30% of patients.[26,395] In the young, rare causes of SCA territory stroke include SCA dissection and fibromuscular dysplasia,[387,555] migraine,[125,700] and transcardiac embolism via a patent foramen ovale during Valsalva maneuver.[31]

EDEMATOUS CEREBELLAR INFARCTIONS PRESENTING AS SPACE-OCCUPYING MASS. Although benign forms of cerebellar infarcts are much more frequent than lethal infarctions, the possibility of rapidly progressive cerebellar swelling with acute hydrocephalus and death must be kept in mind because surgery in this situation may be life saving. This form was first described by Menzies[485] in 1893. However, Fairburn and Oliver[223] and Lindgren[450] deserve considerable credit because they showed, 40 years ago, that total recovery could be obtained with surgical treatment. They emphasized the clinical findings in patients with these infarcts. Edema leads to cerebellar swelling, raised pressure in the posterior fossa, and brain stem compression. Aqueductal or fourth ventricle displacement or occlusion leads to obstructive hydrocephalus and acute intracranial hypertension. Cerebellar swelling may cause downward tonsillar herniation through the foramen magnum and transtentorial upward herniation of the culmen of the vermis.

Involved artery territories and mechanisms in patients with pseudotumoral cerebellar infarcts. In autopsy series, pseudotumoral infarctions involved the PICA territory,[676] SCA territory, or both.[25] In clinical series, the PICA territory is more frequently involved than the SCA territory.[395] Swelling of the cerebellum seems to be related to at least four factors: (1) mainly the large size of the infarction with involvement of more than one-third of the cerebellar hemisphere volume,[676]; (2) the site of the embolic occlusion, with disease at the rostral end of the basilar artery affecting the SCA ostia or with bilateral VA occlusions affecting the PICA ostia, as well as the failure of collateral supply[25]; (3) the increase in vasogenic edema with reperfusion after the migration of an embolus[25]; and (4) the presence of a massive SCA infarction, the particular location for which favors the development of hydrocephalus and edema.[25]

The mechanisms of deterioration vary considerably. Distortion of the fourth ventricle, or less often the sylvian aqueduct, can lead to hydrocephalus, thus further increasing intracranial contents and pressure. The brain stem can be compressed directly from the posterolateral direction. The tegmentum of the pons or medulla is directly compressed, but the basis pontis and ventral brain stem are also pressed against the clivus. Laterally placed lesions cause midline shifts with lateral segmental direct compression also with contralateral changes. Cerebellar tonsillar herniation through the foramen magnum can cause compression of the lower medulla and rostral spinal cord. Upward herniation of the rostral cerebellum through the tentorial incisura causes distortion of the midbrain and aqueduct of Sylvius with buckling of the quadrigeminal plate.[168] In addition, the hemispheral branches of the SCA can be compressed, causing an extension of cerebellar infarction.[168]

Clinical pictures. The clinical presentation is similar to that of cerebellar hemorrhage, but unenhanced CT readily allows distinction between the two conditions.[275,344,540] Acute vertigo, vomiting, headache, dysarthria, and unsteadiness of gait are the key presenting symptoms. The major signs include ataxia of gait and trunk, or ipsilateral axial lateropulsion, or both, which usually prevent standing in the upright position, nystagmus, dysarthria, and ipsilateral limb dysmetria. Delayed alteration of consciousness characterizes 90% of these edematous infarctions. The clouding of consciousness appears from a few hours to 10 days after the onset of other symptoms (mean of 5 days).[25,344,435,676] Altered consciousness occurs either in isolation or together with worsening of other neurologic signs and symptoms. It can progress over the course of a few days or a few hours. Isolated supratentorial hydrocephalus, or disappearance of the fourth ventricle, or both, on CT suggests an edematous cerebellar infarction despite the occasional lack of a cerebellar hypodensity.[457] MRI is usually positive in such cases.

The clinical findings in patients with space-occupying cerebellar infarcts have recently been analyzed by Hornig and colleagues.[365] They collected and analyzed 52 patients with pseudotumoral infarcts studied during a 10-year period. Following the classification suggested by Heros,[344] they divided the clinical course into three phases. Initial clinical symptoms and signs that involved dysfunction were directly related to ischemic cerebellar and brain stem structures. The second phase was characterized by reduced consciousness and new signs of brain stem dysfunction due to compression. During the final third phase, patients became comatose and developed respiratory and cardiovascular dysfunction, the latter most often related to medullary compression. Impaired consciousness, at first drowsiness and later stupor, as well as new brain stem signs, developed most often in this series during the third day after stroke onset.[365] The time interval between

the occurrence of decreased consciousness or brain stem signs or both and coma or decerebrate posturing was 24 hours in 14 of 19 patients who became comatose (range, 4 hours to 3 days).[365] Sypert and Alvord[676] in their landmark paper on edematous cerebellar infarctions also emphasized this interval, which they thought provided a window of opportunity for action to prevent death.

The signs that accompany the second stage of brain stem compression vary considerably. As previously suggested, Hornig et al[365] found that the development of new Babinski signs, and new horizontal gaze abnormalities, were the most common signs. When upward transtentorial herniation is present, the clinical signs are different. In the series of seven patients reported by Cuneo et al[168] in whom upward herniation was shown at necropsy, pupillary abnormalities, abnormal vertical gaze, and decerebrate postures were often found when patients deteriorated. Unequal small pupils often became fixed at midposition or dilated as the rostral brain stem was compressed by the upwardly herniating cerebellum.[168] Kanis and colleagues[388] reported on a single patient who had a large PICA cerebellar pseudotumoral infarct as well as lateral medullary infarction confirmed by MRI. As mass effect increased, the patient had more difficulty swallowing and developed an ipsilateral hemiparesis due to compression of the contralateral medullary pyramid against the clivus. Changes in the right pyramid were confirmed at necropsy after death from a pulmonary embolus 4 weeks after successful surgical decompression.[388]

Surgery is necessary when deterioration of consciousness develops. Total recovery is obtained in 63% of published cases after ventricular drainage or opening of the dura mater by occipital craniectomy.[25,511,637] The prognosis, however, depends on whether or not there is an associated brain stem infarction, because a strong correlation exists between the presence of a hemiplegia or tetraplegia and the presence of a massive pontine infarction associated with the cerebellar infarction at autopsy.[25] Thus surgery should be avoided when severe weakness is present. Absence of paramedian pontine hyperintensity on axial MRI should aid in the surgical decision making.

Neuroimaging is essential for the recognition of pseudotumoral infarcts and to identify coexistent brain stem infarction. MRI is clearly superior to CT for this purpose. An important sign of pressure, obliteration of posterior fossa cisterns, may be easier to determine on CT scans. Midline shifts, compression or obliteration of the fourth ventricle, and hydrocephalus should be readily detected on both CT and MRI scans. Upward and downward cerebellar herniation can best be shown on midsagittal MRI sections. T_2-weighted sagittal sections are especially helpful since they usually optimally show the localization of the cerebellar infarcts as well as vertical shifts and herniations. Vascular diagnostic studies such as MRA, TCD, spiral CT, and/or angiography are very helpful in clarifying the etiology of the infarcts and in making therapeutic decisions.

Cerebellar infarction may be found in patients deeply comatose at the first examination in the emergency department and without history. The sudden appearance of coma of unknown cause together with isolated supratentorial hydrocephalus on CT should always suggest to clinicians an edematous cerebellar infarction requiring emergency surgery. Ventricular drainage may be life saving, and the early release of brain stem compression may allow good or total functional recovery even for a deeply comatose patient.[511]

Surgical treatment. Among brain infarctions, the possibility of life-saving surgery is unique to cerebellar strokes, especially when they present as space-occupying lesions with obstructive hydrocephalus.[223,450] The optimal treatment of patients with pseudotumoral infarcts is still unsettled. Before the CT era, a consensus favored suboccipital craniectomy and aspiration of necrotic tissue as the routine approach to cerebellar infarction.[178,229,294,435,531,683,760] With CT monitoring, recovery has been reported after ventricular drainage without surgical resection of the infarcted tissue.[350,404,637]

The best approach is probably an individualized one, taking into account in each case the severity of the neurologic state, particularly impairment of consciousness.[157] If the patient is alert and clinically stable, medical treatment alone is needed. Osmotic agents as well as hyperventilation are useful in decreasing cerebellar edema in patients with slight mass effect. If the patient is alert but the CT shows hydrocephalus or mass effect on the fourth ventricle, medical treatment is also indicated. In such a patient, some authors suggest monitoring the intracranial pressure and performing surgery when pressure is above 350 mmH$_2$O. When deterioration of consciousness appears, ventricular drainage becomes necessary. If it is not rapidly effective, a surgical decompression is urgently required.

Some authors advocate routine surgical resection because of the theoretical risk of upward transtentorial herniation[168] due to ventricular drainage.[397] The main difficulty in the decision regarding surgery is encountered when brain stem signs are present, sometimes making it impossible to determine whether the deterioration in neurologic state is due to direct compression by the swollen cerebellum or to an associated extensive brain stem infarction. It seems reasonable to avoid surgery in the presence of a massive brain stem infarct, particularly if severe hemi- or tetraplegia is present. MRI is very helpful in this situation in imaging the brain stem.

Chen and colleagues[152] reported on a series of 11 patients with large cerebellar infarcts who deteriorated despite vigorous medical treatment. Treatment using temporary external ventricular drainage and suboccipital craniectomy sometimes including the foramen magnum was quite successful without removing brain tissue.[152] Generally decompression of the cerebellum with removal of necrotic tissue has been advocated in patients who become comatose. Rieke et al[587] reviewed the findings and outcomes among 42 patients with pseudotumoral infarcts. They found that monitoring patients using brain stem auditory evoked responses was useful in detecting pressure-related brain stem dysfunction.[587] The authors concluded that "the preliminary data suggest decompressive craniotomy as the most effective therapy in comatose patients."[587] In awake and drowsy patients, the effectiveness of medical therapy, ventricular drainage, and decompressive craniotomy was uncertain. A formal therapeutic trial has begun in Germany and Austria in an attempt to determine optimal therapy.[423]

OCCLUSION OR SEVERE STENOSIS OF THE BASILAR ARTERY

Kubik and Adams,[424] in their landmark description of occlusion of the basilar artery, summarized the findings as follows:

The onset is sudden and not preceded by tangible causal factors. The first symptom is usually headache, dizziness, con-

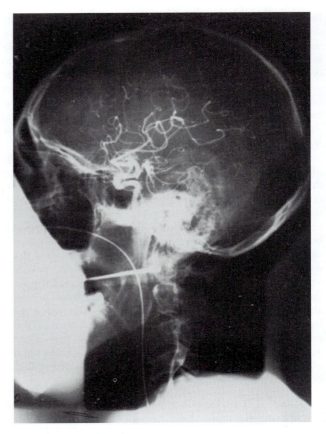

Figure 22.21 Carotid arteriogram demonstrating retrograde filling of the basilar artery and the posterior cerebral and superior cerebellar arteries. Note the midbasilar occlusion.

fusion, or coma. Difficulty in speaking and unilateral paresthesiae occur in a large proportion of the cases. Common findings are pupillary abnormalities, disorders of ocular movement, facial palsy, hemiplegia and/or quadriplegia, and bilateral extensor plantar reflexes. Cranial nerve palsies and contralateral hemiplegia may be combined. . . . It is common for temporary improvement, lasting hours or days, to occur during the course of the illness. In the majority of cases death takes place in from two days to five weeks.

In an angiography study, Archer and Horenstein[35] also found severe deficits in 20 patients with angiographically confirmed basilar artery occlusion: 15 patients died and the other 5 patients were left severely disabled. By contrast, Caplan[110] described four patients among six with verified basilar occlusion who survived the associated acute ischemic event with little (one patient) or no deficit (three patients). Others[36,236,496,515,570] have also noted examples of survival without crippling deficit after basilar artery occlusion, and in fact, Kubik and Adams,[424] in their original paper, mention four patients with clinical findings identical to those with documented basilar occlusion who survived the stroke and were alive months later.

Basilar artery atherosclerotic disease has been recognized at the preocclusive stage of severe stenosis (Fig. 22.21). It is a relatively uncommon lesion compared with basilar artery occlusion. In the Joint Study of Extracranial Arterial Occlusion, basilar artery stenosis was identified in 7.7% of 3,778 patients undergoing four-vessel angiography.[331] In our own survey we identified nine patients with angiographically proven middle or distal segment basilar stenosis, and in reviewing other angiographic and pathologic cases we found that occlusion affected all three basilar artery segments (proximal, middle, and distal) in relatively equal frequencies.[561] TIAs were a common feature of the clinical presentation in patients with basilar artery stenosis, occurring in six of our nine cases. The TIAs usually preceded brain stem stroke, but in two patients they were the sole clinical manifestation. The TIA features included the brief duration of two or more of the following symptoms: dizziness, slurred speech, double vision, dysphagia, and unilateral or bilateral weakness. The TIAs occurred during a period of 1 day to 6 months before stroke. Stroke severity and infarct location varied, but the pons was a frequent locus of injury. The short-term prognosis was good; most patients remained free of symptoms for periods of 1 month to 2 years, usually on anticoagulation or on antiplatelet treatment. Three patients died, one of the original stroke, another from a new basilar territory infarct, and one from unrelated causes.

It should now be quite obvious that no uniform syndrome or outcome is applicable to all patients with basilar artery occlusion. Should this come as a surprise? The situation in the carotid artery is clearly comparable. Sometimes when the ICA is occluded, patients complain of amaurosis fugax followed by symptoms and signs of total ischemia of the anterior and middle cerebral artery branches of the ICA. Such patients are readily diagnosed. Other patients with ICA occlusion have transient or partial deficits, and diagnosis can only be made by laboratory confirmation, usually angiography. There is a wide spectrum of symptomatology, severity of signs, and outcome.[1] The situation in the basilar artery is not very different. Since confirmation of basilar artery occlusion depends on angiography, at present the frequency of this angiographic diagnosis will depend on the indications for angiography in a given institution. Archer and Horenstein[35] angiographically studied severely ill patients; Meyer and colleagues[491] excluded patients with severe brain stem infarction from angiography, but nevertheless identified two patients with unusual basilar artery occlusion. Prognosis depends on the rate and extent of occlusion, presence of collateral circulation, systemic factors (see the section on pathophysiology), and possibly treatment.

Patients with documented severe stenotic lesions of the basilar artery or the ICVAs have a relatively poor prognosis for subsequent brain stem infarction or death.[519] In one series, the stroke rate for such patients was 17 times the expected rate for a matched normal population. Since there is no absolutely uniform syndrome of basilar artery occlusion, this discussion describes common neurologic findings not previously commented on that occur with basilar artery occlusion, characterizes the common patterns of infarction documented at postmortem, and discusses angiographic diagnosis and clinical tempo.

Common Clinical Phenomena

INTERNUCLEAR OPHTHALMOPLEGIA.
In the 1950s Cogan and colleagues[160,161,649] revised the nomenclature and described the usual findings of patients with internuclear ophthalmoplegia. Lutz had originally designated two types of internuclear ophthalmoplegia: an anterior type, in which the internus (i.e., medial rectus) is paralyzed for conjugate movements toward the side of the lesion but functions normally in convergence and the extremus (i.e., lateral rectus) operates normally on lateral gaze, and a posterior type, in which both internal recti function normally on convergence and lateral gaze movements but the extremus on the side of the lesion is paralyzed for voluntary conjugate movements whereas it can function on labyrinthine stimulation. Smith and Cogan[649] said that Lutz's posterior internuclear ophthalmoplegia was merely a partial sixth cranial nerve palsy and these authors proposed a new designation, which is now in common usage. In their terminology, internuclear ophthalmoplegia always involved paralysis of the adducting eye; the posterior type, in their terminology, designates cases in which the medial rectus works normally during convergence, and the anterior type refers to absence of medial rectus function in either convergence or conjugate lateral gaze. In either type nystagmus of the abducting eye occurs, a phenomenon that had led others to designate internuclear ophthalmoplegia as "ataxic nystagmus," a term still used in some regions.[328] Furthermore, analysis of 58 cases (29 unilateral and 29 bilateral) led Smith and Cogan[649] to assert that bilateral internuclear ophthalmoplegia was "invariably indicative of multiple sclerosis" and unilateral internuclear ophthalmoplegia was most commonly vascular in etiology.

Christoff and colleagues,[156] among others, reviewed past examples of clinicopathologic correlation in patients with internuclear ophthalmoplegia and added three examples of their own; they implicated the ipsilateral medial longitudinal fasciculus (MLF) in the production of internuclear ophthalmoplegia. Damage to the right MLF would produce an absence of adduction of the right medial rectus on leftward gaze and abducting nystagmus of the left eye. Vertical nystagmus and skew deviation were frequent concomitant findings. More recently, Gonyea[303] described a number of patients with bilateral internuclear ophthalmoplegia due to vascular disease (only one had documented basilar artery occlusion) and reviewed past examples in the literature; as a result, he took exception to the dictum of Smith and Cogan[649] that bilateral involvement was invariably due to multiple sclerosis. In basilar artery occlusion with extensive pontine infarction, tegmental infarcts are frequently patchy and asymmetric so that unilateral internuclear ophthalmoplegia is more common than the bilateral type. Absence of associated convergence does not necessarily implicate the more rostral midbrain MLF, as Cogan et al[159,160] initially believed.

Although the eyes are generally conjugate at rest in patients with internuclear ophthalmoplegia, some patients have bilateral exotropia; this situation has been referred to as *wall-eyed bilateral internuclear ophthalmoplegia*.[173] Outward deviation of the eyes has been used as evidence of medial rectus nuclear involvement, but Gonyea[303] and Cogan et al[159,160] emphasize that exotropia is to be anticipated with dysconjugate impairment of medial rectus function at any level, including the MLF.

MRI studies of patients with internuclear ophthalmoplegia showed damage of the MLF and adjacent structures.[100] When internuclear ophthalmoplegia was associated with loss of convergence or abnormality of abduction of the contralateral eye, the medial tegmental lesions were usually more extensive than when the only defect was an internuclear ophthalmoplegia.

CONJUGATE HORIZONTAL GAZE PALSY.
Fibers from the frontal eye fields affecting conjugate lateral gaze cross at or near the level of the abducens nucleus in the pons[1] and end in the reticular gray region in the neighborhood of the contralateral abducens nucleus.[167] This region is usually referred to as the paramedian pontine reticular formation (PPRF), or by some as the pontine lateral gaze center. Damage to the abducens nucleus can probably produce an ipsilateral gaze palsy for all lateral eye movements, voluntary and reflex (caloric or vestibulo-ocular).[566]

MRI shows that in patients with a unilateral abduction weakness (sixth cranial nerve palsy), the lesion invariably involves the intrapontine nerve fascicles and not the abducens nucleus.[99] Involvement of the PPRF leads to absence of voluntary lateral gaze to the side of the lesion with preservation of reflex movements.[566] The PPRF also mediates ipsilaterally directed saccades within the contralateral hemifield of movement. Bilateral lesions in the pontine tegmentum involving the abducens nucleus and PPRF produce paralysis of all horizontal eye movements, with sparing of vertical gaze, since this is mediated at a more rostral level. Halsey et al[319] described a patient with subsequently documented basilar artery occlusion and infarction restricted to the basis pontis ventral to the PPRF who had an absence of voluntary lateral gaze. Voluntary vertical gaze was preserved and labyrinthine stimuli produced full conjugate lateral gaze except for absence of adduction of one eye (due to a more rostral MLF lesion). These authors postulate that the descending fibers for voluntary conjugate gaze travel with the corticobulbar and aberrant corticobulbar fibers in the base of the pons in the region of the medial lemniscus. The senior author saw one patient with pontine hemorrhage who was conscious but could not look voluntarily to either side; reflex lateral gaze could be readily evoked by doll's eye maneuver. In unilateral lesions of the PPRF there is often some conjugate deviation of the eyes toward the contralateral side, but this is less than is usually found with supratentorial lesions.

MRI studies of patients with unilateral conjugate gaze palsy show lesions in the paramedian pons, including the abducens nucleus, the nucleus reticularis pontis oralis, and the lateral portion of the nucleus reticularis pontis caudalis. These latter two structures are identified in animals as responsible for lateral gaze and contain burst neurons of the PPRF. In patients with bilateral horizontal gaze palsies there are usually bilateral medial pontine lesions, but some patients have unilateral lesions that include the pontine tegmental raphe.[99] Patients with bilateral horizontal gaze palsies often also have slowness of vertical gaze saccades or limitation of upgaze. Horizontal gaze palsies are common in patients with basilar artery occlusive disease. In one series of 85 patients with proven basilar artery occlusion, 22 had a horizontal gaze palsy.[232]

ONE-AND-A-HALF SYNDROME. Fisher[241] introduced the term one-and-a-half syndrome to refer to "a paralysis of eye movements in which one eye lies centrally and fails completely to move horizontally while the other eye lies in an abducted position and cannot be adducted past the midline." A unilateral pontine lesion involving the PPRF produces an ipsilateral conjugate gaze palsy and also affects the MLF on the same side, leading to paralysis of adduction of the ipsilateral eye on conjugate gaze to the opposite side.[241,566] If normal conjugate gaze to either side is rated 1, full horizontal gaze would score 2. Patients with combined PPRF and MLF lesions on one side only move a single eye in abduction to one side; they are therefore lacking one and one-half components of normal gaze. Others have called this deficit paralytic pontine exotropia because of the deviation of the eye at rest.[634]

OCULAR BOBBING. Fisher[256] introduced the term ocular bobbing to describe an unusual vertical movement of the eyes: "The eyeballs intermittently drip briskly downwards through an arc of a few millimeters and then return to the primary position in a kind of bobbing action." He felt that this was a sign of "advanced pontine disease" and of little diagnostic importance because "the site of the disease process is usually obvious from the other ocular abnormalities" and clinical findings.

Fisher described three examples of bobbing in pontine disease: two patients had pathologic documentation of basilar artery occlusion with extensive infarction of the pontine base and tegmentum; one had a pontine hemorrhage. In the patients with pontine lesions, voluntary and reflex horizontal gaze was lost. The eyes moved conjugately, but the vertical excursion of the bob was only one-fourth to one-third of the normal full voluntary vertical movement. Downward movement was quicker than upward; between downward jerks the eyes rested quietly. Fisher also noted atypical bobbing, either dysconjugate, as in one case of cerebellar hemorrhage, or unilateral. Unilateral bobbing occurred in a patient with a left sixth cranial nerve palsy and consisted of a downward bob of the left eye on attempted left lateral gaze. Nelson and Johnston[528] added four cases of bilateral ocular bobbing, all in patients with pontine hemorrhage, one of whom had a hemorrhage to the tegmentum and fourth ventricle.

The mechanism of bobbing in pontine lesions proposed by Fisher[256] and supported by Nelson and Johnston[528] relates the bobbing to roving eye movements. In patients with coma due to bilateral supratentorial lesions, the eyes rove from side to side freely. In pontine lesions, since horizontal gaze is lost and vertical gaze preserved owing to sparing of the midbrain tegmentum, the vertical vector of gaze is accentuated so that the eyes bob down. In addition, caloric irrigation increases the bobbing, acting as an afferent stimulus to gaze. Similarly, a unilateral bob, when that eye is pointed toward the direction of paralytic lateral gaze, could evoke a downward movement.

Yap and colleagues[764] described two clinical cases of ocular bobbing (one vascular and one probably demyelinative) in which the ocular bobbing occurred synchronously with palatal myoclonus and raised the possibility of an unusual tremor or movement disorder affecting brain stem structures as a mechanism of bobbing. Bosch at al[92] questioned the value of bobbing as a reliable sign of intrapontine disease; they presented a case of "typical ocular bobbing" (referring to bilateral conjugate downward movements) in a patient with a large cerebellar hemorrhage who had no extensive pontine lesion. However, that patient was in deep coma and had distortion of the pons and a small unilateral Duret-type hemorrhage in the adjacent pontine tegmentum. Surely, distortion with physiologic disruption of pontine function was the basis of the bobbing, absent horizontal gaze, and decerebration state.

Others have described bobbing in cerebellar hemorrhage[256,540] and cerebellar infarction.[672] Newman et al[529] described a patient in coma after cranial gunshot wounds. The necrotic temporal lobe was removed, at which time the patient had no spontaneous or reflex oculocephalic eye movements. He became alert after surgery, and ocular bobbing appeared and was accentuated during voluntary eye movements, especially when the patient attempted to gaze into fields of remaining limitations of horizontal eye movements. We have also noted in patients with pontine lesions (hemorrhage or infarction) and preserved consciousness the tendency for bobbing to occur, bilaterally or unilaterally, on attempted voluntary gaze into a field of limited gaze. Newman and colleagues[529] raised the possibility that the vertical vectors could originate inferior to the lesion, for example, in the medulla or vestibular nuclei; they emphasized the possibility of recovery.

Ocular bobbing occurs in a variety of situations in which horizontal gaze is affected despite sparing of vertical gaze capabilities. It usually indicates pontine dysfunction due to an intrinsic pontine lesion or to external pressure, or to toxic or metabolic disruption of function.[265]

OTHER NEURO-OPHTHALMOLOGIC SIGNS.

Ptosis. Ptosis is frequent in patients with basilar artery occlusion and is usually attributed to involvement of the descending sympathetic fibers in the lateral pontine tegmentum. However, even with severe bilateral ptosis, the pupils may not be miotic.[241] Pontine ptosis is often more severe than the ptosis that usually accompanies peripheral Horner syndrome or Horner syndrome found in patients with lateral medullary syndrome. Pontine ptosis is often modified by involvement of the seventh cranial nerve or a hemiparesis.[111] In patients with hemiparesis, whether brain stem or supratentorial, ptosis is often more severe on the hemiparetic side. A peripheral type of facial weakness will diminish the ptosis by paralyzing the orbicularis oculi muscle, widening the palpebral fissure. If basilar artery occlusion produces infarction of a third nerve nucleus, complete bilateral ptosis is the rule.

Pontine pupils. Pontine pupils are frequently pinpoint,[241] but reaction can be seen if a bright light and magnification are used.[569] When pontine and midbrain infarction coexist, the pupils are often at midposition but poorly reactive. Lesions in the midbrain alone, with sparing of the pons, produce fixed dilated pupils. Pupillary constriction is more severe with pontine infarction or hemorrhage than with peripheral Horner syndrome; some have postulated parasympathetic irritation as well as a destructive sympathetic process to explain the pinpoint pupils.

Nystagmus. Nystagmus is common in patients with basilar occlusion but varies, depending on the locus of infarction and the degree of paresis of eye movements. Vertical nystagmus is an important sign of pontine infarction; rhythmic vertical nystagmus does not occur with higher brain stem lesions, although other disorders of vertical gaze are hallmarks of mesencephalic and diencephalic damage.[569]

Skew deviation. Skew deviation refers to an altered vertical position of the eyes, with one eye situated above the other and the vertical displacement remaining nearly constant in all planes of gaze. Skew is quite frequent in patients with brain stem infarction, especially when lesions are asymmetric.

When associated with a unilateral internuclear ophthalmoplegia, the elevated eye is usually ipsilateral to the lesion.[650] Asymmetric lesions in the region of the vestibular nuclei, dorsolateral medulla, brachium pontis, cerebellum, and rostral midbrain may all produce skewing.

PALATAL MYOCLONUS.

Palatal myoclonus is a rhythmic involuntary jerking movement of the soft palate and pharyngopalatine arch, often involving the diaphragm and laryngeal muscles.[679] It usually appears some time after the acute brain stem process, which is most often an infarction. The locus and nature of the responsible vascular lesion have not been analyzed, but the parenchymatous lesion involves the dentate nucleus of the cerebellum, the red nucleus, the inferior olivary nucleus, or their connections (the Guillain-Mollaret triangle). The dentate nucleus and contralateral inferior olive are somatotopically related. Fibers from the dentate nuclei travel in the superior cerebellar peduncle and decussate in the midbrain to the region of the contralateral red nucleus from which the central tegmental tract descends to the inferior olivary nucleus of the same side.[429] The pathologic lesion most often seen in patients with palatal myoclonus is hypertrophic degeneration of the inferior olive, often associated with a lesion of the ipsilateral central tegmental tract or the contralateral dentate nucleus. The olivary lesion includes enlarged neurons, loss of the other neurons, and gliosis, usually with enlargement of the olive; these changes are thought to be trans-synaptic and secondary to lesions of the neuronal system afferent to the inferior olivary nucleus.

The brachial movement may vary in rate (40 to 200/min).[679] The patient may complain of an audible clicking noise due to movement of the eustachian tube or the noise may be heard by the examiner if a stethoscope is applied to the lateral neck. The movements of the pharynx can be readily seen and are often accompanied by a fluttering of the diaphragm, which is usually obvious by chest fluoroscopy. Palatal myoclonus has surprisingly little effect on swallowing.

COMA.

Unresponsiveness to external stimuli occurs in some patients with basilar artery occlusion. Chase et al[148] analyzed 8 of their own cases (7 basilar occlusions, 1 pontine hemorrhage) and 12 prior reports in an attempt to correlate the state of consciousness and electroencephalographic changes with the necropsy findings. Bilateral damage to the medial pontine tegmentum was present in all the comatose patients, whereas of the 11 patients with no more than unilateral tegmental damage, 8 were either alert or only "slightly obtunded." No patient with bilateral tegmental damage was fully alert. There was no reliable relation between the resting electroencephalogram and the size or localization of the lesions, but attempts to activate the electroencephalography by voice or painful cutaneous stimuli were unsuccessful in the unresponsive patient. Lesions of the mesencephalic reticular formation can produce prolonged coma.[376,401,569] In animals, damage to the central tegmental region in the rostral pons, midbrain, and dorsal hypothalamus is associated with unresponsiveness.[569] Lesions below the trigeminal nerve entry zone of the pons usually do not interrupt alertness in the experimental animal.[569]

LOCKED-IN SYNDROME.   Kemper and Romanul[401] described a patient who, although paralyzed and speechless, could move his eyes horizontally and raise his eyebrows. At postmortem, there was extensive destruction of the pontine base and only slight encroachment on the ventral part of the pontine tegmentum unilaterally. They sought to differentiate this paralytic state from akinetic mutism, a condition in which the patient could, under certain circumstances, speak and move. Plum and Posner[569] coined the term *locked-in syndrome* to describe a state in which severe paralysis prevents the usual means of gestural or vocal communication. Usually the patient can communicate by way of vertical eye movements or blinking and can demonstrate full comprehension of his plight and the environment. In some locked-in patients, oral automatisms in the form of chewing and sucking movements can be reflex induced by oral and perioral stimulation, indicating loss of voluntary control over bulbar masticatory function.[59] These patients have been likened to M. Noirtier de Villefort in *The Count of Monte Cristo* by Dumas, who, while encased in armor, could not communicate except with his eyes.

The most common vascular lesion underlying the locked-in syndrome is basilar artery occlusion with extensive destruction of the pontine base. Vertical eye movements are usually spared. Midbrain lesions may also produce a locked-in state. In one such patient, the lesions were confined to the ventral mesencephalon, and eye and lid movement was preserved.[392] In another patient, studied only clinically, bilateral third cranial nerve paralysis, mutism, and quadriplegia were present, but the patient could signal with one hand.[483] Caplan and Zervas[120] described two similar patients with presumed Duret hemorrhages who could communicate by hand signals despite bilateral third cranial nerve paralysis and mutism. The necessary substrate for the locked-in syndrome is bilateral paralysis despite preserved consciousness.

PARESIS.   Some degree of paresis, either transient or persistent, accompanies nearly all cases of basilar artery occlusion. Fisher[264] emphasized that the initial motor weakness can be quite lateralized and referred to this phenomenon as herald hemiparesis of basilar artery occlusion. Fisher[264] described five patients, in four of whom quadriparesis soon developed, and one exhibited jerking of the limbs contralateral to the hemiparesis. Although hemiparesis may occur, the spared side invariably demonstrates some slight paresis, hyperreflexia, and a Babinski sign.[426] It is of practical importance to separate clinically the paramedian penetrating branch lesions with hemiplegia from more serious basilar artery occlusion with bilateral involvement. When basilar occlusion begins with a hemiplegia, the other limbs are generally affected within 24 hours. In one such case, when one of us (L.R.C.) personally examined, with angiographically verified basilar artery occlusion, the patient was hemiplegic when first seen, but the contralateral limbs had episodic shivering movements; the next day he was quadriplegic. At times, the hemiplegia alternates from one side to another. Biemond[70] described a patient who initially developed a right hemiplegia; later, after the right limb weakness had cleared, she became dysarthric and had a left hemiplegia. Right hemiplegia, bilateral tongue and face

weakness, and bilateral extensor plantar responses then developed. At postmortem examination, the left VA was occluded, and the thrombus had extended into the caudal basilar artery. Asymmetries probably depend on VA involvement, adequacy of collaterals on each side, and presence of distal emboli. In the 18 cases carefully studied by Kubik and Adams,[424] one side of the body was generally more affected than the other. Stupor often made precise motor examination difficult. Crossed motor paralysis, ipsilateral facial or conjugate gaze paralysis, and contralateral hemiparesis were found in 4 of the 18 cases of Kubik and Adams. Among the 85 patients of Ferbert et al[232] with angiographically proven basilar artery occlusion, at presentation 31 patients had tetraparesis, 15 had tetraplegia, and 21 had hemiparesis.

DECEREBRATE RESPONSES.   Decerebrate responses are frequent in patients with extensive infarction, although at times the inferior extremity flexes as the arms extend, a response correlated with lesions at the level of the vestibular nuclei in the pontine tegmentum.[569]

SENSORY FINDINGS.   Sensory findings are quite variable and clearly depend on the locus of infarction. Stupor or altered capability of communication often makes determination of sensory abnormalities imprecise. Usually the motor dysfunction far outweighs the sensory signs. Perhaps this is explained by the predominantly medial location of infarction; the more lateral regions, which contain the spinothalamic tracts, and, more rostrally, the main somatosensory lemniscus are supplied by lateral circumferential collaterals and are relatively spared. In the Ferbert et al[232] series, 11 of 85 patients were said to have a hemihypoesthesia. In our experience hemisensory signs usually indicate additional involvement of the medulla (VA) or spread of infarction to the thalamus or PCA territory. Occasional patients with basilar artery disease have bilateral severe, unusual pain sensations in the face. Some patients have likened the feeling to having salt and pepper thrown on their face.[117] This symptom could be due to involvement of crossing fibers crossing the midline from the trigeminal nuclei to join the medial border of the spinothalamic tracts. Alternatively, the symptoms could be explained by involvement of the nucleus raphe magnus in the periaqueductal gray matter. This nucleus had serotonergic projections to the spinal tracts of the fifth cranial nerve and their nuclei.

ATAXIA.   Ataxia is frequently hidden by weakness and has been difficult to analyze, although the location of necropsy findings would predict its presence. Nystagmus is common in patients with tegmental ischemia but may be overshadowed by nuclear, internuclear, or gaze paresis. Vertical nystagmus frequently accompanies internuclear ophthalmoplegia and pontine infarction. Dysarthria, dysphagia, and facile laughing and crying can be due to pseudobulbar paralysis and are present to some degree in most patients with moderate to severe limb paresis.

ABNORMALITIES OF RESPIRATION.   Abnormalities of respiration are also frequent, but their mechanism is difficult to determine because of the extensiveness of the infarction and presence of general medical factors (aspiration, fever, hypoventilation). Apneustic breathing with a hang-up of the inspiratory phase and grossly regular breathing (ataxic respirations) occasionally occur terminally in patients with basilar artery occlusion and carry an ominous prognosis. Fisher[265] and Plum and Posner[569] have outlined other respiratory irregularities and discussed their clinicoanatomic significance. Silverstein[642,643] has outlined the frequency of symptoms and signs in 83 patients with infarction within the "distribution of the basilar artery."

Patterns of Infarction

The regions of infarction in patients with confirmed basilar artery occlusion vary considerably, depending on the portion of the basilar artery occluded. At times the occlusion is quite limited and segmental, whereas in other patients thrombosis can affect multiple segments or even occlude the entire basilar artery and extend into the VA and PCA.[146,426]

Kubik and Adams[424] studied 18 patients with basilar artery occlusion, including six examples of presumed embolic occlusion: eight involved the rostral basilar artery, five the proximal third, two the middle third, and three the entire artery. In their material, the patterns of infarction and vascular occlusion are neatly diagrammed. In the patients with sparing of the rostral tip of the basilar artery, the infarcts were predominantly pontine, usually centering around the midpons. In these cases, the most lateral margins of the basis pontis were often spared and the basis pontis was affected to a far greater degree than the tegmentum. When the basilar tip was occluded, the lesions were predominantly in the midbrain, diencephalon, and rostral pons, and the tegmentum of the pons and midbrain were more often involved than in occlusion of the caudal basilar artery. In one-third of the cases, the infarcts were symmetric, and in many cases the softenings were patchy. The cerebellum was also spared in most cases; the extensive brain stem softening was in striking contrast to the normal or minimally damaged cerebellum.

Silverstein[642] included 11 examples of verified basilar artery occlusion in his series; in 8 patients the lesion included the distal third, in one the proximal third, and in two the middle third. Silverstein remarked, "Embolism was not recorded clinically or pathologically in our series," but three cases had minimal atherosclerosis of the basilar artery, brain stem infarcts, and emboli in various viscera. The infarctions centered around the midpons (again predominantly in a paramedian distribution), were occasionally patchy, and were almost invariably anemic, as opposed to hemorrhagic.

Loeb and Meyer[454] reviewed and tabulated past reports of basilar artery occlusion and the pattern of brain stem infarction. Pontine infarcts always favored median and paramedian zones, with relative sparing of the lateral margins. Biemond[70] noted frequent tegmental sparing and sought to explain it by emphasizing that the tegmentum is mainly supplied by the SCA and its branches. The SCA is the most anatomically constant long circumferential branch vessel and often has a prominent anastomosis with the PCA. Biemond[70] followed small branches of the SCA and found that they formed a corona around the cranial part of the pontine tegmentum and anastomosed with the SCA branches of the opposite side. When a lateral branch of the SCA was injected, the tegmentum was stained bilaterally, but when the basilar artery was injected from the VA, the basis pontis was deeply stained, whereas the tegmentum remained entirely clear. Biemond[70] also obtained

little tegmental staining from injection of the AICA. According to the study of Kubik and Adams,[424] the tegmentum was involved most frequently when the occlusive lesions extended to the basilar tip, thus obstructing the SCA orifices. Our own angiographic material in patients with basilar artery occlusion also demonstrates retrograde filling of the PCA and SCA from carotid injection and the prominence of cerebellar artery anastomotic vessels that fill other lateral circumferential cerebellar artery branches.[138] Tegmental involvement thus depends on the involvement of the distal basilar artery and the adequacy of collaterals. Collateral circulation through the PICA is poor when the VA and basilar artery are both obstructed. Archer and Horenstein[35] wondered whether hypertension, by reducing the number and adequacy of collateral vessels, might considerably affect prognosis.

Angiographic and MRI Diagnosis

Angiography by the standard Seldinger technique or intraarterial digital subtraction angiography have been the principal methods of corroborating the clinical impression of basilar artery occlusive disease. Now MRI can often suggest occlusion by the absence of a signal void in the artery in various slices.[72] MRA shows great promise for allowing corroboration of basilar artery occlusion without invasive catheterization or dye injection.[211,212] TCD is probably accurate in lesions of the proximal basilar artery but to date has not been sensitive to lesions of the mid- and distal basilar artery.[691] Diagnosis of basilar artery occlusion hinges on demonstration of blocked cephalad flow (not simply poor filling or the VA ending in the PICA) and collateral filling of rostral structures. Carotid injection frequently leads to flow through the posterior communicating artery to the PCA, basilar tip, and SCA. Figure 22.21 is an example of such retrograde filling. Even in the presence of a tiny incompetent posterior communicating artery, the PCA may be opacified via anastomosis between posterior branches of the middle cerebral artery and the branches of the PCA with subsequent filling of the distal basilar artery. In addition to the anastomosis between the vermian and hemispheric branches of the PICA, AICA, and SCA, there is also filling via the posterior meningeal branches of the VA and the meningohypophyseal branch of the ICA.[515] Angiographic definition of the disease in the basilar artery can help determine whether long-term warfarin anticoagulation therapy should be used in a patient with slight deficits. Angiography must be done if surgery to create shunts that would increase posterior circulation flow is under consideration. The risk of angiography for posterior circulation disease has been surprisingly low in large centers with trained neuroradiologists and a large number of cases. The CT scan is helpful in documenting cerebellar infarction but to date has been disappointing in defining acute brain stem softenings.

MRI has been a great advance in mapping and defining infarcts in the brain stem and cerebellum. The pattern of brain stem infarction, that is, unilateral or bilateral, tegmental or basal, medial or lateral, rostrocaudal level, can indicate whether the lesion involves the territory of the unilateral or bilateral intracranial VAs, the basilar artery, or single penetrating or circumferential branches. The pattern of cerebellar infarction, most readily seen on T_2-weighted sagittal sections for the vermis and coronal sections for the hemispheres, also helps to define the likely arterial territory and pathology.[15]

Clinical Tempo and Course

Information correlating the usual tempo of neurologic deficit acquisition and the location of vascular occlusion is very scanty. Many studies include patients chosen solely because of the availability of necropsy material, a factor that eliminates the less severely affected patients.[424,642] The clinical studies often lack angiographic or pathologic confirmation.[393,757] Angiographic studies frequently do not detail temporal profiles.[236] Larger series of patients with basilar artery occlusion antedated the widespread use of angiography. Caplan[110] analyzed the clinical course of surviving patients with basilar artery occlusion that have been verified angiographically, but the series was quite small (six cases). TIAs were quite frequent prior to the stroke (four of six cases). The last TIA occurred within 1 month of the stroke in all these patients (within 1 week in three cases). The initial TIA preceded the stroke by a wide range (1 week to 1 year). After onset of a prolonged deficit, five of the six patients had either progression of the deficit over a 2- to 3-day period or fluctuations. Fluctuations occurred over a 2-week period and were sensitive to position in bed.[118] Two patients had sudden-onset deficits, one of which subsequently fluctuated for less than 2 weeks. Only one patient had a progressive course without stabilization or fluctuation over the first 3 days. In another clinical series, Jones et al[384] noted that a temporal profile consisting of an unstable course characterized by progression or remission and relapses was common in patients who had vertebrobasilar system infarction (54%) compared with patients who had carotid system disease (26%). In this series the neurologic deficit in patients with vertebrobasilar disease rarely progressed after 4 days, and most changes occurred within the first 48 hours. Declining consciousness was an ominous sign. Patrick and colleagues[545] also analyzed the temporal profile in their series of 39 cases of clinical vertebrobasilar infarction (7 with angiography). Sudden onset followed by stabilization (12 patients) and gradual onset with later progression (9 patients) were common patterns. Only two patients' deficits progressed after 24 hours, one over 48 hours and the other over 1 week. A total of 13 patients progressed after the original deficit had been stable for 24 hours or more; eight progressed on day 2, two on day 3, and one each on days 4, 6, and 7. Again coma was a poor prognostic sign. These studies indicate that sudden-onset deficits are frequent, a point also emphasized by Kubik and Adams.[424]

Ferbert and colleagues[232] analyzed the early symptoms and course in their 85 patients with angiographically proven basilar artery occlusion. More than half had some premonitory symptoms, usually in the 2 weeks before stroke onset. Vertigo and headache were especially common symptoms. Acute onset of stroke was noted in 31 patients, 11 of whom had TIAs or other prodromal symptoms. In 54 of the 85 patients (64%) the course was progressive with or without prodromal symptoms.

Sudden onset might point to an embolic mechanism (thrombus breaking loose from a more proximal arterial site within the ICVA or the lower basilar artery). Fluctuations and progressions are common but are almost invariably documented only within the first 2 weeks after stroke onset, usually within the first 48 hours; few occur between 1 to 2 weeks. Gradual progression without improvement, especially if stupor develops, is a grave prognostic sign. This evidence, in our view, favors treatment prior to the stroke in those with TIAs and emphasizes treatment

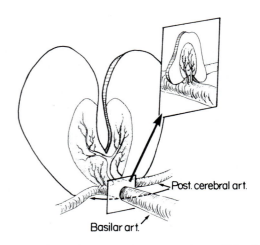

Figure 22.22 Diagrammatic representations of blood supply from the distal basilar artery. Note the single midline vessel supplying the thalamus bilaterally. The area of infarction is shown in gray. (*Insert*) Midbrain with shaded area of infarction.

during the first 1 to 2 weeks after the stroke onset. Vigorous treatment after the deficit is stable, especially after 2 weeks, would not seem to be warranted in patients with basilar artery occlusion because late deficits are rare.

The recent introduction of thrombolytic treatment in patients with basilar artery occlusion has brought new therapeutic promise for treatment of a potentially devastating illness. After angiography has confirmed a basilar artery occlusion, patients have been treated with local infusion by catheter of streptokinase or urokinase[315,771] or recombinant tissue plasminogen activator,[343] and with intravenously administered doses of the latter.[748] The optimum route of administration, optimum dose, and need for and dangers of the concurrent or postinfusion use of platelet antiaggregants, heparin, or warfarin have still to be defined. Endovascular techniques for treatment of basilar artery disease also have untested promise for the future.

Top of the Basilar Artery Occlusion

Occlusive lesions of the rostral tip of the basilar artery lead to bilateral infarction of midbrain, thalamus, and occipital and medial temporal lobes. In this area, in addition to the major tributary branches of the basilar apex, the SCA, posterior communicating artery, and PCA, there are numerous smaller perforating midbrain arteries and vessels that course through the posterior perforating substance to feed the hypothalamus and paramedian diencephalic structures (Fig. 22.22). Atherosclerosis is generally most severe in the proximal basilar artery; as the basilar artery travels cephalad, there is less incidence of atherosclerotic stenosis, and the vessel gradually tapers in size. Occlusions of the basilar apex are generally embolic thrombi originating from the heart or proximal vertebrobasilar system.[21,112] The extent of infarction depends on the size of the thrombus, the length of time it obstructs the main basilar artery, its eventual destination in tributary vessels, and the adequacy of collateral circulation. At times, the ischemic damage is limited to one or both PCA hemispheric territories, and on other occasions the brunt of the damage is to the rostral brain stem structures.

At times the syndrome of rostral basilar territory ischemia follows posterior circulation angiography, usually when the posterior circulation vessels are widely patent and have no important occlusive disease. Cortical blindness, agitated delirium, and an amnesic state are the cardinal features, usually with accompanying headache. The symptoms and signs reverse within 24 hours, leaving a permanent amnesia for the period of the angiography and its sequelae. Mehler[481,482] studied 61 patients with ischemia in the rostral basilar artery territory: 14 patients (23%) had vascular stroke risk factors and prior episodes of vertebrobasilar ischemia and presented with severe bilateral vessel, oculomotor, and behavioral abnormalities. Thrombosis engrafted on atherostenosis and artery-to-artery emboli from the proximal system were common stroke mechanisms in this group; 47 patients had less severe syndromes that were often reversible. Cardiac embolism was more prominent in this group. Among the total group of 61 patients, 28 (46%) were considered to have an embolic etiology (8 intra-arterial, 14 cardiac origin, and 6 unknown source). In situ thrombosis was believed to be responsible in 11 (18%), and 7 patients (11%) had symptoms after angiography, some of whom had documented transient contrast extravasation.

In the following section, we discuss just the findings in those patients with embolism or atherosclerotic occlusions of the basilar artery apex in whom ischemia involved multiple tributaries of the basilar artery. Similar findings, although of more limited extent, can occur in branch occlusions of these basilar apex branches: they have been reviewed above (see midbrain, thalamic, and SCA territory infarcts in the basilar branch occlusion section).

MAJOR CLINICAL SYNDROMES. *Pupillary abnormalities.* When ischemia affects the medial midbrain tegmentum or medial diencephalon, pupillary reactivity is usually abnormal, because the afferent limb of the pupillary reflex arc is interrupted in its course from the optic tract of Edinger-Westphal nucleus. Midbrain pupils are frequently eccentric (corectopia iridis) and may acutely shift position.[631,755] If the lesion only affects the Edinger-Westphal nucleus, the pupils will generally be fixed and dilated, but if, in addition, rostral extension of the lesion occurs with resultant sympathetic paralysis, the deficit will include a midposition, fixed pupil. At times the pupil is oval, a phenomenon that is usually transient and most often found in patients with supratentorial vascular catastrophes that lead to tentorial herniation.[257] Occasionally a pupil will become oval in a patient with midbrain infarction when a third cranial nerve paralysis is developing or recovering.[257] Thalamic infarcts are associated with small, poorly reactive pupils.

Among 61 patients with rostral basilar artery territory infarction Mehler[482] found that 18 (30%) had abnormal pupillary size, shape, or function. Six patients had discrepancies in pupillary reaction between accommodation and light stimuli. Despite abnormal light reactivity, four patients with dorsal midbrain infarcts had constriction on forced lid closure, normal dilatation with psychosensory stimuli, normal-sized pupils, and normal dilatation to drugs applied locally. Two other patients had normal pupillary light reactions but impaired response to convergence accommodation.

Oculomotor dysfunction. Vertical gaze-vertical plane eye movements are voluntarily generated by bilaterally simultaneous activation of the frontal and parietal occipital conjugate gaze centers. Vertical gaze pathways then converge on the periaqueductal region beneath the collicular plate, near the interstitial nucleus of Cajal and the posterior commissure.[484,550,712] In this region in the monkey there is a cluster of neurons important in vertical gaze, which is situated among fibers of the medial longitudinal fasciculus and is generally referred to as the rostral interstitial nucleus of the MLF[105] or the nucleus of the prerubral field.[712] Clinically there is often a disparity between paralysis of voluntary vertical gaze and vertical eye movements reflex-induced by vertical doll's eyes maneuver, bilateral simultaneous caloric stimulation, or Bell's phenomenon, although the anatomic basis for the disparity is not clear. Most commonly, up- and downgazes are affected together. Debate still centers around the question of the need for bilateral lesions, since unilateral stereotactic placed lesions[526] or unilateral vascular[746] and metastatic[38] lesions have on occasion produced upward gaze paralysis. In monkeys and humans, lesions of the pretectum in the posterior commissure region are necessary to produce paralysis of upward gaze.[155,542] Selective paralysis of downward gaze is much rarer; when it occurs, the lesions usually border the red nucleus and lie more ventral and caudal, producing paralysis of upward gaze.[317,378,712]

In one patient with selective downgaze palsy, the lesions were situated bilaterally in the dorsolateral periaqueductal gray, involving the crossing fibers of the commissure of the superior colliculus.[379] The eyes may rest down and are often skewed in asymmetric lesions of the mesodiencephalic junction.[112] Some patients with unilateral lesions of the paramedian midbrain and caudal diencephalon have abnormal control of head and eye posture in the roll plane.[318] Halmagyi and colleagues[318] reported four patients and Mehler[482] reported two patients with ocular tilt reactions. These patients all had a head tilt, conjugate eye torsion, and skewing with hypotropia all to the side ipsilateral or contralateral to the mesodiencephalic lesion. All patients with ocular tilt reactions also had vertical, predominantly upward gaze, palsies. Some patients with mesodiencephalic infarcts have had vertical one-and-a-half syndrome.[87,185] Deleu et al[185] reported a patient in whom all downward saccadic and smooth pursuit eye movements were lost bilaterally, but only a monocular paresis of upgaze was present. The lesion on MRI was confined to the rostral interstitial nucleus of the MLF bilaterally. The authors hypothesized that the lesion affected upgaze premotor fibers in the tracts from these nuclei before or after their decussation in the posterior commissure. Bogousslavsky and Regli[87] reported a patient with a unilateral mesodiencephalic lesion with bilateral upgaze palsy but only monocular paresis of downgaze. Unilateral lesions, by affecting crossing or commissural fibers, can produce bilateral defects in vertical gaze. Among Mehler's[482] series of 61 patients with top of the basilar territory infarction, 47 (77%) had some abnormality of vertical eye position or gaze.

Abnormalities of convergence. Ocular convergence is probably controlled in the medial midbrain tegmentum, although there is considerable debate as to whether a formal nuclear structure, such as the nucleus of Perlia, subserves

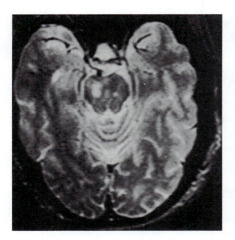
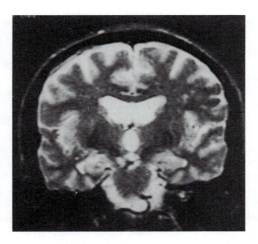

Figure 22.23 T_2-weighted views of pontomesencephalic infarct. (**A**) Axial plane. (**B**) Coronal plane.

this function. One or both eyes may rest in, and convergence vectors are frequently evident on attempted upward gaze. Rhythmic convergence nystagmus may be elicited by following a downgoing optokinetic target. Convergence vectors may also modify lateral gaze. Voluntary lateral movements of the lateral rectus are balanced against convergence vectors, thus limiting abduction and giving the superficial appearance of a sixth cranial nerve palsy (pseudosixth).[112] Lid abnormalities are also a frequent sign of rostral brain stem disease. Unilateral infarction of a third cranial nerve nucleus can lead to complete bilateral ptosis.[111] Retraction of the upper lid, giving the eye a prominent stare (Collier sign) is also frequent in tectal lesions.[162]

Abnormalities of alertness, attention, and behavior.

The medial mesencephalon and diencephalon contain the most rostral portions of the reticular activating system. Infarcts in these regions frequently affect consciousness, sleep, and behavior. Facon and colleagues[222] and later Castaigne et al[144] described patients with basilar apex occlusion in whom prolonged sleep and third cranial nerve palsies were the most prominent features. Segarra[629] later outlined the distribution of the infarction that causes this syndrome, which he believed was due to occlusion of the perforating branches of the mesencephalic artery (the first portion of the PCA as it courses around the midbrain). These vessels have been studied by Foix and Hillemand,[279] Lazorthes,[431] Percheron,[553] and Castaigne and colleagues[145] and are called the paramedian mesencephalic arteries and the anterior and posterior thalamosubthalamic paramedian arteries. They form the most rostral group of vessels in the posterior perforated substance and supply the paramedian midbrain and diencephalon. There is some evidence that a single midline vessel may branch to supply both banks of the third ventricle[145] (Fig. 22.23). Because the reticular gray is adjacent to the third cranial nerve nuclei and the vertical gaze regions near the posterior commissure, somnolence is invariably associated with pupillary abnormalities, third cranial nerve palsies, and defects of vertical gaze, although lateralized motor or sensory signs are often absent. A similar syndrome can occur after herniation, presumably due to extension pressure on these same vascular structures, caused by wedging of the mammillary bodies into the interpeduncular fossa, a situation that causes either median brain stem infarction[449] or Duret[120] hemorrhages. Among our own patients, one with a large putaminal hemorrhage survived the acute stroke but was left with third cranial nerve palsies and slept nearly continuously for 2 years at a nursing home. At postmortem an old slit cavity was found in the putamen and, in addition, butterfly distribution infarctions in the medial midbrain and thalamus developed, probably during the period of herniation. Of 28 patients with rostral brain stem infarcts studied by Castaigne and colleagues,[145] 15 had hypersomnia caused by paramedian tegmental lesions, usually bilateral.

Hallucinations.
Complaints of hallucination are also seen in cases of rostral brain stem infarction and have led to the term peduncular hallucinosis, first used by Jean Lhermitte[445] in 1922 and then by Ludo Van Bogaert.[720,721] All patients described with this phenomenon have had the hallucinations at twilight time or during the night and all have a sleep disorder (nocturnal insomnia or daytime hypersomnolence).[112] The hallucinations are usually vivid, most commonly visual, and contain multiple colors, objects, and scenes. Blood and red hair, horses and green serpents against a red background, and brightly plumed parrots are some examples. Occasionally auditory or tactile hallucinations are associated. Similar hallucinations also accompany sleep deprivation or drug intoxication and may relate to dysfunction of the reticular-activating system. In addition to hallucinations, impulsive reports, which have been called *extraordinary confabulation*, are often made by patients with rostral brain stem infarcts.[665] These consist of descriptions of behavior or present whereabouts that are totally unrealistic. The reports have no approximation to reality and are influenced by surrounding stimuli. For example, a 60-year-old woman was questioned while a newscast of a school incident was on an adjacent television set. She said that she was in school at a lunch bar ready to order English muffins, and if we did not get out of the way she would be late for her next seventh grade class. When asked why she was wearing a nightgown and seemed to be in a hospital bed, she said that she was too lazy that day to get fully dressed and simply came to school in her nightgown in bed. Similarly, others have incorporated into their replies reality items provided by the questioner. Many such patients "dream a lot" and they may be reporting their imaginings as reality.

In most patients with peduncular hallucinations, the lesions have been large, making it difficult to relate the abnormality to any particular anatomic structure. McKee et al[476] reported a single patient with peduncular hallucinations who had very discrete small bilateral lesions in the medial portions of the substantia nigra pars reticulata. Their patient was a diabetic man with prior third cranial nerve palsies that developed 2 years apart, each recovering within 2 months. After a seizure he reported visual hallucinations of animals and people with obscured faces walking across his field of vision. Often the visual hallucinations were preceded by the sensation of being touched on the shoulder or face. The lesions were limited entirely to the pars reticulata and may have affected adjacent fibers of the third cranial nerve just medial to the infarcts, but tegmental structures were completely spared. The pars reticulata has connections with the pedunculopontine nucleus and shows increased discharge during rapid eye movement sleep.

Hemiballism and abnormal movements. It has long been known that involuntary movements occur from deep upper brain stem lesions. In 1927 Martin[467] described a hypertensive man who suddenly developed violent movements of the right limbs associated with facial grimacing, dysarthria, agitation, and finally death. Necropsy revealed a small hemorrhage located in the left subthalamus in the region of the subthalamic nucleus (corpus Luysii). Martin[467] reviewed 12 earlier cases of hemichorea associated with lesions in this region that were verified postmortem; 8 were small hemorrhages, 3 metastases, and 1 unspecified. Whittier[747] later reviewed the subject and attempted to differentiate ballism, that is, incessant violent flinging proximal movements, from other types of adventitious movements such as chorea. Lesions in 30 of the cases he reviewed involved the subthalamic region or "the connections of this region." The most common etiology was hemorrhage, but infarctions in this region were also described. Moersch and Kernohan[503] noted a single patient with hemiballism due to two small adjacent softenings in the subthalamic nucleus but unfortunately did not comment on the offending vascular lesion. More recently, it has become clear from CT correlation that lesions in other sites, especially the striatum and thalamus, can produce a movement disorder difficult to distinguish from that caused by lesions in the subthalamic nucleus.[393] Infarction of the subthalamus can produce a severe movement disorder that is unilateral and characterized by nearly constant flinging and often rotatory proximal arm and leg movements on one side of the body. Frequently a hemiparesis precedes or follows the movement disorder, the movement disappearing as the limbs are paralyzed and returning when the paralysis clears. Unfortunately, the offending vascular lesion in the subthalamus, which is fed by branches of the posterior communicating and posterior choroidal arteries and the PCA, has seldom if ever been characterized.[503] One of us (L.R.C.) has seen a patient in whom unilateral hemiballism was associated with stupor and eye signs typical of basilar apex brain stem infarction (no hemorrhage on CT), but unfortunately the vascular lesion was not verified.

Abnormal movements other than ballistic were present in 7 of 28 rostral brain stem infarcts studied by Castaigne and colleagues.[145] The movements were frequently delayed in onset and had a predilection for the face, arm, and thumb. Clonic, athetoid, and myoclonic movements were described

in patients with bilateral paramedian thalamic infarcts that at times extended to the upper pole of the red nucleus and affected Meynert's tract and the decussation of the brachium conjunctivum. When emboli block the penetrating vessels of the basilar apex, limb paralysis is usually transient or absent. When the most proximal portion of the PCA is affected, a contralateral hemiplegia may occur, at times accompanied by a contralateral third nerve palsy.[359] Often, however, the clinical findings are dominated by unilateral or bilateral posterior cerebral artery territory hemispheral infarction.

Multiple Posterior Circulation Infarcts

Basilar artery occlusion often accompanies ICVA occlusion either on one or both sides with PICA, AICA, SCA, or PCA occlusion due to blockage of their origin by the occlusive thrombus in the parental artery or due to artery-to-artery embolism. Patients with occlusion of the ICVAs and basilar artery and patients with large emboli often have infarcts in multiple cerebellar artery territories. Penetrator branches at various levels (i.e., pontine, midbrain, or thalamosubthalamic level) may also be occluded. Massive multiple infarction may occur when there is no collateral anastomosis involving mainly the cerebellum, ventromedial pons and midbrain, thalamus, and occipitotemporal lobes.

In a pathologic series of 64 patients with cerebellar infarction 13 had cerebellar infarction extended to the territory of more than one artery.[22] These large infarcts all involved the PICA territory (4 bilaterally) together with the SCA territory in 10 cases (3 bilaterally) and AICA territory in 7 cases (1 bilaterally). The full territory of these arteries was usually affected, giving rise to mass effect on the brain stem and tonsillar herniation. They were associated with massive bilateral paramedian pontine infarction in half the patients and were due to basilar artery occlusion in three patients involving either the entire basilar artery or the upper basilar artery with VA occlusion facing the PICA ostium or below it; four patients had unilateral VA occlusion at the PICA ostium, one of whom had a VA occlusion blocking a common trunk of PICA and AICA; two patients had bilateral VA occlusions below the PICA ostia, one of whom had artery-to-artery emboli in one PICA and one PCA; five patients had no occlusion at postmortem examination, two of whom had postangiographic dissection without occlusion, and three others had a cardiac source of embolism. These patients all had signs of massive brain stem infarction and of edematous cerebellar infarction in 70% of cases.[22]

In a clinical series of patients with territorial and small nonterritorial infarcts diagnosed with MRI in most cases, Amarenco and colleagues[28] included four patients with PICA plus SCA infarcts; one was attributed to cardiac embolism, one to ECVA dissection, one to ICVA occlusive disease, and one had no recognized cause. They also included in this series one patient with PICA plus AICA plus SCA infarction who had severe basilar artery disease. Among the clinical series of Tohgi et al,[701] there were eight patients with PICA plus AICA plus SCA infarcts who had angiography; seven severe VA occlusive lesions and four basilar artery occlusive lesions were found at angiography among these eight patients.

In the New England Medical Center registry 37 of the 84

patients (44%) had multiple territory cerebellar infarcts.[126] Others had cerebellar infarcts in one territory but brain stem infarcts in other intracranial territories. The clinical findings can best be thought of as an addition of the findings in each territory. The additional mass of cerebellar infarction has the potential to cause more mass effect than cerebellar infarcts limited to one territory, especially if the full PICA or SCA territory (or both) is included in the lesion.

The multiple territory cerebellar infarcts in the New England Medical Center registry seemed to fall into two groups—those that involved proximal and distal intracranial territories (PICA and SCA) and those that included the middle intracranial territory (PICA and AICA, AICA and SCA, and PICA, AICA, and SCA). The latter group we referred to as middle + territory infarcts. The stroke mechanisms underlying the middle + territory infarcts seemed to be very similar no matter what the configuration of lesions (proximal + middle, middle + distal, proximal + middle + distal). Embolism was the predominant stroke mechanism in patients with proximal and distal territory cerebellar infarction. At times the infarcts were limited to the PICA and SCA cerebellum. The vascular lesion when present was always on the side of the PICA territory infarct since the ECVA and ICVA supply only the ipsilateral PICA but can be the source of embolism to both SCA territories. One patient with severe bilateral ICVA and basilar artery stenosis had bilateral PICA and SCA territory cerebellar infarcts. In most patients, the infarcts also included other noncerebellar structures within the proximal or distal intracranial territories, for example, the medulla, midbrain, thalamus, and PCA hemispheral regions.

Within the proximal + distal group intra-arterial emboli arose from the ECVA in eight patients. Five had VA occlusive disease (three severe atherostenosis, two VAO occlusions), two had ECVA dissections, and one patient had an angiographic complication. Cardiac sources of emboli were cardiomyopathy in two patients and atrial fibrillation, valvular disease, and PFO in one patient each. All the patients with large artery intracranial occlusive disease had severe ICVA disease, bilateral in four patients and at the ICVA/basilar artery junction in the other patient. The pattern in which ICVA lesions caused local proximal territory (medullary or PICA cerebellar, or both) ischemia by hypoperfusion and in addition served as a donor source of embolism to the distal intracranial territory has been discussed in the section on occlusion of the ICVA. In patients with emboli that arose from the heart or ECVAs, the emboli presumably first stopped at the ICVA and then traveled distally, or a part of the embolus broke off and reached the SCA-distal basilar artery region.

In contrast to the proximal + distal territory group of patients with multiple territory infarcts, when the middle territory was involved, the most common cause was large artery intracranial occlusive disease. Ten of the 12 patients with intracranial occlusive disease had severe basilar artery occlusive disease, accompanied by ICVA disease in 7 patients. Embolism was a less common cause, occurring in about one-third of patients. Two patients had only potential cardiac sources of embolism in the form of atrial fibrillation; two had only intra-arterial sources (ECVA dissection and angiographic complication), and two had both potential cardiac and arterial sources—atrial fibrillation and VA occlusion in one patient, and ECVA dissection and a PFO in the other patient. One

patient had severe, presumably migraine-related, vasospasm of both ICVAs and the basilar artery.

In our experience, basilar artery lesions are more often due to in situ occlusive disease of the basilar artery itself or to propagation of thrombus from the ICVA. ICVA and basilar artery occlusive disease often coexist. Since middle territory + infarcts, by definition, must have at some time been related to decreased basilar artery perfusion, the mechanisms of infarction are very similar to those found in patients with basilar artery territory ischemia. By contrast, proximal and distal territory infarcts spare the basilar artery but involve the ICVA supply zone. Their etiology is similar to that found in patients with ICVA disease.

LOW-FLOW STATES WITH RESULTANT BORDER ZONE ISCHEMIA IN THE POSTERIOR CIRCULATION

Occlusion of a blood vessel, whether due to in situ thrombosis or embolus, results in a region of infarction, usually within the center of distribution of that vessel. Collateral circulation is apt to supply the more peripheral zones and thus limit the centrifugal extent of the infarct. When, however, flow is diffusely diminished, for example, during shock due to blood loss or cardiogenic hypotension, the distribution of ischemia more often straddles the border zone regions between major blood vessels. Schneider[773] labeled these border zones *distal fields*, comparable to the far zones of an agricultural irrigation system. Zülch and Behrend,[775] Romanul and Abramowicz,[595,596] Mohr,[504] and Brierley[97] have discussed the localization and pathophysiology of this phenomenon in clinical and experimental hypotension.

Few examples of necropsy-confirmed posterior circulation border zone infarction have been reported. Romanul and Abramowicz[596] described a single patient, a 70-year-old woman, who never awakened from surgical hypotension. Extensive supratentorial and infratentorial boundary zone lesions were found. The posterior circulation lesion was a zone of infarction in the cerebellum at the junction of supply of the inferior cerebellar arteries (AICA and PICA) and the SCA; no brain stem lesion was mentioned. Hutchinson and Yates[372] described four patients with combined vertebral and carotid disease who developed infarction bilaterally in the cerebellum in or adjacent to territory usually supplied by the SCAs after systemic hypotension. In the reported cases, the dominant clinical feature in severe cases was coma, and in milder forms visual agnosia and brachial weakness were due to accompanying supratentorial lesions.

Reports of border zone infarction in the posterior circulation mainly focused on border zone ischemia in the cerebellum, and few reports concentrated on border zone ischemia within the brain stem.

Border Zone Ischemia in the Cerebellum

Certain infarctions have been called watershed, low flow, distal field, border zone, end zone, and nonterritorial cerebellar infarcts. The first two appellations should not be used for the cerebellum because they imply an underlying pathogenetic mechanism that is unproved so far, the other names being better because they describe only an anatomic location. Few pathologic reports on border zone ischemia in the cerebellum exist. In addition to the observations by Zülch[774] and Romanul and Abramowicz[596] cited above, the most important paper was by Rodda in 1971.[593] Macdonell et al[460] also reported pathologic cases. These strokes occurred in boundary zones between the SCA and PICA or between left and right SCAs on the surface of the cortex.[460,593,596,774] The affected area usually measures <2 cm,[593] probably because plentiful anastomoses on the cerebellar cortex limit the extension of infarction. Indeed, in a large pathologic study of patients who had died from systemic shock, Sevestre and his colleagues[633] from La Salpêtrière found only microscopic lesions in the cerebellar cortex. Later CT scan occasionally allowed recognition of these small infarcts either in the distal fields of cerebellar arteries[18] or in the deep small cerebellar white matter.[614] However, only MRI revealed a high frequency of very small cerebellar infarcts <2 cm in extent located in border zone areas. Only two studies are available.[27,28] Among a consecutive series of 115 patients with cerebellar infarcts (diagnosed with MRI in 85% of patients), 36 (31%) had only small border zone infarcts.[28]

These infarcts were usually small and deep or cortical involving the border zones between territories of cerebellar arteries or their branches. The reports sought to identify the stroke mechanisms and clinical findings in these patients with small cerebellar infarcts. Were these lesions the posterior circulation counterpart of cerebral border zone lesions attributable in some patients to systemic hypoperfusion? Could some infarcts represent cerebellar lacunes due to lipohyalinosis, or intracranial branch atheromatous disease, or both? Instead, were the causes of small infarcts identical to those of larger cerebellar infarcts but the small size explained by the rapid development of adequate collateral circulation or by the passage and fragmenting of emboli with fragments blocking small distal arterial branches?

We and others analyzed a series of very small cerebellar infarcts.[27] The material included 47 patients with small infarcts that were found by extensive review of CT and MRI scans of patients with cerebellar infarcts studied at the New England Medical Center (29 patients) and Boston University Medical Center (8 patients) in Boston and at the Hôpital Saint-Antoine in Paris (10 patients). These small cerebellar infarcts accounted for 43%, 26%, and 28% of cerebellar infarcts at these hospitals.[27]

The infarcts seemed to fit five different anatomic patterns (Fig. 22.24). Group I infarcts (29 patients) were cortical and linear and were directed toward the subcortical cerebellar white matter, perpendicular to the cortex and parallel to the penetrating branches. Group II infarcts (15 patients) were very small and were located in the deep white matter. Group

Figure 22.24 Pattern of distribution of cerebellar border zone infarcts.

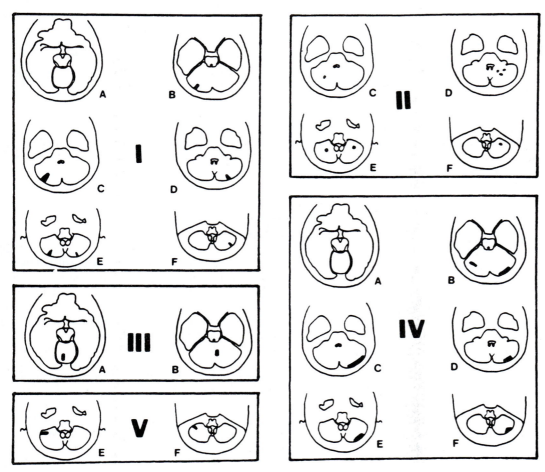

III infarcts (five patients) were located in the rostral and medial cerebellum. Group IV (two patients) infarcts were cortical superficial infarcts. Group V (one patient) infarcts were cortical and ventral and were aligned parallel to penetrating branches. Some patients had more than one type of infarct.[27]

The authors divided the causes of these infarcts into four groups. Group A (two patients) had cardiac arrest or systemic hypoperfusion as the cause of infarction. Group B (nine patients) was considered to have occlusive disease of small penetrating or pial arteries caused by various conditions. In this group, one patient had Wegener's granulomatosis; four had hypercoagulability (two disseminated intravascular coagulation, one thrombocytosis, one polycythemia); in three patients the absence of large artery lesions, the presence of diabetes, and the presence of lacunes suggested disease of small arteries as the cause; and one patient had cholesterol crystal embolism proven by muscle biopsy. Group C, the largest group, contained 27 patients with large artery occlusive disease or brain embolism as the likely cause of their strokes. Sixteen had occlusive lesions, most often involving the VAO, ICVA and basilar artery. Eleven had embolism, nine of cardiac origin and two intra-arterial. In group D, which consisted of nine patients, the cause of the small cerebellar infarcts was unknown mostly because of incomplete evaluation.[27] In this study systemic hypoperfusion was a very rare cause of small infarcts, and very few patients had intrinsic atherostenotic disease of small penetrating or pial arteries as the cause of the small infarcts.[27]

Amarenco et al[28] later prospectively collected patients with territorial and small nonterritorial infarcts studied at the Hôpital Saint-Antoine in Paris during a 6-year period. Thirty-six of the 115 cerebellar infarcts (31%) were small and not localizable readily to one of the cerebellar artery territories. The causes of territorial and small, nonterritorial infarcts were very similar. About one-third of the patients in each group had cardiac sources of embolism; one-fourth had large artery occlusive disease; and in about one-fourth no definite cause could be established. Small artery inflammatory disease and hypercoagulable states were more common in patients with small nonterritorial infarcts than in patients with territorial infarcts.[28] Systemic hypoperfusion and penetrating and pial artery branch disease were not important causes of small infarcts in either series.[28] Infarcts distal to unilateral occlusive lesion of one VA occurred in 18% of patients with territorial cerebellar infarcts and in 5% of patients with small nonterritorial (border zone) infarcts, but this difference was not statistically significant. However, infarcts distal to bilateral vertebral or basilar artery occlusions occurred with a low-flow state at angiography in 14% of patients with nonterritorial (border zone) cerebellar infarcts but in none of the patients with territorial infarcts.

The conclusions of the study were that small nonterritorial infarcts have the same high rate of embolic mechanism (about 50% of cases) as territorial infarcts, have more frequent hypercoagulable states and small artery inflammatory disease than territorial infarcts, and sometimes have a hemodynamic mechanism.[28]

One other study reported eight border zone infarcts among a series of 34 patients diagnosed with MRI, which were attributed to "severe vertebrobasilar atherosclerosis."[56] Mounier-Vehier et al[521] reported a series of 14 consecutive patients with border zone infarcts and confirmed that most of them (9 patients) had a cardioembolic mechanism; three other patients had VA dissections.

Border Zone Ischemia in the Brain Stem

Brain stem lesions due to hypotension have been hypothesized but seldom documented. Romanul[595] identified the medial zone at the tegmentobasal junction of the midpons (the area damaged in central pontine myelinolysis) as a possible zone of vulnerability between medial penetrating branches and tegmental supply from the circumferential cerebellar vessels supplying the tegmentum, but did not refer to necropsy specimens supporting this idea. Jurgensen et al[386] described a 44-year-old epileptic woman who was found to be hypotensive, hypothermic, and comatose after presumed multiple drug injection. At necropsy, there were bilateral, symmetric, round, hemorrhagic infarcts distributed in a columnar fashion in the lateral brain stem tegmentum extending the length of the lower pons and medulla. They were between the short lateral circumferential penetrators and the lateral edge. There were also bilateral hemorrhagic lesions in the lateral putamen. Gilles[297] described isolated necrosis of brain stem nuclei in children after hypotension. The authors have seen two adult patients with a clinical picture following hypotension that closely mimicked pontine hemorrhage: small pupils, absent horizontal gaze, and deep coma. One of these patients had no gross lesion visible at postmortem, but extensive necrosis of brain stem nuclei was seen microscopically, especially in the pons. The other patient had no postmortem examination. Lance and Adams[428] described patients with hypotension who made fine or coarse muscular jerks, especially on conscious attempts at precise movement. They called this phenomenon intention and action myoclonus. Myoclonus was related to probable cerebellum system damage but was not precisely localized. Keane[398] wondered if the sustained upward gaze found in 15 patients who had suffered a cardiorespiratory arrest could be due to "symmetrical cerebellar hypoxic change" that was found at postmortem in the 6 autopsied patients. Downward nystagmus and severe truncal and extremity cerebellar dysfunction was also noted in several patients, leading Keane[398] to suggest a posterior circulation locus for the pathogenic mechanism.

Mechanism of Hypotension-Related Border Zone Ischemia in Posterior Circulation

Hutchinson and Yates[372] and Romanul[595] also speculated that hypotension in patients with pre-existing severe occlusive disease in the VAs may modify the usual locus of infarction. Hinshaw at al,[350] in a radiographic analysis of cerebellar infarcts, described one patient with bilateral border zone lesions in the cerebellum visible on CT scan who had critical stenosis of one VA; the other VA ended in the PICA. We have reported one other observation with cerebellar border zone infarcts and right VA occlusion at the origin with distal reconstitution and retrograde filling via deep cervical anastomoses and, on the left side, tight stenosis of the origin of the VA with distal filling of the left VA via anastomoses with deep cervical arteries[15] (Fig. 22.25). In our series of 47 patients, two had systemic hypotension (cardiac arrest) as the presumed mechanism of their cerebellar border zone infarcts.[27] In both patients these

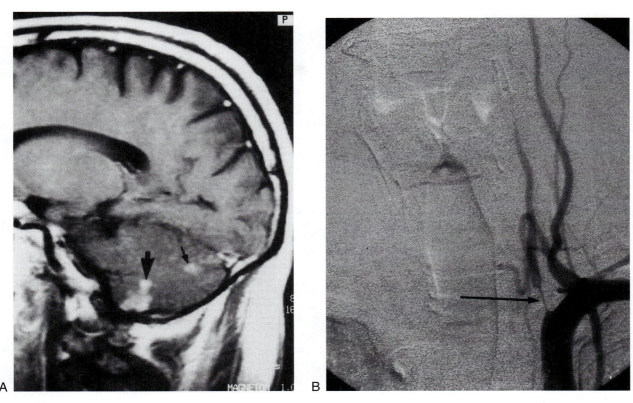

Figure 22.25 (**A & B**) Cerebellar border zone infarcts (*arrows*) and tight stenosis of the left vertebral artery (the right vertebral artery was severely hypoplastic).

infarcts were isolated to the cerebellum, were unilateral, and occurred with severe underlying vertebrobasilar occlusive disease.[27] This is corroborated by the data found in the consecutive series of 115 patients in which we found so-called low-flow infarcts only in patients with bilateral VA occlusive disease or basilar artery occlusion.[28] However, this hypotensive mechanism of border zone ischemia in the cerebellum is probably infrequent, depending on underlying conditions with pre-existing bilateral severe occlusive disease of VAs, or occlusion of basilar arteries without refilling via the posterior communicating arteries because the P1 segments are hypoplastic; most cerebellar border zone infarcts are due to cardiac or artery-to-artery embolism. The site and extent of the cerebellar infarcts simply reflect the size of the embolus causing occlusion: the smaller the embolus, the smaller the recipient artery, and therefore, the more distal the (border zone) infarct. At this time data are insufficient either to specify loci of vulnerability to hypotension in the posterior circulation, especially the brain stem, or to characterize the associated clinical findings.

MIGRAINE

In 1961 Bickerstaff[69] reported a distinct symptom complex occurring in adolescent girls, consisting of repeated episodes of altered vision, vertigo, ataxia, dysarthria, and numbness and tingling of the limbs and sometimes face, followed by headache. The frequent family history of migraine and clearing of ischemic symptoms by the time the headache began stamped the disorder as migrainous for Bickerstaff, and he coined the descriptive term *basilar artery migraine*. Swanson and Vick[673] have corroborated the existence of this syndrome, noted its occasional onset in adult life, and described an occasional familial tendency.[108]

Although traditionally considered a disorder beginning in the first 2 to 3 decades of life, migraine occurring late in life is more frequent than is generally realized. Fisher[253] analyzed the nature of migraine accompaniments and compared their clinical features with a comparable group of patients in whom ischemia was due to verified atherosclerotic occlusive disease. Migrainous deficits developed over a period of 15 to 30 minutes. "Positive" phenomena (for example, scintillations or brightness in the visual sphere or tingling in the tactile sphere) were perceived first and gradually spread within each sensory modality; for example, scintillations traveled gradually across the visual field and paresthesiae spread from one digit to the next and slowly up the limbs. The "positive" phenomena left in their wake "negative" phenomena, for example, blackness or numbness. As positive and later negative phenomena spread within the sensory modality, the earliest affected regions would clear, and finally all symptoms related to that modality would return to normal before a second modality would be affected. Headache would usually, but not always, appear after the deficits has disappeared. Using these clinical criteria and the absence of appropriate angiographic atherosclerotic lesions that might explain the clinical phenomenon, Fisher[267] defined a group of patients whom he believed had transient migrainous spells beginning after the age of 50. Our experience (L.R.C.) with such patients includes those with

(1) a clinical tempo matching that described by Fisher[253]; (2) multiple attacks in a variety of regions; (3) absence of angiographic disease or a source of cerebral emboli; and (4) response to commonly used prophylactic antimigraine agents such as propranolol, phenytoin, and methysergide. In many such patients, attacks are within the distribution of the posterior circulation.

The term basilar artery migraine is perhaps redundant, because it has long been known, but not understood, that migraine tends to involve basilar artery and its branches. Visual scintillations are the most common accompaniments of migraine and are occipital (PCA) in origin. Examples of transient global amnesia are known in migraine, and the pathologic anatomy and physiology of memory suggest a dominant PCA localization.[115] Physiologic studies using xenon-133 have documented oligemia as an early finding or subsequent to focal hyperemia.[644,647] Blood flow changes are maximal in the occipitoparietal regions.[537] Also, angiography performed during the prodromal phase of migraine has demonstrated filling of the PCA from carotid injection, which suggests low pressure in the basilar system. The following example of adult basilar migraine serves to illustrate this problem.

> A 58-year-old physician had no past history of important headache or transient neurologic dysfunction. In January 1980, 5 minutes after intercourse, he noted dizziness and a wobbly, unsteady gait, which was followed by unclear vision and diplopia. An unpleasant dysesthetic feeling was then apparent in his right hand and spread to his right leg and trunk. He became unable to walk and vomited. The attack lasted 20 minutes and left no residue. Subsequently, he had more than 30 nearly identical attacks frequently beginning after intercourse or exertion. During some attacks, his wife noted outward deviation of one eye. Dysphagia, drooling of saliva, and hiccups occasionally accompanied the vertigo, ataxia, diplopia, and right dysesthesia, all of which were invariable features. A neurologist found an internuclear ophthalmoplegia and gait ataxia during one attack and the patient was examined during another attack. He was dysarthric. The right eye was deviated to the right and there was prominent horizontal nystagmus on left gaze. On right gaze he did not adduct the left eye but had abducting nystagmus of the outwardly deviated right eye (internuclear ophthalmoplegia). Gait was grossly ataxic. Spells varied from 15 minutes to 24 hours. Headache was not experienced during or after any attack. Electroencephalography, CT scan with and without contrast, and vertebral angiography were all normal.
>
> Heparin, warfarin, aspirin, and dipyridamole were used sequentially to no avail. After the beginning of phenytoin therapy, there was a transient decrease in the frequency of the attacks, which had by now become very disabling. After methysergide therapy was begun in July 1980, the spells completely disappeared, except for some insignificant intermittent dysesthetic feeling in the physician's right hand. Methysergide therapy was stopped in December 1980, with no further recurrence of the episodes. The tempo of the symptoms, normality of the verte-

brobasilar system angiographically, and response to methysergide strongly suggest a migrainous mechanism, that is, adult basilar migraine. Five years after his last attack, he first noted spells of typical migrainous scintillating scotomas that lasted 20 to 30 minutes without headache.

Some patients who have transient basilar artery territory deficits but normal angiography are, in fact, suffering migrainous spells. Is this more common than we now appreciate? Does physiologic alteration in vascular size with inefficient delivery of blood (spasm?) occur in patients who would not fall within the usually accepted nosology of migraine?[115]

Caplan[125] reviewed his experience with patients who had migraine (classic or common) and posterior circulation ischemic attacks and strokes, who had also had angiography. Nine patients were presented, including the case described above. Men and women of widely varying ages were included. The clinical patterns included patients with just TIAs, single strokes, single stroke followed by attacks, and multiple strokes. In some patients classic migraine developed only months or years later. CT and MRI confirmed infarctions in patients who had strokes with persistent neurologic deficits (seven of nine patients).[125] Angiography showed basilar artery occlusions, severe diffuse narrowing of vertebrobasilar arteries (rather persistent in one patient), or normal posterior circulation vessels. The mechanism of infarction was not elucidated, but clearly vasoconstriction, often protracted, and basilar artery occlusion did occur.[125] The author posited that ischemia was due to protracted vasoconstriction, or to vascular thrombosis precipitated by activation of platelet adhesion and agglutination and activation of the intrinsic and extrinsic coagulation pathways.

Diagnostic Tests

With the advent of high-quality MRI, most regions of infarction can be diagnosed noninvasively, and cerebral angiography, hitherto the principal diagnostic investigation in patients with vertebrobasilar occlusive disease, is relied on less. Use of the studies summarized below is cited widely throughout this chapter. Here attention is briefly paid to general comments concerning the techniques themselves.

COMPUTED TOMOGRAPHY

Although CT is the oldest of the modern brain imaging technologies and has been in general use for about 20 years, it has not been as helpful in evaluating patients with posterior circulation vascular disease when compared with its role in the diagnosis of anterior circulation lesions. Bone-related artifacts, limited views, and suboptimal brain stem resolution limit the utility of CT in imaging acute posterior circulation infarcts. The small size of the brain stem and the dense bony structures surrounding it make visualization of the brain stem, especially the lower pons and medulla, very poor. CT is an excellent modality for detecting significant intraparenchymatous hemorrhage in the brain stem, thalamus, and cerebellum. CT is probably superior to MRI in showing subarachnoid and intraventricular blood, but neither CT nor MRI detects small subarachnoid hemorrhages. Pressure effects on the basal cisterns and hydrocephalus are very well shown by CT.[713] CT can also show the presence of dolichoectatic aneurysmal changes in the basilar artery,[651] and sometimes increased attenuation of the basilar artery on plain, unenhanced CT scans can indicate the likely presence of a thrombus.[290,729] Infarcts in the temporal and occipital lobes in the territory of the PCAs are usually well shown by CT. CT has the advantage of being more widely available, less expensive, and more readily obtainable acutely, especially in an emergency situation outside of regular working hours. CT remains an excellent screening test for hemorrhage and hydrocephalus.

MAGNETIC RESONANCE IMAGING

Even very early studies using first-generation MR scanners showed a dramatic superiority of MR over CT scanning in imaging posterior circulation vascular lesions.[414] Even small infarcts in the medulla, pons, and cerebellum are well shown.[78,284,646] The multiple simultaneous planes of section help to delineate the precise localizations of the lesions in the rostral-caudal, ventral-dorsal, and medial-lateral dimensions. Occlusion of major intracranial arteries can also often be suggested by MRI.[72,622,718] Occluded arteries have high signal intensity on spin-echo sequences, absence of flow void, and no flow enhancement on gradient echo images.[622] Aneurysms and their relation to the brain stem, dolichoectatic arteries, angiomas, and arteriovenous malformations are also frequently well imaged by MRI. The MRI findings do not always match the clinical abnormalities. Biller and colleagues[71] analyzed the clinical and MRI findings in 10 patients with pontine infarction. In one patient, the first MRI at 12 hours after the onset of a left hemiparesis was normal, but 6 days later an infarct was shown in the right basis pontis. In four other patients, the MRI abnormalities were more severe than the clinical findings.[71] So-called silent infarction is very common in other anatomic regions in the brain,[13] so it should come as no surprise that a substantial number of infarcts seem to have no clinical counterpart.[128] The reasons that these infarcts are silent are diverse. There may have been symptoms, but these have been forgotten or considered trivial by the patient. Alternatively, the physician's history may not have been probing or specific enough. The lesion may not produce any clearly abnormal signs.

The finding of infarction on MRI, whether or not the patient describes symptoms or the clinician finds related abnormalities on examination, means that there must have been vascular occlusive lesions at that level at one time. The nonconcordance of MRI and the clinical findings means that clinicians must consider both imaging and clinical findings and in fact add them together to determine the full extent of the ischemic territories. In some patients additional areas of ischemia may be detected by functional testing, as is discussed later.

Localization of the vascular territories of cerebellar infarction is especially important in determining the level of vascular occlusive disease. An infarct in PICA territory means a vascular lesion at the level of the intracranial VA, whereas an AICA territory infarct means a caudal BA lesion, and an SCA territory cerebellar infarct means there must have been a lesion at the rostral end of the BA.[149] Sagittal views of T_2-weighted MRI scans are superior to coronal and axial views in localizing the vascular territory of cerebellar infarcts and should be requested routinely in patients with suspected cerebellar lesions. These sagittal views also show the rostral-caudal location and extent of infarction in the brain stem. Dorsal-ventral (tectal-tegmental-basal) distribution of lesions can also be shown on sagittal and axial sections, whereas medial-lateral distribution is best shown on coronal and axial views.

ULTRASOUND

Ultrasound of the posterior circulation arteries is less familiar to many, although all have had some experience with carotid artery ultrasound evaluation. Clearly, ultrasound is generally underutilized in patients with vertebrobasilar disease.

The difficulty in accessing the VAs in the neck and basilar artery is now reduced by the common use of five somewhat different ultrasound techniques, which obtain maximal information about the posterior circulation: continuous-wave Doppler, B-mode ultrasound and pulsed-wave Doppler (both combined in a *duplex* system), color-flow Doppler, and TCD.

Continuous-wave Doppler remains the first and very important part of ultrasound examination in a patient with suspected vertebrobasilar disease. Retrograde flow in one VA has proved to be a reliable sign of ipsilateral subclavian stenosis or occlusion causing retrograde VA flow. High velocity at the origin of the VA means severe proximal stenosis. The discovery of no velocity or a high-resistance velocity profile on cephalad flow is also a fairly reliable indication of occlusion between the probe and the skull. Normal flow velocity, usually a sign the entire vessel is patent, may be found when the occlusion lies cephalad to the PICA, as flow into this branch often suffices to keep a normal velocity profile in the VA below the occlusion.[685]

Most of the atherosclerosis is at the origin of the VA from the subclavian, which is located in a place at times difficult to insonate with B-mode imaging, behind the clavicle.[75,342] However, color-flow Doppler now images flow direction, turbulence, and velocity in an anatomic image format, and color-flow images are now readily obtained at the VA origin. The ECVAs gain access to the transverse processes at about C6 and course cephalad (where they are accessible to B-mode[704] and color-flow Doppler insonations[709]) after which they cross the narrow spaces bridging the transverse processes. At the skull base, the sharp turns taken by the artery make it difficult to detect and also difficult to follow a stable reflected signal from the blood flowing in the arteries. However, color-flow Doppler images may be obtained at the atlas loop. Even under the best of conditions, quantitative assessments are more often frustrated by the considerable asymmetry in flow velocity and pulsatility in VAs due to asymmetric diameters of both vertebrals and the many variations in the vertebrobasilar circulation. VA calibers are now obtained by B-mode imaging combined with color-flow Doppler at the V1 segment and at the transverse processes.[603,705]

Ackerstaff and colleagues[2] studied 584 arteries by duplex scanning and angiography They were able to distinguish hypoplastic arteries from occlusions. When B-mode images were obtainable, duplex scanning had an 80% sensitivity and a very high specificity (97%). The overall accuracy was 93% for determining stenosis of the proximal VA by 50% or more.[2] Touboul and colleagues[704] studied 100 normal VAs and found that they were able to visualize the pretransverse and C6 to C5, C5 to C4 intertransverse segments in all patients. The VA ostium was visualized in 94% of vessels on the right, but in only 60% of left VAs. The atlas loop of the right ECVA was visualized in all patients, and the left distal ECVA was shown in 90% of patients.[704] In a recent study of 60 patients, color-flow Doppler imaging was more effective than duplex imaging in showing the proximal VAs (88% good visualization of the right VA and 73% of the left VA compared with 80% and 65%, respectively, by duplex sonography).[54] In this study, visualization of the atlas loop of the distal ECVAs was rarely successful using duplex sonography, but 87% of the right and 85% of the left VAs could be imaged in this location using color-flow Doppler imaging.[54] Others have also found a high frequency of diagnostic quality images using color-flow Doppler.[689,709,710]

TCD uses a pulsed-wave Doppler system that operates at low frequencies of 1.5 to 2 MHz and high ultrasound power.[337] The pulses are range gated and have great tissue penetration properties. Insonation through a suboccipital window allows good detection of blood flow velocities in the intracranial VAs and the proximal basilar artery.[107,134,413,691,724] The distal third of the basilar artery is not as well studied.[691] Insonation through temporal windows allows study of flow through the PCA and posterior communicating arteries. More recently color duplex sonography of the intracranial arteries has become available, but the early images do not optimally show long segments of the intracranial arteries. Transcranial duplex color-flow images do, however, allow determination of the angle of insonation, facilitating more precise measurements of blood flow velocities than with conventional TCD ultrasonography.[53,55,390,468,620,714] Basal, temporal, and cerebellar arteriovenous malformations can be successfully imaged by color-Doppler transcranial images. Intravenous boluses of agents that contain microbubbles increase the decibel level of the Doppler spectra and so enhance the color scans. The increased ability to identify the intracranial arteries using color-coded scans allows sonographers to identify, examine, and follow the intracranial arteries more accurately. Also use of so-called three-dimensional scanning, which uses a headpiece apparatus to keep head position constant, aids in analysis of the location of the vessel being insonated. In the three-dimensional system, the 2-MHz probes are fixed in a system of rods that are moved by hand.

Using a transtemporal window, the very distal portion of the basilar artery and the PCAs can often be insonated. Detection of blood flow velocities in the posterior communicating arteries is more difficult because of the course of that artery, which is almost perpendicular to the ultrasonic beam. When this artery serves as a major collateral supply to the distal basilar artery, the vessel is more readily insonated because of the increased flow. Retrograde flow from the ICAs to the posterior communicating arteries to the PCA and then to the distal basilar artery indicates a severe stenosis or occlusion of the basilar artery or the bilateral ICVAs. Monitoring of the PCAs using TCD can also provide evidence of emboli, which are shown as high-intensity transient signals superimposed on the usual background Doppler spectra.[197] These emboli can arise from the heart, the aorta, or the more proximal vertebrobasilar artery system.

MAGNETIC RESONANCE ANGIOGRAPHY

MRA is a functional imaging test that takes advantage of flowing blood to produce signals. The proximal ECVAs are difficult to visualize on MRA, just as they are hard to see on standard arch angiography. Overlapping vessels and shadows and the angulation of the VA origins usually make it difficult to see the ostia unless special views are taken. The second portion of the VAs is well shown, as are usually the atlas loops. Usually films of the ECVAs are taken separately from films of the intracranial, intradural arteries; the very distal ECVAs or the proximal intradural segments of the ICVAs (or both) can be omitted because they are between films. The cranial and cervical arteries are studied separately because of the need to use different head and neck coils for imaging. The looping and kinking of the distal ECVA can produce a false impression of stenosis of that vessel on MRA if the artery goes in and out of the plane of the image. Usually the ICVAs, basilar artery, and proximal portions of the PCAs are well shown. The cerebellar arteries are less reliably shown, but usually the origins of the PICAs, AICAs, and SCAs can be seen. The PICA loops make it impossible to see the full vessel on either anteroposterior or lateral views in the same way that the PICAs are seen on standard angiography. The adequacy of visualization depends heavily on the supervision of the neuroradiologist and the choice of imaging techniques. Some communication between the clinicians and the radiologists before the study is needed to ensure that the radiologists know what information the clinicians seek from the examination.[143]

In one study, MRA results were compared with ultrasound and standard angiography in 41 patients with posterior circulation ischemia.[604] MRA accurately showed all intracranial occlusions and stenoses and one aneurysm of the ICVA. One ICVA dissection was missed. The sensitivity of MRA in this study was 97% and the specificity was 98.9%.[604]

Bogousslavsky and colleagues[85] found intracranial MRA very effective in diagnosing the etiology of posterior circulation infarcts in the Lausanne stroke registry. Among 70 consecutive patients studied with MRA, the commonest lesions shown by MRA were basilar artery stenosis (23 patients), basilar artery occlusion (4 patients), unilateral ICVA stenosis (5 patients), and dolichoectatic intracranial arteries (10 patients). No lesion was found in 26 patients (37%).[85] At the New England Medical Center, we compared TCD and MRA with each other and with standard angiography in 60 patients with vertebrobasilar ischemic symptoms.[599] Standard angiography was available in one-third of the patients. In 170 of 180 (94%) arteries, TCD and MRA agreed on determination of normal versus stenotic versus occluded ICVAs and basilar artery. In five vessels, TCD showed high-grade stenosis, while MRA suggested occlusion. In five other arteries, TCD and MRA did not agree. There was 95% agreement between TCD and MRA and conventional angiography when available. No patient was misdiagnosed when both TCD and MRA were used.[599]

Wentz and colleagues[743] compared MRA with digital intraarterial angiography in 60 patients with vertebrobasilar territory symptoms.[7] MRA showed disease of the ICVAs and basilar artery with 100% sensitivity; stenosis was reliably differentiated from occlusion by MRA, but the severity of stenosis was overestimated in 63% of patients. MRA showed 117 of 120 SCAs and 80 of 90 PICAs, but only 30 of 58 AICAs.[743]

The yield of MRA as a screening procedure is quite high, but the addition of TCD is very helpful. The two studies are complementary. Neck MRA and extracranial ultrasound should always be included, just as both extracranial and intracranial studies are used together in patients with anterior circulation ischemia.

CATHETER X-RAY ANGIOGRAPHY

Angiography as customarily performed using the Seldinger technique of selective arterial catheterization and instillation of contrast is an old and very familiar test that has customarily been considered the gold standard for showing arterial lesions. Documentation and quantification of the nature and severity of arterial lesions are essential for rational therapy. The role of angiography has changed dramatically since the introduction of high-quality noninvasive tests such as ultrasound and MRA, which can adequately screen for the vast majority of occlusive lesions and vascular malformations. When these studies show a vascular lesion or lesions that explain the clinical and imaging results, when the quality of the studies is sufficient, when the studies are all concordant, and when sufficient information has been derived to guide treatment, then catheter angiography is certainly not needed.[143]

Angiography should be done only when (1) the clinical findings are not explained by the results of neuroimaging ultrasound, MRA, and, when indicated clinically, cardiac and hematologic testing; or (2) the quality of the tests is inadequate to exclude severe occlusive disease; or (3) the preliminary tests are quite discordant and do not define the causative process well enough to allow for planning and monitoring of treatment.

OTHER DIAGNOSTIC TESTS

Spiral CT Scanning of the Brain Circulation

Spiral CT is a very new technique for examining the brain and blood vessels. During the examinations, the patient and examining table are moved at a low but accurately controlled speed during continuous scanning, which results in a spiral scanning geometry.[588,772] A distance of 23 cm can be scanned in 24 seconds, and contrast media for vascular imaging can be given in one-fourth to one-sixth the amount used for standard contrast CT. The advantages of spiral CT compared with standard CT are the rapidity of the examination, ability to reconstruct sections using variable table positions, reduced amount of contrast, and less radiation dose. The short time needed for the examination may make spiral CT possible in patients who cannot remain still for MRI/MRA scanning. However, spiral CT imaging takes time for reconstruction, a disadvantage of the technique when compared with MRA.

To date, there are no studies of the utility and accuracy of spiral CT scanning for clarification of arterial disease in pa-

tients with posterior circulation vascular disease. The technique is promising but, like MRA, very dependent on the skill, knowledge, and degree of involvement of the supervising physician.[625]

Functional Tests of Brain Function and Brain Blood Flow

Some tests, such as perfusion MRI, single photon emission computed tomography (SPECT), xenon-enhanced CT, and some positron emission tomography (PET) studies yield information about brain perfusion in the microvasculature.[129] Although these tests of brain function, metabolism, and perfusion have been widely studied in patients with anterior circulation strokes, much less data exist about their utility in patients with vascular disease of the posterior circulation.

SINGLE-PHOTON EMISSION COMPUTED TOMOGRAPHY. This technique uses a variety of different radioisotopes, including ^{133}Xe, iodine-123-iodoamphetamine, and technetium-99M-labeled hexamethylpropyleneamineoxime. SPECT has been used to show diminished perfusion in patients with posterior circulation disease.[163,283] The image resolution of SPECT does not approach that of MRI and so the brain stem cannot be well seen. Abnormalities of perfusion are limited to the cerebellar hemispheres and the temporal and occipital lobe territories supplied by the PCAs. In a single case report, SPECT showed decreased left cerebellar perfusion uptake only after neck turning in a patient with spondylitic compression of the ipsilateral ECVA.[611] In another patient who had proximal VA disease, the authors used an injection of acetazolamide to show abnormal perfusion in the occipital lobes and cerebellum.[184]

SPECT may be useful in some patients in whom there is a mismatch between neuroimaging findings and abnormal signs on examination and in whom the vascular etiology has been clarified.[127] The only regions that can be studied well at present are the cerebellar hemispheres and the posterior poles of the cerebral hemispheres. Because of suboptimal resolution of images, it is presently impossible to visualize or quantitate brain stem perfusion.

POSITRON EMISSION TOMOGRAPHY. PET is now essentially a research technique available only in a few large research centers. PET does have the advantage of yielding metabolic data, information regarding regional cerebral blood flow, and data about the metabolism and uptake of oxygen.[129,573] The oxygen extraction fraction may be a good predictor of tissue viability.[144] Mobilizing PET studies in acute stroke patients has been very difficult.

DIFFUSION-WEIGHTED AND PERFUSION-SENSITIVE MRI. In human stroke patients studied during the first 24 to 48 hours of acute ischemia, diffusion-weighted MRI shows regions of ischemia not found on standard MRI images.[738,739] The results of diffusion-weighted and perfusion studies correlated well with the regions of occlusion shown by MRA. In five patients with posterior circulation occlusions (four basilar artery, one PCA), the dynamic scans showed abnormalities in four, but the scans were not of acceptable quality in the fifth patient, who had a basilar artery occlusion.[739] Perfusion imaging probably depicts well the microvascular flow in various brain regions and so is comparable to PET and SPECT. The image resolution is, however, better with MRI. Diffusion-weighted images allow for early detection of ischemia.

MAGNETIC RESONANCE SPECTROSCOPY. Magnetic resonance spectroscopy also offers promise.[308,366] This technology allows quantification and localization of various biochemical substances within the brain. In regions of brain ischemia, lactate and often N-acetylaspartate accumulate. There are also changes in energy production manifested as abnormal amounts of phosphate moieties (adenosine di- and triphosphate, and so forth). With MR spectroscopy, it may be possible to define and differentiate reversibly injured tissue from an area already infarcted. The clinical utility of MR spectroscopy in patients with posterior circulation disease has not been studied to date.

ELECTROPHYSIOLOGIC TECHNIQUES. Although the brain stem is sometimes difficult to image, the motor, sensory, and reflex functions that occur within the brain stem can be measured by various electrophysiologic techniques. These studies include brain stem auditory evoked responses,[226,627,660,730] masseter and masseter-inhibitory reflexes,[186,538,690] blink reflex,[538] electronystagmography, caloric vestibular testing, and transcranial magnetic stimulation.[233]

CARDIAC EVALUATION. Cardiac evaluation is important in all patients with cerebrovascular disease. About one in five posterior circulation infarcts are caused by cardiac origin embolism.[130,141] In other patients, the aorta may serve as an embolic source. Patients who have cerebrovascular occlusive disease have a high incidence of coexistent coronary artery disease, and subsequent death is more often related to myocardial infarction than recurrent stroke. Transesophageal echocardiography has a definite superiority over transthoracic echocardiography in detecting lesions of the aorta, atrium, and atrial septum.

LUMBAR PUNCTURE. The two most important indications for lumbar puncture are suspected subarachnoid hemorrhage and suspected central nervous system infection, especially meningitis. Small subarachnoid bleeds (so-called warning leaks) may not be sufficient in volume to produce a diagnostic CT scan. Also, if the bleed occurred days previously, CT may be normal despite the presence of subarachnoid blood.[136]

Treatment

Unfortunately not a single definitive study establishes the advantages or disadvantages of a given therapy for patients with well-defined occlusive vascular disease within the posterior circulation. Published studies are either small or not randomized or contain patients lumped together under the general term *vertebrobasilar insufficiency*, often without further definition of the severity and nature of the vascular lesion.

ANTIPLATELET AGENTS

Aspirin and other agents that affect platelet agglutination have been infrequently studied. The Canadian Cooperative Study included 86 patients with vertebrobasilar TIAs and 49 patients with slight nonprogressive vertebrobasilar strokes.[51] Of the 75 posterior circulation patients studied angiographically, 82% had significant appropriately situated lesions.[51] Aspirin reduced the risk of recurrent episodes, stroke, and death in men in both the vertebrobasilar and carotid groups, but not in women. Sulfinpyrazone had no definite effect. The American Aspirin Study excluded patients with only vertebrobasilar attacks.[235] A German study showed a slight statistically insignificant trend favoring a beneficial effect of aspirin in occlusive vertebrobasilar disease.[584]

The European Stroke Prevention Study, which compared treatment with 330 mg aspirin combined in a capsule with 75 mg dipyridamole given three times a day as secondary prevention in patients with TIAs and strokes, did analyze the results by arterial territory.[221,646] Among 356 patients treated with aspirin and dipyridamole, 8.1% had end points (defined as stroke or death) versus 15.5% end points in 355 patients treated with placebo (47.7% reduction).[221] Considering the end point of stroke alone, in the vertebrobasilar group, the stroke incidence was reduced by 65.7% by treatment.[646] These reductions exceeded the effects of the medicines in patients with carotid territory TIAs and strokes. Using the same types of analysis, total end points were reduced 30.5% by treatment in the carotid group versus 51.4% in the vertebrobasilar group, and strokes were reduced by 40% in the carotid territory versus 65.7% in the posterior circulation group.[646]

In the Ticlopidine-Aspirin Stroke Study, 3,069 patients with recent transient ischemia or slight strokes were given either 500 mg ticlopidine or 1,300 mg aspirin to prevent strokes.[330] The results were not reported by vascular territory. Comparing the effectiveness of the two agents in the two territories, ticlopidine was probably equally effective in the carotid and vertebrobasilar ischemic group, whereas aspirin seemed to be more effective in the vertebrobasilar group. In total, fewer patients who had vertebrobasilar ischemia had strokes compared with the carotid territory group. Grotta et al[311] later analyzed the data for vascular territories and commented that patients with carotid symptoms treated with aspirin had the highest incidence of subsequent stroke, whereas those with vertebrobasilar symptoms treated with ticlopidine had the lowest.

ANTICOAGULANTS

Enthusiasm for the use of anticoagulants grew in the 1950s when this form of treatment was being evaluated for vascular disease of all varieties and locations. A number of reports from the Mayo Clinic cerebrovascular department enthusiastically supported the use of anticoagulants for TIA and progressing stroke within the vertebrobasilar system.[495,497,498,640,744] Millikan and colleagues[497] first reported 21 patients who had progressive vertebrobasilar symptoms and were given anticoagulants. Only 14% of these patients died, whereas during this same period 43% of 23 patients who were not treated with anticoagulation and had similar clinical profiles had died. All five patients with intermittent attacks in the vertebrobasilar system had clearing of the attacks. Whisnant[744] collected 140 patients with progressive symptoms due to vertebrobasilar occlusion who were treated with anticoagulants: 12 (8.5%) died, whereas 23 of 59 (58.9%) similar patients not on anticoagulants died. Patients in this study had ischemia that was assumed to be not restricted to a single arterial branch of the vertebral or basilar artery and showed some signs of progressing deficit. The patients were not randomized, the study was retrospective, and most vascular lesions were not verified angiographically. Also, a high percentage of patients with intermittent spells of vertebrobasilar insufficiency had attacks cease after institution of anticoagulant therapy. Following these reports, it became customary in most centers to treat patients who had vertebrobasilar ischemia with anticoagulants, although a true randomized study of anticoagulant treatment has not been performed. Other reports usually contain small numbers of nonrandomized patients. Fazekas et al[228] described 26 patients, of whom 10 had only vertebrobasilar TIAs and 16 had some clinical deficit; 14 were treated with anticoagulants for 6 to 50 months, and the remaining 12 were considered unsuitable for anticoagulant therapy because of "medical or personality disorders." All 26 patients improved; only 3 continued to have episodes (1 on anticoagulants, 2 not), but of decreased frequency. In a series of patients with vertebrobasilar disease seen by Bradshaw and McQuaid,[93] six were treated with anticoagulants. Of these, one with verified basilar occlusion died and five did well, although two had persistent attacks. Of 48 patients with vertebrobasilar disease not treated with anticoagulants, 38 did well.

The use of anticoagulants has been associated with dramatic cessation of attacks or improvement in a progressing vertebrobasilar deficit. Most experienced clinicians will verify their immediate effectiveness in some patients. Heparin and warfarin each have a role to play in patient management, but at present this opinion is conjectural and unproved. In our experience, patients with basilar artery stenosis and transient episodes have responded to warfarin and often have had recurrent spells after cessation of treatment; on the other hand, few patients with vertebral or basilar artery occlusion experience progressive symptoms during the weeks after their stroke, even without anticoagulant.[110] Perhaps these latter patients would be better treated with heparin for 4 weeks or less. Branch disease probably does not warrant use of heparin or warfarin.

A retrospective analysis of the effectiveness of warfarin versus aspirin in patients with symptomatic arterial stenoses in the intracranial posterior circulation found that warfarin was significantly better than aspirin in reducing the rate of stroke.[695] The Warfarin-Aspirin Symptomatic Intracranial Disease Study Group reviewed 68 patients who had 50% to 99% stenosis of the ICVA basilar artery or PCA documented during the evaluation of a stroke or TIA in the territory of the stenosed artery. Forty-two patients were treated with warfarin and 26 were given aspirin. During follow-up, which averaged 13.8 months, 15 of the 68 (22%) patients had a stroke. Patients with bilateral ICVA and basilar artery stenosis had more strokes than patients with unilateral VA, PCA, or PICA disease, and fewer patients receiving warfarin had strokes.[695] This was a retrospective analysis of a small group of patients,

but it does support the possible utility of warfarin in treating patients with large artery stenosis. A prospective trial has begun to compare the two types of agents in prevention of recurrent stroke.[505]

THROMBOLYSIS

The most promising new treatment for recent thromboembolic occlusions of the vertebral and basilar arteries is thrombolytic agents.[103,182,232,315,343,560,648,748,770,771] If the patient has a very recent basilar artery thrombosis, consideration should be given to urgent thrombolytic treatment. Reperfusion offers the patient the best chance of surviving with the least deficit. Hacke and colleagues[315] treated 65 consecutive patients with clinical signs of severe ischemia of the brain stem and thrombotic basilar artery occlusions shown angiographically: 43 were given local intra-arterial thrombolytic therapy (urokinase or streptokinase) within 24 hours of onset, and 22 were given anticoagulants or agents that alter platelet function. Recanalization was shown in 19 of the 43 patients treated with thrombolytic agents. All patients without recanalization died, but 14 of the 19 in whom the artery reopened survived, 10 with a good clinical outcome. Only 3 of 22 patients not treated with thrombolytic agents survived, all with moderately severe deficits. In another large series, 34 patients with basilar artery occlusion were treated with intra-arterial thrombolytic agents within 48 hours, and 6 other patients were treated intravenously.[726] The great majority of patients who did not reperfuse after treatment died (16 of 17 patients) compared with a mortality of 11 of 23 patients who recanalized. There were very few recognized complications of treatment. Patients with embolism fared better than patients with thrombosis engrafted on severe atherostenosis. Site of basilar artery occlusion (proximal, middle, or distal) and extent of collateral blood flow did not affect the outcome.

Systemic intravenous delivery of recombinant tissue plasminogen activator (rtPA) is also feasible and has been effective in a single case report.[748] Intravenous tissue plasminogen activator (tPA) was used by Hennerici and colleagues[339] to treat 10 patients with posterior circulation occlusions (1 bilateral ICVA, 9 basilar artery). Reperfusion was poor: only 2 patients showed complete recanalization, and 3 others had some increase in perfusion after therapy. Only 2 patients recovered, 1 was left severely disabled, and 7 died. Recently the National Institutes of Health tPA stroke trial has reported a 30% reduction in disability in patients receiving 0.9 mg/kg tPA within the 3 hours after onset compared with patients receiving placebo. This was obtained without excess in mortality (<15% in the tPA group compared with the placebo group), but with significantly more symptomatic intracranial hemorrhage in the tPA group than in the placebo group (6.2% versus 0.6%). These results were obtained in both territories, and there was no analysis by vascular territory.[694] The Multicenter Acute Stroke Trial-Italy that included patients with anterior or posterior circulation ischemia treated within 6 hours after onset showed the high risk of intracranial bleeding when using streptokinase intravenously alone or together with aspirin.[523]

A patient treated recently at the New England Medical Center illustrates the potential and problems of thrombolysis.[126] A 17-year-old woman suddenly developed bilateral limb weakness and quickly lapsed into a locked-in state. The etiology was later shown to presumably be a paradoxical embolus through an interatrial septal defect. She was not seen at our hospital until hours after symptom onset. Angiography showed an occlusion of the basilar artery at the level of the AICA branches. She was given an intra-arterial infusion of tPA, and subsequent angiography at the termination of treatment showed a widely patent basilar artery. She was left with some weakness but had major improvement in function. The delay in beginning thrombolysis meant that irreversible ischemia-infarction had occurred before the infusion of tPA. Nevertheless, the recanalization illustrates the great potential of the treatment. Improvement in circulation may have restored areas that were stunned, that is, reversibly ischemic and not functioning normally.

Del Zoppo[182] and Pessin et al[559] recently reviewed the results of thrombolytic therapy in patients with vertebrobasilar occlusive disease. This therapy clearly has promise in selected patients with selected lesions treated quickly, but the ideal agent, route of access, dose, and duration of infusion and the use of anticoagulants have not been determined as yet. New agents that are more fibrin selective are being synthesized and tried. These agents localize at the thrombus region and adhere to fibrin, causing progressive fibrinolysis.[723] If intra-arterial therapy is proved to be superior to intravenous infusion, then only centers with available skilled interventional neuroradiologists will be able to administer treatment.

We believe that, whenever possible, patients with acute basilar artery thrombosis should be treated with thrombolytic agents. The earlier treatment is instituted, the more likely it is to achieve reperfusion before disastrous brain stem infarction occurs. Fresh emboli are more likely to lyse than old thrombi, and embolism probably responds better than in situ occlusion. Occlusive lesions proximal to the basilar artery probably limit the success of thrombolysis, as is the case in anterior circulation disease in which middle cerebral artery thrombi do not lyse well if the ipsilateral carotid artery is occluded or severely stenotic in the neck or carotid siphon. The best agent, best avenue of delivery (intravenous or intra-arterial), best duration of infusion, and best dose are still not known. Local infusion by catheter of recombinant tissue plasminogen activator has also proved effective.[343]

TRANSLUMINAL ANGIOPLASTY

The use of transluminal angioplasty to dilate coronary and renal arteries led to the suggestion that the branches of the aortic arch could be dilated in a similar way. Neurologists feared that fracture of plaques would lead to intracranial arterial embolism and strokes so that the technique has been introduced cautiously. Subclavian, innominate, and proximal VA stenoses have been dilated using transluminal catheters.[382,517,518,590,621,770] Most often the treatment has been performed by general radiologists. The technique is relatively new, and the durability, risk, and complication rate of the procedure are as yet unknown.

Intracerebral transluminal angioplasty is an even newer technique. Sundt and colleagues[668] wrote a preliminary report

in 1980 of successful angioplasty of the basilar artery using a surgical cut-down exposing the distal ECVA at the base of the skull and inserting a catheter from this point distally. In the two patients treated, the technique successfully dilated the basilar artery and the patients did well. In a subsequent report, Piepgras and colleagues[564] described fatal outcomes in two of the four other patients treated by the same technique and called for a moratorium on this treatment. Three of the four patients described in the second report had bilateral VA disease, and the ICVA was the vessel dilated.

More recently, angioplasty of intracranial arteries has become popular and a successful treatment for vasoconstriction following subarachnoid hemorrhage. Interventional neuroradiologists introduce balloon catheters and guide them to the sites of vasoconstriction and then successfully dilate these segments. Stimulated by the success in treating vasoconstriction, more recently neuroradiologists have begun to dilate intracranial regions of stenosis, including those within the posterior circulation.[158,349] The technique is still in a preliminary investigational stage. Stenotic vessels with plaques are clearly very different from smooth arteries that are vasoconstricted. The technique should not be used at present for patients with basilar artery occlusion. We know of anecdotal reports of patients with basilar artery occlusive disease who have done poorly after basilar artery angioplasty. The most tenuous circulation in patients with basilar artery occlusive disease is through the paramedian penetrating arteries. Angioplasty could cause injury to these penetrating arteries when the plaques are stretched and cracked. By contrast, there are fewer penetrators coming from the ICVA; the location of the lateral medullary penetrators, the PICA, and the spinal artery branches can be localized before the procedure and so avoided during angioplasty. In some patients treated to date, technical limitations such as severe tortuosity or narrowing of the ECVA, as well as severe ECVA and/or ICVA stenosis, have limited the ability of the neuroradiologist to place a dilating catheter within the lumen of the stenosed segment. There have been some dramatic successes. The technique is promising in the right patients and with optimal technology and extensive training and experience in the person performing the angioplasty. The early experience of Sundt et al[668] warns that disastrous consequences can occur from fracturing of plaque materials with distal embolization. As in other surgical techniques, the indications for the procedures need to be better defined. Improvement in technology with filters that catch debris distally also would be an important advance.

SURGERY: BYPASS ANASTOMOSES, RECONSTRUCTIONS, AND SHUNTS

Proximal Vertebral Artery Occlusive Disease

For proximal occlusive disease the commonest operative procedure is probably transposition of the VA into the ipsilateral common carotid artery.[190,434,597] When the ipsilateral ICA or common carotid artery is stenosed, carotid endarterectomy is often performed at the same time.

The VA origin in the neck is a relatively small artery. Endarterectomies have been performed in this region but are less common because transposition is easier. Using a technique they referred to as vertebral angioplasty, Imparato et al[375] operated directly on the subclavian-VA origin region using patch grafts, plications, and other techniques to enlarge the arteries and straighten kinks and obstructive lesions.[696]

Occlusive Disease of the Extracranial Vertebral Artery Beyond Its Origin

At times, a bypass can be created by anastomosing external carotid artery branches to the distal ECVA. Fibrous bands, spurs, and other compressive lesions, when present, are removed without opening or anastomosing the ECVA. The usual indication for surgical reconstruction is tight stenosis of the ECVA with symptoms of posterior circulation ischemia. The patency rate in performing reconstructive procedures is high.[66,106,190,373,375,434,597,654]

Occlusive Disease of the Intracranial Vertebral or Basilar Artery

Endarterectomy is also possible on the proximal ICVA after dural penetration, but few such procedures have been performed.[10,34,42,364] Microsurgical techniques make these operations possible, but the exposure is difficult and requires experience.

When intracranial stenosis is present, surgeons have used a number of donor and recipient arteries, depending on the location of the intracranial occlusive disease. Occipital artery to PICA shunts are probably the most common bypass procedures used.[41,363,364,405,601,667,669] The occipital artery can also be anastomosed to the AICA.[39] For more distal basilar artery stenoses, superficial temporal artery to SCA or PCA shunts can be performed.[363,364,670] At times, interposed vein grafts are used. The most common indication for bypass has been persistent attacks of posterior circulation ischemia unresponsive to medical regimens. Enthusiasm for shunts in the anterior circulation was quelled by the Extracranial-Intracranial Bypass Study, which showed in general that bypass was probably inferior to medical treatment.[692]

Some believe[88,282,369] that carotid endarterectomy would be useful in patients with bilateral severe occlusive disease in the posterior circulation, but a formal study showed that the procedure was of little or no benefit.[480]

At present, it seems clear that a variety of surgical procedures can be performed with technical precision, and the patency rate is high. The indications for surgery versus medical treatment are still quite unclear.

References

1. Ackerman E, Levinsohn M, Richards D et al: Basilar artery occlusion in a 10-year-old boy. Ann Neurol 1:204, 1977

2. Ackerstaff RG, Eikelboom BC, Moll FL: Investigation of the vertebral artery in cerebral atherosclerosis. Eur J Vasc Surg 5:229–235, 1991

3. Ackerstaff RG, Hoenefeld H, Slowikowski JM et al: Ultrasonic duplex scanning in atherosclerotic disease of the innominate, subclavian and vertebral arteries: a comparative study with angiography. Ultrasound Med Biol 10: 409, 1984

4. Adams R: Occlusion of the anterior inferior cerebellar artery. Arch Neurol Psychiatry 49:765, 1983

5. Aichner FT, Felber SR, Birhamer GG, Posch A: Magnetic resonance imaging and magnetic resonance angiography of vertebrobasilar dolichoectasia. Cerebrovasc Dis 3:280–284, 1993

6. Alajouanine T, Lhermitte F, Gautier J: Transient cerebral ischemia in atherosclerosis. Neurology (NY) 10:906, 1960

7. Alexander A: The treatment of epilepsy by ligature of the vertebral arteries. Brain 5:170, 1882

8. Alexander C, Burger P, Goree J: Dissecting aneurysms of the basilar artery. Stroke 10:294, 1979

9. Alezais D'Astros L: La circulation artérielle du pédoncule cérébral. J Anat Physiol 28:519–528, 1892

10. Allen G, Cohen R, Preziosi T: Microsurgical endarterectomy of the intracranial vertebral artery for vertebrobasilar transient ischemic attacks. Neurosurgery 81:56, 1981

11. Alom J, Matias-Gurer J, Padeo L et al: Spontaneous dissection of intracranial vertebral artery: clinical recovery with conservative treatment. J Neurol Neurosurg Psychiatry 49:599, 1986

12. Alpert J, Gerson L, Hall R et al: Reversible angiopathy. Stroke 13:100, 1982

13. Amarenco P: Les infarctus du cervelet. Presse Med 18: 909, 1991

14. Amarenco P: The spectrum of cerebellar infarctions. Neurology 41:973–979, 1991

15. Amarenco P, Caplan LR: Vertebrobasilar occlusive disease: review of selected aspects. 3. Mechanisms of cerebellar infarctions. Cerebrovasc Dis 3:66–73, 1993

16. Amarenco P, Chevrie-Muller C, Roullet E, Bousser M-G: Paravermal infarct and isolated cerebellar dysarthria. Ann Neurol 30:211–213, 1991

17. Amarenco P, Cohen A, Tzourio C et al: Atherosclerotic disease of the aortic arch and the risk of ischemic stroke. N Engl J Med 331:1474–1479, 1994

18. Amarenco P, Debroucker T, Cambier J: Dysarthrie et instabilité révélant d'un infarctus distal de l'artère cérébelleuse supérieure gauche. Rev Neurol (Paris) 144: 459–461, 1988

19. Amarenco P, Duyckarets C, Tzourio C et al: The prevalence of ulcerated plaques in the aortic arch in patients with stroke. N Engl J Med 326:221–225, 1992

20. Amarenco P, Hauw J-J, Caplan LR: Cerebellar infarctions. pp. 251–290. In Lechtenberg R (ed): Handbook of Cerebellar Diseases. Marcel Dekker, New York, 1993

21. Amarenco P, Hauw J-J, Gautier J-C: Arterial pathology in cerebellar infarction. Stroke 21:1299, 1990

22. Amarenco P, Hauw J-J, Henin D et al: Les infarctus du territoire de l'artère cérébelleuse postéro-inférieure: étude clinico-pathologique de 28 cas. Rev Neurol 145: 277, 1989

23. Amarenco P, Hauw J-J: Anatomie des artères cérébelleuses. Rev Neurol 145:267, 1989

24. Amarenco P, Hauw J-J: Cerebellar infarction in the territory of the anterior and inferior cerebellar artery. A clinicopathological study of 20 cases. Brain 113:139–155, 1990

25. Amarenco P, Hauw J-J: Infarctus cérébelleux œdémateux. Etude clinico-pathologique de 16 cas. Neurochirurgie 36:234–241, 1990

26. Amarenco P, Hauw J-J: Cerebellar infarction in the territory of the superior cerebellar artery. Neurology (NY) 40:1383, 1990

27. Amarenco P, Kase CS, Rosengart A et al: Very small (border zone) cerebellar infarcts: distribution, mechanisms, causes and clinical features. Brain 116:161–186, 1993

28. Amarenco P, Lévy C, Cohen A et al: Causes and mechanisms of territorial and nonterritorial cerebellar infarcts in 115 consecutive cases. Stroke 25:105–112, 1994

29. Amarenco P, Rosengart A, DeWitt LD et al: Anterior inferior cerebellar artery territory infarcts: mechanisms and clinical features. Arch Neurol 50:154–161, 1993

30. Amarenco P, Roullet E, Chemouilli P, Marteau R: Infarctus pontin inféro-latéral. Deux aspects cliniques. Rev Neurol (Paris) 146:433–437, 1990

31. Amarenco P, Roullet E, Goujon C et al: Infarction in the anterior rostral cerebellum (the territory of the lateral branch of the superior cerebellar artery). Neurology 41:253–258, 1991

32. Amarenco P, Roullet E, Hommel M et al: Infarction in the territory of the medial branch of the posterior inferior cerebellar artery. J Neurol Neurosurg Psychiatry 53:731–735, 1990

33. Amarenco P, Seux-Levieil M-L, Lévy C et al: Carotid artery dissection with renal infarcts. Two cases. Stroke 25:2488–2491, 1994

34. Anson JA, Spetzler RF. Endarterectomy of the intradural vertebral artery via the far lateral approach. Neurosurgery 33:804–811, 1993

35. Archer C, Horenstein S: Basilar artery occlusion: clinical and radiological correlation. Stroke 8:383, 1977

36. Asplund K, Wester P, Fodstad H et al: Long time survival after vertebral/basilar occlusion. Stroke 11:304, 1980

37. Atkinson WJ: The anterior inferior cerebellar artery. J Neurol Neurosurg Psychiatry 12:137, 1949

38. Auerbach S, De Piero T, Romanul F: Sylvian aqueduct syndrome caused by unilateral midbrain lesion. Ann Neurol 11:91, 1982

39. Ausman J, Diaz F, de los Reyes RA et al: Occipital artery to anterior inferior cerebellar artery anastomosis for vertebrobasilar junction stenosis. Surg Neurol 16:99, 1981

40. Ausman J, Lee M, Chater N et al: Superficial artery to superior cerebellar artery anastomosis for distal basilar artery stenosis. Surg Neurol 12:277, 1979

41. Ausman J, Nicoloff D, Chou S: Posterior fossa revascularization anastomosis of vertebral artery to PICA with interposed radial artery graft. Surg Neurol 9:281, 1978

42. Ausman JI, Diaz FG, Pearce JE et al: Endarterectomy of the vertebral artery from C-2 to posterior inferior cerebellar artery intracranially. Surg Neurol 18:400, 1982

43. Awad I, Modic M, Little JR et al: Focal parenchymal lesions in transient ischemic attacks: correlation of computed tomography and magnetic resonance imaging. Stroke 17:399, 1986

44. Awerbuch G, Brown M, Levin JR: Magnetic resonance imaging correlates of internuclear ophthalmoplegia. Int J Neurosci 52:39, 1990

45. Babinski J, Nageotte J: Hémiasynergie, latéropulsion et myosis bulbaire. Nouv Iconog Salpetriere 15:492–512, 1902

46. Babinski J, Nageotte J: Hémiasynergie, lateropulsion et myosis bulbaires avec hémianesthésie et croisées. Rev Neurol 10:358, 1902

47. Baker R, Rosenbaum A, Caplan L: Subclavian steal syndrome. Contemp Surg 4:96, 1974

48. Barbour PJ, Castaldo JE, Rae-Grant AD et al: Internal carotid artery redundancy is significantly associated with dissection. Stroke 25:1201–1206, 1994

49. Barnes KL, Ferrario CM: Role of the central nervous system in cardiovascular regulation. In Furlan A (ed): The Heart and Stroke. Springer Verlag, Heidelberg, 1987

50. Barnes M, Hunt B, Williams I: The role of vertebral angiography in the investigation of third nerve palsy. J Neurol Neurosurg Psychiatry 44:1153, 1981

51. Barnett HJ: The Canadian Cooperative Study of platelet suppressive drugs in transient cerebral ischemia. p. 221. In Price T, Nelson E (eds): Cerebrovascular Disease. Proceedings of the Eleventh Princeton Conference. Lippincott-Raven, Philadelphia, 1979

52. Barrows L, Kubik C, Richardson E: Aneurysms of the basilar and vertebral arteries: a clinicopathologic study. Trans Am Neurol Assoc 81:181, 1956

53. Bartels E: Transkranielle farbkodierte Duplexsonographie moglichkeiten und grenzen der methode im vergleich zur konventionellen transkraniellen Dopplersonographie. Ultraschall Med 14:272–278, 1993

54. Bartels E, Flugel KA: Advantages of color Doppler imaging for the evaluation of the vertebral arteries. J Neuroimag 3:229–233, 1993

55. Bartels E, Flugel KA: Quantitative measurements of blood flow in basal cerebral arteries with transcranial duplex color-flow imaging. J Neuroimag 4:77–81, 1994

56. Barth A, Bogousslavsky J, Regli F: The clinical and topographic spectrum of cerebellar infarcts: a clinical-magnetic resonance imaging correlation study. Ann Neurol 33:451–456, 1993

57. Barth A, Bogousslavsky J, Régli F: Infarcts in the territory of the lateral branch of the posterior inferior cerebellar artery. J Neurol Neurosurg Psychiatry 57:1073–1076, 1994

58. Bassetti C, Bogousslavsky J, Barth A, Regli F: Isolated infarcts of the pons. Neurology 46:165–175, 1996

59. Bauer G, Prugger M, Rumpl E: Stimulus evoked oral automatisms in the locked-in syndrome. Arch Neurol 39:435, 1982

60. Bauer R, Sheehan S, Wechsler N et al: Arteriographic study of sites, incidence and treatment of arteriosclerotic cerebrovascular lesions. Neurology (NY) 12:698, 1962

61. Ben Hamouda-M'Rad I, Biousse V, Bousser M-G et al: Internal carotid artery redundancy is significantly associated with dissection. Stroke 26:1962, 1995

62. Bergan J, MacDonald J: Recognition of cerebrovascular fibromuscular hyperplasia. Arch Surg 98:332, 1969

63. Berguer R, Caplan LR: Panel discussion: Vertigo. p. 165. In Berguer R, Caplan LR (eds): Vertebrobasilar Arterial Disease. Quality Medical Publishing, St. Louis, 1991

64. Berguer R, Feldman AJ: Surgical reconstruction of the vertebral artery. Surgery 93:670, 1983

65. Berguer R, Higgins R, Nelson R: Non-invasive diagnosis of reversal of vertebral artery blood flow. N Engl J Med 302:1349, 1980

66. Berguer R, Kieffer E: Surgery of the Arteries to the Head. Springer-Verlag, New York, 1992

67. Besson G, Bogousslavsky J, Regli F: Posterior choroidal artery infarct with homonymous horizontal sectoranopia. Cerebrovasc Dis 1:117–120, 1991

68. Bewermeyer H, Dreesbach HA, Rackl A et al: Presentation of bilateral thalamic infarction on CT, MRI, and PET. Neuroradiology 27:414–419, 1985

69. Bickerstaff E: Basilar artery migraine. Lancet 1:15, 1961

70. Biemond A: Thrombosis of the basilar artery and the vascularization of the brainstem. Brain 74:300, 1951

71. Biller J, Adams HP, Dunn V et al: Dichotomy between clinical findings and MR abnormalities in pontine infarction. J Comput Assist Tomogr 10:379–385, 1986

72. Biller J, Yuh W, Mitchell GW: Early diagnosis of basilar artery occlusion using magnetic resonance imaging. Stroke 19:297, 1988

73. Biousse V, Chabriat H, Amarenco P, Bousser M-G: Roller-coaster-induced vertebral artery dissection. Lancet 346:767, 1995

74. Bjewer K, Silkerskjold BP: Lateropulsion and imbalance in Wallenberg's syndrome. Acta Neurol Scand 44:91, 1968

75. Bluth EL, Merritt CR, Sullivan MA et al: Usefulness of duplex ultrasound in evaluating vertebral arteries. J Ultrasound Med 8:229, 1989

76. Bogousslavsky J: Thalamic infarcts in lacunar and other subcortical infarcts. pp. 149–170. In Donnan G, Bamford J, Norrving B, Bogousslavsky J (eds): Lacunar Strokes. Oxford University Press, Oxford, 1995

77. Bogousslavsky J, Caplan LR: Vertebrobasilar occlusive disease: review of selected aspects. III. Thalamic infarcts. Cerebrovasc Dis 3:193–205, 1993

78. Bogousslavsky J, Fox AJ, Barnett HJM et al: Clinico-topographic correlation of small vertebrobasilar infarcts using magnetic resonance imaging. Stroke 17:929–938, 1986

79. Bogousslavsky J, Gates PC, Fox AJ et al: Bilateral occlusion of vertebral artery. Neurology (NY) 36:1309, 1986

80. Bogousslavsky J, Khurana R, Deruaz JP et al: Respiratory failure and unilateral caudal brainstem infarction. Ann Neurol 28:668, 1990

81. Bogousslavsky J, Maeder P, Regli F et al: Pure midbrain infarction: clinical syndromes, MRI, and etiologic patterns. Neurology 44:2032–2040, 1994

82. Bogousslavsky J, Miklossy J, Deruaz JP et al: Unilateral left paramedian infarction of the thalamus and midbrain: a clinico-pathological study. J Neurol Neurosurg Psychiatry 49:686, 1986

83. Bogousslavsky J, Regli F, Assal G: The syndrome of unilateral tuberothalamic artery territory infarction. Stroke 17:434, 1986

84. Bogousslavsky J, Regli F, Delaloye B et al: Loss of psychic self-activation with bithalamic infarction. Neurobehavioural, CT, MRI, and SPECT correlates. Acta Neurol Scand 83:309–316, 1991

85. Bogousslavsky J, Regli F, Maeder P et al: The etiology of posterior circulation infarcts: a prospective study using magnetic resonance imaging and magnetic resonance angiography. Neurology 43:1528–1533, 1993

86. Bogousslavsky J, Régli F: Latéro-pulsion axiale isolée lors d'un infarctus cérébelleux flocculo-nodulaire. Rev Neurol (Paris) 140:140–144, 1984

87. Bogousslavsky J, Regli F: Upgaze palsy and monocular paresis of downgaze from ipsilateral thalamo-mesencephalic infarction: a vertical one-and-a-half syndrome. J Neurol 231:43, 1984

88. Bogousslavsky J, Régli F: Vertebrobasilar transient ischemic attacks in internal carotid artery occlusion or tight stenosis. Arch Neurol 42:64–68, 1985

89. Bogousslavsky J, Regli F, Uske A: Thalamic infarcts: clinical syndromes, etiology, prognosis. Neurology 38:837–848, 1988

90. Bollensen E, Buzanoski JH, Prange HW: Brainstem compression by basilar artery anomalies as visualized by MRI. J Neurol 238:49, 1991

91. Borison H, Wang S: Physiology and pharmacology of vomiting. Pharmacol Rev 5:193, 1953

92. Bosch E, Kenlledy S, Aschenbrenner C: Ocular bobbing: the myth of its localizing value. Neurology (NY) 25:949, 1975

93. Bradshaw P, McQuaid P: The syndrome of vertebrobasilar insufficiency. QJ Med 32:279, 1963

94. Brandt T, Dieterich M: Skew deviation with ocular torsion: a vestibular brain stem sign of topographic diagnostic value. Ann Neurol 33:528–534, 1993

95. Breuer R, Marburg O: Zur Klinik und Pathologie der apoplektiformen Bulbärparalyse. Arb Neurol Inst Wien Univ 9:181, 1902

96. Brewster DC, Moncure AC, Darling C et al: Innominate artery lesions: problems encountered and lessons learned. J Vasc Surg 2:99, 1985

97. Brierley JB: The neuropathology of brain hypoxia. p. 243. In Critchley M, O'Leary J, Jennett B (eds): Scientific Foundations of Neurology. FA Davis, Philadelphia, 1972

98. Bright R: Cases illustrative of the effects produced when the arteries and brain are diseased. Guys Hosp Rep 1:9, 1836

99. Bronstein AM, Morris J, DuBoulay G et al: Abnormalities of horizontal gaze: clinical, oculographic and magnetic resonance imaging findings. I. Abducens palsy. J Neurol Neurosurg Psychiatry 53:194, 1990

100. Bronstein AM, Rudge P, Gresty MA et al: Abnormalities of horizontal gaze: clinical, oculographic and magnetic resonance imaging findings. II. Gaze palsy and internuclear ophthalmoplegia. J Neurol Neurosurg Psychiatry 53:200, 1990

101. Brouckaert L, Sieben G, De Reuck J et al: The syndrome

of the anterior inferior cerebellar artery. Acta Neurol Belg 81:65, 1981

102. Browne T, Poskanzer D: Treatment of strokes. N Engl J Med 281:594, 1969

103. Bruckmann H, Ferbert A, del Zoppo G et al: The acute vertebrobasilar thrombosis: angiological clinical comparison and therapeutic implications. Acta Radiol (Stockh), suppl. 369:38, 1986

104. Bull J: Contribution of radiology to the study of intracranial aneurysms. BMJ 2:1701, 1962

105. Buttner-Ennever J, Buttner U, Cohen B et al: Vertical gaze paralysis and the rostral interstitial nucleus of the medial longitudinal fasciculus. Brain 105:125, 1982

106. Callow A: Surgical management of varying patterns of vertebral artery and subclavian artery insufficiency. N Engl J Med 270:546, 1964

107. Cantu C, Yasaka M, Tsuchiya T, Yamaguchi T: Evaluation of the basilar artery flow velocity by transcranial Doppler ultrasonography. Cerebrovasc Dis 2:372–377, 1992

108. Caplan L: A tale of two brothers. Headache 17:49, 1977

109. Caplan L: Bilateral distal vertebral artery occlusion. Neurology (NY) 33:552, 1983

110. Caplan L: Occlusion of the vertebral or basilar artery. Stroke 10:277, 1979

111. Caplan L: Ptosis. J Neurol Neurosurg Psychiatry 37:1, 1974

112. Caplan L: "Top of the basilar" syndrome: selected clinical aspects. Neurology (NY) 30:72, 1980

113. Caplan L: Use of vasodilating drugs in cerebral symptomatology. p. 305. In Miller R, Greenblatt D (eds): Drug Therapy Reviews. Elsevier North-Holland, Amsterdam, 1979

114. Caplan L, Baker R: Extracranial occlusive disease: does size matter? Stroke 11:63, 1980

115. Caplan L, Chedru F, Lhermitte F et al: Transient global amnesia and migraine. Neurology (NY) 31:1167, 1981

116. Caplan L, Goodwin J: Hypertensive lateral tegmental brainstem hemorrhage. Neurology (NY) 32:252, 1982

117. Caplan L, Gorelick P: Salt and pepper in the face pain in acute brainstem ischemia. Ann Neurol 13:344, 1983

118. Caplan L, Sergay S: Positional cerebral ischemia. J Neurol Neurosurg Psychiatry 39:385, 1976

119. Caplan L, Young RR: EEG findings in certain lacunar stroke syndromes. Neurology (NY) 22:403, 1972

120. Caplan L, Zervas N: Survival with permanent midbrain dysfunction after surgical treatment of traumatic subdural hematoma: the clinical picture of a Duret hemorrhage. Ann Neurol 1:587, 1977

121. Caplan LR: Brain embolism, revisited. Neurology 43:1281–1287, 1993

122. Caplan LR: Charles Foix—the first modern stroke neurologist. Stroke 21:348, 1990

123. Caplan LR: Intracranial branch atheromatous disease: a neglected, understudied and underused concept. Neurology (NY) 39:1246, 1989

124. Caplan LR: Lacunar infarction: a neglected concept. Geriatrics 3:71, 1976

125. Caplan LR: Migraine and vertebrobasilar ischemia. Neurology (NY) 41:55, 1991

126. Caplan LR (ed): Posterior Circulation Disease. Blackwell Science, Cambridge, 1996

127. Caplan LR: Question-driven technology assessment: SPECT as an example. Neurology 41:187–191, 1991

128. Caplan LR: Silent brain infarcts. Cerebrovasc Dis, suppl. 1, 4:32–39, 1994

129. Caplan LR: Stroke: A Clinical Approach. pp. 99–150. 2nd Ed. Butterworth-Heinemann, Boston, 1993

130. Caplan LR: The 1991 E. Graeme Robertson lecture: vertebrobasilar embolism. Clin Exp Neurol 28:1–23, 1991

131. Caplan LR: Vertebrobasilar system syndromes. p. 371. In Vinken PJ, Bruyn GW, Klawans HL (eds): Handbook of Clinical Neurology. North-Holland, Amsterdam, 1988

132. Caplan LR, Amarenco P, Rosengart A et al: Embolism from vertebral artery origin occlusive disease. Neurology 42:1505–1512, 1992

133. Caplan LR, Baquis G, Pessin MS et al: Dissection of the intracranial vertebral artery. Neurology (NY) 38:868, 1988

134. Caplan LR, Brass LM, DeWitt LD et al: Transcranial Doppler ultrasound: present status. Neurology (NY) 40:696, 1990

135. Caplan LR, DeWitt LD, Pessin MS et al: Lateral thalamic infarcts. Arch Neurol 45:959, 1988

136. Caplan LR, Flamm ES, Mohr JP et al: Lumbar puncture in stroke. Stroke 18:540A–544A, 1987

137. Caplan LR, Gorelick PB, Hier DB: Race, sex and occlusive cerebrovascular disease: a review. Stroke 17:648, 1986

138. Caplan LR, Rosenbaum A: Role of cerebral angiography in vertebrobasilar occlusive disease. J Neurol Neurosurg Psychiatry 38:601, 1975

139. Caplan LR, Schmahmann JD, Kase CS et al: Caudate infarcts. Arch Neurol 47:133, 1990

140. Caplan LR, Tettenborn B: Embolism in the Posterior Circulation in Vertebrobasilar Disease. p. 52. Quality Medical Publishing, St. Louis, 1991

141. Caplan LR, Tettenborn B: Vertebrobasilar occlusive disease: review of selected aspects. 2. Posterior circulation embolism. Cerebrovasc Dis 2:320–326, 1992

142. Caplan LR, Thomas C, Banks G: Central nervous system complications of addiction to "T's and Blues." Neurology 32:623–628, 1982

143. Caplan LR, Wolpert SM: Angiography in patients with occlusive cerebrovascular disease: a stroke neurologist and a neuroradiologist's views. AJNR 12:593–601, 1991

144. Castaigne P, Buge A, Escourolle R et al: Ramollissement pédonculaire médian, tégmentothalamique avec ophtalmoplégie et hypersomnie. Rev Neurol 106:357, 1962

145. Castaigne P, Lhermitte F, Buge A et al: Paramedian thalamic and midbrain infarcts: clinical and neuropathological study. Ann Neurol 10:127, 1981

146. Castaigne P, Lhermitte F, Gautier J-C et al: Arterial occlusions in the vertebral-basilar system. Brain 96:133, 1973

147. Catsman-Berrevoets CE, Harskamp F: Compulsive presleep behavior and apathy due to bilateral thalamic stroke: response to bromocriptine. Neurology 38:647–649, 1988

148. Chase T, Moretti L, Prensky A: Clinical and electroen-

cephalographic manifestations of vascular lesions of the pons. Neurology (NY) 18:357, 1968

149. Chaves C, Caplan LR, Chung C-S, Amarenco P: Cerebellar infarcts. pp. 143–177. In Appel S (ed): Current Neurology. Vol. 14. Mosby-Year Book, St. Louis, 1994

150. Chaves CJ, Caplan LR, Chung CS et al: Cerebellar infarcts in the New England Medical Center Posterior Circulation Stroke Registry. Neurology 44:1385–1390, 1994

151. Chaves CJ, Pessin MS, Caplan LR et al: Cerebellar hemorrhagic infarction. Neurology 46:346–349, 1996

152. Chen H-J, Lee T-C, Wei C-P: Treatment of cerebellar infarction by decompressive suboccipital craniectomy. Stroke 23:957–961, 1992

153. Chin JH: Recurrent stroke caused by spondylitic compression of the vertebral artery. Ann Neurol 33:558–559, 1993

154. Chiras J, Marciano S, Vega Molina J et al: Spontaneous dissecting aneurysm of the extracranial vertebral artery (20 cases). Neuroradiology 27:327, 1985

155. Christoff N: A clinicopathological study of vertical eye movements. Arch Neurol 31:1, 1974

156. Christoff N, Anderson P, Nathanson M et al: Problems in anatomical analysis of lesions of the medial longitudinal fasciculus. Arch Neurol 2:293, 1960

157. Cioffi FA, Bernini FP, Punzo A, D'Avanzo R: Surgical management of acute cerebellar infarction. Acta Neurochir 74:105–112, 1985

158. Clark WN, Barnwell SL, Young LM, Coull BM: Safety and efficacy of angioplasty for intracranial atherosclerotic stenosis. Stroke 25:155, 1994

159. Cogan D: Internuclear ophthalmoplegia, typical and atypical. Arch Ophthalmol 84:583, 1970

160. Cogan D, Kubik C, Smith WL: Unilateral internuclear ophthalmoplegia. Arch Ophthalmol 44:783, 1950

161. Cogan DG: Supranuclear connections of the ocular motor system. p. 84. In Neurology of the Ocular Muscles. 2nd Ed. Charles C Thomas, Springfield, IL, 1956

162. Collier J: Nuclear ophthalmoplegia with especial reference to retraction of the lids and ptosis and to lesions of the posterior commissure. Brain 50:488, 1927

163. Comerota A, Maurer AH: Surgical correction and SPECT imaging of vertebrobasilar insufficiency due to unilateral vertebral artery stenosis. Stroke 20:952–956, 1989

164. Cornhill J, Akins D, Hutson M et al: Localization of atherosclerotic lesions in the human basilar artery. Atherosclerosis 35:77, 1980

165. Corrin LS, Sandok BA, Houser W: Cerebral ischemic events in patients with carotid artery fibromuscular disease. Arch Neurol 38:616, 1981

166. Cossa P, Richard S: Sur deux cas de syndrome de l'artère cérébelleuse supérieure (ou de ses branches). Rev Neurol (Paris) 633–635, 1955

167. Crosby E, Yoss R, Henderson J: The mammalian midbrain and isthmus regions. II. The fiber connections: D. The pattern for eye movement in the frontal eye fields and the discharge of specific portions of this field to and through midbrain levels. J Comp Neurol 97:357, 1952

168. Cuneo R, Caronna J, Pitts L et al: Upward transtentorial herniation. Arch Neurol 36:618, 1989

169. Currier R, Giles C, Dejong R: Some comments on Wallenberg's lateral medullary syndrome. Neurology (NY) 11:778, 1961

170. Currier R, Giles C, Westerberg M: The prognosis of some brainstem vascular syndromes. Neurology (NY) 8:664, 1958

171. Dadsetan MR, Skeihut HEI: Rotational vertebrobasilar insufficiency secondary to vertebral artery occlusion from fibrous band of the longus coli muscle. Neuroradiology 32:514–515, 1990

172. D'Anglejan-Chatillon J, Ribeiro V, Mas J-L et al: Migraine—risk factor for dissection of cervical arteries. Headache 29:560–561, 1989

173. Daroff R, Hoyt W: Supranuclear disorders of ocular control systems in man. p. 175. In Bach Y, Rita P, Collins C (eds): The Control of Eye Movements. Academic Press, Orlando, FL, 1977

174. Daves J, Treger A: Vertebral grand larceny. Circulation 29:911, 1964

175. Dávila-Román VG, Barzilai B, Wareing TH et al: Atherosclerosis of the ascending aorta. Prevalence and role as independent predictor of cerebrovascular events in cardiac patients. Stroke 25:2010–2016, 1994

176. Davison C: Syndrome of the anterior spinal artery of the medulla oblongata. J Neuropathol Exp Neurol 3:73, 1944

177. Davison C, Goodhart S, Savitsky N: The syndrome of the superior cerebellar artery and its branches. Arch Neurol Psychiatry 33:1143, 1935

178. De Reuck J, Vander Eecken H: Cerebellar infarction and internal hydrocephalus. Acta Neurol Belg 78:129–140, 1978

179. DeBosscher J: Anévrysme de l'artère vertébrale gauche chez un homme 45 ans. Acta Neurol Psychiatr Belg 52:1, 1952

180. Deeb Z, Janetta P, Rosenbaum A et al: Tortuous vertebrobasilar arteries causing cranial nerve syndromes: screening by computed tomography. J Comput Assist Tomogr 3:774, 1965

181. Dejerine J, Roussy G: Le syndrome thalamique. Rev Neurol 14:521, 1906

182. del Zoppo G: Fibrinolytic therapy. pp. 179–192. In Berguer R, Caplan LR (eds): Vertebrobasilar Arterial Disease. Quality Medical Publishing, St. Louis, 1992

183. del Zoppo GJ, Zeumer H, Harker LA: Thrombolytic therapy in stroke: possibilities and hazards. Stroke 17:595, 1986

184. Delecluse F, Voordecker P, Raftopoulos C: Vertebrobasilar insufficiency revealed by xenon-133 inhalation SPECT. Stroke 20:952–956, 1989

185. Deleu D, Buisseret T, Ebinger G: Vertical one-and-a-half syndrome: supranuclear downgaze paralysis with monocular elevation palsy. Arch Neurol 46:1361, 1989

186. Dengler R: The masseter reflex in the topodiagnosis of brainstem lesions. pp. 191–197. In Caplan LR, Hopf HC (eds): Brain-Stem Localization and Function. Springer-Verlag, Berlin, 1993

187. Denny-Brown D: Basilar artery syndromes. Bull N Engl Med Cent 15:53, 1953

188. Denny-Brown D: Recurrent cerebrovascular episodes. Arch Neurol 2:194, 1960

189. Denny-Brown D, Foley J: The syndrome of basilar aneurysm. Trans Am Neurol Assoc 77:30, 1952

190. Deriu GP, Balotta E, Franceschi L et al: Surgical management of extracranial vertebral artery disease. J Cardiovasc Surg 32:413–419, 1991

191. Desmet Y, Brucher JM: L'infarctus bilatéral du territoire latéral du bulbe. Acta Neurol Belg 85:137, 1985

192. Devereaux M, Keane J, Davis R: Automatic respiratory failure associated with infarction of the medulla: report of two cases with pathologic study of one. Arch Neurol 29:46, 1973

193. Devic M, Michel F, Lenglet JP: Nystagmus retractorius, paralysie de la verticalite, areflexie pupillaire et anomalie de la posture du regard par ramollissement dans le territoire de la choroidienne posterieure. Rev Neurol 10:399–404, 1964

194. De Visser B: Afferent limb of the human jaw reflex: electrophysiologic and anatomic study. Neurology (NY) 32:563, 1982

195. DeWitt LD, Buonanno FS, Kistler JP et al: Nuclear magnetic resonance imaging in evaluation of clinical stroke syndromes. Ann Neurol 16:535, 1984

196. Dhamoon SK, Igbal J, Collins GH: Ipsilateral hemiplegia and the Wallenberg syndrome. Arch Neurol 41:179, 1984

197. Diehl RR, Sliwka U, Rautenberg W, Schwartz A: Evidence for embolization from a posterior cerebral artery thrombus by transcranial Doppler monitoring. Stroke 24:606–608, 1993

198. Dieterich M, Brandt T: Ocular torsion and tilt of subjective visual vertical are sensitive brainstem signs. Ann Neurol 33:292–299, 1993

199. Dieterich M, Brandt T: Wallenberg's syndrome: lateropulsion, cyclorotation, and subjective visual vertical in thirty-six patients. Ann Neurol 31:399–408, 1992

200. Diggle FH, Stopford JSB: PICA and vertebral artery thrombosis. Lancet 1:1214–1215, 1935

201. Drayer B, Gur D, Wolfson S et al: Regional blood flow in the posterior fossa: xenon enhanced ET scanning. Acta Neurol Scand, suppl. 2, 60:218, 1979

202. Duffy P, Jacobs G: Clinical and pathologic findings in vertebral artery thrombosis. Neurology (NY) 8:862, 1958

203. Dumenil L: De la paralysie unilatérale du voile du palais d'origine centrale. Arch Gen Med 25:385–401, 1875

204. Dumoulin CL, Hart HR: MR angiography. Radiology 161:717, 1986

205. Duncan G, Parker S, Fisher CM: Acute cerebellar infarction in the PICA territory. Arch Neurol 32:364, 1975

206. Duret H: Recherches anatomiques sur la circulation de l'encéphale. Arch Physiol Norm Pathol 60–91, 316–353, 664–693, 919–957, 1874

207. Duret H: Sur la distribution des artères nourricières du bulbe rachidien. Arch Physiol Norm Pathol 2:97–113, 1873

208. Duvernoy HM: Human Brainstem Vessels. Springer-Verlag, Heidelberg, 1978

209. Easton JD, Sherman DG: Cervical manipulation and stroke. Stroke 8:594, 1977

210. Echiverri HC, Rubino FA, Gupta SR et al: Fusiform aneurysm of the vertebrobasilar arterial system. Stroke 20:1741, 1989

211. Edelman RR, Mattle HP, Atkinson DJ et al: MR angiography. AJR 154:937, 1990

212. Edelman RR, Mattle HP, O'Reilly GV et al: Magnetic resonance imaging of flow dynamics in the circle of Willis. Stroke 21:56, 1990

213. Edwards WH, Mulherin JL: The surgical reconstruction of the proximal subclavian and vertebral artery. In Berguer R, Bauer R (eds): Vertebrobasilar Arterial Occlusive Disease. Lippincott-Raven, Philadelphia, 1984

214. Ekbom K, Grietz T, Kugelberg E: Hydrocephalus due to ectasia of the basilar artery. J Neurol Sci 8:465, 1969

215. Ekestrom S, Eklund B, Liljequist L et al: Noninvasive methods in the evaluation of obliterative disease of the subclavian or innominate artery. Acta Med Scand 206:467, 1979

216. Emanuele M, Dorsch T, Scarff T et al: Basilar artery aneurysm simulating pheochromocytoma. Neurology (NY) 31:1560, 1981

217. Escourolle R, Gautier J-C, Rosa A et al: Anévrysme dissequant vertébrobasilaire. Rev Neurol 128:95, 1972

218. Escourolle R, Hauw J-J, Der Agopian P et al: Les infarctus bulbaires. J Neurol Sci 28:103, 1976

219. Eslinger PJ, Warner GC, Grattan LM, Easton JD: "Frontal lobe" utilization behavior associated with paramedian thalamic infarction. Neurology 41:450–452, 1991

220. Estanol B, Lopez-Rios G: Neuro-otology of the lateral medullary infarct syndrome. Arch Neurol 39:176, 1982

221. European Stroke Prevention Study (ESPS) Group: European stroke prevention study. Stroke 21:1122–1130, 1990

222. Facon E, Steriade M, Werthein N: Hypersomnie prolongée engendrée par des lésions bilatérales du système activateur médial: le syndrome thrombotique de la bifurcation du tronc basilaire. Rev Neurol 98:117, 1958

223. Fairburn B, Oliver LC: Cerebellar softening: a surgical emergency. BMJ 1:1335, 1956

224. Fang H, Palmer J: Vascular phenomena involving brainstem structures. Neurology (NY) 6:402, 1956

225. Fankhauser H, Kamano S, Hanamura T et al: Abnormal origin of the posterior inferior cerebellar artery. J Neurosurg 51:569, 1979

226. Faught E, Oh SJ: Brainstem auditory evoked responses in brainstem infarction. Stroke 16:701–705, 1985

227. Faught E, Trader S, Hanna G: Cerebral complications of angiography for transient ischemia and stroke: prediction of risk. Neurology (NY) 29:4, 1979

228. Fazekas J, Alman R, Sullivan J: Vertebral-basilar insufficiency. Arch Neurol 8:215, 1963

229. Feely MP: Cerebellar infarction. Neurosurgery 4:7–11, 1979

230. Feigin I, Budzilovich G: The general pathology of cerebrovascular disease. p. 128. In Vinken P, Bruyn G (eds): Handbook of Clinical Neurology. Vol. 2. North-Holland, Amsterdam, 1972

231. Feldmann E, Daneault N, Kwan E et al: Chinese-white differences in the distribution of occlusive cerebrovascular disease. Neurology (NY) 40:1541, 1990

232. Ferbert A, Bruckmann H, Drummen R: Clinical features of proven basilar artery occlusion. Stroke 21:1135, 1990

233. Ferbert A, Vielhaber S, Meincke U, Buchner H: Transcranial magnetic stimulation in pontine infarction: correlation to degree of paresis. J Neurol Neurosurg Psychiatry 55:294–299, 1992

234. Field JR, Lee L, McBurney R: Complications of 1000 brachial arteriograms. J Neurosurg 36:324, 1972

235. Fields W, Lemak N, Frankowski R et al: Controlled trial of aspirin in cerebral ischemia. Stroke 8:301, 1977

236. Fields W, Ratinov G, Weibel J et al: Survival following basilar artery occlusion. Arch Neurol 15:463, 1966

237. Fields WS: Collateral circulation in cerebrovascular disease. p. 168. In Vinken P, Bruyn G (eds): Handbook of Clinical Neurology. Vol. 2. North-Holland, Amsterdam, 1972

238. Fields WS: Neurovascular syndromes of the neck and shoulders. Semin Neurol 1:301, 1981

239. Fields WS, Lemak N: Joint study of extracranial arterial occlusion. VII. Subclavian steal. JAMA 222:1139, 1972

240. Fields WS, Lemak NA, Ben-Menachem Y: Thoracic outlet syndrome: review and reference to a stroke in a major league pitcher. AJNR 7:73, 1986

241. Fisher C: Some neuro-ophthalmological observations. J Neurol Neurosurg Psychiatry 30:383, 1967

242. Fisher C, Gore I, Okabe N et al: Atherosclerosis of the carotid and vertebral arteries: extracranial and intracranial. J Neuropathol Exp Neurol 24:455, 1965

243. Fisher CM: A lacunar stroke: the dysarthria clumsy hand syndrome. Neurology (NY) 17:614, 1967

244. Fisher CM: A new vascular syndrome: "the subclavian steal," editorial. N Engl J Med 265:912, 1961

245. Fisher CM: Abulia minor vs agitation behavior. Clinical surgery. p. 9. In Clinical Surgery. Vol. 31. Williams & Wilkins, Baltimore, 1983

246. Fisher CM: Ataxic hemiparesis: a pathologic study. Arch Neurol 35:126, 1978

247. Fisher CM: Bilateral occlusion of basilar artery branches. J Neurol Neurosurg Psychiatry 40:1182, 1977

248. Fisher CM: Cerebral ischemia: less familiar types. Clin Neurosurg 18:267, 1971

249. Fisher CM: Headache in cerebrovascular disease. p. 124. In Vinken P, Bruyn G (eds): Handbook of Clinical Neurology. Vol. 5. North-Holland, Amsterdam, 1968

250. Fisher CM: Is pressure on nerves and roots a common cause of pain? Trans Am Neurol Assoc 97:282, 1972

251. Fisher CM: Lacunar infarct of the tegmentum of the lower lateral pons. Arch Neurol 46:566–567, 1989

252. Fisher CM: Lacunar strokes and infarcts: a review. Neurology (NY) 32:871, 1982

253. Fisher CM: Migrainous accompaniments versus arteriosclerotic ischemia. Trans Am Neurol Assoc 93:211, 1968

254. Fisher CM: Occlusion of the internal carotid artery. Arch Neurol Psychiatry 65:345, 1951

255. Fisher CM: Occlusion of the vertebral arteries. Arch Neurol 22:13, 1970

256. Fisher CM: Ocular bobbing. Arch Neurol 11:543, 1964

257. Fisher CM: Oval pupils. Arch Neurol 37:502, 1980

258. Fisher CM: Pathological observations in hypertensive cerebral hemorrhage. J Neuropathol Exp Neurol 30:536, 1971

259. Fisher CM: Pure motor hemiplegia of vascular origin. Arch Neurol 13:30, 1965

260. Fisher CM: Pure sensory stroke and allied conditions. Stroke 13:434, 1982

261. Fisher CM: Pure sensory stroke involving face, arm, and leg. Neurology (NY) 15:76, 1965

262. Fisher CM: Thalamic pure sensory stroke: a pathologic study. Neurology (NY) 28:1141, 1978

263. Fisher CM: The arterial lesions underlying lacunes. Acta Neuropathol 12:1, 1967

264. Fisher CM: The "herald hemiparesis" of basilar artery occlusion. Arch Neurol 45:1301, 1988

265. Fisher CM: The neurological examination of the comatose patient. Acta Neurol Scand, suppl. 36, 45:1, 1969

266. Fisher CM: The vascular lesion in lacunae. Trans Am Neurol Assoc 90:243, 1965

267. Fisher CM: Transient migrainous accompaniments of late onset. Stroke 10:96, 1979

268. Fisher CM: Vertigo in cerebrovascular disease. Arch Otolaryngol 85:529, 1967

269. Fisher CM, Caplan L: Basilar artery branch occlusion: a cause of pontine infarction. Neurology (NY) 21:900, 1971

270. Fisher CM, Cole M: Homolateral ataxia and crural paresis: a vascular syndrome. J Neurol Neurosurg Psychiatry 28:48, 1965

271. Fisher CM, Karnes W, Kubik C: Lateral medullary infarction: the pattern of vascular occlusion. J Neuropathol Exp Neurol 20:323, 1961

272. Fisher CM, Karnes WE: Local embolism. J Neuropathol Exp Neurol 24:174, 1965

273. Fisher CM, Ojemann RG: A clinico-pathologic study of carotid endarterectomy plaques. Rev Neurol (Paris) 142:573, 1986

274. Fisher CM, Ojemann R, Roberson G: Spontaneous dissection of cervico-cerebral arteries. J Can Sci Neurol 5:9, 1978

275. Fisher CM, Picard E, Polak A et al: Acute hypertensive cerebellar hemorrhage: diagnosis and surgical treatment. J Nerv Ment Dis 140:38, 1965

276. Foix C, Hillemand P: Contribution à l'étude des ramollissements protubérantiels. Rev Med 43:287–305, 1926

277. Foix C, Hillemand P: Irrigation de la protubérance. CR Soc Biol Paris 42:35, 1925

278. Foix C, Hillemand P: Irrigation du bulbe. CR Soc Biol Paris 42:33, 1924

279. Foix C, Hillemand P: Les artères de l'axe encéphalique jusqu'au diencéphale inclusivement. Rev Neurol 32:705, 1925

280. Foix C, Hillemand P, Schalit I: Sur le syndrome latéral due bulbe et l'irrigation du bulbe supérieur: l'artère de la fossette latérale du bulbe, le syndrome de la cérébelleuse inférieure, territoire de ces artères. Rev Neurol 32:160, 1925

281. Ford F, Clark D: Thrombosis of the basilar artery with softenings in the cerebellum and brainstem due to manipulation of the neck. Bull Johns Hopkins Hosp 98:37, 1956

282. Ford JJ, Baker WH, Ehrenhaft JL: Carotid endarterectomy for nonhemispheric transient ischemic attacks. Arch Surg 110:1314–1317, 1975

283. Foster NL, Mountz JM, Bluelein LA et al: Blood flow imaging of a posterior circulation stroke: use of techne-

tium Tc99M hexamethyl-propyleneamine oxime and single photon emission computed tomography. Arch Neurol 45:687–690, 1988

284. Fox AJ, Bogousslavsky J, Carey S et al: Magnetic resonance imaging of small medullary infarctions. AJNR 7: 229–233, 1986

285. Freeman W, Jaffe D: Occlusion of the superior cerebellar artery. Arch Neurol Psychiatry 46:115, 1941

286. French LA, Haines GL: Unilateral vertebral artery ligation. J Neurosurg 7:156, 1950

287. Frens D, Petajan J, Anderson R et al: Fibromuscular dysplasia of the posterior cerebral artery: report of a case and review of the literature. Stroke 5:161, 1974

288. Frisen L, Holmegaard L, Rosencrantz M: Sectorial optic atrophy and homonymous horizontal sectoranopia: a lateral choroidal artery syndrome? J Neurol Neurosurg Psychiatry 41:374–380, 1978

289. Frumkin L, Baloh R: Wallenberg's syndrome following neck manipulation. Neurology 40:611, 1990

290. Gautier JC, Awada A, Majdalani A: Images d'occlusions arterielles intracraniennes aigues obtenues par le scanner X. Rev Neurol 139;12:759–761, 1983

291. Gautier JC, Hauw JJ, Awada A et al: Artères cérébrales dolichoectasiques. Association aux anévrysmes de l'aorte abdominales. Rev Neurol (Paris) 144:437–446, 1988

292. George B, Laurian C: Impairment of vertebral artery flow caused by extrinsic lesions. Neurosurgery 24: 206–214, 1989

293. George B, Laurian C: Vertebro-basilar ischemia with thrombosis of the vertebral artery: report of two cases with embolism. J Neurol Neurosurg Psychiatry 45:91, 1982

294. Géraud G, Guillaume J, Lagarrigue J et al: Les ramollissements pseudo-tumoraux du cervelet. Rev Neurol (Paris) 134:183–195, 1978

295. Gerber N: Congenital atresia of the subclavian artery producing subclavian steal syndrome. Am J Dis Child 113:709, 1967

296. Ghika J, Bogousslavsky J, Regli F: Delayed unilateral akathisia with posterior thalamic infarct. Cerebrovasc Dis 5:55–58, 1995

297. Gilles F: Hypotensive brainstem necrosis. Arch Pathol 88:32, 1969

298. Gillian L: Anatomy and embryology of the arterial system of the brainstem and cerebellum. p. 24. In Vinken P, Bruyn G (eds): Handbook of Clinical Neurology. Vol. 2. North-Holland, Amsterdam, 1972

299. Gillian L: The correlation of the blood supply to the human brainstem with brain stem lesions. J Neuropathol Exp Neurol 23:78, 1964

300. Gillian LA: The arterial blood supply of the human brainstem correlated with vascular lesions. J Neuropathol Exp Neurol 21:303, 1962

301. Girard PF, Bonamour, Garde A, Etienne: Les syndromes de l'oblitération de l'artère cérébelleuse supérieure et du ramollissement global de la calotte protubérantielle dans son tiers supérieur: participation du pathétique. Rev Neurol (Paris) 83:199, 1950

302. Goldstein S: Dissecting hematoma of the cervical vertebral artery. J Neurosurg 56:451, 1982

303. Gonyea E: Bilateral internuclear ophthalmoplegia: association with occlusive cerebrovascular disease. Arch Neurol 31:168, 1974

304. Goodhart S, Davison C: Syndrome of the posterior inferior and anterior inferior cerebellar arteries and their branches. Arch Neurol Psychiatry 35:501, 1936

305. Goodwill J: Temporal arteritis, p. 313. In Vinken P, Bruyn G (eds): Handbook of Clinical Neurology. Vol. 39. North-Holland, Amsterdam, 1980

306. Gorelick PB, Caplan LR, Hier DB et al: Racial differences in the distribution of posterior circulation occlusive disease. Stroke 16:785, 1985

307. Graff-Radford NR, Damasio H, Yamada T et al: Nonhaemorrhagic thalamic infarction. Brain 108:495, 1985

308. Graham GD, Blamire AM, Howseman AM et al: Proton magnetic resonance spectroscopy of cerebral lactate and other metabolites in stroke patients. Stroke 23:333–340, 1992

309. Greenberg J, Skubick D, Shenken H: Acute hydrocephalus in cerebellar infarct and hemorrhage. Neurology (NY) 29:409, 1979

310. Greitz T, Sjögren S: The posterior inferior cerebellar artery. Acta Radiol 1:284, 1963

311. Grotta JC, Norris JW, Kamn A, TASS: Baseline and Angiographic Data Subgroup. Prevention of stroke with ticlopidine: who benefits most? Neurology 42:111–115, 1992

312. Guiang RL, Ellington OB: Acute pure vertiginous disequilibrium in cerebellar infarction. Eur Neurol 16:11, 1977

313. Guillain G, Bertrand L, Péron N: Le syndrome de l'artère cérébelleuse supérieure. Rev Neurol 2:835, 1928

314. Guillard A: Pathologie ischemique cérébrale et anomalie de terminaison intracranienne de l'artère vertébrale. Semin Hop Paris 62:2755, 1986

315. Hacke W, Zeumer H, Ferbert A et al: Intra-arterial thrombolytic therapy improves outcome in patients with acute vertebrobasilar occlusive disease. Stroke 19:1216, 1988

316. Hall AJ, Eaves EC: Posterior inferior cerebellar thrombosis (autopsy). Lancet 2:975–979, 1934

317. Halmagyi G, Evans W, Hallinan J: Failure of downward gaze. Arch Neurol 35:22, 1978

318. Halmagyi MB, Brandt T, Dieterich M et al: Tonic contraversive ocular tilt reaction due to unilateral mesodiencephalic lesion. Neurology (NY) 40:1503, 1990

319. Halsey J, Ceballos R, Crosby E: The supranuclear control of voluntary lateral gaze. Neurology (NY) 17:928, 1967

320. Hamrin B: Polymyalgia arteritica with morphological changes in the large arteries. Acta Med Scand, suppl. 533:4, 1972

321. Handa J, Kamijo Y, Handa H: Intracranial aneurysms associated with fibromuscular hyperplasia of the renal and internal carotid arteries. Br J Radiol 43:483, 1970

322. Hanus S, Homer T, Harter D: Vertebral artery occlusion complicating yoga exercises. Arch Neurol 34:547, 1977

323. Hardin C, Williamson W, Steegman T: Vertebral artery insufficiency produced by cervical osteoarthritic spurs. Neurology (NY) 10:855, 1960

324. Hardin CA, Poser CA: Rotational obstruction of the ver-

tebral artery due to redundancy and extraluminal cervical fascial bands. Ann Surg 158:133–137, 1963

325. Hardy D, Peace D, Rhoton A: Microsurgical anatomy of the superior cerebellar artery. Neurosurgery 6:10, 1980

326. Hari R, Sulkava R, Halti A: Brainstem auditory evoked responses and alpha-pattern coma. Ann Neurol 11:187, 1982

327. Harris TH, Hauser A: Occlusion of the right posterior inferior cerebellar artery and right vertebral artery. Arch Neurol Psychiatry 26:396–400, 1931

328. Harris W: Ataxic nystagmus: a pathognomonic sign in disseminated sclerosis. Br J Ophthalmol 28:40, 1944

329. Hashimoto R, Yoshida M, Tanaka Y: Utilization behavior after right thalamic infarction. Eur Neurol 35:58–62, 1995

330. Hass WK, Easton JD, Adams HP et al: A randomized trial comparing ticlopidine hydrochloride with aspirin for the prevention of stroke in high-risk patients. N Engl J Med 321:501–507, 1989

331. Hass WK, Fields WS, North RR et al: Joint Study of Extracranial Arterial Occlusion. II. Arteriography, technique, sites, and complications. JAMA 203:159, 1986

332. Haughton V, Donegan J, Walsh P et al: Clinical cerebral blood flow measurements with inhaled xenon and ET. AJR 134:281, 1980

333. Hauw J-J, Der Agopian P, Trelles L et al: Les infarctus bulbaires. J Neurol Sci 28:83, 1976

334. Hayem G: Sur la thrombose par artérite du tronc basilaire comme cause de mort rapide. Arch Physiol Norm Pathol 1:270, 1868

335. Helgason C, Caplan LR, Goodwin J et al: Anterior choroidal artery territory infarction: case reports and review. Arch Neurol 3:681, 1986

336. Helgason CM, Wilbur AC: Basilar branch pontine infarction with prominent sensory signs. Stroke 22: 1129–1136, 1991

337. Hennerici M: New technical and clinical aspects for cerebrovascular applications of ultrasound methods. J Neurosci Methods 34:169–177, 1990

338. Hennerici M, Aulich A, Sandmann W et al: Incidence of asymptomatic extracranial arterial disease. Stroke 12: 750, 1981

339. Hennerici M, Hacke W, von Kummer R et al: Intravenous tissue plasminogen activator for the treatment of acute thromboembolic ischemia. Cerebrovasc Dis 1: 124–128, 1991

340. Hennerici M, Klemm C, Rautenberg W: The subclavian steal phenomenon: a common vascular disorder with rare neurologic deficits. Neurology (NY) 38:669, 1988

341. Hennerici M, Rautenberg W, Schwartz A: Transcranial Doppler ultrasound for the assessment of intracranial arterial flow velocity. II. Evaluation of intracranial arterial disease. Surg Neurol 27:523, 1987

342. Hennerici M, Rautenberg W, Sitzer G et al: Transcranial Doppler ultrasound for the assessment of intracranial arterial flow velocity. I. Examination of technique and normal values. Surg Neurol 27:439, 1987

343. Henze T, Boeer A, Tebbe U et al: Lysis of basilar artery occlusion with tissue plasminogen activator. Lancet 2: 1391, 1987

344. Heros R: Cerebellar hemorrhage and infarction. Stroke 13:106, 1982

345. Heros R: Cerebellar infarction resulting from traumatic occlusion of a vertebral artery. J Neurosurg 51:111, 1979

346. Herskovitz S, Lipton RB, Lantos G: Neuro-Behçet's disease. Neurology (NY) 38:1714, 1988

347. Hesselink JR, Teresi L, Davis K et al: Intravenous digital subtraction angiography of arteriosclerotic vertebrobasilar disease. AJR 142:255, 1984

348. Heyman A, Young W, Dillon M et al: Cerebral ischemia caused by occlusive lesions of the subclavian or innominate arteries. Arch Neurol 10:581, 1964

349. Higashida RT, Tsai FY, Halbach VV et al: Transluminal angioplasty for atherosclerotic disease of the vertebral and basilar arteries. J Neurosurg 78:192–198, 1993

350. Hinshaw D, Thompson J, Hasso A et al: Infarction of the brainstem and cerebellum: a correlation of computed tomography and angiography. Radiology 137:105, 1980

351. Hirsch CS, Roessmann U: Arterial dysplasia with ruptured basilar artery aneurysm: report of a case. Hum Pathol 6:749, 1975

352. Hirsh L, Gonzalez C: Fusiform basilar aneurysm simulating carotid transient ischemic attacks. Stroke 10:598, 1979

353. Ho K: Pure motor hemiplegia due to infarction of the cerebral peduncle. Arch Neurol 39:524, 1982

354. Ho K, Meyer K: The medial medullary syndrome. Arch Neurol 38:385, 1981

355. Ho SU, Kim KS, Berenberg RA, Ho HT: Cerebellar infarction: a clinical and CT study. Surg Neurol 16: 350–352, 1981

356. Holmes G: The Cloonian lectures on the clinical symptoms of cerebellar disease and their interpretations. Lancet 1:1177, 1922; 2:59, 1922

357. Holmes G: The symptoms of acute cerebellar injuries due to gunshot wounds. Brain 40:461, 1917

358. Hommel M, Besson G, Le Bas JF et al: Prospective study of lacunar infarction using magnetic resonance imaging. Stroke 21:546–554, 1990

359. Hommel M, Besson G, Pollak P et al: Hemiplegia in posterior cerebral artery occlusion. Neurology (NY) 40: 1496, 1990

360. Hommel M, Bogousslavsky J: The spectrum of vertical gaze palsy following unilateral brainstem stroke. Neurology 41:1229–1234, 1991

361. Hoobler S: The syndrome of cervical rib with subclavian arterial thrombosis and hemiplegia due to cerebral embolism. N Engl J Med 226:942, 1942

362. Hopf HC, Gutmann L: Diabetic 3rd nerve palsy: evidence for a mesencephalic lesion. Neurology 40: 1041–1045, 1990

363. Hopkins LN, Budny JL, Spetzler RF: Revascularization of the rostral brainstem. Neurosurgery 10:364–369, 1982

364. Hopkins LN, Martin NA, Hadley MN et al: Vertebrobasilar insufficiency. II. Microsurgical treatment of intracranial vertebrobasilar disease. J Neurosurg 66:662, 1987

365. Hornig CR, Rust DS, Busse O et al: Space-occupying cerebellar infarction. Clinical course and prognosis. Stroke 25:372–374, 1994

366. Houkin K, Kamada K, Kamiyama H et al: Longitudinal

changes in proton magnetic resonance spectroscopy in cerebral infarction. Stroke 24:1316–1321, 1993

367. Houser OW, Baker H, Sandok B et al: Cephalic arterial fibromuscular dysplasia. Radiology 101:605, 1971

368. Huang CY, Yu YL: Small cerebellar strokes may mimic labyrinthine lesions. J Neurol Neurosurg Psychiatry 48: 263–265, 1985

369. Humphries AW, Young JR, Beven EG et al: Relief of vertebrobasilar symptoms by carotid endarterectomy. Surgery 57:48–52, 1965

370. Hun H: Analgesia, thermic anesthesia, and ataxia, resulting from foci of softening in the medulla oblongata and cerebellum due to occlusion of the left PICA. NY Med J 65:513, 581, 613, 1897

371. Hutchinson E, Yates P: The cervical portion of the vertebral artery: a clinico-pathological study. Brain 79:319, 1956

372. Hutchinson E, Yates P: Carotico-vertebral stenosis. Lancet 1:2, 1957

373. Imparato A: Vertebral artery reconstruction: a nineteen year experience. J Vasc Surg 2:626, 1985

374. Imparato A, Riles T, Kim G et al: Vertebral artery reconstruction. Stroke 12:125, 1981

375. Imparato A, Riles T, Kim G: Cervical vertebral artery angioplasty for brainstem ischemia. Surgery 90:842, 1981

376. Ingvar D, Sourander P: Destruction of the reticular core of the brainstem. Arch Neurol 23:1, 1970

377. Ishikawa K: Natural history and classification of occlusive thromboarteriopathy (Takayasu disease). Circulation 57:27, 1978

378. Jacobs L, Anderson P, Bender M: The lesion producing paralysis of downward but not upward gaze. Arch Neurol 28:319, 1973

379. Jacobs L, Heffner RR, Newman RP: Selective paralysis of downward gaze caused by bilateral lesions of the mesencephalic periaqueductal gray matter. Neurology (NY) 35:516, 1985

380. Jagiella WM, Sung JH: Bilateral infarction of the medullary pyramids in humans. Neurology 39:21–24, 1989

381. Jakob A: Das Kleinhirn. In Von Möllendorff W (ed): Handbuch der mikroskopischen Anatomie des Menschen. Vol. 4. Julius Springer, Berlin, 1928

382. Jensen ME, Mathis JM, DeNardo AJ, Dion JE: Angioplasty of brachiocephalic and cerebral vessels in atherosclerotic disease. Stroke 25:155, 1994

383. Jones EF, Kalman JM, Calafiore P et al: Proximal aortic atheroma. An independent risk factor for cerebral ischemia. Stroke 26:218–224, 1995

384. Jones HE, Millikan C, Sandok B: Temporal profile (clinical course) of acute vertebrobasilar system cerebral infarction. Stroke 11:173, 1980

385. Juge O, Meyer J, Sakai F et al: Critical appraisal of cerebral blood flow measured from brainstem and cerebellar regions after Xe-133 inhalations in humans. Stroke 10: 428, 1979

386. Jurgensen J, Brennan R, Towfighi J: Brainstem arterial end-zone infarction following hypotension in man. Neurology (NY) 31:92, 1981

387. Kalyan-Raman UP, Kowalski RV, Lee RH, Fierer JA:

388. Kanis KB, Ropper AH, Adelman LS: Homolateral hemiparesis as an early sign of cerebellar mass effect. Neurology 44:2194–2197, 1994

389. Kaplan RF, Estol CJ, Damasio H et al: Bilateral polar territory infarcts. Neurology 41:329, 1991

390. Kaps M, Seidel G, Bauer T, Behrman B: Imaging of the intracranial vertebrobasilar system using color-coded ultrasound. Stroke 23:1577–1582, 1992

391. Karalis DG, Chandrasekaran K, Victor MF et al: Recognition and embolic potential of intra-aortic atherosclerotic debris. J Am Coll Cardiol 17:73–78, 1991

392. Karp J, Hurtig H: "Locked-in" state with bilateral midbrain infarcts. Arch Neurol 30:176, 1974

393. Kase C, Maulsby G, De Juan C et al: Hemichoreahemiballism and lacunar infarction in the basal ganglia. Neurology (NY) 31:452, 1981

394. Kase C, Varakis J, Stafford J et al: Medial medullary infarction from fibrocartilaginous embolism to the anterior spinal artery. Stroke 14:413, 1983

395. Kase CS, Norrving B, Levine SR et al: Cerebellar infarction. Clinico-anatomic correlations. Stroke 24:76–83, 1993

396. Kase CS, White JL, Joslyn N et al: Cerebellar infarction in the superior cerebellar artery distribution. Neurology (NY) 35:705, 1985

397. Kase CS, Wolf PA: Cerebellar infarction: upward transtentorial herniation after ventriculostomy. Stroke 24: 1096–1098, 1993

398. Keane J: Sustained up gaze in coma. Ann Neurol 9:409, 1981

399. Keane JR: Locked-in syndrome after head and neck trauma. Neurology (NY) 36:80, 1986

400. Keane JR: Ocular tilt reaction following lateral pontomedullary infarction. Neurology 42:259–260, 1992

401. Kemper T, Romanul F: State resembling akinetic mutism in basilar artery occlusion. Neurology (NY) 17:74, 1967

402. Kerber C, Margolis M, Newton T: Tortuous vertebrobasilar system: a cause of cranial nerve signs. Neurocardiology 4:74, 1972

403. Kertesz A, Black SE, Nicholson L, Carr T: The sensitivity and specificity of MRI in stroke. Neurology (NY) 37: 1580, 1987

404. Khan M, Polyzoidis KS, Adegbite ABO, McQueen JD: Massive cerebellar infarction: conservative management. Stroke 14:745–751, 1983

405. Khodadad G, Singh R, Olinger C: Possible prevention of brainstem stroke by microvascular anastomosis in the vertebrobasilar system. Stroke 8:316, 1977

406. Khurana R: Autonomic dysfunction in pontomedullary stroke. Ann Neurol 12:86, 1982

407. Kieffer SA, Takeya Y, Resch JA et al: Racial differences in cerebrovascular disease: angiographic evaluation of Japanese and American populations. AJR 101:94, 1967

408. Kim J: Pure sensory stroke. Clinical-radiological correlates of 21 cases. Stroke 23:983–987, 1992

409. Kim JS, Lee JH, Im JH, Lee MC: Syndromes of pontine base infarction. A clinical-radiological correlation study. Stroke 26:950–955, 1995

Dissecting aneurysm of superior cerebellar artery. Arch Neurol 40:120–122, 1983

410. Kim JS, Lee JH, Suh DC, Lee MC: Spectrum of lateral medullary syndrome. Correlation between clinical findings and magnetic resonance imaging in 33 subjects. Stroke 25:1405–1410, 1994

411. Kimura K, Yasaka M, Moriyasu H et al: Ultrasonographic evaluation of vertebral artery to detect vertebrobasilar axis occlusion. Stroke 25:1006–1009, 1994

412. Kingsley D, Radue E, DuBoulay E: Evaluation of computed tomography in vascular lesions of the vertebrobasilar territory. J Neurol Neurosurg Psychiatry 43:193, 1980

413. Kinsella, Feldmann E, Brooks JM: The clinical utility of transcranial Doppler ultrasound in suspected vertebrobasilar ischemia. J Neuroimaging 3:115–122, 1993

414. Kistler JP, Buonnano FS, DeWitt LD et al: Vertebral-basilar posterior cerebral territory stroke: delineation by proton nuclear magnetic resonance imaging. Stroke 15:417, 1984

415. Klein R, Hunder G, Stanson A et al: Large artery involvement in giant cell (temporal) arteritis. Ann Intern Med 83:806, 1975

416. Kleineri G, Fazekas F, Kleinert R et al: Bilateral medial medullary infarction: magnetic resonance imaging and correlative histopathologic findings. Eur Neurol 33:74–76, 1993

417. Kommerell G, Hoyt W: Lateropulsion of saccadic eye movements. Arch Neurol 28:313, 1973

418. Koroshetz WJ, Ropper AH: Artery-to-artery embolism causing stroke in the posterior circulation. Neurology (NY) 37:292, 1987

419. Kotila M, Hokkanen L, Laaksonen R, Valanne L: Long-term prognosis after left tuberothalamic infarction: a study of 7 cases. Cerebrovasc Dis 4:44–50, 1994

420. Krayenbüll H, Yasargil M: Radiological anatomy and tomography of the cerebral arteries. p. 65. In Vinken P, Bruyn G (eds): Handbook of Clinical Neurology. Vol. 2. North-Holland, Amsterdam, 1972

421. Krayenbüll H, Yasargil MG: Die vaskulären Erkrankungen im Gebiet der Arteria vertebralis und Arteria basilaris. George Thieme, Stuttgart, 1957

422. Kreuger B, Okazaki H: Vertebral-basilar distribution infarction following chiropractic cervical manipulation. Mayo Clin Proc 55:322, 1980

423. Krieger D, Busse O, Schramm J et al: German-Austrian Space Occupying Cerebellar Infarction Study (GASCIS): study design, methods, patients' characteristics. J Neurol 239:183–185, 1992

424. Kubik C, Adams R: Occlusion of the basilar artery: a clinical and pathologic study. Brain 69:73, 1946

425. Labauge R, Boukobza M, Pages M et al: Occlusion de l'artère vertébrale. Rev Neurol 143:490, 1987

426. Labauge R, Pages M, Marty-Double C et al: Occlusion du tronc basilaire. Rev Neurol 137:545, 1981

427. Lahitte M, Marc-Vergnes J, Rascol A et al: Intravenous angiography of the extracranial arteries. Radiology 137:705, 1980

428. Lance J, Adams R: The syndrome of intention and action myoclonus as a sequel of hypoxic encephalopathy. Brain 86:111, 1963

429. Lapresle J, Ben Hamida M: The dentato-olivary pathway. Arch Neurol 22:135, 1970

430. Lasjaunias P, Guibert-Tranier F, Braun JP: The pharyngo-cerebellar artery or ascending pharyngeal artery origin of the posterior inferior cerebellar artery. J Neuroradiol 8:317–325, 1981

431. Lazorthes G: Vascularisation et Circulation Cérébrales. Masson, Paris, 1961

432. Lazorthes G, Gouazé A, Salamon G, Poulhes J, Espagno J: La vascularisation artérielle du cervelet. pp. 205–219. In Lazorthes G, Gouazé A, Salamon G (eds): La Vascularisation Cérébrale. Masson, Paris, 1978

433. Lechtenberg R, Gilman S: Speech disorders in cerebellar diseases. Ann Neurol 3:285–290, 1978

434. Lee RE: Reconstruction of the proximal vertebral artery. pp. 211–223. In Berguer R, Caplan LR (eds): Vertebrobasilar Arterial Disease. Quality Medical Publishing, St. Louis, 1992

435. Lehrich J, Winkler G, Ojemann R: Cerebellar infarction with brainstem compression: diagnosis and surgical treatment. Arch Neurol 22:490, 1970

436. Lester J, Klee A: Complications of 337 percutaneous vertebral angiographies. Acta Neurol Scand 41:301, 1965

437. Levin B, Margolis G: Acute failure of automatic respirations secondary to a unilateral brainstem infarct. Ann Neurol 1:583, 1977

438. Levine SR, Patel VM, Welch KMA et al: Are heart attacks really brain attacks? In Furlan A (ed): The Heart in Stroke. Springer-Verlag, Heidelberg, 1987

439. Levine SR, Welch KMA: Superior cerebellar artery infarction and vertebral artery dissection. Stroke 19:1431–1434, 1988

440. Levine SR, Welch KMA: Superior cerebellar artery territory stroke, abstracted. Neurology, Suppl. 1, 38:344, 1988

441. Lévy C, Laissy J-P, Raveau V et al: 3D-time-of-flight MR angiography and MR imaging versus angiography in carotid and vertebral artery dissections: a prospective study in 18 patients. Radiology 190:97–103, 1994

442. Levy R, Dugan T, Bernat J et al: Lateral medullary syndrome after neck injury. Neurology (NY) 30:788, 1980

443. Leyden E: Uber die Thrombose der basilar Arterie. Z Klin Med 5:165, 1882

444. Lhermitte F: "Utilization behavior" and its relation to lesions of the frontal lobes. Brain 106:237–255, 1983

445. Lhermitte J: Syndrome de la calotte du pédoncule cérébral: les troubles psycho-sensoriels dans les lesions du mésocéphale. Rev Neurol (Paris) 38:1359–1365, 1922

446. Lhermitte J, Trelles JO: L'artério-sclérose du tronc basilaire et ses conséquences anatomo-cliniques. Jahrbücher Psychiatr Neurol 51:91–107, 1934

447. Lie T: Congenital malformations of the carotid and vertebral arterial systems, including the persistent anastomoses. p. 289. In Vinken P, Bruyn G (eds): Handbook of Clinical Neurology. Vol. 12. North-Holland, Amsterdam, 1972

448. Liljequist L, Ekerstrom S, Nordhus O: Monitoring direction of vertebral artery blood flow by Doppler shift ultrasound in patients with suspected subclavian steal. Acta Chir Scand 147:421, 1981

449. Lindenberg R: Compression of brain arteries as a patho-

genetic factor for tissue necrosis and their areas of prediction. J Neuropathol Exp Neurol 14:223, 1955

450. Lindgren SO: Infarctions simulating brain tumors in the posterior fossa. J Neurosurg 13:575, 1956

451. Lister J, Rhoton A, Matsushima T et al: Microsurgical anatomy of the posterior inferior cerebellar artery. Neurosurgery 10:170, 1982

452. Little JR, St Louis P, Weinstein M et al: Giant fusiform aneurysm of the cerebral arteries. Stroke 12:183, 1981

453. Lochaya S, Kaplan B, Shaffer AB: Pseudocoarctation of the aorta with bicuspid aortic valve and kinked left subclavian artery, a possible cause of subclavian steal. Am Heart J 73:369, 1967

454. Loeb C, Meyer JS: Strokes Due to Vertebro-Basilar Disease. Charles C Thomas, Springfield, IL, 1965

455. Louis-Bar D: Sur le syndrome vasculaire de l'hémibulbe (Wallenberg). Monatsschr Psychiatr Neurol 112:53, 1946

456. Luco C, Hoppe A, Schweitzer M et al: Visual field defects in vascular lesions of the lateral geniculate body. J Neurol Neurosurg Psychiatry 55:12–15, 1992

457. Ludwig B, Swerdlow ML: Lethal cerebellar infarction with normal EMI scan: two cases, abstracted. Neurology 27:402, 1977

458. Luhan J, Pollock S: Occlusion of the superior cerebellar artery. Neurology (NY) 3:77, 1953

459. Lupi-Herrera E, Sanchez-Torres G, Marcushamer J et al: Takayasu's arteritis: clinical study of 27 cases. Am Heart J 93:94, 1977

460. Macdonell RAL, Kalnins RM, Donnan GA: Cerebellar infarction: natural history, prognosis, and pathology. Stroke 18:849–855, 1987

461. Makos MM, McComb RD, Hart MN et al: Alphaglucosidase deficiency and basilar artery aneurysm: report of a sibship. Ann Neurol 22:629, 1987

462. Malamut BL, Graff-Radford N, Chawluk J et al: Memory in a case of bilateral thalamic infarction. Neurology 42:163–169, 1992

463. Mapstone T, Spetzler R: Vertebrobasilar insufficiency secondary to vertebral artery occlusion from a fibrous band. J Neurosurg 56:581, 1982

464. Marburg O: Uber die neuren Fortschritte in der topischen Diagnostic du Pons und Oblongata. Dtsch Z Nervenheilkd 41:41, 1911

465. Margolis MT, Newton TH: The posterior inferior cerebellar artery. pp. 1710–1774. In Newton TH, Poots (eds): Radiology of the Skull and Brain. Angiography. Vol. 68. CV Mosby, St. Louis, 1974

466. Marinesco G, Draganesco S: Hémisyndrome bulbaire relevant d'un ramollissement de l'étage moyen du bulbe, suite de thrombus de l'artère vertébrale droite. Ann Med 13:1–19, 1923

467. Martin JP: Hemichorea resulting from a local lesion of the brain (the syndrome of the body of Luys). Brain 50:637, 1927

468. Martin PJ, Evans DH, Naylor AR: Transcranial color-coded sonography of the basal cerebral circulation. Reference data from 115 volunteers. Stroke 25:390–396, 1994

469. Maruyama K, Tanaka M, Ikeda S et al: A case report of quadriparesis due to compression of the medulla oblon-gata by the elongated left vertebral artery. Rinsho Shinkeigaku 29:108, 1989

470. Maruyama M, Asai T, Kuriyama Y et al: Positive platelet scintigram of a vertebral aneurysm presenting thromboembolic transient ischemic attacks. Stroke 20:687, 1989

471. Mas JL, Bousser MG, Hasboun D et al: Extracranial vertebral artery dissection: a review of 13 cases. Stroke 18:1037, 1987

472. Mas JL, Hénin D, Bousser MG et al: Dissecting aneurysm of the vertebral artery and cervical manipulation: a case report with autopsy. Neurology 39:512–515, 1989

473. Matsumoto S, Okuda B, Imai T et al: A sensory level on the trunk in lower lateral brainstem lesions. Neurology (NY) 38:1515, 1988

474. Matsushita K, Naritomi H, Kazui S et al: Infarction in the anterior inferior cerebellar artery territory: magnetic resonance imaging and auditory brain stem responses. Cerebrovasc Dis 3:206–212, 1993

475. McCusker E, Rudick R, Honch G et al: Recovery from the locked-in syndrome. Arch Neurol 39:145, 1982

476. McKee AC, Levine DN, Kowall NW et al: Peduncular hallucinosis associated with isolated infarction of the substantia nigra pars reticulata. Ann Neurol 27:500, 1990

477. McKissock W, Richardson A, Walsh R: Spontaneous cerebellar hemorrhage: a study of 34 consecutive cases treated surgically. Brain 83:1, 1960

478. McLean CA, Gonzales MF, Dowling JP: Systemic giant cell arteritis and cerebellar infarction. Stroke 24:899–902, 1993

479. McMenemy WH, Lawrence BJ: Encephalomyelopathy in Behçet's syndrome. Lancet 2:353, 1957

480. McNamara J, Heyman A, Silver D et al: The value of carotid endarterectomy in treating transient cerebral ischemia of the posterior circulation. Neurology (NY) 27:682, 1977

481. Mehler MF: The rostral basilar artery syndrome: diagnosis, etiology, prognosis. Neurology 39:9–16, 1989

482. Mehler MF: The neuro-ophthalmologic spectrum of the rostral basilar artery syndrome. Arch Neurol 45:966, 1988

483. Meienberg O, Mumenthaler M, Karbowski K: Quadriparesis and nuclear oculomotor palsy with total bilateral ptosis mimicking coma. Arch Neurol 36:708, 1979

484. Meissner I, Sapir S, Kokmen E et al: The paramedian diencephalic syndrome: a dynamic phenomenon. Stroke 18:380, 1987

485. Menzies WF: Thrombosis of inferior cerebellar artery. Brain 15:436–439, 1893

486. Merkel K, Grinsberg P, Parker J et al: Cerebrovascular disease in sickle cell anemia: a clinical, pathological, and radiological correlation. Stroke 9:45, 1978

487. Merritt H, Finland M: Vascular lesions of the hindbrain (lateral medullary syndrome). Brain 53:290, 1930

488. Mettinger K: Fibromuscular dysplasia and the brain. II. Current concepts of the disease. Stroke 13:53, 1982

489. Meyer J, Hayman L, Amano T et al: Mapping local blood flow of human brain by CT scanning during stable xenon inhalation. Stroke 1:426, 1981

490. Meyer J, Haymann L, Sakai F et al: High-resolution three-dimensional measurement of localized cerebral blood flow by CT scanning and stable xenon clearance:

effect of cerebral infarction and ischemia. Trans Am Neurol Assoc 104:1, 1979

491. Meyer JS, Sheehan S, Bauer R: An arteriographic study of cerebrovascular disease in man: stenosis and occlusion of the vertebral basilar arterial system. Arch Neurol 2: 27, 1960

492. Meyer K, Baloh R, Krohel G et al: Ocular lateropulsion: a sign of lateral medullary disease. Arch Ophthalmol 98: 1614, 1980

493. Milandre L, Bonnefoi B, Pestre P et al: Dolichoectasies artérielles vertébrobasilaires. Complications et pronostique. Rev Neurol (Paris) 147:714–722, 1991

494. Milandre L, Habib M, Hassoun J, Khalil R: Bilateral infarction of the medullary pyramids. Neurology 40:556, 1990

495. Millikan C: Reassessment of anticoagulant therapy in various types of occlusive cerebrovascular disease. Stroke 2:201, 1971

496. Millikan C, Siekert R: Studies in cerebrovascular disease: the syndrome of intermittent insufficiency of the basilar arterial system. Proc Staff Meet Mayo Clin 30:61, 1955

497. Millikan C, Siekert R, Shick R: Studies in cerebrovascular disease: the use of anticoagulant drugs in the treatment of insufficiency or thrombosis within the basilar arterial system. Proc Staff Meet Mayo Clin 30:116, 1955

498. Millikan C, Siekert R, Whisnant J: Anticoagulant therapy in cerebrovascular disease: current status. JAMA 166: 587, 1958

499. Mills CK: Hemianesthesia to pain and temperature and loss of emotional expression on the right side with ataxia of the upper limb on the left. J Nerv Ment Dis 35:331, 1908

500. Mills CK: Preliminary note on a new symptom complex due to lesion of the cerebellum and cerebello-rubro-thalamic system, the main symptoms being ataxia of the upper and lower extremities of one side, and the other side deafness, paralysis of emotional expression in the face, and loss of the senses of pain, heat, and cold over the entire half of the body. J Nerv Ment Dis 39:73–76, 1912

501. Miyashita K, Naritomi H, Sawada T et al: Identification of recent lacunar lesions in cases of multiple small infarctions by magnetic resonance imaging. Stroke 19:834, 1988

502. Mizutani T, Lewis R, Gonatas N: Medial medullary syndrome in a drug abuser. Arch Neurol 37:425, 1980

503. Moersch F, Kernohan J: Hemiballismus, a clinicopathological study. Arch Neurol Psychiatry 41:365, 1939

504. Mohr JP: Neurological complications of cardiac valvular disease and cardiac surgery including systemic hypotension. p. 143. In Vinken P, Bruyn G (eds): Handbook of Clinical Neurology. Vol. 38. North-Holland, Amsterdam, 1979

505. Mohr JP: The Warfarin-Aspirin Recurrent Stroke Study (WARSS) prospective, pp. 443–448. In Moskowitz M, Caplan LR (eds): Cerebrovascular Disease, 19th Princeton Conference. Butterworths-Heinemann, Boston, 1995

506. Mohr JP, Biller J, Hilal SK et al: MR vs CT imaging in acute stroke. In Proceedings of the Seventeenth International Conference on Stroke and the Cerebral Circulation, Phoenix, AZ, 1992

507. Mohr JP, Caplan L, Melski et al: Harvard Cooperative Stroke Registry: a prospective registry. Neurology (NY) 28:754, 1978

508. Mohr JP, Kase C, Meckler R et al: Sensorimotor stroke due to thalamocapsular ischemia. Arch Neurol 34:739, 1977

509. Mokri B, Houser OW, Sandok BA, Piepgras DG: Spontaneous dissections of the vertebral arteries. Neurology 38:880–885, 1988

510. Molnar P, Hegedus K: Direct involvement of intracerebral arteries in Takayasu's arteritis. Acta Neuropathol (Berl) 63:83, 1984

511. Momose KJ, Lehrich JR: Acute cerebellar infarction presenting as a posterior fossa mass. Radiology 109: 343–352, 1973

512. Moosy J: Morphology, sites and epidemiology of cerebral atherosclerosis. Proc Assoc Res Nerv Ment Dis 51:1, 1966

513. Mori E, Yamadori A, Mitani Y: Left thalamic infarction and disturbance of verbal memory: a clinicoanatomical study with a new method of computed tomographic stereotaxic lesion localization. Ann Neurol 20:671, 1986

514. Morrow MJ, Sharpe JA: Torsional nystagmus in the lateral medullary syndrome. Ann Neurol 24:390, 1988

515. Moscow N, Newton T: Angiographic implications in diagnosis and prognosis of basilar artery occlusion. AJR 119:597, 1973

516. Moseley I, Holland I: Ectasia of the basilar artery: the breadth of the clinical spectrum and the diagnostic value of computed tomography. Neuroradiology 18:83, 1979

517. Motarjeme A, Keifer JW, Zuska AJ: Percutaneous transluminal angioplasty of the brachycephalic arteries. AJR 138:457–462, 1982

518. Motarjeme A, Keifer J, Zuska A: Percutaneous transluminal angioplasty of the vertebral arteries. Radiology 139:715, 1981

519. Moufarrij NA, Little JR, Furlan AJ et al: Basilar and distal vertebral artery stenosis: long-term follow-up. Stroke 17:938, 1986

520. Moufarrij NA, Little JR, Furlan AJ et al: Vertebral artery stenosis: long-term follow-up. Stroke 15:260, 1984

521. Mounier-Vehier F, Gedaey I, Leclerc X, Leys D: Cerebellar border zone infarcts are often associated with presumed cardiac sources of ischemic stroke. J Neurol Neurosurg Psychiatry 59:87–89, 1995

522. Mueller S, Sahs A: Brainstem dysfunction related to cervical manipulation. Neurology (NY) 26:547, 1976

523. Multicentre Acute Stroke Trial-Italy (MAST-I) Group: Randomised controlled trial of streptokinase, aspirin, and combination of both in treatment of acute ischaemic stroke. Lancet 346:1509–1514, 1995

524. Naheedy M, Tyler H, Wolf M et al: Diagnosis of thrombotic giant basilar artery aneurysm on computed tomographic scan. Arch Neurol 39:64, 1982

525. Naritomi H, Sakai F, Meyer J: Pathogenesis of transient ischemic attacks within the vertebrobasilar arterial system. Arch Neurol 36:121, 1979

526. Nashold B, Seaber J: Defects of ocular mobility after

stereotactic midbrain lesions in man. Arch Ophthalmol 88:245, 1972

527. Neau J-P, Bogousslavsky J: The syndrome of posterior choroidal artery territory infarction. Ann Neurol 39: 779–788, 1996

528. Nelson J, Johnston C: Ocular bobbing. Arch Neurol 22: 348, 1970

529. Newman N, Gay A, Heilbrun M: Disconjugate ocular bobbing: its relation to midbrain, pontine and medullary function in a surviving patient. Neurology (NY) 21:633, 1971

530. Nishizaki T, Tamikl N, Takeda N: Dolichoectatic basilar artery: a review of 23 cases. Stroke 17:1277, 1986

531. Norris JW, Eisen AA, Branch CL: Problems in cerebellar hemorrhage and infarction. Neurology 19:1043–1050, 1969

532. Norrving B, Cronqvist S: Lateral medullary infarction: prognosis in an unselected series. Neurology 41: 244–248, 1991

533. Norrving B, Magnusson M, Holtas S: Isolated acute vertigo in the elderly; vestibular or vascular disease? Acta Neurol Scand 91:43–48, 1995

534. North R, Fields W, DeBakey M et al: Brachialbasilar insufficiency syndrome. Neurology (NY) 12:810, 1962

535. Oas JG, Baloh RW: Vertigo and the anterior inferior cerebellar artery syndrome. Neurology 42:2274–2279, 1992

536. Obayashi T, Furuse M: The proatlantal intersegmental artery. Arch Neurol 37:387, 1980

537. Olesen J, Larsen B, Lauritzen M: Focal hyperemia followed by spreading oligemia and impaired activation of CBF in classic migraine. Ann Neurol 9:344, 1981

538. Ongerboer de Visser BW, Cruccu G: The masseter inhibitory reflex in pontine lesions. pp. 199–206. In Caplan LR, Hopf HC (eds): Brain-Stem Localization and Function. Springer-Verlag, Berlin, 1993

539. Osborn A, Anderson R: Angiography spectrum of cervical and intracranial fibromuscular dysplasia. Stroke 8: 617, 1977

540. Ott K, Kase C, Ojemann R et al: Cerebellar hemorrhage: diagnosis and treatment. Arch Neurol 31:160, 1974

541. Parkinson D, Reddy V, Ross R: Congenital anastomosis between the vertebral artery and internal carotid artery in the neck. J Neurosurg 51:697, 1979

542. Pasik P, Pasik T, Bender M: The pretectal syndrome in monkeys. I. Disturbance of gaze and body posture. Brain 92:521, 1969

543. Passerini A, Tagliabue G: Aneurysms of the vertebrobasilar system. Radiol Clin Biol 35:257, 1966

544. Patel A, Toole J: Subclavian steal syndrome: reversal of cephalic blood flow. Medicine (Baltimore) 44:289, 1965

545. Patrick B, Ramirez-Lassepas M, Snyder B: Temporal profile of vertebrobasilar territory infarction. Stroke 11: 643, 1980

546. Paulson G, Boesel C, Evans W: Fibromuscular dysplasia. Arch Neurol 35:287, 1978

547. Paulson G, Nashold B, Margolis G: Aneurysms of the vertebral artery. Neurology (NY) 9:590, 1959

548. Paulson GW, Yates AJ, Paltan-Ortiz JD: Does infarction of the medullary pyramid lead to spasticity? Arch Neurol 43:93, 1986

549. Pawl G, Shaw C, Wray L: True traumatic aneurysms of the vertebral artery. J Neurosurg 53:101, 1980

550. Pedersen R, Troost BT: Abnormalities of gaze in cerebrovascular disease. Stroke 12:251, 1981

551. Pelouze GA: Plaque ulcérée de l'ostium de l'artère vertébrale. Rev Neurol 145:478, 1989

552. Percheron G: Les artères du thalamus humain. Rev Neurol (Paris) 132:297–307,309–324, 1976

553. Percheron GMJ: Etude anatomique du thalamus de l'homme adulte et de sa vascularisation artérielle. Thesis, Paris, 1966

554. Peress N, Kane WC, Aronson SM: Central nervous system findings in a tenth decade autopsy population. Prog Brain Res 40:473, 1973

555. Perez-Higueras A, Alvarez-Ruiz F, Martinez-Bermejo A et al: Cerebellar infarction from fibromuscular dysplasia and dissecting aneurysm of the vertebral artery. Report of a child. Stroke 19:521–524, 1988

556. Perneczky A, Perneczky G, Tschabitscher M et al: The relationship between the caudolateral pontine syndrome and the anterior inferior cerebellar artery. Acta Neurochir 58:245, 1981

557. Pessin MS, Chimowitz MI, Levine SR et al: Stroke in patients with fusiform vertebrobasilar aneurysms. Neurology (NY) 39:16, 1989

558. Pessin MS, Daneault N, Kwan E et al: Local embolism from vertebral artery occlusion. Stroke 19:112, 1988

559. Pessin MS, del Zoppo G, Furlan A: Thrombolytic therapy in acute stroke: review and update of selected topics. pp. 409–418. In Moskowitz M, Caplan LR (eds): Cerebrovascular Disease, 19th Princeton Conference. Butterworths-Heinemann, Boston, 1995

560. Pessin MS, del Zoppo GJ, Estol C: Thrombolytic agents in the treatment of stroke. Clin Neuropharmacol 13:271, 1990

561. Pessin MS, Gorelick PB, Kwan ES et al: Basilar artery stenosis: middle and distal segments. Neurology (NY) 37:1742, 1987

562. Peterman A, Siekert R: The lateral medullary (Wallenberg) syndrome: clinical features and prognosis. Med Clin North Am 44:887, 1960

563. Philips PC, Lorenstsen KJ, Shropshire LC, Ahn HS: Congenital odontoid aplasia and posterior circulation stroke in childhood. Ann Neurol 23:410–413, 1988

564. Piepgras DG, Sundt TM, Forbes GS, Smith HC: Balloon catheter transluminal angioplasty for vertebrobasilar ischemia. pp. 215–224. In Berguer R, Bauer R (eds): Vertebrobasilar Arterial Occlusive Disease. Lippincott-Raven, Philadelphia, 1984

565. Pierrot-Deseilligny C, Amarenco P, Roullet E et al: Vermal infarct with pursuit eye movement disorders. J Neurol Neurosurg Psychiatry 53:519, 1990

566. Pierrot-Deseilligny C, Chain F, Serdaru M et al: The one and a half syndrome. Brain 104:665, 1981

567. Pines L, Gilinsky E: Uber die Thrombose der Arteria basilaris und uber die Vascularization de Brucke. Arch Psychiatr 26:380, 1932

568. Pinkerton J, Davidson K, Hibbard B: Primitive hypoglossal artery and carotid endarterectomy. Stroke 6:658, 1980

569. Plum F, Posner J: The Diagnosis of Stupor and Coma. 3rd Ed. FA Davis, Philadelphia, 1980

570. Pochaczevsky R, Uygur Z, Berman A: Basilar artery occlusion. J Can Assoc Radiol 22:261, 1971

571. Pollock M, Blennerhassett J, Clarke A: Giant cell arteritis and the subclavian steal syndrome. Neurology 23:653, 1973

572. Powers SR, Drislane TM, Nevins S: Intermittent vertebral artery compression: a new syndrome. Surgery 49:257–264, 1961

573. Powers WJ, Raichle ME: Positron emission tomography and its application to the study of cerebrovascular disease in man. Stroke 16:361–376, 1985

574. Pratt-Thomas H, Berger K: Cerebellar and spinal injuries after chiropractic manipulation. JAMA 133:600, 1947

575. Pribram H: Complications of cerebral arteriography. p. 184. In Fields W, Sahs A (eds): Intracranial Aneurysms and Subarachnoid Hemorrhage. Charles C Thomas, Springfield, IL, 1965

576. Radner S: Vertebral angiography by catheterization. Acta Radiol [Suppl] (Stockh) 87, 1951

577. Ramsbottom A, Stopford JSB: Occlusion of the PICA. BMJ 1:364–365, 1924

578. Ranalli PJ, Sharpe JA: Contrapulsion of saccades and ipsilateral ataxia: a unilateral disorder of the rostral cerebellum. Ann Neurol 20:311–316, 1986

579. Rao K, Woodlief C: Stimulation of cerebellopontine tumor by tortuous vertebrobasilar artery. AJR 132:602, 1979

580. Reis DJ, Iadecola C, Nakai M: Control of cerebral blood flow and metabolism by intrinsic neural systems in brain. p. 1. In Plum P, Pulsinelli W (eds): Cerebrovascular Diseases. Proceedings of the Fourteenth (Princeton) Conference. Lippincott-Raven, Philadelphia, 1985

581. Reivich M, Holling E, Roberts B et al: Reversal of blood flow through the vertebral artery and its effect on cerebral circulation. N Engl J Med 265:88, 1961

582. Resch JA, Okabe N, Loewenson RB et al: Patterns of vessel involvement in cerebral atherosclerosis: a comparative study between a Japanese and Minnesota population. J Atherosclerosis Res 9:239, 1969

583. Reul GJ, Cooley DA, Olson SK et al: Long-term results of direct vertebral artery operations. Surgery 96:854, 1984

584. Reuther R, Dorndorf W: Aspirin in patients with cerebral ischemia and normal angiograms or nonsurgical lesions: the results of a double-blind trial. p. 97. In Breddin K, Dorndorf W, Loew D et al (eds): Acetylsalicylic Acid in Cerebral Ischemia and Coronary Heart Disease. Schattauer, Stuttgart, 1978

585. Reznik M: Le ramollissement du tronc cérébral. Acta Neurol Belg 81:257, 1981

586. Richter R: Collaterals between the external carotid artery and the vertebral artery in cases of thrombosis of the internal carotid artery. Acta Radiol [Diagn] (Stockh) 40:108, 1953

587. Rieke K, Krieger D, Adams H-P et al: Therapeutic strategies in space-occupying cerebellar infarction based on clinical, neuroradiological and neurophysiological data. Cerebrovasc Dis 3:45–55, 1993

588. Rigauts H, Marchal G, Baert AL, Hupke R: Technical note: initial experience with volume CT scanning. J Comput Assist Tomogr 14:675–682, 1990

589. Ringel S, Harrison S, Norenberg M et al: Fibromuscular dysplasia: multiple "spontaneous" dissecting aneurysms of the major cranial arteries. Ann Neurol I:301, 1977

590. Ringelstein EB, Zeumer H: Delayed reversal of vertebral artery blood flow following percutaneous transluminal angioplasty for subclavian steal syndrome. Neuroradiology 26:189–198, 1984

591. Ringer RA, Culberson JL: Extensor tone disinhibition from an infarction within the midline anterior cerebellar lobe. J Neurol Neurosurg Psychiatry 52:1597–1599, 1989

592. Robertson J: Neck manipulation as a cause of stroke. Stroke 12:1, 1981

593. Rodda R: The vascular lesions associated with cerebellar infarcts. Proc Aust Assoc Neurol 8:101–110, 1971

594. Rogers L, Sweeney P: Stroke: a neurological complication of wrestling. Am J Sports Med 7:352, 1979

595. Romanul F: Examination of the brain and spinal cord. p. 131. In Tedeschi CG (ed): Neuropathology: Methods and Diagnosis. Little, Brown, Boston, 1970

596. Romanul F, Abramowicz A: Changes in brain and pial vessels in arterial boundary zones. Arch Neurol 11:40, 1964

597. Roon A, Ehrenfeld W, Cooke P et al: Vertebral artery reconstruction. Am J Surg 138:29, 1979

598. Ropper A, Fisher CM, Kleinman G: Pyramidal infarction in the medulla: a cause of pure motor hemiplegia sparing the face. Neurology (NY) 29:91, 1979

599. Rosengart A, DeWitt LD, Caplan LR et al: Noninvasive tests in vertebro-basilar occlusive disease. Ann Neurol 32:265, 1992

600. Rosengart A, Hedges TR III, Teal PA et al: Intermittent downbeat nystagmus due to vertebral artery compression. Neurology 43:216–218, 1993

601. Roski R, Spetzler R, Hopkins L: Occipital artery to posterior inferior cerebellar artery bypass for vertebrobasilar ischemia. Neurosurgery 10:44, 1982

602. Ross MA, Biller J, Adams HP et al: Magnetic resonance imaging in Wallenberg's lateral medullary syndrome. Stroke 17:542, 1986

603. Rother J, Schwartz A, Rautenberg W, Hennerici M: Magnetic resonance angiography of spontaneous vertebral artery dissection suspected on Doppler ultrasonography. J Neurol (Germany) 242:430–436, 1995

604. Rother J, Wentz K-U, Rautenberg W et al: Magnetic resonance angiography in vertebrobasilar ischemia. Stroke 24:1310–1315, 1993

605. Rothrock JF, Lyden PD, Hesselink JR et al: Brain magnetic resonance imaging in the evaluation of lacunar stroke. Stroke 18:781, 1987

606. Rubenstein RL, Norman D, Schindler R et al: Cerebellar infarction: a presentation of vertigo. Laryngoscope 90:505, 1980

607. Russel CK: The syndrome of bracchium conjunctivum and the tractus spinothalamicus. Arch Neurol Psychiatry 25:1003–1010, 1931

608. Sacco RL, Bello JA, Traub R et al: Selective propriocep-

tive loss from a thalamic lacunar stroke. Stroke 18:1160, 1987

609. Sacco RL, Freddo L, Bello JA et al: Wallenberg's lateral medullary syndrome. Clinical-magnetic resonance imaging correlation. Arch Neurol 50:609–614, 1993

610. Sackett J, Strother C, Crummy A et al: Computerized fluoroscopic intravenous arteriography of the carotid arteries. Stroke 12:122, 1981

611. Sakai F, Ishii K, Igarashi H et al: Regional cerebral blood flow during an attack of vertebrobasilar insufficiency. Stroke 19:1426–1430, 1988

612. Samson M, Milhout B, Onnient Y et al: Les ramollissements cérébelleux. Données diagnostiques et pronostiques. Semin Hop Paris 62:2766–2769, 1986

613. Samson M, Milhout B, Thiebot J et al: Forme bénigne des infarctus cérébelleux. Rev Neurol 137:373, 1981

614. Savoiardo M, Bracchi M, Passerini A et al: The vascular territories in the cerebellum and brainstem: CT and MR study. AJNR 8:199, 1987

615. Sawada H, Seriu N, Udaka F, Kameyama M: Magnetic resonance imaging of medial medullary infarction. Stroke 21:963–966, 1990

616. Schievink WI, Michels VV, Mokri B et al: A familial syndrome of arterial dissections with lentiginosis. N Engl J Med 332:576–579, 1995

617. Schievink WI, Mokri B: Familial aorto-cervicocephalic arterial dissections and congenitally bicuspid aortic valve. Stroke 26:1935–1940, 1995

618. Schievink WI, Mokri B, O'Fallon WM: Spontaneous recurrent cervical-artery dissection. N Engl J Med 330:393–397, 1994

619. Schievink WI, Mokri B, Piepgras DG, Kuiper JD: Recurrent spontaneous arterial dissections. Risk in familial versus nonfamilial disease. Stroke 27:622–624, 1996

620. Schoning M, Walter J: Evaluation of the vertebrobasilar posterior system by transcranial color Duplex sonography in adults. Stroke 23:1280–1286, 1992

621. Schutz H, Yeung H, Chiu M et al: Dilatation of vertebral artery stenosis. N Engl J Med 304:732, 1981

622. Schwaighofer BW, Klein MV, Lyden PD, Hesselink JR: MR imaging of vertebrobasilar vascular disease. J Comput Assist Tomogr 14:895–904, 1990

623. Schwartz A, Rautenberg W, Hennerici M: Dolichoectatic intracranial arteries: review of selected aspects. Cerebrovasc Dis 3:273–279, 1993

624. Schwartz C, Mitchell J: Atheroma of the carotid and vertebral arterial systems. BMJ 2:1057, 1961

625. Schwartz RB, Jones KM, Chernoff DM et al: Common carotid bifurcation: evaluation with spiral CT. Radiology 185:513–519, 1992

626. Scotti G, Spinnler H, Sterzi R et al: Cerebellar softening. Ann Neurol 8:133, 1980

627. Seales DM, Torkelson RD, Shuman RM et al: Abnormal brainstem auditory evoked potentials and neuropathology in the "locked-in" syndrome. Neurology 31:893–896, 1981

628. Seelig J, Selhorst J, Young H et al: Ventriculostomy for hydrocephalus in cerebellar hemorrhage. Neurology (NY) 31:1537, 1981

629. Segarra J: Cerebral vascular disease and behavior. I. The syndrome of the mesencephalic artery (basilar artery bifurcation). Arch Neurol 22:408, 1970

630. Seldarogiu P, Yazici H, Ozdemir C et al: Neurologic involvement in Behçet's syndrome: a prospective study. Arch Neurol 46:265, 1989

631. Selhorst J, Hoyt W, Feinsod M et al: Midbrain corectopia. Arch Neurol 33:193, 1976

632. Serra Catafan J, Rubio F, Peres Serra J: Peduncular hallucinosis associated with posterior thalamic infarction. J Neurol 239:89–90, 1992

633. Sevestre H, Vercken JB, Hénin D et al: Encéphalopathie anoxique après incompétence cardio-circulatoire. Etude neuropathologique à propos de 16 cas. Ann Med Intern 139:245–250, 1988

634. Sharpe J, Rosenberg M, Hoyt W et al: Paralytic pontine exotropia. Neurology (NY) 24:1076, 1974

635. Sheehan D, Smith G: A study of the anatomy of vertebral thrombosis. Lancet 2:614, 1937

636. Sheehan S, Bauer R, Meyer J: Vertebral artery compression in cervical spondylosis. Neurology (NY) 10:968, 1960

637. Shenkin HA, Zavala M: Cerebellar strokes: mortality, surgical indications, and results of ventricular drainage. Lancet 11:429–431, 1982

638. Sherman D, Hart R, Easton JD: Abrupt change in head position and cerebral infarction. Stroke 12:2, 1981

639. Siekert R, Millikan C, Whisnant J: Reversal of blood flow in the vertebral arteries. Ann Intern Med 61:64, 1964

640. Siekert RG, Whisnant JP, Millikan CH: Surgical and anticoagulation therapy of occlusive cerebrovascular disease. Ann Intern Med 58:637, 1963

641. Silbert PL, Mokri B, Schievink W: Headache and neck pain in spontaneous internal carotid and vertebral artery dissections. Neurology 45:1517–1522, 1995

642. Silverstein A: Acute infarctions of the brainstem in the distribution of the basilar artery. Conf Neurol 24:37, 1964

643. Silverstein A: Pontine infarction. p. 13. In Vinken P, Bruyn G (eds): Handbook of Clinical Neurology. Vol. 12. North-Holland, Amsterdam, 1972

644. Simard D: Cerebral vasomotor paralysis during migraine attack. Arch Neurol 29:207, 1973

645. Simmons Z, Biller J, Adams HP et al: Cerebellar infarction: comparison of computed tomography and magnetic resonance imaging. Ann Neurol 19:291, 1986

646. Sivenius J, Piekkinen PJ, Smets P et al: The European Stroke Prevention Study (ESPS): results by arterial distribution. Ann Neurol 29:596–600, 1991

647. Skinhoj E: Hemodynamic studies within the brain during migraine. Arch Neurol 29:95, 1973

648. Sloan MA: Thrombolysis and stroke: past and future. Arch Neurol 44:748, 1987

649. Smith JL, Cogan D: Internuclear ophthalmoplegia. Arch Ophthalmol 61:687, 1959

650. Smith M, Launa J: Upward gaze paralysis following unilateral pretectal infarction. Arch Neurol 38:127, 1981

651. Smoker WR, Corbett JJ, Gentry LR et al: High-resolution computed tomography of the basilar artery: 2. Vertebrobasilar dolichoectasia: clinical-pathological correlation and review. AJNR 7:61–72, 1986

652. So EL, Toole JF, Dalal P et al: Cephalic fibromuscular

dysplasia in 32 patients: clinical findings and radiologic features. Arch Neurol 38:619, 1981

653. Soffin G, Feldman M, Bender M: Alterations of sensory levels in vascular lesions of lateral medulla. Arch Neurol 18:178, 1968

654. Spetzler RF, Hadley MN, Martin NA et al: Vertebrobasilar insufficiency. I. Microsurgical treatment of extracranial vertebrobasilar disease. J Neurosurg 66:648, 1987

655. Spiller WG: The symptom-complex of occlusion of PICA. J Nerv Ment Dis 35:365–387, 1908

656. Stein B, McCormick W, Rodriques J et al: Incidence and significance of occlusive vascular disease of the extracranial arteries as documented by post-mortem angiography. Trans Am Neurol Assoc 86:60, 1961

657. Steinke W, Sacco RL, Mohr JP et al: Thalamic stroke: presentation and prognosis of infarcts and hemorrhages. Arch Neurol 49:703–710, 1992

658. Stephens R, Stilwell D: Arteries and Veins of the Human Brain. Charles C Thomas, Springfield, IL, 1969

659. Stern B, Krumholz A, Weiss H et al: Evaluation of brainstem stroke using brainstem auditory evoked responses. Stroke 13:705, 1981

660. Stern BJ, Krumholz A, Weiss HD et al: Evaluation of brainstem stroke using brainstem auditory evoked responses. Stroke 13:705–711, 1982

661. Stockard J, Sharbrough F: Unique contributions of short latency auditory and somatosensory evoked potentials to neurologic diagnosis. p. 231. In Desmedt J (ed): Clinical Uses of Cerebral Brainstem and Spinal Somatosensory Evoked Potentials. Karger, Basel, 1980

662. Stopford J: The arteries of the pons and medulla oblongata. I. J Anat Physiol 50:131, 1915

663. Stopford J: The arteries of the pons and medulla oblongata. II. J Anat Physiol 50:255, 1916

664. Struck LK, Biller J, Bruno A et al: Superior cerebellar artery territory infarction. Cerebrovasc Dis 1:71–75, 1991

665. Strukel RJ, Garrick JG: Thoracic outlet compression in athletes: a report of four cases. Am J Sports Med 6:35, 1978

666. Stuss D, Alexander M, Lieberman A: An extraordinary form of confabulation. Neurology (NY) 28:1166, 1978

667. Sundt T, Piepgras D, Houser O et al: Interposition saphenous vein grafts for advanced occlusive disease and large aneurysms in the posterior circulation. J Neurosurg 56:205, 1982

668. Sundt T, Smith H, Campbell J et al: Transluminal angioplasty for basilar artery stenosis. Mayo Clin Proc 55:673, 1980

669. Sundt T, Whisnant J, Piepgras D et al: Intracranial bypass grafts for vertebral basilar ischemia. Mayo Clin Proc 53:12, 1978

670. Sundt TM, Campbell JK, Houser OW: Transpositions and anastomoses between the posterior cerebral and superior cerebellar arteries. Report of two cases. J Neurosurg 55:967–970, 1981

671. Sundt TM, Piepgras D: Occipital to posterior inferior cerebellar artery bypass surgery. J Neurosurg 49:916, 1978

672. Susac J, Hoyt W, Daroff R et al: Clinical spectrum of ocular bobbing. J Neurol Neurosurg Psychiatry 33:771, 1970

673. Swanson J, Vick N: Basilar artery migraine. Neurology (NY) 28:782, 1978

674. Swanson R, Schmidley J: Amnestic syndrome and vertical gaze palsy: early detection of bilateral thalamic infarction by CT and MRI. Stroke 16:823, 1985

675. Symonds C: Two cases of thrombosis of subclavian artery with contralateral hemiplegia of sudden onset, probably embolic. Brain 50:259, 1927

676. Sypert G, Alvord E: Cerebellar infarction: a clinicopathological study. Arch Neurol 32:357, 1975

677. Szdzuy D, Lehman R: Hypoplastic distal part of the basilar artery. Neuroradiology 4:118, 1972

678. Tack KJ, Rhame FS, Brown B, Thompson RC: Aspergillus osteomyelitis. Report of four cases and review of the literature. Am J Med 83:295–300, 1982

679. Tahmoush A, Brooks J, Keltner J: Palatal myoclonus associated with abnormal ocular and extremity movements. Arch Neurol 27:431, 1972

680. Takahashi S: Atlas of Vertebral Angiography. University Park Press, Baltimore, 1974

681. Takahashi S, Goto K, Fukasawa H et al: Computed tomography of cerebral infarction along the distribution of the basal perforating arteries. II. Thalamic arterial group. Radiology 155:119, 1985

682. Tandon P: Vertebrobasilar insufficiency secondary to cervical spondylosis: an overdiagnosed disease. J Indian Med Assoc 74:77, 1980

683. Taneda M, Ozaki K, Wakayama A et al: Cerebellar infarction with obstructive hydrocephalus. J Neurosurg 57:83–91, 1982

684. Tatemichi T, Steinke W, Duncan C et al: Paramedian thalamo-peduncular infarction: clinical syndromes and magnetic resonance imaging. Ann Neurol 32:162–171, 1992

685. Tatemichi TK, Oropeza LA, Sacco RL et al: Doppler diagnosis of vertebral artery occlusion: role of runoff into the posterior inferior cerebellar artery. Ann Neurol 26:158, 1989

686. Tatlow W, Bammer H: Syndrome of vertebral artery compression. Neurology (NY) 7:331, 1957

687. Tatsumi T, Shenkin H: Occlusion of the vertebral artery. J Neurol Neurosurg Psychiatry 28:235, 1965

688. Taveras JM, Wood EH: Diagnostic Neuroradiology. Vol. II. pp. 783–787, 793–796. Williams & Wilkins, Baltimore, 1976

689. Tegeler CH, Kremkau FW, Hitchings LP: Color velocity imaging: introduction to a new ultrasound technology. J Neuroimaging 1:85–90, 1991

690. Tettenborn B, Caplan LR, Kramer G, Hopf HC: Electrophysiology in posterior circulation disease. pp. 124–129. In Berguer R, Caplan LR (eds): Vertebrobasilar Arterial Disease. Quality Medical Publishing St. Louis, 1991

691. Tettenborn B, Estol C, DeWitt LD et al: Accuracy of transcranial Doppler in the vertebrobasilar circulation. J Neurol 237:159, 1990

692. The EC-IC Bypass Study Group: Failure of extracranial-intracranial bypass to reduce the risk of ischemic stroke. N Engl J Med 313:1191–1200, 1985

693. The French Study of Aortic Plaques in Stroke Group: Atherosclerotic disease of the aortic arch as a risk factor for recurrent ischemic stroke. N Engl J Med 334: 1216–1221, 1996

694. The National Institute of Neurological Disorders and Stroke rt-PA Stroke Study Group: Tissue plasminogen activator for acute ischemic stroke. N Engl J Med 333: 1561–1587, 1995

695. The Warfarin-Aspirin Symptomatic Intracranial Disease (WASID) Study Group: Prognosis of patients with symptomatic vertebral or basilar artery stenosis. Stroke 26: 162, 1995

696. Thevenet A: Endarterectomy of the vertebral artery. pp. 224–235. In Berguer R, Caplan LR (eds): Vertebrobasilar Arterial Disease. Quality Medical Publishing, St. Louis, 1992

697. Thomas HM: Symptoms following the occlusion of the PICA. J Nerv Ment Dis 34:48–49, 1907

698. Thompson GN: Cerebellar embolism. Bull Los Angeles Neurol Soc 9:140–155, 1944

699. Thompson JR, Simmons C, Hasso A et al: Occlusion of the intradural vertebrobasilar artery. Neuroradiology 14: 219, 1978

700. Titus F, Montalban J, Molins A et al: Migraine-related stroke: brain infarction in superior cerebellar artery territory demonstrated by nuclear magnetic resonance. Acta Neurol Scand 79:357–360, 1989

701. Tohgi H, Takahashi S, Chibra K et al: Cerebellar infarction. Clinical and neuroimaging analysis in 293 patients. Stroke 24:1697–1701, 1993

702. Tomaszek DE, Rosner MJ: Cerebellar infarction: analysis of twenty-one cases. Surg Neurol 24:223–226, 1985

703. Torma T, Fogelholm M: Complications of cerebral angiography with urograffin. Acta Neurol Scand 43:616, 1967

704. Touboul PJ, Bousser MG, Laplane D et al: Duplex scanning of normal vertebral arteries. Stroke 17:97, 1986

705. Touboul P-J, Mas J-L, Bousser M-G, Laplane D: Duplex scanning in extracranial vertebral artery dissection. Stroke 18:116–121, 1987

706. Tougeron A, Samson Y, Schaison M et al: Syndrome dysarthrie-main malhabile par infarctus cérébelleux. Rev Neurol (Paris) 144:596–597, 1988

707. Toyoda K, Hasegawa Y, Yonehara T et al: Bilateral medial medullary infarction with oculomotor disorders. Stroke 23:1657–1659, 1992

708. Toyoda K, Saku Y, Ibayashi S et al: Pontine infarction extending to the basal surface. Stroke 25:2171–2178, 1994

709. Trattnig S, Hubsch P, Schuster H et al: Color-coded Doppler imaging of normal vertebral arteries. Stroke 21: 1222, 1990

710. Trattnig S, Schwaighofer B, Hubsch P et al: Color-coded Doppler sonography of vertebral arteries. J Ultrasound Med 10:221–226, 1991

711. Trelles J, Trelles L, Urquraga C: Le ramollissement médian du bulbe. Rev Neurol 129:91, 1973

712. Trojanowski J, Wray S: Vertical gaze ophthalmoplegia: selective paralysis of downgaze. Neurology (NY) 30:605, 1980

713. Tsai F, Teal J, Heishima G et al: Computed tomography in acute posterior fossa infarcts. AJNR 3:149, 1982

714. Tsuchiya T, Yasaka M, Yamaguchi T et al: Imaging of the basal cerebral arteries and measurement of blood velocity in adults by using transcranial real-time color flow Doppler sonography. AJNR 12:497–502, 1991

715. Tunick PA, Culliford AT, Lamparello PJ, Kronzon I: Atheromatosis of the aortic arch as an occult source of multiple systemic emboli. Ann Intern Med 114: 391–392, 1991

716. Tunick PA, Kronzon I: Protruding atherosclerotic plaque in the aortic arch of patients with systemic embolization: a new finding seen by transesophageal echocardiography. Am Heart J 120:658–660, 1990

717. Tunick PA, Rosenzweig BP, Katz ES et al: High risk for vascular events in patients with protruding aortic atheromas: a prospective study. J Am Coll Cardiol 23: 1085–1090, 1994

718. Uchino A, Ohnari N, Ohno M: MR imaging of intracranial vertebral artery occlusion. Neuroradiology 31: 403–407, 1989

719. Ueda K, Toole J, McHenry L: Carotid and vertebrobasilar transient ischemia attacks: clinical and angiographic correlation. Neurology (NY) 29:1094, 1979

720. Van Bogaert L: L'hallucinose pedonculaire. Rev Neurol (Paris) 43:608–617, 1927

721. Van Bogaert L: Syndrome inferieure du noyau rouge, troubles psycho-sensoriels d'origine mésocephalique. Rev Neurol (Paris) 40:416–423, 1924

722. Van der Drift J: The EEG in cerebrovascular disease. p. 267. In Vinken P, Bruyn G (eds): Handbook of Clinical Neurology. Vol. 2. North-Holland, Amsterdam, 1972

723. Veistraek M: The search for the ideal thrombolytic agent. J Am Coll Cardiol 10:4B–10B, 1987

724. von Budingen H-J, Staudacher T: Evaluation of vertebrobasilar disease. pp. 167–195. In Newell DW, Aaslid R (eds): Transcranial Doppler. Lippincott-Raven, Philadelphia, 1992

725. von Cramm D, Hebel N, Schieri U: A contribution to the anatomical basis of thalamic amnesia. Brain 108:993, 1985

726. von Kummer R, Brandt T, Muller-Kuypers M et al: Thrombolytic therapy of basilar artery occlusion: preconditions for recanalization and good clinical outcome. pp. 343–348. In Yamaguchi T, Mori E, Minematsu K (eds): Thrombolytic Therapy in Acute Ischemic Stroke III. Springer-Verlag, Berlin, 1995

727. von Reutern GM, Budingen JH: Ultraschalldiagnostik der Hirnversorgenden Arterien. Thieme, Stuttgart, 1989

728. von Reutern GM, Pourcelot L: Cardiac cycle-dependent alternating flow in vertebral arteries with subclavian artery stenoses. Stroke 9:224, 1978

729. Vonofakos D, Marcu H, Hacker H: CT diagnosis of basilar artery occlusion. AJNR 4:525–528, 1983

730. Voordecker P, Brunko E, de Beyl Z: Selective unilateral absence or attenuation of wave V of brainstem auditory evoked potentials with intrinsic brain-stem lesions. Arch Neurol 45:1272–1276, 1988

731. Vuilleumier P, Bogousslavsky J, Regli F: Infarction of the lower brainstem. Clinical, aetiological and MR-topographical correlations. Brain 118:1013–1025, 1995

732. Waither H: Uber einen Dammerzustand mit triebhafter Erregung nach Thalamusschadigung. Monatsschr Psychiatr Neurol 111:1–16, 1945–6

733. Wall M, Slamovits T, Weisberg LA et al: Vertical gaze ophthalmoplegia from infarction in the area of the posterior thalamo-subthalamic paramedian artery. Stroke 17: 546, 1986

734. Wallenberg A: Acute bulbar affection. Arch Psychiatr Nervenheilkd 27:504, 1895

735. Wallenberg A: Anatomischer Befund in einem als "Acute Bulbäraffection (Embolie der art. cerebellar. post. inf. sinistr.?)." Beschriebenem falle. Arch F Psychiatr 34:923–959, 1901

736. Walsh TJ, Hier DB, Caplan LR: Aspergillosis of the central nervous system: clinicopathological analysis of 17 patients. Ann Neurol 18:574–582, 1985

737. Walsh TJ, Hutchins GM, Bukley BH, Mendelsohn G: Fungal infections of the heart: analysis of 51 autopsy cases. Am J Cardiol 45:357–366, 1980

738. Warach S, Chien D, Ronthal M, Edelman RR: Fast magnetic resonance diffusion-weighted imaging of acute human stroke. Neurology 42:1717–1723, 1992

739. Warach S, Li W, Ronthal M, Edelman RR: Acute cerebral ischemia: evaluation with dynamic contrast-enhanced MR imaging and MR angiography. Radiology 182:41–47, 1992

740. Watson AJ: Dissecting aneurysm of arteries other than the aorta. J Pathol Bacteriol 72:439, 1956

741. Weibel J, Fields W: Angiography of the posterior cervicocranial circulation. AJR 98:660, 1966

742. Weinstein M, Modie M, Little J et al: Digital subtraction angiography to evaluate carotid and intracranial arteriosclerotic disease. Stroke 12:123, 1981

743. Wentz K-U, Rother J, Schwartz A et al: Intracranial vertebrobasilar system: MR angiography. Radiology 190: 105–110, 1994

744. Whisnant J: Discussion in cerebral vascular diseases. p. 156. In Millikan C, Siekert R, Whisnant J (eds): Transactions of the Third Princeton Conference on Cerebrovascular Disease. Grune & Stratton, Orlando, FL, 1961

745. Whisnant J, Martin M, Sayre G: Atherosclerotic stenosis of cervical arteries. Arch Neurol 5:429, 1961

746. White DN, Ketelaars EJ, Cledgett PR: Non-invasive techniques for the recording of vertebral artery flow and their limitations. Ultrasound Med Biol 6:315, 1980

747. Whittier J: Ballism and the subthalamic nucleus. Arch Neurol Psychiatry 58:672, 1947

748. Wildemann B, Hutschenreuter M, Kriegtl D et al: Infusion of recombinant tissue plasminogen activator for basilar artery occlusion. Stroke 21:1513, 1990

749. Wilkins R, Brody I: Wallenberg's syndrome. Arch Neurol 22:379, 1970

750. Wilkinson I: The vertebral artery. Arch Neurol 27:392, 1972

751. Wilkinson I, Russel R: Arteries of the head and neck in giant cell arteritis. Arch Neurol 27:378, 1972

752. Williams D: The syndromes of basilar insufficiency. p. 202. In Garland H (ed): Scientific Aspects of Neurology. Williams & Wilkins, Baltimore, 1961

753. Williams D, Wilson T: The diagnosis of the major and minor syndromes of basilar insufficiency. Brain 85:741, 1962

754. Wilson G, Winkelman NW: Occlusion of the PICA. J Nerv Ment Dis 65:125–130, 1927

755. Wilson SAK: Ectopia pupillae in certain mesencephalic lesions. Brain 29:524, 1906

756. Wishart D: Complications in vertebral angiography as compared to nonvertebral cerebral angiography in 447 studies. AJR Radium Ther Nucl Med 113:527, 1971

757. Wolf J: The Classical Brainstem Syndromes. Charles C Thomas, Springfield, IL, 1971

758. Wolman L: Cerebral dissecting aneurysms. Brain 82: 276, 1959

759. Wood D: Cerebrovascular complications of sickle cell anemia. Stroke 9:73, 1978

760. Wood MW, Murphey F: Obstructive hydrocephalus due to infarction of a cerebellar hemisphere. J Neurosurg 30:260–263, 1969

761. Woodhurst W: Cerebellar infarction: review of recent experience. Can J Neurol Sci 7:97, 1980

762. Woolsey R, Chang H: Fatal basilar artery occlusion following cervical spine injury. Paraplegia 17:280, 1979

763. Worster-Drought C, Allen I: Thrombosis of the superior cerebellar artery. Lancet 2:1137, 1929

764. Yap C, Mayo C, Barron K: "Ocular bobbing" in palata; myoclonus. Arch Neurol 18:304, 1968

765. Yates A, Guest D: Cerebral embolism due to an ununited fracture of the clavicle and subclavian thrombosis. Lancet 2:25, 1928

766. Youl BD, Coutellier A, Dubois B et al: Three cases of spontaneous extracranial vertebral artery dissection. Stroke 21:618–625, 1990

767. Young RC, Bennett JE, Vogel CL et al: Aspergillosis: the spectrum of the disease in 98 patients. Medicine (Baltimore) 49:147–173, 1970

768. Yu Y, Moseley I, Pullicino P et al: The clinical pictures of ectasia of the intracerebral arteries. J Neurol Neurosurg Psychiatry 45:29, 1982

769. Zeal AA, Rhoton AL: Microsurgical anatomy of the posterior cerebral artery. J Neurosurg 48:534, 1978

770. Zeumer H: Vascular recanalizing technique in interventional neuroradiology. J Neurol 231:287, 1985

771. Zeumer H, Hacke W, Ringelstein EB: Local intraarterial thrombolysis in vertebrobasilar thromboembolic disease. AJNR 4:401, 1983

772. Zimmerman RA, Gusnard DA, Bilaniuk LT: Pediatric craniocervical spiral CT. Neuroradiology 34:112–116, 1992

773. Zulch K: On circulatory disturbances in borderline zones of cerebral and spinal vessels. In Proceedings of the Second International Congress of Neurology. Excerpta Medica, London, 1955

774. Zülch KJ: The Cerebral Infarct. Springer-Verlag, Berlin, 1986

775. Zülch KJ, Behrend R: The pathogenesis and topography of anoxia, hypoxia, and ischemia of the brain in man. p. 144. In Meyer J, Gastaut H (eds): Cerebral Anoxia and the EEG. Charles C Thomas, Springfield, IL, 1961

Lacunes

J. P. MOHR

JOSÉ-LUIS MARTI-VILALTA

Lacune is a term coined to describe the small cavity remaining in the brain tissue that developed after the necrotic tissue of a deep infarct had been removed (Fig. 23.1). The process is no different from that of any other brain infarcts except that the more common ones affecting the convexity leave a depression or dent in the brain, whereas those confined to the depths must leave a hole, that is, a lacune.

Interest in these lesions arose from their unusual vascular pathology, their rather pure clinical pictures, and their high frequency of presentation in stroke series, about 20% of cerebral infarcts. Little trouble was encountered in separating them from postmortem gas bubble artifacts at autopsy (Fig. 23.2). With improving brain images, some problems have been encountered in trying to determine if the small lesion is an infarct, the late product of a small hemorrhage, or merely an enlarged Virchow-Robin space, but even these problems occur infrequently. In the early years of study, they seemed best explained by a special arteriopathy encountered in hypertension,[52] although other etiologies, including embolism, were also found at autopsy. At first, the clinical syndromes seemed relatively pure since they occurred mainly in the motor pathways or to the thalamus, producing pure motor or pure sensory stroke. Clinical recognition of a small infarct was initially considered important since the hypertensive arteriopathy that affected the vessel feeding a lacune was too small to be seen on angiography, and too little of the brain substance was affected by infarction to disturb the electroencephalogram. Because the arteriopathy was the same as that in hypertensive parenchymatous hemorrhage, anticoagulation was considered too risky to warrant casual use. All told, the recognition of lacunar syndromes in the days before useful brain imaging was both challenging clinically and relevant therapeutically.

The initial concept of lacunes as a set of clinical syndromes with pathologic criteria was soon diluted by new findings. While none of the findings have fundamentally altered the basic concepts, so many exceptions to the basic concepts have appeared that some have challenged their utility. Numerous studies have claimed that the syndromes may have causes other than hypertensive arteriopathy.[52,63,74,146,165] Although the individual reports often contained one or more clinical elements that deviated from the original syndromes, the effect was to blunt the impact of a causal relation of the syndromes

to hypertension. With the introduction of high-quality brain imaging, it was not long before a wider range of locations of small deep infarcts was found, together with an expansion of the syndromes associated with such lesions, now including the brain stem, parts of the thalamus, and other nuclei in the basal ganglia, corona radiata, centrum semiovale, and even some straddling the thalamus and internal capsule; concept was thus expanded to include syndromes overlapping with those caused by Binswanger's disease.[52,120,141,168,192] The earlier insistence on autopsy studies has largely been lost under the weight of publications based entirely on computed tomography (CT) or magnetic resonance imaging (MRI) findings. In recent years, it has been the exception, not the rule, to find a case report with autopsy correlation. Lamentably, the term lacune has passed into common use to refer to any small, deep lesion. Many authors at least attempt to show that its cause is ischemic, but some have exercised no such caution, and the notion has even been introduced that they may come from small hemorrhages. The term lacune is a useful concept when it refers to a lacunar syndrome implying a variety of causes, topographies, and clinical features that need a careful study by the clinician and not a simple diagnosis at the bedside.

Historical Aspects

In 1838 Dechambre[34] used the term *lacune* for the first time with the pathologic criteria mentioned above. From its initial description until the end of the past century, the term lacune was frequently misused in cerebral specimens, and the entity was confused with other cavitary lesions in the brain such as *état criblé* (Fig. 23.3) (small bilateral, multiple lesions in the white matter described by Durand-Fardel in 1842[42], residual necrotic tissue of small infarcts or hemorrhages, enlarged perivascular spaces (Fig. 23.4), and porosis due to postmortem bacterial autolysis. Pierre Marie[127] used lacune as his descriptive term for 50 cases of capsular infarction and clearly established the concept and classification of different small cavities in the brain, ending the period of morphologic confusion. He formulated a syndrome featuring sudden onset of incomplete

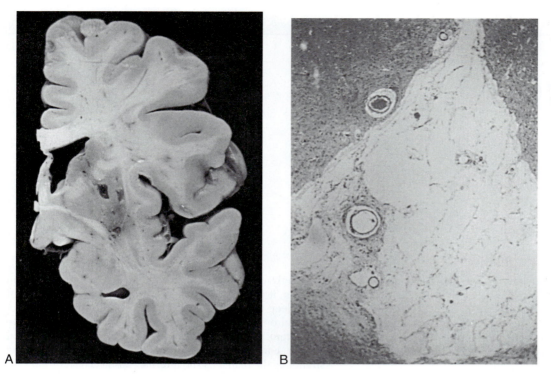

Figure 23.1 Lacunes in the basal ganglia. (**A**) Macroscopic coronal section. (**B**) Microscopic pathology. (H&E stain.)

hemiplegia, unaccompanied by persisting sensory loss, homonymous hemianopia, or permanent aphasia. Considerable improvement in the paralysis occurred within hours to days, but complete recovery was unusual. Walking was disturbed in a special fashion, the patients taking small steps described as *marche à petits pas de Dejerine*. In modern times this latter state has been attributed to patients with many foci of lacunar infarction, the so-called lacunar state. Marie emphasized a capsular and lenticular location for the syndrome. Ferrand[50] later claimed that the same syndrome occurred whether the lesion was capsular or pontine in location. Over 20 years later,

Figure 23.2 Two gas bubble artifacts (arrowheads). Macroscopic coronal section.

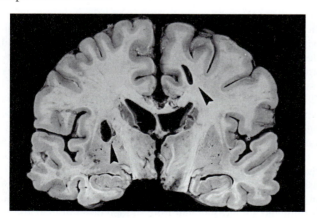

Foix and Levy[68] reiterated these principles, adding the claim that a deep lesion produced a hemiparesis without visual or sensory disturbance, adding the formulation that the hemiparesis affected the arm and leg equally. In another publication, Foix and Hillemand[67] described the effects of a pontine infarction as a "simple" hemiplegia affecting the arm more than the leg, with an associated mild dysarthria. During the first quarter of the present century doubts persisted about the etiology and pathogenesis of lacunes—whether they were ischemic, or hemorrhagic, or inflammatory. The German pathologists Cecil and Oscar Vogt[189] firmly established the ischemic etiology. From the 1930s to the 1960s, only passing references to a capsular lesion producing a pure hemiplegia can be found in most standard textbooks of neurology.[3,195]

Lacunes began their modern comeback almost entirely through the efforts of C.M. Fisher. Largely alone, in a few instances accompanied by or in support of younger colleagues, he described pure motor hemiplegia,[64] pure sensory stroke,[58] homolateral ataxia and crural paresis[63] (known mainly thereafter as ataxic hemiparesis), dysarthria-clumsy hand syndrome,[53] sensorimotor stroke,[142] basilar branch syndromes,[65] and the vascular pathology underlying lacunes.[55] The position was so thoroughly developed that it triggered companion studies, many corroborating,[132,142] and others enlarging on the clinical entities, vascular pathology, and clinicoradiologic correlations.[41,156,193] Other studies attacked the basic principles,[26,168,192] some arguing for other etiologies including embolism,[136] and others recommending that the concepts be abandoned altogether.[112] However, the high frequency of publications worldwide[117] indicates that the subject has be-

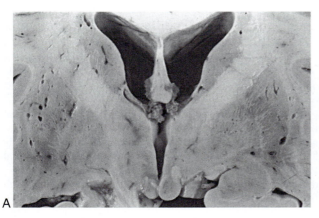 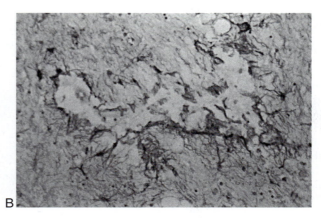

Figure 23.3 État criblé. (**A**) Macroscopic coronal section. (**B**) Microscopic pathology. (GFAP stain.)

come firmly established among the syndromes of stroke. In some countries, notably China, the high frequency of deep infarcts has even been proposed to have a racial or ethnic basis.[33,88]

Definitions

As a term based on neuropathologic findings, lacune refers to a small, deep infarct attributable to a primary arterial disease that involves a penetrating branch of a large cerebral artery (Fig. 23.1). It should not be used to describe lesions of nonvascular origin, nor does it apply to deep infarction that is simply part of a larger stroke affecting the cerebral surface in continuity or separately, such as occurs in embolism affecting the middle cerebral artery. It is also inapplicable to describe deep infarction from disease involving the stems of the large cerebral arteries (such as the middle or anterior cerebral) that affects the penetrating branches.

Figure 23.4 Multiple enlarged perivascular spaces in the putamen of a patient with marked small blood vessel disease. (H&E, ×40.) (From Garcia and Ho,[70] with permission.)

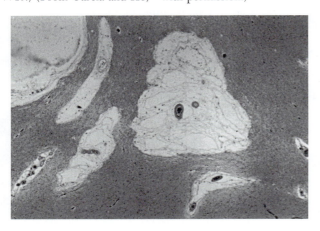

The low frequency of autopsy studies has forced modification of the definitions to include small, deep lesions found by brain imaging, whether CT or MRI. Numerous attempts at definitions have been made, but the most widely seen is the attempt to distinguish among a small, deep infarct, the residue of a small hemorrhage, and dilated Virchow-Robin spaces. For those inclined to use numbers, these are types I, II, and III lacunes, respectively. In an attempt to keep the presentation orderly, emphasis is placed here on the autopsy-based material, followed by those studies based only on brain imaging, and finally on clinical studies alone.

Pathoanatomy

SIZE

Most autopsy-documented lacunar infarcts are small, ranging from 0.2 to 15 mm³ in size.[60] They vary according to the territory supplied by the occluded vessel feeding the infarct. In general, these vessels are 100 to 400 μm[58] in size and serve territories varying from little more than a cylinder the size of the vessel itself to wedges as large as 15 mm on a side. While the smallest infarcts are unresolved by CT scanners, and occasionally even escape detection at autopsy,[156] the largest, the so-called super lacunes are as large as 15 mm³.[60] They are seen as obvious abnormalities at several levels on the CT scan. Thus far few of these super lacunes have been examined at autopsy, and in some that were examined, no detailed search for the underlying vascular pathology was made. Embolism into the stem of the middle cerebral artery with occlusion of several of the lenticulostriates is a possible cause of such infarcts, which do not deserve the name lacune except for their location in the depths of the brain.

LOCATION

Lacunes predominate in the basal ganglia, especially the putamen, the thalamus, and the white matter of the internal capsule and pons and occur occasionally in the white matter of the cerebral gyri. They are rare in the gray matter of the cerebral surface, or in the corpus callosum, visual radiations, centrum semiovale of the cerebral hemispheres, medulla, cerebellum, or spinal cord.[29] In general, the larger the series, the more widespread have been the lesions.[20] In the largest autopsy series thus far reported (169 found among 2,859 patients), 81% of the lacunes seem to have been asymptomatic in life, arguing that many of those seen nowadays in brain imaging are of uncertain clinical significance.

Attempts to include the centrum semiovale and white matter of the temporal lobes in the regions subject to lacunes involves a challenge (thus far not justified by available data) to an important principle long thought important in the production of lacunes: the lack of gradual stepdown in vascular size between the major cerebral artery trunks and the penetrating vessels involved in lacunes. The medullary arteries of the white matter arise from the cortical branches and not directly from the large trunks. If their disease is the same as those of the lenticulostriates and thalamoperforants, it awaits such demonstration.

VASCULAR TERRITORIES INVOLVED

Most lacunes occur in the territories of the lenticulostriate branches of the anterior and middle cerebral arteries, the thalamoperforant branches of the posterior cerebral arteries, and the paramedian branches of the basilar artery. Their occurrence is rare in the territories of the cerebral surface branches.

The lenticulostriates arise from the circle of Willis and the stems of the anterior and middle cerebral arteries to supply the putamen, pallidum, caudate nucleus, and internal capsule. They are comprised of two main groups, those more medial whose lumen is 100 to 200 μm, and those more lateral whose diameters are 200 to 400 μm.[60] The thalamoperforants arise from the posterior half of the circle of Willis and the stems of the posterior cerebral arteries to supply the midbrain and thalamus.[151] Their size varies from 100 to 400 μm. The paramedian branches of the basilar mainly supply the pons. Few branches have been measured, but sizes ranging from 40 to as large as 500 μm have been observed.[55,83] These arteries share in common both a tendency to arise directly from much larger arteries and an unbranching end-artery anatomy. The penetrators are all <500 μm in size and arise directly from the larger 6- to 8-mm internal carotid or basilar artery. Their small size and their point of origin rather proximal in the arterial network are thought to expose these vessels to forces that scarcely reach other similar sized arteries in the cerebral cortex.[72] These latter are apparently protected by a gradual stepdown in size from the 8-mm internal carotid to 3- to 4-mm middle cerebral to 1- to 2-mm surface branches from which the intracortical vessels whose diameters are <500 μm arise. Perhaps this difference explains the low frequency of lacunes in the cerebral surface vessels.[19,25]

The lack of collateral for the penetrators results in an infarct that spreads distally from the point of occlusion through the entire territory of the vessel affected. The exact volume of tissue supplied by each penetrator varies enormously.[55] Some arteries supply little more than the territory

the same diameter as the artery,[60] whereas others arborize widely, and leave an infarct shaped like a wedge or cone.[55] Most capsular infarcts arise from arteries 200 to 400 μm in size and produce infarcts $\geq$2 to 3 mm^3. These small infarcts require 1.5 Tesla MRI to be found regularly, are frequently missed by CT scanning, and are easily overlooked at autopsy.[156]

The arterial occlusion usually occurs in the first half of the course of the penetrating vessel, a location ensuring that most of them will be quite small. These sites are not usually detected by angiography because the course of the individual vessels is difficult to plot to show that one is missing. However, in disease involving the stem of the cerebral artery from which the penetrator arises, or from one of the small number of large penetrators, a bigger infarction results. Occlusions at the ostium of a penetrator where it departs from the parent major cerebral artery may yield a swath of infarction some 15 mm.^{3} These so-called super lacunes[60] are large enough to produce a striking abnormality at several levels on the CT scan. In most instances, however, super lacunes result from occlusions of larger vessels and are not a sign of primary arteriopathy of the penetrating vessels.

ARTEROPATHIES UNDERLYING LACUNES

Microatheroma

Several distinct but related arteriopathies cause lacunes. Microatheroma is believed to be the most common mechanism of arterial stenosis underlying symptomatic lacunes[55,57,60] (Fig. 23.5). The artery is usually involved in the first half of its course. Microatheroma stenosing or occluding a penetrating artery was found in 6 of 11 capsular infarcts in the only published pathologic study on the cause of capsular infarcts,[60] and it was the cause of the only published case of thalamic lacune.[58] The histologic characteristics of the microatheroma are identical with those affecting the larger arteries.

These tiny foci of atheromatous deposits are commonly

Figure 23.5 Intimal deposit of lipid-laden macrophages in a penetrating intracerebral artery that shows partial occlusion of the lumen. (H&E, ×100.) (Courtesy of J.H. Garcia, M.D.)

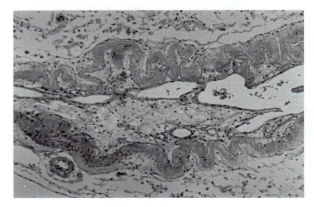

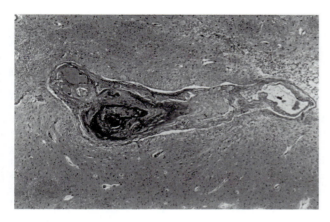

Figure 23.6 Terminal segment of a lenticulostriate artery showing marked mural changes (hyalinization and fibrinoid change) as well as occlusion of the lumen. (H&E, ×60.) (From Garcia and Ho,[70] with permission.)

encountered in chronic hypertension. In the usual nonhypertensive case, atheroma appears mostly in the extracranial internal carotid and basilar arteries, but only rarely in the stems of the major cerebral arteries.[59,66] In hypertension, however, the lesions are not only more advanced for the patient's age, but they are spread more distally in the arterial system, at times involving even some of the cerebral surface arteries. In advanced hypertensives, miniature foci of typical atherosclerotic plaques are found even in arteries as small as 100 to 400 μm in diameter, resulting in a stenosis or occlusion that sets the stage for a lacune.

Lipohyalinosis and Fibrinoid Necrosis

Other arterial disorders seem less common. *Lipohyalinosis*, formerly considered the most frequent cause of lacunes, affects penetrating arteries in a segmental fashion in chronic hypertension.[72] It was the cause attributed to 40 of 50 lacunes studied in serial section by Fisher[55] in four cases of stroke. It seems to occur most often in the smaller penetrating arteries, those below 200 μm in diameter, and accounts for many of the smaller lacunes, especially those that are clinically asymptomatic. Lipohyalinosis has been thought to be an intermediate stage between the fibrinoid necrosis of severe hypertension and the microatheroma associated with more long-standing hypertension.[25,55,83]

Fibrinoid necrosis is a related condition found in arterioles and capillaries of the brain (Fig. 23.6), retina and kidneys in a setting of extremely high blood pressure.[81] It appears histopathologically as a brightly eosinophilic, finely granular, or homogeneous deposit involving the connective tissue of blood vessels.[162] The mechanism is believed to involve disordered cerebrovascular autoregulation[45,180] with a necrotizing consequence.[20] This thesis envisions that the thickened arterial walls are unable to constrict, resulting in a resetting of cerebrovascular autoregulation at higher blood pressure levels. Continued high pressure produces increased capillary hydrostatic pressure and capillary damage. The overdisten-

sion[74,84] of these small arteries occurs in segmental fashion,[73] leading to vascular necrosis,[18–20] which allows red blood cells, plasma, and protein ultrafiltrates into the stretched segments of the wall.[73]

That other vessels are spared such injury is not easily explained. However, the arteriole and capillary necrosis encountered in severe hypertension does not occur in renal arteries, which are protected from hypertension distal to an experimental arterial clamp or to renal arterial stenosis. Larger vessels seem able to absorb enough in the subintima and in their thicker muscularis to resist such change, while the tiny cerebral cortical arteries of a size similar to the deep branches of the circle of Willis are protected by their more distal location.[20,25,74]

Fibrinoid necrosis shares some of the same histochemical, electron microscopic,[74,196] and immunofluorescent[148] characteristics with lipohyalinosis,[49] another cause of lacunes. Both occur in the brain[55,60] in a setting of hypertension, and both occur in a segmental location along the course of the arteries.[55] The two conditions have also been labeled hyalinosis, hyaline fatty change, hyaline arterionecrosis, angionecrosis, fibrinoid arteritis, plasmatic vascular destruction, atherosclerosis of small arteries, and segmental arterial disorganization. Although often considered identical,[55,60] segmental fibrinoid necrosis and lipohyalinosis differ histochemically in that fibrinoid necrosis is said to stain strongly for phosphotungstic acid hematoxylin whereas lipohyalinosis does not.[22,25] Also, lipohyalinosis[55] is found most commonly in a setting of chronic, nonmalignant hypertension,[83] whereas fibrinoid necrosis is said to be found only with extreme blood pressure elevations[25,81] such as occurs in hypertensive encephalopathy[25] and eclampsia.

Charcot-Bouchard Aneurysms

A long-standing, little noted controversy concerns whether lipohyalinosis or microatheroma are the precursor, are the result, or are even related to another commonly encountered arteriopathy in chronic hypertensives, Charcot-Bouchard aneurysms[28,55,56,165] (Fig. 23.7). The controversy also involves

Figure 23.7 A saccular microaneurysm (Charcot-Bouchard) with extravasated erythrocytes and reactive astrocytes. The longitudinally sectioned vessel is seen at the bottom. (H&E, ×33.) (From Garcia and Ho,[70] with permission.)

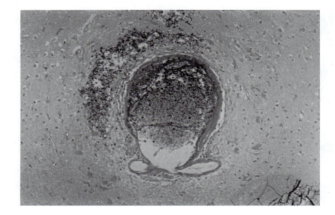

the questions of whether the Charcot-Bouchard arteriopathy represents a true aneurysm formation, or merely a dissection into the wall of a microatheroma, or twists, coils, and loops that are misdiagnosed as aneurysms[23]; whether both lipohyalinosis and Charcot-Bouchard aneurysms deserve consideration as pathologic processes separate from microatheroma of the penetrating arteries; and whether these lesions are simply variants along a spectrum of vascular effects of hypertension. The available evidence suggests that lipohyalinosis is more significant than Charcot-Bouchard aneurysms in the development of lacunes.[55,56] No recent evidence has appeared to support an earlier suggestion that lipohyalinosis is the end stage of an earlier Charcot-Bouchard aneurysm.[165]

Other Causes

Microembolism has been inferred in a few serially sectioned lacunes shown to have normal arteries leading to the infarct.[60] *Macroembolism* is considered elsewhere, but one such case (case 10) is to be found among Fisher and Curry's[64] original descriptions of pure motor stroke (Fig. 23.8). Cholesterol emboli from atheromatous changes in the aortic arch has been shown in pathologic examination, occluding small arteries around multiple lacunar infarcts.[111] Even *polycythemia* has been thought to be a cause of lacunes,[149] the small vessels being obstructed by the sludged blood. Small deep infarcts have been found in patients with antiphospholipid antibodies.[119] Dissection of a tiny artery may occur in the process leading to Charcot-Bouchard aneurysms.[61] Recent attempts have been made[190] to relate severe extracranial carotid stenosis to deep infarcts on a hemodynamic basis, the lacunar infarct being imaged on brain scan. Although the mechanism has been presumed to be perfusion failure in the symptomatic deep territory, the lack of autopsy data leaves the question unsettled of whether such infarction is from embolism from the carotid disease or with associated severe stenosis of a penetrating artery.[123] Amyloid angiopathy related to aging can narrow the lumen of small arteries by deposition of amyloid in the adventitia and media and can produce small infarcts.[122] Varying forms of arteritis may also occur, especially due to chronic meningitis (so-called Heubner's arteritis),[107,134] chronic neurosyphilis,[76,150] any severe granulomatous meningitis, and chronic fibrosing meningitis. Neurocysticercosis,[12] neuroborreliosis,[105] and acquired immunodeficiency syndrome[147] affecting small arteries can produce lacunar infarcts. Arteritis of unknown etiology such as polyarteritis nodosa and granulomatous angiitis, autoimmune disorders like lupus erythematous,[38] or drug abuse, particularly cocaine,[69] may produce small, deep infarcts. Arteritis may have been a major cause of small, deep infarcts[85] when chronic neurosyphilis was in its heyday. However, two major works[32,134] on the subject contain no specific cases, although the authors opined that ". . . they undoubtedly occur."[134] This opinion was not shared by Pentschew,[150] who doubted whether "syphilitic endarteritis" was actually of syphilitic origin.

GENERAL CLINICAL FEATURES

Lacunar infarctions share many risk factors, the most common being hypertension and diabetes mellitus. These two common accompaniments of lacunar disease have been present in comparable degrees in those clinical series exceeding 100 patients collected over the last 20 years: 75% and 29%, respectively, of lacunar cases diagnosed in the Harvard Cooperative Stroke Registry,[141] 74% and 27% of cases in the south Alabama population study,[58] and 72% and 28% of the Barcelona series reported by Arboix et al,[9] in which only 26% had cardiac disease. A high frequency (93%) of hypertension or left ventricular hypertrophy was found by Reimers et al,[158] whereas no clear correlation between blood pressure or hypertension was found in some of the smaller series.[116] The largest currently reported autopsy-based study was that of Tuszynski et al[187] (2,859 patients), who found lacunar infarctions in 169 patients (6%). Hypertension was present in 64%, diabetes in 34%, and smoking in 46%, while there were no known risk factors for cerebrovascular disease in 18%. A correlation was found between high hematocrit and hypertension in the patients with lacunar syndromes in a population-based study.[114] In the Stroke Data Bank project, 337 (27%) of the 1,273 patients diagnosed as having infarction had typical lacunar syndromes. In this large cohort, no striking differences were found among the risk factors for each of lacunar subtypes, but differences were found between lacunar syndrome stroke as a group and other types of infarcts.[130] Lacunar syndrome strokes shared similar risk factors with large vessel infarction except for fewer transient ischemic attacks (TIAs) (13% versus 40%) and prior stroke (19% versus 39%). Compared with cardioembolism, they had more hypertension (75% versus 60%) and diabetes (26% versus 17%) and less cardiac disease (24% versus 77%).[24] They may be more common among blacks.[76]

Atrial fibrillation, one of the hallmarks of embolism, has a low frequency of small, deep infarcts (5%),[7] similar to the frequency in the general population older than 60 years. In a series of patients with atrial fibrillation versus controls neither group known to have symptomatic stroke, Kempster et al[98] found that all infarcts with atrial fibrillation were peripheral and consistent with embolism. In the control group, three asymptomatic infarcts were lacunes.

Figure 23.8 Large, deep infarct reported in the original series of pure motor stroke.

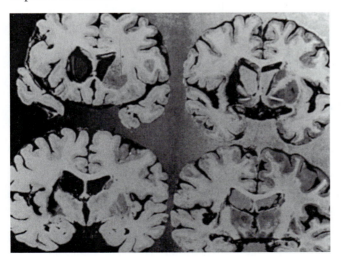

Prior TIAs occur in approximately 20% of cases, a frequency intermediate between embolism (5%) and large artery atherostenosis (40%). No correlation has yet been documented among the type of lacune, severity of the clinical deficit, and occurrence of TIAs. In comparing TIA in lacunar infarcts with TIA in large vessel infarcts, the former presented a higher number of episodes, a longer duration of neurologic deficit in each TIA, and a shorter latency between the first and last TIA and the definitive infarction. Stepwise or stuttering onset is more frequent in lacunar infarcts with TIA than in those without. There is a positive correlation between the number of prior TIAs and the volume of the lacunar infarct.[8]

Compared with the sudden onset more typical of infarction in other territories, a leisurely mode of onset has occurred in many lacunar strokes, delayed over enough time that an opportunity often exists to determine the effects of intervention. In contrast to major atheromatous or embolic stroke, in which a gradual onset is encountered in <5% of cases, as many as 30% of lacunes develop over a period of up to 36 hours.[58,60,90,91] During this time a mild weakness may evolve to total paralysis, usually by intensifying the initial deficit but occasionally by spreading into limbs not affected initially.[58] This smooth onset occurs with equal frequency in all types of lacunar syndromes. Sudden onset occurs in only 40% of cases.[91] The rate of evolution of the stroke appears not to predict the severity of the eventual defect, but this matter has not yet received much detailed study. With respect to the circadian rhythm there is a uniform pattern of onset throughout the 24 hours.[5]

Lacunes typically present with the highly focal symptoms described below, but a few nonfocal symptoms have been reported in clinical series of patients with the typical motor or sensory syndromes. Lability of mood was once taken as a sign of multiple lacunes. This sign occurs in 26% of cases with an equal frequency in single or multiple lacunes visible on CT scan.[37] It may simply be that multiple lacunes are present pathologically but are too small to be seen on CT scan. To date, neither headache (9% to 15%),[108,188] light-headedness, hiccough, or asterixis occur in a predictable manner with a high frequency, nor have they been correlated with the presence of a CT scan abnormality, or with the size or location of the lacunes shown on CT scan. Also, none appear to predict the clinical outcome.

Clinical Syndromes

LACUNAR STATE

For many years, lacunar state was what most clinicians understood was meant by the term lacunes. It was part of the original description by Marie.[127] His syndrome included a progressive decline in neurologic function punctuated by a few episodes of mild hemiparesis followed by the appearance of dysarthria, imbalance, incontinence, pseudobulbar signs, and a short-step gait (described as *marche à petits pas*). It was easy to envision that the small infarcts, widely scattered throughout the deep white matter, might accumulate gradually, each individual infarct inconspicuous but the cumulative effect devastating. Despite a few dissenting voices, matters have remained thus over the years.

Whether because of the effects of antihypertensive treatment or some other undefined cause, the lacunar state is a rarity in modern times. One reason might be that the syndrome had been due to other causes. Fisher[61] has pointed out that symptomatic occult hydrocephalus may have been the more common cause and that Marie's own published cases show such findings. He further noted that most lacunar infarcts are symptomatic and that the number of infarcts is small compared with the greatly deteriorated state of the patients. Earnest et al[44] and Koto et al[106] have observed a correlation between lacunar infarcts and hydrocephalus, suggesting that the former may arise from the pressure on the white matter.

PURE MOTOR STROKE

Pure motor stroke is undoubtedly the most common of any lacunar form, accounting for between one-half and two-thirds of cases, depending on the series.[9,143,158,187] It was the first lacunar syndrome recognized clinically,[64,127] and its features have been the most thoroughly explored.

Clinicoanatomic Correlations

Pure motor stroke, also known as pure motor hemiparesis, has been reported from autopsied cases with focal infarction involving the corona radiata[37] (Fig. 23.9), internal capsule,[60,64] pons,[65] and medullary pyramid.[26,64,117] The most frequent correlations have been with capsular locations. Of the two ends of the capsule, the greatest number have been reported from the posterior limb (Fig. 23.10). *Posterior limb capsular lacunes*[157] usually involve the pallidum and posterior limb of the capsule, which are supplied by the lenticulostriate branches of the middle cerebral artery. The vessels occluded vary in size from small, medially placed penetrators to the larger lateral lenticulostriates. The infarcts range from the genu to the back of the posterior limb. It is in this group that most of the data referable to the classical views of a homunculus in the internal capsule are to be found. Lesions in this region, especially those affecting the corona radiata, have also produced the syndrome of ataxic hemiparesis.

Anterior limb capsular lacunes[156] constitute a smaller number of cases and are smaller sized infarcts that may affect the caudate in addition to the anterior limb of the capsule. Some of them are in the territory of supply of the anterior cerebral artery, including the largest of the penetrating vessel, the recurrent artery of Heubner. Syndromes of hemiparesis comprise only one of the many permutations of anterior capsular infarcts,[157,194] which also include ataxic hemiparesis[93] and some unusual speech and language disorders.[31,145]

Compared with the small number of cases with autopsy correlation, a steadily enlarging group of cases of pure motor stroke have been documented by CT scan alone. One of the larger series, published by Pullicino et al,[156] featured 297 consecutive cases with a CT scan showing one or more foci of low density. Contained in this group were 42 single, small, deep lesions. Hypertension was more prevalent in this group than in the 122 cases with large lesions. Nine of the 42 (21%)

Figure 23.9 Lacune affecting the corona radiata.

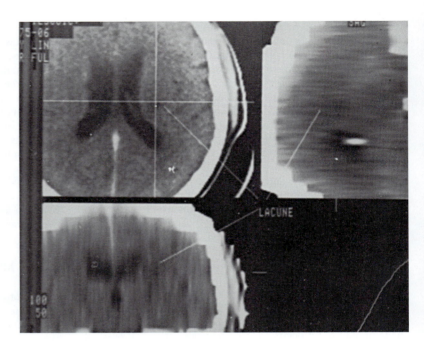

had a pure motor deficit, in contrast to only 10 of 122 (2%) with large lesions, a highly significant difference (P<0.0005). In the NINCDS Pilot Stroke Data Bank project,[142] fully 45 of the 100 cases of lacune were diagnosed by CT scan, most often as instances of pure motor stroke. The pathology in such cases is rarely defined.

Other Causes of Pure Motor Syndromes

Nonlacunar pure motor syndromes have also been described, indicating that the clinical picture alone is not invariably due to deep infarction. Less than a year passed from Marie's de-

Figure 23.10 Axial (**A**)T$_2$- and (**B**)T$_1$-weighted MRI scan showing lacunar infarct in the posterior limb of the internal capsule.

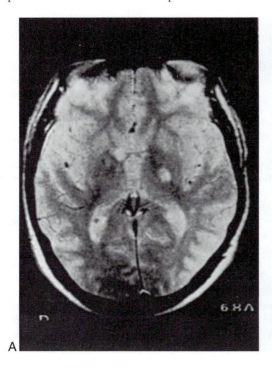

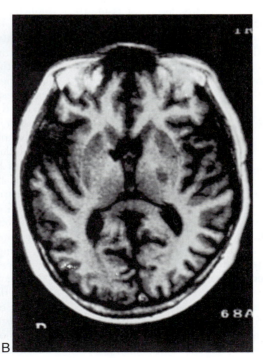

A

B

scription of lacunes before protests against his definitions were lodged. Abadie[1] contrasted the great frequency with which a capsular lesion was diagnosed clinically against the rarity with which such a lesion was found without other complaints accompanying the hemiparesis. His objection set the stage for the many others down through the years.

After Fisher and Curry's report[64] of pure motor stroke, several articles appeared challenging the lacunar origin by detailing a similar syndrome due to a variety of other causes including nocardial abscess of the motor cortex,[192] ischemia-edema after craniotomy for postoperative bleeding,[92] internal carotid artery occlusion in the neck,[2] and cerebral cortical surface infarction. Lesions rostral to the capsule have been described in cases studied only by CT scan,[193] and the syndrome has also been encountered with both deep and superficial low-density lesions on CT inferred to be from infarction.[156] A few such cases have even been reported from hemorrhage.[138,139,157,182]

The clinical picture itself has also come in for criticism. Richter et al[159] studied all cases of stroke that occurred in a single hospital and found that pure motor stroke occurred rarely, was not more prevalent among hypertensives, and did not usually have a good clinical outlook.

However, even the most careful studies exploring the limits of the syndrome and its etiologies have found a remarkably high percentage of cases with a clinical and radiologic picture conforming to the original syndrome described by Fisher and Curry[64]; Pullicino et al[156] studied 297 consecutive patients whose CT scan showed one or more foci of low density and found among them 42 single, small, deep lesions. Hypertension was more prevalent in this group than in the 122 cases with large lesions. Nine of the 42 (21%) had a pure motor deficit, in contrast to only 3 of 122 (2%) with large lesions, a highly significant difference (P <0.0005). Furthermore, in another 13 cases with isolated deep lesions, either the clinical deficit could not be related to the lesion or there was no clinical deficit at all, a point consistent with the observation that deep infarcts may spare the capsule.

Clinical Features

Pure motor stroke is most easily diagnosed when the stroke equally affects the face, arm, and leg on the same side, sparing sensation, vision, language, and behavior.[64] The complete syndrome is somewhat uncommon, however. As a clinical rule, as long as the syndrome is purely motor, such a diagnosis applies when the affected side involves one part more than the other. Some cases have been described in which the face is essentially spared, the one best known being from pyramid infarction.[160] Pure motor monoparesis is almost never due to a lacunar infarct.[133] The term pure motor stroke was initially used to draw attention to the lack of the expected accompanying sensory, visual, or behavior disturbances, especially considering the severity of the weakness. In this sense only is it pure.

Pure motor stroke has been described in both capsular and pontine locations, producing an essentially identical clinical picture as that first suggested by Ferrand.[50] Some reports[54,64] suggested that the capsular infarct case might have an associated conjugate eye movement disturbance that would follow the hemispheral pattern (i.e., deviation of the eyes toward the side of the lesion), whereas those involving the pons

would have the opposite, so-called wrong way eyes. However, this finding occurs too infrequently to serve a useful function.[141]

Despite earlier opinions by Ferrand[50] and by Foix and Levy,[68] it has become clear that pure motor stroke may be associated with considerable variations among the syndromes involving the face, arm, and leg. Fisher and Curry[64] found the arm severely affected in all 50 cases of pure motor stroke, but the lower the lesion occurred in the neuraxis, the less the face was involved.

When the lacune affects the internal capsule and corona radiata, a considerable variety of motor deficits have been encountered, in both severity and formula. Despite the many CT correlations with capsular lesions, only a handful of cases exists with a capsular infarct whose syndrome was fully studied in life. Among this small group, remarkable variations exist. The most compact lesion with a hemiplegia was an autopsied case with an infarct confined to the third quarter of the posterior limb of the internal capsule.[47] This location corresponds to the approximate pathway of the motor fibers as inferred from whole brain anatomic dissections.[164] The clinical deficit had persisted for years, affecting the face, arm, and leg equally. In another autopsied case involving the same site in the posterior limb of the internal capsule, the deficit was less severe. Spastic hemiparesis developed over many hours and lasted for the remaining 9 months of life, paralyzing the tongue, palate, face, arm, and hand, but the leg was only slightly affected.[81] In still another case, ischemia involving the posterior quarter of the internal capsule was associated with a hemiparesis that only slightly affected the face.[141]

Most of the recent studies have been documented by CT scan. Donnan et al[41] found a hemiplegia involving the face, arm, and leg in equivalent fashion in all 36 cases of infarction involving the capsule, but 22 other cases in the same series had incomplete syndromes, the most common being paresis of the arm and leg, sparing the face. The inferred lacune in these latter cases occurred more often in the fibers of the corona radiata, or at extreme ends of the capsule. One lacune with pure facial weakness was located at the genu, whereas another associated with pure leg weakness lay at the extreme posterior end of the capsule. Rascol et al[157] also found a spectrum of syndromes of hemiparesis that varied at one end from equal involvement of the face, arm, and leg to partial syndromes of faciobrachial weakness, in a few cases purely crural[157]; similar incomplete formulas of hemiparesis occurred in the smaller capsulopallidal cases and also in the anterior capsulocaudate infarcts. In the NINCDS Pilot Stroke Data Bank project[143] and in the population-based study of stroke in south Alabama,[78] lacunes located more posteriorly in the capsule produced a deficit greater in the leg than in the arm, but several varieties were encountered, including some whose arm was worse than the leg. Lesions affecting the anterior limb and genu have also been a source of syndromes of partial hemiparesis, in a few cases featuring greater weakness of the face than the leg.[41] For those studied in the Stroke Data Bank, lesions seen in the corona radiata were associated with a hemiparesis that took highly variable forms, whereas those lower in the capsule produced a wide variety of syndromes[24] (Fig. 23.11). Taken together, the CT scan correlations with the syndromes of hemiparesis showed only slight support for the clas-

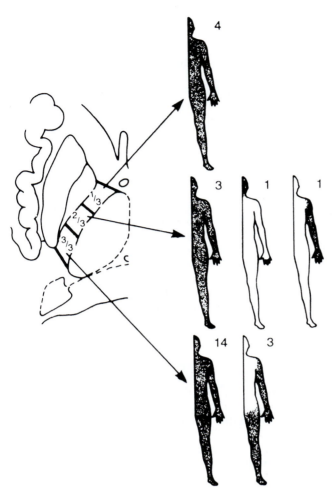

Figure 23.11 Hemiparesis formulas for capsular lesions of the anterior, middle, and posterior thirds of the posterior limb of the internal capsule. (From Chamorro et al,[24] with permission.)

sical view of a homunculus in the internal capsule with the face, arm, and leg displayed in an anteroposterior distribution.

When these findings are taken together, it is no longer possible to infer the exact site and size of the lesion in the motor pathway using the clinical formulation based on the older dogma,[35] that the motor fibers occupy a certain functionally reliable position in the posterior limb of the internal capsule. The case material only vaguely supports the traditional impression of a homunculus whose face is forward, and whose leg is located posteriorly. These findings suggest that even more careful attention to the clinical details in future cases might permit a clearer understanding of the variability and reliability of the pathways that make up the capsule.[9,35,164,168] At the least, the findings thus far indicate that partial syndromes of hemiparesis are common manifestations of lacunar infarction affecting the internal capsule and adjacent territory.

Associated Complaints

Although the main elements of the pure motor stroke syndromes are motor, other complaints are not rare, especially

sensory disturbances, which occur initially in as many as 42% of cases.[41] These complaints usually present as numbness, heaviness, and loss of feeling. Only scant abnormalities are found on clinical examination. Given their vague character, they are all too easily brushed aside or ignored. However, complaints of undue coldness, at times confined to the distal arm, are less easily ignored, and in a few cases personally observed, they have lasted for years.[141] The anatomic pathology of these complaints has not been resolved. These sensory complaints are thought to reflect slight involvement of the projections to the sensory cortex from occlusion of the larger lateral striate vessels, although few such cases have actually been documented by autopsy. When the perception threshold for temperature and thermal pain is measured, a significant thermal hypesthesia on the affected side is found. This semiologic finding has also been reported in pure motor and sensorimotor stroke.[174]

No disturbance in visual field function has been described from such infarcts. Dysphasia, dyspraxia, and other disturbances of higher cerebral function have rarely been described.

Clinical Course

Improvement is the result in a high percentage of cases. It is usually more rapid and more complete than that following cerebral surface infarction with a similar initial motor deficit.[156] The syndromes of partial hemiparesis show the best prognosis, as do those with the smaller infarct size on CT scan, but cases of complete plegia with virtual total recovery has been encountered. Rascol et al[157] found that all their cases regained the ability to walk. Fully 19 of their 30 cases experienced a favorable outcome, whereas another 6 were left with functional incapacity of the upper extremity. Thirty-five of the 42 cases documented in the pilot phase of the NINCDS Stroke Data Bank[142] improved to a functionally useful level within a few months. The improvement occurred regularly in the patients whose initial syndrome was incomplete. Unfortunately, among the seven cases initially paralyzed, only two made much improvement in the first few months, and both of them improved almost to normal.

PURE SENSORY STROKE

Pure sensory stroke is assumed to be due to infarction of the sensory pathway of the brain stem, thalamus, or thalamocortical projections. The thalamus is supplied by very small arteries[151] susceptible to the effects of chronic hypertension. Few autopsy-documented cases have been reported, and the syndrome was not noted in one large autopsy-based series.[187] In this small group, the most common location has been in the thalamus,[51,58,142] mostly in the ventral posterior tier nuclei, the main sensory relay nuclei to the cerebrum.[51] The only autopsied case with pure sensory stroke from a lesion outside the thalamus[77] was a small hemorrhage that involved the corona radiata of the posterior limb of the internal capsule.

CT scan has been the basis of the other sites associated

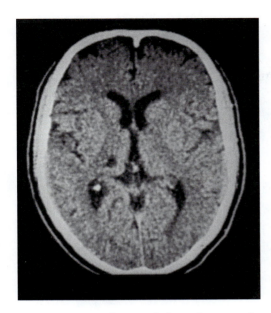

Figure 23.12 CT scan showing thalamic lacunar infarct.

with pure sensory stroke (Fig. 23.12). One case, inferred due to a lacune because of its small size, affected the centrum semiovale, presumably with involvement of the thalamocortical projection area.[163] Caution is necessary in this interpretation, as lacunes in the centrum semiovale are distinctly uncommon in series based on autopsy data.[37,52] Involvement of subthalamic brain stem pathways has not yet been reported to be associated with pure sensory stroke.

Observations on the arterial disease is confined to two cases. In one, a microatheroma was found narrowing the lumen of a small artery to the posterior thalamus,[55] which led to a lacunar infarct. Whether the lacune was symptomatic was unmentioned. In the other, a pure sensory syndrome was described clinically.[58] The 54-year-old patient was recovering from a right-sided pure motor hemiplegia when a feeling of pins and needles developed in the left lower lip, the left side of the mouth, and the fingers of the left hand; the sole of the left foot tingled and felt numb, dull, and swollen many hours later. No sensory deficit was evident on examination. Unpleasant paresthesias affected the left side of the face and the left foot. CT scan was normal on the fourth day. At autopsy 6 months later, a lacune 2 by 2 by 3.7 mm was found in the right ventral posterior nucleus, fed by four tiny arteries that arose from a single artery destroyed by lipohyalinosis.

The lacunes in both of the reported autopsied cases have been quite small. If they are typical, it is easy to understand why many thalamic lacunes have thus far escaped detection by CT scan and require the higher grade image provided by MRI. Larger lesions may be seen by both techniques (Fig. 23.13).

Complete Hemisensory Syndromes

Typically, the disturbance in sensation extends over the entire side of the body, involving the face, proximal as well as distal limbs, and axial structures including the scalp, neck, trunk, and genitalia right to the midline, even splitting the two sides of the nose, tongue, penis, and anus.[51,141] This remarkable midline split, especially when the trunk or abdomen is involved, may be unique to thalamic or thalamocortical pathway lesions. This type of hemisensory syndrome affected one case with a thalamic infarction measuring 4 by 4 by 2 mm.

The earliest reported patient with a complete hemisensory syndrome, but not attributed to lacune,[198] referred to a "plumb-bob" having been dropped down the exact center of the body. In this case, the responsible thalamic infarct was not reported: the main interest to the author was the associated disturbances in higher cerebral function from the remainder of the large left posterior cerebral artery territory infarction. This complaint of total hemisensory loss has also been part of the syndrome in the small number of cases with the syndrome of sensorimotor stroke.

Incomplete Hemisensory Syndromes

Variants in the topography of pure sensory stroke have been reported that involve less than the entire side of the body. One patient, reported with autopsy correlation (case 9 in Fisher's original collection of pure sensory stroke),[51] suffered only TIAs affecting the right fingers, and at another time the right upper and lower lips, right side of the tongue, and the two medial toes of the right foot. At autopsy, a lacune 7 mm in diameter affected the left ventral posterior nucleus. The complaints in other cases, without autopsy documentation, have involved the face, arm, and leg; head, cheek, lips, and hand; unilateral intraoral and perioral sites and fingers, the so-called cheiro-oral syndrome; face, fingers, and foot; shoulder tip and lower jaw; distal forearm alone; fingers alone; and leg alone.[29,51] How many permutations exist is a subject of some interest, since it might serve to determine the organization of a sensory homunculus in the ventral tier nuclei.

Lapresle and Haguenau[113] found partial sensory syndromes involving the face, the arms, the leg, the oral cavity, the peribuccal area and forearm, and the peribuccal area and radial edge of forearm, all from focal thalamic softenings of lacunar size. Fisher's[58] case 9 suffered only TIAs affecting the right fingers, and at another time the right upper and lower lips, the right side of the tongue, and the two medial toes of the right foot. A lacune 7 mm in diameter affecting the left ventral posterior nucleus was found at autopsy. Another case, a 54-year-old patient recovering from a right pure motor hemiplegia, developed a feeling of pins and needles in the left lower lip, the left side of the mouth, and the fingers of the left hand; the sole of the left foot tingled and felt numb, dull, and swollen many hours later. No sensory deficit was evident on examination. Unpleasant paresthesias affected the left side of the face and the left foot. CT scan was normal on the fourth day. At autopsy 6 months later, a 2 by 2 by 3 mm lacune was found in the right ventral posterior thalamus. The complaints in other cases, without autopsy documentation, have involved the face, arm, and leg; head, cheek, lips, and hand; face, fingers, and foot; shoulder tip and lower jaw; distal forearm alone; fingers alone; and leg alone. The full array of permutations has been subject to considerable study recently.[62]

Electrophysiologic studies have found a well-organized topographic arrangement of the ventroposterolateral nucleus

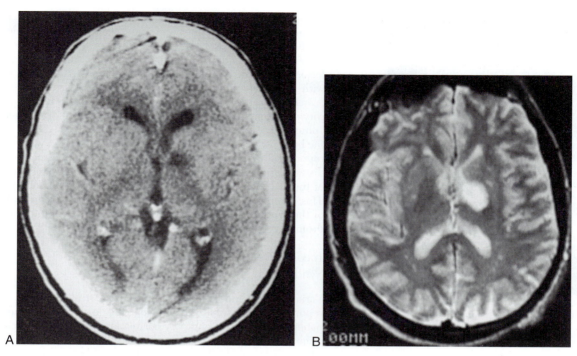

Figure 23.13 Anterior thalamic infarct seen by (**A**) CT and (**B**) MRI scans of the same patient.

of the thalamus in animals, which have been confirmed in humans by single-unit studies of thalamic neurons. The location and size of the receptive field have been mapped, showing a high number of cells concentrated on perioral and digital sensation and only a few for the forearm and upper arm.[118] The organization of the cells is in the sagittal plane with cutaneous and deep stimuli aligned toward one another. The failure of the clinical syndromes from infarction to reflect this type of organization may find its explanation in the vascular anatomy. The small vessels, individually occluded, may cause an infarct that cuts across the functional anatomic fields of somatosensory projections, causing clusters of symptoms and signs from lesions that are at variance with the normal organization.

Nature of the Sensory Complaints

The patients complain of striking alterations in spontaneous sensations.[51,140] The parts feel stretched, hot, sunburned, like pins sticking, larger, smaller, or heavier. Contacts with the skin from eyeglasses, bedclothes, rings, watches, and sheets feel heavier on the affected side and may transiently aggravate the sensory disturbance. The stimulus seems to persist for a few seconds after its removal. In the cases with severe disturbances, the occurrence of a stimulus is better reported than its exact location. In a series of 21 cases, impairment of all sensory types (touch, pinprick, vibration, and position sense) was usually associated with large lacunes in the lateral thalamus; restricted sensory complaints suggest small lacunes at any level of the sensory pathway.[101]

The *Dejerine-Roussy syndrome*,[36] is an uncommon ac-

companiment of lacunar infarction of the thalamus, although dysesthetic accompaniments are common in pure sensory stroke, as outlined above. The full Dejerine-Roussy syndrome was originally described as the effect of occlusion of the thalamogeniculate branch of the posterior cerebral artery, with infarction of the ventral posterolateral and ventral posteromedial nuclei, largely sparing the remaining nuclei of the thalamus. Cases documented only by CT scanning have shown a lesion small enough to qualify for a clinical diagnosis of lacunar infarction.[125] Suffice it to say here that the initial deficit usually includes a hemiparesis and hemisensory syndrome. The pain, which is an inconstant feature in cases with such infarcts, may begin at the onset of the syndrome or appear only later. Delays of up to several months are common. They are intermittent or constant, appear spontaneously, or at other times are provoked by contact with the affected parts. They are usually accompanied by many other disturbances in sensation, including tingling, feelings of excessive weight, and feelings of cold, although a few cases exist in which the sensory function is normal on clinical testing. The special disturbance known as hyperpathia is particularly characteristic but not common: following a sensory stimulus, a disagreeable response occurs that is usually delayed in onset, may spread over a large area, persists after removal of the stimulus, and may even increase in intensity over several seconds. The syndrome may outlast other features of the original stroke syndrome and even become permanent. Amytriptyline has been used with some success, beginning with doses of 10 mg at bedtime and increasing to 25 mg after a week in most patients who tolerate the dry mouth, and to even higher levels in some cases. A month or more may be required to see benefit in those who respond.

Associated Disturbances

Disturbances in motor function, language, and vision might be expected in a setting of thalamic infarction but have thus far been unreported save for a single example of sensorimotor stroke due to thalamic lacune[153] (see below). Given the anatomy of the thalamus and its widely varying projections to the cerebrum, such syndromes should be encountered but have thus far eluded the most careful diagnostic efforts of vascular neurologists.

Clinical Course

Improvement appears to be the rule, often to normal within weeks.[62] The topography of the shrinking deficit may be rather unusual. Improvement in the trunk with persistence in the distal extremities, common in hemispheral disease, is only occasionally encountered. In one case, the deficit shrank to a vertical band from the axilla down the lateral trunk to the thigh,[90] a finding encountered by one of the authors (J.P.M.) in several cases studied in south Alabama.

SENSORIMOTOR STROKE

Three autopsied cases[113,142,182] have been reported to date, only one published under the title sensorimotor stroke.[142] Such cases, although rare, are important since they attest to the occurrence of a combined motor and sensory deficit from a small, deep infarct. Their vascular anatomy also helps to clarify the vascular supply to the thalamus and adjacent internal capsule. The rarity of these cases should obviate any casual assumptions that small, deep infarcts cause most instances of sensorimotor stroke.

The first case report found by one of the present authors (J.P.M.) was published by Garcin and Lapresle[71] as part of a review of sensory disorders from thalamic infarction. The patient was a 65-year-old woman who suddenly developed left hemiparesis and a combination of hypesthesia and dysesthesia in the left peribuccal area and forearm. At autopsy, a small infarct was found straddling the intersection of the ventral posterior lateral and medial nucleus of the right thalamus. Involvement of the internal capsule was not mentioned.

The present senior author's (J.P.M.) patient[142] was a 61-year-old man. The sensory component preceded the motor by several hours. The syndrome evolved smoothly and steadily over approximately a day and then stabilized for many days before beginning to improve. The sensory component involved the entire half of the body, including the neck, ear, and genitalia. The sensory and motor deficits each followed a temporal course and clinical profile typical of pure sensory stroke and pure motor stroke, respectively. Neither deficit faded completely with time, but both underwent considerable improvement. The hemihypalgesia shrank to a vertical band from the axilla down the lateral trunk to the thigh. At autopsy, a well-developed lacune 4 by 4 by 2 mm was present in the ventral lateral nucleus of the thalamus, while the adjacent

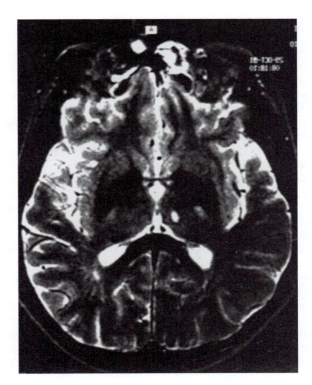

Figure 23.14 MRI scan showing a small thalamic lacune.

internal capsule showed a slight degree of pallor (Fig. 23.14). Efforts to track down the vascular supply to the infarct by means of serial sections were frustrated by the prior gross horizontal section made prior to embedding. The small artery found in the infarct was tracked downward toward its expected source from the posterior cerebral artery. Instead of gradually enlarging, the vessel gradually became smaller and vanished, leaving the authors to infer that its origin was from above the infarct. Efforts to trace the artery upward also proved futile when the serial sections crossed the plane of the original gross section. Here the discontinuity was too great to permit matching of sections to map the course of the artery.

The third patient attracted more interest by his action-induced rhythmic dystonia than by the sensorimotor stroke.[181] The stroke occurred when the patient was age 61, a known diabetic for 4 years. He fell suddenly, with left leg weakness. On examination, he was found to have a left hemiparesis ". . . with loss of all sensory modalities." He improved within a week and was able to walk with support within a month. Involuntary movements began in the left leg by the fourth month. When examined by the authors 4 years after the stroke, he had slight lower facial weakness and slightly exaggerated left-sided reflexes but normal strength and sensation. Autopsy revealed an infarct 3 by 3 by 10 mm involving the ventral posterolateral nucleus of the right thalamus and adjacent internal capsule. No mention was made of the arterial anatomy of the lesion.

The neurovascular issues raised by the case are also of importance. Before such cases were documented, it was believed that the vascular supply to the internal capsule was wholly separate from that to the thalamus. The lenticulostriate branches of the middle cerebral presumably supplied the capsule, while the thalamus was presumed to receive its supply from the perforating branches of the posterior cerebral artery.[153] The extreme posterior nuclei of the thalamus received a few branches from the choroidal arteries.[151] However, three cases now exist showing that a single infarct may involve both the thalamus and the adjacent internal capsule. These cases suffice to overturn earlier claims and reopen the issues of the boundary line between the middle and posterior cerebral artery territories.

At least 13 clinical examples of sensorimotor stroke have been documented by CT scan.[41,80,143,194] In these cases, the lesions have been fairly large. Donnan et al[41] described one extending from the left putamen to the corona radiata, not obviously involving the thalamus. One of the present authors (J.P.M.) encountered two other examples in south Alabama. The first case began as an incomplete pure motor stroke to which the hemisensory component was added within hours. This pattern was the reverse of the author's autopsy-documented case of sensorimotor stroke. In Weisberg's series,[194] eight cases were described with ". . . weakness and sensory disturbance and were found to have a hemiparesis and a decreased appreciation of pinprick, light-touch, vibration, and position sense involving the face, arm, and leg."[194] Large caudatoputaminal infarcts were seen on CT scan. It is presumed that these CT-documented cases affected the thalamocortical projections. However, apart from the cases reported by Groothius et al,[77] no autopsy-documented material has appeared to clarify the course followed by the thalamocortical fibers.

ATAXIC HEMIPARESIS

The syndrome of ataxic hemiparesis[59] has both cerebellar and pyramidal elements. It was initially described as homolateral ataxia with crural paresis,[63,152] its most familiar form. The original authors speculated that the lesion might lie either in the anterior limb of the internal capsule or in the adjacent corona radiata. However, the first autopsied cases showed a pontine lesion of the small size typical of lacunar infarction.[59]

Since these early observations, numerous case reports have shown a low-density CT lesion lying in the corona radiata[89] or the posterior limb of the internal capsule, thalamus, lentiform nucleus, cerebellum, and frontal cortex.[37,59,91,144,171,194] These lesions have not been in the same site in each case and have been encountered as far forward as the head of the caudate and as far posterior as the posterior limb of the internal capsule.[37] As the lesions in all these cases have been documented by CT scan alone, their exact correlation with the syndrome has been called into question by Kistler's disturbing case.[102] This patient had a CT scan showing a corona radiata lesion; a nuclear MR scan revealed a recent pontine lesion that better explained the deficit. The pontine lesion was not seen by CT scan due to the difficulty in averaging the bone densities adjacent to the brain stem. Since this effect prevents all but the largest pontine infarcts from being seen by CT scan, other cases may have had a similar second lesion as well. Although the syndrome is best known from infarction, it has also been reported from tumor,[13] although not in as pure a form, or as intracerebral hemorrhage in the parasagittal part of the precentral area.[185]

The clinical features have been rather similar from case to case. The usual form presents as a mild to moderate weakness of the leg, especially the ankle, with little or no weakness of the upper limb and face accompanied by an ataxia of the arm and leg on the same side. In a few cases,[61,89] a mild and transient hemisensory deficit may initially accompany the motor findings. The syndrome commonly develops only gradually, requiring from hours[89] to a day or more to reach its peak. A few instances of a chronic state exist, but some degree of improvement within days or months is usual. In some cases, the syndrome changes, with the hemiparesis clearing and leaving the ataxia.[89]

Efforts[63,89] to separate hemispheral from brain stem location have met with only limited success: the former are said to have paresthesiae when the lesion is in the thalamus and the latter to have a slightly higher frequency of dysarthria and trigeminal weakness. In most instances, however, no distinctive features separate the cases of capsular or radiation origin from those involving the pons. The extent of weakness accompanying the ataxia is no guide to the location. In both the capsular and pontine cases, weakness may involve more structures than the leg, at times affecting the face and arm almost to the same degree. In all cases, the degree of ataxia is more striking than the weakness and exceeds that attributable to weakness alone.

DYSARTHRIA CLUMSY-HAND SYNDROME

The dysarthria clumsy-hand syndrome has the advantage of emphasizing the distinctive elements of the stroke: in patients presenting with the syndrome, the dysarthria and the ataxia of the upper limb appear to be the prominent components of the clinical deficit, but they do not occur in isolation. The syndrome usually also includes facial weakness, which at times may be profound, dysphagia, and some degree of weakness of the hand and even of the leg. The reflexes on the affected side are usually exaggerated, and the plantar response is extensor. The clinical picture usually develops suddenly. The cases with autopsy correlation have shown no sensory deficit. In one case, the facial weakness was accompanied by impaired strength in opening of the jaw.[172] In the case from pontine hemorrhage, several features occurred that differed from those reported with infarction: vomiting and lethargy occurred at onset; balance was impaired enough that the patient was unable to stand; and the facial weakness was mild. It was only after a week that the persisting deficit was reduced to dysarthria and a clumsy hand.

Some authors have equated the syndrome with ataxic hemiparesis,[186] whereas the originator has come to the view that it is a variant.[61] The best recognized association has been with lacunes of the anterior limb of the internal capsule.[53] Other sites have been reported less often: Spertell and Ransom[179] described a case with a low-density lesion near the genu, and two of Fisher's patients with anterior capsular infarcts had combinations of mild ataxia and dysarthria. In a few other cases, the lesion has been in the basis pontis. The syndrome has also been reported from hemorrhage of the pons.[185]

The outlook for functional recovery is good.

MOVEMENT DISORDERS

Several types of movement disorders have been described with small, deep infarcts. Although the exact vascular occlusion has not been demonstrated in many of these cases, the small size of the infarct and its occurrence in territories fed by small penetrating arteries justify possible inclusion among the lacunar syndromes. The disorder may appear as the only sign of the infarct or may develop later, after an initial syndrome, different in character, has resolved.

Hemichorea-Hemiballismus

Hemichorea-hemiballismus is the most frequently documented form of movement disorder: 68% in a series of 22 patients with movement disorders of vascular origin, lacunar infarcts being the most frequent cause.[40] The infarcts found in different parts of the striatum have been of lacunar size[75,128] including those in the head of the caudate nucleus and adjacent corona radiata,[176] the subthalamic nucleus,[132,135] and the thalamus.[4,90,128] The onset is typically abrupt and is usually unaccompanied by other complaints. The chorea usually involves the forearm, hand, and fingers. In one case, it was accompanied by hemiparesis that faded within 3 months while the chorea persisted unchanged.[176] In some cases, it has been delayed by some weeks or months after the initial occurrence of hemiparesis. One patient familiar to one of the authors (J.P.M.), whose putaminal lesion was documented only by CT scan,[97] suffered choreic movements of the distal parts of the arm and leg that interfered with normal activity and prevented easy walking for over 4 weeks. In this case the chorea improved, only to relapse a few weeks later. Rare ballistic movements were superimposed. The examination revealed normal strength, sensation, and reflexes.

Treatment with haliperidol is a common approach but has not been uniformly effective.[176] Doses as high as 5 mg t.i.d. have been required to suppress the chorea.[97]

Dystonia

Two types of dystonia have been described. *Action-induced rhythmic dystonia* has been documented by an autopsy study. In the case reported,[181] the syndrome began as a sensorimotor stroke. Both these deficits improved within a month. By 3 months, the movement disorder began in the left leg, which had been the most severely affected part in the initial stroke. The disorder spread to involve his entire left side. The fingers of the affected hand became flexed into the palm, leaving only the thumb free. When examined 4 years later, the hand was unchanged, but strength was otherwise normal. Voluntary movements of any parts of the body, including even eye closure, precipitated rhythmic dystonic extension and rotation of the left arm and leg (sparing the trunk) that subsided a few seconds after the voluntary movements ceased. Clonazepam and 5-hydroxytryptophan were successful in suppressing the involuntary movement disorder. At autopsy, an infarct 5 by 1 by 2 mm was found straddling the ventral posterolateral nucleus and the adjacent posterior limb of the internal capsule.

The other type is a *focal dystonia*. One patient has been described whose CT scan showed a low density in the right lenticular nucleus.[169] Like the cases of hemichorea and hemiballism, the deficit appeared abruptly, unaccompanied by weakness or sensory disturbances. Only the distal end of the upper extremity was affected. Although it was described as dystonic, the disorder featured changing postures: "The movements were slow and caused the patient's fingers to assume unusual positions. Activity exacerbated the movements . . . the left hand and forearm showed involuntary movements that produced an unusual posture, with hyperpronation and flexion at the wrist, extension of the fingers, and opposition of the thumb." Haloperidol, 1 mg t.i.d., relieved much of the movement and posture disorder. Attempts to remove the medication >8 months later produced relapse, requiring reinstitution of therapy to suppress the disorder.

Asterixis and Tremor

The unilateral flapping tremor or asterixis affecting an upper extremity may be produced by a lacunar infarct in the basal ganglia, thalamus, internal capsule, or midbrain, although no cases with pathologic images has been published.[129,199] Unilateral tremor can appear several months after the initial lacunar infarction in the caudate nucleus or in thalamus.[39,100]

SPEECH AND LANGUAGE DISORDERS

Mutism, Aphonia, and Anarthria

Bilateral capsular lacunar infarction has been a cause of mutism in the absence of any disturbance in language or praxis. One of Fisher's[60] cases, documented by microscopic vascular pathology, had no difficulty with speech on his first infarct but became mute with the second infarct, involving the left internal capsule. The left capsular lacune was 4 by 4 by 5 mm and lay at the genu. Marie[125] had earlier reported a case of unilateral stroke with "anarthria" and no aphasic symptoms, but the cause of the small, deep lesion was a putaminal hemorrhage.

In subsequent years several such cases have been reported with the lesion documented by brain imaging. None of these bilateral capsular infarct cases have had aphasia apart from the disturbance in articulation. The author's (J.P.M.) collection includes a case of an infarct affecting the posterior limb of the right internal capsule followed by an infarct affecting the left internal capsule at the genu.[143] This last infarct was so small as to be barely visible on CT scan, yet it yielded virtual anarthria, severe dysphonia, and dysphagia but only a mild right arm weakness. Three others have been reported, each with bilateral capsular infarcts, involving the genu or anterior limb of the capsule.[30,110,187]

Disorders of Language

Considerable doubt still remains on whether aphasic disturbances per se occur from lacunes. At least one case[61] indicates that they may. In most instances, the cause is not the primary arteriopathy, but embolism into the stem of the middle cerebral with involvement of many lenticulostriates together. Fisher's is the only autopsy-verified patient to date reported with a language disorder from an infarct involving the territory of a lenticulostriate. The syndrome included a modified pure motor hemiparesis with "motor aphasia." It was attributed to a large infarct involving the genu and anterior limb of the internal capsule and adjacent white matter of the corona radiata. Speech initially was dysarthric, progressed later to mispronunciation of words and then to a state of utterance of single syllable unintelligible sounds, and ended as mutism. Comprehension was reportedly intact. The accompanying weakness severely affected the right side of the face and moderately involved the right hand. This case is important not because of the large size of the infarct but because the underlying lesion was a thrombosis of a lenticulostriate artery.

One case diagnosed by CT scan only has also been associated with a small lesion.[175] It was but one among eight large, deep infarcts attributed to cardiac embolism; the patient presented with an "expressive dysphasia." The disturbance was characterized by ". . . nonfluent conversational speech, naming and reading difficulties, dysgraphia and normal auditory comprehension." The case is of especial interest given the small size of the lesion demonstrated on the CT scan, since a lacunar cause is in the differential diagnosis.

That unilateral, large, deep infarcts may disrupt language function to some degree has never been the subject of serious dispute (Fig. 23.15). Several well-known cases attest to the correlation. However, save for one the case noted above, in each case the infarct has been quite large, of the super lacune category, well beyond the usual limits of the infarcts caused by primary disease of the penetrating arteries. Although it is described in more detail elsewhere in this volume, the subject is touched on here to settle this point of the larger size of the infarcts.

Two famous cases are on record with large infarction documented by autopsy. Bonhoeffer's[16] classic case was associated with a large, deep lesion of the type 1 of Rascol et al,[157] involving the caudate nucleus, internal capsule, and putamen as far laterally as the external capsule. He was unable to speak anything more than a few poorly formed vowels. The cause of the lesion was undetermined, but its large size suggested occlusion of the middle cerebral artery stem. An embolic mechanism was suggested by the second infarct, of fairly large size, affecting almost the entire anterior cerebral artery territory. Kleist[103] reported a case with an infarct of similar size and location (case Bühlmeir) featuring severe dysarthria, rare paraphasias, and only slight disturbance in comprehension. No mention was made of the vascular pathology.

Thirteen others to date have been reported by CT scan, all of whom showed large, deep infarcts.[31,145,175] In Naeser et al's[145] series, at least three had accompanying surface infarcts. That an accompanying surface infarct, which is not obvious on CT scan, might be the cause keeps the value of the reports based entirely on CT scan well below those with autopsy documentation. These cases have been characterized by dysprosody, at times accompanied by dysarthria and a mixture of deficits in syntactic and semantic functions not typical for any of the classical syndromes of dysphasia.

Other Disorders of Higher Cerebral Function

A single instance of pure motor stroke with "confusion" has been recently reported with a 1.2-cm lacune affecting the anterior limb and the anterior portion of the posterior limb of the right internal capsule.[60] The behavior disorder was characterized as ". . . acute onset of confusion and impairment of attention and memory." Recent studies using brain imaging to document the lesion have found a few instances of deep infarction, usually affecting the genu or anterior limb of the internal capsule with greatly reduced level of activity. In a study comparing 11 patients who had multiple lacunes with 11 controls, Wolfe et al[197] found that lacunar patients showed

Figure 23.15 Large anterior capsular infarct with dysnomia.

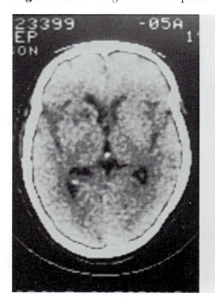 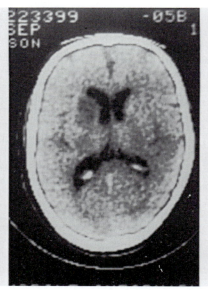 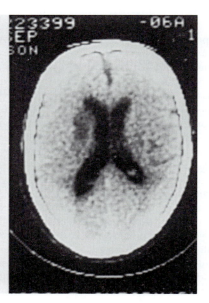

neuropsychological signs of frontal system disturbance, although only 27% met clinical criteria for a diagnosis of dementia. The disturbances were described as ". . . shifting mental set, response inhibition, and executive function . . . [and such patients] . . . were more often rated apathetic on a behavior-rating scale."

Some insight into the underlying mechanisms was provided by the study of one patient by Satomi et al,[177] who performed a single-photon emission computed tomogram (SPECT) study with ^{123}I iodoamphetamine; this study showed decreased vasoreactivity, predominantly to the frontal lobes. Tatemichi et al[183] studied a right-handed man whose infarct was limited to the genu of the capsule in the left hemisphere: they suggested that the impaired SPECT reactivity could be from interruption of thalamofrontal projections passing below the genu, producing a syndrome of frontal lobe dysfunction without direct lesion to the frontal lobe. This patient became the index case of a series subsequently reported sharing similar clinical features.

The literature continues to document disorders of language, memory, orientation, and activity following infarction of the paramedian thalamic nuclei. Save for two reports,[22,154] CT scan has been the basis for the lesion localization. In many of these cases, including some of the autopsied material of Castaigne et al,[22] embolism to the top of the basilar or to the posterior cerebral artery stem or thrombosis of the basilar may have been the cause, not vascular disease of the lacunar type. Given the origin of these cases, the CT scan might not reveal all the foci of infarction, making the correlation with CT findings a bit unreliable.[79,136,178,191] In the few cases with autopsy, the arterial disease has been rather unusual. In the case reported by Poirer et al,[154] a picture of thalamic dementia was encountered. Autopsy showed many small, deep infarcts of lacunar size. The authors formed the impression that the lesion was an angitis hitherto undefined. Among the cases documented only by CT scan, hypertension a normal angiogram, several spells typical of TIAs before the final stroke, and then the emergence of a CT-positive low density have been documented in a few instances, which seems consistent with the course expected from lacunar disease. The patient reported by Michel et al[136] is such an example, described by the authors as having a thalamic lacune. The initial deficit included right hemiparesis with agitation, disorientation, and language disturbances. The language disorder was of the expressive type, with reduction in language, slowness in response, and some verbal paraphasias. Verbal memory was greatly disturbed and was the subject of a special investigation. The presence of the hemiparesis might mean that the scope of the lesion exceeded that seen on CT scan, but this tissue was not settled.

A single case of dysphasia with a small thalamic infarction documented by CT scan has been reported.[56] The size of the infarct was large enough to include the ventral anterior and rostral ventral lateral nucleus, which might be too large for an infarct from primary disease of the thalamoperforant vessels. No cause for the infarct was found. In the other cases in the literature, the infarcts were bilateral or large enough to make it unlikely that they were due to primary arteriopathy of the penetrating vessels. These cases are detailed elsewhere in this volume. The last word has not been written on the syndromes of deep infarction with disturbances in speech and language.

Laboratory Studies

COMPUTED TOMOGRAPHY

Technical limitations of the most modern CT scanners prevent the resolution of most lacunes smaller than 2 mm in the internal capsule and almost all of those in the thalamus and brain stem[155,192] due to obscuring artifact. For the lacunar syndromes in the Stroke Data Bank, a lesion was found in 39% on the first CT scan; most of them were located in the posterior limb of the internal capsule and corona radiata.[24] Repeat CT scan increased the yield to 35%. Brain stem lesions were not often visualized. The mean infarct volume in this cohort was greater in pure motor and sensorimotor stroke syndromes than in ataxic hemiparesis, dysarthria clumsy-hand, and pure sensory stroke syndrome. In those pure motor stroke patients with posterior capsule infarction, there was a correlation between lesion size and hemiparesis severity save for the small number of patients whose infarcts involved the lowest portion of the capsule, supplied by the anterior choroidal artery, where severe deficits occurred without regard for the lesion size. Enhancement of small deep infarcts on CT with intravenous contrast is seen in 13% to 40% of patients, mainly during the second and third week after onset.[115,155]

MAGNETIC RESONANCE IMAGING

MRI has greatly changed the frequency with which small infarcts are demonstrated.[10] Although CT scanning is still used, MRI has now surpassed it in sensitivity for detection of lacunes.[12,86]

In their study of 227 patients with lacunar infarcts, Arboix et al[9] found that CT was positive in 100 patients (44%), whereas MRI was positive in 35 of 45 (78%). MRI was significantly better ($P < 0.001$) than CT for imaging lacunes, especially those located in either the pons ($P < 0.005$) or the internal capsule ($P < 0.001$). Motor stroke, pure or sensorimotor, has the highest positive rate on MRI and pure sensory stroke the lowest. This corresponds with the main volumes of the classical lacunar syndromes on MRI: sensorimotor 1.7 ml; pure motor 1.2 ml; ataxic hemiparesis 0.6 ml; and pure sensory 0.2 ml. Hommel et al[86] used MRI for 100 patients hospitalized with a lacunar infarct syndrome and also found it more sensitive. MRI detected at least one lacune appropriate to the symptoms in 89 patients who had 135 lacunes found by imaging. MRI was more effective when it was performed a few days after the stroke. The superiority of MRI over CT for detection of small lesions now seems generally accepted. Enhancement of small deep infarcts on MRI with intravenous contrast (gadolinium) is seen in 67% during the first week and in 100% by the second week and is useful in differentiating the present lacune from old ones.[139,46] The hyperintense signals on T_2-weighted images in MRI may be either lacunar infarcts, état criblé or dilated perivascular spaces, wallerian degeneration, later stages of small hemorrhages, small artery ectasia, myelin loss, and other incidental white matter lesions, and they must be differentiated.

MR scanners may have a higher yield, as inferred from the experience of Kistler et al[102] and by our experience. To date, only a few lesions seen on MRI have been confirmed by autopsy. Autopsy correlations with CT scanners indicate that CT overestimates lacunar size by as much as 100%.[41] The yield on scans within 2 days of the stroke is very low, but by 10 days over 50% of the lacunes that eventually show on CT scan can be detected.[41,143,156,193,194] The high yield in the study by Rascol et al[157] may have been an artifact of selection, but fully 29 of 30 cases of hemiparesis were documented by CT scan. The population-based study in south Alabama noted that 13% of the strokes were due to lacunes; 40% of these were documented by fourth-generation CT scan.[78] Some of the lesions seen on MRI have been judged to be incidental.[11]

ANGIOGRAM

Similar technical limitations apply to arteriography. Since the artery affected is usually in the range of 100 to 500 μm, conventional angiography does not often demonstrate abnormalities.[56] However, in the case of giant lacunes, stenosis of the middle cerebral artery stem or occasionally one of the larger lateral lenticulostriates may be documented.[157] In a series of young lacunar patients ($\leq$50 years old), conventional angiography was performed in 19, searching for unusual vascular disorders such as vasculitis or extracranial artery dissection; findings were normal in all cases.[123] Ipsilateral extracranial carotid stenosis has a low incidence in lacunar patients and an uncertain relationship.[94] Insufficient cases have been studied to determine how often the angiogram will show major extracranial or intracranial atheroma in classical lacunar syndromes (Fig. 23.16) and what prognostic interaction exists between such findings and the lacunar syndromes. Nowadays angiography by MRI can help in providing the true incidence of abnormalities in large extra- or intracranial vessels in lacunar patients.

NEUROPHYSIOLOGIC STUDIES

Electroencephalogram

The small size prevents most individual lacunes from disrupting enough of the general brain function to produce changes in the conventional electroencephalogram (EEG).[21] In the data from the Pilot Stroke Data Bank, no significant EEG abnormalities were encountered even in cases with a positive CT scan.[143] EEG abnormalities were so infrequent in their 56 lacunar patients that Falcone et al[48] considered a normal EEG a helpful sign suggesting lacune. Quantitative analysis of the different frequencies of the α and μ-rhythms in the EEG has not been useful in the diagnosis and prognosis of lacunar infarcts.[95]

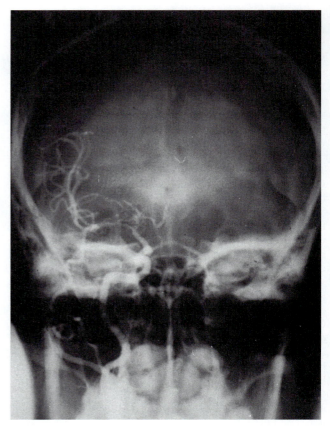

Figure 23.16 Angiographic evidence of middle cerebral artery stem stenosis in a patient with dysnomia. The CT scan of this patient is shown in Figure 23.15.

Evoked Cerebral Responses

A few studies of the somatosensory response have shown alterations in the waveform suggesting a subclinical sensory impairment in clinically pure motor strokes. Efforts to find an abnormality in the sensory evoked potential were disappointing in a personal series studied by us[160]; only those with a large CT lesion and an accompanying motor deficit showed such abnormalities. Other even larger series also failed to show the usefulness of evoked potentials, save for those with the largest lesions and sensorimotor deficits.[109] As a test for brain image-negative lacunes, the evoked potential seems thus far to have little use.

Prognosis

In general the patient with a lacunar infarction has a good prognosis. This was remarked by Pierre Marie and Miller Fisher as one of the characteristics of the lacunes. In comparison with other vascular processes (ischemic or hemorrhagic, hemispheric or in brain stem), lacunes have the best prognosis (not always as good as we expect, however). The prognosis of lacunes is influenced by several factors. The presence of TIAS before the infarct indicates a poor prognosis, more recurrences, and coronary artery disease in the clinical evolution.[8] Generally, when the motor or sensory deficit is complete (affecting the face, arm, and leg), the prognosis is worse than with an incomplete deficit. The size of the lacunar infarction on CT or MRI is usually correlated with prognosis, being better for smaller lesions. Prognosis in such vascular processes as lacunes implies four aspects: survival, recovery of deficits, general or neurologic complications in the acute phase, and recurrences. Survival is the rule in lacunar patients during the acute phase. The possibility of death in this phase is related to other complications rather than lacunar infarct. The risk of death after the acute phase is not different from that in the general population.[137,170] Recovery of deficit is generally good in the first few weeks after onset. Related functional outcome at 6 months[145] to 94% of patients are independent.[14] Complications in the acute phase occur in 18% of patients, urinary infections being the most frequent.[6] The prognosis for recurrence of stroke in lacunar infarcts at 1 year in hospital studies or community series is about 10%. The rate of recurrence in following years is similar.[82,170] The proportion of lacunar infarction has been reported in about one-fourth of recurrences and is especially related to hypertension.[27,170]

Treatment

The patient with a lacunar infarction may have had prior TIAs (20%) close to the infarct onset, or a leisurely mode of onset (30%). In both cases anticoagulant therapy has not proved its efficacy. No specific treatment exists for the necrotic tissue of a small deep infarct, but we can act on its causes and consequences. Atherosclerosis is the most important cause, usually affecting small vessels and less frequently main intracranial or extracranial trunks; the current treatment is directed at correcting vascular risk factors such as hypertension, diabetes mellitus, or cigarette smoking. Specific drugs acting against platelet aggregation such as aspirin or ticlopidine can be used, but their efficacy has not been proved. Extracranial carotid stenosis must be considered as asymptomatic, except in cases in which stenosis is the sole etiologic factor, which could produce lacunes by embolism or hemodynamically.

Hypertension must be treated as in other types of cerebral infarction, that is, not in the first days of the acute phase when figures are greater than 190 to 200 mmHg systolic and 110 to 115 mmHg diastolic. After the acute phase, hypertension[123] must be accurately controlled. Heart diseases (ischemia, atrial fibrillation, or valvulopathy) are considered and treated as risk factors. Similarly, diabetes mellitus must be treated in all patients as a risk factor and occasionally as the etiology.

When an increased hematocrit (> 45%) is the sole cause, phlebotomy could be indicated.[114] When arteritis is the cause of lacunes, as in chronic neurosyphilis, granulomatosis, cysticercosis, or tuberculosis, treatment with penicillin, steroids, praziquantel, or antituberculous drugs is indicated. In relation to the symptoms of lacunar infarct, the treatment can be specific. In all patients with motor deficit, prevention of deep venous thrombosis with low molecular weight heparin (0.2 ml/d SC) is the rule. Motor rehabilitation must be started as soon as possible. When hyperpathia is present in sensory stroke, amitriptyline, carbamazepine, or clonazepam has been used with an irregular response. Movement disorders such as hemichorea-hemiballismus or dystonia can be relieved with haloperidol 1 to 5 mg tid,[74] but this treatment has not always been effective. When motor aphasia is present, speech therapy is started.

Although primary prevention has not been investigated, probably the treatment of hypertension and the other established risk factors (such as diabetes mellitus and cigarette smoking) is the best way to avoid lacunes in the symptomatic or asymptomatic form.

Practical Approach

An acute or stuttering unilateral or focal deficit referable to the brain with motor, sensory, ataxic, or dysarthric deficits in the form of one of the five lacunar syndromes (pure motor, pure sensory, sensorimotor, ataxic hemiparesis, or dysarthria clumsy-hand) suggests the probability of a lacunar infarction. However, this diagnosis is only a possibility that must be confirmed. A patient with a motor deficit must be admitted to the hospital. All cases must be investigated with the aim of confirming the presumed diagnosis, establishing its etiology, and starting the best treatment. The clinical picture can never be considered as synonymous with a lacunar infarction.

The diagnosis of a lacunar syndrome has a 20% possibility of being explained by other processes, vascular or not. The clinical diagnosis of lacunar infarction has a sensitivity between 81% and 95%, that is, the proportion of patients with the same diagnosis at the initial examination and at the end of the study. Specificity, or the proportion of patients with a different final diagnosis who also had other initial diagnoses, is between 81% and 93%.[15,124]

The first step in the study of a patient is to confirm the lacunar infarction and differentiate it from other possible diagnoses. CT scan excludes such other possibilities as tumor, metastasis, subdural hematoma, or abscess, with a positive rate in lacunes of between 15% and 58%,[167,173] but MRI is the best and most useful exploration to confirm lacunar infarction in 74% to 98% of cases[17,166]; MRI can also establish the topography (68%), diagnose silent infarcts (13%) in neurologically normal adults,[104] and differentiate a lacune from other small, deep hyperintensive signals.

Once the lacunar infarct is confirmed by MRI or suspected when the clinical picture is appropriate and MRI is normal, the next step is the etiologic investigation. This is the most important work in the management of a patient with lacunar infarct, and hypertension can never be considered the sole cause of the infarct. Although carotid and other vascular lesions, cardioembolic disease, and hematologic alterations have a low etiologic incidence in patients with lacunar infarct, these must be investigated.[7,87,99,131,184] Etiologic study includes looking for vascular risk factors (mainly hypertension and diabetes mellitus) and trying to find a vascular abnormality by Doppler or MR angiography, a cardioembolic disease by electroencephalogram and echocardiogram, and a hematologic process. Patients with lacunes have a risk of developing dementia in the next 4 years of 23%[121]; because of this it is important to perform a neuropsychological study as a reference point for the follow-up. Treatment of vascular risk factors, other possible etiologies, and the consequences of stroke is the next step.

The evidence is that one in every five ischemic stroke patients has a lacune; such evidence has good sensitivity and specificity in clinical diagnosis and good correlation with lacunar syndromes and with pathologic studies. Thus small vessel disease producing lacunes is a well-established subtype of ischemic stroke; in a recent study at 28 medical centers, small vessel disease was the most common initial diagnosis (38%) in 479 ischemic stroke patients.[124] In spite of this evidence, it is necessary to perform complete investigations in all patients presenting with a lacunar syndrome due to this stroke subtype, as the others have many problematic aspects in terms of etiology, pathology, topography, and treatment that deserve careful and exhaustive clinical study and research.

References

1. Abadie JL: Les localisations functionelles de la capsule interne. Thesis, Bordeaux, 1900
2. Aleksie SN, George AE: Pure motor hemiplegia with occlusion of the extracranial carotid artery. J Neurol Sci 19:331, 1973
3. Alpers BJ: Clinical Neurology. F A Davis Philadelphia, 1958
4. Antin SP, Prockop LD, Cohen SM: Transient hemiballism. Neurology (Minneap) 17:1068, 1967
5. Arboix A, Marti-Vilalta JL: Acute stroke and circadian rhythm. Stroke 21:826, 1990
6. Arboix A, Marti-Vilalta JL: Lacunar syndromes not due to lacunar infarcts. Cerebrovasc Dis 2:287, 1992
7. Arboix A, Marti-Vilalta JL: Presumed cardioembolic lacunar infarcts. Stroke 23:1841, 1992
8. Arboix A, Marti-Vilalta JL: Transient ischemic attacks in lacunar infarct. Cerebrovasc Dis 1:20, 1991
9. Arboix A, Marti-Vilalta JL, Garcia JH: Clinical study of 227 patients with lacunar infarcts. Stroke 21:842, 1990
10. Arboix A, Marti-Vilalta JL, Pujol J et al: Lacunar infarct and nuclear magnetic resonance. A review of sixty cases. Eur Neurol 30:47, 1990
11. Awad IA, Johnson PC, Spetzler RF, Hodak JA: Incidental subcortical lesions identified on magnetic resonance imaging in the elderly. II. Postmortem pathological correlations. Stroke 17:1090, 1986
12. Barinagarrementeria F, Del Brutto OH: Lacunar syndrome due to neurocysticercosis. Arch Neurol 46:415, 1989
13. Bendheim PE, Berg BO: Ataxic hemiparesis from a midbrain mass. Ann Neurol 9:405, 1981
14. Boiten J: Lacunar stroke. A prospective clinical and radiological study. Thesis, Maastricht, 1991
15. Boiten J, Lodder J: Lacunar infarcts. Pathogenesis and validity of the clinical syndromes. Stroke 22:1374, 1991
16. Bonhoeffer K: Klinischer und anatomischer Befund zur Lehre von der Apraxie und der "motorischen Sprachbahn." Monatsschr Psychiatr Neurol 35:113, 1914
17. Brown MM, Hesselink JR, Rothrock JF: MR and CT of lacunar infarcts. AJNR 9:477, 1988
18. Byrom FB: The Hypertensive Vascular Crisis. Grune & Stratton, New York, 1969
19. Byrom FB: The pathogenesis of hypertensive encephalopathy and its relation to the malignant phase of hypertension. Lancet 2:201, 1954
20. Byrom FB, Dodson LF: The causation of acute arterial necrosis in hypertensive disease. J Pathol Bacteriol 60:357, 1948
21. Caplan LR, Young RR: EEG findings in certain lacunar stroke syndromes. Neurology 22:403, 1972
22. Castaigne P, Lhermitte F, Buge A et al: Paramedian thalamic and midbrain infarcts: clinical and neuropathologic study. Ann Neurol 10:127, 1981
23. Challa VR, Moody DM, Bell MA: The Charcot-Bouchard aneurysm controversy: impact of a new histologic technique. J Neuropathol Exp Neurol 51:264, 1992
24. Chamorro AM, Sacco RL, Mohr JP et al: Lacunar infarction: clinical-CT correlations in the Stroke Data Bank. Stroke 22:175, 1991
25. Chester EM, Agamanolis DP, Banker Q, Victor M: Hypertensive encephalopathy: a clinicopathologic study of 20 cases. Neurology 28:928, 1978
26. Chokroverty S, Rubino FA, Haller C: Pure motor hemiplegia due to pyramidal infarction. Arch Neurol 2:647, 1975
27. Clavier I, Hommel M, Besson G et al: Long-term prognosis of symptomatic lacunar infarcts. A hospital-based study. Stroke 25:2005, 1995
28. Cole FM, Yates PO: Pseudo-aneurysms in relationship to massive cerebral haemorrhage. J Neurol Neurosurg Psychiat 30:61, 1967
29. Combarros O, Polo JM, Pascual J et al: Evidence of somatotopic organization of the sensory thalamus based on infarction in the nucleus ventralis posterior. Stroke 22:1445, 1991
30. Croisile B, Henry E, Trillet M, Aimard G: Loss of motivation for speaking with bilateral lacunes in the anterior limb of the internal capsule. Clin Neurol Neurosurg 91:325, 1989
31. Damasio AR, Damasio H, Rizzo M et al: Aphasia with nonhemorrhagic lesions of the basal ganglia and internal capsule. Arch Neurol 39:15, 1982
32. Dattner B, Thomas EW, Wexler G: The Management of Neurosyphilis. Grune & Stratton, New York, 1944
33. Davis LE, Xie JG, Zou AH et al: Deep cerebral infarcts in the People's Republic of China. Stroke 21:394, 1990
34. Dechambre A: Mémoire sur la curabilité du ramollissement cérébral. Gaz Med Paris 6:305, 1838
35. Dejerine J, Dejerine Klumpke H: Anatomie des Centres Nerveux. Vol. 2 Rueff, Paris, 1901
36. Dejerine J, Roussy G: La syndrome thalamique. Rev Neurol (Paris) 14:521, 1906
37. De Reuck J, van der Eecken H: The topography of infarcts in the lacunar state. p. 162. In Meyer JS, Lechner H, Reivich M (eds): Cerebral Vascular Disease. 7th In-

ternational Conference, Salzburg, Thieme Edition/Publishing Sciences Group, New York, 1976

38. Devinsky O, Petito CK, Alonso DR: Clinical and neuropathological findings in systemic lupus erythematosus: the role of vasculitis, heart emboli, and thrombotic thrombocytopenic purpura. Ann Neurol 23:380, 1988

39. Dethy S, Luxen A, Bidaut LM et al: Hemibody tremor related to stroke. Stroke 24:2094, 1993

40. D'Olhaberriague L, Arboix A, Marti-Vilalta JL et al: Movement disorders in ischemic stroke: clinical study of 22 patients. Eur J Neurol 2:553, 1995

41. Donnan GA, Tress BM, Bladin PF: A prospective study of lacunar infarction using computerized tomography. Neurology 32:49, 1982

42. Durand-Fardel M: Mémoire sur une alteration particulière de la substance cérébrale. Gaz Med Paris 10:23, 1842

43. Dustin P Jr: Arteriolar hyalinosis. p. 73. In Richter GU, Epstein MA (eds): International Review Experimental Pathology. Vol. 1. Academic Press, New York, 1962

44. Earnest MP, Fahn S, Karp JH, Rowland LP: Normal pressure hydrocephalus and hypertensive cerebrovascular disease. Arch Neurol 31:262, 1974

45. Ekstrom Jodal B, Haggendal E, Linder LE et al: Cerebral blood flow autoregulation at high arterial pressures and different levels of carbon dioxide tension in dogs. Eur Neurol 6:6, 1972

46. Elster AD: MR contrast enhancement in brainstem and deep cerebral infarction. AJNR 12:1127, 1991

47. Englander RN, Netsky MG, Adelman LS: Location of human pyramidal tract in the internal capsule: anatomic evidence. Neurology 25:823, 1975

48. Falcone N, Fensore C, Lanzetti A et al: Clinical considerations and EEG-CT correlations in lacunar infarcts. Riv Neurol 56:396, 1986

49. Feigin I, Prose P: Hypertensive fibrinoid arteritis of the brain and gross cerebral hemorrhage: a form of "hyalinosis." Arch Neurol 1:98, 1959

50. Ferrand J: Essai sur l'hémiplegie des vieillards, les lacunes de désintegrations cérébrale. Thesis, Rousset, Paris, 1902

51. Fisher CM: Pure sensory stroke involving face, arm and leg. Neurology (Minneap) 15:76, 1965

52. Fisher CM: Lacunes: small deep cerebral infarcts. Neurology (Minneap) 15:774, 1965

53. Fisher CM: A lacunar stroke. The dysarthria clumsy hand syndrome. Neurology (Minneap) 17:614, 1967

54. Fisher CM: Some neuroophthalmologic observations. J Neurol Neurosurg Psychiatry 30:383, 1967

55. Fisher CM: The arterial lesions underlying lacunes. Acta Neuropathol (Berl) 12:1, 1969

56. Fisher CM: Cerebral ischemia: less familiar types. Clin Neurosurg 18:267, 1971

57. Fisher CM: Bilateral occlusion of basilar artery branches. J Neurol Neurosurg Psychiatry 40:1182, 1977

58. Fisher CM: Thalamic pure sensory stroke: a pathologic study. Neurology (NY) 28:1141, 1978

59. Fisher CM: Ataxic hemiparesis. Arch Neurol 35:126, 1978

60. Fisher CM: Capsular infarcts. Arch Neurol 36:65, 1979

61. Fisher CM: Lacunar strokes and infarcts: a review. Neurology (NY) 32:871, 1982

62. Fisher CM: Pure sensory stroke and allied conditions. Stroke 13:434, 1982

63. Fisher CM, Cole M: Homolateral ataxia and crural paresis. A vascular syndrome. J Neurol Neurosurg Psychiatry 28:48, 1965

64. Fisher CM, Curry HB: Pure motor hemiplegia of vascular origin. Arch Neurol (Chic) 13:30, 1965

65. Fisher CM, Caplan, LR: Basilar artery branch occlusion: a cause of pontine infarction. Neurology (Minneap) 21:900, 1971

66. Fisher CM, Gore I, Okabe N, White PD: Atherosclerosis of the carotid and vertebral arteries. Extracranial and intracranial. J Neuropathol Exp Neurol 24:455, 1965

67. Foix C, Hillemand P: Contribution à l'étude des ramollissements protruberantiels. Rev Med 43:287, 1926

68. Foix C, Levy M: Les ramollissements sylviens, Rev Neurol 11:1, 1927

69. Fredericks RK, Leflowitz DS, Challa VR et al: Cerebral vasculitis associated with cocaine abuse. Stroke 22:1437, 1991

70. Garcia JH, Ho KL: Pathology of hypertensive arteriopathy. Neurosurg Clin North Am 3:487, 1992

71. Garcin R, Lapresle J: Syndrome sensitif de type thalamique et etopographie cheiro orale par lesion localisée du thalamus. Rev Neurol 90:124, 1954

72. Gautier JC: Cerebral ischemia in hypertension. p. 181. In Russell R (ed): Cerebral Arterial Disease. Churchill Livingston, London, 1978

73. Giese J: The pathogenesis of hypertensive vascular disease. Dan Med Bull 14:259, 1967

74. Goldblatt H: Studies on experimental hypertension: VII. The production of the malignant phase of hypertension. J Exp Med 67:809, 1938

75. Goldblatt D, Markesbery W, Reeves AG: Recurrent hemichorea following striatal lesions. Arch Neurol 31:51, 1974

76. Gorelick PB, Caplan LR: Racial differences in the distribution of anterior circulation occlusive disease. Neurology 34:54, 1984

77. Groothius DR, Duncan GW, Fisher CM: The human thalamocortical sensory path in the internal capsule: evidence from a capsular hemorrhage causing a pure sensory stroke. Ann Neurol 2:328, 1977

78. Gross CR, Kase CS, Mohr JP, Cunningham SC: Stroke in south Alabama: incidence and diagnostic features. Stroke 15:249, 1984

79. Guberman A, Stuss D: The syndrome of bilateral paramedian thalamic infarction. Neurology (Clevel) 33:540, 1983

80. Gursahani RD, Khadilkar SV, Surya N, Singhal BS: Capsular involvement and sensorimotor stroke with posterior cerebral artery territory infarction. J Assoc Physicians India 38:939, 1990

81. Hanaway J, Young RR: Localization of the pyramidal tract in the internal capsule of man. J Neurol Sci 34:63, 1977

82. Hier DB, Foulkes MA, Swiontoniowski M et al: Stroke recurrence within 2 years after ischaemic infarction. Stroke 22:155, 1991

83. Heptinstall RH: Pathology of the Kidney. 2nd Ed. Vol. 1. p. 121. Little, Brown Company, Boston, 1974

84. Hill GS: Studies on the pathogenesis of hypertensive vascular disease: effect of high pressure intraarterial injections in rats. Circ Res 27:657, 1970

85. Ho KL: Pure motor hemiplegia due to infarction of the cerebral peduncle. Arch Neurol 39:524, 1982

86. Hommel M, Besson G, Le Bas JF et al: Prospective study of lacunar infarction using magnetic resonance imaging. Stroke 21:546, 1990

87. Horwitz DR, Tuhrim S, Weinberger JM: Mechanism in lacunar infarction. Stroke 23:325, 1992

88. Huang CY, Chan FL, Yu YL et al: Cerebrovascular disease in Hong Kong Chinese. Stroke 21:230, 1990

89. Huang CY, Lui FS: Ataxic hemiparesis: localization and clinical features. Stroke 15:363, 1984

90. Hyland HH, Forman DM: Prognosis in hemiballismus. Neurology (Minneap) 7:381, 1957

91. Ichikawa K, Tsutsumishita A, Fujioka A: Capsular ataxic hemiparesis: a case report. Arch Neurol 39:585, 1982

92. Igapashi S, Mori K, Ishijima Y: Pure motor hemiplegia after recraniotomy for postoperative bleeding. Arch Jpn Chir. 41:32, 1965

93. Iragui VJ, McCutchen CB: Capsular ataxic hemiparesis. Arch Neurol 39:528, 1982

94. Kapelle LJ, van Gijn J: Carotid angiography in patients with subcortical ischaemia. p. 80. In Donnan GA, Norrving B, Bamford JM, Bogousslavsky J (eds): Lacunar and Other Subcortical Infarctions. Oxford University Press, Oxford, 1995

95. Kapelle LJ, van Huffelen AC: Electroencephalography in patients with small, deep infarcts. p. 87. In Donnan GA, Norrving B, Bamford JM, Bogousslavsky J (eds): Lacunar and Other Subcortical Infarctions. Oxford University Press Oxford, 1995

96. Kase CS, Levitz SM, Wolinsky JS, Sulis CA: Pontine pure motor hemiparesis due to meningovascular syphilis in human immunodeficiency virus-positive patients [letter]. Arch Neurol 45:832, 1988

97. Kase CS, Maulsby GO, deJuan E, Mohr JP: Hemichorea hemiballism and lacunar infarction in the basal ganglia. Neurology 31:454, 1981

98. Kempster PA, Gerraty RP, Gates PC: Asymptomatic cerebral infarction in patients with chronic atrial fibrillation. Stroke 19:955, 1988

99. Kilpatrick TJ, Matkovic Z, Davis SM et al: Hematologic abnormalities occur in both cortical and lacunar infarction. Stroke 24:1945, 1993

100. Kim JS: Delayed onset hand tremor caused by cerebral infarction. Stroke 23:292, 1992

101. Kim JS: Pure sensory stroke. Clinical-radiological correlates of 21 cases. Stroke 23:983, 1992

102. Kistler JP, Buonanno FS, DeWitt LD et al: Vertebral basilar posterior cerebral territory stroke delineation by proton nuclear magnetic resonance imaging. Stroke 15:417, 1984

103. Kleist K: Gehirnpathologie. p. 930. Barth, Leipzig, 1934

104. Kobayashi S, Okada K, Yamashita K: Incidence of silent lacunar lesion in normal adults and its relation to cerebral blood flow and risk factors. Stroke 22:1379, 1991

105. Kohler J, Kern U, Kasper J et al: Chronic central nervous system involvement in Lyme borreliosis. Neurology 38:863, 1988

106. Koto A, Rosenberg G, Zingesser LH et al: Syndrome of normal pressure hydrocephalus: possible relation to hypertensive and arteriosclerotic vasculopathy. J Neurol Neurosurg Psychiatry 40:73, 1977

107. Kribs M, Kleihues J: The recurrent artery of Heubner. p.40. In Zulch KJ (ed): Cerebral Circulation and Stroke. Springer-Verlag, New York, 1971

108. Kumral E, Bogousslavsky J, Van Melle G et al: Headache at stroke onset: the Lausanne Stroke Registry. J Neurol Neurosurg Psychiatry 58:490, 1995

109. Labar DR, Petty GW, Emerson RG, Mohr JP, Pedley TA: Abnormal somatosensory evoked potentials in patients with motor deficits due to lacunar strokes. Electroencephalogr Clin Neurophysiol 67:74, 1987

110. Laitinen LV: Loss of motivation for speaking with bilateral lacunes in the anterior limb of the internal capsule. Clin Neurol Neurosurg 92:177, 1990

111. Laloux P, Broucher JM: Lacunar infarctions due to cholesterol emboli. Stroke 22:1440, 1991

112. Landau WM: Clinical neuromythology VI. Au clair de lacune: holy, wholly, holey logic. Neurology 39:725, 1989

113. Lapresle J, Haguenau S: Anatomico-clinical correlation in focal thalamic lesions. Z Neurol 205:29, 1973

114. LaRue L, Alter M, Lai SM et al: Acute stroke, hematocrit, and blood pressure. Stroke 18:565, 1987

115. Launay M, N'Diaye M, Bories J: X-ray computed tomography (CT) study of small, deep and recent infarcts (SDRIs) of the cerebral hemispheres in adults. Neuroradiology 27:494, 1985

116. Lazzarino LG, Nicolai A, Poldelmengo P et al: Risk factors in lacunar strokes. A retrospective study of 52 patients. Acta Neurol (Napoli) 11:265, 1989

117. Leestma JE, Noronha A: Pure motor hemiplegia, medullary pyramid lesion, and olivary hypertrophy Arch Neurol 39:877, 1976

118. Lenz FA, Dostrovsky JO, Tasker RR et al: Single unit analysis of the human ventral thalamic nuclear group: somatosensory responses. J Neurophysiol 59:299, 1988

119. Levine SR, Deegan MJ, Futrell N et al: Cerebrovascular and neurologic disease associated with antiphospholipid antibodies: 48 cases. Neurology 40:1181, 1990

120. Loeb C: The lacunar syndromes. Eur Neurol 29:2, 1989

121. Loeb C, Gandolfo C, Croce R et al: Dementia associated with lacunar infarction. Stroke 23:1225, 1992

122. Loeb DJ, Biller J, Yuh WTC et al: Leukoencephalopathy in cerebral amyloid angiopathy. MR imaging in four cases. AJNR 11:485, 1990

123. Luijckx GJ, Boiten J, Lodder J et al: Cardiac and carotid embolism, and other rare definite disorders are unlikely causes of lacunar ischaemic stroke in young patients. Cerebrovasc Dis 6:28, 1996

124. Madden KP, Karanjia PN, Adams HP et al: Accuracy of initial stroke subtype diagnosis in the TOAST study. Neurology 45:1975, 1995

125. Manfredi M, Cruccu G: Thalamic pain revisited. p. 73. In Loeb C (ed): Studies in Cereobrovascular Disease. Masson Italiano Editori, Milano, 1981

126. Marie P: A case of transitory anarthria by lesion of the lenticular zone. Bull Mem Soc Med 23:1291, 1906.

Translated in Cole MF, Cole M: Pierre Marie's Papers on Speech Disorders. Hafner, New York, p. 135–141. 1971

127. Marie P: Des foyers lacunaire de désintegration et de différents autres états cavitaires du cerveau. Rev Med 21:281, 1901

128. Martin JP: Hemichorea (hemiballismus) without lesions in the corpus Luysii. Brain 80:1, 1957

129. Massey EW, Goodman JC, Stewart C et al: Unilateral asterixis: motor integrative dysfunction in focal vascular disease. Neurology 29:1188, 1979

130. Mast H, Thompson JL, Lee SH et al: Hypertension and diabetes mellitus as determinants of multiple lacunar infarcts. Stroke 26:30, 1995

131. Mast H, Thompson JL, Voller H et al: Cardiac sources of embolism in patients with pial artery infarcts and lacunar lesions. Stroke 25:776, 1994

132. Melamed E, Korn Lubetzki I, Reches A et al: Hemiballismus: detection of focal hemorrhage in subthalamic nucleus by CT scan. Ann Neurol 4:582, 1978

133. Melo TP, Bogousslavsky J, Van Melle G et al: Pure motor stroke: a reappraisal. Neurology 42:789, 1992

134. Merritt HH, Adams RD, Solomon HC: Neurosyphilis. Oxford University Press, New York, 1946

135. Meyers R: Ballismus. pp. 476, 490. In Vinken, PJ, Bruyn GW (eds): Handbook of Clinical Neurology. Vol. 6. North Holland, Amsterdam, 1968

136. Michel D, Laurent B, Foyatier N et al: Infarctus thalamique paramedian gauche. Rev Neurol (Paris) 138:6, 1982

137. Millikan C, Futrell N: The fallacy of the lacune hypothesis. Stroke 21:1251, 1990

138. Misra UK, Kalita J: Putaminal haemorrhage leading to pure motor hemiplegia. Acta Neurol Scand 91:283, 1995

139. Miyashita K, Naritomi H, Sawada T et al: Identification of recent lacunar lesions in cases of multiple small infarctions by magnetic resonance imaging. Stroke 19:834, 1988

140. Mohr JP: Lacunes. Neurol Clin North Am 1:201, 1983

141. Mohr JP, Caplan LR, Melski JW et al: The Harvard Cooperative Stroke Registry. Neurology 28:754, 1978

142. Mohr JP, Kase CS, Meckler RJ, Fisher CM: Sensorimotor stroke. Arch Neurol. 34:739, 1977

143. Mohr JP, Kase CS, Wolf PA et al: Lacunes in the NINCDS Pilot Stroke Data Bank, abstracted. Ann Neurol 12:84, 1982

144. Moulin T, Bogousslavsky J, Chopard JL et al: Vascular ataxic hemiparesis: a re-evaluation. J Neurol Neurosurg Psychiatry 58:422, 1995

145. Naeser MA, Alexander MP, Helm Estabrooks N et al: Aphasia with predominantly subcortical lesion sites. Arch Neurol 39:2, 1982

146. Nelson RF, Pullicino P, Kendall BE, Marshall J: Computed tomography on patients presenting with lacunar syndromes. Stroke 11:256, 1980

147. Park YD, Belman AL, Kim TS et al: Stroke in pediatric acquired immunodeficiency syndrome. Ann Neurol 28:303, 1990

148. Paronetto F: Immunocytochemical observations on the vascular necrosis and renal glomerular lesions of malignant nephrosclerosis. Am J Pathol 46:901, 1965

149. Pearce JMS, Chandrasekera CP, Ladusans EJ: Lacunar infarcts in polycythemia with raised packer cell volumes. BMJ 287:935, 1983

150. Pentschew A: Gibt es eine Endarteritis luica der kleinen Hirnrindengefässe (Nissl Alzheimer)? Nervenartz 8:393, 1935

151. Percheron SMJ: Les arteres du thalamus humain. Rev Neurol 132:297, 1976

152. Perman GP, Racey A: Homolateral ataxic and crural paresis: case report. Neurology 30:1013, 1980

153. Plets C, DeReuck J, Vander Ecken H et al: The vascularization of the human thalamus. Acta Neurol Belg 70:685, 1970

154. Poirer J, Barbizet J, Gaston A, Meyrignac C: Démence thalamique. Rev Neurol (Paris) 139:5, 1983

155. Pullicino P, Kendall BE: Contrast enhancement in ischaemic lesions. I. Relationship to prognosis. Neuroradiology 19:235, 1980

156. Pullicino P, Nelson RF, Kendall BE, Marshall J: Small deep infarcts diagnosed on computed tomography. Neurology 30:1090, 1980

157. Rascol A, Clanet M, Manelfe C et al: Pure motor hemiplegia: CT study of 30 cases. Stroke 13:11, 1982

158. Reimers J, de Wytt C, Seneviratne B: Lacunar infarction: a 12 month study. Clin Exp Neurol 24:28, 1987

159. Richter RW, Brust JCM, Bruun B, Shafer SQ: Frequency and course of pure motor hemiparesis: a clinical study. Stroke 8:58, 1977

160. Robinson RK, Richey ET, Kase CS, Mohr JP: Somatosensory evoked potentials in pure sensory stroke and allied conditions, abstracted. Neurology 34:231, 1984

161. Ropper AH, Fisher CM, Kleinman GM: Pyramidal infarction in the medulla: a cause of pure motor hemiplegia sparing the face. Neurology (NY) 29:91, 1979

162. Rosenberg EF: The brain in malignant hypertension. A clinicopathological study. Arch Intern Med 65:545, 1940

163. Rosenberg NL, Koller R: Computerized tomography and pure sensory stroke. Neurology (NY) 31:217, 1981

164. Ross ED: Localization of the pyramidal tract in the internal capsule by whole brain dissection. Neurology (NY) 30:59, 1980

165. Ross Russell RW: Observations on intracerebral aneurysms. Brain 86:425, 1963

166. Rothrock JF, Lyden PD, Hesselink JR et al: Brain magnetic resonance imaging in the evaluation of lacunar infarcts. Stroke 18:781, 1987

167. Rothrock JF, Lyden PD, Yee J et al: "Crescendo" transient ischemic attacks: clinical and angiographic correlations. Neurology 38:198, 1988

168. Rottenberg, DA, Talman W, Chernik NL: Location of pyramidal tract questioned. Neurology (Minneap) 26:291, 1976

169. Russo LS: Focal dystonia and lacunar infarction of the basal ganglia. Neurology (NY) 40:61, 1983

170. Sacco SE, Whisnant JP, Broderick J et al: Epidemiological characteristics of lacunar infarcts in a population. Stroke 22:1236, 1991

171. Sage JI: Ataxic hemiparesis from lesions of the corona radiata. Arch Neurol 40:449, 1983

172. Sakai T, Murakami S, Ito K: Ataxic hemiparesis with trigeminal weakness. Neurology (NY) 31:635, 1981

173. Salgado ED, Weinstein M, Furlan AF et al: Proton magnetic resonance imaging in ischaemic cerebrovascular disease. Ann Neurol 20:502, 1986

174. Samuelsson M, Samuelsson L, Lindell D: Sensory symptoms and signs and results of quantitative sensory thermal testing in patients with lacunar infarct syndromes. Stroke 25:2165, 1994

175. Santamaria J, Graus F, Rubio F et al: Cerebral infarction of the basal ganglia due to embolism from the heart. Stroke 14:911, 1983

176. Saris S: Chorea caused by caudate infarction. Arch Neurol 40:590, 1983

177. Satomi K, Terashima Y, Goto K et al: Capsular pseudobulbar mutism in a patient of lacunar state. Rinsho Shinkeigaku 30:299, 1990

178. Schott B, Maugiere F, Laurent B et al: L'amnésie thalamique. Rev Neurol (Paris) 136:117, 1980

179. Spertell RB, Ransom BR: Dysarthria clumsy hand syndrome produced by capsular infarct. Ann Neurol 6:268, 1979

180. Skinhoj E, Strandgaard S: Pathogenesis of hypertensive encephalopathy. Lancet 1:461, 1973

181. Sunohara N, Mukoyama M, Mano Y, Satoyoshi E: Action induced rhythmic dystonia: an autopsy case. Neurology (Cleve) 34:321, 1984

182. Tapia JF, Kase CS, Sawyer RH, Mohr JP: Hypertensive putaminal hemorrhage presenting as pure motor hemiparesis. Stroke 14:505, 1983

183. Tatemichi TK, Desmond DW, Prohovnik I et al: Confusion and memory loss from capsular genu infarction. A thalamocortical disconnection syndrome? Neurology 42:1966, 1992

184. Tegeler CH, Shi F, Morgan T: Carotid stenosis in lacunar stroke. Stroke 22:1124, 1991

185. Tjeerdsma HC, Rinkel GJE, van Gijn J: Ataxic hemiparesis from a primary intracerebral haematoma in the precentral area. Cerebrovasc Dis 6:45, 1996

186. Tuhrim S, Yang WC, Rubinowitz H, Weinberger J: Primary pontine hemorrhage and the dysarthria clumsy hand syndrome. Neurology (NY) 31:635, 1982

187. Tuszynski MH, Petito CK, Levy DE: Risk factors and clinical manifestations of pathologically verified lacunar infarctions. Stroke 20:990, 1989

188. Vestergaard K, Andersen G, Nielsen MI et al: Headache in stroke. Stroke 24:1621, 1993

189. Vogt C, Vogt O: Zur Lehre der Erkrankungen des striaren Systems. J Psychol Neurol 25:627, 1920

190. Waterston JA, Brown MM, Butler P, Swash M: Small deep cerebral infarcts associated with occlusive internal carotid artery disease. A hemodynamic phenomenon? Arch Neurol 47:953, 1990

191. Wallesch CW, Kornhuber HH, Kunz T, Brunner RJ: Neuropsychological deficits associated with small unilateral thalamic lesions. Brain 106:141, 1983

192. Weintraub MI, Glaser GH: Norcardial brain abcess and pure motor hemiplegia. NY J Med 70:2717, 1970

193. Weisberg LA: Computed tomography and pure motor hemiparesis. Neurology (NY) 29:490, 1979

194. Weisberg LA: Lacunar infarcts. Arch Neurol 39:37, 1982

195. Weschler IS: Textbook of Clinical Neurology. WB Saunders Philadelphia, 1943

196. Wiener J, Spiro D, Lattes RG: The cellular pathology of experimental hypertension: II. Arteriolar hyalinosis and fibrinoid change. Am J Pathol 47:457, 1965

197. Wolfe N, Linn R, Babikian VL et al: Frontal systems impairment following multiple lacunar infarcts. Arch Neurol 47:129, 1990

198. Wyllie J: The Disorders of Speech. p. 340–344. Oliver & Boyd, Edinburgh, 1894

199. Yagnik P, Dhopesh V: Unilateral asterixis. Arch Neurol 38:601, 1981

CHAPTER 24

Cerebral Venous Thrombosis

MARIE-GERMAINE BOUSSER

HENRY J.M. BARNETT

In 1825, Ribes[118] described the clinical history of a 45-year-old man who died after a 6-month history of severe headache, epilepsy, and delirium. Postmortem examination showed thrombosis of the superior sagittal sinus (SSS), the left lateral sinus (LS), and a cortical vein in the parietal region. This was probably the first detailed description of cerebral venous thrombosis (CVT) in a human. Since then, numerous case reports and series have been published, most of them from autopsy material.[8,12,44,61,82,87,107,142,143] They led to the classical description of a rare and severe disease characterized clinically by headache, papilledema, seizures, focal deficits, progressive coma, and death and pathologically by hemorrhagic infarction that was thought to contraindicate the use of anticoagulants.

This early literature and the history of CVT have been extensively covered in two excellent French[61] and English[82] monographs. However, angiography[88,162] and more recently magnetic resonance imaging (MRI)[30,42,43,79, 92,95,96,99,100,108,147,150,151] and magnetic resonance angiography (MRA)[4,30,97,99,100,108,111] have made intra vitam diagnosis possible, and evidence has accumulated that many patients do not fall into this classical description.[3,6,9,10,14,20,29,33,36,47,48,51,63,91, 104,124,135] The recent literature has convincingly shown that

1. CVT is far more common than previously assumed.
2. The spectrum of its clinical presentation is extremely wide.
3. Its mode of onset is highly variable.
4. Its outcome is usually favorable.
5. The treatment of choice is heparin.[20,40,49]

Because of its frequently misleading presentation, its wide variety of causes, its unpredictable course, and its occasional treatment problems, CVT remains a challenge for the clinician.

Relevant Venous Anatomy

Blood from the brain is drained by cerebral veins that empty into dural sinuses, themselves mostly drained by the internal jugular veins.[33,61,69,82]

DURAL SINUSES

The dural sinuses most commonly affected by thrombosis are the SSS, LS, and cavernous sinuses (Figs. 24.1 and 24.2).

Superior Sagittal Sinus

SSS lies in the attached border of the falx cerebri. It starts at the foramen cecum and runs backward toward the occipital protuberance, where it joins with the straight sinus (SS) and LS to form the torcular herophili. Its anterior part is narrow, or sometimes absent, replaced by two superior cerebral veins that join behind the coronal suture.[82] Consequently, the anterior part of the sinus is often poorly visualized on angiography, and its isolated lack of filling is not sufficient to indicate thrombosis.[87,88]

The SSS receives superficial cerebral veins and drains the major part of the cortex. It also receives diploic veins, themselves connected to scalp veins by emissary veins, which explains some cases of SSS thrombosis after cutaneous infections or contusions. The SSS and other sinuses play a major role in cerebrospinal fluid (CSF) circulation because they contain most of the arachnoid villi and granulations (pacchionian bodies) in which much of the CSF absorption takes place. Thus, there is a direct dependency of CSF pressure on the intracranial venous pressure, accounting for the frequency of raised intracranial pressure in SSS or LS thrombosis.

Lateral Sinuses

The LS extend from the torcular herophili to the jugular bulbs and consist of two portions: the transverse portion, which lies in the attached border of the tentorium, and the sigmoid portion, which runs on the inner aspect of the mastoid process and is thereby susceptible to infectious thrombosis in patients with mastoiditis or otitis media. The LS drain blood from the cerebellum, brain stem, and posterior part of the cerebral hemispheres. They also receive some of the diploic veins and some small veins from the middle ear, yet another possible source of septic thrombosis.

623

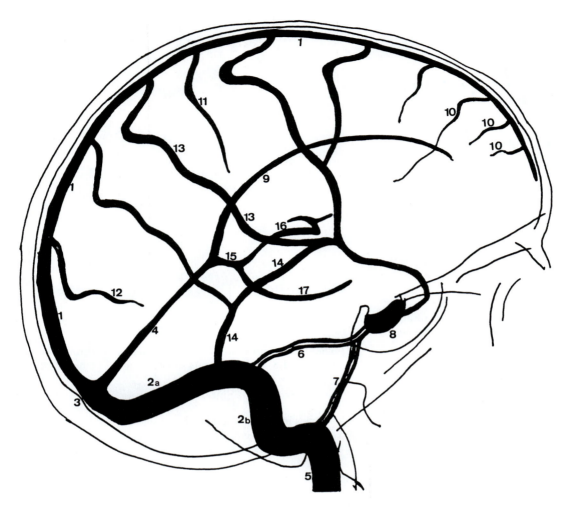

Figure 24.1 Superficial and deep cerebral veins and dural sinuses: *1*, superior sagittal sinus; *2a*, transverse portion of lateral sinus; *2b*, sigmoid portion of lateral sinus; *3*, torcular herophili; *4*, straight sinus; *5*, internal jugular vein; *6*, superior petrosal sinus; *7*, inferior petrosal sinus; *8*, cavernous sinus; *9*, inferior sagittal sinus; *10*, frontal veins; *11*, parietal vein; *12*, occipital vein; *13*, Trolard's vein; *14*, Labbé's vein; *15*, great vein of Galen; *16*, internal cerebral vein; *17*, basal vein.

Numerous LS anatomic variations may be misinterpreted as sinus occlusion on angiography. In particular, the right LS, which is often a direct continuation of the SSS, is frequently larger than the left, which receives most of its supply from the straight sinus. In Hacker's[69] study, the transverse portions were not visualized on ipsilateral carotid angiograms in 14% of cases on the left side and in 3.3% on the right side, whereas sigmoid portions, which may be directly injected via cerebral veins, failed to fill in 4% of cases on the left side and were always demonstrated on the right. An isolated lack of filling of a left transverse sinus is thus more suggestive of hypoplasia than of thrombosis.

Cavernous Sinuses

Cavernous sinuses consist of trabeculated cavities formed by the separation of the layers of the dura and located on each side of the sella turcica, superolaterally to the sphenoid air sinuses. The oculomotor and trochlear cranial nerves, along with the ophthalmic and maxillary branches of the trigeminal nerve, course along the lateral wall of the cavernous sinuses, whereas the abducens nerve and the carotid artery with its surrounding sympathetic plexus are located within the center of the sinus itself.

Cavernous sinuses drain the blood from the orbits through the ophthalmic veins and from the anterior part of the base of the brain by the sphenoparietal sinus and the middle cerebral veins. They empty into both the superior and inferior petrosal sinuses and ultimately into the internal jugular veins. Because of their situation, cavernous sinuses are often thrombosed in relation to infections of the face or sphenoid sinusitis and, in contrast to other varieties of sinus thrombosis, infection is still the leading cause of thrombosis.[40]

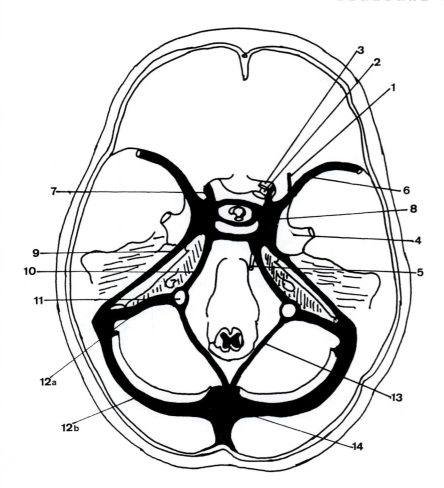

Figure 24.2 Cavernous sinus and dural sinuses: *1*, trochlear cranial nerve; *2*, carotid artery; *3*, optic nerve; *4*, trigeminal nerve; *5*, oculomotor nerve; *6*, sphenoparietal sinus; *7*, ophthalmic vein; *8*, cavernous sinus; *9*, superior petrosal sinus; *10*, inferior petrosal sinus; *11*, internal jugular vein; *12a*, sigmoid portion of lateral sinus; *12b*, transverse portion of lateral sinus; *13*, posterior occipital sinus; *14*, torcular herophili.

Rarely injected on carotid angiograms, cavernous sinuses are now well visualized on computed tomography (CT) and MRI.

CEREBRAL VEINS

The three groups of veins that drain the blood supply from the brain are the superficial cerebral (or cortical), the deep cerebral, and the veins of the posterior fossa (Fig. 24.1).

Superficial Cerebral Veins

Some of the cortical veins—the frontal, parietal, and occipital superior cerebral veins—drain the cortex ascendingly into the SSS, whereas others, mainly the middle cerebral veins, drain descendingly into the cavernous sinuses. These veins are linked by Trolard's great anastomotic vein, which connects the SSS to the middle cerebral veins, which are themselves connected to the LS by Labbé's vein. These cortical veins present some peculiarities[82] that are important to know for understanding some of the clinical features of CVT. They have thin walls, no muscle fibers, and no valves, thereby permitting both their dilatation and the reversal of the direction of blood flow when the sinus in which they drain is occluded. They are linked by numerous anastomoses, allowing the development of a collateral circulation (angiographically visible as corkscrew vessels), which probably explains the good prognosis of some CVTs. The number and location of cortical veins are inconstant, which makes the angiographic diagnosis of isolated cortical vein thrombosis extremely difficult. This anatomic variability, together with the possibility of flow reversal and development of collateral circulation, accounts for the absence of well-delineated venous territories and consequently of well-defined clinical syndromes of cortical vein thrombosis.

Deep Cerebral Veins

Blood from the deep white matter of the cerebral hemispheres and from the basal ganglia is drained by internal cerebral and basal veins that join to form the great vein of Galen, which drains into the straight sinus. In contrast to the superficial veins, the deep system is constant and always visualized at angiography, so that its thrombosis is easily recognized.

Veins of the Posterior Fossa

Posterior fossa veins may be divided into three groups[76,77]: superior veins draining into the galenic system, anterior veins draining into the petrosal sinuses, and posterior veins draining into the torcular and neighboring SS and LS. They are variable in course, and angiographic diagnosis of their occlusion is extremely difficult.

Pathology

Pathologic findings have been extensively described.[61,82,142] They vary, depending on the site of thrombosis and the interval between the onset of symptoms and death.

The *thrombus* itself is like other venous thrombi elsewhere in the body: when it is fresh, it is rich in red blood cells and fibrin and poor in platelets; when it is old, it is replaced by fibrous tissue (Fig. 24.3), sometimes showing recanalization. Its formation is due to the usual pathogenetic factors: venous stasis, increased clotting tendency, changes in the vessel wall, and, less frequently, embolization. Its location and extension are variable. In autopsy series,[12,44,82] extensive thrombosis of the SSS and tributary veins is the most frequent finding, but we will see that this pattern of involvement no longer reflects the common expresion of clinically diagnosable CVT.

The consequences of CVT on the brain are again highly variable; massive brain edema can be the only consequence in thrombosis restricted to the SSS,[82] whereas occlusion of cerebral veins usually leads to infarction. Venous infarcts affect the cortex and adjacent white matter and are often hemorrhagic, which explains the possibility of associated subarachnoid hemorrhage and subdural or intracerebral hematomas. The classical anatomic presentation is that of extensive bilateral hemorrhagic infarcts, located in the superior and internal part of both hemispheres, due to thrombosis of the SSS and its tributary cortical veins (Fig. 24.4).

Incidence

The true incidence of CVT is totally unknown in the absence of epidemiologic studies specifically devoted to this subject. In most autopsy series, the incidence was extremely low. Ehlers and Courville[44] found only 16 SSS thromboses in a series of 12,500 autopsies, and Barnett and Hyland[12] found only 39 noninfective CVTs in 20 years. Kalbag and Woolf[82] indicated that CVT was the principal cause of death in only 21.7 persons/year in England and Wales between 1952 and 1961. By contrast, Towbin[148] found CVT in 9% of 182 consecutive autopsies, and Averback,[6] in a series of 7 cases, insists that primary CVT in young adults is an "under-recognized disease." The more recent publication of large clinical series[3,9,10,20,29,33,36,47,48,51,87,104,124,147] suggests that the true incidence is much higher than that thought from autopsy series, possibly 10 times higher because of a present mortality rate of approximately 10%.[20,147] Three to four new cases are encountered each year in a neurology department in a general hospital. All age groups—from the neonate to the very old—may be affected by CVT, with a slight preponderance in young females because of specific causes such as oral contraceptives, pregnancy, and puerperium.

Etiology

A host of well-known conditions can cause or predispose to CVT (Table 24.1). They include all known surgical, gynecoobstetric, and medical causes of deep vein thrombosis as well as a number of local or regional causes, either infective or

Figure 24.3 Old SSS thrombosis.

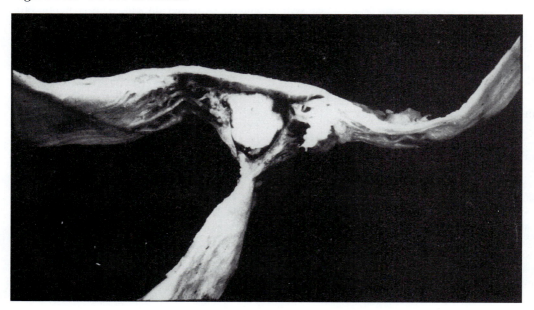

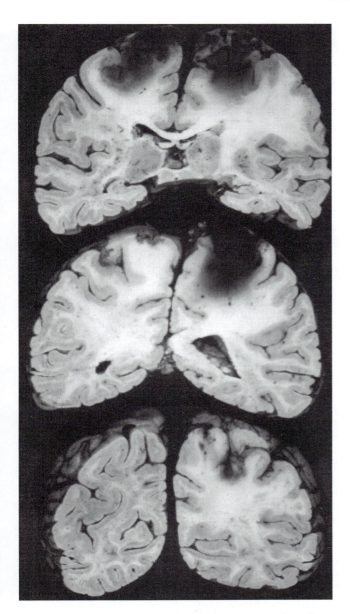

Figure 24.4 Bilateral hemorrhagic infarcts in SSS thrombosis.

Table 24.1 Cerebral Venous Thrombosis: Recognized Causes or Predisposing Conditions

Infectious causes
  Local
    Direct septic trauma[61,82]
    Intracranial infection: abscess, empyema, meningitis,[20,61,82,87,113] syphilitic osteitis[50]
    Regional infections: otitis, tonsillitis, sinusitis, stomatitis, skin[61,82,87,142,143]
  General
    Bacterial: septicemia,[61,82,87] endocarditis,[61,82,87] typhoid,[61] tuberculosis,[107]
    Viral: measles,[82] hepatitis,[107] encephalitis[82] (herpes, HIV),[102] CMV,[102]
    Parasitic: malaria,[33] trichinosis,[56]
    Fungal: aspergillosis[130]
Noninfectious causes
  Local
    Head injury (open or closed, with or without fracture)[12,20,61,82,85,107,147]
    Neurosurgical operation[61,82,107]
    Cerebral infarcts and hemorrhages[12,82]
    Tumors (meningioma, metastasis, glomus tumor, medulloblastoma)[24,61,82,107]
    Porencephaly, arachnoid cysts[20,33,61]
    Dural arteriovenous malformations[89,90,115]
    Infusions into the internal jugular vein[139]
  General
    Surgical: any surgery (with or without deep vein thrombosis)[3,12,33]
    Gynecoobstetric
      Pregnancy and puerperium[3,9,20,29,33,61,82,88,107,124]
      Oral contraceptives (estrogens, progestogens)[3,10,20,55,57,104,124]
    Medical
      Cardiac: congenital heart disease,[33] cardiac failure,[12,61,82,87,107] pacemaker[64]
      Malignancies: visceral carcinomas,[3,12,73,135,137] lymphomas,[40,69] leukemias,[33,40] L-asparaginase therapy,[77] carcinoid[76]
      RBC disorders: polycythemia,[12] posthemorrhagic anemia,[62] sickle cell disease and trait,[59] paroxysmal nocturnal hemoglobinuria,[2,63,130] iron deficiency anemia[3]
      Thrombocythemia (primary or secondary)[3,20,56]
      Coagulation disorders: AT,[125] protein C,[145] and protein S[53] deficiencies, increased resistance to activated protein C,[37,94,166] circulating anticoagulants,[37,90] disseminated intravascular coagulation,[137] heparin or heparinoid induced thrombocytopenia,[80] plasminogen deficiency,[127] epsilon aminocaproic acid treatment[1]
      Severe dehydration of any cause[14,61,62,82,107]
      Digestive: cirrhosis,[33,61] Crohn's disease,[23] ulcerative colitis[163]
      Connective tissue: systemic lupus,[90,57] temporal arteritis,[33] Wegener's granulomatosis,[103] Sjögren syndrome[153]
      Venous thromboembolic disease,[3] Hughes Stovin syndrome[145]
      Others: Behçet's disease,[19,165] sarcoidosis,[3,28] nephrotic syndrome,[15] neonatal asphyxia,[62] parenteral injections,[46] androgen therapy,[133] "ectasy,"[122] homocystinuria,[32] thyrotoxicosis,[134] electrocution[110]
Idiopathic

Abbreviations: HIV, human immunodeficiency virus; CMV, cytomegalovirus; RBC, red blood cells; AT, antithrombin.

noninfective, such as head trauma, brain tumors, and arterial infarcts.

Although infection still constitutes the major identifiable cause in some recent series, it is well established that the incidence of septic CVT has been greatly reduced in developed countries since the introduction of antibiotics. In our own series of 38 cases published in 1985,[20] there were only 4 septic cases, and in our present series of 135 cases, there are only 9 cases (6.6%). Cavernous sinus thrombosis remains the most common form of septic thrombosis, usually following an infection of the middle third of the face due to *Staphylococcus aureus*. Other sites of infection include sphenoid or ethmoid sinusitis, dental abscess, and, less often, otitis media. In chronic forms, gram-negative rods and fungi such as *Aspergillus* species are more commonly isolated.[40,130] Among general causes, parasitic infections such as trichinosis[56] and more recently human immunodeficiency virus and cytomegalovirus infections[10] have been added to the long list of infective conditions possibly leading to CVT.[102]

In young women, CVT occurs more frequently during puerperium than during pregnancy[12,20,33,55,88] and remains very common in developing countries,[9,29] whereas in developed countries, the role of oral contraceptives[3,10,20,25,55,57,104,124] is more important. In our series of 135 cases, oral contraceptive use was the only etiologic factor in 14 patients (10%). This led us, as it did many others,[20,25,57,124] to stop the oral contraceptive and promptly look for CVT (now with MRI) in women presenting with any of the neurologic manifestations compatible with this condition. However, oral contraceptive use was also found together with other conditions, such as systemic lupus or Behçet's disease, in 15 of our patients, stressing the need for an extensive etiologic workup, even in young women taking oral contraceptives.

Among the numerous noninfective medical causes of CVT, congenital thrombophilia is the most frequent, particularly increased resistance to activated protein C with factor V Leiden mutation,[17,35] which has recently been found in 10%,[37] 21%,[166] and 20%[94] of cases in three large series of 40, 19, and 25 patients, respectively, with CVT. Other varieties of congenital thrombophilia such as antithrombin,[125] protein C,[145] and protein S[53] deficiencies are far less frequently involved, with about 40 cases reported altogether. The detection of congenital thrombophilia should be systematic in CVT since it potentiates the risk of venous thrombosis associated with other conditions, including oral contraceptives or puerperium. It is also important for the long-term prevention of venous thrombosis in high-risk situations, both for the patient and for the affected members of the family. Among the other conditions listed in Table 24.1,[1,2,7,15,19,23,24,28,32,46,50,58,59,62,64,73,78,85,89,90,101,103,105,109,110,113,115,122,127,133,134,137,139,153,156,157,163,165] malignancies[7,58,73,101,137] and inflammatory diseases such as Behçet's disease[19,165] and systemic lupus[90,157] are the most frequent.

Despite the continuous description of new causes, the proportion of cases of unknown etiology remains high in recent series, between 20% and 35%[3,10,29,36,47,48,51,104] (21.5% in our series of 135 patients). The search for a cause thus remains one of the most vexing problems in CVT. It necessitates an extensive initial workup and, when no cause is found,

a long follow-up with repeated investigations. In some cases initially interpreted as idiopathic, a general disease can be discovered some months later.[3,20]

Clinical Aspects

Cerebral venous thrombosis presents with a remarkably wide spectrum of symptoms and signs, as illustrated in Table 24.2. Headache is in all series the most frequent symptom, present in about 80% of cases. It is also the earliest symptom in two-thirds of cases.[3] It has no specific features. It is mostly diffuse, progressive, and permanent, but it can be misleading, mimicking migraine or the typical headache of subarachnoid hemorrhage. It is almost invariably associated with other neurologic signs such as papilledema, focal deficits, or seizures. The frequency of papilledema is highly variable, from 7%[150] to 80%[36] in recent series. It can be associated with transient visual obscurations indicating a high-grade papilledema and threatened vision. Focal deficits are inaugural in 15% of cases[29] and are present at some time during the course of the disease in about 50% of patients (Table 24.2). The type of deficit varies with the site and extent of thrombosis; the most frequent are motor and sensory deficits, usually unilateral and often predominating in the leg. Other symptoms include aphasia, cranial nerve palsies, and, more rarely, hemianopia. Seizures are inaugural in 12% to 15% of cases[29] and are present at some time during the course of CVT in about 40% of cases (Table 24.2). Seizures are about equally divided between focal and generalized, and the association of both types is very common. They are infrequent and usually generalized when patients present with isolated intracranial hypertension; by contrast, they are frequent and often partial in patients who have focal deficits. Status epilepticus may occur and can be difficult to control. Alteration of consciousness is present in about half the patients (Table 24.2). It is rarely inaugural and is usually a late sign. Other signs such as cerebellar incoordination or psychiatric disturbances may occur. It should be noted that the classical picture of SSS thrombosis with its bilateral or alternating deficits and/or seizures is a very late pattern of presentation that is now rarely encountered (5 of our 135 patients).

Table 24.2 Main Clinical Signs in Recent Series of Patients with Cerebral Venous Thrombosis[a]

Sign	Einhäupl et al[49] (1990) (n = 71)	Bousser (1997) (n = 135)	Cantu and Barrinagarrementeria[29] (1993) Puerperal (n = 67)	Cantu and Barrinagarrementeria[29] (1993) Nonpuerperal (n = 46)	Daif et al[36] (1995) (n = 40)
Headache	91	78	88	70	82
Papilloedema	27	49	40	52	80
Focal deficits	66	41	79	76	27
Seizures	48	41	60	63	10
Altered consciousness	56	28	63	59	10

[a] Data are percentages.

The mode of onset of symptoms is also highly variable: in our series of 135 patients, it was acute (<48 hours) in 37 patients (27%), of whom 31 had focal signs; it was subacute (>48 hours but <30 days) in 67 (50%), of whom 38 had focal signs; and it was chronic (>30 days) in 31 (23%), of whom 12 had focal signs.

With such a wide spectrum of neurologic signs and modes of onset, the clinical presentation of CVT is extremely variable. It can be separated into five groups: those with isolated intracranial hypertension, those with focal cerebral signs, those with the cavernous sinus syndrome, those with a subacute encephalopathy, and those with unusual presentations.

ISOLATED INTRACRANIAL HYPERTENSION

Isolated intracranial hypertension with headache, papilledema, and sixth nerve palsy, mimicking benign intracranial hypertension (pseudotumor cerebri), is the most homogeneous pattern, accounting for up to 40% of our patients.[3] It can evolve over days, months,[20] or even years.[11] Even though SSS and LS thrombosis have long been recognized as one of the leading causes of benign intracranial hypertension,[20,143] this syndrome is still often subjected only to clinical, CSF, and CT investigation. Since CVT can mimic all the features of benign intracranial hypertension,[3,20,146,147] normal four-vessel angiography or normal MRI and MRA should be added to the classical diagnostic criteria of this syndrome.[146]

FOCAL CEREBRAL SIGNS

Focal signs characterized the second (and largest) group, accounting for roughly 75% of published cases, but the clinical picture is heterogeneous, depending on the mode of onset of focal signs, their nature (deficits, seizures, or both), and their possible association with altered consciousness. Acute cases with, for instance, a sudden hemiplegia, simulate an arterial stroke, but the unusual severity or isolated occurrence of leg involvement, the presence of seizures, and the absence of a well-defined arterial syndrome should alert one to the possibility of CVT, particularly if the patient deteriorates steadily. Chronic cases simulate tumors, whereas subacute cases mimic brain abscesses, particularly in patients with fever, increased erythrocyte sedimentation rate, and CSF pleocytosis.[3,20]

CAVERNOUS SINUS THROMBOSIS

Cavernous sinus thrombosis has a distinctive clinical picture[33,34,40,61,62,91] that includes, in the classical acute cases, chemosis, proptosis, and painful ophthalmoplegia, initially unilateral but frequently becoming bilateral. Dramatic complications can occur such as extension to other sinuses[40] and stenosis (with a mycotic aneurysm in one case) of the intracavernous portion of the internal carotid arteries.[34] However, cavernous sinus thrombosis is not always acute but can also take a more indolent form (either spontaneously or because of the masking effect of an inadequate antibiotic regimen), with an isolated abducens nerve palsy and only mild chemosis and proptosis leading to great diagnostic difficulties.[40]

SUBACUTE ENCEPHALOPATHY

Subacute encephalopathy is the fourth pattern of presentation (i.e., a generalized encephalopathic illness without localizing signs or recognizable features of raised intracranial pressure). The patients are often either very old or very young and are suffering from cachexia or malignant or cardiac diseases: the cerebral thrombosis is often a terminal event.[12] A depressed level of consciousness is the most constant finding, varying from drowsiness to deep coma. This type of presentation is extremely misleading. The differential diagnosis includes encephalitis, disseminated intravascular coagulation, marantic endocarditis, and cerebral vasculitis.

UNUSUAL PRESENTATIONS

The grouping of signs of CVT into the foregoing four main patterns (isolated intracranial hypertension, focal signs, cavernous sinus syndrome, and subacute encephalopathy) does not account for every case. Some rare cases initially present with isolated intracranial hypertension and later develop focal neurologic signs.[3,11,20,59] Some patients may initially present with isolated headache, which can, for instance, be mistaken for a postdural puncture headache after delivery or for migraine, in the presence of aura-like phenomena.[3] Others present with transient ischemic atacks[20] or with grand mal seizures and headache mimicking eclampsia. Psychiatric disturbances (irritability, lack of interest, anxiety, depression) are sometimes the prevailing symptoms. They are particularly misleading during the postpartum period, when they raise the possibility of postpartum psychosis. Other cases present with headache of sudden onset, neck stiffness, and CT scan or lumbar puncture evidence of subarachnoid hemorrhage simulating a ruptured intracranial aneurysm.[3,20] Finally, CVT may be so insidious that it can be totally asymptomatic[66] or discovered at postmortem, particularly in elderly patients dying of congestive heart failure.[12] It is clear from the above description that signs and symptoms of CVT are extremely variable and often misleading. One must consider CVT in all the above-mentioned clinical presentations and make the appropriate investigations to reach the diagnosis. Another important general principle in arriving at the diagnosis is to think about CVT as a possibility in any condition that raises the suspicion of the more common phenomenon of crural and pelvic vein thrombosis (e.g., puerperium, postoperative, and post-traumatic conditions, cardiac failure, and wasting conditions).

NEONATES

In neonates the most frequent presentation is that of an acute illness with seizures,[14] and it has been suggested that CVT is an important and underrecognized cause of seizures in the first 2 weeks of life in term infants.[131] In older children the presentation resembles that of CVT in adults.

Topographic Diagnosis

The relative distribution of sites of CVT is indicated in Table 24.3. This distribution should be considered as a rough estimate, particularly for cortical vein involvement, which is often missed at angiography. Furthermore, it is uncommon for thrombosis to be confined to a single vessel. Thus, in about 75% of cases, multiple veins or sinuses are involved.[3,20,29] This frequent multiple vein involvement, the variability of the cortical venous system, and the rapid development of collateral circulation explain the lack of well-defined topographic clinical syndromes similar to those described in arterial occlusion. There are broad patterns according to the site of venous occlusion, but at present, topographic diagnosis is usually not important for the management of CVT; the crucial step is to recognize CVT itself.

The vessel most commonly affected is SSS: 72% in Ameri and Bousser's[3] series, 70% in our present series, 85% in Daif et al[36] series, (42), and 92% in Cantu and Barinagarrementeria's[1,29] series. The SSS was involved alone in a minority of cases (13%, 55%, 15%, and 29%, respectively, in the four series cited). The LS is almost as often affected as the SSS in some series (70% for Ameri and Bousser[3]) but far less frequently in others (38%) for Cantu and Barinagarrementeria.[29] Its isolated involvement is rare, 9% and 2%, respectively. Cerebral veins are affected in about 40% of cases, but this is probably an underestimation given the much higher frequency of focal clinical signs. Thrombosis of the galenic system is rare, with some 60 reported cases. Only a few cases have been described of petrosal sinus, isolated cortical, or cerebellar vein thrombosis, but these conditions are also likely to be underdiagnosed because of the extreme difficulty of their diagnosis.

SUPERIOR SAGITTAL SINUS THROMBOSIS

When thrombosis is restricted to the SSS, the clinical presentation is that of isolated intracranial hypertension, as described above. In Ameri and Bousser's[3] series, 33% of 79 cases of SSS thrombosis presented as benign intracranial hypertension. Grand mal seizures and psychiatric disturbances occasionally occur in pure SSS thrombosis. In most cases, thrombosis also involves one or both LS, with again intracranial hypertension as the main clinical presentation. Extension to cortical veins, particularly the rolandic and parietal veins, is frequent and is characterized by the acute or progressive onset of a focal motor or sensory deficit, classically more marked in the leg and associated with focal or generalized seizures.

LATERAL SINUS THROMBOSIS

Like SSS thrombosis, LS thrombosis has a variable presentation. Although it can be asymptomatic, isolated LS thrombosis usually manifests as raised intracranial pressure, hence the term *otitic hydrocephalus* coined by Symonds[143] to describe the effects of LS thrombosis secondary to an active or latent ear infection. LS thrombosis frequently extends to other sinuses and veins, especially to the SSS, presenting again as isolated intracranial hypertension. Focal signs occur when thrombosis extends to superior or inferior petrosal sinuses with 5th and 6th cranial nerve involvement, respectively, to the straight sinus and deep venous system (see below), to adjacent cortical veins with aphasia in left LS thrombosis (see below), and to the jugular bulb with involvement of the 9th, 10th, and 11th cranial nerves.

CORTICAL VEIN THROMBOSIS

Any cortical vein can be the seat of thrombosis, but the most often involved are the superior cerebral veins (rolandic, pa-

Table 24.3 Distribution of Venous Thrombosis in Recent Series of Patients with Cerebral Venous Thrombosis

Veins	Milandre et al[104] (1988) (n = 20)	Bousser (1997) (n = 135)	Cantu and Barinagarrementeria[29] (1993) Puerperal (n = 67)	Nonpuerperal (n = 46)	Tsai et al[150] (1995) (n = 29)	Daif et al[36] (1995) (n = 40)
SSS	13 (4)	95 (20)	60 (22)	45 (11)	19 (11)	34 (22)
LS	2	93 (23)	23 (1)	20 (1)	15 (9)	14 (4)
SS	5	18 (1)	0	0	3	3
CS	1	3 (0)	0	0	0	
CV	10 (2)	36 (4)	13	14	1	4
DVS	1 (1)	9 (1)	17 (4)	10		
Association[b]	12	86	39	34	9	26

Abbreviations: SSS, superior sagittal sinus; LS, lateral sinus; SS, straight sinus; CS, cavernous sinus; CV, cortical or cerebellar veins; DVS, deep venous system.

[a] *Data represent numbers of patients. Numbers in parentheses indicate cases in which the venous structure alone was involved.*

[b] *More than one structure involved.*

rieto-occipital, and posterior temporal), which drain into the SSS. The consequences of a cortical vein thrombosis are variable; in an unknown proportion of cases, collateral circulation develops rapidly, and there is no parenchymal lesion. In other cases, an area of localized edema appears that can still be asymptomatic. At a further stage, neurons become edematous or partially ischemic, but this injury is mostly reversible, as judged by the frequency of totally regressive focal deficits. Even when an infarct occurs, confirmed at neuroimaging, it is remarkable that clinical recovery can still be complete in some cases.

Isolated cortical vein thrombosis is extremely rare, with an overall frequency of about 2%.[3,47] It presents with focal deficits or seizures of sudden or progressive onset (or both), mimicking a stroke or a space-occupying lesion. In most cases, thrombosis extends to the SSS with signs of raised intracranial pressure and occasionally to cortical veins on the opposite side, leading to the classical picture of a bilateral parasagittal infarct.

THROMBOSIS OF THE DEEP VENOUS SYSTEM

The clinical presentation of thrombosis of the Galenic system is highly variable. The classic picture is that of a child with an acute coma associated with decerebration, decortication, extrapyramidal hypertonia, signs of raised intracranial pressure, pupillary changes, and rise in blood pressure leading to death in a few hours or days.[44,45,81] Similar cases have been reported in adults. When patients survive, severe sequelae are frequent, such as akinetic mutism, mental retardation, dementia, bilateral athetoid movements, hemiparesis, vertical gaze palsy, and dystonia.[18,44,82,107] Recent reports have illustrated the possibility of benign forms of galenic system thrombosis. The most regular symptoms are headache, nausea and vomiting, gait ataxia, neuropsychological deficits, and drowsiness of a variable degree.[16,18,45,70,84] Other signs are unusual and include impaired upward conjugate gaze, vertical nystagmus, hemiparesis, which may be bilateral or alternating, limb or axial rigidity, tremor, seizures, and signs of raised intracranial pressure. Neuropsychological disturbances with impaired anterograde memory are constant and sometimes severe, resembling Korsakoff's psychosis,[70] but they are usually mild or moderate.[16]

CEREBELLAR VEIN THROMBOSIS

Cerebellar venous infarction is extremely rare and until recently was not recognized during life.[107] Isolated cerebellar vein thrombosis has not been reported, and in all published cases there was an associated sinus thrombosis, mainly the LS.[3,20,52,106,123]

The clinical presentation is variable. The most frequent signs are headache, vomiting, ataxia, and unilateral dysmetria.[20,52,106,123] They are usually of acute onset, but subacute[123] and even chronic cases[20] have been reported. There is early

decrease in conscious level and frequent papilloedema indicating obstructive hydrocephalus.[123] Cranial nerve palsies can occur,[20] and the involvement of the 9th and 10th nerves may suggest propagation of thrombosis to the internal jugular vein.

THROMBOSIS OF THE SUPERIOR AND INFERIOR PETROSAL SINUSES

Thrombosis of the superior and inferior petrosal sinuses is usually a sequel of cavernous sinus thrombosis or infection in the temporal bone with LS thrombosis. Mainly described in the old literature, it is characterized by cranial nerve palsies: the fifth for the superior sinus and the sixth for the inferior.[61,142,143]

INTERNAL JUGULAR VEIN THROMBOSIS

Internal jugular vein thrombosis is frequently initiated by cannulae used for long-term venous access, or it may spread there from the sigmoid sinus. There may be obvious signs of local infection with pain and swelling in the mastoid region and a palpable tender thrombosed vein. Other signs include a jugular foramen syndrome if the infection involves the skull base. There is a risk of venous thromboembolism to the lungs and, in rare instances, there may be widespread propagation of thrombus to the superior vena cava and subclavian veins.

Investigations

COMPUTED TOMOGRAPHY

CT scan with and without contrast injection is usually the first neuroimaging examination carried out in patients with headache, focal deficits, or seizures, particularly on an emergency basis. CT scan is extremely useful to rule out the many conditions that CVT can mimic. It can occasionally detect lesions that can themselves cause CVT, such as meningiomas, abscesses, sinusitis, or mastoiditis. CT scan is also useful in showing brain or sinus changes suggestive of CVT.

CT findings have been described in detail in numerous reports[5,21,23,26,27,31,38,60,66,86,111,116,129,132,152,160,161] and are now well established. They can be divided into direct and indirect signs.

Direct Signs of Cerebral Venous Thrombosis

Three abnormalities are considered direct signs of CVT: the cord sign, the dense triangle, and the delta or empty triangle sign.

The *cord sign*, visible on unenhanced CT scans, repre-

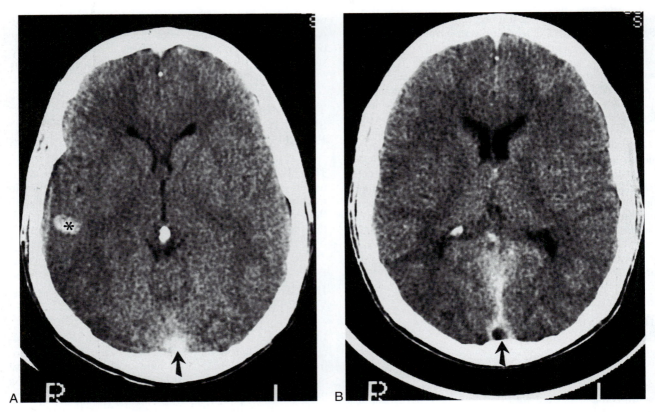

Figure 24.5 (**A**) Unenhanced CT scan. Dense triangle in a recent SSS thrombosis (arrow) with a small cortical hemorrhage (asterisk). (**B**) Enhanced CT scan in the same patient 10 days later. Empty delta sign (arrow).

sents the spontaneous visualization of a thrombosed cortical vein[26,60,116]; it is extremely rare (1 in 116 cases in our series), and its diagnostic value is debated. It can also be seen in internal cerebral veins and vein of Galen thrombosis.[152]

The *dense triangle* also reflects spontaneous SSS opacification by freshly congealed blood[27,111] (Fig. 24.5A); it is a very early sign, again extremely rare, present in less than 2% of cases. It is difficult to assess, particularly in other sinuses (LS and SS), which can be spontaneously hyperdense in normal children or in patients with hemoconcentration.

The *empty delta sign*, described by Buonanno et al,[26] appears after contrast injection and reflects the opacification of collateral veins in the SSS wall contrasting with the noninjection of the clot inside the sinus (Fig. 24.5B). It is the most frequent direct sign, present in approximately 35% of published cases.[5,27,116,161] However, it is absent when thrombosis does not affect the posterior third of the SSS, or when CT scan is performed in the first 5 days after onset of symptoms or more than 2 months later.[132] Its sensitivity and specificity are increased with some technical refinements such as orthogonal sectioning, different window and level settings, and multiplanar reformations.[21,60,66,116,129] These reasons probably explain why the empty delta sign is only found in 10% to 20% of CT scans performed routinely to rule out other conditions in patients suspected to have CVT.[31] Furthermore, it is not pathognomonic, since the early division of the SSS can be responsible for a false delta sign.

Indirect Signs of Cerebral Venous Thrombosis

Indirect and nonspecific abnormalities are more frequent. Intense contrast enhancement of the falx and tentorium[26,27,116] is present in some 20% of cases[31] (Fig. 24.6). It is easily recognized in the tentorium but can be difficult to assess in the falx, particularly in aged patients. It indicates venous stasis or hyperemia of the dura mater. Tentorial enhancement is usually thought to suggest SS thrombosis,[116] but it is not rare in SSS thrombosis.[20,31] It can be associated with dilated transcerebral medullary veins, indicating a major venous status, usually in relation to an extensive SSS thrombosis.[5,101]

A common finding is the presence of small ventricles with swelling and sometimes diffuse low density suggestive of edema.[20,26,31,86,116] Although reported in 20% to 50% of cases, it is not a useful sign because it is nonspecific and is frequently difficult to differentiate from normal brain, particularly in the young. In some cases the cerebral swelling can be confirmed by the later increase in size of ventricles, which were initially small.[86] However, the opposite finding (i.e., enlarged ventricles) is a possibility, particularly in cerebellar vein thrombosis[36,118] and therefore does not exclude the diagnosis.

White matter hypodensity without contrast enhancement suggestive of cerebral edema is present in up to 75% of cases.[60] It can be diffuse or localized and is sometimes associated with a mass effect. It is usually associated with abnormali-

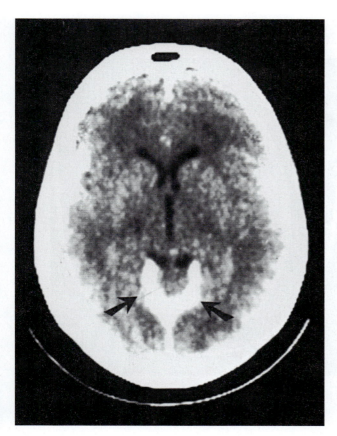

Figure 24.6 Enhanced CT scan. Intense tentorial enhancement in a patient with SSS and thrombosis of both LS (arrow).

ties suggestive of a venous infarct, but it can occasionally be the only sign of CVT.

Usually described by pathologists as hemorrhagic, venous infarcts on CT scan present with a spontaneous hyperdensity in 10% to 50% of cases.[20,23,27,31,116] Two main aspects are encountered: large subcortical often multifocal hematomas[31,55] and petechial hemorrhages within large hypodensities[31] (Fig. 24.7). In rare instances, there is an associated subarachnoid hemorrhage or a subdural hematoma, which can even be the only signs of CVT.[31] Nonhemorrhagic venous infarcts are almost as frequent. They are protean in appearance[31,116]: focal hypodensity with gyral enhancement, areas of hypodensity without enhancement, or isolated gyral enhancement (Fig. 24.8). Hemorrhagic or nonhemorrhagic infarcts can be unilateral or bilateral, single or multiple.[20,26,27,31,116] They are seen superficially in the hemispheres in SSS thrombosis and within the basal ganglia in deep venous system thrombosis.

Cavernous Sinus Thrombosis

The CT scan can sometimes be useful in demonstrating cavernous sinus thrombosis,[34,38] showing on postcontrast CT as multiple irregular filling defects with bulging cavernous sinuses and enlarged orbital veins.[38] The presence of air, seen on coronal sections has been reported in septic thrombosis.[34]

Normal Scan

In 10% to 20% of cases, CT scan is normal in patients with proven CVT, more frequently so (up to 50%) in patients presenting with isolated intracranial hypertension than in those with focal signs (<10%).[31,111]

Summary

The place of CT scan in the diagnostic strategy of CVT is mainly to rule out other conditions such as arterial stroke, abscess, tumors, and subarachnoid hemorrhage on an emergency basis. It should be performed at first without contrast, and, in the absence of hemorrhagic infarct, with contrast. In a minority of cases, it will show the direct pathognomonic signs of CVT, but more frequently only indirect signs are present and MRI or angiographic confirmation should be obtained.

ANGIOGRAPHY

Intra-arterial Angiography

Angiography has been the key procedure in diagnosis of CVT for many years and still remains the method of reference for evaluation of new methods. It requires a perfect technique: four-vessel angiography (conventional or digitalized intra-arterial) with visualization of the entire venous phase on at least two projections (frontal and lateral) and three if possible, oblique views being the best for visualization of the entire SSS.[3,20,69,88,160,162]

The partial or complete lack of filling of veins or sinuses is the best angiographic sign of CVT. Easily recognized when it affects the posterior or whole SSS (Fig. 24.9), both LS (Fig. 24.10), or the deep venous system (Fig. 24.11), it may be more difficult to interpret in other locations such as the anterior third of the SSS or the left LS, where it can be confused with hypoplasia.[69] For occlusion of the anterior part of the SSS to be established, it is necessary to have either involvement of another sinus or nonequivocal indirect signs of CVT, such as delayed emptying and dilated collateral veins. For LS thrombosis the main argument is the absence of filling of the whole sinus or of its sigmoid portion, contrasting with the presence of the sinus groove and normality of the jugular foramen on plain radiographs of the skull. However, in some cases such signs are lacking, and MRI is required to differentiate between thrombosis and hypoplasia[95] (Fig. 24.12).

The absence of a cortical vein is difficult and sometimes impossible to detect except when the vein is partly visualized but stops suddenly and is surrounded by dilated collateral veins (Fig. 24.9). Other angiographic findings include delayed emptying; collateral venous pathways are found in about 50% of cases and almost invariably indicate SSS thrombosis. Dilated and tortuous cortical collateral veins with a corkscrew appearance are much more frequent (Fig. 24.9) than transcerebral or intradural collaterals.[20,69,88,160,162] An important mass effect is extremely rare and has only been reported in a few cases.[20,160]

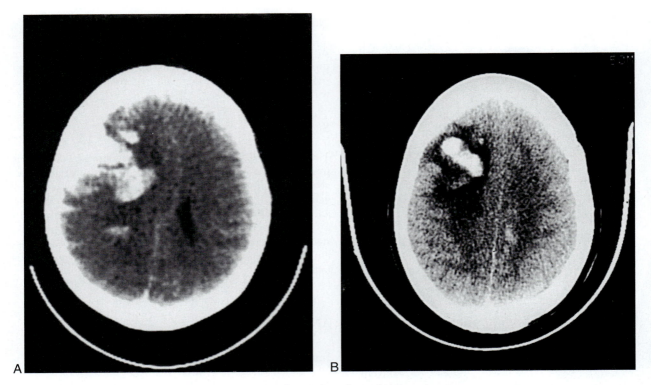

Figure 24.7 Unenhanced CT scans in two patients with SSS thrombosis. (**A**) Spontaneous hyperdensity with severe mass effect suggestive of a hemorrhagic infarct. (**B**) Bilateral hemorrhagic infarct.

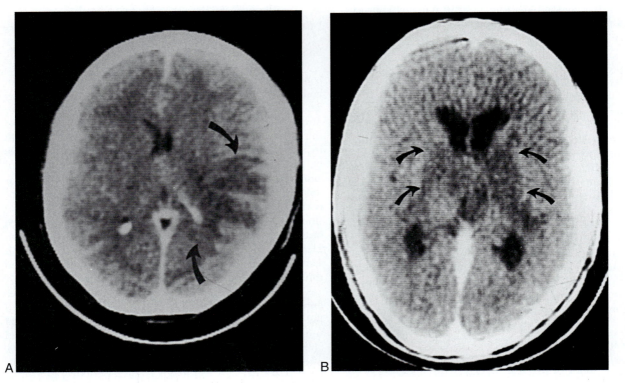

Figure 24.8 Enhanced CT scans. (**A**) Large area of corticosubcortical hypodensity with mass effect on the lateral ventricle in a patient with SSS thrombosis. (**B**) Bilateral basal ganglia hypodensity in a patient with deep cerebral vein thrombosis.

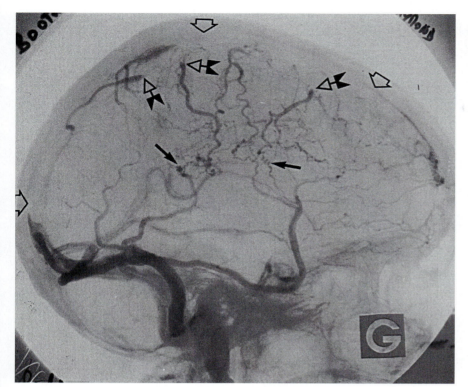

Figure 24.9 Left carotid angiogram. Total SSS occlusion (white arrows) with occlusion of frontoparietal veins (tailed arrows) and anastomotic cortical veins with a corkscrew appearance (straight arrows).

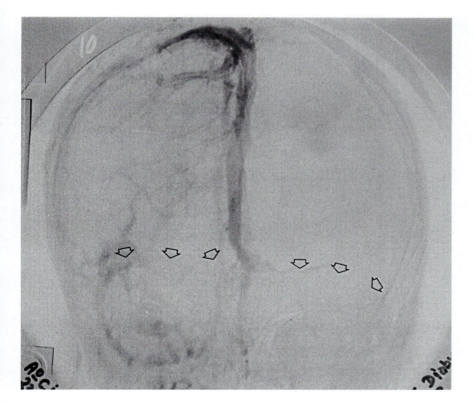

Figure 24.10 Right carotid angiogram. Lack of filling of both LS (white arrows). (From Bousser et al,[20] with permission.)

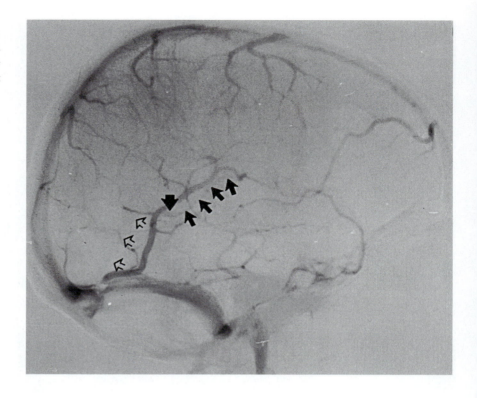

Figure 24.11 Right carotid angiogram. Poor filling of internal cerebral vein (thin black arrows) and vein of Galen (wide black arrow) and lack of filling of straight sinus (white arrows).

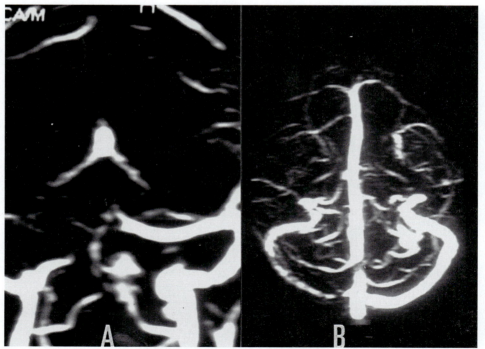

Figure 24.12 MRA (phase contrast). SSS thrombosis (**A**) before and (**B**) 7 days after heparin (recanalization). (Courtesy of Dr. Beyssac, Toulon, France.)

Magnetic Resonance Angiography

The tendency now is to use MRA to replace intra-arterial angiography for the diagnosis of CVT. Several methods can be used: two-dimensional time-of-flight (TOF), three-dimensional TOF, and phase contrast.[4,30,97,98,108,119,150,151] Two-dimensional TOF is the most commonly used, with 1.5- and 3-mm-thick slices in the coronal and axial planes.[30] As with intra-arterial angiography, the typical appearance of CVT on MRA is the absence of flow, indicating a complete thrombosis (Fig. 24.12). Specific limitations exist for each of the MRA techniques as well as the limitations common to all varieties of angiography in CVT: the difficulty in diagnosing partial thrombosis, the inability to differentiate hypoplasia and thrombosis, and the poor yield for cortical vein and cavernous sinus thrombosis. However, MRA has the advantages of being easily repeatable and noninvasive. In most cases it is combined with MRI, this association now being the best diagnostic tool in CVT.

MAGNETIC RESONANCE IMAGING

Thrombosis Imaging

MRI offers major advantages for the evaluation of possible CVT: sensitivity to blood flow, ability to visualize the thrombus itself, and noninvasiveness. A variety of MR findings have been described, mainly relating to the evaluation of thrombosis.[30,42,43,79,92,95,96,99,100,147] At a very early stage, flow void is absent, and the occluded vessel appears isointense on T_1-weighted images and hypointense on T_2-weighted images. The diagnosis at that stage is often impossible on MRI alone. Angiography (or MRA) is required to demonstrate the absence of flow in the thrombosed vessel.

A few days later, the absence of flow void persists, but the thrombus becomes hyperintense, initially on T_1- and then on T_2-weighted images[30] (Fig. 24.13). In large vessels these changes start in the periphery and proceed toward the center. They represent the aging of the thrombus with biochemical conversion of oxyhemoglobin to methemoglobin, rather than extension of thrombosis. This intermediate pattern (increased signal on T_1- and T_2-weighted images) is diagnostic of CVT and is by far the most frequent. It is usually found between days 4 or 5 and days 30 to 35 of the onset of symptoms.[3,42] Late changes (approximately 2 to 4 weeks after onset) can reveal the beginning of vascular recanalization with the resumption of flow void in the previously thrombosed vessel. However, at 6 months, more than two-thirds of cases still have some heterogeneous localized signal abnormalities, which can persist for years and should not be mistaken for a recurrent acute CVT.[42,96] MRI can thus not only reveal venous thrombosis but also the natural history of the thrombotic process (Fig. 24.13). MRI diagnosis is particularly easy in SSS thrombosis,[3,42,92,138,147] but convincing images have also been obtained in cases of thrombosis involving the LS (Fig. 24.14), the SS (Fig. 24.15), the internal cerebral veins and vein of Galen (Fig. 24.15), the cavernous sinus, and the cortical veins.[3,42,92,99,126,138]

In some cases, however, interpretation of MRI images is not easy because of false-negative and false-positive images. False negatives are rare and mostly correspond to very early or very late stage or to isolated cortical vein thrombosis. Most false positives are created by slowly flowing blood. Repositioning the patient, repeating the sequence in a different plane, using at least two sequences, and sometimes obtaining specialized acquisitions are helpful to eliminate these artifacts.[30,42,92,99,126,138,144,147]

Parenchymal Lesions

Besides visualizing the thrombus itself, MRI detects its parenchymal consequences: brain swelling with mass effect and cortical sulcal effacement, increased signal on T_2-weighted images with iso- or hyposignal on T_1-weighted images suggestive of edema, and increased signal on both T_1- and T_2-weighted images, indicating hemorrhagic component.[42,65] These images are nonspecific, but their diagnosis is easy because of the associated MRI signs of sinus thrombosis. The main difficulty is again with isolated cortical vein thrombosis, which can be mistaken for a tumor unless there is a typical stop sign with corkscrew collateral veins on angiography.

Summary

The combination of noncontrast MRI plus MRA is nowadays the best method for the diagnosis and follow-up of CVT. It should be performed as a first-line investigation in case of high clinical suspicion. Its use is limited in certain situations such as deeply comatose subjects requiring artificial ventilation. In such patients, as well as in dubious cases—such as isolated cortical vein thrombosis—intra-arterial angiography may still be required.

OTHER NEUROLOGIC INVESTIGATIONS

Other investigations were most useful in the pre-CT scan era. *Electroencephalogram* changes are constantly found in SSS thrombosis with extension to cortical veins; they are present in roughly 75% of all CVT cases.[20,47] They are nonspecific; the most common pattern is a severe generalized slowing more marked on one side, with frequent superimposed epileptic activity. In some patients with focal symptoms, a generalized slowing indicates a more diffuse lesion than clinically suspected.

Isotope brain scanning with ^{99m}T or ^{111}In labeled platelets has been used to detect sinus thrombosis,[11,22,65] but it has now been supplanted by MRI.

CSF examination is still a useful diagnostic tool since it is very rarely (10%) entirely normal, in composition or in pressure.[3,20,33,48,61,82,87] Abnormalities in composition include raised protein content as well as the presence of red blood cells (in two-thirds of cases) and pleocytosis (in one-third). Mainly seen when focal signs are present, pleocytosis and the presence of red blood cells can also be found in patients presenting with benign intracranial hypertension, indicating that these abnormalities should suggest sinus thrombosis as the

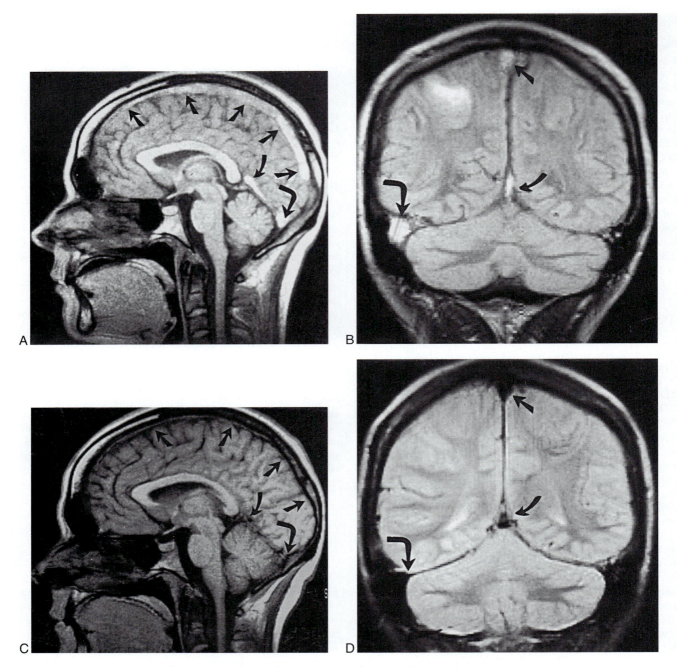

Figure 24.13 MRI, T_1-weighted images. (**A & B**) Hypersignal indicating SSS (straight arrows) LS (angle arrows), and SS (curved arrows) thrombosis. (**C & D**) Same patient 3 months later. Normal flow void in previously thrombosed sinuses.

possible cause of this syndrome. CSF examination is crucial to rule out meningitis, which is extremely difficult to exclude on clinical grounds alone. Although in the CT scan and MRI era, CSF study has become obsolete in most cases of nonseptic CVT presenting with focal signs, it remains crucial in patients with isolated intracranial hypertension to rule out meningitis, to measure CSF pressure, and to remove CSF when the patient's vision is threatened. *Transcranial Doppler* has recently been used to detect massive SSS thrombosis, and it might be

useful to provide day-to-day monitoring of those severe cases that cannot be studied by MRI.[154,164]

GENERAL INVESTIGATIONS

After CVT has been established, investigations should be directed toward demonstrating the underlying etiology. Because of the multiplicity of etiologies, this is a long and difficult task

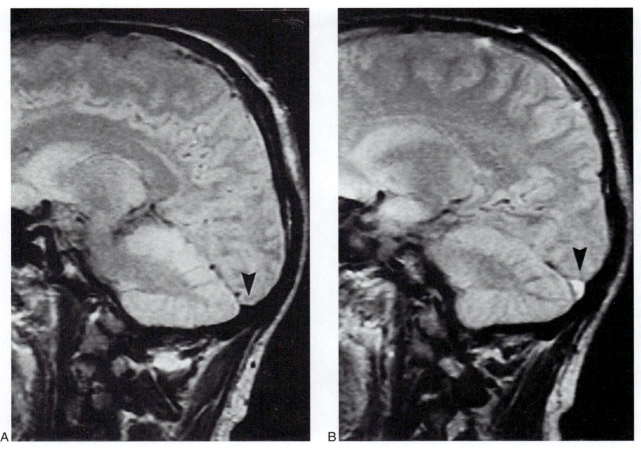

Figure 24.14 MRI, T$_2$-weighted images. (**A**) Lateral sinus hypoplasia (arrowhead). (**B**) Lateral sinus thrombosis (arrowhead).

whenever the cause is not clinically evident. Fever, increased erythrocyte sedimentation rate, or raised polymorphonuclear white blood cell count point to infective, inflammatory, or malignant causes. However, even with such underlying diseases, these abnormalities are sometimes lacking; by contrast, they are occasionally found in idiopathic cases.[20] Their presence is particularly useful as an indication of CVT in patients presenting with benign intracranial hypertension.

Detailed coagulation studies have only rarely been performed in series of CVT, and their results have been conflicting. Some have found hypercoagulability state,[114] an increase in platelet adhesiveness and aggregability,[9] and a decrease in fibrinolytic activity,[9] but this was during pregnancy and puerperium or in women taking oral contraceptives. Others did not confirm these results[55] or found an increased platelet aggregation with the lowest dose of epinephrine as the only abnormality.[20] On the whole, there is no consistent abnormality indicating the presence of a thrombotic process. The main interest of coagulation studies is to detect possible causative conditions such as increased resistance to activated protein C (factor V Leiden), which is present in 10% to 20% of CVT.[37,94,166] This and other varieties of congenital thrombophilia should be systematically looked for in patients with CVT, whether or not other potential causes are present, because they imply a systematic family study, and they modify

the long-term management of the patients (see Etiology section).

Outcome

SHORT-TERM OUTCOME

Mortality

Before the introduction of angiography, CVT was mainly diagnosed at autopsy and was therefore thought to be usually lethal.[61,82,107] In early angiographic series, mortality still ranked between 30% and 50%,[87] but in more recent series, it was lower (38%,[121] 23%,[10] 10% to 15%,[36,147,161] and 6%[3]) (Table 24.4).

There are three main causes of death in CVT: the brain lesion itself, particularly when a massive hemorrhagic infarct is present; intercurrent complications such as sepsis, uncontrolled seizures, and pulmonary embolism, present in 11% of 203 published cases reviewed by Diaz et al,[39] with a mortality rate of 94% and the underlying condition, such as carcinomas,

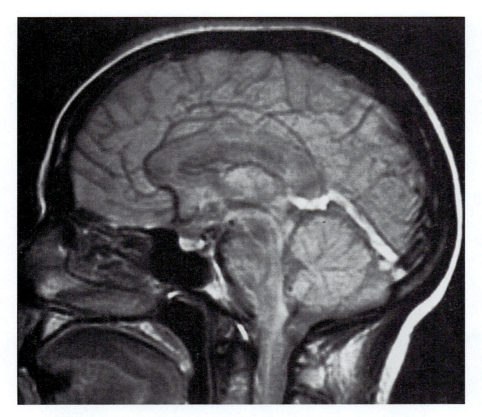

Figure 24.15 MRI, T_2-weighted image (first echo); (TR 2,000 TE 40) hypersignal indicating vein of Galen and SSS thrombosis.

septicemias, leukemias, and paroxysmal nocturnal hemoglobinuria.[3,10,20,121]

Factors classically considered to suggest a bad prognosis are the rate of evolution of thrombosis,[82] the age of the patient (with a high mortality rate in infancy and in the aged[9]), an infectious etiology,[10,40,47] focal symptoms and coma,[3,10,20,61,82] the presence of a hemorrhagic infarct, and an empty delta sign on CT scan.[161] The topography of the cerebral veins involved is also an important prognostic factor, deep cerebral vein thrombosis and cerebellar vein thrombosis carrying a much higher risk than cortical vein thrombosis.[18,44,45,61,87]

Among the underlying conditions, the postpartum state is a favorable one, with a survival of 90% in most recent series.[29]

Functional Recovery

It has long been recognized that if survival occurs in CVT, the prognosis for recovery of function is much better than in arterial thrombosis,[3,20,47,142]; a minority (15% to 25%) of patients are left with disabling sequelae such as optic atrophy or focal deficits.[3,33,47,147,161] Any combination of neurologic signs can persist, according to the site, extent, and severity of

Table 24.4 Outcome in Recent Series of Patients with Cerebral Venous Thrombosis

				Cantu and Barinagarrementeria[29] (1993)			
Outcome	Milandre et al[104] (1988) (n = 20)	Einhäupl et al[49] (1990) (n = 71)	Bousser (1997) (n = 135)	Puerperal (n = 67)	Nonpuerperal (n = 46)	Tsai et al[150] (1995) (n = 29)	Daif et al[36] (1995) (n = 40)
Total recovery	6 (30)	42 (59)	101 (75)	36 (53.7)	24 (52)	22 (71)	29 (72)
Minor sequelae	8 (40)	13 (18.5)	16 (12)	19 (28.3)	3 (6.5)	0	3 (8)
Major sequelae	3 (15)	6 (8.5)	12 (8)	6 (9)	4 (9)	1 (3.5)	4 (10)
Death	3 (15)	10 (14)	6 (5)	6 (9)	15 (33)	6 (21)	4 (10)

a Data represent numbers of patients, with percentages in parentheses.

the parenchymal lesion and to the degree of raised intracranial pressure. In neonates, the functional outcome is usually normal in the absence of associated asphyxia but is frequently abnormal in preterm neonates who have suffered asphyxia.[131]

It is thus apparent that, although CVT is less severe than classically thought, the natural history and prognosis are highly variable. Some patients with acute cases can have a fulminating course leading to death in a few days, whereas others recover rapidly and completely, and still others are left with sequelae. Some patients with chronic disease progressively worsen, and sequelae develop, whereas others recover spontaneously. In extremely benign forms symptoms are limited to transient ischemic attacks, headache, or epilepsy; these patients recover spontaneously and are probably still underrecognized. On the whole, isolated sinus thrombosis carries a good prognosis, provided intracranial hypertension is controlled; however, sinus thrombosis can extend to cerebral veins at any moment, leading to death or sequelae, although this is a minority of cases.

LONG-TERM OUTCOME

Little is known about the long-term outcome of patients with CVT. A few reports suggest that LS thrombosis can later induce arteriovenous malformations affecting the transverse sinus.[3,20,74,96] Residual epilepsy has been reported in 10% to 30% of patients who had seizures during the acute stage.[104,115] Seizures usually occur in the first year and are easily controlled with antiepileptic drugs. In a recent study, no seizures were observed during long-term follow-up in patients who did not have focal signs and did not suffer seizures at the acute stage.[115] The frequency of long-term epilepsy is also low in neonates who suffer CVT without associated asphyxia.[131]

Recurrence of CVT seems infrequent: 11.7% in a recent series of 77 patients followed for a mean of 77.8 months.[115] Recurrences have been reported in cases with a known prothrombotic condition but also in idiopathic cases. The risk of recurrence during a later pregnancy is poorly known but seems low: none in 16 pregnancies in Preter et al's[115] recent series.

Treatment

Because CVT is an uncommon disease with great variability in the natural history, treatment is still controversial. It is based on a combination of symptomatic, etiologic, and antithrombotic medications on a case-by-case basis.

SYMPTOMATIC TREATMENT

As far as anticonvulsant treatment is concerned, some favor its systematic use,[47,82,159] whereas others restrict it to patients who present with seizures.[3,20] Any of the major antiepileptic drugs can be used. The question of the duration of treatment remains open: in our series, anticonvulsants were progres-

sively discontinued 1 year after CVT in patients with a normal electroencephalogram and no recurrent seizures.[115]

Opinions are more divergent on reducing intracranial pressure, and diverse approaches have been used: steroids, mannitol, glycerol, dextran,[3,20,33,59,91,104,124,147] acetazolamide,[20,33,59,124] lumbar punctures,[20,33,59] shunting,[20,53] barbiturate-induced coma,[59,66,72] LS venous bypass, or even surgical decompression.[117,124] The choice among these methods depends on the individual clinical situation. Minor brain swelling often needs no specific treatment. In a patient with isolated intracranial hypertension, particularly if vision is threatened, we favor one lumbar puncture before starting heparin. If vision continues to deteriorate or if consciousness becomes abnormal, mannitol is usually added.[159] In the very rare resistant cases, intracranial pressure monitoring is necessary, and drastic methods such as shunting or barbiturate-induced coma might be required.[59,72]

ETIOLOGIC TREATMENT

Whenever possible, the cause of the CVT should be treated. This applies particularly to septic thrombosis, which requires wide-spectrum combination antibiotics, associated in some cases with surgical treatment of the primary site of infection. It also applies to all the general conditions that can promote CVT and must be specifically treated: malignancies, connective tissue diseases, hematologic disorders, and so forth.

ANTITHROMBOTIC TREATMENT

Although jugular vein ligation and surgical thrombectomy have been performed in the past,[55,117] these surgical methods have been abandoned. Antithrombotic treatment is primarily based on anticoagulants and secondarily on antiplatelet drugs and thrombolytics.

Anticoagulants

Although the use of heparin has been advocated for more than 50 years,[93,141] some authors are still skeptical about its value,[83,140] for two main alleged reasons: the risk of intracerebral bleeding, particularly in an already hemorrhagic infarct, and the lack of enough evidence of efficacy. It is remarkable that the risk of intracerebral bleeding has been emphasized again and again,[12,25,61,63,124] although hardly any undisputable cases have been reported. The two most often quoted cases are those of Gettelfinger and Kokmen,[63] but one worsened after heparin *and* urokinase, and the other suffered paroxysmal nocturnal hemoglobinuria, a notoriously severe underlying condition with an increased hemorrhagic risk. It is clear that the risk of hemorrhage has been overestimated, an impression confirmed by the large number of cases and case series in which heparin has been given without deleterious effects.[3,20,47,48,57,71,82,87,88,147,159] In our first series of 23 heparin-treated patients, there was no worsening, and all survived.[20] This has been prospectively extended to 82 patients[3] and now to 106 patients, all treated with heparin without ill effects. It should be emphasized that even in the 25 patients who had a hemorrhagic infarct, heparin had no harmful effect, as already stressed by Einhaupl et al.[49]

Evidence of the efficacy of heparin in CVT is based on illustrative cases, on retrospective and prospective series, and on one randomized trial. A number of well-documented cases have been reported in which a dramatic improvement occurred shortly after the initiation of heparin in patients who had previously been deteriorating steadily.[3,20,57,67,71,147] Moreover, some of these patients worsened when heparin was changed to oral anticoagulants and rapidly improved again after heparin was resumed.[57,147] Although the value of single case reports is limited, it is impressive that the number of well-documented cases of dramatic improvement shortly after initiation of heparin by far exceeds that of documented cases of hemorrhagic complications.

Heparin has been used in many cases and series with apparently good results.[3,20,47,49,57,67,71,147,159] Thus, in German and French series combined,[158] 143 patients received heparin, and only 4 of them died. This could be difficult to interpret, since CVT patients can recover spontaneously, and it and also could be argued that the most severe cases were excluded.[140] However, this was not the case since the German and the French groups have used heparin in all their CVT patients during the last 10 years. An important contribution has been made by Diaz et al,[39] who reviewed 203 CVT cases reported between 1942 and 1990 and compared the outcome of patients treated[56] and not treated (149) with heparin: 91% survived in the first group compared with 36% in the second.

The best evidence in favor of the efficacy of heparin was brought by one randomized study performed by Einhäupl et al[49] in Germany; high-dose intravenous heparin was compared with placebo in patients with angiographically proved CVT. The study had to be stopped after the first 20 patients because of a statistically significant difference in favor of heparin ($P<0.05$). After 3 months, all 10 heparin-treated patients had either completely recovered or were left with a slight neurologic deficit, whereas in the control group, four patients died or had severe sequelae.

There is thus good evidence that the benefit/risk ratio of heparin is favorable in patients with CVT, but there is still disagreement on the best indications. All would agree that heparin is indicated in patients with coexistent pelvic or deep leg vein thrombosis and pulmonary embolism, or in conditions with an increased thrombotic tendency, such as activated protein resistance, antithrombin, protein C, or protein S deficiencies, or the presence of lupus anticoagulant, but such cases are a minority. A still widely held view is that heparin should not be used in patients with a venous hemorrhagic infarct,[40,55,59,62,63,82,83,124] but this is not based on the available literature, which, as we have seen, shows that >50 reported cases of hemorrhagic CVT have been treated with heparin with no deleterious effects.[3,47,49,104,158,159] Some authors (including ourselves in early reports)[20] recommend the use of heparin only when patients continue to deteriorate despite symptomatic treatment.[10,29] Such an attitude allows a number of cases to recover spontaneously, but it does not face the problem of sudden extension of thrombosis, and it delays the use of heparin until a major brain lesion exists, a situation in which heparin might be more deleterious. Our policy over the last 10 years, which is also that of the German

group,[3,20,47,158,159] has been to anticoagulate with heparin all patients with demonstrated CVT, irrespective of the clinical presentation, etiology, and CT findings (provided no general contraindication to the use of heparin exists). This applies to adults and children but not to neonates, for whom most authors agree that anticoagulation is not necessary.[14,120]

Anticoagulation guidelines are essentially similar to those of deep vein thrombosis of the legs, except that the duration of heparin treatment is longer: heparin can be given with either a continuous intravenous infusion or with subcutaneous injections, aiming at an activated partial thromboplastin time of 2 to 2.5 as the control value. Low molecular weight heparin might prove as effective as conventional heparin, but it has not been properly tested in CVT. There is no fixed duration for heparin treatment, but empirically it is prolonged until the patient improves or at least stabilizes.[158,159] It is then replaced by oral anticoagulants (warfarin), adjusted to obtain an international normalized ratio between 2.5 and 3.5. Duration of treatment is not fixed, but warfarin is usually maintained for at least 3 months. More prolonged treatment is warranted whenever a prothrombotic situation exists such as lengthy immobilization, malignancy, inflammatory disease (Behçet's disease, systemic lupus), inherited thrombophilia, or a history of recurrent venous thrombosis. As far as later pregnancies are concerned, preventive heparin should be used whenever a thrombophilic state exists. In other cases, there are two approaches: either systematic heparin treatment, or no treatment but extremely close follow-up and appropriate investigations and treatment if CVT occurs. Low-dose prophylactic heparin during the postpartum period is a reasonable approach in women with previous postpartum CVT.

Antiplatelet Drugs

The use of aspirin or dipyridamole has been advocated but never properly evaluated. Furthermore, it seems illogical since antiplatelet drugs are of no proven value in the acute treatment of venous thrombosis and are not devoid of hemorrhagic risk.

Thrombolytics

Vines and Davis[160] in 1971 were the first to report on the use of urokinase in CVT, followed 10 years later by Di Rocco et al,[41] who successfully treated five patients with urokinase and heparin. Since then thrombolytic use has been reported in some 50 cases of CVT, either locally or intravenously.[13,54,68,75,112,128,136,155] The results have been favorable, but it is too early to assess precisely the benefit/risk ratio of this treatment and to determine the indications, since, first, it was usually given in combination with heparin and, second, it was often used before other treatments had been adequately tried.[75] The clinical effectiveness and tolerability of thrombolytics in CVT need to be confirmed in larger series. We still favor the use of heparin because of its efficacy, which has been established on a much wider experience, and because of its lower risk of intracerebral bleeding. There is a good argument for trying local urokinase (via the internal jugular route) in patients who worsen despite optimal symptomatic and heparin treatments.

SUMMARY

Treatment of CVT should be started as early as possible. It is based primarily on heparin followed by warfarin. Other modalities of antithrombotic treatment are at present anecdotal. Heparin should be associated, whenever necessary, with symptomatic treatment (anticonvulsants and reduction of raised intracranial pressure) and, whenever possible, with etiologic treatment such as antibiotics in septic cases.

References

1. Achiron A, Gornish M, Melamed E: Cerebral sinus thrombosis as a potential hazard of antifibrinolytic treatment in menorrhagia. Stroke 21:817, 1990
2. Al Hakim M, Katirji MB, Osorio I, Weisman R: Cerebral venous thrombosis in paroxysmal nocturnal hemoglobinuria: report of two cases. Neurology 43:742, 1993
3. Ameri A, Bousser MG: Cerebral venous thrombosis. Neurol Clin 10:876, 1992
4. Anderson CM, Edelman RR, Turski PA: Magnetic resonance venography and cerebral venous thrombosis. p. 289. Anderon CM, Edelman RR, Turski PA (eds): In Clinical Magnetic Resonance Angiography. Vol. 1. Lippincott-Raven, Philadelphia, 1993
5. Anderson SC, Shah CP, Murtagh FR: Congested deep subcortical veins as a sign of dural venous thrombosis: MR and CT correlations. J Comput Assist Tomogr 11:1059, 1987
6. Averback P: Primary cerebral venous thrombosis in young adults. The diverse manifestations of an underrecognized disease. Ann Neurol 3:81, 1978
7. Azzarelli B, Itani AL, Catanzaro PT: Cerebral phlebothrombosis. A complication of lymphoma. Arch Neurol 37:126, 1980
8. Bailey OT, Hass GM: Dural sinus thrombosis in early life, clinical manifestations and extent of brain injury in acute sinus thrombosis. J Pediatr 11:755, 1937
9. Bansal BC, Gupta RR, Prakash C: Stroke during pregnancy and puerperium in young females below the age of 40 years as a result of cerebral venous/sinus thrombosis. Jpn Heart J 21:171, 1980
10. Barinagarrementeria F, Cantu C, Arredondo H: Aseptic cerebral venous thrombosis: proposed prognostic scale. J Stroke Cerebrovasc Dis 2:34, 1992
11. Barnes BD, Winestock DP: Dynamic radionuclide scanning in the diagnosis of thrombosis of the superior sagittal sinus. Neurology 27:656, 1977
12. Barnett HJM, Hyland HH: Noninfective intracranial venous thrombosis. Brain 76:36, 1953
13. Barnwell SL, Higashida RT, Halbach VV et al: Direct endovascular thrombolytic therapy for dural sinus thrombosis. Neurosurgery 28:135, 1991
14. Barron TF, Gusnard DA, Simmermann RA, Clancy RR: Cerebral venous thrombosis in neonates and children. Pediatr Neurol 8:112, 1992
15. Barthelemy M, Bousser MG, Jacobs C: Thrombose veineuse cérébrale au cours d'un syndrome néphrotique. Nouv Presse med 9:367, 1980
16. Baumgartner RW, Landi T: Venous thalamic infarction. Cerebrovasc Dis 2:353, 1992
17. Bertina RM, Koeleman BPLC, Koiser T et al: Mutation in blood coagulation factor V associated with resistance to activated protein C. Nature 369:64, 1994
18. Bots GAM: Thrombosis of the galenic system veins in the adult. Acta Neuropathol 17:227, 1971
19. Bousser MG, Bletry O, Launay M et al: Thrombose veineuse cérébrale au cours de la maladie de Behçet. A propos de deux cas. Revue Neurol (Paris) 136:753, 1980
20. Bousser MG, Chiras J, Sauron B et al: Cerebral venous thrombosis. A review of 38 cases. Stroke 16:199, 1985
21. Brant-Zawadzki M, Chang GY, McCarty GE: Computed tomography in dural sinus thrombosis. Arch Neurol 39:446, 1982
22. Bridgers SL, Strauss E, Smith EO et al: Demonstration of superior sagittal sinus thrombosis by indium 111 platelet scintigraphy. Arch Neurol 43:1079, 1986
23. Brismar J: Computed tomography in superior sagittal sinus thrombosis. Acta Radiol (Stockh) 21:321, 1980
24. Brown MT, Friedeman HS, Oakes WJ et al: Sagittal sinus thrombosis and leptomeningeal medullobastoma. Neurology 41:455, 1991
25. Buchanan DS, Brazinsky JH: Dural sinus and cerebral venous thrombosis. Incidence in young women receiving oral contraceptives. Arch Neurol 22:440, 1970
26. Buonanno F, Moody DM, Ball MR, Laster DW: Computed cranial tomographic findings in cerebral sino-venous occlusion. J Comput Assist Tomogr 2:281, 1978
27. Buonanno FS, Moody DM, Ball RM: CT scan findings in cerebral sinovenous occlusion. Neurology 12:288, 1982
28. Byrne JV, Lawton CA: Meningeal sarcoidosis causing intracranial hypertension secondary to dural sinus thrombosis. Br J Radiol 56:755, 1983
29. Cantu C, Barinagarrementeria F: Cerebral venous thrombosis associated with pregnancy and puerperium; review of 67 cases. Stroke 24:1880, 1993
30. Chelly D, Levy C, Ameri A, Brunereau L: Imagerie des thrombophlébites cérébrales. Ann Radiol 37:108, 1994
31. Chiras J, Bousser MG, Meder JF et al: CT in cerebral thrombophlebitis. Neuroradiology 27:145, 1985
32. Cochran FB, Packman S: Homocystinuria presenting as sagittal sinus thrombosis. Eur Neurol 32:1, 1992
33. Coquillat G, Warter JM: grave accut Thromboses Veineuses Cérébrales. Rapport de neurologie présenté au Congrès de Psychiatrie et de Neurologie de Langue Française. Vol. 1. Masson, Paris, 1976
34. Curnes JT, Creasy JL, Whaley RL, Scatliff JH: Air in the cavernous sinus thrombosis [letter]. AJNR 8:176, 1987
35. Dahlback B, Carlsson M, Svensson PJ: Familial thrombophilia due to a previously unrecognized mechanism characterized by poor anticoagulant response to activated protein C. Proc Natl Acad Sci USA 90:1004, 1993
36. Daif A, Awada A, Al-Rajeh S et al: Cerebral venous thrombosis in adult. A study of 40 cases from Saudi Arabia. Stroke 26:1193, 1995
37. Deschiens MA, Conard J, Horellou MH et al: Coagulation studies, factor V Leiden, antiphospholipid antibod-

ies in 40 cases of cerebral venous thrombosis. Stroke 27:1724, 1996

38. De Slegte RGM, Kaiser MC, van der Baan S, Smit L: Computed tomographic diagnosis of septic sinus thrombosis and their complications. Neuroradiology 30:160, 1988

39. Diaz JM, Schiffman JS, Urban ES, Maccario M: Superior sagittal sinus thrombosis and pulmonary embolism: a syndrome rediscovered. Acta Neurol Scand 86:390, 1992

40. Dinubile MJ: Septic thrombosis of the cavernous sinuses. Neurological review. Arch Neurol 45:567, 1988

41. DiRocco C, Lanelli A, Leone G et al: Heparin-urokinase treatment in a septic dural sinus thrombosis. Arch Neurol 38:431, 1981

42. Dormont D, Anxionnat R, Evrard S et al: MRI in cerebral venous thrombosis. J Neuroradiol 21:81, 1994

43. Dormont D, Sag K, Biondi A et al: Gadolinium-enhanced MR of chronic dural sinus thrombosis. AJNR 16:1347, 1995

44. Ehlers H, Courville CB: Thrombosis of internal cerebral veins in infancy and childhood. Review of literature and report of five cases. J Pediatr 8:600, 1936

45. Eick JJ, Miller KD, Bell KA, Tutton RH: Computed tomography of deep cerebral venous thrombosis in children. Radiology 140:399, 1981

46. Eikmeier G, Kuhlmann R, Gastpar M: Thrombosis of cerebral veins following intravenous application of clomipramine. J Neurol Neurosurg Psychiatr 52:1461, 1989

47. Einhäupl KM, Masuhr F: Cerebral venous and sinus thrombosis. An update. Eur J Neurol 1:109, 1994

48. Einhäupl KM, Villringer A, Habert RL et al: Clinical spectrum of sinus venous thrombosis. In Einhäupl KM, Kempski O, Baethmann A (eds): Cerebral Sinus Thrombosis: Experimental and Clinical Aspects. p. 149. Plenum Press, New York, 1990

49. Einhäupl KM, Villringer A, Meister W et al: Heparin treatment in sinus venous thrombosis. Lancet 338:597, 1991

50. El Alaoui Faris M, Birouk N, Slassi I et al: Thrombose du sinus longitudinal supérieur et ostéite cranienne syphilitique. Rev Neurol 148:783, 1992

51. Enevoldson TP, Ross Russell RW: Cerebral venous thrombosis. New causes for an old syndrome. Q J Med 77:1255, 1990

52. Eng LJ, Longstreth WT, Shaw CM et al: Cerebellar venous infarction: case report with clinicopathologic correlation. Neurology 40:837, 1990

53. Engesser L, Broekmans AW, Briet E et al: Hereditary protein S deficiency. Clinical manifestations. Ann Intern Med 106:31, 1987

54. Eskridge JM, Wessbecher FW: Thrombolysis for superior sagittal sinus thrombosis. J Vasc Interv Radiol 2:89, 1991

55. Estanol B, Rodriguez A, Conte G et al: Intracranial venous thrombosis in young women. Stroke 10:680, 1979

56. Evans RW, Patten BM: Trichinosis associated with superior sagittal sinus thrombosis. Ann Neurol 11:216, 1982

57. Fairburn B: Intracranial venous thrombosis complicating oral contraception: treatment by anticoagulant drugs. BMJ 2:647, 1973

58. Feinberg WM, Swenson MR: Cerebrovascular complications of L-asparaginase therapy. Neurology 38:127, 1988

59. Feldenzer JA, Bueche MJ, Venes JL, Gebarski SS: Superior sagittal sinus thrombosis with infarction in sickle cell trait. Stroke 18:656, 1987

60. Ford K, Sarwar M: Computed tomography of dural sinus thrombosis. AJNR 2:539, 1981

61. Garcin R, Pestel M: Thrombophlébites Cérébrales. Masson, Paris, 1949

62. Gates PC: Cerebral venous thrombosis: a retrospective review. Aust NZ J Med 16:766, 1986

63. Gettelfinger DM, Kokmen E: Superior sagittal sinus thrombosis. Arch Neurol 34:2, 1977

64. Girard DE, Reuler JB, Mayer BS et al: Cerebral venous sinus thrombosis due to indwelling transvenous pacemaker catheter. Arch Neurol 37:113, 1980

65. Go RT, Chiu CL, Neuman LA: Diagnosis of superior sagittal sinus thrombosis by dynamic and sequential brain scanning. Report of one case. Neurology 23:1199, 1973

66. Goldberg AL, Rosenbaum AE, Wang H et al: Computed tomography of dural sinus thrombosis. J Comput Assist Tomogr 10:16, 1986

67. Greitz T, Link H: Aseptic thrombosis of intracranial sinuses. Radiol Clin Biol 35:111, 1966

68. Griesemer DA, Theodorou AA, Berg RA, Spera TD: Local fibrinolysis in cerebral venous thrombosis. Pediatr Neurol 10:78, 1994

69. Hacker H: Normal supratentorial veins and dural sinuses. In Newton TH, Potts DG (eds): Radiology of the Skull and Brain. Angiography. CV Mosby, St. Louis, 1974

70. Haley EC, Brasmear HR, Barth JT et al: Deep cerebral venous thrombosis. Clinical, neuroradiological and neuropsychological correlates. Arch Neurol 46:337, 1989

71. Halpern JP, Morris JGL, Driscoll GL: Anticoagulants and cerebral venous thrombosis. Aust NZ J Med 14:643, 1984

72. Hanley DF, Feldman E, Borel CO et al: Treatment of sagittal sinus thrombosis associated with cerebral hemorrhage and intracranial hypertension. Stroke 19:903, 1988

73. Hickey WF, Garnick MB, Henderson JC, Dawson DM: Primary cerebral venous thrombosis in patients with cancer—a rarely diagnosed paraneoplastic syndrome. Am J Med 73:740, 1982

74. Houser OW, Campbell JK, Campbell RJ, Sundt TM: Arteriovenous malformation affecting the transverse dural venous sinus. An acquired lesion. Mayo Clin Proc 54:651, 1979

75. Horowitz M, Purdy P, Unwin H et al: Treatment of dural sinus thrombosis using elective catheterization and urokinase. Ann Neurol 38:58, 1995

76. Huang YP, Wolf BS: Veins of posterior fossa-superior or galenic draining group. AJR Radiat Ther Nucl Med 95:808, 1965

77. Huang YP, Wolf BS, Antin SP, Okudera T: The veins of the posterior fossa-anterior or petrosal draining group. AJR Radiat Ther Nucl Med 104:36, 1968

78. Hughes JP, Stovin PG: Segmental pulmonary artery an-

eurysms with peripheral venous thrombosis. Br J Dis Chest 53:19, 1959

79. Isensee CH, Reul J, Thron A: Magnetic resonance imaging of thrombosed dural sinuses. Stroke 25:29, 1994

80. Jacquin V, Salama J, Leroux G, Delaporte P: Thromboses veineuses cérébrales et des membres supérieurs associées à une thrombopénie, induites par le polysulfate de Pentosane. Ann Med Intern 139:194, 1988

81. Johnsen S, Greenwood R, Fischman MA: Internal cerebral vein thrombosis. Arch Neurol 28:205, 1973

82. Kalbag RM, Woolf AL: Cerebral Venous Thrombosis. Vol. 1. Oxford University Press, Oxford, 1967

83. Kaplan JM, Biller J, Adams HP: Outcome in nonseptic spontaneous superior sagittal sinus thrombosis in adults. Cerebrovasc Dis 1:231, 1991

84. Kim KS, Walczak TS: Computed tomography of deep cerebral venous thrombosis. J Comput Assist Tomogr 10:386, 1986

85. Kinal ME: Traumatic thrombosis of dural venous sinuses in closed head injuries. J Neurosurg 27:142, 1967

86. Kingsley DPE, Kendall BE, Moseley LF: Superior sagittal sinus thrombosis, an evaluation of the changes demonstrated on computed tomography. J Neurol Neurosurg Psychiatry 41:1065, 1978

87. Krayenbühl H: Cerebral venous and sinus thrombosis. Clin Neurosurg 14:1, 1967

88. Krayenbühl H: Cerebral venous thrombosis. The diagnostic value of cerebral angiogaphy. Schweiz Arch Neurol Neurochir Psychiatr 74:261, 1954

89. Kutluk K, Schumacher M, Mironov A: The role of sinus thrombosis in occipital dural arteriovenous malformations. Development and spontaneous closure. Neurochirurgia 34:144, 1991

90. Levine SR, Kieran S, Puzio K et al: Cerebral venous thrombosis with lupus anticoagulants. Report of 2 cases. Stroke 18:801, 1987

91. Levine SR, Twyman RE, Gilman S: The role of anticoagulation in cavernous sinus thrombosis. Neurology 38:517, 1988

92. Macchi PJ, Grossman RI, Gomori JM et al: High field MR imaging of cerebral venous thrombosis. J Comput Assist Tomogr 10:10, 1986

93. Martin JP, Sheenan HL: Primary thrombosis of cerebral veins (following childbirth) BMJ 1:349, 1941

94. Martinelli I, Landi G, Merati G et al: Factor V gene mutation is a risk factor for cerebral venous thrombosis. Thromb Haemost 75:393, 1996

95. Mas JL, Meder JF, Meary E, Bousser MG: Magnetic resonance imaging in lateral sinus hypoplasia and thrombosis. Stroke 21:1350, 1990

96. Mas JL, Meder JF, Meary E: Dural sinus thrombosis: long term follow-up by magnetic resonance imaging. Cerebrovasc Dis 2:137, 1992

97. Mattle H, Edelkman RR, Reis MA, Atkinson DJ: Flow quantification in the superior sagittal sinus using magnetic resonance. Neurology 40:813, 1990

98. Mattle HP, Wentz KU, Edelman RR et al: Cerebral venography with MR. Radiology 178:453, 1991

99. McMurdo SK, Brant-Zawadzki M, Bradley WG et al: Dural sinus thrombosis study using intermediate field strength MR imaging. Radiology 161:83, 1986

100. Medlock MD, Olivero WC, Hanigan WC et al: Children with cerebral venous thrombosis diagnosed with magnetic resonance imaging and magnetic resonance angiography. Neurosurgery 31:870, 1992

101. Meininger V, James JM, Rio B, Zittoun R: Occlusions des sinus veineux de la dure-mère au cours des hémopathies. Rev Neurol (Paris) 141:228, 1985

102. Meyohas MC, Roullet E: Cerebral venous thrombosis and dural primary infection with human immuno-deficiency virus and cytomegalovirus. J Neurol Neurosurg Psychiatry 52:1010, 1989

103. Mickle JP, McLennan JE, Lidden CW: Cortical vein thrombosis in Wegener's granulomatosis. J Neurosurg 46:248, 1977

104. Milandre L, Gueriot C, Girard N et al: Les thromboses veineuses cérébrales de l'adulte. Ann Med Intern 139:544, 1988

105. Murphy MF, Clarke CRA, Brearley RL: Superior sagittal sinus thrombosis and essential thrombocythaemia. BMJ 287:1344, 1983

106. Nayak AK, Karnad D, Mahajan MV et al: Cerebellar venous infarction in chronic suppurative otitis media. A case report with review of four other cases. Stroke 25:1958, 1994

107. Noetzel H, Jerusalem F: Die Hirnvenen und sinusthrombosen. Monographien aus dem Gesamtgebiete der Neurologie und Psychiatrie 106:1, 1965

108. Padayachee TS, Bingham JB, Grave MJ et al: Dural sinus thrombosis. Diagnosis and follow-up by magnetic resonance angiography and imaging. Neuroradiology 33:165, 1991

109. Patchell RA, Posner JB: Neurologic complications of carcinoid. Neurology 36:745, 1986

110. Patel A, Lo R: Electric injury with cerebral venous thrombosis. Case report and review of the literature. Stroke 24:903, 1993

111. Patronas NJ, Duda EE, Mirfakhraee M, Wollmann RL: Superior sagittal sinus thrombosis diagnosed by computed tomography. Surg Neurol 15:11, 1981

112. Persson L, Lilja A: Extensive dural sinus thrombosis treated by surgical removal and local streptokinase infusion. Neurosurgery 26:117, 1990

113. Pfister HW, Borasio GD, Dirnagl V et al: Cerebrovascular complications of bacterial meningitis in adults. Neurology 42:1497, 1992

114. Poltera AA: The pathology of intracranial venous thrombosis in oral contraception. J Pathol 106:209, 1972

115. Preter M, Tzourio C, Ameri A, Bousser MG: Long term prognosis in cerebral venous thrombosis. A follow up of 77 patients. Stroke 27:243, 1996

116. Rao KCVG, Knipp HC, Wagner EJ: CT findings in cerebral sinus and venous thrombosis. Radiology 140:391, 1981

117. Ray BS, Dunbar HS: Thrombosis of dural venous sinuses as cause of "pseudotumor cerebri." Ann Surg 134:376, 1951

118. Ribes MF: Des recherches faites sur la phlébite. Revue Médicale Française et Etrangère et Journal de Clinique de l'Hôtel-Dieu et de la Charité de Paris 3:5, 1825

119. Rippe DJ, Boyko OB, Spritzer CE et al: Demonstration

of dural sinus occlusion by the use of MR angiography. AJNR 11:199, 1990

120. Rivkin MJ, Anderson ML, Kaye EM: Neonatal idiopathic cerebral venous thrombosis: an unrecognized cause of transient seizures or lethargy. Ann Neurol 32: 51, 1992

121. Rondepierre P, Hamon M, Leys D et al: Thromboses veineuses cérébrales: étude de l'évolution. Rev Neurol (Paris) 151:100, 1995

122. Rothwell PM, Grant R: Cerebral venous sinus thrombosis induced by "ectasy." J Neurol Neurochir Psychiatr 56:1035, 1993

123. Rousseaux M, Lesoin F, Barbaste P, Jomin M: Infarctus cérébelleux pseudo-tumoral d'origine veineuse. Rev Neurol (Paris) 144:209, 1988

124. Rousseaux P, Bernard MH, Scherpereel B, Guyot JF: Thrombose des sinus veineux intra-crâniens (à propos de 22 cas). Neurochirurgie 24:197, 1978

125. Sauron B, Chiras J, Chain G, Castaigne P: Thrombophlébite cérébelleuse chez un homme porteur d'un déficit familial en antithrombine III. Rev Neurol (Paris) 138:685, 1982

126. Savino PJ, Grossman RI, Schatz NJ et al: High field magnetic resonance imaging in the diagnosis of cavernous sinus thrombosis. Arch Neurol 43:1081, 1986

127. Schutta HS, Williams EC, Baranski BG, Sutula TP: Cerebral venous thrombosis with plasminogen deficiency. Stroke 22:401, 1991

128. Scott JA, Pascuzzi RM, Hall PV, Becker GJ: Treatment of dural sinus thrombosis with local urokinase infusion. J Neurosurg 68:284, 1988

129. Segall HD, Ahmadi J, McComb JG et al: Computed tomographic observations pertinent to intracranial venous thrombotic and occlusive disease in childhood. Radiology 143:441, 1982

130. Sekhar LN, Dujovny M, Rao GR: Carotid cavernous sinus thrombosis caused by *Aspergillus fumigatus*. J Neurosurg 52:120, 1980

131. Shevell MI, Silver K, O'Gorman AM et al: Neonatal dural sinus thrombosis. Pediatr Neurol 5:161, 1989

132. Shinohara Y, Yosmitoshi M, Yoshii F: Appearance and disappearance of empty delta sign in superior sagittal sinus thrombosis. Stroke 17:1282, 1986

133. Shiozawa Z, Yamada H, Mabuchi C et al: Superior sagittal sinus thrombosis associated with androgen therapy for hypoplastic anaemia. Ann Neurol 12:578, 1982

134. Siegert CEH, Smelt AHM, De Bruin TWA: Superior sagittal sinus thrombosis and thyrotoxicosis. Possible association in two cases. Stroke 26:496, 1995

135. Sigsbee B, Deck MDF, Posner JB: Nonmetastatic superior sagittal sinus thrombosis complicating systemic cancer. Neurology 29:139, 1979

136. Smith TP, Higashida R, Barnwell S et al: Treatment of dural sinus thrombosis by urokinase infusion. AJNR 15: 801, 1994

137. Smith WDF, Sinar J, Carey M: Sagittal sinus thrombosis and occult malignancy. J Neurol Neurosurg Psychiatry 46:187, 1983

138. Snyder TC, Sachdev HS: MR imaging of cerebral dural sinus thrombosis. J Comput Assist Tomogr 10:889, 1986

139. Souter RG, Mitchell A: Spreading venous cortical

thrombosis due to infusion of hyperosmolar solution into the internal jugular vein. BMJ 285:935, 1982

140. Stam J: Treatment of cerebral venous thrombosis Cerebrovasc Dis 3:329, 1993

141. Stansfield FR: Puerperal cerebral thrombophlebitis treated by heparin. BMJ 1:436, 1942

142. Symonds CP: Cerebral thrombophlebitis. BMJ 2:348, 1940

143. Symonds CP: Hydrocephalic and focal cerebral symptoms in relation to thrombophlebitis of the dural sinuses and cerebral veins. Brain 60:531, 1937

144. Sze G, Simmons B, Krol G et al: Dural sinus thrombosis: verification with spin echo techniques. AJNR 9:679, 1988

145. Tarras S, Gadia C, Mester L et al: Homozygous protein C deficiency in a newborn. Clinicopathologic correlation. Arch Neurol 45:214, 1988

146. Tehindrazanarivelo AD, Evrard S, Schaison M et al: Prospective study of cerebral sinus venous thrombosis in patients presenting with benign intracranial hypertension. Cerebrovasc Dis 2:22, 1992

147. Thron A, Wessel K, Linden D et al: Superior sagittal sinus thrombosis: neuroradiological evaluation and clinical findings. J Neurol 233:283, 1986

148. Towbin A: The syndrome of latent cerebral venous thrombosis: its frequency and relation to age and congestive heart failure. Stroke 4:419, 1973

149. Tsai FY, Higashida RT, Matovich V, Alfieri K: Acute thrombosis of the intracranial dural sinus: direct thrombolytic treatment. AJNR 13:1137, 1992

150. Tsai FY, Wang AM, Matovich V et al: MR staging of acute dural sinus thrombosis: correlation with venous pressure measurements and implications for treatment and prognosis. AJNR 16:1021, 1995

151. Tsuruda JS, Shimakawa A, Pecl NJ, Saloner D: Dural sinus occlusions. Evaluation with phase sensitive gradient echo MR imaging. AJNR 12:481, 1991

152. Ur Rahman N, Al-Tahan AR: Computed tomographic evidence of an extensive thrombosis and infarction of the deep venous system. Stroke 24:744, 1993

153. Urban E, Jabbari B, Robles H: Concurrent cerebral venous sinus thrombosis and myloradiculopathy in Sjögren syndrome. Neurology 44:554, 1994

154. Valdueza JM, Schultz M, Harms L, Einhäupl KM: Venous transcranial Döppler ultrasound monitoring in acute dural sinus thrombosis. Report of two cases. Stroke 26:1196, 1995

155. van Dyke DC, Eldalah MK, Bale JF et al: *Mycoplasma pneumoniae*-induced cerebral venous thrombosis treated with urokinase. Clin Pediatr (Phila) 31:501, 1992

156. Van Vleymen B, de Haenne I, van Hoof A, Pattyn G: Cerebral venous thrombosis in paroxysmal nocturnal haemoglobinuria. Acta Neurol Belg 87:80, 1987

157. Vidailhet M, Piette JC, Wechsler B et al: Cerebral venous thrombosis in systemic lupus erythematosus. Report of 6 cases and review. Stroke 21:1226, 1990

158. Villringer A, Bousser MG, Einhäupl KM: Cerebral sinus venous thrombosis. p. 654. In Hacke W (ed). Neurocritical Care. Vol. 1. Springer-Verlag, Berlin, 1994

159. Villringer A, Meraein S, Einhäupl KM: Treatment of

sinus venous thrombosis—beyond the recommendation of anticoagulation. J Neuroradiol 21:72, 1994

160. Vines FS, Davis DO: Clinical radiological correlation in cerebral venous occlusive disease. Radiology 98:9, 1971

161. Virapongse C, Cazenave C, Quisling R et al: The empty delta sign: frequency and significance in 76 cases of dural sinus thrombosis. Radiology 162:779, 1987

162. Yasargil MG, Damur M: Thrombosis of the cerebral veins and dural sinuses. In Newton TH, and Potts DG (eds): Radiology of the Skull and Brain. Angiography. CV Mosby, St. Louis, 1974

163. Yerby MS, Bailey GM: Superior sagittal sinus thrombosis 10 years after surgery for ulcerative colitis. Stroke 11:294, 1980

164. Wardlaw JM, Vaughan GT, Steers AJW, Sellar RJ: Transcranial Döppler ultrasound findings in venous sinus thrombosis. J Neurosurg 80:332, 1994

165. Wechsler B, Vidailhet M, Piette JC et al: Cerebral venous thrombosis in Behçet's disease: clinical study and long-term follow-up of 25 cases. Neurology 42:614, 1992

166. Zuber M, Toulon P, Marnet L, Mas JL: Factor V Leiden mutation in cerebral venous thrombosis. Stroke 27:1721, 1996

CHAPTER 25

Intracerebral Hemorrhage

CARLOS S. KASE

J. P. MOHR

LOUIS R. CAPLAN

Epidemiology

Intracerebral hemorrhage (ICH) occurs as a result of bleeding from an arterial source directly into the brain substance. Although its relative frequency in patients with stroke is subject to geographic and racial variations, figures between 5% and 10% are most commonly quoted.[203,241,298,341] In a consecutive series of 938 stroke patients entered into the NINCDS Stroke Data Bank, primary ICH accounted for 10.7% of the cases.[202] Similar figures were obtained in population studies from Denmark (10.4%),[155] Holland (9%),[163] the midwestern United States (10%), and southern Alabama (8%).[144] The incidence of ICH increases with advancing age,[29,298] a feature that applies to all types of stroke, both ischemic and hemorrhagic. The incidence rates are relatively constant in predominantly white populations, with rates between 7 and 11 cases per 100,000[33,81,301,308] (Table 25.1). The figures were higher in a U.S. population (southern Alabama) with a mixture of whites and blacks, since the former had an incidence rate of 12/100,000, whereas in blacks the rate was 32/100,000.[144] Similar comparisons between whites and blacks in Cincinnati, Ohio, yielded an overall age- and sex-adjusted incidence of ICH that was 1.4-fold higher in blacks.[29] The difference in ICH incidence was even higher (2.3-fold) for blacks in the younger than 75 years of age group. Also, a Hispanic population in New Mexico had a high incidence of ICH (34.9/100,000) whereas non-Hispanic whites from the same population had an incidence rate (16.6/100,000) comparable to that of whites in other geographic locations.[34] Some series from Oriental countries, such as that from Shibata, Japan,[328] report a several-fold increase (61/100,000 population) in incidence rates of ICH. Along with these differing incidence rates from various geographic locations, a general trend toward declining rates of ICH has been detected in recent decades, starting with the initial observation in Göteborg, Sweden,[8] subsequently

confirmed in the U.S. in the population of Rochester, Minnesota.[122,124] From analysis of data encompassing a 32-year period (1945 to 1976), Furlan et al[122] showed a significant decrease in incidence between the first and second parts of this period: 13.3/100,000 for 1945 to 1960 and 6.7/100,000 for 1961 to 1976. These figures correlated with a similar decline in the frequency and severity of hypertension in the population studied. A similarly declining trend in the incidence of ICH has been reported from Hisayama, Japan,[347] where it was also related to a decrease in the frequency of hypertension.

The role of *hypertension* as a leading risk factor is well established, and its frequency has been estimated to be between 72%[241] and 81%.[122] The causative role of hypertension is supported by the high incidence of left ventricular hypertrophy in autopsy cases of ICH[26,250,319] and the significantly higher admission blood pressure readings in ICH patients compared with those with other forms of stroke.[260] The autopsy study of McCormick and Rosenfield[227] challenged the view that hypertension represents the main causative factor in ICH. Their series included a large number of cases of ICH due to blood dyscrasias, vascular malformations, and tumors, and hypertension was regarded as the sole basis for the bleeding in only 25% of the total. This discrepancy with most reported series of ICH may reflect in part a referral pattern bias, as well as more stringent criteria in establishing a causal relationship between hypertension and ICH. However, clinical series[33,301] have also questioned the validity of the concept of ICH as a condition most commonly related to hypertension: Brott et al[33] found a history of hypertension in only 45% of 154 patients, a figure that rose to only 56% when electrocardiographic or chest radiographic data of cardiomegaly were added as criteria for the diagnosis of hypertension. Similarly, Schütz et al[301] labeled only 59% of their ICH cases as due to hypertension. These data suggest that a sizable proportion of ICH cases are due to nonhypertensive mechanisms.

In addition to advancing age, hypertension, and race, a

Table 25.1 Incidence of Intracerebral Hemorrhage in Studies from Various Geographic Locations

Location	Ref.	No. of Cases	Rate[a]
Rochester, Minnesota	81	81	7
Framingham,		58	
Massachusetts	298		10
Southern Alabama	144	13	12
Cincinnati, Ohio	33	154	11
Giessen, Germany	301	100	11
Shibata, Japan	328	97	61
Bernalillo Co., New Mexico	34		
Non-Hispanic whites		47	17
Hispanics		39	35

[a] Per 100,000 population.

number of other risk factors have been evaluated, including cigarette smoking, alcohol consumption, and serum cholesterol levels. Abbott et al[1] showed an increased risk of intracranial hemorrhage (both ICH and subarachnoid hemorrhage [SAH]) in *cigarette-smoking* Hawaiian men of Japanese ancestry. The risk of "hemorrhagic stroke" was 2.5 times higher in smokers, an effect that was independent of other risk factors. However, the diagnosis of ICH was often made on clinical grounds, without verification by imaging or autopsy findings. In a recent study based on computed tomography (CT) diagnosis of ICH in Finland, Juvela et al[177] found that smoking was not an independent risk factor for ICH. The series reported by Donahue et al[78] and Juvela et al[177] documented an increased risk of ICH in relation to *alcohol ingestion*, an effect that operated independently from other risk factors. Both studies[78,177] showed a strong dose-response relationship between alcohol use and ICH. The series of Juvela et al[177] documented a similar effect for alcohol ingestion within 24 hours from ICH onset and within 1 week from onset. *Low serum cholesterol* level, defined as serum cholesterol below 160 mg/dl, has been shown to be associated with an increased risk of ICH in Japanese men,[328] as well as in Hawaiian men of Japanese origin.[348] Other risk factors have been suggested in some studies. *Cirrhosis* was highly represented (15.5%) in the autopsy series of Boudouresques et al[23] but its significance could not be assessed, since no comparison was available with a control autopsy series of the general population. This factor is regarded as of no significance by most epidemiologic studies[2] and autopsy series of ICH.[250,319] The occasional association of ICH with cirrhosis has been linked to thrombocytopenia and other abnormalities in coagulation.[228] The role of *aspirin use* and risk of ICH is controversial. The Physicians' Health Study,[318] which evaluated the effect of low-dose aspirin (325 mg every other day) against placebo in the primary prevention of coronary events, documented a borderline significant increase in relative risk of hemorrhagic stroke (ICH and SAH) in the aspirin group. Similarly, the SALT (Swedish Aspirin Low-Dose Trial)[336] secondary stroke prevention trial documented a significant increase in the frequency of hemorrhagic stroke in the group assigned to aspirin (75 mg/day), compared with placebo. These data contrast with those from other sec-

ondary stroke prevention trials,[24,40,332,333,349] in which even higher doses of aspirin were used without resulting in an increased risk of ICH.

Pathologic Features and Pathogenesis

Spontaneous ICH occurs predominantly in the deep portions of the cerebral hemispheres. Its most common location is the putamen; this site accounts for 35% to 50% of the cases.[110,122,186,202,241,372] The second site of preference varies in different series; in some it is the subcortical white matter,[122,186,241,250] in others the cerebellum,[166] with frequencies of 30% and 16% respectively. The thalamus follows, with a uniform frequency of 10% to 15%.[109,119,122,186,202,241,361,372] Pontine hemorrhage accounts for 5% to 12% of ICH cases.[109,122,186,202,241] The distribution figures in a series of 100 unselected cases of ICH are shown in Table 25.2.

The hemorrhages of putaminal, thalamic, and pontine location occur in the vascular distribution of small, perforating intracerebral arteries, the lenticulostriate, thalamoperforating, and basilar paramedian groups, respectively. Cerebellar hemorrhage occurs in the area of the dentate nucleus,[75,115] which is supplied by small branches of both the superior and the anterior-inferior cerebellar arteries.[45,75] Thus most ICHs originate from the rupture of small, deep arteries,[106] of diameters between 50 and 200 μm. These same arteries are recognized to be those occluded in cases of lacunar infarcts,[111] a form of stroke correlated with chronic hypertension.[101,104] Thus it is apparent that these various groups of small arteries, located in well-defined anatomic areas, become the target of chronic hypertension, and the result can be either occlusion or rupture, leading to lacunar infarcts or ICH, respectively.

VASCULAR RUPTURE

The actual mechanism of vascular rupture leading to ICH has been the subject of considerable interest, and several detailed pathologic studies[60,62,292] have addressed this point. Because

Table 25.2 Distribution by Site of 100 Cases of Intracerebral Hemorrhage at the University of South Alabama Medical Center

Type	No. of Cases
Putaminal	34
Lobar	24
Thalamic	20
Cerebellar	7
Pontine	6
Miscellaneous	
Caudate	5
Putaminothalamic	4

hypertension is one of its main causative factors,[63] arterial changes associated with it have been commonly implicated in its pathogenesis. Since Charcot and Bouchard[49] described "miliary aneurysms" in brain specimens from hypertensive ICH cases, these lesions have been the subject of extensive interest. Initially, they were thought to represent true dilatations of the arterial wall,[115] and their preferential location deep in the hemispheres lent support to their pathogenic role. However, with the use of a more precise histologic technique, Ellis[90] was able to show that miliary aneurysms represented "false aneurysms" and were actually made of blood collected outside the vessel wall, as "masses of blood" surrounded by either "remains of the vessel wall" or fibrin. His view of the pathogenesis of ICH implied a primary intimal lesion, with or without secondary involvement of the media and adventitia, the former often leading to passage of blood into the vessel wall, with formation of a dissecting aneurysm. Either form of vascular abnormality (dissecting aneurysm or simple "weakening" of the vessel wall by the primary intimal lesion extending into the media and adventitia) would then be responsible for rupture and hemorrhage.

Over the following years, miliary aneurysms in the brain of hypertensives were shown by the use of thick frozen sections[137] and x-ray imaging of brain specimens injected with radiopaque media.[294] Green's study[137] showed three such lesions, two of which were associated with a fresh hemorrhage in the pons and frontal lobe. His view was that these lesions were mainly related to atherosclerosis and that they "may be responsible for some cases of cerebral hemorrhage." However, the definitive work that established the relationship between hypertension and miliary aneurysms was performed by Ross Russell,[294] with the use of postmortem angiography combined with routine histologic study of brain specimens. He found miliary aneurysms in 15 of 16 brains of hypertensive patients and in 10 of 38 normotensive patients. They were mostly found in the basal ganglia, internal capsule, and thalamus, and less commonly in the centrum semiovale and cortical gray matter. He regarded these lesions as most likely acquired, strongly related to hypertension, and, possibly causally related to ICH. He rejected the notion that they may be a consequence rather than a cause of ICH, as they were present in brains of hypertensives without ICH.

This study was followed by a series of observations reported by Cole and Yates[60–62] in a systematic analysis of 100 brains from hypertensive patients and an equal number of brains from normotensive persons. Miliary aneurysms were found in 46% of hypertensives, but only in 7% of normotensives; furthermore, they occurred in 85% of the cases of hypertensives with massive ICH, and in all those with small "slit" hemorrhages, which suggested that small hemorrhages probably result from microaneurysmal "leaks."[60] However, these authors did not establish a relationship between microaneurysms and bleeding sites, thereby failing to prove that these "leaks" had a causal role in ICH.

In 1971, Fisher[106] reported the study of two brains containing three ICHs, one pontine and two putaminal, by serial sections of blocks of tissue containing the hemorrhage. In both putaminal hemorrhages the primary arterial bleeding sites were identified along with multiple sites of secondary bleeding. The latter were thought to result from mechanical disruption and tearing of smaller vessels at the periphery of the enlarging hematoma. In the pontine case only the secondary bleeding sites were recognized. No instances of microaneurysm formation were found in immediate relationship to the hematomas, whereas "lipohyalinosis" was a frequent abnormality of the walls of small arteries harboring the bleeding sites. Miliary aneurysms were identified in both hemorrhages, although not in relation to the bleeding points. Fisher[106] regarded them as an unlikely source of major hemorrhage, but rather as the end result of old small sites of arterial rupture ("the end stage of a limited extravasation"). Following this study, Fisher[102] reported in 1972 a detail of the types of microaneurysms found in brains of hypertensives. He described "saccular," "lipohyalinotic," and "fusiform" varieties of microaneurysms and suggested that the lipohyalinotic form may be the process underlying ICH (as well as lacunar infarcts). He regarded the saccular and fusiform varieties as less likely to be important factors in the pathogenesis of ICH. On the basis of these two studies,[102,106] Fisher concluded that hypertensive ICH most likely results from rupture of one or two lipohyalinotic arteries, followed by secondary arterial ruptures at the periphery of the enlarging hematoma in a cascade or avalanche fashion.

ACTIVE BLEEDING

Early studies[162] prior to the wide availability of CT scanning suggested that the period of active bleeding in ICH is rather brief (<1 hour),[260] and the observation of clinical deterioration after admission was frequently attributed to the effects of brain edema,[162,241] although instances of continuous bleeding were occasionally reported.[191] A number of recent CT studies of the early phases of ICH have helped to clarify these concepts.

Broderick et al[30] evaluated eight patients with ICH by CT within 2½ hours from onset, and again several hours later (within 12 hours from onset in seven patients), documenting a substantial increase in hematoma size (mean percentage increase: 107%) (Fig. 25.1). This increase in the volume of the hemorrhage was accompanied by clinical deterioration in six of the eight patients, all of whom had a 40% increase in hematoma volume. In five of them the clinical deterioration occurred with blood pressure measurements of ≥195 mmHg. The authors suggested that a prolongation of active bleeding for several hours (up to 5 or 6) from onset may not be uncommon as a mechanism of early clinical deterioration in ICH. Similarly, Fehr and Anderson[97] reviewed 56 cases of hypertensive ICH in the basal ganglia and thalamus and documented enlargement of the hematoma by CT in 4 (7%); in 2 of them the increase in hematoma size was documented within 24 hours from onset, in the other 2 on days 5 and 6. Three of these patients had neurologic deterioration: in two who deteriorated within 24 hours, it occurred in the setting of poorly controlled hypertension, whereas the others had adequate blood pressure control; one of the latter two patients was a chronic alcoholic, leading the authors to suggest that this may be a risk factor for delayed progression of ICH.

In recent studies, Fujii et al,[120] Kazui et al,[188] and Brott et al[32] have further clarified the patterns of early enlargement of ICH. Fujii et al[120] studied 419 patients with ICH, in whom they performed the first CT within 24 hours of onset, and the follow-up CTs within 24 hours of admission, showing hematoma enlargement in 60 patients (14.3%). Kazui et al[188] conducted sequential CT evaluations in 204 patients with acute ICH, docu-

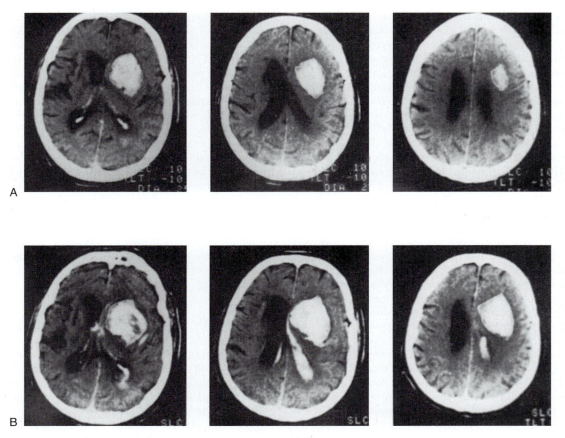

Figure 25.1 Enlargement of left putaminal hemorrhage (**A**) from 25 ml on CT performed 35 minutes after onset, to (**B**) 44 ml on CT done 70 minutes later (105 minutes after onset). (From Broderick et al,[30] with permission.)

menting enlargement of at least 12.5 cm³ or by 40% of the original volume in 20% of the cases. The highest frequency of detection of hematoma enlargement corresponded to patients who had the initial CT scan performed within 3 hours of stroke onset (36%), the detection of enlargement declining progressively as the time from ICH onset to first CT increased, with no documentation of enlargement in those first scanned after 24 hours from onset. These observations suggest that the period of hematoma enlargement can extend for a number of hours from onset as a result of active bleeding, a phenomenon that is frequently, but not always, associated with clinical deterioration. The study of Brott et al[32] included 103 patients first scanned within 3 hours of ICH onset, with subsequent follow-up CT scans 1 hour and 20 hours after the initial one. ICH enlargement (>33% volume increase) was detected in 26% of patients at the 1-hour follow-up scan, and an additional 12% showed enlargement between the 1-hour and 20-hour CT. The change in hematoma volume was often associated with clinical deterioration, but there were exceptions. These authors found no predictors of ICH enlargement, including age, hemorrhage location, severity of initial clinical deficit, systolic and diastolic blood pressure at onset or history of hypertension, use of antiplatelet drugs, platelet counts, prothrombin time, and partial thromboplastin time.

Further studies are needed to identify potential risk factors of early ICH enlargement, to attempt to prevent its associated neurologic morbidity and mortality. Such studies should be facilitated with the use of easy to apply techniques of hematoma volume measurement.[28,199,212] The so-called ABC method uses the formula ABC/2 in which A is the largest diameter of the hematoma in the CT slice with the largest area of ICH, B is the largest diameter of the hemorrhage perpendicular to line A, and C is the number of slices with hematoma times the slice thickness, resulting in the hematoma volume in cm³ (Fig. 25.2). The use of these volumetric measurements of ICH should improve our understanding of the clinical consequences of early changes in hematoma size and their risk factors, to better define clinical and CT patterns of ICH evolution. This should, in turn, serve as the background for new strategies of management of ICH and their eventual testing in randomized clinical trials.

GROSS PATHOLOGIC ANATOMY

The gross pathologic anatomy of ICH includes a number of features peculiar to the various locations of the hematomas. The common *putaminal* variety originates at the posterior

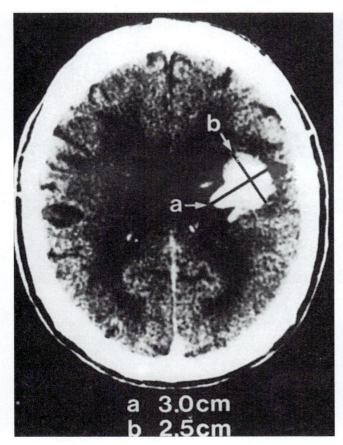

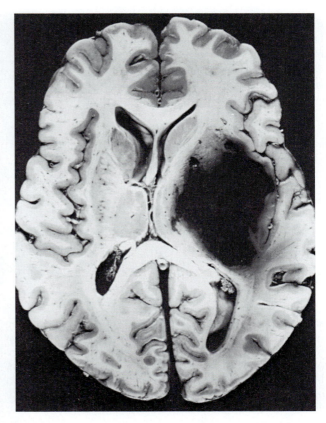

Figure 25.2 Method of calculating hematoma volume on CT, where a is the largest diameter, b is the largest diameter perpendicular to a, and c is the number of 1-cm-thick slices. The formula a × b × c/2 gives the hematoma volume in milliliters. (From Broderick et al,[28] with permission.)

Figure 25.3 Massive right putaminal hemorrhage involving the posterior half of the putamen, globus pallidus, posterior limb of the internal capsule, and claustral area. Effacement of the ipsilateral lateral ventricle, and midline shift is present.

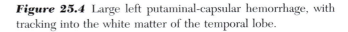

Figure 25.4 Large left putaminal-capsular hemorrhage, with tracking into the white matter of the temporal lobe.

angle of this nucleus and spreads in a concentric fashion, but generally extends more in the anteroposterior than the transverse diameter.[109] This results in an ovoid mass of maximal anteroposterior diameter collected in the putamen and the structures located laterally to it, the external capsule and claustrum. As a result, the insular cortex is pushed laterally, whereas the internal capsule is either displaced medially or directly involved by the hematoma (Fig. 25.3). The origin of this form of ICH in the lateral-posterior aspect of the putamen results from bleeding from a lateral branch of the striate arteries.[109] These laterally placed middle cerebral artery perforating branches have lumens between 200 and 400 μm wide on their entry to the brain,[294] and they supply the putamen, internal capsule, and head of the caudate nucleus. From its initial putaminal-claustral location, a sufficiently large hematoma may extend to other structures in the vicinities: medially into the internal capsule and lateral ventricle, superiorly into the corona radiata, and inferiorly-laterally into the white matter of the temporal lobe (Fig. 25.4). These variations in the pattern of extension result in clinical variants of putaminal hemorrhage. The extension of the hemorrhage from its site of origin can follow several patterns, the most common being dissection

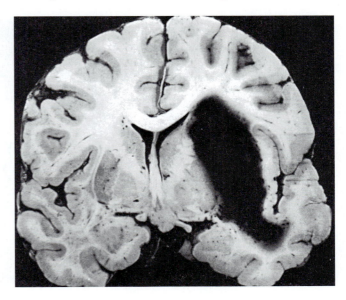

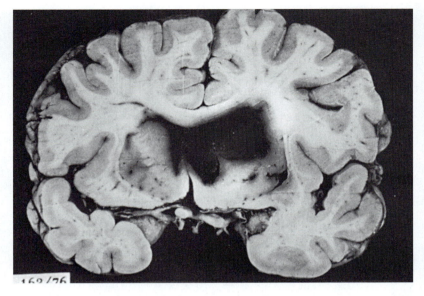

Figure 25.5 Hemorrhage originating from the head of the left caudate nucleus, with involvement of the anterior limb of the internal capsule, and direct ventricular extension with formation of a ventricular cast.

along the course of adjacent white matter fibers. The common medial extension of the hematoma results in communication with the lateral ventricle, through a process of slow leakage of blood rather than as direct communication between active bleeding site and ventricular system.[109] Direct communication of the hematoma with the ventricular system, at times with associated hydrocephalus, is more likely to result from bleeding at sites adjacent to the ventricular space, such as the thalamus[110] or the head of the caudate nucleus.[320] A putaminal hematoma that directly extends into the ventricle is usually of large size, and is then associated with high mortality.[167]

A variant of striatal hematomas is that occurring in the head of the *caudate* nucleus. Although the bleeding source is thought to be the same as in putaminal hemorrhage (the lateral group of striate arteries), this form of ICH is less common.[320] The recognized low frequency of this type of striatal hemorrhage in hypertensive patients leads the clinician to a search for a different underlying cause, such as an arteriove-

nous malformation (AVM) or aneurysm. This variation in the frequency of two types of striatal bleeding (putaminal and caudate) from the same arterial source is unexplained and may reflect a higher frequency of arterial rupture at the more proximal segments of these arteries. This, in turn, may correlate with a higher frequency of "lipohyalinosis" or "microatheroma" at the more proximal segments of these vessels, as shown by Fisher[100] in serial studies of the underlying vascular lesions in cases of capsular infarcts. As it has been implied that the same basic vascular abnormality ("lipohyalinosis," "microatheroma") may be the basis for both lacunar infarcts and ICH in hypertensive patients,[109] the predominantly proximal location of these lesions could explain the low frequency of caudate hemorrhage, as it originates from the distal ends of these lateral striate branches. Caudate hemorrhage occurs most commonly in the head of this nucleus (Fig. 25.5), and ventricular entry is an early event; this component sometimes exceeds by many times the size of the parenchymal hema-

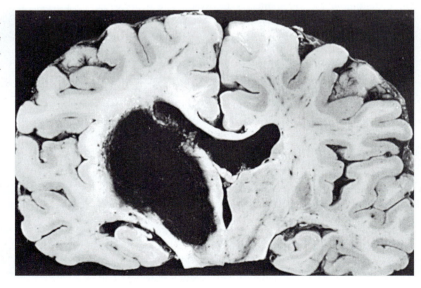

Figure 25.6 Right thalamic hemorrhage, involving most of this nucleus, with extension into the corona radiata, as well as inferiorly into the subthalamic area, with compression of the dorsal midbrain.

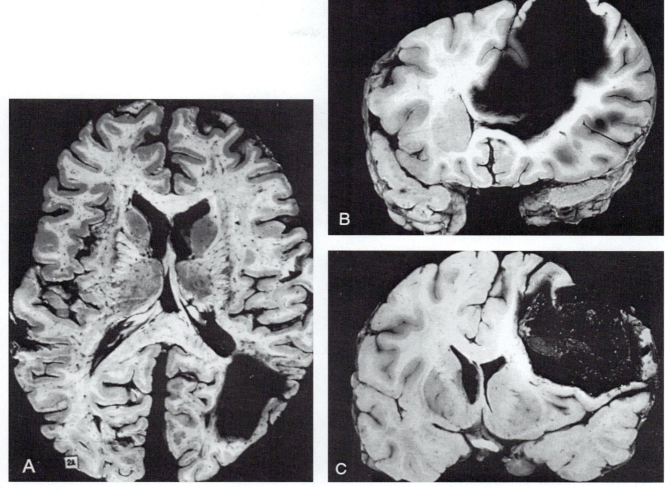

Figure 25.7 (**A**) Right subcortical (white matter) occipital lobe hemorrhage, without extension into the ventricular system or midline shift. (**B**) Large left frontal subcortical hemorrhage, with extension into the lateral ventricle and marked midline shift. (**C**) Large left frontoparietal lobar hemorrhage, with cortical involvement and communication with the subarachnoid space; marked mass effect and midline shift.

toma.[320] Involvement of the anterior limb of the internal capsule is the rule.

Thalamic hemorrhages can involve most or all of this nucleus, and their extension is mostly in the transverse direction, into the third ventricle medially and the posterior limb of the internal capsule laterally (Fig. 25.6). As commonly as the hemorrhage extends transversely, it produces pressure effect or directly extends inferiorly into the tectum and tegmentum of the midbrain. Moderate-sized and large thalamic hematomas will often extend superiorly into the corona radiata and parietal white matter, following the orientation of their fibers.

White matter (*lobar*) hematomas collect along the fiber bundles of the cerebral lobes, most commonly at the parietal and occipital levels[121,186,260,291] (Fig. 25.7). Blood usually collects between the cortex and underlying white matter, separating them and often extending along the white matter path-

ways. These hematomas are close to the cortical surface, at a distance from the ventricular system and midline structures and usually not in direct contact with deep hemispheric structures (internal capsule, basal ganglia).

Cerebellar hemorrhage usually occurs on one hemisphere, and it originates in the area of the dentate nucleus[75,115] (Fig. 25.8). From here it extends into the hemispheric white matter, as well as the cavity of the fourth ventricle. The adjacent brain stem (pontine tegmentum) is rarely involved directly by the hematoma, but is often compressed by it, at times with resultant pontine necrosis. A variant of cerebellar hemorrhage, the midline hematoma originating from the cerebellar vermis is virtually always in direct communication with the fourth ventricle through its roof, and frequently extends into the pontine tegmentum bilaterally. The bleeding artery in this variety usually corresponds to distal branches of the superior cerebellar

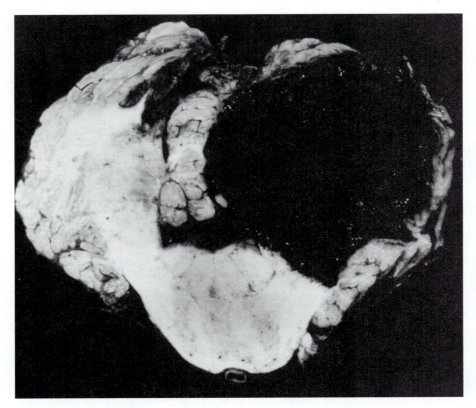

Figure 25.8 Left cerebellar hemorrhage with mass effect on the pontine tegmentum. (From Kase,[180a] with permission.)

artery. These two forms of cerebellar hemorrhage have distinct clinical and prognostic differences.

In *pontine* hemorrhage, the bleeding sites correspond to small paramedian basilar perforating branches.[106] This produces a medially placed hematoma, which extends symmetrically to involve the basis pontis bilaterally, with variable degrees of tegmental extension (Fig. 25.9). Tracking of the hematoma into the middle cerebellar peduncle is rarely seen. A partial unilateral variety of pontine hematoma, predominantly tegmental in location, is recognized clinically and documented by CT scan.[42,182] These hypertensive hemorrhages result from rupture of distal tegmental segments of long circumferential branches of the basilar artery.[42] The hematomas usually communicate with the fourth ventricle, and they extend laterally and ventrally into the tegmentum and upper part of the basis pontis on one side.

The ICH of hypertensive patients is typically a one-time event: in a group of 101 patients with ICH entered into the NINCDS Stroke Data Bank,[202] history of a prior hemorrhage was documented in only one instance. Long-term follow-up studies in patients with ICH have documented a low frequency of recurrent bleeding,[98] which clearly differentiate these cases from those due to aneurysms and AVMs, in which rebleeding is a prominent feature. Occasionally, multiple simultaneous ICHs can occur.[166,366] In a series of 600 consecutive cases of ICH diagnosed by CT scan, Weisberg[366] found 12 instances (2%) of multiple hematomas. These double lesions were probably simultaneous (because of equal CT atten-

uation values) in 11 instances, and they occurred in the same intracranial compartment (supratentorial or infratentorial) in all instances but 1, in which a thalamic and cerebellar hematoma coexisted. The incidence of hypertension was unusually low (2 of 12 patients) in his series, suggesting that cases of

Figure 25.9 Massive midline basal pontine hemorrhage, with destruction of basis and tegmentum bilaterally.

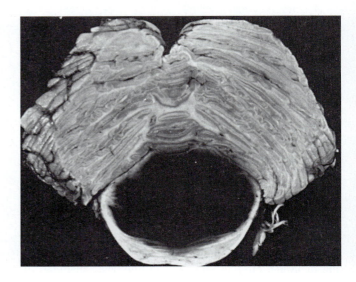

multiple spontaneous ICHs may be frequently due to other causative factors. Similarly, Hickey et al[166] reported two instances of double ICHs in nonhypertensive patients, in whom pathologic brain examination failed to provide the mechanism for the hemorrhages.

HISTOPATHOLOGIC STUDIES

The studies on the histopathology of ICH have been mostly concerned with pathogenic issues. However, the main features on the microscopic anatomy of ICH and its changes with time are well documented. The initial arterial rupture leads to local accumulation of blood, which in part destroys the parenchyma locally, displaces nervous structures in the vicinities, and dissects at some distance from the initial focus. The bleeding sites are at times difficult to locate, and serial sections are necessary to show them.[106] The bleeding sites appear as round collections of platelets admixed with and surrounded by concentric lamellae of fibrin, the so-called bleeding globes[225] or fibrin globes.[106] These fibrin or bleeding globes at the primary and secondary sites are histologically identical, except for the larger size of the former.[106] The bulk of the hematoma is formed by a compact mass of red blood cells, and the bleeding sites are characteristically found at its periphery.

The sequential histologic changes that take place in the hematoma have been recently described in detail by García and colleagues.[123] After hours or days, extracellular edema develops at the periphery of the hematoma, resulting in pallor and vacuolation of myelin sheaths. After 4 to 10 days, the red blood cells begin to lyse, eventually turning into an amorphous mass of methemoglobin. Cellular infiltrates by polymorphonuclear leukocytes appear at the periphery of the hematoma as early as 2 days after onset, and their numbers peak at 4 days.[176] This is followed by the arrival of microglial cells, which become foamy macrophages after the ingestion of cellular debris, including products of disintegration of myelin as well as blood-derived pigments, especially hemosiderin. The final stages of this process are completed by the proliferation of astrocytes at the periphery of the hematoma, where these cells become enlarged and display prominent eosinophilic cytoplasm (gemistocytes), which at times contains hemosiderin granules. Once the chronic stage of hematoma reabsorption and repair has been reached, the astrocytes become replaced by abundant glial fibrils.

This sequential histologic process is correlated with macroscopic changes in the hematoma, which initially becomes a soft, spongy mass of brick-red altered blood (Fig. 25.10). After many months of slowly progressing phagocytosis, the residual of the hematoma is confined to a flat, collapsed cavity lined by reddish-orange discoloration resulting from the accumulation of hemosiderin-laden macrophages[319] (Fig. 25.11).

NONHYPERTENSIVE CAUSES OF INTRACEREBRAL HEMORRHAGE

There are a number of instances in which ICH occurs in the absence of a history of long-standing hypertension. These mechanisms of ICH are (1) small vascular malformations, (2)

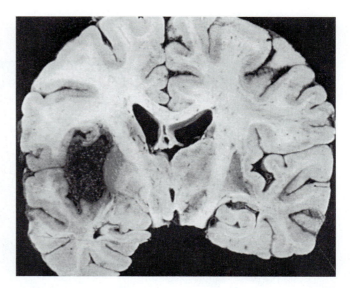

Figure 25.10 A 2-month-old right putaminal-insular hemorrhage, with partial cavitation, good demarcation from the adjacent parenchyma, and lack of signs of mass effect.

sympathomimetic drugs, (3) cerebral amyloid angiopathy, (4) brain tumors, (5) anticoagulants, (6) fibrinolytic agents, and (7) vasculitis.

Small Vascular Malformations

Small vascular malformations, also referred to as angiomas, are frequently implicated in cases of ICH, especially in those of lobar location. The study of Margolis et al[220] first called attention to these lesions when they reported four cases of fatal ICH in young patients, in whom pathologic examination disclosed small vascular malformations, one of which was arteriovenous, two venous, and one probably cavernous. Two other cases with incidentally found (not associated with ICH) malformations were added: a cavernous angioma and a telangiectasis. These authors stressed the need to consider these lesions in cases of nonhypertensive ICH, especially in the young. Since then, several authors have shared this point of view.[64,109,201,297] Fisher[109] recorded 17 such lesions in his series of ICH, and suggested that the hemorrhages they produce are less massive or slower to develop than most hypertensive ones. Russell and coworkers[64,29] reported 21 examples of ICH due to small vascular malformations, 20 of which were arteriovenous, and only 1 a cavernous angioma.[297] The 20 arteriovenous lesions were located in the cerebral convexity (10 cases), deep portions of the hemispheres (4 cases), and cerebellum (6 cases).[64] Because of their small size and the difficulties in diagnosing them in life, the term *cryptic* was proposed for these malformations.[55] However, this term has become obsolete since the introduction of CT and especially magnetic resonance imaging (MRI), as these small lesions, previously undetectable by cerebral angiography, are currently routinely shown by the latter technique. In recent years, multiple series have documented instances of ICH due to rupture of small vascular malformations that occur either sporadically[16,201,288,359] or on a familial basis.[19,57,187]

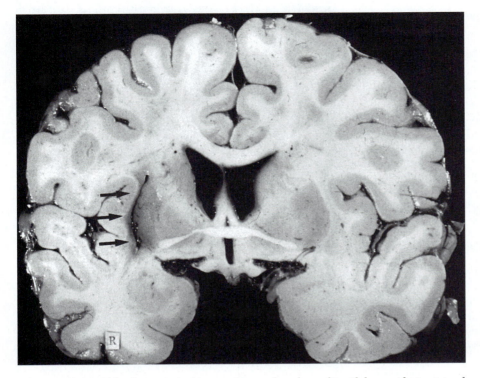

Figure 25.11 Old right putaminal hemorrhage reduced to a slit with hemosiderin-stained edges (*arrows*). (From García et al,[123] with permission.)

Figure 25.12 Incidentally found cavernous angioma in the subcortical white matter of the left frontal lobe, showing widely separated vascular channels with primitive walls, without intervening brain parenchyma. Areas of calcification are shown in the right lower corner. (Hematoxylin and eosin, × 48.)

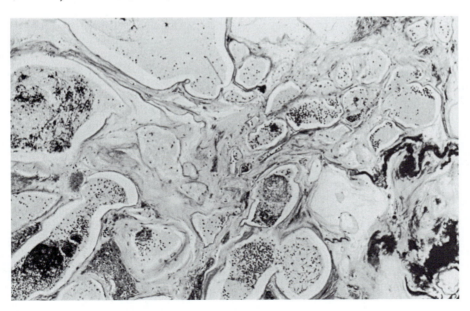

In the series of 18 cases of Becker et al,[16] the hemorrhages were predominantly lobar, reflecting the usually cortical location of the malformations. These authors found a mean age of 23 years in their series, and documented a 2.5:1 female/male ratio, similar to the sex distribution of 42 cases previously reported in the literature. Recent data have added further to the notion that small vascular malformations need to be considered in the differential diagnosis of ICH in the young: in a study of patients between 15 and 45 years of age with nontraumatic ICH, Toffol et al[344] documented ruptured AVM as the most common mechanism, amounting to 38% of the 55 patients in whom a cause for the ICH could be determined.

Cavernous angiomas (Fig. 25.12) are thought to have a generally lower bleeding potential than the arteriovenous variety. However, they occasionally lead to progressive, subacute deficits that result from protracted bleeding or recurrent small hemorrhages, mimicking either brain stem tumors[288] or even multiple sclerosis.[315] Recent data suggest that bleeding from cavernous angiomas may be more common than previously recognized: Weber et al[364] documented intracranial hemorrhage in 3 of 34 (9%) cases of cavernous angioma, 2 of them with meningocerebral hemorrhage and the other case with purely SAH. Simard et al[311] reviewed 138 cases of cavernous angiomas, 40 (29%) of which produced acute intracranial bleeding, in a recurrent pattern in 7 of them. Similarly, other clinical series have documented ICH as the form of presentation of cavernous angiomas in 10% to 33% of the cases.[286,327,351,377]

The current availability of MRI has greatly facilitated the diagnosis of cavernous angiomas (Fig. 25.13). They characteristically appear, on T_2-weighted sequences, as irregular lesions with a central core of mixed (high and low) signal, surrounded by a halo of hypodensity corresponding to hemosiderin deposits, which represent previous episodes of bleeding around the malformation.[281,286,382] Although these lesions generally occur in isolation and with a preference for the cortical and subcortical regions of the cerebral hemispheres and the pons,[281,311] occasional examples are multiple,[286] in which case a familial occurrence is likely.[287] The latter appears to be particularly common among individuals of Mexican-American descent,[187,287] in whom cavernous angiomas are inherited as an autosomal dominant pattern linked to a mutation that has recently been mapped to the short arm of chromosome 7.[128,148]

On the basis of the above reports, it now seems well established that small vascular malformations, both arteriovenous and cavernous, are likely to bleed, and may be responsible for cases of nonhypertensive ICH. The frequency of this occurrence is difficult to establish, but one figure is available from the autopsy study of Russell,[297] in which 21 cases were obtained from a total of 461 cases of ICH, a frequency of 4.5%.

Sympathomimetic Drugs

ICH related to the use of *amphetamines* has been documented in several publications.[71,82,156,215] The preparation most commonly implicated has been intravenous methamphetamine,[71] but cases related to intranasal[156] or oral[82] use of this drug and amphetamine have also been reported. Another sympathomimetic drug, *pseudoephedrine*, has been associated with one reported instance of ICH.[215] These

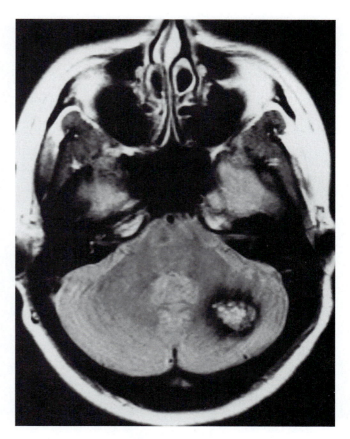

Figure 25.13 MRI (T_2-weighted) of left cerebellar cavernous angioma, with mixed-signal central core and peripheral low-signal hemosiderin ring. (Courtesy of Elias R. Melhem, MD, Division of Neuroradiology, Boston Medical Center, Boston, MA.)

patients have developed the ICHs usually within minutes (20 to 40) to a few hours (4 to 6) after the use of the drug, frequently representing an established pattern of drug abuse for months prior to the ICH, while at times ICH has followed their first-time use.[82] An association with transiently elevated blood pressure has been noticed in about 50% of the cases, and most of the hematomas have been of lobar location.[156,215] Their pathogenesis has been related to either transient drug-induced elevation in blood pressure[82] or an arteritis-like vascular change histologically similar to periarteritis nodosa.[56] The latter is considered to be either a direct "toxic" effect of the drug on cerebral blood vessels, or a hypersensitivity reaction to the drug or its vehicle. The cerebral "arteritis" related to use of these drugs is characterized angiographically by beading (multiple areas of focal arterial stenosis or constriction) of medium-sized and large intracranial arteries,[156,215,221,296,379] an effect that has been shown to be reversible, following use of steroids and discontinuation of drug abuse.[379] However, it is likely that these reversible vascular changes do not correspond to a true vasculitis but rather to a nonspecific phenomenon of multifocal spasm related to the effects of the sympathomimetic drug on the vessel wall. In isolated instances, intravenous use of methamphetamine precipitated an ICH from

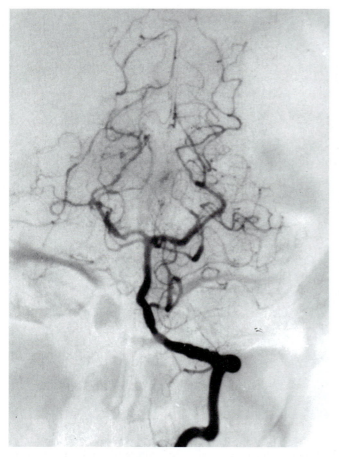

Figure 25.14 Multifocal areas of arterial constriction and dilatation ("beading") in the vertebrobasilar system following an episode of severe headache and transient hypertension (200/110), shortly after the ingestion of a PPA-containing nasal decongestant. (From Kase et al,[181] with permission.)

one instance of documentation of changes consistent with vasculitis.[130] The pathogenesis of these PPA-related hemorrhages is obscure. Although rare patients have been previously hypertensive, about 50% of the reported cases have had transient hypertension at presentation with ICH.[181] This suggests that a possible mechanism of vascular rupture is drug-induced transient hypertension associated with multifocal arterial changes due to vasospasm or, less commonly, vasculitis.

Cocaine is being increasingly reported as a cause of cerebral hemorrhage in young individuals, especially in its precipitate form known as crack. Instances of ICH and SAH have occurred within minutes to 1 hour from use of crack cocaine.[209] The ICHs are either lobar or deep ganglionic (Fig. 25.15), occasionally with multiple hemorrhages in both locations.[138] The mechanism of these ICHs is unclear, although they are in many respects similar to those related to amphetamine and PPA use; the angiographic beading that characterizes the latter two is relatively uncommon in cocaine-related ICHs, which, in turn, have shown a higher association with AVMs or aneurysms as the bleeding mechanism.[209] This suggests that the hypertensive response that frequently follows cocaine use may act in some instances as a precipitant of ICH in pre-existing vascular malformations. In one instance, ICH after cocaine use was related

Figure 25.15 Left putaminal hemorrhage secondary to use of crack cocaine. (Courtesy of Susan S. Pansing, MD, Boston VA Medical Center, Boston, MA.)

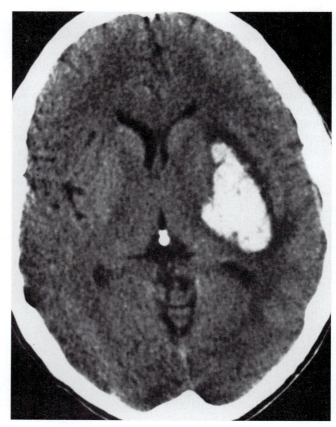

a sylvian-region AVM,[216] and oral use of dextroamphetamine was associated with SAH in the presence of a small middle cerebral artery aneurysm.[225] Most other reports of amphetamine-related ICH and SAH have failed to document preexisting vascular malformations or mycotic aneurysms.

Other sympathomimetic agents have been related to episodes of ICH. *Phenylpropanolamine* (PPA), which is contained in more than 70 over-the-counter nasal decongestants and appetite supressants,[247] has been associated with at least 20 reported instances of ICH and SAH. Most affected patients have been young (median age in the 30s), women more often than men, and generally lacking other risk factors for intracranial hemorrhage.[181] The hemorrhages have occurred within short periods from PPA ingestion, most between 1 and 8 hours.[11,18,93,181,194,323] The ICHs were most commonly of lobar location, and about two-thirds of the cases that underwent angiography showed widespread beading of intracranial arteries (Fig. 25.14), without documentation of other vascular lesions responsible for bleeding, such as AVM or aneurysm. Histologic examination of blood vessels from biopsy material has been nondiagnostic except for to pathologically documented vasculitis of a small intraparenchymal artery.[329]

Cerebral Amyloid Angiopathy

Cerebral amyloid angiopathy (CAA) or congophilic angiopathy, is a unique form of cerebral angiopathy characterized by amyloid deposits in the media and adventitia of medium-sized and small cortical and leptomeningeal arteries.[127,126,174,219,261,280,353] The condition is not associated with systemic vascular amyloidosis, and its most common form of clinical presentation is ICH. CAA virtually always occurs sporadically, but it has been described as a familial condition with autosomal dominant transmission in Iceland[146] and in the Netherlands,[363] where the instances of ICH have occurred at an early age (in the third and fourth decades in the Icelandic cases,[146] in the fifth and sixth decades in the Dutch cases[363]). This angiopathy characteristically affects elderly individuals, its incidence in autopsy series rising steeply with age: 8% in the seventh decade,[340] 23% to 42.8% in the eighth decade, 37% to 46.4% in the ninth decade, and 57% to 58% in persons older than 90.[125,354] The condition has rarely been reported before age 55.[179] CAA is associated with a progressive senile dementia in about 30% of the cases,[127] and histopathologic features of Alzheimer's disease (neuritic plaques and neurofibrillary degeneration) are documented in about 30% of the cases. Hypertension has been infrequently associated with ICH in patients with CAA: only 2 of 9 cases with large ICHs were hypertensive in the series of Okazaki et al,[261] 3 of 7 in the Wagle et al report,[357] 3 of 11 in the series of Gilbert and Vinters,[125] 2 of 11 in the series of Gilles et al,[127] and 2 of 17 in the series of Vonsattel et al.[355]

The Congo red-positive amyloid deposits occur in the media and adventitia of small and medium-sized cortical and leptomeningeal arteries, which also show characteristic birefringence under polarized light (Fig. 25.16). Under the electron microscope, these lesions contain typical nonramified amyloid fibrils, 90 to 110 Å diameter,[127,280] that are identical to those found in systemic amyloidosis and in the central cores of the neuritic plaques of Alzheimer's disease.[262] The amyloid

Figure 25.16 (**A**) Arteries in leptomeninges (*large arrows*) and upper cortical layers (*small arrows*) with amyloid deposits in the vessel wall. (Congo red, × 48.) (**B**) Same field as in Figure A under polarized light showing birefringence of amyloid deposits in the vessel wall. (Congo red, × 48.) (Histologic materials used for this figure were kindly provided by Dr. Jean-Paul Vonsattel, Neuropathology Laboratory, Massachusetts General Hospital, Boston, MA.)

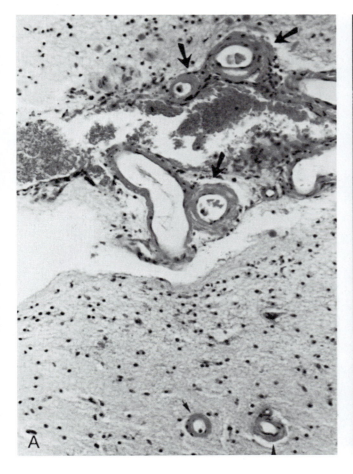
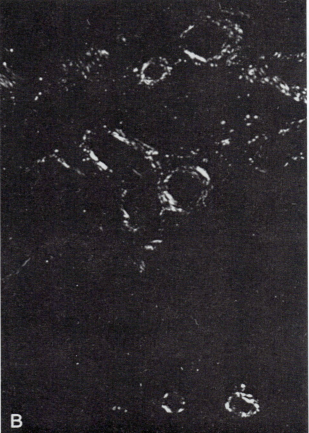

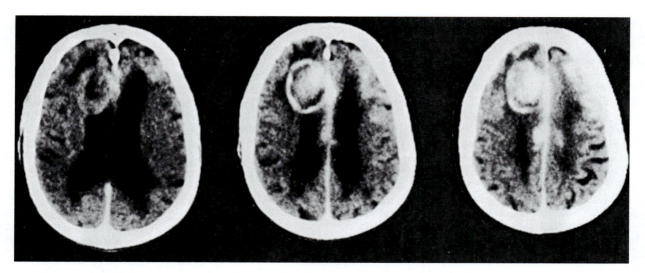

Figure 25.17 Right subcortical frontal hematoma, of 10 to 12 days' duration, with post-contrast ring enhancement. Biopsy specimen of surgically drained hematoma demonstrated widespread amyloid deposits in cortical and leptomeningeal arteries.

deposits in the arterial wall frequently lead to stenosis of the arterial lumen, as well as thickening of the basement membrane, fragmentation of the internal elastic lamina, and loss of endothelial cells.[262,280] An association with fibrinoid necrosis of affected vessels has been occasionally documented,[174,175,218,261,280] followed rarely by microaneurysm formation.[261] Vonsattel et al[355] reported the results of a comparative histologic study of brains with CAA with and without ICH. They found that the features most consistently associated with the occurrence of ICH were a severe degree of vascular amyloid deposit and the coexistence of fibrinoid necrosis, with or without microaneurysm formation. Another factor potentially associated with the pathogenesis of CAA-related ICH is the presence of the $\epsilon 4$ allele of apolipoprotein E (apoE). Greenberg et al[140] have recently reported a significant correlation between the presence of the $\epsilon 4$ allele of circulating apoE and risk of lobar ICH in patients with CAA. Furthermore, the presence of the allele was found to be associated with a significantly earlier age of onset of ICH in its carriers, compared with the age of presentation of CAA-related ICH in individuals without the circulating allele.

Cerebral infarcts and, especially, hemorrhages are the common consequences of CAA, both of which occur in superficial locations, since the angiopathy typically spares the deep white matter and basal ganglionic areas.[125,127,174,219,261,280] As a result, most instances of ICH have occurred as subcortical, lobar hemorrhages,[99,125,268,280,346,355] more often affecting the occipital and parietal lobes, where the angiopathy tends to predominate.[125,261,340] However, examples affecting the frontal subcortical white matter are not uncommon (Fig. 25.17), and Vinters and Gilbert[354] found ICH occurring more often in the frontal and frontoparietal areas than in the occipital or parietal lobes. An additional characteristic of these ICHs has been the tendency to recur over periods of months to years,[99,127,280,346] occasionally occurring simultaneously (Fig. 25.18).[127,268]

In recent years, it has become apparent that patients with CAA not infrequently present with transient episodes of uni-

Figure 25.18 Bilateral lobar hemorrhages secondary to cerebral amyloid angiopathy. (Courtesy of Elias R. Melhem, MD, Division of Neuroradiology, Boston Medical Center, Boston, MA.)

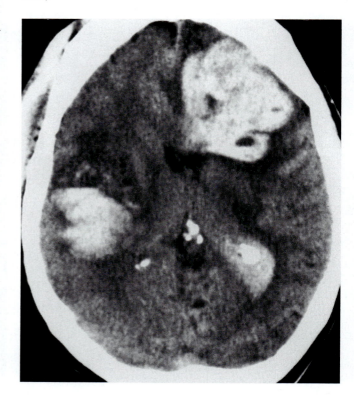

lateral neurologic symptoms, at times labeled as transient ischemic attacks (TIAs).[313] Greenberg at al[141,142] have pointed out that the unilateral symptoms are often sensory or motor, with a characteristic spreading to contiguous parts of the body over periods of minutes, at times encompassing more than one vascular territory, in a manner unlike that of TIAs. A frequent correlate to this presentation has been the detection, with gradient-echo MRI technique, of small cortical-subcortical hemorrhagic lesions in the site appropriate to the presenting symptoms. Furthermore, such transient events frequently appear to precede episodes of major lobar ICH due to CAA. These observations suggest that small cortical-subcortical hemorrhages, which are often multiple and can be easily documented with gradient-echo MRI technique, can be symptomatic with transient unilateral neurologic symptoms prior to the occurrence of major lobar ICH. This raises the disturbing issue of their diagnosis as TIAs and potential management with antiplatelet or, especially, anticoagulant agents, which can be associated with promoting or worsening an episode of bleeding in the setting of CAA, perhaps underscoring the value of MRI imaging in the workup of patients presenting with transient neurologic symptoms.

In conclusion, CAA appears to be an important causative factor for ICH in normotensive, elderly, and at times demented individuals, in particular in the event of subcortical (lobar) hemorrhage, at times in a recurrent pattern. The actual contribution of this factor in ICH in general will need to be determined by systematic search for this form of angiopathy in autopsy studies of ICH, as well as biopsy material obtained from the walls of surgically drained hematomas.

Intracranial Tumors

Intracranial tumors are a well-recognized but uncommon cause of ICH. Underlying tumors have accounted for 1% to 2% of ICH cases in autopsy series,[250] while figures of 6% to 10% have been found in clinical-radiologic series.[213,302] The great majority of the underlying neoplasms have been malignant, either primary or metastatic, but rarely meningiomas[240] or oligodendrogliomas[213] have presented with ICH. An example of a generally benign tumor with relatively high tendency to bleed is pituitary adenoma, which was associated with bleeding in 15% of the cases in one large series of brain tumors.[358] Among the primary malignant brain tumors causing ICH, glioblastoma multiforme predominates,[213] while the metastatic ones have corresponded to melanoma, choriocarcinoma, renal cell, and bronchogenic carcinoma.[126,149,217,302,352] The frequency of hemorrhagic metastases was estimated at 60% for germ-cell tumors, 40% for melanoma, and 9% for bronchogenic carcinoma.[136] The bleeding tendency in neoplasms is thought to be directly related to the richness of their vascular components and their pathologic, neoplastic character.[384] In the case of metastatic choriocarcinoma these features are enhanced by the normal biologic tendency of trophoblastic tissue to invade the walls of blood vessels.[149,307] The location of the hemorrhage relates to some extent to the type of neoplasm involved: those occurring in glioblastoma multiforme are frequently deep into the hemispheres, basal ganglia, or corpus callosum,[213] whereas metastatic ones occur more often in the subcortical white matter[126] (Fig. 25.19) since metastatic nodules frequently deposit at the gray-white matter junction. In approximately one-half of the reported instances of ICH within intracerebral tumors, this event corresponded to the first clinical manifestation of the neoplasm. The radiologic diagnosis by CT can be established easily in instances of multiple metastatic lesions,[126] but cases of ICH into single tumors can be more difficult to diagnose. They should be suspected with the finding of large areas of low-density edema surrounding the hematoma, or in the presence of an area of postcontrast enhancement at the periphery of the hematoma,

Figure 25.19 Large hemorrhage into a metastatic lesion (from bronchogenic carcinoma) in the right frontal subcortical white matter. A second, nonhemorrhagic, metastasis is present in the white matter of the left frontal lobe.

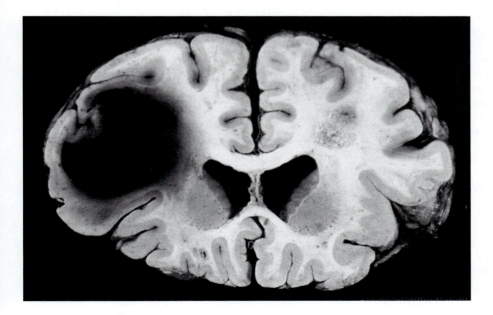

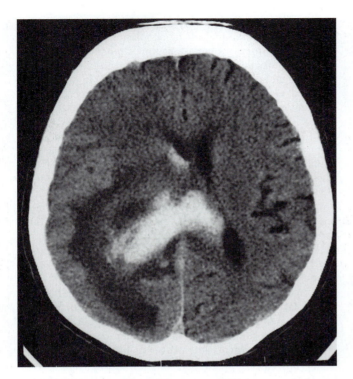

Figure 25.20 CT of hemorrhage into glioblastoma multiforme, with bleeding into the corpus callosum and adjacent thalamus and deep parietal lobe, with extensive surrounding low-density edema.

frequently forming a ring pattern on initial presentation with ICH.[126,213] Since ring enhancement is not expected on presentation of spontaneous, hypertensive ICH,[164,368,381] its presence should strongly suggest the possibility of an underlying, previously asymptomatic primary or metastatic brain tumor. Other features suggesting ICH into a brain tumor include[179] (1) finding of papilledema at presentation with acute ICH; (2) atypical location of the ICH, in areas such as the corpus callosum, which is rarely the site of "spontaneous" ICH and is commonly involved by malignant gliomas (Fig. 25.20); (3) a ring-like high-density area corresponding to blood around a low-density center, resulting from bleeding by tumor vessels at the junction of tumor and adjacent brain parenchyma. In addition, Iwama et al[172] have suggested that a low-density indentation of the periphery of an ICH should raise the suspicion of an underlying tumor nodule on CT. These clinical and radiologic features should prompt a search for a primary or metastatic brain tumor, with MRI and cerebral angiography. If the results of these tests are inconclusive, biopsy of the hematoma cavity should be considered to establish the diagnosis of an underlying brain tumor, since the therapeutic options and prognosis are radically different in comparison with non-tumoral ICH.

Anticoagulants

Long-term oral anticoagulation with warfarin is often listed among the causes of ICH. In our consecutive series of 100 cases of ICH observed over a 3-year period, warfarin anticoag-

ulation was a factor in 9% of the cases.[185] In the autopsy series of 500 cases of intracranial hemorrhage reported by Boudouresques et al,[23] anticoagulation was implicated in 11% of the ICH cases. Rådberg et al[279] documented an anticoagulant-related mechanism in 14% of 200 consecutive patients with ICH, excluding cases due to trauma, ruptured aneurysm, or concomitant brain tumor. Furthermore, anticoagulation follows hypertension as a causative factor in series of cerebellar[266] and lobar[291] locations. Long-term oral anticoagulation has been shown to increase by 8 to 11 times the risk of ICH in comparison with patients of similar age not receiving anticoagulants.[116,157,371,375]

The incidence of ICH in patients receiving warfarin after myocardial infarction is approximately 1% a year.[157] A number of factors are known to contribute to an increased risk of ICH in these patients, including advanced age (>70 years of age)[171,206]; hypertension[13,69,171,185,375]; and concomitant use of aspirin, which has been estimated to double the rate of ICH in comparison with individuals on oral anticoagulants alone.[157,158]

Other features related to ICH on anticoagulants include

1. *Duration of anticoagulation prior to ICH onset*: in two series, most ICHs (70%,[185] 54%[279]) occurred during the first year after treatment onset, while only one-third occurred after that period of time in another report,[116] the other two-thirds being scattered between 2 and 18 years from treatment onset.

2. *Relationship between intensity of anticoagulant effect and ICH risk*: it is now well established that excessive anticoagulant effect is a powerful risk factor for ICH[13,171,185,206,314,375]; Hylek and Singer,[171] reporting data from an anticoagulant therapy unit, showed that the risk of ICH doubled with each 0.5 increase in the prothrombin time ratio above the recommended limit of 2.0; recent data from the Stroke Prevention in Reversible Ischemia Trial,[4,336a] a secondary stroke prevention trial in which patients with TIA or minor ischemic stroke were randomized to either aspirin (30 mg/day) or warfarin (to an international normalized ratio [INR] of 3.0 to 4.5), add further weight to the impact of excessive anticoagulation effect and frequency of ICH: the trial was stopped early, after the occurrence of 24 ICHs (14 fatal) in the warfarin group in comparison with 3 ICHs (1 fatal) in the aspirin group; there was a strong relationship between bleeding complications and increase of INR values.

3. *Location of ICH*: a high frequency of cerebellar location was found in some studies,[185,279,324] whereas others[116,157,375] found no differences in location between anticoagulated and non-anticoagulated patients.

Characteristics of these hemorrhages include a tendency to occur in the absence of signs of systemic bleeding, lack of relationship of ICH with preceding cerebral infarction, frequent leisurely progression of the focal neurologic deficits, at times over periods as long as 48 or 72 hours, and high mortality (46% to 68%) related to hematoma sizes that are, in general, larger than the hypertensive varieties.[116,157,279]

The actual mechanism of ICH in anticoagulated patients is unknown, in part due to the lack of adequate pathologic studies with serial histologic sections aimed at identifying the type of bleeding vessel and the histopathologic abnormality at the bleeding site. Such studies should determine whether anticoagulant-related ICHs have a different microscopic pathology from spontaneous ICH, in terms of the type of affected vessel, as well as the eventual presence of local vascular pathology (microaneurysm, fibrinoid necrosis, lipohyalinosis, CAA) at the rupture site as a possible substrate for this complication of warfarin anticoagulation. It has been hypothesized[157] that ICH in anticoagulated patients could result from enlargement of small, spontaneous hemorrhages that would otherwise occur without clinical consequence in individuals with normal coagulation function. The contributing role of local vascular disease, such as CAA[232] or the vasculopathy of diffuse white matter abnormalities,[157] remains to be determined.

The occurrence of ICH during intravenous *heparin* anticoagulation represents a different situation, since this complication generally occurs in the setting of a preceding acute cerebral infarction (as ICH is extremely uncommon in patients receiving intravenous heparin for noncerebrovascular indications, such as deep vein thrombosis and myocardial infarction[80,153]). Thus, a recent cerebral infarction with local ischemic blood vessels is a likely site for the occurrence of secondary ICH, especially in embolic infarcts, that tend to become hemorrhagic as part of their natural history.[113] ICH in this setting occurs within 24 to 48 hours from onset of heparin treatment,[39] and excessive prolongation of the activated partial thromboplastin time (aPTT) is frequently present.[9,48] In addition to excessive prolongation of aPTT, other risk factors for ICH in the setting of intravenous heparin therapy for acute cerebral infarction include infarcts of large size and uncontrolled hypertension (blood pressure above 180/100).[47] This has led to recommendations to limit the immediate use of intravenous heparin anticoagulation in acute nonseptic cerebral infarction to those cases with subtotal infarcts in a given vascular territory, without uncontrolled hypertension (i.e., blood pressure < 180/100), while maintaining close adherence to a prolongation of the aPTT within the recommended therapeutic range (one and one-half times the control value).[48]

Fibrinolytic Agents

Fibrinolytic agents, including streptokinase, urokinase, and tissue-type plasminogen activator (tPA) are increasingly being used in the treatment of coronary and arterial and venous thrombosis in the limbs and pulmonary circulation. The ability of these agents to produce clot lysis and a relatively low degree of systemic hypofibrinogenemia makes them ideal choices for the treatment of acute thrombosis. However, the major complication, although relatively infrequent, continues to be hemorrhage, in particular ICH. ICH has been reported in 0.4% to 1.3% of patients with acute myocardial infarction (MI) treated with the single-chain tPA alteplase.[339] The clinical and CT features of ICHs related to coronary thrombolysis with tPA have been extensively reviewed.[133,183,184,258,312] The hemorrhages tend to occur early after onset of tPA treatment: in one study 40% of them started during the infusion, and another 25% occurred within 24 hours from onset of treatment.[133] In 70% to 90% of the cases, the hemorrhages are lobar, with virtually no examples of deep ganglionic hemorrhages (Fig. 25.21). In about 30% of the cases the hemorrhages are multiple,[183] and their mortality is high (44% to 66%).[133,183,184,258]

The mechanism of bleeding in this setting is unknown. On several occasions[183,184,258] patients have had excessively prolonged aPTTs at the time of onset of intracranial hemorrhage as a result of the use of intravenous heparin (aimed at preventing reocclusion of reperfused coronary arteries). Other factors suggested as significant in increasing the risk of ICH after the use of tPA in acute MI have included old age (> 65 years), history of hypertension, and pre-tPA use of aspirin,[258] but they were not found to be significantly different in comparison with the nonbleeders in one study.[184] A possible role for local cerebral vascular pathology has been considered, since examples of pretreatment head trauma[184] and concomitant CAA[270,312,373] have been documented in association with ICH after use of tPA. Other coagulation defects related to this treatment, such as hypofibrinogenemia and thrombocytopenia, have not been found to correlate with this complication.

In addition to their established role in the treatment of acute MI, thrombolytic agents have been extensively tested in the management of acute ischemic stroke. Initial pilot studies with the use of intra-arterial agents, mainly urokinase and tPA, yielded encouraging rates of reperfusion, in the order of 55% of patients treated, with hemorrhagic complications (hemorrhagic infarction, ICH) with neurologic deterioration in about 11% of patients.[273] In recent years, attention has been directed to the less invasive administration of intravenous tPA and streptokinase. Initial experience with intravenous tPA administered within 8 hours of stroke onset resulted in angiographically documented rates of reperfusion of a disappointingly low level, in the 26% to 38% range.[72] Despite this low level of recanalization, hemorrhagic changes with neurologic deterioration occurred in 9% of patients. In addition, this study showed that the rate of hemorrhagic complications increased significantly when tPA was administered after 6 hours of stroke onset, in comparison with patients entered into the trial within 6 hours from onset.[376] Other potential risk factors for intracranial hemorrhage after use of tPA in acute ischemic stroke are less clearly defined. In an exploratory analysis of their pilot experience with intravenous tPA given within 3 hours of stroke onset, Levy et al[210] found diastolic hypertension and a tPA dose of 0.95 mg/kg or higher associated with an increased risk of ICH.

Recent nonangiographic studies of intravenous tPA in acute stroke, the European Cooperative Acute Stroke Study[150] and the NINDS rt-PA Stroke Study,[335] used entry windows of 6 hours and 3 hours, respectively, and doses of alteplase of 1.1 mg/kg (to a maximum of 100 mg) and 0.9 mg/kg (to a maximum of 90 mg), respectively. Both studies yielded positive results, especially the NINDS study, which showed an improved functional outcome at 3 months in the group treated with tPA, without an increased mortality due to hemorrhagic complications. Despite a 10-fold increase in symptomatic ICH during the first 36 hours in patients treated with tPA (6.3% versus 0.6% for the placebo group), a net benefit accrued for the tPA-treated group as measured by three functional scales at 3 months from treatment. The intracranial hemorrhages in the tPA group occurred in both the lobar white matter and the deep gray nuclei, and they carried a high mortality (45%). The experience with intravenous streptokinase in acute is-

Figure 25.21 Location of intracranial hemorrhage in nine patients treated with tPA for acute myocardial infarction. (**A**) Left temporal lobar hematoma (left panel), and chronic and acute subdural hematoma (*arrow*) (right panel). (**B**) Right parasagittal frontoparietal lobar hemorrhage. (**C**) Bilateral multiple occipital lobar hematomas. (**D**) Left frontal and occipital hematomas (*arrows*). (**E**) Right cerebellar hemorrhage (*arrows*) (right panel), with extension to the vermis and 4th ventricle (left panel). (**F**) Left posterior temporal lobar hematoma. (**G**) Left frontoparietal lobar hematoma with ventricular extension. (**H**) Small right posterior parietal parasagittal hematoma. (**I**) Left temporoparietal lobar hemorrhage. (From Kase et al,[184] with permission.)

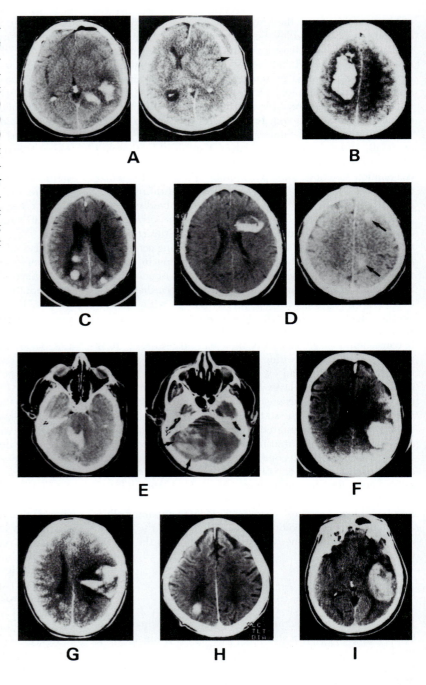

chemic stroke has revealed an alarmingly high rate of ICH and mortality in recently reported results of three clinical trials.[79,249,334] The use of 1.5 million IU of streptokinase within 4[79] or 6[249,334] hours from stroke onset resulted in rates of symptomatic ICH between 6%[249] and 21.2%,[334] with mortality rates of 19%[249] and 34%[334] (at 10 days) and 43.4%[79] (at 90 days), resulting in the termination of the trials. It is possible that the higher rates of ICH after streptokinase than after tPA in acute ischemic stroke may reflect a dose of streptokinase that is too high for this indication (as opposed to its safer profile in the treatment of patients with acute MI[145]). Additional reasons for such observation may include a more pro-

nounced and longer lasting systemic fibrinolytic effect with streptokinase than with tPA.[58]

Vasculitis

The cerebral vasculitides generally result in arterial occlusion and cerebral infarction, and are only rarely responsible for ICH. Most of these unusual examples of ICH secondary to cerebral arteritis have been secondary to *granulomatous angiitis of the nervous system* (GANS).[197] This primary cerebral vasculitis occurs in the absence of systemic involvement, and histologically it is characterized by mononuclear inflammatory exudates with giant cells in the media and adventitia of small and medium-sized arteries and veins. This is occasionally associated with the formation of microaneurysms. The cerebral disease evolves with chronic headache, progressive cognitive decline, seizures, and recurrent episodes of cerebral infarction.[245] Due to its primary cerebral location, systemic features such as malaise, fever, weight loss, arthralgias, myalgias, anemia, and elevated sedimentation rate are absent.[154,245] The diagnosis is favored by lymphocytic cerebrospinal fluid (CSF) pleocytosis with elevated protein, and angiography may show a beading pattern in multiple medium-sized and small intracranial arteries. The instances of ICH reported in patients with GANS have occurred in the setting of progressive encephalopathy or myelopathy,[59,74] although occasionally ICH has been the first manifestation of the condition.[20] The hemorrhages have had a predominantly lobar location, and in rare instances histologic examination of cerebral vessels has shown the association of GANS with CAA,[278,306] suggesting that either vascular lesion could have been responsible for the episode of ICH.

Brain Imaging

COMPUTED TOMOGRAPHY SCAN

CT has had an impact on several aspects of the diagnosis of ICH. This noninvasive test not only allows a precise localization of the hemorrhage and its effects (midline shift, surrounding edema, ventricular extension),[195,303,381] but also provides rapid diagnosis of small or clinically atypical hemorrhages that in the past either were misdiagnosed as infarcts or required extensive invasive diagnostic efforts. This impact is reflected in several modern series of ICH that show lower mortality figures than in the past,[167,295,368,372] a difference largely due to the CT diagnosis of small (usually nonfatal) hemorrhages that were not detected in pre-CT series. The widespread use of this technique has also resulted in an apparent increase in the incidence of ICH in some areas, where the rise in hospital admissions for ICH has paralleled an increase in the use of CT.[295] In addition, the use of contrast infusion in CT in ICH offers the possibility of diagnosing an underlying cause in nonhypertensive or atypically located hematomas. An AVM can be suspected when postcontrast scans show the characteristic pattern of enlarged arteries or veins, or both, seen in as many as two-thirds of the cases.[193] However, delayed scans may be necessary for the diagnosis of an underlying AVM in ICH, since the lesion can be missed in the acute phase, presumably as a result of its compression by the adjacent clot.[291] Finally, bleeding into an unsuspected tumor can be detected with CT scan by the presence of postcontrast enhancement in the area of the ICH,[126] a change not expected in the acute stages of primary ICH.[164]

The characteristic CT aspect of ICH within 4 hours from onset (hyperacute stage[83]) is an area of increased attenuation in the parenchyma, with absorption values in the range of 40 to 90 Hounsfield units.[303] This high attenuation value of

hematomas is mainly due to the hemoglobin protein (globin) contained in the extravasated blood.[255] This raises the possibility that ICH in anemic patients may not show as an area of increased CT attenuation, but rather as an isodense or hypodense area.[255] One such instance was reported by Kasdon et al,[178] in a severely anemic patient (hematocrit of 20%) with a surgically and pathologically proven cerebellar hematoma with an attenuation value of 17 Hounsfield units. In another instance, Jacome[173] reported two recurrent isodense cerebellar hematomas in a patient with a small AVM of the cerebellum. The reason for the lack of the characteristic CT hyperdensity was not found.

On occasion, a hyperacute hematoma, which contains blood that has been extravasated but is not yet clotted,[83] will appear on CT as showing a fluid-blood level (Fig. 25.22). This finding may reflect a CT that is done very early after ICH onset, showing a sedimentation effect in a still unclotted hematoma,[380] whereas at other times it is observed in patients with anticoagulant-related ICH[370] or as a result of bleeding into a pre-existing cavity or cyst.[121]

The acute hematoma is commonly surrounded by a thin halo of low absorption in the adjacent parenchyma, representing edema[254] or extruded serum.[83] After 7 to 10 days, the high attenuation values of the hematoma start to decrease, always from the periphery into the center.[164,254] Depending on its size, the whole hematoma will become isodense in 2 to 3

Figure 25.22 CT of acute ICH in left frontal white matter, with blood-fluid level. (Courtesy of Richard E. Whitehead, M.D., Division of Neuroradiology, Boston Medical Center, Boston, MA.)

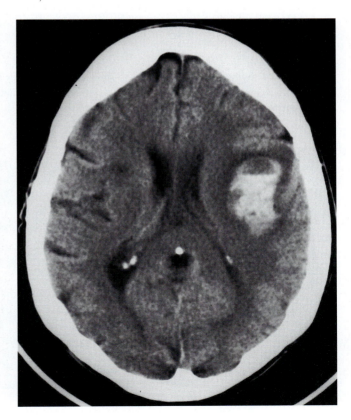

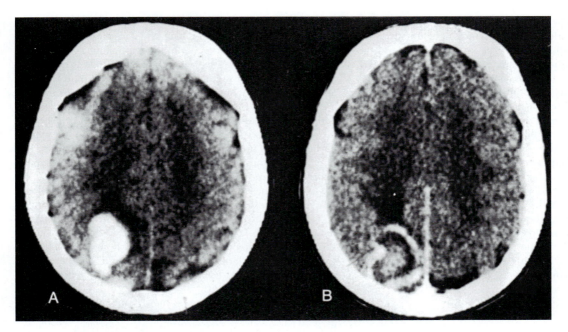

Figure 25.23 (**A**) Right occipital hematoma shown on day 1 as a well-circumscribed homogeneous high-density lesion. (**B**) Repeat CT scan 3 weeks later shows marked reduction in the size and density of the central high-density component, with a well-developed ring following intravenous contrast infusion.

weeks if small or in 2 months if large,[254] and 2 to 4 months later the result will be an area of decreased density indicative of cavity formation.[36] The reduction in size and attenuation values in ICH has been shown to occur at a rate of 0.65 mm and 1.4 Hounsfield units a day, respectively.[77] The mass effect lags behind these two variables in its rate of resolution,[164]

starting to decline after an average of 16.7 days after ictus.[77] This finding reflects the fact that the early signs of CT resolution (judged by reduction in size and attenuation values) merely represent changes in the physical properties of the extravasated blood, rather than actual reduction in hematoma size.

Figure 25.24 Right thalamic hemorrhage shown in three stages of evolution, from the initial homogeneous high-density lesion (*left*), through an intermediate stage of ring enhancement following contrast infusion (*center*), into the chronic stage of cavity formation (*right*).

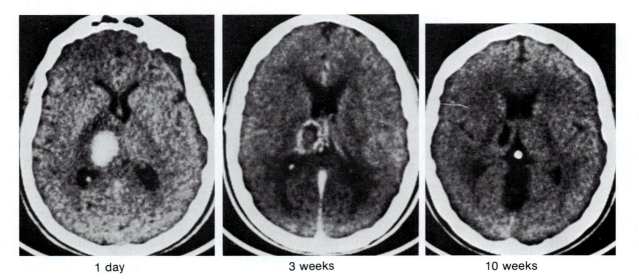

| 1 day | 3 weeks | 10 weeks |

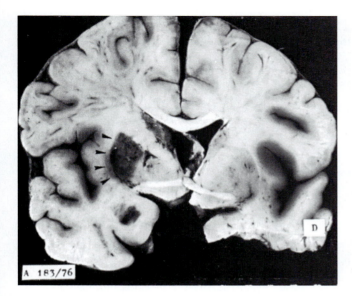

Figure 25.25 Hemorrhagic infarction at the level of the left putamen, shown as an irregularly hemorrhagic area (*arrowheads*), without mass effect.

In addition to these changes, resolving hematomas frequently show the appearance of ring enhancement after contrast infusion[164,381] (Fig. 25.23). This change can appear between 1 and 6 weeks from the onset,[368] can be abolished by administration of steroids,[372] and often disappears after 2 to 6 months.[381] This pattern is recognized as part of the natural CT course of ICH and needs to be differentiated from the similar change observed in cerebral abscess.[381] The mechanism of production of ring enhancement in ICH is unclear. It has been suggested that it is due to hypervascularity at the periphery of the resolving hematoma[381] and/or disruption of the blood-brain barrier at this level, akin to that observed in cerebral infarction,[76] in which postcontrast enhancement occurs regularly.

The final stage in the CT evolution of an ICH represents the complete absorption of the necrotic and hemorrhagic tissue, leaving a residual cavity often ovoid or slit-like in shape (Fig. 25.24). This stage is reached after periods between 8 and 10 weeks from the initial hemorrhage. At times, the residual cavity from old ICH can be indistinguishable from that of old cerebral infarction.

A difficult differential diagnosis involves the differentiation between ICH and hemorrhagic infarction. The latter is a pathologic process of primary embolic ischemic necrosis with secondary aggregation of microspheres of red blood cells spread throughout the area of infarction[113] (Fig. 25.25). This aggregation of petechiae into the infarcted area results in a change of the gross pathologic aspect of the infarct from pale to hemorrhagic. In instances of sparse accumulation of petechiae, their number may not be sufficient to change the attenuation values in the area of infarction by CT, and the lesion will be indistinguishable from a pale, nonhemorrhagic infarction.[68] On the other hand, a densely confluent aggregation of petechiae can result in a homogeneously high-density CT lesion that may not be possible to differen-

tiate from a primary ICH.[68,168] These high-density CT lesions corresponding to densely hemorrhagic infarctions usually show some degree of postcontrast enhancement. In instances when it is difficult to separate densely hemorrhagic infarctions from ICHs, a combination of clinical, CT, MRI, and angiographic features usually allows for their differentiation (Table 25.3). The clinical differences stem from the fact that hemorrhagic infarction almost always (except in instances of venous infarction) results from arterial occlusion by an embolic mechanism, whereas ICH is a classic mass lesion associated with increased intracranial pressure. The differential criteria on CT include the morphology of the high-attenuation lesion (mottled or spotted in hemorrhagic infarction [Fig. 25.26] and dense in ICH), presence or absence of mass effect, topography (subcortical versus corticosubcortical), distribution within or beyond arterial territories, pattern of postcontrast enhancement ("gyral" versus "ring") and presence or absence of blood in the ventricular system. These CT criteria can be further enhanced by MRI and angiographic data. Among these criteria, those that strongly point to ICH are mass effect and presence of intraventricular blood. Features suggestive of hemorrhagic infarction are areas of high density in the brain parenchyma that follow anatomic patterns of arterial distribution, in addition to lack of mass effect.

Figure 25.26 CT aspect of hemorrhagic infarction, shown as irregular mottled areas of high density superimposed on a background of low density corresponding to ischemic infarction.

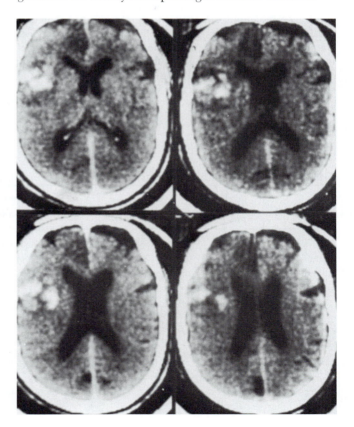

Table 25.3 Hematoma and Hemorrhagic Infarction: Distinguishing Features

	Intracerebral Hematoma	***Hemorrhagic Infarction***
Clinical		
Deficit	Sudden → progression	Maximal from onset
ICP	Increased	Normal
CT scan		
High attenuation	Dense, homogeneous	Spotted, mottled
Mass effect	Prominent	Absent or minimal
Location	Subcortical	Cortex > subcortical white matter
Distribution	Beyond arterial territories	Along branch distribution
Late enhancement	Ring	Gyral
Intraventricular blood	Yes, frequent	Absent
MRI[a]		
Hypointense blood (T_2)	Homogeneous	Patchy, mottled
Hyperintense edema (T_2)	Thin peripheral halo	Extensive, in vascular territory
Angiogram/MRA	Avascular mass effect	Branch occlusion

Abbreviations: ICP, intracranial pressure; CT, computed tomography; MRI, magnetic resonance imaging; T_2, T_2-weighted sequence; MRA, magnetic resonance angiography.

[a] MRI depicts the same features as CT scan in regard to mass effect, location, distribution, late enhancement, and ventricular blood. The table lists only the features that MRI adds to those provided by CT scan.

MAGNETIC RESONANCE IMAGING

MRI has become invaluable in the diagnosis of ICH. This technique not only separates hemorrhage from cerebral infarct, but also provides accurate information on the evolution of intracerebral hematoma, to a more precise degree than that obtained with CT scanning. The ability of MRI to distinguish among acute, subacute, and chronic hematomas is based primarily on its detection of the various chemical changes undergone by the hemoglobin molecule within the substance of the hemorrhage. In addition, the associated features of mass effect and perilesional edema can be further correlated with the hemoglobin changes to provide a precise picture of the evolution of ICH. Furthermore, the use of different MRI sequences, including the T_1-weighted, T_2-weighted, proton density, and gradient-echo images, provides a predictable change in signal intensity within the mass of the hemorrhage, in correlation with the specific time-dependent biochemical changes in the hemoglobin molecule, adding further precision to the estimated age of an intracerebral hematoma. These changes in the MRI characteristics of ICH are summarized in Table 25.4

The MRI characteristics of *hyperacute* ICH include mild hypointensity to isointensity in T_1-weighted images, with high signal intensity in T_2-weighted images.[385]

In the *acute* stage of ICH, which is considered to be between onset and 1 week from onset, the mass of the hemorrhage is rich in oxygen-saturated hemoglobin (oxyhemoglobin). However, within short periods (hours from onset),

Table 25.4 Hemoglobin and MRI Evolution in Hematoma

Stage	Time	Hb Form	Magnetic Property	Hematoma SI T_1	Hematoma SI T_2	Hemosiderin Rim (SI T_2)	Edema (SI T_2)
Hyperacute	Hours	Oxyhemoglobin	Diamagnetic	= or ↓	↑	—	↑↑
Acute	Days	Deoxyhemoglobin	Paramagnetic	= or ↓	↓↓	—	↑↑
Subacute							
Early	Weeks	Methemoglobin (intracellular)	Paramagnetic	↑	↓	↓↓	↑↑
Late	Weeks–months	Methemoglobin (extracellular)	Paramagnetic	↑↑	↑↑	↓↓	—
Chronic	Months–years	Hemosiderin	Paramagnetic	= or ↓	↓↓	↓↓	—

Abbreviations: Hb, hemoglobin; SI, signal intensity relative to normal gray matter; T_1, T_1-weighted sequences; T_2, T_2-weighted sequences; ↓, hypointense relative to brain; ↓↓, markedly hypointense to brain; ↑, hyperintense to brain; ↑↑, markedly hyperintense to brain.

(From Dul and Drayer,[83] with permission.)

oxygen is released from the hemoglobin molecule, and the mass of the hematoma increases its contents of deoxyhemoglobin, which is the predominant biochemical form of hemoglobin during the acute phase of ICH. Gomori et al[132] have postulated that at this early stage of the evolution of a hematoma, its central portion is made of mostly intact red blood cells that contain high concentrations of intracellular deoxyhemoglobin. The change from oxyhemoglobin to deoxyhemoglobin takes place in the central portions of the hemorrhage and then proceeds gradually toward its periphery, thus resulting in a typical aspect on T_2-weighted images of a hypointense central area, frequently surrounded by a rim of high signal change, the latter corresponding to surrounding edema[132] (Fig. 25.27). This central hypointensity on T_2-weighted images correlates well with the hyperintensity of acute hematomas on CT scan.[132] The aspect of the acute hematoma on T_1-weighted images is less characteristic, since it can be either hypointense or isointense, in comparison with the adjacent gray matter.[132]

In the *subacute* stage of ICH, which encompasses the period between 1 and 4 weeks from onset, the main biochemical change is the progressive transformation of deoxyhemoglobin into methemoglobin. This change tends to occur first at the periphery of the hematoma, and it then gradually progresses

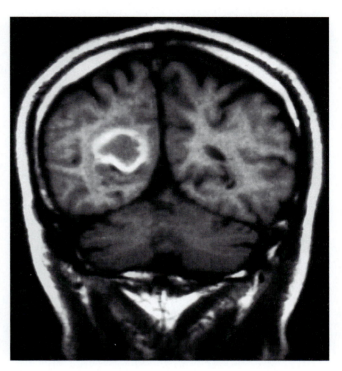

Figure 25.28 Spin-echo sequence, T_1-weighted (TR = 600 ms, TE = 15 ms), of right medial occipital hematoma with central isointense core, surrounded by hyperintense halo. (Courtesy of Dr. Jared K. Thomas, Division of Neuroradiology, Boston Medical Center, Boston, MA.)

Figure 25.27 Spin-echo sequence, T_2-weighted (TR = 3,000 ms, TE = 90 ms), of right occipital hematoma with hypointense center and hyperintense halo of surrounding edema. (Courtesy of Dr. Jared K. Thomas, Division of Neuroradiology, Boston Medical Center, Boston, MA.)

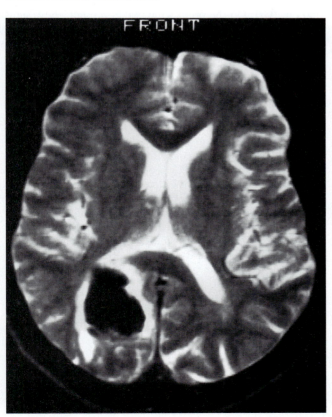

centrally. As a result, the presence of methemoglobin produces a characteristic high signal change in T_1-weighted images at the periphery of the hematoma, a change that subsequently involves the body of the hematoma further as the biochemical change progresses centrally[132] (Fig. 25.28). At this stage, T_2-weighted images are typically hypointense, whereas in the later stages of the subacute phase of the hematoma the T_2-weighted images become progressively more hyperintense; thus both T_1 and T_2 sequences have the same signal characteristic at the late subacute stages.

The *chronic* stage of intracerebral hematoma includes the period beyond 1 month from onset, at which time the hemoglobin molecule is progressively changing into hemosiderin, located primarily inside macrophages. This biochemical change correlates with marked hypointensity on T_2-weighted images[132] (Fig. 25.29). The hypointensity will be more diffuse the more chronic the hematoma, whereas in the early phases of the chronic stage there may be a residual hyperintense center due to the presence of methemoglobin that has not yet changed into hemosiderin. The changes on T_1-weighted images are basically the same as those described for the T_2-weighted sequences. In a study of experimental ICH in rats, Thulborn et al[337] reported the finding of ferritin, as well as hemosiderin, as the predominant iron-storage substances in chronic hematomas. These authors suggested that both compounds are responsible for the MRI changes observed at the late stage of evolution of intracerebral hematomas.

Although these MRI features of ICH are generally accurate, one has to be aware of a certain variability in the characteristics

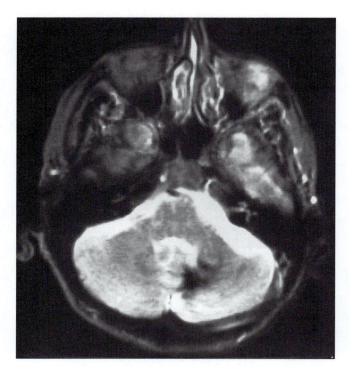

Figure 25.29 Spin-echo sequence, T$_2$-weighted (TR = 2,500 ms, TE = 90 ms), of old left cerebellar hemorrhage showing diffuse hypointensity, with no surrounding edema. (Courtesy of Dr. Jared K. Thomas, Division of Neuroradiology, Boston Medical Center, Boston, MA.)

of the hematomas, in particular in their subacute and chronic stages. This relates primarily to the fact that the changes in the hemoglobin molecule take place gradually, and at times there may be mixture of the various components; for instance, residual methemoglobin may persist in the chronic stage, making the signal characteristics deviate partially from the schematic sequence depicted in Table 25.4.

In addition to its ability to determine the approximate age of the hematoma, MRI has the additional advantage of suggesting at times the mechanism of a nonhypertensive form of ICH. Among these are included (1) the demonstration of an adjacent vascular malformation (AVM or cavernous angioma) in the vicinities of an intracerebral hematoma, the vascular malformation being suggested by the presence of either a serpentine flow void or a round, at times calcified, vascular structure; and (2) the documentation of an underlying brain tumor, either primary or metastatic, adjacent to an acute ICH.

General Clinical and Laboratory Features

The different forms of ICH share a number of clinical features that result from the progressive accumulation of a mass of blood in the parenchyma. These features include mode of

onset, as well as clinical manifestations reflecting increased ICP. ICH occurs characteristically during activity,[106,115] and onset during sleep is extremely rare.[103] It occurred in only one instance in Fisher's series,[103] and in only 3% of ICH cases included in the NINCDS Stroke Data Bank.[202] The type of onset was studied in 70 cases of ICH prospectively included in the Harvard Cooperative Stroke Registry,[241] and was found to be one of gradual and smooth progression in two-thirds of the cases, the deficit being maximal from the onset in the remainder. No cases showed a regressive course in the acute phase, which supports the clinical dictum that a definite improvement in the early hours of a stroke syndrome rules out ICH.[260] Along with a gradual onset over periods of 5 to 30 minutes, patients with ICH frequently show some degree of decreased alertness at the time of admission, as a consequence of increased ICP. The frequency and severity of this sign vary to some extent according to the location of the hemorrhage, but when all forms are considered, it is present in at least 60% of the cases,[167,241] in two-thirds of them to a level of coma.[241,372] Coma has been correlated with ventricular extension of the hemorrhage,[103,372] large size of the hematoma,[167] and poor vital prognosis.[167,277,342,372]

Clinical features of ICH associated with increased ICP are headache and vomiting. Although they also vary widely in their frequency, depending on the location of the hemorrhage, their overall importance at the onset of ICH is limited.[241] Of 54 patients alert enough to report the symptom, only 36% reported headache in the series of Mohr et al.[241] Aring's[5] series disclosed a frequency of headache of 23%. The reporting of vomiting at onset follows similar frequencies, of 44%[241] and 22%[5] in these two series. These findings stress the important clinical point that absence of headache or vomiting does not rule out ICH. On the other hand, when present, these signs suggest ICH (or SAH) as the most likely diagnosis, since occlusive strokes show them in < 10% of cases.[241]

Seizures at the onset of ICH are uncommon. They have been reported at rates as low as 7%,[241] 11%,[122] and 14%[5] when all forms of ICH are considered together. In some groups such as in those with lobar hemorrhages, seizures have been reported in as many as 32% of patients.[186]

In the general physical examination, a frequent abnormality is hypertension, found in as many as 91% of the cases in some series.[241] The high frequency of elevated blood pressure on admission in all forms of ICH correlates with other physical signs indicative of hypertension, such as left ventricular hypertrophy[2] and hypertensive retinopathy.[103] The examination of the ocular fundi in a case of suspected ICH serves the dual purpose of detecting signs of hypertensive retinopathy and allowing careful search for subhyaloid hemorrhages. These represent blood collections in the preretinal space, and their presence is virtually diagnostic of SAH,[260] since they rarely occur in primary ICH.[260,266,291] Although an occasional case of massive primary ICH will show this sign,[360] its presence has a high correlation with ruptured aneurysm as the cause of the intracranial hemorrhage. The findings on neurologic examination permit the differentiation of the different topographic varieties of ICH (see below).

The most reliable general laboratory examination for the diagnosis of ICH is examination of the CSF. Communication of the hematoma with the ventricular space accounts for the presence of bloody or xanthochromic CSF in 70% to 90%

of cases.[5,103,122,241,251,266,372] A somewhat lower frequency of bloody CSF (63%) has been reported in hematomas of lobar location,[291] probably reflecting the less frequent communication with the ventricular system[186] due to the subcortical location of the hematoma. The small percentages of cases with clear CSF in all series of ICH reflect hematomas of small size that do not reach the ventricular system, despite being at times located close to it. Furthermore, on account of their smaller size, the clinical presentation may not be clearly indicative of an ICH, as signs of increased ICP may be lacking making the differential diagnosis with ischemic stroke difficult. It is in this particular group of strokes that CT scan has had its most dramatic impact.

In addition to simple inspection of the CSF for bloody or xanthochromic aspect, spectrophotometric CSF analysis can disclose blood products in virtually 100% of cases.[196] However, this technique is not currently used as the widely available anatomic means of diagnosis (CT and MRI) has made CSF examination unnecessary in establishing the presence of an ICH. Moreover, the uncommon but well-recognized precipitation of uncal or tonsillar herniation by lumbar puncture in supratentorial ICH[109,260,276] has contributed to the abandonment of this test for the diagnosis of ICH.

The value of angiography in the evaluation of ICH cases has similarly declined since the introduction of CT and MR scanning. Most commonly, it shows the nonspecific signs of mass effect at the site of the hematoma,[331] and occasionally extravasation of contrast medium has been detected.[200,237] The study of Mizukami et al[238] correlated the angiographic pattern of displacement of the lenticulostriate arteries with functional prognosis in putaminal hemorrhage. The obvious advantages of CT and MRI in disclosing most of the anatomic features of ICH has rendered angiography a procedure now used only in selected instances. Its main role at present is in the evaluation of nonhypertensive forms of ICH, multiple ICHs, or those located in atypical sites (hemispheral white matter, head of caudate nucleus), to look for possibilities of AVM, aneurysm, or tumor as the cause of the hemorrhage. Even this role is steadily diminishing with improvement in noninvasive brain imaging.

Supratentorial Intracerebral Hemorrhage

Most cases of intracerebral hemorrhage occur in the supratentorial compartment, mostly involving the deep structures of the cerebral hemispheres, the basal ganglia, and the thalamus.[110,122,186,241,259,372] In addition, a substantial number of hemispheral ICHs occur at the level of the subcortical white matter of the cerebral lobes, the so-called lobar hemorrhages.[186,291] These various forms of ICH have distinctive features in terms of clinical presentation, CT aspects, course, and therapy.

PUTAMINAL HEMORRHAGE

Putaminal hemorrhage is the most common form of ICH and has several clinical subtypes determined by the size and pattern of extension of the hematoma. Each of these variables

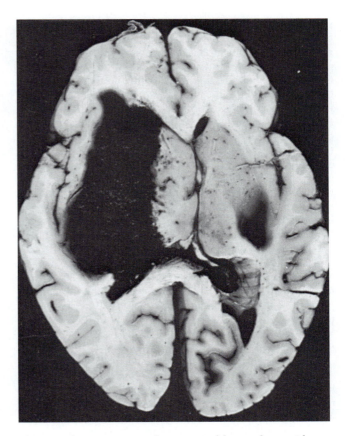

Figure 25.30 Massive right putaminal hemorrhage with ventricular extension. Incidental finding of small hemorrhage on the posterior corner of the contralateral (left) putamen.

independently determines the prognosis. Overall, a mortality of 37% is expected,[167] a figure that is far lower than those quoted in the pre-CT literature,[233] which did not include the undiagnosed smaller cases.

The classical presentation of putaminal hemorrhage described the massive hemorrhages (Fig. 25.30), with rapidly evolving unilateral weakness accompanied by sensory, visual, and behavioral abnormalities. Headache is common, as is vomiting, within a few hours from onset.[241] Although the onset is abrupt, there is often a gradual worsening of both the focal deficit and the level of consciousness in the following minutes or hours.[103,260] A "maximal from the onset" deficit is uncommon. Whether sudden or gradual in evolution, medium-sized or large hematomas are invariably accompanied by a decreased level of alertness correlated with hematoma size. Once the syndrome is well developed, neurologic examination shows a dense flaccid hemiplegia with a hemisensory syndrome and homonymous hemianopia, with global aphasia in dominant hemisphere hematomas, or hemi-inattention in nondominant lesions.[103,260] A horizontal gaze palsy, with the eyes conjugately deviated toward the side of the lesion, is usually found, which can be reversed momentarily by doll's head maneuver or ice-water caloric testing.[276] The pupillary size and reactivity are normal unless uncal herniation has occurred, in which case signs of an ipsilateral third cranial nerve palsy will be present.[103] These abnormalities in oculomotor function have a poor prognosis.[167] Total unilateral motor deficit, coma, and clinical progression following admission all correlate with large hematoma size and poor functional and vital prognosis, as does ventricular extension of the hematoma by CT scan.[167] In all probability, the increased mortality reflects the large size of the hematoma required to dissect a course from the laterally placed original site of bleeding into the paramedian ventricular wall, rather than any primary independent effects of blood entering the ventricular system.[320] Further support of this point is the occurrence of ventricular extension in other varieties of ICH, such as caudate ICH,[320] which has an excellent vital prognosis (see below).

The presence of two hypertensive putaminal hemorrhages, one recent and one old, has been described in pathologic material,[106,119,228,250,341] but the occurrence of simultaneous fresh bilateral putaminal hemorrhages (Fig. 25.30) is distinctly uncommon: it was observed in only 2 of 86 cases in Fisher's series,[110] and in none of 42 hypertensive ICH cases from McCormick and Schochet's series.[228] Multiple ICHs are rare unless due to bleeding diathesis associated with thrombocytopenia,[110,308] metastatic tumor,[126] or cerebral amyloid angiopathy.[127]

Syndromes of Smaller Hematomas

Although many variants of putaminal hemorrhage are recognized, few are well known clinically. Most of the tiny putaminal hemorrhages in pathologic material have occurred along with large hematomas that have dominated the clinical picture.[106] The smallest examples reported by Hier et al[167] (cases 1 through 6), showed motor deficits in a level of hemiparesis rather than hemiplegia, contralateral hemisensory deficits, and normal extraocular movements; five of six had full visual fields and were alert. They all survived and left the hospital with mild functional disability. Rarely, syndromes of pure hemiparesis have been described from a small putaminal hemorrhage.[257,330] Their rarity suggests that a putaminal hemorrhage large enough to compress or destroy the adjacent internal capsule is likely to involve the sensory capsular or paracapsular pathways, leading to a combined sensorimotor syndrome.

Signs of good functional and vital prognosis in putaminal hemorrhage include partial motor deficit, alert mental status, normal extraocular movements, and full visual fields.[167] Mizukami and colleagues, who analyzed the prognosis for recovery in relationship to angiographic[238] and CT[239] findings, found the angiographic pattern of displacement of the lenticulostriate arteries in the anteroposterior views correlated with prognosis; a pattern of medial displacement of the distal branches of these arteries was a poor prognostic sign, as it indicated medial extension of the hematoma into the posterior limb of the internal capsule, frequently transecting it. The preservation of the normal configuration of these arteries was associated with a better functional prognosis. From CT scan, the main prognostic feature was the upward extension of the hematoma: patients with hematomas restricted to a CT level corresponding to the posterior limb of the internal capsule had in general better functional prognosis than those in whom the hematoma was also visible on higher cuts.[239]

Partial capsular involvement by a small adjacent putaminal hematoma could result in a sensorimotor deficit, with marked

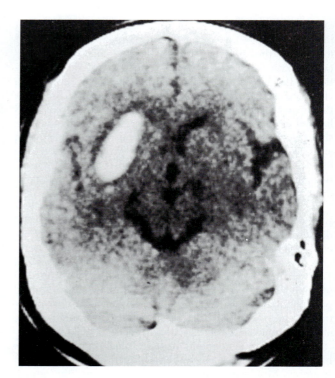

Figure 25.31 Moderate-sized right putaminal hemorrhage with mild effacement of the frontal horn of the lateral ventricle.

dissociation between upper and lower limb involvement, but instances of upper or lower limb monoparesis or monoplegia have thus far not been documented in putaminal hemorrhage,[103] probably on account of the closely packed arrangement of corticospinal fibers in the internal capsule,[91,152,208,293] which make selective fiber involvement by a lesion of expanding character difficult to achieve.

Between the extreme varieties of putaminal hemorrhage lies the common type of medium-sized hematoma (Fig. 25.31). This intermediate variety is characterized by moderate to severe sensorimotor deficit, with minimal or no involvement of oculomotor, visual, or language functions, and is at times associated with remarkably rapid and complete recovery of function. These cases with good prognosis usually compress but do not destroy the internal capsule, by remaining confined to the putaminoclaustral area, without extending medially into the ventricular system.[167]

Patterns of Extension from the Putamen

Extension laterally or superiorly from the putamen greatly increases the severity of the syndrome, even when the hematoma remains small. Lateral extension into the dominant frontotemporal white matter leads to aphasia,[5] and the nondominant parietal lobe produces hemi-inattention and neglect.[260,350] Of interest concerning the aphasia theory, lateral extension into the arcuate fasciculus is thought to be the cause of conduction aphasia,[17] yet such extension, common in putaminal hemorrhage,[3,260] has not caused this syndrome, as global aphasia,[167,243] or relatively nonspecific aphasia with fluent, poorly articulated speech, prominent paraphasias, and relatively spared repetition[3] are the rule.

When a putaminal hematoma expands vertically it collects along the white fiber tracts of the corona radiata and centrum semiovale. This extension into the nondominant frontal and parietal lobes results in prominent inattention and neglect syndromes,[167] which at times may acquire more relevance than the sensorimotor deficit.

CAUDATE HEMORRHAGE

This variety of ICH has been rarely reported in the literature, since it is usually included with putaminal hemorrhage as an example of basal ganglia hematoma.[119,297] Caudate hemorrhage represents approximately 5% to 7% of cases of ICH[320] (Table 25.2), a frequency similar to that of cerebellar hemorrhage.[115,266] Most cases in the literature have been isolated instances reported because of unusual etiologic factors such as eclampsia or vascular malformations of arteriovenous[16,46] or cavernous type.[226] However, as in all varieties of ICH, its most common etiology has been hypertension.[320] The bleeding vessels correspond to deep penetrating branches of the anterior and middle cerebral arteries, vessels of diameter similar to those that supply the putamen and thalamus.[322] Due to its paraventricular location, the caudate also receives blood supply from ependymal arteries that flow outward from the ventricular surface into the parenchyma. These arteries originate beneath the ependymal surface as terminal branches of the anterior choroidal artery, posterior choroidal artery, and striatal rami of the middle cerebral artery.[35]

A number of reported cases of spontaneous hemorrhage in the caudate nucleus has delineated a relatively consistent clinical picture.[14,37,114,320,367] The onset has generally been abrupt, with headache and vomiting commonly followed by variable degrees of decreased level of consciousness. Seizures at onset have been rarely reported,[16] and were not encountered in the series of 12 patients reported by Stein et al.[320] Consistent findings in the physical examination have included neck stiffness and various types of behavioral abnormalities, the latter most often in the form of disorientation and confusion, occasionally accompanied by a prominent short-term memory defect.[52,320] All these features tend to be temporary.[320] The clinical picture is similar to that of SAH from ruptured aneurysm.

In approximately 50% of the cases the common clinical features are accompanied by others, most often taking the form of transient gaze paresis and contralateral hemiparesis, a rare case showing elements of an ipsilateral Horner syndrome.[320] The abnormalities described in gaze mechanisms have most often been horizontal gaze palsies with conjugate deviation or preference toward the side of the hemorrhage, with full correction by oculocephalic maneuvers. Less commonly, vertical gaze palsy has been described, either combined with a horizontal gaze palsy or, more commonly, as an isolated phenomenon. Occasionally, the motor deficit is accompanied by a transient hemisensory syndrome. In those instances in which hemiparesis is a feature, the weakness tends to be slight (never to a degree of hemiplegia) and transient, resolving within days from the onset.[14,114,320]

In typical cases, CT scan shows a hematoma located in the area of the head of the caudate nucleus (Fig. 25.32). Ventricular extension into the frontal horn of the ipsilateral ventricle is an invariable feature.[320] In approximately 75% of cases, mild to moderate hydrocephalus of the body and temporal horns of the lateral ventricles has been present.

Hemorrhages of medium and large size are frequently accompanied by transient gaze palsies and hemiparesis, and those featuring an ipsilateral Horner syndrome have a more inferior and lateral extension of the hemorrhage. Occasionally, the hematomas extend from the region of the head of the caudate nucleus into the anterior portions of the thalamus (Fig. 25.33). In those instances,[52,320] the clinical syndrome has featured a prominent but transient short-term memory defect. Prior to the introduction of CT scan, these cases of caudate ICH with consistent extension into the ventricular system may have been diagnosed as cases of "subarachnoid hemorrhage with negative arteriography," or even as cases of "primary intraventricular hemorrhage."[35] The latter is probably a rare condition,[259] in most instances reflecting a lack of documentation of the parenchymal or meningeal (in cases of ruptured aneurysm) site of origin of the hemorrhage, rather than a hemorrhage truly confined to the ventricular space.

Caudate hemorrhage can be separated from putaminal and thalamic hemorrhage clinically and radiographically. Headache, nausea, vomiting, and stiff neck regularly accompany caudate hemorrhage,[320] but are less common manifestations in putaminal hemorrhage.[167] Disorders of language are regular features of putaminal and thalamic hemorrhage in the dominant hemisphere,[167,244,361] whereas hemorrhages that remain confined to the caudate nucleus have not been associated with aphasia.[320] Furthermore, caudate hemorrhages in the nondominant hemisphere do not show the behavioral abnormalities of hemi-inattention and anosognosia associated with thalamic[38,300,362] and putaminal[167] hemorrhages in that hemisphere. Caudate hemorrhage also needs to be distinguished from anterior communicating artery aneurysms that bleed into the brain parenchyma. In primary caudate hemorrhage there is no accumulation of blood in the interhemispheric fissure, and most of the blood is located in the lateral ventricle adjacent to the involved caudate nucleus. In addition, extension of the hemorrhage into the basal frontal region, a feature invariably seen when hemorrhage into the parenchyma results from ruptured anterior communicating aneurysm, is rarely present in caudate ICH.[320]

The outcome in caudate hemorrhage is usually benign, and most patients recover fully, without permanent neurologic deficits.[320] The accompanying hydrocephalus characteristically tends to disappear as the hemorrhage resolves, and ventriculoperitoneal shunting for persistent hydrocephalus is rarely required.[320] This generally benign outcome in caudate ICH occurs despite the almost constant ventricular extension of the hemorrhage, stressing the fact that the latter in itself is not necessarily a bad prognostic sign in hemorrhages originating in the vicinities of the ventricular system, such as in caudate and thalamic ICH. The documented poor prognostic value of this feature in putaminal ICH[167] reflects the required large size of a laterally originated putaminal hematoma to be able to extend enough medially to open into the ventricular system.

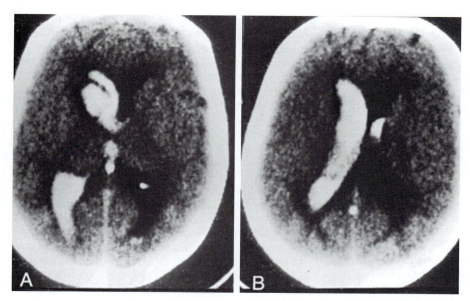

Figure 25.32 (**A**) Hemorrhage originating in the head of the right caudate nucleus with extension into the anterior limb of the internal capsule and into the lateral ventricle and third ventricle. (**B**) Extensive amount of intraventricular blood in the body of the lateral ventricles, primarily on the right side, associated with moderate hydrocephalus.

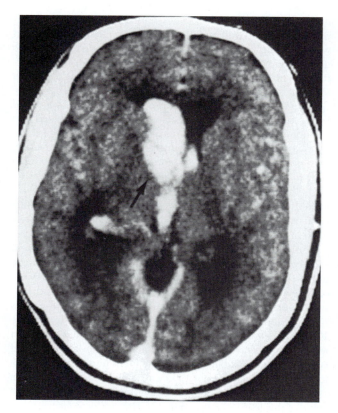

Figure 25.33 Hemorrhage originating from the head of the left caudate nucleus with extension into the anterior-dorsal aspect of the thalamus (*arrow*), lateral ventricle, and third ventricle.

THALAMIC HEMORRHAGE

The thalamic form of ICH accounts for 10% to 15% of parenchymatous hemorrhage.[110,119,121,186,202,241,361,372] Its clinical and pathologic characteristics are well recognized, and the spectrum of clinical variations reflects the size and pattern of extension of the hematoma. The mass originates in the thalamus and, if it enlarges, extends laterally (into the internal capsule), medially (into the third ventricle), or inferiorly (into the subthalamus and dorsal midbrain).[260] Even upward extension into the parietal white matter can occur in the larger examples.

The clinical picture has several distinctive features. These are shown in Table 25.5, which includes a total of 41 patients from two series.[12,361] A typical mode of presentation features a rapid onset of unilateral sensorimotor deficit, frequent occurrence of vomiting (about half of the cases), but a low frequency of headache (less than one-third of the cases). In some the onset was as coma.[96,361] A slowly progressive initial course with headache preceding the focal deficits is distinctly uncommon,[260] and only 4 of 13 patients in the series of Walshe et al[361] evolved with symptoms for 1 to 2 hours before developing hemiparesis. Few present initially with unilateral sensory symptoms (numbness) preceding the onset of hemiparesis and stupor.[96,356,361]

The physical findings (Table 25.5) include hemiparesis or hemiplegia in 100% of the cases,[12,96,361] virtually all of them with an associated severe hemisensory syndrome. The latter usually occurs as a decrease or loss of all sensory modalities over the contralateral limbs, face, and trunk,[260] but small hematomas have affected superficial sensation in a partial distribution in some cases.[320] The motor deficit is severe and equal in arm and leg, but at times the leg has been relatively less affected.[320] The severity and distribution of the motor and

Table 25.5 Clinical Features of Thalamic Hemorrhage

	Walshe et al[361] (N = 18)	Barraquer-Bordas et al[12] (N = 23)
History		
Age (mean)	64	68
Headache	22%	30%
Vomiting	77%	48%
Physical findings		
Level of consciousness		
Alert	6%	21%
Drowsy	33%	40%
Stuporous	33%	18%
Comatose	28%	21%
Hemiplegia-hemiparesis	100%	100%
Hemisensory deficit	100%	100%
Homonymous hemianopia	—	18%
Aphasia	4/7[a]	4
Mutism	1	1
Anosognosia	2/3[a]	2
Upward gaze palsy	94%	35%
Horizontal ocular deviation		
Toward side of lesion	6	3
Opposite side of lesion	3	6
Pupillary abnormalities		
Miosis	100%	70%
Absent light reflex	62%	13%
Mortality	50%	39%

[a] Number of patients with deficit/number of patients tested.

sensory symptoms are similar to those of putaminal hemorrhage, therefore not serving as useful differential points. A homonymous hemianopia is an uncommon finding, and tends to be transient,[103,109] probably reflecting the location of the lateral geniculate body below and lateral to the hematoma. This sign would be expected in large hemorrhages with extrathalamic extension, but those, in addition, affect consciousness severely, precluding the detection of the visual field defect.

The clinical presentation of thalamic hemorrhage has distinctive oculomotor findings. The most characteristic combination is one of upward gaze palsy with miotic unreactive pupils,[12,96,103,109,361] elements of Parinaud syndrome, caused by the enlarging mass exerting effects on the upper midbrain. The upward gaze palsy determines the ocular position at rest of conjugate downward deviation, sometimes associated with convergence, as if the eyes were peering at the tip of the nose.[109] In addition, nystagmus retractorius on attempted upward gaze, and skew deviation are frequently present.[103,109,260] Other less common oculomotor abnormalities reported in thalamic hemorrhage include downward gaze palsy[103,109] anisocoria with ipsilateral miosis, sometimes associated with palpebral ptosis;[103] transient opsoclonus;[190] ipsilateral[12,361] or contralateral[12,189,320] horizontal ocular deviation.

The classical combination of upward gaze palsy with miotic unreactive pupils has high diagnostic value, and it is due to compressive or destructive effects of the thalamic hematoma on the underlying midbrain tectum.[12,103,109,320] The precise anatomic structures involved in these oculomotor abnormalities have been delineated by experimental studies in monkeys[73,267] and a number of observations in humans.[54,55,253] The experimental observations of Pasik et al[267] established that involvement of the posterior commissure and the "nucleus interstitialis of the posterior commissure" was consistently associated with upward gaze palsy. Areas that were not essential for the development of the gaze palsy included the superior colliculi, nuclei of Cajal and Darkschewitsch, and the medial thalamus. The observations of Christoff et al[53,54] in human clinicopathologic material concluded that most lesions producing upward gaze palsy required bilateral or midline involvement of the midbrain tectum, particularly when loss of pupillary light reflex coexisted.[54] However, Denny-Brown and Fischer[73] performed unilateral midbrain tegmental lesions in monkeys, which resulted in upward gaze palsy, skew deviation (with the ipsilateral eye in a higher position than the contralateral eye), and head tilt. In addition, after unilateral stereotactic lesions of the dorsolateral midbrain tegmentum performed in humans for the treatment of pain syndromes, Nashold and Seaber[253] recorded symmetric upward gaze palsy in 13 of 16 subjects. In 10 subjects, downward gaze was impaired as well, but never without upward gaze palsy. Of the 16 patients, 15 had miotic nonreactive pupils, 11 had convergence paralysis, and 10 showed skew deviation, two-thirds with the ipsilateral eye in a lower position.

In summary, virtually all the oculomotor findings observed in thalamic hemorrhage have been described after unilateral tegmental midbrain lesions in humans. This supports the view that the oculomotor findings in this condition are due to compression or extension of the hemorrhage into the midbrain tegmentum. However, other observations[129,283,356] suggest that CSF hypertension and hydrocephalus associated with the hemorrhage may play an additional role in the production of the oculomotor findings, as ventricular shunting has been shown to reverse these manifestations. In conclusion, a compressive effect upon the tegmental-tectal portion of the midbrain, either directly by unilateral compression by the hematoma or indirectly through hydrocephalus, results in the classical oculomotor and pupillary abnormalities of thalamic hemorrhage.

Contralateral Conjugate Eye Deviation

In some instances, thalamic hemorrhage cases may show horizontal eye deviation, with or without the characteristic downward deviation at rest. This horizontal eye deviation is more commonly ipsilateral (toward the side of the lesion),[361] as is routinely observed in putaminal hemorrhage, but a contralateral conjugate deviation (toward the side of the hemiplegia) occasionally occurs.[12,361] This eye deviation occurs in the direction opposite that expected in a supratentorial lesion, thus being labeled the wrong-way eye deviation.[108] Although this peculiar sign has been recorded in an instance of unilateral subarachnoid-sylvian hemorrhage with frontal and insular extension,[272] most reported cases have occurred in association with thalamic hemorrhage.[108,189] The mechanism of the sign is obscure. Post-decussation involvement of horizontal oculomotor pathways by dissection of the hematoma into the ipsilateral brain stem has been suggested, but pathologic studies have failed to confirm it.[108,189,272] Furthermore, this ocular deviation usually behaves as a supratentorial gaze palsy, as oculocephalic and icewater caloric testing produces full excursion in both horizontal directions.[189,272,276]

Aphasia in Dominant Hemisphere Thalamic Hemorrhage

Occasionally, left thalamic hemorrhages have been associated with a peculiar form of language disturbance.[3,12,103,361] Its relatively low reported frequency is probably because its detection is restricted to cases of small dominant hemisphere hemorrhages, as large ones are likely to be accompanied by stupor or coma.[283] A detailed analysis of three cases by Mohr et al[244] stressed the main feature of this syndrome: fluctuating performance in language function from an almost normal one to a profusely paraphasic fluent speech akin to a delirium. The almost "uncontrollable" character of the paraphasias, in conjunction with intact repetition, led the authors to postulate the removal by the thalamic lesion of a controlling influence of that structure over the intact cerebral surface speech areas. Similar clinical observations were reported by Reynolds et al.[283] These authors commented on the frequency of aphasic abnormalities after left stereotactic thalamotomy and suggested that the language disorders following acute thalamic lesions may to some extent be mediated by disturbances in attention and recent memory. The study of Alexander and LoVerme[3] included nine cases of aphasia in left thalamic hematomas, and the speech profile was a fluent, relatively well-articulated speech with poor naming, relatively good repetition, and prominent paraphasias. These authors commented on the lack of distinctive features in aphasias from putaminal and thalamic hemorrhage. They also suggested a prominent role for memory and attention deficits in the production of the language disturbances.

Neglect in Nondominant Thalamic Hemorrhage

Syndromes of hemineglect are classically associated with destructive lesions of the nondominant parietal lobe.[65,159] Other areas, such as the frontal lobe, have rarely given rise to a similar set of symptoms. Among ICHs, the putaminal location can be associated with this syndrome.[167] This occurrence in thalamic hemorrhage is rare: Walshe et al[361] and Barraquer-Bordas et al[12] each described two patients with anosognosia from right thalamic hemorrhage. Watson and Heilman[362] described hemineglect in three cases of right thalamic hemorrhage. These patients exhibited prominent anosognosia and hemispatial agnosia, and cases 1 and 2 showed limb akinesia, manifested as lack of spontaneous movements of the left limbs despite only mild weakness. These patients, in particular cases 1 and 2, had relatively small thalamic hemorrhage that disrupted sensation only partially in case 1 and affected motor function partially, to a level of weakness only, in cases 1 and 2. Case 3 had a larger hemorrhage associated with arm paralysis,

marked leg weakness, absent sensation, bilateral Babinski signs, and drowsiness, while the other two patients were alert and cooperative. These cases illustrated a neglect syndrome similar to that observed in nondominant cortical surface disease, from documented medium-sized and small right thalamic hematomas.

Unusual Sensory Syndromes

Unusual sensory syndromes are infrequently encountered. The best recognized is the thalamic pain syndrome of Dejerine and Roussy,[70] which is usually regarded as a feature of thalamic infarction in the distribution of the perforating branches of the posterior cerebral artery.[271,374] The profoundly distressing dysesthesias and spontaneous pain characteristically arise with a latency of days to weeks from the onset.[70] Its occurrence after thalamic hemorrhage is probably rare: the 8-month follow-up information in the nine survivors from the series of Walshe et al[361] did not mention this sequela. However, Alexander and LoVerme[3] commented on the presence of a central pain syndrome in six of their nine patients with thalamic hemorrhage. The relative rarity of this syndrome in the setting of hemorrhage has suggested that partial thalamic lesions of a precise lateral-posterior location are necessary to produce it.[374] This is in agreement with the finding of this syndrome in two of four cases of CT-documented lacunar infarcts of the posterolateral thalamus reported by Robinson et al.[289] This sensory syndrome is an uncommon feature of the usually more massive thalamic destruction due to hematoma. However, the diagrams of the three original cases of Dejerine and Roussy[70] show old posterolateral thalamic lesions extending laterally well beyond the thalamic boundaries, into the posterior limb of the internal capsule and slightly into the caudal putamen. As the latter areas are outside the territory of supply of the posterior cerebral perforating branches,[213] it is conceivable that they may have represented old hemorrhages rather than infarcts, as the lesions seem to have straddled across two neighboring vascular territories.

A second unusual sensory syndrome is a form of pure sensory stroke, classically associated with small (lacunar) thalamic infarcts,[107] which thus far has not been described in hemorrhage confined to the thalamus. The only instance of a small hemorrhage in that area detected by CT scan occurred in the subthalamic region, and the clinical presentation was hemiballismus.[231] In another single report, Groothuis et al[143] documented in a patient with a pure sensory stroke a small hemorrhage in the posterior limb of the internal capsule rather than in the thalamus. It is conceivable, however, that a small thalamic hemorrhage will eventually be documented in the setting of pure sensory stroke.

The CT aspects of thalamic hemorrhage are shown in Table 25.6. Of interest are the high frequency of ventricular extension (reflecting the location of the hematoma immediately adjacent to the third ventricle), and the resulting high frequency (about 25%)[12,36] of hydrocephalus. As already mentioned, the latter may allow a successful therapeutic intervention in thalamic hemorrhage.[129,283,356] In addition, the CT information on the size of the hematoma has useful prognostic significance: hematomas > 3.3 cm were uniformly fatal in two series,[12,361] and all cases with hematomas < 2.7 cm survived in the report of Walshe et al.[361] Piepgras and Rieger[274] described two patients in their series who survived with hematomas of > 4.0 cm diameter. In addition to the diameter or volume of the hemorrhage, the level of consciousness on admission and the presence of hydrocephalus have a strong relationship to outcome, whereas the age of the patient, side of the hematoma, ventricular extension, and midline shift have shown no prognostic significance.[204,274] The mortality figures in thalamic hemorrhage (Table 25.5) have been slightly higher than in putaminal hemorrhage[361] in some series and comparable in others.[12] In summary, the CT information in thalamic hemorrhage does not only have value in diagnosis, but also gives useful prognostic information and suggests the need for some forms of early surgical intervention.

WHITE MATTER (LOBAR) HEMORRHAGE

The main clinical features of lobar hemorrhage were defined only in the last decade,[186,223,291] and reliable criteria for a choice of therapy are still not available.[222]

Anatomy

Lobar hemorrhages occur in the subcortical white matter of the cerebral lobes, usually extending longitudinally in a plane parallel to the overlying cortex. As they attain larger sizes, their shape changes into the more common oval or round one. They occur in all cerebral lobes but have a predilection for the parietal, temporal, and occipital lobes[121,186,291] (Table 25.7). This predilection for the posterior half of the brain in lobar ICH is unexplained and is probably not a reflection of differences in relative lobe size, as the ratio of 3:1 between parieto-temporo-occipital and frontal hematomas[186] is larger than the anatomic volumetric ratio of 2:1 or 3:2 between these two areas. A possible explanation for this finding is the predilection of intracerebral microaneurysms for the parieto-occipital area found by Cole and Yates.[61] These authors found that the junction of cortical gray and white matter contained about 30% of the microaneurysms, and the diagrams included in their paper show a higher concentration of these lesions on the parieto-occipital areas, and proportionately smaller num-

Table 25.6 Computed Tomography Aspects of Thalamic Hemorrhage

	Walshe et al[361] (N = 18)	Barraquer-Bordas et al[12] (N = 23)
Side of hematoma		
Right/left	8/10	17/6
Size of hematoma		
<3.3 cm	11	—
>3.3 cm	7	—
Ventricular extension	66%	50%
Hydrocephalus	27%	21%

Table 25.7 Location of Lobar Intracerebral Hematomas

Location	No.	
Frontal	4	
Parietal	3	
Temporo-parietal	8	
Parieto-occipital	2	18 (82%)
Parieto-temporo-occipital	1	
Parieto-frontal	2	
Occipital	2	
Total	22	

(From Kase et al,[186] with permission.)

bers of them in the frontal and temporal poles. Although the causal relationship between microaneurysms and ICH has not been established,[105] these anatomic correlations in lobar ICH lend some support to it.

Etiology

The etiologic factors in lobar ICH may be somewhat different than those of other forms of ICH, in particular with regard to a less significant role of hypertension.[186,227,250,291,368] Ropper and Davis[291] reported chronic hypertension in only 31% of their cases of lobar ICH, and in our series[186] only 50% of the cases had elevated blood pressure on admission, half of whom had documented high blood pressure anteceding the hemorrhage. In Weisberg's[368] series only 33% of the cases with lobar ICH were hypertensive, whereas this factor was present in 81% of the deep (ganglionic-thalamic) group of ICH. However, data reported by Broderick et al[31] suggest that hypertension contributes to lobar hemorrhage as much as it does to deep hemispheric, cerebellar, or pontine hemorrhage. These authors found hypertension to be the likely explanation of the ICH in 67% of patients with lobar ICH and in 73% with deep hemispheric, 73% with cerebellar, and 78% with pontine hemorrhage. This predominance of the hypertensive mechanism in lobar ICH remained unchanged with advancing age, arguing against the notion that nonhypertensive mechanisms such as CAA may be the predominant cause of lobar ICH in the elderly.

Etiologic factors other than hypertension that are relevant in lobar ICH include: AVMs, which occur in frequencies between 7% and 14%, tumors in 7% to 9%, and blood dyscrasias or anticoagulation in 5% to 20%[60,103,118] of the hemorrhages, leaving a large group (22% in one series[186]) in whom the mechanism for the ICH remains unknown. This raises the possibility that this variety of ICH may have some etiologic factors that are more common than in other forms of ICH. One such factor may be CAA, which is being increasingly recognized as the substrate of recurrent, sometimes multiple ICH in elderly nonhypertensive individuals.[99,125,127,268,280,346,357]

Clinical Features

The clinical manifestations of lobar ICH have been extensively analyzed,[186,223,291,369] and a number of differences from other types of ICH have been noted. The circumstances at onset

Table 25.8 Comparison of Clinical Features of Lobar ICH with All Forms of ICH

Feature	All Forms of ICH (%)		Lobar ICH (%)			
	HCSR[241]	Lausanne[21]	Kase et al[186]	Ropper and Davis[291]	Weisberg[369]	SDB[223]
Hypertension						
History	72		22	31	30	55
On admission	91	55[b]	66	46	56	?
Headache	33	40	61	46	72	60
Vomiting	51	?	33	61	32	29
Seizures	6	7	33	0	28	16
Coma	24	22	18	0.4	?	19

Abbreviations: HCSR, Harvard Cooperative Stroke Registry; SDB, Stroke Data Bank; ?, information not provided.

[a] Percentages rounded to the closest whole number (decimals from the original omitted).

[b] Not specified whether hypertension was diagnosed by history or at entry examination.

(From Kase,[180] with permission.)

---

are depicted in Table 25.8, comparing series of lobar ICH with those considering all forms of ICH together. The distinguishing features of lobar ICH are lower frequency of hypertension and coma on admission, with higher frequency of headache and seizures. The higher frequency of headache at onset may reflect the larger number of patients who are awake and can give a history in lobar ICH. Ropper and Davis[291] described the headaches in and around the ipsilateral eye in occipital hematomas, around the ear in temporal hemorrhages, bilateral anteriorly in frontal hemorrhage, and anterior temporal (temple) in location in parietal lobe hematomas. The low incidence of coma on admission in lobar ICH is probably related to the peripheral location of the hematoma, at a distance from midline structures.[291]

Seizures as a frequent event at the onset of lobar ICH have been well documented.[95,186,211,223,325,369] The mechanism of seizures in lobar hematomas may reflect the location of the hemorrhage in the gray matter–white matter interface, creating a situation similar to the surgical isolation of cortex by subcortical injury that results in sustained paroxysmal activity from the isolated cortex.[89]

The neurologic deficits on lobar ICHs depend on the location and size of the hematoma[291]: sudden hemiparesis, worse in the arm, with retained ability to walk, in frontal hematoma; combined sensory and motor deficits, the former predominating, and visual field defects in parietal hemorrhage; fluent paraphasic speech with poor comprehension and relatively spared repetition in left temporal lobe hematomas; and homonymous hemianopia, occasionally accompanied by mild sensory changes (extinction to double simultaneous stimulation), in occipital lobe hemorrhages. In our group of 24 patients,[186] hemiparesis and visual field defects were the most common abnormality, found in 60% and 30% of those patients who were not comatose on admission, respectively. Those cases in whom both signs coexisted represented larger and more anteriorly placed hematomas, whereas those with hemianopia and no hemiparesis had a posterior location. From these data, the clinical picture of the patient with a lobar parieto-occipital hematoma emerges as one of sudden onset of headache, sometimes associated with vomiting, not uncommonly associated with seizure activity, with state of consciousness in the alert or obtunded level, associated with mild contralateral hemiparesis and visual field defect. The specific deficits in speech and spatial function will be added when the hematomas are of dominant fronto-temporal or nondominant parietal location, respectively, mimicking those of infarction.[242,252]

Prognosis

The prognosis in lobar hematomas is usually less grave than in other forms of ICH. The mortality figures reported have been 11.5%,[291] 13%,[321] 14%,[284] 20%,[368] 24%,[161] and 29%,[186] all below the mortality rates of each of the other varieties of ICH. A low frequency of 6% has been reported in an autopsy series,[119] whereas in clinical series they represent between 10% and 32% of the cases.[186,291,368] In addition, the functional outcome for survivors is generally better than in the deep hemispheric ICHs, with good outcome reported in 57% to 85% of patients.[161,284,321]

Computed Tomography Aspects

Ropper and Davis[291] provided two-dimensional measurements of 26 hematomas and commented on their tendency to enlarge mostly in the transverse and anteroposterior planes of the CT section. In Weisberg's[368] series of 45 cases of lobar ICH, 10 were found to have intraventricular extension, a factor that did not affect the mortality rates in his group. The CT aspects of our 22 cases[186] are shown in Table 25.9. The volume of the hematoma fell into three main groups, which in turn correlated with the presence of mass effect. Ventricular extension was a factor that correlated with location (proximity to ventricular system) rather than size of the hematoma. The outcome was in part a function of hematoma size, as no patient with a hematoma > 60 cm^3 survived, whereas all those with small hematomas (< 20 cm^3) survived. In the group of intermediate size hematoma, 75% survived, and the functional level was in general poorer than in the group with small hematomas. These figures, in addition, provide some indication of the possible role of surgical drainage as a therapeutic option

Table 25.9 Computed Tomography Aspects and Outcome of Lobar Intracerebral Hematomas

Hematoma Size	No. Cases	Midline Shift	Ventricular Extension	Outcome/Operated
Small (<20 ml)	5	1	0	5 improved/0
Moderate (20–40 ml)	7	6	1	6 improved/3 1 died/0
Massive (>40 ml)	10	10	7	4 improved/2 6 died/1
Total	22	17	8	

(From Kase et al,[186] with permission.)

in lobar ICH. In some series of lobar ICH it has been stated that surgery offers no advantage over medical therapy,[229,291] whereas in our uncontrolled study[186] a trend toward improved outcome following surgery was suggested. This option for lobar hematomas is further encouraged by the superficial location of the hemorrhage, which makes it more easily accessible.[66] This form of therapy is particularly indicated in patients with medium-sized or large hematomas who show signs of progressive neurologic deterioration following diagnosis.[186,259]

Hemorrhage Affecting the Brain Stem and Cerebellum

CEREBELLAR HEMORRHAGE

Early morphologists were aware of apoplectic hemorrhage into the cerebellum and reported single instances in the early 19th century. In 1875 Carion[44] described seven examples of cerebellar hemorrhage in a doctoral thesis and noted some of the major clinical features. Childs[51] reported the first American patient in 1858, a 19-year-old who became ill while shaking her head to amuse a child. Starr[316] analyzed American necropsy cases up to 1906, and Guillain et al[147] reviewed the major clinical features of cerebellar hemorrhage in 1923. In 1932, Michael[235] reported 10 of his own patients and provided a literature review. He divided patients according to their clinical course, that is, fulminating, grave, or benign. Headache, vertigo, and asthenia developed quickly, and he suggested that "antemortem localization is practically impossible in these cases," an opinion shared by McKissock and colleagues[230] in 1960, who described 34 instances of cerebellar hemorrhage, among which were 6 angiomas and 2 aneurysms. The authors commented, "The neurological signs presented by these patients were in the main singularly unhelpful. Localizing signs could not be elicited in those patients who were unconscious except most of them had constricted and nonreactive pupils and periodic respirations. The signs of cerebellar dysfunction were present in less than half."[230]

In a landmark paper in 1959, Fisher and colleagues[115] responded to this challenge in their analysis of the clinical features. Especially important in diagnosis were the inability to walk, gaze palsy without hemiplegia, and the absence of unilateral limb paresis. They found that surgical decompression could be lifesaving, occasionally even in patients in deep coma prior to surgery. More important, patients who had been treated surgically were often able to return to active lives without the overwhelming disability often retained by survivors of basal ganglionic hemorrhage. Although these diagnostic formulations were initially subject to dispute, CT scanning has made the detection of smaller cerebellar hematomas possible[214,248] and has essentially confirmed them and the clinical spectrum of the disease.

Cerebellar hemorrhage appears with a frequency variously quoted as between 5% and 15%.[41,75,110,117,170,236,282,285] The average frequency is about 10%, approximating the relative percentage of weight of the cerebellum in reference to the entire brain. Although this represents a relatively low frequency, the importance of establishing this diagnosis resides in its good prognosis after prompt surgical treatment.[25,110,266] Cerebellar hemorrhage usually occurs in one of the hemispheres, generally originating in the region of the dentate nucleus, probably from distal branches of the superior cerebellar artery[115] or occasionally the posterior-inferior cerebellar artery.[117] In the series of Fisher et al,[115] the left hemisphere was affected twice as often as the right. McKissock et al[230] also commented on a left cerebellar predominance. Most other series do not report hemorrhage laterality.

The hematoma collects around the dentate and spreads into the hemispheral white matter (Fig. 25.34), frequently extending into the cavity of the fourth ventricle as well. The adjacent brain stem (pontine tegmentum) is rarely involved directly by the hematoma, but is often compressed by it, at times resulting in pontine necrosis. The midline variant of cerebellar hemorrhage originates from the vermis, and represents only about 5% of the cases.[115] It virtually always directly communicates with the fourth ventricle through its roof, and frequently extends into the pontine tegmentum bilaterally (Fig. 25.35). The bleeding vessel in this variety usually corresponds to distal branches of the superior or the posterior-inferior cerebellar artery. These two forms of cerebellar hemorrhage have distinctive clinical and prognostic features.

Etiologic factors have a similar distribution to other forms of ICH, hypertension being the leading cause.[115,266] AVMs are said to be frequent in the cerebellum;[230,282] they accounted for 5 of 15 cerebellar hematomas in the autopsy series of McCormick and Rosenfield.[227] In other series[266] a lower fre-

Figure 25.34 Large dentate area cerebellar hemorrhage.

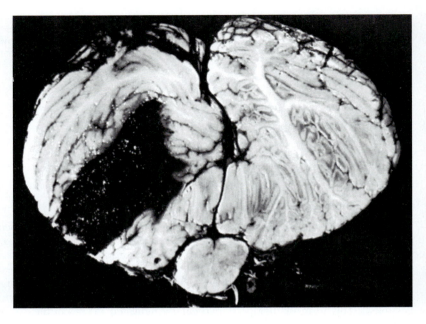

quency of AVMs has been reported (4%), a rate similar to that in other sites of ICH.[291] Anticoagulation is an important etiologic factor in cerebellar hemorrhage and was the second most frequent cause reported by Ott et al.[266] Among 24 cases of ICH in patients on oral anticoagulants,[185] 9 hematomas occurred in the cerebellum. Three of these were of the less common vermian or midline variety. Fisher et al.[115] commented on a relative female preponderance in their series: 13:8; but in other series the female/male ratios were 26:30,[266] 6:6,[75] 1:9,[235] 5:14,[256] and 17:17.[230]

Symptoms usually develop during the working day while

Figure 25.35 Vermian cerebellar hemorrhage with pressure on the pontine tegmentum.

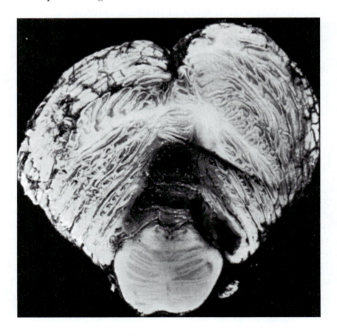

the patient is active. Occasionally a single prodromal episode of dizziness or facial numbness may precede the hemorrhage. The most constant symptom is *an inability to stand or walk*. In many patients this has been dramatic. One man leaned against a fence while painting and could not right himself; another bumped downstairs on his bottom to call for help. Crawling or propelling oneself prone on the floor to get to the bathroom to vomit have been mentioned. Rare patients maintain their ability to walk a few steps, but scarcely any patient with a sizable hemorrhage (> 2 cm) walks into the emergency ward or office. *Vomiting* is also very frequent and was present in 42 of 44 patients in the series of Ott et al,[266] and 12 of 12 patients[25] and 14 of 18 patients[115] in other series. Vomiting usually occurs soon after the onset in cerebellar and subarachnoid hemorrhage but often develops later, following other symptoms, in patients with putaminal hemorrhage. *Dizziness* is also common, occurring in 24 of 44 patients,[266] 8 of 21 patients,[115] and 4 of 12 patients.[25] More often the feeling is one of insecurity, a "drunken feeling," or wavering rather than true rotational vertigo. *Headache* is also very common and occurred in 32 of 44 patients,[266] 10 of 21 patients,[115] and 12 of 12 patients.[75] Most often the pain is occipital, but occasionally it can occur on the side of the head or frontally. At times the headache is abrupt and excruciating, closely mimicking SAH. In other patients the pain can be primarily in the neck or shoulder. An early case described by Thyne[338] developed severe neck stiffness resembling meningitis. Dysarthria, tinnitus, and hiccups occur, but are less frequent. Loss of consciousness at onset is distinctly unusual,[112,266] and by the time the patient reaches the hospital only one-third are obtunded.[266] Most patients gradually worsen over a period of 1 to 3 hours, as in other forms of ICH.[41,43,241]

The physical findings are classically those of a combination of a unilateral cerebellar deficit with variable signs of ipsilateral tegmental pontine involvement. These are detailed in Table 25.10, from an analysis of 38 noncomatose patients from the series of Ott et al.[266] Appendicular and gait ataxia occurred

Table 25.10 Neurologic Findings in Cerebellar Hemorrhage for Noncomatose Patients

Neurologic Finding	No.	%
Appendicular ataxia	17/26	65
Truncal ataxia	11/17	65
Gait ataxia	11/14	78
Dysarthria	20/32	62
Gaze palsy	20/37	54
Cranial nerve findings		
Peripheral facial palsy	22/36	61
Nystagmus	18/35	51
Miosis	11/37	30
Decreased corneal reflex	10/33	30
Abducens palsy	10/36	28
Gag reflex loss	6/30	20
Skew deviation	4/33	12
Trochlear palsy	0/36	—
Hemiparesis	4/35	11
Extensor plantar response	23/36	64
Respiratory irregularity	6/28	21
Nuchal rigidity	14/35	40
Subhyaloid hemorrhage	0/34	—

(From Ott et al,[266] with permission.)

in 65% and 78% of the cases, respectively, among the patients who were alert enough to cooperate for cerebellar function testing. Other patients lean to the side when placed upright. On the side of the hemorrhage there usually is overshoot or inability to brake the limb quickly. This sign is more common than finger-to-nose or finger-to-object ataxia. Signs of involvement of the ipsilateral pontine tegmentum include peripheral facial palsy, ipsilateral horizontal gaze palsy, sixth cranial nerve palsy, depressed corneal reflex, and miosis. In some patients the hemorrhage presses laterally in the area of the cerebellopontine angle, producing peripheral facial palsy, deafness, and diminished corneal response.

From analysis of the relative frequency of signs in noncomatose patients, a characteristic triad of appendicular ataxia, ipsilateral gaze palsy, and peripheral facial palsy was suggested,[266] since at least two of the three signs were present in 73% of those patients tested for all three signs. Skew ocular deviation is also common.[117] Additional findings useful in differential diagnosis are hemiplegia and subhyaloid hemorrhages, both being uncommon enough in cerebellar hemorrhage that their presence essentially rules out the diagnosis.[266] The frequency of unilateral limb weakness in cerebellar hemorrhage has been a matter of controversy. In the series of Fisher et al,[115] hemiplegia was observed only in the setting of a prior stroke, and similar findings were recorded by Ott et al.[266] However, in two autopsy series[25,282] hemiplegia was reported in 50% and 20% of the cases, respectively, and Richardson[285] noted contralateral hemiplegia in > 50% of the cases in his clinical series. Although in some instances reports of ipsilateral hemiplegia may have corresponded to decreased mobility of grossly ataxic limbs or decreased spontaneous movement, a contralateral hemiplegia cannot be explained on those bases, and one

has to assume involvement of the corticospinal tract in the ipsilateral basis points.

Other findings on neurologic examination add little specific diagnostic data: the pupils are commonly small and reactive to light, dysarthria is present in two-thirds of the cases, and the respiratory rhythm is usually unaffected.[266] Unilateral involuntary eye closure has been occasionally observed,[108,234] the involved eye usually being contralateral to the hematoma. This sign has been interpreted as eye closure for avoidance of diplopia, but this is probably not always the case, as it occurs in the absence of diplopia, in both infratentorial and supratentorial strokes.[108] Other less common oculomotor abnormalities, such as ocular bobbing, have occasionally been reported in cerebellar hemorrhage,[22,105,266] but with a lower frequency than in pontine hemorrhage or infarction. Some patients have a head tilt. Neck stiffness and unwillingness to move the head or neck either actively or passively probably signify increased pressure in the posterior fossa. Along with these focal manifestations on neurologic examination, patients with cerebellar hemorrhage may present with variable degrees of decreased alertness. Of the 56 cases reported by Ott et al,[266] 14 (25%) were alert, 22 (40%) drowsy, 5 (9%) stuporous, and 15 (26%) comatose. That two-thirds of the patients are responsive (alert or drowsy) on admission justifies the intensive efforts at diagnosing this condition early, as the surgical prognosis is largely dependent on the preoperative level of consciousness.

The clinical course in cerebellar hemorrhage is notoriously unpredictable: patients who are alert or drowsy on admission can deteriorate suddenly to coma and death without warning,[115,266] while others in a similar clinical status have an uneventful course with complete recovery of function. Of those patients who were not comatose on admission, only 20% had a smooth, uneventful recovery in the series of Ott et al,[266] whereas 80% deteriorated to coma, one-fourth of them within 3 hours from the onset (Fig. 25.36). A similar frequency was observed in the series of Fisher et al,[115] where only 2 of 18 patients had a benign course, the other 16 deteriorating to

Figure 25.36 Coma in patients with cerebellar hemorrhage as a function of time after onset. (From Ott et al,[266] with permission.)

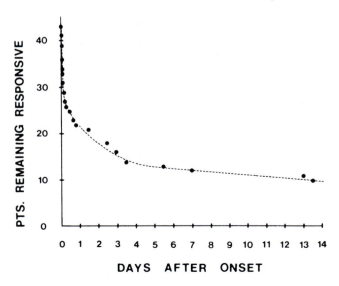

coma at variable intervals, mostly within a few hours after onset. Although most cases deteriorate early in the course, occasional patients have shown fatal decompensations at a later stage, even a month later, although they were stable in the interim.[27] Since prediction of the clinical course cannot be made based on clinical parameters on admission, the recommendation followed that surgical evacuation of the hematoma should be undertaken whenever the diagnosis is made within 48 hours from the onset.[266] The need for prompt diagnosis and emergency surgery had its justification in the documented poor surgical outcome with worsening preoperative mental status, the surgical mortality being 17% for responsive and 75% percent for unresponsive patients.[266] These figures have proved generally accurate, despite occasional reports of good surgical results in comatose patients.[378]

The use of CT scan in cerebellar hemorrhage has permitted the recognition of many different aspects of these lesions, some of which are useful early predictors of clinical course.[139,214,248] Little et al[214] reported two groups of patients with cerebellar hemorrhage: one group had abrupt onset, a more severely depressed level of consciousness, and a tendency toward progressive deterioration, while the other group had a more benign, stable course. The first group required surgical treatment, whereas the second group did well on a medical program. CT scans of the first group showed hematomas of $\geq$ 3 cm in diameter, obstructive hydrocephalus, and ventricular extension of the hemorrhage, whereas these features were absent in the second group of patients, all of whom had hematomas of < 3 cm in diameter. These observations and others[160] have identified a group of cerebellar hemorrhages with a benign course, and accurate predictions may be possible by the combined analysis of clinical and CT data at the time of onset. Especially important is careful monitoring of the status of the patient. The development of obtundation and extensor plantar responses is ominous and is virtually always followed by a fatal outcome without surgery. Heros[165] has outlined the course of the progression.

The uncommon variety of midline (vermian) cerebellar hematoma still represents a serious diagnostic challenge, and its outcome is generally poor. Its frequency in autopsy series has been 6% of all cerebellar hemorrhages.[75] Our experience has documented syndromes featuring relatively acute onset of coma, ophthalmoplegia, and respiratory abnormalities, with variable degrees of bilateral limb weakness. Early extension of the vermian hematoma into the midline pontine tegmentum is probably responsible for the abrupt onset of coma and bilateral oculomotor signs, which can mimic a picture of barbiturate intoxication. This variant of cerebellar hematoma carries a poor prognosis, similar to that of primary pontine hemorrhage. At times, a relatively small hematoma in this location results in fatal brain stem compression.

MIDBRAIN HEMORRHAGE

Spontaneous, nontraumatic mesencephalic hemorrhage is rare. In most instances the hemorrhage dissects down from the thalamus or putamen, or is part of a lesion originating in the cerebellum or pons, or arises from blood dyscrasias or AVMs. From frequency data alone, this subject could be

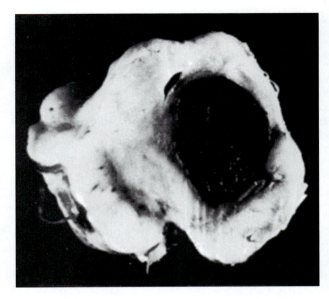

Figure 25.37 Midbrain hemorrhage in patient with bleeding diathesis.

placed at the end of the chapter but is placed here, ahead of the more common problem of pontine hemorrhage, to conform to an orderly anatomic description of brain stem hemorrhage.

Mesencephalic AVMs generally produce a stepwise progressive deterioration. Ataxia and ophthalmoplegia (especially third cranial nerve paralysis and paralysis of upward gaze) are common. Aqueductal or third ventricular blockage or distention often leads to hydrocephalus. Bleeding diathesis can lead to isolated midbrain hemorrhage, as is seen in Figure 25.37 from an elderly leukemic woman who developed a third cranial nerve palsy and contralateral intention tremor shortly before death. Hypertensive primary mesencephalic hemorrhage is very rare but does occur. One might predict that the hemorrhage would be in the tegmentum in the territory supplied by branches of the superior cerebellar arteries, as in the hypertensive patients of Roig et al,[290] Durward et al,[88] and Morel-Maroger et al.[246] The details of these cases follow.

Durward and colleagues[88] described two patients with mesencephalic hematomas. Their first patient was a 71-year-old hypertensive man (blood pressure 230/130) who suddenly could not stand or open his eyes. Signs included bilateral third cranial nerve paralysis, bulbar weakness, and extensor plantar responses. CT scan revealed a 1-cm hematoma in the ventral tegmentum of the midbrain with rupture into the third ventricle. He developed obstructive hydrocephalus, treated by a ventriculoperitoneal shunt, and survived with bilateral third cranial nerve palsies and poor balance with a tendency to fall backward. Arteriography was normal. Although there was no pathologic confirmation, this case may represent a primary hypertensive mesencephalic tegmental hematoma. The second patient was a normotensive young man who developed Weber syndrome (crossed third cranial nerve palsy and hemiparesis) after a week of prodromal headache. The CT scan showed a right midbrain hematoma. After further deterioration the hematoma was surgically decompressed, and microscopic examination of the wall of the hematoma revealed an AVM. This patient survived but was grossly ataxic.

Morel-Maroger and colleagues[246] describe a patient with midbrain hemorrhage caused by hypertension. A 71-year-old patient treated for hypertension for 5 years suddenly lost consciousness and awakened confused and dizzy. He had a diffuse headache and vomited. Findings included a right third cranial nerve palsy, left hemiparesis, and a cerebellar-type ataxia of the right limbs. Blood pressure was 290/110. CT scan documented a 12 × 16 mm hematoma in the right superior cerebellar peduncle. The patient recovered after antihypertensive therapy without surgical intervention.

Roig et al[290] described two patients with hypertensive mesencephalic hematomas detected by CT scan. In one patient there was an ipsilateral third cranial nerve paralysis, and contralateral hemihypesthesia and limb ataxia. The hyperdense lesion was high in the right mesencephalic tegmentum near the midline, probably draining into the third ventricle. Vertebral angiography was normal. A second patient had a right third cranial nerve palsy and left hemiparesis. The lesion was high in the right side of the midbrain. Both patients survived.

Humphreys[169] reported a 10-year-old boy who suddenly developed a right hemiparesis and confusion. Neuro-ophthalmologic findings were not given in detail. CT scan showed a large hematoma in the basis pedunculi extending into the interpeduncular fossa. The lesion was drained surgically and contained nuclear debris. The nature of the lesion is unknown, but it was likely a hemorrhage into an AVM or a benign tumor.

LaTorre et al[205] described a 38-year-old woman who, after complaining of headache and intermittent diplopia for 2 years, vomited and developed bilateral sixth cranial nerve palsies and paralysis of upward gaze. The spinal fluid was bloody, and ventriculography visualized a beaded aqueduct and hydrocephalus. Exploration of the midbrain revealed an AVM of the quadrigeminal plate with a blood clot embedded in the sylvian aqueduct.

Scoville and Poppen[304] also reported a single patient, a 44-year-old woman, who developed an ataxic right hemiparesis in stepwise fashion during 1½ years. Vomiting, bilateral third cranial nerve paralysis, stupor, and pinpoint pupils suddenly supervened. A blood clot was drained from the left cerebral peduncle, and she awakened. Normal blood pressure and coagulation studies and the gradual onset favored an AVM in this patient.

PONTINE HEMORRHAGE

Pontine hemorrhage was recognized as a postmortem finding by morphologists early in the 19th century. As early as 1812, Cheyn[50] cited an example of pontine hemorrhage, as did Serres and Burdach several years later. Gowers,[135] in his 1893 textbook, included a picture of a typical large pontine hemorrhage (Fig. 25.38). By the early years of the 20th century, the usual findings of pontine hemorrhage were recognized.[135]

In 1903, Dana[67] described the syndrome as follows:

1. Headache, malaise, vomiting

2. Sudden and profound coma

3. Twitching of the face and limbs or both

4. Miosis and convergent strabismus or conjugate deviation away from the side of the lesion

5. Slow irregular breathing

6. Irregular pulse

7. Dysphagia

8. Paralysis of limbs or crossed paralysis and exaggerated reflexes

9. Gradual rise of temperature, sometimes to high point

10. Death inside of 24 hours

The works of Oppenheim,[265] in 1905, who reviewed the literature, and Attwater,[7] in 1911, who analyzed 77 examples of pontine hemorrhage found at necropsy, led to the separation of primary hemorrhage from those secondary to sudden increases in intracranial pressure. Attwater[7] postulated that some pontine hemorrhages could be due to "an increase in intracranial tension produced by the rapid entry of blood into the closed cranial cavity." Duret[87] elaborated these ideas several years later in a monograph, having previously described some details of the blood supply of the brain stem.[84–86]

In the second half of the 20th century, clinicians extended the observations, invariably focusing on patients with large pontine hemorrhages found at autopsy. Steegmann[317] described 17 patients, noting that death was usually not instantaneous, no patients dying in less than 22 hours. Pinpoint pupils were very common. All patients had bulbar paralysis, and most had some irregular limb movements. He attributed the "shaking of the limbs, twisting all over and trembling" to abnormal motor phenomena and did not believe, as had earlier authors, that the movements represented true epileptiform convulsions. He also emphasized the frequency of respiratory abnormalities. Five of his 17 patients had respiratory "failure," four had slow labored breathing, and some patients had shallow gasping and increased or irregular respirations. Epstein[92] reviewed a 33-year experience and found 7 patients with pontine hemorrhage among 74 autopsied ICHs (9.1%). Most patients

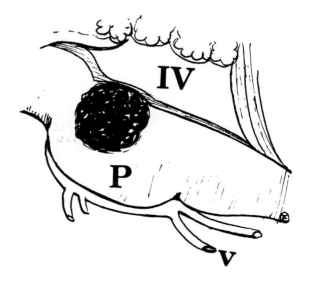

Figure 25.38 Artist's rendition of illustration of pontine hemorrhage in Gowers' textbook. (From Gowers,[135] with permission.)

had severe hypertension before the hemorrhage. Fang and Foley[94] and later Dinsdale[75] reviewed the necropsies at Boston City Hospital and found 511 ICHs among 19,093 autopsies, of which 30 were pontine (6%). Two-thirds of the patients were comatose when first seen, 13% vomited, and 78% were dead within 48 hours. One patient who survived for 23 days had a small hemorrhage in the right pontine tegmentum. All the remainder had massive hemorrhage, usually in the midpons at the junction of the basis pontis and tegmentum, that frequently spread rostrally into the midbrain; the hemorrhages almost never spread caudally to the medulla but frequently ruptured into the fourth ventricle.

In 1971 Fisher,[106] using serial sections from a patient with a massive fatal pontine hemorrhage, identified numerous small vessels with "fibrin globes," which he thought were related to the vascular rupture causing the hemorrhage: "From the gaping end of each of these torn vessels there protruded a large mass of platelets partially encircled by thin concentric layers of fibrin." He suggested that the primary hemorrhage led to pressure on surrounding vessels with subsequent rupture of them, causing a cascade or avalanche effect producing gradual enlargement of the hematoma. Ross Russell[294] had demonstrated large asymptomatic fusiform enlargements on the penetrating vessels of the pons in patients with "atherosclerosis" and hypertensive vascular disease. Cole and Yates,[60] Rosenblum,[292] Fisher,[106] and Caplan[41] all explained bleeding in hypertensive patients as leakage from tiny penetrating vessels damaged by lipohyalinosis and containing small microaneurysms. Kornyey[198] reported a patient whose pontine hemorrhage occurred under clinical observation; the slow march of signs was similar to the pattern of development seen in ganglionic and thalamic hemorrhages, and he provided evidence to support Fisher's postulation of the slowly evolving avalanche. Kornyey's patient was a 39-year-old man referred for admission because of malignant hypertension. While his admission history was being taken, he complained of numb hands, weakness, and dizziness. The blood pressure was 245/170. He became restless and apprehensive and complained

that he could not hear and had difficulty swallowing and breathing. He developed a bilateral sixth cranial nerve palsy and dilated pupils, and his corneal reflexes disappeared. Speech became "bulbar," he was deaf, and he could not move his left leg. Within 15 minutes he was comatose; the pupils were small, and the eyes were converged. There was bilateral bulbar palsy, stiff limbs with exaggerated reflexes, and extensor plantar responses. Two hours after onset he died. A large hemorrhage in the tegmentum of the pons, with some spread into the right basis pontis was found at necropsy.[198] In other patients observed during the onset of pontine hemorrhage, development of the deficit usually evolved gradually over minutes (1 to 30 minutes) and was not as instantaneous as is aneurysmal subarachnoid hemorrhage.

In the pons, the largest penetrating arteries enter medially, arise perpendicular to the basilar artery, and course from the base to the tegmentum. Other small penetrating arteries originate from the short and long circumferential vessels and enter more laterally, also coursing from base to tegmentum. Some arteries enter the tegmentum laterally and course horizontally across it.[42] Since vessels in all of these sites are potentially susceptible to hypertensive damage and lipohyalinosis, they could theoretically also be sites for pontine bleeding. Silverstein[309,310] reviewed the pathologic material from the Philadelphia General Hospital and corroborated that these sites (Fig. 25.39) were the usual regions of pontine hemorrhage. Of 50 cases, 28 were massive central hemorrhages presumably arising from large paramedian penetrators; 11 were more lateralized, usually spreading from base to tegmentum; and 11 had a tegmental location, 4 remaining unilateral and 7 involving the tegmentum bilaterally. Not until the mid-1970s when CT became available, was it possible to diagnose smaller nonfatal pontine hemorrhages accurately and to separate them positively from pontine infarction during life. The clinical correlation of the various sites of hemorrhage predicted from anatomic studies and found by Silverstein was now possible. However, the clinicopathologic correlation of these smaller lateral basal and tegmental hemorrhages is still evolving.

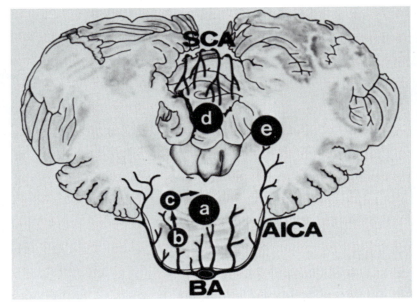

Figure 25.39 Schematic representation of common sites of hypertensive pontine and cerebellar hemorrhages. (**a**) Massive, paramedian pontine. (**b**) Basal pontine. (**c**) Lateral tegmental pontine. (**d**) Cerebellar vermian. (**e**) Cerebellar hemispheral. *Abbreviations:* SCA, superior cerebellar artery; AICA, anterior-inferior cerebellar artery; BA, basilar artery.

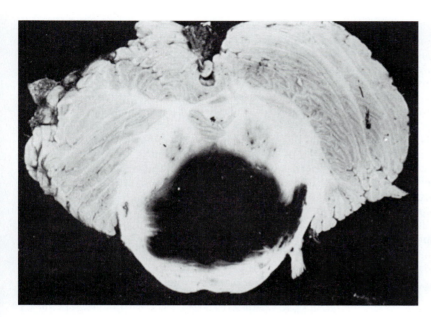

Figure 25.40 Massive pontine hemorrhage with dissection into brachium pontis and fourth ventricle.

Large Paramedian Pontine Hemorrhage

Massive pontine hemorrhage results from rupture of parenchymal midpontine branches originating from the basilar artery. The bleeding vessel is thought to be a paramedian perforator in its distal portion,[75] causing initial hematoma formation at the junction of tegmentum and basis pontis,[75,310] from which the mass grows into its final round or oval shape and replaces most of both subdivisions of the pons (Fig. 25.40). The lesion usually begins in the middle of the pons and extends along the longitudinal axis of the brain stem into the lower midbrain. The hematoma may track into the middle cerebellar peduncles but usually does not extend caudally beyond the pontomedullary junction.[75] In the process of rapid hematoma expansion, destruction of tegmental and ventral pontine structures results, with the classical combination of signs caused by involvement of cranial nerve nuclei, long tracts, autonomic centers, and structures responsible for maintenance of consciousness. Large pontine hematomas also regularly rupture into the fourth ventricle.[75,309,310]

The classical form of pontine hemorrhage, bilateral and massive, is almost exclusively of hypertensive origin. Other etiologies such as cryptic vascular malformation account for ≤10% of the cases in most series.[75,310] Russell[297] regarded pontine hemorrhage as a form of ICH most likely to occur in patients with malignant hypertension or hypertension associated with chronic nephropathy. Clinical presentation is characteristically one of rapid development of coma (80% of cases) without warning signs. Dana[67] recognized that some patients were conscious when first examined: in three different series, 4 of 19 (22%),[94] 10 of 30 (33.3%),[75] and 5 of 50 (10%)[309,310] patients were alert when initially seen. By 48 hours, approximately 80% were dead.[75,94] In some patients (30%) a complaint of severe occipital headache preceded by minutes the catastrophic onset of coma.[263,309] Vomiting was noted in 4 of 30 (13%)[75] and 4 of 19 (22%)[94] patients and occasionally was a prominent early symptom. The frequency of seizures at the onset, estimated to be as high as 22%,[309] probably represents a combination of true convulsive phenomena in rare instances, along with episodes of spasmodic decerebrate posturing, and even the sometimes violent shivering associated with autonomic dysfunction and rapidly evolving hyperthermia. Some patients will present prior to the development of coma with focal pontine signs, such as facial or limb numbness, deafness, diplopia, bilateral leg weakness, or progressive hemiparesis. Physical examination often reveals an abnormal respiratory rhythm or apnea.[75,310,317] Steegmann[317] analyzed these respiratory abnormalities in detail and reported a variety of abnormal respiratory patterns, including "inspiratory gasps of apneustic respiration," Cheyne-Stokes rhythm, slow and labored respirations, "gasping" respiration, and apnea. Two-thirds of his 17 cases exhibited either apnea or severely abnormal patterns of hypoventilation. Hyperthermia frequently coexisted, with temperatures above 39°C in more than 80% of the cases,[263] in one-fourth of whom it reached levels of 42° to 43°C,[309] usually in the preterminal stages. Neurologic examination findings characteristically result from involvement of cranial nerve nuclei and long tracts: quadriplegia with decerebrate posturing, bilateral Babinski signs, absent corneal reflexes, pinpoint miotic pupils, and various forms of ophthalmoplegia.[42,263,317]

The oculomotor findings include the following.

1. *Miotic pinpoint pupils.* These are usually about 1 mm in diameter. They react to light if a strong light source is used, with a tiny constriction detected with a magnifying lens.[108,112] Pontine hemorrhage can be confused with opiate poisoning.[317] The pupillary abnormality probably results from bilateral interruption of descending sympathetic pupillodilator fibers.[108,112] Since in Kornyey's patient pupillary dilatation preceded miosis,[198] it is possible that early stimulation of these fibers could lead to transient pupillary dilatation.

2. *Absent horizontal eye movements.* Their absence by reflex testing with the doll's head maneuver or ice-water caloric stimulation reflects bilateral injury of the paramedian pontine reticular formation. This sign occurs in partial forms or variants such as the "one-and-a-half syndrome,"[108] also referred to as "paralytic pontine exotropia,"[305] which represents a combination of unilateral horizontal gaze palsy plus ipsilateral internuclear ophthalmoplegia, resulting in one immobile eye with only abduction preserved in the contralateral one. It is more commonly seen in the smaller unilateral lesions from infarcts,[108,305] partial hematomas,[15,182,275] AVMs,[305] or tumors,[305] which result in unilateral involvement of the paramedian pontine reticular formation and the dorsally located ipsilateral medial longitudinal fasciculus. In one of our patients with a hematoma limited to the basis pontis, there was no voluntary horizontal gaze, but reflex movements were preserved. This situation has been described by Halsey et al[151] and reflects damage to supranuclear fibers traveling with corticobulbar fibers in the pontine basis before they reach the tegmental paramedian pontine reticular formation.

3. *Ocular bobbing.* Described by Fisher,[105] the term denotes brisk movements of conjugate ocular depression, followed within seconds by a slower return to midposition. It occurs most commonly from a pontine lesion, either hemorrhage or infarction, although it has also been described in cerebellar hemorrhage.[105,165,266,326] Typically, it affects both eyes simultaneously and is accompanied by bilateral paralysis of horizontal gaze.[105] Atypical varieties include unilateral or markedly asymmetric forms, and those occurring when horizontal eye movements are still present.[105,326] The latter form is less strictly localizing to pontine disease, as it can be seen in cerebellar hemorrhage, SAH, and even coma of nonvascular mechanism.[105]

Weakness of pontine and bulbar musculature is invariable in the larger median hemorrhages but is difficult to assess, since patients with bilateral tegmental damage are always comatose. Puffing of the cheeks with expiration, diminished eyelid tone, and pooling of secretions in the oropharynx are commonly observed signs. Deafness, dysarthria, dizziness, and facial numbness occasionally precede the development of coma. Facial weakness is often asymmetric and may be associated with a crossed hemiplegia at the time the patients are first seen.[134]

Limb motor abnormalities are also always present in large tegmental-basal hemorrhages, usually quadriplegia with stiffness of all limbs. Hemiplegia was noted in 4 of 15 tegmental-basal hemorrhages by Goto et al,[134] but was present in only 3 of 28 of Silverstein's bilateral hemorrhages.[309,310] The motor abnormality is usually bilateral with minor asymmetries. Asymmetries in decerebrate posturing, reflexes, or clonus are commonly detected. Tremor, shivering, restless limb movements, and dystonic postures have been common in our experience; patients may suddenly stiffen, giving the false impression of convulsive phenomena. Shivering occurs as the patient is worsening and can be indicative of failing motor function. Decerebrate posturing was noted in 12 of 15 of the patients of Goto et al.[134] Surprisingly, only 2 of 28 of Silverstein's series of large bilateral pontine hematomas were reported to have decerebrate rigidity,[309,310] but 13 had flaccid quadriplegia and 10 "generalized flaccidity."

Massive pontine hemorrhages are always fatal, although death does not come instantaneously. Steegmann[317] noted no deaths among 17 patients in less than 2 hours. Death usually occurs between 24 and 48 hours.[75,94,310,317] Survival for 2 to 10 days is not unusual and depends on the vigor of nursing and supportive care and the presence of complicating respiratory or urinary sepsis. Some patients with medium size hemorrhages survive.[269] On rare occasions a patient has survived the surgical removal of a pontine and fourth ventricular clot,[15,264] usually due to bleeding from a pontine AVM. Since the development of the lesion is so rapid, it is unlikely that surgical treatment could be provided early enough in the larger hemorrhages to be helpful. No other medical or surgical therapy seems likely to help these grave lesions.

Unilateral Basal or Basotegmental Hemorrhages

Unilateral basal or basotegmental hemorrhages are less common than the large paramedian lesions already discussed. In his autopsy-based series, Silverstein[310] described 11 (22%) such lesions; 3 were limited to the base and 8 were basotegmental. The larger lesions ruptured into the fourth ventricle. Reports based on CT scan have shown more restricted syndromes,[248,383] increasing the range of causes of a pure motor syndrome.[365] Gobernado et al[131] described a hypertensive woman with the gradual development over a 3-day period of a pure motor hemiplegia affecting the right arm and leg, sparing the face. CT scan defined a small hematoma limited to the base of the left pons. Another patient with a small hematoma confined to the right basis pontis had an "ataxic hemiparesis" of his left limbs.[299] Small unilateral hematomas limited to the base present with syndromes indistinguishable from lacunar infarction in the same region. Tuhrim et al[343] reported a patient with dysarthria, limb ataxia and extensor plantar response due to a small basal pontine hematoma; although the authors labeled this case dysarthria-clumsy hand syndrome, it more closely resembles ataxic hemiparesis.[101]

Bleeding originating from a pontine penetrating artery may start in the basis pontis, but also frequently dissects dorsally into the tegmentum. When the lesion spreads to the tegmentum, an ipsilateral facial palsy and conjugate gaze or sixth cranial nerve palsy often accompany the contralateral hemiplegia.[118] Larger unilateral lesions may rupture into the fourth ventricle after spreading within the tegmentum (Fig. 25.41). In Silverstein's series[310] these larger unilateral basal tegmental lesions usually lead to hemiplegia, coma, and death.

Lateral Tegmental Brain Stem Hematomas

Lateral tegmental brain stem hematomas usually originate from vessels penetrating into the brain stem from long circumferential branches. They enter the tegmentum laterally and course medially. Small hematomas remain confined to the lateral tegmentum, while larger lesions spread across to the opposite side and can destroy the entire tegmentum. Neurologic examination reveals a predominantly unilateral tegmental lesion with variable degrees of basilar involvement.[42,182]

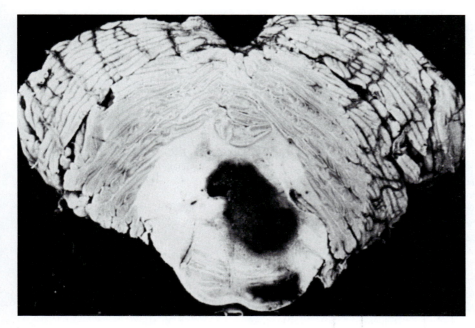

Figure 25.41 Unilateral basotegmental pontine hemorrhage with rupture into fourth ventricle.

Oculomotor abnormalities, especially the "one-and-a-half syndrome," horizontal gaze palsy, internuclear ophthalmoplegia, partial involvement of vertical eye movements, and ocular bobbing have been described.[42,118,182,269,345] The tegmental location of the spinothalamic tract makes sensory symptoms common. Ataxia, either unilateral or bilateral, may also accompany the oculomotor signs.[42,182] Action tremor has developed as the transient hemiparesis improves, possibly explained by involvement of the red nucleus or its connections.[42] Facial numbness, ipsilateral miosis, and hemiparesis also have been noted.[42,182] Two patients[182] developed Cheyne-Stokes respirations, one of the short-cycle type,[112,276] the other of the classical variety. Table 25.11 reviews some reported examples of tegmental pontine hematomas.

We examined two patients with tegmental pontine hemorrhage, and Lawrence and Lightfoote[207] studied a patient with a pontine AVM; all three patients showed vertical pendular ocular oscillations with dizziness and vertical oscillopsia weeks after the hemorrhage. Delayed pain in the contralateral limbs, as in the thalamic pain syndrome, began during recovery from a unilateral tegmental hemorrhage in an additional patient. We have also observed "palatal myoclonus" as a sequela of lateral tegmental hematomas.

MEDULLARY HEMORRHAGE

Hemorrhage into the medulla oblongata is even more rare than hemorrhage into the midbrain.

Arseni and Stanciu[6] described a 40-year-old woman with dizziness, vomiting, and headache with diplopia and right limb paresthesias. She suddenly became somnolent and ataxic with a stiff neck, left hemiparesis, diminished pain and temperature sensation on the left side of the face, left limb ataxia, nystagmus, dysphonia, and dysphagia. Surgical exploration found a hematoma on the floor of the fourth ventricle laterally. After drainage of the clot the patient was said to do well.

Kempe[192] described a similar patient who developed a lateral medullary hematoma. A 25-year-old woman noted diminished hearing on the left and then suddenly became ill with headache, vomiting, vertigo, and hiccups. She was ataxic and fell to the left. Findings included left nystagmus, diminished pain and temperature sensation on the left side of the face, and left facial weakness; the left ear was deaf and unreactive to caloric stimuli. After pneumoencephalogram documented a defect in the rhomboid fossa of the fourth ventricle, exploration revealed a clot bulging through the floor of the fourth ventricle medial to the restiform body. Both of these patients had findings similar to patients with lateral medullary infarcts, and each had a stepwise course. Arteriography was not performed, and CT and MRI were not available. We suspect the underlying process was a cavernous angioma in both instances.

In another patient[276] the explanation was AVM. At age 37, this woman developed weakness and decreased position sense in her left limbs. Right vocal cord and hypoglossal paralysis developed at age 60, and 2 years later she became gradually and then abruptly worse and was hypertensive. Necropsy revealed a hemorrhage in the medial medullary tegmentum with spread into the dorsal medulla and right lateral medulla.

Mastaglia et al,[224] reported two instances of medullary hemorrhage with quite different clinical features. An 87-year-old hypertensive woman was found unconscious with a right gaze palsy, right facial weakness, and left hemiplegia. The hemorrhage was largest in the lateral pons and descended into the medullary pyramid. This case seems to have been a pontine basal-tegmental hemorrhage with unusual caudal dissection, but it did not differ from the clinical picture already described in unilateral pontine hemorrhage. The other patient was hypertensive and had been on warfarin anticoagulation. She de-

Table 25.11 Tegmental Pontine Hemorrhages

Author	EOMs	Motor	Sensory	Other CN	Cerebellar
CT diagnosis					
Caplan and Goodwin[42]	No vertical, R gaze, R 6th, bilat. INO	L ↑ toe	L ↓ pin	R 7th, dysarthria, ptosis	Ataxia R > L
Caplan and Goodwin[42]	"1 ½", vertical nystagmus	L hemip, ↑↑ toes	L ↓ pin	R 7th, 8th, ptosis, dysarthria	Ataxia L > R
Müller et al[248]	R INO	L hemip, ↑↑ toes	L ↓ pin	R 5th, 7th	—
Kase et al[182]	"1 ½", No ↑ gaze,	R hemip	R ↓ pin and JPS	Dysarthria, L 7th	Ataxia L
Kase et al[182]	L INO and 6th, R 4th, bobbing	R hemip	R ↓ pin	Dysphagia, L 7th	Ataxia R & L
Autopsy cases					
Caplan and Goodwin[42]	"1 ½", bobbing, OD ↓ & inward	L hemip, Babinski	L ↓ pin	Dysarthria	Ataxia R > L
Tyler and Johnson[345]	No horizontal or ↑ gaze, bobbing, skew	L hemip, ↑↑ toes	L ↓ pin	R 5th, 7th, dysarthria, dysphagia, ptosis	R tremor
Dinsdale[75]	R gaze palsy	L hemip	L ↓ pin	R 7th, 8th	—
Silverstein[310]	R gaze palsy	L hemip, ↑↑ toes	L ↓ pin	R 7th, ptosis, dysphagia	—
Pierrott-Deseilligny et al[275]	"1 ½"	L hemip, ↑↑ toes	L hemis	R 7th, 5th, 8th	Ataxia R arm

Abbreviations and symbols: CT, computed tomography; INO, internuclear ophthalmoplegia; ↑upward, ↓decreased; 1 1/2, the "one-and-a-half" syndrome; hemip, hemiparesis; JPS, joint position sense; hemis, hemisensory syndrome; CN, cranial nerve; R, right; L, left; OD, right eye; EOM, extraocular movements.

veloped an unusual clinical picture with markedly decreased postural sensation and incoordination of her left limbs, diminished left arm reflexes, numbness over the right eye, and subjective numbness of the right limbs. Autopsy revealed a hemorrhage into the rostral spinal cord with dissection rostrally into the left medullary pyramid. The most likely etiologic factor in this patient was anticoagulation, perhaps compounded by hypertension.

There is one well-documented case of medullary hemorrhage due to hypertension, but it is not certain whether the hemorrhage arose in the medulla or in the caudal pontine tegmentum and dissected into the medulla.[246] A 56-year-old, previously hypertensive man developed difficulty swallowing, and examination revealed paralysis of the left side of the face, soft palate, vocal cord, and tongue. A left Horner syndrome, deafness in the left ear, and paresthesias of the right limbs were also found. CT scan showed a left medullary tegmental hematoma, but the signs of deafness and facial palsy might indicate some pontine involvement.

A recent report by Barinagarrementeria and Cantú[10] included four cases of their own, with a review of 12 others from the literature. The characteristic profile was one of sudden onset of headache, vertigo, dysphagia, dysphonia or dysarthria, and limb incoordination. Frequent findings on examination included palatal weakness (88%), nystagmus and/or cerebellar ataxia (75%), limb weakness (68%), and hypoglossal nerve palsy (56%). Less common signs were facial palsy and Horner syndrome. The mechanism of the medullary hemorrhage could be determined in only 7 of the 16 patients, corresponding to ruptured vascular malformation (3), hypertension (3), and anticoagulant treatment (1). The mortality for the group was 19% (3 of 16), and most of the survivors had either mild (56%) or no residual neurologic deficits (19%).

References

1. Abbott RD, Yin Y, Reed DH, Yano K: Risk of stroke in male cigarette smokers. N Engl J Med 315:717, 1986
2. Abu-Zeid HAH, Choi NW, Maini KK et al: Relative role of factors associated with cerebral infarction and cerebral hemorrhage. Stroke 8:106, 1977
3. Alexander MP, LoVerme SR: Aphasia after left hemispheric intracerebral hemorrhage. Neurology (NY) 30:1193, 1980
4. Algra A: SPIRIT: bleeding complications in patients after cerebral ischemia treated with anticoagulant drugs, abstracted. Stroke 28:231, 1997
5. Aring CD: Differential diagnosis of cerebrovascular stroke. Arch Intern Med 113:195, 1964
6. Arseni C, Stanciu M: Primary hematomas of the brain stem. Acta Neurochir 28:323, 1973
7. Attwater H: Pontine hemorrhage. Guys Hosp Rep 65:339, 1911
8. Aurell M, Head B: Cerebral hemorrhage in a population after a decade of active anti-hypertensive treatment. Acta Med Scand 176:377, 1964
9. Babikian VL, Kase CS, Pessin MS et al: Intracerebral hemorrhage in stroke patients anticoagulated with heparin. Stroke 20:1500, 1989

10. Barinagarrementeria F, Cantú C: Primary medullary hemorrhage: report of four cases and review of the literature. Stroke 25:1684, 1994

11. Barinagarrementeria F, Méndez A, Vega F: Hemorragia cerebral asociada al uso de fenilpropanolamina. Neurología 5:292, 1990

12. Barraquer-Bordas L, Illa I, Escartin A et al: Thalamic hemorrhage: a study of 23 patients with a diagnosis by computed tomography. Stroke 12:524, 1981

13. Barron KD, Fergusson G: Intracranial hemorrhage as a complication of anticoagulant therapy. Neurology (NY) 9:447, 1959

14. Beck DW, Menezes AH: Intracerebral hemorrhage in a patient with eclampsia. JAMA 246:1442, 1981

15. Becker DH, Silverberg GD: Successful evacuation of an acute pontine hematoma. Surg Neurol 10:263, 1978

16. Becker DH, Townsend JJ, Kramer RA, Newton TH: Occult cerebrovascular malformations: a series of 18 histologically verified cases with negative angiography. Brain 70:530, 1979

17. Benson DF, Sheremata WA, Bouchard R et al: Conduction aphasia: a clinicopathological study. Arch Neurol 28:339, 1973

18. Bernstein E, Diskant BM: Phenylpropanolamine: a potentially hazardous drug. Ann Emerg Med 11:311, 1982

19. Bicknell JM, Carlow TJ, Kornfeld M et al: Familial cavernous angiomas. Arch Neurol 35:746, 1978

20. Biller J, Loftus CM, Moore SA et al: Isolated central nervous system angiitis first presenting as spontaneous intracranial hemorrhage. Neurosurgery 20:310, 1987

21. Bogousslavsky J, Van Melle G, Regli F: The Lausanne Stroke Registry: analysis of 1,000 consecutive patients with first stroke. Stroke 19:1083, 1988

22. Bosch EP, Kennedy SS, Aschenbrener CA: Ocular bobbing: the myth of its localizing value. Neurology (NY) 25:949, 1975

23. Boudouresques G, Hauw JJ, Meininger V et al: Étude neuropathologique des hémorragies intracraniennes de l'adulte. Rev Neurol 135:197, 1979

24. Bousser MG, Eschwege E, Haguenau M et al: "AICLA" controlled trial of aspirin and dipyridamole in the secondary prevention of atherothrombotic cerebral ischemia. Stroke 14:5, 1983

25. Brennan RW, Bergland RM: Acute cerebellar hemorrhage: analysis of clinical findings and outcome in 12 cases. Neurology (NY) 27:527, 1977

26. Brewer DB, Fawcett FJ, Horsfield GI: A necropsy series of non-traumatic cerebral haemorrhages and softenings, with particular reference to heart weight. J Pathol Bacteriol 96:311, 1968

27. Brillman J: Acute hydrocephalus and death one month after non-surgical treatment for acute cerebellar hemorrhage. J Neurosurg 50:374, 1979

28. Broderick J, Brott TG, Duldner JE et al: Volume of intracerebral hemorrhage: a powerful and easy-to-use predictor of 30-day mortality. Stroke 24:987, 1993

29. Broderick J, Brott T, Tomsick T et al: The risk of subarachnoid and intracerebral hemorrhages in blacks as compared with whites. N Engl J Med 326:733, 1992

30. Broderick JP, Brott TG, Tomsick T et al: Ultraearly evaluation of intracerebral hemorrhage. J Neurosurg 72:195, 1990

31. Broderick J, Brott T, Tomsick T, Leach A: Lobar hemorrhage in the elderly: the undiminishing importance of hypertension. Stroke 24:49, 1993

32. Brott T, Broderick J, Kothari R et al: Early hemorrhage growth in patients with intracerebral hemorrhage. Stroke 28:1, 1997

33. Brott T, Thalinger K, Hertzberg V: Hypertension as a risk factor for spontaneous intracerebral hemorrhage. Stroke 17:1078, 1986

34. Bruno A, Carter S, Qualls C et al: Incidence of spontaneous intracerebral hemorrhage among Hispanics and non-Hispanic whites in New Mexico. Neurology 47:405, 1996

35. Butler AB, Partian RA, Netsky MG: Primary intraventricular hemorrhage: a mild and remediable form. Neurology (NY) 22:675, 1972

36. Butler JF, Cancilla PA, Cornell SH: Computerized axial tomography of intracerebral hematoma: a clinical and neuropathological study. Arch Neurol 33:206, 1976

37. Cambier J, Elghozi D, Strube E: Hémorragie de la tête du noyau caudé gauche. Rev Neurol (Paris) 135:763, 1979

38. Cambier J, Elghozi D, Strube E: Trois observations de lésions vasculaires du thalamus droit avec syndrome de l'hémisphère mineur: discussion du concept de négligence thalamique. Rev Neurol (Paris) 136:105, 1980

39. Camerlingo M, Casto L, Censori B et al: Immediate anticoagulation with heparin for first-ever ischemic stroke in the carotid artery territories observed within 5 hours of onset. Arch Neurol 51:462, 1994

40. Canadian Cooperative Study Group: A randomized trial of aspirin and sulfinpyrazone in threatened stroke. N Engl J Med 299:53, 1978

41. Caplan LR: Intracerebral hemorrhage. p. 185. In Tyler HR, Dawson DM (eds): Current Neurology. Vol II. Houghton Mifflin, Boston, 1979

42. Caplan LR, Goodwin JA: Lateral tegmental brainstem hemorrhages. Neurology (NY) 32:252, 1982

43. Caplan LR, Mohr JP: Intracerebral hemorrhage: an update. Geriatrics 33:42, 1978

44. Carion F: Contribution à l'Étude Symptomatique et Diagnostique de l'Hémorragie Cérébelleuse. Adrien Delhaye, Paris, 1875

45. Carpenter MB: Human Neuroanatomy. p. 23. 7th Ed. Williams & Wilkins, Baltimore, 1976

46. Carton CA, Hickey WC: Arteriovenous malformation of the head of the caudate: report of a case of total removal. J Neurosurg 12:414, 1955

47. Cerebral Embolism Study Group: Immediate anticoagulation of embolic stroke: brain hemorrhage and management options. Stroke 15:779, 1984

48. Chamorro A, Villa N, Saiz A et al: Early anticoagulation after large cerebral embolic infarction: a safety study. Neurology 45:861, 1995

49. Charcot JM, Bouchard C: Nouvelles recherches sur la pathogénie de l'hémorragie cérébrale. Arch Physiol Norm Pathol 1:110, 1868

50. Cheyn J: Cases of Apoplexy and Lethargy with Observa-

tions upon the Comatose Diseases. Thomas Underwood, London, 1812

51. Childs T: A case of apoplexy of the cerebellum. Am Med Month (NY) 9:1, 1858

52. Choi D, Sudansky L, Schachter S et al: Medial thalamic hemorrhage with amnesia. Arch Neurol 40:611, 1983

53. Chokroverty S, Rubino FA, Haller C: Pure motor hemiplegia due to pyramidal infarction. Arch Neurol 32:647, 1975

54. Christoff N: A clinicopathologic study of vertical eye movements. Arch Neurol 31:1, 1974

55. Christoff N, Anderson PJ, Bender MB: A clinicopathologic study of associated vertical eye movements. Trans Am Neurol Assoc 87:184, 1962

56. Citron BP, Halpern M, McCarron M et al: Necrotizing angiitis associated with drug abuse. N Engl J Med 283: 1003, 1970

57. Clark JV: Familial occurrence of cavernous angiomata of the brain. J Neurol Neurosurg Psychiatry 33:871, 1970

58. Clark WM, Lyden PD, Madden KP et al: Thrombolytic therapy in acute ischemic stroke, letter. N Engl J Med 336:65, 1997

59. Clifford-Jones RE, Love S, Gurusinghe N: Granulomatous angiitis of the central nervous system: a case with recurrent intracerebral hemorrhage. J Neurol Neurosurg Psychiatry 48:1054, 1985

60. Cole FM, Yates PO: Intracranial microaneurysms and small cerebrovascular lesions. Brain 90:759, 1967

61. Cole FM, Yates PO: The occurrence and significance of intracerebral microaneurysms. J Pathol Bacteriol 93:393, 1967

62. Cole FM, Yates PO: Pseudo-aneurysms in relationship to massive cerebral hemorrhage. J Neurol Neurosurg Psychiatry 30:61, 1967

63. Cole FM, Yates PO: Comparative incidence of cerebrovascular lesions in normotensive and hypertensive patients. Neurology (NY) 18:255, 1968

64. Crawford JV, Russell DS: Cryptic arteriovenous and venous hamartomas of the brain. J Neurol Neurosurg Psychiatry 19:1, 1956

65. Critchley M: The Parietal Lobes. p. 326. Hafner, New York, 1966

66. Crowell RM, Ojemann RG: Surgery for brain hemorrhage. p. 233. In Moossy J, Reinmuth OM (eds): Cerebrovascular Diseases. Twelfth Research Conference. Lippincott-Raven, Philadelphia, 1981

67. Dana C: Acute bulbar paralysis due to hemorrhage and softening of the pons and medulla. Med Rec 64:361, 1903

68. Davis KR, Ackerman RH, Kistler JP, Mohr JP: Computed tomography of cerebral infarction: hemorrhagic, contrast enhancement, and time of appearance. Comput Tomogr 1:71, 1977

69. Dawson I, van Bockel JH, Ferrari MD et al: Ischemic and hemorrhagic stroke in patients on oral anticoagulants after reconstruction for chronic lower limb ischemia. Stroke 24:1655, 1993

70. Dejerine J, Roussy G: Le syndrome thalamique. Rev Neurol (Paris) 12:521, 1906

71. Delaney P, Estes M: Intracranial hemorrhage with amphetamine abuse. Neurology (NY) 30:1125, 1980

72. del Zoppo GJ, Poeck K, Pessin MS et al: Recombinant tissue plasminogen activator in acute thrombotic and embolic stroke. Ann Neurol 32:78, 1992

73. Denny-Brown D, Fischer EG: Physiological aspects of visual perception. II. The subcortical visual direction of behavior. Arch Neurol 33:228, 1976

74. De Reuck J, Crevits L, Sieben G, DeCoster W: Granulomatous angiitis of the nervous system: a clinicopathological study of one case. J Neurol 227:49, 1982

75. Dinsdale HB: Spontaneous hemorrhage in the posterior fossa: a study of primary cerebellar and pontine hemorrhage with observations on the pathogenesis. Arch Neurol 10:200, 1964

76. Dolinskas CA, Bilaniuk LT, Zimmerman RA et al: Computed tomography of intracerebral hematomas. II. Radionuclide and transmission CT studies of the perihematoma region. AJR 129:689, 1977

77. Dolinskas CA, Bilaniuk LT, Zimmerman RA, Kuhl DE: Computed tomography of intracerebral hematomas. I. Transmission CT observations on hematoma resolution. AJR 129:681, 1977

78. Donahue RP, Abbott RD, Reed DM, Yanko K: Alcohol and hemorrhagic stroke: the Honolulu Heart Program. JAMA 255:2311, 1986

79. Donnan GA, Davis SM, Chambers BR et al: Trials of streptokinase in severe acute ischaemic stroke, letter. Lancet 345:578, 1995

80. Drapkin A, Merskey C: Anticoagulant therapy after acute myocardial infarction: relation of therapeutic benefit to patient's age, sex, and severity of infarction. JAMA 222:541, 1972

81. Drury I, Whisnant JP, Garraway WM: Primary intracerebral hemorrhage: impact of CT on incidence. Neurology (NY) 34:653, 1984

82. D'Souza T, Shraberg D: Intracranial hemorrhage associated with amphetamine use, letter. Neurology (NY) 31: 922, 1981

83. Dul K, Drayer BP: CT and MR imaging of intracerebral hemorrhage. p. 73. In Kase CS, Caplan LR (eds): Intracerebral Hemorrhage. Butterworth-Heinemann, Boston, 1994

84. Duret H: Etudes Expérimentales et Cliniques sur les Traumatisms Cérébraux. Adrien Delhaye, Paris, 1873

85. Duret H: Recherches anatomiques sur la circulation de l'encéphale. Arch Physiol Norm Pathol 6, 1:60, 919, 1874

86. Duret H: Sur la distribution des artères nourricières du bulbe rachidien. Arch Physiol Norm Pathol 5:97, 1873

87. Duret H: Traumatismes Cranio-cérébraux. Librairie Felix Alcan, Paris, 1919

88. Durward QJ, Barnett HJM, Barr HWK: Presentation and management of mesencephalic hematoma. J Neurosurg 56:123, 1982

89. Echlin FA, Arnett V, Zoll J: Paroxysmal high voltage discharges from isolated and partially isolated human and animal cerebral cortex. EEG Clin Neurophysiol 4: 147, 1952

90. Ellis AG: The pathogenesis of spontaneous cerebral hemorrhage. Proc Pathol Soc (Phila) 12:197, 1909

91. Englander RN, Netsky MG, Adelman LS: Location of human pyramidal tract in the internal capsule: anatomic evidence. Neurology (Minneap) 25:823, 1975

92. Epstein AW: Primary massive pontine hemorrhage. J Neuropathol Exp Neurol 10:426, 1951

93. Fallis RJ, Fisher M: Cerebral vasculitis and hemorrhage associated with phenylpropanolamine. Neurology (NY) 35:405, 1985

94. Fang HCM, Foley JM: Hypertensive hemorrhages of the pons and cerebellum. Arch Neurol Psychiatry 72:638, 1954

95. Faught E, Peters D, Bartolucci A et al: Seizures after primary intracerebral hemorrhage. Neurology 39:1089, 1989

96. Fazio C, Sacco G, Bugiani O: The thalamic hemorrhage: an anatomo-clinical study. Eur Neurol 9:30, 1973

97. Fehr MA, Anderson DC: Incidence of progression or rebleeding in hypertensive intracerebral hemorrhage. J Stroke Cerebrovasc Dis 1:111, 1991

98. Fieschi C, Carolei A, Fiorelli M et al: Changing prognosis of primary intracerebral hemorrhage: results of a clinical and computed tomographic follow-up study of 104 patients. Stroke 19:192, 1988

99. Finelli PF, Kessimian N, Bernstein PW: Cerebral amyloid angiopathy manifesting as recurrent intracerebral hemorrhage. Arch Neurol 41:330, 1984

100. Fisher CM: Capsular infarcts. Arch Neurol 36:65, 1979

101. Fisher CM: Cerebral ischemia—less familiar types. Clin Neurosurg 18:267, 1971

102. Fisher CM: Cerebral miliary aneurysms in hypertension. Am J Pathol 66:313, 1972

103. Fisher CM: Clinical syndromes in cerebral hemorrhage. p. 318. In Fields WS (ed): Pathogenesis and Treatment of Cerebrovascular Disease. Charles C Thomas, Springfield, IL, 1961

104. Fisher CM: Lacunes: small, deep cerebral infarcts. Neurology (Minneap) 15:774, 1965

105. Fisher CM: Ocular bobbing. Arch Neurol 11:543, 1964

106. Fisher CM: Pathological observations in hypertensive cerebral hemorrhage. J Neuropathol Exp Neurol 30:536, 1971

107. Fisher CM: Pure sensory stroke involving face, arm and leg. Neurology (Minneap) 15:76, 1965

108. Fisher CM: Some neuro-ophthalmological observations. J Neurol Neurosurg Psychiatry 30:383, 1967

109. Fisher CM: The pathologic and clinical aspects of thalamic hemorrhage. Trans Am Neurol Assoc 84:56, 1959

110. Fisher CM: The pathology and pathogenesis of intracerebral hemorrhage. p. 295. In Fields WS (ed): Pathogenesis and Treatment of Cerebrovascular Disease. CC Thomas, Springfield, IL, 1961

111. Fisher CM: The arterial lesions underlying lacunes. Acta Neuropathol 12:1, 1969

112. Fisher CM: The neurological examination of the comatose patient. Acta Neurol Scand, suppl. 45:1, 44, 1969

113. Fisher CM, Adams RD: Observations on brain embolism with special reference to the mechanism of hemorrhagic infarction. J Neuropathol Exp Neurol 10:92, 1951

114. Fisher CM, Curry HB: Pure motor hemiplegia of vascular origin. Arch Neurol 13:30, 1965

115. Fisher CM, Picard EH, Polak A et al: Acute hypertensive cerebellar hemorrhage: diagnosis and surgical treatment. J Nerv Ment Dis 140:38, 1965

116. Franke CL, deJonge J, van Swieten JC et al: Intracerebral hematomas during anticoagulant treatment. Stroke 21:726, 1990

117. Freeman RE, Onofrio BM, Okazaki H, Dinapoli RP: Spontaneous intracerebellar hemorhage. Neurology (NY) 23:84, 1973

118. Freeman W, Ammerman HH, Stanley M: Syndromes of the pontile tegmentum, Foville's syndrome: report of 3 cases. Arch Neurol Psychiatry 50:462, 1943

119. Freytag E: Fatal hypertensive intracerebral haematomas: a survey of the pathological anatomy of 393 cases. J Neurol Neurosurg Psychiatry 31:616, 1968

120. Fujii Y, Tanaka R, Takeuchi S et al: Hematoma enlargement in spontaneous intracerebral hemorrhage. J Neurosurg 80:51, 1994

121. Fujimoto M, Yoshino E, Ueguchi T et al: Fluid blood density level demonstrated by computerized tomography in pituitary apoplexy: report of two cases. J Neurosurg 55:143, 1981

122. Furlan AJ, Whisnant JP, Elveback LR: The decreasing incidence of primary intracerebral hemorrhage: a population study. Ann Neurol 5:367, 1979

123. García JH, Ho KL, Caccamo DV: Intracerebral hemorrhage: pathology of selected topics. p. 45. In Kase CS, Caplan LR (eds): Intracerebral Hemorrhage. Butterworth-Heinemann, Boston, 1994

124. Garraway WM, Whisnant JP, Drury I: The continuing decline in the incidence of stroke. Mayo Clin Proc 58:520, 1983

125. Gilbert JJ, Vinters HV: Cerebral amyloid angiopathy: incidence and complications in the aging brain. I. Cerebral hemorrhage. Stroke 14:915, 1983

126. Gildersleve N, Koo AH, McDonald CJ: Metastatic tumor presenting as intracerebral hemorrhage. Radiology 124:109, 1977

127. Gilles C, Brucher JM, Khoubesserian P, Vanderhaeghn JJ: Cerebral amyloid angiopathy as a cause of multiple intracerebral hemorrhages. Neurology (NY) 34:730, 1984

128. Gil-Nagel A, Dubovsky J, Wilcox KJ et al: Familial cerebral cavernous angioma: a gene localized to a 15-cM interval on chromosome 7q. Ann Neurol 39:807, 1996

129. Gilner LI, Avin B: A reversible ocular manifestation of thalamic hemorrhage: a case report. Arch Neurol 34:715, 1977

130. Glick R, Hoying J, Cerullo L, Perlman S: Phenylpropanolamine: an over-the-counter drug causing central nervous system vasculitis and intracerebral hemorrhage. Neurosurgery (NY) 20:969, 1987

131. Gobernado JM, Fernandez de Molina AR, Gimeno A: Pure motor hemiplegia due to hemorrhage in the lower pons. Arch Neurol 37:393, 1980

132. Gomori JM, Grossman RI, Goldberg HI et al: Intracranial hematomas: imaging by high-field MR. Radiology 157:87, 1985

133. Gore JM, Sloan M, Price TR et al: Intracerebral hemorrhage, cerebral infarction, and subdural hematoma after acute myocardial infarction and thrombolytic therapy in the Thrombolysis in Myocardial Infarction Study: Thrombolysis in myocardial infarction, phase II, pilot and clinical data. Circulation 83:448, 1991

134. Goto N, Kaneko M, Hosaka Y, Koga H: Primary pontine

hemorrhage: clinicopathologic correlations. Stroke 11: 84, 1980

135. Gowers WR: A Manual of Diseases of the Nervous System. 2nd Ed. Vol. II. p. 395. JA Churchill, London, 1893

136. Graus F, Rogers LR, Posner JB: Cerebrovascular complications in patients with cancer. Medicine 64:16, 1985

137. Green FHK: Miliary aneurysms in the brain. J Pathol Bacteriol 33:71, 1930

138. Green RM, Kelly KM, Gabrielsen T et al: Multiple intracranial hemorrhages after smoking "crack" cocaine. Stroke 21:957, 1990

139. Greenberg J, Skubick D, Shenkin H: Acute hydrocephalus in cerebellar infarct and hemorrhage. Neurology (NY) 29:409, 1979

140. Greenberg SM, Briggs ME, Hyman BT et al: Apolipoprotein E ϵ4 is associated with the presence and earlier onset of hemorrhage in cerebral amyloid angiopathy. Stroke 27:1333, 1996

141. Greenberg SM, Edgar MA: Case records of the Massachusetts General Hospital (Case 22-1996). N Engl J Med 325:189, 1996

142. Greenberg SM, Vonsattel JP, Stakes JW et al: The clinical spectrum of cerebral amyloid angiopathy: presentations without lobar hemorrhage. Neurology 43:2073, 1993

143. Groothuis DR, Duncan GW, Fisher CM: The human thalamocortical sensory path in the internal capsule: evidence from a small capsular hemorrhage causing pure sensory stroke. Ann Neurol 2:328, 1977

144. Gross CR, Kase CS, Mohr JP et al: Stroke in south Alabama: incidence and diagnostic features—a population based study. Stroke 15:249, 1984

145. Gruppo Italiano per lo Studio della Sopravivenza nell' Infarto Miocardico: GISSI-2: a factorial randomised trial of alteplase versus streptokinase and heparin versus no heparin among 12,490 patients with acute myocardial infarction. Lancet 336:65, 1990

146. Gudmundsson G, Hallgrimsson J, Jonasson TA, Bjarnason O: Hereditary cerebral haemorrhage with amyloidosis. Brain 95:387, 1972

147. Guillain G, Alajouanine T, Marquezy R: Hémorragie cérébelleuse avec spasms toniques et attitude de rigidité des membres inférieures. Bull Mem Soc Med Hôp Paris 47:1120, 1923

148. Günel M, Awad IA, Finberg K et al: A founder mutation as a cause of cerebral cavernous malformation in Hispanic Americans. N Engl J Med 334:946, 1996

149. Gurwitt LJ, Long JM, Clark RE: Cerebral metastatic choriocarcinoma: a postpartum cause of "stroke." Obstet Gynecol 45:583, 1975

150. Hacke W, Kaste M, Fieschi C et al: Intravenous thrombolysis with recombinant tissue plasminogen activator for acute hemispheric stroke: the European Cooperative Acute Stroke Study (ECASS). JAMA 274:1017, 1995

151. Halsey JH, Ceballos R, Crosby EC: The supranuclear control of voluntary lateral gaze. Neurology (NY) 17:928, 1967

152. Hanaway J, Young RR: Localization of the pyramidal tract in the internal capsule of man. J Neurol Sci 34:63, 1977

153. Handley AJ, Emerson PA, Fleming PR: Heparin in the prevention of deep vein thrombosis after myocardial infarction. BMJ 2:436, 1972

154. Hankey GJ: Isolated angiitis/angiopathy of the central nervous system. Cerebrovasc Dis 1:2, 1991

155. Hansen BS, Marquardsen J: Incidence of stroke in Frederiksberg, Denmark. Stroke 8:663, 1977

156. Harrington H, Heller HA, Dawson D et al: Intracerebral hemorrhage and oral amphetamine. Arch Neurol 40: 503, 1983

157. Hart RG, Boop BS, Anderson DC: Oral anticoagulants and intracranial hemorrhage. Stroke 26:1471, 1995

158. Hart RG, Pearce LA: In vivo antithrombotic effect of aspirin: dose versus nongastrointestinal bleeding. Stroke 24:138, 1993

159. Heilman JM, Valenstein E: Frontal lobe neglect in man. Neurology (Minneap) 22:660, 1972

160. Heiman TD, Satya-Murti S: Benign cerebellar hemorrhages. Ann Neurol 3:366, 1978

161. Helweg-Larsen S, Sommer W, Strange P et al: Prognosis for patients treated conservatively for spontaneous intracerebral hematomas. Stroke 15:1045, 1984

162. Herbstein DJ, Schaumburg HH: Hypertensive intracerebral hematoma: an investigation of the initial hemorrhage and rebleeding using chromium Cr 51-labeled erythrocytes. Arch Neurol 30:412, 1974

163. Herman B, Schulte BPM, Van Luijk JH et al: Epidemiology of stroke in Tilburg, The Netherlands: the population-based stroke incidence register. 1. Introduction and preliminary results. Stroke 11:162, 1980

164. Herold S, von Kumer R, Jaeger CH: Follow-up of spontaneous intracerebral haemorrhage by computed tomography. J Neurol 228:267, 1982

165. Heros RC: Cerebellar hemorrhage and infarction. Stroke 13:106, 1982

166. Hickey WF, King RB, Wang A-M, Samuels MA: Multiple simultaneous intracerebral hematomas: clinical, radiologic, and pathologic findings in two patients. Arch Neurol 40:519, 1983

167. Hier DB, Davis KR, Richardson EP, Mohr JP: Hypertensive putaminal hemorrhage. Ann Neurol 1:152, 1977

168. Houser OW, Campbell JK: Computed tomography in cerebrovascular disease: influences of morphology, topography, clinical factors, and temporal profile. p. 181. In Moossy J, Reinmuth OM (eds): Cerebrovascular Diseases. Proceedings of the Twelfth Research Conference. Lippincott-Raven, Philadelphia, 1981

169. Humphreys RP: Computerized tomographic definition of mesencephalic hematoma with evacuation through pedunculotomy. J Neurosurg 49:749, 1978

170. Hyland HH, Levy D: Spontaneous cerebellar hemorrhage. Can Med Assoc J 71:315, 1954

171. Hylek EM, Singer DE: Risk factors for intracranial hemorrhage in outpatients taking warfarin. Ann Intern Med 120:897, 1994

172. Iwama T, Ohkuma A, Miwa Y et al: Brain tumors manifesting as intracranial hemorrhage. Neurol Med Chir 32: 130, 1992

173. Jacome DE: Isodense cerebellar hematoma. Neurology (Cleve) 33:1201, 1983

174. Jellinger K: Cerebrovascular amyloidosis with cerebral hemorrhage. J Neurol 214:195, 1977

175. Jellinger K: Cerebral hemorrhage in amyloid angiopathy, letter. Ann Neurol 1:604, 1977

176. Jenkins A, Maxwell W, Graham D: Experimental intracerebral hematoma in the rat: sequential light microscopic changes. Neuropathol Appl Neurobiol 15:477, 1989

177. Juvela S, Hillbom M, Palomaki H: Risk factors for spontaneous intracerebral hemorrhage. Stroke 26:1558, 1995

178. Kasdon DL, Scott RM, Adelman LS, Wolpert SM: Cerebellar hemorrhage with decreased absorption values on computed tomography: a case report. Neuroradiology 13:265, 1977

179. Kase CS: Intracerebral hemorrhage: non-hypertensive causes. Stroke 17:590, 1986

180. Kase CS: Lobar hemorrhage. p. 363. In Kase CS, Caplan LR (eds): Intracerebral Hemorrhage. Butterworth-Heinemann, Boston, 1994

180a. Kase CS: Cerebellar hemorrhage. p. 425. In Kase CS, Caplan LR (eds): Intracerebral Hemorrhage. Butterworth-Heinemann, Boston, 1994

181. Kase CS, Foster TE, Reed JE et al: Intracerebral hemorrhage and phenylpropanolamine use. Neurology (NY) 37:399, 1987

182. Kase CS, Maulsby GO, Mohr JP: Partial pontine hematomas. Neurology (NY) 30:652, 1980

183. Kase CS, O'Neal AM, Fisher M et al: Intracranial hemorrhage after use of tissue plasminogen activator for coronary thrombolysis. Ann Intern Med 112:17, 1990

184. Kase CS, Pessin MS, Zivin JA et al: Intracranial hemorrhage following coronary thrombolysis with tissue plasminogen activator. Am J Med 92:384, 1992

185. Kase CS, Robinson RK, Stein RW et al: Anticoagulant-related intracerebral hemorrhage. Neurology (NY) 35:943, 1985

186. Kase CS, Williams JP, Wyatt DA, Mohr JP: Lobar intracerebral hematomas: clinical and CT analysis of 22 cases. Neurology (NY) 32:1146, 1982

187. Kattapong VJ, Hart BL, Davis LE: Familial cerebral cavernous angiomas: clinical and radiologic studies. Neurology 45:492, 1995

188. Kazui S, Naritomi H, Yamamoto H et al: Enlargement of spontaneous intracerebral hemorrhage: incidence and time course. Stroke 27:1783, 1996

189. Keane JR: Contralateral gaze deviation with supratentorial hemorrhage: three pathologically verified cases. Arch Neurol 32:119, 1975

190. Keane JR: Transient opsoclonus with thalamic hemorrhage. Arch Neurol 37:423, 1980

191. Kelley RE, Berger JR, Scheinberg P, Stokes N: Active bleeding in hypertensive intracerebral hemorrhage: computed tomography. Neurology (NY) 32:852, 1982

192. Kempe LG: Surgical removal of an intramedullary hematoma simulating Wallenberg's syndrome. J Neurol Neurosurg Psychiatry 27:78, 1964

193. Kendall BE, Claveria LE: Vascular conditions. p. 161. In du Boulay GH, Moseley IF (eds): Computerized Axial Tomography in Clinical Practice. Springer-Verlag, Berlin, 1977

194. Kikta DG, Devereaux MX, Chandar K: Intracranial hemorrhages due to phenylpropanolamine. Stroke 16:510, 1985

195. Kistler JP, Hochberg FH, Brooks BR et al: Computer-ized axial tomography: clinicopathologic correlation. Neurology (NY) 25:201, 1975

196. Kjellin KG, Soderstrom CE: Cerebral haemorrhages with atypical clinical patterns: a study of cerebral hematomas using CSF spectrophotometry and computerized transverse axial tomography ("EMI scanning"). J Neurol Sci 25:211, 1975

197. Kolodny EH, Rebeiz JJ, Caviness VS, Richardson EP: Granulomatous angiitis of the central nervous system. Arch Neurol 19:510, 1968

198. Kornyey S: Rapidly fatal pontile hemorrhage: clinical and anatomic report. Arch Neurol Psychiatry 41:793, 1939

199. Kothari RU, Brott T, Broderick JP et al: The ABCs of measuring intracerebral hemorrhage volumes. Stroke 27:1304, 1996

200. Kowada M, Yamaguchi K, Matsuoka S, Ito Z: Extravasation of angiographic contrast material in hypertensive intracerebral hemorrhage. J Neurosurg 36:471, 1972

201. Krayenbühl H, Siebenmann R: Small vascular malformations as a cause of primary intracerebral hemorrhage. J Neurosurg 22:7, 1965

202. Kunitz SC, Gross CR, Heyman A et al: The Pilot Stroke Data Bank: definition, design and data. Stroke 15:740, 1984

203. Kurtzke JF: Epidemiology of Cerebrovascular Disease. Springer-Verlag, Berlin, 1969

204. Kwak R, Kadoya S, Suzuki T: Factors affecting the prognosis in thalamic hemorrhage. Stroke 14:493, 1983

205. LaTorre E, Delitala A, Sorano V: Hematoma of the quadrigeminal plate. J Neurosurg 49:610, 1978

206. Landefeld CS, Goldman L: Major bleeding in outpatients treated with warfarin: incidence and prediction by factors known at the start of outpatient therapy. Am J Med 87:144, 1989

207. Lawrence WH, Lightfoote WE: Continuous vertical pendular eye movements after brainstem hemorrhage. Neurology (NY) 25:896, 1975

208. Leestma JE, Noronha A: Pure motor hemiplegia, medullary pyramid lesion, and olivary hypertrophy. J Neurol Neurosurg Psychiatry 39:877, 1976

209. Levine SR, Brust JCM, Futrell N et al: Cerebrovascular complications of the use of the "crack" form of alkaloid cocaine. N Engl J Med 323:699, 1990

210. Levy DE, Brott TG, Haley EC Jr et al: Factors related to intracranial hematoma formation in patients receiving tissue-type plasminogen activator for acute ischemic stroke. Stroke 25:291, 1994

211. Lipton RB, Berger AR, Lesser ML et al: Lobar vs thalamic and basal ganglion hemorrhage: clinical and radiographic features. J Neurol 234:86, 1987

212. Lisk DR, Pasteur W, Rhoades H et al: Early presentation of hemispheric intracerebral hemorrhage: prediction of outcome and guidelines for treatment allocation. Neurology 44:133, 1994

213. Little JR, Dial B, Bellanger G, Carpenter S: Brain hemorrhage from intracranial tumor. Stroke 10:283, 1979

214. Little JR, Tubman DE, Ethier R: Cerebellar hemorrhage in adults: diagnosis by computerized tomography. J Neurosurg 48:575, 1978

215. Loizou LA, Hamilton JG, Tsementzis SA: Intracranial

hemorrhage in association with pseudoephedrine overdose. J Neurol Neurosurg Psychiatry 45:471, 1982

216. Lukes SA: Intracerebral hemorrhage from an arteriovenous malformation after amphetamine injection. Arch Neurol 40:60, 1983

217. Mandybur TI: Intracranial hemorrhage caused by metastatic tumors. Neurology (NY) 27:650, 1977

218. Mandybur TI: Cerebral amyloid angiopathy: possible relationship to rheumatoid vasculitis. Neurology (NY) 29: 1336, 1979

219. Mandybur TI, Bates SRD: Fatal massive intracerebral hemorrhage complicating cerebral amyloid angiopathy. Arch Neurol 35:246, 1978

220. Margolis G, Odom GL, Woodhall B, Bloor BM: The role of small angiomatous malformations in the production of intracerebral hematomas. J Neurosurg 8:564, 1951

221. Margolis MT, Newton TH: Methamphetamine ("speed") arteritis. Neuroradiology 2:179, 1971

222. Masdeu JC, Rubino FA: Management of lobar intracerebral hemorrhage, medical or surgical. Neurology (Cleve) 34:381, 1984

223. Massaro AR, Sacco RL, Mohr JP et al: Clinical discriminators separate lobar and subcortical hemorrhage: the Stroke Data Bank. Neurology (NY) 41:1881, 1991

224. Mastaglia FL, Edis B, Kakulas BA: Medullary hemorrhage: a report of two cases. J Neurol Neurosurg Psychiatry 32:221, 1969

225. Matick H, Anderson D, Brumlik J: Cerebral vasculitis associated with oral amphetamine overdose. Arch Neurol 40:253, 1983

226. McConnell TH, Leonard JS: Microangiomatous malformations with intraventricular hemorrhage. Neurology (NY) 17:618, 1967

227. McCormick WF, Rosenfield DB: Massive brain hemorrhage: a review of 144 cases and an examination of their causes. Stroke 4:946, 1973

228. McCormick WF, Schochet SS: Atlas of Cerebrovascular Disease. p. 328. WB Saunders, Philadelphia, 1976

229. McKissok W, Richardson A, Taylor J: Primary intracerebral hemorrhage: a controlled trial of surgical and conservative treatment in 180 unselected cases. Lancet 2: 221, 1961

230. McKissock W, Richardson A, Walsh L: Spontaneous cerebellar hemorrhage: a study of 34 consecutive cases treated surgically. Brain 83:1, 1960

231. Melamed E, Korn-Lubetzki I, Reches A, Siew F: Hemiballismus: detection of focal hemorrhage in subthalamic nucleus by CT scan. Ann Neurol 4:582, 1978

232. Melo TP, Bogousslavsky J, Regli F, Janzer R: Fatal hemorrhage during anticoagulation of cardioembolic infarction: role of cerebral amyloid angiopathy. Eur Neurol 33:9, 1993

233. Meritt HH: A Textbook of Neurology. p. 160. 6th Ed. Lea & Febiger, Philadelphia, 1979

234. Messert B, Leppik IE, Sato Y: Diplopia and involuntary eye closure in spontaneous cerebellar hemorrhage. Stroke 7:305, 1976

235. Michael JC: Cerebellar apoplexy. Am J Med Sci 183: 687, 1932

236. Mitchell N, Angrist A: Spontaneous cerebellar hemorrhage: report of 15 cases. Am J Pathol 18:235, 1942

237. Mizukami M, Araki G, Mihara H et al: Arteriographically

visualized extravasation in hypertensive intracerebral hemorrhage: report of seven cases. Stroke 3:527, 1972

238. Mizukami M, Araki G, Mihara H: Angiographic sign of good prognosis for hemiplegia in hypertensive intracerebral hemorrhage. Neurology (NY) 24:120, 1974

239. Mizukami M, Nishijima M, Kin H: Computed tomographic findings of good prognosis for hemiplegia in hypertensive putaminal hemorrhage. Stroke 12:648, 1981

240. Modesti LM, Binet EF, Collins GH: Meningiomas causing spontaneous intracranial hematomas. J Neurosurg 45:437, 1976

241. Mohr JP, Caplan LR, Melski JW et al: The Harvard Cooperative Stroke Registry: a prospective registry. Neurology (NY) 28:754, 1978

242. Mohr JP, Pessin MS, Finkelstein S et al: Broca aphasia: pathologic and clinical aspects. Neurology (Minneap) 28: 311, 1978

243. Mohr JP, Sidman M: Aphasia: behavioral aspects. p. 279. In Reiser MF (ed): American Hand-book of Psychiatry. Basic Books, New York, 1975

244. Mohr JP, Watters WC, Duncan GW: Thalamic hemorrhage and aphasia. Brain Lang 2:3, 1975

245. Moore PM, Cupps TR: Neurological complications of vasculitis. Ann Neurol 14:155, 1983

246. Morel-Maroger A, Metzger J, Bories J et al: Les hématomes benins du tronc cérébral chez les hypertendus artériels. Rev Neurol (Paris) 138:437, 1982

247. Mueller SM: Phenylpropanolamine: a non-prescription drug with potentially fatal side effects, letter. N Engl J Med 308:653, 1983

248. Müller HR, Wüthrich R, Wiggli U et al: The contribution of computerized axial tomography to the diagnosis of cerebellar and pontine hematomas. Stroke 6:467, 1975

249. Multicentre Acute Stroke Trial—Italy (MAST-I) Group: Randomised controlled trial of streptokinase, aspirin, and combination of both in treatment of acute ischaemic stroke. Lancet 346:1509, 1995

250. Mutlu N, Berry RG, Alpers BJ: Massive cerebral hemorrhage: clinical and pathological correlations. Arch Neurol 8:74, 1963

251. Myoung CL, Heany LM, Jacobson RL, Klassen AC: Cerebrospinal fluid in cerebral hemorrhage and infarction. Stroke 6:638, 1975

252. Naeser MA, Hayward RW: The resolving stroke and aphasia: a case study with computerized tomography. Arch Neurol 36:233, 1979

253. Nashold BS, Seaber JH: Defects of ocular motility after stereotactic midbrain lesions in man. Arch Ophthalmol 88:245, 1972

254. New PFJ: Computed tomography in the diagnosis of hemorrhagic stroke. p. 145. In Thompson RA, Green JR (eds): Advances in Neurology. Lippincott-Raven, Philadelphia, 1977

255. New PFJ, Aronow S: Attenuation measurements, of whole blood and blood fractions in computed tomography. Radiology 121:635, 1976

256. Norris JW, Eisen AA, Branch CL: Problems in cerebellar hemorrhage and infarction. Neurology (NY) 19:1043, 1969

257. Obeso JA, Marti-Masso JF, Carrera N, Astudillo W: Pure

motor quadriplegia secondary to bilateral capsular hematomas. Arch Neurol 37:248, 1980

258. O'Connor CM, Aldrich H, Massey EW et al: Intracranial hemorrhage after thrombolytic therapy for acute myocardial infarction: clinical characteristics and in-hospital outcome, abstracted. J Am Coll Cardiol 15:213A, 1990
259. Ojemann RG, Heros RC: Spontaneous brain hemorrhage. Stroke 14:468, 1983
260. Ojemann RG, Mohr JP: Hypertensive brain hemorrhage. Clin Neurosurg 23:220, 1976
261. Okazaki H, Reagan TJ, Campbell RJ: Clinicopathologic studies of primary cerebral amyloid angiopathy. Mayo Clin Proc 54:22, 1979
262. Okoye MI, Watanabe I: Ultrastructural features of cerebral amyloid angiopathy. Hum Pathol 13:1127, 1982
263. Okudera T, Uemura K, Nakajima K et al: Primary pontine hemorrhage: correlations of pathologic features with postmortem microangiographic and vertebral angiography studies. Mt Sinai J Med 45:305, 1978
264. O'Laoire SA, Crockard HA, Thomas DGT, Gordon DS: Brain-stem hematoma. J Neurosurg 56:222, 1982
265. Oppenheim H: Trattato della Malattie Nervose. Vol II. S.E.I., Milano, 1905
266. Ott KH, Kase CS, Ojemann RG, Mohr JP: Cerebellar hemorrhage: diagnosis and treatment. Arch Neurol 31:160, 1974
267. Pasik P, Pasik T, Bender MB: The pretectal syndrome in monkeys. I. Disturbances of gaze and body posture. Brain 92:521, 1969
268. Patel DV, Hier DB, Thomas CM, Hemmati M: Intracerebral hemorrhage secondary to cerebral amyloid angiopathy. Radiology 151:397, 1984
269. Payne HA, Maravilla KR, Levinstone A et al: Recovery from primary pontine hemorrhage. Ann Neurol 4:557, 1978
270. Pendlebury WW, Iole ED, Tracy RP, Dill BA: Intracerebral hemorrhage related to cerebral amyloid angiopathy and t-PA treatment. Ann Neurol 29:210, 1991
271. Percheron SMJ: Les artères du thalamus humain. Rev Neurol (Paris) 132:297, 1976
272. Pessin MS, Adelman LS, Prager RJ et al: "Wrong-way eyes" in supratentorial hemorrhage. Ann Neurol 9:79, 1981
273. Pessin MS, del Zoppo GJ, Estol CJ: Thrombolytic agents in the treatment of stroke. Clin Neuropharmacol 13:271, 1990
274. Piepgras U, Riger P: Thalamic bleeding: diagnosis, course and prognosis. Neuroradiology 22:85, 1981
275. Pierrott-Deseilligny C, Chain F, Serdaru M et al: The "one-and-a-half" syndrome: electro-oculographic analysis of five cases with deductions about the physiological mechanisms of lateral gaze. Brain 104:665, 1981
276. Plum F, Posner JB: The Diagnosis of Stupor and Coma. 3rd Ed. FA Davis, Philadelphia, 1980
277. Portenoy RK, Lipton RB, Berger AR et al: Intracerebral hemorrhage: a model for the prediction of outcome. J Neurol Neurosurg Psychiatry 50:976, 1987
278. Probst A, Ulrich J: Amyloid angiopathy combined with granulomatous angiitis of the central nervous system: report on two patients. Clin Neuropathol 4:250, 1985
279. Rådberg JA, Olsson JE, Rådberg CT: Prognostic parameters in spontaneous intracranial hematomas with special reference to anticoagulant treatment. Stroke 22:571, 1991
280. Regli F, Vonsattel J-P, Perentes E, Assal G: L'Angiopathie amyloïde cérébrale: une maladie cérébro-vasculaire peu connue—étude d'une observation anatomo-clinique. Rev Neurol (Paris) 137:181, 1981
281. Requena I, Arias M, Lopez-Ibor L et al: Cavernomas of the central nervous system: clinical and neuroimaging manifestations in 47 patients. J Neurol Neurosurg Psychiatry 54:590, 1991
282. Rey-Bellet J: Cerebellar hemorrhage: a clinicopathologic study. Neurology 10:217, 1960
283. Reynolds AF, Harris AB, Ojemann GA, Turner PT: Aphasia and left thalamic hemorrhage. J Neurosurg 48:570, 1978
284. Richardson A: Spontaneous intracerebral and cerebellar hemorrhage. p. 210. In Russell RWR (ed): Cerebral Arterial Disease. Churchill-Livingstone, New York, 1976
285. Richardson AE: Spontaneous cerebellar hemorrhage. p. 54. In Vinken PJ, Bruyn GW (eds): Handbook of Clinical Neurology. Vol. 12. North-Holland Publishing, Amsterdam, 1972
286. Rigamonti D, Drayer BP, Johnson PC et al: The MRI appearance of cavernous malformations (angiomas). J Neurosurg 67:518, 1987
287. Rigamonti D, Hadley MN, Drayer BP et al: Cerebral cavernous malformations: incidence and familial occurrence. N Engl J Med 319:343, 1988
288. Roberson GH, Kase CS, Wolpow ER: Telangiectases and cavernous angiomas of the brainstem: "cryptic" vascular malformations. Neuroradiology 8:83, 1974
289. Robinson RK, Richey ET, Kase CS, Mohr JP: Somatosensory evoked potentials in pure sensory stroke and related conditions. Stroke 16:818, 1985
290. Roig C, Carvajal A, Illa I et al: Hémorragies mésencephaliques isolées. Rev Neurol (Paris) 138:53, 1982
291. Ropper AH, Davis KR: Lobar cerebral hemorrhages: acute clinical syndromes in 26 cases. Ann Neurol 8:141, 1980
292. Rosenblum WI: Miliary aneurysms and "fibrinoid" degeneration of cerebral blood vessels. Hum Pathol 8:133, 1977
293. Ross ED: Localization of the pyramidal tract in the internal capsule by whole brain dissection. Neurology (NY) 30:59, 1980
294. Ross Russell RW: Observations on intracerebral aneurysms. Brain 86:425, 1963
295. Rowe CC, Donnan GA, Bladin PF: Intracerebral haemorrhage: incidence and use of computed tomography. BMJ 297:1177, 1988
296. Rumbaugh CL, Bergeron RT, Fang HCH, McCormick R: Cerebral angiographic changes in the drug abuse patient. Radiology 101:335, 1971
297. Russell DS: The pathology of spontaneous intracranial haemorrhage. Proc Soc Med 47:689, 1954
298. Sacco RL, Wolf PA, Bharucha NE et al: Subarachnoid and intracerebral hemorrhage: natural history, prognosis, and precursive factors in the Framingham Study. Neurology (NY) 34:847, 1984

299. Schnapper RA: Pontine hemorrhage presenting as ataxic hemiparesis. Stroke 13:518, 1982

300. Schott B, Laurent B, Mauguiere F, Chazot G: Négligence motrice par hématome thalamique droit. Rev Neurol (Paris) 137:447, 1981

301. Schütz H, Bödeker R-H, Damian M et al: Age-related spontaneous intracerebral hematoma in a German community. Stroke 21:1412, 1990

302. Scott M: Spontaneous intracerebral hematoma caused by cerebral neoplasms: report of eight verified cases. J Neurosurg 42:338, 1975

303. Scott WR, New PFJ, Davis KR, Schnur JA: Computerized axial tomography of intracerebral and intraventricular hemorrhage. Radiology 112:73, 1974

304. Scoville WB, Poppen JL: Intrapeduncular hemorrhage of the brain. Arch Neurol Psychiatry 61:688, 1949

305. Sharpe JA, Rosenberg MA, Hoyt WF, Daroff RB: Paralytic pontine exotropia: a sign of acute unilateral pontine gaze palsy and internuclear ophthalmoplegia. Neurology (NY) 24:1076, 1974

306. Shintaku M, Osawa K, Toki J et al: A case of granulomatous angiitis of the central nervous system associated with amyloid angiopathy. Acta Neuropathol 70:340, 1986

307. Shuangshoti S, Panyathanya R, Wichienkur P: Intracranial metastases from unsuspected choriocarcinoma: onset suggestive of cerebrovascular disease. Neurology (NY) 24:649, 1974

308. Silverstein A: Intracranial hemorrhage in patients with bleeding tendencies. Neurology (NY) 11:310, 1961

309. Silverstein A: Primary pontile hemorrhage. Conf Neurol 29:33, 1967

310. Silverstein A: Primary pontine hemorrhage. p. 37. In Vinken PJ, Bruyn GW (eds): Handbook of Clinical Neurology. Vol. 12, Part II. North-Holland Publishing, Amsterdam, 1972

311. Simard JM, Garcia-Bengochea F, Ballinger WE et al: Cavernous angioma: a review of 126 collected and 12 new clinical cases. Neurosurgery 18:162, 1986

312. Sloan MA, Price TR, Petito CK et al: Clinical features and pathogenesis of intracerebral hemorrhage after rt-PA and heparin therapy for acute myocardial infarction: the Thrombolysis in Myocardial Infarction (TIMI) II pilot and randomized clinical trial combined experience. Neurology 45:649, 1995

313. Smith DB, Hitchcock M, Philpott PJ: Cerebral amyloid angiopathy presenting as transient ischemic attacks: case report. J Neurosurg 63:963, 1985

314. Snyder M, Renaudin J: Intracranial hemorrhage associated with anticoagulation therapy. Surg Neurol 7:31, 1977

315. Stahl SM, Johnson KP, Malamud N: The clinical and pathological spectrum of brainstem vascular malformations: long-term course simulates multiple sclerosis. Arch Neurol 37:25, 1980

316. Starr M: Cerebellar apoplexy. Med Rec 69:743, 1906

317. Steegmann AT: Primary pontile hemorrhage. J Nerv Ment Dis 114:35, 1951

318. Steering Committee of the Physicians' Health Study Research Group: Final report on the aspirin component of the ongoing Physicians' Health Study. N Engl J Med 321:129, 1989

319. Stehbens WE: Pathology of the Cerebral Blood Vessels. CV Mosby, St. Louis, 1972

320. Stein RW, Kase CS, Hier DB et al: Caudate hemorrhage. Neurology (NY) 34:1549, 1984

321. Steiner I, Gomori JM, Melamed E: The prognostic value of the CT scan in conservatively treated patients with intracerebral hematoma. Stroke 15:279, 1984

322. Stephen R, Stillwell D: Arteries and Veins of the Human Brain. Charles C Thomas, Springfield, IL, 1969

323. Stoessl AJ, Young GB, Feasby TE: Intracerebral haemorrhage and angiographic beading following ingestion of catecholaminergics. Stroke 16:734, 1985

324. Stroke Prevention in Atrial Fibrillation Investigators: Warfarin versus aspirin for prevention of thromboembolism in atrial fibrillation. Lancet 343:687, 1994

325. Sung C-Y, Chu N-S: Epileptic seizures in intracerebral hemorrhage. J Neurol Neurosurg Psychiatry 52:1273, 1989

326. Susac JO, Hoyt WF, Daroff RB, Lawrence W: Clinical spectrum of ocular bobbing. J Neurol Neurosurg Psychiatry 33:771, 1970

327. Tagle P, Huete I, Méndez J et al: Intracranial cavernous angioma: presentation and management. J Neurosurg 64:720, 1986

328. Tanaka H, Ueda Y, Date C et al: Incidence of stroke in Shibata, Japan, 1976–1978. Stroke 12:460, 1981

329. Tapia JF, Golden JA: Case records of the Massachusetts General Hospital (Case 27-1993). N Engl J Med 329:117, 1993

330. Tapia JF, Kase CS, Sawyer RH, Mohr JP: Hypertensive putaminal hemorrhage presenting as pure motor hemiparesis. Stroke 14:505, 1983

331. Taveras JM, Wood EH: Diagnostic Neuroradiology. 2nd Ed. Vol. 2. p. 1018. Williams & Wilkins, Baltimore, 1976

332. The American-Canadian Co-Operative Study Group: Persantine aspirin trial in cerebral ischemia. Part II: Endpoint results. Stroke 16:406, 1985

333. The ESPS Group: The European stroke prevention study (ESPS): principal end-points. Lancet 2:1351, 1987

334. The Multicenter Acute Stroke Trial—Europe Study Group: Thrombolytic therapy with streptokinase in acute ischemic stroke. N Engl J Med 335:145, 1996

335. The National Institute of Neurological Disorders and Stroke rt-PA Stroke Study Group: Tissue plasminogen activator for acute ischemic stroke. N Engl J Med 333:1581, 1995

336. The SALT Collaborative Group: Swedish aspirin low-dose trial (SALT) of 75 mg aspirin as secondary prophylaxis after cerebrovascular ischaemic events. Lancet 338:1345, 1991

336a.The Stroke Prevention In Reversible Ischemia Trial (SPIRIT) Study Group: A randomized trial of anticoagulants versus aspirin after cerebral ischemia of presumed arterial origin. Ann Neurol 42:857, 1997

337. Thulborn KR, Sorensen AG, Kowall NW et al: The role of ferritin and hemosiderin in the MR appearance of cerebral hemorrhage: a histopathologic biochemical study in rats. AJNR 11:291, 1990

338. Thyne W: A case of cerebellar hemorrhage presenting with well marked opisthotonus and Kernig sign. Lancet 79:397, 1901

339. TIMI Study Group: Comparison of invasive and conservative strategies after treatment with intravenous tissue plasminogen activator in acute myocardial infarction: results of the Thrombolysis in Myocardial Infarction (TIMI) phase II trial. N Engl J Med 320:618, 1989

340. Tomonaga M: Cerebral amyloid angiopathy in the elderly. J Am Geriatr Soc 29:151, 1981

341. Toole JF, Patel AN: Cerebrovascular Disorders. 2nd Ed. p. 335. McGraw-Hill, New York, 1967

342. Tuhrim S, Dambrosia JM, Price TR et al: Prediction of intracerebral hemorrhage survival. Ann Neurol 24:258, 1988

343. Tuhrim S, Yang WC, Rubinowitz H, Weinberger J: Primary pontine hemorrhage and the dysarthria clumsy hand syndrome. Neurology (NY) 32:1027, 1982

344. Toffol GJ, Biller J, Adams HP: Nontraumatic intracerebral hemorrhage in young adults. Arch Neurol 44:483, 1987

345. Tyler HR, Johnson PC: Case records of the Massachusetts General Hospital (Case 36-1972). N Engl J Med 287:506, 1972

346. Tyler KL, Poletti CE, Heros RC: Cerebral amyloid angiopathy with multiple intracerebral hemorrhages. J Neurosurg 57:286, 1982

347. Ueda K, Omae T, Hirota Y et al: Decreasing trend in incidence and mortality from stroke in Hisayama residents, Japan. Stroke 12:154, 1981

348. Ueshima H, Iida M, Shimamoto T et al: Multivariate analysis of risk factors for stroke: eight-year follow-up of farming villages in Akita, Japan. Prevent Med 9:722, 1980

349. UK-TIA Study Group: United Kingdom transient ischaemic attack (UK-TIA) aspirin trial: interim results. BMJ 296:316, 1988

350. Valenstein E, Heilman KM: Unilateral hypokinesia and motor extinction. Neurology (NY) 31:445, 1981

351. Vaquero J, Salazar J, Martínez R et al: Cavernomas of the central nervous system: clinical syndromes, CT scan diagnosis, and prognosis after treatment in 25 cases. Acta Neurochir 85:29, 1987

352. Vaughan HG, Howard RG: Intracranial hemorrhage due to metastatic chorionepithelioma. Neurology (NY) 12:771, 1962

353. Vinters HV: Cerebral amyloid angiopathy: a critical review. Stroke 18:311, 1987

354. Vinters HV, Gilbert JJ: Cerebral amyloid angiopathy: incidence and complications in the aging brain. II. The distribution of amyloid vascular changes. Stroke 14:924, 1983

355. Vonsattel JPG, Myers RH, Hedley-Whyte ET et al: Cerebral amyloid angiopathy without and with cerebral hemorrhages: a comparative histological study. Ann Neurol 30:637, 1991

356. Waga S, Okada M, Yamamoto Y: Reversibility of Parinaud syndrome in thalamic hemorrhage. Neurology (NY) 29:407, 1979

357. Wagle WA, Smith TW, Weiner M: Intracerebral hemorrhage caused by cerebral amyloid angiopathy: radiographic pathologic correlation. AJNR 5:171, 1984

358. Wakai S, Yamakawa K, Manaka S, Takakura K: Spontaneous intracranial hemorrhage caused by brain tumors: its incidence and clinical significance. Neurosurgery 10:437, 1982

359. Wakai S, Ueda Y, Inoh S et al: Angiographically occult angiomas: a report of thirteen cases with analysis of the cases documented in the literature. Neurosurgery 17:549, 1985

360. Walsh FB, Hoyt WK: Clinical Neuro-ophthalmology. 3rd Ed. p. 1786. Williams & Wilkins, Baltimore, 1969

361. Walshe TM, Davis KR, Fisher CM: Thalamic hemorrhage: a computed tomographic-clinical correlation. Neurology (NY) 27:217, 1977

362. Watson RT, Heilman KM: Thalamic neglect. Neurology (NY) 29:690, 1979

363. Wattendorff AR, Bots GTAM, Went LN, Endtz LJ: Familial cerebral amyloid angiopathy presenting as recurrent cerebral haemorrhage. J Neurol Sci 55:121, 1982

364. Weber M, Vespignani H, Bracard S et al: Les angiomes caverneux intracérébraux. Rev Neurol 145:429, 1989

365. Weintraub MI, Glaser GH: Nocardial brain abscess and pure motor hemiplegia. NY State J Med 70:2717, 1970

366. Weisberg L: Multiple spontaneous intracerebral hematomas: clinical and computed tomographic correlations. Neurology (NY) 31:897, 1981

367. Weisberg LA: Caudate hemorrhage. Arch Neurol 41:971, 1984

368. Weisberg LA: Computerized tomography in intracranial hemorrhage. Arch Neurol 36:422, 1979

369. Weisberg LA: Subcortical lobar intracerebral haemorrhage: clinical-computed tomographic correlations. J Neurol Neurosurg Psychiatry 48:1078, 1985

370. Weisberg LA: Significance of the fluid-blood interface in intracranial hematomas in anticoagulated patients. Comput Radiol 11:175, 1987

371. Whisnant JP, Cartlidge NEF, Elveback LR: Carotid and vertebral-basilar transient ischemic attacks: effect of anticoagulants, hypertension, and cardiac disorders on survival and stroke occurrence in a population study. Ann Neurol 3:107, 1978

372. Wiggins WS, Moody DM, Toole JF et al: Clinical and computerized tomographic study of hypertensive intracerebral hemorrhage. Arch Neurol 35:832, 1978

373. Wijdicks EFM, Jack CR: Intracerebral hemorrhage after fibrinolytic therapy for acute myocardial infarction. Stroke 24:554, 1993

374. Wilkins RH, Brody IA: The thalamic syndrome (Neurological Classics 18). Arch Neurol 20:559, 1969

375. Wintzen AR, de Jonge H, Loeliger EA, Bots GTAM: The risk of intracerebral hemorrhage during oral anticoagulant treatment: a population study. Ann Neurol 16:553, 1984

376. Wolpert SM, Bruckmann H, Greenlee R et al: Neuroradiologic evaluation of patients with acute stroke treated with recombinant tissue plasminogen activator: the rt-PA Acute Stroke Study Group. AJNR 14:3, 1993

377. Yamasaki T, Handa H, Yamashita J et al: Intracranial and orbital cavernous angiomas: a review of 30 cases. J Neurosurg 64:197, 1986

378. Yoshida 5, Sasaki M, Oka H et al: Acute hypertensive cerebellar hemorrhage with signs of lower brainstem compression. Surg Neurol 10:79, 1978

379. Yu YJ, Cooper DR, Wellenstein DE, Block B: Cerebral angiitis and intracerebral hemorrhage associated with methamphetamine abuse. J Neurosurg 58:109, 1983

380. Zilkha A: Intraparenchymal fluid-blood level: a CT sign of recent intracerebral hemorrhage. J Comput Assist Tomogr 7:301, 1987

381. Zimmerman RD, Leeds NE, Naidich TP: Ring blush associated with intracerebral hematoma. Radiology 122:707, 1977

382. Zimmerman RS, Spetzler RF, Lee KS et al: Cavernous malformations of the brain stem. J Neurosurg 75:32, 1991

383. Zuccarello M, Iavicoli R, Pardatscher K et al: Primary brain stem hematomas, diagnosis and treatment. Acta Neurochir 54:45, 1980

384. Zülch KJ: Neuropathology of intracranial haemorrhage. Prog Brain Res 30:151, 1968

385. Zyed A, Hayman LA, Bryan RN: MR imaging of intracerebral blood: diversity in the temporal pattern at 0.5 and 1.0 T. AJNR 12:469, 1991

Intracranial Aneurysms

J. P. MOHR*

J. PHILIP KISTLER†

Epidemiology

Rupture of an intracranial saccular aneurysm is the most common cause of subarachnoid hemorrhage, exceeding that of ruptures from such as mycotic or myxomatous aneurysms, from other anomalies, or from arteriovenous malformations. Some 80% of nontraumatic subarachnoid hemorrhages are a result of aneurysmal rupture.[126] Although often described as subarachnoid hemorrhage, aneurysmal rupture can also affect the brain substance, the ventricular system, or the subdural space.[21,122,131,159,185,190]

Clinically, the incidence of ruptured aneurysms has ranged from as low as 3.9/100,000/year,[157] a median value of 11/100,000/year,[160] to as high as 17.5[150] to 19.4/100,000/year.[69] Of all strokes entered in the Harvard Cooperative Stroke Registry between 1972 and 1976, subarachnoid hemorrhage from ruptured saccular aneurysm accounted for 6%.[192] In 1981, the Cooperative study estimated the incidence in the United States at 26,000 cases per year,[176] a higher figure than the 20,000 figure cited by Sypert in 1978, who estimated that 400,000 adults in the U.S. harbor unruptured aneurysms, and that every year 5% of these people undergo a major neurologic catastrophe.[211] The peak age for aneurysm rupture is between 55 and 60 years of age.[177] Intracranial aneurysms are somewhat uncommon in children or young adults as revealed by angiogram or postmortem examination. In this group, bleeding from an arteriovenous malformation (AVM) is the more common cause (Fig. 26.1). There seems to be a constancy in the incidence of aneurysmal rupture.[232] This point seems supported by the most recent such study, a 1996 population-based study from Canada, which showed an age-adjusted incidence rate of 7.2/100,000/year (6.2 for men, 8.1 for women) with a mean age of rupture of 46.6 years.[115]

Although the incidence of other forms of stroke and generalized cardiovascular disease appears to be declining, subarachnoid hemorrhage is apparently not following this pattern.[145] Pregnancy seems to increase the risk of subarachnoid hemorrhage, aneurysms predominating over arteriovenous malformations.[171] Intracranial aneurysmal rupture is often cited as a factor in 12% to 25% of maternal deaths, one series reporting it as contributing to 80% of maternal mortality.[81]

PREVALENCE

The true prevalence of intracranial aneurysms remains difficult to ascertain. From autopsy studies roughly 5% of the population is thought to harbor one or more aneurysms.[38,40,43,92,103,204,221,225] No agreement has been reached about the size at which an arterial defect should be designated an aneurysm. McCormick and Acosta-Rua demonstrated that manual perfusion of unruptured aneurysms with saline under a pressure of 70 mmHg caused the size to increase by 30% to 60%,[120] a finding that indicates many smaller aneurysms may be overlooked at autopsy. If aneurysms as small as 2 mm are considered, 17% of routine autopsies reveal an unruptured intracranial aneurysm.[84] If only those lesions larger than 3 mm are included, the incidence in autopsy series will still be less than 4%.[200] Magnetic resonance (MR) scanning is providing a new data base: an eastern Finland study of 21 of 91 families selected randomly from this stable population found 11 of 110 members studied harbored 16 asymptomatic aneurysms, the highest incidence thus far reported.[173]

FATALITY RATE

The fatality rate in aneurysmal rupture remains high. Since many of the studies of subarachnoid hemorrhage are from referral institutions, the referral bias to those surviving the

---

* Supported in part by a gift from the Horace W. Goldsmith Foundation.

† Supported in part by the Eliot B. Shoolman Fund and by Vera and J. W. Gilliland.

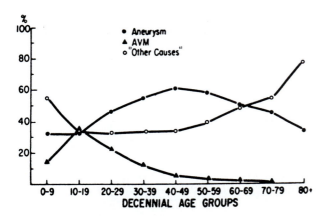

Figure 26.1 Relative probability of major causes of subarachnoid hemorrhage in each decade of life. AVM, arteriovenous malformation. (From Sahs et al,[177] with permission.)

reported to die within the first 3 months. Those entering a hospital with a giant aneurysm or with a neurologic deficit have a particularly bad outcome.[57]

DISABILITY

Beyond the issue of case fatality is *disability*. For more than half of the survivors, it is major. Moreover, fully 64% of those patients well enough to be discharged home after neurosurgical obliteration of the aneurysm never achieve the quality of life they enjoyed before the rupture.[174]

Anatomy and Histopathology

initial rupture may lead to a falsely low reporting rate. In the 1980 population study of south Alabama, Mohr and Kase[132] found an incidence of death above 50%, much of it early in the course (Fig. 26.2), when those diagnosed within 24 hours of rupture were also included. In some locations rates have been as high as 68%.[128] Between 45% and 49%[69] have been

Cerebral aneurysms are classified as saccular, mycotic, traumatic, dissecting, neoplastic, and arteriosclerotic. We use the term *saccular aneurysm* to include all arterial outpouchings of an unknown origin that are not associated with inflammation or tumor, and reserve the term arteriosclerotic aneurysm for the unusual, tortuous, dolichoectatic aneurysm that is asso-

Figure 26.2 Course of acute subarachnoid hemorrhage in a population study. (From Mohr and Kase,[132] with permission.)

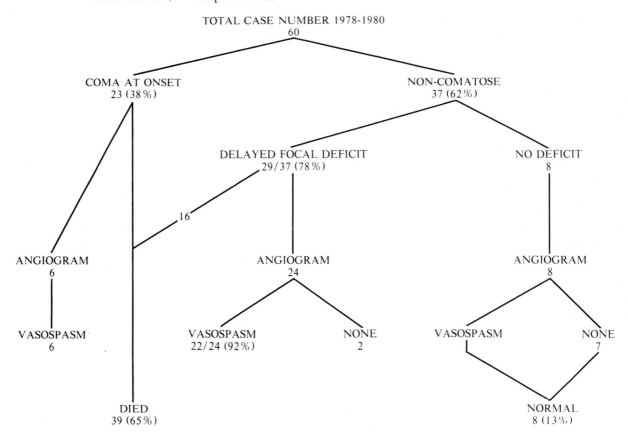

ciated with severe, widespread, atheromatous vascular disease.

SACCULAR ANEURYSMS

Saccular aneurysms most frequently occur at the bifurcations of the large arteries at the base of the brain and rupture into the subarachnoid space of the basal cisterns (Fig. 26.3). Approximately 85% occur in the anterior circulation,[151,152] the usual sites being the junction of the anterior communicating artery with the anterior cerebral artery, the junction of the posterior communicating artery with the internal carotid, and the bifurcation of the middle cerebral artery. In the posterior fossa, the favored sites are the top of the basilar; the junction of the basilar artery and the superior cerebellar artery; or the anterior, inferior cerebellar artery or the junction of the vertebral artery and the posterior inferior cerebellar artery.[91] Of these saccular aneurysms, 12% to 31% are multiple,[179] particularly in mirror locations (9% to 19%).[191]

The pathogenesis of cerebral aneurysms remains controversial[38] but can be condensed to three major hypotheses. The most popular theory is that aneurysms arise from congenital defects in the muscular layer of the cerebral arteries.[22,40,70] A second theory suggests that degenerative changes within the vessel wall eventually result in damage to the internal elastic membrane, creating a local weakness that allows formation of an aneurysm.[77,200,201,204] The third postulates that aneurysms are never a result of developmental deficiencies or

Figure 26.3 A drawing of the arteries at the base of the brain showing the location of 429 saccular aneurysms in 316 consecutive patients with aneurysms on an autopsy service. Approximately 90 percent of the aneurysms occur on the anterior cerebral circulation. Aneurysms are slightly more common on the right side of the intracranial vessels than on the left for reasons that are not apparent. (From McCormick,[119a] with permission.)

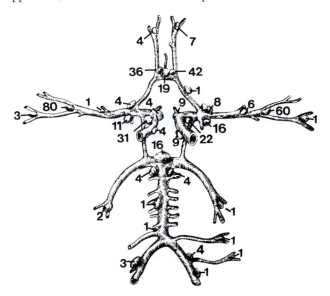

degenerative changes alone, but are always due to the combined effects of these two processes.[32,185]

Aneurysms typically grow out from a base on the arterial wall at the point of a bifurcation, forming a neck with a dome on top.[187] The thickness and length of this neck and the size of the dome vary greatly, making the surgeon's task in approaching each lesion difficult. An internal elastic lamina is not found at the origin of the neck. The normal vascular media is thin and smooth muscle cells are replaced by collagenous connective tissue. At the site of rupture, most often thought to be the dome, the wall may be thinner than 0.3 mm. Although it is easy to imagine that the dome is the site of rupture, rare instances have been reported where the site of rupture was actually at the base.[66] In this case, a small fibrin-filled gap measuring 0.5×0.14 mm marked the site of rupture. Although small, it allowed enough blood to escape into the subarachnoid space to engulf the middle cerebral artery stem and the A1 segment of the anterior cerebral artery. This rupture site was on the neck proximal to the usual site of clip placement. This case could explain how some aneurysms rupture after what seemed to be successful clipping. Studies of the wall pressure at the base of an aneurysm have shown it to be more than twice normal.[20]

What form the defects in the media take is still unclear.[187] Small gaps in the musculature of the media at the points of bifurcation of the cerebral vessels of the circle of Willis were first reported by Forbus in 1930.[70] He postulated that these defects were an important factor in the development of noninflammatory aneurysms. In 1940, Glynn[77] found these "medial defects" in 80% of the bifurcations of cerebral arteries in both aneurysmal and control cases. After observing that vessels with an intact internal elastic membrane tolerated pressures in excess of 600 mmHg without deformity, he concluded that degeneration of the elastic layer was crucial to the genesis of cerebral aneurysms. Glynn suggested that the greater frequency with which aneurysms occur in the arteries of the circle of Willis was probably due to a difference in the elastic tissue. The most readily detected difference is one of position: In the cerebral vessel the elastic tissue is concentrated in the internal elastic lamina. By virtue of its position it was probably more susceptible to injury and degeneration than if it were more widely distributed through the media and adventitia as in other vessels.

In 1963, Stehbens[201] reported studies differentiating the congenital medial defects described by Forbus from those lesions that develop later, apparently on a degenerative basis: funnel-shaped dilatations, areas of thinning, and small outpouchings that probably signify the first stages of aneurysmal formation were described at vessel forks. Severe histologic degenerative changes and fragmentation of the internal elastic lamina were apparent at these points of thinning and evagination, and were thought the result of hemodynamic stress. He supported the hypothesis that aneurysms result from acquired degenerative processes. In 1975, in an electron microscopic examination of five cerebral aneurysms, three preaneurysmal lesions, and three AVMs,[204] he observed that these vascular lesions were remarkably similar to one another and also to the degenerative changes he had previously described in experimental AVMs. Since aneurysmal dilatation and degenerative changes can be induced hemodynamically,[202,203] he reasoned that hemodynamic stress plays a major role in the development of cerebral aneurysms. Hydrodynamic studies using both rigid and elastic models have also demonstrated that the greatest point of stress in the vasculature occurs at the forks of arterial branches.[70,84]

Hereditary factors may also play a role, especially a familial occurrence which suggests genetic factors in the development of these defects.[2,19,27,80] Infundibular widening at the origin of the posterior cerebral artery was documented in 8 of 11 members of one family, 5 of whom also developed frank saccular aneurysms.[59] Aneurysms have been reported at the same site in twins.[32,61,80,148] Intracranial aneurysms are also commonly associated with certain congenital malformations such as polycystic kidneys,[50] AVMs,[14,164,208] moyamoya disease,[138] coarctation of the aorta,[121] Ehlers-Danlos syndrome,[15,79,175] fibromuscular hyperplasia,[23,236] and possibly other connective tissue diseases.[123,158] Certain arterial anomalies of the circle of Willis are also more frequently found in patients harboring aneurysms. The most commonly encountered anomaly is hypoplasia of one or both proximal anterior cerebral arteries in association with an anterior cerebral aneurysm. Of these various associations, only those for polycystic kidney disease, coarctation of the aorta, and fibromuscular hyperplasia are known to be statistically significant. However, since each of these disorders may present with early onset of hypertension, there is reason to question whether the pathogenesis for the increased occurrence of cerebral aneurysms is a function of hereditary or congenital factors or hypertensive degeneration.

The role of systemic arterial hypertension in the genesis of intracranial aneurysms or in their subsequent rupture remains unsettled. While many authors[29,56–58] have favored a role for hypertension, others disagree.[122] Andrews and Spiegel found that hypertension was not significantly more prevalent in the aneurysm population than in the age-matched general population, except for females under 55 years of age.[15]

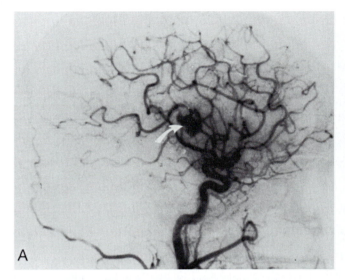

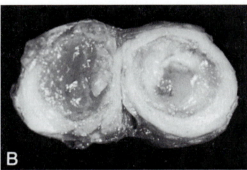

Figure 26.4 Angiographic (**A**) and gross pathologic (**B**) appearance of mycotic middle cerebral artery in a middle-aged male who presented with signs and symptoms of subacute bacterial endocarditis, fever, chills, and grade V/VI holosystolic murmur.

ARTERIOSCLEROTIC ANEURYSMS

These lesions, rather large (hence their name, dolichoectatic), occur most frequently along the basilar artery, but are also found in the internal carotid, middle cerebral, and anterior cerebral arteries.[74] The affected artery is tortuous, widened, and elongated and causes symptoms from compression, embolic phenomenon, or the obstruction of cerebrospinal fluid pathways. Subarachnoid hemorrhage is an uncommon presentation. Arteriosclerosis and hypertension are unquestionably of paramount importance in the etiology of these aneurysms, as they occur almost entirely in patients who have widespread arteriosclerotic disease.

MYCOTIC ANEURYSMS

Mycotic aneurysms typically are located in the distal cerebral circulation as might be expected from their microembolic origin (Fig. 26.4A,B). They may be caused by extension of infection from emboli lodged in the arterial lumen, bacterial embolism of the vasa vasorum, or a combination of these two factors.[137,145,192] Once established, the infective process leads to septic degeneration of the elastic lamina and muscular coats of the vessel wall with resultant rupture and subarachnoid hemorrhage.

They constitute approximately 5% of all cerebral aneurysms, primarily as a complication of subacute bacterial endocarditis (SBE), obvious clinically or occult, and from natural or artificial valve surfaces. Some 15% to 20% of all mycotic aneurysms are in the brain, ranking below only the aorta and its major abdominal and peripheral branches.[192] For patients with bacterial endocarditis, about 17% have been reported to have symptoms of cerebral embolization,[39,83] and mycotic cerebral aneurysms are demonstrated in approximately 4%.[135]

Angiography has been recommended for all patients with embolic symptoms to identify aneurysms prior to the occurrence of subarachnoid hemorrhage, but this policy has never been widely adopted. Those who harbor an aneurysm can be treated with high doses of the appropriate antibiotic and the aneurysm followed with repeat angiograms. If the aneurysm thromboses, no further treatment is necessary. However, if it enlarges, it should be clipped.[137]

DISSECTING ANEURYSMS

Dissecting intracranial aneurysms were once believed to be quite rare and are included here only because of the name "aneurysm." Prior to 1960 there was a total of only 10 pathologically verified cases in the world's literature. In recent years, there has been a great increase in the number of case reports, sufficient to justify its own chapter in this book (see Ch. 29).

TRAUMATIC ANEURYSMS

True traumatic intracranial aneurysms are rare. Aneurysms of the meningeal vessels and false aneurysms have also been reported as a complication of major head trauma. When trauma produces disruption of an artery, a hematoma forms around it, producing a false aneurysm. When, however, only the internal elastic lamina is damaged, the intima may herniate through this defect, producing a true aneurysm. Mixed types may also occur. Traumatic intracranial aneurysms occur most commonly on the internal carotid artery, the middle cerebral artery in relation to bony fractures and penetrating trauma, and the anterior cerebral artery in relation to the falx. Rupture resulting in death occurs in 50% of the reported cases, suggesting that operative management, when clinically feasible, is the therapy of choice (Fig. 26.5).[25,179]

NEOPLASTIC ANEURYSMS

Emboli from an atrial myxoma may lodge in cerebral arteries, invade the arterial wall, and lead to the formation of a neoplastic aneurysm. Cardiac myxomas are benign intracavitary tumors, constituting about 50% of primary cardiac tumors. Approximately 75% of these tumors arise in the left atrium. Systemic emboli have been reported in up to 45% of patients with this tumor type, and about one-half of these are cerebral. Angiographic abnormalities include irregular filling defects in major and minor cerebral artery branches, fusiform and saccular aneurysms, and occlusion of vessels[142] (Fig. 26.6). Tumor emboli apparently remain viable, and can penetrate the endothelium at the site of lodgement, grow subintimally, and eventually infiltrate and destroy the arterial wall.[142]

MULTIPLE AND INCIDENTAL ANEURYSMS

Unruptured multiple aneurysms may occur in up to 13% of cases.[179] The incidental aneurysms are at risk of rupture. This risk seems to be in the range of 1% to 3% per year for each year of survival.[87] While it would appear that aneurysms under 5 mm in diameter are at lower risk for subsequent rupture,[111,120] it is not possible to separate angiographically or clinically those lesions that will remain stable from those that will continue to grow or rupture spontaneously, with devastating consequences to the patient.[5] The operative risks for the elective surgical management of unruptured aneurysms are extremely favorable. Usually there is no mortality and little operative morbidity.

GIANT ANEURYSMS

The term *giant aneurysm* refers here to lesions exceeding 25 mm in greatest diameter. This coincides with the largest size (group 5) in the Cooperative study.[111] In the literature lesions of this size make up about 5% of all intracranial aneurysms, and are unusual in that most (approximately 80%) present with symptoms of mass effect or embolic phenomenon rather than subarachnoid hemorrhage.[136] Giant aneurysms often have such a wide neck and/or become so large that obliteration of the sac becomes impossible (Fig. 26.7A,B). Furthermore, in some cases, calcifications and partial thrombosis make mobilization of these aneurysms extremely hazardous. Despite advances in anesthesia and the development of microsurgical techniques, the risk of dealing directly with giant intracranial aneurysms remains high.[154] The surgical management of these aneurysms presents special problems that will be discussed at length in the section on operative treatment.

Natural History

UNRUPTURED ANEURYSMS

There is relatively little information available to determine the possibility of an asymptomatic aneurysm rupturing in the future. Data from a small number of patients in the Cooperative study[111] and from 65 patients with unruptured aneurysm from the Mayo Clinic[207] suggest that aneurysmal size is the only important variable associated with subsequent rupture. In the 65 patients with unruptured aneurysms followed at the Mayo Clinic, 8 of 29 aneurysms larger than 1 cm ruptured, whereas none of 44 aneurysms 1 smaller than 1 cm ruptured over a mean follow-up interval of 98.5 months. This set of observations still holds. Microsurgical obliteration of asymptomatic aneurysms larger than 7 mm remains a common plan.[152]

SUBARACHNOID HEMORRHAGE

Save for the benefits from early surgery, ample data indicate a high death rate in the week following subarachnoid hemorrhage. The Cooperative study indicated the mortality rate during the first week after subarachnoid hemorrhage could be as high as 27%.[111] Three patient groups have been defined: (1) a high-risk group of 9% of the population, whose average survival after the first subarachnoid hemorrhage is 18 hours; (2) an intermediate group of 47% of the population, whose average survival is about 2 weeks; and (3) a "low-risk" group of 43% of the population, who tolerate the initial hemorrhage quite well and appear to have a low

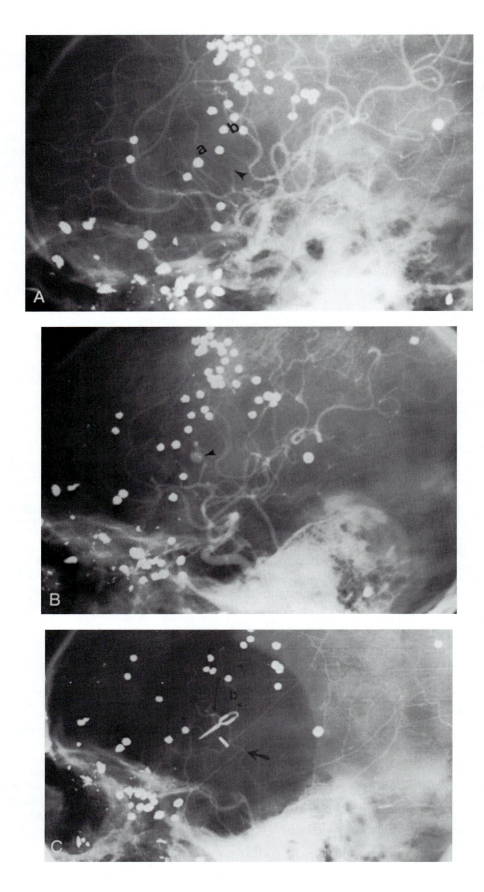

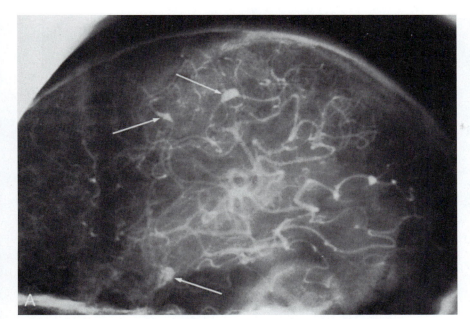

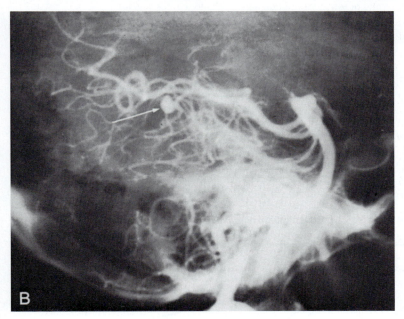

Figure 26.6 (A) Internal carotid artery and (B) posterior cerebral artery angiograms demonstrating multiple neoplastic aneurysms in a 30-year-old female who presented with a history of transient cerebral ischemic events. Echocardiogram demonstrated a large atrial myxoma, which was surgically removed.

Figure 26.5 A 20-year-old patient was hospitalized after sustaining a close-range shotgun blast to the left side of the face. (A) Left common carotid artery angiogram demonstrated spasm (*arrowhead*) at the location where an aneurysm was later demonstrated to arise. The two vessels irrigated by that branch of the middle cerebral artery are labeled *a* and *b*. (B) Repeat common carotid artery angiogram 5 days after the initial study reveals an aneurysm (*arrowhead*). (C) A left external carotid artery angiogram 2 weeks after clipping of the traumatic aneurysm. Obliteration of the aneurysm. Obliteration of the aneurysm necessitated occlusion of the parent vessel. Therefore, the superficial temporal artery (*arrow*) was anastomosed to a distal cortical segment of the occluded artery to ensure adequate arterial flow. The site of anastomosis (*arrow*) and perfusion of middle cerebral artery vessels *a* and *b* via the bypass are demonstrated. (From Spetzler and Owen,[199] with permission.)

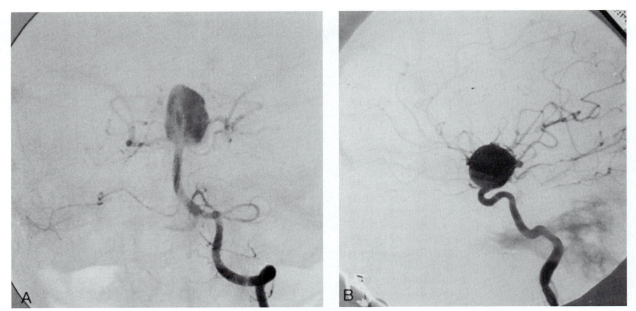

Figure 26.7 (**A**) Anteroposterior view of left vertebral angiogram demonstrates a giant aneurysm of the basilar artery. (**B**) Lateral view of internal carotid artery angiogram showing a giant aneurysm in the same patient.

Figure 26.8 Survival rates of patients admitted at varying intervals after their initial subarachnoid hemorrhage (conservative medical therapy). Note that the curves all parallel each other. In effect, one can restart the natural history by raising the probability of survival to 100 percent at the time of observation, and allowing the patients' probability of future survival to fall parallel with the original line. (From Alvord et al,[13] with permission.)

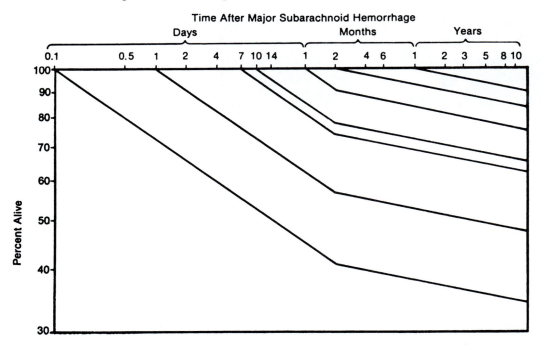

rate of subsequent late hemorrhage. Roughly 90% of the patients dying within 72 hours of hemorrhage harbor an associated intracerebral, intracerebellar, or subdural hematoma and are the more severely affected. These depressing rates have been only slightly improved upon from series reported from the early 1980s, when 3% to 5% died for delayed surgery in the group with the best preoperative clinical state versus 21% to 25% for those in the worst.[97]

Rebleeding is a major cause of morbidity and mortality in the untreated patient. The risk of rebleeding within 1 month is approximately 33%, and the mortality rate from this second hemorrhage is 42%.[111] The risk is greatest between the fifth and ninth days, with 22% of all rebleeding episodes occurring within the first 2 weeks after hemorrhage. Contrast leakage during angiography is thought to be an especially grave prognostic sign.[237] The risk of rebleeding diminishes after the first month but is never gone. Long-term survivors suffer a 3% annual hemorrhage risk.[275]

In the days before early surgery, Alvord and colleagues calculated the probabilities of future survival[13] in their analysis of the natural history of this disease (Fig. 26.8). The parallel curves in Figure 26.8 mathematically define the expected survival for groups of patients (all grades) admitted to study at particular times after subarachnoid hemorrhage. To define the probability of survival for patients of a specific clinical grade, the authors applied the percentages of survival reported for conservative treatment in each of the clinical grades used by the Cooperative study group; proportionately, a grade 1 patient who has survived only 1 day after rupture has by this calculation only a 65% probability of surviving for the same period. The particular advantage of an analysis such as this is that it readily permits the comparison of various reports in the literature and allows a physician to evaluate the results of his own medical or surgical treatments. Obviously, any new therapy would have to improve on these survival probabilities to be justified.

BRAIN INFARCTION

Uncommonly, thrombosis may occur in an aneurysm with extension into nearby healthy vessels. This was the case of Brownlee et al, who had a patient with an anterior communicating artery aneurysm that thrombosed, extending thrombus into each adjacent anterior cerebral artery trunk with infarction. The thrombus was confirmed by autopsy.[34] Infarction with vasospasm, a separate subject, is described below.

Prodromal Symptoms of Aneurysmal Rupture

ENLARGING ANEURYSM

Surgery is increasingly being recommended if there is clinical evidence that a saccular aneurysm is enlarging.[151,152] The onset of a third nerve palsy, particularly when associated with pupillary dilatation and loss of light reflex, is highly suggestive

of an expanding aneurysm at the junction of the posterior communicating artery and the distal internal carotid artery. The motor palsy of the lid and extraocular muscles may precede pupillary dilatation and loss of light and accommodation reflexes. In some instances aneurysmal dilatation thus mimics diabetic third nerve palsy.[50] A mass large enough to cause retrobulbar optic atrophy has been described, initially diagnosed as idiopathic retrobulbar neuritis.[125]

Facial pain or pain around the eye is another possible indication of an expanding aneurysm. In 74 cases of prospectively studied[195] expanding unruptured posterior communicating aneurysms, painful third nerve palsy occurred in 59. The pain typically occurred above the brow and radiated back to the ear. It occurred in episodes of increasing intensity. With each attack of pain the incidence of rupture increased. Without a third nerve palsy, up to seven attacks of pain occurred before rupture in their series. When a third nerve palsy was present, however, no more than three attacks of pain occurred before rupture. In order for a third nerve palsy to occur, the aneurysm at the origin of the posterior communicating artery has to be 7 mm in size. If the third nerve palsy is present for more than 10 days, its chances of recovering are remote.[195]

Other cranial nerve palsies suggesting aneurysmal expansion include sixth nerve palsy in giant cavernous aneurysms and visual field defects of an expanding supraclinoid carotid aneurysm. In some cases focal headache involves the occipital and posterior cervical region when a posterior inferior cerebellar artery (PICA) or anterior/inferior cerebellar artery (AICA) aneurysm expands. Pain in or behind the eye and in the low temple can occur with middle cerebral aneurysm expansion. These complaints may also indicate arterial dissection and are not unique for aneurysm.

WARNING LEAKS

Warning leaks of an aneurysm may cause focal frontal or occipital headache and stiff neck. Sudden headache with pain between the shoulder blades or at the back of the neck accompanied by nausea and vomiting is among the important symptoms. While these are often confused with migrainous headaches, patients usually state that they differ from their usual migraine headache. Computed tomography (CT) or MR scan may be of diagnostic value without contrast to show blood in the subarachnoid space, after which contrast may show filling of the aneurysm. More often than not, however, the amount of blood from a warning leak will not be sufficient to be identified by either form of scan.

When suspicion of a warning leak arises and the patient has no focal neurologic signs that might indicate a mass effect, lumbar puncture is a safe and effective means of making the diagnosis. This should be done any time suspicion of a warning leak arises because of the devastating effects of major aneurysmal rupture. Auer[17] found that half of his patients with major hemorrhage (52 of 238, or 22%) had warning leaks. A variety of syndromes have been described.[4,101,119,153,225]

Subarachnoid Hemorrhage

INITIAL CLINICAL PRESENTATION

At the moment of aneurysmal rupture, intracranial pressure approaches the mean arterial pressure and cerebral perfusion pressure falls.[146] This sudden surge in pressure and intracranial volume may account for the sudden but transient loss of consciousness which occurs in 45% of cases. Whereas a brief moment of excruciating headache may occur just before loss of consciousness, the headache is usually reported upon regaining consciousness. In 10% of cases aneurysmal bleeding may be severe enough to cause loss of consciousness for up to several days.[63] In 45%, severe headache without loss of consciousness occurs as a presenting complaint.[63] Vomiting is another prominent symptom when the patient is awake, but does not correlate well with headache severity. Rarely, a few cases may develop lightheadedness followed by syncope within seconds without headache; we have seen two such patients.

Several risk factors for rupture have long been recognized, but there is remarkably little data on any one factor. Weightlifting has recently been implicated as one of the risk factors for rupture, especially when repetitive upper or lower extremity weight lifts are associated with strenuous Valsalva maneuver.[85] Electroconvulsive therapy may not be the risk it was once taken to be.[18] Pregnancy, often avoided in patients with known aneurysm, has only occasionally been reported with rupture. The recent report of three cases, all near term, points to the paucity of this literature.[105] Seasonal variation has been suggested, men suffering subarachnoid hemorrhage more often in late fall, women in late spring.[41]

Focal Deficits

Among cranial neuropathies, unilateral third nerve palsy after aneurysmal rupture suggests a posterior communicating aneurysm, while sixth nerve palsy has no special localizing value. Hemiparesis, aphasia of the dominant hemisphere, anosognosia (hemineglect) of the nondominant hemisphere, memory loss, and abulia are the more common hemispheric neurologic deficits. An aneurysm located at the bifurcation of the middle cerebral artery may rupture out into the temporal lobe and up into the frontal and parietal lobes (Fig. 26.9), less often into the frontal or parietal region, and occasionally be mistaken for primary parenchymatous hemorrhage.[47]

In many cases there is no adequate explanation for the initial neurologic deficits. The deficits can often be seen gradually to improve over a matter of days. The reason for improvement is uncertain, but may be due to transient interruption of cerebral circulation in a given arterial territory during and immediately after aneurysmal rupture followed by recirculation, something equivalent to a transient ischemic attack.

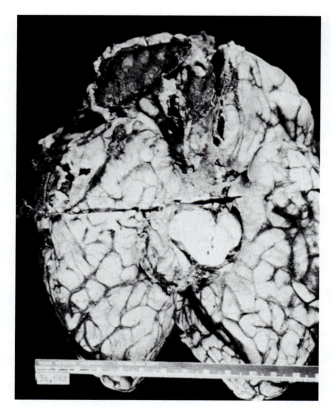

Figure 26.9 Autopsy photograph of base of frontal lobe and circle of Willis showing diffuse subarachnoid hemorrhage and gross hemorrhage into frontal lobe.

Grading Systems

The clinical grading system as modified by Botterell et al,[30] Hunt and Hess,[93] and others has been widely used to categorize the clinical status of patients. It is reviewed in the chapters on medical and surgical management.

INITIAL LABORATORY EVALUATION

Because saccular aneurysms that give rise to subarachnoid hemorrhage are located at the branch points of the large intracranial extracerebral arteries at the base of the brain, blood from the ruptured aneurysm is deposited locally, or sometimes widely, in the basal cisterns, as free or coarsely clotted blood (Fig. 26.10). The specific location of the aneurysm and the severity and magnitude of the rupture determine the location and amount of blood in the various cisterns and fissures of the subarachnoid space.

CT Scan Versus Lumbar Puncture

About 75% of cases will have evidence of subarachnoid clot on non-contrast CT scan if the scan is obtained within the first 48 hours of aneurysmal rupture.[152] Furthermore, the ex-

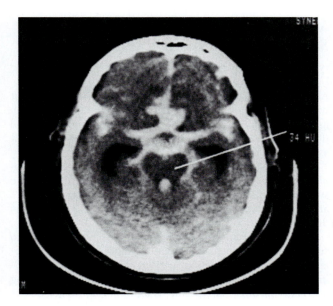

Figure 26.10 Extensive subarachnoid hemorrhage shown on non-contrast CT scan, flooding basilar cisterns with acute ischemic infarction of the midbrain. The patient died shortly thereafter.

tent and location of subarachnoid blood as seen on non-contrast CT scan may give useful information as to the location of the aneurysm and the cause of the initial neurologic deficit. Such scans have been a useful means to predict those patients destined to develop delayed neurologic deficits because of symptomatic cerebral vasospasm[102,103] in the study by Ohman et al, the most important in a logistic regression model.[149] Using the high-resolution CT scan after contrast, aneurysms down to 3 mm in size have been reported in 87% of 76 cases.[184] They are not as easily seen in the supraclinoid portion of the carotid and when bony or movement artifacts are present. In cases where the diagnosis of subarachnoid hemorrhage is uncertain, non-contrast scans should be done first, since contrast scans may show arterial enhancement in the basal cisterns that could be mistaken for clotted blood. AVMs and mycotic aneurysms usually present with parenchymatous blood or subarachnoid blood located over the hemisphere rather than in the basal cistern.

Magnetic Resonance Imaging

MR imaging has been found as useful as CT for the diagnosis of subarachnoid hemorrhage.[115] MR has more recently been able to detect aneurysms 0.5 mm or greater. MR angiography, once considered unsuitable, is now a common means to detect aneurysms and even to make a rough estimate on vasospasm. With the increasing use of nonferrous clips, the former concern of dislodging clips from MR has subsided considerably. Advanced three-dimensional imaging can assist in planning surgery.[106]

Angiography

Cerebral angiography remains the crucial step in diagnosis. With the widespread use of early surgery, angiography has become common on the first day of symptoms. It is mandatory for diagnosis of intracerebral hematoma when emergency surgical evacuation is planned, as an occult aneurysm would be a disagreeable surprise to the surgical team evacuating an acute hematoma.

Where possible, selected angiography should be performed just prior to planned surgery, not only to localize the aneurysm, but also to document its exact anatomy for approach. In one series, rerupture occurred in 2 (1.4%) of 144 cases; all studies were performed through a transaortic approach.[181] Rarely, despite the most thorough studies, a neck cannot be found suitable for clip placement or a tightly looped vessel misleads the team into a diagnosis of aneurysm.

Until the advent of transcranial Doppler MRI, conventional angiography was the only means to diagnose and follow the course of vasospasm.[65] Transcranial Doppler studies (see below) have greatly altered this approach. When angiography is used, angiographic evidence of severe vasospasm (i.e., middle cerebral stem or A1 segment of the anterior cerebral artery less than 1 mm or distal branch of the middle cerebral and anterior cerebral artery at less than 0.5 mm) is present when symptoms of delayed ischemia occur in the territory of the internal carotid artery.[64]

If no aneurysm is found on the initial selected cerebral angiogram, the chance for repeat subarachnoid hemorrhage is quite low (1% to 2%).[26,84,157] Because selected cerebral angiography can miss a subtle aneurysm, particularly of the anterior communicating artery or in the posterior circulation, repeat four-vessel angiography is still a common practice after a week or so. However, recent challenges to this time-honored program have been made, citing the very low frequency of subsequent positive findings if an initial angiogram, in the absence of spasm, has shown no aneurysm.[42,76,86,101,112] Where no aneurysm is found it has been suspected that the aneurysm has obliterated itself in the clot after rupture. Other explanations of subarachnoid hemorrhage include rupture of a small superficial cortical artery,[90] spinal cord AVM,[72,188] an extramedullary aneurysm of the spinal cord (i.e., a cervical radicular artery or an anterior spinal artery aneurysm),[91] or an artery of Adamkiewicz aneurysm. Although they are rare, both a spinal cord AVM and an aneurysm of a cervical artery may appear together. In most cases back pain with minimal headache and subarachnoid blood suggests the diagnosis.

Transcranial Doppler

Transcranial Doppler, a handy bedside and laboratory technique, has become a mainstay in the management of aneurysms, if for no other reason than it offers an excellent means of demonstrating the presence and severity of vasospasm.[127] The details of the technique are found in Chapter 14.

An excellent correlation has been found for angiographic evidence of spasm and Doppler velocities above 100 cm/sec[44] to 120 mg/sec.[194] The first appearance of increased velocity is typically on the fourth day after hemorrhage. Studies seeking signs of earlier or transient spasm have thus far been negative.[172] Flow velocities typically peak on the eleventh and eighteenth day and normalize by the third to fourth week.[188,194] The increase in velocities usually occurs before the appearance of delayed ischemic defects and mirrors the increase in angiographically evident vasospasm. Normal Doppler velocities have been shown associated with no spasm in the vessels insonated.

Vasospasms within the territory of the middle cerebral artery can be detected reliably while those in the anterior cerebral artery to the anterior communicating artery are usually undetected because of the sharp angulation of the artery out of the plane easily insonated by the Doppler.[107] For the same reason, the Doppler has also had difficulty identifying spasm in vessels distal to the circle of Willis and middle cerebral stem.[143]

The Doppler velocity is inversely proportional to the concentration of formed elements in the blood, the hematocrit being the best biologic marker of the number of circulating formed elements. Volume expansion therapy to reduce spasm may result in hemodilution which may reduce the density of circulating particles, improving flow but producing a rise in Doppler velocity due to reduced hematocrit that could be misinterpreted as increasing spasm.[31]

Cerebral Blood Flow, Single-Photon and Positron Emission Tomography

These techniques have had limited application because the patient must usually be transported from an intensive care unit and hold still for long periods of time. Although the application of the technology is difficult, when used they have correlated well with angiographic evidence of vasospasm and revealed evidence of tissue hypoperfusion in advance of symptoms.[52,95,197]

Routine Laboratory Tests

Baseline electrocardiograms (ECGs) are of value because ECGs (peaked P waves, prolonged QT interval, tall T waves) are reported in patients with subarachnoid hemorrhage.[33,77] These changes have been linked to elevated catecholamine blood and urine levels and to hypothalamic dysfunction.[28,48,124,140] These authors hypothesize that α-adrenergic receptors in the myocardium and coronary arteries are stimulated by norepinephrine-containing nerve terminals or circulating epinephrine and result in prolonged muscle fiber contraction which leads to myofibrillar necrosis. The α-adrenergic receptors that exist on the large coronary arteries could occasion coronary spasm and lead to ischemic myocardial damage similar to Prinzmetal angina.[78]

The clinical course correlates with body temperature and the white blood count (WBC).[229] One explanation could be neurogenic hyperthermia.[193] Another is a system effect. An admission WBC above 15,000 or body temperature above 37.5°C had a 55% to 60% mortality compared with 25% to 35% for lower values, in both instances related to high frequencies of vasospasm. Baseline electrolytes have been of little predictive value for outcome[55] but are of value because hyponatremia may develop later in the course, secondary to inappropriate antidiuretic hormone (ADH) secretion or an unknown factor, causing loss of salt and water in the urine with subsequent volume depletion and dilutional hyponatremia. Platelet counts, bleeding time, and other clotting parameters should be documented. Serum viscosity increases with a hematocrit above 40% and a serum-fibrinogen level above 250 mg%. High osmolality has also been related to poor outcome.[55]

Medical Complications of Subarachnoid Hemorrhage

Although many medical complications can arise from a patient who is put to bed following subarachnoid hemorrhage, such as thrombophlebitis with pulmonary embolism and perforated duodenal ulcer, two specific medical complications stand out as being related to subarachnoid hemorrhage.

The first includes ECG changes suggestive of myonecrosis and/or coronary arterial ischemia.[35,49,78,82] Here, the sympathetic nervous system is thought to be overactive[141,147] and myofibrillar degeneration in focal areas of the myocardium has been documented.[163]

The second medical complication specifically related to subarachnoid hemorrhage is hyponatremia[141] either from inappropriate ADH secretion or from secretion of atrial natriuretic hormone.[55] Restriction of free water, while maintaining adequate intravascular volume, is an important management point.

Subarachnoid hemorrhage in patients on anticoagulants conferred a relative risk of death or dependency of 1.9 (95% CI 1.5 to 2.4) on the 15 patients on anticoagulants compared with the 126 not on anticoagulants as recently reported by Rinkel et al.[168]

Delayed Neurologic Deficits

There are three major causes of delayed neurologic deficits (i.e., those following stabilization or improvement of the initial neurologic symptoms or deficits after aneurysmal rupture): rebleeding, hydrocephalus, and cerebral vasospasm. Recognition of the onset, cause, and severity of each of these delayed neurologic deficits will be greatly aided by a precise knowledge of the cause and extent of the initial neurologic deficit and symptoms following subarachnoid hemorrhage. An accurate assessment of ventricular size and the extent and location of subarachnoid blood on early CT scan (24 to 48 hours after the hemorrhage) will be of great value in firmly establishing the diagnosis of each of these three complications.

REBLEEDING

While rerupture of an aneurysm is generally heralded by a sudden severe increase in headache and may be associated with nausea and vomiting, loss of consciousness, and new neurologic deficits, a sudden moderate to severe increase in headache is not in itself diagnostic. Repeat CT or MR scan demonstrating an increase in the amount of blood in the subarachnoid space or a lumbar puncture showing new blood is essential to confirm the diagnosis.[81] Repeating a lumbar puncture in patients who have an increase in headache, however, may present some hazard and should only be done if the diagnosis of rebleed is mandatory. At present, it seems likely that increased morbidity of an aneurysmal rerupture is likely only if the CT scan shows new blood in the cisterns.[81]

The incidence of rebleeding may be as high as 30% of all cases.[144,235] Furthermore, rerupture carries a significant morbidity and mortality. Sixty-two percent of patients studied at the Mayo Clinic who were drowsy or had headache but no other neurologic deficit sustained a major neurologic dysfunction upon rebleeding, and 31% of those patients died as a result of the rebleed.[207] The incidence of rerupture is highest in the first 3 weeks following aneurysmal rupture. By 6 months following aneurysmal rupture the rebleed rate has been estimated to be at 2% to 3% per year.[96]

Because of the high early rebleeding rate and significant morbidity and mortality associated with it, considerable investigative interest has been directed toward the use of antifibrinolytic agents in the preoperative period. Ramirez-Lassepas, in an extensive review of the subject some years ago,[161] pointed out that out of 25 published studies only 13 were controlled and 9 were randomized. The results of all these studies are inconclusive. ϵ-Aminocaproic acid has been studied with conflicting results.[3,75,144,183,189] A recent effort[109] indicates that it may reduce the incidence of rebleeding but may do so at the expense of a higher incidence of ischemic complications than those of controls. Similar experience has been had with a second antifibrinolytic agent, tranexamic acid (the transisomer of α-methyl-cyclohexane carboxylic acid).[75,99,117,222] An accurate diagnosis of rerupture for the purpose of any study is difficult.

To establish firmly that a major rerupture has occurred, a worsening of the clinical status associated with an increased amount of blood seen on CT scan or evidence of an increased amount of blood in the CSF on lumbar puncture must be evident. Such strict criteria would undoubtedly exclude minor moderate rebleeding episodes. To include all patients with an increase in headache without laboratory confirmation of increased blood would result in an overdiagnosis of recurrent hemorrhage. Prophylaxis with ϵ-aminocaproic acid has fallen out of favor.[117]

Negative Angiographic Findings and Rebleeding

Hayward[86] estimated that in 9% of cases of subarachnoid hemorrhage, no aneurysm is found even with repeated four-vessel angiography. The incidence of rebleeding in these cases is low. Of the 41 patients with subarachnoid hemorrhage and no evidence of aneurysm on four-vessel angiography, none had evidence of rebleeding in a follow-up period from 3 months to 2.5 years. It is possible that some of these patients had subarachnoid hemorrhages from causes other than rupture of a saccular aneurysm—for example, rupture of a small superficial artery.[90] The implication from the study by Hayward is that either most of the patients may have thrombosed their aneurysm, or the aneurysm was so small that it was destroyed at the time of rupture.[86]

For perimesencephalic hemorrhage found on CT scan, the benign outlook seems especially clear: none of the 37 patients studied by Rinkel et al[168] rebled over the 18-month to 7-year follow-up.

When the initial angiogram fails to reveal an aneurysm, it seems prudent to keep the patient at rest for from 1 to 3 weeks after the initial hemorrhage, then to repeat the angiogram (an opinion no longer shared by all workers). If aneurysm is not found then, the patient may be mobilized. However, the utility of the bed rest program has not been adequately tested.

HYDROCEPHALUS

Communicating hydrocephalus with dilatation of the lateral ventricles and third and fourth ventricles may occur any time after aneurysmal rupture. In general, however, it occurs between 4 and 20 days following subarachnoid hemorrhage. Ventricular hemorrhage is a major cause, the problem more properly being considered hemocephalus. This effect is usually self-limiting. Vasospasm seems unrelated to hydrocephalus or the need for shunt.[205]

Hydrocephalus may cause no detectable neurologic change if it is mild. Mild drowsiness, urinary incontinence, and inability to move the eyes above the equator are associated with early mild-to-moderate hydrocephalus. More severe hydrocephalus has been associated with profound stupor developing in as short a time as a matter of hours.

Hydrocephalus is often transient and may not require specific surgical intervention. In the past, frequent lumbar puncture was used in hopes of tiding the patient over a critical period until hydrocephalus subsides; at present, repeated lumbar puncture is considered hazardous because of the risk of rerupture, particularly with aneurysms lying in the posterior fossa. Obviously, when supratentorial mass effect exists, lumbar puncture is contraindicated. If significant neurologic deterioration occurs and lumbar puncture is felt to be unsafe, then ventricular drainage or ventricular atrial shunting is advisable.

CEREBRAL VASOSPASM

Narrowing of the caliber of the arteries at the base of the brain frequently follows subarachnoid hemorrhage and can lead to cerebral ischemia and infarction.[67] Compared to the other complications, vasospasm remains the most frightening and devastating, even with advances in prevention and treatment. Literature reviews appear often,[234] but with the wide application of calcium antagonists and vasodilators, and the common practice of early surgery, the literature on this subject has been declining steadily in recent years.

Incidence and Prevalence

Vasospasm is the major cause of delayed serious morbidity and death.[65] Its severity and location are all important in determining whether and where cerebral ischemia and/or cerebral infarction will develop. Its onset is delayed 3 to 21 days after the initial hemorrhage, occurring most often between 4 and 14 days.[65,67,102]

The reports of the incidence of vasospasm in subarachnoid hemorrhage varies widely. At one end of the spectrum is an incidence as low as 15%.[180] The range of 30% to 40% is common,[81,86,89,160] while a few studies showed higher values.[6] Population studies have reported higher values, one at 76%.[144,237] It has proved difficult to account for this wide variation in the incidence. Some of it might reflect patterns of referral but some could be from differences in medical treatment programs.

A separate matter is the incidence and nature of delayed focal ischemic deficits attributed to vasospasm. In most patients there is a period of neurologic improvement or a period of clinical stability between the initial aneurysmal rupture and the onset of symptomatic vasospasm.

Timing of Vasospasm

The onset and duration of vasospasm appears to follow a regular timetable. Reports utilizing angiogram,[96,180,196] or Doppler both show the temporal course of vasospasm to be the same whether or not the vasospasm is later associated with delayed neurologic deficits.

Vasospasm has been documented seconds or minutes following vessel rupture in the experimental animal model but only rarely so reported in humans. One case among the 5,484 cases of subarachnoid hemorrhage was reported in the Cooperative study.[178] Wilkins et al[233] found a mere 32 such cases in the literature and in 13 of these most of the evidence suggested the cause was prior subarachnoid hemorrhage. Liliequist et al[108] described a case in which acute spasm was documented on serial frames of an angiogram that documented acute rupture of the aneurysm during the procedure. Taneda et al found a similar case angiogrammed within 12 hours of the initial rupture who ruptured during the study with sudden spasm that disappeared on repeat study after 14 minutes.[214]

Mohr and Kase[132] had a single case of a patient suffering a syndrome consistent with a transient ischemic attack during the initial phase of aneurysm rupture. Their community-based study also showed vasospasm in 6 of the 20 angiograms done within the first 2 days after onset of subarachnoid hemorrhage severe enough to plunge the patient into coma. Others with extensive experience with community cases have had similar experiences. However, the vast majority of cases referred to a major medical center for surgery do not show these findings *before the third day* after a subarachnoid hemorrhage.[65,228,277] This late occurrence of the first signs of vasospasm has also been reported based on Doppler studies.[172]

Irrespective of the time of onset, the duration of vasospasm may extend beyond 3 weeks. However, if vasospasm has not appeared by the end of the second week, there is little likelihood it will occur or be of clinical significance.[229] Once vasospasm begins to subside, its recurrence in a given portion of an artery is not expected.[183]

Very late appearance of spasm, 7, 14, and 52 weeks after initial subarachnoid hemorrhage, has been described in rare instances.[103] In addition, transient spasm unexplained by ruptured aneurysm has also been described.[36]

Distribution of Vasospasm

The topography varies somewhat, but usually affects the circle of Willis and stems of the major cerebral arteries.[114,160,191,233] In almost all instances the vasospasm begins in the proximal vessels, and spreads distally along the major CSF cylinders passing over the convexity in the general direction of the superior sagittal sinus.

This proclivity of vasospasm to affect the larger vessels may be a result of the differential responsiveness of larger vessels to sympathetic stimulation,[10] a result that is assumed to occur with subarachnoid hemorrhage. The spread of vasospasm through the arterial tree is controlled by factors not currently understood, but the process at least seems to develop in a centrifugal fashion.

Types of Vasospasm

Diffuse, segmental, and local forms of vasospasm have been described. In diffuse spasm, most of the arteries are affected by nearly uniform narrowing for long distances from their origin.[46] Segmental spasm presents with sausagelike bands of varying length. Local spasm is the short segments of narrowing seen in arteries in the vicinity of the aneurysm itself. Some surgeons argue[197] that the presence of the segmental or local varieties in the later stages of vasospasm is not a contraindication to surgery. However diffuse vasospasm has been thought to have a more serious prognosis.[182,206,225]

Predictors of Vasospasm

The incidence, severity, and location of cerebral vasospasm in patients following subarachnoid hemorrhage can be predicted by clotted blood in specific amounts at specific sites in the basal cisterns and fissures of the subarachnoid space as seen on conventional scanning.[67,103,130,132] Vasospasm severe enough to produce symptoms has frequently occurred when the early CT scan shows globular subarachnoid clots larger than 5 × 3 mm in the basal cisterns or layers of blood 1 mm thick or greater in the cerebral fissures.

The location of the clot seen on scan also carries a good correlation with the location of the spasm in the artery enveloped in the clot.[102] This correlation applies only for CT scans obtained later than 24 hours after the hemorrhage. Subarachnoid blood seen in the basal cisterns less than 24 hours after the rupture may dissipate during the 24- to 48-hour period following rupture. Because blood becomes attenuated over time, scans obtained more than 96 hours (4 days) after the rupture may not be reliable. These observations prompted some of the work on clot dispersion done mechanically[220] or with tissue plasminogen activator (TPA)[227] in animals.

Takemae et al[212] were the first to indicate a correlation between high-density CT scan findings and subsequent vasospasm, a study that was updated and enlarged to 177 cases by Mizukami et al.[130] In this latter report, 85% of cases showing high density on the CT scan within 4 days of onset developed vasospasm, compared with none of eight whose CT scan was negative for high density during this period ($P < 0.01$), regardless of the location of the aneurysm. This correlation did not apply for patients whose scans were performed 5 days after onset. Fisher et al[67] independently quantitated the severity of the hemorrhage with the severity of the later vasospasm. Of their 47 cases, the CT scan showed either no evidence of blood or its diffuse distribution in 18 cases; only one experienced severe vasospasm. However, ". . . in the presence of subarachnoid blood clots larger than 5 × 3 mm or layers of blood 1 mm or more thick in fissures and vertical cisterns, severe vasospasm followed almost invariably (23 of 24 cases)." When these CT scan criteria were applied prospectively to 50 cases, a strong correlation existed between extent and location of supratentorial subarachnoid blood and the location and severity of vasospasm and related symptoms. Mohr and Kase[132] had similar experience: all 15 of the angiogrammed cases among the 38 with massive bleeding shown on CT scan had vasospasm, among whom 6 were admitted in coma and angiogrammed the first day.

The occurrence of vasospasm was also significantly correlated with increased intracranial pressure ($P < 0.0001$) in the findings of the Cooperative study.[178] Although the number of cases was too small for detailed analysis, local vasospasm occurred with equal frequency in cases with normal or increased intracranial pressure (3 of 14 versus 14 of 48), while diffuse vasospasm occurred only in those with increased intracranial pressure (0 of 13 versus 12 of 48).

A similar explanation probably applies to the relationship between vasospasm and the severity of the clinical picture. Although the incidence of vasospasm was rather low throughout the data of the Cooperative study,[178] the small group of 63 cases with severe neurologic deficits had a remarkably high incidence of vasospasm.

Proposed Mechanisms of Vasospasm

Work continues on the cause of cerebral vasospasm, but not at the pace prior to the mid-1990s. The numerous candidates for vasospasm seem partly to have discouraged any hope a single cause would be found. The list is long. Among the endogenous substances[196,224] are serotonin,[11,162] prostaglandins,[54,195,271] catecholamines,[22,24,71] angiotensin,[16] and histamine.[10,231] Few of them occur at concentrations high enough to achieve sustained spasm in natural subarachnoid hemorrhage. Prolonged spasm has been produced by a variety of blood preparations including local hemostasis,[229] incubated whole blood,[60] fresh whole blood,[1] blood hemosylate, hemoglobin,[290] oxyhemoglobin,[100,217,219] bilirubin,[126] and low levels of α 1-antitrypsin (α 1-AT), an inhibitor of the enzyme elastase,[216] but not platelet-rich plasma alone.[156]

Some work attributes vasospasm to alteration in the contents of adrenergic fibers in the adventitia. These contain dense core vesicles in their terminal varicosities,[60] which synthesize norepinephrine and disappear after subarachnoid hemorrhage.[71] Pre-depletion of substance P before injection of cisternal blood in the animal model has also been found to prevent vasospasm. Neuropeptide Y has been found in CSF at very high levels in a setting of spasm, and far lower in normals.[1] At the vascular level, vasoconstrictor products of the lipoxygenase, especially hydroperoxyeicosatetraenoic acids (HPETEs), have also been shown to be produced by cerebral vessels and their release could play a role in spasm. A role has even been proposed for substance P.[53] The powerful vasoconstrictor polypeptide endothelin (as ET-1 and ET-3), thought by some to play a role in spasm, has been found only in a very low percentage of cases of subarachnoid hemorrhage, but its cisternal levels have not proved temporally correlated with spasm.[73]

Much of the animal work has been based on the recognition that persistence of the large subarachnoid clot is associated with spasm. The coating of blood has been postulated to lead to local tissue acidosis and an anaerobic state, with inhibition of arterial wall synthesis of prostacyclin and overproduction of thromboxane-A, resulting in vasospasm and platelet hyperaggregation.[210]

At the cellular muscle level, under normal conditions, both contraction and relaxation of smooth muscle is an active process depending on the phosphorylation on a myosin light chain kinase that is activated by binding a complex formed by calcium and calmodulin, a calcium-binding regulatory protein.[128] When the calcium concentration in the sarcoplasma is greater than 10^{-5} U or less than 10^{-7} U the muscle is respectively fully contracted or relaxed when these protein enzymes are available. Phosphorylation of myosin light chain responsible for muscle contraction is also dependent upon a cyclic adenosine monophosphate (AMP)-dependent protein kinase.[45] β-Adrenergic stimulation of the β-adrenergic receptor in the cell membrane increases the availability of cyclic AMP in the sarcoplasma. This in turn decreases the affinity of the myosin light chain kinase for calcium/calmodulin binding and reduces its ability to phosphorylate myosin light chains and to stimulate contraction. For relaxation to occur, the calcium ion concentration must decrease in the sarcoplasma, and must be transported across the cell membrane into the extracellular space or into the intracellular organelles. This active process requires high energy phosphate metabolism to be operational. Only when the calcium concentration in the sarcoplasma is reduced can there be disruption of the actin-myosin cross-bridges responsible for contracting utility. A reciprocal interaction has been shown between calcium and magnesium, by which increased calcium or decreased magnesium causes constriction, while increased magnesium causes relaxation.[12] The increase in the calcium:magnesium ratio from the usual 1:1 in spinal fluid to 3:1 after subarachnoid hemorrhage provides a basis for speculating on a role for calcium in vasospasm, against which the calcium antagonist nimodipine is directed. Inhibition of phosphodiesterase, which plays a role in calcium-mediated smooth muscle contraction, has been a basis for the use of papaverine, and, more recently, for a new inhibitor, amrinone.[238]

Histology of Spasm

Although popular, the term vasospasm has been questioned as the proper term to characterize the vascular changes that reduce lumen diameter. Alksne and Greenhoot,[7,8] Fein et al,[62] and Mizukami et al[129] independently demonstrated fragmentation of myofilaments, destruction of the sarcolemma, and lipid inclusions within abnormal smooth muscle cells in the media close to the internal elastic lamina. Alksne and Branson[9] also documented endothelial cell loss and proliferation in chronic arteriopathy in a monkey and dog model. Other work has shown corrugation of the endothelium with desquamation of endothelial cells but no changes in the media,[189] whereas other investigators show it to involve both endothelium and media,[62] and still others have evidence for involvement of all layers of the vascular wall.[118]

Arterial constriction is favored by many. Canine basilar arteries in spasm between 2 and 28 days after subarachnoid injection of autogenous fresh blood showed no significant change in the radius or wall thickness when tested by strain gauge at various pressures, a finding that indicated that vascular smooth muscle constriction, not irreversible organic changes in the wall, were responsible for the luminal narrowing in vivo.[139]

Clinical Syndromes of Vasospasm

A relationship between vasospasm and delayed clinical deficits was already widely accepted when Millikan,[128] after an extensive literature review, reported no acceptable clinical data bearing on the subject, and found no difference in the incidence of neurologic deficits between cases with vasospasm and those without in his series of 198 consecutive cases of subarachnoid hemorrhage from the Mayo Clinic. In the 81 with spasm, 48 (59%) showed neurologic abnormalities, among them 27 (33%) with focal signs. However, among the other 117 who showed no vasospasm, 83 (71%) had neurologic deficits, 44 (38%) of which were focal.

Although the overall thrust of Millikan's argument came under heavy criticism, his detailed literature review (up to 1975) documented a remarkable paucity of clinical deficits attributable to vasospasm. He cited 45 publications involving over 2,000 clinical cases from 1938 to 1974, and 198 cases in his own series. His clinical material contained 14 cases with hemiparesis-hemiplegia and 8 with dysphasia-aphasia present in the preoperative state at the time the angiogram showed spasm. In 5 of the cases with motor deficit and all of those with dysphasia-aphasia, the onset of the symptoms occurred 24 to 48 hours after the subarachnoid hemorrhage. Of the remaining cases, 3 were described in clinical sketches featuring sudden onset of focal symptoms with angiographic evidence of spasm. But the angiograms also showed occlusions attributed to emboli that involved branches serving the focally symptomatic territories of the middle cerebral artery. Disturbances of consciousness, another type of disorder considered linked to vasospasm, was more frequent in the cases without vasospasm.

The findings of this paper sharpened interest in the subject[64,207] and in its therapy.[2,33] Fisher et al[65] focused their 50 cases on the correlation between vasospasm severity and clinical deficits: of the 25 (50%) with delayed neurologic deficits, all showed severe vasospasm (3 to 4+ on his scale of severity). Another 19 had no focal signs. In all of these cases the angiograms showed only 0 to 2+ spasm. Fisher et al concluded that ". . . blood localized in the subarachnoid space in sufficient amounts at specific sites is the only important etiologic factor in vasospasm." The clinical deficits attributed to vasospasm were described in some detail. Among the 50 cases, right hemiplegia with aphasia occurred in 10; 4 had right hemiparesis without aphasia; 5 had left hemiplegia; 2 each had right and left hemiplegia, aphasia, or initial paralysis of both legs. Signs referable to the middle cerebral artery on one or both sides were the most frequent, while in 8 the presence of abulia and leg weakness suggested that the anterior cerebral artery was affected.

In the years since then, clinical deficits have often been tabulated but syndromes have only occasionally been described. Suzuki et al[209] reported 20 cases of subarachnoid hemorrhage, of whom 9 had angiographic evidence of vasospasm. Two of the 9 ". . . displayed mild ischemic symptoms." Similarly, Sano and Saito[182] reported 68 of 443 cases with angiographic evidence of vasospasm at some point during the preoperative period. The clinical deficits included "disturbance of consciousness" in 58, "motor disturbance" in 40, and 24 with "mental changes." A strong correlation existed between the location of severe vasospasm and the cerebral arterial territory in which delayed ischemic deficit occurred. The neurologic deficits in that study included hemiparesis with or without aphasia when the dominant middle cerebral territory was involved and the middle cerebral stem or its immediate distal branches, upper and lower divisions, were involved. Hemiparesis with or without anosognosia and apractagnosia was present when the nondominant middle cerebral territory was involved. Anterior cerebral territory ischemic deficits were recognized as representing a quiet abulic state in which the patient may be awake but lies quietly with his eyes closed responding to commands with delay. Such a patient may offer no spontaneous conversation, but is able to answer questions with short phrases in a whispered voice, again often after a delay. Food is chewed for a prolonged period of time and often held between the cheek and gum. This state was associated with severe spasm in the A1 or A2 segment of the anterior cerebral artery. Homonymous hemianopic field defects have been seen in patients with severe spasm of the posterior cerebral artery. Focal brain stem dysfunction has been observed with severe spasm of the vertebral basilar artery, but that is rare. These focal neurologic symptoms have been observed to occur gradually over a few days or presented abruptly, coming to their full extent within a matter of minutes or an hour. They have been attributed to reduced blood flow in the arterial territory evolved. This has been amply documented along with an increase in blood volume.[134]

In earlier times, the appearance of these syndromes was taken as a sign of irreversible ischemic deficits and surgery was often delayed or canceled. Rare surprising examples of desperation therapy with extreme increases in blood pressure followed by dramatic reversal of what looked like permanent deficits were too infrequent to be considered typical of the chances for functional recovery. Yet recent work with angioplasty may be revising some of these notions. In some instances, stupor has been reversed by successful angioplasty,[104] as have some other neurologic deficits, raising hopes some deficits may prove reversible. But fatalities have been documented.[110]

If the brain becomes infarcted in a large enough area, cerebral edema may ensue and result in a fatal rise in intracranial pressure. Suggestion of such a severe outcome (i.e., the entire middle cerebral artery territory becoming ischemic and infarcted), can be inferred from the early CT scan when a large clot is noted in the stem of the sylvian fissure and/or sylvian cistern and a second significant clot is noted in the basal frontal inner hemispheric fissure.[102]

Simultaneous clots in these areas correlated well with severe spasm both in the middle cerebral stem and/or middle cerebral bifurcation and the corresponding anterior cerebral artery. Thus, when severe middle cerebral stem spasm reduced flow in that arterial territory, the chance for adequate collateral over the cortical surface into the distal middle cerebral branches from the anterior cerebral artery is eliminated. Likewise, a single large clot in the stem of the sylvian fissure or at the sylvian cistern where the middle cerebral stem bifurcates may ensure severe spasm in the middle cerebral artery stem or at its bifurcation. However, without a significant clot in the basal frontal inner hemispheric fissure, the proximal anterior cerebral artery would not be expected to develop severe vasospasm. Therefore, there would be a chance for adequate collateral flow to develop from the distal anterior cerebral branches into the middle cerebral artery territory. Patients with this particular location of subarachnoid blood may escape the development of ischemic middle cerebral territory symptoms or such symptoms may not be severe and may only be transient.[102]

In the series reported by Mohr and Kase,[132] delayed deficits attributed to vasospasm occurred in 29 of 37 patients (78%). The possibility of delayed ischemic syndromes could not be evaluated in another 23 patients who developed coma at onset and died without regaining consciousness. In only one of their cases was spasm documented angiographically in the absence of a delayed neurologic deficit: a woman with a 6 × 9 mm middle cerebral aneurysm with local spasm of the middle cerebral stem seen on angiogram performed 6 days later; she underwent surgery the seventh day and at no time pre- or postoperatively did a focal deficit occur. The mode of onset (whether sudden or gradual) in 19 of the 37 cases was imprecisely understood, since it developed to its fullest extent during a period between clinical observations. Yet at the most only a few hours lapsed between examinations. In another 7 instances, a sudden onset of the deficit was clearly documented, since two observers encountered the patient within minutes of one another, and in every instance no further progression of the deficit occurred. In 4 others, the syndrome worsened gradually, stretching over a period of several days. In all cases, some focal deficit was present on admission. It remained unchanged until the second to sixth day when other focal deficits made their appearance and the level of consciousness began to sink, first to obtundation, then to coma, over the following 2 to 3 days.

The clinical deficits we personally encountered and those reported in the literature range among surface branch syndromes that could be due to emboli, "distal field" or "watershed" infarcts attributable to perfusion failure, and huge infarcts encompassing both the deep and superficial portions of an entire arterial territory. It may be important that isolated deep infarcts of the lacunar type have not been encountered clinically nor seen on CT scan personally, although they have been mentioned in the autopsy literature (16 isolated caudate infarcts in 119 described by Crompton[47]). The apparent infrequency of such infarcts is especially interesting considering the high incidence of vasospasm confined to the stem of the anterior and middle cerebral arteries.

Autopsy reports have emphasized a variety of findings, but it has proved difficult to correlate specific ischemic lesions with the clinical picture because of the changing nature of the clinical course. The study by Suzuki et al[210] correlated microvascular thromboses with focal infarcts but not with syndromes.

The incidence of ischemic infarcts varies from 25%[165] to as high as 78%.[218] Most infarcts affected the arterial territory of the aneurysm, but also involved others. Some of the reports described widespread ischemic changes of the cerebrum, including the hypothalamus.[47] Others reported similar widespread neuronal loss with white matter edema, but no distinct large foci of infarction, and lesions more proximal than the "watershed" regions. Ischemic zones ranged in size from small cortical foci to large infarcts in arterial territories distal to the

site of the aneurysm,[169,186,218] usually with patent arteries.[97] Thrombi and emboli have been described in some reports and their potential role for symptoms attributable to vasospasm has been the source of considerable speculation.[128,140,169,186] Whether or not an embolic mechanism is frequent, its documentation has proved difficult and its occurrence seems intimately related to the process known as vasospasm. The possibility that emboli might arise from the intima of an artery in "vasospasm" is consistent with the hypothesis that endothelial thrombus formation set in motion by acidosis and platelet aggregation has a more important role in symptoms than does spasm of the arteries.[209,210,230,231] However, Nagasawa et al[139] found no thrombus within any of the freshly removed canine basilar arteries in spasm from 2 through 28 days. All the angiographic studies of Fisher et al failed to demonstrate the mechanism.[65,66]

Outcome Long After Hemorrhage or Surgery

Cognitive deficits have been a nagging problem and are often mentioned by family more than they seem recognized by the professional staff. Detailed testing is uncommon. In Richardson's study of 76 cases,[166] a moderate impairment was found 6 weeks after hospitalization, unrelated to the site of aneurysm rupture but especially common in patients who had experienced generalized vasospasm. By 6 months, the findings had mostly reverted to normal.

References

1. Abel PW, Han C, Noe BD, McDonald JK: Neuropeptide Y: vasoconstrictor effects and possible role in cerebral vasospasm after experimental subarachnoid hemorrhage. Brain Res 463:250, 1988
2. Acosta-Rua GJ: Familial incidence of ruptured intracranial aneurysms. Arch Neurol 35:675, 1978
3. Adams HP: Current status of antifibrinolytic therapy for treatment of patients with aneurysmal subarachnoid hemorrhage. Stroke 13:256, 1982
4. Adams H, Jergenson DD, Kassell NF, Sahs AL: Pitfalls in the recognition of subarachnoid hemorrhage. JAMA 244:794, 1980
5. Allcock JM, Canham PB: Angiographic study of the growth of intracranial aneurysms. J Neurosurg 45:617, 1976
6. Allcock JM, Drake CG: Ruptured intracranial aneurysms: the role of arterial spasm. J Neurosurg 22:21, 1965
7. Alksne JF: Myonecrosis in chronic experimental vasospasm. Surgery 76:1, 1974
8. Alksne JF, Greenhoot JH: Experimental catecholamine induced chronic cerebral vasospasm myonecrosis in vessel walls. J Neurosurg 41:440, 1974
9. Alksne JF, Branson PJ: A comparison of intimal proliferation in experimental subarachnoid hemorrhage and atherosclerosis. Angiology 12:712, 1976
10. Allen GS, Henderson LM, Chow NS, French LA: Cere-

bral arterial spasm. I. In vitro contractile activity of vaso-active agents on canine basilar and middle cerebral arteries. J Neurosurg 40:433, 1974

11. Allen GS, Gross CJ, Henderson LM, Chou SN: Cerebral arterial spasm—Part 4: in vitro effects of temperature, serotonin analogues, large non-physiological concentrations of serotonin and extracellular calcium and magnesium on serotonin induced contractions of the canine basilar artery. J Neurosurg 44:585, 1976

12. Altura BT, Altura BM: Magnesium deficiency induces cerebral vasospasm, abstracted. Stroke 12:118, 1981

13. Alvord EC Jr, Loeser JD, Bailey WL et al: Subarachnoid hemorrhage due to ruptured aneurysms: a simple method for estimating prognosis. Arch Neurol 27:273, 1972

14. Anderson RMD, Blackwood W: The association of arteriovenous angioma and saccular aneurysms of the arteries of the brain. J Pathol Bacteriol 77:101, 1959

15. Andrews RJ, Spiegel PK: Intracranial aneurysms. Age, sex, blood pressure and multiplicity in an unselected series of patients. J Neurosurg 51:27, 1979

16. Andrews P, Papadokis N, Garras H: Reversal of experimental acute cerebral vasospasm by angiotensin converting enzyme inhibition. Stroke 13:480, 1982

17. Auer LM: Unfavorable outcome following early surgical repair of ruptured cerebral aneurysms—a critical review of 238 patients. Surg Neurol 35:152, 1991

18. Bader GM, Silk KR, Dequardo JR, Tandon R: Electroconvulsive therapy and intracranial aneurysm. Convulsive Therapy 11:139, 1995

19. Bannerman RM, Ingall GB, Graf CJ: The familial occurrence of intracranial aneurysms. Neurology 20:283, 1970

20. Banerjee RK, Gonzalez CF, Cho YI, Picard L: Hemodynamic changes in recurrent intracranial terminal aneurysm after endovascular treatment. Academic Radiology 3:202, 1996

21. Basset RC, Lemmen LJ: Subdural hematoma associated with bleeding intracranial aneurysms. J Neurosurg 9:443, 1952

22. Baumbach G, Heistad D: Effect of sympathetic nerves on segmental resistance of cerebral vessels. (Presented at the Seventh Joint Meeting on Stroke and Cerebral Circulation, New Orleans, Louisiana, 19–20 February 1982, abstracted.) Stroke 13:5, 1982

23. Belber CJ, Hoffman RB: The syndrome of intracranial aneurysm associated with fibromuscular hyperplasia of the renal arteries. J Neurosurg 28:556, 1968

24. Bendict CR, Loach AB: Sympathetic nervous system activity in patients with subarachnoid hemorrhage. Stroke 9:237, 1978

25. Benoit BG, Wortman G: Traumatic cerebral aneurysms. J Neurol Neurosurg Psychiatr 36:127, 1973

26. Bequelin C, Seiler R: Subarachnoid hemorrhage with normal cerebral panangiography. Neurosurgery 13:409, 1983

27. Beumont PJV: The familial occurrence of berry aneurysms. J Neurol Neurosurg Psychiatr 31:399, 1968

28. Birse SH, Tom MI: Incidence of cerebral infarction associated with ruptured intracranial aneurysms. Neurology 10:101, 1960

29. Black BK, Hicks S: The relation of hypertension to arterial aneurysms of the brain. US Armed Forces Med J 3:1813, 1952

30. Botterell EH, Lougheed WM, Scott JW et al.: Hypothermia, and interruption of carotid, or carotid and vertebral circulation, in the surgical management of intracranial aneurysm. J Neurosurg 13:1, 1956

31. Brass LM, Pavlakis S, Mohr JP: Transcranial Doppler measurements of the middle cerebral artery: the effect of hematocrit. Stroke 19:1446, 1988

32. Brisman R, Abbassioun K: Familial intracranial aneurysms. J Neurosurg 34:678, 1971

33. Brown FD, Hanlon K, Mullan S: Treatment of aneurysmal hemiplegia with dopamine and mannitol. J Neurosurg 49:525, 1978

34. Brownlee RD, Tranmer BI, Sevick RJ: Spontaneous thrombosis of an unruptured anterior communicating artery aneurysm. An unusual cause of ischemic stroke. Stroke 26:1945, 1995

35. Byer E, Ashman R, Toth LA: Electrocardiograms with large upright T waves and long QT intervals. Am Heart J 33:796, 1947

36. Call GK, Fleming MC, Sealfon S et al: Reversible cerebral segmental vasoconstriction. Stroke 19:1159, 1988

37. Candia CJ, Heros RC, Lavyne MH et al: Effects of intravenous sodium nitroprusside on cerebral blood flow and intracranial. Neurosurgery 3:50, 1978

38. Carmichael R: The pathogenesis of non-inflammatory cerebral aneurysms. J Pathol Bacteriol 62:1, 1950

39. Cates JE, Christ RV: Subacute bacterial endocarditis. Q J Med 20:93, 1951

40. Chason JL, Hindman WM: Berry aneurysms of the circle of Willis. Neurology 8:41, 1958

41. Chyatte D, Chen TL, Bronstein K, Brass LM: Seasonal fluctuation in the incidence of intracranial aneurysm rupture and its relationship to changing climatic conditions. J Neurosurg 82:912, 1995

42. Cioffi F, Pasqualin A, Cavazzani P, DaPian R: Subarachnoid haemorrhage of unknown origin: clinical and tomographical aspects. Acta Neurochir (Wien) 97:31, 1989

43. Cohen MM: Cerebrovascular accidents: a study of two hundred cases. Arch Pathol 60:296, 1955

44. Compton JS, Redmond S, Symon L: Cerebral blood velocity in subarachnoid haemorrhage: a transcranial Doppler study. J Neurol Neurosurg Psychiatry 50:1499, 1987

45. Conti MA, Adelstein RS: Phosphorylations by cyclic adenosine 3',5'-monophosphate-dependent protein kinase regulates myosin light chain kinase. Fed Proc 39:1569, 1980

46. Conway LW, McDonald LW: Structural changes of the intradural arteries following subarachnoid hemorrhage. J Neurosurg 37:715, 1972

47. Crompton MR: Intracerebral hematoma complicating ruptured cerebral berry aneurysm. J Neurol Neurosurg Psychiatr 25:378, 1962

48. Crompton MR: Cerebral infarction following the rupture of cerebral berry aneurysms. Brain 87:263, 1964

49. Cruickshank, JW, Neil-Dwyer G, Stott AW: Possible role of catecholamines, corticosteroids, and potassium in production of electrocardiographic abnormalities associated with subarachnoid hemorrhage. Br Heart J 36:697, 1974

50. Cullom ME, Savino PJ, Sergott RC, Bosley TM: Relative pupillary sparing third nerve palsies. To arteriogram or not? J Neuro-Ophthalmol 15:136, 1995
51. Dalgaard OZ: Bilateral polycystic disease of the kidneys: A follow-up of 284 patients and their families. Acta Med Scand (suppl) 328:186, 1957
52. Davis S, Andrews J, Lichtenstein M et al: A single photon emission computed tomography study of hypoperfusion after subarachnoid hemorrhage. Stroke 21:252, 1990
53. Delgado-Zygmunt TJ, Arbab MA, Edvinsson L et al: Prevention of cerebral vasospasm in the rat by depletion or inhibition of substance P in conducting vessels. J Neurosurg 72:917, 1990
54. Denton IC, Jr, White RP, Robertson JT: The effects of prostaglandins E A F2 on the cerebral circulation of dogs and monkeys. J Neurosurg 36:34, 1972
55. Diringer MN, Lim JS, Kirsch JR, Hanley DF: Suprasellar and intraventricular blood predict elevated plasma atrial natriuretic factor in subarachnoid hemorrhage. Stroke 22:577, 1991
56. Disney L, Weir B, Grace M, Roberts P: Trends in blood pressure, osmolality and electrolytes after subarachnoid hemorrhage from aneurysms. Can J Neurol Sci 16:299, 1989
57. Drake CG: Management of cerebral aneurysms. Stroke 12:273, 1981
58. DuBoulay GH: Some observations on the natural history of intracranial aneurysms. Br J Radiol 38:721, 1965
59. Edelsohn L, Caplan L, Rosenbaum AE: Familial aneurysms and infundibular widening. Neurol 22:1056, 1972
60. Edvinsson L, Owman CH, Sjoberg N: Autonomic nerves, mast cells and amine receptors in human brain vessels: A histochemical and pharmacological study. Brain Res 115:377, 1976
61. Fairbaum B: "Twin" intracranial aneurysms causing subarachnoid hemorrhage in identical twins. Br Med J 1:210–211, 1973
62. Fein JM, Flor WJ, Cohan SL, Parkhurst J: Sequential changes of vascular ultrastructure in experimental vasospasm. J Neurosurg 41:49, 1974
63. Findlay JM, Weir BK, Kanamaru K, Espinosa F: Arterial wall changes in cerebral vasospasm. Neurosurgery 25:736, 1989
64. Fisher CM: Clinical syndromes in cerebral thrombosis, hypertensive hemorrhage and ruptured saccular aneurysm. Clin Neurosurg 22:117, 1975
65. Fisher CM, Roberson GH, Ojemann RG: Cerebral vasospasm with ruptured saccular aneurysm—the clinical manifestations. Neurosurg 1:245, 1977
66. Fisher CM, Ojemann RG: Basal rupture of cerebral aneurysm—a pathological case report. J Neurosurg 48:642, 1978
67. Fisher CM, Kistler JP, Davis JM: Relation of cerebral vasospasm to subarachnoid hemorrhage visualized by computerized tomographic scanning. J Neurosurg 6:1, 1980
68. Fodstad H, Liliequist B, Schannong M, Thulin CA: Tranexamic acid in the preoperative management of ruptured intracranial aneurysms. Surg Neurol 10:9, 1978
69. Fogelholm R: Subarachnoid hemorrhage in middle Finland: incidence, early prognosis and indications for neurosurgical treatment. Stroke 12:296, 1981
70. Forbus WD: On the origin of miliary aneurysms of the superficial cerebral arteries. Bull Johns Hopkins Hosp 47:239, 1930
71. Fraser RAR, Stein BM, Barrett RE, Pool JL: Noradrenergic mediation of experimental cerebrovascular spasm. Stroke 1:356, 1970
72. Garcia CA, Dulcey S, Dulcey J: Ruptured aneurysm of the spinal artery of Adamkiewicz during pregnancy. Neurology 29:394, 1979
73. Gaetani P, Rodriguez Y Baena R, Grignani G et al: Endothelin and aneurysmal subarachnoid haemorrhage: a study of subarachnoid cisternal cerebrospinal fluid. J Neurol Neurosurg Psychiatr 57:66, 1994
74. Gautier JC, Hauw JJ, Awada A et al: Arteres cerebrales dolichoectasiques. Association aux anevrysmes de l'aorte abdominale. Rev-Neurol (Paris) 144:437, 1988
75. Gibbs JR, O'Gorman, P: Fibrinolysis in subarachnoid hemorrhage. Postgrad Med J 43:779, 1967
76. Gilbert JW, Lee C, Young B: Repeat cerebral panangiography in subarachnoid hemorrhage of unknown etiology. Surg Neurol 33:19, 1990
77. Glynn LE: Medical defects in the circle of Willis and their relation to aneurysm formation. J Pathol Bacteriol 51:213, 1940
78. Goldman MR, Rogers EL, Rogers MC: Subarachnoid hemorrhage associated with unusual electrocardiographic changes. JAMA 234:957, 1975
79. Gomez PA, Lobato RD, Rivas JJ et al: Subarachnoid haemorrhage of unknown aetiology. Acta Neurochir (Wien) 101:35, 1989
80. Graf CJ: Spontaneous carotid cavernous fistula: Ehlers-Danlos syndrome and related conditions. Arch Neurol 13:662, 1965
81. Gurus IN, Ghe MT, Richardson AE: The value of computerized tomography in aneurysmal subarachnoid hemorrhage. J Neurosurg 60:763, 1984
82. Hammermeister KE, Reichenbach DD: QRS changes, pulmonary edema and myocardial necrosis associated with subarachnoid hemorrhage. Am Heart J 78:94, 1969
83. Harrison MJG, Hampton JR: Neurologic presentation of bacterial endocarditis. Br Med J 2:148, 1967
84. Hassler O: Morphological studies on the large cerebral arteries with references to aetiology of subarachnoid hemorrhage. Acta Psychiatr Scand (Suppl) 154:1, 1961
85. Haykowsky MJ, Findlay JM, Ignaszewski AP: Aneurysmal subarachnoid hemorrhage associated with weight training: three case reports. Clin J Sport Medicine 6:52, 1996
86. Hayward RD: Subarachnoid hemorrhage of unknown aetiology. A clinical and radiological study of 51 cases. J Neurol Neurosurg Psychiatr 40:926, 1977
87. Heiskanen O: Risk of bleeding from unruptured aneurysms in cases with multiple intracranial aneurysms. J Neurosurg 55:524, 1981
88. Herdt D Jr, Chiro G, Doppman JL: Combined arterial and arteriovenous aneurysms of the spinal cord. Radiology 99:589, 1971
89. Heros RC, Zervas NT, Lavyne MH, Pickren KS: Rever-

sal of experimental cerebral vasospasm by intravenous nitroprusside therapy. Surg Neurol 6:227, 1976

90. Hochberg FH, Fisher CM, Roberson GH: Subarachnoid hemorrhage caused by rupture of a small superficial artery. Neurology 24:319, 1974

91. Hopkins CA, Wilkie FL, Vovis DC: Extramedullary aneurysm of the spinal cord. J Neurosurg 24:1021, 1966

92. Housepian EM, Pool JL: A systematic analysis of intracranial aneurysms from the autopsy file of the Presbyterian Hospital, 1914 to 1956. J Neuropathol Exp Neurol 17:409, 1958

93. Hunt WE, Hess RM: Surgical risk as related to time of intervention in the repair of intracranial aneurysms. J Neurosurg 28:14, 1968

94. Hunt WE, Kosnik EJ: Timing and perioperative care in intracranial aneurysm surgery. Clin Neurosurg 21:79, 1974

95. Jakobsen M, Overgaard J, Marcussen E, Enevoldsen EM: Relation between angiographic cerebral vasospasm and regional CBF in patients with SAH. Acta Neurol Scand 82:109, 1990

96. Kassell NF, Peerless SJ, Durward QJ et al: Treatment of ischemic deficits from vasospasm with intravascular volume expansion and induced arterial hypertension. Neurosurgery 11:337, 1982

97. Kassell NF: Aneurysmal rebleeding: a preliminary report from the cooperative aneurysm study. Neurosurgery 13:479, 1983

98. Kassell NF, Torner JC, Jane JA, Haley EC Jr, Adams HP: The International Cooperative Study on the Timing of Aneurysm Surgery Part 2: Surgical results. J Neurosurg 73:37, 1990

99. Kaste M, Ramsay M: Tranexamic acid in subarachnoid hemorrhage, a double-blind study. Stroke 10:519, 1979

100. Kawakami M, Kodama N, Toda N: Suppression of the cerebral vasospastic actions of oxyhemoglobin by ascorbic acid. Neurosurgery 28:33, 1991

101. Kawamura S, Yasui N: Clinical and longterm followup study in patients with spontaneous subarachnoid haemorrhage of unknown aetiology. Acta Neurochir (Wien) 106:110, 1990

102. Kistler JP, Crowell RM, Davis KR et al: The relation of cerebral vasospasm to the extent and location of subarachnoid blood visualized by CT scan. Neurology 433:424, 1983

103. Kistler JP: Management of subarachnoid hemorrhage from ruptured saccular aneurysm. p 175. In Ropper AH et al (eds): Neurological and Neurosurgical Intensive Care. University Park Press, Baltimore, 1983

104. Konishi Y, Maemura E, Sato E et al: A therapy against vasospasm after subarachnoidal haemorrhage: clinical experience of balloon angioplasty. Neurol Res 12:103, 1990

105. Kriplani A, Relan S, Misra NK, Mehta VS, Takkar D: Ruptured intracranial aneurysm complicating pregnancy. Int J Gynaecol Obstet 48:201, 1995

106. Kurihara N, Takahashi S, Higano S et al: Evaluation of large intracranial aneurysm with three-dimensional MRI. J Comput Assist Tomogr 19:707, 1995

107. Lennihan L, Petty GW, Mohr JP et al: Transcranial

108. Liliequist B, Lindqvist M, Probst F: Rupture of intracranial aneurysm during carotid angiography. Neuroradiology 11:185, 1976

109. Lindsay KW, Vermulen M, Murray G et al: Antifibrinolytic therapy in subarachnoid hemorrhage: reduction of rebleeding without benefit to outcome. Paper 5. Handbook of the American Association of Neurological Surgeons Annual Meeting 1984, pp. 9–10

110. Linskey ME, Horton JA, Rao GR, Yonas H: Fatal rupture of the intracranial carotid artery during transluminal angioplasty for vasospasm induced by subarachnoid hemorrhage. case report. J Neurosurg 74:985, 1991

111. Locksley HB: Natural history of subarachnoid hemorrhage, intracranial aneurysm and arteriovenous malformation. Based on 6368 cases in the cooperative study. Parts I and II. p. 370. In Sahs HL, Perrett GE, Locksley HB, Nishioka H (eds): Intracranial Aneurysms and Subarachnoid Hemorrhage. A Cooperative Study. Lippincott-Raven, Philadelphia, 1969

112. Loiseau H, Castel JP, Stoiber HP: Aspects clinique, neuroradiologiques et evolutifs du syndrome d' "hemmoragie meninges benigne idiopathique." Neurochirurgie 35: 2228, 1989

113. Martelli N, Colli BO, Assirati Jr JA, Machado HR: Cerebromeningeal hemorrhage. Analysis of autopsies performed over a 10 year period. Arq Neuropsiquiatr 46:166, 1988

114. Maspes PE, Marini G: Intracranial arterial spasm related to supraclinoid ruptured aneurysms. Acta Neurochirurg 10:630, 1902

115. Mathieu J, Perusse L, Allard P et al: Epidemiological study of ruptured intracranial aneurysms in the Saguenay-Lac-Saint-Jean region (Quebec, Canada). Can J Neurol Sci 23:184, 1996

116. Matsumura K, Matsuda M, Handa J, Todo G: Magnetic resonance imaging with aneurysmal subarachnoid hemorrhage: comparison with computed tomography scan. Surg Neurol 34:71, 1990

117. Maurice-Williams, RS: Prolonged antifibrinolysis: An effective nonsurgical treatment for ruptured intracranial aneurysm? Br Med J 1:945, 1978

118. Mayberg MR, Okada T, Bark DH: The significance of morphological changes in cerebral arteries after subarachnoid hemorrhage. J Neurosurg 72:626, 1990

119. Mayberg MR: Warning leaks and subarachnoid hemorrhage. West J Med 153:549, 1990

119a.McCormick WF: Vascular diseases. p 38. In Rosenberg RN, et al (eds): The Clinical Neurosciences. vol. 3. Churchill-Livingstone, New York, 1983

120. McCormick WF, Acosta-Rua GJ: The size of intracranial saccular aneurysms: an autopsy study. J Neurosurg 33:422, 1970

121. McCormick WF, Rosenfield DB: Massive brain hemorrhage. A review of 144 cases and an examination of their courses. Stroke 4:946, 1973

122. McCormick WF, Schmalotieg EJ: The relationship of arterial hypertension to intracranial aneurysms. Arch Neurol 34:285, 1977

Doppler detection of anterior cerebral artery vasospasm. Stroke 20:151, 1989

123. McCussick VA: Heritable disorders of connective tissue. C V Mosby, St. Louis, 1972

124. Melville KI, Blum B, Shister HL, Silver MD: Cardiac ischemic changes and arrhythmias induced by hypothalamic stimulation. Am J Cardiol 12:781, 1963

125. Miller NR, Savino PJ, Schneider T: Rapid growth of an intracranial aneurysm causing apparent retrobulbar optic neuritis. J Neuro-Ophthalmol 15:212, 1995

126. Miao FJ, Lee TJ: Effects of bilirubin on cerebral arterial tone in vitro. J Cereb Blood Flow Metab 9:666, 1989

127. Miller JD, Smith RR: Transcranial Doppler sonography in aneurysmal subarachnoid hemorrhage. Cerebrovasc Brain Metab Reviews 6:31, 1994

128. Millikan CH: Cerebral vasospasm and ruptured intracranial aneurysm. Arch Neurol 32:433, 1975

129. Mizukami M, Kin H, Araki G et al: Is angiographic spasm real spasm? Acta Neurochirurg 34:247, 1976

130. Mizukami M, Takemae T, Tazawa T et al: Value of computed tomography in the prediction of cerebral vasospasm after aneurysm rupture. Neurosurg 7:583, 1980

131. Mohr JP, Caplan LR, Melski JS et al: The Harvard Cooperative Stroke Registry: a prospective registry. Neurology 28:754, 1978

132. Mohr JP, Kase CS: Cerebral vasospasm. Rev Neurol 139:99, 1989

133. Molinari GF, Smith L, Goldstein MN et al: Pathogenesis of cerebral mycotic aneurysms. Neurology 23:325, 1973

134. Montgomery EB Jr, Grubb RL, Raichle ME: Cerebral hemodynamics and metabolism in postoperative cerebral vasospasm and treatment with hypertensive therapy. Ann Neurol 9:502, 1981

135. Morgan WL, Bland EF: Bacterial endocarditis in the antibiotic era. Circulation 19:753, 1959

136. Morley TP, Barr HWK: Giant intracranial aneurysms: diagnosis, course and management. Clin Neurosurg 16:73, 1968

137. Moskowitz MA, Rosenbaum AE, Tyler HR: Angiography monitored resolution of cerebral mycotic aneurysms. Neurology 24:1103, 1974

138. Nagamine Y, Takahashi S, Sonobe M: Multiple intracranial aneurysms associated with moyamoya disease. Case report. J Neurosurg 54:673, 1981

139. Nagasawa S, Handa H, Naruo Y et al: Experimental cerebral vasospasm arterial wall mechanics and connective tissue composition. Stroke 13:595, 1982

140. Neil-Dwyer N, Cruickshank J, Doshi A, Walter P: Systemic effects of subarachnoid hemorrhage. p. 256. In Wilkins RH (ed): Cerebral Arterial Spasm. Williams & Wilkins, Baltimore, 1980

141. Nelson PB, Seif SM, Maroon JC, Robinson AG: Hyponatremia in intracranial disease perhaps not the syndrome of inappropriate secretion of antidiuretic hormone (SAIDH). J Neurosurg 55:938, 1981

142. New PFJ, Price DL, Carter B: Cerebral angiography in cardiac myxoma. Radiology 96:335, 1970

143. Newell DW, Grady MS, Eskridge JM, Winn HR: Distribution of angiographic vasospasm after subarachnoid hemorrhage: implications for diagnosis by transcranial Doppler ultrasonography. Neurosurgery 27:574, 1990

144. Nibbelink DW, Tormer JC, Henderson WG: Intracranial aneurysms and subarachnoid hemorrhage. A co-operative study. Antifibrinolytic therapy in recent onset of subarachnoid hemorrhage. Stroke 6:622, 1975

145. Nicholls ES, Johansen HL: Implications of changing trends in cerebrovascular and ischemic heart disease mortality. Stroke 14:152, 1983

146. Nornes, H, Magnaes B: Intracranial pressure in patients with ruptured saccular aneurysm. J Neurosurg 36:536, 1972

147. Norris JW: Effects of cerebrovascular lesions on the heart. Neurol Clin 1:87, 1983

148. O'Brien JG: Subarachnoid hemorrhage in identical twins. Br Med J 1:607, 1942

149. Ohman J, Servo A, Heiskanen O: Risk factors for cerebral infarction in good grade patients after aneurysmal subarachnoid hemorrhage and surgery: a prospective study. J Neurosurg 74:14, 1991

150. Ohno K, Suzuki R, Masaoka H et al: A review of 102 consecutive patients with intracranial aneurysms in a community hospital in Japan. Acta Neurochir (Wien) 94:23, 1988

151. Ojemann RG: Management of the unruptured intracranial aneurysm. N Engl J Med 304:725, 1981

152. Ojemann RG, Crowell RM: Intracranial aneurysms and subarachnoid hemorrhage: incidence, pathology, clinical features and medical management. p 128. In Surgical Management of Cerebrovascular Disease. Williams & Wilkins, Baltimore, 1983

153. Okawara SH: Warning signs prior to rupture of an intracranial aneurysm. J Neurosurg 38:575, 1973

154. Onuma T, Suzuki J: Surgical treatment of giant intracranial aneurysms. J Neurosurg 51:33, 1979

155. Penmink, M, White RP, Cockavell JR: Role of prostaglandin F2 in the genesis of experimental cerebral vasospasm. Angiographic study in dogs. J Neurosurg 37:398, 1972

156. Peterson JW, Roussos L, Kwun BD et al: Evidence of the role of hemolysis in experimental cerebral vasospasm. J Neurosurg 72:775, 1990

157. Phillips LH, Whisnant JP, O'Fallon MW, Sundt TM: The unchanging pattern of subarachnoid hemorrhage in a community. Neurology 30:1034, 1980

158. Pope FM, Nichols AC, Narcisi P et al: Some patients with cerebral aneurysms are deficient in Type III collagen. Lancet 1:973, 1981

159. Post KD, Flamm ES, Goodgold A, Ransahoff J: Ruptured intracranial aneurysms: case morbidity and mortality. J Neurosurg 46:290, 1977

160. Pritz MB, Giannotta SL, Kindt GW et al: Treatment of patients with neurological deficits associated with cerebral vasospasm by intravascular volume expansion. Neurosurgery 3:364–368, 1978

161. Ramirez-Lassepas, M: Antifibrinolytic therapy in subarachnoid hemorrhage caused by ruptured intracranial aneurysm. Neurology 31:316, 1981

162. Raynor RB, McMurtry JS, Pool JL: Cerebrovascular effects of topically applied serotonin in the cat. Neurology 11:190, 1961

163. Reichembach DD, Benedict EP: Catecholamines and cardiomyopathy: the pathogenesis and potential importance of myofibrillar degeneration. Hum Pathol 1:125, 1970

164. Reigh EE, Lemmen LJ: Cerebral aneurysms with other intracranial pathology. J Neurosurg 17:469, 1960

165. Reynolds AF, Shaw C-M: Bleeding patterns from ruptured intracranial aneurysms: an autopsy series of 205 patients. Surg Neurol 15:232, 1981

166. Richardson JT: Cognitive performance following rupture and repair of intracranial aneurysm. Acta Neurol Scand 83:110, 1991

167. Rinkel GJ, Wijdicks EF, Vermeulen M et al: Outcome in perimesencephalic (nonaneurysmal) subarachnoid hemorrhage: a follow-up study in 37 patients. Neurology 40:1130, 1990

168. Rinkel GJ, Prins NE, Algra A: Outcome of aneurysmal subarachnoid hemorrhage in patients on anticoagulant treatment. Stroke 28:6, 1997

169. Robertson EG: Cerebral lesions due to intracranial aneurysms. Brain 72:150, 1949

170. Robinson JL, Hall CS, Sedzimir CB: Arteriovenous malformations, aneurysms and pregnancy. J Neurosurg 41: 63, 1974

171. Robinson RG: Coarctation of the aorta and cerebral aneurysm. Report of two cases. J Neurosurg 26:527, 1967

172. Romner B, Ljunggren B, Brandt L, Saveland H: Transcranial Doppler sonography within 12 hours after subarachnoid hemorrhage. J Neurosurg 70:732, 1989

173. Ronkainen A, Hernesniemi J, Ryynanen M et al: A ten percent prevalence of asymptomatic familial intracranial aneurysms: preliminary report on 110 magnetic resonance angiography studies in members of 21 Finnish familial intracranial aneurysm families. Neurosurgery 35:208, 1994

174. Ropper AH, Zervas NT: Outcome one year after subarachnoid hemorrhage from cerebral aneurysm. J Neurosurg 60:909, 1984

175. Rubenstein MK, Cohen NH: Ehlers-Danlos syndrome associated with multiple intracranial aneurysms. Neurology 14:125, 1964

176. Sahs AL: Preface. p xvii. In Sahs AL, Nibbelink DW et al (eds): Aneurysmal Subarachnoid Hemorrhage. Report of the Cooperative Study. Urban and Schwarzenberg, Baltimore, 1981

177. Sahs AL, Perret GE, Lockesley HB et al: Intracranial aneurysms and subarachnoid hemorrhage. Lippincott-Raven, Philadelphia, 1969

178. Sahs AL, Nibbelink DW, Torner JC: Aneurysmal Subarachnoid Hemorrhage: Report of the Cooperative Study. Urban & Schwarzenberg, Baltimore, 1981

179. Sakoda K, Uozumi T, Oki S et al: A study of the treatment of multiple aneurysms. Hiroshima J Med Sci 38: 151, 1989

180. Saito I, Sano K: Vasospasm following rupture of cerebral aneurysms. Neurol Med Chir (Tokyo) 19:103, 1979

181. Saitoh H, Hayakawa K, Nishimura K: Rerupture of cerebral aneurysms during angiography. Am J Neuroradiol 16:539, 1995

182. Sano K, Saito I: Timing and indication of surgery for ruptured intracranial aneurysms with regard to cerebral vasospasm. Acta Neurochir 41:49, 1978

183. Schucart WA, Hussain SK, Cooper PR: Epsilon-Aminocaproic acid and recurrent subarachnoid hemorrhage. A clinical trial. J Neurosurg 53:28, 1980

184. Schmid UD, Steiger HJ, Huber P: Accuracy of high resolution computed tomography in direct diagnosis of cerebral aneurysms. Neuroradiology 29:152, 1987

185. Schmidt M: Intracranial aneurysms. Brain 53:489, 1930

186. Seifert V, Stolke D, Reale E: Ultrastructural changes of the basilar artery following experimental subarachnoid haemorrhage. A morphological study on the pathogenesis of delayed cerebral vasospasm. Acta Neurochir (Wien) 100:164, 1989

187. Sekhar LN, Heros RC: Origin, growth, and rupture of saccular aneurysms: a review. Neurosurgery 8:248, 1981

188. Sekhar LN, Wechsler LR, Yonas H et al: Value of transcranial Doppler examination in the diagnosis of cerebral vasospasm after subarachnoid hemorrhage. Neurosurgery 22:813, 1988

189. Senguptu RP, So SC, Villarego Ortega FJ: Use of epsilon aminocaproic acid (EACA) in the preoperative management of ruptured intracranial aneurysms. J Neurosurg 44:479, 1976

190. Senter HJ, Sarwar M: Nontraumatic dissecting aneurysm of the vertebral artery. Case Report. J Neurosurg 56:128, 1982

191. Shepherd RH: Prognosis of spontaneous nontraumatic subarachnoid hemorrhage of unknown cause. A personal series 1958–1980. Lancet i:777, 1984

192. Shnider BI, Cotsonas NJ Jr: Embolic mycotic aneurysms, a complication of bacterial endocarditis. Am J Med 16:246, 1953

193. Simpson RK Jr, Fischer DK, Ehni BL: Neurogenic hyperthermia in subarachnoid hemorrhage. South Med J 82:157, 1989

194. Sloan MA, Haley EC Jr, Kassell NF et al: Sensitivity and specificity of transcranial Doppler ultrasonography in the diagnosis of vasospasm following subarachnoid hemorrhage. Neurology 39:1514, 1989

195. Soni RC: Aneurysm of the posterior communicating artery and oculomolar paresis. JNNP 37:475, 1974

196. Sonobe M, Suzuki J: Vasospasmogenic substance produced following subarachnoid haemorrhage, and its fate. Acta Neurochir (Wien) 44:97, 1978

197. Soucy JP, McNamara D, Mohr G et al Evaluation of vasospasm secondary to subarachnoid hemorrhage with technetium 99m hexamethylpropyleneamine oxime (HMPAO) tomoscintigraphy. J Nucl Med 31:972, 1990

198. Sparrow MP, Mrwa U, Hofmann H, Ruegg JC: Calmoduline is essential for smooth muscle contraction. FEBS Letters 125:141, 1981

199. Spetzler RF, Owen MP: Extracranial intracranial arterial bypass to a single branch of the middle cerebral artery in the management of a traumatic aneurysm. Neurosurgery 4:334, 1979

200. Stehbens WE: Intracranial arterial aneurysms. Aust Ann Med 3:214, 1954

201. Stehbens WE: Histopathology of cerebral aneurysms. Arch Neurol 8:272, 1963

202. Stehbens WE: Haemodynamic production of lipid deposition, intimal tears, mural dissection, and thrombosis in the blood vessel wall. Proc R Soc Lond (Biol) 185:357, 1974

203. Stehbens WE: The ultrastructure of the anastomosed

vein of experimental arteriovenous fistulae in sheep. Am J Pathol 76:363, 1974

204. Stehbens WE: Ultrastructure of aneurysms. Arch Neurol 32:798, 1975

205. Steinke D, Weir B, Disney L: Hydrocephalus following aneurysmal subarachnoid haemorrhage. Neurol Res 9: 3, 1987

206. Stornelli SA, French JD: Subarachnoid hemorrhage: factors in prognosis and management. J Neurosurg 21:769, 1964

207. Sundt, RM, Whisnant JP: Subarachnoid hemorrhage from intracranial aneurysms. N Engl J Med 299:116, 1978

208. Suzuki J, Onuma T: Intracranial aneurysms associated with arteriovenous malformations. J Neurosurg 50:742, 1979

209. Suzuki J, Sobata E, Iwabuchi T: Prevention of cerebral ischemic symptoms in cerebral vasospasm with trapidil, an antagonist and selective synthesis inhibitor of thromboxane A$_2$. Neurosurgery 9:679, 1981

210. Suzuki S, Kimura M, Souma M et al: Cerebral microthrombosis in symptomatic cerebral vasospasm: a quantitative histological study in autopsy cases. Neurol Med Chir (Tokyo) 30:309, 1990

211. Sypert GW: Intracranial aneurysm: natural history and surgical management. Compr Ther 4:64, 1978

212. Takemae T, Mizukami M, Kin H et al: Computed tomography of ruptured intracranial aneurysms in acute stage: relationship between vasospasm and high density on CT scan. No To Shinkei 30:861, 1978

213. Tanabe Y, Sakata K, Yamada H et al: Cerebral vasospasm and ultrastructural changes in cerebral arterial wall. J Neurosurg 49: 229, 1978

214. Taneda M, Otsuki H, Kumura E, Sakaguchi T: Angiographic demonstration of acute phase of intracranial arterial spasm following aneurysm rupture. Case report. J Neurosurg 73:958, 1990

215. Tannenbaum H, Nadjmi M, Gruss P: Therapeutic considerations in the treatment of vasospasm in aneurysms. Acta Neurochir 52:158, 1980

216. Tartara F, Gaetani P, Tancioni F et al: Alpha 1-antitrypsin activity in subarachnoid hemorrhage. Life Sciences 59:15, 1996

217. Toda N, Kawakami M, Yoshida K: Constrictor action of oxyhemoglobin in monkey and dog basilar arteries in vivo and in vitro. Am J Physiol 260:420, 1991

218. Tomlinson BE: Brain changes in ruptured intracranial aneurysm. J Clin Path 12:391, 1959

219. Tsuji T, Weir BK, Cook DA: Time-dependent effects of extraluminally applied oxyhemoglobin and endothelial removal on vasodilator responses in isolated, perfused canine basilar arteries. Pharmacology 38:101, 1989

220. Tsuji T, Cook DA, Weir BK, Handa Y: Effect of clot removal on cerebrovascular contraction after subarachnoid hemorrhage in the monkey: pharmacological study. Heart Vessels 11:69, 1996

221. Turnbull HM: Intracranial aneurysms. Brain 41:50, 1918

222. Van Rossum J, Wintzen AR, Endtz LJ et al: Effect of tranexamic acid on re-bleeding after subarachnoid hemorrhage: a double-blind controlled clinical trial. Ann Neurol 2:242, 1977

223. von Baumgarten FJ, Burkhard G, Englert D et al: Local hemostasis in subarachnoid hemorrhage. Eur Neurol 27: 149, 1987

224. von Essen C: Effects of dopamine on the cerebral blood flow in the dog. Acta Neurol Scand 50:39, 1974

225. Waga S, Ohtsubo K, Handa H: Warning signs in intracranial aneurysms. Surg Neurol 3:15, 1975

226. Waga S, Fijimato K, Morooka Y: Dissecting aneurysms of the vertebral artery. Surg Neurol 10:237, 1978

227. Tsuji T, Cook DA, Weir BK, Handa Y: Effect of clot removal on cerebrovascular contraction after subarachnoid hemorrhage in the monkey: pharmacological study. Heart Vessels 11:69, 1996

228. Weir B, Grace M, Hansen J, Rothberg C: Time course of vasospasm in man. J Neurosurg 48:173, 1978

229. Weir B, Disney L, Grace M, Roberts P: Daily trends in white blood cell count and temperature after subarachnoid hemorrhage from aneurysm. Neurosurgery 25:161, 1969

230. Wellum GR, Irvine TW, Zervas NT: Cerebral vasoactivity of heme proteins in vitro. J Neurosurg 56:777, 1982

231. White RP, Hagen AA, Morgan H et al: Experimental study on the genesis of vasospasm. Stroke 6:52, 1975

232. Wiebers DO, Whisnant JP, O'Fallen WM: The natural history of unruptured intracranial aneurysms. N Engl J Med 304:696, 1981

233. Wilkins RH, Alexander JA, Odom GL: Intracranial arterial spasm; a clinical analysis. J Neurosurg 29:12 1968

234. Wilkins RH: Cerebral vasospasm. Crit Rev Neurobiol 6:51, 1990

235. Winn HR, Richardson AE, Jane JA: The long-term prognosis in untreated cerebral aneurysms: 1. The incidence of late hemorrhage in cerebral aneurysm: A 10-year evolution of 364 patients. Ann Neurol 1:358, 1977

236. Wyllie E, Binkley FM, Palubinska AS: Extrarenal fibromuscular hyperplasia. Am J Surg 112:149, 1966

237. Yasui T, Kishi H, Komiyama M et al: Very poor prognosis in cases with extravasation of the contrast medium during angiography. Surg Neurol 45:560, 1996

238. Yoshida K, Watanabe H, Nakamura S: Intraarterial injection of amrinone for vasospasm induced by subarachnoid hemorrhage. Am J Neuroradiol 18:492, 1997

Arteriovenous Malformations and Other Vascular Anomalies

J.P. MOHR

JOHN PILE-SPELLMAN

BENNETT M. STEIN

Arteriovenous malformations (AVMs) are the most commonly recognized of the vascular malformations of the brain lesions because of their clinical and therapeutic implications. The other malformations are not easily visualized on an angiogram and have only recently attracted more attention because of the ability of magnetic resonance angiography to show the lesions.

Arteriovenous Malformations

AVMs are by definition congenital, but some fistulas that have the same appearance may arise from trauma or from venous occlusion. They are composed of a coiled mass of arteries and veins partially separated by thin islands of sclerotic tissue, lying in a bed formed by displacement rather than invasion of normal brain tissue.[110] Although they are congenital, usually many years elapse before they become clinically apparent. Some are more active than others, drawing to them huge collaterals, while others seem almost dormant.

CLASSIFICATION

Many complex, sometimes confusing, schemes of classification for AVMs are in common use. McCormick[107] and McCormick and Schochet[111] have developed a useful and practical

system based on pathology, and Spetzler and Martin[172] have proposed a system based on risks of mortality and morbidity associated with operative intervention.

Lesions not often recognized by clinicians including cavernous angiomas, telangiectasies, and venous malformations are more frequent in routine autopsy evaluations even though it is the AVM that attracts more clinical attention. A category of cryptic malformation is included, which is a clinically invisible form of AVM. This type of malformation is thought to give rise to subcortical hemorrhage in young individuals, which may destroy the original tangle of blood vessels and prevent it from appearing on angiography.[13,23,25,75,109] Telangiectases occur more often in the brain stem, cerebellum, or diencephalon than in the hemisphere or subcortical region.[36,109] Venous malformations are frequently noted in the cerebral white matter against the ventricular wall,[133] but they also occur in the posterior fossa, usually the cerebellum. They have a characteristic angiographic appearance of vessels spreading away from the center like a caput medusa. Their clinical significance is poorly understood because of the low frequency of clinical reports.[162,197]

AVMs are singled out for special attention by the clinician because of their frequent presentation in a young to middle-age group (Table 27.1) and the gross effects produced by hemorrhage or recurrent seizure disorder. They usually occur in isolation, unrelated to other disease states, but a few have been associated with the Weber-Osler-Rendu syndrome, most of them small.[68,155] In one recent large study,[155] 31 of 136

Table 27.1 Age of Onset of Symptoms

			Decade in Life						
Year	**Author**	**Ref.**	**<10**	**<20**	**<30**	**<40**	**<50**	**<60**	**<70**
1980	Parkinson & Bachers	142	4	10	7	15	10	4	2
1980	Nornes & Grip	130	4	18	10	9	11	6	2
1979	Pertuiset et al	149	10	27	43	44	21	15	5
1974	Pia et al	151	11	17	18	23	15	10	3
1970	Moody & Poppen	119	12	15	27	21	16	12	2
1966	Perret & Nishioka	147	15	56	66	70	48	39	10
1965	Svien & McRae	181	13	22	26	19	11	4	
1958	Dinsdale		5	8	11	12	8	5	1
1956	Paterson & McKissock	143	11	38	26	23	7	4	
1953	Mackenzie	96	5	24	6	9	5	1	
1948	Olivecrona & Riives	136	4	14	13	6	6		

cases from a hereditary hemorrhagic telangiectasia clinic were inferred to have cerebral AVMs on magnetic resonance imaging (MRI). Eighteen of these patients underwent angiogram; all were positive and seven had multiple (three or more) AVMs. The AVMs varied in size from 3 to 25 mm in maximal dimension. AVMs have also been described in the Wyburn-Mason syndrome.[198]

AVMs are made up of a tangle of vascular channels, some recognizable as arteries or veins, many merely twisted and convoluted vascular spaces. A characteristic histologic feature is the absence of capillaries[107,177,178] (Fig. 27.1). The arteries leading to veins draining from the malformation seem normal histologically, blending into the malformation near the fistula. The exact margin of the lesion is not often appreciated by angiography and sometimes cannot be discerned even at operation. AVMs vary in size from tiny, so-called cryptic, malformations to massive anomalies that encompass a number of cerebral lobes (Fig. 27.2). On the convexity AVMs are most frequently wedge-shaped with the apex of the wedge directed toward the ventricular system. However, these lesions may assume cylindrical or globoid forms in the white matter (Fig. 27.3). The arterial supply also varies enormously, from the extremes of all major cerebral, brain stem, or cerebellar arterial systems to a single artery to the fistula drained by a single vein. The feeding arteries in the larger malformations are frequently abnormally enlarged and ectatic, reflecting the large loads they carry. Deep arterial feeders often feed the malformation as well. These deep vessels usually arise from branches or main trunks of the major cerebral arteries in the lenticulostriate, choroidal, or thalamoperforant arteries (Fig. 27.4) and reach the AVM after passing through healthy tissues. In the scant studies performed on feeding arteries, the muscularis and elastica are attenuated and perhaps nonfunctional, leading to the loss of autoregulation.[125] There is some evidence that the reactivity of the nutrient arteries is abnormal for a considerable distance proximal to the malformation proper.

The venous drainage of AVMs eventually reaches recognizable venous channels, usually appearing abnormally distended by the large volumes of blood flow through the shunt. The veins follow two basic routes, the most common by superficial drainage coursing over the cortex directly to the major sinuses or collateral venous channels that lead to the major sinuses. The other route is through deep venous channels that reach the ependymal surface of the ventricular system and drain via the deep venous system. In the larger lesions there is often a dual venous network of drainage comprising both superficial and deep veins.

Histologic evaluation of AVMs demonstrates that the large cavernous components of the malformation are mostly devoid of elastica or significant muscularis in the walls[107,109] (Fig. 27.5). Within the malformation, the arteries show endothelial thickening, medial hypertrophy, and occasionally thrombosis; the veins are thin-walled and vary in size, with poorly developed muscular and elastic components. Spontaneous thrombosis may be seen within the confines of the malformation. Some vascular channels show hyalinization of the blood vessel wall with a deposit of collagenous tissue, probably related to spontaneous thrombosis and perhaps recanalization within the confines of the malformation. The exact site of

Figure 27.1 Corrosion specimen of an arteriovenous malformation obtained after the injection of acrylate into the malformation and dissolution of the soft tissue by potassium hydroxide. The specimen reveals the three-dimensional anatomy of the malformation and the configuration of the large venous sinusoids.

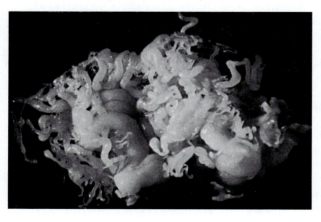

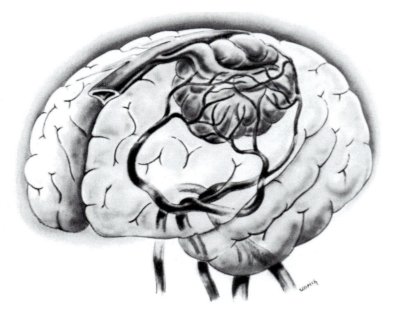

Figure 27.2 Drawing of an arteriovenous malformation located in an eloquent area of the brain and supplied by the three major intracranial vascular systems.

Figure 27.3 Cylinder-shaped arteriovenous malformation located in the frontal region and extended deep to the ventricle with a large vein draining to the ependyma (*arrow*).

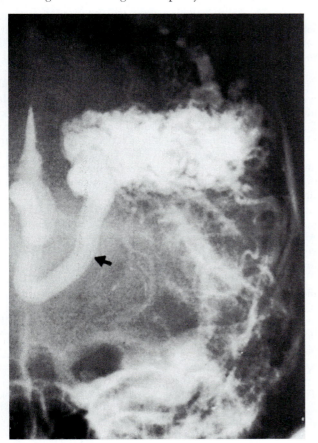

Figure 27.4 Example of a large arteriovenous malformation with a component of deep arterial feeders (*arrows*).

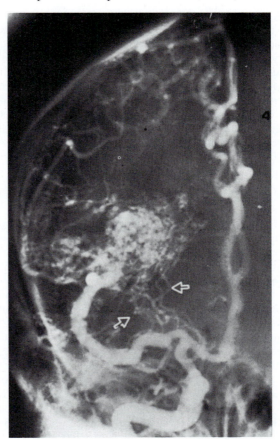

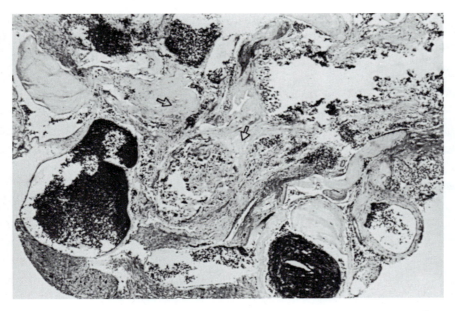

Figure 27.5 Photomicrograph of an arteriovenous malformation at low power demonstrating areas of gliosis (*arrows*) between large thin-walled cavernous sinuses.

the hemorrhage has never been demonstrated histologically. Where hemorrhage has occurred, hemosiderin-laden macrophages are found. Areas of gliosis surrounding old hemorrhagic cleavage planes and other evidence of previous hemorrhage are frequent findings.

Histologic studies of corrosion preparation of AVMs injected with inert substances after removal of the brain at autopsy have shown that there is virtually no normal cerebral tissue within the confines of an AVM (Figs. 27.1 and 27.5). The intense gliosis suggests that the neurons captivated within the margins of a malformation are probably nonfunctional. These findings support traditional views that these lesions are congenital and grow with the brain. Presumably, cerebral function that should be located in the brain occupied by the malformation is displaced to the margin of the malformation.[21]

LOCATION

No method has been generally agreed on for defining the epicenter of an AVM. The huge size of the arterial and venous channels may dwarf whatever fistula can be found and make it absurd to speak of a precise center of the malformation, yet some fistulas are discrete enough to determine if they are lobar, deep, and so forth. When a center is said to be found, it is most often frontoparietal but recent work is documenting the occurrence of brain stem and cerebellar AVMs more frequently.[11,167] Careful volumetric studies suggest there is no special predilection for AVMs in any part of the brain. The locations encountered seem simply to reflect the relative volume of the brain represented by a given region. The frontal lobe, occupying 30% of the brain volume, is shown to have 30% of the AVMs. The posterior fossa, at 12% of brain volume, has some 12% to 14% of the malformations.[6] Location has not had a bearing on the tendency for hemorrhage, growth, regression, vascular complexity, or size.

Enough clinical experience with AVMs is accumulating that some series have appeared describing AVMs in a given location. AVMs arising in the large lobes (e.g., frontal, occipital) seem to have about the same frequency of presentation with headaches, seizures, and hemorrhage, the focal syndrome reflecting the brain region involved. The 70 cases of occipital lobe AVM reported by Kupersmith et al[78] exemplify this point: 39 had headache, 20 had seizures, and hemorrhage occurred in 26, most of these presenting with visual field disturbances.

Among the hitherto less well described locations are the brain stem,[182] corpus callosum, choroidal artery territory, and anterior dura. Picard et al[152] described a series of 43 AVMs affecting the corpus callosum. The lesions were distributed fairly evenly through the callosum, almost half posteriorly. Over 20% had multiple foci. Callosal AVMs have feeders from any (and many from several) of the major cerebral arteries and drain to both superficial and deep venous networks. Several from Picard et al's[152] series were described as giant and diffuse, an appearance we have also encountered.

Choroidal AVMs are infrequently reported. Santoreneos et al[163] reported four cases and undertook a literature review. All their cases originated in the choroid plexus of the lateral ventricle. Such single-vessel origins tax the current, unsatisfactory embryologic theories of AVM formation (see below).

Dural AVMs, often arising from venous occlusion, have most often been reported posteriorly, but a few recent cases have been described in an inferior frontal location with a history of head trauma, the authors indicating their belief in a link between the trauma and the the origin of the dural lesion.[64,69]

NUMBER

The vast majority of AVMs are single, but there has been an increasing frequency of cases with multiple AVMs[34,164,198] (Fig. 27.6). One series of 203 patients reported a frequency of 19 (9%).[198] When multiple, the lesions are usually small.

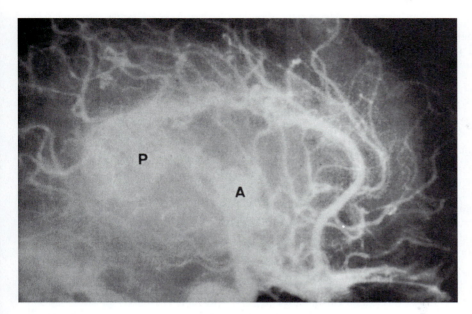

Figure 27.6 Tandem arteriovenous malformations involving the anterior third ventricle (A) and the roof structures of the posterior third ventricle (P). Even though the draining vein is common to these two malformations, they are distinctly separate.

ANGIOGRAPHIC FEATURES

AVMs may also be classified by their angiographic appearance. Pertuiset et al.[148,149] devised a scheme of identifying AVMs according to the territories of their nutrient arteries. Luessenhop and Gennarelli[93] used their location and blood supply. The latter categorization relates an AVM to the three major arterial systems (anterior, middle, and posterior cerebral arteries), taking account of a dual or triple arterial supply, and whether the malformation is primarily superficial or deep in the hemisphere. Spetzler and Martin[172] suggested a classification based on surgical approach. All three systems are useful in determining the operability of these lesions. Some doubts have been raised regarding the adequacy of grading systems, especially in the assessment of interobserver agreements.[80] However, Hamilton and Spetzler[54] have reported that their 5-point AVM grading system has had useful predictive value for neurologic morbidity after embolization or surgery; of 120 cases treated overall, grades I to III showed no impairments, whereas those in grade IV had 21.9% and grade V 16.7%.

For this presentation, we have enlarged the five-category scheme suggested by Parkinson and Bachers[142] in several directions, including features that take into account (1) lesion size; (2) arterial supply and venous drainage; (3) whether the supply is from deep or superficial vessels, or both; (4) whether draining veins are single or multiple, and widely patent or stenotic; (5) whether aneurysms affect the feeding arteries or are found within the nidus; (6) the number of arteries supplying the nidus and veins draining it; (7) whether the nidus appears to be the termination of the feeding arteries or whether they also pass beyond the AVM (en passage); (8) whether the AVM can be considered to arise along the course of an artery or the artery only feeds a focal nidus; (9) whether the lesion is deep, in the subcortical white matter, or confined to the brain surface; (10) whether, if a multiple-feeder AVM, it lies in a border zone shared by major arteries, territories, or vessels from one or more territories appearing to cross anatomic border zones to supply the AVM; and (11) whether feeders also include dural arteries.

TYPES

Deep and Superficial Supply (Multiple Unit Type)

In the multiple unit type, the fistula is fed by vessels that originate separately from the brain surface or from deeper structures (e.g., in the cerebrum, the basal ganglia or diencephalon; in the posterior fossa, the brain stem). In some cases, the deep feeders are difficult to define angiographically and may be obscured by the initial flush of contrast material from the surface feeders. The feeding arteries are branches of a major parent cerebral artery, arising in the usual fashion and then progressively changing in size, direction, and tortuosity as they approach the fistula. Usually the fistula is drained by more than one vein. The venous drainage develops in two major directions, one involving ependymal veins of the ventricle and the other via the deep white matter to the cortex. The larger the AVM, the more numerous the feeders from both the deep and superficial arteries. The more branches of one cerebral artery that feed the fistula, the more likely that similar branches from adjoining major cerebral arteries will also feed the fistula. This latter effect depends on the location of the main fistula: the closer to the arterial border zones, the greater the probability of such feeders. AVMs of this type usually have a pyramidal shape (i.e., on the surface or subsurface) and penetrate deep into the hemispheral white matter. In the largest malformations, most of the hemisphere can be made up of these tortuous vessels, whereas in midline lesions the supply may be drawn from branches of both carotids and the basilar artery.

Single Vessel Source (Single Unit Type)

In the infrequent (3% to 5% of cases) single unit type of AVM, a single arterial feeder, arising from a surface vessel or a deep vessel, empties into a fistula drained by a single vein, a so-called straight line AVM. The fistula may be so small that only the abnormal size of the artery and vein arouse suspicion. In others, the vein is aneurysmal, the best known being the vein of Galen malformation. This group is thought to be more easily approached surgically and may have a lower risk of hemorrhage.

Cerebral and Extracerebral

Cerebral and extracerebral AVMs, varying in reported incidence from 3% to over 20%, have become increasingly recognized in recent years. Separate injection of the external carotid artery is required to demonstrate the extracranial feeders, a step not always taken in earlier days. Some feeders arise from muscular branches of the vertebral arteries. Such feeders are more often found in cerebellar or posterior fossa AVMs, but the extracerebral and transdural supply to the fistula may be over the cerebrum, especially in those cases arising from trauma.

Venous Wall

Venous Wall AVMs represent an arterial supply directly to the venous sinus, in which case the arteries are usually extracerebral in origin and drain directly into the wall of one of the venous sinuses.[83,191]

EMBRYOLOGY

Although some lesions are acquired, it has long been accepted that AVMs represent a disorder of embryogenesis. What kind of disorder and how truly embryologic in origin they are has been a subject of disagreement, with recent studies showing lesions developing over time.[84]

Anomalies of the major extracranial and intracranial vessels are uncommon in patients with AVMs, forcing much of the histologic work to be done on the AVM vessels themselves. AVMs are presumed to result from ". . . incomplete and abnormal resolution of the embryologic vascular network."[140] If this claim is true, some AVMs must represent static anomalies, whereas others have the potential to grow. What relation these two alternatives have to the risk of bleeding or progressive neurologic deficit is unknown. Some clues as to the significance of the various unusual angiographic findings known clinically as AVMs might be found in the details of vascular embryology as it applies to the cerebral circulation. However, despite the progress in understanding of the embryogenesis

of other vascular systems, remarkably little is known of the details as they apply to the surface and deep vessels of the cerebrum.

Standard studies of embryology focused on the development of the major extracranial arteries with only limited information on intracranial arteries with respect to the formation of the circle of Willis and its immediate branches. Until recent years only passing mention has been made of the growth of the branches of the major cerebral arteries and the vascular systems of the cortex and cerebral white matter. Moffat[116] made reference only to a capillary plexus in the 3.7-mm rat embryo. Mall's[98] eight embryo brains showed little development of the arteries in specimens of <4 weeks, but those older showed components of the circle of Willis and all the major vessels over the brain. He noted that all the brain vessels arose at intervals so regular that they appeared segmental. Klosovskii[74] limited remarks on vascular malformations to a few cryptic statements under the heading "Fundamental Facts," and observed that primitive arteriovenous units began their penetration into the developing cerebrum in the second intrauterine month. The units penetrating the brain were tightly looped with the artery and vein more or less parallel. Tiny buds developed from the sides of the loop like tentacles, fusing with others from adjacent vessels to form the capillary bed. "The arteriovenous loops penetrate into the brain from the surface toward the germinal layer in radial fashion," while these same arteriovenous units were cross-linked, at right angles to the penetrating arteriovenous units, by the developing capillary system. These links created a net of vessels parallel to the plane of the cerebral surface. As development proceeds, the capillary network in the developing gray matter becomes more elaborate than that in the white matter. The author did not elaborate on what role, if any, these embryogenic principles might play in the development of AVMs.

The well-known work of Padget[140,141] was mainly devoted to the embryology of the major arteries and veins. However, in one publication[141] some reference was made to a possible embryologic basis of AVMs. The author speculated that both the deep and superficial AVMs had the same embryonic derivation, which

> . . . primarily involves abnormal arterial influx into a relatively large vein on the neural tube . . . . Presuming an arteriovenous (AV) fistula between a definitive artery and vein, the sequence of resulting dilatations, namely veins-to-capillaries-to-arteries, seems clear. The identity, size, and connections of the venous channels present, the subsequent development of veins and the amount of arterial influx may chiefly determine whether the resulting dilated coils are relatively localized or gradually spread to more remote parts.

The process could conceivably be set in motion at any point where the primitive arteries and veins cross one another. It should be possible to use embryologic observations to predict the spectrum of AVMs that could occur.

If this assumption is accepted, two broad categories of AVM are possible. In one form the abnormality would continue to evolve, drawing to it collateral vessels, ever enlarging and eventually rupturing. In another, the disorder might be static, conceivably even capable of regressing with time. Although such possibilities are easily envisioned, no useful criteria have as yet emerged to separate AVMs into these two classifications.

Within the last decade, other workers have added new ideas.[8,14,31,157] Bär[8] found that the extrastriatal vessels of the mouse cortex passed completely through the parenchyma of the telencephalon to the ventricle and were at first simple channels with no media. With the steady outward growth of the telencephalon, the transcerebral vascular trunks elongated but remained connected to the ventricle, while later vessels, increasingly appearing more like arteries, arose from the cortical mantle to penetrate roughly the same depth as did the original primitive vessels. However, this depth brought the vessel to the ventricular wall but left it in the centrum semiovale instead. With each new set of vessels, penetration became progressively less into the white matter, and last of all appeared to arborize entirely within the surface gray matter. Kuban and Gilles[77] observed that some transcerebral vessels originating in the operculum curved over the striatal vascular territories to reach the ventricular wall, arguing that the transcerebral and lenticulostriate systems had no real linkage to one another.

To date no classification of AVMs has been developed according to their presumed disordered embryogenesis. This disappointing state of affairs may be preventing an understanding of the overall problem of the AVMs, or our separation of those representing mere static anomalies from those destined to rupture.

Some studies have suggested a molecular biologic basis for the development of AVMs in disturbances of vascular endothelial growth factor and basic fibroblast growth factor.[159] The former was found to be considerably increased in surgical specimens from patients whose AVMs recurred versus those not associated with regrowth.[171] The number of observations was small, but the suggestions warrant further study. Another group of observations indicates that AVM vessels are deficient in calcitonin gene-related peptide-like, neuropeptide Y-like, and vasoactive intestinal peptide-like immunoreactivity in the circle of Willis, suggesting that faulty neurogenic control of vessels may underlie the development of AVMs.

ACQUIRED ARTERIOVENOUS FISTULAS

Some arteriovenous fistulas that appear angiographically to be AVMs arise from trauma and thrombosis of large veins or sinuses. Two major causes have been identified, trauma and venous thrombosis.

Trauma

Trauma to the brain surface[47] from closed head injury presumably may join or enlarge the existing arteriovenous shunts roughly 90 μm in size near the superior sagittal sinus, and possibly in other sites. Once linked or enlarged, such fistulas would presumably lose their autoregulation and be subject to the same enlargement typical of any arteriovenous link. Such cases should have a history or show evidence of prior head injury and should be confined to the brain surface. To date, no ready classification for these lesions has been developed.

Venous Thrombosis

Thrombosis of a large vein or sinus[47,83,181] may create a high enough resistance to normal arterial flow as to force creation of new pathways. The angiogram usually shows delayed filling of the carotid or vertebrobasilar arteries and those branches having access to a patent vein or sinus, such as the meningeal and other dural arteries, which dilate and convolute in a manner seen in congenital AVMs. These shunts can develop in a fairly short time, possibly months. If sinus thrombosis occurs, a major hemorrhagic lesion may follow.[114] It is still unknown whether the hypertrophied channels become independent of autoregulation or can be expected to subside if the venous obstruction is relieved, nor is it understood whether they have certain theoretic limits in size and extent or continue to develop until they hemorrhage. Lastly, it is unclear whether their proper treatment is ligation or neglect.

Moya-moya and High-Flow Angiopathy

Increasing awareness of a relationship between AVMs and high-grade intracranial stenoses has left unsettled which of the two processes begins first. Some investigators envision a so-called high-flow angiopathy with the development of lesions to the intima in vessels feeding an AVM, the lesions building to the point of causing severe stenosis and occlusion of feeding arteries.[152] Another thesis is that the underlying process of severe stenosis known as moya-moya triggers sufficient vasodilatation in distal vessels as to cause arteriovenous links, which take on a life of their own and have the angiographic appearance of AVMs. Further work is in order on these points.

PHYSIOLOGIC STUDIES

Physiologic evaluation of vascular malformations has been centered around the study of AVMs.[37,129,133,135,168,196] Cerebral blood flow (CBF) recordings indicate a varying degree of arteriovenous blood shunting within an AVM. This shunting depends on the ratio of the feeding arteries to draining veins, the size of the lesion, and the number of shunts within the lesion. When shunting is great enough, left ventricular cardiac failure can occur, as has been seen in children with larger AVMs. Early intraoperative studies by Nornes and Grip[130] underscore the dynamic changes that occur in blood flow through these malformations during occlusion of the various nutrient arteries and with systemic changes of blood pressure and flow. The fall in pressures proceeds in an orderly manner from the parent artery through branches leading finally to the AVM, where pressures may be quite low; by inference, pressures are also low in normal adjacent brain supplied by these same branches.[40] Remarkably, little difference is found in the shear forces in vessels involved in an AVM compared with healthy vessels.[169]

Evidence is now clear that the large feeding arteries lack autoregulation. Tarr et al[184] found four types of responses in CBF to challenge with acetazolamide (Diamox): (1) normal baseline and normal augmentation of CBF; (2) normal baseline and decreased augmentation; (3) low baseline; and (4) low baseline CBF and normal augmentation with acetazolamide. The largest number of patients fell in this last group, and these data were interpreted to mean decreased cerebral blood flow demand but with a normal vascular reserve. None of the patients studied showed abnormalities of the brain vasculature remote from the AVM.

Angiographic signs of disordered autoregulation postoperatively include enlargement of an artery proximal to an AVM in the days after the malformation is occluded by either embolization or surgical ligation (Fig. 27.7). This postocclusion ectasia remains for days to weeks (Fig. 27.8). Persistent ectasia leads to decreased flow and stasis in the arterial system proximal to the AVM. Young et al[203] studied 26 patients by CBF before and after total AVM resection. There were no differences in baseline CBF and CO_2 reactivity between the AVM and six spinal surgical patients in a control group. CBF increased significantly but did not show a hemispheric difference, indicating that obliteration of the shunt results in global increase in blood flow.

In the postoperative state, arterial stasis, even vein thrombosis and venous infarction in the normal brain, has been described.[174,177] The pressure in the feeding arteries postoperatively is high initially and may lead to hemorrhagic complications described by Spetzler et al[174] as "perfusion pressure breakthrough." The pressure and flow that drives the nutrient blood to an AVM is thought to be redirected to the normal circulation following the obliteration of an AVM. This rerouted blood pressures the local arteries beyond their capacities, resulting in edema and then hemorrhage in the area. Postoperative stasis, high arterial pressures, and/or hemorrhagic complications have been described by others as well.[11,81,121,123] Muraszko et al[125] found support for this concept in their *in vitro* study of feeding vessels removed at surgery. In 24 patients four

nutrient vessels taken from the feeding vessels near the AVM showed no spontaneous activity in the perfusion chamber. The authors found that those with unreactive vessels had more postoperative edema and hemorrhage, suggesting that these vessels were subject to normal perfusion pressure breakthrough. The highest CBF increases in the study by Young et al[203] were associated with postoperative brain swelling in one patient and fatal intracerebral hemorrhage in another. Both patients had normal CO_2 reactivity before excision. Similar experiences were reported by Batjer et al.[11]

Recent studies from our institution have indicated a shift of the autoregulation limits toward lower pressures, preserved responsiveness to CO_2, and pharmacologically induced vasodilatation in arteries adjacent to AVMs.[39,204]

Former assumptions of perfusion defects associated with AVMs have proved difficult to certify. In a study of 11 cases of hemispheral AVM, single-photon emission tomography was used to compare the regions of the AVM with a matching contralateral site, before and after acetazolamide administration. The defects in flow surrounding the AVM lesions were found to be related to the size of the AVM, not to any effects explained by local arterial pressure.[53] Preservation of cerebrovascular reserve was also evident, arguing against a specific defect in perfusion around an AVM such as that postulated for steal.

INCIDENCE AND PREVALENCE

In the Cooperative Study of Subarachnoid Hemorrhage,[146,147] still the largest such series to date, symptomatic AVMs were found in 549 of 6,368 cases, representing an incidence of 8.6%

Figure 27.7 (A) Large arteriovenous malformation (AVM) fed by a posterior cerebral artery (*arrowhead*). (B) Enlargement of the posterior cerebral artery (*arrowhead*) after successful embolic occlusion of portions of the AVM and feeding artery with marked reduction of flow through the arteriovenous malformation, but with enlargement of the feeding artery.

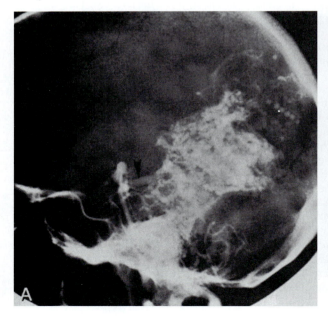
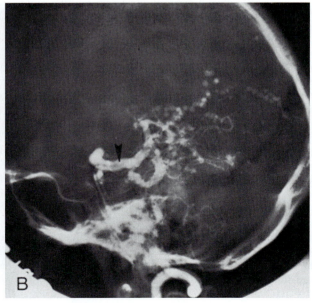

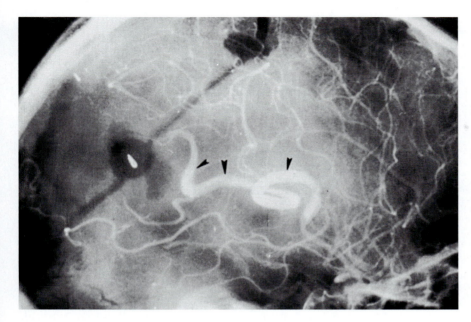

Figure 27.8 Residual ectasia of an artery (*arrowheads*) feeding a malformation after successful obliteration of the malformation. This ectatic state of the feeding artery may remain for many weeks following surgery.

of subarachnoid hemorrhages. Since subarachnoid hemorrhage accounts for roughly 10% of strokes, AVMs make up approximately 1% of all strokes. These incidence figures for AVM are reflected in a population-based prospective study of stroke, one carried out in south Alabama. In an eligible population of 100,000 studied over a period of 3 years, 9 AVMs occurred among 494 stroke cases, yielding an incidence of 1.8%.[51]

Data on the prevalence of AVMs are more difficult to obtain but are equally important, especially in efforts to assess the risk of stroke in asymptomatic cases.[70,117] A high ratio of asymptomatic to symptomatic cases might encourage a less aggressive management for such cases, which are being encountered with increasing frequency. Because of brain imaging awareness of AVMs has increased over the past few decades.[88] The early studies suggested a very low prevalence. These figures were upgraded by McCormick and Rosenfield,[110] who uncovered 196 AVMs among 4,530 consecutive autopsies, an incidence of 4.3%. While not from a population-based study, these data are of special interest since they represent a careful autopsy-based effort to document the prevalence of AVMs, symptomatic or asymptomatic. Only 24 of the McCormick's 196 (12.2%) cases had been symptomatic from their AVMs. This figure yields a symptomatic stroke incidence of 0.52% in this autopsied population, which is in the range of the 1% incidence found in purely clinical studies. Among the 24 symptomatic cases, 21 had suffered hemorrhage, 16 massive, and the remainder had epilepsy or steal phenomena. The distribution of AVMs in cerebral hemispheres was 118 (60%), 28 (14%) affected the brain stem, and the spinal cord was the site in 5 (3%). These distributions closely approximate those in clinically symptomatic series. Given the patterns of case referral, it is no surprise that the

larger series of cases of AVMs come mainly from surgical clinics. The low frequency of the disorder prevents all but a few interested physicians and surgeons from having any but a passing encounter with such cases. In one report of 100 patients angiogrammed for tandem lesions in a setting of high-grade carotid stenosis, two AVMs were found.[49]

The largest single series comprises the 549 cases reported by the Cooperative Study,[146,147] itself a pooled effort involving many centers and the published series of AVMs uncovered in a literature survey carried back over almost half a century. Scarcely more than a dozen publications describe more than 100 cases a series.[26,42,58,61,137,143,148,181,186,195] The period required for each of the major contributors to accumulate such experience has usually been measured in decades. As referring physicians have become more aware that definitive therapy is possible, the database on the patient population for some of the clinical features has changed.

The presumably congenital nature of AVMs might be expected to yield many cases with a family history, but the familial incidence appears quite rare.[9,17,30,45,170] Only seven families had been reported through 1990, involving 15 people in all. The mode of inheritance is uncertain. In contrast to the male preponderance in general for AVMs reported in clinical surgical services, the sexes are equally represented in the scanty family history data (Table 27.2). This constant is not easily explained by patterns of referral and is probably a reliable finding. With a greater awareness of the successes in surgery, efforts at diagnosis have increased in the older population. In large centers modern efforts at diagnosis have shifted the age of onset upward. Given that assumption, AVM is no longer to be considered a diagnosis mainly involving the young, even though most hemorrhages occur in the younger

Table 27.2 Sex

Year	Author	Male	>	Female	Ratio
1981	Guidetti and DeLitala[52]	89		56	1.59
1979	Pertuiset et al[148]	102		60	1.70
1979	Nornes and Grip[130]	40		23	1.74
1973	Morello and Broghi[120]	88		66	1.33
1972	Forster et al.[42]	99		51	1.94
1970	Moody and Poppen[119]	65		40	1.63
1966	Cooperative Study[146]	236		217	1.09
1958	Tönnis	88		46	1.91
1956	Paterson and McKissock[143]	63		47	1.34

age group. Dural and extracerebral AVMs are the only types thought to be usually acquired from trauma.

NATURAL HISTORY AND CLINICAL PRESENTATION

Many retrospective studies of AVMs have afforded us some insight into the clinical presentation of these lesions, but no definitive data are available on the natural history of a large group of AVMs obtained through prospective studies.[19,24,42,58,61,137,143,148,181,186,195] This situation exists because these lesions are generally rare and, when symptomatic, are treated by the various therapeutic modalities that we now have available. Therefore, comments on the natural history of these disorders are anecdotal and are generally based on patients who are not suitable candidates for any form of treatment, yet the clinical experience painstakingly accumulated at a few large centers is the only information available.

As the experience has accumulated, the remarkable variation of clinical material from center to center has become apparent, and with it a hesitancy to offer such experience for publication. In any uncommon condition, it is most important to have data available on the natural history of the condition to discuss risky and sometimes radical forms of treatment with the patient and relatives. Unfortunately, the rarity of these lesions has precluded any definitive prospective study of the natural history. Furthermore, the clinical picture of many of these lesions spans years if not decades. It has therefore been difficult for any one center to accumulate an untreated group of patients who have AVMs in various forms and locations and who have been followed with arteriography for at least 1 to 2 decades.[65]

Anecdotal retrospective evaluations of a moderate number of patients, however, would indicate that these lesions are congenital and, like many congenital lesions, do not manifest until the middle decades, when they are associated with a high incidence of incapacitating or fatal hemorrhages, perhaps as high as 40% to 50% as measured over the normal life expectancy of a young individual. Another small group of individuals presents with a seizure or hemorrhage in the fifth and sixth decades. These individuals have been asymptomatic up to the event and in this context must be viewed in a different light than younger individuals. In the older individual who has lived asymptomatically with the malformation for many decades,

caution is recommended against risky or radical forms of treatment. The overall risk is naturally diminished by the limitation in life expectancy after 50 years.

Estimates of the risk of first hemorrhage depend on the source of the clinical series. Ondra et al[137] obtained a mean follow-up time of 23.7 years for 160 of 166 (96%) symptomatic patients who had not undergone operation and demonstrated a combined rate of mortality and major morbidity of 2.7% a year. The rate of rebleeding was 4% a year and that of mortality 1%. The rates seemed fairly constant from year to year. Horton et al[61] estimated a risk of 0.031/patient-year based on the course of 540 patients seen in referral at a major hospital. Crawford and Russell[25] reported a 42% risk of rehemorrhage in 10.4 years and a slightly higher risk for smaller lesions. In all experienced groups, recurrent hemorrhage within hours to weeks seems quite rare, in contrast to that associated with aneurysms.

On the basis of available information and our own personal experience, young individuals are told that they have a 40% to 50% risk of some major incapacitating or fatal hemorrhage from an AVM in their projected life span. This projection is made regardless of whether the patient presents with hemorrhage, seizure, migraine, or unrelated symptoms. With the frequent utilization of imaging, these lesions may be discovered quite by accident. The fate of a treated AVM seems highly dependent on the form of treatment. Once an AVM has been removed (as proved by postoperative angiography), recurrent hemorrhage should not occur. Therefore, in discussions with the patient and the relatives, the surgical risk should be documented and the fact stressed that if the lesion can be removed the patient is cured. Treatments that fall short of total obliteration of the AVM include embolization,[43] radiotherapy,[73] and partial surgical procedures[62] that have no valid statistical analysis documenting the degree of protection they offer. For embolization, Luessenhop and Presper[95] have stated the generally accepted view that short of total obliteration of the malformation, embolization provides little protection from recurrent hemorrhage or progressive neurologic deficit. They note that seizures are easier to control following embolization, but this may be a factor of closer scrutiny of the patient rather than a direct effect of the embolization. We have a large series of patients who have only been embolized; unfortunately, a large number of these have not been followed for a sufficiently long period to draw any conclusions. It is our clinical impression that embolization affords some protection and amelioration of symptoms when there is a significant reduction in the AVM. Therefore, in frank discussions with the patient, the detriment of any form of incomplete therapy should be stressed and balanced with the risk of that therapy as against the presumed natural risk of the malformation. In good faith, a physician could then recommend a form of incomplete therapy that has minimal risk even though it might have little or no therapeutic effect for the patient, whereas any form of incomplete obliteration associated with a significant risk should be recommended with great reluctance. The risk of surgery as related to the configuration, location, and size of the malformation is discussed in the therapeutic section. Suffice it to say that in our large series of AVMs for which an operation was performed, the risk factors are <2% for mortality and 5% for significant morbidity, with 12% for minor morbidity following total obliteration of the lesion. Radiotherapy is becoming increasingly popular and has been shown to obliterate some of the smaller lesions,[73] but higher doses are required for the larger lesions, raising concern for radiation necrosis[176] and uncertainty of success. The course of the lesions has been shown by repeat angiograms in only a few studies. Growth of the AVM has been documented, as has stability and even regression.[112,113,173,177,178] Minakawa et al[113] repeated the angiogram 5 to 28 years after first discovery or treatment in 20 patients, 16 of whom were untreated while the remaining were residual. The AVM was unchanged in eight, larger in four, smaller in four, and had disappeared in four. The AVMs that disappeared were relatively small and fed by a single feeder or a few feeders. It remains to be seen whether such findings will be reproduced by others, but the possibility of estimation of AVM size by MR should stimulate such studies in the future.

CLINICAL SYNDROMES

Hemorrhage

The vast majority of AVMs that become symptomatic present with hemorrhage.[19,96,101,120,178,187,194] Hemorrhage can be parenchymatous and subarachnoid. Unlike cerebral aneurysms, with which these lesions are often compared, the hemorrhage into the subarachnoid space is generally confined to local subarachnoid spaces and does not spread widely into the large cisterns.

The major clinical presentation is related to a parenchymal hemorrhage with focal neurologic deficits. Approximately half of the clinical presentations of AVMs are intracranial hemorrhage.[19,60,73,75,117,147] Primarily parenchymatous hemorrhage occurs most often (63% of cases), while subarachnoid occurs in 32%, and ventricular least often, at 6%.[60] Among 106 cases seen in 1 year at our institution, 40% had hemorrhage documented by imaging at some time in the course of their illness. Although the malformation itself occupies space, it does not frequently present as a mass lesion in the absence of hemorrhage. In cases of stroke due to causes other than AVM, the brain tissue is essentially healthy and normal before its disruption. Stroke from AVMs is different; the lesion is embedded in the brain, surrounded by healthy tissue, and its disordered vessels may draw circulation from healthy brain or provide blood to healthy brain distal to the malformation. The degree of neurologic deficit depends on the location and size of the hemorrhage.

Those lesions located in polar regions of the brain may become apparent in the face of massive hemorrhage with little more than headache and nonfocal symptoms related to the mass effect and rise of intracranial pressure. However, those lesions located in deep structures such as the diencephalon, basal ganglion, or motor, sensory, and speech areas may present with devastating neurologic deficits secondary to involvement of these areas. Since the hemorrhages are often subcortical and extend into the white matter, there is frequently a separation of the fibers without lasting impairment of function. Many of these patients may make remarkable and often complete recovery from the initial hemorrhage although it may be massive. Unfortunately, a group of patients has fixed and sometimes catastrophic neurologic deficits following the initial hemorrhage, and these remain for the life of the patient. As noted, the degree of subarachnoid blood varies and depends for the most part on two factors, the extent of the hemorrhage and the relationship of the AVM to large cisterns or to the ventricles. Many of the larger malformations project in a wedge-shaped fashion to the ventricle, where the dilated tortuous loops of veins may lie free without ependymal covering. This is a source of hemorrhage in such malformations and may lead to massive amounts of intraventricular blood with acute hydrocephalus and spread of the blood throughout the cerebrospinal fluid.

Settings for the rupture may include the familiar exertional states commonly encountered with other causes of hemorrhage. However, a few authors have found no correlation with activity,[143] a point against advising asymptomatic patients to live a completely sedentary life. Pregnancy was once cautioned against and still remains a management conundrum,[82] but the bleeding rates of 0.031/patient-year during pregnancy compare favorably with the 0.031 risk/patient-year for nonpregnant females,[61] indicating that pregnancy is not a greater risk for those without prior hemorrhage. It was thought that pregnancy, especially during the first trimester, held a greater risk of AVM hemorrhage and some observers suggested cesarean section as a prudent measure to avoid complications during delivery.[61,72] There appears to be no greater risk to the mother during the various phases of pregnancy, and there seems to be no justification for abortion.

A long-standing impression exists that the smaller AVMs appear more prone to hemorrhage than do the very large lesions.[25,27,42,43,58] In Morello and Boroghi's[120] series, rupture had occurred in 86% of the small AVMs, in 75% of those of medium size, but in only 46% of the giant AVMs. These findings are consistent with those in other series and suggest that the larger the lesion, the longer it has been present, and the less likely it is to rupture. At least 10% of AVMs show evidence of prior bleeding at surgery, more often encountered in the smaller AVMs.[52,120] This high prevalence of prior hemorrhage clearly indicates that many are small enough to escape clinical detection. In our own institutional study, predictors for first hemorrhage were deep venous drainage, small AVM size, and high feeding artery pressures.[67]

In some cases, the hemorrhagic onset of symptoms related to these lesions is not recognized by the patient or the treating physician. It may be passed off as a migraine type of headache or severe tension headache, or, when accompanied by a seizure, obscured. In a large series of AVMs for which an operation was performed, we have found approximately 15% with asymptomatic hemorrhages, identified by cystic encephalomalacia with pigmentation surrounding the site of hemorrhage and a review of the clinical history, which bore no indication of previous hemorrhage. None of these hemorrhages has been documented by CT scan or lumbar puncture. This significant incidence of clinically silent hemorrhage raises a question about the authenticity of statements indicating that AVMs are only dangerous if they had previously hemorrhaged.

Multiple hemorrhages associated with untreated AVMs are common.[52] However, the time interval between these hemorrhages may span years or even decades.

Experience (few prospective studies exist) dictates that the hemorrhages do not recur in the short time frame usually associated with the rupture of a cerebral aneurysm. The course of recidivous hemorrhages is unpredictable. A recent report suggests that the risk of hemorrhage may be as high as 6% in the first year.[86] The evaluation of these patients may be carried out at a measured pace and there is rarely the necessity for emergency operation on an AVM to protect against recurrent hemorrhage. Patients frequently inquire about the urgency of the treatment. No ready answer is available, but we say to the patients that these are congenital lesions, they have existed with for a number of years until the time of the hemorrhage, and practical experience would indicate that they are unlikely to rerupture in a relatively brief time frame. Therefore, the workup need not be completely predicated on the fear of recurrent hemorrhage.

Regardless of how close the frequency of AVM hemorrhage approximates that of aneurysms, there is a growing awareness that the severity of the effect of the hemorrhage may be far milder. In a prospective study done at our institution to date, 33 patients enrolled in the Columbia Presbyterian Medical Center AVM database who suffered a spontaneous recurrent hemorrhage showed a less severe syndrome than has traditionally been assumed to occur.[118] None of them died, and only eight (24%) had disabling neurologic deficits. Although the numbers were small, patients with purely intraventricular or subarachnoid hemorrhages seemed to have the best prognosis. A larger prospective study of this subject is clearly in order.

Because hemorrhages from AVMs differ markedly from those of aneurysm and hypertension, it has long been believed they should be easily differentiated from one another clinically. Although AVMs are buried in the brain, they are usually in continuity with the ventricle or cerebral surface. Thus they can produce parenchymatous as well as subarachnoid, or intraventricular hemorrhage, or both. Since they are arteriovenous, the hemorrhage is less violent than that from aneurysm, and it evolves over a longer period than the usual few seconds characteristic of aneurysmal rupture. Since the hemorrhage arises in a malformation, it has a less disruptive impact on cerebral function than does the hypertensive hemorrhage. Vasospasm, that discouraging accompaniment of ruptured aneurysms, is less prevalent since the subarachnoid hemorrhage of an AVM is located away from the base of the brain and is accompanied by a smaller volume of blood injected into the subarachnoid space.[7]

In our own experience, three distinct forms of hemorrhage are encountered:

1. The AVM bleeds mainly into the ventricular system, producing hemocephalus rather than parenchymatous damage (Fig. 27.9). About 10% have this picture. An unrelenting course over minutes from the onset of headache to stupor was the typical presenting picture.

2. The hemorrhage affects the subarachnoid space in a fashion similar to ruptured aneurysm, potentially including severe vasospasm (Fig. 27.10). About 10% have this presentation, some on several occasions.

3. A deficit due to a parenchymatous hemorrhage occurs followed by a satisfactory remission (Fig. 27.11). This condition is decidedly uncommon save in the cases of lobar hemorrhage whose diagnosis as hemorrhage is increasingly documented by imaging, after which they are not left alone to pursue their natural course.

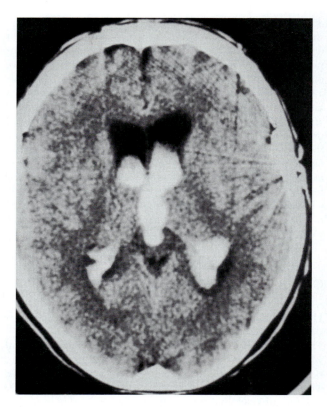

Figure 27.9 Massive intraventricular hemorrhage observed on CT scan following the rupture of a dural posterior fossa arteriovenous malformation.

Little information can be found in the literature to corroborate these syndromes. However, a few cases are described well enough to create a characteristic clinical picture of AVM rupture. Mackenzie[96] stated that "in most cases there has been nothing remarkable about the history, the incident being simply one of sudden onset of severe headache, accompanied by neck stiffness, vomiting, and perhaps pyrexia." Deep hematomas in the basal ganglia[44] have been described with the same smooth onset, hemiparesis, sensory disturbance, ocular motility disorders, and language and mental defects that are encountered in hypertensive hemorrhage.[59] Three such cases in the series of Wilson et al[199] were diagnosed only by surgical exploration, a finding that resurrects McCormick and Nofzinger's[109] long-standing contention that cryptic AVMs are more frequent than has been supposed. Data showing that AVMs cause as few as 10%[59] of parenchymatous hematomas may give some comfort to the physician faced with an etiologic diagnosis. Frequencies as high as 35% to 44%[147] in other series should promptly eliminate any complacency in attempts to make an etiologic diagnosis on clinical grounds alone. In Pia et al's[151] series, among 16 patients with hematomas of 100 to 250 ml size, only 1 died, and 14 fully regained functional capacity. Four had slight to moderate hemiparesis, and two were asymptomatic.

A few other reports have detailed patients who made remarkable functional improvements despite hemorrhage and extensive surgery. Garrido and Stein[44] described a 29-year-old man who had an extensive AVM fed by the lenticulostriate

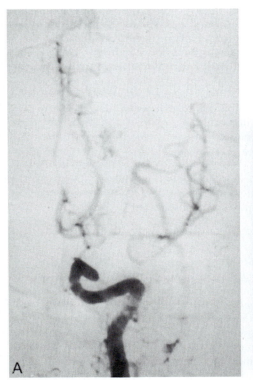

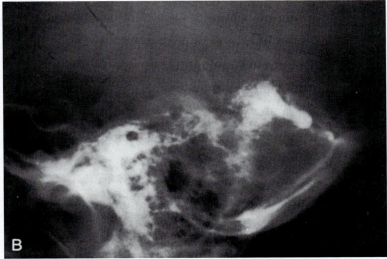

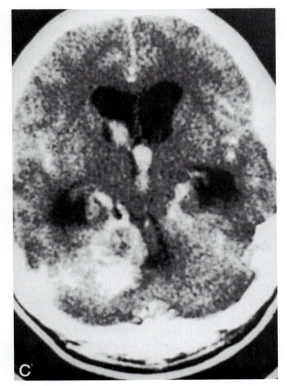

Figure 27.10 (**A**) Intense vasospasm observed following (**B**) the rupture of a posterior fossa arteriovenous malformation (**C**) with massive outpouring of blood into the basal cisterns and ventricles.

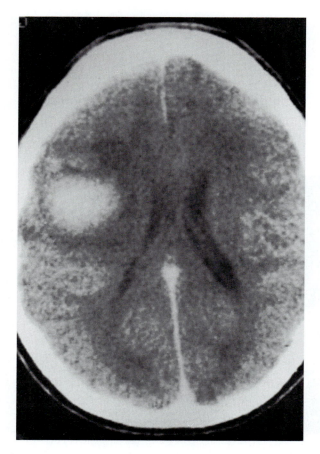

Figure 27.11 CT scan demonstrating parenchymatous hemorrhage following the rupture of a previously unsuspected arteriovenous malformation.

arteries. He developed a hemorrhage with left hemiparesis, hemianopia, and memory impairment. Following removal of this deep-seated lesion, he eventually improved enough to return to work. Other similar cases[62] have been described in which deep hemorrhages and the causative AVM have been removed with good results. However, the outlook may not be as encouraging for all hematoma syndromes: Pertuiset et al[149] found that 19 of their cases with aphasia preoperatively made no postoperative improvement. It might be speculated that AVMs should have a better outlook since some of the bleeding occurs into devitalized tissue. However, it may be premature to consider that such improvements are unique to hematomas from AVMs. Similar improvements have been shown with deep hypertensive hematomas if the size is small, as noted by Hier et al.[59] Ruff and Arbit[161] reported a single instance of acute minor motor aphasia precipitated by a hemorrhage from an AVM affecting the inferior frontal region of the dominant hemisphere. The clinical features and time course for improvement mimicked those documented in cases of infarction. As yet no study has compared the outlook for hematomas of the same size from AVMs and other causes. In the limited experience with lobar hemorrhage[70] and caudate hemorrhage,[179] those due to AVM had features identical to those attributed to other causes. However, should AVMs have a

better clinical outlook, more effort might be appropriate to deal aggressively with such hematomas than is routinely the case in many institutions.

Once hemorrhage has occurred, the risk of rehemorrhage is known to increase, but the extent and the timing are uncertain: in 81 cases of rehemorrhage in the Cooperative Study,[146] 13 were third hemorrhages and 4 were fourth. In a separate study, Krayenbühl and Yasargil[75] found that 12 of 53 recurrent hemorrhages had occurred more than once. Graf et al[48] reviewed the records of 191 patients with AVMs, but the mean period of follow-up was a relatively short 2- to 5-year period. Nevertheless, there was a high rate of initial hemorrhage in the 11- to 35-year-old age group, and the rate of rebleeding was about 2% a year. Smaller lesions were more prone to hemorrhage, and approximately 13% of the patients died as a result of the hemorrhage. It is a generally accepted anecdote that approximately 15% of operated AVMs show evidence of prior but asymptomatic hemorrhage.[75]

Vasospasm

The rarity of vasospasm, symptomatic or merely as an angiographic finding, has been a source of special commentary.[57,87] Although it is generally said that AVMs are associated with a smaller incidence of cerebral vasospasm than cerebral aneurysms, this statement may be based on artifact. The reasons are that these lesions hemorrhage with less frequency into the large basal cisterns than aneurysms, they are less frequent than cerebral aneurysms, and they may be evaluated in the acute stage by arteriography, whereas spasm is generally seen on follow-up arteriography done a few days from the subarachnoid hemorrhage to evaluate the progress of a cerebral aneurysm or its readiness for surgery. Such is not commonly the course of action taken with AVMs once they are identified. Anecdotal cases have certainly been observed in which delayed cerebral vasospasm has been intense following the rupture of an AVM; this spasm may go on to produce death or severe neurologic abnormalities[7] (Fig. 27.10). It is our impression that cerebral vasospasm, when the quantity of blood is sufficient within the entire subarachnoid space, is probably of the same incidence following rupture of a cerebral AVM as in a comparable situation with cerebral aneurysm, but most AVMs do not rupture in ways that bring large amounts of blood into the basal cisterns. If present, vasospasm should be treated vigorously by whatever techniques are currently popular.

Aneurysms

In approximately 10% of the cases, AVMs are associated with cerebral aneurysms.[57,115,138] It is important to recognize this possibility and to perform a complete angiography on all these patients (Fig. 27.12). The question then arises as to which lesion has created the hemorrhage. It used to be thought that it was usually the AVM, but current experience would indicate the cerebral aneurysm. From an anatomic standpoint, the aneurysms are usually located on the feeding arteries proximal to an AVM and are often thin-walled and tenuous, not only at the dome, but also the neck. They apparently arise from abnormalities in the artery wall associated with the high flow and pressure related to the nourishment of an AVM. Rarely

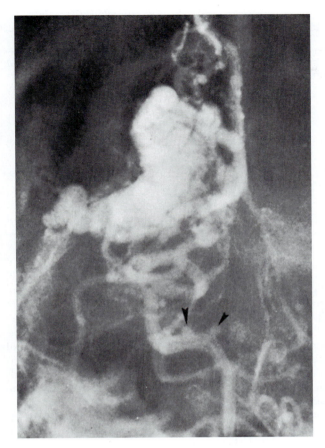

Figure 27.12 Arteriovenous malformation associated with proximal aneurysms (*arrowheads*).

are the aneurysms located on an arterial network distant and unrelated to the AVM. CT or MR scanning, when the site of the hemorrhage is visible, will indicate which lesion has bled. Otherwise, it is pure speculation.

Sometimes the aneurysms are multiple. Which lesion to be operated on first will be discussed under treatment. Clinically, hemorrhage from cavernous and venous malformations is not as frequent as are hemorrhages from AVMs.[46,133,160,162,192] However, as these heretofore obscure conditions are recognized with increasing frequency by CT scans, it is realized that they can be the source of parenchymal and ventricular hemorrhage. Hemorrhages from telangiectasis are rarely recognized by the clinician although some of these cases may fall under the category of hemorrhage from cryptic malformations.[109] On the other hand, pathologists have recognized a high incidence of microscopic hemorrhages associated with cavernous, venous, and telangiectatic malformations.

Seizures

Seizures have attracted special attention because they may alert the physician to an AVM before rupture.[33,139,149,194,196] Some form of seizure disorder affected 32% of the cases of AVMs in our own series. In a study of 35 patients with AVM imaged by MR, the epileptogenic AVM seemed more superfi-

cial in the cortex, had bled before, and was somewhat larger than the non-epileptogenic AVM.[188] The available literature documents a remarkable variation in incidence (Table 27.3). As a presenting feature of AVM, the incidence varies from 28% (Cooperative Study) to 67%.[147] Reports vary over too wide a range to be able to consider that the severity,[90] ease of control with medication, or prognosis for hemorrhage are fully understood. The frequency of seizures correlates so poorly with AVM location that at present no specific relationships can be claimed. None was found among our material.

The type of seizure is often unreported. Several types of attacks labeled as seizures occur. Among these are typical focal epilepsy not associated with loss of consciousness. Others have been of the jacksonian type, with or without the loss of consciousness. Finally, several patients have experienced only a sudden loss of function, without tonic-clonic activity and without headache or loss of consciousness. Whether this latter group represents epilepsy per se is difficult to determine. When attacks have been described, focal spells predominate, varying from 45% to 59%.[147] In the Cooperative Study,[147] 102 cases had seizures, 45% of which were focal, 42% generalized, 8% psychomotor, and 7% unspecified. Ozer et al[139] were unable to distinguish focal AVM seizures from those of other etiology in their 14 cases of seizure among 65 AVMs. Earlier, Olivecrona and Ladenheim[136] were of the opinion that there was more variation in type and frequency of attacks in AVM seizures than in cryptogenic or traumatic epilepsy. Mackenzie[96] made three special observations: in all but 1 of 16 cases the attacks displayed focal features at some time or other; focal seizures had a wide periodicity of up to 20 years, and when they were initially generalized, no remission for longer than 3 years was observed.

A small but separate literature applies to the occipital AVMs. Troost and Newton[185] reported 5 of 26 cases of occipital AVM with focal seizures. The aura varied widely, including "sudden dimming of everything in the right side of vision," "swirling spots of brightly colored lights," "dimming of vision," "red spots," and "frosted glass." Several were followed by generalized seizure. The subject is of interest since some of these attacks mimic the aura often encountered in migraine syndromes. Our experience includes six cases whose seizures have had unusual manifestations. In these cases, in addition to the more common grand mal and focal motor epilepsy, dystonic posturing of a limb (usually the arm) has occurred in brief episodes, affecting the limb(s) at other times by more conventional tonic-clonic epileptiform activity. In another three, the episodes took the form of sudden weakness, lasting between 30 seconds and many minutes. Whether these attacks represent ischemia (see below) or are examples of epilepsy is difficult to determine.

Only limited information exists on anatomic factors that can be identified as risk factors for seizures. Turjman et al[190] used 15 angioarchitectural characteristics of AVMs for correlations with AVMs. These included cortical location, middle cerebral artery feeders, absence of aneurysms, and the presence of a varix or varices in the venous drainage.

The incidence of seizures alone compared with seizures in association with hemorrhage varies from 36.3% to 7.4%, 25.3% to 12.3%, 20.1% to 14.9%, and 40.1% to 10.5%, as is shown in Table 27.3. In the few reports that bear on the subject, the correlation is frequent in the AVMs involving the

Table 27.3 Seizures

Year	Author	No. of Cases	Seizures as First Sign of AVM in % Cases				
			Total	**Alone**	**+ Hemorrhage**	**Generalized**	**Focal**
1980	Stein and Wolpert[177,178]	121	43.8	36.3	7.4		
1980	Parkinson and Bachers[142]	100	67				
1979	Pertuiset et al[149]	162	37.6	25.3	12.3	41	59
1973	Morello and Broghi[120]	154	35.0	20.1	14.9		
1970	Troupp et al[186]	138	26				
1966	Cooperative Study[146]	406	28				
1956	Paterson and McKissock[143]	110	46.4				
1970	Moody and Poppen[119]	105	50.5	40	10.5	55	45
1967	Tönnis	215	48.3				
1959	Krayenbühl and Yasargil[76]	608	41.2				

surface of the brain, especially the centroparietal area[44,47,147] but is unusual for deep AVMs. Hemorrhage occurred within 1 year in only 15% of 90 cases of seizure in the Cooperative Study. Whether the character of the seizure differs when it is associated with hematoma is not certain.

Headaches

AVMs are unusual forms of stroke in that they have been associated with premonitory symptoms and signs, the most common of which is headache. Because headache is such a common complaint in the population at large, it has proved difficult to determine if the headache associated with AVMs is unique to the condition.[2,27,32] The two most common claims for association are with migraine and with unilateral headache. Headache was a presenting complaint in roughly 10% of our patients.

Headaches with migrainous features are common among AVM patients. Mackenzie[96] emphasized the tendency of the headaches to occur before the aura and for the aura to persist beyond the few minutes that typifies migraine, a finding not confirmed by others. One of the earliest reported cases had atypical migraine. The patient reported by Hyland and Douglas[63] in 1930 experienced attacks over a period of 4 years. The attacks followed exertion, each commencing with numbness starting in the hands and spreading up the arms to the chest and neck. Then consciousness would be lost about 10 minutes after the onset. When she regained consciousness, she felt weak and drowsy.

Headaches identical to migraine also occur, sometimes in the same patients who experience atypical migraine in other attacks.[63,91,139] Similar experiences were documented in the early literature. Ennoksson and Bynke[32] described a case with "... luminous crosses replaced by curved flashing lights with convexity upward." Dinsdale described cases with flickering lights. Similarly, Lees[91] described cases with "flashing lights" and "flashes with black spots." These and our own experiences force us to disagree with the opinion of Troost and Newton[185] that AVM headaches are unassociated with the angular, scintillating figures typical of migraine. The association may well be purely coincidental. Paterson and McKissock[143] reviewed a series of AVMs with headache and suggested that the occurrence of migraine in AVMs was simply the incidence of the

disorder in the normal population, and classic migraine in 2%, figures that approximate those with AVM. Some of the more recent authors have not been able to show any correlation between headache and AVMs.[52,91]

That recurrent unilateral headache should arouse suspicion of an ipsilateral AVM is an old concept. The notion of an ipsilateral feature to the AVM headache may have started with Northfield,[131] whose 1940 report stated that the headache "... may affect only one side of the head, usually the side on which the angioma is situated." Very little evidence supports this claim. Based on their experience with 100 cases, Parkinson and Bachers[142] found no evidence that the incidence of headache has a specific relation to location of the AVM. Mackenzie[96] described 12 cases that were persistently unilateral, but other focal neurologic signs were present as well. Likewise, Lees[91] had only three cases whose headache was ipsilateral to the AVM among the 11 headache cases in his series of 70 AVMs. None of them had the alternating headaches typical of migraine. Unilateral headache as a sign of AVM has not been borne out by the authors' experience.

The yield for AVMs in a workup for headache seems quite low. In a lengthy review, Evans,[35] surveying reports on brain imaging done for headache and normal neurologic examination in 3,026 brain scans, found that 0.2% were associated with AVM.

The disappearance of the migraine headaches postoperatively is not unusual and may occur following any type of operation. Disappearance of migraine after operation was a common feature of the early literature, which was made up mostly of single case reports. The question is now raised as to whether all patients with migraine should be evaluated for an AVM. At the very least, CT scan with large bolus contrast should be carried out in these individuals. If anything suspicious is noted, then MR scan should be performed.

Mass Lesion

Although AVMs occupy space they do not act as tumors, and their bulk effect (creating pressure on the brain) is only recognized in terms of massive, distended draining veins. This phenomenon is most commonly noted in those malformations that occupy a site adjacent to the aqueduct of Sylvius. In such instances, the distended veins may block the aqueduct, leading

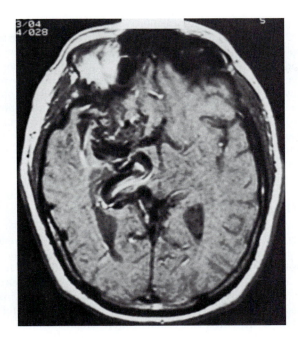

Figure 27.13 Axial MRI showing the large feeding artery and draining vein from an arteriovenous malformation acting as a mass and displacing the midbrain.

to hydrocephalus. In other instances, there is indirect evidence of a mass effect through the development of a raised intracranial pressure perhaps similar to that seen with otitic hydrocephalus where the venous system is obstructed or carrying a higher pressure than it normally accommodates. Although rare, cases have been reported in which papilledema and raised intracranial pressures are a prominent part of the syndrome. Interestingly, this problem does not regress rapidly following the removal of the shunt. Nevertheless, there is a gradual resolution of the increased intracranial pressure and remission of the papilledema so that removal of the AVM to correct this dangerous state should be strongly considered.

Rarely, a large AVM may be placed close enough to the brain that symptoms arise from displacement of healthy tissue or hemorrhage into it. We saw a 44-year-old printer with progressive dystonia and myoclonus whose midbrain was rotated and compressed by the large size of the feeding artery; there had been no hemorrhage (Fig. 27.13). Nishino et al[127] described a 64-year-old man with hemorrhage whose angiogram and MR scan showed that part of the drainage from the AVM was a "varix" embedded in the pons. They found another 26 cases in the literature.

Syndromes of Ischemia: So-Called Steal Syndromes

Clinical information on the subject of steal syndromes is still in the anecdotal stage. In suspect cases, it is presumed that the blood shunting through the fistula results in relative underperfusion of the adjacent brain, leading to focal or generalized symptoms. It is beyond doubt that shunting occurs. It has been amply documented by CBF,[15] by radionuclide brain

scanning,[37] by the preferential path of silastic ball emboli,[177] and by the improved post-treatment perfusion of contrast to branches poorly filled pretreatment.[178] It is also apparent that the neuropathologic study of cases of AVM reveals many foci of infarction, suggesting that the shunting may lead to ischemic necrosis of tissue. Our own experience with cerebral steal approximates the findings reported in the literature. Roughly 6% have some focal deficits of gradual onset. In most, the neurologic deficit is limited to the region of the brain served by the AVM, and no instance occurred with neurologic deficits attributed to sites far distant to that of the AVM. In all cases, the AVM had been fed by both deep and superficial vessels and was quite large. The syndromes evolved over periods as short as 3 years or as long as 10 years. During this time the worsening occurred without notable sudden drops in function or obvious instances of hemorrhage. Some degree of hemiatrophy was present on examination in all cases; except for one patient, who also had a visual field disturbance with a large parietal AVM, the main complaints were motor. Sensory disturbance accompanied the motor in three instances, but language, memory, praxis, and other functions were normal.

In a report comprising large numbers, Paterson and McKissock[143] encountered 8 cases among 110 AVMs with insidious deficits. The remaining literature represents isolated case reports. In a description of seven cases of large, deep AVMs, Luessenhop and Mujica[94] described one patient who had developed a slowly progressing hemiparesis 4 years before her first subarachnoid hemorrhage. A spastic left hemiplegia with no voluntary movements of the hand or ankle, hemihypesthesia, and hemianopia were prominent clinical findings. Two sessions of multiple embolization separated by an interval of approximately 2 weeks were necessary to obstruct the supply to the deep AVM from deep penetrating branches of the circle of Willis arising from anterior, middle, and posterior cerebral arteries. At first no changes occurred, but by 3 weeks she ". . . could walk with a foreleg brace, and recovered voluntary flexion and extension of the fingers of her left hand." By 8 months "she was able to walk rapidly with a cane and had isolated movements of the wrist and fingers of the left hand which she could use for grasping and assisting." Sensory function was improved, but not fully restored.

Kusske and Kelly[79] reported on two patients who were inferred to suffer symptoms of cerebral steal. One was a 43-year-old woman who suffered daily to weekly focal seizures and postictal left arm weakness. Atrophy of the left arm, palsy of the left face, and dysarthria were present prior to therapeutic embolization with silastic balls for a right rolandic AVM. Postembolization, the seizure frequency declined to monthly intervals, and the left arm paresis improved. By 2 years, she had full use of the left hand, normal left facial strength, and improved speech. A second patient, a 45-year-old man with progressive mental deterioration, incomplete hemiparesis, and aggression had an AVM of the sylvian region. After embolization for the AVM, the hemiparesis improved, the visual deficit regressed, the memory and personality changes reversed, and the patient returned to work. In Norlen's[129] case, a 19-year-old man had presented with left-sided spastic hemiparesis following hemorrhages 3 years and 1 year previously. Within 2 months following operative excision of the AVM, there was ". . . pronounced improvement in the paresis and the patient was in good condition." He returned to regular work 2 years later. These dramatic cases leave little doubt that the steal phenomenon exists and may to some degree be reversible. However, much work needs to be done to delineate the spectrum of syndromes that may prove reversible. Attempts to use the Luria battery[24] pre- and postoperatively are quantitative steps in the right direction. Amaurosis fugax has also been reported from a dural AVM,[16] but whether it is attributable to steal is unsettled.

De Reuck et al,[29] using positron emission tomography steady-state techniques with ^{15}O, found major increases in oxygen extraction adjacent to two "huge" AVMs, findings that they argued meant some form of steal can occur in AVM.

Despite these individual reports and efforts to delineate clinical features distinctive for steal, the actual frequency of this form of clinical disorder may have been greatly exaggerated in the past. A recently completed prospective study of AVMs found so few examples of progressing syndrome as to call into question the concept of steal.[103] In this study of 152 cases, of the 13 examples of focal neurologic deficits unrelated to hemorrhage, 11 were static and nonprogressive, and only 12 (1.3%) were progressive. This study had a mean observation time of 17 months, ample time for worsening to be documented. A similar lack of support was found in a neuropsychological study of 31 cases of hemispheral AVM[175] and in a study of measurement of feeding arterial pressure in 32 cases.[128] The frequency seems extremely low, too low to make steal a common occurrence in AVMs and, despite some protests,[22] possibly no longer a high enough frequency to demand separate discussion comparable to that of hemorrhage, seizures, or headache.

Other Vascular Malformations

CAVERNOUS MALFORMATIONS (ANGIOMAS)

Because of their characteristic appearance on MR scan (less so on a CT scan), cavernous malformations are becoming more and more the subject of reports in the literature.[56,109,189,192] These lesions rarely occupy a clinically significant amount of space in the brain but may be located in clinically important cortical or subcortical regions and are occasionally multiple. Although they are masses, they do not produce displacements commensurable to that of a neoplasm. They are composed of cavernous channels with multiple areas of thrombosis. The flow through these lesions is minimal, and therefore they are rarely seen on angiograms. They are recognized by contrast enhancement on CT scans and their characteristic configuration. They are frequently associated with headache and seizures and occasionally with hemorrhage. While not readily identified on CT scan, the distinctive cat's eye appearance on MR has made the diagnosis more frequent since the introduction of MR scanning. This appearance is no longer considered pathognomonic for cavernous angiomas, as it once was.[156]

Their clinical importance is unclear except in a differential diagnosis with tumor and other contrast-enhancing masses. Cavernous malformations usually present with a seizure disorder and the same may be said for venous malformation.[7,38,46,120,131,154,194] These lesions may also be seen with headaches, which may or may not be related to the lesion. It is very often difficult to determine a one-to-one relationship between lesion and symptoms. The lesions may occur anywhere including the cortical surface or deep in the brain stem. MRI has allowed study of family members, which in a small series of cases has suggested a hereditary basis for some instances of multiple cavernous malformations.[30,158] A predominance among Hispanics has been suggested.[71]

TELANGIECTASIS

Telangiectases are uncommon anomalies composed of small clusters of capillary-like vessels located in the brain stem or cerebellum.[33,108,109] They are often deep and multiple. Their clinical significance is dubious. They may rarely be the source of a large hemorrhage, which if located in a critical area may cause death. Mostly they are curiosities noted at postmortem. Although they frequently demonstrate small microhemorrhages on histologic examination, the size of the hemorrhage does not appear to be massive enough to create a clinical syndrome. When associated with the Weber-Osler-Rendu syndrome, the telangiectasis is recognized elsewhere in the body. Rapid advances in genetics are shedding light on the chromosomal aberrations that underlie these anomalies. For the autosomal dominant disorder that is hereditary hemorrhagic telangiectasia, linkage studies have recently implicated chromosome 12.[66]

The telangiectases have long been considered curiosities for the pathologist to describe, with only rare clinical significance,[36] but recent advances suggest otherwise.[155] Prior to high-field MRI, they were most frequently found only at postmortem.

When presenting clinically, hemorrhage is the common syndrome, most often in the white matter of the brain stem, cerebellum, and diencephalic regions, their usual sites of occurrence. Rarely, the hemorrhages may be incapacitating or fatal, and postmortem examination may uncover the lesion as a thrombosed telangiectasia. The venous malformations are often deep within the white matter, but they may extend to the cortical surface, presumably causing seizures.

VENOUS MALFORMATIONS (ANGIOMAS)

These lesions have come under increasing scrutiny because of the use of CT scans and sophisticated angiography.[38,122,132,133,160,162,197] They are represented by a deep prominent vein that shows late on the venous phase of an arteriogram and is associated with a finger-like projection from the main vein. This appearance is characteristic on an arteriogram. Arterial fistulaization may occur.[124] Pathologically, few studies have been done on these lesions, but they appear to be abnormally distended veins located in an abnormal location (i.e., deep in the white matter). Some evidence shows that they represent anomalous venous drainage, which compensates for the absence of normal venous conduits. These lesions rarely hemorrhage. Very few have been resected, and intraoperative studies show that they are devoid of arterial blood. Curiously, they appear to be associated with headaches and occasionally with seizures.

Laboratory Diagnosis

Because the clinical syndromes of AVM are not distinctive for the causes like those of subarachnoid hemorrhage from aneurysm, laboratory studies, especially brain imaging, play an important role. In approximately 10% of the patients, the diagnosis is discovered in a serendipitous fashion.

COMPUTED TOMOGRAPHY

In 85% of AVMs diagnosis can be made by CT scan,[88] a great improvement over the now outmoded radionuclide scanning.[72] The CT scan done with contrast shows an enhancing lesion that is usually at the cortical level extending deep, whose margins are irregular and when viewed with the most sophisticated CT scanners may be associated with serpentine vascular channels (Fig. 27.14). Large hemorrhages from one of these

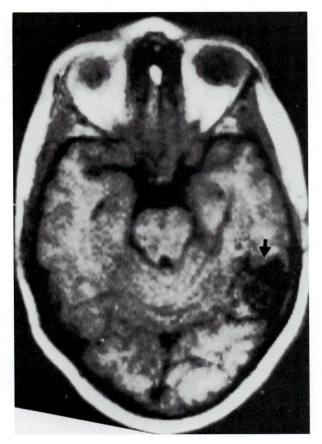

Figure 27.15 Nuclear magnetic resonance evaluation of an arteriovenous malformation. The black areas represent an arteriovenous malformation (*arrow*) with rapid blood flow.

Figure 27.14 CT scan with contrast enhancement demonstrating the serpentine channels characteristic of an arteriovenous malformation (*arrows*).

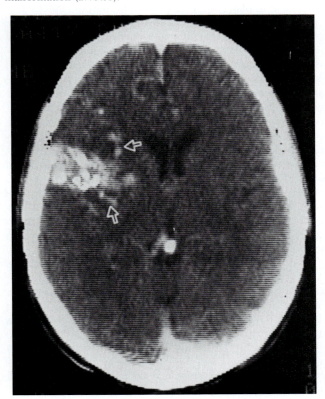

malformations can be recognized on the noncontrast scan, and these may be demonstrated in the ventricular system or in the subarachnoid cisterns at the base of the brain. A hemorrhage may partially obscure the malformation, which, however, should show up as an additional area of enhancement on the enhanced scan. When the malformation contains distended veins related to the aqueduct, hydrocephalus may be present. In those patients who have had previous hemorrhages that are now resolved, the CT scan will often show an area of encephalomalacia, a cleavage area between the nidus of the malformation and the normal brain. Calcium may occasionally be present along with the AVM or associated with the encephalomalacia. Such areas of infarction or encephalomalacia may be extensive, with minimal neurologic abnormalities. The more sophisticated current CT and MR scanners are most important in identifying the exact location of the principal portion of the AVM and its relationship to brain components such as the cortex, ventricular system, brain stem, and diencephalic regions (Fig. 27.15). These relationships are identified as small pinpoint contrast-enhanced areas surrounded by cystic encephalomalacia on an enhanced CT scan (Fig. 27.16). They have a highly characteristic appearance and often lie in a subcortical position. It should be emphasized that all these lesions may be mistaken for other types of pathology, most

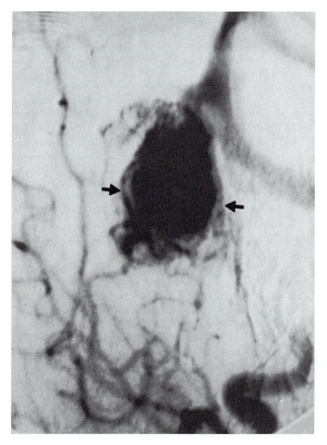

Figure 27.16 Digital subtraction study demonstrating the anatomy of an arteriovenous malformation (*arrows*) of the temporal lobe.

commonly tumors, and therefore angiography is definitive in establishing a diagnosis and identifying the anatomy of the contributing arteries.

MAGNETIC RESONANCE IMAGING

In the last 25 years, MRI has almost eclipsed angiogram and far surpassed CT scanning for the diagnosis of AVM. MRI has yet to replace angiography for the fine details needed by the surgeon, but for routine diagnosis and management planning, it can now be relied on as the first line of diagnosis. Early reports with low field magnets[89,165] showed the high-flow vascular channels of an AVM as dark areas or regions of reduced signal (Fig. 27.15). The intensity of the signal void is related to the flow rates, a finding that offers the opportunity to calculate blood flow noninvasively. As opposed to angiogram, which reveals nothing of the brain parenchyma, MR shows the relationships to surrounding brain well and has proved superior to angiography in defining the nidus.[134] Evidence of prior hemorrhage and its source,[105] the size of the nidus, the source of flow to the lesion, the course of draining veins, and the relation of the malformation to normal brain

structures are now regularly shown. A central focus of high signal surrounded by hypointensity, once thought pathognomonic of cavernous angiomas, has been found due to AVM in five of nine operated cases[156] and to neoplasm in 18 of 24 patients.

Increasing use is being made of functional MR (see also Ch. 12) to identify functionally important tissue in or near the AVM. Many clinics now use this information in planning embolization, surgery, or radiotherapy.[85,97,200]

REGION CEREBRAL BLOOD FLOW

Pre- and postoperative regional (rCBF) studies in some centers are used to evaluate the flow patterns in AVMs. Intraoperative rCBF evaluations have demonstrated that this technique may help in predicting those patients at risk of delayed complications, presumably due to perfusion pressure breakthrough.[203] Positron emission tomography has also recently found an application in localizing the nidus of an AVM. The initial experiences of Leblanc et al,[90] who described the first case in 1990, have recently been expanded to a larger series.

DOPPLER INSONATION

Transcranial Doppler technology has increased the range of investigations for AVMs because the methodology has easy bedside use. Barely a decade old, the techniques for insonation of the intracranial vessels are now well described.[1,92] Using this method, investigations have demonstrated the principal sources of flow to the lesion.[18,50,166] Doppler has also been used to plan and evaluate embolization therapy.[150] It is being used in investigations of perfusion breakthrough. In our experience, the pattern of low resistance to arterial flow typical of AVMs has successfully predicted all angiographically obvious AVMs involving the cerebrum, missing only a handful of AVMs whose shunts required careful examination of the angiogram for their detection, or whose small feeders were exclusively from the anterior choroidal territory. In a recent report from our center,[102] 114 consecutive cases of AVM were compared with 22 non-AVM hemorrhage cases and 52 normals. Medium- to large-size AVMs were easily detected, but 62% of small ones (requiring angiogram for documentation of most of them) were not. Transcranial Doppler was also highly sensitive (80%) in a group of five AVM patients with acute hemorrhage. No relationship was found between flow velocities and whether or not hemorrhage occurred (mean velocities being around 110 to 114 cm/s in both groups). No support was found for the notion of steal.

Impaired CO_2 reactivity is typical of vessels feeding the AVMs and is not seen in those not feeding the malformation, save for the posterior cerebral arteries: some cases have been reported in which the posterior cerebral artery not feeding the AVM has also shown impaired reactivity; the reasons are not known.[102]

Color-coded transcranial Doppler is only now making an appearance, but some of the experience to date has been encouraging; the larger lesions may actually be imaged as well as insonated.[12]

ANGIOGRAPHY

In spite of advances in other forms of diagnostic imaging, arteriography remains the foundation of the diagnosis of vascular abnormalities and has proved superior to MR in defining the details of the vascular supply.[134] However, a few examples of thrombosed, nonhemorrhagic AVMs have been found by brain imaging that were not shown by angiogram.[56,189]

Angiography plays a major role in preparing the patient for therapy. Full documentation of the lesion involves rapid sequence filming, magnification of certain arterial territories, separate injection of the extracerebral vessels, and stereoangiography done in the lateral series. Rapid sequence filming at rates of five to six per second assists in the analysis of arterial supply in terms of number, source, and size of the feeding arteries. This demonstration is especially important when the artery feeding the malformation also feeds healthy cerebrum in its more distal branches. It is recognized that the arterial contributions to an AVM are numerous, and not all may be identified by an angiogram; however, the major ones playing a role in embolization or surgery of an AVM may be identified by conventional angiography. To provide the information of greatest help to the surgeon, stereoscopic angiograms should be obtained. This is carried out simply by performing an x-ray tube shift in an anteroposterior direction while performing the lateral angiogram. These paired angiograms can be visualized with or without the help of a stereoscopic viewer. The resultant stereoscopic image gives a more precise identification of the three-dimensional anatomy of an AVM and is extremely helpful in planning and carrying out an operative approach to these malformations. Modern computer processing is allowing detailed three-dimensional maps of AVMs from multiple images.[41,202] Other techniques that have proved useful are magnification angiography and large injections of contrast material with a prolonged venous phase. In terms of magnification angiography, there are disadvantages to be considered. The malformation and its components are visualized in a somewhat distorted view, which makes exact measurements and the study of relationships difficult. However, magnification angiography will demonstrate small feeders to the malformation, which may not be identified on standard angiography.

All forms of angiography should be as selective as possible. For practical purposes this means injection of the vertebral or internal carotid arteries since techniques for injection directly into the distal feeding vessels of a vascular malformation are cumbersome and not yet readily available. External carotid injection is essential to document dural feeders, which are found the more they are sought, especially in posterior hemispheral and posterior fossa AVMs. Angiotomography and cineangiography have not been of significant use in the evaluation of the more common vascular anomalies such as AVMs. Digital subtraction angiography, especially with arterial injection, provides a good survey but does not give sufficient detail of these lesions to be of major help in planning an operation. Although multiple AVMs are infrequent,[129] the association with aneurysms is well recognized so that comprehensive four-vessel angiography should be carried out in all patients. If severe arterial vasospasm is present once the lesion has been identified, the remainder of the arteriographic study should be deferred to a later date. The high volume injection of contrast agent and a prolonged venous phase are essential in identifying the somewhat ubiquitous and obscure venous malformations. Cavernous malformations rarely show at angiography since their arterial feeders are small and infrequent.

In planning embolization it is frequently necessary to use a different catheter system for diagnosis than for interventional neuroradiology.[43,79,94] In such cases, angiography will be repeated at the time of embolization once this is selected as the course of treatment. Intraoperative arteriography is a difficult procedure that delays an already long operation and has thus far had limited use.

References

1. Aaslid R, Markwalde T-M, Nornes H: Noninvasive transcranial Doppler ultrasound recording of blood flow in basal cerebral arteries. J Neurosurg 57:769, 1982
2. Adie WJ: Permanent hemianopsia in migraine and subarachnoid hemorrhage. Lancet 219:237, 1930
3. Agnoli AL: Extracranial and extra-intracranial arteriovenous angiomas. p. 66. In Pia HW, Gleave JRW, Grote E et al (eds): Cerebral Angiomas. Advances in Diagnosis and Therapy. Springer-Verlag, New York, 1975
4. Almeida GM, Shibata MK, Nakagawa EJ: Contralateral parafalcine approach for parasagittal and callosal arteriovenous malformations. Neurosurgery 14:744, 1984
5. Aminoff MJ: Vascular anomalies in the intracranial dura mater. Brain 96:601, 1973
6. Andoh T, Sakai N, Yamada H et al: Cerebellar AVM: clinical analysis of 14 cases. No To Shinkei 42:913, 1990
7. Arutinov AI, Baron MA, Majorova NA: Experimental and clinical study of the development of spasm of the cerebral arteries related to subarachnoid hemorrhage. J Neurosurg 32:617, 1970
8. Bär T: The vascular system of the cerebral cortex. Adv Anat Embryol Cell Biol 59:1, 1980
9. Barre RG, Suter GS, Rosenblum WI: Familial vascular malformations or chance occurrence? Neurology (NY) 28:98, 1978
10. Batjer H, Samson D: Arteriovenous malformations of the posterior fossa. J Neurosurg 64:849, 1986
11. Batjer HH, Devous MD Sr, Meyer YJ et al: Cerebrovascular hemodynamics in arteriovenous malformation complicated by normal perfusion pressure breakthrough. Neurosurgery 22:503, 1988
12. Baumgartner RW, Mattle HP, Schroth G: Transcranial colour-coded duplex sonography of cerebral arteriovenous malformations. Neuroradiology 38:734, 1996
13. Becker DH, Townsend JJ, Kramer RA, Newton TH: Occult cerebrovascular malformations: a series of 18 histologically verified cases with negative angiography. Brain 102:249, 1979
14. Bergh van den R, Eecken van der H: Anatomy and embryology of the cerebral circulation. Prog Brain Res 30:1, 1968
15. Bessman AN, Hayes GJ, Alman RW, Fazekas JR: Cerebral hemodynamics in cerebral arteriovenous vascular anomalies. Med Ann Dist Columbia 21:422, 1952

16. Bogousslavsky J, Vinuela F, Barnett HJM, Drake CG: Amaurosis fugax as the presenting manifestation of dural arteriovenous malformation. Stroke 16:891, 1985

17. Boyd MC, Steinbok P, Paty DW: Familial arteriovenous malformations. J Neurosurg 62:597, 1985

18. Brass LR, Prohovnik I, Pavlakis S, Mohr JP: Transcranial Doppler examination of middle cerebral artery velocity versus xenon rCBF: two measures of cerebral blood flow. Neurology 37:85, 1987

19. Brown RD Jr, Wiebers DO, Torner JC, O'Fallon WM: Frequency of intracranial hemorrhage as a presenting symptom and subtype analysis: a population-based study of intracranial vascular malformations in Olmsted County, Minnesota. J Neurosurg 85:29, 1996

20. Bruce DA: Surgery of the vein of Galen arteriovenous malformation. Contemp Neurosurg 3:1, 1981

21. Burchiel KJ, Clarke H, Ojemann GA et al: Use of stimulation mapping and corticography in the excision of arteriovenous malformations in sensorimotor and language related neocortex. Neurosurgery 24:322, 1989

22. Carter LP, Gumerlock MK: Steal and cerebral arteriovenous malformations. Stroke 26:1215, 1995

23. Cohen HCM, Tucker WS, Humphreys RP, Perrin RJ: Angiographically cryptic histologically verified cerebrovascular malformations. Neurosurgery 10:704, 1982

24. Conly FK, Moses JA, Helle TL: Deficits in higher cerebral function in two patients with posterior parietal arteriovenous malformations. Neurosurgery 7:230, 1980

25. Crawford JV, Russell DS: Cryptic arteriovenous and venous hamartomas of the brain. J Neurol Neurosurg Psychiatry 19:1, 1956

26. Crawford PM, West CR, Chadwick DW, Shaw MDM: Arteriovenous malformations of the brain: natural history in unoperated patients. J Neurol Neurosurg Psychiatry 49:1, 1986

27. Dandy WE: Arteriovenous aneurysm of the brain. Arch Surg (Chicago) 17:190, 1928

28. Debrun GM, Lacour P, Caron JP et al: Detachable balloon and calibrated-leak balloon techniques in the treatment of cerebral vascular lesions. J Neurosurg 49:635, 1978

29. De Reuck J, De la Meilleure G, Boon P et al: Comparison of cerebral haemodynamic and oxygen metabolic changes due to cavernous angiomas and arteriovenous malformations of the brain. A positron emission tomography study. Acta Neurol Belg 94:239, 1994

30. Dobyns WB, Michels VV, Groover RV et al: Familial cavernous malformations of the central nervous system and retina. Ann Neurol 21:578, 1987

31. Duckett S: The establishment of internal vascularization in the human telencephalon. Acta Anat 80:107, 1971

32. Ennoksson P, Bynke H: Visual field defects in arteriovenous aneurysms of the brain. Acta Ophthalmol 36:586, 1958

33. Epstein N, Epstein F: Arteriovenous malformation presenting as a first seizure in a 13-year-old child: surgical indications. Neurosurgery 7:391, 1980

34. Ericson K, Soderman M, Karlsson B et al: Multiple intracranial arteriovenous malformations: a case report. Neuroradiology 36:157, 1994

35. Evans RW: Diagnostic testing for the evaluation of headaches. Neurol Clin 14:1, 1996

36. Farrell DF, Forno LS: Symptomatic capillary telangiectasis of the brain stem without hemorrhage. Report of an unusual case. Neurology 20:341, 1970

37. Feindel W, Yamamoto YL, Hodge CP: Red cerebral veins and the cerebral steal syndrome: evidence from fluorescein angiography and microregional blood flow by radioisotopes during excision of an angioma. J Neurosurg 35:167, 1971

38. Fierstein SB, Pribam HW, Hieshima G: Angiography and computed tomography in the evaluation of cerebral venous malformations. Neurology 17:137, 1979

39. Fogarty-Mack P, Pile-Spellman J, Hacein-Bey L et al: Superselective intraarterial papaverine administration: effect on regional cerebral blood flow in patients with arteriovenous malformations. J Neurosurg 85:395, 1996

40. Fogarty-Mack P, Pile-Spellman J, Hacein-Bey L et al: The effect of arteriovenous malformations on the distribution of intracerebral arterial pressures. AJNR 17:1443, 1996

41. Foroni R, Giri MG, Gerosa MA et al: A heuristic approach to the volume reconstruction of arteriovenous malformations from biplane angiography. Stereotact Funct Neurosurg 64:134, 1995

42. Forster DMC, Steiner L, Hakanson S: Arteriovenous malformations of the brain. A long-term clinical study. J Neurosurg 37:562, 1972

43. Fox JL, Al Mefty O: Embolization of an arteriovenous malformation of the brain stem. Surg Neurol 8:7, 1977

44. Garrido E, Stein BM: Removal of an arteriovenous malformation from the basal ganglion. J Neurol Neurosurg Psychiatry 41:992, 1978

45. Gerosa M, Cappellotto P, Licata C et al: Cerebral arteriovenous malformations in children (56 cases). Childs Brain 8:356, 1981

46. Giombini S, Morello G: Cavernous angiomas of the brain. Account of fourteen personal cases and review of the literature. Acta Neurochir (Wien) 40:61, 1978

47. Graeb DA, Dolman CL: Radiological and pathological aspects of dural arteriovenous fistulas. J Neurosurg 64:962, 1986

48. Graf CJ, Perret GE, Torner JC: Bleeding from cerebral arteriovenous malformations as part of their natural history. J Neurosurg 58:331, 1983

49. Griffiths PD, Worthy S, Gholkar A: Incidental intracranial vascular pathology in patients investigated for carotid stenosis. Neuroradiology 38:25, 1996

50. Grolimund P, Seiker RW, Aaslid R et al: Evaluation of cerebrovascular disease by combined extracranial and transcranial Doppler sonography. Experience in 1039 patients. Stroke 18:1018, 1987

51. Gross CR, Kase CS, Mohr JP et al: Stroke in south Alabama: incidence and diagnostic features in a population study. Stroke 15:249, 1984

52. Guidetti B, DeLitala A: Intracranial arteriovenous malformations. Conservative and surgical treatment. J Neurosurg 53:149, 1980

53. Hacein-Bey L, Nour R, Pile-Spellman J et al: Adaptive changes of autoregulation in chronic cerebral hypotension with arteriovenous malformations: an acetazol-

amide-enhanced single-photon emission CT study. AJNR 16:1865, 1995

54. Hamilton MG, Spetzler RF: The prospective application of a grading system for arteriovenous malformations. Neurosurgery 34:2, 1994

55. Harders A, Bien S, Eggert HR et al: Haemodynamic changes in arteriovenous malformations induced by superselective embolization: transcranial Doppler evaluation. Neurol Res 10:239, 1988

56. Hashim ASM, Asakura T, Kiochi U et al: Angiographically occult arteriovenous malformations. Surg Neurol 16:431, 1985

57. Hayashi S, Arimoto T, Itakura T et al: The association of intracranial aneurysms and arteriovenous malformation of the brain. J Neurosurg 55:971, 1981

58. Henderson WR, Gomez R: Natural history of cerebral angiomas. BMJ 4:571, 1967

59. Hier DB, Davis KR, Richardson EP, Mohr JP: Hypertensive putaminal hemorrhage. Ann Neurol 1:152, 1977

60. Höök O, Johanson C: Intracranial arteriovenous aneurysms. A follow-up study with particular attention to their growth. Arch Neurol Psychiatry 80:39, 1958

61. Horton JC, Chambers WA, Lyons SL et al: Pregnancy and the risk of hemorrhage from cerebral arteriovenous malformations. Neurosurgery 27:867, 1990

62. Hosobuchi Y: Electrothrombosis of carotid-cavernous fistula. J Neurosurg 42:76, 1975

63. Hyland HH, Douglas RP: Cerebral angioma arteriale. A case in which migrainous headache was the earliest manifestation. Arch Neurol Psychiatry 40:1220, 1938

64. Ishikawa T, Houkin K, Tokuda K et al: Development of anterior cranial fossa dural arteriovenous malformation following head trauma. Case report. J Neurosurg 86:291, 1997

65. Jane JA, Kassell NF, Torner JC, Winn HR: The natural history of aneurysms and arteriovenous malformations. J Neurosurg 62:321, 1985

66. Johnson DW, Berg JN, Gallione CJ et al: A second locus for hereditary hemorrhagic telangiectasia maps to chromosome 12. Genome Res 5:21, 1995

67. Kader A, Young WL, Pile-Spellman J et al: The influence of hemodynamic and anatomic factors on hemorrhage from cerebral arteriovenous malformations. Neurosurgery 34:801, 1994

68. Kadoya C, Momota Y, Ikegami Y et al: Central nervous system arteriovenous malformations with hereditary hemorrhagic telangiectasia: report of a family with three cases. Surg Neurol 42:234, 1994

69. Kaplan SS, Ogilvy CS, Crowell RM: Incidentally discovered arteriovenous malformation of the anterior fossa dura. Br J Neurosurg 8:755, 1994

70. Kase CS, Williams JP, Wyatt DA, Mohr JP: Lobar intracerebral hematomas: clinical and CT analysis of 22 cases. Neurology (NY) 32:1146, 1982

71. Kattapong VJ, Hart BL, Davis LE: Familial cerebral cavernous angiomas: clinical and radiologic studies. Neurology 45:492, 1995

72. Kelly DL, Alexander E, Davis CH, Maynard DC: Intracranial AVMs: clinical review evaluation of brain scans. J Neurosurg 31:422, 1969

73. Kjellberg RN, Hanamura T, Davis KR et al: Bragg-Peak proton beam therapy for arteriovenous malformations of the brain. N Engl J Med 5:269, 1983

74. Klosovskii N: The Development of the Brain and Its Disturbance by Harmful Factors. Macmillan, New York, 1963

75. Krayenbühl H, Siebenmann R: Small vascular malformations as a cause of primary intracerebral hemorrhage. J Neurosurg 22:7, 1965

76. Krayenbühl H, Yasargil G: L'Aneurismo Cerebral. Documenta Geigy, Series Chirurgica 4. Geigy, Basel, 1959

77. Kuban KCK, Gilles FH: Human telencephalic angiogenesis. Ann Neurol 17:539, 1985

78. Kupersmith MJ, Vargas ME, Yashar A et al: Occipital arteriovenous malformations: visual disturbances and presentation. Neurology 46:953, 1996

79. Kusske JA, Kelly WA: Embolization and reduction of the "steal" syndrome in cerebral AVMs. J Neurosurg 40:313, 1974

80. Kuwayama N, Pile-Spellman J, Hacein-Bey L et al: Intraobserver correlation and interobserver reliability of AVM grading systems, abstracted. The International Congress on Interventional Neuroradiology and Intravascular Surgery. November 19–22, 1995, Kyoto, Japan

81. Kvam DA, Michelsen WJ, Quest DO: Intracerebral hemorrhage as a complication of artificial embolization. Neurosurgery 7:491, 1980

82. Lanzino G, Jensen ME, Cappelletto B, Kassell NF: Arteriovenous malformations that rupture during pregnancy: a management dilemma. Acta Neurochir 126:102, 1994

83. Lasjaunias P, Chiu M, Ter Brugge K et al: Neurological manifestations of intracranial dural arteriovenous malformations. J Neurosurg 64:724, 1986

84. Lasjaunias P, Ter Brugge K: Vascular Diseases in Children. Springer-Verlag, New York, 1996

85. Latchaw RE, Hu X, Ugurbil K et al: Functional magnetic resonance imaging as a management tool for cerebral arteriovenous malformations. Neurosurgery 37:619, 1995

86. Lawton MT, Spetzler RF: Surgical management of acutely ruptured arteriovenous malformations. p. 511. In Welch KMA, Caplan LR, Reis DJ et al (eds): Primer on Cerebrovascular Diseases. Academic Press, San Diego, 1997

87. Lazar ML, Watts CC, Kilgore B, Clark K: Cerebral angiography during operation for intracranial aneurysms and arteriovenous malformations: technical note. J Neurosurg 34:706, 1971

88. Leblanc R, Ethier R, Little JR: Computerized tomography findings in arteriovenous malformations of the brain. J Neurosurg 51:765, 1979

89. Leblanc R, Levesque M, Comair Y, Ethier R: Magnetic resonance imaging of cerebral arteriovenous malformations. Neurosurgery 21:15, 1987

90. Leblanc E, Meyer E, Zatorre R et al: Functional PET scanning in the preoperative assessment of cerebral arteriovenous malformations. Stereotact Funct Neurosurg 65:60, 1995

91. Lees F: The migrainous symptoms of cerebral angiomata. J Neurol Neurosurg Psychiatry 25:45, 1962

92. Lindegaard KF, Grolimund R, Asslid R, Nornes H: Eval-

uation of cerebral AVMs using transcranial Doppler ultrasound. J Neurosurg 65:335, 1986

93. Luessenhop AJ, Gennarelli TA: Anatomical grading of supratentorial arteriovenous malformations for determining operability. J Neurosurg 1:30, 1975

94. Luessenhop AJ, Mujica PH: Embolization of segments of the circle of Willis and adjacent branches for management of certain inoperable cerebral arteriovenous malformations. J Neurosurg 54:573, 1981

95. Luessenhop AJ, Presper JH: Surgical embolization of cerebral arteriovenous malformations through internal carotid and vertebral arteries. Long-term results. J Neurosurg 42:443, 1975

96. Mackenzie I: The clinical presentation of cerebral angioma. A review of 50 cases. Brain 76:184, 1953

97. Maldjian J, Atlas SW, Howard RS 2nd et al: Functional magnetic resonance imaging of regional brain activity in patients with intracerebral arteriovenous malformations before surgical or endovascular therapy. J Neurosurg 84:477, 1996

98. Mall FP: On the development of the blood-vessels of the brain in the human embryo. Am J Anat 4:1, 1905

99. Margolis G, Odom GL, Woodhall B: Further experiences with small vascular malformations as a cause of massive intracerebral bleeding. J Neuropathol Exp Neurol 20:161, 1961

100. Marks MP, Lane B, Steinberg G, Chang P: Vascular characteristics of intracerebral arteriovenous malformations in patients with clinical steal. AJNR 12:489, 1991

101. Maspes PE, Marini G: Results of the surgical treatment of intracranial arteriovenous malformations. Vasc Surg 4:164, 1970

102. Massaro AR, Young WL, Kader A et al: Characterization of arteriovenous malformation feeding vessels by carbon dioxide reactivity. AJNR 15:55, 1994

103. Mast H, Mohr JP, Osipov A et al: 'Steal' is an unestablished mechanism for the clinical presentation of cerebral arteriovenous malformations. Stroke 26:1215, 1995

104. Mast H, Mohr JP, Thompson JL et al: Transcranial Doppler ultrasonography in cerebral arteriovenous malformations. Diagnostic sensitivity and association of flow velocity with spontaneous hemorrhage and focal neurological deficit. Stroke 26:1024, 1995

105. Mawad ME, Hilal SK, Silver AJ, Sane P: High resolution, high field MR imaging of cerebral arteriovenous malformations. Radiology 153:143, 1984

106. Maynard KI, Ogilvy CS: Patterns of peptide-containing perivascular nerves in the circle of Willis: their absence in intracranial arteriovenous malformations. J Neurosurg 82:829, 1995

107. McCormick WF: The pathology of vascular ("arteriovenous") malformations. J Neurosurg 24:807, 1966

108. McCormick WF, Hardman JM, Boulter TR: Vascular malformations ("angiomas") of the brain with special reference to those occurring in the posterior fossa. J Neurosurg 28:241, 1968

109. McCormick WF, Nofzinger JD: "Cryptic" vascular malformations of the central nervous system. J Neurosurg 24:865, 1966

110. McCormick WF, Rosenfield DB: Massive brain hemorrhage: a review of 144 cases and an examination of their causes. Stroke 4:946, 1973

111. McCormick WF, Schochet SS Jr: Atlas of Cerebrovascular Disease. WB Saunders, Philadelphia, 1976

112. Mendelow AD, Erfurth A, Grossart K, MacPherson P: Do cerebral arteriovenous malformations increase in size? J Neurol Neurosurg Psychiatry 50:980, 1987

113. Minakawa T, Tanaka R, Koike T et al: Angiographic follow up study of cerebral arteriovenous malformations with reference to their enlargement and regression. Neurosurgery 24:68, 1989

114. Mineta T, Fukuyama K, Koga H et al: Dural arteriovenous malformation associated with occlusion of the superior sagittal sinus: case report. Neurol Med Chir (Tokyo) 31:41, 1991

115. Miyasaka K, Wolpert SM, Prager RJ: The association of cerebral aneurysms, infundibula, and intracranial arteriovenous malformations. Stroke 2:196, 1982

116. Moffat DB: The embryology of the arteries of the brain. Ann R Coll Surg Engl 30:368, 1962

117. Mohr JP, Caplan LR, Melski JW et al: The Harvard 81 Cooperative Stroke Registry. Neurology 28:754, 1978

118. Mohr JP, Mast H, Osipov A et al: Mortality, neurologic impairment and disability following hemorrhage in the course of cerebral arteriovenous malformations, abstracted. Neurology suppl. 48:A371, 1997

119. Moody RA, Poppen JL: Arteriovenous malformations. J Neurosurg 32:503, 1970

120. Morello G, Boroghi GP: Cerebral angiomas. A report of the 154 personal cases and a comparison between the results of surgical excision and conservative management. Acta Neurochir (Wien) 28:135, 1973

121. Morgan MK, Johnston I, Besser M, Baines D: Cerebral arteriovenous malformations, steal and the hypertensive breakthrough threshold. J Neurosurg 66:563, 1987

122. Moritake K, Handa H, Mori K et al: Venous angiomas of the brain. Surg Neurol 14:95, 1980

123. Mullan S, Brown FD, Patronas NJ: Hyperemic and ischemic problems of surgical treatment of arteriovenous malformations. J Neurosurg 51:757, 1979

124. Mullan S, Mojtahedi S, Johnson DL, Macdonald RL: Cerebral venous malformation-arteriovenous malformation transition forms. J Neurosurg 85:9, 1996

125. Muraszko K, Wang HH, Pelton G, Stein BM: A study of the reactivity of feeding vessels to arteriovenous malformations: correlation with clinical outcome. Neurosurgery 26:190, 1990

126. Newton TH, Troost BT: Arteriovenous malformation and fistula. p. 2490. In Newton TH, Potts DG (eds): Radiology of the Skull and Brain: Angiography. Vol. 2. CV Mosby, St. Louis, 1974

127. Nishino A, Sakurai Y, Takahashi A et al: Superior petrosal sinus dural arteriovenous malformation with varix indenting brain stem: report of a case and review of the literature. No To Shinkei 43:62, 1991

128. Norbash AM, Marks MP, Lane B: Correlation of pressure measurements with angiographic characteristics predisposing to hemorrhage and steal in cerebral arteriovenous malformations. AJNR 15:809, 1994

129. Norlen G: Arteriovenous aneurysms of the brain: report

of ten cases of total removal of the lesion. J Neurosurg 6:475, 1949

130. Nornes H, Grip A: Hemodynamic aspects of cerebral arteriovenous malformations. J Neurosurg 53:456, 1980

131. Northfield DWC: Angiomatous malformations of the brain. Guys Hosp Rep 90:149, 1940

132. Numaguchi Y, Kishikawa T, Fukui M et al: Prolonged injection angiography for diagnosing intracranial cavernous hemangiomas. Radiology 131:137, 1979

133. Numaguchi Y, Kitamura K, Fukui M et al: Intracranial venous angiomas. Surg Neurol 18:193, 1982

134. Nussel F, Wegmuller H, Huber P: Comparison of magnetic resonance angiography, magnetic resonance imaging and conventional angiography in cerebral arteriovenous malformation. Neuroradiology 33:56, 1991

135. Okabe T, Meyer JS, Okayasu H et al: Xenon-enhanced CT CBF measurements in cerebral AVMs before and after excision. Contribution to pathogenesis and treatment. J Neurosurg 59:21, 1983

136. Olivecrona H, Ladenheim J: Congenital Arteriovenous Aneurysms of the Carotid and Vertebral Systems. Springer-Verlag, Berlin, 1957

137. Ondra SL, Troupp H, George ED, Schwab K: The natural history of symptomatic arteriovenous malformations of the brain: a 24-year follow up assessment. J Neurosurg 73:387, 1990

138. Ostergaard JR: Association of intracranial aneurysm and arteriovenous malformation in childhood. Congress of Neurological Surgeons. Neurosurgery 3:358, 1984

139. Ozer MN, Sencer W, Block J: A clinical study of cerebral vascular malformations: the significance of migraine. J Mt Sinai Hosp 31:403, 1964

140. Padget DH: The development of the cranial arteries in the human embryo. Carnegie Inst Wash Pub. 575. Contrib Embryol 32:205, 1948

141. Padget DH: The cranial venous system in man in reference to development, adult configuration, and relation to the arteries. Am J Anat 98:307, 1956

142. Parkinson D, Bachers G: Arteriovenous malformations. Summary of 100 consecutive supratentorial cases. J Neurosurg 53:285, 1980

143. Paterson JH, McKissock W: A clinical survey of intracranial angiomas with special reference to their mode of progression and surgical treatment: a report of 110 cases. Brain 79:233, 1956

144. Patronas NJ, Marx WJ, Duda EE, Mullan JJ: Microvascular embolization of arteriovenous malformations: predicting success by cerebral angiography. AJNR 1:459, 1980

145. Pellettieri L: Surgical versus conservative treatment of intracranial arteriovenous malformations. A study in surgical decision-making. Acta Neurochir suppl. 29:1, 1979

146. Perret G: The epidemiology and clinical course of arteriovenous malformations. p. 21. In Pia HW, Gleave JRW, Grote E, Zierski J (eds): Cerebral Angiomas: Advances in Diagnosis and Therapy. Springer-Verlag, New York, 1975

147. Perret G, Nishioka H: Report on the cooperative study of intracranial aneurysms and subarachnoid hemorrhage. Section VI. Arteriovenous malformations. J Neurosurg 25:467, 1966

148. Pertuiset B, Ancri D, Clergue F: Preoperative evaluation of hemodynamic factors in cerebral arteriovenous malformations for selection of a radical surgical tactic with special reference to vascular autoregulation disorders. Neurol Res 4:209, 1982

149. Pertuiset B, Sichez JP, Philippon J et al: Mortalité et morbidité après exerèse chirurgicale totale de 162 malformations artérioveineuses intracraniennes. Rev Neurol 1979

150. Petty GW, Tatemichi TK, Mohr JP et al: Transcranial Doppler changes after treatment for arteriovenous malformations. Stroke 21:260, 1990

151. Pia HW, Gleave JRW, Grote E et al: Cerebral Angiomas: Advances in Diagnosis and Therapy. p. 285. Springer-Verlag, New York, 1975

152. Picard L, Miyachi S, Braun M et al: Arteriovenous malformations of the corpus callosum—radioanatomic study and effectiveness of intranidus embolization. Neurol Med Chir 36:851, 1996

153. Pile-Spellman JM, Baker KF, Liszczak TM et al: High-flow angiopathy: cerebral blood vessel changes in experimental chronic arteriovenous fistula. AJNR 7:811, 1986

154. Pool JL, Potts DG: Aneurysms and Arteriovenous Anomalies of the Brain. Diagnosis and Treatment. p. 463. Harper & Row, New York, 1965

155. Putman CM, Chaloupka JC, Fulbright RK et al: Exceptional multiplicity of cerebral arteriovenous malformations associated with hereditary hemorrhagic telangiectasia (Osler-Weber-Rendu syndrome). AJNR 17:1733, 1996

156. Rapacki TF, Brantley MJ, Furlow TW Jr et al: Heterogeneity of cerebral cavernous hemangiomas diagnosed by MR imaging. J Comput Assist Tomogr 14:18, 1990

157. Rhodes AJ, Hyde JB: Postnatal growth of arterioles in the human cerebral cortex. Growth 29:173, 1965

158. Rigamonti D, Hadley MN, Drayer BP et al: Cerebral cavernous malformations: incidence and familial occurrence. N Engl J Med 319:343, 1988

159. Rothbart D, Awad IA, Lee J et al: Expression of angiogenic factors and structural proteins in central nervous system vascular malformations. Neurosurgery 38:915, 1996

160. Rothfus WE, Albright A, Casey KF et al: Cerebellar venous angioma: "benign" entity? AJNR 5:61, 1984

161. Ruff RL, Arbit E: Aphemia resulting from a left frontal hematoma. Neurology (NY) 31:353, 1981

162. Saito Y, Kobayashi N: Cerebral venous angiomas. Radiology 139:87, 1981

163. Santoreneos S, Blumbergs PC, Jones NR: Choroid plexus arteriovenous malformations. A report of four pathologically proven cases and review of the literature. Br J Neurosurg 10:385, 1996

164. Schlachter LB, Fleischer AS, Faria MA, Tindall GT: Multifocal intracranial arteriovenous malformations. Neurosurgery 7:440, 1980

165. Schoerner W, Bradac GB, Treisch J et al: Magnetic resonance imaging (MRI) in the diagnosis of cerebral arteriovenous angiomas. Neuroradiology 28:313, 1986

166. Schwartz A, Hennerici M: Noninvasive transcranial Doppler ultrasound in intracranial angiomas. Neurology 36:626, 1986

167. Senegor M, Dohrmann GJ, Wollman RL: Venous angiomas of the posterior fossa should be considered anomalous venous drainage. Surg Neurol 19:26, 1983

168. Shenkin HA, Spitz EB, Grant FC, Kety SS: Physiologic studies of arteriovenous anomalies of the brain. J Neurosurg 6:165, 1948

169. Sheth RD, Bodensteiner JB: Progressive neurologic impairment from an arteriovenous malformation vascular steal. Pediatr Neurol 13:352, 1995

170. Snead OC III, Acker JD, Morawetz R: Familial arteriovenous malformation. Ann Neurol 5:585, 1979

171. Sonstein WJ, Kader A, Michelsen WJ et al: Expression of vascular endothelial growth factor in pediatric and adult cerebral arteriovenous malformations: an immunocytochemical study. J Neurosurg 85:838, 1996

172. Spetzler RF, Martin NA: A proposed grading system for arteriovenous malformations. J Neurosurg 65:476, 1986

173. Spetzler RF, Wilson CB: Enlargement of an AVM documented by angiography: case report. J Neurosurg 43:767, 1975

174. Spetzler RF, Wilson CB, Weinstein P et al: Normal perfusion pressure breakthrough theory. Clin Neurosurg 25:651, 1978

175. Stabell KE, Nornes H: Prospective neuropsychological investigation of patients with supratentorial arteriovenous malformations. Acta Neurochir 131:32, 1994

176. Statham P, Macpherson P, Johnston R et al: Cerebral radiation necrosis complicating stereotactic radiosurgery for arteriovenous malformation. J Neurol Neurosurg Psychiatry 53:476, 1990

177. Stein BM, Wolpert SM: Arteriovenous malformations of the brain I: Current concepts and treatment. Arch Neurol 37:1, 1980

178. Stein BM, Wolpert SM: Arteriovenous malformations of the brain II: Current concepts and treatment. Arch Neurol 37:69, 1980

179. Stein RW, Kase CS, Hier DB et al: Caudate hemorrhage. Neurology (NY) 34:1549, 1984

180. Sundt TF Jr, Piepgras DG: The surgical approach to arteriovenous malformations of the lateral and sigmoid dural sinuses. J Neurosurg 59:32, 1983

181. Svien HJ, McRae JA: Arteriovenous anomalies of the brain. Fate of patients not having definitive surgery. J Neurosurg 23:23, 1965

182. Symon L, Tacconi L, Mendoza N, Nakaji P: Arteriovenous malformations of the posterior fossa: a report on 28 cases and review of the literature. Br J Neurosurg 9:721, 1995

183. Sze G, Harper PS, Galicich JH et al: Hemorrhagic neoplasms: MR mimics of occult vascular malformations. Am Soc Neuroradiol May 10–15: 125, 1987

184. Tarr RW, Johnson DW, Rutigliano M et al: Use of acetazolamide challenge xenon CT in the assessment of cerebral blood flow dynamics in patients with arteriovenous malformations. AJNR 11:441, 1990

185. Troost BT, Newton TH: Occipital lobe arteriovenous malformation. Arch Ophthalmol 93:250, 1975

186. Troupp H, Marttila I, Halonen V: Arteriovenous malformations of the brain: prognosis without operation. Acta Neurochir 22:125, 1970

187. Trumpy JH, Eldevik P: Intracranial arteriovenous malformations: conservative or surgical treatment? Surg Neurol 8:171, 1977

188. Trussart V, Berry I, Manelfe C et al: Epileptogenic cerebral vascular malformations and MRI. J Neuroradiol 16:273, 1989

189. Tsitsopoulos P, Andrew J, Harrison MJG: Occult cerebral arteriovenous malformations. J Neurol Neurosurg Psychiatry 50:218, 1987

190. Turjman F, Massoud TF, Sayre JW et al: Epilepsy associated with cerebral arteriovenous malformations: a multivariate analysis of angioarchitectural characteristics. AJNR 16:345, 1995

191. Vinuela F, Fox AJ, Pelz DM, Drake CG: Unusual clinical manifestations of dural arteriovenous malformations. J Neurosurg 64:554, 1986

192. Voigt K, Yasargil MG: Cerebral cavernous haemangiomas or cavernomas. Incidence, etiology, localization, diagnosis, clinical features and treatment. Review of the literature and report of an unusual case. Neurochirurgia 19:59, 1976

193. Wallace JM, Nashold BS Jr, Slewka AP: Hemodynamic effects of cerebral arteriovenous aneurysms. Circulation 31:696, 1965

194. Walter W: The influence of the type and localization of the angioma on the clinical syndrome. p. 271. In Pia HW, Gleave JRW, Grote E, Zierski J (eds): Cerebral Angiomas: Advances in Diagnosis and Therapy. Springer-Verlag, New York, 1975

195. Waltimo O: The change in size of intracranial arteriovenous malformations. J Neurol Sci 19:21, 1973

196. Waltimo O: The relationship of size, density, and localization of intracranial arteriovenous malformations to the type of initial symptom. J Neurol Sci 19:13, 1973

197. Wendling LR, Moore JS, Kieffer SA et al: Intracerebral venous angioma. Radiology 119:141, 1976

198. Willinsky RA, Lasjaunias P, Ter Brugge K, Burrows P: Multiple cerebral arteriovenous malformations (AVMs). Review of our experience from 203 patients with cerebral vascular lesions. Neuroradiology 32:207, 1990

199. Wilson CB, U HS, Dominque J: Microsurgical treatment of intracranial vascular malformations. J Neurosurg 51:446, 1979

200. Witt TC, Kondziolka D, Baumann SB et al: Preoperative cortical localization with functional MRI for use in stereotactic radiosurgery. Stereotact Funct Neurosurg 66:24, 1996

201. Yamada S: Arteriovenous malformations in the functional area: surgical treatment and regional cerebral blood flow. Neurol Res 4:283, 1982

202. Yeung D, Chen N, Ferguson RD et al: Three-dimensional reconstruction of arteriovenous malformations from multiple stereotactic angiograms. Med Phys 23:1797, 1996

203. Young WL, Prohovnik I, Ornstein E et al: The effect of arteriovenous malformation resection on cerebrovascular reactivity to carbon dioxide. Neurosurgery 27:257, 1990

204. Young WL, Pile-Spellman J, Prohovnik I et al: Evidence for adaptive autoregulatory displacement in hypotensive cortical territories adjacent to arteriovenous malformations. Neurosurgery 34:601, 1994

C H A P T E R   2 8

Spinal Cord Ischemia

OSCAR BENAVENTE

HENRY J. M. BARNETT

Spinal cord infarction, although rare compared with cerebral stroke, continues to be a diagnostic puzzle with a dismal prognosis. Its incidence is unknown, and no epidemiologic study has been conducted. An upsurge of interest in the subject has replaced the neglect of former years. This has been due in part to the increased accidental production of cord infarct by modern cardiovascular surgery and to the advances in imaging techniques, including computed tomography (CT) and magnetic resonance imaging (MRI).[19,28,45] These have allowed better visualization of the spinal cord and improved the accurate localization, diagnosis, and management of vascular lesions.[21,67,73]

Blackwood[8] reviewed the records of 3,737 autopsies conducted over 50 years; only five cases of spinal cord infarction were found. Surprisingly, no cases were due to atherosclerosis or hypertensive vascular disease, or both. On the other hand, Slager and Webb[93] found microinfarcts of the spinal cord in 3% of 200 consecutive autopsies performed in asymptomatic patients. Recently Sandson and Friedman[88] described eight cases of spinal cord infarction representing roughly 1.2% of all admissions for stroke in that center. Despite numerous well-documented case reports of spinal cord infarction, misconceptions still exist regarding its pathogenesis and clinical course.

Studies in animals reported more than 100 years ago showed that aortic clamping resulted in paralysis. Clinically, paraparesis as a result of aortic obstruction was recognized at the end of the last century.[31] Bastian[5] in 1882 suggested that spinal cord softening may be the result of vascular occlusion; however, it was not until 1904 that Preobrashenski[80] described the syndrome of anterior spinal artery infarct.

The spinal cord, like the brain, may be subject to thrombotic, embolic phenomena or hemorrhage. For a better understanding of the clinical findings, it is worthwhile to review the vascular anatomy and regulation of the blood flow of the spinal cord.

Blood Supply of the Spinal Cord

The basic pattern of the arterial blood supply to the spinal cord consists of three longitudinal vessels that arise rostrally from the cervical region and descend as far as the conus me-

dullaris, plus numerous feeder arteries and radicular vessels. Anastomoses between the descending and segmentally oriented vessels occur on the surface of the spinal cord, which results in the formation of a rich vascular plexus from which medullary vessels penetrate both the white and the gray matter. These vessels are end arteries and do not anastomose further.[28]

LONGITUDINAL ARTERIES

There are three longitudinal arteries: the anterior spinal artery and the two posterior spinal arteries. The anterior spinal artery forms rostrally from the union of the two anterior spinal branches of each vertebral artery at the level of the foramen magnum. From this site, it descends up to the tip of the conus medullaris. It lies in relation to the anterior median sulcus[37,49] (Fig. 28.1). The caliber of the artery is widest in the lumbosacral region and narrowest in the thoracic region, which has been considered a vulnerable zone for ischemia.

The anterior spinal artery is reinforced by successive contributions of feeder arterial branches, which enter the artery in a caudal direction and supply the spinal cord below the point of their entry. At the conus medullaris and along the filum terminale, the anterior spinal artery communicates by anastomotic branches with the posterior spinal artery.[37,49]

The two posterior spinal arteries originate directly from the vertebral arteries (Fig. 28.2). Each vessel descends on the posterior surface of the spinal cord along the posterolateral sulcus. A common finding is that the arteries are discontinuous, and sometimes one artery moves across to supply the other side.[49] Throughout its course, each posterior spinal artery gives off branches that penetrate the cord to supply the posterior columns, dorsal gray matter, and superficial dorsal aspect of the lateral columns.

RADICULAR TRIBUTARY ARTERIES

Thirty-one pairs of radicular arteries penetrate the spinal canal through the intervertebral foramina. Approximately 7 or 8 of these 62 radicular branches contribute to the vascularization

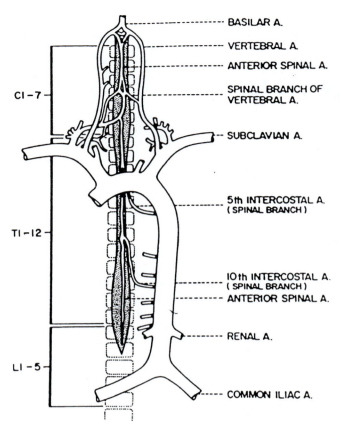

CI – 7

TI – 12

LI – 5

BASILAR A.

VERTEBRAL A.

ANTERIOR SPINAL A.

SPINAL BRANCH OF VERTEBRAL A.

SUBCLAVIAN A.

5th INTERCOSTAL A. (SPINAL BRANCH)

10th INTERCOSTAL A. (SPINAL BRANCH)

ANTERIOR SPINAL A.

RENAL A.

COMMON ILIAC A.

Figure 28.1 Extrinsic vascular supply of the spinal cord. Schematic representation of the anterior spinal artery. (Adapted from Gray[37]; from Benavente and Barnett,[6] with permission.)

of the spinal cord and define three major spinal arterial territories: cervicothoracic, midthoracic, and thoracolumbar.[61,67]

The cervicothoracic territory includes the cervical spinal cord, its brachial plexus enlargement, and the first two or three thoracic segments. This territory is richly supplied by the anterior spinal artery arising from the intracranial vertebral arteries, the midcervical radicular branches of the vertebral artery, and the branches of the costocervical trunk.

In the midthoracic territory, the radicular arteries supplying the middle and lower thoracic cord are less prominent.[89] This territory is usually supplied by a radicular branch arising at about the T7 level; it comprises the fourth to eighth segments of the thoracic cord.

The thoracolumbar territory includes, in addition to the lower thoracic segments, the lumbar enlargement, which relates to the lumbosacral plexus. This segment receives its blood supply from a single artery, called the artery of Adamkiewicz. This artery typically originates from the left 9th, 10th, 11th, or 12th intercostal arteries.[67] This irregular augmentation of the anterior spinal artery system results in watershed areas that may be vulnerable to hypoperfusion, most marked in the thoracic area.[89] These radicular tributaries may be subdivided into two groups according to their origin. The first group consists of those derived from the subclavian artery; the second group is supplied directly from the aorta. At the level of the second thoracic spinal cord segment, there is a

change of arterial supply from a subclavian supply to a direct aortic supply.[15]

Intrinsic Blood Supply of the Cord

When the radicular arteries reach the surface of the spinal cord, they form two distinct systems of intrinsic blood supply (Figs. 28.3 and 28.4). The first is the posterolateral and peripheral plexus formed by the two posterior spinal arteries, which are interconnected by anastomotic channels.[34] This is a centripedal vascular territory and is formed by radial arteries directed inward as branches from the coronal arterial plexus surrounding the spinal cord. It supplies from one-third to one-half of the outer rim of the cord, including the lateral and ventral spinothalamic tracts. These radial arteries are longer in the posterior white columns than in the anterior and lateral columns. This could explain the size and localization of pathologic changes related to vascular disorders.[49]

The second arterial system to the spinal cord is a centrifugal system formed by the sulcal arteries, which arise from the anterior spinal artery and pass backward in the anterior medial sulcus. These arteries enter the gray commissure and, turning left or right, supply the gray matter and adjacent white matter. The corticospinal tract is nourished by both systems.[49]

Both arterial systems are interconnected by a capillary anastomosis in the spinal cord. The number of sulcal arteries supplying each segment of the spinal cord varies with the region of the cord. They are most numerous in the thoracolumbar segment and least numerous in the upper thoracic segment.[110]

Venous System

Two intrinsic systems and one extrinsic system drain the spinal cord.[34,35,61,102,110]

INTRINSIC VENOUS SYSTEM

The anterior median group (central veins) collects blood from both halves of the medial aspects of the anterior horns, anterior gray commissure, and white matter of the anterior funiculus. The central veins also drain adjacent levels above and below through intersegmental anastomoses. They frequently anastomose with other veins within the fissure. Finally, the central veins empty into the anterior median spinal vein.

The other group consists of radial veins that arise from capillaries near the periphery of the gray matter or from the white matter. They are radially oriented and directed outward toward the surface of the spinal cord, where they join the superficial plexus of veins surrounding the cord and form a venous vase corona or corona plexus. These veins are more numerous in the white matter of the posterior and lateral

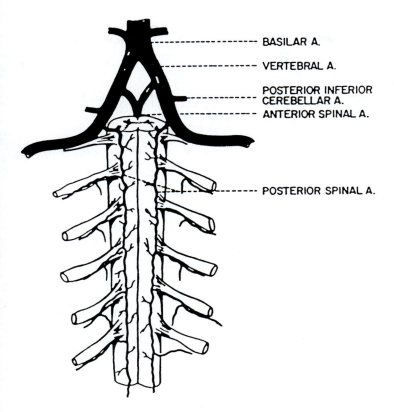

BASILAR A.

VERTEBRAL A.

POSTERIOR INFERIOR CEREBELLAR A.

ANTERIOR SPINAL A.

POSTERIOR SPINAL A.

Figure 28.2 Extrinsic vascular supply of the spinal cord. Schematic representation of the posterior spinal arteries. (Adapted from Gray[37]; from Benavente and Barnett,[6] with permission.)

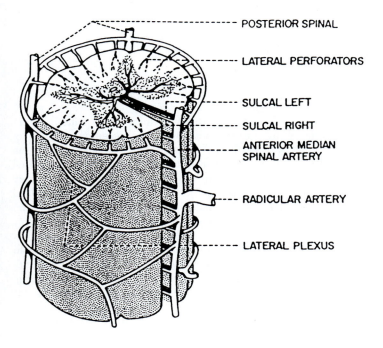

POSTERIOR SPINAL

LATERAL PERFORATORS

SULCAL LEFT

SULCAL RIGHT

ANTERIOR MEDIAN SPINAL ARTERY

RADICULAR ARTERY

LATERAL PLEXUS

Figure 28.3 Intrinsic vascular supply of the cord. The central sulcal is supplied from the anterior median artery, and the lateral is supplied from the anterior and posterior spinal arteries, forming the vasa corona. (From Buchan and Barnett,[15] with permission.)

Figure 28.4 Cross-sectional diagrammatic representation of the territories of the anterior and posterior spinal arteries. (From Mawad et al,[67] with permission.)

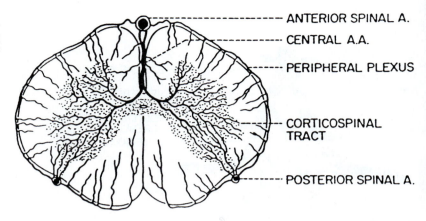

ANTERIOR SPINAL A.

CENTRAL A.A.

PERIPHERAL PLEXUS

CORTICOSPINAL TRACT

POSTERIOR SPINAL A.

funiculi, but they are also found in the anterior funiculus. The radial veins are more prominent at certain cervical and thoracic levels; they drain laterally from the gray matter of the lateral horns as well as posteriorly from the dorsal nucleus of Clark.

EXTRINSIC VENOUS SYSTEM

The extrinsic venous system is very conspicuous on the posterior aspect of the spinal cord and is especially prominent in the lumbosacral region. There is a rich anastomosis between the large venous trunks. The median posterior spinal vein descends in the region of the posterior median septum. This vessel drains blood from the posterior white columns and the end of the posterior horns.

The anterior spinal vein accompanies the anterior spinal artery and receives the sulcal veins. Both the anterior spinal veins and the median posterior spinal vein empty into the radicular veins, which accompany the anterior or posterior spinal roots. These radicular veins drain into the paravertebral and intervertebral plexuses, and then into the azygos and pelvic venous systems.[49] The absence of venous valves may allow infections in the abdominal cavity to spread to the spinal cord. They also render the spinal veins susceptible to Valsalva maneuvers, increasing the intra-abdominal pressure.

Physiology of Spinal Cord Blood Flow

The regulation of spinal cord blood flow is similar to that of brain blood flow. The spinal cord blood vessels are affected by changes in PCO_2 and hypoxia. Hypercapnia increases blood flow. Autoregulation keeps the regional as well as the total spinal cord blood flow constant. As in the brain, there is a high blood flow requirement and metabolic rate in the gray matter.[65,87]

The total cerebral blood flow of the human brain is 50 ml/min/100 g. Spinal cord flow varies, depending on the species and the area of cord studied.[74,87] In monkeys, total flow in

cervical, upper trunk, and lumbar areas is 15, 10, and 20 ml/min/100 g, respectively.[74] The intrinsic blood supply of the cord is directly proportional to the area of gray matter, this being most abundant in the thoracolumbar segment.[98] Consequently this segment may be more vulnerable to hypoperfusion. Another important consideration is that the cord is contained within the spinal canal, which has fixed dimensions. Any changes in contents occurs at the expense of cerebrospinal fluid (CSF), blood, or spinal tissue; if the intraspinal canal pressure rises, this causes a slowing of the spinal cord blood flow and consequent hypoxia.[15]

The blood flow of the spinal cord has a different pattern in the anterior and posterior systems. Flow in the anterior spinal artery is mainly caudal and unidirectional. Flow in the posterior spinal arteries is bidirectional: caudal in the cervical and thoracic regions and rostral in the lumbosacral region.[49]

Pathology of Spinal Cord Infarction

Spinal cord infarction results from interference with the circulation of the cord secondary to a generalized or localized reduction of blood flow. The locations of disease or obstruction that may lead to ischemia of the cord are the aorta, vertebral arteries, intercostal and lumbar arteries, radicular tributary arteries, anterior and posterior spinal arteries, small spinal vessels, and veins.[49] Heart disease leading to hypoperfusion and blood disorders may also interfere with the blood supply to the cord.[15]

The cellular events in spinal cord infarction are similar to those seen in cerebral infarction. According to the intensity of tissue damage, the infarct can be complete or incomplete. In the former, all cellular elements die. In an incomplete infarction, some of the elements survive, especially blood vessels and to a lesser extent astrocytes. Also, the damage can be only "cellular," being confined largely to neurons.

Initially, the infarcted area appears pale and swollen, with reduced consistency. In the central portion of the infarct, the neurons show ischemic changes (eosinophilic cytoplasm) (Fig. 28.5). The earliest change may be present after 6 hours. Astro-

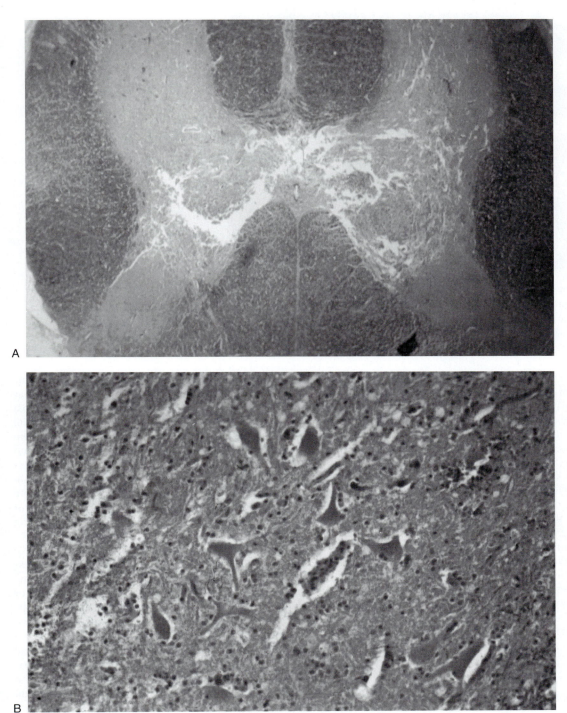

Figure 28.5 (**A**) Transverse section of the lumbar spinal cord showing an infarct involving mainly the gray matter. (H&E/SCR, × 1.) (**B**) Section from the anterior horn showing numerous ischemic neurons with dense eosinophilic cytoplasm. (H&E/SCR, × 25.) The patient suffered ischemic injury of the cord secondary to profound hypotension. (From Benavente and Barnett,[6] with permission.)

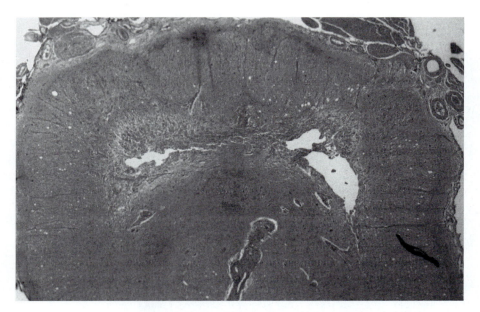

Figure 28.6 Thoracic spinal cord (transverse section) with a large infarct in the territory of the anterior spinal artery, with cavitation and vacuolation of the neuropil. (H&E, × 1.) The patient suffered a rupture of an aortic abdominal aneurysm. (From Benavente and Barnett,[6] with permission.)

cytes, oligodendroglial cells, and microglial cells, along with myelinated axons, disintegrate and give a granular appearance to the neuropil. These changes are followed by neovascularization, with endothelial hyperplasia and fragmentation of the tissue. In the following 2 to 3 weeks, the infarcted area is invaded by phagocytes. These cells liquefy the necrotic tissue, and cavitation occurs (Fig. 28.6). Finally the astrocytes proliferate at the edges of the cavitation.[75]

Because of the tight arrangement of the pathways in the cord, small infarcts are usually associated with more obvious symptoms and signs than similar lesions in the brain.[71] Involvement of spinal cord blood vessels by atherosclerosis or thrombosis is uncommon. This contrasts with the high frequency of similar vascular diseases affecting the cerebral vessels.[49,54,75] Perhaps this discrepancy can be explained by the fact that the blood pressure in the spinal arteries is lower than in other parts of the vascular system. This idea is supported by the occurrence of increased vascular pathology in the cords of patients with coarctation of the aorta, in which there is high blood pressure in the spinal cord system.[49]

Clinical Presentation of Spinal Cord Infarction

Spinal cord infarction has many similarities to cerebral infarction. In both, the clinical picture may be extremely diverse. It depends on the vascular territory involved, the size of the lesion, its cause, and the status of the collateral circulation. The same terms used to describe the pattern of duration of cerebrovascular disease can be applied to the spinal cord.

In older patients, the sudden onset of neurologic symptoms and signs related to the spinal cord strongly suggests vascular disease. If the neurologic manifestations are attributable to a specific arterial territory, the diagnosis is almost certain. Motor, sensory, and autonomic signs may be present. The findings may include paraparesis, tetraparesis, paraplegia, and loss of sphincter control, reflecting the level, vascular territory involved, and extension of the infarct.[71] If these signs remain for more than 24 hours, the event is referred to as a complete infarct. The same type of vascular event can be intermittent or less abrupt in onset, depending mainly on the underlying mechanism and on the presence of collateral circulation.

Transient ischemic attacks (TIAs) can theoretically involve the spinal cord. These focal neurologic deficits that last less than 24 hours rarely precede spinal cord infarctions.[15] Spinal TIAs are probably due to emboli arising from the heart or aorta, the site of ulcerative atherosclerotic disease, plus perhaps a combination of focal atherosclerotic stenosis and systemic hypotension.[89] It is surprising that spinal TIAs are not frequently diagnosed, since ulcerated atheromas and mural thrombi are common findings in the aortas of elderly patients.[71] Ischemic attacks may also occur in coarctation of the aorta due to the steal phenomenon.[56] Spinal TIAs have been reported in patients with spinal arteriovenous malformations (AVMs). The underlying mechanism is either the steal phenomenon, in which blood is shunted through a low-pressure AVM, or the vascular malformation compressing the cord.[99]

The term claudication of the cord was introduced by Dejerine; it was thought to be a result of impaired blood flow secondary to arterial stenosis.[111] It refers to transitory symptoms in the legs associated with exercise and disappearing with rest. Many of the early cases were attributed to syphilitic arteritis of the radicular arteries. Today spinal AVMs are one of the most common causes of this syndrome.[99] Other reported causes are atherosclerosis and pronounced lumbar spondylosis or thoracic disc protrusion.[7,82] Intermittent spinal symptoms have also been described in patients with thoracolumbar spinal cord stenosis, in which the episodic neurologic dysfunction is presumably of vascular origin.[22,108]

The initial symptoms are heaviness in one or both legs that presents during activity and is relieved by rest. Also, sensory symptoms, pain, or sphincter disturbances have been noted. At rest, the neurologic examination generally discloses no significant abnormalities. After exercise, weakness of one or both legs, with hyper-reflexia and extensor plantar responses, has been found.[17,30,82] Transient cord ischemia does not always preclude an infarction, but over long periods a progressive reduction in exercise tolerance occurs, until a permanent deficit develops.[3]

The same pattern of presentation can be applied to the cauda equine. Intermittent claudication of the cauda equina is more common in males, characterized by pain, numbness, and paresthesias with exercise and relief with rest. Symptoms begin in the lower back and buttocks and spread down the legs. Examination at rest is generally normal, but after exercise, minor motor and sensory disturbances may be found. The syndrome of cauda equine claudication has been associated with narrowing of the lumbar spinal canal,[14] disc protrusion, and achondroplasia.[9,39] Symptoms develop with actions or postures that involve extension of the lumbar spine. Relief occurs when the patient leans forward or squats. In a few patients, the precipitation of symptoms relates to exercise of the extremities, perhaps as a result of ischemia of cauda equina roots during exercise. It therefore seems that the syndrome of cauda equina claudication relates to exercise. This may be due to impaired blood flow through radicular arteries at points of constriction. Consequently, the blood supply cannot increase sufficiently during activity.[3,9,24]

In 1926, Foix and Alajouanine[25] described a syndrome of subacute or chronic progressive myelopathy. It was attributed to chronic ischemia of the spinal cord secondary to atherosclerosis, but this has been a subject of recurrent debate.[54] Many other conditions have been implicated in the etiology of this entity. Recently a venous infarction of the spinal cord resulting in a subacute progressive myelopathy was reported.[18] The clinical picture consists of atrophy of the small muscles of the hands with hyperactive reflexes. These patients tend to have a history of hypertension and systemic atherosclerosis. The pathologic changes mainly involve the anterior horns and consist of small cavities or lacunes, plus rarefaction of the neuropil. These types of changes have been observed mainly in the lower cervical cord.

Anterior Spinal Artery Syndrome

The territory supplied by the anterior spinal artery is the most common location of ischemic lesions of the spinal cord. The first clinicopathologic description of anterior spinal artery syndrome was by Spiller[95] in 1909. The underlying cause was syphilitic arteritis. Occlusion of this artery results in infarction of the anterior two-thirds of the spinal cord. Involved structures are the anterior horns of the gray matter, the spinothalamic tracts, and the pyramidal tracts. The level of ischemia may be cervical, thoracic, or lumbosacral.[46,48]

CLINICAL MANIFESTATIONS

Involvement of the vertebral arteries may produce infarction of the cervical level.[51] This syndrome is characterized by the sudden onset of radicular or diffuse neck pain, followed by quadriparesis. Because of spinal shock, the paraplegia may remain flaccid for several days to weeks, with absence of reflexes. Disturbances in the control of vesical and rectal sphincters commonly occur. The sensory loss is marked and involves pain, temperature, pinprick, and light-touch sensation below the segmental or dermatomal level of the lesion. However, proprioception, light touch, and vibration senses are almost always spared. The upper extremities may develop motor neuron signs, and spasticity of the legs may occur, with hyper-reflexia and extensor plantar responses.[26,104] Proprioception and vibration sense may be affected with higher cervical lesions due to involvement of the medial lemniscus.[88]

Infarction of the spinal cord is most common in the thoracic level, due to the presence of a watershed area in the midthoracic region.[49,88] The territory of the anterior spinal artery at this level can be infarcted by aortic or radicular artery disease. The typical thoracic infarction presents with pain in the interscapular region, followed by paraparesis or paraplegia with the arms spared, urinary and rectal incontinence or retention, and a sensory loss to pain and temperature most common at the T4 level. Again, the initial spinal shock gives way to hypertonia, hyper-reflexia, and extensor plantar responses below the level of the lesion.

Infarction of the lumbosacral region in the territory supplied by the anterior spinal artery may be caused by disease or obstruction of the radicular artery of Adamkiewicz. If the lesion is extensive, the patient presents with a flaccid paraplegia due to damage of the large area of gray matter and, consequently, the motor neurons of the anterior horns. Autonomic dysfunction occurs; later, wasting of the legs associated with areflexia may be present.

Occlusion of a central sulcal artery produces small lesions in half the spinal cord.[49,88,97] This can present as an incomplete Brown-Séquard syndrome or a suspended dissociated sensory loss: impairment of pain and temperature sensation over the segment affected by the infarct, with preserved sensation above and below the lesion. This is a rare phenomenon, attributed to embolic or thrombotic occlusion of the perforating branches of sulcal arteries, which produces a localized infarction while the anterior spinal artery is intact (Table 28.1).[20,31,76]

ETIOLOGY

Infarction of the spinal cord involving the territory supplied by the anterior spinal artery may result from interruption of the blood supply due to obstruction of the lumen of any vessel

Table 28.1 Anterior Spinal Artery Syndrome

Back or neck pain of sudden onset
Rapidly progressive paraplegia
Flaccid paraplegia that soon becomes spastic
Areflexia at onset, which becomes hyper-reflexia with extensor plantar response
Sensory level for pain and temperature
Preserved propioception, light touch, and vibration sense
Urinary incontinence
Painful burning dysesthesias below the level of cord injury (during chronic phase)

from the aorta to the intramedullary vasculature, systemic hypoperfusion, or a combination of both[88] (Table 28.2).

Syphilitic arteritis was the most common cause of spinal cord infarction in the prepenicillin era[88]; this was replaced by atherosclerosis of the aorta and spinal arteries before the increased trend in surgery for aortic aneurysm reconstruction. Today, cardiovascular surgery for aortic aneurysm is the leading cause of spinal cord ischemia. Infarction of the spinal cord secondary to emboli has been described in association with bacterial endocarditis,[40,48] atrial myxoma,[44] mitral valve disease,[107] and paradoxical embolism secondary to patent foramen ovale.[72] Fibrocartilaginous emboli (FCE) from herniated intervertebral discs is also a rare but well-recognized phenomenon causing spinal infarction. The mechanisms for this are poorly understood. Srigley and coworkers[96] suggested that fragments of disc material are traumatically forced into bone marrow vertebral plexus and arterial channels. The patient usually experiences sudden onset of back or neck pain, which is followed by progressive and usually permanent spinal cord or brain stem dysfunction. A history of minor head or neck injury and lifting a heavy load at the onset of symptoms is common. The infarction is typically central, with major involvement of the anterior and lateral horns.

The diagnosis is generally made at autopsy or from surgical specimens, when emboli histologically identical to the fibrocartilage of the nucleus pulposus are identified in arteries or veins, or both, of the spinal circulation.[16,96] Tose et al[101] reviewed 32 cases of histologically confirmed FCE and found a high incidence in young women (69%), with only a temporal relation to significant trauma in a minority of patients. In most of the cases (70%) embolization occurred in the cervical cord, in some extending to lower medulla and upper thoracic segments. Infarction was localized to the anterior spinal artery territory in most of the patients. The clinical course in this series showed some distinctive features; first, all patients suffered sudden onset of pain. Second, the interval from onset of pain to maximal neurologic deficit ranged from 15 minutes to 48 hours. On the other hand, in cases of thrombotic infarction neurologic deficits may appear first and in most cases present abruptly accompanied by pain. A third distinguishing feature of infarction secondary to thrombosis was that no case of FCE showed significant improvement of neurologic deficit during the first 48 hours. Finally, the findings in the MRI of cord swelling and increased T_2 signal, plus a collapsed intervertebral disc space at the appropriate level, strongly suggested FCE.

Spinal cord ischemia associated with decompression sickness (caisson disease) has also been described and is the result of circulating nitrogen bubbles that block small spinal arteries.[43] Primary thrombosis of the anterior spinal artery as a cause of spinal infarction has not been well documented and is considered rare. Foo and Rossier,[26] reviewing 60 cases of anterior spinal artery syndrome, found six patients in whom thrombosis of this vessel was the cause. However, in five, the thrombosis could not be considered primary.[26,88]

Dissection of Aortic Aneurysm

Aortic aneurysm is a serious vascular disorder with a lifetime incidence of 2% to 6% and a 1-year mortality rate of 75% in untreated patients.[19] Neurologic complications of aortic aneu-

Table 28.2 Etiology of Spinal Cord Ischemia

Vasculitis
    Polyarteritis nodosa[107]
    Behçet's syndrome[91]
    Giant cell arteritis[33]
Embolic causes
    Atrial myxoma[44]
    Mitral valve disease[107]
    Bacterial endocarditis[40]
    Patent foramen ovale[72]
    Fibrocartilaginous emboli from herniated discs[96,101]
Systemic hypoperfusion
    Cardiorespiratory arrest[2,4,53,81]
    Traumatic rupture of aorta[55]
    Dissection of aortic aneurysm[100,106,112]
    Coarctation of aorta[101]
Iatrogenic causes
    Thoracolumbar sympathectomy[52]
    Surgical correction of scoliosis[64]
    Cardiac catheterization[10]
    Aortography[57]
    Renal artery embolization[29]
    Umbilical artery catheterization[60]
    Vertebral angiography[26,63]
    Aortic surgery[19,45]
    Surgical repair of coarctation of aorta[13]
    Retroperitoneal lymph node dissection[59]
Infectious causes
    Syphilitic arteritis[93]
    Mucormycosis[105]
    Bacterial meningitis[66]
Miscellaneous causes
    Sickle cell anemia[85]
    Cocaine abuse[90]
    Decompression sickness[86]
    Antiphospholipid antibody syndrome[41]
    Crohn's disease[94]
    Cervical subluxation[38]
    Atherosclerosis and thrombosis of aorta[51]

rysms occur at different levels of the nervous system, but most studies focus on spinal cord damage.[84] Aortic dissection is one of the complications of aortic aneurysms and is characterized by hemorrhage into the tunica media of the aorta, separating the aortic wall into two layers. The dissection may extend up or down along the media, involving the innominate, carotid, or femoral arteries, narrowing the lumen of these arteries, and impairing blood flow. This condition is most commonly associated with arteriosclerosis, in which hypertension and aneurysmal dilatation of the aorta predispose to dissection.[12] Less often, dissecting aortic aneurysms occur in Marfan syndrome, pregnancy, aortic stenosis, and hypothyroidism.[49] Dissecting aortic aneurysms can produce spinal cord ischemia when an important intercostal or lumbar artery is sheared or occluded at its origin. Hughes[49] reviewed the literature of 11 cases of aortic dissection with spinal infarction confirmed by autopsy. The spinal damage was more extensive in some cases than in others. The dissection may involve one or several of the intercostal and lumbar arteries. The degree of impairment of blood flow determines the extent of spinal infarction. The other factor of importance is whether a large or small tributary artery is affected.

In general, the mid- and lower thoracic cord is the region most often damaged, because it is supplied by the intercostal arteries that are most frequently affected by aortic dissection.[98] If the artery of Adamkiewicz is involved, the area of maximal damage will be from the T10 to L1 level. The midthoracic cord suffers the maximum insult because it is a watershed zone (T4 to T6) between the blood supply of the upper and lower cord.[43,79,106] The upper part of the cord, which is supplied from branches of the vertebral arteries, is rarely involved. The lumbosacral cord could be damaged if the dissection extends caudally. Necrosis involves gray matter and adjacent white matter, but the white matter at the periphery is sometimes spared. In severe cases, the total cross section of the cord may be necrotic.[49] Acute onset of paraplegia or paraparesis with a thoracic sensory level can be a dramatic presentation in dissection of the aorta. Dissection is usually heralded by the sudden onset of severe pain in the chest or back, or in both regions. However, a few cases of spinal cord infarction have been associated with painless dissecting aneurysms.[32] A review of the literature showed that of 1805 patients with aortic dissection, 4.2% presented with symptoms or signs of spinal cord damage.[112] Among patients with aortic aneurysms, those with thoracoabdominal dilatations tend to have a higher incidence of spinal infarction.[62]

Coarctation of the Aorta

Coarctation of the aorta is a congenital stenosis of the isthmus of the aorta. Coarctation has been divided in two types: infantile and adult. In the infantile form, there is a small segment of narrowing that can occur before, at, or (most frequently) beyond the origin of the left subclavian artery. In the adult type, there is a vast anastomotic circulation between the arteries of the upper trunk and limbs and those beyond the stenosis in the lower trunk and legs. Arteries from the spinal cord form

an important part of this anastomosis. Consequently, spinal complications occur in the adult type of coarctation.

The spinal cord can be affected by ischemia secondary to hypotension. The caudal part of the cord is the most vulnerable, since it is supplied by arteries originating from the aorta distal to the narrowed segment. Symptoms and signs of paresis and sensory and sphincter disturbances have been noted. These symptoms may sometimes be related to activity. In addition, the cord may be damaged as a result of hypertension in the anastomotic system. In this circumstance, the anterior spinal artery becomes enlarged and tortuous and compresses the spinal cord. However, the most frequent mechanism that leads to damage of the cord is ischemia.[103]

Systemic Hypoperfusion

A profound and sustained fall in perfusion pressure may lead to an ischemic myelopathy involving primarily the watershed area of the midthoracic cord. Sandson and Friedman[88] reviewed 14 cases of spinal infarction secondary to hypoperfusion. All had paraplegia with areflexia and urinary dysfunction. In 13 patients, a sensory level was present in the thoracic region. Spinal cord infarction secondary to hypoperfusion occurs most often in the midthoracic region, with predominant involvement of gray matter.[2,90] Azzarelli and Roessmann[4] studied 16 patients who suffered from anoxic episodes (12 cardiorespiratory arrests and 4 pulmonary diseases) and concluded that the spinal cord was most vulnerable to hypoperfusion in the lumbosacral region. All the lesions were symmetric and limited to the gray matter.

Iatrogenic Ischemia of the Spinal Cord

Due to the increased frequency of cardiovascular surgery and invasive diagnostic procedures, iatrogenic spinal cord infarction is encountered more than it used to be. Spinal cord ischemia has been associated with a number of surgical and diagnostic procedures, including thoracolumbar sympathectomy,[52] pneumonectomy,[43] and correction of scoliosis.[64] In these surgical procedures, the ligation of an intercostal or lumbar artery probably causes spinal ischemia. Cardiac catheterization,[10] aortography,[57] and vertebral angiography have also been associated with cord infarction.[26,63]

The replacement, by grafts, of segments of the thoracic or abdominal aorta and its transitory clamping have resulted in ischemic complications of the spinal cord. The anterior spinal artery syndrome is the most common neurologic complication following aortic surgery and was first reported by Mehrez and coworkers[68] in 1962. Paraplegia associated with unruptured aortic aneurysm repair was present in 5% of 101 patients who underwent elective surgery.[45] Crawford and associates[19] also found that 6% of patients developed permanent paraparesis or paraplegia following surgery. The development of ischemic

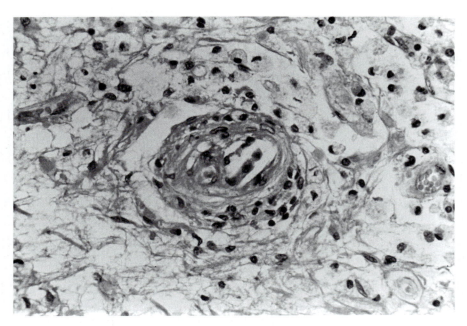

Figure 28.7 Atheromatous debris material including cholesterol clefts obstructing a small medullary artery within the spinal cord. The material came from a severely diseased thoracic aorta removed surgically following aneurysmal rupture. Many similar lesions, found at postmortem, caused this patient's total paraplegia at the T8 level.

myelopathy was dependent on the extent of the aneurysm (higher incidence of paraplegia in large ruptured aneurysms), the presence of previous dissection or rupture, and time of clamping, which is longer in complicated cases.[19] The cord may be damaged during surgery as a result of ligation, resection, or embolization of the artery of Adamkiewicz[83] or most frequently because of sustained hypotension during clamping.[19] Other authors assert that the postoperative paraplegia is due in part to increased intracranial pressure and impairment of spinal blood perfusion during aortic cross-clamping.[70] Showers of atheromatous debris may obstruct a number of intraspinal arterioles precipitated by the surgical handling of an ulcerated atherosclerotic plaque in the aorta (Fig. 28.7).

Surgical repair of coarctation of the aorta also carries a risk of spinal cord injury, but the incidence of paraplegia following surgery is extremely low (0.4%). Curiously, neither the number of intercostal arteries involved during surgery nor the length of clamping has been correlated with the incidence of spinal cord ischemia.[13]

Posterior Spinal Artery Syndrome

Posterior spinal artery infarctions are less common than anterior infarctions, but they do occur.[40] The lesion mainly involves posterior columns and extends to the posterior horns. This manifests as a suspended pattern of total anesthesia at the affected level. There is abolition of tendon and cutaneous reflexes for that specific spinal segment. Vibration and position senses are impaired below the affected level out of proportion to other sensory alterations. Paralysis, if present, is minimal and transient.[49] This syndrome has been described in association with atheromatous embolization,[78] intrathecal injection of phenol,[47] trauma, and syphilitic arteritis[48] (Table 28.3).

Venous Infarction

Venous infarction of the spinal cord is less common than arterial infarction, with most being diagnosed postmortem.[50] The most common causes of venous infarction in the spinal cord are vascular malformations of the spinal cord and acute compression by epidural processes such as hematomas and abscess. Venous infarctions can be classified as hemorrhagic or nonhemorrhagic. The clinical features and the pathologic

Table 28.3 Posterior Spinal Artery Syndrome

Sensory loss for proprioception, vibration, and light touch sensations; with sensory level

Preserved pain and temperature sensation, except at the level of the affected cord segment, where there is suspended global anesthesia

Motor function preserved

Loss of deep tendon and cutaneous reflexes at the level of the affected cord segment findings are remarkably constant. The hemorrhagic type has a sudden onset, with severe pain in the back and sometimes in the legs and abdomen. This is followed by lower extremity weakness, producing a flaccid paraplegia or quadriplegia. The paralysis may be progressive over hours or days. Sensation is impaired in the legs and may involve the trunk or upper limbs, depending on the extent of the lesion. Bowel and bladder dysfunction invariably occur.

The pathologic findings consist of a spinal cord disrupted by the hemorrhagic necrosis, which involves the central gray matter. This type of infarct tends to be more extensive in longitudinal and cross-sectional areas than anterior cord infarctions. The spinal veins are distended and obstructed. Hughes[50] reported seven cases of acute venous spinal cord infarction associated with acute thrombophlebitis; the most common underlying condition was systemic sepsis. Hemorrhagic venous infarction has also been associated with thrombophlebitis migrans, acute myelogenous leukemia, and tuberculosis.[58]

Nonhemorrhagic infarctions evolve slowly, with a clinical onset of as long as 1 year. Leg paralysis, sphincter dysfunction, and sensory loss without back pain are present. Survival time is longer than in hemorrhagic infarction. These types of infarctions are commonly associated with an underlying vascular malformation. This subacute neurologic syndrome, also called subacute necrotic myelitis, is attributed to intramedullary hypertension secondary to a spinal arteriovenous fistula.[50] The nonhemorrhagic infarctions tend to be at the T3 level or below; hemorrhagic infarctions have a more rostral location. Nonhemorrhagic infarctions have been also associated with polycythemia, thrombophlebitis, chronic meningitis, decompression sickness, leg vein thrombosis, and following sclerotherapy for esophageal varices.[42,58]

Differential Diagnosis

The differential diagnosis of spinal cord infarction is broad and includes all conditions that can present as an acute-incomplete myelopathy. These are compressive lesions, spinal cord trauma, transverse myelitis, multiple sclerosis, intramedullary tumor, hematomyelia, and necrotizing myelitis.[88] In middle-aged or elderly patients with slowly progressive paraparesis, the diagnosis of vascular or arteriosclerotic myelopathy should be viewed with suspicion, since many other diseases are more likely, including motor neuron disease, vitamin B_{12} deficiency, cervical spondylosis, and, less commonly, neoplasms, multiple sclerosis, or human T-cell leukemia-1 myelopathy (Table 28.4).

Diagnostic Tests

Sudden neurologic deficit of spinal cord origin requires immediate investigation. Although ischemic disorders of the cord are uncommon, they must be diagnosed by exclusion, and initial investigations must be designed to rule out a compres-

Table 28.4 Differential Diagnosis of Spinal Cord Ischemia

Compressive myelopathy (tumor, epidural or subdural hematoma)
Traumatic myelopathy, including central cord syndrome
Disc herniation
Primary transverse myelitis
Transverse myelitis secondary to multiple sclerosis, Devic syndrome, systemic lupus
Acute necrotizing myelitis
Intramedullary spinal cord tumor
Arteriovenous malformation
Acute polyneuropathy
    Guillain-Barré syndrome
    Porphyria
    HIV-related neuropathy (inflammatory demyelinating polyneuropathy)
    Thallium

Abbreviation: HIV, human immunodeficiency virus.

sive myelopathy. The most important diagnostic aids in assessing vascular disease of the cord are CT, alone or with myelography, and MRI. CT and MRI techniques have reduced the necessity of using plain radiographs, myelography, selective spinal angiography, and CSF surveys. CT scan may show spinal cord swelling, but due to its poor spatial discriminations has not contributed very much to diagnostic imaging of cord ischemia. Hemorrhagic infarctions are clearly visualized by CT. However, MRI produces more detailed and useful images (Fig. 28.8).

MRI has become the method of choice for diagnosing spinal cord ischemia, since it reliably excludes other causes of myelopathy such as compressive lesions, intramedullary neoplasms, or cavitations. On MRI, the infarcted cord can have an increased diameter. Infarcts can first be seen on T_2-weighted images as high-signal lesions during the acute phase. However, in the first hours after the damage, even T_2 images can remain normal. Once the blood-cord barrier becomes affected, enhancement of the ischemic or infarcted tissue can be seen after administration of gadolinium. In the subacute phase, high-intensity lesions are seen on T_2-weighted images. Sometimes the infarcts can be better visualized on contrast-enhanced T_1-weighted images.[1,21,23,67,73] Fortuna et al[27] reviewed 61 cases of cord infarction diagnosed by MRI (T_1-weighted images) during the acute phase; they identified enlargement of the affected cord in about 50% and isodensity in most of the cases (70%). On T_2-weighted images hyperintensity was noted in 90% of the cases. During later states of the cord infarction, T_2-weighted images showed hyperintensity in most of the cases (86%).

The presence of concomitant hyperintensity of the vertebral body immediately below the spinal cord lesion on T_2-weighted images is suggestive of cord ischemia. This has been observed in ischemia secondary to occlusion of the aorta and fibrocartilaginous emboli.[69] Although MRI is a highly sensitive tool for detecting infarction of the spinal cord, a definitive diagnosis is not always possible, since the presence of other conditions such as transverse myelitis, intramedullary tumors, or multiple sclerosis cannot be entirely excluded. MRI should be routinely

Figure 28.8 Sagittal T$_2$-weighted image of the cervical cord shows an abnormal signal hyperintensity within the spinal cord (C2 to C3), without mass effect, consistent with cord infarction. (From Benavente and Barnett,[6] with permission.)

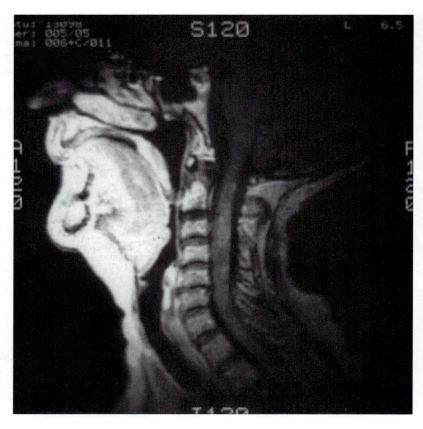

performed in every patient with a clinical picture suggestive of spinal cord infarction.

Treatment and Prognosis

No data are available regarding specific therapeutic regimens in patients who have suffered spinal cord ischemia or infarction. Preventing prolonged and profound hypotension during aortic surgery is essential for reducing the incidence of perioperative cord ischemia. The use of spinal somatosensory evoked potentials during surgery for a thoracoabdominal aneurysm has been shown to be a valuable guide in detecting whether or not the spinal cord is at risk, and measures can be taken to prevent cord ischemia.[36] In experimental animal models, selective hypothermia has proved to be efficacious in reducing paraplegia after prolonged aortic clamping; however, at the present time data in humans are lacking to support this intervention.[109] Correction of underlying pathogenic factors and modification of the usual risk factors such as hypertension, heart disease, and diabetes mellitus are important.[89] If the source is embolic, the use of anticoagulant or antiplatelet drugs should be considered.[15] Treatment is supportive, and special attention must be given to bowel and bladder function and skin integrity. Recent evidence has shown that methylprednisolone reduces the extent of disability after spinal cord trauma and will lead to consideration for its use immediately after a diagnosis of cord ischemia has been established.[11]

There are no case series of spinal ischemia to rely on, but its empirical use may be a reasonable decision.

The prognosis of spinal cord infarction is variable and depends on the degree of parenchymal damage and the etiology. The prognosis seems to be worse in cases due to FCE.[101] Overall, about 24% of patients who suffered cord ischemia experience no improvement; the rest have some degree of functional improvement, and only 20% will have a good recovery with minimal disability.[17] The presence of chronic pain is a disabling feature for these patients in the long term.[77] The duration of dysfunction is useful in determining prognosis, and recovery may be complete. Unless significant recovery occurs in the first 24 hours, however, the chances of major improvement are low.[31]

References

1. Aichner F, Poewe W, Rogalsky W et al: Magnetic resonance imaging in the diagnosis of spinal cord diseases. J Neurol Neurosurg Psychiatry 48:1220, 1985
2. Albert ML, Greer WER, Kantrowitz W: Paraplegia secondary to hypotension and cardiac arrest in a patient who has had previous thoracic surgery. Neurology 19:915, 1969
3. Aminoff MJ: Vascular disorders of the spinal cord. pp. 259–297. In Davidoff RA (ed): Handbook of the Spinal Cord. 1st Ed. Vol. 4. Marcel Dekker, New York, 1987

4. Azzarelli B, Roessmann U: Diffuse "anoxic" myelopathy. Neurology 27:1049, 1977

5. Bastian HC: Spinal cord softening. pp. 1479–1483. In Quain R (ed): Dictionary for Medicine. 1st Ed. London, 1882

6. Benavente OR, Barnett HJM: Spinal cord infarction. pp. 1229–1240. In Carter LP Spetzler RF (eds): Neurovascular Surgery. McGraw-Hill, New York, 1995

7. Bergmark G: Intermittent spinal claudication. Acta Med Scand Suppl 246:30, 1950

8. Blackwood W: Discussion on vascular disease of the spinal cord. Proc R Soc Med 51:543, 1958

9. Blan JN, Logue K: Intermittent claudication of the cauda equina. An unusual syndrome resulting from central protrusion of a lumbar intervertebral disk. Lancet 1:1081, 1961

10. Blankenship JC: Spinal cord infarction resulting from cardiac catheterization. Am J Med 87:239, 1989

11. Bracken MB, Shepard MJ, Holford TR et al: Methylprednisolone administered for 24 or 48 hours, or 48 hours tirilazad mesylate, in the treatment of acute spinal cord injury; results of the third National Acute Spinal Cord Injury randomized controlled trial. JAMA 277:1597–1604, 1997

12. Braunstein H: Pathogenesis of dissecting aneurysm. Circulation 28:1071, 1963

13. Brewer LA, Fosburg RG, Mulder GA, Verska JJ: Spinal cord complications following surgery for coarctation of the aorta. J Thorac Cardiovasc Surg 64:368, 1972

14. Brish A, Lerner MA, Braham J: Intermittent claudication from compression of cauda equina by a narrowed spinal canal. J Neurosurg 21:207, 1964

15. Buchan AM, Barnett HJM: Infarction of the spinal cord. pp. 709–716. In Barnett HJM, Mohr JP, Stein BM, Yatsu FM (eds): Stroke Pathophysiology Diagnosis and Management, Vol. 2. Churchill Livingstone, New York, 1986

16. Case records of the Massachusetts General Hospital. Case 5. N Engl J Med 324:322, 1991

17. Cheshire WP, Santos CC, Massey EW et al: Spinal cord infarction: etiology and outcome. Neurology 47:321–330, 1996

18. Clark CE, Cumming WJK: Subacute myelopathy caused by spinal venous infarction. Postgrad Med J 63:669, 1987

19. Crawford ES, Crawford JL, Safi HJ et al: Thoracoabdominal aortic aneurysms: preoperative and intraoperative factors determining immediate and long-term results of operations in 605 patients. J Vasc Surg 3:389, 1986

20. Decroix JP, Ciaudo-Lacroix C, Lapresle J: Syndrome de Brown-Séquard du à un infarctus spinal. Rev Neurol (Paris) 140:585, 1984

21. Di Chiro G, Doppman JL, Dwyer AJ et al: Tumors and arteriovenous malformations of the spinal cord: assessment using MR. Radiology 156:689, 1985

22. Editorial: Neurogenic intermittent claudication. BMJ 1:662, 1969

23. Elksnis SM, Hogg JP, Cunningham ME: MR imaging of spontaneous spinal cord infarction. J Comput Assist Tomogr 15:228, 1991

24. Evans JG: Neurogenic intermittent claudication. BMJ 2:985, 1964

25. Foix C, Alajouanine T: La myelite necrotique subaige. Rev Neurol 36:601, 1926

26. Foo D, Rossier AB: Anterior spinal artery syndrome and its natural history. Paraplegia 21:1, 1983

27. Fortuna A, Ferrante L, Acqui M, Trillo G: Spinal cord ischemia diagnosed by MRI. J Neuroradiol 22:115–122, 1995

28. Friedman SG, Moccio CG: Spinal cord ischemia following elective aortic reconstruction. Ann Vasc Surg 2:295, 1988

29. Gang DL, Dole KB, Adelman LS: Spinal cord infarction following therapeutic renal artery embolization. JAMA 237:2841, 1977

30. Garcin R, Godlewski S, Rondot P: Etude clinique de medullopathies d'origine vasculaire. Rev Neurol (Paris) 106:558, 1962

31. Geldmacher DS, Nager BJ: Spinal cord vascular disease. pp. 983–988. In Bradley WG, Daroff RB, Fenichel GM, Marsden CD (eds): Neurology in Clinical Practice. Vol. 2. Butterworth-Heinemann, Boston, 1991

32. Gerber O, Heyer EJ, Vieux U: Painless dissections of the aorta presenting as acute neurologic syndromes. Stroke 17:644, 1986

33. Gibb WRG, Urry PA, Lees AJ: Giant cell arteritis with spinal cord infarction and basilar artery thrombosis. J Neurol Neurosurg Psychiatry 48:945, 1985

34. Gillian L: The arterial supply of the human spinal cord. J Comp Neurol 1958

35. Gillilan LA: Veins of the spinal cord. Anatomic details; suggested clinical complications. Neurology 20:860, 1970

36. Grabitz K, Sandmann W, Stuhmeier K, Mainzer B et al: The risk of ischemic spinal cord injury in patients undergoing graft replacement for thoracoabdominal aortic aneurysms. J Vasc Surg 23:230–240, 1996

37. Gray H: Developmental and gross anatomy of the central nervous system. pp. 933–1035. In Clemente CD (ed): Anatomy of the Human Body. 30th Ed. (American Ed.). Lea & Febiger, Philadelphia, 1984

38. Grinker RR, Guy CC: Sprain of cervical spine causing thrombosis of anterior spinal artery. JAMA 88:1140, 1927

39. Hancock DO, Phillips DG: Spinal compression in achondroplasia. Paraplegia 3:23, 1965

40. Harrington AW: Embolism of the spinal cord. Glasgow Med J 103:28, 1925

41. Hasegawa M, Yamashita J, Yamashima T et al: Spinal cord infarction associated with primary antiphospholipid syndrome in a young child. J Neurosurg 79:446–450, 1993

42. Heller SL, Meyer JR, Russell EJ: Spinal cord venous infarction following endoscopy sclerotherapy for esophageal varices. Neurology 47:1081–1085, 1996

43. Henson RA, Parsons M: Ischaemic lesions of the spinal cord: an illustrated review. Q J Med 35:205, 1966

44. Hirose G, Kosoegowa H, Takado M: Spinal cord ischemia and left atrial myxoma. Arch Neurol 24:228, 1971

45. Hollier LH, Symmonds JB, Pairolero PC et al: Thoracoabdominal aortic aneurysm repair: analysis of postoperative morbidity. Arch Surg 123:871, 1988

46. Hughes JT: The pathology of vascular disorders of the spinal cord. Paraplegia 2:207, 1965

47. Hughes JT: Thrombosis of the posterior spinal arteries. Neurology 20:659, 1970

48. Hughes JT: Vascular disorders. p. 61. In Pathology of the Spinal Cord: Major Problems in Pathology. 2nd Ed. Vol. 6. WB Saunders, Philadelphia, 1978

49. Hughes JT: Vascular disorders of the spinal cord. pp. 95–106. In Vinken PJ, Bruyn GW, Klawans HL (eds): Handbook of Clinical Neurology. Vol. 55. Elsevier, Amsterdam, 1989

50. Hughes JT: Venous infarction of the spinal cord. Neurology 21:794, 1971

51. Hughes JT, Brownell B: Spinal cord ischemia due to arteriosclerosis. Arch Neurol 15:189, 1966

52. Hughes JT, Macintyre AG: Spinal cord infarction occurring during thoraco-lumbar sympathectomy. J Neurol Neurosurg Psychiatry 26:418, 1963

53. Imaizumi H, Ujike Y, Asai Y et al: Spinal cord ischemia after cardiac arrest. J Emerg Med 12:789–793, 1994

54. Jellinger K: Spinal cord arteriosclerosis and progressive vascular myelopathy. J Neurol Neurosurg Psychiatry 30:195, 1967

55. Keith WS: Traumatic infarction of the spinal cord. Can J Neurol Sci 1:124, 1974

56. Kendall BE, Andrew J: Neurogenic intermittent claudication associated with aortic steal from the anterior spinal artery complicating coarctation of the aorta. J Neurosurg 37:89, 1972

57. Killen DA, Foster JH: Spinal cord injury as a complication of aortography. Ann Surg 152:211, 1960

58. Kim RC, Smith HR, Henbest ML, Choi BH: Nonhemorrhagic venous infarction of the spinal cord. Ann Neurol 15:379, 1984

59. Leibovitch I, Nash PA, Little JS et al: Spinal cord ischemia after postchemotherapy retroperitoneal lymph node dissection for nonseminomatous germ cell cancer. J Urol 155:947–951, 1996

60. Lemke RP, Idiong N, Al-Saedi S et al: Spinal cord infarct after arterial switch associated with an umbilical artery catheter. Ann Thorac Surg 62:1532–1534, 1996

61. Lozarthes G, Govaze A, Zadeh JO: Arterial vascularization of the spinal cord. J Neurosurg 35:253, 1971

62. Lynch DR, Dawson TM, Raps EC, Galetta SL: Risk factors for the neurologic complications associated with aortic aneurysms. Arch Neurol 49:284, 1992

63. Lyon LW: Transfemoral vertebral angiography as cause of an anterior spinal artery syndrome. J Neurosurg 35:328, 1971

64. MacEwen GD, Bunnell WP, Siram K: Acute neurological complications in the treatment of scoliosis. J Bone Joint Surg 57:404, 1975

65. Marcus ML, Heistad DD, Ehrhardt JC, Abboud FM: Regulation of total and regional spinal cord blood flow. Circ Res 41:128, 1977

66. Mathew P, Todd NV, Hadley DM, Adams JH: Spinal cord infarction following meningitis. Br J Neurosurg 7:701–704, 1993

67. Mawad ME, Rivera V, Crawford S et al: Spinal cord ischemia after resection of thoracoabdominal aortic aneurysms: MR findings in 24 patients. AJNR 155:987, 1990

68. Mehrez IO, Nabseth DC, Hogan EL: Paraplegia following resection of abdominal aortic aneurysm. Ann Surg 156:890, 1962

69. Mikulis DJ, Ogilvy CS et al: Spinal cord infarction and fibrocartilagenous emboli. AJNR 13:155–160, 1992

70. Miyamoto K, Keno A, Wada T, Kimoto S: A new and simple method of preventing spinal cord damage following temporary occlusion of the thoracic aorta by draining the cerebrospinal fluid. J Cardiovasc Surg 16:188, 1960

71. Moossy J: Vascular disease of the spinal cord. pp. 1–17. In Joynt RJ (ed): Clinical Neurology. Vol. 3. Lippincott-Raven, Philadelphia, 1991

72. Mori S, Sadoshima S, Tagawa K et al: Massive spinal cord infarction with multiple paradoxical embolism: a case report. Angiology 44:251–256, 1993

73. Nagashima C, Nagashima R, Morota N, Kobayashi S: Magnetic resonance imaging of human spinal cord infarction. Surg Neurol 35:368, 1991

74. Nystrom B, Stjernschantz J, Smedegard G: Regional spinal cord blood flow in the rabbit, cat and monkey. Acta Neurol Scand 70:307, 1984

75. Okazaki H: Cerebrovascular disease. pp. 27–94. In Okazaki H (ed): Fundamentals of Neuropathology. 2d Ed. Igaku-Shoin, New York, 1989

76. Paine RS, Byers RK: Transverse myelopathy in childhood. Am J Dis Child 85:151, 1953

77. Pelser H, van Gijn J: Spinal infarction: a follow-up study. Stroke 24:896–898, 1993

78. Perier O, Demanet JC, Henneaux J, Vincent AN: Existe-il un syndrome des artères spinales postérieures? À propos de deux observations anatomocliniques. Rev Neurol 103:396, 1960

79. Prendes JL: Neurovascular syndromes of aortic dissection. Am Fam Physician 23:175, 1981

80. Preobrashenski PA: Syphilitic paraplegia with dissociated disturbance of sensation. J Nevropat I Psikhiat 4:394–433, 1904

81. Rajan RK: Ischemic myelopathy following cardiac arrest. Am Fam Physician 29:221, 1984

82. Reichert FL, Rytand DA, Bruck EL: Arteriosclerosis of the lumbar segmental arteries producing ischemia of the spinal cord and consequent claudication of the thighs. A clinical syndrome with experimental confirmation. Am J Med Sci 187:794 1934

83. Reuh MP: Paraplegia following resection of abdominal aortic aneurysm: report of a case of atheromatous embolization to the anterior spinal artery. Vasc Surg 1968

84. Ross RT: Spinal cord infarction in disease and surgery of the aorta. Can J Neurol Sci 12:289, 1985

85. Rothman SM, Nelson JS: Spinal cord infarction in a patient with sickle cell anemia. Neurology 30:1072, 1980

86. Rudar M, Urbanke A, Radonic M: Occlusion of the abdominal aorta with dysfunction of the spinal cord. Ann Intern Med 56:490, 1962

87. Sandler AN, Tator CH: Regional spinal blood flow in primates. J Neurosurg 1976

88. Sandson TA, Friedman JH: Spinal cord infarction. Report of 8 cases and review of the literature. Medicine 68:282, 1989

89. Satran R: Spinal cord infarction. Stroke 19:529, 1988
90. Sawaya GR: Spinal cord infarction after cocaine use. South Med J 83:601, 1990
91. Shakir RA, Sulaiman K, Kahn RA, Rudwan M: Neurological presentation of neuro-Behçet's syndrome: clinical categories. Eur Neurol 30:249, 1990
92. Silver JR, Buxton PH: Spinal stroke. Brain 97:539, 1974
93. Slager UT, Webb AT: Pathologic findings in the spinal cord. Arch Pathol 96:388, 1973
94. Slot WB, Van Kasteel V, Coerkamp EG et al: Severe thrombotic complications in a postpartum patient with active Crohn's disease resulting in ischemic spinal cord injury. Dig Dis Sci 40:1395–1399, 1995
95. Spiller WG: Thrombosis of the cervical anterior median spinal artery; syphilitic acute anterior poliomyelitis. J Nerv Ment Dis 36:601, 1909
96. Srigley JR, Lambert CD, Bilbao JM, Pritzker KPH: Spinal cord infarction secondary to intervertebral disc embolism. Ann Neurol 9:296, 1981
97. Steegmann AT: Syndrome of the anterior spinal artery. Neurology 2:15, 1952
98. Such TH, Alexander L: Vascular system of the human spinal cord. Arch Neurol Psychiatry 41:660, 1939
99. Taylor JR, Van Allen MW: Vascular malformation of the cord with transient ischemic attacks. J Neurosurg 31:576, 1969
100. Thompson GB: Dissecting aortic aneurysm with infarction of the spinal cord. Brain 79:111, 1956
101. Tosi L, Rigoli G, Beltramello A: Fibrocartilaginous embolism of the spinal cord: a clinical and pathogenetic reconsideration. J Neurol Neurosurg Psychiatry 60:55–60, 1996
102. Turnbull IM: Blood supply of the spinal cord. pp. 478–491. In Vinken PJ, Bruyn GN (eds): Handbook of Clinical Neurology. Vol. 12. Elsevier, Amsterdam, 1972
103. Tyler HR, Clark OB: Neurological complications in patients with coarctation of aorta. Neurology 8:712, 1958
104. Van Wieringen A: An unusual cause of occlusion of the anterior spinal artery. Eur Neurol 1:363, 1968
105. von Pohle WR: Disseminated mucormycosis presenting with lower extremity weakness. Eur Respir J 9:1751–1753, 1996
106. Waltimo O, Karli P: Aortic dissection and paraparesis. Eur Neurol 19:254, 1980
107. Whiteley AM, Hauw JJ, Escourolle R: A pathological survey of 41 cases of acute intrinsic spinal cord disease. J Neurol Sci 42:229, 1979
108. Wilson CB: Significance of the small lumbar spinal canal: cauda equina compression syndromes due to spondylosis. III. Intermittent claudication. J Neurosurg 31:449, 1969
109. Wisselink W, Becker MO, Nguyen JH et al: Protecting the ischemic spinal cord during aortic campling: the influence of selective hypothermia and spinal cord perfusion pressure. J Vasc Surg 19:788–796, 1994
110. Woollam DHM, Millen JW: The arterial supply of the spinal cord and its significance. J Neurol Neurosurg Psychiatry 18:97, 1955
111. Zulch KJ, Kurth-Schumacher R: The pathogenesis of "intermittent spinovascular insufficiency" ("spinal claudication of Dejerine") and other vascular syndromes of the spinal cord. Vasc Surg 4:116, 1970
112. Zull DN, Cydulka R: Acute paraplegia: a presenting manifestation of aortic dissection. Am J Med 84:765, 1988

SECTION IV

Specific Medical Diseases and Stroke

J. P. MOHR

The chapters in this section focus on the individual diseases responsible for stroke. Here the emphasis is less on the clinical picture than on the mechanism of disease, epidemiology, laboratory features, and, where unusual or highly specific, also on the clinical syndromes.

Because the book is organized into sections on laboratory science, diagnostic studies, clinical sciences, and therapy, specific comments on the management of the diseases in this section are deferred, where possible, to the more general discussion of therapy in the last section of the book.

The chapters continue to be updated to reflect work completed since the second edition. The impact of current work is reflected in several chapter titles having been condensed, new ones added on new subjects (e.g., CADASIL, aortic arch atheroma), and upgrading to chapter status some titles previously contained within other chapters (e.g., patent cardiac foramen ovale). New authors have taken up some of the subjects.

CHAPTER 29

Dissections and Trauma of Cervicocerebral Arteries

JEFFREY L. SAVER

J. DONALD EASTON

Cervicocerebral arterial dissections occur when blood extrudes into the wall of an artery supplying the brain. The resulting intramural hematoma may compromise the lumen or cause an aneurysmal dilatation (dissecting aneurysm), or both. Dissections are an uncommon cause of cerebral ischemia, except in young adults. They usually occur spontaneously or are associated with trivial trauma to the artery. Major, nonpenetrating trauma of the cervical carotid and vertebral arteries may induce thrombosis, with or without associated dissection. Spontaneous dissection involving extracranial or intracranial arteries, and traumatic arterial injuries, have distinct features that warrant their separate consideration. Data from case series and reports totaling over 1,000 patients were abstracted for this chapter and define the clinical spectrum of these arteriopathies. The natural history of milder cases may not be adequately reflected, as many likely go unrecognized or unreported.

Extracranial Carotid Artery Dissection

The cervical internal carotid artery is the most frequently reported site of cervicocerebral dissection. A community-based population study found an annual incidence among persons 20 years and older of 3.5 per 100,000.[163] Two to four cases per year are reported from large academic centers,[20,22,52,59,131,145] and in one hospital-based series, cervical carotid dissections accounted for 2.5% of all first cerebral infarcts.[25] Overall, these dissections account for perhaps 1% to 2% of cerebral ischemia. Cervical carotid dissection occurs predominantly in the middle adult years: 70% of patients are between ages 35 and 50, with a mean age of 44 years.[79] There is no sex predilection.

The major presenting features are stroke or transient ischemic attack associated with pain in the ipsilateral neck, face, or head. Clinical, radiologic, and prognostic features from 635 cases in the literature are summarized in Table 29.1. Transient monocular blindness constitutes approximately 35% of all transient ischemic attacks.[22,25,59,167] An ipsilateral oculosympathetic paresis (partial Horner syndrome) occurs in one third of patients, due to compression of sympathetic fibers of the internal carotid plexus running along the distended vessel wall. Pulsatile tinnitus or a subjective bruit are prominent complaints in one fourth of patients. Headache or neck pain often precedes the onset of ischemic symptoms, by several hours to 4 weeks, with most cerebral ischemic events occurring within 1 week of onset of local signs.[22] The headache may be pounding, but more often it is nonthrobbing and severe, and ipsilateral scalp tenderness may occur.[21,58] Ipsilateral cranial nerve palsies are occasionally present, most often nerve XII producing lingual paresis, followed in frequency by nerves IX, X, XI, and V. Lower cranial nerve compromise usually arises from expansion of subadventitial dissection to encroach on the upper cervical parapharyngeal space.[61,72,138,178,185] Although individual features are nonspecific, constellations of these symptoms and signs, which are relatively unusual in atheroem-

Table 29.1 Clinical Features
of Extracranial Carotid Dissection

No. of cases	635
Age	44.4 yr (mean), range 4–74
Sex	
Male	53%
Female	47%
Laterality	
Unilateral	86%
Left	60%
Right	40%
Bilateral	14%
Major presenting complaint[a]	
Cerebral infarction	46%
Transient ischemic attack	30%
Neck or head pain	21%
Pulsatile tinnitus only	2%
Asymptomatic bruit only	2%
Associated features at diagnosis	
Symptoms	
Neck pain	20%
Headache	64%
Neck or head pain	67%
Tinnitus or subjective bruit	3%
Signs	
Partial Horner syndrome	32%
Cervical bruit	18%
Lingual paresis	6%
Early outcome	
Angiographic	
Normal or mildly stenotic vessel	
on follow-up imaging	70%
Clinical	
Neurologically normal	50%
Mild deficits only	21%
Moderate to severe deficits	25%
Death	4%

[a] *Major presenting complaint leading to evaluation, not necessarily the initial symptom.*

(Data from references 8, 39, 53, 129, 149a, 157, 161, 176, 181.)

bolic ischemia, are present in about three fourths of the patients with a cervical carotid dissection. Undue headache or neck pain in patients with cerebral ischemia is often the initial clue suggesting a dissection.

Cervical carotid dissection may present with unilateral neck, face, or head pain and oculosympathetic paresis without ischemic symptoms, and thus may mimic an initial episode of Raeder paratrigeminal syndrome or a migraine variant.[21,39,187]

There is an impressive temporal relationship of dissections to minimal neck torsion or trauma in many patients. If such activities as bowling or coughing can precipitate carotid dissections, perhaps few are truly spontaneous, and, for practical purposes, "spontaneous" dissection and dissection related to trivial trauma may be considered as one entity. Types of trivial trauma reported to antedate dissection include almost all varieties of sports activity, violent coughing, vigorous nose-blowing, sexual activity, chiropractic manipulation, anesthesia administration, and neck-turning while leading a parade.[27,74,79,108] Cervical rotation or extension can compress the cervical carotid artery against the transverse processes of the upper cervical vertebrae, and this may precipitate a dissection in the predisposed person.[177,193] (Fig. 29.1). The frequent location of the hematoma in the posterior wall of the distal extracranial cervical internal carotid artery supports the role of mechanical injury.[79]

Spontaneous cervical carotid dissection usually occurs in otherwise healthy people. However, fibromuscular dysplasia is found in about 15% of patients, with a female preponderance.[6,21,25,52,63,79,102,121,152,179] Surprisingly, simultaneous bilateral carotid involvement accounts for 14% of all reported cases of cervical carotid dissection, at least half of which have associated fibromuscular dysplasia.[79,112,117,123] One large tertiary referral series found an incidence of 28%.[160] Cervical carotid dissections have occasionally been associated with additional arteriopathies, including Ehlers-Danlos disease, Marfan syndrome, α_1-antitrypsin deficiency, type I collagen point mutation, systemic lupus erythematosus, and atheromatous plaques.[9,43,46,59,114,119,133,140,159,165] Internal carotid artery redundancies—coils, kinks, and loops—are strongly associated with dissection.[10,77] A history of migraine is present in one fourth of patients.[22,125,182] and one case-controlled investigation showed migraine, as well as oral contraceptives, to be an independent risk factor for dissection.[42] Hypertension is reported in about one fourth of patients.[182] An association of systemic infection and cervical carotid dissection has been attributed to both inflammatory and mechanical (coughing, vomiting) arterial insults.[73] Dissections in more than one family member have been observed on at least four occasions, as well as familial aggregation of dissection and intracranial aneurysm.[109,123] In one series, siblings of patients with cervical artery dissection had a sixfold elevated prevalence of cervical dissections or cerebral aneurysms, 3.5% versus 0.53%.[109]

Early histopathologic reports emphasized the association of these dissections with cystic medial necrosis, and O'Connell et al[134] found an underlying arteriopathy in 10 of 16 published cases. Nevertheless, dissection is reported to occur frequently in microscopically normal arteries or in arteries with minimal disorganization of elastic fibers.[30,54,59,108,135,183] We suspect that most patients who have a dissection in the absence of substantial neck trauma have as-yet ill-defined underlying arteriopathies.[29,80,189] The spectrum of identified arteriopathic substrates of dissection may confidently be predicted to expand with further advances in pathologic and biochemical diagnosis.

Anatomic specimens of cervical carotid dissection often show hemorrhage into subintimal, medial, and, less often, subadventitial layers of the artery[63,134] (Fig. 29.2). Subintimal hemorrhage tends to result in luminal stenosis, while a hematoma in the outer media and subadventitia causes arterial dilatation (aneurysm).[108,134,140] Tortuous or coiled segments may be more susceptible to aneurysm formation.[140] It is unclear whether a primary intimal tear allows dissection of blood to proceed from the lumen into the arterial wall or whether a primary intramedial hematoma secondarily ruptures into the

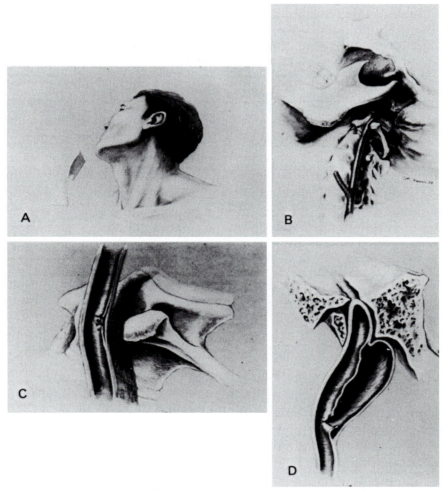

Figure 29.1 Presumed mechanism of carotid injury induced by neck rotation. (**A**) Direction of hyperextension. (**B**) Impingement of artery on the process of the vertebra. (**C**) Intimal tear caused by impingement. (**D**) Progression of intimal tear to dissection. (From Stringer and Kelly,[177] with permission.)

true lumen. It is possible that both mechanisms occur. The former is probably more common. In some patients, no communication between the dissection cavity and the lumen can be demonstrated, while in others an intimal tear is present near the proximal extent of the dissection.

Cervical carotid dissection sometimes results in cerebral ischemic symptoms owing to hemodynamic compromise from stenosis or occlusion, but more often to embolism of thrombotic fragments distally.[25,30,130] Disruption of the endothelial surface exposes thromboplastin and other highly thrombogenic elements to the blood. The importance of embolism is attested to by the occurrence of ischemic symptoms when stenosis is hemodynamically insignificant, by arteriographic evidence of distal emboli, and by the presence of friable intraluminal thrombus seen arteriographically and at surgery.

The diagnosis of cervical carotid dissection is based on a compatible clinical picture coupled with characteristic imaging findings. Arteriography has been the standard imaging technique[28,59,66,87,167] (Figs. 29.3 to 29.5), but is increasingly made unnecessary by evolving noninvasive modalities. Dissection usually begins 2 cm or more distal to the origin of the internal carotid artery and extends rostrally for a variable distance. It usually terminates before entry of the artery into the petrous bone, where mechanical support appears to limit further dissection in all but exceptional cases. Irregular narrowing of the artery is the most frequent arteriographic finding, resulting in a "wavy ribbon" appearance, or a "string sign" if severe (Fig. 29.5). A tapered occlusion beginning distal to the carotid sinus is less specific, but occurs in about 20% of cases. Intimal flaps may be seen near the proximal margin of the dissection. An extraluminal pouch (dissecting aneurysm) may be visualized distally, usually near the base of the skull. Fibromuscular dysplasia of the contralateral carotid artery and embolic occlusion of intracranial arteries are sometimes seen. In rare cases, dissections begin in the common carotid artery or extend distally to involve the intracranial carotid and middle cerebral arteries (Fig. 29.6). Multiple dissections are more likely to be associated with fibromuscular dysplasia.[79,112,117,123]

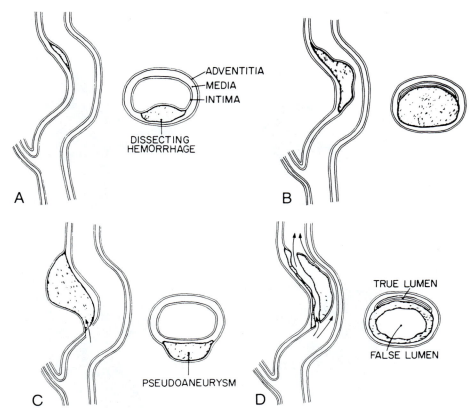

Figure 29.2 Anatomy of dissections. (**A**) Lateral (*left*) and cross-sectional (*right*) schematic views of internal carotid artery demonstrate initial phase of intramedial and subintimal dissecting aneurysm; the three basic arterial layers (intima, media, and adventitia) are delineated. (**B**) Comparable views of progression of intramedial hemorrhage; arterial lumen is reduced in size. (**C**) Comparable views of an intramedial hemorrhage that dissects into the subadventitial, rather than the subintimal plane, as in **A** and **B**; large pseudoaneurysm results. (**D**) Dissecting hemorrhage ruptures through the intima, establishing communication with the true lumen; recanalization may occur, enlarging true and/or false lumen. (From Friedman et al,[63] with permission.)

Noninvasive imaging techniques, including ultrasound, computed tomography (CT) and magnetic resonance (MR), facilitate diagnosis of carotid dissection in several clinical settings. They may confirm clinically suspected dissection without exposing the patient to the minor risks of arteriography, suggest previously unsuspected dissection in clinically atypical cases, supplement diagnosis in angiographically confirmed dissection, and permit serial monitoring of lesion evolution. Extracranial carotid duplex studies interrogate the carotid bifurcation proximal to the level of most dissections. Consequently, duplex studies most commonly provide only indirect evidence of more distal stenosis or occlusion due to dissection, demonstrating reduced or bidirectional internal carotid artery flow without evidence of atheroma.[47,52,55,129,153,176,179] Less often, B-mode gray-scale imaging directly displays a tapering stenosis of the internal carotid artery lumen, and infrequently an intimal flap is directly visualized.[47,176,179] Placement of the ultrasound probe over the retromandibular (high cervical) region often permits direct insonation of a distal stenotic segment.[129,179] Transcranial Doppler sonography delineates intracranial circulation consequences of carotid pathology, including reduced velocities, collateral flow patterns, and distal emboli.[100,174,179] Multimodal ultrasound studies demonstrate up to 95% sensitivity for carotid dissection, and are particularly helpful for serial monitoring of lesion evolution.[179] Ultrasonography's limitations include only moderate specificity of findings and inability to reliably detect dissecting aneurysms.

The role of CT in diagnosis is evolving. Several reports have demonstrated the capacity of emerging techniques, including dynamic helical CT angiography, to detect carotid dissections with high sensitivity and specificity.[41,101,194]

MR imaging (MRI) offers several advantages over conventional arteriography. Conventional T_1-weighted and proton density axial MR at high cervical levels depicts the vessel wall in cross-section with excellent contrast between lumen, vessel wall, and surrounding cervical structures, allowing direct visualization of the intramural hematoma. The pathognomonic MRI sign of dissection is an eccentrically narrowed

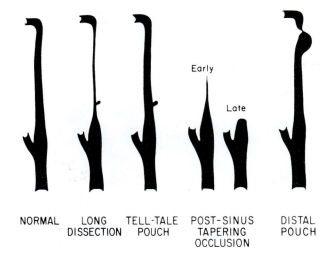

NORMAL   LONG   TELL-TALE   POST-SINUS   DISTAL
          DISSECTION   POUCH   TAPERING   POUCH
                                    OCCLUSION

Figure 29.3 Arteriographic features of carotid dissection. (From Fisher et al,[59] with permission.)

lumen with adjacent semilunar-shaped increased signal (crescent sign), representing extravasated blood in the vessel wall. (Fig. 29.7). Other, less specific findings are (1) an increased signal from the entire vessel, (2) poor or absent visualization of the vessel, and (3) significant compromise of the vessel lumen by adjoining abnormal increased signal tissue.[181] Magnetic resonance angiography (MRA) increases the yield of MR studies, displaying the same vessel silhouette features of dissection as conventional angiography, noninvasively.[96] Taking conventional arteriography as a gold standard, one large series found that MRI exhibited a sensitivity of 84% and a specificity of 99% for diagnosis of carotid dissection, and MRA exhibited a sensitivity of 95% and a specificity of 99%.[103] Several groups have reported dissections diagnosed by MRI that were negative by conventional angiography, occurring when intramural hematomas failed to narrow the arterial lumen detectably.[7,137]

Early reports emphasized major, often fatal, stroke as the sequel of cervical carotid dissection. Recent experience suggests a less serious outcome in most patients, with major stroke occurring in only 20% to 30% of affected individuals (Table 29.1). Prognosis and treatment of carotid and other cervicocephalic dissections are discussed below.

Intracranial Carotid System Dissection

Several clinical features warrant the distinction of dissections involving the intracranial carotid and middle cerebral arteries from those of the extracranial carotid artery. Intracranial dissections are infrequently reported.[13,191] Because specific angiographic and noninvasive imaging features are lacking for these dissections, reliance on pathologic diagnosis has likely resulted in their under-recognition, especially of nonfatal cases. The age profile is younger than for cervical dissection. In a review of 59 reported cases, the mean age of onset was 30 years, and a slight male preponderance was noted.[13] Perhaps half of the patients are under age 16. Ipsilateral headache,

usually severe, immediately precedes or coexists with the onset of neurologic deficit in almost all patients. Major stroke has been the rule, with evolution often occurring over several days. Seizure or syncope can be the initial symptom, and one half of patients have early alteration of consciousness. Aggregate reports show fatal outcome in three fourths of reported cases, with moderate to severe residual neurologic deficits in one half of survivors. Autopsied cases dominate the literature, however, and milder forms may be unrecognized. Subarachnoid hemorrhages, produced when subadventitial hematomas erupt through the external vessel wall, are associated with these dissections in one fifth of cases.[2,13,110] A relationship of intracranial arterial dissection to antecedent intense physical exertion or trivial trauma is noted in one fourth of cases.

The usual site of dissection is the intracranial carotid artery or middle cerebral artery stem, affected in three fourths of cases. The restricted mobility of the distal intracranial internal carotid artery and the middle cerebral artery trunk likely render them vulnerable to shear forces during acceleration-deceleration head movements. Intracranial extension of an extracranial dissection is rare. Bilateral intracranial carotid dissection has also been reported, separated by 6 weeks to 18 months, but less frequently than in the extracranial circulation.[3,36,110,132] The usual plane of intracranial anterior circulation dissection is subintimal, with subadventitial dissections that predispose to subarachnoid hemorrhage in about one fifth of cases. Intracranial arteries are more susceptible to rupture as they lack well-developed external elastic membranes, and their muscularis and adventitial layers are only two-thirds as thick as extracranial arteries.

Arteriograms typically reveal nonspecific stenosis or occlusion, but occasionally suggest dissection by demonstrating irregular, scalloped stenosis of the arteries, resembling a string of beads, or total occlusion following irregular, tapering narrowing.[13,79,131] A double lumen is infrequently demonstrated but is specific for dissection. Intracranial dissection usually involves the middle cerebral artery or the supraclinoid carotid artery, and the latter occasionally extends into the anterior cerebral artery. Dissecting aneurysms are rarely seen in intracranial dissections, possibly due to the subintimal location of most hemorrhages. Arteriographic findings are usually nonspecific, and arteritis, moyamoya, embolic occlusion, and fibromuscular dysplasia are often initial radiologic considerations. The co-appearance of subarachnoid blood, intracranial arterial stenosis, and an aneurysm originating at a nonbifurcation location is highly suggestive of intracranial dissection, but uncommon. MR may demonstrate intramural hemorrhage, enabling more definitive diagnosis.[31,69]

Most affected patients are healthy, without evident arteriopathy. Risk factors, including hypertension, migraine, oral contraceptives, and recreational drug use, have been reported sporadically.[13,173] In isolated cases, intracranial carotid dissection has been associated with cystic medial necrosis, fibromuscular dysplasia, moyamoya, atherosclerosis, homocystinuria, polyarteritis nodosa, and meningovascular syphilis.[13,31,56,57,131,134,139,141] Microscopic intimal abnormalities, presumably developmental, have been recognized in some pathologic studies of intracranial dissection.[50,82,106,131,141,190] These intimal changes may reflect a spectrum of developmental irregularities that underlie dissections, moyamoya, and fibromuscular dysplasia. Despite the potential developmental pre-

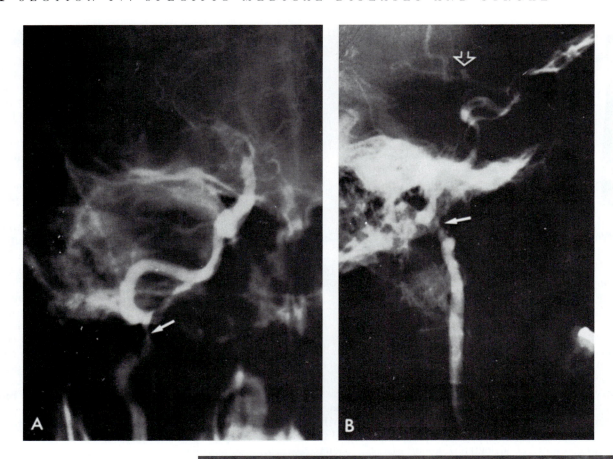

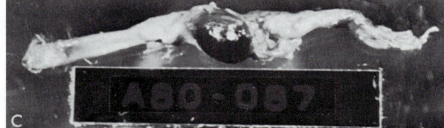

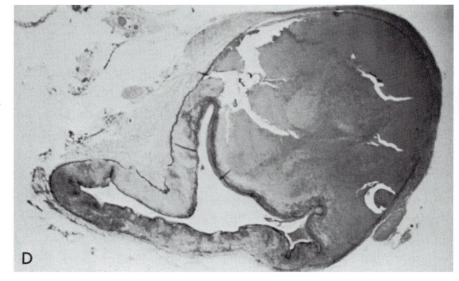

Figure 29.4 Cervical carotid dissection in a 37-year-old man. Severe headache followed a basketball game, with hemiplegia developing several hours later. (**A**) Arteriogram (anterior view) showing stenosis with scalloped borders involving the distal cervical carotid (*arrow*). (**B**) Lateral arteriographic view showing distal stenosis (*closed arrow*) of the cervical carotid with delayed visualization of intracranial vessels (*open arrow*). (**C**) Postmortem revealed a 1.5-cm pseudoaneurysm of the distal cervical carotid. (**D**) Microscopic section of hematoma of the media; there was no intimal tear.

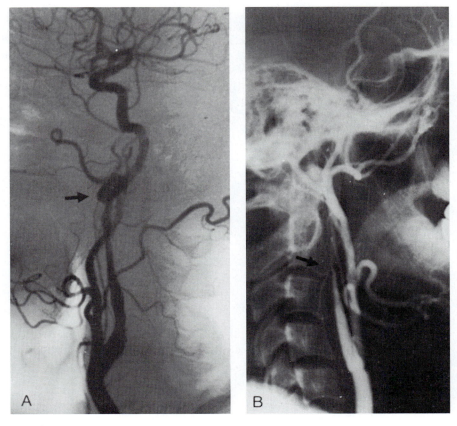

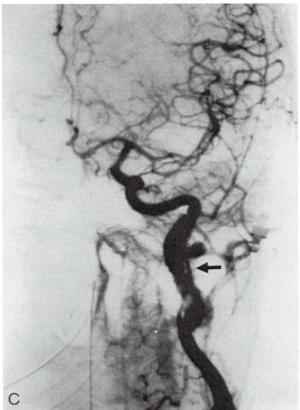

Figure 29.5 Arteriographic features of cervical carotid dissection. (**A**) Pseudoaneurysm (*arrow*) of the distal cervical carotid with proximal luminal narrowing. (**B**) Tapered occlusion (*arrow*) beginning distal to the carotid sinus. (**C**) Double-lumen (*arrow*) with irregularity of the entire lumen.

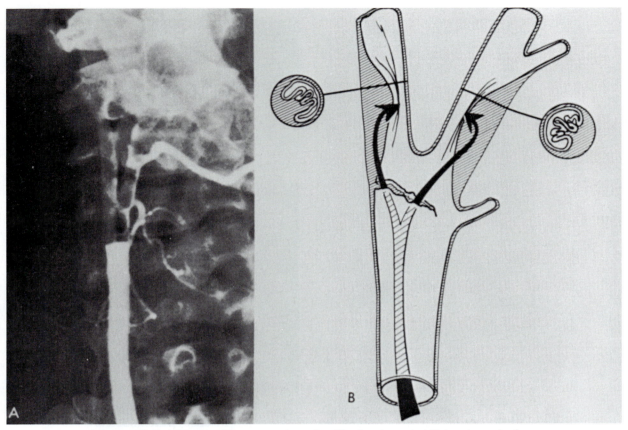

Figure 29.6 A 32-year-old man experienced sudden hemiparesis. (**A**) Arteriography demonstrates a sharp cutoff of contrast at the common carotid bifurcation, with faint visualization of distal vessels. Exploration revealed a transverse intimal tear with subintimal dissection of blood. (**B**) Artist's concept of intimal tear with subintimal dissection of blood and occlusion of the lumen. The insets of the internal and external carotid arteries in cross-section graphically depict luminal compromise. (From Moore,[127] with permission.)

disposition, familial clustering has not been reported. Hypoperfusion as a direct result of luminal obstruction at the dissection site appears to be the usual mechanism of ischemia.

Extracranial Vertebral Artery Dissection

The extracranial vertebral artery is the second most common site of spontaneous or minimally traumatic cervicocerebral arterial dissection, accounting for 15% of cases in the literature. Clinical features and course in 174 cases collected from the literature are summarized in Table 29.2. Dissection of the cervical vertebral artery is characterized by the sudden onset of pain, frequently severe and localized to the neck or head, often the occiput, followed by the immediate, delayed, or progressive onset of ischemic symptoms. Cerebral ischemia is almost universal among reported cases, with infarction in over 70% and transient ischemic attacks in many of the remainder. Dissections producing headache alone undoubtedly occur frequently but usually go unrecognized.

Extracranial vertebral artery dissections may be divided into those related to minor antecedent physical insults and those occurring spontaneously, with overlapping but distinctive clinical features. Minimally traumatic cervical vertebral artery dissections are somewhat more common, and are most often related to sudden mechanical injury of the artery from rotational forces (Fig. 29.8).[64a,65,113,169,170] Most cases have been associated with chiropractic or other neck manipulation, but minor falls, automobile accidents, ceiling painting, yoga, trampoline exercise, vigorously spanking a child, archery practice, throwing the head back to drink from a shotglass, and sudden head-turning have all resulted in vertebral artery dissections.[76,91,147,169] Patient ages have ranged from the first through the seventh decades, with a mean age of 39 years. Females are affected more often than males.[64a,84] Narrowing or occlusion of the vessel, with associated dissecting aneurysm formation, is typically demonstrated at angiography. The vertebral artery is most mobile, and most susceptible to mechanical injury, at the C1–C2 level as it leaves the transverse foramen of the axis and abruptly turns to enter the intracranial cavity (the V3 segment). The C1 to C2 site is involved in 80% to 90% of rotation-related dissections.[64a,84,90]

Extracranial vertebral artery dissections unrelated to sudden cervical rotation are somewhat less frequent.[20,34,38,84,111,122] One fifth to one third of cases exhibit possible predisposing factors of hypertension, migraine, or, in women, oral contraceptive use.[42,182] An association of these spontaneous dissections with a variety of frank arteriopathies has been reported, including cystic medial degeneration, arteritis, fibromuscular dysplasia, elastorrhexis, systemic lupus erythematosus, Ehlers-Danlos syndrome type IV, and Marfan syndrome.[23,38,84,90,113,119,133,151,168,175,192] Fibromuscular dysplasia accounts for one fifth of extracranial vertebral dissections (Table 29.2). Spontaneous cervical vertebral dissections occur

Figure 29.7 Right internal carotid artery dissection in a 30-year-old woman. (**A**) Arteriogram demonstrates stenosis of the distal right internal carotid artery (*arrowheads*). (**B**) Axial T_2-weighted MRI (TE 95 ms, TR 2,000 ms) shows crescentic high-intensity signal (*arrowhead*) from intramural hematoma surrounding the residual lumen of the right internal carotid artery. Compare with normal signal void from opposite, left internal carotid artery (*arrow*).

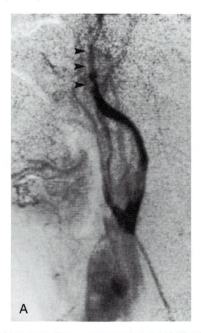

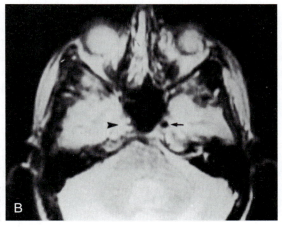

Table 29.2 Clinical Features of Extracranial Vertebral Dissection

No. of cases	174
Age	38.9 yr (mean), range 3–67
Sex	
Male	43%
Female	57%
Laterality	
Unilateral	69%
Left	56%
Right	44%
Bilateral	31%
Clinical features at presentation[a]	
Cerebral infarction	75%
At onset	17%
Delayed	83%
Transient ischemic attack	25%
Neck pain	55%
Headache	53%
Neck or head pain	75%
Lateral medullary symptoms	33%
Associated conditions	
Hypertension	25%
Migraine	13%
Oral contraceptives (among women)	24%
Fibromuscular dysplasia	17%
Early outcome	
Angiographic	
Normal or mildly stenotic vessel on follow-up imaging	78%
Clinical	
Neurologically normal or mild deficits only	83%
Moderate-severe deficits	11%
Death	6%

[a] *Major presenting complaint leading to evaluation, not necessarily the initial symptom.*

(Data from references 48, 147, 157, 182.)

in women 2.5 times more frequently than men.[84] Dissection may affect the artery at any site, but the C1–C2 level is most frequently involved, suggesting that mechanical factors may play a role even in cases with no apparent history of rotation or injury.[34,38,84,122]

The course and prognosis of extracranial vertebral artery dissections are variable. Nearly three fourths of patients suffer delayed or progressive infarction early in their course. The most frequent presentation is a partial or complete lateral medullary syndrome, and is observed in one third of cases. Cerebellar stroke syndromes are the next most common, with occipital, pontine, and midbrain infarcts, and admixtures also seen. Because unilateral vertebral artery occlusion, especially if proximal, may not cause ischemia, due to adequate contralateral vertebral flow, it seems likely that unilateral vertebral artery dissections are under-recognized, explaining the surprisingly high prevalence in the literature of simultaneous bi-

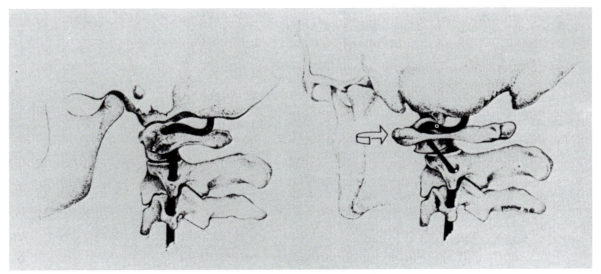

Figure 29.8 Vertebral artery injury with abrupt cervical rotation. The vertebral artery is subject to stretch and mechanical trauma between C1 and C2 when the neck is vigorously rotated and extended. (From Barnett,[11] with permission.)

lateral vertebral dissections and concurrent vertebral and carotid dissections, accounting for one half of all reported cases.[78] As experience with noninvasive ultrasound and MR diagnosis of vertebral artery dissection increases, a greater proportion of mildly symptomatic cases may be recognized.[148]

The angiographic spectrum of extracranial vertebral artery dissections encompasses the same set of patterns as extracranial carotid artery dissections. The most frequent angiographic finding is an irregularly tapering stenosis, present in almost three fourths of cases.[182] Findings of double lumen or intimal flap are more specific, but less common. MRI and ultrasound are less sensitive in detecting vertebral than carotid dissection,[103,147] suggesting a lower clinical threshold be employed for proceeding to conventional angiography. In a small recent series, MRI detected vertebral artery dissection with a sensitivity of 60% and a specificity of 98%, and MRA with a sensitivity of 20% and a specificity of 100%, compared with standard angiography.[103] The smaller size and broad variation in normal caliber of vertebral arteries render them more sensitive to technical artifact on MR. Similarly, extracranial duplex sonography exhibits fair sensitivity and specificity for demonstrating hemodynamic evidence of cervical vertebral artery stenosis due to dissection, but is hampered by limited ability to directly insonate the distal extracranial vertebral artery.[12,48,180]

Intracranial Vertebral Artery Dissection

Intracranial posterior circulation dissections are uncommon, accounting for roughly 5% of reported cervicocerebral dissections. The mean age tends to be in the late 40s in isolated intracranial vertebral artery dissection, slightly older than in dissections at other sites.[33,92,94,155] Among patients with intracranial vertebral dissections that extend to involve the basilar artery, the mean age is somewhat younger, in the late 30s. In contrast to extracranial carotid and vertebral artery dissections, intracranial vertebral artery dissections are more common in men than in women.[24,33] The frequent occurrence of subarachnoid hemorrhage, present in more than one half of reported cases, distinguishes the clinical picture from that of extracranial vertebral artery dissection.[18,33,62,75,94,155,171,184] Brain stem, cerebellar, or hemispheric infarction is the presenting feature in one third of patients, and one tenth present with both subarachnoid hemorrhage and cerebral infarction. Occasional patients present with aneurysms acting as mass lesions, compressing the brain stem and lower cranial nerves.[49,120] Prodromal headaches are exceptional among patients with subarachnoid hemorrhage; most often the initial headache occurs concurrent with massive symptomatic subarachnoid hemorrhage at onset. The most common site for dissection is at or near the origin of the posterior inferior cerebellar artery. At this level the artery may be compressed during head maneuvers, the media and adventitia diminish in size and elastic components, and the external elastic lamina terminates. Pathologic examination reveals subadventitial or transmural dissection with aneurysm formation in most cases of subarachnoid hemorrhage, while subintimal dissection with luminal compromise is more characteristic among the less frequent cases presenting with ischemia.

MRI imaging may demonstrate a pathognomonic crescent sign of high-intensity signal within the vessel wall, representing intramural hematoma. Transcranial Doppler may detect luminal stenosis if present.[47] Angiography is most reliable, although definitive findings of double lumen or intimal flap are rare. Indirect angiographic signs of dissection with luminal compromise may be present, including string sign, string and pearl sign, and wavy ribbon sign. Aneurysmal dilatation of the vertebral artery is often demonstrated. Findings at angiography may be difficult to distinguish from a saccular aneurysm of the posterior inferior cerebellar artery, although irregular lumen contour and early appearance of vessel narrowing usually indicate dissection rather than vasospasm. Not infrequently, the diagnosis of dissection is made unexpectedly at surgery for presumed saccular aneurysm.

Basilar Artery Dissection

Primary dissections of the basilar artery are rare, with only approximately 40 cases reported.[2,5,19,24,57,81,99,143] The mean age of patients is 35 years, and males and females are equally affected.[24] The typical course is abrupt onset of severe brain stem ischemia leading rapidly to coma. The plane of dissection is usually subintimal, although subadventitial and transmural hematomas may occur, producing subarachnoid bleeding and large dissecting aneurysms.[2,5,57,86,191] A small group of patients present with sluggish evolution of recurrent transient ischemic attacks, small infarcts, and/or subarachnoid hemorrhage. Death resulted in more than 60% of cases in the literature. Hypertension is present in more than one third, and association with migraine has been reported.[5,24] Underlying vasculopathies have included defects in the internal elastic lamina, polycystic kidney disease, and homocystinuria.[24,99] Dissections may arise in patients with basilar fusiform aneurysms and dolichoectasia.[143,172]

Traumatic Injury of the Cervical Carotid and Vertebral Arteries

Major nonpenetrating trauma can damage the carotid artery either directly or by a rotational-stretch injury involving the upper cervical vertebra.[15,35,44,45,71,89,97,121,154,193] (Fig. 29.1). Intimal or medial disruption may then result in thrombosis, with or without dissection.[60,158,177] Major nonpenetrating carotid injuries are most often associated with motor vehicle accidents, but bar fights, chiropractic manipulation, falls, strangulation, and hanging have also caused traumatic carotid artery injury.[35,118,146,154,177] Although there may be associated subcutaneous hematomas, or fractures of the mandible or cervical spine, in about one half of patients there is no evidence of neck injury.[35,177] In children, nonpenetrating carotid injury is frequently due to intraoral trauma during falls with blunt objects (e.g., toothbrushes, pencils) in the mouth, contusing the artery in the peritonsillar region.[16,60,142] An 0.08% incidence of carotid dissection was reported in a retrospective review of 15,935 blunt trauma patients.[45]

Frequently, nonpenetrating carotid artery injury occurs in association with a cerebral concussion or contusion, and the onset of symptoms is difficult to discern. Ipsilateral headache and neck pain are common. However, like spontaneous dissections, a lucid interval is the rule, with focal deficits occurring several hours to a few days after the trauma. Often, carotid occlusion or dissection is an unexpected finding in patients who deteriorate after head trauma and in whom a subdural hematoma or delayed intracerebral hematoma is suspected. Based on the frequent finding of apparent embolic occlusion of distal vessels, embolism of thrombus from the site of injury is believed to be a common mechanism of cerebral ischemia in these dissections. Delayed embolism may explain the lucid interval. Oculosympathetic paresis is common and, when present in obtunded trauma patients, should suggest traumatic carotid injury.

Angiography in patients with nonpenetrating carotid injury usually demonstrates occlusion of the distal cervical carotid artery, but the characteristic features of dissection may occasionally be present.[44] Intimal flaps and dissecting aneurysms may be more frequent with traumatic carotid dissections than with their spontaneous counterpart.[121,146,177] In a minority of cases, intrapetrous carotid occlusion occurs, usually associated with basilar skull fractures.[1,4,40] Major stroke is the most commonly reported neurologic sequel of carotid artery trauma, possibly due to under-recognition of less afflicted patients. In a recent large series of patients with blunt internal and common carotid artery traumatic injury, 56% had stroke and 7% a fatal outcome.[149]

The optimal therapy of this disorder is controversial. Arteriotomy with thombectomy and repair of intimal flaps has been advocated, especially in patients with submassive neurologic deficits.[35,136,146,149] An initial medical approach, using anticoagulation and follow-up arteriography, is a reasonable alternative.[93,177,186,193] For surgically inaccessible intrapetrous and other high internal carotid artery injuries, endovascular detachable balloon or coil occlusion has been recommended.[149]

Penetrating injury to the carotid artery is more frequently reported than nonpenetrating trauma.[35,45,71,149] Most such injuries are caused by gunshot or knife wounds and result in tangential laceration of the carotid artery, with simultaneous involvement of the internal jugular vein in about one fourth of patients. The carotid artery is also occasionally injured as an iatrogenic complication of local surgical procedures. Tonsillectomy, trans-sphenoidal pituitary surgery, radical neck dissection, and percutaneous radio frequency trigeminal rhizolysis have all been associated with symptomatic carotid injury. Penetrating carotid injuries may cause cerebral ischemia by either interruption of flow or distal embolism of thrombi. Resulting neck hematomas can cause tracheal compression. Brachial plexus injury, ipsilateral tongue weakness from hypoglossal nerve involvement, and oculosympathetic paresis may coexist. Formation of dissecting aneurysms and arteriovenous fistulas may result. In hemodynamically unstable patients with suspected penetrating carotid injury, immediate surgical exploration should be undertaken. Hemodynamically stable patients may be assessed by angiography, and possibly by ultrasound or MRI.[32,98,126,150] Primary arterial repair, with or without patch grafts, has supplanted carotid ligation as the preferred treatment.[98,105]

Until recently, the frequency of traumatic injuries of the cervical vertebral artery was underappreciated. However, prospective angiographic series have now demonstrated vertebral artery occlusion or dissection in 46% to 75% of consecutive patients with traumatic cervical spine facet joint dislocation or fracture.[107,188] Similarly, in an autopsy series of patients with fatal cervical spine injuries from falls, motor vehicle accidents, or suicidal hanging, 37% showed vertebral artery rupture, intimal disruption, or subintimal bleeding.[156] Facet dislocation excessively stretches the vertebral artery passing between two adjacent transverse foramina, and fractures may produce direct trauma to the vessel wall. Neurologic sequelae are less common than with carotid injury, as a patent contralateral vertebral artery usually fills the intracranial portion of the occluded vertebral artery, the basilar artery, and the posterior cerebral arteries.[188] However, immediate or delayed vertebrobasilar ischemia can occur. Proximal and distal ligation or endovascular balloon or coil occlusion is often recommended for penetrating injury of the cervical vertebral artery to prevent emboli.[116,188] Medical management with anticoagulation is a reasonable treatment option when not contraindicated by systemic traumatic injuries.

Recurrent Dissection and Late Strokes in Spontaneous Extracranial Artery Dissection

In spontaneous or minimally traumatic cervical artery dissections, the risk of recurrent dissection in the initially dissected artery is low, the risk of subsequent dissection in another cervicocerebral vessel slightly higher.[157] In a Mayo Clinic series of 200 patients with cervical arterial dissections followed for over 7 years, the recurrence rate was 2% in the first month and 1% yearly thereafter.[154] The cumulative rate of recurrent dissection over 10 years was 12%. All recurrent dissections occurred in arteries not involved by the initial dissection, other cervical arteries in 87%, and renal arteries in 13%. A family history of dissection was the only significant predictor associated with dissection recurrence.[162] Recurrence was equally frequent among individuals whose initial dissection involved a single vessel as among those with multiarterial dissection. In a collaborative European study of 105 patients, the rate of recurrent dissection also approximated 1% yearly over 10 years.[104] However, all recurrent dissections in this study occurred at the site of the initially dissected vessel, and all patients with recurrence had an underlying frank arteriopathy, either Ehlers-Danlos syndrome or fibromuscular dysplasia. A large prospective Swiss series similarly found a recurrent dissection rate of 4% over a mean 34-month follow-up.[14] Across these series, dissection recurrence rates were similar for carotid and vertebral arteries, with recurrent dissections appearing in 15 of 303 patients with initial internal carotid artery dissections and 5 of 108 patients with initial vertebral artery dissections. The mean time to recurrence was 4.1 years, with a range of 2 days to 8.6 years.

Late strokes—infarctions occurring more than 2 weeks after diagnosis of dissection—are infrequent among both extracranial carotid and vertebral dissections. Among 503 cases with long-term follow-up (mean, 3.4 years) reported in the literature, fewer than 1.6% experienced late cerebral infarction, and most of these occurred in the first year (annualized late stroke rate of 0.4%).[48,104,182] This rate does not reflect the true natural history, as patients in these series were frequently treated with a variety of antithrombotics, and is probably higher than might otherwise be expected in this relatively young population. Nonetheless, this late stroke rate is low enough to cloud the prospect of a randomized clinical trial ever providing definitive information about the proper postacute treatment of arterial dissections. Even if the stroke rate were as high as 5% in the first year after dissection, a sample size of approximately 1,600 patients would be required to compare two treatments with an 80% chance of detecting a 50% reduction in events ($\alpha = 0.05$, 2-tailed). It seems unlikely that such a randomized trial will be carried out.

Treatment

The proper management of extracranial cervicocerebral dissections is controversial. Several medical and surgical treatments have been used in cervical carotid dissection, but randomized controlled clinical trials are lacking, precluding more than a general comparison of outcomes (Table 29.3). Most

Table 29.3 Survey of the Literature on Outcome of Management in 100 Patients

	Patients' Outcomes		
Presenting Feature[a]	Normal	Minor Deficit[b]	Major Deficit or Death
Major stroke (18 cases)			
No Rx or APT	0/13	1/13	12/13
Anticoagulant	1/4	2/4	1/4
Surgery	0	1/1	0
Single TIA or minor stroke (45 cases)			
No Rx or APT	15/17	2/17	0
Anticoagulant	14/16	1/16	1/16
Surgery	6/12	5/12	1/12
Multiple TIA (15 cases)			
No Rx or APT	6/6	0	0
Anticoagulant	5/5	0	0
Surgery	3/4	1/4	0
Other (pain, tinnitus) (22 cases)			
No Rx or APT	18/20	1/20	1/20
Anticoagulant	2/2	0	0
Surgery	0	0	0
Total (in %)	70%	14%	16%

Abbreviations: Rx, medical therapy; APT, antiplatelet therapy; TIA, transient ischemic attack.

[a] Major complaint on presentation to physician, not necessarily the initial symptom.

[b] Nondisabling deficit, residual Horner syndrome considered normal.

(Data from 100 cases from English-language literature since 1975 on extracranial carotid artery dissection. Data from Hart and Easton[79] plus references 17, 26, 66, 88, and 112.)

patients do well, either because of or despite treatment. While the use of anticoagulation might seem contraindicated in a disorder defined by hemorrhage into the arterial wall, most cerebral injury appears to result from secondary thrombotic and embolic complications of the dissection. Thus, anticoagulation, with heparin or low molecular-weight heparins followed by warfarin, is often recommended.[37,59,115,174]

In the patient with cervical artery dissection presenting within 3 to 6 hours of onset of ischemic symptoms, intra-arterial thrombolytic therapy may be considered. Because of the theoretical risk of provoking recurrence or extension of dissecting hemorrhage, we generally avoid systemically administered thrombolytics. Intra-arterial administration of thrombolytics by superselective catheterization directly onto a distal thrombus, beyond the dissection site, may have a lower risk of worsening the dissection while providing beneficial reperfusion.

The time course of healing of the vessel wall guides the duration of anticoagulant therapy. In extracranial internal carotid artery dissections, collating large series, approximately 85% of stenoses, 51% of occlusions, and 43% of aneurysms are found to have improved or returned to normal at follow-up angiography. Serial ultrasound studies show that the median time to resolution of carotid dissections is 6 weeks, most arteries recover by 3 months, and vessels that fail to reconstitute a normal lumen by 6 months are highly unlikely to improve thereafter.[25,51,52,59,67,68,83,108,135,144,176,179] This time course of lesion evolution suggests the following therapeutic algorithm for extracranial carotid dissection. Anticoagulation with heparin or low molecular weight heparin and then with warfarin is recommended. Platelet antiaggregates are recommended for those patients with strong contraindications to anticoagulation. Repeat vessel imaging is recommended 3 months after onset. MRI and MRA imaging is preferred, but combinations of transcranial Doppler, spiral CT, and/or conventional angiography may also be employed. If 3-month imaging shows the dissection has largely resolved with a smooth lumen residua, anticoagulation is generally discontinued and antiplatelet therapy or no antithrombotics begun. If only mild luminal irregularities persist, long-term antiplatelet therapy generally is initiated. If 3-month imaging shows a persisting complete occlusion with smooth origin and terminus, antiplatelet therapy is substituted for anticoagulation. If 3-month imaging shows persisting severe luminal stenosis and irregularity, anticoagulation is continued, and follow-up imaging repeated at 6 months. When 3-month imaging shows a dissecting aneurysm, anticoagulation typically is continued, and serial imaging to monitor lesion evolution is pursued. Extracranial internal carotid artery dissecting aneurysms rarely, if ever, rupture, but they do serve as nidi for thromboembolism.[128]

Surgery is reserved for patients with localized, accessible lesions who experience further ischemia despite medical therapy, and for patients with progressive cranial nerve dysfunction from an enlarging dissecting aneurysm. Aneurysm resection and carotid reconstruction is the most common surgical strategy.[164] For poorly accessible aneurysms of the very distal internal carotid artery, carotid ligation or coil or balloon occlusion may be performed if collateral circulation is adequate, but may increase the risk of cerebral ischemia and intracranial aneurysms later in life.

Activities predisposing to abrupt cervical rotation should probably be avoided in survivors of dissection. Estrogen compounds, which are associated with fibromuscular and intimal arterial proliferation, are empirically discontinued. Vigorous control of hypertension appears prudent.

We apply these same principles to patients with extracranial vertebral artery dissection. The less extensive data available suggest that the natural history of these dissections roughly parallels extracranial carotid dissections, with a broadly similar time-course of vessel recovery or stabilization within 3 months, low incidence of late cerebral ischemia, and low incidence of recurrent dissection.[12,48,104,147] We anticoagulate patients acutely. In the minority whose dissections extend intracranially, we first obtain CT and lumbar puncture to rule out subarachnoid hemorrhage. Follow-up imaging at 3 months determines the choice of (1) continued anticoagulation if severe luminal irregularities persist, (2) antiplatelet therapy for mild luminal abnormalities or occlusion, and (3) antiplatelet therapy or discontinuation of antithrombotics when the vessel appears normal. Aneurysms are serially monitored, and treated surgically or by endovascular techniques if ischemia recurs or local cranial nerve compression ensues. The prognosis for extracranial vertebral dissection tends to be favorable, with approximately 80% having a normal outcome or mild residual deficits, versus 70% for cervical internal carotid artery dissection (Tables 29.1 and 29.2).

In treating *intracranial* dissections, the frequent occurrence of subarachnoid hemorrhage suggests caution in the early use of anticoagulation. However, in situ thrombus propagation and artery-to-artery embolization of thrombi are causes of deterioration in these patients, possibly preventable by anticoagulation. For intracranial carotid artery dissections producing ischemia, immediate anastomosis of the superficial temporal artery to middle cerebral artery branches has been proposed, but also is of unproved value.

Our management approach is tailored to the individual presentation. Patients are divided into those presenting with ischemic symptoms alone, and those presenting with subarachnoid hemorrhage demonstrated by CT or lumbar puncture. In patients with cerebral ischemia without subarachnoid bleeding, a quiet environment and moderation of severe elevations in blood pressure to reduce the chance of delayed subarachnoid hemorrhage is a prudent initial strategy. If the clinical course and angiography suggest recurrent artery-to-artery embolization or a large burden of acute thrombus, early anticoagulation is generally undertaken, or surgical or endovascular vessel occlusion may be pursued. If clinical evolution suggests progressive hemodynamic ischemia unresponsive to moderate hypervolemic therapy, surgical bypass procedures are considered. Serial angiographic studies in patients without subarachnoid hemorrhage typically demonstrate resolution or stabilization of vessel lesions over 2 to 6 months.[95]

Subarachnoid hemorrhage is most commonly a presenting management problem in intracranial vertebral artery dissection. Rebleeding occurs in about one fourth of these patients if the dissecting aneurysm is not directly addressed. The fusiform morphology of dissecting pseudoaneurysms precludes clipping of an aneurysmal neck. If the affected vessel is the nondominant vertebral artery, the contralateral vessel frequently can supply the entire posterior circulation. In these patients, prompt surgical intervention with clip occlusion or endovascular intervention with coil or balloon occlusion has been recommended.[33,62,75,78,92,94,184] Endovascular therapy may be particularly useful for less surgically accessible dissecting aneurysms distal to the posterior inferior cerebellar artery. For dissection in a dominant vertebral artery, surgical wrapping has been advocated, but also is of uncertain value. Test balloon occlusion of a dominant vertebral artery, followed by permanent occlusion if well tolerated, has been successful. Data on recurrent bleeding rates in anterior intracranial circulation dissections presenting with subarachnoid hemorrhage are sparse. Both initial conservative management or test balloon occlusion with permanent occlusion, if well tolerated, are reasonable treatment options. Delayed vasospasm may develop following dissection-related subarachnoid hemorrhage, and is managed according to standard principles.

References

1. Aarabi B, McQueen JD: Traumatic internal carotid occlusion at the base of the skull. Surg Neurol 10:233, 1978
2. Adams HP Jr, Aschenbrener CA, Kassell NF et al: Intracranial hemorrhage produced by spontaneous dissecting intracranial aneurysm. Arch Neurol 39:773, 1982
3. Adelman LS, Doe FD, Samat HB: Bilateral dissecting aneurysms of the internal carotid arteries. Acta Neuropathol (Berl) 29:93, 1974
4. Ajir F, Tibbetts JC: Post-traumatic occlusion of the supraclinoid internal carotid artery. Neurosurgery 9:173, 1981
5. Alexander CB, Burger PC, Goree JA: Dissecting aneurysms of the basilar artery in 2 patients. Stroke 10:294, 1979
6. Anderson CA, Collins GJ Jr, Rich NM et al: Spontaneous dissection of the internal carotid artery associated with fibromuscular dysplasia. Am Surg 4:263, 1980
7. Assaf M, Sweeney PJ, Komorsky G et al: Horner's syndrome secondary to angiogram negative, subadventitial carotid artery dissection. Can J Neurol Sci 20:62, 1993
8. Ast G, Woimant F, Georges B et al: Spontaneous dissection of the internal carotid artery in 68 patients. European J Med 2:466, 1993
9. Austin MG, Schaefer RF: Marfan's syndrome, with unusual blood vessel manifestations. Arch Pathol Lab Med 64:205, 1957
10. Barbour PJ, Castaldo JE, Rae-Grant AD et al: Internal carotid artery redundancy is significantly associated with dissection. Stroke 25:1201, 1994
11. Barnett HJM: Progress towards stroke prevention. Robert Wartenberg Lecture. Neurology (NY) 30:1212, 1980
12. Bartels E, Flugel KA: Evaluation of extracranial vertebral artery dissection with duplex color-flow imaging. Stroke 27:290, 1996
13. Bassetti C, Bogousslavsky J, Eskenasy-Cottier AC et al: Spontaneous intracranial dissection in the anterior circulation. Cerebrovasc Dis 4:170, 1994
14. Bassetti C, Carruzzo A, Sturzenegger M et al: Recurrence of cervical artery dissection. Stroke 27:1804, 1996
15. Batzdorf U, Bentson JR, Machleder HI: Blunt trauma to the high cervical carotid artery. Neurosurgery 5:195, 1979
16. Belfer RA, Ochsenschlager DW, Tomaski SM: Penetrating injury to the oral cavity: a case report and review of the literature. J Emerg Med 13:331, 1995
17. Benoit BG, Russell NA, Grimes JD et al: Spontaneous dissection of carotid and vertebral arteries; management considerations. Can J Neurol Sci 11:328, 1984
18. Berger MS, Wilson CB: Intracranial dissecting aneurysms of the posterior circulation. J Neurosurg 61:882, 1984
19. Berkovic SF, Spokes RL, Anderson RM et al: Basilar artery dissection. J Neurol Neurosurg Psychiatry 46:126, 1983
20. Biller J, Hingtgen WL, Adams HP Jr et al: Cervicocephalic arterial dissections: a ten-year experience. Arch Neurol 43:1234, 1986
21. Biousse V, D'Anglejean-Chatillon J, Massiou H, Bousser M-G: Head pain in non-traumatic carotid artery dissection: a series of 65 patients. Cephalalgia 14:33, 1994
22. Biousse V, D'Anglejean-Chatillon J, Touboul P-J et al: Time course of symptoms in extracranial carotid artery dissections. Stroke 26:235, 1995
23. Bladin PF: Dissecting aneurysm of carotid and vertebral arteries. Vasc Surg 8:203, 1974
24. Bogousslavsky J: Dissections of the cerebral arteries: clinical effects. Curr Opin Neurol Neurosurg 1:63, 1988
25. Bogousslavsky J, Despland PA, Regli F: Spontaneous carotid dissection with acute stroke. Arch Neurol 44:137, 1987
26. Bogousslavsky J, Regli F, Despland PA: Aneurysmes disséquants spontanes de l'artère carotide interne. Rev Neurol (Paris) 11:625, 1984
27. Bostrom K, Liliequist B: Primary dissecting aneurysm of the extracranial part of the internal carotid and vertebral arteries. Neurology 17:179, 1967
28. Bradac GB, Kaernbach A, Bolk-Weischedel D et al: Spontaneous dissecting aneurysm of cervical cerebral arteries. Neuroradiology 21:149, 1981
29. Brandt T, Orberk E, Hausser I et al: Ultrastructural aberrations of connective tissue components in patients with spontaneous cervicocerebral artery dissections. Neurology 46:A193, 1996
30. Brice JG, Crompton MR: Spontaneous dissecting aneurysms of the cervical internal carotid artery. BMJ 2:790, 1964
31. Brugieres P, Castrec-Carpo A, Heran F et al: Magnetic resonance imaging in the exploration of dissection of the internal carotid artery. J Neuroradiol 16:1, 1989
32. Bula WI, Loes DJ: Trauma to the cerebrovascular system. Neuroimag Clin North Am 4:753, 1994
33. Caplan LR, Baquis GD, Pessin MS et al: Dissection of the intracranial vertebral artery. Neurology 38:868, 1988
34. Caplan LR, Zarins CK, Hemmati M: Spontaneous dissection of the extracranial vertebral arteries. Stroke 16:1030, 1985
35. Chandler WF, Coon JV, Ericus MS: Carotid Artery Injuries. Futura, Mt. Kisco, NY, 1982
36. Chang V, Rewcastle NB, Harwood-Nash DCF et al: Bilateral dissecting aneurysms of the intracranial internal

carotid arteries in an 8-year-old boy. Neurology (NY) 25:573, 1975

37. Chapleau CE, Robertson JT: Spontaneous cervical carotid artery dissection: outpatient treatment with continuous heparin infusion using a totally implantable infusion device. Neurosurgery 8:83, 1981

38. Chiras J, Marciano S, Vega Molina J et al: Spontaneous dissecting aneurysm of the extracranial vertebral artery (20 cases). Neuroradiology 27:327, 1985

39. Cox LK, Bertorini T, Laster RE: Headaches due to spontaneous internal carotid artery dissection. Headache 31:12, 1991

40. Crissy MM, Bernstein EF: Delayed presentation of carotid intimal tear following blunt craniocervicocerebral trauma. Surgery 75:543, 1974

41. Dal Pozzo G, Mascalchi M, Fonda C et al: Lower cranial nerve palsy due to dissection of the internal carotid artery: CT and MR imaging. J Comput Assist Tomogr 13:989, 1989

42. D'Anglejean-Chatillon J, Ribeiro V, Mas JL et al: Migraine—a risk factor for dissection of cervical arteries. Headache 29:560, 1989

43. D'Anglejean-Chatillon J, Ribeiro V, Mas JL et al: Dissection de l'artère carotide interne extracranienne: soixante-deux observations. Presse Med 19:661, 1990

44. Davis JM, Zimmerman RA: Injury of the carotid and vertebral arteries. Neuroradiology 25:55, 1983

45. Davis JW, Holbrook TL, Hoyt DB et al: Blunt carotid artery dissection: incidence, associated injuries, screening and treatment. J Trauma 30:1514, 1990

46. De Baets P, Delanote G, Jackers G et al: Atherosclerotic dissection of the cervical internal carotid artery—a case report. Angiology 41:161, 1990

47. de Bray JM, Lhoste P, Dubas F et al: Ultrasonic features of extracranial carotid dissections: 47 cases studied by angiography. J Ultrasound Med 13:659, 1994

47a. de Bray JM, Missoum A, Dubas F et al: Doppler transcranial ultrasonography in carotid and vertebral dissections: 36 cases involving angiography. J Maladies Vasc 19:35, 1994

48. de Bray JM, Penisson-Besnier L, Dubas F et al: Extracranial and intracranial vertebrobasilar dissections: diagnosis and prognosis. J Neurol Neurosurg Psychiat 63:46, 1977

49. De Busscher J: Aneurysme de l'artère vértebrale gauche chez un homme 45 ans. Acta Neurol Belg 52:1, 1952

50. Deck JHN: Pathology of spontaneous dissection of intracranial arteries. Can J Neurol Sci 14:88, 1987

51. Deramond H, Remond A, Rosat P et al: Spontaneous evolution of nontraumatic dissecting aneurysms of the cervical portion of the internal carotid artery. J Neuroradiol 17:167, 1980

52. Desfontaines P, Despland PA: Dissection of the internal carotid artery: aetiology, symptomatology, clinical and neurosonological follow-up, and treatment in 60 consecutive cases. Acta Neurol Belg 95:226, 1995

53. Early TF, Gregory RT, Wheeler JR et al: Spontaneous carotid dissection: duplex scanning in diagnosis and management. J Vasc Surg 14:391, 1991

54. Ehrenfeld WK, Wylie EJ: Spontaneous dissection of the internal carotid artery. Arch Surg 111:1294, 1976

55. Eljamel MSM, Humphrey PRD, Shaw MDM: Dissec-

tion of the cervical internal carotid artery: the role of Doppler/duplex studies and conservative management. J Neurol Neurosurg Psychiatry 53:379, 1990

56. Eskenasy-Cottier AC, Leu HJ, Bassetti C et al: A case of dissection of intracranial cerebral arteries with segmental mediolytic "arteritis." Clin Neuropathol 13:329, 1994

57. Farrell MA, Gilbert JJ, Kaufmann JC: Fatal intracranial arterial dissection: clinical pathological correlation. J Neurol Neurosurg Psychiatry 48:111, 1985

58. Fisher CM: The headache and pain of spontaneous carotid dissection. Headache 22:60, 1982

59. Fisher CM, Ojemann RG, Robertson GH: Spontaneous dissection of cervico-cerebral arteries. Can J Neurol Sci 5:9, 1978

60. Fleming JFR, Petrie D: Traumatic thrombosis of the internal carotid artery with delayed hemiplegia. Can J Surg 11:166, 1968

61. Francis KR, Williams DP, Troost BT: Facial numbness and dysesthesia: new features of carotid artery dissection. Arch Neurol 44:345, 1987

62. Friedman AH, Drake CG: Subarachnoid hemorrhage from intracranial dissecting aneurysm. J Neurosurg 60:325, 1984

63. Friedman WA, Day AL, Quisling RG Jr et al: Cervical carotid dissecting aneurysms. Neurosurgery 7:207, 1980

64. Friedman DP, Flanders AE: Unusual dissection of the proximal vertebral artery: description of three cases. AJNR 13:283, 1991

64a. Frisoni GB, Anzola GP: Vertebrobasilar ischemia after neck motion. Stroke 22:1452, 1991

65. Frumkin LR, Baloh RW: Wallenberg's syndrome following neck manipulation. Neurology (NY) 40:61 1990

66. Garcia-Merino JA, Gutierrez JA, Lopez-Lozano JJ: Double-lumen dissecting aneurysms of the internal carotid artery in fibromuscular dysplasia: a case report. Stroke 14:815, 1983

67. Gauthier G, Rohr J, Wildi E et al: L'hématome disséquant spontane de l'artère carotide interne. 136:53, 1985

68. Gee W, Kaupp HA, McDonald KM et al: Spontaneous dissection of internal carotid arteries: spontaneous resolution documented by serial ocular pneumoplethysmography and angiography. Arch Surg 115:944, 1980

69. Gelbert F, Assouline E, Hodes JE et al: MRI in spontaneous dissection of vertebral and carotid arteries. Neuroradiology 33:111, 1991

70. Gelbert F, Assouline E, Hodes JE et al: MRI in spontaneous dissection of vertebral and carotid arteries. Neuroradiology 33:111, 1991

71. George SM Jr, Croce MA, Fabian TC et al: Cervicothoracic arterial injuries: recommendations for diagnosis and management. World J Surg 15:134, 1991

72. Goodman JM, Zink WL, Cooper DF: Hemilingual paralysis caused by carotid artery dissection. Arch Neurol 40:653, 1983

73. Grau AJ, Buggle F, Steichen-Wiehn C et al: Clinical and biochemical analysis in infection-associated stroke. Stroke 26:1520, 1995

74. Gould DB, Cunningham BS: Internal carotid artery dissection after remote surgery: iatrogenic complications of anesthesia. Stroke 25:1276, 1994

75. Halbach VV, Higashida R, Dowd C et al: Endovascular

treatment of vertebral artery dissections and pseudoaneurysms. J Neurosurg 79:183, 1993

76. Haldeman S, Kohlbeck F, McGregor M: Risk factors for vertebrobasilar artery dissection following cervical spine manipulation: a review of 60 cases. Neurology 46:A440, 1996

77. Hamouda-M'Rad B, Biousse V, Bousser M-G et al: Internal carotid artery redundancy is significantly associated with dissection. Stroke 26:1962, 1995

78. Hart RG: Vertebral artery dissection. Neurology (NY) 38:987, 1988

79. Hart RG, Easton JD: Dissections of cervical and cerebral arteries. Neurol Clin 1:155, 1983

80. Hartman JD, Eftychiadis AS: Medial smooth-muscle cell lesions and dissection of the aorta and muscular arteries. Arch Pathol Lab Med 114:50, 1990

81. Hayman JA, Anderson RM: Dissecting aneurysm of the basilar artery. Med J Aust 2:360, 1966

82. Hegedüs K: Reticular fiber deficiency in the intracranial arteries of patients with dissecting aneurysm and review of the possible pathogenesis of previously reported cases. Eur Arch Psychiatry Clin Neurosci 235:102, 1985

83. Hennerici M, Steinke W, Rautenberg W: High-resistance Doppler flow pattern in extracranial carotid dissection. Arch Neurol 46:670, 1989

84. Hinse P, Thie A, Lachenmayer L: Dissection of the extracranial vertebral artery: report of four cases and review of the literature. J Neurol Neurosurg Psychiatry 54:863, 1991

85. Hoffman M, Sacco RL, Chan S et al: Noninvasive detection of vertebral artery dissection. Stroke 24:815, 1993

86. Hosoda K, Fujita S, Kawaguchi T et al: Spontaneous dissecting aneurysms of the basilar artery presenting with subarachnoid hemorrhage. J Neurosurg 75:628, 1991

87. Houser OW, Mokri B, Sundt TM Jr et al: Spontaneous cervical cephalic arterial dissection and its residuum: angiographic spectrum. AJNR 5:27, 1984

88. Jackson MA, Hughes RC, Ward SP, McInnes EG: Head-banging and carotid dissection. BMJ 287:1262, 1983

89. Janjua KJ, Goswami G, Sagar G: Whiplash injury associated with acute bilateral carotid artery dissection. J Trauma 40:456, 1996

90. Josien E: Extracranial vertebral artery dissection: nine cases. J Neurol 239:327, 1992

91. Katirji MB, Reinmuth OM, Latchaw RE: Stroke due to vertebral artery injury. Arch Neurol 42:242, 1985

92. Kawaguchi S, Sakaki T, Tsunoda S et al: Management of dissecting aneurysms of the posterior circulation. Acta Neurochir (Wien) 131:26, 1994

93. Kestenberg WL: Review of intimal arterial injuries: surgery versus conservative management. Ann Surg 56:504, 1990

94. Kitanaka C, Sasaki T, Eguchi T et al: Intracranial vertebral artery dissections: clinical, radiological features, and surgical considerations. Neurosurg 34:620, 1994

95. Kitanaka C, Tanaki JI, Kuwahara M et al: Nonsurgical treatment of unruptured intracranial vertebral artery dissection with serial follow-up angiography. J Neurosurg 80:667, 1994

96. Klufas RA, Hsu L, Barnes PD et al: Dissection of the carotid and vertebral arteries: imaging with MR angiography. AJR 164:673, 1995

97. Krajewski LP, Hertzer NR: Blunt carotid artery trauma: report of two cases and review of the literature. Ann Surg 191:341, 1980

98. Kuehne JP, Weaver FA, Papanicolaou G et al: Penetrating trauma of the internal carotid artery. Arch Surg 131:942, 1996

99. Kulla L, Deymeer F, Smith TW et al: Intracranial dissecting and saccular aneurysms in polycystic kidney disease. Arch Neurol 39:776, 1983

100. Lash S, Newell D, Mayberg M et al: Artery-to-artery cerebral emboli detection with transcranial Doppler: analysis of eight cases. J Stroke Cerebrovasc Dis 3:15, 1993

101. Leclerc X, Godefroy O, Salhi A et al: Helical CT for the diagnosis of extracranial internal carotid artery dissection. Stroke 27:461, 1996

102. Lederman RJ, Salanga V: Fibromuscular dysplasia of the internal carotid artery—a cause of Raeder's paratrigeminal syndrome. Neurology (NY) 26:353, 1976

103. Levy C, Laissy JP, Raveau V et al: Carotid and vertebral dissections: three dimensional time-of-flight MR angiography and MR imaging versus conventional angiography. Radiology 190:97, 1994

104. Leys D, Moulin T, Stojkovic T et al: Follow-up of patients with history of cervical artery dissection. Cerebrovasc Dis 4:43, 1995

105. Liekweg WG Jr, Greenfield LJ: Management of penetrating carotid arterial injury. Ann Surg 188:587, 1978

106. Linden MD, Chou SM, Furlan AJ, Conomy JP: Cerebral arterial dissection: a case report with histopathologic and ultrastructural findings. Cleve Clin J Med 54:105, 1987

107. Louw JA, Mafoyane NA, Small B et al: Occlusion of the vertebral artery in cervical spine dislocations. J Bone Joint Surg 72B:679, 1990

108. Luken MG, Ascherd GF Jr, Correll JW et al: Spontaneous dissecting aneurysms of the extracranial internal carotid artery. Clin Neurosurg 26:353, 1979

109. Majamaa K, Portimojarvi H, Sotaniemi KA et al: Familial aggregation of cervical artery dissection and cerebral aneurysm. Stroke 25:1704, 1994

110. Manz HJ, Vester J, Lavenstein B: Dissecting aneurysm of cerebral arteries in childhood and adolescence. Virchows Arch 384:325, 1979

111. Mas J-L, Bousser M-G, Hasboun D, Laplane D: Extracranial vertebral artery dissections: a review of 13 cases. Stroke 18:1037, 1987

112. Mas J-L, Goeau C, Bousser M-G et al: Spontaneous dissecting aneurysms of the internal carotid and vertebral arteries—two case reports. Stroke 16:125, 1985

113. Mas J-L, Henin O, Bousser M-G et al: Dissecting aneurysm of the vertebral artery and cervical manipulation: a case report with autopsy. Neurology (NY) 39:512, 1989

114. Mayer SA, Rubin BS, Starman BJ, Byers PH: Spontaneous multivessel cervical artery dissection in a patient with a substitution of alanine for glycine (G13A) in the α1(I) chain of type I collagen. Neurology 47:552, 1996

115. McNeill DH Jr, Dreisback J, Marsden RJ: Spontaneous dissection of the internal carotid artery: its conservation

management with heparin sodium. Arch Neurol 37:54, 1980

116. Meier DE, Brink BE, Fry WJ: Vertebral artery trauma: acute recognition and treatment. Arch Surg 116:236, 1981

117. Milandre L, Perot S, Salamon G, Khalil R: Spontaneous dissection of both extracranial internal carotid arteries. Neuroradiology 31:435, 1989

118. Milligan N, Anderson M: Conjugal disharmony as a hitherto unrecognized cause of strokes. BMJ 281:421, 1980

119. Mitsias P, Levine SR: Large cerebral vessel occlusive disease in systemic lupus erythematosus. Neurology 44:385, 1994

120. Miyazaki S, Yamaura A, Kamata K et al: A dissecting aneurysm of the vertebral artery. Surg Neurol 21:171, 1984

121. Mokri B: Traumatic and spontaneous extracranial internal carotid artery dissections. J Neurol 237:356, 1990

122. Mokri B, Houser OW, Sandok BA et al: Spontaneous dissection of the vertebral arteries. Neurology (NY) 38:880, 1988

123. Mokri B, Houser OW, Stanson AW: Multivessel cervicocephalic and visceral arterial dissections: pathogenic role of primary arterial disease in cervicocephalic arterial dissections. J Stroke Cerebrovasc Dis 1:117, 1991

124. Mokri B, Piepgras DG, Wiebers DO, Houser OW: Familial occurrence of spontaneous dissection of the internal carotid artery. Stroke 18:246, 1987

125. Mokri B, Sundt TM, Houser OW, Piepgras DG: Spontaneous dissection of the cervical internal carotid artery. Ann Neurol 19:126, 1986

126. Montalvo BM, LeBlang SD, Nunez DB et al: Color Doppler sonography in penetrating injuries of the neck. Am J Neuroradiol 17:943, 1996

127. Moore WS: Pathology of extracranial cerebrovascular disease. p. 1206. In Rutherford RB (ed): Vascular Surgery. WB Saunders, Philadelphia, 1984

128. Moreau P, Albat B, Thevenet A: Surgical treatment of extracranial internal carotid artery aneurysm. Ann Vasc Surg 8:409, 1994

129. Mullges W, Ringelstein EB, Leibold M: Non-invasive diagnosis of internal carotid artery dissections. J Neurol Neurosurg Psychiatry 55:98, 1992

130. Mullges W, Ringelstein EB, Weiller C et al: Dissections of the internal carotid artery—new diagnostic and pathogenetic aspects. Fortschr Neurol Psychiatr 59:12, 1991

131. Muzutani T, Goldberg HI, Parr J et al: Cerebral dissecting aneurysm and intimal fibroelastic thickening of cerebral arteries. J Neurosurg 56:571, 1982

132. Nass R, Hays A, Chutorian A: Intracranial dissecting aneurysms in childhood. Stroke 13:204, 1982

133. North KN, Whiteman DAH, Pepin MG, Byers PH: Cerebrovascular complications in Ehlers-Danlos syndrome type IV. Ann Neurol 38:960, 1995

134. O'Connell BK, Towfighi J, Brennan RW et al: Dissecting aneurysms of head and neck. Neurology (NY) 35:993, 1985

135. O'Dwyer JA, Moscow N, Trevor R et al: Spontaneous dissection of the carotid artery. Radiology 137:379, 1980

136. Oragon R, Saranchak H, Lakin P et al: Blunt injuries to the carotid and vertebral arteries. Am J Surg 141:497, 1981

137. Ozdoba C, Sturzenegger M, Schroth G: Internal carotid artery dissection: MR imaging features and clinical-radiologic correlation. Radiology 199:191, 1996

138. Panisset M, Eidelman BH: Multiple cranial neuropathy as a feature of internal carotid artery dissection. Stroke 21:141, 1990

139. Pessin MS, Adelman LS, Barbas NR: Spontaneous intracranial carotid artery dissection. Stroke 20:1100, 1989

140. Petro GR, Witwer GA, Cacayorin ED et al: Spontaneous dissection of the cervical internal carotid artery: correlation of arteriography, CT, and pathology. Am J Radiol 148:393, 1987

141. Pilz P, Hartjes HJ: Fibromuscular dysplasia and multiple dissecting aneurysms of intracranial arteries: a further cause of moyamoya syndrome. Stroke 7:393, 1976

142. Pitner SE: Carotid thrombosis due to intraoral trauma: an unusual complication of a common childhood accident. N Engl J Med 274:764, 1966

143. Pozzati E, Andreoli A, Padovani R et al: Dissecting aneurysms of the basilar artery. Neurosurgery 36:254, 1995

144. Pozzati E, Gaist G, Poppi M: Resolution of occlusion in spontaneously dissected carotid arteries. J Neurosurg 56:857, 1982

145. Pozzati E, Giuliani G, Acciarri N, Nuzzo G: Long-term follow-up of occlusive cervical carotid dissection. Stroke 21:528, 1990

146. Pretre R, Reverdin A, Kalonji T et al: Blunt carotid artery injury. Surgery 115:375, 1994

147. Provenzale JM, Morgenlander JC, Gress D: Spontaneous vertebral dissection: clinical, conventional angiographic, CT, and MR findings. J Comput Assist Tomogr 20:185, 1996

148. Quint DJ, Spickler EM: Magnetic resonance imaging demonstration of vertebral artery dissection: report of 2 cases. J Neurosurg 72:964, 1990

149. Ramadan F, Rutledge R, Oller D et al: Carotid artery trauma: a review of contemporary trauma center experiences. J Vasc Surg 21:46, 1995

149a. Ramadan NM, Tietjen GE, Levine SR, Welch KM: Scintillating scotomata associated with internal carotid artery dissection. Neurology 41:1084, 1991

150. Rao PM, Ivatury RR, Sharma P, et al: Cervical vascular injuries: a trauma center experience. Surgery 114:527, 1993

151. Ringel SP, Harrison SH, Norenberg MD et al: Fibromuscular dysplasia: multiple "spontaneous" dissecting aneurysms of the major cervical arteries. Ann Neurol 1:301, 1977

152. Rossillon R, Six C, Dardenne G: Dysplasie et dissection spontanée bilatérale des carotides internes: à propos d'un cas intérêt du traitement chirurgical. Acta Chir Belg 90:97, 1990

153. Rothrock JF, Lim V, Press G et al: Serial magnetic resonance and carotid duplex examinations in the management of carotid dissection. Neurology (NY) 39:686, 1989

154. Sanzone AG, Torres H, Doundoulakis SH: Blunt trauma to the carotid arteries. Am J Emerg Med 13:327, 1995

155. Sasaki O, Ogawa H, Koike T et al: A clinicopathologic

study of dissecting aneurysms of the intracranial vertebral artery. J Neurosurg 75:874, 1991

156. Saternus KS, Burtscheidt FG: Zur topographie der verletzungen der A vertebralis. p. 61. In Gutmann G (ed): Arteria Vertebralis. Springer-Verlag, Berlin, 1985

157. Saver JL, Easton JD, Hart RG: Dissections and trauma of cervicocerebral arteries. p. 67. In Barnett HJM, Mohr JP, Stein BM, Yatsu FM (eds): Stroke: Pathophysiology, Diagnosis and Management. 2nd ed. Churchill Livingstone, New York, 1992

158. Scherman BM, Tucker WS: Bilateral traumatic thrombosis of the internal carotid arteries in the neck: a case report with review of the literature. Neurosurgery 10:751, 1982

159. Schievink WI, Limburg M, Dorthuys JW et al: Cerebrovascular disease in Ehlers-Danlos syndrome type IV. Stroke 21:626, 1990

160. Schievink WI, Mokri B, O'Fallon M: Recurrent spontaneous cervical-artery dissection. New Engl J Med 330:393, 1994

161. Schievink WI, Mokri B, Piepgras DG: Spontaneous dissections of cervicocephalic arteries in childhood and adolescence. Neurology 44:1607, 1994

162. Schievink WI, Mokri B, Piepgras DG et al: Recurrent spontaneous arterial dissections: risk in familial versus nonfamilial disease. Stroke 27:622, 1996

163. Schievink WI, Mokri B, Whisnant JP: Internal carotid artery dissection in a community: Rochester, Minnesota, 1987–1992. Stroke 24:1678, 1993

164. Schievink WI, Piepgras DG, McCaffrey TV et al: Surgical treatment of extracranial internal carotid artery dissecting aneurysms. Neurosurgery 35:809, 1994

165. Schievink WI, Prakash UBS, Piepgras DG et al: α-Antitrypsin deficiency in intracranial aneurysms and cervical artery dissection. Lancet 343:452, 1994

166. Schulze H-E, Ebner A, Besinger UA: Report of dissection of the internal carotid artery in three cases. Neurosurg Rev 15:61, 1992

167. Sellier N, Chiras J, Benhamou M et al: Spontaneous dissection of the internal carotid artery: clinical, radiological and evolutive features: a study of 46 cases. J Neuroradiol 10:243, 1983

168. Senter HJ, Sarwar M: Nontraumatic dissecting aneurysm of the vertebral artery. J Neurosurg 56:128, 1982

169. Sherman DG, Hart RG, Easton JD: Abrupt change in head position and cerebral infarction. Stroke 12:2, 1981

170. Sherman MR, Smialek JE, Zane WE: Pathogenesis of vertebral artery occlusion following cervical spine manipulation. Arch Pathol Lab Med 111:851, 1987

171. Shimoji T, Bando K, Nakajima K et al: Dissecting aneurysm of the vertebral artery: report of seven cases and angiographic findings. J Neurosurg 61:1038, 1984

172. Shokumbi TN, Vinters HV, Kaufmann GCE: Fusiform intracranial aneurysms. Surg Neurol 29:263, 1988

173. Sinclair W Jr: Dissecting aneurysm of the middle cerebral artery associated with migraine syndrome. Am J Pathol 29:1083, 1953

174. Srinivasan J, Newell DW, Sturzenegger M et al: Transcranial Doppler in the evaluation of internal carotid artery dissection. Stroke 27:1226, 1996

175. Stanley JC, Fry WJ, Seeger JF et al: Extracranial internal carotid and vertebral artery fibrodysplasia. Arch Surg 109:215, 1974

176. Steinke W, Rautenberg W, Schwartz A et al: Noninvasive monitoring of internal carotid artery dissection. Stroke 25:998, 1994

177. Stringer WL, Kelly DL Jr: Traumatic dissection of the extracranial internal carotid artery. Neurosurgery 6:123, 1980

178. Sturzenegger M, Huber P: Cranial nerve palsies in spontaneous carotid artery dissection. J Neurol Neurosurg Psychiatry 56:1191, 1993

179. Sturzenegger M, Mattle HP, Rivoir A, Baumgartner RW: Ultrasound findings in carotid artery dissection: analysis of 43 patients. Neurology 45:691, 1995

180. Sturzenegger M, Mattle HP, Rivoir A et al: Ultrasound findings in spontaneous extracranial vertebral artery dissection. Stroke 24:1910, 1993

181. Sue DE, Brant-Zawadzki MN, Chance J: Dissection of cranial arteries in the neck: correlation of MRI and arteriography. Neuroradiology 34:273, 1992

182. Takis C, Saver JL: Cervicocephalic carotid and vertebral artery dissection: management. p. 385. In Batjer HH, Caplan LR, Friberg L et al (eds): Cerebrovascular Disease. Lippincott-Raven, Philadelphia, 1997

183. Thapedi IM, Ashenhurst EM, Rozdilsky B: Spontaneous dissecting aneurysm of the internal carotid artery in the neck. Arch Neurol 23:549, 1970

184. Tsukahara, T, Wada H, Satake K et al: Proximal balloon occlusion for dissecting vertebral aneurysms accompanied by subarachnoid hemorrhage. Neurosurgery 36:914, 1995

185. Waespe W, Niesper J, Imhof H-G, Valavanis A: Lower cranial nerve palsies due to internal carotid dissection. Stroke 19:1561, 1988

186. Watridge CB, Mulbauer MS, Lowery RD: Traumatic carotid artery dissection: diagnosis and treatment. J Neurosurg 71:854, 1989

187. West TET, Davies RJ, Kelly RE: Horner's syndrome and headache due to carotid artery disease. BMJ 1:818, 1976

188. Willis BK, Greiner F, Orrison WW et al: The incidence of vertebral artery injury after midcervical spine fracture or dislocation. Neurosurgery 34:435, 1994

189. Wirth FP, Miller WA, Russell AP: Atypical fibromuscular hyperplasia: report of two cases. J Neurosurg 54:685, 1981

190. Yamashita M, Tanaka K, Matsuo T et al: Cerebral dissecting aneurysms in patients with moyamoya disease. J Neurosurg 58:120, 1983

191. Yonas H, Agamanolis D, Takaoka Y et al: Dissecting intracranial aneurysms. Surg Neurol 8:407, 1977

192. Youl BD, Coutellier A, Dubois B et al: Three cases of spontaneous extracranial vertebral artery dissection. Stroke 21:618, 1990

193. Zelenock GB, Kasmers A, Whitehouse WM Jr et al: Extracranial internal carotid artery dissections. Arch Surg 117:425, 1982

194. Zuber M, Meary E, Meder J-F, Mas J-L: Magnetic resonance imaging and dynamic CT scan in cervical artery dissections. Stroke 25:576, 1994

CHAPTER 30

Stroke in the Setting of Collagen Vascular Disease

GEORGE W. PETTY

J.P. MOHR

Giant Cell Arteritis

Giant cell arteritis, also known as temporal arteritis, cranial arteritis, or Horton's disease, is an inflammatory disease that affects the medium- and large-sized arteries throughout the body, including the aorta and most of its major branches. Inflammation of the arteries of the head and neck is responsible for the major neurologic symptoms of headache and visual loss. Stroke, although uncommon, is a well-documented and potentially fatal complication.

INCIDENCE

Giant cell arteritis is not a rare disease. The age- and sex-adjusted incidence of giant cell arteritis per 100,000 population, age 50 years or older, in Olmsted County, Minnesota, from 1950 to 1985, was 17.0.[292] There is a dramatic increase in incidence with age. The incidence in Olmsted County was only 2.6 per 100,000 for those in the 50- to 59-year age group, but this increased to 44.6 per 100,000 in those older than age 80 years.[292] There is a threefold greater incidence in women than in men.[292] The incidence of giant cell arteritis may be up to 7 times higher among whites than among blacks,[422] possibly related to the lower frequency of HLA-DR4 (D-related human leukocyte antigen) among blacks than whites.[285] The incidence of giant cell arteritis increased with time in the Olmsted County study, a phenomenon attributed in part to increased awareness on the part of clinicians of the disease and its varied manifestations.[292]

PATHOLOGY

Giant cell arteritis primarily affects the medium and large elastic arteries, sparing the capillaries and veins. Although involvement of the temporal arteries is emphasized in clinical descriptions, the aorta and its branches are commonly involved as well;[279,292,345] in one study, 34 of 248 patients had evidence of large artery involvement.[256] The arterial wall is infiltrated with mononuclear cells (lymphocytes and plasma cells) and, to a lesser extent, with eosinophils and neutrophils predominantly in the media near the internal elastic lamina. Granulomas composed of multinucleated or foreign-body giant cells are found along with the inflammatory cells, but are not invariably present. The vessel may be necrotic in areas, especially in the media. Fibrinoid necrosis usually is not present.[87,212,379] Intimal proliferation and fibrosis may result in lumen narrowing and thrombosis. The exact mechanism of thrombosis in temporal arteritis is uncertain. Anticardiolipin antibodies are detected in some patients with giant cell arteritis and may predict more severe vascular complications.[67]

The etiology of giant cell arteritis is unknown, but there is evidence that immunologic mechanisms are involved. Park et al[350] and Papaioannou et al[349] demonstrated circulating immune complexes in the sera of patients with biopsy-proven giant cell arteritis. Immunoglobulin has been found deposited in the temporal arteries.[44,71,276,350] Several studies have demonstrated an increased frequency of certain histocompatibility antigens, including HLA-B8 and HLA-DR4, among patients with giant cell arteritis,[17,57,191] although others have not.[214] Machado et al[292] noted that the highest incidence rates have been reported from regions with similar ethnic backgrounds: northern Europe and Minnesota.[31,40] Familial and conjugal cases have been reported.[140,442]

787

GENERAL CLINICAL FEATURES

If not known for any other feature, giant cell arteritis would be recognized for the wide variety of syndromes it produces. Headache is the most common presentation in most series.[156,178,191,193,216,233] It is usually constant, said to be especially common at night, and interferes with sleep. The headache is located predominantly in the temporal area, but it may radiate to the scalp, face, jaw, or occiput.[119,178,311] Scalp tenderness is a frequent complaint, and many patients—but by no means all—have swollen, nodular, or pulseless temporal arteries.[191,217,391] Some patients may have jaw claudication.[205] Other prominent symptoms include fever, weight loss, fatigue, and malaise. Many patients have arthralgias, but frank arthritis is uncommon.[178] Dementia, confusion, and psychiatric symptoms, such as depression, have been reported.[61,156,460]

Polymyalgia rheumatica is a syndrome of limb girdle muscle pain and stiffness accompanied by systemic symptoms, including malaise, fever, weight loss, anorexia, and depression. Most patients with giant cell arteritis have symptoms of polymyalgia rheumatica for weeks to months before headache, jaw claudication, or visual loss develop.[3,32,119,217,346] Jones and Hazleman[234] found that 44% of patients who present with polymyalgia rheumatica alone develop overt giant cell arteritis, and 23% develop serious ophthalmologic or neurologic complications, such as visual loss, ophthalmoplegia, or stroke. Alestig and Barr,[3] Bengtsson and Malmvall,[31] and Fauchald et al[119] demonstrated that patients with the clinical diagnosis of polymyalgia rheumatica frequently have giant cell arteritis on temporal artery biopsy. These findings support the notion that polymyalgia rheumatica and giant cell arteritis are not two distinct nosologic entities but rather "facets of a common disease spectrum."[454]

OPHTHALMOLOGIC COMPLICATIONS

Visual loss is the most feared complication of giant cell arteritis. Anterior ischemic optic neuropathy is the most common cause of visual loss in giant cell arteritis. It is a result of thrombosis of the involved posterior ciliary arteries.[31,192,202] Posterior ischemic optic neuropathy and central retinal artery occlusion also may cause visual loss in giant cell arteritis, but less frequently than does anterior ischemic optic neuropathy.[31,41,59,76,83,202] Homonymous hemianopia and cortical blindness may occur as a result of posterior circulation infarction (see below). Once established, the visual loss caused by giant cell arteritis rarely improves, despite treatment with corticosteroids.[192,202,233]

Large series report visual loss in 40% to 50% of patients with giant cell arteritis.[163,178,202,217,391] Hollenhorst et al[202] noted loss of vision within 2 to 3 months of onset of giant cell arteritis symptoms in one-third of patients, and all of the remainder destined to have this symptom suffered loss of vision within 10 months after the onset of other symptoms.

Visual loss typically occurs suddenly, although 10% to 20% of patients with giant cell arteritis experience transient loss of vision (transient monocular blindness, amaurosis fugax) before fixed visual deficits develop.[61,202,217,233,391] It is usually monocular, but bilateral involvement occurred in 33% of patients with visual loss reported by Jonasson et al.[233] Visual loss in the second eye occurred simultaneously or within 24 hours after visual loss in the first eye in 36% of these patients, between the 2nd and 7th day in 36%, and between 1 week and 1 month in the remainder. Monocular or binocular positive visual phenomena ("scintillating scotoma") have been reported.[61]

Visual acuity is usually reduced to hand motion or light perception, and most patients have reduced color perception. The disc is swollen and usually pale, flame hemorrhages may be seen, and disc atrophy subsequently develops. Afferent pupillary defects are common. Field defects are usually altitudinal and inferior, although inferior nasal defects, arcuate defects, and scotomas may be seen.[192,315,470]

Diplopia or ophthalmoplegia, usually transient, occurs in 10% to 15% of patients with giant cell arteritis.[163,202,217,311,391] Hollenhorst et al[202] reported that weakness of an extraocular muscle was demonstrable in only 10 of 22 patients who had complained of double vision; the 10 diplopic patients eventually lost vision in one or both eyes, and 2 others had amaurosis fugax. Dimant et al[100] found that 7 of 14 patients with biopsy-proven giant cell arteritis had ophthalmoplegia on examination, but only 1 complained of diplopia. Only one of their patients had a pattern of ophthalmoplegia that was compatible with a single nerve lesion (cranial nerve III). The other patients had patterns of ophthalmoplegia that did not conform to a lesion of a single nerve. Impairment of upward gaze was common.[100] Large clinical series have indicated that cranial nerve III palsies and cranial nerve VI palsies occur with roughly equal frequency in patients with giant cell arteritis.[163,311,391] Meadows[311] noted that, in his patients with ophthalmoplegias conforming to cranial nerve III paresis, the pupils were spared.

In reviewing the subject of ophthalmoplegia in giant cell arteritis, Fisher[129] noted that ptosis was common and that ophthalmoplegia may be the only neurologic complication in some patients with the disease. He suggested that ophthalmoplegia in giant cell arteritis is caused by damage to the nerves supplying the extraocular muscles, a view shared by others[311] and supported by reports of oculomotor synkinesis[417] and tonic pupil[89] in the condition. However, in an autopsy study of a patient with giant cell arteritis and bilateral ophthalmoplegia, Barricks et al,[27] who documented ischemic necrosis of the extraocular muscles, could find no lesion in the nerves to these muscles. They concluded that extraocular muscle ischemia, as opposed to nerve ischemia, is the mechanism of ophthalmoplegia in giant cell arteritis. Giant cell arteritis may also cause "orbital infarction syndrome," in which orbital pain, blindness, ophthalmoplegia, and anterior and posterior segment ischemia occur as a result of global orbital ischemia.[47]

STROKE IN GIANT CELL ARTERITIS

Stroke is an uncommon but potentially lethal complication of giant cell arteritis.[54,59,70,83,85,115,150,166,180,181,195,206,227,241,260,279,301,312,344–346,391,412,428,445,469,481,484] Although epidemiologic studies have not demonstrated an increased incidence of stroke among patients with giant cell arteritis,[32,217,233] studies from referral centers suggest that patients with giant cell arteritis may be at higher risk for stroke during the active phase of their disease. Paulley and Hughes[355] reported that 8 of 76 patients with giant cell arteritis presented with stroke. Graham[163] found that, of the 8 patients who died within 6 weeks of diagnosis of giant cell arteritis, 4 had stroke.

Stroke caused by giant cell arteritis may occur as the first indication of the disease. In several well-documented autopsy-proven cases, stroke occurred on presentation, without known prior symptoms of giant cell arteritis.[42,78,344,398,484] Usually, however, the more easily recognized other symptoms, such as fever, weight loss, headache, and visual disturbance, precede giant cell arteritis–related stroke for periods of weeks to months.[147,195,398,481,484] The erythrocyte sedimentation rate (ESR) is usually increased in patients with stroke caused by giant cell arteritis, but temporal artery examination and biopsy results may be normal.[206] It is worrisome that several patients had strokes despite therapy with corticosteroids,[54,147,195,398,445,484] sometimes within 2 weeks of initiation of treatment, and some have had stroke despite normalization of the ESR.[484]

Stroke in patients with giant cell arteritis may occur in the carotid or vertebrobasilar circulation. Postmortem examination in such patients most often documents giant cell arteritis involving the extradural segments of the vessels only (Fig. 30.1),[42,78,150,195,206,346,398,481,484] although some have had evi-

Figure 30.1 Pattern of involvement of giant cell arteritis in head and neck arteries. Note high incidence of involvement of vertebral artery (V), superior temporal artery (ST), ophthalmic artery (O), and posterior ciliary artery (PC). Intracranial arteries are rarely involved. CR, central retinal artery; EC, external carotid artery; IC, internal carotid artery. (From Wilkinson and Russell,[484] with permission.)

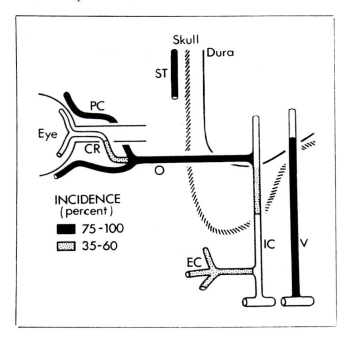

dence of intradural involvement as well.[147,169,226,254,317,322,398,445,460]

In a brief report of a necropsy series, Missen[317] noted that obstruction of the arterial lumen due to giant cell arteritis was "3 times as frequent in the vertebral arteries as in the internal carotids" and that "infarction was found more often in the hind-brain than in the forebrain." In the series by Graham,[163] the four patients who died with stroke soon after the diagnosis of giant cell arteritis all had brain-stem infarction. In autopsy-proven cases of posterior circulation infarction caused by giant cell arteritis, the mechanism of stroke is arteritic involvement of the vertebral arteries with thrombosis and secondary infarction (frequently multifocal) in the vertebrobasilar territory due to local propagation of thrombus[195,484] or artery-to-artery embolus.[195,484]

Clinical syndromes may include unilateral or bilateral occipital infarction, sometimes with top-of-the-basilar syndrome or cortical blindness from embolic occlusion of the distal basilar artery or posterior cerebral arteries.[54,195,481,484] Others have had progressive and fatal infarction of the lower brain stem,[398,484] sometimes heralded by initial development of a lateral medullary syndrome (Wallenberg).[78]

Thrombotic occlusion due to arteritis in the internal carotid arteries, sometimes bilateral,[150,206] has also been described in several autopsy-proven cases.[54,484] In each, the thrombus was found distal to the bifurcation. Sometimes the involved cavernous segments are completely occluded by thrombus, resulting in border zone "distal field" infarction.[150,484] Others have had artery-to-artery embolism with hemorrhagic infarction[54] in the corresponding intracranial arterial territories. Bogousslavsky et al[42] reported a case of giant cell arteritis with bilateral internal carotid artery siphon stenosis "related to internal hypertrophy and fibrosis, with infiltration of the media and elastic layer with lymphocytes and many giant cells" associated with infarction in the brain stem without arteritic involvement or thrombosis of the vertebral arteries. They postulated a steal phenomenon as a mechanism.

Pollack et al[366] reported a case of subclavian steal associated with narrowing of a subclavian artery caused by giant cell arteritis. Giant cell arteritis in the ascending aorta can cause mural thrombus, which may result in cerebral embolism.[344] Similarly, giant cell arteritis involving the coronary arteries can result in myocardial infarction, ventricular mural thrombus formation, and brain embolism.[428]

Involvement of intracranial (intradural) vessels by giant cell arteritis is rare. In a detailed autopsy study of the pattern of arterial involvement in four patients with giant cell arteritis, Wilkinson and Russell[484] found that the vertebral arteries and the petrous and cavernous portions of the internal carotid arteries were consistently involved, but the abnormalities consistently ended at or just beyond the point of penetration of the dura, and intradural vessels were not involved (Fig. 30.1). In a brief report of 23 necropsy cases, Missen[317] found that the intracerebral vessels were involved by giant cell arteritis "infrequently," whereas involvement of the vertebral and carotid arteries was "virtually constant."

There are, however, a few autopsy cases that describe giant cell arteritis in the intracranial as well as extracranial vessels.[147,169,226,254,322,378,398,445,460] Gibb et al[147] reported on a 76-year-old man who developed basilar artery thrombosis after presenting with spinal cord infarction. Autopsy demonstrated infarction of the midbrain and pontine tegmentum. The basilar artery "showed damage and reduplication of the internal elastic lamina and a segment of adventitia with chronic inflammatory cell infiltration" and thrombosis near its origin. A paramedian branch of the basilar artery was also said to have been involved. Thystrup et al[445] found arteritis involving the basilar artery in a patient with temporal arteritis and bilateral occipital infarcts. Other cases are atypical in certain respects. In the cases reported by Kjeldsen and Reske-Nielsen[254] and Ritama,[378] involvement of venules was described, which is atypical for giant cell arteritis and is more often seen with granulomatous angiitis of the central nervous system (see below). In cases 1 and 2 from Jellinger,[226] visceral involvement appeared to be extensive.

Reports of giant cell arteritis confined to the intracranial vessels seem especially rare. The cases reported by Enzmann and Scott,[115] Hinck et al,[199] Hirsch et al,[200] and McCormick and Neuberger,[308] and cases 3, 4, and 5 from Jellinger[226] may represent cases of isolated angiitis of the central nervous system. Reports of giant cell arteritis causing multiple intracranial aneurysms may actually be cases of Takayasu's disease or other as yet uncharacterized disease.[262,314]

DIAGNOSIS

The most common laboratory abnormality in patients with giant cell arteritis is a markedly increased ESR. However, a normal ESR does not exclude the diagnosis.[243,491] Most patients have a mild to moderate normochromic or slightly hypochromic anemia. White blood cell counts are normal or moderately increased.[178,191,202,391] Mild abnormalities of liver enzymes have been reported.[98,174]

Temporal artery biopsy is the most helpful diagnostic procedure.[177] Biopsy is recommended for all patients in whom giant cell arteritis is strongly suspected to avoid management dilemmas if patients relapse or complications develop while they are receiving steroid therapy.[176] Yet the segmental nature of the disease means that a normal temporal artery biopsy does not exclude the diagnosis of giant cell arteritis.[255] In one series of biopsy-proven cases, 86% were diagnosed by unilateral biopsy and the remaining 14% diagnosed only after biopsy of the second side.[176] Other types of vasculitis rarely may cause inflammation of the temporal arteries and mimic the disease.[179,321]

Angiographic signs are infrequently present, but the superficial temporal arteriogram may demonstrate areas of dilation and constriction along the length of the artery,[109,149,211] and changes may also be seen in the internal carotid artery siphon segments.[464] Angiographic abnormalities of intracranial arteries are rare and possibly represent cases of isolated granulomatous angiitis of the central nervous system.[115,199,200] Angiographic findings may be nonspecific, and arteriography offers no diagnostic advantage over the simple procedure of temporal artery biopsy.[217]

TREATMENT AND PROGNOSIS

Once the diagnosis of giant cell arteritis is suspected, the patient should be started on steroid therapy, and a temporal artery biopsy should be done as soon as possible. An initial dosage of 40 to 60 mg/day of prednisone is recommended for the first month or until symptoms of the disease are controlled.[216] Symptoms usually respond promptly to steroids, although visual loss and stroke may occur after the initiation of treatment. Steroids may be tapered while monitoring symptoms and the ESR.[216] There is controversy over the duration of therapy. Rapid tapering is thought to lead to relapse more often than slow tapering. Recurrence of symptoms or increase of the ESR after initial control of the disease indicates relapse and should prompt resumption of higher doses of steroids. Relapse after withdrawal from steroids may not necessarily be accompanied by an increase in ESR, however.[468] In one series, the mean duration of steroid therapy was 5.8 years, 12.8 years being the maximum.[15] The relapse rate after withdrawal of treatment was 47%, 46% of these occurring within 1 month and 96% within 1 year after cessation of treatment. The relapse rate after withdrawal of steroid therapy bore little relationship to the duration of treatment.[15] Alternate-day treatment regimens are thought to be less effective than daily administration of steroids.[213] Some have advocated hospitalization and treatment with high-dose, pulsed intravenous administration of methylprednisolone for patients with acute visual loss.[385]

Giant cell arteritis may cause death by stroke, myocardial infarction, or aortic rupture.[33,279,398] Epidemiologic studies and large clinical series, however, have not demonstrated that patients with giant cell arteritis have decreased survival.[31,191,233]

Isolated Granulomatous Angiitis of the Central Nervous System

Isolated granulomatous angiitis of the central nervous system is an inflammatory arterial disease restricted to the cerebral circulation.[34,37,46,51,52,55,56,60,64,65,72,82,86,88,107,115,118,122, 124,134, 151,154,170, 183,189,199,200, 209,224,226,228, 240,242,258,259, 263,278,288,303, 308,319,327,332,338,343,356,363,367,372,376,392–394,401,405,408,411,416, 456–458,463,467,494,496,498] Unlike giant cell arteritis, isolated granulomatous angiitis of the central nervous system afflicts patients of any age, is characterized by neurologic disease out of proportion to systemic illness, preferentially involves smaller arteries and veins, and responds poorly or not at all to steroids alone.

PATHOLOGY

Like giant cell arteritis, the pathologic process is segmental. Any of the vessels of the brain and spinal cord may be involved, but most reports have noted a predilection for the small leptomeningeal vessels. The precapillary arterioles are most often affected. Some reports, however, have noted a predominance of venular involvement.[51,258] Occasionally the process may be quite focal, involving only one vessel or group of vessels.[35,303,416,496] The inflammatory infiltrate is composed of lymphocytes, plasma cells, granulomas with multinucleated giant cells, and occasionally neutrophils and eosinophils.[86,88] These infiltrates may involve any portion of the vessel wall. Some have noted more inflammation in the intima and adventitia than in the media.[51,82] Occasionally, thrombosis of larger intracranial arteries (internal carotid artery siphon, anterior cerebral, middle cerebral, posterior cerebral, basilar) is found.[18,303,327] Small aneurysms have also been reported.[199,394,416]

The etiology of granulomatous angiitis of the central nervous system is unknown. The available evidence suggests that an infectious agent or an immunologic mechanism may be involved. A necrotizing angiitis of the central nervous system has been observed in brains of turkeys infected with *Mycoplasma gallisepticum*.[73,444] "Virus-like" and "mycoplasma-like" particles in the brain and vascular lesions have been identified by electron microscopy, but no organisms have been cultured.[18,376] Other cases have been reported in association with Hodgkin's lymphoma, acquired immunodeficiency syndrome (AIDS), primary intracerebral lymphoma, varicella encephalitis, leukemia, sarcoid, cerebral amyloid angiopathy, or following varicella zoster infection, including herpes zoster ophthalmicus.[39,46,58,131,148,165,167,219,228,266,275,283,295,299,343,369,371,383,384,386,421,462,494,498] In one report of isolated angiitis of the nervous system in association with cerebral amyloid angiopathy, the giant cells contained congophilic material immunoreactive for the Alzheimer A4 peptide, leading the authors to speculate that the disease may be due to a foreign body reaction to A4 amyloid deposition in some patients.[165] The frequent association with another underlying disease and the pathologic heterogeneity of the lesions have led some to conclude that isolated angiitis of the central nervous system is a "nonspecific reaction, not a unique disease."[498]

CLINICAL AND PATHOLOGIC FEATURES AND AUTOPSY FINDINGS

Despite the hope authors usually entertain to present readers with a dependable "formula" for safely arriving at the diagnosis of the disease in question, examination of numerous histopathologically proven cases of isolated granulomatous angiitis of the central nervous system reveals a discouragingly heterogeneous profile of clinical and diagnostic features with few reliable clues to the diagnosis short of brain biopsy or autopsy.[14,18,37,51,52,55,60,64,65,82,118,122,134,154,189,199,209,224,226,229,240,258,259,278,303,308,327,338,367,372,374,376,392,394,416,456,467,496,498,500]

Patients range in age from 3 years to 96 years. The duration of illness is quite variable. Death may occur within days after presentation in some patients,[327] whereas others have indolent[229,367,500] or benign[34,35] courses lasting for years.

Headache, nausea, vomiting, dementia, amnesic states, disorientation, confusion, somnolence, encephalopathy, or coma occurs early in the course of the disease in many patients. Sometimes the initial presentation may be that of brain tumor. Systemic symptoms, such as fever and weight loss, are uncommon.

Multifocal neurologic symptoms and signs develop in a stepwise progression, with episodes of quantitative and qualitative worsening, usually occurring after variable periods of stabilization (days, weeks, months, or sometimes years). Seizures are common. Ischemic or hemorrhagic stroke (or transient ischemic attack) is a presentation in only a minority of cases.[37,52,259,327,416,467] Many patients develop hemiplegia or extensor plantar responses, and some patients have spinal cord involvement (either alone or in association with brain involvement), including progressive or acute myelopathy with incontinence and paraplegia.[55,154,219,278] Papilledema is common.

The ESR is usually not increased, and when abnormal, it is not as high as in giant cell arteritis. Blood cell counts, electrolytes, and serologic tests for collagen vascular disease are usually normal.

The most consistent spinal fluid abnormality is an increase in protein (frequently over 100 mg/dl), although occasionally spinal fluid may be normal. Increased immunoglobulin values are occasionally reported. Varying numbers of red cells are frequently present. Opening pressure is increased in some but normal in others. Many patients have a moderate lymphocytic pleocytosis (usually less than 150 cells/μl). Isolated angiitis of the central nervous system may therefore appear at presentation as "chronic meningitis."[14,374]

Computed tomography (CT) scan findings may be remarkably heterogeneous, including single or multiple infarcts, single or multiple hemorrhages, tumor with mass effect, tumor with hemorrhage, ring-enhancing lesions suggestive of abscess, and multiple areas of increased attenuation with surrounding decreased attenuation suggestive of multiple metastatic lesions. Brain magnetic resonance (MR) findings are equally heterogeneous and nonspecific for the diagnosis of isolated angiitis of the central nervous system and may include any combination of the following: multiple and bilateral white and gray matter infarcts, either sweeping and confluent or multiple and small white matter lesions with increased signal on T_2-weighted images, diffuse nodular gadolinium enhancement, intraparenchymal hemorrhage, or gadolinium enhancement of the meninges with little or no change in the brain parenchyma.[60,107,168,330] Some of these abnormalities may mimic multiple sclerosis, central nervous system lymphoma, or retinocochleocerebral vasculopathy. Cerebral angiographic results are usually abnormal, with alternating segments of concentric arterial narrowing and dilatation (beading). However, patients may have normal cerebral angiograms at some time during their course.

Autopsy examination of visceral structures is usually normal but rarely may reveal small discrete foci of angiitis.[18,52,64,65,134,374] The most common neuropathologic finding is multiple small foci of infarction, followed by multiple foci of hemorrhage ("brain purpura," "petechiae"). Large infarcts[37,51,52,258,259,327,394] and, less often, large confluent intraparenchymal hemorrhages[37,65,118] may be present. Large- or medium-vessel arterial occlusion by thrombus is uncommon.[18,303,327] Subarachnoid blood[65,394,398,416] and small aneurysms[199,394,496] are encountered rarely. Herniation (uncal or cerebellar) may occur secondary to massive edema or hemorrhage.

DIAGNOSIS

None of the standard laboratory tests are diagnostic for granulomatous angiitis, and normal findings do not exclude the diagnosis. Angiograms, in particular, may be normal;[408] a pattern of alternating dilation and constriction ("beading") is a non-specific sign that may be seen in various vasculitides (including those due to sarcoid, infection, and amphetamine-like drugs) and other noninflammatory conditions (such as intracranial atherosclerosis, especially in diabetic patients).[127,146,215, 269,389,425,426,441] Laboratory tests may include blood cultures, spinal fluid cultures, viral titers (including human immunodeficiency virus), serologic tests for syphilis, drug or toxicology screens, coagulation studies (prothrombin time, partial thromboplastin time, lupus anticoagulant), anticardiolipin antibodies, antinuclear antibodies, rheumatoid factor, complement, cryoglobulins, immunofixation electrophoresis, and antineutrophil cytoplasmic autoantibodies (polyarteritis nodosa, Wegener's granulomatosis). Diagnostic studies or biopsies to exclude sarcoid, lymphoma, or systemic vasculitis should be performed as indicated. Brain biopsy usually is necessary to distinguish among tumor (especially lymphoma or intravascular malignant lymphomatosis),[450] infection, and vasculitis. Because isolated granulomatous angiitis of the central nervous system has a predilection for leptomeningeal vessels, the procedure should include a leptomeningeal biopsy as well as a parenchymal biopsy. However, even these efforts are occasionally unrewarded: the biopsy has been negative in several subsequently autopsy-proven cases.[51,64,189,199,209,498]

TREATMENT

There is no standard treatment. Progression of the disease and death have frequently occurred despite treatment with high-dose steroids.[18,189,226] Remissions have been reported using a combination of prednisone and cyclophosphamide.[88,319] In one patient with Hodgkin's disease, stabilization of granulomatous angiitis of the central nervous system occurred after treatment of the lymphoma.[167]

Takayasu's Arteritis

Takayasu's arteritis (pulseless disease, idiopathic aortitis) is a large-vessel granulomatous arteritis that affects the aorta, its main branches, and occasionally the pulmonary artery. Although pathologic changes in the arteries are similar to those found in giant cell arteritis,[329] Takayasu's arteritis tends to affect younger people, particularly women. Most cases have been reported from Asia, but the disease is found worldwide.[175] Like giant cell arteritis, constitutional symptoms (malaise, weight loss, fever) and increased ESR are common.[175] Symptoms of arm claudication and syncope occur more frequently than retinal or cerebral ischemia.[175] Brachial pressures and pulses are frequently asymmetric, and there may be asymmetry between pressures in the arms and legs.[175]

Cerebrovascular complications occur in patients with more advanced disease, particularly in patients with retinopathy, hypertension secondary to renal artery stenosis, aortic regurgitation, and aortic aneurysms.[223] Cerebral infarction and retinal ischemia may occur consequent to stenosis or occlusion of the carotid or vertebral arteries, but the intracranial

arteries are rarely, if ever, involved.[329] Subclavian steal may also occur, but this physiologic phenomenon is not always accompanied by symptoms of vertebrobasilar ischemia.[495] Intracerebral hemorrhage is usually related to hypertension.[222,465] Aneurysmal subarachnoid hemorrhage has been reported, although this could be a chance association in some cases. In one case, subarachnoid hemorrhage was attributed to an aneurysm of the distal intracranial segment of one of the vertebral arteries.[307]

Treatment may include corticosteroids, cytotoxic agents (cyclophosphamide), surgery, or a combination of these modalities.[411] Regression of carotid stenosis has been reported after administration of corticosteroids.[223] Various surgical reconstructive and bypass procedures have been used[136,152,380,493] with apparent success in some patients, although postsurgical anastomotic stenoses may occur.[152] Some have advised delaying operation until after the inflammatory process can be controlled with corticosteroids,[175] while others have not found this to be problematic.[411] Some patients acquire unusual anastomotic vascular collateral patterns even without surgery, including collaterals from the right coronary artery to both vertebral arteries and the left internal carotid arteries.[306]

Herpes Zoster Ophthalmicus and Delayed Contralateral Hemiparesis

A small number of patients with herpes zoster involving the first division of the trigeminal nerve (herpes zoster ophthalmicus) subsequently develop contralateral hemiparesis weeks to months later.[446] The onset of hemiparesis may be acute and indistinguishable from stroke syndromes caused by more conventional mechanisms, although some patients have more global mental status changes that suggest an underlying meningoencephalitic process.[141,198] Occasionally, the hemiparesis may progress or may recur after a period of improvement.[198] Central retinal artery occlusion,[487] optic neuritis,[92] and orbital pseudotumor syndrome[275] have been reported. Spinal fluid examination may disclose a mild to moderate pleocytosis and increased protein.[198]

CT scans have demonstrated large infarctions ipsilateral to the involved trigeminal nerve, most often in the lenticulostriate territory of the middle cerebral artery, involving the capsule, striatum, and corona radiata.[198,264,459] Cerebral angiography (including MR angiography) may be normal or document segmental narrowing or occlusion in the ipsilateral supraclinoid internal carotid artery siphon segment, middle cerebral artery M1 segment, anterior cerebral artery A1 segment, and anterior cerebral artery A2 segment beneath the genu of the corpus callosum (pericallosal).[48,137,196,198, 293,395] On rare occasions, the ipsilateral posterior cerebral artery P1 segment and contralateral anterior cerebral artery A1 segment have been involved.[48,196,395] Mycotic aneurysms and subarachnoid hemorrhage have been reported.[339] One patient developed aneurysmal dilatation of the intrapetrosal segment of the left internal carotid artery associated with ipsilateral Horner's syndrome, hearing loss, and ear pain.[162] The predilection for involvement of the ipsilateral intracerebral arteries at the base of the brain has led some to suggest that the process may be due to viral spread to the involved arteries by route of the intracranial branches of the ophthalmic division of the trigeminal nerve,[294] but the exact pathogenesis remains unproved.[304]

Postmortem examinations have often documented cerebral infarction in the ipsilateral carotid or middle cerebral artery territory secondary to a necrotizing (not granulomatous) arteritis with or without thrombosis,[102,141,198] although diffuse granulomatous angiitis of the central nervous system may follow herpes zoster ophthalmicus as well.[275] One report has documented an occlusive thrombotic vasculopathy without frank vasculitis.[108] One patient had cerebellar infarction ipsilateral to the involved trigeminal nerve, with a mild mononuclear infiltrate documented in the adventitia of the thrombosed superior cerebellar artery.[128] Large hematomas were found in the two cases reported by Mackenzie et al.[294] Swelling and lymphocytic infiltration of the ipsilateral trigeminal ganglion and nerve trunk have also been noted.[102,141,294] Herpes-like virions have been identified in middle cerebral artery smooth muscle.[102]

Therapy has included corticosteroids, acyclovir, and anticoagulants,[102,198,293] although recovery without treatment has been reported.

Polyarteritis Nodosa

Polyarteritis nodosa is a necrotizing angiitis of the medium to small muscular arteries throughout the body. The peripheral nervous system is more commonly involved than the central nervous system, but in the series by Ford and Siekert,[130] 46% of patients had symptoms and signs referable to the central nervous system. Central nervous system complications tend to occur late in the course of the disease in the setting of renal failure, fever, and other systemic manifestations, and central nervous systemic involvement is not an independent predictor of death.[130,171] Diffuse or multifocal cerebral syndromes, such as headache, confusion, psychiatric syndromes, dementia, lymphocytic meningitis,[184] and generalized or focal seizures are more frequent than stroke. However, 13% of the patients in the series by Ford and Siekert[130] had cerebral infarction or hemorrhage. Cerebral angiography in patients with central nervous system manifestations may demonstrate multiple saccular-shaped aneurysms, similar to those visualized on visceral angiography.[29,449]

Necropsy has demonstrated the necrotizing vasculitic changes in large cerebral arteries (internal carotid, middle cerebral, posterior cerebral),[63,248,351,352] small meningeal arteries,[66,248,297,351,352] or both.[351,352] The size of the associated cerebral infarctions in these cases paralleled the size of the artery involved. In a particularly detailed study presented by Castaigne et al,[63] arteritic involvement of one of the vertebral arteries resulted in thrombosis and infarction in the brain stem and cerebellum. Subarachnoid hemorrhage has been reported,[29] and in one instance necropsy demonstrated massive subarachnoid hemorrhage in the region of the anterior cerebral and anterior communicating artery, with dissection into

the frontal lobe and rupture into the ventricular system.[145] A fusiform arteriosclerotic aneurysm of the anterior communicating artery was noted, but this was not the site of hemorrhage. Instead, the bleeding had emanated from a "longitudinal tear" in an arteritically involved segment of the right anterior cerebral artery.[145] Necropsy-proven cases of cerebral infarction associated with necrotizing arteritis of the cerebral arteries have been reported in the setting of polyarteritis nodosa associated with hepatitis B antigenemia.[410] The spinal cord may also be involved.[173,342]

Diagnostic studies in patients suspected of having polyarteritis nodosa should include serologic tests for hepatitis B and antineutrophil cytoplasmic autoantibody (ANCA) and may include visceral or cerebral angiography[449] or biopsy of an organ system suspected of involvement.[77] Treatment consists of corticosteroids and cyclophosphamide.[121,270] Infantile polyarteritis nodosa, a disease thought to be distinct from the adult form and possibly related to Kawasaki's disease, may cause stroke (infarction, aneurysmal subarachnoid hemorrhage) in children.[113]

Wegener's Granulomatosis

Wegener's granulomatosis is a necrotizing granulomatous vasculitis involving the upper and lower respiratory tract and other organ systems in association with glomerulonephritis.[120] Nervous system complications include peripheral neuropathy and mononeuritis multiplex,[13,103] central nervous system infection,[13] local invasion by destructive granulomatous lesions causing cranial nerve palsies,[13,103,407] and central nervous system vasculitis.[13,103,313,397] Necrotizing granulomatous meningitis with leptomeningeal vasculitis may produce predominantly meningeal and encephalopathic syndromes or multiple cranial neuropathies, sometimes with prominent meningeal enhancement and confluent bifrontal white matter increased T_2-signal abnormalities on brain MR imaging.[331,335,447,477] Pathologically proven cerebrovascular complications have included infarction, hemorrhage (including subarachnoid hemorrhage), and cerebral venous thrombosis.[103,112,135,287,290,313,397,453] These complications typically occur in the setting of well-established extracranial disease, although stroke may rarely be the presenting manifestation of the disease.[334] In one autopsied case reported by Drachman,[103] interhemispheric subarachnoid hemorrhage and cerebral infarction in the distribution of the anterior cerebral artery occurred consequent to panarteritic involvement of this artery. Lucas et al[287] reported a patient who died of caudate hemorrhage with intraventricular rupture. At postmortem examination the hemorrhage appeared to originate from vessels affected by necrotizing vasculitis. The case reported by Satoh et al[397] was a 67-year-old man who developed a clinical syndrome consistent with bifrontal infarction. At autopsy, the medium to large branches of the anterior cerebral artery were thrombosed and fibrinoid necrosis was noted. Necrotizing vasculitis and granulomatous lesions were present in the small arteries and veins in the frontal areas of the base of the brain where a suppurative meningitis was also noted. Necrotizing cerebral thrombophlebitis accounted for cortical vein thrombosis in the patient reported by Mickle et al.[313] Cavernous sinus invasion may occur, and internal carotid artery occlusion has been documented in one such case.[155]

The presence of antineutrophil cytoplasmic autoantibodies (ACPA, ANCA) may facilitate diagnosis of Wegener's granulomatosis.[427] Central nervous system complications may have become less frequent with the advent of protocols combining cyclophosphamide and corticosteroids, which appear to be more effective than corticosteroids alone.[69,120]

Occasional reports of amaurosis fugax, ischemic optic neuropathy,[479] subarachnoid hemorrhage,[274] and stroke-like syndromes[488] have been reported in patients with various forms of necrotizing "allergic" angiitis. In one patient, subarachnoid hemorrhage was caused by vasculitis involving the choroid plexus documented at autopsy.[69]

Lymphomatoid Granulomatosis

Lymphomatoid granulomatosis is an "angiocentric and angiodestructive lymphoreticular proliferative and granulomatous disease" that primarily involves the lungs and may involve the central nervous system in approximately 20% of cases.[282] The disease may mimic Wegener's granulomatosis,[281] and sometimes progression to lymphoma has occurred.[282] Clinical manifestations of central nervous system involvement usually consist of subacute, progressive syndromes of focal brain parenchymal or cranial nerve involvement that mimic neoplasm, encephalitis, or multiple sclerosis, but rarely cerebrovascular disease.[12,201,203,221,238,249,354,480] Primary central nervous system involvement has been reported.[257,400]

Systemic Lupus Erythematosus

Reports on the neurologic and neuropathologic manifestations of systemic lupus erythematosus (SLE) have long emphasized the high frequency of central nervous system complications. However, specific clinical syndromes and pathophysiologic mechanisms of cerebrovascular disease in the setting of SLE have until recently largely remained obscure.[138] This has been the result, in part, of the tendency in older clinical series to either lump stroke under broad categories along with other central nervous system manifestations (neuropsychiatric disturbances, neurologic lesions) or to split neurologic manifestations into various signs and symptoms (hemiplegia, cranial nerve deficits, aphasia).[138,139] Pathologic series have documented various cerebrovascular lesions, but findings in the brain and cerebral vessels at autopsy infrequently correlate with clinical syndromes before death.[95] Several clinical and pathologic reports have called attention to potential embolic and prothrombotic mechanisms of stroke in SLE that were heretofore unrecognized or underemphasized.[95,132,138,160,]

[187,253] These findings may have important therapeutic implications for some patients with SLE and stroke.[138]

The percentage of patients with SLE in whom stroke develops is difficult to estimate from clinical series that often originate from referral centers. In a prospective series of 150 patients followed at Columbia-Presbyterian Medical Center, Estes and Christian[116] mentioned 4 patients who had fatal stroke. Feinglass et al[125] reported that 5 of their 140 SLE patients had "typical cerebrovascular accidents." Other reports have documented clinical syndromes of cerebrovascular disease in 5.6% to 15%,[138,253] and about 6% of patients with SLE die from cerebrovascular disease.[471] Certainly stroke is not the most common central nervous system manifestation of SLE. In the series by Feinglass et al,[125] stroke occurred one-third as often as seizures and one-fifth as often as "psychiatric illness." According to two series, stroke may be more likely to occur during the first 5 years after diagnosis of SLE.[138,253] Kitagawa et al[253] found renal involvement, hypertension, and high titers of anti-DNA antibodies significantly more frequently in SLE patients with stroke than in those without stroke. In their series, Futrell and Millikan[138] found a high risk of stroke (87%) among SLE patients with cardiac valvular disease. Few data exist on recurrence rates in patients with stroke in the setting of SLE, but in the series by Futrell and Millikan,[138] it was alarmingly high—64%.

MECHANISMS OF CEREBROVASCULAR DISEASE IN PATIENTS WITH SYSTEMIC LUPUS ERYTHEMATOSUS

Vasculitis

The sudden occurrence of central nervous system symptoms in a patient with SLE usually arouses diagnostic suspicions of "vasculitis" or "lupus cerebritis." However, if the numerous studies on the central nervous system complications of SLE published over the years have one feature in common, it is the strikingly low frequency of documented vasculitic changes in the vessels on postmortem examination.[95,110,138,231] Johnson and Richardson[231] documented a high frequency of destructive and proliferative lesions in arterioles and capillaries associated with microinfarction and hemorrhage, but vasculitis was found in only 3 of their 24 cases and was thought to be either focal or reactive. Ellis and Verity[110] found vasculitis in only 7% of 57 cases studied from 1955 to 1977. Hanly et al[182] found evidence of "healed vasculitis" in only 1 of 10 brains of SLE patients. Devinsky et al[95] documented not a single instance of vasculitis involving the cerebral vessels among 50 autopsied patients with SLE.

Cerebral Infarction

In the necropsy series reported by Johnson and Richardson,[231] widespread microinfarction in the cortex and brain stem occurred in the vast majority of patients (20 of 24 cases, 83%). This was thought to correlate with the predominant clinical features: seizures, "disturbances of mental function," and cranial nerve abnormalities. In contrast, macroscopically apparent areas of cerebral infarction, which would be expected to correlate with clinical stroke syndromes, occurred in only four cases (17%). The mechanisms of infarction in their few cases of macroscopic infarction were not apparent.[231] In the necropsy series by Ellis and Verity,[110] only 12% had large infarcts (greater than 1 cm) and these were "usually found in the distribution of the middle cerebral artery." Interestingly, in only one patient were they able to identify thrombosis in the responsible artery. Angiographic studies have documented occlusions of large intracranial vessels (internal carotid artery, middle cerebral artery, anterior cerebral artery).[125,419,451] In Trevor's[451] first case, a "rounded filling defect" was demonstrated in the supraclinoid segment of the right internal carotid artery, which 3 years later had recanalized. Other patients have had tapering occlusions of the middle cerebral artery or internal carotid artery, a finding that was thought to indicate arteritis, but no histologic confirmation was available.[451]

In their early communication describing an "atypical verrucous endocarditis" in patients with SLE (Fig. 30.2), Libman and Sacks[277] suspected that cerebral embolism may have occurred in one of their patients (the brain was not examined at necropsy). However, only recently has attention been called to the possibility that cardiogenic brain embolism (with or without associated Libman-Sacks endocarditis) may be an important mechanism of stroke in patients with SLE.[95,132,138,160,253] In a necropsy series of 50 patients with

SLE, Devinsky et al[95] documented embolic brain infarcts in 10 patients (20%), cardiac sources being Libman-Sacks endocarditis in 5 patients, chronic valvulitis in 2 patients, and mural thrombus in 2 patients. Some patients with verrucous endocarditis also have antiphospholipid antibodies.[90,326,497] Documentation of cardiac sources of emboli in patients with SLE and stroke might prompt treatment with anticoagulants.[138]

Thrombotic thrombocytopenic purpura (thrombocytopenia, microangiopathic hemolytic anemia, fever, renal failure, central nervous system signs) may be an important but underdiagnosed mechanism of stroke in the terminal stages of SLE. Thrombotic thrombocytopenic purpura was documented in 7 of the 50 patients (14%) in the necropsy series by Devinsky et al.[95] Retrospectively, they found that 14 (28%) of their patients had a "clinical profile consistent" with thrombotic thrombocytopenic purpura during the terminal stages of the disease, but this diagnosis was made antemortem in only 1 patient.

Antiphospholipid antibodies, including anticardiolipin antibodies and the so-called lupus anticoagulant, are a class of autoantibodies that bind to negatively charged phospholipid molecules.[144] Bowie and colleagues[49] noted the association of thrombotic events with the presence of the "circulating anticoagulant" in patients with lupus 30 years ago, but it has been in only the last decade that attention has been called to the association of antiphospholipid antibodies with cerebrovascular disease, systemic thrombotic events, spontaneous abortion, and thrombocytopenia.[16,22,50,80,81,99,142,187,188,208,]

Figure 30.2 Libman-Sacks endocarditis involving the mitral valve in a patient with systemic lupus erythematosus. (Courtesy of William D. Edwards M.D., Department of Laboratory Medicine and Pathology, Mayo Clinic, Rochester, MN.)

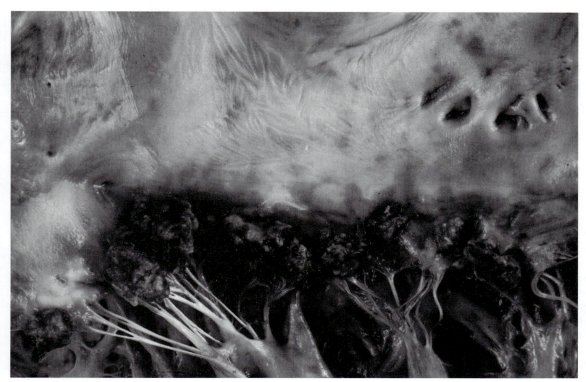

[271,325] These phenomena may be associated with antiphospholipid antibodies either in the setting of SLE or as a "primary" antiphospholipid syndrome.[20] In one series,[253] the lupus anticoagulant was detected in 38% and anticardiolipin antibody in 43% of SLE patients with stroke who were investigated for these abnormalities. Documentation of a procoagulant state due to antiphospholipid antibodies in a patient with SLE and stroke may have important treatment implications, anticoagulants having been recommended by some.[19,50,271] Vasculitis has only rarely been documented in patients with antiphospholipid antibodies.[16,271,280,448]

Confluent white matter increased T_2-signal abnormalities on brain MR imaging in some patients with SLE and dementing illness may represent perivascular demyelination rather than infarction.[245,252]

Hemorrhage

Hemorrhage as a cause of stroke in patients with SLE is well documented clinically but appears to occur less often than infarction.[138,253,268] Intracerebral hemorrhage is sometimes, but not always, associated with hypertension and thrombocytopenia.[138,253,452] For example, in the series by Johnson and Richardson,[231] three patients died from intracerebral hemorrhage, but only one had hypertension, and none had thrombocytopenia. They could not establish the exact mechanism of hemorrhage in these three cases, but they did note that the hemorrhages were lobar, not in the typical location of hypertensive hemorrhage. Small hemorrhages were much more common in their series. The more recent necropsy series by Devinsky et al[95] did not document large intracerebral hematoma. Subarachnoid hemorrhage is frequently found at autopsy, but this may often be in association with intraparenchymal hemorrhage.[110] Some patients with SLE do develop clinical syndromes of subarachnoid hemorrhage. In some instances, the subarachnoid hemorrhage has been secondary to rupture of a berry aneurysm,[116,190,452] a possible chance association. On rare occasions, subarachnoid hemorrhage has occurred secondary to rupture of a fusiform aneurysm with associated transmural angiitis documented at necropsy.[247] In other instances of "primary subarachnoid hemorrhage," neither angiitis nor berry aneurysm has been documented.[253] Subdural hematoma has also been reported, but the mechanisms involved are uncertain.[95,126]

Cerebral Venous Thrombosis

Cerebral venous thrombosis is an uncommon but well-documented cerebrovascular complication in SLE.[112,272,415,461] The mechanism of venous thrombosis in these patients may be multifactorial, lupus anticoagulant and anticardiolipin antibody having been detected in some, but not in all.[272,461] Clinical syndromes have included focal cerebral signs, including alternating hemiparesis, hemiplegia, and aphasia, but clinicians should be particularly alert to the fact that some patients have presented with headache, papilledema, and no focal neurologic signs ("pseudotumor cerebri").[461] Cerebral angiography, MR imaging, or MR angiography may be necessary to confirm this diagnosis.

Scleroderma

Scleroderma (progressive systemic sclerosis) rarely directly causes central nervous system manifestations.[23,159] Convulsions, stroke, and pathologic findings of arterial changes in the brains of patients with scleroderma are frequently the result of hypertension as a consequence of renal disease.[159] Six percent of patients with scleroderma in the series by Averbuch-Heller et al[23] had cerebrovascular disease, but the mechanisms involved were obscure. However, the patient of Lee and Haynes[267] sustained a cerebral infarction associated with arteritic involvement of the ipsilateral internal carotid artery. She had a 10-year history of weight loss, intermittent fever, skin tightening, dysphagia, and Raynaud's phenomenon, and a right hemiparesis and subsequent seizure developed. Blood pressure was normal on admission. A left carotid arteriogram demonstrated long segmental narrowing of the interosseous segment of the internal carotid artery siphon and occlusion of the anterior and middle cerebral arteries. At autopsy, the left carotid artery intima was thickened due to "fibrous proliferation." Muscle fibers in the media were "disorganized and indistinct." The vasa vasorum and medium-sized arteries in the adventitia were surrounded by "inflammatory cells," and a few examples of "fibrinoid change" were seen. Examination of the brain demonstrated a large left cerebral hemisphere infarction with occlusion of the left anterior cerebral artery with recent thrombus and recanalized thrombus in the left middle cerebral artery. Degenerative changes attributable to scleroderma were not documented in these intracranial arteries, but the "surrounding connective tissue . . . showed inflammatory and degenerative changes similar to those in the carotid sheath." The angiographic appearance of "cerebral arteritis" associated with mild cerebrospinal fluid pleocytosis, increased cerebrospinal fluid protein, and increased cerebrospinal fluid opening pressure has been reported in a patient with scleroderma and seizures.[117] Antiphospholipid antibodies have been detected in a patient with scleroderma and cerebral and retinal ischemia.[482]

Rheumatoid Arthritis

Central nervous system manifestations of rheumatoid arthritis are rare and tend to occur in the setting of long-established disease, with either clinical (fever, weight loss, active arthritis) or laboratory (increased rheumatoid factor titer, increased ESR) evidence of disease activity. Rheumatoid meningitis ("pachymeningitis") has been reported as an asymptomatic finding at autopsy[429] or may cause central nervous system symptoms and signs, including headache, visual loss, seizures, altered mental status, aphasia, memory loss, hemiparesis, and spinal cord compression.[28,172,225,239,250,251,302,429] Findings at autopsy include thickening and distension of the meninges with a proteinaceous fluid.[225,429] The dura and leptomeninges demonstrate foci of inflammatory mononuclear cells and multinucleated giant cells.[225,250,251,302,429] Rheumatoid nodules similar to those found elsewhere in the body have been described in the meninges and the choroid plexus.[225,250,251]

Central nervous system vasculitis, either isolated[298,347,431,473] or in association with systemic rheumatoid vasculitis,[230,370,382,420] has been documented on rare occasions. Some of these cases had associated pachymeningitis. Usually the small vessels of the leptomeninges are affected by fibrinoid necrosis, perivascular nodule formation (similar to polyarteritis nodosa), and "onion skin" proliferation. Small infarcts are the usual associated parenchymal findings,[420] although hematoma formation has been associated with necrotizing vasculitis involving the small- and medium-sized arteries in at least one case,[473] and "patchy" subdural and subarachnoid hemorrhage was found in another instance, presumably related to vasculitis involving small vessels in the subarachnoid space.[431] Usually these patients have had encephalopathic syndromes, including seizures and altered mental status,[30,298,347,370,382] although the patient of Watson and co-workers[473] presented with acute signs and symptoms of stroke involving both the left frontal lobe and left pons, subsequently documented to be secondary to hematomas at autopsy.

One of the most feared neurologic complications of rheumatoid arthritis is compressive myelopathy secondary to C1–C2 vertebral subluxation. A well-documented and equally disastrous complication of C1–C2 subluxation is massive vertebrobasilar territory infarction as a result of vertebral artery thrombosis.[235,474] In two autopsy studies, patients presented with occipital headache and episodic vertigo with neck flexion or rotation or with "occasional blackouts."[235,474] The patient of Jones and Kaufmann[235] subsequently had an episode of unconsciousness, disorientation, nystagmus, bilateral extensor plantar responses, and bilateral leg weakness. He became comatose with decerebrate posturing and Cheyne-Stokes respirations, and gradually a coma vigil ensued before death. The patient of Webb et al[474] had occipital headaches and occasional blackouts before being found unconscious with a flaccid left hemiparesis and bilateral extensor plantar responses. She died within 30 hours of onset of coma. Vertebral artery thrombosis was thought to have resulted from pinching of the vertebral artery between the odontoid and rim of the foramen magnum[235] or stretching of the vertebral arteries between the transverse foramina of the C1 and C2 vertebrae.[474] Precipitation of vertebrobasilar ischemic symptoms has been associated with neck flexion, extension, or rotation in patients with C1–C2 subluxation.[207,235,381,474] Some have had angiographic documentation of narrowing or occlusion of the vertebral arteries with these maneuvers.[207,381] Vertebral artery pseudoaneurysm formation has also been reported.[123]

Instances of cerebral and ocular ischemia in the setting of rheumatoid arthritis have been associated with thrombocytosis[106,365] and hyperviscosity syndromes secondary to polyclonal gammopathy.[396]

Sjögren Syndrome

Sjögren syndrome (xerostomia and keratoconjunctivitis sicca) is frequently diagnosed in conjunction with other collagen vascular diseases that may result in central nervous system complications. Anti-Ro (SSA) antibodies are often present in patients with Sjögren syndrome.[185] There is considerable uncertainty and controversy over the definition of Sjögren syndrome and the frequency and severity with which central nervous system complications occur in patients with the primary form of the disease (i.e., Sjögren syndrome not associated with another collagen vascular disease).[4,5,9,10,38,316,320,324,336,337] Multiple sclerosis-like,[8] stroke-like,[10] and dementing[62] syndromes have been reported, along with various CT and MR findings.[6] However, histopathologic documentation of the mechanisms involved has not been apparent in some reports. Postmortem brain examination of three patients with primary Sjogren syndrome demonstrated "diffuse polymorphous meningitis" in three patients, associated with microhemorrhages in two patients, but antemortem clinical correlations were uncertain.[94] Necrotizing arteritis and spinal subarachnoid hemorrhage have been reported in one patient with Sjögren syndrome and cryoglobulinemia.[7] Giordano et al[153] found vasculitis in the basilar artery and vasocentric leptomeningeal infiltrates on postmortem examination of a patient with Sjögren syndrome, positive antinuclear antibody results, aseptic meningitis, and subarachnoid hemorrhage. Perivascular lymphocytic inflammation in leptomeningeal and parenchymal vessels was found in one patient with dementia, Sjögren syndrome, and increased rheumatoid factor.[62]

Sneddon Syndrome

Livedo reticularis is a cutaneous condition characterized by a fixed, deep bluish red, reticulated pattern caused by impaired superficial venous drainage of the skin[368] (Fig. 30.3). This cutaneous sign is found in several diseases, including polyarteritis nodosa, SLE, rheumatoid arthritis, dermatomyositis, and cryoglobulinemia.[368] Cerebrovascular disease in association with livedo reticularis is known as Sneddon syndrome.[68,424] Sneddon's original description also included hypertension as part of a triad.[424] Many, but not all, of these patients have antiphospholipid antibodies[21,164,232,236,273] or antiendothelial cell antibodies.[133] Familial cases have also been reported.[143,284,359]

Livedo reticularis usually precedes neurologic involvement in these patients, but many present with stroke.[236] The most common cerebrovascular manifestation in this syndrome is recurrent cerebral infarction.[236,373,390,402,432,443] Transient ischemic attack, seizures, and dementia (possibly related to multiple infarctions) have been reported.[373,390,432] Various clinical stroke syndromes have been documented, frequently with prominent cortical signs.[373,390,432] The mechanism of infarction in these patients is for the most part unknown. Brain CT and MR imaging frequently document infarction involving the cortex or white matter[143,359,373,390,432,434,443] (Fig. 30.4). Angiograms are either normal or demonstrate narrowing or occlusion of medium-sized arteries and their branches, sometimes with moyamoya-type collateral networks.[143,357,359,373,390,424,432] Asherson et al[21] found "heart valve lesions" in more than a third of patients with livedo reticularis associated with positive anticardiolipin antibodies. Skin biopsies have usually demonstrated "an occlusive and noninflammatory" vasculopa-

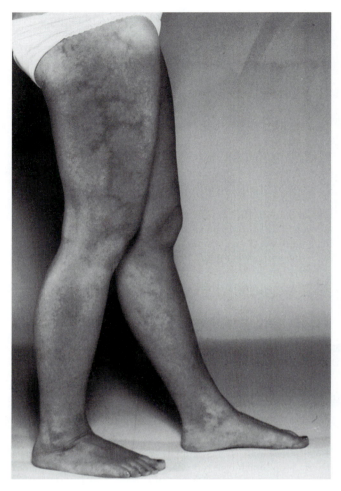

Figure 30.3 Livedo reticularis in a patient with Sneddon syndrome. (Courtesy of Department of Dermatology, Mayo Clinic.)

thy involving the medium-sized arteries with focal and segmental intimal hyperplasia due to fibroelastic proliferation or subendothelial cell proliferation but no evidence of vasculitis.[284,373] Some have found inflammatory changes of the endothelium.[434,435] Brain specimens have demonstrated "vasculopathy with musculoelastic hyperplasia" (Pinol Aquade quoted by Quimby and Perry[368]) or thrombotic vasculopathy[143] with no vasculitis. One patient had nonvasculitic granulomatous changes in the leptomeninges.[45] Various treatments have included antiplatelet agents, warfarin,[273] and plasmapheresis.[402] In view of the occlusive and ischemic nature of the disease and presence of antiphospholipid antibodies and valvular abnormalities in many patients with Sneddon syndrome, warfarin seems to be especially indicated. However, instances of brain hemorrhage have also been reported.[105,455]

Malignant Atrophic Papulosis

Malignant atrophic papulosis (Degos' disease, Köhlmeier-Degos' disease) is a progressive vasculopathy that affects the skin, cerebral circulation, and other organ systems.[93] Charac-

teristic skin lesions consist of umbilicated raised papules with a white center (Fig. 30.5). The appearance of cutaneous lesions usually precedes neurologic manifestations, sometimes by years.[204,489] In some patients, however, neurologic manifestations may precede or accompany the development of cutaneous lesions.[309,405] Bowel perforations may occur.[26,437]

Neurologic complications are varied. In some patients, the initial neurologic manifestations have been symptoms and signs of transient ischemic attack[489] or stroke.[91] Others have had progressive focal or multifocal deficits with stepwise quantitative and qualitative worsening.[84,309,358,406,489] Still others have had evidence of spinal cord involvement.[204,265,309,489] Angiographic findings have included multiple branch occlusions and alternating segmental constriction and dilatation.[358,406] CT scans have demonstrated multifocal areas of infarction, hemorrhage, hemorrhagic infarction, and even subdural hemorrhage.[53,358]

Pathologic examination of brain vessels has documented a peculiar "fibrous intimal proliferation" or "deposition of fibrous material" between endothelium and internal elastic lamina,[53,91,204,265,309,406,489] similar to vascular lesions in the skin. This may be accompanied by thrombosis. Sparse lymphocytic vasculitis and perivascular lymphocytic infiltration were reported in one patient's brain on postmortem examination.[53] The small meningeal arteries are frequently involved,[309] but medium and even large arteries may also be affected.[204,489] Multiple small infarcts, either hemorrhagic or bland, are often found.[53,84,265,309,406,489] These small infarcts may be confluent[472] and involve the cortex[309] or cortex and deeper structures.[204] Less often, large infarction with shift and herniation is documented.[26,406] Venous thrombosis and hemorrhagic venous infarction have been reported.[53] Small parenchymal hemorrhages[91,204] and subarachnoid hemorrhage[309] are occasionally documented.

The exact etiology of this proliferative and occlusive vasculopathy has not been established. Some have reported increased platelet adhesiveness and aggregation,[104] although others have found no coagulation abnormalities.[296] The presence of anticardiolipin antibodies and lupus anticoagulant has been reported in at least one patient with Degos' disease.[114] Various therapies have been used, usually ineffectively, including antiplatelet agents, anticoagulants, corticosteroids, and plasmapheresis.[265,309,413,489]

Behçet's Disease

Behçet's disease is an inflammatory condition of unknown etiology that is clinically typified by the triad of oral aphthous ulcers, genital ulcers, and uveitis. Other manifestations include arthritis, cutaneous vasculitis, thrombophlebitis, colitis, and central nervous system disease.[340,341] Central nervous system complications usually occur in patients who have established cutaneous or ocular disease, but there are well-documented instances of neurologic presentation,[101,220,261,438] and some may have ocular and neurologic manifestations without oral or genital lesions.[289] Neurologic manifestations are varied, and few clinical features point to the underlying diagnosis in the absence of the cutaneous or ocular manifestations. Many

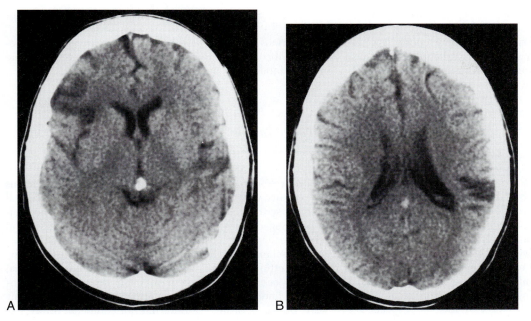

Figure 30.4 Computed tomogram demonstrates infarction in a patient with Sneddon's syndrome. (**A**) Right frontal cortex. (**B**) Left parietal cortex. (Courtesy of Dr. H. S. Luthra, Dr. A. J. D. Dale, Dr. J. Huston, and Department of Diagnostic Radiology, Mayo Clinic Rochester, MN.)

Figure 30.5 Skin lesions of malignant atrophic papulosis (Degos' disease). (Courtesy of Department of Dermatology, Mayo Clinic.)

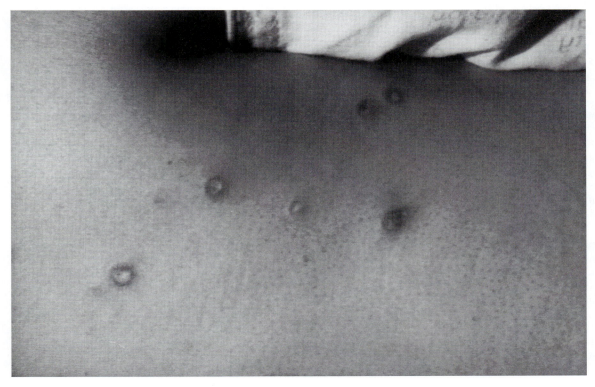

patients present with a syndrome of aseptic meningitis or meningoencephalitis with fever and headache, with or without associated focal neurologic signs.[340,387] Many reports have emphasized a fluctuating course with exacerbations and remissions that are atypical for cerebrovascular disease.[244,286,340,388,490] Corticospinal tract signs, frequently bilateral, are common. Symptoms and signs of brain-stem involvement and pseudobulbar palsy are frequently reported.[286,310,340,388,404,438] Less often, neurologic presentations may be sudden in onset and suggest stroke.[101,111,220,244,261] Some patients have presented with symptoms and signs of increased intracranial pressure, occasionally with minimal or no focal findings, due to angiographically documented cerebral venous sinus thrombosis.[24,74,186,218,348,387,433,476,483] Retinal ischemia and retinal "vasculitis" are also reported.[2,36,220,387]

Spinal fluid examination frequently demonstrates a moderate pleocytosis, predominantly lymphocytic, as well as increased protein, usually less than 100 mg/dl.[340,387] Anticardiolipin antibodies have been reported in patients with Behçet's disease, especially in patients with retinal ischemia or retinal "vasculitis."[210] Brain imaging with CT, and more recently MR imaging, has demonstrated lesions that, in some respects, are atypical for more routine mechanisms of vascular disease.[2,25,197,246,323,353,485] CT scans demonstrate focal and circumscribed regions of decreased density that may enhance after administration of contrast medium.[197,353,485] Findings on MR imaging usually consist of increased signal intensity on T_2-weighted images.[2,323,353] These lesions usually are found in the deep structures, including brain stem, deep nuclei, and hypothalamus and also in the hemispheric white matter and may enhance.[2,25,197,246,323,353,475,476,485] Herskovitz et al[197] have pointed out that, unlike vascular lesions, these findings tend to resolve over time after treatment and frequently do not conform to a single arterial territory. These features, as well as leptomeningeal enhancement in some,[96] might be more suggestive of an inflammatory process as opposed to vascular occlusion.[197] Cerebral hemorrhage has been reported, but the mechanisms involved are unclear.[11,328] Cerebral angiograms have usually been normal,[340] but occasional patients with a "vasculitic appearance" have been reported.[499] There is also a report of a large aneurysmal abnormality of the cervical segment of the internal carotid artery.[97]

The leptomeninges are frequently thickened and opacified.[286,310,388,438] Small regions of softening are most often found in the brain stem and basal ganglia, less often in the deep white matter, and least often in the cortex.[286,310,388,414,438,492] Gliosis has been prominent in some reports.[310,388,438,492] Many patients have had varying degrees of lymphocytic perivascular infiltration, usually mild to moderate,[310,388,414,438,492] sometimes perivenular.[333] Small areas of perivascular necrosis and "scarring" are found, particularly in the brain stem, diencephalon, internal capsule, and basal ganglia.[388] Most reports have emphasized the paucity of arterial lesions and thromboses.[286,388,404,438] Small hemorrhages are also uncommonly documented.[244,328,404] Some reports have emphasized demyelination, perivenular and diffuse.[286,333,414,438,492] On rare occasions, large areas of infarction, either in the cortex or basal ganglia, with "endarteritis and post-thrombotic recanalization" have been reported.[310] Granulomatous or necrotizing angiitis does not appear to be a commonly documented mechanism of central nervous system involvement in Behçet's

disease.[333] Some patients may have antiphospholipid antibodies.[210]

Various therapies have been used, including corticosteroids, anticoagulants (for venous thrombosis), cyclophosphamide, azathioprine, and chlorambucil.[341,476]

Cryoglobulinemia

There are rare reports of central nervous system complications in patients with mixed cryoglobulinemia.[1,360,375,377] Central nervous system manifestations have included diffuse encephalopathic syndromes with focal signs, seizures, myelopathy, and occasionally ischemic stroke.[1,360,375,377] Two patients with cerebral ischemia due to an occlusive intracranial vasculopathy in the setting of hepatitis C virus infection, cryoglobulemia, and hypocomplementemia have been reported.[360] Angiographic findings have included narrowing of the vertebral artery, occlusion of the posterior inferior cerebellar artery, occlusion of the left middle cerebral artery, and progressive stenosis of the distal internal carotid, anterior cerebral, and middle cerebral arteries with development of a moyamoya collateral pattern.[1,360] The exact underlying pathophysiologic mechanisms of vascular occlusions in these patients are unknown, and vasculitis has been documented only rarely.[161,409]

Retinocochleocerebral Vasculopathy (Susac Syndrome)

Retinocochleocerebral vasculopathy is an unusual syndrome of small-vessel occlusions in the retina, cochlea, and brain affecting predominantly young women.[43,79,157,194,237,291,300,305,318,361,362,364,403,439,440] Fewer than 30 cases have been reported. Extracerebral clinical manifestations have included multiple episodes of visual loss related to retinal arteriolar occlusions, sensorineural hearing loss, and tinnitus. Funduscopic examination demonstrates occlusion of multiple retinal arterioles with peculiar "long columns of white material" oscillating with the pulse.[318,364] Neurologic manifestations include encephalopathy with prominent disturbances in cognition, memory and behavior, dysarthria, pseudobulbar affect, ataxia, vertigo, hemiparesis, and hemisensory loss.[43,79,194,305,318,362,440] Spinal fluid examinations may demonstrate a mild pleocytosis (predominantly lymphocytic) and increased concentration of protein.[43,79,305,318,362,440] Cerebral angiograms are usually normal.[43,362,440] CT scans are usually normal, but MR imaging is almost always abnormal and demonstrates increased signal abnormalities on T_2-weighted images in the white matter[43,305,318,362] or white matter and deep gray matter (Fig. 30.6).[362] Brain biopsy has demonstrated gliosis, microinfarcts, small-vessel "sclerosis," or "healed arteritis."[362] Tests for anticardiolipin antibody, lupus anticoagulant, protein C

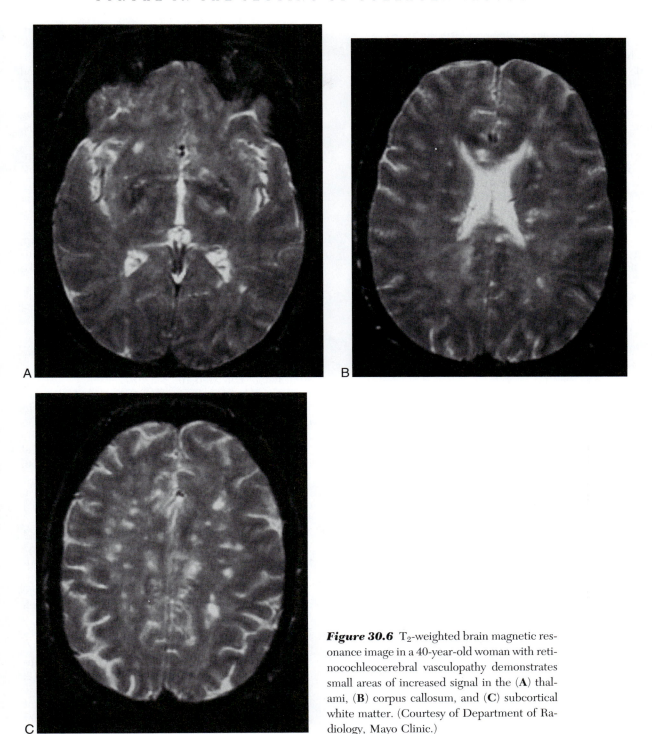

Figure 30.6 T_2-weighted brain magnetic resonance image in a 40-year-old woman with retinocochleocerebral vasculopathy demonstrates small areas of increased signal in the (**A**) thalami, (**B**) corpus callosum, and (**C**) subcortical white matter. (Courtesy of Department of Radiology, Mayo Clinic.)

deficiency, protein S deficiency, and antithrombin III deficiency have been negative.[361,362] No definite underlying connective tissue disease has been identified in these patients. Other patients with partial syndromes of characteristic retinal arteriolar occlusions and cerebral manifestations without cochlear or vestibular symptoms have been reported.[361,362] The etiology remains obscure. Some patients have appeared to respond to steroids and immunosuppressants,[318,440] and oth-

ers have progressed despite these treatments.[43,361,362] The documentation of microangiopathic involvement of muscle in some patients[361,362] suggests that retinocochleocerebral vasculopathy may actually be a systemic disease. The predominance of retinal, cerebral, and cochlear symptoms and signs may indicate preferential involvement of these organs or may simply reflect the eloquence of these structures compared with other organ systems.[361,362] Several arteritides can also be associated with retinal vasculitis, including polyarteritis nodosa, SLE, Wegener's granulomatosis, and Behçet's disease,[430] but the systemic manifestations of these diseases should distinguish them from retinocochleocerebral vasculopathy. Retinocochleocerebral vasculopathy should also be distinguishable from Cogan syndrome,[75] which may produce visual loss due to interstitial keratitis as well as vestibulocochlear symptoms, but rarely central nervous system involvement.[466] Anterior chamber inflammation, which is characteristic in Cogan syndrome, is not seen in retinocochleocerebral vasculopathy. Acute posterior placoid pigment epitheliopathy is a retinal disease characterized by cream-colored posterior pole lesions[418,423,436,478,486] that may also occasionally be associated with cerebral vasculitis. The posterior pole lesions characteristic of this disorder are not seen in patients with retinocochleocerebral vasculopathy. Eales' disease produces visual loss in young men due to retinal vasculitis or periphlebitis and retinal hemorrhage and may also be associated with stroke.[158,399] Retinocochleocerebral vasculopathy is not typically associated with retinal venulitis or hemorrhage, however.

References

1. Abramsky O, Slavin S: Neurologic manifestations in patients with mixed cryoglobulinemia. Neurology (NY) 24: 245, 1974

2. Al Kawi MZ, Bohlega S, Banna M: MRI findings in neuro-Behçet's disease. Neurology 41:405, 1991

3. Alestig K, Barr J: Giant-cell arteritis: a biopsy study of polymyalgia rheumatica, including one case of Takayasu's disease. Lancet 1:1228, 1963

4. Alexander E, McFarland H: Sjögren's syndrome mimicking multiple sclerosis (Letter). Ann Neurol 17:586, 1990

5. Alexander EL: Neurologic disease in Sjögren's syndrome: mononuclear inflammatory vasculopathy affecting central/peripheral nervous system and muscle. A clinical review and update of immunopathogenesis. Rheum Dis Clin North Am 19:869, 1993

6. Alexander EL, Beall SS, Gordon B et al: Magnetic resonance imaging of cerebral lesions in patients with the Sjögren syndrome. Ann Intern Med 108:815, 1988

7. Alexander EL, Craft C, Dorsh C et al: Necrotizing arteritis and spinal subarachnoid hemorrhage in Sjögren syndrome. Ann Neurol 11:632, 1982

8. Alexander EL, Malinow K, Lejewski JE et al: Primary Sjögren's syndrome with central nervous system disease mimicking multiple sclerosis. Ann Intern Med 104:323, 1986

9. Alexander EL, Ranzenbach MR, Kumar AJ et al: Anti-Ro (SS-A) autoantibodies in central nervous system disease associated with Sjögren's syndrome (CNS-SS): clinical, neuroimaging, and angiographic correlates. Neurology 44:899, 1994

10. Alexander GE, Provost TT, Stevens MB, Alexander EL: Sjögren syndrome: central nervous system manifestations. Neurology (NY) 31:1391, 1981

11. Altinörs N, Senveli E, Arda N et al: Intracerebral hemorrhage and hematoma in Behçet's disease: case report. Neurosurgery 21:582, 1987

12. Amin SN, Gibbons CM, Lovell CR et al: A case of lymphomatoid granulomatosis with a protracted course and prominent CNS involvement. Br J Rheumatol 28:77, 1989

13. Anderson JM, Jamieson DG, Jefferson JM: Non-healing granuloma and the nervous system. Q J Med 41:309, 1975

14. Anderson NE, Willoughby EW, Synek BJL: Leptomeningeal and brain biopsy in chronic meningitis. Aust N Z J Med 25:703, 1995

15. Andersson R, Malmvall BE, Bengtsson BA: Long-term corticosteroid treatment in giant cell arteritis. Acta Med Scand 220:465, 1986

16. Antiphospholipid Antibodies in Stroke Study Group: Clinical and laboratory findings in patients with antiphospholipid antibodies and cerebral ischemia. Stroke 21:1268, 1990

17. Armstrong RD, Behn A, Myles A et al: Histocompatibility antigens in polymyalgia rheumatica and giant-cell arteritis. J Rheumatol 10:659, 1983

18. Arthur G, Margolis G: Mycoplasma-like structures in granulomatous angiitis of the central nervous system: case reports with light and electron microscope studies. Arch Pathol Lab Med 101:382, 1977

19. Asherson RA, Chan JKH, Harris EN et al: Anticardiolipin antibody, recurrent thrombosis, and warfarin withdrawal. Ann Rheum Dis 44:823, 1985

20. Asherson RA, Khamashta MA, Ordi-Ros J et al: The "primary" antiphospholipid syndrome: major clinical and serological features. Medicine (Baltimore) 68:366, 1989

21. Asherson RA, Mayou SC, Merry P et al: The spectrum of livedo reticularis and anticardiolipin antibodies. Br J Dermatol 120:215, 1989

22. Asherson RA, Mercey D, Phillips G et al: Recurrent stroke and multi-infarct dementia in systemic lupus erythematosus: association with antiphospholipid antibodies. Ann Rheum Dis 46:605, 1987

23. Averbuch-Heller L, Steiner I, Abramsky O: Neurologic manifestations of progressive systemic sclerosis. Arch Neurol 49:1292, 1992

24. Bank I, Weart C: Dural sinus thrombosis in Behçet's disease. Arthritis Rheum 27:816, 1984

25. Banna M, el-Ramahl K: Neurologic involvement in Behçet disease: imaging findings in 16 patients. AJNR 12: 791, 1991

26. Barlow RJ, Heyl T, Simson IW, Schulz EJ: Malignant atrophic papulosis (Degos' disease): diffuse involvement of brain and bowel in an African patient. Br J Dermatol 118:117, 1988

27. Barricks ME, Traviesa DM, Glaser JS, Levy IS: Ophthalmoplegia in cranial arteritis. Brain 100:209, 1977

28. Bathon JM, Moreland LW, DiBartolomeo AG: Inflammatory central nervous system involvement in rheumatoid arthritis. Semin Arthritis Rheum 18:258, 1989

29. Beattie DK, Hellier WP, Powell MP: Stroke-induced cardiovascular changes: a rare cause of death from polyarteritis nodosa. Br J Neurosurg 9:223, 1995

30. Beck DO, Corbett JJ: Seizures due to central nervous

system rheumatoid meningovasculitis. Neurology (NY) 33:1058, 1983

31. Bengtsson BA, Malmvall BE: The epidemiology of giant cell arteritis including temporal arteritis and polymalgia rheumatica. Arthritis Rheum 24:899, 1981

32. Bengtsson BA, Malmvall BE: Prognosis of giant cell arteritis including temporal arteritis and polymyalgia rheumatica. Acta Med Scand 209:337, 1981

33. Bengtsson BA, Malmvall BE: Giant cell arteritis. Acta Med Scand (suppl) 658:1, 1982

34. Beresford HR, Hyman RA, Shorer L: Self-limited granulomatous angiitis of the cerebellum. Ann Neurol 5:490, 1979

35. Berger JR, Romano J, Menkin M, Norenberg M: Benign focal cerebral vasculitis: case report. Neurology 45:1731, 1995

36. Besana C, Comi G, Del Maschio A et al: Electrophysiological and MRI evaluation of neurological involvement in Behçet's disease. J Neurol Neurosurg Psychiatry 52:749, 1989

37. Biller J, Loftus CM, Moore SA et al: Isolated central nervous system angiitis first presenting as spontaneous intracranial hemorrhage. Neurosurgery 20:310, 1987

38. Binder A, Snaith ML, Isenberg D: Sjögren's syndrome: a study of its neurological complications. Br J Rheumatol 27:275, 1988

39. Blue MC, Rosenblum WI: Granulomatous angiitis of the brain with herpes zoster and varicella encephalitis. Arch Pathol Lab Med 107:126, 1983

40. Boesen P, Sorensen SF: Giant cell arteritis, temporal arteritis, and polymyalgia rheumatica in a Danish county: a prospective investigation, 1982–1985. Arthritis Rheum 30:294, 1987

41. Boghen DR, Glaser JS: Ischaemic optic neuropathy. Brain 98:689, 1975

42. Bogousslavsky J, Deruaz JP, Regli F: Bilateral obstruction of internal carotid artery from giant-cell arteritis and massive infarction limited to the vertebrobasilar area. Eur Neurol 24:57, 1985

43. Bogousslavsky J, Gaio JM, Caplan LR et al: Encephalopathy, deafness and blindness in young women: a distinct retinocochleocerebral arteriolopathy? J Neurol Neurosurg Psychiatry 52:43, 1989

44. Bonnetblanc JM, Adenis JP, Queroi M, Rammaert B: Immunofluorescence in temporal arteritis. N Engl J Med 298:458, 1978

45. Boortz-Marx RL, Clark HB, Taylor S et al: Sneddon's syndrome with granulomatous leptomeningeal infiltration. Stroke 26:492, 1995

46. Borenstein D, Costa M, Jannotta F, Rizzoli H: Localized isolated angiitis of the central nervous system associated with primary intracerebral lymphoma. Cancer 62:375, 1988

47. Borruat FX, Bogousslavsky J, Uffer S et al: Orbital infarction syndrome. Ophthalmology 100:562, 1993

48. Bourdette DN, Rosenberg NL, Yatsu FM: Herpes zoster ophthalmicus and delayed ipsilateral cerebral infarction. Neurology (NY) 33:1428, 1983

49. Bowie EJW, Thompson JH, Jr, Pascuzzi CA, Owen CA, Jr: Thrombosis in systemic lupus erythematosus despite circulating anticoagulants. J Lab Clin Med 62:416, 1963

50. Briley DP, Coull BM, Goodnight SH Jr: Neurological disease associated with antiphospholipid antibodies. Ann Neurol 25:221, 1989

51. Budzilovich GN, Feigin I, Siegel H: Granulomatous angiitis of the nervous system. Arch Pathol Lab Med 76:250, 1963

52. Burger PC, Burch JG, Vogel FS: Granulomatous angiitis: an unusual etiology of stroke. Stroke 8:29, 1977

53. Burrow JN, Blumbergs PC, Iyer PV, Hallpike JF: Kohlmeier-Degos disease: a multisystem vasculopathy with progressive cerebral infarction. Aust N Z J Med 21:49, 1991

54. Butt Z, Cullen JF, Mutlukan E: Pattern of arterial involvement of the head, neck, and eyes in giant cell arteritis: three case reports. Br J Ophthalmol 75:368, 1991

55. Caccamo DV, Garcia JH, Ho KL: Isolated granulomatous angiitis of the spinal cord. Ann Neurol 32:580, 1992

56. Calabrese LH, Mallek JA: Primary angiitis of the central nervous system: report of 8 new cases, review of the literature, and proposal for diagnostic criteria. Medicine (Baltimore) 67:20, 1988

57. Calamia KT, Moore SB, Elveback LR, Hunder GG: HLA-DR locus antigens in polymyalgia rheumatica and giant cell arteritis. J Rheumatol 8:993, 1981

58. Caplan L, Corbett J, Goodwin J et al: Neuro-ophthalmologic signs in the angiitic form of neurosarcoidosis. Neurology (NY) 33:1130, 1983

59. Cardell BS, Hanley T: A fatal case of giant-cell or temporal arteritis. J Pathol 63:587, 1951

60. Case records of the Massachusetts General Hospital: Weekly clinicopathological exercises. Case 33-1995. Progressive neurologic deterioration with unusual findings on magnetic resonance imaging in a 43-year-old man treated for demyelinating disease. N Engl J Med 333:1135, 1995

61. Caselli RJ, Hunder GG, Whisnant JP: Neurologic disease in biopsy-proven giant cell (temporal) arteritis. Neurology (NY) 38:352, 1988

62. Caselli RJ, Scheithauer BW, Bowles CA et al: The treatable dementia of Sjögren's syndrome. Ann Neurol 30:98, 1991

63. Castaigne P, Cambier J, Escourolle R, Brunet P: Les manifestations nerveuses centrales de la périartérite noueuse: à propos d'une observation anatomo-clinique. Ann Med Interne 121:375, 1970

64. Castleman B, McNeely BU: Case records of the Massachusetts General Hospital: case 41152. N Engl J Med 252:634, 1955

65. Castleman B, McNeely BU: Case records of the Massachusetts General Hospital: case 14-1967. N Engl J Med 276:741, 1967

66. Castleman B, McNeely BU: Case records of the Massachusetts General Hospital: case 26-1967. N Engl J Med 276:1432, 1967

67. Chakravarty K, Pountain G, Merry P et al: A longitudinal study of anticardiolipin antibody in polymyalgia rheumatic and giant cell arteritis. J Rheumatol 22:1694, 1995

68. Champion RH, Rook A: Livedo reticularis. Proc R Soc Med 53:961, 1960

69. Chang Y, Kargas SA, Goates JJ, Horoupian DS: Intraventricular and subarachnoid hemorrhage resulting from

necrotizing vasculitis of the choroid plexus in a patient with Churg-Strauss syndrome. Clin Neuropathol 12:84, 1993

70. Chasnoff J, Vorzimer JJ: Temporal arteritis: a local manifestation of a systemic disease. Ann Intern Med 20:327, 1944

71. Chess J, Albert DM, Bhan AK et al: Serologic and immunopathologic findings in temporal arteritis. Am J Ophthalmol 96:283, 1983

72. Clifford-Jones R, Love S, Gurusinghe N: Granulomatous angiitis of the central nervous system: a case with recurrent intracerebral haemorrhage. J Neurol Neurosurg Psychiatry 48:1054, 1985

73. Clyde WA, Thomas L: Pathogenesis studies in experimental mycoplasma disease: *M. gallisepticum* infections of turkeys. Ann NY Acad Sci 225:413, 1973

74. Cobby M, Hall CL, Higgs CMB: Behçet's syndrome presenting as intracranial hypertension in a Caucasian. J R Soc Med 81:478, 1988

75. Cogan DG: Syndrome of nonsyphilitic interstitial keratitis and vestibuloauditory symptoms. Arch Ophthalmol 33:144, 1945

76. Cohen DN, Damaske MM: Temporal arteritis: a spectrum of ophthalmic complications. Ann Ophthalmol 7:1045, 1975

77. Cohen RD, Conn DL, Ilstrup DM: Clinical features, prognosis, and response to treatment in polyarteritis. Mayo Clin Proc 55:146, 1980

78. Collado A, Santamaria J, Ribalta T et al: Giant-cell arteritis presenting with ipsilateral hemiplegia and lateral medullary syndrome. Eur Neurol 29:266, 1989

79. Coppeto JR, Currie JN, Monteiro MLR, Lessell S: A syndrome of arterial-occlusive retinopathy and encephalopathy. Am J Ophthalmol 98:189, 1984

80. Coull BM, Bourdette DN, Goodnight SH Jr et al: Multiple cerebral infarctions and dementia associated with anticardiolipin antibodies. Stroke 18:1107, 1987

81. Coull BM, Goodnight SH: Antiphospholipid antibodies, prethrombotic states, and stroke. Stroke 21:1370, 1990

82. Cravioto H, Feigin I: Non-infectious granulomatous angiitis with a predilection for the nervous system. Neurology (NY) 9:599, 1959

83. Crompton MR: The visual changes in temporal (giant cell) arteritis. Brain 82:377, 1959

84. Culicchia CF, Gol A, Erickson EE: Diffuse central nervous system involvement in papulosis atrophicans maligna. Neurology (NY) 12:503, 1962

85. Cull RE: Internal carotid artery occlusion caused by giant cell arteritis. J Neurol Neurosurg Psychiatry 42:1066, 1979

86. Cupps TR, Fauci AS: Central nervous system vasculitis: the vasculitides. Major Probl Intern Med 21:123, 1981

87. Cupps TR, Fauci AS: Giant cell arteritides: the vasculitides. Major Probl Intern Med 21:99, 1981

88. Cupps TR, Moore PM, Fauci AS: Isolated angiitis of the central nervous system. Am J Med 74:97, 1983

89. Currie J, Lessell S: Tonic pupil with giant cell arteritis. Br J Ophthalmol 68:135, 1984

90. D'Alton JG, Preston DN, Bormanis J et al: Multiple transient ischemic attacks, lupus anticoagulant and verrucous endocarditis. Stroke 16:512, 1985

91. Dastur DK, Singhal BS, Shroff HJ: CNS involvement in malignant atrophic papulosis (Kohlmeier-Degos disease): vasculopathy and coagulopathy. J Neurol Neurosurg Psychiatry 44:156, 1981

92. Deane JS, Bibby K: Bilateral optic neuritis following herpes zoster ophthalmicus (letter). Arch Ophthalmol 113:972, 1995

93. Degos R, Delort J, Tricot R: Dermatite papulosquameuse atrophiante. Bull Soc Franc Dermat Syph 49:148, 1942

94. de la Monte SM, Hutchins GM, Gupta PK: Polymorphous meningitis with atypical mononuclear cells in Sjögren's syndrome. Ann Neurol 14:455, 1983

95. Devinsky O, Petito CK, Alonso DR: Clinical and neuropathological findings in systemic lupus erythematosus: the role of vasculitis, heart emboli, and thrombotic thrombocytopenic purpura. Ann Neurol 23:380, 1988

96. Devlin T, Gray L, Allen NB et al: Neuro-Behçet's disease: factors hampering proper diagnosis. Neurology 45:1754, 1995

97. Dhobb M, Ammar F, Bensaid Y et al: Arterial manifestations in Behçet's disease: four new cases. Ann Vasc Surg 1:249, 1986

98. Dickson ER, Maldonado JE, Sheps SG, Cain JA: Systemic giant-cell arteritis with polymyalgia rheumatica: reversible abnormalities of liver function. JAMA 224:1496, 1973

99. Digre KB, Durcan FJ, Branch DW et al: Amaurosis fugax associated with antiphospholipid antibodies. Ann Neurol 25:228, 1989

100. Dimant J, Grob D, Brunner NG: Ophthalmoplegia, ptosis, and myosis in temporal arteritis. Neurology (NY) 39:1054, 1980

101. Dobkin BH: Computerized tomographic findings in neuro-Behçet's disease. Arch Neurol 37:58, 1980

102. Doyle PW, Gibson G, Dolman CL: Herpes zoster ophthalmicus with contralateral hemiplegia: identification of cause. Ann Neurol 14:84, 1983

103. Drachman DA: Neurological complications of Wegener's granulomatosis. Arch Neurol 8:145, 1963

104. Drucker CR: Malignant atrophic papulosis: response to antiplatelet therapy. Dermatologica 180:90, 1990

105. Dupont S, Fénelon G, Saiag P, Sirmai J: Warfarin in Sneddon's syndrome, letter. Neurology 46:1781, 1996

106. Ehrenfeld M, Penchas S, Eliakim M: Thrombocytosis in rheumatoid arthritis: recurrent arterial thromboembolism and death. Ann Rheum Dis 36:579, 1977

107. Ehsan T, Hasan S, Powers JM, Heiserman JE: Serial magnetic resonance imaging in isolated angiitis of the central nervous system. Neurology 45:1462, 1995

108. Eidelberg D, Sotrel A, Horoupian DS et al: Thrombotic cerebral vasculopathy associated with herpes zoster. Ann Neurol 19:7, 1986

109. Elliott PD, Baker HL, Brown AL: The superficial temporal artery angiogram. Radiology 102:635, 1972

110. Ellis SG, Verity MA: Central nervous system involvement in systemic lupus erythematosus: a review of neuropathologic findings in 57 cases, 1955–1977. Semin Arthritis Rheum 4:253, 1979

111. Emura A, Takeuchi A, Hashimoto T et al: A case of

Behçet's disease with Weber's syndrome. J Rheumatol 13:459, 1986

112. Enevoldson TP, Russell RW: Cerebral venous thrombosis: new causes for an old syndrome? Q J Med 77:1255, 1990

113. Engel DG, Gospe SM Jr, Tracy KA et al: Fatal infantile polyarteritis nodosa with predominant central nervous system involvement. Stroke 26:699, 1995

114. Englert HJ, Hawkes CH, Boey ML et al: Degos' disease: association with anticardiolipin antibodies and the lupus anticoagulant. BMJ 289:576, 1984

115. Enzmann D, Scott WR: Intracranial involvement of giant-cell arteritis. Neurology (NY) 27:794, 1977

116. Estes D, Christian CL: The natural history of systemic lupus erythematosus by prospective analysis. Medicine (Baltimore) 50:85, 1971

117. Estey E, Lieberman A, Pinto R et al: Cerebral arteritis in scleroderma. Stroke 10:595, 1979

118. Faer MJ, Mead JH, Lynch RD: Cerebral granulomatous angiitis: case report and literature review. AJR 129:463, 1977

119. Fauchald P, Rygvold O, Oystese B: Temporal arteritis and polymyalgia rheumatica: clinical and biopsy finding. Ann Intern Med 77:845, 1972

120. Fauci AS, Haynes BF, Katz P, Wolff SM: Wegener's granulomatosis: prospective clinical and therapeutic experience with 85 patients for 21 years. Ann Intern Med 98:76, 1983

121. Fauci AS, Katz P, Haynes BF, Wolff SM: Cyclophosphamide therapy of severe systemic necrotizing vasculitis. N Engl J Med 301:235, 1979

122. Feasby TE, Ferguson GG, Kaufman JCE: Isolated spinal cord vasculitis. Can J Neurol Sci 2:143, 1975

123. Fedele FA, Ho G, Jr, Dorman BA: Pseudoaneurysm of the vertebral artery: a complication of rheumatoid cervical spine disease. Arthritis Rheum 29:136, 1986

124. Feinberg SB: Giant cell arteritis of the central nervous system: the place of roentgen diagnosis. Minn Med 47:656, 1964

125. Feinglass EJ, Arnett FC, Dorsch CA et al: Neuropsychiatric manifestations of systemic lupus erythematosus: diagnosis, clinical spectrum, and relationship to other features of the disease. Medicine (Baltimore) 55:323, 1976

126. Feit H, Frenkel EP, Dunn BR et al: Acute subdural hematomas with lupus anticoagulant (procoagulant inhibitor). Neurology (NY) 34:519, 1984

127. Ferris H: Cerebral arteritis: classification. Radiology 109:327, 1973

128. Filloux F, Townsend J: Herpes zoster ophthalmicus with ipsilateral cerebellar infarction. Neurology (NY) 35:1531, 1985

129. Fisher CM: Ocular palsy in temporal arteritis. Minn Med 42:1258, 1959

130. Ford RG, Siekert RG: Central nervous system manifestations of periarteritis nodosa. Neurology (NY) 15:114, 1965

131. Fountain NB, Eberhard DA: Primary angiitis of the central nervous system associated with cerebral amyloid angiopathy: report of two cases and review of the literature. Neurology 46:190, 1996

132. Fox IS, Spence AM, Wheelis RF, Healey LA: Cerebral embolism in Libman-Sacks endocarditis. Neurology (NY) 30:487, 1980

133. Francés C, Le Tonquéze M, Salohzin KV et al: Prevalence of anti-endothelial cell antibodies in patients with Sneddon's syndrome. J Am Acad Dermatol 33:64, 1995

134. Frayne JH, Gilligan BS, Essex WB: Granulomatous angiitis of the central nervous system. Med J Aust 145:410, 1986

135. Fred HL, Lynch EC, Greenberg SD, Gonzalez-Angulo A: A patient with Wegener's granulomatosis exhibiting unusual clinical and morphologic features. Am J Med 37:311, 1964

136. Friedrich H, Laas J, Walterbusch G, Rickels E: Extra-intracranial bypass procedure with saphenous vein grafts. Thorac Cardiovasc Surg 34:57, 1986

137. Fryer DG, Crane R, Margolis MT: Angiographic changes in intracranial arteritis of ophthalmic herpes zoster. Ann Neurol 15:311, 1984

138. Futrell N, Millikan C: Frequency, etiology, and prevention of stroke in patients with systemic lupus erythematosus. Stroke 20:583, 1989

139. Futrell N, Schultz LR, Millikan C: Central nervous system disease in patients with systemic lupus erythematosus. Neurology 42:1649, 1992

140. Galetta SL, Raps EC, Wulc AE et al: Conjugal temporal arteritis. Neurology (NY) 40:1839, 1990

141. Gasperetti C, Son SK: Contralateral hemiparesis following herpes zoster ophthalmicus. J Neurol Neurosurg Psychiatry 48:338, 1985

142. Gastineau DA, Kazmier FJ, Nichols WL, Bowie EJW: Lupus anticoagulant: an analysis of the clinical and laboratory features of 219 cases. Am J Hematol 19:265, 1985

143. Geschwind DH, FitzPatrick M, Mischel PS, Cummings JL: Sneddon's syndrome is a thrombotic vasculopathy: neuropathologic and neuroradiologic evidence. Neurology 45:557, 1995

144. Gharavi AE, Harris EN, Asherson RA, Hughes GRV: Anticardiolipin antibodies: isotype distribution and phospholipid specificity. Ann Rheum Dis 46:1, 1987

145. Gherardi GJ, Lee HU: Localized dissecting hemorrhage and arteritis: renal and cerebral manifestations. JAMA 199:187, 1967

146. Giang DW: Central nervous system vasculitis secondary to infections, toxins, and neoplasms. Semin Neurol 14:313, 1994

147. Gibb WRG, Urry PA, Lees AJ: Giant cell arteritis with spinal cord infarction and basilar artery thrombosis. J Neurol Neurosurg Psychiatry 48:945, 1985

148. Gilbert GJ: Herpes zoster ophthalmicus and delayed contralateral hemiparesis: relationship of the syndrome to central nervous system granulomatous angiitis. JAMA 229:302, 1974

149. Gillanders LA, Strachan RW, Blair DW: Temporal arteriography. Ann Rheum Dis 28:267, 1969

150. Gilmour JR: Giant-cell chronic arteritis. J Pathol 53:263, 1941

151. Ginsberg L, Geddes J, Valentine A: Amyloid angiopathy and granulomatous angiitis of the central nervous system: a case responding to corticosteroid treatment. J Neurol 235:438, 1988

152. Giordano JM, Leavitt RY, Hoffman G, Fauci AS: Experience with surgical treatment of Takayasu's disease. Surgery 109:252, 1991

153. Giordano MJ, Commins D, Silbergeld DL: Sjögren's cerebritis complicated by subarachnoid hemorrhage and bilateral superior cerebellar artery occlusion: case report. Surg Neurol 43:48, 1995

154. Giovanini MA, Eskin TA, Mukherji SK, Mickle JP: Granulomatous angiitis of the spinal cord: a case report. Neurosurgery 34:540, 1994

155. Goldberg AL, Tievsky AL, Jamshidi S: Wegener granulomatosis invading the cavernous sinus: a CT demonstration. J Comput Assist Tomogr 7:701, 1983

156. Goodman BW: Temporal arteritis. Am J Med 67:839, 1979

157. Gordon DL, Hayreh SS, Adams HP Jr: Microangiopathy of the brain, retina, and ear: improvement without immunosuppressive therapy. Stroke 22:933, 1991

158. Gordon MF, Coyle PK, Golub B: Eales' disease presenting as stroke in the young adult. Ann Neurol 24:264, 1988

159. Gordon RM, Silverstein A: Neurologic manifestations in progressive systemic sclerosis. Arch Neurol 22:126, 1970

160. Gorelick PB, Rusinowitz MS, Tiku M et al: Embolic stroke complicating systemic lupus erythematosus. Arch Neurol 42:813, 1985

161. Gorevic PD, Kassab HJ, Levo Y et al: Mixed cryoglobulinemia: clinical aspects and long-term follow-up of 40 patients. Am J Med 69:287, 1980

162. Görsoy G, Aktin E, Bahar S et al: Post-herpetic aneurysm in the intrapetrosal portion of the internal carotid artery. Neuroradiology 19:279, 1980

163. Graham E: Survival in temporal arteritis. Trans Ophthalmol Soc UK 100:108, 1980

164. Grattan CEH, Burton JL, Boon AP: Sneddon's syndrome (livedo reticularis and cerebral thrombosis) with livedo vasculitis and anticardiolipin antibodies. Br J Dermatol 120:441, 1989

165. Gray F, Vinters HV, Le Noan H et al: Cerebral amyloid angiopathy and granulomatous angiitis: immunohistochemical study using antibodies to the Alzheimer A4 peptide. Hum Pathol 21:1290, 1990

166. Greaves DP: Ophthalmic manifestations of giant cell arteritis. Trans Ophthalmol Soc UK 81:427, 1961

167. Greco FA, Kolins J, Rajjoub RK, Brereton HD: Hodgkin's disease and granulomatous angiitis of the central nervous system. Cancer 38:2027, 1976

168. Greenan TJ, Grossman RI, Goldberg HI: Cerebral vasculitis: MR imaging and angiographic correlation. Radiology 182:65, 1992

169. Greenfield JG: Giant cell arteritis. Proc R Soc Med 44:855, 1951

170. Griffin J, Price DL, Davis L, McKhann GM: Granulomatous angiitis of the central nervous system with aneurysms on multiple cerebral arteries. Trans Am Neurol Assoc 98:145, 1973

171. Guillevin L, Lhote F, Gayraud M et al: Prognostic factors in polyarteritis nodosa and Churg-Strauss syndrome. A prospective study in 342 patients. Medicine (Baltimore) 75:17, 1996

172. Gutman L, Hable K: Rheumatoid pachymeningitis. Neurology (NY) 13:901, 1963

173. Haft H, Finneson BE, Cramer H, Fiol R: Periarteritis nodosa as a source of subarachnoid hemorrhage and spinal cord compression. J Neurosurg 14:608, 1957

174. Hall GH, Hargreaves T: Giant cell arteritis and raised serum alkaline phosphate levels (letter). Lancet 2:48, 1972

175. Hall S, Barr W, Lie JT et al: Takayasu arteritis: a study of 32 North American patients. Medicine (Baltimore) 64:89, 1985

176. Hall S, Hunder GG: Is temporal artery biopsy prudent? Mayo Clin Proc 59:793, 1984

177. Hall S, Lie JT, Kurland LT et al: The therapeutic impact of temporal artery biopsy. Lancet 2:1217, 1983

178. Hamilton CR, Shelley WM, Tumulty PA: Giant cell arteritis: including temporal arteritis and polymyalgia rheumatica. Medicine (Baltimore) 50:1, 1971

179. Hammoudeh M, Khan M: Cranial arteritis as the initial manifestation of malignant histiocytosis. J Rheumatol 9:443, 1982

180. Hamrin B: Polymyalgia arteritica. Acta Med Scand (suppl) 533:1, 1972

181. Hamrin B, Jonsson N, Hellsten S: "Polymyalgia arteritica": further clinical and histopathological studies with a report of six autopsy cases. Ann Rheum Dis 27:397, 1968

182. Hanly JG, Walsh NM, Sangalang V: Brain pathology in systemic lupus erythematosus. J Rheumatol 19:732, 1992

183. Harbitz F: Unknown forms of arteritis with special reference to their relation to syphilitic arteritis and periarteritis nodosa. Am J Med Sci 163:250, 1922

184. Harle JR, Disdier P, Ali Cherif A et al: Démence curable et panartérite noueuse. Rev Neurol (Paris) 147:148, 1991

185. Harley JB, Alexander EL, Bias WB et al: Anti-Ro (SS-A) and anti-La (SS-B) in patients with Sjögren's syndrome. Arthritis Rheum 29:196, 1986

186. Harper CM Jr, O'Neill BP, O'Duffy JD, Forbes GS: Intracranial hypertension in Behçet's disease: demonstration of sinus occlusion with use of digital subtraction angiography. Mayo Clin Proc 60:419, 1985

187. Harris EN, Gharavi AE, Asherson RA et al: Cerebral infarction in systemic lupus: association with anticardiolipin antibodies. Clin Exp Rheumatol 2:47, 1984

188. Harris EN, Hughes GRV, Gharavi AE: Antiphospholipid antibodies: an elderly statesman dons new garments. J Rheumatol, suppl. 13, 14:208, 1987

189. Harrison PE: Granulomatous angiitis of the central nervous system. J Neurol Sci 29:335, 1976

190. Hashimoto N, Handa H, Taki W: Ruptured cerebral aneurysms in patients with systemic lupus erythematosus. Surg Neurol 26:512, 1986

191. Hauser WA, Ferguson RH, Holley KE, Kurland LT: Temporal arteritis in Rochester, Minnesota, 1951 to 1967. Mayo Clin Proc 46:597, 1971

192. Hayreh SS: Anterior ischemic optic neuropathy. Arch Neurol 38:675, 1981

193. Healey LA, Wilske KR: Manifestations of giant cell arteritis. Med Clin North Am 61:261, 1977

194. Heiskala H, Somer H, Kovanen J et al: Microangiopathy

with encephalopathy, hearing loss and retinal arteriolar occlusions: two new cases. J Neurol Sci 86:239, 1988

195. Heptinstall RH, Porter KA, Barkley H: Giant cell (temporal) arteritis. J Pathol 67:507, 1954

196. Herkes GK, Storey CE, Joffe R, Mackenzie RA: Herpes zoster arteritis: clinical and angiographic features. Clin Exp Neurol 64:169, 1987

197. Herskovitz S, Lipton RB, Lantos G: Neuro-Behçet's disease: CT and clinical correlates. Neurology (NY) 38:1714, 1988

198. Hilt DC, Buchholz D, Krumholz A et al: Herpes zoster ophthalmicus and delayed contralateral hemiparesis caused by cerebral angiitis: diagnosis and management approaches. Ann Neurol 14:543, 1983

199. Hinck VC, Carter CC, Rippey GG: Giant cell (cranial) arteritis: a case with angiographic abnormalities. AJR 92:769, 1964

200. Hirsch M, Mayersdorf A, Lehman E: Cranial giant cell arteritis. Br J Radiol 47:503, 1974

201. Hogan PJ, Greenberg MK, McCarty GE: Neurologic complications of lymphomatoid granulomatosis. Neurology (NY) 31:619, 1981

202. Hollenhorst RW, Brown JR, Wagener HP, Shick RM: Neurologic aspects of temporal arteritis. Neurology (NY) 10:490, 1960

203. Hood J, Wilson ER, Jr, Alexander CB et al: Lymphomatoid granulomatosis manifested as a mass in the cerebellopontine angle. Arch Neurol 39:319, 1982

204. Horner FA, Myers GJ, Stumpf DA et al: Malignant atrophic papulosis (Kohlmeier-Degos disease) in childhood. Neurology (NY) 26:317, 1976

205. Horton BT: Complications of temporal arteritis. BMJ 1:105, 1966

206. Howard GF, Ho SU, Kim KS, Wallach J: Bilateral carotid occlusion resulting from giant cell arteritis. Ann Neurol 15:204, 1984

207. Howell SJL, Molyneux AJ: Vertebrobasilar insufficiency in rheumatoid atlanto-axial subluxation: a case report with angiographic demonstration of left vertebral artery occlusion. J Neurol 235:189, 1988

208. Hughes GRV, Asherson RA, Khamashta MA: The antiphospholipid syndrome—from theory to discovery. Postgrad Med J 65:691, 1989

209. Hughes JT, Brownell B: Granulomatous giant celled angiitis of the central nervous system. Neurology (NY) 16:293, 1966

210. Hull RG, Harris N, Gharavi AE et al: Anticardiolipin antibodies: occurrence in Behçet's syndrome. Ann Rheum Dis 43:746, 1984

211. Hunder GG, Baker HL, Rhoton AL et al: Superficial temporal arteriography in patients suspected of having temporal arteritis. Arthritis Rheum 15:561, 1972

212. Hunder GG, Hazleman BL: Giant cell arteritis and polymyalgia rheumatica. In Kelly WN, Harris ED Jr, Ruddy S, Sledge CB (eds): Textbook of Rheumatology. WB Saunders, Philadelphia, 1981

213. Hunder GG, Sheps SG, Allen GL, Joyce JW: Daily and alternate-day corticosteroid regimens in treatment of giant cell arteritis: comparison in a prospective study. Ann Intern Med 82:613, 1975

214. Hunder GG, Taswell HF, Pineda AA, Elveback LR:

215. Hurst RW, Grossman RI: Neuroradiology of central nervous system vasculitis. Semin Neurol 14:320, 1994

216. Huston KA, Hunder GG: Giant cell (cranial) arteritis: a clinical review. Am Heart J 100:99, 1980

217. Huston KA, Hunder GG, Lie JT et al: Temporal arteritis: a 25-year epidemiologic, clinical and pathologic study. Ann Intern Med 88:162, 1978

218. Imaizumi M, Nukada T, Yoneda S, Abe H: Behçet's disease with sinus thrombosis and arteriovenous malformation in brain. J Neurol 222:215, 1980

219. Inwards DJ, Piepgras DG, Lie JT et al: Granulomatous angiitis of the spinal cord associated with Hodgkin's disease. Cancer 68:1318, 1991

220. Iraguli VJ, Maravi E: Behçet syndrome presenting as cerebrovascular disease. J Neurol Neurosurg Psychiatry 49:838, 1986

221. Ironside JW, Martin JF, Richmond J, Timperley WR: Lymphomatoid granulomatosis with cerebral involvement. Neuropathol Appl Neurobiol 10:397, 1984

222. Ishikawa K: Natural history and classification of occlusive thromboaortopathy (Takayasu's disease). Circulation 57:27, 1978

223. Ishikawa K, Yonekawa Y: Regression of carotid stenoses after corticosteroid therapy in occlusive thromboaortopathy (Takayasu's disease). Stroke 18:677, 1987

224. Iwata K, Misu N, Nara Y: Granulomatous angiitis of the central nervous system—a case with recurrent intracerebral hemorrhage. Neurol Med Chir (Tokyo) 32:834, 1992

225. Jackson CG, Chess RL, Ward JR: A case of rheumatoid nodule formation within the central nervous system and review of the literature. J Rheumatol 11:237, 1984

226. Jellinger K: Giant cell granulomatous angiitis of the central nervous system. J Neurol 215:175, 1977

227. Jennings GH: Arteritis of the temporal vessels. Lancet 1:424, 1938

228. Johnson M, Maciunas R, Dutt P et al: Granulomatous angiitis masquerading as a mass lesion: magnetic resonance imaging and stereotactic biopsy findings in a patient with occult Hodgkin's disease. Surg Neurol 31:49, 1989

229. Johnson MD, Maciunas R, Creasy J, Collins RD: Indolent granulomatous angiitis. Case report. J Neurosurg 81:472, 1994

230. Johnson RL, Smyth CJ, Holt GW et al: Steroid therapy and vascular lesions in rheumatoid arthritis. Arthritis Rheum 2:224, 1959

231. Johnson RT, Richardson EP: The neurological manifestations of systemic lupus erythematosus: a clinical-pathological study of 24 cases and review of the literature. Medicine (Baltimore) 47:337, 1968

232. Jonas J, Kölble K, Völcker HE, Kalden JR: Central retinal artery occlusion in Sneddon's disease associated with antiphospholipid antibodies. Am J Ophthalmol 102:37, 1986

233. Jonasson F, Cullen JF, Elton RA: Temporal arteritis: a 14-year epidemiological, clinical and prognostic study. Scott Med J 24:111, 1979

234. Jones JG, Hazleman BL: Prognosis and management of polymyalgia rheumatica. Ann Rheum Dis 40:1, 1981

235. Jones MW, Kaufmann JCE: Vertebrobasilar artery insufficiency in rheumatoid atlantoaxial subluxation. J Neurol Neurosurg Psychiatry 39:122, 1976

236. Kalashnikova LA, Nasonov EL, Kushekbaeva AE, Gracheva LA: Anticardiolipin antibodies in Sneddon's syndrome. Neurology (NY) 40:464, 1990

237. Kaminska EA, Sadler M, Sangalang V et al: Microangiopathic syndrome of encephalopathy, retinal vessel occlusion and hearing loss (abstract). Can J Neurol Sci 2: 241, 1990

238. Kapila A, Gupta KL, Garcia JH: CT and MR of lymphomatoid granulomatosis of the CNS: report of four cases and review of the literature. AJNR 9:1139, 1988

239. Karam NE, Roger L, Hankins LL, Reveille JD: Rheumatoid nodulosis of the meninges. J Rheumatol 21:1960, 1994

240. Kasantikul V, Kasantikul D: Localized necrotizing arteritis of the central nervous system. Surg Neurol 43:510, 1995

241. Katelaris CH, Walls RS: Fatal neurological complications in temporal arteritis: an unusual case. Aust NZ J Med 12:299, 1982

242. Kattah JC, Cupps TR, Di Chiro G, Manz HJ: An unusual case of central nervous system vasculitis. J Neurol 234: 344, 1987

243. Kausu T, Corbett JJ, Savino P, Schatz NJ: Giant cell arteritis with normal sedimentation rate. Arch Neurol 34:624, 1977

244. Kawakita H, Nishimura M, Satoh Y, Shibata N: Neurological aspects of Behçet's disease: a case report and clinico-pathological review of the literature in Japan. J Neurol Sci 5:417, 1967

245. Kaye BR, Neuwelt CM, London SS, DeArmond SJ: Central nervous system systemic lupus erythematosus mimicking progressive multifocal leucoencephalopathy. Ann Rheum Dis 51:1152, 1992

246. Kazui S, Naritomi H, Imakita S et al: Sequential gadolinium-DTPA enhanced MRI studies in neuro-Behçet's disease. Neuroradiology 33:136, 1991

247. Kelley RE, Stokes N, Reyes P, Harik SI: Cerebral transmural angiitis and ruptured aneurysm: a complication of systemic lupus erythematosus. Arch Neurol 37: 526, 1980

248. Kernohan JW, Woltman HW: Periarteritis nodosa: a clinicopathologic study with special reference to the nervous system. Arch Neurol Neurosurg Psychiatry 39:655, 1938

249. Kerr RSC, Hughes JT, Blamires T, Teddy PJ: Lymphomatoid granulomatosis apparently confined to one temporal lobe: case report. J Neurosurg 67:612, 1987

250. Kim RC: Rheumatoid disease with encephalopathy. Ann Neurol 7:861, 1980

251. Kim RC, Collins GH, Parisi JE: Rheumatoid nodule formation within the choroid plexus: report of a second case. Arch Pathol Lab Med 106:83, 1982

252. Kirk A, Kertesz A, Polk MJ: Dementia with leukoencephalopathy in systemic lupus erythematosus. Can J Neurol Sci 18:344, 1991

253. Kitagawa Y, Gotoh F, Koto A, Okayasu H: Stroke in systemic lupus erythematosus. Stroke 21:1533, 1990

254. Kjeldsen MH, Reske-Nielsen E: Pathological changes of the central nervous system in giant cell arteritis. Acta Ophthalmol Scand 46:49, 1968

255. Klein RG, Campbell RJ, Hunder GG, Carney JA: Skip lesions in temporal arteritis. Mayo Clin Proc 51:504, 1976

256. Klein RG, Hunder GG, Stanson AW, Sheps SG: Large artery involvement in giant cell (temporal) arteritis. Ann Intern Med 83:806, 1975

257. Kokmen E, Billman JK Jr, Abell MR: Lymphomatoid granulomatosis clinically confined to the CNS. Arch Neurol 34:782, 1977

258. Kolodny EK, Rebeiz JJ, Caviness VS, Richardson EP: Granulomatous angiitis of the central nervous system. Arch Neurol 19:510, 1968

259. Koo EH, Massey EW: Granulomatous angiitis of the central nervous system protean manifestations and response to treatment. J Neurol Neurosurg Psychiatry 51: 1126, 1988

260. Kott HS: Stroke due to vasculitis. Primary Care 6:771, 1979

261. Kozin F, Haughton V, Bernhard GC: Neuro-Behçet disease: two cases and neuroradiologic findings. Neurology (NY) 27:1148, 1977

262. Kozula S, Iguchi I, Furuse M et al: Cerebral granulomatous angiitis with atypical features. J Neurol 231:38, 1984

263. Kristoferitsch W, Jellinger K, Bock F: Cerebral granulomatous angiitis with atypical features. J Neurol 231:38, 1984

264. Kuroiwa Y, Furukawa T: Hemispheric infarction after herpes zoster ophthalmicus: computed tomography and angiography. Neurology (NY) 31:1030, 1981

265. Label LS, Tandan R, Albers JW: Myelomalacia and hypoglycorrhachia in malignant atrophic papulosis. Neurology (NY) 33:936, 1983

266. Le Coz P, Mikol J, Ferrand J et al: Granulomatous angiitis and cerebral amyloid angiopathy presenting as a mass lesion. Neuropathol Appl Neurobiol 17:149, 1991

267. Lee JE, Haynes JM: Carotid arteritis and cerebral infarction due to scleroderma. Neurology (NY) 17:18, 1967

268. Lee P, Urowitz MB, Bookman AAM et al: Systemic lupus erythematosus: a review of 110 cases with reference to nephritis, the nervous system, infections, aseptic necrosis and prognosis. Q J Med 181:1, 1977

269. Leeds NE, Goldberg HI: Angiographic manifestations in cerebral inflammatory disease. Radiology 98:595, 1971

270. Leib ES, Restivo C, Paulus HE: Immunosuppressive and corticosteroid therapy of polyarteritis nodosa. Am J Med 67:941, 1979

271. Levine SR, Deegan MJ, Futrell N, Welch KMA: Cerebrovascular and neurologic disease associated with antiphospholipid antibodies: 48 cases. Neurology (NY) 40: 1181, 1990

272. Levine SR, Kieran S, Puzio K et al: Cerebral venous thrombosis with lupus anticoagulants: report of two cases. Stroke 18:801, 1987

273. Levine SR, Langer SL, Albers JW, Welch KMA: Sneddon's syndrome: an antiphospholipid antibody syndrome? Neurology 38:798, 1988

274. Lewis IC, Philpott MG: Neurological complications in the Schönlein-Henoch syndrome. Arch Dis Child 31: 369, 1956

275. Lexa FJ, Galetta SL, Yousem DM et al: Herpes zoster ophthalmicus with orbital pseudotumor syndrome complicated by optic nerve infarction and cerebral granulomatous angiitis: MR-pathologic correlation. AJNR 14: 185, 1993

276. Liang GC, Simkin PA, Mammik M: Immunoglobulins in temporal arteritis. Ann Intern Med 81:19, 1974

277. Libman E, Sacks B: A hitherto undescribed form of valvular and mural endocarditis. Arch Intern Med 33:701, 1924

278. Lie JT: Primary (granulomatous) angiitis of the central nervous system: a clinicopathologic analysis of 15 new cases and a review of the literature. Hum Pathol 23:164, 1992

279. Lie JT: Aortic and extracranial large vessel giant cell arteritis: a review of 72 cases with histopathologic documentation. Semin Arthritis Rheum 24:422, 1995

280. Lie JT, Kobayashi S, Tokano Y, Hashimoto H: Systemic and cerebral vasculitis coexisting with disseminated coagulopathy in systemic lupus erythematosus associated with antiphospholipid syndrome. J Rheumatol 22:2173, 1995

281. Liebow AA: Pulmonary angiitis and granulomatosis. Am Rev Respir Dis 108:1, 1973

282. Liebow AA, Carrington CRB, Friedman PJ: Lymphomatoid granulomatosis. Hum Pathol 3:457, 1972

283. Linneman CCJ, Alvira MM: Pathogenesis of varicella-zoster angiitis in the central nervous system. Arch Neurol 37:239, 1980

284. Lossos A, Ben-Hur T, Ben-Nariah Z et al: Familial Sneddon's syndrome. J Neurol 242:164, 1995

285. Love DC, Rapkin J, Lesser GR et al: Temporal arteritis in blacks. Ann Intern Med 105:387, 1986

286. Lu AT, Barasch S: Neurological involvement in Behçet's syndrome: a case report with neuropathological data and a summary of the reported autopsied cases. Bull Los Angeles Neurol Soc 28:85, 1963

287. Lucas FV, Benjamin SP, Steinberg MC: Cerebral vasculitis in Wegener's granulomatosis. Cleve Clin J Med 43: 275, 1976

288. Ludmerer KM, Kissane JM: Chronic meningitis in a 68-year-old man. Am J Med 85:407, 1988

289. Lueck CJ, Pires M, McCartney AC, Graham EM: Ocular and neurological Behçet's disease without orogenital ulceration? J Neurol Neurosurg Psychiatry 56:505, 1993

290. MacFadyen DJ: Wegener's granulomatosis with discrete lung lesions and peripheral neuritis. Can Med Assoc J 83:760, 1960

291. MacFadyen DJ, Schneider RJ, Chisholm IA: A syndrome of brain, inner ear and retinal microangiopathy. Can J Neurol Sci 14:315, 1987

292. Machado EBV, Michet CJ, Ballard DJ et al: Trends in incidence and clinical presentation of temporal arteritis in Olmsted County, Minnesota, 1950–1985. Arthritis Rheum 31:745, 1988

293. Mackenzie RA, Forbes GS, Karnes WE: Angiographic findings in herpes zoster arteritis. Ann Neurol 10:458, 1981

294. Mackenzie RA, Ryan P, Karnes WE, Okazaki H: Herpes zoster arteritis: pathological findings. Clin Exp Neurol 23:219, 1987

295. Magidson MA, Rajendran MM, Leutcher WM: Granulomatous angiitis of the central nervous system with an unusual angiographic feature. Surg Neurol 10:355, 1978

296. Magrinat G, Kerwin KS, Gabriel DA: The clinical manifestations of Degos' syndrome. Arch Pathol Lab Med 113:354, 1989

297. Malamud N, Foster DB: Periarteritis nodosa: a clinicopathologic report, with special reference to the central nervous system. Arch Neurol Psychiatr 47:828, 1942

298. Mandybur TI: Cerebral amyloid angiopathy: possible relationship to rheumatoid vasculitis. Neurology (NY) 29: 1336, 1979

299. Mandybur TI, Balko G: Cerebral amyloid angiopathy with granulomatous angiitis ameliorated by steroid-cytoxan treatment. Clin Neuropharmacol 15:241, 1992

300. Manor RS, Ouaknine L, Ouaknine G: Susac-Red-M syndrome (abstract). Proceedings of the Meeting of the International Neuro-Ophthalmological Society. Freiburg, Germany, June 1994

301. Manschot WA: A fatal case of temporal arteritis, with ocular symptoms. Ophthalmologica 149:121, 1965

302. Markenson JA, McDougal JS, Tsairis P et al: Rheumatoid meningitis: a localized immune process. Ann Intern Med 90:786, 1979

303. Marsden HB: Basilar artery thrombosis and giant cell arteritis (abstract). Arch Dis Child 49:75, 1974

304. Martin JR, Mitchell WJ, Henken DB: Neurotropic herpesviruses, neural mechanisms and arteritis. Brain Pathol 1:6, 1990

305. Mass M, Bourdette D, Bernstein W, Hammerstad J: Retinopathy, encephalopathy, deafness associated microangiopathy (the RED M syndrome): three new cases (abstract). Neurology (NY), suppl. 1, 38:215, 1988

306. Masugata H, Yasuno M, Nishino M et al: Takayasu's arteritis with collateral circulation from the right coronary artery to intracranial vessels—a case report. Angiology 43:448, 1992

307. Masuzawa T, Shimabukuro H, Furuse M et al: Pulseless disease associated with a ruptured intracranial vertebral aneurysm. Neurol Med Chir 24:490, 1984

308. McCormick HM, Neuberger KT: Giant cell arteritis involving small meningeal and intracerebral vessels. J Neuropathol Exp Neurol 17:471, 1958

309. McFarland HR, Wood WG, Drowns BV, Meneses ACO: Papulosis atrophicans maligna (Köhlmeier-Degos disease): a disseminated occlusive vasculopathy. Ann Neurol 3:388, 1978

310. McMenemey WH, Lawrence BJ: Encephalomyelopathy in Behçet's disease: report of necropsy findings in two cases. Lancet 2:353, 1957

311. Meadows SP: Temporal or giant cell arteritis. Proc R Soc Med 59:329, 1966

312. Meneely JK, Bigelow NH: Temporal arteritis. Am J Med 14:46, 1953

313. Mickle JP, McLennan JE, Chi JG, Lidden CW: Cortical vein thrombosis in Wegener's granulomatosis: case report. J Neurosurg 46:248, 1977

314. Milgram JW, Stecher K: Idiopathic arteritis with multiple intracranial aneurysms. Angiology 25:89, 1974

315. Miller NR: Anterior ischemic optic neuropathy: diagnosis and management. Bull NY Acad Med 56:643, 1980

316. Miró J, Peña-Sagredo JL, Berciano J et al: Prevalence of primary Sjögren's syndrome in patients with multiple sclerosis. Ann Neurol 27:582, 1990

317. Missen GA: Involvement of the vertebrocarotid arterial system in giant cell arteritis. J Pathol 106:ii, 1972

318. Monteiro MLR, Swanson RA, Coppeto JR et al: A microangiopathic syndrome of encephalopathy, hearing loss, and retinal arteriolar occlusions. Neurology (NY) 35:1113, 1985

319. Moore PM: Diagnosis and management of isolated angiitis of the central nervous system. Neurology (NY) 39:167, 1989

320. Moore PM, Lisak RP: Multiple sclerosis and Sjögren's syndrome: a problem in diagnosis or in definition of two disorders of unknown etiology? Ann Neurol 27:585, 1990

321. Morgan GJ Jr, Harris ED Jr: Non-giant cell temporal arteritis. Arthritis Rheum 21:362, 1978

322. Morrison AN, Abitol M: Granulomatous arteritis with myocardial infarction. Ann Intern Med 42:691, 1955

323. Morrissey SP, Miller DH, Hermaszewski R et al: Magnetic resonance imaging of the central nervous system in Behçet's disease. Eur Neurol 33:287, 1993

324. Moutsopoulos HM, Sarmas JH, Talal N: Is central nervous system involvement a systemic manifestation of primary Sjögren's syndrome? Rheum Dis Clin North Am 19:909, 1993

325. Mueh JR, Herbst KD, Rapaport SI: Thrombosis in patients with the lupus anticoagulant. Ann Intern Med 92:156, 1980

326. Murphy JJ, Leach IH: Findings at necropsy in the heart of a patient with anticardiolipin syndrome. Br Heart J 62:61, 1989

327. Nagaratnam N, James WE: Isolated angiitis of the brain in a young female on the contraceptive pill. Postgrad Med J 63:1085, 1987

328. Nagata K: Recurrent intracranial haemorrhage in Behçet disease. J Neurol Neurosurg Psychiatry 48:190, 1985

329. Nasu T: Takayasu's truncoarteritis in Japan: a statistical observation of 76 autopsy cases. Pathol Microbiol 43:140, 1975

330. Negishi C, Sze G: Vasculitis presenting as primary leptomeningeal enhancement with minimal parenchymal findings. AJNR 14:26, 1993

331. Newman NJ, Slamovits TL, Friedland S, Wilson WB: Neuro-ophthalmic manifestations of meningocerebral inflammation from the limited form of Wegener's granulomatosis. Am J Ophthalmol 120:613, 1995

332. Newman W, Wolf A: Non-infectious granulomatous angiitis involving the central nervous system. Trans Am Neurol Assoc 77:114, 1952

333. Nishimura M, Satoh K, Suga M, Oda M: Cerebral angio- and neuro-Behçet's syndrome: neuroradiological and pathological study of one case. J Neurol Sci 106:19, 1991

334. Nishino H, Rubino FA, DeRemee RA et al: Neurological involvement in Wegener's granulomatosis: an analysis of 324 consecutive patients at the Mayo Clinic. Ann Neurol 33:4, 1993

335. Nishino H, Rubino FA, Parisi JE: The spectrum of neurologic involvement in Wegener's granulomatosis. Neurology 43:1334, 1993

336. Noseworthy JH, Bass BH, Vandervoort MK et al: The prevalence of primary Sjögren's syndrome in a multiple sclerosis population. Ann Neurol 25:95, 1989

337. Noseworthy JH, Bass BH, Vandervoort MK et al: Reply (letter). Ann Neurol 27:587, 1990

338. Nurick S, Blackwood W, Mair WGP: Giant cell granulomatous angiitis of the central nervous system. Brain 95:133, 1972

339. O'Donohue JM, Enzmann DR: Mycotic aneurysm in angiitis associated with herpes zoster ophthalmicus. AJNR 8:615, 1987

340. O'Duffy JD, Goldstein NP: Neurologic involvement in seven patients with Behçet's disease. Am J Med 61:170, 1976

341. O'Duffy JD, Robertson DM, Goldstein NP: Chlorambucil in the treatment of uveitis and meningoencephalitis of Behçet's disease. Am J Med 76:75, 1984

342. Ojeda VJ: Polyarteritis nodosa affecting the spinal cord arteries. Aust NZ J Med 13:287, 1983

343. Ojeda VJ, Peters DM, Spagnolo DV: Giant cell granulomatous angiitis of the central nervous system in a patient with leukemia and cutaneous herpes zoster. Am J Clin Pathol 81:529, 1984

344. Ostberg G: Temporal arteritis in a large necropsy series. Ann Rheum Dis 30:224, 1971

345. Ostberg G: Morphological changes in the large arteries in polymyalgia arteritica. Acta Med Scand (suppl) 533:135, 1972

346. Ostberg G: On arteritis with special reference to polymyalgia arteritica. Acta Pathol Microbiol Scand (suppl A) 237:1, 1973

347. Ouyang R, Mitchell DM, Rozdilsky B: Central nervous system involvement in rheumatoid disease: report of a case. Neurology (NY) 17:1099, 1967

348. Pamir MN, Kansu T, Erbengi A, Zileli T: Papilledema in Behçet's syndrome. Arch Neurol 38:643, 1981

349. Papaioannou CC, Gupta RC, Hunder GG, McDuffie FC: Circulating immune complexes in giant cell arteritis and polymyalgia rheumatica. Arthritis Rheum 23:1021, 1980

350. Park JR, Jones JG, Harkniss GD, Hazleman BL: Circulating immune complexes in polymyalgia rheumatica and giant cell arteritis. Ann Rheum Dis 40:360, 1981

351. Parker HL, Kernohan JW: The central nervous system in periarteritis nodosa. Trans Am Neurol Assoc 72:54, 1947

352. Parker HL, Kernohan JW: The central nervous system in periarteritis nodosa. Mayo Clin Proc 24:43, 1949

353. Patel DV, Neuman JM, Hier DB: Reversibility of CT and MR findings in neuro-Behçet disease. J Comput Assist Tomogr 13:669, 1989

354. Patton WF, Lynch JP, III: Lymphomatoid granulomatosis: clinicopathologic study of four cases and literature review. Medicine (Baltimore) 61:1, 1982

355. Paulley JW, Hughes JP: Giant cell arteritis or arteritis of the aged. Br Med J 2:1562, 1960

356. Peison B, Padlechas R: Granulomatous angiitis of the nervous system. IMJ 126:330, 1964

357. Pellat J, Perret J, Pasquier B et al: Etude anatomoclinique et angiographique d'une observation de thromboangiose disséminée a manifestations cérébrales prédominantes. Rev Neurol (Paris) 132:517, 1976

358. Petit WA, Jr, Soso MJ, Higman H: Degos disease: neurologic complications and cerebral angiography. Neurology (NY) 32:1305, 1982

359. Pettee AD, Wasserman BA, Adams NL et al: Familial Sneddon's syndrome: clinical, hematologic, and radiographic findings in two brothers. Neurology 44:399, 1994

360. Petty GW, Duffy J, Huston J, III: Cerebral ischemia in patients with hepatitis C virus infection and mixed cryoglobulinemia. Mayo Clin Proc 71:671, 1996

361. Petty GW, Engel AG: Microangiopathic involvement of muscle in patients with retinocochleocerebral vasculopathy (abstract). Neurology 45, suppl, 4:A312, 1995

362. Petty GW, Engel AG, Younge BR et al: Retinocochleocerebral vasculopathy. Medicine, 1998 (in press)

363. Pezeshkpour G, Stuart TD, Estridge MN: Crystalline encephalopathy: cerebral immunoprotein deposits and isolated angiitis. Ann Neurol 17:96, 1985

364. Pfaffenbach DD, Hollenhorst RS: Microangiopathy of the retinal arterioles. JAMA 225:480, 1973

365. Pines A, Kaplinsky N, Olchovsky D et al: Recurrent transient ischemic attacks associated with thrombocytosis in rheumatoid arthritis. Clin Rheumatol 1:291, 1982

366. Pollack M, Blennerhasset JB, Clarke AM: Giant cell arteritis and the subclavian steal syndrome. Neurology (NY) 23:653, 1973

367. Probst A, Ulrich J: Amyloid angiopathy combined with granulomatous angiitis of the central nervous system: report on two patients. Clin Neuropathol 4:250, 1985

368. Quimby SR, Perry HO: Livedo reticularis and cerebrovascular accidents. J Am Acad Dermatol 3:377, 1980

369. Rajjoub RK, Wook JH, Ommaya AK: Granulomatous angiitis of the brain. A successfully treated case. Neurology (NY) 27:588, 1977

370. Ramos M, Mandybur TI: Cerebral vasculitis in rheumatoid arthritis. Arch Neurol 32:271, 1975

371. Rawcastle NB, Tom MI: Non-infectious granulomatous angiitis of the nervous system associated with Hodgkin's disease. J Neurol Neurosurg Psychiatry 25:51, 1962

372. Rawlinson DG, Braun CW: Granulomatous angiitis of the nervous system first seen as relapsing myelopathy. Arch Neurol 38:129, 1981

373. Rebollo M, Val JF, Garijo F et al: Livedo reticularis and cerebrovascular lesions (Sneddon's syndrome): clinical, radiological and pathological features in eight cases. Brain 106:965, 1983

374. Reik L, Grunnett ML, Spencer RP, Donalson JO: Granulomatous angiitis presenting as chronic meningitis and ventriculitis. Neurology (NY) 33:1609, 1983

375. Reik L Jr, Korn JH: Cryoglobulinemia with encephalopathy: successful treatment by plasma exchange. Ann Neurol 10:488, 1981

376. Reyes MG, Fresco R, Chokroverty S, Salud EQ: Virus-like particles in granulomatous angiitis of the central nervous system. Neurology (NY) 26:797, 1976

377. Ristow SC, Griner PF, Abraham GN, Shoulson I: Reversal of systemic manifestations of cryoglobulinemia: treatment with melphalan and prednisone. Arch Intern Med 136:467, 1976

378. Ritama V: Temporal arteritis. Ann Med Fenn 40:63, 1951

379. Robbins SL, Cotran RS: Blood vessels. p. 614. In Pathological Basis of Disease. 2nd Ed. WB Saunders, Philadelphia, 1979

380. Robbs JV, Human RR, Rajaruthnam P: Operative treatment of nonspecific aortoarteritis (Takayasu's arteritis). J Vasc Surg 3:605, 1986

381. Robinson BP, Seeger JF, Zak SM: Rheumatoid arthritis and positional vertebrobasilar insufficiency: a case report. J Neurosurg 65:111, 1986

382. Rodman GP: Clinical pathological conference. J Rheumatol 11:855, 1984

383. Rosenblum WI, Hadfield MG: Granulomatous angiitis of the nervous system in cases of herpes zoster and lymphosarcoma. Neurology (NY) 22:348, 1972

384. Rosenblum WI, Hadfield MG, Young HF: Granulomatous angiitis with preceding varicellazoster. Ann Neurol 3:374, 1978

385. Rosenfeld SI, Kosmorsky GS, Klingele TG et al: Treatment of temporal arteritis with ocular involvement. Am J Med 80:143, 1986

386. Rottino A, Hoffman G: A sarcoid form of encephalitis in a patient with Hodgkin's disease: case report with review of the literature. J Neuropathol Exp Neurol 9:103, 1950

387. Rougemont D, Bousser MG, Wechsler B et al: Manifestations neurologiques de la maladie de Behçet: vingt-quatre observations. Rev Neurol (Paris) 138:493, 1982

388. Rubinstein LJ, Urich H: Meningo-encephalitis of Behçet's disease: case report with pathological findings. Brain 86:151, 1963

389. Rumbaugh CL, Bergeron RT, Fang HC, McCormick R: Cerebral angiographic changes in the drug abuse patient. Radiology 101:335, 1971

390. Rumpl E, Neuhofer J, Pallua A: Cerebrovascular lesions and livedo reticularis (Sneddon's syndrome): a progressive cerebrovascular disorder? J Neurol 231:324, 1985

391. Russell RWR: Giant-cell arteritis: a review of 35 cases. Q J Med 28:471, 1959

392. Russi E, Kraus-Ruppert R, Mummenthaler M: Intracranial giant cell arteritis. J Neurol 221:219, 1979

393. Sabharwal UK, Keogh LH, Weiaman MH, Zvaifler NJ: Granulomatous angiitis of the nervous system: case report and review of the literature. Arthritis Rheum 25:342, 1982

394. Sandhu R, Alexander S, Hornabrook RW, Stehbens WE: Granulomatous angiitis of the CNS. Arch Neurol 36:433, 1979

395. Sarazin L, Duong H, Bourgouin PM et al: Herpes zoster vasculitis: demonstration by MR angiography. J Comput Assist Tomogr 19:624, 1995

396. Sarnat RL, Jampol LM: Hyperviscosity retinopathy secondary to polyclonal gammopathy in a patient with rheumatoid arthritis. Ophthalmology 93:124, 1986

397. Satoh J, Miyasaka N, Yamada T et al: Extensive cerebral infarction due to involvement of both anterior cerebral arteries by Wegener's granulomatosis. Ann Rheum Dis 47:606, 1988

398. Säve-Söderbergh J, Malmvall BO, Andersson R, Bengtsson BA: Giant cell arteritis as a cause of death: report of nine cases. JAMA 255:493, 1986

399. Sawhney IM, Chopra JS, Bansal SK, Gupta AK: Eales' disease with myelopathy. Clin Neurol Neurosurg 88:213, 1986

400. Schmidt BJ, Meagher-Villemure K, Del Carpio J: Lymphomatoid granulomatosis with isolated involvement of the brain. Ann Neurol 15:478, 1984

401. Schraeder PL, Lubar HS, Thorning DR, Dudley AW: Granulomatous arteritis presenting as an acute transverse myelopathy. Wis Med J 73:32, 1974

402. Schulze-Lohff E, Krapf F, Bleil L et al: IgM-containing immune complexes and antiphospholipid antibodies in patients with Sneddon's syndrome. Rheumatol Int 9:43, 1989

403. Schwitter J, Agosti R, Ott P et al: Small infarctions of cochlear, retinal, and encephalic tissue in young women. Stroke 23:903, 1992

404. Scott D: Mucocutaneous-ocular syndrome (Behçet's syndrome) with meningoencephalitis: report of a case with autopsy. Acta Med Scand 161:397, 1958

405. Scully RE, Galdabini JJ, McNeely BU: Case records of the Massachusetts General Hospital: case 43–1976. N Engl J Med 295:944, 1976

406. Scully RE, Galdabini JJ, McNeely BU: Case records of the Massachusetts General Hospital: case 44-1980. N Engl J Med 303:1103, 1980

407. Scully RE, Mark EJ, McNeely WF, McNeely BU: Case records of the Massachusetts General Hospital: case 12–1988. N Engl J Med 318:760, 1988

408. Scully RE, Mark EJ, McNeely WF, McNeely BU: Case records of the Massachusetts General Hospital: case 8–1989. N Engl J Med 320:514, 1989

409. Serena M, Biscaro R, Moretto G, Recchia E: Peripheral and central nervous system involvement in essential mixed cryoglobulinemia: a case report. Clin Neuropathol 10:177, 1991

410. Sergent JS, Lockshin MD, Christian CL, Gocke DJ: Vasculitis with hepatitis B antigenemia: long-term observations in nine patients. Medicine (Baltimore) 55:1, 1976

411. Shelhamer JH, Volkman DJ, Parrillo JE et al: Takayasu's arteritis and its therapy. Ann Intern Med 103:121, 1985

412. Shillingford JP, Heard BE: A case of temporal arteritis: demonstrated at the Postgraduate Medical School of London. Br Med J 2:287, 1960

413. Shimazu S, Imai H, Kokubu S et al: Long-term survival in malignant atrophic papulosis: a case report and review of the Japanese literature. Nippon Geka Gakkai Zasshi 89:1748, 1988

414. Shimizu T, Ehrlich GE, Inaba G, Hayashi K: Behçet's disease (Behçet syndrome). Semin Arthritis Rheum 8:223, 1979

415. Shiozawa Z, Yoshida M, Kobayashi K et al: Superior sagittal sinus thrombosis and systemic lupus erythematosus. Ann Neurol 20:272, 1986

416. Shuangshoti S: Localized granulomatous (giant cell) an-giitis of brain with eosinophil infiltration and saccular aneurysm. J Med Assoc Thai 62:281, 1979

417. Sibony PA, Lessell S: Transient oculomotor synkinesis in temporal arteritis. Arch Neurol 41:87, 1984

418. Sigelman J, Behrens M, Hilal S: Acute posterior multifocal placoid pigment epitheliopathy associated with cerebral vasculitis and homonymous hemianopia. Am J Ophthalmol 88:919, 1979

419. Silverstein A: Cerebrovascular accidents as the initial major manifestation of lupus erythematosus. NY State J Med 5:2942, 1963

420. Singleton JD, West SG, Reddy VV, Rak KM: Cerebral vasculitis complicating rheumatoid arthritis. South Med J 88:470, 1995

421. Sipe JC, Rosenberg JH: Granulomatous giant cell angiitis of the central nervous system. West J Med 127:215, 1977

422. Smith CA, Fidler WJ, Pinals RS: The epidemiology of giant cell arteritis: report of a ten year study in Shelby County, Tennessee. Arthritis Rheum 26:1214, 1983

423. Smith CH, Savino PJ, Beck RW et al: Acute posterior multifocal placoid pigment epitheliopathy and cerebral vasculitis. Arch Neurol 40:48, 1983

424. Sneddon IB: Cerebro-vascular lesions and livedo reticularis. Br J Dermatol 77:180, 1965

425. Sole-Llenas J, Mercader JM, Mirosa F: Cerebral arteritis: angiographic and pathologic study. Angiology 29:713, 1978

426. Sole-Llenas J, Pons-Tortella E: Cerebral angiitis. Neuroradiology 15:1, 1978

427. Specks U, Wheatley CL, McDonald TJ et al: Anticytoplasmic autoantibodies in the diagnosis and follow-up of Wegener's granulomatosis. Mayo Clin Proc 64:28, 1989

428. Spencer WH, Hoyt WF: A fatal case of giant cell arteritis (temporal or cranial arteritis) with ocular involvement. Arch Ophthalmol 64:862, 1962

429. Spurlock RG, Richman AV: Rheumatoid meningitis: a case report and review of the literature. Arch Pathol Lab Med 107:129, 1983

430. Stanford MR, Graham EM: Systemic associations of retinal vasculitis. Int Ophthalmol Clin 31:23, 1991

431. Steiner JW, Gelbloom AJ: Intracranial manifestations in two cases of systemic rheumatoid disease. Arthritis Rheum 2:537, 1959

432. Stephens WP, Ferguson IT: Livedo reticularis and cerebro-vascular disease. Postgrad Med J 58:770, 1982

433. Stern JM, Kesler SM: Raised intracranial pressure in a 16-year-old boy: report of a case of Behçet's disease. S Afr Med J 75:243, 1989

434. Stockhammer G, Felber SR, Zelger B et al: Sneddon's syndrome: diagnosis by skin biopsy and MRI in 17 patients. Stroke 24:685, 1993

435. Stockhammer GJ, Felber SR, Aichner FT et al: Sneddon's syndrome and antiphospholipid antibodies: clarification of a controversy by skin biopsy (letter)? Stroke 23:1182, 1992

436. Stoll G, Reiners K, Schwartz A et al: Acute posterior multifocal placoid pigment epitheliopathy with cerebral involvement. J Neurol Neurosurg Psychiatry 54:77, 1991

437. Strole WE Jr, Clark WH Jr, Isselbacher KJ: Progressive

arterial occlusive disease (Köhlmeier-Degos): a frequently fatal cutaneosystemic disorder. N Engl J Med 276:195, 1967

438. Strouth JC, Dyken M: Encephalopathy of Behçet's disease: report of a case. Neurology (NY) 14:794, 1964

439. Susac JO: Susac's syndrome: the triad of microangiopathy of the brain and retina with hearing loss in young women. Neurology 44:591, 1994

440. Susac JO, Hardman JM, Selhorst JB: Microangiopathy of the brain and retina. Neurology (NY) 29:313, 1979

441. Tabbaa MA, Snyder BD: Vasospasm versus vasculitis in cases with "isolated benign cerebral vasculitis." Ann Neurol 21:109, 1987

442. Tanenbaum M, Tenzel J: Familial temporal arteritis. J Clin Neuro-ophthalmol 5:244, 1985

443. Thomas DJ, Kirby JDT, Britton KE, Galton DJ: Livedo reticularis and neurological lesions. Br J Dermatol 106:711, 1982

444. Thomas L, David S, McClusky RT: Studies of PPLO infection. I. The production of cerebral polyarteritis by *Mycoplasma gallispeticum* in turkeys, the neurotoxic property of the *Mycoplasma*. J Exp Med 123:897, 1966

445. Thystrup J, Knudsen GM, Mogensen AM, Fledelius HC: Atypical visual loss in giant cell arteritis. Acta Ophthalmol (Copenh) 72:759, 1994

446. Tien RD, Felsberg GJ, Osumi AK: Herpes virus infections of the CNS: MR findings. AJR 161:167, 1993

447. Tishler S, Williamson T, Mirra SS et al: Wegener granulomatosis with meningeal involvement. AJNR 14:1248, 1993

448. Toussirot E, Figarella-Branger D, Disdier P et al: Association of cerebral vasculitis with a lupus anticoagulant. A case with brain pathology. Clin Rheumatol 13:624, 1994

449. Travers RL, Allison DJ, Brettle RP, Hughes GRV: Polyarteritis nodasa: a clinical and angiographic analysis of 17 cases. Semin Arthritis Rheum 8:184, 1979

450. Treves TA, Gadoth N, Blumen S, Korczyn AD: Intravascular malignant lymphomatosis: a cause of subacute dementia. Dementia 6:286, 1995

451. Trevor RP, Sondheimer FK, Fessel WJ, Wolpert SM: Angiographic demonstration of major cerebral vessel occlusion in systemic lupus erythematosus. Neuroradiology 4:202, 1972

452. Tsokos GC, Tsokos M, le Riche NGH, Klippel JH: A clinical and pathologic study of cerebrovascular disease in patients with systemic lupus erythematosus. Semin Arthritis Rheum 16:70, 1986

453. Tuhy JE, Maurice GL, Niles NR: Wegener's granulomatosis. Am J Med 25:638, 1958

454. Turnbull J: Temporal arteritis and polymyalgia rheumatica: nosographic and nosologic considerations. Neurology 46:901, 1996

455. Uitdehaag BM, Scheltens P, Bertelsmann FW, Bruyn RP: Intracerebral haemorrhage in Sneddon's syndrome (letter). J Neurol Sci 11:227, 1992

456. Urich H: Neurosarcoidosis or granulomatous angiitis: a problem of definition. Mt Sinai J Med 44:718, 1977

457. Valvanis A, Feiede R, Schubiger O, Hayek J: Cerebral granulomatous angiitis simulating brain tumor. J Comput Assist Tomogr 3:536, 1979

458. Vanderzant C, Bromberg M, MacGuire A, McCune J: Isolated small-vessel angiitis of the central nervous system. Arch Neurol 45:683, 1988

459. Vecht CJ, Sande JJ: Hemispheric infarction after herpes zoster ophthalmicus. Neurology (NY) 32:914, 1982

460. Verker R: Psychiatric aspects of temporal arteritis. J Mental Sci 98:280, 1952

461. Vidailhet M, Piett JC, Wechsler B et al: Cerebral venous thrombosis in systemic lupus erythematosus. Stroke 21:1226, 1990

462. Vilchez-Padilla JJ: CNS varicella-zoster vasculitis (letter). Arch Neurol 39:785, 1982

463. Vincent FM: Granulomatous angiitis. N Engl J Med 296:452, 1977

464. Vincent FM, Vincent T: Bilateral carotid siphon involvement in giant cell arteritis. Neurosurgery 18:773, 1986

465. Vinijchaikul K: Primary arteritis of the aorta and its main branches (Takayasu's arteriopathy): a clinicopathologic autopsy study of eight cases. Am J Med 43:15, 1967

466. Vollertsen RS, McDonald TJ, Younge BR et al: Cogan's syndrome: 18 cases and a review of the literature. Mayo Clin Proc 61:344, 1986

467. Vollmer TL, Guarnaccia J, Harrington W et al: Idiopathic granulomatous angiitis of the central nervous system. Diagnostic challenges. Arch Neurol 50:925, 1993

468. Von Knorring J: Treatment and prognosis in polymyalgia rheumatica and temporal arteritis: a ten-year survey of 53 patients. Acta Med Scand 205:429, 1975

469. Wadman B, Werner I: Thromboembolic complications during corticosteroid treatment of temporal arteritis. Lancet 1:907, 1972

470. Walsh FB, Hoyt WF: p. 213. In Miller NR (ed): Walsh and Hoyt's Clinical Neuro-Ophthalmology. 4th Ed. Vol. 1. Williams & Wilkins, Baltimore, 1982

471. Ward MM, Pyun E, Studenski S: Causes of death in systemic lupus erythematosus. Long-term follow-up of an inception cohort. Arthritis Rheum 38:1492, 1995

472. Warot P, Caron JC, Lehembre P, Houcke M: Maladie de Degos à forme cérébrale. Rev Neurol (Paris) 133:353, 1977

473. Watson P, Fekete J, Deck J: Central nervous system vasculitis in rheumatoid arthritis. Can J Neurol Sci 4:269, 1977

474. Webb FWS, Hickman JA, Brew DSJ: Death from vertebral artery thrombosis in rheumatoid arthritis. Br Med J 2:537, 1968

475. Wechsler B, Dell'lsola B, Vidailhet M et al: MRI in 31 patients with Behçet's disease and neurological involvement: prospective study with clinical correlation. J Neurol Neurosurg Psychiatry 56:793, 1993

476. Wechsler B, Vidailhet M, Piette JC et al: Cerebral venous thrombosis in Behçet's disease: clinical study and long-term follow-up of 25 cases. Neurology 42:614, 1992

477. Weinberger LM, Cohen ML, Remler BF et al: Intracranial Wegener's granulomatosis. Neurology 43:1831, 1993

478. Weinstein JM, Bresnick GH, Bell CL et al: Acute posterior multifocal placoid pigment epitheliopathy associated with cerebral vasculitis. J Clin Neuroophthalmol 8:195, 1988

479. Weinstein JM, Chui H, Lane S et al: Churg-Strauss syndrome (allergic granulomatous angiitis): neuro-ophthal-

mologic manifestations. Arch Ophthalmol 101:1217, 1983

480. Whelan HT, Moore P: Central nervous system lymphomatoid granulomatosis. Pediatr Neurosci 13:113, 1987

481. Whimster WF: Two neurological cases: demonstration at the Royal College of Physicians of London. Br Med J 1:727, 1979

482. Whittaker R, Barnett A, Ryan P: Antiphospholipid syndrome in scleroderma. J Rheumatol 20:1598, 1993

483. Wilkins MR, Gove RI, Roberts SD, Kendall MJ: Behçet's disease presenting as benign intracranial hypertension. Postgrad Med J 62:39, 1986

484. Wilkinson IMS, Russell RWR: Arteries of the head and neck in giant cell arteritis: a pathological study to show the pattern of arterial involvement. Arch Neurol 27:378, 1972

485. Willeit J, Schmutzhard E, Aichner F et al: CT and MR imaging in neuro-Behçet disease. J Comput Assist Tomogr 10:313, 1986

486. Wilson CA, Choromokos EA, Sheppard R: Acute posterior multifocal placoid pigment epitheliopathy and cerebral vasculitis. Arch Ophthalmol 106:796, 1988

487. Wilson CA, Wander AH, Choromokos EA: Central retinal artery obstruction in herpes zoster ophthalmicus and cerebral vasculopathy. Ann Ophthalmol 22:347, 1990

488. Winkelmann RK, Ditto WB: Cutaneous and visceral syndromes of necrotizing or "allergic" angiitis: a study of 38 cases. Medicine (Baltimore) 43:59, 1964

489. Winkelmann RK, Howard FM, Jr, Perry HO, Miller RH: Malignant papulosis of skin and cerebrum: a syndrome of vascular thrombosis. Arch Dermatol 87:94, 1963

490. Wolf SM, Schotland DL, Phillips LL: Involvement of nervous system in Behçet's syndrome. Arch Neurol 12:315, 1965

491. Wong RL, Korn JH: Temporal arteritis without an elevated erythrocyte sedimentation rate: case report and review of the literature. Am J Med 80:959, 1986

492. Yamamori C, Ishino H, Inagaki T et al: Neuro-Behçet disease with demyelination and gliosis of the frontal white matter. Clin Neuropathol 13:208, 1994

493. Yamamoto S, Nozawa T, Aoki H, Isobe Y: Femoro-internal carotid artery bypass for cerebral ischemia in Takayasu's arteritis. Arch Surg 119:1426, 1984

494. Yankner BA, Skolnik PR, Shoukimas GM et al: Cerebral granulomatous angiitis associated with isolation of human T-lymphotropic virus type III from the central nervous system. Ann Neurol 20:362, 1986

495. Yoneda S, Nukada T, Kunihiko T et al: Subclavian steal in Takayasu's arteritis: a hemodynamic study by means of ultrasonic Doppler flowmetry. Stroke 8:264, 1977

496. Yoong MF, Blumbergs PC, North JB: Primary (granulomatous) angiitis of the central nervous system with multiple aneurysms of spinal arteries. Case report. J Neurosurg 79:603, 1993

497. Young SM, Fisher M, Sigsbee A, Errichetti A: Cardiogenic brain embolism and lupus anticoagulant. Ann Neurol 26:390, 1989

498. Younger DS, Hays AP, Brust JCM, Rowland LP: Granulomatous angiitis of the brain: an inflammatory reaction of diverse etiology. Arch Neurol 45:514, 1988

499. Zelenski JD, Capraro JA, Holden D, Calabrese LH: Central nervous system vasculitis in Behçet's syndrome: angiographic improvement after therapy with cytotoxic agents. Arthritis Rheum 32:217, 1989

500. Zimmerman RS, Young HF, Hadfield MG: Granulomatous angiitis of the nervous system: a case report of long-term survival. Surg Neurol 33:206, 1990

CHAPTER 31

Moyamoya Disease

JUNICHI MASUDA

JUN OGATA

TAKENORI YAMAGUCHI

Moyamoya disease is an unusual form of chronic cerebrovascular occlusive disease that is characterized by angiographic findings of bilateral stenosis or occlusion at the terminal portion of the internal carotid artery together with the abnormal vascular network at the base of the brain (Fig. 31.1).[17] The first report of a patient with this disease was published in 1957 by Takeuchi and Shimizu under a diagnosis of bilateral hypoplasia of the internal carotid arteries.[94] This patient was a 29-year-old man who had been suffering from visual disturbance and hemiconvulsive seizures since he was 10 years old, and Takeuchi and Shimizu considered this arterial occlusion to be congenital hypoplasia different from the atherosclerotic lesion based on the histologic findings of a branch of the external carotid artery. Since then, similar cases have been reported, mainly among the Japanese, and a variety of names such as "cerebral juxta-basal telangiectasia" by Sano,[87] "cerebral arterial rete" by Handa,[28] "rete mirabile" by Weidner,[101] and "cerebral basal rete mirabile" by Nishimoto[74] have been applied to this condition. The terms "spontaneous occlusion of the circle of Willis" used by Kudo,[57] or "moyamoya disease" are now commonly used in the literature. The latter term *moyamoya disease* was proposed by Suzuki[92] from the angiographic findings of an abnormal vascular network at the base of the brain, which characterizes this disease category because the Japanese word *moyamoya* means "vague or hazy puff of smoke" in appearance.

Extensive investigations on patients with this characteristic angiographic finding have been conducted mainly by Japanese neurosurgeons over the past 30 years. As a result, the clinical entity of this disease and its concept have now been established. It is well-known for example that progression of stenosis or occlusion of the intracranial major arteries including distal ends of the internal carotid arteries is the primary lesion of this disease, and that the abnormal vascular network (moyamoya vessels) at the base of the brain is their collateral secondary to brain ischemia, although this finding on angiography characterizes the clinical category (Fig. 31-1).[17,50,91,114]

The guideline for the diagnosis of moyamoya disease was established and has been revised by the research committee on spontaneous occlusion of the circle of Willis, organized by the Ministry of Health and Welfare, Japan (MHWJ).[17] The guideline has been published not only in annual reports of the research committee but in some textbooks written in English.[50,114] These publications help advocate this disease as a clinical entity, and it is now known that moyamoya disease is widely distributed all over the world.[25,81] The epidemiology of moyamoya disease is discussed below.

Since the clinical features and radiologic findings have been sufficiently described in the previous edition of this textbook[114] and others,[26,50,91] we shall use the present chapter to summarize the pathology and recent progress on the etiology and pathogenesis of this disease. The recent revision of the guideline for diagnosis in relation to magnetic resonance imaging (MRI) and angiography (MRA) is also addressed.

Guideline for the Diagnosis of Moyamoya Disease

The guideline for the diagnosis of moyamoya disease was developed by the research committee on spontaneous occlusion of the circle of Willis of MHWJ, and was revised recently in 1995[17] (Tables 31.1 and 31.2).

The guideline prior to this latest revision stated that cerebral angiography is indispensable for the diagnosis in all but the autopsied cases.[114] During the last several years, however, the research committee conducted comparative studies to examine whether the MRI and MRA could be substituted for conventional cerebral angiography.[19,35,105] As the quality of the images has been improved, the committee reached the conclusion in 1995 that the diagnosis of moyamoya disease can be made without the conventional cerebral angiography if the MRI and MRA clearly demonstrate all the findings that indicate moyamoya disease, and if the diagnostic criteria applied to the MRI and MRA were added as a supplemented reference in the revision.[17] This revision (Table 31.2), which admits the inclusion of noninvasive methods substituting for invasive angiography in the diagnostic guideline, is expected to become helpful for patients, especially children.

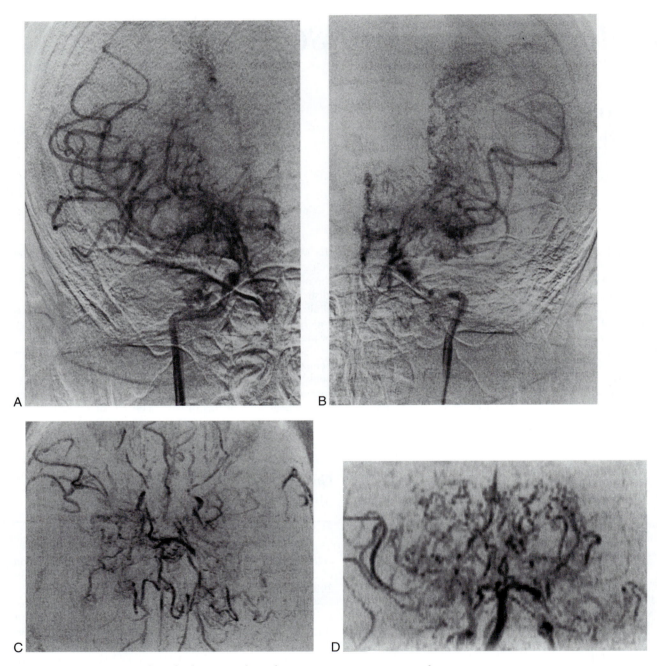

Figure 31.1 Conventional cerebral angiography and magnetic resonance angiography in a 10-year-old boy with moyamoya disease. Anteroposterior views of conventional angiography show (**A**) severe stenosis of the right MCA and (**B**) nearly complete occlusion of the left MCA. Well-developed basal moyamoya vessels are also seen. Magnetic resonance angiography of this patient shows findings similar to those observed by conventional angiography. (**C**) Basal view. (**D**) Anteroposterior view. (From Houkin et al,[35] with permission.)

Table 31.1 Guideline for the Diagnosis of Moyamoya Disease

I. 1. a. Age of onset varies, but is more prevalent in children and in females. Familial occurrence is occasionally present.
   b. Clinical symptoms and manners of progression are variable; asymptomatic, transient, and persistent neurologic deficits of mild to severe.
   c. Cerebral ischemia is frequently observed in the children, and intracranial hemorrhage in the adults.
2. In the children, hemiparesis, monoparesis, sensory disturbance, involuntary movement, headache, and convulsion appear episodically and repetitively, sometimes on alternating sides. Mental retardation or persistent neurologic deficits are also observed. The hemorrhagic episode is rare, unlike the adult type.
3. In the adults, symptoms similar to those observed in the children may appear, but most of them have a sudden onset of intraventricular, subarachnoid, or intracerebral hemorrhage. Patients usually recover from the bleeding with or without persistent neurologic deficits, but some patients follow an unfavorable outcome and die.

II. Angiography is indispensable for the diagnosis. The following findings are observed.
1. Stenosis or occlusion is observed at the terminal portions of the intracranial internal carotid arteries and at the proximal portion of the anterior cerebral arteries and the middle cerebral arteries.
2. Abnormal vascular networks are observed in the vicinity of the occlusive (or stenotic) lesions in the arterial phase.
3. These two findings are found bilaterally. (See the supplemented reference [Table 31.2] when MRI and MRA are available.)

III. Etiology is unknown, and the patients with similar cerebral vascular lesions associated with the following disorders are excluded; atherosclerosis, autoimmune disorders, meningitis, brain tumor, Down syndrome, von Recklinghausen disease, head trauma, postirradiation state, and so forth.

Diagnostic criteria: The patients are diagnosed by reference to I, II, and III, and divided into one of two groups.
1. Definite cases: fulfill all the findings listed in II and III. The children who fulfill II-1, II-2 on one side and have a stenosis on the other side are included.
2. Probable cases: fulfill all the findings listed in II-1, II-2, and III, but not II-3.

IV. In autopsied cases in which cerebral angiography was not performed, diagnosis of moyamoya disease may be done by reference to the following pathologic findings.
1. Intimal thickenings which cause luminal stenosis or occlusion are observed at the intracranial terminal portions of the internal carotid arteries, usually bilaterally. They are sometimes associated with lipid deposition.
2. In the arteries of the circle of Willis and the major arteries, various degrees of stenosis and occlusion are observed in association with intimal fibrous thickening with duplication of the internal elastic lamina in wavy appearance and attenuation of the tunica media.
3. Many small vascular channels (perforators and anastomosing branches) are observed around the circle of Willis.
4. Small vessels forming networks are observed in the pia mater.

(From Fukui,[17] with permission.)

Table 31.2 Supplemented Reference for the Diagnosis of Moyamoya Disease by MRI and MRA

I. The diagnosis of moyamoya disease can be made without conventional cerebral angiography if the MRI and MRA clearly demonstrate all the findings described below that correspond to the diagnostic criteria on conventional cerebral angiography.
1. Stenosis or occlusion is observed at the terminal portions of the intracranial internal carotid arteries and at the proximal portions of the anterior communicating arteries and the middle cerebral arteries on MRA.
2. Visualization of abnormal vascular networks in the basal ganglia on MRA, or demonstration of moyamoya vessels as at least two apparent signal voids in the ipsilateral side of the basal ganglia on MRI.
3. These two findings are found bilaterally.

II. Imaging methods and limitations.
1. The use of magnetic resonance machine with a static magnetic field strength of 1.0 tesla or stronger is recommended.
2. Any method for obtaining the images of MRA can be used.
3. A static magnetic field strength, the imaging method, and the use of contrast medium should be written on the registration card for the patients with spontaneous occlusion of the circle of Willis.
4. To avoid the inclusion of false-positive patients by over- or underestimation of the lesion, only the definite cases should be diagnosed and registered.

III. The diagnosis based on MRI and MRA is recommended for children only, because similar vascular lesions secondary to other disorders may be included in adults.

IV. Films of the MRI and MRA or their copies should be submitted to the research project on therapeutics for specific selected diseases establishing final diagnosis.

(From Fukui,[17] with permission.)

In this revision, autoimmune disorders were added to the list of disorders that should be excluded from moyamoya disease[17] to avoid confusing moyamoya disease with other disorders that can form vascular lesions resembling those of moyamoya disease.

Epidemiology

The incidence and prevalence of moyamoya disease in the Japanese have been surveyed by collaborative studies conducted by research committees on the epidemiology of intractable diseases or on the spontaneous occlusion of the circle of Willis organized by MHWJ in 1984, 1989, and 1994.[100] The estimated number of the patients treated in Japan in 1994 was 3,900 (95% confidence interval: 3,500 to 4,400). The corresponding value surveyed in 1989 was 3,300, but small hospitals (<200 beds) were not included, so the number of the patients in 1994 was recalculated excluding small hospitals, and reestimated as 3,200. Therefore, the prevalence is considered unchanged from 1989 to 1994, and the annual prevalence and incidence is calculated to be 3.16 and 0.35 per 100,000 population, respectively. Female predominance has been re-

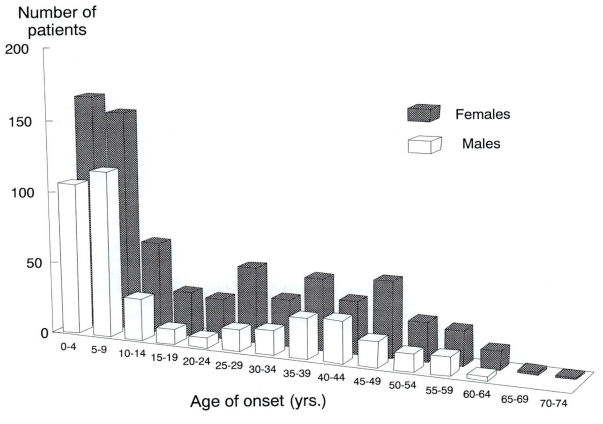

Figure 31.2 Distribution of age-at-onset and sex of the patients with moyamoya disease. (Data from Wakai et al,[100] with permission.)

ported,[114] and was also confirmed in the patient survey of 1994 with a sex ratio of 1.8 (female/male).[100] The peaks of age distribution of the patients were observed in 10 to 14 years old, with a smaller peak in the 40s. The age-at-onset was "under 10 years old" in 47.8% of the patients (childhood moyamoya) although some had developed the disease between the ages of 25 to 49 years (adult-type moyamoya) (Fig. 31.2).

Evidence of the familial occurrence of this disease has been accumulating in medical literature.[48,49,50,103,114] According to the above mentioned nationwide survey, family histories of moyamoya disease were found to be present in 10% of the patients, and 13 pairs of monovular twins were registered as having the disease.[100] The contribution of hereditary factors to the occurrence of moyamoya disease is discussed below in the section on Etiology and Pathogenesis.

Although regional predilection has never been reported within Japan, there are remarkable regional differences in the frequencies of reported moyamoya patients in the world.[25,81,114] After the reports of Taveras in 1969,[97] reports of moyamoya disease have been increasing among non-Japanese people, including whites and blacks, although Caucasian patients are rare. None of the races have as frequent an incidence as the Japanese, but relatively large numbers of patients have been found in Korea[12] and China.[10,11] Korean neurosurgeons performed the first nationwide cooperative survey of moyamoya disease in their country in 1988, and 289 patients were

registered.[12] The reported clinical features of these patients, however, were different from those of Japanese patients. Therefore, it is important to examine whether this heterogeneity suggests racial and regional differences, or whether it is related to any differences in the criteria used for diagnosis of moyamoya disease between the two countries. In 1995, the Japanese neurosurgeons Ikezakai and Fukui organized the collaborative study with Han, the Korean neurosurgeon, and analyzed the patients registered in Korea based on questionnaires about the angiographic findings.[39,40] As the guideline established by the research committee of MHWJ has not been strictly applied to the diagnosis of moyamoya disease in Korea, Ikezakai and Fukui reevaluated the registration records and divided the 451 registered Korean patients into definite (296) cases, probable (103) cases, and unlikely (52) cases. Analysis of the definite cases showed that the clinical features of the Korean patients were similar to those of the Japanese.[39] The pattern of age distribution of the onset showed two peaks ("under 10 years old," and "25 to 49") the same as that of the Japanese, although the adult population was 20% higher in the Korean sample than in the Japanese. There was a slight female predominance ratio 1:3), and the incidence of hemorrhage was significantly higher in the Korean than in the Japanese sample. In the probable cases, on the other hand, more adult cases were included in the Korean cases than in the Japanese, and the clinical features were very different from the definite or probable cases of the Japanese patients.[40]

From these results, the higher incidence of hemorrhage and adult-type moyamoya patients are suggested to be the features of moyamoya disease in Korean patients, but the diagnostic criteria and the interpretation of the angiography by neuroradiologists should be standardized between both countries, and atherosclerotic cerebrovascular stenosis and occlusion should be excluded more carefully in the Korean patients before final conclusions are drawn. Such studies should be undertaken not only in Japan and Korea, but also in Western and other Asian countries, in addition to further investigation in Japan and Korea.

Pathology

Pathologic observations of approximately 100 autopsy cases of moyamoya disease revealed various forms of cerebrovascular lesions encountered in the brain, and their macroscopic and microscopic findings have been accumulated and described in the literature.[27,28,31,33,34,62,63,79,110] The lesion that is observed most frequently at autopsy is intracranial hemorrhage, which is a major cause of death for patients with moyamoya disease.[79] Massive parenchymatous hemorrhage (intracerebral hemorrhage) occurs frequently in the basal ganglia, thalamus, hypothalamus, cerebral peduncle, and midbrain, and often extends and ruptures to the intraventricular spaces.[79] Subarachnoid hemorrhage (SAH) also occurs, but primary SAH caused by rupture of aneurysms seems to be not so frequent as described previously, and many appear to be a secondary extension of parenchymatous hemorrhage.[114] In addition, old brain infarction and focal cortical atrophy of the brain are not uncommon findings and are often found in multiple.[79,110] Furthermore, the infarcts are mostly small and localized in the basal ganglia, internal capsule, thalamus, and the subcortex. The large and arterial territorial infarcts[65] are rare in moyamoya disease, although the occlusion of the intracranial major arteries is present. This may suggest the function of moyamoya vessels as a collateral pathway of arterial occlusion. The frequency and distribution of intracranial hemorrhage and infarction at autopsy may not represent those of patients with moyamoya disease, and the pathologic specimens obtained from the circle of Willis and moyamoya vessels are biased by the unavoidable clinical modifications related to their deaths. Nevertheless, the histologic and immunohistochemical analysis of the postmortem materials have provided a significant amount of valuable information relating to the etiology and pathogenesis of the lesion formation of this disease, and are summarized herein.

THE CIRCLE OF WILLIS AND THE MAJOR BRANCHES

In the guideline for the diagnosis of moyamoya disease, the pathologic findings of intracranial arteries of the autopsied patients are included as an aid for the diagnosis on the autopsied patients without angiography (Table 31.1).[17] The histologic appearance of the circle of Willis and the major branches of the patients with moyamoya disease are characteristic, but

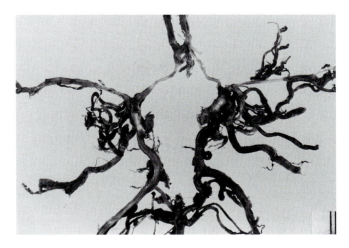

Figure 31.3 Macroscopic appearance of the circle of Willis of a 66-year-old woman with moyamoya disease at autopsy. Tapering of anterior and middle cerebral arteries can be seen bilaterally with network formation of dilated arteries (basal moyamoya vessels).

not peculiar to this disease.[33,34,110] Therefore, it is not always possible to diagnose the patient as having moyamoya disease based solely on pathologic findings.

In macroscopic observation, the circle of Willis and the major branches are tapered and narrowed entirely or partially with overgrown and dilated arteries branching from the circle of Willis (Fig. 31.3). The degree of tapering of arteries and network formation of dilated arteries (moyamoya vessels) and their distributions are variable among the cases. The distal ends of the internal carotid arteries are affected by severe narrowing or occlusion.

In conventional stainings of the specimens obtained from the circle of Willis or its major branches with lesion involvement, the arterial lumen is severely narrowed or occluded by fibrocellular intimal thickening[33,34,63,110] (Fig. 31.4A and Fig. 31.5A). The thickened intima appears to be in a laminated structure with duplication or triplication of internal elastic lamina having a wavy appearance. These features closely resemble the structure noted focally at arterial branching portions in normal controls, the so-called "intimal cushion." The outer diameter of the affected artery usually becomes smaller, and the underlying media are markedly attenuated. These histologic features are common to any site of the lesions, although the degree of intimal thickenings and the distribution in the circle of Willis are variable among the cases.

The recent immunohistochemical staining of this lesion demonstrated that the thickened intima is composed mainly of smooth muscle cells (SMCs) (Fig. 31.5B) that are phenotypically modulated from the contractile type to the synthetic.[63] With this immunohistochemical study, some of the SMCs in the intima were stained positively with the antibody for proliferating cell nuclear antigen (Fig. 31.5C), and thereby were revealed to be proliferating. This evidence strongly suggests that SMC proliferation and phenotypic modulation contribute to the formation of fibrocellular intimal thickening in the circle of Willis of the patients with moyamoya disease. Lipid deposition and lipid-containing macrophages (foam cells) have been found in some autopsy cases,[33,34,110] but are now considered to be an overlapping of atherosclerosis.

Mural thrombi are often found in the stenotic lesions of the circle of Willis and the major branches (Fig. 31.4B), but their frequencies vary among the reports.[33,34,63,109] Judging from their histology, the organization of the thrombi appears to contribute to the pathogenesis of fibrocellular intimal thickening, and this aspect is discussed in the section, Etiology and Pathogenesis.

Aneurysm formation, a relatively common finding in the circle of Willis of the patients with moyamoya disease, and its pathology are summarized below.

PERFORATING ARTERIES (MOYAMOYA VESSELS)

The vascular network at the base of the brain consists of dilated medium- or small- sized muscular arteries branching off the circle of Willis, anterior choroidal arteries, intracranial portions of internal carotid arteries and posterior cerebral arteries. These arteries form complex channels that usually connect to the distal portion of the anterior and middle cerebral arteries. Numerous small dilated and tortuous vessels originating from these channels enter into the base of the brain, and correspond to be lenticulostriate and thalamoperforate arteries.

In microscopic observations, these perforating arteries in the brain parenchyma show various histologic changes. According to the morphometric analysis performed by Yamashita et al,[110] the perforating arteries within the basal ganglia, thalamus, and internal capsule in patients with moyamoya disease can be divided into the following two groups: one is a dilated artery with a relatively thin wall, and the other is a thick-walled artery showing luminal stenosis. Dilatation of the arteries is more prominent in young patients than in adults. The majority of dilated arteries show fibrosis and marked attenuation of

the media with occasional segmentation of the elastic lamina. With hemodynamic stress or aging, the dilated arteries with attenuated walls may predispose to focal protrusion (microaneurysm formation) of the arterial wall, and its rupture is considered one of the mechanisms leading to the parenchymatous hemorrhage in patients with moyamoya disease (Fig. 31.6). The involvement by fibrinoid necrosis of the perforating arteries in the process of aneurysm formation has been shown in the hypertensive parenchymatous hemorrhage, but it has never been confirmed pathologically in patients with moyamoya disease.

By contrast, the stenotic vessels are less frequent in young patients.[110] These stenotic vessels show concentric thickening of the intima with duplication of the elastic lamina and fibrosis of the tunica media (Fig. 31.6). Partial dilatation with discontinuity of the elastic lamina and the occluding thrombus formation with its organization and recanalization are occasionally found. The presence of these histologic changes in the perforating arteries indicates that the arterial obstructive changes of the patients with moyamoya disease are not limited to the circle of Willis and their major branches.

LEPTOMENINGEAL VESSELS

The leptomeningeal anastomoses among the three main cerebral arteries and transdural anastomoses from the external carotid arteries are frequently observed as an abnormal vascular network on cerebral angiograms in patients with moyamoya disease (so-called "vault moyamoya").[50,53,91] Histopathologic and morphometric study of the leptomeningeal vessels was carried out by Kono et al in autopsied brains with moyamoya disease and compared with age-matched controls.[56] They clarified that such anastomoses are not newly formed vessels but merely dilated preexisting ones both in arteries and veins. The attenuation or disruption of the internal elastic

Figure 31.4 Microscopic appearance of the circle of Willis of patients with moyamoya disease at autopsy. (**A**) Intracranial portion of right internal carotid artery of a 60-year-old woman. (Elastica van Gieson Stain.) (**B**) Main trunk of the right middle cerebral artery of a 36-year-old man. Arrows indicate mural fibrin thrombi with its organization. (Mallory's phosphotungstic acid-hematoxylin (PTAH) stain.)

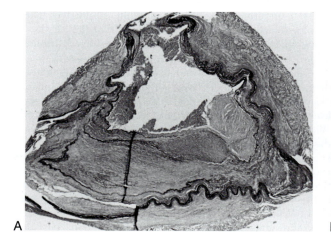
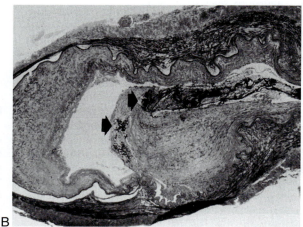

A   B

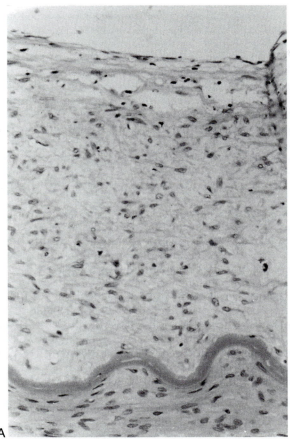

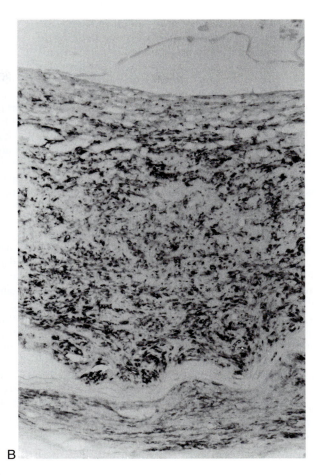

A

B

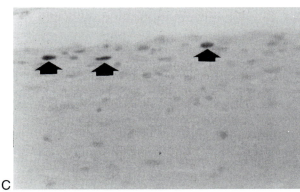

C

Figure 31.5 Microscopic appearances of the basilar artery of a 14-year-old girl with moyamoya disease at autopsy. (**A**) H&E stain, immunohistochemical stain for (**B**) muscle actin, (**C**) proliferating cell nuclear antigen (PCNA). Arrows in Fig. C indicate the nuclei stained positively for PCNA. (Figs. A and B from Masuda et al,[63] with permission.)

lamina is remarkable in the patients with short history of the illness and fibrous intimal thickening is more prominent in the patients who have a longer history of the illness. These structural adaptations in the vascular walls of the leptomeningeal vessels suggest their participation in the collateral circulation at the cerebral cortical surfaces.

ANEURYSM FORMATION

Intracranial aneurysms are frequently associated with moyamoya disease.[30,54,55,72] Such association is far from coincidental since the frequency of aneurysms in patients with moya-

moya disease is higher than in the general population. Intracranial aneurysms are of two types: major artery aneurysms (MAAs) developing from the circle of Willis, and peripheral artery aneurysms (PAAs) located on the moyamoya vessels, choroidal arteries, or any other peripheral arteries serving as collaterals.[30] SAH is caused by rupture of MAAs, whereas parenchymatous hemorrhage or intraventricular hemorrhage is caused by the rupture of PAAs in some cases.

MAAs are found frequently in the arterial complex of anterior communicating artery–anterior cerebral artery in patients with unilateral moyamoya (probable cases), and in the basilar artery in patients with bilateral moyamoya[30] (Fig. 31.7). MAAs are fourfold higher in the unilateral patients than in bilateral patients. Such anatomical distribution of MAAs could be explained if the aneurysms are formed as a result of an increased blood flow through the relatively spared route of cerebral circulation as the stenotic process progresses. This increased blood flow exerts high pressure on the arterial wall, and results in aneurysm formation in susceptible places such as branching sites. Histologically, the aneurysmal wall consists of endothelium with adventitial layers and a disappearance of internal elastic lamina and media, which is not different from saccular aneurysms seen in commonly observed SAH patients. The autopsy cases of aneurysms formed by dissection of the intima from the media are also reported.[66,112]

PAAs are speculated to be responsible for parenchymatous hemorrhage, and two types of aneurysms are reported in histology: saccular (true) aneurysms and pseudoaneurysms consisting of fibrin and erythrocytes, which might be the result of rupture.[116] According to Herreman et al[30] the mean size of PAAs is half that of MAAs, and may not be visualized angiographically in many cases. Thus, PAAs detected in angiography may represent only a subset of those that are larger in size. One third of angiographically visualized PAAs are reported to disappear spontaneously during the follow-up period, and we recently reported the histology of a sclerosed PAA without rupture in an autopsy case[75] and suggested the pathologic processes by which the aneurysms disappear.

EXTRACRANIAL CERVICAL ARTERIES AND SYSTEMIC ARTERIES

The luminal stenosis due to fibrocellular intimal thickening has been described not only in intracranial arteries but also in extracranial arteries including carotid arteries, renal arteries, pulmonary arteries, coronary arteries, and others in patients with moyamoya disease.[38,96] Yamashita et al reported the autopsy case of a 7-year-old Japanese girl with moyamoya disease associated with renovascular hypertension.[111] The histologic study showed systemic involvement of concentric fibrocellular intimal thickening consisting of smooth muscle cells and elastic fibers in intracranial and extracranial carotid, coronary, and renal arteries, and their histologies were similar to those of fibromuscular dysplasia (FMD), the intimal hyperplasia type. Several cases of renovascular hypertension associated with moyamoya disease have been reported in the literature,[13,23,24,108] many of which showed the angiographic or pathologic appearance of FMD. Therefore, it is postulated that the systemic involvement of FMD or FMD-like vascular lesions is present as moyamoya disease, and hypertension may be a result of systemic involvement of the arterial lesions.

Ikeda measured the intimal thickness in the various sites of the extracranial arteries of the autopsy cases with moyamoya disease and compared them with those of age- and sex-matched controls.[38] According to the report, the intimal thickening of the extracranial arteries is generally advanced in moyamoya disease compared with the control cases, and mural thrombi formation and its organization are also present in the extracranial arteries in moyamoya disease. Therefore, the intracranial lesion of moyamoya disease might be one of the manifestations of systemic illness, but there are no pathognomonic changes that suggest any specific disease or etiologic factors of the illness, and thus, the implication of these systemic changes is limited at present.

Etiology and Pathogenesis

There has been serious and continuing debate concerning whether moyamoya disease is acquired or congenital, and none of the proposed hypotheses concerning the pathogenesis

Figure 31.6 Microscopic appearance of the perforating arteries of patients with moyamoya disease at autopsy. (**A**) The artery in the right caudate nucleus of a 60-year-old woman with parenchymatous hemorrhage shows marked dilatation with rupture. (Elastica van Gieson stain.) (**B**) Some of the arteries in the left thalamus of a 39-year-old woman show luminal stenosis due to fibrous and edematous intimal thickening. (Hematoxylin and eosin stain.)

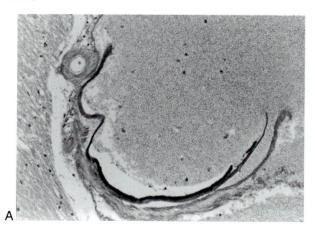
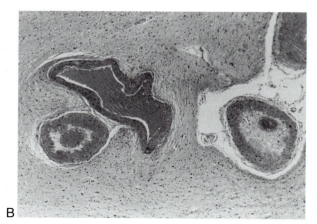

A   B

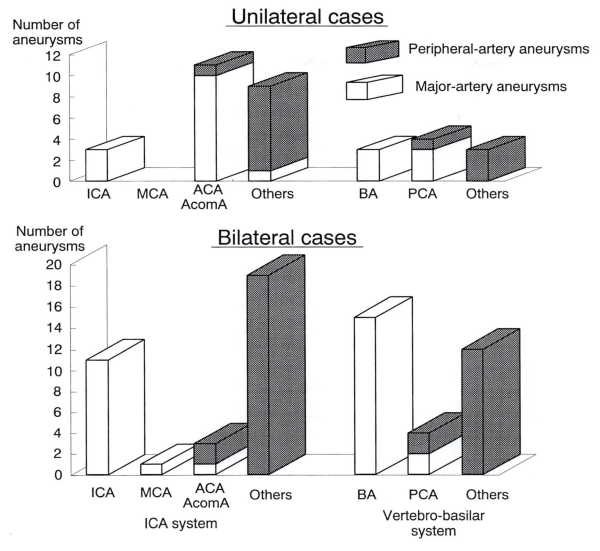

Figure 31.7 Aneursym locations in patients with moyamoya disease. ICA, internal carotid artery; MCA, middle cerebral artery; ACA, anterior cerebral artery; AcomA, anterior communicating artery; BA, basilar artery; PCA, posterior cerebral artery. (Data from Herreman et al,[30] with permission.)

of this disease have resolved to a general agreement.[50,114] Therefore, the etiology still remains unknown at present. Neverthless, moyamoya disease is established as a clinical disease entity, and extensive clinical and pathological studies have been conducted. As a result of this research, the following considerations are now generally accepted: (1) the progression of stenosis or occlusion of the circle of Willis and the major branches including distal ends of the internal carotid arteries is the primary lesion of this disease; (2) an abnormal vascular network (moyamoya vessels) at the base of the brain is collateral secondary to brain ischemia; (3) clinical symptoms and signs are the manifestations of cerebrovascular events secondary to the above-mentioned vascular lesions, including intracranial hemorrhage, infarct, and TIA; and (4) the major cellular components of the thickened intima formed in arteries of

the circle of Willis and the major branches are smooth muscle cells, and proliferation and migration of smooth muscle cells in the intima, induced by unknown mechanisms, may lead to the intimal thickening in association with morphologic and biochemical alteration of extracellular matrix components including elastin, collagen, and other proteoglycans.

By contrast the mechanisms responsible for inducing smooth muscle cell proliferation and migration in the arterial intima of the patients are not yet identified. Furthermore, the reason the intimal thickening occurs in the limited arteries such as the circle of Willis is unknown. As stated above in the section on Epidemiology, hereditary factors have been suggested for a long time to play an important role in the etiology of moyamoya disease, as indicated by the high incidence among the Japanese,[25] occasional familial occurrence,[48] and association with other congenital diseases such as sickle cell anemia,[89] von Recklinghausen disease[60] and Down syndrome.[70] Fukuyama et al suggested a multifactorial mode of inheritance from the genetic study of the patients of familial occurrence.[20,22] The majority of moyamoya patients, however, are sporadic cases. Therefore, DNA typing of human leukocyte antigen (HLA) class II of moyamoya patients is now in progress, and the preliminary data suggest possible association of some subtypes of HLA class II to moyamoya patients, although this is not yet conclusive.[6,88] However, this association (if present) seems to signal a simple DNA marker and may not be linked to any abnormalities of immunological functions of the patients.

Although hereditary factors may be involved in the occurrence of moyamoya disease or its susceptibility, the manner of the clinical manifestations and disease progression is not congenital. Through the accumulation of patient registration and analysis of clinical data, acquired factors are suggested in the occurrence and progression of moyamoya disease, and many hypotheses have been proposed. They include vasculitis with or without autoimmune mechanism,[46,91,92] infection (virus,[104] anaerobic bacteria such as *Propionibacterium acnes*[102] and others), thrombosis,[33,34,109] juvenile atherosclerosis,[33,34] cranial trauma,[16] abnormalities of sympathetic nerve ending,[46] postirradiation state,[8,82] and others.

As noted in the section on Pathology, microthrombi are frequently formed in the vasculature of the patients with moyamoya disease.[33,34,63,109] It appears to contribute to pathogenesis of the fibrocellular intimal thickening through its organization, and this hypothesis is suitable to explain the lamellated structure of the thickened intima of the lesions. If endothelial injury really occurs as the initiation of the lesion formation, it is feasible to speculate that smooth muscle cell migration and proliferation in the intima are induced following the injury. There has been substantial evidence that endothelial injury provokes phenotypic modulation and proliferation of smooth muscle cells and leads to neointima formation, not only in experimental animals[7,64,84,85] but also in patients of angioplasty restenosis.[9,98] In moyamoya disease, however, it is unclear to what extent this process is responsible for the lesion formation. Furthermore, microthrombus is a nonspecific finding and reveals none of any specific etiologic factors for the endothelial injury. None of the factors causing endothelial injury are identified in moyamoya disease.

To examine disturbances in integrity and function of the endothelium, Ikeda and Hosoda immunostained the functional markers (thrombomodulin and the von Willebrand factor) of the endothelial cells covering the thickened intima, but no definite conclusion could be drawn from the studies.[37] Among the hypotheses concerning the mechanisms of arterial injury, chronic arteritis due to immunologic reactions may be implicated.[46] Previous histologic studies did not emphasize the presence of inflammatory cells in the lesions. With cell-type-specific immunohistochemistry, we recently demonstrated the presence of macrophages and T cells in the lesions, especially in the superficial layer of the thickened intima.[63] Infiltration of inflammatory cells observed in patients aged younger than 50 years may be related to the pathological process of moyamoya disease, although the complete exclusion of a concomitant progression of juvenile atherosclerosis or other nonspecific changes unrelated to moyamoya disease is impossible. As this is the case, it is not always easy to separate the histopathology of moyamoya disease from other pathologic changes including atherosclerosis and various forms of arteritis.

In addition to the possible proliferation and migration of smooth muscle cells suggested in the genesis of intimal thickening and moyamoya vessel formation, many researchers have focused their attention on the growth factors and cytokines, and their receptors such as basic fibroblast growth factor (b-FGF),[32,90] platelet-derived growth factor (PDGF),[5] and IL-8. The immunohistochemical stainings[32,90] and measurements of these proteins in the cerebrospinal fluid[3,93] have been attempted in patients with moyamoya disease. These approaches may help to introduce methods of molecular biology and cell biology that are now in rapid progress in relation to the problem of angioplasty restenosis.[9,84,85,98]

Clinical Symptoms and Signs

Clinical symptoms and signs are manifested as a result of the cerebrovascular events that occur in relation to pathologic changes of cerebral arteries in patients with moyamoya disease. Initial symptoms occur abruptly as attacks of cerebrovascular events including transient ischemic attack (TIA), brain infarction, and intracranial hemorrhage, or occasionally as epileptic seizures. There have been some patients without any overt symptoms, who are diagnosed from the angiography performed in asymptomatic cases because of the familial occurrence of this disease.[19] The research committee of MHWJ has defined four clinical types classified according to the initial attacks of the symptoms, and their frequencies are as follows; ischemic (63.4%), hemorrhagic (21.6%), epileptic (7.6%), and others (7.5%) in the registered patients accumulated until 1995.[18]

The ischemic type dominates in childhood moyamoya patients representing 69% of those under 10 years old; TIA occurs in 40% and infarction in 29% manifesting a variety of symptoms including motor paresis, disturbances of consciousness, speech disturbances, sensory disturbances, and others.[29] The course is sometimes repetitive and progressive, and may result in cortical blindness, motor aphasia, or even a vegetative state within several years after onset. These ischemic symptoms such as transient weakness or pareses are provoked by some conditions of hyperventilation, such as blowing wind instruments, blowing to cool something hot, or crying. They are considered to be induced by decreased cerebral blood flow (CBF) due to decreased $PaCO_2$.[26,77] Ischemic deterioration is often precipitated by infection of the upper respiratory tract. Mental retardation and a low intelligence quotient (IQ) during the long follow-up is another important problem for the children, and this is discussed below in the section on Disease Progression and Prognosis.

The hemorrhagic type is prevalent in the adult patients, occurring in 66%, with a predominance of the hemorrhagic type in females.[29] Headache, disturbances of consciousness, and motor paresis are frequently encountered in the hemorrhagic type. Events triggering the bleeding are not identified, but hypertension and aging may be suggested as such factors. Bleeding occurs often in multiple and repetitive intervals from several days to 10 years, and massive bleeding often leads to death.

Epilepsy was observed in about 5% of all patients, more than 80% of whom were children under 10 years old.[29]

Laboratory Findings

Many reports have attempted to establish a diagnostic laboratory test pathognomonic for moyamoya disease, but none of these tests proved successful. Some reports, however, showed fragments of data that provided valuable information concerning the etiology and pathogenesis of this disease. Infection of anaerobic bacteria such as *Propionibacterium acnes*,[102] cytomegalovirus, and Epstein-Barr virus,[104] for example, have been examined by Yamada et al with screenings of the specific antibodies and viral DNAs amplified with polymerase chain reaction, and the reported data suggest positive correlation with moyamoya disease.

Anticardiolipin antibody, an autoantibody against phosphatidyl-glycerol, a component of cell membrane phospholipid, was recently measured in the serum of patients with moyamoya disease (including two cases of postirradiation moyamoya phenomenon), and this antibody showed higher percentages in the patients with moyamoya disease than in the control cases. Also, the titers in positive cases were higher than those in the controls.[106] These data are very interesting, and suggest the possible linkage of inflammation and thrombosis, since this antibody has been suggested to play an important role in arterial thrombi formation in brain infarction.[36,61]

Radiologic Findings

ANGIOGRAPHY

The fundamental angiographic finding of moyamoya disease is bilateral stenosis or occlusion at the intracranial portion of the internal carotid arteries together with a retiform arteriolar network (moyamoya vessels) at the base of the brain (Figs. 31.1A and 31.1B). The stenotic or occlusive changes often extend along the arteries of the circle of Willis and their main branches. The vertebrobasilar system, however, has rarely been reported to be involved in this disease.[91,92,114] Leptomeningeal collateral formation, especially from the branches of the posterior cerebral artery, is frequently noted. Also usually present are transdural anastomoses via the ophthalmic artery, external carotid artery, and vertebral artery.

Suzuki and Takaku divided the phases of disease progression into six stages based on angiographic findings as follows: [91,92] (1) the narrowing of the carotid forks, (2) the initial appearance of moyamoya vessels, (3) the intensification of moyamoya vessels, (4) the minimization of moyamoya vessels (5) the reduction of moyamoya vessels, and (6) the disappearance of moyamoya vessels and collateral circulation only from the external carotid arteries. Kitamura et al confirmed these

chronologic changes of angiographic findings in their follow-up patients; i.e., as the narrowing of the main arteries advances, the moyamoya vessels increase in number, and they are later reduced when transdural anastomoses develop as disease progresses.[51]

As noted above, aneurysm formation is frequently noted in patients with moyamoya disease.

COMPUTED TOMOGRAPHIC SCAN

The findings of moyamoya disease in CT scan are variable according to the clinical types of the patients. The most striking finding in the conventional CT scan is high-density areas (HDAs) that are observed in the basal ganglia and thalamus, ventricular system, and subarachnoid spaces of the patients of hemorrhagic type.[107,114] The HDAs resemble the topography of the hematoma in the internal type of hypertensive intracerebral hemorrhage.

In the ischemic type, there are low-density areas (LDAs) that are relatively small and usually confined to the cerebral cortex and subcortex and dilatation of cortical sulci and ventricles.[107,114] Lacunar infarctions located in the basal ganglia and thalamus are sometimes seen in the adult patients, but are rare in the young patients. Up to 40% of the ischemic-type patients, however, show no abnormalities in a conventional CT scan.[107,114] Contrast study often visualizes tortuous and curvilinear vessels in the basal ganglia, which indicate the presence of moyamoya vessels. The most proximal segment of the anterior and middle cerebral arteries are often poorly opacified.

MAGNETIC RESONANCE IMAGING AND ANGIOGRAPHY

Since MRI and MRA are noninvasive techniques that can visualize various pathologic changes of the brain and the arterial tree, they have a big advantage compared with conventional angiography. MRI can demonstrate small subcortical lesions undetectable by CT scan. Brain infarctions in patients with moyamoya disease are usually small and located in the subcortex, and are often multiple and bilateral. Brain atrophy and slight ventricular dilatation are associated.[19,35,105] Stenotic or occlusive lesions at the distal ends of the internal carotid arteries can be demonstrated by MRA in most patients with this disease (Figs. 31.1C and 31.1D). Apparent moyamoya vessels can be visualized as fine unusual vessels on MRA (Figs. 31.1C and 31.1D) and also as a signal void on the MRI (Fig. 31.8), particularly in the children with moyamoya disease. Small moyamoya vessels, however, are poorly visualized on both MRI and MRA, particularly in adults.

As described in the "Guideline for the Diagnosis of Moyamoya Disease," the research committee recently concluded that diagnosis of this disease can be done without conventional angiography if MRI and MRA visualize the above-mentioned findings bilaterally. To meet this agreement, the guideline was

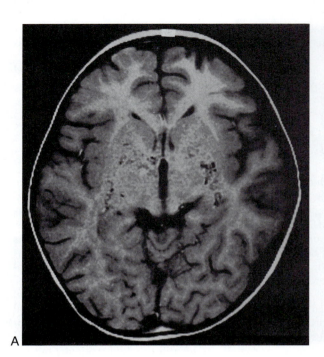
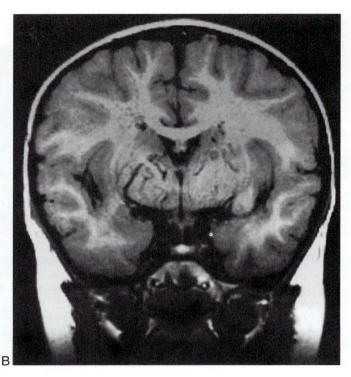

Figure 31.8 Typical magnetic resonance images of moyamoya vessels. (**A**) Axial image reveals multiple signal void in the basal ganglia. (**B**) Coronal image reveals well-developed basal moyamoya vessels in the bilateral basal ganglia. Houkin et al,[35] with permission.

revised in 1995, and the diagnostic criteria on MRI and MRA were supplemented as shown in Table 31.2.[17]

ELECTROENCEPHALOGRAM

Abnormal electroencephalogram (EEG) findings are more frequently found in childhood patients than in adults, and they are related to permanent or transient ischemic changes due to a $PaCO_2$ variation, which is not specific for moyamoya disease.[50,52,91,114] Yoshii and Kudo summarized the EEG findings as follows: (1) diffuse and bilateral abnormal low-voltage or slow waves and spike waves, (2) "buildup" with the appearance of delta waves during hyperventilation, and (3) no effect on photic stimulation.[52,115]

OTHER CLINICAL EXAMINATIONS

Since the symptoms of the ischemic type and epileptic type are caused by impairment of the cerebral blood flow due to arterial stenosis or occlusion, the regional cerebral blood flow and metabolic distribution have been measured by Xe inhalation, and visualized with computer-assisted tomographic methods including stable Xenon-enhanced computed tomography, dynamic computed tomography, positron emission computed tomography (PET), and single photon emission computed tomography. Measurements of these physiological and morphological parameters have been useful for the follow-up of the patients, and the effects of medical and surgical treatment and prognosis of the patients have been evaluated.[26,41,42,59,73,76,77,95]

Disease Progression and Prognosis

As regards disease progression and the prognosis of moyamoya disease, there are remarkable differences between the childhood patients and the adults. In the children, angiographic changes progress with time and sometimes rapidly,[1,15] and the formation of abnormal vascular networks at the base of the brain progresses from unilateral to bilateral during the follow-up.[47,48] However, the prognosis for activity in daily life (ADL) and life expectancy in the childhood moyamoya patients is generally fair, since the irreversible ischemic and hemorrhagic complications are rarely encountered. More than 80% are in good health or in a state of independence, irrespective of treatment received. Recently, however, many children are reported to be not well accommodated in social or school life due to poor intellectual ability, psychological impairment, and personality changes.[2,21,58,68,80] In general, the earlier the onset of the disease and the longer the period of suffering, the lower the mental function and quality of intelligence.[71]

In adults, on the other hand, the progression of angiographic changes is uncommon. Prognosis in ADL and life expectancy, however, is poor since multiple and repetitive intracranial hemorrhages occur in many patients.

Treatment

The majority of the patients (77%) have been surgically treated by any of the revascularization operations, and patients with mild and transient symptoms only tend to be followed in conservative treatment.[18] The surgical treatment is more effective for the improvement in cerebral blood flow than for conservative treatment, according to the physiological parameters revealed by regional CBF measurement and PET studies, and is generally believed to have an advantage for the prediction of better prognosis.[41]

MEDICAL TREATMENT

Vasodilators, antiplatelet agents, antifibrinolytic agents, and fibrinolytic agents are used for the patients with moyamoya disease, and other medications, including anticonvulsants and steroids, are also used for the epileptic type and for patients with increased cranial pressure, respectively.[29,107]

Steroids are considered to be effective in certain cases, especially (1) in cases with involuntary movements and (2) in the active phase of recurrent ischemic or hemorrhagic attacks. This effect is presumed to be related to influences of steroids on edema, regional CBF, and vasculitis.

Antiplatelet agents, acetylsalicylic acid, and ticlopidine chloride may also be prescribed to prevent recurrence of ischemic attacks and thrombosis of the circle of Willis and the main branches, which is thought to play an important role in the progression of moyamoya disease. Other drugs, such as vasodilators, antifibrinolytics, and fibrinolytics are occasionally used for similar purposes. The efficacy of these drugs, however, has never been tested thoroughly in clinical trials on patients with moyamoya disease.

SURGICAL TREATMENT

Surgical revascularizations are classified into three categories of surgical procedures: direct bypass surgery, indirect bypass surgery, and their combinations (Fig. 31.9).[99] This surgical revascularization has been performed to give additional collateral flow to the ischemic brain and thereby to improve regional CBF and to prevent or minimize the irreversible brain damage

Figure 31.9 Selection of surgical revascularization procedures for the patients with moyamoya disease according to the types of initial attacks. (Data from Fukui et al.[18])

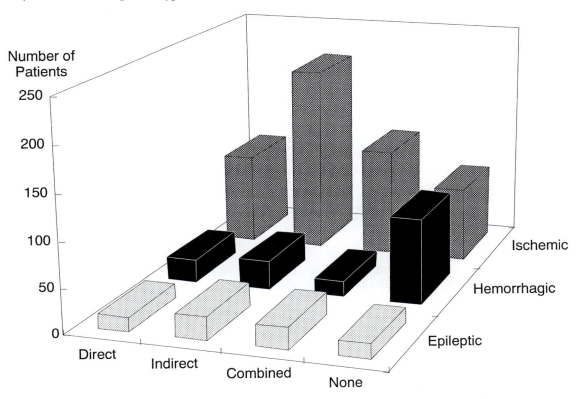

during the follow-up. Also, collateral flow through the bypass is expected to have some effects reducing hemodynamic stress on the moyamoya vessels, and eventually to prevent the occurrence of hemorrhagic events. The evacuation of hematoma and ventricular drainage is performed in the acute stage of the hemorrhagic complication of moyamoya disease.

Superficial temporal artery–middle cerebral artery (STA-MCA) bypass is a direct revascularization surgery that was pioneered by Yasargil and his colleagues,[113] and was applied to moyamoya disease by Karasawa and Kikuchi,[43] and by Reichman et al[83] independently. It is now generally accepted that this direct revascularization surgery seems to provide the patients a remarkable improvement in CBF and a better prognosis than conservative treatment.[41,67] This technique, however, needs the skill of microvascular surgery, and it is not always possible to find a cortical branch suitable for anastomoses. Furthermore, careful intraoperative monitoring of blood pressure and $PaCO_2$ is necessary; otherwise, there is a risk of the ischemic complication perioperatively.[42]

Indirect revascularizations are the surgical procedures that aim to introduce external carotid flow into the internal carotid system via newly developed vascularization through the sutured tissues. Encephaloduroarteriosynangiosis (EDAS)[69] and encephalomyosynangiosis (EMS)[44] are the two representative procedures most commonly applied to patients with moyamoya disease. Other operative methods such as encephaloarteriosynangiosis (EAS), durapexy, and omentum transplantation[45] also belong in this category. These operations can be done on patients who do not have a cortical branch suitable for anastomoses, although revascularization is not always sufficient to give a collateral flow enough to prevent ischemic symptoms. Therefore, the neurosurgeons often perform a combination of direct and indirect revascularization to obtain a better collateral flow.[67]

These surgical revascularizations are frequently performed in the ischemic type of patient (Fig. 31.9), and the effect of surgery on improvement in regional CBF has been proved.[41,42,67] According to the follow-up study of registered patients who received surgery, surgical revascularization seems to be effective for the prevention of ischemic events and for improvement in ADL and intellectual activity of the patients, if the surgical procedures should be chosen properly and performed successfully.[18,68,86] There is a controversy as to whether the introduction of collateral flow by revascularization increases the risk of hemorrhagic events,[4] and therefore the bypass surgery is not commonly performed in the hemorrhagic type of the patients (Fig. 31.9).[18] During the follow-up study after surgery, however, moyamoya vessels actually diminish and often disappear. The data that have been accumulated by the research committee of MHWJ seem to suggest a preventive effect on the recurrence of hemorrhagic events, and this effect seems to be more prominent in direct revascularization than in indirect revascularization or a combination of the two.[18]

It has been very difficult to conduct randomized study in patients with moyamoya disease who are mostly children. Therefore, the long-term effects of the revascularization surgery on the prognosis, including prevention of relapse of the hemorrhagic events and the improvement in ADL and intelligence, have never been evaluated accurately, and the natural course of the patients with this disease remains to be clarified.

Conclusion and Future Directions

As a result of the extensive investigation since the first report of this disease in 1957, the concept of moyamoya disease is now recognized as a disease entity all over the world. Angiographic findings and pathophysiologic features of this disease are well characterized, and the guideline for the diagnosis of this disease is also established including MRI and MRA.[17] Data concerning epidemiology and the long-term effects of medical and surgical treatments on their prognosis have been accumulating, and thus, need to be analyzed carefully and accurately.

As regards the etiology and pathogenesis of this disease, great advances have been achieved during recent years, and such data are expected to provide important clues to solve the genesis of this mysterious disorder. New advanced techniques including molecular genetics, cell biology, and experimental pathology should be applied vigorously. The establishment of an experimental animal model of this disease is expected to become extremely valuable.

Acknowledgments

The authors express their gratitude to Professor M. Fukui, Chairman of the research committee of spontaneous occlusion of the circle of Willis (supported by the Ministry of Health and Welfare, Japan) for providing the new information and data accumulated by the committee. Gratitude is extended to Drs. K. Houkin and Y. Yonekawa for their generous permission to reproduce their data, and to Drs. C. Yutani, M. Nishikawa, and T. Suzuki for allowing us to examine their autopsy cases. Thanks also to Ms. K. Tanaka for her excellent secretarial assistance. This work was partly supported by a grant from the research committee on spontaneous occlusion of the circle of Willis, Ministry of Health and Welfare, Japan.

References

1. Abe H, Houkin K, Yoshimoto T: Angiographical analysis of moyamoya disease. p. 7. In Fukui M (ed): Annual Report (1995) by Research Committee on Spontaneous Occlusion of the Circle of Willis (Moyamoya Disease). Ministry of Health and Welfare, Japan, 1996

2. Abe H, Kamiyama H, Takigawa S et al: Intellectual development of children with moyamoya disease. p. 126. In Yonekawa Y (ed): Annual Report (1989) by Research Committee on Spontaneous Occlusion of the Circle of

Willis (Moyamoya Disease). Ministry of Health and Welfare, Japan, 1990

3. Abe H, Yoshimoto T, Houkin K, et al: Evaluation of cytokine in CSF of the patients with moyamoya disease. Part 2. p.111. In Fukui M (ed): Annual Report (1995) by Research Committee on Spontaneous Occlusion of the Circle of Willis (Moyamoya Disease). Ministry of Health and Welfare, Japan, 1996

4. Aoki N: Cerebrovascular bypass surgery for the treatment of moyamoya disease: unsatisfactory outcome in the patients presenting with intracranial hemorrhage. Surg Neurol 40:372, 1993

5. Aoyagi M, Fukui N, Sakamoto H et al: Altered cellular responses to serum mitogens, including platelet-derived growth factor, in cultured smooth muscle cells derived from arteries of patients with moyamoya disease. J Cell Physiol 147:191, 1991

6. Aoyagi M, Ogami K, Matsushima Y et al: Human leukocyte antigen in patients with moyamoya disease. Stroke 26:415, 1995

7. Bai H-Z, Masuda J, Sawa Y et al: Neointima formation after vascular stent implantation. Spatial and chronological distribution of smooth muscle cell proliferation and phenotypic modulation. Arterioscler Thromb 14:1846, 1994

8. Bitzer M, Topka H: Progressive cerebral occlusive disease after radiation therapy. Stroke 26:131, 1995

9. Casscells W: Migration of smooth muscle and endothelial cells: critical events in restenosis. Circulation 86:723, 1992

10. Chen ST, Liu YH, Hsu CY et al: Moyamoya disease in Taiwan. Stroke 19:53; 1988

11. Cheng MK: A review of cerebrovascular surgery in the People's Republic of China. Stroke 13:249, 1982

12. Choi KS: Moyamoya disease in Korea—a cooperative study. p. 107. In Suzuki J (ed): Advances in Surgery for Cerebral Stroke. Springer-Verlag, Tokyo, 1988

13. Ellison PH, Largent JA, Popp AJ: Moyamoya disease associated with renal artery stenosis. Arch Neurol 38:467, 1981

14. Erickson RP, Wooliscroft J, Allen RJ: Familial occurrence of intracranial arterial occlusive disease (moyamoya) in neurofibromatosis. Clin Genet 18:191, 1980

15. Ezura M, Yoshimoto T, Fujiwara S et al: Clinical and angiographic follow-up of childhood-onset moyamoya disease. Childs Nerv Syst 11:591, 1995

16. Fernandes-Alvares E, Pineda M, Royo C et al: Moyamoya disease caused by cranial trauma. Brain Dev 1:133, 1979

17. Fukui M (Chairman): Guideline for the diagnosis of spontaneous occlusion of the circle of Willis. p.136. In Fukui M (ed): Annual Report (1994) by Research Committee on Spontaneous Occlusion of the Circle of Willis (Moyamoya Disease). Ministry of Health and Welfare, Japan, 1995

18. Fukui M, Kawano T: Follow-up study of registered cases in 1995. p. 12. In Fukui M (ed): Annual Report (1995) by Research Committee on Spontaneous Occlusion of the Circle of Willis (Moyamoya Disease). Ministry of Health and Welfare, Japan, 1996

19. Fukui M, Mizoguchi M, Matsushima T et al: MR angiography in the families of moyamoya patients. p. 102. In Fukui M (ed): Annual Report (1994) by Research Committee of Spontaneous Occlusion of the Circle of Willis (Moyamoya Disease). Ministry of Health and Welfare, Japan, 1995

20. Fukuyama Y, Kanai N, Osawa M: Clinical genetic analysis on moyamoya disease. p. 141. In Yonekawa Y (ed): Annual Report (1991) by Research Committee on Spontaneous Occlusion of the Circle of Willis. Ministry of Health and Welfare, Japan, 1992

21. Fukuyama Y, Mitsuishi Y, Umezu R: Intellectual prognosis of children with TIA type of spontaneous occlusion of the circle of Willis: with special reference to Wechsler's intelligence test and Benton's visual attention test. p. 43. In Handa H (ed): Annual Report (1986) of Research Committee on Spontaneous Occlusion of the Circle of Willis. Ministry of Health and Welfare, Japan, 1987

22. Fukuyama Y, Sugahara N, Osawa M: A genetic study of idiopathic spontaneous multiple occlusion of the circle of Willis. p. 139. In Yonekawa Y (ed): Annual Report (1990) by Research Committee on Spontaneous Occlusion of the Circle of Willis. Ministry of Health and Welfare, Japan, 1991

23. Godin M, Helias A, Tadie M, et al: Moyamoya syndrome and renal artery stenosis. Kidney Int 15:450, 1978

24. Goldberg HJ: Moyamoya associated with peripheral vascular occlusive disease. Arch Dis Child 49:964, 1974

25. Goto Y, Yonekawa Y: Worldwide distribution of moyamoya disease. Neurol Med Chir (Tokyo) 32:883, 1992

26. Gotoh F, Ebihara S, Hata T et al: Local cerebral blood flow and CO_2 responsiveness in patients with "moyamoya disease." p. 97. In Meyer JS, Lechner H, Reivich M (eds): Cerebral Vascular Disease 6. Elsevier Science Publishers, Amsterdam, 1987

27. Hanakita J, Kondo A, Ishikawa J et al: An autopsy case of moyamoya disease. Neurol Surg 1982:10:531, 1982

28. Handa H, Tani K, Kajikawa H et al: Clinicopathological study on an adult case with cerebral arterial rete. No To Shinkei 21:181, 1969

29. Handa H, Yonekawa Y, Goto Y et al: Analysis of the filing data bank of 1500 cases of spontaneous occlusion of the circle of Willis and follow-up study of 200 cases for more than 5 years. p. 14. In Handa H (ed): Annual Report (1984) by Research Committee on Spontaneous Occlusion of the Circle of Willis, Ministry of Health and Welfare, Japan, 1985

30. Herreman F, Nathal E, Yasui N et al: Intracranial aneurysm in moyamoya disease: report of ten cases and review of the literature. Cerebrovasc Dis 4:329, 1994

31. Hirayama A, Kowada M, Fukasawa H et al: Cerebrovascular moyamoya disease: a case report and review of 12 autopsy cases in Japan. No To Shinkei 26:1215, 1974

32. Hoshimaru M, Takahashi JA, Kikuchi H et al: Possible roles of basic fibroblast growth factor in the pathogenesis of moyamoya disease: an immunohistochemical study. J Neurosurg 75:267, 1991

33. Hosoda Y: A pathomorphological analysis of so-called "spontaneous occlusion of the circle of Willis" (cerebrovascular moyamoya disease). No To Shinkei 26:471, 1974

34. Hosoda Y: Pathology of so-called 'spontaneous occlusion of the circle of Willis.' Pathol Annu 19:221, 1984

35. Houkin K, Aoki T, Takahashi A et al: Diagnosis of moya-moya disease with magnetic resonance angiography. Stroke 25:2159, 1994

36. Hughes GRV. The antiphospholipid syndrome: ten years on. Lancet 342:341, 1993

37. Ikeda E, Maruyama I, Hosoda Y: Expression of thrombomodulin in patients with spontaneous occlusion of the circle of Willis. Stroke 24:657, 1993

38. Ikeda E: Systemic vascular changes in spontaneous occlusion of the circle of Willis. Stroke 22:1358, 1991

39. Ikezaki K, Fukui M, Inamura T et al: Epidemiological survey of moyamoya disease in Korea. Part 1. Definite cases. Comparison with Japanese cases. p. 17. In Fukui M (ed): Annual Report (1995) by Research Committee on Spontaneous Occlusion of the Circle of Willis (Moyamoya Disease). Ministry of Health and Welfare, Japan, 1996

40. Ikezaki K, Fukui M, Inamura T et al: Epidemiological survey of moyamoya disease in Korea. Part 2. Probable and unlikely cases. Comparison with Japanese cases. p. 26. In Fukui M (ed): Annual Report (1995) by Research Committee on Spontaneous Occlusion of the Circle of Willis (Moyamoya Disease). Ministry of Health and Welfare, Japan, 1996

41. Ikezaki K, Matsushima T, Kuwabara Y et al: Cerebral circulation and oxygen metabolism in childhood moyamoya disease: A perioperative positron emission tomography study. J Neurosurg 81:843, 1994

42. Iwama T, Hashimoto N, Yonekawa Y: The relevance of hemodynamic factors to perioperative ischemic complications in childhood moyamoya disease. Neurosurgery 38:1120, 1996

43. Karasawa J, Kikuchi H, Furuse S et al: Treatment of moyamoya disease with STA- MCA anastomosis. J Neurosurg 49:679, 1978

44. Karasawa J, Kikuchi H, Furuse S: A surgical treatment of moyamoya disease. Encephalomyosynagiosis. Neurol Med Chir (Tokyo) 17:29, 1977

45. Karasawa J, Touhou H, Ohnishi H et al: Cerebral revascularization using omental transplantation for childhood moyamoya disease. J Neurosurg 79:192, 1993

46. Kasai N, Fujiwara S, Kodama N et al: The experimental study on causal genesis of moyamoya disease: correlation with immunological reaction and sympathetic nerve influence for vascular changes. No Shinkei Geka 10:251, 1982

47. Kawano T, Fukui M, Hashimoto N et al: Follow-up study of patients with "unilateral" moyamoya disease. Neurol Med Chir (Tokyo) 34:744, 1994

48. Kitahara T, Ariga N, Yamamura A et al: Familial occurrence of moyamoya disease: report of three Japanese families. J Neurol Neurosurg Psychiatry 42:208, 1979

49. Kitahara T, Okumura K, Semba T et al: Genetic and immunologic analysis of moyamoya disease. J Neurol Neurosurg Psychiatry 45:1048, 1982

50. Kitamura K, Fukui M, Oka K et al: Moyamoya disease. p. 293. In Toole JF (ed): Handbook of Clinical Neurology. Vol. 11 (55). Vascular Diseases. Part III. Elsevier, Amsterdam, 1989

51. Kitamura K, Kishikawa T, Numaguchi Y et al: Reevaluation of radiological diagnosis of the occlusion of the circle of Willis. p. 72. In Gotoh F (ed): Annual Report (1978) by Research Committee on Spontaneous Occlusion of the Circle of Willis (Moyamoya Disease). Ministry of Health and Welfare, Japan, 1979

52. Kodama N, Aoki Y, Hiraga H et al: Electroencephalographic findings in children with moyamoya disease. Arch Neurol 36:16, 1979

53. Kodama N, Fujiwara S, Horie Y et al: Transdural anastomosis in moyamoya disease: vault moyamoya. No Shinkei Geka 8:729, 1980

54. Kodama N, Suzuki J: Moyamoya disease associated with aneurysm. J Neurosurg 48:565, 1978

55. Konishi Y, Kadowaki C, Hara M et al: Aneurysms associated with moyamoya disease. Neurosurgery 16:484, 1985

56. Kono S, Oka K, Sueishi K: Histopathologic and morphometric studies of leptomeningeal vessels in moyamoya disease. Stroke 21:1044, 1990

57. Kudo T: Spontaneous occlusion of the circle of Willis: a disease apparently confined to Japanese. Neurology 18:485, 1968

58. Kurokawa T, Tomita S, Ueda K et al: Prognosis of occlusive disease of circle of Willis (moyamoya disease) in children. Pediatr Neurol 12:288, 1969

59. Kuwabara Y, Ichiya Y, Otsuka M et al: Cerebral hemodynamic changes in the child and adult with moyamoya disease. Stroke 21:272, 1990

60. Lamas E, Diez Lobato R, Cabello A et al: Multiple intracranial arterial occlusions (moyamoya disease) in patients with neurofibromatosis: one case report with autopsy. Acta Neurochir (Wien) 45:133, 1978

61. Levine SR, Welch KMA: Cerebrovascular ischemia associated with lupus anticoagulant. Stroke 18:257, 1987

62. Maki Y, Nakata Y: Autopsy of a case with an anomalous hemangioma of the internal carotid artery at the skull base. No To Shinkei 17:764, 1965

63. Masuda J, Ogata J, Yutani C: Smooth muscle cell proliferation and localization of macrophages and T-cell in the occlusive intracranial major arteries in moyamoya disease. Stroke 24:1960, 1993

64. Masuda J, Tanaka K: A new model of cerebral arteriosclerosis induced by intimal injury using a silicone rubber cylinder in rabbits. Lab Invest 51:475, 1984

65. Masuda J, Yutani C, Ogata J et al: Atheromatous embolism in the brain: A clinicopathologic analysis of 15 autopsy cases. Neurology 44:1231, 1994

66. Matsuo T, Yokoyama K, Fujii T et al: Cerebral dissecting aneurysms in patients with moyamoya disease. Report of two cases. J Neurosurg 58:120, 1983

67. Matsushima T, Inoue T, Suzuki SO et al: Surgical treatment of moyamoya disease in pediatric patients—comparison between the results of indirect and direct revascularization procedures. Neurosurgery 31:401, 1992

68. Matsushima Y, Aoyagi M, Nariai T et al: Long-term intelligence outcome of childhood moyamoya patients who underwent EDAS more than 9.5 years before. II. Patients with preoperative WISC-TIQ above 70. p. 39. In Fukui M (ed): Annual Report (1995) by Research Committee on Spontaneous Occlusion of the Circle of Willis (Moyamoya Disease). Ministry of Health and Welfare, Japan, 1996

69. Matsushima Y, Inaba Y: Moyamoya disease in children and its surgical treatment. Introduction of a new surgical procedure and its follow-up angiograms. Childs Brain 11:155, 1984

70. Mito T, Becker LE: Vascular dysplasia in Down syndrome: a possible relationship to moyamoya disease. Brain Dev 14:248, 1992

71. Moritake K, Handa H, Yonekawa Y et al: Follow-up study on the relationship between age at onset of illness and outcome in patients with "moyamoya disease." Neurol Surg 14:957, 1986

72. Nagamine Y, Takahashi S, Sonobe M: Multiple intracranial aneurysms associated with moyamoya disease: case report. J Neurosurg 54:673, 1981

73. Nariai T, Suzuki R, Hirakawa K, et al: Vascular reserve in chronic cerebral ischemia measured with acetazolamide challenge test: comparison with positron emission tomography. AJNR 16:563, 1995

74. Nishimoto A, Takeuchi S: Abnormal cerebrovascular network related to the internal carotid arteries. J Neurosurg 29:255, 1968

75. Ogata J, Masuda J, Nishikawa M, et al: Sclerosed peripheral-artery aneurysm in moyamoya disease. Cerebrovasc Dis 6:248, 1996

76. Ogawa A, Yoshimoto T, Suzuki J, et al: Cerebral blood flow in moyamoya disease. Part 1: Correlation with age and regional distribution. Acta Neurochir (Wien) 105:30, 1990

77. Ogawa A, Nakamura N, Yoshimoto T, et al: Cerebral blood flow in moyamoya disease. Part 2: Autoregulation and CO_2 response. Acta Neurochir (Wien) 105:107, 1990

78. Ohmoto T, Hirotsune N, Meguro T et al: Long-term follow-up study of patients with unilateral moyamoya disease. p. 66. In Fukui M (ed): Annual Report (1995) by Research Committee on Spontaneous Occlusion of the Circle of Willis (Moyamoya Disease). Ministry of Health and Welfare, Japan, 1996

79. Oka K, Yamashita M, Sadoshima S et al: Cerebral hemorrhage in moyamoya disease at autopsy. Virchows Arch 392:247, 1981

80. Osawa M, Imaizumi T: Long-term prognosis of pediatric moyamoya a patients followed up to adulthood. p. 46. In Fukui M (ed): Annual Report (1995) by Research Committee on Spontaneous Occlusion of the Circle of Willis (Moyamoya Disease). Ministry of Health and Welfare, Japan, 1996

81. Picard L, Levesque M, Crouzet G et al: The moyamoya syndrome. J Neuroradiol 1:47, 1974

82. Rajakulasingam K, Cerullo LJ, Raimondi AJ: Childhood moyamoya syndrome: postradiation pathogenesis. Childs Brain 5:469, 1979

83. Reichmann O, Anderson RE, Roberts TC et al: The treatment of intracranial occlusive cerebrovascular disease by STA-cortical MCA anastomosis. p. 31. In Handa H (ed): Microneurosurgery. Igaku Shoin, Tokyo, 1975

84. Reidy MA, Fingerle J, Lindner V: Factors controlling the development of arterial lesions after injury. Circulation, 86(suppl III):1845, 1992

85. Ross R: The pathogenesis of atherosclerosis: a perspective for the 1990s. Nature 362:801, 1993

86. Sakurai Y, Arai H: Long-term follow up of pediatric moyamoya disease after surgical revascularization. p. 5. In Fukui M (ed): Annual Report (1995) by Research Committee on Spontaneous Occlusion of the Circle of Willis (Moyamoya Disease). Ministry of Health and Welfare, Japan, 1996

87. Sano K: Cerebral juxta-basal telangiectasia. No To Shinkei 17:748, 1965

88. Sasazuki T: Analysis of HLA class II genes in Moyamoya disease p. 14. In Fukui M (ed): Annual Report (1995) by Research Committee on Spontaneous Occlusion of the Circle of Willis (Moyamoya Disease). Ministry of Health and Welfare, Japan, 1996

89. Seeler RA, Royal JE, Powe L et al: Moyamoya disease in children with sickle cell anemia and cerebrovascular occlusion. J Pediatr 93:808, 1978

90. Suzui H, Hoshimaru M, Takahashi JA, et al: Immunohistochemical reactions for fibroblast growth factor receptor in arteries of patients with moyamoya disease. Neurosurgery 35:20, 1994

91. Suzuki J, Kodama N: Moyamoya disease: a review. Stroke 14:104, 1983

92. Suzuki J, Takaku A: Cerebrovascular "Moyamoya disease": a disease showing abnormal net-like vessels in base of brain. Arch Neurol 20:288, 1969

93. Takahashi A, Sawamura Y, Houkin K, et al: The cerebrovascular fluid in patients in moyamoya disease contains a high level of basic fibroblast growth factor. Neurosci Lett 160:214, 1993

94. Takeuchi K, Shimizu K: Hypoplasia of the bilateral internal carotid arteries. No To Shinkei 9:37, 1957

95. Taki W, Yonekawa Y, Kobayashi A, et al: Cerebral circulation and metabolism in adult's Moyamoya disease—PET study. Acta Neurochir (Wien) 100:150, 1989

96. Tanaka K, Oka K, Yamashita M: Intracranial and systemic vascular lesion and intracranial hemorrhage in spontaneous occlusion of the circle of Willis. p. 86. In Goth F (ed): Annual Report (1981) of the Research Committee on Spontaneous Occlusion of the Circle of Wills. Ministry of Health and Welfare, Japan, 1981

97. Taveras JM: Multiple progressive intracranial arterial occlusion: a syndrome of children and young adults. AJR 106:235, 1969

98. Ueda M, Becker AE, Tsukada T et al: Fibrocellular tissue response after percutaneous transluminal coronary angioplasty: an immunocytochemical analysis of the cellular composition. Circulation 83:1327, 1991

99. Ueki K, Meyer JB: Moyamoya disease: the disorder and surgical treatment. Mayo Clin Proc 69:749, 1994

100. Wakai K, Tamakoshi A, Ohno Y et al: Epidemiology of moyamoya disease in Japan: findings from a nationwide survey. p. 33. In Fukui M (ed): Annual Report (1995) by Research Committee on Spontaneous Occlusion of the Circle of Willis (Moyamoya Disease). Ministry of Health and Welfare, Japan, 1996

101. Weidner W, Hanafee W, Markham C: Intracranial collateral circulation via leptomenigeal and rete mirabile anastomosis. Neurology 15:39, 1965

102. Yamada H, Deguchi K, Sakai N et al: Relationship between moyamoya disease and anaerobic bacterium propionibacterium acnes infection. p. 33. In Handa H (ed):

Annual Report (1987) by Research Committee on Spontaneous Occlusion of the Circle of Willis. Ministry of Health and Welfare, Japan, 1988

103. Yamada H, Nakamura S, Kageyama N: Moyamoya disease in monovular twins: case report. J Neurosurg 53: 109, 1980

104. Yamada H, Tanigawara T, Iwamura M et al: Studies on cytomegalovirus and Epstein-Barr virus infection in moyamoya disease. p. 136. In Fukui M (ed): Annual Report (1995) by Research Committee on Spontaneous Occlusion of the Circle of Willis (Moyamoya Disease). Ministry of Health and Welfare, Japan, 1996

105. Yamada I, Suzuki S, Matsushima Y: Moyamoya disease: comparison with MR angiography and MR imaging versus conventional angiography. Radiology 196:221, 1995

106. Yamada K, Fuse T, Takagi T: Analysis of anticardiolipin antibody in moyamoya disease. p. 116. In Fukui M (ed): Annual Report (1995) by Research Committee on Spontaneous Occlusion of the Circle of Willis (Moyamoya Disease). Ministry of Health and Welfare, Japan, 1996

107. Yamaguchi T, Tashiro M, Hasegawa Y: Collective analysis of the patients with spontaneous occlusion of the circle of Willis in Japan, registered from 1977 to 1982. p. 15. In Gotoh F (ed): Annual Report (1982) by Research Committee on Spontaneous Occlusion of the Circle of Willis (Moyamoya Disease). Ministry of Health and Welfare, Japan, 1983

108. Yamano T, Onouchi Z, Shimada M: Moyamoya disease and renal hypertension: a case probably caused by fibromuscular dysplasia. Brain Dev 6:184, 1974

109. Yamashita M, Oka K, Tanaka K: Cervico-cephalic arterial thrombi and thromboemboli in moyamoya disease—possible correlation with progressive intimal thickening in the intracranial major arteries. Stroke 15: 264, 1984

110. Yamashita M, Oka K, Tanaka K: Histopathology of the brain vascular network in moyamoya disease. Stroke 14: 50, 1983

111. Yamashita M, Tanaka K, Kishikawa T et al: Moyamoya disease associated with renovascular hypertension. Hum Pathol 15:191, 1984

112. Yamashita M, Tanaka K, Matsuo T et al: Cerebral dissecting aneurysms in patients with moyamoya disease. Report of two cases. J Neurosurg 58:120, 1983

113. Yasargil MG: Microsurgery Applied to Neurosurgery. Thieme, Stuttgart, 1969

114. Yonekawa Y, Goto Y, Ogata N: Moyamoya disease: diagnosis, treatment, and recent achievement. p. 721. In Barnett HJM, Mohr JP, Stein BM, Yatsu FM (eds): Stroke: Pathophysiology, Diagnosis, and Management. 2nd Ed. Churchill Livingstone, New York, 1992

115. Yoshii N, Kudo T: Electroencephalographical study on occlusion of the Willis arterial ring. Rinsho Shinkeigaku 8:301, 1968

116. Yuasa H, Tokito S, Izumi K, et al: Cerebrovascular moyamoya disease associated with an intracranial pseudoaneurysm: case report. J Neurosurg 56:131, 1982

CHAPTER 32

Cerebrovascular Fibromuscular Dysplasia

EDWARD B. HEALTON

J. P. MOHR

Definition and Historical Review

Fibromuscular dysplasia (FMD) is an uncommon, idiopathic, systemic vascular disease characterized by nonatherosclerotic abnormalities of smooth muscle and fibrous and elastic tissue in small and medium-sized arteries. FMD is multifocal, affecting renal, cephalic, visceral, iliac, femoral, axillary, subclavian, and internal mammary arteries and the aorta[102,184] There has been only one report of venous involvement[147] but FMD changes have been documented in the venous side of some instances of polytetrafluorethylene (Gore-Tex) grafts in patients whose graft was placed for renal dialysis.[173] The changes have been attributed in part to shear-induced injuries of the intima and upstream release of platelet-derived growth factor. Cephalic vessels are affected in 25% of reported cases of FMD, the most common location after the renal arteries.[106] Although FMD may be widespread and involve the iliac artery,[174] subclavian artery,[25] upper limb arteries,[74] and gastric arteries,[86] one or two arterial territories are usually involved in each patient.

In 1938, Leadbetter and Burkland[100] first described the condition in a 5-year-old hypertensive boy with renal artery stenosis caused by a "smooth muscle plug." Subsequent investigators reported patients with similar renal artery lesions and introduced the terms *fibromuscular hyperplasia*[112] and, later, *fibromuscular dysplasia*,[65,94] to describe the proliferative, disruptive arterial changes. In these early reports,[93,130,186] FMD was established as a unique radiologic and pathologic entity and an important, surgically curable cause of hypertension, but it was believed to be confined to the renal artery.

In 1964, Palubinskas and Ripley[129] first reported angiographic and histologic evidence of FMD outside the renal arteries. One of these patients, an apparently asymptomatic woman, had angiographic "changes in the extracranial internal carotid artery indistinguishable from the classical appearance of fibromuscular hyperplasia." FMD was histologically proven in the internal carotid artery 1 year later,[30,76] and subsequently described in the vertebral, external carotid, and intracranial arteries. Angiographic criteria for distinguishing this disease from other extracranial and intracranial arterial abnormalities were also established.[16,79,124,127,128,183]

There was disagreement, however, about the relationship between FMD and neurologic symptoms. Some authors believed that FMD was usually diagnosed coincidentally and caused neurologic abnormalities infrequently. Others attributed focal or generalized neurologic symptoms to FMD and advocated surgical treatment. In 1965, Connett and Lansche[30] first reported surgical resection of internal carotid artery FMD in a patient with cerebral infarction. Graduated intraluminal dilation was introduced 3 years later and has become the most frequently used surgical procedure.[120]

Although there are now over 600 reported cases of cerebrovascular FMD, the etiology, frequency and pathogenesis of clinical symptoms, and the proper management of this disease remain controversial.[2,7,8,10,14,20,24,37,43,53,80,81,92,107,109,116,131,139,171,188]

Epidemiology

The true incidence of cephalic FMD in the general population is unknown. In 819 consecutive autopsies, FMD of the renal artery occurred in 1.1%[73]; a similar study of cerebrovascular FMD has not been reported. In several large retrospective reviews of consecutive angiograms (totaling approximately 22,000 studies),[31,67,124,162,166] FMD was diagnosed in less than

1% of cases (range: 0.25% to 0.61%). In another review of 936 cephalic angiograms, the incidence of internal carotid artery FMD was 3.7%.[180] In study, a frequency of 10% was cited.[26]

FMD is considerably more common among women, constituting up to 85% of those with cerebrovascular FMD. FMD also may be more common among white ethnic groups.[163] Although it has occurred in patients aged 2 to 83 years, cerebrovascular FMD is usually diagnosed in the fourth or fifth decade and rarely occurs in children.[6,42,101,136,159,177]

Etiology

Ultrastructural studies of FMD have shown that, independent of histologic type, arterial lesions are identical at the subcellular level and "differ only in their intensity and localization."[22,58] Smooth muscle transformation into fibroblast-like cells (myofibroblasts) and increased collagen synthesis are fundamental processes in the morphogenesis of these lesions. The etiology of this process and the stimulus for smooth muscle differentiation are unknown, but several hypotheses have been proposed. Genetic factors in FMD have been suggested in reports of familial FMD among siblings or identical twins.[62,64,108,119,125] The mode of inheritance was consistent with an autosomal dominant trait with reduced penetrance in males.[57,114,151] In some of these studies, however, relatives with only a history of unexplained hypertension, stroke, or acute myocardial infarction were considered to have FMD. Only a few families with angiographic or histologic confirmation of FMD have been reported.[125] Because of an association between FMD and skeletal deformities or features of Ehlers-Danlos syndrome in a few patients, a hereditary mesenchymal defect has been proposed.[152,153] Because renal angiograms have been normal up to 12 years before diagnosis of renal FMD,[11,12] a hereditary abnormality must be associated with other factors to account for the delayed expression in some patients.

Because of the predominance of FMD in women and the stimulatory effect of estrogen on smooth muscle cells, hormonal influences are probably important.[85,148,149,165] Ischemia of the arterial wall also may cause dysplastic abnormalities in humans.[133] Lesions very similar to human FMD have been produced in dogs by experimental occlusions of the vasa vasorum,[121,164] and the renal and internal carotid arteries receive fewer of these nutrient branches than other muscular arteries of similar caliber. Vascular lesions resembling FMD have also been reported in ergotism.[44,45,134]

Because there are vessel wall abnormalities associated with the rubella syndrome, and a disease similar to FMD occurs in domestic turkeys,[87] a viral etiology has been proposed. Stretch-traction stresses on the arterial wall have also been considered, but not uniformly supported[33,103] by experimental evidence.[150]

FMD may have several different etiologies, each acting on vulnerable areas of the arterial wall in hereditarily predisposed individuals when there is hormonally conducive environment.

Pathology and Anatomic Distribution of Lesions

The pathology of FMD is characterized by smooth muscle hyperplasia or thinning, elastic fiber destruction, fibrous tissue proliferation, and arterial wall disorganization.[65,66,167] Inflammation, necrosis, lipid accumulation, and calcification are absent. Although there is not complete agreement about terminology, FMD can be classified into three histologic types based on the arterial layer in which lesions predominate.[66,167] Medial FMD occurs in 90% to 95% of cases, much more commonly in women. Concentric rings of fibrous proliferation or smooth muscle hyperplasia cause medial thickening and destruction of the internal or external elastic lamina. These fibromuscular ridges can occur singly, extend for a variable length along the artery, or alternate sequentially with areas of medial thinning and arterial dilatation. Based on location within the media and the predominant histologic abnormality, medial FMD has been subdivided into medial or perimedial fibroplasia and medial hyperplasia.[71]

Intimal fibroplasia is present in approximately 5% of cases and occurs equally between men and women[172]; fibrous tissue proliferation causes intimal thickening and destruction of the internal elastic lamina. In periarterial (adventitial) fibroplasia, the least common histologic type, there is fibrosis of the adventitia and surrounding periarterial tissue.

Regarding the vessels of neurologic interest, the internal carotid artery is affected in approximately 95% of patients with cephalic FMD, and is bilateral in 60% to 85% of affected individuals.[28,50,106,124,162] The abnormalities characteristically occur in the midportion of the artery, opposite the second cervical vertebra, and they extend 0.5 cm to 7 cm proximally or distally, usually sparing the proximal 2.5 cm. Only 17 patients have been reported with proximal internal carotid artery disease,[118] and FMD of the common carotid artery has been reported in three patients.[182] FMD has occasionally involved the intraosseous carotid artery, either alone or as an extension of cervical abnormalities.[162,182,189] External carotid artery FMD has also been reported.[27,46]

The incidence of vertebral artery FMD is uncertain because complete angiography has not always been performed in patients with cephalic FMD. For this reason, the reported incidence of vertebral artery FMD has varied from 12% to 43% of affected patients, usually in association with internal carotid artery disease.[80,115] Vertebral artery FMD is also commonly located opposite the second cervical vertebra and may extend for 1 cm to 2 cm. There are no reports of FMD at the origin of the vertebral artery.

Intracranial FMD is uncommon. Angiographic abnormalities consistent with FMD have been identified in the intracranial segments of the internal carotid and vertebral arteries, and the anterior cerebral, middle cerebral, posterior cerebral, basilar and anterior inferior, and superior cerebellar arteries, but the abnormalities rarely have been verified histologically.[1,5,41,49,59,157,160,175] In some, it has been associated with moyamoya disease.[11] All but four patients with intracranial disease also had extracranial FMD.

Table 32.1 Neurologic Diagnoses in Patients with Cerebrovascular Fibromuscular Dysplasia[a]

Ref.	Total Patients	Method of Patient Selection	Asymptomatic Bruit	Cerebral Infarction	Transient Ischemic Attack	Unilateral Facial Pain or Horner Syndrome	Nonlocalizing Neurologic Symptoms[b]	Intracranial Aneurysm	Coincidental Fibromuscular Dysplasia[c]
31	79	[e]	8 (10.1)[d]	7 (8.9)	6 (7.6)	0 (0)	3 (3.8)	10 (12.7)	45 (56.9)
115	37	[f]	1 (2.7)	3 (8.1)	4 (10.8)	3 (8.1)	0 (0)	19 (51.4)	7 (18.9)
180	30	[g]	5 (16.7)	3 (10)	16 (53.3)	0 (0)	4 (13.3)	0 (0)	2 (6.7)
178	17	[h]	2 (11.7)	0 (0)	9 (52.9)	0 (0)	6 (35.4)	0 (0)	0 (0)
163	32	[i]	2 (6.3)	9 (28.1)	9 (28.1)	3 (9.4)	4 (12.5)	5 (15.6)	0 (0)
170	49	[i]	11 (22.4)	3 (6.1)	17 (34.7)	0 (0)	15 (30.6)	7 (14.3)	3 (6.1)
36	86	[j]	7 (8.1)	19 (22.1)	58 (67.5)	0 (0)	2 (2.3)	0 (0)	0 (0)
168	40	[k]	6 (15.0)	4 (10.0)	11 (27.5)	0 (0)	19 (47.5)	0 (0)	0 (0)
29	18	[l]	0 (0)	3 (16.7)	6 (33.3)	0 (0)	9 (50.0)	0 (0)	0 (0)
166	15	[m]	1 (6.7)	1 (6.7)	3 (20.0)	0 (0)	2 (13.4)	4 (26.6)	4 (26.6)
124	25	[m]	0 (0)	6 (24.0)	8 (32.0)	0 (0)	2 (8.0)	9 (36.0)	0 (0)

[a] Reported series of 10 or more patients (English language).

[b] Dizziness, vertigo, syncope, generalized seizure, scintillating scotomata, or unspecified.

[c] Head trauma, intracranial mass lesion, or unspecified.

[d] Numbers in parentheses indicate percent.

[e] Review of 13,955 consecutive cerebral angiograms.

[f] Review of 4,000 consecutive cerebral angiograms.

[g] Review of 936 consecutive angiograms.

[h] Review of "radiographic and clinical records."

[i] Review of "medical records and cerebral angiographic registry."

[j] Surgical series: all patients had surgery.

[k] Surgical series: 25 of 40 patients had surgery.

[l] Surgical series: 13 of 18 patients had surgery.

[m] Uncertain.

The histologic abnormalities may cause three patterns of pathology of the arterial wall.[31,79,124] Multifocal stenoses, alternating with mural dilatations (beaded appearance), is the most common pattern and occurs in 80% to 90% of patients. In 6% to 12% of patients, there is a longitudinal stenosis (tubular appearance). When FMD involves the arterial wall in a noncircumferential manner, there may be an outpouching or diverticulum of the wall (4% to 6% of patients) or, rarely, an asymmetrical septal appearance, leading to a weblike stenosis. Lesions with a septal appearance have occurred only in the proximal internal carotid artery, and there have been only three histologically proven cases.[118]

Vessels affected by FMD may become very elongated or kinked. Severe stenosis is uncommon in cephalic FMD, and complete occlusion has been reported in only 14 patients.[3]

Progressive disruption of the arterial wall by FMD may lead to several complications. FMD-related arterial disease has been reported in up to 20% of cervical carotid artery dissections[4,23,39,47,68,117,156] may also underlie arterial dissection in the vertebral, middle cerebral, anterior cerebral, or superior cerebellar arteries and may be the cause of unexplained "spontaneous" dissection in some patients.[61,82,89,111] Multiple arterial dissections associated with FMD have also been reported.[68,146]

Expansion of a dilated arterial segment may cause local saccular or giant aneurysms reported in the midcervical, skull base, or cavernous sinus portions of the internal carotid artery.[17,72,91,189] Similarly, carotid-cavernous sinus and vertebral-perivertebral vein arterial venous fistulas also have been caused by FMD.[55,75]

Intracranial "berry" aneurysms in association with cerebrovascular FMD have been reported in 21% to 51% of affected patients, depending on the completeness of cerebral angiography.[63,77,88,114,124] These aneurysms have the same arterial distribution and histology as in patients without FMD. There has been one report of FMD associated with a cerebral arterial venous malformation.[90]

Cerebrovascular and renal FMD may coexist in as many as 50% of patients when complete angiography is performed.[38,110,124]

Clinical Features and Pathogenesis of Symptoms

Neurologic abnormalities associated with cerebrovascular FMD (Table 32.1) have been attributed to focal cerebral ischemia, global cerebral hypoperfusion, and the direct compressive or disruptive effects of the arterial wall lesion. Focal neurologic abnormalities such as hemiparesis, hemisensory impairment, aphasia, or neglect have usually been attributed to transient cerebral ischemia or cerebral infarction.[155] A causal relationship between FMD and focal cerebral ischemia has been established in a minority of patients, however. In some patients there was severe stenosis or occlusion of the internal carotid artery or vertebral artery.[1,3,9,69,80,145] In others there was nonocclusive thrombus formation at the site of internal carotid artery FMD or distal intracranial or retinal artery branch occlusions, and cerebral embolization seemed likely.[13,29,84,114] Cerebral embolization may be more likely in patients with septal lesions involving the proximal internal carotid artery.[118] In other patients with cephalic FMD and transient ischemic attacks or cerebral infarction, there was dissection of the internal carotid, vertebral, or intracranial arteries.[68] Head-turning precipitated transient ischemic attacks in one patient with internal carotid artery FMD,[142] and neck trauma preceded cerebral infarction in three others.[105,115,187] Focal and generalized neurologic abnormalities also have been reported in patients with cerebrovascular FMD following a subarachnoid hemorrhage because of the association between intracranial aneurysms and FMD.

In most patients with cerebrovascular FMD and symptoms of focal cerebral ischemia, however, the relationship between the two conditions is uncertain. In various reports, therefore, the initial incidence of stroke or transient ischemic attacks was zero to 20% and 7% to 67%, respectively (Table 32.1). In these reports the authors understandably reached widely divergent conclusions regarding the relationship between FMD and focal cerebral ischemia, indicating that it occurred commonly, infrequently, or that the relationship between the two conditions was usually coincidental. This discrepancy is explained in part by the methods of patient selection. In some studies all patients with FMD diagnosed in consecutive angiograms were reviewed, including cases in which FMD was a coincidental abnormality. The incidence of stroke and transient ischemic attack was low in these reports. Other studies have been more selective, excluding patients with coincidental FMD or including predominantly patients with surgical treatment. In some reports, selection criteria were not clearly stated.

In most reports, moreover, it is uncertain how carefully other causes of focal neurologic symptoms were sought. Some patients with stroke or transient ischemic attack and FMD were taking birth control pills, including two patients with cerebral infarction and complete thrombotic occlusion of the internal carotid artery or vertebral artery.[69,145] Carotid artery or vertebral artery atherosclerosis coexisted with FMD in 12% to 35% of patients with symptoms of cerebral ischemia.[29,31,36,180] In a few of these patients, recurrent transient ischemic attacks stopped after surgical resection of an atherosclerotic plaque.[78]

FMD should be considered, therefore, in the differential diagnosis of stroke or transient ischemic attack, especially in young or middle-aged patients, but other more common causes also must be excluded.

Syncope, generalized convulsions, episodic dizziness, vertigo, and scintillating scotomata in patients with cerebrovascular FMD have been attributed to global cerebral hypoperfusion. A few of these patients had bilateral internal carotid artery FMD and syncope, dizziness, or vertigo following head-turning.[98,122,142,176] These positional symptoms presumably were caused by temporary occlusion of the carotid artery or vertebral artery, further compromising cerebral perfusion already reduced by FMD-related stenosis. In most reports, however, the mechanism of cerebral hypoperfusion is unclear, and the causal relationship between these nonfocal neurologic symptoms and FMD is unproven.

Neurologic abnormalities also may be caused by the direct effect of the arterial wall lesions or their associated complications. Cervical bruits caused by turbulent flow through affected arteries are sometimes the only neurologic abnormality. Bruits are frequently audible to the patient and may be reported as troublesome pulsatile tinnitus.[32] Arterial dilatation and disruption of sympathetic nerve fibers may cause anterior cervical pain or tenderness, unilateral facial pain, Horner syndrome, or a fully developed Raeder syndrome.[135,162] Giant internal carotid artery aneurysms caused by FMD have been reported in the cavernous sinus in association with cavernous sinus syndrome, at the base of the skull in patients with lower cranial nerve impairment, and in the midcervical area in one patient with an enlarging neck mass.[72,97,99,143] A cavernous sinus syndrome has also been caused by cartoid-cavernous sinus fistulae in patients with intracavernous carotid FMD.[75,91,189] Vertebral artery-paravertebral venous fistulas have been reported in patients with progressive cervical myelopathy and in two patients with only a cervical bruit.[19,55,144]

Finally, cerebrovascular FMD has also been diagnosed coincidentally in patients with neurologic symptoms associated with head trauma, neoplasm, or other mass lesion.

A few patients with FMD have had associated pes cavus, pectus excavatum, scoliosis, hallux valgus, endocardial fibroelastosis, otosclerosis, and retinal degeneration.[5,51,114] There was no evidence, however, that these abnormalities were other than coincidental.

Angiography and Other Diagnostic Tests

The angiographic appearance of affected vessels is based on the arterial wall morphology previously described.[21] In the most common pattern, irregularly spaced areas of sharply localized concentric narrowing usually reduce the lumen caliber less than 40% and alternate with areas of dilatation, which are always wider than the normal lumen (Fig. 32.1). This appearance, termed the "string of beads," occurs in 80% to 90% of patients. Other less common patterns are tubular stenosis (Fig. 32.2), diverticulum (Fig. 32.3), and, rarely, weblike ste-

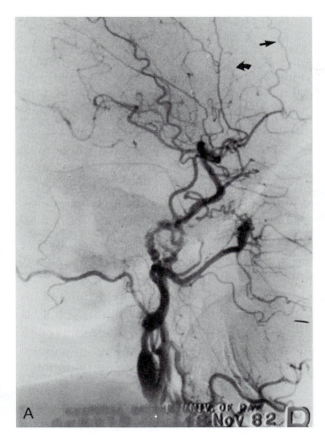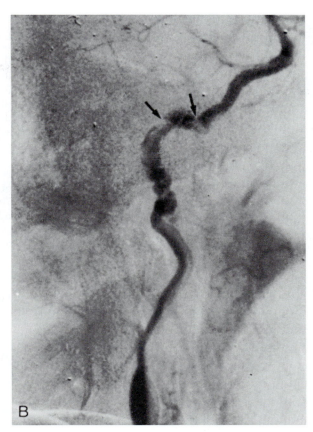

Figure 32.1 Hemodynamically significant fibromuscular dysplasia in the distal cervical segment of internal carotid artery and petrous portion. (**A**) Lateral head and neck projection of carotid angiogram demonstrates typical "string of beads" configuration of fibromuscular dysplasia in the distal cervical and proximal petrous portion of internal carotid artery. Circulation in distal branches of superficial temporal artery (straight arrow) leads circulation in middle cerebral artery branches (curved arrow) indicating hemodynamic significance of carotid stenosis. (**B**) Delayed lateral carotid angiogram shows close-up view of internal carotid artery. Several severe bandlike regions of narrowing (arrows) are present between the dilated regions of fibromuscular dysplasia.

nosis (septum). Severe stenosis is uncommon. When FMD is bilateral, the angiographic pattern occasionally may be different on the two sides.

Angiography may also identify arterial complications of FMD: embolic occlusion of distal vessels, local saccular or giant aneurysms, and arterial dissections. The typical angiographic appearance of dissection is severe linear narrowing (string sign), but complete occlusion and "double barrel" lumen (when the dissecting channel reenters the lumen) have also been described in FMD. A basal "moyamoya" angiographic pattern has been reported in two patients with internal carotid artery and proximal middle cerebral artery stenosis caused by FMD.[126,138]

The angiographic appearance of cerebrovascular FMD must be differentiated from similar arterial patterns: carotid artery stationary arterial waves produced by distal arterial occlusion, increased intracranial pressure, or subarachnoid hemorrhage; arterial spasm or circular spastic contractions at the site of catheterization; Takayasu arteritis; arterial hypoplasia resembling tubular stenosis; posttraumatic or atherosclerotic aneurysm of the internal carotid; and, in intracranial FMD, cerebral vasculitis.[56,60,80,95,124]

When FMD involves the proximal segments of the internal carotid artery, the arterial abnormalities must be differentiated from atherosclerotic cerebrovascular disease. When FMD is diagnosed, full cerebral angiography should be performed.

Magnetic resonance angiography carries some risk of misdiagnosis.[117a] Doppler ultrasonography and B-mode echotomography can detect carotid artery FMD and differentiate these abnormalities from atherosclerosis in some patients.[18,34,96,158] Although reported infrequently, noninvasive hemodynamic studies have been normal or consistent with mild stenosis in most patients.[29,48,178] Superficial temporal artery biopsy may show diagnostic dysplastic abnormalities.[5,101,140]

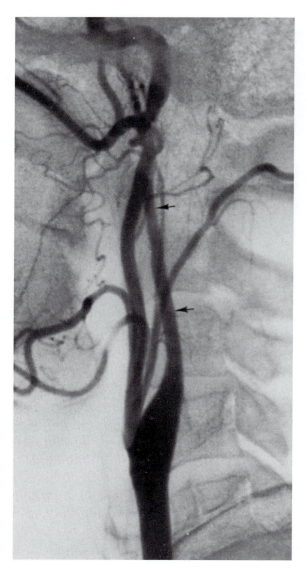

Figure 32.2 Internal carotid artery fibromuscular dysplasia: tubular stenosis (arrows). (From Osborne and Anderson,[124] with permission.)

Treatment Considerations

Because there has been no prospective study of the natural history of untreated cerebrovascular FMD, there is limited information available about anatomic or clinical progression in untreated patients. In renal artery FMD, anatomic progression of arterial lesions has been reported in 8.3% to 37.5% of patients when serial angiographic studies were performed 6 months to 8 years after the initial diagnosis, but progression was usually mild.[15,40,113] A limited number of studies have reported serial angiography in patients with cerebrovascular FMD for whom the angiogram was repeated because of recurrent symptoms or other uncertain reasons. In 31 such selected patients with repeat angiography 3 months to 7 years after

the initial diagnosis, there was no anatomic progression in 18 patients, and progressive stenosis of mild to moderate degree occurred in 7.[4,80,170,178,179] Other abnormalities reported were the development of FMD in the contralateral carotid artery in 1, aneurysm formation at the site of a diverticulum related to FMD in 1, and resolution of spontaneous carotid artery dissection in 3. Progression of cerebrovascular FMD lesions, defined as increasing stenosis or anatomic complication of the arterial lesion, does occur, therefore, in a minority of selected patients.

Information regarding the clinical natural history of FMD is also limited. In two retrospective clinical outcome studies, prognosis was usually benign.[31,178] In the largest such series, 79 patients with FMD diagnosed in association with focal cerebral ischemia (13), intracranial mass lesion (29), intracranial aneurysm (10), or miscellaneous disorders (27) were followed for an average of 5 years. There was no treatment in 64 cases.

Figure 32.3 Internal carotid artery fibromuscular dysplasia: diverticulum (arrow). (From Osborne and Anderson,[124] with permission.)

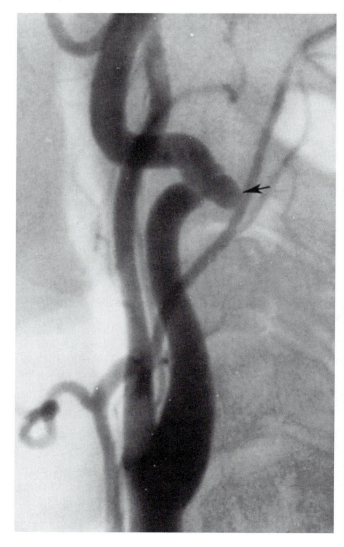

Antiplatelet therapy or anticoagulation was started in 11 patients, and 3 patients had surgical treatment. In the untreated group, one patient, aged 71, had a stroke in the same vascular territory as the fibromuscular dysplastic lesion 216 months after diagnosis. A stroke occurred in two other patients in that group (aged 65 and 75) 50 and 136 months after diagnosis, but the clinical symptoms did not correspond with the FMD lesion. Stroke or transient ischemic attack did not occur in the treated group. In a smaller, study of 17 patients with cerebrovascular FMD followed for an average of 3.8 years, 9 patients were not treated, 7 patients received anticoagulation or antiplatelet therapy, and 1 patient had surgery. In two untreated patients (aged 60 and 79) with severe cerebral atherosclerosis, cerebral infarction occurred 18 months and 5 years after diagnosis.

In untreated patients, therefore, the incidence of stroke or transient ischemic attack clearly related to cephalic FMD appears to be quite low.

Medical treatment using antiplatelet medication or anticoagulation and surgical therapy has been advocated in the initial management of cerebrovascular FMD. Graduated intraluminal dilation has been the most frequently performed surgical procedure, but some patients have had percutaneous transluminal angioplasty, resection of the FMD lesion, arterial bypass, extraction of stenotic rings, or incision of adventitial fibrosis.[52,70,104,161] Because of the frequent association of FMD with atherosclerosis, endarterectomy has also been performed together with these surgical procedures. A controlled trial of medical or surgical therapy has not been performed, and retrospective uncontrolled studies have provided conflicting results. For example, in a retrospective study of 30 patients with cerebrovascular FMD in association with focal cerebral ischemia (19), global or unlocalized neurologic symptoms (4), or no neurologic symptoms (7), followed for an average of 21.5 months (range 1 to 96 months), there was significant benefit to arterial dilation or antiplatelet therapy when compared with no therapy in patients with focal neurologic symptoms.[180] There was also a trend in favor of surgical intervention, but the overall results did not achieve statistical significance. In another report of 45 patients with angiographically proven cerebrovascular FMD, cerebral or retinal infarction did not occur in the 35 patients treated with antiplatelet therapy or followed without therapy.[169] In two of these patients, graduated intraluminal dilation was performed because of persistent nonfocal neurologic symptoms (syncope and vertigo). Stroke also did not occur in the 10 other patients in whom graduated intraluminal dilation was carried out because of persistent neurologic symptoms.

Overall, however, aggregate data from other reports indicate that the incidence of subsequent stroke or transient ischemic attack in medically treated patients is 0% to 4%[31,132,170,178] Operative mortality for patients treated with graduated intraluminal dilation has been zero or not reported, but operative and perioperative morbidity has ranged from 3% to 6%.[106,170] In two studies with long-term follow-up after surgery, there was a 5% to 8% incidence of stroke when perioperative morbidity was included.[29,36,170]

Because of the low incidence of stroke, transient ischemic attack, or other serious outcome in untreated or medically managed patients, a conservative approach to treatment has been recommended, and seems warranted, based on available information.[154] Prior to therapy, all patients with neurologic symptoms should be carefully evaluated for etiologies other than FMD. Patients with associated atherosclerosis should receive appropriate medical or surgical management as indicated for that disorder. Patients with no neurologic symptoms, a cervical bruit alone, or nonlocalizing neurologic abnormalities should receive antiplatelet therapy only. Most patients with stroke or transient ischemic attack attributed to FMD also should receive antiplatelet therapy, which carries less risk than surgery. Patients with focal ischemic symptoms and a high-grade hemodynamically significant stenosis or recurrent symptoms while medically treated may require surgery. Surgical treatment has also been recommended for patients with proximal septal lesions because of the possibly increased risk of thromboembolism.[118]

Management of dissecting aneurysms is difficult because both spontaneous aneurysm resolution and recurrent ischemic symptoms have occurred in untreated patients. An initial trial of antiplatelet therapy or anticoagulation followed by surgery if symptoms continue has been recommended.

Finally, all patients with cephalic FMD should have complete cerebral angiography to identify all FMD lesions and associated intracranial aneurysms. Antiplatelet therapy or anticoagulation should be avoided in patients with aneurysms until appropriate management is completed. All patients should also have long-term blood pressure monitoring and angiographic investigation for renal artery FMD if hypertension occurs.[83,185]

References

1. Abdul-Rahman AM, Abu-Salih Brun A et al: Fibromuscular dysplasia of the cervicocephalic arteries. Surg Neurol 9:217, 1978
2. Alvarez-Amandi MR, Berciano-Blanco JA, Combarros-Pascual O et al: Fibromuscular dysplasia of the cervicocephalic arteries: report of two cases and review of the literature. Med Clin (Barc) 74:98, 1980
3. Andersen CA, Collins GJ, Rich NM et al: Internal carotid artery occlusions associated with fibromuscular dysplasia. Vasc Surg 13:349, 1979
4. Andersen CA, Collins GJ, Rich NM et al: Spontaneous dissection of the internal carotid artery associated with fibromuscular dysplasia. Am Surg 46:263, 1980
5. Andersen PE: Fibromuscular hyperplasia of the carotid arteries. Acta Radiol 10:90, 1970
6. Andersen PE: Fibromuscular hyperplasia in children. Acta Radiol 10:203, 1970
7. Angelini C, Brunoro N, Gallucci V: Report of two patients with fibromuscular dysplasia of the internal carotid artery. Riv Patol Nerv Ment 101:139, 1981
8. Antunes ACM, Borges ACG, DaCosta JC et al: Dysplasia fibromuscular de vasos cerebrais. Arq Neuropsiquiatr 32:118, 1974
9. Appleberg M: Graduated internal dilatation in the treatment of fibromuscular dysplasia of the internal carotid artery. S Afr Med J 51:244, 1977
10. Arnott G, Clarisse J, Houcke M et al: Dysplasia fibro-

musculaire d'artéres cervicales et encéphaliques (a'propos d'un cas d'hémorragie cérébroméningée par rupture d'anévrysme intra-carnien dysplasique). Lille Med 21: 308, 1976

11. Ashleigh RJ, Weller JM, Leggate JR: Fibromuscular hyperplasia of the internal carotid artery—further cause of the "moyamoya" collateral circulation. Br J Neurosurg 6:269, 1992.

12. Aurell M: Fibromuscular dysplasia of the renal arteries. Br Med J 1:1180, 1979

13. Balaji MR, DeWeese JA: Fibromuscular dysplasia of the internal carotid artery. Arch Surg 115:984, 1980

14. Barbizet J, Debrun G, Brunet P et al: Hyperplasie fibromusculaire de la carotide interne. Ann Med Interne (Paris) 122:537, 1971

15. Belan A, Vesela M, Vanek I et al: Percutaneous transluminal angioplasty of fibromuscular dysplasia of the internal carotid artery. Cardiovasc Intervent Radiol 5:79, 1982

16. Bergan JJ, MacDonald JR: Recognition of cerebrovascular fibromuscular hyperplasia. Arch Surg 98:332, 1969

17. Bergentz SE, Ericsson BF, Olivecrona H: Bilateral fibromuscular hyperplasia in the internal carotid arteries with aneurysm formation. Acta Chir Scand 142:501, 1976

18. Boespflug OJ: Ultrasonography of supraaortic trunks. Neuroradiology 27:544, 1985

19. Bonduelle M, Ruscalleda J, Zalzal P: Dysplasie fibromusculaire avec fistule arterioveineuse de l'artére vertébrale extracranienne. Rev Neurol (Paris) 128:204, 1973

20. Boudin G, Guillard A, Romion A: Dysplasies fibromusculaires des artéres carotides et vertébrales. Ann Med Interne 125:863, 1974

21. Bradac GB, Haymat F: Considerations concerning a case of fibromuscular hyperplasia of the carotid arteries. Neuroradiology 1:217, 1970

22. Bragin MA, Cherkasov AP: On the morphogenesis of fibrous-muscular dysplasia of renal arteries (an ultrastructural study). Arkh Patol 41:46, 1979

23. Brown OL, Arnitage JL: Spontaneous dissecting aneurysms of the cervical internal carotid artery. Am J Radiol 118:648, 1973

24. Caes F, Van der Niepen P, Cham B: Fibromuscular dysplasia of the internal carotid artery. Acta Chirurg Belg 86:153, 1986

25. Chambers JL, Neale ML, Appleberg M: Fibromuscular hyperplasia in an aberrant subclavian artery and neurogenic thoracic outlet syndrome: an unusual combination. J of Vasc Surg 20:834, 1994

26. Chiras J, Bories J, Barth MO, Aymard A, Poirier B: Cerebral angiography in ischemic strokes. Neuroradiol 27: 521, 1985

27. Cina C, Williamson C, Ameli FM: Fibromuscular dysplasia of the posterior auricular artery: an unusual aneurysmal lesion. J Cardiovasc Surg (Torino) 29:56, 1989

28. Claiborne TS: Fibromuscular hyperplasia: report of a case with involvement of multiple arteries. Am J Med 49:103, 1970

29. Collins GJ, Rich NM, Clagett GP et al: Fibromuscular dysplasia of the internal carotid arteries: clinical experience and follow-up. Ann Surg 194:89, 1981

30. Connett MC, Lansche JM: Fibromuscular hyperplasia

of the internal carotid artery: report of a case. Ann Surg 162:59, 1965

31. Corrin LS, Sandok BA, Houser OW: Cerebral ischemic events in patients with carotid artery fibromuscular dysplasia. Arch Neurol 38:616, 1981

32. Dufour JJ, Layigne F, Plante R: Pulsatile tinnitus and fibromuscular dysplasia of the internal carotid. J Otolaryngol 14:293, 1985

33. Duncan CE, Buck K, Lynch A: The effect of pressure and stretching on the passage of labeled albumin into canine aortic wall. J Atheroscler Res 5:69, 1965

34. Edell SL, Huang P: Sonographic demonstration of fibromuscular hyperplasia of the cervical internal carotid artery. Stroke 12:518, 1981

35. Effeney DJ, Ehrenfeld WK, Stoney RJ et al: Fibromuscular dysplasia of the internal carotid artery. World J Surg 3:179, 1979

36. Effeney DJ, Ehrenfeld WK, Stoney RJ et al: Why operate on carotid fibromuscular dysplasia? Arch Surg 115: 1261, 1980

37. Ehrenfeld WK, Stoney RJ, Wylie EJ: Fibromuscular hyperplasia of the internal carotid artery. Arch Surg 95: 284, 1967

38. Ehrenfeld WK, Wylie EJ: Fibromuscular dysplasia of the internal carotid artery: surgical management. Arch Surg 109:676, 1974

39. Ehrenfeld WK, Wylie EJ: Spontaneous dissection of the internal carotid artery. Arch Surg 111:1294, 1976

40. Ekelund L, Gerlock J, Molin J et al: Roentgenologic appearance of fibromuscular dysplasia. Acta Radiol 19: 433, 1978

41. Elias WS: Intracranial fibromuscular hyperplasia. JAMA 218:254, 1971

42. Emparanza JI, Aldamiz-Echevarria L, Perez-Yarza E: Ischemic stroke due to fibromuscular dysplasia. Neuropediatrics 20:181, 1989

43. Ennis JT, Bateson EM: Fibromuscular dysplasia of the internal carotid arteries: a report of three cases. Br J Radiol 43:452, 1970

44. Fievez M: Relations ergotisme—hyperplasie fibromusculaire. Nouv Presse Med 4:1753, 1975

45. Fievez M, Koerperich G, Dulieu J: Arterial fibromuscular dysplasia and ergotism. Ann Anat Pathol 20:357, 1975

46. Fiore DL, Pardatscher K, Fiore D et al: Persistant dorsal ophthalmic artery: report of a case with associated fibromuscular hyperplasia of the extracranial internal carotid artery and multiple cerebral aneurysms. Neurochirurgia (Stuttg) 24:106, 1981

47. Fisher CM, Ojemann RG, Roberson GH: Spontaneous dissection of cervico-cerebral arteries. Can J Neurol Sci 5:9, 1978

48. Fitzer PM, Rinaldi I: Abnormal radionuclide angiogram in proven intracranial fibromuscular dysplasia: case report. J Nucl Med 17:190, 1975

49. Frens DB, Petajan JH, Anderson R et al: Fibromuscular dysplasia of the posterior cerebral artery: report of a case and review of the literature. Stroke 5:161, 1974

50. Galligioni F, Iraci G, Marin G: Fibromuscular hyperplasia of the extracranial internal carotid artery. J Neurosurg 34:647, 1971

51. Garcia-Merino JA, Gutierrez JA, Lopez-Lozano JJ et al:

Double lumen dissecting aneurysm of the internal carotid artery in fibromuscular dysplasia: case report. Stroke 14:815, 1983

52. Garrido E, Montoya J: Transluminal dilatation of internal carotid artery in fibromuscular dysplasia: a preliminary report. Surg Neurol 16:469, 1981

53. Gee W, Burton R, Stoney RJ: Atypical fibromuscular hyperplasia involving the internal carotid artery. Ann Surg 7:136, 1974

54. George B, Zerah M, Mourier KL et al: Ruptured intracranial aneurysms: the influence of sex and fibromuscular dysplasia upon prognosis. Acta Neurochir (Wien) 97:20, 1989

55. Geraud J, Manelfe C, Caussanel JP et al: Fistule arterioveineuse spontaneé del artére-vertébrale: role eventuel de la dysplasie fibromusculaire dans sa pathogeneie. Rev Neurol (Paris) 128:206, 1973

56. Gibbons RB, Ashton AL: Buerger's disease and multicentric fibromuscular hyperplasia mimicking Takayasu's arteritis. Arthritis Rheum 23:1067, 1980

57. Gladstein K, Rushton AR, Kidd KK: Penetrance estimates and recurrence risks for fibromuscular dysplasia. Clin Genet 17:115, 1980

58. Golosovskaia MA, Spiridonov AA, Cherkasov AP: Fibromuscular dysplasia of the renal arteries. Arkh Patol 39:19, 1977

59. Green PM, Letellier MA: Fibromuscular dysplasia of the infratentorial circulation: discussion of two cases and treatment. Wis Med J 77:99, 1978

60. Grollman JH, Lecky JW, Rosch J: Miscellaneous diseases of arteries, or all arterial lesions aren't fatty. Semin Roentgenol 5:306, 1970

61. Grotta JC, Ward RE, Flynn TC et al: Spontaneous internal carotid artery dissection associated with fibromuscular dysplasia. J Cardiovasc Surg (Torino) 23:512, 1982

62. Halpern HH, Sanford HS, Viamonte M: Renal artery abnormalities in three hypertensive sisters. JAMA 194:124, 1965

63. Handa J, Kamijyo Y, Handa H: Intracranial aneurysm associated with fibromuscular hyperplasia of renal and internal carotid arteries. Br J Radiol 43:483, 1970

64. Hansen J, Holter C, Thorberg JV: Hypertension in two sisters caused by so-called fibromuscular hyperplasia of the renal arteries. Acta Med Scand 178:461, 1965

65. Harrison EG, Hunt JC, Bernatz PE: Morphology of fibromuscular dysplasia of the renal artery in renovascular hypertension. Am J Med 43:97, 1967

66. Harrison EG, McCormack LJ: Pathologic classification of renal arterial disease in renovascular hypertension. Mayo Clin Proc 46:161, 1971

67. Harrington OB, Crosby VG, Nicholas L: Fibromuscular hypertension of the internal carotid artery. Ann Thorac Surg 9:516, 1970

68. Hart RG, Easton JD: Dissections. Stroke 16:925, 1985

69. Hartman JD, Young I, Bank A et al: Fibromuscular hyperplasia of internal carotid arteries. Arch Neurol 25:295, 1971

70. Hasso AN, Bird CR, Zinke DE et al: Fibromuscular hyperplasia of the internal carotid artery: Percutaneous transluminal angioplasty. Am J Neuroradiol 2:175, 1981

71. Hata J, Hosoda Y: Perimedial fibroplasia of the renal artery: a light and electron microscopic study. Arch Pathol Lab Med 103:220, 1979

72. Havelius U, Hindfelt B, Brismar J et al: Carotid fibromuscular dysplasia and paresis of lower cranial nerves (Collect-Sicard syndrome): case report. J Neurosurg 56:850, 1982

73. Heffelfinger MJ, Holley KE, Harrison EG et al: Arterial fibromuscular dysplasia studied at autopsy. Am J Clin Pathol 54:274, 1970

74. Herpels V, Van de Voorde W, Wilms G, et al: Recurrent aneurysms of the upper arteries of the lower limb: an atypical manifestation of fibromuscular dysplasia—a case report. Angiology 38:411, 1987

75. Hieshima GB, Cahan LD, Mehringer CM et al: Spontaneous arteriovenous fistulae of cerebral vessels in association with fibromuscular dysplasia. Neurosurgery 18:454, 1986

76. Hill LD, Antonius JI: Arterial dysplasia: an important surgical lesion. Arch Surg 90:585, 1965

77. Hirsch CS, Roessman U: Arterial dysplasia with ruptured basilar artery aneurysm: report of a case. Hum Pathol 6:749, 1975

78. Hooshmand H, Boykin ME, Vines FS et al: Fibromuscular dysplasia of the extracranial internal carotid arteries associated with an ulcerative plaque. Stroke 3:67, 1972

79. Houser OW, Baker HL Jr: Fibromuscular dysplasia and other uncommon disease of the cervical carotid artery: angiographic aspects. AJR Am J Roentgenol 104:201, 1968

80. Houser OW, Baker HL, Jr, Sandok BA et al: Fibromuscular dysplasia of the cephalic arterial system. p. 366. In Vinken PJ, Bruyn GW (eds): Handbook of Clinical Neurology. Vol. 11. North-Holland Publishing, Amsterdam, 1972

81. Huber P, Fuchs WA: Gibt es eine fibromuskuläre hyperplasie zerebraler arterien? Fortschr Rontgenstr 107:119, 1967

82. Hugenholtz H, Pokrupa R Montpetit VJA et al: Spontaneous dissecting aneurysm of the extracranial vertebral artery. Neurosurgery 10:96, 1982

83. Hunt JC, Harrison EG, Kincaid OW et al: Idiopathic fibrous and fibromuscular stenoses of the renal arteries associated with hypertension. Mayo Clin Proc 37:181, 1962

84. Iosue A, Kier EL, Ostrow D: Fibromuscular dysplasia involving the intracranial vessels. J Neurosurg 37:749, 1972

85. Irey NS, Manion WC, Taylor HB: Vascular lesions in women taking contraceptives. Arch Pathol 89:1, 1970

86. Jabbari M, Cherry R, Lough JO, et al: Gastric antral vascular ectasia: the watermelon stomach. Gastroenterology 87:1165, 1984

87. Julian LM: The occurrence of fibromuscular dysplasia in the arteries of domestic turkeys. Am J Pathol 101:415, 1980

88. Kalyan-Raman UP, Elwood PW: Fibromuscular dysplasia of intracranial arteries causing multiple intracranial aneurysms. Hum Pathol 11:481, 1980

89. Kalyan-Raman UP, Kowalski RV, Lee RH et al: Dissecting aneurysm of superior cerebellar artery: its associ-

ation with fibromuscular dysplasia. Arch Neurol 40:120, 1983

90. Kaufman HH: Fibromuscular hyperplasia of the carotid artery in a case associated with an arteriovenous malformation. Arch Neurol 22:299, 1970

91. Kaufman HH, Lind TA, Mullan S: Spontaneous carotid-cavernous fistula with fibromuscular dysplasia. Acta Neurochir (Wien) 40:123, 1978

92. Kelly TF, Morris GC, Jr: Arterial fibromuscular disease: observations on pathogenesis and surgical management. Am J Surg 143:232, 1982

93. Kincaid OW, Davis GD: Renal arteriography in hypertension. Mayo Clin Proc 36:689, 1961

94. Kincaid OW, Davis GD, Hallermann FJ et al: Fibromuscular dysplasia of the renal arteries: arteriographic features, classification, and observations on natural history of the disease. Am J Roentgenol 104:271, 1968

95. Kishore PRS, Lin JP, Kricheff II: Fibromuscular hyperplasia and stationary waves of the internal carotid artery. Acta Radiol 11:619, 1971

96. Kliewer MA, Carroll BA: Ultrasound case of the day: internal carotid artery web (atypical fibromuscular dysplasia). Radiographics 11:504, 1991

97. Kramer W: Hyperplasie fibromusculaire et anévrisme extracranien de la carotide interne avec syndrome parapharyngien typique. Rev Neurol (Paris) 120:239, 1969

98. Lamis PA, Carson WP, Wilson JP et al: Recognition and treatment of fibromuscular hyperplasia of the internal carotid artery. Surgery 69:498, 1971

99. Lane RJ, Weisman RA, Savino PJ et al: Aneurysm of the internal carotid artery at the base of the skull: an unusual cause of cranial neuropathies. Otolaryngol Head Neck Surg 88:230, 1980

100. Leadbetter WF, Burkland CE: Hypertension in unilateral renal disease. J Urol 39:611, 1938

101. Lemahieu SF, Marchau MM: Intracranial fibromuscular dysplasia and stroke in children. Neuroradiology 18:99, 1979

102. Letsch R, Kantartzis M, Sommer T et al: Arterial fibromuscular dysplasia: report of a case with involvement of the aorta and review of the literature. Thorac Cardiovasc Surg 28:206, 1980

103. Leung DYM, Glagov S, Mathews MB: Cyclic stretching stimulates synthesis of matrix components by arterial smooth muscle cells in vitro. Science 191:475, 1976

104. Levin SM, Sondheimer F: Surgical technique in fibromuscular disease of the carotid arteries. Angiology 22:463, 1971

105. Llorens-Terol J, Sole-Llenas J, Lura A: Stroke due to fibromuscular hyperplasia of the internal carotid artery. Acta Paediatr 72:299, 1983

106. Luscher TF, Stanson AW, Hauser OW et al: Arterial fibromuscular dysplasia. Mayo Clin Proc 62:931, 1987

107. Maiuri F, Gallicchio B, Gangemi M: Fibromuscular dysplasia of the carotid arteries. Clin Neurol Neurosurg 90:57, 1988

108. Major P, Genest J, Cartier P et al: Hereditary fibromuscular dysplasia with renovascular hypertension. Ann Intern Med 86:583, 1977

109. Manelfe C, Clairesse J, Fredy D: Dysplasies fibromuscu-laires des arteres cervicocephalique. J Neuroradiol 1:149, 1974

110. Manns RA, Nanda KK, Mackie G: Fibromuscular dysplasia of the cephalic and renal arteries. Clin Radiol 38:427, 1987

111. Mas JL, Bousser MG, Hasboun D et al: Extracranial vertebral artery dissections: a review of 13 cases. Stroke 18:1037, 1987

112. McCormack LJ, Hazard JB, Poutasse EF: Obstructive lesions of the renal artery associated with remediable hypertension. Am J Pathol 34:582, 1958

113. Meaney TF, Dustan HP, McCormack LJ: Natural history of renal arterial disease. Radiology 91:881, 1968

114. Mettinger KL: Fibromuscular dysplasia and the brain: current concepts of the disease. Stroke 13:53, 1982

115. Mettinger KL, Erickson K: Fibromuscular dysplasia and the brain: observations on angiographic, clinical, and genetic characteristic. Stroke 13:46, 1982

116. Momose KJ, New PFJ: Non-atheromatous stenosis and occlusion of the internal carotid artery and its main branches. AJR 118:550, 1973

117. Monfort JC, Degos JO, Eizenbaum JF et al: Dissecting aneurysm of the carotid artery in a patient with angiographic evidence of fibromuscular dysplasia. Ann Med Interne 132:333, 1981

118. Morgenlander JC, Goldstein LB: Recurrent transient ischemic attacks and stroke in association with an internal carotid artery web. Stroke 22:94, 1991

119. Morimoto S, Kuroda M, Uchida K et al: Occurrence of renovascular hypertension in two sisters. Nephron 17:314, 1976

120. Morris GC, Lechter A, Debakey ME: Surgical treatment of fibromuscular disease of the carotid arteries. Arch Surg 96:636, 1968

121. Nakata Y: An experimental study on the vascular lesions caused by obstruction of the vasa vasorum. Jpn Circ J 31:275, 1967

122. Nunn DB: Fibromuscular hyperplasia of the internal carotid artery. Am Surg 40:309, 1974

123. Nguyen Bui L, Brant-Zawadzki M, Verghese P, Gillan G: Magnetic resonance angiography of cervicocranial dissection. Stroke 24:126, 1993

124. Osborne AG, Anderson RE: Angiographic spectrum of cervical and intracranial fibromuscular dysplasia. Stroke 8:617, 1977

125. Ouchi Y, Tagawa H, Yamakado M et al: Clinical significance of cerebral aneurysm in renovascular hypertension due to fibromuscular dysplasia: two cases in siblings. Angiology 40:581, 1989

126. Overgaard J, Laursen B, Ingstrup HM: Oligophrenia in a case of late onset in cerebral fibromuscular hyperplasia. Dan Med Bull 17:19, 1970

127. Palubinskas AJ, Perloff P, Newton TH: Fibromuscular hyperplasia: an arterial dysplasia of increasing clinical importance. AJR 98:907, 1966

128. Palubinskas AJ, Newton TH: Fibromuscular hyperplasia of the internal carotid arteries: Radiol Clin Biol 34:365, 1965

129. Palubinskas AJ, Ripley HR: Fibromuscular hyperplasia in extra-renal arteries. Radiology 82:451, 1964

130. Palubinskas AJ, Wylie EJ: Roentgen diagnosis of fibro-

muscular hyperplasia of the renal arteries. Radiology 76: 634, 1961

131. Pappada G, Panzarasa G, Sani R: Intracranial fibromuscular dysplasia: report of two cases and review of the literature. J Neurosurg Sci 31:13, 1987

132. Patman RD, Thompson JE, Talkington CM: Natural history of fibromuscular dysplasia of the carotid artery. Stroke 11:135, 1980

133. Paule WJ, Zemplenyi TK, Rounds DE et al: Light and electronmicroscopic characteristics of arterial smooth muscle cell cultures subjected to hypoxia or carbon monoxide. Atherosclerosis 25:111, 1976

134. Paulson GW: Fibromuscular dysplasia antiovulent drugs and ergot preparations (letter). Stroke 9:172, 1978

135. Paulson GW, Boesel CP, Evans WE: Fibromuscular dysplasia. Arch Neurol 35:287, 1978

136. Perez-Hiqueras A, Alvarez-Ruiz F, Martinez-Bermejo A et al: Cerebeller infarction from fibromuscular dysplasia and dissecting aneurysm of the vertebral artery: report of a child. Stroke 19:521, 1988

137. Perry DO: Fibromuscular disease of the carotid artery. Surg Gynecol Obstet 134:57, 1972

138. Pilz P, Hartjes HJ: Fibromuscular dysplasia and multiple dissecting aneurysms of intracranial arteries: a further cause of moyamoya syndrome. Stroke 7:393, 1976

139. Polin SG: Carotid artery fibromuscular hyperplasia: three cases and review of the literature. Am Surg 35: 501, 1969

140. Pollock M, Jackson BM: Fibromuscular dysplasia of the carotid arteries. Neurology (NY) 21:1226, 1971

141. Probst C: Fibromuscular hyperplasia of cerebral arteries in childhood. Monatsschr Kinderheilkd 119:604, 1971

142. Rainer WG, Cramer GG, Newby JP et al: Fibromuscular hyperplasia of the carotid artery causing positional cerebral ischemia. Ann Surg 167:444, 1968

143. Rebello M, Quintana F, Combarros O et al: Giant aneurysm of the intracavernous carotid artery and bilateral carotid fibromuscular dysplasia (letter). J Neurol Neurosurg Psychiatry, 46:284, 1983

144. Reddy SVR, Karnes WE, Earnest F et al: Spontaneous extracranial vertebral arteriovenous fistula with fibromuscular dysplasia. J Neurosurg 54:399, 1981

145. Rinaldi I, Harris WO, Kopp JE et al: Intracranial fibromuscular dysplasia: report of two cases, one with autopsy verification. Stroke 7:511, 1976

146. Ringel SP, Harrison SH, Norenberg MD et al: Fibromuscular dysplasia: multiple "spontaneous" dissecting aneurysms of the major cervical arteries. Ann Neurol 1: 301, 1977

147. Rosenberger A, Alder O, Lichtig H: Angiographic appearance of the renal vein in a case of fibromuscular dysplasia of the artery. Radiology 118:579, 1976

148. Ross R, Klebanoff SJ: Fine structural changes in uterine smooth muscle and fibroblasts in response to estrogen. J Cell Biol 32:155, 1967

149. Ross R, Klebanoff SJ: The smooth muscle cell. I. In vivo synthesis of connective tissue proteins. J Cell Biol 50: 159, 1971

150. Rothfield NJH: Experimental fibromuscular arterial dysplasia. Radiology 93:1291, 1969

151. Rushton AR: The genetics of fibromuscular arterial dysplasia. Arch Intern Med 140:233, 1980

152. Russo LS Jr: Fibromuscular hyperplasia of the extracranial arteries: report of a case associated with intracranial aneurysm and skeletal deformities and a brief review of the literature. Mt. Sinai J Med (NY) 40:60, 1973

153. Sanchez-Torres G, Contreras R: Fibromuscular dysplasia: a genetic entity related to Ehlers-Danlos syndrome. Arch Inst Cardiol Mex 44:571, 1974

154. Sandok BA: Fibromuscular dysplasia of the internal carotid artery. p. 17. In Barnett HJM (ed): Neurology Clinics. Vol. 1. WB Saunders, Philadelphia, 1983

155. Sandok BA, Houser OW, Baker HL Jr et al: Fibromuscular dysplasia: Neurologic disorders associated with disease involving the great vessels in the neck. Arch Neurol 24:462, 1969

156. Sato S, Hata J: Fibromuscular dysplasia: its occurrence with a dissecting aneurysm of the internal carotid artery. Arch Pathol Lab Med 106:332, 1982

157. Saygi S, Bolay H, Tekkok IH et al: Fibromuscular dysplasia of the basilar artery: a case with brainstem stroke. Angiology 41:658, 1990

158. Schlagenhauff RE, Khatri A: Fibromuscular dysplasia of internal carotid arteries with Doppler ultrasonic studies. NY State J Med 83:234, 1983

159. Shields WD, Ziter FA, Osborn AG et al: Fibromuscular dysplasia as a cause of stroke in infancy and childhood. Pediatrics 59:899, 1977

160. Slagsvold JE, Bergsholm P, Larsen JL: Fibromuscular dysplasia of intracranial arteries in a patient with multiple enchondromas (Ollier disease). Neurology (NY) 27: 1168, 1977

161. Smith LL, Smith DC, Killen JD et al: Operative balloon angioplasty in the treatment of internal carotid artery fibromuscular dysplasia. J Vasc Surg 6:482, 1987

162. So EL, Toole JF, Dalal P et al: Cephalic fibromuscular dysplasia in 32 patients. Arch Neurol 38:619, 1981

163. So EL, Toole JF, Moody DM et al: Cerebral embolism from fibromuscular dysplasia of the common carotid artery. Ann Neurol 6:75, 1979

164. Sottiurai V, Fry WJ, Stanley JC: Ultrastructural characteristics of experimental arterial medical fibroplasia induced by vasa vasorum occlusion. J Surg Res 24:169, 1978

165. Sottiurai VS, Fry WJ, Stanley JC: Ultrastructure of medial smooth muscle and myofibroblasts in human arterial dysplasia. Arch Surg 113:1280, 1978

166. Stanley JC, Fry WJ, Seeger JF et al: Extracranial internal carotid and vertebral artery fibrodysplasia. Arch Surg 109:215, 1974

167. Stanley JC, Gewertz BL, Bove EL et al: Arterial fibrodysplasia: histopathologic character and current etiologic concepts. Arch Surg 110:561, 1975

168. Starr DS, Lawrie GM, Morris GC, Jr: Fibromuscular dysplasia of carotid arteries: long-term results of graduated internal dilation. Stroke 12:196, 1981

169. Stewart DR, Price RA, Nebesar R et al: Progressive peripheral fibromuscular hyperplasia in an infant: a possible manifestation of the rubella syndrome. Surgery 73: 374, 1973

170. Stewart MT, Moritz MW, Smith RB et al: The natural

history of carotid fibromuscular dysplasia. J Vasc Surg 3:305, 1986

171. Strian F, Backmund H: Fibromusculäre Dysplasie der Carotiden: neurologische and atiologische Aspekte. Nervenarzt, 43:557, 1972

172. Sukoff MH, Dorsey TJ, Johnson DA et al: Intimal fibroplasia of the internal carotid arteries. Stroke 2:483, 1971

173. Swedberg SH, Brown BG, Sigley R, et al: Intimal fibromuscular hyperplasia at the venous anastomosis of PTFE grafts in hemodialysis patients: clinical, immunocytochemical, light and electron microscopic assessment. Circulation 80:1726, 1989

174. Thevenet A, Latil JL, Albat B. Fibromuscular disease of the external iliac artery. Ann Vasc Surg 6:19, 1992

175. Tomasello F, Cioff FA, Albanese V: Fibromuscular dysplasia of the basilar artery. Neurochirurgie 19:29, 1976

176. Upson J, Raza ST: Fibromuscular dysplasia of internal carotid arteries: graduated internal dilatation by arterial Fogarty catheter. NY State J Med 76:972, 1976

177. Vies JS, Hendriks JJ, Lodder J et al: Multiple vertebrobasilar infarctions from fibromuscular dysplasia related dissecting aneurysm of the vertebral artery in a child. Neuropediatrics 21:104, 1990

178. Wells RP, Smith RR: Fibromuscular dysplasia of the internal carotid artery: a long term follow-up. Neurosurgery 10:39, 1982

179. Welsh P, Pradier R, Repetto R: Fibromuscular dysplasia of the distal cervical internal carotid artery. J Cardiovasc Surg (Torino) 22:321, 1981

180. Wesen CA, Elliot BM: Fibromuscular dysplasia of the carotid arteries. Am J Surg 151:448, 1986

181. Wing RJ, Waugh RC, Harris JP: Treatment of fibromuscular hyperplasia of the external iliac artery by percutaneous transluminal angioplasty. Australas Radiol 37:223, 1993

182. Wirth FP, Miller WA, Russell AP: Atypical fibromuscular hyperplasia: report of two cases. J Neurosurg 54:685, 1981

183. Wylie EG, Binkley FM, Palubinskas AJ: Extrarenal fibromuscular hyperplasia. Am J Surg 112:149, 1966

184. Wylie EJ, Perloff D, Wellington JS: Fibromuscular hyperplasia of the renal arteries. Ann Surg 156:592, 1962

185. Wylie EJ, Wellington JS: Hypertension caused by fibromuscular hyperplasia of the renal arteries. Am J Surg 100:183, 1960

186. Yamamoto I, Kageyama N, Usui K et al: Fibromuscular dysplasia of the internal carotid artery: unusual angiographic changes with progression of clinical symptoms. Acta Neurochir 50:293, 1979

187. Young PH, Smith KR, Crafts DC et al: Traumatic occlusion in fibromuscular dysplasia of the carotid artery. Surg Neurol 16:432, 1981

188. Zeumer H, Hauke R, Kotlarek F: Fibromuscular dysplasia of the internal carotid and intracerebral arteries. Dtsch Med Wochenschr 100:132, 1975

189. Zimmerman R, Leeds NE, Naidich TP: Carotid-cavernous fistula associated with intracranial fibromuscular dysplasia. Radiology 122:725, 1977

CHAPTER 33

Migraine and Stroke

K. M. A. WELCH

T. K. TATEMICHI (deceased)

J. P. MOHR

Migraine is an episodic headache that is unilateral or bilateral in location, pulsating in quality, moderate to severe in intensity, and exacerbated by physical activity. Associated symptoms include nausea or vomiting, photophobia, and phonophobia. In the United States, migraine occurs in 18% of females and 6% of males.[1] The prevalence of migraine with aura (which includes hemiplegic migraine) is lower, around 4%.[158] Various forms of migraine are recognized, generally classified according to the transient, though sometimes persistent, neurologic deficits that may precede, accompany, or outlast the headache phase. The most accepted current classification was put forward in 1988 by the International Headache Society (IHS) (Table 33.1).

A number of these clinical syndromes may mimic conventional cerebrovascular syndromes, and a number may induce stroke or are associated with an increased stroke risk. These include migraine with aura of different types, retinal or ocular migraine, ophthalmoplegic migraine, familial hemiplegic migraine, and basilar artery migraine.[142,181,182] Each may be transient, prolonged, or persistent.[65] When the deficit of a migraine attack remains, *migraine-induced stroke* is suspected, which should prompt attempts to exclude other causes. The clinical features that often mimic stroke are described below.

Clinical Features

The most prevalent migraine syndromes include typical headache without aura of neurologic deficit (previously termed *common migraine*; IHS classification 1.1), and headache associated with aura of neurologic deficit (previously termed *classic migraine*; IHS classification 1.20).[92] Visual disturbances account for well over half the transient neurologic manifestations. Most frequently, these consist of positive phenomena such as stars, spark photopsia, complex geometric patterns, and fortification spectra. These positive phenomena may leave in their wake negative phenomena such as scotoma or hemianopia. The symptoms are characteristically slow in onset and slow in progression, although occasionally the onset is more abrupt and may be confused with amaurosis fugax. Visual symptoms sometimes progress to visual distortion or misperception, such as micropsia or dysmetropsia. The patterns of symptoms indicate the spread of neurologic dysfunction from the occipital cortex into the contiguous regions of the temporal or parietal lobes. It is critical in making the differential diagnosis from stroke to establish that the neurologic deficit crosses arterial territories. The second most common symptoms are somatosensory and characteristically hand and lower face (cheio-oral) in distribution. Less frequently, the symptoms include aphasia, hemiparesis, or clumsiness of one limb. Mostly, a slow, marchlike progression is characteristic.

Epidemiology

A review of mostly uncontrolled hospital-based studies conducted before 1989 of patients under 50 years of age with a diagnosis of stroke showed that between 1% to 17% were attributed to migraine; in two-thirds of these the diagnosis was made in 1% to 8% of patients and 11% to 17% in one-third.[4] Our own compilation of studies revealed a prevalence of 4% attributed to migraine in 448 total stroke cases, 31% of which had an unknown cause (Table 33.2). In general, stroke was more common in patients with migraine with aura[14,165] and in patients with posterior cerebral artery strokes.[20] In a controlled study, no differences in stroke risk factors were found in migraine sufferers compared with controls without stroke, although those with migraine were more likely to have recurrent stroke, which suggests that migraine may be an independent stroke risk factor (see below).[165] In support, another controlled study of migraine with aura reported that 91% of patients who had stroke during an attack had no arterial lesions, as opposed to 9% of migraine with aura patients who suffered stroke remote from a migraine attack and 18% of patients with stroke without a migraine

Table 33.1 Classification of Migraine Subtypes

IHS Terminology[a] (Previously Used Terms)	Main Features
Migraine without aura (common migraine)	Headache without focal neurologic symptoms
Migraine with aura	Headache with attacks of neurologic symptoms localizable to cerebral cortex or brain stem, developing gradually over 5–20 minutes and lasting <1 hour
Migraine with typical aura (ophthalmic, hemiparesthetic, hemiparetic, hemiplegic, or aphasic migraine, migraine accompaignée)	Aura consisting of homonymous visual disturbances, hemisensory symptoms, hemiparesis or dysphasia, or combinations thereof
Migraine with prolonged aura (complicated migraine, hemiplegic migraine)	Aura symptoms lasting >1 hour and ±7 days with normal brain imaging
Familial hemiplegic migraine[102]	At least one first-degree relative has identical attacks
Basilar migraine (basilar artery migraine, Bickerstaff's migraine, syncopal migraine)	Aura symptoms originate from brain stem or both occipital lobes
Migraine aura without headache (migraine equivalents, acephalalgic migraine)	Aura unaccompanied by headache; when the onset is after 40 years, distinction from transient ischemic attacks may be difficult
Migraine with acute-onset aura	Aura developing fully in <5 minutes
Ophthalmoplegic migraine	Repeated attacks of headache associated with paresis of one or more ocular cranial nerves
Retinal migraine	Repeated attacks of monocular scotomata or blindness lasting <1 hour with headache
Childhood periodic syndromes that may be precursors to or associated with migraine	Poorly defined disorders of childhood, including benign paroxysmal vertigo and alternating hemiplegia
Complications of migraine Status migrainosus	Headache lasting >72 hours with or without treatment and headache-free interval <4 hours
Migrainous infarction (complicated migraine)	Aura symptoms not fully reversible lasting 7 days, and/or associated infarct on brain imaging

[a] From the Headache Classification Committee of the International Headache Society[92]

Table 33.2 Frequency of Cerebral Infarction in Young Adults Associated with Migraine and Occurring During the Course of Migraine

Author (Ref.)	Total Cases	Age Range	History of Migraine N (%)	Stroke During Migraine Attack N (%)
Hindfelt & Nilsson, 1977	64	16–40	7 (11)	4 (6)
Grindal et al., 1978	58	15–40	0 (0)	0 (0)
Snyder & Ramirez-Lassepas, 1980	61	16–49	(2)	NS
Marshall, 1982	114	10–49	0 (0)	0 (0)
Hart & Miller, 1983	100	<40	5 (5)	NS
Hillbom & Kaste, 1983	100	15–55	24 (24)	9 (9)
Spaccavento & Solomon, 1984[171a]	15	20–40	4 (27)	3 (20)
Milton-Jones & Warlow, 1985	75	±45	10 (13)	9 (12)
Adams et al., 1986	144	15–45	20 (14)	4 (3)
Bogousslavsky & Regli, 1987[14]	41	16–29	6 (15)	6 (15)
Alvarez et al., 1989[4]	386	<50	19 (5)	19 (5)
Gautier et al., 1989	112	9–45	16 (14)	NS
Sacquena et al., 1989	61	±40	6 (10)	6 (10)
Bevan et al., 1990	48	15–45	1 (2)	1 (2)
Federico et al., 1990	56	17–45	10 (18)	2 (4)
Milandre et al., 1990	100	16–45	2 (2)	NS
Lisovoski & Rousseaux, 1991	145	5–40	25 (17)	3 (2)
Totals (average %)	1,680		156 (10)	66 (7)

Abbreviation: NS, not specified in report.

history.[15] In some instances, however, stroke risk factors increased stroke risk in migraine with aura.

The overall incidence of "migrainous infarction" has been estimated at 3.36 per 100,000 population per year (95% CI: 0.87 to 4.8) but in the absence of other stroke risk factors becomes 1.44 per 100,000 population per year (95% CI: 0.00 to 3.07).[95] This rate is similar to that reported later in subjects under 50;[20] migrainous infarction accounted for 25% of cerebral infarcts. To place these data in context, the overall incidence of ischemic stroke under age 50 ranges from 6.5 per 100,000[116] to 22.8 per 100,000.[108,121]

Epidemiologic studies that have addressed an association between migraine and stroke have been few. In a retrospective study of parents of migraine sufferers, no increased risk of stroke was found, but the frequency of hypertension was 1.7 times greater in persons with migraine than in those without.[117] In an inconclusive study, the Collaborative Group for the Study of Stroke in Young Women found that the relative risk of thrombotic stroke was twofold higher, greater for women with migraine compared with a neighbor but not with hospital controls.[84] A hospital-based controlled study of 89 cases found that ischemic stroke was increased more than twofold in patients with migraine with aura,[94] but when stroke risk factors were excluded in this group, there was no longer a statistically significant association.

In a case-controlled study, there was no overall association between migraine and ischemic stroke, but among women aged less than 45, migraine and stroke were significantly associated; there was approximately a fourfold increased risk, more so in women who smoked.[183] When this study was extended to a larger population, the results were confirmed and strengthened.[184] The risk of stroke was 3 times control for migraine without aura and 6 times the risk of controls for migraine with aura. Further, young women with migraine who smoked increased their stroke risk to approximately 10 times control, more than 3 times greater than young women without migraine who smoked. For young women with migraine on oral contraceptives the risk of stroke was 14 times control, and 4 times the risk for young women on contraceptives who did not suffer from migraine. There was a dose-effect relationship between risk of stroke and the dose of estrogen: the odds ratio was 4.8 for pills containing 50 μg of estrogen, 2.7 for 30 to 40 μg, 1.7 for 20 μg, and 1 μg for progestogen. In none of these cases was the stroke induced by the migraine attack. In a recently published case-controlled study of 308 patients with either transient ischemic attacks (TIAs) or stroke, a history of migraine was more frequent than controls (14.9% versus 9.1%).[33a] Migraine was the only significant risk factor (odds ratio 3.7) in women below 35 years of age. Although these risk figures appear startlingly high in both studies, it must be remembered that the absolute risk of stroke for this patient population translates to around 19 per 100,000 per year, which is a low rate.

Past Concepts

Clinical and autopsy evidence accrued over the years is persuasive of the existence of migraine-related infarction of the cerebral hemispheres, retina, and brain stem. A survey of the past literature identified cases of persisting neurologic sequelae attributed to migraine, in which the diagnosis was supported by pathologic studies or laboratory investigation. These cases provide a historical review that traces the conceptual evolution of the mechanisms of the disorder.

In 1881, Fere,[59] working with Charcot at the Salpêtrière hospital, provided one of the earliest comprehensive descriptions of the problem. He reviewed 12 patients suffering from classic migraine who also experienced language and sensorimotor symptoms. Fere later reported Charcot's fatal case of a 53-year-old man with classic migraine since adolesence who developed permanent aphasia and right faciobrachial paralysis, offering the following explanation[60]:

> Dans la migraine il existe une constriction passagère d'abord des vaisseaux sous l'influence d'un trouble du système nerveux sympathique; peu à peu la constriction devient permanente et arrive jusqu'à l'oblitération prèsque complète des vaisseaux et determine une thrombose d'ou résulte la mort des tissus compris dans le térritoire vasculaire atteint.

Charcot again emphasized this notion of cerebral ischemia as a result of vasospasm in his discussion of a case of ophthalmoplegic migraine.[37]

AUTOPSY STUDIES

Among the fatal cases of migrainous cerebral infarction that have been studied at autopsy, characteristic pathologic changes have not been consistently identified. In one instance the brain was normal, and in another nonspecific changes were reported.[135] In seven other cases, various abnormalities were found, suggesting several possible mechanisms involved in the pathogenesis of this cerebrovascular syndrome. These publications have been reviewed recently by Mitsias and Ramadan in the historical section of the journal *Cephalalgia*.[131a]

THE CONCEPT OF VASOSPASM

Buckle et al reported a fatal case in which an angiogram just prior to death showed widespread narrowing[26]: A 16-year-old girl had a 4-month history of episodic unresponsiveness during which she was restless, pale and cold, and experienced a dull headache on regaining consciousness. She was admitted because of progressive lethargy over 4 days. She vomited on the day of admission and became comatose shortly thereafter. The exam showed spontaneous writhing movements of all limbs and teeth grinding; no focal abnormalities were detected. Lumbar puncture was normal except for a protein of 125 mg/dl. She developed, 3 hours later, decerebrate rigidity with eye deviation to the right. Right carotid angiography was performed, about 25 hours after the onset of coma, and showed severe narrowing of the supraclinoid carotid and the anterior, middle, and posterior cerebral arteries. The cavernous and extracranial carotid was normal in caliber. The left anterior and middle cerebral arteries were visualized with cross-compression and found to be narrowed. No aneurysm was seen. The patient became hypotensive and died 7 hours later. At necropsy the brain was swollen with evidence of central and uncal herniation. No aneurysm was found nor was there blood clot in relation to any of the major cerebral vessels. No evidence of primary vascular disease was seen in the vessels of the white matter or cortex. All areas of the cerebral cortex were severely ischemic. The underlying white matter showed swollen, irregular axons. The cerebellum and brain stem were free of pathologic changes. Although the exact clinical diagnosis was not firm, alternative explanations were lacking and the authors considered the previous attacks possibly migrainous. The neuropathologic changes were not considered attributable to hypotension, which more characteristically produces laminar necrosis.

ARTERIOPATHY INCLUDING VASCULAR HYPERPLASIA

Oppenheim's case[146] as cited by Hunt[101] was that of a 35-year-old woman who had suffered from migraine since childhood. Four months after giving birth to a child she had an attack of migraine accompanied by transient aphasia, followed subsequently by four similar accompanied attacks. During the last and fatal episode, she was aphasic and delirious with a right hemiplegia. The autopsy showed infarction of the left cerebral hemisphere, produced by thrombosis of the left internal carotid near the origin of the sylvian artery. Microscopic examination of the vessel wall showed a distinct endarteritis, with thickening of the adventitia. Hunt considered this case an example of a pre-existing organic defect in the vessel wall that could not withstand the acute vascular disturbances associated with an attack of migraine.

An unusual constellation of symptoms, collectively referred to as the "malignant migraine syndrome" consisting of classical migraine, occipital seizures, and alternating strokes were reviewed recently by Dvorkin et al.[52] Eight patients were reported, of whom four died because of intractable seizures. The one autopsied case showed cortical infarcts, and the pathologic studies of cerebral biopsies revealed normal large vessels and focal cortical lesions with vascular hyperplasia.

The only other instance demonstrating a possible vasculopathy was a patient with familial hemiplegic migraine who died following a respiratory arrest. Neligan et al[141] reported the case of a 41-year-old woman who, since the age of 9, suffered from episodes of unilateral frontal headache followed after 5 minutes by numbness and weakness of the contralateral face and limbs, accompanied by dysphasia. The episodes lasted for about 1 hour. Thirty-six hours before admission she awoke with severe right temporal headache followed within minutes by left arm weakness. On admission she was drowsy, irritable, and photophobic with a stiff neck and a moderate left hemiparesis. She developed frequent seizures. Spinal fluid exam and bilateral cerebral angiography were normal. She remained in a persistent vegetative state until her death 4

months later. At autopsy, cystic infarcts in the head of the left caudate nucleus and putamen and a granular infarct in the head of the right caudate nucleus were found. Histologic examination confirmed the varying ages of the infarcts. Most of the small arteries were normal, but some within or near the infarcts were thick walled and variably showed subintimal hyperplasia and reduplication of elastic lamina in vessel walls. Examination of the heart and extracranial arteries was unremarkable. The deep microinfarcts were considered to be related to the previous attacks of migrainous hemiplegia, again presumed to have occurred as a result of spasm.

These reports raise the possibility that repeated attacks of severe migraine presumably accompanied by vasospasm may lead to focal arterial injury, whether an "endarteritis" or intimal proliferation and media myonecrosis, comparable with that observed as a result of spasm induced by subarachnoid hemorrhage.[42,58,99] These arterial changes may, in turn, predispose to thrombosis or, in some cases, distal embolization. The autopsied case of familial hemiplegic migraine is exceptional for its demonstration of small deep infarcts, a distinctly uncommon site of migrainous cerebral infarction, indicating that lenticulostriate arteropathy may be one mechanism, a hypothesis favored by Bruyn.[23–25]

THE CONCEPT OF EMBOLISM

Cases clinically resembling cerebral embolism from a cardiac source have been amply described, in many instances with acute hemiplegia so swift in onset that patients reported falling.[11,38,195] The clinical-pathologic features of the patients reported by Guest and Wolf[85] and Polyak[153] are certainly not incompatible with such a mechanism. A frequently cited example of the malignant consequences of migraine, Guest and Wolf's case was a 28-year-old man with a 2-year history of severe headaches associated with nausea but unaccompanied by neurologic symptoms. While eating a meal he suddenly became unresponsive and had right-sided weakness. He died 20 hours after the onset of coma. At autopsy the cortex of the left superior and middle frontal convolutions were stippled with petechial hemorrhage and microscopically showed ischemic changes. Widespread ischemic changes were also seen in the left insula, paracentral lobule, and postcentral gyrus. Patchy areas of ischemic changes were found in the brain stem including the substantia nigra, both pontine reticular nuclei, and the spinal tract of the fifth nerve. The left internal carotid artery was patent up to its bifurcation; the left anterior and middle cerebral arteries were also normal. Guest and Wolf concluded that infarction occurred in the territory of the left anterior cerebral artery presumed due to migrainous vasospasm with no evident structural abnormality of the blood vessels, although an embolism of obscure origin, with the subsequent fragmentation of a clot, is an alternative possibility.

Another example of pathologically verified cerebral infarction associated with migraine, but clinically compatible with embolism, is Polyak's report[153] of the case of Dr. Frank B. Mallory. In his late 20s the patient began to suffer recurrent attacks of scintillating scotoma in the left visual field, sometimes accompanied by nausea.

> At the approximate age of forty-seven, on a Sunday in the summer of 1910 while at dinner, immediately after the reflection from a white surface of bright sunlight into the patient's eyes, he began to complain of brilliant flashes recurring at very frequent intervals, leaving within a few hours—at any rate in less than a day—a visual field defect. The defect, according to the patient's estimate, was at first large, but subsequently it "cleared." The duration of this attack was approximately from 20 to 40 minutes.
> One year after this episode an ophthalmologist, consulted for another reason, found a large hemianopic scotoma in the left upper field. At the age of 71 another ophthalmological exam disclosed an absolute left upper homonymous quadrantic defect extending from the fixation point along the vertical meridian for 10° and along the horizontal meridian for 20°. The brain at autopsy showed an old infarct confined to the lower calcarine lip on the right. Serial sections of the main stem of the calcarine artery and its continuation revealed no occlusions.

Despite the lack of pathologically verified arterial thromboembolism in either of these two cases, the abrupt onset during activity with no premonitory headache and the presence of hemorrhagic infarction in one case support this possibility.

INTRACRANIAL ARTERIAL DISSECTION

Sinclair[169] reported the fatal case of a 27-year-old migraineur with a nontraumatic dissecting aneurysm of the middle cerebral artery that Sinclair ascribed to migraine in the absence of pathologic evidence for congenital vascular anomaly, arteriosclerosis, arteritis, or cystic medial necrosis. The patient had been affected for several years with episodes of right-sided facial and retro-ocular pain refractory to ergot medication. At 16 hours before admission she experienced her usual headache followed 8 hours later by paresthesias of all limbs, weakness of both hands, and tongue numbness. Initially she was lethargic and confused without lateralizing signs, but within 24 hours she developed a flaccid left hemiplegia and died 3 days later. At autopsy the right frontal and parietal lobes showed evidence of recent infarction. The right middle cerebral artery 1 cm from its origin showed dark-red discoloration for a 2 cm distance and was enlarged, firm, and stiff. Microscopically there was dissection of the media with no medial necrosis, an intact elastic lamina, and no intimal tear. Sinclair considered that the local vascular alterations in the course of a migraine attack, in particular the vasodilatory phase as suggested by early experimental studies,[179] contributed to the development of dissection.

CLINICAL STUDIES WITH LABORATORY INVESTIGATIONS

Scattered clinical examples were reported prior to the 1950s describing serious neurologic consequences of migraine, usually permanent visual field defects,[29,88,101,147,160,162,178,191,199]

suspected but not documented to be ischemic in origin. Not only was thrombosis related to vasoconstriction considered a sequela of migraine, but also intracerebral and subarachnoid hemorrhage, presumed related to repeated vasodilatation were recorded,[51,78] in some instances documented by autopsy.[2,32,46,151] Despite demonstration of aneurysm in some of these latter reports, the association linking migraine with hemorrhage is presently considered a curious coincidence, having little biologic plausibility and no support from large series defining the prevalence of migraine among patients with documented aneurysm[187] or angioma.[12] Clinical reports in the last 50 years, however, have provided more convincing evidence for the association between migraine and cerebral infarction, especially those cases documented with the use of angiography, computed tomography (CT) scanning, positron emission tomography (PET), and, most recently, magnetic resonance imaging (MRI). Little corroborating evidence has been accrued to support any of the possible mechanisms raised by autopsy studies discussed above.

Symonds[177] described two cases with hemiplegia and one with persisting hemianopia. The patient, a 54-year-old man with a history of classic migraine since childhood, awoke with a typical visual aura consisting of wavy lines in the right visual field. Instead of spreading across the whole field, the lines remained confined to the right and persisted for 6 months. Unlike the usual spells, no headache ensued in the acute phase of the deficit. When carotid and vertebral angiography was performed at 6 months, no abnormality was evident.

In 1954 Brain described five cases with permanent hemianopia attributed to migraine among a total of 200 patients admitted to the hospital with a stroke syndrome.[18] In one case, not described clinically, an angiogram showed a posterior cerebral artery occlusion.

One of the rare cases of presumed migrainous cerebral infarction subjected to craniotomy was reported by Murphy.[138] A 36-year-old woman had suffered from migraine attacks since childhood, consisting of scintillating scotoma or dimness of vision affecting the left eye followed by left hemicranial headache. She suddenly experienced complete amblyopia, global aphasia, and right hemiplegia preceded by a bout of recurrent, unusually severe headache. The spinal fluid was under an opening pressure of 180 mmHg with a protein of 49, the electroencephalogram (EEG) showed left frontotemporal slowing, and a left carotid arteriogram revealed occlusion of the left anterior cerebral artery with mass effect evident by displacement of the middle cerebral artery. The patient underwent left frontotemporal craniotomy 4 days after admission. "The brain was of normal appearance externally; nonetheless, the cortex was transected and the region of the internal capsule was approached. Just external to the head of the caudate nucleus the white matter was soft and slightly yellow in color. A biopsy specimen obtained was reported as normal cerebral tissue."

Heyck[97] alluded to another patient who had a craniotomy, but no details are given. Swollen cerebral cortex was viewed through a craniotomy defect in another case, although the cerebral tissue was not examined.[5]

In 1962, Connor[41] reported a series of 18 cases, recognizing three groups of patients with complicated migraine, a term he originated and used in the title of his article. Of these patients, 5 had retinal deficits, 10 had hemispheral deficits, and 3 had deficits localized to the brain stem. Among the hemispheral cases, 8 patients were studied by angiography, and 2 showed abnormalities. One of these latter cases is instructive. A 26-year-old man suffered attacks of vertigo, teichopsia, frontal headache, and vomiting. On one occasion he experienced left focal paresthesias with weakness. After a week-long period of constant headache, he developed giddiness and abrupt left hemiplegia. The examination also revealed a left homonymous hemianopia. Angiography of the carotid and vertebral arteries failed to fill the right posterior cerebral artery. When he was admitted 7 months later for attacks of focal motor epilepsy, there were residual sensorimotor deficits on the left and an incomplete left field defect. Angiography on this occasion showed normal filling of both posterior cerebral arteries (PCAs). No history of or investigation for cardiac disease was mentioned. Among the remaining cases most developed a defect (7 of 10) during the course of a migrainous attack and most (7 to 10) had had preceding transient neurologic dysfunction in a topography similar to the persisting deficit. Connor observed,[41] as others prior to him had marked, that there was a predilection for occipital cortex involvement (6 to 10). In only 1 case was the use of ergotamine considered a possible causative factor in the focal deficit.

The largest series of cases, numbering 40, was reported several years later by Pearce and Foster.[149] Specific investigations were performed in 82% for various indications, including persisting visual field or sensorimotor disturbances, ophthalmoplegia, recurrent unilateral headaches confined to the same side, presence of carotid or intracranial bruit, and meningeal symptoms or epilepsy occurring during an attack. Hemispheral symptoms occurred in 19 patients, 12 of whom had deficits persisting beyond 24 hours. Only two vascular malformations were detected among 29 angiograms performed, but these cases had unusual features, including loss of consciousness and seizures. Visual symptoms were present in 10 patients, and 6 had field defects consistent with occipital ischemia. The clinical details of some of these patients were the subject of a later report.[148] This series of cases established the rarity of vascular anomalies in patients with persisting deficits, suggesting that such sequelae are more likely due to infarction. Like Connor,[41] these authors concluded with suggestions compatible with what is now common neurologic practice: angiography should be pursued in cases of persisting migrainous deficits when epilepsy or meningeal symptoms occur, or possibly in any patient more than 35 years old.

Myhrman's case[139] was subjected to angiography on two separate occasions, once after the initial deficit and then a year later when the patient presented with generalized seizures. In both instances the study was normal. The patient, a 37-year-old woman, had a 15-year history of common migraine. During a bout of severe headache she experienced scintillating scotoma in the left visual field. An inferior quadrantic defect was discovered, prompting the initial evaluation. The deficit was persistent for at least a year, when she again came to clinical attention because of an epileptic attack.

Angiography

In a study focusing on the correlation between angiographically defined arterial occlusions in the posterior cerebral artery territory and permanent visual field defects, Kaul et al[107] reported a series of 19 patients, 4 of whom had syndromes attributed to migraine. One patient, a 42-year-old woman, had an occlusion of the main trunk of the PCA presenting with right hemianopia, hemianesthesia, spontaneous pain, transient amnesia, and dysphasia. The remaining 3 had branch occlusions of the calcarine artery, producing pure quadrantic defects. In each case, a prominent though transient visual disturbance was a feature of the previous migraine attacks, and the permanent deficit occurred during the course of a severe migraine.

Despite the increasing refinement in angiographic techniques, the report by Boisen[13] demonstrates the difficulty of interpreting abnormal radiographic findings in the context of permanent migrainous deficits. A 47-year-old patient had carotid stenosis and migraine attacks that improved with anticoagulation, and another patient had vertebral artery occlusion in the setting of thrombocytosis. Similarly, among the nine cases presented by Davis-Jones et al,[47] a 40-year-old hypertensive woman with visual spells developed aphasia with angiography showing a left middle cerebral artery occlusion; no cardiac evaluation was specified.

Rare instances of vasospasm documented by arteriography have been published, the first in 1964 by Dukes and Vieth.[50] A 44-year-old man suffered from accompanied migraine consisting of left hemianopia with numbness of the left side of the body, followed by a throbbing right hemicranial headache. Admitted to the hospital for evaluation of these headaches, the patient underwent arteriography at a time when he had no symptoms or signs. Following the injection for the lateral right carotid views and before the first anteroposterior (AP) films were obtained, he developed scotoma in both visual fields. The visual disturbance reached a peak at 15 minutes but was not accompanied by a sensory disturbance. At that point, a second set of AP films was made. Over the ensuing 30 minutes the symptoms cleared completely supervened by a typical right hemicranial headache, at which time a third set of AP films was obtained. In 15 minutes, he developed a left hemiplegia which cleared after 1 hour. Prior to the focal deficit, the carotid and vertebral system filled well. The first and second sets of AP films demonstrated increasingly poor filling of the intracranial internal carotid system, at a time when the focal deficit was maximal. During the headache phase, good intracranial filling of the internal carotid was observed.

An anomalous finding was reported by Masuzawa et al[122] whose patient, a 27-year-old postpartum migraineur, was studied because of severe recurrent headache with vomiting. The results of the neurologic exam were normal. Arteriography on the right revealed widespread vasodilatation of the intracranial internal carotid system, but no abnormalities of the external carotid. A repeat exam, when the headache had subsided, showed segmental narrowing of the anterior and middle cerebral arteries.

Garnic and Schellinger[74] recounted their unusual experience when demonstrating vasospasm-induced headache in a 33-year-old woman they considered to have cluster headaches. She had severe, sharp, brief retro-orbital pain unaccompanied by autonomic symptoms. Vertigo and nystagmus were present on right lateral gaze. After four vessel-selective injections were performed without event, a repeat right internal carotid injection led to spasm of the internal, middle, and anterior cerebral arteries accompanied by retro-orbital pain. Although intriguing, these findings add little to the understanding of the mechanisms involved in the permanent cerebral injury related to migraine.

Scanning

The widespread use of CT scanning beginning in the mid-1970s permitted documentation of lesions compatible with cerebral infarction, in many cases correlated with arteriography. Single cases were reported by Julien et al,[106] Moorehead et al,[134] and Romain,[163] and a small series of cases by Burns et al,[28] Saudeau et al,[166] and Crowell et al.[45] In each instance CT showed a low-density lesion of the cortex, most commonly in the occipital lobe. Stone and Burns[174] identified 15 patients with a mean age of 33 who had persisting focal deficits that they attributed to migraine, after a retrospective chart review failed to reveal conventional causes for cerebral infarction. Of these, 8 had a past history of migraine; of the 14 who underwent CT scanning, 9 showed evidence of cerebral infarction.

In a radiologic series of selected migrainous patients with or without focal neurologic deficits, the prevalence of CT scan abnormalities ranged from 34% to 71% (Table 33.3). Cala and Mastaglia[30] reported a large series, examining 94 patients with a history of "recurrent migrainous headaches" of whom 6 showed evidence of cerebral infarction. Of these patients, 4 had fixed visual field defects with mesial occipital low densities. Cerebral edema particularly in the periventricular white matter was evident in another 6 patients. These authors had emphasized the prevalence of cerebral edema in an earlier report.[30] Of the 49 migrainous patients studied, 21 had evidence of low attenuation in the white matter, most extensive in the hemisphere on the side of the headache and contralateral to the sensory aura or signs. This finding corroborated the initial report by Baker,[5] who described diffuse low-density zones during a migraine attack which disappeared on subsequent CT examination.

Hungerford et al[100] studied 53 patients who had "exceptionally severe" migraine or serious clinical complications including hemiplegia. The most frequently encountered abnormality was cerebral atrophy, seen in 14 patients, of whom 8 showed focal changes. Well-defined hemispheric low-density lesions indicating infarction were seen in 6 patients. Among 13 patients who had permanent neurologic deficits, 11 had abnormal scans. In the series reported by Mathew et al[123] 12 of 31 patients with various migraine types and an average duration of illness of 11.3 years had abnormal scans. Of the 3 with common migraine, 1 had evidence of multiple infarction and 2 showed mild to moderate hydrocephalus. Of the 3 patients with classic migraine 2 showed focal cortical atrophy and 1 had mild ventricular enlargement. Both of the 2 patients with vertebrobasilar migraine showed moderately severe hydrocephalus and 1 of them also showed multiple infarction. All 4 patients with migraine and hemiparesis showed low-density lesions in regions of the cerebral cortex consistent with their clinical syndrome.

Perhaps the most convincing reports of migrainous cerebral infarction documented by CT scanning, angiography, and, where appropriate, a cardiac and hematologic evaluation appeared in 1979 by Dorfman et al[49] and Rascol et al.[155] In the first series, 4 adults ranging in age from 16 to 32 years were evaluated among 66 cases of CT-confirmed cerebral infarction. One case, a 25-year-old man with a 5-year history of right-sided or bitemporal headaches associated with left visual obscuration, is especially well documented. Following the onset of an episode with characteristic photophobia and right temporal headaches, he went to sleep and awoke 2 hours later, noticing weakness and numbness of the limbs on the left and visual difficulty to the left. Examination showed no behavioral disturbance except mild irritability, a left hemianopia, and a mild left sensorimotor deficit. The cerebrospinal fluid (CSF) was normal. An EEG showed posterior slowing on the right. A CT scan 4 days after onset revealed a low density in the posterior medial portion of the right temporal lobe, becoming less prominent with enhancement. Cerebral arteriography showed a branch occlusion of the right posterior cerebral artery, and no other abnormalites in the remaining intracranial or extracranial system. The results of laboratory studies including echocardiography, collagen vascular screening, routine coagulation profile, and blood cultures were all negative. CT

Table 33.3 Frequency of Computed Tomography Scan Abnormalities in Migraineurs

Author (Ref.)	Total Cases	Migraine Type	Focal or Diffuse Atrophy N (%)	Low-Density Regions N (%)	Cerebral Edema N (%)	Other N (%)
Baker, 1975[5]	11	NS	2 (18)	0 (0)	2 (2)	0 (0)
Cala and Mastaglia, 1976[30]	49	NS	8 (16)	6 (12)	21 (43)	2 (4)
Hungerford et al., 1976[100]	53	± Aura	14 (26)	6 (11)	1 (2)	5 (9)
Mathew, 1978[124]	31	± Aura	11 (35)	6 (19)	0 (0)	0 (0)
Cala and Mastaglia, 1980[31]	94	NS	11 (12)	6 (6)	6 (6)	2 (2)
Ruiz et al., 1982[165a]	22	± Aura	8 (36)	0 (0)	0 (0)	0 (0)
Sargent and Solbach, 1983[165b]	88	± Aura	10 (11)	2 (2)	0 (0)	2 (2)
du Boulay et al., 1983[47a]	53	± Aura	36 (68)	4 (8)	0 (0)	3 (6)
Cuetter and Aita, 1983[45a]	435	± Aura	0 (0)	0 (0)	0 (0)	1 (0.2)
Totals (average %)	836		100 (12)	30 (4)	30 (4)	15 (2)

Abbreviations: NS, not specified in report; ± Aura, with and without aura.

scanning in the remaining 3 patients showed a large, deep infarct in one, an enhancing insular cortex lesion and a presumed hemorrhagic infarct in the third.

Rascol et al[155,156] reported 10 cases of patients with a mean age of 33 years and CT-confirmed cerebral infarction occurring in the course of a migrainous attack. These authors required that three conditions be fulfilled before making a diagnosis of complicated migraine or migrainous cerebral infarction: (1) there must be a previous history of migraine attacks conforming to the Ad Hoc Committee's definition; (2) there must be a close chronologic relationship between the migraine attack and the prolonged or persisting neurologic disorder; (3) other vascular diseases or predisposing disorders must be excluded, such as vascular malformation, atherosclerotic risk factors (e.g., hypertension, diabetes, hyperlipidemia) or atherosclerotic lesions on cerebral angiography, exposure to oral contraceptives, signs of ergotism, and infectious, inflammatory, hematologic, or immunologic diseases that might be associated with cerebral thrombosis. Of the 10 patients, 6 had syndromes referable to the middle cerebral artery, while the remaining 4 had hemianopic defects due to posterior cerebal artery territory infarctions. Arteriography, performed in each patient sometime between 2 days and 6 months from stroke onset, gave an abnormal result in 9, showing internal carotid artery occlusion in 1, middle or posterior cerebral artery stem occlusion in 4, and branch occlusions in the remaining 4 patients.

Castaigne et al[35] reviewed their experience over a 10-year period, during which they encountered 23 patients ranging in age from 15 to 67 (mean, 37 years) who presented with focal neurologic disturbance related to migraine. In 6 patients, all of whom complained of a headache during the course of the stroke, the deficit was persistent. Angiography was performed in 15, all of whom were normal except 1, showing an internal carotid dissection. Among the 5 who had CT scans, 1 showed an infarct.

Migrainous cerebral infarction is not confined to the adult population. Ment et al[128] reported three children of ages 8 to 14 who developed stroke syndromes attributed to migraine in which headache was a prominent feature. One patient studied angiographically had an occlusion of the PCA. The patient reported by Castaldo et al[36] was a 7-year-old boy who presented with a gradually progressive syndrome consisting of dysphasia and right hemiplegia preceded by severe headaches. An occlusion of the middle cerebral artery was visualized on angiography.

Although cerebral edema has been invoked as one cause of transient focal deficits related to migraine,[89,124] these cases demonstrating infarcts and arterial occlusions should dispel any lingering doubts about the pathologic process involved in permanent focal deficits. Bousser et al[16] provided confirmatory and novel evidence for an ischemic process using PET in their study of a 45-year-old man with a long history of classic migraine. In this instance the focal deficit, a pure right hemianopia, occurred on awakening followed by severe generalized headache. The CT scan showed a contrast-enhancing low-density lesion in the left occipital lobe and an unenhanced lesion in the left temporal cortex, the latter suggesting a subclinical old infarct. Cerebral angiography, performed 21 days after onset, was normal. Cerebral blood flow (CBF) and oxygen extraction measured by the oxygen-15 inhalation technique were both reduced in the left occipital cortex, typical of recent infarcts, while in the temporal lobe, CBF was increased with a normal oxygen extraction. The former finding was considered compatible with luxury perfusion and the latter with reactive hyperemia. Unexplained supernormal oxygen extraction occurred in the asymptomatic right occipital lobe.

As is strongly apparent from the foregoing case descriptions, the coincidence of migraine and stroke has proved to be one of the most intriguing and perplexing problems for the diagnostician. These cases must, however, be considered in the light of current concepts of the mechanisms of migraine and classification of migraine-related stroke.

Current Concepts of Migraine and Vascular Pain Pathogenesis

MIGRAINE AURA

Migraine, according to the theory of Wolff,[201] is a primary defect of central nervous system (CNS) vasculature. He postulated that the neurologic features of the aura were due to vasospasm producing ischemia. Subsequently, brain acidosis caused cerebral vasodilatation which was painful. Points put forward in favor of the vascular concept were that the headache associated with migraine has a pulsating quality similar to the headaches secondary to stroke, arteritis, and hypertension. Also, blood vessels are predominantly the pain-sensitive structures in the brain. The drugs used to treat migraine produce vasoconstriction, for example, ergotamines. Vasodilatation (10% carbon dioxide and 90% oxygen) was considered to prevent headache and abort the aura by increasing blood to the brain regions undergoing vasospasm. Methysergide, a serotonin antagonist, prevents vasospasm induced by serotonin and, since it is highly effective in preventing migraine, this linked serotonin release to the triggering of attacks of vasospasm and hence aura.

This model of vasospasm giving way to vasodilatation to explain both the aura and headache still has its supporters. CBF measurements performed by earlier methods certainly supported this notion, and a critical appraisal of more recent CBF studies argues in favor of a primary ischemic basis for the aura.[170] Nevertheless, the clinical features of the aura are distinctly unlike those of acute ischemia due to cerebral vascular disease. For this and other reasons discussed later, this hypothesis is currently less favored than others.

In 1944, Leao reported an experimental phenomenon in rodent brain and retina that has come to be known as spreading depression (SD),[115] although it could also be termed spreading activation. Neuronal depolarization is followed by suppression of neuronal activity in a wave that spreads slowly across the surface of the brain. Two mechanisms have been proposed for SD, one based on the release of K^+ from neural tissue[80] and the other on release of the excitatory amino acid glutamate.[185] The migraine aura, exemplified by an expanding visual scotoma (a suppressive, negative symptom) with preceding peripheral scintillations (a stimulative, positive symptom), was proposed as the clinical counterpart of SD many years ago[111,131] and is now considered by most as a plausible explanation for the migraine aura.[193] Investigation of this model in humans, however, remains very far from complete and has not yet served to establish SD as the mechanism of aura. Most investigations have been limited to the indirect measure of blood flow, facilitated in migraine subjects by the development of noninvasive imaging techniques. CBF falls but only to oligemic values in posterior regions of the cortex in some patients during attacks of migraine with aura.[113] During these studies it was also noted that the regional hypoperfusion developed before and outlasted the focal symptoms. Focal hyperemia, possibly related to neuronal depolarization, was also seen initially, followed by spreading oligemia.[144] The oligemia could be secondary to neuronal suppression which progressively involves larger areas of the brain spreading at a rate similar to experimental SD.[112] For the most part these CBF changes have been demonstrated in migraine with aura (MA) and not in migraine without aura (MO).

Recently a brief report of an ongoing study by Sorensen et al[171] investigated spontaneous migraine with aura with diffusion-weighted (DWI) and perfusion-weighted MRI (PWI). They imaged patients during the aura phase and during the headache phase. Of the five patients imaged, four had significant (20% to 37%) decreases in regional perfusion and (1.5% to 15%) regional cerebral blood volume (rCBV). They exhibited no change on DWI. Headache phase imaging did not reveal any consistent perfusion abnormalities. This again supports the concept that the hypoperfusion seen in migraine aura may not be secondary to ischemia but to primary neuronal dysfunction.

One recent case report of dynamic blood flow measurements with PET and oxygen-15-labeled water demonstrated bilateral hypoperfusion that started in the occipital lobes and spread anteriorly.[203] In this case the patient had migraine without aura suffering only minor visual blurring well into the attack of headache when CBF reduction was well established. Therefore, migraine with and without aura could share a similar pathophysiology.

The most appropriate techniques to indicate SDs are electrophysiologic, but because of limitations of EEG techniques, spontaneous SD has not been recorded previously in migraine sufferers. Magnetoencephalographic (MEG) DC activity supports SDs occurring during an attack.[6] Long duration DC shifts and suppression of neuronal signal occur during the migraine aura and headache that were not found in patients with other forms of headache or in normal subjects. The DC shifts and neuronal symptoms are consistent with SD measured by electrocorticography and MEG in experimental animals.[73]

Migraine Headache

Release of peptides from sensory axons (involving an axon reflex) of the trigeminal nerve supply to certain extracranial arteries, meningeal tissues, dural arteries, and the dural sinuses sets up a pain-sensitive state (neurogenic inflammation) and promotes local vasodilatation, a state postulated to resem-

ble that in pain-sensitive cranial structures during headache of the migraine attack.[136] In support of this model, calcitonin-gene related peptide (CGRP) is released into jugular venous blood during a migraine attack,[77] and this release is blocked by sumatriptan.[168] Sumatriptan is a selective agonist of the D subtype of 5-HT receptors located on peripheral trigeminal nerve terminals that supply pain-sensitive vascular and meningeal structures and is an effective migraine therapy.

Recently Weiller et al investigated whether the activation of brain stem nuclei could be visualized with PET during acute migraine attacks.[190] Compared with the headache-free interval, rCBF was greater in medial brain stem structures and persisted even after complete symptom relief, possibly reflecting a brain stem headache "generator." The region of maximum increase coincided with the anatomic location of the dorsal rapine nuclei and locus ceruleus, structures involved in antinociception and intracerebral vascular control.

HEADACHE OF VASCULAR DISEASE

Not surprisingly, a major difficulty in differential diagnosis is that the symptom of head pain occurs in various forms of acute cerebrovascular disease, including ischemic stroke. The landmark experiments of Ray and Wolff[159] demonstrated that sensitivity to pressure, traction, and faradization occurred in the intracranial internal carotid artery, the first 1 to 2 cm of the MCA stem, the first several centimeters of the anterior cerebral artery just beyond the A2 segment and 1 to 2 cm of the vertebral, anterior and posterior inferior cerebellar, and pontine arteries. These sensitive structures, when electrically stimulated, provoke pain that is localized to specific areas of the scalp and face.

Fisher's clinical-pathologic observations[62,64,68] extended these findings. A study of the headache syndromes due to ischemic cerebrovascular disease showed that most complained of the symptom at the onset of a persisting neurologic deficit, though in some cases headache was premonitory or accompanied TIAs, findings also noted by others.[55,82,127,140,194] The headache was usually not throbbing, often localized, and frequently lateralized ipsilateral to the presumed arterial occlusion; it was occasionally severe. Of special interest was the relatively high frequency of headache in PCA territory infarctions compared with that seen in carotid or basilar disease. Headache was the exception in lacunar strokes with pure motor or pure sensory syndromes, and none occurred in any of the 58 patients with transient monocular blindness. Overall, the frequency of headache was 31% in carotid and 42% in vertebrobasilar disease. Other series, less detailed in the classification of vessel topography, have reported headache with a frequency as low as 9% for anterior and posterior circulations[145] and as high as 50% for vertebrobasilar ischemia in two studies.[56,140] Mitsias and Ramadan have extensively reviewed the literature on this topic up to 1997.[131a]

The possible mechanisms of headache due to thromboembolism have intrigued authors dating from the time of Willis,[200] including Symonds,[176] to the contemporary authorities such as Fisher[64] and Edmeads.[55] Of the prevailing views, dilatation of collaterals, focal distention of the artery,[194] local ischemia of the arterial muscle, and irritation of pain-sensitive arterial wall by atheroma[19] may remain relevant. Currently, the role of serotonin and other vasoactive peptides released from the junctional elements of the trigeminovascular system are the focus of attention.[55] Mitsias and Ramadan also reviewed contemporary concepts of the mechanisms of pain in cerebrovascular disorders.[131a]

Current Concepts of Classification

One drawback in understanding the dilemma that faces the diagnostician has been a lack of consistency in the definition of migraine-related stroke in the studies conducted so far. Strict definition of terms is essential for future comprehensive epidemiologic studies. After a review of the preceding information discussed above, three major issues emerge:

1. Does stroke occur in the course of the migraine attack, causing true migraine-induced cerebral infarction?

2. Does migraine cause stroke because other risk factors for stroke are present to interact with the migraine-induced pathogenesis?

3. Can stroke present as a migraine syndrome, that is, symptomatic migraine?

Recent developments serve to clarify the association between migraine and stroke. First, the IHS classification has led to improved definitions of migraine and migraine-induced stroke in a more specific comprehensive classification.[92] Second, new techniques of brain imaging have provided new insights into the relationship of the disorder by improved diagnosis.

Migrainous cerebral infarction (IHS 1.6.2) is described in the IHS classification as follows: one or more migrainous aura symptoms not fully reversible within 7 days and/or associated with neuroimaging confirmation of ischemic infarction: (1) patient has previously fulfilled criteria for migraine with neurologic aura; (2) the present attack is typical of previous attacks, but neurologic deficits are not completely reversible within 7 days and/or neuroimaging demonstrates ischemic infarction in the relevant area; (3) other causes of infarction ruled out by appropriate investigations. Table 33-1 presents an extended classification of stroke in association with migraine or migraine-related stroke. Included in this classification is migrainous infarction for which we propose the more precise term *migraine-induced stroke*.

COEXISTING STROKE AND MIGRAINE

Definition: *A clearly defined clinical stroke syndrome must occur remotely in time from a typical attack of migraine.*

Stroke in the young is rare and migraine is common. Clearly, the two conditions can coexist without migraine being a contributive factor to stroke. When the two conditions coex-

ist in the young, the true pathogenesis of stroke may be difficult to elucidate. A comorbidity of stroke risk in migraine sufferers seems apparent from the case-controlled series reviewed in a previous section, where none of the strokes were induced by the migraine attack. This increases the clinical significance of coincident stroke and should serve to raise clinical consciousness to the need for stroke risk factor awareness in all migraine sufferers.

The following case is extracted from a prior publication to illustrate the complexity of coexisting cardiac disorder in a migraineur that may serve as a source of embolism causing a focal deficit indistinguishable from accompanied migraine.

> A 42-year-old man had, since the age of 15, suffered bilateral central scotomas, scintillating phenomena, and occipital headache diagnosed as migraine with neurologic aura. He suffered an acute episode of aphasia with right-hand weakness and headache with clinical features unlike his episodes of migraine. He was found to have a mitral valve prolapse. Cerebral angiography revealed an occlusion of the left middle cerebral artery branch.

There is no established association between migraine and mitral valve prolapse (MVP), but evidence is sufficient to suggest that probably all patients with migraine with neurologic symptoms should be evaluated for the presence of this valvular abnormality. There is no clear evidence that migraineurs with MVP may be especially stroke prone.

STROKE WITH CLINICAL FEATURES OF MIGRAINE

Definition: *A structural lesion unrelated to migraine pathogenesis that presents with clinical features typical of migraine.* Symptomatic: In these cases, established structural lesions of the central nervous system or cerebral vessels episodically causes symptoms typical of migraine with neurologic aura. Such cases should be termed symptomatic migraine. Cerebral arteriovenous malformations frequently masquerade as migraine with aura.

Migraine Mimic: In this category, stroke due to acute and progressing structural disease is accompanied by headache and a constellation of progressive neurologic signs and symptoms indistinguishable from those of migraine. This might best be termed a migraine mimic.

The diagnostic discrimination of a migraine mimic can be most difficult to define in patients with established migraine. Many of the cases described in the above section on the conceptual evolution of migraine-related stroke were likely migraine mimics, the diagnosis being hampered by limitation in investigative tools and uncertainty in the knowledge of migraine pathogenesis. The following case report, extracted from a previous publication, illustrates the complexity of the diagnostic situation.

> A 46-year-old woman suffered from migraine without aura for many years, generally worse 1 week prior to menstruation. The pain was always localized, right-sided, and retro-orbital without visual change.

Twenty years previously, oral contraceptives were prescribed, which she took for up to 10 years. There was a family history of migraine. She presented with headache identical with her usual migraine. The head pain persisted, however, increasing in intensity over a period of 1 month and was totally resistant to all prescribed antimigraine medications. She then suddenly became aphasic, and right hemiplegia developed. Cerebral angiography revealed left internal carotid and middle cerebral artery dissection.

This case raised the issue of a pre-existing arteriopathy of 20 years or more presenting with localized arterial pain mimicking migraine. Could repeated migraines have induced a localized arteriopathy secondary to the migrainous process itself that later resulted in dissection?

The issue of spontaneous carotid artery dissection is very relevant because patients with migraine are at increased risk of dissection MGB and the occurrence of dissection as a typical migraine mimic has been reported.[154] Although the mechanism of pain production is not clearly understood, the occurrence of headache is an expected finding, present in 60% of patients,[90] and probably greater in vertebral dissection, along with a variable incidence of ischemic complications, a combination that may mimic accompanied migraine. Fisher[63] analyzed 21 selected cases of angiographically documented cervical carotid dissection, observing that almost all patients (19 of 21) had ipsilateral pain in one or more regions of the head, including forehead, orbit, temple, retro-orbit, side of head, and the frontal region. In addition, 12 patients had neck pain, usually in the upper neck and localized to a region including the mastoid, upper carotid, behind or below the angle of the jaw, and along the sternocleidomastoid muscle. The pain was usually severe, often sudden in onset, described equally as steady or throbbing, and occasionally accompanied by alterations in ipsilateral scalp sensation. The duration ranged from several hours to 2 years, with most lasting no longer than 3 to 4 weeks. About three-fourths of Fisher's patients experienced ischemic complications, and in half the headache preceded the ischemic event by a few hours to four days. Other common diagnostic findings were Horner's syndrome, subjective bruit, dysgeusia, and visual scintillations. Given this clinical picture, it is difficult to avoid considering the possibility that cases formerly diagnosed as carotidynia,[75,157] paratrigeminal syndrome,[69] or migraine cluster with miosis or transient focal deficits,[58,109] may have been instances of carotid dissection. The topic of dissection and migraine has been recently reviewed.[133]

MIGRAINE-INDUCED STROKE

Definition: *Migraine-induced stroke must meet the following criteria: (1) the neurologic deficit must exactly mimic the migrainous symptoms of previous attacks, (2) the stroke must occur during the course of a typical migraine attack, and (3) all other causes of stroke must be excluded, although stroke risk factors may be present.*

Special note: The major problem with this definition is that the IHS classification does not permit the diagnosis of migraine-induced stroke in patients with migraine without aura (see definition). Perhaps, however, migraine without aura begins in "silent" brain areas and has the same pathogenesis as migraine with aura! There is clearly a need for rigorous analysis of patients with migraine-related stroke without aura and more pathophysiologic information on the latter to refine the IHS classification of this subtype.

Without stroke risk factors: The following case, also extracted from a prior publication, satisfies the above criteria without identifiable stroke risk.

A 34-year-old woman had suffered a complex of twice yearly episodes of right homonymous hemianopia, right cheiro-oral numbness, and confusion followed by left hemicranial head pain typical of migraine with aura. In one episode, the neurologic deficit persisted throughout and after the headache. Examination revealed a right homonymous hemianopia and hemiparesis with Babinski's sign were noted. Only the right hemianesthesia persisted 6 weeks later. An electroencephalogram revealed slow activity in the left occipital and posterior temporal regions. Cerebral blood flow was in the oligemic range in the temporo-occipital and parieto-occipital cortex. Magnetic resonance imaging revealed a left thalamic infarct. Cerebral angiography showed fusiform dilatation of the left posterior cerebral artery with narrowing of arterial caliber proximal and distal to the dilatation. No penetrating branches of the posterior cerebral artery were visualized. Repeated angiography 6 weeks later was normal. No stroke risk factors could be elicited.

The arterial lesion in this case clearly involved the posterior cerebral artery and its branches, although the precise arterial pathologic appearance is uncertain. No unequivocal radiographic evidence of dissection, fibromuscular disease, or premature atherosclerosis was present, and the subsequent radiographic appearance of the artery was normal. Similar arteriographic findings have been reported—migraine with an in situ thrombus positioned in the fusiform dilatation.[2] The impaired filling of small penetrating branches supports intravascular thrombus formation. Any large thrombus, if present, might have undergone dissolution by the time of arteriography 48 hours after the event. The transient left-sided neurologic deficit could be explained by compressive edema, occlusion of the top of the basilar penetrating branch, or diaschisis. Study of this case and others like it has produced insight into the pathogenesis of both migraine and the process leading to stroke.

With stroke risk factors: Previous publications that addressed criteria for true migrainous stroke do not include the modifying statement of risk factors in the definition. This subclassification may be important to understanding mechanisms. For example, oral contraceptives are recognized to increase stroke risk in migraine sufferers[184] and may cause coexisting stroke and migraine. In some instances, however, stroke occurs during the migraine attack, and the medication may have increased the risk of coagulopathy but may not have induced stroke in the absence of the migrainous process. The following intriguing question arises: does migraine cause stroke only because risk factors, as yet unknown, are present to interact with the pathophysiologic mechanisms of the migraine attack? Oral contraceptive use may not only exacerbate pre-existing migraine,[48,152,197] but also contribute to the stroke risk in young women with migraine. The Cooperative Study Group in Young Women used a case-control method to evaluate the risk of cerebrovascular disease in users of oral contraceptives[40] and later reported the effect of other risk factors, including hypertension, smoking, and migraine.[183] The risk of cerebral thrombosis among women using oral contraceptives was 9.5 times greater than among nonusers. The role of migraine was assessed in both users and nonusers of contraceptives. Among migraineurs not exposed to birth control pills, the risk of stroke was equivocal, depending on the control group used for comparison. The use of oral contraceptives in combination with migraine, however, increased the relative risk for thrombotic stroke from 2.0 to 5.9. More recent studies reviewed in the epidemiologic section extend this risk to 13 times that of subjects not on oral contraceptives.[184] Of particular interest in relation to the interactive role of migraine is the pathologic finding of intimal hyperplasia associated with thrombosis in three fatal cases of stroke in young women exposed to contraceptives.[138]

UNCERTAIN CLASSIFICATION

Complex or multiple factors: Many migraine-related strokes cannot be categorized with certainty.

> A 37-year-old woman presented with stuttering onset of left hemiparesis and left homonymous hemianopia not accompanied by headaches. She had an established history of migraine with visual aura. Three years previously she sustained the sudden onset of left-sided weakness 15 minutes after taking a second, 2-mg dose of ergotamine 30 to 60 minutes into a typical migraine headache. Opercular branches of the middle cerebral artery were occluded on angiography, and the CT scan showed a right frontal infarct. She was using oral contraceptives and smoked 20 cigarettes daily for 20 years. Investigation at the time also revealed false-positive results from a VDRL test and positive test results from rheumatoid factor. Investigation of the most recent stroke revealed positive anticardiolipin antibody test results with high IgG titers.

Migraine-related stroke associated with ergot therapy is appropriate in this category because it is impossible to confidently exclude an interaction of the drug with the migrainous process to induce stroke. The mechanism of action of 5HT-1D agonists such as ergotamine or sumatriptan may be neurogenic or vasoconstrictive; recorded cases have been associated with excessive dosage of the drug, presumably causing vasospasm.[17] Even allowing for ergot therapy, the case above could not be included in the category of migraine-induced stroke because of the complex factors that might have caused the stroke. Although the second stroke in this case can be categorized as coexisting migraine and stroke, the risk factors of ergot therapy, oral contraceptives, smoking, and the anticardiolipin antibody positivity all could have interacted with the migraine

mechanisms to produce the prior stroke in the process of the migraine attack.

Ergot therapy even in therapeutic doses may produce, although rarely, focal and diffuse cerebral dysfunction. The peripheral vascular and CNS effects of ergot alkaloids in toxic doses have long been recognized, consisting of gangrene, seizures, encephalopathy, and coma. The mechanism responsible for diffuse cerebral dysfunction is not settled and may be the result of either a direct CNS toxic effect or severe cerebral vasoconstriction, although in therapeutic doses ergotamine usually has no effect on cerebral blood flow.[57,86] Scattered reports have appeared, linking ergotamine use to focal disturbances in the ophthalmic and cerebral circulations, manifested by transient monocular blindness, bilateral papillitis, and sensorimotor deficits.[21,129,161,167] Since the recent introduction of sumatriptan there have also been scattered reports of strokelike events, but so far none that have been convincing of primary involvement of the drug or can exclude its use in an event that mimics migraine.

Angiography: The precipitation of migraine-like signs and symptoms during cerebral angiography is not uncommon and can potentially progress to stroke, although not all observers agree.[168] Angiography performed during migraine carries risk because of potential interaction with the migraine mechanism. Nevertheless, because arteriography can be complicated by stroke in all patients, the true pathogenesis of stroke cannot be attributed with certainty to migraine.

Transient focal neurologic events and late-onset migraine accompaniments: Headache is not an invariable occurrence in migraine. Adding to the potential for diagnostic confusion is the occurrence of migraine attacks consisting of visual disturbances or focal deficits not accompanied by typical headache, often termed "migraine sine hemicrania." Charcot[37] identified an incomplete form of ophthalmic migraine as "migraines ophtalmiques frustes" consisting only of "les troubles oculaires."

More controversial has been the entity of accompanied migraine without headache, originally described by Whitty.[196] Fisher[65,66] emphasized that the migrainous syndrome, despite the absence of headache, could be diagnosed on the basis of characteristic clinical features. Since then, painless transient and persistent migraine accompaniments have become more widely recognized. The cause of late-onset migraine accompaniments has not been established.[66] As the name of the syndrome suggests, the clinical features are essentially indistinguishable from migraine without headache. Brain imaging and cerebral arteriography do not reveal accountable structural lesions.

Transient focal neurologic events have recently been extensively analyzed by Teijen et al. Many of these events have features of migraine with aura, especially visual features.[178a] The study by Tzourio et al reviewed in the epidemiologic section found an association with such events and an increased risk for stroke.[183] These studies emphasize the wisdom of thorough evaluation for stroke risk of patients suffering such symptoms.

Miscellaneous: There are rare reports of migraine-like syndromes associated with other manifestations of neurologic disease that are of uncertain pathogenesis and that make the classification of these curiosities uncertain. Occasional reports of cases with migraine-like symptoms and persistent neurologic deficit associated with high CSF protein values and pleocytosis are to be found in the literature. Cerebral vasculitis or focal encephalitis, although unproven, have been proposed in the pathogenesis. Exceptionally, cases of well-documented migraine with aura will show evidence of similar CSF abnormality. Other rare syndromes associated with migraine-related stroke include migraine associated with mitochondrial encephalopathies[53] and "migraine coma."[70]

Hemorrhage: Cases of intracerebral hemorrhage because of migraine have been reported rarely and have been recently reviewed.[33] In our view, investigations have failed to establish true migraine-induced hemorrhage, most cases likely being symptomatic migraine (class IIA) or migraine mimics (class IIB). From the viewpoint of pathogenesis, however, it is not unreasonable that ischemic softening of tissue during true migraine-induced cerebral infarction might become hemorrhagic, so dogmatism must be avoided. Experience with this entity in the context of the current IHS classification is awaited.

Retinal or ocular migraine: This group of disorders is designated as uncertain in classification because of limited clinical information, most clinical case reports or series having been communicated prior to the development of contemporary advanced neurologic investigation. While transient homonymous scintillations or fortification scotoma are well-recognized cortical migrainous phenomena, monocular visual loss due to retinal involvement is less often a manifestation of migraine,[43] although still a differential diagnostic point in the patient presenting with amaurosis fugax.[76] Since both retinal and ciliary circulations may be affected, the term *ocular migraine* is preferred[43] and should be distinguished from the term *ophthalmic migraine*, which refers to any migrainous disturbance of vision whether ocular or cortical.[123,142] To include instances of optic nerve dysfunction that may occur as well, Troost[181] has suggested the broader term *anterior visual pathway migraine*.

Carroll[34] considered the syndrome of retinal migraine an uncommon disorder, usually occurring in a young adult who experiences recurrent and unaccompanied episodes of visual loss or dimness in one or both eyes almost never exceeding 10 minutes in duration, but rarely persisting for an hour or more. He emphasized the usual absence of preceding fortification spectra, the invariable absence of headache, and the nearly invariable return to normal visual function, although with repeated attacks a permanent visual defect may develop. While typical attacks of classic or common migraine occasionally occur at other times, the visual disturbance without headache may be the predominant or sole manifestation of a migrainous disorder.

Subsequent reports have generally corroborated these points; the co-occurrence of headache or the presence of scintillations in other cases have helped to stamp the disorder as migrainous. In children, Hachinski et al[87] encountered 7 out of 100 cases with monocular symptoms in the setting of headache. Except for their unilateral occurrence, the visual disturbances consisted of obscurations and scotomas similar to those in patients with binocular symptoms. Among a group of older adults, Hedges[93] identified 33 cases with ophthalmic symptoms. Interestingly, when followed for periods of between 5 and 10 years, the patients with monocular symptoms had a 45% incidence of vascular complications (not further specified), in contrast to 13% seen in the group with homonymous complaints. This observation serves as a cautionary note: while migrainous transient monocular blindness may occur for the first time in a patient more than 50 years old, carotid atherosclerosis is probably the more likely cause.[1]

The pathophysiology of transient monocular visual loss occurring in the setting of migraine is poorly understood, although investigative efforts in this direction may very well have an impact on our understanding of migrainous disorders in general, comparable with the clarification of the mechanisms of transient hemispheral attacks resulting from the study of amaurosis fugax due to carotid artery disease.[67] Walsh and Hoyt[186] are often cited as recognizing that "the eye itself can be involved in the angiospastic circulatory disturbance of a migraine attack." Only two examples of funduscopic abnormalities photographed *during* an episode of transient monocular visual loss have been reported. Wolter and Burchfield[202] observed disc hyperemia and diffuse retinal opacity with a cherry-red macular spot considered to represent retinal edema. Moreover, although the authors did not believe that a change in vessel caliber had occurred, Troost[181] felt that there was *venous* vasoconstriction, based on his review of the fundus photographs. Kline and Kelly[109] documented transient funduscopic changes occurring in a 48-year-old man with a long-standing history of cluster headaches and recurrent transient monocular visual reduction lasting for 1 to 2 minutes. They observed *venous* narrowing during an attack and subsequent venous dilatation; no retinal arteriolar vasospasm or embolic material was evident. Despite prompt filling of two cilioretinal vessels seen on fluorescein angiography, there was a delay in the appearance of dye in branches of the central retinal artery. In addition, during an attack, pattern-reversal visually evoked potentials showed diminution of amplitude with only a small effect on latency. The authors interpreted the retinal venous narrowing as a phenomenon secondary to reduced arterial flow, although "venous spasm" is an alternative explanation.[3]

Another case, photographed after the episode of amaurosis, also appeared to show retinal *arteriolar* narrowing.[193] Reports of funduscopic examination during an attack have confirmed the observation of arteriolar spasm,[83,164,186,188,198] despite one negative report of five patients, most having binocular visual symptoms.[104] In Fisher's seminal report[67] on transient monocular blindness, 26 cases in the literature of ophthalmoscopically observed narrowing of retinal vessels were reviewed, some of which were quite likely of migrainous origin.

Of the cases in the literature prior to the new IHS classification in 1988, defects in vision included central or centrocecal scotomas, altitudinal defects, monocular constriction, and complete blindness. The mean age of the patients was 37 years, with four times as many women as there were men. The presence of a family history of migraine was variable. The mean duration of migraine was 13 years with diverse migraine subtypes, the most frequent being classic migraine (11 cases), followed by retinal migraine unaccompanied by headache (10 cases). Other headache types included retinal migraine with headache (3 cases), common migraine (3 cases), retinal and classic migraine (1 case), and cluster headache (1 case). The visual loss almost always occurred abruptly, usually in the setting of a headache that appeared as often before or following the onset of the visual disturbance. In a few cases local eye pain was a prominent symptom. A variety of funduscopic abnormalities were reported, as reviewed below. In the four instances where carotid angiography was performed, no abnormalities were evident. Only a small number of cases were fully investigated to exclude alternative causes of abrupt visual loss, although most cases appeared to fulfill the requirements of a prior history of migraine and abrupt visual loss occurring in the context of a migrainous headache.

Many of the cases cited here were reported before modern diagnostic techniques were available, particularly to pursue an embolic etiology, and before the recognition of prothrombotic disorders such as antiphospholipid antibody syndromes that often affect the eye. These are probably the causes most likely to confound a diagnosis of permanent visual loss resulting from retinal migraine. Transient or permanent monocular visual obscurations of migrainous origin, even when accompanied by specific funduscopic abnormalities, is not a syndrome clinically distinguishable from amaurosis fugax or retinal infarction due to embolism. Goodwin et al[79] concluded after a review of 170 attacks in 32 patients with angiographically proved carotid artery disease or cardiogenic emboli that the clinical syndrome of amaurosis fugax was sufficiently variable to preclude definitive distinction from migraine. Other authors have concurred with this view,[43,54] although Corbett has suggested that one clinical subtype of amaurosis is characteristic of ocular migraine. A specific instance is described as follows: gradual monocular constriction beginning as spotty darkening in the periphery, later coalescing into a ring followed by more spots in the darkened area until only small clear spots remain in the center. The eye remains blind for 1 to 2 minutes with clearing from the periphery to the center. This pattern of lobular constriction appears conveniently explained by ischemia in the choroidal circulation which Hayreh[91] has shown to have a segmental, cobblestone architecture.

Galezowski[72] was the first to describe *central retinal artery occlusion* as a consequence of migrainous attacks. At the time of his report he had seen 76 cases of "ophthalmic megrim" and detailed the features of 4 cases, 2 of which involved central retinal artery occlusion. A single case reported briefly by Crowell et al[45] is worthy of mention because of its atypical features and the failure of an extensive evaluation to reveal a nonmigrainous cause. In only 2 other cases[41,138] have ocular and cerebral deficits occurred in the same patient closely linked in time. Ordinarily such a combination, though uncommon, can be considered a sign highly predictive for carotid atherostenosis.[150]

Several examples of *branch retinal arterial occlusions* have been reported.[47,72,81,83,101,189] Gronvall's case[83] of an 18-year-old woman is particularly well documented. Typical attacks began with a sensation of dimness before her eyes consisting of grayish-white patches with a colored margin superimposed on an intact background visual field. After 1 to 2 minutes, a boring pressure in one temple supervened, sometimes accompanied by nausea and vomiting. During one such attack with the usual spots, she experienced sudden right monocular blindness. She was able 10 minutes later to see in the lower half of the visual field, vision returning in the course of a half-minute, but a greyish-black defect persisted in the superior half. An ophthalmologic exam 24 hours later showed a complete upper nasal defect extending into an upper temporal crescent. A patch of retinal edema was evident inferior to the macula, and the inferior temporal artery was threadlike. The results of a routine cardiac exam and hematologic studies were normal.

Brown et al[22] studied 27 patients under 30 years of age with central or branch arterial occlusions. The most common associated finding was a history of migraine, occurring in 8 patients. All had a previous history of scintillating scotomas associated with headaches usually unilateral but not consistently lateralized to the side of the affected eye. Only 1 patient experienced a headache at the time of the occlusion.

Central retinal vein occlusion has been less frequently encountered. Lohlein[120] and Wegner[189] followed the disturbing developments in the case of a 46-year-old man with a 25-year history of migraine who suffered recurrent amaurosis in either eye. He sustained permanent visual loss on three occasions associated with hemorrhage into the optic nerve head on the left, retinal venous occlusions on the right, and later central retinal artery occlusion also on the right. Friedman's single case[71] of central retinal venous occlusions occurred during the course of a severe migraine headache; no abnormalities were found on carotid arteriography.

The recognition of *ischemic optic neuropathy* as a complication of migraine has served to broaden our concept of the presumed site of microcirculatory disturbance in ocular migraine. Seven cases with a mean age of 44 years are known in the literature,[17,101,126,192] each presenting with abrupt visual loss in the form of a central scotoma or arcuate defect occurring during the course of a typical headache. Disc swelling, in some cases accompanied by peripapillary hemorrhages was seen acutely, while optic disc pallor occurred in the later stages; in either situation, the funduscopic appearance was indistinguishable from cases of idiopathic ischemic optic neuropathy. The two patients reported by Weinstein and Feman[192] appear the most exhaustively investigated, revealing no other apparent causative factor including temporal arteritis, collagen vascular disease, syphilis, hyperviscosity or hypercoagulable states, multiple sclerosis, or a compressive nerve lesion. Neither patient had hypertension and in the one patient undergoing carotid angiography, no abnormalities were detected. Fluorescein angiography, performed acutely in the one patient reported by McDonald and Sanders,[126] showed normal arterial filling but a delay in filling of the peripapillary plexus in the upper pole and in the venous phase, dilatation of the superficial peripapillary plexus.

Ischemic susceptibility of the prelaminar portion of the optic nerve might be considered a reflection of its "watershed" position between the retinal and choroidal systems. While the surface of the optic disc derives its blood supply primarily from branches of the central retinal artery, the prelaminar and laminar portions are supplied through an anastomotic arterial circle receiving contributions from the posterior ciliary arteries, pial vessels, and choroidal arterioles.[91,118] Microcirculatory disturbances affecting any of these three vascular sources can be implicated in the pathogenesis of migrainous ischemic optic neuropathy. Endowed with a muscular coat, the short posterior ciliary arteries have been favored as the site of vasoconstriction producing impaired perfusion of the optic nerves.[118] However, there is little doubt that the choroidal circulation may be affected, given the evidence from fluorescein angiography, and the demonstration of *retinal pigmentary changes*. Among Connor's five cases[41] with permanent retinal lesions, two patients with hemicranial headache accompanied by teichopsia developed monocular visual loss with retinal pigment having "the appearance and distribution of that found in retinitis pigmentosa."

MIGRAINE THAT MIMICS STROKE

Hemiplegic Migraine

Liveing,[119] in 1873, first described transient hemiparesis associated with a migraine attack. In 1910, Clarke[38] published the first report of hemiplegic migraine occurring in a family. Whitty[195] classified the disorder into hemiplegic migraine with a family history of migraine with or without aura and familial hemiplegic migraine (FHM) in which attacks occur with stereotypic features in family members, often with severe and longlasting hemiparesis or other persistent aura symptoms, and an autosomal dominant inheritance pattern.

Heyck's monograph in 1956,[96] Bradshaw and Parsons' clinical study in the *Quarterly Journal of Medicine*,[17] and Bruyn's review in the *Handbook of Clinical Neurology*[24] are milestone clinical references. Hemiplegic migraine also has been described in children,[27,98,102] including FHM.[38]

The IHS[92] classifies hemiplegic migraine under migraine with typical aura (IHS 1.2.1) or prolonged aura (IHS 1.2.2.). FHM is classified as a subgroup of migraine with aura (IHS 1.2.3). The working definition includes the criteria for migraine with aura (1.2.1., 1.2.2.) with hemiplegic features that may be prolonged and at least one first-degree relative with identical attacks. As noted above, the overall prevalence of migraine with aura is around 4%; this figure includes hemiplegic migraine. There is no specific information associated with a migraine attack. Clarke[38] published the point that the latter is rare.

Hemiplegic migraine attacks are characterized by hemiparesis or hemiplegia.[24,40,96] The arm and leg are involved in the majority of attacks, often combined with face and hand paresis. Less often, isolated facial and arm paresis occurs. The progression of the motor deficit is slow with a spreading or marching quality. In most cases symptoms are accompanied by homolateral sensory disturbance, particularly cheiro-oral in distribution, again with a slowly spreading or marching quality. Infrequently, the hemiparesis may alternate from side to side, even during an attack. Myoclonic jerks have been reported but are rare. They have been described as Jacksonian, although there is some resemblance to the limb jerking associated with carotid or basilar artery ischemia. Visual disturbance, which takes the form of hemianopic loss or typical visual aura, is common. Homolateral or contralateral localization of the visual disturbance is often obscure, however. When dysphasia occurs, it is more often expressive than receptive. The

neurologic symptoms last 30 to 60 minutes and are followed by severe pulsating headache, hemicranial or whole head in distribution. Nausea, vomiting, photophobia, and phonophobia are associated features. In severe cases, the aura can persist throughout the headache phase.

Manifestations of severe hemiplegic migraine attacks include fever, drowsiness, confusion, and coma, all of which can be prolonged from days to weeks.[137] Severe hemiplegic migraine may lead rarely to persistent minor neurologic deficit, in which the cumulative effect of repeated attacks progresses to profound multifocal neurologic deficit, even dementia.[177]

FHM is characterized by the neurologic deficit described above that is identical in at least one other first-degree relative.[92] There is an autosomal dominant inheritance pattern of the disorder. Other neurologic deficits have been described in association with FHM. Most frequent is a syndrome of progressive cerebellar disturbance, dysarthria, nystagmus, and ataxia.[39,143] Retinitis pigmentosa, sensory neural deafness, tremor, dizziness, and oculomotor disturbances with nystagmus have also been described.[204,205] These neurologic deficits are present between attacks and are not part of the aura. Hemiplegic migraine attacks also may be part of other familial disorders affecting other systems, for example MELAS and CADASIL. Attacks of hemiplegic migraine are less likely to be stereotyped in family members with these conditions, however, because the migraine attack is probably "symptomatic" of the underlying brain disorder.

A recent breakthrough in establishing the cause of FHM was achieved during the clinical investigation of a disease condition termed cerebral autosomal dominant arteriopathy with stroke and ischemic leukoencephalopathy (CADASIL).[8,180] This is characterized by recurring small deep infarcts, dementia, and leukoencephalopathy. Some patients also experience recurrent attacks of severe migraine-like headache with aura symptoms that include transient headache and hemiparesis. Joutel et al[105] studied two large family pedigrees satisfying the IHS criteria for FHM, one with cerebellar signs and the other without. Linkage analysis was performed with a set of DNA markers spanning the most probable location for CADASIL which was mapped recently to chromosome 19. FHM did indeed map to chromosome 19, the most likely location for the gene being a 30 cM interval between D19S216 and D19S215, which encompasses the probable position of the CADASIL locus. But FHM usually has a younger age of onset, only rarely a history of stroke and dementia, no white matter abnormalities on MRI, and a good prognosis. Most recently, Ophoff et al[145] have isolated, on chromosome 19p13.1, a gene encoding the alpha-1 subunit of a brain-specific voltage-gated P/Q type neuronal calcium channel (CACNL1A4) from patients with FHM.

Four different missense mutations were identified in five unrelated FHM families. The investigators also detected premature stops mutations predicted to disrupt the reading frame of CACNL1A4 in two unrelated patients with episodic ataxia type-2 (EA-2). Thus FHM and EA-2 can be considered as allelic channelopathies but of differing molecular mechanism, the former involving a gain of function variant of the Ca^{2+} channel subunit and the latter a decrease in channel density. The results also indicate that different mutations in a single gene may cause phenotypic heterogeneity.

Since this report the same French group identified 10 different missense mutations in the Notch 3 genes of 14 unrelated families with CADASIL. The Notch genes are intimately involved in intercellular signaling during development. Proteins belonging to the Notch family are transmembrane receptors. Nine of the ten mutations either added or mutated a cysteine residue in one of the epidermal growth factor (EGF)-like repeats; EGF-like motifs are to be found in the extracellular domain. It is likely that this mutation strongly affects protein conformation, although how this leads to CADASIL remains to be established. Possibly though, membrane instability and abnormality of cell signaling could be the underlying basis of the migraine attacks in this disorder. The generalizability of the genetic findings in FHM, one of the rarest subtypes of migraine, to the more prevalent migraine subtypes remains to be established. It must be noted that cases of nonfamilial hemiplegic migraine studied by Ophoff et al[145] failed to show mutations. Also, the same group has suggested that chromosome 19 is the locus for migraine with and without aura[125] but review of other studies suggests that this may be controversial.[130] Further, the distribution of the abnormal calcium channel identified is densely cerebellar,[172] a structure not obviously involved in the initiation of a migraine attack. This point is of interest, nevertheless, in view of the occurrence of cerebellar atrophy in a small number of FHM families.[143] It is tempting to speculate that cerebellar atrophy might be explained by abnormal release of excitatory amino acids such as glutamate, which has cytotoxic consequences.

Basilar Migraine

The concept of basilar artery migraine was first proposed by Bickerstaff[9,10] (IHS 1.2.4). The diagnostic criteria include those for migraine with aura plus two or more aura symptoms of the following types: visual symptoms in both the temporal and nasal fields of both eyes, dysarthria, vertigo, tinnitus, decreased hearing, double vision, ataxia, bilateral paresthesias, bilateral paresis, and decreased level of consciousness. The absence of consistent evidence for basilar artery spasm during migraine attacks, and uncertainty about the origin of the mechanisms of the symptoms, prompted the IHS classification committee to remove the word "artery" from the terminology.

Reviewing a personal series of 300 cases, Bickerstaff noticed 34 patients whose attacks were usually heralded by visual disturbances: either complete visual loss or positive phenomena such as teichopsia so dazzling as to obscure the entire field of vision.[9] Other basilar symptoms followed, including dizziness or vertigo, gait ataxia, dysarthria, tinnitus, bilateral acral, perioral, and lingual numbness, or paresthesias. These symptoms persisted for 2 to 60 minutes, ending abruptly, although the visual loss generally recovered more gradually. After the premonitory phase subsided, a severe throbbing occipital headache supervened and was accompanied by vomiting.

These patients recovered completely, and between such attacks many had episodes of classic migraine. Typically affected were adolescent girls. Attacks were usually infrequent strongly related to menstruation. In Bickerstaff's series, all but 2 patients were below 23 years of age and 26 of 34 were girls.[9]

A clear-cut family history of migraine in close relatives was obtained in 82% of cases.

Lapkin et al,[110] encountered this entity in a younger population, reporting a group of 30 children with a mean age at onset of 7 years (range 7 months to 14 years). The duration of episodes ranged from minutes to many hours; one patient was symptomatic for nearly 3 days. Unlike the adolescent cases, the commonest complaint was vertigo (73%), while visual disturbances occurred in 43% of cases. In children more severely affected, pyramidal tract dysfunction was observed as well as cranial nerve abnormalities, including internuclear ophthalmoplegia and facial nerve paresis. A family history of migraine was obtained in 86% of patients. During the follow-up period of 6 months to 3 years, none of the patients showed signs of progressive neurologic dysfunction, although 1 child was mentioned as having developed a permanent oculomotor nerve paralysis. In the majority of cases, the aura lasts between 5 to 60 minutes, but can extend up to 3 days. Visual symptoms commonly occur first, predominantly in the temporal and nasal fields of vision. The visual disturbance may consist of blurred vision, teichopsia, scintillating scotoma, greying of vision, or total loss of vision. The features may start in one visual field and then spread to become bilateral. Bickerstaff pointed out that when vision is not completely obscured, diplopia may occur usually as a sixth nerve weakness. Some form of diplopia may occur in up to 16% of cases.[175] Vertigo and gait ataxia are the next most common symptoms, each occurring in 63% of one series.[175] The ataxia can be independent of vertigo. Tinnitus may accompany vertigo. Dysarthria is as common as ataxia and vertigo. Tingling and numbness, in a typical cheiro-oral spreading pattern seen in migraine with aura, occurs in over 60% of cases. This is usually bilateral and symmetric but may alternate sides with a hemidistribution. Occasionally dysesthesias extend to the trunk. Bilateral motor weakness occurs in more than 50% of cases.

The syndrome of basilar artery migraine (BAM) was later expanded to include alteration in consciousness. Bickerstaff cited four cases in detail and recorded a total of 8 among 32 patients with previously diagnosed BAM.[10] The onset of impaired consciousness occurred in the context of other basilar symptoms with a leisurely onset, not causing the patient to fall or incur self-injury, and was sometimes preceded by a dreamlike state. Ranging from drowsiness to stupor, the altered consciousness was akinetic and usually brief, lasting up to several minutes and not accompanied by rigidity, posturing, tongue biting, urinary incontinence, or changes in the respiratory pattern. Like the usual BAM, a throbbing headache occurred on recovery. Laboratory investigations were generally unrevealing with normal CSF and EEG results. Lee and Lance[115a] encountered seven patients with a similar syndrome of altered consciousness, using the term *migraine stupor*. Unlike the brief episodes observed by Bickerstaff, the duration of stupor ranged from 2 hours to 5 days. Four patients showed aggressive and hysteric behavior during the attacks, leading to initial psychiatric diagnoses. Although impairment of consciousness in some form is common,[175] this progresses to stupor and prolonged coma.[61,114] Other forms of altered consciousness include amnesia and syncope. Drop attacks are rare.

Headache occurs in almost all patients. It has an occipital location in the majority and a throbbing, pounding quality and is accompanied by severe nausea and vomiting. It is unusual for the headache to be unilateral or localized to the more anterior parts of the cranium. Photophobia and phonophobia occur in one-third to one-half of the patients. As with other forms of migraine, the symptoms may occur without headache, but this is usually in no more than 4% of cases.[175] Seizures have been observed in association with basilar migraine.[7] EEG changes without seizures occurring with attacks of typical BAM also have been described. In all, EEG abnormalities are detected in less than one-fifth of cases with basilar migraine[103] and are mostly independent of any clinical manifestation of the disorder.

The EEG findings between attacks are usually spike and wave or spike and slow wave complexes. During an attack, there are diffuse high-voltage slow waves and associated spikes with sharp waves and diffuse beta activity. There is controversy as to whether the association between seizures and basilar migraine are primarily migraine syndromes with secondary epileptic features resulting from functional or ischemic change caused by repeated migraine auras or whether these cases are primarily basilar migraine that evokes epileptogenic features on the EEG and clinical seizures. Permanent brain stem deficits occurring as a result of BAM have been reported rarely. None of Bickerstaff's cases had persisting neurologic disturbances; indeed, he stressed return to complete normality as a criterion for the diagnosis. Among the cases of migraine-associated stroke uncovered in the literature, only four of the five have occurred in the vertebrobasilar territory, excluding the posterior cerebral artery. In Connor's presentation[41] of 18 cases of complicated migraine, 3 were considered to have lesions in the brain stem. In no instance did the transient episodes clearly resemble BAM as defined above. The 1 case described in the text was of a 42-year-old man whose attacks consisted of "right-sided teichopsia, hemianopia, frontal headache and sickness which had occurred every 3 months for 4 years." During the course of an unusually severe attack lasting 2 days, he experienced paresthesias in all limbs. On admission to the hospital, he had a temperature of 104°F, complete ophthalmoplegia, palatal weakness, and left hemiataxia, but normal sensation. CSF was acellular with a protein of 86 mg/dl. An EEG, a pneumoencephalogram, and carotid and vertebral angiograms were all normal. The second patient, a 36-year-old man who had teichopsia, visual loss, hemiparesis, and vomiting during his transient attacks was left with nystagmus on lateral gaze and a sensorimotor deficit following a migraine attical seizure. Angiography was normal. The third patient, a 35-year-old woman who had a 12-year history of headaches with vomiting, presumably common migraine, developed left facial palsy and right hemiparesis during the course of an attack. Angiography in this case was also normal.

Spaccavento and Solomon reported an unusual patient, an otherwise healthy 21-year-old man who had a 2-year history of occipital headaches preceded by ataxia, vertigo, and visual disturbances.[171a] Treatment with propranolol led to an "excellent response." Following discontinuation of this medication, the patient experienced a recurrence of BAM attacks. At some point after the second attack, he abruptly developed vertigo, nausea, and gait ataxia. The neurologic examination revealed a complete lateral medullary syndrome. Blood pressure and routine laboratory studies were unremarkable. Angiography revealed a total occlusion of the left vertebral artery. "The

tapering of the vessel just proximal to the obstruction was considered highly suggestive of vasospasm" according to the authors, but the published angiogram pictures are more consistent with arterial dissection. The patient reported by Cohen and Taylor[39a] suffered a series of devastating strokes in both carotid and vertebrobasilar territories. At the age of 20, he developed episodic throbbing occipital headache preceded by diplopia, dysarthria, perioral and left arm numbness, left arm paresis and scotoma lasting for 2 hours. The first episode of prolonged neurologic dysfunction occurred at the age of 29, when he presented with left hemiparesis, hemianesthesia, hemiataxia, tinnitus, and dysarthria accompanied by headache, nausea, and vomiting. The blood pressure was 236/142 and the EEG showed evidence of an old inferior wall myocardial infarction. The hemiparesis disappeared in several weeks. Four-vessel arteriography was normal. Seventeen months later, he had an episode of left hemiparesis, slurred speech, photophobia, and occipital headache. Blood pressure was 140/100 and he had minimal left-sided incoordination. He was treated with propranolol. After 16 months, 2 days after the propranolol dosage was reduced, he experienced a 1-hour episode of perioral paresthesia and photophobia; 1 month later, he abruptly developed left hemiplegia, sensory loss, and hemianopia. The blood pressure was 170/100. CT scan revealed nonenhancing low densities in the left frontal, left cerebellar, and right parieto-occipital areas on the first day, with enhancement of the latter lesion on the eighth day. A four-vessel angiogram performed on the seventh hospital day was again normal. Laboratory studies for hypercoagulability, vasculitis, homocystinuria, sickle cell disease, and hyperlipidemia were all unremarkable.

Cerebral infarction specifically affecting the brain stem circulation territory understandably has been offered as evidence for a primary vascular cause of basilar migraine. Skinhoj and Paulson in studies performed during the migraine aura found, despite reduction of CBF, that angiography was normal except for impaired filling in the top of the basilar artery.[169a] Frequin et al have provided a dramatic angiographic illustration of basilar artery spasm obtained from a 28-year-old male with basilar migraine complicated by coma.[70a] Cerebral angiography can itself precipitate migraine aura, however, albeit after a time lag of hours. Nevertheless, the combination of the clinical features plus the arteriographic studies mentioned above, emphasizes a primary vascular alternative for the cause of basilar migraine. Cerebrovascular disease is the most serious differential diagnosis of basilar migraine.

Ischemic stroke in the brain stem and posterior cortical regions, either due to cerebral embolism or thrombosis, presents with a constellation of neurologic symptoms and signs of brain stem and posterior circulation defects accompanied in approximately one-third of cases by headache. Basilar artery occlusive disease can, therefore, mimic basilar migraine. Another basilar migraine "mimic" and for which migraine patients are at increased risk is vertebral artery dissection (see above).

The clinical features of embolic and thrombotic infarction in the PCA syndrome have been elegantly described by C. M. Fisher.[65] The warning features of PCA ischemia include photopsia with single and formed visual hallucinations, hemianopic visual loss, transient numbness, episodic light headedness, confusional spells, tinnitus and headache. When stroke becomes established, however, visual complaints are the most dominant. Of importance in the differential diagnosis of basilar migraine, scintillations or shimmering brightness in the visual fields did not occur during transient ischemia, but did occur after occipital lobe infarction was established. Thus, PCA ischemia alone can mimic basilar migraine.

Transient ischemic attacks involving any part of the vertebrobasilar territory must figure largely in the differential diagnosis, particularly if basilar migraine presents for the first time in later years of life. Certain familial disorders present with neurologic deficit in which attacks of hemiplegic or basilar migraine may be part of the symptom complex. This group includes CADASIL, MELAS, and variants of MELAS that are associated with seizures, particularly occipital in origin.[53]

Mechanisms

From the above review it should be apparent that migraine can mimic cerebrovascular disorders, especially ischemic stroke, and stroke can mimic migraine. This poses diagnostic problems for the clinician that in most cases will be resolved. It is uncertain how much of the past literature on migraine-induced stroke described cerebrovascular disorders that were mistaken for migraine. This is not to criticize these earlier reports but to recognize that they were communicated at a time when diagnostic tools were less well developed and that concepts of migraine mechanisms have changed. It remains to be determined how a migraine attack can induce permanent neurologic deficit and brain damage. Perhaps even more intriguing, what constitutes the comorbid increased risk for stroke between attacks? The latter is the most difficult to speculate on because, although comorbid factors may be present (such as increased platelet aggregation or mitral valve prolapse) many are uncertain risk factors for stroke. Indeed, when definite risk factors for stroke are present in migraine sufferers then the stroke is attributed to this cause and not to migraine. On the basis of the epidemiologic data described, however, there must be stroke risk factors yet to be identified that are comorbid with migraine. With regard to the mechanisms whereby stroke is induced during a migraine attack, there is information that provides some limited understanding. The current literature on CBF was reviewed above. To summarize, spreading cortical depression of Leao may induce short-lived increases in CBF followed by a more profound oligemia. Ischemic foci, however, may occasionally occur during attacks of migraine with aura. Possibly, SD is also associated with depolarization of intrinsic neurons that also supply intraparenchymal resistance microvessels, leading to constriction and a consequent flow reduction below the threshold for K^+ release from the neuron. Increased extracellular K^+ then might precipitate depolarization of contiguous cortical neurons. Alternatively, the decreased extracellular space and brain swelling that accompanies spreading cortical depression and possibly migraine could increase microvascular resistance by mechanical compression. Thus, low flow in major intracerebral vessels may be due to increased downstream resistance, not major intracranial arterial vasospasm. Essentially, a low cerebral blood flow and sluggish flow in large intracerebral vessels dur-

ing the aura of migraine when combined with factors predisposing to coagulopathy, could lead, although rarely, to intravascular thrombosis and, thus, migraine-induced cerebral infarction. Release of vasoactive peptides, endothelin, activation of cytokines, and upregulation of adhesion molecules during the neurogenically mediated inflammatory response that may be responsible for headache also may induce intravascular thrombosis. This could explain why migraine-induced stroke usually respects intracranial arterial territories although the aura involves more widespread brain regions. In addition, frequent aura, if due to spreading depression, could induce cytotoxic cell damage and gliosis based on glutamate release or excess intracellular calcium accumulation. This could explain persistent neurologic deficit without evidence of ischemic infarction on the basis of selective neuronal necrosis. Increased extracellular K^+ that might precipitate rarely during episodes of migraine probably relates to variability in the coagulation status, degree of the neuronal and hemodynamic changes, and the interaction of each during the course of the migraine attack.

References

1. Adams HP, Putnam SF, Corbett JJ et al: Amaurosis fugax: the results of arteriography in 59 patients. Stroke 5:742, 1983
2. Adie WJ: Permanent hemianopia in migraine and subarachnoid hemorrhage. Lancet 2:237, 1930
3. Aellig WH: Agonists and antagonists of 5-hydroxytryptamine on veno-motor receptors. Adv Neurol 33:321, 1982
4. Alvarez J, Matias-Guiu J, Sumalla J et al: Ischemic stroke in young adults 1. Analysis of the etiological subgroups. Acta Neurol Scand 80:28, 1989
5. Baker HL: Computerized transaxial tomography (EMI scan) in the diagnosis of cerebral vascular disease. Experience at the Mayo Clinic. p. 195. In Whisnant JP (ed): Cerebral Vascular Diseases. Ninth Conference. Grune & Stratton, Orlando, FL, 1975
6. Barkley GL, Tepley N, Simkins RT et al: Neuromagnetic fields in migraine: preliminary findings. Cephalalgia 10: 171, 1990
7. Basser LS: The relation of migraine and epilepsy. Brain 92:285, 1969
8. Baudrimont M, Dubas F, Joutel A et al: Autosomal dominant leukoencephalopathy and subcortical ischemic stroke: a clinicopathological study. Stroke 24:122, 1993
9. Bickerstaff ER: Basilar artery migraine. Lancet 15, 1961a
10. Bickerstaff ER: The basilar artery and migraine-epilepsy syndrome. Proc R Soc Med 55:167, 1962
11. Blau JN, Whitty CWM: Familial hemiplegic migraine. Lancet 2:1115, 1955
12. Blend R, Bull JWD: The radiological investigation of migraine. p. 1. In Smith RA (ed): Background to Migraine. First Migraine Symposium. William Heinemann Medical Books, London, 1967

13. Boisen E: Strokes in migraine: report on seven strokes associated with severe migraine attacks. Dan Med Bull 22:100, 1975

14. Bogousslavsky J, Regli F: Ischemic stroke in adults younger than 30 years of age. Cause and prognosis. Arch Neurol 44:479, 1987

15. Bogousslavsky J, Regli F, Van Melle G et al: Migraine stroke. Neurology 38:223, 1988

16. Bousser MG, Baron JC, Iba-Zizen MT et al: Migrainous cerebral infarction: a tomographic study of cerebral blood flow and oxygen extraction fraction with the oxygen-15 inhalation technique. Stroke 11:145, 1980

17. Bradshaw P, Parsons M: Hemiplegic migraine: a clinical study. Q J Med 34:65, 1965

18. Brain R: Cerebral vascular disorders. Lancet 2:831, 1954

19. Bright R: Cases illustrative of the effects produced when the arteries of the brain are diseased. Selected chiefly with a view to the diagnosis in such affections. Guy's Hospital Reports 1 (Senes 1):9, 1836

20. Broderick JP, Swanson JW: Migraine-related strokes: clinical profile and prognosis in 20 patients. Arch Neurol 44:868, 1987

21. Brohult J, Forsberg O, Hellstrom R: Multiple arterial thrombosis after oral contraceptives and ergotamine. Acta Med Scand 181:453, 1967

22. Brown GC, Magargal LE, Shields JA et al: Retinal arterial obstruction in children and young adults. Ophthalmology 88:18, 1981

23. Bruyn GW: Cerebral cortex and migraine. Adv Neurol 33:151, 1982

24. Bruyn GW: Complicated migraine. p. 59. In Vinken PJ, Bruyn GW (eds): Handbook of Clinical Neurology. Vol 5. North Holland Publishing Co., Amsterdam, 1968

25. Bruyn GW, Weenink HR: Migraine accompagnee. A critical evaluation. Headache 6:1, 1966

26. Buckle RM, Du Boulay G, Smith B: Death due to vasospasm. J Neurol Neurosurg Psychiatr 27:440, 1964

27. Burke EC, Peters GA: Migraine in childhood: a preliminary report. AJDC 92:330, 1956

28. Burns RJ, Blumbergs PC, Sage MR: Brain infarction in young men. Clin Exp Neurol 16:69, 1979

29. Butler TH: Scotoma in migrainous subjects. Br J Ophthalmol 17:83, 1933

30. Cala LA, Mastaglia FL: Computerized axial tomography findings in patients with migrainous headaches. Br Med J 2:149, 1976

31. Cala LA, Mastaglia FL: Computerized tomography in the detection of brain damage. 2. Epilepsy, migraine, and general medical disorders. Med J Aust 2:616, 1980

32. Caldwell A, Kennedy R: Migraine headaches with pre-headache retinal and visual disturbances in a case of congenital vascular anomaly and subarachnoid hemorrhage. Arch Neurol Psychiatry 61:397, 1953

33. Caplan L: Intracerebral hemorrhage revisited. Neurology 38:624, 1988

33a. Carolei A, Marini C, De Matteis G: History of migraine and risk of cerebral ischaemia in young adults. The Italian National Research Council Study Group on Stroke in the Young. Lancet 347:1503, 1996

34. Carroll D: Retinal migraine. Headache 10:9, 1970

35. Castaigne P, Brunet P, Peirrot-Deseilligny C, Roullet E: Accidents deficitaires neurologiques centraux et migraine. Ann Med Interne 134:306, 1983

36. Castaldo JE, Anderson DMS, Reeves AG: Middle cerebral artery occlusion with migraine. Stroke 13:308, 1982

37. Charcot JM: Sur un cas de migraine ophtalmologique (paralysie oculomotrice periodique). Progr Med 18:83, 1890

38. Clarke JM: On recurrent motor paralysis in migraine, with a report in which recurrent hemiplegia accompanied the attacks. Br Med J 2:1534, 1910

39. Codina A, Acarini PN, Miguel F: Migraine hemiplegique associee a un nystagmus. Rev Neurol 124:526, 1971

39a. Cohen RJ, Taylor JR: Persistent neurologic sequelae of migraine: a case report. Neurology 29:1175, 1979

40. Collaborative Group for the Study of Stroke in Young Women: Oral contraception and increased risk of cerebral ischemia or thrombosis. N Engl J Med 288:871, 1973

41. Connor RCR: Complicated migraine. A study of permanent neurological and visual defects caused by migraine. Lancet 2:1072, 1962

42. Conway LW, McDonald LW: Structural changes of the intradural arteries following subarachnoid hemorrhage. J Neurosurg 37:715, 1972

43. Corbett JJ: Neuro-ophthalmic complications of migraine and cluster headaches. p. 973. In Packard, RC: Neurologic Clinics. Vol 1. WB Saunders, Philadelphia, 1983

44. Cowan CL, Knox DL: Migraine optic neuropathy. Ann Ophthalmol 14:164, 1982

45. Crowell GF, Carlin L, Biller J: Neurologic complications of migraine. Am Fam Physician 26:139, 1982

45a. Cuetter AC, Aita JF: CT scanning in classic migraine. Headache 23:195, 1983

46. Dassen R: Jacqueca oftalmoplejica con paralisis recidivante del III par craneano: muerte en el segundo ataque: necropsia. Semana Med 1:1049, 1931

47. Davis-Jones A, Gregory MC, Whitty CWM: Permanent sequelae in the migraine attack. p. 25. In Cummings JN (ed): Background to Migraine (Fifth Symposium). Springer-Verlag, New York, 1972

47a. du Boulay GH, Ruiz JS, Rose FC, Stevens JM, Zilkha KJ: CT changes associated with migraine. Am J Neuroradiol 4:472, 1983

48. Desrossiers JJ: Headaches related to contraceptive therapy and their control. Headache 13:117, 1973

49. Dorfman LJ, Marshall WH, Enzmann DR: Cerebral infarction and migraine: clinical and radiologic correlations. Neurology 29:317, 1979

50. Dukes HT, Vieth RG: Cerebral arteriography during migraine prodrome and headache. Neurology 14:636, 1964

51. Dunning HS: Intracranial and extracranial vascular accidents in migraine. Arch Neurol Psychiatry 48:392, 1942

52. Dvorkin G, Andermann F, Melancank D et al: Malignant migraine syndrome: classical migraine, occipital seizures, and alternating strokes, abstracted. Neurology 34:245, 1984

53. Dvorkin GS, Andermann F, Carpenter S et al: Classical migraine, intractable epilepsy, and multiple strokes: a syndrome related to mitochondrial encephalomyopathy. pp. 203–232. In Andermann F, Lugaresi E (eds): Migraine and Epilepsy. Butterworth, Stoneham, MS, 1987

54. Edmeads J: Complicated migraine and headache in cerebrovascular disease. Neurol Clin 1:385, 1983

55. Edmeads J: The headaches of ischemic cerebrovascular disease. Headache 19:127, 1979

56. Edmeads J, Barnett HJM: La cephalea en las affeciones cerebrovasculares occlusivas. p. 89. In Friedman AP, Poch GF (eds): Cephaleas Y Jacquecas. Eudeba, Buenos Aires, Argentina, 1973

57. Edmeads JG, Hachinski VC, Norris JW: Ergotamine and the cerebral circulation. Hemicrania 7:6, 1976

58. Fein JM, Flor WJ, Cohan SL, Parkhurst J: Sequential changes of vascular ultrastructure in experimental cerebral vasospasm. J Neurosurg 41:49, 1974

59. Fere C: Contribution a l'etude de la migraine ophtalmique. Rev Med Paris 1:40, 1881

60. Fere C: Note sur un cas de migraine ophtalmique a access repetes suivis de mort. Rev Med Paris 3:194, 1883

61. Ferguson KS, Robinson SS: Life-threatening migraine. Arch Neurol 39:374, 1982

62. Fisher CM: Clinical syndromes in cerebral arterial occlusion. p. 126. In Fields WS (ed): Pathogenesis and Treatment of Cerebrovascular Disease. Charles C Thomas, Springfield, IL, 1961

63. Fisher CM: The headache and pain of spontaneous carotid dissection. Headache 22:60, 1982

64. Fisher CM: Headache in cerebrovascular disease. p. 124. In Vinken PJ, Bruyn GW (eds): Handbook of Clinical Neurology. Vol 5. North-Holland Publishing Co., Amsterdam, 1968

65. Fisher CM: Late-life migraine accompaniments as a cause of unexplained transient ischemic attacks. Can J Med Sci 7:9, 1980

66. Fisher CM: Migraine accompaniments versus arteriosclerotic ischemia. Trans Am Neurol Assoc 93:211, 1968

67. Fisher CM: Observations of the fundus oculi in transient monocular blindness. Neurology 9:333, 1959

68. Fisher CM: Occlusion of the internal carotid artery. Arch Neurol Psychiatry 65:346, 195

69. Fisher CM: Reader's benign paratrigeminal syndrome with dysgeusia. Trans Am Neurol Assoc 96:234, 1972

70. Fitzsimons R, Wolfenden WH: Migraine coma: meningetic migraine with cerebral edema associated with a new form of autosomal dominant cerebellar ataxia. Brain 108:555, 1985

70a. Frequin ST, Linssen WH, Pasman JW, et al: Recurrent prolonged coma due to basilar artery migraine. A case report. Headache 31:75, 1991

71. Friedman MW: Occlusion of the central retinal vein in migraine. Arch Ophthalmol 45:678, 1951

72. Galezowski X: Ophthalmic megrim. Lancet 1:176, 1882

73. Gardner-Medwin AR, Tepley N, Barkley GL et al: Magnetic fields associated with spreading depression in anesthetized rabbits. Brain Res 562:153, 1991

74. Garnic JD, Schellinger D: Arterial spasm as a finding intimately associated with onset of vascular headache. Neuroradiology 24:273, 1983

75. Gelmers HJ: The pericarotid syndrome. A combination of hemicrania, Horner's syndrome, and internal carotid artery wall lesion. Acta Neurochirurgica 57:37, 1981

76. Glaser JS: Neuro-ophthalmology. Vol 2. Harper & Row, New York, 1978

77. Goadsby PJ, Edvinsson L, Ekman R: Release of vasoactive peptides in the extracerebral circulation of men and the cat during activation of the trigeminovascular system. Ann Neurol 23:193, 1988

78. Goldflamm S: Beitrag zur Aetiologie und Symptomatologie der spontanen subarachnoidealen Blutungen. Disch Z Neervenheilk 76:158, 1923

79. Goodwin JA, Gorelick P, Helgason C: Transient monocular visual loss: amaurosis fugax or migraine, abstracted. Neurology 34(Suppl. 1):246, 1984

80. Graftstein B: Mechanism of spreading cortical depression. J Neurophysiol 19:154, 1956

81. Graveson GS: Retinal arterial occlusion in migraine. Br Med J 2:838, 1949

82. Grindal A, Toole J: Headache and transient ischemic attacks. Stroke 5:603, 1975

83. Gronvall H: On changes in the fundus oculi and persisting injuries to the eye in migraine. Acta Ophthalmol 16(Suppl 14–16):602, 1938

84. Group for the Study of Stroke in Young Women: Oral contraceptives and stroke in young women. JAMA 231:718, 1975

85. Guest IA, Wolf AL: Fatal infarction of the brain. Br Med J 1:225, 1964

86. Hachinski VC, Norris JW, Cooper PW, Edmeads JG: Ergotamine tartrate and cerebral blood flow. Can J Neurol Sci 2:333, 1975

87. Hachinski VC, Porchawka J, Steele JC: Visual symptoms in the migraine syndrome. Neurology 23:570, 1973

88. Harrington DO: Ophthalmoplegic migraine. A discussion of its pathogenesis: report of the pathological findings in a case of recurrent oculomotor palsy. Arch Ophthalmol 49:643, 1953

89. Harrison MJG: Hemiplegic migraine (letter). J Neurol Neurosurg Psychiatry 44:652, 1981

90. Hart RG, Easton JD: Dissection of cervical and cerebral arteries. Neurol Clin 1:155, 1983

91. Hayreh SS: Pathogenesis of visual field defects: role of ciliary circulation. Br J Ophthalmol 54:289, 1970

92. Headache Classification Committee of the International Headache Society: Classification and diagnostic criteria for headache disorders, cranial neuralgias, and facial pain. Cephalalgia 8:27, 1988

93. Hedges TR: An ophthalmologist's view of headache. Headache 19:151, 1979

94. Henrich JB, Horowitz RI: A controlled study of ischemic stroke risk in migraine patients. J Clin Epidemiol 42:773, 1989

95. Henrich JB, Sandercock PAG, Warlow CP, Jones LN: Stroke and migraine in the Oxfordshire Community Stroke Project. J Neurol 233:257, 1986

96. Heyck H: Neue Beitrage zur Klinik und Pathogenese der Migrane. G. Thieme Verlag, Stuttgart, Germany, 1956

97. Heyck H: Pathogenesis of migraine. Res Clin Stud Headache 2:1, 1969

98. Holguin J, Fenichel G: Migraine. J Pediatrics 70:290, 1967

99. Hughes JT, Schianchi M: Cerebral artery spasm. A histological study at necropsy of the blood vessels in cases of subarachnoid hemorrhage. J Neurosurg 48:515, 1978

100. Hungerford GD, Du Boulay GH, Zilkha KJ: Computer-

ized axial tomography in patients with severe migraine: a preliminary report. J Neurol Neurosurg Psychiatry 39: 990, 1976

101. Hunt JR: A contribution to the paralytic and other persistent sequelae of migraine. Am J Med Sci 150:313, 1915

102. Isler W: Acute hemiplegia and hemisyndromes in childhood. In Clinics in Developmental Medicine. Heinemann Medical, London, 1971. pp. 41–42

103. Jacome DE: EEG features in basilar artery migraine. Headache 27:80, 1987

104. Joffe SN: Retinal blood vessel diameter during migraine. The Eye, Ear, Nose and Throat Monthly 52:338, 1973

105. Joutel A, Bousser M-G, Biousse V et al: A gene for familial hemiplegic migraine maps to chromosome 19. Nature Genetics 5:4045, 1993

106. Julien J, Laguey A, Darriet D: Infarctus cerebral au cours d'un acces migraineux. Sem Hop Paris 55:810, 1979

107. Kaul SN, du Boulay GH, Kendall BE, Russel WR: Relationship between visual field defect and arterial occlusion in the posterior cerebral circulation. J Neurol Neurosurg Psychiatry 37:1022, 1974

108. Kittner SJ, McCarer RJ, Sherwin RW et al: Black-white differences, in stroke risk among young adults. Stroke 24 (Suppl 1):113, 1993

109. Kline LB, Kelly CL: Ocular migraine in a patient with cluster headaches. Headache 20:253, 1980

110. Lapkin ML, French JH, Golden GS: The EEG in childhood basilar artery migraine. Neurology 27:580, 1977

111. Lashley K. Patterns of cerebral integration indicated by the scotomas of migraine. Arch Neurol Psychiatry 46: 333, 1941

112. Lauritzen M: Links between cortical spreading depression and migraine: clinical and experimental aspects. In Olesen J (ed): Migraine and Other Headaches: the Vascular Mechanism. Vol. 1. Raven Press, New York, 1991. pp. 143–151

113. Lauritzen M, Olsen TS, Lassen NA, Paulson OB: The role of spreading depression in acute brain disorders. Ann Neurol 14:569, 1983

114. Lawall JS, Oommen JK: Basilar artery migraine presenting as conversion hysteria. J Nerv Ment Dis 166:809, 1978

115. Leao AAP: Spreading depression of activity in cerebral cortex. J Neurophysiol 7:379, 1944

115a. Lee CH, Lance JW: Migraine stupor. Headache 17:32, 1977

116. Leno C, Berciano J, Combarros O et al: A prospective study of stroke in young adults in Cantabria, Spain. Stroke 24:792, 1993

117. Leviton A, Malvea B, Graham JR: Vascular disease, mortality, and migraine in the parents of migraine patients. Neurology 24:669, 1975

118. Lieberman MF, Maumenee AE, Green RW: Histologic studies of the vasculature of the anterior optic nerve. Am J Ophthalmol 82:405, 1968

119. Liveing E: On megrim, sick-headache, and some allied disorders: a contribution to the pathology of nerve-storms. J & A Churchill, London, 1873

120. Lohlein W: Erblindung durch Migrane. Dtsch Med Wehnsche 48:1408, 1922

121. Marini C, Carolei A, Roberts RS et al: Focal cerebral ischemia in young adults: a collaborative case-control study. Neuroepidemiol 12:70, 1993

122. Masuzawa T, Shinoda S, Furuse M et al: Cerebral angiographic changes on serial examination of a patient with migraine. Neuroradiology 24:277, 1983

123. Mathew NT: Complicated migraine and differential diagnosis of migraine. p. 9. In Mathew RJ (ed): Treatment of Migraine. Pharmacological and Biofeedback Considerations. Spectrum Publications, New York, 1981

124. Mathew NT: Computerized axial tomography in migraine. p. 63. In Greene R (ed): Current Concepts in Migraine Research. Lippincott-Raven, Philadelphia, 1978

125. May A, Ophoff RA, Terwindt GM et al: Familial hemiplegic migraine locus on 19p13 is involved in the common forms of migraine with and without aura. Hum Genet 96:604, 1995

126. McDonald WI, Sanders MD: Migraine complicated by ischemic papillopathy. Lancet 1:521, 1971

127. Medina J, Diamond S, Rubino S: Headaches in patients with transient ischemic attacks. Headache 15:194, 1975

128. Ment LR, Duncan CC, Parcells PR, Collins FC: Evaluation of complicated migraine in childhood. Child's Brain 7:261, 1980

129. Merhoff GC, Porter JM: Ergot intoxication: historical review and description. Ann Surg 180:773, 1974

130. Merikangas KR: Genetics of migraine and other headache. Curr Opin Neurol 9:202, 1996

131. Milner PM: Note on a possible correspondence between scotomas of migraine and spreading depression of Leao. Electroencephalogr Clin Neurophysiol 910:705, 1958

131a. Mitsias P, Ramadan NM: Headache in ischemic cerebrovascular disease. Part I: Clinical features. Part II: Mechanisms and predictive value. Cephalalgia 12:269, 341, 1992

132. Moen M, Levine SR, Newman DS et al: Bilateral posterior cerebral artery strokes in a young migraine sufferer. Stroke 19:525, 1988

133. Mokri B: Spontaneous dissections of cervicocephalic arteries. In Welch KMA, Caplan LR, Peis DJ et al (eds): Primer on Cerebrovascular Disease. Academic Press, San Diego, 1997. pp. 390–396

134. Moorehead MT, Movius HJ, Moorehead JR et al: Classic migraine with cerebral cortical infarction causing permanent hemianopsia. South Med J 72:821, 1979

135. Morenas L, Dechaume J: Migraine aphasique et monoplegique. Etude anatomo-clinique. Les rapports de la migraine avec l'epilepsie. J Med Lyon 10:259, 1929

136. Moskowitz, MA: The neurobiology of vascular head pain. Ann Neurol 16:157, 1984

137. Munte TJ, Muller-Vahl H: Familial migraine coma: a case study. J Neurol 237:59, 1990

138. Murphy JP: Cerebral infarction in migraine. Neurology 5:359, 1955

139. Myhrman G: Migrainous attacks with persistent brain lesions. Acta Medica Scand 181:583, 1967

140. Nappi G, Bono G: Headaches and transient cerebral ischemia: comments on Welch's report. Adv Neurol 33: 41, 1982

141. Neligan P, Harriman DGF, Pearce J: Respiratory arrest

in familial hemiplegic migraine: a clinical and neuro-pathological study. Br Med J 2:732, 1977

142. O'Connor PJ: Strokes in migraine. p. 40. In Cummings JN (ed): Background to Migraine (Fifth Symposium). Springer-Verlag, New York, 1972

143. Ohta M, Araki S, Kuroiwa Y: Familial occurrence of migraine with a hemiplegic syndrome and cerebellar manifestations. Neurology 17:813, 1967

144. Olesen J, Larsen B, Lauritzen M: Focal hyperemia followed by spreading oligemia and impaired activation of RCBF in classic migraine. Ann Neurol 9:344, 1981

145. Ophoff RA, Terwindt GM, Vergouwe MN et al: Familial hemiplegic migraine and episodic ataxia type-2 are caused by mutations in the Ca^{+2} channel gene CAC-NL1A4. Cell 87:543, 1996

146. Oppenheim H: Casuistischer Beitrag zur Prognose der Hemikranie. Charite-Annalen, 15:298, 1890

147. Ormond AW: Two cases of permanent hemianopsia following severe attacks of migraine. Ophthalmol Rev 32:192, 1913

148. Pearce J: The ophthalmological complications of migraine. J Neurol Sci 6:73, 1968

149. Pearce JMS, Foster JB: An investigation of complicated migraine. Neurology 15:323, 1965

150. Pessin MS, Duncan GW, Mohr JP, Poskanzer DC: Clinical and angiographic features of carotid transient ischemic attacks. N Engl J Med 296:358, 1977

151. Peters R: Todliche gehirnblutung bei menstrueller migrane. Beitr Pathol 93:209, 1934

152. Phillips BM: Oral contraceptives and migraine. Br Med J 2:99, 1968

153. Polyak S: The Vertebrate Visual System. University of Chicago Press, Chicago, 1957

154. Ramadan NM, Tietjen GE, Levine SR, Welch KMA: Scintillating scotoma associated with internal carotid artery dissection. Neurology 41:1084, 1991

155. Rascol A, Cambier J, Guiraud B et al: Accidents ischemiques cerebraux au cours de crises migraineuses. A propos des migraines compliquees. Rev Neurol (Paris) 135:867, 1979

156. Rascol A, Clanet M, Rascol O: Cerebrovascular accidents complicating migraine attacks. p. 110. In Rose FC, Amory WK (eds): Cerebral Hypoxia in the Pathogenesis of Migraine. Pitman Books Limited, London, 1982

157. Raskin NE, Prusiner S: Carotidynia. Neurology 27:43, 1977

158. Rasmussen J, Olesen J: Migraine with aura and migraine without aura: an epidemiological study. Cephalalgia 12:221, 1992

159. Ray BS, Wolff HG: Experimental studies on headache. Pain-sensitive structures of the head and their significance in headache. Arch Surg 41:813, 1940

160. Rich WM: Permanent quadrantanopsia after migraine. Br Med J 116:592, 1948

161. Richter AM, Banker VP: Carotid ergotism. Radiology 106:339, 1973

162. Robinson BE: Permanent homonymous migrainous scotomata. Arch Ophthalmol 53:566, 1955

163. Romain LF: Stroke as a complication of migraine disease. J Ind State Med Assoc 74:506, 1981

164. Rosenstein AM: Beitrag Zu den beiderseitigen Verdun-

kelungen des Sehvermogens mit vorübergehenden ophthalmoskopischen Befund bei Herzklappenfehler. Klin Mbl Augenheilk 75:357, 1925

165. Rothrock J, North J, Madden K et al: Migraine and migrainous stroke: risk factors and prognosis. Neurology 43:2473, 1993

165a.Ruiz JS, du Boulay GH, Zilkha KJ, Rose FC: The abnormal CT scan in migraine patients. In Rose FC, Amory WK (eds): Cerebral Hypoxia in the Pathogenesis of Migraine. Pitman Books Limited, London, 1982

165b.Sargent JD, Solbach P: Medical evaluation of migraineurs: review of the value of laboratory and radiologic tests. Headache 23:62, 1983

166. Saudeau D, Larmande P, Odier F, Autret A: Migraine compliquee, epilepsie et hypodensite tomodensitometrique. Rev Neurol (Paris), 138:787, 1982

167. Senter HJ, Lieberman AN, Pinto R: Cerebral manifestations of ergotism. Report of a case and review of the literature. Stroke 7:88, 1976

168. Shuaib A, Hachinski VC: Migraine and the risks from angiography. Arch Neurol 45:911, 1988

169. Sinclair W: Dissecting aneurysm of the middle cerebral artery associated with migraine syndrome. Am J Pathol 29:1083, 1953

169a.Skinhoj E, Paulson OB: Regional blood flow in internal carotid distribution during migraine attack. Br Med J 6:569, 1969

170. Skyhoj-Olsen TS, Friberg L, Lassen NA: Ischemia may be the primary cause of the neurologic deficits in classic migraine. Arch Neurol 44:156, 1987

171. Sorensen AG, Cutrer FM, Moskowitz MA, Rosen BR: Investigation of Spontaneous Migraine Aura in Humans Using Functional MRI. Proceedings of the International Society for Magnetic Resonance in Medicine, 4th Annual Meeting and Exhibition, New York 1:282, 1996

171a.Spaccavento LJ, Solomon GD: Migraine as an etiology of stroke in young adults. Headache. 24:19, 1984

172. Starr TVB, Prystay W, Snutch TP: Primary structure of a calcium channel that is highly expressed in the rat cerebellum. Proc Natl Acad Sci U S A 88:5623, 1991

173. Stewart WF, Lipton RB, Celentano DD, Reed ML: Prevalence of migraine headache in the United States. JAMA 267:64, 1992

174. Stone GM, Burns RJ: Cerebral infarction caused by vasospasm. Med J Aust 1:556, 1982

175. Sturzenegger MH, Meienberg O: Basilar artery migraine: a follow-up study of 82 cases. Headache 25:408, 1985

176. Symonds C: The circle of Willis. Br Med J 1:119, 1956

177. Symonds C: Migrainous variants. Trans Med Soc Lond 67:237, 1952

178. Thomas JJ: Migraine and hemianopsia. J Nerv Ment Dis 34:153, 1907

178a.Tietjen GE, Levine SR, Brown E, et al: Factors that predict antiphospholipid immunoreactivity in young people with transient focal neurological events. Arch Neurol 50:833, 1993

179. Torda C, Wolff HG: Experimental studies on headache: transient thickening of walls of cranial arteries in relation to certain phenomena of migraine headache and action

of ergotamine tartrate on thickened walls. Arch Neurol Psychiatry 53:329, 1945

180. Tournier-Lasserve E, Iba-Zizen MT, Romero N, Bousser MG: Autosomal dominant syndrome with stroke-like episodes and leukoencephalopathy. Stroke 22:1297, 1991

181. Troost BT: Migraine. In Glaser JS (ed): Neuro-ophthalmology, Vol 2. Harper & Row, New York, 1978

182. Troost BT: Migraine and facial pain. p. 288. In Lessell S, Van Dalen JTW (eds): Neuro-ophthalmology. Vol 2. Excerpta Medical, Princeton, NJ, 1982

183. Tzourio C, Iglesias S, Hubert J-B et al: Migraine and risk of ischemic stroke: a case-controlled study. Br Med J 307:289, 1993

184. Tzourio C, Tehindrazanarivelo A, Iglesias S et al: Case-control study of migraine and risk of ischaemic stroke in young women. Br Med J 310:830, 1995

185. Van Harreveld A: The nature of the chick's magnesium-sensitive retinal spreading depression. J Neurobiol 15:333, 1984

186. Walsh WB, Hoyt WF: Clinical Neuro-ophthalmology. Vol. 2. Williams & Wilkins, Baltimore, 1969

187. Walton JN: Subarachnoid Hemorrhage. Livingstone Ltd., London, 1956

188. Weber LW, Runge W: Storungen und Verandewnger des Sehappartas bei Psychosen und Neurosen. p. 800. In Schieck R, Bruckner A (eds): Kurzes Handbuch der Ophthalmologie. Vol. 6. Julius Springer, Berlin, 1931

189. Wegner W: Augenspiegelbefunde bei Migrane. Klin Monatsbl Augenh 76:194, 1926

190. Weiller C, May A, Limmroth V et al: Brainstem activation in human migraine attacks. Nat Med 1:658, 1995

191. Weiner A: A case of permanent homonymous hemianopia following an attack of migraine. Med Record 99:849, 1921

192. Weinstein JM, Feman SS: Ischemic optic neuropathy in migraine. Arch Ophthalmol 100:1097, 1982

193. Welch KMA: Migraine is a biobehavioural disorder. Arch Neurol 44:323, 1987

194. Wells C: Premonitory symptoms in cerebral embolism. Arch Neurol 5:490, 1961

195. Whitty CWM: Familial hemiplegic migraine. J Neurol Neurosurg Psychiatry 16:172, 1953

196. Whitty CWM: Migraine without headache. Lancet 2:283, 1967

197. Whitty CWM, Hockaday JM, Whitty MM: The effect of oral contraceptives in migraine. Lancet 1:856, 1966

198. Wilbrand H, Saenger A: Neurologic des Auges. Vol. 3. JF Bergmann, Weisbaden-Munchen, 1906

199. Williams TA: Variable migrainous recurrent paralyses followed by permanent incomplete lateral homonymous hemianopsia. 99:187, 1911

200. Willis T: Cerebri anatome, cui accessit nervorum descripto et usus. London, 1664. (As translated by Samuel Pordage, 1681, and reproduced in facsimile in Willis T: The Anatomy of the Brain and Nerves. McGill University Press, Montreal, 1965)

201. Wolff, HG: Headache and Other Head Pain. Oxford University Press, New York, 1963

202. Wolter JR, Burchfield WJ: Ocular migraine in a young man resulting in unilateral transient blindness and retinal edema. J Pediatr Ophthalmol 8:173, 1971

203. Woods RP, Lacoboni M, Mazziotta JC: Bilateral spreading cerebral hypoperfusion during spontaneous migraine headache. N Engl J Med 331:1689, 1994

204. Young GF, Leon-Barth CA, Green J: Familial hemiplegic migraine, retinal degeneration, deafness, and nystagmus. Arch Neurol 23:201, 1970

205. Zifkin B, Andermann E, Andermann F, Kirkham T: An autosomal dominant syndrome and hemiplegic migraine, nystagmus, and tremor. Ann Neurol 8:329, 1980

Hypertensive Encephalopathy

HENRY B. DINSDALE

J.P. MOHR

The term *hypertensive encephalopathy* refers to an acute cerebral syndrome precipitated by sudden, severe hypertension.[33] It is a medical emergency requiring prompt, effective treatment. Its incidence has declined in recent years, presumably because of improved treatment of hypertension, but this makes it even more important for clinicians to be alert to the condition, as it may be fatal if undiagnosed. Hypertensive encephalopathy is not to be confused with uremic encephalopathy or the various cerebrovascular complications of chronic, sustained hypertension[18]; indeed, it develops more easily in patients who are normotensive before the acute hypertensive episode.

Pathogenesis

Cerebral blood flow remains constant under normal circumstances, despite wide variations of systemic blood pressure. This autoregulation depends primarily on a myogenic response of brain resistance vessels to elevations in arterial pressure and is essentially independent of control by the autonomic nervous system in normal circumstances. The mean systemic arterial blood pressure in a healthy adult is 90 mmHg, and the lower limit of normal autoregulation is approximately 60 mmHg. Long-standing hypertension causes a shift of the cerebral blood flow/blood pressure curve to the right due presumably to thickening vessel walls and diminished responsiveness of resistance vessels.[48] Therefore, sudden elevations to relatively higher blood pressure levels are required to produce hypertensive encephalopathy in a patient with chronic hypertension, as compared to a normotensive person. Children may have the curve shifted to the left,[20] leaving them more at risk for the development of hypertensive encephalopathy. Adults rarely develop hypertensive encephalopathy at levels below 250/150 mmHg unless they were previously normotensive. The rate and the extent of rise of blood pressure are the most important factors determining the development of hypertensive encephalopathy, but it is difficult clinically and experimentally to evaluate them independent of each other.

Some patients show a "breakthrough of autoregulation" when systemic blood pressure is raised suddenly by angiotensin infusion, and it is suggested this results from forced dilatation of cerebral resistance vessels.[25] However, animal studies, which allow more detailed examination of regional cerebral blood flow, demonstrate that patterns of blood flow with acute hypertension are complex with both low and high flow areas coexisting in adjacent cortical regions.[6] Numerous studies have documented surface pial artery behavior in response to systemic hypertension with emphasis on regions either of vascular narrowing (spasm)[41] or dilatation.[15] During initial blood pressure elevation there is a generalized decrease in diameter of surface cerebral arteries and maintenance of autoregulation, but when mean systemic arterial pressure exceeds 170 mmHg, dilatation accompanied by a focal increase in cerebral blood flow is seen in some arteries that had resting diameters 100 μm or less. The largest component of cerebrovascular resistance is provided by penetrating, parenchymal arterioles, which are unavailable for in vivo visual inspection. Less is known about their physiologic behavior, but in some circumstances they show changes in flow and caliber opposite to that found in surface vessels.[16]

Retinal vessels possess interendothelial tight junctions and a blood-retinal barrier, providing a model for comparison with cerebral vessels. Experiments in monkeys demonstrate that when systolic pressure becomes greater than 150 mmHg, retinal precapillary arterioles are markedly constricted with focal leakage of fluorescein.[11] Maximal vascular reactivity in response to hypertension is observed in the small precapillary arterioles, some of which become narrowed due to fibrin deposition in their walls. Dilatated necrotic arterioles are uncommon.

Brain swelling, occasionally sufficient to cause herniation of cerebellar tonsils through the foramen magnum, is well

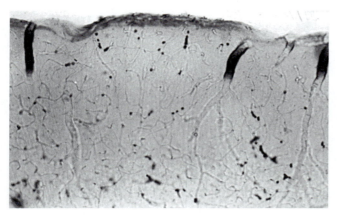

Figure 34.1 Rat cerebral cortex 90 seconds after onset of hypertension. Horseradish peroxidase is present in the walls of three penetrating arterioles at level of lower portion of molecular layer and 2nd and 3rd cortical layers. (× 80.) (Courtesy of Dr. S. Nag.)

documented at autopsy in patients dying during the hypertensive crisis[1,4] and in animal models of hypertensive encephalopathy.[2] Brain weight is increased, gyri are flattened and ventricles compressed, with microscopic examination revealing both generalized and patchy areas of edema,[1] providing autopsy confirmation of the computed tomographic (CT) appearance of areas of diminished density in the white matter in patients with hypertensive encephalopathy.[38]

Hypertensive permeability changes in penetrating cerebral vessels have been carefully studied by Nag et al.[31] Within 90 seconds of angiotensin-induced hypertension, penetrating cerebral arterioles show abnormal permeability to protein-bound dyes and swelling of astrocytes limited to permeable regions. These changes are most pronounced at the level of the second and third cortical cell layers (Fig. 34.1) and are mediated by enhanced pinocytosis, which provides a means of rapid transport of macromolecules from blood through vessel walls to the neuropil. Pinocytosis is probably an important mechanism leading to the extravasation of protein-rich fluid into brain and the subsequent development of brain edema. Structural damage to cerebral vessels is not necessary for the production of brain edema, but vascular permeability presumably is increased further in the presence of the frequently associated findings of acute fibrinoid change of vessel walls, thrombosis, and microinfarction. In addition to osmotic changes, hydrostatic factors may alter the water content of the brain; central noradrenergic mechanisms, neuropeptides,[37] and sympathetic stimulation[14] have been shown to influence brain water permeability.

Extensive fibrin deposits (fibrinoid necrosis) are found in medium- and small-sized arteries throughout the brain. Similar vascular lesions are common in the kidney and retina. If hypertensive encephalopathy develops in a patient with long-standing hypertension, a variety of additional hypertensive cerebrovascular changes may be found, including medial atrophy, hyperplasia, hyalinization, microinfarcts, and microaneurysms.

Epidemiology

Hypertensive encephalopathy is only infrequently described in the current literature, making estimations of incidence difficult to determine. In one recent study, the incidence of acute hypertensive emergencies in a 12-month period were recorded in a major center.[55] Fully 24% of all medical emergencies were described as having hypertension as a clinically presenting feature. Neurologic deficits occurred in 21%, headache in 22% of cases. Diastolic blood pressures for the group overall was 130 ± 15. However, hypertensive encephalopathy was present in only 16% of total cases, making this diagnosis as uncommon as many clinicians believe is the case. Its occurrence is more common in the pediatric age group, but even in this age group only 12 examples were encountered in a large outpatient department (Iowa) in a 15-year period ending in 1994.[54]

Diseases associated with hypertensive encephalopathy are well known. Sometimes the syndrome will develop in a setting of acute or chronic renal disease including glomerulonephritis,[42] disseminated vasculitis (e.g., polyarteritis nodosa), pheochromocytoma,[34] and the immediate postoperative phase of carotid endarterectomy.[21]

Other less common but well-documented causes include autonomic stimulation secondary to bladder or gastrointestinal distention in patients with spinal cord injuries and rebound hypertension with substantial elevation of plasma catecholamines following discontinuation of clonidine[39] or other antihypertensive drugs. Rebound hypertension causing hypertensive encephalopathy has also been reported in children after withdrawal of minoxidil, especially if withdrawal was rapid and the total cumulative dose of the drug relatively high.[28] Patients taking monoamine oxidase inhibiting drugs may induce a hypertensive crisis if they ingest food high in tyramine content. Hypertensive encephalopathy can develop in infants with renal artery stenosis, thrombosis, or coarctation of the aorta.[27] Systemic arterial hypertension sufficient to cause hypertensive encephalopathy is a well-documented complication of thermal injury in children, particularly in males, and increases with the magnitude of the thermal injury. Scorpion envenomation is another rare but well-documented cause.[46]

Clinical Features

Hypertensive encephalopathy may present at any age from the newborn[27] to the elderly but is most common in the second to fourth decades of life. The most important diagnostic factor is awareness by the responsible clinician of the association between severely elevated blood pressure and the patient's neurologic status.

Hypertension accompanies many types of cerebrovascular disease, and the diagnosis of cerebral infarction, cerebral hemorrhage, or subarachnoid hemorrhage is considered in some patients with hypertensive encephalopathy, but the degree of elevation of blood pressure in hypertensive encephalopathy is usually much greater than that encountered with other cerebrovascular events. The diagnosis of hypertensive encephalopathy is supported by the absence of computed tomographic evidence of cerebral hemorrhage or infarction and the resolution of the neurologic syndrome when blood pressure is returned to normal.

Severe acute hypertension can produce symptoms of headache, nausea, and vomiting within a few hours, presumably as the result of increasing intracranial pressure. There may be a variety of visual symptoms, including blurring or dimness, scintillating scotomata, or visual loss. Cortical blindness, color blindness, and dyslexia have been documented.[22] In the early stages of encephalopathy, patients may be anxious, agitated, and complaining of headache, while others are drowsy, confused, or disoriented. Generalized or focal convulsions or both may occur early, especially in children.[35] Blood pressure is elevated to high levels. Bradycardia may reflect increasing intracranial pressure. A variety of changes of respiratory rhythm can develop, especially if the patient is showing neurologic deterioration. Optic disc swelling can reflect either increasing intracranial pressure or local ischemia of the nerve head, which can occur with normal intracranial pressure, progress to optic nerve infarction, and leave a permanent visual field defect. Visual acuity may be impaired because of subhyaloid hemorrhages or bullous retinal detachment.[49] Initial swelling of the optic disc can be masked by retinal edema. Fibrinoid necrosis of retinal arterioles may produce focal hemorrhage and serosanguinous exudates. Retinal ischemia leads to focal edema and collections of swollen neurons that appear as cotton-wool spots.

Although casual reference is often made to diffuse or focal "narrowing" or "spasm" of retinal arteries, there are few convincing reports of such "spasm" in hypertensive encephalopathy, especially with return to normal diameter following treatment. Vessel narrowing noted on funduscopic examination usually results from the structural changes of arteriosclerosis.

Generalized hyperreflexia is a common early finding. Focal or lateralizing motor or sensory signs are sometimes present, which may be postictal or reflect focal cerebral ischemia. If hypertensive encephalopathy goes undiagnosed and untreated, the patient's condition may deteriorate within a few hours, with stupor progressing to coma and death.

Lumbar puncture should be avoided. Eclampsia can be considered a special example of hypertensive encephalopathy. Hypertension is a complication of 5 to 7% of pregnancies.[36] Approximately one-fourth of patients with essential hypertension who become pregnant develop superimposed preeclampsia as defined by the development, after the 24th week of pregnancy, of blood pressure greater than 145/90 mmHg, proteinuria, and persisting peripheral edema. If hypertension is not managed carefully, the patient will enter the eclamptic phase, with weight gain and increasing ankle and pretibial edema. The patient becomes restless, complains of headache and visual blurring, and often has an epileptic convulsion at home, after which she is brought to the hospital. Convulsions develop before labor in 50 percent of eclamptic patients, during labor in 25 percent, and within 24 hours of delivery in the remainder.[52]

Laboratory Studies

CT may show regions of decreased density in the cerebral or cerebellar white matter that disappear with reduction of blood pressure, suggesting reversal of cerebral edema.[23] In a few cases, signs of ischemia have also been documented.

Magnetic resonance imaging (MRI) provides even better documentation of these changes.[17] Recent studies have expanded the database for the changes distinctive for hypertensive encephalopathy.[53] In four reported pediatric cases, low signal on T_2-weighted MRI is most frequently seen in the parieto-occipital regions, typically found not only in the white matter but also in the surface gray matter within 24 hours of the onset of symptoms, resolving within a month from onset.[44] In some instances, these lesions have been correlated with the transient syndrome of cortical blindness.[29]

A small number of cases have been studied by transcranial Doppler (TCD).[56] In one case, suffering the form of hypertensive encephalopathy with eclampsia, TCD velocities in the middle cerebral artery were increased in the days before cesarean section and continued for some days afterwards. No definite cause was found, but it was assumed to be related to arterial spasm.

Treatment

The Joint National Committee on Detection, Evaluation and Treatment of High Blood Pressure in its 1984 report[24] divided the treatment of severe hypertension into two categories: (1) hypertensive emergencies in which severe elevation of blood pressure results in acute end organ damage and represents an acute threat to vital organs or to the patient's survival, and (2) hypertensive urgencies in which severe elevation of blood pressure represents a potential threat, but acute end organ damage is not present. The patient with hypertensive encephalopathy belongs in the first category and must be treated in the hospital where blood pressure, seizures, level of consciousness, and airway patency can be monitored closely.

Under normal conditions, symptoms of cerebral hypoperfusion develop when mean arterial pressure is reduced to 40% of baseline levels. Therefore, a patient with a blood pressure of 225/150 mmHg will have a reduction of cerebral blood flow if pressure is lowered to 140/100 mmHg, and develop symptoms of cerebral anoxia if pressure drops to 110/70 mmHg or less. Patients with chronic hypertension have their lower limit of autoregulation set at a higher level than normotensive patients,[26,48] which may explain reports of boundary zone infarction after rapid treatment of chronic hypertension.[12]

Overzealous treatment of hypertension in a setting of acute stroke—separate from hypertensive encephalopathy—is now recognized as carrying some risk of intensifying the ischemic process, so that a clear diagnosis should be made before proceeding with aggressive therapy.[47]

An ideal drug to lower blood pressure rapidly in an emergency would have rapid reversible action that is predictable and controlled, low toxic-to-therapeutic ratio, and no depressant effects on the central nervous system. Such an ideal drug is not yet available, but those currently favored are the vasodilators nitroprusside, diazoxide, and hydralazin. Vasodilators elevate intracranial pressure in some circumstances depending upon the extent of brain swelling, level of preexisting blood pressure, $PaCO_2$, and method of administration.[5,30,50,51] Concern has therefore been expressed that vasodilators might be harmful by increasing intracranial pressure; however, clinical experience strongly suggests that the benefits of prompt reduction of blood pressure outweigh other considerations. Some authors advocate the continuous monitoring of intracranial pressure throughout treatment.[13]

Sodium nitroprusside is given intravenously (0.5 to 0.8 μ/kg/min) and requires skillful and constant supervision. The rate of infusion is adjusted according to response, and its hypotensive effect is potentiated by a head-up tilt of the patient. Its effect is seen within a few minutes through venous relaxation and increased venous capacitance while maintaining an unchanged cardiac output.

Diazoxide must be given rapidly intravenously, but the effect is less predictable and controlled than with sodium nitroprusside. The recommended dose is 150 mg given in 15 to 30 seconds. This usually produces a dramatic lowering of blood pressure within 1 to 2 minutes. It causes sodium retention and also interferes with carbohydrate metabolism, which could be a disadvantage as suggested by evidence of increased CNS damage in the presence of hyperglycemia.[45]

Hydralazine may increase cardiac work and therefore must be given cautiously to patients with coronary artery disease. It increases heart rate, stroke volume, and cardiac output and appears to be less effective than sodium nitroprusside or diazoxide in treating encephalopathy.

Captopril, an angiotensin-converting enzyme inhibitor, is effective in acutely reducing blood pressure and reversing encephalopathy in some patients treated under carefully controlled conditions.[3] Recent reports of intravenous enalaprilat found rapid clinical effects were as easily achieved at doses of 0.625 as were obtained at higher doses.[19] Stable reduction in blood pressure to values below 95 mmHg occurred within 45 minutes of onset.

Oral drugs lower blood pressure less rapidly than parenteral drugs and may be used in urgent situations to treat patients who have not yet developed encephalopathy or severe cardiac complications. Nifedipine, an oral calcium channel blocking agent,[8] has been compared with intravenous sodium nitroprusside in patients with severe (diastolic blood pressure greater than 130 mmHg) uncomplicated (free of focal neurologic signs or coma) hypertension.[10] Treatment with nifedipine resulted in less time in the intensive care unit for the patient without an increase in morbidity or mortality. Nifedipine was administered as a 10-mg oral dose and repeated within 2 hours if diastolic blood pressure had not fallen below 120 mmHg. The average total dose required was 20 mg with the onset of effect within 1 hour and peak effect at 1.5 or 2 hours following the initial dose. Blood pressure was lowered immediately with sodium nitroprusside, but it took longer to stabilize the diastolic blood pressure at an acceptable lower level. Nifedipine is effective in the treatment of hypertensive urgencies and some emergencies, but caution is required using this medication in the elderly, those with coronary dis-

ease, and in patients whose volume is depleted because of vomiting.[32] Absorption of nifedipine from the oral cavity is slow and incomplete. The capsule should be bitten and the contents swallowed if a rapid effect is required. Similar experiences have been reported with nicardipine.[43]

During the acute phase of hypertensive encephalopathy it may be necessary to attempt to lessen cerebral edema directly, in addition to lowering blood pressure. Dexamethasone 4 to 6 mg intramuscularly every 4 to 6 hours reduces cerebral edema.[40] Steroids probably have multiple modes of action on central nervous system function, including effects on neurotransmitters and other systems,[9] as well as restoring normal permeability to cerebral vessels. Hyperosmolar agents such as mannitol or glycerol may also be given to treat cerebral edema in the absence of renal disease.

Anticonvulsants will usually be required from the outset. Intravenous administration ensures rapid loading doses of drugs such as phenytoin. Diazepam is much favored as an anticonvulsant drug in emergency situations, but its central depressant action, including the risk of respiratory arrest, dictates that it be used with caution. The hypotensive effect of diazepam can also complicate assessment of the efficacy of other hypotensive agents.

Parenteral agents can be discontinued and oral antihypertensive drugs commenced when blood pressure is reduced to target levels, which will be slightly higher for patients with long-standing hypertension than for normotensives. Treatment with a diuretic is often combined with a β-blocker such as propanolol. If there is impairment of renal function, a loop diuretic such as furosemide will be required.

Eclamptic patients require stabilization of vital signs achieved by controlling convulsions, lowering blood pressure, and maintaining renal output. Pregnancy can then be terminated, at which time one may have to treat hypovolemia, disseminated microvascular coagulation, and the cumulative effects of various medications.

There is a general clinical impression that patients who survive hypertensive encephalopathy make a complete neurologic recovery. A minority of patients, however, are left with focal neurologic deficits such as occipital lobe infarction. It is also possible that general disturbances might remain due to multiple small infarcts of the cerebral cortex and white matter. A multicenter follow-up study with careful neurologic and psychometric evaluation would help to determine the long-term consequences of this illness, but with improved treatment of hypertension it is unlikely that any single hospital will develop a sizeable number of such patients in the future.

The quality of follow-up care and treatment of blood pressure in patients with hypertensive encephalopathy has been demonstrated to be as poor as the management of hypertension in the general population.[7]

References

1. Adams RD, VanderEecken HM: Vascular diseases of the brain. Annu Rev Med 4:213, 1953
2. Byrom FB: The pathogenesis of hypertensive encephalopathy and its relation to the malignant phase of hyper-

tension: experimental evidence from the hypertensive rat. Lancet 2:201, 1954

3. Case DB, Atlas SA, Sullivan PA, Laragh JH: Acute and chronic treatment of severe and malignant hypertension with the oral angiotensin converting enzyme inhibitor captopril. Circulation 64:765, 1981

4. Chapmen K, Karimi R: A case of postpartum eclampsia of late onset confirmed by autopsy. Am J Obstet Gynecol 117:858, 1978

5. Cottrell JE, Patel K, Turndorf H, Ransohoff J: Intracranial pressure changes induced by sodium nitroprusside in patients with intracranial mass lesions. J Neurosurg 48:329, 1978

6. Dinsdale HB, Robertson DM, Haas RA: Cerebral blood flow in acute hypertension. Arch Neurol 31:80, 1974

7. Dollery CT: The care of patients with malignant hypertension in London 1974–1975. p. 37. In McLachlan G (ed): A Question of Quality. Oxford University Press, London, 1976

8. Ellrodt AG, Ault MJ, Riedinger MS, Murata GH: Efficacy and safety of sublingual nifedipine in hypertensive emergencies. Am J Med 79:19, 1985

9. Fishman RA: Steroids in the treatment of brain edema. N Engl J Med 306:359, 1982

10. Franklin C, Nightingale S, Mamdani B: A randomized comparison of nifedipine and sodium nitroprusside in severe hypertension. Chest 90:500, 1986

11. Garner A, Ashton N, Tripathi R et al: Pathogenesis of hypertensive retinopathy: an experimental study in the monkey. Br J Ophthalmol 59:3, 1975

12. Graham DI: Ischaemic brain damage of cerebral perfusion type after treatment of severe hypertension. Br Med J 4:739, 1975

13. Griswold WP, Viney J, Mendoza SA, James HE: Intracranial pressure monitoring in severe hypertensive encephalopathy. Crit Care Med 9:573, 1981

14. Grubb RL, Raichle ME, Eichling JO: Peripheral sympathetic regulation of brain water permeability. p. 264. In Ingvar DH, Lassen NA (eds): Cerebral Function, Metabolism and Circulation. Munksgaard, Copenhagen, 1977

15. Haggendal E, Johansson B: On the pathophysiology of the increased cerebrovascular permeability in acute arterial hypertension in cats. Acta Neurol Scand 48:265, 1972

16. Harper AM, Deshmukh VD, Rowen JO, Jennett WB: The influence of sympathetic nervous activity on cerebral blood flow. Arch Neurol 27:1, 1972

17. Hauser RA, Lacey M, Knight MR: Hypertensive encephalopathy: magnetic resonance imaging demonstration of reversible cortical and white matter lesions. Arch Neurol 45:1078, 1988

18. Healton EB, Brust JC, Feinfeld DA, Thomson GE: Hypertensive encephalopathy and the neurologic manifestations of malignant hypertension. Neurology (NY) 32:127, 1982

19. Hirschl MM, Binder M, Bur A et al: Clinical evaluation of different doses of intravenous enalaprilat in patients with hypertensive crises. Arch Intern Med 13:2217, 1995

20. Hulse JA, Taylor DSI, Dillon MJ: Blindness and paraplegia in severe childhood hypertension. Lancet 2:553, 1979

21. Ille O, Woimant F, Pruna A et al: Hypertensive encepha-

lopathy after bilateral carotid endarterectomy. Stroke 26: 488, 1995

22. Jellinek EH, Painter M, Prineas J, Ross Russell RW: Hypertensive encephalopathy with cortical disorders of vision. QJ Med 33:239, 1964

23. Jespersen CM, Rasmussen D, Hennild V: Focal intracerebral oedema in hypertensive encephalopathy visualized by computerized topographic scan. J Intern Med 225:349, 1989

24. Joint National Committee on Detection, Evaluation and Treatment of High Blood Pressure: The 1984 Report of the Joint National Committee. Arch Intern Med 144: 1045, 1984

25. Lassen NA, Agnoli A: Scand J Clin Lab Invest 30:113, 1972

26. Ledingham JGG, Rajagopalan B: Cerebral complications in the treatment of accelerated hypertension. QJ Med 48: 25, 1979

27. Mace S, Hirschfeld S: Hypertensive encephalopathy. Am J Dis Child 137:32, 1983

28. Makker SP, Moorthy B: Rebound hypertension following minoxidil withdrawal. J Pediatr 96:762, 1980

29. Marra TR, Shah M, Mikus MA: Transient cortical blindness due to hypertensive encephalopathy. Magnetic resonance imaging correlation. J Clin Neuro-Ophthalmol 13: 35, 1993

30. Marsh ML, Shapiro HM, Smith RW, Marshall LF: Changes in neurologic status and intracranial pressure associated with sodium nitroprusside administration. Anesthesiology 51:336, 1979

31. Nag S, Robertson DM, Dinsdale HB: Cerebral cortical changes in acute experimental hypertension: an ultrastructural study. Lab Invest 36:150, 1977

32. O'Mailia J, Sander G, Giles T: Nifedipine-associated myocardial ischemia or infarction in the treatment of hypertensive urgencies. Ann Intern Med 107:85, 1987

33. Oppenheimer BS, Fishberg AM: Hypertensive encephalopathy. Arch Intern Med 41:264, 1928

34. Phillips DJ, Davies AH, Bliss BP. Hypertensive encephalopathy secondary to a phaeochromocytoma: the cause of death after carotid endarterectomy. Case report. J Cardiovasc Surg 35:533, 1994

35. Popp MB, Friedberg DL, MacMillan BG: Clinical characteristics of hypertension in several children. Ann Surg 191:473, 1980

36. Pritchard JA, MacDonald PC: Hypertensive disorders in pregnancy. p. 666. In Williams: Obstetrics. 16th Ed. Appleton & Lange, E. Norwalk, CT, 1980

37. Raichle ME, Grubb RL, Eichling JO: Central neuroendocrine regulation of brain water permeability. Ciba Found Symp 56:219, 1977

38. Rail DL, Perkin GD: Computerized tomographic appearance of hypertensive encephalopathy. Arch Neurol 37: 310, 1980

39. Reid JL, Wing LMH, Dargie HJ et al: Clonidine withdrawal in hypertension: changes in blood pressure and plasma and urinary noradrenaline. Lancet 1:1171, 1977

40. Reulen HJ, Hadjidimos A, Shermann K: The effect of dexamethasone on water electrolyte content and on rCBF in perifocal brain edema in man. p. 239. In Reulen HJ,

Shermann K (eds): Steroids and Brain Edema. Springer-Verlag, New York, 1972

41. Rodda R, Denny-Brown D: The cerebral arteries in experimental hypertension. Vol. I. The nature of arteriolar constriction and its effects on the collateral circulation. Am J Pathol 49:53, 1966

42. Saatci I, Topaloglu R: Cranial computed tomographic findings in a patient with hypertensive encephalopathy in acute poststreptococcal glomerulonephritis. Turkish J Pediatr 36:325, 1994

43. Sabbatini M, Strocchi P, Amenta F: Nicardipine and treatment of cerebrovascular diseases with particular reference to hypertension-related disorders. Clin Experim Hypertension 17:719, 1995

44. Sebire G, Husson B, Lasser C et al: Encephalopathie induite par l'hypertension arterielle: aspects cliniques, radiologiques et therapeutiques. Arch Pediatrie 2:513, 1995

45. Siemkowicz E, Hansen AJ: Brain extracellular ion composition and EEG activity following 10 minutes ischemia in normotensive and hyperglycemic rats. Stroke 12:236, 1981

46. Sofes S, Gueron M: Vasodilators and hypertensive encephalopathy following scorpion envenomation in children. Chest 97:118, 1990

47. Strandgaard S, Olesen J, Skinhoj E, Lassen NA: Autoregulation of brain circulation in severe arterial hypertension. Br Med J 1:507, 1973

48. Strandgaard S, Paulson OB: Cerebrovascular damage in hypertension. J Cardiovasc Risk 2:34, 1995

49. Stropes LL, Luft SC: Hypertensive crisis with bilateral bullous retinal detachment. JAMA 238:1948, 1977

50. Stullken EH Jr, Sokoll MD: Intracranial pressure during hypotension and subsequent vasopressor therapy in anesthetized cats. Anesthesiology 42:425, 1975

51. Turner JM, Powell D, Gibson RM, McDowall DJ: Intracranial pressure changes in neurosurgical patients during hypotension induced with sodium nitroprusside or trimethaphan. Br J Anaesth 49:419, 1977

52. Vliegen JH, Muskens E, Keunen RW et al: Abnormal cerebral hemodynamics in pregnancy-related hypertensive encephalopathy. Eur J Obstetr Gyn & Reproduct Biol 49:198, 1993

53. Weingarten K, Barbut D, Filippi C, Zimmerman RD: Acute hypertensive encephalopathy: findings on spin-echo and gradient-echo MR imaging. AJR. Amer J Roentgenol 162:665, 1994

54. Wright RR, Mathews KD: Hypertensive encephalopathy in childhood. J Child Neurol 11:193, 1996

55. Zampaglione B, Pascale C, Marchisio M, Cavallo-Perin P: Hypertensive urgencies and emergencies. Prevalence and clinical presentation. Hypertension 27:144, 1996

56. Zunker P, Ley-Pozo J, Louwen F: Cerebral hemodynamics in pre-eclampsia/eclampsia syndrome. Ultrasound in Obst Gyn 6:411, 1995

Multi-Infarct Dementia

PABLO MARTINEZ-LAGE
VLADIMIR HACHINSKI

Vascular Cognitive Impairment: a New Starting Point

If therapy and prevention are the essence and the justification of medicine, the study of disease should focus on its initial stages, when the pathologic process might be stopped, slowed, or, ideally, reversed. This is particularly true for diseases of the nervous system, where tissue does not regenerate, and especially in the aged nervous system, when plasticity, compensatory capacities, and functional reserve are seriously limited. The concept of dementia, historically and conventionally, applies to a syndrome characterized by the loss of intellectual abilities to a point where the subject is no longer able to cope with occupational, social, or routine daily activities.[2] It obviously implies such a degree of severity and brain damage that in most instances it proves irreversible. Psychiatrists, neurologists, geriatricians, and least of all patients and families, cannot afford to wait until this "point of no return" has been reached to establish a diagnosis, the first step of treatment. Regardless of the etiology or pathophysiology, the clinical picture of dementia must be understood merely as a stage, a severe one, of a brain disease.[81] Dementia is the result of a pathologic process that starts with the presence of a particular combination of risk factors or genetic susceptibility, or both, and is followed by a so-called asymptomatic, preclinical or silent stage in which the brain damage is already present but no symptoms are noticed and signs may not be elicited. Subsequently, as the brain damage progresses and the "functional reserve" of the brain becomes exhausted, the first cognitive complaints start to appear, but they are so mild that patients, families, and even general physicians are not alarmed. It is only when the picture of dementia starts to bloom fully that specialized medical attention is sought. At this stage, little can be done in terms of therapy or prevention. It could be argued, however, that early detection of dementing illnesses is futile if no effective treatments are available. But the opposite is also true: no effective treatments will be available if they are not tested in the initial, presymptomatic, or early symptomatic stages. While this statement is applicable to all types of de-

mentia, it deserves particular emphasis in cerebrovascular disease. Several prophylactic measures, from diet and lifestyle to vascular surgery, have been proved effective in the prevention of stroke.[153] Since dementia from vascular causes shares, by definition, many etiologic mechanisms with stroke, it is potentially preventable.[84] Unfortunately, vascular dementia is, also by definition, untreatable, if by the time it can be diagnosed the vascular damage to the brain is so extensive that it cannot be reversed. The relevance of early detection of cognitive changes related to vascular disease is thus self-evident.

The concept of vascular cognitive impairment (VCI) has been suggested to encompass all different degrees of intellectual decline related to ischemic cerebrovascular disease as the afore-described continuum, emphasizing the importance of early detection.[83] The definition of VCI appears as a new and necessary starting point to move away from the old concept of vascular dementia and the great confusion it brings. The best index of this confusion is probably the fact that, despite several attempts, no reliable and reproducible diagnostic criteria have been developed so far.[215] The idea of dementia included in the old concept of vascular dementia (VD) has been traditionally identified and extracted from the clinical picture of Alzheimer's disease (AD), and has been artificially based on preformed and untested hypotheses.[82] Taking AD as the standard model for the definition of dementia has led to the inclusion of memory impairment as a sine qua non requirement to diagnose dementia. Vascular disease, however, is more likely to affect other areas of cognition, such as executive functions or language, especially in early cases. Personality changes and behavioral or affective disorders may prove to be much more prominent than memory impairment in patients with cerebrovascular disease. Even when memory is affected, the pattern of amnestic deficits may prove to be different from those present in AD patients if adequate tests are applied. Direct involvement of the hippocampus, one of the hallmarks of AD pathology, is rarely caused by vascular mechanisms. Prospective collaborative studies are then needed to investigate which cognitive syndromes result from which vascular changes. New diagnostic criteria should be based on the results of these studies. The current strategy of diagnosing patients on the basis of an untested idea of what the cognitive picture has to be will surely exclude many patients who do not have memory deficits. Besides, if dementia is defined similarly for AD and VD, a differential diagnosis based on clinical symptoms is impossible. Apart from severity and memory impairment requirements, other aspects of current diagnostic criteria for VD, such as the presence of focal signs, the chronologic progression of the disease, the amount of clinical or radiologic evidence of stroke required, have not been formally tested in clean, unbiased samples of cerebrovascular patients. The lack of etiologic categorization is also difficult to accept. Only when VCI is recognized, diagnosed, and investigated in its earliest stages will questions be solved regarding its neuropsychological features and distinction from other forms of cognitive decline (AD), etiologic categorizations and interactions, neuroimaging characteristics, epidemiology and risk factors, prevention, and treatment.

Pathological Substrate: Focal Vascular Brain Damage Not Chronic Ischemia

Cognition or intelligence has been defined as "the aggregate or global capacity of the individual to act purposefully, to think rationally, and to deal effectively with the environment.[214] This simple definition, which implicitly describes the four major classes of cognitive functions—receptive, memory and learning, thinking, and expressive functions—highlights the term *global* and implies the brain working "as a whole" as the anatomic and physiologic substrate. Therefore, after excluding those areas of the nervous system related to the maintenance of vigilance, vegetative control, and primary sensory and motor functions, it is understandable that any lesion in areas of the brain rostral to the upper brain stem can potentially affect cognition. A discussion about the anatomic substrate of cognition is out of the scope of this chapter; however, when dealing with cerebral ischemic disease, it is important to bear in mind the model of anatomic correlations of complex functions based on large-scale neurocognitive networks reviewed by Mesulam.[135,136] According to this model: (1) Components of a single function are represented in different interconnected locations throughout the brain; (2) individual cortical or subcortical areas may belong to different overlapping networks and participate in several complex functions; (3) lesions confined to a single region may result in multiple deficits; (4) impairment of an individual complex function usually requires simultaneous involvement of several regions to be severe and persisting; (5) the same cognitive function may be affected by a lesion in different brain areas. Hence, in a simplistic, but useful conception, cerebrovascular disease can affect cognition (VCI) by destroying the neural components (cortical areas) of the networks, or their connections (white matter disease, subcortical relay centers). Within this model, both size and location of infarcted tissue are important regarding clinical manifestations, and no assumptions are made as to which cognitive functions are to be impaired.

In the definition of VCI, cognitive refers to all levels of intellectual decline, of any nature and severity, and vascular points to all causes of ischemic cerebrovascular disease.[16]

Hence, the anatomopathologic substrate of VCI is ischemic infarction. Intracerebral and subarachnoid hemorrhages, although englobed by the broadness of the term *vascular*, must be excluded from the concept of VCI on methodologic and pragmatic grounds. On the one hand, they constitute easily recognizable entities with well-known risk factors, manifestations, and therapy; on the other, they very rarely cause progressive cognitive decline leading to dementia, an idea which is inherent to the concept of VCI.

Historically, chronic cerebral ischemia was claimed to be the underlying mechanism of VD.[59] This idea, which even conceptually is difficult to sustain, that ischemia maintained over time usually leads to infarction, was based on the observation of arteriosclerosis in the cerebral arteries of patients with "chronic brain failure."[1,11] Some of these patients had developed dementia in the course of repeated spells of clinical symptomatology (the so-called postapoplectic dementia), whereas others declined progressively. Some of them showed multiple areas of cerebral softening, while in others only brain atrophy and diffuse neuronal loss, which Alzheimer had described as "cortical decay," was observed. The general hypothesis that prevailed during the first half of the century was that aging might be accompanied by a gradual narrowing of cerebral arteries which led to decreased cerebral blood flow and diffuse "nutritional disturbance," and then to atrophy, neuronal loss, and dementia. After the works of Miller Fisher[60] and Tomlinson et al,[201] the concept of postapoplectic dementia was recovered, and brain infarction, rather than chronic ischemia, started to be recognized as the true mechanism of intellectual decline. The old terminology of arteriosclerotic dementia was substituted by the more descriptive term of *multi-infarct dementia* (MID).[80] Nonetheless, chronic ischemia continued to be advocated after evidence was provided that cerebral blood flow decreased prior to the development of the clinical syndrome in patients with multi-infarct dementia.[170] Of note in this study, all patients showed infarcts, but longitudinal neuroimaging studies were not performed. It is not known, then, whether the presence of multiple infarcts also preceded the onset of dementia. Besides, all patients had a history of multiple strokes, transient ischemic attacks, or reversible ischemic neurologic signs, suggesting that reduced cerebral blood flow might be the consequence of multiple infarctions. The same authors later reported that cognition and cerebral blood flow fluctuated together in patients with MID and related such changes to the presence of focal infarcts.[137] Further evidence against the plausibility of chronic ischemia as a mechanism underlying intellectual decline related to vascular disease has been provided from two different sources. On the one hand, attempts to restore normal cerebral blood flow by carotid endarterectomy or extracranial-intracranial bypass surgery have not been translated in better neuropsychological outcome.[5] On the other hand, studies where cerebral blood flow and oxygen metabolism measurements are coupled show that reduced flow is not accompanied by an increased oxygen extraction fraction,[24,62] thus providing evidence that it is the decrease in neuronal function that primarily causes changes in blood flow, and not the opposite. Such reduction in cortical function must certainly be related to focal cerebral infarction either locally or remotely in other cortical, subcortical, or white matter areas.

Vascular Mechanisms

Assuming that focal cerebral ischemic infarction is the pathoanatomic substrate of VCI might lead to misinterpretation. It could be argued that if ischemic stroke is the cause of cognitive decline, then all efforts should be invested in the study of stroke. Any attempt to define new entities such as VCI or even vascular dementia would be unnecessary and confusing. However, the concept of ischemic infarction, far from being restrictive, should be understood in its broadest terms considering its multiple etiologies, its heterogeneous clinical manifestations, and its multiple and varied radiologic correlates.

While the prevalence of cognitive impairment among patients with ischemic stroke is 35.2%, 10 times higher than in control subjects,[194] not all patients presenting with stroke develop intellectual decline. Similarly, the incidence of dementia among these patients is nine times higher than that in controls.[195] Several studies have looked at possible differential traits that would characterize which stroke patients develop dementia. Some authors have emphasized the presence of bilateral lesions[51,117] while others highlight the importance of dominant hemispheric infarction.[73,122,144,197] Some studies show no effect of infarct location or even clinical severity on the rate of dementia.[144] The importance of lacunar over cortical infarcts is reported in some studies,[43,140,161,197,220] but not all.[73,115,125] Interestingly, cerebral and ventricular atrophy have been repeatedly reported in association with dementia.[37,73,96,117,125,198] Data regarding the presence or absence of vascular risk factors among stroke patients with and without dementia are also controversial.[96,117,125,144,197,198] In conclusion, the above-mentioned stroke-related variables are insufficient to explain why some patients with stroke develop dementia while others do not. The problem remains unsolved even when white matter lesions are taken into consideration[17,122,204] (see below). By contrast, there is growing recognition that cognitive changes attributable to vascular causes occur in the absence of a clinical stroke.[22,44,132] In all likelihood, a better understanding of the intrinsic cellular and molecular mechanisms by which ischemia leads to brain damage will help to solve this question. Recent advances in the molecular biology of brain ischemia suggest that the current conception of ischemic infarction should be expanded far beyond that of the classical necrotic cavitary lesion.

The concept of *incomplete infarction* was originally used by Lassen[118] to describe focal ischemic lesions with necrosis but not "emollision." A few years later it was applied to designate vascular changes in the white matter (loss of myelin, axons, and oligodendrocytes; glial reaction) of presumed ischemic origin and comparable to those occurring in the "transitional zone surrounding many complete infarctions."[27] More recently, the term has been reviewed and recovered to identify areas of brain damage, including the cortex, caused by reversible ischemia of moderate severity.[66] Histologically, these lesions are characterized by selective neuronal death with little or no glial reaction. Such neuropathologic changes are well known to occur in relation with global cerebral ischemia, but they also appear in the periphery of classical cavitary infarcts. Experimental and clinical evidence has been provided to suggest that they can occur in cases of focal ischemia in the absence of necrotic lesions.[66] While the term *incomplete* is unfortunate, the importance of the concept resides in the fact that such lesions would not be detected with conventional neuroimaging techniques.

Together with this form of neuronal selective "necrosis," another important aspect of ischemia-induced brain damage is that of apoptosis.[20] Experimental studies have shown that cerebral ischemia leads to DNA fragmentation and protein synthesis inhibition, and these findings have been interpreted as signs of "programmed" cell death or apoptosis.[121] The question of whether such process might lead to delayed, or even progressive, cell loss remains open. Of special interest in this respect are the profound changes that ischemia induces in the modulation and regulation of the expression of certain gene families such as the "immediate early genes" (c-*fos*, c-*jun*) and those related to the stress response.[3,36,90] Such changes at the gene expression level occur in both global and transient or prolonged focal ischemia models and have been related to the mechanisms of excitotoxicity, neuronal death, as well as with mechanisms of neuroprotection. Remarkably, in models of focal ischemia changes in gene expression may explain delayed neuronal changes in remote areas outside the cerebral ischemic focus.[113]

Lastly, of exceptional relevance is the increasingly recognized role that non-neuronal cell populations play in the production of tissue damage induced by ischemia.[68] Oligodendrocytes are particularly sensitive to ischemia, which might explain the development of white matter changes with ischemic insults that are otherwise insufficient to cause cavitary infarctions.[217] On the other hand, astrocytes and microglia are rapidly activated by ischemic insults and breakdown of the blood-brain barrier. Astrocytes are actively involved in several neuroprotective mechanisms such as the maintenance of extracellular fluid homeostasis, scavenging of oxygen free radicals, reuptake of excytotoxic neurotransmitters, or release of trophic factors. Distortion of these responses, or overactivation and proliferation of astrocytes surviving an ischemic insult, may result in an inflammatory response with overexpression of nitric oxide synthetase, sustained production of nitric oxide, release of glutamate and cytokines, overproduction of free radicals, phagocytic behavior, contributing to neuronal death postischemia. A similar reaction involves the microglia with overexpression and production of mediators of the inflammatory response and acute phase proteins.[71] Of particular interest is the fact that one of the proteins overexpressed is the amyloid precursor protein (APP), which places cerebral ischemia as a potential triggering factor of β-amyloid deposition and development of neuropathologic changes of the Alzheimer type.[68] In experimental models of focal cerebral ischemia, the microglial response occurs not only at the primary ischemic lesion, but also in other ipsilateral and contralateral brain regions days or even weeks after the original insult.[145]

In summary, not only are the pathophysiologic mechanisms leading to cerebral ischemia multiple and varied, but the anatomic and cellular expression of ischemia-induced brain damage may occur in different ways (Fig. 35.1). The classical, clinically defined, computed tomography (CT) or magnetic resonance imaging (MRI) detectable infarct would represent only one of these ways, certainly an important and frequent one. In such a scenario, the clinical relevance of short-lived, moderately severe ischemic insults, insufficient to cause rec-

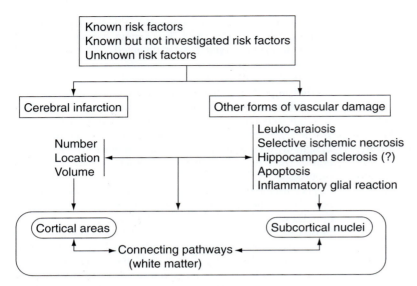

Figure 35.1 Etiology of vascular cognitive impairment.

ognizable symptoms or cavitary infarcts, whether embolic, thrombotic, or hemodynamic in origin, might be more important than traditionally believed. Future research will focus in the development of diagnostic tools, such as functional neuroimaging (functional MRI, receptor-oriented positron emission tomography (PET), and single photon emission computed tomography (SPECT) or analytical measurements of the inflammatory response, that will prove useful in the detection of cellular and subcellular changes induced by brain ischemia.

White Matter Vascular Damage

The relevance of white matter ischemic disease as one of the anatomopathologic substrates of cognitive impairment was initially emphasized in the original descriptions of "arteriosclerotic dementia."[1,11] With the introduction of CT imaging, the presence of white matter "rarefaction," described as decreased radiologic density in the periventricular regions and centrum semiovale, was reported in 1.7% to 14% of the adult population.[74,109,203] Such changes were soon related to the presence of cognitive changes, dementia,[77,149,167,187,188] as well as to a higher incidence of vascular risk factors.[55,69,92] Pathologic correlations showed that areas of white matter rarefaction, as seen on CT, corresponded to demyelination, white matter infarcts, lacunes, or dilated perivascular spaces, and, in the majority of cases, arteriosclerosis was present.[74,128,147] Not a few authors hurried to name this combination of dementia, vascular risk factors, and white matter changes as *Binswanger's disease* (BD) or *subcortical arteriosclerotic encephalopathy* (SAE), a term that had been recovered some years before by Caplan and Schoene.[29] An "epidemic" of this previously rare disease[157] subsequently invaded the literature.[28,109,171] It was already known, however, that not all the

white matter changes seen on CT were caused by arteriosclerosis. Some studies had reported the presence of ependymal disruption and periventricular gliosis, as well as hydrocephalus, edema or dilated perivascular Virchow-Robin spaces, as alternative explanations.[128,167] In patients with Alzheimer's disease, white matter changes were described as incomplete infarction[27] and were associated with the presence of amyloid angiopathy.[95] To emphasize such heterogeneity and avoid any presumption about etiology or neuropathology, the term *leukoaraiosis* (LA) was suggested[78] and became widely used.

Far from solving the questions surrounding the "matter of white matter," the introduction of MRI brought confusion and led to skepticism. The extremely high sensitivity of MRI was accompanied by very low specificity. Initial studies reported some degree of leukoaraiosis in up to 80% to 90% of healthy subjects over the age of 60.[33,57,222] Contrary to what had been described with CT, leukoaraiosis on MRI was not correlated with cognitive changes.[87,91,142,165,178,202] One study showed that leukoaraiosis on MRI did not correlate with that seen on CT, and only the latter was associated with cognitive dysfunction.[112] The higher sensitivity of MRI was the most likely explanation for these contradictory results. Pathologic correlations provided evidence that, in fact, some of the hyperintense "lesions" seen on MRI corresponded to normal structures or age-associated atrophic changes. Hyperintensities adjacent to the frontal horns of the lateral ventricles corresponded to the subcallosal fascicle and the hyperintense thin area that surrounded the lateral ventricular wall, termed "rims" or "halos," was caused by ependymitis granularis.[192] Similarly, some of the small punctate hyperintense lesions were shown to represent enlarged Virchow-Robin spaces filled with cerebrospinal fluid (CSF) and not infarcts.[8,18]

The distinction of periventricular (PVH) and deep white matter hyperintensities (DWMH), including small punctate, early confluent, and diffuse changes, as well as the use of quantitative or semiquantitative approaches to grade the severity of the findings,[54] markedly improved the specificity of MRI. While some degree of white matter change was detected in more than 80% of elderly subjects, the prevalence of moderate to severe changes (periventricular hyperintensities extending into the deep white matter, or subcortical patchy, confluent, or diffuse changes) was shown to be less than 20%.[23,54,130] Several studies showed a correlation of leukoaraiosis with neuropsychological dysfunction, specifically with attention deficits, speed of information processing and other fronto-subcortical functions, only when distribution and severity of the white matter changes were taken into account.[14,21,65,101,107,134,179,219] Moderate to severe white matter changes were described in 26% to 70% (periventricular) and 20% to 25% (subcortical) of patients with Alzheimer's disease, and in 80% (periventricular) and 50% (subcortical) of cases with vascular dementia.[139,177]

With respect to risk factors for leukoaraiosis, the association with advancing age has been a universal finding in every study. The significant effect of cerebrovascular risk factors has been reported in numerous studies,[6,23,54,70,108,130,191,193] but not all.[87,165] Of note, the association of leukoaraiosis and vascular risk factors is stronger for subcortical than for periventricular lesions. In general, a history of stroke and hypertension shows the most consistent association, with diabetes, cardiac disease, increased fibrinogen levels or carotid atherosclerosis on ultrasound being less frequently reported.

The etiology of leukoaraiosis is still a question of open debate. Several neuropathologic studies on brains subjected to pre- or postmortem MRI have shown that punctate hyperintensities are caused by either perivascular demyelination and gliosis, dilated Virchow-Robin spaces, or small lacunes.[18,34,56,131,148] More diffuse patchy or confluent MRI lesions are associated with ischemic infarction,[131] areas of myelin pallor and axonal loss[34,76,119] multiple lacunes,[56,166] diffuse vacuolation and decreased density of glial cells,[148] or multiple sclerosis.[119] In many instances, the term *incomplete infarction* has been used to describe the presence of myelin and axonal loss with astrocytic gliosis but without necrosis or cavitation, as suggested by Brun and Englund.[27] Studies using postmortem MRI have also confirmed that periventricular rims, thin caps, and halos correspond to subependymal glial accumulations associated with loss of the ependymal lining,[34,56] and only when they extend into the subcortical white matter are they accompanied by vascular ischemic changes.[119] Several etiologic mechanisms have been hypothesized to explain these radiologic and neuropathologic changes. Lacunes and other infarcts probably account for an important proportion of the lesions, as shown by pathologic studies. That leukoaraiosis is associated with small-vessel disease is supported by both clinical and neuropathologic evidence.[56,206] It is the mechanism by which arteriolopathy, either in the form of arteriosclerosis or amyloid angiopathy, leads to white matter rarefaction that remains to be elucidated. Some authors have rescued the old concept of chronic ischemia, and decreased cerebral blood flow has been described in the white matter of patients with leukoaraiosis.[55,112] However, no evidence showing that reduction of blood flow is the cause, and not the consequence, of white matter lesions has been provided.[88] The causative role of episodic systemic hypotension which, in combination with narrowing of the vessel lumen, might lead to distal vascular insufficiency in the territory of the nonanastomotic vessels supplying the white matter, and eventually to infarction was suggested by Brun and Englund[27] and emphasized by Wallin and Blennow.[211] Repeated ischemic insults not reaching ne-

crotic or infarction thresholds could, however, damage more vulnerable cell groups such as oligodendrocytes[217] or trigger an astrocytic gliotic reaction.[147] An alternative hypothesis that explains the perivascular changes and the frequent absence of cavitary infarcts relates leukoaraiosis to a breakdown in the blood-brain barrier. Leakage and extravasation of serum proteins could take place in arteriosclerotic vessels, especially under ischemic conditions, and would lead to astrocytic activation, gliosis, release of vasoactive peptides, and further ischemia.[9,79,211]

Categorization

One of the most important sources of confusion and misunderstanding in the field of VD is the fact that it has traditionally been considered a single condition, irrespective of etiology or pathogenetic mechanisms.[82] While there is no doubt that VD is produced by ischemic infarction, this can only be understood as the final common pathway or common pathologic substrate where multiple pathophysiologic mechanisms concur.[212] This has been ignored by all available sets of diagnostic criteria,[35,172] which not only explains part of their poor reproducibility,[126,207,215] but also prevents their accurate application in the investigation of risk factors, etiology and, ultimately, prevention and treatment of VD.[16] The concept of dementia itself leads to the avoidance of such a crucial question. Given the degree of severity required by the time a diagnosis of dementia can be established, enough time has been allowed for different vascular mechanisms to concur and contribute to the clinical manifestations. In such a setting, the exact role of each factor cannot be discerned. The proposed concept of VCI will probably shed light on this area. Early recognition of cognitive changes related to cerebrovascular disease will help establish more accurate correlations between a particular cause and its clinical or radiologic manifestations. Also, a better understanding of the etiologic interactions of different vascular mechanisms will be reached. Ideally, a diagnosis of VCI should always be followed by a statement regarding the etiology, along with its likelihood (i.e., probable, possible, or associated with).

The different etiopathogenic and anatomopathologic categories of vascular mechanisms leading to cognitive decline and dementia have been extensively reviewed.[49,67,147,156,199] Numerous attempts to classify and categorize VD are available in the literature.[40,52,89,123,124,138,143,172,173,199,210] Unfortunately, most of them mix anatomic and pathophysiologic criteria, and only a few are based on clinical manifestations.[40,52,143,199] Etiologic classifications usually consist of mere listings of causes of stroke and are of limited value. Besides, many concepts are still poorly defined and remain confusing. The term *multi-infarct dementia* is often used to describe cases where the clinical picture of dementia results from the accumulation of several infarcts in the territory of large- or medium-sized arteries. Such a conception is usually applied in two senses. On the one hand, multi-infarct and single infarct dementia are considered separate entities.[172,210] While the distinction is academically laudable, both entities would necessarily fall together in a classification based on etiology or pathophysiology. On the other hand, the distinction between cases of "multi-infarct" dementia and those related to a hemodynamic mechanism might lead to misinterpretation since both entities result from the accumulation of multiple infarcts. In this case, the categorization is necessary, but the terminology is unfortunate. Terms like *chronic hypoperfusion*, *hemodynamic vascular dementia*, or *misery perfusion* are vaguely used and erroneously taken as synonyms of chronic ischemia. Brun has clearly stated how it is episodic hypoperfusion leading to infarction (surrounded by "incomplete infarction") and not chronic hypoperfusion itself that causes dementia.[26] In general, the concept *multi-infarct dementia* was conceived as a general term to emphasize that it was the accumulation of infarcts and not chronic ischemia that caused VD. In this sense, it would encompass all forms of vascular dementia once hemorrhages have been excluded. Today, the use of *multi-infarct dementia* is restricted to the aforementioned subtype of VD, and the general term has been substituted for ischemic vascular dementia. However, the reasons that justified its coining still exist and that is how the title of this chapter is meant to be understood.

Any classification of VCI should be based on etiology and pathophysiology. The different subtypes resulting from such categorization should be supported by pathologic data and, more important, should be clinically recognizable. Pathologic studies describe three main types of ischemic lesions in patients with dementia and no other neurodegenerative findings: arterial infarcts, lacunes, and subcortical leukoencephalopathy (white matter rarefaction, selective incomplete white matter ischemia, white matter gliosis or demyelination).[43,67,147,156] Other pathologic findings, less conspicuously described, include granular cortical atrophy (cortical microinfarcts), ischemic sclerosis (hippocampal or subicular sclerosis), laminar necrosis, perivascular protein deposits, and incomplete infarction. The question arises as to whether a *pathologic diagnosis* can be reached from clinical and paraclinical data, and how this can be related to a particular *etiologic diagnosis*. Is the traditional clinical method of neurology the best method for classifying VCI?

The first step consists in the recognition of cognitive symptoms and signs and their combination into clinical syndromes. A thorough characterization of the different patterns of cognitive deficits would facilitate an approximation to a topographic and subsequently an etiologic diagnosis. Vascular cognitive deficits, more precisely VD, have traditionally been classified as cortical or subcortical.[40,52] Such clinicotopographic division has always brought some etiologic implications. Cortical forms would be associated with large/medium-sized arterial infarcts while lacunar infarcts and white matter disease (often termed as Binswanger's disease) would manifest as subcortical dementias. Nevertheless, this distinction is based on the concept of dementia and excludes not only mild early cases, but also patients with cognitive decline without memory impairment.

SYNDROMES RESTRICTED TO ONE AREA OF COGNITION

Any clinical classification of VCI should provide information about what and how many areas of cognition are affected without preformed ideas. Focal syndromes with only one cognitive

domain affected should be distinguished from those in which the clinical picture includes deficits in two or more areas. That cerebrovascular disease can cause intellectual deficits confined to a single cognitive area is known since the work of Broca. The challenge for modern neurology is to recognize which patients will continue to develop further cognitive decline, ultimately dementia, and which are the mechanisms underlying such process. Certain clinicotopographic correlations may be considered when dealing with circumscribed cognitive deficits. In general, confined disturbances of language (aphasia), praxis (apraxia), or recognition (agnosia) will usually result from cortical lesions.[105] Exceptions include cases of transcortical aphasia or hemineglect syndromes caused by subcortical lesions involving the thalamus or basal ganglia.[42,213] In the majority of cases, however, an atheroembolic or cardioembolic infarct will be the underlying lesion. In some instances, watershed infarcts will manifest with an isolated transcortical aphasia or visuospatial disturbance.[4,61] Impairment of memory functions as a consequence of vascular lesions will rarely occur in an isolated fashion. Such cases have been described in relation to bilateral temporal lobe ischemia after episodes of global hypoxic ischemia.[163,209] This entity, known as hippocampal or subicular sclerosis, has been related to a vascular mechanism,[39] but the evidence is not conclusive. Dickson et al[45] found 13 cases among 81 autopsies performed on subjects who were 80 years of age or older and had been recruited in longitudinal studies of aging and dementia. While risk factors for cerebral hypoperfusion were common, clinical cardiovascular measures were not significantly different from patients without hippocampal sclerosis. Four patients had other neuropathologic findings, such as ballooned neurons or argyrophilic grains, suggestive of a neurodegenerative disorder. In the series of Knopman et al[111] 10 of 14 patients with so-called dementia without distinctive histopathological features had hippocampal sclerosis together with neurodegnerative findings in the frontoparietal cortices. After a thorough review of clinical and pathologic data from 8 patients with hippocampal sclerosis, 7 of which had a cardiac disorder, Corey-Bloom et al[38] concluded that "the relationship to cardiovascular disease remains unclear." They also found a decrease in neocortical synaptic density in these patients. Whether there is a connection between this finding and previous episodes of ischemia-hypoxia is also unclear. Consequently, while hippocampal sclerosis with selective neuronal loss and gliosis in the vulnerable regions has been related to global hypoperfusion, a history of episodic hypoxia cannot always be elicited, and in some cases a neurodegenerative disease cannot be ruled out. Whether hippocampal sclerosis can be diagnosed on the basis of neuroimaging findings has not been determined. Memory impairment may also occur in relation to deep infarcts involving the thalamus, basal ganglia, or anterior basal forebrain, but it is usually accompanied by other cognitive, affective, or personality changes.[64] Disturbance of executive functions may prove to be one of the hallmarks of cognitive impairment resulting from vascular causes. In patients with established dementia, impairment with executive functions helps to distinguish patients with VD from those with AD.[106,186,208] Describing an "isolated" compromise of executive functions may, however, be imprecise since different tasks, such as attention, planning, programming, anticipation, set shifting, or memory search strategies, are included under this heading.

The anatomic substrate for these abilities relies in complex and extensive neural networks including prefrontal cortical regions, basal ganglia, thalamus, and white matter connecting pathways that can be damaged by different vascular lesions in various locations.[41] Dysexecutive syndromes may follow small discrete lesions involving the paramedian thalamic nuclei[162] or the thalamocortical pathways that travel in the caudal capsular genu.[196] Patients with multiple frontal atheroembolic or lacunar infarcts as well as patients with extensive white matter damage may also present impaired executive functions.[12] Infarcts in the territory of the anterior cerebral artery or the anterior branches of the middle cerebral artery may result in impaired executive syndromes, disturbances of motivation or drive, and personality changes, depending on whether the dorsolateral prefrontal, the anterior cingular, or the lateral orbital cortices are predominantly affected. Similar symptoms have been described in patients with infarcts in the territory of the deep penetrating arteries supplying the caudate nucleus.[30]

FOCAL LESIONS CAUSING SYNDROMES INVOLVING MORE THAN ONE COGNITIVE AREA

Clinicotopographic correlations are more difficult to establish in patients presenting with two or more affected areas of cognition. The crucial step is to determine if the combination of cognitive deficits is the consequence of a single, strategically placed infarct or whether an accumulation of vascular lesions is taking place. Lesions in the angular gyrus, unilateral or bilateral thalamic infarctions, basal forebrain infarcts, and capsular genu infarctions are classic examples of clinically diagnosable dementia syndromes caused by strategically placed vascular injuries. Aphasia, alexia, visuoconstructional disturbances, and Gerstmann syndrome are the predominant manifestations of the angular gyrus syndrome resulting from infarcts in the posterior territory of the middle cerebral artery.[40] Various combinations of memory deficits, aphasia, frontal-like symptoms, apraxia, agnosia, mood and behavioral changes may result from unilateral or bilateral thalamic infarcts.[31,162] While most clinical series describe atherothrombotic or cardioembolic mechanisms for paramedian thalamic infarctions, some neuropathologic studies have emphasized the role of thalamic lacunes in the development of dementia in patients with cerebrovascular disease.[43] Basal forebrain lesions causing amnesia, dysexecutive symptoms, and behavioral changes are usually related to anterior communicating artery aneurysm rupture or surgery, and less frequently to infarcts in the territory of the penetrating branches of the anterior cerebral artery or the artery of Heubner.[64] Similar symptoms may result from small infarcts in the caudal capsular genu. In these cases, a lacunar mechanism is postulated.[196] Other lesions, such as those occurring in the territory of the posterior cerebral artery, which may cause different combinations of memory loss, aphasia, reading or writing disturbances, or visual agnosia, may also be considered strategic infarct dementia as a separate entity. However, the mechanisms leading to these types of lesions are varied, and the category would disappear if etiopathogenic criteria are to prevail in the categorization of VCI.

Most of the aforementioned categories of VCI are clinically recognizable, and their etiopathogenic implications may be effortlessly deciphered. It is important, however, to identify these entities as they may represent potential targets not only for preventive measures, but also for longitudinal studies to investigate the mechanisms by which cognitive impairment develops and progresses in the direction of dementia. The importance of recognizing these clinical syndromes of circumscribed or focal cognitive deficits and classifying them as VCI resides in the fact that cognitive impairment may continue to progress, increase in severity, or involve other areas of cognition. As previously mentioned, the idea of progression is inherent to the concept of VCI. Information regarding the mechanisms by which such progression takes place is surprisingly scarce, and it is extremely difficult to identify stroke patients at risk of developing further cognitive decline. Longitudinal studies are urgently needed in this field. The same statement applies for cases of cognitive impairment involving two or more areas of cognition which cannot be explained by a single infarct.

SYNDROMES INVOLVING MULTIPLE COGNITIVE AREAS

In all probability, this will prove to be the most common clinical presentation of VCI. As in all the examples described above, a thorough characterization of the neuropsychological deficits will be essential for classification. While prospective studies on VCI are performed, it can be hypothesized that most patients will fall into any of three possible cognitive models, that is, cortical, subcortical, and white matter deficits, or a combination of these.

Cortical VCI

Various combinations and degrees of fluent or nonfluent aphasia, alexia, agraphia, ideational or ideomotor apraxia, visuoconstructional or visuospatial deficits, agnosia, apperceptive or associative agnosia, or acalculia will characterize cortical syndromes, for which the accumulation of multiple cortical infarcts in the territory of large- or medium-sized arteries is considered the most frequent mechanism.[52] Cortical deficits would also be expected in cases of granular cortical atrophy, a rare neuropathologic entity that has been described in the context of amyloid angiopathy, generalized microembolic occlusion of cortical vessels, or hemodynamic disorders.[212] The concept of incomplete or selective ischemic necrosis, which substitutes the confusing term of *incomplete infarction*, is gaining acceptance as a form of vascular cortical damage that can potentially cause cognitive decline.[66] Selective neuronal death without cavitation occurs in certain vulnerable brain areas after global ischemia and has been described in the periphery of cavitary infarcts. It has been postulated that short episodes of ischemia might be severe enough to cause neuronal death but too short to induce glial destruction and cavitation. These lesions would not be detected by structural neuroimaging techniques, except for the presence of atrophy, and would be ignored in studies aiming to correlate infarct volume and severity of cognitive decline. The possibility that areas of selective necrosis may be detected with functional neuroimaging methods (PET or SPECT) and the investigation of whether these pathologic changes may be responsible of cognitive changes in patients with cerebrovascular disease opens a field for future research.[141,151] Selective ischemic neuronal loss in cortical regions has also been presented as a possible explanation for cognitive decline occurring in patients with internal carotid artery occlusion. Instead of cortical atrophy, callosal atrophy may represent a more reliable neuroradiologic correlate in these cases.[218]

Subcortical VCI

Patients with subcortical patterns of cognitive deficiencies should be carefully evaluated. Classic, well-established classifications of VD have identified subcortical forms of dementia with small-vessel disease in the form of either lacunar state or Binswanger's disease.[52,89,123,173] This traditional and generally accepted notion needs reconsideration. First, subcortical deficits may be caused by single or multiple atheroembolic infarcts, as described above. Second, the boundary between lacunar states and Binswanger's disease is not well established. Patients with dementia and multiple lacunes show white matter rarefaction in most cases[204] and lacunes are "very commonly found in the basal grey nuclei, thalami, pons, and cerebral white matter" in patients with Binswanger's disease.[28] Patients with lacunes and cognitive impairment have more severe white matter changes and a higher number of lacunes than lacunar patients with normal cognition. Both entities coincide in clinical manifestations, risk factors, and neuroradiologic findings, and it is not surprising that some authors have described them as "closely related"[152] or even "probably identical."[171] In a recent review, several pathologic conditions, including hypertension, amyloid angiopathy, hypercoagulable states, pseudoxanthoma elasticum, or syphilis, have been associated with clinical or even neuropathologic pictures diagnosed as Binswanger's disease.[28] This is probably the most important consideration, the syndrome that combines clinical strokes, subcortical cognitive deficits, gait disturbance, pyramidal and extrapyramidal signs, pseudobulbar syndrome with radiologic findings of white matter rarefaction, multiple lacunar infarcts and ventricular dilatation that progresses gradually or stepwise with periods of stabilization, is in fact a syndrome with different etiologies and pathogeneses. If this is kept in mind, terms like Binswanger's syndrome, or subcortical VCI might be more appropriate so long as they are followed by a statement about etiology. A label like "subcortical arteriosclerotic encephalopathy" would apply only to cases involving arteriolosclerosis, a descriptive "noncommittal" pathologic concept[147] with an excessively broad etiologic meaning. Arteriolosclerosis or lipohyalinosis of small muscular arteries and arterioles, characterized by vessel wall thickening, fibrous proliferation of the subendothelium, degeneration of the intima, endothelial swelling, intramural edema, presence of erythrocytes and lipid-laden macrophages with occasional fibrinoid necrosis, is related to hypertension but may be present in normotensive subjects[169] and has been described in hereditary forms of VD,[185] as well as in association with amyloid

angiopathy.[48] The NINDS-AIREN group used the term *small-vessel disease with dementia* to include lacunes and white matter lesion as causes of subcortical vascular dementia.[172] According to their description, Binswanger's disease would combine both lacunes and leukoencephalopathy and cerebral amyloid angiopathy or hypoperfusion are recognized as possible causes of white matter lesions. Wallin, Brun, and Gustafson[210] presented Binswanger's disease and lacunar state as synonyms. Brun's statement, according to which Binswanger's disease is the name given to a lacunar state that causes dementia, is very descriptive.[25] Wallin and Blennow[212] had previously tried to separate hyalinosis-associated forms of small-vessel dementia from other vessel-wall disorders such as amyloid angiopathy. In their classification, lacunar dementia, Binswanger's disease, and subcortical white-matter dementia are presented as different entities but when detailed descriptions are attempted, the overlap supported the conclusion that "subcortical white-matter dementia may be considered a combination of Binswanger's disease and lacunar dementia." One of the important contributions of these authors is the hypothesis (plausible but yet to be consistently proven) that hemodynamic-hypoxic mechanisms play an important role in the pathogenesis of white-matter vascular damage. The role of hypotension as an etiopathogenic factor for vascular dementia had already been highlighted by Sulkava and Erkinjuntti.[190] Therefore, cardiac arrhythmia, hypotension, anesthesia, sleep-apnea, and other disorders inducing cerebral hypoperfusion-hypoxia associated or not to other occlusive vasculopathies should be added to the list of causes or contributing factors of the Binswanger syndrome. Cerebral hypoxic and ischemic injury resulting from systemic illnesses is in fact a significant risk factor for the development of dementia after stroke.[146] Another entity that has to be added to the list of causes of subcortical forms of VCI is the more and more recognized hereditary form named cerebral autosomal dominant arteriopathy with subcortical strokes and ischemic leukoencephalopathy (CADASIL).[32] The disease is characterized by the combination of migraine with aura, mood disturbances, transient ischemic attacks and strokes at an unusual young age, pseudobulbar palsy, gait disturbances with pyramidal signs, and subcortical dementia with predominance of frontal-like symptoms in the members of the same family. Except for the absence of hypertension or other vascular risk factors, the clinical features are strikingly similar to those described in patients given a diagnosis of Binswanger's disease.[15] The resemblance persists in MRI findings as patients with CADASIL show small infarcts and extensive areas of abnormal signal in the periventricular and deep white matter as well as in the basal ganglia and brain stem.[175] Histologically, apart from white matter changes and lacunes, small arteries in the leptomeninges, white matter and deep gray structures show concentric thickening with splitting of the lamina elastica interna, hyalinosis of the media, and deposits of a granular PAS-positive material replacing the smooth muscle cells.[100] Similar changes have been described in muscle and skin vessels in some patients.[174] The prevalence of this disease is unknown but it may be more frequent than initially presumed. There were 25 families reported in Europe by 1993[15] and this number doubled in two years.[32] Genetic linkage studies had located the responsible gene in chromosome 19, and the critical region has already been mapped with mutations described in the Notch-3 gene.[99]

Genetic tests will probably be available soon, and this will allow studies to investigate whether cases of so-called Binswanger's disease are in fact CADASIL sporadic patients.

As can be appreciated, there is too much confusion surrounding subcortical VCI. Terminology has hidden ignorance for years and has prevented progress in the understanding of etiology and risk factors for the different types of this condition. Fortunately, some authors have already suggested separating lacunar states and Binswanger's disease from subcortical syndromes caused by CADASIL, amyloid angiopathy or coagulopathies.[124] However, the former terms are still maintained. Lacunar state and Binswanger's disease are probably two different ways to designate the same clinicoradiologic picture, and their use presumably contributes to increasing the confusion surrounding this matter as patients with different etiologies are grouped together under the same heading. The term *subcortical VCI* is suggested here to elude misconceptions regarding pathophysiology and emphasize the multiple etiologic nature of the clinical picture of subcortical cognitive deficits caused by small infarcts and white matter damage. CADASIL or amyloid angiopathy may be easy to recognize when certain clinical circumstances such as family history or lobar hemorrhage concur. For the remaining cases, laboratory investigation may reveal a hypercoagulable state such as hyperfibrinogenemia. An elevated number of patients will still remain etiologically undiagnosed but with all likelihood, hypertension will be the cause in an important proportion. Therefore, dividing these cases into hypertensive and nonhypertensive groups may facilitate further research in this field.

White Matter VCI, the Loss of Brain Connectivity

There is little doubt that white matter damage occurs and causes cognitive decline in patients without stroke. Moreover, pathologic studies show that leukoaraiosis is not always associated with lacunar infarcts suggesting that lacunes and white matter changes may correspond to different mechanisms in some patients.[58,74,128,206] While the pathogenesis of leukoaraiosis is still obscure, a vascular mechanism, such as infarction, increased permeability of white matter vessels, ischemic loss of vulnerable oligodendrocytes, or self-perpetuated glial inflammatory reactions induced by ischemia, can be claimed in the majority of cases. Therefore, these patients need to be recognized as a subtype of VCI despite the absence of a clinical history of stroke or radiologic evidence of infarction. Whether patients with leukoaraiosis with and without lacunar infarcts can be distinguished on a clinical basis requires prospective studies. Subjects with white matter hyperintensities and "no other focal MRI changes" perform poorly on tasks measuring speed of mental processing such as the trail-making test or an assembly procedure of the Purdue pegboard test while memory, attention, and conceptualization performance is similar to those without leukoaraiosis.[179] After excluding stroke patients and those with definite, well-demarcated white matter infarction, Boone and colleagues[14] reported low scores on attention, speed of information processing, and tests measuring frontal lobe functions among patients with severe white matter lesions. Ylikoski and colleagues[219] found significant negative correlation between severity of leukoaraiosis and attention and mental processing speed scores but not with memory, verbal, or constructional functions. Similar results were reported by Junqué and colleagues[101] in a sample of patients with minor stroke, including lacunar syndromes. Patients with subcortical infarctions display a similar pattern of frontal lobe dysfunction[216] but disturbances of memory and visuospatial abilities are also present.[37,204] The hypothesis is, therefore, that isolated white matter damage produces similar but more restricted cognitive deficits than lesions involving subcortical gray structures. Following Mesulam's model, lesions affecting the connecting components of neurocognitive networks cause different symptoms and signs than those directly involving subcortical relay centers. The distinction is important if etiopathogenic mechanisms and risk factors are different for isolated white matter damage from those for white matter rarefaction associated to small subcortical infarcts.

Categorization of VCI is complex and laborious. Clinical, etiologic, and pathogenic criteria should guide clinicians and researchers when classifying patients in homogeneous groups so that useful meaningful conclusions can be reached regarding risk factors, preventive or therapeutic measures.

Epidemiology

VCI exists only as a concept and its prevalence and incidence will remain unknown until valid diagnostic criteria are available. The Canadian Study on Health and Aging (CSHA) evaluated over 10,000 elderly subjects of whom 18.1% showed some degree of cognitive impairment as measured with the modified mini-mental scale. Among the subjects, 861 presented cognitive decline without dementia and of these, 149 (17.3%) had a vascular cause for their cognitive impairment.[47] VCI was the second cause of cognitive decline without dementia in this study, after age-associated memory impairment. If patients with vascular dementia and mixed dementia (AD with a vascular component) are considered, it can be said that 4.8% of the population evaluated in the CSHA had some degree of VCI.[180] It is likely, however, that this figure underestimates the contribution of vascular causes to cognitive decline in the general population, since no neuroimaging evaluation was required in this survey.

VASCULAR RISK FACTORS AND COGNITION

There is sufficient evidence that vascular factors play a significant role in the development of cognitive decline in nondemented subjects. Breteler and colleagues[45] have demonstrated that the presence of electrocardiographic signs of myocardial infarction, peripheral arterial disease, or carotid atheromatous changes doubles the proportion of subjects falling below the cut-off score of 24 points in the Mini-Mental State (MMS) Examination. History of stroke multiplied this proportion by 3. When demented patients are excluded from a representative cohort of the elderly population, vascular risk factors such as hypertension or diabetes are significant predictors of lower scores in cognitive tests such as the Cambridge

Cognitive Examination (CAMCOG).[132] This effect appears to be independent of the presence of stroke. Newly diagnosed hypertensives show poor performance on tests measuring attention and reaction times as compared with controls.[13] Similar results were reported by van Swieten et al[205] who found that elderly hypertensives performed worse on tests measuring frontal functions and speed of mental processes (trail-making tests, stroop test) than nonhypertensives, an effect that was explained by the presence of moderate to severe confluent white matter lesions. Cognitive deficits associated to hypertension have been described in many other studies. Diabetes and hypercholesterolemia were independent correlates of abstract reasoning/visuospatial deficits and memory dysfunction, respectively, in 249 stroke-free patients after adjusting for age, education, and occupation.[44] The effect of hypercholesterolemia on memory deficits might be explained by an association with the presence of the allele ϵ4 of the apolipoprotein E (apo E) and hence to early Alzheimer's changes, but a vascular mechanism seems plausible for the effect of diabetes. Whether all these forms of cognitive impairment herald dementia remains unknown, as they go undetected in the population. Recent reports from different longitudinal epidemiologic surveys have shown that both hypertension[46,181] and diabetes[120,158] are significant risk factors for dementia, including VD and AD.

COGNITION IN STROKE

The proportion of stroke patients classified as cognitively impaired varies depending on which diagnostic tool is used and what cut-off points are selected. Mori et al[144] found that 51% of their 300 stroke patients (including 76 with hemorrhages) had some abnormalities in the Hasegawa dementia rating scale, which is similar to the MMS. Moderate or severe deficits were found in 15% of cases. Using the CAMCOG, Kwá et al[116,187] detected some degree of cognitive impairment in 47 of 129 stroke patients, including 12 with severe aphasia. Grace et al[75] found that 29% of their 70 patients with stroke scored 24 or less in the Folstein MMS, while 43% fell below the cut-off of 79 in the modified MMS (3MS). The difference can be explained by the fact that the 3MS adds items exploring cued recall, semantic fluency, and abstract thinking. Deficits in these areas are expected in cerebrovascular disease and are not detected by the MMS. The 3MS had a stronger relationship with a functional independence measure than the MMS. However, both tests showed low sensitivity rates to detect stroke-related cognitive impairment in this study. Patients were classified as cognitively impaired when they scored 2SDs below the norm in two or more cognitive domains in a neuropsychological battery including tests for mental control, orientation, language, visuospatial abilities, verbal fluency, and memory. Using these criteria, 32 patients (46%) were impaired, 56% of these patients scored higher than 24 in the MMS, and 31% obtained more than 79 points in the 3MS. Tatemichi and colleagues[194] administered a 17-item neuropsychological battery assessing memory, orientation, language, visuospatial ability, abstract reasoning, and attention to a sample of 227 consecutive patients with stroke. Using the 5th percentile scores of control subjects as the cut-off point, 35.2% failed four or more items and were considered cogni-

tively impaired. Stroke was more likely to be associated with deficits in visual recognition, orientation, category fluency, repetition and attention. More importantly, cognitive impairment was associated with functional impairment and dependent living, even after adjusting for physical disability.

DEMENTIA AFTER STROKE

It is now well demonstrated that having a stroke is a significant risk factor for dementia. Numerous studies have shown that the prevalence of dementia among patients with stroke is much higher than would be expected for populations of the same age. Ladurner et al[117] evaluated a series of 71 stroke patients. It is not clear whether they were consecutive cases, but using the Wechsler Adult Intelligence Scale (WAIS) they found that 40 (56%) patients had cognitive deterioration severe enough to qualify as early dementia. Hypertension, bilateral lesions, general atrophy and thalamic infarcts were more frequent among the demented group. Kotila and colleagues[115] followed a sample of 52 stroke patients for 4 years. They observed that 35% showed some deterioration in their verbal or performance IQ. Three patients (6%) developed dementia, a number which is not that low as only subjects younger than 65 were recruited. Studying consecutive patients with multiple infarcts, Loeb et al[125] found dementia in 55% of their 98 cases, as defined by the Blessed dementia score. After excluding 14 patients with possible mixed dementia, dementia was associated with multiple lesions in thalamic and cortical areas, as well as with brain atrophy. The study by Babikian et al[7] was also focused on patients with two or more infarcts. They used an extensive neuropsychological battery and found some degree of cognitive impairment in "virtually every patient," but "only" seven patients (30% of their sample) were demented according to their MMS score. As mentioned, the frequency of dementia in all these samples of patients with stroke is much higher than expected. However, the number of patients included in these studies might be too small and no control groups were used for comparison. To confirm these findings, Tatemichi and colleagues[195] Carried out a prospective study in which the frequency of dementia was evaluated in 251 patients with stroke and compared to that in a control sample of 249 stroke-free subjects. Using DSM-III-R criteria 66 patients from the stroke sample (26.3%) were demented while only 8 controls (3.2%) fulfilled these criteria. After adjusting for age and education, the odds ratio for stroke was 9:4. Interestingly, the frequency of AD aggravated by stroke was 10% in the stroke sample, higher than the frequency of all dementias in the control group. The same group of investigators studied the incidence of dementia in 185 stroke patients and 241 age-matched controls after a follow-up of 1 to 4 years. Incidence rates were 8.4 and 1.3 per 100 person-years, respectively. The relative risk for dementia associated with stroke was 5.5. When the mechanisms for dementia were analyzed, it was found that 12 patients had not presented any obvious precipitating event such as new focal or global ischemia. Either silent progressive cerebrovascular disease or occult AD were claimed as possible explanations for the development of dementia in these cases. The authors hypothesized that stroke not only increases the risk for VD but may also enhance the cognitive consequences of aging or aggravate the effects of AD. This conclusion has been confirmed to a certain extent by the findings of the longitudinal study on dementia after ischemic stroke performed in Rochester, Minnesota.[114] In this study, 196 out of 971 nondemented stroke patients developed dementia after 6,782 person-years of observation. The incidence of dementia during the first year after stroke was nine times higher than that in the general population. When only AD was analyzed, the incidence was approximately twice that in the community.

PREVALENCE OF VASCULAR DEMENTIA

Despite the extensive literature on this matter, a similar statement as that for VCI could be formulated regarding the prevalence of VD. The concept of prevalence is based on the premise that a population can be divided into cases and controls or noncases. This is particularly complicated for a disease such as VD, which is chronic, is in need of reliable diagnostic markers or diagnostic criteria, and shares so many features with other conditions that affect the same age groups such as stroke or AD. It is not surprising that prevalence figures for VD dance from one study to another depending on the sample under survey (autopsy series, general hospital samples, stroke patients, population-based studies) or the diagnostic tool applied (pathology, clinical criteria, clinical and neuroimaging data).

The largest autopsy series in the literature included 675 demented subjects from three different sources: a psychiatric hospital (137 patients), a general hospital (230 patients), and a geriatric hospital (308 patients).[97] The overall frequency of VD was 15.7%. Among patients with AD (60%) a total of 56 (8.3%) patients had vascular lesions and 53 additional patients (7.9%) received the diagnosis of mixed dementia. This diagnosis of mixed dementia was defined by the presence of sufficient lesions to fulfil both AD and VD pathologic criteria. The lowest rate of VD was obtained in the psychiatric population (9.5%) and the highest in the autopsy population from the general hospital (18.3%). Frequency numbers reported in other studies with much smaller sample sizes are highly variable from 0% to 19%. Autopsy series have the highest diagnostic accuracy, but samples are inevitably biased and all published series are focused on demented patients and not on consecutive series of autopsies. The frequency of VD among patients with a clinical diagnosis of AD is 2.3% (3.5% if hippocampal sclerosis is included) when autopsy diagnosis is performed.[110] Moreover, 30% to 40% of patients with a pathologic diagnosis of AD, not mixed dementia, have one or more infarcts (see below).

Hospital-based series should offer a reasonable diagnostic accuracy if detailed cognitive and clinical examinations are performed and adequate neuroimaging techniques are used, but these studies are also subjected to significant referral bias. Series of patients referred for dementia or memory problems will be biased toward AD, and those referred for stroke or general medicine will probably include a higher proportion of VCI. The problem of referral or selection bias is easily avoided if population-based designs are chosen, but then other methodologic difficulties arise. Most epidemiologic studies do

not include neuroimaging evaluation. This will necessarily lead to an underestimation of VD, as not all patients suffer a clinical stroke. In the study by Skoog et al,[182] 10 patients received a diagnosis of VD only after CT was evaluated. Community or population-based studies may also suffer from two types of selection biases. On the one hand, a significant bias may be introduced by nonresponders if they have a higher incidence of vascular disease, as might be expected. On the other, the majority of studies follow a double-phase design in which a population is first screened for the presence of dementia and those screening positive are then clinically evaluated. Patients with vascular disease are more likely to die or abandon the study between the first and second phase of the study than those without. Exclusion of institutionalized patients may also leave many VD patients out of the studies.[53] All these circumstances will probably lead to a significant underestimation of vascular causes of dementia. However, these sources of bias are easy to be controlled and accounted for if adequate methodologies are applied. Hébert and Brayne[86] have reviewed 10 prevalence studies. All were performed on representative samples of the reference populations, applied the same diagnostic criteria (DSM-III) and reported specific data on VD.[19,63,85,104,154,168,180,189,200,221] Prevalence rates varied form 1.2% to 5.6%. The two studies using CT evaluation reported higher prevalence figures. Lower rates were obtained in those studies that excluded institutionalized subjects, despite the fact that two of them counted cases of mixed dementia as VD. Prevalence of VD increased with age in eight studies but followed a linear trend rather than the exponential increase described in AD. No significant differences were observed between men and women. The prevalence of total dementia was similar for the 10 studies; however, the proportion of cases with VD varied from 24% to 48%. As expected, it was higher in the Japanese surveys. Among the European studies only the one from Italy showed an AD/VD ratio lower than one. Not surprisingly, it was the only study that included CT as part of the clinical evaluation. Apart from this, one of the most important determinants of distortions in prevalence figures of VD is how mixed dementia is diagnosed and classified. Skoog et al included mixed dementia cases as VD, obtaining a prevalence rate of 13.9% for VD.[53] Prevalence of VD in the Rotterdam study was 1%. AD accounted for 72% of dementias in this survey, but this figure included patients with mixed dementia.[159] These numbers are obviously misleading if the contribution of vascular causes to the prevalence of dementia is to be estimated. Unfortunately the diagnosis of mixed dementia does not differentiate cases in which stroke is just accompanying AD from those patients that would not be demented had they not presented any cerebrovascular disease. The diagnostic category of possible AD introduced by the NINCDS-ADRDA criteria does not solve this question. The concept of mixed dementia should be reviewed and redefined (see below).

RISK FACTORS FOR VASCULAR COGNITIVE IMPAIRMENT

As has been mentioned, investigation of potential risk factors or markers for VCI will only be feasible when reliable diagnostic criteria are available. If attention is focused on VD, it can also be said that risk factors remain unknown. Research and literature in this area is somewhat scarce and there are three main questions that have not yet been answered:

Are risk factors for VD the same as for stroke?, What should be the control population with which to compare VD patients?

What putative risk factors should be investigated?

From what has been written in this chapter, the reader will understand that the answer to the first question will only be reached if different types of VD are considered separately. Stroke-related variables alone (number, volume, location) are possibly not sufficient to explain all cases of VD. Cases in which VD is the consequence of the accumulation of atherothrombotic or cardioembolic infarcts will surely respond to the same risk factors as for carotid disease or cardiopathy. However, other types of vascular damage to the brain such as leukoaraiosis, selective ischemic necrosis, or atrophy are probably important in a number of cases. Whether risk factors for the development of these type of lesions are the same as those for stroke requires further research. A similar approach is needed to answer the second question. The investigation of risk factors requires that cases and noncases be clearly separated. In the field of VD the presence of certain risk factors has been used to establish such distinction and this diagnostic bias has led to the assumption that vascular risk factors are indeed risk factors for VD. A more appropriate setting is probably that in which cases and noncases are separated on the basis of the presence of dementia for each category of cerebrovascular disease. Patients with lacunes and dementia should be compared to lacunar patients with no cognitive decline. The third question is crucial. To date, only the presence or absence of traditional vascular risk factors has been investigated. The effect of whether these factors were treated or adequately controlled has not been evaluated. Other potential factors such as hypotension, hypoxic conditions, hypercoagulable states, or markers of acute phase reactions have received little attention. Genetic factors and family history have been only partially assessed. Family history of leukoaraiosis, for instance, is difficult to investigate, and the importance of the presence of migraine with aura or psychiatric disorders in the family should be evaluated in the light of the new findings on CADASIL.

When neurologically normal controls are chosen for comparison, it is not surprising that known vascular risk factors such as hypertension, heart disease, diabetes, smoking and carotid bruits are significantly more frequent among patients with "multi-infarct dementia," especially if diagnosis is made on the basis of the ischemic score.[140] Katzman et al[103] used a nonselected sample of controls to investigate the distribution of vascular risk factors in patients with "multi-infarct and mixed dementia." A history of prior stroke and diabetes was significantly more frequent among cases. The proportion of hypertensives was even higher in the control group, but left ventricular hypertrophy was observed more frequently in patients with dementia. These differences were not significant. Epidemiologic works using this type of community or population-based designs for the investigation of risk factors for VD are unfortunately scarce in the literature. Yoshitake et al[220] followed up a representative sample of 828 nondemented subjects older than 65. After 7 years, 103 subjects developed dementia and either CT or autopsy findings were available in 89 of them. Using the NINDS-AIREN criteria, VD was diagnosed in 50 cases (48.5%). The most frequent type of VD was that resulting from multiple lacunar infarcts and, as the authors emphasize, half of these patients lacked a history of stroke. Univariate analysis showed that age, alcohol intake, diabetes, history of stroke, systolic and diastolic blood pressure, and increased hematocrit were significant risk factors for VD. Low educational level did not have a significant effect. When these variables were entered in a multivariate analysis only age, systolic blood pressure, alcohol intake, and history of stroke at entry remained significant, even when occurrence of stroke during follow-up was considered. The question of whether risk factors for VD are the same as those for stroke has been analyzed in several studies confronting samples of patients with stroke with and without dementia. Methodologic differences regarding sample sizes, inclusion criteria, or diagnostic criteria for VD are probably responsible for the variability of results across studies and prevents their comparison. Ladurner et al[117] compared 40 patients with stroke and early dementia, defined by the WAIS scores, with 31 nondemented stroke patients. Only hypertension was found to be more frequent among the demented patients. The prevalence of hypertension, cardiopathy, and of "associated hypertension, cardiopathy and diabetes" was found to be significantly higher in the group of patients with dementia that Loeb et al[125] included in their study. Dementia was diagnosed according to the Blessed dementia score and only patients with multiple infarcts were included. Analysis of data collected from the Stroke Data Bank Cohort[198] revealed that myocardial infarction and history of previous stroke, but not hypertension, diabetes, atrial fibrillation, or antiplatelet or anticoagulant therapies were significantly associated with prevalent dementia (including AD). Educational level only showed a nonsignificant trend of association. When incident cases were analyzed, previous stroke and cortical atrophy were the only important predictors. The population-based study of Rochester[114] included 971 patients with a first-ever stroke; 196 patients became demented. Age, male sex, having a second stroke, and mitral valve prolapse were the only variables with a significant effect on the incidence of dementia. In their prospective study on dementia after stroke, Tatemichi et al found that age, education, race, history of prior stroke, and diabetes mellitus were independently associated with dementia.[197] The presence of race among the significant factors might suggest a role for genetic factors; however, this variable lost significance when patients with suspected AD and stroke were excluded. Gorelick and colleagues[72] carried out a similar study on consecutive patients with stroke, but only patients with two or more cerebral infarcts were recruited. Among 147 patients, 61 had multi-infarct dementia. Age, hypertension, proteinuria, myocardial infarction, smoking, and systolic blood pressure were significant predictors of dementia in a multivariate analysis. However, hypertension and proteinuria, which might have reflected systemic damage from diabetes, lost significance when education was included in the multiple logistic regression model. Interestingly, the effect of systolic blood pressure was "protective" with an OR of 0.91 for a 1-unit increase. As previously mentioned, the results of these studies are too varied to draw any conclusions. Similarly to AD, it appears that any analysis on risk factors for VD should be adjusted for both age and educational level. Among the cardiovascular variables, repetitive stroke is the only consistent factor across different studies. Apart from methodologic differences, it would be of interest to analyze the proportion of cases with lacunar or atherothrombotic infarcts, or that of patients with or without white matter changes, but this information is not provided in all studies. Another important point is that in all the mentioned studies, only traditional vascular risk factors were investigated. Some authors have suggested that other factors such as increased platelet activation,[93,133] increased fibrinogen,[128] and/or immunologic abnormalities[127] might be related to VD. Also, clinical events leading to cerebral hypoperfusion or hypoxia may facilitate the development of dementia in stroke patients.[146] Some reports have described an increased proportion of the allele ∈4 of apo E in patients with VD, but neuropathologic studies have not confirmed this association.[10] Careful analysis of all these data—together with the fact that despite intensive control of vascular risk factors in the last decades incidence of VD has not changed significantly—reveals that further research in this area is urgently needed.

Vascular Pathology in Alzheimer's Disease: What Is Mixed Dementia?

Tomlinson, Blessed, and Roth[201] applied the concept of mixed dementia to describe four brains from patients with dementia that showed AD-type neurodegenerative changes and "cerebral softenings." Both types of changes were severe enough to have caused dementia had they been on their own. However, they did not exactly know how to classify five additional demented cases that had senile plaques counts and volumes of cerebral softening in the upper limit of that observed in controls. The absence of neocortical neurofibrillary changes was striking in these patients. With some reserves they used the term *probable mixed dementia*.

Brains from patients with AD show three types of vascular changes: amyloid angiopathy, white matter lesions, and infarcts. Amyloid angiopathy is present in 80% of patients and is moderate to severe in one- to two-thirds of them.[48,211] The severity of the angiopathy is associated with the apo E polymorphism. It has been shown that the proportion of apo E/∈4 carriers is increased in those with amyloid angiopathy and the degree of severity is higher in monozygotes.[102] On the other hand, the presence of amyloid angiopathy increases the risk of having a vascular ischemic or hemorrhagic lesion at autopsy by a factor of 3. Interestingly enough, the risk increases 14 times if both hypertension and amyloid angiopathy are associated in the same individual.[155] White matter lesions (leuko-araiosis) on CT or MRI of the brain in patients with AD may be detected in 30% to 90% of cases, depending on the criteria, but they are moderate to severe in only 20% to 30%. One study has shown that leukoaraiosis is not more frequent in early AD patients than in controls if both groups are adjusted for age and presence of vascular risk factors.[50] Whether the presence of white matter lesions worsens the

cognitive deficit is difficult to evaluate. As previously described, the pathophysiology of white-matter vascular damage has been related with distal ischemia (amyloid angiopathy), hypotension, increased vascular permeability, or inflammatory astrocytic reactions. The presence of ischemic infarcts in the brains of patients with neuropathologically confirmed AD (not mixed dementia) is by no means infrequent. Zubenko et al[223] found at least one infarct in 20 of their 91 patients with AD diagnosed according to the criteria of Kachaturian. Among the 190 brains diagnosed with AD according to the CERAD criteria evaluated by Premkumar et al,[164] 36% of cases had vascular lesions (recent or chronic infarcts, multiple microinfarcts, leukoaraiosis, or haemorrhagic infarcts). The proportion of apo E/∈4 carriers was significantly higher in those with vascular lesions. Similar findings have been reported in other studies.[168,216]

The question arises if the presence of these vascular lesions is just coincidental. Existing evidence suggests that this is not the case and that vascular lesions might play a significant pathophysiologic role and contribute to the development of dementia in this "subtype" of AD. On the one hand, when vascular lesions are present, age of onset of dementia is significantly delayed for at least 6 years[48,176] (Bowler, personal communication). Besides, the density of neurofibrillary changes is significantly lower in AD patients with vascular lesions.[150] Sabbagh et al found that one half of their "plaque-only" AD cases had vascular pathology.[176] Patients with vascular dementia may have higher densities of senile plaques than subjects with vascular lesions and no dementia.[43] Moreover, Nagy et al analyzed the association of pathologic findings with cognitive scores. In their "pure" AD cases, CAMCOG scores correlated significantly with neurofibrillary tangle and neuritic plaque density while in AD patients with vascular disease cognitive scores correlated with total and neuritic plaque density but not with neurofibrillary tangle density.[150] Epidemiologic studies have also provided valuable information regarding the contribution of vascular factors to AD. Hypertension has been shown to be a significant risk factor not only for VD but also for AD in two different studies.[46,181] A similar role has been confirmed for diabetes[120,158] and atrial fibrillation.[160] New data supporting the role of ischemic lesions in the development of dementia in patients with AD have been reported by Snowdon et al.[184] According to them, in subjects with neuropathologic changes consistent with AD, the risk of having presented dementia in life increases 20 times if lacunar infarcts are present in the basal ganglia, thalamus, or white matter. Molecular or genetic epidemiology and neuropathologic studies have also shown that apo E/∈4 increases the risk not for VD, but for mixed dementia.[10,183] Finally, it should not be overlooked that similarly to brain trauma, cerebral ischemia may upregulate the amyloid precursor protein in the experimental animal and facilitate the deposition of β-amyloid in the human brain.[68,98]

Mixed dementia represents an important proportion of cases and its study has been systematically avoided. Cerebrovascular disease can precipitate the appearance of intellectual decline when the brain is challenged by the presence of early degenerative changes and vice versa. Also, a question may be formulated as to whether cerebral ischemia can play a role as a triggering factor of cellular and subcellular changes ultimately leading to neurodegeneration. Attention to all these matters and recognition of this potentially preventable and treatable component of Alzheimer's disease will undoubtedly help a high number of patients.

Conclusions and Perspectives

The concept of VCI is formulated as a necessary starting point for the progress on the field of cerebrovascular disease and cognition. It should not be understood as a new entity, but rather as a new tool, a new way of approaching a problem that remains tied to old, preformed, untested, or unproven concepts that impede further progress. As has been suggested,[82,84] an International Data Bank of prospectively collected and longitudinally followed cases will be invaluable in this field. Information collected for each patient should include a minimally agreed upon set of diagnostic instruments. Clinical data on age and symptoms at onset, pattern of progression, cerebrovascular events, family history, as well as demographic data are essential. Results from neurologic and cardiovascular examinations should be collected in a simple and standardized format. Information on risk factors should be carefully gathered, including data on treatment and the extent to which they are efficiently controlled. Investigation of risk factors may include laboratory tests for homocysteine, antiphospholipid antibodies, fibrinogen, platelet activation, or acute phase reaction proteins. Genetic testing for apo E status is recommended for any research project on cognitive decline and dementia. Besides, DNA should be collected and stored for every patient, as it is conceivable that new susceptibility genes will be discovered soon for AD, VD, or both. Basic quantitative and comparable information on cognition is imperative. The Folstein Mini-Mental State Examination is probably the most widely used instrument, and normative data adjusted for age and education are already available in several populations. However, short mental status tests have proved efficient to detect dementia, although their validity as screening instruments for early cognitive changes has not been fully tested. Therefore, a comprehensive, complete battery of indispensable neuropsychologic tests should be included whenever possible. Different cognitive screening scales could then be analyzed for sensitivity and specificity. Neuroimaging data should provide information on type, number, and location of infarcts. White matter changes should be classified regarding type, location, and degree of severity on the basis of agreed upon and standardized scales. The role of functional imaging needs to be adequately assessed. Other investigations including echocardiogram, carotid ultrasound, Holter-ECG, blood pressure monitoring, autonomic function tests, tests for sleep-apnea, or vasculitis screening, may prove useful in selected cases. Finally, the combination of clinical and neuroimaging data should be translated in an attempt of etiological diagnosis where probable or possible etiopathogenic mechanisms should be defined. Only when data are collected in this systematized manner may cases be reclassified as soon as new advances are achieved in the understanding of the vascular mechanisms and causes of cognitive impairment. Once diagnostic criteria for VCI are developed, early detection and diagnosis will soon be followed by a better understanding of its pathogenic mechanisms and etiologies; its distinctive clinical manifestations will be more accurately characterized; the role of known vascular risk factors will be reassessed and new risk factors will be recognized. Understandably, the field for a better management of patients will be sown and fertilized. Patients will be classified in different stages—the "brain at risk" stage characterized by the presence of risk factors, the "predementia stage" where the first cognitive symptoms appear, and the dementia stage—for which potential therapeutic interventions are already available.

Acknowledgments

Dr. Martinez-Lage is supported by Grant #95/5551 from the Fondo de Investigación Sanitaria of the Ministry of Health of Spain. This work has been partially supported by Dr. Hachinski's Trillium Clinical Scientist Award.

References

1. Alzheimer A: Die seelenstoerungen auf arteriosclerotischer grundlage. Allg Z Psychiat Gericht Med 59:695, 1902

2. American Psychiatric Association: Diagnostic and Statistical Manual of Mental Disorders. 4th Ed. American Psychiatric Press, Washington DC, 1994

3. An G, Lin T-N, Liu J-S, et al: Expression of c-*fos* and c-*jun* family genes after focal cerebral ischemia. Ann Neurol 33:457, 1993

4. Arboix A, Martí-Vilalta JL: Manifestaciones clínicas de los infartos isquémicos cerebrales de los "territorios frontera." p. 33. In Matías-Guiu J, Martinez-Vila E, Martí-Vilalta JL (eds): Isquemia cerebral global. JR Prous Editores, Barcelona, 1992

5. Asken MJ, Hobson RW: Intellectual change and carotid endarterectomy, subjective speculation or objective reality: a review. J Surg Res 23:367, 1977

6. Awad IA, Johnson PC, Spetzler RF et al: Incidental subcortical lesions identified on magnetic resonance imaging in the elderly. Vol. 1. Correlations with age and cerebrovascular risk factors. Stroke 17:1084, 1986

7. Babikian VL, Wolfe N, Linn R et al: Cognitive changes in patients with multiple cerebral infarcts. Stroke 21:1013, 1990

8. Ball MJ: Leuko-araiosis explained. Lancet 1:612, 1989

9. Baloh RW, Vinters HV: White matter lesions and disequilibrium in older people. Arch Neurol 52:975, 1995

10. Betard C, Robitaille Y, Gee M et al: ApoE allele frequencies in Alzheimer's disease, Lewy body dementia, Alzheimer's disease with cerebrovascular disease and vascular dementia. Neuroreport 5:1893, 1994

11. Binswanger O: Die abgrenzung der allgemeinen progressive paralyse. Berl Klin Wochschr 31:1103, 1894

12. Bogousslavsky J, Brunasconi A, Kumral E: Acute multi-

ple infarction involving the anterior circulation. Arch Neurol 53:50, 1996

13. Boller F, Vrtunski PB, Mack JL et al: Neuropsychological correlates of hypertension. Arch Neurol 34:701, 1977

14. Boone KB, Miller BL, Lesser IM et al: Neuropsychological correlates of white matter lesions in healthy elderly subjects: a threshold effect. Arch Neurol 49:549, 1992

15. Bousser MG, Tournier-Lasserve E: Summary of the proceedings of the first International Workshop on CADASIL. Paris, May 19-21, 1993. Stroke 25:704, 1994

16. Bowler JV, Hachinski VC: History of the concept of vascular dementia. Two opposing views on current definitions and criteria for vascular dementia. p. 1. In Prohovnik I, Wade J, Knezevic S et al (eds): Vascular dementia: a review of concepts and ideas. John Wiley & Sons, Chichester, 1996

17. Bracco L, Campani D, Baratti E et al: Relation between MRI features and dementia in cerebrovascular disease patients with leukoaraiosis: a longitudinal study. J Neurol Sci 120:131, 1993

18. Braffman BH, Zimmerman RA, Trojanowski JQ et al: Brain MR: pathologic correlation with gross and histopathology. vol. 1. Lacunar infarction and Virchow-Robin spaces. AJNRR 9:621, 1988

19. Brayne C, Calloway P: An epidemiologic study of dementia in a rural population of elderly women. Br J Psychiatry 155:214, 1989

20. Bredesen DE: Neural apoptosis. Ann Neurol 38:839, 1995

21. Breteler MMB, van Amerongen NM, van Swieten JC et al: Cognitive correlates of ventricular enlargement and cerebral white matter lesions on magnetic resonance imaging. The Rotterdam study. Stroke 25:1109, 1994

22. Breteler MMB, Claus JJ, Grobbee DE et al: Cardiovascular disease and distribution of cognitive function in elderly people: the Rotterdam study. BMJ 308:1604, 1994

23. Breteler MMB, van Swieten JC, Bots ML et al: Cerebral white matter lesions, vascular risk factors, and cognitive function in a population-based study: the Rotterdam Study. Neurology 44:1246, 1994

24. Brown WD, Frackowiak SFJ: Cerebral blood flow and metabolism studies in multiinfarct dementia. Alzheimer Dis Assoc Disord 5:131, 1991

25. Brun A: Vascular dementia: pathological findings. p. 653. In Burns A, Levy R (eds): Dementia. Chapman & Hall, London, 1994

26. Brun A: Pathology and pathophysiology of cerebrovascular dementia: pure subgroups of obstructive and hypoperfusive etiology. Dementia 5:145, 1994

27. Brun A, Englund E: A white matter disorder in dementia of the Alzheimer type: a pathoanatomical study. Ann Neurol 19:253, 1986

28. Caplan LR: Binswanger's disease—revisited. Neurology 45:626, 1995

29. Caplan LR, Schoene WC: Clinical features of subcortical arteriosclerotic encephalopathy (Binswanger disease). Neurology 28:1206, 1978

30. Caplan LR, Schmahmann JD, Kase CS et al: Caudate infarcts. Arch Neurol 47:133, 1990

31. Castaigne P, Lhermitte F, Buge A et al: Paramedian thalamic and midbrain infarcts: clinical and neuropathological study. Ann Neurol 10:127, 1981

32. Chabriat H, Vahedi K, Iba-Zizen MT et al: Clinical spectrum of CADASIL: a study of 7 families. Lancet 346:934, 1995

33. Chimowitz MI, Awad IA, Furlan AJ: Periventricular lesions on MRI. Facts and theories. Stroke 20:963, 1989

34. Chimowitz MI, Estes ML, Furlan AJ et al: Further observations on the pathology of subcortical lesions identified on magnetic resonance imaging. Arch Neurol 49:747, 1992

35. Chui HC, Victoroff JI, Margolin D et al: Criteria for the diagnosis of ischemic vascular dementia proposed by the State of California Alzheimer's disease diagnostic and treatment centers. Neurology 42:473, 1992

36. Collaço-Moraes Y, Aspey BS, de Beleroche JS et al: Focal ischemia causes an extensive induction of immediate early genes that are sensitive to MK-801. Stroke 25:1855, 1994

37. Corbett A, Bennett H, Kos S: Cognitive dysfunction following subcortical infarction. Arch Neurol 51:999, 1994

38. Corey-Bloom J, Sabbagh MN, Bondi MW et al: Hippocampal sclerosis contributes to dementia in the elderly. Neurology 48:154, 1997

39. Crystal HA, Dickson DW, Sliwinski MJ et al: Pathological markers associated with normal aging and dementia in the elderly. Ann Neurol 34:566, 1993

40. Cummings JL, Benson DF: Vascular dementias. p. 153. In Cummings JL, Benson DF (eds): Dementia: A Clinical Approach. 2nd Ed. Butterworth-Heinemann, Boston, 1992

41. Cummings JL: Frontal-subcortical circuits and human behavior. Arch Neurol 50:873, 1993

42. Damasio AR, Damasio H, Rizzo M et al: Aphasia with nonhemorrhagic lesions of the basal ganglia and internal capsule. Arch Neurol 39:15, 1982

43. del Ser T, Bermejo F, Portera A et al: Vascular dementia. A clinicopathological study. J Neurol Sci 96:1, 1990

44. Desmond DW, Tatemichi TK, Paik M et al: Risk factors for cerebrovascular disease as correlates of cognitive function in a stroke-free cohort. Arch Neurol 50:162, 1993

45. Dickson DW, Davies P, Bevona C et al: Hippocampal sclerosis: a common pathological feature of dementia in very old (≥ 80 years of age) humans. Acta Neuropathol 88:212, 1994

46. Duara R, Barker W, Harwood D et al: Risk factors for Alzheimer's disease in women. Ann Neurol 40:500A, 1996

47. Ebly E, Hogan D, Parhad I: Cognitive impairment in the nondemented elderly. Arch Neurol 52:612, 1995

48. Ellis RJ, Olichney JM, Thal LJ et al: Cerebral amyloid angiopathy in the brains of patients with Alzheimer's disease: the CERAD experience, part XV. Neurology 46:1592, 1996

49. Erkinjuntti T, Hachinski VC: Rethinking vascular dementia. Cerebrovasc Dis 3:3, 1993

50. Erkinjuntti T, Gao F, Lee DH et al: Lack of difference in brain hyperintensities between patients with early Alzheimer's disease and control subjects. Arch Neurol 51:260, 1994

51. Erkinjuntti T, Ketonen L, Sulkava R et al: CT in the differential diagnosis between Alzheimer's disease and vascular dementia. Acta Neurol Scand 75:262, 1987

52. Erkinjuntti T: Types of multi-infarct dementia. Acta Neurol Scand 75:391, 1987

53. Evans DA, Funkenstein HH, Albert MS et al: Prevalence of Alzheimer's disease in a community population of older persons. Higher than previously reported. JAMA 262:2551, 1989

54. Fazekas F, Schmidt R, Offenbacher H et al: Prevalence of white matter and periventricular magnetic resonance hyperintensities in asymptomatic volunteers. J Neuroimag 1:27, 1991

55. Fazekas F, Niederkorn K, Schmidt R et al: White matter signal abnormalities in normal individuals: correlation with carotid ultrasonography, cerebral blood flow measurements, and cerebrovascular risk factors. Stroke 19: 1285, 1988

56. Fazekas F, Kleinert R, Offenbacher H et al: Pathologic correlates of incidental MRI white matter signal hyperintensities. Neurology 43:1683, 1993

57. Fazekas F: Magnetic resonance signal abnormalities in asymptomatic individuals: their incidence and functional correlates. Eur Neurol 29:164, 1989

58. Ferrer I, Bella R, Serrano MT et al: Arteriolosclerotic leucoencephalopathy in the elderly and its relation to white matter lesions in Binswanger's disease, multi-infarct encephalopathy, and Alzheimer's disease. J Neurol Sci 98:37, 1990

59. Ferszt R, Cervós-Navarro J: Cerebrovascular pathology—aging and brain failure. p. 133. In Cervós-Navarro J, Sarkander HI (eds): Brain Aging and Neuropharmacology. Vol. 21. Raven Press, New York, 1983

60. Fisher CM: Dementia in cerebrovascular disease. p. 232. In Toole JF, Siekert RG, Whisnant JP (eds): Cerebral Vascular Disease. Transactions of the Sixth Princeton Conference. Grune & Stratton, New York, 1986

61. Fisher M, McQuillen JB: Bilateral cortical border-zone infarction. Arch Neurol 38:62, 1981

62. Frackowiak RSJ, Possilli C, Legg NJ et al: Regional cerebral oxygen supply and utilization in dementia: a clinical and physiological study with oxygen-15 and positron tomography. Brain 104:753, 1981

63. Fratiglioni L, Grut M, Forsell Y et al: Prevalence of Alzheimer's disease and other dementias in an elderly population: Relationship with age, sex, and education. Neurology 41:1886, 1991

64. Freeman R, Bear D, Greenberg MS: Behavioral disturbances in cerebrovascular disease. p. 137. In Toole JF (ed): Handbook of Clinical Neurology, Vol. 11. Vascular Diseases, Part III. Elsevier Science Publishers, Amsterdam, 1989

65. Fukui T, Sugita K, Sato Y et al: Cognitive functions in subjects with incidental cerebral hyperintensities. Eur Neurol 34:272, 1994

66. Garcia JH, Lassen NA, Weiller C et al: Ischemic stroke and incomplete infarction. Stroke 27:761, 1996

67. Garcia JH, Brown GG: Vascular dementia: Neuropathologic alterations and metabolic brain changes. J Neurol Sci 109:121, 1992

68. Gehrmann J, Banati RB, Wiessnert C et al: Reactive microglia in cerebral ischaemia: an early mediator of tissue damage? Neuropathol Appl Neurobiol 21:277, 1995

69. George AE, de León MJ, Gentes CI et al: Leukoencephalopathy in normal and pathologic aging: 1. CT of brain lucencies. AJNR 7:561, 1986

70. Gerard G, Weisberg LA: MRI periventricular lesions in adults. Neurology 36:998, 1986

71. Giulian D, Vaca K: Inflammatory glia mediate delayed neuronal damage after ischemia in the central nervous system. Stroke, suppl. I:I–84, 1993

72. Gorelick PB, Brody J, Cohen D et al: Risk factors for dementia associated with multiple cerebral infarcts. A case-control analysis in predominantly African-American hospital-based patients. Arch Neurol 50:714, 1993

73. Gorelick PB, Chatterjee A, Patel D et al: Cranial computed tomographic observations in multi-infarct dementia. Stroke 23:804, 1992

74. Goto K, Ishii N, Fukasawa H: Diffuse white-matter disease in the geriatric population. Radiology 141:687, 1981

75. Grace J, Nadler JD, White DA et al: Folstein vs Modified Mini-Mental State Examination in geriatric stroke. Stability, validity, and screening utility. Arch Neurol 52:477, 1995

76. Grafton ST, Sumi SM, Stimac GK et al: Comparison of post mortem magnetic resonance imaging and neuropathologic findings in the cerebral white matter. Arch Neurol 48:293, 1991

77. Gupta SR, Naheedy NH, Young JC et al: Periventricular white matter changes and dementia. Clinical, neuropsychological, radiological and pathological correlation. Arch Neurol 45:637, 1988

78. Hachinski VC, Potter P, Merskey P: Leuko-araiosis: an ancient term for a new problem. Arch Neurol 44:21, 1987

79. Hachinski VC, Munoz DG: Leuko-araiosis: an update. Bull Clin Neurosci 56:24, 1991

80. Hachinski VC, Lassen NA, Marshall J: Multi-infarct dementia: a cause of mental deterioration in the elderly. Lancet 2:207, 1974

81. Hachinski V: New concepts of vascular dementia. p. 237. In Boccalon H (ed): Vascular medicine. Proceedings of the 16th World Congress of the International Union of Angiology, Paris 13–18 September. Elsevier Scientific Publishers, Amsterdam, 1992

82. Hachinski V: Vascular dementia: a radical redefinition. Dementia 5:130, 1994

83. Hachinski VC, Bowler JV: Vascular dementia. Neurology 43:2159, 1993

84. Hachinski VC: Preventable senility: a call for action against vascular dementias. Lancet 340:645, 1992

85. Hasegawa K: The clinical issues of age-related dementia. Tohoku J Exp Med, suppl. 161:29, 1990

86. Hébert R, Brayne C: Epidemiology of vascular dementia. Neuroepidemiology 14:240, 1995

87. Hendrie HC, Farlow MR, Austrom MG et al: Foci of increased T_2 signal intensity on brain MR scans of healthy elderly subjects. AJNR 10:703, 1989

88. Herholz K, Heindel W, Rackl A et al: Regional cerebral blood flow in patients with leuko-araiosis and atherosclerotic carotid artery disease. Arch Neurol 47:392, 1990

89. Hershey LA, Olszewski WA: Ischemic vascular dementia. p. 335. In Morris JC (ed): Handbook of dementing illnesses. Marcel Dekker, New York, 1994

90. Higashi T, Nishi S, Nakai A et al: Regulatory mechanisms of stress response in mammalian nervous system during cerebral ischaemia or after heat shock. Neuropathol Appl Neurobiol 21:471, 1995

91. Hunt AL, Orrison WW, Yeo RA et al: Clinical significance of MRI white matter lesions in the elderly. Neurology 39:1470, 1989

92. Inzitari D, Diaz F, Fox A et al: Vascular risk factors and leuko-araiosis. Arch Neurol 44:42, 1987

93. Iwamoto T, Kubo H, Takasaki M: Platelet activation in the cerebral circulation in different subtypes of ischemic stroke and Binswanger's disease. Stroke 26:52, 1995

94. Janota I: Dementia, deep white matter damage and hypertension: Binswanger's disease. Psychol Med 11:39, 1981

95. Janota I, Mirsen TR, Hachinski VC et al: Neuropathologic correlates of leuko-araiosis. Arch Neurol 46:1124, 1989

96. Jayakumar PN, Taly AB, Shanmugam V et al: Multi-infarct dementia: a computed tomographic study. Acta Neurol Scand 73:292, 1989

97. Jellinger K, Danielczyk W, Fischer P et al: Clinicopathological analysis of dementia disorders in the elderly. J Neurol Sci 95:239, 1990

98. Jendroska K, Poewe W, Daniel SE et al: Ischemic stress induces deposition of amyloid β immunoreactivity in human brain. Acta Neuropathol 90:461, 1995

99. Joutel A, Corpechot C, Ducros A et al: Notch 3 mutations in CADASIL, a hereditary adult-onset condition causing stroke and dementia. Nature 383:707, 1996

100. Jung HH, Bassetti C, Tournier-Lasserve E, et al: Cerebral autosmal dominant arteriopathy with subcortical infarcts and leucoencephalopathy: a clinicopathological and genetic study of a large Swiss family. J Neurol Neurosurg Psychiatry 59:138, 1995

101. Junqué C, Pujol J, Vendrell P et al: Leuko-araiosis on magnetic resonance imaging and speed of mental processing. Arch Neurol 47:151, 1990

102. Kalaria RN, Cohen DL, Premkumar DRD: Apolipoprotein E alleles and brain vascular pathology in Alzheimer's disease. Ann NY Acad Sci 777:266, 1996

103. Katzman R, Aronson M, Fuld P et al: Development of dementing illnesses in an 80-year-old volunteer cohort. Ann Neurol 25:317, 1989

104. Kawano H, Ueda K, Fijishima M: Prevalence of dementia in a Japanese community (Hisayama): Morphological reappraisal of the type of dementia. Jpn J Med 29:261, 1990

105. Kertesz A: Localization and Neuroimaging in Neuropsychology. Academic Press, San Diego, 1994

106. Kertesz A, Clydesdale S: Neuropsychological deficits in vascular dementia vs Alzheimer's disease. Arch Neurol 51:1226, 1994

107. Kertesz A, Polk M, Carr T: Cognition and white matter changes on magnetic resonance imaging in dementia. Arch Neurol 47:387, 1990

108. Kertesz A, Black SE, Tokar G et al: Periventricular and subcortical hyperintensities on magnetic resonance imaging. 'Rims, caps, and unidentified bright objects.' Arch Neurol 45:404, 1988

109. Kinkel RW, Jacobs L, Polachini H et al: Subcortical arteriosclerotic encephalopathy (Binswanger's disease). Arch Neurol 42:951, 1985

110. Klatka LA, Schiffer RB, Powers JM et al: Incorrect diagnosis of Alzheimer's disease. A clinicopathological study. Arch Neurol 53:35, 1996

111. Knopman DS, Mastri AR, Frey WH II et al: Dementia lacking distinctive histologic features: a common non-Alzheimer degenerative dementia. Neurology 40:251, 1990

112. Kobari M, Meyer JS, Ichijo M et al: Leukoaraiosis: correlation of MR and CT findings with blood flow, atrophy, and cognition. AJNR 11:273, 1990

113. Kogure K, Kato H: Altered gene expression in cerebral ischemia. Stroke 24:2121, 1993

114. Kokmen E, Whisnant JP, O'Fallon WM et al: Dementia after ischemic stroke: a population-based study in Rochester, Minnesota. Neurology 46:154, 1996

115. Kotila M, Waltimo O, Niemi M-L et al: Dementia after stroke. Eur Neurol 25:134, 1986

116. Kwá VIH, Limburg M, Voogel AJ et al: Feasibility of cognitive screening of patients with ischaemic stroke using the CAMCOG. A hospital-based study. J Neurol 243:405, 1996

117. Ladurner G, Iliff LD, Lechner H: Clinical factors associated with dementia in ischaemic stroke. J Neurol Neurosurg Psychiatry 45:97, 1982

118. Lassen NA: Incomplete cerebral infarction-focal incomplete ischemic tissue necrosis not leading to emollision. Stroke 13:522, 1982

119. Leifer D, Buonanno FS, Richardson EP: Clinicopathologic correlations of cranial magnetic resonance imaging of periventricular white matter. Neurology 40:911, 1990

120. Leisbon C, Rocca W, Hanson V: Risk of dementia associated with diabetes mellitus. Am J Epidemiol 145:301, 1997

121. Li Y, Sharov VG, Jiang N et al: Ultrastructural and light microscopic evidence of apoptosis after middle cerebral artery occlusion in the rat. Am J Pathol 146:1045, 1995

122. Liu CK, Miller BL, Cummings JL et al: A quantitative MRI study of vascular dementia. Neurology 42:138, 1992

123. Loeb C: Vascular dementia: terminology and classification. p. 79. In Chopra JS, Jagannathan K, Sawhney IMS et al (eds): Progress in Cerebrovascular Disease. Current Concepts in Stroke and Vascular Dementia. Elsevier Science Publishers, Amsterdam, 1991

124. Loeb C, Meyer JS: Vascular dementia: still a debatable entity? J Neurol Sci 143:31, 1996

125. Loeb C, Gandolfo C, Bino G: Intellectual impairment and cerebral lesions in multiple cerebral infarcts. A clinical-computed tomography study. Stroke 19:560, 1988

126. Lopez OL, Larumbe MR, Becker JT et al: Reliability of NINDS-AIREN criteria for the diagnosis of vascular dementia. Neurology 44:1240, 1994

127. Lopez OL, Rabin BS: Alteraciones immunológicas de la demencia vascular. p. 91. In Lopez Pousa S, Manubens JM, Rocca WA (eds): Epidemiología de la Demencia

Vascular. Controversias en Su Tratamiento. JR Prous Editores, Barcelona, 1992

128. Lotz PR, Ballinger WE, Quisling RG: Subcortical arteriosclerotic encephalopathy: CT spectrum and pathologic correlation. AJNR 7:817, 1986

129. Mahler ME, Cummings JL: Behavioral neurology of multi-infarct dementia. Alzheimer Dis Assoc Disord 5: 122, 1991

130. Manolio TA, Kronmal RA, Burke GL et al: Magnetic resonance abnormalities and cariovascular disease in older adults. The cardiovascular Health Study. Stroke 25:318, 1994

131. Marshall VG, Bradley WG, Marshall ChE et al: Deep white matter infarction: Correlation of MRI imaging and histopathologic findings. Radiology 167:517, 1988

132. Martinez-Lage P, Manubens JM, Martinez-Lage JM et al: Vascular risk factors and cognitive performance in a non-demented elderly population. Neurology, suppl. 1: A289, 1996

133. Martinez-Vila E, Martinez-Lage P, Rocha E et al: β-Thromboglobulin, platelet factor 4, and circulating platelet aggregates in Alzheimer's disease and multi-infarct dementia. p. 43. In Culebras A, Matías-Guiu J, Román CG (eds): New Concepts in Vascular Dementia. Prous Science Publishers, Barcelona, 1993

134. Matsubayashi K, Shimada K, Kawamoto A et al: Incidental brain lesions on magnetic resonance imaging and neurobehavioral functions in the apparently healthy elderly. Stroke 23:175, 1992

135. Mesulam MM: A cortical network for directed attention and unilateral neglect. Ann Neurol 10:309, 1981

136. Mesulam MM: Large-scale neurocognitive networks and distributed processing for attention, language, and memory. Ann Neurol 28:597, 1990

137. Meyer JS, Rogers RL, Judd BW et al: Cognition and cerebral blood flow fluctuate together in multi-infarct dementia. Stroke 19:163, 1988

138. Meyer JS, Rogers RL, Mortel KF: Multi-infarct dementia: Demography, risk factors, and therapy. p. 199. In Ginsberg MD, Dietrich WD (eds): Cerebrovascular Diseases. Lippincott Raven Press, New York, 1989

139. Meyer JS, Kawamura J, Terayama Y: White matter lesions in the elderly. J Neurol Sci 110:1, 1992

140. Meyer JS, McClintic K, Rogers LG et al: Aetiological considerations and risk factors for multi-infarct dementia. J Neurol Neurosurg Psychiatry 51:1489, 1988

141. Mielke R, Herholz K, Grond M et al: Severity of vascular dementia is related to volume of metabolically impaired tissue. Arch Neurol 49:909, 1992

142. Mirsen TR, Lee DH, Wong CJ et al: Clinical correlates of white matter changes on magnetic resonance imaging of the brain. Arch Neurol 48:1015, 1991

143. Mirsen T, Hachinski VC: Epidemiology and classification of vascular and multi-infarct dementia. p. 61. In Meyer JS, Lechner H, Marshal J, Toole JF (eds): Vascular and Multi-infarct Dementia. Future Publishing, Mount Kisco, 1988

144. Mori S, Sadoshima S, Ibayashi S et al: Relation of cerebral blood flow to motor and cognitive function in chronic stroke patients. Stroke 25:309, 1994

145. Morioka T, Kalehua AN, Streit WJ: Characterization of microglial reaction after middle cerebral artery occlusion in the rat brain. J Comp Neurol 327:123, 1993

146. Moroney JT, Bagiella E, Desmond DW et al: Global hypoxic-ischemic events increase the risk of dementia after stroke. Ann Neurol 38:290, 1995

147. Munoz DG. The pathological basis of multi-infarct dementia. Alzheimer Dis Assoc Disord 5:77, 1991

148. Muñoz DG, Hastak SM, Harper B et al: Pathologic correlates of increased signals of the centrum ovale on magnetic resonance imaging. Arch Neurol 50:492, 1993

149. Naeser MA, Gebhardt C, Levine H: Decreased computerized tomography numbers in patients with presenile dementia. Detection in patients with otherwise normal scans. Arch Neurol 37:401, 1980

150. Nagy Z, Esiri MM, Jobst KA et al: The effects of additional pathology on the cognitive deficit in Alzheimer disease. J Neuropathol Exp Neurol 56:165, 1997

151. Nakagawara J, Sperling B, Lassen NA: Incomplete infarction of reperfused cortex may be quantitated with iomazenil. Stroke 28:124, 1997

152. Nichols FT III, Mohr JP: Binswanger's subacute arteriosclerotic encephalopathy. p. 875. In Barnett HJM, Mohr JP, Stein BM, Yatsu FM (eds): Stroke: Pathophysiology, Diagnosis, and Management. Churchill Livingstone, New York, 1986

153. Norris JW, Hachinski VC: Prevention of Stroke. Springer-Verlag, New York, 1991

154. O'Connor DW, Pollitt PA, Hyde JB et al: The prevalence of dementia as measured by the Cambridge Mental Disorders of the Elderly Examination. Acta Psychiatr Scand 79:190, 1989

155. Olichney JM, Hansen LA, Hofstetter R et al: Cerebral infarction in Alzheimer's disease is associated with severe amyloid angiopathy and hypertension. Arch Neurol 52:702, 1995

156. Olsson Y, Brun A, Englund E: Fundamental pathological lesions in vascular dementia. Acta Neurol Scand, suppl. 168(suppl.):31, 1996

157. Olzewsky J: Subcortical arteriosclerotic encephalopathy: review of the literature on the so-called Binswanger's disease and presentation of two cases. World Neurol 3: 359, 1962

158. Ott A, Stolk RP, Hofman A et al: Association of diabetes mellitus and dementia. The Rotterdam Study. Diabetologia 39:1392, 1996

159. Ott A, Breteler MMB, van Harskamp F et al: Prevalence of Alzheimer's disease and vascular dementia: association with education. The Rotterdam Study. BMJ 310: 970, 1995

160. Ott A, Breteler MMB, de Bruyne MC et al: Atrial fibrillation and dementia in a population based study. The Rotterdam Study. Stroke 28:316, 1997

161. Parnetii L, Mecocci P, Santucci C et al: Is multi-infarct dementia representative of vascular dementias? A retrospective study. Acta Neurol Scand 81:484, 1990

162. Pepin EP, Auray-Pepin L: Selective dorsolateral frontal lobe dysfunction associated with diencephalic amnesia. Neurology 43:733, 1993

163. Petito CK, Feldemann E, Pulsinelli WA et al: Delayed hippocampal damage in humans following cardiorespiratory arrest. Neurology 37:1281, 1987

164. Premkumar DRD, Cohen DL, Hedera P et al: Apolipoprotein E-є4 alleles in cerebral amyloid angiopathy and cerebrovascular pathology associated with Alzheimer's disease. Am J Pathol 148:2083, 1996

165. Rao SM, Mittenberg W, Bernardin L et al: Neuropsychological test findings in subjects with leukoaraiosis. Arch Neurol 46:40, 1989

166. Révész T, Hawkins CP, du Boulay EPGH et al: Pathological findings correlated with magnetic resonance imaging in subcortical arteriosclerotic encephalopathy (Binswanger's disease). J Neurol Neurosurg Psychiatry 52:1337, 1989

167. Rezek DL, Morris JC, Fulling KH et al: Periventricular white matter lucencies in senile dementia of the Alzheimer type and in normal aging. Neurology 37:1365, 1987

168. Rocca WA, Bonaiuto S, Lippi A et al: Prevalence of clinically diagnosed Alzheimer's disease and other dementing disorders: a door-to-door survey in Appignano, Macerata Province, Italy. Neurology 40:626, 1990

169. Rockwood K, Ebly E, Hachinski H et al: Presence and treatment of vascular risk factors in patients with vascular cognitive impairment. Arch Neurol 54:33, 1997

170. Rogers RL, Meyer JS, Mortel KF et al: Decreased cerebral blood flow precedes multi-infarct dementia, but follows senile dementia of the Alzheimer type. Neurology 36:1, 1986

171. Román GC: Senile dementia of the Binswanger type. A vascular form of dementia in the elderly. JAMA 258:1782, 1987

172. Román GC, Tatemichi TK, Erkinjuntti T et al: Vascular dementia: diagnostic criteria for research studies. Report of the NINDS-AIREN International Workshop. Neurology 43:250, 1993

173. Ross GW, Cummings JL: Vascular dementias. p. 271. In Thal LJ, Moos WH, Gamzu ER (eds): Cognitive Disorders. Pathophysiology and Treatment. Marcel Dekker, New York, 1992

174. Ruchoux MM, Chabriat H, Bousser MG et al: Presence of ultrastructural arterial lesions in muscle and skin vessels of patients with CADASIL. Stroke 25:2291, 1994

175. Sabbadini G, Francia A, Calandriello L et al: Cerebral autosomal dominant arteriopathy with subcortical infarcts and leucoencephalopathy (CADASIL). Clinical, neuroimaging, pathological, and genetic study of a large Italian family. Brain 118:207, 1995

176. Sabbagh MN, Corey-Bloom J, Salmon D et al: Alzheimer's disease without neocortical tangles: a second look. Ann Neurol 40:500A, 1996

177. Schmidt R: Comparison of magnetic resonance imaging in Alzheimer's disease, vascular dementia and normal aging. Eur Neurol 32:164, 1992

178. Schmidt R, Fazekas F, Offenbacher H et al: Magnetic resonance imaging white matter lesions and cognitive impairment in hypertensive individuals. Arch Neurol 48:417, 1991

179. Schmidt R, Fazekas F, Offenbacher H et al: Neuropsychologic correlates of MRI white matter hyperintensities: a study of 150 normal volunteers. Neurology 43:2490, 1993

180. Shibayama H, Kasahara Y, Kobayashi H et al: Prevalence of dementia in a Japanese elderly population. Acta Psychiatr Scand 74:144, 1986

181. Skoog I, Lernfelt B, Landahl S et al: 15-year follow-up study of blood pressure and dementia. Lancet 347:1141, 1996

182. Skoog I, Nilsson R, Palmertz B et al: A population-based study of dementia in 85-year-olds. N Engl J Med 328:153, 1993

183. Slooter AJ, Tang M-X, van Duijn CM et al: Apolipoprotein E epsilon 4 and the risk of dementia with stroke. JAMA 277:818, 1997

184. Snowdon DA, Greiner LH, Mortimer JA et al: Brain infarction and the clinical expression of Alzheimer's disease. JAMA 277:813, 1997

185. Sourander P, Wåhlinder J: Hereditary multi-infarct dementia. Acta Neuropathol 39:247, 1977

186. Starkstein S, Sabe L, Vázquez S et al: Neuropsychological, psychiatric, and cerebral blood flow findings in vascular dementia and Alzheimer's disease. Stroke 27:408, 1996

187. Steingart A, Hachinski VC, Lau C et al: Cognitive and neurological findings in demented patients with diffuse white matter lucencies on computed tomographic scan (leuko-araiosis). Arch Neurol 44:36, 1987

188. Steingart A, Hachinski VC, Lau C et al: Cognitive and neurological findings in subjects with diffuse white matter lucencies on computed tomographic scan (leuko-araiosis). Arch Neurol 44:32, 1987

189. Sulkava R, Wikström J, Aromaa A et al: Prevalence of severe dementia in Finland. Neurology 35:1025, 1985

190. Sulkava R, Erkinjuntti T: Vascular dementia due to cardiac arrhythmias and hypotension. Acta Neurol Scand 76:123, 1987

191. Sullivan P, Pary R, Telang F et al: Risk factors for white matter changes detected by magnetic resonance imaging in the elderly. Stroke 21:1424, 1990

192. Sze G, de Armond SJ, Brandt-Zawadzki M et al: Foci of MRI signal (pseudo lesions) anterior to the frontal horns: histologic correlations of a normal finding. AJNR 7:381, 1986

193. Tarvonen-Schröder S, Röyttä M, Rähä I et al: Clinical features of leuko-araiosis. J Neurol Neurosurg Psychiatry 60:431, 1996

194. Tatemichi TK, Desmond DW, Stern Y et al: Cognitive impairment after stroke: frequency, patterns, and relationship to functional disabilities. J Neurol Neurosurg Psychiatry 57:202, 1994

195. Tatemichi TK, Desmond DW, Mayeux R et al: Dementia after stroke: baseline frequency, risks, and clinical features in a hospitalized cohort. Neurology 42:1886, 1992

196. Tatemichi YK, Desmond DW, Prohovnik I et al: Confusion and memory loss from capsular genu infarction: A thalmocortical disconnection syndrome? Neurology 42:1966, 1992

197. Tatemichi TK, Desmond DW, Paik M et al: Clinical determinants of dementia related to stroke. Ann Neurol 33:568, 1993

198. Tatemichi TK, Foulkes MA, Mohr JP et al: Dementia in stroke survivors in the Stroke Data Bank Cohort. Prev-

alence, incidence, risk factors, and computed tomographic findings. Stroke 21:858, 1990

199. Tatemichi TK, Sacktor N, Mayeux R: Dementia associated with cerebrovascular disease, other degenerative diseases, and metabolic disorders. p. 123. In Terry RD, Katzman R, Bick KL (eds): Alzheimer's Disease, Lippincott Raven Press, New York, 1994

200. The Canadian Study of Health and Aging: Study methods and prevalence of dementia. Can Med Assoc J 150:899, 1994

201. Tomlinson BE, Blessed G, Roth M: Observations on the brains of old demented people. J Neurol Sci 11:205, 1970

202. Tupler LA, Coffey E, Logue PE et al: Neuropsychological importance of subcortical white matter hyperintensity. Arch Neurol 49:1248, 1992

203. Valentine AR, Moseley IF, Kendall BE: White matter abnormality in cerebral atrophy: clinicoradiological correlations. J Neurol Neurosurg Psychiatry 43:139, 1980

204. van Swieten JC, Staal S, Kappelle LJ et al: Are white matter lesions directly associated with cognitive impairment in patients with lacunar infarcts? J Neurol 243:196, 1996

205. van Swieten JC, Geyskes GG, Derix MMA et al: Hypertension in the elderly is associated with white matter lesions and cognitive decline. Ann Neurol 30:825, 1991

206. van Swieten JC, van den Hout HW, van Ketel BA et al: Periventricular lesions in the white matter on magnetic resonance imaging in the elderly. A morphometric correlation with arteriolosclerosis and dilated perivascular spaces. Brain 114:761, 1991

207. Verhey FRJ, Lodder J, Rozendaal N et al: Comparison of seven sets of criteria used for the diagnosis of vascular dementia. Neuroepidemiology 15:166, 1996

208. Villardita C: Alzheimer's disease compared with cerebrovascular dementia. Neuropsychological similarities and differences. Acta Neurol Scand 87:299, 1993

209. Volpe BT, Petito CK: Dementia with bilateral medial temporal lobe ischemia. Neurology 35:1793, 1985

210. Wallin A, Brun A, Gustafson L: Swedish consensus on dementia diseases. Classification and nosology. Acta Neurol Scand, suppl 157:8, 1994

211. Wallin A, Blennow K: Pathogenetic basis of vascular dementia. Alzheimer Dis Assoc Disord 5:91, 1991

212. Wallin A, Blennow K: Heterogeneity of vascular dementia: Mechanisms and subgroups. J Geriatr Psychiatry Neurol 6:177, 1993

213. Watson RT, Valenstein E, Heilman KM: Thalamic neglect. Possible role of the medial thalamus and nucleus reticularis in behavior. Arch Neurol 38:501, 1981

214. Weschler D: The Measurement of Adult Intelligence. 3rd Ed. Williams & Wilkins, Baltimore, 1944

215. Wetterling T, Kanitz R-D, Borgis K-J: Comparison of different diagnostic criteria for vascular dementia (ADTCC, DSM-IV, ICD-10, NINDS-AIREN). Stroke 27:30, 1996

216. Wolfe N, Linn R, Babikian VL et al: Frontal systems impairment following multiple lacunar infarcts. Arch Neurol 47:129, 1990

217. Yamanouchi H: Loss of white matter oligodendrocytes and astrocytes in progressive subcortical vascular encephalopathy of Binswanger type. Acta Neurol Scand 83:301, 1991

218. Yamauchi H, Fukuyama H, Nagahama Y et al: Atrophy of the corpus callosum associated with cognitive impairment and widespread cortical hypometabolism in carotid occlusive disease. Arch Neurol 53:1103, 1996

219. Ylikoski R, Ylikoski A, Erkinjuntti E et al: White matter changes in healthy elderly persons correlate with attention and speed of mental processing. Arch Neurol 50:818, 1993

220. Yoshitake T, Kiyohara Y, Kato I et al: Incidence and risk factors of vascular dementia and Alzheimer's disease in a defined elderly Japanese population: The Hisayama Study. Neurology 45:1161, 1995

221. Zhang M, Katzman R, Salmon D et al: The prevalence of dementia and Alzheimer's disease in Shanghai, China: Impact of age, gender, and education. Ann Neurol 27:428, 1990

222. Zimmerman RD, Fleming CA, Lee BCP et al: Periventricular hyperintensity as seen by magnetic resonance: prevalence and significance. AJNR 7:13, 1986

223. Zubenko GS, Stiffler S, Stabler S et al: Association of the apolipoprotein E ε4 allele with clinical subtypes of autopsy confirmed Alzheimer's disease. Am J Med Genet 54:199, 1994

CHAPTER 36

Atherosclerotic Disease of the Aortic Arch

PIERRE AMARENCO

ARIEL COHEN

Anatomically, the arch of the aorta is a precerebral artery. Therefore, complicated atherosclerotic plaques of this artery located proximal to the ostium of the left subclavian artery may constitute a threat for the brain. Atherosclerotic plaques in the aortic arch are common in individuals over 60 years of age. These plaques frequently ulcerate with subsequent formation of superimposed mural thrombi as a natural healing process (see Fig. 36.9). Mural thrombi can occasionally be exuberant, loosely adherent, and mobile and may give rise to cruoric emboli distally in the brain or peripheral arteries. Ulcerated plaques not yet covered by mural thrombi may release atheromatous material contained within the plaque, with cholesterol emboli to the brain, retina, kidney, lower limbs, or other peripheral organs.

In vascular neurology, the most commonly recognized site of atherosclerosis causing brain infarction is the origin of the internal carotid artery (ICA). These lesions are easily diagnosed by ultrasound testing and are accessible to surgery. The reports by Fisher in 1951[37] reemphasized the relationship between extracranial carotid stenosis or occlusion and ipsilateral hemispheral infarction, and the occurrence of intra-arterial embolism as a very important cause of brain ischemia. He pointed out that these lesions could be recognizable before the completed ischemic event by identifying transient ischemic attacks in the days or weeks before.[36,37] Then the first successful carotid endarterectomy by DeBakey in 1953,[85] which introduced a possible therapeutic prevention of this problem by a surgical procedure, stimulated considerable efforts during the following 40 years toward diagnosing clinically, angiographically, noninvasively, and preventing this condition.

Other potential sites of atherosclerosis or sources of arteroarterial embolism have thus been understudied or even neglected.[17,18] However, prospective registries such as the Stroke Data Bank have shown that significant high-grade stenosis of the ICA is the cause of an ipsilateral brain infarct in fewer than 15% of cases.[1] In more than 20% of cases, the cause is cardioembolic, and in 25% of cases an arteriosclerotic disease causes a lacunar stroke.[78] Thus, in up to 40% of cases,

the exact cause of brain infarction is unknown, and by default a diagnosis of moderate ICA stenosis (<70%) or minor cardiac abnormalities such as patent foramen ovale is accepted.[78] These patients may also have risk factors for atherosclerotic disease that could be located in other, unexplored arteries. Similarly, it has been shown that patients with asymptomatic cholesterol emboli in a retinal artery do not have more frequent ipsilateral carotid stenosis than do controls,[13] and hence the source of retinal embolism should be located further down in the arterial tree.

However, until now, in patients with brain infarct of unknown cause or with retinal cholesterol emboli, complicated atherosclerotic disease of the aortic arch has not been routinely considered as a possible cause. Nowadays, the advent of transesophageal echocardiography has allowed clinicians to detect plaques and thrombi in the aortic arch.[47,90,100,101] Several recent works have definitively established a statistical association between the presence of atherosclerotic disease in the aortic arch and ischemic stroke.[2,3,27,31,40,45,61,84,92,93] If one accepts that a causal link between brain infarcts and complicated plaques with highly mobile thrombi within the aortic arch lumen is likely, other plaques without mobile components could conceivably be markers for diffuse atherosclerosis and hence for the true cause of ischemic stroke and for future systemic ischemic events.

Aortic Arch Plaques As Risk Factors

FREQUENCY OF ATHEROSCLEROTIC DISEASE OF THE AORTA IN THE GENERAL POPULATION

All available data are from autopsy and echocardiography studies. At autopsy, patients with no cerebrovascular disease but with other neurologic disease had ulcerated plaques in

Table 36.1 Prevalence and Risk of Ischemic Stroke in the Presence of Large Protruding Plaques in the Aortic Arch in Case Control Studies

Case Control Studies		N	Patients (%)	Controls (%)	Adjusted Odds Ratio
Autopsy					
Amarenco et al[3] Ulcerated plaques (UP)		239	28	5	4.0 (95% CI, 2.1–7.8)
Khathibzadeh et al[50] UP, thrombi, debris		40	68	34	5.8 (95% CI, 1.1–31.7)
Transesophageal echocardiography					
Tunick et al[92]	P1 ≥5 mm	122	27	9	3.2 (95% CI, 1.6–6.5)
Amarenco et al[2]	P1 ≥4 mm	250	14.4	2.0	9.1 (95% CI, 3.3–25.2)
Jones et al[45]	P1 ≥5 mm	215	21.4	3.5	8.2 (95% CI, 3.0–22.4)
Nihoyannopoulos et al[65]	P1 not measured	42	48	22	Not done
Stone et al[82]	P1 ≥5 mm	49	32.7	7	Not done
Di Tullio et al[31]	P1 ≥5 mm	106	26	13	2.6 (95% CI, 1.1–5.9)
Intraoperative epiaortic echo					
Dávila-Román et al[27]	P1 ≥3 mm	158	26.6	18.1[a]	1.65 (95% CI, 1.1–2.4)

[a] Of patients in this study, 88.3% underwent coronary artery bypass grafting explaining this high rate of aortic plaques in the control group.

the aortic arch in 5% of cases.[3] Patients with cerebral hematoma had ulcerated plaques in 20% of cases. By comparison, patients with brain infarcts had ulcerated plaques in 28% of cases.[3] Ulcerated plaques in the aortic arch seem mainly to involve patients aged 60 years or more and hypertensive patients. Ulcerations were noted under the age of 60 in only 1% of patients, and their frequency increased with aging. In patients with brain infarcts, ulcerated plaques were found in 21% of those between 60 to 69 years, 31% of those between 70 to 79, and 36% of those over 80.[3] In a group of patients who have had transesophageal echocardiography, Karalis et al found 7% of large aortic arch atherosclerotic disease.[47] Finally, in a population-based study of healthy volunteers, Jones et al found a frequency of simple atheroma in the aortic arch of 22% of participants and complicated plaques (>5 mm in thickness or "irregular surface suggesting ulceration") in 4% of participants.[45]

CASE-CONTROL STUDIES

Atherosclerosis in the aortic arch is obviously a marker of generalized atherosclerosis. Several recent studies reinforce the notion that plaques in the aortic arch are independent risk factors for brain ischemia (Table 36.1). In our autopsy study performed in the Laboratory of Neuropathology at La Salpêtrière hospital in 500 consecutive patients, we and others found ulcerated plaques in the aortic arch in 28% of patients with cerebrovascular disease and in only 5% of patients with other neurologic disease (Fig. 36.1).[3] This difference was very significant and after adjustment for age, sex, and hypertension, we found an odds ratio of 4.0 (95% confidence interval [CI] to 2.1 to 7.8). When we compared the frequency of ulcerated plaques in the aortic arch in patients with brain infarct of unknown cause with those suffering infarcts of known etiology we also found a highly significant difference (61% versus 28%, adjusted odds ratio 5.7; 95% CI, 2.4 to 13.6). The presence of ulcerated plaques in the aortic arch was not correlated to

the presence of internal carotid artery stenosis or atrial fibrillation.[3] These two last points suggest that ulcerated plaques in this autopsy series may have been causally related to some brain infarction of unknown etiology. One other observation was that among the 75 patients with ulcerated plaques in the aortic arch only 2 were less than 60 years and 73 (97%) were 60 years or older.

Recently Khathibzadeh et al[50] studied 120 consecutive autopsies, 40 of whom had cerebral, visceral, or lower limb embolisms at pathologic examination. They were able to confirm an association between ulcerated plaques, mural thrombi, or both in the aortic arch and arterial embolism. Ulcerated plaques, mural thrombi, or both in the aortic arch or in the descending aorta were found in 25 patients (69%) with cerebral infarction. Among the 12 patients with cerebral infarction that had not been diagnosed clinically, 9 had ulcerated plaques in the aortic arch, and 28 had silent visceral embolisms at pathologic examination.

In 1991, Tunick and colleagues[92] reported a retrospective study based on the recruitment of their echocardiography laboratory comparing the frequency of plaques ≥5 mm in thickness in the thoracic aorta in 12 patients referred for discovering the source of emboli and in 12 patients referred for other cardiologic reasons.[92] They found such large plaques in 27% of the patients who had an embolic event and in 9% of those who had no emboli. After adjustment for principal risk factors, the odds ratio was 3.2 (95% CI, 1.6 to 6.5).[92] However, because this study was retrospective and the results were not adjusted for the presence of other potential cause of brain infarction or peripheral emboli, the question of aortic plaques as markers remained incompletely answered.

In a prospective case-control study using transesophageal echocardiography (TEE) in 250 consecutively admitted patients over 60 years of age with brain infarcts (Fig. 36.2), we and our colleagues found a frequency of plaques in the aortic arch significantly different from that of controls[2] (Table 36.2). We found that the risk of brain infarction associated with aortic arch plaques located proximal to the left subclavian artery

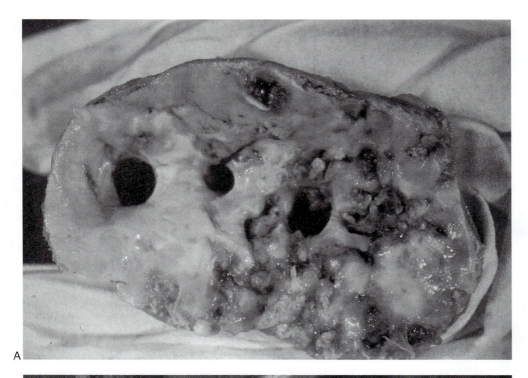

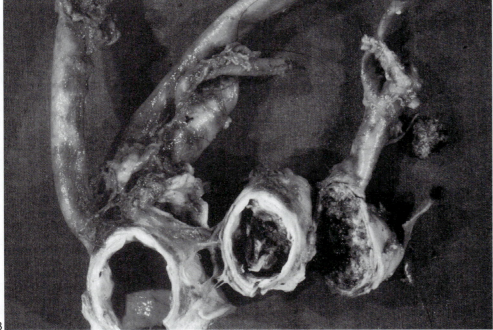

Figure 36.1 Aortic arch at autopsy. (**A**) Ulcerated plaques in the aortic arch all around the origin of the cerebral arteries. (**B**) Aortic arch cut into three parts: the first part is free of severe atheroma; in the second, a large atherosclerotic plaque with superimposed thrombus protrudes into the lumen, with a 70%–80% stenosis, located just after the take-off of the left common carotid artery; in the third, this very large plaque involves the origin of the left subclavian artery, which is occluded.

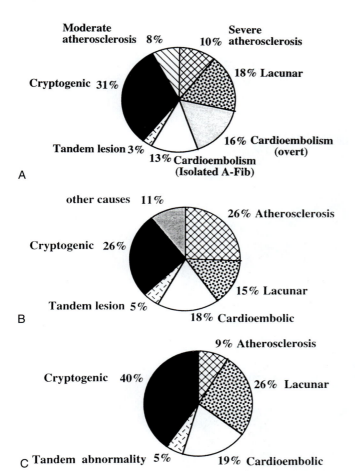

Figure 36.2 Frequency of stroke subtypes in three series of consecutive patients: (**A**) 250 consecutive patients ≥60 years old; (**B**) the Lausanne Stroke Registry (891 consecutive brain infarcts); (**C**) the Stroke Data Bank (1,273 consecutive brain infarcts). (Fig. A from Amarenco et al[12]; Fig. C from Sacco et al,[78] with permission.)

ostium was significant for plaques >1 mm in thickness, and the risk remained almost the same for plaques between 1 and 3.9 mm in thickness. However, this finding did not establish a causal link. Indeed, plaques that were from 1 to 3.9 mm in thickness were frequently associated with carotid stenosis, which may have been the actual source of the brain emboli.

On the contrary, with plaques ≥4 mm, a causal link seemed possible for several reasons. First, the odds ratio for the risk of stroke increased sharply from less than 5 to more than 13 when the thickness of plaques is ≥4 mm (Table 36.2). This large increase was observed only for lesions of ≥4 mm located proximal to the left subclavian artery ostium in the ascending aorta or proximal arch, not for those distal to the left subclavian artery ostium in the distal arch or descending aorta. Second, the high increase in the risk of ischemic stroke associated with plaques of ≥4 mm in the proximal arch was independent of the presence of the two major risk factors for stroke in the elderly: carotid stenosis and atrial fibrillation. We found that the frequency of plaques of ≥4 mm in the proximal arch did not differ according to the degree of carotid stenosis, and that the frequency of such plaques was lower in patients with atrial fibrillation than in those without atrial fibrillation. Third, plaques ≥4 mm in thickness located proximal to the left subclavian artery ostium were also associated with an abrupt increase in the risk of stroke among patients who had ischemic strokes with no apparent cause (Table 36.3). Furthermore, the presence of a mobile component of the plaque was associated with a risk ratio of 14 among patients with ischemic stroke of unknown cause.

This clear-cut difference in the risk of stroke between patients with plaques <4 mm thick and those with plaques ≥4 mm thick may be related to the composition of the larger lesions in the aortic arch. Lesions ≥4 mm thick may contain thrombotic material superimposed on ulcerated plaques, as Culliford et al observed at surgery.[25] This superimposed thrombotic material, as well as what should be the actual plaque, may be included within the measurement of the "plaque thickness" made at TEE and could account for the high increased risk. The presence of a thrombus may also explain the more frequent mobile component in patients with plaques ≥4 mm in thickness.[2]

Table 36.2 Risk of Cerebral Infarct as a Function of Thickness of Atherosclerotic Plaques in the Ascending Aorta and Proximal Arch

Wall Thickness	Patients % (n)	Controls % (n)	Crude OR (95% CI)	Adjusted OR[a] (95% CI)	P
<1 mm[b]	39.6 (99)	75.6 (189)	1	1	—
1 to 1.9 mm[c]	11.2 (28)	6.4 (16)	3.3 (1.7; 6.5)	4.4 (2.1–8.9)	<0.001
2 to 2.9 mm[c]	22.4 (56)	10.4 (26)	4.1 (2.4; 7.0)	5.0 (2.7–9.0)	<0.001
3 to 3.9 mm[c]	12.4 (31)	5.6 (14)	4.2 (2.2; 8.3)	3.4 (1.5–7.4)	<0.001
≥4 mm	14.4 (36)	2.0 (5)	13.8 (5.2; 36.1)	9.1 (3.3–25.2)	<0.001

Abbreviations: CI, confidence interval; OR, odds ratio.

[a] After controlling for age, sex, hypertension, cigarette smoking, high serum cholesterol, diabetes, past myocardial infarction, and atrial fibrillation.

[b] Reference category.

[c] The adjusted risk of plaques 1–3.9 mm is 4.4 (95% confidence interval, 2.8 to 6.8).

(From Amarenco et al[2] with permission.)

Table 36.3 Comparison of the Frequency of Plaques ≥4mm in the Ascending Aorta and Proximal Arch in 250 Consecutive Patients with Ischemic Stroke Older than 60 and According to the Stroke Etiology

Patient Group	No. of Patients	Patients with Plaques ≥4 mm in the Ascending Aorta and Proximal Arch Number (%)	Adjusted[a] Odds Ratio (95% CI)
Other likely cause (carotid stenosis ≥70% and definite cardiac source of embolism)	74	4 (5.4)	7.8 (2.5–24.7)
Presumed lacunar infarct	44	4 (9.1)	4.5 (1.4–14.7)
Other possible cause (carotid stenosis 31%–69% and isolated atrial fibrillation)	54	6 (11.1)	3.1 (1.2–8.4)
No other imputable lesion	78	22 (28.2)[b]	—

Abbreviation: CI, confidence interval.

[a] Comparison between patients with no culprit lesion and those with a likely or possible cause or a lacunar infarct; covariates for adjustment were the same as in Table 36.2.

[b] The odds ratio was 4.7 (95% confidence interval, 2.2 to 10.1) for the comparison between patients with no other culprit lesion with the whole group of 172 patients with a likely or possible cause or a lacunar infarct.

(From Amarenco et al,[2] with permission.)

These results were strengthened by another case control study performed the same year in Australia by Jones and colleagues who found a 7.1-fold increase in the risk of ischemic stroke in the presence of "complex atheroma" in the aortic arch. The singularity of this study was that the authors compared patients with brain infarcts or transient ischemic attacks (TIAs) with a population-based control group including only healthy volunteers.[45] Among 304 consecutive patients with a first-ever ischemic stroke, they included 215 (of whom 20 had only TIAs), and 202 healthy volunteers for TEE examination; 94% of patients with ischemic stroke and 78% of control subjects also had carotid imaging. They found "simple" plaques >5 mm thick and smooth in the ascending aorta and aortic arch in 33% of patients and 22% of controls, and "complex" plaques ≥5 mm thick or any plaques with irregular surface or with mobile component in 22% of patients and 4% of controls. In a further analysis using a more objective measure of atheroma severity than plaque morphology, comparing patients and controls with plaques ≥5 mm thick or <5 mm thick rather than "simple" and "complex" plaques, they found an adjusted odds ratio of 8.2 (95% CI, 3.0 to 22.4) for plaques ≥5 mm thick and 2.2 (95% CI, 1.2 to 4.1) for plaques <5 mm. They also found mobile protruding atheroma in the aortic arch in 11 patients and in only 1 control subject (crude OR, 10.8; 95% CI, 1.4 to 84.7). However, they did not confirm a significant association between complex aortic arch plaques and ischemic stroke of unknown origin (20% in patients with stroke of unknown origin and 23% in patients with ischemic stroke with a known cause).[45]

Dávila-Román and colleagues studied a consecutive series of 1334 cardiac patients 50-years-old or older who were undergoing open heart surgery.[27] This study used an intraoperative epiaortic ultrasonography device (not TEE), that allows the assessment of the entire length of the ascending aorta from the root of the aorta to the level of the proximal arch, a region that is difficult to image with TEE (which shows mainly the aortic arch). The ascending aorta is also more likely to be a donor site for brain embolism than more distal regions of the aorta. Among 1,200 patients who underwent epiaortic ultrasonography, 158 had a previous embolic event and 1,042 were free of embolic event. They found plaques ≥3 mm in the ascending aorta in 26.6% of patients who had a previous neurologic event and in 18.1% in the "control" subjects who were free of neurologic event. Most of these patients (88.3%) were undergoing coronary artery bypass grafting, which easily explains the high rate of protruding plaques in the control group. Multivariate analysis showed that significant predictors of previous neurologic ischemic events were hypertension (OR = 1.81), ascending aorta atherosclerosis (OR = 1.65), atrial fibrillation (OR = 1.54), and, in the subset of 789 patients evaluated for carotid artery disease with ultrasound, severe carotid stenosis (OR = 2.7).

Nihoyannopoulos et al[65] prospectively studied the aorta of 152 consecutive patients older than 40 years referred to look for atherosclerosis of the thoracic aorta. Lesions in the aorta were classified into fixed atherosclerotic lesions and mobile lesions. In addition, duplex ultrasound of carotid arteries was performed in all patients with distinction between obstructive lesion (stenosis >50%) and nonobstructive lesion (stenosis <50%). Among the whole group of 152 patients, 44 (29%) had at least one major atheromatous lesion in the thoracic aorta. Atherosclerotic plaques were located in the horizontal portion of the aortic arch in 20 of these 44 patients (45%), in the ascending aorta in 7 patients (16%), and in the descending aorta in 17 patients (39%). All but 2 patients with major atherosclerotic lesions in the descending aorta also had other smaller lesions at the horizontal portion. Only 3 of the 44 (8%) patients had mobile lesions. Atherosclerotic plaques in the thoracic aorta were present in 20 of 42 (48%) patients with embolic event, and in 24 of 110 (22%) patients without embolic event (P < 0.001). Among the 152 patients, 26 had atherosclerotic lesions in the carotid arteries, including 7 with <50% stenosis, all of them associated with extensive atherosclerotic disease in the thoracic aorta, 19 with >50% stenosis, 16 with plaques in the aorta, and 3 without plaque.

Stone et al[82] have studied with TEE 49 consecutive patients ≥40 years of age with ischemic stroke and 57 age-matched control subjects without stroke. They found protruding plaque ≥5 mm in 16 (32.7%) patients and 4 (7%) control subjects. Interestingly, they tried to distinguish ulceration within plaques and adherent mobile debris by using video calipers. Using multiplane transducers ulcers were defined as craters ≥2 mm in depth and width. The 49 patients were divided into 23 with unexplained ischemic stroke and 26 with a known cause. Ulcerated plaques were significantly more frequent in patients with unexplained ischemic stroke (39%) than in patients with a known cause (8%) and the control subjects (7%) with $P < 0.001$.[82] This study was the first attempt to determine the clinical importance of what can be interpreted as ulceration at TEE examination. Although numbers were small, the authors believed that these results concurred with what has been found at autopsy with ulcerated plaques in the same groups of patients with brain infarcts of unknown cause.[3]

More recently Di Tullio and colleagues[31] studied 106 patients and 114 stroke-free control subjects and found more frequently large (≥0.5 cm) protruding atheroma in the proximal aortic arch in the stroke patients than in controls (26% versus 13%), particularly in patients ≥60 years or older with unexplained stroke than in controls (22% versus 8%). After multivariate analysis, proximal aortic atheroma was found independently associated with stroke (adjusted odds ratio 2.6, 95% CI 1.1 to 5.9). As Stone et al[82] found, Di Tullio et al[31] noted that ulcerated (using the same definition for ulceration) and mobile atherosclerotic lesions were also more frequent in patients than in controls (12% versus 5%; $P < 0.06$). They also found that differences were entirely attributable to patients 60 years or older, and concluded that the absence of carotid stenosis does not exclude aortic atheromas as a potential cause for ischemic stroke.[31]

ATHEROSCLEROTIC DISEASE OF THE AORTIC ARCH AS A MARKER FOR NEW ISCHEMIC EVENTS

Plaques ≥4 mm Thick Predict a High Risk of Recurrent Brain Infarction

The therapeutic implications of this new finding of transesophageal echocardiography must be defined with the knowledge of the event rates of recurrent brain infarcts and other cardiovascular events (Table 36.4). Tunick et al[93] have found an annual event rate of 33% in 42 patients who had protruding plaques ≥5 mm in the thoracic aorta as compared with 7% in 42 matched controls. However, this study did not focus on plaques that were located only in the aortic arch but in the entire thoracic aorta, and the difference between the two groups was not significant concerning brain and retinal emboli only (seven versus three events in patients and controls, respectively).[93]

The French Study of Aortic Plaques in Stroke (FAPS) study group prospectively followed 331 consecutive patients admitted for brain infarction for 2 to 4 years.[84] All patients had transesophageal echocardiography at presentation. The incidence of recurrent brain infarction was 11.9 per 100 person-years of follow-up in 45 patients with aortic arch plaques ≥4 mm as compared with 3.5 in 143 patients with plaques from 1 to 3.9 mm and with 2.8 in 143 patients with no plaque (wall thickness <1 mm). In patients with brain infarction of unknown cause at entry and with plaques ≥4 mm in thickness,

Table 36.4 Risk of New Vascular Events in Patients with Large Protruding Plaques as Compared with Control Subjects

Follow-up Studies	*Patients*	*Controls*	*Relative Risk*
Tunick et al[93] 42 pts	Pl ≥5 mm	No atheroma	
Mean follow-up 14 months			
Stroke + MI + peripheral emboli	33% at 2 yrs	7% at 2 yrs	4.3 (95% CI, 1.2–15.0)
Stroke + retina	16% at 2 yrs	7% at 2 yrs	
FAPS study[84a] 331 pts	Pl ≥4 mm	No atheroma	
788 person-years of follow-up			
Stroke + MI + peripheral emboli	26 p.100 p-y	5.9 p.100 p-y	3.5 (95% CI, 2.1–5.9)
Stroke	11.9 p.100 p-y	2.8 p.100 p-y	3.8 (95% CI, 1.8–7.8)
Mitusch et al[61] 183 pts			
241 person-years of follow-up	Pl ≥5 mm or	Pl <5 mm	
	Mobile thrombi		
Stroke + peripheral emboli	13.8 p.100 p-y	4.1 p.100 p-y	4.3 (95% CI, 1.5–12.0)
Previously symptomatic patients:			
Stroke + peripheral emboli	15.9 p.100 p-y	7.1 p.100 p-y	
Dávila-Román et al[102] 1800 pts	11 ≥5 mm	No atheroma	
All events	30% at 1 yr	9% at 1 yr	1.7 (95% CI, 1.6–2.0)
Neurological events	11% at 1 yr	3% at 1 yr	1.6 (95% CI, 1.2–3.2)

a For the estimated risk at 1, 2, 3, and 4 years, see the Kaplan-Meier curve and make projections on y axis (Figs. 36.3 and 36.4).

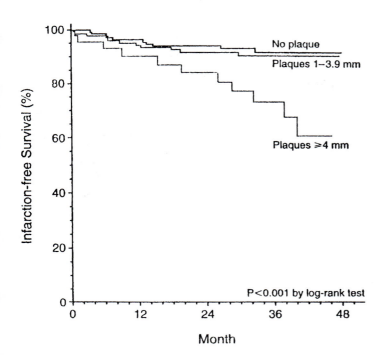

Figure 36.3 Risk of recurrent brain infarct. (From The French Study,[84] with permission.)

the event rates was 16.4 per 100 person-years of follow-up for recurrent brain infarction.

Multivariate analysis showed that aortic arch plaques ≥4 mm in thickness were significant predictors of new brain infarcts, independently from the presence of carotid stenosis, atrial fibrillation and peripheral artery disease, with a relative risk of 3.8 (95% CI, 1.8 to 7.8; $P < 0.002$). The significant difference observed between the three Kaplan-Meier curves (Figs. 36.3 and 36.4) according to the aortic plaque thickness is a further strong argument for a causality link between plaques ≥4 mm in thickness and brain infarcts in some of these patients.

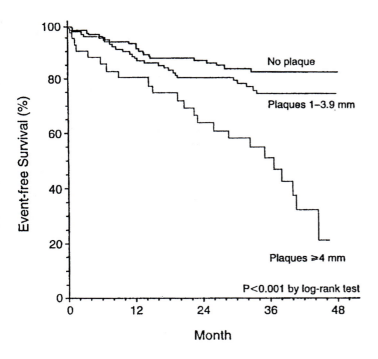

Figure 36.4 Risk of new vascular events (combining brain infarcts, myocardial infarctions, peripheral events, and vascular deaths). (From The French Study,[84] with permission.)

Plaques ≥4 mm Thick Predict a High Risk of New Vascular Events

The FAPS study also showed that the presence of plaques ≥4 mm in thickness in the aortic arch is a strong and independent predictor of all vascular events with a relative risk of 3.5 [95% confidence interval, 2.1 to 5.9; $P < 0.001$].[84] The incidence of all vascular events (combining stroke, myocardial infarction, peripheral emboli, and vascular death) was 26 per 100 person-years of follow-up as compared with 9.1 and 5.9, in the groups with plaques ≥4 mm thick, 1 to 3.9 mm thick, and no plaque, respectively. These observations led the FAPS investigators to the conclusion that plaques ≥4 mm in thickness in the aortic arch are above all good markers for generalized atherosclerosis that could be used to select patients at high vascular risk in therapeutic trial.

More recently, Mitusch and colleagues followed a selection of 183 symptomatic and asymptomatic patients who had transesophageal echocardiography examination and in whom plaques were detected in the aortic arch.[61] The patients were divided into 136 with raised plaques <5 mm thick (including 71 symptomatic patients) and 47 with protruding plaques ≥5 mm thick or with mobile components (including 33 symptomatic patients). During a follow-up of 241 person-years, if only previously symptomatic patients are considered, the incidence of new vascular events was 7.1 per 100 person-years of follow-up in 71 patients with aortic arch plaques less than 5 mm, and 15.9 in 33 patients with plaques more than 5 mm thick or with mobile components. In a multivariate analysis, plaques ≥5 mm thick or with mobile component were found to be independent predictors of vascular events with a relative risk of 4.3 (95% CI, 1.5 to 12.0; $P < 0.006$), as was a history of previous embolism or of coronary artery disease with a relative risk of 4.0 each. In this study, however, not all patients had a detection of carotid stenosis; thus, the multivariate analysis did not take into account this important potential source of embolism. Moreover, multivariate analysis has not been performed in symptomatic patients only, probably because of the lack of power.

Montgomery and colleagues followed 33 patients with aortic arch plaques ≥5 mm thick or with mobile component. In this study, the Kaplan-Meier risk of all deaths at 18 months was 33%.[64]

Thus, plaques in the aortic arch ≥4 mm thick as detected with TEE are markers for a high risk of recurrent brain infarcts and even more prominently for other cardiovascular events. The relative benefits and risks of therapeutic interventions should now be evaluated in these patients. As far as causal relationship between aortic plaques and ischemic stroke is concerned, the following observation shows how difficult the relationship is to define.

A 66-year-old man, a heavy smoker with arterial hypertension and hypercholesterolemia, had a sudden left-sided brachiofacial hemiparesis resulting from right MCA infarction. Diagnostic work-up found a right internal carotid artery stenosis of 40% at the origin, atrial fibrillation without thrombus or spontaneous echocontrast at transesophageal echocardiography, and a severe atherosclerotic plaque with a mobile debris in the thoracic aorta after the take-off of the left subclavian artery (Fig. 36.5A). Atrial fibrillation was thought to be the probable cause and the patient was treated with warfarin.

Three months later, he presented with the blue toe syndrome involving both feet (Fig. 36.4B). The angiography showed a severely stenosed and ulcerated abdominal aorta (Fig. 36.4C), while transesophageal echocardiography showed the mobile debris in the same position and extent (which led us to conclude that it was probably not a thrombus but a ruptured plaque), and ultrasound examination, MR angiography, and spiral-CT angiography showed that the right carotid stenosis had progressed to 90% stenosis (Fig. 36.4D). Warfarin therapy was discontinued and switched to aspirin.

We concluded from this case that the pedunculated and mobile debris in the thoracic aorta was a mere marker for a generalized and particularly severe atherosclerotic disease and that the true cause of the brain infarct likely was the right carotid stenosis. Unfortunately, we did not perform a TCD monitoring on this patient.

This observation is interesting because it illustrates how difficult it is to establish a causal relationship between aortic arch debris (in cases where it is located in the aortic arch proximal to the ostium of the left subclavian artery) and an ischemic stroke. Nevertheless, these lesions are strong predictors of new vascular events and of recurrent brain infarcts, and this is the only important thing from a therapeutic point of view when a medical treatment with antithrombotic drugs is planned.

Aortic Arch Plaques as Markers for Coronary Artery Disease

In 1988, Tobler and Edwards studied at autopsy 97 specimens of ascending aorta from adults who had clinically symptomatic coronary heart disease.[86] All these patients had myocardial infarction, and most of them had had coronary artery bypass grafting. They found that 38% of these patients had atherosclerotic plaques greater than 8 mm in thickness in the ascending aorta. This result showed that the association between plaques in the ascending aorta and symptomatic coronary artery plaques may be stronger than that observed between ulcerated plaques in the aortic arch and ischemic stroke in another pathologic study in which only 26% of patients with ischemic stroke had ulcerated plaques in the aortic arch.[3]

Later in the Framingham cohort, Witteman et al[98] found that the presence of calcified thoracic aortic plaques on chest x-ray film was associated with an increased risk of cardiovascular death. Using transesophageal echocardiography for the detection of aortic plaques in 600 consecutive examinations of patients seen in their echocardiography laboratory or in the operating room, Fazio et al[33] selected 61 patients who had previously had coronary angiography for various cardiologic reasons within one year of TEE examination. They found a coronary artery obstruction in at least one vessel in 41 patients and atherosclerotic plaques of the aorta in 39 patients. Atherosclerotic plaques in the thoracic aorta were present in 37 of the 41 (90%) patients with coronary artery obstruction as compared with 2 of the 20 (10%) patients without coronary artery obstruc-

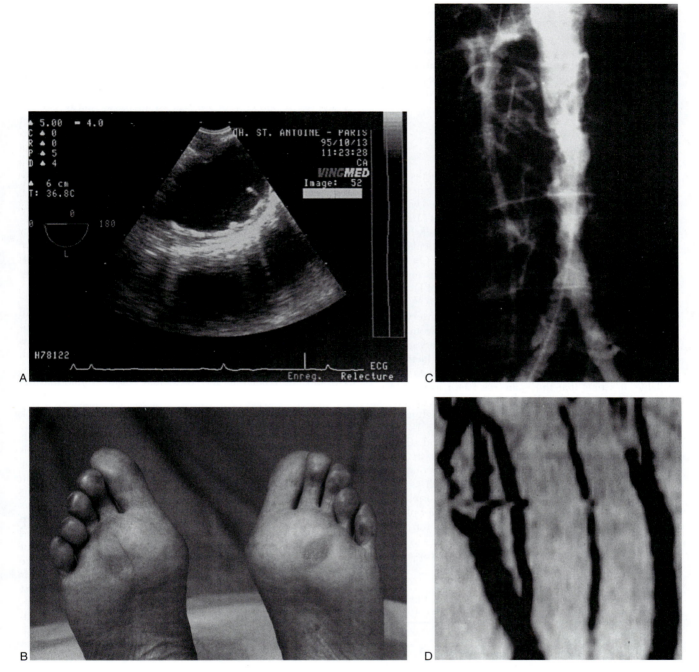

Figure 36.5 Patient who had a right-sided brain infarct, with an ipsilateral 40% stenosis of the internal carotid artery and atrial fibrillation. (**A**) Mobile debris in the thoracic aorta. (**B**) Blue toe syndrome 3 months later. (**C**) Aortography showing severely ulcerated abdominal aorta. (**D**) Ninety percent stenosis of the right internal carotid artery at the time the blue toe syndrome developed.

tion, with a sensitivity of 90% and a specificity of 90% for angiographically proved obstructive coronary artery disease. The positive predictive value for obstructive coronary artery disease was 95% and the negative predictive value was 82%. In a study with a similar design, Tribouilloy et al[88] found that thoracic aortic plaques had a negative predictive value of 99% for significant

coronary obstructive disease. Despite evident bias of recruitment, these studies quite convincingly showed that atherosclerotic aortic plaques appear to be sensitive and specific predictors of obstructive coronary artery disease.

The FAPS investigators followed 331 consecutive patients with a previous ischemic stroke during 788 person-years.[84] The incidence of myocardial infarction and sudden death was 9 per 100 person-years of follow-up in patients with plaques in the proximal aortic arch ≥4 mm thick, 4.2 per 100 person-years in patients with plaques 1 to 3.9 mm thick, and 1.4 per 100 person-years in patients with no plaques in the aortic arch. These results clearly show that aortic arch plaques are good markers for future coronary artery events, at least in patients with previous ischemic stroke.

Aortic Arch Plaques and Other Markers for Atherosclerosis

Among risk factors such as hypertension, diabetes mellitus, hypercholesterolemia, and cigarette smoking, cigarette smoking seems to be the strongest risk factor associated with severe aortic arch atherosclerosis in case control studies (Table 36.5). Hypertension[3] and diabetes mellitus[45] occasionally have been found associated with aortic arch plaques, particularly those ulcerated at autopsy. Hypercholesterolemia has been found to be associated with severe aortic arch plaques in only one case control study with a mean total cholesterol level of 218 ± 48 mg/dl versus 210 ± 47 mg/dl ($P < 0.030$).[27] This case control study included patients with coronary artery disease. It is well known that the main risk factor for carotid stenosis is hypertension, the main risk factor for coronary artery disease is hypercholesterolemia, and the main risk factor for peripheral arterial disease is smoking. From the data currently available, it seems that the main risk factor associated with aortic arch atherosclerotic disease is smoking. Indeed, in these studies, peripheral arterial disease was also strongly associated with aortic arch disease (Table 36.5).

The relation between aortic arch and carotid atherosclerosis have been more debated. In our autopsy study, there was a proportion of carotid stenosis ≥75% as frequent in patients with ulcerated plaques in the aortic arch as in those without. Similarly, carotid stenosis <75% or normal carotid artery was as frequent in patients with ulcerated plaques in the aortic arch as in patients without.[3] In our further case-control study using TEE in living patients, there was a significant relation between the severity of carotid stenosis and aortic

arch plaques 1 mm to 3.9 mm thick, but we confirmed the lack of association between carotid stenosis and plaques ≥4 mm thick. We indeed found plaques ≥4 mm thick in 14% of patients with no carotid stenosis, 15% of patients with moderate (<70%) carotid stenosis, and in 15% of patients with severe (≥70%) carotid stenosis. Dávila-Román et al[27] had similar findings. They reported the presence of severe carotid stenosis in 4% of patients with no atheroma and in 6.5% of patients with atherosclerosis of the ascending aorta. In another study of 100 patients undergoing cardiac surgery using epiaortic ultrasonography and carotid ultrasound, Dávila-Román et al[26] found that the 10 patients with severe atherosclerosis in the ascending aorta were well distributed in the group of patients with mild carotid stenosis <50% (4 patients), with moderate carotid stenosis 50% to 79% (3 patients), and severe carotid stenosis 80% to 99% (3 patients).

On the contrary, Di Tullio et al[31] found that the frequency of large atheromas in the aortic arch increased with the degree of carotid stenosis: 6% in patients with no carotid stenosis, 29% in patients with <60% carotid stenosis, and 40% in patients with ≥60% carotid stenosis. However, the positive predictive value of a ≥60% carotid stenosis was only 16% for large aortic atheroma. Moreover, 36% of patients with mild or no carotid stenosis had large or complex aortic arch atherosclerosis.[31] Jones et al[45] reported similar results. There was a significant association between the severity of aortic arch atherosclerosis and the severity of carotid stenosis; however, as in the Di Tullio et al[31] study, Jones et al[45] found that the presence of carotid disease was not a reliable predictor of aortic atherosclerosis (positive predictive value, 57%; negative predictive value, 73%).

Desmopoulos et al[30] compared the frequency of protruding aortic arch atheroma in 45 patients with carotid stenosis ≥50% and ischemic stroke and in 45 patients with ischemic stroke without carotid stenosis. Aortic plaques were found in 17 (38%) and 7 (16%) patients, respectively. Mobile lesions were found almost exclusively in patients with carotid stenosis (13% versus 2%). However, in selecting as "control" group 45 patients without carotid stenosis, the authors likely selected patients referred to them for discovery of cardiac source of emboli, that is, mainly those with atrial fibrillation or embolic brain infarct of unknown source. They therefore biased their study toward patients with atherosclerotic disease in the first group and without atherosclerotic disease in the second group. In the FAPS study,[84] which included consecutive patients with ischemic stroke, 13.3% of patients with carotid stenosis ≥70% and 11.8% of patients with carotid stenosis ≥30% had plaques ≥4 mm.

Aortic Arch Plaques As Causal Factors for Brain Infarction

ATHERO (CHOLESTEROL CRYSTAL) EMBOLI

Cholesterol Emboli to the Brain

Ulcerated plaques in the aortic arch were first recognized pathologically as potential donor sites of cholesterol crystal emboli (atheroemboli) to the brain, retina, peripheral organs

Table 36.5 Association Between Smoking, Peripheral Arterial Disease and Severe Aortic Arch Atherosclerosis

	No Aortic Arch Atheroma	*Large AA Plaques*[a]	*P v*
FAPS study[84]			
Smoking	39.9%	57.8%	0.03
Peripheral vascular disease	7%	24.4%	0.003
Dávila-Román et al[27]			
Smoking	46.4%	61.3%	<0.001
Peripheral vascular disease	6.8%	19.5%	<0.001
Jones et al[45]			
Smoking	11%	24%	0.01

[a] *Corresponds to plaques ≥4 mm thick in the FAPS study, ≥3 mm thick in the Dávila-Román et al study, and ≥5 mm thick in the Jones et al study*

such as kidneys, and distal lower limb arteries with the blue toe syndrome. These crystals only block distal arteriolar vessels and may only cause very small cortical or subcortical infarctions. Most frequently they are asymptomatic as routinely found in retinal arteries,[69] in muscle biopsy when performed,[1] or in small arteries of abdominal viscera at autopsy.[22] Panum is generally acknowledged the first to have proposed, as early as in 1862, that ulcerated atherosclerotic plaques could give rise to artery-to-artery emboli.[68] In 1945, Flory pointed out embolization of the systemic arterial system from atherosclerotic plaques of the aorta as probably more frequent than is generally realized.[38] Winter reported in 1957 two observations of patients with multiple cerebral infarctions resulting from cholesterol emboli from eroded atheromata of the ascending segment of the aorta.[97]

> The first patient was a 67-year-old syphilitic man who had sudden onset of aphasia, mental confusion, and right hemiparesis. During the five months he was hospitalized, the hemiparesis improved almost completely, but abnormal restlessness and agitation characterized his behavior during the last months. He showed a gradual mental and physical deterioration until his death. At autopsy he had a large syphilitic aneurysm of the innominate artery. The intimal surface of the aneurysm, as well as the ascending aorta and the remainder of the aorta, was covered by innumerable atheromata, most of which were eroded and partly calcified. Soft thrombi, containing cholesterol crystals, were adherent to many. No thrombi were found in the heart, and the carotid bulb was patent. No emboli were found in any of the viscera. However, there were multiple old cortical infarcts, the largest of these measuring 4 × 2 cm. The majority of infarcts were much smaller, varying from few millimeters to 2 cm, and generally confined to the cortex. . . . At microscopic examination, the multiple infarcts involved both the cerebral and cerebellar hemispheres, and both the cortex and subcortical white matter. . . . The lumen of arterial branches were occluded by one or more cholesterol crystals, often surrounded by foreign-body giant cells. . . . Occasionally, the crystals were seen protruding through the vessel wall, covered outside by a thin layer of adventitia. . . . Some of the arteries were occluded by amorphous material staining like fibrin but showing organization.[97]

Winter found that no vessels larger than 83 μm and none smaller than 8 μm contained cholesterol emboli. He believed that the sudden lodgment of the cholesterol crystals in the cerebral vessels induces arterial spasm with resulting damage to the nerve cell, and that contraction of the artery forces the crystal deeper into the media, inducing persistent spasm. He thought that when cholesterol crystals emboli are embedded in a mass of fibrin and atheromatous debris, complete obliteration of the lumen may easily occur, as in any other true embolus.

Then Sturgill and Netsky reported another case with multiple small old cortical infarcts measuring 1 cm or less, infarcts in the caudate nucleus and cerebellar hemisphere and severe erosive atherosclerosis of the entire aorta.[83] Soft brown grumous material in the eroded regions was scraped away with ease. Friable atheromatous material was present at the origin of the arteries arising from the aortic arch. Aortic plaques contained innumerable cholesterol slits. Leptomeningeal arteries containing cholesterol slits were seen adjacent to zones of cortical infarction. The cholesterol crystals were either in the lumen or in the media, and the wall of the affected vessels were fibrotic, especially the adventitia.

Gore and Collins reported 16 cases of atheroembolism and noted that the patients were all 60 years of age or older.[41] Among the 13 cases who came to autopsy, 12 involved multiple sites, 12 the kidneys (with infarcts in 4 cases), 10 the pancreas (with pancreatitis in one case) and spleen (with 3 infarcts), 4 the prostate and gastrointestinal tract, 3 the liver and adrenal glands, 2 the brain (with 3 infarcts), heart (with 2 infarcts) and bone marrow, and 1 the testis and lower extremities. Brain infarcts resulted in "encephomalacia" attributable to atheromatous emboli in branches of the cerebral arteries. They noted that the aorta was the principal source of origin for the embolic material.[41]

In 1964, Saloway and Aronson found 16 cases of atheromatous embolism to the brain among 6,685 consecutive adult autopsies performed during 5 years in their institution, and found 14 previously published cases in the literature.[81] Six patients had cerebral vascular disease prior to the terminal episode. Lateralizing signs (mostly hemiplegia) were noted in 6 patients, and nonlateralizing signs (depression of consciousness or unresponsiveness) in 4; 2 patients died shortly after admission; interestingly 3 had no apparent counterpart to the underlying encephalomalacia. Three patients developed acute vascular insufficiency of the distal portion of an extremity during the terminal phase of their illness. The presence of aortic atherosclerosis was noted in each of the 16 cases. The majority of the supratentorial malacic lesions were located in the lateral cortical and subcortical cerebral tissues, as well as in the basal ganglia. The infarcts often varied in age, suggesting an intermittent release of emboli. None of the infarcts in the brain stem was proved to be a direct result of atheromatous embolism since the demonstrable emboli were found only in terminal leptomeningeal branches of the cerebral hemispheres as well as the cerebellum. Atheromatous emboli were of small size and arrested in vessels with diameters less than 200 μm. In their discussion, the authors emphasized that any trauma, surgical manipulation of aortic aneurysm, carotid angiography, or carotid thromboendarterectomy significantly increased the hazard of atheroembolism to the kidneys or brain.

Several case reports have shown the difficulties of the diagnosis of such multiple brain infarcts because of recurrent cholesterol crystal embolism from extreme ulcerative atheroma commencing in the ascending aorta. This condition, as in the case reported by McDonald, causes fluctuating, but also progressive, cerebral symptoms including confusion, disorientation, variable and asymmetrical weakness of limbs, and plastic rigidity of all four limbs.[57] Other peripheral organ involvement is very helpful for the correct diagnosis, especially renal infarcts, pancreatitis, intestinal infarcts, and purple toes.[19,20] Sweeney in a case record of the Massachusetts General Hospital first reported the very frequent watershed or border zone distribution of cerebral infarction in case of multiple recurrent cholesterol emboli.[20] Beal et al[7] reported the unique observation of one patient who had innumerable TIAs lasting 3 to 8 minutes during a 3-year-period then developed progressive left arm weakness. At that time he had a right carotid endarterectomy, but postoperatively the left leg gradually became paralyzed, with lateral gaze palsy to the left; then he remained drowsy and disoriented and died from renal failure, gastrointestinal bleeding, and empyema. At pathologic examination he had severe ulcerative atherosclerosis of the thoracic aorta, with multiple infarcts in the adrenal glands, spleen, pancreas, kidney, and brain. Brain infarctions were mainly distributed to the cortical border zone areas on each side. Many small (15 to 120 μm) arteries adjacent to the infarcts were occluded by cholesterol crystals.[7]

A frequent feature is the occurrence of several focal ischemic episodes involving the retina and brain, and then a progressive encephalopathy develops with confusional state and astasia. Skin and muscle biopsies may show typical cholesterol crystals.[15] Rare clinical presentations may be falsely diagnosed as panarteritis nodosa.[73,22]

Cholesterol Emboli to Retinal Artery

Another frequent feature of atheromatous cholesterol emboli is retinal infarction, amaurosis fugax, or asymptomatic bright plaques discovered at funduscopy.[43,69,77] Recently Bruno and

colleagues studied 70 consecutive men with asymptomatic retinal cholesterol emboli seen in an eye clinic and 21 men without cholesterol emboli randomly selected from the same clinic.[13] They found carotid stenosis ipsilateral to embolus in 13% of patients and in none of the control subjects (P = 0.18). Heterogeneous or echolucent plaque on either side was present in 95% of patients and 60% of controls ($P < 0.001$). The authors concluded that cholesterol emboli indicate systemic atherosclerosis rather than ipsilateral carotid artery stenosis.[13] One can suggest that the source of embolism, if not in the carotid, should be located farther down in the aortic arch. Bruno et al[12] followed these 70 patients and 70 controls during a mean of 3.4 years. The annual event rate for ischemic stroke was 8.5% in patients as compared with 0.8% in controls (relative risk 9.9; 95% CI, 2.3 to 43.1). Myocardial infarction or vascular death occurred with an annual event rate of 7.7% as compared with 4.9% in controls. This study showed that retinal cholesterol emboli are an important risk factor for brain infarction independently of common vascular risk factors.

Atheroemboli and Cardiac Surgery

Atheromatous emboli from the aortic arch also have been recognized the cause of brain infarction in patients undergoing cardiac surgery. Price and Harris in 1970[70] and then McKibbin et al[58] in 1976 both reported the clinical and ne-

Figure 36.6 Usual distribution of cholesterol emboli to the brain in the border zone area (end zone territories): diagrammatic views of basal, superior, and lateral surface of the brain. Area of infarction stippled. (From Price and Harris,[70] with permission.)

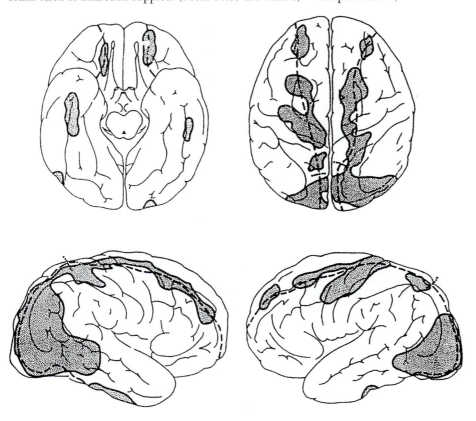

cropsy findings of one patient who had atheroemboli during cardiac surgery under retrograde aortic perfusion. Price and Harris observed that the aorta was studded with calcified atherosclerotic plaques. Embolic arterial occlusions were found in the heart, kidney, spleen, pancreas, and brain. The majority of occluded vessels had an inner diameter of less than 200 μm (range 54 to 384 μm). In these vessels, there were the biconvex, needle-shaped crystals characteristic of atheromatous embolism. The cerebral arteries were moderately atherosclerotic. The distribution of infarction was mostly in border zone areas (Fig. 36.6).[70] In the case reported by McKibbin et al,[58] postmortem examination showed multiple infarcts in the brain, eyes, and spleen resulting from emboli of cholesterol crystals and other atheromatous debris from a ruptured plaque in the ascending aorta at the site of the aortotomy.

In 1985, Gardner and colleagues identified risk factors for perioperative strokes in 3,279 consecutive patients undergoing coronary artery bypass grafting.[40] They made a case-control study of 56 patients who had perioperative stroke and 112 control patients. They identified increased age, pre-existing stroke (20% versus 8%), protracted cardiopulmonary bypass time, and severe perioperative hypotension (23% versus 4%) as significant risk factors for perioperative stroke. Severe atherosclerotic disease of the ascending aorta (14% versus 3%) was also found a very significant predictor of perioperative stroke.

Indeed, the landmark autopsy study published in 1992 by Blauth and colleagues showed a close relation between severe atherosclerosis of the ascending aorta, atheroembolism, and age in patients who died after cardiac surgery for myocardial revascularization or valve operations.[11] Among 221 patients who died, embolic disease was identified in 69 patients, and atheroemboli in 48 patients. Of these 48 patients, 46 (95.8%) had severe atherosclerosis of the ascending aorta at autopsy. Conversely, among 123 patients who had severe atherosclerosis in the ascending aorta, 46 (37.4%) had pathologic evidences of atheroembolic events, but only 2 (2%) showed evidence among the 98 patients without significant atherosclerosis in the ascending aorta.

Cholesterol Embolization and Antithrombotic Treatments

Treatments for this condition have been controversial. There has been a temporal association of cholesterol emboli with both warfarin and streptokinase therapy.[34,59,67] Cholesterol emboli may occur because antithrombotic effects prevent thrombosis over an ulcerated plaque.[63] Bruns et al[14] have reported on a patient who developed livedo reticularis, confusion, transient monocular blindness, pancreatitis, and renal failure while on warfarin for phlebitis. A renal biopsy showed cholesterol emboli. After discontinuation of the anticoagulant, the patient was asymptomatic and renal function improved. Only antiplatelet therapy seems reasonable in these cases.

THROMBOEMBOLI TO THE BRAIN

Various circumstances have suggested that thromboemboli to the brain can originate from the aortic arch resulting in territorial brain infarction (Fig. 36.7).

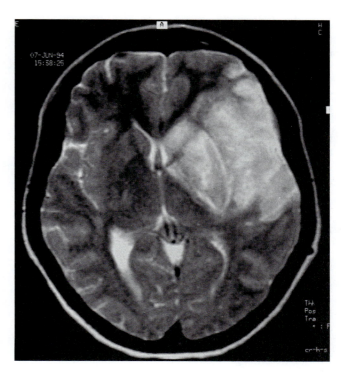

Figure 36.7 Embolic infarction in the middle cerebral artery territory in a patient with large mobile atherothrombotic lesion in the aorta.

Frequency of Mural Thrombi in the Aorta

Studying the heart, aorta, peripheral, extracranial, and intracranial arteries of 178 consecutive autopsies, Fisher et al found 42 mural thrombi. One-half of them were in the thoracic aorta, one-third intracardiac, and only 3 in iliofemoral arteries.[35] Gagliardi et al[39] reported that mural thrombi were present in nearly 4% of the nonaneurysmal aortoiliac lesions they managed during a 9-year period. In the series of Mitchell et al,[60] mobile thrombi in the aortic arch accounted for 5 patients among 600 (0.8%) consecutive intraoperative TEE. These patients had no symptoms of ischemia that could be related to these lesions before and after the surgical procedure (coronary artery bypass graft). The authors concluded that even large mobile lesions in the thoracic aorta may exist for at least several months without producing systemic embolic events.[60] However, one can argue that the same evolution has occasionally been noted for mural thrombi in the atrium, left ventricle, or internal carotid artery origin. With an incidence estimated at 0.5% of all 10,671 autopsies performed during a 28-year period in another study,[55] the clinical relevance of such mural thrombi has indeed been debated.[38,49,60,66,96] Nowaday, this is no longer a matter of controversy since we have data on the prevalence and the high risk of recurrence of such lesions in patients with stroke or peripheral embolism. Associated factors that favor the thrombus formation are not well known. Plaque rupture, hypercoagulable state,[91,80] systemic fungal infections,[16,46] or lupus anticoagulant could be involved. Occasionally, thrombi may develop upon calcified plaques at the site of the ligamentum arteriosum, at the junction between the inferior surface of the aortic arch and the beginning of the descending aorta, as reported by Laperche and his colleagues.[54] The ligamentum arteriosum is the remnant of the fetal ductus arteriosus. The other reported conditions that favored aortic thrombosis were chest trauma[21] and thoracic gunshot wound.[10]

Culliford et al have reported 12 patients with large protruding plaques in the aortic arch with mobile component in the lumen that have been operated on. All patients had mural thrombi superimposed upon ulcerated plaques in the aortic arch.[25]

Mobile Aortic Arch Plaques and Intra-arterial Procedures

As soon as cerebral angiography, aortography, coronarography, cardiac catheterization, and percutaneous coronary angioplasty were performed, cerebral ischemic complications were reported by the time of or after the procedure.[71,94] It has been suggested that the catheter can dislodge a piece of atheroma or a thrombus involving the dome of the aortic arch.

Mobile Aortic Arch Plaques and Cardiac Surgery

Intra- or postoperative ischemic strokes are major causes of morbidity of cardiac surgery with the use of cardiopulmonary bypass. Among the numerous etiologies of these complications, atheroma of the ascending aorta is recognized as one of the main risk factors.[40,58] Cardiac surgeons routinely search for atheroma in this part of the aorta with manual palpation, or better with intraoperative echography to prevent consequences of the manipulation of the artery.[28,56]

Dávila-Román et al[26] studied the ascending aorta using epiaortic ultrasonography intraoperatively in 100 consecutive patients. Atherosclerosis was classified mild (intimal thickening <3 mm) in 33% of patients, moderate (intimal thickening >3 mm) in 19% of patients, and severe (intimal thickening >3 mm throughout the entire circumference in all three segments of the ascending aorta) in 10% of patients. In 17% of these patients with moderate or severe plaques, the ultrasonographic findings in the ascending aorta altered the operative procedure with mainly relocation of the aortic cannula or aortic clamp, or with distal aortic or femoral cannulation to avoid embolization.[26] Ribakove et al[72] studied with TEE 97 patients prior to surgery under cardiopulmonary bypass. Among these patients, 10 had mobile lesions in the aortic arch. Four of them were treated with hypothermic circulatory arrest and aortic arch debridement, and none suffered strokes. The other 3 patients were treated with standard techniques and 3 had strokes. Katz et al[48] from the same institution reported the unique observation of a patient who had the transesophageal probe in place when the aorta was cannulated for the cardiopulmonary bypass. This intraoperative echocardiography showed the disappearance of previously mobile protruding material in the aortic arch upon cannulation of the aorta. The patient awoke from operation with hemiplegia. The study by Katz and colleagues on 130 patients found that 3 of the 12 patients (25%) with a mobile atheroma in the aortic arch had

a postoperative stroke as compared with 2 of 118 (2%) without a mobile component (P <0.001).[48] Thus, mobile aortic arch plaques are associated with a high risk of postoperative stroke in patients undergoing cardiac surgery with cardiopulmonary bypass, and the authors were able to show that modifications of surgical techniques of cannulation in patients with previously recognized protruding atheroma in the aortic arch can significantly reduce the frequency of postoperative neurologic complications.[48,72]

To avoid embolization to the brain from the undersurface of the arch, the tip of the cannula is placed beyond the orifice of the left subclavian artery.[24] Barzilai and colleagues have also reported using intraoperative epiaortic echography that in 8 (24%) of the 33 patients they studied, the composition, severity, and location of plaques delineated ultrasonically led to the selection of alternate cannulation sites without resultant embolism.[6] Summarizing their experience on 1,200 patients having cardiac operations, Wareing et al[95] from the same institution found 231 patients with moderate (plaque thickness 3 to 5 mm; 168 patients) or severe (plaque thickness >5 mm protruding, mobile, or ulcerated; 63 patients) atherosclerosis of the ascending aorta. The stroke rate was 1.1% in patients with no or mild atherosclerosis of the ascending aorta. It was zero among 27 patients with moderate or severe aortic plaques who had ascending aortic replacement. The stroke rates were higher for the 111 patients with moderate or severe ascending aortic disease who had only minor modifications of the technique to avoid potential sources of embolization (6.3%).

Mobile Thrombi in the Lumen of the Aortic Arch and Embolic Brain Infarction of Unknown Source

The presence of ulcerated plaques in the aortic arch has been acknowledged as a rare causative factor in strokes,[7,19,20,41,43, 69,76,81,83,97] likely because in the past there was no way to diagnose it during life.[7,76,81] Most reports were isolated and mainly concerned cholesterol emboli instead of thromboemboli, complications of cardiac surgery, aortography, and anticoagulant treatment.[14,34,63,67] In 1986, we found several cases of thromboembolic brain infarcts thoroughly studied during life and at autopsy with no other potential causes than ulcerated plaques in the aortic arch, and we wondered if these lesions could have been causal.[4,5] This question formed the basis for our autopsy study.[3] Sadony et al[79] in 1988 reported recurrent embolism in a patient who had a free-floating thrombus diagnosed by angiography. Several papers since 1990 have reported the TEE recognition of aortic arch debris as the only potential source of emboli in patients with unexplained stroke or peripheral emboli.

Tunick and his colleagues reported in 1990 the first observations of large protruding plaques in the thoracic aorta diagnosed by TEE in three patients who had recurrent brain and peripheral emboli and no other source of emboli.[90]

The first patient was a 68-year-old woman with atrial fibrillation and bilateral carotid bruit. She had an episode of transient dysarthria and an embolus to one toe. At TEE examination there was no thrombus in cardiac cavities, but in the aortic arch and descending thoracic aorta there were large protruding plaques with superimposed mobile echoes in the lumen. The second patient was a 77-year-old woman who had unstable angina. She had cardiac catheterization showing mainly a severe obstruction of the circumflex coronary artery. At the end of the procedure she had a cerebellar infarction. Carotid and cardiac cavity explorations were normal, but TEE showed a large protruding atherosclerotic plaque in the aortic arch with a small mobile component. The third patient was a 70-year-old man who had unexplained posterior circulation symptoms and was referred to their laboratory to look for a cardiac source of embolism. The TEE showed neither thrombus in the left cavities nor atrial septal abnormality, but again there were very large and protruding atherosclerotic plaques in the aortic arch and descending thoracic aorta with mobile components. Neck ultrasound examination also showed an occlusion of the right internal carotid artery and a 90% stenosis of the left internal carotid artery stenosis, which were obviously not the explanation of the posterior circulation symptoms.

In the Karalis et al series of 556 echocardiographic examinations, 11 (31%) out of 36 patients with atheroma in the thoracic aorta had systemic emboli, and this occurred mainly with pedunculated and mobile (8 of 11 patients) rather than layered and immobile aortic debris (3 of 25 patients; $P < 0.002$).[47] Then Rubin et al,[75] Toyoda et al,[87] Horowitz et al,[44] and Dee et al.[29] reported a high frequency of large protruding plaques, occasionally with a mobile component, in the thoracic aorta in patients with unexplained systemic or brain emboli. The frequency of mobile lesions in the aortic arch in various series is summarized in Table 36.6. Rubin et al[75] reported TEE examination in 64 patients with embolic stroke in whom intra-aortic debris was found in about one-sixth of patients. Toyoda and colleagues also examined with TEE 62 patients with presumed embolic stroke and found 26 patients (42%) with "complicated" aortic arch plaques (>3 mm in thickness with markedly irregular surface).[87] One particularity of this study is that the authors first performed a comparison between histopathologic changes in the aorta and TEE examination done after death in 5 patients who died from cardiovascular disease (see below) in order to validate their TEE criteria of significant (complicated) lesions: localized raised lesion of more than 3 mm thick with a markedly irregular surface or broad acoustic shadow. Among their 62 patients, 52 had other potential embolic sources in the heart or cervical arteries, and in the remaining 10 patients with unexplained embolic stroke, 3 had significant lesions in the aortic arch.[87]

Horowitz and her colleagues evaluated 183 patients with brain ischemia for an embolic source and found 7 (4%) patients with mobile, frond-like projections of aortic plaque at TEE examination.[44] Among these 7 patients, 1 had a significant ipsilateral carotid artery stenosis, 1 had a thrombus in the atrial appendage, and 1 had a recent myocardial infarction with left ventricular dilatation and apical dyskinesia, but no evidence of intracardiac thrombus. Of the 4 remaining patients, 2 had small deep infarcts, one in association with diabetes mellitus, the other with hypertension, therefore with a strong suspicion of penetrating branch atherosclerotic occlu-

Table 36.6 Prevalence of Mobile Thrombi in the Lumen of the Aortic Arch in Consecutive Series

Origin of Series	*Sample Size*	*Mobile Thrombi*	*Percentage of Mobile Thrombi*
Consecutive ischemic stroke pts			
Toyoda et al[87] 1992 (embolic stroke)	62	3	4.8%
Nihoyannopoulos et al[65] 1993	152	3	2.0%
Jones et al[45] 1994 (unselected pts)	202	11	5.4%
Amarenco et al[2] 1994 (unselected pts)	250	7	2.8%
Stone et al[82] 1995 (unselected pts)	49	2	4.1%
Consecutive TEE performed in an echolab			
Tunick et al[92] 1991	122	11	9.0%
Karalis et al[47] 1991	556	11	2.0%
Mitchell et al[60] 1992	600	5	0.8%
Mitusch et al[62] 1995	335	8	2.4%
Embolic events or unexplained brain infarction			
Tunick et al[92] 1991 (embolic events)	122	11	9.0%
Karalis et al[47] 1991 (embolic events)	44	11	25.0%
Horowitz et al[44] 1992 (embolic stroke)	183	7	4.0%
Nihoyannopoulos et al[65] 1993 (embolic events)	42	3	7.1%
Amarenco et al[2] 1994 (unexplained brain infarct)	78	6	7.7%
Stone et al[82] 1995 (unexplained brain infarct)	23	2	8.7%
Mitusch et al[62] 1995 (embolic events)	80	5	6.3%

Figure 36.9 (**A**) TEE imaging of a broad-based proximal and distal hyperechogenic aortic arch plaque. The plaque thickness is measured perpendicularly to the far wall, as the distance between the medial-adventitial interface and the internal side of the lesion. The largest thickness is 4.9 mm. (**B**) Multiplane TEE imaging of the aortic arch showing two mobile thrombi in the lumen located both on the proximal and far wall (arrows). Note also the increased wall thickness in the distal arch. (**C**) Multiplane TEE imaging of the ascending aorta and aortic arch showing a huge and mobile thrombus (maximal length 61 mm) attached to the wall of the ascending aorta about 2 cm superior to the level of the aortic cusps. Patient was operated on: the cannula was inserted between the right femoral artery and right atrium. A 60 × 30 mm thrombus was removed from the anterior wall of the ascending aorta, which included several distal mobile components. The ascending aorta was replaced using a Dacron graft. Histopathologic examination found an ulceration with superimposed thrombus.

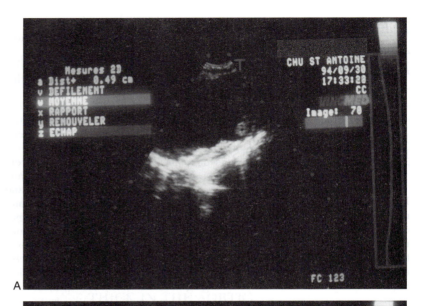

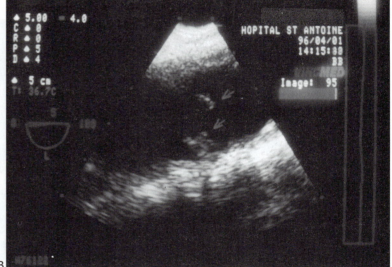

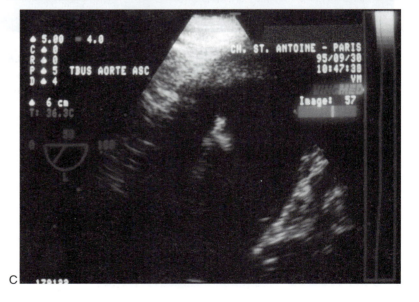

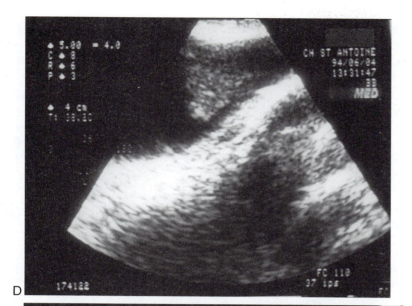

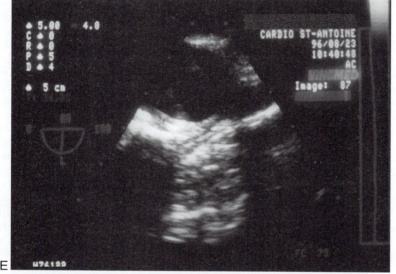

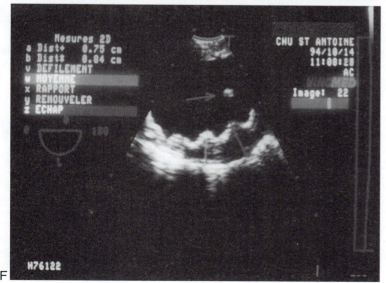

Figure 36.9 *(Continued)* (**D**) Off-axis TEE imaging obtained with a multiplane probe of a fresh thrombus located at the origin of the left subclavian artery in a young woman who had a severe cerebral infarction just after a cerebral angiography. Note the absence of any atherosclerotic lesion in the aortic wall. (**E**) Transverse TEE imaging of the aortic arch obtained with a multiplane probe showing a complex hyperechogenic plaque in front of the origin of the left subclavian artery. The presence of a superimposed hypoechoic mass suggests it was a thrombus. (**F**) Multiplane TEE imaging of the distal aortic arch showing heterogeneous plaque with surface irregularities that may suggest ulceration. The plaque thickness is measured perpendicularly to the far wall, at two different levels (8.4 mm and 7.5 mm). Note the presence of a mobile thrombotic component (arrow).

Table 36.7 Risk of Brain Infarct as a Function of Morphologic Characteristics of Atherosclerotic Plaques in the Ascending Aorta and Proximal Arch

Wall Thickness	Crude OR (95% CI)	P value	Adjusted OR[a] (95% CI)	P
Calcifications	2.9 (2.1; 4.2)	<0.001	2.3 (1.6; 3.3)	<0.001
Irregular surface	4.3 (2.5; 7.1)	<0.001	3.4 (2.0; 5.7)	<0.001
Thickness ≥4 mm	7.6 (3.4; 17.2)	<0.001	5.4 (2.3; 12.4)	<0.001
Thickness ≥4 mm with calcifications	6.9 (3.0; 15.9)	<0.001	2.2 (0.8; 5.9)	=0.095
Thickness ≥4 mm with irregular surface	11.3 (4.0; 32.2)	<0.001	7.4 (2.6; 21.8)	<0.001
Thickness ≥4 mm without calcifications	∞ (7.0; ∞)	<0.001		

Abbreviations: CI: Confidence interval; OR: Odds ratio.

[a] Adjusted for age, sex, peripheral vascular diseases, tobacco consumption, and hypertension.

As mentioned above, Toyoda et al published an important paper on the comparison between histopathologic changes in the aorta and TEE examination.[87] They were able to correlate TEE images and pathology. Five patients who had died from cerebrovascular or cardiovascular disease had TEE examination of the thoracic aorta immediately after death. The thoracic aorta was soaked in physiological saline solution. Forty areas of these aortas were analyzed with special attention paid to the intimal-medial thickness, presence or absence of surface irregularity, and acoustic shadow. A significant lesion at TEE was defined as a localized raised lesion of more than 3 mm thick with a markedly irregular surface. Among the 40 areas screened, the echocardiographer found 18 areas with significant (complicated) lesions.

Then the pathologist, blinded from the result of TEE findings, found complicated lesions (i.e., ulceration of the luminal surface [14 lesions], massive calcification [8 lesions], or both) in 23 of the 40 areas examined. These 23 pathologically complicated lesions included 17 of the 18 "complicated" lesions diagnosed at TEE, and 6 of the 22 areas diagnosed as normal by the echocardiographer; these 6 areas had small ulcerations or small patchy calcifications at pathological examination, and were classified by the pathologist as complicated lesions. Two areas diagnosed by the echocardiographer as complicated with a string-like lesion swinging into the lumen were found by the pathologist severely ulcerated with a peeled surface. The authors concluded that the sensitivity of TEE detection of complicated lesions was 74% and the specificity 94%.[87]

Surface irregularities, calcifications, hypoechoic plaques (suggestive of thrombus), and mobile thrombus floating in the lumen of the aortic arch have been shown to be reliably diagnosed by intraoperative TEE compared with pathologic material removed at surgery in 31 patients.[103]

PLAQUE MORPHOLOGY AND RISK OF ISCHEMIC STROKE

The nature of the material seen with transesophageal echocardiography is now more clear. Videopathologic correlations, besides those of Toyoda et al,[87] in patients who had endarterectomy of their aortic arch lesions have shown that large pro-

truding hypoechogenic lesions seen at TEE correspond pathologically with thrombi superimposed upon ulcerated plaques (Fig. 36.8).[27,54,89,91] As opposed to what is commonly found when coronary and iliac arteries are stenosed, in the aorta there is no compensatory arterial remodeling consisting in enlargement in relation to the plaque area.[53] One explanation for this lack of compensatory remodeling of the aorta may lie in the fact that the material bulging into the lumen is thrombus instead of protruding plaque. In a case control study in the FAPS cohort, we found that thrombus in the aortic arch as detected by TEE is more frequent than in controls with an odds ratio of 11.1 (95% CI, 3.3 to 36.7). Multivariate analysis (Table 36.7) showed that calcifications, irregularities of plaques, plaques ≥4 mm in thickness as seen at TEE in the aortic arch were independently associated with brain infarcts, but also that this association was even more important with plaques ≥4 mm in thickness with irregular surface. Maybe more interesting and intriguing is the strong association between brain infarcts and plaques ≥4 mm in thickness when plaques are not calcified. Furthermore, the relative risk for recurrent brain infarction and new vascular events is much higher in patients with plaques ≥4 mm and noncalcified plaques than in patients with plaques ≥4 mm and plaque calcification (Table 36.8). This may indicate that plaques ≥4 mm are heterogeneous markers and that those with non-calcified plaques have a much higher risk than those calcified. These points should be taken into account in future therapeutic trials.

Table 36.8 Risk of New Vascular Events (Brain Infarction, Myocardial Infarction, Peripheral Emboli, or Vascular Death) in Patients with Plaques ≥4 mm in the Aortic Arch Proximal to the Take-off of the Left Subclavian Artery, According to the Presence or the Lack of Calcification of Plaques

	Odds Ratio	P
New vascular events		
Calcifications	4.1 (2.0–8.5)	<0.001
No calcifications	9.6 (3.9–24.0)	<0.001

NATURAL HISTORY OF PLAQUES IN THE THORACIC AORTA

The evolution of plaques ≥4 mm in thickness in the aortic arch is poorly understood. Montgomery and colleagues studied the natural history of severe atherosclerotic disease of the thoracic aorta.[64] Thirty patients had follow-up TEE, including 10 patients who had mobile lesion in the aorta at the first examination; 8 had atheroma ≥5 mm thick, and 12 had atheroma <5 mm thick. Of the 18 patients with mobile lesions or lesions ≥5 mm thick, 11 (61%) had formation of new mobile lesions. Conversely, of the 10 patients with previously mobile lesion, 7 (70%) had resolution of the mobile component, and 7 had new mobile lesions. Overall, among the 30 patients, 20 (66%) had no change in atherosclerotic severity grade.[64]

In a study of 21 patients with aortic arch plaques ≥4 mm with a follow-up TEE done at day >60, the status of the wall thickness was unchanged in 15%, increased in 30%, and decreased in 55% (Blanchard, Cohen et al, unpublished data). Of the 18 patients who had a mobile component, 11 (61%) no longer had mobile component at follow-up TEE, and this persisted in 7 (39%). A better characterization of plaque component such as thrombus, fat, calcification, and fibrous tissue, should undoubtedly be possible in the future, with a better image resolution, magnetic resonance imaging, and MR angiography or spiral-CT angiography.

RELATION BETWEEN COMPLEX INTRA-AORTIC DEBRIS AND MITRAL ANNULAR CALCIFICATION

In a recent prospective study from the Framingham cohort, mitral annular calcifications (MAC) have been recognized as marker for new brain infarction independently from the traditional stroke risk factors including atrial fibrillation, coronary artery disease, and risk factors for atherosclerosis.[9] In this study, MAC conferred an excess of ischemic stroke in patients with carotid stenosis as compared with patients with similar carotid stenosis but without MAC. These data may suggest that MAC plays a role as an embolic source of ischemic stroke. Alternatively, an unidentified confusion factor may serve as the true source of emboli in patients with MAC, which should then be considered as surrogate markers for embolic sources. Indeed, Rubin et al[74] have found a close association between the presence of MAC and those of complex intra-aortic debris. In 85 consecutive TEE examinations of patients who previously had transthoracic echocardiography for various indications, they found 7 patients with MAC and 8 with complex (protruding plaques ≥7 mm thick, >5 mm in thickness and irregular surface, or plaque with mobile echo density in the lumen) intra-aortic debris. Complex intra-aortic debris was found in 3 of the 7 patients (43%) with MAC and in only 5 of the 78 (6%) without MAC (P <0.01). Although the sample size was small, the authors concluded that complex intra-aortic debris could explain some of the emboli in patients with MAC who have had no other source of emboli identified, as well as explain the increased risk of stroke in patients with carotid stenosis and MAC over those with carotid stenosis alone.[74]

The FAPS investigators also assessed the presence of MAC (unpublished data) in 338 consecutive patients with ischemic stroke and 311 control subjects who had TEE for various cardiologic reasons. After review of videotapes, information about the presence of MAC was available in 301 patients and 270 control subjects. In these 571 subjects, we found MAC in 179 and protruding plaques ≥4 mm thick in the aortic arch in 46 patients. Plaques ≥4 mm thick were found in 16 of the 179 (8.9%) patients with MAC and in 30 of the 392 (7.7%) patients without MAC. If only the group of patients with ischemic stroke was considered, we found plaques ≥4 mm thick in the aortic arch in 14 of the 103 (13.6%) patients with MAC and in 27 of the 198 (13.6%) patients without MAC (unpublished data). We also found mobile debris in the aortic arch in 4 of the 103 (3.9%) patients with MAC and in 4 of the 198 (2%) of patients without MAC. Finally, in the subsample of 103 patients with unexplained ischemic stroke, we found plaques ≥4 mm thick in 9 of the 26 (34%) patients with MAC and in 14 of the 65 (21.5%) patients without MAC. These data do not support the hypothesis of Rubin et al.[74] Therefore, further studies are needed.

Treatment

Not a single definitive study establishes the advantages or disadvantages of a given therapy for patients with well-defined large protruding sessile or mobile plaques in the lumen of the aortic arch. Any therapeutic strategy thus remains empirical. Craig et al[23] reported in an abstract form a series of 29 patients who had systemic embolism (27 cerebral and 2 peripheral) and mobile plaques in the aortic arch found by TEE examination; 19 patients received warfarin and 10 either aspirin (7) or no treatment (3). The morphology of plaques was similar in both groups. During a mean follow-up of 13 ± 12 months there were 6 events in the nonanticoagulated group, while no event occurred in the warfarin group.[23] These results should be taken cautiously because this is a nonrandomized study and the presentation was preliminary. In the FAPS cohort,[64] as well as in Mitusch et al[61] follow-up study, no difference in event rates was found in patients treated with anticoagulant or antiplatelet agents. However, in the subset of patients with mobile thrombus in the lumen of the aortic arch, anticoagulant therapy seems logical, although this awaits confirmation in a randomized study. Meanwhile, in our opinion, in the presence of thrombi in the aortic arch (especially mobile thrombi in the lumen), a short-term anticoagulant therapy should be considered. In other cases, only antiplatelet therapy seems to be needed.

Nevertheless, anticoagulant therapy has been acknowledged as the cause of recurrent cholesterol emboli in patients with severe aortic atherosclerosis.[14] In these cases, recurrent emboli stopped with discontinuation of warfarin therapy. Koren et al[51] followed a cohort of 78 patients with protruding plaques ≥5 mm in thickness for an average of 29 weeks treated with anticoagulant or antiplatelet agents. Among 38 patients on heparin or warfarin, 4 subsequently had a blue toe syndrome associated with progressive renal insufficiency, an increased frequency of transient ischemic attacks, or both. On the other hand, there was no blue-toe syndrome among the 40 patients on antiplatelet agents. The two groups of patients were similar in regard to age and vascular risk factors. The blue toe syndrome may represent accelerated embolization of cholesterol. The hypothesis is that anticoagulation prevents thrombus formation on ulcerated plaques, allowing the release of atheromatous material contained in the plaques. However, there are suggestions that the risk of anticoagulation-induced embolization is probably not that great. In our autopsy study, we found that 28% of unselected consecutive patients with ischemic stroke had ulcerated plaques in the aortic arch.[3] If such figures are extrapolated to everyday practice, high rates of cholesterol embolization would be expected, given the extensive use of anticoagulants. This does not seem to be the case and has not been reported in large trials of warfarin in patients with atrial fibrillation and previous stroke.[32] In the future, however, well-designed trials should evaluate the frequency of such adverse events.

Because of the high risk of larger plaques in the aortic arch, the new possibilities of intra-arterial therapy as well as surgery could probably be evaluated in the future in scientific protocols. But at the present time there is no sufficient level of evidence to routinely use such empirical therapies, although this is feasible and can be justified on a case-by-case basis, as reported by Belden, Caplan and their colleagues.[8]

> These authors reported the observation of a 61-year-old hypertensive hypercholesterolemic woman who had multiple brain emboli within 10 months of follow-up. After the first cerebral event, she was started on warfarin. Despite INRs between 1.5 and 3.5, she had three new posterior circulation infarcts. Repeat TEE again showed a large, broad-based aortic atheroma with an attached echogenic mass. At surgical exploration, there were extensive plaque and thrombus extending into the lumen of the aorta and proximal arch vessels precluding thrombus removal. The ascending and transverse aorta and roots of the proximal great vessels were resected and replaced with a synthetic graft. After surgery she had no new neurologic deficits and has done well after 5 months of follow-up.[8]

As the authors concluded, this case illustrates that aggressive surgical management in selected cases is feasible. Others have reported endarterectomy of the aortic arch in patients with recurrent systemic emboli uncontrolled by anticoagulant or antiplatelet agents. Tunick et al reported two patients who no longer had recurrent systemic embolism after the surgical procedures.[89,91]

> The first patient[89] was a 53-year-old woman who had surgery for a right femoral embolus. After surgery, she had a right hemispheric stroke. Subsequently, she lost her right radial pulse, then had an acute ischemia of the left leg. She was operated with removal of a large thrombus in the left femoral artery. TEE showed a large mass in the aortic arch protruding into the lumen with small mobile components. The left atrium and atrial appendage were free of thrombi. Carotid ultrasound were normal. Surgery of this aortic arch lesion was decided because of the recurrent emboli. "An aortotomy was made from the mid-portion of the ascending aorta to past the left subclavian artery. Beneath the origin of the innominate artery there was an ulceration measuring 2 cm

by 3 cm. There was no debris or clot (sic) within the crater and it was removed with endarterectomy. Opposite the origin of the left subclavian artery, there was a large, mobile plaque measuring 3 cm by 4 cm, which projected into the lumen. The plaque was removed by endarterectomy (Fig. 36.8). An additional 3.5 cm mass was removed from the lumen of the aorta. The patients had an excellent recovery without subsequent emboli." A repeat TEE two months later showed normal aortic arch. Pathologic examination confirmed that the material removed was ulcerated plaques with superimposed thrombi.

> The second patient[91] was a 43-year-old man with a history of embolism in the right leg requiring a right above-the-knee amputation in 1982. Then he had an embolus to the left arm treated by embolectomy in 1983. He was treated with warfarin until left lower-extremity intermittent claudication developed in 1991 despite a correct prothrombin time. Angiography showed an occlusion of the femoral artery. TEE showed a protruding mass in the distal arch with a large, mobile component moving freely with the blood flow. The heart was normal. Surgery was decided because of recurrent embolization while on anticoagulant. "The patient had exploration of the aortic arch under profound hypothermia and circulatory arrest, and left leg embolectomy. In the distal arch there was an ulcerated atherosclerotic plaque with a loosely adherent mass 3 to 4 cm in length and 1 cm in diameter. The mass was removed and the plaque was treated by endarterectomy. . . . The material removed from the aortic arch and from the leg was found to be an old and recent thrombus on pathologic examination. Repeat TEE showed a normal aorta." In addition, this patient had a hypercoagulable state.

However, these most unusual observations by Belden et al[8] and Tunick et al[89,91] cannot be generalized to everyday practice because the patients were younger than the mean age of patients with aortic atherosclerosis. Surgery has potentially a high morbidity in patients with severe aortic arch atherosclerosis, who are frequently older than 75 years. Culliford, Tunick, and their colleagues reported in an abstract their preliminary experience with 12 patients who had aortic arch endarterectomy, 5 for recurrent embolisms presumably because of large and mobile atheroma, and 7 during previously planned heart surgery.[25] Among the 12 patients, 1 died of aortic dissection, and 1 had parietal infarct on CT with regressive confusion. The 11 survivors were followed during a mean of 12 months under treatment with anticoagulant or antiplatelet agents. One patient died at 8 months, and one other had a peripheral embolus to toes at 3 months. This preliminary series (not yet published) shows that the benefits and risks of surgical procedures should be clearly evaluated in the future.

Thrombolysis has proved to be successful in one case, but again an anecdotal report is of limited clinical use,[42] and thrombolysis has also been suspected as the cause of cholesterol embolization.[59] On the basis of the natural history of these lesions, we believe it is now time for randomized therapeutic trials including patients with brain infarcts of unknown cause and plaques $\geq$4 mm thick in the aortic arch proximal to the left subclavian artery ostium.

The Missing Link

Aortic arch atherosclerotic disease is probably an underestimated source of brain and retinal emboli, particularly when moving thrombi are present in the lumen. It may account for a part of brain infarcts of unknown etiology, with no carotid or cardiac source of emboli. Clinicians should be aware that this location of atherosclerotic disease is rare under 60 years of age,[3,31] although it may be encountered (23 patients aged 26 to 61 among 27,855 TEE examinations performed in 15 academic centers in 4 years).[101] It mainly involves patients older than 60 years of age and is actually frequent in those 80 or older. Transesophageal echocardiography is accurate, safe, and well tolerated for the examination of the aortic arch, even in very old patients. These findings have important practical implications for patients and for future clinical trials.

References

1. Amarenco P, Cohen A, Baudrimont M, Bousser M-G: Transesophageal echocardiographic detection of aortic arch disease in patients with cerebral infarction. Stroke 23:1005–1009, 1992
2. Amarenco P, Cohen A, Tzourio C et al: Atherosclerotic disease of the aortic arch and the risk of ischemic stroke. N Engl J Med 331:1474–1479, 1994
3. Amarenco P, Duyckaerts C, Tzourio C et al: The prevalence of ulcerated plaques in the aortic arch in patients with stroke. N Engl J Med 326:221–225, 1992.
4. Amarenco P, Hauw J-J, Gautier J-C: Arterial pathology in cerebellar infarction. Stroke 21:1299–1305, 1990
5. Amarenco P: Les Infarctus Cérébelleux. Etude Anatomo-Clinique de 64 Cas et Revue de la Littérature. (MD Thesis). University of Paris Nord, Paris, 1986
6. Barzilai B, Marshall WG, Saffitz JE, Kouchoukos N: Avoidance of embolic complications by ultrasonic characterization of the ascending aorta. Circulation 80(suppl I):I-275–I-279, 1989
7. Beal MF, Williams RS, Richardson EP, Fisher CM: Cholesterol embolism as a cause of transient ischemic attacks and cerebral infarction. Neurology 31:860–865, 1981
8. Belden JF, Caplan LR, Bojar R et al: Treatment of multiple brain emboli from an ulcerated, thrombogenic aorta with aortectomy and graft replacement. Neurology 49:621–622, 1997
9. Benjamin EJ, Plehn JF, D'Agostino RB et al: Mitral annular calcification and the risk of stroke in an elderly cohort. N Engl J Med 327:374–379, 1992
10. Bergin PJ: Aortic thrombosis and peripheral embolization after thoracic gunshot wound diagnosed by transesophageal echocardiography. Am Heart J 119:688–690, 1990
11. Blauth CI, Cosgrove DM, Webb BW et al: Atheroembolism from the ascending aorta. An emerging problem in cardiac surgery. J Thorac Cardiovasc Surg 103:1104–1112, 1992
12. Bruno A, Jones WL, Austin JK et al: Vascular outcome in men with asymptomatic retinal cholesterol emboli. A cohort study. Ann Intern Med 122:249–253, 1995
13. Bruno A, Russell PW, Jones WL et al: Concomitants of asymptomatic retinal cholesterol emboli. Stroke 23:900–902, 1992
14. Bruns FJ, Segel DP, Adler S: Control of cholesterol embolization by discontinuation of anticoagulant therapy. Am J Med Sci 275:105–108, 1978
15. Buge A, Vincent D, Rancurel G et al: Embolies rétiniennes, musculaires et cutanées de cholestérol. Encéphalopathie progressive. Rev Neurol (Paris) 142:577–581, 1985
16. Byard RW, Jimenez CL, Carpenter BF, Hsu E: Aspergillus-related aortic thrombosis. Can Med Assoc J 136:155–156, 1987
17. Caplan LR: Brain embolism, revisited. Neurology 43:1281–1287, 1993
18. Caplan LR: Intracranial branch atheromatous disease: a neglected, understudied and underused concept. Neurology 39:1246–1250, 1989
19. Case Records of the Massachusetts General Hospital (Case: 21–1972). N Engl J Med 286:1146–1153, 1972
20. Case Records of the Massachusetts General Hospital (Case: 25–1967). N Engl J Med 276:1368–1377, 1967
21. Chan KL: Usefulness of transesophageal echocardiography in the diagnosis of conditions mimicking aortic dissection. Am Heart J 122:495–504, 1991
22. Chomette G, Auriol M, Tranbaloc P et al: Les embolies cholestéroliques. Incidence anatomique et expressions cliniques. Ann Méd Interne 131:17–21, 1980
23. Craig WR, Dressler FA, Vaughn LM et al: Patients presenting with systemic emboli are often found to have mobile plaque in the aortic arch by transesophageal echocardiography (TEE). J Am Coll Cardiol 23:400A [Abstract], 1995
24. Culliford AT, Colvin SB, Rohrer K et al: The atherosclerotic ascending aorta and transverse arch: a new technique to prevent cerebral injury during bypass: experience with 13 patients. Ann Thorac Surg 41:27–35, 1986
25. Culliford AT, Tunick PA, Katz ES et al: Initial experience with removal of protruding atheroma from the aortic arch: diagnosis by transesophageal echo, operative technique, and follow-up, abstracted. J Am Coll Cardiol 21:342A, 1993
26. Dávila-Román VG, Barzilai B, Wareing TH et al: Intraoperative ultrasonographic evaluation of the ascending aorta in 100 consecutive patients undergoing cardiac surgery. Circulation 83 (suppl III):III47–III53, 1991
27. Dávila-Román VG, Barzilai B, Wareing TH et al: Atherosclerosis of the ascending aorta. Prevalence and role as independent predictor of cerebrovascular events in cardiac patients. Stroke 25:2010–2016, 1994
28. Dávila-Román VG, Barzilai B: Insight on aortic atheroembolism from transesophageal and intraoperative echocardiography. Current Opinion in Cardiology 8:808–813, 1993
29. Dee W, Geibel A, Kasper W et al: Mobile thrombi in atherosclerotic lesions of the thoracic aorta: the diagnos-

tic impact of transesophageal echocardiography. Am Heart J 126:707–710, 1993

30. Demopoulos LA, Tunick PA, Bernstein NE et al: Protruding atheromas of the aortic arch in symptomatic patients with carotid stenosis. Am Heart J 129:40–44, 1995

31. Di Tullio MR, Sacco RL, Gersony D et al: Aortic atheromas and acute ischemic stroke: a transesophageal echocardiographic study in an ethnically mixed population. Neurology 46:1560–1566, 1996

32. EAFT (European Atrial Fibrillation Trial) Study Group: Secondary prevention in non-rheumatic atrial fibrillation after transient ischaemic attack or minor stroke. Lancet 342:1255–1262, 1993

33. Fazio GP, Redberg RF, Winslow T, Schiller NB: Transesophageal echocardiographically detected atherosclerotic aortic plaques is a marker for coronary artery disease. J Am Coll Cardiol 21:144–150, 1993

34. Feder W, Auerbach R: "Purple toes": an uncommon sequela of oral coumadin drug therapy. Ann Intern Med 55:911–917, 1961

35. Fisher CM, Gore I, Okabe N, White PD: Atherosclerosis of the carotid and vertebral arteries—extracranial and intracranial. J Neuropathol Exp Neurol 24:455–476, 1965

36. Fisher CM: Occlusion of the carotid arteries. Arch Neurol Psychiatry 72:187–204, 1954

37. Fisher CM: Occlusion of the internal carotid artery. Arch Neurol Psychiatry 65:346–377, 1951

38. Flory CM: Arterial occlusions produced by emboli from eroded aortic atheromatous plaques. Am J Pathol 21:549–565, 1945

39. Gagliardi JM, Batt M, Khodja RH, Le Bas P: Mural thrombus of the aorta. Ann Vasc Surg 2:201–204, 1988

40. Gardner TJ, Horneffer PJ, Manolio TA et al: Stroke following coronary artery bypass grafting: a ten-year study. Ann Thor Surg 40:574–580, 1985

41. Gore I, Collins DP: Spontaneous atheromatous embolization. Review of the literature and a report of 16 additional cases. Am J Clin Pathol 33:416–426, 1960

42. Hausmann D, Gulba D, Bargheer K et al: Successful thrombolysis of an aortic arch thrombus in a patient after mesenteric embolism. N Engl J Med 327:500–501, 1992

43. Hollenhorst RW: Vascular status of patients who have cholesterol emboli in the retina. Am J Ophth 61:1159ff, 1966

44. Horowitz DR, Tuhrim S, Budd J, Goldman ME: Aortic plaque in patients with brain ischemia: diagnosis by transesophageal echocardiography. Neurology 42:1602–1604, 1992

45. Jones EF, Kalman JM, Calafiore P et al: Proximal aortic atheroma. An independent risk factor for cerebral ischemia. Stroke 26:218–224, 1995

46. Kalayjian RC, Herzig RH, Cohen AM, Hutton MC: Thrombosis of the aorta caused by mucormycosis. South Med J 81:1180–1182, 1988

47. Karalis DG, Chandrasekaran K, Victor MF et al: Recognition and embolic potential of intraaortic atherosclerotic debris. J Am Coll Cardiol 17:73–78, 1991

48. Katz ES, Tunick PA, Rusinek H et al: Protruding aortic atheromas predict stroke in elderly patients undergoing cardiopulmonary bypass: experience with intraoperative

transesophageal echocardiography. J Am Coll Cardiol 20:70–77, 1992

49. Kempczinski RF: Lower-extremity arterial emboli from ulcerating atherosclerotic plaques. JAMA 241:807–810, 1979

50. Khathibzadeh M, Mitusch R, Stierle U et al: Aortic atherosclerotic plaques as a source of systemic embolism. J Am Coll Cardiol 27:664–669, 1996

51. Koren MJ, Bryant B, Hilton TC: Atherosclerotic disease of the aortic arch and the risk of ischemic stroke [letter]. New Engl J Med 332:1237, 1994

52. Laloux P, Brucher J-M: Lacunar infarctions due to cholesterol emboli. Stroke 22:1440–1444, 1991

53. Lanza GM, Zabalgoitia-Reyes M, Frazin L et al: Plaque and structural characteristics of the descending thoracic aorta using transesophageal echocardiography. J Am Soc Echo 4:19–28, 1991

54. Laperche T, Sarkis A, Monin J-L et al: The ligamentum arteriosum: an unreported origin of peripheral emboli diagnosed by transesophageal echocardiography. Am Heart J 124:222–223, 1992

55. Machleder HI, Takiff H, Lois JF, Holburt E: Aortic mural thrombus: an occult source of arterial thromboembolism. J Vasc Surg 4:473–478, 1986

56. Marshall WG, Barzilai B, Kouchoukos NT, Saffitz J: Intraoperative ultrasonic imaging of the ascending aorta. Ann Thorac Surg 48:339–344, 1989

57. McDonald WI: Recurrent cholesterol embolism as a cause of fluctuating cerebral symptoms. J Neurol Neurosurg Psychiatry 30:489–496, 1967

58. McKibbin DW, Bukley BH, Green WR et al: Fatal cerebral atheromatous embolization after cardiopulmonary bypass. J Thorac Cardiovasc Surg 71:741–745, 1996

59. Mendia R, Cavaliere G, Sparacio F et al. Does thrombolysis produce cholesterol embolisation? Lancet 339:562, 1992

60. Mitchell MM, Frankville DD, Weinger MB, Dittrich HC: Detection of thoracic atheroma with transesophageal echocardiography in patients without symptoms of embolism. Am Heart J 122:1768–1771, 1991

61. Mitusch R, Doherty C, Wucherpfennig H et al: Vascular events during follow-up in patients with aortic arch atherosclerosis. Stroke 28:36–39, 1997

62. Mitusch R, Stierle U, Kummer-Kloess D et al: Systemic embolism in aortic arch atheromatosis. Eur Heart J 15:1373–1380, 1994

63. Moldveen-Geronimus M, Merriam JC: Cholesterol embolization, from pathological curiosity to clinical entity. Circulation 35:946–953, 1967

64. Montgomery DH, Ververis JJ, McGorisk G et al: Natural history of severe atheromatous disease of the thoracic aorta: a transesophageal echocardiographic study. J Am Coll Cardiol 27:95–101, 1996

65. Nihoyannopoulos P, Joshi J, Athanasopoulos G, Oakley CM: Detection of atherosclerotic lesions in the aorta by transesophageal echography. Am J Cardiol 71:1208–1212, 1993

66. Oliver DO: Embolism from mural thrombus in the thoracic aorta. Br Med J 3:655–656, 1967

67. Oster P, Rieben FW, Waldherr R, Schettler G: Blood

clotting and cholesterol crystal embolization. JAMA 242: 2070–2071, 1979

68. Panum LP: Experimentelle beiträge zur lehre von der embolie. Virchow's Arch Path Anat 25:308–310, 1862

69. Pfaffenbach DD, Hollenhorst RW: Morbidity and survivorship of patients with embolic cholesterol crystals in the ocular fundus. Am J Ophthalmol 75:66–72, 1973

70. Price DL, Harris J: Cholesterol emboli in cerebral arteries as a complication of retrograde aortic perfusion during cardiac surgery. Neurology 20:1209–1214, 1970

71. Ramirez G, O'Neill WM, Lambert R, Bloomer A: Cholesterol embolization, a complication of angiography. Arch Intern Med 138:1430–1432, 1978

72. Ribacove GH, Katz ES, Galloway AC et al: Surgical implications of transesophageal echocardiography to grade the atheromatous aortic arch. Ann Thorac Surg 53: 758–763, 1992

73. Richards AM, Eliot RS, Kanjuh VI et al: Cholesterol embolism: a multisystem disease masquerading as polyarteritis nodosa. Am J Cardiol 15:696–707, 1965

74. Rubin DC, Hawke MW, Plotnick GD: Relation between mitral annular calcium and complex intraaortic debris. Am J Cardiol 71:1251–1252, 1993

75. Rubin DC, Plotnick GD, Hawke MW: Intra-aortic debris as a potential source of embolic stroke. Am J Cardiol 69:819–820, 1992

76. Russell R: Less common varieties of cerebral arterial disease: Cerebral atheroembolism. pp. 394–395. In Russell RWR (ed): Vascular disease of the central nervous system. 2nd ed. Churchill Livingstone, Edinburgh, 1983

77. Russell RWR: Atheromatous retinal embolism. Lancet ii:1354–1356, 1963

78. Sacco RL, Ellenberg JH, Mohr JP et al: Infarcts of undetermined cause: the NINCDS stroke data bank. Ann Neurol 25:382–390, 1989

79. Sadony V, Walz M, Löhr E et al: Unusual cause of recurrent arterial embolism: floating thrombus in the aortic arch surgically removed under hypothermic cardiocirculatory arrest. Eur J Cardio-thor Surg 2:469–471, 1988

80. Shapiro ME, Rodvien R, Bauer KA, Salzman EW: Acute aortic thrombosis in antithrombine-III deficiency. JAMA 245:1759–1761, 1988

81. Soloway HB, Aronson SM: Atheromatous embolism to central nervous system. Arch Neurol 11:657–667, 1964

82. Stone DA, Hawke MW, LaMonte M et al: Ulcerated atherosclerotic plaques in the thoracic aorta are associated with cryptogenic stroke: a multiplane transesophageal echocardiographic study. Am Heart J 130:105–108, 1995

83. Sturgill BC, Netsky MG: Cerebral infarction by atheromatous emboli. Arch Pathol 76:189–196, 1963

84. The French Study of Aortic Plaques in Stroke Group: Atherosclerotic disease of the aortic arch as a risk factor for recurrent ischemic stroke. N Engl J Med 334; 1216–1221, 1996

85. Thompson JE: The evolution of surgery for the treatment and prevention of stroke. The Willis lecture. Stroke 27:1427–1434, 1996

86. Tobler HG, Edwards JE: Frequency and location of atherosclerotic plaques in the ascending aorta. J Thorac Cardiovasc Surg 96:304–306, 1988

87. Toyoda K, Yasaka M, Nagata S, Yamaguchi T: Aortogenic embolic stroke: a transesophageal echocardiographic approach. Stroke 23:1056–1061, 1992

88. Tribouilloy C, Shen WF, Peltier M, Lesbre JP: Noninvasive prediction of coronary artery disease by transesophageal echocardiographic detection of thoracic aortic plaque in valvular heart disease. Am J Cardiol 74: 258–260, 1994

89. Tunick PA, Culliford AT, Lamparello PJ, Kronzon I: Atheromatosis of the aortic arch as an occult source of multiple systemic emboli. Ann Intern Med 114: 391–392, 1991

90. Tunick PA, Kronzon I: Protruding atherosclerotic plaque in the aortic arch of patients with systemic embolization: a new finding seen by transesophageal echocardiography. Am Heart J 120:658–660, 1990

91. Tunick PA, Lackner H, Katz ES et al: Multiple emboli from a large aortic arch thrombus in a patient with thrombotic diathesis. Am Heart J 124:239–241, 1992

92. Tunick PA, Perez JL, Kronzon I: Protruding atheromas in the thoracic aorta and systemic embolization. Ann Intern Med 115:423–427, 1991

93. Tunick PA, Rosenzweig BP, Katz ES et al: High risk for vascular events in patients with protruding aortic atheromas: a prospective study. J Am Coll Cardiol 23: 1085–1090, 1994

94. Wang SP, Chiang BN: Thrombus formation in the ascending aorta: a complication of angiography. Cathet Cardiovasc Diagn 13:50–53, 1987

95. Wareing TH, Dávila-Román VG, Daily BB et al: Strategy for the reduction of stroke incidence in cardiac surgical patients. Ann Throac Surg 55:1400–1408, 1993

96. Williams GM, Harrington D, Burdick J, White RI: Mural thrombus of the aorta: frequently neglected cause of large peripheral emboli. Ann Surg 194:737–744, 1981

97. Winter WJ. Atheromatous emboli: a cause of cerebral infarction. Arch Pathol 64:137–142, 1957

98. Witteman JCM, Kannel WB, Wolf PA et al: Aortic calcified plaques and cardiovascular disease (Framingham Study). Am J Cardiol 66:1060–1064, 1990

99. Zabalgoitia M, Gandhi DK, Evans J et al: Transesophageal echocardiography in the awake elderly patient: its role in the clinical decision-making process. Am Heart J 120:1147–1153, 1990

100. Pop G, Sutherland GR, Koudstaal PJ, Sit TW, de Jong G, Roelandt JRTC: Transoesophageal echocardiography in the detection of intracardiac embolic sources in patients with transient ischemic attacks. Stroke 21: 560–565, 1990

101. Laperche T, Laurian C, Roudaut R et al: Mobile thromboses of the aortic arch without aortic debris. A transesophageal echocardiographic finding associated with unexplained arterial embolism. Circulation 96:288–294, 1997

102. Dávila-Román et al: Atherosclerosis of the ascending aorta: independent predictor of neurologic events and long-term mortality. Circulation 94:I–391, 1996

103. Vaduganathan V, Ewton A, Nagueh SF et al: Pathologic correlates of aortic plaques, thrombi and mobile "aortic debris" imaged in vivo with transesophageal echocardiography. J Am Coll Cardiol 30:357–363, 1997

CHAPTER 37

Binswanger's Disease

J. P. MOHR

H. MAST

Binswanger's disease, currently also known as subacute arteriosclerotic encephalopathy, refers to a particular form of cerebrovascular disease that has its onset between the ages of 50 and 65, is associated with recurrent brief focal neurologic deficits, and features a progressive dementia. The exact cause of this process still remains uncertain, but some authors consider it attributable to selective arteriosclerotic changes in the penetrating vessels of the deep white matter of the cerebral hemispheres with resultant subcortical infarction.

Despite the use of the term, it remains unclear whether Binswanger's disease encompasses several different clinical and pathologic disorders, and its underlying pathology remains unsettled. The scanty pathologic documentation of the disorder since Binswanger's original description might have sufficed to keep it among the obscure forms of cerebrovascular disease were it not for the recent surge of interest because findings on computed tomographic (CT) and magnetic resonance (MR) scans are not easily explained by conventional concepts of atherothrombosis or embolism. The many instances of low densities in the white matter found in routine CT or high signal on T_2-weighted MR requiring explanation and the attractiveness of the eponym disease keep it popular. Several reports have claimed a characteristic CT picture, one encountered in up to 3% to 4% of cranial CTs of elderly patients. Whether merely rarely diagnosed in the past or eventually understandable in different terms than at present, a review of the status of Binswanger's disease seems worthy of treatment in this text chapter form.

Original Observations

OTTO BINSWANGER

In a now-famous lecture in 1894, before the Jahresversammlung des Vereins Deutscher Irrenärzte (Annual Meeting of the German Psychiatrists) in Dresden, Otto Binswanger set forth his concept of vascular dementia.[3] Later published in three parts in the Berliner Klinische Wochenschrift, the lecture Binswanger gave delineated a heterogeneity of four dementia syndromes of vascular origin, starting with the then best-understood cause of dementia, syphilis (synonym "progressive paralysis"). The other three were to have a major effect in thinking about vascular disease and dementia in the century that followed.

Encephalitis subcorticalis chronica progressiva (ESCP) was the first of these subtypes, only later labeled "Binswanger's disease" and not always with the same elements described by Binswanger. He cited its rarity—he had seen only 8 cases in the prior 11 years—and summarized the macroscopic pathology with special emphasis on the severe white matter atrophy (WMA), which he found most pronounced in the occipital and temporal lobes. The atrophy was associated with ventricular enlargement, mainly of the inferior and posterior horns: "the main sites of the disease are the posterior brain segments." He found the cortex only slightly narrowed, and noted it was otherwise not involved. The clinical picture featured gradual intellectual decline and focal signs such as aphasia, hemianopia, hemiparesis, and hemisensory loss. The severity of the focal syndromes could fluctuate at the onset of the disease process but reached a stable state toward the end. Seizures also occurred. He offered the opinion that ESCP usually started around age 50 but one case was 72 at onset. The course went on for 10 or more years. Periods of clinical stability lasting several years were noted. Death was the result of secondary causes (infection, cardiac failure) or "apoplectiform attacks."

Binswanger followed his general remarks with the only detailed clinicopathologic case report he was ever to publish. Using a purely macroscopic evaluation of the brain, he described the autopsy as revealing an asymmetric hemispheral WMA of the lower parietal as well as the upper and lateral temporal lobes. Measurements of both hemispheres after a coronal section through the posterior sylvian fissure showed a width of 8.7 cm of the right compared to 7.3 cm of the left hemisphere. The ventricles were enlarged, especially the lower horns. The frontal gray matter was described as only slightly narrowed. Contrary to his postulates as to the pathophysiology of ESCP being from arteriosclerosis, his only detailed case showed no arteriosclerotic changes in the basal arteries. The smaller vessels were not described. Cavitary lesions were not mentioned (an important point differing from findings of subsequent authors—see below), and Binswanger explicitly stated there were ". . . nowhere signs of focal disease." The spinal cord showed diffuse pathologic changes throughout.

The patient had suffered for several years from "dizziness" (not further specified by Binswanger), visual decline of the right eye interpreted as "choreoiditis disseminata," and "ptyalism." Beginning in his late 40s, he suffered severe left-sided headache, paresthesias of the right arm and leg, fine motor disturbance of the right hand, and the complaint of "missing words," together with episodes of sudden loss of memory for remote events. More recent events were well-remembered. Calculation was impaired. Further symptoms were a depressed mood and—being fully aware of his state—a fear of becoming insane. No detailed neurologic examination was documented, but Binswanger stated that the strength of the right-sided extremities and sensory testing were normal. (It remains unclear whether the initial history was taken by Binswanger himself or cited from notes of other physicians.) Because of a syphilitic infection acquired 26 years before, an "antiluetic" treatment was initiated and believed to result in an incomplete remission of the syndrome.

The patient returned to his previous professional activity but never regained his previous level of intellectual performance. Instead, a gradual decline occurred, with increasing forgetfulness (especially for recent events) and paraphasic errors. Confusional states began about 5 years after the initial event and finally mandated hospital admission. The neurologic examination at that time showed a minimal right-sided central facial paresis and slight tongue deviation to the right. The pupils were normal in size and shape and reacted normally to light. Hearing was intact. No motor deficit was found in the arms, but the legs showed mild bilateral weakness, more pronounced on the right. The patient could walk normally. Sensory testing showed normal pain perception. Other sensory qualities could not be evaluated reliably. The patient's speech, apparently fluent, was severely disturbed with a "completely meaningless stringing of words." A *spoon* was called *school* (the corresponding German words "Löffel" and "Schule" being phonetically farther apart than their English translation); a watch (or clock): "that is . . . I really don't know now—Erfurt—in Erfurt." (Erfurt: a German city); a hat: "a hat"; a ring: "That is also a hat." After offering the correct term for spoon, the patient immediately agreed and mumbled repetitively "Löffel." Repetition was intact. Simple commands (showing the tongue, lifting the right or left hand) were followed correctly, but errors emerged in more complex tasks (picking the wrong verbally named object, drawing a ring in the air, whereas the investigator asked "show me my ring"). Reading and writing were also grossly impaired. The patient's behavior was "quite correct" and he struggled unsuccessfully to communicate his problems.

In the following four years, nocturnal episodes of confusion and agitation became an increasing problem and the neuropsychological deficits progressed. Stereotype rubbing movements of the hands on the thighs and two generalized seizures were noted. The patient finally died in the course of an infection.

Binswanger then described two additional syndromes. *Arteriosclerotic brain degeneration (ABD)* was considered separate from ESCP. The anatomic features were summarized as widespread large-artery arteriosclerosis affecting the brain vessels as well as other organs with subsequent severe cardiac and renal changes. The weight of the brains in these cases was markedly reduced. He noted that, "generally, the vessel-holes are very enlarged. Already by macroscopic inspection, in the vicinity of the vessels in many areas of the cortex and the white matter, the brain parenchyma is discolored light gray to red-brown and slightly sunken in, especially in the area of the basal ganglia and internal capsule an état criblé is prominent." The white matter was discolored throughout, the cortex pale but only slightly narrowed, and the ventricles showed enlargement. "Miliary apoplexies" surrounding the arteriosclerotic vessels were pointed out. Microscopy revealed "simple atrophic or fatty degenerative" changes in small cortical and white matter arteries (and veins), in some "larger ones" with luminal narrowing (no specific microscopy had been described for ESCP). In the area surrounding these vessels, neuronal and glial cell decline was found. The cortex showed a "degenerative-atrophic process" affecting cortical neurons. Myelinated cortical fibers were reduced in number.

In ABD the intellectual deficit was characterized by a more remittent course than in the ESCP cases. Patients with ABD could show almost complete remission of memory deficits and fluctuated more than their generally stable or relentlessly progressing ESCP counterparts. A variety of intermittent focal neurologic syndromes (attributable to small, deep infarcts?) and episodes of loss of consciousness (seizures?) were also seen. Stable focal deficits as in ESCP were not listed. Binswanger further commented that "the close relationship" of ESCP and ABD allowed for intermediate forms that blurred clinical discrimination.

Finally, in addition to these disseminated in situ arterial pathologies, Binswanger noted "embolic and thrombotic" large artery occlusions leading to cerebral infarcts. This third form of vascular dementia he called "dementia post apoplexiam" with acute onset ("apoplectical insult") of intellectual and focal deficits with a stable nonremittent course. He gave no further anatomical details and cited no literature. Other nonvascular dementia forms like "simple, presenile dementia" (the precursor of today's Alzheimer's disease) and alcoholic dementia were also discussed by Binswanger, but are not discussed further here. Although he promised future detailed descriptions, namely of ESCP, Binswanger did not write further on the topic.

ALOIS ALZHEIMER

Some years after Binswanger, Alois Alzheimer published a series of articles also based primarily on lectures. The one given in 1902 before the same Jahresversammlung des Vereins Deutscher Irrenaerzte summarizes his and Binswanger's work eight years after the first presentation.[1] He began by stating that he and Binswanger were the first in Germany to work and lecture on "arteriosclerotic brain atrophy" in detail, but he also emphasized the contribution of Klippel, and pointed out the proposal of other French authors to name the syndrome "Maladie de Klippel." Alzheimer noted that in addition to ". . . arteriosclerotic brain atrophy Binswanger also described an Encephalitis subcorticalis chronica diffusa which he says shows a strong arteriosclerosis of the brain arteries." Alzheimer thus made the assumption conceivable that Binswanger (and he) thought the subcortical fiber atrophy was the result of a nutritional disturbance based on arteriosclerosis. He then noted that "Binswanger's Encephalitis subcorticalis [is] as the anatomical investigation shows only a subform of arteriosclerotic brain atrophy." In neither this nor his later citations of Binswanger in the context of ESCP (slightly renamed by Alzheimer) did his writing contain any suggestion that the syndrome be named "Binswanger's disease." Instead, his use of the phrase "Binswanger's encephalitis" can also be read as indicating disagreement with Binswanger's view that ESCP deserved the status of a distinct syndrome.

Nevertheless, Alzheimer offered a separate description of ESCP, without clear reference to the origin of his data, leaving unsettled whether he was citing from Binswanger's work or his own observations. He mentioned having seen "three cases." Autopsy showed a "severe arteriosclerotic disease of the long vessels of the deep white matter" with highly atrophic hemispheral white matter, sparing the U fibers in "typical cases." He also noted an association with severe arteriosclerosis of the vessels serving the basal ganglia and the medulla oblongata ("arteriosclerotic bulbar paralysis"), and, like Binswanger, he also noted that the focal softenings typical of infarction were absent. Microscopy of ESCP—which was not presented by Binswanger—showed numerous "foci" (Herde) throughout the white matter with localized and also diffuse glial proliferation. Similar microscopical "foci" were noticed in the internal capsule, nucleus lentiformis, thalamus, and pons. Otherwise, Alzheimer's presentation, including the clinical syndrome, added little to Binswanger's initial report on ESCP. The most important additional information offered by Alzheimer on ESCP was the presence of severe arteriosclerotic changes involving lenticulostriate vessels and the microscopic finding of focal glial proliferation and neuronal decline in the white matter and elsewhere.

Alzheimer used another term, *arteriosclerotic brain degeneration*, as a general heading embracing all types of vascular dementia. He provided clinical and anatomic descriptions, again without reference to the number of cases and source of his observations. The autopsy findings showed marked reductions of brain weight, enlarged ventricles, only slight narrowing of the cortical convolutions, and severe atheromatosis of the macroscopically visible arteries. After cutting the brain, "enormously enlarged vessel spaces," a rigid and discolored hemispheric white matter with grayish discoloration along the course of the vessels, and occasional miliary softenings and small capillary aneurysms were seen. The areas of the basal ganglia and the internal capsule displayed an *état criblé*, the latter term left unexplained by Alzheimer and Binswanger (enlarged perivascular spaces in the original definition by Durand-Fardel).[15] The corpus dentatum was regularly degenerated. Microscopy revealed arteriosclerotic foci scattered throughout the cortex, white matter, and basal ganglia. In the center of these foci, a highly degenerated vessel was found. The degree of degenerative changes within the foci varied from slight glial proliferation to a complete decline of neuronal tissue being replaced by a rigid glial scar. When the diseased small vessel was cut longitudinally, the surrounding focus ran

along the course of the artery. The perivascular spaces were enlarged. Next to these focal pathologies, diffuse changes of glial cell proliferation and "fatty, pigmentous" ganglia cell degeneration throughout all parts of the hemispheres were noted.

The clinical presentation of ABD was characterized by remission and relapses in the initial phase and in later stages by a relentlessly progressive course of intellectual decline. Reversible focal events occurred with a broad variety of symptoms, some of them suggesting seizures. Stable focal signs as in ESCP were at least less common, but hemipareses in the wake of "small capsular foci" were recognized, and aphasia was a common finding. Coexisting renal and cardiac diseases were identified as one of the major causes of death.

In addition to the subcortical variant of small vessel disease of the brain, Alzheimer also postulated a cortical small vessel pathology, which he termed *senile cortical atrophy* (using the word "senile" because of the preferred occurrence in very old age classes and its combination with "senile dementia"). Typical of this subform were small wedge-shaped cortical infarcts composed of a dense glial scar with occasional softenings confined to few convolutions. The foci appeared sunken under the niveau of the cortex and the "severely atrophic convolutions show numerous punctate indentations." No information was provided on the localization of these findings on the cortex (border zones?), but reference was made to an underlying pathology of a "larger artery" (contradicting his initial remark that this subform was based on cortical small vessel pathology).

Alzheimer also addressed other forms of dementia, which, in his opinion, were based on large vessel arteriosclerosis, described as "perivascular gliosis": A severe narrowing of a major cerebral artery with subsequent hemodynamic failure and chronic ischemia in its supply territory was termed *perivascular gliosis*. Neuronal tissue that "obviously poses the highest demand on nutrition" suffered most whereas the glia was proliferating. The anatomic picture was a focal distribution of these changes confined to the given arterial territory affecting the cortex as well as deep structures of one or more convolutions. Alzheimer pointed out that a complete occlusion owing to thrombosis of the same vessel could result in a large softening (infarct) instead of leading to "chronic degenerative decline."

Dementia post apoplexiam received only brief mention. "The basal ganglia and the region of the internal capsule are a preferred site of atheromatous vessel disease, especially also for bleedings. [. . .] Histology teaches that for the dementia [post apoplexiam] not the apoplex as such, but hemispheric arteriosclerotic foci are responsible." Cases with findings of dementia symptoms before the bleed were cited in support. This and the described progressive course of "dementia post apoplexiam" is at odds with Binswanger's view.

Summarizing his presentation, Alzheimer stated that "there are typical cases of the described forms, but also mixed cases." Why in a given situation of severe brain vessel arteriosclerosis one case developed only cortical changes whereas another showed lesions confined to the white matter remained to be clarified. "We have seen that arteriosclerotic brain disease without macroscopically visible foci can cause the most numerous and severe focal symptoms." In his view on the mechanisms of ischemic damage to brain tissue, he characterized chronic ischemic lesions as a form of "incomplete softening" leading to rigid scars, whereas thrombosis (and embolism) resulted in acute colliquation necrosis, the former being the main cause of vascular dementia. The possibility of overlapping events in individual patients was well noticed.

OTHER AUTHORS

Following the lead of Alzheimer, almost all subsequent articles note the occurrence of *multiple lacunes* in the basal ganglia and the thalamus, findings contrary to those in Binswanger's original case. Most authors have also commented on the presence of *arteriosclerotic changes* in basal arteries of the brain as well as in the penetrating vessels of the white matter, findings also not included in Binswanger's original case.

Separate from the nature of the underlying vascular disease, most authors concur that the main weight of the lesions falls on the white matter. Virtually all authors have described the relative sparing of the cortical gray matter and the subcortical U fibers, emphasizing the main involvement in the centrum semiovale and deeper fiber systems. There is some inconsistency in the descriptions of the myelin disorder in the white matter. Although small cystic lesions have been commonly noted, and the term *demyelination* has been used frequently, the nature of the demyelination seems different in many of the reports. Some authors emphasize sparing of the axons, others comment on small or large areas of demyelination, and some note destruction of both the axons and the myelin. The literature is briefly summarized here, with emphasis on any findings that add to or change the concepts explaining Binswanger's disease.

Bucholz, in 1905, described five cases,[7] and Ladame, in 1912, one case, of Binswanger's ESCP.[31] Both authors concurred that the disease was a severe form of cerebral atherosclerosis. Few details were given. In 1920, Nissl described the brain of a patient with a progressive mental deterioration punctuated by episodes of dysfunction attributable to numerous focal changes in the white matter, in the surface convolution as well as deep in the hemispheres, varying in size, associated with arteriosclerotic vessels of various calibers.[44] He described vascular changes that consisted of severe and often extreme thickening of the vascular walls to such an extent that the distinction between the artery, vein, and capillary was not possible. The thickening was caused by concentric lamellae arranged in onionskin pattern. He did not note a predilection of the lesions for the posterior half of the brain, and no focal lesions were described in the subcortical gray matter or in the brain stem. The work of Farnell and Globus in 1932 echoed the previous descriptions, added no new data, and served mainly to continue earlier trends.[17] Davison, in 1942, reported a very atypical case referred to as Binswanger's disease, which included swelling of the patchily involved white matter as well as some involvement of the overlying gray matter.[12] Although atheromatous changes were seen in the small blood vessels of the white matter, it is unclear whether this case should be included among those referred to as Binswanger's disease. Neuman's 1947 case is usually listed in the Binswanger's disease literature but is also so atypical in its course and pathologic findings that it is more likely to be some type of other

myelinoclastic disorder, and is not further considered in our evaluation.[42]

In 1962, Olszewski published an important review of the tiny world literature to that time and added two cases of his own.[46] In this article he published the translations of Binswanger's, Alzheimer's, and Nissl's descriptions of the disease. Olszewski took the position that the condition was an arteriosclerotic process preferentially affecting the vessels of the subcortical gray matter and the white matter and proposed the term *subcortical arteriosclerotic encephalopathy* (Binswanger's type), now also known as SAE. He attributed the demyelination to multiple areas of infarction with disruption of long tracts. In this article the original observations of Binswanger's case were largely set aside, and little attention was paid to issues of chronic ischemia and syndromes representing disease of the white matter.

Jelgersma described a case of SAE in 1964 that resembled previous cases clinically and pathologically.[29] The vascular changes included relatively severe hyalinosis, hypertrophy of the media, atherosclerosis of the cerebral vessels, and etat lacunaire of the basal nuclei; both the myelin sheaths and the axons had evidence of degeneration; the cortex and U fibers were normal. Although noting the vascular abnormalities, he took the relative sparing of the cortex and U fibers to argue against a vascular process. Few authors have followed this lead of a nonvascular cause of the disorder, but Jelgersma's work represents one definite etiological path parallel with those for vascular disease.

Pathology and Brain Imaging

The development of brain imaging (i.e., CT and MR) has added another dimension of observations, spreading the literature in several directions. One has been the continuation of the neuropathologically based observations, from many countries and continents, with some reference to imaging findings; another has been the collection of patients whose anatomic findings are based mainly on imaging data, supported by a smaller number of autopsies; and a third is the mainly imaged-based attempts to characterize the clinical picture, assuming the imaging finding represents the autopsy not done. The latter two provide an overlap with the disorder known as leukoariosis,[51] itself a descriptive term arising from observations of CT (and more recently, of MR) scans. Considering the nonuniformity of definitions and extent of evaluations of these patients, some unavoidable overlap with leukoariosis is to be expected in the present review, but it is not intentional.

In 1970, Biemond added two cases to the literature and concurred with most previous opinions that this was a vascular process.[2] He also noted patchy demyelination of the white matter. He appears to have been the first to suggest the possibility of diagnosing this condition antemortem based on the typical clinical syndrome described by Binswanger. In 1974, preceding the first imaging studies, DeLong et al discussed the clinicopathologic correlations in a case of Binswanger's disease, and briefly reviewed the literature to that point. The various theories regarding the possible causes were cited, but no new theories were advanced. Burger et al[8] presented a patient in 1976 who appeared to have Binswanger's disease. They noted that his ventricles were large and that he had an abnormal radioactive Iodinated serum albumin (RISA) which suggested the diagnosis of normal pressure hydrocephalus (NPH). The patient did not respond to shunting. He subsequently developed a subdural hematoma that required surgical drainage. In the last stages of his disease, he had myoclonic jerks, and demonstrated triphasic waves on his electroencephalogram (EEG). Electrolyte levels were reported to be normal. Results of neuropathologic examination were not consistent with Creutzfeldt-Jakob disease, but were more in line with Binswanger's disease. This case is somewhat atypical because of the presence of the myoclonic jerks and the triphasic waves. White subsequently reported another case with triphasic waves; his case also was atypical in that the patient had a remarkably short course of 6 weeks.[56] Autopsy revealed large basilar territory infarct. The comments in the section on neuropathologic findings include the discovery of multiple lacunar infarctions in the subcortical white matter; no comments are made about the presence of other possible causes of triphasic waves.

In 1978, Caplan and Schoene described the pathologic findings in five cases and extended these observations to six living patients in an effort to diagnose this disease antemortem.[9] Neuropathologic examination revealed that all of the patients had multiple lacunar infarcts (a finding that was not cited in Binswanger's initial contribution). Diffuse loss of nerve fibers and dense gliosis were seen in the white matter. Thickening of the intrinsic arteries and arterioles was noted in all the patients. The authors formulated a syndrome using the combination of hypertension, repeated acute focal neurologic deficits, periods of clinical plateau or even improvement, asymmetrical weakness with pseudobulbar palsy, and hydrocephalus (ex vacuo) by pneumoencephalography (PEG). CT scanning, then only recently on the scene, was cited as a possible tool for the diagnosis because of its easy detection of hydrocephalus. They differentiated SAE from état lacunaire by the subacute progression of deficits in the former compared with the isolated small discrete strokes typical of the latter. Rosenberg added a case in 1979 in which the patient also had multiple lacunar infarcts.[50] He ascribed loss of myelinated fibers with relative preservation of axons except in the circumscribed zones of subtotal necrosis scattered throughout the centrum semiovale, and mild gliosis in the central convolutional white matter of the hemispheres. He also discussed the bilateral white matter lucencies seen on CT, noting that this change was not special.

Janota described seven cases said to be Binswanger's, with two cases that had been diagnosed as Alzheimer's disease during life in a 1981 report.[28] He believed the pathologic changes found in the white matter were typical of those seen in infarction. He noted that all of the patients had hypertension, and the cerebral arteries had thickening and fibrosis in their walls. He discussed previous observations on Binswanger's disease and emphasized the presence of hypertension in most reports. He then cited a study by Valentine that had noted that 1.6% of patients with cerebral atrophy had low attenuation of the deep white matter; none of these cases had had pathologic examination. Lacking any pathologic data, Valentine thought that this condition was probably état criblé.[54] Janota sought to join this observation with his own, and suggested that these cases represented Binswanger's disease. This led him to the conclusion that Binswanger's disease was a much more common clinical and pathologic entity than had been believed and that it had been undiagnosed prior to the availability of CT. He concluded that SAE appeared to be more common than previously thought. Several authors have followed Janota's example and have concluded that the changes seen on CT are specific for Binswanger's disease, relying on single autopsied cases in each series to support their contention.[35]

Okeda noted that the media of the medullary arteries was significantly thicker in patients with either SAE or hypertensive hemorrhage than in controls.[45] He postulated that the severe hypertrophy of the media was the result of pathologic hyperreactivity to hypertension. He felt that this structural alteration impaired autoregulation, exposing the deep white matter more directly to fluctuations of blood pressure, so that decrease in blood pressure produced a "counter-steal" with ischemia of the more distal white matter, and increases in blood pressure caused edema of the deep white matter. He also commented that changes in the vessels of patients with SAE were more pronounced than those observed in other hypertensive individuals. Another possible explanation is that some of the cases are in fact dysmyelinating diseases, and the cases reported as having little gliosis represent another, nonvascular, disease.

The relationship between vascular disease and central white matter histopathologic findings has been the subject of several studies. In 1985, Dubas et al[14] reported 17 cases of leukoencephalopathy attributed to vascular disease. The white matter findings in all cases featured diffuse demyelination, none involving the U fibers, corpus callosum, or internal capsule (in agreement with Binswanger's observations). Blood vessel walls were found thickened and hyalinized, typical of cerebral amyloid angiopathy. Hypertension was common to some of the cases as were basal ganglia lacunes (not noted by Binswanger). The authors proposed the mechanism for this leukoencephalopathy to be hypoperfusion of the distal white matter and alteration of the blood brain barrier. Similar findings were made on 12 patients by Gray et al[23] who also had amyloid angiopathy. Three of the patients had CT scanning, which showed white matter hypodensities. A diffuse bilateral loss of hemispheral white matter myelin, sparing U fibers, was found to have a predominance in the periventricular areas. The histopathology in these cases featured edematous lesions showing spongiosis, swollen oligodendroglia, and widening of the perivascular spaces, but did not prominently feature infarction. The authors suggested that a common mechanism of hypoperfusion of the distal white matter causes the leukoencephalopathy.

Inzitari et al[27] noted a difference between the histopathology of what they decided was leukoaraiosis and what they characterized as Binswanger's subcortical arteriosclerotic encephalopathy. The findings in the first group did not seem to have a vascular basis, while those in the latter did. This study is a bit at odds with some of the other case series reported, adding to the difficulties in settling the mechanisms of disease at work in this cohort.

Furuta et al[21] in 1991 reported vascular changes seen in the medullary arteries (mainly those of the centrum semiovale in 110 cases said to be non-neuropsychiatric patients, mostly old, but some in their 20s, comparing the findings with those of 20 cases having subcortical arteriosclerotic encephalopathy

(Binswanger's disease), and 20 having Alzheimer's disease. The authors found a prominent fibrohyaline thickening of the arterial walls, proportional in severity to the age in decades. The findings were the most prominent in descending sequence from the frontal, parietal, occipital, and temporal lobes, and were present in both the "non-neuropsychiatric" and demented groups. The intensity of the sclerotic changes correlated with the degree of ischemic white matter changes as well as with blood pressure. It may be important to note that the distribution of the vascular changes noted in their material was in the opposite order to that stressed by Binswanger (the latter stressing parietal-occipital predominating), so it is not certain that these findings are the same or different from those from Binswanger. Nontheless, these authors pointed to a correlation between the severity of the vascular changes and those of the white matter disease. Similar findings were reported by Tomonaga et al[53] in their hypertensive populations.

A similar view that severe arteriosclerotic changes underlie the white matter findings was put forward by Zeumer et al[57] in presenting the findings of one patient with status lacunaris. A patchy, diffuse white matter involvement was found with total or partial myelin sheath destruction, comparatively minor injury to the axons, and considerable astroglial proliferation. They formulated a correlation with the syndrome and the CT scan showing moderately dilated ventricles; symmetrical, diminished density of the white matter without signs of space-occupying lesion; and microinfarctions in the basal ganglia. They used these criteria to diagnose 47 other elderly patients thought to have Binswanger's disease on the basis of CT findings of periventricular white matter low attenuation.

Lacunes and Binswanger's Disease

It should be clear from this review of the clinical course of lacunar infarctions that some patients with multiple lacunar infarctions will resemble the clinical state described as typical for Binswanger's disease. Most cases that have been described as Binswanger's disease also had lacunar infarctions in the basal ganglia, despite Binswanger having made no such notation. Assuming for the purpose of the current discussion that small, deep infarcts are part of Binswanger's disease, the issue of lacunar infarcts in the central white matter has been the subject of reviews[35] and justifies further discussion.

In 1980, De Reuck et al equated the infarcts in the centrum semiovale with those known in deeper sites as lacunes.[13] They described four patients, three of whom had clinical histories very atypical for Binswanger's disease, having cystic or lytic lesions in the periventricular white matter (not noted by Binswanger in his own case) surrounded by variable degrees of demyelination. They also had lacunes in the thalamus and basal ganglia (lacking in Binswanger's case). Despite some of the atypical features, the neuropathologic changes were said to be the same as those seen in subacute arteriosclerotic encephalopathy. De Reuck expressed the opinion that these changes were the result of disease involving the lenticulostriate and medullary cerebral arteries. The sparing of the U fibers was ascribed to their blood supply being derived directly from the cortical vessels and not from the medullary, penetrating arteries. He equated the lesions in the white matter with those of the lacunes seen in the basal ganglia. However, the authors did not believe that a primary arteriopathy such as that usually

responsible for lacunes was the sole factor necessary for the development of Binswanger's disease. They expressed the view that the periventricular white matter is a watershed area, supplied by end arteries, the medullary arteries. They proposed that the combination of the severe penetrating vessel disease with hypoperfusion in the watershed area produced the pathologic picture of Binswanger's disease. The argument used had been articulated years before by Lindenberg and Spatz: demyelination in this area was the result of poor perfusion of these watershed areas during periods of hemodynamic crisis resulting in distal field infarction in the immediate periventricular area and less severe ischemic injury producing demyelination more proximally in the course of the medullary arteries.[34]

C. M. Fisher proposed a process of multiple lacunar infarcts as the morphologic basis underlying "subcortical arteriosclerotic encephalopathy (Binswanger's type)."[20] This observation is at odds with his earlier work indicating only a low frequency of lacunar lesions in the centrum semiovale. Further, a central thesis for lacunes was that they occur mainly in the territories of very small vessels (e.g., thalamoperforants, lenticulostriates, paramedian branches of the basilar artery), which arise from very large ones, thus not being buffered from the effects of hypertension.

Prior Editions of This Book

The opinions on the existence and nosology of Binswanger's disease continue to change. A dubious approach was promulgated in the first edition of this book.[43] In the second edition, Bogousslavsky took a middle ground, describing Binswanger's disease as diffuse white matter pathology linked with "some infarcts, usually deep, but sometimes involving the cortex" with the internal capsule being "markedly spared."[4]

Brain Imaging

Many studies have focused mainly on the CT or MR scan, with the autopsy and histopathologic details given less attention. Figure 37.1 is an example of the abnormalities found. Lotz et al performed a case-control study[36] for the 82 patients having a CT scan prior to autopsy. Twenty of them had CT findings the authors took to represent changes consistent with subacute arteriosclerotic encephalopathy (SAE—as noted, often considered the same as Binswanger's disease). Microscopy was said to have confirmed the diagnosis in 18 of them. A point of special interest was similar histologic vascular findings among 10 control patients showing normal cerebral white matter by CT scan, although the authors considered the findings less severe than those for patients with SAE.

Mather et al reviewed their experience with 20 cases showing white matter changes on CT scan, which suggested a diagnosis of Binswanger's disease.[37] They concluded that Binswanger's disease is probably due to chronic or acute-on-chronic white matter ischemia. They also noted the occurrence of lacunar infarctions in this group. They differentiated Binswanger's disease clinically from multi-infarct dementia[26] by its time course.

Leifer et al[33] reported their imaging and pathologic correlations for seven patients with MR. Apart from the periventricular findings, the extensive subcortical changes on MR were explained by multiple sclerosis in one case and by subcortical

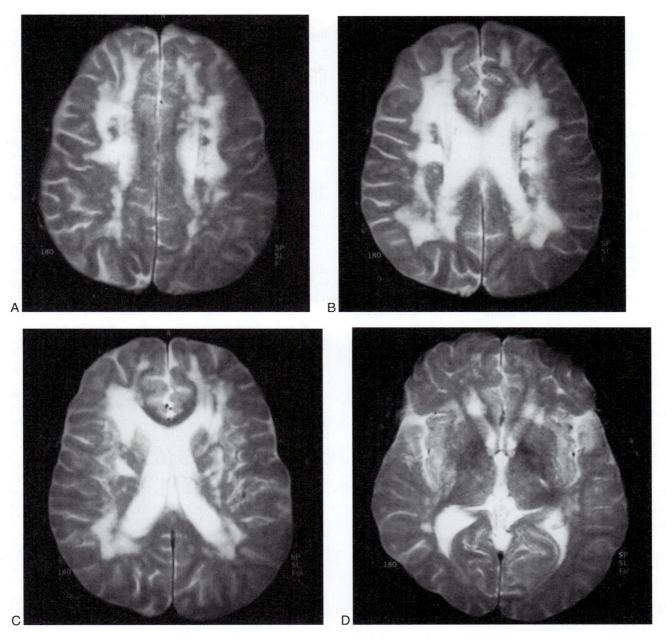

Figure 37.1 (A–D) T$_2$-weighted MR showing high-signal changes in the centrum semi-ovale and corona radiata in a 35-year-old man with recurrent strokes and positive family history of early strokes. There is relative sparing of the basal ganglia and capsular structures.

arteriosclerotic encephalopathy (again equated with Binswanger's disease) in another, the latter showing widespread fiber loss and lacunar changes. Likewise, Revesz et al[49] reported on four cases described as subcortical arteriosclerotic encephalopathy. They considered a "firm" diagnosis was made clinically and pathologically, and a good correlation was observed between the extent and severity of the abnormal MRI signal and the pathologic changes. Microscopic signs of axonal and myelin loss with gliosis were found in the areas with signal abnormalities on MR. The subcortical U fibers were spared. They attributed the abnormal MR signal to increased tissue water attributable to gliosis and an expanded extracellular space.

Acceptability of Binswanger's Disease as an Entity

Few authors expressed concerns that the literature left unsettled the ambiguities of whether a Binswanger disease could actually be said to exist. Clearly, the generally accepted altered definitions of "Binswanger's disease" are in line with the notions of ABD or the combined disease category offered by Binswanger and Alzheimer. If matters are to remain in this state, the Binswanger eponym is a misnomer and should be replaced by the names of other authors (Klippel, Conso, Pactet, Marie, even Alzheimer) who contributed more to ABD. Acceptance of the current view supports notions that infarction, not chronic ischemia, underlies the clinical syndromes. Hachinski has taken the strong position that Binswanger's is neither a disease nor deserves his name,[25] and Pantoni and Garcia have also concluded that Binswanger's original case description is insufficient to justify a disease entity.[47] The points raised by Binswanger over a century ago warrant further consideration.

The lengthy review already undertaken above was intended to put in at least one place as many of the pubished observations as we could find. Sadly, no distinctive picture emerges as to lesion size, topography, severity, or underlying cause. If an attempt is made to preserve the concept of Binswanger's disease based on the elements in his original case, it is necessary to separate the actual findings (white matter atrophy, more posterior than frontal; no large artery disease; no deep focal infarcts of the lacunar type) of Binswanger's only case from the opinions he offered as to the disease process (arteriosclerosis).

Alzheimer's contribution relates to this dichotomy mainly by his separation of Binswanger's ESPC from those that Alzheimer attributed to more visible arteriosclerosis. Many of Alzheimer's observations on "senile cortical atrophy" seem consistent with modern-day interpretations of distal field infarction from large carotid artery or middle cerebral artery stenosis or occlusion. His notion of small cortical wedge-shaped scars, which he attributed to arteriosclerosis of the small cortical vessels, resembles Pozzi's "granular cirrhosis of the brain"[48] and the old Winniwarter-Buerger concept of selective vulnerability to disease of vessels in the arterial border zones.

Subsequent authors have tended more to "lump" rather than "split" the differing findings, but more recent studies have impacted on two mechanisms of ischemic stroke that differ somewhat from older formulations.

Reports on "true" ESCP cases are rare. In only 1 out of 84 autopsies of demented patients Brun and Englund[5] found diffuse white matter atrophy with underlying fibrohyalinosis of the small penetrating arteries and arteriosclerosis of larger vessels. Lacunes, larger infarcts, or findings consistent with Alzheimer's disease were not seen in this case.

NONVASCULAR THESES

A few authors have been dissatisfied with the explanation that the demyelination occurred on a vascular basis and proposed other causes. Feigen and Popoff proposed that both vessel wall changes and the demyelination were the late effects of cerebral edema initiated by hypertensive disease.[18] Although they commented that there was relatively little glial reaction in the areas of demyelination, they do not give any details about their cases, so it is difficult to interpret this remark. No data were offered to support this theory. Jellinger and

Neumayer thought there may have been an associated nutritional disturbance with organic damage of the blood vessels.[30]

BINSWANGER'S DISEASE AS CADASIL

Much of the haggling over Binswanger's disease can be set aside as tiresome arguments as to the completeness of the original observations by Binswanger and the subsequent interpretations by Alzheimer. Less easily set aside is the predominance of the lesions in the centrum semiovale, a site not typically affected by hypertension-related lacunes (see above) and often spared even in convexity infarction associated with large-artery stenosis or occlusion of the internal carotid and major branches of the circle of Willis.

CADASIL is a condition that has among its features a disproportionate involvement of the centrum semiovale; sparing of U fibers; relative infrequency of small, deep infarcts; minor impact from hypertension, and heavy involvement of the transcerebral vessels.[10] A rare disease, only recently recognized, and even more recently explained as a genetic disorder, it has become important enough to warrant its own chapter (see Chapter 38). Some authors have described members of families sharing a dominant inheritance with findings taken as typical for Binswanger's disease.[24]

It would be no shame to Binswanger to have failed to make such a diagnosis based on one case seen over a century ago, so whether his original case was CADASIL can never be known. Still, he paused to reflect on some unusual features of his case before concluding it must be a special form of the then-known arteriosclerosis. Perhaps not. Instead, it can be hoped that the existence of CADASIL, whether or not the explanation for Binswanger's case, will attract new attention to the basic biology of vascular beds that are often considered one functional system. Instead, there appear to be several within the central nervous system, each set perhaps subject to its own diseases.

Syndrome Effects of Predominantly Centrum Semiovale Infarction

Apart from the disease underlying the centrum semiovale lesions, Binswanger's disease as a clinical entity prompts consideration of what is known of the effects of such lesions in the centrum semiovale on disturbances of higher cerebral function.[52] The problem bears on whether the lesions (whether from ischemia or infarction) serve mainly to reduce the number of fibers in a fashion attributed to the volume effect attributed a generation ago to Lashley,[32] produce specific syndromes supporting the older connectionist model of linkages between certain "centers,"[22] or can be explained by yet other effects, such as injury to neurotrasmitter pathways serving the likes of vasoreactivity.[52]

It is a source of frustration that this field is plagued by

problems segregating one from another of the many coexisting disease entities in this mainly elderly population. The frequent coexistence of focal ischemic lesions, leukoaraiosis, and histopathologic markers for Alzheimer's and Lewy Body disease complicates the issue, and few attempts to analyze the independent effects of diffuse and focal lesions in demented patients have been made.

Differential effects from various diseases aside, the effect of focal ischemic lesions in the context of dementia remains largely unsettled. Lumping under the unsatisfactory term *dementia* all disturbances in behavior, histopathologic investigations have suggested a rough relationship between sum-loss of brain tissue and dementia.[6] However, aggregate infarct volume studies based on brain imaging have failed to show a strong association.[52] Volume estimates in the latter studies included lacunes as well as large infarcts, so whatever role small, deep infarcts play could weigh toward or against a relationship between lesion volume and dementia in imaging studies, making them differ from those for histopathologic studies.

Similar problems in correlating infarcts with dementia arise when the number of infarcts is taken into account. A clear correlation between multiple lacunar infarcts and dementia has not been established and the concept of multi-infarct dementia (MID) is further obscured by its unclear definition. Some authors equated MID with multiple lacunes/ état lacunaire, while others have used multifocal thrombotic and/or embolic infarcts as the characterizing elements, or proposed a combination of the two. The finding of coexisting pathologic markers for nonvascular dementias (Alzheimer's disease, Lewy Body disease) in many patients with vascular changes further complicates the issue, often making it impossible to assign the syndrome to one cause or the other.

Putting aside pure aggregate lesion volume, many investigations have had difficulty correlating dementia with the number and size of centrum semiovale lesions. In a controlled, prospective clinical and histopathologic study,[11] leukoencephalopathy alone was not significantly associated with dementia, but multiple lacunes and a sum-loss of more than 50 ml of brain tissue by small and/or larger infarcts was more common among the demented cases, suggesting that leukoaraiosis has a less prominent role than focal lesions in the etiology of dementia. Likewise, no matter how multi-infarct dementia is defined (a process of multiple lacunes, multiple nonlacunar infarcts,[19] or a combination of both lesion types),[39] convincing evidence has not yet been put forward to correlate the number of infarcts with dementia.

The lack of better confirmation of the importance of vascular lesions in dementia might be the result, in part, of failing to take into account the cerebral site of lesions. Damage to the temporo-occipital or thalamic territory of the posterior cerebral artery, the basal ganglia bilaterally, the frontal brain in the anterior cerebral artery territory, and the caudate nucleus (see Chapter 23) has all been shown to induce dementia, but most of this evidence stems from acute stroke, where such correlations are well-established. Binswanger and Alzheimer referred only in passing to acute dementia syndromes, and their work did not address specific brain areas carrying functions important for memory and cognition. The importance of these sites in progressive dementia has yet to be established, but an active literature is developing under the term *specific*

infarct dementia (SID).[52] This subject is further discussed in Chapter 23. In passing, it should be noted that any dementia attributed to deep lesions would run at odds with the single case described by Binswanger, where no such findings were noted.

Chronic Ischemia

Apart from deciding if there is a Binswanger's disease and how the white matter disease influences dementia, few authors have addressed or admitted the possibility of a chronic ischemia, a concept that was central to the theses of Binswanger and Alzheimer. All through their work is a tacit assumption that diseased small vessels can cause a nutritional disorder, which leads to atrophy, gliosis, and other injuries to the cerebrum, whether or not gross macroscopic or microscopic signs of infarction are found. This concept is at odds with much of the modern emphasis on energy failure thresholds, the two notions perhaps contrasting metaphorically as an incandescent light versus fluorescent light model of ischemia and infarction.

The importance of chronic ischemia may be supported by several studies, which, however, are not restricted to dementia cases. Using positron emission tomography (PET), Meguro et al found a reduction in cerebral blood flow in patients with diffuse white matter ischemic changes.[38] The trend toward rising oxygen extraction fractions was consistent with chronic hypoperfusion. The finding of patch-like ischemic lesions in the periventricular regions and the centrum semiovale has led to the thesis of "incomplete ischemia" from hypoperfusion in the distal fields of the long, medullary branches.[13] Histopathologic investigations have shown hyalinization and concentric thickening of the media with proliferation and fibrosis of the intima[53] resulting in luminal narrowing especially involving the medullary arteries supplying the periventricular white matter.[21] In a combined MRI and histopathologic examination of arteriosclerotic vascular changes and white matter alterations, demyelination and astrogliosis correlated with white matter patches on MRI, and was regularly associated with an increased ratio of wall thickness to the external diameter of arterioles.[55] Angioarchitectural studies support the concept of zones of vulnerability in specific white matter regions related to aging effects and the pattern of collateral pathways.[40] Further pathologic studies have established that tortuosity, coiling, and spiraling of the perforating cortical arterioles occur commonly with aging, extending through the thickness of the cerebral cortex to the subcortical white matter.[16] The effect of increasing arterial tortuosity with age has been analyzed by computer modeling, an effort that has suggested that resistance to flow is markedly elevated, thus raising the threshold of minimum pressure required for perfusion.[41] The long course of the medullary arteries already results in a large pressure drop, greater than that along short arterioles (which supply the cortex and corpus callosum). Thus, tortuosity and other arteriosclerotic changes further exacerbate this pressure drop, increasing the susceptibility of the centrum semiovale to chronic ischemic damage.

These findings suggest that there may be more to the

concept of chronic ischemia than has been appreciated heretofore. In the end, Binswanger and Alzheimer might have made a greater contribution to pathophysiology in the notion of chronic ischemia than to any disease bearing either of their names.

References

1. Alzheimer A: Neuere Arbeiten über die Dementia senilis und die auf atheromatöser Gefäßerkrankung basierenden Gehirnkrankheiten. Monatsschr Psychiatr Neurol 3:101, 1898

2. Biemond A: On Binswanger's subcortical arteriosclerotic encephalopathy and the possibility of its clinical recognition. Psychiatr Neurol 73:413, 1970

3. Binswanger O: Die Abgrenzung der allgemeinen progressiven Paralyse. Berl Klin Wochschr 31:1103–1105, 1137–1139, 1180–1186, 1894

4. Bogousslavsky J: Binswanger's disease. pp. 805–819. In Barnett HJM, Mohr JP, Stein BM, Yatsu FM (eds): Stroke: Pathophysiology, Diagnosis, and Management. 2nd Ed. Churchill Livingstone, New York, 1992

5. Brun A, Englund E: A white matter disorder in dementia of the Alzheimer type: a pathoanatomical study. Ann Neurol 19:253, 1986

6. Brust JCM: Dementia and cerebrovascular disease. pp. 131–147. In Mayeux R, Rosen WG (eds): The Dementias. Lippincott-Raven, Philadelphia, 1983

7. Buchholz: Ueber die Geistesstörungen bei Arteriosklerose und ihre Beziehungen zu den psychischen Erkrankungen des Seniums. Arch Psychiatr Nervenkr 39:499, 1905

8. Burger PC, Burch JG, Kunze U: Subcortical arteriosclerotic encephalopathy (Binswanger's disease)—a vascular etiology of dementia. Stroke 7:626, 1976

9. Caplan LR, Schoene WC: Clinical features of subcortical arteriosclerotic encephalopathy (Binswanger disease). Neurology 28:1206–1215, 1978

10. Chabriat H, Tournier-Lasserve E, Vahedi K et al: MRI features of cerebral autosomal dominant arteriopathy with subcortical infarcts and leukoencephalopathy. Neurology 46:A212, 1996

11. Crystal HA, Dickson DW, Sliwinski MJ et al: Pathological markers associated with normal aging and dementia in the elderly. Ann Neurol 34:566–573, 1993

12. Davison C: Progressive subcortical encephalopathy. J Neuropathol Exp Neurol 1:42, 1942

13. De Reuck J, Crevits L, DeCoster W et al: Pathogenesis of Binswanger's chronic subcortical encephalopathy: A clinical and radiological investigation. Neurology 30: 920–928, 1980

14. Dubas F, Gray F, Roullet E, Escourolle R: Lencoencephalopathies arteriopathiques (17 cas anatomo-cliniques). Rev Neurol 141:93, 1985

15. Durand-Fardel M: Memoire sur une alteration particulière de la substance cerebral. Gaz Med Paris 10:23, 1842

16. Fang HCH. Observations on aging characteristics of cerebral blood vessels, macroscopic and microscopic features.

pp. 155–166. In Terry RD, Gershon S (eds): Neurobiology of Aging. Lippincott-Raven Press, Philadelphia, 1976

17. Farnell FJ, Globus JH: Chronic progressive vascular subcortical encephalopathy. Arch Neurol Psychiatr 27:593, 1932

18. Feigen I, Popoff N: Neuropathological changes late in cerebral edema: the relationship to trauma, hypertensive disease, and Binswanger's encephalopathy. J Neuropathol Exp Neurol 22:500, 1963

19. Fields WS: Multi-infarct dementia. Neurologic Clinics 74: 405–413, 1986

20. Fisher CM: Binswanger's encephalopathy: a review. J Neurol 236:65–79, 1989

21. Furuta A, Ishii N, Nishihara Y, Horie A: Medullary arteries in aging and dementia. Stroke 22:628:7–11, 1991

22. Geschwind N: Disconnection syndromes in animals and man. Brain. 88:237, 1965

23. Gray F, Dubas F, Roullet E, Escourolle R: Leukoencephalopathy in diffuse hemorrhagic cerebral amyloid angiopathy. Ann Neurol 18:54, 1985

24. Gutierrez-Molina M, Caminero-Rodriguez A, Martina Garcia C et al: Small arterial granular degeneration in familial Binswanger's syndrome. Acta Neuropath 87:98, 1994

25. Hachinski V. Binswanger's disease: neither Binswanger's nor a disease [editorial]. J Neurol Sci 103:1, 1991

26. Hachinski VC, Lassen NA, Marshall J. Multi infarct dementia. A cause of mental deterioration in the elderly. Lancet 2:207–210, 1974

27. Inzitari D, Mascalchi M, Giordano GP et al: Histopathological correlates of leukoaraiosis in patients with ischemic stroke. Eur Neurol 29:23, 1989

28. Janota I: Dementia, deep white matter damage and hypertension: "Binswanger's disease." Psychol Med 11:39, 1981

29. Jelgersma HC: A case of encephalopathia subcorticalis chronica (Binswanger's disease). Psychiatr Neurol Basel 147:81, 1964

30. Jellinger K, Neumayer E: Progressive subcorticale vasculare Encephalopathie Binswanger. Eine Klinischneuropathologische Studie. Arch Psychiatr Nervenkr 205:523, 1964

31. Ladame C: Encephalopathie sous-corticale chronique. Encephale 7:13, 1912

32. Lashley K: Brain Mechanisms and Intelligence. University of Chicago Press, Chicago, 1929

33. Leifer D, Buonanno FS, Richardson EP Jr: Clinicopathologic correlations of cranial magnetic resonance imaging of periventricular white matter. Neurology. 40:911, 1990

34. Lindenberg R, Spatz F: Ueber die Thromboendarteritis Obliterans der Hirngefässe. Virchows Arch Pathol Anat 305:531, 1940

35. Loeb C: Dementia due to lacunar infarctions: a misnomer or a clinical entity? Europ Neurol 35:187, 1995

36. Lotz PR, Ballinger WE Jr, Quisling RG: Subcortical arteriosclerotic encephalopathy: CT spectrum and pathologic correlation. Am J Roentgenol 147:1209, 1986

37. Mathers SE, Chambers BR, Merory JR, Alexander I: Subcortical arteriosclerotic encephalopathy: Binswanger's disease. Clin Exp Neurol 23:67, 1987

38. Meguro K, Hatazawa J, Yamaguchi T: Cerebral circula-

tion and oxygen metabolism associated with subclinical periventricular hyperintensity as shown by magnetic resonance imaging. Ann Neurol 28:378–383, 1990

39. Meyer JS, McClintic KL, Rogers RL et al: Aetiological considerations and risk factors in multi-infarct dementia. J Neurol Neurosurg Psychiat 51:1489–97, 1988

40. Moody DM, Bell MA, Challa VR: Features of the cerebral vascular pattern that predict vulnerability to perfusion or oxygenation deficiency: an anatomical study. AJNR 11:431–439, 1990

41. Moody DM, Santomore WP, Bell MA: Does tortuosity in cerebral arterioles impair down-autoregulation in hypertensives and elderly normotensives? A hypothesis and computer model. Clin Neurosurg 37:372–387, 1991

42. Neumann MA: Chronic progressive subcortica encephalopathy—report of a case. J Gerontol 2:57, 1947

43. Nichols FT, Mohr JP: Binswanger's subacute arteriosclerotic encephalopathy. pp. 875–885. In Barnett HJM, Mohr JP, Stein BM, Yatsu FM (eds): Stroke Pathophysiology, Diagnosis, and Management. Vol. II. Churchill Livingstone, New York, 1986

44. Nissl: Zur Kasuistik der arteriosklerotischen Demenz (ein Fall von sog. "Encephalitis subcorticalis"). Ges Neurol 19:438, 1920

45. Okeda R: Morphometrische Vergeichsuntersuchungen an Hirnarterien bei Binswanger Encephalopathie und Hochdruckencephalopathie. Acta Neuropathol 26:23, 1973

46. Olszewski J: Subcortical arteriosclerotic encephalopathy. Review of the literature on the so-called Binswanger's disease and presentation of two cases. World Neurol 3:359, 1962

47. Pantoni L, Garcia JH: The significance of cerebral white matter abnormalities 100 years after Binswanger's report. A review. Stroke 26:1293, 1995

48. Pozzi S: Sur un cas de cirrhose atrophique granuleuse disseminée des circonvolutions cerebrales. Encephale 3:155, 1883

49. Revesz T, Hawkins CP, du Boulay EP et al: Pathological findings correlated with magnetic resonance imaging in subcortical arteriosclerotic encephalopathy (Binswanger's disease). J Neurol Neurosurg Psychiatr 52:1337, 1989

50. Rosenberg GA, Kornfeld M, Stovring J, Bicknell JM: Subcortical arteriosclerotic encephalopathy (Binswanger): computerized tomography. Neurology 29:1102, 1979

51. Tarvonen-Schroder S, Roytta M, Raiha I et al: Clinical features of leuko-araiosis. J Neurol Neurosurg Psychiatr 60:431, 1996

52. Tatemichi TK: How acute brain failure becomes chronic. A view of the mechanisms and syndromes of dementia related to stroke. Neurology 40:1652–1659, 1990

53. Tomonaga M, Yamanouchi H, Tohgi H, Kameyama M: Clinicopathologic study of progressive subcortical vascular encephalopathy (Binswanger type) in the elderly. J Amer Geriat Soc 30:524, 1982

54. Valentine AR, Moseley IF, Kendall BE: White matter abnormalities in cerebral atrophy: clinicoradiological correlations. J Neurol Neurosurg Psychiatr 43:139, 1980

55. van Swieten JC, van den Hout JHW, van Ketel BA et al: Periventricular lesions in the white matter on magnetic resonance imaging in the elderly: a morphometric correlation with arteriosclerosis and dilated perivascular spaces. Brain 114:761–771, 1991

56. White JC: Periodic EEG activity in subcortical arteriosclerotic encephalopathy (Binswanger's type). Arch Neurol 36:485, 1979

57. Zeumer H, Hacke W, Kolmann HL, Ringelstein EB: Subcortical arteriosclerotic encephalopathy (Binswanger's disease). Exp Brain Res. Suppl 5:272, 1982

CADASIL (Cerebral Autosomal Dominant Arteriopathy with Subcortical Infarcts and Leukoencephalopathy)

H. CHABRIAT

A. JOUTEL

K. VAHEDI

E. TOURNIER-LASSERVE

MARIE-GERMAINE BOUSSER

CADASIL is a newly identified cause of stroke and vascular dementia.[55] It is an inherited arterial disease of mid-adulthood resulting from mutations of the *Notch3* gene on chromosome 19.[29] The disease was first reported in European families.[6] Since 1993, CADASIL has been diagnosed in American, African, and Asiatic pedigrees, suggesting that the condition might be found all over the world and is not limited to Caucasian pedigrees. In 1996, the disease remains largely underdiagnosed.

History

In 1955, Van Bogaert reported two sisters belonging to a family originating from Belgium having a "subcortical encephalopathy of Binswanger's type of rapid course" with onset during mid-adulthood.[58] Their clinical presentation included dementia, gait disturbances, pseudobulbar palsy, seizures, and focal neurologic deficits. Two other sisters died at age 36 and 43 years after a progressive dementia. The father had a stroke at age 51 and died after a myocardial infarct. Pathologic examination revealed widespread areas of white-matter rarefaction in the brain associated with multiple small infarcts located mainly in the white matter and basal ganglia.[58] These lesions were thought to be secondary to a familial arteriosclerosis of the brain similar to that reported by Mutrux et al a few years before.[36] In 1977, Sourander and Walinder called "hereditary multi-infarct dementia" a familial condition observed in a Swedish pedigree and characterized by dementia associated with pseudobulbar palsy occurring 10 to 15 years after recurrent stroke-like episodes.[49,50] The age of onset was between 29 and 38 years, and the age at death varied from 30 to 53. The authors reported three cases of brain lesions identical to those observed by Van Bogaert and also caused by a small vessel disease. The wall of the small arteries was thickened causing a reduction of their lumen. Atherosclerosis of basal arteries was found in only one family member. In the pedigree, the condition followed an autosomal dominant pattern of transmission. Up to 1993, several families having a close presentation were reported using numerous eponyms:

933

Chronic familial vascular encephalopathy,[52] Familiäre zerebrale arteriosklerose,[23] Familiäre zerebrale Gefäßerkrankung,[14] Hereditary Multi-infarct Dementia,[48] Démence sous-corticale familiale avec leucoencéphalopathie artériopathique,[16] Familial disorder with Subcortical ischemic strokes, dementia and leukoencephalopathy,[34] and Slowly progressive familial dementia with recurrent strokes and white-matter hypodensities on CT scan.[44] In 1976, we had a patient who was 50 years old with a clinical history of recurrent lacunar infarcts who presented with a widespread hypodensity of the white matter on CT scan. He had no vascular risk factor, in particular no hypertension. Ten years later, his daughter came to see us for a long history of attacks of migraine with aura and transient ischemic attacks and for a recent minor stroke. Her CT scan and MRI showed lesions in the white matter identical to those observed in her father. These two observations were the basis of the extensive clinical MRI, and genetic study of over 50 subjects from this very large family originating from the western part of France called Loire-Atlantique. The data were first presented as "Recurrent strokes in a family with diffuse white matter and muscular lipidosis—a new mitochondrial cytopathy?"[7] then as "Autosomal dominant syndrome with stroke-like episodes and leukoencephalopathy,"[54] and later as "Autosomal dominant leukoencephalopathy and subcortical ischemic strokes."[3]

Because of the confusion raised by all these different names, we proposed in 1993, when we demonstrated that the gene was located on chromosome 19, the acronym CADASIL (Cerebral Autosomal Dominant Arteriopathy with Subcortical Infarcts and Leukoencephalopathy) to designate this disease and highlight its main characteristics.[55] The location on chromosome 19 found in our initial family was immediately confirmed in a second French pedigree.[34,55] The gene mapping was essential to define the natural history of the disease. Since this date, CADASIL has been recognized in about 120 families, first in Europe and more recently in the U.S. and North Africa. The genetic analysis of additional families allowed us to show the genetic homogeneity of the disease and to refine the genetic mapping within a 2 cM interval on chromosome 19 in 1995.[19] In 1996, we demonstrated that various mutations of the Notch 3 gene were responsible for the disease.[29] This recent finding is a major step in the history of CADASIL. As a consequence, genetic testing could be now used for diagnosis. Also, this discovery is important to understand the pathophysiology of the disease, which is essential to open therapeutic avenues.

Clinical Presentation

After the gene mapping in 1993, the study of families with proven linkage to the CADASIL locus allowed us to draw the natural history of the disease and to recognize its clinical spectrum.

CADASIL is a disease of mid-adulthood. The mean age at the onset of symptoms is 45 years in the largest series of families linked to chromosome 19 so far reported.[13] It can vary from 4 to 68 years among the different pedigrees and within families.[13,16,19] These large variations are due in part to the fact that migraine with aura, one of the first symptoms of the disease, was inconstantly recognized as a clinical manifestation of CADASIL. The age of onset does not significantly differ according to sex[13,56] and, when considering the two most frequent symptoms of the disease, strokes and/or dementia, it does not differ either between the different generations in a given family.[56] The duration of the disease varies between 10 and 30 years.[13] Mean age at death is about 65 years, but it varies from 30 to 80 years in the reported affected pedigrees.

Stroke is the most frequent clinical manifestation of the disease. About 85% of symptomatic subjects suffer transient ischemic attacks or completed strokes.[13] Most frequently, they occur in the absence of vascular risk factors. Within 45 affected subjects, Chabriat et al found only 3 with hypertension and 10 smokers.[13] The frequency of stroke or transient ischemic attacks (TIAs) among the affected members within a given family varies from 0% to 100%. However, the absence of stroke in all the symptomatic members was observed in only one family.[12] The ischemic events occur at a mean age of 49 years with a large range from 27 to 65 years.[13,56] All of the temporal profiles of ischemic manifestations are observed: TIA, reversible ischemic neurologic deficits, and completed strokes. The ischemic deficits are of the subcortical type. Two-

Figure 38.1 Natural history of CADASIL summarized showing the different mean ages of occurrence of each symptom in the disease.

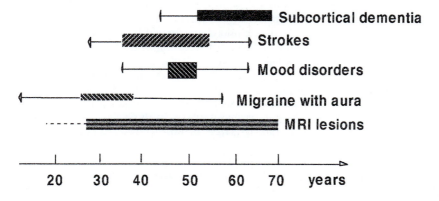

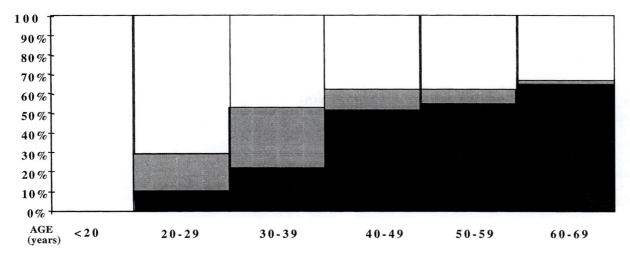

Figure 38.2 MRI results of subjects born of an affected subject according to age. About 50% of subjects born of affected patients presented with signal abnormalities at MRI examination after 30 years of age suggesting the complete penetrance of the disease. After 60 years of age, all subjects with abnormal MRI presented with neurologic symptoms. Open bars, normal MRI; gray bars, asymptomatic with WMA; black bars, symptomatic with WMA.

thirds of them are classical lacunar syndromes: pure motor stroke, ataxic hemiparesis, pure sensory stroke, sensory motor stroke. Other focal neurologic deficits of abrupt onset are less frequently observed: dysarthria either isolated or associated with motor or sensory deficit, monoparesis, paresthesias on one limb, isolated ataxia, nonfluent aphasia, hemianopia. These latter signs can also be secondary to lacunar infarcts. We are aware of only two patients over age 60 with a cortical infarct in large artery territories associated with lacunar lesions.[11] The ischemic manifestations are isolated in 40% of cases, particularly at the onset of the disease. More frequently, they are associated with other symptoms of the disease such as mood disturbances or dementia.[6,13,56] Some episodes of focal deficits occur in association with headache.[49,54] When they are transient, they can be difficult to distinguish from attacks of migraine with aura.[54] In the largest series of affected families, among subjects with ischemic events, 40% had TIAs, 70% had completed strokes, and 10% had both. During the course of the disease, the number of TIAs varies from one to tens and in most cases, the number of completed strokes is between 2 and 5.[3,13,39,54,59]

Dementia, the second most frequent clinical manifestation of CADASIL, is reported in one-third of symptomatic patients.[13] It is observed at a mean age of 60 years and it is present in 90% of patients before death.[13] Over age 65, 80% of CADASIL patients are demented. The age at the onset of dementia varies from 40 to 70 years.[56] The exact onset of cognitive impairment in CADASIL is more difficult to ascertain precisely. Recently, Taillia et al showed that two non-demented symptomatic patients, the younger of whom was aged 35 years, could also have altered performances using the Wisconsin Card Sorting test, a task very sensitive to frontal dysfunction.[53] In 90% of cases, the cognitive impairment occurs step by step and is associated with recurrent stroke

events. The dementia satisfies the NINDS-AIREN and DSM IV diagnostic criteria for vascular dementia.[18,40] The cognitive deficit is of the subcortical type with predominating frontal symptoms (apragmatism and apathy) and memory impairment.[15] Aphasia, apraxia, or agnosia are rare or observed only at the end course of the disease.[15,44] Dementia is always associated with pyramidal signs, pseudobulbar palsy, gait difficulties, and/or urinary incontinence.[6] The severity of the lesions and particularly their location could be determining for the occurrence of the cognitive impairment in the disease. In a positron emission tomography study of one demented patient and of his cousin who was totally asymptomatic, both with equally widespread white matter lesions at MRI examination, we recently found a decrease of cortical metabolism only in the demented subject who had the most severe basal ganglia lesions.[10] In the absence of cortical lesions, these findings suggested the presence of remote metabolic effects of basal ganglia infarcts (diaschisis) causing dementia in CADASIL. Cortical lesions of Alzheimer's disease associated with typical subcortical lesions of CADASIL have been reported only in one case with a rapidly progressive and massive deterioration leading to a vegetative state at age 49.[24] In 10% of cases, the neuropsychological decline is isolated, mimicking the course of Alzheimer's disease.[12,59]

Twenty percent to 30% of affected subjects suffer attacks of migraine with aura.[13] This symptom is present in 40% of CADASIL families, but its frequency varies from 0% to 85% of the patients within the affected pedigrees.[56,59] Migraine with aura is the earliest clinical manifestation of the disease, occuring at a mean age of 30 years[56] but occasionally before the age of 20 years.[27,59] In a given subject, the frequency of attacks also is highly variable, from one attack in life to several per month.[13] As usually observed in migraine with aura, the most frequent neurologic symptoms associated with headache are visual and/or sensitive. However, the frequency of attacks with basilar, hemiplegic, or prolonged aura, according to IHS diagnosis criteria, is noticeably high.[13,28,56,59] A few patients have been reported with severe attacks[12] including unusual symptoms such as confusion, fever, or coma.[20,21] Migraine with aura is usually associated with the other symptoms of CADASIL. However, particularly at onset of the disease, attacks of migraine with aura can be isolated. In a few families, migraine with aura appears as the main and sole symptom of the disease in several family members.[12,59]

Nearly 20% of CADASIL patients present with severe mood disturbances.[13] The frequency of such manifestations is widely variable between families.[56] Most patients have a severe depression of the melancholic type sometimes alternating with typical manic episodes.[13,59] The diagnosis of bipolar mood disorder was indeed considered in some subjects until the MRI examination was performed.[53] Thus, the differential diagnosis with a psychiatric disease can be difficult, particularly when such mood disturbances are inaugural and isolated. The late onset of recurrent depressive episodes or of bipolar

disorders; their poor response to treatment; their association with a cognitive impairment; and even the sole presence of a family history of stroke, migraine with aura, or dementia should lead to the performance of an MRI of the brain in these subjects.[13,54] The association of any of these symptoms with WMA at MRI is strongly suggestive of CADASIL and should prompt a genealogical study including all first- and second-degree relatives. The exact cause of mood disturbances in CADASIL remains undetermined. The location of ischemic lesions in basal ganglia or in frontal white matter may play a key role in their occurrence.[1,4]

Other neurologic manifestations have occasionally been reported in CADASIL. Focal or generalized seizures have been reported in 6% to 7% of cases.[13] Deafness of acute or progressive onset has been observed in two cases[13] and one personal case. The absence of cranial nerve palsy, spinal cord disease (except in one case[27]) and of symptoms of muscular origin is noteworthy in CADASIL. The cause of the radiculopathy reported in one case by Ragno et al has not been detailed.[23]

Figure 38.3 MRI of two affected subjects (**A** & **B**): Symptomatic patient with stroke and dementia. (**C** & **D**) Asymptomatic patient. (From Tournier-Lasserve et al,[54] with permission.)

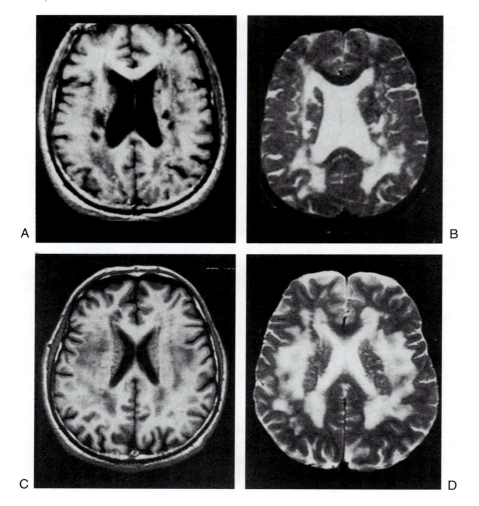

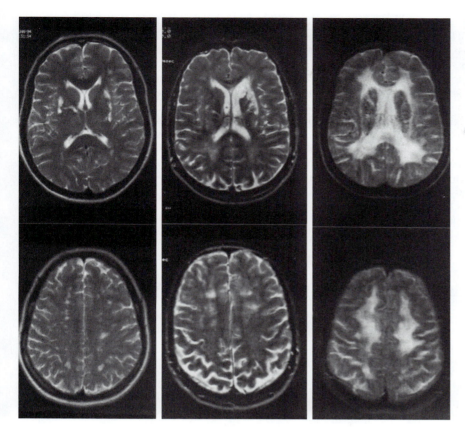

Figure 38.4 MRI of 3 subjects (right, middle, left) with CADASIL showing signal abnormalities on T_2-weighted images located in basal ganglia and white matter of various severity. (From Leys and P. Scheltens,[32] with permission.)

Finally, the natural history of the disease is summarized in Figure 38.1. CADASIL starts between 20 and 30 years in one-fifth of the patients with attacks of migraine with aura. Ischemic manifestations observed in 4/5 patients mainly occur during the fourth and fifth decades. They are sometimes associated with severe mood disturbances. Dementia occurs between 50 and 60 years and is found nearly constantly before death, which occurs at a mean age of 65 years. The course of the disease can widely vary among the affected family members between and within concerned pedigrees.

Neuroimaging

MRI is essential for the diagnosis of CADASIL. It is always abnormal in symptomatic patients.[6,55] The signal abnormalities can be detected during a presymptomatic period of variable duration. MRI signal abnormalities are observed as early as 20 years of age.[13,56] After 35, all subjects having the affected gene have an abnormal MRI.[11,13,55] The study of asymptomatic subjects with abnormal MRI allowed us to increase the number of informative subjects for genetic linkage analysis.[3,54] The percentage of asymptomatic subjects with abnormal MRI decreases progressively with aging among the gene carriers but does not reach 0% after 60 years (Fig. 38.2).

MRI shows on T_1-weighted images punctiform or nodular hyposignals in basal ganglia and white matter. T_2-weighted images show hypersignals in the same regions often associated with widespread areas of increased signal in the white matter (Figs. 38.3 and 38.4).[6,46] The severity of the signal abnormalities is variable. These lesions dramatically increase with age in affected patients.[11] In subjects under 40 years, T_2 hypersignals are usually punctate or nodular with a symmetrical distribution, and predominate in periventricular areas and in the centrum semi-ovale. Later in life, white-matter lesions are diffuse and can involve the whole of the white matter including the U fibers under the cortex.[11] The scores evaluating the severity of the lesions based on a semiquantitative rating scale significantly increase with age not only in white matter but also in basal ganglia and brain stem. The frontal and occipital periventricular lesions are constant when MRI is abnormal. The frequency of signal abnormalities in the external capsule (2/3 of the cases) and in the anterior part of the temporal lobes (40%) is noteworthy.[6,11,46] Brain stem lesions are mainly observed in the pons. The mesencephalon and medulla are usually spared. Cortical or cerebellar lesions are exceptional. They have been observed in only two cases older than 60 years.[11] CT scan can reveal the white matter and basal ganglia lesions but is much less sensitive than MRI.[3]

Other Investigations

Cerebral angiography obtained in 14 patients belonging to seven affected families was normal except in one case with a detectable narrowing of small arteries.[13] Recently, Weller et al reported a worsening of the neurologic status in two CA-DASIL patients after angiography.[61] One of them had a severe headache, vomiting, confusion, somnolence, and a grand mal seizure that resolved within several hours. The examination was found normal with only a limited vasospasm in one.[61] Ultrasound studies and echocardiography are usually normal. No biological or muscular markers of mitochondrial diseases have been observed in CADASIL [34,54] despite the occasional presence of a severe muscular lipidosis.[54] CSF examination is usually normal, but oligoclonal bands with pleocytosis have been reported.[13] Electromyogram is essentially normal. A monoclonal immunoglobulin was detected in two cases of our first family[54] but not in the other affected pedigrees.[13] The ultrastructural studies of skin and muscle with electron microscopy revealed the arterial abnormalities typical of CADASIL (see pathology).[41]

Pathology

Macroscopic examination of the brain shows a diffuse myelin pallor and rarefaction of the hemispheric white matter sparing the U fibers (Fig. 38.5).[26] Lesions predominate in the periventricular areas and centrum semi-ovale. They are associated with lacunar infarcts located in the white matter and basal ganglia (lentiform nucleus, thalamus, caudate).[42] The most severe hemispheric lesions are the most profound.[3,16,42] In the brain stem, the lesions are more marked in the pons and are similar to the pontine rarefaction of myelin of ischemic origin described by Pullicino et al.[38] The macroscopic study of the cortex is essentially normal, but a case has recently been reported in a women with diffuse brain lesions, including microlacunar infarcts (diameter less than 200 microns) within the cortex, mainly in layer 6 adjacent to the white matter.[42] No territorial or border-zone infarct has been so far reported.

Microscopic investigations show that the wall of cerebral and leptomeningeal arterioles is thickened and that their lumen is significantly reduced.[3] Such abnormalities can also be detected by leptomeningeal biopsy.[36] Some inconstant features are similar to those reported in patients with hypertensive encephalopathy:[3,39] duplication and splitting of internal elastic lamina, adventitial hyalinosis and fibrosis, hypertrophy of the media. However, a distinctive feature is the presence of a granular material within the media extending into the adventitia.[39] The periodic acid-Schiff (PAS) positive staining suggests the presence of glycoproteins (Fig. 38.6). Staining for amyloid substance and elastin is negative.[26,42] Immunohistochemistry does not support the presence of immunoglobulins. By contrast, the endothelium of the vessels is usually spared. On electron microscopy, the smooth muscle cells appear swollen and often degenerated, some of them with multiple nuclei. Sometimes they are not detectable and are replaced by collagen fibers. The media contain a granular, electron-dense, osmiophilic material,[3,42] which consists of granules of about 10 nm to 15 nm in diameter. It is localized close to the cell membrane of the smooth vessel cells (Fig. 38.7). The smooth vessel cells are separated by large amounts of this unidentified material. In a single case, these vascular abnormalities were found associated with typical lesions of Alzheimer's disease.[24]

Recently, Ruchoux et al made the crucial observation that the vascular abnormalities observed in the brain were also detectable in other organs.[41,42] The granular and osmiophilic material surrounding the smooth muscle cells as seen with electron microscopy is also present in the media of arteries located in the spleen, liver, kidneys, muscle, and skin[42] as well as in the wall of carotid and aortic arteries. The presence of this material in the skin and muscle vessels now allows us to confirm the intra vitam diagnosis of CADASIL, although sensitivity and specificity have not yet been rigorously assessed.[42,43] These vascular lesions can also be detected by nerve biopsy.[45]

Genetics

The study of our first very large French family allowed us to map the affected gene on chromosome 19.[55] A crucial step for this mapping was the use of the neuroimaging results for genetic linkage analysis. Thus, asymptomatic family members

Figure 38.5 Pathologic examination of one deceased patient with CADASIL showing the diffuse myelin loss and pallor sparing the U fibers in the frontal white matter. (Loyez stain, × 0.75.) (From Bandrimont et al,[3] with permission.)

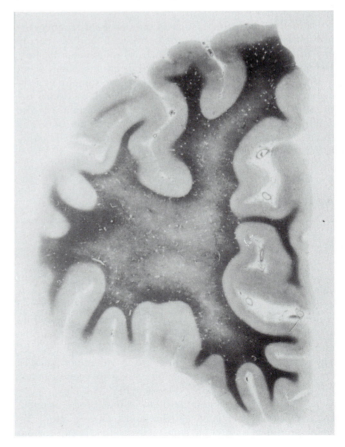

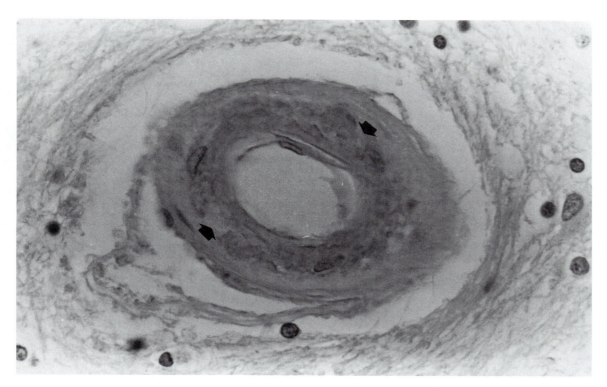

Figure 38.6 Eosinophilic material in the media (arrow) of a perforating artery in the white matter. (H&E stain, × 284.) (From Baudrimont et al,[3] with permission.)

having white-matter signal abnormalities at MRI examination were considered as affected, whereas asymptomatic family members with a normal MRI were considered as not affected if they were above 35 and of unknown status if they were below 35 for the genetic study.[55] A systematic screening of the genome was then performed and the responsible gene was located on chromosome 19. This mapping was immediately confirmed in a second French family.[55] Since this date, the genetic linkage to the corresponding locus has been confirmed in numerous families. All of those individuals with a sufficient number of informative meiosis were found to be linked to chromosome 19, suggesting the genetic homogeneity of CADASIL.[19] The single exception so far is the family reported by St. Clair et al who used less precise diagnostic criteria.[51] Analysis of additional pedigrees with new microsatellite markers allowed us to refine the locus assignment to within a 2-cm interval.[29] Eventually, mutations of the *Notch3* gene were demonstrated to cause CADASIL.[21] The identification of *Notch3* mutations causing the disease will now allow the performance of individual genetic testing. Yet this finding raises important ethical problems very similar to those encountered in families with Huntington's disease. In the absence of any efficient treatment, genetic counseling and testing should be performed only in specific and trained centers.

Diagnosis

The diagnosis of CADASIL should be raised in adult patients with TIAs or strokes, severe mood disorders, attacks of migraine with aura or dementia, whenever their MRI discloses widespread signal abnormalities in the subcortical white matter and basal ganglia. This association should prompt a genealogical study of the family including all first- and second-degree relatives. Clinical and/or neuroimaging data obtained from these latters are crucial to confirm the hereditary origin of the disease. The diagnosis can be confirmed by electron microscopy study of vessels in muscle or skin biopsies. If the diagnosis is impossible or remains uncertain, genetic testing might be used in the future for confirmation.

A crucial step for diagnosis is also to differentiate CADASIL from other diseases with a similar presentation. Particularly, the clinical and MRI features of CADASIL are very close to that of Binswanger's disease (BD) but the two conditions differ on three major points; conversely to CADASIL, BD occurs most often in hypertensive patients, is not associated with migraine with aura, and is not recognized as an autosomal dominant condition.[2] However, it should be noted that the familial character has not been systematically evaluated in most cases of BD and that the two cases of BD reported in sisters by Van Bogaert are possibly cases of CADASIL.[58] Other causes of vascular leukoencephalopathies are easier to recognize. Amyloid angiopathies of hereditary origin can present with ischemic strokes and MRI white-matter signal abnormalities but are essentially characterized by recurrent lobar cerebral hemorrhages and the presence of amyloid deposits within the wall of brain vessels.[8,25] The mitochondrial encephalomyopathy with lactic acidosis and stroke-like episodes (MELAS) often occurs in children or in early adult life. It is responsible for cortical and subcortical infarcts of asymmetrical distribution, sometimes outside of a vascular territory, and is often associ-

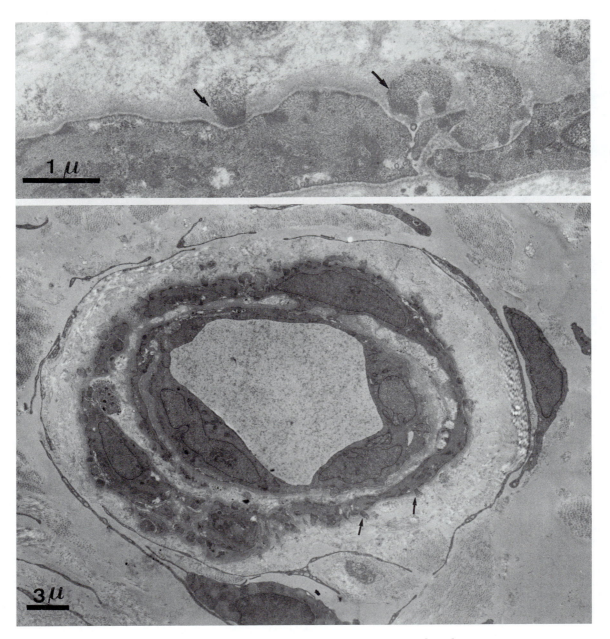

Figure 38.7 Electron microscopy revealing granular material (arrows) surrounding the smooth muscle cells within the media of a skin artery in CADASIL. (Courtesy of M.M. Ruchoux, Service de Neuropathologie, CHRU Lille, France.)

ated with ragged-red muscle fibers. The disease is transmitted following a maternal inheritance.[35] The "familial young-onset arteriosclerotic leukoencephalopathy" reported in Japanese pedigrees is an autosomal recessive condition associated with alopecia and skeletal abnormalities, secondary to a thickening of the intima of small cerebral vessels.[22] The hereditary leukoencephalopathy reported recently by Lossos et al, a disorder with increased skin collagen content, leads to a progressive dementia and is associated with palmoplantar keratoderma.[33] CADASIL, particularly at onset, can be difficult to differentiate from multiple sclerosis. The

autosomal dominant pattern of transmission of the disease, the absensce of optic nerve or spinal cord involvement and the symmetrical distribution of white-matter signal abnormalities often associated with basal ganglia infarcts at MRI examination are the most helpful signs to recognize the disease.[57] Also, adrenoleukodystrophy, an X-linked metabolic disorder with accumulation of very long chain fatty acids, can be observed in adults, but, conversely to CADASIL, it does not involve basal ganglia; the cerebral disease is progressive and associated with spinal cord and peripheral nerve demyelination.[60]

Conclusion

CADASIL is a newly recognized hereditary vascular disease. In 1996, the disease remained largely undiagnosed although it is not a rare condition. We are aware of at least 100 affected families mainly in Europe and in increasing amounts of families diagnosed in other continents. The characterization of the disease is an important step in the understanding and classification of vascular dementias.[9,13] Moreover, this will question the place of Binswanger's disease within the group of vascular leukoencephalopathies. Also, this finding will bring new insights into the pathophysiology of leukoaraiosis so frequently associated with stroke and into the very unclear field of migraine or mood disturbances associated with MRI white-matter abnormalities.[37,47]

The identification of *Notch3* mutations in CADASIL is a crucial step in understanding the molecular mechanisms leading to the vascular alterations in this disease. The gene identification will now allow the development of individual genetic testing, raising new ethical problems in the field of vascular dementia. This result is also essential to understand the pathophysiology of the disease before opening therapeutic avenues.

ACKNOWLEDGMENTS

Clinical work on CADASIL was supported in part by grants from Assistance Publique/Hôpitaux de Paris (Réseau EMUL 93704), AFM (Association Française contre les Myopathies), Synthelabo France (Division Cardiovasculaire), La Fondation de France and Foundation Sanofi Thrombose. MRI studies were made possible with the help of the Association pour la Recherche sur la Sclérose en Plaques (ARSEP). Gene identification was made possible thanks to support from INSERM, BioMérieux, Association Francaise contre les Myopathies, Fondation de France, Ministère de la Recherche.

We thank all the members of the families who participated to this research. We are grateful to all the members of the "Reseau EMUL CADASIL" for their help and collaboration.

References

1. Aylward ED, Roberts-Willie JV, Barta PE, Kumar AJ et al: Basal ganglia volume and white matter hyperintensities in patients with bipolar disorder. Am J Psychiatry 5: 687–693, 1994
2. Babikian V, Ropper AH: Binswanger's disease: a review. Stroke 18:2–12, 1987
3. Baudrimont M, Dubas F, Joutel A et al: Autosomal dominant leukoencephalopathy and subcortical ischemic strokes: a clinicopathological study. Stroke 24:122–125, 1993
4. Bhatia KP, Marsden CD: The behavioural and motor consequences of focal lesions of the basal ganglia in man. Brain 117:859–876, 1994
5. Bonthius DJ, Mathews KD, Adams HP: CADASIL in a North American family: linkage to chromosome 19. Neurology 46:A211–A212, 1996
6. Bousser MG, Tournier Lasserve E: Summary of the first international workshop on CADASIL. Stroke 25: 704–770, 1994
7. Bousser MG, Tournier-Lasserve E, Aylward R et al: Recurrent strokes in a family with diffuse white-matter abnormalities—a new mitochondrial cytopathy. J Neurol 235(suppl 1):S4–S5, 1988
8. Bornebrock M, Haan J, Van Buchem MA et al: White-matter lesions and cognitive deterioration in presymptomatic carriers of the amyloid precursor protein gene codon 693 mutation. Arch Neurol 53:43–48, 1996
9. Bowler JV, Hachinski V: Progress in the genetics of cerebrovascular disease: inherited subcortical arteriopathies. Stroke 25:1696–1698, 1994
10. Chabriat H, Bousser MG, Pappata S: Cerebral autosomal dominant arteriopathy with subcortical infarcts and leukoencephalopathy: a positron emission tomography study in two affected family members. Stroke 26:1729–1730, 1995
11. Chabriat H, Taillia H, Iba-Zizen MT et al: MRI features of cerebral autosomal dominant arteriopathy with subcortical infarcts and leukoencephalopathy. Neurology 46: A212, 1996
12. Chabriat H, Tournier-Lasserve E, Vahedi K et al: Autosomal dominant migraine with MRI abnormalities mapping to the CADASIL locus. Neurology 45:1086–1091, 1995
13. Chabriat H, Vahedi K, IbZizen MT et al: Clinical spectrum of CADASIL: a study of 7 families. Lancet 346: 934–939, 1995
14. Colmant HJ: Familiäre zerebrale Gefäberkrankung. Zbl Allgemein Pathologie Bd 124:163, 1980
15. Davous P, Bequet D: CADASIL. Un nouveau modèle de démence sous-corticale. Rev Neurol 151:634–639, 1995
16. Davous P, Fallet-Bianco C: Démence sous-corticale familiale avec leucoencéphalopathie artériopathique. Observation clinicopathologique. Rev Neurol (Paris) 5: 376–384, 1991
17. De Silva R, Bone RIB, Behan P: Cerebral autosomal dominant arteriopathy with subcortical infarcts and leukoencephalopathy in context: data from two Scottish pedigrees. Ann Neurol 40:531, 1996
18. Diagnostic and Statistical Manual of Mental Disorders; DSMIV; 4th Ed. of the American Psychiatric Association, Washington D.C., 1991
19. Ducros A, Nagy T, Alamowitch S et al: CADASIL, genetic homogeneity and mapping of the locus within a 2 cm interval. Am J Hum Genet 58:171–181, 1996
20. Fitzimons RB, Wolfenden WH: Migraine coma. Meningitic migraine with cerebral oedema associated with a new form of autosomal dominant cerebellar ataxia. Brain 108: 555–577, 1991
21. Frequin STFM, Linssen WHJP, Pasman JW et al: Recurrent prolonged coma due to basilar artery migraine. A case report. Headache 31:75–81, 1991
22. Fukutake T, Hirayama K: Familial young-onset arterio-

sclerotic leukoencephalopathy with alopecia and lumbago without arterial hypertension. Eur Neurol 35:69–79, 1995

23. Gerhard: Familiäre zerebrale Arteriosklerose. Zbl Allg Path Bd 124:163, 1980

24. Gray F, Robert F, Labrecque R et al: Autosomal dominant arteriopathic leukoencephalopathy and Alzheimer's disease. Neuropath Applied Neurobiol 20:22–30, 1994

25. Greenberg SM, Vonsattel JPG, Stakes JW et al: The clinical spectrum of cerebral amyloid angiopathy. Neurology 43:2073–2079, 1993

26. Gutierrez-Molina M, Caminero-Rodriguez A, Martinez Garcia C: Small arterial granular degeneration in familial Binswanger's syndrome. Acta Neuropath 87:98–105, 1994

27. Hutchinson M, O'Riordan J, Javed M et al: Familial hemiplegic migraine and autosomal dominant arteriopathy with leukoencephalopathy (CADASIL). Ann Neurol 38:817–824, 1995

28. International Headache Society: Classification and diagnostic criteria for headache disorders, cranial neuralgias and facial pain. Cephalalgia suppl 7:8, 1988

29. Joutel A, Corpechot C, Ducros A et al: Notch 3 mutations in CADASIL, a hereditary adult-onset condition causing stroke and dementia. Nature 383:707–710, 1996

30. Jung HH, Basseti C, Tournier-Lasserve E et al: Cerebral autosomal dominant arteriopathy with subcortical infarcts and leukoencephalopathy: a clinicopathological and genetic study of a Swiss family. J Neurol Neurosurg Psychiatry 59:138–143, 1995

31. Lammie GA, Rakshi J, Rossor MN et al: Cerebral autosomal dominant arteriopathy with subcortical infarcts and leukoencephalopathy (CADASIL)—confirmation by biopsy in 2 cases. Clin Neuropath 14:201–206, 1995

32. Leys D, Schettens P: Vascular Dementia. Dordrecht, Netherlands

33. Lossos A, Cooperman H, Soffer D et al: Hereditary leukoencephalopathy and palmoplantar keratoderma. A new disorder with increased skin collagen content. Neurology 45:331–337, 1995

34. Mas JL, Dilouya A, De Recondo J: A familial disorder with subcortical ischemic strokes, dementia and leukoencephalopathy. Neurology 42:1015–1019, 1992

35. Matthews PM, Tampieri D, Berlovic SF et al: Magnetic resonance imaging shows specific abnormalities in the MELAS syndrome. Neurology 41:1043–1046, 1991

36. Mutrux S: Etude d'un cas familial de paralysie pseudobulbaire à forme pontocerebelleuse. Monatschr Psych U Neurol 122;6:349–385, 1951

37. Osborn RE, Alder DC, Mitchell CS: MR Imaging of the brain in patients with migraine headaches. AJNR 12:521–524, 1991

38. Pullicino P, Ostow P, Miller L et al: Pontine ischemic rarefaction. Ann Neurol 37:460–466, 1995

39. Ragno M, Tournier-Lasserve E, Fiori M et al: An Italian kindred with cerebral autosomal dominant arteriopathy with subcortical infarcts and leukoencephalopathy (CADASIL). Ann Neurol 38:231–236, 1995

40. Roman GC, Tatemichi TK, Erkinjuntti T et al: Vascular dementia: diagnostic criteria for research studies—report of the NINDS-AIREN International Workshop. Neurology 43:250–260, 1993

41. Ruchoux MM, Chabriat H, Bousser MG et al: Presence of ultrastructural arterial lesions in muscle and skin vessels of patients with CADASIL. Stroke 25:2291–2292, 1994

42. Ruchoux MM, Guerrouaou D, Vandehaute B et al: Systemic vascular smooth muscle cell impairment in cerebral autosomal dominant arteriopathy with subcortical infarcts and leukoencephalopathy. Acta Neuropathol 89:500–512, 1995

43. Sabbadini G, Francia A, Calandriello L et al: Cerebral autosomal dominant arteriopathy with subcortical infarcts and leukoencephalopathy (CADASIL). Clinical, neuroimaging, pathological and genetic study of a large Italian family. Brain 118:207–215, 1995

44. Salvi F, Michelucci R, Plasmati R et al: Slowly progressive familial dementia with recurrent strokes and white matter hypodensities on CT scan. Ital J Neurol Sci 13:135–140, 1992

45. Schroder JM, Sellhaus B, Jörg J: Identification of the characteristic vascular changes in a sural nerve biopsy of a case with cerebral autosomal dominant arteriopathy with subcortical infarcts and leukoencephalopathy (CADASIL). Acta Neuropathol (Berl) 89:116–121, 1995

46. Skehan SJ, Hutchinson M, MacErlaine DP: Cerebral autosomal dominant arteriopathy with subcortical infarcts and leukoencephalopathy: MR findings. Am J Neuroradiol 16:2115–2119, 1995

47. Soges LJ, Cacayorin ED, Petro GR Ramachandran TS: Migraine evaluation by MR. AJNR 9:425–429, 1988

48. Sonninen V, Savontaus ML: Hereditary multi-infarct dementia. Eur Neurol 27:209–215, 1987

49. Sourander P, Walinder J: Hereditary multi-infarct dementia. Lancet 7:1015, 1977

50. Sourander P, Walinder J: Hereditary multi-infarct dementia. Morphological studies of a new disease. Acta Neuropathol (Berl) 39:247–254, 1977

51. St Clair D, Bolt J, Morris S, Doyle D: Hereditary multi-infarct dementia unlinked to chromosome 19q12 in a large Scottish pedigree: evidence of probable locus heterogeneity. Med Genet 32:57–60, 1995

52. Stevens DL Hewlett RH, Brownell, B: Chronic familial vascular encephalopathy. Lancet 2:1364–1365, 1977

53. Taillia H, Chabriat H, Kurtz A et al: Neuropsychological alterations in CADASIL (cerebral autosomal dominant arteriopathy with subcortical infarcts and leukoencephalopathy): a study of 10 patients. Cerebrovascular Dis 6(suppl 2):122, 1996

54. Tournier-Lasserve E, Iba-Zizen MT, Romero N, Bousser MG: Autosomal dominant syndrome with stroke-like episodes and leukoencephalopathy. Stroke 22:1297–1302, 1991

55. Tournier-Lasserve E, Joutel A, Melki J et al: Cerebral autosomal dominant arteriopathy with subcortical infarcts and leukoencephalopathy maps on chromosome 19q12. Nature Genetics 3:256–259, 1993

56. Vahedi K, Chabriat H, Ducros A et al: Analysis of CADASIL clinical natural history in a series of 134 patients belonging to 17 families linked to chromosome 19. Neurology 46: A211, 1996

57. Valk J, Van Der Knaap MS: White-matter disorders. Current Opinion Neurol Neurosurg 4:843–851, 1991

58. Van Bogaert L: Encephalopathie sous-corticale progressive (Binswanger) à évolution rapide chez deux soeurs. Med Hellen 24:961–972, 1955
59. Verin M, Rolland Y, Landgraf F et al: New phenotype of CADASIL with migraine as prominent clinical feature. J Neurol Neurosurg Psychiat 59:579–585, 1995
60. Weller M, Liedtke W, Petersen D et al: Very late onset adrenoleukodystrophy. Possible precipitation of demyelination by cerebral contusion. Neurology 42:367–370, 1992
61. Weller M, Petersen D, Dichgans J, Klockgether T: Cerebral angiography complications link cerebral autosomal dominant arteriopathy with subcortical infarcts and leukoencephalopathy to familial hemiplegic migraine. Neurology 46:844, 1996
62. Wieelard R, Bornebroek M, Ophoff RA et al: A four generation Dutch family with cerebral autosomal dominant arteriopathy with subcortical infarcts and leukoencephalopathy (CADASIL), linked to chromosome 19p13. Clin Neurol Neurosurg 97:307–313, 1995

CHAPTER 39

Cerebral Amyloid Angiopathy

HARRY V. VINTERS

Cerebral amyloid angiopathy (CAA), synonymous with cerebral congophilic angiopathy (CCA) and cerebrovascular amyloidosis, defines and describes a group of clinicopathologic entities, a common feature of which is infiltration of cerebral and cerebellar (including leptomeningeal) microvessel walls (arterioles, venules, and capillaries) by a hyaline eosinophilic substance with characteristic staining properties.[12,95,106] It has been recognized in various forms for several decades, but its significance as a *nosologic* entity has emerged within the past two or three decades for several reasons. It is recognized as a relatively common cause of primary intracerebral/intraparenchymal brain hemorrhage, particularly in elderly and demented individuals. CAA is now also recognized as one of the microscopic lesions characteristic of brain morphologic changes that evolve in the course of Alzheimer's disease/senile dementia of Alzheimer type (AD/SDAT).

CAA is implicated as the cause of primary nontraumatic intracerebral hemorrhage in as many as 10% to 15% of patients over the age of 60 years, and almost 20% of patients over the age of 70 years. Its association with ischemic lesions is less clearly defined. Unfortunately, at the present time, CAA is refractory to therapeutic intervention, but novel insights into its pathogenesis and biochemical/immunohistochemical features are providing important clues to possible treatment of this entity in the future. Several reviews place CAA in its proper context as the cause of hemorrhagic and ischemic stroke.[27,39,94,95,107] The recognition that CAA is an important component of the neuropathologic changes that occur with AD/SDAT has led to important insights into the evolution and pathogenesis of this microangiopathy, although, as will be discussed, its precise relationship to the other microscopic brain lesions that are found in excess in the brains of patients with AD/SDAT is not fully understood. Several reviews have summarized the morphologic, immunohistochemical, and biochemical/molecular findings that have emerged from numerous studies on CAA and related brain amyloids.[9,48,77,81,82,106] Essentially, any disorder in which an amyloid is found to be deposited in the central nervous system (CNS) is one that can be expected to have CAA as a component. CAA-related *stroke* in these various disorders, however,

is extremely variable. Although detailed discussion of the molecular genetics/molecular biology of amyloidoses in general and AD amyloid in particular is beyond the scope of this chapter, several excellent reviews summarize key findings and historical milestones in this field.[48,52,75,81,82] Emphasis in this chapter will be placed on the most common form of CAA encountered, namely that associated with brain aging and AD/SDAT.

Clinicopathologic Features

AD/SDAT OR AGE-RELATED CAA

Clinical Features

Although most frequently CAA (of variable degrees) is found at autopsy in elderly individuals or patients with AD/SDAT, in a small number of such patients it can produce stroke.[99] Usually this takes the form of cerebral parenchymal hemorrhage.[27,95] Hemorrhages related to CAA are usually peripherally placed within the brain or "lobar" rather than being in the brain stem or basal ganglia, and generally involve the cortex and subcortical white matter, reflecting the fact that CAA as a microvascular lesion is almost exclusively confined to neocortical and adjacent leptomeningeal microvessels.[27,95,99] Primary cerebellar hematomas resulting from CAA have rarely been documented.[97] Demographic characteristics of patients shown to have well-documented CAA-related brain hemorrhage are summarized in Table 39.1, as are associated major neuropathologic findings.[95]

CAA-related intracerebral hemorrhage (ICH) is noted most commonly in the elderly; most cases are reported in individuals in the seventh or later decades of life. No sex preponderance exists among affected patients, and hemorrhage tends to occur at the same age in males and females, the mean

Table 39.1 Neuropathologic Features
of CAA-Associated Encephalic Hematomas

	Percentage (approx)
Location	
Frontal lobe	35
Temporal lobe	14
Parietal lobe	26
Occipital lobe	19
Deep central gray matter	3–4
Cerebellum	<2
Corpus callosum	Rare
Sex distribution	51.4 female, 48.6 male
Associated features	
Hypertension	
By clinical history	32
Evidence at autopsy	11
Dementia	
Clinical	40
AD/SDAT changes at autopsy	44

Abbreviation: AD/SDAT, Alzheimer's disease/senile dementia of Alzheimer type.

(Adapted from Vinters,[95] with permission.)

age of hemorrhage being in the early seventies. In the brains of patients who come to autopsy, frequently "mixed microangiopathy," with features of both hypertensive and amyloid angiopathy, are found—not surprising when one considers that a significant proportion of patients with CAA-related intraparenchymal hemorrhage are elderly and likely to have had hypertension during life. In some patients, morphologic correlates of hypertension (left ventricular hypertrophy, cardiomegaly) are found at autopsy even when clinical hypertension has not been documented during the patient's life. Almost half of patients with CAA-related ICH summarized in one review[95] were noted to show some degree of dementia during life, and at least a similar proportion showed histopathologic changes of AD at autopsy. However, not infrequently CAA-related brain hemorrhage may be the initial manifestation of the patient's cerebral amyloidosis, which may be "unmasked" by the hemorrhagic stroke.

Over time, CAA-related ICH may involve several lobes on both sides of the brain. Rarely, multiple simultaneous ICHs result from CAA. Hemorrhage may extend directly into the subarachnoid space or into the ventricular system (Figs. 39.1 and 39.2). Although most CAA-related cerebral hemorrhages are large, "miliary" and petechial bleeds may be noted within affected brain matter, and associated scattered microinfarcts may be present.[68,95,106] Despite the well-established association between CAA and primary ICH, the actual site of bleeding from an amyloid-infiltrated arteriole is rarely identified unless serial histologic sections adjacent to a hematoma are carefully examined.[107]

Recently, useful criteria for the diagnosis of CAA-associated ICH have been defined by the Boston Cerebral Amyloid Angiopathy Group.[37] According to this group, the diagnosis

of definite CAA can be established only by full autopsy examination demonstrating lobar (cortical or subcortical) hemorrhage and severe CAA in the absence of another diagnostic lesion. The diagnosis of probable CAA with supporting pathologic evidence is made based on clinical data and pathologic tissue (evacuated hematoma or cerebral cortical biopsy specimen) showing all three of the following: lobar, cortical or subcortical hemorrhage, some degree of CAA in the brain biopsy specimen, and absence of another diagnostic lesion. The diagnosis of probable CAA is made when clinical data and neuroimaging findings demonstrate all of the following: patient age of 60 years of older, multiple hemorrhages restricted to characteristic sites, described above, and absence of another cause of ICH (e.g., anticoagulation, head trauma, vascular malformation, blood dyscrasia). The diagnosis of possible CAA is based on the patient being 60 years of age or older, having a characteristically located ICH without another etiologic explanation, or multiple hemorrhages with a possible but not a definite cause or some hemorrhages in an atypical location (e.g., the brain stem). These criteria will need to be validated prospectively, but provide a valuable framework within which a neurologist or neurosurgeon can make the diagnosis of CAA-related ICH with varying degrees of certainty. They also highlight the importance of the neuropathologist's paying particularly close attention to evacuated hematoma material, particularly from an elderly individual. Frequently, careful examination of evacuated clot can yield an etiologic diagnosis that explains a patient's cerebral hemorrhage, whether the result of CAA or some other cause (e.g., neoplasm, vascular malformation).

Patients with CAA are also at increased risk for primary ICH when thrombolytic agents or anticoagulants are administered.[37] Controversy has surrounded the relative merits of confirming the diagnosis of CAA-related ICH and/or treating the patient by, respectively, brain biopsy or evacuation of the clotted blood. Early reports based on small numbers of patients suggested that neurosurgical procedures might eventuate in subsequent massive CAA-related brain hemorrhage. Subsequent investigations have suggested that, with modern neurosurgical and neuroanaesthetic techniques, individuals with CAA-related brain hemorrhage may safely undergo operative procedures, and individuals who present with CAA-related ICH may improve neurologically following clot evacuation.[40]

The association between CAA and cerebral ischemic lesions/encephalomalacia within the brain is much less clearly established than that between CAA and primary ICH.[1,13,106] Cerebral infarcts are relatively common in the brains of patients with CAA. This may relate to the more frequent occurrence of CAA at advanced age (i.e., affected patients are also prone to show the complications of hypertensive microvascular disease and atherosclerosis). One retrospective postmortem analysis of 25 patients with CAA in the setting of AD/SDAT showed that seven patients experienced clinically significant cerebral infarcts or hemorrhages or both.[20] However, there did not appear to be a statistically significant difference in the incidence of infarcts or hemorrhages in hypertensive as opposed to normotensive individuals. Thus, hypertension did not appear to be an additional risk factor in the causation of cerebral infarct or hemorrhage associated with CAA of AD. Transient ischemic attacks (TIAs) have been described in patients with CAA, though the association is largely anecdotal.[86]

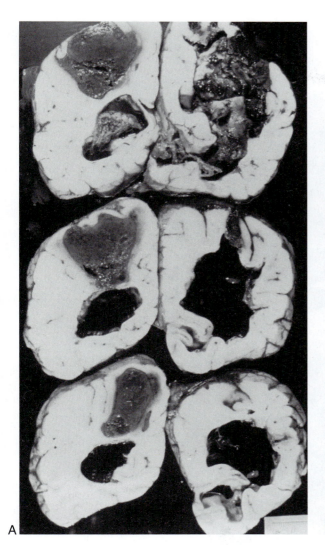
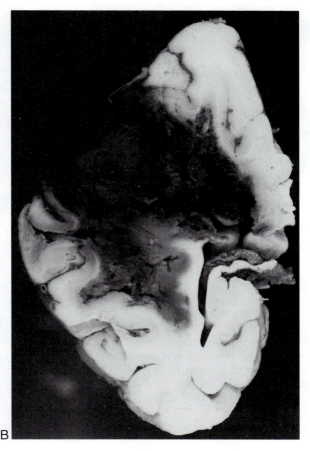

Figure 39.1 (**A**) Multiple bilateral cerebral hematomas related to CAA in an elderly demented patient have extended into both the subarachnoid space and the lateral ventricles. (**B**) Massive left parietal hematoma in a 72-year-old woman with SDAT, showing prominent extension into the subarachnoid space. (Fig. A from Vinters and Mah,[16] with permission; Fig. B from Ferreiro et al,[20] with permission.)

One study has shown an association between severe CAA and cerebral infarct in AD patients.[69a]

The precise relationship of CAA to dementia, particularly dementia of the Alzheimer type (AD/SDAT) is more puzzling.[28,29] CAA occurs commonly in the brains of AD patients, though it also frequently occurs in the CNS of individuals of advanced age with no neurologic deficit.[4,30,56,99] CAA is recognized as one of the four primary microscopic hallmarks by which the clinical diagnosis of AD is confirmed with neuropathologic studies.[9,48,81,82,100] Various investigators have estimated the frequency of CAA in AD as being from 75% to 100%.[17] Of the other neuropathologic features of Alzheimer's disease (senile/neuritic plaques, granulovacuolar degeneration, neurofibrillary tangles), senile plaques are biochemically most closely linked to CAA. In the author's experience, approximately 10% to 15% of brains from patients with the clini-

cal diagnosis of AD/SDAT show severe amyloid angiopathy as the most significant or predominant microscopic abnormality within the brain at autopsy, although usually significant numbers of senile plaques and neurofibrillary tangles (within either the neocortex or the hippocampus) are also found. At the present time, there is no way to clinically distinguish patients with AD and unusually severe CAA from those with negligible CAA unless such patients develop CAA-related ICH. Indeed, it is likely that the neuropathologic substrates of AD/SDAT are heterogeneous,[5] i.e., some patients have a pronounced degree of microvascular amyloid, whereas many others have extensive cortical and hippocampal neurofibrillary tangles and senile plaques in the presence of scant CAA. The role (if any) of CAA in the causation of multi-infarct dementia (MID) remains to be defined.

Other clinicopathologic entities are much less commonly

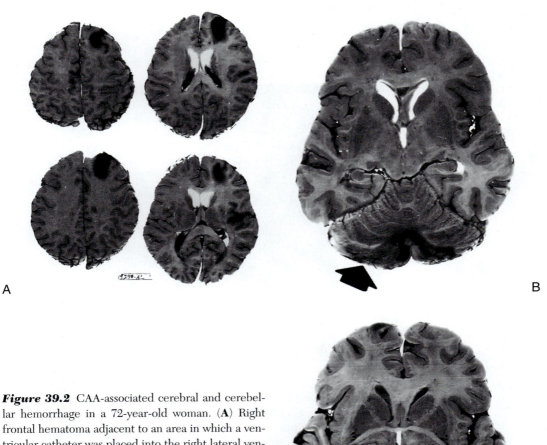

Figure 39.2 CAA-associated cerebral and cerebellar hemorrhage in a 72-year-old woman. (**A**) Right frontal hematoma adjacent to an area in which a ventricular catheter was placed into the right lateral ventricle. The presence of CAA may have led to large size of the hemorrhage. (**B**) Horizontal section through upper cerebellum, demonstrating scar of remote hematoma in the left cerebellum (arrow) and a more recent (3-week-old) hemorrhage extending from right cerebellar hemisphere across the vermis. (**C**) Lower horizontal cut, revealing inferior extension of hemorrhage into the right cerebellum. (Case reviewed by courtesy of Dr. Francoise Robert, Montreal, Canada, who generously provided the photographs.)

associated with CAA. Greenberg et al[39] described three patients in whom dementia developed within an unusually rapid time course, progressing from intact baseline to profound dementia within a few days to 24 months. Pathologic abnormalities in these patients included patchy white matter demyelination and "tissue loss," petechial cortical hemorrhages and cortical infarcts as well as various numbers of senile plaques and neurofibrillary tangles. Other individuals have reported differing forms and degrees of leukoencephalopathy in patients with diffuse CAA.[35] Very rarely, CAA may present as a mass lesion[7] or with primary subarachnoid hemorrhage,[67] though as a cause of subarachnoid hemorrhage, CAA must be considered extraordinarily rare in comparison to berry/saccular aneurysms or vascular malformations of the brain. Though CAA is almost always restricted to the brain, rare cases of spinal cord vascular and leptomeningeal amyloid protein

deposition in the context of hemorrhagic CAA have been described.[90] Angiitis or vasculitis as a manifestation of CAA will be described below.

Neuropathologic, Immunohistochemical, and Biochemical Features

The existence of CAA must be suspected in any individual who comes to autopsy with the diagnosis of AD/SDAT or dementia. If such an individual has a superimposed lobar cerebral hemorrhage, the likelihood of finding CAA becomes much greater. The characteristic features of CAA-related brain hemorrhage have been discussed above and are illustrated in Figures 39.1 and 39.2. It must be re-emphasized that, given the large number of patients who have the clinico-pathologic features of AD/SDAT, the percentage of these individuals likely to experience a CAA-related brain hemorrhage is extraordinarily small.[12,95,106] Nevertheless, in the appropriate clinical context CAA becomes a much more likely diagnostic consideration.

Histopathologic confirmation of CAA is easily made on paraffin section of the brain. Even on routine (H&E-stained) sections, CAA can be detected as a hyaline eosinophilic material replacing the normal smooth muscle cell media component of cortical arterioles. Venules may also be involved by CAA. There may be some value in distinguishing involvement of different types and sizes of vessels by CAA, because only patients with extensive arteriolar amyloid deposition are likely to develop brain hemorrhage. Capillary amyloid deposits are frequently, though not invariably associated with adjacent senile plaques containing amyloid cores.[3] In leptomeningeal vessels, the amyloid deposition is less commonly found in the media of arterioles and larger arteries, but more frequently involves their adventitia. All forms of CAA can be confirmed in brain tissue examined at biopsy or necropsy by Congo-red staining and polarization microscopy (Fig. 39.3).

A key question becomes: Given the frequency of even relatively severe forms of CAA, especially in patients with AD/SDAT why do only a small percentage of affected individuals develop ICH? While amyloid usually infiltrates the media and adventitia of severely involved vessels, luminal stenosis is not always present, although it is observed in a small number of unusually severe cases. Small arteries may show associated fibrinoid necrosis of the vessel wall and the formation of miliary aneurysms that resemble more traditionally defined Charcot-Bouchard aneurysms, classically described with hypertensive cerebral microvascular disease (Fig. 39.4). These latter microvascular abnormalities may increase the propensity for ICH, especially if, during life, rapid changes in systemic blood pressure have occurred. Mandybur[55] has described a series of CAA-associated vasculopathies (Fig. 39.5). These changes include clustering of multiple arteriolar lumina or glomerular formations, aneurysmal dilatation of vessels, and obliterative intimal changes, as well as double barreling or "lumen within a lumen" appearance of affected arterioles, which may also show degenerative vessel wall changes. Chronic inflammatory perivascular infiltrates may be seen (see discussion of vasculitis below). The deposition of fibrillar amyloid within the vessel wall may lead to injury or separation of smooth muscle cells, rendering the affected vessel weak and thus prone to rupture-producing hemorrhage. However, the elastica in larger (meningeal) vessels involved by CAA is often remarkably well preserved. Ultrastructural analysis of CAA shows the expected presence of characteristic 7-nm to 9-nm filaments that are

Figure 39.3 Routine histologic study of CAA. (**A**) Brain biopsy from an elderly patient with lobar cerebral hemorrhage. Congo-red stained section shows thickened arterioles (arrows), viewed without polarized light. (**B**) Same section viewed *with* polarized light shows birefringent vessel walls (arrows) but virtually no parenchymal amyloid deposits. (× 95.)

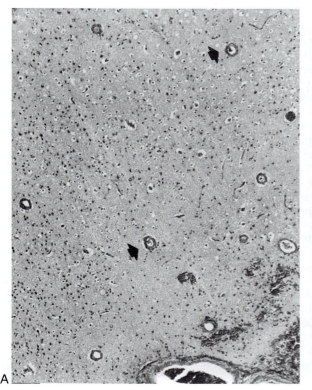
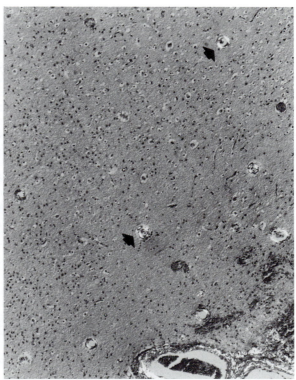

A   B

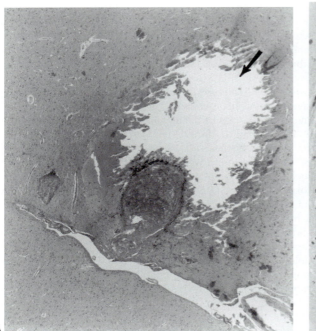
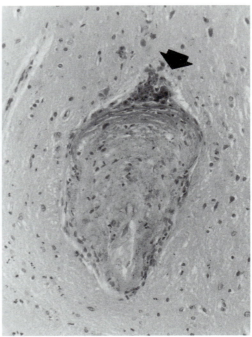

Figure 39.4 CAA-associated microaneurysms resembling typical Charcot-Bouchard type aneurysms. The larger of the two aneurysms (**A**) is surrounded by old and recent (arrow) hemorrhage. Smaller aneurysm (**B**) shows old hemorrhage (arrowhead) surrounding adventitia. (H&E; Fig. A × 25, Fig. B × 165.)

seen in disorganized skeins and random or haphazard arrangements, and scattered medial smooth muscle cells or the debris of necrotic/apoptotic smooth muscle cells.[105] In arteriolar CAA, however, the endothelium is frequently surprisingly well preserved, as is the junction between CAA-affected microvessels and the surrounding brain parenchyma.[105] However, in examples of severe capillary amyloid deposition, endothelial injury or necrosis has occasionally been identified.[116]

An important study by Vonsattel et al[107] has examined CAA with and without ICH in autopsy material. As expected, CAA was more severe in the brains of patients with ICH than in those without, and, of interest, fibrinoid necrosis of arterioles was seen only in the brains of patients with cerebral hemorrhage. Microaneurysms occurred only in the presence of severe CAA. In the brains of two patients with ICH, fibrinoid necrosis, microaneurysms, and vascular rupture were seen in close association with the cerebral hemorrhage. This group has also proposed a system whereby the severity of CAA can be graded in a given vessel (Fig. 39.6) and have highlighted the patchy nature of amyloid deposition in longitudinal segments of affected vessels; i.e., regions of affected arteriole may show focally accentuated mural amyloid deposits. This can be dramatically illustrated in thick sections of brain matter stained with appropriate techniques (Fig. 39.7).

A major advance in our current understanding of the biochemistry and molecular biology of CAA and related brain amyloids occurred with the isolation and characterization of cerebral microvascular amyloid from patients with AD and Down syndrome (DS) by Glenner's group in 1984.[31,32] Though Glenner utilized leptomeningeal microvessels, amy-

loid-laden microvessels were subsequently isolated from the neocortex of a patient with AD using comparable biochemical techniques.[71] Both microvascular and senile plaque core amyloid were eventually found to be composed of a polypeptide with a molecular weight of approximately 4,200, showing a unique amino acid composition and sequence that differed substantially from that of other known amyloid proteins.[9,48,52,75,77,81,82] This protein is now referred to as the Alzheimer beta/A4 peptide. It originates from a much larger molecule, the amyloid precursor protein (APP), a membrane-spanning protein encoded by a gene on chromosome 21. Alternately spliced transcripts of the APP gene encode APP isoforms of varying lengths (695, 751, or 770 amino acids), described as APP_{695}, APP_{771} or APP_{770}.[33,48,52,75,81,82] The largest of these transcripts (APP_{751} and APP_{770}) contains a roughly 60 amino acid segment with pronounced hemology to Kunitz serine protease inhibitors. Beta/A4 peptide represents the near-C-terminal portion of APP, including 28 amino acids immediately external to the transmembrane domain together with the first 12 to 15 residues of the transmembrane domain. Details of the biochemical and molecular processing of APP are to be found in several reviews.[42,48,52,58,64,75,81,82,87]

Numerous monoclonal and polyclonal antibodies to beta/A4 and APP have now been developed and are routinely used to demonstrate protein deposition in vessel walls and brain parenchyma by means of immunohistochemical approaches at the light and electron microscopic levels.[15,44,46,54,57,77,101,103,104,112] These provide a much more accurate and specific way to detect CAA and related brain amyloids than previous cytochemical methods (e.g., Congo red, thioflavin S or T), although the latter techniques can still be used as a screening tool, particularly in laboratories where beta/A4 or APP antibodies are not available. The anti-beta/A4 immunoreagents usually work extremely well in paraffin sections and many are available from commercial sources. Results of studies using anti-beta/A4 or anti-APP antibodies show that such antibodies routinely label senile plaques (SPs) of various configurations, and demonstrate beta/A4 protein in a subpial "band-like" distribution, as well as in the cerebellum. Such antibodies also usually effectively demonstrate CAA associated with aging or AD/SDAT, including arterial or capillary forms (Fig. 39.8). Not infrequently, perivascular halos of beta/A4 immunoreactivity are seen around CAA microvessels. Beta/A4 immunoreactivity can often be highlighted using antigen unmasking techniques including pretreatment of tissue sections with formic acid.[51,102] Beta/A4 amyloid is by no means the only molecular component of CAA or senile plaques, e.g., proteoglycans have been immunolocalized to both structures and may interact with beta/A4 to determine the evolution of lesion development in specific loci, e.g., the microvessel wall or brain parenchyma.[88] Furthermore, cystatin C or gamma-trace, a molecule important in the pathogenesis of Icelandic CAA (see

below), has been found to localize within AD/SDAT brain microvascular amyloid.[101,104] The implications of these various biochemical and immunohistochemical observations for approaches to making the diagnosis of brain amyloidosis, including CAA, during life are discussed below.

Molecular Pathogenesis

To some extent, the pathogenesis of CAA cannot be separated from the evolution of SPs, given that both have a major biochemical component of beta/A4 protein. However, sensitive biochemical assays have indicated that SP and vascular beta/A4 amyloid are probably chemically distinct; i.e., vascular beta/A4 contains 39 amino acid residues, whereas SP beta/A4 has 42 or 43.[74] This suggests that tissue-specific endopeptidases may determine differential processing of APP in the brain parenchyma and microvessel wall. Microglial or pericyte function or dysfunction may also play a role in plaque formation, as well as the genesis of vessel wall amyloid. Early ultrastructural studies of SPs in relation to cerebral microvessels suggested that all SPs were found in close proximity to brain capillaries.[61,62] This led to the hypothesis that capillary degen-

Figure 39.5 CAA-associated secondary vascular changes. (**A**) Cortical parenchymal vessel shows hyaline (amyloidotic) thickening of vessel wall. Note poorly defined intimal thickening on luminal aspect of the amyloid, and hemosiderin-containing macrophages around the vessel and in adjacent brain parenchyma. (**B**) Focal thickening of amyloidotic vessel wall by foamy histiocytes (arrows). (H&E, × 190.)

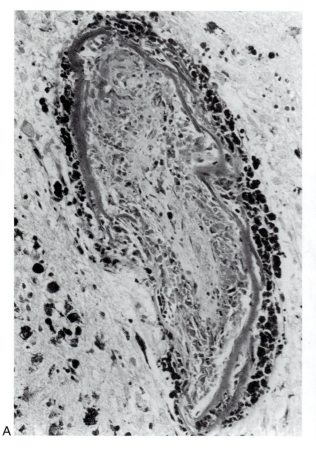

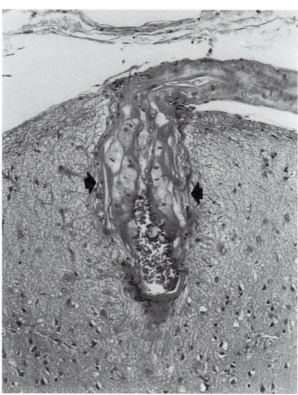

A

B

eration leading to the formation or deposition of amyloid fibrils might be a primary pathogenic event in development of the SP. Some cortical parenchymal amyloid deposits in many AD brains are certainly associated with capillaries and structural abnormalities of the cerebral capillary endothelium (i.e., site of the blood-brain barrier [BBB]) suggest "leakiness" or dysfunction of the BBB in AD CNS.[10,89] However, double- and triple-label immunohistochemical studies show that capillary degeneration probably plays only a limited role, if any, in the formation of most SPs.[50]

More recent studies have specifically addressed the pathogenesis of CAA (as distinct from SPs) in AD patients with severe CAA. Some immunohistochemical studies with antibodies to beta/A4 and various segments of APP show that anti-beta/A4 recognizes primarily extracellular amyloid deposits in blood vessel walls.[49] Conversely, anti-APP antibodies tend to immunolabel smooth muscle (sm) cells, which suggests that beta/A4 in blood vessel walls may derive from degenerating APP-containing sm cells. Immunocytochemical studies at the ultrastructural level show that vascular amyloid fibrils may initially form within abluminal basement membrane (i.e., in an extracellular location).[118] The basement membrane may sequester beta/A4-containing APP segments that are then processed further by local proteases to yield segments that are amyloidogenic. Other studies have shown that CAA may result from proliferating and degenerating sm cells of the vascular media, whereas microglia/macrophages seem not to be involved in the process.[114] One group has found sm cytoplasmic immunoreactivity for beta/A4 rather than simply APP, small

beta/A4 immunoreactive deposits that are not yet fibrillar, and monomeric and oligomeric forms of beta/A4.[23] Ultrastructural studies of brain biopsy material from patients with severe CAA support the occurrence of sm cell degeneration within arteriolar media unrelated to specific abnormalities of adjacent brain parenchyma or microvascular endothelium.[105]

Recently, sensitive immunoassays have confirmed that beta/A4 of 42 (1–42) rather than 40 amino acid length constitute the principal biochemical component of both intracerebral and meningeal CAA blood vessels, but this is essentially undetectable in extracranial vasculature.[78,85] In Down syndrome patients, cortical beta/A4 1–42 (43) deposition precedes the deposition of beta/A4 1-40.[45] Finally, tissue culture studies of cerebrovascular sm cells from dogs have demonstrated that such cells accumulate beta/A4 at early passages, shortly after isolation from brain parenchyma, that sm from "younger" cerebral and extracerebral arteries can be induced to deposit intracellular fibrillar and nonfibrillar beta/A4, and that proliferation of sm cells diminished when significant amounts of beta/A4 had accumulated.[22,113] Freshly solubilized beta/A4 1-42 may cause cultured sm cells to undergo degeneration and an increase in levels of cellular APP and soluble beta/A4. However, preaggregation of the beta/A4 1-42 abolishes these in vitro effects.[14] Despite their inherent limitations, tissue culture studies of cerebral endothelium and smooth muscle may be able to address the different biologic phenomena that appear to determine parenchymal and microvessel wall deposition of beta/A4 protein.

In view of the discovery within the last several years that

Figure 39.6 Grading system to describe severity of CAA in a given artery/arteriole using light microscopic criteria. Diagram is based on criteria defined by Vonsattel et al.[107] Diagram by Ms. Toni King.

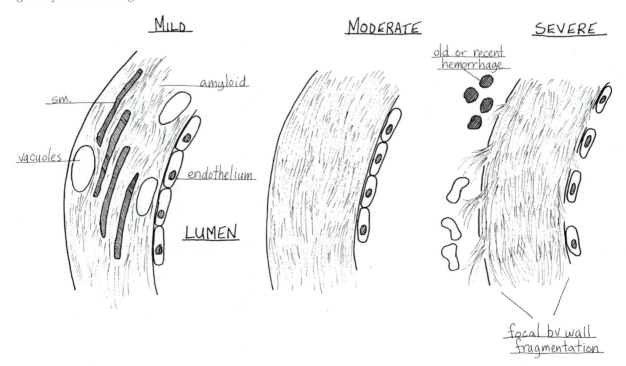

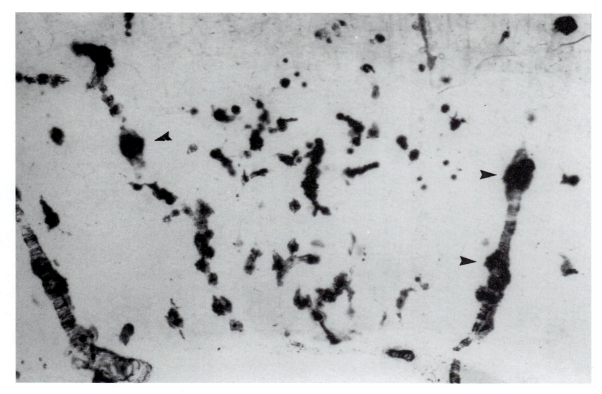

Figure 39.7 Polyethylene glycol embedded brain, 100 μm thick section stained using the Campbell-Switzer technique. Note both capillary and arteriolar amyloid. The arteriolar amyloid shows "tuft-like" areas of focal accentuation with extension of amyloid into brain parenchyma, probably corresponding to Vonsattel "severe" grade (arrows).

apolipoprotein E ϵ4 (apo E4) gene dose is a major risk factor for late onset AD,[11,79] there has been interest in whether Apo E isoforms are over-represented in patients with unusually severe CAA. One group has found evidence for Apo E4 as an independent risk factor for CAA and CAA-related brain hemorrhage.[38] However, analysis of Apo E genotypes in another large series of patients with autopsy-proven CAA-associated ICH has shown a relatively high frequency of Apo E2 in this population.[66]

Making the Diagnosis of CAA Antemortem

Being able to predict which patients, with or without AD/SDAT, carry a significant burden of CAA would be of obvious value to clinicians. Unfortunately, the diagnosis of CAA in an aging or demented patient is almost impossible to make using computerized tomographic (CT) or magnetic resonance imaging (MRI) scanning techniques, though the finding of an atrophic brain in a patient who has experienced a slowly progressive dementing illness implies that some degree of CAA will be present within the patient's brain. If CAA declares its presence by producing ICH, the probable or possible diagnosis of CAA becomes much more straightforward (see criteria described above). The neuropathologic features of CAA-related ICH predict the antemortem radiographic findings.[98] CAA-related hemorrhages are usually visualized as peripheral or lobar hemorrhages (Fig. 39.9), with or without mass effect. Hemorrhage may be seen in an otherwise atrophic brain. Rarely, CAA-related hemorrhages occur in unusual locations such as the corpus callosum. Otherwise, superficial location of the hematoma, irregular borders, and surrounding edema are characteristic features on CT scanning, and ring enhancement is sometimes seen.[98] The size of vessels involved by CAA is usually too small to be visualized by conventional cerebral angiography.

Other approaches to indirect, noninvasive methods for making the diagnosis of CAA or brain amyloid in general have included: (1) performing a biopsy of an extra-cerebral site at which beta/A4 is demonstrable, and potentially quantifiable, using immunohistochemistry; (2) measuring beta/A4 or APP levels or other informative proteins within plasma or cerebrospinal fluid (CSF); (3) finding a means by which cerebral beta/A4 could specifically be imaged during life. In order to test specific hypotheses relevant to such detection systems for intracerebral amyloid, including CAA, a reliable animal model for CNS beta/A4 deposition would be valuable. For instance, transgenic mice may eventually be available routinely to assist with such studies, though most transgenic mouse models that have been used to study the evolution of AD/SDAT-related changes in the brain show relatively minimal microvascular amyloid deposition.[24,43] Although beta/A4 deposits can be detected in the brains of many species of aged animals, relatively few of these (e.g., some simians) show progressive accumula-

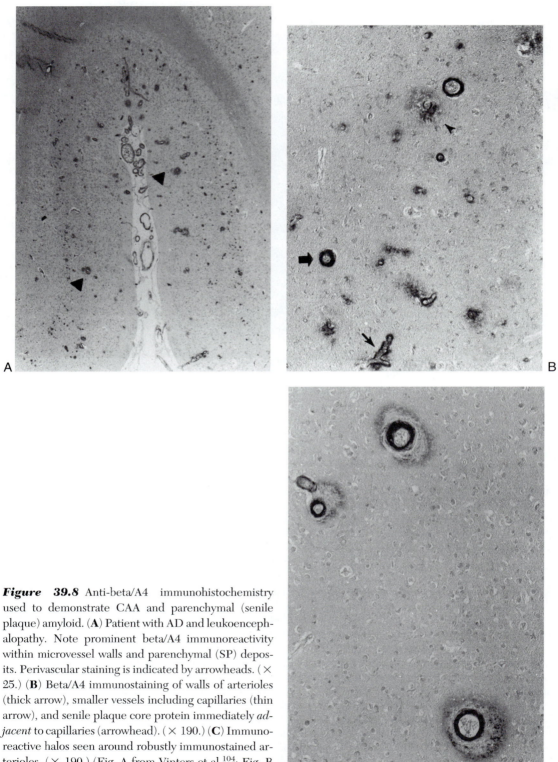

***Figure* 39.8** Anti-beta/A4 immunohistochemistry used to demonstrate CAA and parenchymal (senile plaque) amyloid. (**A**) Patient with AD and leukoencephalopathy. Note prominent beta/A4 immunoreactivity within microvessel walls and parenchymal (SP) deposits. Perivascular staining is indicated by arrowheads. (× 25.) (**B**) Beta/A4 immunostaining of walls of arterioles (thick arrow), smaller vessels including capillaries (thin arrow), and senile plaque core protein immediately *adjacent* to capillaries (arrowhead). (× 190.) (**C**) Immunoreactive halos seen around robustly immunostained arterioles. (× 190.) (Fig. A from Vinters et al.[104]; Fig. B from Vinters et al.[101a] reproduced with permission.)

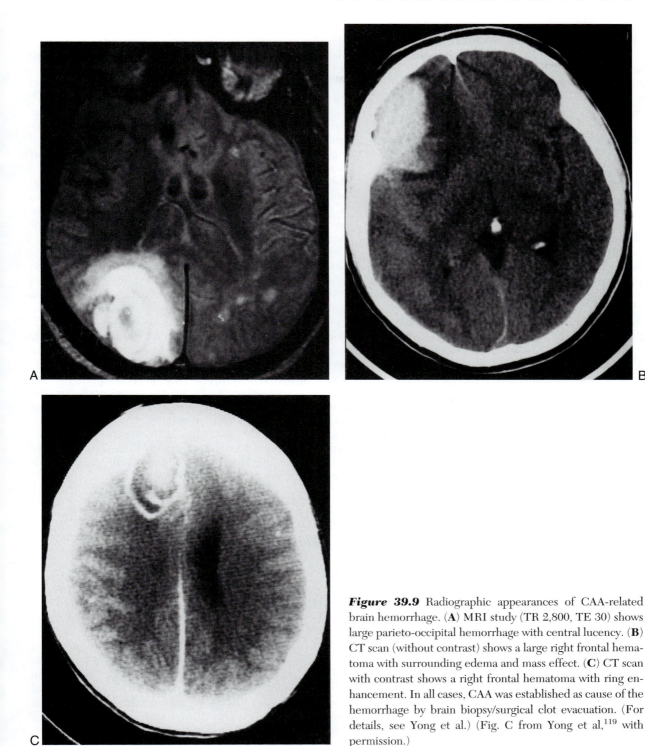

Figure 39.9 Radiographic appearances of CAA-related brain hemorrhage. (**A**) MRI study (TR 2,800, TE 30) shows large parieto-occipital hemorrhage with central lucency. (**B**) CT scan (without contrast) shows a large right frontal hematoma with surrounding edema and mass effect. (**C**) CT scan with contrast shows a right frontal hematoma with ring enhancement. In all cases, CAA was established as cause of the hemorrhage by brain biopsy/surgical clot evacuation. (For details, see Yong et al.) (Fig. C from Yong et al,[119] with permission.)

tion of the protein in a predictable fashion.[83] The squirrel monkey is one species that develops beta/A4 amyloid deposition in cerebral and meningeal arteries in a pattern resembling human CAA,[108] though usually without associated stroke.

Vascular and nonvascular beta/A4 immunoreactive deposits have been detected within the skin and gastrointestinal tract of patients with AD and some aged, neurologically nor-mal individuals.[47] However, the changes within peripheral sites are not predictive of amyloid burden within the brain of affected patients; thus, biopsy of peripheral tissues does not provide a "window" on the severity or extent of CNS amyloid-osis. Many laboratories have developed assays for beta/A4 and APP within CSF and plasma.[63,65,70,73] Levels of beta/A4 have been found to be elevated in the CSF of patients with early-onset AD in one study,[65] whereas they have been found by others to be either decreased (especially beta/A4 1–42) in clinically diagnosed AD patients or show no significant differences between AD patients and those who have other neurodegenerative diseases or are neurologically intact.[63,91] APP levels may also be decreased in patients with probable AD.[92] One difficulty with these investigations is that AD/SDAT is a neuropathologically heterogeneous condition, and many of the studies describing beta/A4 and APP levels are performed on patients with clinically diagnosed disease only. Optimally, assays of beta/A4 and APP should be standardized, to the extent possible, against autopsy findings in patients whose CSF or plasma has been assayed shortly before death. One such study indicates that CSF beta/A4 levels are decreased in patients with marked CAA but do not correlate with numbers of amyloid plaques.[72] Decreased CSF levels of cystatin C appear to correlate with the presence of CAA-related intracerebral hemorrhage,[84] a finding that is especially intriguing in view of the colocalization of gamma-trace/cystatin C with beta/A4 in arterial lesions of patients with stroke-prone CAA.[101,104]

Novel neuroimaging approaches to detecting beta/A4 within the CNS are being developed and are potentially of immense clinical and biologic value. Studies in aged primates have used intracisternal injections of anti-beta/A4 antibody one day prior to sacrifice, followed by immunohistochemical localization of the primary antibody in postmortem brain.[109] A small fraction (no more than 15%) of the cerebral amyloid deposits and especially those near the cortical surface were labeled using this in vivo technique. A vector-mediated BBB drug transport system has also been used to allow for delivery of ^{125}I-labeled beta/A4 1–40 into rat brain.[80] Labeling of AD brain amyloid deposits by the tagged beta/A4 was demonstrated. Further exploitation of this strategy shows immense potential for allowing effective in vivo imaging of CNS amyloid burden, including the extent and severity of CAA. Obviously, this may allow for eventual monitoring of the effects of drugs that have the potential to remove amyloid from the CNS or inhibit its formation therein.

DUTCH HEREDITARY CEREBRAL AMYLOID ANGIOPATHY

Hereditary cerebral hemorrhage with amyloidosis (primarily CAA) has been described in a small number of patients living in a coastal region of the Netherlands. Study of this relatively small group of patients is of potentially immense biological importance, since the predominant cerebral microvascular lesions show a molecular kinship to AD/SDAT-related CAA, though patients in general do not develop extensive neurofibrillary tangle pathology characteristic of AD/SDAT.[8] The condition, described as hereditary cerebral hemorrhage with amyloidosis-Dutch type (HCHWA-D) is inherited as an autosomal dominant disease that results from deposition of beta/A4-amyloid within meningeal and cortical parenchymal arteries and arterioles.[60] Brain tissue also shows "preamyloid" deposits and beta/A4 immunoreactive plaques in the brain parenchyma (Plate 39.1). HCHWA-D results from a point

mutation at codon 693 of the amyloid precursor protein (APP) gene on chromosome 21, leading to a substitution of glutamine for glutamic acid at residue 22 of beta/A4.[115] The existence of this well-defined point mutation allows for presymptomatic testing of patients at risk and genetic counseling. Affected patients develop recurrent strokes and dementia. Of interest, the dementia may be "unmasked" by the first stroke, but may also precede any evidence of cerebrovascular disease. Radiographic features of affected patients show the presence of focal lesions that include hemorrhages, hemorrhagic and nonhemorrhagic infarcts. MRI studies clearly show diffuse whitematter damage visualized as areas of incomplete infarction with demyelination.[41] Diffuse white-matter hyperintensities on MRI are an early symptom of HCHWA-D since they have been found on MRI scans of patients who have not yet experienced evidence of stroke.[8]

Histopathologically, the CAA associated with HCHWA-D shows important similarities to and differences from AD-related CAA. In HCHWA-D, beta/A4 peptide deposition in affected arterioles and arteries appears to begin at the junction of the media and adventitia and proceeds to involve the entire media, causing sm cell degeneration in affected vessel walls.[60] Cortical arterioles often show one or two layers of radially oriented beta/A4 immunoreactive deposits around a layer of homogeneous beta/A4 that replaces the media. Degenerating neuronal process (neurites), as well as reactive astrocytes and microglia, may surround affected arterioles, capillaries, and cortical plaques.[59] This has been hypothesized to represent (in part) a reaction to invasion of the perivascular neuropil by beta/A4 fibrils.[60] Cystatin C and APP colocalize with vascular beta/A4 protein. Affected microvessels often show structural changes, including loss of SM cells, dramatically demonstrable using antibodies to alpha-smooth muscle actin.

ICELANDIC CEREBRAL AMYLOID ANGIOPATHY

The condition described as hereditary cerebral hemorrhage with amyloidosis of Icelandic type (HCHWA-I) is of interest for its morphologic similarities to both HCHWA-D and AD/SDAT-related CAA, at the same time as HCHWA-I shows important biochemical dissimilarities with the Dutch and Alzheimer conditions. Icelandic CAA is increasingly coming to be described as hereditary cystatin C amyloid angiopathy (HCCAA), in view of the biochemical lesion that is associated with the clinicopathologic entity. This is also an autosomal dominant disorder that causes fatal cerebral hemorrhage in normotensive individuals. Affected patients are usually much younger than those affected by HCHWA-D, i.e., brain hemorrhage occurs frequently in the third and fourth decades of life.[69] The condition results from a mutation in the gene encoding the cysteine protease inhibitor, cystatin C or gammatrace. A single nucleotide is substituted in codon 68 (A for T), resulting in the replacement of leucine by glutamine in the protein sequence. This point mutation results in a gammatrace/cystatin C protein that shows increased tendency to aggregate and causes deposits of amyloid in the walls of small arteries and arterioles in the neocortex and leptomeningeal vessels. Just as amyloid deposition in HCHWA-D and some cases of AD-related CAA produces cerebral hemorrhage, so the CAA in Icelandic patients frequently results in fatal ICH. Amyloid protein deposition and CAA can be demonstrated using antibodies to cystatin C.[69,101] Using single- and double-label immunohistochemistry, cystatin C immunoreactivity has been found to localize to the media of parenchymal microvessels and the adventitia of leptomeningeal vessels.[110] Immunohistochemical findings suggest progressive loss of arteriolar sm cells as cystatin C accumulates. However, in less severely affected CAA vessels, cystatin C was present in cells that clearly had the phenotype of sm, suggesting that sm cells synthesize or process cystatin C; note the analogy to beta/A4 deposition or processing within arteriolar media in Alzheimer or age-related CAA. Measurement of cystatin C levels in CSF samples obtained from HCCAA patients shows that levels of this protein are significantly lower than in control patients, allowing for a minimally invasive diagnostic test for HCCAA that has relatively high predictive value.[69]

Two recent findings in non-Icelandic patients relevant to cystatin C are particularly intriguing. Graffagnino et al have described a patient with sporadic CAA that caused ICH in an elderly Croatian male, in whom a mutation in cystatin C identical to that found in HCCAA was demonstrated.[34] Even more significant for possible experimental studies of CAA in experimental animals, CAA in aged simians including squirrel and rhesus monkeys (known to be immunoreactive with anti-beta/A4 antibodies) has also been shown to be immunolabeled with antibodies to cystatin C.[111] Furthermore, cystatin C cDNA from the simians, especially the squirrel monkeys, which are particularly prone to develop CAA, showed several amino acid substitutions in the predicted cystatin C sequence, including the mutation that is thought to be causal for HCCAA.[69,111] This important study indicates that alterations in cystatin C may influence the extent or severity of amyloid deposition in the walls of cerebral parenchymal microvessels.

CAA IN SPONGIFORM ENCEPHALOPATHIES

Various spongiform encephalopathies and associated neurodegenerative disorders are now commonly referred to as prion protein diseases, since the prion protein (PrP) plays an essential role in their pathogenesis. In these diseases, PrP undergoes conformational change from an alpha-helix to a beta-sheet structure. Brain parenchymal amyloid deposition is a component of some of these disorders, in particular Gerstmann-Sträussler-Scheinker disease (GSSD), though it is *not* found uniformly in all other spongiform encephalopathies. A form of prion protein cerebral amyloid angiopathy (PrP-CAA) has also been described.[26] Both GSSD and PrP-CAA are associated with well-defined mutations of the gene that encodes prion protein, *PRNP*. Despite the relative prominence of CAA in some of these conditions, stroke is not a major clinical finding in affected individuals, who more commonly experience a wide range of clinical manifestations including ataxia, spastic paraparesis, extrapyramidal signs, and dementia.[26] However, understanding the molecular pathogenesis of PrP-CAA may facilitate an understanding of mechanisms common to the etiopathogenesis of other forms of CAA described above.

OCULOLEPTOMENINGEAL AMYLOIDOSIS

Oculoleptomeningeal amyloidosis (OLAM), described in small numbers of patients in Japan, North America, and Europe, is characterized by widespread deposition of amyloid within the vitreous and retinal vessels, usually with meningovascular amyloid deposition adjacent to the brain and sometimes within it. Various vascular tissues throughout the body are also infiltrated by amyloid, and there may be associated peripheral nerve degeneration. Patients frequently experience seizures, cerebral infarcts, and, rarely, cerebral hemorrhage. The strokes are thought to result from adventitial infiltration of meningeal vessels with associated intimal thickening or weakening of the vessel wall. Biochemically, the amyloid has been found to represent transthyretin or prealbumin. In a syndrome of meningocerebrovascular amyloidosis discovered in Hungary, a mutation at codon 18 of the gene encoding transthyretin has been discovered.[25,93] This mutation (TTRD18G) is associated primarily with CNS deposition of amyloid proteins, particularly centered on blood vessel walls. Subpial and subependymal regions also showed amyloid deposition. This represents yet another hereditary condition in which CNS amyloidosis, including CAA, is a major pathologic component.

VASCULITIS ASSOCIATED WITH CAA

Rarely, CAA, usually of a severe degree, is associated with vasculitis, which primarily affects amyloid-laden microvessels. This is an extraordinarily rare concurrence of neuropathologic entities, and at present its pathogenesis is unknown despite careful clinicopathologic analysis of several cases.[2,21,36,76,117] Usually the vasculitis takes the form of a chronic granulomatous angiitis, with prominent multinucleated foreign body-type giant cells. Although most examples of CAA with chronic granulomatous angiitis (CAA/CGA) occur in the more common aging or AD-associated form of CAA, rarely, multinucleated giant cells are seen in reaction to microvascular amyloid in patients with HCHWA-D. Clinical presentation is extremely variable, but sometimes relates to CNS hemorrhage, which usually occurs in the presence of CAA without CGA. The age range of patients affected is substantial; virtually all reported examples have occurred in patients from 40 to 85 years, with a slight male preponderance. Survival is extremely variable, and there is anecdotal evidence that some patients improve with steroid therapy.

Histopathologic findings are, as expected, those of chronic granulomatous angiitis superimposed on CAA. Involvement of meningeal or cortical vessels may predominate, although in some instances both parenchymal and meningeal arterioles are involved. Even in the absence of grossly visible bleeding in affected brains, there is often microscopic evidence of old and recent cortical hemorrhage, sometimes with associated infarcts. Very commonly, multinucleated giant cells are seen aligned adjacent to beta/A4 immunoreactive microvascular amyloid deposits present in the walls of vessels,[106] suggesting that the giant cell arteritis is a response to the presence of amyloid in vessels walls, rather than a *cause* of amyloid deposition in vessel walls.[2,36]

Accepting the hypothesis that the vascular deposits of CAA in most patients with CAA/CGA elicit a perivascular inflammatory response including multinucleated giant cells, one must explain what is unique about these individuals, as the vast majority of patients with CAA fail to show any significant inflammatory response to the microangiopathy. It is conceivable that beta/A4 or cystatin C protein in the vessel walls is altered, perhaps by association with a carbohydrate moiety or other antigen, or that genes encoding CAA proteins might have aberrant gene sequences, possibly as a result of somatic mutation, since CAA/CGA is usually not a familial condition. At present, there is no evidence for such a mutation based on analysis of APP- or cystatin C-specific gene sequence DNA examined from affected brain specimens.[2] Some studies suggest that CAA/CGA may result from the absence of amyloid P component (AP) in affected vessel walls; i.e., the suggestion has been made that amyloid P component is somehow protective against recognition of the amyloid as being foreign, with the resultant induction of phagocytic activity and granulomatous inflammatory response.[117] However, some cases of CAA/CGA occur in the presence of immunohistochemically demonstrable amyloid P component. Otherwise, CAA/CGA shows the presence of a mixture of CD4$^+$ and CD8$^+$ T-cells together with multinucleated giant cells (histiocytes) in the granulomatous inflammatory foci. The study of this extraordinarily rare coincidence of lesions, i.e., CAA and CGA, brings up the much more important issue of what response within brain parenchyma, if any, might be elicited by the presence of amyloid that is confined to microvessel walls. Initial immunohistochemical studies that have addressed this issue suggest that CAA amyloid deposition is associated with an increase or activation of monocyte/macrophage lineage cells.[117] Clearly, studies of relatively "pure" forms of CAA, specifically HCHWA-D and HCHWA-I, will be informative in answering questions related to the effects of CAA on surrounding brain parenchyma.

Future Prospects

Approaches to understanding the pathophysiology and clinicopathologic manifestations of CAA will require the skills of multidisciplinary investigators, ranging from clinical neuroscientists to molecular geneticists. Particularly important questions relevant to the pathogenesis of CAA include the following:

1. What effects, if any, on brain parenchyma result from the relatively "pure" deposition of amyloid proteins in the walls of cerebral microvessels?

2. Is the evolution of CAA, or indeed progression of cerebral amyloidosis, especially in AD/SDAT, amenable to intervention by a therapeutic process that can remove amyloid from the brain substance or microvessel wall once it has been deposited there? Can the formation and deposition of amyloid within CNS be predicted and prevented?

3. What are the precise cellular events that contribute to amyloid protein or precursor protein (APP, cystatin C) processing in the sm cells of cerebral arteriolar walls? To what extent can amyloid deposition be conceived of in physicochemical terms?[18,19,53]

4. How do amyloid protein molecules interact with nonamyloid protein molecules (e.g., proteoglycans) to result in amyloid deposition in microvessel walls?

5. Are CAA and AD/SDAT two diseases or one?[26,96]

At the same time as basic neuroscientists address the fundamental cellular and molecular biology relevant to the pathogenesis of CAA, clinicians might shortly have the opportunity to attempt interventional procedures aimed at diminishing amyloid load in CAA or preventing the development of CAA altogether. In order for this to be effective, adequate means to reliably image brain amyloid, including CAA, will need to be developed. Unfortunately, at present, the extent and severity of CAA can only be assessed most accurately at autopsy, though the severity of vascular change in a given brain region can be substantially estimated from a generous brain biopsy. Iatrogenic manipulation of the cellular processes that lead to CAA will require a detailed understanding of the molecular pathogenesis of CAA, as well as the use of novel methods of drug delivery to the brain that allow for their penetration across the BBB and arteriolar endothelium, into the arteriolar media and brain parenchyma itself. Development of therapeutic strategies to attack CAA is of key importance, given that with the aging population this form of microangiopathy is very likely to increase in prevalence. It is likely to become an even more important cause of stroke than it is at present.

Acknowledgments

Work in the author's laboratory was supported by P30 AG10123 and P01 AG12435. Benjamin Chen and Annetta Pierro assisted with manuscript preparation.

References

1. Anders KH, Secor DL, Vinters HV: Cerebral amyloid angiopathy (CAA) associated with ischemic necrosis, abstracted. J Neuropathol Exp Neurol 52:275, 1993
2. Anders KH, Wang ZZ, Kornfeld M et al: Giant cell arteritis in association with cerebral amyloid angiopathy: Immunohistochemical and molecular studies. Hum Pathol (in press)
3. Bell MA, Ball MJ: Neuritic plaques and vessels of visual cortex in aging and Alzheimer's disease. Neurobiol Aging 11:359, 1990
4. Bergeron C, Ranalli PJ, Miceli PN: Amyloid angiopathy in Alzheimer's disease. Can J Neurol Sci 14:564, 1987
5. Bird TD, Sumi SM, Nemens EJ et al: Phenotypic hetero-

geneity in familial Alzheimer's disease: a study of 24 kindreds. Ann Neurol 25:12, 1989

6. Blumenthal HT, Premachandra BN: The aging-disease dichotomy. Cerebral amyloid angiopathy—an independent entity associated with dementia. J Am Ger Soc 38:475, 1990

7. Briceno CE, Resch L, Bernstein M: Cerebral amyloid angiopathy presenting as a mass lesion. Stroke 18:234, 1987

8. Bornebroek M, Hann J, Maat-Schieman MLC et al: Herediatary cerebral hemorrhage with amyloidosis—Dutch type (HCHWA-D): I—A review of clinical, radiologic and genetic aspects. Brain Pathol 6:111, 1996

9. Castaño EM, Frangione B: Human amyloidosis, Alzheimer disease and related disorders. Lab Invest 58:122, 1988

10. Claudio L: Ultrastructural features of the blood-brain barrier in biopsy tissue from Alzheimer's disease patients. Acta Neuropathol 91:6, 1996

11. Corder EH, Saunders AM, Strittmatter WJ et al: Gene dosage of apolipoprotein E type 4 allele and the risk of Alzheimer's disease in late onset families. Science 261:921, 1993

12. Coria F, Rubio I: Cerebral amyloid angiopathies. Neuropathol Appl Neurobiol 22:216, 1996

13. Crooks DA: Cerebral amyloid angiopathy. J Neurol Neurosurg Psychiatry 57:1457, 1994

14. Davis-Salinas J, Van Nostrand WE: Amyloid beta-protein aggregation nullifies its pathologic properties in cultured cerebrovascular smooth muscle cells. J Biol Chem 270:20887, 1995

15. Delaère P, Duyckaerts C, He Y et al: Subtypes and differential laminar distributions of betaA4 deposits in Alzheimer's disease: relationship with the intellectual status of 26 cases. Acta Neuropathol 81:328, 1991

16. Duckett S (ed): The Pathology of The Aging Human Nervous System. Lea & Febiger, Philadelphia, 1991

17. Ellis RJ, Olichney JM, Thal LJ et al: Cerebral amyloid angiopathy in the brains of patients with Alzheimer's disease: the CERAD experience, part XV. Neurology 46:1592, 1996

18. Esler WP, Stimson ER, Ghilardi JR et al: *In vitro* growth of Alzheimer's disease beta-amyloid plaques displays first-order kinetics. Biochemistry 35:749, 1996

19. Esler WP, Stimson ER, Ghilardi JR et al: Point substitution in the central hydrophobic cluster of a human beta-amyloid congener disrupts peptide folding and abolishes plaque competence. Biochemistry 35:13914, 1996

20. Ferreiro JA, Ansbacher LE, Vinters HV: Stroke related to cerebral amyloid angiopathy: the significance of systemic vascular disease. J Neurol 236:267, 1989

21. Fountain NB, Eberhard DA: Primary angiitis of the central nervous system associated with cerebral amyloid angiopathy: report of two cases and review of the literature. Neurology 46:190, 1996

22. Frackowiak J, Mazur-Kolecka B, Wisniewski HM et al: Secretion and accumulation of Alzheimer's beta-protein by cultured vascular smooth muscle cells from old and young dogs. Brain Research 676:225, 1995

23. Frackowiak J, Zoltowska A, Wisniewski HM: Non-fibrillar beta-amyloid protein is associated with smooth mus-

cle cells of vessel walls in Alzheimer disease. J Neuropathol Exp Neurol 53:637, 1994

24. Games D, Adams D, Alessandrini R et al: Alzheimer-type neuropathology in transgenic mice overexpressing V717F beta-amyloid precursor protein. Nature 373:523, 1995

25. Garzuly F, Wisniewski T, Brittig F, Budka H: Familial meningocerebrovascular amyloidosis, Hungarian type, with mutant transthyretin (TTR Asp18Gly). Neurology 47:1562, 1996

26. Ghetti B, Piccardo P, Frangione B et al: Prion protein amyloidosis. Brain Pathol 6:127, 1996

27. Gilbert JJ, Vinters HV: Cerebral amyloid angiopathy: incidence and complications in the aging brain. I. Cerebral hemorrhage. Stroke 14:915, 1983

28. Glenner GG: Alzheimer's disease: the commonest form of amyloidosis. Arch Pathol Lab Med 107:281, 1983

29. Glenner GG: On causative theories in Alzheimer's disease. Hum Pathol 16:433, 1985

30. Glenner GG, Henry JH, Fujihara S: Congophilic angiopathy in the pathogenesis of Alzheimer's degeneration. Ann Pathol 1:120, 1981

31. Glenner GG, Wong CW: Alzheimer's disease and Down's syndrome: sharing of a unique cerebrovascular amyloid fibril protein. Biochem Biophys Res Commun 122:1131, 1984

32. Glenner GG, Wong CW: Alzheimer's disease: initial report of the purification and characterization of a novel cerebrovascular amyloid protein. Biochem Biophys Res Commun 120:885, 1984

33. Golde TE, Estus S, Usiak M et al: Expression of beta amyloid protein precursor mRNAs: recognition of a novel alternatively spliced form and quantitation in Alzheimer's disease using PCR. Neuron 4:253, 1990

34. Graffagnino C, Herbstreith MH, Schmechel DE et al: Cystatin C mutation in an elderly man with sporadic amyloid angiopathy and intracerebral hemorrhage. Stroke 26:2190, 1995

35. Gray F, Dubas F, Roullet E, Escourolle R: Leukoencephalopathy in diffuse hemorrhagic cerebral amyloid angiopathy. Ann Neurol 18:54, 1985

36. Gray F, Vinters HV, Le Noan H et al: Cerebral amyloid angiopathy and granulomatous angiitis: Immunohistochemical study using antibodies to the Alzheimer A4 peptide. Hum Pathol 21:1290, 1990

37. Greenberg SM, Kunz DP, Hedley-Whyte ET et al: Weekly clinicopathological exercises. Case: 22–1996. N Engl J Med 335:189, 1996

38. Greenberg SM, Rebeck GW, Vonsattel JPG et al: Apolipoprotein E epsilon4 and cerebral hemorrhage associated with amyloid angiopathy. Ann Neurol 38:254, 1995

39. Greenberg SM, Vonsattel JPG, Stakes JW et al: The clinical spectrum of cerebral amyloid angiopathy: presentations without lobar hemorrhage. Neurology 43:2073, 1993

40. Greene GM, Godersky JC, Biller J et al: Surgical experience with cerebral amyloid angiopathy. Stroke 21:1545, 1990

41. Haan J, Roos RAC, Algra PR et al: Hereditary cerebral haemorrhage with amyloidosis—Dutch type. Magnetic

resonance imaging findings in 7 cases. Brain 113:1251, 1990

42. Haas C, Selkoe DJ: Cellular processing of beta-amyloid precursor protein and the genesis of amyloid beta-peptide. Cell 75:1039, 1993

43. Hsiao K, Chapman P, Nilsen S et al: Correlative memory deficits, Abeta elevation, and amyloid plaques in transgenic mice. Science 274:99, 1996

44. Ikeda S-I, Allsop D, Glenner GG: Morphology and distribution of plaque and related deposits in the brains of Alzheimer's disease and control cases. An immunohistochemical study using amyloid beta-protein antibody. Lab Invest 60:113, 1989

45. Iwatsubo T, Mann DMA, Odaka A et al: Amyloid beta protein (Abeta) deposition: Abeta42 (43) precedes Abeta40 in Down syndrome. Ann Neurol 37:294, 1995

46. Joachim C, Games D, Morris J et al: Antibodies to non-beta regions of the beta-amyloid precursor protein detect a subset of senile plaques. Am J Pathol 138:373, 1991

47. Joachim CL, Mori H, Selkoe DJ: Amyloid beta-protein deposition in tissues other than brain in Alzheimer's disease. Nature 341:226, 1989

48. Joachim CL, Selkoe DJ: The seminal role of beta-amyloid in the pathogenesis of Alzheimer disease. Alz Dis Assoc Disorders 6:7, 1992

49. Kawai M, Kalaria RN, Cras P et al: Degeneration of vascular muscle cells in cerebral amyloid angiopathy of Alzheimer disease. Brain Research 623:142, 1993

50. Kawai M, Kalaria RN, Harik SI, Perry G: The relationship of amyloid plaques to cerebral capillaries in Alzheimer's disease. Am J Pathol 137:1435, 1990

51. Kitamoto T, Ogomori K, Tateishi J, Prusiner SB: Formic acid pretreatment enhances immunostaining of cerebral and systemic amyloids. Lab Invest 57:230, 1987

52. Kosik KS: Alzheimer's disease: A cell biological perspective. Science 256:780, 1992

53. Maggio JE, Mantyh PW: Brain amyloid—a physicochemical perspective. Brain Pathol 6:147, 1996

54. Mak K, Yang F, Vinters HV et al: Polyclonals to beta-amyloid (1–42) identify most plaque and vascular deposits in Alzheimer cortex, but not striatum. Brain Research 667:138, 1994

55. Mandybur TI: Cerebral amyloid angiopathy: the vascular pathology and complications. J Neuropathol Exp Neurol 45:79, 1986

56. Mandybur TI: The incidence of cerebral amyloid angiopathy in Alzheimer's disease. Neurology 25:120, 1975

57. Mann DMA, Jones D, Prinja D, Purkiss MS: The prevalence of amyloid (A4) protein deposits within the cerebral and cerebellar cortex in Down's syndrome and Alzheimer's disease. Acta Neuropathol 80:318, 1990

58. Marotta CA, Majocha RE, Tate B: Molecular and cellular biology of Alzheimer amyloid. J Mol Neurosci 3:111, 1992

59. Maat-Schieman MLC, Radder CM, van Duinen SG et al: Hereditary cerebral hemorrhage with amyloidosis (Dutch): a model for congophilic plaque formation without neurofibrillary pathology. Acta Neuropathol 88:371, 1994

60. Maat-Schieman MLC, van Duinen SG, Bornebroek M

et al: Hereditary cerebral hemorrhage with amyloidosis—Dutch type (HCHWA-D): II—A review of histopathological aspects. Brain Pathol 6:115, 1996

61. Miyakawa T, Shimoji A, Kuramoto R, Higuchi Y: The relationship between senile plaques and cerebral blood vessels in Alzheimer's disease and senile dementia. Virchows Arch [Cell Pathol] 40:121, 1982

62. Miyakawa T, Uehara Y: Observations of amyloid angiopathy and senile plaques by the scanning electron microscope. Acta Neuropathol 48:153, 1979

63. Motter R, Vigo-Pelfrey C, Kholodenko D et al: Reduction of beta-amyloid peptide$_{42}$ in the cerebrospinal fluid of patients with Alzheimer's disease. Ann Neurol 38:643, 1995

64. Murphy M: The molecular pathogenesis of Alzheimer's disease: clinical prospects. Lancet 340:1512, 1992

65. Nakamura T, Shoji M, Harigaya Y et al: Amyloid beta protein levels in cerebrospinal fluid are elevated in early-onset Alzheimer's disease. Ann Neurol 36:903, 1994

66. Nicoll JAR, Burnett C, Love S et al: High frequency of apolipoprotein E epsilon2 in patients with cerebral hemorrhage due to cerebral amyloid angiopathy. Ann Neurol 39:682, 1996

67. Ohshima T, Endo T, Nukui H et al: Cerebral amyloid angiopathy as a cause of subarachnoid hemorrhage. Stroke 21:480, 1990

68. Okazaki H, Reagan TJ, Campbell RJ: Clinicopathologic studies of primary cerebral amyloid angiopathy. Mayo Clin Proc 54:22, 1979

69. Ólafsson Í, Thorsteinsson L, Jensson Ó: The molecular pathology of hereditary cystatin C amyloid angiopathy causing brain hemorrhage. Brain Pathol 6:121, 1996

69a. Olichney JM, Hansen LA, Hofstetter CR, Grundman M, Katzman R, Thal LJ: Cerebral infarction in Alzheimer's disease is associated with severe amyloid angiopathy and hypertension. Arch Neurol 52:702, 1995

70. Pardridge WM, Buciak JL, Yang J et al: Measurement of amyloid peptide precursor of Alzheimer disease in human blood by double antibody immunoradiometric assay. Alz Dis Assoc Disorders 5:12, 1991

71. Pardridge WM, Vinters HV, Yang J et al: Amyloid angiopathy of Alzheimer's disease: amino acid composition and partial sequence of a 4,200-Dalton peptide isolated from cortical microvessels. J Neurochem 49:1394, 1987

72. Pirttilä T, Mehta PD, Soininen H et al: Cerebrospinal fluid concentrations of soluble amyloid beta-protein and apolipoprotein E in patients with Alzheimer's disease. Correlations with amyloid load in the brain. Arch Neurol 53:189, 1996

73. Podlisny MB, Mammen AL, Schlossmacher MG et al: Detection of soluble forms of the beta-amyloid precursor protein in human plasma. Biochem Biophys Res Commun 167:1094, 1990

74. Prelli F, Castaño E, Glenner GG, Frangione B: Differences between vascular and plaque core amyloid in Alzheimer's disease. J Neurochem 51:648, 1988

75. Price DL, Sisodia SS, Gandy SE: Amyloid beta amyloidosis in Alzheimer's disease. Cur Opin Neurol 8:268, 1995

76. Rhodes RH, Madelaire NC, Petrelli M et al: Primary angiitis and angiopathy of the central nervous system

and their relationship to systemic giant cell arteritis. Arch Pathol Lab Med 119:334, 1995

77. Roberts GW, Lofthouse R, Allsop D et al: CNS amyloid proteins in neurodegenerative diseases. Neurology 38: 1534, 1988

78. Roher AE, Lowenson JD, Clarke S et al: Beta-amyloid-(1–42) is a major component of cerebrovascular amyloid deposits: Implications for the pathology of Alzheimer disease. Proc Natl Acad Sci USA 90:10836, 1993

79. Roses AD: Apolipoprotein E affects the rate of Alzheimer disease expression: beta-amyloid burden is a secondary consequence dependent on APOE genotype and duration of disease. J Neuropathol Exp Neurol 53:429, 1994

80. Saito Y, Buciak J, Yang J, Pardridge WM: Vector-mediated delivery of ^{125}I-labeled beta-amyloid peptide Abeta$^{1-40}$ through the blood-brain barrier and binding to Alzheimer disease amyloid of the Abeta$^{1-40}$/vector complex. Proc Natl Acad Sci USA 92:10227, 1995

81. Selkoe DJ: Alzheimer's disease: A central role for amyloid. J Neuropathol Exp Neurol 53:438, 1994

82. Selkoe DJ: The molecular pathology of Alzheimer's disease. Neuron 6:487, 1991

83. Selkoe DJ, Bell DS, Podlisny MB et al: Conservation of brain amyloid proteins in aged mammals and humans with Alzheimer's disease. Science 235:873, 1987

84. Shimode K, Fujihara S, Nakamura M et al: Diagnosis of cerebral amyloid angiopathy by enzyme-linked immunosorbent assay of cystatin C in cerebrospinal fluid. Stroke 22:860, 1991

85. Shinkai Y, Yoshimura M, Ito Y et al: Amyloid beta-proteins 1–40 and 1–42 (43) in the soluble fraction of extra- and intracranial blood vessels. Ann Neurol 38:421, 1995

86. Smith DB, Hitchcock M, Philpott PJ: Cerebral amyloid angiopathy presenting as transient ischemic attacks. Case report. J Neurosurg 63:963, 1985

87. Snow AD, Malouf AT: *In vitro* and *in vivo* models to unravel the potential roles of beta/A4 in the pathogenesis of Alzheimer's disease. Hippocampus 3:257, 1993

88. Snow AD, Mar H, Nochlin D et al: Early accumulation of heparin sulfate in neurons and in the beta-amyloid protein-containing lesions of Alzheimer's disease and Down's syndrome. Am J Pathol 137:1253, 1990

89. Stewart PA, Hayakawa K, Akers M-A, Vinters HV: A morphometric study of the blood-brain barrier in Alzheimer's disease. Lab Invest 67:734, 1992

90. Tokuda T, Ikeda S, Maruyama K et al: Spinal cord vascular and leptomeningeal amyloid beta-protein deposition in a case with cerebral amyloid angiopathy. Acta Neuropathol 84:207, 1992

91. van Gool WA, Kuiper MA, Walstra GJM et al: Concentrations of amyloid beta protein in cerebrospinal fluid of patients with Alzheimer's disease. Ann Neurol 37:277, 1995

92. Van Nostrand WE, Wagner SL, Shankle WR et al: Decreased levels of soluble amyloid beta-protein precursor in cerebrospinal fluid of live Alzheimer disease patients. Proc Natl Acad Sci USA 89:2551, 1992

93. Vidal R, Garzuly F, Budka H et al: Meningocerebrovascular amyloidosis associated with a novel transthyretin mis-sense mutation at codon (TTRD18G). Am J Pathol 148:361, 1996

94. Vinters HV: Amyloid and the central nervous system: the neurobiology, genetics and immunocytochemistry of a process important in neurodegenerative diseases and stroke. p. 55. In Cancilla PA, Vogel FS, Kaufman N (eds): Neuropathology. Williams & Wilkins, Baltimore, 1990

95. Vinters HV: Cerebral amyloid angiopathy. A critical review. Stroke 18:311, 1987

96. Vinters HV: Cerebral amyloid angiopathy and Alzheimer's disease: two entities or one? J Neurol Sci 112:1, 1992

97. Vinters HV: Cerebral amyloid angiopathy. p. 821. In Barnett HJM, Mohr JP, Stein BM, Yatsu FM (eds): Stroke. Pathophysiology, Diagnosis, and Management. 2nd Ed. Churchill Livingstone, New York, 1992

98. Vinters HV, Duckwiler GR: Intracranial hemorrhage in the normotensive elderly patient. Neuroimaging Clin North America 2:153, 1992

99. Vinters HV, Gilbert JJ: Cerebral amyloid angiopathy: incidence and complications in the aging brain. II. The distribution of amyloid vascular changes. Stroke 14:924, 1983

100. Vinters HV, Miller BL, Pardridge WM: Brain amyloid and Alzheimer disease. Ann Intern Med 109:41, 1988

101. Vinters HV, Nishimura GS, Secor DL, Pardridge WM: Immunoreactive A4 and gamma-trace peptide colocalization in amyloidotic arteriolar lesions in brains of patients with Alzheimer's disease. Am J Pathol 137:233, 1990

101a. Vinters HV, Pardridge WM, Secor DL, et al. p. 213. In Ginsberg MD, Dietrich WD (eds): Cerebrovascular Diseases. 16th Research (Princeton) Conference. Raven Press, New York, 1989

102. Vinters HV, Pardridge WM, Secor DL, Ishii N: Immunohistochemical study of cerebral amyloid angiopathy. II. Enhancement of immunostaining using formic acid pretreatment of tissue sections. Am J Pathol 133:150, 1988

103. Vinters HV, Pardridge WM, Yang J: Immunohistochemical study of cerebral amyloid angiopathy: use of an antiserum to a synthetic 28-amino-acid peptide fragment of the Alzheimer's disease amyloid precursor. Hum Pathol 19:214, 1988

104. Vinters HV, Secor DL, Pardridge WM, Gray F: Immunohistochemical study of cerebral amyloid angiopathy. III. Widespread Alzheimer A4 peptide in cerebral microvessel walls colocalizes with gamma trace in patients with leukoencephalopathy. Ann Neurol 28:34, 1990

105. Vinters HV, Secor DL, Read SL et al: Microvasculature in brain biopsy specimens from patients with Alzheimer's disease: an immunohistochemical and ultrastructural study. Ultrastruct Pathol 18:333, 1994

106. Vinters HV, Wang ZZ, Secor DL: Brain parenchymal and microvascular amyloid in Alzheimer's disease. Brain Pathol 6:179, 1996

107. Vonsattel JPG, Myers RH, Hedley-Whyte ET et al: Cerebral amyloid angiopathy without and with cerebral hemorrhages: a comparative histological study. Ann Neurol 30:637, 1991

108. Walker LC, Masters C, Beyreuther K, Price DL: Amyloid in the brains of aged squirrel monkeys. Acta Neuropathol 80:381, 1990

109. Walker LC, Price DL, Voytko ML, Schenk DB: Labeling of cerebral amyloid *in vivo* with a monoclonal antibody. J Neuropathol Exp Neurol 53:377, 1994

110. Wang ZZ, Jensson O, Thorsteinsson L, Vinters HV: Microvascular degeneration in hereditary cystatin C amyloid angiopathy of the brain. APMIS 105:41, 1997

111. Wei L, Walker LC, Levy E: Cystatin C Icelandic-like mutation in an animal model of cerebrovascular beta-amyloidosis. Stroke 27:2080, 1996

112. Wisniewski HM, Bancher C, Barcikowska M, et al: Spectrum of morphological appearance of amyloid deposits in Alzheimer's disease. Acta Neuropathol 78:337, 1989

113. Wisniewski HM, Frackowiak J, Mazur-Kolecka B: In vitro production of beta-amyloid in smooth muscle cells isolated from amyloid angiopathy-affected vessels. Neurosci Lett 183:120, 1995

114. Wisniewski HM, Fraçkowiak J, Zóltowska A, Kim KS: Vascular beta-amyloid in Alzheimer's disease angiopathy is produced by proliferating and degenerating smooth muscle cells. Amyloid: Intl J Exp Clin Invest 1:8, 1994

115. Wisniewski T, Frangione B: Molecular biology of Alzheimer's amyloid–Dutch variant. Mol Neurobiol 6:75, 1992

116. Wisniewski HM, Wegiel J, Wang KC, Lach B: Ultrastructural study of the cells forming amyloid in the cortical vessel wall in Alzheimer's disease. Acta Neuropathol 84:117, 1992

117. Yamada M, Itoh Y, Shintaku M et al: Immune reactions associated with cerebral amyloid angiopathy. Stroke 27:1155, 1996

118. Yamaguchi H, Yamazaki T, Lemere CA et al: Beta amyloid is focally deposited within the outer basement membrane in the amyloid angiopathy of Alzheimer's disease. An immunoelectron microscopic study. Am J Pathol 141:249, 1992

119. Yong WH, Robert ME, Secor DL et al: Cerebral hemorrhage with biopsy-proved amyloid angiopathy. Arch Neurol 49:51, 1992

CHAPTER 40

Coagulation Abnormalities in Stroke

BRUCE M. COULL

THOMAS G. DeLOUGHERY

WILLIAM M. FEINBERG

In normal circumstances the coagulation system is balanced between maintaining flowing blood in the vessels and stemming any leaks from disruptions in vessel integrity. However, many factors can upset that balance and result in thrombosis. Activation of blood coagulation with thrombosis is an obligatory event in almost all ischemic strokes. The formation of thrombus most often ensues from the sudden and pathologic activation of the hemostasis that may be found with endothelial injury within an atherosclerotic precerebral artery or within the heart. Whereas many well-defined defects in hemostasis are associated with hemorrhagic stroke, most coagulation disorders that favor ischemic stroke remain less well characterized. A predisposition to thrombotic events is often termed a hypercoagulable state by clinicians, but a better terminology when thrombosis is favored is a prethrombotic state, which may involve activated blood coagulation, increased platelet reactivity, or impaired fibrinolysis.

Pathogenesis of Thrombosis

VASCULAR INJURY

As shown in Figure 40.1, prevention of intravascular thrombosis involves a dynamic interplay between the normal blood vessel and certain plasma proteins, platelets, fibrin formation, and fibrinolysis. Interactions among multiple plasma proteins, protein C, protein S, antithrombin III (ATIII), tissue factor pathway inhibitor, and normal vascular endothelial cells form an important barrier to thrombosis. A key protein, thrombomodulin, is expressed on the endothelial surface and promotes the activation of protein C. When combined with another natural anticoagulant, protein S, this complex can rapidly inactivate activated factors V and VIII. By suppression of thrombin activation of thrombin-inducible fibrinolytic inhibitor, activated protein C may also have an indirect fibrinolytic effect. Protein S is found in the plasma as both an active (free) and an inactive (C4b binding protein bound) form. A glycosaminoglycan, heparan, is also widely distributed on the normal endothelial surface. Heparan binds and enhances the anticoagulant function of ATIII. Once bound to endothelial heparan, ATIII rapidly neutralizes the clotting enzyme thrombin, as well as activated factor X and other prothrombotic serine proteases.[28,55,56]

Vascular endothelial cells also inhibit platelet adhesion and platelet aggregation. When the endothelium is activated by local injury, inflammation, or other thrombogenic stimuli, prostacyclin (PGI_2) is released. PGI_2 leads to vasodilatation and inhibits platelet plug formation. Blood vessels may also markedly enhance local fibrinolysis via the synthesis and release of tissue plasminogen activator (tPA). Endothelium can synthesize and release nitric oxide, which has potent platelet inhibitory activity.[19,204]

Although usually a barrier against thrombosis, the normal vascular endothelium may become a potent prothrombotic surface when injured. Mediators of inflammation such as interleukin-1, tumor necrosis factor, and immune complexes may induce endothelial cells to express the prothrombotic tissue factor, expose binding sites for clotting factors, and downregulate thrombomodulin expression. With severe injury, endothelial cells may be lost from the vascular surface alto-

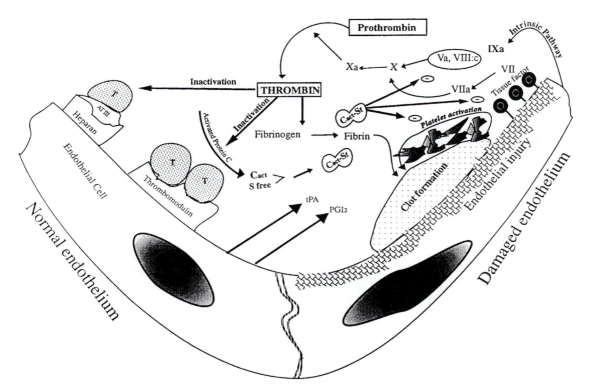

Figure 40.1 When vascular endothelium is injured, clot formation is instigated by expression of tissue factor and activation of platelets and the coagulation pathways. The pivotal reaction is transformation of prothrombin to thrombin (T) with cleavage of fibrinogen to fibrin. The normal endothelium limits thrombosis by inactivating thrombin and by releasing prostacyclin (PGI_2), and tissue plasminogen activator (tPA). Activated protein C (Cact) when complexed with free protein S (S free) antagonizes platelet and factor X activation. See text for details.

gether.[77,171] Brain vascular endothelium may not be as effective a barrier against thrombosis as vascular endothelium in other tissues. Some but not all studies suggest that the expression of thrombomodulin by brain vascular endothelium varies regionally within the brain and is limited in amount when compared with systemic vessels.[18,187]

In established atherosclerosis other prothrombotic factors also play a role. The atheromatous "gruel" that composes the inside of the plaque is rich in both tissue factor and lipids, which support coagulation reactions. For example, the rupture of an atherosclerotic plaque within a carotid or vertebral artery may expose the thrombogenic surface, which promotes mural thrombus formation. In addition, potent platelet activating surfaces are exposed that lead to platelet deposition.

FACTOR V LEIDEN, ANTITHROMBIN III, PROTEIN C, AND PROTEIN S DEFICIENCIES

Hereditary Deficiencies

By far the most common inherited defect leading to venous thrombosis is the clinical syndrome of hereditary resistance to activated protein C caused by the mutation in factor V

(factor V Leiden), which renders activated factor V unable to be cleaved by activated protein C. This defect is present in 1% to 9% of normal populations, 20% of patients suffering from their first episode of deep venous thrombosis, and 60% of patients with recurrent venous thromboses due to hypercoagulable states. Several case-control and prospective studies have failed to find evidence of an important contribution of the factor V Leiden mutation in arterial stroke.[152,162]

Much less common are deficiencies or defects in protein C, protein S, and ATIII (approximately 1:1,000 to 5,000 people). People who carry these defects have a higher incidence of thrombosis than people with factor V Leiden.[67] Unlike ATIII deficiency, protein C and protein S deficiencies can be associated with superficial thrombophlebitis.[147] The cerebral event most often associated with defects in these anticoagulant systems, including factor V Leiden, is cerebral vein thrombosis, which may occur in 1% to 3% of affected patients, many of whom are young adults with these defects.[22,25,48,50,93,203] The clinical presentation is distinct from children who have cerebral vein thrombosis due to ear infections or dehydration. In the absence of an established explanation, patients with cerebral vein thrombosis should receive testing for these coagulation abnormalities.

Although patients with arterial strokes are often screened for defects in natural anticoagulants, hypercoagulable states such as protein C deficiency have never been convincingly shown to be associated with premature atherosclerosis, and family studies do not reveal an overabundance of arterial events in patients with protein C, protein S, or ATIII deficiency.[133,144,162] The high prevalence of factor V Leiden has allowed testing of the hypothesis that this defect is associated with arterial stroke. In a group of well-defined patients no increased risk was seen.[152] This has been verified in several other populations.[162] Two studies, one of them retrospective, have failed to document deficiencies in the natural anticoagulant proteins in most patients who experience stroke. A prospective study did find free protein S deficiency in 23% of young patients with stroke of uncertain cause.[85] However, a more recent case-control study found that low protein S levels were common in hospitalized patients.[133] C4b binding protein is an acute-phase reactant. This higher level of C4b binding protein binds and reduces levels of free protein S. In another prospective study D'Angelo and colleagues[42] reported that a reduced protein C level measured at the time of acute stroke was correlated with a poor outcome, but no differences in ATIII levels were found between survivors and nonsurvivors of stroke. However, levels of these natural anticoagulants can be decreased in any acute inflammatory situation and these results must be viewed with this perspective.

The laboratory tests one should choose for measuring these factors are activity assays. Ten percent of defects are in the functional aspect of the molecule and will be missed with antigen assays. In addition, 60% of protein S is bound to C4b binding protein. The most common defect in protein S is a normal total protein S level but decreased free levels of protein S.[35] Thus, if one only assays total protein S levels, many patients with defects will be missed. Two clinical assays for factor V Leiden are available. The activated protein C resistance test is a coagulation-based test that measures the ability of added activated protein C to prolong the activated partial thromboplastin time (aPTT). This is compared with a control and a ratio determined. Although inexpensive and relatively easy, this test suffers from several problems. One problem is that normal patients with high levels of factor VIII may have ratios sufficiently low to overlap with the abnormal range. This can be seen with pregnant patients. Secondly, some patients with ratios in the low normal range will have the defect on genetic analysis. This test is also affected by heparin, warfarin, and lupus inhibitors. A newer testing methodology is being developed to overcome some of these problems.

More than 95% of patients with resistance to activated protein C have the ARG506GLN mutation defect, which is readily identifiable by polymerase chain reaction technology. This allows definitive diagnosis and determination of heterozygote and homozygote states.

Acquired Deficiencies

Acquired deficiencies of ATIII and proteins C and S have also been reported to produce a prethrombotic state related to brain infarction. Although extensive epidemiologic studies have not yet been performed, acquired anticoagulant protein deficiencies are usually associated with stroke in special clinical settings. Many of these clinical situations are outlined in

Table 40.1 Acquired Deficiencies of Antithrombin III and Proteins C and S

Consumption coagulopathy
Disseminated intravascular coagulation (shock, sepsis)
Surgery
Pre-eclampsia
Liver dysfunction
Acute hepatic failure
Cirrhosis
Renal disease
Nephrotic syndrome
Hemolytic-uremic syndrome
Malignancies
Leukemia (acute promyelocytic leukemia)
Malnutrition or gastrointestinal loss
Vascular reconstruction (diabetes, age)
Protein-calorie deprivation
Inflammatory bowel disease
Drugs
Estrogens-progestins
Heparin
L-asparaginase
Other
Vasculitis (? systemic lupus erythematosus)
Infection—neutropenia
Hemodialysis
Plasmapheresis

Table 40.1. Reduced levels of the anticoagulant proteins have been found in perioperative settings in women who are pregnant or taking oral contraceptives, and in patients with malignancies, hepatic failure, or the nephrotic syndrome. Acute fluctuations of anticoagulant protein levels can also follow plasmapheresis and hemodialysis. When transient ischemic attacks (TIAs), stroke, or amaurosis fugax are encountered in patients with any of these conditions, careful evaluation may uncover one of these prethrombotic states.

ACTIVATION OF HEMOSTASIS AND FIBRIN FORMATION

Simple assays are now available for measuring specific activation and breakdown products of coagulation.[119,169] When prothrombin is cleaved by factor Xa to form thrombin, the activation peptide ($F_{1.2}$) is cleaved off. The plasma levels of $F_{1.2}$ reflect ongoing activation of hemostasis. The conversion of fibrinogen to cross-linked fibrin clot is a complex multistep process that is mediated by thrombin. In the first step thrombin cleaves off fibrinopeptides A and B to form circulating fibrin monomers. The circulating fibrin monomer is then covalently cross-linked by thrombin-activated factor XIII. When the fibrin clot is lysed via fibrinolysis, specific breakdown products form. These include either nonspecific fibrin(ogen) degradation products or D-dimer that is specific to fibrin degradation.[4,141,143]

During the acute phase of ischemic stroke the intense activation of coagulation produces elevated levels of hemostatic markers including fibrinopeptide A, prothrombin activation fragment $F_{1,2}$, and thrombin-antithrombin complex.[42, 61,63,68,99,180,181,184] These markers decline slowly, but elevated levels may persist for weeks to months,[61,181] and some studies have found persistent elevation in these markers in patients with chronic stroke compared with controls.[184,185,205] One possible conclusion from these data is that there is an underlying prothrombotic state in patients with cerebrovascular disease. However, prospective data from large patient cohorts are lacking to support this notion. Elevated levels of hemostatic markers have been found in patients with atrial fibrillation.[10,60,86,114] The levels of these markers are reduced by anticoagulation[62,111,125] and have been reported to decline after cardioversion.[123] To date, levels of these hemostatic markers have not been correlated prospectively with stroke risk.

Fibrinogen itself is a strong independent risk factor for myocardial infarction and stroke.[36,52,54,105,123,127,155,202,206] Fibrinogen levels increase after stroke,[38] and elevated fibrinogen levels are associated with an increased risk of further cardiovascular events in stroke survivors.[38,158] Patients who have infection-associated stroke have higher levels of fibrinogen after stroke than those without a recent infection.[5] Possible mechanisms for the increased risk of stroke include activation of hemostasis, increased blood viscosity, a reflection of underlying inflammation, and decreased cerebral blood flow.[53,155] Fibrinogen also plays a critical role in platelet activation through binding to platelet glycoprotein IIb-IIIa membrane receptors,[29] which might be another mechanism favoring thrombosis. Although there is a strong statistical association between fibrinogen levels and stroke risk, the utility of monitoring fibrinogen levels in individual patients as a marker of stroke risk is unproved.

FIBRINOLYSIS

Homeostasis depends on the balance between clot formation and clot degradation or fibrinolysis. Depression of fibrinolytic activity can tip the balance toward thrombosis. The fibrinolytic system is equilibrated between tPA and its primary inhibitor, plasminogen activator inhibitor type one (PAI-1). Either reduced levels of tPA or elevated levels of PAI-1 can inhibit fibrinolysis and predispose to thrombosis. Both of these mechanisms have been suggested in venous thrombosis[101] but have not been comprehensively studied in stroke. However, several rare inherited conditions are associated with depressed fibrinolysis including plasminogen deficiency, qualitative plasminogen abnormalities, plasminogen activator deficiency, elevation of PAI-1, dysfibrinogenemia, and factor XII/prekallikrein deficiency.[16,47,73,75,89,100,140] These disorders usually present with venous thrombosis, but cases of arterial thrombosis including stroke have been described.

Fibrinolytic degradation products such as cross-linked D-dimer are increased after stroke[58,61,68,181,184] and levels are correlated with stroke size, severity, and subsequent mortality.[63] Peak levels of D-dimer occur later than the peak of fibrin markers, suggesting a relative excess of fibrin formation over

fibrin(ogen)olysis in the acute phase of stroke. Functional assays have shown decreased stimulatable fibrinolytic activity after stroke.[79,107]

Although elevated levels of both tPA antigen and PAI-1 antigen have been observed after stroke,[27,122,131,185] the elevated levels of tPA antigen do not necessarily indicate elevated plasma fibrinolytic activity, since much of the tPA may be bound to PAI-1. Prospective population studies have demonstrated the seemingly paradoxical finding that elevated tPA antigen levels are associated with an increased risk of myocardial infarction and stroke.[44,160,161] Elevated tPA antigen levels are also associated with the degree of carotid atherosclerosis.[166] Elevated tPA levels do not necessarily denote increased fibrinolytic activity, but instead may indicate an ongoing response to atherosclerosis and thrombosis and increased clot formation rather than a more effective fibrinolytic response. Furthermore, like the increase in PGI_2 seen in patients with atherosclerosis, elevated tPA may be just a marker for ongoing endothelial damage.[142] These markers may eventually provide additional information for identifying patients at high risk of stroke.

At least one lipoprotein, lipoprotein (a) [Lp(a)], can inhibit fibrinolysis in vitro and may have a similar important effect in vivo.[172] Lp(a) has substantial homology to plasminogen, the precursor to plasmin.[135] Lp(a) also stimulates the release of PAI-1 from endothelial cells and effectively competes with plasminogen for binding either to fibrin or to the surface of vascular endothelial cells, inhibiting fibrinolysis.[57,87] Lp(a) levels have recently been found to be elevated in selected populations with cerebrovascular disease, and most, but not all, studies have shown elevated levels of Lp(a) to be a potent risk factor for stroke, especially in young patients.[72, 102,117,170,176,207] However, Lp(a) levels do not appear to be associated with stroke characteristics, recurrence, or prognosis.[163,195] Unfortunately there is no established treatment for increased Lp(a) levels and management consists of aggressively controlling other risk factors, especially lowering the low density lipoprotein (LDL) cholesterol to <100.

INCREASED PLATELET REACTIVITY

The concept that increased platelet reactivity may contribute to stroke is reasonable but has not been thoroughly tested, in part because of a lack of sensitive and specific laboratory assays for platelet activity. Increased platelet aggregation after stroke and TIA has been demonstrated by elevated levels of platelet release proteins[58,61,63,68,69,173,182] and more recently by urinary metabolites of thromboxane.[113,194] However, a chronic state of increased platelet reactivity is difficult to demonstrate. Patients with extensive peripheral atherosclerosis or marked hypercholesterolemia also exhibit similar evidence of enhanced platelet activation,[70] but these observations have not been prospectively correlated with stroke risk. Several small series using in vitro platelet aggregation have been said to show "aspirin non-responders,"[1,90] but this technique has technical limitations.

In contrast to the uncertain role of platelet reactivity in most patients with ischemic stroke, patients with myeloproliferative disease (MPD) including polycythemia vera rubra (PV) and essential thrombocythemia (ET) have increased platelet reactivity, increased platelet counts, and large, dysfunctional platelets, which are strongly associated with stroke.[9,97,138,168] Thrombosis occurs more frequently in PV and ET than in acute myelocytic leukemia or chronic granulocytic leukemia and is a major cause of morbidity and mortality in patients with these myeloproliferative disorders. Up to 40% of patients with PV or ET will experience a thrombotic episode, and the incidence of thrombosis could be as high as 75%/year. Arterial occlusions are more common than venous events,[34,98,139,164,168,192] and stroke is often the presenting feature of both PV and ET. At the time of diagnosis, 25% of patients with myeloproliferative syndromes manifest atherosclerosis, and one study showed 50% of patients with evidence of carotid intimal thickening. Increasing age, elevated hematocrit, and treatment with phlebotomy in PV all predispose to thromboembolism. Importantly, the magnitude of the elevation of the platelet count does not correlate with the risk of thrombosis. In a recent study the average platelet count at the time of stroke was 600,000, but two thirds of patients had counts <400,000. In the absence of MPD, secondary thrombocytosis is an occasional but much less common cause of stroke.[41,167]

Antiplatelet therapy, usually with aspirin, is recommended for treatment of patients with cerebral, coronary artery, or peripheral vascular thrombosis. Platelet inhibitors usually suppress the platelet hyper-reactivity associated with MPD and can increase the usually shortened mean platelet survival time.[193] Lower doses of aspirin (e.g., <80 mg daily) should probably be avoided because these doses may not suppress platelet function in some patients. In addition to its antithrombotic effects, aspirin may also inhibit platelet secretion of vascular growth factors and inflammatory cytokines, thereby reducing chronic vascular damage.

In addition to pharmacologic antithrombotic measures, lowering of elevated platelet counts should be considered in patients with MPD and a history of thrombosis. Hydroxyurea (e.g., 1 g daily to start) has been shown in a randomized trial to prevent thrombotic complications in patients with essential thrombocytosis.[193] A platelet count of 250,000 to 450,000/cm is an appropriate target. The use of anagrelide to lower platelet counts should be considered if patients become refractory to hydroxyurea or are unable to tolerate the drug.[193] α-Interferon has also been reported to be effective.

HEPARIN-INDUCED THROMBOCYTOPENIA

Heparin-induced thrombocytopenia (HIT) is an immune-mediated process in which antibodies against heparin are directed toward platelets, causing increased platelet activation.[14,109] Two classes of HIT have been described. Type I is relatively common, occurring 1 to 5 days after exposure to heparin. The platelet count may be as low as 50,000/mm^3, but the syndrome is clinically benign. It is thought to arise directly from heparin-mediated platelet aggregation.[14,109] Type II occurs 6 to 10 days after heparin exposure and is associated with a high risk of thrombotic events including stroke.[6,13–15,109,110] HIT may provide some insight into immune mechanisms that

promote thrombosis.[12,109] The HIT antibodies are IgG antibodies that bind to a complex of heparin and platelet factor 4.[96] HIT antibodies may also bind to heparan on the surface of endothelial cells and stimulate the production of tissue factor on the endothelial cell surface.[31]

The incidence of thromboembolism in patients receiving heparin has been estimated to be as high as 1% to 2%,[14] although 5% to 10% of patients may develop thrombocytopenia. Recent studies have shown that the incidence of HIT is considerably decreased with low molecular weight heparin.[201] A recent 14-year retrospective review found that patients identified with isolated HIT had a 30-day risk of thrombosis of 53%.[200] Most thromboses were venous. Although platelet counts in HIT may fall as low as 20,000/mm^3, hemorrhagic complications are uncommon. HIT is often seen in postsurgical settings, perhaps due to the combined influence of surgery-induced inflammation and heparin exposure. Atkinson and colleagues[13] have emphasized the relationship between HIT and ischemic stroke after endarterectomy. Becker and Miller[14] reviewed 29 patients with HIT-related stroke from the literature. They found that few patients had previous cerebrovascular disease and that most patients either died (25%) or were left disabled from their strokes. HIT has also been associated with cerebral venous thrombosis.[115] Prevention of HIT is the best management strategy, and patients on heparin should have platelet counts closely monitored. Once HIT is recognized, heparin should be promptly discontinued. Since low molecular weight heparin will cross-react with antiheparin antibodies, once cannot use these agents for anticoagulation in patients with HIT. Currently a heparanoid, ORG10172 (Organon), is approved for use in patients with HIT.

ANTIPHOSPHOLIPID ANTIBODIES

Antiphospholipids (aPLs) are polyclonal, polyclass antibodies directed against certain phospholipids.[49,81,118,128,174] They are produced in a variety of clinical situations and are important to recognize because in certain patients aPLs are associated with a hypercoagulable state characterized by thrombocytopenia, fetal loss, stroke, dementia, optic changes, Addison's disease, and skin rashes. aPLs were first described by Conley in the 1950s when it was noted that patients with systemic lupus erythematosus (SLE) often had prolonged aPTTs. Soon after an association with false-positive Venereal Disease Research Laboratory (tests) (VDRLs) was noted. Despite the elevation of the aPTT it was observed that these patients did not develop hemorrhagic complications unless they also had hypoprothrombinemia or thrombocytopenia. Bowie first described the association of aPL and thrombosis in 1964. Feinstein and Rapaport in a 1972 review called this phenomenon the lupus anticoagulant. Harris, recognizing that cardiolipin is a major component of the VDRL test, developed and popularized the anticardiolipin (aCL) antibody test in the mid-1980s. In the 1980s it become well recognized that patients did not have to have SLE to have symptomatic disease from aPL.

Semantically, patients with aPL and one major clinical

criterion are said to have the aPL syndrome. The major clinical criteria include venous or arterial thrombosis (including neurologic disease), thrombocytopenia, or frequent miscarriages. Clinical criteria in patients with aPL who do not have lupus or other rheumatologic or autoimmune disorders define the primary antiphospholipid antibody syndrome (PAPS). In distinction to SLE-aPL patients, patients with PAPS are more often male and typically have low- or normal-titer antinuclear antibodies and no other criteria for SLE. In SLE and related rheumatic illnesses aPLs impart an increased risk of thrombosis similar to that observed in PAPS.[80,95,186] In one series of more than 1,000 patients with SLE, neurologic disorders were strongly associated with the presence of either the lupus anticoagulant (LA) or aCL.[126] The terms lupus anticoagulant and lupus inhibitor are used interchangably for aPLs that prolong the aPTT. Studies have established that aCLs and LAs are quite distinct in their epitope specificity and differ in their thrombogenic potential. Certain aPLs also require a cofactor termed apolipoprotein H or β_2-glycoprotein-I for epitope binding, and not all aPLs that are detected with enzyme-linked immunosorbent assay (ELISA) methods are thrombogenic.[64] These observations may help to clarify much of the confusion about the role of differing aPLs in stroke. One recent observation that will require further study is the finding that antibodies that react to oxidized LDL can cross-react with cardiolipin. Thus, the aCLs often seen in older stroke patients may be a manifestation of underlying oxidized LDL-induced atherosclerosis and not a true aPL syndrome.[191]

The prevalence of aPLs in healthy adults increases with age and is estimated to be 2% to 12%, depending on which tests are used for detection.[64,66,175] As evidenced by the Physicians Health Study, patients with aPL most often experience venous thrombosis, but an association with stroke and TIA is particularly well established in subjects with high levels of IgG aCL or those with an LA.[26,64,78,120] Case-control studies indicate that certain aPLs represent an independent risk factor for stroke. This association of aPL with ischemic events is strongest among young individuals, with a reported prevalence as high as 46%.[25] Hess and colleagues,[92] in a prospective hospital-based study of 110 patients (average age 58 years) admitted with a diagnosis of stroke or TIA, found an 8.2% prevalence of IgG aCL, compared with 1.6% in age-matched healthy blood donors. Stroke recurrence or mortality rates in subjects with aPL have been estimated from a few studies with limited numbers of patients. In a prospective study of 81 patients with aPL of the IgG class who presented with a first stroke or TIA, 31% experienced recurrent stroke with an average recurrence rate of 0.41 events/subject/yr (41% incidence).[120] The highest event rate was seen in patients with the highest levels of IgG aCL. Taken together, these reports suggest that aPL may be present in roughly 10% of all strokes and that the association is greater for stroke in the young, and especially in subjects with unexplained recurrent stroke.

The clinical presentation of stroke and TIA associated with aPL has few distinguishing features. Both large and small cerebral arterial occlusions in either the anterior and posterior circulations as well as venous occlusions are all reported to occur. Amaurosis fugax, retinal vein or artery occlusion, ischemic retinopathy, ophthalmoplegia from a cranial neuropathy, and migraine-like positive or negative visual phenomena, with or without headache, have been emphasized in some case reports. Although deep lacunar infarctions and isolated white matter signal-enhancing lesions on magnetic resonance imaging (MRI) and large brain infarctions occur, most strokes are relatively small and involve cortex and subadjacent white matter. No single mechanism for stroke associated with aPL has been established, but a few pathologic reports have demonstrated nonspecific microvascular platelet-fibrin plugs, suggesting possible thrombosis in situ. However, cardiac lesions, including mitral valve degeneration and nonbacterial thrombotic endocarditis, often accompany the aPL syndrome and could be responsible for these lesions as well.[20,94]

Sneddon syndrome, with stroke and livedo reticularis of the skin in the absence of systemic disease is a commonly encountered aPL relationship.[39,121,177] Besides livedo reticularis, some patients report Raynaud phenomenon and demonstrate acrocyanosis. Sneddon syndrome is more common in women than in men and has been linked to tobacco use. Skin biopsy demonstrates focal epidermal ulceration with chronic inflammatory infiltrates in the dermis, without evidence of vasculitis.[121] Vascular dementia, presumably from recurrent stroke, often ensues in patients with this syndrome. Although not all subjects with Sneddon syndrome harbor aPL, it appears likely that aPLs augur a worse prognosis among persons with Sneddon syndrome.[103] Patients with Sneddon syndrome are typically younger and have fewer stroke risk factors than older individuals with stroke but many Sneddon syndrome patients report migraine-like headaches and have hypertension. Progressive cognitive deterioration in the absence of a history of stroke-like episodes and despite antithrombotic therapy may occur. This clinical course is reminiscent of the insights of both Sneddon[177] and Rebello et al,[157] who emphasized that stroke with Sneddon syndrome often left little neurologic deficit but the patients gradually became demented nonetheless. Unfortunately, except for the possible relationship to high aCL levels and an LA, no specific findings identify those subjects who are likely to experience recurrent ischemic events and progressive dementia. Many patients with Sneddon syndrome eventually develop complex partial seizures. Generalized seizures and status epilepticus are also the cardinal feature of the syndrome of ischemic encephalopathy, which includes altered mental status, diffuse systemic involvement of pulmonary and cardiac function, and dermatologic manifestations.[11,26]

Myelopathy, especially in patients with SLE, has been associated with the aPL syndrome. Since the clinical presentation can be indistinguishable from the myelopathic form of multiple sclerosis, the term *lupoid sclerosis* has been suggested for this entity.[132] One peculiar form of dermatologic disease associated with myelopathy, brain infarction, and dementia is the Kohlmeier-Degos syndrome.[45,51] The vascular pathology appears to be identical to that described in Sneddon and other aPL syndromes: the skin signs are characterized by papules with a porcelain white center distributed over the trunk and extremities. This illness has a predilection for men, unlike Sneddon syndrome, and may frequently involve the gastrointestinal tract as well as the central nervous system.

A satisfactory explanation is lacking for the apparent prothrombotic state with aPL, but data from coagulation studies and the results of experiments with cultured vascular endothelial cells provide evidence that some aPLs interfere with the vascular endothelial anticoagulant functions, whereas others directly activate endothelial thrombogenic mechanisms. Membranes of circulating white blood cells and platelets have also been implicated as a target for prothrombotic binding of aPLs. The thrombogenicity of aPLs may stem from the targeting by aPLs of prothrombin on damaged membrane surfaces and the interference with the activated protein C pathway. aPls can interfere with thrombomodulin-induced protein C activation and also with protein S cofactor function for protein C. The importance of platelet activation in the process is supported by analysis of brain tissue removed from patients with aPL-related stroke in which small arteries and microvessels are occluded by platelet fibrin plugs. Thrombocytopenia is frequently noted during thrombotic episodes associated with aPL.[64] A possible explanation for this observation is that platelet membranes are rich in phospholipids upon which the prothrombinase complex can assemble.

The thorough evaluation of patients suspected of having aPL often requires multiple testing procedures because unfortunately no one test can adequately screen a patient for aPL.[81,188] An effective initial screen is the hexagonal phospholipid assay and the aCL assay. If these are negative but clinical suspicion remains high then further tests include (1) kaolin clotting time, (2) dilute Russell viper venom time (dRVVT), and (3) lupus inhibitor screen (different aPTT reagents). One caveat in testing is that levels of aPL may fall during thrombotic events and tests may need to be repeated in a steady state.

The two main groups of assays for aPLs include testing for the presence of antibodies to cardiolipin and the coagulation-based tests for aPL.

Coagulation-Based Tests

Since by definition aPLs react with phospholipids, and phospholipids are used in coagulation tests to provide a surface for the coagulation reaction to occur, all the coagulation tests are based on the premise that if there are antibodies binding to the phospholipid, the coagulation reaction will be slowed and the clotting time prolonged. For positive tests, verification that an elevated aPTT is due to an inhibitor is accomplished by demonstrating that the aPTT does not correct with a 50:50 mix. This involves performing an aPTT on an equal mixture of the patient's and normal pooled plasma. The mixture is incubated for 30, 60, and 120 minutes and aPTTs are done at each time point. For the three major diagnostic considerations, the aPTT behaves differently when the 50:50 mix is used:

1. Factor deficiency. aPTT will correct to normal at time 0 and stay in the normal range at each of the time points.

2. aPL. aPTT does not correct to normal (may partially correct) at time 0 or any time point; it may actually prolong further (lupus cofactor effect).

3. Factor inhibitors. aPTT corrects to normal at time 0 but then prolongs at the next time points.

Once it is established that the prolongation of the clotting time is due to an inhibitor, the dependence of the inhibitor on phospholipids should be demonstrated. To do this, phospholipids derived from platelets or hexagonal phase phospholipids (named for the shape they assume in suspension) are added to the patient's plasma. Since aPLs bind avidly to both platelet and hexagonal phase phospholipids, the addition of these lipids will correct the prolonged coagulation tests. Factor inhibitors will not correct with platelet phospholipids. Thus, suspect aPLs are identified with coagulation-based tests that demonstrate a prolonged clotting time; when a test is positive, a 50:50 mix is used to prove an inhibitor is the cause. Platelet membrane or hexagonal phospholipids are employed to correct the abnormal clotting time and thereby show phospholipid dependency. Tests for aPLs are as follows:

1. aPTT. This is only sensitive to 30% of aPLs. Sensitivity can be increased by using different reagents. Many patients with aPLs will have normal aPTTs and therefore this test alone cannot exclude aPLs.

2. dRVVT. This test is highly sensitive to interference with aPLs because very little phospholipid is added to the reaction. The test is performed by initiating the coagulation cascade with Russell viper venom.

3. Kaolin clotting time. This test uses no added phospholipid and is the most sensitive to aPL but is a very demanding technique.

4. Platelet neutralization test. When the coagulation reaction that is prolonged by a plasma sample does not correct with a 50:50 mix, extracts of platelet membranes are added to the reaction. If the coagulation time corrects to normal this is very specific for aPL.

5. Hexagonal phase phospholipids. This test follows the same principle as the platelet neutralization test but utilizes hexagonal phase phospholipids. This testing method may be used in the presence of therapeutic anticoagulants and other factor deficiencies. This is the only valid test for lupus inhibitors when patients are on anticoagulants.

Anticardiolipin Antibody Tests

An ELISA test is used for detecting antibodies to cardiolipin. Unlike the coagulation-based tests, ELISA can be performed on plasma that has been anticoagulated. Test results are reported either in standard deviation (SD) of optical density with >3 SD abnormal or in arbitrary units. Tests are also reported as specific isotype (IgG, IgA, IgM). It is still debatable whether specific isotypes are associated with different patterns of disease. The antibodies that react with cardiolipin on ELISA differ from those that cause the lupus inhibitor effect on coagulation tests. Only 60% of patients with aPLs will have both aCLs and lupus inhibitors. Consequently it is necessary to assay for both types of antibodies in assessing patients for aPLs. Recently it has been discovered that aCLs actually react with a complex of a cardiolipin and a protein known as β_2-glycoprotein I. ELISA tests utilizing this complex are being investigated to see if they provide more clinical information than the routine aPL ELISA.

Unfortunately, well-designed prospective studies to define effective treatment algorithms for most patients with aPL have not been performed. To prevent the high incidence of recurrent thrombotic events in certain patients, anecdotal evidence based on clinical case reports has advanced the notion that warfarin in doses sufficient to increase the international normalized ratio (INR) above 3 may be required and that ASA or warfarin at lower INRs is ineffective.[108] This approach is reasonable for treating patients who experience multiple thromboses or recurrent events, such as subjects with the Sneddon syndrome. Subjects with minimal symptoms or a single mild event may be given ASA, although the optimal dose is unknown. Coexisting risk factors, such as hypertension and cigarette smoking, should be aggressively treated since these risk factors are directly injurious to vascular endothelium. While it is possible to suppress the LA with prednisone, this treatment, except as indicated for coexisting SLE or other connective tissue diseases, has not been effective in the aPL syndrome.[64] For subjects who experience acute encephalopathy, seizures, or disseminated intravascular coagulation, plasmapheresis and immunosuppression therapy have been effective for short-term management in a few instances.[11,64]

Homocystinuria and Homocysteinemia

The 20-fold or more increases in plasma homocysteine, homocystine, cysteine-homocysteine, and related mixed disulfides (together termed homocyst(e)ine [Hcy] that typify homocystinuria produce premature atherosclerosis that is frequently complicated by early stroke or other large arterial occlu-

sions.[137] Homocystinuria is a metabolic consequence of one of several inborn errors of metabolism that impair cystathionine β-synthase (CBS) or several other enzyme systems important for methionine metabolism (Fig. 40-2). These are autosomal recessive traits, and persons homozygous for CBS deficiency often develop atherosclerosis and thromboembolic complications including stroke by age 30. The classic phenotype of children with homocystinuria includes ocular, vascular, skeletal, and nervous system abnormalities. Affected individuals may have a marfanoid habitus with arm spans greater than body height, setting-sun lenticular dislocations, and cognitive impairment. A malar flush and livedo reticularis are sometimes present, but the phenotypic expression varies considerably, and some individuals with homocystinuria exhibit none of these characteristics. About 0.3% to 1.5% of the general population may be heterozygous for CBS deficiency, with the estimated incidence of homocystinuria approximately 1 in 332,000 live births. In obligate heterozygotes, CBS activity is reduced by 50% but it is not known for certain whether these individuals are at increased risk of stroke.

In contrast to the striking plasma elevations found in homocystinuria, even modest elevations in plasma Hcy and related metabolites are now recognized as independent risk factors for ischemic stroke and related forms of atherosclerotic vascular disease.[21,71,82] Case-control studies suggest that as many as 30% of subjects with ischemic stroke have plasma levels of Hcy approximately 1.5 times higher than levels mea-

Figure 40.2 Methionine metabolism and homocysteinemia. Plasma homocysteine levels may increase because of genetic or acquired metabolic deficiencies in pathways of methionine metabolism. The principal causes include dysfunction of the cystathionine β-synthase enzyme system for cysteine metabolism and because of dysfunction of remethylation tetrahydrofolate (THF) pathway, as may occur with folate or vitamin B_{12} deficiencies. See text for details. N^5-MTHF, methyltetrahydrofolate.

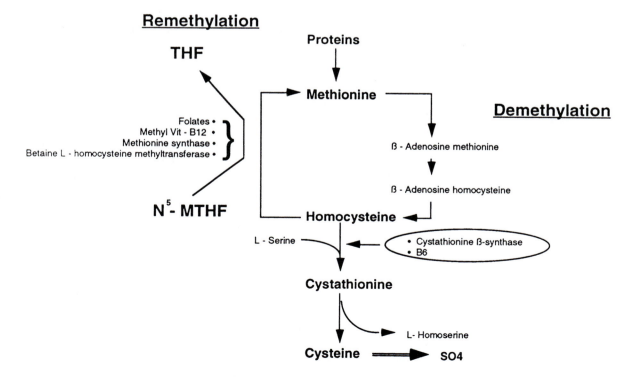

sured in healthy individuals of similar age and sex.[17,23,40] Plasma Hcy is lower in premenopausal women than in men of similar age, but levels increase with age and after menopause gender differences disappear altogether. Clarke et al[32] found plasma Hcy levels to be inversely related to red-cell folate and serum vitamin B_2 levels. Others have found a direct relationship between plasma Hcy levels and serum uric acid concentration.[40] However, the association of plasma Hcy with other stroke risk factors such as hypertension or diabetes mellitus is weak, and the current consensus is that elevated plasma Hcy is an independent risk factor for stroke.[21,148] Malinow and colleagues[130] found that modest rises of Hcy (>10.5 μmol/L) in asymptomatic adults increased the odds of carotid intimal thickening over threefold when compared with subjects with plasma Hcy levels <5.88 μmol/L. For elderly subjects, plasma Hcy levels of 14 to 16 μmol/L signify a relative risk of stroke of approximately 2.8 compared with subjects with levels <10 μmol/L. Prospective and case-control studies have found that the incidence of stroke increased with increasing Hcy levels.[130,148] Based on these findings, the attributable risk of stroke due to such modest increases in Hcy could be very significant because of the high prevalence of this mild degree of Hcy elevation.

The range of normal for serum Hcy is controversial. Given that folate deficiency raises Hcy levels and that almost 90% of the population does not ingest the minimal 400 μg/day of folate to maximally decrease folate levels, using population-based ranges of normal may underestimate the burden of excess Hcy. In metabolic ward studies in which subjects had Hcy measured after folate loading, the range of normal was 4 to 8 μmol/L.[189] These levels are lower than levels reported for some so called normal elderly populations.[40,196]

Besides certain genetic predispositions, many individuals are at risk of hyperhomocysteinemia because of acquired defects in methionine metabolism. As shown in Figure 40.2, decreased CBS activity and reduced remethylation of Hcy may produce hyperhomocysteinemia via abnormalities in folate-, cobalamine-, or betaine-dependent metabolic pathways. Data from case-control studies of normal subjects as well as those with vascular disease indicate that an inverse relationship exists between plasma folate and vitamin B_{12} levels and plasma Hcy concentration. This observation may partially explain the results from follow-up of 2,006 subjects in the First National Health and Nutrition Examination Survey Follow-up Study in which a serum folate of <9.2 nmol/L was associated with slightly increased risk of stroke (relative risk 1.37).

Recently a mutation in methylenetetrahydrofolate reductase (MTHFR) in the folate pathway has been correlated with an increase in plasma Hcy and may possibly be a cardiovascular disease risk factor.[104] The common thermolabile MTHFR variant results from a C- to T-point mutation at nucleotide 677 (changing Ala to Val), which significantly reduces the enzyme's basal activity.[74] This mutation is prevalent in the population, with the frequency of heterozygotes being 40% to 50% and homozygotes 5% to 15% in several populations. Its presence has been associated with increased plasma Hcy and possibly an increase in myocardial infarctions.[76,112] Studies on the T667C mutation as a risk factor for myocardial infarctions and other vascular disease have given variable results. Kluijtmans et al[112] reported an odds ratio of 3 to 1 for premature myocardial infarction with the T667C mutation in a select group of patients. Gallagher and colleagues[76] also reported an increased risk in both heterozygous and homozygous patients for the T667C mutation. However, other studies have not shown an association between T667C and myocardial infarction and other vascular diseases.[46] Data are currently lacking for support of this mutation as a risk factor in stroke.

Numerous studies indicate that homocysteinemia promotes the development of premature atherosclerosis, and the vascular pathology of large arteries from subjects with homocysteinemia demonstrates features typical of atherosclerosis such as fibrous intimal plaques, medial fibrosis, and disruption of the internal elastic membranes.[134] Accumulation of lipids is less conspicuous in affected arteries, and despite the documentation of premature atherosclerosis, the vascular occlusive events appear to be disproportionate to the severity of arterial pathology. Converging lines of evidence from experimental studies have demonstrated a damaging effect of Hcy on vascular endothelial cells and interference with the regulatory functions of endothelial cells on coagulation and nitric oxide generation.[88,190]

Probably all young persons with unexplained stroke and especially those with atherosclerosis should have Hcy levels measured.[71] A single plasma determination is probably an effective screen, but some have advocated that giving a methionine load beforehand could increase the number of subjects testing positive by up to 30%. If elevated levels are detected, first-degree family members should also receive testing. Since hyperhomocysteinemia is not limited to young individuals, elderly patients with stroke and TIA due to atherosclerosis should be considered for testing if an obvious cause for the atherosclerosis is lacking. As indicated in Figure 40.2, when an elevated level of Hcy is detected, serum folate and vitamin B_{12} levels should also be measured. Establishing the presence of hyperhomocysteinemia has clinical utility, since even in the absence of low serum folate or B_{12}, plasma homocysteine may be lowered by giving dietary supplements of folic acid, biotin, and vitamins B_{12} and B_6.[71,129]

Sickle Cell Disease

A critical single-point mutation that causes the substitution of valine for glutamic acid in the hemoglobin b chain underlies sickle cell anemia (SSA) and its consequent disease (SSD). Biochemically, because the solubility of deoxyhemoglobin S is lower than normal hemoglobin, HbS polymerization occurs when SSA erythrocytes are exposed to acidotic or hypoxic environments.[85,106] The extremely rigid sickled erythrocyte produces a tremendous increase in blood viscosity that contributes to red blood cell sludging in the microcirculation during sickle crises. Even in the absence of crisis, SSA frequently causes a progressive systemic vasculopathy involving many organs including the brain.[165] Fortunately, this untoward result only happens in about 30% of patients with SSA. Individuals with SSD experience vascular occlusive events, often recurrent, which include catastrophic stroke as well as infarctions of the kidney, lungs, bone, skin, and eye. Symptoms usually begin in early childhood, but occasionally persons with SSA may live into early or middle adulthood before manifesting adverse effects.

The prevalence of sickle trait (HbSA) in black Americans is estimated to be about 8.5%, with hemoglobin HbSS occurring in up to 0.16% and the variant HbSC in 0.21% of black Americans. Roughly 10% of individuals with HbSS and 2% to 5% of those with HbSC will experience symptomatic stroke, but based on results from asymptomatic subjects with SSA who underwent brain MRI scanning, an additional 13% may develop asymptomatic stroke.[136] Unlike SSD, stroke with sickle trait usually occurs in circumstances that cause severe hypoxia, heat stress, or dehydration.[156,159]

As SSD develops, there is a progressive segmental narrowing of the distal internal carotid artery and portions of the circle of Willis and proximal branches of the major intracranial arteries.[179] Pathologically this large vessel arteriopathy demonstrates intimal proliferation and an increase in fibroblasts and smooth muscle cells within the arterial wall. The progressive nature of this occlusive arteriopathy is evidenced by the occasional development of the moyamoya phenomenon. Besides large arterial pathology, sickled cell plugging of the microcirculation and cerebral veins is also well documented.[150] These alterations of arterial, capillary, and venous circulation increase the risk of both brain infarction and intracerebral hemorrhage (ICH). The incidence of brain infarction peaks around age 10 and outnumbers ICH, which occurs more often in older subjects, by a ratio of 3 to 1. Typically, infarctions include both deep and subcortical structures, but brain stem, spinal cord, and retinal infarctions as well as dural sinus thrombosis have all been reported. Pavlakis and colleagues[145] have emphasized the occurrence of watershed or borderzone infarctions particularly in territories of the middle cerebral artery. They speculate that a combination of occlusive arteriopathy and perfusion failure produces watershed strokes. ICH in SSD can result either from medial necrosis of cerebral arterioles with subsequent vascular rupture, or from venous thrombosis. Increased cerebral blood flow, only partially explained by the underlying anemia, and increased cerebral blood volume may contribute to the predisposition to ICH.[153]

Mean blood velocities increase within the circle of Willis and middle cerebral artery as the cerebral arteriopathy in SSD develops. This observation has led to the increasingly widespread use of transcranial Doppler and cerebral MRI for the early detection of children with SSA who are at risk of stroke from SSD.[2,3,197] Besides helping to identify presymptomatic individuals, these techniques also effectively identify individuals with asymptomatic stroke or vasculopathy who may benefit from therapeutic intervention. Careful monitoring with transcranial Doppler is particularly useful for following patients who have already had a stroke and are receiving ongoing treatments.

Although some asymptomatic persons with SSA may tolerate HbS of up to 50%, the mainstay of treatment for SSD is repeated exchange transfusion to maintain the concentration of HbSS at <30%. This treatment is highly effective for reducing the risk of stroke in SSD.[146] For children with previous stroke, the risk of stroke recurrence is exceedingly high if HbS levels are not suppressed. Powars et al[151] reported a 67% recurrence in untreated persons, compared with a 10% incidence of recurrent stroke in those receiving repeated transfusions.

Table 40.2 Patients with Ischemic Stroke in Whom Additional Screening for Coagulopathies May Be Appropriate

Under age 50 with no obvious cause for stroke
Multiple unexplained strokes
Prior history of venous thrombosis
Family history of thrombosis
Abnormalities on routine screening coagulation tests

Chronic transfusion therapy should be maintained long term, since one study showed that even after 10 years of treatment the risk of stroke recurrence was 50% a year if transfusions were withheld.[2,43,199] Bone marrow transplantation is used to avoid the complications of repeated transfusions, but patients receiving this treatment are reported with stroke and other neurologic complications especially during the phase of profound thrombocytopenia.[198] The timing of bone marrow transplantation is controversial as one would like to transplant before end-stage organ damage occurs yet limit transplant to those patients destined to get these complications. There is as of yet no satisfactory answer to this dilemma.[149] The use of hydroxyurea has markedly decreased the incidence of sickle cell crisis in adults and children with severe disease.[30,33] However, it is too early to know if the use of hydroxyurea will decrease the incidence of vascular complication.

Screening of Stroke Patients for Coagulopathies

There is no simple answer to the question of which patients with stroke should receive additional testing for coagulation abnormalities.[83,89,183] Stroke patients in whom the yield of screening is likely to be highest are young patients, those with repeated unexplained strokes, and those with a prior history of thrombosis (particularly venous). Patients with unexplained cerebral venous thrombosis (cortical vein or sagittal sinus thrombosis) should be investigated for hypercoagulable condi-

Table 40.3 Laboratory Screening Tests for Coagulopathies in Selected Patients

Protein C, protein S, and antithrombin III levels by functional assay
Free protein S antigen
Anticardiolipin antibody assay by ELISA
Functional assay for lupus anticoagulant
Hemoglobin electrophoresis (especially in black Americans)
Homocyst(e)ine level
Lipoprotein(a)
Factor V Leiden by polymerase chain reaction, or functional assay for activated protein C resistance
Thrombin time for dysfibrinogenemia

Abbreviation: ELISA, enzyme-linked immunosorbent assay.

tions, especially APC-R. Patients with livedo reticularis and left heart valvular abnormalities and women with a history of spontaneous abortion should be screened for antiphospholipid antibodies. A hemoglobin electrophoresis should be considered in young black American patients. A suggested approach is summarized in Tables 40.2 and 40.3.

References

1. Ackerman RH, Newman KL: Incomplete antiplatelet effects in patients on aspirin compounds, abstracted. Ann Neurol 28:224, 1990

2. Adams RJ: Sickle cell disease and stroke [editorial; comment]. J Child Neurol 10:77, 1995

3. Adams RJ, Nichols FT, Figueroa R et al: Transcranial Doppler correlation with cerebral angiography in sickle cell disease. Stroke 23:1073, 1992

4. Alkjaersig N, Fletcher A: Catabolism and excretion of fibrinopeptide A. Blood 60:148, 1982

5. Ameriso SF, Wong VLY, Quismorio FP, Fisher M: Immunohematologic characteristics of infection-associated cerebral infarction. Stroke 22:1004, 1991

6. Ansell J, Deykin D: Heparin-induced thrombocytopenia and recurrent thromboembolism. Am J Hematol 8:325, 1980

7. The Antiphospholipid Antibodies and Stroke Study (APASS) Group: Anticardiolipin antibodies are an independent risk factor for first ischemic stroke. Neurology (NY) 43:2069, 1993

8. Antiplatelet Trialists Collaboration: Collaborative overview of randomized trials of antiplatelet therapy. I. Prevention of death, myocardial infarction, and stroke by prolonged antiplatelet therapy in various categories of patients. BMJ 308:81, 1994

9. Arboix A, Besses C, Acin P et al: Ischemic stroke as first manifestation of essential thrombocythemia. Report of six cases. Stroke 26:1463, 1995

10. Asakura H, Hifumi S, Jokaji H et al: Prothrombin fragment F1 + 2 and thrombin-antithrombin complex are useful markers of the hypercoagulable state in atrial fibrillation. Blood Coagul Fibrinolysis 3:469, 1992

11. Asherson RA, Piette JC: The catastrophic antiphospholipid syndrome 1996: acute multi-organ failure associated with antiphospholipid antibodies: a review of 31 patients. Lupus 5:414, 1996

12. Aster R: Heparin-induced thrombocytopenia: understanding improves but questions remain [editorial]. J Lab Clin Med 127:418, 1996

13. Atkinson JL, Sundt Jr TM, Kazmier FJ et al: Heparin-induced thrombocytopenia and thrombosis in ischemic stroke. Mayo Clin Proc 63:353, 1988

14. Becker PS, Miller VT: Heparin-induced thrombocytopenia. Stroke 20:1449, 1989

15. Bell WR: Heparin-associated thrombocytopenia and thrombosis. J Lab Clin Med 111:600, 1988

16. Berdeaux D, Marlar R: Report of an American family with elevated PAI-1 as a cause of multiple thromboses

17. responsive to prednisone, abstracted. Thromb Haemost 65:1044, 1991

18. Boers GHJ, Smals AGH, Trijbels FJM et al: Heterozygosity for homocystinuria in premature peripheral and cerebral occlusive arterial disease. N Engl J Med 313:709, 1985

19. Boffa MC: Thrombomodulin in human brain microvasculature [letter]. Lupus 4:165, 1995

20. Bombeli T, Mueller M, Haeberli A: Anticoagulant properties of the vascular endothelium. Thromb Haemost 77:408, 1997

21. Bouillanne O, Millaire A, De Groote P et al: Prevalence and clinical significance of antiphospholipid antibodies in heart valve disease: a case-control study. Am Heart J 132:790, 1996

22. Boushey CJ, Beresford SAA, Omenn GS, Motulsky AG: A quantitative assessment of plasma homocysteine as a risk factor for vascular disease—probable benefits of increasing folic acid intakes. JAMA 274:1049, 1995

23. Bousser MG, Chiras J, Bories J, Castaigne P: Cerebral vein thrombosis—a review of 38 cases. Stroke 16:199, 1985

24. Brattstrom LE, Israelsson B, Jeppson J-O, Hultberg BL: Folic acid—an innocuous means to reduce plasma homocysteine. Scand J Clin Lab Invest 48:215, 1988

25. Brey RL, Coull BM: Cerebral venous thrombosis—role of activated protein C resistance and factor V gene mutation. Stroke 27:1719, 1996

26. Brey RL, Hart RG, Sherman DG, Tegeler CH: Antiphospholipid antibodies and cerebral ischemia in young people. Neurology (NY) 40:1190, 1990

27. Briley DP, Coull BM, Goodnight SH Jr: Neurological disease associated with antiphospholipid antibodies. Ann Neurol 25:221, 1989

28. Brockman MJ, Schwendemann G, Stief TW: Plasminogen activator inhibitor in acute stroke. Mol Chem Neuropathol 14:143, 1991

29. Broze GJ Jr: Tissue factor pathway inhibitor and the revised theory of coagulation. Annu Rev Med 46:103, 1995

30. Cahill M, Mistry R, Barnett DB: The human platelet fibrinogen receptor: clinical and therapeutic significance. Br J Clin Pharmacol 33:3, 1992

31. Charache S, Terrin ML, Moore RD et al: Multicenter Study of Hydroxyurea SCA. Effect of hydroxyurea on the frequency of painful crises in sickle cell anemia. N Engl J Med 332:1317, 1995

32. Cines DB, Tomasaki A, Tannenbaum S: Immune endothelial cell injury in heparin-associated thrombocytopenia. N Engl J Med 316:581, 1987

33. Clarke R, Daly L, Robinson K et al: Hyperhomocysteinemia: an independent risk factor for vascular disease. N Engl J Med 324:1149, 1991

34. Claster S, Vichinsky E: First report of reversal of organ dysfunction in sickle cell anemia by the use of hydroxyurea: splenic regeneration. Blood 88:1951, 1996

35. Colombi M, Radaelli F, Zocchi L, Maiolo AT: Thrombotic and hemorrhagic complications in essential thrombocythemia: a retrospective study of 103 patients. Cancer 67:2926, 1991

36. Comp PC, Doray D, Patton D, Esmon CT: An abnormal

distribution of protein S occurs in functional protein S deficiency. Blood 67:504, 1986

36. Cook NS, Ubben D: Fibrinogen as a major risk factor in cardiovascular disease. TIPS Rev 11:444, 1990

37. Cortelazzo S, Finazzi G, Ruggeri M et al: Hydroxyurea for patients with essential thrombocythemia and a high risk of thrombosis. N Engl J Med 332:1132, 1995

38. Coull B, Beamer N, de Garmo P et al: Chronic blood hyperviscosity in subjects with acute stroke, transient ischemic attack, and risk factors for stroke. Stroke 22:162, 1991

39. Coull BM, Bourdette DN, Goodnight SH et al: Multiple cerebral infarctions and dementia associated with anticardiolipin antibodies. Stroke 18:1107, 1987

40. Coull BM, Malinow MR, Beamer N et al: Elevated plasma homocyst(e)ine concentration as a possible independent risk factor for stroke. Stroke 21:572, 1990

41. Crowley JJ, Hannigan M, Daly K: Reactive thrombocytosis and stroke following cardiopulmonary bypass surgery: case report on three patients. Eur Heart J 15:1144, 1994

42. D'Angelo A, Landi G, D'Angelo SV et al: Protein C in acute stroke. Stroke 19:579, 1988

43. Davies SC, Olatunji PO: Blood transfusion in sickle cell disease. Vox Sang 68:145, 1995

44. de Bono D: Significance of raised plasma concentrations of tissue-type plasminogen activator and plasminogen activator inhibitor in patients at risk from ischaemic heart disease. Br Heart J 71:504, 1994

45. Degos R, Kalis B: La papulose atrophiante maligne. Rev Pract 19:4335, 1969

46. DeLoughery TG, Evans A, Sadeghi A et al: Common mutation in methylenetetrahydrofolate reductase—correlation with homocysteine metabolism and late-onset vascular disease. Circulation 94:3074, 1996

47. Dolan G, Greaves M, Cooper P, Preston FE: Thrombovascular disease and familial plasminogen deficiency: a report of three kindred. Br J Haematol 70:417, 1988

48. Dulli DA, Luzzio CC, Williams EC, Schutta HS: Cerebral venous thrombosis and activated protein C resistance. Stroke 27:1731, 1996

49. Emlen W: Antiphospholipid antibodies: new complexities and new assays. Arthritis Rheum 39:1441, 1996

50. Enevoldson TP, Russel RWR: Cerebral vein thrombosis: new causes for an old syndrome? Q J Med 77:1255, 1990

51. Englert H, Hawkes CH, Boey ML et al: Degos' disease: association with anticardiolipin antibodies and the lupus anticoagulant. BMJ 289:576, 1984

52. Ernst E: Plasma fibrinogen—an independent cardiovascular risk factor. J Intern Med 227:365, 1990

53. Ernst E: Fibrinogen as a cardiovascular risk factor—interrelationship with infections and inflammation. Eur Heart J (suppl K) 14:82, 1993

54. Ernst E, Resch KL: Fibrinogen as a cardiovascular risk factor: a meta-analysis and review of the literature. Ann Intern Med 118:956, 1993

55. Esmon CT: Molecular events that control the protein C anticoagulant pathway. Thromb Haemost 70:29, 1993

56. Esmon CT: Thrombomodulin as a model of molecular mechanisms that modulate protease specificity and function at the vessel surface. FASEB J 9:946, 1995

57. Etingin OR, Hajjar DP, Hajjar KA et al: Lipoprotein(a) regulates plasminogen activator inhibitor-1 expression in endothelial cells: a potential mechanism in thrombogenesis. J Biol Chem 266:2459, 1991

58. Feinberg WM, Bruck DC: Time course of platelet activation following acute ischemic stroke. J Stroke Cerebrovasc Dis 1:124, 1991

59. Feinberg WM, Bruck DC, Jeter MA, Corrigan JJ: Fibrinolysis after acute ischemic stroke. Thromb Res 64:117, 1991

60. Feinberg WM, Bruck DC, Pearce LA: Intravascular coagulation in patients with atrial fibrillation, abstracted. Neurology (NY) 41:298, 1991

61. Feinberg WM, Bruck DC, Ring ME, Corrigan JJ: Hemostatic markers in acute stroke. Stroke 20:592, 1989

62. Feinberg WM, Cornell ES, Nightingale SD et al: Relationship between prothrombin activation fragment F1.2 and international normalized ratio (INR) in patients with atrial fibrillation. Stroke 28:1101, 1997

63. Feinberg WM, Erickson LP, Bruck D, Kittelson J: Hemostatic markers in acute ischemic stroke. Association with stroke type, severity, and outcome. Stroke 27:1296, 1996

64. Feldmann E, Levine SR: Cerebrovascular disease with antiphospholipid antibodies: immune mechanisms, significance, and therapeutic options. Ann Neurol, suppl. 1, 37:S114, 1995

65. Ferster A, Vermylen C, Cornu G et al: Hydroxyurea for treatment of severe sickle cell anemia: a pediatric clinical trial. Blood 88:1960, 1996

66. Fields RA, Toubbeh H, Searles RP et al: The prevalence of anticardiolipin antibodies in a healthy elderly population and its association with antinuclear antibodies. J Rheumatol 16:623, 1989

67. Finazzi G, Barbui T: Different incidence of venous thrombosis in patients with inherited deficiencies of antithrombin III, protein C and protein S. Thromb Haemost 71:15, 1994

68. Fisher M, Francis R: Altered coagulation in cerebral ischemia. Platelet, thrombin, and plasmin activity. Arch Neurol 47:1075, 1990

69. Fisher M, Levine PH, Fullerton A et al: Marker proteins of platelet activation in patients with cerebrovascular disease. Stroke 39:692, 1982

70. Fitzgerald G, Smith B, Pedersen A, Brash A: Increased prostacyclin biosynthesis in patients with severe atherosclerosis and platelet activation. N Engl J Med 310:1065, 1984

71. Fortin IJ, Genest J Jr: Measurement of homocyst(e)ine in the prediction of atherosclerosis. Clin Biochem 28:155, 1995

72. Franceschini G, Cofrancesco E, Safa O et al: Association of lipoprotein(a) with atherothrombotic events and fibrinolytic variables. A case-control study. Thromb Res 78:227, 1995

73. Francis R: Clinical disorders of fibrinolysis: a critical review. Blut 59:1, 1989

74. Frosst P, Blom HJ, Milos R et al: A candidate genetic risk factor for vascular disease: a common mutation in methylenetetrahydrofolate reductase [letter]. Nature Genet 10:111, 1995

75. Furlan A, Lucas F, Craciun R, Wohl R: Stroke in a young adult with familial plasminogen disorder. Stroke 22:1598, 1991

76. Gallagher PM, Meleady R, Shields DC et al: Homocysteine and risk of premature coronary heart disease—evidence for a common gene mutation. Circulation 94:2154, 1996

77. Gimbrone MA Jr: Vascular endothelium: an integrator of pathophysiologic stimuli in atherosclerosis. Am J Cardiol 75:67B, 1995

78. Ginsburg KS, Liang MH, Newcomer L et al: Anticardiolipin antibodies and the risk for ischemic stroke and venous thrombosis. Ann Intern Med 117:997, 1992

79. Glueck C, Rorick M, Scherler M et al: Hypofibrinolytic and atherogenic risk factors for stroke. J Lab Clin Med 125:319, 1995

80. Goldstein R, Moulda JM, Smith CD, Sengar DP: MHC studies of the primary antiphospholipid antibody syndrome and of antiphospholipid antibodies in systemic lupus erythematosus. J Rheum 23:1173, 1996

81. Goodnight SH: Antiphospholipid antibodies and thrombosis. Curr Opin Hematol 1:354, 1994

82. Graham IM, Daly LE, Refsum HM et al: Plasma homocysteine as a risk factor for vascular disease. JAMA 277:1775, 1997

83. Greaves M: Coagulation abnormalities and cerebral infarction. J Neurol Neurosurg Psychiatry 56:433, 1993

84. Green D, Otoya J, Oriba H, Rovner R: Protein S deficiency in middle-aged women with stroke. Neurology (NY) 42:1029, 1992

85. Green MA, Noguchi CT, Marwah SS et al: Polymerization of sickle cell hemoglobin at arterial oxygen saturation impairs erythrocyte deformability. J Clin Invest 81:1669, 1988

86. Gustafsson C, BlombSck M, Britton M et al: Coagulation factors and the increased risk of stroke in nonvalvular atrial fibrillation. Stroke 21:47, 1990

87. Hajjar KA, Gavish D, Breslow JL, Nachman RL: Lipoprotein(a) modulation of endothelial cell surface fibrinolysis and its potential role in atherosclerosis. Nature 339:303, 1989

88. Harpel PC, Zhang X, Borth W: Homocysteine and hemostasis: pathogenic mechanisms predisposing to thrombosis. J Nutr suppl. 4, 126:1290S, 1996

89. Hart RG, Kanter MC: Hematologic disorders and ischemic stroke. A selective review. Stroke 21:1111, 1990

90. Helgason CM, Tortorice KL, Winkler SR et al: Aspirin response and failure in cerebral infarction. Stroke 24:345, 1993

91. Hess DC: Models for central nervous system complications of antiphospholipid syndrome. Lupus 3:253, 1994

92. Hess DC, Krauss J, Adams RJ et al: Anticardiolipin antibodies: a study of frequency in TIA and stroke. Neurology (NY) 41:525, 1991

93. Hoffman CJ, Miller RH, Hultin MB: Correlation of factor VII activity and antigen with cholesterol and triglycerides in healthy young adults. Arterioscler Thromb 12:267, 1992

94. Hojnik M, George J, Ziporen L, Shoenfeld Y: Heart valve involvement (Libman-Sacks endocarditis) in the antiphospholipid syndrome. Circulation 93:1579, 1996

95. Horbach DA, vai Oort E, Donderse RC et al: Lupus anticoagulant is the strongest risk factor for both venous and arterial thrombosis in patients with systemic lupus erythematosus. Comparison between different assays for the detection of antiphospholipid antibodies. Thromb Haemost 76:916, 1996

96. Horsewood P, Warkentin TE, Hayward CP, Kelton JG: The epitope specificity of heparin-induced thrombocytopenia. Br J Haematol 95:161, 1996

97. Jabaily J, Iland HJ, Laszlo J et al: Neurologic manifestations of essential thrombocythemia. Ann Intern Med 99:513, 1983

98. Johnson M, Gernsheimer T, Johansen K: Essential thrombocytosis: underemphasized cause of large-vessel thrombosis. J Vasc Surg 22:443, 1995

99. Jones SL, Close CF, Mattock MB et al: Plasma lipid and coagulation factor concentrations in insulin dependent diabetics with microalbuminuria. BMJ 298:487, 1989

100. Jorgenson M, Bonnevie-Nielsen V: Increased concentration of the fast-acting plasminogen activator inhibitor in plasma associated with familial venous thrombosis. Br J Haematol 65:175, 1987

101. Juhan-Vague I, Valdier J, Alessi M et al: Deficient t-PA release and elevated PA inhibitor levels in patients with spontaneous or recurrent deep venous thrombosis. Thromb Haemost 57:67, 1987

102. Jürgens F, Költringer P: Lipoprotein(a) in ischemic cerebrovascular disease: a new approach to the assessment of stroke. Neurology (NY) 37:513, 1987

103. Kalashnikova LA, Nasonov EL, Kushakhaeva AE, Grecheva LA: Anticardiolipin antibodies in Sneddon's syndrome. Neurology (NY) 40:464, 1990

104. Kang SS, Passen EL, Ruggie N et al: Thermolabile defect of methylenetetrahydrofolate reductase in coronary artery disease. Circulation 88:1463, 1993

105. Kannel WB, Wolf PA, Castelli WP, D'Agostino RB: Fibrinogen and risk of cardiovascular disease: the Framingham study. JAMA 258:1183, 1987

106. Keidan AJ, Sowter MC, Johnson CS et al: Effect of polymerization tendency of hematological, rheological and clinical parameters in sickle cell anemia. Br J Haematol 71:551, 1989

107. Kempter B, Peinemann A, Biniasch O, Haberl RL: Decreased fibrinolytic stimulation by short-term venous occlusion test in patients with cerebrovascular disease. Thromb Res 79:363, 1995

108. Khamashta MA, Cuadrado MJ, Mujic F et al: The management of thrombosis in the antiphospholipid-antibody syndrome. N Engl J Med 332:993, 1995

109. Kibbe MR, Rhee RY: Heparin-induced thrombocytopenia: pathophysiology. Semin Vasc Surg 9:284, 1996

110. King DJ, Keltron JG: Heparin-associated thrombocytopenia. Ann Intern Med 100:535, 1984

111. Kistler JP, Singer DE, Millenson MM et al: Effect of low-intensity warfarin anticoagulation on level of activity of the hemostatic system in patients with atrial fibrillation. Stroke 24:1360, 1993

112. Kluijtmans LAJ, Van den Heuvel LPWJ, Boers GHJ et al: Molecular genetic analysis of mild hyperhomocysteinemia: a common mutation in the methylenetetrahy-

drofolate reductase gene is a genetic risk factor for cardiovascular disease. Am J Hum Genet 58:35, 1996

113. Koudstall P, Ciabattoni G, van Gijn J et al: Increased thromboxane biosynthesis in patients with acute cerebral ischemia. Stroke 24:219, 1993

114. Kumagai K, Fukunami M, Ohmori M et al: Increased intravascular clotting in patients with chronic atrial fibrillation. J Am Coll Cardiol 16:377, 1990

115. Kyritsis AP, Williams EC, Schutta HS: Cerebral venous thrombosis due to heparin-induced thrombocytopenia. Stroke 21:1503, 1990

116. Landi G, D'Angelo A, Boccardi E et al: Venous thromboembolism in acute stroke: prognostic importance of hypercoagulability. Arch Neurol 49:279, 1992

117. Lassila R, Manninen V: Hypofibrinolysis and increased lipoprotein(a) coincide in stroke [editorial]. J Lab Clin Med 125:301, 1995

118. Leéon-Velarde F, Ramos MA, Hernández JA: The role of menopause in the development of chronic mountain sickness. Am J Physiol 272:R90, 1997

119. Leroy-Matheron C, Lamare M, Levent M, Gouault-Heilmann M: Markers of coagulation activation in inherited protein S deficiency. Thromb Res 67:607, 1992

120. Levine SR, Brey RL, Sawaya KL et al: Recurrent stroke and thrombo-occlusive events in the antiphospholipid syndrome. Ann Neurol 38:119, 1995

121. Levine SR, Langer SL, Albers JW, Welch KMA: Sneddon's syndrome: an antiphospholipid antibody syndrome? Neurology (NY) 38:798, 1998

122. Lindgren A, Lindoff C, Norrving B et al: Tissue plasminogen activator and plasminogen activator inhibitor-1 in stroke patients. Stroke 27:1066, 1996

123. Lip GY: Fibrinogen and cardiovascular disorders. Q J Med 88:155, 1995

124. Lip GY, Rumley A, Dunn FG, Lowe GD: Plasma fibrinogen and D-dimer in patients with atrial fibrillation: effects of cardioversion to sinus rhythm. Int J Cardiol 51:245, 1995

125. Lip GYH, Lip PL, Zarafis J et al: Fibrin D-dimer and β-thromboglobulin as markers of thrombogenesis and platelet activation in atrial fibrillation. Effects of introducing ultra-low-dose warfarin and aspirin. Circulation 94:425, 1996

126. Love PE, Santoro SA: Antiphospholipid antibodies: anticardiolipin and the lupus anticoagulant in systemic lupus erythematosus (SLE) and in non-SLE disorders. Ann Intern Med 112:682, 1990

127. Lowe GD, Lee AJ, Rumley A et al: Blood viscosity and risk of cardiovascular events: the Edinburgh Artery Study. Br J Haematol 96:168, 1997

128. Mackworth-Young CG: The Michael Mason Prize Essay (1994). Antiphospholipid antibodies and disease. Br J Rheumatol 34:1009, 1995

129. Malinow MR: Plasma homocyst(e)ine: a risk factor for arterial occlusive diseases. J Nutr suppl. 4, 126:1238S, 1996

130. Malinow MR, Nieto FJ, Szklo M et al: Carotid artery intimal-medial wall thickening and plasma homocyst(e)ine in asymptomatic adults. The Atherosclerosis Risk in Communities Study. Circulation 87:1107, 1993

131. Margaglione M, Di Minno G, Grandone E et al: Abnormally high circulation levels of tissue plasminogen activator and plasminogen activator inhibitor-1 in patients with a history of ischemic stroke. Arterioscler Thromb Vasc Biol 14:1741, 1994

132. Marullo S, Clauvel JP, Intrator L et al: Lupoid sclerosis with antiphospholipid and antimyelin antibodies. J Rheum 20:747, 1993

133. Mayer SA, Sacco RL, Hurlet-Jensen A et al: Free protein S deficiency in acute ischemic stroke: a case-control study. Stroke 24:224, 1993

134. McCully KS: Vascular pathology of homocysteinemia: implications for the pathogenesis of atherosclerosis. Am J Pathol 56:111, 1969

135. McLean JW, Tomlinson JE, Kuang WJ et al: cDNA sequence of human apolipoprotein (a) is homologous to plasminogen. Nature 330:132, 1987

136. Moser FG, Miller ST, Bello JA: The spectrum of brain abnormalities in sickle-cell disease: a report from the Cooperative Study of Sickle Cell Disease. AJNR 17:965, 1996

137. Mudd SH, Levy HL, Skouby F: Disorders of transsulfuration. p. 693. In Scriver C, Beaudet AL, Sly WS, Valle D (eds): The Metabolic Basis of Inherited Disease. 6th Ed. Vol. 1. McGraw-Hill, New York, 1989

138. Murphy S, Iland H, Rosenthal D, Laszlo J: Essential thrombocythemia: an interim report from the Polycythemia Vera Study Group. Semin Hematol 23:177, 1986

139. Murphy S, Peterson P, Iland H, Laszlo J: Experience of the Polycythemia Vera Study Group with essential thrombocythemia: a final report on diagnostic criteria, survival, and leukemic transition by treatment. Semin Hematol 34:29, 1997

140. Nagayama T, Shinohara Y, Nagayama M et al: Congenitally abnormal plasminogen in juvenile ischemic cerebrovascular disease. Stroke 24:2104, 1993

141. Nossel H: Relative proteolysis of fibrin B chain by thrombin and plasmin as a determinant of thrombosis. Nature 291:165, 1981

142. Oates JA, FitzGerald GA, Branch RA et al: Clinical implications of prostaglandin and thromboxane A2 formation. N Engl J Med 319:689, 1988

143. Owen J, Kvam D, Nossel H et al: Thrombin and plasmin activity and platelet activation in the development of venous thrombosis. Blood 60:476, 1983

144. Pabinger I, Schneider B, GTH Study Group Natural Inhibitors: Thrombotic risk of women with hereditary antithrombin III-, protein C- and protein S-deficiency taking oral contraceptive medication. Thromb Haemost 71:548, 1994

145. Pavlakis SG, Bello J, Prohovnik I et al: Brain infarction in sickle cell anemia: magnetic resonance imaging correlates. Ann Neurol 23:125, 1988

146. Pegelow CH, Adams RJ, McKie V et al: Risk of recurrent stroke in patients with sickle cell disease treated with erythrocyte transfusions. J Pediatr 126:896, 1995

147. Permpikul P, Rao LVM, Rapaport SI: Functional and binding studies of the roles of prothrombin and β-2-glycoprotein I in the expression of lupus anticoagulant activity. Blood 83:2878, 1994

148. Perry IJ, Refsum H, Morris RW et al: Prospective study

of serum total homocysteine concentration and risk of stroke in middle-aged British men. Lancet 346:1395, 1995

149. Platt OS, Guinan EC: Bone marrow transplantation in sickle cell anemia—the dilemma of choice. N Engl J Med 335:426, 1996

150. Portnoy BA, Herion JC: Neurological manifestations in sickle cell disease. Ann Intern Med 76:643, 1972

151. Powars D, Wilson B, Imbus C et al: The natural history of stroke in sickle cell disease. Am J Med 65:461, 1978

152. Press RD, Liu XY, Beamer N, Coull BM: Ischemic stroke in the elderly—role of the common factor V mutation causing resistance to activated protein C. Stroke 27:44, 1996

153. Prohovnik I, Pavlakis SG, Piomelli S et al: Cerebral hyperemia, stroke and transfusion in sickle cell disease. Neurology (NY) 39:334, 1989

154. Provenzale JM, Barboriak DP, Allen NB, Ortel TL: Patients with antiphospholipid antibodies: CT and MR findings of the brain. AJR 167:1573, 1996

155. Qizilbash N: Fibrinogen and cerebrovascular disease. Eur Heart J suppl. A, 16:42, 1995

156. Radhakrishnan K, Thacker AK, Maloo JC, El-Mangoush MA: Sickle cell trait and stroke in the young adult. Postgrad Med J 66:1078, 1990

157. Rebello M, Val JF, Garijo F et al: Livido reticularis and cerebrovascular lesions (Sneddon's syndrome). Brain 106:965, 1983

158. Resch KL, Ernst E, Matrai A, Paulsen HF: Fibrinogen and viscosity as risk factors for subsequent cardiovascular events in stroke survivors. Ann Intern Med 117:371, 1992

159. Reyes MG: Subcortical cerebral infarctions in sickle cell trait. J Neurol Neurosurg Psychiatry 52:516, 1989

160. Ridker PM: Plasma concentration of endogenous tissue plasminogen activator and the occurrence of future cardiovascular events. J Thromb Thrombol 1:35, 1994

161. Ridker PM, Vaughan DE, Stampfer MJ et al: Endogenous tissue-type plasminogen activator and risk of myocardial infarction. Lancet 341:1165, 1993

162. Ridker PM, Hennekens CH, Lindpaintner K et al: Mutation in the gene coding for coagulation factor V and the risk of myocardial infarction, stroke, and venous thrombosis in apparently healthy men. N Engl J Med 332:912, 1995

163. Ridker PM, Stampfer MJ, Hennekens CH: Plasma concentration of lipoprotein (a) and the risk of future stroke. JAMA 273:1269, 1995

164. Riuniti O, Barbui T, Finazzi G et al: Polycythemia vera: the natural history of 1213 patients followed for 20 years. Ann Intern Med 123:656, 1995

165. Rothman SM, Fulling KH, Nelson JS: Sickle cell anemia and central nervous system infarction: a neuropathological study. Ann Neurol 20:684, 1986

166. Salomaa V, Stinson V, Kark JD et al: Association of fibrinolytic parameters with early atherosclerosis. The ARIC Study. Atherosclerosis Risk in Communities Study. Circulation 91:284, 1995

167. Saxena VK, Brands C, Crols R et al: Multiple cerebral infarctions in a young patient with secondary thrombocythemia. Acta Neurol 15:297, 1993

168. Schafer AI: Bleeding and thrombosis in the myeloproliferative disorders. Blood 64:1, 1984

169. Schoene NW: Design criteria: tests used to assess platelet function. Am J Clin Nutr suppl. 65:1665S, 1997

170. Schreiner PJ, Chambless LE, Brown SA et al: Lipoprotein(a) as a correlate of stroke and transient ischemic attack prevalence in a biracial cohort: the ARIC study. Ann Epidemiol 4:351, 1994

171. Schved JF, Gris JC, Ollivier V: Procoagulant activity of endotoxin or tumor necrosis factor activated monocytes is enhanced by IgG from patients with lupus anticoagulant. Am J Hematol 41:92, 1992

172. Scott J: Lipoprotein(a): thrombogenesis linked to atherosclerosis at last? Nature 341:22, 1989

173. Shah AB, Beamer N, Coull BM: Enhanced in vivo platelet activation in subtypes of ischemic stroke. Stroke 16:643, 1985

174. Shapiro SS: The lupus anticoagulant antiphospholipid syndrome. Annu Rev Med 47:533, 1996

175. Shi W, Krilis SA, Chong BH et al: Prevalence of lupus anticoagulant and anticardiolipin antibodies in a healthy population. Aust NZ J Med 20:231, 1990

176. Shintani S, Kikuchi S, Hamaguchi H, Shiigai T: High serum lipoprotein(a) is an independent risk factor for cerebral infarction. Stroke 24:965, 1993

177. Sneddon IB: Cerebrovascular lesions and livedo reticularis. Br J Dermatol 77:180, 1965

178. Sohngen D, Wehmeier A, Specker C, Schneider W: Antiphospholipid antibodies in systemic lupus erythematosus and Sneddon's syndrome. Semin Thromb Hemost 20:55, 1994

179. Stockman JA, Nigro MA, Mishkin NM et al: Occlusion of large cerebral vessels in sickle cell anemia. N Engl J Med 287:846, 1972

180. Takano K, Yamaguchi T, Kato H, Omae T: Activation of coagulation in acute cardioembolic stroke. Stroke 22:12, 1991

181. Takano K, Yamaguchi T, Uchida K: Markers of a hypercoagulable state following acute ischemic stroke. Stroke 23:194, 1992

182. Taomoto K, Asada M, Kanazaua Y, Matsumoto S: Usefulness of the measurement of plasma-thromboglobulin (B-TG) in cerebrovascular disease. Stroke 14:518, 1983

183. Tatlisumak T, Fisher M: Hematologic disorders associated with ischemic stroke. J Neurol Sci 140:1, 1996

184. Tohgi H, Kawashima M, Taa K, Suzuki H: Coagulation-fibrinolysis abnormalities in acute and chronic phases of cerebral thrombosis and embolism. Stroke 21:1663, 1990

185. Tohgi H, Takahahi H, Chiba K, Tamura K: Coagulation-fibrinolysis system in poststroke patients receiving antiplatelet medication. Stroke 24:801, 1993

186. Toubi E, Khamashta MA, Panarra A, Hughes GR: Association of antiphospholipid antibodies with central nervous system disease in systemic lupus erythematosus. Am J Med 99:397, 1995

187. Tran ND, Wong VL, Schreiber SS et al: Regulation of brain capillary endothelial thrombomodulin mRNA expression. Stroke 27:2304, 1996

188. Triplett DA: Antiphospholipid-protein antibodies: labo-

ratory detection and clinical relevance. Thromb Res 78: 1, 1995

189. Ubbink JB, Becker PJ, Vermaak WJH, Delport R: Results of B-vitamin supplementation study used in a prediction model to define a reference range for plasma homocysteine. Clin Chem 41:1033, 1995

190. Upchurch GR Jr, Welch GN, Loscalzo J: Homocysteine, EDRF, and endothelial function. J Nutr suppl. 4, 126: 1290S, 1996

191. Vaarala O, Mänttäri M, Manninen V et al: Anti-cardiolipin antibodies and risk of myocardial infarction in a prospective cohort of middle-aged men. Circulation 91: 23, 1995

192. Vadher BD, Machin SJ, Patterson KG et al: Life-threatening thrombotic and haemorrhagic problems associated with silent myeloproliferative disorders. Br J Haematol 85:213, 1993

193. Van Genderen PJJ, Mulder PGH, Waleboer M et al: Prevention and treatment of thrombotic complications in essential thrombocythaemia: efficacy and safety of aspirin. Br J Haematol 97:179, 1997

194. Van Kooten F, Ciabattoni G, Patrono C et al: Evidence for episodic platelet activation in acute ischemic stroke. Stroke 25:278, 1994

195. Van Kooten F, van Krimpen J, Dippel DWJ et al: Lipoprotein(a) in patients with acute cerebral ischemia. Stroke 27:1231, 1996

196. Verhoef P, Hennekens CH, Malinow MR et al: A prospective study of plasma homocyst(e)ine and risk of ischemic stroke. Stroke 25:1924, 1994

197. Verlhac S, Bernaudin F, Tortrat D et al: Detection of cerebrovascular disease in patients with sickle cell disease using transcranial Doppler sonography: correlation with MRI, MRA and conventional angiography. Pediatr Radiol suppl. 1, 25:S14, 1995

198. Walters MC, Patience M, Leisenring W et al: Bone marrow transplantation for sickle cell disease. N Engl J Med 335:369, 1996

199. Wang WC, Kovnar EH, Tonkin IL et al: High risk of recurrent stroke after discontinuance of five to twelve years of transfusion therapy in patients with sickle cell disease. J Pediatr 118:377, 1991

200. Warkentin T, Kelton J: A 14-year study of heparin-induced thrombocytopenia. Am J Med 101:502, 1996

201. Warkentin TE, Levine MN, Hirsh J et al: Heparin-induced thrombocytopenia in patients treated with low-molecular-weight heparin or unfractionated heparin. N Engl J Med 332:1330, 1995

202. Wilhelmsen L, Svardsudd K, Korsan-Bengtsen K: Fibrinogen as a risk factor for stroke and myocardial infarction. N Engl J Med 311:50, 1984

203. Wintzen AR, Broekmans AW, Bertina RM et al: Cerebral haemorrhagic infarction in young patients with hereditary protein C deficiency: evidence for "spontaneous" cerebral venous thrombosis. BMJ 290:350, 1985

204. Wu KK, Thiagarajan P: Role of endothelium in thrombosis and hemostasis. Annu Rev Med 47:315, 1996

205. Yamazaki M, Uchiyama S, Maruyama S: Alterations of haemostatic markers in various subtypes and phases of stroke. Blood Coagul Fibrinolysis 4:707, 1993

206. Yarnell JWG, Baker IA, Sweetnam PM et al: Fibrinogen, viscosity, and white blood cell count are major risk factors for ischemic heart disease. Circulation 83:836, 1991

207. Zenker G, Költringer P, Boné G et al: Lipoprotein(a) as a strong indicator for cerebrovascular disease. Stroke 17: 942, 1986

CHAPTER 41

Stroke and Substance Abuse

JOHN C. M. BRUST

According to the World Health Organization, drug dependence is "a state of psychic or physical dependence, or both, on a drug, arising in a person following administration of that drug on a periodic or continuous basis."[130] Drug abuse, on the other hand, implies a social judgment, whether or not the substance is taken continuously, periodically, or infrequently, and whether or not it is legally available. When alcohol and tobacco are included, millions of Americans are substance abusers, and many of them are at increased risk of stroke, occlusive or hemorrhagic.[63,270,384] Mechanisms vary, including an increased incidence of atherosclerotic infarction in alcohol drinkers, cerebral complications of endocarditis common in parenteral drug abusers, and vasculitides affecting users of particular substances.[61,62]

Opiates

There are currently about half a million heroin abusers in the United States,[59] whose commonest causes of death are violence, overdose, acute adverse reactions, and AIDS.[58,60,194] Other medical complications include stroke. Heroin is usually taken parenterally (and in addicts more than once a day), and so infectious endocarditis is common,[21,82,319,386,387,415] especially with *Staphylococcus aureus* and *Candida*.[496] It affects in equal frequency the mitral, aortic, and tricuspid valves,[218] and cerebral emboli are common.

Stroke may be occlusive or hemorrhagic. Infarction follows embolic vessel occlusion or, less often, bacterial or fungal meningitis. Cerebral or subarachnoid hemorrhage usually follows rupture of a septic ("mycotic") aneurysm.[12,153,229] Unlike saccular ("berry") aneurysms, septic aneurysms are more likely to present with subtle or insidiously progressive neurologic or systemic symptoms (e.g., headache, fever, syncope, hemiparesis, aphasia) than with a sudden onset suggesting subarachnoid hemorrhage; and cerebrospinal fluid (CSF) white cell pleocytosis may occur in asymptomatic endocarditis patients days before a mycotic aneurysm ruptures.[64] The infrequency with

which these aneurysms spontaneously disappear during antimicrobial therapy, the high mortality associated with their rupture, and the relative ease (compared to berry aneurysms) of surgical removal support the view that cerebral angiography should be performed in endocarditis patients with either unexplained neurologic symptoms or abnormal CSF, and that, once found, most mycotic aneurysms should be promptly excised.[69,139] Mycotic aneurysms in heroin users have also occurred on the carotid[295] and subclavian arteries.[173]

Heroin abusers may also have hemorrhagic stroke secondary to hepatitis, liver failure, and deranged clotting, or to heroin nephropathy with uremia or malignant hypertension. Nine heroin addicts were reported from Harlem Hospital Center with stroke unassociated with endocarditis.[66] In three, age 41 to 45, the relation of stroke to heroin was uncertain: one, while using heroin, had an intracerebral hemorrhage in the presence of probable heroin nephropathy and malignant hypertension; another, normotensive, had a basal ganglia hemorrhage 3 days after beginning methadone detoxification; the third, mildly hypertensive, had a probable capsular infarct 6 weeks after starting methadone maintenance. In six other patients, age 25 to 38, heroin appeared more directly causal. Four, all normotensive, had probable cerebral infarcts in association with loss of consciousness after intravenous heroin. Cerebral angiography in one of these was normal but in another showed stenosis of the internal carotid artery at the siphon and of the early anterior cerebral artery, plus occlusion of the middle cerebral artery; the changes suggested primary vessel disease more than emboli. Cerebral infarctions occurred in two other patients who were using heroin at the time, although the strokes were not related to overdose, nor did they follow a recent injection. In one of these patients, who was normotensive, cerebral angiography suggested widespread small vessel arteritis. None of these patients was using oral contraceptives or had other illnesses that would predispose to stroke. Consistent with hypersensitivity, one patient had 10% eosinophilia, serum hypergammaglobulinemia, and a positive direct Coombs test, and another had an ESR of 94 mm and two positive latex fixation tests. Except for cocaine in one patient (whose stroke followed an acute reaction to heroin), no other drugs were being used.

Other reports of stroke in heroin abusers include that of a 19-year-old man who had taken heroin intravenously weekly for a year, plus intermittent lysergic acid diethylamide (LSD), and developed sudden global aphasia;[313] cerebral angiography suggested diffuse angiitis. A 21-year-old woman developed hemiparesis 2 weeks after starting daily heroin use and 6 hours after an intravenous injection.[527] Symptoms began with vomiting, headache, sweating, and shortness of breath, suggesting anaphylaxis, and cerebral angiography showed narrowing and irregularity of the distal internal carotid artery, suggesting arteritis. Eosinophilia and the fact that her husband had shared her heroin were consistent with hypersensitivity to heroin or an adulterant. A normotensive 20-year-old man who had used heroin occasionally for 2 years took his first intravenous injection in 8 months and developed sudden left homonymous hemianopia and incoordination; cerebral angiography showed "beading" of the right posterior cerebral artery.[259] Occlusive stroke has also followed heroin sniffing[27] in one such case, involving a 34-year-old man, cerebral angiography was normal.[203] Within minutes of intravenous heroin a young German had an intracerebral hemorrhage.[268]

Heroin could cause stroke by a number of possible mechanisms.[66,75] Following heroin overdose, hypoventilation and hypotension have produced permanent brain damage with bilateral cerebral leukoencephalopathy,[154] and hemiplegia has appeared upon awakening from nalorphine-responsive coma.[66] Delayed postanoxic encephalopathy has also occurred.[95,399,403] Bilateral globus pallidus infarction, commonly associated with shock, has been reported in over 270% of heroin addict autopsies[387,476] and hemichorea was present in one patient with heroin stroke.[66] In no stroke patient has hypotension been documented, however, nor has any had bibracheal palsy or other signs suggestive of borderzone ("watershed") infarction.[3,56]

Direct toxic injury from either heroin or an adulterant is another possibility. Heroin is usually mixed with quinine and lactose or mannitol, as well as, on occasion, talc, starch, curry powder, Ajax, Vim, caffeine, or even strychnine.[75] Quinine caused amblyopia in a heroin addict,[65] and may contribute to acute adverse reactions with pulmonary edema or sudden death following parenteral injection.[19,302] There is no evidence linking quinine to stroke, however.

Embolization of foreign material to the brain has not been observed in parenteral heroin users (even though the jugular vein is frequently used, with occasional accidental arterial injection), but has been documented at autopsy in abusers of other agents,[17,348,444] including opiates. Probably because of restricted heroin supply, pentazocine (Talwin) and tripelennamine (Pyribenzamine) ("Ts and Blues") were widely abused in Chicago and other midwestern cities during the 1970s.[285,508] Oral tablets were crushed, suspended in water, passed through cotton or a cigarette filter, and injected intravenously, and cerebral infarcts and hemorrhages occurred in users.[77] Common at autopsy was pulmonary arteriolar occlusion by microcrystalline cellulose[215] or particulate magnesium silicate (talc),[478] used to bind pentazocine and tripelennamine. Such microemboli also reached the brain, especially when multiple lung emboli produced pulmonary hypertension and opened "functional pulmonary arteriovenous shunts."[75] "Beaded arteries" were seen at cerebral angiography in Ts and Blues stroke patients, consistent with vasculitis, in turn

secondary to "a granulomatous or immune process provoked by the injection of foreign material."[75]

Talc microemboli were also found at autopsy in the liver, spleen, and central nervous system of a parenteral paregoric abuser.[70] A young man who several times a day injected pulverized unfiltered meperidine tablets intravenously had occasional seizures following injection and then developed difficulty concentrating, impaired memory, and visual blurring; fundal hemorrhages and areas of arterial occlusion were seen, and his symptoms improved with abstinence.[296]

Posterior cerebral artery occlusion followed intravenous injection of a melted hydromorphone (Dilaudid) suppository; the authors speculated that the mechanism was paradoxical fat embolism of the product's cocoa butter content.[41]

Some heroin strokes have followed the first injection in weeks or months, and laboratory studies have further suggested an immunologic cause. Heroin nephropathy may be immunologically mediated;[101,144,172,257] the C3 component of complement is reduced in patients with heroin pulmonary edema; and heroin addicts frequently have hypergammaglobulinemia[28,387] (including elevated IgM independent of IgG and IgA levels[102,219,364,374]), circulating immune complexes,[374] antibodies to smooth muscle and lymphocyte membranes,[219] false-positive serology,[28,45] and lymph node hypertrophy.[75] Opium, morphine, codeine, and meperidine, moreover, have caused urticaria, angioneurotic edema, and anaphylaxis.[450] Whether the offending antigen is the opiate or a contaminant is unclear, but morphine binding by gamma globulin has been reported in addicts[414,437] and experimental animals.[38,419,503]

Relevant to heroin stroke and its possible mechanisms is heroin myelopathy. Acute paraparesis, sensory loss, and urinary retention have been reported in at least 16 heroin users, occurring shortly after injection and frequently following a period of abstinence.[299,388,415,416,421,449,487] In some, symptoms were present upon awakening from coma. Proprioception and vibratory sense were often preserved relative to loss of spinothalamic sensory modalities, suggesting infarction in the territory of the anterior spinal artery.[115,149,199,499] Autopsy in one patient showed necrosis "confined almost entirely" to the upper thoracic spinal cord gray matter and in another demonstrated additional involvement of the anterior aspect of the posterior columns and a pyramidal tract in the lower thoracic cord. If these lesions were cord infarcts, their possible causes, as with cerebral stroke in heroin users, include "watershed" infarction during a period of coma, hypoventilation, and hypotension,[199] as well as hypersensitivity reaction. Consistent with the latter, a young man, remaining conscious, had several episodes of numbness and weakness of both legs for a few minutes after injection.[416] An adolescent developed, 11 days after injection, a rash on the chest and feet and then, 6 days later, became paraplegic following a second injection.[449] Cord biopsy in another patient, moreover, showed vasculitis affecting mainly small arteries and arterioles, with "double refractile fragments" in inflamed tissue, including vessel walls.[233] (Such foreign particles have also been seen in the skin of heroin addicts.[212]) A patient at Harlem Hospital had heroin injected into a vessel over his midthoracic spine and within 30 minutes developed paraparesis and then urinary retention and sensory loss below that level. Myelography was normal. Whether the vessel injected was arterial or venous, the common intercostal origins of the posterior cutaneous and spinal arteries or veins would have allowed access of injected material directly to the spinal cord,[14,397] but that would not explain whether the damage was direct toxicity, hypersensitivity, or embolism of foreign material.

A man using intravenous heroin for the first time in 2 years became comatose and apneic; receiving nalorphine, he developed over several hours quadriplegia, anarthria, dysphagia, and sensory loss consistent with a ventral pontine lesion.[178] Recovery was partial, and whether or not the lesion was vascular was not determined.

A heroin addict with unexplained clotting abnormalities was found to have high circulating levels of heparin, presumably added to her drug mixture;[332] if heparin becomes a common adulterant, addicts will obviously be at increased risk for hemorrhagic stroke.

Amphetamine and Related Agents

Although their manufacture was greatly reduced after the 1972 Controlled Substances Act, amphetamine and similar stimulants are still produced in huge quantities.[492] There are two patterns of abuse. Housewives, truck drivers, or students may take it orally, often with sedatives or alcohol. Addicts more often take it intravenously, sometimes in doses of up to 300 mg every few hours over days. Strokes common to any parenteral drug abuse are therefore encountered. There are also strokes that may be unique to these agents.

Acutely, amphetamine can cause excitement, hypertension, and a rectal temperature of over 109°F, followed by coma, vascular collapse, and death;[38,170,231,308,402,538] at autopsy there are diffuse cerebral edema and petechiae, without large infarcts or hematomas.[38,48,189,231,538] In dogs[537] or rabbits[249] given lethal doses of amphetamine there was severe hyperpyrexia and, at autopsy, subendocardial and epicardial hemorrhage, myocardial fiber necrosis, and, in the brain, neuronal degeneration in the cerebral cortex and cerebellum.[249,536,537] Curare prevented the fever and the fatal course, suggesting that the hyperpyrexia was secondary to muscle hyperactivity and that death was secondary to heat stroke. Fever may have also contributed to similar brain pathological findings in cats receiving chronic methedrine over 2 weeks, although in that study neuronal catecholamine depletion was suspected as the primary cause.[102,126]

Significant brain hemorrhage was not present in these experimental animals but has been found, along with focal neurologic signs, in animal and human cases of heat stroke,[89,135,142,283] often with severe clotting abnormalities, including decreased prothrombin activity, thrombocytopenia, hypofibrinogenemia, and fibrinolysis.[455] Hyperpyrexia and disturbed clotting have not been reported, however, with intracranial hemorrhage after amphetamine use. Over 30 patients have been reported, aged 16 to 60.[71,86,94,109,125,131,151,160,176,186,240,254,315,316,322,325,333,338,372,400,458,489,517,530,531,533,534] Eighteen had taken the drug orally, nine intravenously, two orally and intravenously, one nasally and intravenously,

five by inhalation, and two by uncertain route. Most were chronic users, but in five patients stroke followed a first exposure. The dose was usually unknown, but in one case was as low as 80 mg. Except for one instance each of diethylpropion and pseudoephedrine, all took amphetamine or methedrine; seven also took methylphenidate, LSD, dimethoxymethylamphetamine ("STP"), cocaine, heroin, or barbiturates. Severe headache usually occurred within minutes of drug use. Blood pressure was elevated in 15 of the 26 in whom it was recorded, with diastolic pressures as high as 120 mmHg in 5. Eight patients died, usually soon after admission. Computed tomography (CT), done on 14 patients, showed, variably, intracerebral hemorrhage (frequently lobar), subarachnoid hemorrhage, or no abnormality. In 12 patients at angiography, irregular narrowing ("beading") of distal cerebral arteries suggested vasculitis; three of these patients had taken the drug only orally. Such vessel changes were present at autopsy in three (including one whose angiogram showed only an avascular mass). In another patient a cerebral vascular malformation was seen by both angiography and CT.

Thus, some of these amphetamine-induced intracranial hemorrhages seem to have been secondary to acute hypertension, some to cerebral vasculitis, and some to a combination of the two, but in others neither feature was apparent. While acute hypertension secondary to amphetamine could be causal, in some patients it might have been a transient result of the stroke.[108] Conversely, in others, fleeting blood pressure elevations could have been missed.

Amphetamine-induced cerebral vasculitis, which has caused occlusive as well as hemorrhagic strokes, appears to be of more than one type. Necrotizing angiitis, sometimes affecting the nervous system, occurred in 14 Los Angeles abusers of multiple drugs, including amphetamine, methedrine, barbiturates, chlordiazepoxide, diazepam, marijuana, hydroxyzine, LSD, heroin, meperidine, mescaline, oxycodone, oxymorphone, dimethoxymethylamphetamine, and strychnine.[87] All but 2 patients used intravenous methedrine, and one used it exclusively. Five patients were asymptomatic, and in the others there was fever, weight loss, malaise, weakness, skin rash, pneumonitis, pulmonary edema, hematuria, proteinuria, renal failure, abdominal pain, pancreatitis, gastrointestinal hemorrhage, arthralgia, myalgia, peripheral neuropathy, anemia, leukocytosis, and hemolysis. One patient had renal failure, severe hypertension, papilledema, retinal detachment, "progressive encephalopathy," and, at autopsy, vasculitis affecting pontine arterioles. Another, with "mental obtundation" and hypertension, had at autopsy "recent and resolving cerebral and pontine infarction," "marked cerebellar hemorrhage," and vasculitis in the cerebrum, cerebellum, and brain stem. Vessel lesions consisted acutely of fibrinoid necrosis of the media and intima, with infiltration by neutrophils, eosinophils, lymphocytes, and histiocytes; later there was destruction of muscular and elastic components, replacement by collagen, and often "a nodular (nodose) bulge with nearly aneurysmal dilatation." The authors considered these lesions, which affected only muscular arteries and arterioles, typical for polyarteritis nodosa and distinguished them from hypersensitivity angiitis, which involves small arteries, capillaries, and venules. They further noted that more than one drug or adulterant could have caused them, and that, in contrast to polyarteritis nodosa,[155,156] they were not associated with the presence of Australia antigen.[88]

While such brain lesions have been found pathologically in other polydrug (including amphetamine) abusers,[51,254] in some, cerebral arteritis has been presumed on the basis of cerebral angiography,[71,86,131,333,432,434, 530,534] and sometimes the relation to amphetamine abuse has been tenuous. In a report of three young men who developed ischemic strokes in association with intranasal methamphetamine, cerebral angiography revealed in one supraclinoid beading of the internal carotid artery, in another occlusion of the internal carotid artery near its origin, and in the third supraclinoid occlusion of the internal carotid artery.[427] In another report, thalamic infarction followed intranasal methamphetamine use, but angiography was not performed.[442] A radiographic study of 19 young drug abusers, most taking intravenous methedrine and hospitalized for coma or stroke, revealed widespread segmental constrictions of large and medium sized cerebral arteries and stenosis or occlusion of many penetrating arterioles, consistent with either multiple emboli or vasculitis and thrombosis.[432] The same authors then gave rhesus monkeys intravenous methedrine, 1.5 mg/kg (considered the lower limit of dosage for most abusers), and did serial cerebral angiograms for 2 weeks.[433] Several animals studied 10 minutes after receiving the drugs showed irregularly decreased caliber of small cerebral vessels, with a return to normal at 24 hours. In others these changes occurred in both small and large vessels and persisted for the 2-week period, in one actually worsening. Clinically there was hypertension and behavioral change. Postmortem examination at 2 weeks revealed subarachnoid hemorrhage in some animals, with numerous brain petechial hemorrhages, infarcts, edema, microaneurysms, and perivascular white blood cell cuffing. In a later study monkeys received intravenous methedrine three times weekly.[435] After either a month or a year serial angiograms showed occlusions and slow blood flow in small cerebral arteries, and at autopsy there were attenuated and fragmented brain arterioles and capillaries, microaneurysms, dilated venules, petechiae, neuronal loss, and gliosis. Talc crystals were present in capillaries (the drug was given as crushed methamphetamine hydrochloride [Desoxyn] tablets); but against such particles playing a critical role in the vasculitis was the fact that in the animals receiving crushed placebo tablets containing all the ingredients of Desoxyn except methedrine vasculitis was minimal or absent.

In rats receiving 2 weeks of intravenous methedrine, brain capillaries had, by electron microscopy, abnormal "budding" from the luminal walls of endothelial cells and vesicles within the endothelial cell cytoplasm.[435] These changes affected vessels smaller than 100 μm and would therefore be missed angiographically. (The vulnerability of small vessels might be related to their separate innervation: large cerebral vessels are innervated by the peripheral sympathetic nervous system, but nerve terminals on smaller arteries appear to be from central noradrenergic neurons.)[188]

Of three monkeys receiving intravenous methylphenidate (Ritalin) for a month, all had "a moderate degree of vascular change" angiographically, but only one had "some chromatolysis" histologically.[347] Rats receiving methylphenidate, however, had the same severe degree of histologic brain damage as those receiving methedrine.

These lesions are different from polyarteritis nodosa, in which elastic arteries, capillaries, and veins are spared. Whether they are the result of direct toxicity or of hypersensitivity is unclear, nor can the possibility be excluded that the early angiographic findings are secondary to subarachnoid hemorrhage (although beading of distal pial arteries in subarachnoid hemorrhage is rare[86]). In an adolescent amphetamine abuser with mononeuritis multiplex, sural nerve biopsy showed apparent hypersensitivity angiitis of medium and small muscular arteries, arterioles, venules, and veins, with fibrinoid necrosis and infiltration by polymorphonuclear leukocytes, lymphocytes, eosinophils, and plasma cells.[467] The central nervous system was clinically unaffected, however.

Federal restrictions on amphetamine do not apply to phenylpropanolamine (PPA), a similar but less potent drug found, sometimes with ephedrine or caffeine, in over-the-counter decongestants (e.g., Contac) and diet pills (e.g., Dexa-diet, Dexatrim, Anorexin, Maxi-slim), as well as in drugs made deliberately to resemble amphetamine ("look-alike pills").[44,358] Although the FDA has restricted over-the-counter combinations of PPA, ephedrine, and caffeine, an estimated 5 billion doses of PPA are used in the United States annually.[294] Acute hypertension, severe headache, psychiatric symptoms, seizures, and hemorrhagic stroke have occurred in users.[39,138,239,258,321,358–360,375,435,447,519] A case reported as "cerebral arteritis" in a PPA user was based simply on angiographic "beading."[438] PPA with caffeine, from a commercial diet preparation, produced subarachnoid hemorrhage in rats receiving it intraperitoneally in three to six times the recommended dose.[359]

Ephedrine and pseudoephedrine are present in over-the-counter decongestants and bronchodilators. Complications have included headache, tachyarrhythmia, hypertensive emergency, and hemorrhagic and occlusive stroke.[57,148,316,334, 390,473] Occlusive stroke was reported in two users of the anorexiant phentermine; one patient also used phendimetrazine.[271] Occlusive stroke also occurred in a young man after intranasal use of amphetamine combined with caffeine.[287] Middle cerebral artery occlusion was reported in a young man 36 hours after recreational use of 3,4-methylenedioxymethamphetamine ("ecstasy").[329]

A young man who had previously used "speed" and LSD had a subarachnoid hemorrhage within an hour of ingesting pills that turned out to be ephedrine.[528] Cerebral angiography was initially normal but a week later showed beading and branch occlusions suggesting arteritis; a biopsy from grossly normal skin showed deposits of IgM and the C3 component of complement periluminally in dermal vessels, consistent with circulating immune complexes.

A young woman who injected crushed methylphenidate tablets into her jugular veins developed immediate right hemiplegia after a left injection and two months later left hemiplegia after a right injection; presumably the injections were inadvertently into the carotid artery, but the exact mechanism of stroke was not determined.[83] Intraretinal talc microemboli have been seen in the fundi of intravenous methylphenidate abusers.[17,495] In some there were retinal vascular and choroidal abnormalities, neovascularization, and vitreous hemorrhage,[495] and in one, who had not had a clinical stroke, talc and cornstarch emboli were also present in arterioles, capillaries, and veins of brain and lung.[17] Infarction of the medial medulla in a young woman occurred a few minutes after intravenous methylphenidate; at autopsy there was systemic granulomatosis due to talc and talc deposits in small vessels around the medullary infarct.[348]

Mycotic subclavian and carotid aneurysms developed following inadvertent intra-arterial injection of the diet compound phentermine.[180]

Death has followed parenteral[13] or oral[418] abuse of propylhexedrine from "Benzedrex" inhalers; stroke has not yet been reported in such patients, and the cause of death has been uncertain.

Cocaine

In the 1980s cocaine use became widespread in the United States. In 1982 it was estimated that 28% of people aged 18 to 25 had used cocaine hydrochloride, usually intranasally but often parenterally (including cocaine-heroin mixtures—so-called speedballs).[62] In 1985 the appearance of commercially prepared alkaloidal cocaine ("crack") led to acceleration of the epidemic, with increasing addictive use and widespread illegal trafficking and social disruption. Smokable "crack" produces a psychological "high" even more intense than that which follows intravenous cocaine hydrochloride and is taken in larger and more frequent doses. The result has been increasing morbidity and mortality, including stroke.[238,518]

Parenteral cocaine users are at risk for stroke related to infection, including endocarditis, AIDS, and hepatitis. They also develop strokes caused directly by the drug itself, whether taken intranasally, intravenously, or intramuscularly or smoked as "crack."[303] The first report of a cocaine-related stroke was in 1977: a middle-aged, mildly hypertensive man injected cocaine intramuscularly after drinking a bottle of wine and an hour later abruptly developed aphasia and right hemiparesis; CSF was normal, and cerebral angiography was refused.[67] The same year fatal rupture of a cerebral saccular aneurysm occurred in a young man sniffing cocaine.[326] Further cases were not reported until the mid-1980s, but by the early 1990s over 300 cases of stroke had been described, about half occlusive and half hemorrhagic.[6,22,76,78,80,81,97,98,103,104, 107,111–113,122,132,140,157,169,174,177,179,187,193,196,216,225,237,252,267, 274,275,277,280,281,301,306,307,309,310,323,330,335,345–348,353,357,363,366, 367,369,392,393,396,405,406,411,422,428,429,446,448,452,460–463,466,484,492, 504,513,523]

Ischemic strokes have included transient ischemic attacks and infarction of cerebrum, thalamus, brain stem, spinal cord, and retina.[112,281,349] Infarction has occurred in newborns whose mothers used cocaine shortly before delivery[81] and in pregnant women.[112,281,303,349] In some cases cerebral infarction has been attributed to vasculitis on the basis of angiographic findings;[252] such changes, however, may have represented vasospasm following undiagnosed subarachnoid hemorrhage.[304] Autopsies have usually shown histologically normal cerebral vessels,[303,307,366] although in five cases mild cerebral vasculitis was observed at biopsy or autopsy.[78,140,281,356] In these cases cerebral angiography was negative. Conversely, a man with multiple cerebral infarcts clinically and by magnetic resonance imaging had "multifocal areas of segmental stenosis and dilatation" by angiography, yet brain

biopsy revealed no evidence of vasculitis.[335] A young crack smoker had middle cerebral artery branch occlusion, cardiomyopathy, and a left atrial thrombus.[396] A 20-year-old with no other risk factors had superior cerebellar artery occlusion 6 months after last use, raising the possibility of delayed effects.[111] In a 27-year-old occasional cocaine sniffer with "heaviness and paresthesias" in the legs and occasional "forgetfulness," magnetic resonance imaging revealed multiple periventricular white matter lesions.[513]

Intracerebral or subarachnoid hemorrhage has occurred during or within hours of cocaine use or has had less clear temporal relationship. In some instances there has been other substance use, especially ethanol. Nearly half of those undergoing angiography have had saccular aneurysms or vascular malformations. Other hemorrhages have included bleeding into embolic infarction or glioma.[523] Cerebral hemorrhages have occurred in newborns and postpartum women.[196,303,345] In a patient with multiple cerebral hemorrhages after smoking crack, autopsy revealed histologically normal cerebral vessels.[169]

The mechanisms of cocaine-related stroke are unclear.[423] Striking, considering that cocaine and amphetamine have similar actions and effects, are the high frequency of underlying aneurysm or vascular malformation in hemorrhagic strokes of cocaine users compared to amphetamine users and, conversely, the frequency of vasculitis in amphetamine users compared to cocaine users. Cocaine hydrochloride is more often associated with hemorrhagic than occlusive stroke, whereas hemorrhagic and occlusive strokes occur with roughly equal frequency in "crack" users, but the rising prevalence of stroke since the appearance of "crack" is probably attributable to wider use and higher dosage rather than to a peculiarity of "crack" itself. By blocking re-uptake of norepinephrine from sympathetic nerve endings (and probably also by affecting calcium flux) cocaine is a vasoconstrictor.[217,223,275] Acute hypertension can result, leading to intracranial hemorrhage, especially in subjects with underlying aneurysms or vascular malformations.[366] Coronary artery vasoconstriction has been documented during cardiac catheterization,[84,291,352] and there are numerous reports of angina pectoris and myocardial infarction during or following cocaine use.[84,464] Cocaine also causes cardiac arrhythmia and cardiomyopathy, which, like myocardial infarction, carries the potential risk for embolic stroke.[85,248,512] Cerebral vasoconstriction may cause occlusive stroke, and it is possibly significant that cocaine metabolites, which in some chronic users are detectable in urine for weeks, have also been reported to cause cerebral vasospasm.[401,516] The situation is complex, however, for cerebral and peripheral vessels frequently respond differently to similar stimuli. Whereas intraluminal cocaine constricted cat and rat pial vessels in vitro, topical cocaine dilated pial vessels in living cats,[118,217,401] and in rabbits intravenous cocaine has produced both vasoconstriction and vasodilatation of cerebral vessels.[114,267,510] In swine cocaine given intravenously caused carotid artery constriction, but in vitro there was no response, suggesting that at least in that species the vasoconstriction effect was indirect, through "release of humoral and/or neural vasoactive substances."[368]

In vitro studies with platelets have been conflicting. Cocaine reportedly enhanced the response of platelets to arachidonic acid, thereby promoting aggregation.[491] It also directly inhibited fibrinogen binding to activated platelets and caused dissociation of preformed platelet aggregates.[230] In rabbits repeated cocaine injections caused arteriosclerotic aortopathy.[292] In a cocaine user with symptoms of coronary artery disease protein C and antithrombin III were depleted and returned to normal, with clearing of symptoms, when use was discontinued.[85]

Ethanol reportedly enhances cocaine toxicity; in the presence of ethanol cocaine is metabolized to cocaethylene, which, perhaps even more powerfully than cocaine itself, binds to the synaptic dopamine transporter and blocks reuptake.[408] Cocaine and ethanol synergistically depress myocardial contraction.[522] The relevance of these observations to stroke in users of both cocaine and ethanol is uncertain.

It is controversial whether cocaine (or other psychostimulants) causes lasting mental abnormalities and, if so, whether they are a consequence of cerebrovascular disease. Human studies using controls suggest that chronic cocaine use produces subtle cognitive impairment,[373,514] and a CT study found significant degrees of cerebral atrophy in habitual cocaine users compared to first-time users and nonusers.[383] Studies with positron emission tomography (PET) and single photon emission tomography (SPECT) in chronic cocaine users found irregularly decreased blood flow in the cerebral cortex; some of these subjects had normal CT or MRI scans, and in some (but not all), PET and SPECT abnormalities were associated with deficits on psychometric testing.[214,474,497,505]

It is also controversial how cocaine affects the fetus. Perinatal and neonatal strokes—both occlusive and hemorrhagic—may be underrecognized in newborns exposed to cocaine in utero.[117,461] Cerebral blood flow studies during the first few days of life in cocaine-exposed neonates are consistent with persisting vasoconstriction.[260] Some investigators have speculated that cocaine-induced vasospasm during the first trimester is responsible for CNS malformations (including encephalocele, holoprosencephaly, and hypoplastic cerebellum).[193] Others have doubted such causality.[506]

Phencyclidine

Phencyclidine (PCP, "angel dust") became a widely abused American street drug in the 1970s; it can be smoked, eaten, or injected, and is often misrepresented as marijuana or mescaline. One to 5 mg produce euphoria, emotional lability, and a feeling of diffuse numbness; 5 to 15 mg cause confusion, excitation, decreased sensory perception, and body distortion; higher doses cause psychosis, myoclonus, nystagmus, seizures, coma, and sometimes fatal respiratory and circulatory collapse.[60,68,253,341,365] Hypertension can occur both early and late during intoxication[99,129,341] and may be related to enhancement of the action of catecholamines and serotonin.[221] However, contractile responses to PCP of isolated basilar and middle cerebral arteries were not prevented or reversed by methysergide, phentolamine, atropine, diphenhydramine, or indomethacin, raising the possibility of PCP receptors on cerebral blood vessels.[7]

A 13-year-old boy became comatose after taking PCP; admission blood pressure was normal, and he became more alert, but 3 days later his condition deteriorated with a blood pressure of 220/130 mmHg. At autopsy there was an intracerebral hemorrhage.[129] A 6-year-old boy became unresponsive with seizures and right hemiparesis; urine contained PCP. CT demonstrated left parieto-occipital lucency and vessel enhancement suggesting a vascular malformation. He recovered, and cerebral angiography was not done.[99] A young man collapsed after smoking PCP; blood pressure was 180/100 mmHg, and at autopsy there was subarachnoid hemorrhage without parenchymal hematoma. A 17-year-old-boy with PCP in his blood died following perforation of the ventral surface of his basilar artery.[53] Hypertensive encephalopathy followed PCP ingestion in a young woman with systemic lupus erythematosus and a history of migraine.[69]

LSD

Lysergic acid diethylamide (LSD) in high doses causes severe hypertension, obtundation, and convulsions.[52,93,471] In vitro spasm of cerebral vessel strips immersed in LSD-containing solution was prevented or reversed by methysergide.[6] Following ingestion of four LSD capsules, a 14-year-old boy developed seizures and, 4 days later, left hemiplegia; carotid angiography showed progressive narrowing of the internal carotid artery from its origin to the siphon, with occlusion at its bifurcation.[465] A young woman developed sudden left hemiplegia a day after oral LSD; angiography showed marked constriction of the internal carotid artery at the siphon; 9 days later the vessel was occluded at that level.[312] A 19-year-old with acute aphasia and cerebral angiographic findings consistent with arteritis had used both LSD and heroin, and the time relationship of either drug to the stroke was not stated.[313] Another patient with angiographic evidence of vasculitis had used both LSD and "diet pills."[432]

Marijuana

Because marijuana is the most widely used illicit drug in the United States, it is hardly surprising that occlusive stroke affects its users; causality is another matter. In fact, the diagnosis of stroke in some reports is dubious. Two young men had only conjugate deviation of the eyes for days or weeks after marijuana use,[26,350] and another young man awoke with dysarthria and hemiparesis the morning after smoking marijuana.[92] In none of these patients was imaging performed. Two young men, both hypertensive cigarette smokers, developed hemiparesis during marijuana smoking, and CT showed cerebral infarction.[535] Another young smoker of tobacco and marijuana had three possible transient ischemic attacks and then hemiparesis and aphasia; CT showed a striatocapsular infarct.[25] Proposed mechanisms for alleged marijuana-induced stroke include systemic hypotension and cerebral vasospasm, but neither has been documented in clinical reports. In rats, delta-9-tetrahydrocannabinol (the psychoactive ingredient of marijuana) has vasoconstrictor action on systemic vessels.[4] In humans, marijuana has unpredictable effects on cerebral blood flow, either increasing or decreasing it.[339]

Barbiturates

Usually abused orally, barbiturates and other sedatives and tranquilizers can cause cerebral infarction in association with overdose and diffusely decreased brain perfusion, but occlusive or hemorrhagic stroke has not otherwise been reported. A 20-year-old man taking orally a combination of secobarbital and strychnine ("M and Ms") became comatose with right hemiplegia, and cerebral angiography showed widespread segmental vascular irregularity consistent with arteritis; he had been taking other drugs as well for at least 10 years.[434] Cerebral vasculitis was also found in four other barbiturate abusers; two also abused chlorpromazine, one took other unidentified drugs, and the fourth apparently used only barbiturates, but whether orally or parenterally was not revealed.[432]

Monkeys receiving dissolved secobarbital (Seconal) capsules, 1.5 mg/kg intravenously three times a week for a year, had narrowing of small arteries at cerebral angiography. Histologically there were scattered talc crystals in brain capillaries, without cellular reaction; one animal had a frontal lobe microinfarct.[434]

Inhalants

Inhalation of vapors to achieve euphoric intoxication is common in the United States, especially among children. Substances include aerosals, enamels, paint thinners, lighter fluid, cleaning fluid, glues, cements, gasoline, and anesthetics. Death results from violence, accidents, suffocation, aspiration, or cardiac arrhythmia. Clinical stroke has not been reported, but radioisotope brain scan in a boy with status epilepticus after toluene sniffing showed several wedge-shaped areas of increased uptake in both cerebral hemispheres, consistent with infarcts.

Alcohol

Coronary artery disease and myocardial infarction may be less prevalent in those who drink alcohol than in those who do not.[5,354] The increased risk of coronary artery disease in heavy drinkers becomes an indirect risk for cardioembolic stroke secondary to cardiac wall hypokinesia or arrhythmia. Alcohol intoxication and withdrawal are also directly associated with cardiac arrhythmia ("holiday heart"),[133,324,488] and thromboembolism is a prominent feature of alcoholic cardiomyopathy.[76]

A large literature has addressed whether acute or chronic alcohol use is a risk factor for stroke independent of its cardiac effects or other risk factors.[20,251,262,281,297,370,425] Retrospective studies, most notably from Finland, have found an association between recent heavy alcohol use and both occlusive and hemorrhagic stroke.[205,207–209,477] The Finnish studies, however, used population prevalence data as controls, and other similarly designed analyses have either not found such an association,[211] or, as in the NINCDS Data Bank, only for intracerebral hemorrhage.[355] A study from Chicago found that the association between alcohol intoxication and stroke disappeared when corrected for cigarette smoking.[166,167]

Numerous case-control and cohort studies have addressed the relationship of stroke to chronic alcohol use.[31,54,100,146,192,162,159,183,201,255,266,300,311,371,378,380,385,420,438,445,454,470,485,503] Contradictory findings are not surprising, for studies have differed in endpoints chosen (e.g., total stroke, occlusive stroke, hemorrhagic stroke, or stroke mortality), amount and duration of alcohol consumption, correction for other risk factors (especially hypertension and smoking), ethnicity and socioeconomics of populations being studied, and selection of controls. Drinkers tend to be overrepresented among hospitalized controls, leading to the impression that alcohol is protective against stroke; they tend to be underrepresented among community controls identified by a questionnaire, leading to the impression that alcohol is a risk factor for stroke.[36]

Among cohort studies, the Yugoslavia Cardiovascular Disease Study found increased stroke mortality among drinkers, and, although the association was especially strong for hypertensives, it persisted with adjustment for blood pressure.[278,279] A reduced risk was found for modest drinkers. In the Honolulu Heart Study heavy drinkers had an increased risk of hemorrhagic stroke independent of other risk factors including hypertension and smoking.[42,123,235,479] There was no comparable risk for occlusive stroke. Early reports from the Framingham Study found both positive[526] and negative[163,242,246,247] associations; a later report described lower than expected stroke incidence among "moderate" drinkers and higher rates in both heavy drinkers and nondrinkers.[525] In the Nurses' Health Study independent of smoking and hypertension there was an inverse association between modest alcohol intake (less than two drinks daily) and occlusive stroke, with a positive association at higher intake; subarachnoid hemorrhage was associated with both low and high alcohol intake.[468] In the Lausanne Stroke Registry severity of internal carotid artery stenosis inversely correlated with "light-to-moderate" alcohol intake; there were too few patients to assess heavy intake.[46] The Japanese Hisayama Study initially reported positive correlations;[250] later it found no independent association between alcohol and occlusive or hemorrhagic stroke after adjusting for other variables,[500] still later it found that heavy drinking conferred increased risk for cerebral hemorrhage in hypertensives, whereas light alcohol consumption reduced the risk of cerebral infarction.[261] A study of Japanese physicians found a positive association between stroke mortality and alcohol intake.[272,273] Three other Japanese studies found either independent associations between alcohol and hemorrhagic but not occlusive stroke,[481] no association between alcohol and hemorrhagic or occlusive stroke,[206] no association between alcohol and occlusive stroke,[480] and a "J-shaped relationship" between alcohol intake and occlusive stroke: drinkers of less than 42 g/d ethanol had a lower risk and heavy drinkers a higher risk than "never drinkers."[224]

In a review of 62 epidemiologic studies that examined the relation between stroke and "moderate" alcohol consumption (less than two drinks, or 1 oz. of absolute ethanol) it was concluded that ethnicity played a role in the disparate results.[72] Among whites, moderate doses of alcohol seemed to protect against ischemic stroke, whereas higher doses increased risk. (This pattern is similar to that for alcohol and coronary artery disease.) Among the Japanese, little association seemed to exist between alcohol and ischemic stroke. In both populations all doses of alcohol seemed to increase the risk of both intracerebral and subarachnoid hemorrhage. Some studies have suggested that the risk of hemorrhagic stroke declines with abstinence, but the evidence is insufficient to draw an association between stroke and recent intoxication per se.

An Australian case control study found that low doses of ethanol (less than 20 g/d) were protective against "all strokes, all ischemic strokes, and primary intracerebral hemorrhage."[227] A British case control study found that the protective effect of "light or moderate" drinking compared to nondrinking disappeared when corrected for exercise and obesity.[457] An Italian case control study found that the role of alcohol as a risk factor for stroke "was practically lost" after correction for previous strokes, hypertension, diabetes, obesity, and hyperlipidemia.[30,31] A study from northern Manhattan found "ethanol abuse" to be an independent risk factor for recurrent stroke.[439] A study from Denmark found that moderate wine drinking reduced the likelihood of stroke, moderate drinking of "spirits" increased the likelihood, and moderate drinking of beer had no effect in either direction.[173]

Studies with duplex ultrasound and angiography have shown that heavy ethanol consumption increases the risk of carotid artery atherosclerosis, whereas low ethanol intake has a beneficial effect.[381] Similarly, a study using CT scanning found that one to five drinks daily reduced the risk of leukoaraiosis in stroke patients, whereas heavier alcohol consumption increased the risk.[232] The Japanese Hisayama study found alcohol to be an independent risk factor for "vascular dementia."[532]

As with coronary artery disease, several mechanisms might explain the association between alcohol and stroke. Alcohol acutely and chronically raises blood pressure,[29,32,42, 55,127,228,245,264,278,314,327,328,336,337,407,436,486] perhaps related to increased adrenergic activity and to increased blood levels of cortisol, renin, aldosterone, and vasopressin.[164] Corticotropin-releasing hormone is sympatho-excitatory when administered centrally; in normal subjects dexamethasone blocked the increased sympathetic discharge and the increased blood pressure induced by intravenous ethanol. The systolic blood pressure decline during the first week following a stroke is greater in heavy drinkers than in light drinkers or abstainers,[185] and with abstinence, blood pressure may become normal.[317]

Perhaps related to its protective effects, alcohol lowers blood levels of low-density lipoproteins and elevates levels of high-density lipoproteins.[23,73,79,191] One study found that alcohol seemed preferentially to protect large vessels from atherosclerosis, perhaps accounting for ethnic differences in patterns of protection or risk.[410] The relationship is uncertain, however, for alcohol may not raise blood levels of the more protective HDL-2 subfraction.[18,165]

Alcohol acutely decreases fibrinolytic activity, increases factor VIII, increases platelet reactivity to ADP, and shortens bleeding time.[204,210,290,298,343] In one study moderate ethanol consumption was associated with elevated endogenous tissue plasminogen activator.[417] Ethanol reportedly decreases plasma fibrinogen levels,[116] increases levels of prostacyclin,[226,289] decreases platelet function,[96,134,192,241,389,404, 413,475] and stimulates release of endothelin from endothelial cells.[494] In chronic alcoholics, decreased levels of clotting factors, excessive fibrinolysis, and platelet abnormalities appear to be secondary to liver disease.[147,164] During or following ethanol withdrawal "rebound thrombocytosis" and platelet hyperaggregability have been observed.[190,220] In rats this rebound followed withdrawal in animals receiving ethanol or white wine but not in those receiving red wine, possibly reflecting a protective effect of red wine tannins.[431]

Acute alcohol intoxication had been accompanied by cerebral vasodilatation[342,545] and blood-brain barrier leakage of albumin,[391] perhaps contributing to the severity of traumatic intracerebral hemorrhage during drinking.[36,459] Increased cerebral blood flow has also been observed during alcohol withdrawal.[195] Chronic drinking is associated with reduced cerebral blood flow, mainly from reduced cerebral metabolism.[37] Alcohol-related hemoconcentration may also contribute to reduced cerebral blood flow.[164]

In vitro studies involving a variety of mammals have shown ethanol to be a potent vasoconstrictor of basilar and middle cerebral artery segments, and in living rats ethanol caused vasoconstriction of cerebral arterioles[161] and blocked the vasodilatation produced by acetycholine, histamine, and ADP but not the vasodilatation produced by nitroglycerin or the vasoconstriction produced by a thromboxane analog.[474] In cultured canine vascular smooth muscle cells, ethanol exposure caused depletion of intracellular magnesium ion.[11] Such an effect could lead to calcium ion overload, causing both hypertension and cerebral vasoconstriction, and, indeed, pretreatment of animals with magnesium ion prevents ethanol-induced stokes.[8,10]

Some investigators believe that snoring and sleep apnea are risk factors for stroke. To the extent that ethanol contributes to these conditions, it would be increasing that risk.[382]

Tobacco

Epidemiologic studies have shown smoking to be a major risk factor for coronary artery and peripheral vascular disease.[15,120,243,379] Although a few reports have been negative or demonstrated only insignificant trends toward increased risk of stroke among smokers,[105,200,244] most case control and cohort studies have shown that smoking does increase the risk for both occlusive and hemorrhagic stroke.[12,43,49,50,74, 110,119,167,181,182,184,202,234,236,269,284,286,300,320,351,376,377,426,443,456, 498,526] In women smokers the risk of occlusive and hemorrhagic stroke is greater in those taking oral contraceptives.[91,141,158,394,430] In a prospective cohort study of middle-aged women smoking increased stroke risk in a dose-dependent fashion; for those smoking 25 or more cigarettes daily, the relative risk for all stroke was 3.7 and for subarachnoid hemorrhage 9.8 independent of other risk factors, including oral contraceptives, hypertension, and alcohol.[90] In another report smoking in hypertensive men and women carried a 15-fold risk for subarachnoid hemorrhage and was a greater risk than hypertension itself.[49] In another study the treatment of hypertension reduced stroke incidence in nonsmokers but not in smokers.[344] In the Honolulu Heart Program stroke risk was independent of coronary artery disease.[1] The Framingham Study found smoking to be a risk factor for subarachnoid hemorrhage and, independent of age and hypertension, for both occlusive and hemorrhagic stroke; this risk was dose-dependent and disappeared when smoking ceased.[441,524] Others have confirmed reduction of risk with cessation of smoking.[269,426,511]

Among smokers the risk of stroke mortality is reduced among those smoking cigarettes with lower tar yield.[482] On the other hand, stroke was reported following application of a nicotine patch.[398]

Several possible mechanisms could underlie tobacco's risk for stroke. Smoking aggravates atherosclerosis; in a study of identical twins discordant for smoking, carotid plaques were significantly more prominent in the smokers, and in other reports smoking correlated in dose-related fashion with severity of extracranial carotid atherosclerosis.[46,175,520] The reversibility of stroke risk with cessation of smoking is against such a mechanism being paramount, however.[361,424,524] Smoking one cigarette causes transient increases in arterial wall stiffness that increase the likelihood of plaque formation.[276] Carbon monoxide in cigarette smoke reduces blood's oxygen carrying capacity, and nicotine constricts coronary arteries.[35,331] Coronary artery constriction and increased myocardial oxygen demand induced by cocaine are exacerbated by concomitant tobacco smoking.[352] In animals nicotine damages endothelium, and increased numbers of circulating endothelial cells are found in smokers.[106,539] Smoking acutely raises blood pressure, systole more than diastole; cerebral blood flow is reduced even after such acute effects have worn off.[282,318] Smoking is not a risk factor for chronic hypertension, but it accelerates the progression of chronic hypertension to malignant hypertension.[168,222] Smokers become tachycardic, and atrial fibrillation has followed nicotine gum chewing.[35] Smoking increases platelet reactivity and inhibits prostacyclin formation.[33,361,362,412,453] It also raises blood fibrinogen, a linkage noted in several stroke studies, and polycythemia secondary to smoking increases blood viscosity.[451] The increased risk of subarachnoid hemorrhage in smokers has been blamed on increased elastolytic activity in the serum.[137]

Progressive multifocal symptoms occurred in four young women who smoked and used oral contraceptives. Cerebral angiography demonstrated moyamoya, and abnormal studies included elevated ESR, positive antinuclear antibodies, and elevated CSF IgG. Disease progression ceased with discontinuation of oral contraceptives and reduction in smoking.[305]

References

1. Abbott RD, Reed DM, Yano K: Risk of stroke in male cigarette smokers. N Engl J Med 315:717, 1986
2. Abu-Zeid HAH, Choi NW, Maini KK et al: Relative role of factors associated with cerebral infarction and cerebral hemorrhage: a matched pair case-control study. Stroke 8:106, 1977
3. Adams JH, Brierley JB, Connor RCR, Treip CS: The effects of systemic hypotension upon the human brain: clinical and neuropathological observations in 11 cases. Brain 89:235, 1966
4. Adams MD, Earnhardt JT, Dewcy WL, Harris LS: Vasoconstrictor actions of delta-8- and delta-9-tetrahydrocannabinol in the rat. J Pharmacol Exp Ther 196:649, 1976
5. Ahlawat SK, Siwach SB: Alcohol and coronary artery disease. Int J Cardiol 44:157, 1994
6. Altes-Capella J, Cabezudo-Artero JM, Forteza-Rei J: Complications of cocaine abuse. Ann Intern Med 107:940, 1987
7. Altura B, Altura BM: Phencyclidine, lysergic acid diethylamide, and mescaline: cerebral artery spasms and hallucinogenic activity. Science 212:1051, 1981
8. Altura BM, Altura BT: Role of magnesium and calcium in alcohol-induced hypertension and strokes as probed by in vivo television microscopy, digital image microscopy, optical spectroscopy, 31P-NMR spectroscopy and a unique magnesium ion-selective electrode. Alcoholism Clin Exp Res 18:1057, 1994
9. Altura BM, Altura BT, Gebrewold A: Alcohol-induced spasms of cerebral blood vessels: relations to cerebrovascular accidents and sudden death. Science 220:331, 1983
10. Altura BM, Gebrewold A, Altura BT, Gupta RK: Role of brain [Mg2+] in alcohol-induced hemorrhagic stroke in a rat model: a 31P-NMR in vivo study. Alcohol 12:131, 1995
11. Altura BM, Zhang A, Cheng TP, Altura BT: Ethanol promotes rapid depletion of intracellular free Mg in cerebral vascular smooth muscle cells: possible relation to alcohol-induced behavioral and stroke-like effects. Alcohol 10:563, 1993
12. Amine AB: Neurosurgical complications of heroin addiction: brain abscess and mycotic aneurysm. Surg Neurol 7:385, 1977
13. Anderson RJ, Garza H, Garriott JC, Dimaio V: Intravenous propylhexedrine (Benzedrex) abuse and sudden death. Am J Med 67:15, 1979
14. Anson BJ: p. 728. Morris's Human Anatomy: McGraw-Hill, New York, 1966
15. Aronow WS, Kaplan NM: Smoking. p. 50. In Kaplan NM, Stamler J (eds): Prevention of Coronary Heart Disease. Philadelphia, WB Saunders, 1983
16. Ashley MJ: Alcohol consumption, ischemic heart disease, and cerebrovascular disease. J Stud Alcohol 43:869, 1982
17. Atlee W: Talc and cornstarch emboli in eyes of drug abusers. JAMA 219:49, 1972
18. Avogaro P, Cazzolato G, Belussi F, Bittolo Bon G: Altered apoprotein composition of HDL-2 and HDL-3 in chronic alcoholics. Artery 10:317, 1982
19. Baden MM: Pathology of the addictive states. p. 189. In Richter RW (ed): Medical Aspects of Drug Abuse. Harper & Row, Hagerstown, MD, 1975
20. Balow J, Alter M, Resch J: Cerebral thromboembolism:

a clinical appraisal of 100 cases. Neurology (NY) 16:559, 1966

21. Banks T, Fletcher R, Ali N: Infective endocarditis in heroin addicts. Am J Med 55:444, 1973

22. Baquero M, Alfaro A: Progressive bleeding in spontaneous thalamic hemorrhage. Neurologia 9:364, 1994

23. Barboriak JJ, Anderson AJ, Hoffman RG: Interrelationships between coronary artery occlusion, high-density lipoprotein cholesterol, and alcohol intake. J Lab Clin Med 94:348, 1979

24. Barenek JT: Morphine binding by serum globulins from morphine-treated rabbits. Fed Proc 33:474, 1974

25. Barnes D, Palace J, O'Brien MD: Stroke following marijuana smoking. Stroke 9:1381, 1992

26. Barrett CP, Braithwaite RA, Teale JD: Unusual case of tetrahydrocannabinol intoxication confirmed by radio-immunoassay. Br Med J 2:166, 1977

27. Bartolomei F, Nicoli F, Swiader L, Gastaut JL: Accident vasculaire cerebral ischemique apres prise nasale d'heroine. Une nouvelle observation. Presse Med 21:983, 1992

28. Becker C: Medical complications of drug abuse. Adv Intern Med 24:183, 1979

29. Beevers DG: Alcohol and hypertension. Lancet 2:114, 1977

30. Beghi E, Bogliun G, Cosso P et al: Cerebrovascular disorders and alcohol intake: preliminary results of a case-control study. Ital J Neurol Sci 13:209, 1992

31. Beghi E, Bogliun G, Cosso P et al: Stroke and alcohol intake in a hospital population. A case-control study. Stroke 26:1691, 1995

32. Beilin LJ: Alcohol and hypertension. Clin Exp Pharmacol Physiol 22:185, 1995

33. Belch JJ, McArdle BM, Burns P et al: The effects of acute smoking on platelet behavior, fibrinolysis, and haemorheology in habitual smokers. Thromb Haemost 51:6, 1984

34. Bement CL, Cohen L, Nielson SW, Langner RO: Arterial injury in rabbits following alternate day injections of cocaine. FASEB J 3:A297, 1989

35. Benowitz NL: Pharmacologic aspects of cigarette smoking and nicotine addiction. N Engl J Med 319:1318, 1988

36. Ben-Shlomo Y, Markowe H, Shipley M, Marmot MG: Stroke risk from alcohol consumption using different control groups. Stroke 23:1093, 1992

37. Berglund M: Cerebral blood flow in chronic alcoholics. Alcoholism Clin Exp Res 5:295, 1981

38. Bernheim J, Cox JN: Heat stroke and amphetamine intoxication in a sportsman. Schweiz Med Wochenschr 90: 322, 1960

39. Bernstein E, Diskant B: Phenylpropanolamine, a potentially hazardous drug. Ann Emerg Med 11:315, 1982

40. Besson HA: Intracranial hemorrhage associated with phencyclidine abuse. JAMA 248:585, 1982

41. Biter S, Gomez CR: Stroke following injection of a melted suppository. Stroke 24:741, 1993

42. Blackwelder WC, Yano K, Rhoads GC et al: Alcohol and mortality: the Honolulu Heart Study. Am J Med 68:164, 1980

43. Bloch C, Richard JL: Risk factors for atherosclerotic diseases in the Prospective Parisian Study. I. Comparison with foreign studies. Rev Epidemiol Sante Publique 33: 108, 1985

44. Blum A: Phenylpropanolamine: an over-the-counter amphetamine? JAMA 245:1346, 1981

45. Boak RA, Carpenter CM, Miller JN: Biologic false-positive reactions for syphilis among narcotic addicts: a report on the incidence of BFP reactions as measured by the TPI test. JAMA 175:326, 1961

46. Bogousslavsky J, Van Melle G, Despland PA, Regli F: Alcohol consumption and carotid atherosclerosis in the Lausanne Stroke Registry. Stroke 21:715, 1990

47. Bohmfalk GL, Story JL, Wissinger JP, Brown WE: Bacterial intracranial aneurysm. J Neurosurg 48:369, 1978

48. Bonhoff C, Lewrenz H: Über Werkamine. p. 144. Springer-Verlag, Berlin, 1954

49. Bonita R: Cigarette smoking, hypertension, and the risk of subarachnoid hemorrhage: a population-based case-control study. Stroke 17:831, 1986

50. Bonita R, Scragg R, Stewart A et al: Cigarette smoking and risk of premature stroke in men and women. Br Med J 293:6, 1986

51. Bostwick DG: Amphetamine induced cerebral vasculitis. Hum Pathol 12:1031, 1981

52. Bourne PG: Acute Drug Abuse Emergencies. Academic Press, San Diego, CA, 1976

53. Boyko OB, Burger PC, Heinz ER: Pathological and radiological correlation of subarachnoid hemorrhage in phencyclidine abuse: case report. J Neurosurg 67:446, 1987

54. Boysen G, Nyboe J, Appleyard M et al: Stroke incidence and risk factors for stroke in Copenhagen, Denmark. Stroke 19:1345, 1988

55. Brackett, DJ, Gauvin DV, Lerner MR et al: Dose- and time-dependent cardiovascular responses induced by ethanol. J Pharmacol Exp Ther 268:78, 1994

56. Brierley JB: The neuropathology of brain hypoxia. p. 243. In Critchley M, O'Leary JL, Jennett B (eds): Scientific Foundations of Neurology. Heinemann, London, 1972

57. Bruno A, Nolte KB, Chapin J: Stroke associated with ephedrine use. Neurology 43:1313, 1993

58. Brust JCM: Drug abuse and nervous system toxins. p. 540. In Rosenberg R (ed): Neurology. Vol. 5: The Science and Practice of Clinical Medicine. Dietschy JM (ed-in-chief). Grune & Stratton, Orlando, FL, 1980

59. Brust JCM: The non-impact of opiate research on opiate abuse. Neurology (NY) 33:1327, 1983

60. Brust JCM: Neurology and drug abuse. Neurology and Neurosurgery Update Series 4/29:1, 1983

61. Brust JCM: Stroke and drugs. p. 517. In Toole JF (ed): Vascular Diseases, Part III, Vol 55 of Handbook of Clinical Neurology, Rev Series II. Elsevier, Amsterdam, 1989

62. Brust JCM: Drug dependence. In Joynt RJ (ed): Clinical Neurology. Harper & Row, New York, 1991

63. Brust JCM: Neurological Aspects of Substance Abuse. Butterworth-Heinemann, Newton, MA, 1993

64. Brust JCM, Dickinson PCT, Hughes JEO, Holtzman RNN: The diagnosis and treatment of cerebral mycotic aneurysms. Ann Neurol 27:238, 1990

65. Brust JCM, Richter RW: Quinine amblyopia related to heroin addiction. Ann Intern Med 74:84, 1971

66. Brust JCM, Richter RW: Stroke associated with addiction to heroin. J Neurol Neurosurg Psychiatry 39:194, 1976

67. Brust JCM, Richter RW: Stroke associated with cocaine abuse? NY State J Med 77:1473, 1977

68. Burns RS, Lerner SE: Causes of phencyclidine-related deaths. Clin Toxicol 12:463, 1978

69. Burns RS, Lerner SE: The effects of phencyclidine in man: a review. p. 449. In Domino EF (ed): PCP (Phencyclidine): Historical and Current Perspectives. NPP Books, Ann Arbor, MI, 1981

70. Butz WC: Disseminated magnesium and silicate associated with paregoric addiction. J Forensic Sci 15:581, 1970

71. Cahill DW, Knipp H, Mosser J: Intracranial hemorrhage with amphetamine abuse. Neurology (NY) 31:1058, 1981

72. Camargo CA: Moderate alcohol consumption and stroke: the epidemiologic evidence. Stroke 20:1611, 1989

73. Camargo CA, Williams PT, Vranizan KM et al: The effect of moderate alcohol intake on serum apolipoproteins A-I and A-II: a controlled study. JAMA 253:2854, 1985

74. Candelise L, Bianchi F, Galligoni F et al: Italian multicenter study on cerebral ischemic attacks. III. Influence of age and risk factors on cerebral atherosclerosis. Stroke 15:379, 1984

75. Caplan LR, Hier DB, Banks G: Stroke and drug abuse. Stroke 13:869, 1982

76. Caplan LR, Hier DB, DeCruz I: Cerebral embolism in the Michael Reese Stroke Registry. Stroke 14:530, 1983

77. Caplan LR, Thomas C, Banks G: Central nervous system complications of addiction to "T's and Blues." Neurology (NY) 32:623, 1982

78. Case records of the Massachusetts General Hospital. N Engl J Med 329:117, 1993

79. Castelli WP, Gordon T, Hjortland MC et al: Alcohol and blood lipids: the Cooperative Lipoprotein Phenotying Study. Lancet 2:153, 1977

80. Chadan N, Thierry A, Sautreaux JL et al: Rupture aneurysmale et toxicomanie á la cocaine. Neurochirurgie 37:403, 1990

81. Chasnoff IJ, Bussey ME, Savich R, Stack CM: Perinatal cerebral infarction and maternal cocaine use. J Pediatr 108:456, 1986

82. Cherubin CE: The medical sequelae of narcotic addiction. Ann Intern Med 67:23, 1967

83. Chillar RK, Jackson AL: Reversible hemiplegia after presumed intracarotid injection of Ritalin. N Engl J Med 304:1305, 1981

84. Chokshi SK, Miller G, Rongione A, Isner JM: Cocaine and cardiovascular disease: the leading edge. Cardiology 3:1, 1989

85. Chokshi SK, Moore R, Pandian NG, Isner JM: Reversible cardiomyopathy associated with cocaine intoxication. Ann Intern Med 111:1039, 1989

86. Chynn KY: Acute subarachnoid hemorrhage. JAMA 233:55, 1973

87. Citron BP, Halpern M, McCarron M et al: Necrotizing angiitis associated with drug abuse. N Engl J Med 283:1003, 1970

88. Citron BP, Peters RL: Angiitis in drug abusers. N Engl J Med 284:112, 1971

89. Clowes GHA, O'Donnell TF: Heat stroke: N Engl J Med 291:564, 1974

90. Colditz GA, Bonita R, Stampfer MJ et al: Cigarette smoking and risk of stroke in middle-aged women. N Engl J Med 318:937, 1988

91. Collaborative Group for the Study of Stroke in Young Women: Oral contraception and increased risk of cerebral ischemia or thrombosis. N Engl J Med 288:871, 1973

92. Cooles P: Stroke after heavy cannabis smoking. Postgrad Med J 63:511, 1987

93. Corales RL, Maull KI, Becker DP: Phencyclidine abuse mimicking head injury. JAMA 243:2323, 1980

94. Coroner's Report: Amphetamine overdose kills boy. Pharm J 198:172, 1967

95. Courville CN: The process of demyelination in the central nervous system. IV. Demyelination as a delayed residual of carbon monoxide asphyxia. J Nerv Ment Dis 125:534, 1957

96. Cowan DH: Effect of alcoholism on hemostasis. Semin Hematol 17:137, 1980

97. Cregler LL, Mark H: Medical complications of cocaine abuse. N Engl J Med 315:1495, 1986

98. Cregler LL, Mark H: Relation of stroke to cocaine abuse. NY State J Med 87:128, 1987

99. Crosley CJ, Binet EF: Cerebrovascular complications in phencyclidine intoxication. J Pediatr 94:316, 1979

100. Cullen K, Stenhouse NS, Wearne KL: Alcohol and mortality in the Busselton study. Int J Epidemiol 11:67, 1982

101. Cunningham EE, Brentjens JR, Zielezny MA et al: Heroin nephropathy: a clinicopathologic and epidemiologic study. Am J Med 68:47, 1980

102. Cushman P, Grieco MH: Hyperimmunoglobulinemia associated with narcotic addiction: effects of methadone maintenance treatment. Am J Med 54:320, 1973

103. Daras M, Tuchman AJ, Koppel BS et al: Neurovascular complications of cocaine. Acta Neurol Scand 90:124, 1994

104. Daras M, Tuchman AJ, Marks S: Central nervous system infarction related to cocaine abuse. Stroke 22:1320, 1991

105. Davanipour Z, Sobel E, Alter M et al: Stroke/transient ischemic attack in the Lehigh Valley: evaluation of smoking as a risk factor. Ann Neurol 24:130, 1988

106. Davis JW, Shelton L, Eigenberg DA et al: Effects of tobacco and non-tobacco cigarette smoking on endothelium and platelets. Clin Pharmacol Ther 37:529, 1985

107. DeBroucker T, Verstichel P, Cambier J, De-Truchis P: Accidents neurologiqes après prise de cocaine. Presse Med 18:541, 1989

108. Delaney P: Intracranial hemorrhage associated with amphetamine use. Neurology (NY) 31:923, 1981

109. Delaney P, Estes M: Intracranial hemorrhage with amphetamine abuse. Neurology (NY) 30:1125, 1980

110. Department of Health and Human Services: The Health Consequences of Smoking: Nicotine Addiction. A Report of the Surgeon General. (DHHS Publ No [CDC] 88-8406.) US Government Printing Office, Washington, DC, 1988

111. Deringer PM, Hamilton LL, Whelan MA: A stroke associated with cocaine use. Arch Neurol 47:502, 1990

112. Devenyi P, Schneiderman JF, Devenyi RG, Lawby L: Cocaine-induced central retinal artery occlusion. Can Med Assoc J 138:129, 1988

113. Devore RA, Tucker HM: Dysphagia and dysarthria as a result of cocaine abuse. Otolaryngol Head Neck Surg 98:174, 1988

114. Diaz-Tejedor E, Tejada J, Munoz J: Cerebral arterial changes following cocaine IV administration: an angiographic study in rabbits. J Neurol 239 (suppl 2):S38, 1992

115. DiChiro G, Fried LC: Blood flow currents in spinal arteries. Neurology (NY) 21:1088, 1971

116. DiMinno G, Mancini M: Drugs affecting plasma fibrinogen levels. Cardiovasc Drugs Ther 6:25, 1992

117. Dixon SD, Bejar R: Echoencephalographic findings in neonates associated with maternal cocaine and methamphetamine use: incidence and clinical correlates. J Pediatr 115:770, 1989

118. Dohi S, Jones D, Hudak ML, Traystman RJ: Effects of cocaine on pial arterioles in cats. Stroke 21:1710, 1990

119. Doll R, Gray R, Hafner B et al: Mortality in relation to smoking: twenty-two years observations on female British doctors. Br Med J 1:967, 1980

120. Doll R, Hill AB: Mortality of British doctors in relation to smoking: observations on coronary thrombosis. Natl Cancer Inst Monogr 19:205, 1966

121. Doll R, Peto R: Mortality in relation to smoking: 20 year's observations on male British doctors. Br Med J 2:1525, 1976

122. Dominguez R, Vila-Coro AA, Slopis JM, Bohan TP: Brain and ocular abnormalities in infants with in utero exposure to cocaine and other street drugs. Am J Dis Child 145:688, 1991

123. Donahue RP, Abbott RD, Reed DM, Yano K: Alcohol and hemorrhagic stroke: the Honolulu Heart Study. JAMA 255:2311, 1986

124. Doyle JT, Heslin AS, Hilleboe HE et al: A prospective study of degenerative cardiovascular disease in Albany: report of three years' experience. 1. Ischemic heart disease. Am J Public Health 47:25, 1957

125. D'Souza T, Shraberg D: Intracranial hemorrhage associated with amphetamine use. Neurology (NY) 31:922, 1981

126. Duarte Escalante O, Ellinwood EH: Central nervous system cytopathological changes in cats with chronic methedrine intoxication. Brain Res 21:151, 1970

127. Dyer A, Stamler J, Paul O et al: Alcohol consumption, cardiovascular risk factors, and mortality in two Chicago epidemiologic studies. Circulation 56:1067, 1977

128. Dyer AR, Stamler J, Paul O et al: Alcohol consumption and 17-year mortality in the Chicago Western Electric Company. Prev Med 9:78, 1980

129. Eastman JW, Cohen SN: Hypertensive crisis and death associated with phencyclidine poisoning. JAMA 231:1270, 1975

130. Eddy NB, Halbach H, Isbell H, Seevers MH: Drug dependence: its significance and characteristics. Bull WHO 32:721, 1965

131. Edwards K: Hemorrhagic complications of cerebral arteritis. Arch Neurol 34:549, 1977

132. Engstrand BC, Daras M, Tuchman AJ et al: Cocaine-related ischemic stroke. Neurology (NY), suppl 1. 39: 186, 1989

133. Ettinger PO, Wu CF, DeLa Cruz C et al: Arrhythmias and the "holiday heart": alcohol-associated cardiac rhythm disorders. Am Heart J 95:555, 1978

134. Fenn CG, Littleton JM: Inhibition of platelet aggregation by ethanol: the role of plasma and platelet membrane lipids. Br J Pharmacol 73:305P, 1981

135. Ferris EB, Blankenhorn MA, Robinson HW et al: Heat stroke: clinical and chemical observations on 44 cases. J Clin Invest 17:249, 1938

136. Flamm ES, Demopoulos HB, Seligman ML et al: Ethanol potentiation of central nervous system trauma. J Neurosurg 46:328, 1977

137. Fogelholm R: Cigarette smoking and subarachnoid hemorrhage: a population-based case-control study. J Neurol Neurosurg Psychiatry 50:78, 1987

138. Forman HP, Levin S, Stewart B et al: Cerebral vasculitis and hemorrhage in an adolescent taking diet pills containing phenylpropanolamine: case report and review of the literature. Pediatrics 83:737, 1989

139. Frazee JG, Cahan LD, Winter J: Bacterial intracranial aneurysms. J Neurosurg 53:633, 1980

140. Fredericks RK, Lefkowitz DS, Challa VER, Troost BT: Cerebral vasculitis associated with cocaine abuse. Stroke 22:1437, 1991

141. Frederiksen H, Ravenholt RT: Thromboembolism, oral contraceptives, and cigarettes. Public Health Rep 85: 197, 1970

142. Freeman W, Dumoff S: Cerebellar syndrome following heat stroke. Arch Neurol Psychiatry 51:67, 1944

143. Friberg L, Cederlof R, Lorich U et al: Mortality in twins in relation to smoking habits and alcohol problems. Arch Environ Health 27:294, 1973

144. Friedman EA, Sreepada Rao TK, Nicastri AD: Heroin-associated nephropathy. Nephron 13:421, 1974

145. Friedman GD, Dales LG, Ury HK: Mortality in middle-aged smokers and non-smokers. N Engl J Med 300:213, 1979

146. Fuchs CS, Stampfer MJ, Colditz GA et al: Alcohol consumption and mortality among women. N Engl J Med 332:1245, 1995

147. Fujii Y, Takeuchi S, Tanaka R et al: Liver dysfunction in spontaneous intracerebral hemorrhage. Neurosurgery 35:592, 1994

148. Garcia-Albea E: Subarachnoid hemorrhage and nasal vasoconstrictor abuse. J Neurol Neurosurg Psychiatry 46: 875, 1983

149. Garland H, Greenburg J, Harriman DGF: Infarction of the spinal cord. Brain 89:645, 1966

150. Gay GR, Inaba DS, Sheppard CW et al: Cocaine: history, epidemiology, human pharmacology, and treatment: a perspective on a new debut for an old girl. Clin Toxicol 8:149, 1975

151. Gericke OL: Suicide by ingestion of amphetamine sulfate. JAMA 128:1098, 1945

152. Gill JS, Zezulka AV, Shipley MJ et al: Stroke and alcohol consumption. N Engl J Med 315:1041, 1986

153. Gilroy J, Andaya L, Thomas VJ: Intracranial mycotic aneurysms and subacute bacterial endocarditis in heroin addiction. Neurology (NY) 23:1193, 1973

154. Ginsberg MD, Hedley-Whyte ET, Richardson EP: Hypoxic-ischemic leukoencephalopathy in man. Arch Neurol 33:5, 1976

155. Gocke DJ, Christian CL: Angiitis in drug abusers. N Engl J Med 284:112, 1971

156. Gocke DJ, Morgan C, Lockshin M et al: Association between polyarteritis and Australia antigen. Lancet 2: 1149, 1970

157. Golbe LI, Merkin MD: Cerebral infarction in a user of free-base cocaine ("crack"). Neurology (NY) 36:1602, 1986

158. Goldbaum GM, Kendrick JS, Hogelin GC, Gentry EM: The relative impact of smoking and oral contraceptive use on women in the United States. JAMA 258:1339, 1987

159. Goldberg RJ, Burchfiel CM, Benfante R et al: Lifestyle and biologic factors associated with atherosclerotic disease in middle-aged men. 20-year findings from the Honolulu Heart Program. Arch Intern Med 155:686, 1995

160. Goodman SJ, Becker DP: Intracranial hemorrhage associated with amphetamine abuse. JAMA 212:480, 1970

161. Gordon EL, Nguyen TS, Ngai AC, Winn HR: Differential effects of alcohols on intracerebral arterioles. Ethanol alone causes vasoconstriction. J Cerebral Blood Flow Metab 15:532, 1995

162. Gordon T, Doyle JT: Drinking and mortality: the Albany Study. Am J Epidemiol 125:263, 1987

163. Gordon T, Kannel WB: Drinking habits and cardiovascular disease: the Framingham Study. Am Heart J 105: 667, 1983

164. Gorelick PB: Alcohol and stroke. Stroke 18:268, 1987

165. Gorelick PB: The status of alcohol as a risk factor for stroke. Stroke 20:1607, 1989

166. Gorelick PB, Rodin MB, Langenberg P et al: Is acute alcohol ingestion a risk factor for ischemic stroke?—results of a controlled study in middle-aged and elderly stroke patients at three urban medical centers. Stroke 18:359, 1987

167. Gorelick PB, Rodin MB, Langenberg P et al: Weekly alcohol consumption, cigarette smoking, and the risk of ischemic stroke: results of a case-control study at three urban medical centers in Chicago, Illinois. Neurology (NY) 39:339, 1989

168. Green MS, Jucha E, Luz Y: Blood pressure in smokers and non-smokers: epidemiologic findings. Am Heart J 111:932, 1986

169. Green R, Kelly KM, Gabrielson T et al: Multiple intracerebral hemorrhages after smoking "crack" cocaine. Stroke 21:957, 1990

170. Greenwood R, Peachey RS: Acute amphetamine poisoning: an account of three cases. Br Med J 1:742, 1957

171. Grieg M, Pemberton J, Hay I, MacKensie G: A prospective study of the development of coronary heart disease in a group of 1202 middle-aged men. J Epidemiol Community Health 34:23, 1980

172. Grishman E, Churg J, Porush JG: Glomerular morphology in nephrotic heroin addicts. Lab Invest 35:415, 1976

173. Gronback M, Deis A, Sorensen TI et al: Mortality associated with moderate intakes of wine, beer, or spirits. BMJ 10:1165, 1995

174. Guidotti M, Zanasi S: Cocaine use and cerebrovascular disease: two cases of ischemic stroke in young adults. Ital J Neurol Sci 11:153, 1990

175. Haapanen A, Koskenvuo M, Kaprio J et al: Carotid arteriosclerosis in identical twins discordant for cigarette smoking. Circulation 80:10, 1989

176. Hall CD, Blanton DE, Scatliff JH, Morris CE: Speed kills: fatality from the self administration of methamphetamine intravenously. South Med J 66:650, 1973

177. Hall JAS: Cocaine-induced stroke: first Jamaican case. J Neurol Sci 98:347, 1990

178. Hall JH, Karp HR: Acute progressive ventral pontine disease in heroin abuse. Neurology (NY) 23:6, 1973

179. Hamer JJ, Kamphuis DJ, Rico RE: Cerebral hemorrhages and infarcts following use of cocaine. Ned Tijdschr Geneeskd 135:333, 1991

180. Hamer R, Phelp D: Inadvertent intra-arterial injection of phentermine: a complication of drug abuse. Ann Emerg Med 10:148, 1981

181. Hammond EC: Smoking in relation to mortality and morbidity: finding in the first 34 months of follow-up in a prospective study started in 1959. JNCI 32:1161, 1964

182. Hammond EC: Smoking in relation to death rates of 1 million men and women. Natl Cancer Inst Monogr 19: 127, 1966

183. Hansagi H, Romelsjo A, Gerhardsson de Verdier M, Andreasson S, Liefman A: Alcohol consumption and stroke mortality. 20 year follow-up of 15,077 men and women. Stroke 26:1768, 1995

184. Harmsen P, Rosengren A, Tsipogianni A, Wilhelmsen L: Risk factors for stroke in middle-aged men in Göteborg, Sweden. Stroke 21:223, 1990

185. Harper G, Castleden CM, Potter JF: Factors affecting changes in blood pressure after acute stroke. Stroke 25: 1726, 1994

186. Harrington H, Heller HA, Dawson D et al: Intracerebral hemorrhage and oral amphetamine. Arch Neurol 40: 503, 1983

187. Harruff RC, Phillips AM, Fernandez GS: Cocaine-related deaths in Memphis and Shelby County. Ten-year history, 1980–1989. J Tenn Med Assoc 84:66, 1991

188. Hartman BK, Zide D, Udenfriend A: The use of dopamine beta-hydroxylase as a marker for the central noradrenergic nervous system in rat brain. Proc Natl Acad Sci USA 69:2722, 1972

189. Harvey JK, Todd CW, Howard JW: Fatality associated with Benzedrine ingestion: a case report. Del Med 21: 111, 1949

190. Haselager EM, Vreeken J: Rebound thrombocytosis after alcohol abuse: a possible factor in the pathogenesis of thromboembolic disease. Lancet 1:774, 1977

191. Haskell WJ, Camargo C, Williams PT et al: The effect of cessation and resumption of moderate alcohol intake on serum high-density lipoprotein subfractions: a controlled study. N Engl J Med 310:805, 1984

192. Haut MJ, Cowan DH: The effect of ethanol on hemostatic properties of human blood platelets. Am J Med 56:22, 1974

193. Heier LA, Carpanzano CR, Mast J et al: Maternal cocaine abuse: the spectrum of radiologic abnormalities in the neonatal CNS. AJR 157:1105, 1991

194. Helpern M, Rho Y-M: Deaths from narcotism in New York City. NY State J Med 66:2391, 1966

195. Hemmingsen R, Barry DL, Hertz MM, Klinken L: Cerebral blood flow and oxygen consumption during ethanol withdrawal in the rat. Brain Res 173:259, 1979

196. Henderson CE, Torbey M: Rupture of intracranial aneurysm associated with cocaine use during pregnancy. Am J Perinatol 5:142, 1988

197. Hennekens CH, Rosner B, Cole DS: Daily alcohol consumption and fatal coronary heart disease. Am J Epidemiol 107:196, 1978

198. Hennekens CH, Willett W, Rosner B et al: Effects of beer, wine, and liquor in coronary deaths. JAMA 242:1973, 1979

199. Henson RA, Parsons M: Ischemic lesions of the spinal cord: an illustrated review. Q J Med 36:205, 1967

200. Herman B, Leyten ACM, van Luuk JH et al: An evaluation of risk factors for stroke in a Dutch community. Stroke 13:334, 1982

201. Herman B, Schmintz PIM, Leyten ACM et al: Multivariate logistic analysis of risk factors for stroke in Tilburg, the Netherlands. Am J Epidemiol 118:514, 1983

202. Herrschaft H: Prophylaxe zerbraler Durchblutungsstörungen. Fortschr Neurol Psychiatr 53:337, 1985

203. Herskowitz A, Gross E: Cerebral infarction associated with heroin sniffing. South Med J 66:778, 1973

204. Hillbom M, Kangasaho M, Kaste M et al: Acute ethanol ingestion increases platelet reactivity: is there a relationship to stroke? Stroke 16:19, 1985

205. Hillbom M, Kaste M: Does ethanol intoxication promote brain infarction in young adults? Lancet 2:1181, 1978

206. Hillbom M, Kaste M: Does alcohol intoxication precipitate aneurysmal subarachnoid hemorrhage? J Neurol Neurosurg Psychiatry 44:523, 1981

207. Hillbom M, Kaste M: Ethanol intoxication: a risk factor for ischemic brain infarction in adolescents and young adults. Stroke 12:422, 1981

208. Hillbom M, Kaste M: Alcohol intoxication: a risk factor for primary subarachnoid hemorrhage. Neurology (NY) 32:706, 1982

209. Hillbom M, Kaste M: Ethanol intoxication: a risk factor for ischemic brain infarction. Stroke 14:694, 1983

210. Hillbom M, Kaste M, Rasi V: Can ethanol intoxication affect hemocoagulation to increase the risk of brain infarction in young adults? Neurology (NY) 33:381, 1983

211. Hilton-Jones O, Warlow CP: The cause of stroke in the young. J Neurol 232:137, 1985

212. Hirsch CS: Dermatopathology of narcotic addiction. Hum Pathol 3:37, 1972

213. Ho K, Rassekh Z: Mycotic aneurysm of the right subclavian artery: a complication of heroin addiction. Chest 74:116, 1978

214. Holman BL, Carvalho PA, Mendelson J et al: Brain perfusion is abnormal in cocaine-dependent polydrug users: a study using technetium-99m-HMPAO and ASPECT. J Nucl Med 32:1206, 1991

215. Houck RJ, Bailey G, Daroca P et al: Pentazocine abuse. Chest 77:227, 1980

216. Hoyme HE, Jones KL, Dixon SD et al: Prenatal cocaine exposure and fetal vascular disruption. Pediatrics 85:743, 1990

217. Huang QF, Gebrewold A, Altura BT, Altura BM: Cocaine-induced cerebral vascular damage can be ameliorated by Mg^{2+} in rat brain. Neurosci Lett 109:113, 1990

218. Hubbell G, Cheitlin MD, Rapaport E: Presentation, management, and follow-up evaluation of ineffective endocarditis in drug addicts. Am Heart J 102:85, 1981

219. Husby G, Pierce PE, Williams RL: Smooth muscle antibody in heroin addicts. Ann Intern Med 83:801, 1975

220. Hutton RA, Fink FR, Wilson DT, Marjot DH: Platelet hyperaggregability during alcohol withdrawal. Clin Lab Haematol 3:223, 1981

221. Illett KF, Jarrott B, O'Donnell SR et al: Mechanism of cardiovascular actions of 1-(1-phenylcyclohexyl) piperidine hydrochloride (phencyclidine). Br J Pharmacol Chemother 28:73, 1966

222. Isles C, Brown JJ, Cumming AM et al: Excess smoking in malignant phase hypertension. Br Med J 1:579, 1979

223. Isner JM, Chokshi SK: Cocaine and vasospasm. N Engl J Med 321:1604, 1989

224. Iso H, Kitamara A, Shimamoto T et al: Alcohol intake and the risk of cardiovascular disease in middle-aged Japanese men. Stroke 26:767, 1995

225. Jacobs IG, Roszler MH, Kelly JK et al: Cocaine abuse: neurovascular complications. Radiology 170:223, 1989

226. Jakubowski JA, Vaillancourt R, Deykin D: Interaction of ethanol, prostacyclin, and aspirin in determining human platelet reactivity in vitro. Arteriosclerosis 8:436, 1988

227. Jamrozik K, Broadhurst RJ, Anderson CS, Stewart-Wynne EG: The role of lifestyle factors in the etiology of stroke. A population-based case-control study in Perth, Western Australia. Stroke 25:51, 1994

228. Janssens E, Mounier-Vehier F, Hamon M, Leys D: Small subcortical infarcts and primary subcortical hemorrhages may have different risk factors. J Neurol 242:425, 1995

229. Jara FM, Lewis JF, Magilligan DJ: Operative experience with infective endocarditis and intracerebral mycotic aneurysm. J Thorac Cardiovasc Surg 80:28, 1980

230. Jennings LK, White MM, Sauer CM et al: Cocaine-induced platelet defects. Stroke 24:1352, 1993

231. Jordan SC, Hampson F: Amphetamine poisoning associated with hyperpyrexia. Br Med J 2:844, 1960

232. Jorgensen HS, Nakagama H, Raaschou HO, Olsen TS: Leukoaraiosis in stroke patients. The Copenhagen Stroke Study. Stroke 26:588, 1995

233. Judice DJ, LeBlanc HJ, McGarry PA: Spinal cord vasculitis presenting as spinal cord tumor in a heroin addict. J Neurosurg 48:131, 1978

234. Juvela S, Hillbom M, Numminen H, Koskinen P: Cigarette smoking and alcohol consumption as risk factors for aneurysmal subarachnoid hemorrhage. Stroke 24:639, 1993

235. Kagan A, Popper JS, Rhoads GG, Yano K: Dietary and other risk factors for stroke in Hawaiian Japanese men. Stroke 16:390, 1985

236. Kahn HA: The Dorn study of smoking and mortality among US veterans: report on 8½ years of observations. Natl Cancer Inst Monogr 19:i, 1966

237. Kaku DA, Lowenstein DH: Recreational drug use: a growing risk factor for stroke in young people. Neurology (NY), 39(suppl 1):16, 1989

238. Kaku DA, Lowenstein DH: Emergence of recreational drug abuse as a major risk factor for stroke in young adults. Ann Intern Med 113:821, 1990

239. Kane FJ, Greene BQ: Psychotic episodes associated with the use of common proprietary decongestants. Am J Psychiatry 123:484, 1966

240. Kane FJ, Keeler MH, Reifler CB: Neurological crisis following methamphetamine. JAMA 210:556, 1969

241. Kangasaho M, Hillbom M, Kaste M, Vapaatalo H: Effects of ethanol intoxication and hangover on plasma levels of thromboxane B_2 and 6-keto-prostaglandin $F_1\alpha$ and on thromboxane B_2 formation by platelets in man. Thomb Haemost 48:232, 1982

242. Kannel WB: Current status of the epidemiology of brain infarction associated with occlusive arterial disease. Stroke 2:295, 1971

243. Kannel WB, D'Agostino RB, Belanger AL: Fibrinogen, cigarette smoking, and risk of cardiovascular disease: insights from the Framingham Study. Am Heart J 113:1006, 1987

244. Kannel WB, Dawber TR, Cohen ME et al: Vascular disease of the brain-epidemiologic aspects: the Framingham Study. Am J Public Health 55:1355, 1965

245. Kannel WB, Sorlie P: Hypertension in Framingham. p. 553. In Paul O (ed): Epidemiology and Control of Hypertension. Symposia Specialists, Miami, 1975

246. Kannel WB, Wolf PA, Dawber TR: An evaluation of the epidemiology of atherothrombotic brain infarction. Milbank Mem Fun Q 53:405, 1975

247. Kannel WB, Woosley P: Alcohol and cardiovascular risk. Circulation, 52(suppl II):200, 1975

248. Karch SB, Billingham ME: The pathology and etiology of cocaine-induced heart disease. Arch Pathol Lab Med 112:225, 1988

249. Kasirsky G, Zaidi IH, Tansy MF: LD50 and pathologic effects of acute and chronic administration of methamphetamine HCl in rabbits. Res Commun Chem Pathol Pharmacol 3:215, 1972

250. Katsuki S: Hisayama study. Jpn J Med 10:167, 1971

251. Katsuki S, Omae T: Stroke prone profiles in the Japanese. p. 215. In Engel A, Larsson T (eds): First Thule International Symposium on Stroke, 1966. Nordiska Bokhandein, Stockholm, 1967

252. Kaye BR, Fainstat M: Cerebral vasculitis associated with cocaine abuse. JAMA 258:2104, 1987

253. Kessler GF, Demers LM, Brennan RW: Phencyclidine and fatal status epilepticus. N Engl J Med 291:979, 1974

254. Kessler JT, Jortner BS, Adapon BD: Cerebral vasculitis in a drug abuser. J Clin Psychiatry 39:559, 1978

255. Khaw AL, Barrett-Connor E: Dietary potassium and stroke-associated mortality: a 12-year prospective study. N Engl J Med 316:235, 1987

256. Kiechl S, Willeit J, Egger G et al: Alcohol consumption and carotid atherosclerosis: evidence of dose-dependent atherogenic and antiatherogenic effects. Results from the Bruneck Study. Stroke 25:1593, 1994

257. Kilkoyne MM, Daly JJ, Gocke DJ et al: Nephrotic syndrome in heroin addicts. Lancet 1:17, 1972

258. King J: Hypertension and cerebral hemorrhage after Trimolers ingestion. Med J Aust 2:258, 1979

259. King J, Richards M, Tress B: Cerebral arteritis associated with heroin abuse. Med J Aust 2:444, 1978

260. King TA, Perlman JM, Laptook AR et al: Neurologic manifestations of in utero cocaine exposure in near-term and term infants. Pediatrics 96:259, 1995

261. Kiyohara Y, Kato I, Iwamoto H et al: The impact of alcohol and hypertension on stroke incidence in a general Japanese population. The Hiseyama Study. Stroke 26:368, 1995

262. Klassen AC, Loewenson RB, Resch JA: Cerebral atherosclerosis in selected chronic disease states. Atherosclerosis 18:321, 1973

263. Klatsky AJ, Friedman GD, Siegelaub AB: Alcohol consumption before myocardial infarction: results from the Kaiser-Permanente epidemiologic study of myocardial infarction. Ann Intern Med 81:294, 1974

264. Klatsky AL, Friedman GD, Siegelaub AB et al: Alcohol consumption and blood pressure: Kaiser-Permanente Multiphasic Health Examination data. N Engl J Med 296:1194, 1977

265. Klatsky AJ, Friedman GD, Siegelaub AB: Alcohol use, myocardial infarction, sudden cardiac death, and hypertension. Alcoholism Clin Exp Res 3:33, 1979

266. Klatsky AL, Friedman GD, Siegelaub AB: Alcohol and mortality: a ten-year Kaiser-Permanente experience. Ann Intern Med 95:139, 1981

267. Klonoff DC, Andrews BT, Obana WG: Stroke associated with cocaine use. Arch Neurol 46:989, 1989

268. Knoblauch AL, Buchholz M, Koller MG, Kistler H: Hemiplegie nach Injektion von Heroin. Schweiz Med Wochenschr 113:402, 1983

269. Koch A, Reuther R, Boos R et al: Risikofactoren bei cerebralen Durchblutungsesstörungen. Verh Dtsch Ges Inn Med 83:1773, 1977

270. Kokkinos J, Levine SR: Stroke. In Brust JCM (ed): Neurologic Complications of Drug and Alcohol Abuse. Neurol Clin 11:577, 1993

271. Kokkinos J, Levine SR: Possible association of ischemic stroke with phentermine. Stroke 24:310, 1993

272. Kono S, Ikeda M, Ogata M et al: The relationship between alcohol and mortality among Japanese physicians. Int J Epidemiol 12:437, 1983

273. Kono S, Ikeda M, Tokudome S et al: Alcohol and mortality: a cohort study of male Japanese physicians. Int J Epidemiol 15:527, 1986

274. Konzen JP, Levine SR, Charbel FT, Garcia JH: The mechanisms of alkaloidal cocaine-related stroke. Neurology 42(suppl 3):249, 1992

275. Konzen JP, Levine SR, Garcia JH: Vasospasm and thrombus formation as possible mechanisms of stroke related to alkaloidal cocaine. Stroke 26:1114, 1995

276. Kool MJ, Hoeks AP, Struijker Boudier HA et al: Short and long-term effects of smoking on arterial wall properties in habitual smokers. J Am Coll Cardiol 22:1881, 1993

277. Koppel BS, Kaunitz AM, Daras M et al: Cocaine-associated stroke during pregnancy. Ann Neurol 32:239, 1992

278. Kozaravic D, McGee D, Vojvodic N et al: Frequency of alcohol consumption and morbidity and mortality: the Yugoslavia cardiovascular disease study. Lancet 1:613, 1980

279. Kozarevic DJ, Vodvodic N, Gordon T et al: Drinking

habits and death: the Yugoslavia Cardiovascular Disease Study. Int J Epidemiol 12:145, 1983

280. Kramer LD, Locke GE, Ogunyemi A, Nelson L: Neonatal cocaine-related seizures. J Child Neurol 5:60, 1990

281. Krendel DA, Ditter SM, Frankel MR, Ross WK: Biopsy-proven cerebral vasculitis associated with cocaine abuse. Neurology (NY) 40:1092, 1990

282. Kubota K, Yamaguchi T, Abe Y: Effects of smoking on regional cerebral blood flow in neurologically normal subjects. Stroke 14:720, 1983

283. Kumar P, Rathore CK, Nagar AM et al: Hyperpyrexia with special reference to heat stroke: an analysis of 108 cases. J Indian Med Assoc 43:213, 1964

284. Kurtzke JF: Epidemiology of Cerebrovascular Disease. Springer-Verlag, New York, 1969

285. Lahmeyer HW, Steingold RG: Pentazocine and tripelennamine: a drug abuse epidemic? Int J Addict 15:1219, 1980

286. Lakier JB: Smoking and cardiovascular disease. Am J Med 93:8S, 1992

287. Lambrecht GL, Malbrain ML, Chew SL et al: Intranasal caffeine and amphetemine causing stroke. Acta Neurol Belg 93:146, 1993

288. Lamont CM, Adams FG: Glue-sniffing as a cause of a positive radio-isotope brain scan. Eur J Nucl Med 7:387, 1982

289. Landolfi R, Steiner M: Ethanol raises prostacyclin in vivo and in vitro. Blood 64:679, 1984

290. Lang WE: Ethyl alcohol enhances plasminogen activator secretion by endothelial cells. JAMA 250:772, 1983

291. Lange RA, Cigarroa RG, Yancy CW et al: Cocaine-induced coronary artery vasoconstriction. N Engl J Med 321:1557, 1989

292. Langner RO, Bement CL, Perry LE: Arteriosclerotic toxicity of cocaine. Natl Inst Drug Abuse Res Monogr Ser 88–1585:325, 1987

293. LaPorte RE, Cresanta JL, Kuller LH: The relationship of alcohol consumption to atherosclerotic heart disease. Prev Med 9:22, 1980

294. Lasagna L: Phenylpropanolamine: A Review. Wiley, New York, 1988

295. Ledgerwood AM, Lucas CE: Mycotic aneurysm of the carotid artery. Arch Surg 109:496, 1974

296. Lee J, Sapira JD: Retinal and cerebral microembolization of talc in a drug abuser. Am J Med Sci 265:75, 1973

297. Lee K: Alcoholism and cerebral thrombosis in the young. Acta Neurol Scand 59:270, 1979

298. Lee K, Nielsen JD, Zeeberg I, Gormsen J: Platelet aggregation and fibrinolytic activity in young alcoholics. Acta Neurol Scand 62:287, 1980

299. Lee MC, Randa DC, Gold LH: Transverse myelopathy following the use of heroin. Minn Med 59:82, 1976

300. Lee TK, Huang ZS, Ng SK et al: Impact of alcohol consumption and cigarette smoking on stroke among the elderly in Taiwan. Stroke 26:790, 1995

301. Lehman LB: Intracerebral hemorrhage after intranasal cocaine use. Hosp Physician 7:69, 1987

302. Levine LH, Hirsch CS, White LW: Quinine cardiotoxicity: a mechanism for sudden death in narcotic addicts. J Forensic Sci 18:167, 1973

303. Levine SR, Brust JCM, Futrell N et al: Cerebrovascular complications of the use of the "crack" form of alkaloidal cocaine. N Engl J Med 323:699, 1990

304. Levine SR, Brust JCM, Welch KMA: Cerebral vasculitis associated with cocaine abuse or subarachnoid hemorrhage. JAMA 259:1648, 1988

305. Levine SR, Fagan SC, Floberg J et al: Moya-moya, oral contraceptives, and cigarette use. Ann Neurol 24:155, 1988

306. Levine SR, Washington JM, Jefferson MF et al: "Crack" cocaine-associated stroke. Neurology (NY) 37:1849, 1987

307. Levine SR, Welch KM: Cocaine and stroke. Stroke 19:779, 1988

308. Lewis E: Hyperpyrexia with antidepressant drugs. Br Med J 2:1671, 1965

309. Libman RB, Masters SR, de Paola A, Mohr JP: Transient monocular blindness associated with cocaine abuse. Neurology 43:228, 1993

310. Lichtenfield PJ, Rubin DB, Feldman RS: Subarachnoid hemorrhage precipitated by cocaine snorting. Arch Neurol 41:223, 1984

311. Lieber CS: To drink (moderately) or not to drink. N Engl J Med 310:846, 1984

312. Lieberman AN, Bloom W, Kishore PS, Lin JP: Carotid artery occlusion following ingestion of LSD. Stroke 5:213, 1974

313. Lignelli GJ, Buchheit WA: Angiitis in drug abusers. N Engl J Med 284:112, 1971

314. Lip GY, Beevers DG: Alcohol, hypertension, coronary disease, and stroke. Clin Exp Pharmacol Physiol 22:189, 1995

315. Lloyd JTA, Walker DRH: Death after combined dexamphetamine and phenylzine. Br Med J 2:168, 1995

316. Loizou LA, Hamilton JG, Tsementzis SA: Intracranial hemorrhage in association with pseudoephedrine overdose. J Neurol Neurosurg Psychiatry 45:471, 1982

317. Longstreth WT, Koepsell TD, Yerby MS, van Belle G: Risk factors for subarachnoid hemorrhage. Stroke 16:377, 1985

318. Longstreth WT, Swanson PD: Oral contraceptives and stroke. Stroke 15:747, 1984

319. Louria DB, Hensle T, Rose J: The major medical complications of heroin addiction. Ann Intern Med 67:1, 1967

320. Love BB, Biller J, Jones MP et al: Cigarette smoking. A risk factor for cerebral infarction in young adults. Arch Neurol 47:693, 1990

321. Lovejoy FH: Stroke and phenylpropanolamine. Pediatr Alert 12:45, 1981

322. LoVerme S: Complications of amphetamine abuse. p. 5. In Culebras A (ed): Clini-Pearls. Vol. 2, No. 8. Creative Medical Publications, Syracuse, NY, 1979

323. Lowenstein DH, Massa SM, Rowbotham MC et al: Acute neurologic and psychiatric complications associated with cocaine abuse. Am J Med 83:841, 1987

324. Luck JC: Arrhythmias and social drinking. Ann Intern Med 93:253, 1983

325. Lukes SA: Intracerebral hemorrhage from an arteriovenous malformation after amphetamine injection. Arch Neurol 40:60, 1983

326. Lundberg GD, Garriott JC, Reynolds PC et al: Cocaine-related death. J Forensic Sci 22:402, 1977

327. MacMahon S: Alcohol consumption and hypertension. Hypertension 9:111, 1987

328. MacMahon SW, Norton RN: Alcohol and hypertension: implications for prevention and treatment. Ann Intern Med 105:124, 1986

329. Manchanda S, Connolly MJ: Cerebral infarction in association with Ecstasy abuse. Postgrad Med J 69:874, 1993

330. Mangiardi JR, Daras M, Geller ME et al: Cocaine-related intracranial hemorrhage: report of nine cases and reviews. Acta Neurol Scand 77:177, 1988

331. Maouad J, Fernandez F, Barrillon A et al: Diffuse or segmental narrowing (spasm) of coronary arteries during smoking demonstrated on angiography. Am J Cardiol 53:354, 1984

332. Maqbool Z, Billett HH: Unwitting heparin abuse in a drug addict. Ann Intern Med 96:790, 1982

333. Margolis MT, Newton TH: Methamphetamine ("speed") arteritis. Neuroradiology 2:179, 1971

334. Mariani PJ: Pseudoephedrine-induced hypertensive emergency: treatment with labetalol. Am J Emerg Med 4:141, 1986

335. Martin K, Rogers T, Kavanaugh A: Central nervous system angiopathy associated with cocaine abuse. J Rheumatol 22:780, 1995

336. Mathews JD: Alcohol use, hypertension, and coronary heart disease. Clin Sci 51:661, 1976

337. Mathews UD: Alcohol and hypertension. Aust NZ J Med 9:158, 1979

338. Matick H, Anderson D, Brumlik J: Cerebral vasulitis associated with oral amphetamine overdose. Arch Neurol 40:253, 1983

339. Mathew RJ, Wilson WH: Substance abuse and cerebral blood flow. Am J Psychiatry 148:292, 1991

340. Mayhan WG: Responses of cerebral arterioles during chronic ethanol exposure. Am J Physiol 262:H787, 1992

341. McCarron MM, Schultze BW, Thompson GA et al: Acute phencyclidine intoxication: incidence of clinical findings in 1000 cases. Ann Emerg Med 10:237, 1981

342. McQueen JD, Sklar FK, Posey JB: Autoregulation of cerebral blood flow during alcohol infusion. J Stud Alcohol 39:1477, 1978

343. Meade TW, Chakrabarti R, Haines AP et al: Characteristics affecting fibrinolytic activity and plasma fibrinogen concentrations. Br Med J 1:153, 1979

344. Medical Research Council Working Party: MRC Trial of treatment of mild hypertension: principle results. Br Med J 291:97, 1985

345. Mercado A, Johnson G, Calver D, Sokol RJ: Cocaine, pregnancy, and postpartum intracerebral hemorrhage. Obstet Gynecol 73:467, 1989

346. Meza I, Estrad CA, Montalvo JA et al: Cerebral infarction associated with cocaine use. Henry Ford Hosp Med J 37:50, 1989

347. Mittleman RE, Wetli CV: Cocaine and sudden "natural" death. J Forensic Sci 32:11, 1987

348. Mizutami T, Lewis R, Gonatas N: Medial medullary syndrome in a drug abuser. Arch Neurol 37:425, 1980

349. Mody CK, Miller BL, McIntyre HB et al: Neurologic complications of cocaine abuse. Neurology (NY) 38:1189, 1988

350. Mohan H, Sood GC: Conjugate deviation of the eyes after cannabis intoxication. Br J Ophthalmol 48:160, 1964

351. Molgaard CA, Bartok A, Peddercord KM et al: The association between cerebrovascular disease and smoking: a case-control study. Neuroepidemiology 5:88, 1986

352. Moliterno DJ, Willard JE, Lange RA et al: Coronary vasoconstriction induced by cocaine, cigarette smoking, or both. N Engl J Med 330:454, 1994

353. Moore PM, Peterson PL: Nonhemorrhagic cerebrovascular complications of cocaine abuse. Neurology (NY), 39(suppl 1):302, 1989

354. Moore RD, Pearson TA: Moderate alcohol consumption and coronary artery disease: a review. Medicine (Baltimore) 65:242, 1986

355. Moorthy G, Price TR, Tuhrim S et al: Relationship between recent alcohol intake and stroke type?—the NINCDS Stroke Data Bank. Stroke 17:141, 1986

356. Morris JN, Kagan A, Pattison DC et al: Incidence and prediction of ischemic heart disease in London busmen. Lancet 2:553, 1966

357. Morrow PL, McQuillen JB: Cerebral vasculitis associated with cocaine abuse. J Forensic Sci 38:732, 1993

358. Mueller SM: Neurologic complications of phenylpropanolamine use. Neurology (NY) 33:650, 1983

359. Mueller SM, Ertel PJ: Subarachnoid hemorrhage associated with over-the-counter diet medications. Stroke 14:16, 1983

360. Mueller SM, Solow EB: Seizures associated with a new combination "pick-me-up" pill. Ann Neurol 11:322, 1982

361. Murchison LE, Fyfe T: Effects of cigarette smoking on serum lipids, blood glucose, and platelet adhesiveness. Lancet 2:182, 1966

362. Nadler JL, Velasso JS, Horton R: Cigarette smoking inhibits prostacyclin formation. Lancet 1:1248, 1983

363. Nalls G, Disher A, Darabagi J et al: Subcortical cerebral hemorrhages associated with cocaine abuse: CT and MR findings. J Comput Assist Tomogr 13:1, 1989

364. Nickerson DS, Williams RL, Boxmeyer M et al: Increased opsonic capacity of serum in chronic heroin addiction. Ann Intern Med 72:671, 1970

365. Noguchi TT, Nakamura GR: Phencyclidine-related deaths in Los Angeles County, 1976. J Forensic Sci 23:503, 1978

366. Nolte KB, Brass LM, Fletterick CF: Intracranial hemorrhage associated with cocaine abuse: a prospective autopsy study. Neurology 46:1291, 1996

367. Nolte KB, Gelman BB: Intracerebral hemorrhage associated with cocaine abuse. Arch Pathol Lab Med 113:812, 1989

368. Nunez BD, Miao L, Ross JN et al: Effects of cocaine on carotid vascular reactivity in swine after balloon vascular injury. Stroke 25:631, 1994

369. Nwosu CM, Nwabueze AC, Ikeh VO: Stroke at the prime of life: a study of Nigerian Africans between the ages of 16 and 45 years. East Afr Med J 69:384, 1992

370. Okada H, Horibe H, Ohno Y et al: A prospective study of cerebrovascular disease in Japanese rural communities, Akabane and Asahi. I: Evaluation of risk factors in the occurrence of cerebral hemorrhage and thrombosis. Stroke 7:599, 1976

371. Oleckno WA: The risk of stroke in young adults: an analysis of the contribution of cigarette smoking and alcohol consumption. Public Health 102:45, 1988

372. Olsen ER: Intracranial hemorrhage and amphetamine usage. Angiology 28:464, 1977

373. O'Malley S, Adamse M, Heaton RK, Gawin FH: Neuropsychological impairment in chronic cocaine abusers. Am J Drug Alcohol Abuse 18:131, 1992

374. Ortona L, Laghi V, Cauda R: Immune function in heroin addicts. N Engl J Med 300:45, 1979

375. Ostern S, Dodson WH: Hypertension following Ornade ingestion. JAMA 194:472, 1965

376. Paffenbarger RS Jr, Wing AL: Chronic disease in former college students. XI. Early precursors of nonfatal stroke. Am J Epidemiol 94:524, 1971

377. Paffenbarger RS Jr, Wing A: Characteristics in youth predisposing to fatal stroke in later years. Lancet 1:753, 1967

378. Paganini-Hill A, Ross RK, Henderson BE: Post-menopausal oestrogen treatment and stroke: a prospective study. Br Med J 297:519, 1988

379. Palmer JR, Rosenberg, Shapiro S: "Low yield" cigarettes and the risk of nonfatal myocardial infarction in women. N Engl J Med 320:1569, 1989

380. Palomaki H, Kaste M: Regular light-to-moderate intake of alcohol and the risk of ischemic stroke. Is there a beneficial effect? Stroke 24:1828, 1993

381. Palomaki H, Kaste M, Raininko R et al: Risk factors for cervical atherosclerosis in patients with transient ischemic attack or minor ischemic stroke. Stroke 24:970, 1993

382. Palomaki H, Partinen M, Erkinjuntti T, Kaste M: Snoring, sleep apnea syndrome, and stroke. Neurology 42(suppl 6):75, 1992

383. Pascual-Leone A, Dhuna A, Anderson DC: Cerebral atrophy in habitual cocaine abusers: a planimetric CT study. Neurology 41:34, 1991

384. Patel AN: Self-inflicted strokes. Ann Intern Med 76:823, 1972

385. Peacock PB, Riley CP, Lampton TD et al: The Birmingham stroke, epidemiology, and rehabilitation study. p. 231. In Stewart G (ed): Trends in Epidemiology: Applications to Health Service Research and Training. Charles C Thomas, Springfield, IL, 1972

386. Pearson J, Richter RW: Neuropathological effects of opiate addiction. p. 308. In Richter RW (ed): Medical Aspects of Drug Abuse. Harper & Row, Hagerstown, MD, 1975

387. Pearson J, Richter RW: Addiction to opiates: neurologic aspects. p. 365. In Vinken PJ, Bruyn GW (eds): Handbook of Clinical Neurology. Vol. 37: Intoxications of the Nervous System. North-Holland, Amsterdam, 1979

388. Pearson J, Richter RW, Baden MM et al: Transverse myelopathy as an illustration of the neurologic and neuropathologic features of heroin addiction. Hum Pathol 3:109, 1972

389. Pennington SN, Smith CP: The effect of ethanol on thromboxane synthesis by blood platelet. Prostaglandins 2:43, 1979

390. Pentel P: Toxicity of over-the-counter stimulants. JAMA 252:1898, 1984

391. Persson LI, Rosengren LE, Johansson BB, Hansson HA: Blood brain barrier dysfunction to peroxidase after air embolism, aggravated by acute ethanol intoxication. J Neurol Sci 42:65, 1979

392. Peterson PL, Moore PM: Hemorrhagic cerebrovascular complications of crack cocaine abuse. Neurology (NY), suppl 1. 39:302, 1989

393. Peterson PL, Roszler M, Jacobs I, Wilner HI: Neurovascular complications of cocaine abuse. J Neuropsychiatr 3:143, 1991

394. Pettiti DB, Wingerd J: Use of oral contraceptives; cigarette smoking, and risk of subarachnoid hemorrhage. Lancet 2:234, 1978

395. Petitti DB, Wingerd J, Pellegrin F, Ramcharan S: Risk of vascular disease in women: smoking, oral contraceptives, non-contraceptive estrogens, and other factors. JAMA 242:1150, 1979

396. Petty GW, Brust JCM, Tatemichi TK, Barr ML: Embolic stroke ofter smoking "crack" cocaine. Stroke 21:1632, 1990

397. Pick TP, Howden R: Gray's Anatomy. p. 548. Running Press, Philadelphia, 1974

398. Pierce JR: Stroke following application of a nicotine patch. Ann Pharmacol 28:402, 1994

399. Plum F, Posner JB, Hain RF: Delayed neurologic deterioration after anoxia. Arch Intern Med 110:18, 1962

400. Poteliakhoff A, Roughton BC: Two cases of amphetamine poisoning. Br Med J 1:26, 1956

401. Powers RH, Madden JA: Vasoconstrictive effects of cocaine, metabolites and structural analogs on cat cerebral arteries. FASEB 4:A1095, 1990

402. Pretorius HPJ: Dexedrine intoxication of children: two cases, one fatal. S Afr Med J 27:945, 1953

403. Protass LM: Delayed postanoxic encephalopathy after heroin use. Ann Intern Med 74:738, 1971

404. Quintana RP, Lasslo A, Dugdale ML et al: Effects of ethanol and of other factors on ADP-induced aggregation of human blood platelets in vitro. Thromb Res 20:405, 1980

405. Qureshi AI, Safdar K, Patel M et al: Stroke in young black patients. Risk factors, subtypes, and prognosis. Stroke 26:1995, 1995

406. Ramadan J, Levine SR, Welch KMA: Pontine hemorrhage following "crack" cocaine use. Neurology 41:946, 1991

407. Ramsey LE: Liver dysfunction in hypertension. Lancet 2:111, 1977

408. Randell T: Cocaine, alcohol mix in body to form even longer lasting, more lethal drug. JAMA 267:1043, 1992

409. Randin D, Vollenweider P, Tappy L et al: Suppression of alcohol-induced hypertension by dexamethasone. N Engl J Med 332:1733, 1995

410. Reed DM, Resch JA, Hayashi T et al: A prospective study of cerebral artery atherosclerosis. Stroke 19:820, 1988

411. Reeves RR, McWilliams ME, Fitzgerald MJ: Cocaine-induced ischemic cerebral infarction mistaken for a psychiatric syndrome. South Med J 88:352, 1995

412. Renaud S, Blache O, Dumont E et al: Platelet function after cigarette smoking in relation to nicotine and carbon monoxide. Clin Pharmacol Ther 36:389, 1984

413. Rhoads GG, Blackwelder WC, Stemmerwan GN et al: Coronary risk factors and autopsy findings in Japanese-American men. Lab Invest 38:304, 1978

414. Richter RW, Pearson J: Heroin addiction related neurological disorders. p. 320. In Richter RW (ed): Medical Aspects of Drug Abuse. Harper & Row, Hagerstown, MD, 1975

415. Richter RW, Pearson J, Bruun B et al: Neurological complications of addiction to heroin. Bull NY Acad Med 49: 3, 1973

416. Richter RW, Rosenberg RN: Transverse myelitis associated with heroin addiction. JAMA 206:1255, 1968

417. Ricker PM, Vaughn DE, Stampfer MJ et al: Association of moderate alcohol consumption and plasma concentration of endogenous tissue-type plasminogen activator. JAMA 272:929, 1994

418. Riddick L, Reisch R: Oral overdose of pro-pylhexedrine. J Forensic Sci 26:834, 1981

419. Ringle DA, Herndon BL: In vitro morphine binding by sera from morphine-treated rabbits. J Immunol 109:174, 1972

420. Rodgers H, Aitken PD, French JM et al: Alcohol and stroke. A case-control study of drinking habits past and present. Stroke 24:1473, 1993

421. Rodriguez E, Smokvina M, Sokolow J, Grynbaum BB: Encephalopathy and paraplegia occurring with use of heroin. NY State J Med 71:2879, 1971

422. Rogers JN, Henry TE, Jones AM et al: Cocaine-related deaths in Pima Country, Arizona, 1982–1984. J Forensic Sci 31:1404, 1986

423. Rogers KJ, Nahorski SR: Depression of cerebral metabolism by stimulant doses of cocaine. Brain Res 57:255, 1973

424. Rogers RL, Meyer JS, Shaw TG et al: Cigarette smoking decreases cerebral blood flow suggesting increased risk for stroke. JAMA 250:2796, 1983

425. Ramanova MV, Romanov NS: Cerebral circulation disturbance in patients with chronic alcoholism. Sov Med 7:148, 1978

426. Rogot E: Smoking and General Mortality Among US Veterans, 1954–1969. National Heart and Lung Institute, Bethesda MD, 1974

427. Rothrock JF, Rubenstein R, Lyden PD: Ischemic stroke associated with methamphetamine inhalation. Neurology (NY) 38:589, 1988

428. Rowbotham MC: Neurologic aspects of cocaine abuse. West J Med 149:442, 1988

429. Rowley HA, Lowenstein DH, Rowbotham MC, Simon RP: Thalamomesencephalic strokes after cocaine abuse. Neurology (NY) 39:428, 1989

430. Royal College of General Practitioners: Oral Contraceptives and Health. Pitman, London, 1974

431. Ruf JC, Berger JL, Renaud S: Platelet rebound effect of alcohol withdrawal and wine drinking in rats. Relation to tannins and lipid peroxidation. Arterioscler Throm Vasc Biol 15:140, 1995

432. Rumbaugh CL, Bergeron RT, Fang HCH, McCormick R: Cerebral angiographic changes in the drug abuse patient. Radiology 101:335, 1971

433. Rumbaugh CL, Bergeron T, Scanlon RL et al: Cerebral vascular changes secondary to amphetamine abuse in the experimental animal. Radiology 101:345, 1971

434. Rumbaugh CL, Fang HCH: The effects of drug abuse on the brain. p. 37s. Med Times, March, 1980

435. Rumbaugh CL, Fang HCH, Higgins RE et al: Cerebral microvascular injury in experimental drug abuse. Invest Radiol 11:282, 1976

436. Russell M, Cooper ML, Frone M et al: Drinking patterns and blood pressure. Am J Epidemiol 128:917, 1988

437. Ryan JJ, Parker CW, Williams RL: Gamma-globulin binding of morphine in heroin addicts. J Lab Clin Med 80:155, 1972

438. Ryu SJ, Lin SK: Cerebral arteritis associated with oral use of phenylpropanolamine: report of a case. J Formos Med Assoc 94:53, 1995

439. Sacco RL: Risk factors and outcomes for ischemic stroke. Neurology 45(suppl 1):S10, 1995

440. Sacco RL, Shi T, Zamanillo MC, Kargman DE: Predictors of mortality and recurrence after hospitalized cerebral infarction in an urban community: the Northern Manhattan Stroke Study. Neurology 44:626, 1994

441. Sacco RL, Wolf PA, Bharucha NE et al: Subarachnoid and intracerebral hemorrhage: natural history, prognosis, and precursive factors in the Framingham Study. Neurology (NY) 34:847, 1984

442. Sachdeva K, Woodward KG: Caudal thalamic infarction following intranasal methamphetamine use. Neurology 39:305, 1989

443. Salonen JT, Puska P, Tuomilehto J et al: Relation of blood pressure, serum lipids, and smoking to the risk of cerebral stroke: a longitudinal study in eastern Finland. Stroke 13:327, 1982

444. Sapira JD: The narcotic addict as a medical patient. Am J Med 45:555, 1968

445. Sasaki S, Zhang XH, Kesteloot H: Dietary sodium, potassium, saturated fat, alcohol, and stroke mortality. Stroke 26:783, 1995

446. Sauer CM: Recurrent embolic stroke and cocaine-related cardiomyopathy. Stroke 22:1203, 1991

447. Schaffer CB, Pauli MW: Psychotic reaction caused by proprietary oral diet agents. Am J Psychiatry 137:1256, 1980

448. Schwartz ICA, Cohen JA: Subarachnoid hemorrhage precipitated by cocaine snorting. Arch Neurol 41:705, 1984

449. Schein PS, Yessayun L, Mayman CI: Acute transverse myelitis associated with intravenous opium. Neurology (NY) 21:101, 1971

450. Schoenfeld MR: Acute allergic reactions to morphine, codeine, meperidine hydrochloride, and opium alkaloids. NY State J Med 60:2591, 1960

451. Schwarcz TH, Hogan LA, Endean ED et al: Thromboembolic complications of polycythemia: polycythemia vera versus smokers' polycythemia. J Vasc Surg 17: 518, 1993

452. Seaman ME: Acute cocaine abuse associated with cerebral infarction. Ann Emerg Med 19:34, 1990

453. Seiss W, Lorenz R, Roth P, Weber PC: Plasma catecholamines, platelet aggregation and associated thromboxane formation after physical exercise, smoking, or norepinephrine infusion. Circulation 66:44, 1982

454. Semenciw RM, Morrison MI, Mao Y et al: Major risk factors for cardiovascular disease mortality in adults: results from the Nutrition Canada Survey Study. Int J Epidemiol 17:317, 1988

455. Shibolet S, Coll R, Gilat T, Sohar E: Heatstroke: its clinical picture and mechanism in 36 cases. Q J Med 36:525, 1967

456. Shinton R, Beevers G: Meta-analysis of relation between cigarette smoking and stroke. Br Med J 298:789, 1989

457. Shinton R, Sagar G, Beevers G: The relation of alcohol consumption to cardiovascular risk factors and stroke. The West Birmingham stroke project. J Neurol Neurosurg Psychiatry 56:458, 1993

458. Shukla D: Intracranial hemorrhage associated with amphetamine use. Neurology (NY) 32:917, 1982

459. Simonsen J: Traumatic subarachnoid hemorrhage in alcohol intoxication. J Forensic Sci 8:97, 1963

460. Simpson RK, Fischer DK, Narayan RK et al: Intravenous cocaine abuse and subarachnoid hemorrhage: effect on outcome. Br J Neurosurg 4:27, 1990

461. Singer LT, Yamashita TS, Hawkins S et al: Increased incidence of intraventricular hemorrhage and developmental delay in cocaine-exposed, very low birth weight infants. J Pediatr 124:765, 1994

462. Sloan MA, Kittner SJ, Rigamonti D, Price TR: Occurrence of stroke associated with use/abuse of drugs. Neurology 41:1358, 1991

463. Sloan MA, Mattioni TA: Concurrent myocardial and cerebral infarctions after intranasal cocaine use. Stroke 23:427, 1992

464. Smith HWB, Liberman HH, Brody SL et al: Acute myocardial infarction temporally related to cocaine use: clinical, angiographic, and pathophysiologic observations. Ann Intern Med 107:13, 1987

465. Sobel J, Espinas OE, Friedman SA: Carotid artery obstruction following LSD capsule ingestion. Arch Intern Med 127:290, 1971

466. Spires MC, Gordon EF, Choudhuri M, Maldonado E, Chan R: Intracranial hemorrhage in a neonate following prenatal cocaine exposure. Pediatr Neurol 5:324, 1989

467. Stafford CR, Bogdanoff BM, Green L, Spector HB: Mononeuropathy multiplex as a complication of amphetamine angiitis. Neurology (NY) 25:570, 1975

468. Stamfer MJ, Coditz GA, Willett WC et al: A prospective study of moderate alcohol consumption and the risk of coronary disease and stroke in women. N Engl J Med 319:267, 1988

469. Stason WB, Neff RK, Miettinen OS, Jick H: Alcohol consumption and nonfatal myocardial infarction. Am J Epidemiol 104:603, 1976

470. Stemmermann GN, Hayashi T, Resch JA et al: Risk factors related to ischemic and hemorrhagic cerebrovascular disease at autopsy: the Honolulu Heart Study. Stroke 15:23, 1984

471. Stimmel B: Cardiovascular Effects of Mood-Altering Drugs. Raven Press, New York, 1979

472. St. Leger AS, Cochrane AL, Moore F: Factors associated with cardiac mortality in developed countries with particular reference to the consumption of wine. Lancet 1:1017, 1979

473. Stoessl AJ, Young G, Feasby TE: Intracerebral hemorrhage and angiographic beading following ingestion of catecholaminergics. Stroke 16:734, 1985

474. Strickland TL, Stein R: Cocaine-induced cerebrovascular impairment: challenges to neuropsychological assessment. Neuropsychol Rev 5:69, 1995

475. Stuart M: Ethanol inhibited platelet prostaglandin synthesis in vitro. J Stud Alcohol 40:1, 1979

476. Sturner WQ, Stressman G, Helpern M: Bilateral symmetrical encephalomalacia in the globus pallidus in drug addicts. Paper read at the meeting of the American Academy of Forensic Sciences, Chicago, February, 1968

477. Syrjanen J, Valtonen VV, Ivananainen M et al: Association between cerebral infarction and increased serum bacterial antibody levels in young adults. Acta Neurol Scand 73:273, 1986

478. Szwed JJ: Pulmonary angiothrombosis caused by "blue velvet" addiction. Ann Intern Med 73:771, 1970

479. Takeya Y, Popper JS, Shimizu Y et al: Epidemiologic studies of coronary heart disease and stroke in Japanese men living in Japan, Hawaii, and California: incidence of stroke in Japan and Hawaii. Stroke 15:15, 1984

480. Tanaka H, Hayaski M, Date C et al: Epidemiologic studies of stroke in Shibata, a Japanese provincial city: preliminary report on risk factors for cerebral infarction. Stroke 16:773, 1985

481. Tanaka H, Ueda Y, Hayashi M et al: Risk factors for cerebral hemorrhage and cerebral infarction in a Japanese rural community. Stroke 13:62, 1982

482. Tang JL, Morris JK, Wald NJ et al: Mortality in relation to tar yield of cigarettes: a prospective study of four cohorts. BMJ 311:1530, 1995

483. Tarasyuk IK: The effect of alcohol misuse on the development and course of acute brain circulation disorders. Zh Nevropatol Psikhiatr 76:1777, 1976

484. Tardiff K, Gross E, Wu J et al: Analysis of cocaine-positive fatalities. J Forensic Sci 34:53, 1989

485. Taylor JR, Combs-Orme T: Alcohol and strokes in young adults. Am J Psychiatry 142:116, 1985

486. Tell GS, Rutan GH, Kronmal RA et al: Correlates of blood pressure in community-dwelling older adults. The Cardiovascular Health Study. Hypertension 23:59, 1994

487. Thompson WR, Waldman MB: Cervical myelopathy following heroin administeration. J Med Soc NJ 67:223, 1970

488. Thornton JR: Atrial fibrillation in healthy non-alcoholic people after an alcoholic binge. Lancet 2;1013, 1984

489. Tibbetts JC, Hinck VC: Conservative management of a hematoma in the fourth ventricle. Surg Neurol 1:253, 1973

490. Tibblin G, Wilhelmsen L, Werko L: Risk factors for myocardial infarction and death due to ischemic heart disease and other causes. Am J Cardiol 35:514, 1975

491. Togna G, Tempesta E, Togna AR et al: Platelet responsiveness and biosynthesis of thromboxane and prostacyclin in response to in vitro cocaine treatment. Haemostasis 15:100, 1985

492. Toler KA, Anderson B: Stroke in an intravenous drug user secondary to the lupus anticoagulant. Stroke 19:274, 1988

493. Treffert DA, Joranson D: Restricting amphetamines. JAMA 245:1336, 1981

494. Tsaji S, Kawano S, Michida T et al: Ethanol stimulates immunoreactive endothelin-1 and -2 release from cultured human unbilical vein endothelial cells. Alcohol Clin Exp Res 16:347, 1992

495. Tse DT, Ober RR: Talc retinopathy. Am J Ophthalmol 90:624, 1980

496. Tuazon CU, Sheagren JN: Staphylococcal endocarditis in parenteral drug abusers: source of the organism. Ann Intern Med 82:788, 1975

497. Tumeh SS, Nagel JS, English RJ et al: Cerebral abnormalities in cocaine abusers: demonstration by SPECT perfusion brain scintigraphy. Radiology 176:821, 1990

498. Tuomilehto J, Bonita R, Stewart A et al: Hypertension, cigarette smoking, and the decline in stroke incidence in eastern Finland. Stroke 22:7, 1991

499. Turnbull IM: Microvasculature of the human spinal cord. J Neurosurg 35:141, 1971

500. Ueda K, Hasuo Y, Kiyohara Y et al: Hisayama: incidence, changing pattern during long-term follow up, and related factors. Stroke 19:48, 1988

501. US National Institute on Alcohol Abuse and Alcoholism: Alcohol and health. Second special report to the Congress. DHEW Pub No ADM 75–212, US Government Printing Office, Washington, DC, 1975

502. Van Dyuke C, Byck R: Cocaine. Sci Am 246:128, 1982

503. Van Vanukis H, Wasserman E, Levine L: Specificities of antibodies to morphine. J Pharmacol Exp Ther 180: 514, 1972

504. Vivancos F, Diez-Tejedor E, Martinez N et al: Stroke due to abuse of cocaine. J Neurol 24(suppl 1):S39, 1994

505. Volkow ND, Fowler JS, Wolf AP, Gillespi A: Metabolic studies of drugs of abuse. In Harris L (ed): Problems of Drug Dependence, 1990. Washington DC: NIDA Research Monograph 105, DHHS, 1991:47

506. Volpe BJ: Effect of cocaine use on the fetus. N Engl J Med 327:399, 1992

507. Von Arbin M, Britton M, De Faire U, Tisell A: Circulatory manifestations and risk factors in patients with acute cerebrovascular disease and in matched controls. Acta Med Scand 218:373, 1985

508. Wadley C, Stillie GD: Pentazocine (Talwin) and tripelennamine (Pyribenzamine): a new drug abuse combination or just a revival? Int J Addict 15:1285, 1980

509. Walbran BB, Nelson JS, Taylor JR: Association of cerebral infarction and chronic alcoholism: an autopsy study. Alcoholism 5:531, 1981

510. Wang A-M, Suojanen JN, Colucci VM: Cocaine- and methamphetamine-induced acute cerebral vasospasm: an angiographic study in rabbits. Am J Neuroradiol 11: 1141, 1990

511. Wannamethee SG, Shaper AG, Whincup PH, Walker M: Smoking cessation and the risk of stroke in middle-aged men. JAMA 274:155, 1995

512. Weiner RS, Lockhart JT, Schwartz RG: Dilated cardiomyopathy and cocaine abuse: report of two cases. Am J Med 81:699, 1986

513. Weingarten KO: Cerebral vasculitis associated with cocaine abuse or subarachnoid hemorrhage? JAMA 259: 1658, 1988

514. Weinrieb RM, O'Brien CP: Persistent cognitive deficits attributed to substance abuse. In Brust JCM (ed): Neurologic Complications of Drug and Alcohol Abuse. Neurol Clin 11:663, 1993

515. Weiss MH, Craig JR: The influence of acute ethanol intoxication on intracranial physical dynamics. Bull Los Angeles Neurol Soc 43:1, 1978

516. Weiss RD, Gawin FH: Protracted elimination of cocaine metabolities in long-term, high-dose cocaine abusers. Am J Med 85:879, 1988

517. Weiss SR, Raskind R, Morganstern NL et al: Intracerebral and subarachnoid hemorrhage following use of methamphetamine ("speed"). Int Surg 53:123, 1970

518. Wetli C, Wright RK: Death caused by recreational cocaine use. JAMA 241:2519, 1979

519. Wharton BK: Nasal decongestants and paranoid psychosis. Br J Psychiatry 117:429, 1970

520. Whisnant JP, Homer D, Ingall TJ et al: Duration of cigarette smoking is the strongest predictor of severe extracranial carotid atherosclerosis. Stroke 21:707, 1990

521. Wilhelmsen L, Svardsudd K, Korsan-Bengsten K et al: Fibrinogen as a risk factor for stroke and myocardial infarction. N Engl J Med 311:501, 1984

522. Wilson LD, Henning RJ, Suttheimer C et al: Cocaethylene causes dose-dependent reductions in cardiac function in anesthetized dogs. J Cardiovasc Pharmacol 26: 965, 1995.

523. Wojak JC, Flamm ES: Intracranial hemorrhage and cocaine use. Stroke 18:712, 1987

524. Wolf PA, D'Agostino RB, Kannel WB et al: Cigarette smoking as a risk factor for stroke: the Framingham Study. JAMA 259:1025, 1988

525. Wolf PA, D'Agostino RB, Odell P et al: Alcohol consumption as a risk factor for stroke: the Framingham Study. Ann Neurol 24:177, 1988

526. Wolf PA, Kannel WB, Verter J: Current status of risk factors for stroke, p. 317. In Barnett HJM (ed): Neurologic Clinics. Vol. 1: Symposium on Cerebrovascular Disease. WB Saunders, Philadelphia, 1983

527. Woods BT, Strewler GJ: Hemiparesis occurring six hours after intravenous heroin injection. Neurology (NY) 22: 863, 1972

528. Wooten MR, Khangure MS, Murphy MJ: Intracerebral hemorrhage and vasculitis related to ephedrine abuse. Ann Neurol 13:337, 1983

529. Yano K, Rhoads GG, Kagan V: Coffee, alcohol and risk of coronary heart disease among Japanese men living in Hawaii. N Engl J Med 297:405, 1977

530. Yarnell PR: "Speed" headache and hematoma. Headache 17:69, 1977

531. Yatsu FM, Wesson DR, Smith DE: Amphetamine abuse. p. 50. In Richter RW (ed): Medical Aspects of Drug Abuse. Harper & Row, Hagerstown, MD, 1975

532. Yen DJ, Wong SJ, Ju TH et al: Stroke associated with methamphetamine inhalation. Eur Neurol 34:16, 1994

533. Yoshitake T, Kiyohara Y, Kato I et al: Incidence and risk factors of vascular dementia and Alzheimer's disease in a defined elderly Japanese population: the Hisayama Study. Neurology 45:1161, 1995

534. Yu YJ, Cooper DR, Wellenstein DE, Block B: Cerebral angiitis and intracerebral hemorrhage associated with methamphetamine abuse: case report. J Neurosurg 58: 109, 1983

535. Zachariah SB: Stroke after heavy marijuana smoking. Stroke 22:406, 1991

536. Zalis EG, Kaplan G, Lundberg GD, Knutson RA: Acute lethality of the amphetamines in dogs and its antagonism with curare. Proc Soc Exp Biol Med 18:557, 1965

537. Zalis EG, Lundberg GD, Knutson RA: The pathophysiology of acute amphetamine poisoning with pathologic correlation. J Pharmacol Exp Ther 158:115, 1967

538. Zalis EG, Parmley LF: Fatal amphetamine poisoning. Arch Intern Med 112:822, 1963

539. Zimmerman M, McGreachie J: The effect of nicotine on aortic endothelium: a quantitative ultrastructural study. Atherosclerosis 63:33, 1987

540. Zhang A, Altura BT, Altura BM: Ethanol-induced contraction of cerebral arteries in diverse mammals and its mechanism of action. Eur J Pharmacol 248:229, 1993

Stroke in Young Adults

SERGE BLECIC

JULIEN BOGOUSSLAVSKY

In the Western world, stroke is the third cause of death after cardiovascular disorders and cancer, and is considered mainly a disease of the middle-aged or elderly. Nevertheless, young adults are also affected by cerebrovascular disease.[1,3,6,12,20,35,52,57,61,67,70,79,81,98] Although the frequency of stroke death is lower than in the general stroke population, stroke is particularly dramatic in younger patients because it involves a previously healthy adult and sometimes leads to serious sequelae for the rest of the patient's life. The burden is also extremely heavy on spouse, family and society.[1,3,6,12,20,35,52,57,67,70,79,81,98]

It is now well known that stroke in young adults is not a rare event.[1,3,6,12,20,35,52,57,63,67,70,79,81,98] Reports from the neurological departments in Lausanne, Switzerland (Lausanne Stroke Registry) and in Brussels, which survey stroke patients admitted to a population base primary care center, show that, respectively, 225 (13.5%) of 1,661 patients and 116 (11.4%) of 1,017 patients with first-ever stroke were not older than 45 years.

Stroke in young patients constitutes a challenge because of its social impact and also because of the large variety of associated diagnostic and etiologic problems[1,3,6,12,20,35,52,57,67,70,79,81,98] (Table 42.1).

Epidemiology

The annual incidence of stroke in people between 15 and 49 years varies greatly. In the Stockholm county of Sweden, a 5-year survey suggested an annual stroke incidence of 34/100,000 in adults younger than 55 years. Estimates from the Mayo Clinic gave, in 1970, an annual incidence of stroke of 10.4/100,000 in women between 15 and 29 years of age.

In previously published studies, most strokes in young adults were shown to be of ischemic origin. Actually, hemorrhage is relatively rarer in young than in older patients, and only one study published in 1984 disclosed a higher frequency of hemorrhage in young patients.[87] Indeed, in the Lausanne and Brussels registries, respectively, 5% and 7% percent of stroke in persons under 30 years of age and 12% and 13% of stroke in persons between 30 and 45 years of age were hemorrhages. These proportions do not differ from those encountered in the general stroke population.[1,3,6,12,20,35,52,57,67,70,78,81,98]

In previously published studies transient ischemic attacks (TIAs) represented one-third of ischemic events.[1,3,6,12,20,35,52,57,67,70,78,81,98] It seems that TIAs in young patients may constitute a different group with a very low risk of developing permanent stroke,[79] as shown in a study from Tronsø, Norway, which showed that all patients with TIA were stroke free for 55 months.[67]

The mortality rate is not well known.[1,3,6,12,35,52,57,63,67,70,79,81,98] Overall death during the acute phase may vary from 1.5% to 7.3%. One study of young patients with acute stroke showed a mortality rate at 1 month of 6.6%, which is less than in the general stroke population.[67]

The sex ratio most frequently shows a female predominence in adults under 30 years while a male predominance emerges over 30 years.[1,3,6,12,35,52,57,63,67,70,79,81,87,98]

It is extremely difficult to assess the real frequency of stroke etiology in young adults, because most patients are hospitalized in secondary or tertiary care centers and the findings are biased towards rare causes. Table 42.2 shows different frequencies and etiologies of stroke observed in recent literature.[1,3,6,12,35,52,57,67,79,81,87,98]

However, the frequency of stroke etiology in young adults remains extremely variable in studies previously published. The frequency of arteriopathy varies from 11% to 17% while cardiac emboli account for 11% to 35% of cases.[1,3,6,12,20,35,52,57,67,70,78,81,98] Other etiologies are rarer and may depend on environmental factors such as alcohol or drug consumption,[33,53,68,75,80] the advent of AIDS-related diseases,[11,90] or, in developing countries, other infections.[106]

Arteriopathies

Arteriopathies in young adults can be classified in two main categories: atherosclerotic and nonatherosclerotic.

ATHEROSCLEROSIS

The prevalence of atherosclerosis increases with age and, obviously, it is more frequent in patients older than 30 years (Fig. 42.1). Overall, atherosclerosis, including large and small

Table 42.1 Potential and Possible Causes of Ischemic Stroke in the Young

Arterial Disease
    Atherosclerosis
        Large artery atherosclerosis (including postactinic disease and cholesterol embolism)
        Small artery disease (hypertension associated)
    Nonatherosclerotic disease
Noninflammatory
    Dissection, fibromuscular dysplasia, moyamoya and variants, neoplastic angioendotheliosis, Bürger's disease, neurofibromatosis, Kohlmeyer-Degos disease, AIDS, homocytinuria, Marfan syndrome, Fabry's disease, Sneddon syndrome, Van Bogaert-Divry syndrome, pseudoxanthoma elasticum, dolichoectasia, Grönblad-Strandberg disease, contraceptive-induced hyperplasia, reversible cerebral angiopathies (toxemia, peripartum, some toxic angiopathies, subarachnoid hemorrhage vasospasm, paroxysmal hypertension, hyperparathyroidism, idiopathy)
Inflammatory
    Takayasu's disease, granulomatous arteritides, aortoarteritis, infective arteritis (syphilis, tuberculosis, rickettsiosis, neuroborreliosis, brucellosis, mycoses, AIDS, herpes zoster, mycoplasma pneumoniae, malaria), Eales disease, some toxic angiopathies, systemic arteritides (Wegener syndrome, rheumatoid arthritis, sarcoidosis, collagen disease, polyarteritis nodosa, Behçet's disease, relapsing polychondritis, ulcerative colitis)
Migraine Stroke
Trauma (dissection, in situ thrombosis)
Venous Thrombosis
Hematologic Conditions
    Hyperviscosity (myeloproliferative syndromes, dysproteinemia)
    Coagulopathy (Moschcowitz disease, disseminated intravascular coagulation, paraneoplastic, paroxysmal nocturnal hemoglobinuria, thrombocytosis, sickle cell disease, hemoglobin sickle cell disease, thalassemia, hemoglobin C disease, protein C deficiency, resistance to activated protein C, factor V Leyden deficiency, protein S deficiency, antithrombin III deficiency, prekallikrein deficiency, factor XII deficiency, heparin cofactor II deficiency, C2 deficiency, antiphospholipid syndrome, alcohol intoxication, platelet hyperaggregability, vitamin K or antifibrinolytic therapy, snake bite)
    Anemia
Heart Disease
    Valvular (mitral stenosis, prosthetic valve, infective endocarditis, marantic endocarditis, Libman-Sacks endocarditis, mitral annulus calcification, mitral valve prolapse, rheumatic heart disease)
    Atrial fibrillation and sick sinus syndrome
    Acute myocardial infarction, left ventricular akinesia/aneurysm, atrial septal aneurysm
    Left (right) atrial myxoma, cardiac rhabdomyoma (tuberous sclerosis), cardiac papillary fibroelastoma, left ventricular cavernous angiectasia
    Dilated cardiomyopathy (with/without myopathy)
    Chagas disease
    Cardiac surgery/catheterism
    Atrial (including patent foramen ovale) and ventricular septal defects with shunt (paradoxical embolism); Chiari network
Pulmonary Disease
    Arteriovenous malformations/fistula, Rendu-Osler-Weber syndrome
    Pulmonary vein thrombosis
Other Embolic Phenomena
    Fat embolism, fibrocartilaginous embolism, air embolism (divers), foreign particle embolism (iatrogenic), embolism distal to saccular aneurysm, tumor embolism
Other Disorders
    Neuroleptic malignant syndrome
    Congenital odontoid aplasia, atlantoaxial subluxation
    Mediastinal mass (tumor, thyroid mass)
    Osteopetrosis
    MELAS (mitochondrial encephalomyopathy with lactic acidosis and strokelike episodes) syndrome

artery disease, has been considered the cause of stroke in 7% to 30% of patients younger than 50 years. In a recent study from Brussels, 47 (41%) of 117 patients below 50 years had stroke due to atherosclerosis. It is not surprising to see that these patients were significantly older than other young patients with stroke of other origin, and indeed, this proportion fell to 11% when only young adults below 35 years were considered (Fig. 42.1). The risk factors were identical to those found in the general population with stroke, being mainly arterial hypertension, hyperlipidemia, cigarette smoking, alcohol consumption,[1,3,6,12,20,35,39,50,52,53,61,67,70,79,80,81,87,98] and ischemic cardiopathy. Arterial hypertension was found in roughly 60% of the Brussels patients. More than 50% of the patients had two or more risk factors for atherosclerosis. The most frequent association was hypertension and hyperlipidemia, mainly hypertriglyceridemia, confirming the previous findings, which emphasized the causal role of hypertriglyceridemia rather than hypercholesterolemia in these pa-

Table 42.2 Frequency and Etiology of Stroke in Different Series

Study	Upper Age Limit	Percent of All Strokes	Stroke Etiology (%)				
			Cardio-embolism	Athero-sclerosis	Nonathero-sclerotic Arteriopathies	Miscellanous Coag. Disorders Toxics	Uncertain Etiology
Marshall (1981)	49	—	12	—	—	15	29
Adams (1986)	45	3	24	27	27	—	7
Radhakrishnan (1986)	40	19	21	—	—	—	—
Bogousslavsky (1987)	30	—	29	5	26	—	11
Gautier (1989)	45	3	12	15	45	29	9
Alvarez (1989)	50	—	18	56	15.3	15	10
Bevan (1990)	45	8.5	35	31	19	19	4
Love (1990)	45	—	22	27	26	13	12
Awada (1992)	45	25	18	30	26	26	29
Carolei (1993)	44	—	19	33	12.6	12.6	25
Leno (1993)	50	—	17	—	—	—	—
Kapelle (1994)	45	4	21	31	31	31	16
Kittner (1995)	45	12.3	26	26	12	37	—

tients.[7,45,62] The roles of hyperlipidemia type IIb and of congenital hyperlipidemia have also been demonstrated.[7,62]

NONATHEROSCLEROTIC ARTERIOPATHIES

Nonatherosclerotic arteriopathies are numerous, but their role in stroke genesis is crucial. In Brussels, 35 (30%) of 117 patients had stroke due to nonatherosclerotic arteriopathies.

Interestingly, this proportion reached 51% in patients younger than 35 years. Table 42.1 summarizes these arteriopathies.

Arterial Dissection

A dissection is produced by the subintimal penetration of blood in a cervicocephalic vessel with subsequent longitudinal extension of intramural hematoma for a distance between its layers; it is usually associated with intimal tears (Fig. 42.2). Worldwide, it is probably the most common nonatheroscle-

Figure 42.1 Etiology of cerebral infarct based on 117 patients under 50 years of age. (**A**) Patients under 35 years of age (n = 55). (**B**) Patients over 35 years of age (n = 62). (1) atherosclerosis, (2) nonatherosclerotic arteriopathies, (3) coagulation and hematologic disorders, (4) miscellaneous (toxins, etc.), (5) uncertain or unknown causes, (6) cardioembolism.

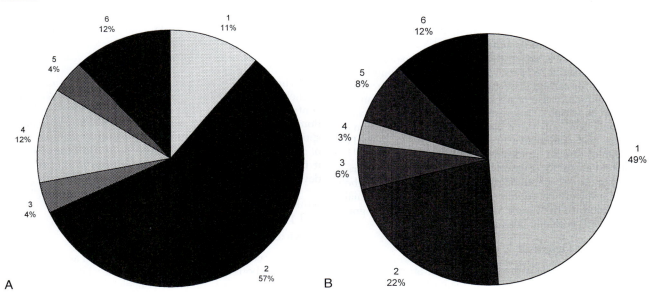

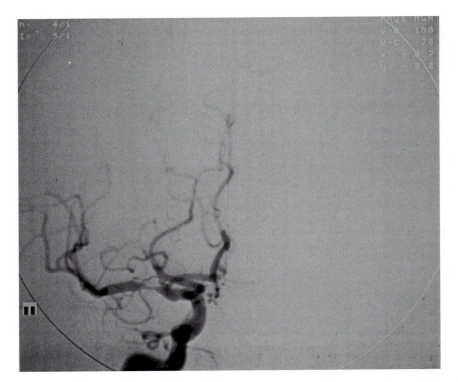

Figure 42.4 Reversible angiopathy. Segmental narrowing of the proximal part of the right middle cerebral artery in a 19-year-old cocaine addict.

methylamphetamine, and phenylpropanolamine. In the idiopathic form, spontaneous vasoconstriction may occur in adults without risk factors for stroke. The spontaneous form is more common in women, and many of these patients have a history of migraine.[18,23,64,100]

In all patients, neurologic deficits are preceded by severe headaches, nausea, and vomiting, mimicking the symptoms of classical migraine or subarachnoid hemorrhage. Less often, patients have epileptic seizures at onset. Frequently, the neurologic deficits are transient, lasting from 7 days to 6 months. Few patients remain handicapped or die. Cerebral hemorrhage can occur, in relation to reperfusion.[18,23,29,51,64,73,88,100,102,103]

The classical pattern on cerebral angiography is multiple narrowings of the arteries arising at the circle of Willis, which generally disappear within a few days to several months after onset. Transcranial Doppler can be useful for the follow-up and the assessment of vasoconstriction.[18] Cerebrospinal fluid examination is often normal, but more rarely it can show a slight pleiocytosis.

The pathologic processes underlying reversible cerebral angiopathy remain unclear. In several cases, severe acute arterial hypertension at onset was suspected to be the direct cause of arterial vasoconstriction.[23]

Homocystinuria

Homocystinuria is an autosomal recessive disease that includes three distinct entities, which differ clinically and biochemically.[96] However, they have in common the increase of homocysteine and methionine in blood and urine.

The most common form corresponds to a decrease in cystathionine-β-synthase activity, which is a pyridoxine-dependent enzyme crucial for the transfer of the sulfur atom from methionine to cysteine.[36,41,96] The two other forms are associated with a decrease in the conversion of homocysteine to cysteine due to impairment of methyl-tetrahydrofolate methyl-transferase enzyme activity or to a decrease of the blood concentration of methyl-tetrahydrofolate and methyl-cobalamine, two cofactors of the former reaction.[36,41,96]

Deficiency in cystathionine-β-synthase is the most frequent form, which leads to an increase of methionine and homocysteine in both blood and urine, and therefore to a decrease in blood cysteine concentration.[16,36,41,46,74,96,120] Cystathionine-β-synthase deficiency is rare, estimated at 1/200,000 inhabitants with a peak incidence rate in Ireland. The homozygotes are clinically involved and have an enzyme activity around 1% to 5%, while the heterozygotes are generally clinically spared, although enzyme activity is biochemically impaired (40% to 60% of the normal value). However, it has been suggested that even in heterozygotes, a slight increase in homocysteine could be an independent risk factor for stroke, inducing early atherosclerosis in these patients.[16,36,41,46,74,120]

Homocysteine in excess disturbs collagen metabolism and induces several systemic and neurologic disorders.[16,36,41,46,74,96,120]

Vascular events, either thrombosis or emboli, result from degenerative lesions involving medium-sized arteries. They occur in the early stages of life, frequently before the age of 20 years.[16,36,96] Premature atherosclerosis and thrombosis have also been observed.[16]

Moyamoya Disease

Moyamoya disease is a clinical entity that was first described in Japan by Takeuchi and Shimizu in 1957. They reported a 27-year-old man who had bilateral cerebral infarcts due to bilateral hypoplasia of the internal carotid arteries.[108]

The majority of patients with moyamoya are found in Asia, especially in Japan, although several patients have been reported elsewhere in the world. The Japanese term "moyamoya" means obscure or vague and therefore the name "moyamoya disease" was proposed because of the unusual, smoke appearance of the vascular network found in these patients.[25,43,47,98,108,109] The annual incidence rate is estimated at 0.1 in 100,000 inhabitants.[48] It affects children most frequently, with a maximal peak in frequency over the age of 6 years. Clinical presentation is varied, and repeated TIAs can be observed, mainly at the onset of the disease; ischemic strokes are more common than intracranial hemorrhage. The latter are assumed to be due to an increase of blood pressure on the small perforators or into the anastomotic network as a consequence of the occlusions of middle-sized arteries. The disease is frequently accompanied by partial or generalized seizures.[25,43,47,48] The etiology of this disease remains unknown.

Cerebral angiography is the best means of investigating patients with moyamoya. Bilateral occlusions or, less frequently, stenosis of the cavernous part of the internal carotid arteries, associated with a puffy, cloudy-appearing arteriolar network at the bases of the skull are usually found.[47] This network depends on several collateral anastomoses, such as leptomeningeal anastomoses with the anterior and the posterior vascular systems, intradural anastomoses, and anastomoses of external carotid or ophthalmic arteries with anterior cerebral arteries. This pattern can evolve, and anastomoses can increase or disappear.[43,47,48,109]

Currently, the advent of MR angiography allows a good estimation of the vascular network in patients suspected to have moyamoya.[25,47,48] In addition, the combination of classical magnetic regonance imaging (MRI) and MRA allows a better definition of the collateral network and of potential small infarcts in the deep perforator territory.

Cerebral Autosomal Dominant Arteriopathy with Subcortical Infarcts and Leucoencephalopathy

Cerebral autosomal dominant arteriopathy with subcortical infarcts and leukoencephalopathy, best known under its acronym CADASIL, is characterized by recurrent subcortical ischemic strokes and, finally, dementia.[84,111,112]

The etiology of CADASIL is an autosomal dominant arteriopathy, distinct from atherosclerotic and amyloid arteriopathies. It generally involves patients younger than in classical arteriosclerotic arteriopathy. The name *CADASIL* was first used by Mas et al in 1992, who, studying a French family, demonstrated a genetic disorder characterized by recurrent brain infarction starting in mid-adult life. In these patients and in their asymptomatic relatives, magnetic resonance imaging disclosed leukoencephalopathy and small deep infarcts. Mas et al thought that the pedigree pattern suggested autosomal

dominant inheritance.[84] Finally, about 71 patients belonging to two different families were studied.

An autopsy study, performed on one patient, showed multiple small subcortical infarcts, diffuse myelin loss, hemispheric hematoma, and pallor of the white matter. Microscopically, this pathologic process involved mainly small and medium-sized arteries and consisted of thickening of the arterial wall with deposit of nonfibrinoid eosinophilic material in the media. In this case, the elastic layer was fragmented and reduplicated.

Using linkage analysis on lymphoblastoid cells, Tournier-Lasserve et al in 1993 demonstrated that the most likely location for the CADASIL gene was assigned on the 19th chromosome between D19S221 and D19S222 sites.[101]

Cardioembolism

Cardioembolism is probably the etiology that clinicians should rule out first in a young adult with ischemic stroke. In fact, the high rate of recurrence and the possibility of avoiding this by appropriate treatment make cardioembolism the first etiology to determine. In the literature, cardioembolism has been found to be the cause of 10% to 40% of stroke in young adults.[39,42,66,101,112] This variable rate could be explained by variable diagnostic criteria for cardioembolism and by potential geographic variations. Actually, rheumatic heart disease, which was frequent at the beginning of the century in Western countries, is now much more prevalent as a cause of stroke in developing countries. Conversely, in Europe and North America, valvular disease, patent foramen ovale, and arrhythmia are considered the most common causes or mechanisms of cardioembolism. Since the eradication of infectious diseases such as group B β-hemolytic streptococcus, the frequency of cardiopathy and of cardioembolism has decreased.[9,38,42,66,101] In a study from Brussels, definite cardioembolism accounted for only 12% of young patients with stroke (Fig. 42.1). Valvulopathies, associated or not with arrhythmia, were the most common finding. Concerning valvulopathies, it has become obvious that very strict criteria should be used for the diagnosis of pathologic mitral valve prolapse, and it is likely that the morphology of the valves is also important. In our experience, mitral valvular pathologies are the most common. Aortic valve disease was rare and, when found, associated with other valvular pathologies. In young patients, arrhythmia was never found in isolation but always associated with mitral valve involvement.

Patent foramen ovale is frequently found; its prevalence is estimated at 20% to 25% of healthy adults and 35% to 45% of unselected young adults with ischemic stroke.[8,9,38,58,72,95,118]

The classical situation of paradoxical embolism from the venous bed is rarely proven.[58,95,99] Other situations, such as the association of patent foramen ovale with interatrial septal aneurysm or isolated patent foramen ovale without evidence for venous thrombosis, are more frequent.[10,28,65] In a recent study of patients below 60 years included in the Lausanne Stroke Registry, patent foramen ovale and interatrial septum aneurysm were associated in 25% of the cases.[19] Conversely,

References

1. Adams HP, Butler MJ, Biller J et al: Nonhemorrhagic cerebral infarction in young adults. Arch Neurol 43:793, 1986
2. Alarcon-Segovia D, Délézé M, Oria C et al: Antiphospholipid antibodies and the antiphospholipid syndrome in systemic lupus erythematosus. A prospective analysis of 500 consecutive patients. Medicine 66:353, 1989
3. Alvarez J, Matias-Guiu J, Sumalla J et al: Ischemic stroke in young adults. I. Analysis of the etiological subgroups. Acta Neurol Scand 80:28, 1989
4. Amarenco P, Duyckaerts C, Tzourio C et al: The preva-

stroke. Neurology 38:223, 1988
22. Brey RL, Hart RG, Sherman DG, Tegeler CH: Antiphospholipid antibodies and cerebral ischemia in young people. Neurology 40:1190, 1990
23. Brick JF: Vanishing cerebrovascular disease of pregnancy. Neurology 38:804, 1988
24. Broekmans AW: Hereditary protein C deficiency. Haemostasis 15:233, 1985
25. Bruno A, Adams HP, Biller J et al: Cerebral infarction due to Moyamoya disease in young adults. Stroke 19:826, 1988
26. Bruno A, Nolte KB, Chapin J: stroke associated with ephedrine use. Neurology 43:1313, 1993
27. Bruyn RPM, Van Der Veen JPW, Donker AJM et al:

the clinical evidence for deep venous thrombosis or existence of Valsalva maneuver before or at onset of stroke was present in only one-sixth of the patients. Other rare causes can be associated with patent foramen ovale (Table 42.1).

Nevertheless, and because of the relatively high frequency of recurrence in cases of cardioembolism, occult cardiac abnormality should be ruled out early after stroke in young adults.[117] Echocardiography is a useful screening procedure in young adults with stroke, but any potentially pathologic finding should be carefully assessed before attributing stroke to cardioembolism. Transthoracic echocardiography should be the first step. It could rule out left ventricle dysfunction, mitral valve prolapse, left ventricular thrombus, and pat-

lished, particularly in systemic lupus erythematosis. However, few studies have reported a high frequency of antiphospholipid antibodies (APA) in stroke patients who were not suffering from clinical autoimmune disease.[22] Although many thrombogenic mechanisms for stroke have been proposed in patients with elevated APA, no clear relationship between the presence of APA and stroke has been demonstrated.[2,5,22,37,49,50,69,93,94]

Migraine Stroke

Table 43.1 Relationship of Cryptogenic Stroke with PFO

Study	N[a] (patients)	Age	PFO (Cryptogenic)	PFO (Control)	P
Younger patients					
Lechat[49]	26	<55	54% (14/26)	10% (10/100)	<0.001
Webster[90]	34	<40	56% (19/34)	15% (6/40)	<0.001
Cabanes[11]	64	<55	56% (36/64)	18% (9/50)	<0.0001
De Belder[19b]	39	<55	13% (5/39)	3% (1/39)	—
Di Tullio[23]	21	<55	47% (10/21)	4% (1/24)	<0.001
Hausmann[36]	18	<40	50% (9/18)	11% (2/18)	<0.05
			46% (93/202)	11% (29/271)	
Older patients					
De Belder[19b]	64	>55	20% (13/64)	5% (3/56)	<0.001
Di Tullio[23]	24	>55	38% (9/24)	8% (6/77)	<0.001
Hausmann[36]	20	>40	15% (3/20)	23% (23/98)	NS
Jones[44]	57	>50	18% (10/57)	16% (29/183)	NS
			21% (35/165)	15% (61/414)	

[a] Cryptogenic stroke.

[b] Includes different stroke subtypes.

tack) (TIA) (44 patients), ischemic stroke (52 patients), or peripheral artery embolism (9 patients) using contrast TT and transesophageal (TE) echocardiography.[19] This was compared to the PFO prevalence by contrast TE echocardiography in 94 controls. When the patients were divided by age, in patients younger than 55, PFO was seen in 13% with ischemic events, compared to 3% in the controls. Among the patients older than 55, PFO was seen in 20% of the patients compared to 5% in the control group.

Di Tullio et al performed contrast TTE in 146 consecutive patients with acute ischemic stroke.[23] According to National Institute of Neurological Disorders and Stroke (NINDS) Stroke Data Bank Criteria, patients were categorized into those with defined cause of stroke and those with cryptogenic stroke. Among the 146 patients studied, 101 (69%) were diagnosed with strokes of determined cause and 45 (31%) with cryptogenic strokes. A PFO was detected in 42% of patients with cryptogenic stroke compared with 7% in those with determined cause of stroke. This was observed both in the younger (47% compared with 4%) and in the older (38% compared with 8%) age subgroups. The adjusted odds ratios for PFO and cryptogenic stroke diagnosis were 9.8 for the entire study group, 20.9 for younger patients, and 7.1 for the older patients.

On the other hand, the association of PFO with cryptogenic stroke in older population was not seen by several studies. In Hausmann's study, of 18 patients younger than 40 with unexplained cerebral embolic event, 50% had PFO compared to 11% in the control group confirming the previous findings.[36] However, in 20 older patients, the frequency of PFO was 15% compared to 23% in the control group. Jones et al also found that in 57 cryptogenic stroke patients older than 50, the prevalence of PFO was 18%, not significantly different from 16% seen in the controls.[44] Therefore, although the association between cryptogenic stroke and PFO is established in the younger population, in the older population this is as yet not clearly es-

tablished. Table 43.1 summarizes the results of the studies discussed in this section.

Technical Aspects of Contrast Echocardiography

CONTRAST ECHOCARDIOGRAPHY

TTE and TEE with saline contrast injection are the most widely used techniques for PFO detection. Agitated saline is prepared by mixing 0.5 to 1.0 ml of air with 10 ml of normal saline through two syringes connected by a stopcock. While imaging the heart in four-chamber view, this mixture is injected through a peripherally placed intravenous line. A PFO is judged to be present if any microbubble is seen in the left-sided cardiac chambers within three cardiac cycles from the maximum right atrial pacification. Using TTE imaging, Figure 43.1 shows the appearance of microbubbles in the left-sided cardiac chambers after the venous injection of contrast material.

The amount of air used does not appear to influence the sensitivity of this technique. When either 0.2 ml of air or 1.0 ml of air was used, there was no difference in the detection rate of PFO.[80] In a consecutive series of 75 patients, the detection rate was identical (9.3%) with 0.2 ml of air, producing $34 \pm 9/mm^3$ microbubbles or 1.0 ml of air producing $152 \pm 79/mm^3$ microbubbles. Injection is performed with and without Valsalva maneuver. In two series, amongst the stroke population, Valsalva maneuver increased the sensitivity from

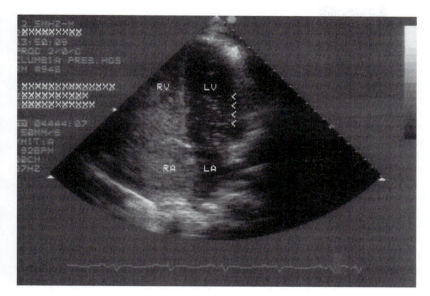

Figure 43.1 Transthoracic echocardiographic view of the heart with the appearance of microbubbles in left atrium (LA) and left ventricle (LV) demonstrated after saline contrast injection in a patient with PFO. Arrows (<) point to the microbubbles. RA, right atrium; RV, right ventricle.

30% to 40% in one series and from 30% to 50% in another.[49,90] Coughing during injection may further increase the sensitivity.[83]

Saline contrast injection as described can be performed while imaging the heart with a TEE probe. Again, PFO is judged to be present with the visualization of microbubbles in the left atrium within three cardiac cycles from the right atrial opacification. Figure 43.2 demonstrates the passage of microbubbles from right atrium into the left atrium through PFO as demonstrated by TEE. Similarly, as noted in the section "TCD in PFO Detection," contrast injection can be performed while the flow is being monitored in the cerebral circulation using transcranial Doppler (TCD) ultrasound. Valsalva maneuver can also be performed with either TEE or TCD contrast studies to increase the sensitivity of the technique.

Doppler color-flow detection of PFO is possible with TE. However, this technique is not as sensitive as the ones using contrast injection.[3]

SAFETY OF TEE STUDIES

TEE is a safe procedure. Daniel et al reviewed 10,419 TEEs from 15 centers, of which 9,240 (88.7%) were in conscious patients.[17] In 201 (1.9%), insertion of the probe was unsuccessful. In 90 of 10,128 cases with successful probe insertion, the examination had to be interrupted because of the patient's intolerance of the procedure. There was one death (mortality rate 0.0098%). Its safety has also been shown in patients aged over 70 years.[59]

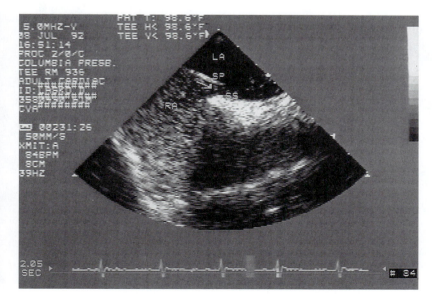

Figure 43.2 Vertical transesophageal echocardiographic view of fossa ovalis area demonstrating the passage of microbubbles through PFO (arrow) from right atrium (RA) into left atrium (LA). Separation of septum primum (SP) from septum secundum (SS) is clearly visualized.

SAFETY OF CONTRAST INJECTION

Saline contrast injection, used in conjunction with echocardiography or with TCD is also a safe procedure. This procedure is routinely performed safely in children with known right-to-left shunt without side effects. Van Hare et al performed saline contrast echocardiography in 889 children without any side effects.[89] The American Society of Echocardiography also supports the safety of this technique.[6] None of the studies using this technique for PFO detection in stroke patients reports side effects. Furthermore, even in many cases in which TCD documented the delivery of microbubbles to the brain, there were no known side effects.

Embolic Material Delivery to the Brain

TCD IN PFO DETECTION

Paradoxical embolization through a PFO is considered to be the mechanism for stroke associated with PFO. In support, direct demonstration of embolism through a PFO to the central circulation is shown in Figure 43.3 comparing the baseline flow pattern obtained by TCD in the middle cerebral artery with that seen after saline contrast injection in a patient with PFO.

Teague et al performed TCD with saline contrast injection in 46 patients with stroke and documented delivery of microbubbles in the central circulation in 19.[86] Di Tullio et al performed TCD simultaneously with contrast TTE in 80 stroke patients.[24] In 14 of the 80 patients, contrast TTE study was positive, of which all and an additional 7 were detected by TCD. Jauss et al performed contrast TEE and TCD studies simultaneously and noted the appearance of microbubbles in the cranial circulation in 14 of the 15 patients in whom TEE detected a PFO.[42] Karnik et al performed contrast TEE and TCD in 36 patients. Fifteen had positive contrast TEE study. Of these, TCD detected embolic material in the middle cerebral artery in 13 of 15.[45] Job et al performed contrast TEE and TCD in 137 patients, noting that TEE detected PFO in 65, of which TCD detected 58.[43] Klötzsch et al also performed contrast TEE and TCD in 111 patients, noting that TCD detected 42 of 46 shunts noted by TEE.[47]

Several studies performed contrast TTE, TEE and TCD in the same patient group to compare the sensitivity of the techniques. Nemec et al performed contrast TTE as well as TEE studies along with contrast TCD in 32 patients. TEE diagnosed right-to-left intracardiac shunt in 13 patients, of which all were identified by TCD.[57] By contrast, TTE contrast study identified only 7 of 13. Di Tullio et al performed TTE, TEE and TCD with saline contrast injection in 49 patients and noted positive TEE study in 19, among which 13 were detected by TCD and 9 by TTE study.[22] Studies discussed in this section are summarized in Table 43.2.

It can be clearly seen that TEE contrast study is the most sensitive method available for the detection of PFO, followed by TCD and TTE contrast studies. However, it must be recog-

Figure 43.3 (**A**) Baseline TCD pattern of middle cerebral artery. (**B**) Signals detected after microbubbles reach the central circulation in a patient with PFO.

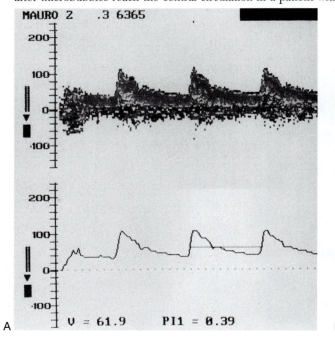

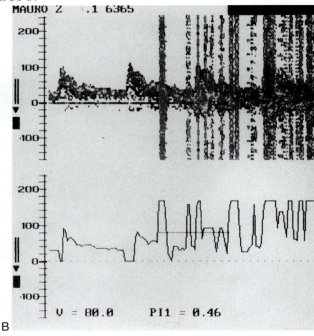

Table 43.2 Comparison of Techniques for PFO Detection

Study	N	TTE	TCD	TEE
Teague[86]	46	26% (12/46)	41% (19/46)	—
Di Tullio[24]	80	18% (14/80)	26% (21/80)	—
Jauss[42]	50	—	28% (14/50)	30% (15/50)
Karnik[45]	36	—	36% (13/36)	42% (15/36)
Job[43]	137	—	42% (58/137)	47% (65/137)
Klötzsch[47]	111	—	38% (42/111)	41% (46/111)
Nemec[57]	32	23% (7/32)	41% (13/32)	41% (13/32)
Di Tullio[22]	49	18% (9/49)	27% (13/49)	38% (19/49)
		20% (42/207)	36% (193/541)	42% (173/415)

Abbreviations: TCD, transcranial Doppler; TEE, transesophageal echocardiography; TTE, transthoracic echocardiography.

nized that detection of microbubbles in the central circulation does not need to be limited to that caused by PFO. Any right-to-left shunt, such as that due to ventricular septal defect or intrapulmonary shunt, may result in the delivery of microbubbles to the central circulation and thus detection by TCD. As a result, TCD will not identify the site of right-to-left shunt whereas TTE or TEE studies will provide this information. When one compares the characteristics of PFO detected by TEE study alone to PFO detected by both TEE and TTE studies, it is noted that PFO detectable only by TEE study is significantly smaller than that detected by both TEE and TTE studies.[91]

THROMBUS LODGED IN PFO

In support of PFO as a conduit for paradoxical embolization, there are a significant number of case reports demonstrating venous thrombi trapped in PFO in patients with central or systemic embolization. Since the widespread use of two-dimensional echocardiography became prevalent in 1980s, numerous case reports of thrombus trapped in PFO have been published supporting the role of PFO as a conduit for paradoxical embolization.[41,54–56,60,76,82] Figure 43.4 demonstrates a TEE echocardiographic view of a thrombus trapped in PFO in a patient with stroke and peripheral embolization at our center. This was successfully surgically removed.

Factors Associated with Paradoxical Embolization

SIZE OF PFO

A large number of autopsy studies are available to demonstrate the prevalence of PFO in the general population. When the published studies are combined, as shown in Table 43.3, the prevalence of PFO is approximated at

Table 43.3 Autopsy Prevalence of PFO

Study	N	Prevalence (%)
Parsons[63]	399	26
Fawcett[27]	306	32
Scammon[71]	809	29
Patten[64]	4,083	25
Seib[78]	500	17
Wright[93]	492	23
Schroeckenstein[77]	144	35
Sweeney[85]	64	31
Hagen[31]	965	27
Thompson[87]	1,000	29
Penther[66]	500	15
Total	9,262	26

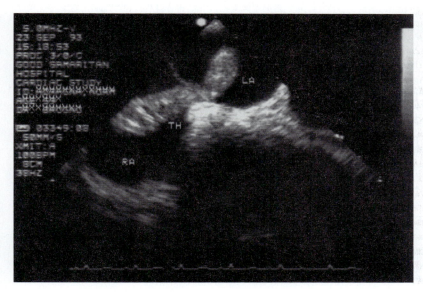

Figure 43.4 Transesophageal echocardiographic view of a thrombus (TH) trapped in PFO. LA, left atrium; RA, right atrium.

26%.[31,63,64,66,71,77,78,85,87,93] It is also noted in one study that the prevalence of PFO changes with age. Overall, Hagen et al noted the prevalence was 27.3%.[31] Among those aged 0 to 39 years, it was 34.3%, for 40 to 89 years old 24.4% and for those above 90 years 20.2%. Another study noted that the orifice size varies among patients with PFO. Thompson et al noted that 29% of the specimens had orifice size of 0.2 to 0.5 cm (probe patent), and 6% had orifice size 0.6 to 1.0 cm (pencil patent).[87]

Given the high prevalence of PFO in the general population and variability in the size of PFO, its size may be a critical factor in determining the importance of an individual PFO to act as a conduit for paradoxical embolization. Using contrast TTE, Webster et al observed that when the appearance of microbubbles was compared in young stroke patients to the controls, the stroke patients had more microbubbles entering the left-sided chambers compared to the controls.[90] Van Camp et al, using contrast TEE, compared the degree of shunt and the morphological appearance of PFO in 29 patients with cryptogenic stroke and in 28 controls.[88] They demonstrated a larger shunt through PFO of cryptogenic stroke patients compared to that through the PFO of the control group.

The morphological appearance of a PFO in cryptogenic stroke patients is also reported to be different from that found in the controls. Bridges et al measured the size of PFO by visualizing the balloon size across the PFO on fluoroscopy.[8] This was significantly larger in patients with PFO and presumed paradoxical embolism compared to that predicted from an autopsy series.

Homma et al assessed the degree of shunt though PFO in stroke patients using contrast TE and demonstrated that there is a large variability in the degree of right-to-left shunt.[39] Furthermore, the size of defect and the degree of shunt were significantly larger in cryptogenic stroke patients compared to those with known cause of stroke. In 16 cryptogenic stroke patients, the separation of septum primum from septum secundum measured 2.1 ± 1.7 mm versus 0.57 ± 0.78 mm ($P < 0.01$) in 7 patients with known cause of stroke. The number of microbubbles seen in left atrium was also significantly larger in cryptogenic stroke patients compared to those with known cause of stroke: 13.9 ± 10.7 versus 1.6 ± 0.8 ($P < 0.0005$).

Using contrast TCD, Job et al noted that massive paradoxical embolism through a PFO was identified significantly more frequently in patients with cryptogenic stroke than in patients with known cause of stroke or in the normal controls.[43] Also, Hausmann et al studied 78 patients with PFO detected by contrast TEE. They noted that the patients with unexplained arterial ischemic events and clinical evidence for paradoxical embolism had significantly larger shunt and PFO compared to the patients in whom PFO was an incidental finding.[37] Therefore, it appears that the morphological characteristics of PFO may play a role in its becoming a likely conduit for paradoxical embolization and may possibly modify the risk of initial or recurrent stroke.

DEEP VENOUS THROMBOSIS

For paradoxical embolization to occur, there needs to be a source of embolus. Since a significant stroke can result from an embolic occlusion by an embolus as small as 1 mm in diameter,[30] this may be harbored in a variety of locations in the body. Stöllberger et al performed venogram in patients with PFO.[84] In their study, 13 of 24 patients with PFO and documented leg vein thrombosis had history of suspected paradoxical embolism compared to 1 out of 8 patients with PFO without leg vein thrombosis having history of paradoxical embolism. This study demonstrated that patients with PFO who have paradoxical embolization may harbor the source of embolus in the lower extremities. It is notable that this study used venogram rather than ultrasound studies, which are routinely used, but have a much lower sensitivity for detecting venous thrombi, particularly in calf veins.[38] It is entirely possible that small thrombi that can serve as a source for paradoxical embolism are not detectable by ultrasound-based studies.

On the other hand, Ranoux et al, also using venogram, noted that only 1 of 13 patients with cryptogenic stroke had DVT.[67] Gautier et al, performing venography in 23 cryptogenic stroke patients with PFO, detected only three patients with DVT.[29] Therefore, the frequency of DVT in cryptogenic stroke patients with PFO is not clearly defined although the most recent series indicates that it is increased.

CHIARI'S NETWORK

Chiari's network is a network of threads and fibers in right atrium considered to represent congenital remnants of the right valve of the sinus venosus. This structure is generally considered not to be clinically significant. However, by preferentially directing the blood from inferior vena cava towards the fossa ovalis area, this structure may contribute to persistence of a PFO and development of an atrial septal aneurysm (ASA). Schneider et al reviewed 1,436 TEE studies and noted 29 patients with Chiari's network.[73] Patent foramen ovale was seen in 83% of these patients. Furthermore, intense right-to-left shunting occurred significantly more frequently in patients with Chiari's network than in control patients. Chiari's network was also frequently associated with ASA.

Thus, it appears that patients with large PFO, with evidence for DVT, and the presence of Chiari's network may be at a higher risk for cerebral ischemia from paradoxical embolization.

Atrial Septal Aneurysm

ASA is a redundancy of interatrial septum detected most commonly by TTE or TEE studies. It is detected significantly more frequently using TEE study compared to TTE study. The prevalence from autopsy series is estimated at 1% (16 of 1,578).[81] Most commonly, on TTE study, it is defined as 15 mm protrusion or excursion of interatrial septum with base of 15 mm.[32] On TEE study, it is defined as more than 10 mm protrusion beyond the plane of the septum into left or right atrium.[53] Although the definition varies somewhat in various series, using TTE the prevalence is estimated at 0.23% (Table

Table 43.4 Prevalence of ASA by TTE Study

Study	ASA Patients	Percent
Hanley[32]	80/36,200	0.22
Gallet[28]	10/4,840	0.21
Longhini[50]	23/4,000	0.57
Bewick[4]	6/4,700	0.12
Wolf[92]	12/724	1.7
Belkin[2]	36/6,979	0.5
Brand[67]	35/3,500	1.0
Roudant[69]	44/62,540	0.08
Katayama[46]	26/2,074	1.2
Oneglia[61]	38/4,031	0.94
Schneider[73]	20/12,137	0.16
Total	330/141,725	0.23%

Abbreviations: ASA, atrial septal aneurysm; TTE, transthoracic echocardiography.

Table 43.5 Prevalence of ASA by TEE Study

Study	Prevalence	Percent
Schneider[73]	23/765	3.0
Schreiner[75]	7/340	2.1
Zabalgoitia-Reyes[94]	20/199	10
Pearson[65]	32/410	7.8
Mirode[52]	32/751	4.2
Total	114/2,465	4.6

Abbreviations: ASA, atrial septal aneurysm; TEE, transesophageal echocardiography.

43.4).[2,4,28,32,46,50,61,67,69,73,92] A considerably higher prevalence of 4.6% is noted among those referred for TEE (Table 43.5).[52,65,73,75] Figure 43.5 demonstrates the TEE view of ASA.

ASA is associated with embolic events. In a consecutive series of 410 patients undergoing TEE, Pearson et al noted that the prevalence of ASA was 15% in those with stroke, but only 4% in the control group.[65] As shown in Table 43.6, when the published studies are combined, the prevalence of ASA in patients with cerebral-systemic embolic events is high and reaches 13%.[1,10–13,20,48,52,62]

The mechanism for ASA's association with embolic events is not well defined. However, it is well known that ASA is associated with PFO. Table 43.7 describes the prevalence of PFO among patients with ASA. It can be seen that approximately 60% of the patients with ASA also have PFO. Thus, the relationship of ASA with embolic events is most likely based on its association with PFO. Since ASA is usually highly mobile, protruding from right to left atrium, it is unlikely that a thrombus forms in the ASA itself. This is corroborated by Mügge's series of 195 patients with ASA which only documented two possible thrombi at the site of ASA.[53]

Stroke Recurrence Prevention

The yearly incidence of cryptogenic stroke and the prevalence of PFO in both the general population and the population with cryptogenic stroke can be used to estimate the number of strokes attributable to PFO.[25] The yearly incidence of stroke in the U.S. is estimated at 400,000 to 500,000[9,58] and approximately 40% are cryptogenic. If one uses Lechat et al's findings[49] and assumes that the prevalence of PFO in the general population detected by TTE is 10% versus 40% in cryptogenic stroke patients, then up to 48,000 strokes each year may be attributable to the presence of a PFO.

At the present time, treatment for patients with cryptogenic

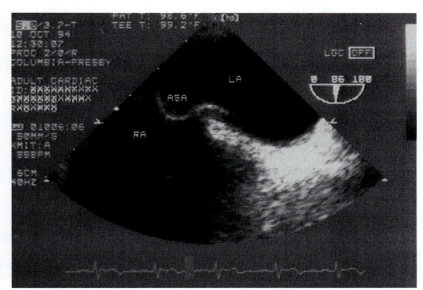

Figure 43.5 Transesophageal echocardiographic view of ASA. LA, left atrium; RA, right atrium.

Table 43.6 TEE Defined ASA in Patients with Cerebral-Systemic Embolization

Study	Prevalence	Percent
Cabanes[11]	28/100	28
Mirode[52]	16/191	8.4
Cohen[13]	20/214	9.3
Catapano[12]	8/51	16
Decoodt[20]	29/301	9.6
Bussiere[10]	4/46	8.7
Ostoic[62]	9/118	7.6
Labovitz[48]	40/270	15
Albers[1]	31/145	21
	185/1,436	13

Abbreviations: ASA, atrial septal aneurysm; TEE, transesophageal echocardiography.

stroke and PFO is undefined. Several potential modalities can be considered. These are medical therapy with warfarin or one of the available antiplatelet agents, percutaneous PFO closure, and surgical PFO closure. Each of these modalities is discussed in the following sections. In the past, ligation of inferior vena cava (IVC) or Greenfield filter placement has been attempted in order to prevent paradoxical embolization. However, Greenfield filter allows for passage of thrombus up to 3 mm in diameter, certainly large enough to cause significant stroke, and IVC ligation results in unacceptable lower extremities edema.[16] Therefore, IVC ligation is not used in the cryptogenic stroke patients with PFO for stroke recurrence prevention.

MEDICAL THERAPY

Recurrence on medical therapy may be high. Sharma et al report experience in 17 patients with ASA and PFO with 12 months follow-up.[79] They found that although there was no recurrence in patients treated with warfarin, there was 50% incidence of recurrence in those treated with aspirin. Comess et al report on 33 patients with PFO with a mean recurrent

Table 43.7 PFO Prevalence among Patients with ASA

Study	Method	Prevalence
Silver[81]	Autopsy	50% (8/16)
Hanley[32]	TTE	49% (24/49)
Mügge[53]	TEE	54% (106/195)
Schneider[73]	TEE	77% (17/22)
Zabalgoitia-Reyes[94]	TEE	85% (17/20)
Pearson[65]	TEE	69% (20/29)
		58% (192/331)

Abbreviations: PFO, patent foramen ovale; TEE, transesophageal echocardiography; TTE, transthoracic echocardiography.

event of 16% per year compared to 7% in the control population.[15] However, some studies demonstrate low recurrence. Hanna et al report no neurologic event recurrence among 13 medically treated stroke patients with PFO, with follow-up to 41 months.[33] More recently, Mas et al retrospectively studied 132 patients with stroke or TIA with PFO or ASA under 60 years old. Over the mean follow-up of 22.6 months, they report 6 with stroke or TIA with actuarial risk of 6.4% at 2 years.[51] Bogousslavsky et al report on 92 patients treated with aspirin and 37 with anticoagulant, followed for a mean of 36 months. There were 8 patients with recurrent stroke and 8 with TIA at 36 months follow-up.[5] The relatively low risk seen in the last two series may have been due to the patient selection criteria, which only included those under age 60. As a result of conflicting reports, at this time the efficacy of medical therapy remains unclear for prevention of recurrent neurologic events in patients with PFO.

Currently, the PFO in Cryptogenic Stroke Study (PICSS) is underway. This is an NIH-supported multicenter study to assess the efficacy of medical therapy for cryptogenic stroke patients with TEE defined PFO. This study derives from the patients from the Warfarin Aspirin Recurrent Stroke Study (WARSS) and is expected to be completed in the year 1999.

PERCUTANEOUS CLOSURE OF PFO

Since PFO represents a possibly repairable lesion, interest in closing them is high. Bridges et al report on transcatheter PFO closure in 36 patients with presumed paradoxical embolism with mean age of 39 years, followed for a mean duration of 8.4 months.[8] There was no recurrent stroke. More recently, Ende reports on the experience of 10 patients with mean age of 40 years with presumed paradoxical embolism followed for a mean of 32 months.[26] He also reports no recurrence of neurologic events. Schräder et al also report no recurrence in 23 patients with a mean follow-up of 1 to 24 months.[74] However, mechanical failure of the devices has been reported and its long-term efficacy and durability remain inconclusively defined.[68]

SURGICAL CLOSURE OF PFO

Surgical closure has been attempted with mixed results. Harvey et al report no recurrence in four patients with mean age of 35 years followed for 7 to 21 months.[35] Zhu et al report two patients with recurrence amongst 6 patients with mean age of 35 years with a mean follow-up of 3.9 years.[95] Homma et al[40] report on 9 patients with a mean follow-up of 12 months with no recurrence. Figure 43.6A demonstrates the PFO seen at the time of surgery, and demonstrates the same area after repair. More recently, Duvuyst et al report no recurrence in 30 patients younger than 60 years followed for a mean of 2 years,[21] and Dearani et al report one recurrence in 24 patients younger than 50, with a mean follow-up of 2.9 years.[18]

The number of patients in each one of the series is small for both percutaneous and surgical closure. Also, the selection criteria vary among the studies, and the patients included in

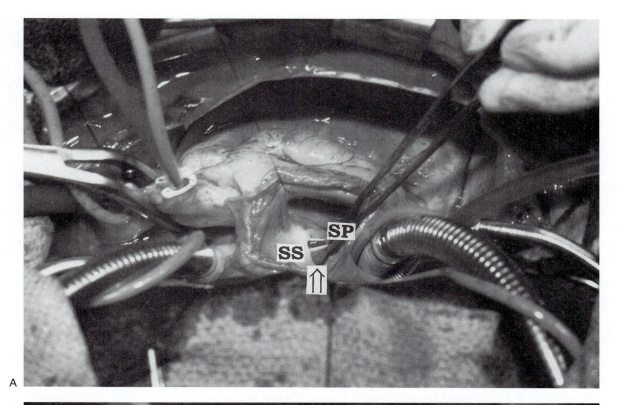

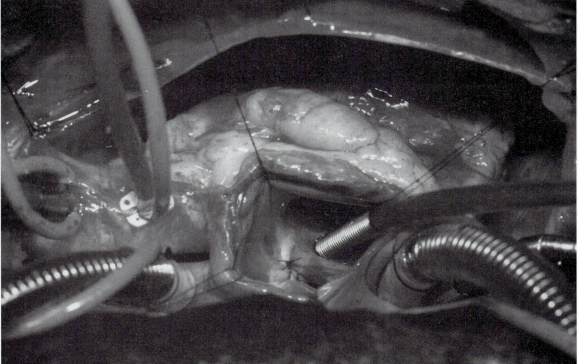

Figure 43.6 Intraoperative view of fossa ovalis area. (**A**) PFO before repair. Septum primum (SP) is pulled away from septum secundum (SS) by forceps revealing PFO. (**B**) Fossa ovalis area after repair.

them are young. Consequently, the efficacy of percutaneous or surgical PFO closure remains undefined and is best reserved for young patients able to undergo medical therapy.

References

1. Albers GW, Comess KA, DeRook FA et al: Transesophageal echocardiographic findings in stroke subtypes. Stroke 25:23–28, 1994

2. Belkin RN, Waugh RA, Kisslo J: Interatrial shunting in atrial septal aneurysm. Am J Cardiol 57:310–312, 1986

3. Berkompas DC, Sagar KB: Accuracy of color Doppler transesophageal echocardiography for diagnosis of patent foramen ovale. J Am Soc Echo 7:253–256, 1994

4. Bewick DJ, Montague TJ: Atrial septal aneurysm: spectrum of clinical and echocardiographic presentations. Canadian Med Assoc J 136:609–611, 1987

5. Bogousslavsky J, Garazi S, Jeanrenaud X et al: Stroke recurrence in patients with patent foramen ovale. Lausanne Stroke Registry Group. Neurology 46:1301–1305, 1996

6. Bommer WJ, Shah PM, Allen H et al: The safety of contrast echocardiography: report of the committee on contrast echocardiography for the American Society of Echocardiography. J Am Coll Cardiol 3:6–13, 1984

7. Brand A, Keren A, Branski D et al: Natural course of atrial septal aneurysm in children and the potential for spontaneous closure of associated septal defects. Am J Cardiol 64:996–1001, 1989

8. Bridges ND, Hellengrand W, Latson L et al: Transcatheter closure of patent foramen ovale after presumed paradoxical embolism. Circulation 86:1902–1908, 1992

9. Broderick JP, Phillips SJ, Whisnant JP et al: Incidence rates of stroke in the eighties: The end of the decline in stroke? Stroke 20:577–582, 1989

10. Bussiere JP, Bonnet D, Renard JL et al: Apport de l'echocardiographie trans-oesophagienne a l'exploration de l'etage auriculaire au cours d'emlolies systemiques. Ann Med Interne (Paris) 143:5–10, 1992

11. Cabanes L, Mas JL, Cohen A et al: Atrial septal aneurysm and patent foramen ovale as risk factors for cryptogenic stroke in patients less than 55 years of age. A study using transesophageal echocardiography. Stroke 24:1865–1873, 1993

12. Catapano O, Oldani A, Milandri M et al: Valutazione ecocardiografica transesofagea dell'aneurisma del setto interatriale nelli'ischemia cerebrale cardioembolica. Cardiologia (Italy) 37:859–864, 1992

13. Cohen A, Roudant R, Cormier B: Is transesophageal echocardiography mandatory in young patients without left heart disease and significant cerebrovascular atherosclerosis? J Am Coll Cardiol 19:32A, 1992

14. Cohnheim J: Thrombose und Embolie. Vorlesungen Uber Allgemenie Pathologie. col I. Hirschwald, Berlin, 1877

15. Comess KA, DeRook FA, Beach KW et al: Transesophageal echocardiography and carotid ultrasound in patients with ischemic stroke: prevalence of findings and recurrent stroke. J Am Coll Cardiol 23:1958–1963, 1994

16. Dalman R, Kohler TR: Cerebrovascular accident after Greenfield filter placement for paradoxical embolism. J Vasc Surg 9:452–454, 1989

17. Daniel WG, Erbel R, Kasper W et al: Safety of transesophageal echocardiography: a multicenter survey of 10,419 patients. Circulation 83:817–821, 1991

18. Dearani JA, Morris JJ, Click RL et al: PFO closure to prevent recurrent stroke or TIA in young adults. J Am Coll Cardiol 27:409A, 1996

19. De Belder MA, Tourikis L, Leach G, Camm J: Risk of patent foramen ovale for thromboembolic events in all age groups. Am J Cardiol 69:1316–1320, 1992

20. Decoodt P, Kacenelenbogen R, Noel P et al: Possible mechanisms of embolization associates with an atrial septal aneurysm. Circulation 86:I–145, 1992

21. Devuyst G, Bogousslavsky J, Rouchat P et al: Prognosis after stroke followed by surgical closure of patent foramen ovale: a prospective follow-up study with brain MRI and simultaneous transesophageal and transcranial Doppler ultrasound. Neurology 47:1162–1166, 1996

22. Di Tullio MR, Sacco RL, Venketasubramanian N, et al: Comparison of diagnostic techniques for the detection of a patent foramen ovale in stroke patients. Stroke 24:1020–1024, 1993

23. Di Tullio MR, Sacco RL, Gopal A et al: Patent foramen ovale as a risk factor for cryptogenic stroke. Ann Intern Med 117:461–465, 1992

24. Di Tullio MR, Sacco RL, Massaro A et al: Transcranial Doppler with contrast injection for the detection of patent foramen ovale in stroke patients. Int J Card Imaging, 9:1–5, 1993

25. Ellenberg JH: The extrapolation of attributable risk to new populations. Stat Med 7:717–725, 1988

26. Ende DJ, Chapra S, Rao S: Transcatheter closure of atrial septal defect or patent foramen ovale with the buttoned device for prevention of recurrence of paradoxic embolism. Am J Cardiol 78:233–236, 1996

27. Fawcett E, Blachford JV: The frequency of an opening between the right and left auricles at the seat of the foetal foramen ovale. J Anat Physiol 35:67–70, 1900

28. Gallet B, Malergue MC, Adam C et al: Atrial septal aneurysm—a potential cause of systemic embolization. Br Heart J 53:292–297, 1985

29. Gautier JC, Dürr A, Koussa S et al: Paradoxical cerebral embolism with a patent foramen ovale. Cerebrovascular Dis 1:193–202, 1991

30. Gibo H, Carver CC, Rhoton AL et al: Microsurgical anatomy of the middle cerebral artery. J Neurosurg 54:151–169, 1981

31. Hagen PT, Scholz DG, Edwards WD: Incidence and size of patent foramen ovale during the first 10 decades of life. Mayo Clin Proc 59:17–20, 1984

32. Hanley PC, Tajik AJ, Hynes JK et al: Diagnosis and classification of atrial septal aneurysm by two-dimensional echocardiography: report of 80 consecutive cases. J Am Coll Cardiol 6:1370–1382, 1985

33. Hanna JP, Sun JP, Furlan AJ et al: Patent foramen ovale and brain infarct. Echocardiographic predictors, recurrence and prevention. Stroke 25:782–786, 1994

34. Hart RG, Miller VT: Cerebral infarctions in young adults: a practical approach. Stroke 14:110–145, 1983

35. Harvey JR, Teague SM, Anderson JL et al: Clinically silent atrial septal defects with evidence for cerebral embolization. Ann Int Med 105:695–697, 1986
36. Hausmann D, Mügge A, Becht I, Daniel WG: Diagnosis of patent foramen ovale by transesophageal echocardiography and association with cerebral and peripheral embolic events. Am J Cardiol 70:668–672, 1992
37. Hausmann D, Mügge A, Daniel WG: Identification of patent foramen ovale permitting paradoxic embolism. J Am Coll Cardiol 26:1030–1038, 1995
38. Hirsh J, Hull RD, Raskob GE: Clinical features and diagnosis of venous thrombosis. J Am Coll Cardiol 8: 114B–127B, 1986
39. Homma S, Di Tullio MR, Sacco RL et al: Characteristics of patent foramen ovale associated with cryptogenic stroke, a biplane transesophageal echocardiographic study. Stroke 25:582–586, 1994
40. Homma S, Di Tullio MR, Sacco RL et al: Surgical closure of patent foramen ovale in selected patients with cryptogenic stroke: a preliminary study. Stroke 26:172, 1995
41. Hust MH, Staiger M, Braun B: Migration of paradoxic embolus through a patent foramen ovale diagnosed by echocardiography: successful thrombolysis. Am Heart J 129:620–622, 1995
42. Jauss M, Kaps M, Keberle M et al: A comparison of transesophageal echocardiography and transcranial Doppler sonography with contrast medium for detection of patent foramen ovale. Stroke 25:1265–1267, 1994
43. Job FP, Ringelstein EB, Grafen Y et al: Comparison of transcranial contrast Doppler sonography and transesophageal contrast echocardiography for the detection of patent foramen ovale in young stroke patients. Am J Cardiol 74:381–384, 1994
44. Jones EF, Calafiore P, Donnan GA, Tonkin AM: Evidence that patent foramen ovale is not a risk factor for cerebral ischemia in the elderly. Am J Cardiol 74: 596–599, 1994
45. Karnik R, Stöllberger C, Valentin A et al: Detection of patent foramen ovale by transcranial contrast Doppler ultrasound. Am J Cardiol 69:560–562, 1992
46. Katayama H, Mitamura H, Mitani K et al: Incidence of atrial septal aneurysm: echocardiographic and pathologic analysis. J Cardiol (Japan) 20:411–421, 1990
47. Klötzsch C, Janßen G, Berlit P: Transesophageal echocardiography and contrast TCD in the detection of a patent foramen ovale: experiences with 111 patients. Neurology 44:1603–1606, 1994
48. Labovitz AJ, Camp A, Castello R et al: Usefulness of transesophageal echocardiography in unexplained cerebral ischemia. Am J Cardiol 72:1448–1452, 1993
49. Lechat P, Mas JL, Lascault G et al: Prevalence of patent foramen ovale in patients with stroke. N Engl J Med 318: 1148–1152, 1988
50. Longhini C, Brunazzi MC, Musacci G et al: Atrial septal aneurysm: echopolycardiographic study. Am J Cardiol 56: 653–656, 1985
51. Mas JL, Zuber M et al: Recurrent cerebrovascular events in patients with patent foramen ovale or atrial septal aneurysm, or both and cryptogenic stroke or TIA. French Study Group on Patent Foramen Ovale and Atrial Septal Aneurysm. Am Heart J 140:1083–1088, 1995
52. Mirode A, Tribouilloy C, Boey S et al: Aneurysmes du septum interauriculaire. Apport de l'echographie transoesophagienne. Relation avec les accidents systemiques emboliques. Ann Cardiol Angeiol (Paris) 42:7–12, 1993
53. Mügge A, Daniel WG, Angermann C et al: Atrial septal aneurysm in adult patients. A multicenter study using transthoracic and transesophageal echocardiography. Circulation 91:2785–2792, 1995
54. Mügge A, Daniel WG, Haverich A, Lichtlen PR: Diagnosis of noninfective cardiac mass lesions by two-dimensional echocardiography. Comparison of the transthoracic and transesophageal approaches. Circulation 83:70–78, 1991
55. Nagelhout DA, Pearson AC, Labovitz AJ: Diagnosis of paradoxic embolism by transesophageal echocardiography. Am Heart J 21:1552–1554, 1991
56. Nellessen U, Daniel WG, Matheis G et al: Impending paradoxical embolism from atrial thrombus: correct diagnosis by transesophageal echocardiography and prevention by surgery. J Am Coll Cardiol 5:1024–1044, 1985
57. Nemec JJ, Marwick TH, Lorig RJ et al: Comparison of transcranial Doppler ultrasound and transesophageal contrast echocardiography in the detection of interatrial right to left shunts. Am J Cardiol 68:1498–1502, 1991
58. 1992 Heart and Stroke Facts. American Heart Association, Dallas, 1991
59. Ofili EO, Rich MW: Safety and usefulness of transesophageal echocardiography in persons aged > 70 years. Am J Cardiol 66:1279–1280, 1990
60. Ofori CS, Moore LC, Helper G: Massive cerebral infarction caused by paradoxical embolism: detection by transesophageal echocardiography. J Am Soc Echo 8:563–566, 1995
61. Oneglia C, Faggiano P, Sabatini T et al: Aneurisma del setto atriale ed anomalie associate. Esperienza personale su 38 casi. Minerva Cardioangiol (Italy) 41:95–100, 1993
62. Ostoic T, Helgason C, Hoff J, Devries S: Determining the source of stroke: evaluation of the findings with transesophageal echocardiography in the context of coexistent carotid artery disease. Circulation 88:I–223, 1993
63. Parsons FG, Keith A: Seventh report of the Committee of Collective Investigation of the Anatomical Society of Great Britain and Ireland, for the years 1896–1897. J Anat Physiol 32:164–186, 1897
64. Patten BM: The closure of the foramen ovale. Am J Anat 48:19–44, 1931
65. Pearson AC, Nagelhout D, Castello R et al: Atrial septal aneurysm and stroke: a transesophageal echocardiographic study. J Am Coll Cardiol 18:1223–1229, 1991
66. Penther P: Le foramen ovale permeable: etude anatomique. A propos de 500 autopsies consecutives. Archives des maladies du coeur et des vaisseax 87:15–21, 1994
67. Ranoux D, Cohen A, Cabanes L et al: Patent foramen ovale: is stroke due to paradoxical embolism? Stroke 24: 31–34, 1993
68. Rocchini AP: Transcatheter closure of atrial septal defects, past, present and future. Circulation 82:1044–1045, 1990
69. Roudant R, Gosse P, Chague F et al: Clinical and echocardiographic features of the aneurysm of the atrial septum

in infants and adults: experience with 44 cases. Echocardiography 6:357–362, 1989

70. Sacco RL, Ellenberg JH, Mohr JP et al: Infarcts of undetermined cause: the NINCDS Stroke Data Bank. Ann Neurol 25:382–390, 1989

71. Scammon RE, Norris EH: On the time of the post-natal obliteration of the fetal blood-passages (foramen ovale, ductus arteriosus, ductus venosus). Anat Rec 15:165–180, 1918

72. Schneider B, Hanrath P, Vogel P, Meinertz T: Improved morphologic characterization of atrial septal aneurysm by transesophageal echocardiography: relation to cerebrovascular events. J Am Coll Cardiol 16:1000–1009, 1990

73. Schneider B, Hofmann T, Justen MH, Meinertz T: Chiari's network: normal anatomic variant or risk factor for arterial embolic events? J Am Coll Cardiol 26:203–210, 1995

74. Schräder R, Steinke W, Nacimiento W et al: Cerebrovasc Dis 6:16, 1996

75. Schreiner G, Erbel R, Mohr-Kahaly S et al: Nachweis von aneurysmen des vorhofseptums mit hilfe der transösophagealen echokardiographie. Z Kardiol 74:440–444, 1985

76. Schreiter SW, Phillips JH: Thromboembolus traversing a patent foramen ovale: resolution with anticoagulation. J Am Soc Echo 7:659–662, 1994

77. Schroeckenstein RM, Wasenda GJ, Edwards JE: Valvular competent patent foramen ovale in adults Minn Med. 55: 11–13, 1972

78. Seib GA: Incidence of the patent foramen ovale cordis in adult American whites and American negroes. Am J Anat 55:511–525, 1934

79. Sharma AK, Ofili E, Castello R et al: Effect of treatment on recurrent embolic events with atrial septal aneurysm and associated right to left shunting. J Am Soc Echo 4: 294, 1991

80. Sherman D, Di Tullio M, Marboe C et al: Effect of air contrast dose on the echocardiographic detection of patent foramen ovale. J Stroke Cerebrovasc Dis Suppl S582, 1992

81. Silver MD, Dorsey JS: Aneurysms of the septum primum in adults. Arch Pathol Lab Med 102:62–65, 1978

82. Silverman M: Paradoxical embolus. N Engl J Med. 329: 930, 1993

83. Stoddard MF, Keedy DL, Dawkins PR: The cough test is superior to the Valsalva maneuver in the delineation of right-to-left shunting through a patent foramen ovale during contrast transesophageal echocardiography. Am Heart J 125:185–189, 1993

84. Stöllberger C, Slany J, Schuster I et al: The prevalence of deep venous thrombosis in patients with suspected paradoxical embolism. Ann Intern Med 119:461–465, 1993

85. Sweeney LJ, Rosenquist GC: The normal anatomy of the atrial septum in the human heart. Am Heart J 98: 194–199, 1979

86. Teague SM, Sharma MK: Detection of paradoxical cerebral echo contrast embolization by transcranial Doppler ultrasound. Stroke 22:740–745, 1991

87. Thompson T, Evans W: Paradoxical embolism. Quart J Med 23:135–150, 1930

88. Van Camp G, Schulze D, Cosyns B, Vandenbossche JL: Relation between patent foramen ovale and unexplained stroke. Am J Cardiol 71:596–598, 1993

89. Van Hare GF, Silverman NH: Contrast two-dimensional echocardiography in congenital heart disease: technique, indications and clinical utility. J Am Coll Cardiol 13: 673–686, 1989

90. Webster MW, Chancellor AM, Smith HJ et al: Patent foramen ovale in young sroke patients. Lancet 2:11–12, 1988

91. Weslow RG, Di Tullio MR, Sacco RL et al: Morphological and functional characteristics of patent foramen ovale identifiable only by transesophageal echocardiography. Stroke 26:173, 1995

92. Wolf WJ, Casta A, Sapire DW: Atrial septal aneurysms in infants and children. Am Heart J 113:1149–1153, 1987

93. Wright RR, Anson BJ, Cleveland HC: The vestigial valves and the interatrial foramen of the adult human heart. Anat Rec 100:331–335, 1948

94. Zabalgoitia-Reyes M, Herrera C, Ghandi DK et al: A possible mechanism for neurologic ischemic events in patients with atrial septal aneurysm. Am J Cardiol 66: 761–764, 1990

95. Zhu WX, Khandheria BK, Warnes CA et al: Closure of patent foramen ovale for cryptogenic stroke in young patients: long-term follow-up. Circulation 86:I–147, 1992

SECTION V

Stroke Therapy

HENRY J. M. BARNETT
BENNETT M. STEIN

The Preface to the third edition of this volume devoted to cerebrovascular disease pointed out that a major leap forward has occurred in the understanding, prevention, and treatment of stroke. Therapy has begun to enjoy a high profile, and an aura of fresh excitement is sweeping over the field of stroke neurology. This is simply a reflection of the newer understandings in pathophysiologic mechanisms, in biochemical and molecular changes in ischemia, and in imaging of the brain and blood vessels, and of a surge in pharmaceutical inquiry making genuine differences in the short-term and long-term management of patients at the bedside, in the clinic, and in the community.

This section describes in detail the state of the art of stroke prevention and, most excitingly, of stroke treatment. New knowledge about the value of anticoagulants is available and is described here. New platelet inhibitors have been introduced. Their benefits and shortcomings are reviewed. Prevention still may be claimed to have made the most important contributions to care to date, but the early breakthroughs in thrombolytic therapy vindicate the opinions of those who have maintained that cerebral ischemia is not untreatable.

Surgical therapy for cerebrovascular disease has been studied in major clinical trials involving patients on both sides of the Atlantic and the Pacific, as well as in Africa and Australia. We are close to being able to identify the full gamut of patients with symptomatic disease who will and will not benefit from carotid endarterectomy. The story on asymptomatic disease remains unclear, but work continues.

Surgical therapy has been complemented by endovascular procedures in the management of vascular malformations. It is being extensively studied in cerebral aneurysms, and by the time the next edition of this book is written, we should know with reasonable certainty whether this technology can be extended to stenosing lesions extracranially and possibly even intracranially.

The intent of the following chapters is to apprise readers fully about the prevention and treatment of cerebrovascular disorders as seen in late 1997. The millennium has not yet arrived for stroke victims, but the problems are beginning to yield to the pressures of basic and clinical scientific research.

Principles of Hemostasis and Antithrombotic Therapy

MARK A. CROWTHER

JEFFREY GINSBERG

Fundamentals of Anticoagulant Action and Administration

Antithrombotic therapy is an accepted part of both the acute and chronic management of patients with cerebrovascular disease.[6,13,99] Such therapy reduces the risk of cardioembolic events,[6,9,27] is effective in the management of acute ischemic syndromes,[67] and may reduce long-term morbidity of cerebral ischemia.[8,50,97] In addition, antithrombotic agents may modulate the development of atherosclerotic vascular disease, the cause of the majority of ischemic cerebrovascular disorders.[77] Recent developments in this field include an increase in the number of available antithrombotic agents, many with different mechanisms of action, and in the number of indications for their use. Particularly exciting are the clinical trials demonstrating the efficacy of low molecular weight heparin and thrombolytics in the setting of acute ischemic stroke.

In this chapter we review (1) the hemostatic system and its regulation and discuss the coagulation cascade, and (2) most of the classes of antithrombotic agents currently available. We do not review, in detail, studies examining the clinical utility of each of these agents or the antiplatelet agents, because these topics are covered elsewhere in the text.

Currently available antithrombotics are broadly divided into five classes: anticoagulants, thrombolytic agents, defibrinogenating agents, direct thrombin inhibitors, and antiplatelet agents. Drugs from each of these classes have been studied in patients with stroke; the first four of these will be reviewed in this chapter.

Hemostasis

The hemostatic system is composed of a highly regulated series of both procoagulant and anticoagulant zymogens and cofactors. Hemostasis (the physiological response to vascular injury) and thrombosis (the pathological formation of thrombus) are both the result of activation of this system. Thrombosis is due to an imbalance between endogenous procoagulant and fibrinolytic systems.[59] Thrombi are composed of a fibrin network, within which platelets, red blood cells, white blood cells, and protein constituents of blood are found.[30] Contents of a thrombus vary depending on the conditions under which it forms: arterial emboli are rich in platelets and fibrin whereas venous thrombi contain fewer platelets and more red blood cells.[65] Thrombi change dynamically[24] due to incorporation of both procoagulant and anticoagulant proteins into the clot structure.[66,123] As thrombi age they organize, platelets are removed, and the fibrin network stabilizes as a result of migration of fibroblasts and smooth muscle cells into the thrombus. Dependent on the activity of the fibrinolytic system, thrombi may lyse, embolize, or be incorporated into the vessel wall.

Thrombosis is triggered as a result of one or more of a triad of abnormalities, first described by Virchow: stasis,

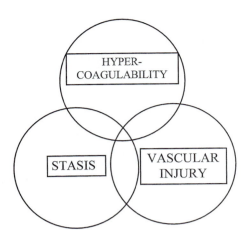

Figure 44.1 Virchow's triad. Virchow originally described the classic triad of stasis, hypercoagulability and vascular injury, which contribute to most, if not all, cases of thrombosis.

hypercoagulability, and vascular injury (Fig. 44.1). Thus, arterial thrombosis occurs at sites of arterial narrowing with endothelial damage and turbulent blood flow (as are found at atherosclerotic plaques). Venous thrombosis, such as superior sagittal sinus thrombosis, may be secondary to a congenital hypercoagulable state, a reversible prothrombotic condition, local infection or trauma, or it may be idiopathic.

THE COAGULATION CASCADE AND THROMBUS FORMATION

Hemostasis depends on a system of interdependent plasma proteins and blood cellular elements (Fig. 44.2). Coagulation factors circulate in plasma in inactive, zymogen forms. Thrombosis is initiated by a combination of endothelial injury and exposure of subendothelial protein matrix to circulating blood. Exposure of subendothelium results in platelet adhesion and

activation, mediated primarily by platelet Ib/IX receptors. As a result, platelets undergo shape change and degranulate. Platelet fibrinogen receptors (GP IIb/IIIa) then undergo a conformational change resulting in fibrinogen binding to the platelet and tethering of additional platelets to the developing thrombus. Simultaneously, endothelial cells expose tissue factor to which circulating activated factor VII adheres. The tissue factor-factor VIIa complex initiates coagulation by activating coagulation factors X and IX. Factor IXa binds factor VIIIa (its coenzyme) on a phospholipid surface and, in the presence of calcium, forms the Xase complex. This complex then activates factor X; factor Xa then assembles on a phospholipid surface with factor Va (its coenzyme), to form the "prothrombinase complex" that activates prothrombin to thrombin. Thrombin (1) cleaves fibrinopeptide A and B from fibrinogen, thus forming fibrin, (2) activates factor XIII, which crosslinks assembled fibrin polymers, (3) activates further factor Va, VIIIa, Xa, and IXa, which results in the autocatalytic production of additional thrombin, and (4) activates platelets, which results in further thrombus growth.[30]

Once a thrombus is formed, it grows until it either occludes a vessel or embolizes or, alternatively, a balance between procoagulant and anticoagulant forces is achieved and thrombus growth is arrested. Nonocclusive thrombi, which are seen relatively more frequently in high-flow vessels (such as the carotid artery), can embolize or become organized and incorporated into a vessel wall, accelerating development of a local atherosclerotic lesion.

There are relatively few laboratory tests assessing in vivo activity of the coagulation cascade. The bleeding time is sensitive to reductions in platelet numbers and to quantitative platelet defects; however, it does not predict hemorrhage accurately in high-risk patients. Because of a lack of in vivo tests to assess activity of the coagulation system, a variety of in vitro techniques have been developed.

The integrity of the coagulation cascade is assessed using assays that time thrombus formation within a sample of patient plasma. These tests [which include the activated partial thromboplastin time (APTT), prothrombin time (PT) and thrombin clotting time (TCT)] are sensitive to significant deficiencies of the functional activity of one or more coagulation factors

Figure 44.2 The coagulation cascade. In vivo activation of coagulation is dependent upon the generation of factor VIIa/tissue factor at sites of vascular injury, with subsequent generation of thrombin. Although other coagulation factors (such as factor XII) are assessed by commonly employed coagulation tests (such as the aPTT), their role in physiological coagulation is unclear.

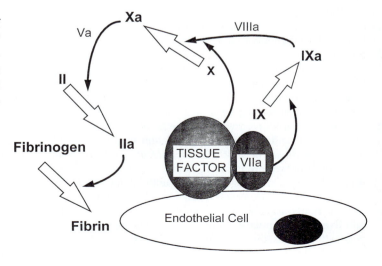

Table 44.1 Tests Commonly Employed in the Assessment of Coagulation

Test	Purpose	Utility
Activated partial thromboplastin time (aPTT)	Assesses the intrinsic and common pathways of the coagulation cascade (factors XII, XI, X, IX, VII, V, II, and fibrinogen)	Used to monitor heparin therapy Prolonged with factor depletion (i.e., hemophilia)
Prothrombin time (PT)	Assesses the extrinsic and common pathways of the coagulation cascade (factors VII, X, V, II, and fibrinogen)	Used to monitor warfarin therapy Most commonly prolonged in liver disease or vitamin K depletion
Thrombin clotting time (TCT)	Assesses the functional activity of fibrinogen	Used to monitor heparin therapy Most commonly prolonged in hypofibrinogenemic states

(Table 44.1). These tests do not reflect the activity of some antithrombotics (e.g., the low molecular weight heparins), and they do not quantitate the levels of antithrombotic drugs. In addition, abnormalities in these tests are nonspecific; a prolonged aPTT may be due to hemophilia, heparin therapy, disseminated intravascular coagulation, or a lupus anticoagulant. To overcome these limitations, additional assays (including clot-based, chromogenic, and immunologic assays) have been developed and are now employed in most routine coagulation laboratories. These assays can be used to monitor the anticoagulant effect of medications (such as the low molecular weight heparins), to determine whether patients have a prothrombotic state (i.e., factor V Leiden mutation testing), to determine antithrombotic drug levels (i.e., chromogenic or immunologic testing of hirudin levels), and to determine the concentrations of coagulation factors (i.e., factor VIII levels in patients with hemophilia).

Testing the activity of the coagulation system in vivo is difficult because activated coagulation factors have extremely short half-lives and are rapidly inactivated by circulating inhibitors. However, a variety of assays that measure activated coagulation factors complexed to their specific inhibitors or activation peptides of specific coagulation factors have been developed. These plasma tests allow direct assessment of in vivo activity of the coagulation system and include prothrombin fragment (F1.2), thrombin-antithrombin complexes (TAT) and fibrinopeptide A (FPA) (Table 44.2). F1.2 and TAT are surrogates for thrombin generation, whereas FPA levels reflect the catalytic activity of unregulated thrombin.[14]

Similarly, with the exception of the bleeding time, there are no tests that assess in vivo platelet function. In vitro platelet function is assessed using aggregometry, whereas plasma levels of β_2 thromboglobulin are markers of systemic platelet activation.

When monitoring is necessary, one of several coagulation assays is usually performed to monitor anticoagulant drug therapy. The most appropriate test depends upon which coagulation factors are most affected by the anticoagulant. Thus, unfractionated heparin is usually monitored by the APTT. Low molecular weight heparins, which do not significantly prolong the APTT or TCT, are usually given in a fixed dose without monitoring. However, low molecular weight heparin levels can be monitored by antifactor Xa heparin levels. Warfarin therapy, which reduces the functional levels of four coagulation factors (factors II, VII, IX and X), produces a prolongation in the PT, which is sensitive to reductions in the activity of factors II, VII, and X. Although the PT is an effective way to monitor warfarin, variability in the sensitivity of different prothrombin time reagents to the anticoagulant effect of warfarin is marked. This variability means that a fixed dose of warfarin, in a given patient, will produce different prothrombin times when patients' plasmas are assayed using different PT reagents. In order to overcome this variability, the PT is converted to an international normalized ratio (INR), which is calculated as follows:

$$INR = \left(\frac{PT\ patient}{PT\ control}\right)^{ISI^b}$$

where ISI is the international sensitivity index and reflects the sensitivity of the PT reagent. This conversion standardizes results and reduces variability in intensity of anticoagulant therapy among different centers.[58]

Table 44.2 Markers of Activation of the Coagulation System

Name		Significance
Prothrombin fragment	F1.2	Reflects systemic thrombin generation
Thrombin-antithrombin complex	TAT	Reflects systemic thrombin activity
Fibrinopeptide A	FPA	Reflects unopposed thrombin activity
D-dimer	DD	Reflects systemic fibrinolysis

ENDOGENOUS REGULATORS OF COAGULATION

Coagulation factors are tightly regulated by a series of control mechanisms that are built into each stage of the coagulation cascade to limit the extent of thrombus formation. The tissue factor-factor VIIa complex is rapidly inactivated by formation of a quaternary complex with tissue factor pathway inhibitor (TFPI) and factor Xa. This reaction effectively "turns off" one

Figure 44.3 The activated protein C pathway. Thrombin binds with thrombomodulin on the surface of endothelial cells. This complex activates protein C to activated protein C (APC), a potent anticoagulant. APC inactivates factors Va and VIIIa, thus "turning off" the coagulation cascade.

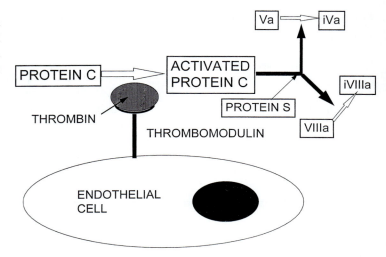

THE FIBRINOLYTIC SYSTEM

Plasmin is the principal fibrinolytic enzyme. It is produced when tissue-plasminogen activator (tPA), released by endothelial cells, cleaves plasminogen to plasmin. Plasmin is found both in fluid phase and bound to fibrin, although fluid phase plasmin is rapidly inactivated by α_2-antiplasmin (α-AP). In turn, tPA is inhibited by plasminogen-activator inhibitor-1 (PAI-1). Plasmin that escapes regulation degrades fibrin and fibrinogen by proteolytic cleavage. This process releases fibrin(ogen) degradation products, including D-dimer. Congenital deficiency of plasminogen is associated with a thrombotic diathesis, whereas deficiency of α_2-AP is associated with a congenital hemorrhagic state.[37,69] Systemic fibrin(ogen)olysis occurs when plasmin escapes regulation by α_2-AP.[126] Circulating plasmin degrades both fibrin and fibrinogen, resulting in systemic hypofibrinogenemia,[82] and might, therefore, account for the bleeding complications that are associated with thrombolytic therapy.[47,73]

The activity of the fibrinolytic system is best assessed using ex vivo clot-based assays. These include the euglobulin clot lysis time and the urea clot lysis time. Antigen levels and the functional activity of plasminogen (as well as its inhibitors) can be determined using immunological and functional testing, respectively.

of the initiating mechanisms of the coagulation cascade.[45] In addition, thrombin down-regulates its own production by a number of mechanisms. When present in high concentration, thrombin lyses factors Va and VIIIa. In addition, it binds to thrombomodulin, a cell surface glycoprotein, forming a complex that activates protein C. Activated protein C (APC) is a potent anticoagulant protein, which acts in concert with its cofactor, protein S, to degrade factors Va and VIIIa.[83] Activated protein C may also stimulate fibrinolysis[39] (Fig. 44.3). Antithrombin III, a circulating plasma protein, rapidly inactivates fluid phase thrombin as well as factors IXa and Xa. This inactivation is accelerated several thousandfold by unfractionated and low molecular weight heparin.[72,98] The clinical importance of the plasma inhibitors of coagulation is supported by the fact that congenital deficiency of protein C, protein S, or antithrombin III is associated with a lifelong predisposition to venous thrombosis.[124] The liver removes activated circulating coagulation factors[36]; therefore, patients with liver disease who receive activated coagulation factors for treatment of hemophilia are predisposed to acute disseminated intravascular coagulation.[11]

Thrombin binds to fibrin within a thrombus and remains catalytically active, maintaining its ability to generate fibrin (through cleavage of fibrinogen) and to up-regulate its own production (through generation of factors Va and VIIIa). Fibrin-bound thrombin is not effectively inactivated by heparin-antithrombin III complexes, because the heparin binding site on thrombin is blocked when thrombin is fibrin bound. Thus, fibrin-bound thrombin is resistant to inactivation by heparin and related compounds.[125] Fibrin-bound thrombin may be responsible for extension or recurrence of thrombosis in patients who are adequately anticoagulated or in patients whose thrombi recur early after discontinuation of anticoagulants. Therefore, agents that inactivate fibrin-bound thrombin may be more effective than heparin or related compounds in lowering the risk of thrombotic recurrence. Newer antithrombotics, particularly direct thrombin inhibitors (see later section), are able to inactivate fibrin-bound thrombin directly and may thus be more effective than heparin for the treatment of patients with acute venous thromboembolic disorders.[2]

PHYSIOLOGIC MECHANISMS TO PREVENT UNWANTED THROMBUS FORMATION

The prevention of pathological thrombus formation is critical; mechanisms to prevent pathological thrombosis include blood flow rheology, potent inhibitors of coagulation in the circulation, and the antithrombotic nature of the endothelium. Laminar flow of blood through vessels prevents platelet adhesion to endothelium. If turbulence occurs in a vessel, however, platelet adherence rises dramatically.[118] Normal endothelial surfaces are nonthrombogenic and react with neither platelets nor blood components.[118] Intact endothelial cells are negatively charged, and as such, repel cellular elements of blood. Endothelial cells produce prostacyclin (PGI_2), which is a powerful inhibitor of platelet aggregation.[38] In addition, intact endothelial cells express both thrombomodulin and heparan sulphate. As discussed above, thrombomodulin, in concert with thrombin, can activate protein C. Endothelial heparin sulfate, a cell surface glycosaminoglycan, catalyzes circulating antithrombin III to inactivate coagulation factors IIa, IXa, Xa and XIa.[111] Furthermore, endothelial cells are primary sources of tPA, which initiates the fibrinolytic pathway.

SUMMARY

The balance between the coagulation cascade and the fibrinolytic pathway determines the rate of formation and dissolution of thrombus; however, at any point in time, both processes are active within a thrombus. Inhibition of coagulation (through use of anticoagulants), inhibition of platelet activity (through use of antiplatelet agents), or potentiation of fibrinolysis (through use of thrombolytics) form the basis for the pharmacological treatment of patients with thrombosis.

Principles of Anticoagulant Action

The antithrombotic drugs used in clinical practice either increase the activity of endogenous anticoagulant or fibrinolytic systems, or reduce functional levels of coagulation factors. Selective inhibition of coagulation results in a decrease in fibrin generation and/or increase in fibrinolysis. Antithrombotic agents (such as heparin) do not potentiate the fibrinolytic system; however, by preventing further fibrin deposition, they do accelerate thrombolysis.

SPECIFIC AGENTS

Heparins and Related Compounds

Unfractionated heparin is a heterogeneous mixture of polysulphated glycosaminoglycans of variable molecular weights (3,000 to 20,000 D). Heparin is derived from porcine intestinal mucosa or bovine lung. It is not absorbed after oral administration, and is thus given parenterally. It is marketed as either a sodium or calcium salt for intravenous or subcutaneous administration. The pharmacokinetics of unfractionated heparin vary widely among individuals, due primarily to differences in the amount of soluble and cell surface protein binding of heparin.[130,131] The half-life of heparin increases in proportion to the infused dose,[17,18] with the majority of heparin being cleared by reticuloendothelial uptake or renal clearance. After bolus injection, heparin is initially cleared by a saturable mechanism with a short half-life (approximately 10 minutes), followed by a more gradual clearance with a longer half-life.[17,18] Very large boluses, such as those used in aortocoro-

nary bypass, overwhelm the clearance mechanisms, resulting in excretion of intact heparin in the urine.[34]

Heparin has an immediate anticoagulant effect after intravenous injection. After subcutaneous injection, the peak anticoagulant effect occurs at three to four hours, with a sustained anticoagulant effect up to 12 hours after injection.[92]

Protamine sulphate reverses the anticoagulant effect of heparin. One milligram of protamine inactivates approximately 100 IU of heparin activity. Thus, assuming a heparin half-life of 30 minutes, 25 mg of intravenous protamine should inactivate a 5,000-unit intravenous heparin bolus, if administered 30 minutes after the heparin dose. The half-life of protamine is shorter than that of heparin, and, therefore, rebound anticoagulation may occur due to persistent heparin effect after the protamine effect has been lost.[112]

Heparin catalyses antithrombin III-mediated inactivation of factors IIa, IXa, Xa, XIa, XIIa. Antithrombin III forms a covalent complex with the activated coagulation factor and is consumed in the reaction, whereas heparin, acting as a catalyst, is not consumed. Although, in the absence of heparin, antithrombin III inactivates these clotting factors, heparin accelerates the reactions several thousandfold. The heparin-antithrombin III complex is ineffective at inactivating fibrin-bound thrombin (see above).

In high dose, heparin also inactivates thrombin by catalyzing heparin cofactor II (HC II). Like antithrombin III, HC II inactivates thrombin by forming a covalent complex. The rate of this reaction is accelerated by heparin and by agents, such as danaparoid (see below), that contain dermatan sulphate.

The antithrombotic effect of heparin is usually monitored using the APTT, which is sensitive to therapeutic levels of unfractionated heparin. The two-unit TCT can also be used to monitor heparin therapy; however, it is more difficult to standardize than the APTT. Heparin levels can be measured using factor Xa inhibition (anti-Xa heparin level), which quantifies the inhibition of factor Xa by heparin in the plasma. Similar antifactor IIa assays are also available. Protamine sulphate neutralization of heparin can be used to monitor heparin levels, although this technique is cumbersome.

Two recently identified problems exist in monitoring heparin therapy. The first is the use of a target APTT, which is a fixed ratio of 1.5 to 2.5 times the patient's baseline APTT, because in patients with a short baseline APTT, a target range that includes 1.5 times baseline may result in an APTT that is only slightly above the upper limit of normal, likely resulting in underdosing of heparin. Second, the degree of APTT prolongation of a plasma sample in a heparin-treated patient is a reflection of both the plasma heparin level in the patient and the sensitivity of the APTT reagent to heparin. The latter is important because there is considerable reagent-to-reagent variability in the sensitivity to heparin. In order to establish uniform heparin levels, the therapeutic range for each APTT reagent should be established by determining the APTT range that corresponds to ex vivo antifactor Xa heparin levels of 0.35 to 0.70 units/ml. In most cases, this will result in a therapeutic APTT of 60 to 85 seconds, although there can be dramatic variability among APTT reagents.[23]

Heparin should be administered intravenously or subcutaneously. Intravenous heparin is usually administered with an initial bolus followed by a continuous infusion. The APTT should be determined 6 hours after the bolus, and the heparin infusion adjusted to achieve a therapeutic APTT. Based on the response of the patient, the frequency of monitoring and dose adjustments should be individualized, but for most patients once daily monitoring is sufficient. Administration of heparin is facilitated by use of a heparin dosing nomogram.[31] In patients requiring large doses of heparin (more than 35,000 units of intravenous heparin per day) anti-Xa heparin levels more accurately reflect the antithrombotic effect of heparin than does the APTT. This effect occurs primarily because some patients have elevated levels of factor VII, which can result in a blunting of the APTT response to heparin.[75] Heparin can be given by intermittent intravenous injection, but this results in an increased risk of bleeding.[46,100]

Subcutaneous heparin is effective and is widely used for the prevention of venous thromboembolism and is safe and effective for the treatment of patients with venous thromboembolism.

Low Molecular Weight Heparin

Low molecular weight heparins have been designed to overcome the limitations of standard heparin and are produced by enzymatic or chemical depolymerization of standard heparin. The mean molecular weight of unfractionated heparin is approximately 15,000 D, whereas the mean molecular weight of the low molecular weight heparins is approximately 5,000 D. Several low molecular weight heparins have been evaluated in large clinical trials and are available for clinical use.

Low molecular weight heparins do not bind avidly to plasma or cell surface proteins, and therefore they have more predictable pharmacokinetic profiles than standard heparin.[16,20,21,42,52,54,57,130,131] As a result, they can be administered subcutaneously without laboratory monitoring.[70,74] These agents, which are cleared primarily by the kidneys, produce their peak anticoagulant effect two to six hours after subcutaneous injection.

Low molecular weight heparins catalyze antithrombin III. Because of their short chain length, they are relatively ineffective inhibitors of thrombin, but are effective inhibitors of factor Xa. When administered in therapeutic doses, low molecular weight heparins do not reliably prolong the APTT. Anticoagulant monitoring of low molecular weight heparins is not usually required; however, it can be performed, if needed, using anti-Xa heparin levels; the optimal therapeutic range for low molecular weight heparins (i.e., the range in which the optimal antithrombotic to hemorrhagic ratio is achieved) is unknown, but it is likely in the range of 0.5 to 1.5 anti-Xa units/ml.

The usual dose of low molecular weight heparins for the treatment of patients with venous thromboembolic disease is 100 anti-Xa heparin units/kg subcutaneously twice daily. In the largest trial of these agents in patients with acute ischemic stroke, doses of 4,100 anti-Xa units once or twice daily were employed, with the twice-daily dose being more effective.[67]

The primary complication of low molecular weight heparin therapy is hemorrhage. The incidence of hemorrhage with low molecular weight heparin is probably lower than that of unfractionated heparin, particularly if the unfractionated heparin and low molecular weight heparin are given in doses that produce an equivalent antithrombotic effect. In addition, low molecular weight heparins have a lower risk of heparin-associated thrombocytopenia[121] than unfractionated heparin.

Because of their predictable pharmacokinetics, their favorable hemorrhagic/therapeutic ratio and their proven efficacy in many clinical situations,[67,70,74,85,86] low molecular weight heparins are being used with increasing frequency and might eventually replace unfractionated heparin in many clinical situations.

Oral Anticoagulants

Oral anticoagulants were first isolated after it was noted that animals consuming improperly cured sweet clover hay suffered a hemorrhagic diathesis, which was improved by transfusion of whole blood from unaffected animals.[108] A variety of oral anticoagulant medications are now available. Warfarin (4-hydroxycoumarin) is the most widely used in North America. It is available for either intravenous or oral use; however, the intravenous form is rarely used. Warfarin is a racemic mixture of R and S enantiomers, with the R enantiomer having a longer serum half-life than the S enantiomer (46 versus 32 hours).[91] After absorption, 99% of warfarin in circulation is bound to albumin. Free or unbound warfarin is metabolically active. Displacement of warfarin from albumin, coupled with reduced enteric production of vitamin K, is responsible for the enhanced anticoagulant effect of warfarin seen in patients receiving antibiotics, particularly sulfonamides.

Warfarin blocks the cyclic interconversion of vitamin K and its 2,3-epoxide,[56] which results in reduced posttranslational modification of the procoagulant factors II, VII, IX, and X and the anticoagulant proteins, protein C and protein S. As a result, these factors are dysfunctional and do not participate in coagulation.[79] The degree of impairment of coagulation is proportional to the reductions in levels of these coagulation factors, although there is experimental evidence to support the hypothesis that reductions in the levels of factors II and X are more important than reductions in the levels of factor VII for the antithrombotic effects of warfarin.[55,128,133] Administration of vitamin K by the oral, intravenous, or subcutaneous route reverses the anticoagulant effects of warfarin, usually within 24 hours of their administration.[94,103,110] In an emergency, factors II, VII, IX and X can be replaced using plasma products. Human plasma should only be used to reverse the anticoagulant effect of warfarin in emergency situations.

The anticoagulant response to a given dose of warfarin varies widely among individuals, due to variations in warfarin bioavailability, rates of warfarin metabolism, and levels of vitamin K. Many medications and foods interact with warfarin, either by changing bioavailability of vitamin K or warfarin, or by modifying metabolic clearance of warfarin.[56,127] Drugs that increase warfarin's metabolic clearance (i.e., carbamazepine)[53] or reduce its bioavailability (i.e., cholestyramine)[63] decrease the anticoagulant response to warfarin, whereas drugs that inhibit clearance of warfarin (i.e., erythromycin)[122] or displace it from albumin (i.e., sulfonamides)[90] increase the anticoagulant response to a given warfarin dose.

The anticoagulant effect of warfarin is monitored using a one-stage prothrombin time (PT).[96] The PT is sensitive to reductions in levels of three of four vitamin K-dependent procoagulant factors (factors II, VII, and X). Due to variations in the sensitivity of prothrombin time reagents and automated coagulation machines to warfarin,[95] the international normalized ratio (INR), rather than the PT, should be used to monitor warfarin therapy.[56] Using this system, the target INR for most indications is 2.0 to 3.0.[56]

The most frequent complication of warfarin therapy is bleeding. Major hemorrhage occurs infrequently; in patients less than 70 years old receiving warfarin for atrial fibrillation, the rate of major hemorrhage is 1.7% per year, rising to 4.2% per year in patients over the age of 70,[4] rates that are significantly greater than those seen with aspirin therapy. More than one-third of major bleeds are intracranial.[4] Warfarin is teratogenic when taken during the first trimester. Teratogenic effects of warfarin include midline facial defects and central nervous system malformations.[61] Because of the risk of embryopathy, warfarin should not be used in pregnant patients, and patients should be counseled against becoming pregnant while taking warfarin. Rare complications of warfarin include skin necrosis,[68] dermatitis, and a syndrome of painful, blue toes.

Warfarin therapy is effective in prevention of venous thromboembolism in high-risk patients,[109] in prevention of arterial embolism in patients with atrial fibrillation,[9] and myocardial infarction,[104] and in treatment of patients with acute venous thromboembolism.[60]

Danaparoid (Orgaran)

Danaparoid is derived from porcine and bovine mucosa and is a heterogeneous mixture of heparan sulfate, dermatan sulphate, and chondroitin sulphate, all of which are polysulphated glycosaminoglycans with structural similarities to heparin. Danaparoid has been studied in the treatment and prophylaxis of venous thromboembolic disease.[1,28,35,44] Although the antibody that has been implicated in the pathogenesis of heparin-induced thrombocytopenia cross-reacts with danaparoid in about 10% of cases,[26,78] the clinical relevance of this is uncertain, since danaparoid has been shown to be a safe and effective antithrombotic in patients with this condition.[48,49] The drug is not well absorbed after oral administration; therefore, it must be given parenterally. It is available for subcutaneous and intravenous administration. After intravenous injection, the peak anticoagulant effect of danaparoid is achieved within minutes. After subcutaneous administration, the peak anticoagulant effect is delayed, although bioavailability is nearly 100%.[32] Orgaran has a biological half-life unlike that seen with other antithrombotics; components of its antithrombotic activity persist for varying lengths of time. Thus, the half-life of its antithrombin effect is 4.3 hours, whereas its anti-Xa activity has a half-life of 24.5 hours.[32] Renal excretion accounts for 40% to 50% of plasma clearance of the anti-Xa activity of danaparoid[32] and its pharmacokinetics are not affected by hepatic disease.[33] When administered after an intravenous bolus of danaparoid, protamine sulphate will partially reverse its anti-IIa effect, but does not affect the anti-Xa anticoagulant effect.[106]

The principal anticoagulant effect of danaparoid is due to heparan sulphate, which catalyzes antithrombin III-mediated inactivation of thrombin and factor Xa. About 10% of the anticoagulant effect of the drug is due to dermatan sulphate-mediated catalysis of thrombin by heparin cofactor II. In addi-

tion, the low affinity fraction of heparan sulphate produces an anticoagulant effect through an unknown mechanism. Danaparoid has less platelet inhibitory effect than heparin, which may account for its favorable antithrombotic to hemorrhagic ratio when compared to unfractionated heparin.[87]

Danaparoid is usually administered in a weight-adjusted dose without laboratory monitoring, although its anticoagulant activity can be measured using anti-Xa heparin levels. The usual prophylactic dose of danaparoid is 750 to 1,000 anti-Xa units subcutaneously twice daily, a dose that has been shown to significantly reduce the risk of both proximal and total deep vein thrombosis when compared with unfractionated heparin in patients with thrombotic stroke.[115] For treatment of patients with acute thrombosis, danaparoid is usually administered in a dose of 1,250 to 2,000 anti-Xa units subcutaneously twice daily; in one study, the latter regimen was significantly more effective than unfractionated heparin in treatment of patients with deep vein thrombosis.[35] If anti-Xa heparin levels are monitored, a therapeutic level similar to that required for low molecular weight heparins (i.e., 0.5 to 1.5 anti-Xa U/ml) should be employed.

The principal complication of danaparoid therapy is bleeding: danaparoid appears to cause less bleeding than standard heparin in animal models in which equivalent antithrombotic doses of heparin and danaparoid are administered[87]; however, studies of sufficient power to verify this finding in patients receiving danaparoid have not been performed.[101]

Direct Thrombin Inhibitors

Direct thrombin inhibitors are a new class of drugs that have been designed to inactivate thrombin via specific, high-affinity interactions with the catalytic site on the thrombin molecule. Two types of direct thrombin inhibitors are currently in clinical trials: polypeptide congeners of the leech anticoagulant (hirudins) and synthetic arginine derivatives (argatroban). Only the hirudins will be discussed in this chapter.

Hirudin is the principal anticoagulant in the saliva of the medicinal leech, *Hirudo medicinalis*. Recombinant hirudin (r-hirudin) is now available in sufficient quantities for clinical evaluation. Hirudin is not absorbed after oral administration and must be given parenterally. The drug is currently being evaluated in several phase III trials, for patients with ischemic coronary disease, and for the prophylaxis and treatment of deep vein thrombosis and heparin-induced thrombocytopenia.

The direct thrombin inhibitors have predictable pharmacokinetics when compared with unfractionated heparin,[119,132] a finding that is presumably due to their lack of plasma and cell surface protein binding. This allows weight-based dosing and may allow these agents to be administered with little or no monitoring of their anticoagulant effect. The lack of protein binding also suggests that direct thrombin inhibitors are not inactivated at the site of thrombus formation, by locally released proteins, such as platelet factor IV. These proteins, which are released in the vicinity of a thrombus by platelets, bind to and reduce the local antithrombotic effect of heparin and related compounds.

After intravenous injection, the plasma half-life of r-hirudin is 2.8 hours. Intravenous infusion of r-hirudin produces steady-state plasma concentrations proportional to the infused dose.[25,80] Clearing of r-hirudin is mainly by the kidneys; its half-life is markedly prolonged in patients with renal failure and patients on dialysis.[89]

The anticoagulant effect of hirudin is maximal within minutes of intravenous injection; the peak effect is delayed several hours after subcutaneous injection. Hirudin does not require plasma cofactors, such as antithrombin III or heparin cofactor II, for its antithrombotic effect.[64] Unlike heparin and related compounds, direct thrombin inhibitors are not catalysts and are therefore consumed on a mole-to-mole basis as they inhibit thrombin.[41] Thus, to be effective, direct thrombin inhibitors must be present in sufficient quantities at the site of a thrombus to inhibit thrombin activity and must be continually delivered to the thrombus to replace the drug that is consumed when it binds to thrombin.

Plasma r-hirudin levels can be determined using a chromogenic assay[51,76,105,120] or one of several immunoassays.[62] Hirudin produces dose-dependent prolongation of thrombin-dependent clotting tests and, therefore, its anticoagulant activity can be monitored using these tests. The activated partial thromboplastin time (APTT) and APTT ratio (measured APTT/baseline APTT) appear to correlate well with plasma levels of hirudin.[22,80,102,119] Thrombin clotting times (TCT) are sensitive to low levels of hirudin, but are not useful for measuring higher levels.[80,102]

The major side effect of r-hirudin is bleeding and there is no specific antidote for the anticoagulant effect of this direct thrombin inhibitor.[40] Reversal of the anticoagulant effect of r-hirudin has been attempted using protein C-depleted activated prothrombinase complex[107] or dDAVP;[19] however, neither has been adequately studied in patients receiving clinically relevant doses of r-hirudin. Hirudin is not effectively removed by hemodialysis.[117] Therefore, bleeding complications can be difficult to manage, particularly when amounts of drug that produce a marked anticoagulant effect are administered. The hemorrhagic effects of direct thrombin inhibitors are clinically relevant; excess major bleeding in patients receiving r-hirudin has been seen in three trials of the drug in patients with coronary artery disease.[7,12,88] However, r-hirudin does not potentiate heparin-induced thrombocytopenia, nor is it known to cause osteoporosis, two well-documented complications of unfractionated heparin.

Hirudin is a foreign protein and is therefore immunogenic. Thus, patients can develop neutralizing antibodies, or antibodies that can cause allergic reactions. The formation of neutralizing antibodies has the potential to limit the number of times direct thrombin inhibitors can be used in an individual patient.

Defibrinogenating Snake Venoms

Snake venoms contain a variety of potent activators of the human coagulation system. Clinical experience is greatest with ancrod, a salivary enzyme of the Malayan pit viper, which produces its anticoagulant effect by cleaving fibrinopeptide A from fibrinogen, producing fibrin monomer. This fibrin monomer then self-associates to form a fibrin polymer.[43] Unlike thrombin, ancrod does not activate factor XIII, which would normally cross-link fibrin polymer. Thus, the fibrin polymer that results from ancrod cleaving fibrinogen is easily disrupted by the endogenous fibrinolytic system and cleared

by the reticuloendothelial system.[93] Reductions in fibrinogen levels lead to both a reduced risk of thrombosis and a reduction in blood viscosity, which may increase flow rates, further decreasing the risk of thrombosis and increasing perfusion to ischemic areas.

Ancrod is administered parenterally, either by intermittent intravenous injection or by subcutaneous injection.[54] Its plasma half-life is 3.5 hours; however, its defibrinogenating effect may last for several days. After an intravenous infusion of 0.5 to 1.0 unit/kg (which must be given over at least 6 hours), the plasma fibrinogen level will usually fall over a period of hours to levels less than 1 g/L. Once daily intravenous or subcutaneous administration is required to maintain the fibrinogen level at less than 1 g/L. Reversal of the anticoagulant effect of ancrod is effected with a solution of polyclonal antiancrod antibodies. In addition, the fibrinogen level can be increased by administration of cryoprecipitate. Ancrod prolongs the thrombin clotting time proportionately to the fall in fibrinogen level.

The primary complication of ancrod therapy is hemorrhage. Additional complications include allergic reactions and the potential to cause thrombosis[71]; this latter complication may occur because ancrod does not inhibit the formation or activity of thrombin. In some patients with impaired fibrinolysis, fibrin polymer may spontaneously cross-link, forming a thrombus.

Ancrod is currently being evaluated in a large randomized trial in patients with acute ischemic stroke.[3]

Thrombolytic Agents

In contrast to anticoagulants, thrombolytic agents produce their effect by activating the endogenous fibrinolytic system. This results in thrombus dissolution and restoration of blood flow. The thrombolytic agents currently available for clinical use are enzymes that convert plasminogen to plasmin, which then cleaves fibrin to form fibrin degradation products. After systemic administration, thrombolytics induce a systemic fibrinolytic state, due to the generation of plasmin that escapes regulation.[81]

The three commonly used thrombolytic agents are tissue plasminogen activator (tPA), streptokinase, and urokinase. Streptokinase is a bacterial enzyme isolated from culture and purified for clinical use; tPA and urokinase, which are produced by recombinant techniques, are enzymes normally produced within endothelial cells and maintain the normal "antithrombotic" properties of intact endothelium. All three of these thrombolytics produce similar clinical effects when administered to patients with acute thrombosis, although tPA produces less fibrinogenolysis than the other two. They are administered by intravenous infusion or intravenous bolus; streptokinase produces dose-dependent hypotension and thus should be given over at least 60 minutes. A modified form of streptokinase (acyl-plasminogen streptokinase activator complex, APSAC) has been produced that does not cause hypotension after bolus intravenous injection.

All three agents are rapidly cleared from the circulation after intravenous injection; their anticoagulant effect is prolonged because of (1) systemic depletion of fibrinogen; (2) an acquired "dysfibrinogenemia" secondary to the inhibitory effects of fibrin and fibrinogen degradation products they produce; (3) plasmin generation, which escapes regulation because of antiplasmin depletion[126]; and (4) a qualitative platelet defect.[113] Although traditionally administered as boluses followed by infusions, these agents are now usually given as single injections over 30 to 90 minutes. In patients with pulmonary embolism, prolonged infusions of thrombolytics are no more effective than bolus infusions and may be associated with an increased risk of hemorrhage.[5]

The thrombolytics produce their antithrombotic effect through plasmin generation. Streptokinase binds to circulating plasminogen, forming a complex that then catalyzes the formation of additional plasmin. This free, circulating plasmin complexes with its primary inhibitor, α-2 antiplasmin. Systemic fibrino(geno)lysis occurs when α_2 antiplasmin levels are depleted. In theory, and in experimental models, both tPA and single-chain urokinase (scu-PA) have a significant advantage over streptokinase; they exhibit "fibrin specificity," that is, they bind first with fibrin and then activate plasminogen. This produces thrombolysis that is localized to the vicinity of the thrombus without the production of a systemic fibrinolytic state.[15,116] In addition, fibrin-bound plasmin is resistant to inhibition by α-2 antiplasmin.[129] However, when given in clinically relevant doses, the thrombolytic effect of tPA is not localized. Thus, tPA (and scuPA) produces a systemic fibrinolytic state, similar to that seen with SK, secondary to systemic depletion of α_2 antiplasmin.[29,114]

Monitoring the anticoagulant effects of thrombolytic agents is not usually performed because of their immediate onset of action and the fact they are given in a fixed or weight-based dose by short intravenous infusion. For the reasons discussed above, the anticoagulant effect of the thrombolytics persist until well after their disappearance from the circulation. Therefore, monitoring of patients who have received thrombolytics is complicated; the dysfibrinogenemia and qualitative platelet defect found in patients who have received thrombolytics are particularly difficult to detect and quantify.

The major complication of thrombolytic therapy is bleeding. Major bleeding, including intracerebral hemorrhage, occurs in up to 4.2% of patients receiving thrombolytic therapy for acute myocardial infarction.[81] In a recent randomized, placebo-controlled trial, tPA in patients with acute ischemic stroke was associated with a rate of symptomatic intracerebral bleeding of 6.4%, a 10-fold increase compared with patients who did not receive thrombolytics.[10] In addition, conversion of nonhemorrhagic to hemorrhagic stroke occurred significantly more frequently in patients receiving thrombolytics than in those who did not.[8,10]

Reversal of the anticoagulant effect of the thrombolytics can be achieved quickly with administration of cryoprecipitate (until the fibrinogen level is 1 g/L or greater), ϵ-amino caproic acid (given as a bolus of 5 gm IV over 30 to 45 minutes followed by an infusion as indicated by laboratory testing), and, if bleeding persists, platelets.

Other complications of thrombolytics include allergic reactions. Streptokinase is a foreign protein and, therefore, antibody generation may lead to neutralizing antibodies, or to anaphylactic reactions. Because of this, repeated administration of streptokinase should ordinarily be avoided. tPA and UK are not immunogenic.

SUMMARY

Cerebral ischemia is due, in many cases, to embolic or *in situ* thrombosis in the cerebral arterial circulation. Antithrombotic agents are effective at preventing cardioembolic cerebral ischemia (in patients with atrial fibrillation and myocardial infarction). In addition, there is emerging evidence that thrombolytics, if administered immediately after the onset of cerebral ischemia, reduce long-term morbidity from stroke. However, complications of therapy, including intracerebral hemorrhage and systemic bleeding, occur with increased frequency. Therefore, identification of high-risk subgroups for these complications should be developed.

Recent developments in antithrombotic drugs (particularly the low molecular weight heparins, the thrombolytics, and the direct thrombin inhibitors) as well as the development of better laboratory techniques to monitor antithrombotic therapy will all increase the utility of antithrombotic therapy in patients with stroke.

Acknowledgments

Dr. Crowther is the recipient of a Medical Research Council of Canada Fellowship. Dr. Ginsberg is the recipient of a Heart and Stroke Foundation of Ontario Research Scholarship.

References

1. Agnelli G, Cosmi B, Di Filippo P et al: A randomised, double-blind, placebo-controlled trial of dermatan sulphate for prevention of deep vein thrombosis in hip fracture. Thromb Haemost 67:203–208, 1992
2. Agnelli G, Renga C, Weitz JI et al: Sustained antithrombotic activity of hirudin after its plasma clearance: comparison with heparin. Blood 80:960–965, 1992
3. Anonymous: Ancrod for the treatment of acute ischemic brain infarction. Ancrod Stroke Study Investigators. Stroke 25:1755–1759, 1994
4. Anonymous: Bleeding during anithrombotic therapy in patients with atrial fibrillation. Arch Intern Med 156:409–416, 1996
5. Anonymous: National Institutes of Health Consensus Panel: Thrombolytic therapy in thrombosis. Ann Intern Med 93:141–144, 1980
6. Anonymous: Optimal oral anticoagulant therapy in patients with nonrheumatic atrial fibrillation and recent cerebral ischemia. European Atrial Fibrillation Trial Study Group. N Engl J Med 333:5–10, 1995
7. Anonymous: Randomized trial of intravenous heparin versus recombinant hirudin for acute coronary syndromes. The Global Use of Strategies to Open Occluded Coronary Arteries (GUSTO) IIa Investigators. Circulation 90:1631–1637, 1994
8. Anonymous: Randomised controlled trial of streptoki-

nase, aspirin, and combination of both in treatment of acute ischaemic stroke. Multicentre Acute Stroke Trial—Italy (MAST-I) Group. Lancet 346:1509–1514, 1995

9. Anonymous: Risk factors for stroke and efficacy of antithrombotic therapy in atrial fibrillation. Analysis of pooled data from five randomized controlled trials. Arch Intern Med 154:1449–1457, 1994

10. Anonymous: Tissue plasminogen activator for acute ischemic stroke. The National Institute of Neurological Disorders and Stroke rt-PA Stroke Study Group. N Engl J Med 333:1581–1587, 1995

11. Anonymous: Thrombogenic materials in prothrombin complex concentrates. Ann Intern Med 81:766–770, 1974

12. Antman EM: Hirudin in acute myocardial infarction. Safety report from the Thrombolysis and Thrombin Inhibition in Myocardial Infarction (TIMI) 9A Trial. Circulation 90:1624–1630, 1994

13. Barnett HJ, Eliasziw M, Meldrum HE: Drugs and surgery in the prevention of ischemic stroke. N Engl J Med 332:238–248, 1995

14. Bauer K, Weitz JI: Laboratory markers of coagulation and fibrinolysis. p. 1197. In Colman RW, Hirsh J, Marder VJ, Salzman EW (eds): Hemostasis and Thrombosis: Basic Principles and Clinical Practice. 3rd ed. Lippincott-Raven, Philadelphia, 1994

15. Bergmann SR, Fox KA, Ter-Pogossian MM et al: Clot-selective coronary thrombolysis with tissue-type plasminogen activator. Science 220:1181–1183, 1983

16. Boneu B, Buchanan MR, Caranobe C et al: The disappearance of a low molecular weight heparin fraction (CY 216) differs from standard heparin in rabbits. Thromb Res 46:845–853, 1987

17. Boneu B, Caranobe C, Cadroy Y et al: Pharmacokinetic studies of standard and unfractionated heparins, and low molecular weight heparins in the rabbit. Semin Thromb Hemost 14:18–27, 1988

18. Boneu B, Caranobe C, Gabaig AM et al: Evidence for a saturable mechanism of disappearance of standard heparin in rabbits. Thromb Res 46:835–844, 1987

19. Bove CM, Casey BC, Marder VJ: DDAVP reduces bleeding during continued hirudin administration in the rabbit. Thromb Haemos 75:471–475, 1996

20. Bratt G, Tornebohm E, Widlund L, Lockner D: Low molecular weight heparin (KABI 2165, Fragmin): pharmacokinetics after intravenous and subcutaneous administration in human volunteers. Thromb Res 42:613–620, 1986

21. Briant L, Caranobe C, Saivin S et al: Unfractionated heparin and CY 216: pharmacokinetics and bioavailabilities of the antifactor Xa and IIa effects after intravenous and subcutaneous injection in the rabbit. Thromb Haemos 61:348–353, 1989

22. Bridey F, Dreyfus M, Parent F et al: Recombinant hirudin (HBW 023): biological data of ten patients with severe venous thrombo-embolism. Am J Hematol 49:67–72, 1995

23. Brill-Edwards P, Ginsberg JS, Johnston M, Hirsh J: Establishing a therapeutic range for heparin therapy. Ann Intern Med 119:104–109, 1993

24. Cade J, Hirsh J, Regoeczi E: Mechanisms for elevated fibrin/fibrinogen degradation products in acute experimental pulmonary embolism. Blood 45:563–568, 1975

25. Cardot JM, Lefevre GY, Godbillon JA: Pharmacokinetics of rec-hirudin in healthy volunteers after intravenous administration. J Pharmacokinet Biopharm 22:147–156, 1994

26. Chong BH, Magnani HN: Orgaran in heparin-induced thrombocytopenia. Haemostasis 22:85–91, 1992

27. Cleland J, Cowburn PJ, Falk RH: Should all patients with atrial fibrillation receive warfarin? Eur Heart J 17:674–681, 1996

28. Cohen AT, Phillips MJ, Edmondson RA et al: A dose ranging study to evaluate dermatan sulphate in preventing deep vein thrombosis following total hip arthroplasty. Thromb Haemost 72:793–798, 1994

29. Collen D, Topol EJ, Tiefenbrunn AJ et al: Coronary thrombolysis with recombinant human tissue-type plasminogen activator: a prospective, randomized, placebo-controlled trial. Circulation 70:1012–1017, 1984

30. Colman RW, Marder VJ, Salzman EW et al In: Overview of hemostasis. p. 3. In Colman RW, Hirsh J, Marder VJ, Slazman EW (eds): Hemostasis and Thrombosis: Basic Principles and Clinical Practice. 3rd ed. Lippincott-Raven, Philadelphia, 1994

31. Cruickshank MK, Levine MN, Hirsh J et al: A standard heparin nomogram for the management of heparin therapy. Arch Intern Med 151:333–337, 1991

32. Danhof M, de Boer A, Magnani HN, Stiekema JC: Pharmacokinetic considerations on Orgaran (Org 10172) therapy. Haemostasis 22:73–84, 1992

33. de Boer A, Stiekema JC, Danhof M, Breimer DD: The influence of Org 10172, a low molecular weight heparinoid, on antipyrine metabolism and the effect of enzyme induction on the response to Org 10172. Br Clin Pharmacol 32:23–29, 1991

34. deSwart CAM, Nijmeyer B, Roelofs JMM, Sixma JJ: Kinetics of intravenously administered heparin in normal subjects. Blood 60:1251–1258, 1982

35. de Valk HW, Banga JD, Wester JW et al: Comparing subcutaneous danaparoid with intravenous unfractionated heparin for the treatment of venous thromboembolism. A randomized controlled trial. Ann Intern Med 123:1–9, 1995

36. Deykin D: The role of liver in serum induced hypercoagulability. J Clin Invest 45:256–263, 1966

37. Dolan G, Preston FE: Familial plasminogen deficiency and thromboembolism. Fibrinolysis (suppl.) 22:26, 1988

38. Ehrman ME, Jaffe EA: Prostacyclin (PGI2) inhibits the development in human platelets of ADP and arachidonic acid-induced shape change and procoagulant activity. Prostaglandins 20:1103–1116, 1980

39. Esmon CT, Comp PC: Generation of fibrinolytic activity by infusion of activated protein C into dogs. J Clin Invest 68:1221–1228, 1981

40. Fareed J, Walenga JM, Pifarre R et al: Some objective considerations for the neutralization of the anticoagulant actions of recombinant hirudin. Haemostasis suppl 21 1:64–72, 1991

41. Fenton JW II, Villanueva GB, Ofosu FA, Maraganore

JM: Thrombin inhibition by hirudin: how hirudin inhibits thrombin. Haemostasis suppl 21 1:27–31, 1991

42. Frydman AM, Bara L, Le Roux Y et al: The antithrombotic activity and pharmacokinetics of enoxaparine, a low molecular weight heparin, in humans given single subcutaneous doses of 20 to 80 mg. J Clin Pharmacol 28: 609–618, 1988

43. Gaffney PJ, Brasher M: Mode of action of ancrod as a defibrinating agent. Nature 251:53–54, 1974

44. Gallus A, Cade J, Ockelford P et al: F. Orgaran (Org 10172) or heparin for preventing venous thrombosis after elective surgery for malignant disease? A double-blind, randomised, multicentre comparison. ANZ-Organon Investigators' Group. Thromb Haemost 70: 562–567, 1993

45. Girard TJ, Warren LA, Novotny WF et al: Functional significance of the Kunitz-type inhibitory domains of lipoprotein-associated coagulation inhibitor. Nature 338: 518–520, 1989

46. Glazier RL, Crowell EB: Randomized prospective trial of continuous vs intermittent heparin therapy. JAMA 236:1365–1367, 1976

47. Gore JM, Granger CB, Simoons ML et al: Stroke after thrombolysis. Mortality and functional outcomes in the GUSTO-I trial. Global Use of Strategies to Open Occluded Coronary Arteries. Circulation 92:2811–2818, 1995

48. Greinacher A, Eckhardt T, Mussmann J, Mueller-Eckhardt C: Pregnancy complicated by heparin associated thrombocytopenia: management by a prospectively in vitro selected heparinoid (Org 10172). Thromb Res 71: 123–126, 1993

49. Greinacher A, Philippen KH, Kemkes-Matthes B et al: Heparin-associated thrombocytopenia type II in a patient with end-stage renal disease: successful anticoagulation with the low-molecular-weight heparinoid Org 10172 during haemodialysis. Nephrol Dial Transplant 8: 1176–1177, 1993

50. Hacke W, Kaste M, Fieschi C et al: Intravenous thrombolysis with recombinant tissue plasminogen activator for acute hemispheric stroke. European Cooperative Acute Stroke Study (ECASS). JAMA 274:1017–1025, 1995

51. Hafner G, Fickenscher K, Friesen H et al: Evaluation of an automated chromogenic substrate assay for the rapid determination of hirudin in plasma. Thromb Res 77:165–173, 1995

52. Handeland GF, Abildgaard U, Holm HA, Arnesen KE: Dose adjusted heparin treatment of deep venous thrombosis: a comparison of unfractionated and low molecular weight heparin. Eur J Clin Pharmacol 39:107–112, 1990

53. Hansen JM, Siersboek-Nielsen K, Skovsted L: Carbamazepine-induced acceleration of diphenylhydantoin and warfarin metabolism in man. Clin Pharmacol Ther 12:539–543, 1971

54. Harker LA, Maraganore JM, Hirsh J: Novel antithrombotic agents. p. 1638. In Colman RW, Hirsh J, Marder VJ, Salzman EW (eds): Hemostasis and Thrombosis: Basic Principles and Clinical Practice. 3rd ed. Lippincott-Raven, Philadelphia, 1994

55. Hellemans J, Vorlat M, Verstraete M. Survival time of prothrombin and factors VII, IX, X after complete synthesis blocking doses of coumarin derivatives. Br J Haematol 9:506–512, 1963

56. Hirsh J, Dalen JE, Deykin D et al: Oral anticoagulants: mechanism of action, clinical effectiveness, and optimal therapeutic range. Chest 108(4):231–46, 1995

57. Hirsh J, Levine MN: Low molecular weight heparin. Blood 79:1–17, 1992

58. Hirsh J, Poller L. The international normalized ratio. A guide to understanding and correcting its problems. Arch Intern Med 154:282–288, 1994

59. Hirsh J, Salzman EW, Marder VJ et al: Overview of the thrombotic process and its therapy. p. 1151. In Colman RW, Hirsh J, Marder VJ, Salzman EW (eds): Hemostasis and Thrombosis: Basic Principles and Clinical Practice. 3rd ed. Philadelphia, Lippincott-Raven, 1994

60. Hull R, Delmore T, Genton et al: Warfarin sodium versus low-dose heparin in the long-term treatment of venous thrombosis. N Engl J Med 301:855–858, 1979

61. Iturbe-Alessio I, Fonesca MC, Mutchinik O et al: Risks of anticoagulant therapy in pregnant women with artificial heart valves. N Engl J Med 315:1390–1393, 1986

62. Iyer L, Adam M, Amiral J et al: Development and validation of two enzyme-linked immunosorbent assay (ELISA) methods for recombinant hirudin. Semin Thromb Hemost 21:184–192, 1995

63. Jahnchen E, Meinertz T, Gilfrich HJ et al: Enhanced elimination of warfarin during treatment with cholestyramine. Br J Clin Pharmacol 5:437–440, 1978

64. Jakubowski JA, Maraganore JM: Inhibition of coagulation and thrombin-induced platelet activities by a synthetic dodecapeptide modeled on the carboxy-terminus of hirudin. Blood 75:399–406, 1990

65. Jorgensen L. Experimental platelet and coagulation thrombi. A histological study of arterial and venous thrombi of varying age in untreated and heparinized rabbits. Acta Pathol Microbiol Scand [A] 62:189, 1964

66. Kaminski M, McDonagh J: Studies on the mechanism of thrombin: interaction with fibrin. J Biol Chem 258: 10530–10535, 1983

67. Kay R, Wong KS, Yu YL et al: Low-molecular-weight heparin for the treatment of acute ischemic stroke. N Engl J Med 333:1588–1593, 1995

68. Kock-Weser J: Coumarin necrosis. Ann Intern Med 68: 1365–1367, 1968

69. Koie K, Kamiya T, Ogata K, Takamatsu J: Alpha-2-plasmin-inhibitor deficiency 7 (Miyasato disease). Lancet 2:1334–1336, 1978

70. Koopman MMW, Prandoni P, Piovella F et al: Treatment of patients with proximal-vein thrombosis with intravenous unfractionated heparin in hospital compared with subcutaneous low-molecular-weight heparin out of hospital or with early discharge. N Engl J Med 334: 682–687, 1996

71. Krishnamurti C, Bolan CD, Reid TJ III, Alving BM: Pharmacology and mechanism of action of ancrod: potential for inducing thrombosis. Blood 79:2492, 1992

72. Kurachi K, Fujikawa K, Schmier G, Davie EW: Inhibition of bovine factor IXa and Xa by antithrombin III. Biochemistry 15:373–377, 1976

73. Lauer JE, Heger JJ, Mirro MJ: Hemorrhagic complica-

tions of thrombolytic therapy. Chest 108:1520–1523, 1995

74. Levine M, Gent M, Hirsh J et al: A comparison of low-molecular weight heparin administered primarily at home with unfractionated heparin administered in the hospital for proximal deep-vein thrombosis. N Engl J Med 334:677–681, 1996

75. Levine MN, Hirsh J, Gent M et al: A randomized trial comparing activated thromboplastin time with heparin assay in patients with acute venous thromboembolism requiring large daily doses of heparin. Arch Intern Med 154:49–56, 1994

76. Longstaff C, Wong MY, Gaffney PJ: An international collaborative study to investigate standardisation of hirudin potency. Thromb Haemost 69:430–435, 1993

77. Loscalzo J: The relation between atherosclerosis and thrombosis. Circulation 86(suppl. 6): III95–III99, 1992

78. Magnani HN: Heparin-induced thrombocytopenia (HIT): an overview of 230 patients treated with orgaran (Org 10172). Thromb Haemost 70:554–561, 1993

79. Malhotra OP, Nesheim ME, Mann KG: The kinetics of activation of normal and gamma-carboxyglutamic acid-deficient prothrombins. J Biol Chem 260:279–287, 1985

80. Marbet GA, Verstraete M, Kienast J et al: Clinical pharmacology of intravenously administered recombinant desulfatohirudin (CGP 39393) in healthy volunteers. J Cardiovasc Pharmacol 22:364–372, 1993

81. Marder VJ, Hirsh J, Bell WR: Rationale and practical basis of thrombolytic therapy. p. 1514. In Colman RW, Hirsh J, Marder VJ, Salzman EW (eds): Hemostasis and Thrombosis: Basic Principles and Clinical Practice. 3rd ed. Lippincott-Raven, Philadelphia, 1994

82. Marder VJ, Rothbard RL, Fitzpatrick PG, Francis CW: Rapid lysis of coronary artery thrombi with APSAC: treatment by bolus intravenous injection. Ann Inter Med 104:304–310, 1986

83. Marlar RA, Kleiss AJ, Griffin JH: Human protein C: inactivation of factors V and VIII in plasma by the activated molecule. Annals NY Acad Sci 370:303–310, 1981

84. Matzsch T, Bergqvist D, Hedner U, Ostergaard P: Effects of an enzymatically depolymerized heparin as compared with conventional heparin in healthy volunteers. Thromb Haemost 57:97–101, 1987

85. Melandri G, Semprini F, Cervi V et al: Benefit of adding low molecular weight heparin to the conventional treatment of stable angina pectoris. A double-blind, randomized, placebo-controlled trial. Circulation 88:2517–23, 1993

86. Menzin J, Colditz GA, Regan MM. Cost-effectiveness of enoxaparin vs low-dose warfarin in the prevention of deep-vein thrombosis after total hip replacement surgery. Arch Intern Med 155:757–764, 1995

87. Meuleman DG: Orgaran (Org 10172): its pharmacological profile in experimental models. Haemostasis 22:58–65, 1991

88. Neuhaus KL, von Essen R, Tebbe U et al: Safety observations from the pilot phase of the randomized r-Hirudin for Improvement of Thrombolysis (HIT-III) study. A study of the Arbeitsgemeinschaft Leitender Kardiologischer Krankenhausarzte (ALKK). Circulation 90:1638–1642, 1994

89. Nowak G, Bucha E, Goock T et al: Pharmacology of r-hirudin in renal impairment. Thromb Res 66:707–715, 1992

90. O'Reilly RA: The pharmacodynamics of the oral anticoagulant drugs. Prog Hemost Thromb 2:175–213, 1974

91. O'Reilly RA: Vitamin K and the oral anticoagulant drugs. Ann Rev Med 27:245–261, 1976

92. O'Sullivan EF, Hirsh J, McCarthy RA, de Gruchy GC, Heparin in the treatment of venous thrombo-embolic disease: administration, control and results. Med J Aus 2:153–159, 1968

93. Pizzo SV, Schwartz ML, Hill RL, McKee PA: Fibrin destruction by arvin: the mechanism of arvin anticoagulation. Clinical Research 20:46, 1972

94. Pengo V, Banzato A, Garelli E, et al: Reversal of excessive effect of regular anticoagulation: low oral dose of phytonadione (vitamin K1) compared with warfarin discontinuation. Blood Coag Fibrinolysis 4:739–741, 1993

95. Poller L, Taberner DA: Dosage and control of oral anticoagulants: an international survey. Br J Haematol 51:479–485, 1982

96. Quick AJ: The prothrombin time in haemophilia and obstructive jaundice. J Biol Chem 109:73–74, 1935

97. Rabbani LE, Loscalzo J: Recent observations on the role of hemostatic determinants in the development of the atherothrombotic plaque. Atherosclerosis 94:1–7, 1994

98. Rosenberg RD: Actions and interactions of antithrombin and heparin. N Engl J Med 292:146–151, 1975

99. Rothrock JF, Hart RG: Antithrombotic treatment of cerebrovascular diseases. p. 1438. In Colman RW, Hirsh J, Marder VJ, Salzman EW (eds): Hemostasis and Thrombosis: Basic Principles and Clinical Practice. 3rd ed. Lippincott-Raven, Philadelphia, 1994

100. Salzman EW, Deykin D, Shapiro RM, Rosenberg RD: Management of heparin therapy. N Engl J Med 292:1046–1050, 1975

101. Scheffler E, Aulmann M, Remppis A: Successful use of a heparinoid (danaparoid sodium) for heparin-induced thrombocytopenia type II in aortic valve reoperation. Z Kardiol 84:565–568, 1995

102. Schiele F, Vuillemenot A, Kramarz P et al: A pilot study of subcutaneous recombinant hirudin (HBW 023) in the treatment of deep vein thrombosis. Thromb Haemost 71:558–562, 1994

103. Shetty HG, Backhouse G, Bentley DP, Routledge PA: Effective reversal of warfarin-induced excessive anticoagulation with low dose vitamin K1. Thromb Haemost 67:13–15, 1992

104. Smith P: Long-term anticoagulant treatment after acute myocardial infarction. The Warfarin Re-Infarction Study. Ann Epidemiol 2:549–552, 1992

105. Spannagl M, Bichler H, Lill H, Schramm W: A fast photometric assay for the determination of hirudin. Haemostasis suppl 21 1:36–40, 1991

106. Stiekema JC, Wijnand HP, ten Cate H et al: Partial in vivo neutralisation of plasma anticoagulant effects of Lomoparan (Org 10172) by protamine chloride. Thromb Res 63:157–167, 1991

107. Stuever T, Iqbal O, Hoppensteadt D et al: Protein C depleted activated prothrombin complex neutralizes the

bleeding associated with hirudin. Thromb Haemost 73: 1454, 1995

108. Suttie JW: Vitamin K antagonists. p. 1562. In Colman RW, Hirsh J, Marder VJ, Salzman EW (eds): In Hemostasis and Thrombosis: Basic Principles and Clinical Practice. 3rd ed. Lippincott-Raven, Philadelphia, 1994

109. Taberner DA, Poller L, Burslem RW, Jones JB: Oral anticoagulants controlled by the British comparative thromboplastin versus low-dose heparin in prophylaxis of deep vein thrombosis. Br Med J 1:272–274, 1978

110. Taberner DA, Thomson JM, Poller L: Comparison of prothrombin complex concentrate and vitamin K1 in oral anticoagulant reversal. Br Med J 76:83–85, 1976

111. Teien AN, Abildgaard U, Hook M: The anticoagulant effect of heparan sulfate and dermatan sulfate. Thromb Res 8:859–867, 1976

112. Teoh KH, Young E, Bradley CA, Hirsh J: Heparin binding proteins. Contribution to heparin rebound after cardiopulmonary bypass. Circulation 88:II420–11425, 1993

113. Terres W, Umnus S, Mathey DG, Bleifeld W: Effects of streptokinase, urokinase, and recombinant tissue plasminogen activator on platelet aggregability and stability of platelet aggregates. Cardiovasc Res 24:471–477, 1990

114. Topol EJ, Bell WR, Weisfeldt ML: Coronary thrombolysis with recombinant tissue-type plasminogen activator. A hematologic and pharmacologic study. Ann Intern Med 103:837–843, 1985

115. Turpie AG, Levine MN, Hirsh J et al: Double-blind randomised trial of Org 10172 low-molecular-weight heparinoid in prevention of deep-vein thrombosis in thrombotic stroke. Lancet 1:523–526, 1987

116. Van de Werf F, Bergmann SR, Fox KA et al: Coronary thrombolysis with intravenously administered human tissue-type plasminogen activator produced by recombinant DNA technology. Circulation 69:605–610, 1984

117. Vanholder RC, Camez AA, Veys NM et al: Recombinant hirudin: a specific thrombin inhibiting anticoagulant for hemodialysis. Kidney Int 45:1754–1756, 1994

118. Vasiliev JM, Gelfand IM: Mechanisms of non-adhesiveness of endothelial and epithelial surfaces. Nature 274: 710–711, 1978

119. Verstraete M, Nurmohamed M, Kienast J et al: Biologic effects of recombinant hirudin (CGP 39393) in human volunteers. European Hirudin in Thrombosis Group. J Am Coll Cardiol 22:1080–1088, 1993

120. Wagenvoord RJ, Hendrix HH, Kolde HJ, Hemker HC: Development of a rapid and sensitive chromogenic heparin assay for clinical use. Haemostasis 23:26–37, 1993

121. Warkentin TE, Levine MN, Hirsh J et al: Heparin-induced thrombocytopenia in patients treated with low-molecular-weight heparin or unfractionated heparin. N Engl J Med 332:1330–1335, 1995

122. Weibert RT, Lorentz SM, Townsend RJ et al: Effect of erythromycin in patients receiving long-term warfarin therapy. Clin Pharm 8:210–214, 1989

123. Weisel JW, Nagaswami C, Korsholm B et al: Interactions of plasminogen with polymerizing fibrin and its derivatives, monitored with a photoaffinity cross-linker and electron microscopy. J Mol Biol 235:1117–1135, 1994

124. Weitz JI, Brain MC, Carbone PP et al (eds): Antithrombin III, Protein C, and Protein S deficiency. In Current Therapy. p. 201. Hematology-Oncology. 5th ed. Mosby, Toronto, 1995 p. 201.

125. Weitz JI, Hudoba M, Massel D et al: Clot-bound thrombin is protected from inhibition by heparin-antithrombin III but is susceptible to inactivation by antithrombin III-independent inhibitors. J Clin Invest 86:385–391, 1990

126. Weitz JI, Leslie B, Ginsberg JS: Soluble fibrin degradation products potentiate tissue plasminogen activator-induced fibrinogen proteolysis. J Clin Invest 87: 1082–1090, 1991

127. Wells PS, Holbrook AM, Crowther NR, Hirsh J: Interactions of warfarin with drugs and food. Ann Intern Med 121:676–683, 1994

128. Wessler S, Gitel SN: Warfarin. From bedside to bench. N Engl J Med 311:645–652, 1984

129. Wiman B, Collen D: Molecular mechanism of physiological fibrinolysis. Nature 272:549–550, 1978

130. Young E, Cosmi B, Weitz J, Hirsh J: Comparison of the non-specific binding of unfractionated heparin and low molecular weight heparin (Enoxaparin) to plasma proteins. Thromb Haemost 70:625–630, 1993

131. Young E, Wells P, Holloway S et al: Ex-vivo and in-vitro evidence that low molecular weight heparins exhibit less binding to plasma proteins than unfractionated heparin. Thromb Haemost 71:300–304, 1994

132. Zammit A, Pepper DS, Dawes J: Interaction of immobilised unfractionated and LMW heparins with proteins in whole human plasma. Thromb Haemost 70:951–958, 1993

133. Zivelin A, Rao LV, Rapaport SI: Mechanism of the anticoagulant effect of warfarin as evaluated in rabbits by selective depression of individual procoagulant vitamin K-dependent clotting factors. J Clin Invest 92: 2131–2140, 1993

Platelet Function and Antiplatelet Agents

BABETTE B. WEKSLER

Cerebral ischemia most frequently results from occlusive thrombi that form in carotid, vertebrobasilar, or intracerebral arteries. Local activation of blood platelets along the walls of diseased arteries is an important initiating step in thrombus formation under condition of high flow; this catalyzes local thrombin generation, further amplifying thrombotic potential. Platelet thrombi forming on atherosclerotic plaque may occlude a vessel directly, or may embolize into intracerebral endarteries, occluding them and producing ischemic neurologic dysfunction.[2,44] Because platelet activation is directly linked to cerebral arterial ischemia, therapy directed against the early, platelet-dependent steps of hemostasis rather than anticoagulation has proved useful in preventing episodes of cerebral ischemia in patients with atherosclerosis.[4,37] By contrast, venous thrombi that form under condition of vascular stasis are more independent of platelet activation and contain mainly fibrin and erythrocytes. Such thrombi are better prevented by anticoagulation than by antiplatelet agents. These distinctions of arterial versus venous thrombi are far from absolute, and combinations of antiplatelet plus anticoagulant therapy are being tested at the present time for possible improved antithrombotic efficacy in arterial disease, although increased risk of bleeding from the combination therapy is a major concern.

Platelets are not always major components of occluding arterial emboli. Emboli consisting of cholesterol crystals released from ulcerated plaques or fibrin from intracardiac mural thrombus or heart valve vegetations comprise about 15% of cerebral ischemic episodes. Control of these types of emboli is better achieved by anticoagulation than by antiplatelet therapy.[6,43]

It should be stressed that cerebral arterial or venous thrombosis tends to occur on abnormal vascular surfaces, since the normal vascular endothelial lining of blood vessels is thromboresistant.[2] The abnormalities leading to thrombogenesis on the vascular surface may or may not involve morphologically detectable changes. Direct trauma and surgical interventions mechanically damage endothelium, producing a highly thrombogenic surface by exposing subendothelial components. However, factors such as turbulent blood flow,

inflammatory changes, oxidant stress, the interaction of endothelium with microbes or tumor cells, or involvement with atherosclerotic disease causes endothelial dysfunction that is prothrombotic, even though the endothelial monolayer remains intact.

Effective prevention and treatment of platelet-related cerebral ischemia requires understanding the contributions of endothelial function, platelet reactivity, hemostatic abnormalities, and participation of other blood cells in platelet-vascular interactions. Abnormalities in any one (or more) of these components may predispose to cerebral ischemia or may alter the functioning of the other key components in a prothrombotic direction.

Role of Vascular Endothelium in Platelet Function and Thrombosis

The vascular endothelium has been termed the "ideal blood-compatible container" because of its normal lack of interaction with blood cells. Indeed, a normal endothelial surface facing the blood does not activate hemostasis. The absence of interaction between normal endothelium and blood cells or coagulant factors or both is far from a passive process. The endothelium actively promotes the fluidity of the blood and keeps leukocytes and platelets unreactive with each other or with endothelial cells by numerous mechanisms[14] (Fig. 45.1).

ANTITHROMBOTIC AND ANTIPLATELET FUNCTIONS OF NORMAL ENDOTHELIUM

First, endothelial cells are negatively charged and repel the adhesion of negatively charged platelets, red cells, and leukocytes. Next, endothelium secretes antiplatelet substances with

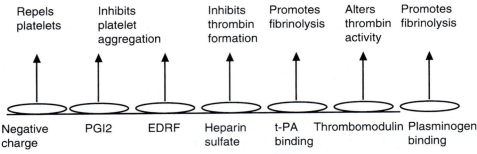

Figure 45.1 Functions of normal vascular endothelium that contribute to nonthrombogenicity: these include effects on platelets, blood coagulation, and fibrinolysis.

vasodilating properties such as prostacyclin, nitric oxide (the endothelial-derived relaxing factor),[123] and adenosine diphosphate-metabolizing enzymes (ADPases).[66] Endothelium also provides several mechanisms for controlling thrombin generation that bear importantly on platelets, because thrombin is a potent platelet activator, and activated platelets, in turn, strongly promote localized generation of thrombin.[88] Thus, the lumenal surface of endothelial cells is rich in heparan sulfate proteoglycans that activate antithrombin III, a natural plasma inhibitor of thrombin and other serine protease procoagulant factors. Next, endothelial cells synthesize thrombomodulin, a membrane protein that binds thrombin and alters its enzymatic activity so that it no longer cleaves fibrinogen but instead activates protein C, a natural anticoagulant that blocks further thrombin generation. Furthermore, endothelium produces tissue factor pathway inhibitor, a key control in the extrinsic pathway of coagulation. The extrinsic pathway forms thrombin through tissue factor-factor VII activation of the tenase complex that is efficiently activated on platelet surfaces.

In addition, normal endothelium actively participates in localizing and potentiating fibrinolysis, the process of clot dissolution. Components of the fibrinolytic enzyme cascade are assembled on the endothelial surface by binding to specific receptors.[45,46,81] The bound fibrinolytic factors are protected from inactivation by plasma inhibitors and, at the same time, the biologic activity of the bound fibrinolytic components is amplified consequent to their localization on endothelium. Moreover, endothelial cells secrete both plasminogen activators (favoring fibrinolysis) and plasminogen activator–inhibitors (inhibiting fibrinolysis); the balance of their synthesis and release is regulated by thrombin and by endothelial growth factors. Normal profibrinolytic activity of the vascular endothelium is an important component of the control of thrombosis, and appears to take place continuously, favoring the clearance of incipient thrombi and activated coagulation activities.

PROTHROMBOTIC FUNCTIONS OF ABNORMAL ENDOTHELIUM: INTERACTION WITH PLATELETS

Under conditions of turbulent blood flow, oxidant stress, ischemia, atherosclerosis or inflammation, normal endothelium loses many of the above-mentioned thromboresistant proper-

ties. Production of thrombomodulin, nitric oxide, and prostacyclin are suppressed, and the capacity of the endothelium to metabolize ADP to adenosine decreases. Increased plasminogen activator inhibitor-1 is produced, and the activated endothelium supports the binding and activation of plasma procoagulant factors.[103] One of the earliest alterations of endothelial function during activation by the conditions mentioned previously involves the development of adherent properties for leukocytes or for platelet-leukocyte aggregates. These changes involve the display of specific adhesion receptors on the endothelial surface, particularly P-selection (CD62). Activated platelets are another source of P-selectin, which is translocated to the platelet surface where it mediates adhesion and rolling of neutrophils and lymphocytes along activated endothelium.[28]

Receptors for coagulation factors appear on intact endothelial cells both after exposure to cytokines, such as tumor necrosis factor (TNF), endotoxin or interleukin-1 (IL-1) and after exposure to thrombin;[104] these cells also produce IL-1. These inflammatory stimuli induce production of tissue factor by endothelium, thus activating the extrinsic pathway of coagulation on the endothelial surface.[22,23] Thus, activated endothelial cells generate fibrin on their lumenal surface but still resist platelet aggregation.[102] However, the subendothelial matrix produced by activated endothelial cells has enhanced capacity to attract platelet aggregation and to generate fibrinopeptides via the extrinsic pathway components tissue factor and factor VIIa.[124] Fibrin deposition on subendothelial matrix derived from activated endothelium is particularly pronounced at low shear rates, suggesting that turbulent flow or stasis further enhances thrombosis on exposed subendothelium in the vicinity of activated endothelial cells.

How Normal Hemostatic Functions of Platelets Can Contribute to Cerebral Ischemia

Blood platelets circulate in the blood for 7 to 10 days, even though they lack nuclei and are almost incapable of protein synthesis. While they are packed with potentially vasoactive substances, circulating platelets normally remain unreactive with other platelets or with the vascular endothelium as they travel through the bloodstream. Only when specifically activated—for example, upon encountering a break in endothelial continuity—do platelets adhere to surfaces, change shape from flat discs to spiny spheres, spread out along the damaged surface, aggregate into clumps that directly occlude small wounds, and release their vasoactive contents. Most important, upon activation, platelets serve to initiate, augment, and localize fibrin formation by activating thrombin on their surface membranes, and thus to participate in forming a stable clot.

The major signal for physiological platelet activation is disruption of endothelium with exposure of prothrombotic components in the subendothelial matrix. These prothrombotic substances include collagen and adhesive molecules such as von Willebrand factor, thrombospondin, and fibronectin. However, as mentioned previously, more subtle endothelial dysfunction produced by turbulent flow, hyperlipidemia, or inflammation, can also activate platelets. Platelet activation comprises a sequence of steps, each sensitive to different pharmacologic interventions. Recent understanding of the biochemistry and physiology of these steps, gained in part through molecular studies of rare inherited platelet dysfunctions, has permitted development of new therapies targeted to key steps in the activation sequence.

The many stimuli for platelet activation include vasoactive nucleotides, amines, enzymes lipids, and microorganisms. Some of the agonists, such as adenosine diphosphate (ADP), epinephrine, and serotonin, are released by platelets themselves, while others are present in the blood plasma (e.g. vasopressin), subendothelium (e.g., collagen) or are formed upon platelet activation (thrombin, TXA_2). Pathologic stimuli that activate platelets include turbulent flow, hypotonicity, foreign surfaces (including prosthetic grafts and intravascular catheters), tumor cells, viruses, and bacteria. Weak stimuli such as serotonin or epinephrine, or low concentrations of ADP cause reversible platelet aggregation unaccompanied by release of platelet contents. Strong stimuli such as thrombin, collagen, or high concentrations of ADP directly cause irreversible platelet aggregation, the release of platelet granule contents, and the synthesis of thromboxane A_2 (TXA_2), a very potent platelet agonist and vasoconstrictor. During platelet activation, released ADP and serotonin further promote platelet aggregation. Combinations of stimuli, which probably occur normally under physiologic conditions, act synergistically.

Platelet Membrane Proteins Mediating Platelet Activation

Platelet adhesion receptors mediate the attachment of platelets to substrate proteins. Adhesion receptors that are important in normal hemostasis and represent potential therapeutic targets for preventing thrombosis include the following glycoproteins (GP): GPIa, a collagen receptor; GPIb, a receptor for von Willebrand factor; the GPIIb/IIIa complex, a major receptor for fibrinogen, fibronectin, and von Willebrand fac-

tor; GPIV, a receptor for thrombospondin, a glycoprotein crucial for irreversible platelet activation; and $\alpha_v\beta_3$, a receptor for several adhesive proteins including fibrinogen, fibronectin, and vitronectin. Many of the adhesive glycoproteins that are ligands for these receptors share the peptide sequence RGD [arginine (R), glycine (G), aspartic acid (D)] that is directly involved in cell-cell adhesion. All of these receptors are functional on resting platelets except for GPIIb/IIIa, which requires platelet activation to undergo a conformational change in order to bind its ligand, fibrinogen.[20,99]

PLATELET ADHESION

Platelet adhesion to other platelets, to activated endothelium, and to subendothelium exposed after injury is the first major step in the sequence of platelet activation. GPIb-IX is the major platelet membrane molecule that mediates platelet adhesion to the subendothelium, and is a receptor for matrix-bound von Willebrand factor at high shear rates as well as a binding site for thrombin. At low shear, the GPIIb/IIIa complex also participates in platelet adhesion to surfaces through binding fibrinogen.

The GPIb-V-IX complex is a receptor for von Willebrand factor and amplifies the platelet response to thrombin. It is particularly involved in platelet activation that is caused by abnormal shear stress, as found in arteries narrowed by arteriosclerosis, and its activation during shear stress in a thromboxane-independent manner accounts for part of the resistance to aspirin that is observed in connection with increased atherosclerotic risk factors. Changes in conformation of GPIbα or vWF can induce interaction between these two molecules. The binding to collagen of vWF induces small conformational changes that permit its binding to GPIb. Shear stress in the presence of vWF can also induce calcium transients in platelets and induce phosphorylation of tyrosine residues. The binding of vWF to GPIb involves redistribution of the GPIb-V-IX complex to the surface-connected canalicular system, linking the complex to the membrane-associated cytoskeleton via the actin-binding protein, filamin, and also activating PI3kinase and pp60 c-src, while phosphorylation of GPIb helps regulate actin polymerization and the activation of GPIIb/IIIa. Theoretically, inhibition of platelet adhesion should be antithrombotic, and peptides that block GPIb-IX function are under development as antithrombotic agents. Absence or dysfunction of GPIb is characteristic of Bernard-Soulier syndrome, a rare platelet disorder characterized by bleeding.

PLATELET AGGREGATION

Platelet aggregation is the step in platelet activation most relevant to the pathogenesis of occlusive vascular events in an oxygen-sensitive vascular bed. In this process, activated platelets group together atop an adherent layer of platelets at the site of injury or disease to form "white thrombi" that may either be transient or may become reinforced with fibrin as the nidus of a stable clot. These platelet plugs normally halt bleeding from injured microvessels, but when formed pathologically or excessively in the cerebral microcirculation can produce transient ischemic attacks or stroke.

Role of Glycoprotein Receptors

Initial contact of agonists with platelets bind specific glycoprotein receptors present on the platelet membrane and transduce activating signals. These receptors include heterodimeric glycoproteins of the integrin superfamily that bind a variety of adhesive proteins. Similar (but not identical) receptors are shared by other cell types such as endothelium and leukocytes.[19] Integrins mediate many of the interactions among different cell types that participate in thrombosis as well as adhesive interactions between cells and the extracellular matrix, and thereby link the processes of hemostasis, inflammation, and immune recognition.

The most important platelet integrin is GPIIb/IIIa, a bimolecular complex uniquely found on platelets and megakaryocytes. Platelet aggregation by all known pathways depends upon the activation of GPIIb/IIIa by platelet agonists. Therefore, activation of this complex is a crucial step in platelet hemostatic and thrombotic functions. Because of the central role of GPIIb/IIIa in platelet aggregation, the development of specific inhibitors of GPIIb/IIIa is a major goal of current antiplatelet therapy. The GPIIb/IIIa protein complex is present on resting platelets in an inactive state. When platelet agonists such as ADP activate the complex by inducing a conformational change, GPIIb/IIIa markedly increases the binding of fibrinogen, becomes associated with cytoskeletal proteins and with enzymes such as kinases (pp60, c-src) involved in signalling, forms receptor clusters, and becomes phosphorylated.[20,21] Both outside-inside signalling (i.e., agonist-driven) and inside-outside signalling (i.e., kinase/phosphatase-driven) are involved in this activation process. Inhibitors of thromboxane synthesis, such as aspirin, do not block GPIIb/IIIa activation. However, drugs that block GPIIb/IIIa have profound effects upon platelet activity. The development of specific monoclonal antibodies or peptides that block GPIIb/IIIa function has already led to novel approaches to antiplatelet therapy to treat acute vascular events and prevent reocclusion.

Arachidonic Acid Pathway

Platelet aggregation is mediated by several different biochemical pathways that are separately regulated and are differentially responsive to antiplatelet drugs. One major pathway involves the metabolism of arachidonic acid. Receptor-mediated activation of platelets by agonists activates phospholipase C, initiating formation of a cascade of intracellular second messengers (Fig. 45.2). Cleavage of membrane-bound phosphati-

Figure 45.2 Pathways leading to platelet aggregation. Stimulation of specific receptors on platelet surface activate the arachidonic acid pathway, phosphatidyl inositol hydrolysis, or granule release singly or in combination. The products synthesized or released further augment activation. Not shown here is the activation of the glycoprotein (GP) IIb-IIIa receptor on the platelet surface by epinephrine, collagen, thrombin, or thromboxane (TX) A_2. Inhibition of platelet activation results from (1) blocking expression of GPIIb-IIIa receptors, (2) arachidonic acid conversion by cyclooxygenase, (3) TXA_2 production, (4) TXA_2 receptor function, (5) raising cAMP.

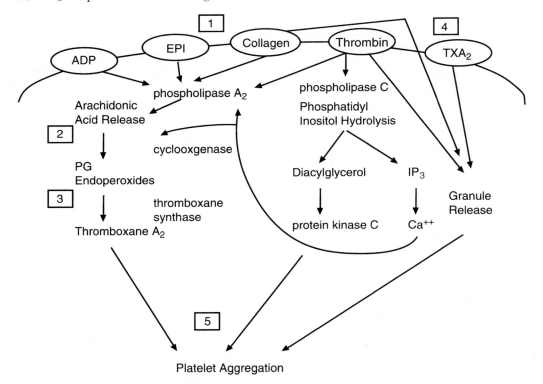

dyl inositol yields inositol 1,4,5-triphosphate (IP_3) and diacylglycerol. IP3 releases stored Ca^{2+}, permitting activation of phospholipase A_2, which in turn releases arachidonic acid from membrane lipids. The enzyme cyclooxygenase rapidly catalyzes oxygenation of the arachidonic acid to produce unstable prostaglandin endoperoxides that are further converted to TXA_2, a potent platelet agonist and vasoconstrictor (Fig. 45.2). TXA_2 diffuses out of the platelet and then binds to its own specific membrane receptor, which activates phospholipase C, producing more IP3 and diacylglycerol, and further stimulating platelet activation. Meanwhile, diacylglycerol activates protein kinase C which translocates to the plasma membrane and triggers activation of GPIIb-IIIa (by exposing the fibrinogen binding site), permitting platelet aggregation and release of platelet granule contents. Both secreted ADP and TXA_2 are platelet agonists that recruit nearby unactivated platelets and enhance further platelet aggregation. This pathway of platelet activation depends upon normal activation of the cyclooxygenase-mediated generation of TXA_2. This pathway is blocked by aspirin and nonsteroidal anti-inflammatory drugs that inhibit cyclooxygenase activity and, therefore prevent production of TXA_2 and TXA_2-mediated platelet release.

Other Pathways

Platelet aggregation that depends upon ADP derived from extraplatelet sources such as red cells can operate directly without requiring release or thromboxane generation. This pathway of platelet aggregation continues in the presence of aspirin.

Thrombin activates phospholipase C and produces irreversible platelet aggregation and release independently of arachidonic acid metabolism or TXA_2; thus thrombin-mediated platelet aggregation is not blocked by aspirin even when TXA_2 is not produced. Similarly, platelet activation by the phosphorylcholine derivative, platelet activating factor (PAF) produced by leukocytes or disturbed endothelial cells is also aspirin-insensitive. The existence of these separate pathways for platelet aggregation might be regarded as evolutionary fail-safe mechanisms to prevent hemorrhage.

Physiologic Limitations to Platelet Activation

In practical therapeutics, these multiple pathways of platelet aggregation mean that drugs capable of inhibiting only one of the pathways—for example, aspirin as an inhibitor of thromboxane production—can be expected to inhibit platelet activation only in situations where that pathway is important. Natural mechanisms to control platelet activation include (1) plasma ADPases and endothelial ecto-ADPases that break down released ADP to form adenosine, an inhibitor of platelet activation, (2) prostacyclin released by endothelial cells, which stimulates adenylate cyclase and raises platelet cyclic AMP levels, resulting in a block of calcium release and inhibition of platelet aggregation and secretion, (3) production of NO via NO synthases in platelets, endothelial cells and monocytes, which in turn stimulates platelet guanylate cyclase levels[82] thus inhibiting platelet activation. NO is formed from L-arginine; this amino acid has been shown to inhibit platelet aggre-

gation, whereas inhibitors of NO synthase potentiate the effects of L-arginine.

At the present time, the only agents capable of inhibiting all three major pathways of platelet activation are those that block GPIIb-IIIa, the membrane receptor necessary for fibrinogen binding and platelet aggregation.[21]

Platelet Release Reaction

The platelet release reaction normally accompanies and augments platelet aggregation and its consequences (i.e., the acceleration of localized clot formation and the release of vasoactive factors that favor vascular occlusion). During the release reaction, preformed mediators are released into the blood or displayed on the surface membrane of platelets. Additional short-lived mediators are synthesized and released at this same time.

Platelets contain several types of granules rich in substances that participate in blood coagulation, cell-cell interactions and wound repair, including coagulation factors, cellular adhesion molecules, calcium, vasoactive amines, growth factors and nucleotides. The different types of platelet granules are functionally distinguished by contents and ease of release and consist of dense granules, alpha granules, lysosomes, and peroxisomes. The contents of dense granules—ADP, ATP, serotonin, and calcium—are released upon platelet exposure to weak stimuli.

By contrast, strong stimuli are required for release of alpha granule contents, namely, fibrinogen, fibronectin, von Willebrand factor, thrombospondin, coagulation factors V and XI, platelet-derived growth factor (PDGF), epidermal growth factor (EGF), transforming growth factor-β (TGF-β), the antiheparin, platelet factor 4 (PF4), and beta thromboglobulin. Alpha granules also contain albumin, immunoglobulins, antibacterial proteins, and a complement inhibitor. Moreover, the membrane of alpha granules contains P-selectin and beta-amyloid precursor protein, and upon platelet activation, P-selectin is translocated to the platelet plasma membrane where it mediates cell-cell interactions with leukocytes and plays an important role in inflammatory reactions. Platelet lysosomes contain acid hydrolases, neutral proteases, elastase, complementing activating enzymes, and a heparitinase. Peroxisomes contain catalase. Release of dense and alpha granule components usually accompanies platelet aggregation; release may also occur from platelets adherent to damaged endothelium or subendothelium.

PLATELET SYNTHESIS OF VASOACTIVE LIPID MEDIATORS

By contrast to these preformed proteins, vasoactive lipid mediators associated with platelets are not stored in granules. Instead, vasoactive lipids are rapidly synthesized and immediately released by platelets during platelet activation. Most of these substances are oxygenated metabolites of arachidonic acid. Platelet agonists release arachidonic acid from stored ester forms via activation of phospholipase A_2, and the released arachidonate serves as substrate for formation of several eicosanoids and hydroxylated fatty acids. TXA_2 is a major platelet product of arachidonic acid oxygenation by the cyclooxygenase pathway. As mentioned, cyclooxygenase catalyzes the addition of molecular oxygen to arachidonic acid to yield endoperoxide intermediates, which are then converted to TXA_2 by a specific TXA_2 synthetase or to prostaglandins by specific isomerases. The synthesis and release of TXA_2 occurs very rapidly upon platelet activation. G-protein linked, 7-membrane spanning receptors for TXA_2 are present on platelets, leukocytes, and vascular cells. These receptors bind not only TXA_2 but also endoperoxide precursors of TXA_2 that have similar vasoconstricting properties. Signal transduction via the TXA_2 receptor initiates platelet activation and causes constriction of vascular cells. Aspirin irreversibly acetylates cyclooxygenase near its active site, inactivating the cyclooxygenase function and blocking formation of endoperoxides from arachidonic acid. This effect accounts for the profound inhibition by aspirin of TXA_2 synthesis in platelets and its depression of platelet function.

Platelets also synthesize hydroxyeicosatetraenoic acid (12-HETE) from arachidonic acid via the lipoxygenase pathway. By contrast to TXA_2 synthesis, which occurs in a rapid burst, 12-HETE is synthesized continuously over a long period. 12-HETE is an inflammatory mediator that is chemotactic for leukocytes and can be converted to additional bioactive products by leukocytes. Leukocytes can transform platelet 12-HETE into several different di-HETEs. 12-HETE stimulates vascular smooth muscle proliferation and can contribute to progression of atherosclerosis. It is of interest that activated platelets also release cholesterol that may be incorporated into the atherosclerotic plaque. Aspirin has no effect on HETE formation.

Interactions among different cell types within blood vessels can modulate the formation of arachidonic acid products in several ways. These interactions are a form of transcellular metabolism, yielding products that may not be made by one cell type alone. Arachidonic acid is released by activated platelets (aspirin treated or not) and can be transformed into other vasoactive substances by leukocytes or endothelial cells that are in close proximity. Endothelial cells can convert platelet-derived arachidonic acid into prostacyclin (PGI_2), an antiplatelet and vasodilating product. Similarly, endoperoxides released by endothelial cells can be converted into TXA_2 by adjacent aspirin-treated platelets.[53]

How Platelet Activation Promotes Blood Coagulation

The result of the release of granule contents by platelets responding to strong agonists such as collagen, TXA_2 or thrombin, is acceleration of primary hemostatic plug formation and efficient catalysis of blood coagulation on the surface of the activated platelets. By providing specific sites, receptors, and lipid cofactors for the assembly of the key complex of procoagulant enzymes, and additional procoagulant factors, the activated platelet membrane enhances the rate of thrombin generation 200,000-fold over the reaction rate in the fluid phase.

Since thrombin is itself a strong stimulus for platelet activation, for the release reaction, and for TXA_2 formation, the initial production of traces of thrombin at the injury site further enhances platelet activation and promotes coagulation.

THE RELEASE REACTION AS A LINK BETWEEN HEMOSTASIS AND INFLAMMATION

Platelets are instrumental in the recruitment of leukocytes to the injury site. Several substances released by platelets are chemotactic for neutrophils (e.g., 12-HETE, PF4, PDGF). Moreover, platelet proteases can cleave the complement protein C5 to release a chemotactic fragment C5a and potentiate C3 activation, augmenting leukocyte function. Platelet P-selectin, displayed on the plasma membrane of activated platelets, mediates interactions between platelets and leukocytes including leukocyte-aggregate rolling on vascular endothelium; leukocyte activation can also be mediated by platelet P-selectin. While activated endothelial cells also display P-selectin on their lumenal surface, this is a transient phenomenon, whereas activated platelets remain P-selectin coated.

Adhesive proteins released by platelets play numerous roles in both hemostasis and inflammation, and therefore contribute to thrombosis. Fibrinogen is necessary for platelet-platelet interaction; von Willebrand factor is crucial for normal primary hemostasis in high-flow systems such as arteries. Thrombospondin is important in stabilizing platelet aggregates. In addition, activated platelets are a rich source for growth factors affecting the activities of vascular cells and fibroblasts. PDGF and EGF are mainly released during platelet aggregation but can be released upon platelet adhesion alone. These factors are chemotactic for leukocytes, smooth muscle cells, and fibroblasts, as well as stimulating cell division of smooth muscle cells and fibroblasts during wound healing. In addition to its chemotactic and mitogenic roles, PDGF is a vasoconstrictor.[9] A major source of TGF-β in blood is release by activated platelets. TGF-β stimulates the synthesis of matrix proteins. These growth factors released by platelets are all stable polypeptides that adhere well to the subendothelial matrix where they persist in an active state. It is clear that when these factors are inappropriately released, for example, from hyperreactive platelets, they are capable of promoting atherosclerosis. Therefore, antiplatelet therapy that depresses the release of platelet granule contents, has potential antiatherosclerotic value.

MIXED ROLES OF PLATELETS IN FIBRINOLYSIS AND THROMBOLYSIS

Blood clots are resolved by fibrinolysis, a process involving generation of the protease plasmin, which fragments insoluble fibrin. Platelets contribute to fibrinolysis and can be activated or inhibited during this process. Platelets participate both in promoting and in inhibiting fibrinolysis. Platelets can bind plasminogen and plasminogen activators (both urokinase and tissue type activators) by mechanisms involving the integrin GPIIb/IIIa.[70] Activated platelets display thrombospondin on their membranes (released from α-granules); thrombospondin binds plasminogen[81] and enhances its activation. Therefore, platelets act to localize plasminogen and its activation in a way similar to their localization and activation of plasma procoagulants. Platelet-bound plasminogen is more readily activated by tissue plasminogen activator and streptokinase, suggesting that platelets can enhance local fibrinolysis. In turn, plasmin at low concentrations enhances and at high concentrations, depresses platelet activation.[93]

Platelets also participate in limiting fibrinolysis, since they contain and secrete two fibrinolytic antagonists, plasminogen activator inhibitor-1 (PAI-1) and α_2-antiplasmin. Platelets release factor XIII, the fibrin-stabilizing factor that crosslinks newly formed fibrin strands to enhance clot stability. The net effect of these different platelet activities seems to be that platelet-rich thrombi resist thrombolysis and that platelets become activated during therapeutic thrombolysis.[34]

Specific Roles for Platelets in Cerebrovascular Disease

The normal participation of platelets in hemostasis following vascular injury contributes to the exaggerated platelet activation in patients with atherosclerosis or vascular diseases marked by a thrombotic diathesis, such as collagen vascular disease. Thus, the interaction between normally functioning platelets and abnormal vascular surfaces may suffice to potentiate thrombosis.

PLATELET HYPERACTIVITY IN CARDIOVASCULAR AND CEREBROVASCULAR DISEASE

The overall process of platelet activation appears to be enhanced in numerous situations where an acute cardiovascular or cerebrovascular event has recently occurred, for example shortly after a stroke, myocardial infarction, or episode of unstable angina. Whether or not a chronic state of platelet hyperactivity exists is unclear. Attempts to document pre-existing hyper-reactivity of platelet function in patients with atherosclerosis or patients at risk of repeated episodes of cerebral ischemia have given quite variable results.[32,39,55,77,118] Multiple mechanisms for this variability are now recognized. Clinical studies have often used platelet aggregation patterns as a marker for platelet activation. Many factors enhance platelet aggregability, including stress, elevated plasma lipids and free fatty acids, inflammatory states, and smoking. Increased circulating catecholamines, while weak direct platelet agonists, augment platelet aggregability by other agonists, oppose the effects of natural antiplatelet factors such as prostacyclin, and

can offset some of the antiplatelet efficacy of aspirin. Clinical settings marked by stress, in which catecholamine levels are increased, show increases in plasma fibrinogen and factor VIII-vWF, both important factors favoring platelet activation.[68] Increased plasma fibrinogen has been observed to be an independent risk factor for stroke, perhaps in part through its stimulatory effect on platelet aggregation.[32] High levels of platelet activation markers, such as plasma levels of PF4 and β-thromboglobulin, are associated with carotid artery wall thickening.[39]

ENVIRONMENTAL EFFECTS ON PLATELET REACTIVITY

A circadian rhythm in the incidence of acute myocardial infarction, stroke, and sudden death has been observed, with the highest incidences in the morning shortly after rising.[68,110] Investigation of the pathophysiology of these events indicates that platelet aggregability is highest soon after rising and correlates with increases in plasma catcholamine and free fatty acid levels.[110] Aspirin administration has been shown to ablate the morning excess of myocardial infarctions and sudden death; specific studies in stroke have not been done, but it is logical to postulate a similar mechanism. Numerous studies have documented that circulating platelet aggregates are increased during the first days after an episode of acute cerebral ischemia.

Documentation of platelet activation associated with cerebral ischemia or risk of cerebral ischemia is difficult.[55] Because of the localized nature of atherosclerosis, overall platelet function and survival often appear normal in patients with cardiovascular or cerebrovascular disease, since only a small percentage of platelets may be activated at a particular time in the locally diseased vascular bed. Moreover, activated platelets may be rapidly cleared from the circulation, limiting their detectability. Measurement of platelet aggregation thresholds, circulating platelet aggregates, circulating activated platelets, or increased levels in blood or urine of platelet release products have all been used to try to distinguish platelet-related risks for occlusive cerebrovascular events. Each of these techniques tends to show a correlation between increased platelet activation and recent cerebral ischemia when measured in small research studies. However, sensitivity is poor, and artifactual activation of platelets during specimen procurement is a major problem. In many instances, traces of platelet activation or hypercoagulability persist for many months after an episode of cerebral ischemia.

Measurement of platelet-specific urinary TXA_2 metabolites has been used to document episodic platelet activation in acute ischemic stroke,[57,118] but direct correlation with neurologic symptoms during the study period was not achievable. Flow cytometric techniques that are highly sensitive to small populations of activated cells have been used to detect platelet activation or platelet-leukocyte interaction,[69] and may be of value in monitoring effects of antiplatelet therapies under research conditions. The clinical ideal of predictively identifying patients at risk of cerebral ischemia due to platelet hyper-reactivity is unlikely to be achieved by presently available methods.

Platelet counts alone do not necessarily represent a risk

factor. However, elevated platelet counts in a setting of myeloproliferative disease are associated with increased risk of thrombosis including cerebral thrombosis, and lowering the platelet count by chemotherapy appears to decrease stroke and thrombotic risk in these diseases.[24] In myeloproliferative diseases, platelets are often very large, and platelet mass is increased disproportionately to platelet count, so that platelet numbers underestimate total platelet mass. This disproportion probably contributes to thrombotic risk. Aspirin is also beneficial in reducing stroke risk in these patients, especially if the platelet count has been normalized.[24] By contrast, secondary thrombocytosis, for example, occurring after removal of the spleen for any reason, is not associated with increased thrombotic risk in general or stroke risk in particular.

In situations where platelet destruction is enhanced, a compensatory increase in megakaryocyte size may result in release of platelets that are "younger" and more hemostatically active than usual. These platelets might augment the process of atheroma formation.[38] Young platelets have been found to be larger than average, to produce more prothrombotic factors and to aggregate in response to lower concentrations of agonists. Large platelets are a risk factor for death and recurrent vascular events following myocardial infarction. Patients with acute stroke have increased platelet volume compared with age- and sex-matched control subjects and the high platelet volume may persist for months.[77] It is known that blood concentration of PDGF is elevated in young patients with coronary atherosclerosis or hypercholesterolemia.[75] The source of the PDGF is not clearly defined since it could represent platelets, or, alternatively, activated vascular cells and monocytes, all of which produce this factor. In any case, it is likely that the increased blood concentrations of such mitogens contribute to progression of atherosclerosis.

Pharmacologic Bases for Use of Platelet Inhibitory Drugs in the Prevention of Cerebral Ischemia

Drugs that inhibit platelet function are employed to prevent acute occlusive events in many types of vascular disease settings in addition to cerebral ischemia, including myocardial infarction, unstable and chronic angina pectoris, peripheral vascular disease, arterial grafting, and coronary artery surgery. Numerous large, well-controlled clinical trials have demonstrated that use of antiplatelet drugs significantly lowers the risk of subsequent vascular occlusive events in patients who have had a prior occlusive event, and extensive meta-analyses of these studies have been published and updated.[4] In all of these clinical settings, about 25% to 30% risk reduction is observed using currently available drugs. A summary of pharmacologic rationales for antiplatelet drug use appears in Table 45.1. A discussion of the well established drugs used to prevent

recurrent cerebral ischemia together with new pharmacologic approaches follows.

ASPIRIN

Effects on Hemostatic Parameters and Eicosanoid Production

Aspirin has long been known to prolong bleeding time. This prolongation involves decreased platelet aggregation. Aspirin was first shown in 1971 to affect platelet function by irreversible acetylation of the platelet enzyme cyclooxygenase (prostaglandin endoperoxide synthase), rendering that enzyme incapable of catalyzing the attachment of molecular oxygen to arachidonic acid to form prostaglandin endoperoxides G2 and H2.[102,116] Platelets thus cannot produce endoperoxides and therefore production of eicosanoid metabolites by platelets from these key intermediates is inhibited. Therefore, synthesis of TXA_2 is completely blocked in aspirin-treated platelets. The peroxidase function of the cyclooxygenase, which is not involved in prostanoid synthesis, is unaffected by aspirin. Even low doses of aspirin rapidly (within minutes) and effectively block platelet cyclooxygenase in vivo. Certain peculiarities of platelet kinetics favor this profound and long-lasting effect of aspirin. First, while platelets circulate for 7 to 10 days, they do not synthesize new cyclooxygenase, and once exposed to aspirin are therefore permanently unable to produce TXA_2. Second, while aspirin is rapidly deacetylated in the liver, because platelets circulate, their cyclooxygenase can be efficiently acetylated or inactivated in the preportal circulation during contact with freshly absorbed aspirin. Therefore high, persistent blood levels of aspirin are not required for the inhibitory effect on platelet function (see the following discussion).

Since TXA_2 is a major eicosanoid produced by blood platelets and a strong stimulus for platelet aggregation and release, as well as a powerful vasoconstrictor, inhibition of its synthesis by aspirin markedly impairs one major pathway of platelet activation, and decreases platelet activation induced by ADP, epinephrine or collagen, as well as decreasing platelet release of preformed vasoactive substances. In contrast, platelet activation by thrombin is not inhibited by aspirin, since thrombin activates platelets by a pathway independent of cyclooxygenase. However, aspirin administration (325 to 500 mg/d) has been reported to decrease platelet-dependent thrombin generation in vitro and in vivo.[106] The inhibitory effect of aspirin on thrombin generation is weaker in patients with hypercholesterolemia, who are known to have increased hypercoagulability and often show enhanced platelet TXA_2 generation.[107] Increased fibrinogen also decreases an aspirin effect.[31] It is postulated that the antithrombinogenic effect of aspirin may involve acetylation of platelet membrane proteins, but the mechanism is not yet clear. The clinical relevance of aspirin-induced impairment of thrombin generation remains to be assessed.

While aspirin has a permanent effect on platelet cyclooxygenase, other cell types such as vascular endothelium, kidney or lung epithelium, or monocytes, are capable of rapid resynthesis of cyclooxygenase. As a result, the inhibitory effect of

Table 45.1 Mechanisms of Actions of Antiplatelet Drugs

Action	Effects on Platelets	Drug
Inhibition of membrane receptor	Prevent ADP and fibrinogen binding; block adhesion or aggregation	Ticlopidine, clopidigrel[a] Abciximab, antibodies to GPIIb/IIIa[b] RGD peptide analogs[b]
	Prevent thrombin binding	Disintegrins[b]
Alter arachidonic acid metabolism	Blocks cyclooxygenase, PG endoperoxide and TXA_2 synthesis; inhibits platelet aggregation and secretion	Aspirin, NSAIDs Sulfinpyrazone[a] Fish oils, ω-3 fatty acids[a]
	Inhibits TXA_2 synthesis alone	TXA_2 synthetase inhibitors[b]
Inhibit TXA_2 receptors	Prevents TXA_2 and PG endoperoxide binding	TXA_2 receptor antagonists[b]
Increase cyclic AMP	Stimulate adenylate cyclase; lower intracellular Ca^{2+}; block aggregation and secretion	PGI_2 and analogs (iloprost)[b] PGE_1, PGD_2
	Maintain raised cAMP	Dipyridamole[a] Methylxanthines[a] Phosphodiesterase inhibitors[a]
Increase cyclic GMP	Stimulate platelet NO synthesis; block aggregation and secretion	L-arginine[b] Nitroprusside[a]
Inhibit calcium channels	Decrease aggregation and secretion	Ca^{2+} channel blockers[a] Local anesthetics[a] Beta blockers[a]
Inhibit thrombin generation or action	Inhibit aggregation and secretion; block thrombus formation	Heparin, LMW heparin Antithrombin peptides[b] Hirudin[b], hirulog[b] Abciximab[b]

Abbreviations: ADP, adenosine diphosphate; cAMP, cyclic adenosine monophosphate; GP, glycoprotein; cGMP, cyclic guanosine monophosphate; NO, nitric oxide; TXA_s, thromboxane A_2; PGI_2, prostacyclin; NSAIDs, nonsteroidal antiinflammatory drugs.

[a] Limited or adjunct therapeutic effects.

[b] Under development for clinical use.

aspirin on eicosanoid synthesis in these tissues is much briefer than the prolonged inhibitory effect on platelets, which persists for the lifespan of the platelets. Moreover, these other tissues synthesize cyclooxygenase-2, a second form of the enzyme which is inducible by inflammatory stimuli and cytokines to a high concentration. Cyclooxygenase-2 is also inhibited by aspirin, but its rapid resynthesis in many cell types (monocytes, vascular endothelium, and smooth muscle, but not including platelets) makes eicosanoid production by these cells less easily inhibited by aspirin. Therefore, intermittent dosage with aspirin can achieve selective inhibition of platelet function without impairing the production of vasoprotective prostaglandins such as prostacyclin or PGE_2.

Aspirin has little or no effect upon the lipoxygenase pathway of arachidonic acid metabolism and thus 12-HETE production by platelets is not altered.

Pharmacokinetics of Aspirin Effects on Platelets and Hemostasis

Aspirin is rapidly absorbed after oral administration and reaches a peak plasma level within 30 minutes of a single dose. The drug is rapidly deacetylated in the liver to form salicylate, which has little or no antiplatelet efficacy, so that 3 hours after a single dose of aspirin, plasma levels of acetylsalicylic acid are negligible. However, since platelet cyclooxygenase is inactivated by aspirin within minutes, even a brief exposure to aspirin produces a maximal inhibitory effect on platelets. It has been demonstrated that administration of a very low dose of aspirin (1 mg/h orally) which is fully deacetylated on first pass through the liver, completely inactivates platelet cyclooxygenase in vivo within a few hours, because the cyclooxygenase in platelets passing through the preportal circulation is acetylated (thus inactivated) by the newly absorbed, intact aspirin molecules before reaching the liver.[79] In this setting, cyclooxygenase in peripheral tissues exposed to the systemic circulation containing only salicylate is virtually unaffected. Thus low-dose or slow-release oral aspirin has good antiplatelet potency.

Dose Considerations

In clinical studies it has been recognized that, for maintenance of antiplatelet effects in vivo, only small daily doses of aspirin (20 to 325 mg/d) were required both in normal individuals and atherosclerotic subjects[60,121,122] since platelet inhibition is cumulative over time. Higher or more frequent doses of aspirin may inhibit prostacyclin formation in blood vessels, but in many clinical settings this is physiologically unimportant. However, the incidence of gastric distress and gastrointestinal bleeding increase with increasing aspirin dose. For maximal inhibition of platelet aggregation during aspirin therapy, TXA_2 synthesis must be decreased by 95%[79]; 160 to 325 mg of aspirin daily appears to produce the desired level of platelet inhibition, except for individuals who have a very rapid rate of platelet turnover.

At these doses, aspirin tends to prolong the bleeding time by about twofold over baseline in at least 60% of individuals; larger doses of aspirin do not further prolong bleeding time. Very high doses, indeed, may slightly shorten the bleeding time, presumably because of inhibition of vascular cyclooxygenase. Prolongation of bleeding time by aspirin correlates poorly with either gastric irritation or gastrointestinal bleeding. After aspirin is stopped, bleeding time returns to normal within 1 to 2 days, and regardless of the dose administered, platelet aggregation and formation of TXA_2 return to predosing levels within 7 to 10 days, following a linear recovery pattern starting after a 1- to 2-day initial lag that probably indicates acetylation of megakaryocyte cyclooxygenase by aspirin. Alcohol ingestion will slow down recovery from aspirin-induced prolongation of bleeding time by several days; this may contribute to incidence of gastrointestinal bleeding in aspirin users. Enteric-coated aspirin has antiplatelet effects equivalent to those of plain aspirin.[1]

Aspirin has been reported to have effects upon fibrinolysis in addition to its effects on platelet activation.[22,72] Chronic aspirin administration is associated with shortening of the plasma clot lysis time, perhaps by acetylation of fibrinogen that impedes factor XIII-induced fibrin cross linking, permitting fibrinolysis to occur more easily.[11] Large doses of aspirin may inhibit the release of tissue plasminogen activator from venous endothelium following venous occlusion, without altering the release of PAI-1.[64] The predicted result would be inhibition of fibrinolysis, but whether or not the net effects of aspirin on fibrinolysis are clinically relevant has not been established.

At high concentrations, such as those used to treat rheumatic fever or rheumatoid arthritis, aspirin can produce hypoprothrombinemia and inhibit synthesis of vitamin K–dependent clotting factors. These effects are most likely due to salicylate, not to acetylsalicylate, and can be reversed by vitamin K. At usual antiplatelet doses of aspirin, there is no significant depression of vitamin K–dependent clotting factors.

Clinical Evidence for Antithrombotic Effects of Aspirin

Aspirin was approved by the FDA in 1980 for prevention of transient ischemic attacks and stroke and in 1985 for prevention of unstable angina and secondary prevention of myocardial infarction. The standard recommended dose is 325 mg/d. In numerous controlled clinical trials of aspirin therapy, the overall decrease in incidence of these vascular endpoints has ranged from about 20% to 25% for stroke[3,13,15] or myocardial infarction to 40% to 50% for progression of unstable angina to myocardial infarction or sudden death.[4] In addition, aspirin treatment has decreased the incidence of pulmonary embolism after hip surgery and the rate of coronary artery

reocclusion following bypass graft surgery. Major meta-analyses have confirmed this interpretation of risk reduction for multiple types of vascular event endpoints including stroke, and have shown that risk reduction by antithrombotic therapy is similar for both sexes.[4]

For ischemic stroke or TIA, aspirin was beneficial in the elderly as well as in younger patients[100]; however for prevention of embolic stroke in subjects more than 75 years with atrial fibrillation, anticoagulation was more effective.[87,105] A similar extent of clinical benefit has been documented over a dose range between 160 mg/d and 1,300 mg/d in numerous studies without head-to-head dose comparisons.[4] In the Dutch study in secondary prevention of stroke that compared two low doses of aspirin, 30 or 283 mg/d, both doses appeared to have similar efficacy.[29] However, considerable controversy remains over the optimum dose of aspirin to use for prevention of cerebral ischemia in high-risk patients, and many neurologists feel that 1,300 mg/d is needed, although to date there are no reported controlled clinical trials of stroke prevention comparing this dose level with low doses such as those successfully used in the ISIS study of acute myocardial infarction.[7,48,80,111]

Data from primary prevention studies supporting beneficial effects of aspirin are less clear.[15] Although some of the earliest trials showing aspirin to be antithrombotic were those dealing with secondary prevention of TIA and stroke in patients who previously had experienced an episode of cerebral ischemia, the Physicians Health Study of aspirin in primary prevention of myocardial infarction in over 20,000 healthy males suggested no reduction in stroke risk in this group and, indeed, a slight increase in hemorrhagic strokes was observed.[103] This study used an aspirin dose of 325 mg every other day.

Aspirin has been studied in patients with asymptomatic carotid artery stenosis of 50% or more to ascertain if ischemic events (TIA, stroke, MI, unstable angina or death) could be prevented. A total of 372 patients were randomly assigned to 325 mg/d of aspirin or identically appearing placebo for a median follow-up of 2.3 years. The rate per year of ischemic events or death was 12.3% for the placebo group and 11.0% for the aspirin group ($P = 0.61$). The conclusion was that aspirin did not protect asymptomatic patients with high-grade carotid stenosis from stroke.[25] Because this was a small study, a modest benefit from aspirin therapy might have been inapparent (β error). A larger trial would be needed to verify whether or not there was a true treatment effect.

Platelet Functions Unaffected by Aspirin

The limited efficacy of aspirin in preventing occlusive vascular events such as stroke relates to its restricted effects on platelet function. In contrast to its inhibition of platelet aggregation and TXA_2 synthesis, aspirin does not decrease platelet adhesion, does not prolong abnormally short platelet survival, fails to decrease secretion of vascular growth factors from platelets (especially when secretion is induced by thrombin) and does not block thrombin-induced platelet activation. In the presence of high fibrinogen concentrations, antiplatelet effects are diminished.[31] The platelet release reaction induced by high concentrations of ADP is also not decreased by aspirin.[89]

Shear-induced platelet aggregation can be aspirin independent, and is mediated by large vWF multimers.[86] Thus, platelet activation is only partially inhibited by aspirin. While this fact most likely limits the severity of the bleeding tendency induced by aspirin, it also accounts for the limitations of the antithrombotic effects of the drug in clinical practice. Therefore, while aspirin markedly depresses cyclooxygenase-related platelet functions, it does not prevent the progression of atherosclerosis or the occurrence of restenosis after a vascular procedure.[47,65] Thus, in clinical trials aspirin therapy failed to alter restenosis rates after coronary or peripheral angioplasty,[97,83] graft patency after coronary artery surgery[40] or stroke or restenosis after carotid endarterectomy.[47,65] However, one study of the growth of carotid artery plaques measured by ultrasound indicated that the progression of the plaques was slower when patients were treated with 900 mg/d of aspirin compared to 50 mg/d aspirin.[84] Whether or not this reflects an anti-inflammatory effect of the larger dose of aspirin has not been clearly determined.

Another reason for a lack of aspirin effect on progression of atherosclerosis may be the way in which aspirin affects cyclooxygenase-2 in monocytes and vascular tissues. Platelets contain only cyclooxygenase-1, which is fully inhibited by aspirin. Resting monocytes and vascular cells contain cyclooxygenase-1 but high levels of cyclooxygenase-2 are induced during activation, especially due to inflammatory stimuli. Aspirin alters the enzymatic activity of cyclooxygenase-2 instead of simply inhibiting it, by binding near the active site and altering its conformation.[62] As a result, arachidonic acid is metabolized by aspirinated cyclooxygenase-2 into 15-hydroperoxyeicosatetraenoic acid (15-HPETE). This unstable intermediate then forms 15-HETE, a chemotactic end product that is mitogenic for vascular smooth muscle cells and fibroblasts, and thus promotes atherosclerosis.[62] In theory, this effect of aspirin on the induced high amounts of cyclooxygenase-2 found in damaged or inflamed arteries could account for the lack of inhibitory effect of aspirin on progression of atherosclerosis.

Aspirin Nonresponders

The limited effects of aspirin in reducing risk of cerebral ischemia have raised the question whether some patients might be nonresponders to aspirin therapy. Unlike the situation in patients with unstable angina or prior myocardial infarction, where a low dose of aspirin appears to offer benefit equal to a higher dose, controversy remains unresolved about the optimal dose for stroke-prone patients.[7,48,80] A proportion of patients receiving aspirin therapy after a first episode of cerebral ischemia presents with recurrent stroke.[42] In one recent study, 129/2231 (5.7%) of consecutive admissions for ischemic stroke were classified as aspirin failures, since patients were taking aspirin at the time of admission. Pertinent characteristics of these patients included significant hyperlipidemia, ischemic heart disease, and lower dose of aspirin, suggesting that individuals with greater risk factors for occlusive vascular disease might benefit less from aspirin.[12]

In a separate study, designed to test if patients with cerebral ischemia develop "aspirin resistance" over time, patients with history of previous ischemic stroke who were prescribed aspirin were repeatedly tested at 6-month intervals for aspirin effects on platelet aggregation.[50] Testing at outset, using ara-

chidonate, epinephrine, ADP, and collagen to stimulate aggregation, revealed that 228 of 306 patients had complete aspirin effects and 78 had partial inhibition of platelet aggregation. Upon repeat testing, 33% of those initially showing complete inhibition had lost part of the antiplatelet effect of aspirin. In patients whose initial testing showed only a partial aspirin effect, escalation of aspirin dose (by increments of 325 mg/d) achieved complete inhibition in 35 of 52, but 8 of these same patients later reverted to partial inhibition. The question of compliance was addressed only by reminding the patients to take a dose of aspirin on the morning of testing. Overall about 8% of patients showed aspirin resistance even at 1,300 mg/d. Eight patients had recurrent stroke during the study and at admission each had an incomplete inhibition pattern. No clear reason for a diminished aspirin effect was found; the patients were not taking other nonsteroidal anti-inflammtory drugs that can interfere with platelet acetylation by aspirin. Hyperlipidemia, which is associated with a lesser aspirin effect, was not evaluated in this study. Another recent study indicated that about 10% of outpatients prescribed aspirin or ticlopidine as antiplatelet therapy were noncompliant with medication and showed a decreased inhibition of platelet aggregation on repeat testing.[56]

OTHER NONSTEROIDAL ANTI-INFLAMMATORY DRUGS

Aspirin belongs to a large class of nonsteroidal anti-inflammatory drugs (NSAIDs) that inhibit eicosanoid synthesis by blocking cyclooxygenase function. Aspirin is distinctive as it is the only member of this class of drugs that is an irreversible rather than a competitive inhibitor of cyclooxygenase.[91] Other NSAIDs such as indomethacin, ibuprofen, or indobufen are more potent inhibitors of cyclooxygenase than aspirin on a molar basis, but because they act competitively, the inhibitory effect lasts only while a critical blood level of drug is maintained. Neither salicylate nor any of the nonaspirin NSAIDs can acetylate cyclooxygenase. This means that the antiplatelet effects of most NSAIDs require high, continuous blood levels of drug and that their overall antiplatelet efficacy is of shorter duration than that of aspirin, since cyclooxygenase is not permanently inactivated. Thus, most NSAIDs must be given in multiple daily doses for clinical antiplatelet effect, a scenario that makes compliance a problem. However, in certain settings, their competitive inhibitory effect can be used to advantage. For example, in preparing for surgery, where a short scheduled interruption of the antiplatelet activity during the surgical procedure is desirable, preoperative treatment with NSAIDs such as ibuprofen may be useful because of the limited duration of the antiplatelet action. The competitive blockade of cyclooxygenase by NSAIDs has a second clinical consequence that should be remembered in patients taking multiple drugs: NSAIDs taken shortly before a dose of aspirin can block the aspirin's irreversible inactivation of cyclooxygenase on a steric basis, since aspirin is rapidly deacetylated in the liver. Therefore, patients using a daily aspirin as an antiplatelet drug while being treated with other NSAIDs for anti-inflammatory effects should take their aspirin about an hour in advance of their next dose of NSAID so that acetylation of platelet cyclooxygenase is complete before a competitive inhibitor is given.

INHIBITORS OF THROMBOXANE SYNTHESIS OR THROMBOXANE RECEPTORS OR BOTH

Imidazole analogs and other chemical species that block activity of thromboxane synthase have been developed and tested in experimental models for their capacity to interrupt platelet activation by preventing thromboxane formation from endoperoxides while favoring increased production of vascular prostacyclin from these same intermediates. While model systems indicate that these antithrombotic goals can be achieved, preliminary clinical trials of these agents have been disappointing for two reasons. First, inhibition of thromboxane synthesis is only transient since these drugs are competitive inhibitors of thromboxane synthase, and second, prostaglandin endoperoxides bind to and activate thromboxane receptors to promote platelet aggregation and vasoconstriction.

Further development has concentrated on combining inhibition of thromboxane synthesis with blockade of thromboxane-endoperoxide receptors in the same compound. Early trials suggested that these combination inhibitors reduced experimental coronary thrombosis in animals and prevented reperfusion-induced arrhythmias, enhanced coronary thrombolysis, and improved outcome in experimental carotid artery thrombosis.[90,115] However, clinical trials with these inhibitors have not yielded very encouraging results.[33] In one trial, vapiprost, a TXA receptor antagonist, failed to decrease the incidence of restenosis after coronary angioplasty.[98] The Ridogrel Versus Aspirin Patency Trial (RAPT) compared ridogrel, another combination inhibitor, to aspirin in patients with acute myocardial infarction who underwent thrombolysis with streptokinase.[85] Vessel patency at 1 to 2 weeks was similar in both treatment groups, but there were fewer new ischemic events including ischemic strokes in the ridogrel group, leading to the conclusion that ridogrel was not more effective than aspirin in enhancing fibrinolysis but might be better at preventing new ischemic events. One limitation of thromboxane synthase inhibitor-thromboxane receptor blockade is that their therapeutic effects result in part from redirection of platelet prostaglandin endoperoxide metabolism to vasodilatory prostaglandins (by transcellular metabolism). This implies that the combined TXA_s inhibitors will be less effective in patients taking aspirin, in whom platelet endoperoxide production is blocked.[96]

PROSTACYCLIN AND ITS ANALOGS

Epoprostenol (prostacyclin, PGI_2) and PGE_1 are direct inhibitors of platelet aggregation by virtue of their stimulation of adenylate cyclase, producing increased platelet cAMP, activating cAMP-dependent protein kinases and enhancing uptake of Ca^{2+} into intracellular storage pools. The resulting low platelet Ca^{2+} levels maintain platelets in a resting state and inhibit platelet activation. Oral preparations of PGI_2 are not yet available, and intravenous PGI_2 is a potent vasodilator at the concentrations required to inhibit platelet aggregation; thus efficacy is limited by hypotension as well as by the instability of the drug under physiologic conditions. In addition, PGI_2 receptors may become desensitized or down-regulated by the drug (or by increased endogenous PGI_2 production) leading to enhanced platelet adhesion to endothelium. PGI_2 or synthetic congeners such as iloprost have been successfully used to support hemodialysis in bleeding patients where heparin could not be given and as a substitute for heparin during cardiac surgery. However, PGI_2 did not affect restenosis rates after angioplasty in a controlled clinical trial in which patients were also receiving aspirin.[38] Possibly, longer-acting congeners now under development might be more effective.

FISH OILS AND POLYUNSATURATED FATTY ACIDS

Interest in antiplatelet and antithrombotic effects of dietary modification, outside of cholesterol, has focused on the effects of highly polyunsaturated fatty acids present in oils of coldwater fish like salmon or mackeral that are rich in eicosapentaenoic and docosahexaenoic acids. These fatty acids compete with arachidonic acid as substrates for cyclooxygenase and form eicosanoids of the ω-3 series (an extra double bond in the fatty acid chain is located 3 carbons from the carboxy terminus) in place of the ω-6 eicosanoids formed from arachidonate. The product PGI_3 is similar to prostacyclin in antiaggregatory and vasodilatory activity, whereas TXA_3 is a very weak platelet agonist. Administration of fish, fish oil, or the ω-3 fatty acids has been shown to decrease platelet aggregation, prolong bleeding time and to decrease TXA_2 production, while vascular prostacyclin levels increase.[27,61] In addition, ω-3 fatty acids have anti-inflammatory effects on neutrophil and monocyte functions. Diets including regular intake of fish have been associated with decreased coronary artery disease mortality.[59,61] However, no association has been found between fish intake and stroke incidence in several epidemiologic studies.[73,78] A possible explanation for the difference between effects of ω-3 fatty acids in coronary disease and in cerebrovascular disease might reside in the antiarrhythmic effects of these fatty acids.[10]

AGENTS TRIED HISTORICALLY THAT HAVE NOT PROVED EFFECTIVE ANTIPLATELET DRUGS

Sulfinpyrazone, a uricosuric agent related to phenylbutazone, but possessing little anti-inflammatory activity, is a weak competitive inhibitor of cyclooxgyenase. In experimental models, sulfinpyrazone was shown to decrease platelet adhesion to subendothelium or to artificial surfaces and to have endothelial protective activity possibly related to scavenging of oxygen-free radicals. Although one early study suggested that sulfin-pyrazone was useful in preventing sudden death in patients with myocardial ischemia, the drug has not been shown to decrease rates of vascular reocclusion in patients with unstable angina or stroke (either alone or in combination with aspirin, and it is no longer used for antithrombotic purposes.[16]

Dipyridamole, a pyrimidopyrimidine derivative, has been tested as antithrombotic drug in a number of model systems based on its properties as a phosphodiesterase inhibitor and inhibitor of adenosine uptake by cells. In theory, as a phosphodiesterase inhibitor, dipyridamole should raise platelet cAMP levels, potentiate prostacyclin, and prevent platelet activation. These effects, however, cannot be demonstrated in vitro nor in vivo, at concentrations that are clinically achievable. A number of clinical trials have examined whether dipyridamole potentiates the effects of aspirin or anticoagulation, another pharmacologically attractive hypothesis. Early small trials had suggested, for example, that dipyridamole decreased fistula thrombosis in dialysis patients with arteriovenous fistulas, and decreased cardioembolic stroke in patients who continued to embolize despite anticoagulation.[35] However, in large controlled, double-blind trials, no significant benefit has been demonstrated when dipyridamole was added to other antiplatelet agents or anticoagulants.[3,35] Dipyridamole is a vasodilator, acting through its inhibition of cellular adenosine uptake to raise plasma adenosine values, as adenosine is vasodilatory. Thus, its chief side effect is vascular headache. There seems to be no reason to prescribe dipyridamole as an antiplatelet, antithrombotic drug for stroke prevention.

Intravenous *dextran* infusion has been used prophylactically to prevent pulmonary embolism after hip surgery, a setting where anticoagulation was historically considered undesirable because of hematoma formation. Dextran can inhibit platelet function and prolong bleeding time, probably by binding to platelet membranes and preventing platelet-platelet interactions or platelet binding to von Willebrand factor. It is rarely used today, in part because it has been replaced by drugs that have less potential for causing anaphylaxis.

DRUGS THAT BLOCK ADP-MEDIATED PLATELET ACTIVATION

Ticlopidine (5,-[O-chlorobenzyl]-4,5,6,7-tetrahydrothieno-[3,2,-c]pyridine hydrochloride) is an antithrombotic thieno-pyridine, chemically unrelated to other antiplatelet drugs. Ticlopidine blocks ADP-mediated platelet activation processes. Because ADP is widely involved in the early step in most pathways of activation that enables platelets to bind fibrinogen, ticlopidine has much broader inhibitory effects on platelet function than does aspirin.[92,95]

The effects of ticlopidine ingestion on platelet function include decreased binding of ADP and fibrinogen to platelet membranes, decreased platelet adhesion to artificial surfaces, the lengthening of abnormally short platelet survival toward normal, and a marked, dose-dependent increase in the bleeding time. By contrast, ticlopidine does not affect arachidonic acid metabolism by platelets and does not alter TXA_2 synthesis. Bleeding time is much more prolonged by ticlopidine than by aspirin, and prolongation depends on the ticlopidine dose.

When the two drugs are given together, their effects on bleeding time are additive. Ticlopidine also decreases blood viscosity, decreases fibrinogen levels and enhances red cell deformability, suggesting possibly beneficial rheologic properties. In many different experimental thrombosis systems, ticlopidine has been shown to decrease thrombosis and to improve outcome whether or not platelets are important in the pathogenesis of the thrombosis. Ticlopidine appears similarly effective in both men and women.

Ticlopidine itself is a prodrug, with little activity in vitro. It must be metabolized in the liver to a still unidentified metabolite to develop in vivo activity. Thus, normal platelets incubated directly with ticlopidine behave normally, whereas platelets incubated with plasma from persons taking ticlopidine show inhibited ADP-related functions. Once platelets are affected by the drug, they remain so. Demonstration of in vivo antiplatelet activity requires several days after starting oral administration, and it takes about a week to reach a steady state. The active metabolite also is slowly cleared, so that antiplatelet effects are prolonged for some days after the ingestion of drug is stopped. As a result, ticlopidine should be considered an effective steady-state antiplatelet agent but not a drug that acts acutely.

Clinical Studies with Ticlopidine

Relatively few controlled clinical studies using ticlopidine as a major antiplatelet agent are available. Two major studies of ticlopidine in the prevention of stroke after previous transient cerebral ischemia or previous stroke have been published. In the Canadian American Ticlopidine Study (CATS) of patients with prior stroke, ticlopidine was shown to effectively reduce recurrent TIA or stroke when compared to placebo.[36] In the Ticlopidine-Aspirin Stroke Study (TASS), ticlopidine appeared to be slightly more effective (20%) than aspirin in preventing TIA, stroke, or death following an initial TIA or reversible stroke.[49] Maximum benefit occurred during the first year of treatment and the difference between groups remained, but diminished, over time. Subgroup analysis of TASS suggested that patients who first presented with a reversible cerebral ischemic event and took ticlopidine, rather than aspirin, had significantly even greater reduction of risk for another TIA-RIND or a reversible cerebral ischemic event, stroke, or death.[8] A second subgroup analysis of TASS data indicated that nonwhite patients had a 48% reduction in risk of nonfatal stroke or death with ticlopidine and a 60% risk reduction in fatal or nonfatal stroke.[120] The validity of such ex post facto subgroup analyses has been strongly criticized, however, and independent studies of similar types of patients treated prospectively, have not been carried out.[117] Ticlopidine has also been reported to reduce neurologic deficit after subarachnoid hemorrhage without directly affecting incidence of vasospasm. Other studies have shown ticlopidine to reduce risk of myocardial infarction in patients with unstable angina and to decrease restenosis after CABG,[5] and to decrease MI and stroke in patients with peripheral vascular disease.[52]

Combinations of Antiplatelet Agents

Since aspirin and ticlopidine have quite different modes of action, there has been considerable interest in combining these drugs to improve antiplatelet activity. Serious concerns yet to be resolved involve whether increased risk of bleeding induced by the combination of ticlopidine and aspirin is clinically tolerable, and whether the marked prolongations of bleeding time resulting from the drug combination predict such an increased bleeding risk. One small study in patients with cerebral ischemia compared the combination of low dose ticlopidine (100 mg/d) plus low-dose aspirin (81 mg/d) with either drug alone or placebo, and showed that the drug combination markedly inhibited platelet aggregation by ADP, arachidonate and PAF, and reduced plasma concentrations of platelet factor 4 and beta-thromboglobulin, two markers of platelet activation-release in vivo.[114] Only the combination of both drugs prolonged platelet survival. The bleeding time was prolonged significantly more by the drug combination than by either drug alone. The cardiologic experience with combined ticlopidine and aspirin suggests good efficacy and reasonable safety. Recently, this combination has been used short term to prevent thrombosis in vascular stents placed after coronary angioplasty, with encouraging success; outcomes are improved over anticoagulation plus aspirin.[94] Among 517 patients assigned ticlopidine plus aspirin, or anticoagulation plus aspirin after placement of Palmaz-Schatz coronary artery stents, the risk of myocardial infarction was 82% lower and the need for repeated intervention 78% lower in the group receiving ticlopidine (250 mg/bid) plus aspirin (100 mg/bid). Hemorrhagic complications occurred only in the anticoagulant therapy group (6.5%), who also received aspirin 100 mg bid.[93] Stenting after atherectomy has potential also in severe carotid artery disease, and trails of similar antiplatelet regimens are likely to be undertaken, based on the cardiologic experience.

Limitations of Ticlopidine Use

At the customary clinical dose for antiplatelet therapy (250 mg bid), ticlopidine has several significant negative side effects including rash, diarrhea and sudden, unpredictable neutropenia and agranulocytosis. In published studies of ticlopidine prophylaxis for cerebral ischemia, almost 50% of treated subjects discontinued their treatment before the end of the study because of side effects, necessity for other treatment modalities, or cerebral ischemic events.[36,49] Severe neutropenia has been consistently reported in 1% to 2% of subjects taking ticlopidine; this complication usually occurs during the first 3 months of therapy and is usually reversible if the drug is stopped. Therefore, careful frequent monitoring of the blood count during early months of treatment is imperative, since the onset of life-threatening neutropenia can be very rapid. A few cases of fatal bone marrow depression have been reported. Thrombocytopenia and rarely, thrombotic thrombocytopenic purpura have also been observed.

Because of the very prolonged bleeding time that may be produced by the drug, hemorrhage may occur and patients have been cautioned to avoid taking nonsteroidal anti-inflammatory drugs together with ticlopidine because of the possibility of increasing hemorrhagic risk. This makes the coadministration of ticlopidine and aspirin problematic, despite encouraging results from the combination drug studies detailed above. In emergency situations, for example, when urgent surgery is required in a patient taking ticlopidine, the prolonged bleeding time can be reversed by desmopressin or by a bolus dose of dexamethasone (20 mg), but the antiplatelet

effects of the drug are not altered by this treatment. Several small clinical studies have suggested that surgery can safely follow without enhanced bleeding risk. In a patient already taking ticlopidine who presents with recurrent TIAs or progressive stroke, in whom heparinization is desired, administration of dexamethasone to improve bleeding time should be considered to decrease concern about hemorrhagic risk. The untoward side effects and need for intensive monitoring of blood count during the first 3 months of therapy have made ticlopidine a problematic drug, and considerable effort has been undertaken to find safer analogs. *Clopidogrel*, a single isomer thienopyridine closely related to ticlopidine, has antiplatelet activity in animal models and is currently being evaluated for its antithrombotic effects in cerebrovascular and cardiovascular disease in the hope that the active isomer will lack the hematologic toxicity of ticlopidine, which is a racemic mixture.[95] The CAPRIE study, comparing aspirin with clopidogrel in over 19,000 patients with prior myocardial infarction, stroke or peripheral vascular disease, reported an 8.7% relative-risk reduction in combined endpoint events in favor of clopidogrel, without any of the marrow toxicity previously found with ticlopidine.[18] This suggests that clopidogrel, when available clinically, will provide safer antithrombotic efficacy than ticlopidine and will be a satisfactory alternative to aspirin.

DRUGS AFFECTING PLATELET ACTIVATION RECEPTORS

Platelet membrane glycoproteins participate in key interactions between platelets and other cells and are involved in signalling that activates platelet responses. Two major membrane receptor complexes are involved, GPIb-IX and GPIIa/IIIb. As detailed earlier, the GPIb/X complex mediates platelet adhesion via von Willebrand factor. While peptides that interfere with GPIb function are being studied experimentally as potential antithrombotic substances, there is considerable concern that inhibition of GPIb mediated platelet function might produce a severe bleeding tendency. GPIIa/IIIb, by contrast, mediates platelet aggregation induced by all physiologic agonists without affecting platelet adhesion. This suggests that blocking GPIIa/IIIb might be antithrombotic while sparing hemostasis.[22] Compounds that block GPIIa/IIIb function are currently receiving much attention in prevention of cardiovascular ischemic events.

Recent development and clinical testing of such drugs represent a novel therapeutic approach to platelet-dependent pathologic processes, different from all previously available antiplatelet therapy. To date, most of the information obtained about GPIIb/IIIa antagonists has been obtained in the acute cardiovascular setting, where blockade of the receptor markedly reduces thrombosis and restenosis after angioplasty.[30] But, in view of the observation that patients with inherited defects in GPIIb/IIIa function (Glanzmann's thrombasthenia) have mainly mucocutaneous bleeding and rarely central nervous system bleeding, it is hoped that GPIIb/IIIa antagonists can be used in prevention of stroke as well. Clinical trials with this objective have not yet been done, but trials in cardiovascular disease are very promising. Two treatment approaches have been used to block critical sites on the GPIIb/IIIa complex, (1) monoclonal antibodies, or (2) "disintegrins" from snake venom, peptides containing the RGD motif, or peptidomimetics.

The humanized monoclonal antibody c7E3, known as abciximab, binds to and blocks GpIIb/IIIa.[20,22] In the EPICS trial (Evaluation of c7E3Fab in the Prevention of Ischemic Complications), bolus, or 12-hour infusion of abciximab was given to over 2,000 patients undergoing coronary angioplasty or atherectomy.[30] Patients receiving abciximab infusion had a 35% reduction in endpoint events of myocardial infarction and need for emergent revascularization, and furthermore, after 6 months of follow-up, the rate of clinically significant restenosis was decreased 26% compared to placebo or bolus drug alone.[112] Positive results required blockade or more than 80% of GPIIb/IIIa receptors. Aspirin and heparin were also given. Major risks of this therapy include enhanced bleeding risk and production of antimouse IgG antibodies.

These results imply that a short-term decrease in platelet reactivity could produce an acute antithrombotic effect as well as long-term benefits of preventing late reocclusion of damaged coronary arteries.[54] Recent evidence further broadens the direct antithrombotic effects of abciximab by demonstrating that it inhibits thrombin formation triggered by tissue factor.[88] In a platelet-dependent model system, blockade of GPIIb/IIIa and the vitronectin receptor $\alpha_v \beta_3$ by abciximab not only inhibited thrombin generation by 50% but also inhibited the formation of thrombin-antithrombin complexes (TAT), generation of prothrombin F1 + 2, release of PDGF and platelet factor 4 from platelets, incorporation of thrombin into clots, and formation of procoagulant platelet microparticles. These observations suggest that blockade of platelet integrins leads to a decrease in most of the indicators of hypercoagulability that have been described as markers of acute or chronic cerebral ischemia. To date, no trials of abciximab to treat cerebral ischemia or to prevent stroke in high risk patients have been undertaken, and whether the antithrombotic effects observed in the heart can be transferred to the cerebral circulation without incurring excess bleeding has not been determined. However, in the EPICS trial, no excess of strokes or cerebral hemorrhage was observed among abciximab-treated patients.[30]

Similarly, studies in cardiovascular settings using the synthetic disintegrin, Integrelin, or a nonpeptide GPIIb/IIIa antagonist, Lamifiban, showed decrease in acute ischemic endpoints.[108,109] Theoretical advantages of such peptides, peptidomimetics, or nonpeptide RGD mimetics—especially recently developed oral preparations—include ease of administration and possibility of use over prolonged periods as preventive therapy.[26] No results with these agents in clinical trials in cerebral ischemia have been published.

DIRECT THROMBIN INHIBITORS

Thrombin is the most potent physiologic platelet activator, and thrombin bound to the surface of a clot is not readily inactivated by heparin, so that platelets localized to thrombi are particularly resistant to aspirin- or heparin-based antithrombotic therapies. Direct antithrombin agents appear a reasonable approach for treatment of thrombin-mediated, platelet-dependent occlusive events taking place on diseased arteries.[63] How to target

platelet recruitment to ongoing arterial thrombus without impairing normal hemostasis is a difficult task and hemorrhagic complications, particularly hemorrhagic strokes, have halted some clinical trials such as GUSTO, and TIMI 9, which employed hirudin, a direct thrombin inhibitor.[96]

The major approaches that are being studied use several antithrombin peptides. Recombinant hirudin, a 57 amino-acid polypeptide cloned from the medicinal leech, is a direct and irreversible inhibitor of thrombin that can block platelet deposition and platelet-dependent thrombosis formation in experimental models. However, hirudin also blocks hemostasis at antithrombotic concentrations and is antigenic. Antithrombin peptides containing D-Phe-Pro-Arg sequences interact with the catalytic site of thrombin and block thrombin-induced platelet aggregation and fibrinogen cleavage in vitro and in vivo. A bifunctional antithrombin peptide (Hirulog) that combines part of the hirudin sequence with the active site inhibitory peptide (Hirulog) is also being tested, as are benzamidine-based compounds, and oral antithrombins. To date, antithrombotic efficacy can easily be detected but in general the concentrations needed to achieve this also increase risks of hemorrhage. Clinical trials of Hirulog mainly in angioplasty models and of argipidine (argatroban) are in process. Possible development of specific inhibitors for extrinsic pathway or tissue factor-mediated thrombus formation may yield the antithrombotic specificity required, sparing hemostasis.

COMBINATIONS OF ANTIPLATELET AGENTS AND ANTICOAGULANTS

Anticoagulation has been traditionally used to prevent cardioembolic stroke in patients with atrial fibrillation. The SPAF (Stroke Prevention in Atrial Fibrillation) trials have compared both efficacy and safety of aspirin and warfarin. SPAF I suggested that warfarin was more effective but the overall number of events was small, making interpretation difficult.[87] SPAF II examined age effects of these two regimens (warfarin to maintain INR 2.0–4.5 or aspirin 325 mg/d) in patients less than and more than 75 years old in prevention of ischemic stroke and systemic embolism.[105] The absolute rate of the primary events varied with age. In treated low-risk patients younger than 75, the primary event rate per year was 1.3% for those taking warfarin and 1.9% for those taking aspirin (RR 0.67, $P = 0.24$). In treated patients older than 75, the primary event rate was 3.6% per year with warfarin and 4.8% with aspirin (RR 0.73, $P = 0.39$). However, the rate per year of all stroke (ischemic plus hemorrhagic) with residual deficit was 4.6% with warfarin and 4.3% with aspirin. Thus, while warfarin may be more effective than aspirin for preventing ischemic stroke in fibrillating older patients or high-risk young patients, the overall rate of stroke in warfarin-treated patients remains high, reflecting bleeding complications due to the intervention itself. These results in patients with atrial fibrillation are similar to those from the Sixty Plus Reinfarction Study in which elderly patients anticoagulated after one myocardial infarction were observed to have fewer ischemic strokes but more hemorrhagic strokes, resulting in no net benefit in terms of stroke prevention although the incidence of recurrent myocardial infarction was clearly decreased.[99,101]

The combination of anticoagulants with antiplatelet drugs has been examined in several clinical settings that do not directly involve the cerebral circulation: heart valve replacements, coronary stents thrombolysis; and angioplasty.[17] Benefit in terms of reduced mortality, especially from vascular causes, and decreased embolic rates, without severe increase in bleeding was achieved in the heart valve patients.[113] The combination of ticlopidine and aspirin appears superior to anticoagulation in maintaining patency of coronary artery stents.[94] A comparison of the results of four separate trials of heart valve patients treated with aspirin (between 75 and 000 mg/d combined with moderate anticoagulation (INR 1.5 to 4.5) suggested that the rate of bleeding complications correlated with increased aspirin dose rather than INR level, suggesting that aspirin dose should be kept low if the combination were to be used.[41]

ANTIPLATELET AGENTS IN THROMBOLYTIC COMBINATION THERAPY

There has been a long interest in using fibrinolytic agents such as streptokinase and tissue plasminogen activator to treat occlusive stroke. The use of antiplatelet agents during coronary thrombolysis has improved outcome by decreasing early reocclusion rates, although the tradeoff risk is that of bleeding.[30,34,41] However, attempts to utilize thrombolytic therapy to prevent cerebral damage after stroke have been frustrated by an unacceptably high incidence of bleeding complications and excess mortality therefrom, even when thrombolysis is applied very early after onset of cerebral ischemia. Of five recent clinical trials of thrombolytic therapy in patients with acute stroke, only one, using tissue plasminogen activator within 3 hours of onset of ischemic symptoms, did not report increased mortality.[76] Indeed, the most recent trial of thrombolytic therapy for stroke, using streptokinase, was terminated early for this reason.[51,74] It must be concluded that the risks accompanying thrombolysis differ widely in different parts of the vascular system, and that the combinations of thrombolytic, anticoagulant and antiplatelet drugs that currently give best resolution of thrombus in the coronary bed or peripheral circulation do not appear to be tolerated in the cerebral circulation.[119] In this regard, it is of interest that the single clinical trial of thrombolysis for stroke that gave positive results was one in which antiplatelet therapy with aspirin was not given in conjunction with the fibrinolytic agents.[76]

Acknowledgments

This study was supported by a National Institutes of Health SCOR in Thrombosis HL 18828.

References

1. Ali M, McDonald JWD, Thiessen JJ, Coates PE: Plasma acetylsalicylate and salicylate and platelet cyclooxygenase activity following plain and enteric-coated aspirin. Stroke 11:9, 1980

2. Amarenco P, Cohen A, Tzourio C et al: Atherosclerotic disease of the aortic arch and the risk of ischemic stroke. N Engl J Med 331:1474, 1994

3. American-Canadian Co-operative Study Group: Persantine Aspirin Trial in cerebral ischemia, part II: endpoint results. Stroke 16:418, 1985

4. Antiplatelet Trialists' Collaboration: Collaborative overview of randomised trials of antiplatelet therapy. I. Prevention of death, myocardial infarction and stroke by prolonged antiplatelet therapy in various categories of patients. Br Med J 308:8, 1994

5. Balsano F, Rizzon P, Violi F et al and the STA I Group: Antiplatelet treatment with ticlopidine in unstable angina, a controlled multicenter trial. Circulation 82:17, 1990

6. Barnett JHM, Eliasziw M, Meldrum HE: Drugs and surgery in the prevention of ischemic stroke. N Engl J Med 332:238, 1995

7. Barnett JHM, Kaste M, Meldrum H, Eliasziw M: Aspirin dose in stroke prevention: beautiful hypotheses slain by ugly facts. Stroke 27:588, 1996

8. Bellavance A: Efficacy of ticlopidine and aspirin for prevention of reversible cerebrovascular ischemic events. The Ticlopidine Aspirin Stroke Study. Stroke 24:1452, 1993

9. Berk BC, Alexander RW, Brock TA et al: Vasoconstriction: a new activity for platelet-derived growth factor. Science 232:87, 1986

10. Billman GF, Hallaq A, Leaf A: Prevention of ischemia-induced ventricular fibrillation by ω-3 fatty acids. Proc Natl Acad Sci USA 91:4427, 1994

11. Bjornsson TD, Schneider DE, Berger H Jr: Aspirin acetylates fibrinogen and enhances fibrinolysis: fibrinolytic effect is independent of changes in plasminogen activator levels. J Pharm Exp Therap 250:154, 1989

12. Bornstein NM, Kakrpov VG, Aronovich BD et al: Failure of aspirin treatment after stroke. Stroke 25:275, 1994

13. Bousser MG, Eschwege E, Haguenau M et al: "AICLA" controlled trial of aspirin and dipyridamole in the secondary prevention of atherothrombotic cerebral ischemia. Stroke 14:5, 1983

14. Brenner BM, Troy JL, Balterman BJ: Endothelium-dependent vascular responses: mediators and mechanisms. J Clin Invest 84:1373, 1989

15. Bronner LL, Kanter DS, Manson JE: Primary prevention of stroke. N Engl J Med 333:1392, 1995

16. Canadian Cooperative Study Group: A randomized trial of aspirin and sulfinpyrazone in threatened stroke. N Engl J Med 299:53, 1978

17. Cappelleri JC, Fiore LD, Brophy MT et al: Efficacy and safety of combined anticoagulant and antiplatelet therapy versus anticoagulant monotherapy after mechanical heart-valve replacement: a metaanalysis. Am Heart J 130:547, 1995

18. CAPRIE Steering Committee: A randomised, blinded trial of clopidogrel versus aspirin in patients at risk of ischaemic events (CAPRIE). Lancet 348:1329, 1996

19. Cheresh DA, Berliner SA, Vincente V. Ruggeri ZM: Recognition of distinct adhesive sites on fibrinogen by related integrins on platelets and endothelial cells. Cell 58:945, 1989

20. Coller BS: A new murine monoclonal antibody reports an activation-dependent change in the conformation and/or microenvironment of the platelet glycoprotein IIb/IIIa complex. J Clin Invest 76:101, 1985
21. Coller BS: Platelets and thrombolytic therapy. N Engl J Med 322:33, 1990
22. Coller BS, Anderson K, Weisman HF: New antiplatelet agents: Platelet GPIIb/IIIa antagonists. Thrombosis and Haemostasis 74:302, 1995
23. Colluci M, Balconi G, Lorenzet R et al: Cultured human endothelial cells generate tissue factor in response to endotoxin. J Clin Invest 71:1893, 1983
24. Cortelazzo S, Finazzi G, Ruggeri M et al: Hydroxyurea for patients with essential thrombocythemia and a high risk of thrombosis. N Engl J Med 332:1132, 1995
25. Cote R, Battista RN, Abrahamowicz M et al: Lack of effect of aspirin in asymptomatic patients with carotid bruits and substantial carotid narrowing. The Asymptomatic Cervical Bruit Study Group. Ann Int Med 123:649, 1995
26. Coutre S, Leung L: Novel antithrombotic therapeutics targeted against platelet glycoprotein IIb/IIIa. Ann Rev Med 46:257, 1995
27. DeCaterina R, Giannessi D, Mazzone A et al: Vascular prostacyclin is increased in patients taking fish oil n-3 polyunsaturated fatty acids prior to coronary bypass surgery. Circulation 82:428, 1990
28. Diacovo TG, Puri KD, Warnock RA et al: Platelet-mediated lymphocyte delivery to high endothelial venules. Science 273:252, 1996
29. The Dutch TIA Trial Study Group: A comparison of two doses of aspirin (30 mg vs 283 mg a day) in patients after a transient ischemic attack or minor ischemic stroke. N Engl J Med 325:1261, 1991
30. The EPICS Investigators: Use of a monoclonal antibody directed against the platelet glycoprotein IIb/IIIa receptor in high-risk coronary angioplasty. N Engl J Med 330:956, 1994
31. Ernst E, Resch KL: Fibrinogen as a cardiovascular risk factor: a metaanalysis and review of the literature. Ann Int Med 118:956, 1993
32. Feinberg WM, Erickson LP, Bruck D, Kittelson J: Hemostatic markers in acute ischemic stroke; association with stroke type, severity and outcome. Stroke 27:1296, 1996
33. Fiddler GI, Lumley P: Preliminary clinical studies with thromboxane synthase inhibitors and thromboxane receptor blockers: a review. Circulation 81(suppl I):169, 1990
34. Fitzgerald DJ, Wright F, FitzGerald GA: Increased thromboxane biosynthesis during coronary thrombolysis: evidence that platelet activation and thromboxane A2 modulate the response to tissue-type plasminogen activator in vivo. Circ Res 65:83, 1989
35. FitzGerald GA: Dipyridamole. N Engl J Med 316:1247, 1987
36. Gent M, Easton JD, Hachinski VC et al: The Canadian-American Ticlopidine Study (CATS) in thromboembolic stroke. Lancet 1:1215, 1989
37. Genton E, Barnett JJ, Fields WS et al: Cerebral ischemia: the role of thrombosis and of antithrombotic therapy: study group on antithrombotic therapy. Stroke 8:150, 1977
38. Gershlick AH, Spriggins D, Davies SW et al: Failure of epoprostenol (prostacyclin, PGI$_2$) to inhibit platelet aggregation and to prevent restenosis after coronary angioplasty; results of a randomised placebo controlled trial. Br Heart J 71:7, 1994
39. Ghaddar HB, Cortes J, Salomaa V et al: Correlation of specific platelet activation markers with carotid arterial wall thickness. Thromb Haemost 74:943, 1995
40. Goldman S, Copeland J, Moritz T et al: Long term graft patency (3 years) after coronary artery surgery: effects of aspirin. Results of a VA Cooperative study. Circulation 89:1138, 1994
41. Goodnight, S: Antiplatelet therapy with aspirin: from clinical trials to practice. Thromb Haemost 74:401, 1995
42. Grotemeyer KH, Schorafinski HW, Husstedt IW: 2-year followup of aspirin responders and aspirin non-responders—a pilot study including 180 post-stroke patients. Thromb Res 71:397, 1993
43. Grotta JC: Current medical and surgical therapy for cerebrovascular disease. N Engl J Med 317:1505, 1987
44. Gunning AJ, Pickering GW, Robb-Smith AH, Russell RR: Mural thrombosis of the internal carotid artery and subsequent embolization. Quart J Med 33:155, 1964
45. Hajjar KA: Cellular receptors in the regulation of plasmin generation. Thromb Haemost 74:294, 1995
46. Hajjar KA, Nachman RL; Endothelial cell mediated conversion of glu-plasminogen to lys-plasminogen: further evidence for assembly of the fibrinolytic system on the endothelial cell surface. J Clin Invest 82:1769, 1988
47. Harker LA, Bernstein EF, Dilley RB et al: Failure of aspirin plus dipyridamole to prevent restenosis after carotid endarterectomy. Ann Intern Med 116:731, 1992
48. Hart RG, Harrison MJG: Aspirin wars: the optimal dose of aspirin to prevent stroke. Stroke 27:585, 1996
49. Hass WK, Easton JD, Adams HP et al for the Ticlopidine Aspirin Stroke Study Group: A randomized trial comparing ticlopidine hydrochloride with aspirin for the prevention of stroke in high-risk patients. N Engl J Med 321:501, 1989
50. Helgason CM, Bolin KM, Hoff JA et al: Development of aspirin resistance in persons with previous ischemic stroke. Stroke 25:2331, 1994
51. Hommel M, Boissel JP, Cornu C et al: Termination of trial of streptokinase in severe acute ischemic stroke. Lancet 345:57, 1995
52. Janzon I, Bergquist D, Boberg J et al: Prevention of myocardial infarction and stroke in patients with intermittent claudication: effects of ticlopidine. Results from the STIMS, the Swedish Ticlopidine Multicentre Study. J Int Med 227:301, 1990
53. Karim S, Habib A, Levy-Toledano S, Maclouf J: Cyclooxygenase-2 increases the potential of endothelial cells to provide prostaglandin H2 to aspirinated platelets for the synthesis of thromboxane. Thromb Haemost 73:212, 1995
54. Kleiman NS, Ohman ME Califf RM et al: Profound inhibition of platelet aggregation with monoclonal antibody 7E3 Fab following thrombolytic therapy: results of the TIMI 8 pilot study. J Am Coll Cardiol 22:381, 1993

55. Knapp HR, Reilly IA, Alessandrini P, FitzGerald GA: In vivo indexes of platelet function and vascular function in patients with atherosclerosis. N Engl J Med 314:937, 1986

56. Komiya T, Kudo M, Urabe T, Mizuno Y: Compliance with antiplatelet therapy in patients with ischemic cerebrovascular disease. Assessment by platelet aggregation testing. Stroke 25:2337, 1994

57. Koudstaal PJ, Ciabattoni G, van Gijn J et al: Increased thromboxane synthesis in patients with acute cerebral ischemia. Stroke 24:219, 1993

58. Kristensen SD, Roberts KM, Kishk YT, Martin JF: Accelerated atherogenesis occurs following platelet destruction and increases in megakaryocyte size and DNA content. Eur J Clin Invest 20:239, 1990

59. Kromhout D, Bosschieter EB, deLezenne Coulander C: The inverse relation between fish consumption and mortality from coronary artery disease. N Engl J Med 312:1205, 1985

60. Kyrle PA, Eichler HG, Jager U, Lechner K: Inhibition of prostacyclin and thromboxane A_2 generation by low-dose aspirin at the site of plug formation in man in vivo. Circulation 75:1025, 1987

61. Leaf A: Cardiovascular effects of n-3 fatty acids. N Engl J Med 318:549, 1988

62. Lecomte M, Laneuville O, Ji C et al: Acetylation of human prostaglandin H synthase-2 (cyclooxygenase-2) by aspirin. J Biol Chem 269:13207, 1994

63. Lefkowitz J, Topol EJ: Direct thrombin inhibitors in cardiovascular medicine. Circulation 90:1522, 1994

64. Levin RI, Harpel PC, Harpel JG, Recht PA: Inhibition of tissue plasminogen activator activity by aspirin in vivo and its relationship to levels of tissue plasminogen activator antigen, plasminogen activator inhibitor and their complexes. Blood 74:1635, 1989

65. Lindblad B, Persson NH, Takolander R, Bergqvist D: Does low-dose acetylsalicylic acid prevent stroke after carotid surgery? A double-blind, placebo-controlled randomized trial. Stroke 24:1125, 1993

66. Marcus AJ, Safier LB, Hajjar KA et al: Inhibition of platelet function by an aspirin-insensitive endothelial cell ADPase. Thromboregulation by endothelial cell. J Clin Invest 88:1690, 1991

67. Markwardt F: The development of hirudin as an antithrombotic drug. Thromb Res 74:1, 1994

68. Marler JR, Price TR, Clark GL et al: Morning increase in onset of ischemic stroke. Stroke 20:473, 1989

69. Michelson AD: Flow cytometry: a clinical test of platelet function. Blood 87:4925, 1996

70. Miles LA, Ginsberg MH, White JG, Plow EF: Plasminogen interacts with human platelets through two distinct mechanisms. J Clin Invest 77:2001, 1986

71. Moake JL, Turner NA, Stathopoulos NA et al: Shear-induced platelet aggregation can be mediated by vWF released from platelets, as well as by endogenous large or unusually large vWF multimers, requires adenosine diphosphate and is resistant to aspirin. Blood 71:1366, 1988

72. Moroz L: Increased blood fibrinolytic activity after aspirin ingestion. N Engl J Med 296:525, 1977

73. Morris M, Manson, J, Rosner B et al: Fish consumption and cardiovascular disease in the Physicians Health Study: a prospective study. Am J Epidemiol 142:166, 1995

74. The Multicenter Acute Stroke Trial—Europe Study Group (MAST-E): Thrombolytic therapy with streptokinase in acute ischemic stroke. N Engl J Med 335:145, 1996

75. Nilsson J, Svensson J. Hamsten A, deFaire U: Increased platelet-derived mitogenic activity in plasma of young patients with coronary atherosclerosis. Atherosclerosis 61:237, 1986

76. The National Institute of Neurological Disorders and Stroke rt-PA stroke Study Group. Tissue plasminogen activator for acute ischemic stroke. N Engl J Med 333:1581, 1995

77. O'Malley T, Langhorne P, Elton RA, Stweart MD: Platelet size in stroke patients. Stroke 26:995, 1995

78. Orencia AJ, Daviglus M, Dyer AR et al: Fish consumption and stroke in men: 30-year findings of the Chicago Western Electric Study. Stroke 27:204, 1996

79. Patrono C: Aspirin as an antiplatelet drug. New Engl J Med 330:1287, 1994

80. Patrono C, Roth GJ: Aspirin in ischemic cerebrovascular disease: how strong is the case for a different dosing regimen? Stroke 27:756, 1996

81. Plow EF, Felez J, Miles LA: Cellular regulation of fibrinolysis. Thromb Haemost 66:32, 1991

82. Radomski MW, Palmer RM, Moncada S: An L-arginine/nitric oxide pathway present in human platelets regulates aggregation. Proc Natl Acad Sci USA 87:5193, 1990

83. Ranke C, Creutzig A, Luska G et al: Controlled trial of high versus low-dose aspirin treatment after percutaneous transluminal angioplasty in patients with peripheral vascular disease. Clin Invest 72:673, 1994

84. Ranke C, Hecker H, Creutzig A, Alexander K: Dose-dependent effect of aspirin on carotid atherosclerosis. Circulation 87:1873, 1993

85. The RAPT Investigators: Randomized trial of ridogrel, a combined thromboxane/endoperoxide receptor antagonist and thromboxane A2/prostaglandin endoperoxide receptor antagonist, versus aspirin as adjunct to thrombolysis in patients with acute myocardial infarction. Circulation 89:588, 1994

86. Ratnatunga CP, Edmondson SF, Rees GM, Kovacs IB: High-dose aspirin inhibits shear-induced platelet reaction involving thrombin generation. Circulation 85:1077, 1992

87. Report of the Stroke Prevention in Atrial Fibrillation study. N Engl J Med 322:863, 1990

88. Reverter JC, Beguin S, Kessels H et al: Inhibition of platelet-mediated, tissue factor-induced thrombin generation by the mouse/human chimeric 7E3 antibody. Potential implications for the effect of c7E3 Fab treatment on acute thrombosis and clinical restenosis. J Clin Invest 98:863, 1996

89. Rinder CS, Student LA, Bonan H et al: Aspirin does not inhibit adenosine diphosphate induced platelet alpha granule release. Blood 82:505, 1993

90. Rose WF, Mu DX, Lucchesi BR: Thromboxane antagonism in experimental canine carotid artery thrombosis. Stroke 24:820, 1993

91. Roth GJ, Stanford N, Majerus PW: Acetylation of prostaglandin synthetase by aspirin. Proc Natl Acad Sci USA 72:3073, 1975

92. Saltiel E, Ward A: Ticlopidine: a review of the pharmacodynamic and pharmacokinetic properties and therapeutic efficacy in platelet-dependent disease states. Drugs 34: 222, 1987

93. Schafer AI, Adelman B: Plasmin inhibition of platelet function and of arachidonic acid metabolism. J Clin Invest 75:456, 1985

94. Schomig A, Neumann F-J, Kastrati A et al: A randomized comparison of antiplatelet and anticoagulant therapy after the placement of coronary artery stents. N Engl J Med 334:1084, 1996

95. Schror K: The basic pharmacology of ticlopidine and clopidogrel. Platelets 4:252, 1991

96. Schror, K: Antiplatelet drugs: A comparative review. Drugs 50:7, 1995

97. Schwartz L, Lesperance J, Bourassa MG et al: The role of antiplatelet agents in modifying the extent of restenosis after percutaneous transluminal coronary angioplasty. Am Heart J 119:232, 1990

98. Serruys PW, Rutsch W, Heyndrickx GR et al: Prevention of restenosis after percutaneous transluminal coronary angioplasty with thromboxane A2 receptor blockade: a randomized, double-blind, placebo-controlled trial. Circulation 84:1568, 1991

99. Shattil SJ, Brass LP: Induction of the fibrinogen receptor on human platelets by intracellular mediators. J Biol Chem 262:992, 1987

100. Sivenius J, Riekkinen PH, Laakso M et al: European Stroke Prevention Study (ESPS): antithrombotic therapy is also effective in the elderly. Acta Neurol Scand 87:111, 1993

101. The Sixty Plus Reinfarction Study Research Group: A double blind trial to assess long-term oral anticoagulant treatment in elderly patients after myocardial infarction. Lancet ii:989, 1980

102. Smith JB, Willis AL: Aspirin selectively inhibits prostaglandin production in human platelets. Nature 231:235, 1971

103. Steering Committee of the Physicians' Health Study Research Group: Final report on the aspirin component of the ongoing Physicians' Health Study. N Engl J Med 321: 129, 1989

104. Stern DM, Nawroth PP: Modulation of endothelial cell hemostatic properties by tumor necrosis factor. J Exp Med 153:740, 1986

105. Stroke Prevention in Atrial Fibrillation Investigators: Warfarin versus aspirin for prevention of thromboembolism in atrial fibrillation: Stroke Prevention in Atrial Fibrillation II study. Lancet 343:687, 1994

106. Szeczklik A, Krzanowski M, Gora P, Radwan J: Antiplatelet drugs and generation of thrombin in clotting blood. Blood 80:2006, 1992

107. Szeczeklik A, Musial J, Undas A et al: Aspirin inhibits thrombinogenesis in normocholesterolemic but not in hypercholesterolemic man. Thomb Haemost 69:798, 1993

108. Tcheng JE, Harrigton RA, Kottke-Marchant K et al for the IMPACT investigators: Multicenter, randomized, double-blind, placebo-controlled trial of the platelet integrin glycoprotein IIb/IIIa blocker Integrelin in elective coronary intervention. Circulation 91:2151, 1995

109. Theroux P, Kouz, D, Knudtson ML: A randomized double-blind controlled trial with the non-peptide platelet GP IIb/IIIa antagonist R044–9883 in unstable angina. Circulation 90:I-232, 1994

110. Tofler GH, Brezinski D, Schafer AI et al: Concurrent morning increase in platelet aggregability and the risk of myocardial infarction and sudden cardiac death. N Engl J Med 316:1514, 1987

111. Tohgi H, Konno S, Tamura K et al: Effect of low-to-high doses of aspirin on platelet aggregability and metabolites of thromboxane A2 and prostacyclin. Stroke 23:1400, 1993

112. Topol EJ, Califf RM, Weisman HF et al: Randomized trial of coronary intervention with antibody against platelet IIb/IIIa integrin for reduction of clinical restenosis: results at six months. Lancet 343:881, 1994

113. Turpie AGG, Gent M, Laupacis A et al: A comparison of aspirin with placebo in patients treated with warfarin after heart-valve replacement. N Engl J Med 329:524, 1993

114. Uchiyama S, Yamazaki M, Maruyama S et al: Shear induced platelet aggregation in cerebral ischemia. Stroke 25:1547, 1994

115. Vandeplassche G, Hermans C, Somers Y et al: Combined thromboxane A2 synthase inhibition and prostaglandin endoperoxide receptor antagonism limits myocardial infarct size after mechanical coronary occlusion and reperfusion at doses enhancing coronary thrombolysis by streptokinase. J Am Coll Cardiol 21:1269, 1993

116. Vane JR: Inhibition of prostaglandin synthesis as a mechanism of action for aspirin-like drugs. Nature 231:232, 1971

117. van Gijn J, Algra A: Ticlopidine, trials and torture. Stroke 25:1097, 1994

118. van Kooten F, Ciabattoni G, Patrono C et al: Evidence for episodic platelet activation in acute ischemic stroke. Stroke 25:278, 1994

119. Wardlaw JM, Warlow CP, Counsell C. Systematic review of evidence on thrombolytic therapy for acute ischemic stroke. Lancet 350:607, 1997

120. Weisberg LA: The efficacy and safety of ticlopidine and aspirin in non-whites: analysis of a patient subgroup from the Ticlopidine Aspirin Stroke Study. Neurology 43:27, 1993

121. Weksler BB, Kent JL, Rudolph D et al: Effects of low dose aspirin on platelet function in patients with recent cerebral ischemia. Stroke 16:5, 1985

122. Weksler BB, Tack-Goldman K, Subramanian VA, Gay WA Jr: Cumulative inhibitory effect of low dose aspirin on vascular prostacyclin and platelet thromboxane production in patients with atherosclerosis. Circulation 71: 332, 1985

123. Yao S-K, Ober JC, Krishnaswami A et al: Endogenous nitric oxide protects against platelet aggregation and cyclic flow variations in stenosed and endothelium-injured arteries. Circulation 86:1302, 1992

124. Zwaginga JJ, Sixma JJ, DeGroot PG: Activation of endothelial cells induces platelet thrombus formation on their matrix. Arteriosclerosis 10:49, 1990

Antithrombotic Therapy in Diseases of the Cerebral Vasculature

HENRY J.M. BARNETT

HEATHER E. MELDRUM

MICHAEL ELIASZIW

Most vascular strokes are accompanied by thrombosis, with or without an embolic component. It was natural that the discovery and introduction of agents that alter coagulation—heparin and Warfarin—would stimulate attempts to use them for the prevention and treatment of ischemic strokes. Three decades after these anticoagulants were discovered, a new series of drugs was identified that affects the process of thrombosis by altering platelet aggregation, and these drugs have also been evaluated in stroke prevention.

This chapter examines the rapid progress that has been made in determining the role of the antithrombotic strategies in stroke prevention and reviews what has been learned of their value in patients with recent strokes. The disciplined randomized clinical trial has replaced the flawed methods of reaching therapeutic conclusions from anecdotal observations or from case-series using historical controls. Conclusive evidence from clinical trials has become available in a number of areas of stroke prevention. Within the foreseeable future, the complete spectrum of usefulness of anticoagulants and of platelet inhibitors should come into sharp focus.

Anticoagulants

Anticoagulants have been investigated in several circumstances: transient ischemic attacks (TIAs) and nondisabling strokes of atherothrombotic origin, progressing stroke, com-

pleted stroke, cardiogenic stroke, and other uncommon conditions. Some of these conditions have been investigated with appropriately strict trial methodology. Others still await such rigorous investigation.

TRANSIENT ISCHEMIC ATTACKS AND NONDISABLING STROKE

The efficacy and usefulness of anticoagulants remain uncertain in the prevention of stroke in patients with TIAs or nondisabling stroke resulting from atherothrombotic disease in the major cerebral arteries.

A few small, randomized studies were conducted in the 1950s and 1960s, and an aggregate of 185 patients drawn from four studies, totaling 90 in the treated category and 95 in the control category, was studied for an average of 19 and 21 months, respectively.[9,10,11,67] During this time, 18 strokes occurred, 10 in the placebo group and 8 in the warfarin-treated groups. Death was more frequent in the warfarin-treated than in the placebo groups (15 versus 10); cerebral hemorrhage was the explanation for the increased risk of death in the warfarin-treated group. These early randomized evaluations were flawed in many ways. The major faults resulted from the immaturity of the disciplined design and execution of clinical trials: the entry characteristics were not precise by today's standards; a variety of ischemic events of varying pathogenesis undoubtedly were included; definition and evaluation of end points were vague; the mix of patients represented a mixture of atherothrombotic and cardiogenic stroke; imperfect attention was paid to risk factors, particularly hypertension; strict concern was not shown for compliance and contaminating therapy; there was inadequate strictness of follow-up, and avoidance of crossover. All of these factors were reported in less detail than would be demanded today, and the dose was not regulated as well as required by today's standards. No attempt was made to blind the investigators. The most obvious flaws were in the sample size: by modern biostatistical calculations, the aggregate of patients entered into all the anticoagulant studies represents a sampling that falls short of the ideal by approximately 95%.[86]

No modern trial of appropriate size has specifically been designed to address the efficacy of anticoagulants in TIA or nondisabling stroke presumed to be arising in the cerebral arteries. This is remarkable in view of the fact that warfarin has been employed empirically for 50 years with varying degrees of enthusiasm for symptoms in the carotid and vertebral-basilar artery territories. A few small trials, too small to give important answers, have compared anticoagulants and aspirin.

One of the contemporary ongoing trials in acute stroke is randomizing a subset of patients with TIA, provided they have computed tomography (CT) evidence of a brain infarction in the territory of the symptoms.[94] This study will shed some light on the enigma of Warfarin in TIA due to large artery disease. The results may not be generalizable. A retrospective study from seven centers of 151 patients with ischemic events resulting from stenosis of the internal carotid artery reported fewer major vascular events including strokes in those patients treated with Warfarin than with aspirin.[30] A randomized trial called Warfarin versus Aspirin in Symptomatic Intracranial Disease (WASID) planned as a sequel to these observations will provide definitive answers (Chimowitz M, personal communication, 1997). Again, it will be focused on a very specific entity, and the generalizability of the findings will be uncertain.

In conclusion, it is reasonable to recommend for the time being that patients with TIA or nondisabling stroke resulting from atherothrombotic disease of the carotid or vertebral basilar arteries be given warfarin when platelet antiaggregants fail to reduce the ischemic attacks or are not tolerated and when carotid endarterectomy is not indicated. This pragmatic approach can be justified when clinical trials are not available and the patients in question are threatened with serious and distressing illness such as disabling stroke.

PROGRESSING STROKE (STROKE IN EVOLUTION)

Common practice considers that heparin followed by warfarin is indicated if observation provides clear evidence of recognizable worsening of an ischemic neurologic disability.[10,29] This practice has been based on incomplete and largely anecdotal data. Many of the reports have not included a strict definition of progressing stroke. Adding to the confusion of decision-making in this condition is the inability to determine, in a particular patient with progressing stroke, the cause of the progression. The incidence of progressing stroke needs to be clarified; the pathogenesis requires further study.

Diagnostic tests to clarify the mechanism of stroke progres-

sion in any given patient are imperfect. Stroke in evolution is by no means synonymous with thrombosis in evolution. If a subgroup could be identified with exactitude in which progressing thrombus formation or thromboembolic phenomena were recognizable by objective study, the rationale for a trial of anticoagulant therapy would be on firm ground. Progression of a stroke in a stepwise fashion is easier to regard as a stroke due to repeated episodes of thromboembolism than is an indolently progressive stroke. Patients exhibiting stepwise progression may speculatively be considered as likely to benefit from anticoagulation. Conversely, patients who are adding to their neurologic deficit in a nonstepwise progressing fashion probably are not exhibiting continuing thrombus formation. Accumulation of excitatory neurotoxins probably accounts for most of the progression in this common situation. The edema and the herniations resulting from this ischemic cascade are identifiable by CT examination. Neurotoxin accumulation and brain edema will not be expected to respond to anticoagulants. Until effective measures are available to correct the cellular and molecular abnormalities accompanying ischemia, many patients with an infarction, whether edematous or not, will continue to experience this type of worsening for several days after an ictus.

Before considering any treatment for the progressing stroke patient, a CT examination is essential. The examination will identify the presence of substantial edema and ensure the recognition of intracerebral hemorrhage: hemorrhagic infarction and intracerebral hematoma. Intracerebral hemorrhage undoubtedly often went unrecognized in the past and contaminated the early studies of anticoagulant therapy administered for progressing stroke patients.

Two studies of later date, one randomized, one observational, have been neither conclusive nor encouraging in regard to the indications for anticoagulants in progressing stroke. The randomized trial involved 225 patients with recent onset of ischemic stroke.[34] As many patients went on to progress in the heparin-treated group as in the placebo group. In the observational trial, half of the 36 patients with progressing symptoms deteriorated despite receiving heparin.[49]

The use of heparin followed by Warfarin in patients with progressing stroke is an empirical strategy. It is a reasonable, but not a proven therapy. Once initiated, the duration of anticoagulant therapy is unknown. A few weeks is a rational period because this is the time when worsening is common. The dangers of anticoagulants influence the recommendation that warfarin should be used only for a limited time. In some patients with progressing stroke, antifibrinolysins will be considered before anticoagulant therapy.

COMPLETED STROKE

Making the distinction between a progressing stroke and a completed stroke may be difficult. If no worsening occurs over several hours, the term "completed stroke" is in general use.

Anticoagulants serve no purpose and certainly carry a decided risk after a large infarction has produced a disabling stroke.[42] It is known, however, that a patient with a more modest ischemic disability of recent origin could subsequently experience a more damaging and disabling additional infarction. The WARSS trial is designed to determine differential benefit between Warfarin and aspirin in patients who have suffered an ischemic stroke within 30 days.[94] The results of this study will be available in 1999.

The large International Stroke Trial (IST) recruited 19,436 patients who had experienced a stroke within 48 hours of commencing therapy and compared the benefit of aspirin, low-dose heparin, or medium-dose heparin in a factorial design.[76] Results suggest no significant benefit for heparin in reducing deaths within 14 days or for reducing early recurrence of stroke. The low-dose heparin regimen was ineffective and the medium dose was hazardous because of intracranial and major extracranial hemorrhage. Aspirin given to 9,674 individuals and 9,657 controls yielded an absolute reduction of deaths of 3 per 1,000 patients and of recurrent stroke of 7 per 1,000.[55]

Low-molecular-weight heparin was tested in a randomized trial of 312 patients within 48 hours of an ischemic stroke.[56] Despite the fact that the high-dose group, the low-dose group, and the placebo group did not show differences at 10 days, the number who died or were dependent at 6 months was 65% in the placebo group, 52% in the low-dose group, and 45% in the high-dose group. This result is encouraging from a well-designed and well-conducted study, but confirmation from another trial is needed.

In the early stages of the development of cerebral ischemia, the distinction between a stroke in evolution and a completed stroke is often uncertain. In the era of recognized benefit from tPA as an antifibrinolysin, patients with stroke in evolution must be evaluated as potential candidates for this therapy (see Ch. 51). Even though worsening is apparent if the ischemic symptoms are of less than 3 hour duration, they may still be candidates for tPA. If tPA proves not to be indicated, the guidelines for a progressing stroke or a completed stroke will be applicable.

THROMBI VISIBLE IN EXTRACRANIAL CEREBRAL ARTERIES AND CAROTID STUMPS

Patients under investigation for TIA or partial stroke commonly are submitted to angiography. On infrequent occasions, a thrombus is seen in the carotid or vertebral arteries appropri-

Figure 46.1 (**A**) A thrombus (arrow) streaming up an internal carotid artery beyond stenosis of terminal common carotid and proximal internal carotid artery segments. External carotid artery is occluded. (**B**) The same patient with simultaneous occurrence of thrombus (arrow) in cavernous sinus portion of the internal carotid artery. The patient received anticoagulation therapy, had no further ischemic events, and refused further investigation. (Fig. A from Barnett et al,[15] with permission.)

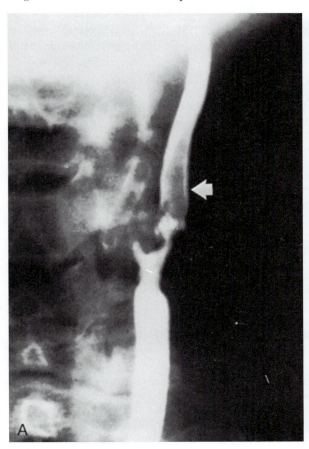
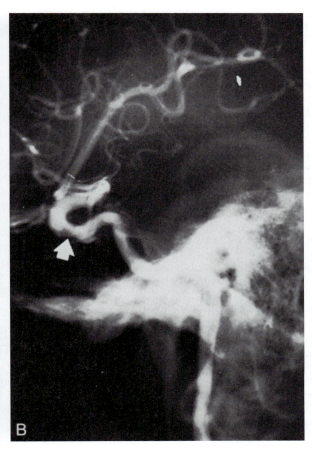

ate to the ischemic events. Many of the recognized examples have been detected in association with tight stenoses of the involved arteries. Animal studies have demonstrated that thrombus develops beyond experimental arterial stenosis.[46] On the other hand, patients may have no detectable underlying disease in the artery containing the thrombus. Systemic disorders or the use of drugs and other substances, including the contraceptive pill, which alter coagulation account for most of the intra-arterial thrombi visualized in otherwise normal arteries.[13]

Some regard the finding of an intraluminal thrombus as an indication for emergency endarterectomy. This is an uncertain strategy for a variety of reasons. There is an increased hazard in the management of this condition by thromboendarterectomy. Of 29 patients recognized with thrombus in the extracranial portion of stenosed carotid arteries, a worsening of the previous ischemic deficit was detected in 25% of those submitted to urgent surgery.[24] No worsening was seen in those receiving anticoagulant or platelet antiaggregant therapy alone. Four other reports of small series of intraluminal thrombi have corroborated the fact that this is a dangerous lesion and that the perioperative complication rate is between 18 and 25%.[21,45,59,68] The surgical creation of a denuded endothelium over a long extent of the artery and the operative release of thromboplastin may add to the possibility of further and extending thrombosis. There are examples where thrombus is visible in the artery in the neck coexisting with thrombus within the cavernous portion of the same internal carotid artery (Fig. 46.1). Any attempt to remove the thrombus from the neck will not improve the likelihood of lysis of the intracranial thrombus. It is improbable that a thrombotic tendency with a so-called hypercoagulable state will benefit from the isolated surgical removal of one thrombus located in an otherwise normal artery. It is known that such thrombi are subject to spontaneous lysis; disappearance of thrombi in these locations have been observed to occur on a number of occasions without progression of the neurologic deficit. This observation has been made on patients with and without stenosing lesions.

The empirical recommendation for patients in whom a thrombus is radiologically visible in an extracranial artery is for 4 to 6 weeks of anticoagulant therapy, beginning with heparin and proceeding with the simultaneous and subsequent administration of Warfarin. When the international normalized ratio (INR) is at acceptable levels, the heparin will be discontinued. In patients with a thrombus beyond carotid stenosis, after 4 to 6 weeks of anticoagulation therapy, a repeat angiogram should be performed as a prelude to the carotid endarterectomy. In those with systemic or iatrogenic disorders, the decision to continue anticoagulation treatment will be dependent upon the ability of the physician to alter these abnormal coagulation processes.

A variant of the situation in which intraluminal thrombi are visualized in the stenosed internal carotid artery occurs when such clots are identified in the "stump" of the totally occluded internal carotid artery[14] (Fig. 46.2). Thrombi in the stump may be carried up in the collateral channels supplying the brain through the external carotid artery. These lesions are an uncommon but proven cause of ischemic events beyond an artery known to be occluded.

The recognition of these thrombi present two difficulties. First, because a stump is common, occurring in two-thirds of

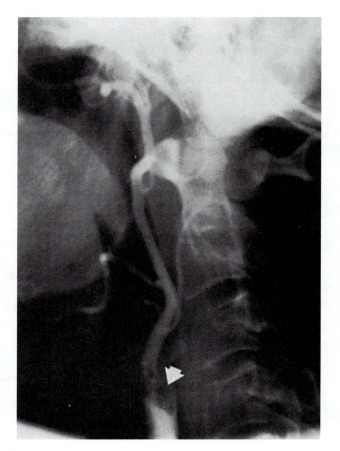

Figure 46.2 Thrombus within "stump" of internal carotid artery (arrow). Some thrombus visible in irregular lumen of external carotid artery.

the patients who have occluded an internal carotid artery, it is important to be as certain as possible that the stump is not incidental but is the cause of the continuing ischemic events in a given patient. Second, the angiographic visualization of thrombus may be very difficult, and its existence is no more than by inference when an irregular stump or a stump with changing length or shape, or a stump with a central shadow intruding into the contrast, suggests the presence of a thrombus. When the stump syndrome was recognized initially, it was recommended that patients with these findings should be considered for stump obliteration.[14] Subsequent experience has identified this as a high-risk procedure. A total of 4 to 6 months of anticoagulant treatment, followed by an indefinite period of aspirin treatment, is preferred.[16,83]

CEREBRAL VEIN AND SINUS THROMBOSIS

Cerebral vein and sinus thrombosis has been dealt with completely in Chapter 24. The original recommendation for therapy was to avoid anticogulants because of the nature of the infarction found in these patients. Subsequent case-series and a randomized trial have proven this speculation to be erroneous. Patients treated with heparin have a lower mortality rate and experience fewer instances of progressing disability than those not treated with heparin. Progression of the ischemic process in these patients, unlike arterial lesions producing infarction, appears to be due to progressive thrombogenesis.

CARDIOEMBOLIC STROKE

The use of anticoagulants for cardioembolic stroke is covered in Chapter 48.

SUMMARY

A summary of the recommended uses for anticoagulants in cardiac and noncardiac disorders is presented in Table 46.1. Most of the indications are based on empirical decisions not supported by randomized studies. All have been discussed above except for the coagulation abnormalities (Ch. 44), venous and sinus disease (Ch. 24) and cerebral emboli from pulmonary vein thrombosis. The latter is a rare complication of severe chest trauma or pulmonary sepsis. When this condition is clinically identified, anticoagulants are indicated until the primary process is controlled. Anticoagulants for patients with cerebral ischemic events related to cardiac conditions are discussed in Chapter 48, but the recommendations are summarized in Table 46.1.

Platelet Antiaggregants

A description of the physiology, pathophysiology, and pharmacologic responses of the platelets is given in Chapter 45.

Interest in platelet antiaggregants in stroke prevention began at about the time that the intensive search for the pathogenesis of transient cerebral and retinal ischemic events had narrowed to define the two causative mechanisms: those of a hemodynamic nature and those related to thromboembolic events. For the latter, the more common mechanism, the platelet inhibitor appeared as an important therapeutic prospect. Studies of platelet physiology were focusing attention on the importance of the platelet in initiation of thrombosis in fast-flowing arterial systems. Experimental studies determined that the platelets adhered to irregular surfaces, discharged their contents, and thereby triggered aggregation with the attraction of other platelets, the addition of fibrin, and the formation of a whitish-gray platelet-fibrin thrombus. Clinical observations were made of material passing through the retinal arterioles in a few patients with monocular amaurosis fugax, and it was hypothesized that the material was platelet-fibrin in nature.[41,48] Eventually, by fortuitous postmortem study, this speculation was proved to be correct.[8] Such material has since been observed at surgical procedures, passing through cortical branches of the middle cerebral artery at craniotomy (Fig. 46.3).

Nonsteriodal anti-inflammatory drugs that alter platelet function were identified: within 2 years, sulfinpyrazone, aspi-

Table 46.1 Recommended Use of Anticoagulants in Cerebral Vascular Disease

Indication	Basis of Recommendation	Heparin	Warfarin	Duration of Warfarin	Remarks
Nonvalvular atrial fibrillation	7 randomized trials	Not recommended	INR 2.0–3.0	Indefinite	Mandatory age 60–75; exceptions apply <60 years and >75 years
Thrombi left ventricle	Single randomized trial, Many case-series	Initially	INR 2.0–3.0	3–6 months	Longer duration if fibrillation develops
Rheumatic valve disease	Case-series	Not recommended	INR 2.0–3.0	Indefinite	Convincing historical controls
Prosthetic heart valves	Small randomized trials, Case-series	Not recommended	INR 2.5–3.5	Indefinite	Mandatory with mechanical discretionary with bioprosthetic
Cerebral vein and sinus thrombosis	Small randomized trial, Case-series	Initially	INR 2.0–3.0	3 months	Despite hemorrhagic nature of infarcts
Thrombi in cerebral arteries, in symptomatic "stumps" of ICA	Case-series	Initially	INR 2.0–3.0	1 month	Follow with ASA 650–975 mgm
Recurrent ischemic events despite platelet inhibitors	Case reports	Not recommended	INR 3.0–3.5	3 months	No good data Use and duration empirical
Progressing stroke	Single negative randomized trial, Case-series	Not recommended	INR 2.5–3.5	1 month	Data not convincing
Pulmonary vein thrombosis	Case reports	Not recommended	INR 2.0–3.5	1 month	Complication of chest injuries and infection

Abbreviations: ICA, internal carotid artery; INR, international normalized ratio.

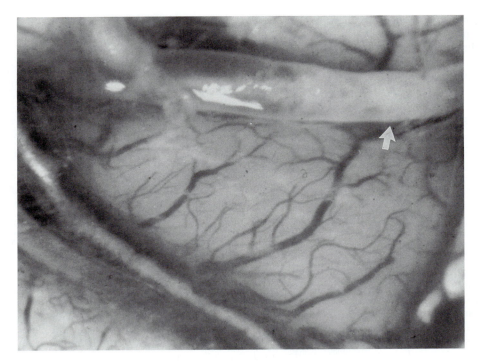

Figure 46.3 White platelet-fibrin material (arrow) in the cortical branch of the middle cerebral artery flowing from left to right and exposed at craniotomy in a patient undergoing superficial anastomosis between the temporal and middle cerebral arteries. The patient had symptoms related to intracranial stenosis of the internal carotid artery. The platelet-fibrin origin of some transient ischemic attacks in the hemisphere due to proximal major vascular disease is confirmed by such chance observations. ($\times$ 10.) (Photograph provided by Dr. H. Reichman, Loyola University.) (From Barnett et al,[17] with permission.)

rin, and dipyridamole were all discovered to have such properties.[37,62,79,96] Their mechanisms of action differed, but all were submitted to experimental evaluation in situations involving arterial thrombosis. They appeared to be worthy of clinical studies in patients with stroke-threatening symptoms. The initial anecdotal observations, made in patients with frequent recurrent events of amaurosis fugax, with and without thrombocytosis, were exciting and led to clinical trials.[12,50]

The first clinical trial involved a heterogeneous group of patients, probably with a variety of pathogenic mechanisms.[1] It included 169 patients with transient cerebral ischemia (TIA) and stroke, used dipyridamole in moderate and then in large daily dosage, but showed negative results after an average of 25 months of treatment.

The first trial launched to evaluate aspirin against placebo in stroke prevention in TIA and nondisabling stroke patients was designed in 1970 and began in 1971. The trial was a factorial design and in the two arms which included aspirin, a benefit in stroke and death was observed. The benefit was only detected in males (Fig. 46.4). By modern standards, this seminal aspirin trial did not enter a sufficient numbers of patients to allow any credible subgroup analyses. The lack of female responsiveness, not observed in subsequent trials, is most likely explained by the fact that only 200 women were studied. Not recognized until later was the fact that women with TIA and nondisabling stroke are at lower risk than men. Ideally the study should have included more women than men.[35]

Six platelet inhibiting drugs have been subjected to clinical trials in patients with TIA or stroke of noncardiac origin: dipyridamole, aspirin, sulfinpyrazone, suloctidil, ticlopidine, and clopidogrel.[1,5,22,23,28,38,40,43,44,47,52,57,75,80,84,90] Sulfinpyrazone, suloctidil, and possibly dipyridamole are of no value in stroke prevention. Trials testing for benefit of combinations of sulfinpyrazone or dipyridamole with aspirin did not detect significant benefit for the combination over that of aspirin alone.[17]

The data on the benefit from platelet inhibition in stroke reduction are definite. Meta-analyses, not including ticlopidine or clopidogrel, but involving more than 100,000 patients in 145 clinical trials, have examined the benefit of platelet inhibitors in patients with all vascular disorders prone to occlusive events.[6] Vascular events were reduced 25%. In patients with previous nondisabling strokes or TIAs, the odds reduction was 22% for vascular events and 23% for nonfatal strokes.

A meta-analysis was performed of all trials in which aspirin alone was compared with placebo in patients with TIA or nondisabling, noncardiac strokes. The outcome events were stroke, fatal stroke, or death from a vascular cause; nonfatal myocardial infarctions were not counted.[17] Unlike previous meta-analyses, this review was confined to patients presenting with cerebral ischemic events. It was reasoned that an agent that is effective in reducing the risk of myocardial infarction due to coronary artery disease may not be equally effective in reducing the risk of stroke due to cerebral artery disease.

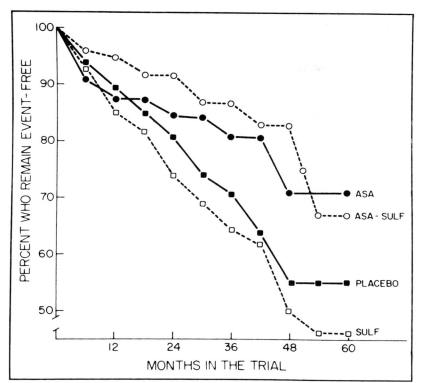

Figure 46.4 Lack of benefit of sulfinpyrazone, benefit of ASA ($p < 0.005$) and lack of synergism or antagonism of combination in male patients. (From the Canadian Medical Association Journal, with permission.)[26]

Differences are known to be present in the vascular reactivity and thrombus formation in various circulatory beds.[7,65,88]

From this group of patients, no single trial determined that aspirin alone in high doses (900 to 1,300 mg daily) or low doses (75 to 300 mg daily) was significantly more effective than placebo in preventing strokes in this group of patients (Fig. 46.5). The trend was towards benefit in all of these trials, although the overall reduction in the relative risk of stroke associated with high-dose or low-dose aspirin was modest. Aspirin combined with dipyridamole or sulfinpyrazone was significantly more effective than placebo, but there was no difference between combined therapy and aspirin alone (Fig. 46.6).

These indirect comparisons raise the question of a possible synergistic effect between aspirin and other antiplatelet agents, but meta-analyses cannot directly test for a statistically significant drug interaction. A large randomized trial should be conducted to establish the role of aspirin combined with other platelet inhibitors and the optimal dose of aspirin in patients with TIAs or strokes of arterial origin.

Ticlopidine

Ticlopidine is an effective platelet inhibitor that reduces the risk of stroke in TIA and ischemic stroke patients. It inhibits platelet aggregation by a different mechanism than aspirin. It acts by altering the platelet membrane and interfering with the membrane-fibrinogen interaction and thereby blocks the platelet glycoprotein IIb/IIIa receptors.[33,74] Unlike aspirin, where the maximal effect occurs after 20 minutes, ticlopidine's effect is maximal at 24 to 48 hours. Bleeding time is more prolonged than with aspirin and normalizes within 1 week.

Ticlopidine has been evaluated in two stroke-threatened populations: 3,069 patients with TIA or recent nondisabling stroke were given 250 mg of ticlopidine twice daily or aspirin 1,300 mg daily by random assignment in the Ticlopidine Aspirin Stroke Study (TASS).[52] The risk of nonfatal stroke or death from any cause at 3 years was 17% in the ticlopidine group and 19% in the aspirin group (relative risk reduction with ticlopidine 12%, absolute reduction 2%). The 3-year risk of fatal or nonfatal stroke was 10% in the ticlopidine and 13% in the aspirin groups, respectively, for a relative risk reduction of 21% and an absolute risk reduction of 3% favoring ticlopidine.

In the Canadian-American Ticlopidine Study (CATS), 1,072 patients were given, by random assignment, either 250 mg of ticlopidine twice daily or placebo.[44] Patients were required to have experienced a major stroke within 1 to 16 weeks prior to entering the trial. A relative risk reduction of 30% favored ticlopidine when the combined yearly rates of stroke, myocardial infarction, and deaths from vascular causes were analyzed. These combined outcomes occurred in 15% of the placebo group and 11% of the ticlopidine group. This was the first trial in which entry did not include patients with only TIA. Exclusive benefit attributable to ticlopidine for patients with stroke has been claimed. This is a misleading claim. It overlooks the fact that many of the aspirin trials included patients with strokes as well as with TIA. Both the ticlopidine and the aspirin trials involved patients whose stroke was not sufficiently disabling to prevent return visits to clinics.

The side effects of ticlopidine range from inconvenient to

Trial Name	Dose* (mg)	Sample Size†	Strokes‡ (n)	Strokes & VD§ (n)	Stroke RR Reduction¶	Stroke & VD RR Reduction	Stroke RR Reduction (CI)	Stroke & VD RR Reduction (CI)
(A) HIGH DOSE ASPIRIN versus PLACEBO								
AITIA[40]	A: 1300	A: 88 *(126)*	11	13	34%	39%		
		P: 90 *(106)*	14	18				
Canadian[25]	A: 1300	A: 144 *(312)*	22	26	- 6%	11%		
		P: 139 *(300)*	20	28				
French[47]	A: 900	A: 147 *(368)*	8	*11*	23%	28%		
		P: 155 *(388)*	*11*	*16*				
AICLA[22]	A: 990	A: 198 *(486)*	17	20	42%	37%		
		P: 204 *(517)*	31	34				
Danish Co-op[80]	A: 1000	A: 101 *(210)*	17	20	-57%	-28%		
		P: 102 *(213)*	11	16				
Swedish Co-op[84]	A: 1500	A: 253 *(506)*	32	51	1%	- 8%		
		P: 252 *(504)*	32	47				
UK-TIA[90]	A: 1200	A: 815 *(3428)*	101	*156*	11%	6%		
		P: 814 *(3581)*	119	*173*				
Overall¥					11%	9%		
(B) LOW DOSE ASPIRIN versus PLACEBO								
SALT[75]	A: 75	A: 676 *(1724)*	93	125	16%	17%		
		P: 684 *(1734)*	112	152				
UK-TIA[90]	A: 300	A: 806 *(3516)*	100	*154*	14%	9%		
		P: 814 *(3581)*	119	*173*				
Overall#					15%	13%		

-100 -50 0 50 100   -100 -50 0 50 100

Aspirin Worse — Aspirin Better   Aspirin Worse — Aspirin Better

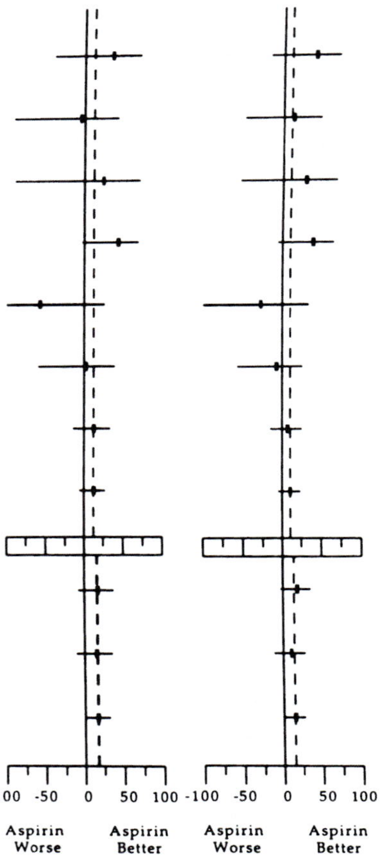

* A = Aspirin. P = Placebo.
† Number of subjects per group *(Estimated person-years of follow-up)*.
‡ Includes all fatal and non-fatal strokes. *Figures in italics are estimates.*
§ VD = Vascular death.
¶ A negative number indicates an increase in risk.
¥ 95% CI: Overall stroke (-7% to 26%), p-value = 0.205; Overall stroke & VD (-6% to 22%), p-value = 0.230.
95% CI: Overall stroke (-2% to 30%), p-value = 0.079; Overall stroke & VD (-1% to 26%), p-value = 0.076.
Test for heterogeneity among the RR reductions in each analysis was statistically non-significant. All p-values are two-tailed.

Figure 46.5 Reduction in the relative risk of the combined outcome of fatal or nonfatal stroke and death from a vascular cause associated with high-dose or low-dose aspirin as compared with placebo in patients with transient ischemic attacks or stroke of noncardiac origin. High doses of aspirin ranged from 900 mg to 1,300 mg/day, and low doses from 75 mg to 300 mg/day. Each tick mark represents the reduction in the relative risk of stroke or vascular death, and each horizontal line the corresponding 95% confidence interval. The broken vertical lines represent the overall relative-risk reduction. The overall reduction in the relative risk associated with high-dose aspirin was 11% (95% confidence interval, −7 to 26; P = 0.20) for stroke and 9% (95% confidence interval, −6 to 22; P = 0.23) for stroke or vascular death. The overall reduction in the relative risk associated with low-dose aspirin was 15% (95% confidence interval, −1 to 26; P = 0.08) for stroke and 13% (95% confidence interval, −1 to 26; P = 0.08) for stroke or vascular death. A negative number indicates an increase in risk. All values are two-tailed. The result of a test for heterogeneity in the relative-risk reduction for each group of trials was not statistically significant. The numbers in parentheses are estimated person-years of follow-up. AITIA denotes Aspirin in Transient Ischemic Attacks trial, A aspirin, P placebo, AICLA Accidents Ischémiques Cérébraux Liés l'Atherosclerose, UK-TIA United Kingdom Transient Ischaemic Attack trial, and SALT Swedish Aspirin Low-Dose Trial. (From Barnett et al,[17] with permission.)

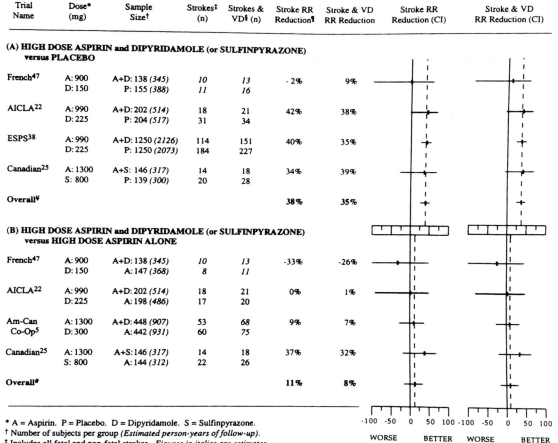

Trial Name	Dose* (mg)	Sample Size†	Strokes‡ (n)	Strokes & VD§ (n)	Stroke RR Reduction¶	Stroke & VD RR Reduction	Stroke RR Reduction (CI)	Stroke & VD RR Reduction (CI)
(A) HIGH DOSE ASPIRIN and DIPYRIDAMOLE (or SULFINPYRAZONE) versus PLACEBO								
French[47]	A: 900 D: 150	A+D: 138 (345) P: 155 (388)	10 11	13 16	− 2%	9%		
AICLA[22]	A: 990 D: 225	A+D: 202 (514) P: 204 (517)	18 31	21 34	42%	38%		
ESPS[38]	A: 990 D: 225	A+D: 1250 (2126) P: 1250 (2073)	114 184	151 227	40%	35%		
Canadian[25]	A: 1300 S: 800	A+S: 146 (317) P: 139 (300)	14 20	18 28	34%	39%		
Overall¥					38%	35%		
(B) HIGH DOSE ASPIRIN and DIPYRIDAMOLE (or SULFINPYRAZONE) versus HIGH DOSE ASPIRIN ALONE								
French[47]	A: 900 D: 150	A+D: 138 (345) A: 147 (368)	10 8	13 11	−33%	−26%		
AICLA[22]	A: 990 D: 225	A+D: 202 (514) A: 198 (486)	18 17	21 20	0%	1%		
Am-Can Co-Op[5]	A: 1300 D: 300	A+D: 448 (907) A: 442 (931)	53 60	68 75	9%	7%		
Canadian[25]	A: 1300 S: 800	A+S: 146 (317) A: 144 (312)	14 22	18 26	37%	32%		
Overall#					11%	8%		

* A = Aspirin. P = Placebo. D = Dipyridamole. S = Sulfinpyrazone.
† Number of subjects per group *(Estimated person-years of follow-up)*.
‡ Includes all fatal and non-fatal strokes. *Figures in italics are estimates.*
§ VD = Vascular death.
¶ A negative number indicates an increase in risk.
¥ 95% CI: Overall stroke (24% to 49%), p-value = 0.000002; Overall stroke & VD (22% to 45%), p-value < 0.000001.
95% CI: Overall stroke (-17% to 32%), p-value = 0.418; Overall stroke & VD (-17% to 28%), p-value = 0.479.
Test for heterogeneity among the RR reductions in each analysis was statistically non-significant. All p-values are two-tailed.

Figure 46.6 Reduction in the relative risk of the combined outcome of fatal or nonfatal stroke and death from a vascular cause associated with high-dose aspirin and dipyridamole (or sulfinpyrazone) as compared with placebo or high-dose aspirin alone in patients with transient ischemic attacks or strokes of noncardiac origin. The doses used were 900 mg to 1,300 mg/day of aspirin, 150 mg to 300 mg/day of dipyridamole, and 800 mg/day of sulfinpyrazone. Each tick mark represents the reduction in the relative risk of stroke or vascular death, and each horizontal line the corresponding 95% confidence interval. The broken vertical lines represent the overall relative-risk reduction. The overall relative-risk reduction associated with high-dose aspirin and dipyridamole as compared with placebo was 38% (95% confidence interval, 24 to 49; $p < 0.001$) for stroke and 35% (95% confidence interval, 22 to 45; $p < 0.001$) for stroke or vascular death; the overall relative-risk reduction associated with high-dose aspirin and dipyridamole as compared with high-dose aspirin alone was 11% (95% confidence interval, − 17 to 32; P = 0.42) for stroke and 8% (95% confidence interval, − 17 to 28; P = 0.42) for stroke or vascular death. A negative number indicates an increase in risk. All P values are two-tailed. The result of a test for heterogeneity in the relative-risk reduction for each group of trials was not statistically significant. The numbers in parentheses are estimated person-years of follow-up. A denotes aspirin, D dipyridamole, P placebo, AICLA Accidents Ischémiques Cérébraux Liés l'Atherosclerose, ESPS European Stroke Prevention Study, S sulfinpyrazone and ACCS American-Canadian Co-operative Study. (From Barnett et al,[17] with permission.)

disastrous. Approximately 5% of patients stop therapy because of persistent diarrhea. Transient diarrhea is more common and was encountered in 22% of the patients in CATS. Rash was twice as common in the TASS trial with ticlopidine as with aspirin. Bone marrow suppression during the trials was always reversible with the cessation of the drug. Neutropenia in both trials was reported at about 1%. Subsequently, the situation has not been so optimistic. Of the 640 instances of bone marrow suppression reported to the manufacturers of ticlopidine, 16% had fatal outcomes.[18,64,78] Some of these patients, monitored in the recommended manner after the institution of therapy, were found early to have suppressed bone marrow function, but failed to respond to appropriate therapy.

Unsettled Issues in the Use of Platelet Inhibitors

Aspirin and ticlopidine are effective in stroke prevention. The relative risk reduction of stroke and vascular death varies between 7% and 42%. Translated into absolute risk reduction, their benefit is modest. There are unsettled problems in the use of platelet inhibitors.

THE OPTIMAL DOSE OF ASPIRIN

The earliest trial of aspirin as an antithrombotic drug, the Canadian Aspirin Study, utilized 1,300 mg/day. This dose was selected empirically because no evidence of the mode of action on the platelet enzyme components was known and the concept of an antithrombotic substance generated by the endothelial cell had not been conceived. In time, it became known that the cyclooxygenase enzyme of the platelet was essential to the formation of thromboxane A_2 with the triggering of platelet-generated thrombosis. The same enzyme in the endothelial cell was essential for the formation of prostacyclin, a powerful antiaggregant. Aspirin was found to inhibit cyclooxygenase function and to do so in both the platelet and the endothelial cell, thus interfering with the production of thromboxane A_2 and of prostacyclin. It was hypothesized that the benefit of inhibiting the platelet activity might be overwhelmed by the coincidental inhibition of the endothelial cell function and that larger doses of aspirin would not be as effective as smaller doses and might actually provoke thrombosis and increase the number of clinical events.

This putative increase in the number of clinical events has not been found. It is even possible to speculate that the variability in the relative risk reduction of stroke and vascular death in series of stroke-threatened patients may be dose-related. Series with higher relative risk reduction were taking 975 to 1,300 mg/day, while the lower levels of relative risk reduction were in the series of patients taking less.[36] One thing is certain: there is no evidence to substantiate the postulate that less aspirin is more likely to reduce the risk of stroke than does more aspirin.[27]

Thirty-six randomized trials designed to compare different doses of aspirin against placebo were reviewed and the conclusions were: "For all patients and for subgroups of patients with previous vascular conditions, there was no relationship between dose and vascular events."[27]

Aspirin prolongs the bleeding time and has been associated with bruising, gastrointestinal hemorrhage, wound hematoma, and possibly an increased risk of hemorrhagic infarction. The concern has been that there was a major dose-dependancy for the gastrointestinal hemorrhage. From the randomized trials included in the Anti-Platelet Trialists Collaboration, the pooled odds ratios of gastrointestinal bleeding (hematemesis, meleno), peptic ulcer, and upper gastrointestinal symptoms all varied between 1.3 and 2.0 and were said to be suggestively dose-related. Nevertheless, the conclusion was reached that "there is no significant difference between the three clinical categories (gastrointestinal hemorrhage, ulcer, upper gastrointestinal symptoms) for those taking 1,200 or 300 mg daily." Fatal gastrointestinal hemorrhages were described as "very rare."[73]

Other meta-analyses have been done involving large numbers of patients taking aspirin in clinical trials of cardiac and stroke-threatened patients taking various doses of aspirin for prolonged periods.[27,58] To quote directly from Cappelleri et al, once again from their review of 36 published trials, in what they described as a major metaregression analysis: "For all patients, a dose-response relation was not found with gastrointestinal hemorrhage and hemorrhagic stroke."[27] In the NASCET trial, in which 2,325 patients took varying doses of aspirin (325 up to 1,300 mg per day), neither the incidence of serious wound hematoma at the endarterectomy site nor the incidence of serious gastrointestinal bleeding nor the occurrence of intracerebral hematoma or hemorrhagic infarction was dose-related.[61] (Figs. 46.7 and 46.8). Thus, the second major hypothesis leading to the espousal of a low dose of aspirin has not been proven to be of major consequence when submitted to clinical observation. Three additional considerations further reduce concern about dose-related complication. First, the knowledge that peptic ulcer results from an antibiotic-sensitive organism must not be overlooked. Second, enteric coating of aspirin substantially reduces, although it does not completely eliminate, gastrointestinal blood loss.[77] More important than dose of aspirin in aggravating gastric or duodenal bleeding has been the concurrent use of non-aspirin, nonsteriodal anti-inflammatory drugs.[95]

The question then arises about the importance of picking an optimum dose. Many are content to accept the benefit that a low dose will confer in patients with any type of thrombotic vascular lesion and with the assumption that there are no substantial differences between arterial beds, whether they be coronary, peripheral, or cerebral.[51] Others are convinced that low-dose aspirin is the only appropriate therapeutic strategy.[4,66] These conclusions are difficult to accept at the present time.[19] Many considerations make it safer to conclude that the optimal dose of aspirin for stroke prevention in stroke-threatened patients is not known:

1. There are patients known to be "nonresponders" as measured by platelet function to low dose, some of whom will respond in the higher therapeutic range.[2,53] Platelet aggregation in response to collagen may vary according to the dose of aspirin.[63]

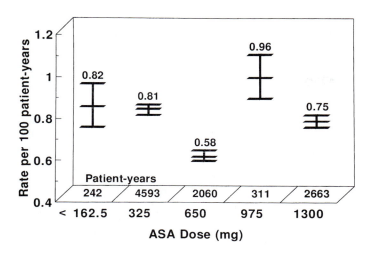

Figure 46.7 Dose-specific rates of bleeding complications as a function of actual patient-year exposure to various dosages of aspirin during follow-up in the NASCET. The upper and lower horizontal lines represent 95% confidence intervals about the rate. The patient-years of exposure are given along the horizontal axis.

2. There are mechanisms other than through the cyclo-oxygenase system whereby aspirin alters thrombus formation and to interfere with some of them, a larger dose is required. The arterial systems are not homogeneously responsive.[7,88]

3. In experimental arterial injury, dose-dependent variations in inhibition of thrombus formation and on the number of emboli and the timing of emboli have been reported.[3,20,54,60,70,72,85,89,91,92,93,97]

4. In the Physician's Health Study, a low-dose regimen (325 mg every other day) was effective in reducing myocardial infarction, but not stroke. Because there were nearly 200 stroke outcome events, it would be improbable that a benefit was present and overlooked. It raises the question of the propriety of equating the effect of aspirin on different arterial systems.

5. The North American Symptomatic Carotid Endarterectomy Trial (NASCET) collaborators reported a fivefold increase in post-endarterectomy strokes in the patients taking 325 mg or less at the time of surgery compared with those taking 650 to 1,300 mg. There is a study now underway to confirm or deny the hypothesis that there is less risk of postop-

erative stroke with moderate- to high-dose aspirin than with low-dose aspirin.[87]

6. If there is a proven therapeutic advantage to a particular dose of aspirin, it should become widely accepted. A daily dose of 325 mg is commonly recommended as the right dose even though scientific data indicating it to be optimum is lacking. Therapeutic trials of new platelet inhibitors or other agents, old or new, deemed capable of reducing the risk of stroke will continue to be against aspirin. To test any preparation against a suboptimal dose of aspirin could misrepresent the value of the alternative agent.

7. In the ESPS-2 trial, dypyridamole was evaluated against a minidose of aspirin (50 mg). The very large International Stroke Trial (IST) evaluated a small dose of aspirin (325 mg daily) against heparin and an ongoing trial Warfarin Aspirin Recurrent Stroke Study (WARSS) is evaluating 325 mg of aspirin against Warfarin. TASS tested ticlopidine against 1,300 mg of aspirin. Unexpectedly, the clopidogrel investigators evaluating the potential successor to ticlopidine decided to use 325 mg of aspirin. The unanswered question is whether or not 50 to 325 mg is the optimal aspirin dose. The problem of the dose of aspirin will haunt the results of studies in which aspirin is the standard until a direct-comparison dose trial of aspirin has established equivalence of low and higher dose in stroke prevention.

Tolerance for aspirin is largely tied to gastrointestinal distress, and there is no doubt that with ordinary aspirin this is dose-related. This dose-related intolerance is greatly ameliorated for most people by the use of an enteric-coated variety of aspirin. This variety of coating has been shown to have the same platelet inhibiting properties as the usual compressed tablet.[39] There is a delay of several hours after initiating therapy in platelet inhibition; thereafter, the activity remains constant. Enteric-coated aspirin is the preparation of first choice.

PLATELET INHIBITORS IN PRIMARY STROKE PREVENTION

Only aspirin has been studied in primary vascular disease prevention. No trial has been designed to determine specifically whether or not there is benefit from platelet inhibitors in

Figure 46.8 Incidence of wound hematomas at the carotid endarterectomy site in the NASCET patients. The number of patients at each of the four doses of aspirin is 607, 245, 29, and 276, respectively.

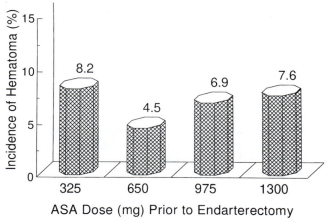

preventing stroke in populations without any evidence of symptomatic vascular disease. The design of the two primary prevention trials that have been completed was ideal to evaluate benefit for myocardial infarction or peripheral vascular disease. The outcome of stroke was reported, but the age of the population studied averaged a decade below that of the average age of occurrence of stroke.

Stroke was not reduced in the two large primary prevention population studies conducted in the United States and Great Britain. In the American male doctors study, 325 mg of aspirin was administered every other day to 22,071 normal individuals.[81] In the British male doctors study, 500 mg daily was given to 5,139 individuals.[69] The American trial raised the possibility of an increase in the number of hemorrhagic strokes related to aspirin use. Editorial commentary warned of this risk of brain hemorrhage.[71] When the longer follow-up was reported one year later, this trend to hemorrhage was less impressive.[82] A similar concern about hemorrhagic stroke was raised in the British primary prevention trial. Nine hemorrhagic strokes occurred in the patients in the aspirin group, compared with one hemorrhagic stroke in those receiving the placebo. The unsatisfactory part of these reports is that in neither instance were the definitions and criteria of cerebral hemorrhage identified, nor was the mode of determining the presence of hemorrhage disclosed. No indication was given as to the confirmatory use or otherwise of CT scanning to validate the hemorrhage.

The failure to identify reduction in stroke despite a reduction in myocardial infarction in the American primary prevention trial is of great interest. It may be explained in two ways. First, it might be speculated that the dose of 325 mg every other day was adequate to prevent myocardial infarction, but inadequate to prevent stroke. The assumption that the primary vascular processes are identical in ischemic stroke and ischemic heart disease may be incorrect. Second, the trials involved populations at risk for myocardial infarction, but on average they were a decade younger than is known to be the peak age incidence for stroke expectancy. As a low-risk group, the benefit may simply have been missed. A trial of platelet inhibitors designed and conducted specifically to evaluate the possible benefit of aspirin in primary stroke prevention with dose variations of aspirin and studying an older age group should be considered.

One trial has studied aspirin in the prevention of vascular events in patients known to have asymptomatic ≥ 50% carotid artery stenoses.[31] The trial was negative. After a mean follow-up of 2.3 years, stroke and death occurred in 12% of the placebo group and 11.0% of the aspirin group. Benefit may have been present and missed for several reasons. The dose may have been too low at only 325 mg per day. The total number of individuals in the trial was small with only 372 individuals. Only 21 outcome events of stroke occurred. This study failed to detect the significant benefit of reduction in myocardial infarction (MI) seen in the Physician's Health Study. There were 7 MIs in the aspirin group and 4 in the placebo group. This paradox may be explained on the basis of the small population studied.

CLOPIDOGREL

Clopidogrel is a thienopyridine derivative closely related to ticlopidine, which blocks the aggregation of platelets by adenosine diphosphate (ADP), inhibiting the binding of ADP to

its platelet receptor and thereby interfering with platelet-fibrinogen reactions.[28] Its antithrombotic activity was found to be greater than ticlopidine in animal models. A large trial of 19,185 patients afflicted with recent ischemic stroke, recent MI, or symptomatic peripheral vascular disease tested 325 mg of aspirin against the new compound. A nonsignificant benefit for stroke reduction (relative reduction 7.3%) favored clopidogrel. Adding MI, ischemic stroke, and vascular death together, the relative risk reduction was 9.4% (Figs. 46.9 and 46.10).

The only adverse effect from clopidogrel rated as "severe" was skin rash. This occurred in 0.3% of the subjects compared with 0.1% of those taking aspirin. For rash, 0.9% of those on clopidogrel stopped the drug compared with 0.4% for those taking aspirin. Severe gastrointestinal bleeding occurred in 0.7% of those taking aspirin compared with 0.5% of those taking clopidogrel. Neutropenia was equally uncommon in the two treatment groups, being less than 0.2%.

In terms of stroke prevention, clopidogrel is not likely to replace aspirin as the platelet inhibitor of choice. The lurking doubt remains that the result of the clopidogrel trial was dependent on the use of a dose of aspirin that was too low (325 mg daily). No one knows what the results in stroke prevention would have been in the aspirin arm of the trial with a larger dose. It is disappointing, too, that after 17,000 patient-years of follow-up, the risk of stroke was not significantly reduced. After an aggregate of 6,000 patient-years of follow-up in the group with cerebral ischemic symptoms, in the clopidogrel group, there were 298 strokes, of which 17 were fatal, and in the aspirin group, there were 322 strokes, of which 16 were fatal.

Clopidogrel will likely be accepted as a replacement for ticlopidine and become the platelet inhibitor of second choice to be given to patients threatening with a stroke as a result of recent TIA or nondisabling ischemic stroke. Once it has passed the regulating agencies, it will be recommended when patients are intolerant of aspirin or when events continue despite aspirin in adequate dose. The reported low incidence of reversible neutropenia, only 10% of that observed with ticlopidine, coming from such a large sample of patients, is reassuring. It is presumed that there will be a requirement imposed by the licensing bodies for blood counts for the first few months of therapy for each patient. This will add to the cost and inconvenience of substituting this drug for aspirin.

IS THERE A PLACE FOR DIPYRIDAMOLE

This question has been raised despite early disappointing results from all trials of dipyridamole in preventing stroke. Neither alone in one trial nor in conjunction with 900 to 1,300 mg of aspirin in three separate trials was there a benefit against placebo in the first instance nor against aspirin alone in the three factorial-design studies. A large factorial-design trial of 6,602 patients tested 50 mg of aspirin against the standard dose of 400 mg daily of dipyridamole, the combination of both, and against placebo. The conclusions were that stroke or death was reduced in relative terms by 13% with 50 mg of aspirin, by 16% with dipyridamole, and by 37% with the combination. There was no treatment arm which included the larger dose

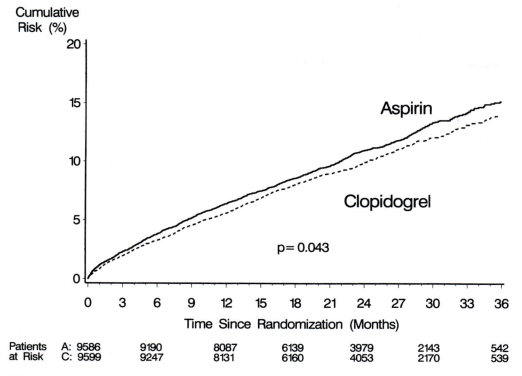

Patients   A: 9586   9190   8087   6139   3979   2143   542
at Risk   C: 9599   9247   8131   6160   4053   2170   539

Figure 46.9 Cumulative risk of ischemic stroke, myocardial infarction, or vascular death. A, aspirin; C, clopidogrel. (From CAPRIE Steering Committee[27] with permission.)

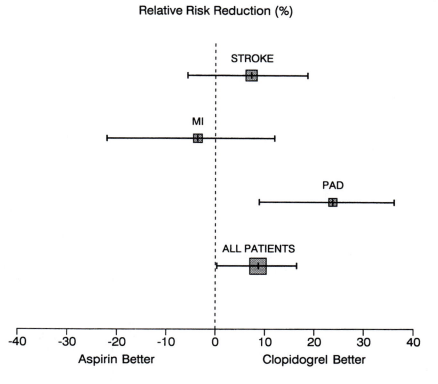

Figure 46.10 Relative-risk reduction and 95% CI by disease subgroup. MI, myocardial infarction; PAD, peripheral arterial disease. (From CAPRIE Steering Committee,[27] with permission.)

Table 46.2 Recommended Use of Platelet Inhibitors in Cerebral Artery Disorders

Indications	Basis of Recommendation	First Choice Suggested Dose[b]	Second Choice	Duration	Remarks
Ischemic events from large artery disease (TIA, nondisabling stroke)	Clinical randomized trials	Aspirin[a] 650–975 mg/day	Ticlopidine when ASA not tolerated or events continue despite ASA	Indefinite	With ticlopidine, regular blood counts required
Recent completed ischemic stroke	Single clinical trial (IST)	Aspirin[a] 650–975 mg/day	None	Indefinite	Further trials needed
Nonvalvular atrial fibrillation	Randomized trial	Aspirin[a] 650–975 mg/day	None tested	Indefinite	<60 years with low risk profile; >75 years if rigid regulation uncertain
Ischemic events with mitral valve prolapse, mitral annulus calcification	Case-series	Aspirin[a] 650–975 mg/day	None tested	Indefinite	Treatment not indicated without retinal or cerebral ischemic events
Perioperative period-carotid endarterectomy	Data generated from NASCET	Aspirin[a] 650–975 mg/day	None tested	30 days perioperative. Then indefinite	ACE trial will pinpoint correct dose
Dissection cerebral artery	Empirical	Aspirin[a] 650–975 mg/day	None tested	3 months	Data very uncertain
Asymptomatic carotid stenosis	Single small negative trial— low dose	Aspirin[a] 650–975 mg/day	Ticlopidine if ASA not tolerated	Indefinite	Larger study needed
Primary prevention	Negative clinical trials—low dose	Aspirin[a] 650 mg/day	None tested	Indefinite	Needs a trial before universal adoption

Abbreviations: TIA, transient ischemic attack; ASA, acetylsalicylic acid; IST, International Stroke Trial; NASCET, North American Symptomatic Carotid Endarterectomy Trial; ACE, Aspirin and Carotid Endarterectomy Trial

[a] Enteric-coated aspirin recommended

[b] Dose empirical choice of authors

of aspirin used in the previous negative studies. The problem with acceptance of these results rests in part upon the comparison with the very small dose which has never before been evaluated in a stroke prevention trial. A remarkable deviation from customary practice was the request of the patients in the trial to forego active treatment of known benefit. One-fourth of the patients took only placebo.[32]

CONCLUSIONS

It has been established in stroke prevention that there are specific circumstances in which platelet inhibitors are to be preferred to anticoagulants. The recommendations for their use are set out in Table 46.2. Aspirin remains the platelet inhibitor of first choice. Ticlopidine is the next choice when aspirin is not tolerated or when ischemic events continue despite aspirin. Clopidogrel may replace ticlopidine when and

if it becomes generally available. The use of dipyridamole cannot be recommended on the strength of present data.

References

1. Acheson J, Danta G, Hutchinson EC: Controlled trial of dipyridamole in cerebral vascular disease. BMJ 1:614, 1969
2. Ackerman RH, Newman KL: Incomplete antiplatelet effects in patients on aspirin compounds. Abstracted Ann Neurol 28:224, 1990
3. Akopov SS, Grigorian GS, Gabrielian ES: Dose-dependent aspirin hydrolysis and platelet aggregation in patients with atherosclerosis. J Clin Pharmacol 32:133, 1992
4. Algra A, Van Gijn: Aspirin at any dose above 30 mg offers only modest protection after cerebral ischaemia. J Neurol Neurosurg Psychiatry 60:197, 1996

5. The American-Canadian Co-Operative Study Group: Persantine Aspirin Trial in cerebral ischemia: endpoint results. Stroke 16:406, 1985

6. Antiplatelet Trialists' Collaboration: Collaborative overview of randomised trials of antiplatelet therapy. I: Prevention of death, myocardial infarction, and stroke by prolonged antiplatelet therapy in various categories of patients. BMJ 308:81, 1994

7. Antonov AS, Key NS, Smirnov MD, et al: Prothrombotic phenotype diversity of human aortic endothelial cells in culture. Thromb Res 67:135, 1992

8. Ashby BM, Oakley N, Lorentz I, Scott D: Recurrent monocular blindness. BMJ 2:894, 1963

9. Baker RN: An evaluation of anticoagulant therapy in the treatment of cerebrovascular disease: report of the Veterans Administration Cooperative Study of Atherosclerosis. Neurology (NY) 11:132, 1961

10. Baker RN, Broward JA, Fang HC et al: Anticoagulant therapy in cerebral infarction: report on cooperative study. Neurology (NY) 123:823, 1962

11. Baker RN, Schwartz WS, Rose AS: Transient ischemic strokes: a report of a study of anticoagulant therapy. Neurology (NY) 16:841, 1966

12. Barnett HJM: Transient cerebral ischemia: pathogenesis, prognosis and management. Ann R Coll Physicians Surgeons Can 7:153, 1974

13. Barnett HJM: Platelet and coagulation function in relation to thromboembolic stroke. p.45. In Thompson RA, green JR (eds): Advances in Neurology. Lippincott-Raven, Philadelphia, New York, 1977

14. Barnett HJM, Peerless SJ, Kaufmann JCE: "Stump" of internal carotid artery—a source for further cerebral embolic ischemia. Stroke 9:48, 1978

15. Barnett HJM: Problems in the therapy of stroke prevention-antithrombotic drugs and surgical considerations. p.243. In Barnett HJM, Paoletti P, Flamm ES, Brambilla G (eds): Cerebrovascular Diseases: New Trends in Surgical and Medical Aspects. Elsevier Biomedical, North Holland, Amsterdam, 1981.

16. Barnett HJM: The stump syndrome. In Smith R (ed): Stroke and the Extracranial Vessels. Lippincott-Raven, Philadelphia, 1984

17. Barnett HJM, Eliasziw M, Meldrum HE: Drugs and surgery in the prevention of ischemic stroke. N Engl J Med 332:238, 1995

18. Barnett HJM, Eliasziw M, Meldrum HE: Prevention of ischemic stroke (Reply). NEJM 333:460, 1995

19. Barnett HJM, Kaste M, Meldrum HE, Eliasziw M: Aspirin dose in stroke prevention: beautiful hypotheses slain by ugly facts. Stroke 27:588, 1996

20. Bernhardt J, Konstantin R, Luscher TF et al: Acetylsalicylic acid, at high concentrations, inhibits vascular smooth muscle cell proliferation. J Cardiovasc Pharmacol 21:973, 1993

21. Biller J, Adams HP, Jr, Boarini D et al: Intraluminal clot of the carotid artery. A clinical-angiographic correlation of nine patients and literature review. Surg Neurol 25:467, 1986

22. Bousser MG, Eschwege E, Haguenau M et al: "AICLA" controlled trial of aspirin and dipyridamole in the secondary prevention of athero-thrombotic cerebral ischemia. Stroke 14:5, 1983

23. Boysen G, Sorensen PS, Juhler M et al: Danish very-low-dose aspirin after carotid endarterectomy trial. Stroke 19:1211, 1988

24. Buchan AM, Gates P, Pelz D, Barnett HJM: Intraluminal thrombus in the cerebral circulation. Stroke 19:681, 1988

25. The Canadian Cooperative Study Group: a randomized trial of aspirin and sulfinpyrazone in threatened stroke. N Engl J Med. 299:53, 1978

26. The Canadian Cooperative Study Group: Randomized trial of therapy with platelet antiaggregants for threatened stroke-1: Design and main results of the trial. CMAJ 1980; 122:295.

27. Cappelleri JC, Lau J, Kupelnick B, Chalmers TC: Efficancy and safety of different aspirin dosages on vascular diseases in high-risk patients: a metaregression analysis. Online J Curr Clin Trials Doc. 174, March 1995

28. CAPRIE Steering Committee: A randomised, blinded, trial of clopidogrel versus aspirin in patients at risk of ischaemic events (CAPRIE). Lancet 348:1329, 1996

29. Carter AB: Use of anticoagulants in patients with progressive cerebral infarction. Neurology (NY) 11:601, 1961

30. Chimowitz MI, Kokkinos J, Strong J et al: The warfarin-aspirin symptomatic intracranial disease study. Neurology 45:M88, 1995

31. Côté R, Battista RN, Abrahamowicz M: Lack of effect of aspirin in asymptomatic patients with carotid bruits and substantial carotid narrowing. Ann Intern Med. 123:649, 1995

32. Diener HC, Cunha L, Forbes C, Sivenius J, Smets P, Lowenthal A: European Stroke Prevention Study 2. Dipyridamole and acetylsalicylic acid in the secondary prevention of stroke. J Neurol Sci 143:1, 1996

33. Di Minno G, Cerbone AM, Mattioli PL et al: Functionally thrombasthenic state in normal platelets following the administration of ticlopidine. J Clin Invest. 75:328, 1985

34. Duke RJ, Bloch RF, Turpie AGG et al: Intravenous heparin for the prevention of stroke progression in acute partial stable stroke: a randomized controlled trial. Ann Intern Med 105:825, 1986

35. Dyken ML: Antiplatelet aggregating agents in transient ischemic attacks and the relationship of risk factors. p.141. In Breddin K, Loew D, Uberla K et al (eds) Prophylaxis of Venous, Peripheral, Cardiac and Cerebral Vascular Diseases with Acetylsalicylic Acid. Schattauer Verlag, Stuttgart, Germany, 1981

36. Dyken ML: Controversies in stroke: past and present: the Willis Lecture. Stroke 24:1251, 1993

37. Emmons PR, Harrison MJ, Honour AJ, Mitchell JR: Affect of a pyrimido pyrimidine derivative on thrombus formation in the rabbit. Nature 208:255, 1965

38. ESPS Group: European Stroke Prevention Study. Stroke 21:1122, 1990

39. Faigel DJ, Jakubowski JA, Stampfer MJ et al: Multiple doses of regular and enteric-coated aspirin produce equivalent platelet inhibitory effects. Curr Ther Res 39:519, 1986

40. Fields WS, Lemak NA, Frankowski RF, Hardy RJ: Controlled trial of aspirin in cerebral ischemia. Stroke 8:301, 1977

41. Fisher CM: Observations of the fundus oculi in transient monocular blindness. Neurology (NY) 9:333, 1959

42. Genton E, Barnett HJM, Fields WS et al: Cerebral ischemia: the role of thrombosis and of anti-thrombotic therapy. Stroke 8:150, 1977

43. Gent M, Blakely JA, Hachinski V et al: A secondary prevention, randomized trial of suloctidil in patients with a recent history of thromboembolic stroke. Stroke 16:416, 1985

44. Gent M, Blakely JA, Easton JD et al: The Canadian American Ticlopidine Study (CATS) in thromboembolic stroke. Lancet 1:1215, 1989

45. Gertler JP, Blankensteijn JD, Brewster D et al: Carotid endarterectomy for unstable and compelling neurologic conditions: do results justify an aggressive approach? J Vasc Surg. 19:32, 1994

46. Grady PA, Blaumanis OR: Arterial wall changes in experimental stenosis. p. 347. In Reivich M, Hurtig HD (eds). Cerebrovascular Diseases. Lippincott-Raven, Philadelphia, 1983

47. Guiraud-Chaumeil B, Rascol A, David JL et al: Prévention des récidives des accidents vasculaires cérébraux ischémiques par les anti-agrégants plaquettaires: résultats d'un essai thérapeutique contrôlé de 3 ans. Rev Neurol (Paris) 138:367, 1982

48. Gunning AJ, Pickering GW, Robb-Smith AHT, Russell RR: Mural thrombosis of the internal carotid artery and subsequent embolism. Q J Med 33:155, 1964

49. Haley EC, Kassell NF, Torner JC: Failure of heparin to prevent progression in progressing ischemic infarction. Stroke 19:10, 1988

50. Harrison MJG, Marshall J, Meadows JC, Ross Russell RW: Effect of Aspirin in Amaurosis Fugax. Lancet 2(727), 1971

51. Hart RG, Harrison MJG: Aspirin wars: the optimal dose of aspirin to prevent stroke. Stroke 27:585, 1996

52. Hass WK, Easton JD, Adams HP Jr et al: A randomized trial comparing ticlopidine hydrochloride with aspirin for the prevention of stroke in high-risk patients. N Engl J Med. 321:501, 1989

53. Helgason CM, Tortorice KL, Winkler SR et al: Aspirin response and failure in cerebral infarction. Stroke 24:345, 1993

54. Hormes JT, Austin JH, James G et al: Toward an optimal 'antiplatelet' dose of aspirin: preliminary observations. J Stroke Cerebrovasc Dis 1:27, 1991

55. International Stroke Trial Collaborative Group: The International Stroke Trial (IST): a randomised trial of aspirin, subcutaneous heparin, both, or neither among 19435 patients with acute ischaemic stroke. Lancet 1997;349:1569–81.

56. Kay, R, Sing Wong K, Ling Yu Y et al: Low-molecular-weight heparin for the treatment of acute ischemic stroke. N Engl J Med 333:1588, 1995

57. Lindblad B, Persson NH, Takolander R, Bergqvist D: Does low-dose acetylsalicylic acid prevent stroke after carotid surgery? A double-blind, placebo-controlled randomized trial. Stroke 24:1125, 1993

58. Matchar DB, McCrory DC, Barnett HJM, Feussner JR: Medical treatment for stroke prevention. Ann Intern Med 121:41, 1994 [Erratum. Ann Intern Med 121:470, 1994]

59. McCrory DC, Goldstein LB, Samsa GP et al: Predicting complications of carotid endarterectomy. Stroke 24:1285, 1993

60. Mickelson JK, Hoff PT, Homeister JW et al: High dose intravenous aspirin, no low dose intravenous or oral aspirin, inhibits thrombus formation and stabilized blood flow in experimental coronary vascular injury. J Am Coll Cardiol 21:502, 1993

61. Munson RJ, Sharpe BL, Finan JW et al: for the North American Symptomatic Carotid Endarterectomy Trial (NASCET) Group: The NASCET Experience of Bleeding Complications of Patients on Aspirin. Abstract presented at the 22nd International Joint Conference on Stroke and Cerebral Circulation, February 6–8, 1997

62. Mustard JF, Rowsell HC, Smythe HA et al: The effect of sulfinpyrazone on platelet economy and thrombus formation in rabbits. Blood 29:859, 1967

63. O'Brien JR: How much aspirin? Thromb Haemost 64:486, 1990

64. Oh PI, Lanctôt KL, Naranjo CA, Shear NH: Fatal aplastic anemia associated with ticlopidine therapy—approaches to an adverse drug reaction. Can J Clin Pharmacol 2:19, 1995

65. Page C, Rose M, Yacoub M, Pigott R: Antigenic heterogeneity of vascular endothelium. Am J Pathol. 141:673, 1992

66. Patrono C, Roth GJ: Aspirin in ischemic cerebrovascular disease: how strong is the case for a different dosing regimen? Stroke 27:756, 1996

67. Pearce JMS, Gubbay SS, Walton JN: Long-term anticoagulant therapy in transient cerebral ischaemic attacks. Lancet 1:6, 1965

68. Pelz DM, Buchan A, Fox AJ et al: Intraluminal thrombus of the internal carotid arteries: angiographic demonstration of resolution with anticoagulant therapy alone. Radiology. 160:369, 1986

69. Peto R, Gray R, Collins R et al: Randomized trial of prophylactic daily aspirin in British male doctors. Br Med J 296:313, 1988

70. Ratnatunga CP, Edmondson SF, Rees GM, Kovacs IB: High-dose aspirin inhibits shear-induced platelet reaction involving thrombin generation. Circulation 85:1077, 1992

71. Relman AS: Aspirin for the primary prevention of myocardial infarction. (Editorial) N Engl J Med. 318:245, 1988

72. Roald HE, Orvium U, Bakken IJ et al: Modulation of thrombotic responses in moderately stenosed arteries by cigarette smoking and aspirin ingestion. Arterioscler Thromb 14:617, 1994

73. Roderick PJ, Wilkes HC, Meade TW: The gastrointestinal toxicity of aspirin: an overview of randomised controlled trials. Br J Clin Pharmac 35:219, 1993

74. Saltiel E, Ward A: Ticlopidine: a review of its pharmacodynamic and pharmacokinetic properties, and therapeutic efficacy in platelet-dependent disease states. Drugs 34:222, 1987

75. The SALT Collaborative Group: Swedish Aspirin Low-dose Trial (SALT) of 75 mg aspirin as secondary prophylaxis after cerebrovascular ischaemic events. Lancet. 338:1345, 1991

76. Sandercock P: International Stroke Trial (IST)—Main. Stroke 27:1931, 1996

77. Savon JJ, Allen ML, DiMarino AJ et al: Gastrointestinal

blood loss with low dose (325 mg) plain and enteric-coated aspirin administration. Am J Gastroenterol 90:581, 1995

78. Shear NH: Prevention of ischemic stroke (Letter to the editor). N Engl J Med 333:460, 1995

79. Smythe HA, Ogryzlo MD, Murphy EA, Mustard JF: Effect of sulfinpyrazone (Anturan) on platelet economy and blood coagulation in man. JAMA 92:818, 1965

80. Sorensen PS, Pedersen H, Marquardsen J et al: Acetylsalicylic acid in the prevention of stroke in patients with reversible cerebral ischemic attacks: a Danish Cooperative Study. Stroke 14:15, 1983

81. Steering Committee of the Physician's Health Study Research Group: Special report: preliminary report: findings from the aspirin component of the ongoing physician's health study. N Engl J Med 318:262, 1988

82. Steering Committee of the Physician's Health Study Research Group: Final report on the aspirin component of the ongoing physician's health study. N Engl J Med 321:129, 1989

83. Sundt TM, Jr, Dyken ML, Jr: Surgical treatment for ischemic vascular disease. In Harrison MJG, Dyken ML (eds). Cerebral Vascular Disease. Butterworth, London, 1983

84. The Swedish Cooperative Study: High-dose acetylsalicylic acid after cerebral infarction. Stroke 18:325, 1987

85. Szezeklik A, Krzanaowski M, Gora P, Radwan J: Antiplatelet drugs and generation of thrombin in clotting blood. J Blood 80:2006, 1992

86. Taylor DW, Sackett DL, Haynes RB: Sample size for randomized trials in stroke prevention: how many patients do we need? Stroke 15:968, 1984

87. Thorpe KE, Taylor DW, for the North American Symptomatic Carotid Endarterectomy Trial Collaborators. ASA and Carotid Endarterectomy. Abstract presented at the 22nd International Joint Conference on Stroke and Cerebral Circulation, February 6–8, 1997

88. Turner RR, Beckstead JH, Warnke RA, Wood GS: Endothelial cell phenotypic diversity: in situ demonstration of immunologic and enzymatic heterogeneity that correlates with specific morphologic subtypes. Am J Clin Pathol 87:569, 1987

89. Uchiyama S, Yamazaki M, Maruyama S et al: Shear-induced platelet aggregation in cerebral ischemia. Stroke 25:1547, 1994

90. UK-TIA Study Group: The United Kingdom transient ischaemic attack (UK-TIA) aspirin trial: final results. J Neurol Neurosurg Psychiatry 54:1044, 1991

91. VanPampus ECM, Huijgens PC, Zevenbergen A et al: Influence of aspirin on human megakaryocyte prostaglandin synthesis. Eur J Haematol 50:264, 1993

92. Vesvres MH, Doutremepuich F, Lalanne MCI, Doutremepuich CH: Effects of aspirin on embolization in an arterial model of laser-induced thrombus formation. Haemostasis 23:8, 1993

93. Walters TK, Mitchell DC, Wood RF: Low-dose aspirin fails to inhibit increased platelet reactivity in patients with peripheral vascular disease. Br J Surg 80:1266, 1993

94. WARSS, APASS, PICSS, HAS and GENESIS Study Groups: The feasibility of a collaborative double-blind study using an anticoagulant. Cerebrovascular Diseases 7:100, 1997

95. Weil J, Colin-Jones D, Langman M et al: Prophylactic aspirin and risk of peptic ulcer bleeding. BMJ 310:827, 1995

96. Weiss HJ, Aledort LM: Impaired platelet connective-tissue in man after aspirin ingestion. Lancet 2:495, 1967

97. Winocour PD, Watala C, Perry DW, Kiniough-Rathbone RL: Decreased platelet membrane fluidity due to glycation or acetylation of membrane proteins. Thromb Haemost 68:577, 1992

Pharmacologic Modification of Acute Cerebral Ischemia

JAMES C. GROTTA

DAVID CHIU

The concept of neuroprotection relies on the principle that delayed neuronal injury occurs after ischemia. Neurons suffer irreversible damage after only a few minutes of complete cessation of blood flow. Such a condition might exist during cardiac arrest. In most instances of acute focal brain ischemia, however, a state of zero blood flow occurs only in the core of the ischemic region. The larger surrounding penumbral area receives reduced blood flow which causes loss of normal function that may lead to permanent cellular damage if uncorrected, but allows for recovery if blood flow is restored.

Because ischemia is clearly a process and not an instantaneous event, the potential exists for modifying the process after the clinical ictus and altering the final outcome. It is equally apparent from experimental models that if neuroprotective treatments are to succeed, they must be instituted within a few minutes after the onset of ischemia. Previous clinical trials of neuroprotection may have failed because treatment was delayed and therefore unlikely to render a benefit.

The concept of cytoprotection is not new in the clinical domain. It has been known for years that hypothermia reduces ischemic neuronal injury. Accidental hypothermia can protect a drowning victim from otherwise fatal hypoxic-ischemic brain damage. Animal stroke models confirm the beneficial effects of hypothermia (Fig. 47.1). Its mechanism of action is uncertain but probably related to decreased presynaptic release of various neurotransmitters including glutamate. Therapeutic cooling of the brain is under evaluation in head trauma[8] but has yet to be evaluated in stroke. Nevertheless, a rule of management of the acute stroke patient is that fever should be aggressively treated. Hyperbaric oxygen was not effective in small pilot studies in human stroke.

Ischemic Cascade

A major accomplishment of in vivo and in vitro model systems of cerebral ischemia is an understanding of the *ischemic cascade*. Each step along this cascade might be a target for therapeutic intervention. Several variables exist that may affect the ischemic cascade and consequently the severity of stroke, most important the depth of blood flow reduction, its duration before reperfusion occurs, its distribution (i.e., global or focal), and the adequacy of reperfusion, assuming it does occur. However, many of the events that have been described seem to follow in a fairly predictable order.[4,8,11,15,22]

First there is reduction of blood flow, followed rapidly by inhibition of protein synthesis, depletion of intracellular energy stores, membrane depolarization, and release of extracellular potassium. This is accompanied by an initial increase in oxygen extraction and glucose metabolism, and lactic acidosis. Membrane depolarization causes opening of voltage-operated calcium channels, allowing disruption of tightly regulated neuronal calcium homeostasis. Glutamate is released from presynaptic stores, and in the presence of glycine activates the N-methyl-D-aspartate receptor. The immediate consequence is increased sodium permeability and cellular swelling, but the more damaging event is further elevation of intracellular calcium through the NMDA-associated ion channel. Further perturbations in ion flux occur as a result of glutamate's effect on the α-amino-3-hydroxy-5-methyl-4-isoxazole propionic acid (AMPA) and metabotropic receptors. Documented increases in other neurotransmitters such as γ aminobutyric acid (GABA), dopamine, and norepinephrine may also be damaging.

Increased intracellular calcium activates a large number of damaging enzymatic pathways. Calcium (through calmodulin)

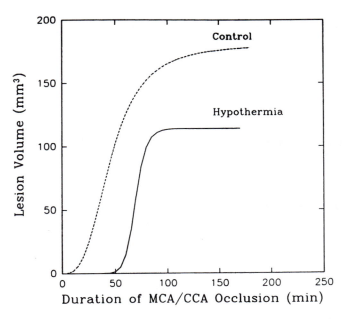

Figure 47.1 The effect of hypothermia (30°) on an animal model of stroke. Long-Evans rats were exposed to transient tandem CCA/MCA occlusion for variable intervals (x axis), and infarct volume measured after 24 hours (y axis). Note that hypothermia (begun 15 minutes after the onset of ischemia) both reduced lesion volume and prolonged the time of ischemia before damage appeared.[37]

activates protein kinases such as Cam-kinase II and protein kinase C, which may imbalance neuronal homeostasis by causing protein phosphorylation. Other pivotal enzyme systems activated by calcium include the proteases such as calpain, which causes cytoskeletal proteolysis; lipases, such as phospholipase A, which leads to production of arachidonic acid and free radical formation; phospholipase C, which results in release of intracellular calcium stores; and nitric oxide synthase (NOS), resulting in increased nitric acid (NO). The consequences of free radical production and these enzyme perturbations are widespread, including disruption of neuronal (and endothelial) membrane and cytoskeletal integrity and damage to mitochondrial function.

Increased gene expression in ischemic regions, possibly induced by spreading depolarizations after ischemia, has many damaging consequences. Cytokines such as tumor necrosis factor (TNF) and interleukin-1(IL-1) result in tissue inflammation, and adhesion molecules such as intercellular adhesion molecule (ICAM)-1 result in white blood cell interaction with vascular endothelium to produce blood brain barrier damage and may also plug up the microcirculation resulting in "no reflow." Growth factors such as nerve growth factor (NGF) basic fibroblast growth factor (bFGF) may result in increased production of NO and also have been reported to be protective when exogenously administered.[23]

Neuroprotective therapy is directed at these biochemical events that occur consequent to arterial occlusion. Numerous preclinical studies in animal models of global and focal ischemia have shown efficacy by targeting each of the steps along this ischemic cascade. Rather than enumerating each of these studies, it is probably more useful to describe the broad lessons from these studies that can be applied to clinical trials. Because these drugs interrupt the ischemic cascade in tissue that is not yet dead, they have been shown to be most effective in animal models of focal cerebral ischemia where there is an extensive ischemic penumbra or relatively mild ischemic injury. Because their effect is primarily on penumbral regions, we can expect relatively modest benefit by using any one of these drugs alone. Furthermore, in our animal models, we have found that neuroprotective therapies, when started after the onset of ischemia but prior to reperfusion, can augment the beneficial effect of reperfusion and can also extend the time window for starting reperfusion therapy. However, none of these drugs when used alone provides substantial reduction of infarct volume unless they are started within 1 hour of the onset of ischemia.

Multimodality Therapy

An understanding of the ischemic cascade has enabled us to design neuroprotective therapy aimed at each of these steps. This has led to the emerging concept that multimodality therapy may be necessary to maximize a therapeutic attack on acute ischemic stroke. A therapy targeting only one of these processes is unlikely to result in a therapeutic "home run." We would make the analogy that these events are like the invading hordes; stop only the first wave and the reinforcements in the subsequent waves will get you; and bombarding the reinforcements without turning back the first attack will also do no good. Carrying this analogy further at the risk of oversimplification, reduction of cerebral blood flow (CBF) can be equated with the first wave, release of neurotransmitters the second, calcium entry the third, enzyme activation the fourth, NO and free radical production the fifth, gene expression the sixth, microvascular white blood cell (WBC), adhesion the seventh, and apoptosis the eighth. Reperfusion strategies are directed at the first wave, and various "neuroprotective" strategies at the second through eighth.

Combinations of reperfusion and neuroprotective strategies have been shown to be effective in several laboratories. Uematsu[32] found that neuronal calcium signal increased after MCA occlusion in rats and that this was not attenuated by reperfusion. The noncompetitive NMDA ion channel blocker MK-801 administered during ischemia was able to attenuate intracellular calcium and increased the amount of neuronal salvage over that achieved only by reperfusion. The addition of the dihydropyridine voltage-operated calcium channel antagonist nimodipine to MK-801 augmented the beneficial effect on both calcium and neuronal necrosis.[32]

Zivin and Mazzarella[35] found a positive effect of the thrombolytic tissue plasminogen activator (TPA) in a rabbit autologous clot embolism model. While MK-801 had no beneficial effect by itself in this model, when added to TPA it was able to increase efficacy by approximately 33% over that achieved by TPA alone. More recently, the same group found an additive effect of anti-ICAM-1 to TPA.[6]

In our laboratory, we were unable to find any additive effect of combining a voltage-operated calcium channel antagonist

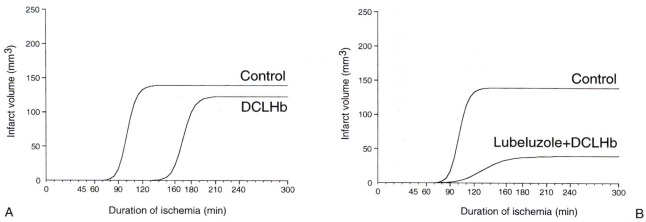

Figure 47.2 (**A**) The effect of hemodilution to HCT = 30 by DCLHb begun 15 minutes after the onset of ischemia on an animal model of stroke analyzed as in Figure 47.1. Note that DCLHb both reduced lesion volume and prolonged the time of ischemia before damage appeared. (**B**) The combined effect of DCLHb and lubeluzole.[3]

(nicardipine) to a competitive antagonist of glutamate at the NMDA receptor (CGS-19755). Both were modestly effective alone.[20] This finding has reinforced in our minds the necessity of including an attack on the "first wave," i.e., reduced CBF, in any combination strategy.

More recently, we have studied blood substitutes as reperfusion agents, and combined one of these with a promising neuroprotective drug. DCLHb (diaspirin cross-linked hemoglobin) is derived from human erythrocytes and has the same oxygen dissociation characteristics as normal hemoglobin in human red cells. Therefore, it is an ideal hemodiluting agent; it can be given as an intravenous solution, resulting in hemodilution without loss of oxygen carrying capacity. A postischemic exchange and top load of DCLHb, lowering rat hematocrit from 50% to 30% reduced infarct volume and almost doubled the duration of MCA occlusion that could be tolerated before neuronal necrosis began to be seen.

Lubeluzole is a sodium and calcium channel blocker which may have an effect on glutamate induced NO production.[12] We have found that postischemic administration of this drug also reduces infarct volume, but does not prolong the duration of MCA occlusion tolerated. The combination of DCLHb and lubeluzole had an additive effect reducing ischemic damage to less than 33% of that measured in controls, while at the same time prolonging to over 2 hours the duration of MCA occlusion that could be tolerated before any permanent neuronal necrosis was produced (Fig. 47.2).[3]

Reperfusion Injury

There is considerable debate as to whether or not reperfusion itself has damaging effects. Certainly, if there is disruption of the blood brain barrier, reperfusion can be associated with cerebral edema and hemorrhage. However, even in the absence of such gross abnormalities, reperfusion after a period

of occlusion long enough to produce cellular injury may result in increased production of free radicals, gene expression, and inflammatory events which may augment cellular damage. Recent experimental evidence has shown greater histologic damage particularly in cortex after temporary middle cerebral artery (MCA) occlusion lasting 3 hours compared to permanent MCA occlusion.[34,36] The effect of neuroprotective therapies on reperfusion injury deserves greater attention.

Clinical Status of Neuroprotective Therapy

To date, seven classes of neuroprotective drugs have reached the stage of pivotal phase III efficacy trials in acute stroke patients based on published phase II data (Table 47.1). They are the calcium channel antagonist nimodipine, the glutamate antagonists, lubeluzole, the free radical scavenger tirilizad, anti-ICAM-1 antibody, GM_1 ganglioside, and cytidine-5'-diphospho(CDP)-choline. These, as well as promising therapeutic approaches still in phase II testing, are discussed in detail below.

CALCIUM ANTAGONISTS

The first practical pharmacologic agents to be clinically evaluated for cytoprotection in cerebral ischemia were the calcium channel antagonists. There are several classes of calcium channels that play a role in brain ischemia. The presynaptic N-type calcium channels are voltage-gated and regulate neurotransmitter release. The voltage-gated L-type calcium channels are sensitive to the dihydropyridine compounds, of which

Table 47.1 Status of Clinical Testing of
Cytoprotective Agents

Agent	Clinical Testing in Stroke Completed or in Progress
Hypothermia	?[a]
Hyperbaric oxygen	Phase II
Calcium antagonists	
Nimodipine	Phase III
Nicardipine	Phase II
NMDA antagonists	
Selfotel	Phase III
Dextrorphan	Phase II
Cerestat	Phase III
Eliprodil	Phase III
Magnesium	Phase II
Lamotrigine	?
Glycine site antagonists	Phase II
Fosphenytoin	Phase II/III
Glutamate release inhibitors	?
AMPA antagonists	?
Adenosine agonists	?
GABA agonists	Phase III
Kappa-selective opioid antagonists	Phase II
Lubeluzole	Phase III
Nitric oxide synthase inhibitors	?
Free radical scavengers	Phase III
Anti-ICAM antibody	Phase III
GM-1 ganglioside	Phase III
Calpain inhibitors	[b]
Basic fibroblast growth factor	[b] Phase III
CDP-choline	Phase III
DCLHb	Phase II
Combined cytoprotective strategies	?
Cytoprotection plus thrombolysis	[b] Phase II

Abbreviations: NMDA, N methyl D aspartate; AMPA, adenosine mono-
phosphatase; GABA, γ aminobutyric acid; ICAM, intercellular adhesion
molecule; GM, monosialoganglioside; CDP, cytidine 5'-diphosphocholine;
DCLHb, diaspirin cross-linked hemoglobin.

[a] *No known human studies in stroke*

[b] *Human testing planned*

nimodipine and nicardipine are examples. Calcium influx through NMDA receptor-mediated channels is both ligand- and voltage-dependent. Other classes of calcium channels have distinct activation or inactivation characteristics, or resemble L-type channels, but are insensitive to dihydropyridines.

The calcium channel antagonist that has undergone the most extensive investigation in stroke is nimodipine. The cytoprotective effect of nimodipine results from its ability to block calcium influx and prevent the increase of intracellular calcium. Nimodipine has been studied in experimental models of cerebral ischemia and in clinical trials in subarachnoid hemorrhage, head injury, and cardiac arrest, as well as acute focal ischemia (see reference 17 for review and references).

Several randomized controlled clinical studies have conclu-sively demonstrated the effectiveness of nimodipine in preventing ischemic neurologic deficits secondary to aneurysmal subarachnoid hemorrhage. Prophylactic therapy with nimodipine is now standard treatment in subarachnoid hemorrhage. The usual dose is 60 mg orally every 4 hours for 21 days, but a lower dose or a more frequent dosing schedule may be used if hypotension is limiting. Although it is uncertain whether nimodipine has its primary effect in this clinical setting as a neuroprotective drug or as a vasodilator, the use of nimodipine does not result in angiographically evident improvement of vasospasm.

Nimodipine was studied in cardiac resuscitation in a randomized placebo-controlled trial in Finland.[17] Patients who were resuscitated after ventricular fibrillation in the field received a bolus dose of nimodipine or placebo immediately after resuscitation, followed by a 24-hour infusion. There was no difference in survival after 1 year in the overall group, but subgroup analysis showed that patients who had a greater than 10-minute delay in resuscitation efforts had a significantly lower mortality when treated with nimodipine.

Finally, oral nimodipine has been investigated in ischemic stroke in at least 10 randomized placebo-controlled trials. These studies enrolled patients with time windows ranging from 12 to 48 hours, used nimodipine doses between 60 and 240 mg/d, and treated for periods of 14 to 28 days. A few of the earlier studies found a significant difference in mortality and neurologic function in favor of nimodipine therapy, but the later, larger studies failed to replicate this result[2] (Fig. 47.3A). One study showed a better outcome in the placebo-treated patients, a finding attributed to hypotension induced by the drug.[33]

In posthoc and meta-analysis, a benefit was found for low to moderate doses of nimodipine (30 mg PO q6h) in the subgroup of patients who were treated earliest (within 12 hours).[26] Nimodipine appeared to prevent the early deterioration seen in many untreated stroke patients (Fig. 47.3B). If "stroke progression" represents conversion of ischemic penumbra into infarction, a logical hypothesis is that nimodipine protects the penumbra by maintaining calcium homeostasis. It follows that prevention of clinical deterioration in the first day or so after stroke provides a useful construct for designing clinical trials of neuroprotective agents.

In summary, given the weight of the evidence, nimodipine cannot be considered generally effective in improving the outcome of ischemic stroke. Nevertheless, there remains the belief that nimodipine may be beneficial in selected patients, an idea bolstered by the data from subarachnoid hemorrhage trials, experimental models of focal ischemia, and subgroup analysis in clinical trials of ischemic stroke. The ideal stroke patient who stands to gain the most from nimodipine therapy is the patient with progressing neurologic deficits whose hemodynamic status is not destabilized by treatment and in whom treatment can be initiated early.

Another dihydropyridine calcium channel antagonist, nicardipine, has been tested in randomized placebo-controlled trials in aneurysmal subarachnoid hemorrhage.[21] Intravenous nicardipine, given as an infusion of .15 mg/kg/hr for up to 14 days following hemorrhage, was shown to decrease the incidence of symptomatic and angiographic vasospasm. Nicardipine has also been tested in a pilot stroke study.[29] Hypotension is a frequent, dose-related side effect, however, and could potentially negate the overall benefit of treatment.

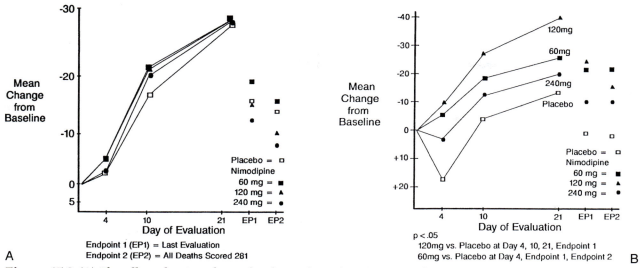

Figure 47.3 (**A**) The effect of various doses of oral nimodipine begun up to 48 hours after the onset of acute ischemic stroke on neurologic function (Toronto Stroke Scale—y axis) (N = 890). (**B**) In patients treated with nimodipine within 12 hours of stroke onset, nimodipine prevented early deterioration (N = 144).

GLUTAMATE ANTAGONISTS AND OTHER NEUROTRANSMITTER MODULATORS

NMDA antagonists are the first class of acute stroke therapeutic agents to proceed from development in the laboratory to testing in humans employing modern principles of clinical trial design, most important relatively early treatment. As such, the results of current clinical trials have been closely scrutinized by basic scientists, preclinical animal modelers, and clinical researchers. The potential utility of NMDA antagonists in stroke was first recognized when it was observed that a hypoxic or ischemic insult results in elevation of brain levels of the excitatory neurotransmitter glutamate. Excessive stimulation of postsynaptic NMDA receptors allows entry of calcium and sodium ions into the cell. Excitotoxic neuronal death is believed to result from at least two mechanisms: first, rapid cell swelling caused by sodium and water influx, and second, intracellular calcium accumulation and consequent activation of proteases, phospholipases, and protein kinases. NMDA receptor activation requires concomitant membrane depolarization and activation by glycine (Fig. 47.4).

Competitive NMDA antagonists bind directly to the glutamate site of the NMDA receptor to inhibit the action of glutamate. Noncompetitive antagonists block the NMDA-associated ion channel in a use-dependent manner. Other designer compounds antagonize the glycine or the polyamine site of the NMDA receptor. Phencyclidine (also known as "angel dust") and the anesthetic agent ketamine are classical NMDA antagonists. Prototypes of competitive and noncompetitive NMDA antagonists are now in phase III clinical trials for the treatment of stroke.

CGS19755 (Selfotel) is a competitive NMDA receptor an-

tagonist that limits neuronal damage in animal stroke models. Selfotel was evaluated in a randomized double-blind placebo-controlled ascending dose phase IIa study to determine its safety and tolerability and obtain pharmacokinetic and preliminary efficacy data. Patients were treated within 12 hours of the onset of ischemic hemispheric stroke.[19]

The serum half-life of a single intravenous dose of 1 to 2 mg/kg was 2 to 3.3 hours. Non-CNS adverse effects were infrequent and not different between the Selfotel and placebo groups. Neuropsychiatric adverse experiences were common, dose-related, and lasted an average of 24 hours. Symptoms

Figure 47.4 The NMDA receptor is activated by glutamate (G). Its activity is also dependent on glycine (Gly) binding. The NMDA receptor operated channel is noncompetitively blocked by magnesium (Mg), Zinc (Zn), and PCP.

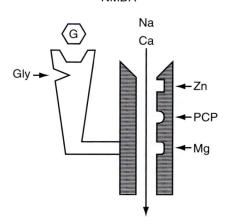

Table 47.2 Adverse Experiences (AEs) to Various Doses of CG S-19755 (Selfotel)

Side Effect	*1.0* mg/kg	*1.5* mg/kg	*1.75* mg/kg	*2.0* mg/kg
Agitation	1/6	1/6	2/6	4/6
Hallucinations	1/6	2/6	3/6	3/6
Confusion	0/6	2/6	1/6	3/6
Paranoia	0/6	0/6	0/6	2/6
Delirium	0/6	0/6	1/6	2/6
	Range		*≈Average*	
Onset time of AE	20 min–22 h		1–3 h	
Duration of AE	2–60 h		24 h	

included hallucinations, agitation, confusion, dysarthria, ataxia, delirium, paranoia, and somnolence (Table 47.2). There were no permanent sequelae. Severe adverse reactions were managed with low doses of intravenous lorazepam or haloperidol. Two doses of 1 mg/kg were well tolerated. However, when the dose was increased to 2 mg/kg given either twice or even once, adverse experiences occurred in all patients. When the dose was decreased to 1.5 mg/kg, mild adverse experiences were noted in some patients, but easily managed with reassurance and low doses of lorazepam. For this reason, 1.5 mg/kg was deemed to be the maximal tolerated dose.

There was no difference in mortality between the Selfotel and placebo groups. The percent change in both the NIH Stroke Scale and the Barthel Index Score showed a trend towards greater improvement in treated patients. The improvement was comparable at all doses of Selfotel. Based on these data, phase III studies of a single dose of 1.5 mg/kg of Selfotel given within 6 hours of the onset of acute hemispheric stroke were begun in the United States and Europe, but recently suspended because of an unfavorable efficacy/toxicity ratio.

The noncompetitive NMDA antagonist dextrorphan has also been evaluated in a recent pilot study.[1] Patients were enrolled in this study within 48 hours of the onset of hemispheric cerebral infarction. Initially, patients were treated with either dextrorphan or placebo using a 1-hour loading dose of 60 to 150 mg followed by a 23-hour ascending-dose maintenance infusion up to a maximal total dose of 3,310 mg. Subsequently, additional patients were treated with dextrorphan in an open-label fashion, using a 1-hour loading dose of 145 to 260 mg followed by an 11-hour infusion of 30 to 70 mg/h.

As with Selfotel, adverse effects of dextrorphan were noted in a dose-dependent fashion. Some side effects were particularly prominent during the loading dose, including nystagmus, somnolence, nausea, and vomiting. Hypotension occurred at the highest loading doses. During the maintenance infusion, the most common side effects were agitation, confusion, hallucinations, and hypertension. There were no apparent differences in the ranges of National Institutes of Health (NIH) Scores in placebo patients or low, medium, or high-dose dex-

trorphan patients. At the present time, no further clinical trials of dextrorphan are in progress.

Finally, a phase IIa dose escalation and tolerability study of the noncompetitive NMDA antagonist CNS1102 (Cerestat) was reported.[25] As with Selfotel and dextrorphan, this was a multicenter placebo-controlled double-blind escalating dose study. Patients with either carotid or vertebral basilar territory stroke within 18 hours of onset were included. Dosing ranged from 30 mg/kg to 150 μg/kg, consisting of a 10- to 30-μg bolus followed by a 4- or 6-hour continuous infusion of 3 to 20 μg/kg/h. Side effects observed were hypertension, headache, sedation, nausea, vomiting, disorientation, and paresthesias. Of 94 patients, only 10 had mild to moderate agitation or confusion, which seemed to be less severe than the side effects seen with Selfotel and dextrorphan. Phase III studies of Cerestat are underway in stroke and head injury. A preliminary report in abstract form suggests possible efficacy with higher dose ranges which produce relatively mild CNS side effects.[14]

In summary, while preclinical studies of competitive and noncompetitive NMDA antagonists suggest that they can effectively protect penumbral regions, clinical studies have thus far been disappointing. This may be in part because phencyclidine-like side effects have limited the dose given to stroke patients so that therapeutic brain levels have not been reached. Consequently, there is great interest in developing strategies for inhibiting glutamate effect while avoiding the side effect profile of direct NMDA receptor antagonism.

A phase III trial of eliprodil, which acts on the polyamine site of the NMDA receptor, is underway in acute stroke patients, although preclinical and phase II clinical data have not been published. Little is known about the properties of this agent. Glycine site antagonists are beginning early clinical evaluation. Two glutamate-inhibiting drugs under evaluation for stroke and currently available on hospital formularies are magnesium and lamotrigine. Magnesium blocks the NMDA-associated ion channel, and a pilot study of magnesium sulfate (8 mmol intravenous loading dose followed by 65 mmol over 24 hours) showed the drug was well tolerated.[27] The antiepileptic drug lamotrigine inhibits glutamate release and has shown beneficial effects in a gerbil model of global cerebral ischemia.

On the horizon are the presynaptic glutamate release inhibitors, AMPA receptor antagonists, adenosine agonists, dopamine D1 antagonists, and GABA agonists. These drugs have shown promise in preclinical studies and are beginning early clinical evaluation. They reduce excitotoxic injury with the advantage of avoiding the side effects of NMDA antagonists. The anticonvulsant clomethiazole is a GABA$_A$ agonist that was recently shown to be neuroprotective in animal models of focal and global ischemia. Clomethiazole is now entering phase III testing in humans. Acadesine, an adenosine-regulating agent, decreased the incidence of perioperative stroke in post hoc analysis in a multicenter trial of patients undergoing coronary artery bypass graft surgery. The kappa-selective opiate antagonist nalmefene is undergoing phase II testing in acute stroke patients. Preliminary data suggest a possible benefit. Naloxone was not effective in pilot clinical studies.

Preclinical studies have shown that phenytoin can reduce neuronal injury, possibly by inhibiting spreading electrical depolarization in penumbral regions and thereby reducing postischemic glutamate release. A combined phase II/III study of fosphenytoin, an aqueous-soluble, rapidly injectable prodrug of phenytoin, is underway for stroke.

LUBELUZOLE

Lubeluzole is a novel benzothiazole compound that has emerged as a neuroprotective agent in animal models of focal ischemia. Blockade of sodium channels may be one of the mechanisms contributing to its neuroprotective effect. Lubeluzole inhibits glutamate release after ischemia and reduces potassium-induced increases of intracellular calcium. Finally, it may prevent glutamate-mediated increases in nitric oxide production.[19]

A phase II clinical trial of lubeluzole in acute ischemic stroke suggested that lubeluzole lowers mortality and disability in some patients.[13] Two dosing regimens were compared to placebo. The low-dose treatment consisted of 7.5 mg of lubeluzole administered intravenously over 1 hour, followed by a continuous infusion of 10 mg per day for 5 days. The high-dose regimen was twice this dose. Subjects diagnosed with acute ischemic stroke in the middle cerebral artery territory were treated within 6 hours of onset of symptoms. Electrocardiographic QT prolongation was observed at plasma concentrations of 100 ng/ml or greater, and there was a higher incidence of ventricular fibrillation in the group that received high-dose lubeluzole. The low-dose lubeluzole group experienced no excess of cardiac arrhythmias compared to placebo. In patients with moderate to large strokes, mortality was 7% in the lower dose lubeluzole patients compared to 20% with placebo (Fig. 47.5). Based on the results of this pilot study, phase III randomized multicenter double-blind placebo-controlled trials of the low-dose lubeluzole regimen in acute ischemic stroke were recently completed in Europe and North America. Results of these studies were conflicting but showed possible benefit. Further studies are underway.

A recently reported pilot study of another ion channel blocker, lifarizine, also suggested reduced mortality and improved outcome,[31] but because the drug causes hypotension, further clinical testing is not planned.

OTHER CYTOPROTECTIVE STRATEGIES

Other strategies of neuroprotection attack later stages of the ischemic cascade.[15,16] Nitric oxide synthesis is induced by stimulation of glutamate receptors, and nitric oxide in turn has a number of complex actions relevant to ischemia and cell injury. Endothelium-derived nitric oxide causes vasodilatation beneficial to ischemic brain, but neuronal nitric oxide generates oxygen free radicals toxic to cells. In animal models of stroke, nitric oxide synthase inhibitors have complex effects befitting the dual role of nitric oxide in cerebral ischemia. The usefulness of nitric oxide modulation in stroke likely will hinge on the ability to favorably manipulate the beneficial and deleterious effects of nitric oxide.

Free radical scavengers affect a late stage of the ischemic process. Tirilazad mesylate, a 21-aminosteroid free radical scavenger, was shown in a randomized double-blind phase II trial to be safe and well tolerated when given at doses up to 6 mg/kg/d for 10 days to patients with aneurysmal subarachnoid hemorrhage. A trend toward improvement of outcome was demonstrated in patients treated with 2 mg/kg/d compared with vehicle. Phase III human testing is in progress in subarachnoid hemorrhage, head injury, and stroke. An initial study of 150 mg bolus within 6 hours of stroke onset followed by 6 mg/d for 3 days suggested possible benefit in men, but not women. A follow-up study using larger doses is underway.[28]

On a more macroscopic scale, clot lysis is clearly advantageous to limiting cellular damage, whether spontaneous or therapeutically achieved, but reperfusion leads to an influx of leukocytes which physically block capillaries and restrict

Figure 47.5 Phase II results of lubeluzole in patients with acute ischemic stroke. European Stroke Scale (ESS) at start: L70.

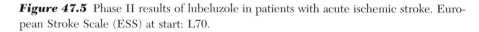

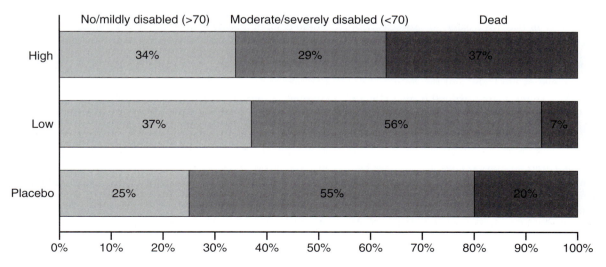

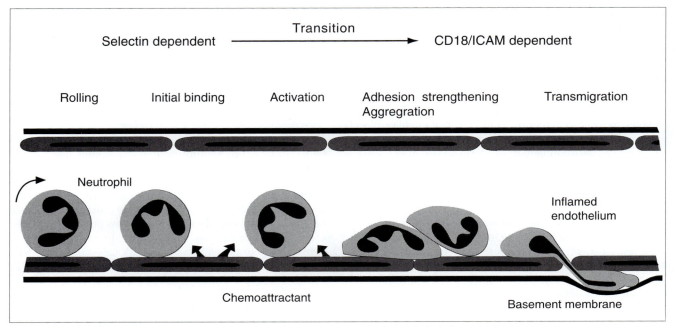

Figure 47.6 Schematic of white blood cell (WBC) adhesion to the vascular endothelial surface (selectin dependent). Interaction between the WBC CD18 receptor and endothelial intercellular adhesion molecule (ICAM) results in transmigration of the WBC through the inflamed endothelium.

reperfusion. The inflammatory cells release cytotoxic products that generate free radicals and damage endothelium. White blood cells also migrate out of the vascular compartment, causing inflammation. In toto, these effects of WBCs are thought to contribute to so-called reperfusion injury (Fig. 47.6). In animal stroke models, monoclonal antibody directed against intercellular adhesion molecule-1 on vascular endothelium prevents leukocyte activation and improves neurologic outcome. A murine anti-ICAM-1 antibody Emlimomab was associated with fewer and worse outcome in phase III testing in stroke patients. Additional studies of anti-WBC therapy will be planned.

The monosialoganglioside GM$_1$ is thought to limit excitotoxicity and facilitate nerve repair and regrowth. In a study of 792 acute stroke patients, there was a nonsignificant trend toward greater recovery in patients treated for 3 weeks with GM-1 compared to placebo.[24] Post hoc analysis showed a statistically significant difference in neurologic outcome favoring GM-1 in the subgroup of patients treated within 4 hours. There was no difference in mortality, and the drug had no significant side effects. To our knowledge, no further studies of gangliosides in acute stroke are planned.

Antagonists of the proteolytic enzyme calpain may be effective in preserving neuronal structural integrity, and basic fibroblast growth factor given intravenously is efficacious in experimental middle cerebral artery occlusion. Both are beginning early testing in humans.

CDP-choline (citicoline) is a precursor of phosphatidyl choline, which is incorporated into the membrane of injured neurons and may prevent membrane breakdown into free radical-generating lipid byproducts. Oral citicoline has few if any side effects. A phase III trial of three different doses of CDP-choline for 6 weeks beginning within 24 hours after acute stroke was recently completed and suggests efficacy.[7] However, a dose response relationship was not found and further studies are underway. In the recently completed study, 259 patients were treated with 500, 1,000, or 2,000 mg daily or placebo for 6 weeks. Both the 500- and 2,000-mg groups demonstrated benefit. In the 500-mg group, which has been chosen for further study, 53% of treated patients were fully independent at 3 months compared to 33% with placebo. Side effects were minor.

BLOOD SUBSTITUTES

These compounds, derived from human hemoglobin, have a dual property: they may be neuroprotective by improving tissue oxygenation, and they may also augment perfusion because of their low viscosity. Several cell-free hemoglobin solutions are under clinical evaluation, but development has been cautious because of concerns about potential allergic and infectious complications, and nephrotoxicity. The agent farthest along in clinical development is diaspirin crossed-linked hemoglobin (DCLHb), which is human hemoglobin derived from banked red blood cells, heat treated, and diaspirin cross-linked to prevent dissociation. It has similar oxygen affinity to that of blood. Probably because hemoglobin binds endothelial NO, it has a slight pressor effect. Studies in animal stroke models have consistently shown improved perfusion of ischemic regions and reduced infarct size.[5,9,10,18] The drug may be particularly effective by maintaining flow and oxygenation in the core of the infarct, thereby maintaining it in a "penumbral" state until definitive reperfusion by spontaneous or therapeutic thrombolysis occurs. In one study, DCLHb was able to double the length of time MCA occlusion could be withstood before ischemic damage appeared[18] (Fig. 47.2). Alone or combined with other neuroprotective drugs, it may be an ideal drug for prehospital administration to prolong the time window for thrombolytic therapy. Early phase II clinical safety trials in stroke patients have begun, but no data are yet available.

In summary, clinicians may soon have at their disposal an armamentarium of treatments for acute stroke. The physician might select from a menu of neuroprotective therapies, each targeting one of the successive waves of the ischemic cascade. For drugs with a large safety margin, and which attack early steps in the ischemic cascade (lubeluzole, DCLHb), treatment might be initiated in the field. After the patient has been admitted to the emergency room, thrombolytic therapy might be implemented along with antiadhesion molecule. A free radical scavenger or other anti-inflammatory agent might also be administered, all within 6 hours of stroke onset. Subsequently, a promoter of neuronal repair is selected. This futuristic model of stroke treatment is fast approaching. In concert with intensive care monitoring in the acute stage and sound traditional management, there is great promise that neuroprotection can make a significant impact on stroke outcome.

Conclusions

1. Increasing knowledge of the "ischemic cascade" is generating new cytoprotective strategies.

2. The complexity of the cascade suggests the limited impact of any one strategy and the advantage of rational combination therapies.

3. Since these drugs affect intracellular processes occurring in normal cellular function and signalling, side effects can be expected.

4. Clinical and laboratory data suggest that the time window for starting cytoprotective therapy is short.

5. No effective cytoprotective drug is currently available clinically.

6. Phase III trials are providing important new data for lubeluzole, anti-ICAM, Cerestat, citicoline, and tirilazad. Others are not far behind.

References

1. Albers GW, Atkinson RP, Kelley RE et al: Safety, tolerability, and pharmacokinetics of the N-Methyl-B aspartate antagonist dextrorphan in patients with acute stroke. Stroke 26:254, 1995
2. The American Nimodipine Study Group: Clinical trial of nimodipine in acute ischemic stroke. Stroke 23:3, 1992
3. Aronowski J, Strong R, Grotta J: Combined neuroprotection and reperfusion therapy for stroke: the effect of lubeluzole and diaspirin cross-linked hemoglobin in experimental focal ischemia. Stroke 27:1571, 1996
4. Aronowski J, Waxham N, Grotta J: Neuronal protection and preservation of calcium/calmodulin-dependent protein kinase II and protein kinase C activity by dextrorphan treatment in global ischemia. J Cereb Blood Flow Metab 13:550, 1993
5. Bowes M, Burhop K, Zivin J: Diaspirin cross-linked hemoglobin improves neurological outcome following reversible but not irreversible CNS ischemia in rabbits. Stroke 25:2253, 1994
6. Bowes M, Rothlein R, Fagan S, Zivin J: Monoclonal antibodies preventing leukocyte activation reduce experimental neurologic injury and enhance efficacy of thrombolytic therapy. Neurology 45:815, 1995
7. Clark W, Warach S, for the Citicholine Study Group: Randomized dose response trial of citicholine in acute ischemic stroke patients. Neurology 49:671, 1997
8. Clifton G, Allen S, Barrodale P et al: A phase II study of moderate hypothermia in severe brain injury. J Neurotrauma 10:263, 1993
9. Cole D, Schell R, Drummond J, Reynolds L: Focal cerebral ischemia in rats: effect of hypervolemic hemodilution with diaspirin crossed-linked hemoglobin versus albumin on brain injury and edema. Anesthesiology 78:335, 1993
10. Cole D, Schell R, Przybelski R et al: Focal cerebral ischemia in rats: effect of hemodilution with cross-linked hemoglobin on CBF. J Cereb Blood Flow Metab 12:971, 1992
11. DeGraba TJ, Ostrow PT, Strong RA et al: The temporal relation calcium-calmodulin binding and neuronal damage after global ischemia. Stroke 23:876, 1992
12. De Ryck M, Scheller D, Clincke G et al: Lubeluzole, a novel benzothiazole protects neurologic function, reduces infarct size and blocks peri-infarct glutamate rise after cerebral thrombotic stroke in rats. Cerebrovasc Dis 5:264, 1995
13. Diener H, Hacke W, Hennerici M et al: Lubeluzole in acute ischemic stroke. A double blind placebo controlled phase II trial. Stroke 27:76, 1996
14. Edwards D, and the CNS 1102-008 Study Group: Cerestat (aptiganel hydrochloride) in the treatment of acute ischemic stroke: results of a phase II trial. Neurology 46:A424, 1996
15. Ginsberg MD: Neuroprotection in brain ischemia: an update (Part I). The Neuroscientist 1:95, 1995
16. Ginsberg MD: Neuroprotection in brain ischemia: an update (Part II). The Neuroscientist 1:164, 1995
17. Grotta JC: Clinical aspects of the use of calcium antagonists in cerebrovascular disease. Clin Neuropharmacol 14:373, 1991
18. Grotta J, Aronowski J: DCLHb for focal ischemia and reperfusion. Cerebrovasc Dis 6:189, 1996
19. Grotta J, Clark W, Coull B et al: Safety and tolerability of the glutamate antagonist CGS 1975 (selfotel) in patients with acute ischemic stroke: results of a phase IIa randomized trial. Stroke 26:602, 1995
20. Grotta JC, Picone CM, Dedman JR et al: Neuronal protection correlates with prevention of calcium-calmodulin binding. Stroke 21 (Suppl III):28, 1990

21. Haley C, Kassel N, Torner J, and the Participants: A randomized controlled trial of high dose intravenous nicardipine in aneurysmal subarachnoid hemorrhage—a report of the Cooperative Aneurysm Study. J Neurosurg 78: 537, 1993

22. Hossmann K: Viability thresholds and the penumbra of focal ischemia. Ann Neurol 36:557, 1994

23. Kirschner P, Henshaw R, Weise J et al: Basic fibroblast growth factor protects against excitotoxicity and chemical hypoxia in both neonatal and adult rats. J Cereb Blood Flow Metab 15:619, 1995

24. Lenzi GL, Grigoletto F, Gent M et al and the Early Stroke Trial Group: Early treatment of stroke with monosialoganglioside GM-1: efficacy and safety results of the early stroke trial. Stroke 25:1552, 1994

25. Minematsu K, Fisher M, Li L et al: Effects of a novel MNDA antagonist on experimental stroke rapidly and quantitatively assessed by diffusion-weighted MRI. Neurology 43:397, 1993

26. Mohr J, Orgogozo J, Harrison M et al: Meta-analysis of oral nimodipine trials in acute ischemic stroke. Cerebrovasc Dis 4:197, 1994

27. Muir KW, Lees KR: A randomized, double-blind, placebo- controlled pilot trial of intravenous magnesium sulfate in acute stroke. Stroke 26:1183, 1995

28. Orgogozo J, Musch B, Peters G and the TESS II Steering Committee: Trial of tirilazad mesylate in acute ischemic stroke (TESS II). Cerebrovasc Dis 6:190, 1996

29. Rosenbaum D, Zabramski J, Frey J et al: Early treatment of ischemic stroke with a calcium antagonist. Stroke 22: 437, 1991

30. Sherman D: Double-blind randomized, placebo-controlled, parallel-group trial of the efficacy and safety of enlimomab (anti-ICAM-1) compared to placebo administered within 6 hours of the onset of symptoms for treatment of acute ischemic stroke. Cerebrovasc Dis 6:189, 1996

31. Squire I, Lees K, Pryse-Phillips W et al, the Lifarizine Study Group: The effects of lifarizine in acute cerebral infarction: a pilot safety study. Cerebrovasc Dis 6:156, 1996

32. Uematsu D, Araki N, Greenberg J et al: Combined therapy with MK-801 and nimodipine for protection of ischemic brain damage. Neurology 41:88, 1991

33. Wahlgren N, MacMahon D, De Keyser J et al: for the INWEST Study Group: Intravenous Nimodipine West European Stroke Trial (INWEST) of nimodipine in the treatment of acute ischemic stroke. Cerebrovasc Dis 4: 204, 1994

34. Yang G, Betz L: Reperfusion-induced injury to the blood-brain barrier after middle cerebral artery occlusion in rats. Stroke 25:1658, 1994

35. Zivin J, Mazzarella V: Tissue plasminogen activator plus glutamate antagonist improves outcome after embolic stroke. Arch Neurol 48:1235, 1991

36. Aronowski J, Strong R, Grotta J: Reperfusion injury: Demonstration of brain damage produced by reperfusion after transient focal ischemia in rats. J Cereb Blood Flow Metab 17:1048, 1997

37. Aronowski J, Ostrow P, Samways E, Strong R, Zivin J, Grotta J: Graded bioassay for demonstration of brain rescue from experimental acute ischemia in rats. Stroke 25: 2235, 1994

Cardiogenic Brain Embolism: Incidence, Varieties, and Treatment

JUDITH A. HINCHEY

ANTHONY J. FURLAN

HENRY J. M. BARNETT

Definitions

Cerebral embolism refers to an obstruction of a blood vessel in the brain by an embolus originating anywhere in the circulatory system. In the National Institute of Neurological Disorders and Stroke (NINDS) classification,[296] *pathologic* sources for arterial embolism include the heart, the great vessels (artery-to-artery), and other sources such as those that produce paradoxical embolism. The cardioembolic category of emboli is distinctly different from artery-to-artery emboli, which are classified in the atherothrombotic category.

Cardiogenic brain embolism, the subject of this chapter, refers to an obstruction in the cerebral arteries by an embolus originating in the heart.

Frequency

A pooling of data from several clinical, epidemiologic, and multicenter projects, although differing in criteria and extent of laboratory workup, indicates that 15% to 20% of all ischemic strokes are cardioembolic.[33,40,52,109,175,275] The prevalence of cardioembolic stroke in patients younger than 45 years of age is much higher, ranging from 23% to 36%.[4,26,53] This is ex-

plained mainly by the lower prevalence of atherothrombotic strokes in this age group, and despite the fact that some of the major cardiac conditions underlying cerebral emboli are more frequent in the elderly.[333] The most common cardiac conditions associated with cerebral emboli are listed in Table 48.1 In older subjects, stenosing cerebral artery lesions and potential sources of cardiac origin for emboli coexist, and care must be taken in the investigation to determine which is the likely cause of the cerebral ischemia.

The relative incidence of the types of stroke keeps changing as technology advances to allow a more precise diagnosis. A good example is the change resulting from the introduction of transesophageal echocardiography. As described in Chapter 36 clinical evidence has accumulated replacing pathological suspicion that emboli from aortic ulcerative atheromatous lesions cause strokes.

General Features of Cerebral Ischemia of Cardioembolic Origin

Traditionally, cardioembolic strokes have been regarded as severe and disabling. Undoubtedly, large cortical infarctions with hemorrhagic transformation are commonly of cardiac ori-

Table 48.1 Most Common Cardiac Conditions Associated with Cerebral Emboli

Source	All Cardiogenic Emboli (%)
Nonvalvular atrial fibrillation	45
Acute myocardial infarction	15
Ventricular aneurysm	10
Rheumatic heart disease	10
Prosthetic cardiac valve	10
Others	10

(Adapted from the Cerebral Embolism Task Force,[52] with permission.)

gin.[105,195,339] These findings result from embolization of sufficiently large quantities of thrombus material or large vegetations, constituting many of the cardiogenic emboli (Tables 48.1 and 48.2). Other cardiogenic emboli are smaller (Table 48.2); the associated hemisphere events may be transient or minor with a small area of infarction,[144,168] or they may be retinal and present as transient monocular blindness or a retinal infarction.[18,39,160,327]

The cerebral circulation absorbs 10% to 15% of the cardiac output.[219] Carotid artery blood flow accounts for approximately 90% of total cerebral blood flow.[138,139] The most common sites for lodgment of cardiac emboli are the main trunk and branches of the middle cerebral artery (MCA). In a careful observational study, balloon emboli placed in the internal carotid artery favored the MCA location and lodged in the anterior cerebral artery only 7% of the time[120] (Fig. 48.1). About 10% of cerebral emboli enter the vertebral-basilar circulation, where they lodge mainly in the top of the basilar artery, or in the main trunk, or in one of the branches of the posterior cerebral arteries.[48,247]

Modern investigative techniques are capable of identifying many sources of smaller cardiogenic emboli. The traditional sources are recognized by the new technology to cause many small, as well as large, lesions.[144,168] Transient ischemic events, both hemispheric and retinal, occur from cardiac sources. In the Oxfordshire Community Stroke Project, TIAs were equally common as a prelude to cardioembolic stroke as they were to large artery or lacunar types of stroke.[325]

Clinical Diagnosis

Many features from the history of onset and physical findings have been claimed to be relatively specific for an embolic stroke, as opposed to a thrombotic stroke. These include

Table 48.2 Embolus Size (with Respect to Origin)

Large	Small
Ventricular thrombus (fibrin-rich)	Calcific material (valvular)
Atrial thrombus (fibrin-rich)	Small vegetations
	Platelet thrombi
Tumor material	Myxomatous material
Large vegetations	Septic material

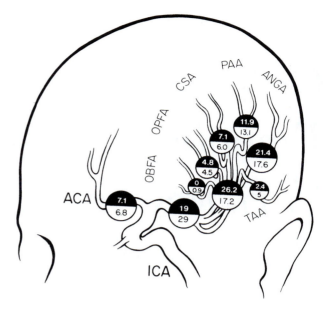

Figure 48.1 "Balloon" catheters lodged in the branches of the internal carotid artery (ICA), in a proportion strikingly similar to the occlusion of branches of the anterior cerebral artery (ACA) and middle cerebral arteries. The lower numbers refer to the percentages of spontaneous occlusions, the upper to the percentages of the total "balloon emboli" that appear at these sites. The highest percentages of both were in the main middle cerebral trunk, the parietal arteries (PAA), and angular arteries (ANGA), with fewer in the central sulcus artery (CSA), operculofrontal artery (OPFA), temporal arteries (TAA), and orbitofrontal artery (OBFA). (Adapted from Gacs et al,[120] with permission.)

the abrupt onset of a maximal deficit in an awake, usually active patient; headache, seizure, or diminished level of consciousness at the onset; and rapid improvement. Important additional features are a history of systemic embolism, the presence of a predisposing heart condition, and the involvement of more than one vascular area in the history or examination of the patient.[49,167,213,215,216]

Conversely, the investigators in the Stroke Data Bank concluded that some clinical features occurred more frequently in patients with infarcts of arterial rather than cardioembolic origin: fractional arm weakness (shoulder more involved than hand), diabetes, hypertension, and male gender.[314]

Emboli tend to occlude individual cortical branches and thus are frequently incriminated as the underlying cause in several distinct clinical syndromes: isolated Wernicke's aphasia,[31,141] Broca's aphasia,[206] global aphasia without hemiparesis,[191] isolated hemianopia, and other features of the posterior cerebral artery syndromes.[31,105,247]

The most specific criteria suggesting cardioembolic sources may be narrowed to (1) abrupt onset, (2) diminished level of consciousness at onset, (3) the history or presence of systemic embolism, and (4) the presence of a heart condition.[31,175,260]

Cardiac Evaluation

With a possible cardiac source in mind, inquiry must be made about rheumatic fever, recent or remote history of myocardial infarction, myocardial revascularization, systemic embolism, and syncope or palpitations either in the past or at the onset of the stroke.

Physical examination must seek the presence of arrhythmia, cardiac valve dysfunction, cardiomegaly, cardiac failure, and any evidence of systemic embolization (petechiae, splinter hemorrhages, Roth's spots, visceral or limb ischemia).

Chest x-ray is used to help diagnose cardiomegaly or congestive heart failure.

A twelve-lead electrocardiogram (ECG) with a rhythm strip is used to detect an acute or old myocardial infarct and the nature of any dysrhythmia (e.g., atrial fibrillation, sick sinus syndrome). A 24-hour Holter monitor is recommended when the suspicion for a dysrhythmia is high and routine ECG is nondiagnostic.[262]

Echocardiography has a major role in the evaluation of patients suspected of a cardiac source for embolism. M-mode and particularly two-dimensional (2D) echocardiography are excellent in showing the spatial and anatomic relationships of the heart, including valve configuration and movement, ventricular wall function, and the detection of masses in its cavities.[254,255]

Transesophageal echocardiography (TEE) is superior for the evaluation of the left atrial appendage, the mitral valve apparatus, and the atrial septum.[68,79,86,189,203,244,253,286,291] It is also superior for detection of mitral valve strands and spontaneous echo contrast, which have been associated with an increased risk of thromboembolism.[189] It is sensitive in detecting atheromatosis of the aortic arch, which has recently been recognized as an occult source of systemic emboli.[7,112,253,317]

Doppler echo is a useful technique for measuring the pressure gradient across a stenotic valve and thus estimating its severity. Color Doppler flow mapping is useful for estimating the degree of valvular regurgitation, and it provides a reasonable correlation with angiographic studies. Its greatest impact is in congenital heart diseases.[293] Contrast echocardiography is mainly used for the detection of intracardiac shunts.

It is beyond the scope of this chapter to provide more technical details and potential pitfalls of echo; several good reviews have been published.[101,254,255,286,293] Echo is excellent in the detection of left ventricular thrombi[85] (Fig. 48.2), mitral valve prolapse,[81,231,342] infective endocarditis,[220,232] patent foramen ovale,[188] atrial septal aneurysm,[283] cardiac myxoma,[204] and possibly left atrial thrombi.[203,290] It may detect very small valvular vegetations, such as occur in nonbacterial thrombotic endocarditis,[196] and may provide prognostic clues in many cardiac conditions. For example, left atrial spontaneous echo contrast was found to be a good indicator for an increased thromboembolic risk in mitral valve disease.[70]

Transcranial Doppler ultrasonography (TCD) detects microemboli made up of air, atheromatous material, platelets, and fibrinogen.[63] It has been shown to be more sensitive than contrast 2D echo in detecting left to right atrial shunts.[310] TCD's ability to distinguish cardiac sources of emboli and their significance remains under investigation.[14,126,134,315]

Other diagnostic techniques include ultrafast cardiac computed tomography (CT) scan, cardiac magnetic resonance imaging (MRI),[243] and isotope-labeled platelet scintigraphy.[92] These are relatively new and expensive, and further experience is needed before their role in the diagnosis of cardiac sources of emboli can be ascertained.

Algorithms for a cardiac workup in patients with acute stroke have been suggested.[79,311] Extensive cardiac evaluation, including TEE, is considered mandatory for young stroke patients unless another pathogenesis is clear. For older patients, some advocate its use only if there is evidence of cardiac disease.[97] The difficulty with this approach is that cerebral embolism may be the presenting complaint in patients with cardiac disease not evident on history or physical examination.[160]

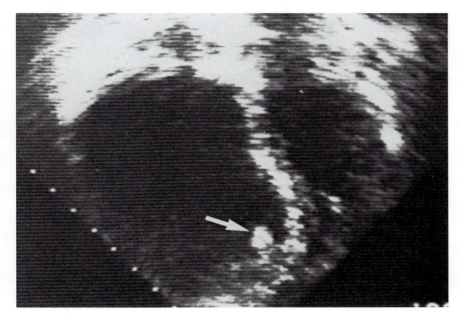

Figure 48.2 Two-dimensional echocardiogram showing a mobile thrombus (arrow) within the left ventricle in a patient with dilated cardiomyopathy.

Hence, echocardiography should be considered in the workup of older patients with threatened or completed stroke in whom noncardiac mechanisms are not apparent.[53] The role of TEE in the evaluation of acute stroke is controversial.[68,79,147] TEE has been shown to be more sensitive in detecting possible sources of emboli in patients with and without clinical or physical evidence of heart disease.[6,68,147,189,245,291] The impact of the results of TEE on patient management has not been shown to be significant.[147,291]

A retrospective analysis of 184 consecutive patients with focal cerebral ischemia admitted to an intensive stroke research unit illustrates the value of careful cardiac study.[262] There were 116 patients with stroke and 68 with transient ischemic attacks; cardiac disease was known by history and examination in 18.4%. An ECG detected cardiac disease in a further 14.1%: 3 additional patients with atrial fibrillation and 23 with silent myocardial infarction, predominantly in diabetics. Two-dimensional echocardiography, performed in approximately two-thirds of the patients, detected potential cardiac sources of emboli in a further 11.9%: 11 patients had dyskinetic segments, 6 had left ventricular thrombi, 1 had endocarditis, and 1 had global left-ventricular dysfunction. All were monitored with continuous ECG recording for 48 hours; four instances of atrial fibrillation not previously suspected were detected. Approximately one-fourth of these patients underwent more prolonged ECG monitoring: two more with atrial fibrillation and with one sick sinus syndrome were diagnosed. In summary, a number of these patients had potential sources of emboli not evident on history and examination; the majority (15.2%) were detected from the use of ECG monitoring and 2D echocardiography.

Radiologic Evaluation

BRAIN COMPUTED TOMOGRAPHY AND MAGNETIC RESONANCE IMAGING

Certain CT findings are fairly characteristic of embolic infarction: (1) the presence of a cortical infarct, especially in the distribution of the middle or posterior cerebral artery territories, (2) the demonstration of multiple infarcts in different territories, (3) an embolus visible in the middle cerebral artery ("hyperdense MCA sign") (Fig. 48.3), and (4) hemorrhage, usually deep within the infarct.[105,143,195] The disintegration of the original embolus and distal migration of embolic fragments result in hemorrhagic transformation.[52,105] The capillary walls, damaged by ischemia, are unable to bear the impact of the restored blood flow (Fig. 48.4). However, some instances of hemorrhagic transformation have been shown by autopsy to have persistent occlusion of the main artery. This suggests that hemorrhagic transformation will occur with obstructive arterial pressure resulting from an early rise in perfusion pressure in the presence of efficient leptomeningeal collaterals.[233]

CT studies that have looked at hemorrhagic infarction immediately after stroke onset report a prevalence of 2% to 4%[50,113]; studies that included serial scans 2 to 4 days after the stroke onset report a prevalence of 10% to 20%.[51,143] A recent study[234] identified hemorrhagic transformation in 6.2% at 1 to 4 days, 27.5% at 10 days, and 40.6% at 1 month. This last figure is similar to the frequency reported in autopsy studies.[105,195] The majority of hemorrhagic transformations are clinically silent.

MRI can better identify multiple embolic infarcts in different territories,[338] adds no distinctive diagnostic features, but may be combined with MR angiography to identify MCA stem embolic occlusions. Proton density-weighted MR may be the earliest imaging technique to detect embolic infarcts.[289]

CEREBRAL ANGIOGRAPHY

Isolated occlusion of the middle cerebral artery, the posterior cerebral artery, or one of their branches in the absence of atherosclerotic changes is highly suggestive of cardiogenic embolism. In a study where angiography was carried out within 6 hours of stroke onset, 15 of the 22 patients who had isolated intracranial occlusion demonstrated a well-defined cardiac source of emboli.[102] Spontaneous recanalization occurs in the majority of patients undergoing serial angiography.[234] In the

Figure 48.3 A noncontrast scan demonstrating the left middle cerebral artery as a high-density structure along with nonhemorrhagic infarction in the distribution of the left middle and posterior cerebral arteries. (From Gacs et al,[121] with permission.)

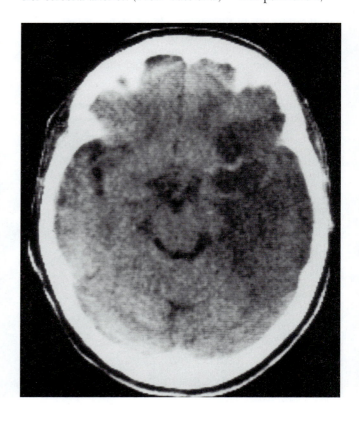

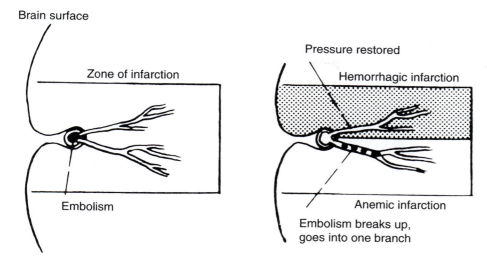

Brain surface

Zone of infarction

Embolism

Pressure restored

Hemorrhagic infarction

Anemic infarction

Embolism breaks up,
goes into one branch

Figure 48.4 Hypothetical mechanism of hemorrhagic transformation caused by distal migration of embolic fragments with reperfusion of infarcted tissue. (Adapted from Toole,[316] with permission.)

era of tPA studies, further evidence of the frequency of intra-arterial thrombi causing ischemic stroke has been studied. The tendency for spontaneous recanalization has been observed frequently.[77]

Cardiac Diseases Causing Cerebral Embolism

Intracardiac thrombi form in the presence of structural abnormalities of the heart valves or its walls or chambers. They develop in the presence of dysrhythmias that cause stasis within the left atrium or in dyskinetic states of the left ventricle. Emboli may arise from valve vegetations, intracardiac tumors, or even from systemic veins when the embolic material traverses the heart through a patent foramen ovale or atrial septal defect (paradoxical embolism). Very rarely do emboli arise from pulmonary veins or from a pulmonary arteriovenous fistula. The mechanisms of these embolic phenomena are shown in Figure 48.5. The cardiac disorders associated with embolism and the location of the sources are listed in Table 48.3.

Cardiac Dysrhythmias and Cerebral Embolism

The two abnormalities of cardiac rhythm most often associated with focal cerebral ischemia are atrial fibrillation and the sick sinus syndrome.

Diffuse *nonfocal* cerebral ischemia (i.e., syncope or Stokes-Adams attacks) may be caused by cardiac dysrhythmias that induce cerebral hypoperfusion. Reduction in cerebral perfusion is usually the result of complete heart block or paroxysmal tachyarrhythmia associated with a rapid ventricular rate of more than 180 beats per minute (e.g., paroxysmal atrial tachycardia, ventricular tachycardia, or ventricular fibrillation). Focal cerebral ischemia is rare with such disturbances of cardiac rhythm. Of 290 patients requiring insertion of a pacemaker for cardiac arrhythmias, 4 had experienced focal cerebral ischemic symptoms, but in only 2 was the focal ischemia related to their cardiac rhythm disturbance.[261]

ATRIAL FIBRILLATION

For many years atrial fibrillation (AF) has been known to be associated with an increased risk of cerebral emboli from thrombus material originating in the left atrium. Older reports included many patients with rheumatic heart disease and concomitant valvular disease carrying an independent risk. In the Framingham study[334] the presence of both carried a 17-fold increase in the risk of stroke as compared to normal controls.

In an autopsy study of 642 patients with atrial fibrillation of various causes, a left atrial thrombus was found in 15.8% as opposed of 1.7% in 642 age- and sex-matched controls. Left ventricular thrombus was encountered in 1% of patients with AF. Cerebral infarction occurred in 32.2% of the patients with AF and in only 11% of the controls. The frequency of cerebral infarction increased with the duration of fibrillation; the most common causes of AF were rheumatic and ischemic heart disease.[3] Patients with idiopathic hypertrophic subaortic stenosis (also called idiopathic hypertrophic cardiomyopathy) are likely to suffer atrial fibrillation.[84,272]

Nonvalvular atrial fibrillation (NVAF) is the term commonly used to specify the group of patients in which the underlying cause is other than valvular disease. NVAF affects 2% to 5% of the general population over the age of 60[166,238]

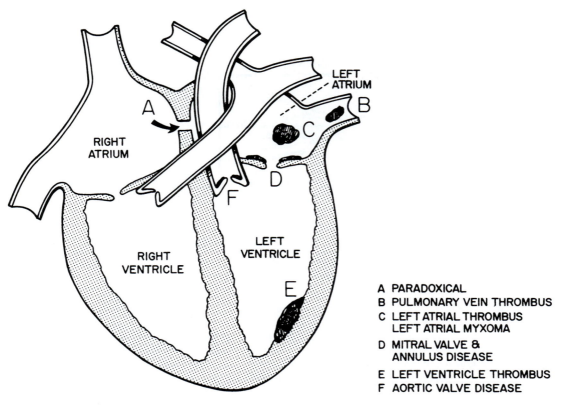

RIGHT ATRIUM

LEFT ATRIUM

RIGHT VENTRICLE

LEFT VENTRICLE

A PARADOXICAL
B PULMONARY VEIN THROMBUS
C LEFT ATRIAL THROMBUS
  LEFT ATRIAL MYXOMA
D MITRAL VALVE &
  ANNULUS DISEASE
E LEFT VENTRICLE THROMBUS
F AORTIC VALVE DISEASE

Figure 48.5 A schematic representation of the heart showing the potential sites of origin of emboli.

Table 48.3 Important Cardiac Sources for Cerebral Ischemia

Disorder	Location of Potentially Embolic Material
Myocardial infarction, recent, with endocardial damage	Endocardial surface left ventricle
Myocardial infarction, old, with akinetic segment or major aneurysmal dilation	Particularly apical, in left ventricle, trapped in trabeculae corneae cordis
Rheumatic mitral stenosis[a]	Auricle or dilated atrium
Rheumatic mitral regurgitation[a]	"Jet" lesions on atrial endocardium
Infective endocarditis	On the valve surface and at its attachment
Nonbacterial thrombotic endocarditis	On the valve surface
Libman-Sacks endocarditis	On the valve surface and less commonly on chordae tendineae, papillary muscles, and mural endocardium
Myxomatous degeneration (mitral valve prolapse)[a]	At atrial site of valve attachment, also on valve surface
Mitral annulus calcification[a]	Attached to valve surface[b]
Calcific aortic stenosis[a]	Calcification begins at base of cusp, but rarely extends to free edge
Prosthetic heart valve[a]	At site of attachment, also on surface of device
Cardiomyopathy	Atrium or ventricle, usually trapped in trabeculae corneae cordis
Atrial myxoma	Tumor usually attached to margin of septum secundum
Atrial fibrillation	Thrombus within the left atrium
Sick sinus syndrome	Thrombus within the left atrium

[a] These are prone to infective endocarditis.

[b] In addition to thrombi, calcific material from the degenerative valve may break off as embolic material.

(Adapted from Barnett,[17] with permission.)

and, within this group, its prevalence increases steeply with advancing age.[166] NVAF is a major cause of cardioembolic stroke[49,52,216] as well as of massive cerebral infarction.[339] The presence of atrial fibrillation in acute stroke patients is associated with a worsened prognosis at 1 and 6 months.[47]

In the Framingham study,[334] NVAF carried a fivefold increased risk for stroke. The frequency of stroke varies depending on the populations under study: as low as 1.7% per year in an outpatient-based study in Olmsted County[74] and as high as 5% to 9% in inpatient-based studies.[103, 270] For a group of nontreated patients with either chronic or intermittent AF, a 6% yearly risk of stroke has been suggested.[305]

NVAF is not a uniform group. The elderly, those with coexisting congestive heart failure or hypertension and those with a past history of stroke, harbor a higher stroke risk. Other risk factors include recent onset of arrhythmia, chronic forms (as opposed to paroxysmal), left ventricular wall abnormalities by echocardiogram, and the presence of left atrial enlargement.[45,107,305,333,335]

A subset of NVAF patients that carries a significantly lower risk of stroke includes patients younger than 60 years who are without definable heart disease. This group of "lone atrial fibrillators" carries a yearly risk of stroke of less than 0.5%.[178,237]

Thyrotoxicosis is complicated by atrial fibrillation in 10% to 30% of patients,[87] but accounts for only 2% to 5% of all NVAF cases.[248] Several reports, however, suggest that if provocative tests to reveal occult thyrotoxicosis are used, this figure may be as high as 30%.[87,109] Whether the risk of stroke in such patients is similar to or higher than other NVAF patients is controversial.[248,256]

Based on the accepted pathogenesis of stroke in most patients with NVAF (i.e., embolus originating from a left atrial thrombus), antithrombotic treatment has been administered and evaluated in eight randomized trials.[35,62,88,98,249,303,304,306] All trials demonstrated a benefit from warfarin compared with both placebo and aspirin. A meta-analysis (Fig. 48.6) carried out with the data from these trials shows an overall relative risk reduction of stroke of 64% (95% confidence interval, 51–74, $P < 0.001$) favoring warfarin over placebo, and 48% (95% confidence interval, 33–60, $P < 0.001$) favoring warfarin over aspirin.[21]

The risk from atrial fibrillation rises above the age of 60, and increases in patients with hypertension, history of recent congestive heart failure, or previous episodes of thromboembolism. Although warfarin is superior to aspirin (Fig. 48.6), aspirin is an acceptable alternative to lifelong therapy with warfarin in patients without these risk factors who are under the age 60 years. There is a higher risk for hemorrhagic complications in patients over 75 years of age, so that some recommend using aspirin rather than warfarin. If used, the older patients must have rigid control of the international normalized ratio (INR), not exceeding 3.0, and blood pressure must be carefully monitored.

Anticoagulant therapy is strongly recommended in patients with AF secondary to mitral valve disease, dilated or hypertrophic cardiomyopathy, in patients with chronic NVAF who are between the age of 60 to 75 years and in patients of any age who have documented systemic embolism, or in those with concomitant congestive heart failure. It is also recommended in patients with newly recognized thyrotoxicosis before a euthyroid state is reached, and before cardioversion in all patients.[87]

SICK SINUS SYNDROME

The term *sick sinus syndrome* (SSS) encompasses any form of sinus node depression, such as marked sinus bradycardia (<50 beats/min), sinus arrest, or sinoatrial block. The SSS occurs throughout life, but is more common in older patients. It may be associated with ischemic heart disease, cardiomyopathies, and neuromuscular disease, but is frequently idiopathic or degenerative in origin. The bradyarrhythmia is often associated with paroxysmal atrial tachyarrhythmia, including supraventricular tachycardia and atrial flutter or fibrillation. Such a combination is often referred to as the tachycardia-bradycardia syndrome.[155]

The clinical manifestations are mainly those produced by transient global cerebral ischemia (i.e., light-headedness and syncope). However, patients with SSS are at high risk for stroke, which is usually massive and presumably of cardiac embolic origin.[1,99,271]

Of a total of 56 patients with SSS, Rubenstein et al[271] described 10 patients with focal cerebral ischemia in whom the bradycardia-tachycardia syndrome was present. Fairfax et al[99] found a significantly higher incidence of embolism (predominantly cerebral) in 100 patients with SSS, compared with 712 age- and sex-matched controls with chronic complete heart block. Their criteria for SSS were unexplained sinus bradycardia with a pulse less than 60, or recurrent sinus arrest with or without supraventricular tachyarrhythmias. Systemic and cerebral embolism occurred in 16% of these patients with SSS, compared to only 1.9% of those with chronic complete heart block ($P < 0.001$). Only 3 patients out of 16 had purely systemic emboli, and in 13 the embolus was to the cerebral or retinal circulation with or without systemic embolism.

The only effective treatment for SSS is pacemaker implantation, but the stroke rate is still high after pacing.[106] There are several types of pacemakers, and reports that analyzed the stroke rate with respect to the type of pacemaker found a higher rate when ventricular demand pacemakers were used, as opposed to those of atrial demand, especially in the elderly.[106,276] Further analysis disclosed a much higher incidence of atrial fibrillation in the patients with ventricular pacemakers, an important factor that can partly explain the higher incidence of stroke in this group. In the majority of patients, chronic AF appeared after pacer implantation. A causal factor may be the development of atrial enlargement in patients with the ventricular pacemaker, caused by atrial contraction against atrioventricular valves closed due to the retrograde ventriculoatrial conduction.[276] Thus, it seems that one of the measures for stroke prevention is to install an atrial demand pacemaker in all suitable candidates.[276] Platelet antiaggregation agents may or may not provide protection against stroke, and the role of anticoagulants has not been thoroughly assessed.[106]

Myocardial Infarction

Acute myocardial infarction (AMI) is complicated by stroke in 2.5% of patients within 2 to 4 weeks of onset.[161,259] Most strokes occur in the presence of left ventricular thrombi

Trial Name	Time Since Last Event	INR Range* (Aspirin Dose)	Sample Size†	Number of Strokes‡	Relative Risk Reduction of Stroke§

(A) WARFARIN versus PLACEBO

AFASAK[249]	1 month	2.8 - 4.2	W: 335 (250)	5	
			P : 336 (382)	18	
BAATAF[35]	6 months	1.5 - 2.7	W: 212 (487)	3	
			P : 208 (435)	13	
CAFA[62]	1 year	2.0 - 3.0	W: 187 (235)	7	
			P : 191 (239)	11	
SPAF-I[306]	2 years	2.0 - 4.5	W: 210 (260)	7	
			P : 211 (244)	18	
VA[98]	91% patients event-free	1.4 - 2.8	W: 281 (489)	9	
			P : 290 (483)	24	
EAFT[88]	Recent event required	2.5 - 4.0	W: 225 (507)	21	
			P : 214 (405)	54	
Overall					

(B) WARFARIN versus ASPIRIN

AFASAK[249]	1 month	2.8 - 4.2 (75 mg)	W: 335 (250)	5	
			A: 336 (364)	17	
SPAF-I[306]	2 years	2.0 - 4.5 (325 mg)	W: 210 (260)	7	
			A: 552 (720)	27	
EAFT[88]	Recent event required	2.5 - 4.0 (300 mg)	W: 225 (507)	21	
			A: 404 (838)	94	
SPAF-II[304]	2 years	2.0 - 4.5 (325 mg)	W: 555 (1493)	41	
			A: 545 (1460)	44	
SPAF-III[303]	1 month	2.0 - 3.0 (325 mg)	W: 523 (581)	14	
			A: 521 (558)	49	
Overall					

```
        -100  -50   0   50  100
```
Warfarin Worse   Warfarin Better

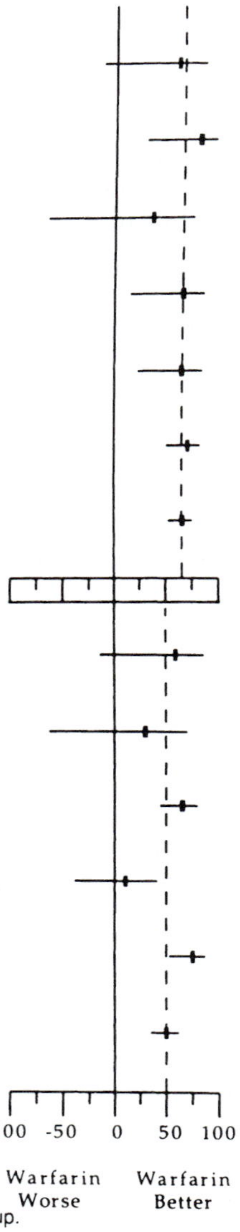

* INR = International Normalized Ratio.
† Number of subjects per group *(Estimated person-years of follow-up)*.
  W = Warfarin. P = Placebo, except for BAATAF that allowed aspirin.
  A = Aspirin, except SPAF-III that combined low-intensity, fixed-dose warfarin (INR 1.2 - 1.5).
‡ Includes all fatal and non-fatal stroke, intracranial hemorrhage, and systemic embolism.
§ Relative risk reduction due to warfarin treatment was calculated using person-years of follow-up.

Figure 48.6 Meta-analyses showing the relative risk reduction of stroke among patients with nonvalvular atrial fibrillation receiving (**A**) warfarin as compared with placebo, and (**B**) warfarin as compared with aspirin. The relative risk reduction is indicated by a solid rectangle, with its corresponding 95% confidence interval as a horizontal line. The overall relative risk reduction is represented by the broken vertical line: (**A**) 64%; 95% confidence interval, 51% to 74%; $P < 0.001$, and (**B**) 48%, 95% confidence interval, 33% to 60%; $P < 0.001$. All *P*-values are two-tailed. Test for heterogeneity among relative risk reductions in each analysis was statistically nonsignificant. (From *New England Journal of Medicine*,[20] with permission.)

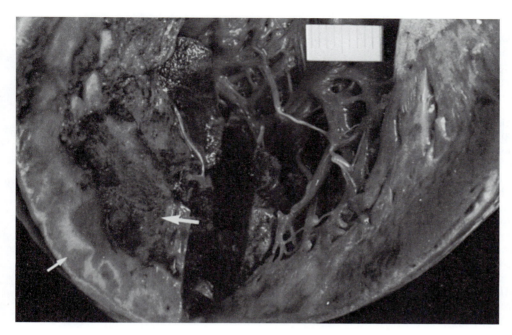

Figure 48.7 Pathologic specimen showing myocardial infarction (small arrow) with superimposed mural thrombosis (large arrow).

(LVT)[161,302,329] (Fig. 48.7), believed to be the underlying cause for the cerebral embolism. Other factors associated with increased risk of thromboembolism include increased age, history of stroke, chronic atrial fibrillation, and serum glutamic oxaloacetic transaminase (SGOT) levels four times normal.[309]

The presence of LVT is best detected with two-dimensional echocardiography, a specific, sensitive technique superior to cardiac ventriculography (Fig. 48.2).[254,255] By this technique, LVT were detected in 30% to 35% of patients sustaining AMI, 2 to 11 days after its onset.[13,185,280,320]

Specific risk factors for LVT include the presence of a hypokinetic or akinetic segment of the ventricular wall, injury to the endocardial surface, or persistently abnormal left ventricular flow patterns.[78,322] Prediction of apical thrombus formation in acute MI based on the left ventricular spatial flow patterns has found only severe wall motion abnormalities predictive of developing LVT. In addition, heparin was found to help prevent LVT formation.[177] These complications are more common in transmural and in anterior wall infarcts. The combination of stasis and thrombogenicity enhances the formation of LVT.[12,118,161,229,329] Echocardiographic follow-up of relatively small numbers of patients with AMI, who had LVT but were treated in a "conservative" way (mini-dose heparin and aspirin), showed resolution of the thrombus in 80% of cases after 1 year, and at 2 years a further disappearance in 20% was documented.[229] In another study,[184,185] where two-thirds of the patients with LVT were anticoagulated, about half the LVTs were resolved by the end of 12 weeks, regardless of treatment. In the anticoagulated group 93% showed either resolution or change in size or shape of the thrombus.[185] A total of 23 patients at high risk for embolization because of mobile or protruding LVT were treated with high dose heparin. Within 1 to 3 weeks of treatment, 83% of thrombi disap-

peared. There were no emboli and only one gastrointestinal hemorrhage requiring only medical treatment.[148]

The risk of clinical cerebral embolism in patients with LVT followed for up to 2 years is between 10% and 15%. The majority of strokes occur during the first 3 months, most within the first 10 days.[89,118,212] Risk factors for embolization include advanced age, as well as protrusion and mobility of the thrombotic mass in the left ventricle.[161,212,323]

In an autopsy study,[214] the prevalence of LVT as detected by echocardiography was confirmed; evidence of cerebral and systemic embolization was higher than suspected clinically. Thrombi in the left heart were found in 35% of patients with a history of myocardial infarction. Patients with acute myocardial infarction had thrombi in the left side of the heart in 40% of instances, compared to only 26% in those with healed myocardial infarction. In patients with acute myocardial infarction with or without mural thrombi, cerebral and systemic arterial occlusions were detected in 35% and 21% respectively. In patients with healed myocardial infarction, arterial occlusions were detected in 26% of patients with and in 28% of patients without mural thrombi.

LVT in healed myocardial infarction are usually associated with a persistent left ventricular dyskinesia or the presence of a left ventricular aneurysm. When these conditions have existed, LVT have been detected by echocardiography in almost half of the patients. The likelihood of emboli occurring has been variable.[118,187,302] In a recent study, where LVT were first detected at a mean of 32 months following an AMI, the embolic rate was 10% during 22 months of follow-up.[302] The embolization rate from left ventricular aneurysms appears to be low at 0.35 per 100 patient years.[187]

Treatment to prevent stroke after AMI is still controversial.[53,89,118,229] Several controlled clinical trials demonstrated beneficial effects of anticoagulant therapy, yet the occurrence of hemorrhagic complications was high.[53] Recently several large controlled studies have demonstrated much more favorable results. The first two studies, including 421 patients, clearly favored heparin anticoagulation. Both studies used subcutaneous (SC) heparin, 12,500 units every 12 hours for 10 days in patients with anterior AMI. The first study compared this regimen to SC heparin in a dose that is given to prevent venous thrombosis (5,000 units bid).[320] The incidence of LVT at day 10 was 11% in the high-dose group compared to 32% in the low-dose group. Nonhemorrhagic infarction occurred in 1% and 4%, respectively. In the second study, the presence of LVT was evaluated by echocardiography before discharge.[280] LVT were present in 36.5% of the controls who received no anticoagulation, as compared to 17.7% of the heparin-treated group. There were two embolic strokes in the control group compared to none in the treatment group.

A third study compared long-term warfarin therapy with placebo[294]: 1,214 patients entered the study at a mean of 27 days following the onset of AMI and were followed for an average of 37 months. The target warfarin range was 2.8 to 4.8 international normalized ratio (INR) yet serious bleeding was noted in only 0.6% per year of the warfarin group. Stroke relative risk reduction was 55% and death and reinfarction risk reductions were 24% and 34% respectively.

Most would agree with high-dose heparin for those with an anterior AMI.[177,142,148,190,321] A meta-analysis of 11 studies reported an odds ratio of 0:14 for preventing embolization in the anticoagulated versus no anticoagulation, with an event difference rate of −0.33.[321]

Antiplatelet agents have usually, but not always, been found ineffective in the prevention/resolution of LVT and subsequent emboli.[162,181,184] In a meta-analysis, antiplatelet agents were not shown to prevent LVT formation.[321] Nevertheless, in a large multicenter trial, the stroke prevalence within 10 days of an AMI was reduced by half in those patients who were treated early with a 160-mg daily dose of aspirin as compared to placebo.[159]

Thrombolytic therapy is of short duration and is usually discontinued before the detection of LVT. Thus, its role in prevention of LVT formation and subsequent stroke is uncertain.[53,89] Some studies show a decrease in LVT formation after streptokinase therapy,[93,150,200,321] others have not.[218] The two most commonly used thrombolytic agents (i.e., streptokinase [SK] and alteplase tissue plasminogen activator [tPA]) are associated with an increased rate of intracerebral hemorrhage.[257] With tPA the risk is lower, but the overall stroke rate is similar because of an apparent excess in ischemic strokes with the use of this agent.[158] Both SK and tPA may increase platelet aggregation, mainly by thrombin activation. This paradoxical hypercoagulable state is not inhibited by aspirin but can be reversed with heparin.[94] The latest large study addressing this controversy[158] compared heparin to placebo subsequent to SK and tPA: heparin was started 12 hours after the administration of the thrombolytic agents. No additional benefit was detected from heparin with respect to stroke prevention or reinfarction, whereas the occurrence of major bleeding was somewhat higher. Thrombolytic therapy has also been shown to cause emboli in patients with preexisting thrombi.[22,240,340]

The recommended treatment policy for patients with acute anterior transmural myocardial infarction includes the use of high-dose heparin, even if thrombolytic therapy is given initially.[89,142,148,151,190,321] Heparin should be given intravenously or subcutaneously in a dose sufficient to maintain a kaolin-cephalin coagulation time between 1.5 to 2.5 times the control. Echocardiography should be performed 5 to 7 days later to detect LVT. If no thrombus or wall motion abnormalities are found, heparin should be discontinued. If LVT or dyskinetic regions are present, warfarin may be started and continued under echocardiographic monitoring. Anticoagulant therapy should be discontinued after 3 to 6 months, even if LVT persists.[53,288,331]

Routine anticoagulation has not been recommended if LVT are detected in an aneurysmal sac at a time remote from AMI.[118] Instead, long-term anticoagulation has been recommended only in patients with cerebral insults attributed to persistent LVT.[53,288] However, this "conservative" approach must be assessed in light of the third study mentioned, which found a significant risk reduction of stroke following long-term warfarin after MI.[294]

Atrial Septal Aneurysm

Atrial septal aneurysm (ASA) has recently been associated with stroke, especially in young patients. It is best detected by TEE.[245] It is speculated that this is a source of embolism,[32,199,225,245] although Burger et al, studying 38 coronary artery bypass patients who had an associated ASA, found no strokes in a mean of 25 months' follow-up.[43] Most patients were on aspirin. In a study of 100 stroke patients up to age 55, an ASA was found in 28% as compared to 8% in the control population. A patent foramen ovale was associated in 71.9% of all cases of ASA, similar to earlier studies.[245] A strong correlation was found between those with cryptogenic stroke and ASA. There was a synergistic effect on the risk of stroke when ASA was associated with a patent foramen ovale,[44] as had been found by others.[61,307] Bogousslavsky et al found a 25% association between ASA and PFO. Looking at stroke recurrence in those with PFO, an associated ASA was not a significant risk factor.[32]

NONISCHEMIC CARDIOMYOPATHIES

This term is used to describe a heterogeneous, relatively rare group of cardiac conditions of different etiologies that result in progressive global cardiac dysfunction. Traditionally, the cardiomyopathies are divided into three types: dilated (formerly called congestive), hypertrophic, and restrictive. The latter is very rare in Western countries, whereas in the tropics it exists mainly as endocardial fibroelastosis. The hypertrophic type (also called idiopathic hypertrophic subaortic stenosis) is seldom associated with intracardiac thrombi or cerebral embolism unless atrial fibrillation coexists.[115,128]

DILATED CARDIOMYOPATHY

Differing causal conditions have been described in relation to this syndrome, including inflammatory processes (such as viral infections, Chagas disease, and other infectious agents), immunologic disorders, toxic agents (mainly alcohol and chemotherapeutic agents such as Adriamycin), nutritional deficiencies, and peripartum cardiomyopathy, as well as several forms of familial cardiomyopathies.[117,157] Unless a specific cause is identified, it is best to refer to most cases as idiopathic. *Idiopathic dilated cardiomyopathy* (IDC) affects predominantly young men. It is a rare disease manifested by progressive heart failure, arrhythmia, or thromboembolism, and its diagnosis is made by exclusion.[2,265,300] Prognosis is very poor and there is a high incidence of sudden death. Arrhythmias are common, either as nonsustained ventricular tachycardia or as chronic atrial fibrillation, which develops in 20% to 30% of the patients.[210,265] This arrhythmia and the high prevalence of left ventricular thrombi found in IDC, as well as in other types of dilated cardiomyopathies, are believed to be the underlying cause for stroke and other embolic complications in these patients. In an autopsy study of 152 IDC patients,[265] ventricular thrombi or mural endocardial plaques (considered to be organized thrombi) were found in up to 78% of cases. The pathogenesis is believed to be chronic intracavitary stasis. Unlike patients after myocardial infarction, there is no aneurysmal sac, and thrombi tend to be relatively small and scattered throughout the cavity with a predilection for the apex, where stasis is maximal[58,130,208] (Fig. 48.8). Echocardiography

Figure 48.8 Thrombus protruding (arrow) from trabeculae carneae cordis in patient with dilated cardiomyopathy. (From Barnett,[17] with permission.)

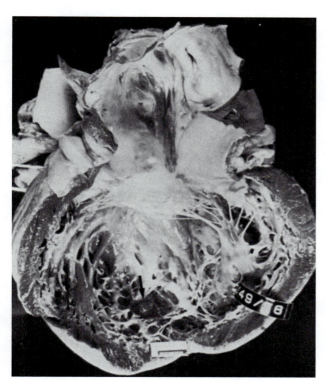

detects the presence of thrombi in 11% to 58% of patients with dilated cardiomyopathy (Fig. 48.2), yet it is not helpful for the detection of patients at high risk for stroke, as no correlation has been found between the detection of thrombi and the presence of emboli.[58,130] The annual frequency of embolic complication varies between 1.4% and 3.5% in different series,[58,117] depending on the presence or absence of anticoagulant therapy and probably also on the severity of the disease. Controversy exists regarding the importance of congestive heart failure, marked cardiac enlargement, and the presence of atrial fibrillation.[58,117,130]

The recommended empirical treatment to reduce the risk of embolization is long-term anticoagulation.[117,288] However, recently it has been reported that most patients do not receive this treatment.[208] This conservative approach may be due to the fact that the benefit of long-term anticoagulation has not been established convincingly or because of the higher risk for bleeding in such patients.[100,300] A plea for a prospective randomized trial of anticoagulation, including low-dose and minidose warfarin, has recently been published.[100]

Cerebral infarction is an uncommon complication in patients with inherited neuromuscular diseases who are prone to develop cardiomyopathies.[28] Cerebral embolization may occur in several specific cardiomyopathies, complicating systemic disease such as sarcoidosis and amyloidosis.[263]

Valvular Heart Disease

In developed countries there has been a dramatic decline in the incidence of rheumatic heart disease. This has partially been offset by the recognition of an association between mitral valve prolapse and other less frequent valvular lesions and cerebral ischemia. Valvular disorders remain significant causes of embolic cerebral ischemia.

RHEUMATIC HEART DISEASE

Clinical embolic events occur in about 20% of patients with rheumatic heart disease (RHD).[65,193] Embolism usually complicates mitral stenosis or mixed stenosis-regurgitation, whereas pure mitral regurgitation or aortic disease less frequently results in embolism.[65,69]

MITRAL STENOSIS

Mitral stenosis is most often of rheumatic origin. Left atrial thrombi (Fig. 48.9) form in a large number of affected patients, particularly in the presence of atrial fibrillation or cardiac failure.[131] Left atrial thrombus is present in 15% to 17% of patients at autopsy, regardless of whether or not there has been a history of embolism.[65] Thrombi may develop in patients with only mild mitral stenosis,[284] explaining why embolism may be a presenting symptom of mitral stenosis. Thrombi

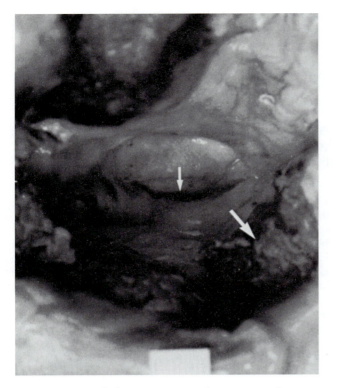

Figure 48.9 Pathologic specimen showing mitral stenosis (small arrow) and left atrial thrombus (large arrow).

may develop on "jet lesions" that can form on the wall of the left ventricle (Fig. 48.10). In patients with mitral stenosis, the annual incidence of all symptomatic emboli is about 4%; more than half are cerebral, but many asymptomatic systemic emboli and occasional asymptomatic cerebral emboli are found at postmortem. Recurrent embolism is common (30% to 75%), usually within 6 to 12 months of the sentinel event,[69,193,308] and the presence of atrial fibrillation increases the risk of embolism fourfold.[65] The risk of embolism also increases with increasing duration of mitral stenosis.[269]

Surgical repair of mitral stenosis, either open or closed commissurotomy, also carries some risk of embolism. Percutaneous valvuloplasty, a technique that was only recently introduced, probably carries the same risk.[72,193,239]

Long-term anticoagulation is recommended for prophylaxis in patients with rheumatic mitral stenosis and coexistent atrial fibrillation, as the combination of both carries a 17-fold increase in stroke risk compared with matched controls.[334] The embolic and recurrent embolic rates are notably reduced with long-term anticoagulation, although long-term therapy is not totally protective.[65,193,308]

MITRAL REGURGITATION

Mitral regurgitation most commonly results from mitral valve prolapse or papillary muscle dysfunction in association with ischemic or rheumatic heart disease. When severe, the incom-

petence produces an ulcerated "jet lesion" on the atrial endocardial surface; left atrial thrombus may form there. This occurs in somewhat less than 10% of patients and almost invariably in the presence of atrial fibrillation.[301] Thromboembolism is a recognized complication of mitral regurgitation.[251] The incidence is low, even though atrial fibrillation is a common accompaniment particularly late in its course.[96,285]

AORTIC STENOSIS

Isolated aortic stenosis is mainly caused by calcification of the valve cusps, a process observed predominantly in elderly people. Until recently, this was considered a relatively benign disorder causing dizziness or syncope. Sudden death was an occasional complication. Most patients seen with cerebral embolism have had multivalvular rheumatic disease or coexistent infective endocarditis.[182] With the introduction of echocardiography, Doppler, and catheterization, it has become evident that calcific aortic stenosis may be responsible for more cerebral vascular insults than previously recognized.[72,153,168] Cerebral vascular events occasionally complicate catheterization or percutaneous balloon valvuloplasty in patients with aortic stenosis.

Figure 48.10 Pathologic specimen showing mitral stenosis resulting from rheumatic heart disease with "jet lesions" (arrows) on the wall of the left ventricle.

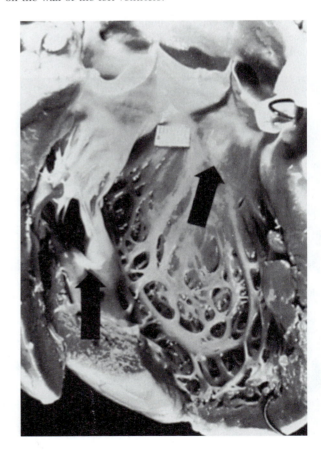

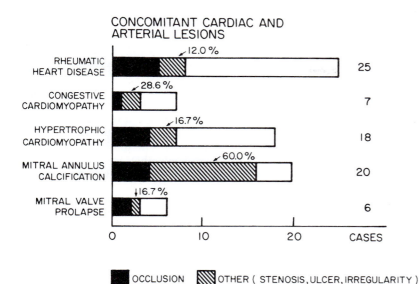

CONCOMITANT CARDIAC AND
ARTERIAL LESIONS

RHEUMATIC HEART DISEASE	12.0 %	25
CONGESTIVE CARDIOMYOPATHY	28.6 %	7
HYPERTROPHIC CARDIOMYOPATHY	16.7 %	18
MITRAL ANNULUS CALCIFICATION	60.0 %	20
MITRAL VALVE PROLAPSE	16.7 %	6

0   10   20   CASES

■ OCCLUSION   ▨ OTHER (STENOSIS, ULCER, IRREGULARITY)

Figure 48.11 A study of 76 patients with a variety of cardiac lesions in association with cerebral ischemic events. Cerebral angiography indicated the highest percentage of concomitant potentially thromboembolic lesions in patients with mitral annulus calcification. (Courtesy of Dr. T. Irino, Osaka, Japan.)

Calcific aortic stenosis is detected by echocardiography in about 1% of consecutive patients with either TIAs or strokes.[230,262] Emboli in these patients usually manifest as transient monocular blindness and retinal strokes.[39] The emboli are small, composed of calcium, and detected by funduscopy. Because of their small size, they may produce no signs or symptoms elsewhere in the brain or in the systemic vasculature.[72] A relatively large autopsy study corroborates this hypothesis,[153] while another is not supportive.[182]

Larger emboli are usually caused by manipulation of the valve either by percutaneous balloon valvuloplasty or by the passage of a catheter.[168] After manipulation, some emboli are clinically silent and detected only by brain CT scan.[72]

Long-term antithrombotic therapy is not recommended in isolated aortic stenosis. Antiplatelet agents may have a place in some symptomatic patients, although the evidence is based on speculation.[52,193]

IDIOPATHIC HYPERTROPHIC SUBAORTIC STENOSIS

Idiopathic hypertrophic subaortic stenosis (IHSS) is felt to carry a low risk of embolism.[115] Atrial fibrillation is often associated in those who do have a presumed cardioembolic source.[84,272]

MITRAL ANNULUS CALCIFICATION

Mitral annulus calcification (MAC) is a process of calcification that afflicts elderly people and is considered to be a degenerative aging process.[179,227,251] Apart from the coexistence of calcific aortic valve, MAC is frequently associated with coronary atherosclerosis, cardiac conduction disturbances, chronic atrial fibrillation, cardiomegaly, congestive heart failure, and carotid artery disease[11,116,179,223,227,230] (Fig. 48.11). Thus, it

is not surprising that MAC is associated with an increased risk of stroke.[11,75,223,230] Caseation of the ring and superimposed thrombus or endocarditis have been detected[194,252] (Fig. 48.12), and a few case reports have provided pathologic evidence of calcific embolic material in patients with MAC.[113,194,264] For the most part, it is to be considered a marker of generalized calcific atherosclerosis, and it may not be an important cause of embolism.[52,116] The significance of this lesion to stroke remains unsettled because it occurs in a population prone to progressive atheroma, and it is difficult to define which of the potential embolic mechanisms are operative in a given patient.

MITRAL VALVE PROLAPSE

Mitral valve prolapse (MVP), first described by Barlow in 1963, is a common cardiac condition that has received considerable attention within the last 3 decades since the discovery that it may harbor several life-threatening complications.[73] Classically, the diagnosis rests on the clinical findings of midsystolic click and late systolic murmur, and it is confirmed by the echocardiographic (M-mode, 2D or both) demonstration of prolapse of the mitral leaflets into the left atrium during systole.[81] However, as MVP may produce no or ambiguous auscultatory findings on the one hand, and yet may be echocardiographically overdiagnosed (based on the less strict criteria of the past)[81], on the other, its prevalence has varied enormously. Even in more recent reports it varies between 3% and 13%[279,326] depending on the population under study. The usually accepted figure today is 4%.[81,205]

MVP is characterized pathologically by mucinous and fibromyxomatous degeneration of the leaflets and the chordae tendineae.[250] Usually an isolated finding, MVP may be an inherited disorder (autosomal dominant) and may be associated with other connective tissue disorders, including Marfan and Ehlers-Danlos syndromes.[81]

Clinically, MVP is commonly silent or associated with non-

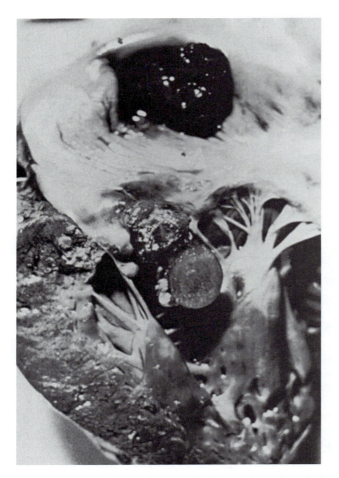

Figure 48.12 Large thrombus attached to mitral annulus calcification: an incidental postmortem finding in an elderly patient. (From Pomerance,[252] with permission. From BMJ Publishing Group.)

specific symptoms.[81] Several serious complications are known[19,80,81,202]: (1) infective endocarditis—the estimated risk is three to eight times higher than in the general population; (2) mitral regurgitation—MVP accounts for 38% to 64% of all cases of severe, pure mitral regurgitation; (3) serious arrhythmias; (4) sudden death (presumably arrhythmic); (5) nonbacterial thrombotic endocarditis (Fig. 48.13); and (6) cerebral and retinal ischemia.

Barnett[18] was the first to report the association between cerebral ischemic events and MVP, and subsequent reports followed.[23,137] Several studies have clearly demonstrated a significantly increased frequency of echocardiographically detectable MVP in patients under the age of 45 with cerebral ischemia, compared to simultaneously studied age-and sex-matched controls.[19,281]

There are several autopsy-proven cases of stroke in association with MVP.[36,64,127,282] In three cases, thrombus was present on the myxomatous mitral valve (Fig. 48.14). Several echocardiographic studies done on patients with MVP who sustained strokes reported the detection of left atrial masses, possibly thrombi, located in the angle formed by the posterior mitral leaflet and the posterior atrial wall, and even of a mobile

mass, that was attached to the prolapsing leaflet.[133,228,267] It is important to ensure that this appearance is not produced merely by the folding of the redundant tissue of the degenerate leaflet. In other patients, embolic material resembling platelets and fibrin has been observed in the fundi[327] (Fig. 48.15). It is presumed that emboli of fibrin and platelets, originating from thrombotic deposits on the valve and its attachment, play a major role in the causation of the cerebral ischemic events.[336]

Cerebral or retinal ischemia may be the presenting complaint, and noncerebral systemic emboli have also been reported in patients with MVP.[36,127,160] Most cerebral events are mild strokes, TIAs, or recurrent amaurosis fugax.[160,174,327,336] Massive infarcts have been described, some reported when atrial fibrillation coexists.[282] Some patients have associated tachyarrhythmias or abnormalities of platelet activity.[281,336] Stroke associated with MVP has been described in women on oral contraceptives.[95]

Several reports detected the presence of MVP in more than 30% of young stroke patients[34,180]; other studies claim that MVP was the putative cause in only 1.7% to 6% of similar patients.[23,91,135,226,268] The difference may be explained by the diligence with which complete cardiac studies are conducted, by the echocardiographic criteria used and by patient selection. By looking only at the data from young patients in whom the stroke remains unexplained despite an extensive search, figures are more consistent and indicate the presence of MVP in about 20%.[336] This is further supported by a recent study[171] that looked at this issue from another perspective: by comparing two groups of age-matched stroke patients with and without MVP but with similar attributes, a significant lack of stroke risk factors was found in the MVP group.

Considerable attention has been focused on the examination of patients with MVP to determine what features, if any, distinguish the majority who will follow a very benign course and the small minority who will suffer serious complications. According to echocardiographic criteria used in a retrospective study,[205] the group of patients with the classical form of MVP (i.e., thickening of the mitral valve leaflets and redundancy) was found to be at a higher risk for infective endocarditis (3% as compared to 0% in the nonclassical group), for moderate to severe mitral regurgitation (12% and 0%), and for the need for mitral valve replacement (6.6% and 0.7%). However, the frequency of stroke was similar (7.5% and 5.8%, respectively).

A prospective study on 237 patients with echocardiographically documented MVP followed for a mean of 6.2 years[231] disclosed two groups of patients. Those with redundant mitral valve leaflets had a complication rate of 10.3% as compared to 0.7% in the "nonredundant" group. The complications included sudden death, infective endocarditis, and cerebral embolic events.

Demographic data indicate that men, and those patients over 45 years of age, are at increased risk of complications—mainly severe mitral regurgitation and infective endocarditis.[80,202]

Reliable predictors of stroke in populations with MVP have not been well defined. Overall, the stroke risk for those who harbor MVP and are followed in cardiac clinics is low, a fact that is discordant with the relatively high prevalence of MVP in younger stroke patients presenting to a neurology service.[10,165,222] The situation here is to be compared to cervical

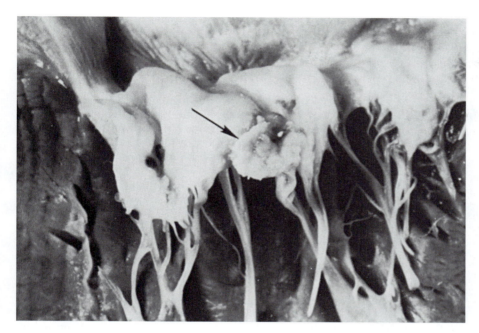

Figure 48.13 Portion of posterior mitral valve leaflet, with largest vegetation (arrow) adherent to atrial surface near margin of closure. There is moderate, diffuse thickening of valve cusps. (From Bramlet et al,[36] with permission.)

spondylosis. This condition is nearly ubiquitous in older patients and very few develop spastic paraparesis. On the other hand, among older subjects with slowly progressive spastic paraparesis, cervical spondylosis is the commonest cause.

Recurrence of cerebral ischemic events may occur; in one report the yearly stroke rate was 7%[16] and in a recent review[236] recurrence has occurred in 20% of patients, mainly months or years apart, and most patients had only recurrent TIAs or showed an almost complete recovery.

In summary, MVP is a common finding in the young, carries a benign course for most individuals, and is an unusual cause of stroke among those harboring MVP (the yearly incidence is 0.02%).[336] It should be considered as the underlying cause for stroke only if extensive search for other causes has been negative.

Prophylactic treatment is unwarranted in individuals with asymptomatic MVP. In patients where cerebral ischemia is attributed to MVP, aspirin therapy is recommended on empirical grounds, and only in treatment failures, when further events occur, should anticoagulants be used[193,336] for periods of 3 to 6 months, followed by aspirin therapy.

Guidelines for subacute bacterial endocarditis (SBE) prophylaxis as well as other conditions in the general management of certain subgroups of MVP patients have been published,[81] but are beyond the scope of this chapter.

MITRAL VALVE STRANDS

Mitral valve strands have been recently associated with cerebrovascular disease. Lee and colleagues[189] identified mobile strands on the mitral valve by TEE in 11 out of 50 patients

(22%) with an unknown source of cerebral embolism. All 50 consecutive patients had a normal transthoracic echocardiogram except for diffuse thickening or calcification of the mitral valve. Mobile strands were seen in 39% of thickened or calcified mitral valves. Tice et al[313] also found an increased incidence of mitral valve strands in patients undergoing TEE looking for a source of embolism. They found MV strands in 15% of those with stroke of unknown etiology.

These strands are filamentous structures seen only by TEE. Lee et al describe the pathology report of strands removed during a valve replacement as Lambl's excrescences, which are filiform processes found on the valves. Whether these strands are a cause of embolism themselves or act as a nidus or marker for potential thrombi is unknown.[60,111,189,313]

PROSTHETIC HEART VALVE

Thromboembolism remains a major cause of morbidity and mortality complicating prosthetic valve implantation despite the introduction of new models of mechanical valves and bioprosthetic valves that have been especially designed to lessen thrombogenicity.[30,89,235,298] The majority of the thromboembolic events are cerebrovascular.[183,235,277]

There are many kinds of mechanical valves, all of which require lifelong anticoagulation therapy to prevent thromboembolism.[122,298] Even with such treatment, patients with mechanical valves experience further embolic events at a rate comparable to nonanticoagulated patients with bioprosthetic valves. The rate of embolism in patients with mechanical mitral valves averages 3% to 4% per year. In the aortic position, the rate is estimated to be lower—averaging 1.2% to 2.2%

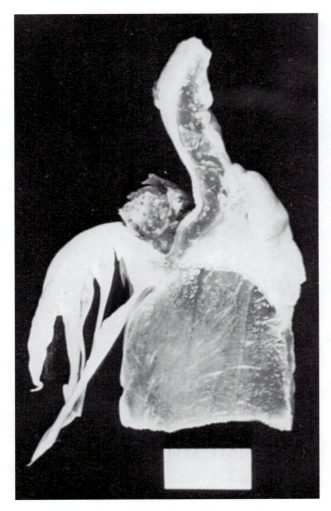

Figure 48.14 Large thrombus attached to prolapsing mitral valve and its attachment to the left atrium. (From Barnett,[16] with permission.)

per year. When a bioprosthetic valve is inserted, long-term anticoagulation is not recommended when other risk factors are absent. The embolic rate for nonanticoagulated patients averages 2% to 4% per year and may be as low as 1.2% per year for the aortic bioprosthetic valve.[30,53,90]

In addition to the site and type of valve used, factors that influence the risk of arterial thromboembolism include the presence of atrial fibrillation, the first 3 postoperative months, left atrial thrombus, previous emboli, and the number of valves replaced.[90,152,235,298]

The presence of one or more of these risk factors usually requires the initiation of anticoagulant therapy. Thus, as many as 80% of these patients will be anticoagulated[152] and exposed to the hazards of bleeding. The incidence of major hemorrhage complicating anticoagulant therapy is estimated at 1% to 2% per year[193] and the combination of thrombotic and bleeding complications account for about 75% of valve-related complications in patients with mechanical valves and for about 50% of the complications in bioprosthetic valves.[30,89,235] The

obvious need to reduce those risks has led to two different approaches:

1. A randomized trial was carried out in Europe, comparing the rate of *late* thromboembolic events in three different mechanical heart valve prostheses. The results showed a better outcome with the Bjork-Shiley valve.[183] Another study compared the latter with porcine bioprosthesis during a mean follow-up of 12 years[30]: survival with an *intact* valve was better with this mechanical valve, whereas bleeding complications were higher. There was no difference in thromboembolic events rate.

2. An attempt is being made to find a better equilibrium between activated procoagulants (initiated by the synthetic material of the prosthetic valve) and the anticoagulant—endogenous or exogenous (warfarin). In two recent prospective randomized studies high-intensity anticoagulation (international normalized ratio [INR] 2:5 to 4:0 or prothrombin time ratio 2.5) was compared to moderate intensity anticoagulation (INR 2.0 to 2.25 or prothrombin time ratio 1:5) in patients with bioprosthetic[319] and mechanical[277] valves. While the rate of thromboembolism remained similar, the risk of bleeding complications was significantly lower in those patients receiving the moderate dose.

Antiplatelet agents alone are much inferior to warfarin in adults with mechanical prosthetic valves and pose unacceptable risks of thromboembolism.[217] A trial of 186 patients with mechanical heart valves or tissue valves with atrial fibrillation were treated with warfarin and randomly assigned to receive aspirin 100 mg per day or placebo. The INR was targeted at 3.0 to 4.5. After 4 years of average follow-up, major systemic embolism occurred in 5 aspirin-treated patients and 13 in the placebo group. Four and 12 events were in the cerebral arteries in the aspirin and placebo groups, respectively.[318] Earlier, smaller studies had suggested the possibility that dipyridamole added to anticoagulants might improve upon the outlook for patients with prosthetic heart valves.[56] However, the recommended therapy is an anticoagulant with aspirin.

In children, because of the difficulty of controlling anticoagulation, several trials have used antiplatelet agents alone and claimed efficacy and safety.[242,330] This issue, however, remains controversial.[209] A recent study utilizing a medium-intensity anticoagulation in pregnant women disclosed a low incidence of thromboembolism or hemorrhage, yet the rate of fetal wastage and neonatal mortality was high.[278]

Prosthetic valve endocarditis is another complication and a potential source of cerebral embolism. Endocarditis has a yearly incidence of about 2.4%[66] in patients with prosthetic valves. Recently a much lower yearly incidence was reported (<1%).[30] The use of newer and more advanced valves may explain this difference. The occurrence of neurologic complications is higher with mechanical valves and when the prosthesis is in the mitral position.[172]

INFECTIVE ENDOCARDITIS

The clinical spectrum of infective endocarditis (IE) has changed in many aspects during the last 25 years. At one time, it was primarily a subacute infection on a preexisting rheu-

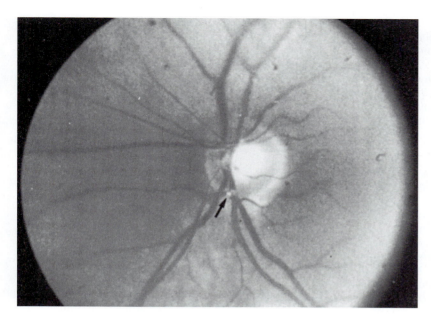

Figure 48.15 Embolus (arrow) to the inferior branch of the central retinal artery in a patient with mitral valve prolapse. (From Watson,[327] with permission.)

matic valvular disease caused by nonvirulent streptococcal species. With the declining incidence of rheumatic heart disease, its incidence has decreased, yet the relative involvement of previously normal cardiac valves has increased, and many cases are detected in young intravenous drug abusers.[156,170] Normal cardiac valves may become infected by virulent organisms, mainly *Staphylococcus aureus*, which is responsible for most cases of acute infective endocarditis.[156]

Neurologic complications contribute to the high mortality of infective endocarditis, and the central nervous system becomes involved in several ways: ischemic and hemorrhagic strokes, multiple microemboli presenting as toxic encephalopathy, meningitis, pyogenic arteritis, mycotic aneurysm, and subarachnoid hemorrhage.[258]

Despite improved antibiotic and surgical therapy, the stroke rate continues to be high, averaging 15% to 20% of all patients with IE.[144,258,274] This unchanged risk can be explained by the following: (1) the majority of strokes occur within the initial 48 hours of presentation and may herald the existence of IE[144,274] and (2) the risk and severity of embolism is higher when the offending organism is *Staphylococcus aureus* or *epidermidis* and with mechanical prosthetic valves,[71,144,172,274] all of which are more prevalent now.

The type and severity of the neurologic manifestations are determined in part by the size of the septic emboli, which are composed mainly of infected vegetations.[220] Attempts to predict the risk of embolism by echocardiographic detection of valvular vegetations have not been proven to be totally reliable,[42,144] and the only measure proven to reduce the rate of stroke is early control of the infection by means of antibiotic therapy.[71,144,241]

As recurrent emboli seldom occur after the infection is controlled,[144,241] anticoagulants are not indicated for patients with native valve endocarditis.[144,193,241] It is normally recommended to continue anticoagulation in patients with prosthetic valve endocarditis unless an embolic stroke develops.[90,172,193,332] Anticoagulant therapy then poses the hazard of intracerebral bleeding. Intracerebral hemorrhages (ICHs)

occur in 7% of native valve endocarditis, mainly in intravenous drug abusers with uncontrolled *Staphylococcus aureus* infection and is presumably the result of pyogenic arteritis.[144,145]

Mycotic aneurysm, an uncommon complication of IE, may be responsible for the ICH. It occurs in all types of endocarditis, usually in distal branches of the middle cerebral artery. Aneurysms, which probably develop as a result of septic embolization to the vasa vasorum, usually are clinically silent and can heal with prolonged antibiotic treatment.[41,258] Rupture occurs unpredictably and, as this carries a high mortality rate, an attempt must be made for their early detection. This complication should be sought in patients with focal neurologic findings, cerebrospinal fluid pleocytosis, and evidence of infarction or ICH on their CT scans.[41] Early four-vessel angiography is indicated in these patients. For those who require long-term anticoagulation, repeat angiography is recommended after completion of antibiotic therapy.[273] Magnetic resonance angiography is not adequate at the present time to replace conventional arteriography in evaluating these patients.

Mural endocarditis is very rare, but may occur either in the presence of a ventricular septal defect, with "jet lesions," with perforation of a cusp, or from rupture of a chordae tendineae in severely debilitated or immunosuppressed patients. The causative organism is usually *Candida albicans*,[292] whereas *Aspergillus* is commonly the underlying cause in patients with prior cardiovascular surgery.[337]

NONBACTERIAL THROMBOTIC ENDOCARDITIS

Nonbacterial thrombotic endocarditis (NBTE) is the name commonly used to describe what was previously referred to as marantic, terminal, and verrucous endocarditis.

Although described in a vast range of disease processes,

especially, those that are chronic and wasting,[46,197] NBTE is most common in patients with cancer: adenocarcinoma of the lung, pancreas, and prostate and hematologic malignancies predominating.[27,197,266]

Cerebral infarction is the second most common neuropathologic finding in patients dying of cancer, and within this group NBTE accounts for more than 25%.[132] Other cancer-related causes of symptomatic infarction include disseminated intravascular coagulopathy (DIC), septic emboli, tumor emboli, and cerebral venous and sinus thrombosis.

As the name implies, NBTE is a noninfectious type of endocarditis mainly found on previously normal cardiac valves, the mitral and aortic valves being the most commonly affected. The vegetations in NBTE are usually small and are composed of platelet and fibrin deposits (Fig. 48.16). The pathogenesis is still uncertain: a deranged valvular surface must precede the formation of NBTE, and a hypercoagulable state is usually present. Whether the latter is a prerequisite for the formation of NBTE and what is the exact mechanism (DIC, tumor mucin, or procoagulant may be contributory in individual patients) for this prothrombotic state is still debatable.[197,266]

Clinically, NBTE is underdiagnosed.[197,266] The main reasons are (1) NBTE is clinically silent in many cases; (2) significant cardiac murmurs are absent in the majority of cases; and (3) the vegetations are usually small, and detection is difficult by both invasive and noninvasive techniques. Two-dimensional echocardiography is a relatively good diagnostic tool,[196] and early cerebral angiography may confirm the presence of multiple arterial branch occlusions reflecting brain emboli.[266] The clinical manifestations of NBTE are those of multiple systemic emboli with neurologic manifestations predominating, usually in the form of acute focal neurologic deficits, suggesting stroke. A diffuse form is suggestive of a metabolic encephalopathy. Embolic myocardial infarction is an occasional serious complication.[197,266]

Treatment is empirical. Most reports have been anecdotal and retrospective. Heparin anticoagulation may be beneficial, especially when there is a recognizable coagulopathy.[266]

SYSTEMIC LUPUS ERYTHEMATOSUS AND RELATED DISEASES

Systemic lupus erythematosus (SLE) is a multisystem autoimmune disease in which neuropsychiatric manifestations are protean, but clinical cardiac disease is considered rare.[5,54,149] Central nervous system (CNS) involvement may manifest as delirium, psychosis, depression, altered consciousness, focal cerebral ischemia, cranial nerve dysfunction, chorea, myelop-

Figure 48.16 Mitral valve vegetation of nonbacterial thrombotic endocarditis (arrow). (From Rogers et al,[266] with permission.)

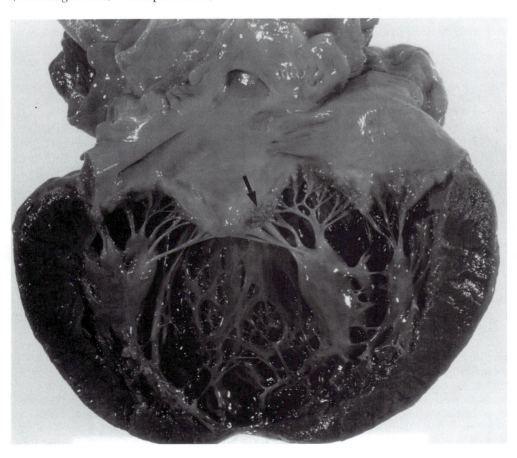

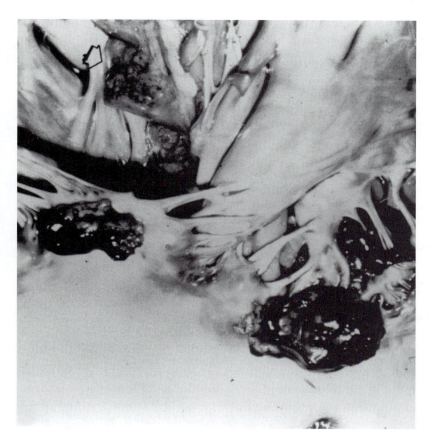

Figure 48.17 Mitral valve area of opened left atrium and ventricle. There are several large vegetations involving both the valvular and the ventricular mural (open arrow) endocardium. (From Fox et al,[110] with permission.)

athy and CNS infection.[5] Cerebral ischemia (usually recurrent episodes) occurs in 15% to 20% of all SLE patients.[82,119]

Until recently most of these CNS disorders were attributed to CNS vasculitis or vascular disorders other than embolism.[163] Atypical verrucous endocarditis (Fig. 48.17) or Libman-Sacks (L-S) endocarditis is a well-known common pathologic finding in SLE patients earlier thought to have no clinical significance.[149] This endocarditis is not confined to valvular surfaces only, and has other features differentiating it from NBTE or rheumatic valvulitis.[110] After reconsidering several pathologic and echocardiographic findings in patients with SLE,[67,82,119,123] several new concepts have emerged.

1. The etiology of strokes and maybe other CNS manifestation in SLE patients are often the result of cardiac emboli (presumably originating from L-S endocarditis) with or without the presence of an antibody mediated hypercoagulable state.

2. Clinically important valvular involvement in SLE is relatively frequent and sometimes requires surgery. This valvular involvement is different from (although perhaps the end stage of) L-S endocarditis and is also associated with an increased risk for stroke. It is referred to as nonspecific (chronic) valvulitis, mainly involving the mitral and aortic valves. Long-standing steroid treatment, known to facilitate scarring and calcification, may play a causal role.

3. Echocardiography is a useful tool in the detection and follow-up of valvular lesion in SLE patients.

4. A hypercoagulable state (induced mainly by antiphospho-

lipid antibodies) is frequently found in SLE patients.[140] Its role in the pathogenesis of stroke in patients with or without cardiac lesion has yet to be determined. Antiphospholipid antibodies may predispose to L-S endocarditis.[12] This hypothesis is supported by recent reports of SLE patients that show a higher frequency of valvular lesions in those possessing antiphospholipid antibodies.[55,125]

Treatment is controversial. Anticoagulant therapy is recommended in patients who have sustained a stroke, as well as for stroke prevention in patients at high risk (i.e., with recognizable cardiac valvular lesions or previous TIA).[119,129,341]

Other autoimmune rheumatic disease can cause central nervous system dysfunction through various mechanisms, including the presence of antiphospholipid antibodies and cardiac involvement. In Sjögren's syndrome, cardioembolic stroke may be attributed to coexistent cardiomyopathy.[236]

ANTIPHOSPHOLIPID ANTIBODIES

The antiphospholipid antibody syndrome is associated with both venous and arterial thrombi. Originally associated with SLE, it is now known to occur without this and is then called the primary antiphospholipid syndrome. Some features of this syndrome include thrombocytopenia, recurrent early fetal loss, livedo reticularis, and deep venous thrombosis, although these are not required for the diagnosis. Elevated antiphospholipid antibodies have been associated with certain cardiac abnormalities, including valvular heart disease, coronary artery disease, cardiomyopathies and, less commonly, thrombi within the ventricles.[169,124] In a study of 128 patients with elevated antiphospholipid antibodies and either ischemic stroke or transient ischemia,[9] 39% of all echocardiograms were abnormal with 22% having mitral valve abnormalities. Specific abnormalities included myxomatous thickening of the mitral valve, mitral valve prolapse, mitral and aortic insufficiency, aortic valve calcification, akinetic wall segments, cardiomyopathy, atrial septal defect and intracardiac thrombi. Sixteen percent of all patients also had SLE. Brenner et al evaluated 34 consecutive patients with primary antiphospholipid syndrome using echocardiographic studies and found that 9 of these patients had either a stroke or a TIA, and 11 patients (32%) had abnormal findings.[38] Of those presenting with arterial thrombosis,[21] which includes all 9 cerebrovascular cases, 64% had abnormal echocardiograms. The most common abnormality was mitral leaflet thickening associated with either mitral regurgitation (MR) or MR and mitral stenosis. Vegetation-like lesions on the mitral or aortic valve were seen in 2 patients. No comment was made on other potential causes for stroke or TIA in these patients. The percentage of abnormal cardiac evaluations in patients with SLE and elevated antiphospholipids is increased compared to those with SLE without elevated antiphospholipids.[173,192] Whether these lesions are the cause of stroke or merely an association is unclear and requires further investigation.

PARADOXICAL EMBOLISM

The name implies that an embolus originating in the venous system finds its way to lodge in the arterial tree, and implies the existence of right to left shunts. Possible shunts incriminated in the pathophysiology of paradoxical embolism include patent foramen ovale (PFO), atrial septal defect (ASD), and pulmonary arteriovenous fistula.[164,198,297]

Previously considered an unusual cause of cerebral embolism,[146,164,211] paradoxical embolism through a PFO has become a more popular explanation for strokes of unknown cause; especially in the young.[188,328] This concept needs to be examined critically.

PFO is found in about 30% of autopsies[136] (Fig. 48.18) and, recently, with the introduction of 2D contrast echocardiography, a physiologic shunt was demonstrated in 10% to 18% of normal people by the use of this noninvasive technique.[188,201,328] By using a transesophageal color-coded Doppler echo, the detection of PFO may be improved.[221]

The presence of PFO by itself cannot explain the occurrence of cerebral embolism. Under normal conditions, the pressure in the right heart is lower than in the left side, the foramen ovale stays closed, and there is no right to left shunt. In pathologic conditions where pulmonary hypertension exists, such shunts do occur,[186] but in the healthy population such shunts may occur only transiently during Valsalva maneuvers.[201]

A major difficulty in the acceptance of paradoxical embolism as the underlying mechanism for a substantial number of the strokes of unknown cause is the absence of venous thrombosis or signs of pulmonary embolism.[164,188,328] In previous reports, the presence of venous thrombosis was considered essential for the diagnosis.[211,312] In making more sweeping claims for its importance, it is being assumed that there is an occult source, as occurs in cases of pulmonary embolism.[299]

The prevalence of PFO demonstrated by contrast echo was found to be much higher in young patients with stroke of unknown cause compared to control groups.[188,328] In the Lechat series[188] the authors referred to MVP as a risk factor only, whereas the PFO was claimed to be causal. There was no evidence for crural vein disease, or pulmonary embolism, nor were the controls contemporary. Recently, transcranial

Figure 48.18 Patent foramen ovale, shown in autopsy specimen from 85-year-old man. (**A**) Right atrial (RA) view shows a probe in foramen ovale, between limbus and valve (V) of fossa ovalis. (**B**) Left atrial (LA) view shows the same probe as in Fig. A exiting through ostium secundum, the prominent fenestration in the valve. Normally, when left atrial pressure exceeds right atrial pressure, the valve of the fossa ovalis impressed against the limbus and thereby closes the foramen ovale. IVC, inferior vena cava; MV, mitral valve; SVC, superior vena cava; TV, tricuspid valve. (From Hagen et al,[136] with permission.)

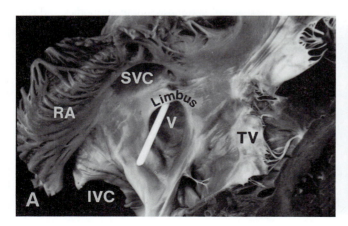
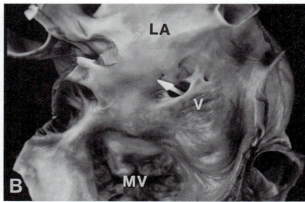

Doppler has been used to clarify the potential cerebral embolic significance of a demonstrated shunt.[57]

Prophylactic treatment in this condition is an unsettled issue. In cases of proven venous thrombosis, the institution of anticoagulant therapy for several months, and other means of therapy, such as caval umbrellas, should be undertaken following the guidelines for the prevention of pulmonary emboli.[154] If the source of embolism is occult, a treatment regimen that includes a short course of anticoagulation followed by aspirin or aspirin alone may be sufficient.[29,188] In some patients, closure of the PFO may be warranted.

CONGENITAL HEART DISEASE

Many congenital heart diseases are complicated by systemic or cerebral embolism. Mechanisms for embolization include cardiac dysrhythmia, paradoxical embolism, and bacterial endocarditis. The majority are in the cyanotic group, in which the blood viscosity is high and there is an increased tendency for venous thrombosis. Emboli are reported mainly in patients with the tetralogy of Fallot, ventricular or atrial septal defect, and transposition of the great vessels.[8,25] In one study in which 124 adults with cyanotic heart disease were followed for an average of 6.1 years, no clinical stroke was detected even in the presence of high hematocrit level.[246] In contrast, clinically silent atrial septal defect was incriminated as an underlying cause for stroke in young adults.[146] Atrial septal aneurysm, a rare congenital condition that is usually associated with an interarterial shunt and sometimes with mitral valve prolapse, has received attention as a possible cause for cardioembolic stroke.[24,83] Two-dimensional echocardiography preferably by the transesophageal route is the imaging technique of choice for the diagnosis of this defect.[283] Possible mechanisms include thrombus formation in the aneurysmal sac or paradoxical embolism.[24]

CARDIAC MYXOMA

Cardiac myxoma, the most common primary heart tumor, is a rare tumor and a very rare cause of stroke. The tumor is usually benign and originates in the left atrium in 75% of cases. Primarily diagnosed in young and middle-aged adults, it may present with either constitutional, cardiac obstructive or embolic symptoms, alone or in combination. Obstructive symptoms are due mainly to an intermittent mitral stenosis. The constitutional symptoms are not specific and may mimic those arising in a variety of malignant, infectious, and immunologic dieases.[204]

Embolic manifestations occur in 20% to 45% of patients, sometimes as the first symptom. Although emboli may lodge in any part of the vascular bed, the central nervous system is involved in up to 50% of cases.[204] The embolic material consists mainly of myxomatous tissue, but occasionally only thrombotic material (originating from an adherent thrombus) can be found. In addition to multiple brain infarctions, tumor emboli cause cerebral aneurysms located on peripheral

branches, which rarely rupture, presenting as an intracranial hemorrhage.[176,204]

Neurologic manifestations consist mainly of acute focal neurologic deficits that may be the initial presentation of the tumor.[176] As the tumor is friable, recurrent cerebral emboli are common prior to its surgical removal. These symptoms rarely recur following successful surgical removal.[176]

Diagnosis rests on the utilization of 2D echocardiography, but cardiac CT or MRI can be added.[176,204] Therapy is surgical, and anticoagulation prior to surgery is not effective.[176]

Cardiac Surgery

Many patients with the cardiac diseases described, of which the most prevalent is coronary artery disease, are subject to surgical procedures. Complicating systemic embolism occurs in all types of cardiac surgery including cardiopulmonary bypass (open heart) done for a variety of reasons, closed heart surgery (for other conditions), and heart transplantation.[224] As many as 5% of patients undergoing coronary artery bypass grafting are afflicted with a stroke.[38] Possible mechanisms include macroembolization of air, valve, and aortic atheroma debris, or left ventricular thrombus as well as microembolization of gas, fat, and aggregates of blood cells, platelets, and fibrin or particles of silicone or polyvinyl chloride tubing.[287] Hypotension, as a mechanism, is less common.[295] Encephalopathy may be a more common sequel based on prospective neuropsychiatric testing. Surgical techniques and equipment are being modified, especially with the help of TCD, to lessen intraoperative emboli.[59] Other techniques to lessen intraoperative emboli include intraoperative ultrasonography of the ascending aorta[224] and retrograde cerebral perfusion.[15,76]

When early heart surgery is performed as a result of cardioembolic stroke, the risk of cerebral complication (mainly hemorrhage) is high (29%), particularly in the presence of infective endocarditis or large infarcts.[207]

LEFT VENTRICULAR ASSIST DEVICES

Left ventricular assist devices (LVAD) are being used more commonly as a bridge to heart transplantation. Their use is often limited by cerebral emboli and the longer patients are kept on LVADs the higher their risk of stroke. Proposed mechanisms of ischemic stroke include alteration of coagulation factors, infection and thrombi formation on the artificial surfaces.[92] Different assist devices are being devised to reduce the thromboembolic risk.

ACUTE TREATMENT OF NONSEPTIC CARDIOGENIC BRAIN EMBOLISM

In general, anticoagulant therapy is recommended for the prevention of nonseptic recurrent emboli in most cases of cardiogenic emboli. It is the therapy shown to be effective in most of these conditions.[53,288,341]

There are two problems that remain to be considered in view of the potential risk of anticoagulant therapy: (1) the optimal dose of anticoagulation to be used, and (2) the optimal time to start anticoagulant treatment. The optimal dosage (i.e., maximal prevention of recurrent emboli with minimal bleeding complications) is currently under intensive investigations for most of the cardiac sources. Generally speaking, a lower dose level of anticoagulation seems to suffice for most patients with emboligenic sources. As in the prevention of pulmonary emboli from deep-vein thrombosis[154] the newly recommended dose for warfarin treatment aims to prolong the prothrombin time to 1.5 times control (INR between 2 and 3).[53] In the future, it is expected that even lower doses may be shown to be adequate. In general, it is recommended that heparin be used for the first few days and then to switch to warfarin.[288]

The optimal time to start treatment is still controversial,[288,341] and the physician faces a dilemma: the risk of recurrent emboli without treatment is about 12% during the first 2 weeks, and under early anticoagulant therapy it will drop to about 4%; yet the risk of therapy related to symptomatic brain hemorrhage and clinical worsening will be 5% for the same period.[52,288] This risk may be much higher in older patients, in those with large infarct size, with elevated blood pressure, and when bolus doses of heparin are given.[51,234] Such patients are excluded from the early treatment group. Keeping in mind that spontaneous hemorrhagic transformation mainly occurs within 48 hours after the stroke onset[143] and that anticoagulants may be hazardous in such patients because they may induce massive hematomas,[53,234] the following strategy is recommended: anticoagulant therapy should be withheld for 48 hours, and then, after obtaining a new CT scan, anticoagulation should be started in younger patients who have nonhemorrhagic infarcts of small or medium size. In other cases (i.e., elderly or hypertensive patients and those with large or hemorrhagic infarcts), it is advisable to withhold treatment for 2 weeks.[53,288]

Acknowledgments

The authors are indebted to Ms. Heather Meldrum for many helpful suggestions about the content and style of this chapter and to Dr. Michael Eliasziw for providing expert biostatistical advice and calculations.

References

1. Abdon NJ, Zettervall O, Carlson J et al: Is occult atrial disorder a frequent cause of non-hemorrhagic stroke? Long-term ECG in 86 patients. Stroke 13:832, 1982

2. Abelmann WH, Lorell BH: The challenge of cardiomyopathy. J Am Coll Cardiol 13:1219, 1989

3. Aberg H: Atrial fibrillation. I. A Study of atrial thrombosis and systemic embolism in a necropsy material. Acta Med Scand 185:373, 1969

4. Adams HP, Jr, Butler MJ, Biller J, Toffol GJ: Nonhemorrhagic cerebral infarction in young adults. Arch Neurol 43:793, 1986

5. Adelman DC, Saltiel E, Klinenberg JR: The neuropsychiatric manifestations of systemic lupus erythematosus: an overview. Semin Arthritis Rheum 15:185, 1986

6. Albers GW, Comess KA, DeRook FA et al: Transesophageal echocardiographic findings in stroke subtypes. Stroke 25:23, 1994

7. Amarenco P, Cohen A, Baudrimont M, Bousser MG: Transesophageal echocardiographic detection of aortic arch disease in patients with cerebral infarction. Stroke 23:1005, 1992

8. Amitai Y, Blieden L, Shemtov A, Neufeld HN: Cerebrovascular accidents in infants and children with congenital cyanotic heart disease. Isr J Med Sci 20:1143, 1984

9. The Antiphospholipid Antibodies in Stroke Study Group: Clinical and laboratory findings in patients with antiphospholipid antibodies and cerebral ischemia. Stroke 21:1268, 1990

10. Appelblatt NH, Willis PW, Lenhart JA et al: Ten- to forty-year follow-up of 69 patients with systolic click with or without apical late systolic murmur. Am J Cardiol 35:119, 1975

11. Aronow WS, Koenigsberg M, Kronzon I, Gutstein H: Association of mitral annular calcium with new thromboembolic stroke and cardiac events at 39-month follow-up in elderly patients. Am J Cardiol 65:1511, 1990

12. Asherson RA, Lubbe WF: Cerebral and valve lesions in SLE: association with antiphospholipid antibodies. J Rheumatol 15:539, 1988

13. Asinger RW, Mikell FL, Elsperger J, Hodges M: Incidence of left ventricular thrombosis after acute transmural myocardial infarction. N Engl J Med 305:297, 1981

14. Babikian VL, Hyde C, Pochay V, Winter MR: Clinical correlates of high-intensity transient signals detected on transcranial Doppler sonography in patients with cerebrovascular disease. Stroke 25:1570, 1994

15. Baker AJ, Naser B, Benaroia M, Mazer CD: Cerebral microemboli during coronary artery bypass using different cardioplegia techniques. Ann Thorac Surg 59:1187, 1995

16. Barnett HJM: Embolism in mitral valve prolapse. Annu Rev Med 33:489, 1982

17. Barnett HJM: Heart in ischemic stroke—a changing emphasis. p. 291. In Barnett HJM (ed): Neurologic Clinics. WB Saunders, Philadelphia, 1983

18. Barnett HJM: Transient cerebral ischemia: pathogenesis, prognosis and management. Ann R Coll Physicians Surg Can 7:153, 1974

19. Barnett HJM, Boughner DR, Taylor WD et al: Further evidence relating mitral-valve prolapse to cerebral ischemic events. N Engl J Med 302:139, 1980

20. Barnett HJM, Eliasziw M, Meldrum, HE: Drug therapy: drugs and surgery in the prevention of ischemic stroke. New England Journal of Medicine 332:238, 1995

21. Barnett HJM, Jones MW, Boughner DR, Kostuk WJ: Cerebral ischemic events associated with prolapsing mitral valve. Arch Neurol 33:777, 1976

22. Bautista RE: Embolic stroke following thrombolytic

therapy for myocardial infarction in a patient with preexisting ventricular thrombi. Stroke 26:324, 1995

23. Beattie BA, Biller J, Adams HP Jr et al: Mitral valve prolapse is an uncommon cause of stroke in young adults, abstracted. Neurology (NY), suppl. I, 39:S183, 1989

24. Belkin RN, Kisslo J: Atrial septal aneurysm: recognition and clinical relevance. Am Heart J 120:948, 1990

25. Berthrong M, Sabiston DC Jr: Cerebral lesions in congenital heart disease: a review of one hundred and sixty-two cases. Bull Johns Hopkins Hosp 89:384, 1951

26. Bevan H, Sharma K, Bradley W: Stroke in young adults. Stroke 21:382, 1990

27. Biller J, Challa VR, Toole SF, Howard VJ: Non-bacterial thrombotic endocarditis: a neurologic perspective of clinicopathologic correlations of 99 patients. Arch Neurol 39:95, 1982

28. Biller J, Ionasescu V, Zellweger H et al: Incidence of cerebral infarction in inherited neuromuscular conditions. Stroke 18:805, 1987

29. Biller J, Johnson MR, Adams HP et al: Further observations on cerebral or retinal ischemia with right-left intracardiac shunts. Arch Neurol 44:740, 1987

30. Bloomfield P, Wheatley DJ, Prescott RJ, Miller HC: Twelve-year comparison of Bjork-Shiley mechanical heart valve with porcine bioprostheses. N Engl J Med 324:573, 1991

31. Bogousslavsky J, Cachin D, Regli F et al: Cardiac sources of embolism and cerebral infarction—clinical consequences and vascular concomitants: the Lausanne Stroke Registry. Neurology (NY) 41:855, 1991

32. Bogousslavsky J, Garazi S, Jeanrenaud X et al: Stroke recurrence in patients with patent foramen ovale: the Lausanne study. Neurology 46:1301, 1996

33. Bogousslavsky J, Melle GV, Regli F: The Lausanne Stroke Registry: analysis of 1000 consecutive patients with first stroke. Stroke 19:1083, 1988

34. Bogousslavsky J, Regli F: Ischemic stroke in adults younger than 30 years of age. Arch Neurol 44:479, 1987

35. The Boston Area Anticoagulation Trial for Atrial Fibrillation Investigators: The effect of low-dose warfarin on the risk of stroke in patients with nonrheumatic atrial fibrillation. N Engl J Med 323:1505, 1990

36. Bramlet DA, Decker EL, Floyd WL: Nonbacterial thrombotic endocarditis as a cause of stroke in mitral valve prolapse. South Med J 75:1133, 1982

37. Brenner B, Blumenfeld Z, Markiewicz W, Reisner SA: Cardiac involvement in patients with primary antiphospholipid syndrome. J Am Coll Cardiol 18:931, 1991

38. Breuer AC, Furlan AJ, Hanson MR: Central nervous system complications of coronary artery bypass graft surgery: prospective analysis of 421 patients. Stroke 14:682, 1983

39. Brockmeier LB, Adolph RJ, Gustin BW et al: Calcium emboli to the retinal artery in calcific aortic stenosis. Am Heart J 101:32, 1981

40. Broderick JP, Phillips SJ, O'Fallon M et al: Relationship of cardiac disease to stroke occurrence, recurrence and mortality. Stroke 23:1250, 1992

41. Brust JCM, Dickinson PCT, Hughes JEO, Holtzman RNN: The diagnosis and treatment of cerebral mycotic aneurysms. Ann Neurol 27:238, 1990

42. Buda AJ, Zotz RJ, Le Mire MS, Buch DS: Prognostic significance of vegetations detected by two-dimensional echocardiography in infective endocarditis. Am Heart J 112:1291, 1986

43. Burger AJ, Jadhav P, Kamalesh M, Stubbe I: Absence of cerebrovascular events in a prospective study of coronary artery bypass patients with atrial septal aneurysms taking aspirin. Am J Cardiol 75:305, 1995

44. Cabanes L, Mas JL, Cohen A et al: Atrial septal aneurysm and patent foramen ovale as risk factors for cryptogenic stroke in patients less than 55 years of age. Stroke 24:1865, 1993

45. Cabin HS, Clubb KS, Hall C et al: Risk for systemic embolization of atrial fibrillation without mitral stenosis. Am J Cardiol 65:1112, 1990

46. Cammarosano C, Lewis W: Cardiac lesions in acquired immune deficiency syndrome (AIDS). J Am Coll Cardiol 5:703, 1985

47. Candelise L, Pinardi G, Morabito A: The Italian Acute Stroke Study Group: Mortality in acute stroke with atrial fibrillation. Stroke 22:169, 1991

48. Caplan LR: Top of the basilar syndrome. Neurology (NY) 30:72, 1980

49. Caplan LR, Hier HB, D'Cruz I: Cerebral embolism in the Michael Reese Stroke Registry. Stroke 14:530, 1983

50. Cerebral Embolism Study Group: Cardioembolic stroke, immediate anticoagulation and brain hemorrhage. Arch Intern Med 147:636, 1987

51. Cerebral Embolism Study Group: Immediate anticoagulation of embolic stroke: a randomized trial. Stroke 14:668, 1983

52. Cerebral Embolism Task Force: Cardiogenic brain embolism. Arch Neurol 43:71, 1986

53. Cerebral Embolism Task Force: Cardiogenic brain embolism: the second report of the cerebral embolism task force. Arch Neurol 46:727, 1989

54. Cervera R, Font J, Pare C et al: Cardiac disease in systemic lupus erythematosus. Prospective study of 70 patients. Ann Rheum Dis 51:156, 1992

55. Chartash EK, Lans DM, Paget SA et al: Aortic insufficiency and mitral regurgitation in patients with systemic lupus erythematosus and the antiphospholipid syndrome. Am J Med 86:407, 1989

56. Chesebro SN, Adams PC, Fuster V: Antithrombotic therapy in patients with valvular heart disease and prosthetic heart valves. J Am Coll Cardiol 8:41B, 1996

57. Chimowitz M, Nemec J, Marwick T et al: Transcranial Doppler ultrasound detects right to left cardiac or pulmonary shunts. Neurology (NY) 41:1902, 1991

58. Ciaccherie M, Castelli Q, Cecchi F et al: Lack of correlation between intracavitary thrombosis detected by cross-sectional echocardiography and systemic emboli in patients with dilated cardiomyopathy. Br Heart J 62:26, 1989

59. Clark RE, Brillman J, Davis DA et al: Microemboli during coronary artery bypass grafting. J Thorac Cardiovasc Surg 109:249, 1995

60. Cohen A, Crassard I, Tzourio C et al: Mitral valve strands

and the risk of brain infarcts: a case control study, abstracted. Stroke 27:180, 1996

61. Comess KA, DeRook FA, Beach KW et al: Transesophageal echocardiography and carotid ultrasound in patients with cerebral ischemia: prevalence of findings and recurrent stroke risk. J Am Coll Cardiol 23:1598, 1994

62. Connolly SJ, Laupacis A, Gent M et al: Canadian atrial fibrillation anticoagulation (CAFA) study. J Am Coll Cardiol 18:349, 1991

63. Consensus Committee of 9th International Cerebral Hemodynamic Symposium: Basic identification criteria of Doppler microembolic signals. Stroke 26:1123, 1995

64. Cook AW, Bird TD, Spence AM et al: Myotonic dystrophy, mitral-valve prolapse, and stroke. Lancet 1:335, 1978

65. Coulshed N, Epstein EJ, McKendrick CS et al: Systemic embolism in mitral valve disease. Br Heart J 32:26, 1970

66. Cowgill LD, Addonizio VP, Hopeman AR: Prosthetic valve endocarditis. Curr Concepts Cardiol 11:623, 1986

67. Crozier IG, Li E, Milne MJ, Nicholls MG: Cardiac involvement in systemic lupus erythematosus detected by echocardiography. Am J Cardiol 65:1145, 1990

68. Cujec B, Polasek P, Voll C, Shuaib A: Transesophageal echocardiography in the detection of potential cardiac source of embolism in stroke patients. Stroke 22:727, 1991

69. Daley R, Mattingly TW, Holt CL et al: Systemic arterial embolism in rheumatic heart disease. Am Heart J 42:566, 1951

70. Daniel WG, Nellessen U, Schroder W et al: Left atrial spontaneous echo contrast in mitral valve disease: an indicator for an increased thromboembolic risk. J Am Coll Cardiol 11:1204, 1988

71. Davenport J, Hart RG: Prosthetic valve endocarditis 1976–1987; antibiotics, anticoagulation, and stroke. Stroke 21:993, 1990

72. Davidson CJ, Skelton TN, Kisslo KB et al: The risk for systemic embolization associated with percutaneous balloon vavuloplasty in adults. Ann Intern Med 108:557, 1988

73. Davies NJ, Montague TJ: Mitral valve prolapse: the cardiac disease of the decade revisited. Ann R Coll Physicians Surg Can 22:307, 1989

74. Davis PH, Dambrosia JM, Schoenberg BS et al: Risk factors for ischemic stroke: a prospective study in Rochester, Minnesota. Ann Neurol 22:319, 1987

75. de Bono DP, Warlow CP: Mitral annulus calcification and cerebral or retinal ischemia. Lancet 2:383, 1979

76. Deeb GM, Jenkins E, Bolling SF et al: Retrograde cerebral perfusion during hypothermic circulatory arrest reduces neurologic morbidity. J Thorac Cardiovasc Surg 109:259, 1995

77. del Zoppo GJ, Poeck K, Pessin MS et al: Recombinant tissue plasminogen activator in acute thrombotic and embolic stroke. Ann Neurol 32:78, 1992

78. Delemarre BJ, Visser CA, Bot H, Dunning AJ: Prediction of apical thrombus formation in acute myocardial infarction based on left ventricular spatial flow pattern. J Am Coll Cardiol 15:355, 1990

79. DeRook FA, Comess KA, Albers GW, Popp RL: Trans-

esophageal echocardiography in the evaluation of stroke. Ann Intern Med 117:922, 1992

80. Devereux RB, Hawkins I, Kramer-Fox R et al: Complications of mitral valve prolapse: disproportionate occurrence in men and older patients. Am J Med 81:751, 1986

81. Devereux RB, Kramer-Fox R, Kligfield P: Mitral valve prolapse: causes, clinical manifestations, and management. Ann Intern Med 111:305, 1989

82. Devinsky O, Petito CK, Alonso DR: Clinical and neuropathological findings in systemic lupus erythematosus: the role of vasculitis, heart emboli, and thrombotic thrombocytopenic purpura. Ann Neurol 23:380, 1988

83. Di Pasquale G, Andreoli A, Grazi P et al: Cardioembolic stroke from atrial septal aneurysm. Stroke 19:640, 1988

84. Di Pasquale G, Urbinati S, Pinelli G, Andreoli A. Risk of stroke in idiopathic hypertrophic subaortic stenosis. Stroke 23:612, 1992

85. Domenicucci S, Bellotti P, Chiarella F et al: Spontaneous morphologic changes in left ventricular thrombi: prospective two-dimensional echocardiographic study. Circulation 75:737, 1987

86. Dressler FA, Labovitz AJ: Systemic arterial emboli and cardiac masses. Association with TEE. Cardiol Clin 11:447, 1993

87. Dunn M, Alexander J, de Silva R, Hildner F: Antithrombotic therapy in atrial fibrillation. Chest 95(suppl.):118S, 1989

88. EAFT (European Atrial Fibrillation Trial) Study Group: Secondary prevention in non-rheumatic atrial fibrillation after transient ischaemic attack or minor stroke. Lancet 342:1255, 1993

89. Editorial: Left ventricular thrombosis and stroke following myocardial infarction. Lancet 335:759, 1990

90. Edmunds LH: Thrombotic and bleeding complications of prosthetic heart valves. Ann Thorac Surg 44:430, 1987

91. Egeblad H, Sorensen PS: Prevalence of mitral valve prolapse in younger patients with cerebral ischaemic attack: a blinded controlled study. Acta Med Scand 216:385, 1984

92. Eidelman BH, Obrist WD, Wagner WR et al: Cerebrovascular complications associated with the use of artificial circulatory support services. Neurology Clinics 11:463, 1993

93. Eigler N, Maurer G, Shah PK: Effect of early systemic thrombolytic therapy on left ventricular mural thrombus formation in acute anterior myocardial infarction. Am J Cardiol 54:261, 1984

94. Eisenberg PR, Sherman LA, Jaffe AS: Paradoxic elevation of fibrinopeptide-A after streptokinase: evidence for continued thrombosis despite intense fibrinolysis. J Am Coll Cardiol 19:527, 1987

95. Elam MB, Viar MJ, Ratts TE, Chesney CM: Mitral valve prolapse in women with oral contraceptive-related cerebrovascular insufficiency. Arch Intern Med 146:73, 1986

96. Ellis LB, Ramirez A: The clinical course of patients with severe "rheumatic" mitral insufficiency. Am Heart J 78:406, 1969

97. Ewy CA, Appleton CP, DeMaria AN et al: ACC/AHA guidelines for the clinical application of echocardiography. Circulation 82:2323, 1990

98. Ezekowitz MD, Bridgers SL, James KE et al: Warfarin

in the prevention of stroke associated with nonrheumatic atrial fibrillation. N Engl J Med 327:1406, 1992

99. Fairfax AJ, Lambert CD, Leatham A: Systemic embolism in chronic sinoatrial disorder. N Engl J Med 295:190, 1976

100. Falk RH: A plea for a clinical trial of anticoagulation in dilated cardiomyopathy. Am J Cardiol 65:914, 1990

101. Felner JM, Blumenstein BA, Schlant RC et al: Sources of variability in echocardiographic measurements. Am J Cardiol 45:995, 1980

102. Fieschi C, Argentino C, Lenzi GL et al: Clinical and instrumental evaluation of patients with ischemic stroke within the first six hours. J Neurol Sci 91:311, 1989

103. Fisher CM: The posterior cerebral artery syndrome. Can J Neurol Sci 13:232, 1986

104. Fisher CM: Reducing risks of cerebral embolism. Geriatrics 34:59, 1979

105. Fisher CM, Adams RD: Observations on brain embolism with special reference to hemorrhagic infarction. p. 17. In Furlan AJ (ed): The Heart and Stroke: Exploring Mutual Cardiovascular Issues. Springer-Verlag, New York, 1987

106. Fisher M, Kase CS, Stelle B, Mills RM, Jr: Ischemic stroke after cardiac pacemaker implantation in sick sinus syndrome. Stroke 19:712, 1988

107. Flegel KM, Shipley MJ, Rose G: Risk of stroke in nonrheumatic atrial fibrillation. Lancet 1:526, 1987

108. Forfar JC, Miller HC, Toft A: Occult thyrotoxicosis: a correctable cause of "idiopathic" atrial fibrillation. Am J Cardiol 44:9, 1979

109. Foulkes MA, Wolf PA, Price TR et al: The stroke data bank design, methods, and baseline characteristics. Stroke 19:547, 1988

110. Fox IS, Spence AM, Wheelis RF, Healey LA: Cerebral embolism in Libman-Sacks endocarditis. Neurology (NY) 30:487, 1980

111. Freedberg RS, Goodkin GM, Perez JL et al: Valve strands are strongly associated with systemic embolization: a transesophageal echocardiographic study. J Am Coll Cardiol 26:1709, 1995

112. The French Study of Aortic Plaques in Stroke Group: Atherosclerotic disease of the aortic arch as a risk factor for recurrent ischemic stroke. N Engl J Med 334:1216, 1996

113. Fulkerson PK, Beaver BM, Auseon JC, Graber HL: Calcification of the mitral annulus. Etiology, clinical associations, complication and therapy. Am J Med 66:967, 1979

114. Furlan AJ, Cavalier SJ, Hobbs RE et al: Hemorrhage and anticoagulation after nonseptic embolic brain infarction. Neurology (NY) 32:280, 1982

115. Furlan AJ, Craciun AR, Raju NR, Hart N. Cerebrovascular complications associated with idiopathic hypertrophic subaortic stenosis. Stroke 15:282, 1984

116. Furlan AJ, Cracuin AR, Salcedo E et al: Risk of stroke in patients with mitral annular calcification. Stroke 15:801, 1984

117. Fuster V, Gersh BJ, Giuliani ER et al: The natural history of idiopathic dilated cardiomyopathy. Am J Cardiol 47:525, 1981

118. Fuster V, Halperin JL: Left ventricular thrombi and cerebral embolism. N Engl J Med 320:392, 1989

119. Futrell N, Millikan C: Frequency, etiology, and prevention of stroke in patients with systemic lupus erythematosus. Stroke 20:583, 1989

120. Gacs G, Merei FT, Bodosi M: Balloon catheter as a model of cerebral emboli in humans. Stroke 13:39, 1982

121. Gacs G, Fox AJ, Barnett HJM, Vinuela F: CT visualization intracranial arterial thromboembolism. Stroke 14:756, 1983

122. Gadboys, HC, Litwak RS, Niemetz J, Wisch N: Role of anticoagulants in preventing embolization from prosthetic heart valves. JAMA 202:134, 1967

123. Galve E, Candell-Riera J, Pigrau C et al: Prevalence, morphologic types, and evolution of cardiac valvular disease in systemic lupus erythematosus. N Engl J Med 319:817, 1988

124. Galve E, Ordi J, Barquinero J et al: Valvular heart disease in the primary antiphospholipid syndrome. Ann Intern Med 116:293, 1992

125. Galve E, Ordi J, Candell-Riera J et al: Valvular heart disease in systemic lupus erythematosus. N Engl J Med 320:740, 1989

126. Georgiadis D, Grosset DG, Kelman A et al: Prevalence and characteristics of intracranial microemboli signals in patients with different types of prosthetic cardiac valves. Stroke 25:587, 1994

127. Geyer SJ, Franzini DA: Myxomatous degeneration of the mitral valve complicated by nonbacterial thrombotic endocarditis with systemic embolization. Am J Clin Pathol 72:489, 1979

128. Glancy DL, O'Brien KP, Gold HK, Epstein SE: Atrial fibrillation in patients with idiopathic hypertrophic subaortic stenosis. Br Heart J 32:652, 1970

129. Gorelick PB, Rusinowitz MS, Tiku M et al: Embolic stroke complicating systemic lupus erythematosus. Arch Neurol 42:813, 1985

130. Gottdiener JS, Gay JA, VanVoorhees L et al: Frequency and embolic potential of left ventricular thrombus in dilated cardiomyopathy: assessment by 2-dimensional echocardiography. Am J Cardiol 52:1281, 1983

131. Graef I, Berger AR, Bunim JJ, de la Chapelle CE: Auricular thrombosis in rheumatic heart disease. Arch Pathol 24:344, 1937

132. Graus F, Rogers LR, Posner JB: Cerebrovascular complications in patients with cancer. Medicine (Baltimore) 64:16, 1985

133. Gross CM, Nichols FT, von Dohlen TW, D'Cruz IA: Mitral valve prolapse and stroke: echocardiographic evidence for a missing causative link. J Am Soc Echo 2:94, 1989

134. Grosset DG, Georgiadis D, Abdullah I et al: Doppler emboli signals vary according to stroke subtype. Stroke 25:382, 1994

135. Hachinski V, Norris JW: The Acute Stroke. p. 141. FA Davis, Philadelphia, 1985

136. Hagen PT, Scholz DG, Edwards WD: Incidence and size of patent foramen ovale during the first 10 decades of life: an autopsy study of 965 normal hearts. Mayo Clin Proc 59:17, 1984

137. Hanson MR, Conomy JP, Hodgman JR: Brain events associated with mitral valve prolapse. Stroke 11:499, 1980

138. Hardesty WH, Roberts B, Toole JF et al: Studies of

carotid-artery blood flow in man. N Engl J Med 263: 944, 1960

139. Hardesty WH, Whitacre WB, Toole JF et al: Studies on vertebral artery blood flow in man. Surg Gynecol Obstet 116:662, 1963

140. Harris EN, Gharavi AE, Hughes GRV: Antiphospholipid antibodies. Clin Rheum Dis 11:591, 1985

141. Harrison MJG, Marshall J: Wernicke aphasia and cardiac embolism. J Neurol Neurosurg Psychiatry 50:938, 1987

142. Hart RG. Cardiogenic embolism to the brain. Lancet 339:589, 1992

143. Hart RG, Easton JD: Hemorrhagic infarcts. Stroke 17: 586, 1986

144. Hart RG, Foster JW, Luther MF, Kanter MC: Stroke in infective endocarditis. Stroke 21:695, 1990

145. Hart RG, Kagen-Hallet K, Joerns SE: Mechanisms of intracranial hemorrhage in infective endocarditis. Stroke 18:1048, 1987

146. Harvey JR, Teague SM, Anderson JR et al: Clinically silent atrial septal defects with evidence of cerebral embolization. Ann Intern Med 105:695, 1986

147. Hata JS, Ayres RW, Biller J et al: Impact of transesophageal echocardiography on the anticoagulation management of patients admitted with focal cerebral ischemia. Am J Cardiol 72:707, 1993

148. Heik SC, Kupper W, Hamm C et al: Efficacy of high dose intravenous heparin for treatment of left ventricular thrombi with high embolic risk. JACC 24:1305, 1994

149. Hejtmancik MR, Wright JC, Quint R, Jennings FL: The cardiovascular manifestations of systemic lupus erythematosus. Am Heart J 68:119, 1964

150. Held AC, Gore JM, Paraskos et al: Impact of thrombolytic therapy on left ventricular mural thrombi in acute myocardial infarction. Am J Cardiol 62:310, 1988

151. Hess DC, D'Cruz IA, Adams RJ, Nichols FT: Coronary artery disease, myocardial infarction, and brain embolism. Neurol Clinics 11:399, 1993

152. Hetzer R, Topalidis T, Borst HG: Thromboembolism and anticoagulation after isolated mitral valve replacement with porcine heterografts. p. 172. In Cohn LH, Gallucci V (eds): Cardiac Prostheses. Yorke, New York, 1982

153. Holley KE, Bahn RC, McGoon DC, Mankin HT: Spontaneous calcific embolization associated with calcific aortic stenosis. Circulation 27:197, 1963

154. Hull R, Hirsh J, Jay R et al: Different intensities of anticoagulation in the long-term treatment of proximal venous thrombosis. N Engl J Med 307:1676, 1982

155. Hurst JW, Schlant RC, Rackley CE et al: The Heart: Arteries and Veins. 7th Ed. McGraw-Hill, New York, 1990, p. 506

156. Hurst JW, Schlant RC, Rackley CE et al: The Heart: Arteries and Veins. 7th Ed. McGraw-Hill, New York, 1990, p. 1230

157. Hurst JW, Schlant RC, Rackley CE et al: The Heart: Arteries and Veins. 7th Ed. McGraw-Hill, New York, 1990, p. 1278

158. International Study Group: In-hospital mortality and clinical course of 20,891 patients with suspected acute myocardial infarction randomized between tissue plas-

minogen activator or streptokinase with or without heparin. Lancet 336:71, 1990

159. ISIS-1 (Second International Study of Infarct Survival) Collaborative Group: Randomized trial of intravenous streptokinase, oral aspirin, both, or neither among 17,187 cases of suspected acute myocardial infarction: ISIS-2. Lancet 2:349, 1988

160. Jackson AC, Boughner DR, Barnett HJM: Mitral valve prolapse and cerebral ischemic events in young patients. Neurology (NY) 34:784, 1984

161. Johannessen KA, Nordrehaug JE, von der Lippe G, Vollset SE: Risk factors for embolization in patients with left ventricular thrombi and acute myocardial infarction. Br Heart J 60:104, 1988

162. Johannessen KA, Stratton JR, Taulow E et al: Usefulness of aspirin plus dipyridamole in reducing left ventricular thrombus formation in anterior wall acute myocardial infarction. Am J Cardiol 63:101, 1989

163. Johnson RT, Richardson EP: The neurological manifestations of systemic lupus erythematosus. Medicine (Baltimore) 47:337, 1968

164. Jones HR Jr, Caplan LR, Come PC et al: Cerebral emboli of paradoxical origin. Ann Neurol 13:314, 1983

165. Jones HR, Jr, Naggar CZ, Seljan MP, Downing LL: Mitral valve prolapse and cerebral ischemic events. A comparison between a neurology population with stroke and a cardiology population with mitral valve prolapse observed for five years. Stroke 13:451, 1982

166. Kannel WB, Abbott RD, Savage DD, McNamara PM: Epidemiologic features of chronic atrial fibrillation: the Framingham study. N Engl J Med 306:1018, 1982

167. Kannel WB, Dawber TR, Cohen MS et al: Vascular diseases of the brain: epidemiologic aspects: the Framingham study. Am J Public Health 55:1355, 1965

168. Kapila A, Hart RG: Calcific cerebral emboli and aortic stenosis: detection by computed tomography. Stroke 17: 619, 1986

169. Kaplan SD, Chartash EK, Pizzarello RA, Furie RA. Cardiac manifestations of the antiphospholipid syndrome. Am Ht J 124:1331, 1992

170. Kaye D: Changing pattern of infectious endocarditis. Am J Med, suppl. 6B:157, 1985

171. Kelly RE, Pina I, Lee SC: Cerebral ischemia and mitral valve prolapse: case-control study of associated factors. Stroke 19:443, 1988

172. Keyser DL, Biller J, Coffman TT, Adams HP Jr: Neurologic complications of late prosthetic valve endocarditis. Stroke 21:472, 1990

173. Khamashta MA, Cervera R, Asherson RA, Font J et al: Association of antibodies against phospholipids with heart valve disease in systemic lupus erythematosus. Lancet 335:1541, 1990

174. Kimball RW, Hedges TR: Amaurosis fugax caused by a prolapsed mitral valve leaflet in the midsystolic click, later systolic murmur syndrome. Am J Ophthalmol 83: 469, 1977

175. Kittner SJ, Sharkness CM, Price TR et al: Infarcts with a cardiac source of embolism in the NINCDS Stroke Data Bank: historical features. Neurology 40:281, 1991

176. Knepper LE, Biller J, Adams HP, Bruno A : Neurologic manifestations of atrial myxoma. Stroke 19:1435, 1988

177. Kontny F Dale J, Nesvold A et al: Left ventricular thrombosis and arterial embolism in acute anterior myocardial infarction. J Int Med 233:139, 1993

178. Kopecky SL, Gerah BJ, McGoon MD et al: The natural history of lone atrial fibrillation. N Engl J Med 317:669, 1987

179. Korn D, DeSanctis RW, Sell S: Massive calcification of the mitral annulus: a clinical pathological study of 14 cases. N Engl J Med 267:900, 1962

180. Kouvaras G, Bacoulas G: Association of mitral leaflet prolapse with cerebral ischemic events in the young and early middle-aged patient. Q J Med 55:387, 1985

181. Kouvaras G, Chronopoulos G, Souffras G et al: The effects of long-term antithrombotic treatment on left ventricular thrombi in patients after an acute myocardial infarction. Am Heart J 119:73, 1990

182. Kumpe CW, Bean WB: Aortic stenosis: a study of the clinical and pathologic aspects of 107 proved cases. Medicine (Baltimore) 27:139, 1948

183. Kuntze CE, Ebels T, Eijelaar A, van der Heide JNH: Rates of thromboembolism with three different mechanical heart valve prostheses: randomized study. Lancet 1:514, 1989

184. Kupper AJF, Verheught FWA, Peels CH et al: Effect of low dose acetylsalicylic acid on the frequency and haematologic activity of left ventricular thrombus in anterior wall acute myocardial infarction. Am J Cardiol 63:917, 1989

185. Kupper AJF, Verheught FWA, Peels CH et al: Left ventricular thrombus incidence and behavior studies by serial two-dimensional echocardiography in acute anterior myocardial infarction: left ventricular wall motion, systemic embolism and oral anticoagulation. J Am Coll Cardiol 13:1514, 1989

186. Lang I, Steurer G, Weissel M, Burghuber OC: Recurrent paradoxical embolism complicating severe thromboembolic pulmonary hypertension. Eur Heart J 9:678, 1988

187. Lapeyre AC 3d, Steele PM, Kazmier FJ et al: Systemic embolism in chronic left ventricular aneurysm: incidence and the role of anticoagulation. J Am coll Cardiol 6:534, 1985

188. Lechat P, Mas JL, Lescault G et al: Prevalence of patent foramen ovale in patients with stroke. N Engl J Med 318:1148, 1988

189. Lee RJ, Bartzokis T, Yeoh TK et al: Enhanced detection of intracardiac sources of cerebral emboli by transesophageal echocardiography. Stroke 22:734, 1991

190. Left ventricular thrombosis and stroke following myocardial infarction. (editorial) Lancet 335:759, 1990

191. Legatt AD, Rubin MJ, Kaplan LR et al: Global aphasia without hemiparesis: multiple etiologies. Neurology (NY) 37:201, 1987

192. Leung WH, Wong KL, Lau CP et al: Association between antiphospholipid antibodies and cardiac abnormalities in patients with systemic lupus erythematosus. Am J Med 89:411, 1990

193. Levine HJ, Pauker SG, Salzman EW: Antithrombotic therapy in valvular heart disease. Chest 95(suppl.):98S, 1989

194. Lin CS, Schwartz IS, Chapman I: Calcification of the mitral annulus fibrosus with systemic embolization. Arch Pathol Lab Med 111:411, 1987

195. Lodder J, Krijne-Kubat B, Broekman J: Cerebral hemorrhagic infarction at autopsy: cardiac embolic cause and the relationship to the cause of death. Stroke 17:626, 1986

196. Lopez JA, Fishbein MC, Seigel RJ: Echocardiographic features of nonbacterial thrombotic endocarditis. Am J Cardiol 59:478, 1987

197. Lopez JA, Ross RS Fishbein MC, Siegel RJ: Nonbacterial thrombotic endocarditis: a review. Am Heart J 113:773, 1987

198. Loscalzo J: Paradoxical embolism: clinical presentation, diagnostic strategies, and therapeutic options. Am Heart J 112:141, 1986

199. Lucas C, Leys D, Mounier-Vehier F et al: Stroke patterns in patients with atrial septal aneurysm and ischemic stroke of unknown cause. Cerebrovasc Dis 4:337, 1994

200. Lupi G, Comenicucci S, Chiarella F et al: Influence of thrombolytic treatment followed by full dose anticaogulation on the frequency of left ventricular thrombi in acute myocardial infarction. Am J Cardiol 64:588, 1989

201. Lynch JJ, Schuchard GH, Gross CM, Wann LS: Prevalence of right-to-left atrial shunting in a healthy population: detection by Valsalva maneuver contrast echocardiography. Am J Cardiol 53:1478, 1984

202. MacMahon SW, Robert JK, Kramer-Fox R et al: Mitral valve prolapse and infective endocarditis. Am Heart J 113:1291, 1987

203. Manning WJ, Weintraub RM, Waksmonski CA et al: Accuracy of transesophageal echocardiography for identifying left atrial thrombi. Ann Intern Med 123:817, 1995

204. Markel ML, Waller BF, Armstrong WF: Cardiac myxoma: a review. Medicine (Baltimore) 66:114, 1987

205. Marks AR, Choong CY, Chir MBB et al: Identification of high-risk and low-risk subgroups of patients with mitral-valve prolapse. N Engl J Med 320:1031, 1989

206. Marsh III EE, Biller J, Tranel D et al: Etiology of stroke in Broca's asphasia. Neurology (NY) 40(suppl. 1):325, 1990

207. Maruyama M, Kuriyama Y, Sawada T et al: Brain damage after open heart surgery in patients with acute cardioembolic stroke. Stroke 20:1305, 1989

208. Maze SS, Kotler MN, Parry WR: Flow characteristics in the dilated left ventricle with thrombus. JACC 13:873, 1989

209. McGrath LB, Gonalez-Levin L, Eldredge WJ et al: Thromboemblic and other events following valve replacement in a pediatric population treated with antiplatelet agents. Ann Thorac Surg 43:285, 1987

210. McKenna WJ, Alfonso F: Arrhythmias in the cardiomyopathies and mitral valve prolapse. p. 59. In Zipes DP, Rowlands DJ (eds): Progress in Cardiology. Lea and Febiger, Philadelphia, 1988

211. Meister SG, Grossman W, Dexter L, Dalen JE: Paradoxical embolism: diagnosis during life. Am J Med 53:292, 1972

212. Meltzer RS, Visser CE, Fuster V: Intracardiac thrombi and systemic embolization. Ann Intern Med 104:689, 1986

213. Meyer JS, Charney JZ, Rivera VM et al: Cerebral embo-

lization: prospective clinical analysis of 42 cases. Stroke 2:541, 1971

214. Miller RD, Jordan RA, Parker RL, Edwards JE: Thromboembolism in acute and in healed myocardial infarction. II. Systemic and pulmonary arterial occlusion. Circulation 6:7, 1952

215. Millkan CH, Bauer RB, Goldschmidt J et al: A classification and outline of cerebrovascular disease: II Stroke 6: 564, 1975

216. Mohr JP, Caplan LR, Melski JW et al: The Harvard cooperative stroke registry: a prospective registry. Neurology (NY) 28:754, 1978

217. Mok CK, Boey J, Wang R et al: Warfarin versus dipyridamole-aspirin and pentoxifylline-aspirin for the prevention of prosthetic heart valve thromboembolism: a prospective randomized clinical trial. Circulation 72:1059, 1985

218. Mooe T, Teien D, Karp K, Eriksson P: Left ventricular thrombosis after anterior myocardial infarction with and without thrombolytic treatment. J Int Med 237:563, 1995

219. Mountcastle VB: Medical Physiology. 13th Ed. Vol. 2. CV Mosby, St. Louis, 1974

220. Mugge A, Daniel WG, Frank G, Lichtlen PR: Echocardiography in infective endocarditis: re-assessment of prognostic implications of vegetation size determined by the transthoracic and the transesophageal approach. J Am Coll Cardiol 14:631, 1989

221. Mugge A, Daniel WG, Klopper JW, Lichtlen PR: Visualization of patent foramen ovale by transesophageal color-coded Doppler echocardiography. Am J Cardiol 62:837, 1988

222. Naggar CZ, Pearson WN, Seljan MP: Frequency of complication of mitral valve prolapse in subjects aged 60 years and older. Am J Cardiol 58:1209, 1986

223. Nair CK, Thomson W, Ryschon K et al: Long-term follow-up of patients with echocardiographically detected mitral annular calcium and comparison with age- and sex-matched control subjects. Am J Cardiol 63:465, 1989

224. Nakatani T, Frazier OH, Lammermeier DE et al: Heterotopic heart transplantation: a reliable option for a select group of high-risk patients. J Heart Transplant 8:40, 1989

225. Nater B, Bogousslavsky J, Regli F, Stauffer JC: Stroke patterns with atrial septal aneurysm. Cerebrovasc Dis 2: 342, 1992

226. Nencini P, Inzitari D, Baraffi MC et al: Incidence of stroke in young adults in Florence, Italy. Stroke 19:977, 1988

227. Nestico PF, Depace NL, Morganroth J et al: Mitral annular calcification: Clinical pathophysiology, and echocardiographic review. Am Heart J 107:989, 1984

228. Nichol P, Kertesz A: Two-dimensional echocardiographic (2DE) detection of left atrial thrombus in patient with mitral valve prolapse and strokes. Circulation 59/60(suppl. 11):18, 1979

229. Nihoyannopoulos P, Smith GC, Maseri A, Foale RA: The natural history of left ventricular thrombus in myocardial infarction: a rationale in support of masterly inactivity. J Am Coll Cardiol 14:903, 1989

230. Nishide M, Irino T, Gotoh M et al: Cardiac abnormalities in ischemic cerebrovascular disease studied by two-dimensional echocardiography. Stroke 14:541, 1983

231. Nishimura RA, McGoon MD, Shub C et al: Echocardiographically documented mitral valve prolapse: long-term follow-up of 237 patients. N Engl J Med 313:1305, 1985

232. O'Brien JT, Geiser EA: Infective endocarditis and echocardiography. Am Heart J 108:386, 1984

233. Ogata J, Yutani C, Imakita M et al: Hemorrhagic infarct of the brain without the reopening of the occluded arteries in cardioembolic stroke. Stroke 20:876, 1989

234. Okada Y, Yamaguchi T, Minematsu K et al: Hemorrhagic transformation in cerebral embolism. Stroke 20:598, 1989

235. Olesen KH, Rygg IH, Wennevold A, Nyboe J: Long-term follow-up in 185 patients after mitral valve replacement with the Lillehei-Kaster prosthesis: overall results and prosthesis-related complications. Eur Heart J 8:680, 1987

236. Olsen ML, Arnett FC, Rosenbaum D et al: Sjögren's syndrome and other rheumatic disorders presenting to a neurology service. J Autoimmun 2:477, 1989

237. Onundarson PT, Thorgeirsson G, Jonmundsson E et al: Chronic atrial fibrillation: epidemiologic features and 14-year follow-up: a case-control study. Eur Heart J 8: 521, 1987

238. Ostrander LD, Brandt RL, Kjelsberg MO, Epstein FH: Electrocardiographic findings among the adult population of a total natural community. Tecumseh, Michigan. Circulation 31:888, 1965

239. Palacois I, Block PC, Brandi S et al: Percutaneous balloon valvotomy for patients with severe mitral stenosis. Circulation 75:778, 1987

240. Pape LA, Love DG. Gore JM: Massive thromboembolic stroke and death after fibrinolytic therapy of St. Jude prosthetic mitral valve thrombosis: documentation by transthoracic Doppler echocardiography. Am Heart J 128:406, 1994

241. Paschalis C, Pugsley W, John R, Harrison MJG: Rate of cerebral embolic events in relation to antibiotic and anticoagulant therapy in patients with bacterial endocarditis. Eur Neurol 30:87, 1990

242. Pass HI, Sade RM, Crawford FA, Hohn AR: Cardiac valve prostheses in children without anticoagulation. J Thorac Cardiovasc Surg 87:832, 1984

243. Paydarfar D, Krieger D, Dib N et al: Magnetic resonance imaging of the cardiac chambers: clinico-pathological correlations, abstracted. Stroke 27:179, 1996

244. Pearson AC, Labovitz AJ, Tatineni S, Gomez CR: Superiority of transesophageal echocardiography in detecting cardiac source embolism in patients with cerebral ischemia of uncertain etiology. J Am Coll Cardiol 17:66, 1991

245. Pearson AC, Nagelhout D, Castello R et al: Atrial septal aneurysm and stroke: a transesophageal echocardiographic study. J Am Coll Cardiol 18:1223, 1991

246. Perloff JK, Rosove MH, Child JS, Wright GB: Adults with cyanotic congenital heart disease: hematologic management. Ann Intern Med 109:406, 1988

247. Pessin MS, Lathi ES, Cohen MB et al: Clinical features and mechanism of occipital infarction. Ann Neurol 21: 290, 1987

248. Petersen P: Thromboembolic complications in atrial fibrillation. Stroke 21:4, 1990

249. Petersen P, Godtfredsen J, Boysen G: Placebo-controlled, randomized trial of warfarin and aspirin for prevention of thromboembolic complications in chronic atrial fibrillation: the Copenhagen AFASAK study. Lancet 1:175, 1989

250. Pomerance A: Ballooning deformity (mucoid degeneration) of atrioventricular valves. Br Heart J 31:343, 1969

251. Pomerance A: Cardiac pathology and systemic murmurs in the elderly. Br Heart J 30:687, 1968

252. Pomerance A: Pathological and clinical study of calcification of the mitral valve ring. J Clin Pathol 23:354, 1970

253. Pop G, Sutherland GR, Koudstaal PJ et al: Transesophageal echocardiography in the detection of intracardiac embolic sources in patients with transient ischemic attacks. Stroke 21:560, 1990

254. Popp RL: Echocardiography. I. Medical progress. N Engl J Med 323:101, 1990

255. Popp RL: Echocardiography: II. Medical Progress. N Engl J Med 323:165, 1990

256. Presti CF, Hart RG: Thyrotoxicosis, atrial fibrillation, and embolism revisited. Am Heart J 117:976, 1989, 1990

257. Price TR: Stroke in patients treated with thrombolytic therapy for acute myocardial infarction: the thrombosis in myocardial infarction clinical trial and a review of placebo-controlled trials. Stroke, 21(suppl. III):8, 1990

258. Pruitt AA, Rubin RH, Karchmer AW, Duncan GW: Neurologic complications of bacterial endocarditis. Medicine (Baltimore) 57:329, 1978

259. Puletti M, Morocutti C, Borgia C et al: Acute myocardial infarction and brain. Ital J Neurol Sci 8:245, 1987

260. Ramirez-Lassepas M, Cipolle RJ, Bjork RJ et al: Can embolic stroke be diagnosed on the basis of neurologic clinical criteria? Arch Neurol 44:87, 1987

261. Reed RL, Siekert RG, Meredith J: Rarity of transient focal cerebral ischemia in cardiac dysrhythmia. JAMA 223:893, 1973

262. Rem JA, Hachinski VC, Boughner DR, Barnett HJM: Value of cardiac monitoring and echocardiography in TIA and stroke patients. Stroke 16:950, 1985

263. Rice GPA, Ebers GC, Newland F, Wysocki GP: Recurrent cerebral embolism in cardiac amyloidosis. Neurology (NY) 31:904, 1981

264. Ridolfi RL, Hutchins GM: Spontaneous calcific emboli from calcific mitral annulus fibrosus. Arch Pathol Lab Med 100:117, 1976

265. Roberts WC, Siegel RJ, McManus BM: Idiopathic dilated cardiomyopathy: analysis of 152 necropsy patients. Am J Cardiol 60:1340, 1987

266. Rogers LR, Cho ES, Kempin S, Posner JB: Cerebral infarction from nonbacterial thrombotic endocarditis: clinical and pathological study including the effects of anticoagulation. Am J Med 83:746, 1987

267. Rothbard RL, Nanda NC, Fleck G, Heinle RA: Mitral valve prolapse and stroke: detection of potential emboli by real-time two-dimensional echocardiography. Circulation, 59/60(suppl. 11):99, 1979

268. Rothrock JF, Dittrich HC, Fleck P et al: Mitral valve prolapse and ischemic stroke in the young. Circulation 78:601, 1988

269. Rowe JC, Bland EF, Sprague HB, White PP: The course of mitral stenosis without surgery: ten- and twenty-year perspectives. Ann Intern Med 52:741, 1960

270. Roy D, Marchand E, Gagne P et al: Usefulness of anticoagulant therapy in the prevention of embolic complications of atrial fibrillation. Am Heart J 112:1139, 1986

271. Rubenstein JJ, Schulman CL, Yurchak PM, De Sanctis RW: Clinical spectrum of the sick sinus syndrome. Circulation 46:5, 1972

272. Russell JW, Biller J, Hajduczok ZD et al: Ischemic cerebrovascular complications and risk factors in idiopathic hypertrophic subaortic stenosis. Stroke 22:1143, 1991

273. Salgado AV, Furlan AJ, Keys TF: Mycotic aneurysm, subarachnoid hemorrhage and indications for cerebral angiography in infectious endocarditis. Stroke 18:1057, 1987

274. Salgado AV, Furlan AJ, Keys TF et al: Neurological complications of native and prosthetic valve endocarditis: a 12-year experience. Neurology (NY) 39:173, 1989

275. Sandercock PAG, Warlow CP, Jone LN: Predisposing factors for cerebral infarction: the Oxfordshire community stroke project. BMJ 298:75, 1989

276. Santini M, Alexidou G, Ansalone G et al: Relation of prognosis in sick sinus syndrome to age, conduction defects and modes of permanent cardiac pacing. Am J Cardiol 65:729, 1990

277. Saour JN, Sieck JO, Mamo LAR, Gallus AS: Trial of different intensities of anticoagulation in patients with prosthetic heart valves. N Engl J Med 322:428, 1990

278. Sareli P, England MJ, Berk MR et al: Maternal and fetal sequelae of anticoagulation during pregnancy in patients with mechanical heart valve prostheses. Am J Cardiol 63:1462, 1989

279. Savage DD, Garrison RJ, Devereaux RD et al: Mitral valve prolapse in the general population. I. Epidemiologic features: the Framingham Study. Am Heart J 106:571, 1983

280. The SCATI (Studio sulla Calciparina nell' angina e nella Trombosi Ventricolare nell'infarto) group: randomized controlled trial of subcutaneous calcium-heparin in acute myocardial infarction. Lancet 2:182, 1989

281. Scharf RE, Hennerici M, Bluschke V et al: Cerebral ischemia in young patients: is it associated with mitral valve prolapse and abnormal platelet activity in vivo? Stroke 13:454, 1982

282. Schnee MA, Bucal AA: Fatal embolism in mitral valve prolapse. Chest 83:285, 1983

283. Schneider B, Hanrath P, Vogel P, Meinertz T: Improved morphologic characterization of atrial septal aneurysm by transesophageal echocardiography: relation to cerebrovascular events. J Am Coll Cardiol 16:1000, 1990

284. Selzer A, Cohn KE: Natural history of mitral stenosis: a review. Circulation 45:878, 1972

285. Selzer A, Katayama F: Mitral regurgitation: clinical patterns, pathophysiology and natural history. Medicine (Baltimore) 51:337, 1972

286. Seward JB, Khandheria BK, Oh JK et al: Transesophageal echocardiography: technique, anatomic correlations, implementation, and clinical applications. Mayo Clin Proc 63:649, 1988

287. Shaw PJ, Bates D, Cartlidge NEF et al: Neurologic and

neuropsychological morbidity following major surgery-comparison of coronary artery bypass and peripheral vascular surgery. Stroke 18:700, 1987

288. Sherman DG, Dyken ML, Fisher M et al: Antithrombotic therapy for cerebrovascular disorders, suppl. Chest 95:140S, 1989

289. Shimosegawa E, Inugami A, Okudera T et al: Embolic cerebral infarction: MR findings in the first 3 hours after onset. AJR 160:1077, 1993

290. Shrestha NK, Morenco FL, Narciso FV et al: Two-dimensional echocardiographic diagnosis of left atrial thrombus in rheumatic heart disease: a clinicopathologic study. Circulation 67:341, 1983

291. Shyu KG, Chen JJ, Huang ZS et al: Role of transesophageal echocardiography in the diagnostic assessment of cardiac sources of embolism in patients with acute ischemic stroke. Cardiology 85:53, 1994

292. Silver MD: Infective endocarditis. p. 517. In Silver MD (ed): Cardiovascular Pathology. Churchill Livingstone, New York, 1983

293. Simpson IA, Camm AJ: Colour Doppler flow mapping: a new dimension for cardiac diagnosis. BMJ 300:1, 1990

294. Smith P, Arnesen H, Holme I: The effect of warfarin on mortality and reinfarction after myocardial infarction. N Engl J Med 323:147, 1990

295. Sotaniemi KA: Long-term neurologic outcome after cardiac operation. Ann Thorac Surg 59:1336, 1995

296. Special Report from the National Institute of Neurological Disorders and Stroke: Classification of cerebrovascular diseases. III. Stroke 21:637, 1990

297. Stagaman DJ, Presti C, Rees C, Miller DD: Septic pulmonary arteriovenous fistula: an unusual conduit for systemic embolization of right-sided valvular endocarditis. Chest 97:1484, 1990

298. Stein PD, Kantrowitz A: Antithrombotic therapy in mechanical and biological prosthetic heart valves and saphenous vein bypass grafts. Chest 95:107S, 1989

299. Stein PD, Willis PW, DeMets DL: History and physical examination in acute pulmonary embolism in patients without preexisting cardiac or pulmonary disease. Am J Cardiol 47:218, 1981

300. Stevenson LW, Perloff JK: The dilated cardiomyopathies: clinical aspects. Cardiol Clin 6:187, 1988

301. Store J, Lisan P, Delmonico JE Jr, Bailey CP: Physiopathological concepts of mitral valvular disease: review of 225 cardiotomies. JAMA 155:103, 1954

302. Stratton JR, Resnick AD: Increased embolic risk in patients with left ventricular thrombi. Circulation 75:1004, 1987

303. Stroke Prevention in Atrial Fibrillation Investigators: Adjusted-dose warfarin versus low-intensity, fixed-dose warfarin plus aspirin for high-risk patients with atrial fibrillation: Stroke Prevention in Atrial Fibrillation III randomised clinical trial. Lancet 348:633, 1996

304. Stroke Prevention in Atrial Fibrillation Investigators: Warfarin versus aspirin for prevention of thromboembolism in atrial fibrillation: Stroke Prevention in Atrial Fibrillation II Study. Lancet 343:687, 1994

305. Stroke Prevention in Atrial Fibrillation Investigators: Design of a multicenter randomized trial for the Stroke Prevention in Atrial Fibrillation Study. Stroke 21:538, 1990

306. Stroke Prevention in Atrial Fibrillation Investigators: Stroke Prevention in Atrial Fibrillation Study: final results. Circulation 84:527, 1991

307. Suber M, Mas JL et al: Risk of recurrent stroke in patients with atrial septal aneurysm or patent foramen ovale: a French multicentric study, abstracted. Cerebrovas Dis 4:247, 1994

308. Szekely P: Systemic embolism and anticoagulant prophylaxis in rheumatic heart disease. Br Med J 1:209, 1964

309. Tanne D, Reicher-Reiss H, Boyko V, Behar S: SPRINT study group. Stroke risk after anterior wall acute myocardial infarction. Am J Cardiol 76:825, 1995

310. Teague SM, Sharma MK: Detection of paradoxical cerebral echo contrast embolization by transcranial Doppler ultrasound: Stroke 22:740, 1991

311. Tegeler CH, Downes TR: Cardiac imaging in stroke. Curr Concepts Cerebrovasc Dis Stroke 26:13, 1991

312. Thompson T, Evans W: Paradoxical embolism. Q J Med 23:135, 1930

313. Tice FD, Slivka AP, Walz ET et al: Mitral valve strands in patients with focal cerebral ischemia. Stroke 27:1183, 1996

314. Timsit SG, Sacco RL, Mohr JP et al: Early clinical differentiation of cerebral infarction from severe atherosclerotic stenosis and cardioembolism. Stroke 23:486, 1992

315. Tong DC, Bolger A, Albers GW: Incidence of transcranial Doppler-detected cerebral microemboli in patients referred for echocardiography. Stroke 25:2138, 1994

316. Toole JF: Cerebrovascular Disorders. 4th ed. p. 245. Lippincott-Raven, Philadelphia, 1990

317. Tunick PA, Culliford AT, Lamparello PJ, Kronzon I: Atheromatosis of the aortic arch as an occult source of multiple systemic emboli. Ann Intern Med 114:391, 1991

318. Turpie AGG, Gent M, Laupacis A et al: A comparison of aspirin with placebo in patients treated with warfarin after heart-valve replacement. N Engl J Med 329:524, 1993

319. Turpie AGG, Gunstensen J, Hirsh J et al: Randomized comparison of two intensities of oral anticoagulant therapy after tissue heart valve replacement. Lancet 1:1242, 1988

320. Turpie AGG, Robinson JG, Doyle DJ et al: Comparison of high-dose with low-dose subcutaneous heparin to prevent left ventricular mural thrombosis in patients with acute transmural anterior myocardial infarction. N Engl J Med 320:352, 1989

321. Vaitkus PT, Barnathan ES: Embolic potential prevention and management of mural thrombus complicating anterior myocardial infarction: a meta-analysis. JACC 22:1004, 1993

322. Van Dantzig JM, Delemarre BJ, Bot H et al: Doppler left ventricular flow pattern versus conventional predictors of left ventricular thrombus after acute myocardial infarction. J Am Coll Card 25:1341, 1995

323. Visser CA, Kan G, Meltzer RS et al: Embolic potential of left ventricular thrombus after myocardial infarction:

a two-dimensional echocardiographic study of 119 patients. J Am Coll Cardiol 5:1276, 1985

324. Wareing TH, Davila-Roman VG, Barzilai B et al: Management of the severely atherosclerotic ascending aorta during cardiac operations. J Thorac Cardiovasc Surg 103: 453, 1992

325. Warlow CP, Dennis MS, van Gijn J et al: What caused this transient or persisting ischaemic event? p. 191. In Stroke: A Practical Guide to Management. Blackwell Scientific Publications, Bath Press, Bath, 1996

326. Warth DC, King ME, Cohen JM et al: Prevalence of mitral valve prolapse in normal children. J Am Coll Cardiol 5:1173, 1985

327. Watson RT: TIA, stroke and mitral valve prolapse. Neurology (NY) 29:886, 1979

328. Webster MWI, Smith HJ, Sharpe DN et al: Patent foramen ovale in young stroke patients. Lancet 2:11, 1988

329. Weinreich DJ, Burke JF, Pauletto FJ: Left ventricular mural thrombi complicating acute myocardial infarction: long-term follow-up with serial echocardiography. Ann Intern Med 100:789, 1984

330. Weinstein GS, Mavroudis C, Ebert PA: Preliminary experience with aspirin for anticoagulation in children with prosthetic cardiac valves. Ann Thorac Surg 33:549, 1982

331. Weintraub WS, Ba'albake HA: Decision analysis concerning the application of echocardiography to the diagnosis and treatment of mural thrombi after anterior wall acute myocardial infarction. Am J Cardiol 64:708, 1989

332. Wilson WR, Geraci JE, Danielson GK et al: Anticoagulant therapy and central nervous system complications in patients with prosthetic valve endocarditis. Circulation 57:1004, 1978

333. Wolf PA, Abbott Rd, Kannel WB: Atrial fibrillation: a major contributor to stroke in the elderly: the Framingham study. Arch Intern Med 147:1561, 1987

334. Wolf PA, Dawber TR, Thomas HE, Kannel WB: Epidemiologic assessment of chronic atrial fibrillation and risk of stroke: the Framingham study. Neurology (NY) 28: 973, 1978

335. Wolf PA, Kannel WB, McGee DL: Duration of atrial fibrillation and imminence of stroke: the Framingham study. Stroke 14:664, 1983

336. Wolf PA, Sila CA: Cerebral ischemia with mitral valve prolapse. Am Heart J 113:1308, 1987

337. Woods GL, Wood RP, Shaw BW Jr: Aspergillus endocarditis in patients without prior cardiovascular surgery: report of a case in a liver transplant recipient and review, abstracted. Rev Infect Dis 2:263, 1989

338. Yadav JS, Kinkel PR, Klee D et al: Small cerebral embolic infarctions: evaluation by magnetic resonance imaging. Neurology (NY), 39(suppl. 1):160, 1989

339. Yamanouchi H, Tomonaga M, Shimada H et al: Nonvalvular atrial fibrillation as a cause of fatal massive cerebral infarction in the elderly. Stroke 20:1653, 1989

340. Yasaka M, Yamaguchi T, Yonehara T, Moriyasu H: Recurrent embolization during intravenous administration of tissue plasminogen activator in acute cardioembolic stroke. Angiology 45:481, 1994

341. Yatsu FM, Hart RG, Mohr JP, Grotta JC: Anticoagulation of embolic strokes of cardiac origin: an update. Neurology (NY) 38:314, 1988

342. Zenker G, Erbel R, Kramer G et al: Transesophageal two-dimensional echocardiography in young patients with cerebral ischemic events. Stroke 19:345, 1988

Medical Complications of Stroke

SANDRA HANSON

THOMAS J. DEGRABA

CARLOS VILLAR-CORDOVA

FRANK M. YATSU

Medical complications associated with strokes are important for two reasons. First, patients suffering strokes, particularly the elderly, frequently have one or more pre-existing medical or psychiatric disorders that must be considered since their deterioration is a constant threat. The most frequent medical or psychiatric problems encountered in these patients are cardiopulmonary disorders and organic brain syndromes with confusion and memory impairment. Second, strokes, by the nature of the patients becoming disabled, confined, and losing a sense of self-esteem, may precipitate medical and psychiatric complications. These latter disorders include cardiopulmonary disorders, such as cardiac arrhythmias, impaired swallowing with potential for aspiration, pulmonary emboli, atelectasis and depression, plus primarily neurological disorders as well. Although neurologic complications of strokes are beyond the scope of this chapter since they will be discussed in the section dealing with neurointensive care, these neurologic disorders relate to increased intracranial pressure, seizures, and organic brain syndrome with confusion, disorientation, agitation, somnolence, and coma. The importance of recognizing medical and neurologic complications of stroke patients is the impact of these complications have on morbidity and mortality. For example, in a study of medical and neurologic complications in a medical intensive care, similar for its intensity of care as a stroke unit, Bleck et al found that in over 1,700 patients, medical and neurologic complications added to the patients' morbidity and mortality significantly.[9]

Listed in Table 49.1 are the various body systems that may be primarily or secondarily aggravated or provoked by strokes. These are divided into the following disorders: (1) cardiopulmonary, (2) psychiatric, (3) nutritional, (4) excretory, (5) neuromuscular and integument, (6) neurologic, and (7) other systemic problems.

Cardiopulmonary Complications

Cardiovascular and pulmonary complications associated with strokes are most commonly due to (1) pre-existing diseases that can be aggravated by stroke, including coronary artery disease, congestive heart failure and chronic obstructive pulmonary disease (COPD); (2) stroke-induced cardiac arrhythmias, neurogenic pulmonary edema, and electrocardiographic (ECG) abnormalities; (3) pulmonary emboli secondary to deep venous thrombosis; and (4) hypertension and the potential problems associated with its aggressive therapy.[8,11,21,42,56,58,67,69,84,85,103,111]

With pre-existing cardiovascular and pulmonary diseases, strokes may worsen the underlying condition because of either neurologic deficits or secondary metabolic derangements.

It has been recognized for years that cerebral vascular events, such as subarachnoid hemorrhage, acute thromboembolic stroke, and cerebral hemorrhage, have been associated with electrocardiographic abnormalities.[13,14,22,26,40] ECG abnormalities and acute cerebral events were found in over 90% of patients in two large studies[26,38] as compared to approximately 40% in the age-matched control population. The most common changes were QT prolongation (up to 45%), ST segment depression or T-wave inversion (35% to 50%), and U waves (up to 28%). Studies have also demonstrated a significant increase in cardiac arrhythmias with ectopic ventricular activity being the most common.[77,79] Myers et al[77] noted that the occurrence of arrhythmias was independent of coexisting heart disease. The importance of the occurrence of these ECG abnormalities was highlighted by Levy et al,[60] who showed

Table 49.1 Medical and Neurological Complications of Stroke: Common Pre-existing Disorders and Their Aggravation by Strokes, Plus Their Precipitation

Pre-existing Disorders	Aggravations
Cardiopulmonary	Cardiac arrhythmias, congestive failure, blood pressure elevations, impaired cardiac output, myocardial infarction, chronic obstructive pulmonary disease, pulmonary embolism, atelectasis, pneumonia, intubation, tracheostomy, sleep apnea
Psychiatric	Depression, confusional states, delirium, agitation, organic brain syndrome, "sundowning," hallucinations & delusions
Nutritional	Adequate nutrition with feedings: oral vs nasogastric vs gastrostomy, body weight and electrolyte balance & metabolism, syndrome of inappropriate antidiuretic hormone secretion, CNS salt losing, salt retention, maintenance of body weight, dehydration, diabetes
Excretory	Bladder: spastic bladder, incontinence, urinary tract infections Bowels: incontinence, constipation
Neuromuscular and cutaneous	From immobility: decubiti and "bed integument sores," contractures, venous thrombosis, pulmonary emboli, atelectasis, increased loss of muscle tone
Neurologic	Increased intracranial pressure from brain edema, seizures, stupor, coma, higher cortical and cognitive deficits, dementia, encephalopathy
Other systemic problems	Hypertension, sepsis, hypercoagulable states, temperature regulation failure, hyper- and hypoglycemia
Miscellaneous issues	Costs, consultations, rehabilitation, OT/PT, DNR, issues of "living will" physician-assisted suicide, use of a stroke unit

Abbreviations: CNS, central nervous system; OT/PT, occupational therapy and physical therapy; DNR, do not resuscitate.

that the prognosis for patient survival was much worse in patients with ischemic changes or arrhythmias on their ECG. In addition, it was noted that outcome was dependent upon ECG changes acquired during the acute stroke period rather than upon pre-existing heart disease.[60] Norris et al[80] demonstrated, in a group of 230 patients with stroke, that serum creatinine kinase (CK-MB) isoenzymes were elevated in 11% of the patients. This CK-MB elevation correlated with evidence of acute myocardial ischemia by ECG and was associated with a 92% incidence of cardiac arrhythmia. Also of note was that progressive ischemic changes on the ECG along with the timing of the CK-MB elevation indicated that the cardiac changes were most likely a result of, and not the cause of, the acute cerebral vascular event. Myers et al[76] demonstrated that patients with ischemic infarcts and TIAs had an elevation of plasma norepinephrine levels as compared to a control population, which indicated that an increase in peripheral sympathetic activity could produce cardiac abnormalities. Studies also demonstrate that elevated plasma norepinephrine concentration correlated with an increase in CK-MB, but not with an increased incidence of cardiac arrhythmias.[77] Again, the significance of elevation of cardiac isoenzymes in the setting of acute cerebral vascular events of more than twofold (66% versus 30%) is an increase in the mortality over those patients with normal cardiac enzymes.[26]

The etiology of these ECG changes and cardiac abnormalities represents a combination of factors. Existence of concomitant underlying coronary artery disease plays a predominant role in the appearance of cardiac abnormalities and mortality.[60] Patients with severe coronary artery disease, subjected to an elevation in sympathetic nervous stimulation due to an intracerebral event, could clearly cause cardiac changes, such as ischemia or arrhythmias, due to increased myocardial oxygen demand. The theory that has gained the widest support is that discharge of catecholaminergic neurotransmitters into the systemic circulation, in association with cerebral infarction, subarachnoid hemorrhage, and increased intracranial pressure, plus increased vagal traffic to the heart, provokes both hypertension and cardiac muscle damage.[78] As a result of the catecholaminergic response to the acute stroke, borderline compensated cardiac function may fail; under these circumstances, measures to improve cardiac output, such as digitalization, are indicated.[31] Particularly vulnerable are patients with massive subarachnoid hemorrhage who may infrequently experience atrial fibrillation and rarely life-threatening ventricular fibrillation.[111] Again, pre-existing cardiac disease in patients with ischemic stroke makes it difficult to know if arrhythmias such as atrial fibrillation preceded or were a result of the stroke.[61]

In addition to the increase in myocardial contractility and heart rate, in general, there is evidence that local discharge of the sympathetic nerve fibers within the ventricular muscle itself lead to a myofibrillar degeneration.[40] The subendocardial changes seen on autopsy studies are characterized by contraction band necrosis, which are concentric around sympathetic nerve terminals, monocyte infiltration, and early calcification (up to 24 hours following tissue injury).[95] These findings correlate with elevations in cardiac enzymes and are histopathologically distinct from ischemic infarctions resulting from coronary artery disease.

In view of the evidence that cerebral vascular events cause serious arrhythmias, myocardial damage, and increased mortality, it is recommended that all patients with stroke be monitored for cardiac arrhythmias[111] in the first 24 to 72 hours after admission, and that serial isoenzymes are obtained on all patients with new ECG abnormalities.

Treatment modalities for these cardiac changes include beta-blockers to inhibit the catecholaminergic output, lidocaine for arrhythmia, and atropine for vagotonia. Type 1A antiarrhythmics, such as quinidine and procainamide, may prolong the QT interval and may not be appropriate in this setting.

It is well accepted that the greatest risk for mortality following a transient ischemic attack (TIA) or stroke is from cardiac causes.[37,104] It is estimated that 33% of patients with TIAs or stroke have symptomatic coronary artery disease.[15,51] Toole et al[104] showed, in a 9-year follow-up study, that greater than 60% of all deaths in patients with TIAs results from myocardial infarctions. Others have echoed the findings that TIAs are not only a warning for future strokes, but point toward coronary artery disease and increased incidence of death resulting from myocardial infarction.[37,75] In light of the data of coronary artery disease existing in patients with thromboembolic stroke and TIA, a unified approach for cardiac monitoring and evaluation of coronary artery disease must be employed. In a prospective study of 506 patients presenting with symptomatic extracranial cerebral vascular disease (n = 288) or asymptomatic carotid bruits (n = 218), 48% of those with clinical symptoms or ECG findings consistent with coronary artery disease and 16% with no suspicion of coronary artery disease had severe coronary stenosis by angiography, warranting a revascularization procedure, or showed an inoperable lesion.[42] The high prevalence of coronary artery disease suggests that patients with symptomatic coronary disease who have TIAs or stroke, requiring extracranial vascular surgery, should undergo coronary angiography. Patients without clinically apparent coronary artery disease should have cardiac screening including ECG stress or stress thallium tests. If these results are positive, coronary angiography should be performed to identify coronary stenosis requiring angioplasty or surgical intervention prior to carotid endarterectomy. Di Pasquale et al[28] support the concept of cardiovascular evaluation. In a prospective study of 83 patients with TIAs or mild stroke without symptoms or ECG signs of ischemic heart disease, they demonstrated a 28% rate of coronary artery disease on exercise ECG tests and exercise thallium 201 myocardial scintigraphy. This is compared to a 6% rate of coronary artery disease seen in an age- and sex-matched control group with no clinical symptoms of cerebrovascular or coronary artery disease. Boucher et al[10] demonstrated the predictive value of a stress thallium test. It was shown that 8 out of 16 patients with no clinical history of coronary artery disease, and who had a positive stress thallium test, went on to have a myocardial infarction (MI) after their revascularization procedure for carotid occlusive disease. None of the 32 patients with normal stress thallium test had an MI after their operation. These data support the contention that presentation of cerebral ischemia should prompt an evaluation of the coronary arteries.

Respiratory compromise is a major source of morbidity and mortality in the post-stroke setting.[7] Coexisting pulmonary diseases such as chronic obstructive pulmonary disease (COPD), as well as perturbations of respiratory mechanisms resulting from stroke, including weakness of respiration muscles due to hemiparesis, impairment of respiration due to brain stem lesions, and inadequate cough and gag leading to aspiration, may embarrass and decompensate borderline pulmonary function. In addition, immobility of extremities due to paralysis with attendant stasis of blood and thrombosis can lead to multiple pulmonary emboli, and generalized immobility can lead to atelectasis resulting in O_2 desaturation, thus threatening further hypoxic brain injury.

Pneumonia occurs in one-third of stroke patients and is associated with significant morbidity and mortality in this population.[45] Major contributory factors for pneumonia include dysphagia, impaired gag or cough reflex, impaired cognitive function, dehydration, immobility and expiratory muscle weakness. Bedside evaluation by a water swallow test[24] or videofluoroscopy can be used to identify dysphagia in patients suspected of having swallowing impairment. Kidd et al[54] reported that loss of pharyngeal sensation can also be a marker for silent aspiration. Holas et al[43] found that the relative risk of pneumonia was 6.95 times greater for those patients who aspirated compared with those who did not, and 5.57 times greater in patients with silent aspiration versus those who cough when aspirating or who did not aspirate at all. Studies have shown that most stroke patients are able to resume oral feeding with rehabilitation techniques that include diet modification and compensatory swallowing exercises.[44,45] Mobilization, incentive spirometry, and aggressive pulmonary toilet, as needed, are effective in reducing the complications of pneumonia. In some cases, if gag and swallowing are severely affected, intubation may need to be instituted to avoid the danger of aspiration. Fevers, mental status changes, and reduction in oxygen saturation by pulse oximetry could all point to the development of pneumonia and atelectasis.

Pulmonary embolism secondary to deep venous thrombosis (DVT) from a paretic limb is another source of pulmonary compromise in the post-stroke setting. Peak incidence occurs in the first week, although the risk of venous thrombosis persists beyond this period with the highest risk in those with limb paralysis who are nonambulatory. In these patients, DVT prophylaxis is recommended and includes low-dose subcutaneous heparin,[19,66] mobilization, and external compression devices such as pneumatic calf compression boots and compression stockings. Studies have also shown that low-molecule-weight heparinoids may be beneficial and safe in the prevention of DVTs.[106,107] In a recent report of interim data from the International Stroke Trials, addition of 12,500 units sc twice daily to aspirin for recurrent stroke prevention resulted in a higher incidence of significant intracerebral and noncerebral hemorrhages.[96] Although the report did not specifically target DVT, the data suggest that use of lower doses of sc heparin (5,000 units twice a day) remains the preferred approach to DVT prophylaxis.

Neurogenic pulmonary edema (NPE) occurs in association with dramatic insults to the central nervous system, such as massive subarachnoid hemorrhage, seizures, or head trauma, although it has occurred with cerebral infarction.[29,92] Although NPE could occur from congestive heart failure resulting from massive and sustained hypertension secondary to catecholaminergic release, the most common mechanism is transudation of serum into lung alveoli.[102,105] In an analysis of 25 hemorrhagic stroke patients, 3 of whom experienced NPE, Touho et al[105] measured pulmonary arterial pressure, pulmonary capillary wedge pressure, central venous pressure, cardiac index, systemic vascular resistance index, pulmonary vascular resistance index, and extravascular lung water using a double-indicator dilution method. The primary disorder found with NPE is the last of increased extravascular lung water. The defect is not explained by left ventricular failure, but by high permeability pulmonary edema. Although α-adrenergic blockade, such as the use of phenoxybenzamine, has been advocated, institution of positive end-expiratory pressure suffices in clearing the patient of NPE.

Psychiatric Complications

Depression is a common complication of stroke with an incidence estimated between 30% to 60% in the 2-year period immediately following the ischemic event.[63] The period of high risk for development of clinically important depression extends for at least 2 years post-stroke.[62,63,86–91] The prevalance of major depression at different time-points post-stroke was studied by Astrom et al in a prospective fashion and reported to be 25% at the acute stage, 31% at 3 months, decreasing to 16% at 12 months, 19% at 2 years, and then increasing to 29% at 3 years.[6] The risk factor most often cited as important for the development of depression is lesion location, specifically the left anterior hemisphere.[6,47,62,86,87,88,89,91] This may be an important risk factor in the early post-stroke period with other factors, such as lack of social support and dependence in activities of daily living, playing the larger role at later time-points.[6] The need for identification and treatment of this problem should not be underestimated, since recovery from stroke may be significantly limited by concurrent depression. Parikh et al reported a disparity in the recovery of activities of daily living in depressed patients compared to nondepressed patients despite otherwise comparable clinical profiles during the acute hospitalization.[83] In their study, this disparity was present later in the patients course even though the depression had remitted. Depressed mood following stroke has also been linked to an increased risk of subsequent mortality.[72] Patients who are both depressed and socially isolated seem to be particularly vulnerable. The pharmacologic treatment of post-stroke depression has been successful with a variety of agents including tricyclic antidepressants,[33,63,59] methylphenidate,[59] and more recently with selective serotonin reuptake inhibitors.[5] The greater potential for side effects with tricyclic antidepressants would tend to favor the class of selective serotonin reuptake inhibitors as a first choice for treatment in this setting.[2,36] Another interesting observation in recent years has been the increased incidence of silent cerebral infarction detected with MRI or CT scans in patients with senile onset depression.[20,32,35,57] It has been suggested that silent cerebral infarction or high signal changes on MRI represent a risk factor for depression and may even be a direct cause of depression in the older population.

Another psychiatric complication of stroke, pathologic emotionalism, has not received as much attention. This problem typically begins within the first 4 to 6 weeks following stroke onset. It is characterized by the sudden onset of weepiness or laughter that cannot be easily controlled. Although it has been described as an emotional response inappropriate to the social situation, House et al found that the emotional outburst followed an appropriate emotional stimulus.[48] Provoking factors for pathologic crying were situations involving sadness and sentimentality, and provoking factors for pathologic laughter were amusing situations. The response, however, was out of proportion to the stimulus. Studies have focused on the location of lesions as the important variable in causation, but the areas implicated have varied widely. In the study by House et al,[48] lesions in the left frontal and temporal regions seemed to confer increased risk for this complication. They also noted that pathologic emotionalism could be associated with symptoms of a more general mood disturbance. Andersen et al studied patients with post-stroke pathological crying with MRI and concluded that damage to the serotonergic raphe nuclei of the brain stem or their ascending projections may be a key factor.[4] Successful approaches to treatment have included tricyclic antidepressants, levodopa, and selective serotonin reuptake inhibitors.[3,97,99,108]

Generalized anxiety disorder has also been described in the post-stroke period. Using DSM III criteria, various studies have estimated the frequency of this diagnosis at 3% to 11%.[17,48,71,100] In a study by Castillo et al, if patients with anxiety disorder also having a comorbid major or minor depression were included, a frequency of 27% in the early post-stroke period and 23% in the late post-stroke period was described. Three-fourths of the patients with anxiety disorder in this study also had major or minor depression. Early-onset anxiety was associated with a previous history of psychiatric disorder. The median duration was 3 months for those with late-onset and 1.5 months for those with early-onset anxiety disorder. They concluded that the presence of anxiety was significantly associated with depression.[18]

Acute confusional state or acute agitated delirium may occur as an acute presentation of stroke without any other localizing features. Symptoms and signs can include disorientation, extreme distractability, incoherent stream of thought, agitation, restlessness, and hyperactivity. This presentation is seen most often in patients with stroke in the right middle cerebral artery vascular territory.[16,70,98] The specific component of agitation is seen most frequently with inferior division right middle cerebral artery lesions with injury to the right temporal lobe.[16,70] Infarction in the posterior cerebral artery territory or rostral basilar artery syndome may also cause an acute confusional syndrome.[25,68] Unfortunately, recognition of the neurologic or vascular cause may be delayed due to the paucity of focal findings or the presence of only subtle focal neurologic deficits which are ignored or impossible to recognize because of the prominence of the confusional state.[68] These behavioral abnormalities have been attributed to psychiatric illness, drug intoxication, alcohol withdrawal, or infection, thus delaying diagnostic studies for stroke. Although resolution of the acute confusional state is common, a chronic confusional state after injuries of this type has been described.[70,74]

Nutritional Complications

Nutrition is a major concern in stroke patients who have disorders related to sensorium, altered thirst mechanisms, dysphagia, or aphasia, wherein body needs cannot be appreciated or expressed. In patients with altered sensorium, such as stupor and coma, assiduous attention must be given to hydration, electrolytes, and nutrition, and in difficult cases of long duration, the specialized training of nutritionists can be invaluable. Similarly, for dysphagia, speech therapists may be needed to guide appropriate planning for feeding, diet, and training. The varieties of dysphagia depend upon multiple factors that cannot be easily reduced to a few principles, such as difficulty with solids or liquids or both. However, in general, if the patient's stroke involves the swallowing mechanisms, such as impairment of the Xth cranial nerve, special precautions should be made to avoid aspiration by avoiding swallowing until adequate mechanisms are demonstrated. In those patients who have persistent dysphagia with the real fear of aspiration, either a nasogastric tube such as a Dobhof for a percutaneous gastrostomy should be used because the amount of caloric needs per day cannot be met by intravenous infusions alone.

For patients who have mild difficulty with slowness of swallowing, for example, use of pureed foods with frequent feeding and even using positions other than the upright position to avoid aspiration can be used along with self-administered suction to minimize saliva and food accumulation in the side and posterior portions of the mouth.

In one study assessing the effects of graded levels of intervention by dysphagia therapists on complications such as pneumonia, dehydration, calorie-nitrogen deficit, recurrent upper airway obstruction, and death following stroke, assessments were randomly made in 115 post-stroke subjects between the ages of 20 and 90 years.[23] These subjects had to have failed the Burke Dysphagia Screening Test, but were excluded with severe dysphagia as gauged by a modified barium swallow test when they would aspirate >50% of the various consistencies. These patients were randomly assigned to three graded levels of a therapist's intervention, including maneuvers used by the patient alone or with the help of family members, in controlling dietary consistency and in reinforcing compensatory swallowing techniques. In measuring the outcomes for these complications, no significant difference between the several treatment strategies was found. These findings suggest that while a dysphagia expert may initiate dysphagia training, patients and family members can adequately follow through with no increase in the occurrence of complications when handled by so-called experts. It should be pointed out, however, that initial instruction from dysphagia experts in training family members is critical in averting complications.[24]

The majority of stroke patients brought into the hospital after a period of time, such as a day, are generally dehydrated from not drinking fluids, and an assessment of the fluid balance should be made with intake and output, along with other indices of dehydration such as skin turgor, hemoconcentration, and urinary concentration. When uncertain, as in patients with depressed sensorium, intake and outputs should be complemented with regular body weights.

Under circumstances of massive strokes, particularly subarachnoid hemorrhage, the syndrome of inappropriate antidiuretic hormone (SIADH) secretion may occur, heralded by mental confusion and correlated with suppressed plasma sodium, usually below 120 mEq/L, although the rapidity of fall is crucial. The usual signs of SIADH should be associated with this diagnosis, which includes low plasma sodium with commensurate plasma hypo-osmolality, paradoxical urinary hyperosmolality, increased urinary secretion of sodium, normal renal and adrenal functions, and restoration of plasma

sodium with fluid restriction. In hyponatremic patients, it should be kept in mind that efforts to restore plasma sodium should proceed slowly at a rate of no more than 12 mEq/L/day. To quantify the total deficit of sodium, it is calculated by taking 70% of the body weight as body water and then multiplying the per liter deficit by the total body water. This total figure for the sodium deficit gives a rough guide for replacement. As a handy rule, if only one-half of that amount is given over the first 24 hours with frequent checks of the electrolytes and osmolality, the potential hazards of pontine and extra-pontine myelinolysis are minimized. Conversely, for the problem of hypernatremia, care must be taken to guard against it, especially in stuporous patients or those with impaired thirst mechanisms who cannot report those symptoms. Concentrations above 154 mEq/L can occur quickly under situations of increased body temperature and external heat when insensible perspiration is excessive. Use of diuretics or dehydrating agents, such as mannitol for cerebral edema, may quickly cause hypernatremia.

Occasionally, hyponatremia is not associated with volume expansion, and the natriuresis can be accounted by the unusual condition of "cerebral salt wasting." This condition has been controversial since many of the features simulate SIADH except for the lack of volume expansion. However, studies showing an increased release of atrial natriuretic peptide (ANP) from the brain, which expresses renin and aldosterone levels, suggest that it is indeed a specific, though rare disorder.[50]

Excretory Complications

Attention to the functions of excretion is as important as the other functions being discussed, again in those patients who are unable to express their needs or desires. Stroke patients with cerebral, brain stem, or spinal lesions are frequently incontinent of urine and feces because of a loss of voluntary control over sphincters or an inability to respond to sensations indicating a full bladder or rectum.[53] Brain stem and spinal cord lesions will, by interfering with both afferent and efferent pathways to the bladder and rectum, lead to either incontinence or retention.

For urinary retention, indwelling catheters should be reserved for the last, although dreaded urinary tract infections can now be treated and prevented more effectively than in the past. For the potential complications of hydronephrosis and hydroureters, constant indwelling catheterization may be necessary. For overflow or autonomous bladders, which account for persistent incontinence, condom catheters for men can be effective in avoiding skin maceration from frequent urination. Since women may experience skin maceration more readily from incontinence, catheterization is justified until bladder function is restored by normal or manual means.

Fecal incontinence can occur under conditions similar to urinary incontinence, and the use of diapers can prevent skin maceration and soiling. Diets high in fiber can reduce the degree of incontinence in patients with loose stools. Fecal impaction can be a serious problem if left untreated, and to avoid this problem, regularity is required with the use of enemas, laxatives, disimpactions, suppositories, and high-fiber diets.

Neuromuscular and Integument Complications

Although trained nursing and rehabilitation personnel are vigilant in avoiding complications related to immobility, daily attention to these areas must be paid since breakdown in management can result in skin sores, decubitus ulcers, and contractures that are difficult to correct once established. In addition to good daily skin care with cleansing and lubrication, movements of joints, both paralyzed and healthy, must be undertaken to avoid contractures, which can develop quickly.

In addition to these complications of immobility, stationary positions for long periods of time may result in venous stasis, venous thrombosis, and pulmonary emboli. To prevent this, use of stockings, pressurized cuffs, and subcutaneous heparin will help reduce the incidence of venous thrombosis. Since muscle tone and mass loss occur quickly, particularly in elderly subjects, both passive and active exercises must begin as soon as feasible following the stroke to maintain muscle tone and strength. Active turning of the paralyzed patient is important to optimize lung ventilation, since static postures can lead to stasis and the occurrence of atelectasis.

As a general rule, active physiotherapy and occupational therapy should begin as soon as possible after the stroke in order to optimize the recovery process. Implementation of these procedures has salutary effects on the patient's psyche as well.

Neurologic Complications

In a study of over 1,700 patients admitted to a medical intensive care unit, Bleck et al[9] found that medical and neurologic complications significantly added to the morbidity and mortality of patients. For example, metabolic encephalopathy, seizures, hypoxic-ischemic encephalopathy, and strokes were common complications that added significantly to morbidity, while sepsis was the commonest cause of encephalopathy, and strokes or seizures. These medical intensive-care data, similar to the experience of an acute stroke unit, emphasize the need to recognize both medical and neurologic complications, since their occurrence adds significantly to the patients' morbidity and mortality.

Because the chapter on neurointensive care will deal with major neurologic problems, this section will only briefly mention them. The major neurologic complications with strokes are seizures, increased intracranial pressure, stupor/coma, higher cortical function impairment, and dementia. Seizures of partial type may occur with any variety of strokes, from ischemic to hemorrhagic, and the onset may be either simultaneous with the stroke or sometime after.[55] The occurrence of seizures does not affect the long-term prognosis for the

stroke patient, and control of the seizures with anticonvulsants is generally excellent.[34] Electroencephalogran (EEG) findings with strokes may be those of periodic lateralized epileptiform discharges (PLEDs) or bilateral independent periodic transients (BIPLEDs), as well as nonperiodic spikes occurring singly or in bursts, sharp waves or sharp and slow waves contralateral to the stroke.[109]

Increased intracranial pressure due to brain edema may be a serious problem since it may lead to one of several herniation syndromes that can be the prelude to death. Although intracranial monitoring with either dural or intraventricular monitoring devices is the only means to measure accurately intracranial pressure, increasing lethargy, somnolence, stupor, and coma are good clinical indicators of a declining sensorium that may, following a stroke, indicate increased intracranial pressure. In addition, with substantial brain edema with midline shifts, particularly >1 cm, the patient will likely become stuporous or comatose.[93] Under these circumstances, measures to reduce intracranial pressure are indicated, such as the use of dehydrating agents, such as mannitol, or of hyperventilation. These measures are short-term, and evidence suggests that the chronic use of these measures may have counterproductive effects. For example, Kaufmann et al have shown in an experimental model of brain edema that repeated use of labeled mannitol resulted in increased brain edema with greater penetration of mannitol in the injured area.[52] Thus, the treating physician must realize that the patient receiving regular infusions of mannitol may, in fact, worsen and will therefore require careful neurologic evaluation. In addition, Muizelaar et al have reported on their studies of hyperventilation in head trauma patients, and found that those patients hyperventilated with a $PaCO_2$ of 25 ± 2 mmHg have a worse outcome than those not hyperventilated or those hyperventilated but treated with a buffering agent.[73] As with the use of dehydrating agents, the use of hyperventilation in stroke patients with increased intracranial pressure may have adverse effects not due to the stroke alone. The attending physician must be cognizant of the potential harm hyperventilation may have and be aware that it may result in a decline in neurological status.

Other Systemic Disorders

Other systemic problems such as fever, sepsis, hypercoagulable states, and impaired temperature regulation may supervene in stroke patients. As with the other medical and neurologic complications, diligent observation of the patient's status including vital signs, laboratory studies, and the neurologic examination should provide clues on the presence of supervening systemic complications. Although fever may be of central origin because of impaired diencephalic function, the burden of proof is on the need to exclude an infectious process. This is particularly important in stroke patients with impaired motor or respiratory functions, since their ability to handle the infection is further impaired.

On occasion, the presence of a hypercoagulable state is not immediately appreciated in cases of either arterial or venous occlusive diseases. When the cause of these cases is not apparent, more detailed investigations for cause is warranted to find a treatable cause, as discussed in the chapters dealing with these conditions. For example, investigations to exclude the antiphospholipid syndrome, presence of antithrombin III, reductions of protein C and S, resistance to protein C activation, and homocyst(e)inemia are warranted, as well as disseminated intravascular coagulation as a converse situation. These complications should be considered since they are treatable conditions.

Miscellaneous Issues

Hypertension in the setting of acute strokes presents several clinical dilemmas. First, in patients with neurologic deficits who display extremely elevated blood pressure (e.g., with diastolic blood pressures > 140 mmHg) the question of hypertensive encephalopathy must be considered.[110] This entity, described initially in 1927 by Fishberg and Oppenheimer,[51] typically presents with encephalopathic symptoms, such as seizures or mental confusion, plus excessive hypertension. Many stroke patients will present with both mental confusion and hypertension. As a result, hypertensive encephalopathy is frequently misdiagnosed. However, if strict clinical criteria are adhered to, the diagnosis can be made readily. First, the blood pressure must be excessively high with diastolic >140 mmHg

(except in pregnant women and children). Second, the CT scan of brain should not show any evidence of strokes. Third, the fundi will almost invariably show grade IV Keith-Wagner funduscopic changes of hypertension with edema, hemorrhage, and exudates. Fourth, patient's sensorium will improve with judicious reductions of blood pressure, i.e., a mean arterial blood pressure decrease of 10% to 15% with medications such as nitroprusside or labetalol. Certain drugs, such as reserpine or nimodipine, should be avoided since the blood pressure will drop precipitously and may cause watershed infarcts from severely reduced cerebral perfusion pressure in defectively autoregulated cerebral vessels.

Hypertension in acute strokes should not be treated unless to a modest degree of 10% to 15% reduction or if the patient has evidence of hypertensive encephalopathy.[12,27,39,49,112] One of the major reasons for not reducing blood pressure is to maintain necessary perfusion pressure of the cerebral circulation to ensure adequate tissue access to obligatory nutrients of oxygen and glucose. Strandgaard et al,[101] in their classic observation on cerebral blood flow in hypertensives, noted that these individuals lose homeostatic control when the mean arterial pressure is reduced to below approximately 125 mmHg. More recently, Hayashi et al[41] investigated stroke patients with increased intracranial pressure using intraventricular recording devices and found that hypotensive agents, such as calcium channel blockers, could produce a profound increase in intracranial pressure due to vasodilatation, while only a trivial reduction in systemic arterial pressure occurred. These studies confirm the long-feared complication of hypo-

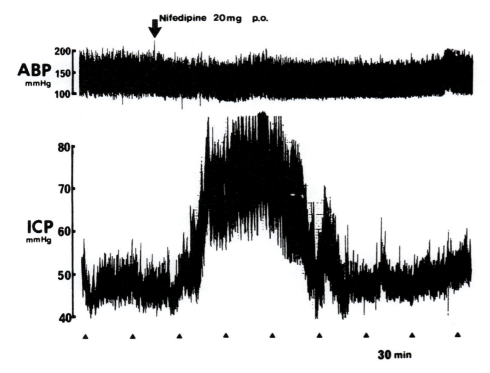

Figure 49.1 Arterial blood pressure (ABP) and intracranial pressure (ICP) after administration of 20 mg sublingual nifedipine. This subject had marked elevation of ICP>40 mmHg. Note that a trivial reduction of ABP is associated with a dramatic, nearly 30 mmHg, rise in intracranial pressure (ICP). (From Hayashi et al,[41] with permission.)

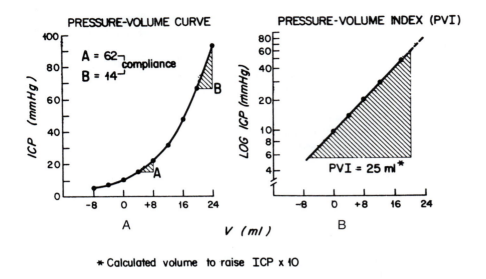

Figure 49.2 (**A**) Relationship between ICP and volume (V) in normal adults. With increases in ICP, small increments in volume (e.g., from edema or hemorrhage) cause progressively greater increases in ICP. For example, with ICP at "A" of 17 mmHg, a volume (V) increase of 4 ml results in an 8 mmHg rise in ICP while with an initial ICP at "B" of 70 mmHg, a similar volume (V) increase of 4 ml provokes a 27 mmHg rise in ICP. Thus, compliance, or the change in ICP for any given increase in volume, is lower at reduced ICPs, such as at "A," than at higher ones, such as at "B." (**B**) Semilogarithmic plot illustrating the pressure-volume index (PVI), the volume required to increase ICP by 1 log or 10 mmHg.[110]

tensive therapy in patients with strokes by compromising the perfusion pressure.[112] (See Figs. 49-1 and 49-2.)

It is a common occurrence with acute strokes that hypertension will be an accompaniment since the secretion of catecholamines will provoke hypertension. Because this response may be temporary to the body's response to stress, it has been argued that the elevated blood pressure is mobilized to ensure an adequate perfusion pressure. Perfusion pressure is defined as the difference between the mean arterial and mean venous (or cerebrospinal fluid [CSF]) pressures. The perfusion pressure should be maintained at >70 mmHg. Since the issues of whether hypertension in the acute stroke situation should be controlled or not is controversial, Lisk and colleagues assessed this issue in a prospective study.[64] They found that no treatment of moderately elevated hypertensive patients with ischemic strokes did as well as patients who had their blood pressures reduced modestly using various antihypertensive agents. As a result, it can be concluded that patients with acute ischemic strokes should not have their hypertensince sive blood pressures reduced unless a question of hypertensive encephalopathy exists. However, it is conceded that since additional bleeding may occur in patients showing intracerebral hemorrhages, provoked by sustained hypertension, the blood pressure can be reduced by 10% to 15%. Further drops in mean arterial pressure should be avoided because these chronically hypertensive patients have their autoregulation of blood flow regulated at a higher level than normal. As a result, a mean arterial pressure of 110 mmHg may be below the level of autoregulation, which results in the blood flow paralleling the blood pressure.

Although the issue of treating hypertension in the acute phases of stroke remains problematic, in the chronic phase beyond the first weeks following a stroke, the hypertensive patient should be treated to normalize the blood pressure to minimize the chances of stroke recurrence. In fact, at this time, every effort should be made to minimize or control all risk factors for stroke related to atherosclerosis. These include control of hypertension (the most important risk factor for strokes), smoking, diabetes mellitus, and elevated lipids, plus others such as obesity, stress, and sedentary life. In a study of 662 stroke patients with a first stroke, the effect of hypertension was evaluated on stroke recurrence.[101] Of this group of stroke patients, nearly 60% had hypertension and 81 of these patients had a second stroke, which was significantly higher than those without hypertension. Diastolic hypertension appeared to be a greater risk, although the importance of either diastolic or systolic hypertension or both varies with individual studies. Of patients with an initial diastolic blood pressure of >95 mmHg, 43% had stroke recurrences by the end of the study compared to 19% below this level, a statistically significant difference. Furthermore, diastolic blood pressure control correlated with a parallel reduction in stroke occurrence. Thus, this study again reinforces the old adage that hypertension control after the acute stroke episode is crucial in minimizing stroke recurrence.

Another factor not frequently discussed is the relative costs related to strokes, both for the patients and their insurance coverages. For example, in patients with lethal strokes in which the chances of recovery are nil, requesting various consultations may be fruitless, since death is inevitable and the various tests and consults only burden the patient's costs. Similar decisions must be considered with various forms of drug treatments, preferably in collaboration with patients and their families. An example of this is the use of antiplatelet drugs to prevent stroke recurrences. Although aspirin is effective and less expensive than ticlopidine, the latter may be more effective though more costly. The question is whether the added cost burden to the patient and expected improved outcome justify the expenditure. While costs for the optimum treatment of stroke should not be considered if maximized outcome is the result, the reality is that cost is a factor to consider, especially for elderly individuals on fixed retirement income, such as Social Security alone. In an effort to develop modeling strategies to predict the outcome of this dilemma, a hypothetical cohort of 100 patients at risk for stroke over the age of 65 was developed.[82] The group was randomly assigned to receive ticlopidine (500 mg daily) or aspirin (1,300 mg daily). From published data, they estimated the incidence of strokes, life expectancy, and lifetime medical care costs associated with each therapy. In their model, two fewer strokes per hundred would occur with ticlopidine than those receiving aspirin, and this difference is concluded to be cost-effective for both the financial costs as well as quality-of-life issues. Although hypothetical modeling may mimic real life, the reality for many fixed-income stroke victims receiving Social Security is that they simply cannot afford to expend their limited resources on more expensive medication. Under those circumstances, the treating physician and the patients would likely opt for the practical choice. On the other hand, with patients for whom cost is not a factor, using more expensive interventions and drugs is a luxury unencumbered by cost constraints.

A similar consideration should be given to patients and the use of rehabilitative services, especially if potential recovery is borderline or nil and if, again, the issue of draining their own resources becomes an issue. Although Medicare will cover short-term rehabilitation, prolonged physiotherapy, which can become costly, becomes an issue. Fortunately, in some cases, patients and their families can frequently rise to the occasion and provide daily care, which they have learned from physiotherapists to enhance recovery of stroke victims.[65] While the use of family members should be optimal, in many cases it is not, but when costs for the family become a burden, the physician must play a role in concert with the physiatrists to teach family members the needed exercises. In the final analysis, it is usually family members that can truly provide the encouragement and motivation for patients to continue their daily routine of exercises. It should be pointed out that during the rehabilitation phase, the family, patient, and treating physician must be cognizant of the medical complications that can supervene, as are addressed in this chapter.[94]

The medical complications noted above can, in fact, be a cause of severe morbidity during rehabilitation as it is during the acute strokes and therefore recapitulates the patients' problems. This is dramatized in a study of medical and neurologic complications during rehabilitation in a group of 100 stroke patients receiving rehabilitation. In a review of 100 such patients, Dromerick and Reding[30] analyzed the medical complications. These included urinary tract infection (44 cases), depression (33), musculoskeletal pain (31), urinary retention (25), falls (25), fungal dermatitis (24), hypotension (19), diabetes mellitus (16), hypertension (15), and other neu-

romedical problems (194). The mean ± SD numbers of medical and neurologic complications per patient were 3.6 ± 2 and 0.6 ± 0.8, respectively. Complications were independent of the severity of strokes and the duration in the rehabilitation hospital stay. Although cardiac impairment correlated with cardiac complications, the patients' age, sex, or type of stroke were not related to the complication rate. Thus, while it might be concluded that the stroke patient is relatively free of medical complications following the acute period and going into rehabilitation, this is not the case for these largely medically compromised patients. These findings reinforce the need to be vigilant with these stroke patients throughout the recovery period.

References

1. Alter M, Friday G, Lai SM et al: Hypertension and risk of stroke recurrence. Stroke 25:1605, 1994
2. Agerholm M: Side effects of nortriptyline treatment for post-stroke depression (letter). Lancet 1:519, 1984
3. Andersen G, Vestergaard K, Riis JO: Citaloparm for post-stroke pathological crying. Lancet 342:837, 1993
4. Andersen G, Ingeman-Nielsen M, Vestergaard K et al: Pathoanatomic correlation between poststroke pathological crying and damage to brain areas involved in serotonergic neurotransmission. Stroke 25:1050, 1994
5. Andersen G, Vestergaard K, Lauritzen L: Effective treatment of poststroke depression with the selective serotonin reuptake inhibitor citalopram. Stroke 25:1099, 1994
6. Astrom M, Adolfsson R, Asplund K: Major depression in stroke patients: a 3-year longitudinal study. Stroke 24: 976, 1993
7. Bamford J, Dennis M, Sandercock P et al: The frequency, cause and timing of death within 30 days of a stroke: the Oxfordshire Community Stroke Project. J Neurol Neurosurg Psych 53:824, 1990
8. Barnett HJ: Heart in ischemic stroke—a changing emphasis. Neurol Clin 1:291, 1983
9. Bleck TP, Smith MC, Pierre-Louis SJ, et al: Neurologic complications of critical medical illnesses. Crit Care Med 21:98, 1993
10. Boucher CA, Brewster DC, Darling RC et al: Determination of cardiac risk by dipyridamole-thallium imaging before peripheral vascular surgery. N Eng J Med 94: 312, 1985
11. Breuer AC, Furlan AJ, Hanson MR et al: Central nervous system complications of coronary artery bypass graft surgery: prospective analysis of 421 patients. Stroke 14:682, 1983
12. Brott T, Reed RL: Intensive care for acute stroke in the community hospital setting. The first 24 hours. Stroke 20:694, 1989
13. Burch GE, Meyers R, Abildskov JA: A new electrocardiographic pattern observed in cerebrovascular accidents. Circulation 9:719, 1954
14. Byer E, Ashman R, Toth LA: Electrocardiogram with

large, upright T-waves and long Q-T intervals. Am Heart J 33:796, 1947

15. Canadian Cooperative Study Group: A randomized trial of aspirin and sulfinpyrazone in threatened stroke. N Eng J Med 299:53, 1978

16. Caplan LR, Kelly CS, Hier DB et al: Infarcts of the inferior division of the right middle cerebral artery: mirror image of Wernicke's aphasia. Neurology 36:1015, 1986

17. Castillo CS, Starkstein SE, Fedoroff JP et al: Generalized anxiety disorder after stroke. J Nerv Ment Dis 181: 100, 1993

18. Castillo CS, Schultz SK, Robinson RG: Clinical correlates of early-onset and late-onset poststroke generalized anxiety. Am J Psychiatry 152:1174, 1995

19. Clagget GP, Anderson F Jr, Levine MN et al: Prevention of venous thromboembolism. Chest 102:3915, 1992

20. Coffey CE, Figiel GS, Djang WT et al: Subcortical hyperintensity on magnetic resonance imaging: a comparison of normal and depressed elderly subjects. Am J Psychiatry 147:187, 1990

21. Cunha BA, Gingrich D, Rosenbaum GS et al: Pneumonia syndromes: a clinical approach in the elderly. Geriatrics 45:49, 1990

22. Davis TP, Alexander J, Lesch M: Electrocardiographic changes associated with acute cerebrovascular disease: A clinical review. Prog Cardiovas Dis 36:245, 1993

23. DePippo KL, Holas MA, Reding MJ et al: Dysphagia therapy following stroke: a controlled trial. Neurology 44:1655, 1994

24. DePippo KL, Holas MA, Reding MJ: Validation of the 3 oz. water swallow test for aspiration following stroke. Arch Neurol 49:1259, 1992

25. Devinsky O, Bear D, Volpe BT: Confusional states following posterior cerebral artery infarction. Arch Neurol 45:160, 1988

26. Dimant J, Grog D: Electrocardiographic changes and myocardial damage in patients with acute cerebrovascular accidents. Stroke 8:448, 1977

27. Dinsdale HB: Hypertensive encephalopathy. Neurol Clin 1:3, 1983

28. DiPasquale GD, Andreoli A, Pinelli G et al: Cerebral ischemia and symptomatic coronary heart disease: a prospective study of 83 patients. Stroke 17:1098, 1986

29. Drislane FW, Samuels MA: How cardiorespiratory problems are caused by neurologic disease. J Respir Dis 9: 31, 1988

30. Dromerick A, Reding M: Medical and neurological complications during inpatient stroke rehabilitation. Stroke 25:358, 1994

31. Eisenberg S, Madison L, Sensenbach W: Cerebral hemodynamic and metabolic studies in patients with congestive failure. Circulation 21:704, 1960

32. Figiel GS, Krishnan KRR, Doraiswamy PM et al: Subcortical hyperintensities on brain magnetic resonance imaging: a comparison between late age onset and early onset elderly depressed subjects. Neurobiol Aging 26: 245, 1991

33. Finklestein SP, Weintraub RJ, Karmouz N et al: Antidepressant drug treatment for poststroke depression: retrospective study. Arch Phys Med Rehabil 68:772, 1987

34. Fish DR, Miller DH, Roberts RC et al: The natural history of late-onset epilepsy secondary to vascular disease. Acta Neurol Scand 80:524, 1989

35. Fujikawa T, Yamawaki S, Touhouda Y: Incidence of silent cerebral infarction in patients with major depression. Stroke 24:1631, 1993

36. Fullerton AG: Side-effects of nortriptyline treatment for post-stroke depression (letter). Lancet 1:519, 1984

37. Goldner JC, Whisnant JP, Taylor WF: Long term prognosis of transient cerebral ischemic attacks. Trans Am Neurol Ass 94:20, 1969

38. Goldstein D: The electrocardiogram in stroke with relationship to pathophysiological type and comparison with prior tracings. Stroke 10:253, 1979

39. Graham DI: Ischemic brain damage following emergency blood pressure lowering in hypertensive patients. Acta Med Scand (Suppl) 678:61, 1982

40. Greenhoot JH, Reichenbach DD: Cardiac injury and subarachnoid hemorrhage: a clinical pathological and physiological correlation. J Neurosurg 30:521, 1969

41. Hayashi M et al: Treatment of systemic hypertension and intracranial hypertension in cases of brain hemorrhage. Stroke 19:314, 1988

42. Hertzer NR, Young JR, Beven EG et al: Coronary angiography in 506 patients with extracranial cerebrovascular disease. Arch Intern Med 145:849, 1985

43. Holas MA, DePippo KL, Reding MJ: Aspiration and relative risk of medical complications following stroke. Arch Neurol 51:1051, 1994

44. Horner J, Buoyer FG, Alberts M et al: Dysphagia following brainstem stroke: clinical correlates and outcome. Arch Neurol 48:1170, 1991

45. Horner J, Massey EW, Riski JE et al: Aspiration following stroke: clinical correlates and outcome. Neurol 38: 1359, 1988

46. House A, Dennis M, Mogridge L et al: Mood disorder in the year after stroke. Br J Psychiatry 158:83, 1991

47. House A, Dennis M, Warlow C et al: Mood disorders after stroke and their relation to lesion location: a CT scan study. Brain 113:1113, 1990

48. House A, Martin D, Molyneux A et al: Emotionalism after stroke. BMJ 298:991, 1989

49. Hund E, Grau A, Hacke W: Neurocritical care for acute ischemic stroke. Neurol Clin 13:511, 1995

50. Ishikawa SE, Saito T, Kaneko K et al: Hyponatremia responsive to fludrocortisone acetate in elderly patients after head injury. Ann Intern Med 106:187, 1987

51. Kannel WB, Wolf PA: Manifestations of coronary disease predisposing to stroke: the Framingham Study. JAMA 250:2942, 1983

52. Kaufmann AM, Cardosa ER: Aggravation of vasogenic cerebral edema by multiple dose mannitol. J Neurosurg 77:584, 1992

53. Kendall AR, Karafin I: Classification of neurogenic bladder disease. Urol Clin North Am 1:37, 1974

54. Kidd D, Lawson J, Nesbitt R et al: Aspiration in acute stroke: a clinical study with videofluoroscopy. Quarterly J Medicine 86:825, 1993

55. Kilpatrick CJ, Davis SM, Tress BM et al: Epileptic seizures in acute stroke. Arch Neurol 47:157, 1990

56. Kolin A, Norris JW: Myocardial damage from acute cerebral lesions. Stroke 15:990, 1984

57. Krishnan KKR, Goli V, Ellinwood EH et al: Leuko-encephalopathy in patients diagnosed as major depressive. Biol Psychiatry 23:519, 1988

58. Lacy PS, Earle AM: Central neural control of blood pressure and cardiac arrhythmias during subarachnoid hemorrhage in rats. Stroke 16:998, 1985

59. Lazarus LW, Moberg PJ, Langsley PR et al: Methylphenidate and nortriptyline in the treatment of poststroke depression: a retrospective comparison. Arch Phys Med Rehabil 75:403, 1994

60. Levy S, Yaar I, Melamed E et al: The effect of acute stroke on cardiac functions as observed in an intensive care unit. Stroke 5:775, 1974

61. Lin HJ, Wolf PA, Benjamin EJ et al: Newly diagnosed atrial fibrillation and acute stroke. The Framingham Study. Stroke 26:1527, 1995

62. Lipsey JR, Robinson RG, Pearlson GD et al: Mood change following bilateral hemisphere brain injury. Br J Psychiatry 143:266, 1983

63. Lipsey JR, Robinson RG, Pearlson GD et al: Nortriptyline treatment of post-stroke depression: a double-blind study. Lancet 1:297, 1984

64. Lisk DR, Grotta JC, Lamki LM et al: Should hypertension be treated after acute stroke? A randomized controlled trial using single photon emissions computed tomography. Arch Neurol 50:855, 1993

65. Lorish TR, Sandin KJ, Roth EJ et al: Stroke rehabilitation. 3. Rehabilitation evaluation and management. Arch Phys Med Rehabil 75:S47, 1994

66. McCarthy ST, Turner JJ, Robertson D et al: Low dose heparin as a prophylaxis against deep venous thrombosis after acute stroke. Lancet 2:800, 1977

67. McMahon SM, Heyman A: The mechanics of breathing and stabilization of ventilation in patients with unilateral cerebral infarction. Stroke 5:518, 1974

68. Mehler MF: Reversible rostral basilar artery syndrome. Arch Intern Med 148:166, 1988

69. Mikel HS, Yashes NV, Kempski O et al: Breathing 100% oxygen after global brain ischemia in Mongolian gerbils results in increased lipid peroxidation and increased mortality. Stroke 18:426, 1987

70. Mori E, Yamadori A: Acute confusional state and acute agitated delirium: occurrence after infarction in the right middle cerebral artery territory. Arch Neurol 44:1139, 1987

71. Morris PL, Robinson RG, Raphael B: Prevalence and course of depressive disorders in hospitalized stroke patients. Int J Psychiatry Med 20:349, 1990

72. Morris PLP, Robinson RG, Andrzejewski P et al: Association of depression with 10-year poststroke mortality. Am J Psychiatry 150:124, 1993

73. Muizelaar JP, Marmarou A, Ward JD et al: Adverse effects of prolonged hyperventilation in patients with severe head injury: a randomized clinical trial. J Neurosurg 75:731, 1991

74. Mullally WJ, Huff K, Ronthal M et al: Chronic confusional state with right middle cerebral artery occlusion. Ann Neurol 32:A96, 1982

75. Muuronen A, Kaste M: Outcome of 314 patients with transient ischemic attacks. Stroke 13:24, 1982

76. Myers MG, Norris JW, Hachinski VC et al: Plasma norepinephrine in stroke. Stroke 12:200, 1981

77. Myers MG, Norris JW, Hachinski VC et al: Cardiac sequelae of acute stroke. Stroke 13:838, 1982

78. Norris JW: Effects of cerebrovascular lesions on the heart. Neurol Clin 1:87, 1983

79. Norris JW, Froggart GM, Hachinski VC: Cardiac arrhythmias in acute stroke. Stroke 9:392, 1978

80. Norris JW, Hachinski VC, Myers MG et al: Serum cardiac enzymes in stroke. Stroke 10:548, 1979

81. Oppenheimer BS, Fishberg AM: Hypertensive encephalopathy. Arch Int Med 41:264, 1928

82. Oster G, Huse DM, Lacey MJ et al: Cost-effectiveness of ticlopidine in preventing stroke in high-risk. Stroke 25:1149, 1994

83. Parikh RM, Robinson RG, Lipsey JR et al: The impact of poststroke depression on recovery in activities of daily living over a 2-year follow-up. Arch Neurol 47:785, 1990

84. Rem JA, Hachinski VC, Boughner DR et al: Value of cardiac monitoring and echocardiography in TIA and stroke patients. Stroke 16:950, 1985

85. Robin ED, Whaley RD, Crump CH et al: Alveolar gas tensions, pulmonary ventilation and blood pH during physiologic sleep in normal subjects. J Clin Invest 37:981, 1958

86. Robinson RG: Depression in aphasic patients: frequency, severity, and clinicopathological correlations. Brain Lang 14:282, 1981

87. Robinson RG, Price TR: Post-stroke depressive disorders: a follow-up study of 103 outpatients. Stroke 13:635, 1982

88. Robinson RG, Szetela B: Mood change following left hemisphere brain injury. Ann Neurol 9:447, 1981

89. Robinson RG, Kubos KL, Starr LB et al: Mood changes in stroke patients: relationship to lesion location. Compr Psychiatry 24:555, 1983

90. Robinson RG, Starr LB, Kubos KL et al: A two-year longitudinal study of post-stroke mood disorders: findings during the initial evaluation. Stroke 14:736, 1983

91. Robinson RG, Kubos KL, Starr LB et al: Mood disorders in stroke; importance of location of lesion. Brain 107:81, 1984

92. Rockoff MA, Kennedy SK: Physiology and clinical aspects of raised intracranial pressure. p. 7. In Ropper AH, Kennedy S, Zervas NT (eds): Neurological and Neurosurgical Intensive Care. University Park Press, Baltimore, 1983

93. Ropper AH: Lateral displacement of the brain and level of consciousness in patients with an acute hemispheral mass. N Eng J Med 314:953, 1986

94. Roth EJ, Noll SF: Stroke rehabilitation. 2. Comorbidities and complications. Arch Phys Med Rehabil 75:S42, 1994

95. Samules MA: Neurogenic heart disease: a unifying hypothesis. Am J Cardiol 60:15J, 1987

96. Sandercock P, for the International Stroke Trial Collaborative Group: IST: Preliminary results: Part I: Effects of aspirin and heparin separately and in combination. Cerebrovasc Dis 6:23, 1996

97. Schiffer R, Herndon R, Rudick R. Treatment of patho-

logic laughing and weeping with amitriptyline. N Engl J Med 312:1480, 1985

98. Schmidley JW, Messing RO: Agitated confusional states in patients with right hemispheric infarctions. Stroke 5:883, 1984

99. Sloan RL, Brown KW, Pentland B: Fluoxetine as a treatment for emotional lability after brain injury. Brain Inj 6:315, 1992

100. Starkstein SE, Cohen BS, Fedoroff P et al: Relationship between anxiety disorders and depressive disorders in patients with cerebrovascular injury. Arch Gen Psychiatry 47:246, 1990

101. Strangaard S, Olesen J, Skinhoj E et al: Autoregulation of brain circulation in severe arterial hypertension. Br Med J 1:507, 1973

102. Theodore J, Robin ED: Pathogenesis of neurogenic pulmonary oedema. Lancet 2:749, 1975

103. Timaris PS: Aging of respiration p. 303. In Timaris PS (ed): Physiological Basis of Geriatrics. Macmillan Publishing Co., New York/London, 1988

104. Toole JR, Yuson CP, Janeway R et al: Transient ischemic attacks: a prospective study of 225 patients. Neurology 28:746, 1978

105. Touho H, Karasawa J, Shishido H et al: Neurogenic pulmonary edema in the acute stage of hemorrhagic cerebrovascular disease. Neurosurgery 25:762, 1989

106. Turpie AG, Levine MN, Hirsh J et al: Double-blind randomized trial of ORG 10172 low-molecular-weight heparinoid in prevention of deep vein thrombosis in thrombotic stroke. Lancet 1:523, 1987

107. Turpie AG, Gent M, Cote R et al: A low-molecular-weight heparinoid compared with unfractionated heparin in the prevention of deep vein thrombosis in patients with acute ischemic stroke. Ann Intern Med 117:353, 1992

108. Udaka F, Yamao S, Nagata H et al: Pathologic laughing and crying treated with levodopa. Arch Neurol 41:1095, 1984

109. Verma NP, Kooi KA: Contralateral epileptiform transients in stroke (CETS). Epilepsia 27:437, 1986

110. Wechsler LR, Ropper AH: Management of stroke in the intensive care unit. Semin Neurol 6:324, 1986

111. Wolf PA, Kannel WB, McGee DL et al: Duration of atrial fibrillation and imminence of stroke: the Framingham Study. Stroke 14:664, 1983

112. Yatsu FM, Zivin J: Hypertension in acute ischemic stroke: not to treat. Arch Neurol 42:999, 1985

CHAPTER 50

The Intensive Care of the Stroke Patient

DERK KRIEGER

WERNER HACKE

The role of neurocritical care medicine in stroke management is threefold: (1) to treat and monitor patients undergoing invasive treatments that are aimed at reversing or ameliorating neurologic deficits, such as thrombolytic therapy and neuroprotective strategies; (2) to provide special interventions directed toward complications of stroke, such as elevated intracranial pressure and seizures; and (3) to provide an appropriate environment for the care of obtunded patients with insecure airways and to carefully monitor and control blood pressure. Beneficial management of acute strokes requires timely coordination of the prehospital phase and emergency assessment, as well as treatment and proficient monitoring and follow-up. Only measures initiated shortly after onset of stroke permit a halt to the progression of brain tissue damage and improve outcome. Success of any therapy will depend greatly on early intervention, but also on the rapid recognition and referral of these patients to institutions offering adequate diagnostic and therapeutic expertise. In this chapter current trends and emerging therapies for neurocritical care of patients with cerebral ischemia will be reviewed.

Emergency Assessment of Severe Stroke Patients

Stroke treatment begins with evaluation of the vital signs that mandate supportive care. After the stroke patient has been medically stabilized with regards to airway, breathing, and circulation, a focused history is taken with special emphasis on vascular risk factors and information that helps to identify potential caveats, including seizures, migraine, drug abuse, or concomitant medical illnesses. The initial management of a stroke patient should focus on airway assessment, conscientious control of blood pressure, and standardized neurologic examination, for example, by using the National Institute of Health Stroke Scale. The initial evaluation includes observa-

tion of breathing pattern and function, determination of blood pressure and heart rate, and assessment of arterial O_2 saturation using pulse oximetry. Simultaneously, blood samples for clinical chemistry, coagulation, and hematology studies are drawn, and a venous line (preferably central) inserted. Standard electrolyte solutions are given until clinical chemistry results are received.

ANCILLARY TESTS AND EARLY NEURORADIOLOGIC EVALUATION

Expedited diagnostic procedures include electrocardiogram (ECG) and laboratory values, including blood chemistry, hematologic and coagulation studies, and urine analysis. Furthermore, neurodiagnostic procedures, including computed tomography (CT), Doppler sonography, and angiography should be available on an emergency basis. CT scanning of the head rapidly excludes hemorrhagic strokes and may identify size and type of stroke. Currently, thrombolytic therapy is not recommended if CT demonstrates early changes of a recent major infarction such as sulcal effacement, mass effect, edema, or possible hemorrhage patients[2] or with initial CT parenchymal hypodensity exceeding one-third of the middle cerebral artery territory.[63] Patients with CT hypodensities exceeding one-half of the middle cerebral artery territory are at significant risk for fatal "malignant" brain edema.[65,93] These thresholds are somewhat arbitrary and may be modified or replaced. In the setting of an acute ischemic stroke it is desirable to establish a vascular diagnosis. Utilization of modern CT techniques such as spiral CT scanning allows for rapid and reliable demonstration of the site and size of a presumed arterial occlusion and state of the collaterals.[134,179] Other current techniques with potential impact on early therapy in acute stroke include transcranial Doppler sonography[96,142] single-photon emission CT,[5] and perfusion and diffusion MRI.[174,175] Patients presenting with large hemispheric strokes and poor collateral blood flow are particularly prone to symptomatic hemorrhagic transformation,[53] and may need to be excluded from systemic thrombolytic therapy. Additionally, demonstration and localization of the vascular lesion may alter therapeutic decisions, such as in the case of a progressive brain stem stroke due to basilar occlusion that requires local intra-arterial rather than IV thrombolysis. Doppler sonography of the internal carotid and vertebral arteries and intracranial vasculature detects occlusions and high-grade stenoses with acceptable reliability and may guide fluid management, institution of anticoagulants, and blood pressure control.[64,95,132,184]

Despite other techniques, selective angiography of the cervical and intracranial vasculature remains the gold standard for the demonstration of arterial stenosis or occlusion. Today, intra-arterial catheter techniques, using digital subtraction angiography (DSA), requiring only small boluses of contrast media, are relatively safe even in the acute stroke setting and can be performed easily. Currently, we consider intra-arterial DSA in all clinically deteriorating patients with cerebrovascular emergencies suitable for endovascular therapy, including basilar occlusion,[66,186,187,189] severe vasospasm after SAH,[75] and intracranial internal carotid artery bifurcation (carotid "T").[80]

Rapidly evolving magnetic resonance tomography (MRT) techniques, such as diffusion-weighted imaging, may identify ischemic tissue as early as 30 minutes after stroke onset and may distinguish between ischemic penumbra and irreversible ischemic brain injury.[15,106–108,175] Perfusion- and diffusion-weighted magnetic resonance imaging (MRI) may also indicate compromise of arterial blood flow prior to initiating potential risky revascularization procedures.[92,136] Routine T_1-weighted MRI sequences may confirm recent arterial dissections in patients with cerebral embolism, demonstrating vessel wall hematoma in the subacute stage. Nuclear magnetic resonance (NMR) spectroscopy allows in vivo quantitation of changing chemical moieties in infarcted brain tissue, including adenosine triphosphate, lactate, and N-acetyl aspartate[49,59]; however, specificity and sensitivity in cerebral ischemia are as yet unexplored. Currently, advanced magnetic resonance (MR) techniques are predominantly used as research instruments because they require excessive time, are in particular susceptible to movement artifacts, and are not readily available for routine use in noncompliant patients in emergency department settings. It is conceivable that rapid development of MR technology will overcome these shortcomings in the near future.

Positron emission tomography (PET) is an established modality to assess brain perfusion and metabolism in stroke patients and to demonstrate a characteristic temporal pattern of changes in evolving cerebral infarction.[14,129] Determinations of cerebral blood flow (CBF), cerebral blood volume (CBV), and cerebral metabolic rate ($CMRO_2$) demonstrate the efficacy of various compensatory mechanisms in occlusive cerebrovascular disease and may discriminate salvageable ischemic areas from irreversible tissue damage in cerebral ischemia.

PET and diffusion/perfusion-weighted MRI data confirm that brain tissue in human stroke is frequently recruited into the volume of infarct over many hours. There is likely considerable variation between individuals and considerable variation between brain regions in a single individual, indicating that the choice of any particular fixed time window of treatment may be too long for some and too short for others. At present, only single photon emission cerebral tomography (SPECT) is readily available in most institutions and can be widely utilized to assess acute stroke patients. Although it can only assess brain perfusion, SPECT depicts the area of ischemia with accuracy and improves the prognostic value of early clinical assessment.[5,6] Demonstration of large perfusion defects in stroke patients increases the likelihood of hemorrhagic complications or massive brain edema formation and thus may alter therapeutic decisions.[102] Therefore, SPECT is potentially useful for selecting or stratifying patients in clinical therapeutic trials.[5,6,67]

ENSURING BEST POSSIBLE QUALITY OF THE ANCILLARY TESTS

As a rule, diagnostic tests must be performed without undue delay and with the *best possible* quality. If no skilled neurosonologist is present in the emergency department, initiation of specific treatment should not be postponed but an alternate diagnostic procedure, such as angiography, may be initiated. Many patients with acute strokes are uncooperative and restless. As a consequence, neuroimaging tests may be artifactual and of low quality. Therefore, it may be appropriate to use short-acting sedative drugs in order to get the best possible test results. Sometimes it may even become necessary to perform an angiogram with general anesthesia to obtain results of appropriate quality. Consequently, in patients who require intubation, sedation, and mechanical ventilation, clinical monitoring may be significantly impaired. Decisions for intubation to undertake a diagnostic test should be made very carefully and only if immediate therapeutic interventions can evolve from the result of the diagnostic test.

Patients with severe strokes who eventually will be admitted to an intensive care unit (ICU) should be continuously accompanied by a physician while diagnostic tests are performed. These patients need supplemental oxygen via a nasal cannula, placement of a Foley catheter, and a nasogastric tube to lessen the chance of aspiration. In the case of swallowing disturbances, frequent oral suctioning is needed. A venous line, preferably a central venous line, should be inserted. Frequent assessment of consciousness and motor impairment allows for early recognition of improvement or deterioration of the clinical state. If for whatever reason a time delay during the diagnostic sequence is foreseen, the patient should be admitted to the ICU for close monitoring in the meantime.

If sedation is required for diagnostic procedures, IV diazepam (5 to 10 mg), midazolam (1 to 5 mg), or repeated doses of propofol (10 to 20 mg) are preferred. During CT- and MRI-scanning, ECG monitoring and, if available, pulse oximetry should be attained. Additionally, video monitoring is available in most MRI units. During neuroimaging procedures a physician should be nearby the angiography suite or in the scanner room at all times. If the patient needs to be intubated, IV anesthesia should be reversed on arrival at the ICU. We recommend IV flumazenil 0.2 mg in repeated doses up to 1 mg within 5 minutes and IV naloxone 0.4 mg up to 5 to 10 mg.

Other Technical Appliances for Intensive Care Stroke Management

INTRACRANIAL PRESSURE MONITORING

Intracranial pressure (ICP) monitoring may provide data for rational treatment of elevated ICP. The discussion of the variety of types of ICP-monitoring devices available is beyond the scope of this chapter. The main categories of ICP measurement include epidural, subdural, intraparenchymal, and intraventricular methods. ICP can be determined via fluid-coupled (ventricular drain) or nonfluid coupled systems (pneumatic devices, fiberoptic strain gauge). Although each method has merits, familiarity on the part of the physician and nursing staff is probably most important for safe and dependable ICP monitoring. Besides unreliable measurements, technical pitfalls include ICP drifting, inadequate implantation, and infectious complications.[149] The overall risk for surgical trauma and hemorrhage varies between 0.3% and 1%, for infection up to 5% in particular with ventricular catheter.[11]

Clear guidelines for instituting ICP monitoring in large hemispheric strokes have not been established. These infarcts are often associated with a decreased level of consciousness and neurologic deterioration within the first few days after onset.[65] CT scans reveal variable degrees of tissue shifts secondary to edema within and adjacent to the infarct. As the edema progresses, the resulting local and hemispheric swelling shifts the midline structures (horizontal shift) and later the medial aspects of the temporal lobe (vertical shift). Eventually, the additional volume of edematous brain cannot be accommodated in the cranial vault without elevating ICP. Therefore, consequences of brain tissue shifts and elevated ICP may both be responsible for neurologic decline. Tissue shifts and their effects have been studied in experimental models.[116,117] Locally increased ICP secondary to mass lesions is compensated up to a point by displacement of cerebrospinal fluid (CSF) and blood without increasing ICP globally. Once that critical point is reached, the global ICP rises dramatically with any increase of mass within the brain. Additionally, hydrocephalus resulting from obstruction of CSF outflow tracts may aggravate cerebral ischemia, resulting in more mass effect in a self-perpetuating cycle.

Although measuring and controlling ICP have not been shown conclusively to change outcome, there is a clear rationale for their use. The presence of elevated ICP is an important prognostic indicator. The Heidelberg group studied 48 patients with hemispheric infarctions that underwent medical ICP management.[150] All ICP sensors were placed on the affected side, in 7 patients on both sides. ICP sensors were placed between day 2 and 3 after stroke onset. Of the 48 patients, 37 had opening pressures of less than 25 mmHg, 8 below 35 mmHg, and only 3 above 35 mmHg. Maximum ICP values during the observation period were able to distinguish between survivors and nonsurvivors. The difference of ICP values in patients undergoing bilateral monitoring ranged between 5 and 15 mmHg with consistently higher values on the affected side. Interestingly, the degree of midline shift as determined by CT was associated neither with outcome nor with concurrent ICP values. Actually, midline shift and ventricular compression preceded the elevation of ICP by hours, sometimes days. There is a close correlation between displacement of the pineal gland from the midline and level of consciousness: 4 to 6 mm is associated with drowsiness, 6 to 8 mm with stupor, and >8.5 mm with coma.[144] ICP monitoring should be considered in (1) patients with deteriorating level of consciousness secondary to edema formation in massive hemispheric stroke; (2) patients with a reasonable chance of recovery as inferred from age and comorbid factors; and (3) with the intention on the part of the physician and the family to use ICP data to initiate alternative therapeutic modalities, such as hemicraniectomy or institution of hypothermia, if standard medical therapy fails.

NEUROPHYSIOLOGIC ASSESSMENT

The main goals of neurophysiologic monitoring techniques are to evaluate CNS function in unresponsive patients and forecast neurologic deficit.[18,27,84] In principle, EEG reflects cortical electrical activity derived from the synergy of cortical and subcortical structures, whereas evoked potentials reflect the summation of electrical responses at various levels of the neuraxis within a particular sensory pathway following repetitive stimuli.

EVOKED POTENTIAL MONITORING

Despite the particularly useful features of evoked potentials in the assessment of unresponsive patients receiving narcotics, analgesics, and agents for elevated ICP, there are several limitations: (1) data acquisition, signal processing, and analysis are critical and require sophisticated machinery and software and a well-trained staff; (2) only short-latency evoked potentials are resistant to external variables, such as anesthetics, barbiturates, and hypothermia; and (3) the specificity of the signal pattern abnormality is low. Evoked potentials can be used continuously or discontinuously (serially). Continuous monitoring is a valuable procedure to detect ischemic tissue damage during vascular neurosurgery, based on the notion that there is reversible loss of cortical somatosensory evoked potentials (SSEP) at local blood flow reduction of approximately 12 to 15 ml/100 g/min.[10,17] The serial use of evoked potentials on the neurocritical care unit is almost exclusively of prognostic value. Interpretation is based on clinical correlative studies. We recommend the use of SSEP and brain stem acoustic evoked potentials (BAEP) in stroke patients for prognostication and assessment of brain stem integrity.

Several studies in nontraumatic coma revealed, with very few exceptions, that the early bilateral absence of cortical SSEP (N20–P25 complex, median nerve) with preserved spinal waves (N13) are associated with death, persistent coma, or the development of a vegetative state.[87–89]

Wave V of the brain stem BAEP, generated in the inferior colliculus, is often diminished in amplitude or lost as tissue shifts around the tentorium with compression of the midbrain. The anatomic level of brain stem destruction,[115–117] brain stem infarction due to basilar artery occlusion,[50,87] and brain stem impairment following massive cerebellar[87,90] and hemispheric infarction[158] have been correlated with abnormal patterns of BAEP. As a consequence, progressive loss of wave V amplitude in serial recordings may indicate impending midbrain distortion from mass effects. Prognostication with BAEP is sometimes hampered by the absence of wave I because of sensorineural hearing loss due to pre-existing deafness, eighth nerve damage, swelling with orotracheal intubation, or hemotympanum. Again, entirely normal BAEP can be associated with persistent coma or a vegetative state, since damage above the inferior colliculus escapes recognition.

EEG MONITORING

Using the international 10–20 System, there exists a reliable relationship between scalp electrode placement and underlying cerebral topography.[77] While its localization value is little compared with CT and MR imaging, EEG allows useful diagnostic inferences at the bedside when transportation of ICU patients for imaging studies is deemed too hazardous. Other well-perceived benefits of EEG include close correlations with the cerebral metabolic rate, sensitivity to hypoxia and ischemia, and detection of seizure activity. Thus, application of EEG monitoring may include: (1) monitoring unstable hemispheric ischemia,[162,181] (2) detecting nonconvulsive seizure activity,[81] and (3) managing medically induced coma.[177]

TRANSCRANIAL DOPPLER ULTRASONOGRAPHY

TCD applies relatively low frequency ultrasonographic waves to record intracranial blood flow velocity (BFV) in basal cerebral arteries. The most commonly used technique is "freehanding" the probe so that the ultrasound beam penetrates one of several "acoustic windows." The technique is highly dependent on examiner skill and requires practice and experience. However, new developments promise reliable documentation using color-coded flow charts of the basal arteries. TCD provides important information concerning the intracranial vasculature, collateral flow, and signal characteristics of the various arteries.[7] We expect further improvement of diagnostic properties with the use of doppler ultrasound contrast agents, which will increase the signal-to-noise ratio significantly and reduce the number of patients without acoustic windows. In the neurocritical care unit, TCD allows bedside examination of basal cranial arteries. With constant flow through a vessel, BFV increases inversely to the vessel's cross-sectional area. There is a strong correlation between TCD BFV and angiographically confirmed stenosis and vasospasm.[96] However, various technical, physiologic, and clinical factors have to be recognized for accurate interpretation. A given BFV value does not predict regional CBF, because TCD cannot determine the actual diameter of the insonated vessel. Bedside TCD can reliably detect cerebral vasospasm in subarachnoid hemorrhage patients and thus guide institution of hypertensive-hypervolemic therapy.[61] In raised ICP there is progressive reduction in end diastolic velocity, reflected in an elevated pulsatility index (PI), calculated by systolic velocity minus diastolic velocity divided by mean velocity. It is noteworthy that PI is not helpful in monitoring intracranial hypertension, since hyperventilation, cerebral vasospasm, and reduced cerebral metabolism also influence pulsatility. A different approach analyzes pulse-wave dynamics by subjecting velocity waveform to Fourier analysis using up to five harmonics, and comparing its deviations from the systemic arterial pulse wave. Correlation of indirect TCD-cerebral perfusion pressure with invasive ICP monitoring was high.[1] Close-meshed intermittent TCD monitoring in acute cerebrovascular occlusions may escort thrombolytic therapy to demonstrate recanalization.[141] Continuous monitoring of cerebral ischemia using TCD probes mounted on a helmet holder or glued on the temporal plane is currently under investigation. Therapeutic decisions toward early surgery in patients with ongoing cerebral embolism, such as in infective endocarditis or hemodynamic compromise of cerebral vasculature in high-grade carotid stenosis or occlusion, may improve outcome in some patients.

CEREBRAL BLOOD FLOW AND METABOLISM

Quantifying CBF at the bedside has been a long-standing goal of neurointensivists. Such data can gauge the presence or risk of cerebral ischemia, restored circulation, and clarify the state of autoregulation. It can also identify cerebral hyperemia, a potential contributor to cerebral edema formation. Unfortunately, procedures that meet accepted standards, such as SPECT and PET are impractical and not applicable to continuous or close-meshed bedside monitoring.

In the future, indirect methods assessing oxygen saturation, using thermal and laser doppler techniques, may serve as substitutes and are under investigation.[33–35] Since there is an ongoing progress among the spectrum of possible approaches, no clear guidelines can be given at the present time. Currently, we employ intraparenchymal fiberoptic devices (determination of tissue oxygenation) in combination with pressure probes (parenchymal ICP) in patients with massive cerebral infarctions prone to edema formation for guiding osmotherapy and timing of decompressive surgery. Near-infrared spectroscopy monitoring devices are currently evaluated for use in neurocritical care patients. At this time, technical limitations and variable readings prevent broader, prospective use. Additionally, new thermo- and color-dilutional techniques for bedside evaluation of CBF are now in pilot phases of clinical application. A drawback of these methods is their invasiveness, requiring jugular vein canulation, and central venous and arterial access.

The roles of brain temperature and tissue oxygenation monitoring are not yet established for neurocritical care patients. These techniques may become increasingly important in the setting of therapeutic hypothermia, since brain temperature differs from core temperature in stroke patients[152] and tissue oxygen concentration may reflect energy metabolism of brain tissue.[171,185]

General Principles of Intensive Care Therapy of Stroke

The majority of stroke patients requiring critical care treatment enter the hospital via the emergency department. A different management strategy is necessary for a patient arriving at the hospital within the first few hours after stroke onset than for patients admitted later, for example 24 hours after stroke. The neurologic examination has to be focused on the severity of deficit, lesion localization, and possible sources of the stroke (Table 50.1). Accompanying conditions, such as hypertensive crisis, hyperglycemia, aspiration, seizures, or cardiac arrhythmia, must be treated simultaneously. Time is critical, since the therapeutic window may be quite narrow in a given patient.

RESPIRATORY FUNCTION

All patients with acute strokes should be monitored by means of capillary oximetry, targeting at oxygenation levels >95%. Increasing the PaO_2 by administration of supplemental oxygen is a simple adjunct, which compensates for possible impairment of respiratory capacity of stroke patients. In addition, it has to be anticipated that peripheral oxygen saturation may not always parallel conditions in the environment of cerebral ischemia, making additional oxygen justified even with normal blood gases. The ischemic stroke patient usually has a stable airway. Some patients with acute intracranial internal carotid artery (ICA) or middle cerebral artery (MCA) embolism may demonstrate early breathing abnormalities due to neurogenic ventilatory dysfunction. A quick physical assessment of respiratory function includes observation of the quality and rate of respiration. Tachypnea may indicate pneumonia, bronchospasm, congestive heart failure, or impending ventilatory failure. The use of accessory respiratory muscles indicates further respiratory compromise. Auscultation of the neck may reveal

Table 50.1 Indications for ICU Treatment of Acute Cerebral Ischemia

Progressing symptoms, crescendo TIA
Fluctuating, hemodynamically induced infarction
Embolic intracranial ICA/MCA occlusion
Endocarditis with septic cerebral emboli
Arterial dissection plus embolism
Thrombolytic or hypertensive-hypervolemic therapy

Abbreviations: ICU, intensive care unit; TIA, transient ischemic attack; ICA, internal carotid artery; MCA, middle cerebral artery.

Table 50.2 Indications for Endotracheal Intubation

$PO_2 < 50–60$ mmHg
$PCO_2 > 50–60$ mmHg
Vital capacity < 500–800 ml
Signs of respiratory distress
Tachypnea > 30
Dyspnea
"Self PEEP" with expiratory grunting
Recruitment of accessory muscles
Respiratory acidosis
Significantly altered mental state
Risk for aspiration
Loss of maintenance of stable airways

the presence of stridor secondary to vocal chord paralysis or poor pharyngeal tone. Unconscious patients should be evaluated for the cough and gag reflex; in the awake patient palatal movement as well as voluntary cough and swallowing may be assessed as well. Ventilatory drive is usually unimpaired for the great majority of acute stroke patients. However, in patients with vertebrobasilar or large MCA infarction, abnormal breathing patterns may occur. Normal arterial PO_2 values are in the 70 to 80 mmHg range for patients over the age of 65. Stroke patients have decreased inspiratory force as compared with normal subjects and also exhibit an impaired response to increases in airway resistance. In addition, ventilation may be particularly compromised during sleep. Continuous transdermal oximetry is warranted but does not necessarily reflect brain tissue oxygenation, particularly within the deep white matter. Another concern is the adequacy of airway protection. Defects in airway protection arise from impaired oropharyngeal motility or sensation and loss of protective reflexes from ischemic or compressive brain stem dysfunction or decreased levels of consciousness. Alternatively, bilateral insular region infarcts may impair airway protection secondary to impaired volitional swallowing. These factors create a high risk for aspiration of stomach contents or oropharyngeal secretions, which often occur already prior to presentation. In questionable cases, frequent oropharyngeal suctioning, or better, endotracheal intubation is warranted to prevent aspiration of gastric contents and provide sufficient ventilation.

In the event of an abnormal respiratory pattern, severe hypoxemia, or hypercarbia, and in the unconscious patients who are at high risk for aspiration pneumonia, early endotracheal intubation is recommended (Table 50.2).

There are several techniques to insert an endotracheal tube. Except in the field, where blind nasotracheal intubation can be performed with only local anesthesia, atraumatic orotracheal intubation under direct laryngoscopy is generally preferred in more controlled environments. Nasotracheal intubation may be better tolerated by patients and makes nursing care of the mouth easier but carries a higher risk of nasal trauma and inflammation of the paranasal sinuses. Therefore, we generally prefer transoral endotracheal intubation for the first few days.

Elective intubation must be performed under optimum conditions. Monitoring should include ECG, sphygmomanometry, and end-expiratory CO_2. However, intubation and mechanical ventilation bear several objections in acute stroke patients: (1) laryngoscopy and intubation may initiate substantial hemodynamic responses and (2) hypnotics may worsen elevated ICP. As a consequence, we recommend intubation carried out only by properly trained physicians and the use of short-acting sedatives with minimal cardiodepressive side effects, such as thiopental (3 to 5 mg/kg), etomidate (0.3 to 0.5 mg/kg), and propofol (0.1 to 0.2 mg/kg/min) in combination with rapidly acting, depolarizing relaxant succinylcholine (1.2 mg/kg). All mentioned hypnotics blunt the ICP response.[109] For maintenance of anesthesia on the respirator, a combination of opioids and benzodiazepines via infusion pump offering additional ICP-lowering effects seems most beneficial.[71,110]

There is controversy whether acute stroke patients should be intubated at all. A recent study reported mortality rates exceeding 90% in intubated and ventilated stroke patients.[46] In contrast, the Houston,[62] and Heidelberg,[159] series explicitly demonstrate that careful patient selection and appropriate treatment are beneficial, allowing survival rates of almost 40% with acceptable outcomes.

BLOOD PRESSURE MANAGEMENT

Antihypertensive drugs should be used only rarely in the emergency department setting. In ischemic stroke, during the first hours after symptom onset as many as 70% of the patients will have a blood pressure of 170/100 or higher,[19] which is not surprising as approximately 50% of stroke patients have a history of hypertension. Increases in adrenergic tone have been documented in the setting of acute stroke and explain, in part, acute transient elevations in arterial blood pressure, which often resolve without pharmacologic treatment. Blood pressure (BP) management is a critical issue in view of recent reports.[95,97,132,184] Antihypertensive therapy administered in the first hours may be dangerous. Pharmacologic effects superimposed on spontaneous blood pressure decline may result in a hazardous hypotension. Rapid decrease of BP in acute stroke patients may be unfavorable for a number of reasons. Provided adequate collateral blood flow, the ischemic penumbra surrounding the profoundly ischemic core may eventually recover over time. However, decrease in BP may promote irreparable injury of the tissue at risk. Another unproved theoretical concern is that blood flow distal to a vessel obstruction is sluggish, and thus, further decrease in blood flow predisposes to thrombus propagation. On the other hand, untreated elevated BP may precipitate secondary hemorrhagic infarction, worsen perifocal edema, and lead to hypertensive encephalopathy. Special attention to BP has to be paid if thrombolytic therapy is envisioned for a given patient. According to the guidelines for thrombolytic therapy, only moderate measures to reduce critically elevated BP should be used. Patients requiring aggressive IV antihypertensive management should be excluded from systemic thrombolytic therapy because of a presumed increased risk for intracerebral hemorrhage. In the absence of end organ dysfunction, in patients without a significant history of hypertension the following approach is

Table 50.3 Antihypertensive Treatment in Acute Ischemic Stroke

Systolic BP 180/230 and/or diastolic BP < 120
    Do not treat unless patient is a candidate for thrombolytic therapy (see text)
Systolic BP > 230 and diastolic BP 120/140 on repeated readings 5 min apart
    Labetalol 10 mg IV
    Nifedipine 10 mg sl, urapidil 12.5 mg IV (see text)
Diastolic BP > 140, systolic BP not significantly elevated on repeated readings 5 min apart
    Sodium nitroprusside 0.5–10 μg/kg/min, double dose after 3–5 min

suggested (Table 50.3). For diastolic blood pressure (DBP) > 140 mmHg on two readings 5 minutes apart, sodium nitroprusside (0.5 to 10 μg/kg/min) is recommended. For systolic blood pressure (SBP) > 230 mmHg and or DBP 121 to 140 mmHg on two readings 20 minutes apart, IV labetalol (10 to 20 mg over 1 to 2 minutes every 10 to 20 minutes) is recommended. If SBP is 180/230 and/or DBP is 105/120, treatment should be deferred unless the patient is a candidate for IV treatment with rt-PA, in which case SBP should be kept <185 mmHg.[2,21] In Europe, nifedipine and urapidil are the drugs of first choice.[64] Nifedipine is commonly used in its parenteral form using small dosages to titrate BP. Overshoot hypotension is rarely a problem with that approach. For isolated elevation of DBP, nitroglycerine (in Europe) and sodium nitroprusside (in North America) are frequently used. For some antihypertensive substances alteration of CBF and ICP have been described.[109]

Hypotension is detrimental in acute stroke patients and should be treated aggressively. It is noteworthy that hypotension in the acute stroke setting suggests the possibility of underlying myocardial ischemia that needs to be ruled out by 12-lead ECG before any volume expansion is initiated. Fluid replacement with normal saline, volume expanders such as colloids or albumin, is the first-line treatment. Pressors such as dopamine or phenylephrine may be necessary but are rarely effective without adequate intravascular volume.

HYPERGLYCEMIA

Increased blood glucose concentrations at the time of stroke appear to be associated with poor outcome.[24] Increased glucose levels in cerebral ischemia lead to increased lactic acid production, worsening acidosis, and subsequent tissue damage. Diabetic patients who are poorly controlled at stroke onset have a particularly poor prognosis.[133] Therefore, efforts should be directed to control blood glucose concentration as quickly as possible in the range of 5.5 to 8 mmol/L (100 to 150 mg/dl) without producing hypoglycemia. Experimental studies on the effects of hyperglycemia on infarct size are conflicting and depend on the model used.[155] It seems that deleterious effects of hyperglycemia depend on the presence of collateral blood supply. Hyperglycemia is associated with worse outcome in a model of focal infarction, where the infarcted zone receives collateral supply.[56] In contrast, hyperglycemia may decrease infarct size in a model of nonanastomosing arterial bed. A possible protective effect of hyperglycemia during focal ischemia is the membrane-stabilizing effect that glucose exerts in the peri-infarct region. This effect prohibits spontaneous potassium depolarization and is associated with decreased regional metabolism.[121,122] Hyperglycemia in the peri-infarct region in a focal ischemic model is associated with normal metabolic rates, whereas normoglycemia increases metabolism and the rate of spontaneous potassium depolarizations in the peri-infarct region.[120] Increases of metabolism in the peri-infarct area have been shown to be associated with selective neuronal necrosis.[123] It is noteworthy that glucose metabolism in the peri-infarct region remains increased in normoglycemic rats whose neuronal activity had been suppressed by inducing barbiturate coma.[122] In conclusion, although the membrane-stabilizing effect of hyperglycemia in the peri-infarct region involves neuronal tissue, the associated increases in regional metabolism do not.

NUTRITION

Careful evaluation of swallowing is recommended before the patient is offered oral nutrition. In patients with impaired swallowing enteral feeding may be established by a nasogastric or, preferably, nasoduodenal/nasojejunal tube. It is important to consider that the presence of a feeding tube or an endotracheal intubation does not categorically prevent aspiration. In some institutions methylene blue is added to tube feedings for easy identification of gastrointestinal tract contents within the patient's expectorate. Depending on the severity and recovery of swallowing deficits, percutaneous gastrostomies or tracheostomies may become necessary. In general, enteral feeding should be instituted as soon as possible and gastrointestinal tolerance carefully monitored. Additionally, recent clinical studies have demonstrated that the enteral route is preferred over the parenteral route.[130,154] Enteral feeding is clearly cheaper and associated with reduced septic morbidity. Critically ill patients with neurologic injury may develop a hypercatabolic state. These patients may require 35 to 40 kcal/kg/d and protein intake of 1.5 to 2.5 g/kg/d.

CARDIAC OUTPUT AND FLUID MANAGEMENT

Circulatory support has long been recognized to be vital in the care of non-neurologic emergencies. Congestive heart failure is uncommon within the first hours after stroke onset. Nonetheless, the physician must carefully exclude acute cardiac disorders, including myocardial infarction, arrhythmias, such as atrial fibrillation, and significant valvular disease. Each of these conditions may predispose to stroke and may jeopardize cardiac function. A significant percentage of elderly stroke patients may have low cardiac output at the time of stroke onset. In the setting of acute cerebral ischemia, cardiac output should be augmented by treating congestive heart failure and correcting fluid overload or dehydration. A large number of patients with acute ischemic strokes are hypovolemic on

presentation and need fluid replacement to increase cerebral perfusion. A central venous catheter is useful for monitoring central venous pressure and administration of fluids, medication, and nutrition. Direct application of a central venous catheter is accomplished through the internal jugular or subclavian veins. Pneumothorax is less frequent using the internal jugular vein, but jugular puncture can impede the drainage of venous blood from the brain (especially in patients with increased ICP) and carries the additional risk of jugular vein thrombosis. Therefore, the subclavian vein approach is often preferred. A central venous catheter with multiple lumens permits uninterrupted therapy and simultaneous monitoring of the central venous pressure (CVP). Only rarely are pulmonary artery catheters necessary to monitor circulation in severe heart failure or in patients requiring aggressive hypervolemic-hypertensive therapy.

Although ECG alterations may accompany acute cerebral ischemia, arrhythmias secondary to stroke are infrequent. Significant alterations of ST segments and/or T waves on ECG may appear in the acute phase mimicking myocardial ischemia. Cardiac embolism secondary to atrial fibrillation requires management of the supraventricular arrhythmia.

Optimal fluid management requires a balance of maintaining adequate hydration to decrease blood viscosity and avoiding excessive, particularly hypotonic, fluids, which can enhance cerebral edema formation. Brain swelling peaks at 48 to 72 hours after stroke onset in large infarctions,[145] but may occur as early as 24 hours after stroke onset.[65] Elderly individuals with pre-existing cerebral atrophy may tolerate brain edema quite well. In contrast, younger individuals with extended early infarct signs are at higher risk of deterioration from brain edema.[93] In this setting, fluid restriction to 1,500 ml/24 h may become necessary, and hypotonic solutions should be strictly avoided.

Central venous lines allow the infusion of higher volumes and higher concentrations of electrolytes, provided that continuous ECG monitoring is available. Serious electrolyte disturbances are rare in stroke. Hyponatremia may occur due to inappropriate antidiuretic hormone secretion (SIADH) or due to excess release of atrial natriuretic factor (ANF). SIADH is managed by fluid restriction or occasionally hypertonic saline, whereas normovolemia should be maintained if excess ANF is suspected. Overly rapid correction of hyponatremia can precipitate central pontine myelinolysis.[125]

NORMOTHERMIA

Elevated body and brain temperature may adversely influence cerebral ischemia. Therefore, temperature control is important, since infection and fever are frequently observed in acute stroke patients. Simple physical measures such as cooling blankets, alcohol wraps, and antipyretic drugs are usually effective in lowering elevated body temperature. If infection is present or aspiration pneumonia suspected, early use of antibiotics is recommended.

DEEP VEIN THROMBOSIS

Pulmonary embolism is a common threat during the recovery period, in particular for bedridden individuals with hemiplegia. Deep vein thrombosis can be prevented by subcutaneous heparin (5,000 IE bid) or more effective and safer by low-molecular-weight heparinoids (adjusted by factor Xa assay).[169] We recommend platelet counts in patients on heparin q 3 days and discontinuation of heparin if platelet count decreases by 30% or below 100,000. Elastic stockings or pneumatic devices also decrease the risk of pulmonary embolism during hospitalization.[153] Prevention of acute pulmonary embolism is of major importance in the care of stroke patients. Pulmonary embolism is the cause of death in up to 25% of patients following ischemic strokes.[157] An evaluation of the lower extremities by Doppler ultrasound and venous compression should be prompted by the suspicion of deep vein thrombosis or pulmonary embolism. Since chest pain and dyspnea will occur in 70% to 80% of those patients with documented pulmonary embolism, nurses and physicians should be attentive to those signs. Oxygen desaturation may be the only and earliest indication of multiple pulmonary emboli. Tachypnea is a sensitive sign of pulmonary embolism (and of pneumonia). Examination of lower extremities should be performed daily to detect signs of deep vein thrombosis. If pulmonary embolism is suspected, a perfusion lung scan should be performed immediately. In selected patients with hemodynamic compromise pulmonary angiography and thrombolysis will be necessary. Anticoagulation is indicated for documented pulmonary embolism with full-dose IV heparin for 5 to 10 days to be followed by warfarin for at least 3 months. An inferior vena cava umbrella can also be used when full-dose heparin is contraindicated (e.g., large hemorrhagic stroke).

INFECTION PREVENTION

Bacterial pneumonia accounts for 15% to 25% of stroke deaths. The majority of the pneumonias are caused by aspiration. Since aspiration may be detected by video fluoroscopy in as many as 50% of patients during the initial days after stroke onset, oral feeding should be withheld until the patient has demonstrated both intact swallowing with small amounts of water and intact coughing to command. Urinary tract infection is the most common medical complication of acute ischemic stroke. It is present, but not causal, in as many as 40% of patients dying from stroke.[157] The majority of hospital-acquired urinary tract infections are associated with the use of indwelling catheters. However, intermittent catheterization or the use of condom catheters is not always feasible in the setting of severe stroke and may contribute to decubital ulcer.

STROKE-ASSOCIATED SEIZURES

Partial (focal) or secondary generalized epileptic attacks may occur in the acute phase of ischemic stroke. Clonazepam (2 mg IV) or diazepam (10 to 20 mg IV) followed by rapid loading with fosphenytoin (loading dose of 10 to 15 mg/kg, followed by 300 to 750 mg daily doses) is the treatment of choice. Myoclonic jerks are treated in the acute phase with clonazepam (approximately 6 to 10 mg daily).

Special Interventions of Intensive Care Therapy of Stroke

The mechanisms of ischemic injury initiated by local impairment of cerebral blood flow are complex and highly variable in time and space among individual patients. Because there is believed to be no proved efficient therapy available, a fatalistic attitude toward stroke management is present among lay people and many medical care providers. Patients are frequently admitted merely for "observation" and to receive physiotherapy and supportive medical care. More recently, special care units dedicated to stroke treatment (stroke units) are increasing in number in parallel with effectiveness of therapy. Due to the nature of the disease, intermediate care facilities attached to ICUs offer logistic advantages with regard to staffing and equipment. The nurse/patient ratio of 1:2 (maximal 1:3) is worthwhile. Given an overall prevalence of approximately 800 ischemic strokes per 100,000 and an incidence of 150 cases per 100,000 each year, we estimate stroke units with 2.5 beds per 100,000 inhabitants and early rehabilitation units offering approximately 10 beds per 100,000 people sufficiently meet the requirements. A recent community-based, prospective, and consecutive study on the effect of stroke units of unselected acute stroke patients could demonstrate a benefit on survival rate, reduced length of hospital stay, and discharge to a nursing home.[82] Rehabilitation, to be optimally successful, should be fully integrated with other therapies. It should be begun as early as possible during the acute phase of the disease. With emerging effective remedies, such as thrombolytics and neuroprotectants, and novel approaches to improve functional outcome of cerebral ischemia, optimal return of the patient to the previous and vocational environment is feasible and a desired goal.[51]

Restoring and Increasing Altered Cerebral Blood Flow

Treatment alternatives to restore following acute stroke include thrombolysis and surgical or interventional radiologic procedures. While anticoagulation and carotid endarterectomy play a definite role in primary and secondary prophylaxis of embolic stroke, their value for treatment of acute strokes is controversial and needs to be established in future trials. This review describes evolving rationales to enhance impaired CBF and summarizes results of current therapeutic trials.

ANTICOAGULATION

In the final stages of thrombotic occlusion of an atheromatous cerebral artery, thrombotic material accumulates at the wall of a severe stenosis until the lumen becomes obstructed. It is believed but unproven that thrombi tethered to the site of the stenosis may extend distally in the bloodstream and at some time become dislodged, causing cerebral embolism. In addition, obstructing thrombi may further diminish blood flow in the affected vascular territory, thus aggravating cerebral ischemia. Cotreatment with full-dose heparin and high-dose (100 mg rt-PA) thrombolysis did not result in increased hemorrhage rates in one study,[92] a finding that was recently supported by a report from Cologne, where they used the National Institute of Neurological Disorders and Stroke (NINDS) protocol,[118] plus immediate full-dose anticoagulation.[60] Both trials were not placebo controlled. The accepted rationale for anticoagulant therapy is to prevent re-embolization. Their usefulness in acute management is unknown.[47] Although heparin is the most commonly prescribed antithrombotic drug, evidence about its safety and efficacy is still limited.[26,44,100] Until recently, no controlled data were available that would have shown a benefit of early anticoagulation on stroke outcome. There is disagreement about the best level of anticoagulation, route of administration, the timing and duration of treatment, or the use of a bolus dose. Currently, physicians are unsure about the severity of stroke or the size of infarction on baseline CT that would contraindicate treatment. Additionally, the influence of vascular distribution or presumed cause of stroke on treatment response is unknown. The International Stroke Trial (IST) testing two doses of subcutaneous heparin, alone or with aspirin in a large placebo-controlled trial, was completed and showed no benefit of antithrombotic treatment. The slight beneficial trend of heparin was leveled out by an increased rate of symptomatic intracerebral hemorrhage. The methodology of this megatrial was criticized, as no data verification was guaranteed and outcome assessment was achieved by telephone interviews.

Low-molecular-weight heparins and heparinoids have potential advantages over heparin. Their more selective antithrombotic actions may improve safety and the risk of a severe, symptomatic autoimmune thrombocytopenia is less. A recent randomized trial revealed positive effects of fraxiparine on stroke outcome after 6 months when administered within 48 hours after stroke onset.[85] The trial of ORG 10172 in acute stroke treatment (TOAST),[3] testing the heparinoid IV against placebo was unable to demonstrate a benefit in improving outcomes following 3 months after stroke onset. Interestingly, this trial revealed an improvement of patients treated with ORG at 7 days but this effect was lost at 3 months follow-up. Additionally, despite an increased risk of bleeding, the overall outcomes were not different. The only subgroup of patients that responded to therapy consisted of persons with stroke secondary to large artery atherosclerosis. Risks of early recurrent stroke and neurologic worsening were relatively low in the entire study population.[168] A European variant of this study, EUROTOAST, is currently recruiting. In this particular trial, different doses of sc heparinoid are compared with IV treatment.

CAROTID ENDARTERECTOMY

Emergency carotid endarterectomy (CEA) early after cerebral infarction is a controversial issue because the operation presumably carries a high risk of perioperative worsening and bleeding complication. Controversy concerning the advisability of carotid endarterectomy in the presence of acute cerebral ischemia is based on the contention that a "pale" infarct may be converted into a hemorrhagic one. This is explainable only in the setting of a major territorial infarction, which is usually only encountered in complete carotid occlusion and insufficient collateral blood flow. With respect to the rate of neurologic decline secondary to hemorrhagic complications with thrombolytic therapy for acute strokes, the clinical consequences of hemorrhagic transformation after restoration of blood flow are probably overestimated.[92,113] Actually, in artery-to-artery embolic stroke, presumably the most important cause of stroke associated with high-grade ICA stenosis, the danger of reperfusion injury due to CEA is probably not a problem. Reperfusion injury, nevertheless, may occur in embolic stroke, caused by spontaneous or induced recanalization of the occluded brain vessel. This is not influenced by CEA. Reperfusion trauma may exist, however, in the rare setting of hemodynamically induced stroke. Although emergency carotid endarterectomy is not safe enough to be generally recommended, it is feasible in selected cases with adequate blood pressure monitoring and performed by experienced vascular surgeons.[173] Surgical recanalization in acute stroke may be indicated in carotid occlusions occurring in the hospital, either spontaneously, during angiography, or immediately after carotid surgery. Patients on adequate anticoagulation with progressive neurologic deficits secondary to high-grade stenosis or floating intraluminal thrombus of the internal carotid artery may also be considered candidates.

ANGIOPLASTY AND STENTING

With recent advances in endovascular therapy, percutaneous transluminal angioplasty and intravascular stenting may serve as a treatment alternative to carotid endarterectomy and may be suitable for surgically inaccessible sites, such as intracranial carotid and middle cerebral artery lesions. Currently, angioplasty and stenting of the supra-aortic vessels are being analyzed to determine their safety, feasibility, and long-term durability. Technical success was reported in 94.6% of 1,971 cases of balloon angioplasty of the carotid, vertebral, innominate, and subclavian arteries summarized in a recent survey.[83] Morbidity results varied in each vascular territory from 0% to 2.1%; severe morbidity was found in 0.9%. No deaths were reported. Similar rates of complication were reported for extracranial balloon angioplasty in a series placing a small distal "protection" balloon above the lesion to trap particles or debris dislodged during the procedure.[164] The recurrence rate was evaluated in a 6- to 12-month follow-up study of 292 symptomatic patients with ≥70% extracerebral stenoses treated with transluminal balloon angioplasty. Recurrent stenoses were found in 8.2% of patients re-evaluated.[76] Intravascular stenting of the carotid artery is reported to have a procedure-related stroke frequency of 2% and patient stents of 94% at a mean follow-up of 25 months.[104] Intracranial angioplasty has also been reported in a small series of 17 highly selected patients who failed maximal medical therapy, including systemic anticoagulation, blood pressure control, and antiplatelet medication.[29] Complications included two strokes (11.8%), which occurred during the procedure. All successfully treated patients at 3- and 6-month follow-up had no further neurologic events and no evidence of restenosis. Symptomatic vasospasm with significant stenosis after subarachnoid hemorrhage is treated by angioplasty with increasing frequency. Several studies have reported marked clinical improvement of ischemic deficits as well as angiographic resolution in patients refractory to standard medical therapy when angioplasty was performed within 6 to 48 hours after onset.[75] To date, transluminal angioplasty and stenting are important considerations for symptomatic, hemodynamically significant stenoses involving coronary, renal, or peripheral vascular territories. Devices specifically designed for the needs of the supra-aortic and cerebral vasculature are still pending, and their safety and efficacy have not been evaluated in clinical trials. No well-controlled long-term trials have thus far provided evidence for the durability of endovascular therapy of stenoses of the extra- or intracranial arteries.

THROMBOLYSIS

Experience with thrombolytic therapy in cerebral artery occlusion dates back to the late 1950s.[163] Controlled clinical studies performed thereafter were unsatisfactory, mainly due to intracerebral hemorrhage, and the treatment modality was rejected for a number of years. Since the early 1980s, local intra-arterial thrombolytic therapy was reintroduced for vertebrobasilar artery occlusions[66,188,189] and the anterior circulation.[39,92,112] Thrombolytic treatment of acute stroke is reviewed in Chapter 51.

HYPERVOLEMIC-HYPERTENSIVE HEMODILUTION

Blood flow in vessels is dependent on the physics of tubular flow and hemorrheology. Blood is a non-newtonian fluid with increased viscosity at lower flow rates. The force required to restore flow after it is interrupted (the yield stress) is proportional to the third power of the hematocrit. Hemodilution for cerebral ischemia has therefore been favored for a long time as a relatively safe and easy concept applicable to an unselected patient population. As with other treatment alternatives, results of clinical trials are equivocal[58,79,148,161] and the theoretic concept for hemodilution in cerebral ischemia, that is, reduction of blood viscosity improves microcirculation in the peri-infarct tissue, has been challenged, since hemoglobin depletion simply reduces oxygen availability in the presence of utmost vasodilation in the ischemic penumbra.

In contrast, hypervolemic-hypertensive hemodilution (HHH) was demonstrated to be beneficial in case series of patients with large vessel obstruction and hemodynamic insufficiency, such as severe vasospasm[128,147] or arterial occlu-

Table 50.4 Hypertensive-Hypervolemic Therapy

High-volume colloidal infusion (hetastarch 500–1,500 ml)
Ringer's solution (5,000–10,000 ml)
Blood transfusions if necessary
Dopamine/dobutamine (10–30 mg/kg/min)

sion,[40,48] (Tables 50.4 and 50.5). Three clinical parameters can be determined to ensure and monitor hypervolemia in stroke patients: (1) cardiac filling pressures (CVP, pulmonary artery diastolic pressure [PADP], pulmonary capillary wedge pressure [PCWP]) should be held at high normal levels, (2) fluid balance should ensure that input is greater than output, and (3) body weight should ensure that no weight loss occurs. Cardiac filling pressures are most often used to follow circulatory hemodynamics in critical stroke patients. However, CVP and PCWP are poor indicators of intravascular volume, and targeting at cardiac output values seems most rational to guide HHH.[8,17]

To date, there have been no prospective, randomized controlled clinical trials establishing the efficacy of hypertensive, hypervolemic, hemodilutional, or hyperdynamic therapy and no data demonstrating that such therapy provides more meaningful clinical benefits, or is more cost effective than standard care. At present, hypervolemic therapy is initiated and applied in an arbitrary fashion. HHH treatment can be applied in a safe fashion; however, it is time consuming and costly because it requires constant monitoring and modification of treatment in an ICU setting.

The ideal substance for hemodilution should be a low-viscosity fluid that also carries oxygen. Recently, a blood substitute consisting of stable nontoxic diaspirin cross-linked hemoglobin (DCLHb) has been developed and shown effective in ameliorating ischemic damage in experimental models and is currently under scrutiny in preliminary clinical trials.[9,31]

NEURONAL PROTECTION

When CBF drops below the threshold of cerebral ischemia, a complex series of events termed ischemic cascade is triggered, eventually leading to ischemic cell death.[10,17,156] Disruption of calcium homeostasis is the central element culminating in

Table 50.5 Required Controls for Hypertensive-Hypervolemic Therapy

Physical examination: edema
Labs including osmolarity of urine and serum
Mean arterial BP ≥ systolic BP: 160/180 mmHg
Central venous pressure
    Increase colloid fluid input to CVP: 10–12 mmHg
Fluid status and weight control ≥ hematocrit: 33%–38%
Daily chest x-ray
Pulmonary artery catheter
    Increase colloid fluid input to PCWP 14–18 mmHg
    Titrate cardiac index (CI) to 3.5–4.5 L/min

cell death, which has led to new treatment strategies that attempt to maintain or restore calcium balance in neurons subjected to significant ischemia.[37] Initially it was hoped that selective dihydropyridine-type calcium entry blockers, such as nimodipine, would provide sufficient neuroprotection; however, in the final analysis only modest benefit can be achieved if oral treatment is initiated within the first 12 hours after onset.[111] Moreover, a placebo-controlled trial of IV nimodipine was halted prematurely because of increased frequency of poorer outcomes among the actively treated patients.[172]

Current attention has focused on the role of excitatory amino acids and radicals,[4,41,86] "oxidative stress," including the role of nitrous oxide,[183] and apoptosis[146] in brain damage after cerebral ischemia. Specific therapeutic trials and current hypothesis of mode of action are addressed in Chapter 47.

Treatment of Raised Intracranial Pressure

The mechanism of neurologic deterioration in patients with large hemispheric infarction with edema ("malignant" middle cerebral artery infarction),[86] involves displacement of the brain stem from pressure gradients developing as the result of mass effect from infarcted and edematous brain tissue. This condition carries a mortality of approximately 80%. In these patients, brain tissue shifts often induce subsequent vascular compromise and infarctions in the anterior and posterior cerebral artery circulation. As a result, a cycle of new infarction and edema is set in motion that most patients do not survive. In posterior fossa mass lesions, occlusive hydrocephalus may be initiated by aqueductal occlusion. Additional damage, either ascending transtentorial herniation or basilar artery compression against the clivus, may occur secondary to massive brain stem compression by acute expanding cerebellar mass lesions. Exact understanding of the pathophysiology of raised intracranial pressure with ischemic stroke allows appropriate management. The Monro-Kellie doctrine holds that the intracranial space is one compartment filled with a relatively incompressible content where the intracranial pressure is equally distributed. This may be the case in global brain injury, such as venous hypertension or metabolic encephalopathies, but does not hold for focal mass lesions. As early as 1885, von Bergmann found that ICP is not always transmitted in equal directions inside the skull.[16] In focal mass lesions, brain tissue shifts secondary to pressure gradients as opposed to intracranial pressure elevation.[20,55,144,176] Recently, the pressure gradients occurring with focal mass lesions of various size have been demonstrated using simultaneous intraparenchymal ICP monitors in a rat experiment.[178] The armamentarium to combat intracranial hypertension is complex and many approaches are simply heuristic. This is in particular due to the lack of understanding how focal or diffuse cerebral lesions exert detrimental effects on brain function. Techniques to monitor continuously metabolic activity and cerebral blood flow have to be applied to determine the urgency and approaches to encounter intracranial hypertension.

Table 50.6 Requirements for Treatment of Elevated Intracranial Pressure in Patients with Massive Hemispheric Strokes

Critical care unit setting
Consulting neurosurgeon
Invasive monitoring
    Arterial line
    ICP monitor
    Central venous line
    Pulmonary artery catheter
Neurophysiologic monitoring
    EEG
    Evoked potentials
    Doppler sonography

In the following we discuss different medical and surgical modalities that are currently in use and may be applied as a stepwise escalation aimed to increase cerebral elastance in patients with focal mass lesions, such as cerebral infarctions (Tables 50.6 and 50.7).

BASIC PROCEDURES

Slight elevation of the head (approximately 20°) without causing jugular obstruction by bending the neck or rotating the head is traditionally regarded as an effective, however unproven, basic maneuver to lower ICP, mainly by optimizing venous return. Recently, this practice has become controversial because the reduction in venous pressure by head eleva-

Table 50.7 Management of Intracranial Hypertension in Stroke

Basic procedures for suspected intracranial hypertension
1. Head elevation, avoid jugular compression by bending the neck or rotating the head
2. Blood pressure control, optional arterial line unless on IV drip for BP control
3. Glycerol[a] 0.25 g/kg q6h
Critically elevated intracranial pressure
1. Endotracheal intubation and mechanical ventilation to keep $PaCO_2$: 28 − 35 mmHg
2. Sedation with short-acting benzodiazepines and/or morphine, propofol
                    if ineffective
1. Mannitol 0.25–0.5 g/kg q4–6h, preferably with furosemide 5–20 mg
2. THAM-buffer 3 mmol/h, pH < 7.55, BE < 10
                    if ineffective
1. Consider pentobarbital to suppress EEG to burst suppression, 0.3–0.6 g bolus, max. 10 g/day or alternative anesthetics (see text)
2. Consider experimental strategies; hemicraniectomy, moderate hypothermia (see text)

[a] Currently not used in North America.

tion at the level of the superior sagittal sinus may be counteracted by the reduction in hydrostatic carotid artery pressure, with subsequent reduction of cerebral perfusion pressure.

OSMOTIC AGENTS AND DIURETICS

Hyperosmolar therapy for raised ICP extracts water and reduces the volume of the normal brain. The latency from administration to ICP reduction is usually several minutes, with maximal reduction occurring at 20 to 60 minutes. Duration and degree of ICP reduction depend on (1) the volume of remaining normal brain that is subject to shrinkage, (2) the proportion of disrupted blood-brain barrier, (3) the initial ICP, and (4) the dose of agent used. The goal of osmotherapy is to increase serum osmolarity to approximately 315 to 320 mOsm/L. Evidently, short rises of osmolality are more suitable and effective than continuous elevation. Glycerol (currently only used in Europe) can be administered enterally or intravenously, being more potent via the enteral route.[119] We recommend 1 g/kg glycerol as 50% solution enterally or alternatively 10% solution via a central venous line. Glycerol has a shorter duration of action than mannitol because of greater brain penetration and tubular reabsorption. Fluid overload, hemolysis, and electrolyte disturbance are adverse effects to consider, however. Dehydration contributing to hypotension is deleterious in acute stroke and may be less pronounced than with mannitol. Other occasional side effects include nausea, vomiting, diarrhea, hemoglobinuria, and bleeding diathesis.

Currently, we recommend the use of mannitol only for more severe cases, such as impending transtentorial herniation, mainly because of a slightly faster onset of action. We use a bolus of 0.5 to 1 g/kg and continue with 0.25 to 0.5 g/kg mannitol (20% solution) every 4 hours, if glycerol fails to control elevated ICP. Once a plateau of osmolarity is reached, transient intravascular fluid overloads may evoke rebound intracerebral hypertension. Therefore, mannitol should be used only briefly, and it is prudent to restrict water intake with mannitol therapy until the underlying cerebral mass lesion subsides and the ICP remains stable.

The role of renal loop diuretics, such as furosemide and ethacrynic acid, is unresolved. The theoretic advantage over osmotic agents is the lack of initial CBF increase, but their sustained effects remain unclear. Currently, renal loop diuretics are probably best suited as adjuncts to other therapies.

STEROIDS

The use of corticosteroids in settings other than decreasing vasogenic cerebral edema adjacent to brain tumors remains controversial. The role in ischemic stroke is even less certain because multiple potential effects have to be considered simultaneously. No study demonstrated a beneficial effect of steroids in this setting.[7,126,127]

Potential benefits are outweighed by hyperglycemia, often caused by high-dose steroid application. With these concerns, we generally avoid steroids in brain edema after stroke.

EXTENSIVE PROCEDURES

The following strategies may be used in combination and require substantial sedation and anesthesia. The inability to evaluate central nervous system function and neuromuscular performance must be weighed against the benefits of such therapies. We recommend further methods only in ICUs equipped with adequate technical appliances and experienced staff. Usually patients need to be intubated and may require ICP monitoring. As for other critical care patients, appropriate sedation in order to optimize management in an intensive care environment is essential for patients with severe strokes. Since preservation and frequent assessment of the neurologic performance is of paramount interest for neurologically ill patients, the following guidelines on sedation are summarized. Prior to initiation of any sedation, important life-threatening disturbances, including infection, metabolic derangement, hypoxia, hypercarbia, acidosis, and hemodynamic shock that may lead to restlessness and agitation, have to be ruled out. Drugs used for sedative purposes affect neurologic performance by their effect on neuronal synaptic activity, cerebral blood flow, metabolism, and intracranial pressure. With the exception of high-dose barbiturate therapy, sedation should be minimized to the smallest dosage required and briefest duration possible. An individual regimen using short-acting sedatives with high therapeutic index, administered by intermittent bolus or IV infusion must be tailored to individual patients.

SEDATION

Stroke patients may not cooperate or misinterpret diagnostic and therapeutic procedures, and thus require sedation to facilitate cooperation and comfort during interventions. Preferable, potent agents with rapid onset and clearance include midazolam 1 to 5 mg, fentanyl 50 to 100 μg, thiopental 25 to 100 mg, and propofol 10 to 20 mg. Longer procedures or transports to the CT or angiography suite require longer acting agents, such as lorazepam 1 to 2 mg, morphine 2 to 7 mg, or droperidol 1 to 5 mg. In these cases, immediate re-evaluation of the neurologic exam can be achieved with flumazenil 0.3 to 1 mg and naloxone 0.4 to 0.8 mg.

Medium-term sedation for stroke patients on intensive care units represents a therapeutic dilemma for several reasons. (1) Obscurity of pertinent clinical findings and respiratory depression is disadvantageous; in contrast, pain and other nociceptive stimuli may be harmful by aggravating the stress response, leading to increased heart rate, blood pressure, brain metabolism, and ICP. (2) Sedation reduces brain metabolism and precipitates struggling and resistance to nursing care, procedures, and mechanical ventilation; in contrast, ablation of the sympathetic drive with pharmacologic sedation may precipitate severe cardiovascular collapse with aggravation of brain ischemia. Prior careful assessment of the volume status and hemodynamic reserve is essential to prevent hazardous arterial hypotension. The use of opioids is advantageous because relief of pain and sedation reduce hyperadrenergic responses without perturbation of intracranial dynamics when ventilation is controlled. Limiting effects of opioids include gastrointestinal hypomotility, compromising attempts at enteral nutrition, and hold-up of the weaning process from mechanical ventilation and successful extubation. Other agents under consideration include barbiturates (i.e., thiopental: bolus: 0.25 to 0.75 mg/kg, infusion: 2 to 3 mg/kg/h) benzodiazepines (i.e., midazolam: bolus: 0.02 to 0.08 mg/kg, infusion: 0.05 to 0.1 mg/kg/h), neuroleptics (i.e., droperidol: bolus: 0.01 to 0.1 mg/kg), and propofol (bolus: 0.1 to 0.3 mg/kg, infusion: 0.6 to 6 mg/kg/h). All of these medications have been shown to reduce cerebral metabolism and blood flow/volume.

BARBITURATE "COMA" AND GENERAL ANESTHESIA

Short-acting barbiturates, such as thiopental, effectively decrease elevated ICP. The effect is presumably mediated through reduction of cerebral blood flow and volume, due partly to a coupled reduction in metabolic rate.[45] In addition to reducing the volume of the normal brain, barbiturates (1) reduce brain swelling, perhaps as a result of mild systemic hypotension and (2) offer free radical scavenger properties with subsequent edema reduction in models of ischemic stroke. The complications of high-dose barbiturate administration (safety limit approximately 10 mg/kg/d) include hypotension, most pronounced at the time of bolus administration,[105] and predisposition to infection and decubital ulcers.[124] Systemic hypotension mainly results from decreased venous tone, baroreflex tone, and sympathetic activity. Cardiovascular side effects may be aggravated by concomitant dehydration induced by osmotherapy and diminished cardiac filling pressures. Maximal reduction in cerebral metabolism is accompanied by electrocerebral silence. Since some tolerance develops with continued barbiturate administration, we prefer the application of multiple small boluses (0.3 to 0.6 mg/kg). For induced barbiturate coma we recommend EEG monitoring to titrate the dosage by achieving continuous burst and suppression pattern.

Other agents with similar effects on intracranial dynamics and metabolism as barbiturates include propofol and ketamine. *Propofol* is an ultrashort-acting alkylphenol with pure sedative-hypnotic and little, if any, analgesic action.[69] Its mechanism of action is still not completely understood, but a recent investigation suggested activation of the alpha-subtype of the GABA receptor-ionophore complex.[68] Besides reduction of systemic vascular resitance, propofol is thought to decrease cerebral metabolism and blood flow in a dose-dependent fashion.[160] Ketamine is a short-acting structural analogue of phencyclidine that induces rapid hypnosis with profound amnesia and also provides excellent analgesia. This drug is also unique among sedative drugs in that it lacks any depressant action on ventilation or circulatory tone. An additional attribute is the potential neuroprotective value via its noncompetitive antagonism at the NMDA receptor.[135] The use of ketamine sedation in patients with massive stroke is nevertheless constrained by a significant increase of CBF and ICP.[182]

HYPERVENTILATION

Hypocarbia causes cerebral vasoconstriction, whereas CBF reduction is almost immediate although peak ICP reduction may take up to 30 minutes after CO_2 is changed.[143] PCO_2 reduction from 35 to 29 mmHg, best achieved by raising the ventilation rate at a constant tidal volume (12 to 14 mg/kg), lowers ICP 25% to 30% in most patients. Failure of elevated ICP to respond to hyperventilation bears a poor prognosis.[101] Vasoconstriction with subsequent CBF reduction seems to be safe above 20 mmHg for stroke patients. In selected patients with poor cerebral compliance, strict hyperventilation may cause paradox ICP elevation by increasing thoracic venous and CSF pressure. The beneficial effect of sustained hyperventilation on ICP is unresolved. In theory, ICP reduction ceases when pH of CSF reaches equilibrium, but in practice this may not occur for many hours. Some authors believe that prolonged hyperventilation has a beneficial effect on brain water volume. As with osmotherapy, adverse rebound effects can occur if normoventilation is resumed too rapidly.[114] We recommend to keep PCO_2 constant between 35 and 30 mmHg until the underlying cerebral mass lesion subsides and the ICP remains stable. Recently, a more restrictive use of hyperventilation has been proposed in the neurosurgical literature because of circulatory side effects of forced hyperventilation ($PaCO_2 < 30$ mmHg). It should be also noted that hyperventilation, like osmotherapy and barbiturates, has only a limited time of efficacy. In most instances the effects exhaust after 1 to 2 days.

MUSCLE RELAXANTS

Neuromuscular paralysis can reduce elevated ICP by preventing increases in intrathoracic and venous pressure associated with coughing, straining, suctioning, or "bucking" the ventilator. Nondepolarizing agents, such as vecuronium (10 μg/h) with only minor histamine liberation and ganglion-blocking effects, are preferred in this situation. We pretreat critical patients with bolus muscle relaxants prior to suctioning and avoid possible hazardous chronic use.

TEMPERATURE CONTROL AND THERAPEUTIC HYPOTHERMIA

Hyperthermia increases cerebral metabolic rate and should be rigorously avoided by employing antipyretics and cooling devices, as well as infection control as necessary. Conversely, hypothermia reduces cerebral metabolism and thus may permit prolonged periods of otherwise inadequate CBF without brain damage.[12,138,190] The concept of induced hypothermia is derived from infants undergoing cardiac surgery in total circulatory arrest with profound hypothermia and no residual neurologic deficit. Body temperature can be decreased by various procedures, including cooling blankets, gastric ice water instillation, peritoneal lavage, and extracorporeal pumps. Beneficial effects of moderate hypothermia (31° to 33°C) on elevated ICP have been shown in traumatic brain injury.[30,99] Currently, efforts are directed toward technical feasibility and applicability of hypothermia in massive brain edema after stroke. Although there is now strong experimental evidence that hypothermia protects against cerebral ischemia, the mechanism of action is not fully understood, but is likely multifactorial. Besides reduction of $CMRO_2$, the mechanism of action may depend on a marked reduction in the release of excitatory neurotransmitters, particularly glutamate and aspartate in the peri- and postischemic period.[13,23,57] Calcium-mediated effects of neuronal injury may be inhibited as a consequence of temperature-induced inactivation of important calcium-dependent enzyme systems including calcium/calmodulin-dependent protein kinase II and protein kinase C.[25,28] Decreasing the brain temperature from 37°C to 27°C decreases cerebral blood flow significantly ($P < .0001$) as determined by xenon-133 washout in adults during cardiopulmonary bypass. Since the decline in blood flow is less than the reduction in CMRO$_2$, an apparent luxuriant cerebral perfusion results.[32] Thus, hypothermia appears to ensure a more than adequate oxygen supply to the brain by providing a relatively high CBF. Hypothermia may also lower the minimum amount of CBF necessary to maintain cell viability, thereby expanding the ischemic penumbra surrounding an infarct.[12] Cerebral edema due to ischemia is generally regarded as initially being cytotoxic, water accumulation within cells, and only later vasogenic, water moving over the blood-brain barrier (BBB) into the interstitial space. Moderate intraischemic hypothermia reduces BBB disruption and subsequent edema and neuronal injury in experimental animals.[42] Given the impressive experimental findings pertaining to the benefit of peri- and postischemic hypothermia and the hyperthermia in hypoxic-ischemic brain injury, the time seems primed for clinical trials using moderate hypothermia in acute cerebral infarctions and global cerebral ischemia. It is also evident from experimental studies that hypothermia should be achieved within the first hours if it is to be of any benefit. Preliminary safety considerations suggest that efficacy of either mild postischemic hypothermia (34°C to 36°C) or prevention of hyperthermia should be tested.[98] The appropriate duration of hypothermia in cerebral ischemia needs to be determined. Pilot studies indicate that periods of up to 196 hours of moderate hypothermia can be managed with relative safety (Fig. 50.1). Effective methods to accomplish rapid cooling remain to be developed, but will probably involve a combination of selective brain cooling, systemic cooling, and pharmacologic manipulation of the temperature control mechanisms. Current protocols are using cooling blankets placed above and below the patient and nasogastric lavage with iced saline. Once rectal temperature reaches 33°C, patients are kept between 32°C and 34°C by adjusting the blanket thermostat. The sedative of choice is propofol in doses up to 50 μg/kg/min. The use of propofol prevents shivering in most instances. However, some patients may require continuous infusions of paralytics (vecuronium, 10 μg/h) and narcotics (fentanyl, 50 to 100 μg/h). For monitoring purposes, ICP sensors equipped with microthermistors to measure brain temperature should be introduced. This is particularly important since temperature gradients between body core and brain have recently been reported in stroke patients.[152] The rewarming interval is critical for patients with increased ICP during hypothermia and should be performed passively over a period of 10 to 12 hours (0.5°C/h[30,99]).

CRANIECTOMY

Since Cushing first described decompressive craniotomy for relief of ICP,[36] surgical decompression has been advocated as a treatment for severe brain edema associated with intracra-

nial hypertension. The effects of craniotomy on the biomechanical properties of the various intracranial compartments have been studied in experimental models. In the normal brain, craniotomy significantly increases the tissue compliance in the cortical gray matter, indicating that brain tissue is compliant in the presence of an open skull. High compliance in the brain tissue, in addition to that of the CSF space, is related to altered pressure-volume relationships within the intracranial cavity. In contrast, in the intact brain the compliance of the intravascular compartment remains constant after craniotomy. As a consequence, formation of brain edema may be facilitated.[72] The biomechanical effects of craniotomy in the normal brain may not be translated into those that occur in focal mass lesions. Decompressive craniotomy in the presence of large cerebral infarctions evidently reduces mortality and size of infarction in experimental animals.[43,54]

In the clinical setting, decompressive surgery may be considered for patients where medical measures fail to reduce ICP or where signs of downward displacement, such as pupillary abnormalities or horizontal shift with the Kernohan-Woltman phenomenon, occur. Decompressive craniectomy was first performed in patients with head-injury-related cerebral edema and has recently regained popularity with favorable results in patients with massive cerebellar and hemispheric infarctions.[38,74,103,131,137,139,140,150] The timing of craniotomy in the treatment of massive cerebral infarcts remains unknown and procedural details need to be investigated. Surgery should not be delayed until irreversible brain stem damage has occurred, as expected with bilateral fixed and dilated pupils. Brain stem acoustic-evoked potentials have been shown useful to assist in decision making toward craniectomy in posterior fossa mass lesions[87,90] and hemispheric mass lesions.[89,158] In a pilot study to determine the beneficial effect of craniotomy on outcome in massive hemispheric infarcts, mortality was decreased from >80% to 35% and among survivors, 65% were moderately and 35% severely disabled[140] (Fig. 50.2). The relation of infarct size and quality of leptomeningeal collaterals in proximal middle cerebral artery and intracranial internal carotid artery bifurcation occlusions raises the question of whether timely surgery in massive hemispheric infarctions may further improve outcome.[80] Effects of decompressive surgery performed at various stages after endovascular middle cerebral artery occlusion in experimental animals have corroborated this hypothesis.[43]

The rationale for decompressive surgery in massive hemispheric infarction is to allow for controlled "extracranial herniation," reduction of intracranial hypertension, and increased perfusion pressure. As a consequence, decompressive surgery should be performed as early as possible in patients who present with massive hemispheric infarcts and progressive decline of consciousness. Decision making for craniectomy is based on age, comorbidity, rapidity of clinical deterioration, extent and mass effect of infarction as demonstrated by CT, and presence of collateral blood flow. ICP monitoring did not prove helpful in management of patients with massive hemispheric stroke.[150] Therefore, we recommend early craniectomy be considered in patients with rapid clinical deterioration and CT signs of hemispheric infarction with midline shift and normal brain stem acoustic-evoked potentials.[140,158]

Recommendations for patients with massive cerebellar masses are similar (Fig. 50.3). Timely surgery is suggested to

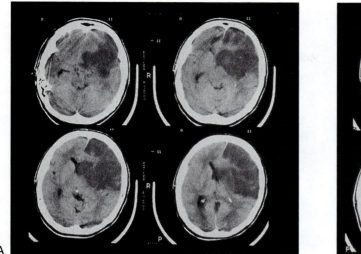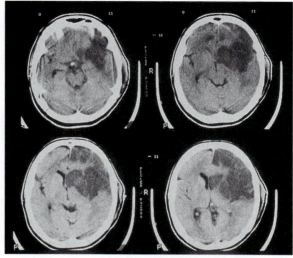

A   B

Figure 50.1 Effects of moderate hypothermia on edema in massive hemispheric stroke. (**A**) Note compression of the lateral ventricle and an anteroseptal shift of 5 mm prior to institution of hypothermia and (**B**) reduction of mass effect and subsequent decrease of anteroseptal shift to 2 mm after 12 hours of moderate hypothermia.

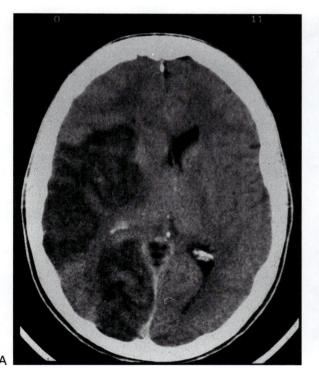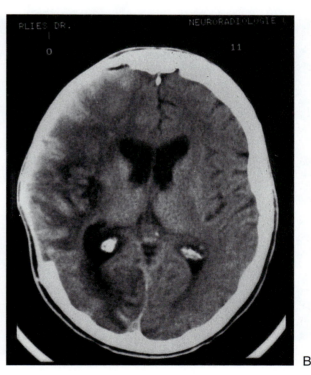

A   B

Figure 50.2 Effects of craniotomy in massive hemispheric stroke. (**A**) Presurgical scan in an obtunded patient with anisocoric pupils 24 hours after stroke onset. Note significant midline shift at the anteroseptal and pineal level. (**B**) Repeat scan was obtained 2 weeks after onset. This patient survived with a significant deficit including dense hemiplegia, left visual field cut and hemineglect, but remained cognitively intact and only occasionally needed assistance for his daily needs.

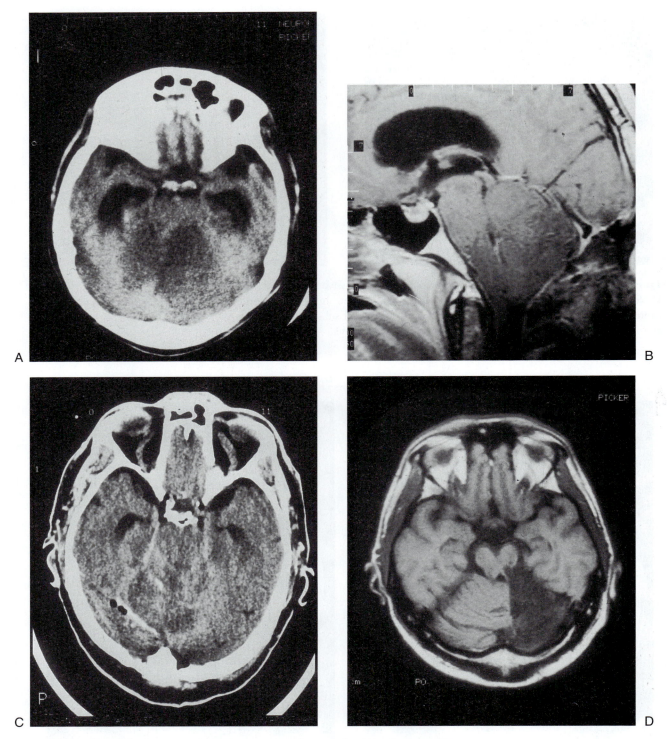

Figure 50.3 Effects of craniotomy in massive posterior fossa stroke. (**A**) Admission CT in a comatose patient reveals posterior fossa hypodensity indicative of a cerebellar stroke with significant brain stem compression and obstructive hydrocephalus. (**B**) Sagittal T₁-weighted MRI indicates severe brain stem compression with barely visible IV ventricle and impending tonsillar as well as upward transtentorial herniation. (**C**) Repeat CT 24 hours after surgical decompression of the posterior fossa and removal of infarcted tissue reveals decreasing hydrocephalus. (**D**) Axial T₁-weighted MRI shows residual tissue defect obtained on day 30.

avoid secondary brain stem injury.[103] Surgical strategies should be based on level of consciousness, CT evidence of hydrocephalus, and results of brain stem acoustic-evoked potentials.[87–89] Conscious individuals with no hydrocephalus can be managed by careful clinical observation and evoked potential studies. This approach is almost always successful when >48 hours have elapsed since the onset of stroke, but until this time, there must be awareness of the possibility of acute deterioration. In patients presenting with signs of hydrocephalus on CT, immediate surgical intervention is advisable.[94,139]

Concluding Remarks

The simultaneous development of understanding the molecular mechanisms underlying cell death, evaluating efficacy of pharmacologic interventions in animal stroke models, and advancements in measuring ischemic injury in patients will revolutionize the treatment of acute stroke. Therefore, neurocritical care for stroke requires adequate personnel and equipment to monitor and affect the anatomic, metabolic, and hemodynamic aspects of brain injury. This review includes the latest interdisciplinary critical care approaches to manage severe stroke. However, it has to be stressed that the time from onset to treatment is the crucial denominator of any therapeutic success. Attempts to institute treatment as early as possible require immediate reliable diagnosis of cerebral ischemia in presumed patients. Since recanalizing techniques can be beneficial only for salvageable neuronal tissue, the combination of immediate neuroprotection and early thrombolysis may augment therapeutic results.

References

1. Aaslid R, Lindegaard KF: Cerebral hemodynamics. pp. 60–85. In Aaslid R (ed): Transcranial Dopplersonography. Springer-Verlag, Vienna, 1986
2. Adams HP, Brott TG, Furlan AJ et al: Guidelines for thrombolytic therapy for acute stroke: a supplement to the guidelines for the management of patients with acute ischemic stroke. Circulation 94:1167–1174, 1996
3. Adams HP, Woolson RF, Clarke WR et al: Design of the trial of ORG 10172 in acute stroke treatment (TOAST). Implications for other trials of treatments of persons with acute ischemic stroke. Controlled Clinical Trials. Neurology, 1996
4. Albers GW, Goldberg MP, Choi DW: N-methyl-D-aspartate antagonists: ready for clinical trial in brain ischemia? *Ann Neurol* 25:398–403, 1989
5. Alexandrov AV, Black SE, Ehrlich LE et al: Simple visual analysis of brain perfusion on HMPAO SPECT predicts early outcome in acute stroke. Stroke 27:1537–1542, 1996
6. Alexandrov AV, Grotta JC, Davis SM, Lassen NA: Brain SPECT and thrombolysis in acute ischemic stroke: time for a clinical trial. *J Nucl Med* 37:1259–1262, 1996
7. Anderson DC, Cranford RE: Corticosteroids in ischemic stroke. Stroke 10:623–628, 1979
8. Archer DP, Shaw DA, Leblanc RL et al: Haemodynamic considerations in the management of patients with subarachnoid haemorrhage. Can J Anaesth 38:454–470, 1991
9. Aronowski J, Strong R, Grotta JC: Combined neuroprotection and reperfusion therapy for stroke. Effect of lubeluzole and diaspirin cross-linked hemoglobin in experimental focal ischemia. Stroke 27:1571–1577, 1996
10. Astrup J: Thresholds in cerebral ischemia—the ischemic penumbra. Stroke 12:723–725, 1981
11. Aucoin PJ, Kotilainen HR, Gantz NM et al: Intracranial pressure monitors: epidemiologic study of risk factors and infections. Am J Med 80:369–376, 1986
12. Baker CJ, Onesti ST, Solomon RA: Reduction by delayed hypothermia of cerebral infarction following middle cerebral artery occlusion in the rat: a time-course study. J Neurosurg 77:438–444, 1992
13. Baker AJ, Zornow MH, Grafe MR et al: Hypothermia prevents ischemia-induced increases in hippocampal glycine concentrations in rabbits. Stroke 22:666–673, 1991
14. Baron JC, von Kummer R, Del Zoppo GJ: Treatment of acute ischemic stroke: challenging the concept of a rigid and universal time window. Stroke 26:2219–2221, 1995
15. Benveniste H, Hedlund LW, Johnson GA: Mechanism of detection of acute cerebral ischemia in rats by diffusion weighted magnetic resonance microscopy. Stroke 23:746–754, 1992
16. Bergmann E Von: Ueber den Hirndruck. Arch Lin Chir 32:705–732, 1885
17. Branstom NM, Symon L, Crockhard HA, Pasztor E: Relationship between the cortical evoked potential and local cortical blood flow following acute middle cerebral artery occlusion in the baboon. Exp Neurol 45:195–208, 1974
18. Britt CW: Nontraumatic "spindle coma": clinical, EEG and prognostic features. Neurology 31:393–397, 1981
19. Britton M, Carlsson A, DeFaire U: Blood pressure course with acute stroke and matched controls. Stroke 17:861–864, 1986
20. Broaddus WC, Pendelton GA, Delashaw JB et al: Differential intracranial pressure recordings in patients with dual ipsilateral monitors. pp. 41–44. In Hoff JT, Betz AL (eds): Intracranial Pressure VIII. Springer-Verlag, Heidelberg, 1989
21. Brott TG, Reed RL: Intensive care for acute stroke in the community hospital setting: the first 24 hours. Curr Concepts Cerebrovasc Dis Stroke 24:1–5, 1989
22. Brown MM, Butler P, Gibbs J et al: Feasibility of percutaneous transluminal angioplasty for carotid artery stenosis. J Neurol Neurosurg Psychiatry 53:238–243, 1990
23. Busto R, Globus My-T, Dietrich WD et al: Effect of mild hypothermia on ischaemia-induced release of neurotransmitters and free fatty acids in rat brain. Stroke 20:904–910, 1989
24. Candelise L, Landi G, Orazio EN et al: Prognostic significance of hyperglycemia in acute stroke. Arch Neurol 42:661–663, 1985

25. Cardell M, Boris-Moeller F, Wieloch T et al: Hypothermia prevents the ischemia-induced translocation and inhibition of protein kinase C in rat striatum. J Neurochem 57:1814–1817, 1991

26. Cerebral Embolism Study Group: Immediate anticoagulation of embolic stroke. A randomized trial. Stroke 14: 668–676, 1983

27. Chiappa KH, Ropper AH: Long-term electrophysiologic monitoring of patients in the neurology intensive care unit. Semin Neurol 4:469–479, 1984

28. Churn SB, Taft WC, Billingsley MS et al: Temperature modulation of ischemic neuronal death and inhibition of calcium/calmodulin-dependent protein kinase II in gerbils. Stroke 21:1715–1721, 1990

29. Clark WM, Barnwell SL, Nesbit G et al: Safety and efficacy of percutaneous transluminal angioplasty for intracranial artherosclerotic disease. Stroke 26:1200–1204, 1995

30. Clifton GL, Allen S, Barrodale P et al: A phase II study of moderate hypothermia in severe brain injury. J Neurotrauma 10:263–271, 1993

31. Cole DJ, Drummond JC, Patel PM et al: Effect of oncotic pressure of diaspirin cross-linked hemoglobin (DCLHb) on brain injury after temporary focal cerebral ischemia in rats. Anesth Analg 83:342–347, 1996

32. Croughwell N, Smith LR, Quill T et al: The effect of temperature on cerebral metabolism and blood flow in adults during cardiopulmonary bypass. J Thorac Cardiovasc Surg 103:549–554, 1992

33. Cruz J: Combined continuous monitoring of systemic and cerebral oxygenation in acute brain injury: preliminary observations. Crit Care Med 21:1225–1232, 1993

34. Cruz J: Jugular venous oxygen saturation monitoring. (letter) J Neurosurg 77:162, 1992

35. Cruz J, Raps EC, Hoffstad OJ et al: Cerebral oxygenation monitoring. Crit Care Med 21:1242–1246, 1993

36. Cushing H: The establishment of cerebral hernia as a decompressive measure for inaccessible brain tumors: with the description of intermuscular methods of making the bone defect in temporal and occipital regions. Surg Gynecol Obstet 1:297–314, 1905

37. DeGraba TJ, Ostrow PT, Grotta JC: Threshold of calcium disturbances after focal cerebral ischemia in rats. Implications of the window of therapeutic opportunity. Stroke 24:1212–1217, 1993

38. Delashaw JB, Broaddus WC, Kassel NF et al: Treatment of right hemispheric cerebral infarction by hemicraniectomy. Stroke 21:874–881, 1990

39. DelZoppo GJ, Ferbert A, Otis S: Local intra-arterial fibrinolytic therapy in acute carotid territory stroke. A pilo study. Stroke 19:307–313, 1988

40. Denny-Brown D: The treatment of recurrent cerebrovascular symptoms and the question of "vasospasm." Med Clin North Am 35:1457–1474, 1951

41. Diener HC, Hacke W, Hennerici M et al: Lubeluzole in acute ischemic stroke: a double-blind, placebo-controlled, phase II trial. Stroke 27:76–81, 1996

42. Dietrich WD, Busto R, Halley M, Valdes I: The importance of brain temperature in alterations of the blood-brain barrier following cerebral ischemia. J Neuropathol Exp Neurol 49:486–497, 1990

43. Doerfler A, Forsting M, Reith W et al: Decompressive craniectomy in a rat model of "malignant" cerebral hemispheric stroke: experimental support for an aggressive therapeutic approach. J Neurosurg 85:853–859, 1996

44. Duke RJ, Block FR, Turpie AGG et al: Intravenous heparin for the prevention of stroke progression in acute partial stable stroke. A randomized clinical trial. Ann Intern Med 45:825–828, 1986

45. Eisenberg HM, Frankowski RF, Contant CF et al: High dose barbiturate control of elevated intracranial pressure in patients with severe head injury. J Neurosurg 69: 15–23, 1988

46. El-Ad B, Bornstein N, Fuchs P, Korczyn AD: Mechanical ventilation in stroke patients—is it worthwhile? Neurology 47:657–659, 1996

47. Estol C, Pessin MS: Anticoagulation: is there still a role in atherothrombotic stroke? Stroke 21:820–824, 1990

48. Farhat SM, Schneider RC: Observations on the effect of systemic blood pressure on intracranial circulation in patients with cerebrovascular insufficiency. J Neurosurg 27:441–445, 1968

49. Felber SR, Aichner FT, Sauter R et al: Combined magnetic resonance imaging and proton magnetic resonance spectroscopy of patients with acute stroke. Stroke 23: 1106–1110, 1992

50. Ferbert A, Buchner H, Brückmann H et al: Evoked potentials in basilar artery thrombosis: correlation with clinical and angiographic findings. Electroenceph Clin Neurophysiol 69:136–147, 1988

51. Fieschi C, Argentino C, Lenzi G et al: Therapeutic window for pharmacological treatment in acute focal cerebral ischemia. Ann NY Acad Sci 522:662–666, 1988

52. Eisher M, Sotak CH, Minematsu K et al: New magnetic resonance techniques for evaluating cerebrovascular disease. Ann Neurol 32:115–122, 1992

53. Forsting M, Krieger D, Von Kummer R et al: The prognostic value of collateral blood supply in acute middle cerebral artery occlusion. pp. 160–167. In DelZoppo GJ, Mori E, Hacke W (eds): Proceedings of the 2nd International Symposium on Thrombolytic Therapy in Acute Ischemic Stroke. Springer-Verlag, Berlin, Heidelberg, New York, 1993

54. Forsting M, Reith W, Schäbitz WR et al: Decompressive craniectomy for cerebral infarction. Stroke 26:259–264, 1995

55. Frank JI: Large hemispheric infarction, deterioration, and intracranial pressure. Neurology 45:1286–1290, 1995

56. Ginsberg MD, Prado R, Dietrich WD et al: Hyperglycemia reduces the extent of cerebral infarction in rats. Stroke 18:570–574, 1987

57. Globus MY-T, Busto R, Dietrich WD et al: Intra-ischaemic extracellular release of dopamine and glutamate is associated with striatal vunerability to ischemia. Neurosci Lett 91:36–40, 1988

58. Goslinga H, Eijzenbach V, Heuvelmans, JHA et al: Custom-tailored hemodilution with albumin and crystalloids in acute ischemic stroke. Stroke 23:181–188, 1992

59. Graham GD, Blamire AW, Howseman AM et al: Proton magnetic resonance spectroscopy of cerebral lactate and

other metabolites in stroke patients. Stroke 23:333–340, 1992

60. Grond M, Rudolf J, Neveling M et al: Immediate heparin after rt-PA therapy does not increase risk of hemorrhage, Abstracted. Stroke 28:266, 1997

61. Grosset DG, Straton J, McDonald I et al: Use of transcranial doppler sonography to predict development of a delayed ischemic deficit after subarachnoid hemorrhage. J Neurosurg 78:183–187, 1993

62. Grotta J, Pasteur W, Khwaja G et al: Elective intubation for neurologic deterioration after stroke. Neurology 45:640–644, 1995

63. Hacke W, Kaste M, Fieschi C et al: Intravenous thrombolysis with recombinant tissue plasminogen activator for acute hemispheric stroke. JAMA 274:1017–1025, 1995

64. Hacke W, Schwab S, DiGeorgia M: Intensive care of acute ischemic stroke. Cerebrovasc Dis 4:385–392, 1994

65. Hacke W, Schwab S, Horn M et al: The "malignant" middle cerebral artery infarction: clinical course and neuroradiological signs. Arch Neurol 53:309–315, 1996

66. Hacke W, Zeumer H, Ferbert A et al: Intra-arterial thrombolytic therapy improves outcome in patients with acute vertebrobasilar occlusive disease, Stroke 19:1216–1222, 1988

67. Hanson SK, Grotta JC, Rhoades H et al: Value of single-photon emission-computed tomography in acute stroke therapeutic trials. Stroke 24:1322–1329, 1993

68. Hara M, Yoshihisa K, Ikemoto Y: Propofol activates $GABA_A$ receptor-chloride ionophore complex in dissociated hippocampal pyramidal neurons in the rat. Anesthesiology 79:781–788, 1993

69. Harris CE, Grounds RM, Murray AM et al: Propofol for long-term sedation in the intensive care unit. Anaesthesia 45:366–372, 1990

70. Hart G: Cardiogenic embolism to the brain. Lancet 339:589–594, 1992

71. Hartmann A, Stingele R, Schnitzer MS: General treatment strategies for elevated intracranial pressure. pp. 101–116. In Hacke W (ed): Neuro Critical Care. Springer-Verlag, New York, 1994

72. Hatashita S, Hoff JT: The effect of craniectomy on the biomechanics of normal brain. J Neurosurg 67:573–578, 1987

73. The Hemodilution in Stroke Study Group: Hypervolemic hemodilution treatment in acute stroke. Results of a randomized multicenter trial using pentastarch. Stroke 20:317–323, 1989

74. Heros R: Cerebellar haemorrhage and infarction. Stroke 13:166–169, 1982

75. Higashida R, Halbach VV, Cahan L et al: Transluminal angioplasty for treatment of intracranial artery vasospasm. J Neurosurg 71:648–653, 1989

76. Higashida RT, Tsai FY, Halbach VV et al: Transluminal angioplasty, thrombolysis, and stenting for extracranial and intracranial cerebral vascular disease. J Intervent Cardiol 9:192–198, 1996

77. Homan RW, Herman J, Purdy P: Cerebral location of international 10–20 system electrode placement. Electroenceph Clin Neurophysiol 66:376–382, 1987

78. Hommel M, Boissel P, Cornu C et al: Termination of trial of streptokinase in severe acute ischaemic stroke. Lancet 345–57, 1995

79. Italian Acute Stroke Study Group: Haemodilution in acute stroke. Lancet i:318–321, 1988

80. Jansen O, Kummer R VON, Forsting M et al: Thrombolytic therapy in acute occlusion of the intracranial internal carotid artery bifurcation. Am J Neuroradiol 16:1977–1986, 1995

81. Jordan KG: Continuous EEG and evoked potential monitoring in the neuroscience intensive care unit. J Clin Neurophysiol 10:445–475, 1993

82. Jorgensen HS, Nakayama H, Raaschou HO et al: The effect of a stroke unit: reduction in mortality, discharge rate to nursing home, length of hospital stay, and cost. A community-based study. Stroke 26:1178–1182, 1995

83. Kachel R: Results of balloon angioplasty in the carotid arteries. J Endovasc Surg 3:22–30, 1996

84. Karnaze DS, Marshall LF, Bickford RG: EEG monitoring of clinical coma: the compressed spectral array. Neurology 32:289–292, 1982

85. Kay R, Wong KS, Yu YL et al: Low-molecular-weight heparin for the treatment of acute ischemic stroke. N Eng J Med 333:1588–1593, 1995

86. Kochhar A, Zivin JA, Lyden PD et al: Glutamate antagonist therapy reduces neurologic deficits produced by focal central nervous system ischemia. Arch Neurol 45:148–153, 1988

87. Krieger D, Adams H-P, Rieke K, Hacke W: Monitoring therapeutic efficacy of decompressive craniotomy in space occupying cerebellar infarcts using brainstem auditory evoked potentials. Electroenceph Clin Neurophysiol 88:261–270, 1993

88. Krieger D, Adams H-P, Rieke K et al: Prospective evaluation of prognostic significance of evoked potentials in acute basilar occlusion. Crit Care Med 21:1169–1174, 1993

89. Krieger D, Adams H-P, Schwarz S et al: Prognostic and clinical relevance of pupillary responses, intracranial pressure monitoring, and brainstem auditory evoked potentials in comatose patients with acute supratentorial mass lesions. Crit Care Med 21:1944–1950, 1993

90. Krieger D, Aschoff A: Evozierte Potentiale vor und nach Dekompressionskraniotomie bei raumforderndem Kleinhirninfarkt. Nervenarzt 60:36–39, 1989

91. Krieger D, Busse O, Schramm J, Ferbert A: German–Austrian Space Occupying Cerebellar Infarction Study (GASCIS): study design, methods, patient characteristics. J Neurol 239:47–49, 1992

92. Kummer R von, Hacke W: Safety and efficacy of intravenous tissue plasminogen activator and heparin in acute middle cerebral artery stroke. Stroke 23:646–652, 1992

93. Kummer R von, Meyding-Lamadé U, Forsting M et al: Sensitivity and prognostic value of early computed tomography in middle cerebral artery trunk occlusion. Am J Neuroradiol 15:9–15, 1994

94. Laun A, Busse O, Calatayud V, Klug N: Cerebellar infarcts in the area of supply of the PICA and their surgical treatment. Acta Neurochir (Wien) 1:295–306, 1984

95. Lavin P: Management of hypertension in patients with acute stroke. Arch Int Med 146:66–68, 1986

96. Ley-Pozo J, Ringelstein EB: Noninvasive detection of

occlusive disease of the carotid siphon and middle cerebral artery. Ann Neurol 28:640–647, 1990

97. Lisk DR, Grotta JC, Lamki LM et al: Should hypertension be treated after stroke? A randomized controlled trial using single photon emission computed tomography. Arch Neurol 50:855–862, 1993

98. Marion DW, Leonov Y, Ginsberg M et al: Resuscitative hypothermia. Crit Care Med, Suppl. 24:S81–S89, 1996

99. Marion DW, Penrod LE, Kelsey SF et al: Treatment of traumatic brain injury with moderate hypothermia. N Engl J Med 336:540–546, 1997

100. Marsh EE, Adams HP, Biller J et al: Use of antithrombotic drugs in the treatment of acute ischemic stroke. A survey of neurologists in practice in the United States. Neurology 64:1631–1634, 1989

101. Marshall LF, Smith RW, Shapiro HM: The outcome of aggressive treatment in severe head injuries: part I. the significance of intracranial pressure monitoring. J Neurosurg 50:20–30, 1979

102. Masdeu JC, Brass LM: SPECT imaging of stroke. J Neuroimaging, suppl. (1995) 5(Suppl 1):14–22.

103. Mathew P, Teasdale G, Bannan A, Oluoch-Olunya D: Neurosurgical management of cerebellar hematoma and infarct. J Neurol Neurosurg Psychiatry 59:287–292, 1995

104. Mathias K: Stent placement in supra-aortic artery disease. pp. 87–92. In Liermann DD (ed): Stents. State of the Art and Future Developments. Polyscience Publication, Inc. Morin Heights, Canada, 1995

105. Metz S, Slogoff S: Thiopental sodium by single bolus dose compared to infusion for cerebral protection during cardiopulmonary bypass. J Clin Anesth 2:226–231, 1990

106. Minematsu K, Fisher M, Li W et al: Effects of a novel NMDA antagonist on experimental stroke rapidly and quantitatively assessed by diffusion-weighted MRI. Neurology 48:397–403, 1993

107. Minematsu K, Li L, Sotak CH et al: Reversible focal ischemic injury demonstrated by diffusion-weighted magnetic resonance imaging in rats. Stroke 23:1304–1311, 1992

108. Minematsu K, Li W, Fisher M et al: Diffusion-weighted magnetic resonance imaging: rapid and quantitative detection of focal brain ischemia. Neurology 42:235–240, 1992

109. Mirski MA, Muffelman B, Ulatowski JA, Hanley DF: Sedation for the critically ill neurologic patient. Crit Care Med 23:2038–2053, 1995

110. Modica PA, Tempelhoff R: Intracranial pressure during induction of anaesthesia and trachael intubation with etomidate-induced EEG burst suppression. Can J Anaesth 39:236–241, 1992

111. Mohr JP, Orgogozo J, Harrison M et al: Meta-analysis of oral nimodipine trials in acute ischemic stroke. Cerebrovasc Dis 4:197–203, 1994

112. Mori E, Tabuchi M, Yoshida T, Yamadori A: Intracarotid urokinase with thromboembolic occlusion of the middle cerebral artery. Stroke 19:802–812, 1988

113. Mori E, Yoneda Y, Tabuchi M et al: Intravenous recombinant tissue plasminogen activator in acute carotid artery territory stroke. Neurology 42:976–982, 1992

114. Muizelaar JP, Marmarou A, Ward JD et al: Adverse effects of prolonged hyperventilation in patients with severe head injury: a randomized trial. Neurosurgery 75:731–739, 1991

115. Nagao S, Kuyama H, Honma Y et al: Prediction and evaluation of brainstem function by auditory brainstem responses in patients with uncal herniation. Surg Neurol 27:81–86, 1987

116. Nagao S, Roccaforte P, Moody RA: Acute intracranial hypertension and auditory brain-stem responses. part I: changes in the auditory brain-stem and somatosensory evoked responses in intracranial hypertensions in cats. J Neurosurg 51:669–676, 1979a

117. Nagao S, Roccaforte P, Moody RA: Acute intracranial hypertension and auditory brain-stem responses. part II: the effects of brain-stem movement on the auditory brain-stem responses due to transtentorial herniation, J Neurosurg 51:846–851, 1979b

118. National Institute of Neurological Disorders and Stroke rt-PA Stroke Study Group: Tissue plasminogen activator for acute ischemic stroke. N Engl J Med 333:1581–1587, 1995

119. Nau R, Prins F, Kolenda H, Prange H: Temporal reversal of serum to cerebrospinal fluid glycerol concentration gradient after intravenous infusion of glycerol, Eur J Clin Pharmacol 42:181–185, 1992

120. Nedergaard M, Astrup J: Infarct rim: effect of hyperglycemia on direct current potential and [C14]2-deoxyglucose phosporylation. J Cereb Blood Flow Metab 6:607–615, 1986

121. Nedergaard N, Jakobsen J, Diemer NH: Autoradiographic determination of cerebral glucose content, blood flow, and glucose utilization in focal ischemia of the rat brain: influence of plasma glucose concentration. J Cereb Blood Flow Metab 8:100–108, 1988

122. Nedergaard N, Diemer NH: Experimental cerebral ischemia: barbiturate resistant increase in regional glucose utilization. J Cereb Blood Flow Metab 8:763–766, 1988

123. Nedergaard N, Diemer NH: Focal ischemia of the rat brain with special reference to the influence of plasma glucose concentration. Acta Neuropathol 73:131–137, 1987

124. Neuwelt EA, Kikuchi K, Hill SA: Barbiturate inhibition of lymphocyte function. Differing effects of various barbiturates used to induce coma. J Neurosurg 56:254–259, 1982

125. Norenberg MD: A hypothesis of osmotic endothelial injury. A pathogenetic mechanism in central pontine myelinolysis. Arch Neurol 40:66–69, 1983

126. Norris JW: Steriod therapy in acute cerebral infarction, Arch Neurol 33:69–71, 1976

127. Norris JW, Hachinski VC: Megadose steroid therapy in ischemic stroke. Stroke 16:150, 1985

128. Orgitano TC, Wascher TM, Reichman OH et al: Sustained increased cerebral blood flow with prophylactic hypertensive hypervolemic hemodilution ("triple-H" therapy) after subarachnoid hemorrhage. Neurosurgery 27:729–739, 1990

129. Paczynski R, Hsu CY, Diringer MN: Pathophysiology of ischemic injury. In Fisher M (ed): Stroke Therapy, pp. 29–64. Butterworth–Heinemann, Boston, 1995

130. Pennington CR, Powell-Tuck J, Shaffer J: Review Arti-

cle: artificial nutritional support for improved patient care. Aliment Pharmacol Ther 9:471–481, 1995

131. Plum F: Critical care and acute severe stroke. Neurology Alert 15:26–28, 1996

132. Powers WJ: Acute hypertension after stroke: the scientific basis for treatment decisions. Neurology 43: 461–467, 1993

133. Pulsinelli WA, Levy DE, Sigsbee B et al: Increased damage after ischemic stroke in patients with hyperglycemia with or without established diabetes, Am J Med 74: 540–544, 1983

134. Puskas Z, Schuierer G: Determination of blood circulation time for optimizing contrast medium administration in CT-angiography. Radiologe 36:750–757, 1996

135. Ransom RB, Waxman SG, Davis PK: Anoxic injury of CNS white matter: protective effect of ketamine. Neurology 40:1399–1403, 1990

136. Reith W, Fisher M: Diffusion-weighted magnetic resonance imaging for acute ischemic stroke. Vasc Med Rev 5:307–317, 1994

137. Rengachary SS, Batnitzky S, Morantz RA et al: Hemicraniectomy for massive cerebral infarction, Neurosurgery 8:321–328, 1981

138. Ridenour TR, Warner DS, Todd MM et al: Mild hypothermia reduces infarct size resulting from temporary but not permanent focal ischemia in rats. Stroke 23: 733–738, 1992

139. Rieke K, Krieger D, Adams H-P et al: Therapeutic strategies in space occupying cerebellar infarction based on clinical, neuroradiological and neurophysiological data. Cerebrovasc Dis 3:45–55, 1993

140. Rieke K, Schwab S, Krieger D et al: Decompressive surgery in space-occupying hemispheric infarction: results of an open prospective trial, Crit Care Med 23: 1576–1587, 1995

141. Ringelstein EB, Biniek R, Weiller C et al: Type and extent of hemispheric brain infarctions and clinical outcome in early and delayed middle cerebral artery recanalization. Neurology 42:289–298, 1992

142. Ringelstein EB, Zeumer H, Poeck K: Non-invasive diagnosis of intracranial lesions in the vertebrobasilar system. A comparison of doppler sonographic and angiographic findings. Stroke 16:848–854, 1985

143. Rockoff MA, Ropper AH: Treatment of intracranial hypertension. In Ropper AH, Kennedy SK, Zervas NT (eds): Neurological and Neurosurgical Intensive Care. pp. 21–38. University Park Press, Baltimore, 1983

144. Ropper AH: Lateral displacement of the brain and level of consciousness in patients with acute hemispheral mass. N Engl J Med 314:953–958, 1986

145. Ropper AH, Shafran B: Brain edema after stroke: clinical syndrome and intracranial pressure, Arch Neurol 41: 26–29, 1984

146. Rosenbaum DM, Michaelson M, Batter DK et al: Evidence for hypoxia-induced, programmed cell death of cultured neurons. Ann Neurol 36:864–870, 1994

147. Rosenwasser RH, Delgado TE, Buchheit WA et al: Control of hypertension and prophylaxis against vasospasm in cases of subarachnoid hemorrhage: a preliminary report. Neurosurgery 12:658–661, 1983

148. Scandinavian Stroke Study Group: Multicenter trial of hemodilution in acute ischemic stroke. I. results in the total patient population, Stroke 18:691–699, 1987

149. Schnitzer MS, Aschoff A: Intracranial pressure monitoring. In Hacke W (ed): Neuro Critical Care. pp. 90–97. Springer-Verlag, Berlin, Heidelberg, New York, 1994

150. Schwab S, Aschoff A, Spranger M et al: The value of ICP monitoring in acute hemispheric stroke. Neurology 47:393–398, 1996

151. Schwab S, Rieke K, Aschoff A et al: Hemicraniectomy in space occupying hemispheric infarction: useful early intervention or desperate activism? Cerebrovasc Dis 6: 325–329, 1996

152. Schwab S, Spranger M, Aschoff A et al: Brain temperature monitoring and modulation in patients with severe MCA infarction. Neurology 48:762–767, 1997

153. Scurr JH, Coleridge-Smith PD, Hasty JH: Regimen for improved effectiveness of intermittent pneumatic compression in deep venous thrombosis prophylaxis. Surgery 102:817–820, 1987

154. Shikora SA, Ogawa AM: Enteral nutrition and the critically ill. Postgrad Med J 72:395–402, 1996

155. Sieber FE, Traystman RJ: Special issues: glucose and the brain. Crit care Med 20:104–114, 1992

156. Siesjö BK: Pathophysiology and treatment of focal cerebral ischemia. Parts I and II: pathophysiology, J Neurosurg 77:169–184, 1992

157. Silver FL, Norris JW, Lewis AJ, Hachinski VC: Early mortality following stroke: a prospective review. Stroke 15:492–496, 1948

158. Steiner T, Krieger D, Jauss M et al: Hemicraniectomy for massive cerebral infarction: presurgical prognostic factors. Stroke 26:172A, 1995

159. Steiner T, Mendoza G, De Georgia M et al: Prognosis of stroke patients requiring mechanical ventilation in a neurological critical care unit. Stroke 28:711–715, 1997

160. Stephan H, Sonntag H, Schenk HD et al: Effects of Disoprivan on cerebral blood flow, oxygen consumption and cerebral vascular reactivity. Anaesthetist 36:60–65, 1987

161. Strand T, Asplund K, Eriksson S et al: A randomized controlled trial of hemodilution therapy in acute ischemic stroke. Stroke 15:980–989, 1984

162. Stringer WA, Hasso AN, Thompson JR et al: Hyperventilation-induced cerebral ischemia in patients with acute brain lesions: demonstration by xenon enhanced CT. Am J Neuroradiol 14:475–484, 1993

163. Sussman BJ, Fitch TSP: Thrombolysis with fibrolysins in cerebral arterial occlusion. J Am Med Assoc 167: 1705–1709, 1958

164. Theron J: Angioplasty of brachiocephalic vessels. In Viñuela V, Halbach VV, Dion JE (eds): Interventional Neuroradiology: Endovascular Therapy of the Central Nervous System. pp. 167–180. Lippincott-Raven, Philadelphia, 1992

165. Théroux P, Ouimet H, Latoor JG et al: Prediction and prevention of myocardial infarction during the acute phase of unstable angina. J Am Coll Cardiol 1989, 13: 192A

166. Thom SR: Functional inhibition of leucocyte B2-integrins by hyperbaric oxygen in carbon monoxide me-

diated brain injury in rats. Toxicol Appl Pharmacol 123: 248–256, 1993

167 Tibbles PM, Perrotta PL: Treatment of carbon monoxide poisoning: a critical review of human outcome studies comparing normobaric oxygen with hyperbaric oxygen. Ann Emerg Med 24:269–276, 1994

168. TOAST-Investigators: Preliminary results of the trial ORG 10172 in acute stroke treatment (TOAST). Presented at the European Stroke Conference, May 29th, 1997, Amsterdam

169. Turpie AGG, Gent M, Cote R et al: A low-molecular-weight heparinoid compared with unfractioned heparin in the prevention of deep vein thrombosis in patients with acute ischemic stroke. A randomized, double-blind study. Ann Intern Med 117:449–456, 1992

170. Vander Ark GD, Pommerantz M: Reversal of ischemic neurological signs by increasing the cardiac output. Surg Neurol 1:257–258, 1979

171. Van Sandbrink H, Maas AJR, Avezaat CJJ: Continuous monitoring of partial pressure of brain tissue oxygenation in patients with severe head injury. Neurosurgery 38: 21–31, 1996

172. Wahlgren NG, MacMahon DG, De Keyser J et al for the INWEST study group: Intravenous Nimodipine West European Stroke Trial (INWEST) of nimodipine in the treatment of acute ischemic stroke. Cerebrovasc Dis 4: 197–203, 1994

173. Walters BB, Ojeman RG, Heros RC: Emergency carotid endarterectomy. J Neurosurg 66:817–823, 1987

174. Warach S, Li W, Ronthal M, Edelman RR: Acute cerebral ischemia: evaluation with dynamic contrast-enhanced MR imaging and MR angiography. Radiology 182:41–47, 1992

175. Warach S, Chien D, Li W et al: Fast magnetic resonance diffusion-weighted imaging of acute human stroke. Neurology 42:1717–1723, 1992

176. Weaver DD, Winn HR, Jane JA: Differential intracranial pressure in patients with unilateral mass lesions. J Neurosurg 56:660–665, 1982

177. Winer J, Rosenwasser R, Jimenez F: Electroencephalographic activity and serum and cerebrospinal fluid pentobarbital levels in determining the therapeutic endpoint during barbiturate coma. J Neurosurg 29:739–742, 1991

178. Wolfla CE, Luerssen TG, Bowman RM, Putty TK: Brain tissue pressure gradients created by expanding frontal epidural mass lesion. J Neurosurg 84:642–647, 1996

179. Wolpert SM, Brückmann H, Greenlee R et al: Neuroradiologic evaluation of patients with acute stroke treated with recombinant tissue plasminogen activator. Am J Neuroradiol 14:3–13, 1993

180. Wong KS, Lam WW, Liang E et al: Variability of magnetic resonance angiography and computed tomography angiography in middle cerebral artery stenosis. Stroke 27:1084–1087, 1996

181. Wood JH, Polyzoidis KS, Epstein CM et al: Quantitative EEG alterations after isovolemic hemodilution augmentation of cerebral perfusion in stroke patients. Neurology 34:764–768, 1984

182. Wyte SR, Shapiro HM, Turner P: Ketamine-induced intracranial hypertension. Anesthesiology 36:174–176, 1972

183. Xue D, Slivka A, Buchan AM: Tirilazad reduces cortical infarction after transient but no permanent focal cerebral ischemia in rats. Stroke 23:894–899, 1992

184. Yatsu FM, Zivin JA: Hypertension in acute ischemic stroke. Not to treat. Arch Neurol 42:999–1000, 1985

185. Zauner A, Bullock R, Di X, Young HF: CO2, pH, and temperature monitoring: evaluation in the feline brain. Neurosurgery 37:1168–1177, 1995

186. Zeumer H, Freitag HJ, Grzyska U, Neunzig HP: Local intra-arterial fibrinolysis in acute vertebrobasilar occlusion. Technical developments and recent results. Neuroradiology 31:336–340, 1989

187. Zeumer H, Freitag HJ, Zanella F et al: Local intra-arterial fibrinolytic therapy in patients with stroke: urokinase versus recombinant tissue plasminogen activator (r-TPA). Neuroradiology 35:159–162, 1993

188. Zeumer H, Hacke W, Kolmann HL, Poeck K: Lokale Fibrinolysetherapie bei Basilaristhrombose. Dtsch Med Wochenschr 107:728–732, 1982

189. Zeumer H, Hündgen R, Ferbert A, Ringelstein EB: Local intraarterial fibrinolytic therapy in inaccessible internal carotid occlusion. Neuroradiology 26:315–317, 1984

190. Zhang RL, Chopp M, Chen H et al: Postischemic (1 hour) hypothermia significantly reduces ischemic cell damage in rats subjected to 2 hours of middle cerebral artery occlusion, Stroke 24:1235–1240, 1993

191. Zivin JA, Grotta JC: Animal stroke models. They are relevant to human disease. Stroke 21:181–188, 1990

Thrombolytic and Defibrinogenating Agents for Ischemic and Hemorrhagic Stroke

THOMAS G. BROTT

WERNER HACKE

Rationale for the Use of Thrombolytic Agents

SELECTED EXPERIMENTAL OBSERVATIONS

The isolation of pharmacologic quantities of tissue plasminogen activator (tPA) and the first use of tPA in animal studies were reported in the 1980s.[90,103] In rabbits improved neurologic outcome was observed in those animals receiving tPA compared with those receiving placebo. Lysis required no longer than 15 minutes, and postembolization was effective for up to 45 minutes but not with treatment delays up to 60 minutes.[104]

Infarct volume and mortality was decreased when tPA was given to rats inflicted with embolic stroke.[81,82] Streptokinase normalized hemispheric blood flow, oxygen consumption, and oxygen extraction at 5 minutes but not at 30 minutes in a dog model.[22] In a baboon model, intracarotid urokinase improved neurologic outcome,[24] but intravenous tPA was ineffective.[23]

EMERGING CLINICAL OBSERVATIONS

Major milestones in the use of thrombolysis in patients with ischemic stroke were reported in 1995. The first encouraging results were reported from a large randomized trial of intravenous tPA conducted by the European Cooperative Stroke Study (ECASS) investigators.[44] This was followed by convincingly positive results from each of the two randomized trials of intravenous tPA carried out by the National Institute of Neurological Disorders and Stroke (NINDS) investigators.[76] Results became available from the three large randomized controlled trials[27,73,74] evaluating intravenous streptokinase as a treatment for acute ischemic stroke.

Intra-arterial strategies have continued to advance. The first randomized controlled trials of intra-arterial thrombolytic therapy were reported in 1996.[25,32] This chapter summarizes the results of these trials and touches on new developments in vascular biology, pharmacology, anatomic and clinical diagnosis, and combination therapies related to the opening of occluded arteries. Contemporary recommendations are presented at the conclusion of the chapter.

Table 51.1 Frequency of Occlusion and Size of Thrombi in Acute Ischemic Stroke

Study	No. of Patients	Time of Angiogram (h)	% with Occlusions[a]	% of Occlusions, ICA[b]	% of Occlusions, MCA stem[b]
Fieschi et al[37]	80	<6	76	23	33
Wolpert[100]	139	<8	81	28	48
del Zoppo et al[25]	80	<6	74	N/A	50 (M1 or M2)

Abbreviations: ICA, internal carotid artery; MCA, middle cerebral artery; PROACT, Prolyse in Acute Thromboembolism Trial.

[a] *Inclusion and exclusion criteria differed among studies (e.g., PROACT study accepted only patients with MCA occlusion).*

[b] *No exclusive category as some patients had tandem occlusions of the ICA and MCA.*

RADIOGRAPHIC IDENTIFICATION OF THROMBUS IN ISCHEMIC STROKE

Thrombolytic agents will be expected to be effective for patients with stroke only when an acute thrombus is present as the cause of the presenting symptoms. Several angiographic studies address the frequency of occluding thrombi.[25,32,37,98] Indirect observations came from the National Institutes of Health (NIH) tPA pilot study[12] (Table 51.1). Approximately 75% of patients with acute ischemic stroke had detectable thrombus. Most thrombi were large, and some were tandem, involving the internal carotid artery (ICA) and its middle cerebral artery (MCA) branch.

Angiography only identifies the major cerebral arteries and their larger branches, so the absence of arterial filling does not indicate absence of acute thrombus. Thrombi large enough in size to result in infarction may not be detected. However, to ensure appropriate patient selection, studies of fibrinolysins have excluded angiogram-negative patients.

The NINDS tPA Stroke Study[76] suggests that thrombosis in situ or acute emboli in small cerebral arteries or arterioles will cause small vessel, lacunar-type infarction. Patients with small vessel infarction receiving tPA had significantly better outcomes at 3 months compared with the placebo patients at 3 months. Similar but not better outcomes were noted in cardioembolic and atherothrombotic-embolic patients. The latter are most closely associated with arteriographically detectable clot.

THE NATURE OF CEREBROVASCULAR THROMBI

Experimentally new thrombi respond better to thrombolytic therapy.[54] Dissolution of platelet-poor thrombi is better than that of platelet-rich thrombi.[19] In the setting of acute stroke the morphology is largely unknown. In a postmortem series, 15 emboli were described by Masuda et al[68] (Fig. 51.1). The ages of these thrombi were not known. They consisted largely of cholesterol crystals, platelets, red blood cells, and fibrin. In another study of 12 patients who died following thrombolytic treatment, 3 patients had fibrin-poor emboli.[84] Studies of reti-

nal embolization demonstrate the heterogeneity of emboli: platelets, fibrin, calcium, and cholesterol emboli are the common types.[17] Bacteria, fat, air, and foreign bodies may also be seen.

In the living brain emboli may be seen with computed tomography (CT). Hyperdensity on CT, which follows the expected contour and position of an intracranial artery, is suggestive of thrombus.[94] Patients with atrial fibrillation have not been reported to have a lower incidence of the dense artery sign than patients with atheroembolic stroke.

THE FATE OF UNTREATED CEREBROVASCULAR THROMBI

Acute thrombi associated with acute stroke commonly recanalize spontaneously in a period of hours or days.[37] The seminal observations of Fieschi et al[37] involved 80 ischemic stroke patients receiving angiography within 6 hours of the onset of symptoms. In 61 of these 80 patients occlusions by thrombi were seen intracranially: in isolated arteries in 22, as plaques in the carotid accompanied by intracranial arterial occlusion in 20, and as ICA occlusion in 19. Repeat angiogram in 8 and transcranial doppler in 7 of the 15 patients with isolated occlusion of the MCA stem demonstrated spontaneous recanalization in 11 patients. The reperfusion occurred within 24 hours in four patients and in the other seven within 1 week. None of these patients showed significant neurologic improvement following recanalization. Several studies of serial angiography have established varying degrees of recanalization. In the study of Mori et al,[71] 2 of 12 patients with carotid territory artery occlusion had partial recanalization; none had full recanalization at 60 minutes. Yamaguchi et al[99] detected complete or partial recanalization in 47 untreated patients. Fourteen percent of patients exhibited spontaneous recanalization in the Prolyse in Acute Thromboembolism Trial (PROACT) study.[25]

The mechanism of spontaneous recanalization is unknown. The current rationale is that endogenous tPA activates fibrin-bound plasminogen on the surface of the thrombus, which then facilitates clot lysis. A relationship of endogenous tPA concentrations to spontaneous lysis has not been studied.

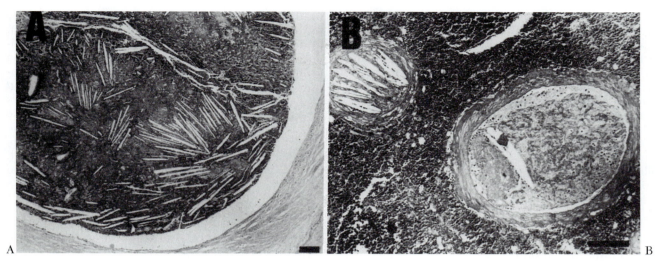

Figure 51.1 Morphologically different emboli, occurring simultaneously, totally occlude cerebral arteries. (**A**) A heterogeneous embolus occludes the right middle cerebral artery trunk. (**B**) Heterogeneous emboli occlude two branch arteries of the right middle cerebral artery. Cholesterol crystals are prominent in two of the three emboli. Scale bars = 100 μm. (From Masuda et al,[68] with permission.)

Thrombolytic Agents

STREPTOKINASE

The foundation of clinical thrombolysis was established in 1933 when Tillet and Garner[92] reported that streptococci released a substance that dissolved blood clots. Streptokinase is a single-chain protein with a molecular weight of 47,000 that exhibits little or no intrinsic enzymatic activity. However, streptokinase combines with plasminogen to form a one-to-one stoichiometric complex that activates plasminogen to plasmin. Streptokinase is not fibrin specific, and high circulating concentrations can result in depletion of plasminogen, fibrinogen, α-II-antiplasmin, and coagulation factors V and VIII. Depletion of these substances characterizes the lytic state, which may result in hemostatic failure. Depletion of platelet-bound fibrinogen, the molecular links of one platelet to another, may also occur and will inhibit platelet aggregation.

UROKINASE

Urokinase is a double-chain serine protease with a total molecular weight of 54,000 that directly activates plasminogen to plasmin.[7] Urokinase is not fibrin specific. It activates circulating plasminogen at rates equal to that of its activation of fibrin-bound plasminogen, hence high concentrations of urokinase may result in depletion of plasminogen, fibrinogen, α-II-antiplasmin, and coagulation factors V and VIII.

PRO-UROKINASE

Pro-Urokinase (pro-UK) is the inactive single-chain precursor of urokinase that has been isolated from urine, plasma, and cultured cells.[52] Pro-UK has intrinsic plasminogen-activating potential, but the efficiency is approximately 100-fold less than that of urokinase. When pro-UK undergoes proteolysis by plasmin or kallikrein, the activated form results. Pro-UK has significant fibrin specificity, which may result from preferential conversion of pro-UK to urokinase at the fibrin surface.[64] Pro-UK is under active clinical investigation, as described below. It is not generally commercially available.

RECOMBINANT TISSUE PLASMINOGEN ACTIVATOR

tPA is the plasminogen activator produced in physiologic concentrations endogenously. tPA is synthesized and secreted by endothelial cells and occurs as either a single- or double-polypeptide chain. The single chain form has a molecular weight of 70,000. The double-chain form results from a proteolytic cleavage of the single-chain form. tPA is relatively fibrin specific.[18] The presence of fibrin enhances the efficacy of plasminogen activation by two or three orders of magnitude.[51] In the absence of fibrin binding, tPA has very limited capability for plasminogen activation in plasma and so consumption of circulating fibrinogen is minimized. Recombinant DNA techniques are used to produce tPA for clinical use. The most widely used preparation is the single-chain form, alteplase. The double-chain form, duteplase, is also under investigation. Rapid clearance of tPA takes place in humans, largely through the liver, and so the serum half-life is approximately 4 to 6 minutes.[42] Importantly, the half-life of tPA in circulation can be greatly extended if tPA is bound to fibrin on clot because the primary inactivating sites are sequestered.

Plasminogen activator inhibitor type 1 (PAI-1) is a protease inhibitor that is the primary regulator of tPA activity. PAI-1 acts to inhibit tPA by forming a stable one-to-one stoichiometric complex. PAI-1 rapidly inhibits tPA in circulation but inhibits fibrin-bound tPA slowly.[97] PAI-1 is a 45,000 molecular weight protein that is synthesized by vascular endothelial cells. PAI-1 is also found in platelets. In platelet-rich clots the magnitude of PAI-1 can be enough to result in significant inhibitory activity at the site of a clot where activated platelets are present. Platelet PAI-1 may be one explanation why platelet-rich arterial thrombi can be resistant to lysis.[63,85]

Intravenous Thrombolysis for Cerebral Infarction

EARLY RANDOMIZED TRIALS OF INTRAVENOUS TISSUE PLASMINOGEN ACTIVATOR

In the late 1980s and early 1990s three small randomized trials of tPA were carried out. Although these studies were not adequately powered to demonstrate efficacy, they did demonstrate the feasibility of randomized study of very early thrombolytic therapy. The results suggested potential benefit and also acceptable safety.

In the study by Mori and colleagues,[71] 31 patients with acute carotid artery territory ischemic stroke who could be treated within 6 hours were randomized in double-blind fashion to receive either tPA (duteplase) or placebo over 60 minutes. Patients were randomized into one of three groups; 20 or 30 mega-international units of duteplase or placebo. Cerebral angiography was carried out before and after treatment. Complete or partial reperfusion was demonstrated for 47% of the tPA-treated patients compared with 17% of the placebo-treated patients. Patients given the higher tPA dose had a higher degree of clinical improvement compared with those treated with placebo. One parenchymal hemorrhage occurred in each of the three groups.

In the study of Yamaguchi and colleagues,[99] patients who could be treated within 6 hours were randomized to receive either 20 mega-international units of tPA (duteplase) or placebo over 60 minutes. Ninety-eight patients were randomized and had cerebral arteriography immediately after treatment. Arterial patency following treatment was significantly better in the tPA-treated patients; 21% had either complete or greater than 50% arterial patency compared with 4% of the placebo-treated patients. Clinically, 16% of the tPA-treated patients had marked improvement compared with 6% of the placebo-treated patients. Hemorrhagic transformation was similar in the two groups, with massive hemorrhage occurring in four of the tPA-treated PA-treated patients and five of the placebo-treated patients.

The smallest randomized trial reported was that of Haley and colleagues,[45] who emphasized time to treatment. Twenty patients were randomized to receive either tPA (alteplase) or placebo within 90 minutes of stroke onset, and an additional seven were randomized between 91 and 180 minutes to receive tPA or placebo. The dose of tPA was 0.85 mg/kg. In the 0- to 90-minute group, six tPA-treated patients improved by four or more points in the NIH Stroke Scale (NIHSS) score at 24 hours compared with one patient in the placebo group ($P < 0.05$). In the 91- to 180-minute group, there was no difference with regard to early improvement. One fatal intracerebral hemorrhage occurred, in the placebo group.

MAJOR RANDOMIZED TRIALS OF INTRAVENOUS TISSUE PLASMINOGEN FACTOR

European Cooperative Acute Stroke Study

ECASS[44] was the first large-scale randomized study of tPA as treatment for stroke. ECASS was a prospective, multicenter, double-blind, placebo-controlled study. Eligible patients with acute ischemic hemispheric stroke who could be treated within 6 hours from the onset of symptoms were randomized to receive 1.1 mg/kg of alteplase or placebo over 60 minutes, 10% given as a bolus. Heparin, oral anticoagulants, hemorheologic agents, and brain protective substances were prohibited during the first 24 hours. Patients were ineligible if they had very severe deficit with impairment of consciousness and/or forced head and eye deviation; had only mild neurologic deficit; or were already improving. In addition, patients with major early infarct signs on the baseline CT scan were to be excluded. If the baseline CT scan showed diffuse sulcal effacement, parenchymal hypodensity, and edema as evidenced by loss of gray-white differentiation involving more than 33% of the MCA territory, the patient was to be ineligible for ECASS. The other inclusion and exclusion criteria have been described.

The first primary hypothesis of ECASS was that there would be a difference between the tPA-treated and the placebo-treated groups in the activities of daily living at 3 months, defined as a difference of 15 points on the Barthel Index. The second primary hypothesis was that there would be a difference between the tPA- and the placebo-treated groups in the global clinical condition at 3 months, defined as a difference of one grade on the Modified Rankin Scale at 90 days after treatment. The primary analysis was to be intent to treat. However, the investigators prospectively anticipated a sizable proportion of protocol violators and so specified a definition of a target population. They also specified prospectively an analysis of that target population that would be performed at the conclusion of the study.

Over approximately 18 months, 620 patients were randomized at 75 centers in 14 European countries. In the intent-to-treat analysis, there was no statistically significant differ-

Table 51.2 Results of European
Cooperative Acute Stroke Study

	Intent to Treat Population (n = 611)		Target Population (n = 511)	
	tPA	Placebo	tPA	Placebo
Barthel Index (median)	85	75	90	80
Modified Rankin Scale Score 0–1 at 3 months (%)	36	29	41[a]	29[a]
Parenchymal hematoma (%)	20[a]	7[a]	19[a]	7[a]
30-Day mortality (%)	18	13	15	12

[a] Statistically significant (P <0.05).

(Data from Hacke et al.[44])

ence in either of the two primary endpoints (Table 51.2). To derive the target population, 109 patients were excluded from the intent-to-treat group; 66 of these exclusions were because of abnormalities on CT scan, 52 with major early infarction, 2 with primary hemorrhage, and 12 with the CT scan being either unavailable or unreadable. For the remaining target population of 511 there was no significant difference in the Barthel Index between the tPA-treated patients and the placebo-treated patients (P = 0.16) at 90 days after treatment (Table 51.2). The difference was significant in favor of the tPA-treated patients as measured by the Modified Rankin Scale. The median score at 90 days was 2 for the tPA-treated patients and 3 for the placebo-treated patients (P = 0.035).

Mortality at 30 days was not statistically different in the two groups, 17.9% for the tPA-treated patients and 12.7% for the placebo-treated patients (P = 0.08). At the end of the 90-day observation period, mortality was 18.9% in the tPA-treated patients compared with 15.8% in the placebo-treated patients (P = 0.04). Parenchymal hematoma was more common in the tPA-treated patients, occurring in 19.8% compared with 6.5% for the placebo-treated patients (P <0.001). With regard to safety, ECASS investigators noted a significant inverse relationship between protocol violation in patients treated with alteplase and 7-day survival (Fig. 51.2). They attributed this relationship in large part to treatment of patients with signs by CT scan of major cerebral infarction, that is, signs of cerebral infarction on the baseline CT scan already involving more than 33% of the MCA territory. This is discussed further below.

The NINDS tPA Stroke Study:
Part 1, Early Improvement

The NINDS tPA Stroke Study[76] was actually two clinical trials. Part I was designed to test early clinical effect. The primary hypothesis was that a greater proportion of patients treated with tPA compared with those treated with placebo would have early improvement (defined as complete resolution of neurologic symptoms at 24 hours or improvement in the NIHSS of 4 points or more). Patients were randomized to receive either 0.9 mg/kg of tPA over 60 minutes with 10% of the dose as a bolus, or placebo. Patients with all types of

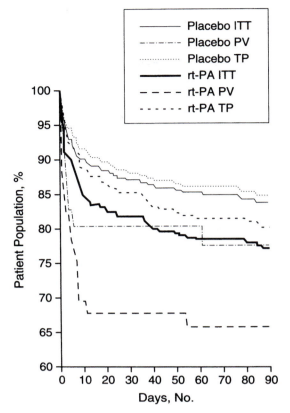

Figure 51.2 Kaplan-Meier curve for patients from the ECASS Trial: placebo intention-to-treat (ITT), placebo protocol violators (PV), placebo target population (TP), rt-PA intention-to-treat, rt-PA protocol violators, and rt-PA target population. Survival at 7 days is significantly lower in patients with protocol violations treated with rt-PA. Differences in survival between the rt-PA-treated patients and placebo groups reached significance only after 90 days in both the TP and ITT groups (note that the y-axis begins at 60%). (From Hacke et al,[44] with permission.)

ischemic stroke were eligible for this study if they could be randomized and treated within 180 minutes of symptom onset. Principal exclusion criteria are listed in Table 51.3. The trial was designed to ensure that approximately half of the patients would be randomized and treated within 90 minutes of symptom onset; the number of patients in the 91- to 180-minute group at a given clinical center could never exceed the number of patients in the 0- to 90-minute group by more than two.

Part 1 included 301 randomized patients. Sixty-seven (47%) of the 144 patients randomized to tPA had early improvement compared with 57 (39%) of the 147 patients randomized to placebo (relative risk, 1.2; P = 0.21). A post hoc comparison of the median NIHSS scores at 24 hours showed a median of 8 (interquartile range, 3 to 17) for the tPA-treated patients and 12 (interquartile range, 6 to 19) for the placebo-treated patients (P <0.02). Symptomatic intracerebral hemorrhage occurred in eight (6%) of the tPA-treated patients compared with none of the placebo-treated patients.

Table 51.3 NINDS rt-PA
Stroke Study Exclusion Criteria

Stroke or head trauma within the preceding 3 months

Major surgery within 14 days

Any history of intracranial hemorrhage

Systolic blood pressure >185

Diastolic blood pressure >110

Rapidly improving or minor symptoms

Symptoms suggestive of subarachnoid hemorrhage

Gastrointestinal hemorrhage or urinary tract hemorrhage within 21 days

Arterial puncture at a noncompressible site within 7 days

Seizure at the stroke onset

Patients taking anticoagulants with a prothrombin time >15 seconds

Patients receiving heparin within 48 hours and an elevated partial thromboplastin time

Platelet count <100,000

Blood glucose <50 mg/dl (2.7 mmol/L)

Blood glucose >400 mg/dl (2.7 mmol/L)

Patients were also excluded if aggressive measures were required to lower blood pressure to within the specified limits; patients responding to a single dose of labetalol were not excluded, but those requiring multiple doses of nitroprusside therapy for blood pressure control were excluded

Abbreviations: rt-PA, recombinant tissue plasminogen activator.

(Data from NINDS rt-PA Stroke Study Group.[76])

The NINDS tPA Stroke Study: Part 2, 3-Month Outcome

At the time of the final interim analysis of the results from Part 1, the Data and Safety Monitoring Committee determined that the prospectively defined 3-month outcome measures for the Part 1 patients favored the tPA group. Accordingly, the Committee recommended that a second trial be performed that should proceed with identical randomization procedures, eligibility criteria, and study logistics but that should address 3-month outcome. The primary hypothesis was that there would be a consistent and persuasive difference between the tPA and placebo groups in the proportion of patients who recovered with minimal or no deficit 3 months after treatment. Recovery with minimal or no deficit was defined as an NIHSS score of 0 or 1, a Barthel Index of 95 or 100, a modified Rankin Scale of 0 or 1, and a Glasgow Outcome Scale of 1. The results of these four scales were also to be combined into a global statistic of 3-month outcome. Three-month outcome measures for Part 2 were determined in a manner identical to that used to determine those measures for Part 1. At the time Part 2 was initiated, the clinical investigators were blinded to all results of Part 1, and they remained blinded to all results until completion of all follow-up for Part 2.

For the 333 patients randomized to receive tPA or placebo in Part 2, outcome at 3 months favored the tPA-treated patients for each of the four outcome measures (Table 51.4). The tPA-treated patients were 32%, 38%, 50%, and 55% more likely than placebo-treated patients to recover with minimal or no deficit by the four measures. The absolute percentage difference in the tPA-treated patients and the placebo-treated patients was 11% to 13%, implying that for every 100 patients treated with tPA, an additional 11 to 13 would recover compared with 100 patients not treated with tPA.

Symptomatic intracranial hemorrhage occurred in 12 (7%) of the tPA-treated patients compared with 2 (1%) of the placebo-treated patients, but early mortality was not higher.

Combined Results of NINDS tPA Trial

For 624 patients in Parts 1 and 2 of the NINDS trial, the benefits of tPA at 3 months were demonstrated for each of the four outcome measures. The relative and absolute differences between the tPA- and placebo-treated patients were nearly identical in Part 1 of the NINDS trial to those shown for Part 2. In this combined analysis, outcome at 3 months did not vary by stroke subtype at baseline. In other words, patients with infarcts thought to be secondary to small vessel occlusive disease benefitted as well as patients with infarcts thought to be secondary to large vessel occlusive disease or cardioembolic disease. The combined analysis revealed an overall symptomatic hemorrhage rate of 6.4% of the tPA-treated patients compared with 0.6% in the placebo-treated patients (P <0.001). However, mortality at 3 months in the combined analysis was not higher for the tPA-treated patients than for the placebo-treated patients (P = 0.30). Furthermore, severe disability and death were not higher in the tPA-treated patients.

RANDOMIZED TRIALS OF INTRAVENOUS STREPTOKINASE

Multicenter Acute Stroke Trial-Italy

The Multicenter Acute Stroke Trial-Italy (MAST-I) was a non-placebo-controlled, randomized trial of intravenous streptokinase for acute ischemic stroke[74] (Table 51.5). Interpretation of the results resulted in "disagreement [among the investigators] so profound that separate interpretations of the same study are required."[93] The clinical investigators reported the design, results, and their interpretation of the study[74] while the principal biostatisticians reported their differing interpretations.[93] The trial was designed to determine whether intravenous streptokinase, aspirin, or the combination of streptokinase and aspirin was superior to the absence of either of those therapies. Patients were eligible if they had symptoms compatible with acute ischemic stroke, could be randomized and treated within 6 hours of symptom onset, had a CT scan showing no evidence for hemorrhage, were not comatose, and did not have rapid resolution of neurologic symptoms. One hundred fifty-seven patients were randomized to receive streptokinase, 153 were randomized to receive aspirin (300 mg daily every day until day 10), 156 were randomized to receive streptokinase plus aspirin, and 156 were randomized to receive neither. Intravenous heparin, oral anticoagulants, and antiplatelet regimens were to be avoided, but subcutaneous heparin up to 15,000 units a day was allowed. A sample size of approximately 500 was anticipated.[65] The Data Monitoring

Table 51.4 Favorable Outcome at 3 Months in the NINDS rt-PA Stroke Study, Part 2[a]

	tPA (%)	Placebo (%)	Absolute % Difference	Odds Ratio (with 95% CI)	P Value
Global test				1.7 (1.2–2.6)	0.008
Barthel Index	50	38	12	1.6 (1.1–2.5)	0.026
Modified Rankin Scale	39	26	13	1.71 (0.1–2.5)	0.019
Glasgow Outcome Scale	44	32	12	1.6 (1.1–2.5)	0.025
NIHSS	31	20	11	1.7 (1.0–2.8)	0.033

[a] *Scores of 95 or 100 on the Barthel index, ≤1 on the NIHSS and Modified Rankin Scale, and 1 on the Glasgow Outcome Scale were considered a favorable outcome by the investigators.*

(Data from NINDS rt-PA Stroke Study Group.[76])

Committee suggested that the study be stopped at 622 patients because of excess early hazard in thrombolytic therapy.

The principal hypotheses of the study were that there would be a significant reduction of 6-month mortality and disability by both streptokinase and aspirin. For streptokinase, 196 of the 313 actively treated patients were dead or disabled at 6 months compared with 200 of the control patients, a negligible difference. For aspirin, 193 of the aspirin-treated patients were dead or disabled at 6 months compared with 203 of the 313 control patients, again a negligible difference. Therefore, the study was negative. Patients treated with streptokinase alone or with aspirin had a higher case fatality than patients treated with aspirin alone or with neither aspirin nor streptokinase (odds ratio, 2.7; 95% confidence interval, 1.7 to 4.3; 2 P <0.001).

Multicenter Acute Stroke Trial-Europe

The Multicenter Acute Stroke Trial-Europe (MAST-E) was a multicenter, placebo-controlled, randomized trial with 48 centers in France and the United Kingdom[73] (Table 51.5). Patients with moderate to severe ischemia in the territory of the middle cerebral artery were randomized to receive either intravenous streptokinase (1.5 million units over 1 hour) or placebo, within 6 hours after the onset of the stroke. The primary efficacy endpoint was combined mortality and severe disability at 6 months (severe disability Rankin Scale score of ≥3). The trial was designed for a population of 600 patients, but the Data Monitoring Committee recommended stopping the trial early when 310 patients had been randomized because of increase in mortality among the streptokinase-treated patients, secondary to intracerebral hemorrhage. At 6 months, 124 (79%) of the streptokinase-treated patients had died or were disabled compared with 126 (82%) of the placebo-treated patients; mortality was 47% for the streptokinase-treated patients at 6 months compared with 38% for the placebo-treated patients (P = 0.06) (Table 51.5). The difference in mortality could largely be attributed to the higher rate of hemorrhagic transformation of cerebral infarction in the streptokinase-treated patients. Symptomatic intracerebral hemorrhage occurred in 21% of the streptokinase-treated patients compared with 2.6% of the placebo-treated patients (P <0.001).

In contrast to the NINDS tPA Stroke Study and ECASS, the use of heparin, oral anticoagulants, or aspirin was not prohibited during the first 24 hours in MAST-E. Thirty-one percent of the streptokinase-treated patients and 12% of the placebo-treated patients received heparin within 12 hours of randomization (P = 0.04), which could have adversely af-

Table 51.5 Randomized Trials of Streptokinase

Study	Time to Treatment (h)	No. of Patients	Treatment Group	Mortality (%)	Intracerebral Hematoma (%)
Multicenter Acute Stroke Trial–Italy[73] (MAST-I)[b]	≤6	622	SK + 300 mg ASA vs	34[a]	10[a]
			SK vs	19	6[a]
			300 mg ASA vs	10	2
			standard therapy	13[a]	0.6[a]
Multicenter Acute Stroke Trial–Europe[74] (MAST-E)[b]	≤6	270	SK vs	35[a]	18[a]
			placebo	18[a]	3[a]
Australian Streptokinase Study[27] (ASK)[b]	<4	340	SK + 100 mg ASA vs	36[a]	13
			placebo + 100 mg ASA	21[a]	3

[a] *P ≤ 0.05.*

[b] *All studies terminated prior to completion due to increased mortality in treatment group.*

fected safety, particularly in the streptokinase-treated patients.

Australian Streptokinase Trial

In the Australian Streptokinase Trial (ASK), patients were randomized earlier, within 4 hours from symptom onset[27] (Table 51.5). In addition, the investigators prospectively planned a comparison of those patients randomized within 3 hours of symptom onset with those patients randomized 3 to 4 hours from symptom onset.

The sample size was designed to be 600,[28] but the Safety Monitoring Committee advised that the trial be suspended because of significantly poorer outcomes among streptokinase-treated patients receiving treatment >3 hours after stroke. The rate of recruitment of patients for randomization <3 hours following symptom onset was thought to be too low to justify continuing the trial for that group alone, and so ASK was terminated. Three hundred forty patients were randomized from 40 centers. The groups were well balanced. The primary outcome measure was the combination of death and disability, with the latter defined as a Barthel Index <60 3 months after the stroke. This unfavorable outcome occurred in 48.3% of the streptokinase-treated patients compared with 44.6% for the placebo-treated patients (the relative risk for an unfavorable outcome following streptokinase treatment was 1.08 [95% confidence interval, 0.74 to 1.86]). A significant difference was seen between the relative risks for early and late treatment outcomes ($P = 0.04$). The relative risk for an unfavorable outcome following streptokinase treatment in patients treated in ≤3 hours was 0.66 (95% confidence interval, 0.28 to 1.58). However, for patients treated beyond 3 hours from stroke onset, the relative risk for an unfavorable outcome in the streptokinase-treated patients was 1.22 (95% confidence interval, 0.80 to 1.86).

This difference with regard to time to treatment was not noted in the incidence of intracerebral hematoma. Overall, hematoma occurred in 13.2% of the streptokinase-treated group (12.6% symptomatic) and in 3% in the placebo-treated group (2.4% symptomatic) ($P < 0.01$). The hematoma rate in patients treated within 3 hours was 9.8% for the streptokinase-treated patients and 0% in the placebo-treated patients.

In addition to intracranial hematoma formation, hypotension was a problem in ASK. A decrease in systolic blood pressure of >20 mmHg within a few minutes of initiation of streptokinase or placebo occurred in 33% of the streptokinase-treated patients compared with 6% in the placebo-treated patients. Four patients (2.2%) had anaphylactic shock.

The differential effect with regard to treatment within 3 hours compared with treatment beyond 3 hours demonstrated in ASK is a finding consistent with but more robust than the time effect reported from the NINDS tPA pilot studies. In addition, when time was used as a continuous variable, there was a trend toward increased death and disability with later streptokinase treatment ($P = 0.10$).

Concerns Regarding the Streptokinase Trials

The negative results from these streptokinase studies are unsettling (Table 51.5). The differences in results from those reported in the NINDS tPA Stroke Study[76] could relate to time of treatment, dose of streptokinase, and difference in the two thrombolytic drugs. In contrast to the NINDS tPA Stroke Study, a small minority of patients in the streptokinase trials were treated in <3 hours of symptom onset. For example, in MAST-I 26% of the patients were randomized within 3 hours. In ASK, 21% of the patients were randomized within 3 hours. In the NINDS tPA Stroke Study, all 624 patients were randomized within 3 hours and 302 (48%) were randomized within 90 minutes. Such very early treatment occurred in only 3 (1%) of the 340 ASK patients. Later treatment may be particularly important if patients with signs of major cerebral infarction by CT scan are not excluded from treatment. These patients had a particularly high rate of adverse outcome in ECASS.[44] The dose of intravenous streptokinase used in the three trials was 1.5 million units, identical to the dose used for myocardial infarction. By contrast, the doses of tPA used in the NINDS trial and ECASS were significantly lower than those used for myocardial infarction (approximately 60% and 77% of the myocardial infarction dose, respectively). The lower dose of tPA used in the NINDS trial was determined as the result of dose escalation safety trials. One pilot trial with 52 patients was performed prior to initiation of the streptokinase trials.[28]

Predictors of Good Outcome Following Intravenous Thrombolysis

Although the NINDS tPA Study was conducted in two parts, the post hoc subgroup analysis combined the results.[79] Variables were chosen for analysis that might influence the outcome regardless of treatment. Twenty-nine baseline variables were examined. In the univariate analysis, race, diabetes, hypertension, baseline mean arterial pressure, and baseline systolic blood pressure showed a significant interaction with tPA treatment. In a reconstructed multivariate model, none of the variables examined significantly interacted with treatment. Patients of a particular age, race, gender, and so forth had neither more nor less likelihood of benefiting from tPA, implying generalized efficacy of tPA for acute ischemic stroke. Whether or not the patients were treated with tPA, diabetes, admission mean arterial pressure by age interaction, thrombus on baseline CT scan, and age by NIHSS score interaction were independently associated with fewer favorable outcomes.

Predictors of good outcome are also being examined by the ECASS investigators.[29] In their initial report, they suggested that age younger than 70 years, treatment with recombinant tPA, a normal initial CT scan, a favorable Scandinavian Stroke Scale score, the absence of diabetes or cardiac conditions, and the absence of hypertension may predict a good outcome. They categorized their MCA territory infarctions into subcortical and combined cortical/subcortical.[16] Because they saw no difference in the number of subcortical infarctions in the tPA group (23%) compared with the placebo group (21%), they hypothesized that thrombolysis does not prevent subcortical infarction.

In the randomized trials of streptokinase (MAST-E,

MAST-I, ASK), subgroup analyses have also been performed in an attempt to generate hypotheses regarding ideal patients for treatment. The MAST-E investigators reported that good outcome, after excluding patients with symptomatic hemorrhage, was only predicted by the unified neurologic score.[50] Subgroup analysis of the MAST-I trial will be more complicated given the factorial design of this study and the absence of a placebo-treated group.[66] The ASK investigators identified time-to-thrombolytic treatment as a significant influence on response to thrombolytic therapy.[20,27] In their study, treatment of acute ischemic stroke with streptokinase was not beneficial. However, poor outcomes were confined to those patients receiving therapy beyond 3 hours after onset; those receiving therapy less at ≤3 hours from symptom onset had improved outcome (odds ratio for a poor outcome, 0.4, 95% confidence interval, 0.1 to 1.0). The ECASS investigators reported no increase in the rate of hemorrhage in the patients in their study treated in <3 hours compared with patients treated 3 to 6 hours after symptom onset. Time to treatment did not seem to be a predictor of hemorrhage in the ASK trial. There was no significant difference in the incidence of either hemorrhagic transformation or hematoma formation between the patients treated within 3 hours and the patients treated after 3 hours.

Adequacy of collateral circulation is also a predictor of good outcome following thrombolysis. Collaterals were not addressed in the large intravenous trials but have been studied as part of intra-arterial thrombolysis case series.[15,38,87] Recently, a prospective study of 77 patients confirmed the relationship of small clot size with lysis mentioned above; results showed that rates of recanalization at 8 hours were 73% for MCA branches, 27% for the MCA stem, and only 14% for the intracranial internal carotid bifurcation. When collaterals were good or scarce, recanalization at <8 hours from symptom onset had no predictive value for good outcome independent of the collaterals. Predictors of poor outcome were parenchymal hypodensity by CT scan at the time of treatment involving ≥50% of the MCA territory ($P = 0.002$), scarce collaterals ($P = 0.009$), and site of occlusion ($P = 0.017$).

Safety of Intravenous Thrombolysis

INTRACRANIAL HEMORRHAGE

Intravenous thrombolytic therapy carries a risk. Intracranial hemorrhage has complicated its use in patients with myocardial and cerebral infarction.

In the NINDS tPA Stroke Study, symptomatic intracranial hemorrhage within 6 hours occurred in 20 (6.4%) of the tPA-treated patients compared with 2 (0.6%) of the placebo-treated patients ($P < 0.001$).[76] Tables 51.2 and 51.5 show the incidence of intracranial hematoma from other intravenous thrombolysis studies. Methodologic differences include inclusion/exclusion criteria, differences in definitions of hematoma, differences in assessment by CT, and differences in the use of heparin. Caution in comparisons is required.

Symptomatic intracerebral hemorrhage in the setting of intravenous thrombolytic therapy[12,26] is similar to that of spontaneous intracerebral hemorrhage.[11] Decline in level of consciousness, headache, nausea and vomiting, abrupt rise in systemic blood pressure, increase in the initial focal neurologic deficit, or the appearance of a new neurologic deficit should prompt an emergency CT scan. The case-mortality rate is also similar to that for spontaneous intracerebral hemorrhage.[10,12,26]

Risk Factors of Intracranial Hemorrhage

Later time to treatment, higher dose of thrombolytic agent, elevated blood pressure, and severity of neurologic deficit have been suggested as potential risk factors. Small numbers make conclusions difficult.

Regarding *time to treatment*, in the Burroughs Wellcome dose-escalation safety study, patients with hemorrhage transformation were treated with tPA later (6.1 ± 1.5 hours) than patients without hemorrhagic transformation (5.3 ± 1.7 hours; $P < 0.05$). In addition, the rate of intracranial hemorrhage in the randomized trials of tPA and streptokinase was lowest in the NINDS tPA trial (6.4%), in which all patients were treated within 3 hours, nearly half within 90 minutes. Nonetheless, a multivariable analysis of intracerebral hemorrhage occurring in patients treated in the NIH tPA pilot studies did not show an association of time to treatment.[63] The rate of symptomatic hemorrhage in the NINDS tPA Stroke Study was not significantly different among patients treated at 0 to 90 minutes compared with patients treated at 90 to 180 minutes.[76]

With regard to *dose of thrombolytic* agent and the occurrence of intracranial hemorrhage, the data are suggestive but not conclusive. In those studies using doses of either tPA[44] or streptokinase[27,73,74] approaching or equivalent to the doses used for myocardial infarction, the rates of intracranial hemorrhage have been higher than in the NINDS trials,[76] in which a dose approximately 75% of that used for myocardial infarction was administered. Other differences in these trials make interpretation difficult. In the NIH tPA pilot studies,[12] intracranial hemorrhage did not occur in patients treated with ≤0.6 mg/kg of tPA, and the multivariable analysis of that patient population showed that dose of tPA was significantly related to the occurrence of intracerebral hematoma.[63] The study of Trouillas and colleagues[95] reported the lowest hematoma rate of any of the late thrombolysis studies, that is, studies treating patients >4 hours and <8 hours after stroke onset. With 0.8 mg/kg of tPA over 90 minutes, the hematoma rate for the 43 treated patients was only 6.9%, essentially identical to that in the NINDS trial, in which the dose was 0.9 mg/kg, but patients were treated earlier and without early heparin.

Severe hypertension has been suspected as a significant predictor of thrombolysis-related intracranial hemorrhage. In the NIH pilot studies, diastolic hypertension was significantly associated with the occurrence of intracranial hemorrhage.[63] However, in the much larger NINDS tPA Stroke Study, neither systolic nor diastolic blood pressure were significantly associated with the occurrence of symptomatic hemorrhage among the tPA-treated patients in the final multivariable model.[78] This model was the primary model for the hemorrhage analysis and included only the 20 symptomatic hemorrhages that occurred in the tPA-treated patients. The small number of hemorrhages limited the predictive power of the model. When the investigators combined symptomatic with asymptomatic hemorrhage in all patients,[78] both the tPA-treated patients and the placebo-treated patients, the final multivariable model included pulse pressure (odds ratio, 1.02 mmHg; 95% confidence interval, 1.004 to 1.035) and minor external bleeding. Because pulse pressure was so highly correlated with other indices of blood pressure such as systolic blood pressure and diastolic blood pressure, those variables too could have been associated with the occurrence of symptomatic or asymptomatic intracranial hemorrhage. Severe hypertension was not reported as a risk factor for hemorrhagic transformation in the ECASS trial,[60] the MAST-E trial,[72] or the MAST-I[67] trial in the analyses published thus far.

Severity of initial neurologic deficit was associated with the occurrence of symptomatic intracranial hemorrhage in the NINDS tPA Stroke Study hemorrhage analysis.[78] Patients with a baseline NIHSS score of >20 (very severe deficit) were 11 times more likely to develop a symptomatic intracranial hemorrhage than patients with an initial NIHSS score of ≤5 (mild deficit). The ECASS investigators used logistic regression models to examine risk factors for hemorrhagic transformation.[60] For hemorrhagic infarction, they found clinical severity of stroke (odds ratio, 2.5) and the presence of early ischemic changes on baseline CT scan (odds ratio, 3.5). The risk factor for parenchymal hematoma was that of advanced age (odds ratio, 1.3 by 10 years of age). The MAST-I investigators[67] reported that neurologic severity at baseline was a significant predictor of subsequent hemorrhagic transformation.

The *baseline CT scan* has been particularly important with regard to predicting subsequent intracranial hemorrhage following thrombolytic therapy. The ECASS investigators were the first to suggest this possibility in their initial report, in which protocol violators who received tPA had a significantly worse outcome than the other patients.[44] They subsequently followed up with an analysis of CT scan and other factors that might predict the subsequent thrombolysis-related intracranial hemorrhage referred to above.[60] A central reading of all the baseline CT scans was carried out by von Kummer and Hacke.[96] They found that the presence of early ischemic changes on the baseline CT scan resulted in an odds ratio of 3.5 ($P = 0.001$) for the occurrence of subsequent hemorrhagic infarction. In the NINDS study, the incidence of early abnormalities, defined as mass effect and edema (acute hypodensity), was low. For symptomatic intracerebral hemorrhages occurring in the tPA-treated patients, the final multivariable model included severity, as mentioned above, but also abnormal baseline CT scan (i.e., the presence of mass effect or brain edema [acute hypodensity]). The odds ratio for the early CT abnormalities and the occurrence of symptomatic hemorrhage was 7.8, with a 95% confidence interval of 2.2 to 27.1. The limitations of the predictive model are considerable. In the MAST-E streptokinase trial, the degree of abnormality on the baseline CT scan was found to be a predictor of hemorrhagic transformation.[72]

Arterial recanalization has been suspected to be a risk factor for hemorrhage. The issue is not settled, given the small numbers of patients in studies in which angiography was required before and after the initiation of thrombolytic therapy.[26,71,99] From these observations, arterial recanalization may not be a risk for hemorrhage.

Minimizing Intracranial Hemorrhage

The lack of definitive information about risk factors limits efforts to prevent thrombolysis-related intracranial hemorrhage. Thrombolytic therapy should be initiated as soon as possible. Pending results from the two ongoing trials of tPA begun 3 to 5 hours after symptom onset, nonprotocol use of tPA should be limited to patients who can be treated within 3 hours. Treatment should be limited to patients with an initial systolic blood pressure of ≤185 mmHg or diastolic blood pressure ≤110 mmHg. Change in level of consciousness, neurologic deterioration, headache, nausea and vomiting, or the development of acute hypertension should be carefully monitored. These developments could herald the beginning of intracranial hemorrhage and should prompt interruption of thrombolytic therapy and performance of an emergency CT scan. As in spontaneous intracerebral hemorrhage, the appropriate treatment of thrombolysis-related intracerebral hemorrhage is not well established.

SYSTEMIC HEMORRHAGE

Systemic hemorrhage is uncommon following intravenous thrombolytic therapy for stroke. In the NIH tPA pilot stroke studies,[46] one case of fatal pericardial tamponade was reported, and a second case was recently reported by the Emergency Management of Stroke (EMS) investigators.[31] In the NINDS tPA Stroke Study,[76] serious systemic bleeding occurred in five of the tPA-treated patients and in none of the placebo-treated patients; none of these events were fatal. In the ECASS investigation,[44] four tPA-treated patients and two placebo-treated patients had systemic bleeding complications, but none required transfusion. The MAST-E investigators[73] and the ASK investigators[27] reported no serious systemic hemorrhagic complications. Systemic bleeding was observed in two patients in the MAST-I receiving streptokinase and in seven patients receiving aspirin.[74] Severe systemic hemorrhage (requiring transfusion) occurred in two patients, one receiving streptokinase and one aspirin.

REPERFUSION INJURY AND EDEMA

Delayed lysis of a thrombus in the stem of the MCA or one of the larger branches following the beginning of substantial irreversible neuronal injury might result in edema, secondary to either breakdown of the blood-brain barrier or the effects of free radical-related amplification of neuronal injury. Cerebral edema increases temporally following the onset of ischemic stroke. It is not possible to separate evolving edema secondary to the primary injury from edema secondary to clot lysis and reperfusion. Two cases suggestive of severe edema have been reported[58] in which the authors suggested reperfusion injury as the mechanism of the edema and clinical deterioration.

ARTERIAL REOCCLUSION

Arterial reocclusion after successful thrombolysis is an important potential complication. It has been reported in 15% or more patients with successful thrombolysis for myocardial infarction.[30,47] Intravenous thrombolysis stroke trials did not allow direct assessment of arterial reocclusion. The five large randomized trials of thrombolytic therapy have identified a potential problem with reocclusion. In the angiographically based series of high-dose tPA discussed above, reocclusion at 24 hours occurred in 1 of 11 patients with complete or partial recanalization at 8 hours. Reocclusion in the setting of cerebral infarction may be less than in myocardial infarction. Most ischemic stroke patients have either a cardioembolic or an atheroembolic mechanism for their stroke. The embolus lodges in a distal normal vessel. With lysis of the clot, no underlying complex atherosclerotic plaque is left behind to trigger acute thrombus formation.

SECONDARY EMBOLIZATION

Most ischemic stroke patients in the thrombolytic trials were thought to have an embolic etiology, either cardioembolic or atheroembolic. The presumed mechanism is that of a thrombus generated either from the surface of an abnormality in the vessel wall or from a pre-existing thrombus. Systemic thrombolysis has the potential to dislodge further embolic material from the source of the original symptom-producing thrombus. Lysis of a pre-existing cardiac, aorta, or cervical thrombus with embolization has been identified.[55] Unintended embolism could result from the therapeutic fragmentation of the original occluding thrombus. For example, when an M1 thrombus is broken up by an intravenous lytic agent, the resulting smaller particles may be large enough to lodge and occlude downstream M2 or M3 branches. This latter circumstance has been documented radiographically in the setting of local intra-arterial thrombolysis. Secondary embolization would be difficult if not impossible to prove in the setting of intravenous thrombolysis.

Data from Selected Case Series

INTERNAL CAROTID ARTERY OCCLUSION

Jansen and colleagues[53] reported recanalization after intravenous tPA in 16 patients (12.5%) with intracranial ICA occlusion. Treatment was administered within 8 hours of the onset of symptoms. Intracranial hemorrhage occurred in 1 of the 16 patients. The clinical outcomes were generally poor. In a dose-escalation safety study of tPA (alteplase), ICA occlusion was identified in 28 of 139 patients with acute stroke within 6 hours of symptom onset.[26] The recanalization rate for intracranial ICA occlusion was 8%.

VERTEBRAL BASILAR INFARCTION

In 51 consecutive patients from Heidelberg, only 6 patients were treated intravenously (70 to 100 mg of tPA), and the results were not reported separately from the total group.[9] Most case series of this lesion report on regional or local intra-arterial therapy. Too few patients with this location of infarction were included in the tPA or streptokinase trials for any conclusions to be drawn.

HIGH-DOSE THROMBOLYSIS

In the NINDS tPA Stroke Study,[76] the dose of tPA was 0.9 mg/kg. In ECASS,[44] the dose was 1.1 mg/kg, and in the case series of Trouillas and colleagues,[95] the dose of tPA was 0.8 mg/kg. The highest dose thus far tested is 100 mg of tPA (alteplase), combined with intravenous heparin.[96]

For the primary goal of safety following high-dose tPA plus heparin,[59] the authors reported three parenchymal hematomas (9%), all fatal, and nine hemorrhagic infarctions (28%), of which four were associated with poor outcome. The recanalization rate at 8 hours for either complete or partial reperfusion was 11 of 32 (34%). At 24 hours, an additional three patients had complete or partial reperfusion. Fourteen of the 32 patients had good outcome (44%), 9 had poor outcome (28%), and 9 died (28%). Reperfusion and effective collateral blood flow were associated with small infarct volume and good clinical outcome.

LOW-DOSE THROMBOLYSIS

Firm evidence is not available to indicate that doses of tPA (or streptokinase) lower than those evaluated in the larger randomized trials are ineffective. In the NINDS dose-escalation pilot studies,[12,46] no dose effect was seen for efficacy (defined as very early improvement), even though a dose effect was identified for intracerebral hemorrhage.[12] For example, 18 patients were treated with ≤0.6 mg/kg of tPA and 6 (33%) of those patients had very early neurologic improvement, a rate not significantly different from that for patients treated with higher doses. Likewise, in the Burroughs Wellcome dose-escalation study,[19,26] a dose effect for efficacy was not noted. A slightly higher dose of tPA, 0.8 mg/kg, was recently reported by Trouillas and colleagues.[95] In an open protocol, they evaluated patients between the ages of 20 and 81 with all types of ischemic stroke in the carotid territory who could be treated within 7 hours of stroke onset. Forty-three consecutive patients were evaluated and treated, with the mean time to treatment being 232 ± 79 minutes. At 3 months, 25 patients (58%) had complete resolution of symptoms, and only 2 patients had died (4.6%). Three patients had post-thrombolysis hematomas (6.9%), and one of these patients died.

These three studies suggest that a dose of tPA lower than the 0.9 mg/kg used in the NINDS tPA Stroke Trial could be effective. A second related hypothesis would be that patients with less severe neurologic deficits, presumably also with smaller occlusive thrombi, could benefit from lower doses of tPA. This hypothesis could be tested in a trial of patients with lacunar syndromes or restricted MCA distribution syndromes (or both), randomized to receive either standard dose tPA at 0.9 mg/kg or a lower dose, possibly 0.6 mg/kg.

Intra-Arterial Thrombolysis for Cerebral Infarction

Thrombolytic agents introduced at or within the occluding thrombus provide a higher concentration of thrombolytic agent where it is needed while minimizing the systemic concentration. The potential exists for greater efficacy with regard to arterial recanalization and greater safety with regard to hemorrhage. Patients previously evaluated and treated with local intra-arterial techniques tended to be those with more severe neurologic syndromes. The technique involves performance of a cerebral arteriogram, location of the occluding clot, and then navigation of a microcatheter to the site of the clot (Fig. 51.3). The clot is usually penetrated, and small amounts of lytic agent are given distal to the clot. The microcatheter is then withdrawn into or just at the proximal end of the clot where further thrombolytic agent is administered, usually over 30 to 120 minutes. The agents most commonly used or under investigation are urokinase, tPA (alteplase), and pro-UK at doses lower than those used in intravenous treatment.

RANDOMIZED TRIALS OF LOCAL THROMBOLYSIS

One randomized trial has been completed, the PROACT.[25] Patients who could be treated within 6 hours with an acute stroke localized to the MCA territory were eligible for angiography if the baseline NIHSS score was >4 and <30. If an M1 or M2 thrombous was identified, then the patient was randomized on a 2:1 basis to receive either 6 mg of pro-UK or placebo. The angiogram was repeated after 60 minutes. Posttreatment NIHSS score assessments were performed, as were CT scans. Preliminary results indicate that 46 patients were randomized and 40 were treated, 26 with pro-UK and 14 with placebo. The baseline NIHSS scores were 17 for the pro-UK patients and 17 for the placebo patients. Partial recanalization was seen in 15 of the 26 pro-UK-treated patients (58%) compared with 2 of the 14 placebo-treated patients (14%) ($P =$ 0.017). Intracranial hemorrhage with deterioration occurred

in 4 of 26 pro-UK patients (15%) and in 2 of 14 placebo-treated patients (14%). Outcomes were not statistically different; five of the pro-UK-treated patients had an NIHSS score of ≤1 compared with one of the placebo-treated patients. Both groups received heparin.

The same investigators are now carrying out PROACT 2. Approximately 60 centers are participating, and it is anticipated that 150 to 200 patients will be randomized on a 2:1 basis to either 9 mg of pro-UK locally administered plus heparin or intravenous control (heparin). The heparin dose for both groups will be a 2,000-unit bolus followed by a 4-hour intravenous infusion at 500 units an hour. The primary outcome will be the percentage of patients at 3 months with a Rankin Scale value of ≤2.

LARGER CASE SERIES OF LOCAL THROMBOLYSIS

The larger case series[3,29,35,48,49,57,59,75,88,89] of intra-arterial thrombolytic therapy are listed in Table 51.6. Most series of patients had carotid distribution of ischemic stroke.

Complete clot lysis is reported for 67 of a total of 174 patients (39%) and partial clot lysis with partial recanalization for 62 patients (36%). The combined partial or complete recanalization rate for these patients was 74%, higher than that of the intravenous studies. It is difficult to make comparisons with regard to the potential advantages and disadvantages of urokinase over tPA.

The patients reported in these series vary greatly in neurologic deficit, angiographic anatomy, time to treatment, and method of neurologic evaluation at follow-up. Conclusions regarding efficacy are not possible, but the results are encouraging.

Intracranial hemorrhage is the most feared complication of local intra-arterial therapy. Reporting methods differ, so interpretation of the reported symptomatic hematoma rate should be made with caution. Symptomatic intracranial hematoma is lower than that reported for intravenous thrombolysis series, occurring in 20 of 469 patients (4%) (Table 51.6). This rate is also lower than that reported in the PROACT randomized trial of intra-arterial pro-UK, in which 24-hour CT scans were performed on all patients, while it was not required in most of the case series.

Other complications of intra-arterial thrombolysis include arterial intracranial embolization, subarachnoid hemorrhage, arterial perforation, secondary embolization, hemorrhagic infarction, groin hematoma, and retroperitoneal hematoma. Such complications are infrequent, <5% in aggregate for all the series.

Neurointerventional techniques have been evolving over the last 5 years. Barnwell and colleagues[3] have reported distal clot lysis, primarily in the M1 segment of the MCA, following penetration of proximal occlusion of the ICA. Local thrombolysis has been reported in association with carotid angioplasty (G. Roubin, personal communication, 1996) and for treatment of thrombotic complications of carotid endarterectomy.[4] Recanalization may be more often achieved when the thrombo-

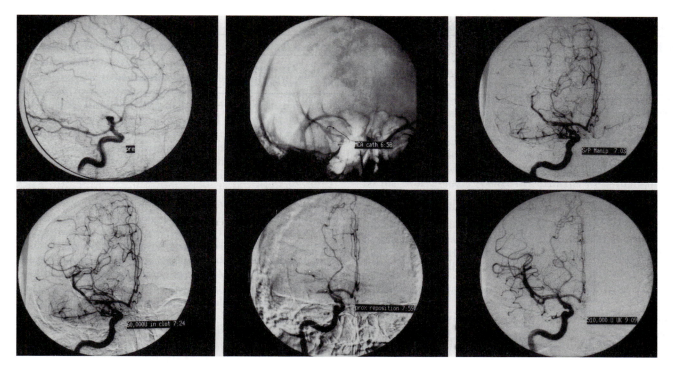

Figure 51.3 Local intra-arterial thrombolysis. A 32-year-old man developed left hemiplegia at approximately 4:00 AM and at 4.30 AM was noted in the Emergency Department to have an NIHSS score of 9. The interventional neuroradiology team was notified shortly before 5:00 AM, the patient's cerebral arteriogram was initiated at approximately 5:45 AM, and an occlusion of the right M1 segment of the middle cerebral artery was identified (upper left). A Tracker-18 microcatheter was placed across the area of suspected clot and then retracted approximately into the area of clot (upper middle). Mechanical manipulation of the acute thrombus was carried out with two passes through the clot (upper right), and partial recanalization was achieved prior to the initiation of urokinase. Following local administration of 60,000 units of urokinase (lower left), further flow was established through the middle cerebral artery stem. However, reocclusion took place (lower middle) requiring reposition of the catheter. Flow was re-established (lower right), and the procedure was discontinued after approximately 2½ hours of infusion with a total urokinase dose of 260,000 units. The post-procedure NIHSS score was 4, and at 2 days the NIHSS score was 0. (Courtesy of James L. Leach, M.D., University of Cincinnati Medical Center, Cincinnati, OH.)

embolism is iatrogenic.[101] In 14 consecutive patients with iatrogenic thromboembolism treated by local intra-arterial thrombolysis, complete recanalization was accomplished in 8 and partial recanalization in 6 patients.[6] All eight of the patients with complete recanalization were asymptomatic at the time of hospital discharge; four of the five patients with partial recanalization had mild or moderate deficits at the time of discharge.

LOCAL THROMBOLYSIS FOR VERTEBRAL BASILAR OCCLUSION

Three large case series of vertebral basilar infarction have been published since 1991[100] (Table 51.7). Most of the 102 patients received local intra-arterial urokinase. No patients were reported in these series as treated within 3 hours of symptom onset; 120 minutes was the median from the beginning of treatment to the time of recanalization.[100] Complete recanalization was reported in 28 patients (48%), and partial recanalization was reported in 21 of 58 patients (36%). For the total group of 102 patients (Table 51.7), complete or partial recanalization was accomplished for 72 (71%). As expected in patients who had either occlusion of a vertebral or the basilar artery, mortality was high: only one-third of patients survived. Good outcome was related to arterial recanalization, collateral circulation, and earlier onset of treatment.

Because good outcomes were achieved in some of the patients reported above and because of the presumed bleak outlook for untreated patients, some investigators favor open therapy. However, Brandt et al[8] recently reported a consecutive angiographic series of 22 patients with angiographically proven occlusions of the caudal vertebral artery or the basilar artery. Twenty did not receive thrombolytic therapy and all 20 survived for more than 1 year. Magnetic resonance imaging scans were performed on 17, and 14 had a brain stem infarct identified.

drug administration was accomplished very early, suggesting the lack of a direct neuronal protective effect. However, when anti-ICAM-1 was given 15 minutes after embolization and tPA was then added 2 hours later, an additive effect on neurologic outcome was documented. Zivin[102] hypothesized that the pre-thrombolytic administration of anti-ICAM-1 provided protection from reperfusion injury. Using an experimental stroke model in rats, a combination of ellipodril, a mixed NMDA receptor/neuronal calcium channel antagonist, plus tPA was studied.[62] Either agent alone decreased the neurologic deficit and the infarct volume by approximately 50%. Combined treatment improved the neurologic deficit by 70% ($P < 0.001$) versus controls and the infarct volume by 89% ($P < 0.01$) versus controls.

Investigation of combination neuronal protection and thrombolysis is now in the planning stages in humans. One plan is to randomize patients who can be treated within 6 hours to standard dose tPA versus standard dose tPA plus the neuronal protectant.

NOVEL PLASMINOGEN ACTIVATORS UNDER CLINICAL INVESTIGATION

E6010

E6010 is the first second-generation tPa to be tested in patients with stroke.[70] The E6010 molecule differs from endogenous tPA in that a cystine moiety is replaced by serine at the 84 position in the epidermal growth factor domain. This alteration results in a prolonged half-life of >20 minutes compared with the much shorter half-life of endogenous tPA. Mori and colleagues[70] performed a multicenter dose-escalation trial with intravenous bolus injections of 0.12 mg/kg and 0.22 mg/kg in patients with carotid artery territory stroke who could be treated in <6 hours after symptom onset. Primary endpoints were recanalization at 60 minutes determined by cerebral angiography and neurologic recovery at 28 days as determined by the Hemispheric Stroke Scale (HSS) score. Twenty-nine patients were studied with low-dose and 30 patients with high-dose E6010. Complete or partial recanalization was achieved for 26% of low-dose patients and 35% of high-dose patients. Improvement by >20 points in the HSS score was obtained in 58% of low-dose and 57% of high-dose patients. Intracranial hemorrhage with neurologic deterioration occurred in 8% of the low-dose patients and in 17% of the high-dose patients. The investigators consider that there is acceptable safety and a promising rate of neurologic recovery and have begun a randomized placebo-controlled trial.

Reteplase

Reteplase (rPA) is a mutant form of endogenous tPA.[77] rPA is less fibrin specific than endogenous tPA but has a longer half-life and may have greater lytic potency.[91] Like TNK-tPA, rPA has been under investigation as intravenous thrombolytic treatment for acute myocardial infarction. No trials have been conducted in stroke patients.

TNK-Tissue Plasminogen Activator

TNK-tPA is a long half-life, fibrin-specific variant of tPA.[56] TNK-tPA has fibrin specificity comparable to that of alteplase for lysis, but it has eightfold less activity in the absence of fibrin compared with tPA.[5] This results in at least an order of magnitude lesser potential for fibrinogen depletion in human plasma compared with tPA. TNK-tPA may also be more potent with regard to lysis. In a rapid arterial-venous shunt model of clot lysis, TNK-tPA was 7.5 to 13.5 times more potent than tPA. TNK-tPA is approximately 90-fold more resistant to the primary inhibitor of tPA, PAI-1.

TNK-tPA is currently under investigation as treatment for acute myocardial infarction. Results from comparison studies against tPA (alteplase) should be available sometime soon.

SPECIAL ROLE OF DIAGNOSTIC STUDIES FOR THROMBOLYSIS

A diagnostic challenge is to develop the capability for rapid detection of clot, cerebral ischemia, and irreversible cerebral injury. Earlier availability of such information allows earlier decisions regarding the potential for benefit and the identification of risk of thrombolytic therapy for the individual. Advances are required in both conventional and helical CT. Improvements are needed in CT, spiral CT, magnetic resource angiography, magnetic resonance imaging, and single-photon emission CT to determine which patients may be treated and with what risks.

Guidelines for the Use of Thrombolytic Therapy

Guidelines for thrombolytic therapy for acute stroke have been developed.[1,2,86]

For intravenous therapy, the following recommendations have been made:

1. Intravenous tPA at 0.9 mg/kg with a maximum of 90 mg with 10% of the dose given as a bolus followed by an infusion lasting for 60 minutes is the recommended treatment with 3 hours of symptom onset for ischemic stroke. This therapy cannot be recommended for use beyond 3 hours after symptom onset.

2. Intravenous administration of streptokinase outside of clinical investigation cannot be recommended as a treatment for ischemic stroke.

3. Thrombolytic therapy cannot be recommended unless the diagnosis is made by a physician with appropriate expertise in the clinical diagnosis of stroke and interpretation of CT of the brain. If the baseline CT demonstrates changes suggestive of major infarction, then thrombolytic therapy should be avoided.

4. Thrombolytic therapy cannot be recommended for patients excluded in the NINDS study (see Table 51.2).

5. Thrombolytic therapy should not be given unless emergency ancillary care and facilities to handle bleeding complications are readily available.

6. Caution is advised before giving tPA to patients with severe stroke, NIHSS score >22.

7. Whenever possible, the risks of potential effects of tPA should be discussed with the patient and family before treatment is initiated.

For intra-arterial therapy, the following recommendations have been made:

1. Further testing of intra-arterial thrombolytic therapy should proceed, but intra-arterial thrombolytic therapy should be considered investigational and only used in the clinical trial setting.

2. Intra-arterial thrombolysis should be performed only by physicians who are experienced in neurointerventional techniques and in centers with neurologic expertise.

Conclusions

Intravenous administration of tPA is the first effective therapy for stroke, with demonstrated benefit and safety for patients who can be treated within 3 hours. The rate of neurologic recovery is improved, and one additional patient with total recovery or near total recovery results from approximately every eight patients treated. The risk of symptomatic intracranial hemorrhage is relatively low, and mortality is not increased. Angiography-based studies of intravenous thrombolytic therapy as well as case series of local intra-arterial therapy document (1) modest rates of arterial recanalization following thrombolytic therapy and (2) extended time to lysis following thrombolytic therapy, suggesting resistance of cerebral clots to thrombolysis with single-agent treatment. Mechanical disruption of the clot, adding antiplatelet agent(s), and the use of second- and third-generation thrombolytic drugs offer promise for the future. Improvements in early diagnostic evaluation of patients, particularly magnetic resonance imaging techniques, hold promise for better patient selection. Finally, the benefits of arterial recanalization may be supplemented by neuronal protection, particularly when both strategies are used simultaneously, and if they can be used very early following the onset of symptoms.

Acknowledgments

The authors are indebted to Heather Meldrum for her insightful content and editorial suggestions.

References

1. Adams HP, Brott TG, Furlan AJ et al: Guidelines for thrombolytic therapy for acute stroke: a supplement to the guidelines for the management of patients with acute ischemic stroke. Stroke 27:1711–1718, 1996

2. Adams HP, Brott TG, Furlan AJ et al: Guidelines for thrombolytic therapy for acute stroke: a supplement to the guidelines for the management of patients with acute ischemic stroke. Circulation 94:1167–1174, 1996

3. Barnwell SL, Clark WM, Nguyen TT et al: Safety and efficacy of delayed intra-arterial urokinase therapy with mechanical clot disruption for thromboembolic stroke. AJNR 15:1817–1822, 1994

4. Barr JD, Horowitz MB, Mathis JM et al: Intraoperative urokinase infusion for embolic stroke during carotid endarterectomy. Neurosurgery 36:606–611, 1995

5. Bennett WF, Paoni NF, Keyt BA et al: High resolution analysis of functional determinants on human tissue-type plasminogen activator. J Biol Chem 266:5191–5201, 1991

6. Berg-Dammer E, Henkes H, Nahser HC, Kuhne D: Thromboembolic occlusion of the middle cerebral artery due to angiography and endovascular procedures: safety and efficacy of local intra-arterial fibrinolysis. Cerebrovasc Dis 6:222–230, 1996

7. Bernik MB, Oller EP: Increased plasminogen activator (urokinase) in tissue culture after fibrin deposition. J Clin Invest 53:823–834, 1973

8. Brandt T, Pessin MS, Kwan ES, Caplan LR: Survival with basilar artery occlusion. Cerebrovasc Dis 5:182–187, 1995

9. Brandt T, von Kummer R, Muller-Kuppers M, Hacke W: Thrombolytic therapy of acute basilar artery occlusion: variables affecting recanalization and outcome. Stroke 27:875–881, 1996

10. Broderick JP, Brott TG, Tomsick TA et al: The risk of subarachnoid and intracerebral hemorrhages in blacks as compared with whites. N Engl J Med 326:733–736, 1992

11. Brott T, Broderick J: Intracerebral hemorrhage. Heart Dis Stroke 2:59–63, 1992

12. Brott T, Haley EC Jr Levy D et al: Urgent therapy for stroke. Part I pilot study of tissue plasminogen activator administered within 90 minutes. Stroke 23:632–640, 1992

13. Brott T, Haley EC Jr, Levy D et al: Strategies for early treatment of acute cerebral infarction. pp. 195–203. In Hacke W et al (eds): Thrombolytic Therapy in Acute Ischemic Stroke. Springer-Verlag, Berlin, 1991

14. Brott TG, Reed RL: Intensive care for acute stroke in the community hospital setting: the first 24 hours. Stroke 20:694–697, 1989

15. Brucker AB, Potuschak H, Laich E et al: Relation of thrombolytic reperfusion and of collateral circulation to outcome in patients suffering cerebral main artery occlusion. pp. 288–293. In del Zoppo GJ, Mori E, Hacke W (eds): Thrombolytic Therapy in Acute Ischemic Stroke II. Springer-Verlag, Berlin, 1993

16. Busse O, von Kummer R, Toni D et al: The risk for cortical versus subcortical infarction after thrombolysis. Cerebrovasc Dis 6:188, 1996

17. Cerebrovascular disease. pp. 2210–2514. In Miller NR (ed): Walsh and Hoyt's Clinical Neuroophthalmology. 4th Ed. Williams & Wilkins, Baltimore, 1991

18. Collen D, Streson JM, Marafino B et al: Biological properties of human tissue-type plasminogen activator ob-

tained by expression of recombinant DNA in mammalian cells. J Pharmacol Exp Ther 231:146–152, 1984

19. Coller BS: Platelets and thrombolytic therapy. N Engl J Med. 322:33–42, 1990

20. Davis S, Donnan G: ASK trial: predictors of good outcome. Cerebrovasc Dis 6:183, 1996

21. Davis SM, Donnan GA, Gerraty RP et al: Australian Urokinase Stroke Trial. Cerebrovasc Dis 6:188, 1996

22. De Ley G, Weyne J, Demeester G et al: Experimental thromboembolic stroke studied by positron emission tomography: immediate versus delayed reperfusion by fibrinolysis. J Cereb Blood Flow Metab 8:539–545, 1988

23. del Zoppo GJ, Copeland BR, Anderchek K et al: Hemorrhagic transformation following tissue plasminogen activator in experimental cerebral infarction. Stroke 21: 596–601, 1990

24. del Zoppo GJ, Copeland BR, Waltz TA et al: The beneficial effect of intracarotid urokinase on acute stroke in a baboon model. Stroke 17:638–643, 1986

25. del Zoppo GJ, Higashada RT, Furlan AJ et al: The Prolyse in Acute Cerebral Thromboembolism Trial (PRO-ACT): results of 6 mg dose tier. Stroke 27:164, 1996

26. del Zoppo GJ, Poeck K, Pessin MS et al: Recombinant tissue plasminogen activator in acute thrombotic and embolic stroke. Ann Neurol 32:78–86, 1992

27. Donnan GA, Davis SM, Chambers BR et al: Streptokinase for acute ischemic stroke with relationship to time of administration. JAMA 276:961–966, 1996

28. Donnan GA, Davis SM, Chambers BR et al: Australian Streptokinase Trial (ASK). pp. 80–85. In del Zoppo GJ, Mori E, Hacke W (eds): Thrombolytic Therapy in Acute Ischemic Stroke II. Springer-Verlag, Berlin, 1993

29. ECASS Trial Group: Predictors of good outcome. Cerebrovasc Dis 6:182, 1996

30. Ellis SG, Topol EJ, George BS et al: Recurrent ischemia without warning: analysis of risk factors for in-hospital ischemic events following successful thrombolysis with intravenous tissue plasminogen activator. Circulation 80: 1159–1165, 1989

31. Emergency Management of Stroke (EMS) Investigators: Combined intra-arterial and intravenous t-PA for stroke. Stroke 28:273, 1997

32. The EMS Bridging Trial Investigators: Combined intravenous and intra-arterial thrombolysis versus intra-arterial thrombolysis alone: preliminary safety and clot lysis. Cerebrovasc Dis 6:184, 1996

33. EMS Bridging Trial Investigators: Combined intravenous/intra-arterial thrombolytic therapy: safety, time-to-treatment, and frequency of clot. Stroke 27:165, 1996

34. The European Ad Hoc Consensus Group: European strategies for early intervention in stroke. Cerebrovasc Dis 6:315–324, 1996

35. Ezura M, Kagawa S: Selective and superselective infusion of urokinase for embolic stroke. Surg Neurol 38: 353–358, 1992

36. Fagan SC, Morgenstern LB, Petitta A et al: rt-PA reduces length of stay and improves disposition following stroke. Stroke 28:272, 1997

37. Fieschi C, Argetino C, Lenzi GL et al: Clinical and instrumental evaluzation of patients with ischemic stroke within the first six hours. J Neurol Sci 91:311–322, 1989

38. Forsting M, Krieger D, von Kummer R et al: The prognostic value of collateral blood flow in acute middle cerebral artery occlusion. pp. 288–293. In del Zoppo GJ, Mori E, Hacke W (eds): Thrombolytic Therapy in Acute Ischemic Stroke II. Springer-Verlag, Berlin, 1993

39. Fox T, Hamann GF, Strittmatter M et al: Local intra-arterial fibrinolysis in vertebro-basilar thrombosis—prognostic criteria. Cerebrovasc Dis 6:186, 1996

40. Freitag HJ, Becker V, Thie A et al: Lys-plasminogen as an adjunct to local intra-arterial fibrinolysis for carotid territory stroke. Neuroradiology 38:181–185, 1996

41. Gallup Poll, June, 1996: Available through the National Stroke Association, Englewood, CO

42. Garabedian HD, Gold HK, Leinbach RC et al: Comparative properties of two clinical preparations of recombinant human tissue-type plasminogen activator in patients with acute myocardial infarction. J Am Coll Cardiol 9:599–607, 1987

43. Grond M, Rudolf J, Neveling M et al: Immediate heparin after rt-PA therapy dose not increase risk of hemorrhage. Stroke 28:272, 1997

44. Hacke W, Kaste M, Fieschi C et al: Intravenous thrombolysis with recombinant tissue plasminogen activator for acute hemispheric stroke. JAMA 274:1017–1025, 1995

45. Haley EC Jr, Brott TG, Sheppard GL et al: Pilot randomized trial of tissue plasminogen activator in acute ischemic stroke. Stroke 24:1000–1004, 1993

46. Haley EC Jr, Levy DE, Brott TG et al: Urgent therapy for stroke: Part II pilot study of tissue plasminogen activator administered 91–180 minutes from onset. Stroke 23:641–645, 1992

47. Heras M, Chesebro JH, Thompson PL, Fuster V: Prevention of early and late rethrombosis and further strategies of coronary reperfusion. pp. 203–229. In Julian D, Kubler W, Norris RM et al (eds): Thrombolysis in Cardiovascular Disease. Marcel Dekker, New York, 1989

48. Higashada RT, Halbach VV, Barnwell SL et al: Thrombolytic therapy for acute stroke. J Endovasc Surg 1:4–15, 1994

49. Hiramoto M, Yoshimizu N, Satoh K, Takamatsu S: Intra-arterial urokinase therapy in thromboembolic stroke, abstracted. Stroke 25:268, 1994

50. Hommel M, Besson G, Serradj AJ, for the MAST-E group: Multicenter Acute Stroke Trial—Europe trial: predictors of good outcome. Cerebrovasc Dis 6:183, 1996

51. Hoylaerts M, Rijken DC, Lijnen HR, Collen D: On the regulation and control of fibrinolysis. J Biol Chem 257: 2912–2919, 1982

52. Husain SS, Gurewich V, Lipinsk B: Purification and partial characterization of a single-chain high-molecular-weight form of urokinase (pro-urokinase) and urokinase from human urine. Arch Biochem Biophys 220:31–38, 1983

53. Jansen O, von Kummer R, Forsting M et al: Thrombolytic therapy in acute occlusion of the intracranial internal carotid artery bifurcation. Stroke 27:785–786, 1996

54. Kanamass K, Watanabe I, Cercek B et al: Selective decrease in lysis of old thrombus after rapid administration

of tissue-type plasminogen activator. J Am Coll Cardiol 14:1359–1364, 1989

55. Keren A, Medina A, Gottlieb S et al: Lysis of mobile left ventricular thrombi during acute myocardial infarction with urokinase. Am J Cardiol 60:1180–1181, 1987

56. Keyt BA, Paoni NF, Refino CJ et al: A faster-acting and more potent form of tissue plasminogen activator. Proc Natl Acad Sci USA 91:3670–3674, 1994

57. Kinoshita Y, Terada T, Nakai E et al: Intra-arterial thrombolytic therapy for acute cerebral occlusion. Stroke 28:234, 1997

58. Koudstaal PJ, Stibbe J, Vermeulen M: Fatal ischemic brain oedema after early thrombolysis with tissue plasminogen activator in acute stroke. BMJ 297:1571–1574, 1988

59. LaMonte MP, Hurst RW, Raps EC et al: Selective intra-arterial thrombolysis for acute cerebral ischemia: a case-control comparison. Neurology (suppl. 4), 45:A469, 1995

60. Larrue V, von Kummer R, Huxter G et al: Predictors of hemorrhagic transformation in the ECASS trial. Cerebrovasc Dis 6:181, 1996

61. Lefkovits J, Plow EF, Topol EJ: Platelet glycoprotein IIb/IIIa receptors in cardiovascular medicine. N Engl J Med 332:1553–1559, 1995

62. Lekieffre D, Nowicki JP, Benavides J, Scatton B: Ellipodril increases the benefit of thrombolysis in an embolic stroke model in rats. Cerebrovasc Dis 6:191, 1996

63. Levy DE, Brott TG, Haley EC Jr et al: Factors related to intracranial hematoma formation in patients receiving tissue-type plasminogen activator for acute ischemic stroke. Stroke 25:291–297, 1994

64. Lijnen HR, Van Hoef B, De Cock F, Collen D: The mechanism of plasminogen activation and fibrin dissolution by single chain urokinase-type plasminogen activator in a plasma milieu in vitro. Blood 73:1864–1872, 1989

65. The MAST-I Collaborative Group: Thrombolytic and antithrombotic therapy in acute ischemic stroke: multicenter acute stroke trial—Italy (MAST-I). pp. 86–94. In del Zoppo GJ, Mori E, Hacke W (eds): Thrombolytic Therapy in Acute Ischemic Stroke II. Springer-Verlag, Berlin, 1993

66. The MAST-I Investigators: Predictors of good outcome in the MAST Italy trial. Cerebrovasc Dis 6:183, 1996

67. The MAST-Italy Investigators: Risk factors in the MAST-Italy trial. Cerebrovasc Dis 6:181, 1996

68. Masuda J, Yutani C, Ogata J et al: Atheromatous embolism in the brain: a clinicopathologic analysis of 15 autopsy cases. Neurology 44:1231–1237, 1994

69. Montrucchi G, Bergerone S, Bussolino F: Streptokinase induces intravascular release of platelet-activating factor in patients with acute myocardial infarction and stimulates its synthesis by cultured human endothelial cells. Circulation 88:1476–1483, 1993

70. Mori E, Takakura K, Yamaguchi T et al: Multicenter trial of a novel modified t-PA, E6010 by i.v. bolus injection in patients with acute carotid artery territory stroke. Cerebrovasc Dis 6:191, 1996

71. Mori E, Yoneda Y, Tabuchi M et al: Intravenous recombinant tissue plasminogen activator in acute carotid artery territory stroke. Neurology 42:976–982, 1992

72. Moulin T, Besson G, Crepin-Leblond T et al: Hemorrhagic transformations in the MAST-E trial: predictive factors. Cerebrovasc Dis 6:182, 1996

73. Multicenter Acute Stroke Trial—Europe Study Group: Thrombolytic therapy with streptokinase in acute ischemic stroke. N Engl J Med 335:145–150, 1996

74. Multicenter Acute Stroke Trial—Italy (MAST-I) Group: Randomized controlled trial of streptokinase, aspirin, and combination of both in treatment of acute ischaemic stroke. Lancet 346:1509–1514, 1995

75. Nakagawara J, Hyogo T, Katsumi S, Nakamura J: A superselective intra-arterial trial using rt-PA for embolic stroke. Cerebrovasc Dis 6:184, 1996

76. The National Institute of Neurological Disorders and Stroke rt-PA Stroke Study Group: Tissue plasminogen activator for acute ischemic stroke. N Engl J Med 333:1581–1587, 1995

77. Neuhaus KL, von Essen R, Vogt A et al: Dose finding with a novel recombinant plasminogen activator (BM 06.022) in patients with acute myocardial infarction: results of the German Recombinant Plasminogen Activator Study. J Am Coll Cardiol 24:55–60, 1994

78. The NINDS t-PA Stroke Study Group: Symptomatic intracerebral hemorrhage after t-PA for stroke. Stroke 28:272, 1997

79. The NINDS t-PA Stroke Study Group: Generalized efficacy of t-PA for acute stroke: subgroup analysis of the NINDS t-PA Stroke Trial. Stroke 28:271, 1997

80. Overgaard K, Meden P, Boysen G: Experimental combined thrombolysis and neuroprotection. Cerebrovasc Dis 6:191, 1996

81. Overgaard K, Sereghy T, Boysen G et al: Reduction of infarct volume and mortality by thrombolysis in a rat embolic stroke model. Stroke 23:1167–1174, 1992

82. Overgaard K, Sereghy T, Boysen G et al: Reduction of infarct volume by thrombolysis with rt-PA in an embolic rat stroke model. Scand J Clin Lab Invest 53:383–393, 1993

83. Pancioli A, Broderick J, Kothari R et al: Public perception of stroke warning signs and potential risk factors. Stroke 28:236, 1997

84. Pilz P, Ladurner G, Griebnitz E: Neuropathological findings after thrombolytic therapy in acute ischemic stroke. pp. 224–227. In Hacke W, del Zoppo GJ, Hirschberg M (eds): Thrombolytic Therapy in Acute Ischemic Stroke. Springer-Verlag, Berlin, 1991

85. Potter van Loon BJ, Rijken DC, Brommer EJP, van der Maas APC: The amount of plasminogen, t-PA and PAI-1 in human thrombi and the relation to ex-vivo lysibility. Thromb Haemost 67:101–105, 1992

86. Quality Standards Subcommittee of the American Academy of Neurology: Practice advisory: thrombolytic therapy for acute ischemic stroke—summary statement. Neurology 47:835–839, 1996

87. Ringelstein EB, Biniek R, Weiller C et al: Type and extent of hemispheric brain infarctions and clinical outcome in early and delayed middle cerebral artery recanalization. Neurology 42:289–298, 1992

88. Sasaki O, Takeuchi S, Koike T et al: Fibrinolytic therapy for acute embolic stroke: intravenous, intracarotid, and

intra-arterial local approaches. Neurosurgery 36: 246–253, 1995

89. Satoh K, Matsubara S, Ueda S, Matsumoto K: Local thrombolytic therapy in 153 cases of acute major cerebral artery occlusion. Cerebrovasc Dis 6:184, 1996

90. Sherry S: The origin of thrombolytic therapy. J Am Coll Cardiol 14:1085–1092, 1989

91. Smalling RW, Bode C, Kalbfleisch J et al: More rapid, complete, and stable coronary thrombolysis with bolus administration of reteplase compared with alteplase infusion in acute myocardial infarction. Circulation 91: 2725–2732, 1995

92. Tillet WS, Garner RL: The fibrinolytic activity of hemolytic streptococci. J Exp Med 58:485–502, 1933

93. Tognoni G, Roncaglioni MC: Dissent: an alternative interpretation of MAST-I. Lancet 346:1515, 1995

94. Tomsick T, Brott T, Barsan W et al: Prognostic value of the hypertense middle cerebral artery sign and stroke scale score before ultraearly thrombolytic therapy. AJNR 17:79–85, 1996

95. Trouillas P, Nighoghossian N, Getenet JC et al: Open trial of intravenous tissue plasminogen activator in acute carotid territory stroke: correlations of outcome with clinical and radiological data. Stroke 27:882–890, 1996

96. von Kummer R, Hacke W: Safety and efficacy of intravenous tissue plasminogen activator and heparin in acute middle cerebral artery stroke. Stroke 23:646–652, 1992

97. Wagner OF, de Vries C, Hohmann C et al: Interaction between plasminogen activator inhibitor 1 (PAI-1) bound to fibrin and either tissue-type plasminogen (t-PA) or urokinase-type plasminogen activator (u-PA). J Clin Invest 84:647–655, 1989

98. Wolpert SM, Bruckman H, Greenlee R et al: Neuroradiologic evaluation of patients with acute stroke treated with recombinant tissue plasminogen activator. AJNR 14:3–13, 1993

99. Yamaguchi T, Hayakawa T, Kiuchi H, for the Japanese Thrombolysis Study Group: Intravenous tissue plasminogen activator ameliorates the outcome of hyperacute embolic stroke. Cerebrovasc Dis 3:269–272, 1993

100. Zeumer H, Freitag JJ, Grzyska V et al: Interventional neuroradiology: local intra-arterial fibrinolysis in acute vertebrobasilar thromboembolic disease. AJNR 4: 401–404, 1983

101. Zeumer H, Grzyska U, Kucinski T, Freitag HJ: Local intra-arterial fibrinolysis: the appropriate aid to treat embolic complications during endovascular procedures. Cerebrovasc Dis 6:184, 1996

102. Zivin JA: Reperfusion injury: treatment after thrombolysis. Cerebrovasc Dis 6:191, 1996

103. Zivin JA, Fisher M, DeGirolami U et al: Tissue plasminogen activator reduces neurological damage after cerebral embolism. Science 230:1289–1292, 1985

104. Zivin JA, Lyden PD, DeGirolami U et al: Tissue plasminogen activator: reduction of neurological damage after experimental embolic stroke. Arch Neurol 45:387–391, 1988

CHAPTER 52

Brachiocephalic Angioplasty and Interventional Thrombolysis

JOHN PILE-SPELLMAN

HOANG DUONG

Brachiocephalic Angioplasty

INTRODUCTION

The treatment options and indications for stenotic disease of the great vessels of the arch causing stroke are changing. Prophylactic surgical endarterectomy for carotid arteries narrowed by more than 70% by atherosclerotic vascular disease significantly decreases the stroke rate.[56] Prophylactic angioplasty for cerebrovascular disease remains uncharted territory. Angioplasty has been performed for vessels of all sizes from those as large as the aorta to those as small as the coronary and tibial arteries. It has been used on systemic and pulmonary arteries, as well as on systemic veins and vein grafts. Angioplasty can be performed in the angiography suite as well as in the operating room. Although results vary, there is every indication that it is a well-tolerated procedure.[23,34,47,59,63,76] Previous experience with angioplasty in the peripheral vascular bed has shown that vascular patency is achieved in more than 85% of patients for more than 3 years with a reasonably low complication rate.

To date, the exact role of angioplasty for stroke prophylaxis is undefined. Case series done so far have been helpful in describing the outcomes in highly selected groups of patients. These studies have been instrumental in standardizing methods and materials and in setting the stage for randomized, controlled clinical trials. (Hobson RW: Carotid revascularization endarterectomy vs. stent trial (crest). Personal communication.) It is hoped that treatment of carefully selected patients in well-controlled studies will make possible successful

intervention and greater understanding of the expanding role of intervention neuroradiology in the treatment of stenotic and occlusive disease. Specific indications for specific diseases with specific interventions will need to be delineated.

In summary, angioplasty of the brachiocephalic arteries is a viable therapeutic option. Concerns regarding distal emboli continue but can be minimized with proper patient selection and technical advances (see contraindications in text following). The rate of restenosis appears higher than with direct surgery, and this limitation is under vigorous study.

CAROTID ANGIOPLASTY

Although carotid disease is far more common than brachiocephalic disease, endovascular methods have been slow to develop because surgery (carotid endarterectomy) is an excellent therapy, with a high success rate and a low complication burden. In spite of this, preliminary experience with carotid angioplasty has been very encouraging.[68] Controlled clinical trials are needed to determine the role of angioplasty in the treatment of stenotic disease.

At present, carotid angioplasty can be considered for restenosis after carotid endarterectomy (Fig. 52.1), for inflammatory carotid disease, for hemodynamically unstable patients, and for patients with strokes in evolution.[36] Angioplasty may also be indicated for surgically inaccessible stenotic lesions (Fig. 52.2), such as in patients with high bifurcation or intrapetrous stenosis. Endovascular treatment for a totally occluded internal carotid artery has also been advocated in the very early stages where there is no thrombus or there

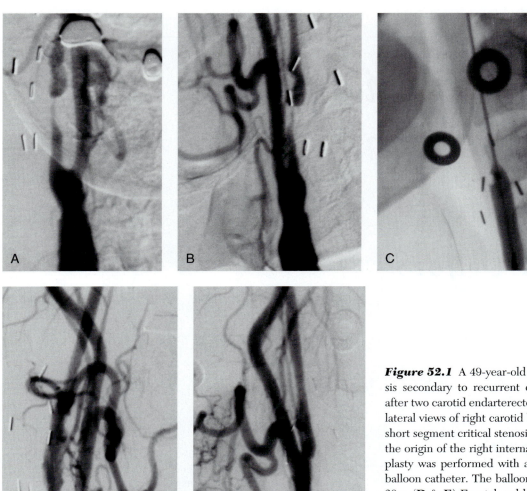

Figure 52.1 A 49-year-old woman with left hemiparesis secondary to recurrent carotid stenosis 18 months after two carotid endarterectomies: (**A & B**.) Frontal and lateral views of right carotid bifurcation demonstrating a short segment critical stenosis approximately 1 cm above the origin of the right internal carotid artery. (**C**) Angioplasty was performed with a 5 mm × 2 cm Meditech balloon catheter. The balloon was inflated to 12 atm for 30 s. (**D & E**) Frontal and lateral views of right carotid bifurcation after angioplasty showing near total reopening of the right internal carotid artery at the site of balloon dilatation.

is a short thrombus that can be evacuated.[44] Angioplasty of recurrent stenosis after endarterectomy has been reported effective, though not without some difficulty.[7]

Carotid angioplasty has been done since the early 1980s and a large number of case series have been reported.[6,39,42,53,66,74] More recent case series with larger numbers of patients have been reported with good results[24,70,77] (Table 52.1). The group from Caen reported a large case series of 259 carotid angioplasties, of which 136 were performed with distal balloon protection.[70] They reported no embolic complications when cerebral protection was used. They also found that stent placement eliminated the risk of immediate dissection and reduced the risk of delayed restenosis.

The Seville group reported 98 symptomatic patients with high-grade carotid stenosis in whom 85 percutaneous transluminal angioplasties were performed. Thirty-day morbidity of disabling strokes was 4.9% and there were no deaths. The mean follow-up period of 18.7 months showed an 86.7% rate of survival without stroke and a 7.4% restenosis rate. The calculated 4-year ipsilateral stroke–free probability was 95.3%.[24]

In a consecutive case series of 107 patients with 126 significant carotid stenoses reported by Yadav et al,[77] angioplasty and stenting were effective, relatively safe, and durable over the time of observation (6 months). The patients had a Mayo Clinic mean risk score of 3.54 ± 1.21. Balloon angioplasty with stenting was ultimately successful in all patients. There was a 7.9% rate in 30-day morbidity/mortality for the combined endpoints of stroke and death (7 minor strokes, 3 major strokes, and 1 death). The 30-day incidence for ipsilateral strokes was 1.6%. There were no strokes in the subsequent 6-month follow-up. Restenosis was seen in 4.9% of the 81 patients who had a second angiogram (Table 52.1).

VERTEBRAL, SUBCLAVIAN, AND BRACHIOCEPHALIC ANGIOPLASTY

Arguably, angioplasty may be the treatment of choice for inflammatory and atherosclerotic stenoses of the main trunks arising from the aortic arch, as well as of the vertebral arter-

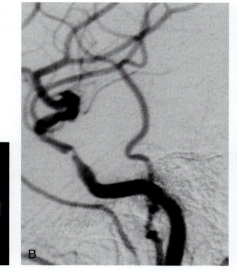

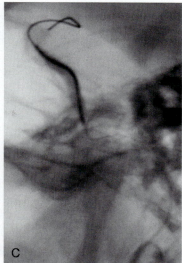

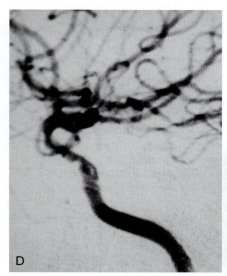

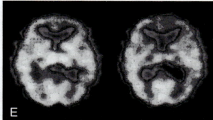

Figure 52.2 A 72-year-old woman with bilateral carotid stenosis and global cerebral hypoperfusion on cerebral SPECT (**A**). Despite maximal medical treatment, she remained with symptoms of lightheadedness and blurred right eye vision. (**B**) Lateral view of right internal carotid arteriogram showing a critical tandem stenotic lesion at the level of the posterior genu of the right cavernous internal carotid artery. (**C**) Angioplasty was performed with a 3 mm × 10 mm Stealth balloon angioplasty catheter. The angioplasty balloon was inflated to 7 atm. (**D**) Moderate improvement in the caliber of the right carotid siphon was achieved after angioplasty. (**E**) Pre- and postangioplasty cerebral 99mTc-HMPAO SPECT scans showing significant improvement in global cerebral perfusion following revascularization.

ies.[6,39,53,66] This argument is the most convincing for symptomatic vertebral artery origin stenosis.[68] In one series of 42 patients with posterior circulation disease,[33] the proximal vertebral artery was involved in 34 cases, the distal vertebral artery in 5, and the basilar artery in 3. The success rate for angioplasty was 98%. Three permanent complications occurred (7.1%). Clinical follow-up examination demonstrated improvement of symptoms in 39 cases (92.9%).

Subclavian angioplasty appears to be a viable option in treating patients with symptomatic stenosis. Angioplasty for subclavian artery stenosis has a relatively high reported success rate, in the range of 90%, with a total complication rate of approximately 8%.[50,73] Occlusions are significantly riskier to treat, with poor patency rates.[62]

The relative efficacy of brachiocephalic angioplasty in preventing strokes associated with symptomatic brachiocephalic stenosis has yet to be determined and will require clinical trials.

The relative indications and contraindications for offering angioplasty have yet to be determined. Extreme caution is advised in those patients with the following:

1. Lesions >3 cm in length, highly ulcerated, or occluded.
2. Large infarcts within the last week with areas of infarction on computed tomography (CT)/magnetic resonance imaging >2.5 cm in diameter.

PRE-ENDOVASCULAR WORKUP AND TREATMENT

The appropriate workup for patients requiring supra-aortic vessel angioplasty has yet to be determined. The workup should address a number of points: (1) identify the offending lesion, (2) assess the severity and extent of associated vascular

Table 52.1 Case Series: Reports for Carotid Angioplasty

Group	Caen, France	Birmingham, AL, U.S.	Seville, Spain	New York, NY, U.S.
Number of patients	259	107	98	16
Patient eligibility for carotid endarterectomy	Yes	Yes	Yes	No
Periprocedural complications:				
Death	0.4%	0.7%	0%	0%
Major stroke	1.2%	1.4%	4.9%	0%
Minor stroke	1.2%	4.8%	—	0%
Success rate	—	99%	92%	93%
Follow-up time	—	291 days	18.7 months	—
Follow-up: major stroke rate	—	1%/yr	5%/4 yr	—
Follow-up: restenosis rate	7.7%	—	7.4%	—
Reference	Theron et al, 1996	Yadav et al, 1997	Gil-Peralta et al, 1996	Hacein-Bey et al, 1997
Comments	ASVD, inflammatory stenosis, stents used in one-half with lower stroke rate	Change in stents to Wallstent with reduction in delayed collapse	30-day morbidity. Similar reporting: as ECST, NASCET, results as good	30-day morbidity. Only severe surgically and medically intractable patients treated

Abbreviations: ASVD, atherosclerotic vascular disease; ECST, European Carotid Surgery Trial; NASCET, North American Symptomatic Carotid Endarterectomy Trial.

pathology, (3) assess cerebrovascular reserve, (4) assess associated comorbidity, and (5) assess the likelihood of effectiveness and risk of all treatment alternatives.

Optimal materials and methods for pre-endovascular workup have yet to be determined. The development of catheters and stents and the need for cerebral protection and anticoagulation are under current investigation.

Catheters

Low-profile, high-pressure, highly trackable balloons are needed. The authors use an Ultrathin ST Balloon Catheter by Meditech (Wavertown, MA). For intracranial angioplasty, the Stealth dilatation catheter (Target, CA) can be navigated around the carotid siphon or through tortuous vertebral arteries.

Stents

Advocates of stents feel that they (1) decrease the risk of dangerous intimal flaps, (2) protect against elastic rebound, and (3) decrease restenosis. Stents can be (1) self-expanding or balloon expandable, (2) metallic, biodegradable, or polymer, or (3) mesh, slotted tube, or coil. No stents have FDA approval for brachiocephalic use.

Three types of stents have reportedly been used in the brachiocephalic circulation:

1. The Wallstent (Schneider) is a self-expanding metallic mesh stent and has been used in most recent series.

2. The Flexstent (Gianturco-Roubin, Cook) is a balloon-expandable, stainless steel, single-wire structure.

3. The Palmaz-Schatz stent (Johnson & Johnson International Systems) is a balloon-expandable, stainless steel, slotted tube.

Other stents include the Wiktor stent (Medtronic Interventional Vascular), the Micro stent (Applied Vascular Engineering Inc.), the Cordis stent (Cordis), and Multi Link stent (Advanced Cardiovascular Systems).

Indications for stenting of the carotid arteries may be similar to coronary stenting, that is: (1) suboptimal angiographic results and (2) abrupt vessel closure during angioplasty.[17]

Cerebral Protection/Monitoring

The angioplasty procedure can be performed without vascular protection or with proximal or distal vascular protection. The need for distal protection from emboli has been considered by many to be critical, and special triple coaxial catheter systems for carotid angioplasty with cerebral protection have been designed.[25,43,67] Many do not routinely use it.

Anticoagulation

Anticoagulation, including heparin and antiplatelet agents, is crucial. The amount of heparin administered varies greatly, and complications may result from both excessive and insufficient anticoagulation.[46] Pretreatment of all lesions with urokinase (UK) may be considered, especially if there is any suspicion that part of the angiographic stenosis is due to the thrombus. Direct intra-arterial calcium channel blockers such as verapamil (1 to 2 mg) may help decrease angioplasty-induced spasm in the more muscular arteries.

Future Directions

Angioplasty for carotid and brachiocephalic vessels is currently under intense investigation and initial results are encouraging. With future development, angioplasty will no doubt play an increasing role in the treatment of carotid and brachiocephalic stenosis. Although patient acceptance for a procedure considered "less invasive" may be higher than for surgery, the relative cost-effectiveness of these treatments may ultimately determine their use. Initial comparisons of angioplasty and stenting with surgery suggest that carotid endarterectomy is more cost-effective.[37] Lower-cost methods and materials for angioplasty will be essential for its full utilization.

Thrombolysis

INTRA-ARTERIAL THROMBOLYSIS

Intravenous thrombolysis (IVT) in patients with stroke has clearly been demonstrated to improve the functional outcome at 6-month follow-up.[9,10,13,19,61,72] The role of intra-arterial thrombolysis (IAT) remains to be clarified despite a number of studies over the last 40 years[2,15,21,27,28,38,51,69,75] (Tables 52.2 and 52.3). Theoretically, IAT results in more rapid lysis and more complete recanalization than intravenous methods.[38,49,54,71,78] The brain's sensitivity to ischemia is the problem.[4,12] Practically, the delay associated with catheter placement needed for IAT in the cerebral circulation is difficult to reduce. IAT indications include (1) emboli that develop in the hospital, particularly in the catheterization laboratory; (2) vertebrobasilar ischemia; and (3) an investigational protocol.[14,16]

Contraindications are similar to those of IVT, including stroke occurring for more than 4 hours, hemorrhagic stroke, recent surgery, bleeding, diathesis, and so forth.

CAROTID ARTERY TERRITORY

Results of case series on thrombolysis in the carotid artery territory have been encouraging, although not convincing even in recent studies. Del Zoppo et al[15] reported 20 patients with angiographically demonstrated acute carotid occlusion. The patients were treated with intra-arterial thrombolytic therapy in two institutions with UK or streptokinase (SK) (6,000 to 7,000 units) within 8 hours and recanalization was achieved in 18 of the 20 (90%) (complete: 15 patients; partial: 3 patients). There was favorable improvement in 12 of the 20, and hemorrhagic transformation was demonstrated in 4 (20%) of the recanalized patients with no clinical deterioration. Of the 20 patients, 3 patients died (recanalized: 2 patients; unrecanalized: 1 patient). One patient death was unrelated to the hemorrhagic transformation.

Mori et al[51] reported 22 patients with acute middle cerebral artery occlusion. They were treated with intra-arterial UK infusion after 0.83 to 12 hours (mean 4.5 hours) from onset. Recanalization occurred in 10 of the 22 cases. Improved neurologic outcome and decreased volume of infarction was demonstrated in the recanalized group versus the unrecanalized group (recanalized: 8 of 10; 80% versus unrecanalized: 4 of 12; 33%). Hemorrhage was observed in 4 cases (18%; recanalized: 1, unrecanalized: 3) In the unrecanalized group 3 patients died of causes unrelated to hemorrhage.

Theron et al[69] also tried intra-arterial SK (50,000 to 150,000 U) infusion in 12 patients with carotid territory occlusion. Of 9 patients without combined surgical intervention, 8 patients (89%) achieved recanalization, and among those 6 favorable outcomes (66%) were observed. Hemorrhage was observed in three cases (33%), all of which occurred in lenticulostriate artery territory after recanalization. One patient died as the result of hemorrhage. The

Table 52.2 Intra-arterial Thrombolytic Therapy for Acute Stroke—Results of Studies

Investigator	No. of Patients	Recanalization	Favorable Outcome	Mortality	Hemorrhagic Infarction
Carotid					
Del Zoppo[15]	20	18 (90%)[a]	12 (60%)	3 (15%)	4 (20%)
			R: 12, U: 0	R: 2, U: 1	R: 4, U: 0
Mori[51]	22	10 (45%)	10 (45%)	3 (14%)	4 (18%)
			R: 8, U: 2	R: 0, U: 3	R: 1, U: 3
Theron[69]	9	8 (89%)	6 (67%)	1 (11%)	3 (33%)
			R: 6, U: 0	R: 1, U: 0	R: 3, U: 0
Vertebrobasilar					
Hacke[27]	43	19 (44%)	10 (24%)	30 (70%)	4 (9%)
			R: 10, U: 0	R: 6, U: 24	R: 2, U: 2
Zeumer[78]	7	7 (100%)	4 (57%)	2 (22%)	1 (14%)
			R: 4, U: 0	R: 2, U: 0	R: 1, U: 0

Abbreviations: R: recanalized; U: unrecanalized.

[a] Figures in parentheses show percent to number of patients in each line.

Table 52.3 Intra-arterial Thrombolytic Therapy for Acute Stroke—Analysis of Results in Relation to Recanalization

		No. of Patients	*Favorable Outcome*	*Mortality*	*Hemorrhagic Infarction*
Carotid		51	28 (55%)[a]	7 (14%)	11 (22%)
	Recanalized	36	26 (72%)	3 (8%)	8 (22%)
	Unrecanalized	15	2 (13%)	4 (27%)	3 (20%)
Vertebrobasilar		50	14 (28%)[b]	32 (64%)[b]	5 (10%)
	Recanalized	26	14 (54%)	8 (31%)	3 (12%)
	Unrecanalized	24	0 (0%)	24 (100%)	2 (8%)
Total		101	42 (42%)[b]	39 (39%)[b]	16 (16%)
	Recanalized	62	40 (65%)	11 (18%)	11 (18%)
	Unrecanalized	39	2 (5%)	28 (72%)	5 (13%)

[a] $p < 0.005$, [b] $p < 0.001$: square test. Figures in parentheses show percent to patients in each line.

author suggested that the risk of basal ganglia hemorrhage is high if treatment is delayed (> 6 hours) in patients with lenticulostriate artery involvement.

VERTEBROBASILAR ARTERY TERRITORY

Vertebrobasilar occlusion has a dismal prognosis. IAT for acute vertebrobasilar occlusion has been attempted by many investigators.[48,51,79] Hacke et al[27] treated 43 patients with vertebrobasilar occlusion presenting with acute (8 of the 43) or progressive (35 of the 43) neurologic deterioration. Treatment with urokinase began within 24 hours after the onset of the stroke in most patients. The results were compared with 22 patients treated by conventional therapy (antiplatelet agents or anticoagulants), retrospectively. Recanalization was obtained in 19 of the 43 (44%) patients, with favorable outcome in 10 patients and death in 6 patients. By contrast, poor clinical outcome with high mortality was evident in 24 of the 43 patients without recanalization (favorable outcome: 0; death: 24), and of all of 22 patients receiving the conventional therapy, only 3 had a favorable outcome; 19 died. Hemorrhage occurred in 4 patients (9%) (recanalized: 2; unrecanalized: 2), with 2 deaths following acute deterioration in the treated group. Of 4 patients who hemorrhaged, 3 had been treated with prolonged low-dose infusion concomitant with heparinization. Zeumer et al[78] reported 7 new patients treated by superselective intra-arterial infusion under the revised protocol. Based on their experience, they recommended high dose with shorter duration of treatment. Recanalization was obtained in all cases (100%) with 4 of the 7 (58%) recovery, 1 of the 7 (14%) locked-in state, and 2 of the 7 (29%) death. Heparinization was started after partial thromboplastin time was shown to be twice or less than the normal value. Small intracerebellar hemorrhage was observed in 1 patient (14%) under heparnization without clinical deterioration. They emphasized the progressive course of acute vertebrobasilar stroke leading to coma, decerebration, and finally death, and suggested that indication for treatment should be determined not by time limit, but by careful neurologic examinations combined with angiographic findings. Furthermore, it was suggested that high-dose local administration with short duration using superselective cath-

eterization technique would decrease the risk of hemorrhage and work more effectively on recanalization (Fig. 52.3).

From these results it appears that the recanalized group has a better clinical outcome than the unrecanalized group after carotid intra-arterial thrombolysis. There is no correlation between recanalization and occurrence of hemorrhagic infarction. In addition, the number of deaths has been significantly decreased after recanalization for acute vertebrobasilar stroke in both anterior and posterior circulations. On the other hand, no correlation is demonstrated between hemorrhagic infarction and outcome or death in the carotid or vertebrobasilar circulation, or both territories.

Secondary hemorrhage in treated patients does not appear to be significantly different than hemorrhage occurring spontaneously after cerebral infarction (hemorrhagic infarction [HI]). The latter is related to increased permeability through ischemic endothelium, reopening of the occluded vessel due to the spontaneous recanalization or migration of the embolus, development of the collateral circulation, or rupture of the vessel secondary to vessel necrosis.[30,31,35,57,65] The secondary hemorrhage varies in size and pattern from a few scattered petechiae within an ischemic/infarcted tissue without mass effect (hemorrhagic transformation) to massive intracerebral hematoma.[14,16] The occurrence is influenced by various factors such as the etiology of the vessel occlusion (thrombus vs. embolus), the size of the infarction, the patient's age and medical condition (e.g., hypertension, coagulopathy, etc.), or concomitant treatment (e.g., thrombolytic, anticoagulant therapy).[14,16,57] The reported incidence of HI has been influenced by the type of the study. In pathologic examinations, the frequency of HI has been reported to be about 30% (18% to 42%), (51% to 71% in embolic strokes, 2% to 21% in nonembolic strokes).[31,57] The clinically or radiologically detectable evidence would be less, and a study showed that HI was observed in 5% of cases within 24 hours and 20% within 2 weeks after the onset of the CT examination.[31,58] In most recent series, the incidence of HI demonstrated in CT scans has been presumed to be 10% or less in the occlusive stroke without anticoagulation treatment.[64]

Hemorrhagic infarction usually occurs within the first 2 weeks, beginning 24 to 48 hours after the onset of symptoms.[35] Significant deterioration associated with HI has been reported in 11 to 15% of cases, most of which are massive

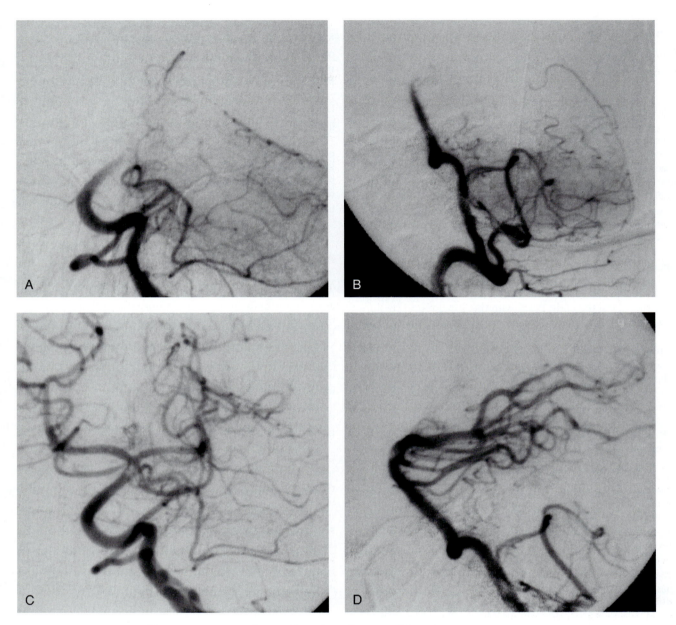

Figure 52.3 A 65-year-old man presenting with acute flaccid quadriparesis, bilateral nonreactive pupils and depressed corneal reflexes. (**A & B**) Frontal and lateral views of left vertebral arteriogram showing complete occlusion of the basilar trunk beyond the origins of the anterior inferior cerebellar arteries. (**C & D**) Successful recanalization of the basilar artery was achieved after intra-arterial infusion of 650,000 U of urokinase. A small fragment of thrombus remained near the basilar tip after thrombolysis. The patient's motor deficit and cranial nerve palsies improved at the end of the procedure.

intracerebral hematomas occurring within 48 hours from the onset of symptoms.[65]

In summary, from published case series, recanalization has been achieved in approximately two-thirds of the patients, with a higher incidence of recanalization being seen in the carotid than in vertebral artery territories. Favorable outcome has been shown in approximately one-half of the carotid territory strokes treated and one-fourth of the vertebrobasilar territory. Mortality is approximately 15% in carotid patients and 65% in patients with the vertebrobasilar disease. Hemorrhagic infarction occurred in approximately 15% (Table 52.3). The logistic difficulties of IAT remain daunting, but controlled clinical trials are underway and will help delineate the uncertainties.

Postsubarachnoid Hemorrhage Cerebral Vasospasm

INTRODUCTION

Despite several recent advances in the treatment of cerebral aneurysms, the morbidity and mortality of aneurysmal subarachnoid hemorrhage remains high, with 50% dying in the first few months and nearly two-thirds of the survivors experiencing reductions in their quality of life.[3,5,26,52,60] One of the reasons for continued poor outcome after bleeding is cerebral vasospasm, which affects nearly one-third of all patients who survive the hemorrhagic ictus.[3,53] While the medical treatment of vasospasm has improved significantly since the introduction of calcium channel blockers (e.g., nimodipine, etc.) and hypertensive-hypervolemic therapy, none of these treatments has proved entirely effective.

Starting in the early 1980s with the initial report by Zubkov, several groups have demonstrated that angioplasty in the setting of medically intractable vasospasm not only is effective in reversing vessel narrowing, but can improve cerebral blood flow and neurologic function.[8,11,22,32,45,56,80] More recently, others have combined the intra-arterial administration of papaverine with angioplasty and achieved similarly encouraging results.[40,41]

The onset of delayed arterial narrowing and resultant cerebral ischemia following subarachnoid hemorrhage usually occurs 4 to 8 days after bleeding. Altered sensorium usually develops, but focal deficits are not uncommon. Patients likely to be affected are those whose initial CT scan demonstrates large amounts of blood in the basal cisterns.[20] Recently, transcranial Doppler (TCD) ultrasonography has allowed for the earlier diagnosis of presymptomatic vasospasm by demonstrating increased velocities and pulsatility indexes in the middle cerebral artery (MCA).[1,29] The normal mean MCA velocity ranges between 30 and 80 cm/sec. In mild vasospasm it increases to 120–200 cm/s. In severe vasospasm it is greater than 200 cm/s. Single photon emission computed tomography (SPECT) can serve as an additional aid by demonstrating regional cerebral perfusion abnormalities. Together, SPECT and TCD allow for the identification of patients at risk for clinical deterioration and who are therefore potentially helped by angioplasty. However, cerebral angiography remains the definitive method for the diagnosis of vasospasm and gives information not only about the degree of arterial narrowing (>50% = significant reduction in cerebral blood flow), but defines the length of the narrowing, which gives information about the reversibility of the process.

PATIENT SELECTION

Patients who become symptomatic while under maximal medical therapy instituted on the basis of noninvasive study with TCD and SPECT are unlikely to improve unless more aggressive management is undertaken.[18] Patients who become symptomatic prior to maximal medical intervention are generally not candidates until these other avenues have been exhausted. Nevertheless, as soon as medical management fails, angioplasty should be performed. It has been the experience of most authors that angioplasty results are best when it is performed within 6 to 12 hours of symptom onset, but complete recoveries have been documented even when performed 48 hours after the initial deterioration.[18,55] Controversy exists as to the value and safety of angioplasty in the setting of hemorrhagic conversion. Eskridge et al have reported that in their experience this is unlikely and that they do not consider such low-density changes to be a contraindication. By contrast, unsecured distal aneurysms do constitute a contraindication, with two out of two patients in their series having succumbed to rebleeding.[18]

ANGIOPLASTY TECHNIQUE

A number of balloons are available for performing intracranial angioplasty for the treatment of vasospasm. Although the original results from Russia were accomplished with a latex balloon, most U.S. groups prefer the newer low-pressure silicone balloons, which elongate with overinflation but do not increase in diameter. This reduces the risk of endothelial damage and vessel rupture. Furthermore, these balloons can be passed intracranially without the aid of guide wires via an introducer catheter placed in the internal carotid or vertebral artery, further reducing endothelial trauma, and allowing for digital subtraction road mapping.

Treatment of the diseased segments is accomplished with repeated rapid inflations of less than 5 seconds, starting proximally and ending distally. Heparinization is maintained throughout the procedure but is reversed with protamine on termination. Technically it is very difficult to dilate vessels more distal than the proximal A1, M1, and P1 segments. For segments distal to these, intra-arterial papaverine has been advocated. Eskridge and others have also maintained that all angiographically involved vessels should be treated during the treatment session, as treatment of the symptomatic territories alone has led to the need for unnecessary repeat treatments.

INTRA-ARTERIAL PAPAVERINE

Papaverine inhibits cAMP/cGMP, thereby directly dilating smooth muscle. First described by Kaku for use in augmenting the effect of angioplasty, especially on distal vessels, this addition has been adopted by other groups.[18,40] The technique involves the infusion of 300 mg of papaverine over 30 minutes into each affected vessel prior to balloon inflation. This controlled rate of infusion limits rapid alterations in systemic blood pressure and increases in intracranial pressure. Intra-arterial papaverine has been used in preparation for angioplasty and alone for less severe narrowing or for hypoplastic A1 and P1 segments too small for angioplasty balloons. Papaverine pretreatment not only makes the placement of the balloon easier but renders the vessel less resistant to dilatation. Especially in the anterior cerebral artery territory, papaverine

Table 52.4 Results of Angioplasty for Cerebral Vasospasm

Series	No. of Patients	Angiographic Improvement	Clinical Improvement	Complications	Outcome
Zubkov[80]	33	99%	Unknown	0%	64% mortality
Newell[55]	10	100%	80%	30%	Unknown
Brothers[8]	4	100%	100%	Unknown	Unknown
Konishi[45]	8	100%	63%	13%	Unknown
Higashida[32]	28	100%	61%	11%	Unknown
Eskridge[18]	60	100%	60%	12%	17% mortality
Fujii[22]	19	83%	63%	Unknown	11% mortality
Coyne[11]	13	Unknown	31%	Unknown	46% mortality
Total	175	97%	60%	9%	11–64% mortality

can be used after balloon angioplasty to further treat still stenotic distal areas.

RESULTS AND COMPLICATIONS

Using the above-mentioned selection criteria, approximately 10% of subarachnoid hemorrhage patients or 30% of patients with symptomatic vasospasm require angioplasty. Of the 48 patients undergoing angioplasty alone and the 12 undergoing angioplasty with papaverine treatment in the Harborview series (97% within 18 hours of symptoms), 66% of the angioplasty patients and 33% of the papaverine/angioplasty patients demonstrated sustained increases of at least 2 points on the Glasgow Coma Scale. Patients treated within 12 hours demonstrated even better responses. Two patients were treated after more than 48 hours of symptoms; 1 showed a complete recovery, and the other died. Interestingly, all vessels ballooned showed angiographic improvement, with no recurrence, while vessels undergoing papaverine infusion alone were improved only half the time, and stenosis recurred in one-third, requiring repeat infusion. Of the patients undergoing angioplasty, 17% died, but 50% were grade 5. Nevertheless, 70% of the mortality was directly related to the angioplasty procedures (four vessel ruptures, one basal ganglia bleed due to papaverine and anticoagulation, and two unsecured aneurysmal reruptures). In those who survived, all are purportedly "doing well" without adverse sequelae secondary to the angioplasty.

To date, more than 200 patients treated with angioplasty for vasospasm have been presented in various peer-reviewed and non–peer-reviewed journals. Together, these series show that angiographic improvement occurs in almost all cases in which angioplasty is performed (93%), with about 60% of patients showing clinical improvement (31% to 100%). Procedural complications occur in 9% (range 0% to 30%), and most of these commonly consist of vessel rupture and rebleeding from unclipped aneurysms. Some series quote dismal outcomes for these patients (11% to 64% mortality), but more recently groups in the U.S. and Japan have shown that with aggressive angioplasty, recalcitrant vasospasm mortality can be reduced to less than 20% (Table 52.4). Timing is also critical, with improved results for patients identified soon after medical management has failed.

References

1. Aaslid R, Huber P, Nornes H: Evaluation of cerebrovascular spasm with transcranial Doppler ultrasound. J Neurosurg 60:37–41, 1984
2. Abe T, Kazawa M, Naito I: Clinical effect of urokinase (60,000 units/day) on cerebral infarction—comparative study by means of multicenter double blind test. Blood Vessels 12:342–358, 1981
3. Allcock JM, Drake CG: Ruptured intracranial aneurysms—the role of arterial spasms. J Neurosurg 22:21–29, 1965
4. Astrup J, Siesjö BK, Symon L: Thresholds in cerebral ischemia—the ischemic penumbra. Stroke 12:723–725, 1981
5. Barker FG, Heros RC: Clinical aspects of vasospasm. Neurosurg Clin North Am 1:277–288, 1990
6. Becker GJ, Katzen BT, Dake MD: Noncoronary angioplasty. Radiology 170:921–940, 1989
7. Bergeon P, Rudondy P, Benichou H et al: Transluminal angioplasty for recurrent stenosis after carotid endarterectomy: prognostic factors and indications. Int Angiol 12:256–259, 1993
8. Brothers MF, Holgate RC: Intracranial angioplasty for treatment of vasospasm after subarachnoid hemorrhage: technique and modifications to improve branch access. AJNR 11:239–247, 1990
9. Brott T, Haley EC, Levy D et al: Safety and potential efficacy of tissue plasminogen activator (tPA) for stroke. Stroke 21:18 1990
10. Brott T, Haley EC, Levy DE et al: Investigational use of tPA for stroke. Ann Emerg Med 17:1202–1205, 1988
11. Coyne TJ, Montanera WJ, Macdonald RL, Wallace MC: Percutaneous transluminal angioplasty for cerebral vasospasm after subarachnoid hemorrhage. Can J Surg 37:391–396, 1994
12. Crowell RM, Olsson Y, Klatzo I, Ommaya A: Temporary occlusion of the middle cerebral artery in the monkey. Stroke 1:439–448, 1970
13. Del Zoppo GJ: Investigational use of tPA in acute stroke. Ann Emerg Med 17:1196–1201, 1988
14. Del Zoppo GJ: Thrombolytic therapy in cerebrovascular disease. Stroke 19:1174–1179, 1988

15. Del Zoppo GJ, Ferbert A, Otis S et al: Local intra-arterial fibrinolytic therapy in acute carotid territory stroke: pilot study. Stroke 19:307–313, 1988

16. Del Zoppo GJ, Zeumer H, Harker LA: Thrombolytic therapy in stroke: possibilities and hazards. Stroke 17: 595–607, 1986

17. Eckhout E, Kappenberger L, Goy JJ: Stents for Intracoronary Placement: Current Status and Future Directions

18. Eskridge JM, Newell DW, Winn HR: Endovascular treatment of vasospasm. Neurosurg Clin North Am 5: 437–447, 1994

19. Executive Committee for the Asymptomatic Carotid Atherosclerosis Study: Endarterectomy for asymptomatic carotid artery stenosis. JAMA 273:1421–1428, 1995

20. Fisher CM, Kistler JP, Davis JM: Relation of cerebral vasospasm to subarachnoid hemorrhage visualized by computerized tomographic scanning. Neurosurgery 6: 1–9, 1980

21. Fletcher AP, Alkjaersig N, Lewis M et al: A pilot study of urokinase therapy in cerebral infarction. Stroke 7: 135–142, 1976

22. Fujii Y, Takahashi A, Ezura M, Mizoi K: Balloon angioplasty immediately after surgical clipping for symptomatic vasospasm on admission: report of four cases. Neurosurg Rev 18:79–84, 1995

23. Gentles TL, Lock JE, Perry SB: High pressure balloon angioplasty for branch pulmonary artery stenosis: early experience. J Am Coll Cardiol 22:867–872, 1993

24. Gil-Peralta A, Mayol A, Gonzalez M et al: Percutaneous transluminal angioplasty of the symptomatic atherosclerotic carotid arteries: results, complications, and follow-up. Stroke 27:2271–2273, 1996

25. Gobin Y, Hassani R, Batellier J et al: Transluminal angioplasty of the brachiocephalic artery with cerebral protection. J Mal Vasc 16:188–190, 1991

26. Graf CJ, Nibbelink DW: Cooperative study of intracranial aneurysms and subarachnoid hemorrhage. Report on a randomized treatment study: 3. intracranial surgery. Stroke 5:557–601, 1974

27. Hacke W, Zeumer H, Ferbert A et al: Intra-arterial thrombolytic therapy improves outcome in patients with acute vertebrobasilar occlusive disease. Stroke 19: 1216–1222, 1988

28. Hanaway J, Torack R, Fletcher AP, Landau WM: Intracranial bleeding associated with urokinase therapy for acute ischemic hemispheral stroke. Stroke 7:143–146, 1976

29. Harders AG, Gilsbach JM: Time course of blood velocity changes related to vasospasm in the circle of Willis measured by transcranial Doppler ultrasound. J Neurosurg 66:718–728, 1987

30. Hart RG, Easton JD: Hemorrhagic infarcts. Stroke 17: 586–589, 1986

31. Henze T, Boeer A, Tebbe U, Romatowski J: Lysis of basilar artery occlusion with tissue plasminogen activator. Lancet ii:1391, 1967

32. Higashida R et al: Transluminal angioplasty for treatment of intracranial arterial vasospasm. J Neurosurg 71: 648–653, 1989

33. Higashida RT, Tsai FY, Halbach VV et al: Transluminal angioplasty for atherosclerotic disease of the vertebral and basilar arteries. J Neurosurg 78:192–198, 1993

34. Hijazi ZM, Fahey JT, Kleinman CS, Hellenbrand WE: Balloon angioplasty for recurrent coarctation of aorta. Immediate and long-term results [see comments]. Circulation 84:1150–1156, 1991

35. Hornig CR, Dorndorf W, Agnoli AL: Hemorrhagic cerebral infarction—a prospective study. Stroke 17:179–185, 1986

36. Inomori S, Fujino H, Yamataki A et al: Percutaneous transluminal angioplasty for multiple brachiocephalic artery stenosis: case report. No Shinkei Geka 18:295–299, 1990

37. Jordan WD Jr, Roye GD, Fisher WS, McDowell HA Jr: A cost comparison of carotid angioplasty and carotid endarterectomy for the treatment of carotid stenosis. Society of Vascular Surgeons, 1997 meeting.

38. Jungreis CA, Wechsler LR, Horton JA: Intracranial thrombolysis via a catheter embedded in the clot. Stroke 20:1578–1580, 1989

39. Kachel R, Endert G, Basche S et al: Percutaneous transluminal angioplasty (dilatation) of carotid, vertebral, innominate artery stenoses. Cardiovasc Intervent Radiol 10: 142–146, 1987

40. Kaku Y, Yonekawa Y, Tsukahara T, Kazekawa K: Superselective intra-arterial infusion of papaverine for the treatment of cerebral vasospasm after subarachnoid hemorrhage. J Neurosurg 77:842–847, 1992

41. Kassell NF, Helm G, Simmons N et al: Treatment of cerebral vasospasm with intra-arterial papaverine. J Neurosurg 77:848–852, 1992

42. Kerber CW, Cromwell LD, Loehden OL: Catheter dilatation of proximal stenosis during distal bifurcation endarterectomy. AJNR 1:348–349, 1980

43. Kinoshita A, Itoh M, Takemoto O: Percutaneous transluminal angioplasty of internal carotid artery: a preliminary report of seesaw balloon technique. Neurol Res 15: 356–358, 1993

44. Komiyama M, Nishio A, Nishijima Y: Endovascular treatment of acute thrombotic occlusion of the cervical internal carotid artery associated with embolic occlusion of the middle cerebral artery: case report. Neurosurgery 34: 359–363, 1994

45. Konishi Y, Maemura E, Shiota M et al: Treatment of vasospasm by balloon angioplasty: experimental studies and clinical experiences. Neurol Res 14:273–281, 1992

46. Lam JY, Chesebro JH, Steele PM et al: Antithrombotic therapy for deep arterial injury by angioplasty. Efficacy of common platelet inhibition compared with thrombin inhibition in pigs. Circulation 84:814–820, 1991

47. Lorenzi G, Domanin M, Constantini A: PTA and laser assisted PTA combined with simultaneous surgical revascularization. J Cardiovasc Surg 32:456–462, 1991

48. Maiza D, Theron J, Pelouze GA et al: Local fibrinolytic therapy in ischemic carotid pathology. Ann Vasc Surg 2: 205–214, 1988

49. Marder VJ, Sherry S: Thrombolytic therapy: current status [Second of two parts]. N Engl J Med 318:1585–1595, 1988

50. Mathias KD, Luth I, Haarmann P: Percutaneous translu-

minal angioplasty of proximal subclavian artery occlusions. Cardiovasc Intervent Radiol 16:214–218, 1993

51. Mori E, Tabuchi M, Yoshida T, Yamadori A: Intracarotid urokinase with thromboembolic occlusion of the middle cerebral artery. Stroke 19:802–812, 1989

52. Mullan S: Conservative management of the recently ruptured aneurysm. Surg Neurol 3:27–32, 1975

53. Mullan S, Duda EE, Patro NAS: Some examples of balloon technology in neurosurgery. J Neurosurg 52: 321–329, 1980

54. National Institutes of Health Consensus Conference: Thrombolytic therapy in treatment. Br Med J 280: 1585–1587, 1988

55. Newell DW, Eskridge JM, Mayberg MR, Winn HR: Angioplasty for the treatment of symptomatic vasospasm following subarachnoid hemorrhage. Neurosurgery 71: 654–660, 1989

56. North American Symptomatic Carotid Endarterectomy Trial: Beneficial effect of carotid endarterectomy in symptomatic patients with high-grade carotid stenosis. New Engl J Med 325:445–453, 1991

57. Okada Y, Yamaguchi T, Minematsu K et al: Hemorrhagic transformation in cerebral embolism. Stroke 20:598–603, 1989

58. Ott BR, Zamani A, Kleefield J, Funkenstein HH: The clinical spectrum of hemorrhagic infarction. Stroke 4: 630–637, 1986

59. Ramsay LE, Waller PC: Blood pressure response to percutaneous transluminal angioplasty for renovascular hypertension: an overview of published series. Br Med J 300:569–572, 1990

60. Ropper AH, Zervas NT: Outcome 1 year after SAH from cerebral aneurysm. Management morbidity, mortality, and functional status in 112 consecutive good-risk patients. J Neurosurg 60:909–915, 1984

61. The rt-PA/Acute Stroke Study Group: An open safety/efficacy trial of rt-PA in acute thromboembolic stroke: final report. Stroke 22:153, 1991

62. Sharma S, Kaul U, Rajani M: Identifying high-risk patients for percutaneous transluminal angioplasty of subclavian and innominate arteries. Acta Radiol 32:381–385, 1991

63. Shoenfeld R, Hermans H, Novick A et al: Stenting of proximal venous obstructions to maintain hemodialysis access. J Vasc Surg 19:532–538, 1994

64. Sloan MA: Thrombosis and stroke: past and future. Arch Neurol 44:748–768, 1987

65. Takahashi A, Sugawara K, Mizoi K et al: Superselective local thrombolysis for acute MCA embolism utilizing tPA. Abstracts of 6th Annual Meeting of the Japanese Society for Intravascular Neurosurgery, 29, 1990

66. Theron J: Angioplasty of brachiocephalic vessels. pp. 167–180. In Viñuela F, Halbach VV, Jaryl ED (eds): Interventional Neuroradiology: Endovascular Therapy of the CNS. Lippincott-Raven, Philadelphia, 1992

67. Theron J, Courtheoux P, Alachkar F et al: New triple coaxial catheter system for carotid angioplasty with cerebral protection. AJNR 11:869–874, 1990

68. Theron J, Courtheoux P, Alachkar F, Maiza D: [Intravascular technics of cerebral revascularization]. [Review] [French]. J Malad Vasc 15:245–256, 1990

69. Theron J, Courtheoux P, Casasco A et al: Local intraarterial fibrinolysis in the carotid territory. AJNR 10:753–765, 1989

70. Theron JG, Payelle GG, Coskun O et al: Carotid artery stenosis: treatment with protected balloon angioplasty and stent placement. Radiology 201:627–636, 1996

71. Thrombolysis in Myocardial Infarction Study Group: The thrombolysis in myocardial infarction (TIMI) trial. N Engl J Med 312:932–936, 1985

72. The tPA-Acute Stroke Study Group: An open multicenter study of the safety and efficacy of various doses of rt-PA in patients with acute stroke: preliminary results. Stroke 21:181, 1990

73. Trinca M, Millaire A, Marache P et al: Angioplasty of the subclavian arteries. Immediate and mid-term results. [Review] [French]. Ann Cardiol D'Angeiol 42:127–132, 1993

74. Tsai FY, Higashida RT, Matovich V et al: Seven year experience with PTA of carotid artery. Neuroradiology, suppl. 33:S397–S398, 1991

75. Tsai F, Shah D, Matovich V, Alfieri K: Intra-arterial therapy for acute cerebral infarction and progressive stroke. Proc ASNR 26:288, 1988

76. Wisselink W, Money SR, Becker MO et al: Comparison of operative reconstruction and percutaneous balloon dilatation for central venous obstruction. Am J Surg 166: 200–204, 1993

77. Yadav JS, Roubin GS, Iyer S et al: Elective stenting of the extracranial carotid arteries. Circulation 95:376–381, 1997

78. Zeumer H, Freitag HJ, Grzyska U, Neunzig HP: Local intraarterial fibrinolysis in acute vertebrobasilar occlusion: technical developments and recent results. Neuroradiology 31:336–340, 1989

79. Zeumer H, Hacke W, Ringelstein EB: Local intraarterial thrombolysis in vertebrobasilar thromboembolic disease. AJNR 4:401–404, 1983

80. Zubkov YN, Nikiforov BM, Shustin VA: Balloon catheter technique for dilatation of constricted cerebral arteries after aneurysmal SAH. Acta Neurochir (Wien) 70:65–79, 1984

Atherosclerotic Disease of the Carotid Arteries

Overview: A Medical Perspective

HENRY J. M. BARNETT

HEATHER E. MELDRUM

MICHAEL ELIASZIW

Early Attempts to Evaluate Carotid Endarterectomy

The first publication in a major English language journal detailing a surgical procedure designed to prevent a threatening stroke in the carotid artery territory came in 1954 from a team of two surgeons (Eastcott and Rob) and a physician (Pickering).[13] Since that time, physicians and surgeons have maintained a mutual interest in the ever-expanding role that carotid endarterectomy has come to play in preventing ischemic stroke arising from the extracranial arteries. Surgeons and neurologists, together with radiologists, subjected carotid endarterectomy to early randomized clinical trials. In 1970 in the first trial, the study design was inadequate by modern standards: there were too few patients (N = 316), entry of many patients without appropriate carotid symptoms, too many lost patients, too many crossovers, and an unacceptably high perioperative complication rate.[21] The second trial in 1984 was much smaller (N = 41) but the perioperative complication rate was excessive.[38] During the ensuing years surgical skills continued to develop, and despite the negative results of the early studies, the procedure was not abandoned. Instead, it was carried out in increasing numbers, not only in symptomatic patients with various degrees of stenosis, but also in patients with stenosis and no symptoms and in patients with stenosis and symptoms that were loosely accepted as related to the stenotic lesion. These nonhemispheric and vertebrobasilar symptoms in all probability were unrelated to the carotid lesions in most if not all instances, and the plaques that were removed were incidental and asymptomatic.

By the mid-1980s two particular concerns emerged that questioned the exponential growth in enthusiasm for endar-terectomy. First, the rising numbers of endarterectomies being done increased the uncertainty that such a large number were indicated and that every patient benefited.[5,43] Second came the disturbing revelation from community studies that the average rate of morbidity and mortality of almost 10% was so high that benefit for the individual patient appeared dubious.[44] With these concerns in mind, further scientific evaluation of carotid endarterectomy began.

Carotid Endarterectomy for Symptomatic Patients with Severe Carotid Stenosis

After a decade of randomized clinical trials a much clearer understanding of the indications for endarterectomy has emerged.[18,29,35] The areas of certainty may now be summarized as follows:

1. Patients with focal hemisphere or retinal ischemic symptoms, either in the form of transient ischemic attacks or as persisting nondisabling deficits, with a 70% to 99% stenosis of the appropriate internal carotid artery have a 17% absolute risk reduction in terms of ipsilateral stroke when treated with the best medical care and carotid endarterectomy compared with the best medical care alone (Fig. 53.1). These patients should be denied this procedure only if they have recently had a disabling stroke or have an illness that makes them too sick to be submitted to endarterectomy.

2. The surgical procedure must be carried out only by surgeons who have a low perioperative complication rate. If this

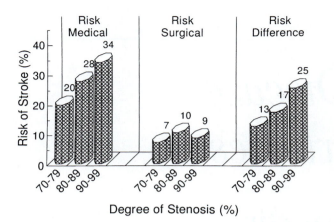

Figure 53.1 Kaplan-Meier estimates of the risk of any ipsilateral stroke at 2 years by degree of angiographically defined stenosis in the symptomatic carotid artery of patients in the North American Symptomatic Carotid Endarterectomy Trial (NASCET). For medically treated patients, the risk of stroke increases with increasing deciles of stenosis, whereas the risk remains similar across all degrees of stenosis for surgically treated patients. The net result, in absolute terms, is that patients with the most severe stenosis receive the greatest benefit from carotid endarterectomy. (From Barnett et al,[4] with permission.)

rate approaches a combined morbidity and mortality of 10%, the benefit of endarterectomy is negated. The patient should be referred to a center and a surgeon with a complication rate in the ≤6% range for any stroke or perioperative death and ≤3% for disabling stroke.

3. The benefit of the procedure has been validated only by conventional angiography, and the measurement of the degree of stenosis utilized the index of the North American Symptomatic Carotid Endarterectomy Trial (NASCET) or its equivalent converted from the European Carotid Surgery Trial (ECST) method (Fig. 53.2).

4. In the presence of a high vascular risk profile, the annual risk of stroke for patients with severe stenosis treated medically is more than double what it is for patients with a low or negligible vascular risk profile. The benefit of surgery is greater for the patients in the high vascular risk profile category (Fig. 53.3). These vascular risks collectively do not add to the hazard of endarterectomy.

5. Two conditions related to the carotid artery impose a definite increase in the risk of endarterectomy. First, there is a doubling of the perioperative stroke and death rate for patients in whom the opposite (usually asymptomatic) carotid artery is occluded.[22] Nevertheless, even at this level of operative risk, surgical treatment in these patients confers a fourfold benefit over medical treatment alone (Fig. 53.4). Second, a large intraluminal thrombus, seen in the angiogram, is an indicator of an immediate risk from endarterectomy of 18% to 22%. These high figures were seen in NASCET as well as in other reported series.[1,7,8,23,30,36] The risk for patients with an intraluminal thrombus treated medically is equally forbidding in the 30-day postdiagnosis period. The empirical treatment of choice is a 30-day period on anticoagulants. If repeat imaging

studies determine the dissolution of the thrombus, the endarterectomy should proceed.

6. The surgical benefit for patients with severe stenosis is durable, up to at least 5 years, as studied in NASCET (Fig. 53.5) and ECST.

7. The risk for medical therapy increases with the degree of stenosis and reaches its maximum at 90% to 94%. Patients with near occlusion of the artery, with or without a string sign, have a risk less than half that observed in the most serious range of all, 90% to 94% (Fig. 53.6). Patients with near-occlusion, with or without a string sign, benefit from endarterectomy. The greatest benefit, with an absolute difference of 26.4%, was seen in those patients at greatest risk in the 90% to 94% group.[31]

8. Patients with readily identifiable ulcerative lesions in the angiogram are at greater risk than those with no such visible ulcerative lesions. The highest risk is in the patients with an ulcerative lesion who are in the 10th decile of stenosis (Fig. 53.7). There is only a minimal increase in the risk of endarterectomy in this latter group of patients. They are all candidates for endarterectomy.[16]

9. The risk of stroke is three times higher in medically treated patients with hemisphere symptoms related to severe stenosis than in similar patients with only retinal ischemic symptoms (Fig. 53.8). Patients in both groups benefit from endarterectomy.[40]

10. The procedure of endarterectomy has only a short-term effect on the baroreceptors in the carotid sinus. A small number of patients experience hypertension or hypotension for a few hours. After 24 hours the level of blood pressure that ensues will be unrelated to the surgical procedure and is identical to that seen in medically treated control patients with the same amount of carotid disease[15] (Fig. 53.9).

11. Carotid endarterectomy for patients with severe carotid disease has been shown to be cost-effective.[28] Only six endarterectomies need be performed in symptomatic patients with a 70% to 99% stenosis of the appropriate carotid artery to prevent one stroke in a 2-year period (Table 53.1). When the stenosis is 90% to 99%, only four symptomatic patients need be submitted to the procedure to prevent one stroke in 2 years.

Persisting Uncertainties about Carotid Endarterectomy

All of the indications for carotid surgical therapy have not been settled. Persisting uncertainties are outlined as follows:

1. Symptomatic patients with an appropriate lesion that produces less than a 70% stenosis are still under study. In early 1998 the final analysis from NASCET will be available to settle finally the issue of benefit or otherwise for these patients. It is possible but still speculative that symptomatic patients in the 50% to 69% stenosis range, especially those with a high risk profile, will be found to benefit from endarterectomy.

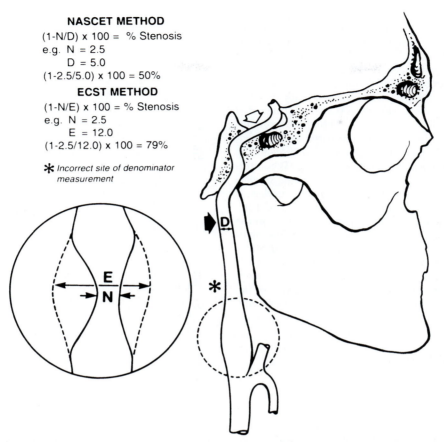

NASCET METHOD

(1-N/D) x 100 = % Stenosis

e.g. N = 2.5

D = 5.0

(1-2.5/5.0) x 100 = 50%

ECST METHOD

(1-N/E) x 100 = % Stenosis

e.g. N = 2.5

E = 12.0

(1-2.5/12.0) x 100 = 79%

✻ *Incorrect site of denominator measurement*

Figure 53.2 The North American Symptomatic Carotid Endarterectomy Trial (NAS-CET) calculates the percentage of stenosis by using the narrowest linear diameter in two (or three planes) as the numerator, and the artery well beyond the carotid bulb (circled) and any poststenotic dilatation as the denominator (closed arrow). Measurement of the artery too close to the bulb produces a misleading denominator (asterisk). NASCET measures were conducted at a site well beyond the usual poststenotic or arteriosclerotic dilatation. The European Carotid Surgery Trial (ECST) used the same numerator but took the imagined site of the wall of the carotid bulb as the denominator. ECST calculations yielded 46% more patients in the "severe" category than those of NASCET. The open arrow points to the common site of stenosing atheroma in the intracranial portion of the internal carotid artery. (From Barnett et al,[6] with permission.)

2. ECST has not found any benefit for symptomatic patients with stenosis that NASCET would measure at <50%.[17] If NASCET's final analyses confirm this negative benefit, these patients will almost certainly be best treated medically.

3. The Asymptomatic Carotid Atherosclerosis Study (ACAS) provided data indicating modest benefit overall for asymptomatic patients with a ≥60% stenosis as measured by ultrasound. There was an absolute stroke risk reduction of 1% at 5 years between the patients given best medical care plus endarterectomy and those given best medical care alone[20] (Fig. 53.10). The investigators were unable to provide data from the 1,659 patients that indicated a benefit for patients in the higher deciles of stenosis compared with the lower deciles of stenosis. There were too few patients and outcome events for subgroup analysis. The observational case series and the prospective observations made on the "asymptomatic other side" mea-sured by angiography in the ECST and the NASCET studies suggest strongly that the asymptomatic patient with a ≥85% stenosis will benefit from endarterectomy[3,9,19,26,34] (Fig. 53.11). When data become available from future studies, it is expected that the greatest benefit from endarterectomy for asymptomatic patients will be for those with the tightest stenosis and a high vascular risk profile (Fig. 53.12).

4. No data exist to support the popular practice of performing endarterectomy on asymptomatic patients as a prelude to other major vascular surgical procedures, such as coronary artery bypass grafting.[25,33] As evidence accumulates, it becomes more likely that the usual cause of ischemic stroke in patients submitted to coronary artery bypass grafting (CABG) is embolization from a diseased aorta into which the shunt for the cardiopulmonary bypass is inserted.

5. The economic benefit and cost-effectiveness of endarterectomy for symptomatic patients with a <70% stenosis is unknown. The economic benefit and cost-effectiveness for screening and submitting asymptomatic patients to endarterectomy is equally uncertain.[37,42] To prevent one stroke in 2 years in asymptomatic patients of the type submitted to endarterectomy in ACAS would require 67 operations[3] (Table 53.2). This is 11 times the number required in symptomatic patients. If the surgical complication rate from ACAS is recalculated based on the number of patients actually submitted to endarterectomy (744), instead of a calculation based on an intention-to-treat of the 845 patients randomized to surgery, the perioperative risk becomes 2.6% instead of 2.3%. When this calculation is done at 2 years, the adjusted risk of surgical treatment is 3.8%. The number needed-to-treat by endarterectomy to prevent one stroke in 2 years increases to 83 patients. If the optimistic interpretation placed by some on the results of the ACAS trial were fully adopted, it has been estimated that there are 2 million people in the United States who could be offered this procedure in the coming year. This is twice as many as have ever been submitted to this procedure worldwide. The identification of a more precise group of patients who will benefit from surgical intervention in the absence of symptoms is urgently required.

The Best Medical Care for Patients with Known Carotid Disease

The best medical care is just as important as the surgical considerations for patients with various degrees of carotid stenosis whether symptomatic or asymptomatic. The evidence that

Figure 53.3 Kaplan-Meier estimates of the average annual risk of ipsilateral stroke related to the number of risk factors present in the medically treated patients of the North American Symptomatic Carotid Endarterectomy Trial (NASCET) symptomatic with a 70% to 99% stenosis of the carotid artery. The list of 16 risk factors that comprise the risk profile has been previously published.[35] The risk of stroke rises with an increasing number of risk factors. (From Barnett et al,[3] with permission.)

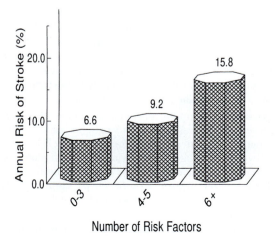

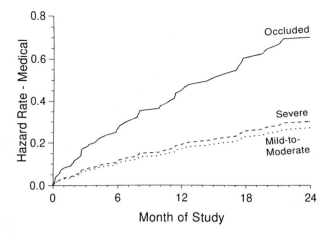

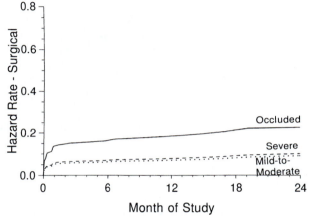

Figure 53.4 (**A**) Cumulative hazard curves showing risk (hazard rate) of ipsilateral stroke for medically treated patients at three degrees of contralateral carotid artery disease. (**B**) Cumulative hazard curves showing risk (hazard rate) of ipsilateral stroke for surgically treated North American Symptomatic Carotid Endarterectomy Trial (NASCET) patients with ≥70% stenosis at at three levels of contralateral carotid artery disease. Severe contralateral stenosis carried the same prognosis as did a mild to moderate stenosis. By contrast, a contralateral occlusion added greatly to the risk in medically treated patients. The surgical risk was double that of patients without contralateral occlusion but substantially less than in those treated medically. (From Gasecki et al,[22] with permission.)

managing vascular risk factors slows the process of arteriosclerotic progression is compelling (see Ch. 1). Patients should be urged strongly to submit to strict control of hypertension and of diabetes. If either of these conditions is out of reasonable control, plans for endarterectomy, even in patients symptomatic with severe disease, should be deferred until these abnormalities are corrected. Uncontrolled hypertension at the time of endarterectomy raises the specter of postoperative intracerebral hematoma. Ischemic stroke complicating the procedure is likely to be more disabling in the presence of hyperglycemia. Evidence has emerged from NASCET centers that carotid endarterectomy in the diabetic, regardless of reg-

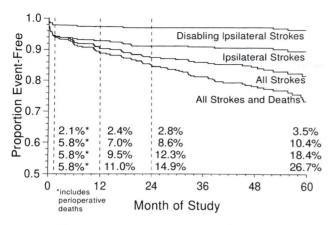

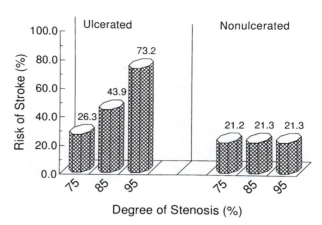

Figure 53.5 Kaplan-Meier curves showing event-free survival after carotid endarterectomy in symptomatic North American Symptomatic Carotid Endarterectomy Trial (NASCET) patients with a 70% to 99% stenosis. The percentages at the bottom are the Kaplan-Meier risk estimates at 30 days and 12, 24, and 60 months, respectively, for three types of stroke and death.

Figure 53.7 Two-year estimates of ipsilateral stroke risk by presence (and absence) of definite plaque ulceration and degree of stenosis for medically treated North American Symptomatic Carotid Endarterectomy Trial (NASCET) patients with a 70% to 99% stenosis, calculated from a Cox proportional hazards regression model. The presence of definite carotid plaque ulceration on an angiogram is a marker for poor prognosis, which is exacerbated by increasing degrees of stenosis. In the absence of plaque ulceration, the risk of stroke remains relatively constant. (From Barnett et al,[4] with permission.)

ulation, carries a higher risk (7.8%) of perioperative stroke than in the nondiabetic patient (3.7%).[41] In the younger patient with carotid disease, the presence of homocystinemia must be investigated and treated for life when detected. Zero tolerance should attend hyperlipidemia and cigarette smoking.

Antithrombotic therapy, in the form of platelet inhibitors, is inferior to endarterectomy, but this does not mean that patients undergoing endarterectomy should not be given platelet inhibitors. The Mayo Asymptomatic Carotid Endarterectomy (MACE) trial is a clear example of the hazard of withholding platelet inhibitors and relying on endarterectomy for stroke prevention alone.[27] The surgical arm was denied the aspirin given in the medical arm. The surfeit of myocardial

and cerebral ischemic events that occurred in the surgical patients in this small randomized trial led to stopping the study.

The accumulated evidence from large numbers of trials of stroke-threatened patients has established that platelet inhibition is beneficial in patients with ischemic symptoms.[2] Aspirin is the drug of choice. This matter is fully discussed in Chapter 46.

Patients in NASCET who were on lower (325 mg or less)

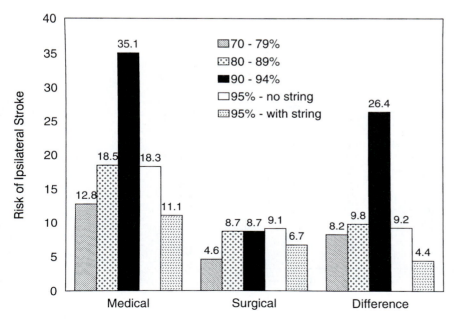

Figure 53.6 Kaplan-Meier estimates of ipsilateral stroke at 1 year according to five subgroups of stenosis. The worst prognosis was for patients with a 90% to 94% stenosis proven by angiography. Conversely, these patients had the most dramatic benefit from endarterectomy (26.4% absolute risk reduction) patients with near occlusion, with and without a string sign benefit from endarterectomy. The outlook for patients with a string sign was better than for patients with an 80% to 94% stenosis. (From Morgenstern,[31] with permission.)

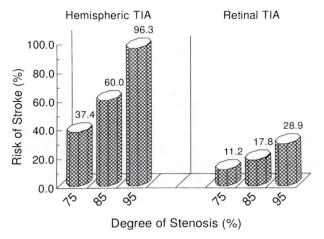

Figure 53.8 Two-year estimates of ipsilateral stroke risk by the type of transient ischemic attack (TIA) and degree of stenosis for medically treated North American Symptomatic Carotid Endarterectomy Trial (NASCET) patients with a ≥70% stenosis, calculated from a Cox proportional hazards regression model. The overall prognosis for patients presenting with a first-ever hemispheric TIA is worse than for patients presenting with a first-ever retinal TIA. In both cases, the outlook is affected by the degree of carotid artery stenosis. (From Barnett et al,[4] with permission.)

Table 53.1 Risk of Ipsilateral Stroke or Any Perioperative Stroke or Perioperative Death (NASCET)[a]

Month of Study	Medical Risk (%)	Surgical Risk (%)	Risk (%) Difference	RRR (%)	NNT
30 days	3.3	5.8	−2.5	—	—
1 year	17.3	7.5	9.8	57	10
2 years	26.0	9.0	17.0	65	6

Abbreviations: RRR, relative risk reduction; NNT, number needed to treat.

[a] *From the North American Symptomatic Carotid Endarterectomy Trial (NASCET). The risk of stroke for 331 medically treated and 328 surgically treated patients with symptoms appropriate to severe stenosis are given at 30 days and 1 and 2 years. To prevent one stroke in 2 years, six patients need to have endarterectomy.*

(From Barnett et al,[3] with permission.)

doses of aspirin at the time of endarterectomy had a fivefold increase of perioperative stroke and death compared with those on 650 mg or more. A trial is ongoing to test this retrospective data-generated hypothesis. It will settle the question of the optimum perioperative dose of aspirin in patients being submitted to endarterectomy.[41]

The two platelet inhibitors in common use, aspirin and ticlopidine, prolong bleeding time and hemorrhagic complica-

Figure 53.9 Mean systolic blood pressure over time for medically and surgically treated patients adjusted for baseline differences. The dotted horizontal line represents the mean pressure at baseline. The percentage of patients on antihypertensive medication at each follow-up clinic visit is represented by a single bar, as there was no difference between the medical and surgical groups. The single-hatched bar indicates the percentage of patients on one medication, whereas the cross-hatched bar indicates the percentage of patients on two or more medications. It would appear that the postrandomization rise seen in both treatment arms was due to a modest reduction in the strictness with which the antihypertensive regimen was managed. (From Eliasziw et al,[15] with permission.)

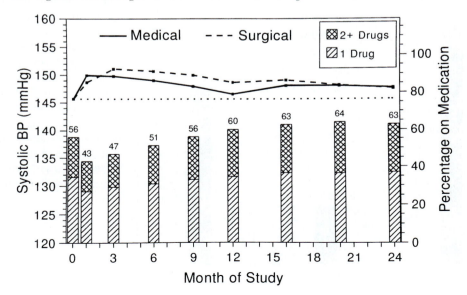

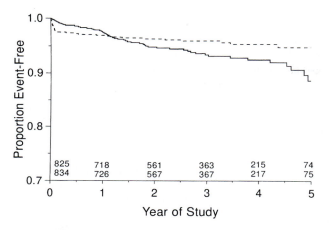

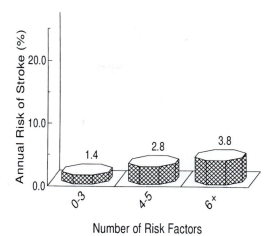

Figure 53.10 Kaplan-Meier curves showing the probability that asymptomatic patients will survive free of a combined outcome of ipsilateral stroke of any severity or any perioperative stroke death by treatment group. The solid line indicates medical patients, and the broken line, surgical patients. The estimated number of patients who remained event-free in each treatment group is shown at the bottom of the graph. (Modified from Executive Committee for the Asymptomatic Carotid Atherosclerosis Study,[20] with permission.)

Figure 53.12 Kaplan-Meier estimates of the average annual risk of ipsilateral stroke by the number of risk factors presented by medically treated patients with an asymptomatic contralateral stenosis in the North American Symptomatic Carotid Endarterectomy Trial (NASCET). The list of 16 risk factors that comprise the risk profile has been previously published.[35] The risk of stroke rises with an increasing number of risk factors. (From Barnett et al,[3] with permission.)

tions. Meticulous surgical technique will obviate the wound hematoma. Evidence suggests that neither this complication nor severe gastrointestinal hemorrhage or intracerebral bleeding is dose-related.[32]

Asymptomatic patients and patients not known to have disease of the carotid arteries have been subjected to inconclu-

sive clinical trials of platelet inhibition. No benefit in stroke reduction was detected in a small trial of 372 patients with asymptomatic carotid stenosis.[12] This may be due to the small sample size, the small number of outcome events, and that only one low dose (325 mg) of aspirin was utilized. The Physicians Health Study found no reduction in stroke, despite a 46% reduction in myocardial infarction in 22,000 male physicians free of known vascular disease.[39] The low dose of aspirin (325 mg every other day) may also have been the reason for lack of any benefit. It would seem wise to recommend 325 mg

Figure 53.11 Average annual risk (hazard rate) of ipsilateral stroke by the degree of stenosis defined by angiography in the asymptomatic carotid artery of patients in the North American Symptomatic Carotid Endarterectomy Trial (NASCET). The curve was generated by fitting a Cox proportional hazards regression model. Only in a >70% stenosis is the annual risk of stroke 3% or more, which approximates the best risk of endarterectomy. (From Barnett et al,[3] with permission.)

Table 53.2 Risk of Ipsilateral Stroke or Any Perioperative Stroke or Perioperative Death (ACAS)[a]

Month of Study	Medical Risk (%)	Surgical Risk (%)	Risk (%) Difference	RRR (%)	NNT
30 days	0.4	2.3	−1.9	—	—
1 year	2.4	3.0	−0.6	—	—
2 years	5.0	3.5	1.5	30	67
5 years	11.0	5.1	5.9	53	17

Abbreviations: RRR, relative risk reduction; NNT, number needed to treat.

[a] From the Asymptomatic Carotid Atherosclerosis Study (ACAS). The risk of stroke is compared between medically and surgically treated patients. To prevent one stroke in 2 years, 67 patients need to have endarterectomy. Adjusting the surgical to include only the patients who had endarterectomy, the 30-day surgical risk becomes 2.6%, the 1-, 2-, and 5-year risks rise to 3.3%, 3.8%, and 5.4% respectively. The number needed to treat to prevent one stroke in 2 years becomes 83.

(From Barnett et al,[3] with permission.)

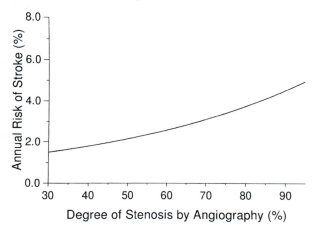

Figure 53.13 Line graph showing the mean peak systolic velocity across time, as measured by ultrasound, for medically and surgically treated patients in the North American Symptomatic Carotid Endarterectomy Trial (NASCET). "Ipsilateral" refers to the recently symptomatic artery for which the patient was randomized into NASCET, and "contralateral" refers to the artery on the patient's other side. Except for the sharp drop in velocity at 30 days, which corresponds to the effectiveness of surgery on the ipsilateral artery, all lines have a similar slope. This suggests that in both the medical and surgical patients the accumulation of atheroma occurs at a similar rate.

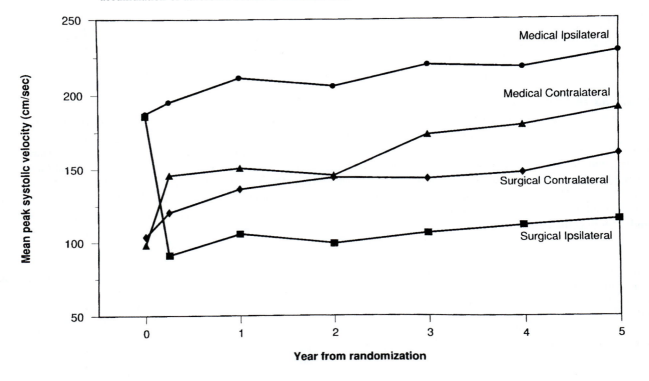

of enteric-coated aspirin twice daily for patients with known asymptomatic carotid disease.

Investigation of Patients Suspected of Carotid Disease

Clinical trials have established the efficacy of endarterectomy for some patients but still leave uncertain the benefit from endarterectomy in other patients. The degree of stenosis and the presence or absence of symptoms will determine the extent of the investigation.

Medical history and investigation must identify whether the episodes are attributable to cardioembolic, lacunar, or large artery causes. A screening by carotid artery ultrasound is recommended for all patients.

If the patient has experienced focal hemispheric or retinal symptoms and the ultrasound suggests a stenosis at or above 70%, taking into consideration the peak systolic volumes and frequencies and the B-mode studies, the patient may be a candidate for endarterectomy. Some surgeons recently have

declared that these individuals can be taken to the operating room without further imaging study.[10] There are several compelling reasons why this is an unwise proposal. It assumes that the ultrasound studies can be accurately correlated to conventional angiography. It assumes that there is no need to image the intracranial circulation. Neither of these assumptions is correct. Of the patients who are claimed by ultrasound to be at or above 70%, 15% will be shown by angiography to have narrowing that is below this.[14] If submitted to endarterectomy, these patients would receive a procedure with a perioperative risk of stroke or death of at least 6%. The evidence that they would benefit when the lesion is <70% is lacking. The condition of the intracranial carotid artery and its major middle cerebral artery trunk and branches are vital to decisions about the potential benefit of endarterectomy. A severe intracranial carotid or middle cerebral artery stenosis will make a cervical carotid endarterectomy of doubtful benefit. The patient with severe carotid intracranial stenosis faces an operative risk known to be double that for patients without intracranial stenosis.[30] Intracranial aneurysms, arteriovenous malformations, and intraluminal thrombi will not be identified by ultrasound alone.

A special problem is posed by the patient whose ultrasound suggests an arterial occlusion in the territory of the symptoms. Frequently these patients do not have a complete occlusion and by angiography have a near-occlusion. They will benefit from endarterectomy and do considerably worse if treated medically. Complete occlusion can be detected with certainty only by conventional angiography.[14]

The noninvasive angiography derived from magnetic resonance images has not been able to avoid the exaggerated measurement in percent stenosis caused by turbulence. This is unfortunate because there is still a small but definite risk from conventional angiography and it would be preferable if it could be avoided. In busy centers where expert neuroradiographers have had their work submitted to prospective independent evaluation, the risk of an ischemic stroke from angiography is 0.4% to 0.5%. Four of five strokes that complicate angiography are nondisabling, with only moderate, mild, or no eventual disability. In NASCET, with a requirement for angiography prior to randomization, nondisabling strokes occurred in 0.62% of 2,887 procedures. Including disabling stroke, the total stroke complication rate is estimated at 0.7%. While this is undesirable, it is a risk only about one-tenth that of endarterectomy. If endarterectomy is done without verified indications, the complications are quite unacceptable and unnecessary.

Carotid stenosis is found very frequently in aging populations in which there has been ultrasound investigation of patients with neck bruits, or from routine use of ultrasound in a general checkup for vascular disease. (See the next part of this chapter.) Angiography leading to endarterectomy is justifiable only for asymptomatic patients with the highest degrees of stenosis. There is a favorable outlook for patients with lesser degrees of stenosis with medical care alone. If symptoms develop, the subsequent studies should include angiography.

As a sequel to endarterectomy, it has been a common practice to keep the patient under surveillance with periodic examinations by ultrasound. Studies from the NASCET patient base have established that the risk of further arterial narrowing is no greater on the side submitted to endarterectomy than it is in the artery on the other side that is neither severely stenosed nor symptomatic. The progression of the arteriosclerotic process, in all but exceptional patients, is at a rate about 4% per year[11] (Fig. 53.13). From these observations and a similar British study, it is difficult to justify the expense of repeated ultrasound examinations.[24] New or recurrent symptoms would immediately change this picture and repeat ultrasound would be required.

References

1. Barnett HJM: Prospective randomized trial of symptomatic patients: results from the NASCET study. pp. 537–539. In Moore WS (ed): Surgery for Cerebrovascular Disease. 2nd WB Saunders, Philadelphia, 1996
2. Barnett HJM, Eliasziw M, Meldrum H: Drug therapy: drugs and surgery in the prevention of ischemic stroke. N Engl J Med 332:238–248, 1995
3. Barnett HJM, Eliasziw M, Meldrum HE, Taylor DW: Do the facts and figures warrant a 10-fold increase in the performance of carotid endarterectomy on asymptomatic patients? Neurology 46:603–608, 1996
4. Barnett HJM, Meldrum HE, Eliasziw M: Lessons from the symptomatic trials for the management of asymptomatic disease. p. 385. In Caplan LR, Shifrin EG, Nicolaides AN, Moore WS (eds): Cerebrovascular Ischaemia Investigation & Management. Med-Orion, Nicosia, Cyprus, 1996.
5. Barnett HJM, Plum F, Walton JN: Carotid endarterectomy: an expression of concern. Stroke 15:941–943, 1984
6. Barnett HJM, Meldrum E, Eliasziw M: The North American Symptomatic Carotid Endarterectomy Trial: further observation. In Veith RJ (ed): Current Critical Problems in Vascular Surgery. Vol. 6. Quality Medical Publishing. St. Louis, MO, 1994
7. Biller J, Adams HP Jr, Boarini D et al: Intraluminal clot of the carotid artery. A clinical-angiographic correlation of nine patients and literature review. Surg Neurol 25:467–477, 1986
8. Buchan A, Gates P, Pelz D, Barnett HJM: Intraluminal thrombus in the cerebral circulation. Stroke 19:681–687, 1988
9. Chan R, Eliasziw M, Sharpe B et al: Asymptomatic internal carotid artery disease. Observations from NASCET. Abstract presented at the 21st International Joint Conference on Stroke and Cerebral Circulation, January 25–27, 1996
10. Chervu A, Moore WS: Carotid endarterectomy without arteriography. Ann Vasc Surg 8:296–302, 1994
11. Cheung RTF, Chan RKT, Eliasziw M et al and the North American Symptomatic Carotid Endarterectomy Trial: Early postoperative carotid artery stenosis and late restenosis. Experience from the North American Symptomatic Carotid Endarterectomy Trial. Abstract presented at the 21st International Joint Conference on Stroke and Cerebral Circulation, January 25–27, 1996
12. Cote R, Battista RN, Abrahamowicz M et al: the Asymptomatic Cervical Bruit Study Group. Lack of effect of aspirin in asymptomatic patients with carotid bruits and substantial carotid narrowing. Ann Intern Med 123:649–655, 1995
13. Eastcott HHG, Pickering GW, Rob CG: Reconstruction of internal carotid artery in a patient with intermittent attacks of hemiplegia. Lancet ii:994–996, 1954
14. Eliasziw M, Rankin RN, Fox AJ et al for the North American Symptomatic Carotid Endarterectomy Trial (NASCET) Group. Accuracy and prognostic consequences of ultrasonography in identifying severe carotid artery stenosis. Stroke 26:1747–1752, 1995
15. Eliasziw M, Spence JD, Barnett HJM for the North American Symptomatic Carotid Endarterectomy Trial (NASCET) Group. Carotid endarterectomy does not affect long-term blood pressure: observations from NASCET. Cerebrovasc Dis (in press)
16. Eliasziw M, Streifler JY, Fox AJ et al for the North American Symptomatic Carotid Endarterectomy Trial: Significance of plaque ulceration in symptomatic patients with high-grade carotid stenosis. Stroke 25:304–308, 1994
17. European Carotid Surgery Trialists' Collaborative Group. Endarterectomy for moderate symptomatic carotid stenosis: interim results from the MRC European Carotid Surgery Trial. Lancet 347:1591–1593, 1996
18. European Carotid Surgery Trialists' Collaborative Group. MRC European Carotid Surgery Trial: interim results for

symptomatic patients with severe (70–99%) or with mild (0–29%) carotid stenosis. Lancet 337:1235–1243, 1991

19. European Carotid Surgery Trialists' Collaborative Group. Risk of stroke in the distribution of an asymptomatic carotid artery. Lancet 345:209–212, 1995

20. Executive Committee for the Asymptomatic Carotid Atherosclerosis Study. Endarterectomy for asymptomatic carotid artery stenosis. JAMA 273:1421–1428, 1995

21. Fields WS, Maslenikov V, Stirling Meyer et al: Joint study of extracranial arterial occlusion. V. Progress report of prognosis following surgery or nonsurgical treatment for transient cerebral ischemic attacks and cervical carotid artery lesions. JAMA 211:1993–2003, 1970

22. Gasecki AP, Eliasziw M, Ferguson GG et al for the North American Symptomatic Carotid Endarterectomy Trial (NASCET). Long-term prognosis and effect of endarterectomy in patients with symptomatic severe carotid stenosis and contralateral carotid stenosis or occlusion: results from NASCET. J Neurosurg 83:778–782, 1995

23. Gertler JP, Blankensteijn JD, Brewster DC et al: Carotid endarterectomy for unstable and compelling neurologic conditions: do results justify an aggressive approach? J Vasc Surg 19:32–42, 1994

24. Golledge J, Cuming R, Ellis M et al: Clinical follow-up rather than duplex surveillance after carotid endarterectomy. J Vasc Surg 25:55–63, 1997

25. Graor RA, Hertzer NR: Management of coexistent carotid artery and coronary artery disease. Stroke 19:1441–1444, 1988

26. Hennerici M, Hulsbomer HB, Hefter H et al: Natural history of asymptomatic extracranial arterial disease: results of a long-term prospective study. Brain 110:777–791, 1987

27. MACE (Mayo Asymptomatic Carotid Endarterectomy) Study Group: Results of a randomized controlled trial of carotid endarterectomy for asymptomatic carotid stenosis. Mayo Clin Proc 67:513–518, 1992

28. Matchar DB, Pauk J, Lipscomb J: A health policy perspective on carotid endarterectomy: cost, effectiveness, and cost-effectiveness. pp. 680–689. In Cerebrovascular Disease. 2nd Ed. Moore WS (ed): Surgery for WB Saunders Philadelphia, Pa., 1996

29. Mayberg MR, Wilson SE, Yatsu F et al: Carotid endarterectomy and prevention of cerebral ischemia in symptomatic carotid stenosis. JAMA 266:3289–3294, 1991

30. McCrory DC, Goldstein LB, Samsa GP et al: Predicting complications of carotid endarterectomy. Stroke 24:1285–1291, 1993

31. Morgenstern LB, Fox AJ, Sharpe BL et al for the North American Symptomatic Carotid Endarterectomy Trial (NASCET) Group: The risks and benefits of carotid endarterectomy in patients with near occlusion of the carotid artery. Neurology, 48:911–915, 1997

32. Munson RJ, Sharpe BL, Finan JW et al for the North American Symptomatic Carotid Endarterectomy Trial (NASCET) Group: The NASCET experience of bleeding complications of patients on aspirin. Abstract presented at the 22nd International Joint Conference on Stroke and Cerebral Circulation, February 6–8, 1997

33. Newman DC, Hicks RG: Combined carotid and coronary artery surgery: a review of the literature. Ann Thorac Surg 45:574–581, 1988

34. Norris JW, Zhu CZ, Bornstein NM, Chambers BR: Vascular risks of asymptomatic carotid stenosis. Stroke 22:1485–1490, 1991

35. North American Symptomatic Carotid Endarterectomy Trial Collaborators: Beneficial effect of carotid endarterectomy in symptomatic patients with high-grade carotid stenosis. N Engl J Med 325:445–453, 1991

36. Pelz DM, Buchan A, Fox AJ et al: Intraluminal thrombus of the internal carotid arteries: angiographic demonstration of resolution with anticoagulant therapy alone. Radiology 160:369–373, 1986

37. Perry JR, Szalai JP, Norris JW for the Canadian Stroke Consortium: Consensus against both endarterectomy and routine screening for asymptomatic carotid artery stenosis. Arch Neurol 54:25–28, 1997

38. Shaw DA, Venables GS, Cartlidge NEF et al: Carotid endarterectomy in patients with transient cerebral ischaemia. J Neurol Sci 64:45–53, 1984

39. Steering Committee of the Physicians' Health Study Research Group: Final report on the aspirin component of the ongoing Physicians' Health Study. N Eng J Med 321:129–35, 1989

40. Streifler JY, Eliasziw M, Benavente OR et al for the North American Symptomatic Carotid Endarterectomy Trial: The risk of stroke in patients with first-ever retinal vs hemispheric transient ischemic attacks and high-grade carotid stenosis. Arch Neurol 52:246–249, 1995

41. Thorpe KE, Taylor DW for the North American Symptomatic Carotid Endarterectomy Trial Collaborators: ASA and carotid endarterectomy. Abstract presented at the 22nd International Joint Conference on Stroke and Cerebral Circulation, February 6–8, 1997

42. Warlow C: Endarterectomy for asymptomatic carotid stenosis? Lancet 345:1254, 1995

43. Warlow CP: Carotid endarterectomy: does it work? Stroke 15:1068–1076, 1984

44. Winslow CM, Soloman DH, Chassin MR et al: The appropriateness of carotid endarterectomy. N Engl J Med 318:721–727, 1988

Medical Considerations

PHILIP A. TEAL

J. W. NORRIS

Since the previous edition of this book, there have been major advances in diagnosis and management of carotid atherosclerosis that have considerably influenced the decision analysis on intervention in asymptomatic carotid stenosis. Fairly extensive community studies of patients with asymptomatic neck bruits and, later, those involving noninvasive imaging clearly indicated that stroke risk was minimal, no more than 1% to 2% per year.

The publication of studies of carotid surgery in symptomatic cases and, more recently, asymptomatic patients with significant carotid stenosis indicated a serious gap in therapeutic benefit. Whereas symptomatic carotid artery stenosis over 90% carries a stroke risk of 15% to 20% per year, even the severest cases of asymptomatic disease are associated with an almost 10-fold lower stroke risk. The significant risk of standard, invasive angiography, on average approximately 1% with individual institutions reporting as low as 0.4% to as high as 4%, coupled with reported perioperative morbidity and mortality of 1% to 5%, makes the case for routine carotid surgery in asymptomatic stenosis hard to justify.

However, as noninvasive neurovascular imaging improves, surgeons place more and more reliance on duplex ultrasound, magnetic resonance angiography, and other methods, either alone or in combination. Soon we may have techniques equal to, or even superior to, standard contrast angiography (Fig. 53.14).

In addition, carotid angioplasty and stenting are becoming recognized techniques (although still experimental) that can destroy or remodel plaques as effectively, and possibly as safely, as open carotid surgery (Fig. 53.15). The optimal management of asymptomatic carotid stenosis discovered in patients scheduled for vascular and general surgery still remains elusive.

All these advances indicate a glimmer, if not a light, at the end of the tunnel that soon there will be effective techniques of screening and low risk approaches for treating patients with asymptomatic carotid stenosis. This may help to answer the challenge to one of nature's most deadly and disabling conditions: stroke.

Prevalence of Carotid Stenosis

Carotid stenosis is a marker for generalized atherosclerosis and thereby serves as a predictor of future cerebrovascular, coronary, and other vascular events. Population-based carotid studies reveal that approximately 4% of asymptomatic middle-aged or elderly adults have ultrasound evidence for carotid stenosis of greater than 50%.[10] The overall incidence of carotid stenosis in patients over age 65 with carotid stenosis was 7% in women and 9% in men based on the Framingham analysis of a cohort of 1,116 members aged 66 to 93.[20] The incidence of high-grade stenosis (>80%) is substantially lower, however, probably less than 1%.[10] Carotid stenosis is age dependent with prevalence rates ranging from about 0.5% in people in their 50s to 10% or more in octogenarians.[60,65,67]

Determinants of Carotid Stenosis

Independent determinants of carotid atherosclerosis include age, male gender, cigarette smoking, elevated systolic and diastolic blood pressure, raised levels of blood cholesterol, and elevated plasma homocysteine levels.[20,76]

Age is the strongest predictor for carotid disease and for stroke in general with a sharp increase in prevalence of both conditions after 70 years of age.[61,90] Gender also plays a major role in the development of carotid disease.[38,60] A community-based stroke prevention study reported prevalence rates for carotid stenosis were higher for men than for women[90] (Table 53.3). The incidence of high grade stenosis (>80%) was twice as frequent in men as in women.

Smoking is a powerful independent factor in the development and progression of carotid atherosclerosis and may be the strongest predictor of severe carotid disease in patients under the age of 45.[68,71,89] In an angiographic study of 752 patients, the duration of smoking was the most significant independent predictor of the presence of severe carotid atherosclerosis exceeding the influence of factors such as age, hypertension, diabetes, and gender.[89] The total amount of cigarettes smoked as measured in pack-years is also a powerful predictor of carotid artery plaque thickness, as demonstrated by ultrasound measurements of carotid wall thickness.[16]

Systolic blood pressure has a significant direct bearing on the degree of carotid stenosis and the risk of stroke.[61,83,90] Diurnal variability in systolic blood pressure may serve as a strong predictor of the development of early carotid atherosclerosis, as measured by intimal to media wall thickness on B-mode ultrasound.[73] The importance of diastolic hypertension is less certain.[20]

The role of hyperlipidemia in stroke is complex. The connection between hyperlipidemia and coronary artery disease is well established, but a less consistent effect has been reported for the presence and severity of carotid artery steno-

Figure **53.14** Three-dimensional, color-coded (color not shown) computed tomography (CT) angiography with carotid plaques clearly visible.

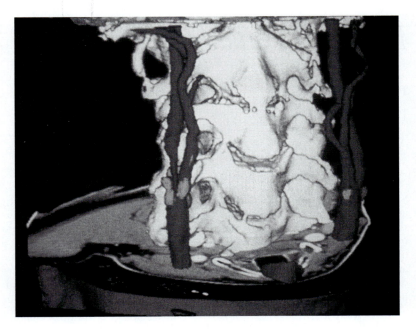

sis.[21,25,85,91] Recent evidence links lipid lowering to the slowing of carotid atherosclerosis, and population studies show that the severity and progression of carotid atheroma are related to circulating blood lipid levels.[1,22,35,53,72] In the Multiple Risk Factor Intervention Trial (MRFIT), patients with cholesterol levels between 6.22 and 7.25 mmol/L had twice the incidence of ischemic stroke than those with cholesterol levels between 5.18 and 6.22 mmol/L.[53]

High plasma homocysteine levels are associated with the development of atherosclerosis and carotid artery disease, but direct causality with stroke has not yet been established. In the Framingham study, the odds ratio for carotid stenosis of ≥25% was 2 for subjects with plasma homocysteine concentrations in the highest quartile (≥14.4 μmol/L) compared with those in the lowest quartile (< 9.1 μmol/L). [76] The British Regional Heart Study reported a graded increase in the relative risk of stroke with increasing levels of homocysteine.[62]

Stroke Risk of Asymptomatic Carotid Stenosis

Asymptomatic carotid stenosis carries a low annual risk of ipsilateral stroke of approximately 2%. This long-held conventional wisdom has been confirmed by prospective data from

Figure **53.15** Placement of stent in a patient with symptomatic carotid stenosis. Note that the ulcer at the carotid bulb is smaller after stenting. The stent is clearly visible in postprocedure figure.

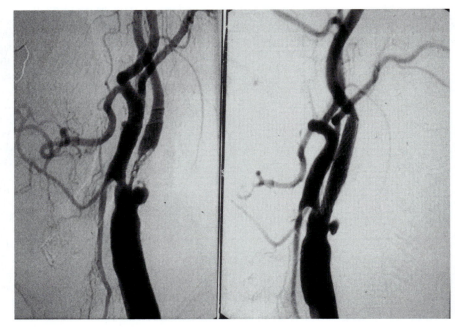

Table 53.3 Prevalence of Carotid Stenosis Based on Age and Gender

	% Prevalence	
Age	Men	Women
40–49	8.2	3.35
50–59	39.7	22.3
60–69	66.4	48.7
70–79	82.5	76.7

(From Willeit and Kicchl,[90] with permission.)

both natural history studies and randomized treatment trials (Table 53.4). In the Toronto study, individuals with greater than 75% stenosis on ultrasound had a 2.5% annual risk of ipsilateral stroke.[9] Remarkably similar stroke risks were reported in patients enrolled in recently reported randomized treatment trials based on angiographic assessment.

The European Carotid Surgery Trial (ECST) reported a 1.9% annual stroke rate in patients with asymptomatic stenosis of greater than 70%.[18] The Asymptomatic Carotid Atherosclerosis Study (ACAS) projected a 2.2% annual risk for any ipsilateral stroke in medically treated patients with greater than 60% stenosis.[19] The risk of major ipsilateral stroke was much lower. In the North American Symptomatic Carotid Endarterectomy Trial (NASCET) study, the annualized stroke rate from the "asymptomatic-other-side" is >4% per year if the stenosis is above 70%, but below 85% the strokes are often due to a cardioembolic or lacunar cause (unpublished data, courtesy of H. J. M. Barnett).

With lesser degrees of carotid stenosis, the annual stroke rate is almost negligible. Ultrasound studies have reported annual stroke risks of 1% to 1.3% for patients with less than 75% stenosis.[14,28,36,48,58] In the ECST study, the annual risk of ipsilateral stroke fell to 0.7% or less in patients with asymptomatic carotid stenosis of less than 70% as measured by their angiographic criteria.

Data regarding the natural history of carotid disease in

Table 53.4 Annual Stroke Rate in Patients with Asymptomatic Carotid Stenosis

Study	n	% Stenosis	Measurement Method	Stroke Risk/Year
Meissner et al[48]	292	≥80	OPG	2.1
Hennerici et al[28]	235	>50%	Ultrasound	1.0
Norris et al[58]	177	75–99	Ultrasound	2.5
	319	<75	Ultrasound	1.3
ECST[18]	127	70–99	Angio	1.9
	843	30–69	Angio	0.7
Hobson et al[32]	233	50–79	Angio	2.3
ACAS[19]	843	60–99	US/angio	2.2
Cote et al.[14]	372	≥50%	Ultrasound	2.3
Johnson et al[36]	232	50–79	Ultrasound	1.6

surgical trials or angiography-based studies must be evaluated cautiously, because of selection bias. Stringent protocols in surgical trials may exclude many patients with carotid stenosis from evaluation. In the ACAS trial, for example, approximately 25 subjects were screened for every patient enrolled.[19] Similarly, angiographic series are unlikely to represent consecutive patients owing to ethical and practical considerations. Nevertheless, all available prospective data support the premise that asymptomatic carotid stenosis imparts only a very modest stroke hazard.

Risk Assessment

Several factors affect the prognosis of individuals with carotid disease. The major determinants of stroke risk are the symptom status of the patient, the severity of carotid narrowing, the rate of disease progression, and the presence of carotid plaque ulceration.[17,18] Male gender, age, and the presence of coexisting medical and other vascular diseases serve as additional risk markers for carotid-associated stroke.[54] Coexisting coronary artery disease may pose a greater health risk.[30] The annual risk of myocardial infarction is 5% to 9% in patients with significant asymptomatic carotid narrowing.[9,28]

The emergence of symptoms in a patient with a previously silent carotid stenosis of ≥70% escalates the annual stroke risk to 13% or more from the asymptomatic base rate of 2% to 2.5% rate. The nature of the symptoms modifies the severity of stroke risk; hemispheric transient ischemic attacks (TIAs) are a more potent predictor of future stroke than retinal symptoms such as amaurosis fugax.[82] Patients with carotid stenosis must be carefully educated about the signs and symptoms of TIAs, as investigation and treatment strategies are more aggressive and urgent once symptoms have been experienced. Unfortunately, stroke, rather than TIA, is the initial neurologic event in up to half of the patients with asymptomatic stenosis.

Risk stratification based on the degree of carotid stenosis has been firmly established for symptomatic patients with greater than 70% narrowing by the results of the NASCET and ECST trials.[18,59] This biologically plausible effect was previously noted in observational studies of asymptomatic carotid stenosis.[9] In the ECST, the annual risk of ipsilateral stroke was 0.6%, 0.7%, and 1.9% for degrees of stenosis <30%, 30% to 69%, and 70% to 99%, respectively. Only when the degree of stenosis exceeded 80% did the risk of stroke increase to a more substantial rate of 3.2% annually, although this observation is based on a relatively small number of patients with high-grade disease. The Toronto study also demonstrated a dichotomy in stroke risk based on severity of stenosis.[9] The annual rate of ipsilateral stroke was 2.5% in patients with greater than 75% carotid stenosis but was only 1.3% in those with lesser degrees of narrowing. In the Veterans Affairs Cooperative Study the annual incidence of ipsilateral stroke was approximately 2.3% in 233 medically treated patients with high-grade stenosis.[32] Unfortunately, the ACAS trial was not powered to detect group differences, and there were too few outcome events in this study to support or dispute the theory of risk stratification based on severity of carotid stenosis.

Rapid progression of carotid stenosis has been associated with an increased risk for TIA and stroke. [9,56,69] A serial ultrasound study of 232 patients who were followed for several years detected progressive stenosis in 23% of patients. [36] Progression to severe stenosis or occlusion was most likely in those patients already established moderate stenosis rather than just mild degrees of narrowing. The estimated risk of stroke due to the occlusion of a progressive stenosis is up to 20% to 30%. [13]

The presence of plaque ulceration and unstable plaque morphology bears directly on the stroke risk in symptomatic carotid stenosis. [81,92] Plaque ulceration may also carry a substantial risk for stroke in asymptomatic patients, although the magnitude of this effect requires further evaluation. Moore et al[52] reported a stroke incidence of 34% in patients with asymptomatic ulcerative lesions of the carotid artery followed over a 5-year period. The presence of plaque ulceration has been associated with formation of luminal thrombus and distal embolization. [81] Plaque rupture and thinning of the fibrous cap may also be important in the production of symptoms in carotid artery stenosis. [6] At present, color-flow Doppler-assisted duplex imaging cannot reliably detect the presence of plaque ulceration in high-grade carotid lesions.

Cholesterol deposition or intraplaque hemorrhage as determined by ultrasound echolucency and plaque heterogeneities may be associated with symptom development. Echolucent plaque morphology is an ultrasound marker for increased stroke risk. [41] In some cases, it is suggested that rapid progression of carotid stenosis is related to intraplaque hemorrhage and the rupture or fissuring of the plaque surface, which exposes collagen and other thrombogenic substances to the blood. [6]

Active, unstable carotid plaques shed microembolic particles that can be recognized on transcranial Doppler as "high intensity transients" (HITS). [4] The occurrence of microemboli is a marker for the presence of ulceration on angiography. [84] The clinical correlates of HITS require further evaluation, but available evidence suggests that these embolic signals are more frequent in symptomatic arteries and in moderate to severe carotid stenosis. [44,79] The detection of microembolic HITS may define a high-risk subgroup of patients with severe asymptomatic carotid stenosis, particularly if the rate of emboli detection is $\geq$2 per hour. [80]

The presence of silent cerebral infarction detected by computed tomography (CT) or magnetic resonance imaging (MRI) scanning may be associated with an increased risk of future stroke. Silent cerebral infarctions are often small and deep. In one study, silent cerebral infarction was found in approximately 20% of 115 asymptomatic patients, and the incidence was higher ipsilateral to the side with carotid stenosis. [57] In the ACAS trial, ipsilateral silent infarctions were detected in 8% to 9% of the 1,528 patients who had baseline CT scans. [19]

The presence of multiple risk factors may identify a high-risk group of patients with asymptomatic carotid stenosis. [5,11] Risk factor profiles have been proposed to triage patients for intervention[11] (Table 53.5). In NASCET the risk of ipsilateral stroke increases with the number of risk factors in both asymptomatic and symptomatic carotid stenosis, although the order of magnitude is almost fivefold greater for high-grade symptomatic stenosis. [5] A multicenter natural history study is underway to evaluate the interplay of risk factors such as the degree

Table 53.5 Risk Profile in Asymptomatic Carotid Stenosis

Risk factors for ischemic events
  Age
  Gender
  Diabetes mellitus
  Peripheral vascular disease
  Cardiac conditions
  Cigarette smoking
  Polycythemia
  Hyperfibrinogenemia
  Hyperlipidemia
Risk factors specific for stroke
  High degree of stenosis (>75%)
  Echolucent lesions
  Ulceration of carotid plaques
  Imperfect collateral anatomy
  Previous carotid endarterectomy
  Asymptomatic cerebral infarcts

(From Consensus Group,[11] with permission.)

of stenosis, plaque echogenicity and ulceration, cerebral vascular reserve, and the presence of silent infarction.

Clinical Detection of Asymptomatic Carotid Stenosis

Asymptomatic carotid stenosis may be clinically suspected owing to the presence of a cervical or orbital bruit, the visualization of a retinal embolus on funduscopic exam, or occasionally because of the subjective awareness of pulse-synchronous tinnitus. Asymptomatic carotid stenosis is frequently detected by ultrasound examination in individuals screened by their physician during investigations for cerebrovascular symptoms in other vascular territories, or in patients undergoing evaluation prior to cardiac surgery or other procedures.

Cervical bruits are present in 3% to 4% of the normal adult population and the prevalence increases with age, reaching 8% of normal people over 75 years, 10% over 85 years, and in 13% of individuals over the age of 95. [31,86] Bruits localized to the mid-cervical region near the angle of the mandible may be due to turbulent blood flow within a stenotic carotid artery. Not all cervical bruits reflect the presence of significant stenosis of the underlying internal carotid artery. In one carotid Doppler study there was a 64% incidence of carotid stenosis ipsilateral to the neck bruit, and a 33% incidence on the contralateral "silent" side. [8] Cervical bruits may be due to stenosis of the external carotid artery, and at times represent the presence of transmitted cardiac murmurs, arterial kinks or coils, or hyperdynamic vascular states, as in thyrotoxicosis or anemia.

Cervical bruits may be inaudible even in the presence of

hemodynamically significant carotid stenosis. In the ACAS trial, bruits were detected in only 75% of patients who had carotid narrowing greater than 60%.[19] A cervical bruit was present in only two-thirds of the patients with high-grade symptomatic stenosis (>70%) in the NASCET study.[59] Carotid bruits may disappear when the stenosis is extreme due to low flow, and up to 30% of patients with severe stenosis will have no detectable bruit.[11] Anatomic variations in the carotid bifurcation, the effects of position and posture, hemodynamic factors, and the skill of the clinician may also determine the presence and detection of a carotid bruit. Orbital bruits suggest increased or turbulent flow through the carotid siphon and occasionally are heard contralateral to a severe carotid stenosis or occlusion, reflecting the presence of augmented flow that serves to provide collateral blood via the anterior communicating artery.

Screening and Investigation of Asymptomatic Carotid Stenosis

Duplex ultrasonography is the primary modality used to screen for the presence of carotid stenosis. The severity of stenosis based on Doppler frequency shift or calculated flow velocities is expressed as a percentage of area reduction, commonly reported in ranges such as 0% to 15%, 16% to 49%, 50% to 79%, and 80% to 99%, or occlusion. Diagnostic criteria for detecting carotid stenosis of greater than 60% have been reported to correlate ultrasound findings with ACAS surgical criteria.[49] Information regarding the nature of the atherosclerotic plaque may be visualized by B-mode ultrasonography. Duplex ultrasonography is low cost and noninvasive and can be used in a serial fashion to evaluate the activity of the carotid plaque over time.

In ultrasound laboratories with high-quality controls, duplex ultrasonography is capable of a high degree of accuracy compared with angiography.[33,64] The addition of color-flow duplex imaging enhances the diagnostic accuracy of carotid ultrasound.[64] The accuracy of ultrasound technology is highly operator-dependent. The angle of insonation of the carotid artery is critical for determination of velocities. Variations in carotid bifurcation anatomy such as a high bifurcation, arterial loops, or the presence of heavy calcification of the plaque may interfere with accurate measurements. Ultrasound may produce a false-positive impression of carotid occlusion. In the ACAS trial, careful standardization and training of the sonographers produced a 93% positive predictive value for ultrasound compared with angiography.[33]

Magnetic resonance angiography (MRA) used alone or in combination with duplex ultrasonography provides another safe, noninvasive method for evaluating carotid stenosis. The reported accuracy of MRA compared with angiography for the measurement of carotid stenosis varies.[42,45] At present, MRA is limited by its tendency to overestimate the degree of stenosis and occasional misdiagnosis of severe stenosis as complete occlusion. However, MRA is complementary to duplex ultrasonography and is able to image the cervical and

intracranial circulation as well as the brain parenchyma during the same study. MRA is an evolving technology and its clinical value in distinguishing between surgical and nonsurgical carotid disease remains undetermined.

Contrast angiography remains the gold standard for the preoperative determination of carotid stenosis. The measurement of stenosis with conventional angiography is, however, also subject to inaccuracies and intraobserver differences, and the criteria for calculating the degree of stenosis vary.[34,55] More important, carotid angiography is expensive and carries a significant risk of stroke. Angiography-related morbidity was 0.7% in the NASCET study and 1.2% in the ACAS trial. These figures are in keeping with the generally recognized risks based on a review of the literature.[27] In the ACAS study, angiography accounted for almost 50% of the surgical morbidity. Complication rates at single centers may be much higher. In one series of 200 consecutive angiograms for symptomatic carotid disease there was a 4% incidence of stroke and a mortality rate of 1%.[15] Such extreme complication rates for a diagnostic procedure are unusual and unacceptable. Hospital audits should ensure that cerebral angiography is competently and safely performed. It has been proposed that stroke risks could be reduced by the selective use of preoperative angiography performed only when the results of noninvasive tests (MRA and/or duplex ultrasonography) are discordant or technically inadequate.[39] Increasingly, many surgeons proceed to surgery for either symptomatic or asymptomatic carotid disease solely on the basis of noninvasive assessments. The scientific validity of this approach has not been verified, although a decision analysis model suggests that the use of preoperative noninvasive tests would result in lower 5-year stroke risk compared with angiography.[39] MRA and ultrasound may overestimate the degree of stenosis and can miss near occlusions. Tandem intracranial stenosis will go undetected if ultrasound is the only modality used to evaluate carotid disease.

Benefits of Screening

Mass screening of the general population for the presence of asymptomatic carotid stenosis cannot be justified on either medical or economic grounds. The absolute risk of stroke is low and the benefits of carotid endarterectomy are modest, even in the best surgical hands. It is estimated that screening just half of the US population older than 60 years of age would cost approximately $7 billion.[46] A population-based screening program and subsequent surgery for patients with carotid stenosis greater than 60% stenosis would prevent only about 4% of first-time strokes, and the overall impact on public health would be negligible.[88]

The benefits of targeted screening of individuals at risk, for example, those with carotid bruits or multiple risk factors, remain uncertain. The cost-effectiveness of screening is determined by the prevalence of disease in the targeted population. The one-time screening of a high-risk population of asymptomatic patients as defined by the history of prior myocardial infarction, peripheral vascular disease, or a carotid bruit may

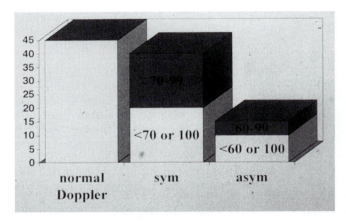

Figure 53.16 Screening carotid Doppler in consecutive patients with proven peripheral vascular disease reveals that 55% have carotid lesions, of which about half are potential candidates for carotid endarterectomy. (From Alexandrova et al,[2] with permission.)

not be cost-effective[63] (Fig. 53.16). Further data are required to better define the subpopulation of patients at high risk of stroke because of asymptomatic carotid stenosis.

Carotid Surgery with Other Operations

The management of carotid stenosis in an asymptomatic patient scheduled for surgery, particularly cardiac surgery, poses a therapeutic challenge. A prospective ultrasound study detected the presence of asymptomatic stenosis of greater than 50% in 130 of 582 (22%) patients scheduled for cardiac surgery[75] and in 30% scheduled for peripheral arterial surgery.[23] The overall stroke risk associated with coronary artery bypass graft (CABG) surgery is approximately 2% with ranges reported from 1% to 6%. Extracranial carotid stenosis has been implicated as a cause of CABG-related stroke as a result of either hemodynamic or embolic mechanisms. Most studies, however, fail to demonstrate an increased rate of stroke ipsilateral to an asymptomatic carotid narrowing.

Intracranial blood flow velocities measured during cardiac surgery are not generally affected by severe carotid stenosis.[87] The majority of perioperative strokes are embolic rather than hemodynamic in nature, including emboli arising from the heart or from atherosclerosis of the aortic arch triggered by cannulation or cross-clamping of the aorta.[37]

At present there are no clearly defined indications or convincing justification for simultaneous carotid and CABG surgery.[51] The majority of CABG-related strokes in this setting are due to embolic mechanisms from noncarotid sources. Some centers will perform unilateral carotid endarterectomy in patients with bilateral severe carotid disease, and evidence suggests that morbidity and mortality are lower when the procedures are staged if carotid endarterectomy is deemed neces-

sary.[24] The decision to proceed with simultaneous carotid endarterectomy and coronary artery bypass grafting in an asymptomatic patient must be tempered by the increased risk of stroke, approximately 5.6%, associated with the combined procedure.

For patients with asymptomatic carotid stenosis undergoing noncardiac surgery, the risk of attributable perioperative stroke is low, and the carotid stenosis may be appropriately dealt with as an independent condition.

Medical Therapy for Stroke Prevention in Asymptomatic Stenosis

Optimal medical treatment is appropriate for all patients with carotid stenosis. Stroke risk factors such as smoking, hypertension, hyperlipidemias, diabetes, and ischemic heart disease should be identified and managed vigorously.

The importance of treating hypertension cannot be overestimated as even seemingly trivial reductions in diastolic blood pressure by an average of 2 mmHg can reduce the incidence of stroke and TIAs by 15%.[12] Sustained reductions in blood pressure by about 6 mmHg reduce the risk of stroke by almost 40%.[43] The Systolic Hypertension in the Elderly Program (SHEP) has shown that treatment of isolated systolic hypertension produces equally significant reductions in the incidence of stroke, even in the elderly.[77] It has been hypothesized that one mechanism by which antihypertensive therapy reduces the risk of stroke is by slowing the progression of atherosclerosis. In the SHEP trial, progression of carotid stenosis occurred in only 14% of patients on active treatment for systolic hypertension versus a 31% rate of progression in those randomized to placebo. Regression of carotid stenosis occurred only in those individuals on active treatment.

Cigarette smoking is an independent risk factor for carotid arterial wall thickening and is a reversible risk factor for stroke. In a recent study and a meta-analysis of observational data, the cessation of smoking decreases the risk of stroke to levels near those of nonsmokers within 2 to 5 years.[40,78] While it is uncertain whether the reductions in attributable stroke risks as a result of smoking cessation are in part due to direct effects on the stability of carotid artery plaque, the end results are highly beneficial.

Cholesterol-lowering medications have been shown to halt the progression of carotid atherosclerosis and occasionally result in the regression of carotid plaques.[1] Overview analysis of cholesterol-lowering trials has not demonstrated a reduction in stroke risk in marked contrast to the decrease in the reduction in deaths due to coronary artery disease.[3,29] Results from the Scandinavian Simvastatin Survival Study (4S) suggest that aggressive reduction in cholesterol levels may reduce stroke risk. In this trial, the rate of stroke and TIA was reduced from 4.3% to 2.7% over a median follow-up of 5.4 years.[74] Further clinical trials are needed to demonstrate the effectiveness and cost benefits of cholesterol reduction in patients with carotid artery disease.

The benefits of aspirin for the primary prevention of

stroke in patients with asymptomatic carotid stenosis have not been established. Aspirin has not been proved to be beneficial for the primary prevention of stroke in low-risk asymptomatic individuals. The presence of asymptomatic carotid stenosis is a marker for generalized atherosclerosis and likely identifies a group with intermediate risks for vascular events, especially cardiac but also for stroke. A randomized study of 372 patients with asymptomatic high-grade ($\geq$50%) carotid stenosis found no long-term protective effect from 325 mg of aspirin given every other day.[14] Aspirin treatment may, however, slow the progression of carotid plaque growth in a dose-dependent fashion.[66] Large-scale trials would be required to evaluate the specific effects and optimal dose of aspirin in asymptomatic carotid disease, although its widespread use is likely to continue based on proved cardiac indications for the prevention of myocardial infarction.

Surgical Therapy for Asymptomatic Carotid Stenosis

In selected patients with asymptomatic stenosis, carotid endarterectomy can be performed with low perioperative morbidity and mortality. Guidelines from the stroke council of the American Heart Association recommend that carotid endarterectomy for asymptomatic stenosis should carry a combined neurologic morbidity and mortality of less than 3%.[51] Recent reviews of published series and pooled data analysis report 30-day morbidity and mortality rates between 2.3% to 3.35%.[70]

RESULTS OF RANDOMIZED TRIALS

The benefit of carotid endarterectomy for asymptomatic stenosis has been evaluated in four randomized controlled trials involving 3,355 patients.[7,28,32,47] The results of these completed trials leave many unanswered questions. The Asymptomatic Carotid Surgery Trial is still in progress.[26]

The Carotid Artery Stenosis with Asymptomatic Narrowing: Operation versus Aspirin (CASANOVA) entered 410 patients with 50% to 90% asymptomatic stenosis.[7] Serious design flaws marred the results of this study. Patients with greater than 90% stenosis were excluded. Several different treatment options were permitted and patients were allowed to cross over from the medical to the surgical arms. No statistically significant benefit was found for surgery. The perioperative mortality and stroke morbidity was 6.9%. The Mayo Clinic Trial was terminated after enrolling only 71 patients due to a significantly higher rate of myocardial infarctions in the surgical arm. The study design permitted the use of aspirin only in the patients in the medical arm. No conclusions regarding the efficacy of carotid endarterectomy can be drawn from this report.[47]

The Veterans Affairs Cooperative Study 167 studied 444 men with greater than 50% stenosis randomized to optimal medical treatment plus carotid endarterectomy or to optimal medical treatment alone.[17] The combined incidence of ipsilateral neurologic events, including TIAs, was 8.0% in the surgical group and 20.6% in the medical group ($P < 0.001$). There was no significant benefit from carotid endarterectomy when TIAs were excluded, and the analysis was restricted to the hard endpoints of stroke or death. The 30-day rate of permanent stroke or death was 4.7% in the surgical group.

ACAS randomized 1,662 patients with asymptomatic carotid stenosis of 60% or greater to aggressive medical management alone or combined with carotid endarterectomy[19] (Table 53.6). The primary outcome measures were ipsilateral stroke or any stroke or death in the perioperative period. The surgical standards in this study were excellent, with a 30-day stroke or death rate of 2.3% or an estimated 2.7% if all surgical patients had undergone angiography. After a median follow-up of 2.7 years, the Kaplan-Meier projections for the 5-year event rate were estimated to be 5.1% for surgical patients and 11.0% for patients treated medically ($P = 0.004$). Carotid endarterectomy resulted in a 5-year relative stroke risk reduction of 53% or an absolute risk reduction of only 5.9% over 5 years. This equates to a reduction in stroke incidence from 2.2%/yr to 1%/yr. The reduction in major ipsilateral stroke or death was 6% in the medical arm versus 3.4% in the surgical arm. This absolute risk reduction for major disabling stroke was less than 0.5% per year and did not reach statistical significance. ACAS failed to identify high-risk patient subsets based on the severity of stenosis, probably owing to the small number of outcome events. Somewhat surprisingly, the benefits of surgery in women remain more uncertain as their absolute and relative 5-year reductions in stroke and death were only 1.4% and 17%, respectively, compared with 8% and 66%, respectively, for men. The reasons for this apparent gender difference are not entirely clear but can be explained in part by the higher perioperative complication rate in women (3.6% in women versus 1.7% in men).

The generalizability of the ACAS results are in doubt. To qualify for this study, 25 individuals were screened for each patient enrolled. During the early organization of this trial,

Table 53.6 Estimated 5-Year Risk of Outcome Events in the ACAS Trial for Patients with Greater Than 60% Asymptomatic Carotid Stenosis

Outcome Event	Surgery	Medical	P Value
Ipsilateral stroke, perioperative stroke, death	5.1%	11.0%	0.004
Major ipsilateral stroke, perioperative stroke, death	3.4%	6.0%	Not significant (NS)
Any major stroke or perioperative death	6.4%	9.1%	NS
Major stroke or death	20.7%	25.5%	NS

Abbreviation: ACAS, Asymptotic Carotid Atherosclerosis Study.

(From Executive Committee for the Asymptomatic Carotid Atherosclerosis Study [ACAS],[19] with permission.)

10% of the surgeons who submitted applications to participate were rejected and seven institutions were found to be unacceptable.[50]

Careful patient selection, good clinical judgment, and superb surgical skills are required to produce a meaningful benefit from endarterectomy in patients who are symptom-free. The 30-day surgical morbidity and mortality must be less than 3% as any potential benefits are easily eliminated by excessive complication rates. Surgeons and institutions must maintain running logs of results to ensure these exacting standards are maintained.

Based on calculations from the ACAS data, 17 patients must undergo carotid endarterectomy to prevent one stroke in 5 years, or 85 operations are needed to prevent one stroke in 1 year. The number of operations needed to prevent one disabling stroke per year is 170.[88]

Summary

The optimal management of asymptomatic carotid stenosis remains undetermined and many unresolved questions remain in the wake of recent trials. The absolute risk of stroke in patients with asymptomatic carotid stenosis is low. While carotid endarterectomy performed on highly selected patients at carefully qualified medical centers by surgeons of exemplary skill resulted in a statistically significant reduction in overall stroke risk, the generalizability, clinical relevance, and cost-effectiveness of this approach remains highly controversial. The uncomfortably thin margin of benefit from surgery would be eliminated if perioperative morbidity and mortality were to exceed the very low 2.3% rate achieved in the ACAS trial. Asymptomatic carotid stenosis can be detected reliably and noninvasively by ultrasound and MRA. Our analysis of currently available data leads us to conclude that the mere presence of carotid stenosis of greater than 60% is not adequate to define a surgical indication. Further efforts are required to define the subgroups of patients at highest risk who are most likely to benefit and least likely to be harmed by surgery. The importance of the degree of stenosis as an independent variable for predicting stroke in asymptomatic patients requires clarification. The importance of plaque characteristics and the predictive value of vascular risk factors and other patient variables including age and gender must be defined.

In the interim, with imperfect data clinicians and surgeons should proceed cautiously. Targeted screening of individuals at high risk for carotid stenosis is rational but mass population screening is not indicated. The application of optimal medical prevention must be sustained and vigilant. Surgery should be offered only to optimal candidates deemed to be at high risk. Technological advances continue to improve the accuracy of noninvasive imaging; nevertheless, conventional angiography remains for now the gold standard for the presurgical assessment of stenosis. Stringent quality control measures are needed to monitor the results of any intervention. The challenge for the future will be to validate scientifically new treatments and technologies such as angioplasty and stenting and to identify patients at risk in a systematic and cost-efficient manner.

References

1. Adams HP, Byington RP, Hoen H: Effect of cholesterol-lowering medications on progression of mild atherosclerotic lesions of the carotid arteries and on the risk of stroke. Cerebrovasc Dis 5:171–177, 1995
2. Alexandrova NA, Gibson WC, Norris JW, Maggisano R: Carotid artery stenosis in peripheral vascular disease. J Vasc Surg 23:645–649, 1996
3. Atkins D, Psaty BM, Koepsell TD et al: Cholesterol reduction and the risk for stroke in men. Ann Intern Med 119:136–145, 1993
4. Babikian VL, Hyde C, Pochay V et al: Clinical correlates of high-intensity transient signals detected on transcranial Doppler sonography in patients with cerebrovascular disease. Stroke 25:1570–1573, 1994
5. Barnett HJM, Eliasziw M, Meldrum HE et al: Do the facts and figures warrant a 10-fold increase in the performance of carotid endarterectomy on asymptomatic patients? Neurology 46:603–608, 1996
6. Carr S, Farb A, Pearce WH et al: Atherosclerotic plaque rupture in symptomatic carotid artery stenosis. J Vasc Surg 23:755–766, 1996
7. The CASANOVA Study Group: Carotid surgery versus medical therapy in asymptomatic carotid stenosis. Stroke 22:1229–1235, 1991
8. Chambers BR, Norris JW: Clinical significance of asymptomatic neck bruits. Neurology 35:742–745, 1985
9. Chambers BR, Norris JW: Outcome in patients with asymptomatic neck bruits. N Engl J Med 315:860–865, 1986
10. Colgan MP, Strode GR, Sommer JD et al: Prevalence of asymptomatic carotid disease: results of duplex scanning in 348 unselected volunteers. J Vasc Surg 8:674–679, 1988
11. Consensus statement on the management of patients with asymptomatic atherosclerotic carotid bifurcation lesions. Consensus Group. International Angiology 14:5–16, 1995
12. Cook NR, Cohen J, Hebert PR et al: Implication of small reductions in diastolic blood pressure for primary prevention. Arch Intern Med 155:701–709, 1995
13. Cote R, Barnett HJM, Taylor DW: Internal carotid occlusion: a prospective study. Stroke 14:898–902, 1983
14. Cote R, Battista RN, Abrahamowicz M et al: Lack of effect of aspirin in asymptomatic patients with carotid bruits and substantial carotid narrowing. Ann Intern Med 123:649–655, 1995
15. Davis KN, Humphrey PR: Complications of cerebral angiography in patients with symptomatic carotid territory ischemia screened by carotid ultrasound. J Neurol Neurosurg Psychiatry 56:967–972, 1993
16. Dempsey RJ, Moore RW: Amount of smoking independently predicts carotid artery atherosclerosis severity. Stroke 23:693–696, 1992
17. Eliasziw M, Streifler JY, Fox AJ et al: Significance of

plaque ulceration in symptomatic patients with high-grade carotid stenosis. Stroke 25:304–308, 1994

18. European Carotid Surgery Trialists' Collaborative Group MRC European Carotid Surgery Trial: interim results for symptomatic patients with severe (70–99%) or with mild (0–29%) carotid stenosis. Lancet 337:1235–1243, 1991

19. Executive Committee for the Asymptomatic Carotid Atherosclerosis Study (ACAS): Endarterectomy for asymptomatic carotid artery stenosis. JAMA 273:1421–1428, 1995

20. Fine-Edelstein JS, Wolf PA, O'Leary DH et al: Precursors of extracranial carotid atherosclerosis in the Framingham study. Neurology 44:1046–1050, 1994

21. Ford CS, Crouse JR, Howard G et al: The role of plasma lipids in carotid bifurcation atherosclerosis. Ann Neurol 17:301–303, 1985

22. Gasecki AP, Eliasziw M, Fox AJ et al: Serum cholesterol level is associated with the severity of carotid stenosis in symptomatic patients: results from NASCET. Cerebrovasc Dis 4:417–420, 1994

23. Gentile AT, Taylor LM, Moneta GL et al: Prevalence of asymptomatic carotid stenosis in patients undergoing infrainguinal bypass surgery. Arch Surg 130:900–904, 1995

24. Giangola G, Migaly J, Riles TS et al: Perioperative morbidity and mortality in combined vs. staged approaches to carotid and coronary revascularization. Ann Vasc Surg 10:138–142, 1996

25. Grotta JC, Yatsu FM, Pettigrew LC et al: Prediction of carotid stenosis progression by lipid and hematologic measurements. Neurology 39:1325–1331, 1989

26. Halliday AW: The Asymptomatic Carotid Surgery Trial (ACST): rationale and design. Euro J Vasc Surg 8:703–710, 1994

27. Hankey GJ, Warlow CP, Molyneux AJ: Complications of cerebral angiography for patients with mild carotid territory ischemia being considered for carotid endarterectomy. J Neurol Neurosurg Psychiatry 53:542–548, 1990

28. Hennerici M, Julsbomer H-B, Hefter H et al: Natural history of asymptomatic extracranial arterial disease. Brain 110:777–791, 1987

29. Herbert PR, Gasiano JM, Hennekens CH: An overview of trials of cholesterol lowering and risk of stroke. Arch Intern Med 155:50–55, 1995

30. Hertzer NR, Beven EG, Young JR et al: Incidental asymptomatic carotid bruits in patients scheduled for peripheral vascular reconstruction. Results of cerebral and coronary angiograph. Surgery 96:535–543, 1984

31. Heyman A, Wilkinson WE, Hey den S et al: Risk of stroke in asymptomatic persons with cervical arterial bruits: a population study in Evans County, Georgia. N Engl J Med 320:838–841, 1980

32. Hobson RW, Weiss DG, Fields WS et al: Veterans Affairs Cooperative Study Group: efficacy of carotid endarterectomy for asymptomatic carotid stenosis. N Engl J Med 328:221–227, 1993

33. Howard G, Cambless LE, Baker WH et al: A multicenter validation study of Doppler ultrasound versus angiogram. J Stroke Cerebrovasc Dis 1:1421–1428, 1991

34. Howard VJ, Toole JF, Grizzle J et al: Comparison of multi-center study designs for investigation of the efficacy of carotid endarterectomy. Stroke 23:583–593, 1992

35. Iso H, Jacobs DR, Wentworth D et al: Serum cholesterol levels and 6 year mortality from stroke in 350,977 men screened for the Multiple Risk Factor Intervention Trial. N Engl J Med 320:904–910, 1989

36. Johnson BF, Verlato F, Berglin RO et al: Clinical outcome in patients with mild and moderate carotid artery stenosis. J Vasc Surg 21:120–126, 1995.

37. Jones EL, Craver JM, Michalik RA et al: Combined carotid and coronary operations: when are they necessary? J Thorac Cardiovasc Surg 87:7–16, 1984

38. Josse MO, Touboul PJ, Mas JL et al: Prevalence of asymptomatic carotid artery stenosis. Neuroepidemiology 6:150–152, 1987

39. Kuntz KM, Skillman JJ, Whittemore AD et al: Carotid endarterectomy in asymptomatic patients—is contrast angiography necessary? A morbidity analysis. J Vasc Surg 22:706–716, 1995

40. Kwachi I, Colditz GA, Stampfer MJ et al: Smoking cessation and decreased risk of stroke in women. JAMA 269:232–236, 1993

41. Langsfeld M, Gray-Weale AC, Lusby RJ: The role of plaque morphology and diameter reduction in the development of new symptoms in asymptomatic carotid arteries. J Vasc Surg 9:548–557, 1989

42. Laster RE, Acker JD, Halford HH et al: Assessment of MR angiography versus arteriography for evaluation of cervical carotid bifurcation disease. AJNR 14:681–688, 1993

43. MacMahon S, Culter JA, Stamler J: Antihypertensive drug treatment. Potential, expected, and observed effects on stroke and on coronary heart disease. Hypertension, 13(suppl 1):S145–150, 1989

44. Markus HS, Thomson ND, Brown MM: Asymptomatic cerebral embolic signals in symptomatic and asymptomatic carotid artery disease. Brain 118:1005–1011, 1995

45. Masaryk AM, Ross JS, Dicello MC et al: 3DTOF MR angiography of the carotid bifurcation: potential and limitations as a screening examination. Radiology 179:797–804, 1991

46. Matcher D: Carotid endarterectomy: decision making and cost analysis. Presented at the Congress of Neurological Surgeons Annual Meeting; October 3, 1994; Chicago, IL

47. Mayo Asymptomatic Carotid Endarterectomy Study Group: Results of a randomized controlled trial of carotid endarterectomy of asymptomatic carotid stenosis. Mayo Clin Proc 67:513–518, 1992

48. Meissner I, Weibers DO, Whisnant JP et al: The natural history of asymptomatic carotid artery occlusive lesions. JAMA 258:2704–2707, 1987

49. Moneta GL, Edwards JM, Papanicolaou G et al: Screening for asymptomatic internal carotid artery stenosis: duplex criteria for discriminating 60% to 90% stenosis. J Vasc Surg 21:989–994, 1995

50. Moore WS: The asymptomatic carotid artery stenosis study (ACAS): In Bernstein EF, Callow AD, Nicolaides AN, Shifrin EG (eds): Cerebral Revascularization. Med-Orion Publishing Co., London, 1993

51. Moore WS, Barnette HJM, Beebe HG et al: Guidelines for carotid endarterectomy. A multidisciplinary consensus

statement from the ad hoc committee, American Heart Association. Circulation 91:566–579, 1995

52. Moore WS, Boren C, Malone JM et al: Natural history of nonstenotic asymptomatic ulcerative lesions of the carotid artery. Arch Surg 113:1352–1359, 1978

53. Neaton JD, Blackburn H, Jacobs D et al: Serum cholesterol level and mortality findings for men screened in the MRFIT trial. Arch Intern Med 152:1490–1500, 1992

54. Nicolaides AN, Barnett HJM, Belcaro GV, for the Consensus Group: Consensus statement on the management of patients with asymptomatic atherosclerotic carotid bifurcation lesions. Int Angio 14:5–23, 1995

55. Norris JW, Alexandrov AV, Bladin CF, Maggisano R: Progress in evaluating carotid artery stenosis. J Vasc Surg 22:637–638, 1995

56. Norris JW, Bornstein NM: Progression and regression of carotid stenosis. Stroke 17:755–757, 1986

57. Norris JW, Zhu CZ: Silent stroke and carotid stenosis. Stroke 23:483–485, 1992

58. Norris JW, Zhu CZ, Bornstein NM et al: Vascular risks of symptomatic carotid stenosis. Stroke 22:1458–1490, 1991

59. North American Symptomatic Carotid Endarterectomy Trial Collaborators: Beneficial effect of carotid endarterectomy in symptomatic patients with high-grade carotid stenosis. N Engl J Med 325:445–453, 1991

60. O'Leary DH, Polak JF, Kronmal RA et al: Distribution and correlates of sonographically detected carotid artery disease in the cardiovascular health study. Stroke 23:1752–1760, 1991

61. Parnetti L, Santucci A, Menculini G et al: Relevance of aging in carotid disease: results of a population survey. Cerebrovasc Dis 5:386–390, 1995

62. Perry IJ, Refsum H, Morris RW et al: Prospective study of serum total homocysteine concentration and risk of stroke in middle-aged British men. Lancet 346:1395–1398, 1995

63. Perry JR, Szalai JP, Norris JW, for the Canadian Stroke Consortium: Consensus against carotid surgery and screening for asymptomatic stenosis. Arch Neurol 54:25–28, 1997

64. Polak JF, Bajakian RL, O'Leary DH et al: Detection of internal carotid artery stenosis: comparison of MR angiography, colour Doppler sonography and arteriography. Radiology 182:35–40, 1992

65. Prati P, Vanuzzo D, Casaroli M et al: Prevalence and determinants of carotid atherosclerosis in a general population. Stroke 23:1705–1711, 1992

66. Ranke C, Heckor H, Creutzig A et al: Dose-dependent effect of aspirin on carotid atherosclerosis. Circulation 87:1873–1879, 1993

67. Ricci S, Flamini FO, Celani MG et al: Prevalence of internal carotid artery stenosis in subjects older than 49 years: a population study. Cerebrovasc Dis 1:16–19, 1991

68. Rodman KD, Furian AJ: Severe extracranial carotid atherosclerosis in young adults. J Stroke Cerebrovasc Dis 2:173–177, 1992

69. Roederer GO, Langlois YE, Jager KA et al: The natural history of carotid disease in asymptomatic patients with cervical bruits. Stroke 15:605, 1984

70. Rothwell PM, Slattery J, Warlow CP: A systemic comparison of the risks of stroke and death due to carotid endarterectomy for symptomatic and asymptomatic stenosis. Stroke 27:266–269, 1996

71. Salonen JT, Seppanon K, Rauramaa R, Salonen R: Risk factors for carotid atherosclerosis: the Kuopio Ischemic Heart Disease Risk Factor Study. Ann Med 21:227–229, 1989

72. Salonen R, Salonen JT: Progression of carotid atherosclerosis and its determinants. A population-based ultrasonography study. Atherosclerosis 81:33–40, 1990

73. Sander D, Klingelhofer J: Diurnal systolic blood pressure variability is the strongest predictor of early carotid atherosclerosis. Neurology 47:500–507, 1996

74. Scandinavian Simvastatin Survival Study Group: Randomized trial of cholesterol lowering in 4444 patients with coronary heart disease: The Scandinavian Simvastatin Survival Study. Lancet 344:1383–1389, 1994

75. Schartz LB, Bridgman AH, Kieffer RW et al: Asymptomatic carotid artery stenosis and stroke in patients undergoing cardiopulmonary bypass. J Vasc Surg 21:146–153, 1995

76. Selub J, Jacques PF, Bostom AG et al: Association between plasma homocysteine concentrations and extracranial carotid-artery stenosis. N Engl J Med 332:286–291, 1995

77. SHEP Cooperative Research Group: Prevention of stroke by antihypertensive drug treatment in older persons with isolated systolic hypertension: final results of the Systolic Hypertension in the Elderly Program (SHEP). JAMA 265:3255–3264, 1991

78. Shinton R, Beevors G: Meta-analysis of relation between cigarette smoking and stroke. Br Med J 298:789–794, 1989

79. Siebler M, Kleinschmidt A, Sitzer M et al: Cerebral microembolism in symptomatic and asymptomatic high-grade internal carotid artery stenosis. Neurology 44:615–618, 1994

80. Siebler M, Nachtmann A, Sitzer M et al: Cerebral microembolism and the risk of ischemia in asymptomatic high-grade internal carotid artery stenosis. Stroke 26:2184–2186, 1995

81. Sitzer M, Muller W, Siebler M et al: Plaque ulceration and lumen thrombus are the main sources of cerebral microemboli in high-grade internal carotid artery stenosis. Stroke 26:1231–1233, 1995

82. Streifler JY, Eliasziw M, Benavente OR: The risk of stroke in patients with first-ever retinal vs hemispheric transient ischemic attacks and high-grade carotid stenosis. Arch Neurol 52:246–249, 1995

83. Sutton-Tyrrell K, Wolfson SK, Kuller LH: Blood pressure treatment slows the progression of carotid stenosis in patients with isolated systolic hypertension. Stroke 25:44–50, 1994

84. Valton L, Larrue V, Arrue P et al: Asymptomatic cerebral embolic signals in patients with carotid stenosis. Stroke 26:813–815, 1995

85. van Merode T, Hick P, Hoeks APG et al: Serum HDL/total cholesterol ratio and blood pressure in asymptomatic atherosclerotic lesions of the cervical carotid arteries in men. Stroke 16:34–38, 1985

86. van Ruiswyk J, Noble H, Sigmann P: The natural history of carotid bruits in elderly persons. Ann Intern Med 112:340–346, 1990

87. von Reutern GM, Hetzl A, Birnbaum D et al: Transcranial Doppler ultrasonography during cardiopulmonary bypass in patients with severe carotid stenosis or occlusion. Stroke 19:674, 1988

88. Warlow C: Surgical treatment of asymptomatic carotid stenosis. Cerebrovasc Dis, Suppl. 6:S7–14, 1996

89. Whisnant JP, Homer D, Ingall TJ et al: Duration of cigarette smoking is the strongest predictor of severe extracranial carotid artery atherosclerosis. Stroke 21:707–714, 1990

90. Willeit J, Kicchl S: Prevalence and risk factors of asymptomatic carotid artery atherosclerosis. Arterioscler Thromb 23:1705–1711, 1992

91. Yasaka M, Yamaguchi T, Shichiri M: Distribution of atherosclerosis and risk factors in atherothrombotic occlusion. Stroke 24:206–211, 1991

92. Zukowski AJ, Nicolaides AN, Lewis RT et al: Incidence of CT scan cerebral infarction in relation to carotid plaque ulceration. J Vasc Surg 1:782–786, 1984

Surgical Considerations in Symptomatic Disease

G. PATRICK CLAGETT
JAMES T. ROBERTSON

Historical Perspective

The history of the surgical treatment of carotid atherosclerosis is marked by collaborative efforts and complementary contributions from surgeons, neurologists, and radiologists.[45,151,152] In 1927, Moniz of Lisbon described the technique of cerebral arteriography that allowed definitive antemortem diagnosis of carotid atherosclerosis. Ten years later, in 1937, Moniz described four patients with symptomatic cerebral ischemia associated with occlusion of the ipsilateral internal carotid artery diagnosed by arteriography. In seminal papers in the early 1950s, Fisher focused attention on the relationship between extracranial carotid disease and cerebral infarction, and made several important observations about the nature of carotid occlusive disease that led directly to the development of the concept of surgical reconstruction of the extracranial vessels.[60,61] He defined the basic nature of the lesion as atherosclerosis of the extracranial vessels, pointing out the predilection for atheroma to occur at the carotid bifurcation in the neck, and he also observed that the internal carotid artery distal to the bifurcation and the intracranial vessels were usually free of disease. To Fisher, these observations not only indicated that extracranial carotid disease was, indeed, an important cause of strokes, but also suggested a possible form of therapy to prevent stroke. He speculated: "It is even conceivable that someday vascular surgery will find a way to bypass the occluded portion of the artery during the period of ominous, fleeting symptoms. Anastomosis of the external carotid artery . . . with the internal carotid artery above the area of narrowing should be feasible."[60,61]

As a result of Fisher's publications, Carrea, Molins, and Murphy performed the first successful surgical reconstruction of the carotid artery in Buenos Aires on October 20, 1951.[152] The patient had stenosis of the left internal carotid artery and had suffered a stroke. They performed the procedure suggested by Fisher and the patient made an uneventful recovery. Also in 1951 Wylie introduced the procedure of thromboendarterectomy for removal of atherosclerotic plaques from the aortoiliac segment. On January 28, 1953, Strully, Hurwitt, and Blankenberg first attempted carotid thromboendarterectomy. Although unsuccessful, they suggested that endarterectomy should be feasible in such cases when the distal vasculature was patent. The first successful carotid endarterectomy was performed by DeBakey on August 7, 1953.[37] The patient had suffered a frank stroke and had total occlusion of the left internal carotid artery. Following the operation, an arteriogram demonstrated the internal carotid artery to be patent in both its extracranial and intracranial portions. The patient lived for 19 years without further strokes and died in 1972 of emphysema. The operation that gave the greatest impetus to development of surgery for carotid occlusive disease was that of Eastcott, Pickering, and Rob, which was performed in London on May 19, 1954.[46] The case was a woman who had recurrent transient ischemic attacks associated with a stenosis of the left carotid bifurcation. She underwent resection of the bifurcation with restoration of blood flow by anastomosis of the internal carotid artery to the common carotid artery. The patient was completely relieved of symptoms, and the operation dramatically demonstrated that removal of carotid bifurcation atherosclerosis could halt transient ischemic attacks and, presumably, prevent stroke.

Carotid Endarterectomy in Modern Times

In the decades following these seminal developments in the 1950s, carotid endarterectomy became one of the most common cardiovascular operations performed. The number of patients undergoing endarterectomy in hospitals in the United States rose from 15,000 in 1971 to 107,000 in 1985. However, the efficacy and appropriateness of carotid endarterectomy sustained severe criticism by neurologists and physicians in the mid-1980s.[10,20,43,44,160,164] Concerns centered on the effectiveness of the operation, and this was reflected in marked geographic variation in rates of endarterectomy.[96] Adding to this uncertainty was the decline in the number of nonfatal and fatal strokes,[16,93] the influence of risk factor management in reducing strokes,[64,91,138] and the emerging recognition of the efficacy of antiplatelet drugs in preventing stroke.[7] Early randomized trials evaluating carotid endarterectomy yielded negative results.[58,137] When a contemporary randomized trial demonstrated that extracranial-intracranial bypass was ineffective in preventing stroke,[47] this presented an opportunity to re-examine the efficacy of carotid endarterectomy, and several randomized trials were begun in both symptomatic and asymptomatic patients.

Doubt and uncertainty were reflected in a dramatic decrease in the number of annual carotid endarterectomies with approximately 70,000 being performed in 1989. At this time, Whisnant and colleagues estimated that approximately 35,000 new patients each year with carotid transient ischemic attacks or recovered stroke with stenosis would be candidates for carotid endarterectomy.[161] If this estimate was correct, the number of carotid endarterectomies each year far exceeded the indications for the procedure in symptomatic patients. In addition, approximately half of the carotid endarterectomies were performed on asymptomatic patients.[20,62,76] In addition to the projected excess number of procedures, critics brought forth the evidence that the surgical risk was too high to justify the operation and that antiplatelet therapy probably had an outcome better than surgical treatment.[7,10,28,44] A statement from the American College of Physicians, concerning the indications for carotid endarterectomy, concluded that surgical mortality rates of less than 1% and stroke-related morbidity of less than 3% in symptomatic patients and stroke mortality plus stroke-related morbidity of less than 2% for patients with asymptomatic carotid disease were the values that must be matched to compete with available medical therapy.[25] A consensus of a selected committee of neurologists, neurosurgeons, and vascular surgeons, recognizing the confusion concerning indications for carotid endarterectomy, recommended that in the absence of definitive data from clinical trials, carotid endarterectomy should be performed with low morbidity and mortality in selected patients with appropriate symptoms and a hemodynamically significant carotid lesion.[12] The limits were categorized by clinical presentation. The com-

bined morbidity and mortality of the procedure should not exceed 3% for asymptomatic lesions, 5% for transient ischemic attacks, and 7% for ischemic stroke. In addition, the 30-day mortality rate from all causes related to endarterectomy should not exceed 2%. Concomitantly, ongoing audits should be performed in an institution where endarterectomy is being performed to ensure adherence to these suggested guidelines.

An exciting scientific landmark and partial resolution to controversies surrounding carotid endarterectomy was announced on February 21, 1991 at the International Stroke Conference of the American Heart Association in San Francisco by Dr. H. J. M. Barnett, the principal investigator of the North American Symptomatic Carotid Endarterectomy Trial (NASCET).[31,141] An interim analysis of 659 patients who had been randomized to either medical or surgical therapy for transient ischemic attack or mild disabling stroke ipsilateral to a 70% to 99% narrowing of the internal carotid artery were unequivocally shown to be treated best by surgical therapy[113] (Fig. 53.17). Among the symptomatic patients with high-grade carotid stenosis, carotid endarterectomy reduced the overall risk of fatal and nonfatal ipsilateral stroke, despite any perioperative risk of stroke or death from any cause. Including perioperative morbidity and mortality or its 32-day equivalent time in the medical group, over 26% of the medical group, but only 9% of the surgical patients, had experienced fatal or nonfatal ipsilateral stroke at 24 months. This represented an absolute risk reduction in favor of surgery of 17% and a relative risk reduction of 65%.

Further analyses were conducted to ascertain the importance of commonly recognized risk factors associated with stroke.[113] These included age (greater than 70 years), sex (male), systolic hypertension (greater than 160 mmHg), diastolic hypertension (greater than 90 mmHg), recentness of onset of symptoms (less than 30 days), type of prior cerebrovascular events (stroke, not TIA), degree of stenosis (greater than 80%), presence of ulceration as determined by arteriography, and a history of smoking, hypertension, myocardial infarction, congestive heart failure, diabetes, intermittent claudication, or elevated blood lipid levels. The proportion of medically treated patients who had an ipsilateral stroke within 2 years was 17% in the low-risk group (0–5 risk factors), 23% in the moderate-risk group (6 risk factors), and 39% in the high-risk group (7 or more risk factors) ($P < 0.001$). The ipsilateral stroke prognosis of surgical patients did not vary according to the number of risk factors present and averaged 9% at 2 years. In other words, after carotid endarterectomy there were no significant increases in event rates among patients with increasing numbers of baseline risk factors. Thus, the degree of benefit that individual patients received from carotid endarterectomy was directly proportional to the risk that they faced without surgery, and those with the highest risk at entry gained the most.

Another secondary analysis showed that the finer divisions of the degree of high-grade stenosis broken down into deciles correlated with degrees of risk reduction after surgery.[113] The absolute risk reduction for all ipsilateral stroke at 2 years was 26% among patients with a stenosis of 90% to 99% at entry, 18% among those with stenosis of 80% to 89%, and 12% with stenosis of 70% to 79%. This decreasing margin of efficacy for carotid endarterectomy suggests that with stenoses less than 50% to 60%, there may be little benefit of

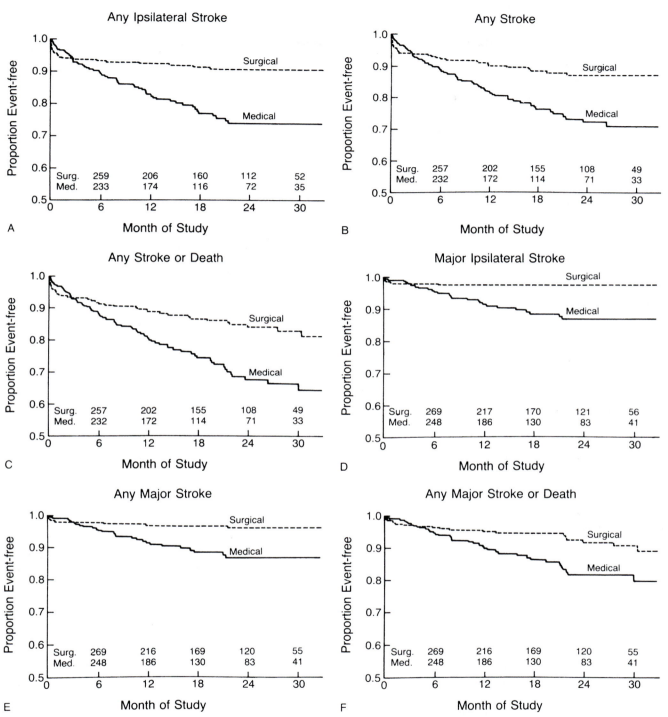

Figure 53.17 (**A–F**) Survival curves for the treatment groups. These Kaplan-Meier survival curves show the probability of surviving six events indicating treatment failure after randomization. The number of patients who remained event-free in each treatment group is shown at 6-month intervals at the bottom of each graph; the numbers at time zero are 328 in the surgical group and 331 in the medical group. The curves of the groups differed significantly (by Mantel-Haenszel chi-square test, $P < 0.001$ for all events except "any major stroke or death," for which $P < 0.01$). (From NASCET Collaborators,[113] with permission.)

carotid endarterectomy because medical treatment would produce equivalent results.

Two other important studies were reported shortly after the NASCET results were announced. In the first, results of the European Carotid Surgery Trial (ECST) demonstrated a clear benefit for carotid endarterectomy in patients with advanced stenoses.[54] This large scale trial uses different methods to measure degree of stenosis than NASCET. ECST uses a method whereby the angiographic point of maximum stenosis is compared with the *estimated* diameter of the carotid bulb at that level. This method gives very similar results to that using the normal common carotid artery diameter. NASCET compares the diameter of the maximum stenosis to the diameter of the distal, nontapering cervical internal carotid artery.[113,141] The two methods do not produce equivalent measurements. For example, a 70% ECST stenosis is equivalent to a 40% NASCET stenosis. These distinctions are important when considering the biologic significance of increasing degrees of stenosis severity in determining prognosis with medical therapy balanced against the risk of endarterectomy.

The third randomized study showing benefit of carotid endarterectomy came from Veterans Administration (VA) hospitals.[102] This was a small study with relatively short follow-up that stopped accruing patients when NASCET and ECST results were announced. Despite premature closure, the VA study demonstrated a significant reduction in the endpoints of stroke and crescendo TIA.

In addition to showing benefit of carotid endarterectomy, the randomized studies have emphasized the alarmingly high rate of stroke encountered in symptomatic patients with high-grade stenosis treated medically. The risk of stroke was severalfold higher than previous estimates based on results from natural history studies and randomized trials assessing the benefit of antiplatelet therapy. There was little attempt to correlate symptoms with carotid pathology in many of these trials and only a small proportion of patients underwent arteriography.[17,23,42,57,73,134,139,149,156,157] In addition, many patients entering the antiplatelet therapy trials had posterior circulation symptoms that may have a different natural history than carotid-based symptoms. The tendency to extrapolate results from antiplatelet therapy trials to patients with focal symptoms and ipsilateral carotid stenosis led to the underestimation of stroke risk and the potential benefit of carotid endarterectomy. NASCET and other studies documented the importance of correlating symptoms with carotid disease morphology and pathology assessed with careful arteriography.

Attention is now focused on determining the benefit of endarterectomy in symptomatic patients with moderate degrees of stenosis.[9] The ongoing NASCET is following two groups of randomized patients, low-moderates (30% to 49% stenosis) and high-moderates (50% to 69% stenosis). ECST results in these groups of patients have recently been published and show no benefit of carotid endarterectomy in high or low patients with moderate symptomatic carotid stenosis.[53] However, these results must be interpreted with caution, since ECST methods of measuring stenosis tend to overestimate severity in comparison with that of the NASCET method. Therefore, it is most likely that ECST patients with moderate stenoses have less advanced disease than patients judged to be moderate by NASCET criteria. Probably even more important, the perioperative major stroke and death rate was 8%

in ECST in comparison with 2.1% in the first phase of NASCET.[113] The more favorable risk/benefit ratio of carotid endarterectomy in NASCET and the relatively greater degree of stenoses with presumably higher stroke risk with medical therapy would suggest the possibility of finding a beneficial effect of carotid endarterectomy for patients with moderate stenosis in NASCET.

While clearly delineating the biologic significance of severity of stenosis in symptomatic patients, NASCET has also determined that other factors are important in determining stroke prognosis with medical therapy and the potential benefit of endarterectomy. Contralateral occlusion,[65] angiographic findings of ulceration,[50,144] and hemispheric, as opposed to retinal, ischemic events,[143] all increase the risk of stroke for a given level of stenosis. In addition, multiple stroke risk factors in combination with these prognostic indicators further elevate this risk. Therefore, all of these factors must be taken into account before recommending carotid endarterectomy in a given patient. While the severity of stenosis may be the most important determinant in selecting patients for surgery, the ultimate threshold may be adjusted upward or downward depending on the absence or presence of other risk factors.

The benefits of carotid endarterectomy will not be realized if perioperative morbidity and mortality is excessive. The reported risk of endarterectomy shows wide variation, and concerns have been raised about whether the results from NASCET and other randomized studies can be extrapolated to the nation as a whole. Two independent studies showed that patients undergoing endarterectomy in the United States in 1981 and 1982 had a perioperative combined major stroke and death rate of 9% to 10%.[44,164] In a more contemporary report, published in 1992, the national mortality for Medicare beneficiaries undergoing carotid endarterectomy was found to be 2.5%.[83] Using ratios derived from NASCET data, one can estimate that the national incidence of combined *major* stroke and death may be 7% to 8% (three times the mortality rate[133]) and the incidence of all strokes (major and minor) and death may be as high as 25% (10 times the mortality rate). If the perioperative morbidity and mortality were this high in NASCET and other trials, these studies would have shown no benefit of carotid endarterectomy. These considerations are disturbing and point to the importance of ongoing quality improvement audits.

In clinical settings where the risk of carotid endarterectomy is acceptably low according to published guidelines, the operation can be recommended in patients with at least a 50% carotid stenosis or a large ulcerative plaque with ipsilateral transient ischemic attacks, amaurosis fugax, a reversible ischemic neurological deficit, or small stroke and selected cases of recurrent, symptomatic carotid stenosis.[107,109] Individualized patients may require surgery for progressing stroke, progressive retinal ischemia, acute carotid occlusion, symptomatic carotid stump syndrome (treated with external carotid reconstruction), global cerebral ischemia due to multiple large vessel occlusive disease, selected tandem lesions where the proximal stenosis is greater than the distal, and in certain cases of symptomatic carotid dissection and true or false aneurysm. The procedure is generally not indicated in patients presenting with vertebrobasilar distribution transient ischemic attacks, multi-infarct dementia, patients with severe neurologic deficits, and those with evidence of intracranial hemorrhage or large infarcts. Medical contraindications include the presence of uncontrolled congestive heart failure, recent myocardial infarction, unstable angina, dementia, advanced malignancy, and uncertain diagnosis.

Operative Planning and Management

PREOPERATIVE EVALUATION

The physician must take whatever measures are necessary to ensure that the carotid lesion is the cause of the patient's symptoms. The best surgical results are in patients operated upon for true transient ischemic attacks or amaurosis fugax. Because evidence from postmortem and stroke registries report that 15% to 25% of ischemic events can be attributed to a cardiac embolic or dysrhythmic source, cardiac evaluation is essential.[24,167] Patients with unstable angina pectoris, a recent myocardial infarction, or uncontrolled congestive heart failure should be treated medically if at all possible. Since postoperative myocardial infarction is a leading cause of death after carotid endarterectomy, patients must have adequate oxygenation and intravascular volume expansion before surgery. The immediate preoperative use of aspirin for platelet inhibition is recommended and data from NASCET suggest that higher dose (650 mg to 1,200 mg daily) aspirin may be more beneficial than low dose (80 mg to 650 mg daily) or no aspirin in the prevention of perioperative thromboembolic complications.[8] Aspirin dosage in the prevention of perioperative complications is the subject of an ongoing trial, the Aspirin in Carotid Endarterectomy (ACE) Trial. If the patient is having active transient ischemic attacks despite aspirin therapy or has preocclusive stenosis, especially when combined with intraluminal clot, intravenous continuous heparin therapy keeping the partial thromboplastin time at one and one-half times control is recommended.[130] Platelet counts should be performed every third day, and if thrombocytopenia occurs, heparin must be stopped to avoid thrombotic complications. If the patient is severely hypertensive, every effort at control of hypertension prior to surgery or heparin treatment is mandated because of the increased risk of operating on patients with uncontrolled blood pressures in excess of 180/110 mmHg. Severe chronic obstructive pulmonary disease may be a relative contraindication to surgery. Preoperative management of pulmonary toilet is recommended in an effort to improve function. Uncontrolled diabetes mellitus must be regulated.

PREPARATION

When the brain is presented with an ischemic insult, the cerebrovascular reactivity or cerebral autoregulation is impaired or lost. The perfusion pressure of the brain depends on the systemic mean arterial pressure and, simultaneously, because of the loss of autoregulation, the brain is extremely vulnerable

to sudden changes in system arterial pressure. The anesthesiologist must be aware of this liability in patients presenting for operation with ischemia and choose appropriate general anesthetic agents or regional local anesthesia.[2,34,135,146] The operating table should be horizontal without head elevation and the head turned partially to the opposite side with modest elevation of the ipsilateral shoulder. Gentle preparation of the operative site avoids the possibility of dislodging fragments from a fragile carotid plaque.

INITIAL DISSECTION

A reverse S-shaped incision is preferred, in order to minimize postoperative wound contracture with discomfort and to afford wide exposure. Alternatively, many surgeons employ a simple oblique incision along the anterior border of the sternocleidomastoid muscle. The incision characteristically begins at the level of the mastoid and extends anteriorly along the anteromedial border of the sternocleidomastoid muscle to about one to two finger-breadths above the sternal notch in the midline. Sharp dissection is essential. The use of an electrocautery knife is preferred by many. After sectioning the platysma muscle vertically, the plane of dissection is anteromedial to the sternocleidomastoid muscle beginning inferiorly and proceeding superiorly. In the upper mid-portion of the incision, the transverse cervical nerve, which is responsible for the skin innervation medial to the incision and along the lower jaw, is divided. The approach to the carotid sheath begins inferiorly along the anterior border of the sternocleidomastoid muscle and proceeds superiorly.

The carotid sheath is a fascial sheath formed by extensions of the deep cervical fascia and prevertebral fascia. The sheath contains the carotid artery, the jugular vein, the vagus nerve, and the deep cervical lymphatic chain. Inferiorly, along the common carotid artery, the carotid sheath is very well-defined, and the thickened sheath overlying the common carotid is best opened vertically; this incision is extended superiorly toward the carotid bifurcation. Dissection of the common carotid artery should proceed along its medial border to prevent injury to the vagus nerve which sometimes is found anteriorly on this vessel. The carotid sheath is less well-defined superiorly because of vascular branches. The sheath may be preserved and tacked up with small sutures attached to the platysma. This allows subsequent closure of the sheath and also tends to elevate the carotid artery. Exposure of the common carotid artery may involve sectioning of the omohyoid muscle. At this point in the operation, many surgeons heparinize the patients with 100 to 150 U/kg.[27] This may inhibit further thromboembolic phenomena during more cephalad dissection.

PREVENTION OF INTRAOPERATIVE EMBOLIZATION

The major danger through this portion of the operation is embolization produced by excessive manipulation of the carotid bifurcation.[130,146] The surgeon must be intensely aware of the fragile nature of an atherosclerotic plaque, particularly with ulceration and/or intraluminal clot. Intraoperative embolization is a major cause of minor or major stroke. A "no touch" technique is employed whereby the common carotid, internal carotid, and external carotid arteries are all exposed and dissected free with minimal manipulation of the disease-bearing carotid bifurcation area. The common facial vein enters the internal jugular vein usually at the level of the bifurcation of the common carotid artery and routinely requires ligation and division. There may be numerous other branches that must be ligated and divided in order to adequately expose the targeted artery.

A major difficulty is encountered in achieving exposure for lesions extending high into the internal carotid artery or patients with high carotid bifurcations. When exposure is required above the second cervical vertebra or a line drawn between the tip of the mastoid and the angle of the mandible, special techniques are required.[104] Anterior subluxation of the mandible can extend the exposure to above the body of the first cervical vertebra.[59] This is almost always accompanied by sectioning of the posterior belly of the digastric muscle and sometimes by styloidectomy. Multiple techniques for mandibular subluxation have been described,[41,95,136] but the most currently favored is that of circummandibular/transnasal wiring manipulations that fix the mandible in a subluxed anterior location for the duration of the operation.[59]

Many surgeons routinely use monitoring with electroencephalography to determine the need for shunting and also to detect intraoperative episodes of ischemia produced by embolic debris or shunt occlusion.[118,130,140] During the operation, if a major unexpected change occurs in the electroencephalogram (EEG), an embolus to the main trunk of the middle cerebral artery must be suspected. If this is a minor embolic episode, the change will frequently reverse, but if major, it may persist, and if it does, the routine recommended by Sundt includes ensuring that heparinization is present by augmenting the original heparin dose if necessary and immediately giving intravenously 3 mg/kg thiopental or more, if necessary, to reach burst suppression of the EEG.[130] Subsequently, the endarterectomy should be completed as quickly as possible, and if the EEG change disappears or is minor, subsequently, the patient is allowed to awaken from anesthesia. If not, on-the-table arteriography is recommended, and if an embolus is found in the middle cerebral artery, some have advocated middle cerebral artery embolectomy or extracranial, intracranial bypass.[130] However, a better option may be regional infusion of fibrinolytic agents such as urokinase. Single case reports have documented lysis of middle cerebral artery emboli and reversal of neurologic deficits.[11,33]

If EEG monitoring is not performed, some surgeons routinely introduce an intra-arterial shunt.[130,147,153] The shunt may be employed as a straight, common carotid-to-internal carotid shunt or an externally looped shunt. Embolus as a result of shunt usage may be produced by intimal injury to the proximal, common, or distal internal carotid arteries or even dissection of the intima. The shunt may undergo occlusion during the procedure, and emboli may be introduced into the shunt at the time of placement. Most surgeons place the shunt into the internal carotid artery first and allow it to backbleed freely before carefully inserting it into the common carotid artery. Some have recommended placement of the shunt first into the common carotid artery, making certain that any embolic material has been flushed from the common carotid artery and the shunt allowed to bleed slightly before placing it into the internal carotid artery.[130] Soaking the shunt in heparinized saline before use may retard thrombus formation within the shunt and prevent air bubbles from forming in the shunt at the time of placement.

Prior to arteriotomy and shunt insertion, Rummel tourniquets are used for vascular control. A large Rummel tourniquet is placed around the common carotid artery and small Rummel tourniquets are placed around the external and internal carotid arteries. Again, manipulation of the disease-bearing segment of the carotid bifurcation is avoided during these maneuvers. Some surgeons temporarily occlude the internal carotid artery with a Silastic vascular loop or a small aneurysm clip. Fine vascular clamps are preferred by some surgeons to obtain proximal and distal control. Whether or not a proximal vascular clamp or Rummel tourniquets are used, every effort should be made to avoid carotid plaque at the bifurcation and to apply these constricting devices on normal artery. All of these maneuvers are designed not only to prevent damage to normal intima, but to prevent fracture of atherosclerotic plaque with subsequent stenosis or subintimal dissection, or a site for thrombus formation with distal embolization intraoperatively or postoperatively.

ENDARTERECTOMY PROCEDURE

The arteriotomy begins in the proximal common carotid artery and extends into the internal carotid artery. A #11 blade is used to open the common carotid artery at the site below the plaque, and then angled Potts scissors are used to incise the artery through the plaque into the normal distal internal carotid artery. Obviously, the occluding clamps and/or loops are tightened prior to the arteriotomy. Some surgeons insist on removing the plaque from the internal carotid artery distally as the initial step. Others will immediately place a shunt in the internal and, subsequently, in the common carotid artery or vice versa as described. Then the plaque is carefully dissected from the arterial wall using a blunt dissector, for example, a Penfield-4. When normal intima is reached in the common carotid artery, the intima is sharply dissected to allow no loose flap. In some cases, the entire common carotid artery has eccentric thickening; this necessitates leaving a small shelf of plaque. The endarterectomy should proceed proximally as far as possible to reach a portion of the vessel where plaque is minimal, and the resulting shelf is small at the point where the endarterectomy ends. On occasion, this requires endarterectomy of the common carotid artery to the level of the clavicle. At the bifurcation, the plaque is peeled from below upward to the external carotid artery, where it is carefully dissected from the external carotid artery by intussusception. As this process proceeds up the external carotid artery, it is wise to release the occluding Rummel tourniquet temporarily to allow the plaque to be carefully removed and to ascertain the backflow from the external carotid artery. It is important to make certain that the external carotid artery is left patent.[108,130] If there is uncertainty, it may be necessary to form a separate arteriotomy on the external carotid artery, remove external carotid artery plaque, and patch the arteriotomy with vein or prosthetic material. Subsequently, the plaque is peeled out of the internal carotid artery, and it will usually peel out quite smoothly distally. If the plaque is removed prior to the insertion of a shunt, less distal artery need be exposed. On the other hand, if normal intima was exposed distal to the plaque prior to the insertion of the shunt, the plaque can quite easily be removed even with the shunt in place.

If the plaque peels out easily and leaves a distal smooth surface, no tacking sutures are necessary. If the distal intima remains thickened and infiltrated with plaque, it is necessary to remove this to the point of normal intima. The technique of nicking the more available thickened intima with the Potts scissors and peeling out the thickened intima circumferentially is recommended.[130] If there is any question about the distal intima's being loose, it should be tacked down with 6-0 double-arm Prolene sutures proceeding from within the artery to the outer wall where the suture is tied. The suture should be placed vertically rather than horizontally to avoid constricting the lumen. Virtually all experienced surgeons recommend visualization of the distal endpoint and the transition area between the endarterectomy site and normal intima. "Blind" endarterectomy may invite distal flaps that can lead to postoperative thromboembolic phenomena.

During dissection of the plaque, the endarterectomy bed is frequently irrigated with heparinized saline. This irrigation allows the identification of loose pieces of debris and plaque that must be meticulously removed from the endarterectomy site to prevent postoperative thrombus formation. If a shunt has been used, it is helpful to place a 4-0 Prolene or 3-0 silk suture around the shunt to allow subsequent ease in removal of the shunt through the small remaining arteriotomy at the time of arterial closure. Other surgeons, to minimize migration of the shunt, will place 5- or 6-0, double-arm Prolene sutures around the shunt and through the arterial wall with a loose tie externally and remove this suture prior to shunt removal.

RECONSTRUCTION OF THE ARTERY

Once the vessel is meticulously cleaned, primary closure or closure with a vein or fabric patch ensues. The available experience in the literature supports the use of a patch over primary closure.[62,76,78] Many report fewer postoperative carotid occlusions or ischemic events with the use of a patch. In addition, the incidence of restenosis may be minimized.[26,36,78] Meticulous placement of sutures to ensure a smooth patch, vein or prosthetic, is essential. A 6-0 Prolene suture is recommended as a running suture. Primary closure of the artery should also be effected using 6-0 Prolene suture. In unusual cases where plaque is focally confined to the carotid bulb with minimal extension into the internal carotid artery, primary closure can be recommended if the arteriotomy does not extend beyond the bulb. Some surgeons have used 5-mm diameter of the internal carotid artery as the threshold to determine the need for patch closure.[26] Just prior to closure, regardless of the closure method, the shunt is removed, all vessels are

allowed to flush, and closure is completed. Flushing is important to remove air and debris. After closure, the external and common carotid arteries are first opened and then the internal carotid artery is opened to minimize air or particulate embolization into the internal carotid artery system. If a fabric patch has been used and was properly preclotted, bleeding is easily controlled by the application of hemostatic agents. Additional arterial sutures may be needed if the initial suture technique did not ensure close and regular placement of the suture, allowing for site bleeding.

Meticulous attention is necessary to avoid damage to the running suture with placement of additional sutures. Some surgeons stress nonreversal of heparin or waiting at least 20 minutes to reverse heparin with protamine sulfate. Studies in animals suggest that this practice reduces thrombus formation at the endarterectomy site. If bleeding is a problem after the first 10 to 20 minutes, the heparin may be reversed in stages. The half-life of heparin is approximately 50 to 60 minutes and this should be taken into account at the time of heparin reversal with protamine sulfate.[27] Generally a 0.5 to 1 mg equivalent reversal dose is used (0.5 to 1 mg of protamine sulfate for every 100 units of heparin).

The arterial wall is then palpated to determine the presence of a thrill, which would indicate a loose intimal flap or some obstructive intraluminal mass. If a thrill is present, an arteriogram should be performed to determine the characteristics of the endarterectomy. If a clot or debris is found inside the lumen, the vessel must be reoccluded and opened, and all debris removed. If there is any question about the patency of the arterial system, an arteriogram should be performed.[39] Operative ultrasound may also be used. If there is evidence of external carotid artery occlusion or obstruction, a clamp should be placed on the proximal external carotid artery, and distal occlusion of the internal carotid artery achieved by placement of Rummel tourniquets or vascular occluding clips or clamps. When the external carotid artery is opened, an intimal flap will almost invariably be found; this should be removed and flow restored in the external carotid. Because the external carotid artery lumen diameter is small with frequent branches, a patch closure is usually necessary to ensure an adequate lumen. Patency of the external carotid artery is important to prevent an occluded stump as a source of embolism postoperatively and also to ensure adequate collateral circulation.

Prior to operation, the surgeon will have determined whether or not the vessels had kinks or loops. After the endarterectomy, it is essential to remove any significant kinks or loops in the internal carotid artery system that are contiguous with the endarterectomy and arteriotomy closure. These can be removed by resection and reanastomosis or plication with 6-0 Prolene suture and subsequent vein or fabric patching.[3]

The overriding surgical principle must be reconstruction of the artery to ensure optimal, unimpaired, well-directed arterial flow.[100] The goal is to operate on the patient safely and not produce the stroke for which the prophylactic operation has been performed. Hertzer's comment, "Few major operations are conceptually so simple, yet technically so unforgiving, as a carotid endarterectomy,"[76] must be remembered. Rather than using confirmatory intraoperative arteriography, many surgeons are now using operative duplex ultrasound to determine the patency and the quality of the reconstructed artery.[90]

This noninvasive procedure deserves further consideration. Subsequent to meticulous hemostasis, the wound is closed. Because most of these patients had been medicated with aspirin, and heparin is sometimes incompletely reversed, wound hematomas are common.[27] While these hematomas are usually minor, airway compromise can occur with large hematomas. It is important to ensure that the field is dry prior to wound closure.

POSTOPERATIVE MANAGEMENT

Hypertension

It is critical that blood pressure be maintained at a level of approximately 150 mmHg systolic as a maximum. This may require the intravenous use of nitroprusside or nitroglycerin. The sudden restoration of high flow, particularly after removal of a very tight stenosis and in the presence of heparin and/or aspirin, may produce intracerebral hemorrhage. The meticulous control of blood pressure is the major way of minimizing hyperperfusion that often occurs following the removal of a high-grade stenosis. Sundt has shown flows to increase over 100% after successful endarterectomy, particularly in patients presenting with strokes, generalized cerebral ischemia, and multiple transient ischemic attacks.[146] Postoperative hypertension is a major treatable and preventable event. The therapy for postoperative hypertension should begin at the point of restoration of flow and be maintained throughout the patient's hospital stay. Fortunately, the postoperative instability in blood pressure usually disappears within 12 to 24 hours.

Hypotension

Postoperative hypotension may be as disastrous as postoperative hypertension. This instability of blood pressure in the postoperative state occurs in at least 50% of patients operated on under general anesthesia, but is unusual in patients operated on under regional anesthesia.[2,135] The instability of blood pressure is due to carotid sinus malfunction.[18] The carotid sinus is a major baroreceptor in normal individuals, and elevation in peripheral perfusion pressure results in stimulation of the receptor, and the afferent limb of the receptor, the glossopharyngeal nerve, conducts the impulse to the medulla, which, through activation of the sympathetic or parasympathetic system, usually the latter, produces a lowering of peripheral vascular tone and blood pressure and slowing of the pulse rate. Patients with atherosclerosis of the carotid body often lose effective baroreceptor action.

Following endarterectomy, the carotid bulb can again distend, and the carotid sinus reflex can overrespond, producing postoperative hypotension. On the other hand, as a result of the surgical procedure the reflex may be abolished, and postoperative hypertension occurs. Significant postoperative hypotension may produce cerebral ischemic complications and can best be treated by placing the patient in a Trendelenburg position, making certain that volume replacement is adequate and using vasopressors. Phenylephrine increases left ventricular work and myocardial oxygen demands and may be associated with unfavorable cardiac events.[128] Dopamine is preferred when a pressor is needed. In an effort to avoid postoperative hypotension, many surgeons routinely section the carotid sinus nerve. Others routinely anesthetize this nerve with local anesthetic; however, this maneuver can result in postoperative hypertension.[51]

Postoperative Complications and Their Management

STROKE OR TRANSIENT NEUROLOGIC DEFICIT

Neurologic deficits within the first 12 hours of operation are almost always due to thromboembolic phenomena stemming from the endarterectomy site or damaged internal common or external carotid arteries. Immediate exploration is indicated without the need for confirmatory arteriography or noninvasive tests.[68,92] Neurologic deficits that begin beyond 12 to 24 hours of operation may be due to thromboembolic phenomena stemming from the endarterectomy site, but may also be caused by postoperative hyperperfusion syndrome or intracerebral hematoma. These latter conditions may be worsened by immediate heparinization and re-exploration. Therefore, deficits occurring beyond 12 to 24 hours should be promptly investigated with a computed tomography (CT) scan and arteriography.

If the patient awakens from anesthesia with a postoperative neurologic deficit, the surgeon is faced with a major catastrophe of the operation.[130,146] If the patient has a profound hemiplegia and aphasia and eye deviation to the side of the lesion, the prognosis is grave but not hopeless. Usually, a much less severe neurologic deficit is present. In the presence of a major deficit, the most likely cause is thrombosis of the internal carotid artery with or without distal embolization. The next most common cause is a distal internal carotid artery or middle cerebral artery embolus. In the face of an immediate significant deficit that is greater than the preoperative deficit, the patient should be given additional heparin to ensure full anticoagulation, and the blood pressure should be elevated with vasopressors. Preparation should be made to immediately return the patient to the operating room. Many surgeons insist that their patients be awakened in the operating room so that immediate neurologic examination can determine whether or not a deficit is present and, thus, minimize time to re-exploration. If upon reopening the wound an excellent pulse is present in the carotid artery and flow is present on Doppler ultrasound examination, an on-the-table arteriogram is performed. If the arteriogram reveals an intimal flap or irregular mural thrombus at the endarterectomy site, then appropriate vessel isolation and reopening of the vessel is indicated. Thrombus is removed and backbleeding is allowed. At this point, the mechanical cause of thrombosis is usually defined as an intimal flap and this is repaired. If on initial inspection of the artery there is no pulse, the vessel is obviously thrombosed, and a preliminary arteriogram is not necessary prior to opening the vessel and extracting the thrombus.

Prior to restoration of flow, an internal carotid arteriogram is done by placing a small catheter into the distal internal carotid artery and injecting 4 to 5 ml of contrast agent to ensure that the distal internal carotid artery is patent and to determine whether there is an embolus in the middle cerebral artery. If the vessel is patent with or without middle cerebral artery embolus, flow can be restored after reconstruction of the vessel. If an embolus exists in the intracranial carotid or middle cerebral artery, the patient's blood pressure may be raised and back-bleeding allowed in the hope that the embolus will flush down the open artery. The arteriogram is repeated, and if the distal internal carotid artery embolus persists, local infusion of thrombolytic agents should be considered.[11,33] Alternatively, craniotomy and embolectomy or extracranial-intracranial bypass surgery should be considered.

If on opening the artery no thrombus is present and no backflow occurs, a #3 Fogarty catheter should be passed distally to the level of the carotid canal and distended gently to remove distal thrombus. A distal thrombus without local operative thrombus would indicate distal intimal damage to the internal carotid artery, probably from dissection produced by shunting or intimal damage produced by forceful clamping. Not infrequently, on returning the patient to the operating room, the artery and arteriogram are normal. In this circumstance, it is presumed that either operative ischemia occurred despite monitoring or shunting or an embolus had occurred and lysed. A distal branch or branches of the middle cerebral artery may be found to contain emboli. Craniotomy with embolectomy, thrombolytic agents, or medical therapy may be the most satisfactory therapy. Generally, the prognosis with a distal embolus in the cortical arteries is not resolvable with surgical therapy.

If angiography demonstrates no cause for the neurologic deficit but shows evidence of a mass lesion, an intracerebral hemorrhage is present. If the arteriogram is normal, a postoperative computed tomography (CT) or magnetic resonance imaging (MRI) scan is indicated to determine the presence of an intracerebral clot or infarction. If an intracerebral hemorrhage is seen, the patient's blood pressure should be maintained at a normal level. The heparin must be reversed with protamine sulfate. If the patient received aspirin, platelet transfusion may be important to reverse the aspirin effect and restore normal hemostasis. Subsequently, surgical evacuation may be lifesaving. Unfortunately, when intracerebral hemorrhage occurs, it is often a massive bleed. If the hemorrhage is extensive and in the major hemisphere, no therapy is probably the most humane in view of the patient's dismal prognosis.

If arteriography confirms an external carotid artery occlusion and an embolus is seen in the internal carotid system or the arteriogram is otherwise normal, the probability is that an embolus arose from the external carotid artery.[108] This patient should have the external carotid artery isolated, opened, and a thrombectomy performed and correction of intimal flap or other technical fault carried out. If a common carotid occlusion is found, one can suspect an intimal lesion with dissection as the cause. This will necessitate extending the arteriotomy proximally beyond the original clamp site with appropriate repair.

OPERATIVE DAMAGE TO NERVES

The sensory branches of the cervical plexus, namely, the transverse cervical nerve and the greater auricular nerve, are frequently severed or injured during the course of carotid endar-

terectomy. The resulting ipsilateral numbness of the upper neck, lower face, and lower ear is vexing to some patients but is generally well-tolerated. Permanent hypesthesia in this area is common after carotid endarterectomy. Of much greater consequence is injury to cranial nerves in the field of dissection, because the resulting neurologic deficits can produce serious complications.[14,55,63,79,150] Fortunately, cranial nerve injury is infrequent and is usually reversible with transient neurologic deficits lasting weeks to months. In one major series, the frequency of clinically significant injury to the recurrent laryngeal nerve was 6%, to the hypoglossal nerve 5%, to the marginal mandibular nerve 2%, and to the superior laryngeal nerve 2%.[79] Some degree of minor injury is probably more common, and studies prospectively assessing patients after endarterectomy for asymptomatic, as well as symptomatic, cranial nerve deficits report a higher frequency.[55,63] In addition to these nerve injuries, damage to the cervical sympathetic chain may produce a complete Horner syndrome or in the case of high dissection of the internal carotid artery an incomplete Horner syndrome.

Meticulous surgical technique and knowledge of the anatomy with application of sharp dissection and routine use of the bipolar cautery will prevent most of these complications, except the loss of the transverse cervical and greater auricular nerves. Advocates of the transverse cervical incision argue that the transverse cervical nerve can be spared and that the postoperative wound is more cosmetic, but the limits of exposure by this approach are a liability.

VAGAL NERVE INJURY

Injury to the main trunk of the vagus nerve is rare.[14,79] The nerve usually runs posterior to the carotid artery between the carotid artery and the internal jugular vein and is covered by a separate fascial sheath. It may be injured in high exposure and by careless use of the cautery. Injury can be minimized by meticulous attention to anatomic detail and the use of the bipolar cautery. On occasion, the vagus nerve may course anterior to the carotid artery on the right. In this circumstance, the recurrent branch of the laryngeal nerve arises at the level of the carotid bifurcation and can be easily sectioned. This anatomic variation is termed a "nonrecurrent" recurrent laryngeal nerve and is almost always associated with an aberrant origin of the right subclavian artery from the distal aortic arch. The identification of this vascular anomaly on preoperative arteriography should alert the surgeon to the presence of an anomalous recurrent laryngeal nerve. Complications can further be avoided by a policy of not sectioning any nerve until its origin is determined. On occasion, an anterior vagus nerve is present and the nerve and its recurrent branch are at jeopardy when mobilizing the common carotid artery. The policy of beginning dissection medially and maintaining circumferential dissection within the periadventitial plane will facilitate displacement and mobilization of the nerve away from the artery. The fibers of the recurrent laryngeal nerve run in the medial aspect of the main trunk of the vagus nerve, and injury to the medial portions of the vagus nerve can result in recurrent laryngeal nerve injury.

The recurrent laryngeal branch can be damaged by placing a self-retaining retractor deep to the level of the trachea. The right nerve arises from the vagus trunk at the root of the neck at about the level of C7–T1 and loops around the subclavian artery. Posterior to the subclavian artery the nerve runs superiorly and medially behind the common carotid artery into the groove between the trachea and the esophagus where it ascends to the lower border of the cricoid cartilage. It becomes the inferior laryngeal nerve and supplies intrinsic muscles of the larynx that control the vocal cord. Damage results in unilateral vocal cord paralysis. This nerve is rarely, if ever, exposed during carotid endarterectomy and is usually damaged by traction or electrocautery. Bilateral recurrent laryngeal nerve injury results in mid-line vocal cord apposition that can severely compromise the airway. Because of this possibility, many recommend indirect laryngoscopy prior to the second stage of bilateral staged carotid endarterectomies.

The superior laryngeal nerve is a branch of the vagus nerve at the lower margin of the first cervical vertebra and runs posteriorly and medially to the internal and external carotid arteries. The nerve divides into an internal and an external branch. The internal branch is responsible for the sensory supply of the epiglottis and the larynx above the vocal cords. The external branch is responsible for the motor supply to the cricothyroid muscle and the inferior pharyngeal constrictor. The nerve is covered by loose fascia posterior and medial to the carotid arteries and can best be seen just medial and deep to the carotid bifurcation. It is usually damaged by careless use of the cautery or direct posterior compression medial to the carotid bifurcation. Meticulous technique will minimize damage to this nerve. It also may be damaged by high exposure of the internal carotid artery at and above C1, so that in high dissection the medial aspect of the vagus nerve must always be respected. Damage to the superior laryngeal nerve is very disabling, because the patient not only has difficulty in swallowing but has loss of sensation in the ipsilateral epiglottis and larynx, allowing food to migrate into the larynx, which produces aspiration and annoying coughing. This most commonly occurs at night.

HYPOGLOSSAL NERVE INJURY

The hypoglossal nerve is responsible for total innervation of the tongue.[14] Paralysis of the nerve produces a slight impairment of speech and deviation of the tongue to the side of the paralysis with subsequent ipsilateral tongue atrophy. The descending hypoglossal branch leaves the nerve usually at its inferior curve and runs anterior and medial to the jugular vein and anterior to the internal carotid artery. Section of the descendens hypoglossi above the cervical branch, which forms the ansa cervicalis, produces no clinical syndrome. This branch, along with the cervical branch, is responsible for the motor supply of the deep strap muscles of the neck. As an external landmark, the hypoglossal nerve is usually found at the level of the occipital artery. It is invariably crossed superiorly by the branch of the occipital artery to the sternocleidomastoid muscle. Occasionally, the nerve is crossed by an aberrant vein, and this vein may be closely adherent to the nerve. The nerve may be injured by direct traction or by injudicious use of electrocautery in areas contiguous for the nerve. With an overlying vein the nerve may be ligated and divided with the vein unless the nerve is meticulously exposed. If the hypoglossal nerve is sectioned, it should be sutured primarily.

FACIAL NERVE INJURY

Total facial nerve paralysis is rare and occurs only when high exposure of the internal carotid artery is required. In order to expose the internal carotid artery at C2 and above, some surgeons recommend extending the incision anterior to the tragus of the ear and reflecting the superficial lobe of the parotid superiorly and anteriorly. In the process of this extensive dissection, traction on the main facial nerve trunk may produce a complete facial nerve paralysis.[104] This potential complication can be avoided by using alternative methods to gain high exposure of the internal carotid artery such as mandibular subluxation.[59]

The more common injury involves that of the marginal mandibular branch of the facial nerve; this usually occurs with anterior and superior retraction along the angle of the mandible where the marginal mandibular branch is vulnerable.[14] Injury to this branch produces asymmetry of the mouth secondary to paralysis of the depressor muscle of the lip. This is annoying to the patient in speech, and when eating, the patient may bite the lower lip. Deficit is usually transient and usually clears within 3 months.

GLOSSOPHARYNGEAL NERVE INJURY

The glossopharyngeal nerve is usually remote from the field of dissection during carotid endarterectomy but may be injured during high exposure of the internal carotid at the base of the skull.[131] It leaves the skull via the jugular foramen and passes between the internal and external carotid arteries just below the stylopharyngeal muscle near its insertion onto the styloid process. This nerve provides sensory fibers to the mucosa of the pharynx and motor fibers to elevate the larynx and pharynx during swallowing. Injury results in defective swallowing with dysphagia and recurrent aspiration. In severe cases, with repeated aspiration, aggressive treatment with tracheostomy and parenteral or enteral feeding must be considered.

SPINAL ACCESSORY NERVE INJURY

This motor nerve is rarely injured during carotid endarterectomy.[14] After exiting the jugular foramen, the nerve lies superficial to the internal jugular vein and courses into the sternocleidomastoid muscle. The nerve is usually injured by misdirected exposure of the carotid artery into the posterior triangle of the neck, or by traction, or by cautery injury in superior exposures of the internal carotid artery. Damage results in complete paralysis of the sternocleidomastoid and trapezius muscles, which causes a dropped shoulder. This can result in discomfort in the neck and shoulder and can be debilitating for active individuals. If the nerve is sectioned and recognized, primary suture should be attempted.

WOUND HEMATOMA, VEIN PATCH RUPTURE, AND OTHER WOUND COMPLICATIONS

Most patients undergoing carotid endarterectomy have been treated with preoperative aspirin and are continued on antithrombotic therapy in the postoperative period. Bleeding complications, particularly wound hematomas, occur in 1.4% to 3% of patients undergoing endarterectomy, and are associated with incomplete reversal with protamine of intraoperative heparin, hypertension, and perioperative antiplatelet therapy.[94,154] If intraoperative heparin is not fully reversed or continuous heparin anticoagulation is administered postoperatively, perioperative aspirin therapy would potentially increase the incidence of hematomas and other bleeding complications.[27]

While most postoperative hematomas are minor and of no clinical consequence, large hematomas cause pain, tracheal deviation, and airway embarrassment and require emergency drainage. An important symptom suggesting the presence of a significant hematoma that may lead to airway compromise is the inability to swallow. Where the airway is severely compromised, the wound must be opened in bed but, if possible, the patient should be returned to the operating room. If the airway is stable, the neck should be prepped and draped and the wound opened under local anesthesia prior to intubation. Often the hematoma can be evacuated without the necessity of general anesthesia. If possible, the rapid induction of general endotracheal anesthesia with respiratory paralysis and an attempt at intubation should be avoided because of major difficulty in placing an endotracheal tube without prior evacuation of the hematoma. If intubation is required, the endotracheal tube probably should be left in place for 2 to 3 days to ensure that the airway is maintained.

Rarely is there rupture of the suture line or vein graft used to close the carotid artery. If there is, extreme emergency exists. The patient's death is imminent unless the airway can be maintained, the bleeding stopped, and shock treated. The major stroke and death rate associated with vein patch rupture is 48%.[85] It may be necessary from a lifesaving standpoint to open the wound in the bed and occlude the carotid artery manually. If possible, the patient should be returned to the operating room, where appropriate exposure and isolation of the carotid artery can be achieved. On occasion, emergency tracheostomy is required, because of the inability to intubate the patient under these circumstances. With resuscitation and control of bleeding, the patient should be immediately anticoagulated with heparin to prevent carotid thrombosis. If a ruptured vein patch is found to be etiologic, this should be replaced with prosthetic material. On rare occasion, suture breakage with dehiscence of the arteriotomy will be present. This requires simple resuture with appropriate material.

The overall incidence of saphenous vein patch rupture is 0.5% and occurs 1 to 7 days after the operation.[85,117,129] There appears to be a higher incidence in females, and is more common when ankle saphenous vein is used. There is a linear correlation between diameter of intact veins and rupture pressure, and biomechanical studies would suggest that saphenous veins less than 4 to 5 mm in diameter should not be used for vein patch reconstruction.[6] This finding may explain the apparent difference in vein patch strength between proximal and distal saphenous veins.

Prevention of hematoma requires meticulous attention to hemostasis during wound closure and the awareness of the liability of using aspirin or not reversing heparin at the end of the procedure. In addition, careful control of blood pressure in the prevention of postoperative hypertension is essential.

Postoperative wound infection is rare. Treatment requires opening the wound, adequate drainage, and antibiotics directed at causative organisms. An overriding concern is arterial disruption in the face of wound infection. This concern is heightened with the use of prosthetic material for patch closure; fortunately, this complication is extremely rare. Individual management is indicated and has included drainage and antibiotics for low virulence infections and resection of the infected artery with vein graft replacement for more serious infections.

On rare occasions, a false aneurysm will occur at delayed intervals following endarterectomy. This is most unusual with primary closure of the arteriotomy and usually occurs with patch angioplasty. It may be secondary to a low-grade infection of a prosthetic patch or partial dehiscence of the suture line. The aneurysm usually presents as a pulsatile neck mass and may be associated with transient ischemic attacks or stroke. Rarely, a hypoglossal or vagal nerve is compressed with resultant clinical symptoms. Surgical repair involves wide exposure with excision of the aneurysm and reconstruction of the artery with vein graft if infection is present. In the absence of infection, prosthetic replacement with ePTFE has been successfully employed.

HYPERPERFUSION SYNDROME AND INTRACEREBRAL HEMATOMA

The incidence of hyperperfusion syndromes following carotid endarterectomy is reported to be between 0.3% and 1%.[114,125,166] The pathophysiology appears to be secondary to paralysis of autoregulation engendered by chronic ischemia.[86,146] Restoration of internal carotid flow leads to hyperperfusion in the ipsilateral cerebrovascular bed. Isotopic regional cerebral blood flow studies and transcranial Doppler examinations have documented marked increases in ipsilateral cerebral blood flow.[86,146] Pathologic changes include a spectrum of findings ranging from mild cerebral edema to petechial hemorrhages to frank intracerebral hemorrhage.[114,166] The syndrome is often heralded by ipsilateral frontal headache within the first week after endarterectomy. However, ipsilateral headache is not specific for hyperperfusion syndrome and, in fact, is not uncommon following endarterectomy. Headache may also be produced by carotid occlusion. If the patient's headache is better in the sitting position, it is most likely secondary to increased flow, whereas if it is worse in the sitting position, it may indicate carotid occlusion. In patients with the hyperperfusion syndrome, headache may be followed by focal motor seizures that are often difficult to control. Even more alarming is the postictal Todd's paralysis that can mimic postendarterectomy stroke from internal carotid thrombosis. Angiography, along with CT or MRI studies, may be necessary to distinguish between these disorders. Risk factors for the hyperperfusion syndrome include a high-grade (greater than 70%) stenosis, poor collateral hemispheric flow, contralateral carotid occlusion, evidence of chronic ipsilateral hypoperfusion, pre- and postoperative hypertension, preexisting ipsilateral cerebral infarction, and preoperative anticoagulation or antiplatelet therapy.[114,166]

Seizures from the hyperperfusion syndrome are usually successfully treated with Dilantin.[89] Aspirin and anticoagulants should be avoided and hypertension carefully controlled. The most catastrophic complication stemming from hyperperfusion is intracerebral hemorrhage that may be massive and fatal. Intracranial hemorrhage has been reported to occur in 0.5% to 0.7% of patients undergoing carotid endarterectomy and may account for up to 20% of perioperative strokes.[122,127] Among the risk factors for hyperperfusion syndrome, recent cerebral infarction and surgical relief of a high-grade stenosis appear to be prominent. Medical treatment and supportive care are important. If the patient has been on aspirin, platelet transfusions may be required to reverse the aspirin effect. Obviously, all heparin should be discontinued and blood pressure controlled at normal levels.

CARDIAC COMPLICATIONS

A leading cause of death after endarterectomy is myocardial infarction, either immediate or, more often, delayed.[101,110] In view of the close association between arteriosclerotic heart disease and carotid atherosclerosis, every patient must be assumed to have coronary artery disease. Unstable angina, congestive heart failure, and significant cardiac arrhythmias are relative contraindications for carotid endarterectomy. They should be corrected or ameliorated as much as possible prior to the operation. All patients undergoing endarterectomy need adequate oxygenation and postoperative cardiac monitoring. Meticulous attention is indicated to avoid fluid overload or congestive heart failure.

Recurrent Carotid Stenosis

Symptomatic recurrent carotid disease occurs in 0.6% to 3% of patients after carotid endarterectomy.[132] Asymptomatic lesions occur with a much greater frequency (6.7% to 49%), depending on the method used in detection.[132] When lifetable methods are used to calculate the recurrence over time, the presence of hemodynamically significant lesions greater than 50% is approximately 25% at 5 years. In reported series, the need for reoperative carotid endarterectomy is 0.5% for asymptomatic lesions and 1.4% for symptomatic lesions.[36,142]

Medical treatment with antiplatelet therapy has no influence on the development of clinical manifestations of recurrent carotid stenosis.[70,72]

The etiology of recurrent disease can be broadly categorized into local or systemic factors. One of the more important local determinants is residual defects at the endarterectomy site.[148] The most important risk factor seems to be the degree of residual plaque left at the time of original endarterectomy.[4] Flaps and other technical defects may also be important.[126] Systemic factors that have been associated with the development of recurrent disease include female gender, continued smoking after endarterectomy, hypercholesterolemia, diabetes mellitus, hypertension, young age at original endarterectomy, and associated severe atherosclerotic disease.[29,35,38,124,159] Female gender is the most consistently reported risk factor for recurrence of disease. The high incidence of recurrence in females may be related to the smaller vessel size in these patients.[74] The histopathology of recurrent lesions is interesting, because late recurrent lesions have atherosclerotic features and are more likely to be symptomatic than earlier lesions which are often bland and asymptomatic. Serial observations in a large number of patients have shown that early and late recurrent lesions are a continuum of atherosclerotic changes.[30] Early lesions (recurrence less than 2 to 3 years) are predominantly neointimal fibromuscular hyperplasia consisting of proliferating smooth muscle cells surrounded by proteoglycans. Late recurrent lesions (recurrence interval greater than 2 to 3 years) tend to have elements of atherosclerosis with foam cells, cholesterol crystals, abundant collagen, and calcium.[30] Late recurrent lesions tend to be easier to endarterectomize in comparison with earlier recurrent lesions.

Reoperation for recurrent carotid disease can be technically challenging; however, the overall incidence of major morbidity and mortality approximates those of primary carotid endarterectomy except for the incidence of cranial nerve injury. In general, the mean risk of stroke with reoperation is approximately 4%, with a death rate of approximately 1.2%, and a cranial nerve injury rate of approximately 12%.[132]

Other Issues

INCREASING THE BENEFIT/COST RATIO OF THE PROCEDURE

In response to increasing costs of health care, physicians have been challenged to conserve hospital resources, minimize costs, and continue to provide quality care. The length of stay following carotid endarterectomy has decreased dramatically and some groups have reported 24-hour admissions for many of their patients undergoing endarterectomy.[32,80] Traditionally, patients have been observed in an intensive care unit (ICU) setting for 12 to 24 hours after the operation. In retrospective analyses, many have pointed out that only 10% to 20% of patients required this expensive monitoring.[116] Predictors of the need for ICU observation include preoperative history of hypertension, myocardial infarction, arrhythmia, recent stroke, and chronic renal failure.[97,116] Patients not having these risk factors have been successfully observed for a short period (2 to 4 hours) in a postanesthetic recovery room setting.[82,103] Following this, patients can be monitored on a standard hospital ward and discharged the next day. Some have pointed out that local anesthesia for the performance of carotid endarterectomy is important in the success of the approach; however, others have used this care algorithm successfully in patients having general anesthesia.[80]

A more controversial cost-saving approach has relied on duplex ultrasonography alone or in combination with magnetic resonance angiography (MRA) and the elimination of contrast angiography in the preoperative workup of patients undergoing endarterectomy.[1,52,120,155] In addition to being expensive, contrast angiography has a 0.5% to 1% incidence of major neurologic complications; this accounted for almost half of the neurologic morbidity observed in the ACAS trial.[56] Angiography also results in complications at the arterial puncture site in approximately 5% of patients as well as contrast-induced renal dysfunction in 1% to 5%.

Several centers have reported the results of carotid endarterectomy performed with duplex examination alone or in combination with MRA.[1,80] All groups advocating the noninvasive approach stress that optimal results can be realized only with a fully equipped vascular laboratory with well-trained personnel and an established quality control record.[1] Although duplex criteria have been modified in order to increase accuracy of diagnosing 70% stenoses as defined by NASCET criteria,[105,115] cutoff points for specific degrees of stenosis should be established by each vascular laboratory. Laboratories should maintain ongoing protocols to correlate angiographic and duplex findings to ensure continued diagnostic accuracy. While committed vascular laboratories may report excellent results, very few prospective studies have been performed with angiographic validation. Furthermore, excellent results reported from single centers cannot be extrapolated to national practice. The ultrasound results from NASCET demonstrated that there was significant underestimation and overestimation of the degree of stenosis in comparison with angiography.[49] The ACAS study also demonstrated significant variability between centers and machinery in the duplex ultrasonographic determination of stenosis severity.[81] Mismanagement of even a small number of patients incorrectly categorized by duplex ultrasonography could have major economic and medical consequences that would quickly abolish the cost-effectiveness of eliminating angiography.[88] As an example, a symptomatic patient with a greater than 70% stenosis identified by duplex ultrasonography as having a low- or moderate-grade stenosis might be denied carotid endarterectomy and be at high risk of stroke with inappropriate medical therapy.

In addition to validation of individual vascular laboratory results with a high degree of accuracy, all experts recommend limiting carotid endarterectomy based on duplex ultrasonography alone or coupled with MRA to patients with clear-cut history and physical findings that correlate with the duplex findings.[1,52,120,155] Furthermore, a CT scan or MRI should be obtained to rule out other intracranial explanations for the patient's symptoms. Indications for adjunctive arteriography under these circumstances include (1) a discrepancy among the history, physical examination, duplex scan, and CT scan;

(2) patients presenting with vertebrobasilar symptoms, since they often have proximal brachiocephalic disease; (3) patients suspected of proximal disease involving branches from the aortic arch (patients with unequal arm blood pressures or duplex ultrasonographic evidence of abnormal flow characteristics of the proximal common carotid arteries); (4) patients with duplex findings suggestive of distal internal carotid artery or carotid siphon disease; (5) patients presenting with focal cerebrovascular symptoms and a stenosis of less than 70% according to duplex criteria because these patients may have an ulcerative plaque or disease in the innominate or intracranial vessels; (6) patients with duplex evidence of total carotid occlusion in the presence of ongoing ipsilateral hemispheric symptoms (patients may have a near total occlusion or a "string sign"); and (7) patients with contralateral carotid occlusion since ipsilateral duplex results are often overestimated because of increased ipsilateral flow velocities.

CLOSURE TECHNIQUE OF CAROTID ARTERIOTOMY

The rationale for vein patch closure following carotid endarterectomy is to improve the safety and durability of the procedure. By increasing lumen size, reconstructing a portion of the endarterectomy site with endothelialized tissue, and altering the hemodynamic configuration of the carotid bifurcation, vein patch closure theoretically should reduce thrombus accumulation and could prevent perioperative stroke and asymptomatic occlusion of the internal carotid artery.[5] Recurrent carotid stenosis also might be prevented or delayed in causing hemodynamically significant compromise because of the increase in lumen size.[78] Despite the attractiveness of these theoretical considerations, vein patch closure has some drawbacks. In addition to increasing operative time, vein patch closure is associated with its own unique set of complications, including patch rupture, false aneurysm formation, and thromboembolism stemming from the dilated aneurysmal reconstructed bifurcation. When prosthetic material is used for the patch, the potential for infection is present, albeit small, and infection may lead to catastrophic complications.

The results from randomized, prospective studies would suggest that the routine use of vein patch closure decreases perioperative stroke morbidity and asymptomatic occlusion only when total stroke morbidity and mortality exceed 5% to 7%.[26,123] In settings where perioperative morbidity and mortality are less than 2% to 3%, there is no significant difference between primary closure and vein or prosthetic patch angioplasty in perioperative morbidity and mortality.[28,87,99,111] In male patients, the use of vein patch closure does not significantly reduce the long-term follow-up incidence of recurrent carotid disease.[28] However, in females, who have a higher incidence of recurrent carotid stenosis, vein patch closure significantly reduces the incidence of this long-term complication.[48]

Considerations bearing on the decision of whether or not to use vein patch closure are broadly categorized into three major groups.[26] First, in clinical settings in which the incidence of perioperative ischemic stroke and carotid thrombosis is unacceptably high, consideration should be given to employing routine vein patch closure. Once again, ongoing quality improvement audits are necessary to define unacceptably high results that trigger reassessment of multiple technical and patient selection factors that may influence these rates. One factor that may reduce these rates is the more liberal use of vein patch closure. Next, local or anatomic risk factors need to be considered. These factors require careful intraoperative assessment. Among these, the size of the internal carotid artery is critical. Some studies have defined 5 mm in external diameter as measured with calipers as being the lower limit acceptable for primary closure.[28] Redundant carotid arteries with loops or kinks that are at or near the site of endarterectomy are also problematic. Resection or imbrication of redundant portions of the vessel are necessary under these circumstances, and the longitudinal arteriotomy should be closed with a vein patch. Vein patch closure is also recommended when extensive disease is present and when a longer arteriotomy in the internal carotid artery is necessary. The need for distal tacking sutures also implies that diseased intima is left behind. In such cases, the arteriotomy is extended well above the diseased intima, and a vein patch closure is used. Likewise, if extensive disease is present in the common carotid artery, extending the arteriotomy proximally and closing with a vein patch may be important to prevent recurrent stenosis at this site. The inability to obtain a smooth transition between an endarterectomized and an unendarterectomized vessel wall, either proximally or distally, may give rise to unstable, nonlaminar flow phenomena that favor thrombogenesis. These transition areas with a pronounced shelf of intima should be covered with a vein patch if the shelf cannot be removed. Other local problems that would be helped with vein patch closure include a crooked or spiral-shaped arteriotomy and failure to obtain precise and even arteriotomy closure.

Systemic risk factors for recurrent carotid disease have already been mentioned. In all major studies, women have been found to have a much higher than expected rate of recurrent carotid stenosis. Vein patch closure is recommended in all women unless the internal carotid artery is greater than 5 mm in diameter and the arteriotomy short and confined to the bulb. In addition, if multiple systemic atherosclerotic risk factors are present in a patient, one should consider using vein patch closure to prevent or delay recurrent carotid disease.

CAROTID SHUNT AND MONITORING

The main benefit of using an internal shunt during carotid endarterectomy is the re-establishment of some blood flow in the minority of patients who might need it.[106] A secondary benefit associated with the use of a shunt comes with closure of the arteriotomy. The shunt may serve as a stent over which the arteriotomy closure, primarily or with a patch, can be facilitated. The principal risk of using a shunt involves technical complications associated with its placement. With increasing familiarity in the use of a shunt, these risks may be reduced. The major risk is the introduction of emboli into the internal carotid artery resulting in cerebral embolization. Careful back-bleeding of the shunt to completely flush air and other debris, along with placement of the shunt proximally

and distally in areas free of gross atherosclerotic debris, minimizes the potential for this complication. The second complication that occurs with the shunt is intimal injury. With soft, plastic materials specifically designed for use in the internal carotid artery and with the availability of different sized shunts, these complications have also been minimized. Another potential complication associated with shunt use is that it may interfere with carotid endarterectomy and prevent the surgeon from visualizing the distal endpoint. When a shunt is in place, a longer arteriotomy is required to ensure adequate visualization of the distal endpoint.

Advocates of routine shunting point to excellent results in large series and argue persuasively that expensive monitoring techniques are unnecessary because facility and familiarity are enhanced by routine shunting.[153] Those who prefer selective shunting point out that only 10% to 15% of patients who are intolerant of temporary carotid clamping will benefit from an internal shunt. The problem comes in identifying these 10% to 15% of patients who might require a shunt.[145] Methods used include monitoring neurologic status during temporary carotid occlusion in an awake patient under local/regional anesthesia,[84] measurement of internal carotid artery back pressure ("stump pressure" of less than 50 mmHg is the generally accepted criterion for need for shunt placement),[71] isotopic regional cerebral blood flow measurements,[145] transcranial Doppler monitoring,[69] and somatosensory evoked potential (SEP) monitoring[119] and EEG monitoring.[162] All of these techniques have their limitations and some are expensive and cumbersome. From data in the literature, patients most vulnerable to an intraoperative cerebral infarct related to hypoperfusion are those who have had prior strokes, those who have a contralateral carotid occlusion, and those who show changes during intraoperative EEG monitoring. A shunt would be necessary in most patients with prior infarcts and/ or contralateral carotid occlusion and mandatory in all who show EEG changes or who develop a neurologic deficit during regional anesthesia. The controversy surrounding selective shunt use based on monitoring versus routine shunt use will continue as long as surgeons perform carotid endarterectomy, and it is unlikely that it will be laid to rest by a randomized trial because of the low incidence of perioperative stroke with either approach. Both approaches are valid and depend primarily upon training and local availability and the expense of monitoring techniques. The only approach that is not valid is routine *nonshunt* use.

TIMING OF OPERATION AFTER STROKE

The early experience with carotid endarterectomy resulted in a generally accepted policy to delay the operation for 4 to 6 weeks in patients diagnosed with acute stroke, regardless of its severity, for fear of clinical deterioration associated with conversion of a bland infarct into a hemorrhagic one.[15,21,165] Recent reports have suggested that an early operation without waiting 4 to 6 weeks is safe in patients with a minor disabling stroke.[98,121,163] On the other hand, a higher incidence of perioperative strokes has been reported in patients undergoing operation within 5 to 6 weeks after presenting stroke.[67] A compelling reason for not delaying the operation is that patients may be placed at risk for a recurrent stroke during the waiting period, particularly in circumstances where the stenosis is advanced or preocclusive.[40] This reasoning is supported by the fact that, in the NASCET, 4.9% of the 103 medically treated patients diagnosed with symptoms of stroke upon entry had a recurrent ipsilateral stroke within 30 days after randomization.[66]

The NASCET database provides further information.[66] Subgroup analysis was carried out of 100 surgical patients with 70% to 99% stenosis who were diagnosed with nondisabling hemispheric stroke at entry into the trial. Of these patients 40% had carotid endarterectomy performed within 30 days and the remainder had their endarterectomy performed at delayed times. There was no significant difference in the perioperative stroke and death rate and delayed stroke and death rate, and no association was found between an abnormal preoperative CT scan result and the subsequent risk of stroke when an early operation was performed. Based on these results, early carotid endarterectomy for severe carotid stenosis after nondisabling stroke can be done with rates of morbidity and mortality comparable with those who receive a delayed operation. Delaying the procedure for 4 to 6 weeks for patients with symptomatic high-grade stenosis exposes them to a risk of recurrent stroke, which may be avoidable by earlier surgery.

SIMULTANEOUS CAROTID ENDARTERECTOMY AND CORONARY ARTERY BYPASS

It is generally accepted that coronary artery disease is highly prevalent in patients presenting with carotid artery atherosclerotic stenoses. Many studies have documented that one-fourth to one-third of patients undergoing carotid endarterectomy have severe underlying coronary artery disease.[77,158] The converse, however, is not true. The incidence of hemodynamically significant carotid artery stenosis in screening studies of patients undergoing coronary artery bypass is 5% to 11%.[13,19] Special problems arise in patients who have advanced disease in both territories. While many centers have reported favorable experiences in combined carotid endarterectomy and coronary artery bypass procedures performed simultaneously,[22,75] others point out that the overall stroke and death rate with this approach is higher than with either procedure alone. It is not clear whether this is due to increased magnitude of the operation or the overall poor risk of such patients with advanced disease in both territories. Simultaneous operation is generally restricted to patients whose carotid lesions appear to present a real threat in the postoperative period after coronary artery bypass. It should be considered in patients with precarious coronary disease such as unstable angina or high-grade left main lesions who have symptomatic high-grade carotid stenoses, bilateral high-grade asymptomatic stenoses, or ipsilateral advanced, asymptomatic stenosis and contralateral occlusion. Staged approaches are appropriate in most patients. Initial carotid endarterectomy followed by coronary artery bypass is frequently applied to patients who present with symptomatic, high-grade carotid lesions who have stable coronary artery disease. In patients undergoing urgent or emergent coronary artery bypass grafting who have advanced carotid disease, a reverse staged approach may be employed, whereby carotid endarterectomy is carried out later. There appears to be an increased morbidity from performing carotid endarterectomy immediately after coronary artery bypass grafting, and available data would suggest that the operation should be delayed for at least 2 weeks.[75] In a unique approach, one group has demonstrated the feasibility of performing carotid endarterectomy with an intra-aortic balloon counter pulsation device in place; this procedure is followed 24 to 48 hours later with coronary artery bypass grafting.[112] Little data exist from prospective studies or randomized trials to guide in the decision making for these complex patients and most require individualized attention.

References

1. Ahn SS, Baker JD, Moore WS: Carotid endarterectomy based on duplex scanning without routine arteriography. Perspectives Vasc Surg 4:109, 1991
2. Allen BT, Anderson CB, Rubin BG et al: The influence of anesthetic technique on perioperative complications after carotid endarterectomy. J Vasc Surg 19:834, 1994
3. Archie JP Jr: Carotid endarterectomy with reconstruction techniques tailored to operative findings. J Vasc Surg 17:141, 1993
4. Archie JP Jr: Early and late geometric changes after carotid endarterectomy patch reconstruction. J Vasc Surg 14:258, 1991
5. Archie JP Jr: Prevention of early restenosis and thrombosis-occlusion after carotid endarterectomy by saphenous vein patch angioplasty. Stroke 17:901, 1986
6. Archie JP Jr, Green JJ Jr: Saphenous vein rupture pressure, rupture stress, and carotid endarterectomy vein patch reconstruction. Surgery 107:389, 1990
7. Barnett HJM, Eliasziw M, Meldrum HE: Drugs and surgery in the prevention of ischemic stroke. N Engl J Med 332:238, 1995
8. Barnett HJM, Kaste M, Meldrum H, Eliasziw M: Aspirin dose in stroke prevention. Beautiful hypotheses slain by ugly facts. Stroke 27:588, 1996
9. Barnett HJM, Meldrum HE: Update on carotid endarterectomy. Curr Opin Cardiol 10:511, 1995
10. Barnett HJM, Plum F, Walton JN: Carotid endarterectomy—an expression of concern. Stroke 15:941, 1984
11. Barr JD, Horowitz MB, Mathis JM et al: Intraoperative urokinase infusion for embolic stroke during carotid endarterectomy. Neurosurg 36:606, 1995
12. Beebe HG, Clagett GP, DeWeese JA et al: Assessing risk associated with carotid endarterectomy. A statement for health professionals by an Ad Hoc Committee on Carotid Surgery Standards of the Stroke Council, American Heart Association. Stroke 20:314, 1989
13. Berens E, Kouchoukos N, Murphy S, Wareing T: Preoperative carotid artery screening in elderly patients undergoing cardiac surgery. J Vasc Surg 15:313, 1992
14. Bergqvist D: Peripheral nerve injuries associated with carotid endarterectomy. Semin Vasc Surg 4:47, 1991

15. Blaisdell WF, Claus RH, Galbraith JG, Smith JA Jr: Joint study of extracranial arterial occlusion IV—a review of surgical considerations. JAMA 209:1889, 1969

16. Bonita R, Stewart A, Beaglehole R: International trends in stroke mortality: 1970–1985. Stroke 21:989, 1990

17. Bousser MG, Eschwege E, Haguenau M et al: AICLA: controlled trials of aspirin and dipyridamole in the secondary prevention of atherothrombotic cerebral ischemia. Stroke 14:5, 1983

18. Bove EL, Fry WJ, Gross WS, Stanley JC: Hypotension and hypertension as consequences of baroreceptor dysfunction following carotid endarterectomy. Surgery 85:663, 1979

19. Brener B, Brief D, Alpert J et al: The risk of stroke in patients with asymptomatic carotid stenosis undergoing cardiac surgery: a follow-up study. J Vasc Surg 5:269, 1987

20. Brott TG, Labutta RJ, Kempczinski RF et al: Changing patterns in the practice of carotid endarterectomy in a large metropolitan area. JAMA 255:2609, 1986

21. Bruetman ME, Fields WS, Crawford ES, Debakey ME: Cerebral hemorrhage in carotid artery surgery. Arch Neurol 9:458, 1963

22. Cambria RP, Ivarsson BL, Akins CW et al: Simultaneous carotid and coronary disease: safety of the combined approach. J Vasc Surg 9:56, 1989

23. Canadian Cooperative Study Group: A randomized trial of aspirin and sulfinpyrazone in threatened stroke. N Engl J Med 299:53, 1978

24. Caplan LR: Diagnosis and treatment of ischemic stroke. JAMA 266:2413, 1991

25. Cebul RD, Whisnant JP: Indications for carotid endarterectomy. Ann Intern Med 111:675, 1989

26. Clagett GP: Vein patch graft closure for carotid endarterectomy. p. 85. In Ernst CB, Stanley JC (eds): Current Therapy in Vascular Surgery. 2nd Ed. BC Decker, Philadelphia, 1991

27. Clagett GP, Krupski WC: Antithrombotic therapy in peripheral arterial occlusive disease. Chest, 108(suppl.):S431, 1995

28. Clagett GP, Patterson CB, Fisher DF Jr et al: Vein patch versus primary closure for carotid endarterectomy. A randomized prospective study in a selected group of patients. J Vasc Surg 9:213, 1989

29. Clagett GP, Rich NM, McDonald PT et al: Etiological factors for recurrent carotid artery stenosis. Surgery 93:313, 1983

30. Clagett GP, Robinowitz M, Youkey RJ et al: Morphogenesis and clinicopathologic characteristics of recurrent carotid disease. J Vasc Surg 3:10, 1986

31. Clinical alert: benefit of endarterectomy for patients with high-grade stenosis of the internal carotid artery. NINDS News Release, February 27, 1991

32. Collier PE: Are one-day admissions for carotid endarterectomy feasible? Am J Surg 170:140, 1995

33. Comerota AJ, Eze AR: Intra-operative high dose regional urokinase infusion for cerebrovascular occlusion following carotid endarterectomy. J Vasc Surg 24:1008, 1996

34. Corson JD, Chang BB et al: The influence of anesthetic choice on carotid endarterectomy outcome. Arch Surg 122:807, 1987

35. Cuming R, Worrell P, Woolcock NE et al: The influence of smoking and lipids on restenosis after carotid endarterectomy. Eur J Vasc Surg 7:572, 1993

36. Das MB, Hertzer NR, Ratliff NB et al: Recurrent carotid stenosis: a five year series of 65 re-operations. Ann Surg 202:2875, 1985

37. DeBakey ME: Successful carotid endarterectomy for cerebrovascular insufficiency. JAMA 233:1083, 1975

38. Dempsey RJ, Moore RW, Cordero S: Factors leading to early recurrence of carotid plaque after carotid endarterectomy. Surg Neurol 42:278, 1995

39. Donaldson MC, Ivarsson BL, Mannick JA, Whittemore AD: Impact of completion angiography on operative conduct and results of carotid endarterectomy. Ann Surg 217:682, 1993

40. Dosick SM, Whalen RC, Gale SS, Brown OW: Carotid endarterectomy in the stroke patient: computerized axial tomography to determine timing. J Vasc Surg 2:214, 1985

41. Dossa C, Shepard AD, Wolford DG et al: Distal internal carotid exposure: a simplified technique for temporary mandibular subluxation. J Vasc Surg 12:319, 1990

42. The Dutch TIA Trial Study Group: A comparison of two doses of aspirin (30 mg v 283 mg a day) in patients after a transient ischemic attack or minor ischemic stroke. N Engl J Med 325:1261, 1991

43. Dyken ML: Carotid endarterectomy studies: a glimmering of science. Stroke 17:355, 1986

44. Dyken ML, Pokras R: The performance of endarterectomy for disease of the extracranial arteries of the head. Stroke 15:948, 1984

45. Eastcott HHG: The beginning of stroke prevention by surgery. Cardiovasc Surg 2:164, 1994

46. Eastcott HHG, Pickering GW, Rob CG: Reconstruction of internal carotid artery in a patient with intermittent attacks of hemiplegia. Lancet ii:994, 1954

47. The EC/IC Bypass Study Group: Failure of extracranial-intracranial arterial bypass to reduce the risk of ischemic stroke: results of an international randomized trial. N Engl J Med 313:1191, 1985

48. Eikelboom BC, Ackerstaff RGA, Hoeneveld H et al: Benefits of carotid patching: a randomized study. J Vasc Surg 7:240, 1988

49. Eliasziw M, Rankin RN, Fox AJ: Accuracy and prognostic consequences of ultrasonography in identifying severe carotid artery stenosis. Stroke 26:1747, 1995

50. Eliasziw M, Streifler JY, Fox AJ et al: Significance of plaque ulceration in symptomatic patients with high grade carotid stenosis. Stroke 25:304, 1994

51. Elliott BM, Collins GJ Jr, Youkey JR et al: Intraoperation local anesthetic injection of the carotid sinus nerve. A prospective, randomized study. Am J Surg 152:695, 1986

52. Erdoes LS, Marek JM, Mills JL et al: The relative contributions of carotid duplex scanning, magnetic resonance angiography, and cerebral arteriography to clinical decision making: a prospective study in patients with carotid occlusive disease. J Vasc Surg 23:950, 1996

53. European Carotid Surgery Trialists' Collaborative Group: Endarterectomy for moderate symptomatic carotid stenosis: interim results from the MRC European Carotid Surgery Trial. Lancet 347:1591, 1996

54. European Carotid Surgery Trialists' Collaborative

Group: MRC European Surgery Trial: interim results for symptomatic patients with severe (70–99%) or with mild (0–29%) carotid stenosis. Lancet 337:1235, 1991

55. Evans WE, Mendelowitz DS, Liapisc J: Motor speech deficit following carotid endarterectomy. Ann Surg 196: 461, 1982

56. Executive Committee for the Asymptomatic Carotid Atherosclerosis Study: Endarterectomy for asymptomatic carotid artery stenosis. JAMA 273:1421, 1995

57. Fields WS, Lemak NA, Frankowski RF et al: Controlled trial of aspirin in cerebral ischemia. Stroke 8:301, 1977

58. Fields WS, Maslenikov V, Meyer JS et al: Joint study of extracranial arterial occlusion. V. Progress report of prognosis following surgery or nonsurgical treatment for transient cerebral ischemic attacks and cervical carotid artery lesions. JAMA 211:1993, 1970

59. Fisher DF Jr, Clagett GP, Parker JI et al: Mandibular subluxation for high carotid exposure. J Vasc Surg 1:727, 1984

60. Fisher M: Occlusion of the carotid arteries. Arch Neurol Psychiatry 72:187, 1954

61. Fisher M: Occlusion of the internal carotid artery. Arch Neurol Psychiatry 65:346, 1951

62. Fode NC, Sundt TM, Robertson JT et al: Multicenter retrospective review of results in complication of carotid endarterectomy in 1981. Stroke 17:370, 1986

63. Forssell C, Takolander R, Bergqvist D et al: Cranial nerve injuries associated with carotid endarterectomy. A prospective study. Acta Chir Scand 151:595, 1985

64. Garraway WM, Whisnant JP: The changing pattern of hypertension and the declining incidence of stroke. JAMA 258:214, 1987

65. Gasecki AP, Eliasziw M, Ferguson GG et al: Long-term prognosis and effect of endarterectomy in patients with symptomatic severe carotid stenosis and contralateral carotid stenosis or occlusion: results from NASCET. J Neurosurg 83:778, 1995

66. Gasecki AP, Ferguson GG, Eliasziw M et al: Early endarterectomy for severe carotid artery stenosis after a nondisabling stroke: results from the North American Symptomatic Carotid Endarterectomy Trial. J Vasc Surg 20:288, 1994

67. Giordano JM, Trout HH III, Kozloff L, DePalma RG: Timing of carotid artery endarterectomy after stroke. J Vasc Surg 2:250, 1985

68. Gray JL, Baker WH: Recognition and management of acute stroke following carotid endarterectomy. p. 73. In Ernst CB, Stanley JC (eds): Current Therapy in Vascular Surgery. 3rd Ed. CV Mosby, St. Louis, 1995

69. Halsey JH Jr: Risks and benefits of shunting in carotid endarterectomy. Stroke 23:1583, 1992

70. Hansen F, Lindblad B, Persson NH, Bergqvist D: Can recurrent stenosis after carotid endarterectomy be prevented by low-dose acetylsalicylic acid? A double-blind, randomised and placebo-controlled study. Eur J Vasc Surg 7:380, 1993

71. Harada RN, Comerota AJ, Good GM: Stump pressure, electroencephalographic changes, and the contralateral carotid artery: another look at selective shunting. Am J Surg 170:148, 1995

72. Harker LA, Bernstein EF, Dilley RB et al: Failure of aspirin plus dipyridamole to prevent restenosis after carotid endarterectomy. Ann Intern Med 116:731, 1992

73. Hass WK, Easton JD, Adams HP Jr et al: A randomized trial comparing ticlopidine hydrochloride with aspirin for the prevention of stroke in high-risk patients. N Engl J Med 321:501, 1989

74. Healy DA, Zierler E, Nicholls SC: Long-term follow-up and clinical outcome of carotid restenosis. J Vasc Surg 10:662, 1989

75. Hertzer N, Loop F, Beven E et al: Surgical staging for simultaneous coronary and carotid disease: a study including prospective randomization. J Vasc Surg 9:455, 1989

76. Hertzer NR: Carotid endarterectomy—a crisis in confidence. J Vasc Surg 7:611, 1988. Presidential Address

77. Hertzer NR, Beven EG, Young JR et al: Coronary artery disease in peripheral vascular patients. A classification of 1,000 coronary angiograms and results of surgical management. Ann Surg 199:223, 1984

78. Hertzer NR, Beven EG, O'Hara PJ et al: A prospective study of vein patch angioplasty during carotid endarterectomy: 3 yr. results for 801 patients and 917 operations. Ann Surg 206:628, 1987

79. Hertzer NR, Feldman BJ, Beven EG, Tucker HM: A prospective study of the incidence of injury to the cranial nerves during carotid endarterectomy. Surg Gynecol Obstet 151:781, 1980

80. Hirko MK, Morasch MD, Burke K et al: The changing face of carotid endarterectomy. J Vasc Surg 23:622, 1996

81. Howard G, Chambless LE, Baker WH et al: A multicenter validation study of Doppler ultrasound versus angiography. J Stroke Cerebrovasc Dis 1:166, 1991

82. Hoyle RM, Jenkins JM, Edwards WH Sr et al: Care management in cerebral revascularization. J Vasc Surg 20:396, 1994

83. Hsia DC, Krushat WM, Moscoe LM: Epidemiology of carotid endarterectomies among Medicare beneficiaries. J Vasc Surg 16:201, 1992

84. Imparato AM, Ramires A, Riles T, Mintzer R: Cerebral protection in carotid surgery. Arch Surg 117:1073, 1982

85. John TG, Bradbury AW, Ruckley CV: Vein-patch rupture after carotid endarterectomy: an avoidable catastrophe. Br J Surg 80:852, 1993

86. Jorgensen LG, Schroeder TV: Defective cerebrovascular autoregulation after carotid endarterectomy. Eur J Vasc Surg 7:370, 1993

87. Katz D, Snyder SO, Gandhi RH et al: Long-term follow-up for recurrent stenosis: a prospective randomized study of expanded polytetrafluoroethylene patch angioplasty versus primary closure after carotid endarterectomy. J Vasc Surg 19:198, 1994

88. Kent KC, Kuntz KM, Patel M et al: Perioperative imaging strategies for carotid endarterectomy. An analysis of morbidity and cost-effectiveness in symptomatic patients. JAMA 274:888, 1995

89. Kieburtz K, Ricotta JJ, Moxley RT: Seizures following carotid endarterectomy. Arch Neurol 47:568, 1990

90. Kinney EV, Seabrook GR, Kinney LY et al: The importance of intraoperative detection of residual flow abnormalities after carotid artery endarterectomy. J Vasc Surg 17:912, 1993

91. Klag MJ, Whelton PK, Seidler AJ: Decline in US stroke mortality: demographic trends and antihypertensive treatment. Stroke 20:14, 1989

92. Koslow AR, Ricotta JJ, Ouriel K et al: Reexploration for thrombosis in carotid endarterectomy. Circulation, suppl. III:III73, 1989

93. Kotila M: Decline in the incidence of stroke. Stroke 19: 1572, 1988

94. Kunkel JM, Gomez ER, Spebar MJ et al: Wound hematomas after carotid endarterectomy. Am J Surg 148:844, 1984

95. Larsen PE, Smead WL: Vertical ramus osteotomy for improved exposure of the distal internal carotid artery: a new technique. J Vasc Surg 15:226, 1992

96. Leape LL, Park RE, Solomon DH et al: Relation between surgeons' practice volumes and geographic variation in the rate of carotid endarterectomy. N Engl J Med 321:653, 1989

97. Lipsett PA, Tierney S, Gordon TA, Perler BA: Carotid endarterectomy—is intensive care unit care necessary? J Vasc Surg 20:403, 1994

98. Little JR, Moufarrij NA, Furlan AS: Early carotid endarterectomy after cerebral infarction. Neurosurgery 24: 334, 1989

99. Lord RSA, Raj TB, Stary DL et al: Comparison of saphenous vein patch, polytetrafluoroethylene patch, and direct arteriotomy closure after carotid endarterectomy. Part I. Perioperative results. J Vasc Surg 9:521, 1989

100. Lusby RJ, Wylie EJ: Complications of carotid endarterectomy. Surg Clin North Am 63:1293, 1983

101. Mackey WC, O'Donnell TF Jr, Callow AD: Cardiac risk in patients undergoing carotid endarterectomy: impact on perioperative and long-term mortality. J Vasc Surg 11:226, 1990

102. Mayberg MR, Wilson SE, Yatsu F et al: Carotid endarterectomy and prevention of cerebral ischemia in symptomatic carotid stenosis. JAMA 266:3289, 1991

103. McConnell DB, Yeager RA, Moneta GL et al: Just in time decision making for ICU care after carotid endarterectomy. Am J Surg 171:502, 1996

104. Mock CN, Lilly MP, McRae RG, Carney WI Jr: Selection of the approach to the distal internal carotid artery from the second cervical vertebra to the base of the skull. J Vasc Surg 13:846, 1991

105. Moneta GL, Edwards JM, Chitwood RW: Correlation of North American Symptomatic Carotid Endarterectomy Trial (NASCET) angiographic definition of 70% to 99% internal carotid artery stenosis with duplex scanning. J Vasc Surg 17:152, 1993

106. Moore WS: Shunting during carotid endarterectomy: always, never, sometimes? Semin Vasc Surg 2:28, 1989

107. Moore WS, Barnett HJM, Beebe HG et al: Guidelines for carotid endarterectomy. A multidisciplinary consensus statement from the Ad Hoc Committee, American Heart Association. Circulation 91:566, 1995

108. Moore WS, Martello JY, Quinones-Baldrich WJ, Ahn SS: Etiologic importance of the intimal flap of the external carotid artery in the development of postcarotid endarterectomy stroke. Stroke 21:1497, 1990

109. Moore WS, Mohr JP, Najafi H et al: Carotid endarterectomy: practice guidelines. Report of the Ad Hoc Committee to the Joint Council of the Society for Vascular Surgery and the North American Chapter of the International Society for Cardiovascular Surgery. J Vasc Surg 15:469, 1992

110. Musser DJ, Nicholas GG, Reed JF III: Death and adverse cardiac events after carotid endarterectomy. J Vasc Surg 19:615, 1994

111. Myers SI, Valentine J, Chervu A et al: Saphenous vein patch versus primary closure for carotid endarterectomy: long-term assessment of a randomized prospective study. J Vasc Surg 19:15, 1994

112. Myers SI, Valentine RJ, Estrera A et al: The intra-aortic balloon pump, a novel addition to staged repair of combined symptomatic cerebrovascular and coronary artery disease. Ann Vasc Surg 7:239, 1993

113. NASCET Collaborators: Beneficial effect of carotid endarterectomy in symptomatic patients with high-grade carotid stenosis. N Engl J Med 325:445, 1991

114. Naylor AR, Ruckley CV: The post-carotid endarterectomy hyperperfusion syndrome. Eur J Vasc Endovasc Surg 9:365, 1995

115. Neale ML, Chambers JL, Kelly AT et al: Reappraisal of duplex criteria to assess significant carotid stenosis with special reference to reports from the North American Symptomatic Carotid Endarterectomy Trial and the European Carotid Surgery Trial. J Vasc Surg 20:642, 1994

116. O'Brien MS, Ricotta JJ: Conserving resources after carotid endarterectomy: selective use of the intensive care unit. J Vasc Surg 14:796, 1991

117. O'Hara PJ, Hertzer NR, Krajewski LP, Beven EG: Saphenous vein patch rupture after carotid endarterectomy. J Vasc Surg 15:504, 1992

118. Ojemann RG, Crowell RM: Cerebral Management of Cerebral Vascular Disease. Williams & Wilkins, Baltimore, 1983

119. Panetta TF, Legatt AD, Veith FJ: Somatosensory evoked potential monitoring during carotid surgery. p. 273. In Greenhalgh RM, Hollier LH (eds): Surgery for Stroke. WB Saunders, London, 1993

120. Patel MR, Kuntz KM, Klufas RA et al: Preoperative assessment of the carotid bifurcation. Can magnetic resonance angiography and duplex ultrasonography replace contrast arteriography? Stroke 26:1753, 1995

121. Piotrowski JJ, Bernhard VM, Rubin JR et al: Timing of carotid endarterectomy after acute stroke. J Vasc Surg 11:45, 1990

122. Pomposelli FB, Lamparello PJ, Riles TS et al: Intracranial hemorrhage after carotid endarterectomy. J Vasc Surg 7:248, 1988

123. Ranaboldo CJ, Barros D'Sa AAB, Bell PRF et al: Randomized controlled trial of patch angioplasty for carotid endarterectomy. Br J Surg 80:1528, 1993

124. Rapp JH, Qvarfordt P, Krupski WC et al: Hypercholesterolemia and early restenosis after carotid endarterectomy. Surgery 101:277, 1987

125. Reigel MM, Hollier LH, Sundt TM Jr: Cerebral hyperperfusion syndrome: a cause of neurologic dysfunction after carotid endarterectomy. J Vasc Surg 5:628, 1987

126. Reilly LM, Okuhn SP, Rapp JH et al: Recurrent carotid

stenosis: a consequence of local or systemic factors? The influence of unrepaired technical defects. J Vasc Surg 11:448, 1990

127. Riles TS, Imparato AM, Jacobowitz GR et al: The cause of perioperative stroke after carotid endarterectomy. J Vasc Surg 19:206, 1994

128. Riles TS, Kopelman I, Imparato AM: Myocardial infarction following carotid endarterectomy: a review of 683 operations. Surg 85:249, 1979

129. Riles TS, Lamparello PJ, Giangola G, Imparato AM: Rupture of the vein patch: a rare complication of carotid endarterectomy. Surgery 107:10, 1990

130. Robertson JT, Auer NJ: Extracranial occlusive disease with carotid artery. p. 1559. In Youmans JR (ed): Neurological Surgery. Vol. 3. WB Saunders, Philadelphia, 1982

131. Rosenbloom M, Friedman SG, Lamparello PJ: Glossopharyngeal nerve injury complicating carotid endarterectomy. J Vasc Surg 5:469, 1987

132. Rossi PJ, Myers SI, Clagett GP: Reoperative approaches for carotid restenosis. Semin Vasc Surg 7:195, 1994

133. Rothwell PM, Slattery J, Warlow CP: A systematic review of the risks of stroke and death due to endarterectomy for symptomatic carotid stenosis. Stroke 27:260, 1996

134. The SALT Collaborative Group: Swedish aspirin low-dose trial (SALT) of 75 mg aspirin as secondary prophylaxis after cerebrovascular ischemic events. Lancet 338: 1345, 1991

135. Shah DM, Darling RC III, Chang BB et al: Carotid endarterectomy in awake patients: its safety, acceptability, and outcome. J Vasc Surg 19:1015, 1994

136. Shaha A, Phillips T, Scalea T et al: Exposure of the internal carotid artery near the skull base: the posterolateral anatomic approach. J Vasc Surg 8:618, 1988

137. Shaw DA, Venables GS, Cartlidge NEF et al: Carotid endarterectomy in patients with transient cerebral ischemia. J Neurol Sci 64:45, 1984

138. Shinton R, Beevers G: Meta-analysis of relation between cigarette smoking and stroke. Br Med J 298:789, 1989

139. Sorenson PS, Pedersen H, Marquardsen J et al: Acetylsalicylic acid in the prevention of stroke in patients with reversible cerebral ischemic attacks: a Danish Cooperative Study. Stroke 13:15, 1983

140. Spetzler RF, Martin N, Hadley MN et al: Microsurgical endarterectomy under barbiturate protection: a prospective study. J Neurosurg 65:63, 1986

141. Steering Committee of NASCET: North American Symptomatic Carotid Endarterectomy Trial: methods, patients characteristics and progress. Stroke 22:711, 1991

142. Stoney RJ, String ST: Recurrent carotid stenosis. Surg 80:705, 1976

143. Streifler JY, Eliasziw M, Benavente OR et al: The risk of stroke in patients with first ever retinal vs hemispheric transient ischemic attacks and high-grade carotid stenosis. Arch Neurol 52:246, 1995

144. Streifler JY, Eliasziw M, Fox AJ et al: Angiographic detection of carotid plaque ulceration: comparison with surgical observations in a multicenter study. Stroke 25: 1130, 1994

145. Sundt TM, Sharbrough FW, Peipgras DG et al: Correla-

tion of cerebral blood flow and electroencephalographic changes during carotid endarterectomy. Mayo Clin Proc 56:533, 1981

146. Sundt TM Jr: Occlusive Cerebral Vascular Disease: Diagnosis and Surgical Management. WB Saunders, Philadelphia, 1987

147. Sundt TM Jr, Ebersold MJ, Sharbrough FW et al: The risk-benefit ratio of intraoperative shunting during carotid endarterectomy: relevancy to operative and postoperative results in complications. Ann Surg 203:196, 1986

148. Sundt TM Jr, Houser OW, Fode NC et al: Correlation of postoperative and two-year follow-up angiography with neurological function in 99 carotid endarterectomies in 86 consecutive patients. Ann Surg 203:90, 1986

149. A Swedish Cooperative Study: High-dose acetylsalicylic acid after cerebral infarction. Stroke 18:325, 1987

150. Theodotou B, Mahaley MS Jr: Injury of the peripheral cranial nerves during carotid endarterectomy. Stroke 16: 894, 1985

151. Thompson JE: Carotid surgery: the past is prologue. J Vasc Surg 25(1):131, 1997

152. Thompson JE: Historical perspective of carotid artery disease. p. 3. In Whittemore AD (ed): Advances in Vascular Surgery. Vol 1. Mosby–Year Book, St. Louis, 1993

153. Thompson JE: Role of shunting during carotid endarterectomy. p. 57. In Ernst CB, Stanley JC (eds): Current Therapy in Vascular Surgery. 3rd Ed. CV Mosby, St. Louis, 1995

154. Treiman RL, Cossman DV, Foran RF et al: The influence of neutralizing heparin after carotid endarterectomy on postoperative stroke and wound hematoma. J Vasc Surg 12:440, 1990

155. Turnipseed WD, Kennell TW, Turski PA et al: Combined use of duplex imaging and magnetic resonance angiography for evaluation of patients with symptomatic ipsilateral high-grade carotid stenosis. J Vasc Surg 17: 832, 1993

156. UK-TIA Study Group: United Kingdom transient ischemic attack (UK-TIA) aspirin trial: interim results. Br Med J 296:317, 1988

157. UK-TIA Study Group: The United Kingdom transient ischemic attack (UK-TIA) aspirin trial: final results. J Neurol Neurosurg Psychiatry 54:1044, 1991

158. Urbinati S, DiPasquale G, Andreoli A et al: Frequency and prognostic significance of silent coronary artery disease in patients with cerebral ischemia undergoing carotid endarterectomy. Am J Cardiol 69:1166, 1992

159. Valentine RJ, Myers SI, Hagino RT, Clagett GP: Late outcome of patients with premature carotid atherosclerosis after carotid endarterectomy. Stroke 27:1502, 1996

160. Warlow C: Carotid endarterectomy: does it work? Stroke 15:1068, 1984

161. Whisnant JP, Fisher L, Robertson JT, Scheinberg P: Carotid endarterectomy decreased stroke and death in patients with transient ischemic attacks. Ann Neurol 22: 72, 1987

162. Whittemore AD, Kauffman JL, Kohler TR, Mannick JA: Routine electroencephalographic (EEG) monitoring during carotid endarterectomy. Ann Surg 197:707, 1983

163. Whittemore AD, Ruby ST, Couch NP, Mannick

JA: Early carotid endarterectomy in patients with small, fixed neurologic deficits. J Vasc Surg 1:795, 1984

164. Winslow CM, Solomon DH, Chassin MR et al: The appropriateness of carotid endarterectomy. N Engl J Med 318:721, 1988

165. Wylie EJ, Hein MF, Adams JE: Intracranial hemorrhage following surgical revascularization for treatment of acute stroke. J Neurosurg 21:212, 1964

166. Youkey JR, Clagett GP, Jaffin JH et al: Focal motor seizures complicating carotid endarterectomy. Arch Surg 119:1080, 1984

167. Zhu CZ, Norris JW: Role of carotid stenosis in ischemic stroke. Stroke 21:1131, 1990

Surgical Considerations in Asymptomatic Disease

ROBERT W. BARNES

JAMES T. ROBERTSON

Patients with asymptomatic carotid disease have three patterns of clinical presentation. Many individuals are discovered to have an incidental cervical bruit on routine examination, or to have an abnormal noninvasive study during screening for carotid disease. A second group of patients are noted to have angiographic evidence of asymptomatic carotid stenosis contralateral to symptomatic disease. Finally, patients may be identified with asymptomatic carotid disease during preoperative workup for major operations, particularly prior to cardiac or vascular procedures. Controversy regarding management of patients with these manifestations of asymptomatic carotid disease is evident in a large number of publications over the past 30 years. A Medline search of the medical literature regarding medical or surgical management of asymptomatic carotid disease revealed 381 citations in English between 1966 and 1996. From this database, the authors reviewed all 211 articles that provided outcome data on more than 19,500 unique patients with asymptomatic carotid disease. Of importance is the fact that there have been only five published randomized clinical trials[7,8,12,18,19] comparing surgical with medical management of asymptomatic carotid stenosis, and all but one of these have been reported in the past 5 years.[7,12,18,19] This chapter will review the evidence supporting treatment options for patients with various clinical patterns of asymptomatic carotid disease. The authors will summarize their recommendations for patient selection, evaluation of comorbidity, diagnostic evaluation, operative management, and follow-up of patients undergoing endarterectomy for asymptomatic carotid stenosis.

Isolated Asymptomatic Carotid Disease

ASYMPTOMATIC CAROTID BRUIT

Patients with asymptomatic cervical bruits are not considered for operation without further diagnostic evaluation to document the presence of "significant" carotid stenosis. The definition of hemodynamically significant carotid stenosis varies among reported series, but many authors accept a ≥50% diameter reduction or a ≥75% area reduction relative to the normal distal internal carotid artery. In models of the circulation, a stenosis of this degree will be associated with a detectable drop in pressure across the narrowing. A review of the literature reveals 19 publications between 1984 and 1995 in which carotid duplex ultrasonography or arteriography has quantified the degree of stenosis in patients with asymptomatic carotid bruits being considered for endarterectomy (see the Suggested Readings). Of the 7,255 patients reported, 2,109, or 29%, had a ≥50% carotid stenosis, while the remainder had lesser degrees of stenosis. Thus, the majority of patients with carotid bruits do not have severe carotid obstruction. On the other hand, patients may have severe carotid stenosis (especially if ≥85%) or occlusion of the internal carotid artery without an audible bruit. These facts must be kept in mind when interpreting the outcomes of patients with cervical bruits (see the Suggested Readings).

ASYMPTOMATIC CAROTID STENOSIS

Nonrandomized Clinical Studies

Between 1971 and 1996, 43 nonrandomized clinical studies have been published that describe unique patients who have been treated medically or surgically for ≥50% asymptomatic carotid stenosis (see the Suggested Readings). The aggregate crude outcomes of these patients are shown in Table 53.7. The number of patients reported in these series has ranged from 12 to 292 for medically treated patients and from 5 to 291 for those treated surgically. Reported lengths of patient follow-up have extended to 96 months for medically treated patients and to 184 months for those undergoing operation, with aggregate mean follow-up reported about 1 year longer

Table 53.7 Aggregate Crude Outcomes of Nonrandomized Studies of Medical and Surgical Therapy of ≥50% Asymptomatic Carotid Stenosis

Treatment	Number of Studies	Number of Patients	Mean Follow-up	Outcome (%)									
				TIA Ipsilateral		TIA Contralateral		Stroke Ipsilateral		Stroke Contralateral		Death	
				Early	Late	Early	Late	Early	Late	Early	Late	Early	Late
Medical	26	2,879	35 mo	—	14.1	—	1.4	—	7.2	—	2.8	—	19.5
Surgical	23	1,997	46 mo	0.9	1.7	0	1.1	2.6	2.0	0.2	3.0	0.7	20.8

for surgically treated patients. In medically managed patients, the late incidence of ipsilateral transient ischemic attack (TIA), 14.1%, was approximately twice that of ipsilateral stroke, 7.1%, with annual rates of 4.8% and 2.5%, respectively. Individual reports of the incidence of ipsilateral TIA and stroke ranged from a low of 1.1% and 0.7% per year, respectively, to a high of 15.7% and 16.7%, respectively. Of all the late strokes in medically treated patients, 28% involved the hemisphere contralateral to the severe carotid stenosis. The late crude death rate was 6.7% per year, where "crude" refers to the number of patients with these outcome events divided by the number of patients under observation.

The incidence of ipsilateral TIA in surgically treated patients was low, 1.7% or 0.4% per year, with more than one-third occurring in the 30-day period after operation. Nearly 40% of the late TIAs occurred in the distribution of the contralateral hemisphere. The aggregate perioperative stroke rate, 2.8%, accounted for more than one-third of all strokes after operation. The late (after the 30-day postoperative period) ipsilateral stroke rate averaged 0.5% per year, whereas the contralateral stroke rate was 0.8% per year. The absolute crude risk reduction for ipsilateral stroke for surgically treated patients compared with those treated medically was 2.6%, with a crude relative risk reduction of 36%. The relative risk reduction for all strokes was 22%. The crude death rate for surgically treated patients was 5.6% per year.

Controversy arises in a subset of patients with a ≥50% asymptomatic carotid stenosis and occlusion of the contralateral internal carotid artery. Between 1967 and 1993, 34 nonrandomized clinical studies reported outcomes of 2,300 patients treated either medically or surgically for this combination of carotid lesions (see the Suggested Readings and Table 53.8). The aggregate crude ipsilateral and total

stroke risks for medically and surgically treated patients were higher than those for patients without contralateral carotid occlusions shown in Table 53.7. The crude annual total stroke rate for medically managed patients was 4.5% per year, and for surgically treated patients the rate was 5.0% per year. These data do not point to significant benefit, and suggest possible adverse effect of surgical intervention on asymptomatic carotid stenosis with contralateral carotid occlusion. The crude annual death rates for medically and surgically treated patients were 7.4% and 6.7%, respectively.

Randomized Clinical Trials

Five prospective randomized clinical trials have been reported comparing carotid endarterectomy with the best medical management of patients with asymptomatic carotid stenosis. The first was a single-center trial reported by Clagett et al[8] in 1984. In the small patient sample (N = 29), no strokes occurred in either medically or surgically treated patients during a mean follow-up of 32 months. When combined with 28 eligible but nonrandomized patients, the incidence of all unfavorable outcomes was significantly greater in patients undergoing operation (31.0%) than in those treated medically (3.6%).

The results of the four other multicenter randomized clinical trials reported in the past 5 years are depicted in Table 53.9. Because of significant differences in study design and patient management, each of these trials will be analyzed separately.

The first reported multicenter randomized clinical trial was the CASANOVA (Carotid Artery Stenosis with Asymptomatic Narrowing: Operation versus Aspirin) study[7] reported in 1991. After screening Doppler ultrasound and subsequent arteriography, 410 patients with an asymptomatic carotid ste-

Table 53.8 Aggregate Crude Outcomes of Nonrandomized Studies of Medical and Surgical Therapy of Patients with ≥50% Asymptomatic Carotid Stenosis and Contralateral Carotid Occlusion

Treatment	Number of Studies	Number of Patients	Mean Follow-up	Outcome (%)					
				Ipsilateral Stroke		Contralateral Stroke		Death	
				Early	Late	Early	Late	Early	Late
Medical	13	1,219	38 mo	—	10.5	—	3.8	—	23.5
Surgical	21	1,081	44 mo	5.6	8.2	1.2	3.2	4.9	20.7

Table 53.9 Crude Outcomes of Multicenter Randomized Clinical Trials Comparing Medical or Surgical Therapy of Patients with Asymptomatic Carotid Stenosis

Trial	Year	Treatment	Stenosis	Number of Patients	Mean Follow-up (mo)	TIA Ipsilateral Early	TIA Ipsilateral Late	TIA Contralateral Early	TIA Contralateral Late	Stroke Ipsilateral Early	Stroke Ipsilateral Late	Stroke Contralateral Early	Stroke Contralateral Late	Death Early	Death Late
CASANOVA	1991	Medical	50–90	204	42	0	8.3	—	—	1.5	8.3	—	—	1.5	17.2
		Surgical	50–90	206	43	1.9	6.3	—	—	3.4	6.8	—	—	1.5	17.5
MACE	1992	Medical	≥50	35	24	—	11.4	—	—	0	0	0	0	—	—
		Surgical	≥50	36	24	2.7	0	0	—	5.6	0	2.7	0	0	—
VA Coop 167	1993	Medical	≥50	233	48	0.4	10.7	0	1.3	0.4	9.0	0	2.6	0.4	33.0
		Surgical	≥50	211	48	0.9	2.4	0	1.4	2.4	2.4	0	3.3	1.9	31.3
ACAS	1995	Medical	≥60	834	32	—	6.0	—	—	0.2	5.9	—	4.1	0.1	10.6
		Surgical	≥60	825	32	—	2.7	—	—	2.1	1.7	—	3.3	0.4	9.7

Abbreviations: TIA, transient ischemic attack; CASANOVA, Carotid Artery Stenosis with Asymptomatic Narrowing: Operation versus Aspirin; MACE, Mayo Asymptomatic Carotid Endarterectomy; VA Coop 167, Veterans Affairs Cooperative Study 167; ACAS, Asymptomatic Carotid Atherosclerosis Study.

nosis of 50% to 90% diameter reduction (relative to the normal distal internal carotid artery) were randomized to one of two groups. Group A consisted of 206 patients with unilateral or bilateral stenosis who were assigned unilateral or bilateral carotid endarterectomy, respectively. Subsequent endarterectomy was recommended for a disease progression to a >50% stenosis of the contralateral carotid or a restenosis of >50%. Group B comprised 204 patients considered to receive "medical therapy." However, this group was designed to receive operation for (1) the more affected side of a bilateral carotid stenosis, (2) progression of a stenosis exceeding 90%, (3) development of a bilateral >50% stenosis (operation on the more severe side), and (4) a TIA appropriate to a >50% stenosis. All patients of both groups received 330 mg acetylsalicylic acid and 75 mg dipyridamole three times daily for the duration of the study. The results of this trial revealed no significant difference between the two groups for the study endpoints of ischemic neurologic deficit exceeding 24 hours or death due to operation or stroke. Of note is the fact that 53 (26%) of group A "surgery" patients and 19 (9%) of group B "medical" patients did not comply with the study protocol. Of group A patients, 46 (22%) did not undergo operation. Of group B patients, 85 (42%) had carotid endarterectomy during the course of follow-up. These methodologic characteristics unique to the trial, along with the exclusion of patients with a >90% stenosis, make it difficult to reach conclusions about the efficacy of surgical versus medical therapy of patients with asymptomatic carotid stenosis based on this study.

The Mayo Asymptomatic Carotid Endarterectomy study[19] (MACE) was carried out at the three Mayo Clinic centers. The study was designed to compare the efficacy of carotid endarterectomy alone with medical treatment with low-dose aspirin (80 mg/day) for patients with an asymptomatic carotid stenosis of ≥50% diameter reduction. Patients were screened for pressure-reducing carotid lesions by ocular pneuomoplethysmography and stenosis documented by duplex ultrasonography or intravenous digital subtraction arteri-

ography. Patients assigned to operation underwent preoperative contrast arteriography. Patients randomized to operation did not receive aspirin. Primary endpoints included any TIA, stroke, or death. Secondary endpoints were myocardial infarction and coronary artery bypass for symptomatic coronary disease. The study was terminated after a mean follow-up of 23.6 months because of an excessive number of secondary endpoints (eight myocardial infarctions) in the 36 patients randomized to operation compared with none in the 35 patients assigned to medical treatment ($P = 0.0037$). There was no significant difference between the groups in the number of total neurologic events (four each, $P = 0.974$) or strokes (0 medical, 3 surgical, $P = 0.0866$). The investigators concluded that the adverse outcomes in the surgical group could be related to the absence of aspirin use and recommended that patients with asymptomatic carotid stenosis should receive aspirin, unless contraindicated, throughout the perioperative period and thereafter. Because of the small size of the trial and its early termination, no conclusions can be drawn from the study regarding the relative value of medical versus surgical therapy of asymptomatic carotid disease.

The Veterans Affairs Cooperative Study 167 Group[18] conducted a multicenter (N = 11) randomized clinical trial of 444 men with asymptomatic carotid stenosis of ≥50% diameter reduction. Patients were screened by ocular pneumoplethysmography or duplex ultrasonography and all underwent contrast arteriography prior to randomization. Patients were randomized to optimal medical therapy including aspirin (625 mg twice daily or, if poorly tolerated, 325 mg daily) plus carotid endarterectomy (surgical group = 211 patients) or to optimal medical therapy alone (medical group = 233 patients). Primary endpoints included TIA, transient monocular blindness, and stroke (fatal and nonfatal). The incidence of these neurologic endpoints for both ipsilateral and contralateral events was significantly lower ($P < 0.002$) in the surgical group, 12.8%, than in the medical group, 24.5% (relative risk 0.51, 95% confidence interval, 0.32 to 0.81). There was an even greater difference between the groups for ipsilateral end-points alone, 8.8% versus 20.6% ($P < 0.001$, relative risk 0.38, 95% confidence interval 0.22 to 0.67). However, there were no significant differences between the two groups in the incidence of ipsilateral stroke, all strokes, or all strokes and deaths. A major criticism of this trial was the combination of TIA and transient monocular blindness with stroke as primary endpoints.[4] The study was designed in an era when all neurologic events, including TIAs, were considered valid endpoints in multicenter trials, including trials evaluating the efficacy of medical therapy such as aspirin.[6,13] Furthermore, the serious prognosis of TIA in the presence of carotid stenosis has been established in many studies, especially the North American Symptomatic Carotid Endarterectomy Trial (NASCET)[24] and the European Carotid Surgery Trial (ECST).[11] Nevertheless, because of the study design and sample size, one cannot conclude from this study that carotid endarterectomy and optimal medical therapy are more effective in preventing stroke than medical therapy alone.

The Asymptomatic Carotid Atherosclerosis Study[12] (ACAS) was the largest and most recent multicenter prospective randomized clinical trial of asymptomatic carotid stenosis to be reported. Over a 5-year period in 39 centers in the United States and Canada, 1,662 patients with an asymptomatic carotid stenosis of $\geq$60% diameter reduction relative to the distal normal internal carotid artery were randomized. Patients were selected by screening duplex ultrasonography with angiographically validated threshold criteria (95% positive predictive value), combined duplex and ocular pneumoplethysmography, or arteriography. All patients randomized to operation required preoperative arteriography. All patients received stroke risk factor modification and 325 mg of aspirin daily. Participating surgeons required credentialing with documented combined neurologic morbidity and mortality rates in 50 previous consecutive carotid endarterectomies of <5.0% for all indications and <3.0% for asymptomatic patients.[22] The initial primary endpoints were ipsilateral TIA, stroke, or any perioperative TIA, stroke, or death. However, after the results of the Veterans Affairs Cooperative Study 167[18] and the initial NASCET report[24] were published, the ACAS Executive Committee and the Data and Safety Monitoring Committee voted to restrict the primary endpoint to stroke and perioperative complications or death. Randomization assigned 825 patients to operation and 834 to medical therapy. Protocol failures occurred in 101 (12%) of surgical patients and 45 (5%) of medical patients. The 30-day combined stroke and mortality rate in surgical patients was 2.3%, which included a preoperative stroke rate from arteriography of 1.2%. After a median of 2.7 years of follow-up, the study achieved its significant boundary. The Kaplan-Meier estimates of ipsilateral stroke and any perioperative stroke or death was 11% for the medical group and 5.1% for the surgical group. The absolute risk reduction in the 5-year ipsilateral stroke risk in the surgical group was 5.9% and the relative risk reduction was 53% (95% confidence interval, 22% to 72%, $P = 0.004$). The difference between the two treatment groups for outcomes of any stroke or any perioperative death and for any stroke or death did not reach statistical significance ($P = 0.09$ and $P = 0.08$, respectively). Unlike the NASCET study, the ACAS results did not demonstrate

increasing stroke risk in medically treated patients with increasing severity of stenosis. The favorable effect of carotid endarterectomy on ipsilateral stroke reduction was primarily evident in men (66% relative risk reduction, 95% confidence interval, 36% to 82%) as compared with women (17% relative risk reduction, 95% confidence interval—96% to 65%), although the difference between genders was not statistically significant ($P = 0.10$). The ACAS study group recognized the relatively low risk of stroke in patients followed medically and that, by using ACAS entry criteria, about 19 carotid endarterectomies are required to prevent one stroke over 5 years. The conclusions of the study emphasized that the results should be applied only to patients with low operative risks and only in centers with documented surgical morbidity and mortality rates of less than 3%.[23] Although the ACAS study design, statistical inferences, and interpretation have been criticized,[3,17,25] the trial remains the most definitive study reported to date suggesting a benefit from carotid endarterectomy in stroke prevention in selected good-risk patients with asymptomatic carotid stenosis.

The Asymptomatic Carotid Surgery Trial[15] (ACST) has been initiated in Europe but the results have not been published. This 5-year study will compare carotid endarterectomy plus the best medical therapy with the best medical therapy alone in preventing stroke and death in asymptomatic patients with asymptomatic carotid stenosis. Unlike the ACAS study, ACST allows considerably greater latitude in patient selection and exclusion at the discretion of the participating investigators, in order to facilitate patient recruitment.

It is of interest to compare the aggregate crude stroke rate (early and late) of all reported nonrandomized studies of medical and surgical therapy of asymptomatic carotid disease (a bruit or a $\geq$ 50% stenosis) with the combined outcomes of the Veterans Affairs Cooperative Study 167[18] and the ACAS trial[12] (Table 53.10). With relatively similar periods of follow-up, the overall stroke rates for the medically and surgically treated patients in the nonrandomized studies (10.9% and 7.8%, respectively) were remarkably similar to the combined

Table 53.10 Aggregate Crude All-Stroke Rate of Medical and Surgical Therapy of Asymptomatic Carotid Disease (Bruit or $\geq$50% Stenosis) of All Reported Nonrandomized Studies and the Combined Results of the VA Cooperative Study 167 and the ACAS Trial

Design	Treatment	No. of Patients	Mean Follow-up	Stroke Rate (%)
Nonrandom	Medical	3,390	40 mo	10.9
(N = 47)	Surgical	1,997	46 mo	7.8
Random	Medical	1,067	40 mo	10.6
(VA + ACAS)	Surgical	1,036	40 mo	7.2

Abbreviations: VA, Veterans Affairs; ACAS, Asymptomatic Carotid Atherosclerosis Study.

stroke rates in the two randomized trials (10.6% and 7.2%, respectively.)

Contralateral Carotid Disease

The second major category of patients presenting with asymptomatic carotid disease includes those who have angiographic evidence of a carotid stenosis contralateral to symptomatic disease. Most patients undergo carotid endarterectomy on the symptomatic lesion. Controversy exists about the best subsequent management for the contralateral asymptomatic stenosis. To date there have not been any prospective randomized clinical trials to address this issue. Another controversy exists about the most appropriate therapy of a subset of patients with contralateral asymptomatic carotid disease, namely, those with ulcerated carotid plaques.

CONTRALATERAL ASYMPTOMATIC CAROTID STENOSIS

Table 53.11 depicts the aggregate crude outcomes of the 22 nonrandomized studies of medical and surgical management of patients with a ≥50% asymptomatic carotid stenosis contralateral to symptomatic carotid disease (see the Suggested Readings). All patients had undergone previous carotid endarterectomy for the symptomatic lesion. The preponderance of studies reported outcomes of nonoperative medical treatment of the contralateral asymptomatic carotid stenosis, with operation reserved for those individuals who developed symptoms of TIA or recovery from stroke. The majority of medically treated patients if they became symptomatic had a TIA as the initial event. The crude late ipsilateral stroke rate of patients treated medically, 3.1%, was less than the early perioperative stroke rate of patients undergoing prophylactic endarterectomy, 3.8%, as well as the combined early and late postoperative stroke rate of surgical patients (6.5%). All reports so far of patients with contralateral asymptomatic carotid disease suggest that medical management carries a prognosis equal to or superior to that of prophylactic carotid endarterectomy of the asymptomatic lesion. Whether this favorable outcome

of medical management is a reflection of successful prior carotid endarterectomy of the opposite symptomatic lesion is conjectural. It is important to recognize that these patients require careful clinical follow-up, because a significant number of patients (10% to 15%) will develop TIAs, which should lead to carotid endarterectomy to minimize the subsequent risk of stroke. However, the literature to date suggests that the incidence of stroke without antecedent TIAs is less than the risk of prophylactic carotid endarterectomy. Recent analysis of the contralateral asymptomatic disease in patients of ECST suggests that, whereas the stroke risk does not warrant prophylactic operation, the risk does increase with increasing severity of the asymptomatic carotid stenosis (see the Suggested Readings).

ASYMPTOMATIC ULCERATED CAROTID PLAQUE

Pathologic examination of excised carotid plaques often reveals gross or microscopic ulceration of the lesion, exposing the content of the atheroma to the flowing blood. This feature is more common in patients with symptoms of TIA or stroke that may be the result of thromboembolism or atheroembolism from the ulcerated plaque. Although gross irregularities of the carotid stenosis on arteriograms are frequently called "ulcerated plaques," subsequent pathologic examination of excised plaques confirms the diagnosis of true ulceration in only about 50% of cases. Nevertheless, the radiographic appearance of "ulcerated plaque" has been thought to potentially increase the risk of stroke associated with asymptomatic carotid lesions. Table 53.12 presents the crude outcomes of three nonrandomized studies[10,14,16] of medically managed patients with asymptomatic "ulcerated" carotid plaques contralateral to previously operated symptomatic disease. The study by Dixon et al,[10] which included patients from the initial report by Moore et al,[20] suggested that patients with an asymptomatic ulcerated carotid plaque were at significant risk of future stroke. However, review of the lifetable curves reveals that most strokes occurred 5 years after a relatively stroke-free period, implying that carotid disease progression might have developed in the interval. The other two studies[14,16] showed a relatively low risk of stroke during medical follow-up of asymptomatic ulcerated carotid plaques. These reports sug-

Table 53.11 Aggregate Crude Outcomes of Nonrandomized Studies of Medical and Surgical Therapy of Patients with ≥50% Asymptomatic Carotid Stenosis Contralateral to Symptomatic Carotid Disease

				Outcome (%)									
				TIA Ipsilateral		*TIA Contralateral*		*Stroke Ipsilateral*		*Stroke Contralateral*		*Death*	
Treatment	*Number of Studies*	*Number of Patients*	*Mean Follow-up*	*Early*	*Late*	*Early*	*Late*	*Early*	*Late*	*Early*	*Late*	*Early*	*Late*
Medical	15	801	48 mo	—	9.6	—	2.5	—	3.1	—	1.7	—	21.5
Surgical	7	299	36 mo	3.9	3.1	0	0	3.8	2.7	0	0	1.0	23.2

Abbreviation: TIA, transient ischemic attack.

Table 53.12 Crude Outcomes of Nonrandomized Clinical Studies of Medical Therapy of Patients with Ulcerated Carotid Plaques Contralateral to Symptomatic Disease

Author	Year	No. of Patients	Mean Follow-up	Outcome (%)				
				TIA Ipsilateral	TIA Contralateral	Stroke Ipsilateral	Stroke Contralateral	Death
Dixon	1982	141	(to 120 mo)	7.1	—	12.1	—	24.8
Harward	1983	79	54 mo	7.6	1.3	2.5	6.3	36.7
Grotta	1984	26	16 mo	3.8	—	3.8	—	—

Abbreviation: TIA, transient ischemic attack.

gest that angiographic evidence of carotid ulceration should not be the basis for surgical intervention for asymptomatic carotid disease.

Asymptomatic Carotid Disease in the Preoperative Patient

The final major category of patients presenting with asymptomatic carotid disease includes those who are candidates for major operation, especially patients undergoing coronary artery bypass or peripheral arterial reconstruction. These patients may manifest asymptomatic carotid bruits or may be screened noninvasively for an asymptomatic carotid stenosis, because of their systemic risk of widespread atherosclerosis. More studies have been published on this group of patients than on any other category of asymptomatic carotid disease. Although some prospective studies have been carried out, there have not been any randomized clinical trials comparing medical with surgical management of asymptomatic carotid stenosis in patients who are candidates for major operation. Most reports have addressed patients undergoing coronary artery bypass grafting. The operation of coronary artery bypass carries an inherent risk of stroke regardless of the presence of concomitant carotid disease. Thrombotic or air emboli associated with cardiopulmonary bypass[5] or atheroembolism from the cannulation site in a diseased ascending aorta[9] may result in a perioperative stroke rate of about 2%. Several strategies are available for managing patients with combined carotid and coronary or peripheral vascular disease. Simultaneous or concomitant operations may be carried out under the same anesthetic. Staged procedures may be performed with initial carotid endarterectomy followed at a subsequent operation for coronary artery bypass or peripheral vascular reconstruction. A reverse-staged procedure involves initial coronary or vascular operation followed subsequently by carotid endarterectomy. Finally, coronary artery bypass or peripheral vascular reconstruction may be carried out alone and the asymptomatic carotid disease may be followed medically, with endarterectomy performed only if future symptoms develop. The aggregate crude outcomes of nonrandomized studies addressing these various therapeutic options for >50% asymptomatic carotid stenosis in preoperative patients with coronary or periph-

eral arterial disease are shown in Table 53.13 (see the Suggested Readings). Most studies have reported only short-term perioperative (30-day) results of these different approaches.

The largest body of literature relates to the performance of concomitant or simultaneous carotid endarterectomy at the time of coronary artery bypass grafting. Although some studies have reported perioperative stroke rates as high as 10% to 15% with combined operations, the aggregate stroke incidence of 3.8% approaches the risk of perioperative myocardial infarction (3.2%) or death (4.6%). The next most frequently recommended strategy of staged carotid endarterectomy followed subsequently by coronary artery bypass is associated with the lowest incidence of perioperative stroke (1.8%). However, this benefit is offset in many series with a higher risk of myocardial infarction (9.1%) and perioperative mortality (6.6%). A few studies have been reported of reverse-staged procedures, with initial coronary artery bypass followed subsequently by carotid endarterectomy. This practice has resulted in perioperative stroke rates (3.2%) no greater than those associated with concomitant procedures, and with a reduced incidence of perioperative myocardial infarction (1.6%) or death (2%). Several studies have reported limiting the operation to the intended coronary or peripheral vascular procedure, with medical management of the associated asymptomatic carotid artery disease. These reports do not suggest a significant increase in perioperative stroke. Indeed, all of the studies of peripheral arterial reconstructions have suggested that the incidence of perioperative stroke is no greater in patients with a ≥50% asymptomatic carotid stenosis (1.1%) than in patients with lesser or no carotid disease (1.2%). Nevertheless, the late follow-up of these patients is important, for a significant number (10% to 20%) will develop TIAs, which should lead to a recommendation for carotid endarterectomy to prevent stroke. In addition, patients undergoing peripheral arterial reconstruction with concomitant asymptomatic carotid disease appear to be at increased risk of perioperative or late myocardial infarction or cardiac-related death.[1,2]

The correlation of cardiac risk with asymptomatic carotid disease can be seen in Table 53.14, which compares the aggregate crude total mortality with cardiac mortality from all of the nonrandomized studies exclusive of those reporting patients undergoing coronary artery bypass. Approximately one-third of the early (30-day) perioperative deaths were due to cardiac cause. Of the late deaths in both medically and surgically managed patients, approximately 50% are the result of coronary artery disease. Thus, asymptomatic carotid disease would ap-

Table 53.13 Aggregate Crude Outcomes of Nonrandomized Studies of Management of >50% Asymptomatic Carotid Artery Stenosis in Preoperative Patients with Coronary or Peripheral Vascular Disease

			Perioperative Outcome (%)		
Treatment	*No. of Studies*	*No. of Patients*	*Stroke*	*Myocardial Infarction*	*Death*
Concomitant CEA/CABG	65	4,016	3.8	3.2	4.6
Staged CEA/CABG	23	850	1.8	9.1	6.6
Reverse staged CABG/CEA	6	248	3.2	1.6	2.0
CABG only	15	894	4.4	—	7.4
Vascular surgery only	6	358	1.1	—	—

Abbreviations: CEA, carotid endarterectomy; CABG, coronary artery bypass graft.

pear to be as much a harbinger of future morbidity or mortality from cardiac disease as it is a risk factor for stroke.

Current Recommendations

Given the aforementioned controversies in the burgeoning literature about asymptomatic carotid disease, what should the clinician recommend for a patient with an asymptomatic carotid bruit or an abnormal noninvasive cerebrovascular test? We believe that the answer lies in the responses to the following four questions:

Does the patient have significant risk factors and comorbidity?

Does the patient have significant carotid stenosis?

Are anesthetic and operative expertise available?

Does the patient (or family) understand the nature and importance of transient ischemic attacks?

First, the clinician must recognize and intervene in important risk factors for stroke. However, in addition to the traditional atherosclerotic risk factors, major operative risk factors such as symptomatic or cryptic coronary artery disease, pulmonary insufficiency, chronic renal disease, and the like must be recognized or uncovered. Because one must operate

Table 53.14 Aggregate Crude Total Mortality and Cardiac Mortality of Nonrandomized Studies of Medical and Surgical Therapy of Patients with ≥50% Carotid Stenosis (Exclusive of Patients Undergoing Coronary Artery Bypass)

	No. of	All Deaths (%)		Cardiac Deaths (%)	
Treatment	*Patients*	*Early*	*Late*	*Early*	*Late*
Medical	4,524	0.8	20.2	0	10.8
Surgical	4,508	1.0	17.4	0.3	8.7

upon about 19 individuals for every stroke prevented over a 5-year period,[12] one must carefully screen out those individuals whose perioperative risk may be double that of the best-reported series of carotid endarterectomy for asymptomatic stenosis (less than 3% combined morbidity and mortality).

Second, the diagnostic evaluation of candidates for carotid endarterectomy of asymptomatic carotid disease should reliably identify those patients with at least 60% diameter reduction at the site of stenosis relative to the distal normal internal carotid artery. In practice, many surgeons have restricted operation for asymptomatic disease to lesions that reduce the carotid diameter by 80% or greater. Unfortunately, no well-designed studies to date, including ACAS, have documented whether this more restrictive policy is valid, but this strategy has been employed by many surgeons for the past 15 years. The authors favor duplex ultrasonography as the best method for noninvasive quantification of the severity of carotid stenosis. It is important for each noninvasive laboratory to validate the accuracy of the duplex threshold criteria, by means of blinded comparison of duplex results with those of carotid arteriograms. Vascular laboratories must not rely on published results of others describing duplex frequency or velocity indices. However, once validated, such duplex criteria can be used in lieu of routine arteriography in selected cases to plan operation. Because of the known risk of arteriography, which in the ACAS study was nearly 50% of the perioperative risk,[12] carotid endarterectomy without preoperative arteriography may decrease the risk/benefit ratio in patients with asymptomatic carotid disease. This practice, however, is feasible only in those centers where the positive predictive value of carotid duplex scanning exceeds the risk of arteriography. In all other instances, preoperative arteriography is probably indicated, especially for patients in whom the duplex results indicate less than an 80% carotid stenosis. The authors have not been impressed that magnetic resonance angiography (MRA) is sufficiently accurate in quantifying stenosis of the carotid bulb to warrant its use in preoperative assessment of patients with carotid disease.

Third, if carotid endarterectomy is chosen, the clinician should refer the patient to a surgeon whose operative outcomes are documented and within the acceptable range of ≤3% combined neurologic morbidity and mortality.[23] Only by unbiased audit can such information be ascertained, and in the future it will be incumbent on surgeons themselves and, indeed, hospital credentialing committees to assure that such outcome criteria are established.[21] If a surgeon's outcomes are in the acceptable range, then the particulars of the procedure, such as the type of anesthesia, methods of cerebral monitoring, use of a carotid shunt, employment of a carotid patch, and monitoring of the integrity of the carotid repair all become of secondary importance.

The final goal of the clinician managing a patient with asymptomatic carotid disease is the careful clinical follow-up for adverse outcomes. Perhaps the most important "risk factor" for future stroke in such a patient is the development of a TIA. Unfortunately, few patients understand the characteristics or the clinical importance of a TIA. It is thus incumbent on all physicians dealing with patients with asymptomatic carotid disease to educate both the patient and the family about the nature of the seemingly trivial manifestations that may herald a future stroke. The authors have emphasized the importance of teaching patients the mnemonic of the 4 S's, namely, disturbances in strength, sensation, sight, or speech, in an effort to increase awareness of TIAs. The reinforcement of these principles when soliciting symptoms at follow-up patient visits is as important as follow-up duplex examinations in managing patients with asymptomatic carotid disease.

Conclusions

Patients with asymptomatic carotid disease may present with an isolated carotid bruit or a stenosis, with angiographic evidence of stenosis contralateral to symptomatic disease, or as asymptomatic disease prior to major cardiovascular operation. In the past 30 years, more than 200 articles have been published on this topic, yet only four multicenter randomized clinical trials have been reported, only two of which have shown some evidence of a favorable effect of carotid endarterectomy on neurologic outcome. The ACAS trial is the first to document the efficacy of carotid endarterectomy plus optimal medical management in reducing estimated 5-year stroke risk in good risk patients with a ≥60% asymptomatic carotid stenosis. This effect was limited primarily to men, and the 53% relative risk reduction from 11% to 5.1% estimated over 5 years of follow-up was achieved only in centers with validated low operative risk of <3%. It is of some historical interest to note that the crude aggregate all-stroke risk of medically and surgically treated patients with asymptomatic carotid disease (10.9% and 7.8%, respectively) is remarkably similar to the combined outcomes of such patients reported in the Veterans Affairs Cooperative Study 167 and the ACAS trial (10.6% and 7.2%, respectively).

Unfortunately, despite a wealth of publications on asymptomatic carotid disease, many questions remain unanswered, particularly by well-designed randomized clinical trials. Patients with an asymptomatic carotid stenosis and a contralateral carotid occlusion are at increased risk of stroke regardless of medical or surgical management. Patients with asymptomatic carotid stenosis contralateral to operated symptomatic carotid disease have a very low rate of future stroke without a warning TIA, and there is no evidence in the literature that prophylactic operation will improve neurologic outcome unless the patient develops symptoms. The greatest number of publications (86) have been devoted to asymptomatic carotid disease in preoper-

ative patients, particularly candidates for coronary artery bypass grafting. Although such patients may be at somewhat greater risk of stroke, there is no evidence in the extensive literature that prophylactic carotid endarterectomy before, at the time of, or after coronary artery bypass grafting can reduce the risk of stroke, myocardial infarction, or death in this patient population.

The clinician is thus left with several dilemmas in managing patients with asymptomatic carotid disease. The authors believe that patients with a severe carotid stenosis, especially with ≥80% diameter reduction, should be considered for prophylactic carotid endarterectomy, but only if no significant comorbidity exists and if surgical expertise is available (documented <3% risk of combined stroke and death). In particular, this decision must be based on avoiding operation in those patients with evident or silent coronary artery disease, because the leading cause of perioperative or late deaths is myocardial infarction. Finally, all clinicians must recognize that the leading predictor ("risk factor") of stroke in patients with asymptomatic carotid disease is a TIA. It is incumbent on physicians to educate patients and their families about the nature and significance of TIAs, which, if they occur, should lead to surgical intervention to reduce stroke risk. For many patients with asymptomatic carotid disease, especially those with comorbid conditions, deferring operation until TIAs develop may prove Amore cost-effective than routine injudicious carotid endarterectomy.

References

1. Barnes RW, Liebman PR, Marszalek PB et al: The natural history of asymptomatic carotid disease in patients undergoing cardiovascular surgery. Surgery 90:1075, 1981
2. Barnes RW, Nix ML, Sansonetti D et al: Late outcome of untreated asymptomatic carotid disease following cardiovascular operations. J Vasc Surg 2:843, 1985
3. Barnett HJM, Eliasziw M, Meldrum HE, Taylor DW: Do the facts and figures warrant a 10-fold increase in the performance of carotid endarterectomy on asymptomatic patients? Neurology 46:603, 1996
4. Barnett HJM, Haines SJ: Carotid endarterectomy for asymptomatic carotid stenosis. N Engl J Med 328:276, 1993
5. Bull DA, Neumayer LA, Hunter GC et al: Risk factors for stroke in patients undergoing coronary artery bypass grafting. Cardiovasc Surg 1:182, 1993
6. Canadian Cooperative Study Group: A randomized trial of aspirin and sulfinpyrazone in threatened stroke. N Engl J Med 299:53, 1978
7. The CASANOVA Study Group: Carotid surgery versus medical therapy in asymptomatic carotid stenosis. Stroke 22:1229, 1991
8. Clagett GP, Youkey JR, Brigham RA et al: Asymptomatic cervical bruit and abnormal ocular pneumoplethysmography: a prospective study comparing two approaches to management. Surgery 96:823, 1984
9. Davila-Roman VG, Barzilai B, Wareing TH et al: Intraoperative ultrasonographic evaluation of the ascending aorta

in 100 consecutive patients undergoing cardiac surgery. Circulation 84, suppl. 3:S47, 1991

10. Dixon S, Pais O, Raviola C et al: Natural history of nonstenotic, asymptomatic ulcerative lesions of the carotid artery: a further analysis. Arch Surg 117:1493, 1982

11. European Carotid Surgery Trialists' Collaborative Group: MCR European Carotid Surgery Trial: interim results for symptomatic patients with severe (70–99%) or with mild (0–29%) carotid stenosis. Lancet 337:1235, 1991

12. Executive Committee for the Asymptomatic Carotid Atherosclerosis Study: Endarterectomy for asymptomatic carotid artery stenosis. JAMA 273:1421, 1995

13. Fields WS, Lemak NA, Frankowski RF, Hardy, RJ: Controlled trial of aspirin in cerebral ischemia. Stroke 8:301, 1977

14. Grotta JC, Bigelow RH, Hu H et al: The significance of carotid stenosis or ulceration. Neurology 34:437, 1984

15. Halliday AW for the steering committee (Halliday A, Thomas D, Mansfield A) and for the collaborators: The asymptomatic carotid surgery trial (ACST): rationale and design. Eur J Vasc Surg 8:703, 1994

16. Harward TRS, Kroener JM, Wickbom IG, Bernstein EF: Natural history of asymptomatic ulcerative plaques of the carotid bifurcation. Am J Surg 146:208, 1983

17. Hertzer NR: A personal view: the asymptomatic carotid atherosclerosis study results—read the label carefully. J Vasc Surg 23:167, 1996

18. Hobson RW II, Weiss DG, Fields WS et al: Efficacy of carotid endarterectomy for asymptomatic carotid stenosis. N Engl J Med 328:221, 1993

19. Mayo Asymptomatic Carotid Endarterectomy Study Group: Results of a randomized controlled trial of carotid endarterectomy for asymptomatic carotid stenosis. Mayo Clin Proc 67:513, 1992

20. Moore WS, Boren C, Malone JM et al: Natural history of nonstenotic, asymptomatic ulcerative lesions of the carotid artery. Arch Surg 113:1352, 1978

21. Moore WS, Treiman RL, Hertzer NR et al: Guidelines for hospital privileges in vascular surgery. J Vasc Surg 10: 678, 1989

22. Moore WS, Vescera CL, Robertson JT et al: Selection process for surgeons in the asymptomatic carotid atherosclerosis study. Stroke 22:1353, 1991

23. Moore WS, Young B, Baker WH et al: Surgical results: a justification of the surgeon selection process for the ACAS trial. J Vasc Surg 23:323, 1996

24. North American Symptomatic Carotid Endarterectomy Trial Collaborators: Beneficial effect of carotid endarterectomy in symptomatic patients with high-grade carotid stenosis. N Engl J Med 325:445, 1991

25. Warlow C: Endarterectomy for asymptomatic carotid stenosis? Lancet 345:1254, 1995

Suggested Readings

NONINVASIVE EVALUATION OF CAROTID BRUITS

AbuRahma AF, Robinson PA: Prospective clinicopathophysiologic follow-up study of asymptomatic neck bruit. Am Surg 56:108, 1990

Aldoori MI, Benveniste GL, Baird RN et al: Asymptomatic carotid murmur: ultrasonic factors influencing outcome. Br J Surg 74:496, 1987

Autret A, Saudeau D, Bertrand PH et al: Stroke risk in patients with carotid stenosis. Lancet 329:888, 1987

Bock RW, Gray-Weale AC, Mock PA et al: The natural history of asymptomatic carotid artery disease. J Vasc Surg 17:160, 1993

Chambers BR, Norris JW: Outcome in patients with asymptomatic neck bruits. N Engl J Med 315:860, 1986

Donaldson MC, Sabine C, Showah AT, Bucknam CA: Recent experience with the asymptomatic cervical bruit. Arch Surg 122:893, 1987

Ellis MR, Franks PJ, Cuming R et al: Prevalence, progression and natural history of asymptomatic carotid stenosis: is there a place for carotid endarterectomy? Eur J Vasc Surg 6:172, 1992

Ellis MR, Greenhalgh RM: Management of asymptomatic carotid bruit. J Vasc Surg 5:869, 1987

Endean ED, Steffen G, Chmura C et al: Outcome of asymptomatic cervical bruits in a veteran population. J Cardiovasc Surg 32:620, 1991

Johnson BF, Verlato F, Bergelin RO et al: Clinical outcome in patients with mild and moderate carotid artery stenosis. J Vasc Surg 21:120, 1995

Johnson JM, Kennelly MM, Decesare D et al: Natural history of asymptomatic carotid plaque. Arch Surg 120:1010, 1985

Meissner I, Wiebers DO, Whisnant JP, O'Fallon WM: The natural history of asymptomatic carotid artery occlusive lesions. JAMA 258:2704, 1987

Moore DJ, Miles RD, Gooley NA, Sumner DS: Noninvasive assessment of stroke risk in asymptomatic and nonhemispheric patients with suspected carotid disease: five-year follow-up of 294 unoperated and 81 operated patients. Ann Surg 202:491, 1985

Norris JW, Zhu CZ, Bornstein NM, Chambers BR: Vascular risks of asymptomatic carotid stenosis. Stroke 22:1485, 1991

O'Holleran LW, Kennelly MM, McClurken M, Johnson JM: Natural history of asymptomatic carotid plaque: five-year follow-up, study. Am J Surg 154:659, 1987

Roederer GO, Langlois YE, Jager KA et al: The natural history of carotid arterial disease in asymptomatic patients with cervical bruits. Stroke 15:605, 1984

Shanik GD, Moore DJ, Leahy A et al: Asymptomatic carotid stenosis: a benign lesion? Eur J Vasc 6:10, 1992

Taylor LM, Loboa L, Porter JM: The clinical course of carotid bifurcation stenosis as determined by duplex scanning. J Vasc Surg 8:255, 1988

Tong Y, Royle J: Outcome of patients with symptomless carotid bruits: a prospective study. Cardiovascular Surgery 4: 174, 1996

ASYMPTOMATIC CAROTID BRUIT

Dorazio RA, Ezzet F, Nesbitt NJ: Long-term follow-up of asymptomatic-carotid bruits. Amer J Surg 140:212, 1980

Heyman A, Wilkinson WE, Heyden S et al: Risk of stroke in asymptomatic persons with cervical arterial bruits: a population study in Evans County, Georgia. N Engl J Med 302: 838, 1980

Wiebers DO, Whisnant JP, Sandok BA, O'Fallon WM: Prospective comparison of a cohort with asymptomatic carotid bruit and a population-based cohort without carotid bruit. Stroke 21:984, 1990

Wolf PA, Kannel WB, Sorlie P, McNamara P: Asymptomatic carotid bruit and risk of stroke: the Framingham study. JAMA 245:1442, 1981

ASYMPTOMATIC CAROTID STENOSIS

(In addition to those listed above) under Noninvasive Evaluation of Carotid Bruits.)

Anderson RJ, Hobson RW II, Padberg FT Jr et al: Carotid endarterectomy for asymptomatic carotid stenosis: a ten-year experience with 120 procedures in a fellowship training program. Ann Vasc Surg 5:111, 1991

Appleberg M, Cottier D, Crozier J et al: Carotid endarterectomy for asymptomatic carotid artery stenosis: patients with severe bilateral disease a high risk subgroup. Aust NZ J Surg 65:160, 1995

Batson RC, Sottiurai VS: Management of asymptomatic carotid artery stenosis. Int Surg 69:239, 1984

Bogousslavsky J, Despland PA, Regli F: Asymptomatic tight stenosis of the internal carotid artery: long-term prognosis. Neurology 36:861, 1986

Brott T, Thalinger K: The practice of carotid endarterectomy in a large metropolitan area. Stroke 15:950, 1984

Caracci BF, Zukowski AJ, Hurley JJ et al: Asymptomatic severe carotid stenosis. J Vasc Surg 9:361, 1989

Deriu GP, Ballotta E, Bonavina L et al: The rationale for patch-graft angioplasty after carotid endarterectomy: early and long-term follow-up. Stroke 15:972, 1984

Easton JD, Sherman DG: Stroke and mortality rate in carotid endarterectomy: 228 consecutive operations. Stroke 8:565, 1977

Freischlag JA, Hanna D, Moore WS: Improved prognosis for asymptomatic carotid stenosis with prophylactic carotid endarterectomy. Stroke 23:479, 1992

Hennerici M, Rautenberg W, Mohr S: Stroke risk from symptomless extracranial arterial disease. Lancet 316:1180, 1982

Hertzer NR, Flanagan RA Jr, O'Hara PJ, Beven EG: Surgical versus nonoperative treatment of asymptomatic carotid stenosis: 290 patients documented by intravenous angiography. Ann Surg 204:163, 1986

Javid H, Ostermiller WE, Hengesh JW et al: Carotid endarterectomy for asymptomatic patients. Arch Surg 102:389, 1971

Libman RB, Sacco RL, Shi T et al: Outcome after carotid endarterectomy for asymptomatic carotid stenosis. Surg Neurol 41:443, 1994

Lindberg B, Norback B, Svendsen P, Synek V: Carotid endarterectomy: a review of 104 operations. J Cardiovasc Surg 16:161, 1975

Mansour MA, Mattos MA, Faught WE et al: The natural history of moderate (50% to 79%) internal carotid artery stenosis in symptomatic, nonhemispheric, and asymptomatic patients. J Vasc Surg 21:346, 1995

Moneta GL, Taylor DC, Nicholls SC et al: Operative versus nonoperative management of asymptomatic high-grade internal carotid artery stenosis: improved results with endarterectomy. Stroke 18:1005, 1987

Moore WS, Boren C, Malone JM, Goldstone J: Asymptomatic carotid stenosis: immediate and long-term results after prophylactic endarterectomy. Amer J Surg 138:228, 1979

Nunn DB: Carotid endarterectomy: an analysis of 234 operative cases. Ann Surg 182:733, 1975

Park Y, El-Bayar H, Hye RJ et al: Safety and long-term benefit of carotid endarterectomy in the asymptomatic patient. Ann Vasc Surg 4:218, 1990

Riles TS, Fisher FS, Lamparello PJ et al: Immediate and long-term results of carotid endarterectomy for asymptomatic high-grade stenosis. Ann Vasc Surg 8:144, 1994

Rosenthal D, Rudderman R, Borrero E et al: Carotid endarterectomy to correct asymptomatic carotid stenosis: ten years later. J Vasc Surg 6:226, 1987

Thompson JE, Patman RD, Talkington CM: Asymptomatic carotid bruit: long-term outcome of patients having endarterectomy compared with unoperated controls. Ann Surg 188:308, 1978

Treiman RL, Cossman DV, Foran RF et al: The risk of carotid endarterectomy for the asymptomatic patient: an argument for prophylactic operation. Ann Vasc Surg 4:29, 1990

CONTRALATERAL CAROTID OCCLUSION

Andersen CA, Rich NM, Collins GJ Jr et al: Unilateral internal carotid arterial occlusion: special considerations. Stroke 8:669, 1977

Baker WH, Dorner DB, Barnes RW: Carotid endarterectomy: is an indwelling shunt necessary? Surgery 82:321, 1977

Bland JE, Chapman RD, Wylie EJ: Neurological complications of carotid artery surgery. Ann Surg 171:459, 1970

Bloodwell RD, Hallman GL, Keats AS, Cooley DA: Carotid endarterectomy without a shunt: results using hypercarbic general anesthesia to prevent cerebral ischemia. Arch Surg 96:644, 1968

Chung WB: Long-term results of carotid artery surgery for cerebrovascular insufficiency. Am J Surg 128:262, 1974

Cote R, Barnett HJM, Taylor DW: Internal carotid occlusion: a prospective study. Stroke 14:898, 1983

Dyken ML, Klatte E, Kolar OJ, Spurgeon C: Complete occlusion of common or internal carotid arteries. Arch Neurol 30:343, 1974

Faught WE, Van Bemmelen PS, Mattos MA et al: Presentation and natural history of internal carotid artery occlusion. J Vasc Surg 18:512, 1993

Fields WS, Lemak NA: Joint study of extracranial arterial occlusion: X. Internal carotid artery occlusion. JAMA 235:2734, 1976

Friedman SG, Riles TS, Lamparello PJ et al: Surgical therapy for the patient with internal carotid artery occlusion and contralateral stenosis. J Vasc Surg 5:856, 1987

Grillo P, Patterson RH Jr: Occlusion of the carotid artery: prognosis (natural history) and the possibilities of surgical revascularization. Stroke 6:17, 1975

Hammacher ER, Eikelboom BC, Bast TJ et al: Surgical treatment of patients with a carotid artery occlusion and a contralateral stenosis. J Cardiovasc Surg 25:513, 1984

Hennerici M, Hulsbomer H-B, Rautenberg W, Hefter H:

Spontaneous history of asymptomatic internal carotid occlusion. Stroke 17:718, 1986

Heyman A, Young WG Jr, Brown IW Jr: Long-term results of endarterectomy of the internal carotid artery for cerebral ischemia and infarction. Circulation 36:212, 1967

Kleiser B, Widder B: Course of carotid artery occlusions with impaired cerebrovascular reactivity. Stroke 23:171, 1992

Lees CD, Hertzer NR: Postoperative stroke and late neurologic complications after carotid endarterectomy. Arch Surg 116:1561, 1981

Ludtke-Handjery A, Debbert R, Gref H et al: The risk of surgical therapy to patients with unilateral stenosis and contralateral occlusion of the carotid artery. Thorac Cardiovasc Surgeon 27:334, 1979

Mackey WC, O'Donnell TF Jr, Callow AD: Carotid endarterectomy contralateral to an occluded carotid artery: perioperative risk and late results. J Vasc Surg 11:778, 1990

Moore DJ, Modi JR, Finch WT, Sumner DS: Influence of the contralateral carotid artery on neurologic complications following carotid endarterectomy. J Vasc Surg 1:409, 1984

Nicholls SC, Kohler TR, Bergelin RO et al: Carotid artery occlusion: natural history. J Vasc Surg 4:479, 1986

Ott DA, Cooley Da, Chapa L, Coelho A: Carotid endarterectomy without temporary intraluminal shunt. Ann Surg 191:708, 1980

Patterson RH Jr: Risk of carotid surgery with occlusion of the contralateral carotid artery. Arch Neurol 30:188, 1974

Persson AV, Griffey EE, Jaxheimer EC, Jewell ER: The natural history of total occlusion of the internal carotid artery. Vasc Diag Ther 5:15, 1984

Phillips MR, Johnson WC, Scott RM et al: Carotid endarterectomy in the presence of contralateral carotid occlusion. Arch Surg 114:1232, 1979

Rautenberg W, Mess W, Hennerici M: Prognosis of asymptomatic carotid occlusion. J Neurol Scs 98:213, 1990

Sachs SM, Fulenwider JT, Smith RB III et al: Does contralateral carotid occlusion influence neurologic fate of carotid endarterectomy? Surgery 96:839, 1984

Sacquegna T, De Carolis P, Pazzaglia P et al: The clinical course and prognosis of carotid artery occlusion. J Neur Neurosurg Psych 45:1037, 1982

Thompson JE, Talkington CM: Carotid endarterectomy. Ann Surg 184:1, 1976

Vermassen F, Flamme A, DeRoose J et al: Long-term results after carotid endarterectomy for carotid artery stenosis with contralateral occlusion. Ann Vasc Surg 4:323, 1990

Waltimo O, Kaste M, Fogelholm R: Prognosis of patients with unilateral extracranial occlusion of the internal carotid artery. Stroke 7:480, 1976

Whittemore AD: Carotid endarterectomy: an alternative approach. Arch Surg 115:940, 1980

Young JR Jr, Humphries AW, Beven EG, de Wolfe VG: Carotid endarterectomy without a shunt: experiences using hyperbaric general anesthesia. Arch Surg 99:293, 1969

CONTRALATERAL CAROTID STENOSIS

Calligaro KD, Hass B, Westcott CJ et al: Risk of prophylactic contralateral carotid endarterectomy. Ann Vasc Surg 6:147, 1992

Durward QJ, Ferguson GG, Barr HWK: The natural history of asymptomatic carotid bifurcation plaques. Stroke 13:459, 1982

The European Carotid Surgery Trialists Collaborative Group: Risk of stroke in the distribution of an asymptomatic carotid artery. Lancet 345:209, 1995

Hatsukami TS, Healy DA, Primozich JF et al: Fate of the carotid artery contralateral to endarterectomy. J Vasc Surg 11:244, 1990

Humphries AW, Young JR, Santilli PH et al: Unoperated, asymptomatic significant internal carotid artery stenosis: a review of 182 instances. Surgery 80:695, 1976

Johnson N, Burnham SJ, Flanigan DP et al: Carotid endarterectomy: a follow-up study of the contralateral non-operated carotid artery. Ann Surg 188:748, 1978

Langsfeld M, Gray-Weale AC, Lusby RJ: The role of plaque morphology and diameter reduction in the development of new symptoms in asymptomatic carotid arteries. J Vasc Surg 9:548, 1989

Levin SM, Sondheimer FK, Levin JM: The contralateral diseased but asymptomatic carotid artery: to operate or not? Am J Surg 140:203, 1980

McKittrick JE, Henrikson J, Iwasiuk GW: Indications for contralateral endarterectomy: role of the noninvasive laboratory. Am J Surg 140:206, 1980

Morrow CE, Espada R, Howell JF: Operative and long-term results of staged contralateral carotid endarterectomy: a personal series. Surgery 103:242, 1988

Naylor AR, John T, Howlett J et al: Fate of the non-operated carotid artery after contralateral endarterectomy. Br J Surg 82:44, 1995

Norrving B, Nilsson B, Olsson JE: Progression of carotid disease after endarterectomy: a Doppler ultrasound study. Ann Neurol 12:548, 1982

Podore PC, De Weese JA, May AG, Rob CG: Asymptomatic contralateral carotid artery stenosis: a five-year follow-up study following carotid endarterectomy. Surgery 88:748, 1980

Riles TS, Imparato AM, Mintzer R, Baumann FG: Comparison of results of bilateral and unilateral carotid endarterectomy five years after surgery. Surgery 91:258, 1982

Roederer GO, Langlois YE, Lusiani L et al: Natural history of carotid artery disease on the side contralateral to endarterectomy. J Vasc Surg 1:62, 1984

Sannella NA: Bilateral severe carotid stenosis or occlusion and computed tomographic scan positive hemispheric stroke with neurologic deficit: immediate contralateral carotid endarterectomy. Ann Vasc Surg 6:252, 1992

Satiani B, Chen TY, Shook L, Finnie K: Contralateral disease progression after carotid endarterectomy. Surgery 114:46, 1993

Schroeder T, Helgstrand UJV, Egeblad MR, Engell HC: Asymptomatic carotid lesions after endarterectomy of contralateral carotid artery: five-year follow-up study and prognosis. Arch Surg 122:795, 1987

Sobel M, Imparato AM, Riles TS, Mintzer R: Contralateral neurologic symptoms after carotid surgery: a nine-year follow-up. J Vasc Surg 3:623, 1986

Sterpetti AV, Schultz RD, Feldhaus RJ: Asymptomatic carotid artery stenosis on the side contralateral to endarterectomy:

a comparison between patients with and those without operation. J Vasc Surg 8:453, 1988

CAROTID STENOSIS IN PREOPERATIVE PATIENTS

Akins CW, Moncure AC, Daggett WM et al: Safety and efficacy of concomitant carotid and coronary artery operations. Ann Thorac Surg 60:311, 1995

Babu SC, Shah PM, Singh BM et al: Coexisting carotid stenosis in patients undergoing cardiac surgery: indications and guidelines for simultaneous operations. Am J Surg 150:207, 1985

Balderman SC, Gutierrez IZ, Makula P et al: Noninvasive screening for asymptomatic carotid artery disease prior to cardiac operation: experience with 500 patients. J Thorac Cardiovasc Surg 85:427, 1983

Barnes RW, Liebman PR, Marszalek PB et al: The natural history of asymptomatic carotid disease in patients undergoing cardiovascular surgery. Surgery 90:1075, 1981

Berens ES, Kouchoukos NT, Murphy SF, Wareing TH: Preoperative carotid artery screening in elderly patients undergoing cardiac surgery. J Vasc Surg 15:313, 1992

Berkoff HA, Turnipseed WD: Patient selection and results of simultaneous coronary and carotid artery procedures. Ann Thorac Surg 38:172, 1984

Bernhard VM, Johnson WD, Peterson JJ: Carotid artery stenosis: association with surgery for coronary artery disease. Arch Surg 105:837, 1972

Brener BJ, Brief DK, Alpert J et al: A four-year experience with preoperative noninvasive carotid evaluation of two thousand twenty-six patients undergoing cardiac surgery. J Vasc Surg 1:326, 1984

Brener BJ, Brief DK, Alpert J et al: The risk of stroke in patients with asymptomatic carotid stenosis undergoing cardiac surgery: a follow-up study. J Vasc Surg 5:269, 1987

Cambria RP, Ivarsson BL, Akins CW et al: Simultaneous carotid and coronary disease: safety of the combined approach. J Vasc Surg 9:56, 1989

Carey JS, Cukingnan RA: Complications of combined brachiocephalic and coronary revascularization. Ann Thorac Surg 25:385, 1978

Carney WI Jr, Stewart WB, De Pinto DJ et al: Carotid bruit as a risk factor in aortoiliac reconstruction. Surgery 81:567, 1977

Carrel T, Stillhard G, Turina M: Combined carotid and coronary artery surgery: early and late results. Cardiology 80:118, 1992

Chang BB, Darling RC III, Shah DM et al: Carotid endarterectomy can be safely performed with acceptable mortality and morbidity in patients requiring coronary artery bypass grafts. Am J Surg 168:94, 1994

Cooperman M, Martin EW Jr, Evans WE: Significance of asymptomatic carotid bruits. Arch Surg 113:1339, 1978

Cosgrove DM, Hertzer NR, Loop FD: Surgical management of synchronous-carotid and coronary artery disease. J Vasc Surg 3:690, 1986

Coyle KA, Gray BC, Smith RB III et al: Morbidity and mortality associated with carotid endarterectomy: effect of adjunctive coronary revascularization. Ann Vasc Surg 9:21, 1995

Craver JM, Murphy DA, Jones EL et al: Concomitant carotid and coronary artery reconstruction. Ann Surg 195:712, 1982

Crawford ES, Palamara AE, Kasparian AS: Carotid and noncornay operations: simultaneous, staged, and delayed. Surgery 87:1, 1980

Dalton ML Jr, Parker TM, Mistrot JJ, Bricker DL: Concomitant coronary artery bypass and major noncardiac surgery. J Thorac Cardiovasc Surg 75:621, 1978

Duchateau J, Nevelsteen A, Sergeant P et al: Combined myocardial and cerebral revascularization: a ten year experience. J Cardiovasc Surg 30:715, 1989

Dunn EJ: Concomitant cerebral and myocardial revascularization. Surg Clin North Am 66:385, 1986

Emery RW, Cohn LH, Whittemore AD et al: Coexistent carotid and coronary artery disease surgical management. Arch Surg 118:1035, 1983

Ennix CL Jr, Lawrie GM, Morris GC Jr et al: Improved results of carotid endarterectomy in patients with symptomatic coronary disease: an analysis of 1,546 consecutive carotid operations. Stroke 10:122, 1979

Evans WE, Cooperman M: The significance of asymptomatic unilateral carotid bruits in preoperative patients. Surgery 77:521, 1978

Faggioli GL, Curl GR, Ricotta JJ: The role of carotid screening before coronary artery bypass. J Vasc Surg 12:724, 1990

Faidutti B, Steichen FM, Thevoz F, Hahn CJ: Coronary artery and associated aortic or major arterial atherosclerosis: one-stage surgical management. Arch Surg 105:71, 1972

Fillinger MF, Rosenberg JM, Semel L et al: Combined carotid endarterectomy and coronary artery bypass in a community hospital. Cardiovasc Surg 1:7, 1993

Fode NC, Sundt TM Jr, Robertson JT et al: Multicenter retrospective review of results and complications of carotid endarterectomy in 1981. Stroke 17:370, 1986

Furlan AJ, Craciun AR: Risk of stroke during coronary artery bypass graft surgery in patients with internal carotid artery disease documented by angiography. Stroke 16:797, 1985

Gerraty RP, Gates PC, Doyle JC: Carotid stenosis and perioperative stroke risk in symptomatic and asymptomatic patients undergoing vascular or coronary surgery. Stroke 24:1115, 1993

Giangola G, Migaly J, Riles TS et al: Perioperative morbidity and mortality in combined vs. staged approaches to carotid and coronary revascularization. Ann Vasc Surg 10:138, 1996

Gravlee GP, Cordell AR, Graham JE et al: Coronary revascularization in patients with bilateral internal carotid occlusions. J Thorac Cardiovasc Surg 90:921, 1985

Gugulakis A, Kalodiki E, Nicolaides AN: Combined carotid endarterectomy and coronary artery bypass grafting: a literature review. Int Angiol 10:167, 1991

Halpin DP, Riggins S, Carmichael JD et al: Management of coexistent carotid and coronary artery disease. Southern Med J 87:187, 1994

Hertzer NR, Loop FD, Beven EG et al: Surgical staging for simultaneous coronary and carotid disease: a study including prospective randomization. J Vasc Surg 9:455, 1989

Hertzer NR, Loop FD, Taylor PC, Beven EG: Combined myocardial revascularization and carotid endarterectomy. J Thorac Cardiovasc Surg 85:577, 1983

Hertzer NR, Loop FD, Taylor PC, Beven EG: Staged and

combined surgical approach to simultaneous carotid and coronary vascular disease. Surgery 84:803, 1978

Ivey TD, Strandness DE, Williams DB et al: Management of patients with carotid bruit undergoing cardiopulmonary bypass. J Thorac Cardiovasc Surg 87:183, 1984

Jausseran JM, Bergeron P, Reggi M et al: Single staged carotid and coronary arteries surgery: indications and results. J Cardiovasc Surg 30:407, 1989

Jones EL, Craver JM, Michalik RA et al: Combined carotid and coronary operations: when are they necessary? J Thorac Cardiovasc Surg 87:7, 1984

Kartchner MM, McRae LP: Carotid occlusive disease as a risk factor in major cardiovascular surgery. Arch Surg 117:1086, 1982

Korompai FL, Hayward RH, Knight WL: Noncardiac operations combined with coronary artery bypass. Surg Clin North Am 62:215, 1982

Kouchoukos NT, Daily BB, Wareing TH, Murphy SF: Hypothermic circulatory arrest for cerebral protection during combined carotid and cardiac surgery in patients with bilateral carotid artery disease. Ann Surg 219:699, 1994

Lefrak EA, Guinn GA: Prophylactic carotid artery surgery in patients requiring a second operation. Southern Med J 67:185, 1974

Lord RSA, Graham AR, Shanahan MX et al: Rationale for simultaneous carotid endarterectomy and aortocoronary bypass. Ann Vasc Surg 1:201, 1986

Lubicz S, Kelly A, Field PL et al: Combined carotid and coronary surgery. Aust NZ J Surg 57:593, 1987

Maki HS, Kuehner ME, Ray JF III: Combined carotid endarterectomy and myocardial revascularization. Am J Surg 158:443, 1989

Matano R, Ascer E, Gennaro M et al: Outcome of patients with abnormal ocular pneumoplethysmographic measurements undergoing coronary artery bypass grafting. Cardiovasc Surg 2:266, 1994

Matar AF: Concomitant coronary and cerebral revascularization under cardiopulmonary bypass. Ann Thorac Surg 41:431, 1986

Mehigan JT, Buch WS, Pipkin RD, Fogarty TJ: A planned approach to coexistent cerebrovascular disease in coronary artery bypass candidates. Arch Surg 112:1403, 1977

Minami K, Gawaz M, Ohlmeier H et al: Management of concomitant occlusive disease of coronary and carotid arteries using cardiopulmonary bypass for both procedures. J Cardiovasc Surg 30:723, 1989

Morris GC Jr, Ennix CL Jr, Lawrie GM et al: Management of coexistent carotid and coronary artery occlusive atherosclerosis. Cleveland Clin Q 45:125, 1978

Newman DC, Hicks RG, Horton DA: Coexistent carotid and coronary arterial disease: outcome in 50 cases and method of management. J Cardiovasc Surg 28:599, 1987

O'Donnell TF Jr, Callow AD, Willet C et al: The impact of coronary artery disease on carotid endarterectomy. Ann Surg 198:705, 1983

Ogren C, Klamer TW, Towne JB, Bandyk DF: The role of noninvasive cerebrovascular testing in patients undergoing coronary artery surgery. Bruit 7:22, 1983

Okies JE, MacManus Q, Starr A: Myocardial revascularization and carotid endarterectomy: a combined approach. Ann Thorac Surg 23:560, 1977

Perler BA, Burdick JF, Minken SL, Williams GM: Should we perform carotid endarterectomy synchronously with cardiac surgical procedures? J Vasc Surg 8:402, 1988

Perler BA, Burdick JF, Williams GM: The safety of carotid endarterectomy at the time of coronary artery bypass surgery: analysis of results in a high-risk patient population. J Vasc Surg 2:558, 1985

Pillai L, Gutierrez IZ, Curl GR et al: Evaluation and treatment of carotid stenosis in open-heart surgery patients. J Surg Res 57:312, 1994

Pome G, Passini L, Colucci V et al: Combined surgical approach to coexistent carotid and coronary artery disease. J Cardiovasc Surg 32:787, 1991

Reichart B, Becker HM, Autenrieth G et al: Stenosis of the supra aortic branches combined with artery disease: one-stage surgical treatment. Thorac Cardiovasc Surgeon 30:269, 1982

Reis RL, Hamner H III: Management of patients with severe, coexistent coronary artery and peripheral vascular disease. J Thorac Cardiovasc Surg 73:909, 1977

Reul GJ Jr, Cooley DA, Duncan JM: The effect of coronary bypass on the outcome of peripheral vascular operations in 1093 patients. J Vasc Surg 3:788, 1986

Rice PL, Pifarre R, Sullivan HJ et al: Experience with simultaneous myocardial revascularization and carotid endarterectomy. J Thorac Cardiovasc Surg 79:922, 1980

Ricotta JJ, Faggioli GL, Castilone A, Hassett JM, for the Buffalo Cardiac Cerebral Study Group: Risk factors for stroke after cardiac surgery: Buffalo Cardiac-Cerebral Study Group. J Vasc Surg 21:359, 1995

Rizzo RJ, Whittemore AD, Couper GS et al: Combined carotid and coronary revascularization: the preferred approach to the severe vasculopath. Ann Thorac Surg 54:1099, 1992

Robertson JT, Fraser JC: Evaluation of carotid endarterectomy with and without coronary artery bypass surgery. Cerebrovascular Diseases, Lippincott-Raven, Philadelphia, 1981

Ropper AH, Wechsler LR, Wilson LS: Carotid bruit and the risk of stroke in elective surgery. N Engl J Med 307:1388, 1982

Rosenthal D, Caudill DR, Lamis PA et al: Carotid and coronary arterial disease: a rational approach. Am Surg 50:233, 1984

Saccani S, Beghi C, Fragnito C et al: Carotid endarterectomy under hypothermic extracorporeal circulation: a method of brain protection for special patients. J Cardiovasc Surg 33:311, 1992

Salasidis GC, Latter DA, Steinmetz OK et al: Carotid artery duplex scanning in preoperative assessment for coronary artery revascularization: the association between peripheral vascular disease, carotid artery stenosis, and stroke. J Vasc Surg 21:154, 1995

Sayers RD, Thompson MM, Underwood MJ et al: Early results of combined carotid endarterectomy and coronary artery bypass grafting in patients with severe coronary and carotid artery disease. J R Col Surg Edinb 38:340, 1993

Schultz RD, Sterpetti AV, Feldhaus RJ: Early and late results in patients with carotid disease undergoing myocardial revascularization. Ann Thorac Surg 45:603, 1988

Schwartz LB, Bridgman AH, Kieffer RW et al: Asymptomatic

carotid artery stenosis and stroke in patients undergoing cardiopulmonary bypass. J Vasc Surg 21:146, 1995

Schwartz RL, Garrett JR, Karp RB, Kouchoukos NT: Simultaneous myocardial revascularization and carotid endarterectomy. Circulation (suppl 1):S66:1–97, 1982

Treiman RL, Foran RF, Cohen JL et al: Carotid bruit: a follow-up report on its significance in patients undergoing an abdominal aortic operation. Arch Surg 114:1138, 1979

Treiman RL, Foran RF, Shore EH, Levin PM: Carotid bruit: significance in patients undergoing an abdominal aortic operation. Arch Surg 106:803, 1973

Turnipseed WD, Berkoff HA, Belzer FO: Postoperative stroke in cardiac and peripheral vascular disease. Ann Surg 192:365, 1980

Urschel HC, Razzuk MA, Gardner MA: Management of concomitant occlusive disease of the carotid and coronary arteries. J Thorac Cardiovasc Surg 72:829, 1976

Vassilidze TV, Cernaianu AC, Gaprindashvili T et al: Simultaneous coronary artery bypass and carotid endarterectomy: determinants of outcome. Texas Heart Inst J 21:119, 1994

Vermeulen F, Hamerlijnck R, Defauw J et al: Combined carotid and coronary revascularization. Acta Chir Belg 93:239, 1993

Wang JS, Laj ST, Yu TJ et al: Synchronous carotid endarterectomy and myocardial revascularization. Chin Med J (Taipei) 54:14, 1994

Weiss SJ, Sutter FP, Shannon TO, Goldman SM: Combined cardiac operation and carotid endarterectomy during aortic cross-clamping. Ann Thorac Surg 53:813, 1992

Medical Management of Aneurysmal Subarachnoid Hemorrhage

HAROLD P. ADAMS, JR.

BETSY B. LOVE

Subarachnoid hemorrhage (SAH) accounts for 5% to 10% of all strokes and has an incidence of 11:19.4/100,000[51] Unlike other types of stroke, the incidence of SAH is not declining. The leading cause of SAH, accounting for approximately 80% of cases, is rupture of an intracranial saccular aneurysm. Patients with bleeding secondary to ruptured saccular aneurysms have a poorer prognosis and present more complicated management problems than those with SAH of other etiologies. The care of patients with SAH not due to a ruptured aneurysm differs from those who have an aneurysm. Outcomes among persons who do not have an aneurysm are usually better. They are less seriously ill, and rebleeding or delayed cerebral ischemia is uncommon.[96] This chapter is restricted to the treatment of SAH secondary to ruptured aneurysms.

Early diagnosis and better medical and surgical care are reducing mortality from SAH.[51] Yet, despite these advances, SAH is a frequent cause of death or disability. In population-based studies, the 30-day mortality of SAH is nearly 50%.[12,51,101,123] Most deaths occur within 1 week of the ictus, 10% die before being able to reach medical attention, and 25% die within 24 hours.[101] Causes of sudden death include a large intraparenchymal hematoma, destruction of brain tissue, acute hydrocephalus, increased intracranial pressure, myocardial ischemia, cardiac arrhythmias, and respiratory failure. In these cases, computed tomography (CT) usually demonstrates massive intracerebral, intraventricular, or subarachnoid hemorrhage. These moribund patients often have ataxic or periodic respirations, suggesting brain stem failure. In these instances, survival is unlikely even with prompt medical care.

Even by excluding terminally ill persons, the natural history of SAH is grim. The 3-month mortality among patients who reach a major medical center is approximately 25%.[3,24] The leading causes of death are sequelae of the initial hemorrhage, recurrent aneurysmal rupture, and vasospasm with ischemic stroke. Another 20% to 40% of hospitalized patients have major neurologic residuals.[95,97,100] The chief reasons for neurologic impairment are the consequences of the initial aneurysmal rupture, vasospasm and ischemia, hydrocephalus, complications of surgery, and complications of medical management. Sequelae include cranial nerve palsies, paralysis, aphasia, mental status changes, behavioral disorders, and psychiatric disturbances that could hamper return to gainful employment or independence.

The two most important factors that influence prognosis after SAH are the interval from SAH and the person's level of consciousness.[100] Most deaths and complications develop within 2 weeks of SAH; patients surviving this period without major complications have a generally favorable prognosis. When examining the possible usefulness of any intervention, the interval from SAH until treatment should be considered. The key test of any medical or surgical therapy is whether it improves outcome among acutely ill patients treated within the first few days after SAH.

The admitting level of consciousness is the most important clinical factor (Table 54.1). The 6-month mortality among comatose patients is 71%, whereas only 11% of initially alert patients die during the same time period.[2] The size of the aneurysm is not a major determinant of prognosis. Although data conflict, aneurysms located on the basilar artery or its branches are associated with a poorer prognosis.[100,101] Patients

Table 54.1 Factors Predicting Less Favorable Outcome after Subarachnoid Hemorrhage

Clinical
  Admitting level of consciousness (coma)
  Interval from subarachnoid hemorrhage (<3 days)
  Age (>65)
  Sex (women)
  Prior hemorrhage or unrecognized warning leak
  Presence of focal neurologic signs on admission
  Presence of major comorbid diseases, including hypertension

Diagnostic tests
  Hyponatremia or hypovolemia
  Abnormal CT scan
    Local, thick, or diffuse collection of subarachnoid blood
    Intracerebral or intraventricular blood
    Mass effect
    Hydrocephalus
  Evidence of additional blood (rebleeding) on sequential CT scan
  Vasospasm on arteriography
  High-flow velocities (vasospasm) detected by transcranial Doppler
  Aneurysm located on anterior cerebral or vertebrobasilar arteries
  Giant aneurysm (25 mm or greater)

Abbreviation: CT, computed tomography.

older than 65 years have a poorer prognosis than younger persons.[100] Favorable outcomes among women are less common than among men.[66,97] Pre-existing medical conditions, such as hypertension and diabetes mellitus, do not have major effects on prognosis. Patients who do not reach medical attention until after a second rupture of the aneurysm have a worse prognosis than those who have a single hemorrhage.[24] LeBlanc[69] reported that the mortality among persons who had a "warning leak" was 52% compared with 23% among persons with a single hemorrhage.

The results of an initial CT examination also provide prognostic clues (Table 54.1).[2,100] In general, CT and clinical findings are parallel and correlate with the time lag from SAH.[2] Patients with CT evidence of hydrocephalus, mass effect, intracerebral hematoma, intraventricular hemorrhage, or diffuse subarachnoid blood have a poorer prognosis than those who have a normal CT or only a minimal amount of subarachnoid blood. Early elevations in thrombin-antithrombin III complex and plasmin α-2-plasmin inhibitor complex are more common among persons who have severe hemorrhages and poor outcomes.[52] Fujii[31] and colleagues confirmed these findings and also detected elevations in d-dimer, which suggests activation of the body's fibrinolytic responses. They found relationships between alternations in these coagulation factors with the amount of subarachnoid blood seen on CT or the presence of a major intraventricular or intracerebral hemorrhage.

The complications of SAH that can lead to death or disability are summarized in Table 54.2. For many years, attention was directed toward the prevention of rebleeding or ischemic complications of cerebral vasospasm. These two conditions account for approximately 60% of unfavorable outcomes. Still, one-third of all patients who die or become disabled after

SAH are injured primarily by the consequences of the initial hemorrhage.[12] As management to prevent rebleeding and vasospasm improves, treatment of these early complications becomes increasingly important.[12]

Therefore, the goals of medical management are (1) to stabilize an acutely ill patient and prevent early complications, (2) to forestall recurrent hemorrhage, and (3) to prevent vasospasm and cerebral ischemia. Treatment is multifactorial and complex; therapy aimed at prevention of one complication might aggravate management of another. Successful management of one complication can leave the patient at risk for another; for example, prevention of early rebleeding in a seriously ill patient means that the person subsequently can develop vasospasm and ischemia. Much of the care of SAH is empirical or is based on anecdotal evidence; several components have not been tested in clinical trials. Thus, some recommendations are based on weak or conflicting scientific evidence.

Diagnosis

The key to successful management of SAH is early treatment, which, in turn, is based on prompt and accurate diagnosis.[24] The drive to popularize stroke as a "brain attack" is, in part, stimulated by the successful early care of persons with ruptured aneurysms.[15] Delayed recognition is a major problem. Approximately 10% of patients do not recognize the nature

Table 54.2 Complications of Aneurysmal Subarachnoid Hemorrhage

Neurologic
  Intraparenchymal hematoma
  Intraventricular hemorrhage
  Brain edema
  Hydrocephalus (acute, subacute, chronic)
  Recurrent hemorrhage
  Vasospasm—ischemic stroke
  Seizures

Nonneurologic
  Arterial hypertension/hypotension
  Myocardial infarction
  Cardiac arrhythmia
  Congestive heart failure
  Neurogenic pulmonary edema
  Adult respiratory distress syndrome
  Atelectasis
  Pneumonia
  Gastrointestinal bleeding
  Anemia
  Venous thromboembolism
  Bleeding disorders
  Hyponatremia/hypernatremia
  Water loss
  Hypokalemia

of their symptoms and do not quickly seek medical attention. More bothersome is that physicians initially diagnose disorders other than SAH in up to 25% of cases.[1,58] Physician misdiagnoses can delay treatment for days.[58] Misdiagnosis is most likely in the least seriously ill patients, ones most likely to be helped by early medical or surgical therapy.

Acute Management

Patients with recent SAH are critically ill; their evaluation and treatment is urgent.[22,74,124] They should be transported rapidly to a medical center that has the capability to treat a patient with a ruptured aneurysm. Acute, potentially life-threatening complications should be anticipated (Table 54.2). Personnel should assess the patient quickly and perform frequent measurements of vital signs, blood pressure, and neurologic status. Heart rate should be monitored. The airway, breathing, and circulation should be supported, and if necessary, supplemental oxygen, endotracheal intubation, or ventilatory assistance should be given.[124] Intravenous access is placed to expedite emergent administration of drugs. Normal saline or 0.45 saline can be given at a slow rate to maintain patency of the line.

Table 54.3 Initial Diagnostic Evaluation of a Patient with a Suspected Subarachnoid Hemorrhage

Cranial CT (without contrast)
Cerebrospinal fluid exam (if CT does not show blood)
Complete blood count
Platelet count
Prothrombin time
Partial thromboplastin time
Serum glucose
Blood urea nitrogen and serum creatine
Serum electrolytes
Serum calcium
Urinalysis
Electrocardiogram
Chest radiograph
Cerebral arteriogram
Optional tests (in selected cases)
Cervical spine radiograph (comatose patient—unwitnessed—to rule out spine injury)
Arterial blood gases
Liver function tests
Bleeding time
Electroencephalogram
Contrast-enhanced CT
Magnetic resonance imaging
Cerebral blood flow study
Transcranial Doppler ultrasonography

Abbreviation: CT, computed tomography.

Table 54.4 Abnormalities Found by Unenhanced Cranial CT in Persons with Recent[a] Subarachnoid Hemorrhage

Abnormality	%
Subarachnoid blood	85–92
Focal, thin collection	
Focal, thick collection	
Diffuse, thin collection	
Diffuse, thick collection	
Intraventricular blood	15–20
Intraparenchymal blood	15–20
Subdural blood	1–2
Hydrocephalus	10–20
Mass effect	5–8
Ischemic lesion	1–2
Aneurysm	5
Normal	5–10

Abbreviation: CT, computed tomography.

[a] Within 3 days, yield highest on day of hemorrhage and then declines.

The initial evaluation should include CT, chest x-ray, electrocardiogram, and blood work (Table 54.3) CT can demonstrate subarachnoid blood and a number of other complications (Table 54.4 and Fig. 54.1). When CT shows intracranial bleeding, a lumbar puncture should be avoided. CT will be normal in approximately 10% of cases. If CT is negative, a cerebrospinal fluid (CSF) specimen should be obtained. Magnetic resonance imaging (MRI) may not be as good as CT for detecting subarachnoid blood (Fig. 54.2). Once the diagnosis of SAH is confirmed, arteriography is required to demonstrate the presence and location of the aneurysm (Fig. 54.3). Both carotid circulations and the entire vertebrobasilar system are examined, although the sequence of the arterial studies is influenced by the findings on CT. If the first study is negative, a second arteriogram is performed approximately 2 weeks after SAH in persons whose bleeding is not in a perimesencephalic pattern. A repeat arteriogram will allow detection of an aneurysm in an additional 1% to 2% of patients.

Patients are admitted to a unit where monitoring equipment and neurologically trained nurses are available. Acute care is divided into general supportive efforts and treatment of specific complications (Table 54.5).[74,124] For the first 24 hours, blood pressure, vital signs, and neurologic assessments are measured hourly. Thereafter, examinations are spaced farther apart in stable patients. Cardiac monitoring and, if necessary, continuous intraarterial or noninvasive blood pressure monitoring is usually extended for at least 24 to 48 hours after admission.

Forced bed rest is a traditional part of management. Visitors and external stimuli are restricted. Passive range of motion exercises and frequent turning are performed. A water mattress or an alternating-pressure pneumatic bed can help reduce the risk of pressure sores or atelectasis. Patients are assisted with self-care activities, such as bathing. Black et al[9] showed that external pneumatic calf compression stockings reduce the inci-

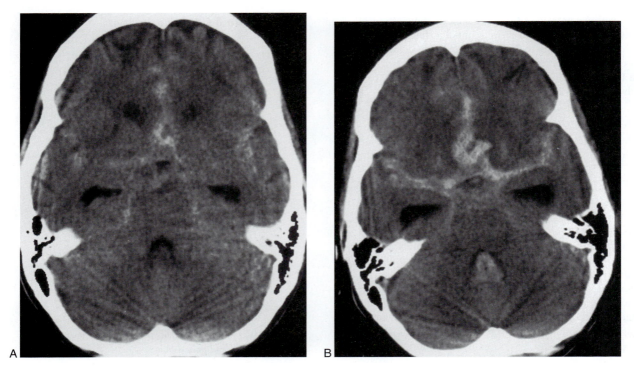

Figure 54.1 Two computed tomographic scans obtained approximately 4 hours apart in a patient who had a recurrent hemorrhage. (**A**) Subarachnoid blood in interhemispheric fissure and basal cisterns is seen. The patient suddenly deteriorated. (**B**) A second study shows additional subarachnoid blood and intraventricular hemorrhage. Hydrocephalus (enlargement of the temporal horns) is also present.

dence of deep vein thrombosis. Subcutaneous heparin as a prophylaxis for deep venous thrombosis should be avoided. Gentle pulmonary toilet and nursing care to avoid pneumonia are important. The value of forced bed rest in preventing rebleeding was tested by the Cooperative Study of Intracranial Aneurysms and Subarachnoid Hemorrhage: the cumulative rate of rebleeding was 25% during the first 14 days after SAH.[86] In general, the prognosis of persons treated only with forced bed rest now represents the natural history of SAH.

Because intravenously administered drugs often are needed, IV access is maintained with an infusion of normal saline. Alert persons are given a soft, high-fiber diet supplemented by stool softeners.[124] Caffeinated and alcoholic beverages are avoided. Stuporous and comatose patients are not fed during the acute treatment period. If a seriously ill person is stable several days after SAH and the airway is secured, nasogastric feedings can be instituted. Parenteral hyperalimentation usually is not required. Multivitamins are added to the diet or IV fluids.

SYMPTOMATIC TREATMENT

Patients often are confused or agitated as the result of brain injury, hydrocephalus, or increased intracranial pressure. Pain or nausea can also lead to irritability. Agitation increases the risk of rebleeding and aggravates increased intracranial pressure. Control of pain or nausea can calm an upset patient. Regular administration of diazepam or phenobarbital may be useful in providing sedation in agitated patients.

The headache of SAH is intense and patients should receive ample medication.[74,124] Most alert persons require frequent doses of analgesics such as codeine, meperidine, or morphine. The drugs usually are given parenterally, in equianalgesic dosages to those administered to other patients with severe pain. These medications can be combined with acetaminophen, hydroxyzine hydrochloride, or promethazine. Some patients will have photophobia and phonophobia; a quiet, dark environment will help relieve some of these symptoms that may aggravate headache. Sedation and sleep also might help control pain.

Aspirin affects platelet aggregation and prolongs the bleeding time. There is concern that aspirin could potentiate rebleeding. Juvela[53] has suggested that aspirin might reduce the risk of delayed ischemic deficits. At present, however, the use of aspirin as an analgesic is avoided until the risk of rebleeding has been eliminated. Severe nausea and intense vomiting are frequent and important complaints, particularly during the first 24 hours after SAH, and nauseated patients should receive antiemetics, such as trimethobenzamide or prochlorperazine, to control these symptoms.

ANTICONVULSANTS

Approximately 25% of patients have seizures, most of which occur within the first 24 hours.[44,111] Hart et al[44] noted that 63% of the seizures happened at the time of aneurysmal rupture. However, some of these "seizures" may not be truly epileptic phenomena but may represent transient decerebrate posturing secondary to increased intracranial pressure.[28,44] There is no correlation between epileptic seizures at the time of aneurysmal rupture and the risk of rebleeding, early mortality, or major morbidity.[44,111] Although seizures after hospitalization are uncommon, they can be associated with recurrent hemorrhage. While physicians do prescribe anticonvulsants to patients who have had a seizure as part of SAH, the prophylactic use of these drugs in persons who have not had a seizure is controversial. The rationale for prophylactic treatment with anticonvulsants is that a seizure is a dangerous event in a person with a recent SAH. Because of the low rate of seizures after admission, Hart et al[44] and Sundaram and Chow[111] doubted the need for routine administration of anticonvulsants to patients with recent SAH. However, others advise regular use of either phenobarbital or phenytoin to reduce the risk of seizures. No trial has tested the value of anticonvulsants in persons with SAH. Pending such a trial, the decision to prescribe anticonvulsants is individualized. The benefit in seizure prophylaxis must be weighed against potential adverse reactions. If a patient is having convulsions, IV doses of anticonvulsants are given.

MYOCARDIAL ISCHEMIA AND CARDIAC ARRHYTHMIA

Cardiac arrhythmias can be detected in almost all patients during the first few hours after SAH, and in approximately 20% the arrhythmias are severe or life-threatening (Table

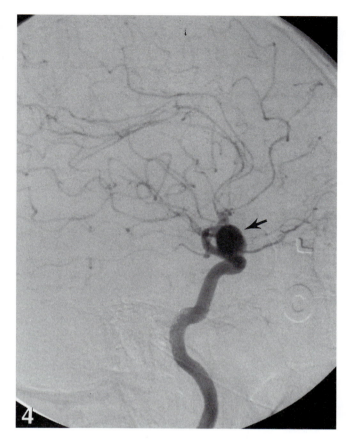

Figure 54.3 Left lateral carotid arteriogram using subtraction technique shows an aneurysm of the internal carotid artery (arrow) in the region of the carotid siphon.

Figure 54.2 T$_1$-weighted magnetic resonance imaging (MRI) demonstrates a large aneurysm (arrow) arising from the right internal carotid artery.

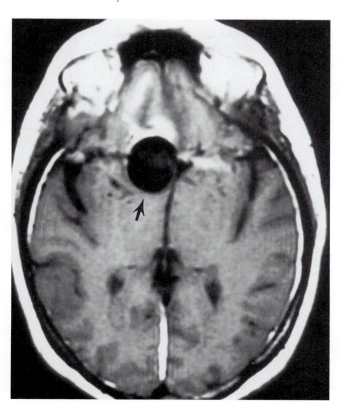

54.6).[21,73,90] Ventricular arrhythmias can be a cause of sudden death after SAH. DiPasquale et al[21] noted torsade de pointes (a chaotic form of ventricular tachycardia with the QRS complexes varying between positive and negative polarity) in 3.8% of 132 patients who had Holter monitoring. Changes resembling those of acute myocardial ischemia can be noted in 50% to 80% of patients.[33] In fact, many persons with SAH have secondary myocardial ischemia and left ventricular dysfunction.[129] Elevations of the cardiac isoenzyme, creatine kinase, also are noted. Subendocardial areas of focal ischemic necrosis are found among patients who died of SAH even when they had no history of coronary artery disease.

The frequency of electrocardiographic changes can be predicted by the severity of bleeding detected by CT and the patient's neurologic status; the changes are most common among seriously ill persons with diffuse subarachnoid blood, intraventricular hemorrhage, or a large intracerebral hematoma.[73] Although Brouwers et al[13] correlated elevated plasma levels of norepinephrine with a poor outcome after SAH, they could not find a relationship of norepinephrine to cardiac ischemia. Still, it is assumed that the release of catecholamines by the posterior hypothalamus is important in the development of cardiac complications. Markedly elevated levels of norepinephrine can lead to hypokalemia, systemic hypertensive effects, left ventricular strain, coronary artery vasospasm,

Table 54.5 Medical Management of Persons with Aneurysmal Subarachnoid Hemorrhage

Emergent treatment
  Support airway
  Supplemental oxygen
  Ventilatory assistance
  Intravenous access—normal saline or 0.45 saline

Other acute treatment
  Close observation
    Cardiac monitoring
    Arterial pressure monitoring
  Bed rest with restricted monitoring
    Passive/active range of motion
    Water/alternating pressure mattress
    Assistance with self-care
    Gentle pulmonary toilet
    Avoidance of indwelling bladder catheter, if possible
  External pneumatic calf compression stockings
  IV saline with multiple vitamins (2–3 L daily)
Alert patients—soft, high-fiber diet
Obtunded patients—nasogastric feedings
Stool softeners
Antacids
Sucralfate

Symptomatic treatment
  Analgesics
    Codeine, meperidine, morphine
    Supplemented by acetaminophen, promethazine, or hydroxyzine
      HCl
  Agitation
    Short-acting benzodiazepine or barbiturates
  Nausea/vomiting
    Trimethobenzamide
    Prochlorperazine
  Seizures
    Phenytoin
    Phenobarbital
  Cardiac arrhythmias
    Propranolol
    Metoprolol
    Calcium channel blockers

Neurogenic pulmonary edema
  Dobutamine
Arterial hypertension
  Oral:
    Propranolol
    Labetalol
    Hydralazine
    Nimodipine
    Nicardipine
  Parenteral:
    Esmolol
    Vasotec
Hyponatremia
  Continue normal saline fluids
  Avoid diuretics
  Modest fluid restriction
  Hyperosmolar sodium fluids
  Fludrocortisone
Increased intracranial pressure
  Intracranial pressure monitoring
  Elevation of head of bed
  Correct metabolic disturbance
  Hyperventilation
  Avoidance of corticosteroids
  Furosemide
  Mannitol
  Intraventricular catheter to drain CSF
  Repeated lumbar punctures
  Surgical decompression
Vasospasm
  Nimodipine
Rebleeding
  Aminocaproic acid/tranexamic acid
  Surgical clipping
  Endovascular obliteration

Abbreviation: CSF, cerebrospinal fluid.

a "stunned" myocardium, or cardiac toxicity.[90,129] Administration of a β-blocker such as propranolol may reduce the number and severity of cardiac sequelae. In a small study, Neil-Dwyer et al[80] noted necrotic myocardial lesions in six patients who died after SAH and who had not taken propranolol. No necrotic lesions were seen among six persons who died but who had taken the drug. Hamann et al[42] gave metoprolol to 11 patients with SAH; no major side effects were noted from the use of this selective agent. Cardiac rhythms remained normal and no additional antihypertensive drugs were needed. Further study is needed on the potential value of a β-blocker or calcium channel blocker in reducing cardiac sequelae of SAH. A particularly vulnerable subgroup of patients may exist. Pending more definitive data, administration of these drugs is decided on a case-by-case basis; there appears little reason

Table 54.6 Electrocardiographic Abnormalities after Subarachnoid Hemorrhage

Prominent P waves	Prominent/inverted U waves
Prolonged/shortened P-R interval	Pathological Q waves
Broad/inverted/flattened T waves	S in V, and R in V_5 combined
Prolonged/shortened Q-T interval	>35
Elevation/depression S-T segment	Rhythm disturbances

to give drugs to all patients routinely. Since the first 24 to 48 hours is the period of highest risk for cardiac complications, there is little justification to initiate treatment with these drugs after that time.

Neurogenic pulmonary edema is a rare, severe complication that usually occurs in critically ill persons. Markedly increased extravascular lung water and an intrapulmonary shunt lead to hypoxia. This complication is frequently ascribed to increased sympathetic activity that leads to a "stunned" myocardium, heart failure, and vascular congestion.[124] Treatment is difficult but includes oxygen and positive pressure ventilatory assistance.[124] Dobutamine (5 to $10\mu g/kg/hr$) increases the cardiac index and left ventricular stroke work index and decreases the total peripheral vascular resistance, leading to a diuresis and a reduction in pulmonary congestion; it is now recommended for the treatment of neurogenic pulmonary edema following SAH.[71,124]

ANTIHYPERTENSIVE TREATMENT

Arterial hypertension is common; it results from elevated catecholamines and renins produced by hypothalamic disturbances (Table 54.5).[81,115] Additionally, elevated intracranial pressure can induce arterial hypertension to maintain adequate cerebral perfusion pressure. Arterial hypertension may also be secondary to seizures, vomiting, agitation, or pain. In addition, a patient may also have pre-existing hypertension.

Hypertension after SAH is correlated with an increased rate of vasospasm and higher mortality.[115] Arterial hypertension also marks patients at high risk for recurrent hemorrhage. Administration of antihypertensive drugs is a traditional component of early management of SAH.[74,124] However, rapid or major reductions in blood pressure may be dangerous. Patients with vasospasm or increased intracranial pressure can have worsening of neurologic deficits or deterioration in consciousnes in conjunction with a drop in blood pressure. Some antihypertensive drugs (nitroglycerin, sodium nitroprusside, apresoline) are vasodilators and secondary enlargement of the cerebral vascular bed might increase intracranial pressure.

Blood pressure often returns to normal after admission to the hospital or when symptoms such as pain are treated; thus, the use of an antihypertensive drug might be avoided. Patients with mild hypertension (mean arterial blood pressure less than 120 mmHg) should not receive antihypertensive drugs. Persons with a mean arterial blood pressure above 120 mmHg or a systolic blood pressure higher than 180 mmHg should be treated. The goal should be to reach blood pressure levels that are normal for the patient and to avoid hypotension.

While alert persons with elevated arterial blood pressure can be given oral medications, parenteral drugs have the advantage of a prompt response. Antihypertensive drugs used prior to SAH usually are continued and should not be stopped abruptly. Short-acting antihypertensive drugs are desirable because of rapid resolution of the unwanted effects of excessive decline in blood pressure. Because persons often are dehydrated or hyponatremic, diuretics are avoided. Propranolol, hydralazine, or labetalol are the most frequently prescribed oral antihypertensives. Nimodipine or nicardipine may be use-

ful antihypertensive agents in persons with recent SAH. Patients with markedly elevated or unstable arterial pressures may warrant a continuous IV infusion of labetalol or sodium nitroprusside. The rate of infusion is adjusted to responses in blood pressure. If the mean arterial blood pressure is >125 mmHg, esmolol IM or vasotec intravenously can be given.[124] Intravenous drugs should be given only if continuous intrarterial or noninvasive blood pressure monitoring can be performed. The dosage of any antihypertensive drug is individualized. Patients often are very sensitive to antihypertensive drugs, and drops in blood pressure can be greater than expected. Required doses may be less than those needed for other hypertensive emergencies.

Drug-induced hypotension might help prevent rebleeding. In a randomized trial, the Cooperative Aneurysm Study compared drug-induced hypotension to forced bed rest.[82] Vigorous use of antihypertensive drugs was associated with a 2-week mortality of 25% and a rebleeding rate of 20%. These rates were similar to those noted with bed rest. However, this study was performed more than 25 years ago, and the antihypertensive drugs tested included diuretics, reserpine, and methyldopa. Newer antihypertensive drugs such as calcium channel blockers, selective β-blockers, or angiotensin-converting enzyme inhibitors might be safer and more effective in lessening the risk of recurrent hemorrhage. Antihypertensive drugs should be discontinued if a patient develops signs of ischemia secondary to vasospasm, to allow for an increase in cerebral perfusion pressure.

MANAGEMENT OF ELECTROLYTES AND FLUIDS

Disturbances in water balance and sodium balance occur in approximately one-third of patients.[126] These complications are most likely to develop in critically ill persons with large hemorrhages. Hyponatremia and volume depletion are correlated with a poor prognosis and the subsequent development of hydrocephalus, vasospasm, and ischemic stroke.[125] Severe hyponatremia can cause convulsions and is one of the causes of coma after SAH. The primary indication for rapid correction of hyponatremia is development of seizures in a patient without neurologic disease; however, this indication becomes blurred in patients with recent SAH. Conventional management of mild to moderate hyponatremia is fluid restriction. More vigorous treatment of hyponatremia consists of IV administration of hypertonic saline combined with a diuretic, such as furosemide, to prevent cardiac failure.

In the past, hyponatremia after SAH was attributed largely to the inappropriate secretion of antidiuretic hormone and was treated with fluid restriction. Recent evidence suggests that both sodium and water are lost.[126,127] Declines in plasma volume, red blood cell mass, and total blood volume occur.[127] A negative sodium balance results from the kidney's inability to conserve sodium (cerebral salt wasting).[23] The mechanism of water and sodium loss after SAH has not been explained. Increased blood levels of atrial natriuretic factor and decreased renins have been implicated. The source of plasma and cerebrospinal fluid (CSF) atrial natriuretic factor is presumably the heart, not the brain. Weinand et al[122] suggest that interplay between antidiuretic hormone and atrial natriuretic factor may differ considerably among patients.

Fluid restriction to control hyponatremia and the development of cerebral edema was tested in a randomized study; no improvement in mortality was found.[83] Recent evidence suggests that strict fluid restriction is dangerous because it leads to contracted blood volume, increased blood viscosity, and hemoconcentration. These changes might increase the risk of ischemia in persons prone to vasospasm.[125]

In contrast to previous attempts to restrict fluids, most patients now are given at least maintenance volumes of colloid and crystalloid solutions. The usual daily administration of liquids, including dietary and intravenous fluids, is at least 2 to 3 L.[124] Adjustments may be required depending upon urinary or insensible water losses. If there is concern about the IV fluids inducing cardiac failure, a solution containing a lower concentration of sodium is used. Placement of a central venous pressure or pulmonary artery wedge pressure line to evaluate the cardiac status of patients given large volumes of fluids may improve safety. Increased volumes of sodium-containing fluids will overcome the volume contraction but may not reverse the hyponatremia.[23] If the serum sodium does not normalize, modest fluid restriction or infusion of a hyperosmolar solution containing sodium can be instituted. Simultaneous use of diuretics is avoided because they induce natriuresis as well as water loss.

Wijdicks et al[127] administered 0.2 mg of fludrocortisone twice a day combined with daily fluid intake of at least 3 L to 39 patients with recent SAH and noted improvements in plasma volume and sodium balance. Wijdicks[124] recommends the addition of fludrocortisone to the regimen when the serum sodium is < 125 mmol/L. Hypokalemia is often noted after SAH. It probably results from vomiting or can be secondary to elevated levels of corticosteroids, renin, or catecholamines. Because hypokalemia is associated with life-threatening cardiac arrhythmias after SAH, it should be corrected rapidly.

MANAGEMENT OF OTHER MEDICAL COMPLICATIONS

Gastrointestinal bleeding can result from hemorrhagic gastritis, stress gastric ulcers, or an esophageal tear secondary to vomiting. Persons should be given antacids every 4 to 6 hours in an effort to reduce the risk of these side effects; dosages can be administered via a nasogastric tube placed in obtunded persons.[74] Wijdicks[124] recently recommended sucralfate to prevent gastrointestinal side effects. Because sucralfate does not have central nervous system side effects, it has potential advantages in critically ill patients prone to depression in consciousness.

Obtunded patients are at high risk for adult respiratory distress syndrome, atelectasis, pulmonary hypoventilation, or aspiration pneumonia. Securing the airway, bronchopulmonary toilet, and ventilatory assistance may be required. Other events such as renal failure, hepatic dysfunction, urinary tract infections, or other illnesses should be treated. Therapy for pre-existing medical conditions is continued.

TREATMENT OF INCREASED INTRACRANIAL PRESSURE

A decline in consciousness is the hallmark of increased intracranial pressure, which, in turn, can result from a large intracerebral or intraventricular hematoma, mass effect of a secondary ischemic lesion, cerebral edema, or hydrocephalus. SAH also causes vasoparalysis and loss of autoregulation; dilated intracranial vessels will aggravate intracranial pressure. Intracranial pressure is elevated markedly within a few minutes of an aneurysmal rupture; it may even transiently equal mean arterial blood pressure. A massive rise in intracranial pressure probably is one of the causes of sudden death after SAH, and is one of the etiologies of several other complications including cardiac arrhythmias. High intracranial pressure may also lead to intracranial circulatory hypoperfusion, which induces ischemia. Prompt, aggressive treatment of increased intracranial pressure is one the keys to successful treatment of SAH.[124]

Several medical and surgical measures are available. Monitoring intracranial pressure is indicated for many patients; the results guide the timing of surgical or medical interventions. Technological advances that permit more accurate measurements include stereotactic placement of microscopic transducers in the brain or ventricles. These measures are not accompanied by prohibitive rates of complications. Continuous intraventricular drainage combined with monitoring is an option, but this technique can be complicated by a sudden reduction in intracranial pressure and changes in transmural pressure may precipitate recurrent aneurysmal rupture. Treatment of increased intracranial pressure includes elevating the head of the bed to promote venous drainage, fluid restriction, correction of hyponatremia, and preventing hypoventilation and secondary hypercarbia. Intubation and hyperventilation are indicated if a patient is deteriorating. There is no evidence that dexamethasone is useful in managing brain edema following intracranial hemorrhage. Because of the lack of established benefit in controlling intracranial hypertension and because of many potential side effects, it should not be given. Furosemide can reduce intracranial pressure by limiting production of CSF, and in an emergency it can be given. However, furosemide's diuretic effects can lead to electrolyte disturbances and hypovolemia. There are no studies testing its value in the management of recent SAH.

Mannitol is an osmotic agent that can be given to control increased intracranial pressure. A response is noted within minutes and the duration of effect is approximately 4 to 6 hours. The drug can be repeated as needed. Secondary dehydration, hyperosmolarity, and a rebound increase in brain edema are possible complications. Repeated measurements of osmolality and serum electrolytes should be done. Measurement of central venous or pulmonary artery wedge pressure also will improve the safety of this treatment.

Emergent evacuation of a large hematoma may be performed. Such hematomas, usually in the basal ganglia and adjacent white matter, are seen most frequently with ruptured aneurysms of the internal carotid or middle cerebral arteries. Surgical removal of the hematoma can be life-saving and is used to treat a rapidly worsening patient. Some patients recover and return to independent activity.[87,108,124] Patients who are in better clinical condition and those with a ruptured aneurysm of the middle cerebral artery are most likely to benefit. Patients with very large hematomas, extensive intraventricular hemorrhage, or shifts of midline structures on CT have the poorest postoperative outcomes. Unfortunately, these patients are most frequently referred for operation. Although the data to support a recommendation for surgical evacuation of a large hematoma are lacking, it is an option in any patient not responding to medical measures. Physicians and families need to be aware that the patient's life can be saved but that the neurologic sequelae of a severe intracerebral hematoma can be considerable.

HYDROCEPHALUS

Hydrocephalus is a frequent complication that results from massive collections of blood that fill the ventricles, block the aqueduct of Sylvius, or obstruct the fourth ventricle. Blood can fill the subarachnoid cisterns or coat the arachnoid villi. The prolonged presence of extensive subarachnoid clots is strongly associated with the appearance of hydrocephalus; thus, an intervention that extends the presence of these clots may promote development of hydrocephalus. Conversely, therapies that stimulate clot lysis may lessen the risk of hydrocephalus.[111]

Hydrocephalus after SAH can be divided into three categories: (1) acute—appearing within hours of aneurysmal rupture, (2) subacute—developing a few days after the ictus, and (3) delayed—ventricular dilatation that is noted weeks to years later.[36,46] Acute hydrocephalus is an important cause of massively increased intracranial pressure and coma. Subacute hydrocephalus is a cause of a gradual decline in consciousness that occurs a few days following the hemorrhage. Intracranial pressure is more modestly elevated. The rate of delayed communicating hydrocephalus after SAH is reported to be 7%. Symptoms of delayed hydrocephalus are subacute dementia, gait apraxia, and bladder incontinence. In this setting, intracranial pressure often fluctuates and may not be consistently elevated.

Depending on the criteria used for the diagnosis of acute hydrocephalus, its incidence varies considerably between series. Based on CT evidence of ventricular enlargement, Black[8] diagnosed the presence of acute hydrocephalus in 63% of patients (Fig. 54.1). Others have reported a frequency of 16% to 34%. Some patients with ventricular enlargement may be asymptomatic. However, most will have decreased consciousness. Besides a decline in alertness, other symptoms of acute hydrocephalus include bilateral motor signs, miosis, and downward deviation of the eyes. Acute hydrocephalus predicts increased mortality and morbidity and is correlated with subsequent development of vasospasm and ischemic stroke.[8] A patient with acute hydrocephalus can be observed, medically managed and followed with sequential CT studies, and treated with repeated lumbar puncture. Although acute hydrocephalus may resolve spontaneously, most patients require placement of a temporary ventriculoperitoneal or ventriculocaval shunt.[36,46] Insertion of a ventricular catheter may be difficult in a patient with an intraventricular clot, because it may occlude the catheter. Inagawa et al[50] used continuous cisternal drainage; this method might relieve intracranial pressure as well as expedite lavage of blood from the subarachnoid space. Placement of a shunt should be recommended for any patient with depressed consciousness and enlarging ventricles. Some patients require only temporary placement; if necessary, the shunt can be made permanent later. Shunting is not always effective. Hasen et al[45] reported a high rate of shunt-related complications, including intracranial infections.

Rebleeding

Recurrent hemorrhage is a feared complication of SAH. It is a leading cause of death and neurologic morbidity during the first 2 weeks after SAH and is often a fatal complication.[3,47,51] In the series of Broderick et al[12] rebleeding accounted for half of the deaths that occurred more than 2 days after SAH. Mortality among patients who have rebleeding is approximately twice that of persons with a single hemorrhage.

Preventing recurrent hemorrhage is a major goal of medical management. Torner et al[116] found that the greatest risk period for rebleeding is during the first 24 hours after the ictus. It peaked at approximately 4% of patients during that time. In a Swedish series 9.6% of all patients admitted within 24 hours of SAH had very early rebleeding; most of these patients died.[47] Steiger et al[109] found a low rate of rebleeding between 5 to 13 days after SAH. The cumulative rate of rebleeding during the first 2 weeks after SAH is approximately 15% to 25%.[116] Edner and Ronne-Engstrom[24] found more than 50% of rebleeding episodes occurred within 1 week of SAH. Thereafter, the risk of rebleeding declines quickly. The rate of rebleeding is 0.5% per day for the time window of 10 to 30 days after SAH. The rate of recurrent hemorrhage after 1 month drops to 2% to 3% year and persists at that level for at least the next 10 years.[116] The early high rate of recurrent hemorrhage has implications for the choice of treatment. Bleeding can recur even before a surgical team can be mobilized or before a drug can reach "therapeutic" levels in blood and CSF.

Several clinical features identify persons at highest risk for early rebleeding. The most important is the admitting level of consciousness; patients in coma are at greatest risk. Rebleeding is also more common among older persons, women, and those with a systolic blood pressure >170 mmHg. The results of baseline CT do not predict rebleeding.

Recurrent hemorrhage usually causes a sudden headache and a rapid change in neurologic condition, including a drop in consciousness. Extensor spasms or posturing are important early signs. A "convulsion" that occurs during the acute period after SAH often marks a recurrent hemorrhage.[44] However, rebleeding in a comatose patient may be overlooked. It may be manifested only by a sudden change in respiratory pattern or vital signs.

Recurrent hemorrhage should be sought in any patient who develops a new headache or worsens after SAH. The differential diagnosis of rebleeding is listed in Table 54.7. The clinical diagnosis of rebleeding can be incorrect in as many as one-third of cases. Other causes of the worsening include seizures, ischemia, or medical complications. The diagnosis of rebleeding should not be made solely on clinical features, as this leads to overdiagnosis. Recurrent hemorrhage can be proved most

Table 54.7 Differential Diagnosis Neurologic
Worsening after Subarachnoid Hemorrhage

Recurrent hemorrhage	Hypotension
Vasospasm—brain ischemia	Hypoxia
Subacute hydrocephalus	Hyperglycemia/hypoglycemia
Seizures	Effects from drugs
Hyponatremia	Effects of medical complications
Hypocalcemia	(pneumonia, renal failure, etc.)

easily by the presence of additional blood on CT (Table 54.7 and Fig. 54.1B). Changes in CSF may be difficult to interpret.

Measures to ameliorate recurrent hemorrhage are not effective; therefore, treatment is aimed at prevention. Choices include prolonged bed rest, drug-induced hypotension, carotid ligation, antifibrinolytic drugs, intracranial clipping of the aneurysm, and endovascular obliteration of the aneurysm. The utility of forced bed rest and drug-induced hypotension in preventing rebleeding have been discussed previously. Steiger et al[109] concluded that nimodipine, given to prevent vasospasm and ischemia following SAH, also lowers the risk of rebleeding. This benefit is probably from its actions on lowering blood pressure. Thie and Heaze[114] treated 111 patients with factor XIII concentrate for 15 days after SAH. No adverse effects were seen and only nine patients had recurrent hemorrhage. No additional clinical studies of this medical therapy are available. Carotid ligation can be performed to prevent rebleeding from aneurysms of the distal internal carotid artery that cannot be approached by an intracranial operation.[92] The goal is to reduce transmural pressure on the aneurysmal wall or thrombosis of the aneurysm and thus lower the risk of recurrent rupture. Because of advances in intracranial operative techniques and development of invasive neuroradiologic procedures, carotid ligation is done rarely.

ANTIFIBRINOLYTIC THERAPY

The rationale for the use of antifibrinolyic therapy (aminocaproic acid or tranexamic acid) is that the perianeurysmal clot formed by the initial hemorrhage abuts and supports the aneurysm, thus helping to prevent rerupture. Treatment would be given before surgery to prevent rebleeding while the patient is recovering from the acute effects of SAH. Antifibrinolytic drugs cross the blood-brain barrier, but peak CSF levels are lower than plasma levels and are also delayed.[117] When these drugs are given as a constant IV infusion, a steady state in CSF is reached only at 36 hours. This means that the possible therapeutic level of drug in CSF may not be achieved during the period of highest risk for recurrent hemorrhage.

The use of antifibrinolytic drugs is controversial. Studies provide conflicting data. A randomized, placebo-controlled trial of tranexamic acid was performed in the United Kingdom and The Netherlands.[121] Mortality was 28% among the 130 persons with aneurysms who were treated with tranexamic acid and 32% among 155 placebo-treated patients who had aneurysms—a result that is not statistically significant. Although rebleeding was reduced considerably with treatment,

the positive effects in preventing recurrent bleeding were negated by a significantly higher rate of ischemic stroke in the actively treated group. Kassell et al[61] compared the results of treatment of 467 patients with aneurysmal SAH seen within 3 days, who had delayed surgery, and who received antifibrinolytic drugs with outcomes in 205 patients who did not receive either tranexamic acid or aminocaproic acid. Although it was not a randomized trial, the two populations were similar. The 14-day rebleeding rate was reduced from 19.4% to 11.7% with treatment. Conversely, ischemic events developed in 32.4% of patients given antifibrinolytic drugs and 22.7% of the controls.

Clinicians are concerned about the safety of antifibrinolytic drugs. Although critically ill persons with SAH are at bed rest for prolonged periods, the frequency of deep vein thrombosis or pulmonary embolism is low among treated patients. A fluminant myopathy, rhabdomyolysis, or myoglobinuria can complicate prolonged administration (more than 2 weeks) of high doses of aminocaproic acid.[14] High doses of aminocaproic acid can increase bleeding by inhibiting platelet function.[35] Antifibrinolytic drugs accentuate the development of hydrocephalus.[36,61]

Ischemic stroke is the most feared potential side effect of antifibrinolytic therapy. The increased risk of ischemia might be the result of (1) a persistent subarachnoid clot that induces vasospasm (2) an intravascular change in coagulation that potentiates intra-arterial thrombosis or embolism, or (3) a change in blood viscosity that impairs perfusion. Using sequential measurements of cerebral blood flow, Tsementzis et al[119] found reductions in flow following the administration of tranexamic acid. This potentiation of hypoperfusion could be an important factor in worsening ischemia in a person with vasospasm. Two large studies, previously described, noted that ischemic events negated the efficacy of antifibrinolytic therapy in preventing rebleeding.[61,121] The risk of ischemia with treatment markedly increases at approximately the seventh day after SAH. Beck et al[7] found that the combination of nicardipine and aminocaproic acid could be given successfully; the rates of both rebleeding and ischemic stroke were low. Additional research is needed to examine the usefulness of the combination of antifibrinolytic and calcium channel blocking drugs. If the risks of both rebleeding and ischemia are reduced, this combined regimen would allow delaying operation until patients are more stable.

Antifibrinolytic drugs are the only effective medical treatment currently available to reduce the risk of early rebleeding following SAH. Using a decision tree analysis, Dippel et al[22] concluded that early treatment with antifibrinolytic drugs and nimodipine followed by delayed operation is the optimal treatment strategy for good condition patients. Antifibrinolytic drugs remain a part of the preoperative care of persons scheduled for delayed surgery. Still, the risks of treatment must be weighed against the potential for preventing recurrent hemorrhage. These drugs should not be given if a large amount of subarachnoid blood is seen on CT because of the high risk of ischemic stroke.[22] The duration of treatment is limited to 10 to 14 days and the drug is stopped 6 to 8 hours before surgery. This therapy should not be started when a patient is scheduled for early operation or in a person who has a delayed diagnosis because persons surviving 7 to 14 days after SAH have already passed the period of highest risk for rebleeding. There is little indication to give these drugs to persons with nonaneurysmal SAH.

INTRACRANIAL OPERATION

Surgery is an important component of management. Indications for surgery include clipping the aneurysm to prevent rebleeding, placement of a shunt to treat hydrocephalus, or evacuation of a hematoma. Most important is the treatment of the aneurysm. Most patients should have surgery. Exceptions are considered on a case-by-case basis; for example, the patient's age, the severity of the neurologic injury, or the presence of serious comorbid diseases may weigh against an intracranial operation. While persons older than 60 years tolerate intracranial operation less well than younger persons, age alone is not a reason for excluding surgery from a treatment regimen.

For most patients, the question is not whether the aneurysm should be clipped but, rather, what is the ideal time for the operation. The optimal time for intracranial operation is not established. Early surgery (within 3 days of SAH) eliminates the risk for rebleeding and could be done before vasospasm appears. The primary reason for delaying surgery has been that a lag permits the patient's condition to improve before being subjected to the stresses associated with and the risk of an intracranial operation. In the past, early intracranial surgery was complicated by high morbidity and mortality. Because surgery performed 10 to 14 days after SAH was associated with much better postoperative results, delayed operation became a standard part of care. Some authors still advocate delayed operation.[22] However, to delay surgery leaves the aneurysm untreated during the period of highest risk for rebleeding. Surgeons rightfully point out that overall results of management, not just postoperative statistics, should be compared. The overall results of early medical care followed by a delayed operation are not satisfactory.[3]

Neurosurgical techniques, including the operating microscope, advances in neuroanesthesia, and improved perioperative care ease early intracranial operation. Several reports have spurred reconsideration of early intracranial surgery (less than 3 days after SAH). Kassel et al[56] noted that the number of medical complications, the frequency of vasospasm, and the length of hospitalization were reduced by early operation. Some investigators suggested that lavage of the subarachnoid space during early operation would prevent vasospasm by removal of clots or that operative clipping of the aneurysm would ease treatment of vasospasm.[56]

Several groups describe favorable results from early surgery combined with a variety of interventions, including therapy with calcium entry blockers or volume expansion and monitoring with transcranial Doppler.[70] Juvela et al[54] concluded that early surgery was associated with a decline in deaths due to either rebleeding or surgery by 32% and in mortality from all causes by 21%.

In a nationwide study in Japan, Nishimoto et al[85] noted that mortality among persons operated on within 48 hours of SAH was not lower than among those who had surgery later. This was not a controlled study and included persons who had surgery to treat a major intracerebral hematoma, but the mortality among persons in good condition who had surgery 24 to 48 hours after SAH was 44%. A small trial in Finland demonstrated improved outcomes with early operation.[88] While the data favor early operation, the results were distorted by

a simultaneous randomization to placebo or active treatment with calcium channel blocking drugs. Miyaoka et al[76] reported better management results with early surgery in good condition patients, while those who were most seriously ill did better with delayed operations.

The influence of the timing of surgery was examined in a large international epidemiologic study that evaluated the outcomes of 3,521 patients hospitalized within 3 calendar days of SAH.[62,63] While not a randomized trial, its large numbers assured that prognostic factors were similar in the groups that had early or delayed surgery. Intracranial clipping of the aneurysm was done in approximately 92% of the 1,600 patients who had surgery planned for days 0 to 3. However, only 76% of persons with surgery planned for days 11 to 14 and 62% of those with surgery planned for 15 + days after SAH actually underwent operation; many patients died or developed major complications that contraindicated operation. Among patients who had surgery, postoperative results were generally superior with delayed operation performed after day 10; good outcomes were noted in 77% of those who had surgery on days 11 to 14 versus 66% of patients who had surgery on days 0 to 3. The rates of favorable outcome were similar among patients operated on each day during the 0- to 3-day interval. The postoperative results were analogous regardless of the patient's age, sex, admitting level of consciousness, or location of the aneurysm. Inclusion of the unfavorable outcomes that occurred while awaiting operation demonstrates that the results of early operation are equal to early medical care and delayed surgery; 62% of patients with surgery on days 11 to 14 and 63% of patients with surgery planned on days 0 to 3 had favorable responses. Early surgery was not associated with a high rate of intraoperative complications, such as rerupture of the aneurysm or worsening of brain edema.

Early operation reduces the mortality and morbidity from rebleeding. However, early operation does not seem to prevent the development of vasospasm or sufficiently ease the treatment of secondary ischemia to lower the morbidity and mortality from this complication. Early operation (less than 3 days of SAH) is effective, but the results of early surgery are not so overwhelming that it should be recommended for all cases. Early operation is not the standard of care. Plans for surgery should continue to be made on a case-by-case basis. For example, Deruty et al[20] restrict early operation only to alert persons who are younger than 50 years. An important consideration is the skill of the neurologic surgeon, who must have demonstrated success in operating on these acutely ill persons. If all these criteria are not met, the patient may not be best served by an early, emergent operation to clip the aneurysm. While the optimal time for surgery is unsettled, the potential benefit from early operation emphasizes the importance of early, accurate diagnosis.

ENDOVASCULAR TREATMENT TO OBLITERATE THE ANEURYSM

Endovascular obliteration of the aneurysm or parent vessel is used to treat aneurysms of the intracavernous or proximal portions of the internal carotid artery, including persons who have a carotid-cavernous fistula.[72,84] Tandem placement of balloons in the parent artery (trapping) can shrink the aneurysm or lead to its occlusion. Larson et al[67] treated 58 patients with aneurysms; they found that proximal occlusion or trapping of the internal carotid artery was relatively effective and the risk of ischemic stroke was low. However, detachable balloons can be difficult to place directly into an aneurysm. The sizes and shapes of the balloons may not correspond to the contour of the aneurysm.[84] Rarely, balloons can be lost and migrate into distal vessels. The balloons can deflate and the aneurysm can recanalize. Finally, balloons might place pressure on the aneurysmal wall and lead to a recurrent rupture.[84]

Development of microendovascular catheters and detachable coils has stimulated greater interest in endovascular occlusion of aneurysms.[75] In particular, aneurysms that are unclippable might be occluded by an endovascular treatment.[75,106] Casasco et al[16] placed coils in 71 aneurysms (43 within 3 days of SAH) primarily located on the vertebrobasilar arteries. Total occlusion was achieved in 84% of cases and outcomes were good in 60. Complications from treatment included occlusion of the parent artery, rerupture of the aneurysm, and heparin-induced bleeding. The usefulness of endovascular placement of coils to occlude a recently ruptured aneurysm has not been established. Neither the safety nor the long-term efficacy of this therapy has been established. Endovascular therapy is probably not as safe as conventional arteriography. It should be done only by skilled interventional neuroradiologists who are adept at the technique. A clinical trial comparing surgical clipping with endovascular occlusion is needed.

Recently, Kinguasa et al[65] reported the success of endovascular placement of a cellulose acetate polymer into recently ruptured aneurysms. Secondary thrombosis led to partial occlusion in 9 of 12 cases. Obliteration of the aneurysmal sac expedited ancillary care to treat vasospasm, and allowed the patients to stabilize before operative repair of the aneurysm. Further research is needed on this therapy.

Vasospasm and Ischemic Stroke

Early intracranial operation and antifibrinolytic drugs reduce the risk of recurrent hemorrhage. Yet, these advances are not accompanied by declines in mortality and morbidity primarily because of vasospasm-induced ischemic stroke. Brain infarction accounts for approximately one-third of all unfavorable outcomes after SAH.[60]

The term *vasospasm* is used to describe the luminal narrowing detected by arteriography performed approximately 1 week after SAH. Abnormalities may be restricted to one artery or involve several vessels. Although it can complicate bleeding from other sources, vasospasm usually is associated with ruptured aneurysms. Autopsy examination of patients dying from the effects of acute vasospasm reveal morphologic changes in capillaries, veins, small arteries, and larger arteries.[60] Changes include disruption of the internal elastic lamina, swelling of the media, smooth muscle necrosis, and infiltration of the adventitia by macrophages, lymphocytes, and plasma cells.

Smith et al[107] noted endothelial desquamation, intimal proliferation, necrosis and fibrosis of the media, and intramural deposits of type V collagen. They concluded that the lumen of the vessel can remain constricted for weeks after SAH. Degenerative changes in the medial and intimal layers can persist for at least 2 weeks.

The amount of blood in the subarachnoid space is correlated with the development of vasospasm.[60] A normal component of blood is presumably released at the time of SAH. This substance or a combination of factors, once liberated into the subarachnoid space, causes the vasospastic process. A large number of constituents of blood have been implicated, but oxyhemoglobin, a principal component of blood, may be the responsible pathogen.[27,79] Vasospasm has been ascribed to a prolonged arterial contraction, a substance that inhibits vasodilatation, an immunoreactive or inflammatory process, a mechanical phenomenon, or depressed arterial metabolism.[60,107] For example, Nagatani et al[79] proposed that the breakdown products of blood lead to impaired mitochondrial function and reduced energy levels in cerebral arteries. Elevations of platelet-activating factors that may mediate inflammatory responses and that are a close link to eicosanoids are common and are linked to infarction after SAH.[48] Findlay et al[27] concluded that vasospasm is related to sustained contraction of the media associated with degenerative changes in both smooth muscle cells and endothelium. Recently, Kasuya et al[64] concluded that vasospasm is the result of an impairment of endothelium-dependent relaxation. Disturbances in arachidonate metabolism and elevations of endothelin, a potent vasoconstrictor, also may be important in the development of vasospasm.[32,94,102] It is likely that vasospasm is the result of a complex, multifactorial process.

The arterial narrowing caused by vasospasm impairs cerebral autoregulation and increases cerebral vascular resistance.[60] Declines in perfusion pressure and blood flow lead to brain ischemia.[60] A low mean arterial pressure, elevated intracranial pressure, or increased viscosity secondary to hemoconcentration or dehydration can aggravate the process. The end result is infarction in the arterial beds of the involved arteries. Infarctions are usually cortical and in border zone regions between the anterior, middle, and posterior cerebral arteries.

Major arterial narrowing can be detected arteriographically at 1 week after SAH in approximately 70% of patients (Figs. 54.4 to 54.6).[60] Vasospasm causes symptoms in approximately 20% to 30% of patients.[60] The severity of the arterial narrowing correlates with the likelihood of ischemic signs and an unfavorable outcome. Vasospasm is seen most frequently in the distal portion of the internal carotid artery and proximal sections of the anterior and middle cerebral arteries. The site of the ruptured aneurysm does not influence the development of vasospasm, but a common location for the narrowing is adjacent to the clot and aneurysm. It also can be generalized or localized to an area of the brain remote from the aneurysm. Vasospasm is detected rarely before 48 hours of SAH, peaks at 5 to 10 days, and usually abates by 14 to 21 days.

Vasospasm is more likely to occur in young patients, women, patients in poor neurologic condition, those with acute hydrocephalus, or those with an abnormal ECG.[8,60] Juvela[53] recently reported that the use of aspirin before SAH can lessen the likelihood of vasospasm and ischemia. The extent of sub-

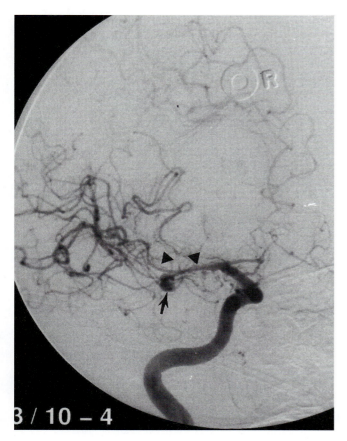

Figure 54.4 Anteroposterior view of a right carotid arteriogram using subtraction technique demonstrates an aneurysm of the right middle cerebral artery (arrow) and vasospasm of the middle cerebral artery (arrowheads).

arachnoid blood as seen on a early CT study is an important predictor.[29] Ischemic complications of vasospasm also are most likely to occur among persons who have hyponatremia, dehydration, or hypotension. The symptoms of vasospasm usually begin insidiously.[30] Findings can wax and wane over several hours or evolve suddenly. Increased headache, low-grade fever, increased meningismus, seizures, and disturbances of consciousness usually are followed by the appearance of focal neurologic deficits that primarily reflect ischemia in the vascular territories of the anterior and middle cerebral arteries. The process can proceed to infarction, leading to neurologic residuals and hypodense lesions detected by CT.

The differential diagnosis of vasospasm as the cause of neurologic worsening after SAH is the same as for rebleeding (Table 54.7). Alternative diagnoses should be excluded before vasospasm-induced ischemia is diagnosed. Arteriography is the most definitive way to establish a firm diagnosis of vasospasm. Cerebral blood flow measurements will detect local or generalized hypoperfusion.

Sequential transcranial Doppler studies are used to monitor for the development of vasospasm.[37,68] Progressive narrowing of the lumen can be accompanied by increased velocity in the arteries. Changes in flow velocity are uncommon during the first 48 hours after SAH.[68] Transcranial Doppler is particularly

useful in persons with narrowing in the middle cerebral artery.[37] Changes in velocity may precede the development of ischemic symptoms, and increases in velocity are highest among persons with ischemic deficits.[37] Disturbances in flow velocity are influenced by the patient's age, the presence of hypertension, or tissue hyperemia.[10,25,34] Flow velocities also can be affected by the extent of peripheral arteriolar resistance vessels, arterial anastomoses, or the use of nimodipine.[110] Although some researchers question the clinical value of transcranial Doppler assessments in management of persons with recent SAH,[16] other physicians routinely use the study to assess patient responses to treatment.[40] Current evidence supports the use of transcranial Doppler as an adjunctive way to monitor persons for the development of vasospasm. With future experience and with refinement and development of this technology, the need for arteriography in time may be eliminated.

PREVENTION AND TREATMENT OF VASOSPASM OR ISCHEMIC STROKE AFTER SUBARACHNOID HEMORRHAGE

A number of therapies that might prevent or reverse vasospasm have been examined. Early intracranial operation and lavage of the subarachnoid space may remove clots. The ra-

Figure 54.5 Lateral view of a vertebral arteriogram shows a lobulated aneurysm at the junction of the vertebral and posterior-inferior cerebellar arteries (large arrow) and vasospasm of the contralateral vertebral artery (small arrows).

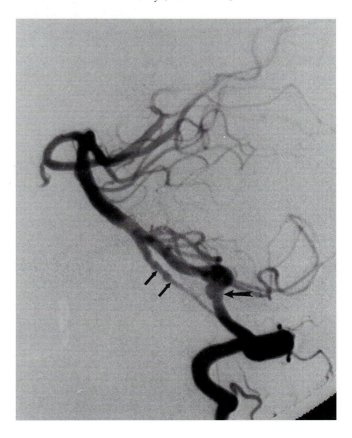

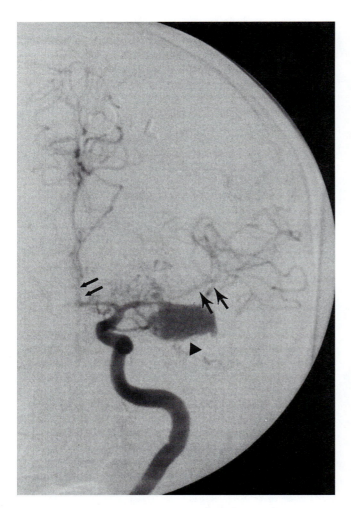

Figure 54.6 Anteroposterior view of a left carotid arteriogram using subtraction technique demonstrates a large fusiform aneurysm arising from the middle cerebral artery (arrowhead). In addition, vasospasm is present in the proximal anterior cerebral artery (small arrows) and middle cerebral artery (larger arrows).

tionale is that evacuation of the clots might prevent the release of the substances that induce vasospasm. However, surgical removal of clots in a critically ill patient can be difficult; some of the collected blood can be far from the operative field. Extensive manipulation of the brain to remove the subarachnoid clots may also injure penetrating vessels leading to ischemic deficits. Despite promising preliminary studies, the International Cooperative Study on the Timing of Aneurysm Surgery did not shown any reduction in the incidence or severity of vasospasm.[62] It appears that vigorous lavage of the subarachnoid space is not a feasible way to prevent vasospasm in most patients.

Several small clinical studies report the potential usefulness of intrathecal thrombolytic therapy in the setting of acute surgical treatment of a ruptured aneurysm.[11,77,99,120] Most studies treated only those patients who were considered at very high risk for vasospasm and ischemia. Outcomes generally were favorable, with ischemic deficits developing less frequently than expected. Major bleeding complications were few. Mizoi

et al[77] compared 30 patients given intrathecal tissue plasminogen activator (up to 2 mg per day for 5 days) to 75 controls. None of the treated patients had delayed ischemic neurologic deficits while 11 controls had ischemic strokes. Sasaki et al[99] performed a phase II clinical study of tissue plasminogen activator in 53 high-risk patients; three different doses of tissue plasminogen activator given three times a day for 5 days were examined. Bleeding complications occurred in four patients. Severe vasospasm was not observed and two-thirds of the patients who received a dose of 0.1 mg had satisfactory lysis of the clots. In a nonrandomized study, Usui et al[120] compared outcomes of patients who received urokinase, tissue plasminogen activator, or no specific treatment. Although intrathecal thrombolytic therapy was safe and promoted more rapid clearance of blood from the subarachnoid space, outcomes were similar at 3 months in all three groups.

Thrombolytic drugs can be instilled into the basal cisterns safely. The risk of major bleeding complications, in particular, brain hemorrhage, appears to be low. The risk of hemorrhage means that thrombolytic drugs should not be given unless the unruptured aneurysm has been clipped or occluded. Because the goal of this treatment is to prevent the development of vasospasm, it should be administered soon after SAH. Thus, the use of thrombolytic drugs is predicated on early surgical repair of the aneurysm. The usefulness of thrombolytic drugs in prevention of vasospasm and ischemic stroke is not established. The optimal timing of treatment, the duration of treatment, the best drug, or the best dose are not known. Considerable research, including prospective controlled trials, is needed before intrathecal thrombolytic therapy is added to the usual care of persons with recently ruptured aneurysms.

CALCIUM CHANNEL BLOCKING DRUGS

Influx of extracellular calcium is an important component in sustaining contraction of smooth muscle and is a critical element in the process of cellular ischemia. A drug that inhibits calcium entry might prevent vasospasm or its cerebral ischemic consequences. The presumed therapeutic benefit is amelioration of cellular ischemia, or affecting platelet aggregation or vascular activity. The dihydropyridine derivatives nimodipine and nicardipine have received the most attention. Nimodipine reduces blood pressure but increases cerebral blood flow. Its hypotensive effects are dose-related. The area of increased blood flow is at the border zone of the ischemic lesion.

The positive results of a small randomized trial done by Allen et al[5] stimulated additional research on nimodipine. Most studies report a reduction in morbidity and mortality due to ischemia but do not show any effect in preventing vasospasm.[89,93] A large trial in the United Kingdom established the usefulness of nimodipine in improving outcome after SAH.[93] Favorable outcomes were increased from 67% to 80.2% with treatment. Two meta-analyses confirm the efficacy of nimodipine in persons with recent SAH.[6,113] In general, nimodipine is safe and complications are few. As with all calcium entry blockers, hypotension is a potential side effect. The discrepancy between the efficacy of nimodipine in forestalling brain infarction following SAH and the lack of efficacy in persons with ischemic stroke from other causes has not been explained. However, nimodipine generally is started as soon as the diagnosis of SAH is confirmed. Thus, it reaches vulnerable areas of the brain before the processes of vasospasm and ischemic stroke have begun. Nimodipine's primary benefit may be as a prophylactic treatment for ischemia.

Patients with recently ruptured aneurysms receive nimodipine as part of their general medical care (Table 54.8).[22,74] If the illness is not diagnosed until 10 to 14 days after SAH, the patient has already survived the period of greatest risk of ischemia and nimodipine probably is not necessary. While the duration of treatment in clinical studies was up to 3 weeks following SAH, a shorter course (10 to 14 days) may be all that is needed. The usual oral dosage of nimodipine is 60 mg every 6 hours. Comatose patients can receive the medication via nasogastric tube. A parenteral form of nimodipine is available in Europe. Hypotensive effects may be prominent in persons receiving intravenous nimodipine.

Nicardipine has similar potential therapeutic action. It was evaluated in a large clinical trial.[39,40] The trial permitted aggressive treatment of symptomatic vasospasm with drug-induced hypertension and hypervolemic hemodilution. At 3 months after SAH, the actively treated and control groups had comparable rates of favorable and unfavorable outcomes. However, the frequency of symptomatic vasospasm was reduced from 46% to 32% with the use of nicardipine.[39] The rate of moderate to severe vasospasm, as judged by increases in flow velocities detected by transcranial Doppler, was reduced with nicardipine.[40] In addition, hypertensive drugs and hypervolemic therapy were prescribed in 38% of controls and 25% of persons given nicardipine. In another study comparing two doses of nicardipine (0.075 or 0.15 mg/kg/h), the same investigators found that the lower dose of nicardipine was associated with a slightly increased rate of severe vasospasm, but overall outcomes were similar to those seen with the larger dose (0.15 mg/kg/h).[41] Shibuya et al[103] gave intrathecal nicardipine to 50 patients with SAH; they noted declines in both symptomatic and angiographic vasospasm. The comparison study of Haley et al[41] also noted that patients who received larger doses of nicardipine had a high rate of prematurely stopping the medication. The results of these studies suggest

Table 54.8 Management Options in Prevention or Treatment of Vasospasm and Brain Ischemia after Subarachnoid Hemorrhage

Prevention
  Nimodipine
  Maintain adequate hydration
  Intrathecal administration or rtPA
  Intrathecal lavage
Symptomatic treatment
    Treat increased intracranial pressure
    Discontinue antihypertensive and antifibrinolytic drugs
    Volume expansion and drug-induced hypertension
      Monitor CVP or PAWP and ECG
      Administer colloid solutions
      Versection
      Titrate arterial pressure
Angioplasty

that nicardipine is effective in preventing the ischemic sequelae of SAH, but the combination of aggressive volume expansion and drug-induced hypertension also is effective. These additional data support the use of calcium channel blockers supplemented by hypervolemic hemodilution and hypertension for prevention of ischemic stroke after SAH.

USE OF OTHER DRUGS IN THE PREVENTION OF VASOSPASM OR ISCHEMIC STROKE

Calcitonin-gene-related peptide (CGRP) is a potent vasodilator that has been tested in patients with recent subarachnoid hemorrhage. A small clinical trial tested CGRP given for up to 10 days after SAH.[26] Hypotension was a common side effect and two-thirds of the treated patients did not complete the treatment. Although this study was reported as negative, largely as the result of its small size, favorable outcomes were noted in 66% of treated patients and 60% of controls. While CGRP has not been established as useful in improving outcomes after stroke, the results are intriguing and additional studies might establish the benefit of this powerful vasodilator.

In an experimental model, nitric oxide increased cerebral blood flow, reduced cerebral vascular resistance, reversed angiographic evidence of vasospasm, and reduced cerebral blood flow velocity.[4] Clinical studies have not been performed. Nonpeptide endothelin receptor antagonists are a potential therapy.[128] While preliminary experimental studies show promise, considerable research is needed. Other possible medical therapies for vasospasm include cyclosporine, actinomycin D, GM1 gangliosides, and 2-chlorodeoxyadenosine.[43,91,98,104]

Pilot clinical studies of supraselective intra-arterial administration of papaverine suggest that this vasodilator may be helpful.[17] Kaku et al[55] found that the drug should be given before the artery loses its ability to respond. Hypotension does not appear to be a complication of local intra-arterial infusions. Although pilot clinical studies show the promise of local intra-arterial infusions of papaverine, considerable research including controlled clinical trials is required.

Corticosteroids can protect against peroxidative and free radical reactions. In experimental models, high doses of methylprednisolone can preserve antioxidant activity. Intravenous methylprednisolone has a vasodilatory effect on vascular smooth muscle. The 21-aminosteroids do not have immunosuppressive and glucocorticoid effects which can limit the use of conventional steroids. These compounds scavenge free radicals and inhibit lipid peroxidation, features that promote stabilization of membranes of ischemic tissues. Clinical trials tested intravenously administered tirilazad given as a supplement to oral nimodipine.[38,57] The rates of favorable outcomes were highest among persons given 6 mg/kg/d.

HYPERVOLEMIC HEMODILUTION AND DRUG-INDUCED HYPERTENSION

Increasing cerebral blood flow can ease ischemic symptoms and prevent permanent neurologic sequelae (Table 54.8).[59,74,78] Reduction in the diameter of the vascular lumen implies that the blood's rheologic characteristics can influence flow. Severe losses of water and sodium result in hemoconcentration, which, in turn, increases viscosity and reduces blood flow. Measures to prevent infarction by correcting the sodium and water losses are initiated upon admission to the hospital. Strict fluid restriction is avoided. Patients are usually prescribed at least 2 to 3 L of fluids daily.[124,125] Metabolic disorders that promote hyperosmolarity are treated.

Because autoregulation is impaired, cerebral blood flow becomes pressure-dependent. Cerebral perfusion pressure is altered by changes in the mean arterial pressure and intracranial pressure. Improvement in venous drainage by positioning and elevation of the head, treatment of brain edema, and control of hydrocephalus will lower intracranial pressure and improve perfusion. When feasible, antihypertensive drugs are avoided. After the diagnosis of symptomatic vasospasm is made, more aggressive treatment of increased intracranial pressure, including hyperventilation and mannitol, might help. Antihypertensive drugs and antifibrinolytic drugs are discontinued.

Several groups report reversal of ischemic symptoms using the combination of volume expansion and drug-induced hypertension.[59,60,78] In some instances, neurologic signs can reappear when the therapy is discontinued.[59] Although no controlled trials of this regimen have been done, the recent trial of nicardipine demonstrates a benefit from this aggressive therapy.[39,40] If an improvement is not observed following volume expansion, a vasopressor (most commonly, dopamine or phenylephrine) is added in an attempt to increase mean arterial pressure and cerebral perfusion pressure. Darby et al[19] noted that the increases in cerebral blood flow following use of dopamine may be independent of changes in blood pressure, the dopamine may have direct cerebrovascular effects.

This regimen is vigorous and patients need intensive observation. Patients should have continuous monitoring of arterial pressure, cardiac rhythm, central venous pressure, or pulmonary artery wedge pressure.[78] Continuous intracranial pressure monitoring also may be needed. Frequent laboratory assessments of serum electrolytes, serum osmolarity, blood gases, and blood counts are needed. Complications of the therapy include congestive heart failure, pulmonary edema, acute myocardial infarction, and cardiac arrhythmias. Worsening of brain edema, hypertensive intracerebral hemorrhage, hemorrhagic transformation of an infarction, and rerupture of the aneurysm also can occur.[112] In one series, rebleeding happened in 3 of 16 patients whose aneurysms had not been operated on.[59] Shimoda et al[105] reported worsening of brain edema in 18 of 94 patients given hypervolemic hemodilution and eight cases of hemorrhagic infarction. They advised not using hypervolemic hemodilution if the patient's CT examination showed an ischemic area in the brain, particularly if the abnormality is seen within 6 days of SAH. Hetastarch used as a volume-expanding drug can be complicated by prolongation of the partial thromboplastin time and bleeding.[118]

TRANSCRANIAL ANGIOPLASTY

Transluminal angioplasty successfully dilates vasospastic arteries.[18] Development of microballoons allows for catheterization in small-to-medium-sized arteries at the base of the brain.

Angioplasty does stretch and disrupt the arterial wall.[49] Pathologic effects occur mainly in the medial layer of the arteries and involve degeneration of muscle elements and proliferation of nonmuscle components. This intervention usually is not prescribed until a patient has not responded to other measures to reverse vasospasm or brain ischemia. Responses have been dramatic in some cases. Reported complications are few. Because transluminal angioplasty now is performed frequently in persons with severe vasospasm, a trial that tests its usefulness is needed.

Conclusions

Considerable progress is being made in the management of SAH. Medical and surgical therapies that effectively prevent rebleeding and vasospasm are reflected by declines in mortality and morbidity. Still, there is considerable room for improvement. Several promising therapies are being tested; one or more of these interventions likely will be shown to further improve outcome of SAH. However, most therapies are based on early treatment. Thus, the medical community needs to increase attention to early diagnosis and acute care of these critically ill persons.

References

1. Adams HP Jr, Jergenson DD, Kassell NF, Sahs AL: Pitfalls in the recognition of subarachnoid hemorrhage. JAMA 244:794, 1980
2. Adams HP Jr, Kassell NF, Torner JC: Usefulness of computed tomography in predicting outcome after aneurysmal subarachnoid hemorrhage: a preliminary report of the Cooperative Aneurysm Study. Neurology 35:1263, 1985
3. Adams HP Jr, Kassell NF, Torner JC et al: Early management of aneurysmal subarachnoid hemorrhage: a report of the Cooperative Aneurysm Study. J Neurosurg 54:141, 1981
4. Afshar JKB, Pluta RM, Boock RJ et al: Effect of intracarotid nitric oxide on primate cerebral vasospasm after subarachnoid hemorrhage. J Neurosurg 83:118,1995
5. Allen AS, Ahn HS, Preziosi TJ et al: Cerebral arterial spasm—a controlled trial of nimodipine in patients with subarachnoid hemmorrhage. N Engl J Med 308:619, 1983
6. Barker FG II, Ogilvy CS: Efficacy of prophylactic nimodipine for delayed ischemic deficit after subarachnoid hemorrhage. A metaanalysis. J Neurosurg 84:405, 1996
7. Beck DW, Adams HP Jr, Flamm ES et al: Combination of aminocaproic acid and nicardipine in treatment of aneurysmal subarachnoid hemorrhage. Stroke 19:63, 1988
8. Black PMcL: Hydrocephalus and vasospasm after subarachnoid hemorrhage from ruptured intracranial aneurysms. Neurosurgery 18:12, 1986

9. Black PMcL, Crowell RM, Abbott WM: External pneumatic calf compression reduces deep venous thrombosis in patients with ruptured intracranial aneurysms. Neurosurgery 18:25, 1986

10. Boecher-Schwarz HG, Ungersboeck K, Ulrich P et al: Transcranial Doppler diagnosis of cerebral vasospasm following subarachnoid haemorrhage. Correlation and analysis of results in relation to the age of patients. Acta Neurochir (Wien) 127:32, 1994

11. Brinker T, Seifert V, Dietz H: Subacute hydrocephalus after experimental subarachnoid hemorrhage. Its prevention by intrathecal fibrinolysis with recombinant tissue plasminogen activator. Neurosurgery 31:306, 1992

12. Broderick JP, Brott TG, Duldner et al: Initial and recurrent bleeding are the major causes of death following subarachnoid hemorrhage. Stroke 25:1342, 1994

13. Brouwers PJAM, Westenberg HGM, van Gijn J: Noradrenaline concentration and electrocardiographic abnormalities after aneurysmal subarachnoid hemorrhage. J Neurol Neurosurg Psychiatry 58:614, 1995

14. Brown JA, Wollmann RL, Mullan S: Myopathy induced by epsilon-aminocaproic acid. J Neurosurg 57:130, 1982

15. Camarata PJ, Heros RC, Latchaw RE: "Brain attack." The rationale for treating stroke as a medical emergency. J Neurosurg 34:144, 1994

16. Casasco AE, Aymard A, Gobin P et al: Selective endovascular treatment of 71 intracranial aneurysms with platinum coils. J Neurosurg 79:3, 1993

17. Clouston JE, Numaguchi Y, Zoarski GH et al: Intraarterial papaverine infusion for cerebral vasospasm after subarachnoid hemorrhage. Am J Neuroradiol 16:27, 1995

18. Coyne TJ, Montanera WJ, Macdonald RL, Wallace MC: Percutaneous transluminal angioplasty for cerebral vasospasm after subarachnoid hemorrhage. Can J Surg 37:391, 1994

19. Darby JM, Yonas H, Marks EC et al: Acute cerebral blood flow response to dopamine-induced hypertension after subarachnoid hemorrhage. J Neurosurg 80:857, 1994

20. Deruty R, Mottolese C, Pecisson-Guyotat I, Soustiec JF: Management of the ruptured intracranial aneurysm. Early surgery, late surgery, or modulated surgery. Acta Neurochir (Wien) 113:1, 1991

21. Di Pasquale G, Pinelli G, Andreoli A et al: Torsade de pointes and ventricular flutter-fibrillation following spontaneous cerebral subarachnoid hemorrhage. Int J Cardiol 18:163, 1988

22. Dippel DWJ, van Crevel H, Lindsay KW et al: Management of subarachnoid hemorrhage. A decision analysis. Cerebrovasc Dis 5:350, 1995

23. Diringer MN, Wu KC, Verbalis VG, Hanley DF: Hypervolemic therapy prevents volume contraction but not hyponatremia following subarachnoid hemorrhage. Ann Neurol 31:543, 1992

24. Edner G, Ronne-Engstrom E: Can early admission reduce aneurysmal rebleeds? A prospective study on aneurysmal incidence, aneurysmal rebleeds, admission and treatment delays in a defined region. Br J Neurosurg 5:601, 1991

25. Ekelund A, Saveland H, Romner B, Brandt L: Transcranial Doppler ultrasound in hypertensive versus normotensive patients after aneurysmal subarachnoid hemorrhage. Stroke 26:2071, 1995

26. European CGRP in Subarachnoid Haemorrhage Study Group: Effect of calcitonin-gene-related peptide in patients with delayed postoperative cerebral ischaemia after aneurysmal subarachnoid haemorrhage. 339:831, 1992

27. Findlay JM, MacDonald RL, Weir BKA: Current concepts of pathophysiology and management of cerebral vasospasm following aneurysmal subarachnoid hemorrhage. Cerebrovasc Brain Metab Reviews 3:336, 1991

28. Fisher CM: Clinical syndromes in cerebral thrombosis, hypertensive hemorrhage and ruptured saccular aneurysm. Clin Neurosurg 22:117, 1975

29. Fisher CM, Kistler JP, Davis JM: Relation of cerebral vasospasm to subarachnoid hemorrhage visualized by computerized tomographic scanning. Neurosurgery 6:1, 1980

30. Fisher CM, Roberson GH, Ojemann RG: Cerebral vasospasm with ruptured saccular aneurysm: the clinical manifestations. Neurosurgery 1:245, 1977

31. Fujii Y, Takeuchi S, Sasaki O et al: Hemostasis in spontaneous subarachnoid hemorrhage. Neurosurgery 37:226, 1995

32. Gaetani P, Rodriguez Y, Baena R et al: Endothelin and aneurysmal subarachnoid hemorrhage. A study of subarachnoid cisternal cerebrospinal fluid. J Neurol Neurosurg Psychiatry 57:66, 1994

33. Gascon P, Ley TJ, Toltzis RJ, Bonow RO: Spontaneous subarachnoid hemorrhage simulating acute transmural myocardial infarction. Am Heart J 105:511, 1983

34. Giller CA, Purdy P, Giller A et al: Elevated transcranial Doppler ultrasound velocities following therapeutic arterial dilation. Stroke 26:123, 1995

35. Glick R, Green D, Tsao CH et al: High dose e-aminocaproic acid prolongs the bleeding time and increases rebleeding and intraoperative hemorrhage in patients with subarachnoid hemorrhage. Neurosurgery 9:398, 1981

36. Graff-Radford NR, Torner JC, Adams HP Jr, Kassell NF: Factors associated with hydrocephalus after subarachnoid hemorrhage: a report of the Cooperative Aneurysm Study. Arch Neurol 46:744, 1989

37. Grosset DG, Straiton J, McDonald I, Bullock R: Angiographic and Doppler diagnosis of cerbral artery vasospasm following subarachnoid hemorrhage. Br J Neurosurg 7:291, 1993

38. Haley EC Jr, Kassell NF, Alves WM et al and the participants: Phase II trial of tirilazad in aneurysmal subarachnoid hemorrhage. A report of the Cooperative Aneurysm Study. J Neurosurg 82:786, 1995

39. Haley EC Jr, Kassell NF, Torner JC and the participants: A randomized controlled trial of high-dose intravenous nicardipine in aneurysmal subarachnoid hemorrhage. A report of the Cooperative Aneurysm Study. J Neurosurg 78:537, 1993

40. Haley EC Jr, Kassell NF, Torner JC and the participants: A randomized trial of nicardipine in subarachnoid hemorrhage. Angiographic and transcranial Doppler ultrasound results. A report of the Cooperative Aneurysm Study. J Neurosurg 78:548, 1993

41. Haley EC Jr, Kassell NF, Torner JC et al and the partici-

pants: A randomized trial of two doses of nicardipine in aneurysmal subarachnoid hemorrhage. A report of the Cooperative Aneurysm Study. J Neurosurg 80:788, 1994

42. Hamann G, Haass A, Schimrigk K: Beta blockade in acute aneurysmal subarachnoid hemorrhage. Acta Neurochir (Wien) 121:119, 1993

43. Handa Y, Hayashi M, Takeuchi H et al: Effect of cyclosporine on the development of cerebral vasospasm in a primate model. Neurosurgery 28:380,1991

44. Hart RG, Byer JA, Slaughter JR et al: Occurrence and implications of seizures in subarachnoid hemorrhage due to ruptured intracranial aneurysms. Neurosurgery 8:417, 1981

45. Hasen D, Vermeulen M, Wijdicks EFM et al: Management problems in acute hydrocephalus after subarachnoid hemorrhage. Stroke 20:747, 1989

46. Heros RC: Acute hydrocephalus after subarachnoid hemorrhage. Stroke 20:715,1989

47. Hillman J, von Essen C, Leszniewski W, Johansson I: Significance of "ultra-early" rebleeding in subarachnoid hemorrhage. J Neurosurg 68:901, 1988

48. Hirashima Y, Endo S, Ohmori T et al: Platelet-activating factor (PAF) concentration and PAF acetylhydrolase activity in cerebrospinal fluid of patients with subarachnoid hemorrhage. J Neurosurg 80:31, 1994

49. Honma Y, Fujiwara T, Irie K et al: Morphological changes in human cerebral arteries after percutaneous transluminal angioplasty for vasospasm caused by subarachnoid hemorrhage. Neurosurgery 36:1073, 1995

50. Inagawa T, Kamiya K, Matsuda Y: Effect of continuous cisternal drainage on cerbral vasaspasm. Acta Neurochir (Wien) 112:128, 1991

51. Ingall TJ, Whisnant JP, Wiebers DO, O'Fallon WM: Has there been a decline in subarachnoid hemorrhage mortality? Stroke 20:718, 1989

52. Itoyama Y, Fujioka S, Takaki S et al: Significance of elevated thrombin-anti-thrombin III complex and plasmin-alpha$_2$-plasmin inhibitor complex in the acute stage of nontraumatic subarachnoid hemorrhage. Neurosurgery 35:1055, 1994

53. Juvela S: Aspirin and delayed cerebral ischemia after aneurysmal subarachnoid hemorrhage. J Neurosurg 82:945, 1995

54. Juvela S, Kaste M, Hillbom M: The effects of earlier surgery and shorter bedrest on the outcome in patients with subarachnoid haemorrhage. J Neurol Neurosurg Psychiatry 52:776, 1989

55. Kaku Y, Yonekawa Y, Tsukahara T, Kazekawa K: Superselective intra-arterial infusion of papaverine for the treatment of cerebral vasospasm after subarachnoid hemorrhage. J Neurosurg 77:842, 1992

56. Kassell NF, Boarini DJ, Adams HP Jr et al: Overall management of ruptured aneurysm: comparison of early and late operation. Neurosurgery 9:120, 1981

57. Kassell NF, Haley EC Jr, Apperson-Hansen C, Alves WM and the participants: Randomized, double-blind, vehicle-controlled trial of tirilazad mesylate in patients with aneurysmal subarachnoid hemorrhage. A cooperative study in Europe, Australia and New Zealand. J Neurosurg 84:221, 1996

58. Kassell NF, Kongable GL, Torner JC et al: Delay in referral of patients with ruptured aneurysms to neurosurgical attention. Stroke 16:587, 1985

59. Kassell NF, Peerless SJ, Durward QJ et al: Treatment of ischemic deficits from vasospasm with intravascular volume expansion and induced arterial hypertension. Neurosurgery 11:337, 1982

60. Kassell NF, Sasaki T, Colohan ART, Nazar G: Cerebral vasospasm following aneurysmal subarachnoid hemorrhage. Stroke 16:562, 1985

61. Kassell NF, Torner JC, Adams HP Jr: Antifibrinolytic therapy in the acute period following aneurysmal subarachnoid hemorrhage: preliminary observations from the Cooperative Aneurysm study. J Neurosurg 61:225, 1984

62. Kassell NF, Torner JC, Haley EC et al: The International Cooperative Study on the Timing of Aneurysm Surgery. I. Overall management results. J Neurosurg 73:18, 1990

63. Kassell NF, Torner JC, Haley EC et al: The International Cooperative study on the timing of aneurysm surgery. II. Surgical results. J Neurosurg 73:34, 1990

64. Kasuya H, Weir BKA, Nakane M et al: Nitric oxide synthase and guanylate cyclase levels in canine basilar artery after subarachnoid hemorrhage. J Neurosurg 82:250, 1995

65. Kinugasa K, Mandai S, Kamata I et al: Prophylactic thrombosis to prevent new bleeding and to delay aneurysm surgery. Neurosurgery 36:661, 1995

66. Kongable GL, Lanzino G, Germansson TP et al and the participants: Gender-related differences in aneurysmal subarachnoid hemorrhage. J Neurosurg 84:43, 1996

67. Larson JJ, Tew JM Jr, Tomsick TA, Van Loveren HR: Treatment of aneurysms of the internal carotid artery by intravascular balloon occlusion. Long-term follow-up of 58 patients. Neurosurgery 36:23, 1995

68. Laumer R, Steinmeier R, Gonner F et al: Cerebral hemodynamics in subarachnoid hemorrhage evaluated by transcranial Doppler-sonography. Part I. Reliability of flow velocities in clinical management. Neurosurgery 33:1, 1993

69. LeBlanc R: The minor leak preceding subarachnoid hemorrhage. J Neurosurg 66:35, 1987

70. LeRoux PD, Elliott JP, Downey L et al: Improved outcomes after rupture of anterior circulation aneurysms. A retrospective 10-year review of 224 good-grade patients. J Neurosurg 83:394, 1995

71. Levy ML, Rabb CH, Zelman V, Giannotta SL: Cardiac performance enhancement from dobutamine in patients refractory to hypervolemic therapy for cerebral vasospasm. J Neurosurg 79:494, 1993

72. Lewis AI, Tomsick TA, Tew JM Jr: Management of 100 consecutive direct carotid-cavernous fistulas. Results of treatment with detachable balloons. Neurosurgery 36:239, 1995

73. Manninen PH, Ayra B, Gelb AW, Pelz D: Association between electrocardiographic abnormalities and intracranial blood in patients with acute subarachnoid hemorrhage. J Neurosurg Anesth 7:12, 1995

74. Mayberg MR, Batjer HH, Dacey R et al: Guidelines for the management of aneurysmal subarachnoid hemorrhage. Circulation 90:2592, 1994

75. McDougall CG, Halbach VV, Dowd CF et al: Endovascular treatment of basilar tip aneurysms using electrolytically detachable coils. J Neurosurg 84:393, 1996

76. Miyaoka M, Sato K, Ishii S: A clinical study of the relationship of timing to outcome of surgery for rupture of cerebral aneurysms. A retrospective analysis of 1,622 cases. J Neurosurg 79:373, 1993

77. Mizoi K, Yoshimoto T, Takahashi A et al: Prospective study on the prevention of cerebral vasospasm by intrathecal fibrinolytic therapy with tissue type plasminogen activator. J Neurosurg 78:430, 1993

78. Mori K, Arai H, Nakajima K et al: Hemorheological and hemodynamic analysis of hypervolemic hemodilution therapy for cerebral vasospasm after aneurysmal subarachnoid hemorrhage. Stroke 26:1620, 1995

79. Nagatani K, Masciopinto J, Letarte PB et al: The effect of hemoglobin and its metabolites on energy metabolism in cultured cerebrovascular smooth-muscle cells. J Neurosurg 82:244, 1995

80. Neil-Dwyer G, Walter P, Cruikshank JM et al: Effect of propranolol and phentolamine on myocardial necrosis after subarachnoid hemorrhage. Br Med J 2:990, 1978

81. Neil-Dwyer G, Walter P, Shaw HJH et al: Plasma renin activity in patients after a subarachnoid hemorrhage: a possible predictor of outcome. Neurosurgery 7:578, 1980

82. Nibbelink DW: Considerations in the treatment of stroke: Cooperative Aneurysm study: antihypertensive and antifibrinolytic therapy following subarachnoid hemorrhage from ruptured intracranial aneurysm. p. 155. In Whisnant JP, Sandok BA (eds): Cerebral Vascular Diseases. Grune & Stratton, Orlando, Florida, 1975

83. Nibbelink DW, Torner JC, Burmeister LF: Fluid resriction in combination with antifibrinolytic therapy. p. 307. In Sahs AL, Nibbelink DW, Torner JC (eds): Aneurysmal Subarachnoid Hemorrhage. Urban & Schwarzenberg, Baltimore, 1981

84. Nichols DA, Meyer FB, Piepgras DG, Smith PL: Endovascular treatment of intracranial aneurysms. Mayo Clin Proc 69:272, 1994

85. Nishimoto A, Veta K, Onbe H et al: Nationwide cooperative study of intracranial aneurysm surgery in Japan. Stroke 16:48, 1985

86. Nishioka H: Report of the Cooperative Study of Intracranial Aneurysms and Subarachnoid Hemorrhage. Section VII, Part I: Evaluation of conservative measurement of ruptured intracranial aneurysms. J Neurosurg 25:574, 1966

87. Nowak G, Schwachenwald R, Arnold H: Early management in poor grade aneurysm patients. Acta Neurochir (Wien) 126:33, 1994

88. Ohman J, Heiskanen O: Timing of operation for ruptured supratentorial aneurysms: a prospective randomized study. J Neurosurg 70:55, 1989

89. Ohman J, Servo A, Heiskanen O: Long-term effects of nimodipine on cerebral infarcts and outcome effects after aneurysmal subarachnoid hemorrhage and surgery. J Neurosurg 74:8, 1991

90. Oppenheimer SM: Neurogenic cardiac effects of cerebrovascular disease. Curr Opin Neurol 7:20, 1994

91. Papo I, Benedetti A, Carteri A et al: Monosialoganglioside in subarachnoid hemorrhage. Stroke 22:22, 1991

92. Perret GE, Nibbelink DW: Randomized treatment study: carotid ligation. p. 121. In Sahs AL, Nibbelink DW, Torner JC (eds): Aneurysmal Subarachnoid Hemorrhage. Urban & Schwarzenberg, Baltimore, 1981

93. Pickard JD, Murray GD, Illingworth R et al: Effect of oral nimodipine on cerebral infarction and outcome after subarachnoid haemorrhage: British Aneurysm Nimodipine Trial. Br Med J 298:636, 1989

94. Pickard JD, Walker V, Brandt L et al: Effect of intraventricular haemorrhage and rebleeding following subarachnoid haemorrhage on CSF eicosanoids. Acta Neurochir (Wien) 129:152, 1994

95. Proust F, Hannequin D, Langlois O et al: Causes of morbidity and mortality after ruptured aneurysm surgery in a series of 230 patients. The importance of control angiography. Stroke 26:1553, 1995

96. Rinkel GJE, Wijdicks EFM, Vermeulen M et al: The clinical course of perimesencephalic non-aneurysmal subarachnoid haemorrhage. Ann Neurol 29:463, 1991

97. Rosenorn J, Eskesen V, Schmidt K: Clinical features and outcome in females and males with ruptured intracranial saccular aneurysms. Br J Neurosurg 7:287, 1993

98. Ryba M, Grieb P, Pastuszko M et al: Successful prevention of neurological deficit in SAH patients with 2-chlorodeoxyadenosine. Acta Neurochir (Wien) 124:61, 1993

99. Sasaki T, Ohta T, Kikuchi H et al: A phase II clinical trial of recombinant human tissue-type plasminogen activator against cerebral vasospasm after aneurysmal subarachnoid hemorrhage. Neurosurgery 35:597, 1994

100. Saveland H, Brandt L: Which are the major determinants for outcome in aneurysmal subarachnoid hemorrhage? Acta Neurol Scand 90:245, 1994

101. Schievink WI, Wijdicks EFM, Parisi JE et al: Sudden death from aneurysmal subarachnoid hemorrhage. Neurology 45:871, 1995

102. Seifert V, Loffler BM, Zimmerman M et al: Endothelin concentrations in patients with aneurysmal subarachnoid hemorrhage. Correlation with cerebral vasospasm delayed ischemic neurologic defects and volume of hematoma. J Neurosurg 82:55, 1995

103. Shibuya M, Suzuki Y, Enomoto H et al: Effects of prophylactic intrathecal administration of nicardipine on vasospasm in patients with severe aneurysmal subarachnoid haemorrhage. Acta Neurochir (Wien) 131:19, 1994

104. Shigeno T, Mima T, Yanagisawa M et al: Prevention of cerebral vasospasm by actinomycin D. J Neurosurg 74: 940, 1991

105. Shimoda M, Oda S, Tsugane R, Sato O: Intracranial complication of hypervolemic therapy in patients with a delayed ischemic deficit attributed to vasospasm. J Neurosurg 78:423, 1993

106. Sinson G, Philips MF, Flamm ES: Intraoperative endovascular surgery for cerebral aneurysm. J Neurosurg 84: 63, 1996

107. Smith RR, Clower BR, Grotendorst GM et al: Arterial wall changes in early human vasospasm. Neurosurgery 16:171, 1985

108. Stachnink JB, Layon AJ, Day AL, Gallagher J: Craniotomy for intracranial aneurysm and subarachnoid hemor-

rhage. Is course, cost or outcome affected by age? Stroke 27:276, 1996

109. Steiger HJ, Fritschi J, Seiler RW: Current pattern of in-hospital aneurysmal rebleeds. Acta Neurochir (Wien) 127:21, 1994

110. Steinmeier R, Laumer R, Bondar I et al: Cerebral hemodynamics in subarachnoid hemorrhage evaluated by transcranial Doppler sonography. Part 2. Pulsatility indices normal reference values and characteristics in subarachnoid hemorrhage. Neurosurgery 33:10, 1993

111. Sundaram MBM, Chow F: Seizures associated with spontaneous subarachnoid hemorrhage. Can J Neurol Sci 13:229, 1986

112. Terada T, Komai N, Hayashi S et al: Hemorrhagic infarction after vasospasm due to ruptured cerebral aneurysm. Neurosurgery 18:415, 1986

113. Tettenborn D, Dycka J: Prevention and treatment of delayed ischemic dysfunction in patients with aneurysmal subarachnoid hemorrhage. Stroke 21 (suppl. IV) IV85, 1990

114. Thie A, Heaze T for the FISAH Study Group: Factor XIII concentrate for prevention of recurrent subarachnoid hemorrhage. Results of a multicenter pilot study. Neurochir 34:107, 1991

115. Toftdahl DB, Torp-Pedersen C, Engel UH et al: Hypertension and left ventricular hypertrophy in patients with spontaneous subarachnoid hemorrhage. Neurosurgery 37:235, 1995

116. Torner JC, Kassell NF, Wallace RB, Adams HP Jr: Preoperative prognostic factors for rebleeding and survival in aneurysm patients receiving antifibrinolytic therapy: report of the Cooperative Aneurysm Study. Neurosurgery 9:506, 1981

117. Tovi D, Thulin CA: Ability of tranexamic acid to cross the blood-brain barrier and its use in patients with ruptured intracranial aneurysms. Acta Neurol Scand 48:257, 1972

118. Trumble ER, Muizelaar JP, Myseros JS et al: Coagulopathy with the use of hetastarch in the treatment of vasospasm. J Neurosurg 82:44, 1995

119. Tsementzis SA, Meyer CHA, Hitchcock ER: Cerebral blood flow in patients with a subarachnoid hemorrhage during treatment with tranexamic acid. Neurochir 35: 74, 1992

120. Usui M, Saito N, Hoya K, Todo T: Vasospasm prevention with postoperative intrathecal thrombolytic therapy. A retrospective comparison of urokinase, tissue plasminogin activator, and cisternal drainage alone. Neurosurgery 34:235, 1994

121. Vermeulen M, Lindsay KW, Murray GD et al: Antifibrinolytic treatment in subarachnoid hemorrhage. N Engl J Med 311:432, 1984

122. Weinand ME, O'Boynick PL, Goetz KL: A study of serum antidiuretic hormone and atrial natriuretic peptide levels in a series of patients with intracranial disease and hyponatremia. Neurosurgery, 25:781, 1989

123. Whisnant JP, Phillips LH II, Sundt TM Jr: Aneurysmal subarachnoid hemorrhage: timing of surgery and mortality. Mayo Clin Proc 57:471, 1982

124. Wijdicks EFM: Worst case scenario. Management in poor-grade aneurysmal subarachnoid hemorrhage. Cerebrovasc Dis 5:163, 1995

125. Wijdicks EFM, Vermeulen M, Hijdra A, van Gijn J: Hyponatremia and cerebral infarction in patients with ruptured intracranial aneurysms: is fluid restriction harmful? Ann Neurol 17:137, 1985

126. Wijdicks EFM, Vermeulen M, Ten Haaf JA et al: Volume depletion and natriuresis in patients with a ruptured intracranial aneurysm. Ann Neurol 18:211, 1985

127. Wijdicks EFM, Vermeulen M, van Brummelen P, van Gijn J: The effect of fludrocortisone acetate on plasma volume and natriuresis in patients with aneurysmal subarachnoid hemorrhage. Clin Neurol Neurosurg 90:209, 1988

128. Willette RN, Zhang H, Mitchell MP et al: Nonpeptide endothelin antagonist. Cerebrovascular characterization and effects on delayed cerebral vasospasm. Stroke 25: 2450, 1994

129. Yuki K, Kodama Y, Onda J et al: Coronary vasospasm following subarachnoid hemorrhage as a cause of stunned myocardiation. J Neurosurg 75:308, 1991

CHAPTER 55

Intracranial Aneurysms

Surgical Management

JOSEPH M. ZABRAMSKI
ROBERT F. SPETZLER

An aneurysm is defined as an abnormally circumscribed dilatation of an artery. In the cerebral circulation, most aneurysms take the form of thin-walled sacs protruding from the arteries of the circle of Willis or its major branches. With few exceptions these lesions make their presence known only after a rupture produces subarachnoid hemorrhage (SAH). Even more rarely, intracranial aneurysms present with the signs and symptoms of a mass lesion or are discovered incidentally when cerebral angiography, computed tomography (CT), or magnetic resonance imaging (MRI) is performed for other diagnostic purposes (Figs. 55.1 and 55.2).

The modern history of intracranial aneurysms began with Charles Symonds,[146] who after suggesting that the diagnosis of SAH could be made during life, investigated the matter at the request of his mentor, Harvey Cushing.[30] Symonds not only coined the term *subarachnoid hemorrhage* and described the use of lumbar puncture for its diagnosis, but also brought to the attention of the medical community the relationship between this finding and rupture of intracranial aneurysms.

The introduction of cerebral angiography by Moniz[92] in 1927 allowed the diagnosis of ruptured cerebral aneurysm to be verified and the lesion to be accurately localized. By 1933, Dott[36] reported the clinical and angiographic findings of eight patients and the operative treatment of two of them. In 1937, Dandy[31] performed the first intracranial clipping of an aneurysm, and with this bold approach opened the doors to the surgical therapy of intracranial aneurysms.

Incidence

Aneurysmal SAH is a major health care problem throughout the world. In the United States and Canada, there are approximately 30,000 new cases per year for an incidence rate of 12 per 100,000 population. Incidence rates vary from 6[78] to 26[61]

per 100,000 population per year, with Finland[75] and Japan[61,102] reporting the highest values. Women outnumber men by a ratio of roughly 1.6:1 in most large series.[50,72,113] Jellinger reviewed 12 postmortem studies, totaling 87,772 examinations, and noted aneurysms in approximately 2% of cases.[65] The frequency varies considerably from one report to another. Much of this variation is the result of a lack of agreement in the medical community about the size at which an arterial defect should be designated an aneurysm. If microaneurysms (2 mm or less) are considered, up to 17% of routine autopsies can be expected to reveal intracranial aneurysms.[52] However, if only lesions larger than 4 mm are considered, the apparent incidence falls to less than 2%. The problem is further complicated by evidence suggesting that aneurysm size may be significantly underestimated during routine autopsy examinations. In an elegant study, McCormick and Acosta-Rua[84] demonstrated that perfusing the intracranial vessels with saline under a pressure of 70 mmHg caused the size of aneurysms to increase from 30% to 60%.

In the United States the peak age for aneurysm rupture is between 40 and 60 years of age.[62,72,80] Intracranial aneurysms are rare in children and adolescents.[80,87,107] In postmortem studies, the prevalence of intracranial aneurysms increases with age and reaches a peak in the fifth to sixth decades of life.[58,62,83] The annual incidence rates for subarachnoid hemorrhage parallel this change in prevalence, increasing from 3 per 100,000 population in the third decade to 30 per 100,000 in the sixth decade.[62,81,112] When intracranial hemorrhage does occur in children, bleeding from an arteriovenous malformation (AVM) is usually the underlying cause; after 20 years of age, hemorrhage is more likely to be the result of a ruptured aneurysm (Fig. 55.3).

SAH during pregnancy is one of the leading causes of maternal mortality in North America.[20,60,90] The incidence is reported to vary between 1 per 2,000 and 1 per 10,000

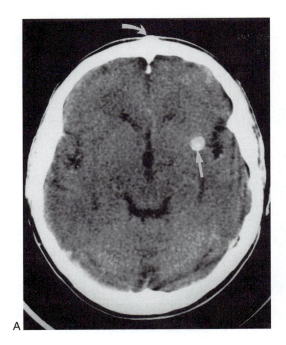

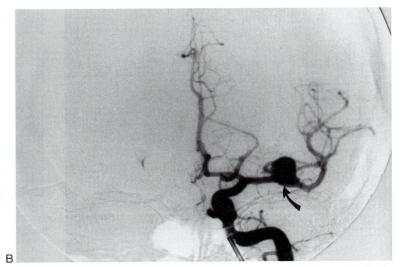

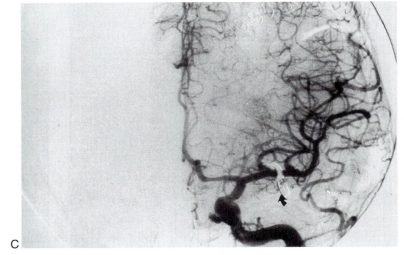

Figure 55.1 A 64-year-old woman sought evaluation by a plastic surgeon for treatment of a bony prominence in the mid-forehead. (**A**) As part of her evaluation, a basic head computed tomography (CT) scan was obtained. CT findings included a focal area of increased density (straight arrow) in the left sylvian fissure compatible with a partially calcified middle cerebral artery aneurysm. There was no history consistent with previous subarachnoid hemorrhage. Note the small bony prominence (curved arrow) in the frontal region. (**B**) Anteroposterior view of the left internal carotid artery angiogram reveals a large, irregularly shaped, left middle cerebral artery aneurysm (arrow). (**C**) A postoperative angiogram demonstrates complete obliteration of the aneurysm with no compromise of the parent vessels. A slightly curved aneurysm clip (arrow) is faintly visible in this subtracted image.

pregnancies, with the cause related to AVMs and aneurysms with about equal frequency.[90,116] AVMs tend to rupture early during pregnancy or during delivery, while aneurysms are reported to rupture most commonly during the third trimester and only rarely during labor.[20,90,115] The evaluation and treatment of SAH during pregnancy should be the same as if the patient were not pregnant. The medical welfare of the mother should never be jeopardized by withholding procedures deemed essential because of the fear of potential detrimental effects on the fetus. Craniotomy and clipping of the aneurysm are the most appropriate forms of therapy.[60,90,115] Prophylactic cesarean section has been recommended for the management of pregnant women with untreated aneurysms, but vaginal delivery with lumbar epidural anesthesia appears to be equally safe and effective and is therefore the method of choice.[60] Cesarean section is recommended if the mother is moribund and the child appears viable.

Distribution

The International Cooperative Study on the Timing of Aneurysm Surgery constitutes the most extensive series that has evaluated patients for the distribution of ruptured aneurysms.[72,73] This study was the collaborative effort of 213 neurosurgeons at 68 medical centers in 15 countries. A total of 3,521 patients with documented aneurysmal SAH was enrolled. In contrast with earlier studies of this type, most pa-

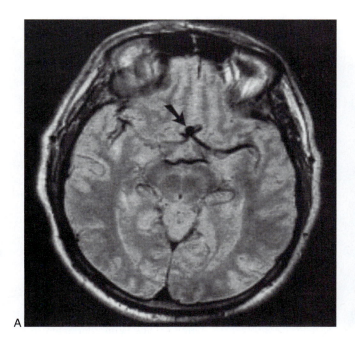

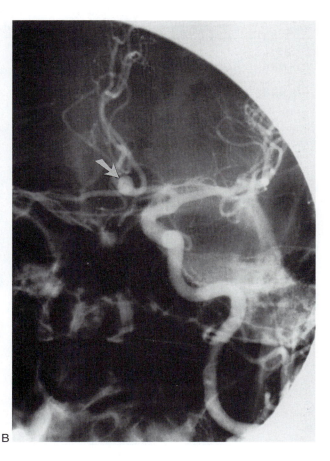

Figure 55.2 A 34-year-old man had severe recurrent headaches following a motor vehicle accident. (**A**) Transverse T_1-weighted magnetic resonance imaging through the base of the brain demonstrates a flow-related vascular defect consistent with an anterior communicating artery aneurysm (arrow). (**B**) Oblique view of the left common carotid artery angiogram confirms the presence of a small, approximately 6-mm, anterior communicating artery aneurysm (arrow). The patient underwent elective clipping of the aneurysm without complication.

Figure 55.3 Relative probability of major causes of subarachnoid hemorrhage in each decade of life. AVM, arteriovenous malformation. (From Locksley[80] with permission.)

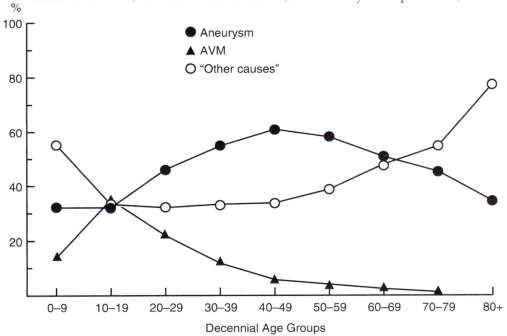

Table 55.1 Distribution of Ruptured Aneurysms

Artery	No. of Cases	(%) Total
Internal Carotid		
Cavernous	11	0.3
Ophthalmic	89	2.5
Posterior Communicating	807	23.0
Carotid Bifurcation	144	4.1
Anterior Cerebral		
Proximal to Anterior Communicating	59	1.7
Anterior Communicating	1,184	34.0
Distal to Anterior Communicating	131	3.7
Middle Cerebral		
Proximal (M1) Segment	101	2.9
At Tri/Bifurcation	662	19.0
Distal to Tri/Bifurcation	23	0.7
Posterior Cerebral		
P1	11	0.3
P2 at Posterior Communicating	10	0.3
Distal Posterior Cerebral	10	0.3
Vertebral		
Posterior Inferior Cerebellar	88	2.5
Vertebral Junction	18	0.5
Basilar		
Trunk	7	0.2
Superior Cerebellar	16	0.4
Bifurcation (Tip)	106	3.0
Other	44	1.2
Total	3,521	

(*Data from Kassel et al.*[72])

tients in this series underwent complete angiographic evaluation, including the posterior fossa vertebrobasilar system.

The distribution of ruptured aneurysms in these patients is presented in Table 55.1. The anterior communicating artery was the most common site of rupture, accounting for 34% of cases. It was followed by the internal carotid artery (30%) and the middle cerebral artery distributions (22%). Aneurysms in the internal carotid artery distribution were most often encountered at the origin of the posterior communicating artery, followed by the carotid bifurcation and the origin of the ophthalmic artery. Aneurysms of the posterior circulation most commonly occurred at the basilar tip, followed by the vertebral origin of the posterior inferior cerebellar artery and the other basilar trunk branches. Overall, aneurysms of the vertebral and basilar artery systems composed 7.6% of the Cooperative Study series.

Multiple aneurysms are found in 20% to 30% of patients with aneurysmal SAH.[6,96,106] When more than one aneurysm is discovered at angiography, the lesion responsible for the hemorrhage must be identified so that it can be treated first. In a retrospective analysis of 205 aneurysms in 69 patients, Nehls et al[96] found that irregularity of contour was the most important factor identifying the site of rupture, although size and location were also helpful. When aneurysms were of similar size, the more irregular of the aneurysms was the site of rupture in 93.3% of cases. In fact, in only one instance did a larger but less irregular aneurysm rupture. When aneurysms have smooth walls, the largest and most proximal aneurysm was the one most likely to rupture. Finally, when all other factors were equal, the most frequent site of rupture was the posterior communicating artery followed by the anterior communicating artery, the middle cerebral artery, and other internal carotid artery branch points. Focal spasm in the area of aneurysm is a rare but highly reliable angiographic sign for localizing the site of rupture. A CT scan can also help identify the aneurysm responsible for hemorrhage. Focal accumulations of subarachnoid blood (e.g., within the interhemispheric or sylvian fissures) are the most indicative signs (Fig. 55.4).

Natural History

Numerous retrospective studies have been conducted in an effort to elucidate the natural history of SAH. Attempts to assemble a representative series have been hampered by the problems of evaluating patients who receive no treatment because of selection criteria and by the lack of angiographic evaluation in many historical studies. Despite these difficulties, various authors have collected valuable data that shed light on the factors affecting the prognosis of patients with ruptured aneurysms. The results of several population studies suggest that at least 15% of patients are found dead after the initial hemorrhage.[26,78,151] For patients who survive the acute hemorrhage, data from multiple Cooperative Studies suggest that the mortality rate during the first 2 weeks is 20% to 30%, with a morbidity of about 20%.[69,72,80] Rebleeding is a major cause of death and disability in the untreated patient. The risk of rebleeding during the first 2 weeks after hemorrhage is approximately 20% and increases to 33% at 1 month and 50% at 6 months.[64,69,80,118] Mortality from this second hemorrhage is 40% to 50%. The risk of rebleeding continues to diminish but does not go to zero. Approximately 3% of long-term survivors can be expected to rebleed annually.[64]

Even considering the limitations of the accumulated data, it is not unreasonable to estimate that left untreated, there is a 45% mortality rate during the first year following rupture of an aneurysm and a significant continuing threat of rebleeding thereafter. It becomes apparent, then, why so many treatment modalities have been applied in attempts to influence the unfavorable prognosis of these patients.

With regard to an individual patient's prognosis and chance of ultimate recovery, the most important factor appears to be the patient's clinical condition at the time treatment is begun. One of the systems most widely used in the grading of a patient's condition is the Hunt and Hess classification (Table 55.2). The scale heavily weighs level of consciousness because this is the most important factor in predicting outcome. In discussing overall management outcome, patients are frequently divided into good grades (Hunt and Hess clinical grades 1, 2 and 3) and poor grades (Hunt and Hess grades 4 and 5).

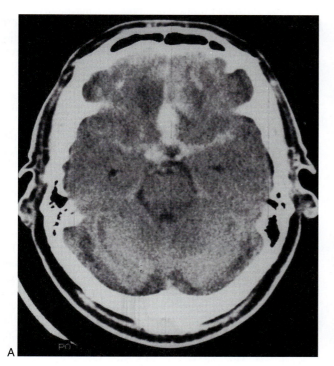

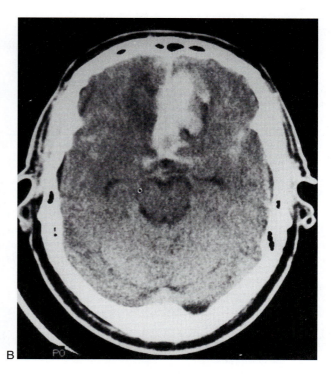

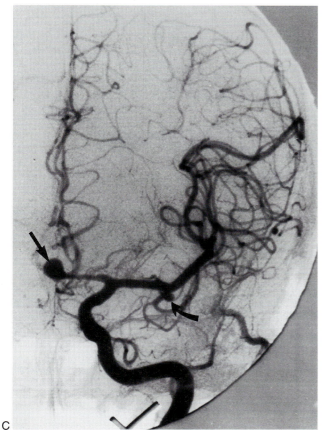

Figure 55.4 A 56-year-old man presented with the sudden onset of severe headache, nausea, and photophobia. On evaluation in the emergency room, the patient was mildly lethargic and confused. (**A & B**) Basic head computed tomography scan images at two levels demonstrate a severe subarachnoid hemorrhage with a large collection of blood within and adjacent to the interhemispheric fissure. Hemorrhage in this distribution is nearly pathognomonic for rupture of an anterior communicating artery aneurysm. (**C**) Anteroposterior view of the left internal carotid artery angiogram reveals an approximately 7-mm anterior communicating artery aneurysm (straight arrow), as well as the presence of a much smaller, incidental left middle cerebral artery aneurysm (curved arrow).

Table 55.2 Hunt and Hess Clinical Grading Scale

Group	Condition
0	Unruptured aneurysm
1	Asymptomatic or minimal headache and slight nuchal rigidity
2	Moderate or severe headache nuchal rigidity; no neurologic deficit other than cranial nerve palsy
3	Drowsiness, confusion, or mild focal deficit
4	Stupor, moderate to severe hemiparesis
5	Deep coma, decerebrate posturing, moribund appearance

Preoperative Management

No discussion of the surgical treatment of patients with aneurysmal subarachnoid hemorrhage would be complete without reviewing preoperative management. The discussion here is limited, as this topic is reviewed thoroughly elsewhere in this text (Ch. 54).

DIAGNOSIS

The usual clinical presentation of patients with aneurysmal hemorrhage is that of an individual seized with a sudden severe headache. If alert, the patient often describes the pain as "the worst headache of my life" or "like something exploded in my head." Nausea, vomiting, stiff neck, and variations in the level of consciousness are also common manifestations. Twenty percent of patients present with a sudden loss of consciousness, which may be accompanied by apnea and circulatory arrest. Patients with less severe symptoms may not recognize the severity of the episode or may be misdiagnosed if they do seek medical evaluation. Careful attention to the history and the hyperacute character of the symptoms readily separates this from other causes of headache.

When the clinical diagnosis of SAH is entertained, an orderly plan for evaluation of the patient, such as that presented below, should be followed.

1. Clinical history
2. General physical and neurologic examination
3. Routine laboratory evaluation
4. CT scan
5. Lumbar puncture (if CT is negative)
6. Four-vessel cerebral angiography

The admission evaluation should include baseline electrocardiogram (ECG), electrolytes, complete blood count, and clotting parameters. ECG changes (peaked P waves, elevated T waves, prolonged QT intervals, depressed ST segments, and other electrical evidence of cardiac stress) have been reported in a large percentage of patients with SAH. These changes have been linked to elevated catecholamine levels and may lead to cardiac ischemia and frank myocardial infarction.

CT has contributed extensively to the diagnostic capabilities of the clinician. It has proved to be a particularly valuable adjunct in the management of the patient with SAH. About 95% of patients with rupture of an intracranial aneurysm will be found to have evidence of hemorrhage on their initial CT scan if the scan is obtained within 24 hours of the bleeding episode.[2] The number of scans positive for blood decreases progressively over the ensuing days to about 75% on day 3 after hemorrhage.

Lumbar puncture remains a valuable aid in the diagnosis of SAH. While CT is well-recognized as the initial procedure of choice for the evaluation of these patients, it should be emphasized that *a negative CT scan does not rule out SAH.* When the CT scan is negative for SAH in a patient with a history suggestive of an aneurysmal bleed, the clinician should proceed to lumbar puncture. A negative CT can occur in the patient who has suffered a small (or warning) hemorrhage and in the patient whose evaluation has been delayed for more than 2 to 3 days after rupture. When CT is unavailable and the patient is alert with no lateralizing signs, lumbar puncture can be performed to evaluate the cerebrospinal fluid (CSF).

CSF soon after rupture of an aneurysm is characterized by a reddish-orange color, xanthochromia, that changes to yellow as oxyhemoglobin is converted to bilirubin. Depending on the severity of the hemorrhage, blood may not be detected in the lumbar CSF until several hours after the rupture of the aneurysm. Evidence of aneurysmal hemorrhage in the CSF often persists for 1 to 2 weeks, again depending on the severity of the bleed. Although the blood from a traumatic tap tends to clear over successive collection tubes, this is not a reliable sign that the patient does not have SAH. The presence of xanthochromia in the spun supernatant of a fresh CSF specimen is diagnostic of SAH, regardless of the cell counts.

The patient with confirmed SAH should undergo cerebral angiography as soon as clinically feasible. Angiography should be performed by an experienced team using biplanar magnification views. The subtraction of critical films can further enhance detail that would normally be hidden by overlying bone. Digital subtraction angiography (DSA) can be useful for obtaining special views. The clinical suspicion regarding the location of the ruptured aneurysm can be used to determine which of the major vessels is to be injected first; however, since 20% to 30% of patients have multiple aneurysms, a complete four-vessel study should be performed unless the patient's condition dictates otherwise.

Occasionally, cerebral angiography fails to demonstrate the source of a documented episode of SAH. In such patients, we recommend repeat angiography after resolution of hemorrhage, usually within 2 to 3 weeks. Because the risk of rebleeding from a ruptured aneurysm is greatest during this same 2- to 3-week interval, early repeat angiography with special views should be undertaken if there is any question regarding the adequacy of the initial study. The sites where aneurysms are most often missed are the anterior communicating artery complex and in the posterior fossa at the origin of the posterior inferior cerebellar artery.

GENERAL CARE

The preoperative care of the patient with aneurysmal SAH is directed toward minimizing the risk of recurrent hemorrhage and accelerating the patient's clinical recovery. Routine management should include admission to an intensive care unit, with cardiac monitoring and placement of an arterial line for the monitoring of blood pressure. Supportive care includes bed rest in a quiet room as well as sedation and pain medication as needed. For sedation and control of pain, we prefer small IV doses of morphine sulfate (1 to 4 mg/hr), which has a short half-life and can be readily reversed if necessary to evaluate apparent changes in mental status.

BLOOD PRESSURE AND FLUID MANAGEMENT

Whether to treat hypertension, the choice of drugs, dosage schedules, and other elements of the management of blood pressure can be complex issues in the patient with aneurysmal SAH. Hypertension may represent a response to increased intracranial pressure (ICP), pain, or anxiety. Blood pressure often returns to a normal range after the patient has been admitted to the hospital and these problems have been addressed.

In general, we do not recommend treatment of hypertension in patients with systolic blood pressures under 160 mmHg. To control blood pressures above this level, we prefer one of the dihydropyridine class of calcium antagonists such as nimodipine or nicardipine. These agents have the advantage that while they lower systemic blood pressure, they tend to increase cerebral blood flow. Nimodipine is the only agent presently approved by the Food and Drug Administration (FDA) for the prevention and treatment of delayed cerebral vasospasm, and is thus started before other antihypertensives are instituted. Treatment with nimodipine (60 mg/4 h, orally) for the first 21 days after hemorrhage has been shown to significantly improve outcome and to decrease the incidence of delayed ischemic deficits in patients with ruptured aneurysms.[16,113,147] We routinely treat all patients with aneurysmal SAH with nimodipine, beginning therapy soon after they are admitted to the intensive care unit. Occasionally patients are markedly sensitive to this agent, particularly the elderly and those on multiple antihypertensive medications. Therefore, we begin nimodipine therapy with 30 mg (orally or via nasogastric tube) every 4 hours and increase this dose to 60 mg every 4 hours if the patient remains clinically stable. If blood pressure remains consistently above 160 mmHg before surgical clipping of the ruptured aneurysm, despite sedation and the initiation of nimodipine, small doses of labetalol or hydralazine-hydrochloride can be given intravenously.

After the aneurysm is clipped, nimodipine is continued, but other antihypertensive agents are held for the first 2 weeks after hemorrhage (when patients are at greatest risk of vasospasm) unless systolic blood pressure exceeds 200 mmHg. Thereafter, routine medical management for hypertension is utilized. Careful monitoring of neurologic function is essential during the administration of antihypertensive agents. If the patient's clinical status deteriorates after receiving antihypertensive medication, vasospasm should be suspected and the blood pressure should be quickly returned to a previously well-tolerated level.

In patients who develop clinically symptomatic vasospasm, fluid therapy should be maximized and the blood pressure pharmacologically elevated. Our protocol for the management of symptomatic spasm is outlined in Table 55.3. It is important to recognize early symptoms of clinically significant vasospasm prior to the onset of severe ischemic deficits. Worsening headache, hyponatremia, and increasing lethargy 5 to 10 days after hemorrhage are the most frequent harbingers of vasospasm.

Fluid and electrolyte management and the treatment of vasospasm are reviewed in detail elsewhere in this text (Ch. 54). In general, we use prophylactic hypervolemic therapy (Table 55.4) for all patients with aneurysmal hemorrhage during the initial 10 to 14 days after hemorrhage; patients without clinical or transcranial Doppler evidence of spasm are then gradually weaned from intravenous fluid therapy.

VENTRICULAR DRAINAGE

Hydrocephalus is a constant threat in the patient with SAH. When CT reveals evidence of hydrocephalus or intraventricular hemorrhage or when the patient has a depressed level of consciousness (i.e., Hunt and Hess grades 3 to 5), an external ventriculostomy drain should be placed. The ventriculostomy is initially closed to drainage and monitored. If the ICP is elevated above 20 mmHg, the drain is opened at a level 15 cm above the external auditory meatus. CSF drainage at these levels maximizes cerebral perfusion and often improves clinical status by one to two grades on the Hunt and Hess scale. Monitoring ICP is also useful in deciding whether to proceed with surgery in poor grade patients (Hunt and Hess grades 4 and 5; see section on Timing of Surgery). Postoperatively, the drain is left open to constant drainage at 10 to 15 cm H_2O, until CSF output falls below 30 to 40 ml per shift, or until the 14th day after hemorrhage when the drain is progressively elevated in an attempt to wean the patient from the ventricu-

---

Table 55.3 Prophylactic Hypervolemic Fluid Therapy

Low-risk vasospasm protocol
(CT scan—Fisher grade 1 or 2)
  Normal saline—150 mL/h
  Serum sodium level daily
    If serum sodium <135 mEq/L, switch to high-risk protocol

High-risk vasospasm protocol
(CT scan—Fisher grade 3)
  Swan-Ganz catheter
    Continuous monitoring of PADP
    Cardiac output and parameters once daily
  Normal saline 150 mL/h
  Plasmanate (5% plasma protein fraction [human], Miles Inc.)
    100 mL/hr prn PADP or PCWP <10 mmHg
  Serum sodium level twice daily
    If serum sodium <135 mEq/L, begin 3% saline solution at
      30–50 ml/hr; hold for PADP >16 mmHg

Abbreviations: CT, computed tomography; PADP, pulmonary artery diastolic pressure; PCWP, pulmonary capillary wedge pressure.

Table 55.4 Hypervolemic-Hypertensive Treatment Protocol for Clinically Symptomatic Vasospasm

Swan-Ganz catheter
   Constant monitoring of PADP
   Cardiac output and parameters at 8-hour intervals
Normal saline—150 mL/h
Plasmanate (5% plasma protein fraction [human], Miles Inc.)
   100 mL/hr prn PADP or PCWP <12 mmHg
DDAVP injection (desmopressin acetate, Rhône-Poulenc Rorer Inc.)
   1 mL IV at 12-hour intervals if urine output >200 mL/h for two consecutive hours
   (hold if PADP >16 mmHg or serum sodium <135)
Neosynephrine infusion (50 mg in 250 mL normal saline)
   Titrate to maintain blood pressure between 180 and 220 systolic and reverse ischemic deficits
   (maintain systemic vascular resistance <1500 dyne/s/m^2)
Dopamine infusion
   Titrate to maintain cardiac output ≥5 L/min
   (hold for heart rate >120 beats/min)
Serum sodium level twice daily
   If serum sodium level <135 mEq/L, begin 3% sodium chloride solution at 30 to 50 ml/h
   (hold for PADP >16 mmHg)

Abbreviations: PADP, pulmonary artery diastolic pressure; PCWP, pulmonary capillary wedge pressure.

lostomy. In our experience, approximately 30% of patients will require a CSF-shunting procedure.

Risk of infection from external ventriculostomy can be minimized by combining meticulous sterile technique during placement of the catheter, with the use of prophylactic antibiotics (we prefer cefuroxime 1.5 g given immediately before placement of the catheter) and routine tunneling of the ventriculostomy catheter a minimum of 4 cm subcutaneously from the insertion site. Finally, it is important that the catheter be connected to a closed drainage system that does not require opening the system directly to air for zeroing or obtaining CSF samples (Becker External Drainage System, PS Medical, Goleta, CA 93117). CSF samples are obtained twice weekly on a routine basis for cell counts, gram stain, and culture. Using this protocol, we have not found it necessary to change the ventriculostomy site every 2 to 3 days as some authors have recommended.[82,160] We routinely leave external ventricular drainage catheters in place for as long as 2 to 3 weeks and have had only a 3% to 5% incidence of infection.

ANTIFIBRINOLYTIC THERAPY

Amicar and other antifibrinolytic agents that were once widely used to reduce the incidence of early rebleeding while patients awaited surgery (usually a period of 10 to 14 days) have fallen into disfavor. One reason for this change is that with modern microsurgical techniques, early clipping of aneurysms can be performed without increased operative morbidity and mortality. More important, however, evidence from a number of studies has demonstrated that while therapy with antifibrino-

lytic agents significantly reduced the risk of early rebleeding by as much as 50%, their use was associated with an equally significant increase in the risk of ischemic complications.[44,71,152,153] In addition, the use of antifibrinolytic agents has been linked to an increased risk of hydrocephalus.[47,71,108,114] Overall, these studies fail to demonstrate any clear benefit associated with antifibrinolytic therapy, and this treatment can no longer be recommended.

Timing of Surgery for Ruptured Aneurysms

Over the last 15 years, there has been a gradual swing in policy regarding the timing of surgery from that of delayed management to minimize the risks of surgical complications to one of early surgery to prevent rebleeding and improve overall outcome. This change reflects a natural evolution associated with developments in the field of neurosurgery.

Prior to the development of microsurgical techniques and modern neuroanesthesia, the risks of early operative intervention for the clipping of ruptured aneurysms outweighed any potential benefit. In the late 1970s and early 1980s, a small number of authors began reporting good outcomes in patients undergoing early surgery for ruptured aneurysms.[59,76,124,157] Simultaneously, the emphasis of outcome studies on aneurysmal SAH shifted from operative morbidity and mortality to overall management outcome.

In a 1981 report, the Cooperative Aneurysm Study Group analyzed the overall results of medical management and delayed surgery for clipping the ruptured aneurysm in 249 patients.[1] The authors reported a favorable outcome in only 46% of patients with a mortality rate of 36.2%. Of patients admitted in good condition with a potential for complete recovery, only 55.7% had a favorable outcome and 28.7% died. Other authors reported similar results with an overall management mortality for delayed surgery of between 40% and 60%.[38,68,88,117] These dismal results considerably heightened interest in whether early surgical intervention could improve outcome.

This issue was addressed by the International Cooperative Study on the Timing of Aneurysm Surgery.[72,73] Between January 1981 and June 1983, 3,521 patients who were hospitalized within 3 days of SAH were enrolled in the cooperative multi-institutional protocol. This was an intention-to-treat study. When the patient was admitted, the surgeon stated the time of scheduled surgery. Results were analyzed on the basis of outcome assessed 6 months after hemorrhage. Intracranial operations were performed in 92% of patients who had surgery planned for days 0 to 3: This number fell to 76% for those patients scheduled for surgery on days 11 to 14, and to 62% for those with surgery scheduled for 15 or more days after hemorrhage. Patients who did not undergo clipping of their aneurysm died or had complications related to rebleeding or vasospasm that contraindicated surgery. Among alert patients, those operated within 48 hours of rupture did as well as those undergoing surgery 2 weeks after hemorrhage. Early operation was not accompanied by a significantly higher rate of surgical complications than those associated with delayed operation. The overall results of management were almost identical in patients with surgery planned within 3 days of hemorrhage and in those with surgery scheduled for 11 to 14 days.

With the demonstration that early surgery could safely eliminate the risk of rebleeding, attention turned to the more aggressive prevention and treatment of delayed ischemic deficits secondary to vasospasm. In good-grade patients (Hunt and Hess grades 1 to 3), multiple groups have reported that early surgery, the use of calcium antagonists, and hypervolemic-hypertensive therapy can reduce overall management mortality to 10% or less, with good outcomes in 75% or more of those who survive.[7,8,77,79,101,125,151]

We reviewed our experience at the Barrow Neurological Institute from 1987 to 1990. Over this 3-year period, we operated early on all patients with documented aneurysmal SAH regardless of their clinical grade (excluding only patients without evidence of brain stem function). Early surgery (within 72 hours of hemorrhage) was performed on 90 patients. All patients were treated with aggressive fluid management, including hypervolemic-hypertensive therapy in those that developed evidence of cerebral vasospasm. At 3-month follow-up, the overall outcome was good in 81% of patients, poor in 8%, and 11% had died. In good-grade patients (Hunt and Hess grades 1 to 3), 88% had a good outcome and only 7% had died. In 23 poor-grade patients (Hunt and Hess grades 4 and 5), 56% had a good outcomes and 26% had died. Severe deficits affected 3 patients and 1 was vegetative.

Based on our own experience and that in the literature, we now recommend surgery on all good-grade patients (Hunt and Hess grades 1 to 3) regardless of the time of presentation. When patients are referred on a delayed basis (4 or more days after hemorrhage) and are neurologically stable, we routinely maximize fluid-volume status and proceed with surgery. Many surgeons will delay surgery in such patients if the initial angiogram shows evidence of vasospasm. Although angiographic vasospasm may affect surgical outcome, its effects on overall management outcome is an issue that has not been addressed in clinical trials. When surgery is delayed because of angiographic evidence of vasospasm, patients are exposed to the risks of rebleeding. Furthermore, if the arterial spasm becomes clinically symptomatic, it cannot be treated safely in an aggressive fashion. Until this issue is more thoroughly studied, we do not believe that angiographic evidence of vasospasm should be considered a contraindication to surgery. Special care should be taken in these patients to limit the risks of ischemic injury; hypovolemia and hypotension should be avoided. Blood pressure should be maintained within 10 to 15 mm of preoperative values. Once proximal control of the aneurysm has been obtained, the surgeon can safely apply papaverine to the exposed vessels to relieve arterial spasm and improve blood flow while the dissection and clipping proceed.

The decision of when and whether to operate on poor-grade patients (Hunt and Hess grades 4 and 5) after aneurysmal hemorrhage is much more controversial. Nevertheless, it is clear that patients admitted in poor condition soon after hemorrhage may have a good outcome. We have developed a protocol for the selection of operative candidates based on CT scan data, ICP measurements, and angiographic findings (Fig. 55.5). Briefly, all patients presenting with SAH in grades 4 and 5 have a ventriculostomy placed except those who show radiographic evidence of irreversible brain destruction. For example, a large hematoma in the dominant basal ganglia

Figure 55.5 Treatment algorithm for the management of poor-grade patients with aneurysmal subarachnoid hemorrhage. CT, computed tomography; SAH, subarachnoid hemorrhage; ICP, intracranial pressure. (Adapted from Bailes et al,[13] with permission.)

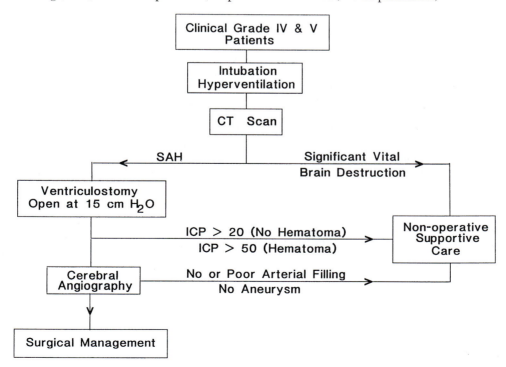

would preclude active treatment. In addition, operative intervention is withheld for three reasons after ventriculostomy: if ICP cannot be controlled below 20 mmHg in the patient without hematoma, if ICP is greater than 50 mmHg in the patient with a hematoma, and if there is poor or absent intracranial filling on angiography. The remaining patients undergo early surgery for aneurysm clipping, irrespective of their neurologic examination. Postoperatively, patients are treated with calcium antagonists and aggressive hypervolemic-hypertensive therapy.

Certainly, patients in worse neurologic condition are expected to have a poorer outcome; however, clinical examination alone soon after aneurysmal hemorrhage is not a good criterion for predicting outcome.[13,56,111] In a prospective study that evaluated our protocol in 54 poor-grade patients, 35 patients (20 grade 4 and 15 grade 5) were selected for active treatment: 19 (54%) had good outcomes at 3 months and were independent for all activities of daily living, 4 (11%) were dependent for some activities but were not housebound, 4 patients were institutionalized with poor outcomes, and 8 (23%) patients had died.[13] There were no survivors in the nonoperative group. Clearly, an aggressive surgical approach based on appropriate selection criteria is warranted in grade 4 and grade 5 patients.

While the decision tree outlined in Figure 5 is helpful in selecting patients for surgery, the decision of whether to operate in the poor-grade patient often rests on associated clinical variables. For example, most surgeons would clip a posterior communicating artery aneurysm in a young Hunt and Hess grade 4 patient with a nondominant temporal lobe hematoma, whereas few would attempt intervention for a deep clot in the dominant hemisphere of an elderly grade 4 patient with a carotid bifurcation aneurysm.

Management of Multiple and Incidental Aneurysms

Multiple aneurysms and aneurysms discovered incidentally are at risk of rupture. Attempts have been made to define a critical size (diameter) below which aneurysms should be observed. Wiebers et al[159] reported on 130 conservatively treated patients with unruptured aneurysms. During an average follow-up of 8.3 years, there were 15 hemorrhages, all in patients with aneurysms greater than 10 mm in diameter (mean diameter, 21.3 mm). By contrast, the mean diameter for ruptured aneurysms seen at the same institution was only 7.5 mm. To explain this discrepancy, the authors postulate that the mean size of aneurysm rupture is smaller if the rupture occurs soon after hemorrhage or, alternatively, that the rupture may be associated with a temporary decrease in the size of the aneurysm. Other studies have not supported these findings.

Juvela et al[67] investigated the natural history of unruptured aneurysms in 142 patients. During a median follow-up of 13.9 years, there were 27 first episodes of hemorrhage for an annual rupture rate of 1.4%. The median diameter of aneurysms at the beginning of the follow-up period was 4 mm in both those with and those without later hemorrhage. In an autopsy series, Cromptom[29] found the critical size for aneu-

rysm rupture to be 4 mm. Similarly, McCormick and Acosta-Rua[84] found 5 mm to be the critical size for rupture. In an analysis of angiograms from 1,093 patients with SAH admitted to the Cooperative Aneurysm Study, Kassell and Torner[70] found that the median diameter for ruptured aneurysms was 7 mm, 71% of the aneurysms were smaller than 10 mm, and 13% were less than 5 mm in diameter. In general, the data from the literature suggest that the critical size for rupture is between 4 and 7 mm.

Some controversy continues about the management of these lesions. A few authors recommend that unruptured aneurysms should not be operated on because the morbidity and mortality of surgery are higher than that associated with their natural history. However, a thoughtful analysis by van Crevel et al[150] suggests otherwise. These authors used modern decision analysis techniques to compare the risks of nonoperative and operative treatment in patients with incidental aneurysms and calculated the break-even age at which patients with incidental aneurysms would no longer benefit from surgery (Fig. 55.6). They pointed out that when an aneurysm ruptures the consequences are often devastating. Population studies suggest that approximately 15% of patients are found dead after their initial hemorrhage,[26,78,151] while 30% to 40% of those who are hospitalized have poor outcomes or die despite aggressive medical and surgical treatment.[26,50,72,78,113,151] A review of the largest natural history studies reveals a risk of rupture for intact aneurysms of 1% to 2% per year.[32,64,67] Using these figures, the estimated combined morbidity and mortality for aneurysm rupture are 1.5% to 3% at 3 years and 2.5% to 5% at 5 years.

Microsurgical techniques and improvements in anesthesia have made the operative risks for the elective management of unruptured aneurysms extremely favorable. Samson et al[123]

Figure 55.6 Age of the patient at which surgery and no surgery have the same expected morbidity and mortality (break-even age) related to management of an incidental aneurysm. Patients are assumed to be good surgical candidates from a medical standpoint. • females; ○ males. (Adapted from van Crevel et al,[150] with permission.)

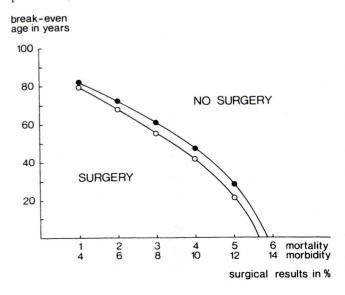

reported no mortality and 6.3% morbidity in 49 patients. Sala-zar[121] had no mortality and 3.4% morbidity in his series. Drake[38] successfully clipped 289 unruptured aneurysms with no mortality and a morbidity of 1.7%.

This analysis indicates that incidental aneurysms are not benign lesions. In experienced hands, these lesions can be surgically treated with a combined morbidity and mortality less than that of their natural history over 3 to 5 years. If an aneurysm is accessible, and the patient is a good operative risk, then surgical treatment is the therapy of choice.

Management of Mycotic Aneurysms

Mycotic aneurysms develop as a result of infection in the arterial wall. The term *mycotic* was coined by Osler in 1885,[105] and although it more properly refers to lesions caused by fungal infections, common usage through the years has applied the term mycotic to aneurysms produced by any infectious agent.

Mycotic aneurysms constitute approximately 5% of cerebral aneurysms. They occur primarily as a complication of subacute bacterial endocarditis (SBE) but are also seen in patients with congenital heart disease and prominent right-to-left shunts. In patients who develop SBE, approximately 17% are reported to have symptoms of cerebral embolization. Clinical and pathologic studies have demonstrated the presence of mycotic aneurysms in approximately 4% of patients with SBE. The aneurysms are believed to result from the direct extension of infection from septic emboli that lodge in the arterial lumen or within the vasovasorum of the vessel wall. Once established, the ensuing infectious process leads to damage of the vessel wall and aneurysmal dilatation. The aneurysms are usually fusiform in shape, but saccular aneurysms do occur. Unlike congenital aneurysms, which are normally located at the proximal branching points of the circle of Willis, mycotic aneurysms typically are located more peripherally (Fig 7).

Considering the evidence that these lesions arise from septic emboli, angiographic evaluation is recommended for patients with SBE and symptoms suggesting cerebral ischemic events. In centers with high-resolution MRI, screening for aneurysms using the combination of MRI of the brain and magnetic resonance angiography (MRA) of the head is a reasonable option; conventional angiography should be used to confirm abnormal findings prior to the institution of treatment.

Patients who harbor an unruptured bacterial aneurysm(s) should be treated with high doses of the appropriate antibiotics, and the aneurysm should be followed with repeat angiography.[21,23,95] Because of the high morbidity and mortality associated with rupture of these lesions, follow-up should be obtained at weekly intervals during the initial stages of treatment. If the aneurysm thromboses or disappears, no further treatment is necessary. However, if the aneurysm enlarges or remains unchanged, it should be treated surgically. Available experience is insufficient to comment on whether fungal aneurysms can be treated successfully without surgery. Because aneurysms associated with fungal infections are most frequently found in patients with severe immunosuppression, the prognosis for this group is generally quite poor.

General Operative Considerations

Although we strongly recommend the early clipping of ruptured aneurysms, we believe that surgery in these difficult cases is best performed by a well-rested, experienced team. At our institution, surgery is usually performed within 12 to 24 hours of admission. This short delay provides adequate time for complete angiographic evaluation and medical stabilization of the patient, including placement of a ventriculostomy, if indicated. In our experience, many poor-grade patients will improve clinically during this period by as much as one to two grades on the Hunt and Hess scale. The patient with an intracerebral or extra-axial hematoma who is deteriorating is an obvious exception and requires emergency surgical intervention.

The anesthesiologist should be experienced in the management of neurosurgical cases and familiar with the surgeon's

Figure 55.7 (**A**) Angiographic and (**B**) gross pathologic appearance of mycotic middle cerebral artery aneurysm (arrow) in a middle-aged male who presented with a history of left-hemisphere transient ischemic attacks, as well as with signs and symptoms of subacute bacterial endocarditis, including dyspnea, fever, chills, and a grade V/VI systolic ejection murmur.

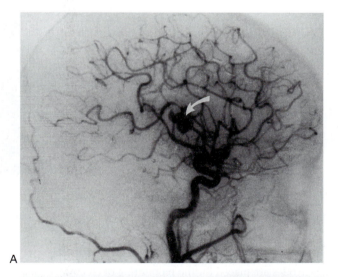

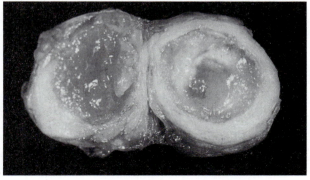

Figure 55.8 (**A&B**) Surface electrode placement for compressed spectral analysis monitoring of electroencephalogram activity and for median nerve somatosensory evoked potentials. The planned craniotomy incision has been outlined with a skin marker.

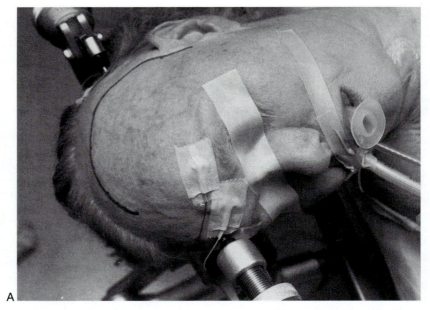

A

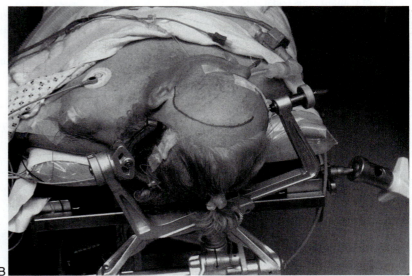

B

preferences for intraoperative management (i.e., use of mannitol, barbiturates; see next section). They should assist with the operative positioning of the patient, including the padding of all pressure points. In all but the most urgent cases, surface electrodes are placed for the monitoring of electroencephalogram (EEG) and somatosensory evoked potentials (Fig. 55.8).

ANESTHESIA FOR ANEURYSM SURGERY

Advances in neuroanesthesia have markedly reduced the preoperative risks of intracranial surgery. Modern anesthetic management begins before the patient is transferred to the surgical suite with a complete review of the patient's history and current medical problems. In the alert patient, mild sedation can reduce stress and blood pressure fluctuations before the induction of anesthesia. Anesthesia is usually induced using a combination of agents with the goal of avoiding significant swings in blood pressure and heart rate. Hypotension in the clinically compromised patient may significantly reduce cerebral blood flow (CBF), while hypertension may increase the risk of recurrent aneurysmal hemorrhage. At our institution, a sedative such as midazolam combined with sodium thiopental and lidocaine is used for induction and is followed by complete neuromuscular blockade prior to any attempt at intubation. The patient is ventilated to maintain the end tidal pCO_2 between 30 and 40 mmHg until brain retraction is begun; it is then lowered to 25 mmHg. Anesthesia is maintained with a combination of inhalational agents such as isoflurane and nitrous oxide, while small intravenous doses of sufentanil (or fentanyl in the patient with cardiac instability) are used to titrate blood pressure and heart rate within 10% of preoperative values. Mannitol (25 to 50 g) is delivered intravenously if the brain is not already slack when the dura is opened. Ventricular drainage and barbiturates are also valuable adjuncts in further reducing brain volume before retraction.

Previously, moderate systemic hypotension was routinely employed by most surgeons to reduce the risks of rupture during the dissection and clipping of aneurysms. This degree of hypotension would normally result in little or no change in CBF; however, in patients with aneurysmal SAH, particularly those with a depressed level of consciousness or vasospasm, impaired cerebral autoregulation can lead to significant, generalized cerebral ischemia.[33,43,55,155] Most authors have abandoned the use of systemic hypotension in favor of short periods of temporary vessel occlusion to reduce the risk of premature aneurysm rupture or to control hemorrhage after rupture.[9,10,63,142] In general, temporary occlusion of the major intracranial vessels is well-tolerated for 10 to 20 minutes.[63,85,91,100,122,142,143,145] Moderate hypothermia (33° to 34°C), common under general anesthesia, also increases the brain's tolerance of ischemia. We routinely combine this degree of hypothermia with deep barbiturate anesthesia. Barbiturates are begun just prior to brain retraction: thiopental is administered as a loading dose of 5 to 10 mg/kg of body weight followed by a continuous infusion titrated to produce 10 to 20 seconds of complete EEG burst suppression (Fig. 55.9). Blood pressure is maintained within 10% of preoperative values with small doses of ephedrine if necessary. Clinical and laboratory evidence suggests that barbiturates reduce the risk of ischemic injury during temporary vessel occlusion.[27,57,85,128–132]

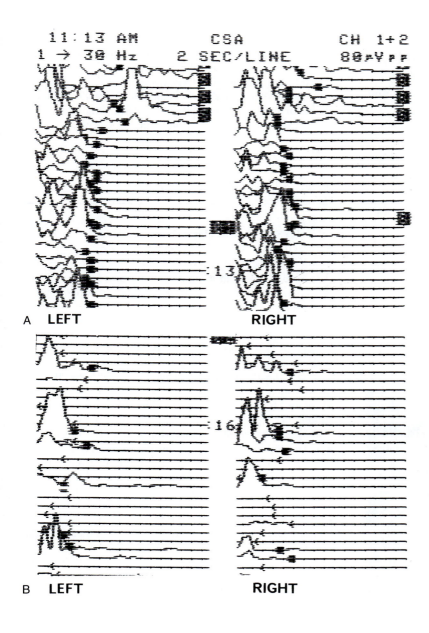

A LEFT   RIGHT

B LEFT   RIGHT

Figure 55.9 Compressed spectral analysis of electroencephalogram (EEG) activity during surgery for elective clipping of an incidental aneurysm. CSA (**A**) before and (**B**) after indication of deep barbiturate coma with EEG burst suppression. Each line of the display represents a 2-second frequency spectrum analysis of EEG activity between 0 and 30 Hz. The flat lines represent periods of complete EEG burst suppression.

DIRECT CLIPPING OF ANEURYSMS

The treatment of choice for most intracranial aneurysms is direct clipping of the neck. Aneurysms that are unsuitable for direct clipping can be approached in the various ways discussed below. Advances in microsurgical technique and the availability of a wide spectrum of aneurysm clips have increased the percentage of aneurysms suitable for direct neck obliteration.

Three types of spring-loaded clips are typically used (Fig. 55.10): (1) clips with parallel blades placed directly across the neck of the aneurysm come in all lengths, curves, and bayonet shapes; (2) circumferential clips that enclose the parent vessel to obliterate the aneurysm neck between the ends of the concave jaws; and (3) clips that combine the parallel, long, thin jaws of the first type with a proximal round aperture through which an artery or nerve may pass. These clips, in combination with the new thin appliers, permit accurate obliteration of the aneurysm neck even in narrow, awkward locations. Special clips with ultralow closing pressures designed to prevent intimal injury are also available for temporary vessel occlusion.

General principles involved in surgical management of acutely ruptured aneurysms are briefly discussed. First and foremost, the operating room staff should be experienced with microsurgical techniques. Exposed surfaces of the brain should be covered (we prefer Telfa strips) and protected from dehydration and trauma. CSF drainage and mannitol can be used to help facilitate brain retraction. The induction of barbiturate burst suppression when the dura is opened will also encourage brain relaxation, increase tolerance to ischemia, and afford a greater margin of safety if temporary vessel occlusion is needed. The approach to a ruptured aneurysm should include early exposure and control of the parent vessel. The

neck of the aneurysm should be completely exposed. With the neck of the aneurysm dissected free, the surgeon should select the appropriate clip and apply it in an unhurried manner. If the clip is not satisfactorily placed, the reapplication of a different clip or the trial of an alternate clip applier should be attempted until perfect clip placement has been achieved. After the surgeon is satisfied that the clip has been appropriately placed, the dome of the aneurysm can be decompressed with a small needle to verify complete neck occlusion. Last and most important, should the aneurysm rupture, the impulse to react quickly and to attempt clip placement hurriedly should be resisted. Instead, a suction must carefully and gently be placed to permit controlled dissection of the aneurysm to continue. Frequently, hemorrhage from the ruptured dome can be controlled by gentle tamponade with a small cotton patty held in place with the sucker tip. At this point, temporary clips can be placed across the parent vessel(s) and dissection completed about the neck of the aneurysm. As discussed above, temporary occlusion of major cerebral vessels under barbiturate protection is well-tolerated for 15 to 20 minutes, assuming systemic pressure has been maintained in a normal range.

In certain broad-necked aneurysms, multiple clips may be necessary. The wide variety of fenestrated Sugita (SIMS Surgical Inc., Keene, NH) and Sundt-Kees (Codman, Johnson & Johnson, Randolph, MA) clips is particularly adaptable to occlusion of an awkward aneurysm neck. Fenestrated, straight, or right-angle clips can be placed serially over the parent vessel to extend the length of neck occlusion (Fig. 55.11).

Specific Operative Techniques

ANEURYSMS OF THE ANTERIOR CIRCULATION

Approximately 85% of intracranial aneurysms involve the anterior circulation. The majority of these aneurysms (95%) is readily treated using the pterional approach. Minor modifications may be helpful for exposing some specific lesions, but the general approach is similar. Because it is the most common approach used for aneurysm surgery, it is presented in some detail.

Following the induction of general anesthesia, the patient's head is positioned using three-point skeletal fixation and rotated from 30° to 60° off midline toward the opposite shoulder. The degree of rotation depends on the specific lesion, being greatest for anterior communicating artery aneurysms and least for those aneurysms involving the posterior communicating artery and the internal carotid artery bifurcation. The skin incision is made from the posterior margin of the zygomatic process and carried forward and superiorly in a gently curving arc to a point just behind the hairline in the middle of the forehead (Fig. 55.12). The scalp and underlying muscle are elevated together with the exception of a small facial cuff along the insertion of the temporalis muscle. This cuff is used during closure to firmly secure the temporalis muscle in its normal anatomic position, helping to reduce postoperative problems with temporal

Figure 55.10 Types of aneurysm clips available to the surgeon. (**A–C**) Clips with parallel blades in various shapes and sizes are placed directly across the aneurysm neck. (**D**) Circumferential clips that enclose the parent vessel completely and obliterate the aneurysm neck between the ends of concave jaws. (**E**) Clips that combine parallel jaws for obliterating the aneurysm neck with a proximal aperture through which an artery or nerve may pass.

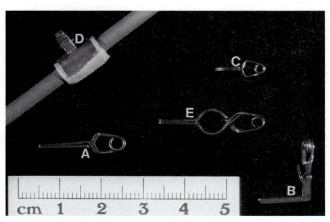

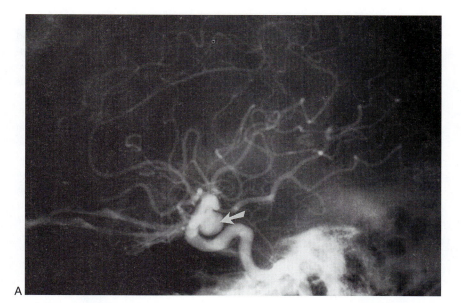

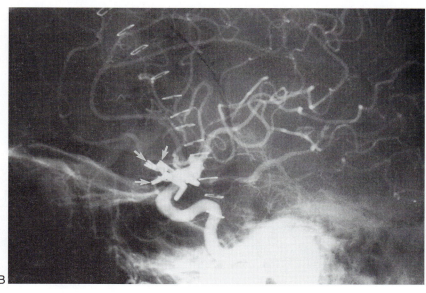

Figure 55.11 A 53-year-old woman was referred for evaluation after experiencing transient ischemic attacks that affected the right upper extremity. (**A**) Lateral view of the left internal carotid artery angiogram demonstrating a large, wide-necked, left internal carotid artery aneurysm (arrow). Cardiac workup and extracranial vascular evaluation were negative for other possible embolic sources. (**B**) Lateral view of the postoperative left internal carotid artery angiogram demonstrating good clipping of the aneurysm. Note that a combination of three clips (arrows) has been used to obliterate the aneurysm neck and reconstruct the parent vessel.

mandibular joint dysfunction and to improve cosmetic appearance (Fig. 55.12).

The soft tissues are retracted, and a free frontotemporal bone flap is turned (Fig. 55.13). Care is taken to bring this flap as close to the frontal fossa floor as possible. With the aid of a high-speed air-drill (Midas Rex Pneumatic Tools, Inc., Fort Worth, TX), bony resection of the lateral frontal wall and pterion is completed, bringing the dissection flush with the frontal fossa floor (Fig. 55.13). This bony removal minimizes the need for brain retraction to expose the basal cisterns. The dura is tacked to the edges of the bony craniotomy at 2- to 3-cm intervals to assure hemostasis. The dura is opened in a semilunar fashion and remains hinged along the floor of the frontal fossa. The dura is elevated and retracted with stay sutures over the muscle to provide maximum direct exposure. The brain should be covered to prevent drying and trauma from retractors and instruments; Telfa strips are a good choice

and can be readily cut to different sizes. The frontal lobe is gently elevated with a self-retaining retractor (Fig. 55.13). If necessary, another small, thin retractor can be placed over the temporal lobe at its junction with the sylvian fissure.

If there is any resistance to retraction, measures to increase relaxation of the brain are instituted as outlined above, including mannitol, barbiturates, and CSF drainage. In the patient without a ventricular catheter, retraction becomes easier once the basal cisterns are opened. Incising the arachnoid around the optic nerve and internal carotid artery provides a pathway for ample CSF drainage. The basal portion of the sylvian fissure is opened to complete exposure of the internal carotid artery. The need for further opening of the sylvian fissure is dictated by the type of aneurysm being approached, being least for anterior communicating artery aneurysms and greatest for those of the middle cerebral artery. By observing the proper arachnoid planes, the proximal middle cerebral

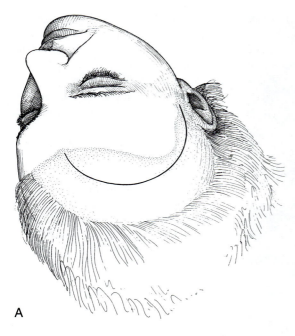

A

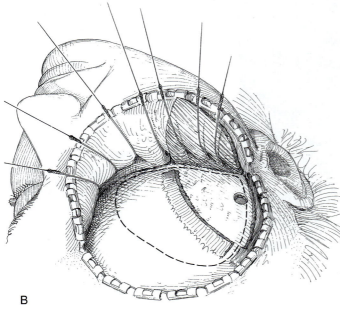

B

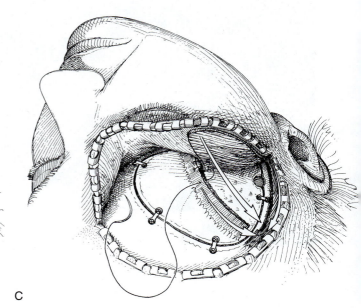

C

Figure 55.12 Pterional approach to anterior circulation aneurysms (see text for details). (**A**) Outline of scalp incision. (**B**) The scalp flap and underlying temporalis muscle have been elevated together with the exception of a small fascial cuff along the insertion of the temporalis muscle (arrows). Fishhooks have been used to retract the scalp and temporalis muscle flaps. Note the outline for the planned bone flap, which is brought to the midpupillary line and as close to the frontal fossa floor as possible. This type of bony dissection helps minimize the degree of brain retraction needed to visualize the basal cisterns. (**C**) The intracranial portion of the procedure has been completed, and the bone flap has been replaced and fixed securely in position with miniplates and screws. The cut edges of the temporalis fascia are being approximated with a running suture. This closure helps to ensure normal anatomic function of the temporalis muscle, as well as to improve the postoperative cosmetic appearance of the temporal fossa region. (Adapted from Spetzler et al,[138] with permission.)

artery and its major trunks can be exposed without dividing any arterial branches (Fig. 55.13).

The dissection and clipping of internal carotid artery and posterior communicating artery aneurysms are also greatly aided by opening the sylvian fissure widely. This is particularly true for carotid artery bifurcation aneurysms where the surgeon must take special care to avoid including any of the numerous small perforating arterial branches that arise from the proximal segments of the anterior cerebral and middle cerebral arteries.

The same general exposure is adequate for approaching anterior communicating artery aneurysms, except that only the basal portion of the sylvian fissure need be opened. Anterior communicating artery aneurysms can be approached directly through the resection of a small portion of the ipsilateral gyrus rectus or by following the proximal portion of the anterior cerebral artery to the communicating artery complex. The advantage of approaching through the gyrus rectus is that the small perforating arteries and recurrent artery of Heubner are exposed to less risk of injury. The surgeon has to recognize the wide variability of the anatomy of the anterior communicating artery region. There may be two or more communicating arteries each with multiple perforating branches. In addition to exposing the anterior communicating artery and its perfora-

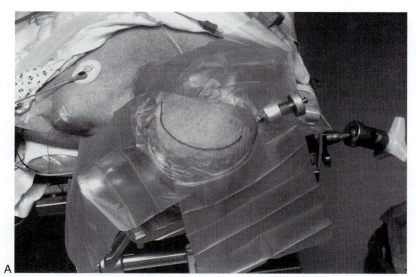

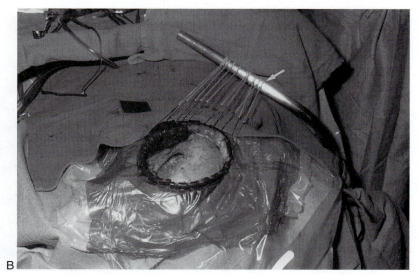

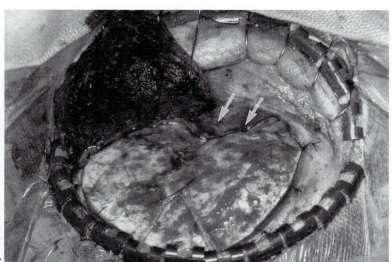

Figure 55.13 Surgical treatment of the incidental left middle cerebral artery aneurysm in the 64-year-old woman presented in Fig. 55.1 (**A**) The patient has been positioned for a pterional craniotomy and the incision outlined. Self-adhering sterile drapes help isolate the field and protect the electrodes used for intraoperative monitoring from moisture. (**B**) The scalp flap has been elevated, and the skin and muscle are being retracted with fishhooks attached to rubber bands, which are, in turn, secured to a Leyla bar (arrow). (**C**) The craniotomy bone flap has been turned and elevated, exposing the underlying dura. Dural tackup sutures have been placed at regular intervals around the margin of the bone flap to control bleeding. The lateral wall of the sphenoid wing has been removed with a high-speed drill to bring the bony dissection flush with the frontal fossa floor (arrows). The removal of bone minimizes the retraction needed to visualize the basal cisterns and aneurysm.

Figure 55.13 (Continued) (**D**) The dura has been opened and retracted with stay sutures. The brain surface is covered with Telfa strips to protect it from drying and trauma. The frontal lobe is being gently elevated to expose the basal cisterns. The pristine white silhouette of the optic nerve (arrow) is faintly visible through an intact vale of arachnoid at the tip of the retractor blade. (**E**) The sylvian fissure has been widely opened and the aneurysm at the middle cerebral artery bifurcation exposed (arrows). Note the marked irregularity of the aneurysm dome. At surgery, blood could be readily visualized swirling through the thinned outpouchings of the aneurysm surface. (**F**) The aneurysm has been dissected free of the surrounding vessels and the neck obliterated with a single clip. The dome of the aneurysm has been punctured and collapsed to ensure that it no longer fills.

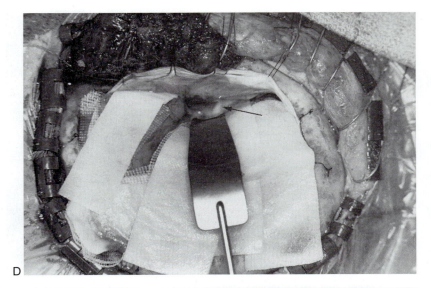

D

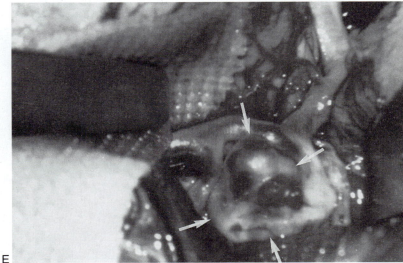

E

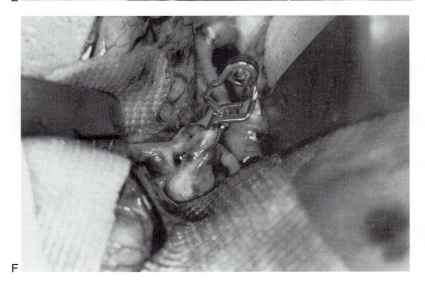

F

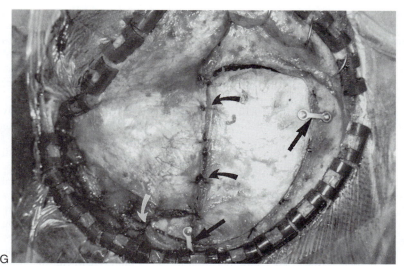

Figure 55.13 *(Continued)* **(G)** The craniotomy bone flap has been replaced and secured in position with miniplates and screws (straight arrows). The cut edges of the temporalis fascia have been reapproximated (curved arrows) and only the scalp closure remains to be completed.

tors, the surgeon must identify the proximal (A_1) and distal (A_2) branches of both anterior cerebral arteries, as well as the frontopolar branches and the recurrent arteries of Heubner to both hemispheres. Failure to protect the multitude of vessels in this area from occlusion can lead to serious neurologic morbidity. The side of approach to these midline lesions is governed by the size of the aneurysm and the anatomy of the feeding vessels. Not infrequently, anterior communicating artery aneurysms are found in patients in whom one of the proximal anterior cerebral arteries is absent or markedly atretic, and the remaining or dominant artery supplies both hemispheres. The aneurysms in such cases tend to occur at the junction of the dominant vessel with the anterior communicating artery, in a direct line with the blood flow. When the aneurysm is large, it may obscure the parent vessels and is best exposed from the side of the dominant anterior cerebral artery. The occurrence of aneurysms in association with vascular anomalies that increase flow and shear stress at branch points argues in favor of the hypothesis that aneurysms are acquired lesions. Other examples would include the common finding of aneurysms on the feeding vessels of AVMs and the frequent association of aneurysms with arterial fenestrations.

Paraclinoid and ophthalmic artery aneurysms that arise from the internal carotid artery as it exits the cavernous sinus are also approached with the pterional approach. Complete exposure of the neck of these aneurysms for clipping commonly requires resection of the anterior clinoid process and roof of the optic foramen. This bony dissection is performed using a high-speed drill with a small diamond-tipped burr. The optic nerve and internal carotid artery can be further mobilized by dividing the dural sleeves that invest these structures.

PERICALLOSAL ANEURYSMS

Pericallosal aneurysms are relatively uncommon, comprising about only 3% of aneurysms in most major series. An intrahemispheric approach is used for exposure. The bone flap should be sufficiently anterior to allow proximal control of the parent vessel prior to visualization of the aneurysm. A bifrontal scalp incision located well behind the hairline provides good exposure. The scalp flap is reflected forward and inferiorly exposing the anterior third of the cranium. A right-sided, nondominant approach is preferred; however, the final decision should be determined from the venous angiogram: the side with the greatest room between draining veins is selected. Tsutsumi et al[148] have recently emphasized the complications associated with sacrificing bridging veins in the intrahemispheric approach to ruptured aneurysms in this area, particularly in the patient with recent SAH. It is relatively unimportant whether the approach is ipsilateral or contralateral. To minimize retraction of the frontal lobe, the bone flap should be carried across the sagittal sinus; the dura is then opened so that it remains hinged along the edge of the sinus and retracted with stay sutures to maximize midline exposure. The parent vessel is exposed proximally and followed until the aneurysm is identified. The aneurysm is clipped in the usual manner.

ANEURYSMS OF THE POSTERIOR CIRCULATION

Basilar Bifurcation Aneurysms

Aneurysms involving the terminal portion of the basilar artery are relatively rare, accounting for only 7% to 8% of cases of aneurysmal SAH. The majority of these lesions arises from the basilar tip and the junction between the superior cerebellar and posterior cerebral arteries. While once considered formidable, advances in microsurgical technique and the availability of a wide variety of clips and appliers have made the approach to these lesions routine at major referral centers. For large or giant aneurysms of the basilar artery, the surgeon may need to consider hypothermic circulatory arrest as an adjunct in clipping; the indications and rationale for this approach are discussed later in this section.

Three approaches are used to expose aneurysms involving the basilar bifurcation: the pterional, subtemporal, and orbitozygomatic approaches. The pterional approach, as described above, provides excellent exposure for small and medium-sized aneurysms that arise from the basilar tip or origin of the superior cerebellar arteries (Figs. 55.12 and 55.13). This approach is particularly useful for those aneurysms that point forward or straight up from the basilar bifurcation. After the carotid artery is exposed, the sylvian fissure is opened widely and the posterior communicating artery is followed to the posterior cerebral artery and the basilar tip.

For large aneurysms and those that point back into the brain stem or that arise from a high basilar bifurcation, the subtemporal (Fig. 55.14) or orbitozygomatic (Fig. 55.15) approach is preferred. The subtemporal approach as first advocated by Drake[39,40] provides an excellent exposure to the terminal portion of the basilar artery. Because of the potential risk of retraction injury to the temporal lobe associated with this exposure, the approach is usually performed from the nondominant (right) side. A modified pterional scalp incision is used with a slight posterior extension to increase the exposure of the anterior temporal lobe. A free frontotemporal bone flap is turned, with care taken to bring the flap as close to the frontal and middle fossae floors as possible. A high-speed drill is used to complete the removal of bone from the lateral wall of the temporal fossa, which usually includes partial resection of the zygomatic root (Fig. 55.14). The importance of bony removal cannot be overemphasized. Any lip of bone remaining above the middle fossa floor will require increased retraction of the temporal lobe. By this approach, the basilar artery is exposed beneath the anterior third of the temporal lobe. The temporal lobe is covered with protective strips and retracted upward to expose the tentorial edge and arachnoid of the prepontine cistern (Fig. 55.14). If there is any resistance to retraction, measures to increase relaxation of the brain should be instituted as outlined above. The arachnoid is opened widely, exposing the full course of the third cranial nerve as well as the ipsilateral superior cerebellar and posterior cerebral arteries. If the basilar artery is not already in view, these vessels can be followed proximally until their juncture with the basilar artery is visible. In the patient with an acutely ruptured aneurysm, swelling and edema increase the risks of temporal lobe retraction and the difficulty of obtaining adequate exposure with this approach. As a result, many advocates of this approach prefer to delay surgery for 2 to 3 weeks after an aneurysm ruptures before attempting surgical clipping.

The adoption of skull base techniques to the management of aneurysms of the vertebrobasilar system reduces the risks of exposing these lesions by substituting bone removal for brain retraction. Since the publication of the second edition of this text in 1992, we have all but abandoned the subtemporal approach to basilar tip aneurysms, preferring now to use the orbitozygomatic approach for these lesions, as well as for most aneurysms involving the upper third of the basilar artery. In addition to reducing the need for brain retraction, the orbitozygomatic approach decreases the distance at which the surgeon must work to reach the upper basilar artery and creates a wide corridor with multiple avenues of exposure. The details of this approach have been published elsewhere.[3,49,86,104] The initial skin incision and exposure are essentially identical to those used for the pterional approach. A frontotemporal bone flap is turned, with care taken to bring the flap as close to the frontal and middle fossae floors as possible. A series of osteotomies are made with a small reciprocating saw, and the superior and lateral walls of the orbit are removed together as a single free bone flap along with the zygomatic bone and arch (Fig. 55.15). A high-speed drill is used to complete bony resection of the medial orbital wall and anterior clinoid process.

The operative approach to the upper basilar artery with the orbitozygomatic approach is between the frontal and temporal lobes. The sylvian fissure is widely split and the temporal lobe is gently retracted along its medial surface to open a corridor to the prepontine cisterns. The arachnoid planes are opened to allow full exposure of the posterior communicating artery, anterior choroidal artery, and the third cranial nerve (Fig. 55.15). If the basilar artery is not already visible, the posterior communicating artery is followed to the posterior cerebral artery and the basilar bifurcation. By changing the angle of the scope, the surgeon can view the aneurysm from anterior and lateral perspectives to ensure that all perforators have been freed from the neck. At this juncture, it is critical to expose the posterior cerebral artery and third cranial nerve on the opposite side. Dissection needs to be sufficient to allow complete visualization of the clip during placement across the aneurysm neck to ensure that it does not incorporate other neural or vascular structures. Perforating branches arising from the proximal posterior cerebral arteries and distal basilar trunk are numerous and important. An otherwise excellent clipping that traps even one of these perforators in the clip blades can cause severe neurologic deficits. Multiple trials of clips, with and without fenestrations, may be necessary to occlude the aneurysm neck safely. Following clipping, the orbitozygomatic bone and pterional bone flaps are replaced; the use of miniplates and screws (Fig. 55.15) ensures anatomic alignment and excellent cosmetic result.

Midbasilar Aneurysms

Aneurysms located along the middle third of the basilar artery from the level of the origin of the anterior inferior cerebellar arteries and above are the most difficult to approach and clip successfully. Fortunately, these lesions make up less than 1% of aneurysms in published series of SAH. Aneurysms in this location are best exposed using a combined supra- and infratentorial skull base approach that involves extensive bony removal of the petrous apex to minimize retraction of the cerebellum and brain stem (Fig. 55.16). This type of complex approach is best accomplished by an experienced neurosurgeon and an otologist with a special interest in temporal bone anatomy.[5,135] Bone removal is the key to minimizing retraction in this type of approach. Removal of even a few millimeters of bone laterally can dramatically improve exposure. Since it is difficult to obtain complete control of the parent vessel in this region, the final stages of dissection and manipulation of the aneurysm prior to clipping may best be performed under total circulatory arrest.

Aneurysms arising in this region often involve significant portions of the wall of the parent vessel and may not be suitable for direct clipping. In such cases, sacrifice of the basilar

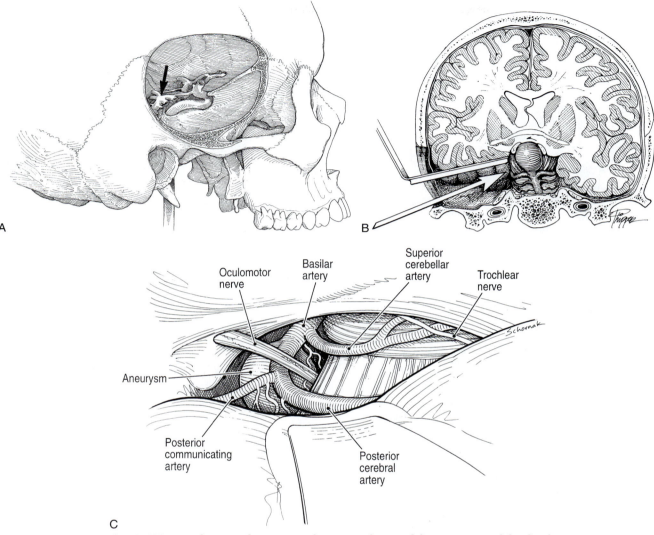

A

B

C

Figure 55.14 Subtemporal exposure. This approach is used for aneurysms of the distal basilar artery including those arising from the superior cerebellar arteries and the basilar artery tip. (**A**) Lateral view of the skull demonstrates the bony dissection for this approach to the upper basilar artery (arrow). The lateral wall of the temporal bone, along with a portion of the root of the zygoma, has been removed with a high-speed drill. Bony removal minimizes the extent of temporal lobe retraction needed for exposure of the basal cisterns. (**B**) Coronal section through the midportion of the temporal fossa illustrates the extent of temporal lobe retraction required for this approach. Because of the potential risks associated with temporal lobe retraction, this approach is usually performed from the nondominant (right) side. (**C**) The pertinent anatomy seen from a right subtemporal exposure for a basilar tip aneurysm. This approach provides good visualization of the perforating branches extending along the posterior surface of the aneurysm. It is particularly well-suited for those aneurysms that angle posteriorly; however, it may be difficult for the surgeon to visualize the contralateral posterior cerebral artery and oculomotor nerve. (Courtesy of the Barrow Neurological Institute.)

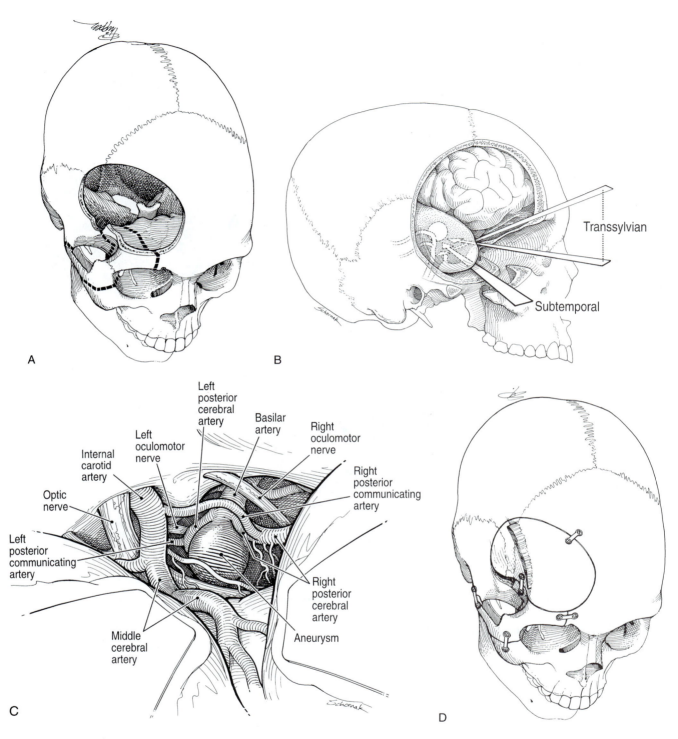

Figure 55.15 Orbitozygomatic approach. This approach is used for aneurysms of the upper third of the basilar artery. (**A**) The exposure begins with a standard pterional craniotomy. The roof and lateral wall of the orbit, along with the zygoma are then removed as one piece using the combination of osteotomies (dashed lines) illustrated in this sketch. (**B**) The extensive bony removal provides a wide corridor of exposure with multiple angles of approach to the upper basilar artery and its branches, including transsylvian and subtemporal routes (arrows). (**C**) The pertinent anatomy seen from a right orbitozygomatic transsylvian approach for a basilar tip aneurysm is illustrated. The sylvian fissure has been widely

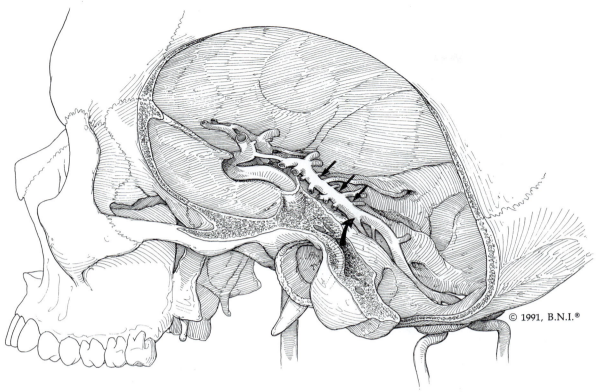

Figure 55.16 Combined subtemporal-suboccipital exposure for approaching aneurysms of the lower two-thirds of the basilar artery (straight arrows) and the vertebrobasilar junction (curved arrow). (Courtesy of the Barrow Neurological Institute.)

artery should be considered either by Hunterian ligation or the use of endovascular techniques.

Vertebral Artery Aneurysms

Aneurysms of the vertebral arteries typically arise at the origins of the posterior inferior cerebellar arteries (PICA) and the junction of the vertebral vessels with the basilar artery. They are relatively uncommon, accounting for only about 2% of cases in major studies. Aneurysms arising from the origin of PICA are best exposed by a far-lateral suboccipital (posterior fossa) approach.

For this approach, the patient is placed in a lateral decubi-tus or park-bench position on the operating room table, and the head is fully flexed and turned 30° from midline to the side of the lesion (Fig. 55.17). We prefer a hockey stick inci-sion that allows lateral bone removal down to the foramen magnum and up to the transverse sinus, as well as removal of the posterior arch of the C1 vertebral body.

Lateral bony removal minimizes the need for cerebellar retraction while increasing the angles for exposure and dis-section. Using a high-speed diamond drill, the posterior arch of C1 is resected to the lateral margin of the foramen transversarium, and the foramen magnum is resected to the edge of the sigmoid sinus and occipital condyle on the side of the aneurysm. The dura is opened in the midline and

opened and dissection extended along the anterior choroidal artery, allowing the anterior tip of the temporal lobe to be retracted laterally. The carotid and middle cerebral arteries are displaced anteriorly to expose the aneurysm. If exposure is limited by the posterior communicating artery, it can be divided between hemostatic clips. This approach allows good visualization of the contralateral posterior cerebral artery and oculomotor nerve. (**D**) Reconstruction and fixation of the orbitozygomatic osteotomy and pterional bone flap with miniplates and screws provide an excellent cosmetic result. (Courtesy of the Barrow Neuro-logical Institute.)

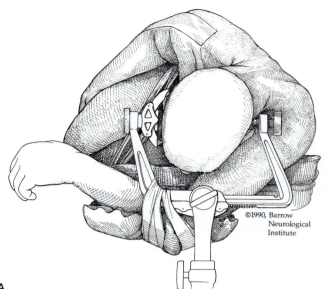

A

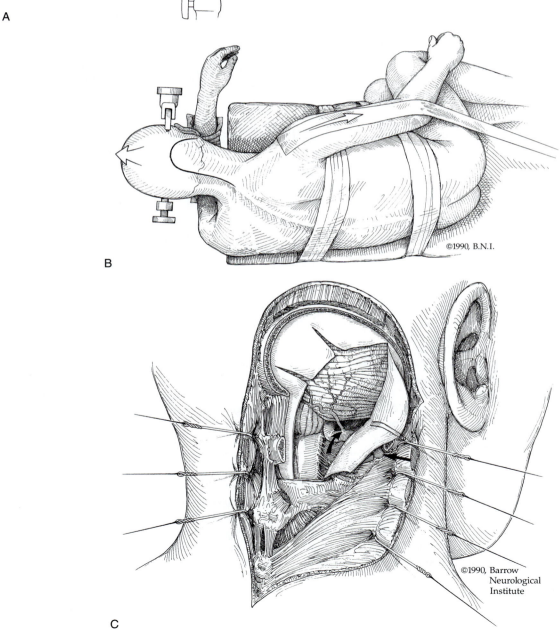

B

C

Figure 55.17 Approach used for exposure of vertebral artery aneurysms. (**A**) The patient is placed in the park-bench position. Care is taken to ensure proper padding of all pressure points. Note the cradle support for the lower arm. (**B**) Surgeon's view of the operative position. The incision for exposing the right vertebral artery is outlined. (**C**) The surgical exposure has been completed. The posterior arch of the first cervical vertebra has been resected laterally on the right side to the edge of the bony foramen of the vertebral artery (straight arrow). The suboccipital bone dissection has been carried to the sigmoid sinus and the medial edge of occipital condyle. The vertebral artery is visible intradurally as it courses medially to give rise to the origin of the posterior inferior cerebellar artery (curved arrow). (Courtesy of the Barrow Neurological Institute.)

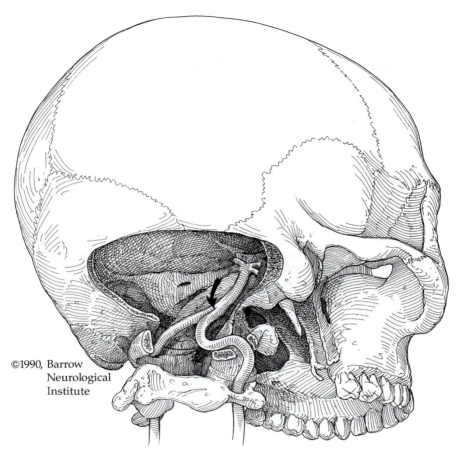

©1990, Barrow Neurological Institute

Figure 55.18 For lateral suboccipital exposure for visualizing aneurysms arising from the vertebrobasilar junction (arrow). The posterior arch of the first cervical vertebra is resected laterally to completely free the vertebral artery from its bony foramen, while the suboccipital bone dissection is carried to the edge of the sigmoid sinus and through the medial third of the occipital condyle. This bony dissection minimizes retraction of the cerebellum and brain stem, which is poorly tolerated. (Courtesy of the Barrow Neurological Institute.)

extended in a cruciate fashion to the edges of the bony dissection. This approach exposes the vertebral artery through the cranial nerves from a lateral and inferior view. The vertebral artery is followed from its entry into the posterior fossa to the aneurysm, which may arise above, below, medial, or lateral to the origin of PICA (Fig. 55.17). The aneurysm can usually be identified and manipulated by working around the intervening cranial nerves. If necessary, the ninth cranial nerve and a few of the upper rootlets of the tenth cranial nerve can be sacrificed. The neck of the aneurysm is carefully dissected free and clipped in the usual fashion. Care must be taken to avoid compromise of PICA and the distal vertebral artery.

By extending the bony dissection even farther laterally to remove the medial third of the occipital condyle (Fig. 55.18), the surgeon can obtain sufficient exposure to approach aneurysms of the vertebrobasilar junction. The details of this so-called extreme far-lateral, or transcondylar, approach are well-described in the literature.[34,12,51,53] Bilateral temporary occlusion of the vertebral arteries can help reduce the risks of rupture during the final stages of dissecting and clipping these rare aneurysms.

Giant Intracranial Aneurysms

In the literature, the term *giant aneurysm* is reserved for lesions greater than 25 mm in diameter.[94] Giant aneurysms occur predominantly in females with a female-to-male ratio of about 3:1.[80,94,158] They most commonly occur in patients 30 to 60 years of age, the same age range at risk for aneurysms in general. The reported incidence of giant aneurysms varies, but they probably constitute no more than 5% of intracranial aneurysms.[80]

The patient with a giant aneurysm may present with signs and symptoms of a mass lesion. Chronic headache, visual impairment, oculomotor palsies, or progressive hemiparesis is common when the aneurysm arises in the anterior circulation[25,37,48,94,134,154,158]; other cranial nerve palsies and signs of brain stem compression may result from giant aneurysms of the vertebrobasilar system.[37,38,93] Embolic symptoms (i.e., transient ischemic attacks [TIAs] and stroke) have also been reported, as many of these giant aneurysms contain extensive intramural thrombus.

Although it is generally believed that giant aneurysms seldom rupture, only a few studies in the literature support this notion. Our own experience and that of others suggest that from 30% to 80% of patients with giant aneurysms present with SAH.[18,37,80,94,103,158] Some patients who present with mass effect or embolic symptoms have evidence of remote hemorrhage on MRI or at surgery.

The evaluation of the patient with a giant aneurysm should include both angiography and CT or MRI. Findings on CT or MRI may be pathognomonic for the diagnosis of giant aneurysms, demonstrating a large basal mass with a variable area of contrast filling associated with a partially enhancing intramural thrombus (Fig. 55.19). In other cases, more extensive thrombosis may result in a nonenhancing mass that can easily be mistaken for tumor. Because of intramural thrombus, the size of giant aneurysms is frequently underestimated when evaluated by angiography alone. The true size of these lesions can often be appreciated only by studying CT scans or MR images.

From the few available reports in the literature, it appears that the prognosis for unoperated giant aneurysms is grim.[28,94] As many as 80% of patients die within a few years of diagnosis,

either from SAH or from increasing mass effect as the aneurysm continues to enlarge.

The management of giant intracranial aneurysms poses special problems. The neck of these lesions may become so wide that it incorporates the origins of adjacent branches making direct obliteration by clipping impossible. In other cases, calcification of the neck or partial thrombosis of the aneurysm makes attempts at clipping extremely hazardous. Finally, the sheer size of the lesion combined with an awkward location may make it impossible to dissect the neck properly. A variety of surgical techniques has been developed to deal with these problems, including ligation or trapping procedures with or without microvascular bypass, partial resection of the aneurysm combined with direct microsurgical repair of the parent vessel, and clipping or direct repair under hypothermic circulatory arrest. The indications and basic principles of these techniques are described below, along with references for the interested reader.

CAROTID ARTERY LIGATION

Carotid artery ligation is performed to protect the aneurysm on the assumption that the reduction of arterial pressure and flow resulting from occlusion will decrease the likelihood of aneurysmal rupture and induce thrombosis of the sac. Physiologically, this approach is supported by the immediate reduction in intravascular pressure that occurs distal to ligation of the internal carotid artery.[14,15,54,99] Serial angiographic studies have shown that carotid ligation can obliterate or reduce the

Figure 55.19 A 56-year-old woman presented with dementia and progressive right-sided weakness. (**A**) Contrast-enhanced head computed tomography scan demonstrates a large, centrally enhancing mass with a thin rim of contrast bordering the lesion, producing the so-called target sign. This picture is nearly pathognomonic for a partially thrombosed giant aneurysm; the nonenhancing portion of the mass (arrow) represents thrombus within the aneurysm dome. (**B**) Lateral view of the left internal carotid artery angiogram in the same patient confirms the diagnosis of a giant internal carotid artery aneurysm (arrow). Note that the size of the aneurysm is grossly underestimated by the angiogram (compare with the computed tomography scan), as only the central portion of the lesion fills with contrast.

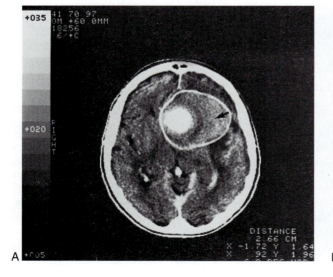
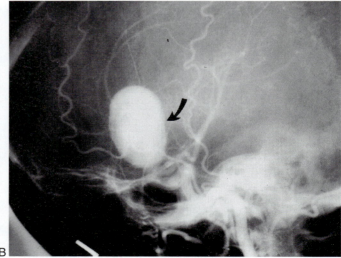

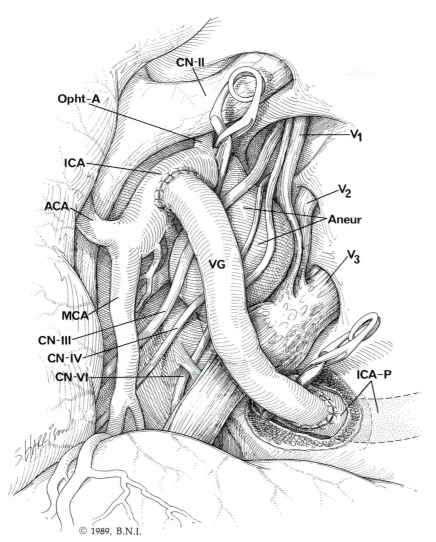

© 1989, B.N.I.

Figure 55.20 Vein graft (VG) from the petrous segment of the internal carotid artery (ICA-P) to the supraclinoid segment of the internal carotid artery (ICA) for the treatment of a giant aneurysm (Aneur) involving the cavernous segment of the internal carotid artery. Note that the aneurysm has been eliminated from the circulation by the placement of proximal and distal clips. For the purpose of illustration the lateral wall of the cavernous sinus has been removed in this drawing to allow visualization of the course of the 3rd, 4th, and 6th cranial nerves (CN), and the 5th cranial nerve (V). Other labeled structures include the ophthalmic artery (Opht-A), anterior cerebral artery (ACA), middle cerebral artery (MCA), and the optic nerve (CN-II). (Adapted from Spetzler et al,[136] with permission.)

size of giant aneurysms.[94,139,140] Because the risk of precipitating cerebral ischemia is considerable, simple carotid ligation has become a less favored alternative for the treatment of these lesions.

Cerebral infarction is a major immediate complication of carotid artery occlusion: Approximately 10% to 20% of patients are unable to tolerate carotid artery occlusion.[74,97,99] In a series of 220 patients, Odom and Tindall[99] reported ischemic complications in 34 patients. Significantly, despite the immediate opening of the carotid artery after the onset of ischemia in this series, only 12 patients recovered completely.

Numerous techniques, including Wada's test, the measurement of carotid artery stump pressures, EEG monitoring, jugular venous blood sampling, gradual occlusion, and CBF measurements, have been proposed to help predict which patients can withstand permanent carotid occlusion. Wada's test, which involves a trial occlusion of the carotid artery (most recently using endovascular balloon techniques)[45,156] as a test of adequate collateral circulation, reduces but does not eliminate ischemic complications, as the onset of ischemic deficits is often delayed for hours to days. The majority of these delayed complications following carotid artery occlusion is most

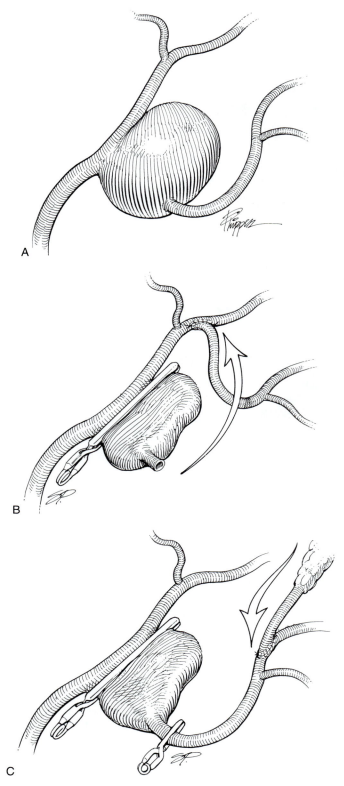

likely caused by embolic propagation rather than low flow rates. Clearly, however, there are patients in whom the limited availability of collateral blood supplies markedly increases the risks of carotid occlusion.

Measurement of regional CBF with the carotid artery open and occluded may be of predictive value in selecting patients who can tolerate carotid occlusion.[42,89] Miller et al[89] used a 25% reduction in CBF following occlusion of the carotid artery as their critical level; patients with reductions in CBF greater than 25% were rejected as candidates for carotid occlusion. Although this method resulted in the rejection of 20% of patients tested, the authors report that it virtually eliminated the incidence of preoperative ischemic complications following carotid artery occlusion.

It has long been recognized that carotid artery occlusion decreases the pressure in the distal internal carotid artery and causes the angiographic obliteration of some intracranial aneurysms. However, it does not completely protect the patient from the risk of rebleeding. Norlen and Olivecrona[98] reported a 10% to 15% incidence of death from recurrent SAH in the long-term follow-up of patients undergoing carotid occlusion. In the report by the Cooperative Study, Nishioka[97] reported an 8% rebleeding rate on long-term follow-up in 39 patients following carotid artery occlusion for the treatment of ruptured aneurysms and noted that repeat hemorrhage led to death in 8%. In this same study, the authors reported a 16% incidence of late TIAs and a 16.6% incidence of delayed stroke ipsilateral to the side of internal carotid occlusion.

The above discussion provides the rationale for our preference of utilizing an arterial bypass or venous jump graft in combination with trapping procedures for those aneurysms in which direct clipping or reconstruction is not possible.

DIRECT CLIPPING

With modern microsurgical techniques, the majority of giant intracranial aneurysms can be directly clipped. Management often requires temporary trapping of the aneurysm. As discussed earlier, temporary vessel occlusion appears to be safe for 10 to 20 minutes, when the patient is under deep barbiturate anesthesia with burst suppression of EEG activity. To enhance the collateral blood supply, the patient should be kept normotensive or mildly hypertensive during temporary vessel occlusion.

Giant aneurysms involving the anterior circulation are approached initially in a standard fashion as described above with the goal of isolating the aneurysm neck. Care must be taken to ensure that all branches and adjacent vessels have been identified and dissected free from the neck before clipping is attempted. Temporary clipping of the parent vessel and major branches decreases the risk of rupture during the

Figure 55.21 Various options available for microvascular reconstruction in the treatment of a giant middle cerebral artery (MCA) aneurysm. (**A**) As an aneurysm enlarges, it may involve the origin of one or more vessels. The treatment of such cases requires a combination of clipping and vascular reconstruction.

The vessel arising from the wall of the aneurysm may either be (**B**) divided near its origin and anastomosed end-to-side (arrow) to another branch of the MCA, or (**C**) occluded at its origin and revascularized distally with a branch of the superficial temporal artery (arrow). (Courtesy of the Barrow Neurological Institute.)

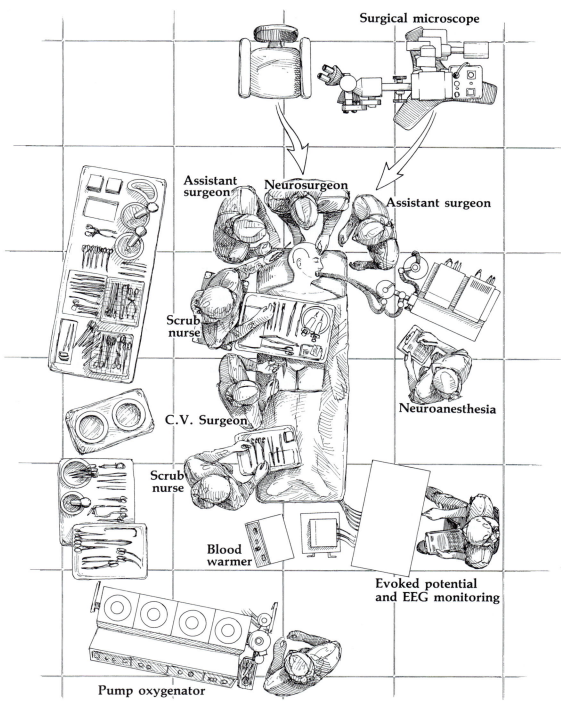

Figure 55.22 Layout of the operating room in neurosurgical cases that involve the use of hypothermic circulatory arrest. (From Blazier et al,[22] with permission.)

final stages of dissection and clipping. If preoperative studies demonstrate extensive thrombus within the aneurysm sac or if the aneurysm is difficult to collapse, the dome can be opened sharply and the thrombus removed manually or with an ultrasonic aspirator. Occasionally, it is necessary to perform a limited endarterectomy to permit clipping of the aneurysm neck without compromise of the parent vessel. If the surgeon is

fully prepared and focused, the neck of the aneurysm can usually be decompressed and prepared for clipping within the safe period of temporary vessel occlusion defined above.

When giant aneurysms involve the supraclinoid portion of the internal carotid artery, proximal control of the artery can be obtained in the neck. Preoperative angiography should include views of the carotid bifurcation to ensure that it is not significantly diseased. To aid in clipping, the aneurysm can be readily collapsed during temporary vessel occlusion by gentle aspiration of blood from a catheter placed in the cervical portion of the internal carotid artery.[17]

BYPASS PROCEDURES

A small minority of giant aneurysms, particularly those involving the cavernous portion of the internal carotid artery, is best managed by combining a trapping procedure with an arterial bypass or venous jump graft.[11,141,144] Although a number of authors have demonstrated that dissection in the cavernous sinus for control of these aneurysms is possible, the risk of ischemic complications and cranial nerve deficits is significant.[34,35,66,109] Knowledge of the anatomy in this region has increased significantly in the last 5 years, primarily as a result of the management of skull base tumors.[110,126,127] Consequently, short venous jump grafts from the petrous portion of the carotid artery to its supraclinoid portion have replaced the much longer grafts from the cervical carotid that were previously necessary for a high-flow bypass (Fig. 55.20) These short venous grafts reduce the risks of late stenosis and offer markedly higher flow than does the superficial temporal artery. Several groups have recently published descriptions of this procedure along with operative results.[35,46,136]

When giant aneurysms arise at the middle cerebral artery trifurcation, the neck often involves one of the major branches such that direct clipping becomes impossible without sacrificing the vessel. In such cases, the involved vessel can be divided at the time of the aneurysm clipping and reanastomosed to one of remaining intact trifurcation branches (Fig. 55.21), or the aneurysm itself can be resected and the vessel wall can be directly reconstructed.[24,140,141] Alternatively, an extracranial-intracranial arterial bypass can be performed (using the superficial temporal artery) to provide the needed collateral blood flow to the involved vessels (Fig. 55.21).[11,141] Using such an approach, the surgeon can eliminate the majority of giant middle cerebral artery aneurysms from the circulation.

HYPOTHERMIC CIRCULATORY ARREST

The surgical management of giant aneurysms of the vertebrobasilar system presents special problems. Because of the awkward location of these lesions, they cannot readily be controlled by temporary clipping of feeding vessels. In addition, these aneurysms are surrounded by numerous small but highly important perforating branches that supply the brain stem and cerebellum. Accurate dissection and clipping of the aneurysm neck with preservation of these perforators are paramount for a good outcome. A useful adjunct for the treatment of these lesions is total circulatory arrest under deep hypothermia. Several groups have reported improved results using this technique in the treatment of giant intracranial aneurysms.[19,41,133,137,149] We reserve the use of this technique for giant aneurysms involving the vertebrobasilar system.

A multispecialty team with good coordination and understanding between its members is essential. The team should include a neurosurgeon, a cardiothoracic surgeon, a pump technician, and an anesthesiologist with experience in both neurologic and cardiovascular surgery. Figure 55.22 illustrates the typical layout of the room and the location of the team members. The aneurysm is exposed using one of the approaches described above depending on its location, and the neck is inspected. Occasionally, the neck of the aneurysm will be free of perforating branches and readily clippable. More commonly, the size of the aneurysm precludes the necessary visualization to allow safe clipping. In such cases, further dissection is delayed while the patient is prepared for circulatory arrest. The femoral vessels are exposed, the patient is fully heparinized, and the femoral artery and vein are cannulated (Fig. 55.23). Extracorporeal circulation is initiated, and the patient is gradually cooled to a core temperature of approximately 15°C. The pump is stopped and the blood is allowed to drain into the bypass pump reservoir, collapsing the aneurysm. Dissection about the neck of the aneurysm is completed, with care being taken to free all perforating vessels and major branches. If the aneurysm contains extensive thrombosis, it can be opened and partially evacuated to enable clipping of the neck.

After clipping of the aneurysm, the pump is restarted

Figure 55.23 Technique used to establish extracorporeal circulation during hypothermic circulatory arrest for intracranial aneurysms. The femoral artery and vein are cannulated in the groin and connected to the pump oxygenator and heat exchanger. This approach allows the cardiovascular and neurosurgical teams to work simultaneously as illustrated in Figure 55.24. CVP, central venous pressure. (From Spetzler et al,[137] with permission.)

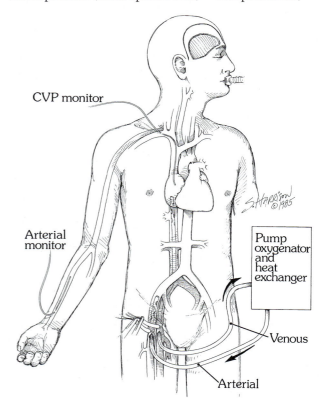

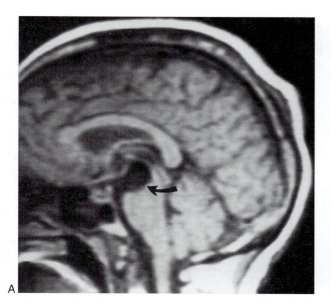

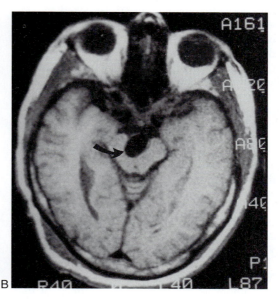

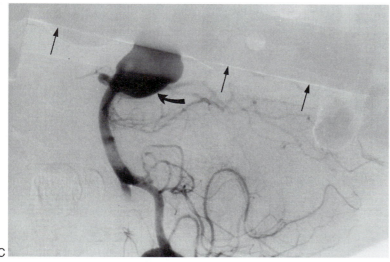

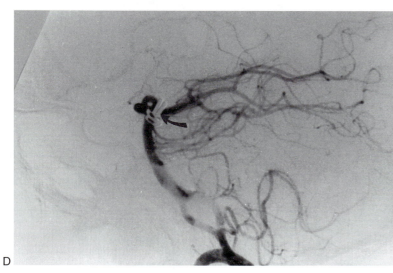

Figure 55.24 A 51-year-old woman sustained a cervical spine fracture and mild head trauma in a motor vehicle accident. Magnetic resonance imaging of the head and neck was performed as part of her initial trauma evaluation. (**A&B**) Sagittal and transverse T_1-weighted images revealed a giant, incidental basilar tip aneurysm (arrows). The cervical spine fracture was treated by immobilizing the patient with a halo vest and ring. (**C**) A lateral view of the vertebral artery angiogram confirmed the diagnosis of a giant basilar tip aneurysm (curved arrow). Artifact from the halo ring is apparent (straight arrows). On both the magnetic resonance images and the angiogram, the aneurysm dome angles up and back, distorting and displacing the brain stem. The cervical spine fracture healed without complication. Four months after her accident, the patient underwent elective clipping of the aneurysm under hypothermic circulatory arrest via a subtemporal approach. The patient's recovery was quick and uneventful. (**D**) Lateral view of the postoperative vertebral angiogram reveals complete obliteration of the aneurysm with preservation of the parent vessels. A single straight clip is faintly visible across the neck of the aneurysm (arrow).

and the patient is gradually rewarmed. The risk of intracerebral hematoma formation is minimized by avoiding any movement of the retractors after the patient has been heparinized and before he or she has been rewarmed and weaned from extracorporeal circulation and the heparin has been reversed. In addition, clotting factors and platelets are replenished by transfusing one to two units of autologous, fresh, whole blood that was removed during the initial exposure of the aneurysm. If necessary, the pump can be primed with one to two units of packed cells to maintain an adequate hemoglobin level.

Using this technique, we have successfully clipped 53 giant basilar artery aneurysms. There were 35 women and 18 men with a mean age of 58.8 years (range, 8 to 77 years). The most common presentation was SAH (n = 26) followed by mass effect (n = 22) and embolism (n = 1). Four patients had incidental lesions found when CT or MRI was performed for other diagnostic purposes (Fig. 55.24). The mean period of circulatory arrest was 21 minutes with a range of 5 to 75 minutes, at a mean temperature of 14.5°C. There were six deaths (11%) in the preoperative period; three deaths were directly related to effects of the initial hemorrhage, two were the result of complications from clipping, and one patient died secondary to a postoperative myocardial infarction. Other surgical complications were transient and related to the manipulation of cranial nerves. At a 6-month follow-up the overall outcome revealed that 30 patients were neurologically intact, 8 had mild deficits (independent), and 2 patients had moderate deficits (some assistance necessary) but were nevertheless leading active lives. The remaining 10 patients had poor outcomes (severe deficits or death). The best predictor of outcome was preoperative clinical status. Thirty-five patients in this series were in good condition prior to surgery (Hunt and Hess grade 0, 1, or 2); at late follow-up (mean, 3.7 years), 26 of the 35 patients (74%) were neurologically intact, and 4 (11%) had minor deficits but were independent. Three patients (9%) in this good-grade group had poor outcomes, compared with 66% in the group of patients who were in poor condition preoperatively.

Summary

Advances in neuroanesthesia, the development of new microsurgical instruments, and the rapid evolution of microvascular techniques have dramatically reduced the operative morbidity and mortality associated with the surgical management of intracranial aneurysms. In patients with acute aneurysmal SAH, early surgical intervention has now virtually eliminated the risk of rebleeding, while changes in preoperative management, including the use of hypervolemic-hypertensive therapy and calcium antagonist, have significantly blunted the devastating effect of vasospasm. In patients admitted in good condition, early surgery and aggressive management have reduced morbidity and mortality to as little as 10% to 15%. The management of patients with giant aneurysms of the vertebrobasilar system remains a significant challenge. Hypothermic circulatory arrest provides a useful adjunct for the treatment of these rare lesions, but innovative new strategies are needed.

References

1. Adams HP, Kassel NF, Torner JC et al: Early management of aneurysmal subarachnoid hemorrhage: a report of the Cooperative Aneurysm Study. J Neurosurg 54:141, 1981
2. Adams HP Jr., Kassell NF, Torner JC et al: CT and clinical correlations in recent aneurysmal subarachnoid hemorrhage: a preliminary report of the Cooperative Aneurysm Study. Neurology 33:981, 1983
3. Alaywan M, Sindou M: Fronto-temporal approach with orbito-zygomatic removal. Surgical anatomy. Acta Neurochir 104:79, 1990
4. Al-Mefty O, Borba LA, Aoki N et al: The transcondylar approach to extradural nonneoplastic lesions of the craniovertebral junction. J Neurosurg 84:1, 1996
5. Al-Mefty O, Fox JL, Rifai A et al: A combined infratemporal and posterior fossa approach for the removal of giant glomus tumors and chondrosarcomas. Surg Neurol 28:423, 1987
6. Andrews RJ, Spiegel PK: Intracranial aneurysms. Age, sex, blood pressure, and multiplicity in an unselected series of patients. J Neurosurg 51:27, 1979
7. Auer LM: Acute operation and preventive nimodipine improve outcome in patients with ruptured cerebral aneurysms. Neurosurgery 15:57, 1984
8. Auer LM, Brandt L, Ebeling U et al: Nimodipine and early aneurysm operation in good condition SAH patients. Acta Neurochir (Wien) 82:7, 1986
9. Ausman JI, Diaz FG, Malik GM et al: Current management of cerebral aneurysms: is it based on facts or myths? Surg Neurol 24:625, 1985
10. Ausman JI, Diaz FG, Malik GM et al: Management of cerebral aneurysms: further facts and additional myths. Surg Neurol 32:21, 1989
11. Ausman JI, Diaz FG, Sadasivan B et al: Giant intracranial aneurysm surgery: the role of microvascular reconstruction. Surg Neurol 34:8, 1990
12. Babu RP, Sekhar LN, Wright DC: Extreme lateral transcondylar approach: technical improvements and lessons learned. J Neurosurg 81:49, 1994
13. Bailes JE, Spetzler RF, Hadley MN et al: Management morbidity and mortality of poor-grade aneurysm patients. J Neurosurg 72:559, 1990
14. Bakay L, Sweet WH: Cervical and intracranial intra-arterial pressures with and without occlusion. Surg Gynecol Obstet 95:67, 1952
15. Bakay L, Sweet WH: Intra-arterial pressures in the neck and brain. Late changes after carotid closure, acute measurements after vertebral closure. J Neurosurg 10:353, 1953
16. Barker FG, Ogilvy CS: Efficacy of prophylactic nimodipine for delayed ischemic deficit after subarachnoid hemorrhage: a metaanalysis. J Neurosurg 84:405, 1996
17. Batjer HH, Samson DS: Retrograde suction decompression of giant paraclinoidal aneurysms. Technical note. J Neurosurg 73:305, 1990
18. Battaglia R, Pasqualin A, Da Pian R: Italian cooperative study on giant intracranial aneurysms: 1. Study design and clinical data. Acta Neurochir Suppl (Wien) 42:49, 1988

19. Baumgartner WA, Silverberg GD, Ream AK et al: Reappraisal of cardiopulmonary bypass with deep hypothermia and circulatory arrest for complex neurosurgical operations. Surgery 94:242, 1983

20. Biller J, Adams HP Jr: Cerebrovascular disorders associated with pregnancy. Am Fam Physician 33:125, 1986

21. Bingham WF: Treatment of myocotic intracranial aneurysms. J Neurosurg 46:428, 1977

22. Blazier CJ, Cavanaugh E, Antonioli L: Surgical treatment of complex cerebrovascular lesions utilizing hypothermia and circulatory arrest: nursing implications. BNI Q 5:33, 1990

23. Bohmfalk GL, Story JL, Wissinger JP et al: Bacterial intracranial aneurysms. J Neurosurg 48:369, 1978

24. Bojanowski WM, Spetzler RF, Carter LP: Reconstruction of the MCA bifurcation after excision of a giant aneurysm. Technical note. J Neurosurg 68:974, 1988

25. Bokemeyer C, Frank B, Brandis A et al: Giant aneurysm causing frontal lobe syndrome. J Neurol 237:47, 1990

26. Bonita R, Thomson S: Subarachnoid hemorrhage: epidemiology, diagnosis, management, and outcome. Stroke 16:591, 1985

27. Branston NM, Hope DT, Symon L: Barbiturates in focal ischemia of primate cortex: effects on blood flow distribution, evoked potential, and extracellular potassium. Stroke 10:647, 1979

28. Bull J: Massive aneurysms at the base of the brain. Brain 92:535, 1969

29. Cromptom MR: Mechanism of growth and rupture in cerebral berry aneurysms. Br Med J 5496:1138, 1966

30. Cushing H: Contributions to the clinical studies of intracranial aneurysms. Guys Hosp Rep 73:159, 1923

31. Dandy WE: Intracranial aneurysm of internal carotid artery cured by operation. Ann Surg 107:654, 1938

32. Dell S: Asymptomatic cerebral aneurysm: assessment of its risk of rupture. Neurosurgery 10:162, 1982

33. Dernbach PD, Little JR, Jones SC et al: Altered cerebral autoregulation and CO_2 reactivity after aneurysmal subarachnoid hemorrhage. Neurosurgery 22:822, 1988

34. Dolenc VV: A combined epi- and subdural direct approach to carotid-ophthalmic artery aneurysms. J Neurosurg 62:667, 1985

35. Dolenc VV: Surgery of vascular lesions of the cavernous sinus. Clin Neurosurg 36:240, 1990

36. Dott NM: Intracranial aneurysms: cerebral arteriradiography: surgical treatment. Tr Med Chir Soc Edinburgh 47:219, 1932

37. Drake CG: Ligation of the vertebral (unilateral or bilateral) or basilar artery in the treatment of large intracranial aneurysms. J Neurosurg 43:255, 1975

38. Drake CG: Progress in cerebrovascular surgery. Management of cerebral aneurysm. Stroke 12:273, 1981

39. Drake CG: The surgical treatment of aneurysms of the basilar artery. J Neurosurg 29:436, 1968

40. Drake CG: Surgical treatment of ruptured aneurysms of the basilar artery. Experience with 14 cases. J Neurosurg 23:457, 1965

41. Drake CG, Barr HKW, Coles JC et al: The use of extracorporeal circulation and profound hypothermia in the treatment of ruptured intracranial aneurysm. J Neurosurg 21:575, 1964

42. Erba SM, Horton JA, Latchaw RE et al: Balloon test occlusion of the internal carotid artery with stable xenon/CT cerebral blood flow imaging. AJNR 9:533, 1988

43. Fein JM, Lipow K, Marmarou A: Cortical artery pressure in normotensive and hypertensive aneurysm patients. J Neurosurg 59:51, 1983

44. Fodstad H: Antifibrinolytic treatment in subarachnoid haemorrhage: present state. Acta Neurochir (Wien) 63:233, 1982

45. Fox AJ, Viñuela F, Pelz DM et al: Use of detachable balloons for proximal artery occlusion in the treatment of unclippable cerebral aneurysms. J Neurosurg 66:40, 1987

46. Fukushima T: Direct operative approach to the vascular lesions in the cavernous sinus: summary of 27 cases. Mt. Fuji Workshop. Cerebrovas Dis 6:169, 1988

47. Graff-Radford NR, Torner J, Adams HP Jr et al: Factors associated with hydrocephalus after subarachnoid hemorrhage. A report of the Cooperative Aneurysm Study. Arch Neurol 46:744, 1989

48. Gross M: Giant middle cerebral aneurysm presenting as hemiparkinsonism [letter]. J Neurol Neurosurg Psychiatry 50:1075, 1987

49. Hakuba A, Liu S, Nishimura S: The orbitozygomatic infratemporal approach: a new surgical technique. Surg Neurol 26:27 1986

50. Haley EC Jr, Kassell NF, Torner JC et al: A randomized controlled trial of high-dose intravenous nicardipine in aneurysmal subarachnoid hemorrhage: a report of the Cooperative Aneurysm Study. J Neurosurg 78:537, 1993

51. Hammon WM, Kempe LG: The posterior fossa approach to aneurysms of the vertebral and basilar arteries. J Neurosurg 37:339, 1972

52. Hassler O: Morphological studies on the large cerebral arteries, with reference to etiology of subarachnoid haemorrhage. Acta Psychiat Scand 154:1, 1961

53. Heros RC: Lateral suboccipital approach for vertebral and vertebrobasilar artery lesions. J Neurosurg 64:559, 1986

54. Heyman A, Tindall GT, Finney WHM et al: Measurement of retinal artery and intracarotid pressures: following carotid artery occlusion with the Crutchfield clamp. J Neurosurg 17:297, 1960

55. Hitchcock ER, Tsementzis SA, Dow AA: Short- and long-term prognosis of patients with a subarachnoid haemorrhage in relation to intra-operative period of hypotension. Acta Neurochir (Wien) 70:235, 1984

56. Hochman MS: Reversal of fixed pupils after spontaneous intraventricular hemorrhage with secondary acute hydrocephalus: report of two cases treated with early ventriculostomy. Neurosurgery 18:777, 1986

57. Hoff JT, Pitts LH, Spetzler RF et al: Barbiturates for protection from cerebral ischemia in aneurysm surgery. Acta Neurol Scand 56:158, 1977

58. Housepian EM, Pool JL: A systematic analysis of intracranial aneurysms from the autopsy file of the Presbyterian Hospital, 1914 to 1956. J Neuropathol Exp Neurol 17:409, 1958

59. Hugenholtz H, Elgie RG: Considerations in early surgery on good-risk patients with ruptured intracranial aneurysm. J Neurosurg 56:180, 1982

60. Hunt HB, Schifrin BS, Suzuki K: Ruptured berry aneurysms and pregnancy. Obstet Gynecol 43:827, 1974

61. Inagawa T, Ishikawa S, Aoki H: Aneurysmal subarachnoid hemorrhage in Izumo City and Shimane Prefecture of Japan. Incidence. Stroke 19:170, 1988

62. Ingall TJ, Whisnant JP, Wiebers DO et al: Has there been a decline in subarachnoid hemorrhage mortality? Stroke 20:718, 1989

63. Jabre A, Symon L: Temporary vascular occlusion during aneurysm surgery. Surg Neurol 27:47, 1987

64. Jane JA, Kassell NF, Torner JC et al: The natural history of aneurysms and arteriovenous malformations. J Neurosurg 62:321, 1985

65. Jellinger K: Pathology and aetiology of intracranial aneurysms. p. 5. In Pia HW, Langmaid C, Zierski J (eds): Cerebral Aneurysms. Advances in Diagnosis and Therapy. Springer-Verlag, New York, 1979

66. Johnston I: Direct surgical treatment of bilateral intracavernous internal carotid artery aneurysms. Case report. J Neurosurg 51:98, 1979

67. Juvela S, Porras M, Heiskanen O: Natural history of unruptured intracranial aneurysms: a long-term follow-up study. J Neurosurg 79:174, 1993

68. Kassell NF, Drake CG: Timing of aneurysm surgery. Neurosurgery 10:514, 1982

69. Kassell NF, Torner JC: The International Cooperative Study on timing of aneurysm surgery—an update. Stroke 15:566, 1984

70. Kassel NF, Torner JC: Size of intracranial aneurysms. Neurosurgery 12:291, 1983

71. Kassell NF, Torner JC, Adams HP Jr: Antifibrinolytic therapy in the acute period following aneurysmal subarachnoid hemorrhage. Preliminary observations from the Cooperative Aneurysm Study. J Neurosurg 61:225, 1984

72. Kassell NF, Torner JC, Haley EC Jr et al: The International Cooperative Study on the timing of aneurysm surgery. Part 1: Overall management results. J Neurosurg 73:18, 1990

73. Kassell NF, Torner JC, Jane JA et al: The International Cooperative Study on the timing of aneurysm surgery. Part 2: Surgical results. J Neurosurg 73:37, 1990

74. Landolt AM, Millikan CH: Pathogenesis of cerebral infarction secondary to mechanical carotid artery occlusion. Stroke 1:52, 1970

75. Linn FH, Rinkel GJ, Algra A et al: Incidence of subarachnoid hemorrhage: role of region, year, and rate of computed tomography: a meta-analysis. Stroke 27:625, 1996

76. Ljunggren B, Brandt L, Kagstrom E et al: Results of early operations for ruptured aneurysms. J Neurosurg 54:473, 1981

77. Ljunggren B, Brandt L, Saveland H et al: Outcome in 60 consecutive patients treated with early aneurysm operation and intravenous nimodipine. J Neurosurg 61:864, 1984

78. Ljunggren B, Saveland H, Brandt L et al: Aneurysmal subarachnoid hemorrhage: total annual outcome in a 1.46 million population. Surg Neurol 22:435, 1984

79. Ljunggren B, Saveland H, Brandt L et al: Early operation and overall outcome in aneurysmal subarachnoid hemorrhage. J Neurosurg 62:547, 1985

80. Locksley HB: Natural history of subarachnoid hemorrhage, intracranial aneurysms and arteriovenous malformations. Based on 6368 cases in the Cooperative Study. J Neurosurg 25:219, 1966

81. Longstreth WT Jr, Nelson LM, Koepsell TD et al: Cigarette smoking, alcohol use, and subarachnoid hemorrhage. Stroke 23:1242, 1992

82. Mayhall CG, Archer NH, Lamb VA et al: Ventriculostomy-related infections. A prospective epidemiologic study. N Engl J Med 310:553, 1984

83. McCormick WF: Problems and pathogenesis of intracranial arterial aneurysms. p. 219. In Moossy J, Janeway R (eds). Cerebral Vascular Disease. Seventh Conference. Grune & Stratton, Orlando, Florida, 1971

84. McCormick WF, Acosta-Rua GJ: The size of intracranial saccular aneurysms: an autopsy study. J Neurosurg 33:422, 1970

85. McDermott MW, Durity FA, Borozny M et al: Temporary vessel occlusion and barbiturate protection in cerebral aneurysm surgery. Neurosurgery 25:54, 1989

86. McDermott MW, Durity FA, Rootman J et al: Combined frontotemporal-orbitozygomatic approach for tumors of the sphenoid wing and orbit. Neurosurgery 26:107, 1990

87. Meyer FB, Sundt TM Jr, Fode NC et al: Cerebral aneurysms in childhood and adolescence. J Neurosurg 70:420, 1989

88. Milhorat TH, Krautheim M: Results of early and delayed operations for ruptured intracranial aneurysms in two series of 100 consecutive patients. Surg Neurol 26:123, 1986

89. Miller JD, Jawad K, Jennett B: Safety of carotid ligation and its role in the management of intracranial aneurysms. J Neurol Neurosurg Psychiatry 40:64, 1977

90. Minielly R, Yuzpe AA, Drake CG: Subarachnoid hemorrhage secondary to ruptured cerebral aneurysm in pregnancy. Obstet Gynecol 53:64, 1979

91. Mizoi K, Yoshimoto T: Permissible temporary occlusion time in aneurysm surgery as evaluated by evoked potential monitoring. Neurosurgery 33:434, 1993

92. Moniz E: L'encephalographie arterielle, son importance dans la localisation des tumeurs cerebrales. Rev Neurol (Par) 2:72, 1927

93. Morgan DW, Honan W: Lateral gaze palsy due to giant aneurysm of the posterior fossa (letter). J Neurol Neurosurg Psychiatry 51:883, 1988

94. Morley TP, Barr HW: Giant intracranial aneurysms: diagnosis, course, and management. Clin Neurosurg 16:73, 1969

95. Moskowitz MA, Rosenbaum AE, Tyler HR: Angiographically monitored resolution of cerebral mycotic aneurysms. Neurology 24:1103, 1974

96. Nehls DG, Flom RA, Carter LP et al: Multiple intracranial aneurysms: determining the site of rupture. J Neurosurg 63:342, 1985

97. Nishioka H: Results of treatment of intracranial aneurysms by occlusion of the carotid artery in the neck. J Neurosurg 25:660, 1966

98. Norlen G, Olivecrona H: Treatment of aneurysms of the circle of Willis. J Neurosurg 10:404, 1953

99. Odom GL, Tindall GT: Carotid ligation in the treatment

of certain intracranial aneurysms. Clin Neurosurg 15: 101, 1968

100. Ogilvy CS, Carter BS, Kaplan S et al: Temporary vessel occlusion for aneurysm surgery: risk factors for stroke in patients protected by induced hypothermia and hypertension and intravenous mannitol administration. J Neurosurg 84:785, 1996

101. Ohman J, Heiskanen O: Timing of operation for ruptured supratentorial aneurysms: a prospective randomized study. J Neurosurg 70:55, 1989

102. Ohno K, Suzuki R, Masaoka H et al: A review of 102 consecutive patients with intracranial aneurysms in a community hospital in Japan. Acta Neurochir 94:23, 1988

103. Onuma T, Suzuki J: Surgical treatment of giant intracranial aneurysms. J Neurosurg 51:33, 1979

104. Origitano TC, Anderson DE, Tarassoli Y et al: Skull base approaches to complex cerebral aneurysms. Surg Neurol 40:339, 1993

105. Osler W: Gulstonian lectures on malignant endocarditis. Lancet 1:393, 1885

106. Ostergaard JR, Hog E: Incidence of multiple intracranial aneurysms. Influence of arterial hypertension and gender. J Neurosurg 63:49, 1985

107. Ostergaard JR, Voldby B: Intracranial arterial aneurysms in children and adolescents. J Neurosurg 58:832, 1983

108. Park BE: Spontaneous subarachnoid hemorrhage complicated by communicating hydrocephalus: epsilon amino caproic acid as a possible predisposing factor. Surg Neurol 11:73, 1979

109. Parkinson D: Carotid cavernous fistula: direct repair with preservation of the carotid artery. Technical note. J Neurosurg 38:99, 1973

110. Paullus WS, Pait TG, Rhoton AL Jr: Microsurgical exposure of the petrous portion of the carotid artery. J Neurosurg 47:713, 1977

111. Petruk KC, West M, Mohr G et al: Nimodipine treatment in poor-grade aneurysm patients. Results of a multicenter double-blind placebo-controlled trial. J Neurosurg 68:505, 1988

112. Phillips LH, Whisnant JP, O'Fallon WM et al: The unchanging pattern of subarachnoid hemorrhage in a community. Neurology 30:1034, 1980

113. Pickard JD, Murray GD, Illingworth R et al: Effect of oral nimodipine on cerebral infarction and outcome after subarachnoid haemorrhage: British aneurysm nimodipine trial. Br Med J 298:636, 1989

114. Pinna G, Pasqualin A, Vivenza C et al: Rebleeding, ischaemia and hydrocephalus following anti-fibrinolytic treatment for ruptured cerebral aneurysms. A retrospective clinical study. Acta Neurochir (Wien) 93:77, 1988

115. Pool JL: Treatment of intracranial aneurysms during pregnancy. JAMA 192:209, 1965

116. Robinson JL, Hall CS, Sedzimir CB: Arteriovenous malformations, aneurysms, and pregnancy. J Neurosurg 41: 63, 1974

117. Ropper AH, Zervas NT: Outcome 1 year after SAH from cerebral aneurysm: management morbidity, mortality and functional status in 112 consecutive good-risk patients. J Neurosurg 60:909, 1984

118. Rosenorn J, Eskesen V, Schmidt K et al: The risk of

119. Roski RA, Spetzler RF, Nulsen FE: Late complications of carotid ligation in the treatment of intracranial aneurysms. J Neurosurg 54:583, 1981

120. Sahs A, Perret GE, Locksley HB et al: Aneurysms and Subarachnoid Hemorrhage. Lippincott-Raven, Philadelphia, 1969

121. Salazar JL: Surgical treatment of asymptomatic and incidental intracranial aneurysms. J Neurosurg 53:20, 1980

122. Samson D, Batjer HH, Bowman G et al: A clinical study of the parameters and effects of temporary arterial occlusion in the management of intracranial aneurysms. Neurosurgery 34:22, 1994

123. Samson DS, Hodosh RM, Clark WK: Surgical management of unruptured asymptomatic aneurysms. J Neurosurg 46:731, 1977

124. Samson DS, Hodosh RM, Reid WR et al: Risk of intracranial aneurysm surgery in the good grade patient: early versus late operation. Neurosurgery 5:422, 1979

125. Saveland H, Ljunggren B, Brandt L et al: Delayed ischemic deterioration in patients with early aneurysm operation and intravenous nimodipine. Neurosurgery 18: 146, 1986

126. Sekhar LN, Schramm VL Jr, Jones NF: Subtemporal-preauricular intratemporal fossa approach to large lateral and posterior cranial base neoplasms. J Neurosurg 67:488, 1987

127. Sekhar LN, Schramm VL Jr, Jones NF et al: Operative exposure and management of the petrous and upper cervical internal carotid artery. Neurosurgery 19:967, 1986

128. Selman WR, Spetzler RF: Therapeutics for focal cerebral ischemia. Neurosurgery 6:446, 1980

129. Selman WR, Spetzler RF, Anton AH et al: Management of prolonged therapeutic barbiturate coma. Surg Neurol 15:9, 1981

130. Selman WR, Spetzler RF, Roessmann UR et al: Barbiturate-induced coma therapy for focal cerebral ischemia: effect after temporary and permanent MCA occlusion. J Neurosurg 55:220, 1981

131. Selman WR, Spetzler RF, Roski RA et al: Barbiturate coma in focal cerebral ischemia: relationship of protection to timing of therapy. J Neurosurg 56:685, 1982

132. Selman WR, Spetzler RF, Zabramski JM: Induced barbiturate coma. p. 343. In Wilkins RH, Rengachary SS (eds): Neurosurgery. McGraw-Hill, New York, 1985

133. Silverberg GD, Reitz BA, Ream AK: Hypothermia and cardiac arrest in the treatment of giant aneurysms of the cerebral circulation and hemangioblastoma of the medulla. J Neurosurg 55:337, 1981

134. Sonntag VKH, Yuan RH, Stein BM: Giant intracranial aneurysms: a review of 13 cases. Surg Neurol 8:81, 1977

135. Spetzler RF, Daspit CP, Pappas CTE: The combined supra- and infratentorial approach for lesions of the petrous and clival region: experience with 46 cases. J Neurosurg 76:588, 1992

136. Spetzler RF, Fukushima T, Martin N et al: Petrous carotid-to-intradural carotid saphenous vein graft for intracavernous giant aneurysm, tumor, and occlusive cerebrovascular disease. J Neurosurg 73:496, 1990

137. Spetzler RF, Hadley MN, Rigamonti D et al: Aneurysms

of the basilar artery treated with circulatory arrest, hypothermia, and barbiturate cerebral protection. J Neurosurg 68:868, 1988

138. Spetzler RF, Lee KS: Reconstruction of the temporalis muscle for the pterional craniotomy. J Neurosurg 73:636, 1990

139. Spetzler RF, Schuster H, Roski RA: Elective extracranial-intracranial arterial bypass in the treatment of inoperable giant aneurysms of the internal carotid artery. J Neurosurg 53:22, 1980

140. Sundt TM Jr, Piepgras DG: Surgical approach to giant intracranial aneurysms. Operative experience with 80 cases. J Neurosurg 51:731, 1979

141. Sundt TM Jr, Piepgras DG, Fode NC et al: Giant intracranial aneurysms. Clin Neurosurg 37:116, 1991

142. Suzuki J: Temporary occlusion of trunk arteries of the brain during surgery. In Suzuki J (ed): Treatment of Cerebral Infarction. Springer-Verlag, New York, 1987

143. Suzuki J, Kuak R, Okudaira Y: The safe time limit of temporary clamping of cerebral arteries in the direct surgical treatment of intracranial aneurysm under moderate hypothermia. p. 326. In Suzuki J (ed): Cerebral Aneurysms. Neuron, Tokyo, 1979

144. Symon L: Management of giant intracranial aneurysms. Clin Neurosurg 36:21, 1990

145. Symon L, Momma F, Murota T: Assessment of reversible cerebral ischaemia in man: intraoperative monitoring of the somatosensory evoked response. Acta Neurochir suppl (Wien) 42:3, 1988

146. Symonds CP: Spontaneous subarachnoid hemorrhage. Q J Med 18:93, 1924

147. Tettenborn D, Dycka J: Prevention and treatment of delayed ischemic dysfunction in patients with aneurysmal subarachnoid hemorrhage. Stroke 21:85, 1990

148. Tsutsumi K, Shiokawa Y, Sakai T et al: Venous infarction following the interhemispheric approach in patients with acute subarachnoid hemorrhage. J Neurosurg 74:715, 1991

149. Uihlein A, MacCarty SC, Michenfelder JD et al: Deep hypothermia and surgical treatment of intracranial aneurysms. A five-year survey. JAMA 195:639, 1966

150. van Crevel H, Habbema JD, Braakman R: Decision analysis of the management of incidental intracranial saccular aneurysms. Neurology 36:1335, 1986

151. Vapalahti M, Ljunggren B, Saveland H et al: Early aneurysm operation and outcome in two remote Scandinavian populations. J Neurosurg 60:1160, 1984

152. Vermeulen M, Lindsay KW, Murray GD et al: Antifibrinolytic treatment in subarachnoid hemorrhage. N Engl J Med 311:432, 1984

153. Vermeulen M, Muizelaar JP: Do antifibrinolytic agents prevent rebleeding after rupture of a cerebral aneurysm? A review. Clin Neurol Neurosurg 82:25, 1980

154. Versavel M, Witmer JP, Matricali B: Giant aneurysm arising from the anterior cerebral artery and causing an isolated homonymous hemianopsia. Neurosurgery 22:560, 1988

155. Voldby B, Enevoldsen EM, Jensen FT: Cerebrovascular reactivity in patients with ruptured intracranial aneurysms. J Neurosurg 62:59, 1985

156. Weil SM, van Loveren HR, Tomsick TA et al: Management of inoperable cerebral aneurysms by the navigational balloon technique. Neurosurgery 21:296, 1987

157. Weir B, Aronyk K: Management mortality and the timing of surgery for supratentorial aneurysms. J Neurosurg 54:146, 1981

158. Whittle IR, Dorsch NW, Besser M: Giant intracranial aneurysms: diagnosis, management, and outcome. Surg Neurol 21:218, 1984

159. Wiebers DO, Whisnant JP, Sundt TM Jr et al: The significance of unruptured intracranial saccular aneurysms. J Neurosurg 66:23, 1987

160. Wyler AR, Kelly WA: Use of antibiotics with external ventriculostomies. J Neurosurg 37:185, 1972

Interventional Neuroradiological Management

FERNANDO VIÑUELA

ALLAN J. FOX

GARY DUCKWILER

The present association of microvascular neurosurgery, interventional neuroradiology, stroke neurology, neurointensivism, and neurorehabilitation has dramatically changed the therapeutic management of ischemic and hemorrhagic stroke.

Subarachnoid hemorrhage (SAH) accounts for about 10% of all strokes and in 50% of cases is related to a ruptured aneurysm. This disease has an immediate 25% mortality and only 10% to 20% of all patients make a good neurologic recovery without treatment.[14]

The etiology of intracranial aneurysms may be congenital, fusiform, mycotic, traumatic, inflammatory, neoplastic, or berry aneurysms. Most ruptured intracranial aneurysms are berry aneurysms and more than 80% of them are in the anterior circulation.[4] Most aneurysms tend to be single, although they can be multiple, and in 7% of cases they may have a familiar incidence.[7,29]

An increased incidence of aneurysm may be associated with polycystic kidney disease, Ehler-Danlos syndrome, Marfan syndrome, moyamoya disease, and hereditary hemorrhagic telangiectasia.[1,8,18,30]

Patients harboring an aneurysm may present with a sudden intracranial hemorrhage, evidences of intracranial mass effect, and, more rarely, with transient ischemic attacks or ischemic stroke. The increased utilization of brain magnetic imaging (MRI) and magnetic resonance angiography (MRA) has also increased the depiction of incidental aneurysms.[5] The therapeutic management of intracranial aneurysms needs a multidisciplinary team led by an expert microvascular neurosurgeon. There is a population of aneurysms that present difficult technical challenges and high morbidity/mortality to neurosurgical techniques alone. New therapeutic alternatives to these cases are now offered by interventional neuroradiology. A dynamic technical and scientific partnership between these two specialties is widening the spectrum of aneurysms that can be obliterated with a lower morbidity/mortality. This spectrum includes difficult aneurysms due to their size (large, giant, or fusiform), due to their location (intracavernous, posterior fossa, superior hypophyseal aneurysms, etc.) or aneurysms in patients in Hunt and Hess grades 3 to 5 or in the elderly population.

Interventional Neuroradiology and Intracranial Aneurysms

The participation of highly sophisticated companies with superb engineering expertise working in close association with interventional neuroradiologists has accelerated the development of endovascular delivery systems that allows safe navigation to the level of and beyond the circle of Willis. Intracranial aneurysms are predominantly located in the circle of Willis, and now they can be safely reached by the endovascular route. The utilization by expert interventional neuroradiologists of this new generation of microcatheters and microguides permits placing these systems in aneurysms and excluding them from the circulation with the delivery of a variety of embolic materials. After the aneurysm has been anatomically excluded, the interventional neuroradiologist can also contribute to the treatment of symptomatic vasospasm by performing endovascular angioplasty of the spastic arteries.

The endovascular neurointerventional techniques for the occlusion of intracranial aneurysms may be divided in two categories:

(1) Techniques of aneurysm obliteration with occlusion of parent artery, and

(2) techniques of aneurysm obliteration with preservation of parent artery.

Techniques of Aneurysm Obliteration with Occlusion of Parent Artery

The endovascular occlusion of an artery related to a skull base or intracranial large or giant aneurysm using detachable balloons is well-described in the literature.[6,9,10,15,38] These aneurysms may be saccular or fusiform, and they may be located in the anterior or posterior circulation. Patients harboring this type of aneurysm may present with mass effect, ischemia, seizures, or intracranial hemorrhage. The presence of wall calcifications or intraluminal thrombi does not preclude the possibility of a devastating intracranial hemorrhage.[11,31,40]

The endovascular occlusion of this type of aneurysm is preceded by diagnostic information upon the *anatomy* of the aneurysm (size, location, calcifications, thrombus formation), the intracranial *collateral circulation* and the *cerebral function and perfusion*.

The anatomic and topographic characteristics of the aneurysm are depicted by computed tomography (CT), MRI, MRA, and cerebral angiography.[2,3] It is mandatory to evaluate the true size of the aneurysm and neck as well as the state of the brain in contact with the aneurysm (atrophy, edema, acute or old hemorrhage, or infarct).

The brain collateral circulation is better evaluated by standard digital cerebral angiography. MRA can give an approximate idea of the anatomic characteristics of the circle of Willis, but has a limited contribution on its dynamic aspects. Mechanical temporary occlusion of the arteries in the neck during cerebral angiography shows the dynamic value of anterior and posterior communicating arteries as sources of collateral circulation to the brain.

The evaluation of the collateral circulation also becomes important as a source of recanalization of a large or giant aneurysm in cases of indiscriminate proximal occlusion of the parent artery. This information is essential in posterior circulation aneurysms and in anterior circulation aneurysms distal to the circle of Willis.[15] The collateral circulation may also be a source of rerupture in dissecting fusiform aneurysms at the vertebrobasilar junction if the aneurysm is not trapped by the endovascular route.

Cerebral function and perfusion may be evaluated by EEG, SPECT, XENON-CT scan, and diffusion and perfusion MR.[12,13,32,33]

The pre-embolization functional evaluation of the brain is mandatory to avoid catastrophic ischemic complication. The parent artery is temporarily occluded with a nondetachable balloon during an average time of 30 minutes while clinical, electrophysiologic (EEG), and hemodynamic (xenon-CT, SPECT) monitoring is performed.

The permanent occlusion of the parent artery may be performed proximal to the location of the giant aneurysm or distal and proximal to it (aneurysm trapping). The advocates of the latter technique fear the possibility of postembolization thromboembolic complications due to intracranial migration of fresh clot after the giant aneurysm is occluded.[15]

Detachable balloons remain the most popular embolic material to achieve a permanent occlusion of a brachiocephalic or intracranial artery related to a giant aneurysm. The procedure is fast, inexpensive, and safe in experienced hands. The balloons most commonly used were developed about two decades ago, are made from both latex and silicone materials, and have been used for aneurysms for many years.[10,15,19] The patient is under neuroleptic anesthesia and systemic heparinization. A pre-embolization complete angiographic evaluation of brain circulation and the circle of Willis is always performed. If the patient tolerates the parent artery temporary balloon occlusion, the balloon is then detached in place. Not unusually, two detachable balloons are placed as security against the possibility of early deflation of one of them. The procedure is followed by a complete cerebral angiography to assess the anatomical status of the aneurysm and the collateral circulation distal to the occlusion of the parent artery.

The availability of a new generation of nondetachable and detachable coils also permits their use as embolic agents to occlude a parent artery. The procedure is slower but also safe and has a good use in dissecting aneurysms. It is possible to pack the dissecting aneurysm with coils as well as the proximal and distal part of the parent artery. This procedure can be safer than balloon placement, because of lower wall tension in the dissected artery, and it has become popular in posterior cerebral and vertebral fusiform aneurysms (Fig. 55.25).

When the collateral circulation distal to a giant saccular of fusiform aneurysm is insufficient, it is necessary to perform an external-to-internal circulation bypass.[36,37] The type of bypass (arterial or venous graft) depends on the patient's vascular anatomy and the type of flow necessary to the brain. The vascular bypass is immediately followed by endovascular occlusion of the giant aneurysm/parent artery in order to create an immediate blood flow demand to the bypass.

Bilateral vertebral artery occlusion has been successfully used without bypass as a treatment for giant saccular or fusiform aneurysms of the vertebrobasilar system.[11,15] The combination of bilateral vertebral artery balloon occlusion following an external carotid-posterior cerebral bypass is also used in giant saccular or fusiform aneurysms when the circle of Willis

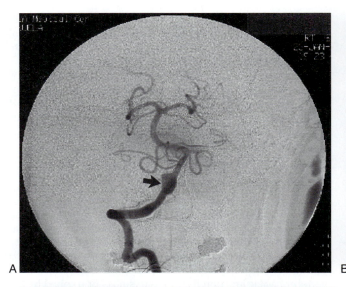

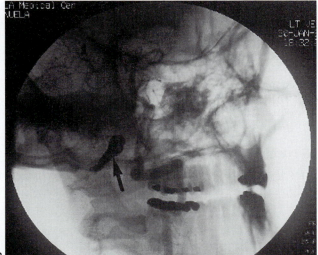

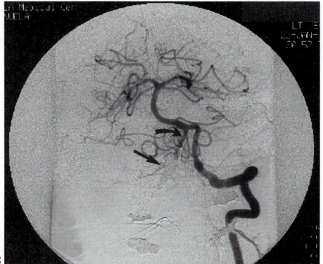

Figure 55.25 GDC Embolization of fusiform dissecting aneurysms. (**A**) Right vertebral angiogram shows a ruptured dissecting aneurysm (arrow) in a patient presenting with acute subarachnoid hemorrhage. (**B**) GDC cast of the dissecting aneurysm (arrow) is seen in a postembolization non-subtracted left vertebral angiogram. (**C**) Postembolization subtracted left vertebral angiogram shows the GDC cast (straight arrows) and retrograde filling of distal right vertebral artery and right PICA (curved arrow). Patient remained neurologically intact.

is insufficient. The balloons may be located proximal or distal to posterior inferior cerebellar artery (PICA) origin. If the balloons are positioned proximal to the origin of well-developed PICAs, they will exert a vascular sump effect that will keep the vascular bypass opened (Jacques Moret's vascular vacuum mechanism).

In limited cases, it is necessary to perform embolization by the Guglielmi detachable coil (GDC) of a large aneurysm before occluding its parent artery. The most classic example is a large or giant carotid-ophthalmic artery. It is necessary to isolate the aneurysm from the ophthalmic and posterior communicating arteries (sources of aneurysms recanalization). This endeavor is difficult to achieve, because a balloon distally placed might compromise the lumen of the anterior choroidal artery. The ostium of the ophthalmic artery may be occluded safely in most cases due to the extensive external carotid-ophthalmic collaterals. In these circumstances, it is better to partially embolize the aneurysm with coils and then block the parent artery with coils or detachable balloons. The partial coil embolization will be enough to promote aneurysm thrombosis without increasing the aneurysm mass effect upon the optic nerve.

The parent artery occlusion in intracranial large or giant aneurysm remains an appropriate technique for those aneurysms with a high surgical morbidity/mortality. Long-term angiographic and CT/MRI follow-ups show successful aneurysm occlusion in many cases and substantial decrease of the size of the aneurysm and improvement of the aneurysm mass effect. The intraluminal embolization of these aneurysms with coils tends to achieve incomplete anatomic results if the neck is wide and may increase the aneurysm mass effect and occasionally precipitate catastrophic intracranial hemorrhage in a nonruptured aneurysm.

Techniques of Aneurysm Obliteration with Preservation of the Lumen of the Parent Artery

This endovascular technology is becoming more popular with the utilization of the GDC.[16,17] The utilization of balloons,[19,20,34,35] pushable nondetachable coils,[22,26] and liquid agents[25,28] to occlude intracranial aneurysms lack sufficient control and predictability to make them safe to occlude an acutely ruptured aneurysm.

The GDC system was developed by Dr. Guglielmi and associates in 1989.[16] It consists of the endovascular catheterization of an aneurysm with a microcatheter and occlusion of it by delivering detachable platinum microcoils (Fig. 55.26). The platinum microcoil is soldered to a stainless steel guidewire that permits accurate delivery, withdrawal, and repositioning of the coil until it is safely anchored in the aneurysm. The platinum coil is detached by using an electric current of 1 mA. Several coils are delivered into the aneurysm through the same microcatheter until the aneurysm is densely packed. Most important in achieving a complete and permanent occlusion of the aneurysm is tight packing of the coils, not the presence of intra-aneurysmal clots (phenomenon of electrothrombosis). The presence of large intraluminal clots in the aneurysm facilitates coil remodeling and aneurysm recanalization.

There is a variety of platinum coils with different diameters and sizes to select from, depending on the size of the aneurysm and its anatomical integrity (ruptured versus unrup-

Figure 55.26 GDC Occlusion of ruptured basilar tip aneurysm. (**A**) Right vertebral angiogram shows a small, pear-shaped saccular basilar tip aneurysm with a narrow neck (open arrows). (**B**) Immediate postembolization right vertebral angiogram shows a dense GDC packing (arrows) occluding the aneurysm lumen. The basilar tip and posterior cerebral arteries origins are preserved.

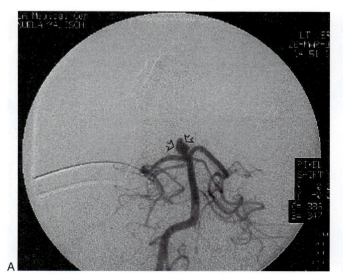
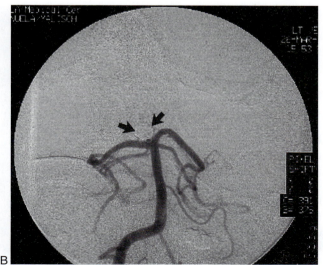

tured). The recent development of a special soft coil has improved the density of the packing and the treatment of the super-hot aneurysm (an aneurysm treated within 24 hours of rupturing). This coil is very delicate and fills the interstices of the regular coils without displacing them or the microcatheter out of the aneurysm.

TECHNICAL CONSIDERATIONS

GDC embolization of intracranial aneurysms requires that appropriate techniques be used by trained interventional neuroradiologists to minimize technical or clinical complications. The techniques discussed here have been adopted by most neurointerventional units around the world, after more than 4,000 intracranial aneurysms have been treated with GDCs.

General anesthesia should be used, unless contraindicated by the patient's medical condition. General anesthesia allows a perfect visualization of the aneurysm catheterization with the microcatheter-guidewire combination under road mapping. The delivery of the GDC coil is performed with accurate visualization of the neck of the aneurysm and surrounding normal vasculature. It also permits immediate patient control in cases of clinical complications, such as aneurysm perforation, thromboembolic complications, or sudden increase in intracranial pressure.

Systemic heparinization is used for most patients. In superacute aneurysms, a bolus of 3,000 to 5,000 units of heparin is delivered intravenously as soon as the dome and body of the aneurysm are occluded with GDC coils. This approach is based on a higher frequency of thromboembolic complications rather than hemorrhagic complications during GDC embolization. The systemic heparinization may or may not be reversed with protamine sulfate at the end of the procedure; this may be immediately complemented with aspirin (325 mg two times a day) in selected cases.

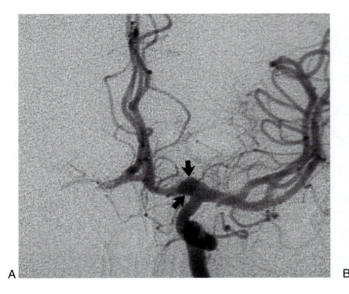

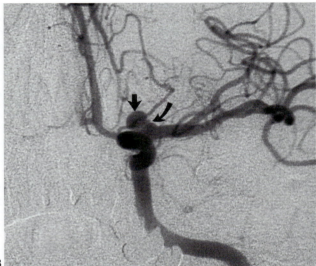

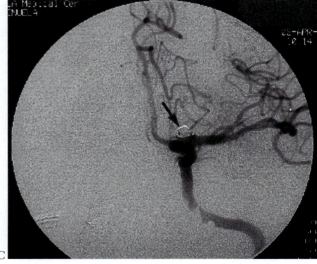

Figure 55.27 Special views for especial aneurysms. (**A**) AP view of left internal carotid angiogram shows a double density (arrows) overlying A1 portion of left anterior cerebral artery, suspicious of an aneurysm. (**B**) A Waters oblique view of the left internal carotid artery shows the body (arrow) and neck (curved arrow) of the aneurysm arising from the left internal carotid artery bifurcation. (**C**) Postembolization angiogram shows a complete, dense GDC packing of the aneurysm (arrow) with preservation of the left internal carotid artery bifurcation.

The angiographic evaluation of the aneurysm is focused on the identification of the best view that separates the neck of the aneurysm from the parent artery and surrounding branches. This view will be used to deliver the GDC coils and to assess immediate and long-term anatomic results. The utilization of standard angiographic views is misleading due to the common superimposition of arteries (Fig. 55.27).

In selected cases such as carotid-ophthalmic and anterior communicating aneurysms, the manual reshaping of the microcatheter, tailored to the arterial geometry, helps to enter the aneurysm and anchor the microcatheter in it. The tailored 3-D shape of the microcatheter keeps the catheter in place, reduces the need of recatheterization of the aneurysm, and improves the density of the GDC packing.

The first coil delivered into an aneurysm should be the largest capable of crossing the aneurysm neck as many times as possible (Fig. 55.28). The success in obtaining an early nest with inclusion of the aneurysm inflow, and in some cases the utilization of a protecting balloon across a wide-neck aneurysm during coil delivery (Jacques Moret reconstructive technique), allows a very dense GDC packing of the aneurysm (Fig. 55.29). The utilization of last generation soft coils has also improved anatomic results and decreased technical complications and morbidity/mortality.

The endovascular exploitation of GDC utilization in aneurysms carries a very low morbidity. To recognize there is a population of aneurysms that cannot be treated by GDC technology is essential. With these types, it is better to discontinue the procedure and consider other therapeutic options instead of pushing the technology to dangerous and nonpredictable circumstances. The future evolution of GDC technology includes 3-D GDC coils and coils with special surface modifications (Yuichi Murayama ionic implantation paper). This new generation of GDC coils will improve immediate and long-term anatomic results by increasing aneurysm packing and eliciting a stronger "scarring" cellular response.

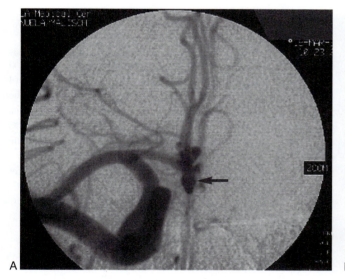

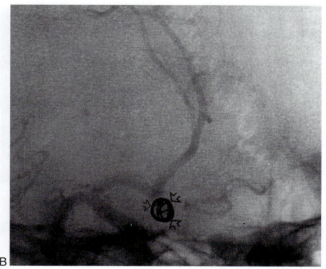

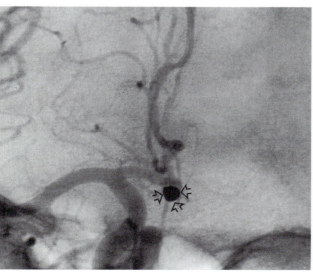

Figure 55.28 Initial GDC framing of an aneurysm. (**A**) Right internal carotid angiogram shows a ruptured, small saccular anterior communicating aneurysm (arrow). (**B**) Initial successful framing of the aneurysm with inclusion of its neck (arrows) by the first GDC coil. (**C**) Dense and complete GDC packing of the aneurysm (arrows) with preservation of the anatomy of the anterior cerebral artery.

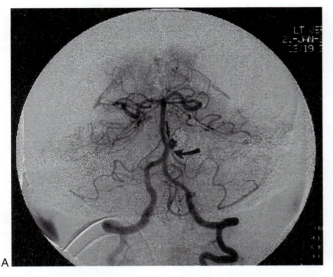

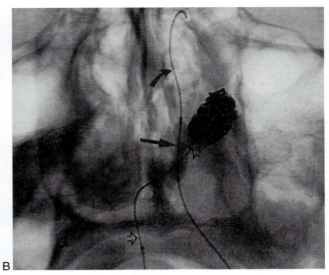

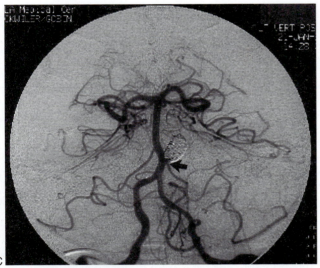

Figure 55.29 GDC embolization and balloon protection. (**A**) Left vertebral angiogram shows partial recanalization (arrows) of a basilar–AICA aneurysm 6 months postembolization. Note the left AICA origin (curved arrow) in close association with the neck of the aneurysm. (**B**) An inflated nondetachable balloon (arrows) anchored by a guidewire (curved arrows) closes the neck of the aneurysm while a GDC coil (open arrow) is delivered in the aneurysm. This maneuver described by Dr. Jacques Moret facilitates a safer and tighter GDC packing in wide neck aneurysms. (**C**) Postembolization left vertebral angiogram shows a complete GDC aneurysm occlusion and preservation of basilar artery and left AICA origin (arrows).

TOPOGRAPHIC DISTRIBUTION AND ANATOMIC RESULTS

The anatomic results of GDC embolization are primarily dependent on the neck size of the aneurysm in relation to the size of its body. The location of the aneurysm and the patient's clinical status play a lesser role in the overall anatomic results.

The best immediate and long-term anatomic results are observed in small saccular aneurysms with a small neck (4 mm or less). Table 55.5 shows the immediate anatomic results in 327 patients with 362 aneurysms treated at the University of California, Los Angeles (UCLA). Of these aneurysms, 57% were in the anterior circulation and 44.1% were in posterior circulation. The higher incidence of posterior circulation aneurysms of this series when compared with the published neurosurgical series is an expression of the inclusion criteria used to select GDC patients. (Anticipated surgical difficulty, attempted surgical clipping, poor neurological status [Hunt and Hess grades 3 to 5], poor medical condition or age.) The most

Table 55.5 GDC Embolization of Intracranial Aneurysms: UCLA Experience in 327 Patients/ 362 Aneurysms—Anatomic Results

Type	Comp (%)	Neck Remn. (%)	Body Fill (%)	Attempt (%)
Small aneurysm/small neck (105 aneurysms)	82.0	6.1	0	1.9
Small aneurysm/large neck (94 aneurysms)	49.0	37.0	1.0	13.0
Large aneurysms (115 aneurysms)	43.6	42.0	6.0	8.4
Giant aneurysm (48 aneurysms)	26.5	53.0	16.5	4.0

Abbreviations: GDC, Guglielmi detachable coil; UCLA, University of California, Los Angeles.

common aneurysms treated in the UCLA series were basilar bifurcation (23%), carotid ophthalmic/paraophthalmic (21%), anterior communicating (12%), posterior communicating (12%), and middle cerebral bifurcation (8%).

The GDC technology can be safely used in the acute phase of subarachnoid hemorrhage. Viñuela et al reported 2.7% technical complications with an immediate 8.9% morbidity and 1.7% mortality related to the technique in 403 patients.[39] Of their aneurysms, 57% were in the posterior circulation, and 43% in the anterior circulation. Also, 20% were in Hunt and Hess grade 1, 26% in grade 2, 30% in grade 3, 17% in grade 4 and 6.5% in grade 5. GDC embolization of the ruptured aneurysm was performed within 48 hours of hemorrhage in 36% of patients, between 3 to 6 days in 38%, 7 to 10 days in 17%, and 11 to 15 days in 7% of patients.

The safety of the GDC technology also allows endovascular occlusion of multiple aneurysms in the same procedure. This is very useful in patients presenting in the acute phase of SAH with the impending risk of developing symptomatic vasospasm. Endovascular occlusion of the ruptured and incidental aneurysms allows the use of an aggressive triple-H (hypertension, hypervolemia, hemodilution) therapy without fearing an intracranial hemorrhage from the incidental aneurysm.

Postembolization cerebral angiography performed 6 months or more after the original procedure demonstrated aneurysm recanalization due to coil compaction in 3.6% of aneurysms with a small neck, in 12.2% in small aneurysms with a wide neck, in 23% of large aneurysms (larger than 10 mm), and in 37% of giant aneurysms (larger than 25 mm).

In 5.2% of all aneurysms, postembolization surgical clipping of the aneurysm was performed. In some patients with acute subarachnoid hemorrhage, a partial GDC occlusion of the ruptured aneurysm was sufficient to avoid a fatal rehemorrhage. A second complete embolization or a complete surgical clipping was performed after the acute phase of SAH had subsided. This combined endovascular-neurosurgical practice appears to be of great value in patients with symptomatic vasospasm.

Endovascular angioplasty of symptomatic vasospasm may be mechanical and/or chemical. Symptomatic patients who do not improve after 4 to 6 hours of intensive triple-H therapy (hypertension, hypervolemia, hemodilution) and intravenous infusion of calcium channel blockers should be taken to the neuroangiography suite for emergency cerebral angiography followed by mechanical and/or chemical angioplasty.

Mechanical balloon angioplasty was originally reported by Zukov[41] in 1984 and later by Higashida,[21] Le Roux,[27] and others. It consists in the dilatation of vasospasm in the arteries of the circle of Willis by using soft balloons. If performed in the early phases of ischemia, it may achieve a dramatic clinical improvement in more than 50% of patients.[27] To improve local circulation and potential collaterals, a complete arterial dilatation of the proximal anterior and posterior circulations may be performed in one sitting.

Mechanical angioplasty has low morbidity and mortality if performed by an experienced interventional neuroradiologist. The most severe technical complication is arterial rupture due to balloon overinflation. This can be avoided by restricting balloon angioplasty to P1, M1, A1, or IC/basilar segments.

Chemical angioplasty is performed by the intracranial infusion of papaverine into the symptomatic arterial territory.[23] Intra-arterial nimodipine also appears to achieve similar anatomic results. It is technically simpler and safer than the mechanical angioplasty although the long-term angiographic results show a higher recurrence rate than the mechanical angioplasty.[24] Papaverine should not be infused with contrast material or heparin, because it precipitates in small crystals. These small crystals may occlude eloquent arteries such as perforating branches of the vertebrobasilar system producing symptoms of posterior fossa ischemia.

In severe cases of diffuse arterial vasospasm, it is appropriate to utilize mechanical angioplasty of the circle of Willis followed by chemical angioplasty of peripheral circulation.

TECHNICAL COMPLICATIONS AND IMMEDIATE MORBIDITY/ MORTALITY

The technical complications most frequently related to GDC use in aneurysms include cerebral embolization (2.7%), aneurysm perforation (2.4%), and parent artery occlusion (clot or coil migration) (2.4% [Table 55.6]).

The use of aggressive systemic heparinization during and immediately after the procedure plus a more sophisticated knowledge of how and when to embolize the neck of the aneurysm have decreased postembolization cerebral embolization.

Table 55.6 GDC Embolization of Intracranial Aneurysms: UCLA Experience in 327 Patients/ 362 Aneurysms—Technical Complications

Aneurysm perforation	8 pts	2.4%
Cerebral embolization	9 pts	2.7%
Parent artery occlusion	8 pts	2.4%
Arterial dissection/neck	2 pts	0.61%
Coil rupture	3 pts	0.9%

Abbreviations: GDC, Guglielmi detachable coil; UCLA, University of California, Los Angeles.

Table 55.7 GDC Embolization of Intracranial Aneurysms: UCLA Experience in 327 Patients/ 362 Aneurysms—Morbidity/Mortality/Hunt and Hess Grading

Grade	*Morbidity*	*Mortality*
1 (44 pts)	2 pts (4.5%)	0%
2 (39 pts)	5 pts (12.0%)	0%
3 (40 pts)	3 pts (7.5%)	1 pt (2.5%)
4 (15 pts)	1 pt (7.0%)	3 pts (20.0%)
5 (11 pts)	1 pt (9.0%)	3 pts (27.0%)

Abbreviations: GDC, Guglielmi detachable coil; UCLA, University of California, Los Angeles.

Table 55.8 GDC Embolization of Intracranial Aneurysms: UCLA Experience in 327 Patients/362 Aneurysms—Morbidity/Mortality/Day of Hemorrhage

Day	Morbidity	Mortality
0–2 (68 pts)	4 pts (5.8%)	3 pts (4.4%)
3–6 (53 pts)	3 pts (5.6%)	4 pts (7.5%)
7–10 (17 pts)	1 pt (5.8%)	0%
11–15 (11 pts)	1 pt (9.0%)	0%
>15 (40 pts)	5 pts (12.0%)	0%

Abbreviations: GDC, Guglielmi detachable coil; UCLA, University of California, Los Angeles.

This complication still remains relatively high in middle cerebral artery aneurysms because of the difficulty in isolating the neck of the aneurysm from surrounding arteries.

The use of the GDC 10 system and the appearance of the soft coils have decreased aneurysm perforation in acutely ruptured aneurysms. This technical complication is seldom observed in unruptured aneurysms.

The development of a wider variety of GDC coils (different in diameter and length) and the use of Moret's reconstructive technique (a protecting nondetachable balloon across the neck of the aneurysm) have decreased parent artery occlusion due to untoward coil migration and have improved the density of the aneurysm GDC packing.

Patients' morbidity/mortality separated by Hunt and Hess grading is shown in Table 55.7. Patients' morbidity/mortality broken down by the day of hemorrhage is shown in Table 55.8. Patient's morbidity/mortality related to the aneurysm topography is shown in Table 55.9.

The rehemorrhage rate was 2.5% (5 of 189 parts) after an average clinical follow-up of approximately 24 months in 189 patients presenting with a ruptured aneurysm. No cases of rehemorrhage were seen in aneurysms with a stable, nonexpanding residual neck. We may summarize our experience with using the GDC technique in intracranial aneurysms by stating that

GDC technology is safe for embolization of intracranial, ruptured, and unruptured aneurysms.

GDC embolization of ruptured aneurysms improves the natural history of the disease by decreasing rehemorrhage and allows an aggressive medical/endovascular balloon angioplasty therapy of symptomatic vasospasm.

The present anatomic results are mostly influenced by the neck size of the aneurysm more than its location or by the patient's clinical status.

Morbidity/mortality is within an acceptable range for the population of patients and aneurysms treated (aneurysms with high surgical morbidity/mortality).

The present anatomic and clinical results will improve with an ascent into the learning curve of the interventional neuroradiologist, with the development of a new generation of GDC (3-D GDC, use of ionic implantation to modify the GDC surface, etc.) and with a better understanding of aneurysm flow dynamics (computer simulation programs to predict flow characteristics).

A critical analysis of long-term anatomic and clinical outcome will determine the efficacy of this technology.

A strict, prospective scientific evaluation of GDC and neurosurgical, anatomic, and clinical outcomes will be necessary to find the appropriate place of this new endovascular technology in the therapeutic management of intracranial aneurysms.

References

1. Adams HP, Kassell NF, Wissoff HS et al: Intracranial saccular aneurysms and moyamoya disease. Stroke 10: 174, 1979
2. Aoki S, Sasaki Y, Machida T et al: Cerebral aneurysms: detection and delineation using 3D CT angiography. Am J Neuroradiol 13:1115–1120, 1992
3. Artmann H, Vonofakos D, Muller H et al: Neuroradiologic and neuropathologic findings with growing giant intracranial aneurysm: review of the literature. Surg Neurol 21:391, 1984
4. Atehbens WE: Aneurysms and anatomical variation of cerebral arteries. Arch Path 75:45, 1963
5. Atlas SW, Grossman RI, Goldberg HI et al: Partially thrombosed giant intracranial aneurysms: correlation of MRI and pathological findings. Radiology 162:111–114, 1987
6. Aymard A, Gobin YP, Hodes JE et al: Endovascular occlusion of vertebral arteries in the treatment of unclippable vertebrobasilar aneurysms. J Neurosurg 74:393–398, 1991
7. Bannerman RM, Ingall GB, Graf CJ: The familial occurrence of intracranial aneurysms. Neurology 20:283, 1970
8. Belber CJ, Hoffman RB: The syndrome of intracranial aneurysms associated with fibromuscular hyperplasia of the renal arteries. J Neurosurg 28:556, 1969
9. Berenstein A, Ranshohoff J, Kupersmith M et al: Transvascular treatment of giant aneurysms in the cavernous carotid and verebral arteries: functional investigation and embolization. Surg Neurol 21:3–12, 1984
10. Debrun G, Fox A, Drake CG et al: Giant unclippable aneurysms: treatment with detachable balloons. Am J Neuroradiol 2:167–173, 1981

Table 55.9 GDC Embolization of Intracranial Aneurysms: UCLA Experience in 327 Patients/362 Aneurysms—Morbidity/Mortality/Aneurysm

Aneurysm	Morbidity	Mortality
Basilar tip (74 pts)	6 pts 8.1%	3 pts 4.0%
Carotid ophthalmic (70 pts)	2 pts 2.8%	0 pts 0%
Posterior comm (39 pts)	2 pts 5.1%	0 pts 0%
Middle cerebral (26 pts)	1 pt s 3.8%	2 pts 7.6%
Anterior comm (41 pts)	3 pts 7.3%	0 pts 0%

Abbreviations: GDC, Guglielmi detachable coil; UCLA, University of California, Los Angeles.

11. Drake CG: Giant intracranial aneurysms: experience with surgical treatment in 174 patients. Clin Neurosurg 26: 12–95, 1979

12. Echard DA, Purdy PD, Bonte FJ et al: Temporary balloon occlusion of the carotid artery combined with brain blood flow imaging as a test to predict tolerance prior to permanent carotid sacrifice. Am J Neuroradiol 13: 1565–1569, 1992

13. Erba SM, Horton JA, Latchaw RE et al: Balloon test occlusion of the internal carotid artery with stable xenon-CT cerebral blood flow imaging. Am J Neuroradiol 9: 533–538, 1988

14. Fisher CM: Clinical syndromes in cerebral thrombosis, hypertensive hemorrhage and ruptured saccular aneurysm. Clin Neurosurg 22:117–124, 1975

15. Fox AJ, Viñuela F, Pelz DM et al: Use of detachable balloons for proximal artery occlusion in the treatment of unclippable cerebral aneurysms. J Neurosurg 66:40–46, 1987

16. Guglielmi G, Viñuela F, Dion J et al: Electrothrombosis of saccular aneurysms via endovascular approach. Part 2. Preliminary clinical experience. J Neurosurg 75:8–14, 1991

17. Guglielmi G, Viñuela F, Duckwiler G et al: Endovascular treatment of posterior circulation aneurysms by electrothrombosis using electrically detachable coils. J Neurosurg 77:515–524, 1992

18. Hatfield PM, Pfister RC: Adult polycystic disease of the kidneys (Potter type 3). JAMA 222:157, 1972

19. Higashida RT, Halbach VV, Barnwell SL et al: Treatment of intracranial aneurysms with preservation of the parent vessel: results of percutaneous balloon embolization in 84 patients. Am J Neuroradiol 11:633–640, 1990

20. Higashida RT, Halbach VV, Cahan LD et al: Detachable balloon embolization therapy of posterior circulation intracranial aneurysms. J Neurosurg 71:512–519, 1989

21. Higashida RT, Halbach VV, Cahan LD et al: Transluminal angioplasty for treatment of intracranial arterial vasospasm. J Neurosurg 71:648–653, 1989

22. Hilal SK, Khandji A, Solomon RW et al: Obliteration of intracranial aneurysms with preshaped highly thrombogenic coils, Abstracted. Radiology, 173(suppl.):S250

23. Kaku Y, Yonekawa T, Tsukahara T et al: Superselective intra-arterial infusion of papaverine for the treatment of cerebral vasospasm after subarachnoid hemorrhage. J Neurosurg 77:842–847, 1992

24. Kassell NF, Helm G, Simmons N et al: Treatment of cerebral vasospasm with intra-arterial papaverine. J Neurosurg 77:848–852, 1992

25. Kinugasa K, Mandai S, Terai Y et al: Direct thrombosis of aneurysms with cellulosa acetate polymer. Part II: Preliminary clinical experience. J Neurosurg 77:501–507, 1992

26. Knuckey NW, Haas R, Jenkins R et al. Thrombosis of difficult intracranial aneurysms by the endovascular placement of platinum-Dacron microcoils. J Neurosurg 77:43–50, 1992

27. Le Roux PD, Newell DW, Eskridge J et al: Severe symptomatic vasospasm: the role of immediate postoperative angioplasty. J Neurosurg 80:224–229, 1994

28. Mandai S, Kinugasa K, Ohmoto T: Direct thrombosis of aneurysms with cellulose acetate polymer. Part 1: Results of thrombosis in experimental aneurysms. J Neurosurg 77:497–500, 1992

29. McKissock W, Richardson A, Walsh L et al: Multiple intracranial aneurysms. Lancet 1:623, 1964

30. McKusik VA: The cardiovascular aspects of Marfan's syndrome: a heritable disorder of connective tissue. Circulation 11:321, 1955

31. Mehdorn HM, Chater NL, Townsend JJ et al: Giant aneurysms and cerebral ischemia. Surg Neurol 13:49–57, 1980

32. Monsein LH, Jeffrey PJ, Van Heerden BB et al: Assessing adequacy of collateral circulation during balloon test occlusion of the internal carotid artery with Tc99m-HMPAO SPECT. Am J Neuroradiol 12:1045,1051, 1991

33. Moody EB, Dawson RC III, Sandler MP: Tc99m-HMPAO SPECT imaging in interventional neuroradiology: validation of balloon test occlusion. Am J Neuroadiol 12:1043–1044, 1991

34. Romodanov AP, Schegelov VI: Intravascular occlusion of saccular aneurysms of the cerebral arteries by means of a detachable balloon catheter. pp. 25–49. In Krayenbuhl H (ed): Advances and Technical Standards in Neurosurgery. Vol 9. Springer-Verlag, New York, 1982

35. Schegelov VI: Endovascular occlusion of saccular intracranial aneurysms: results in 617 patients. In Proceedings from the 27th Annual Meeting of the American Society of Neuroradiology, Orlando, Florida, 1989, p 43

36. Spetzler RF, Carter LP: Revascularization and aneurysm surgery current status. Neurosurgery 16:111–116, 1985

37. Sundt TM Jr, Piepgras DG, Marsh WR et al: Saphenous vein bypass grafts for giant aneurysms and intracranial occlusive disease. J Neurosurg 65:439–450, 1986

38. Taki W, Nishi S, Yamashita K et al: Selection and combination of various endovascular techniques in the treatment of giant aneurysms. J Neurosurg 77:37–42, 1992

39. Viñuela F, Duckwiler G, Mawad M: Guglielmi detachable coil embolization of acute intracrainal aneurysm: perioperative anatomical and clinical outcome in 403 patients. J Neurosurg 86:475–482, 1997

40. Whittle JR, Dorsch NW, Besser M: Giant intracranial aneurysms: diagnosis, management and outcome. Surg Neurol 21:218–230, 1984

41. Zukov YN, Nikiforov BM, Shustin VA: Balloon catheter technique for dilation of constricted cerebral arteries after aneurysmal SAH. Acta Neurochir (Wien) 70:65–79, 1984

Vascular Malformations of the Brain and Dura

BENNETT M. STEIN

JOHN PILE-SPELLMAN

STEVEN R. ISAACSON

Management Decisions

In order to determine the best management for a given disease process, there are certain basic facts that must be considered. These include a knowledge of the natural history of the disease process and the risk/benefit statistics of the various forms of treatment. The problem in dealing with vascular malformations is compounded because of our lack of understanding of the natural history of the various vascular malformations, including arteriovenous malformations (AVMs), telangiectasias, and cavernous and venous malformations.[8,13,14,19,29,35,36,41,46,56,61,81,91,106,110,113,114,150,161,162] Therefore, the liability of a "do nothing" course of action may not be fully appreciated by the medical community. Lack of information occurs because of the uncommon occurrence of these lesions, the fact that they often become apparent in young people but have a clinical course that may span decades.

In dealing with a relatively large group of patients who have had AVMs over the past 20 years, we have been able to review only a handful of them who have had sequential arteriography while their AVMs remain unmolested.[140,141] This group was culled primarily from a Veterans Administration hospital population. The longest interval of follow-up was only 10 years. This small group of patients stressed the variability of these lesions, in that three lesions remained the same, three got bigger, and three got somewhat smaller but did not disappear. The number of case reports documenting spontaneous obliteration of AVMs are few and anecdotal.[142,159] Most articles that speak of the natural history of vascular malformations are retrospective in nature.[13,36,41,46,47,113,114,150] Many of them are tainted by selec-

tion of patients based on age, history, and size and location of malformations or deal with patients who have undergone tentative therapy. Obviously, such reviews give only a glimmer of the true nature of these disorders. Unfortunately, they are the best that we have and currently must be relied on to provide the judgment for successful management of these problems.

The basic methods of therapy include the following alone or in combination: (1) surgery, (2) embolization, and (3) radiation, always with the option of leaving the lesion alone if risk of therapy appears too great. There are strong advocates for each of these methods. Our attitude is toward an aggressive approach, since we regard these lesions as inherently dangerous, occurring in a young and productive age group in which hemorrhage can be severely incapacitating or fatal.

The risks of surgery and embolization are self-evident at the time these procedures are performed whereas the risks of radiotherapy may not be apparent for a number of years after the full course of treatment is rendered. Similarly, the benefit of surgery is evident after the performance of the procedure, since complete proven obliteration of the lesion is the aim and, when accomplished, implies cure of the patient. In terms of modification of a seizure disorder, the beneficial results of surgery may be difficult to determine. When embolization is utilized, rarely producing obliteration of the AVM, the benefits are not immediately apparent. It may take years, if not decades, of follow-up to determine the impact of this treatment on the incidence of recidivous hemorrhages, seizure disorders, or progressive neurologic deficits. In the case of radiotherapy, conventional or focused, the situation is even more nebulous. The changes that occur in an AVM and the surrounding normal brain affected by radiotherapy span years.

Therefore, in the case of risk the answers may not be known for a number of years following the institution of radiotherapy. Proponents of radiation therapy stress that there is a high rate of AVM obliteration at the 2-year interval after therapy.[12,52,68,144]

Other factors that influence the natural history and therapy of these malformations include age, sex, social habits, and anatomic factors such as the size and location of the malformation and prior medical history. Reviewing our cases and considering that 15% of hemorrhages are silent, we feel that a history of hemorrhage is not a major factor in determining the future risk of a malformation. Other neurosurgeons with large series of AVMs, however, disagree and have expressed the opinion that a malformation that has previously hemorrhaged is more dangerous than one that has not.[32,46,78,114,163] Recent reviews of the problem indicate that the incidence of recurrent hemorrhage with serious outcome is 2% per year, and when measured in a young person the risk becomes intolerable.

The premise, therefore, that short-term follow-up will determine the risk after a treatment that is short of complete obliteration is false. Treatment that results in occlusion of portions of the malformation or of the feeding vessels, scarification and thickening of the walls of the vessels, or partial removal of the malformation falls short of complete obliteration of the malformation and therefore must stand the test of time over a considerable follow-up period and cannot be equated with cure.

Surgery

RISK CONSIDERATIONS

Each patient with an AVM must be evaluated on an individual basis in reference to age, previous history, and size and location of the AVM. Locational designations include superficial or deep, hemispheric, basal ganglion, brain stem, posterior fossa, or medial hemisphere.[17,25,30,33,44,71,84,117,132–134,138,140,167,170,171]

In reference to age, a younger person not only is exposed over a longer period to the natural risk from hemorrhage than an older person, but also will exhibit a better tolerance of surgery.[34] Since these AVMs frequently become apparent in the second, third, and fourth decades, it is this group that should be the focus of our concern. In general, patients over the age of 60 years are treated in a less aggressive fashion than younger patients. Other medical conditions such as cardiac abnormalities, presence of aneurysms, and systemic disease have to be considered in establishing risk.

The size of an AVM is considered another major factor in the operability of these lesions. A small lesion located in an accessible region of the brain, for example, the frontal pole, is relatively easy to remove and requires no adjuvant therapy[135,139,142,147] (Fig. 56.1). Larger lesions that involve more than one lobe or the posterior fossa and deep areas of the brain may be inoperable because of their great volume.[136] This would appear to run contrary to the theory that all tissue within the confines of a malformation is nonfunctional; not so:

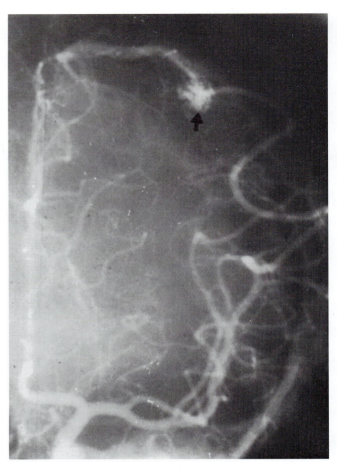

Figure 56.1 Relatively small and circumscribed arteriovenous malformation (arrow) that presents minimal surgical challenge.

the technical difficulties encountered in attempting to remove massive malformations that span lobes of the brain are geometrically increased with size and will then preclude operative intervention (Fig. 56.2). The size and number of arterial to venous shunts must also be taken into account.[115,141,165]

The location of the malformation is one of the most important predictors of operability. Those lesions that are located superficially and in polar regions of the brain may be removed with relative ease.[1,31,32,131,139,163] Eloquent regions of the brain are often the site of AVMs. These may successfully be treated by experienced surgeons.[17,26,30,71,143,167] Malformations located in the diencephalon and basal ganglion are generally considered inoperable (Fig. 56.3), although there are rare reports of such lesions being removed.[44,134,152] Those malformations located in the brain stem—unless dissected by previous hemorrhage, reaching the surface of the brain stem, or lying in the cerebellopontine angle—are generally considered inoperable[30,132] (Fig. 56.4). Malformations located in obscure areas of the brain, such as the medial hemisphere, insula, roof of the third ventricle, and lateral ventricle, may be removed with some difficulty[133,138,170,171] (Fig. 56.5). Cerebellar lesions can be difficult to remove, since many of them are extensive with poorly defined borders. However, many can

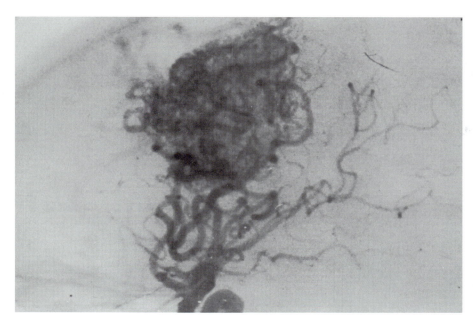

Figure 56.2 Large arteriovenous malformation involving multiple lobes of eloquent brain. This is generally an inoperable lesion.

Figure 56.4 Brain stem arteriovenous malformation (arrows) lying in pia of the brain stem. This lesion is potentially resectable.

Figure 56.3 Large arteriovenous malformation involving the diencephalic area. This is generally an untreatable problem.

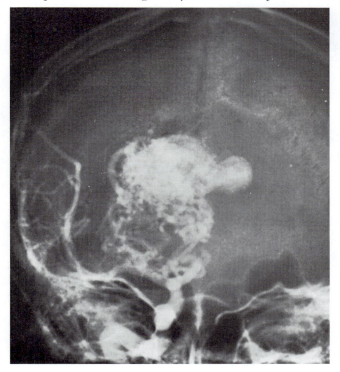

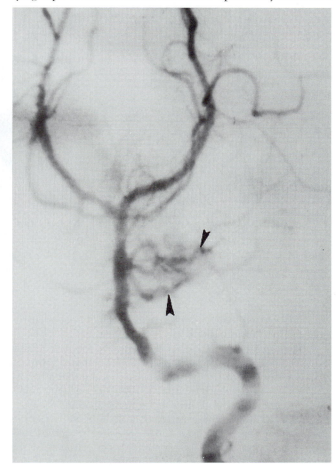

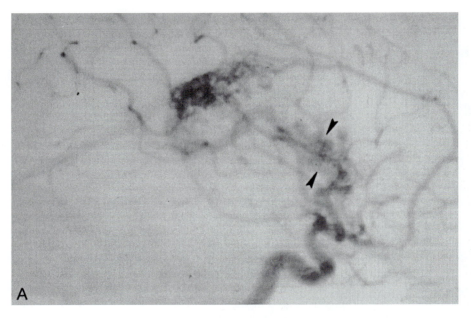

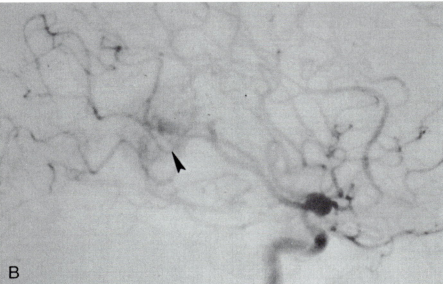

Figure 56.5 (**A**) An arteriovenous malformation located within the anterior third ventricle (arrows) following unsuccessful proton beam therapy. (**B**) Successful removal of the anterior third ventricular arteriovenous malformation. The second malformation (arrow) was resected at a subsequent operation.

be removed, and considering the resiliency of cerebellar tissue, the long-term outlook can be excellent.[33,140]

The weight to be placed on the patient's history is debatable. We consider this factor the least important and approach AVMs regardless of history. Others have stated that a history of hemorrhage demands treatment, other factors being equal.

A detailed review of the arteriographic anatomy is invaluable in determining the exact course of the feeding arteries and draining veins and this is further assisted by stereoscopic lateral angiograms. This materially aids the surgeon in the operative approach and design of the operation. The location

of feeding arteries, the complexity and duplication of the draining venous system and the discreteness of the malformation or definition of its borders are all factors that must be taken into consideration in a general fashion in determining the operability of a lesion. Magnetic resonance imaging (MRI) has been particularly useful in visualizing the configuration as well as relationship to border structures of an AVM.

In general, the determination of operability of a lesion must be made by a neurosurgeon and a neurologist experienced in the management of a large number of AVM patients. The same principles expressed here have relevance to the other less common vascular malformations of the brain that have been previously categorized.

PREOPERATIVE ADJUVANT PROCEDURES

We consider preoperative embolization, performed with a variety of substances, a valuable adjuvant to surgical resection of more complicated AVMs.[60,153] This technique was introduced in a large number of cases by Luessenhop and Spence in 1960 and has since been refined by the neuroradiologist using transfemoral intravascular techniques to deliver the embolic material to the AVM.[11,27,54,156,166] The initial work of Luessenhop and Spence introduced the use of ceramic pellets, later changed to Silastic pellets, which could be introduced directly into the internal carotid circulation if this nourished the area of the AVM.[77] This early work has permitted a significantly long follow-up. The following conclusions were reached in recent articles, surveying more than 200 patients:

1. Recurrent hemorrhage rate and severity were not altered by embolization without obliteration of the AVM.

2. The safety of the procedure, both short term and long term, was verified.

3. Seizure disorder and progressive neurologic deterioration were often improved following successful embolization.

4. Surgery was facilitated by preoperative embolization.

The high-speed selective angiogram is the road map used to guide all treatments. Superselective angiograms of feeding pedicles can be helpful.[155] The angioarchitecture, feeding arteries and draining veins, relative flow rates, associated aneurysms, stenosis, occlusions, shift in watershed, apparent compartments, and degree of ectasia should all be identified prior to formulating an endovascular approach. Stereo views may show the exact configuration of the arteries and veins with the nidus, and can be quite helpful prior to surgery, particularly in the effort to spare normal brain.

Communication in the development and execution of the goals, strategies, and tactics of the treatment is essential if the best result is to be achieved. Going over the plan in detail with the patient allows the patient to participate fully and actively in the healing process and helps avoid confusion and unnecessary suffering. Endovascular treatment of AVMs requires the coordination of a large team to address complex, difficult, and overlapping problems. Active participation from stroke neurologists, cerebral vascular neurosurgeons, radiosurgeons, and interventional neuroradiologists helps immeasurably in addressing complex AVMs. Input from anesthesiologists, nurses, and radiographic technologists is essential for developing tactics and executing a plan.

Neuroradiologists using interventional techniques have utilized particulate emboli or liquid adhesives in the preoperative treatment of AVMs.[76,128,156,166] Previously emboli were made from Silastic, are spherical, and range in size from 1.5 mm to a maximum of 4 mm. The maximum is determined by the lumen of the largest catheter that can be directed via a transfemoral route to either the internal

carotid or vertebrate arteries. Other materials utilized are Gelfoam, isopropyl alcohol fragments, and NBCA (*N*-butyl cyanoacrylate).

Today, embolization is most often carried out with NBCA, a liquid adhesive that polymerizes and solidifies when in contact with blood. The material is injected through a microcatheter placed directly into the AVM nidus.[29,65] The advantage of this technique is that it delivers the material directly to the AVM and fills the interstices. With refinement of intravascular catheters, it is possible to effectively deliver embolic material directly into the AVM. By this technique embolic material is placed into the AVM nidus with some overflow to the venous side, maximizing stasis.[11,37,38,49,111,116,154,156,157] The placement of NBCA into the AVM has prepared the patient best for surgical resection (Fig. 56.6).[23,86,109,142,143,165]

The angioarchitecture is the most important factor in terms of safe embolization. Embolization may also eliminate deep feeding arteries that are relatively inaccessible or represent the final blood supply, an enigma to the surgeon working in the difficult margin around the malformation deep within the brain. Having already occluded arteries such as the lenticulostriate and branches of the posterior cerebral arteries allows the surgeon to approach this treacherous part of the operation with greater confidence (Fig. 56.7).

Staging the embolization allows large hemodynamic changes to be made slowly and compensatory mechanisms to be implemented before additional stress is placed on critical tissue.[63] These factors can be particularly important in eloquent areas such as the motor strip and deep white matter tracts. In large AVMs it is possible to do noncontiguous, noncomplementary areas at the same sitting. This interruption of shunts in a gradual fashion addresses the issue of "perfusion pressure breakthrough."[137] This theory presumes that the sudden removal of a large artery to venous shunt throws an intolerable load on the normal circulation surrounding the AVM and may result in hemorrhage, edema, and infarction of the normal tissue. The situation is similar to congestive heart failure seen after removal of a large artery to venous shunts in the systemic circulation. The suggested abnormalities in the major arteries nourishing an AVM with apparent loss of autoregulation or elastic qualities would support this theory. Successful embolization in a staged fashion permits a gradual reduction in these large shunts.

Endovascular tactics depend on the strategy and the goals. The vascular anatomy, including the size of the vessels, number of loops, collateral flow, watershed anastomosis, anomalies, venous outflow, and functional anatomy, all need to be considered.

Usually it is best to go after the largest macrofistula component of the AVM first to slow the flow down. This permits greater understanding of the remaining AVM and decreases some of the venous hypertension. However, it is most often the deep periventricular feeders that are the most challenging surgically and that are the source of bleeds. Hypotension is often useful to allow more control during embolization and to keep the embolization material from passing into the cranial or systemic venous system. Total flow arrest can also be helpful and can be done by a second catheter with a balloon introduced into the system. Staged embolization should be consid-

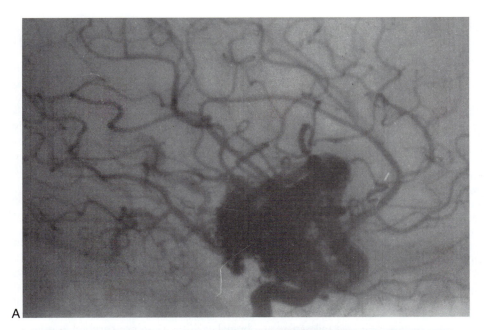

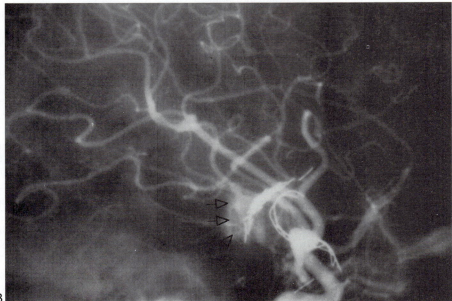

Figure 56.6 (**A**) Lateral arteriogram showing a large temporal arteriovenous malformation. (**B**) Lateral angiogram of the same patient following successful endovascular embolization. The arteriovenous malformation has virtually disappeared. The contrast seen (arrows)
is related to the endovascular material and does not represent residual arteriovenous malformation. The surgery was facilitated by this preoperative embolization.

ered when there are a number of feeders involving eloquent
areas or when normal pressure perfusion breakthrough is a
possibility.

Superselective angiography and Wada testing are extremely useful in limiting postembolization neurologic deficit
even in small AVMs. Superselective amobarbital or sodium
methohexital and lidocaine injections are used for provocative
testing during brain embolotherapy and appear to be both
sensitive and specific in avoiding embolization of important

areas of the brain.[121] They are particularly useful in patients
who have had a previous stroke or embolization. Mean pressure measurements within the feeding arteries give useful information regarding the effectiveness of embolization. Pressure recordings can give information regarding such different
occurrences as kinks in the catheter, hemodynamic changes
during embolization, or risks of bleeding. Our preference for
embolic agents is acrylate: NBCA because it is permanent and
controllable, gives excellent penetration, allows deep penetra-

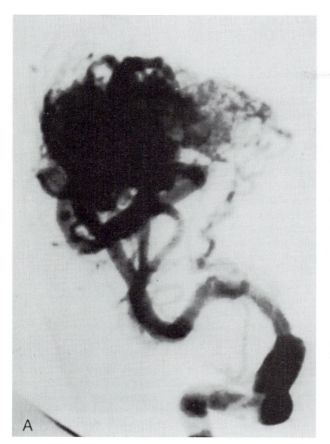

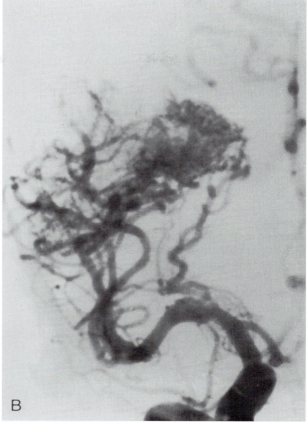

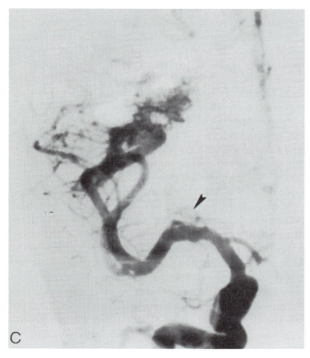

Figure 56.7 (**A**) Large arteriovenous malformation of the frontotemporal region with deep and superficial arterial supply. (**B**) Elimination of much of the superficial blood supply to this malformation following embolization. (**C**) Elimination of the deep arterial supply to the malformation (arrow) by balloon-directed Silastic pellets.

tion into the nidus, can be placed through a tiny catheter, and sets up a reactive scarring. The polymerization time can be altered by adding iodized oil (Lipiodol) or glacial acetic acid.[121,172] PVA and coils can also be used and are preferred by some. Balloons can be helpful in some situations with large fistulas.

If there is major venous occlusion, it is theoretically possible that the malformation could explode. In such cases, an apparently successful embolization may be followed within hours to days by the development of a parenchymal hematoma, in a few cases large enough to be fatal. This complication is rare.[72,75,156,157]

Permanent agents such as NBCA have many advantages over less lasting agents and allow a much wider range of therapeutic options. They give more freedom in the staging of the embolization, allow definitive embolization treatment to be appreciated, and allow radiosurgery to be used on the remaining AVM. The combination of radiosurgery and embolization has been encouraging by some reports. However, the acrylates can recanalize.

Palliative embolization of cerebral AVMs is occasionally indicated and can be quite effective. The indications include (1) progressive neurologic deterioration, (2) medically intractable seizures, (3) dangerous pseudoaneurysms associated with bleeds, (4) intractable headaches, and (5) cardiac failure. Headaches can be associated with a dural component or large venous aneurysm, particularly in the area of the thalamus or incisura. Neurologic changes can occasionally be reversed with embolization.

Aberrant embolic material may lodge in arteries not directly feeding the malformation.[142] This complication, which is nothing short of an iatrogenic embolic stroke, is seen less frequently as angiographers have gained experience (Fig. 56.8). Such complications have led to the establishment of major guidelines for cases suitable for embolization. First, the feeding arteries should "mainline" into the malformation, such as the straighter surface branches of the middle cerebral artery or the posterior cerebral artery. Anterior cerebral and, especially, the acutely angulated anterior choroidal lenticulostriate and thalamoperforating arteries are generally more difficult for reliable embolization. Recently microballoon catheter systems have been used to successfully "divert" emboli at acute angles to the mainstream blood flow.[54,65,156,157] This has opened new vistas in the use of embolization, and even brain stem malformations may be embolized. Second, the flow of emboli to an AVM is favored by large diameters of the feeding arteries. The size ratio between the arteries to be embolized and those to be avoided should be greater than 4.5:1.[166] Taking all into consideration, the serious complication rate in experienced hands is in the range of 2%.

As shown by Luessenhop and Presper, and others,[11,23,37,54,75,157,165] embolization as a primary procedure is rarely successful in totally obliterating the malformation. Obviously, when the shunt becomes successfully reduced by a series of emboli the "sink effect" of the AVM in drawing embolic material toward it decreases. Theoretically, repeated injections of NBCA afford a better opportunity of totally occluding the malformation. Because of these factors, the best use of embolization is as an adjuvant to surgery.

GENERAL SURGICAL TECHNIQUES

Operations on vascular malformations, especially AVMs, are complex procedures that are not commonly performed outside of large centers and are taxing not only to the patient but also to the surgeon. The immediate postoperative results may be devastating to the patient with major neurologic deficits, albeit temporary.[9,32,47,53,93,108,112,119,136,139,142,143,149,162,163] The initial impact, therefore, to the patient's psyche may be severe. Although the majority of patients have experienced the devastating effects of hemorrhage, there is a group of patients who live asymptomatic with their AVMs, not realizing the potential hazard of their lesions. Even those patients who have experienced hemorrhage may have recovered fully and forgotten its devastating effects. Because many of these patients are intact neurologically and able to function in spite of their AVM at the time they consult the neurosurgeon, a discussion in depth about the implications of the malformation, the natural history, and the operative aims and risks should be carried out with the patient and family prior to decision about treatment. The impact of the discussion is often disturbing to the patient, who is left in a quandary deciding what to do about a condition of which he knows little and fears even less, in the face of a dire prognostication by his physicians and the recommendation of a difficult and perhaps risky operation. This impact on the psyche has been noted to take its toll both before and after the operation, the latter in an anticlimactic state when the patient, fearing death or disablement, finds that he is intact and able to function.

Our team has elicited the help of a psychiatrist in interviewing patients prior to operative intervention and during the difficult postoperative period. In some of the patients psychological testing has been carried out prior to operation to determine their ability to withstand the stress and strains of decision making, the operation, and the postoperative convalescence. Often it is beneficial to have the patients discuss their situation with other patients who have undergone surgical treatment for an AVM. For this purpose, there is a national support group composed of patients who are quite willing to discuss the situation with individuals teetering on the edge of what they consider the most important decision of their life. Frequently, there will be a patient who has already undergone operation for an AVM still in the hospital when a patient awaiting AVM surgery is admitted. It is extremely beneficial to have the preoperative patient discuss matters openly and freely with the patient who has already gone through the procedure in the hospital setting. Therefore a wide-ranging discussion should be carried out prior to the surgery, regarding all aspects of the disorder and the diagnostic and therapeutic modalities that are contemplated during the patient's hospitalization. We also encourage patients to take notes, develop questions, and review or seek second opinions. These points cannot be emphasized too greatly, for a patient who is well prepared for surgery, other therapeutic endeavors, and diagnostic procedures both pre- and postoperatively will be able to withstand and understand the operative procedure and get involved vigorously in any rehabilitation that may be required in the postoperative period. If the surgeon contemplates the possibility of residual postoperative defects that may require extensive

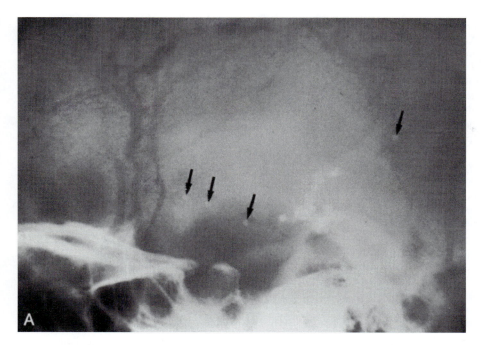

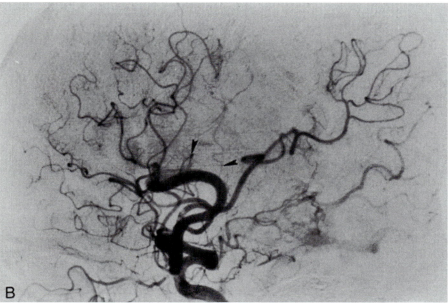

Figure 56.8 (**A**) Aberrant emboli (arrows) during the course of successful reduction in an arteriovenous malformation. (**B**) These emboli block important branches of the middle cerebral artery (arrows). Although these aberrant emboli occluded major arteries, the neurologic deficit was short-lived.

rehabilitation therapy, the various effects of these defects should be explained in detail to the patient, discussing it in terms of the patient's lifestyle, career, and social activities. Our team includes the surgeon, neurologist, psychiatrist, and on occasion other patients in a setting conducive to thoughtful, unhurried, deliberate, and methodic reviews of the problem.

Following admission to the hospital the patient is placed on Decadron (dexamethasone, Merck Sharp & Dohme) therapy, usually 4 mg every 6 hours, antacids to cover the adverse gastric effects of steroid therapy, and an appropriate anticonvulsant if the patient has not already been on an anticonvulsant. Appropriate loading doses must be given, since in many instances the patient is admitted to the hospital shortly prior to the contemplated operative procedure. One of the greatest concerns is for postoperative seizures, especially when operating on superficial supratentorial AVMs. If the patient cannot be loaded properly, a boost of intravenous phenobarbital is given the morning of the surgery as part of the preparation.

In most instances, the patients are not operated on in the acute throes of hemorrhage from an AVM.[117] Generally, we prefer to allow the hemorrhage to absorb and the patient to stabilize with decreased edema around the area of the hematoma cavity prior to operating and removing the AVM. In such cases vigorous supportive measures and dehydrating agents are not needed, as most of these patients are in the middle decades, young and healthy, and have a normal cardiovascular system and cerebral circulation except for the dynamic changes associated with the AVM. The threat of recurrent hemorrhage is far less than seen in intracranial aneurysms, and therefore no special precautions are taken in these patients preoperatively to avert such recurrent hemorrhage.[95,96] Patients are allowed to carry out normal routine daily activities and are only sedated the night before and the morning of the operation.

In the operating room, the patient is placed on the operating table equipped with a heating blanket.[113,114] This prevents heat loss and adverse cooling of the patient during the long operative procedure. The anesthesia team sets up an intravenous catheter system and arterial line, usually in the radial artery, to monitor the blood pressure during induction. As with intracranial aneurysms, severe elevations of blood pressure should be avoided during induction if possible. Following the placement of the arterial line, the patient is then induced, usually by intravenous anesthesia.

After the intubation of the patient and establishment of anesthesia, the patient is turned on the side and a special spinal drainage catheter is inserted via the lumbar spine.[120] This utilizes a 14-gauge needle and an indwelling 5 French catheter. This is a ureteral type of catheter with a blunt tip and side holes. Its large size and multiple holes prevent blockage of this catheter system during the positioning of the patient and the performance of the operation. Generalities of the positioning include generous padding of the patient, especially over bony areas, again because of the length of the operation; rigid fixation of the head is carried out with a pin vise type of headholder. The surface of the malformation should be placed as closely as possible to the horizontal or parallel to the floor. Also, the malformation should be as high as feasible above heart level in order to promote venous drainage and reduce the turgor within the malformation. In most patients, male and female, we remove only enough hair to perform a generous craniotomy around the malformation.

Special positions are used for malformations that are located in somewhat obscure areas.[138] For those malformations located high over the convexity or in the medial hemispheric region a sitting- or semisitting-slouch position is utilized so that the surgeon may work directly toward the malformation (Fig. 56.9). All the interhemispheric malformations may be approached by some version of the sitting position. For those medially placed malformations that are in the region of the uncus or hippocampus, a subtemporal exposure or a sylvian fissure exposure may be utilized. In this case the patient is generally placed supine with the head extended in an attempt to place the malformation in the best perspective for the surgeon and as high as possible above the heart. The lateral or prone position is used for convexity, parietal, or occipital lesions. Those on the under surface or tentorial surface of the occipital lobe are approached best with the patient in a prone

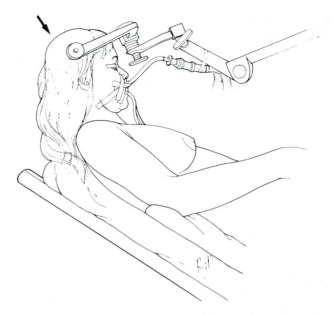

Figure 56.9 The sitting-slouch position used in the interhemispheric approach to medial hemisphere and deep midline arteriovenous malformations.

position. For posterior fossa operations the patient may be in either the sitting, lateral, or the preferred prone position.

Our anesthesia group has been monitoring cerebral blood flow by xenon and transcranial Doppler. This has been useful in alerting us to potential serious circulatory changes during AVM removal.[10,73,97,100,101,105,124,173] The choice of an anesthetic agent is left up to the anesthesiologist; however, we prefer that the anesthesia agenda recognize the need for hypotension, often for prolonged periods, during the operative procedure. As with anesthetic agents, the choice of hypotensive drugs is left to the anesthesiologist. Prolonged periods of blood pressure reduction to 80 to 85 mmHg systolic may be required, and the anesthesiologist is cautioned to use agents that can be given for such prolonged periods of time. Rarely is it necessary to lower blood pressure below 80 mmHg systolic for any prolonged period of time; however, short periods of greater hypotension under one-half hour may be necessary to control deep bleeding from thin-walled vessels, especially in the periventricular area, to which some AVMs extend. In this circumstance, blood pressure should be maintained between 70 and 80 mmHg systolic until the dissection is completed.

Brain relaxation is essential and this is accomplished by spinal drainage of cerebrospinal fluid, attention to the blood gases, especially the Pco_2 level, which should be kept between 25 and 30 mmHg by proper ventilatory adjustments. Rarely should it be necessary to use large doses of dehydrating agents. If the brain is tight and requires vigorous measures for relaxation, the operation should be terminated as early as possible and recognition given to the fact that intracranial pressure is elevated and the patient further evaluated postoperatively, with reoperation carried out when feasible.

The following are some general principles applied to the removal of AVMs, especially those located in relatively accessi-

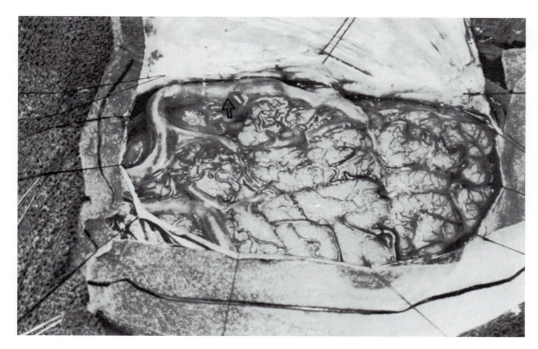

Figure 56.10 Operative photograph showing a large cortical vein (arrow) visible as a definitive landmark guiding the surgeon in resection of an arteriovenous malformation.

ble areas such as the convexities or polar regions of the cerebral hemispheres. The craniotomy should be generous and the dura opened widely so that the surface of the brain may be inspected. Landmarks are identified and correlated with angiogram analysis. Generally, the venous system on the surface of the brain provides the best road map as to the position of the AVM. Normal arteries course in and out in a tortuous fashion from gyri to sulci (Fig. 56.10). In dealing with AVMs where the feeding arteries are enlarged and even more tortuous, the arteries may be difficult to identify at the margin of the malformation; however, the veins generally remain on the surface and can be correlated with the angiogram. In our estimation, the use of stereoscopic angiograms evaluated in the operating room is useful in determining the exact configuration of the malformation. Although the malformation appears to reach the surface as seen in computed tomography (CT) scans and angiograms, in fact, the major portion of the malformation often lies just subcortical and the cortical appearance may not reflect the extent of the malformation under the surface (Fig. 56.11). It is important in such cases to violate as little of the cortex as possible, by making a linear incision, removing a small amount of brain, and relying on retraction of the relaxed brain to visualize the deeper portions of the malformation. Again, evaluation of the angiogram, MRI, and CT scan will give the surgeon a good indication as to what to expect.

In the initial phase of the operation major superficial feeding arteries are sought: the large feeding arteries hidden in sulci may be especially difficult to visualize. It is important to anticipate how deep they are from the surface so that the sulci may be opened and the artery identified and sectioned. Cautery is used for the smaller arteries; cautery plus metallic clipping is used for the larger arteries as they are interrupted.

By the use of bipolar cautery and microdissection under the microscope, the margin of the malformation as it approaches the surface of the brain is gradually circumscribed, with interruption of as many of the feeding arteries as possible. One large draining vein, either deep or superficial, particularly the largest vein, should be left until the final stage of the operation. To interrupt such a large draining system early will cause undue turgor within the malformation and greatly complicate the operative removal of these already treacherous lesions (Fig. 56.12).

Generally, there is a well-defined gliotic plane in which it is easy to dissect between the malformation and the normal brain. Tortuous coils of large corkscrew sinusoids may bulge into this interface and should be circumvented. When some of the major supply to the malformation has been secured, it is possible to gently coagulate, shrink back, and toughen these large venous channels on the periphery of the malformation, further simplifying the removal. However, it is generally impossible to shrink back major portions of the malformation in order to decompress it and attain greater working space between the malformation and the normal brain. This space is narrow and provided by removal of the gliotic area around the malformation and gentle retraction on the relaxed brain as the surgeon works deeper and deeper around the periphery of the malformation. Most of the large feeding arteries terminate in the malformation and may be interrupted at its margin. Others, enlarged and abnormally tortuous, may pass close by the malformation while giving large branches to the malformation. These primary arteries should not be interrupted; rather, their branches should be interrupted as the dissection is carried out. This type of arrangement may be anticipated from close scrutiny of the stereoscopic angiograms. In many cases,

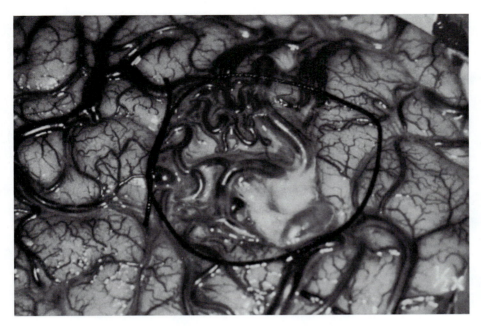

Figure 56.11 Operative photograph with a silk suture designating the major portion of the malformation underlying the cortex and not visible on the cortex.

it may be necessary to dissect an artery in transit off the surface of a malformation. This requires microscopic dissection and exact control of the feeding vessels, with care being taken not to allow cautery to injure the primary vessel in transit.

Gradually, the margin around the malformation is developed deeper and deeper as the surgeon works toward the deep apex of the malformation. In some cases this apex will be found at the ependymal surface of the ventricle. Often there are secondary or primary draining veins at this apex that drain into the ependymal venous system. There may be arteries from the choroid plexus or anomalous periventricular arteries that enter deep portions of the malformation. In the white matter surrounding the malformation at its deeper extent are numerous small, thin-walled arteries carrying blood under high flow. These appear to be aberrant in the white matter and are extremely difficult to control by cautery or clipping because of the diaphanous nature of their walls and the cooling effect of the rapid blood flow on the cautery. These must be treated with great respect and their control is often assisted by hypotensive anesthesia. It is in this area, and not the surface, that the hypotension becomes invaluable. Similarly, the ependymal veins draining the malformation are also treacherous and must be secured, preventing massive hemorrhage into the ventricle and dispersion of blood throughout the cerebrospinal fluid with potential for hydrocephalus or vasospasm. When the choroid plexus supplies deeper portions of the malformation the surgeon may find it extremely difficult to analyze and secure this blood supply. It appears to come from many different directions because of dual supply from the anterior and posterior choroidal arteries, which enter the choroid plexus in opposing directions. In many instances, it may be necessary to resect large portions of the choroid plexus that may be related to the deep portion of the malformation.

Preoperative embolization can be useful in occluding some of the deep arterial supply to apex portions of the malformation. This materially assists the surgeon as this treacherous region deep in the brain along the narrow plane between the malformation and the normal brain is approached. When the major arterial supply has already been occluded by embolization, the task of removing the lipial segment of the malformation is made easier, although not simple. It should be restated that a primary large draining venous system should be left intact until every arterial feeder to the malformation has been secured. It also goes without saying that it is virtually impossible to remove larger malformations piecemeal; however, some of the small malformations measuring under 1 cm may be coagulated and removed piecemeal.

Following the successful resection of the malformation, hemostasis is tested, and residual fragments are searched for by allowing the blood pressure to come back to normotensive levels before hemostatic agents are placed around the area of resection and the wound closed. In some instances, elevation of the blood pressure from previously hypotensive levels to normotensive levels will lead to the disclosure of residual malformation in the periphery of an otherwise clean resection. Residual portions are identified by development of "vascular blisters," red veins in the white matter or the surface of the brain. Resection of these fragments must be accomplished; otherwise postoperative hemorrhage or other problems from residual malformation will plague the surgeon in the postoperative period. We prefer metallic clips only on large feeding arteries and draining veins and rely primarily on cautery. This leaves a cleaner wound that is easier to analyze by CT scan and postoperative angiography. Nothing specific is done with the cavity left by the removal of small or large AVMs. Any opening into the ventricular system should be covered as well as possible, usually with a sheet of Gelfoam, to prevent blood

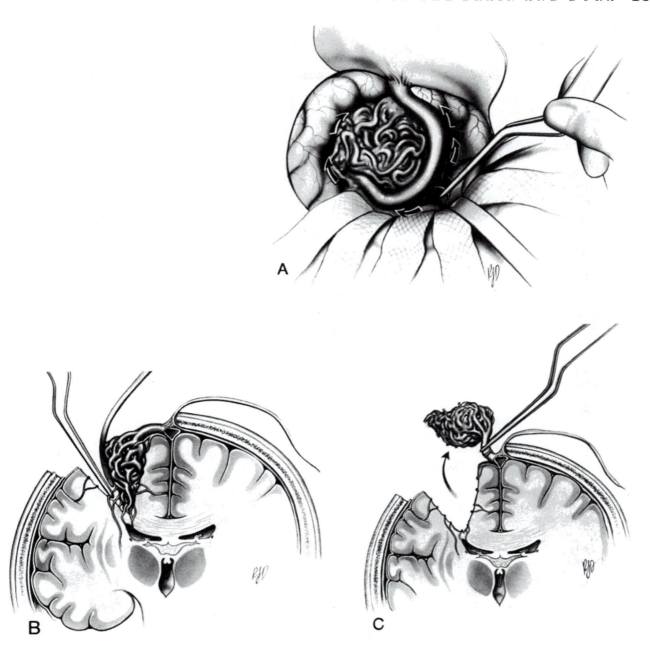

Figure 56.12 The basic technique in the removal of an arteriovenous malformation. (**A**) Circumscription of the initial incision. (**B**) Securing of the deep arterial supply. (**C**) Final interruption of the major draining vein.

from mixing directly with the cerebrospinal fluid of the ventricle. The dura is closed and the bone flap and the rest of the wound are closed in the standard fashion. The patient is extubated and remains in a position similar to the one maintained during the operative procedure. This minimizes elevation of the intracranial venous pressure in the postoperative period and thereby reduces the risk of postoperative hemorrhage. The patient is monitored closely with intra-arterial blood pressure recording in the intensive care unit. In normotensive patients, we keep the systolic pressure below 120 mmHg, primarily through the use of β-blocking agents. To attain lower pressures in an awake young patient is near impossible for a prolonged period.

The two greatest dangers in the postoperative period are hemorrhage and seizures. We have seen the latter occur as soon after the operative procedure as when the patient is being moved from the operating table to the stretcher. Postoperative clots are avoided or minimized by elevation of the head, maintenance of normotension, and minimization of Valsalva maneuvers or other maneuvers that will raise venous pressure.

Some patients become extremely restless in the postoperative period, straining at restraints or attempting to dislodge their support systems. In such cases, it may be necessary to provide sedation, such as intravenous diazepam (Valium), titrated to the patient's need. If there is any hint of something amiss, such as a patient who has wakened from the surgery relatively intact and subsequently deteriorates, a CT scan should be carried out immediately, searching for evidence of intracranial bleeding. We have found that the most likely time for a postoperative hemorrhage is within the first 12 to 24 hours. Delayed hemorrhaging after this period is extremely uncommon. If a postoperative clot is found, then the patient must be returned to the operating room and as much of the clot removed as possible. It may be extremely difficult to identify the bleeding source; however, residual malformation may be suspected in these cases. Perhaps the surgeon has intuition, recalling an area that looked suspicious at the time of closure. It is here that one learns the lesson that inspection and evaluation of the wound at normotensive levels is as important as the time spent during removal of the AVM. It may be impossible to remove all of the clot in the second operation and perhaps unwise to remove the margin of the clot except in the areas that are under suspicion. The time necessary for postoperative arteriography is better spent operating on the patient reducing the intracranial pressure by removing as much clot as possible and searching for residual portions of the malformation at the site of the bleeding point.

Postoperative seizures may be prevented in most cases by the appropriate use of anesthetic and anticonvulsant drugs. Some seizures are probably induced by changes in the cortical veins adjacent to the malformation. These changes are stasis, propagation of cortical vein thrombosis, and other dynamic changes that occur in blood flow within these important veins once the shunt has been removed. If the patient is properly loaded with anticonvulsants prior to surgery and given a boost of phenobarbital at the commencement and termination of the operation, then the incidence of postoperative seizures is markedly reduced. If the patient has a history of seizures, it is prudent to provide dual anticonvulsant coverage in the immediate intra- and postoperative periods. If the initial 12- to 24-hour postoperative period passes uneventfully, the patient is mobilized as rapidly as possible.

Any neurologic deficits are treated as soon as applicable by intensive physiotherapy. On many occasions lesions that involve the sensory cortex of the parietal lobe will lead to severe paralysis because the patient has no stereognostic perception pertaining to these extremities. It is amazing how these patients may thus remain totally "paralyzed" for a week or 10 days and suddenly begin movement as their concept of the motor engram becomes viable again.

Postoperative arteriography is carried out in all cases. This is usually done in the week following operation. We have not done yearly or later arteriography and have had no adult cases of rebleeding when the immediate postoperative angiogram is negative. If a residual is seen, removal should be considered if possible.

The situation in children may be different. Kader et al report five children who had negative (for residual AVM) postoperative angiograms, and later, 1 to 9 years, developed large recurrent AVMs.[62] This strongly suggests the potential, in children, for the regrowth of an AVM removed at surgery. There-fore, children may require follow-up angiograms at a time well removed from the operation.

A word should be said about postoperative deficits and their treatment. The surgeon will generally know whether the operation has gone well and whether the deficit will be a temporary one, perhaps lasting weeks, or whether the deficit is attributable to an intraoperative disaster and will be of a permanent nature. In any event the psychological impact of severe deficits, whether they are temporary or permanent, is unnerving to patients, even though they were coached about this prior to the operative procedure. Therefore, encouragement and the early institution of vigorous rehabilitation are absolutely essential to these patients. Most of them are young and will work eagerly with a well-motivated therapist. Many of these deficits, especially the temporary ones, may be severe, with hemiplegia, hemisensory deficits, and other neurologic deficits of significant nature depending on the locus of the lesion. Because of the striking dynamic changes that occur in the cerebrovascular system following the resection of complicated AVMs, one may anticipate a high incidence of these temporary neurologic deficits postoperatively. In spite of the frequent occurrence of such deficits, there is marked improvement in almost all cases within days to weeks. These events suggest that the vascular changes responsible for these postoperative deficits are not on the basis of arterial occlusion with ischemic infarction but, rather, on the basis of venous stasis or infarction and brain edema, all reversible phenomena.

With removal of the AVM-associated shunts, there is decreased flow in the venous system with stasis and thrombosis. In addition, the vascular dynamics of not only the venous but also the arterial system lead to profound changes in intravascular pressure and flow resulting in brain edema, which is frequently observed on postoperative CT scans. Another consideration is arterial collateralization, which occurs rapidly in these young patients. The removal of large shunts and this collateral phenomenon provide a lush blood supply to the brain. It is presumed that these changes are wholly reversible and responsible for a very singular course of events following the obliteration of an AVM. On the other hand, visual field defects that are complete postoperatively may or may not recover fully or even to a partial degree.[84] It is very difficult to predict the course of these deficits, since the visual system is so intimately involved with many of the malformations, including those that permeate the parietal area, as well as those located directly in or adjacent to the calcarine sulcus. Deficits related to cranial nerve or brain stem involvement by an AVM of the posterior fossa may take much longer to resolve or may never resolve. Resolution is often predicated on the condition of these cranial nerves prior to the operative procedure. Severe cerebellar deficits postoperatively will almost always resolve, depending on the extent of the involvement of the cerebellar structures, especially the deep nuclei.

VASCULAR CHANGES RELATED TO OBLITERATION OF THE ARTERIOVENOUS MALFORMATION

It is a common observation that arteries at a distance from the malformation fill better immediately after the occlusion of the shunt, confirming some of the tenets of the theory of cerebral steal. However, less desirable effects also can occur, including acute cerebral edema, venous congestion, and, occasionally, frank hemorrhage. Using pulsed echo Doppler flowmeters and electromagnetic flow measurement with miniature probes, Nornes and Grip[100] studied the local hemodynamics of AVMs in 16 operated patients. A wide variation was found in the calculated flow in individual arteries, from as little as 3 ml/min to as much as 550 ml/min. The pressure of the arteries at their entrance into the AVM fistula was much reduced (40 to 77 mmHg) compared with systemic pressure, but on temporary occlusion an instant pressure rise to 55 to 95 mmHg occurred. On the venous side, the pressure fell to zero. The pressure drop along arteries leading to the fistula was greatest for the longer feeding arteries. These arteries also shared greater flow velocities and were of larger diameter. The cerebral perfusion pressure was estimated to be lowest in areas fed by these longer, more dilated arteries, whose final output was into the AVM fistula; these same arterial beds experienced the greatest increase in cerebral perfusion pressure after shunt occlusion and the highest incidence of postocclusion vasogenic edema. Presumably, these same arterial beds are more susceptible to "normal perfusion pressure breakthrough."[137] Very short feeding arteries did not show these effects.

A study of progressive postocclusive changes in the arterial networks has proved most instructive. Some feeding arteries undergo rapid reduction in size, but many take weeks to return to normal caliber. These slowly resolving changes suggest defective autoregulation not only within the malformations, but also in the large feeding arteries. This phenomenon may play a role in the perfusion pressure breakthrough theory and in the production of neurologic deficits in the post-treatment phase. In support of defective autoregulation are not only postobliteration ectasias in the feeding arteries, but the work of Nornes et al[100,101] and others[4,6,10,42,50,94,115,124] who demonstrated many of the hemodynamic changes normally associated with autoregulation but lacking in AVMs. Dynamic studies in our laboratory have demonstrated a defective contractile response of large AVM nutrient arteries.[98] Young et al,[172,173] recording blood flow during the removal of AVMs, have demonstrated a marked increase in blood flow, hyperemia, and presumed "congestion" of the brain around the AVM after removal. They have also confirmed the changes in intra-arterial and intravenous pressure that occur with AVM removal.[173] One of our cases is instructive (Fig. 56.13).

CASE STUDY. The patient was a 32-year-old right-handed man. He had a single focal motor seizure progressing to a grand mal convulsion initially involving the right side of the body, hand, arm, and face approximately 5 weeks prior to admission. Evaluation including a CT scan and angiogram demonstrated a left parietal AVM (Fig. 56.13A) and a proximal middle cerebral aneurysm (Fig. 56.13B). There was no evidence of hemorrhage. On April 30, 1984 total excision of the AVM without embolization was carried out (Fig. 56.13C). The major feeding artery was a middle cerebral branch that was markedly enlarged and went directly to the AVM. Postoperatively, the patient had no neurologic deficits and was discharged from the hospital 1 week after the surgery.

The patient was readmitted to the hospital on June 1, 1984, and, without a preliminary angiogram but with normal neurologic examination, the left middle cerebral artery aneurysm was uneventfully clipped. Hypotension to 80 mmHg systolic was used for 10 minutes, during the clip application. There was no evidence of cerebral vasospasm or evidence that this aneurysm had previously hemorrhaged. The patient was slow to awake from the operation, and it was noted that he was paretic on the right side. The arm, in fact, was flaccid and moved only to painful stimulation. He was not speaking and did not understand commands. A cerebral angiogram was immediately carried out. This showed marked vascular changes in the region of the AVM resection without residual AVM (Fig. 56.13D). The arteries proximal to the AVM showed ectasias and pooling of dye, indicating stasis of the contrast media and presumably blood in these vessels. The patient's blood pressure during this postoperative period fluctuated between 120 and 130 mmHg. Approximately 2 hours after the angiogram, he had a major seizure and was given appropriate intravenous anticonvulsants. He was also volume expanded and his blood pressure was maintained at a level of 140 to 150 mmHg systolic with a dopamine infusion; he had no further seizures. Within 24 hours after the operative procedure, he could squeeze the right hand weakly to command, but did not respond to other verbal commands, suggesting an improving dysphasia. The right lower extremity was markedly improved. Approximately 36 hours after the operation the patient was responding to verbal commands and the strength in the right arm was 80% normal. The dopamine drip was gradually reduced and the patient subsequently made a full recovery.

Our theory is that ectatic changes persisted unexpectedly in the large feeding artery to the malformation, even after total removal. At the time of the second operative procedure for the clipping of the aneurysm, brief hypotension was used to a level of 80 mmHg for a period of approximately 10 minutes. With the background of the ectatic changes in the arteries nourishing the parietal temporal region, it would appear that some ischemia resulted and that these arteries were unable to autoregulate. The postoperative dysphasia and paresis cleared rapidly following the institution of volume expansion and hypertensive therapy. It is surprising that these vascular changes had not resolved at a period of 5 weeks from the initial operative procedure. There is strong suggestion that these large arterial feeders proximal to an AVM are abnormal in terms of their contractility and their ability to respond to physiologic changes in blood volume and blood pressure.[10,42,43,50,94,98]

POSTOPERATIVE CARE

All AVM patients are monitored closely in a neurologic intensive care unit (ICU) setting for 24 to 72 hours postoperatively, depending on anticipated complications from surgery. Prevention and recognition of adverse circulatory changes or brain edema is paramount. Anticipation of these events can be gleaned from intraoperative observations and circulatory studies.[8,9,73,115,162] All the usual parameters are measured, including evaluation of cardiopulmonary function via Swan-Ganz catheter. The systolic blood pressure for 24 hours is maintained below 120 mmHg. Anemia is treated and intravenous fluids are limited. In cases of severe brain edema osmotherapy, steroids, and if necessary, intubation with respiratory control and barbiturate coma are instituted.[4]

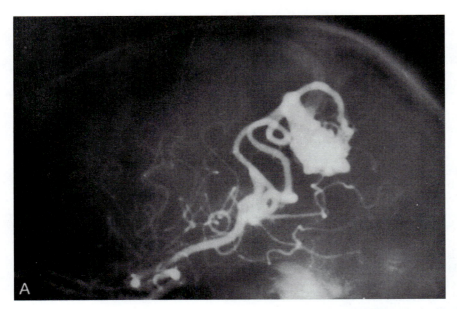

Figure 56.13 (**A**) Angiogram demonstrating a large parietal arteriovenous malformation. (**B**) Arteriogram demonstrating the proximal aneurysm (arrow).

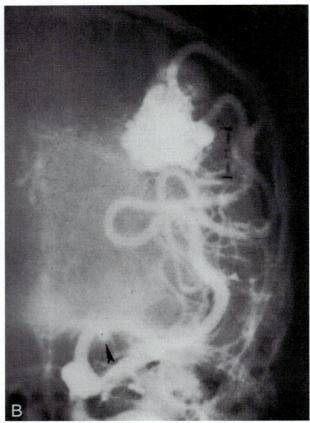

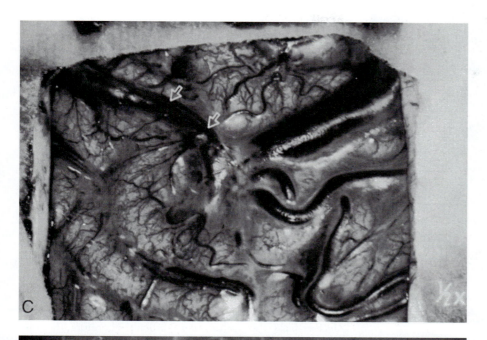

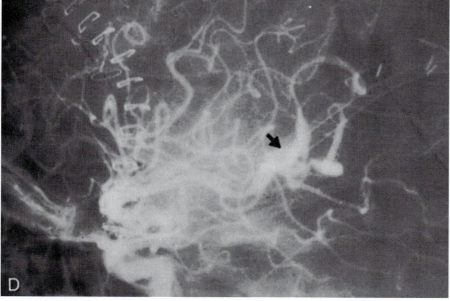

Figure 56.13 (Continued) (**C**) Operative photograph showing the large feeding artery (arrows) demonstrated by arteriography. (**D**) Arteriogram immediately following aneurysm surgery showing ectasia and stasis (arrow) within the middle cerebral artery previously supplying the arteriovenous malformation. The malformation had been resected 5 weeks previously.

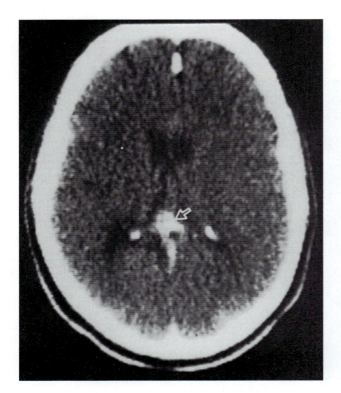

Figure 56.14 A CT scan with contrast performed 2 months following the removal of a posterior third ventricular arteriovenous malformation. This scan suggested residual arteriovenous malformation (arrow), which was shown by subsequent angiography not to be the case.

POSTDISCHARGE CARE

Careful follow-up of the patient after discharge from the hospital is necessary in order to modify anticonvulsant drug regimes and encourage the patient in further rehabilitation therapy or direct the patient back into a normal sociologic environment following these massive operations and psyche-wrenching problems. In our experience, if, in an adult, the malformation has been shown to be totally removed by postoperative arteriography, we have never seen a recurrence of the AVM. We have seen, however, on a number of occasions, CT scans with contrast performed for one reason or another months after successful removal of an AVM that suggest residual or recurrent malformation (Fig. 56.14). In all these cases, repeat arteriography has shown no residual malformation, leading us to assume that the CT scan can be fallaciously positive in the postoperative period. These changes are probably related to hyperemia, hyperperfusion, and gliosis around the resection and show up as "apparent vascular channels" on the postoperative CT scan. Therefore, in terms of false positive findings, we do not consider the CT scan a reliable way to evaluate the patient postoperatively. On the other hand, when scans are negative, this has been well correlated with negative postoperative arteriograms, and, of course, the CT scan is invaluable in showing the gradual reduction of cerebral edema around the margins of the malformation and any

changes in ventricular size. Likewise MRI and magnetic resonance angiography (MRA) are not definitive studies to detect the presence or absence of an AVM. Arteriography is still the gold standard.

SPECIAL CIRCUMSTANCES RELATED TO THE LOCATION OF ARTERIOVENOUS MALFORMATIONS

Posterior Fossa Arteriovenous Malformations

Posterior fossa AVMs deserve special consideration because of their rarity and high mortality and morbidity in terms of surgical resection or natural history.[17,30,33,132] These lesions are about one-tenth as common as supratentorial AVMs. They can be divided into the categories shown in Table 56.1 and Figure 56.15.

These lesions, even the larger ones, appear to have lower flow than their counterparts. They are much more difficult to visualize and analyze by angiography. The overlying bone structures, the lower flow in the vertebral system, and other factors make this analysis more difficult. Therefore, these lesions cannot be approached with the anatomic precision that one utilizes in the supratentorial region. In my (B.M.S.) series of 40 posterior fossa malformations, the age distribution was the same as for other locations; however, virtually all these malformations presented with hemorrhage. In this aspect, these lesions are particularly treacherous because hemorrhages have led to severe brain stem compression and coma in many of the patients. When the lesions involve the cranial nerves, cranial nerve dysfunction may be permanent or prolonged. Similarly, those that involve the intrinsic structure of the brain stem may leave permanent damage as a result of hemorrhage.[17] There is very little margin of error or resiliency in the brain stem, as opposed to some other portions of the brain. All these malformations must be approached with respect. Until recently it has been impossible to embolize these lesions and thereby reduce the shunt and turgor within the malformation prior to operative intervention. Currently, with the balloon-directed embolic technique, it is possible to embo-

Table 56.1 Posterior Fossa Arteriovenous Malformation Categories[a]

Cerebellar
Cerebellar hemisphere
Anterior vermis-midbrain
Posterior vermis-fourth ventricle
Brain stem
Intrinsic
Extrinsic
Cisternal-cerebellopontine angle

[a] *See also Figure 56.15.*

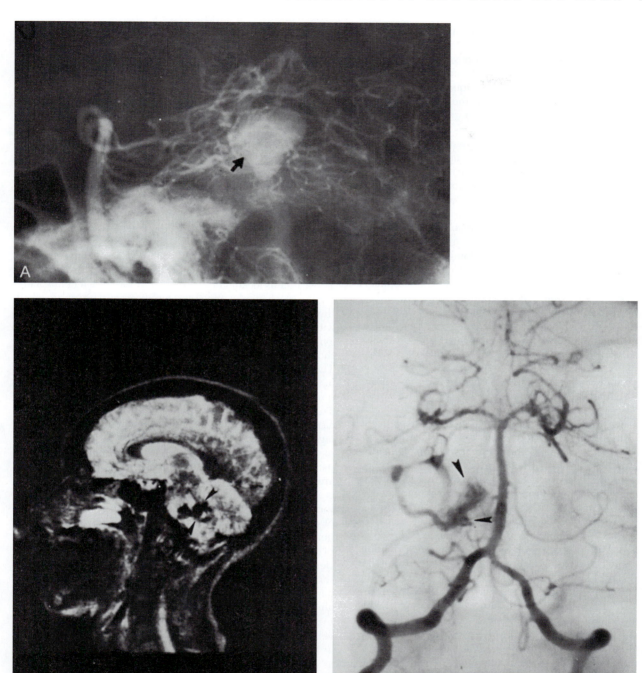

Figure 56.15 Examples of posterior fossa arteriovenous malformations. (**A**) Large anterior cerebellar vermis malformation associated with a venous aneurysm (arrow). (**B**) Nuclear magnetic resonance scan of brain stem arteriovenous malformation located within the substance of the brain stem (arrows) and unsuitable for surgical treatment. (**C**) Cerebellopontine angle arteriovenous malformation (arrows) commencing on the surface of the brain stem and extending deep (this arteriovenous malformation was resected).

lize into the posterior inferior or anterior inferior cerebellar arteries, successfully reducing major arterial contributions to these malformations. The development of small mobile intravascular catheters has made it possible to successfully embolize these obscure malformations with liquid adhesives (Fig. 56.15).[156] It should be understood that these techniques are difficult and have the potential of creating devastating problems should the normal brain stem arteries be compromised.

Operations on these malformations, as elsewhere, require wide exposure. The positioning of the patient is extremely important. For those malformations that lie in the hemispheral or posterior vermis region, the sitting position may be inappropriate, because it is necessary to elevate the cerebellum against gravity to visualize the feeding vessels from the posterior inferior or anterior inferior cerebellar arteries. Furthermore, although the sitting position is desirable in reducing venous tension within the malformation and adding a certain degree of hypotension, it can lead to devastating consequences when air embolism enters these high-flow systems. Also, it appears that induced hypotension may be counterproductive and, in fact, dangerous in those situations where a relative hypotension already exists. Clinical experience suggests that the removal of the shunt results in decrease in flow in the major sinuses of the posterior fossa and that this decrease in flow and resultant stasis are further compounded by the use of hypotension during the operative procedure. At least in one case, this has led to massive progressive thrombosis within these veins, with severe neurologic deficits. There is only one circumstance in which we routinely have the patient in the sitting position, and this is for lesions that are located in the anterior vermis adjacent to the midbrain region. Here the cerebellum falls away from the tentorium and a supracerebellar infratentorial approach may be used to great advantage, undermining and circumscribing the malformation while the feeding arteries, mostly the superior cerebellar and choroidal arteries, are identified and divided. The draining veins are generally to the straight sinus in the midline and these can be avoided during the excision of most of the malformation. In other cases, the lateral or three-quarter prone position has been utilized, although this has the disadvantage of producing somewhat higher venous pressures; however, the ease for the surgeon, retraction of the cerebellum with the aid of gravity, and the avoidance of stasis in the sinuses are all advantageous.

Those malformations that involve the brain stem can be analyzed only at the time of surgery. Unfortunately, angiography is not sophisticated to the point where we can definitely determine how much of these malformations are intrinsic to the brain stem. Generally, they involve surface and superficial portions of the brain stem and can be dissected from these areas, since their feeding arteries come from pial branches of the major arteries of the posterior circulation. The venous drainage is also in the pia, therefore; these important vessels may be identified without entering the substance of the brain stem as the malformation is peeled away from the brain stem. Cranial nerve involvement is another matter. Here, the feeding arteries may also supply the cranial nerves, and the large draining veins may have affected the cranial nerves by contiguous pressure. In the postoperative period one may anticipate significant cranial nerve palsies. These are particularly bothersome when the 9th and 10th cranial nerves are involved. In such cases, even with unilateral involvement, patients have experienced difficulty in swallowing. This problem may last for months and must be managed by the placement of a nasogastric tube or gastrostomy. Tracheotomy over a prolonged period may also be necessary in such cases.

In a series of 40 posterior fossa malformations in our experience, the mortality rate has been 2% and serious morbidity 12% (see later discussion on surgical management).

Medial Hemisphere Arteriovenous Malformations

Medial hemisphere AVMs, often involving portions of the limbic system, constitute a surprisingly high percentage of AVMs—25% in my series.[138] In terms of surgical resection, these deserve special consideration. The location of these malformations can be categorized advantageously (Table 56.2). This categorization has the advantage of localizing the lesion and is a determinant in the surgical approach (Fig. 56.16). Those lesions located in the more anterior medial hemisphere region, involving the uncus and hippocampus, are approached through the sylvian fissure or through a subtemporal approach with varying degrees of resection of the inferior temporal gyrus. The malformations that are most difficult to reach are those located medial to the trigone of the lateral ventricle. These may require a two-stage operation with an initial interhemispheric-parafalx approach followed by an infratemporal-tentorial approach to the residual portion of the malformation. Transcortical incisions via the temporoparietal region have also been recommended;[31] however, these have the disadvantage of not only violating eloquent areas of the brain, especially on the dominant side, but also reaching the malformation at its venous side, which often enters the ventricle, while the arterial supply is most distant from the surgeon. The approach is also relatively blind until the ventricular portion of the malformation is reached and requires a fair amount of retraction of eloquent areas of the brain. The surgeon is assisted when hemorrhage has occurred, and there is softening or cavitation of the overlying white matter and cortex; however, in our experience, this has been uncommon. In most instances in our series, these difficult malformations have been managed by a parafalx-interhemispheric approach. The surgeon may reach almost as far as the peduncle of the midbrain to interrupt feeding arteries to these malformations located medial to the ventricular trigone. Those malformations located posteriorly at the splenium and involving the roof of the third ventricle as well as portions of the cingulate gyrus or the septal regions may be approached by a variety of interhemispheric approaches; the anteroposterior direction is dependent on the location of the malformation. The central area related to the

Table 56.2 Medial Hemisphere Arteriovenous Malformation Regions

Amygdaloid-uncus (anteromedial temporal)
Parahippocampal-fusiform gyrus (medial temporal)
Paratrigonal
Splenial-posterior third ventricle
Cingulate-medial hemisphere
Genu-interhemispheric

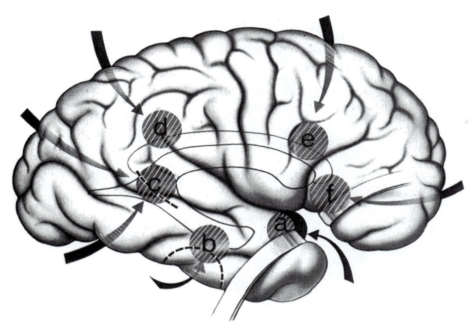

Figure 56.16 The various approaches to arteriovenous malformations of the medial hemisphere. These approaches are cataloged in Table 56.2.

rolandic draining veins and the motor and sensory strip should be spared any retraction.

The interhemispheric approaches, except for the most anterior ones, are effected with the patient in the sitting- or semisitting-slouch position (Fig. 56.9). This significantly reduces venous tension and gives the surgeon the most direct exposure of the surface of the malformation while facilitating control of the feeding arteries, whether they be from the anterior cerebral, posterior choroidal (medial and lateral), the anterior choroidal, or the posterior cerebral arteries. The results of surgery have been excellent, which is ironic, considering the difficulty in removing these lesions and their often obscure location.

Those lesions lying in the diencephalic region may be approached by a variety of routes. Those located in relation to the lenticulostriate arteries, if separable from these arteries, may be approached through a sylvian fissure-splitting incision, with microsurgical removal of the lesion while preserving the important lenticulostriate arteries. The vast majority of thalamic lesions, however, are inoperable or, if operable, are located in the more dorsal aspect of the thalamus or caudate nucleus, often entering the ventricular system. These may then be approached through the same interhemispheric approaches as used for medial hemisphere AVMs or by a route direct to the ventricular system. For those malformations located deep and involving the thalamus and roof of the third ventricle, the deep venous system, including the two important internal cerebral veins and the vein of Galen, should be and can be preserved in the successful removal of these lesions. These lesions are supplied primarily from major branches of the medial posterior choroidal arteries, and to a lesser extent from the lateral posterior choroidal arteries that enter into the glomus of the choroid plexus in the trigone of the lateral ventricle. It may take multiple attempts to remove

these pesky and somewhat obscure malformations that involve regions of the thalamus. Their position is not easily identifiable when one observes the ependyma, even in cases of previous hemorrhage. The malformations seem to be somewhat diffuse and intertwined with portions of the thalamus.

We have found another interesting group of lesions located in the posterior corpus callosum, body of the caudate, and pulvinar region of the dominant hemisphere. Three such cases, all presenting with hemorrhages, were associated with profound recent memory deficits. These lesions have been discrete, and the structures involved were the body and tail of the caudate, portions of the corpus callosum, the left or dominant fornix, and small portions of the pulvinar (Fig. 56.17). We have not observed recent memory loss with similar lesions located in the nondominant hemisphere. The suggestion is that the aforementioned dominant hemisphere structures have some relation to the acquisition of memory.

Aneurysms and Arteriovenous Malformations

In 10% to 15% of AVMs, there may be a tandem lesion of an aneurysm.[24] This frequently occurs proximal to the AVM on the main feeding vessel. The decision as to which lesion should be treated first depends on which is symptomatic. In the face of a hemorrhage, the cause is usually the aneurysm, in which case this should be treated first and the AVM at a future date. If the site of hemorrhage is the AVM or the lesions are asymptomatic, then we prefer to remove the AVM first. There is then the possibility that the aneurysm will regress, and certainly with reduction of blood flow the aneurysm will be easier to treat. If the site of hemorrhage cannot be determined, then the aneurysm, on speculation, should be treated first. In some cases when the lesions are in proximity, it is possible to treat

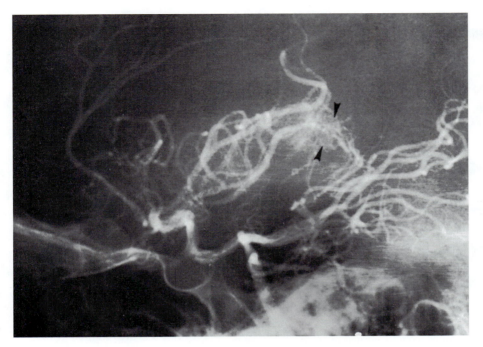

Figure 56.17 Dominant hemisphere arteriovenous malformation (arrows) located in the region of the ventricular trigone, involving the caudate nucleus. fornix, and, to a lesser extent, the corpus callosum.

both at the same operation. In the case of tandem operations, 4 to 6 weeks should elapse between operations.[51,58]

Intraoperative Angiography

Although some have recommended it, we have not found intraoperative angiography useful or practical. It is extremely difficult to obtain quality, and one must also consider the interference of various metallic retractors. This technique also requires prolonged intra-arterial catheterization with heparinization and attendant risks as well as the prolongation of an already lengthy operation. Therefore, we have not recommended or used this procedure, relying more on our experience, judgment, and view through the operating microscope as to the configuration and totality of removal of AVMs.

Radiation Therapy for Arteriovenous Malformations

The technology to perform radiosurgery has been available in the form of the Proton Beam and the Gamma Knife for over two decades. Unfortunately, no rigorous follow-up studies were done on the early patients to prove the effectiveness and analyze the complication rate, long term, of this revolutionary treatment of AVMs. In less than a decade, with the proliferation of linear accelerators and Gamma Knife units, we are beginning to experience follow-up data on a large number of patients, many followed for only a short time. Additionally, in

this era of analysis of the cost-effectiveness of any treatment, we are witnessing reviews comparing microsurgery with radiosurgery in the treatment of AVMs.[103,130] We present a thorough review of the topic in order for the readers to draw their own conclusion.

While microsurgery can be performed on the majority of AVMs with acceptable morbidity and mortality, some lesions, because of location, cannot be operated on with an acceptable risk. In addition, there are some patients who are medically infirm and cannot undergo conventional surgery. In these instances radiosurgery is considered the treatment of choice.

Focused radiation delivered by stereotactic techniques is a useful alternative for those small lesions that are situated deep or in eloquent locations of the brain. Other AVMs that are large may be treated with a combination of embolization and radiosurgery if microsurgery is not an option.

The goal of stereotactically focused radiation, as in any AVM therapy, is the prevention of potentially fatal intracranial hemorrhage by inducing an angiographically confirmed obliteration of the nidus. The process is one of endothelial proliferation, vessel thickening, and eventual luminal obliteration. This ongoing process of obliteration does not, in and of itself, offer protection from hemorrhage. The real risk of intervening hemorrhage in the latency period between radiosurgical treatment and obliteration is one of the major considerations in a decision to apply focused radiation.

Studies of the natural history of AVMs suggest an annual rebleeding rate for an unruptured and untreated lesion of 2% to 4%.[13,22,36,41,46,59,106] Once hemorrhage has occurred, the rebleeding rate may increase from 6% to 18% in the immediate period before gradually returning to the predicted levels of 2% to 4% over the next several years.[36,41,46,59,118] Not present in most radiosurgical series is detailed information about the proximity of radiosurgery to prior hemorrhage. This information would be helpful in discerning the effect of radiosurgery on the natural history of bleeding.

Pollock et al, in a review of the Gamma Knife experience at the University of Pittsburgh, reported that there was no statistically different change in the rate of bleeding AVMs that were not yet obliterated in comparison with their preradiosurgery rate or the natural historical rate of untreated AVMs. Their pretreatment rate was 2.4% while the rebleeding rate was 4.8%, with the total risk for treatment per patient of 7.4% after treatment.[118] Colombo et al, in an update of their linear accelerator data, reported an increased risk of bleeding after treatment. This was attributed to only partially obliterated lesions.[20,21] Both of these studies had significant mortality rates from these new hemorrhages.

Technical factors may influence the rebleeding rate and the obliteration rate. These include the volume of the nidus treated, the dose delivered to the prescription isodose, completeness of coverage by the prescription isodose, and homogeneity of the dose. These physical aspects of treatment are all interrelated. Radiosurgery is reported to obliterate small AVMs with an overall rate of success approximately 80% at a latency of 2 to 3 years.[18,39,40,74,78,118,144–146] Interpretation of these angiographic obliteration rates may be misleading. They do not reflect all lesions at risk but, rather, only the ones that underwent follow-up angiography. However, obliteration rates appear to be remarkably similar across radiation treatment devices and multiple institutions.[12,16,18,20,21,36,39,40,64,70,78,145] The range of obliteration by angiographic follow-up of 70% to 92% may depend not only on the volume treated but the time in allowing the radiobiologic process to mature at 3 years or more.[18,78] It is also important to recognize that there may be no protection against bleeding by partial obliteration of the AVM. The evidence relating to partial obliteration and its effect on protection from hemorrhage is inconclusive.[67,68,145,146] In this circumstance, repeat radiosurgery, surgery, or embolization may help reduce further risk of bleeding.[83,85]

The most rapidly proliferating devices for radiosurgery are the Gamma Knife and linear accelerator. Although both can treat a similar volume, there are significant differences in prescription isodose, maximum dose, and the tolerance of adjacent normal tissue to injury.[82] The influence of volume on obliteration rate is not definite. Recent reports have suggested that success in obliterating AVMs is initially dependent on the volume treated for both the Gamma Knife and linear accelerator.[12,18,21,39,70,78] However, on closer evaluation of these studies, the relationship between volume, dose, and obliteration rate appears overshadowed by the effect of complete coverage of the target nidus by the prescription isodose.[18,20,21,39,40,118,168]

Yamamoto et al reported that there was no statistically different rate of occurrence of postradiosurgical hemorrhage based on the AVM size.[168] This was regardless of whether the AVM had ruptured. In addition in the Mayo Clinic series of 121 patients treated by Gamma Knife therapy, it was a complete coverage of the AVM by the prescription isodose that was essential to a successful obliteration rather than the volume, within general limits.[18,168]

Linear-accelerator-based (LINAC) institutions find that although the smallest volumes obliterated sooner, by 2 to 3 years, the effect of volume on obliteration was not significant. Colombo et al demonstrated an 8.4% first-year bleeding rate and a 4% second-year rate for partially covered lesions. Analysis of these latest data from Colombo from their linear accelerator experience reveals that dose inhomogeneity may have significantly increased the risk of hemorrhage.[21] However, the reason for the apparent failure of obliteration in their large-volume lesions may have been insignificant dose to the periphery and not the diameter of the lesion.

Friedman et al reported that their success with all-size radiosurgical volume may be due to several factors.[39,40] With modern linear accelerator units, treatments have larger collimator capacity. This makes possible the treatment of larger volumes with pure isocenters when used with contemporary dosimetry and treatment planning. The dose delivered is also important. Some have recommended 20 Gy to the periphery of the lesion; this would place larger lesions at risk for the development of radiation-induced complications. While smaller lesions have faster times to obliteration with higher doses, larger lesions also have high obliteration rates, although not until 3 years. It appears that approximately 1,600 cGy to the periphery of the volume in larger lesions is satisfactory in a significant number of cases.[40] Therefore, a 3-year wait, especially for larger volume lesions, before declaring radiosurgery treatment a failure is warranted.[18,168]

The use of radiosurgery is not without its adverse consequences. Acute and late adverse changes have been reported by most groups performing radiosurgery.[20,40,67,68,78,82,83,130,144,145,149] The tolerance of normal brain to conventionally fractionated radiation is traditionally described as being influenced by dose/volume relationships. Radiosurgically delivered therapy is less well delineated by these relationships. At issue are not only the volumes of treatment and the technical differences between delivery modalities but the endpoints used to define tolerance and their clinical and radiographic nature. Caution has been generally exercised in prescribing treatment of larger AVMs because of the volume at risk for injury. However, complication rates for AVMs treated by Gamma Knife at the Mayo Clinic for lesions greater than 10 cm^3 were similar to those for smaller lesions.[18,168] Linear accelerator data support the ability to safely treat larger AVMs with obliteration-successful doses in some cases.[40] While the data of Kjellberg et al provided the early guidelines used to define the doses used in radiosurgery, these may project artificially low endpoints for complications.[67,68,82,83] A review of several radiosurgery series suggests that the observed rate of deleterious reactions after radiosurgery may be as high as 9%.[82,83]

When the diagnosis of an AVM is anticipated from imaging or clinical impressions, a full selective angiogram is performed. Candidacy for radiosurgery will then depend on size, location, presence of aneurysms, drainage patterns, and, to some extent, patient preference. Super-selective embolization is then used to obliterate appropriately sized lesions or maximally reduce moderate to large AVMs. If the obliteration is complete as shown by angiogram, the patient is then observed and nothing more is done. The remaining lesions are then reevaluated for operability by microsurgical technique. With endovascular therapies as an aid, moderate to large AVMs may be reduced to sizes amenable to treatment by microsurgery or radiosurgical techniques available with contemporary treatment planning and delivery systems. The patient is then followed by MRI until obliteration is suggested and at that time an angiogram is performed. If obliteration has taken place, then the patient is followed. Residual nidus may be approached by further embolization, microsurgery, or radiosurgery.[18,85]

Moderate to high degrees of success in treating selected AVMs are possible using radiosurgery. Barring a multi-institutional trial, the decision algorithm for the use of radiosurgery will be influenced by the skills, experience, and prejudices inherent in each multidisciplinary center. Radiosurgery will continue to be a useful complementary therapy to the contemporary microsurgical techniques available for the removal of AVMs.

Results of Surgical Management

The following surgical results are based on a personal series of 470 operated cases of AVMs located in various parts of the brain. The problem presented by AVMs has been approached not only from the surgical viewpoint in this series but also as a team effort. This team includes a neurologist, a neuroradiologist, and a neuroanesthesiologist. The development of a team is consistent with our aim to treat these difficult lesions in the best way possible, including improvement in the surgical mortality and morbidity. This tribunal of physicians interested in AVMs selects patients for operation and rejects other patients who have malformations too large or located in inaccessible areas, which in our experience would result in a surgical morbidity and mortality rate too high to justify operation. Nevertheless, difficult malformations were not excluded if it was felt in each case, on the basis of past experience and location, that these could be resected with low surgical morbidity and mortality. Therefore 40% of the patients had malformations located in the dominant hemisphere and 45% of the patients had malformations located in eloquent portions of the brain, including the motor, sensory, and speech areas. An obscure group of malformations previously described, located on the medial hemisphere, constituted approximately 25% of the cases. Malformations located in the posterior fossa, which in our experience have a higher mortality and morbidity rate than those located elsewhere in the brain, made up approximately 10% of the patients. The malformations had a wide spectrum of features, including (1) age of the patient, (2) size, (3) number and size of feeding arteries, and (4) direction and size of draining veins. All these factors were considered in determining operability.

The overall mortality was 1.5% in the series of personally operated AVMs. Morbidity is categorized as follows: (1) severe neurologic deficits such as hemiparesis, hemisensory loss, and speech deficits (2.5%); (2) moderate neurologic deficits that were not so severe as to impair the patient's functional activity but that limited daily living activities to a modest extent (3.5%); and (3) mild and nonlimiting neurologic deficits. In this last category fall primarily the various visual field defects that occurred in those lesions located in the optic radiations or the primary visual areas. These deficits range from hemianopias to quadrantopias or sector defects and after a period of time were compensated for by the patient so they did not compromise social or work activities. Visual field defects were seen in 12% of the patients. These were the mortality and morbidity figures we aimed for in determining whether a patient's AVM was operable. We feel that these figures justify our approach to selected AVMs.

In this series there were no recurrences of malformations in adults that had been totally resected, as proved by a postoperative angiogram. In only one instance was a postoperative formal angiogram not performed because of extenuating circumstances on behalf of the patient. Additionally, there were no subsequent hemorrhages once the malformation had proved to be removed. In the series there were approximately 10% with aneurysms that occurred, for the most part, on proximal feeding arteries to the malformation. Not all these patients were treated by definitive surgery, that is, clipping of the aneurysm, and to date there has been no bleeding from the remaining aneurysm if it was left in place, which was the case in approximately 20% of those patients who had both aneurysms and AVM, the AVM having been resected.

Outcome from Conservative Management

Experience with conservative management in nonrandomized evaluations has been reported over many years. Troupp et al[150] found neither the size nor the location of the AVM to have predictive value for rupture.

Few studies have yet appeared dealing with the natural history of unruptured AVMs. McCormick and colleagues' autopsy series[88–91] showed that only 12% of their cases had been symptomatic in life. In the few studies in which repeated angiograms have been done, roughly a third of AVMs have been found to enlarge, a third have remained static, and a third have shown regression[34,142,143] without any specific therapy. Whether such cases are exceptional and whether factors can be identified to predict the future course remain unknown at present.

As with intracranial aneurysms, steady advances in surgical technique have encouraged the more experienced surgeons to take on the more challenging cases. A recent series comparing surgical and conservative management is that of 145 cases reported by Guidetti and DeLitala.[47] Based on their experience, these authors recommend surgery. Heros et al[53] have recorded a similar experience.

Other Vascular Malformations

In this section we consider malformations that are more commonly seen by the neuropathologist than are AVMs and that appear to be less commonly seen by the clinician.[88,91] These would include (1) cavernous malformations, (2) venous malformations, (3) telangiectasias, (4) vein of Galen malformations, (5) dural arteriovenous malformations, (6) carotid-cavernous fistulas, and (7) "cryptic malformations." These entities have been alternatively termed angiomas, which is a misnomer. There is no indication that any of these are neoplastic or have the capability of enlargement through proliferation; rather, the term *angioma* should be discarded in favor of *malformation*.

CAVERNOUS MALFORMATIONS

Cavernous malformations of the brain, although occasionally incidental, are increasingly recognized as a heretofore obscure cause of seizures, hemorrhage, and progressive neurologic deficit. This apparent increased incidence can be attributed to the widespread use of contemporary and sophisticated imaging techniques. Although recognized on CT scan as a lesion without contrast, the appearance of cavernous malformations by MRI is virtually pathognomonic. Their nature of repeated small hemorrhages creates the MRI image of various stages of blood breakdown and thereby a variegated well-circumscribed lesion.[19,87,104,123,129,151,158]

Headaches may or may not be related, but the hemorrhages, when they do occur, are related to the malformation. These malformations are made up of a multitude of large cavernous vascular channels that can be identified neither as arteries nor as veins. Major portions are often thrombosed, and whatever portions are patent have such low-flow characteristics that they are generally not visible on angiograms, even with a prolonged venous phase and maximal injection of contrast agent. These lesions are most commonly seen in the cerebral hemispheres, where they may be superficial or deep and, in the latter case, paraventricular. In approximately 20% of cases, they are infratentorially located in the cerebellum or brain stem. In 5% of cases, they are found in the spinal cord. They generally appear as a dense contrast-enhancing area without mass effect. The larger ones may extend from the surface of the brain to the paraventricular region. In the spinal cord, they are intramedullary. Major hemorrhages, when they occur, are rarely fatal and in most cases pursue a benign course with a low incidence of recidivous hemorrhage.

These lesions are commonly mistaken for intracranial tumors, but can be readily identified by the lack of mass effect. When exposed at surgery, they often appear larger than expected from the scan finding.[5] In some cases, the lesions may be encapsulated, with clefts at the margins, the result of old hemorrhage. Their resectability depends on the border between abnormal and normal, which, if indistinct, precludes excision. In most cases, symptomatic or asymptomatic, surgery is advised. This is based on the natural history. Many of the hemorrhages are presumed to be asymptomatic. In addition, the buildup of scar around the lesion from repeated hemosiderin deposition is felt to be a process leading to intractable seizures. Cavernous malformations of the brain stem generally have a more progressive and disastrous course. To date there is no evidence that radiosurgery plays a definitive role in the treatment of these lesions; in fact, it may be contraindicated.[69,160] One of our cases is illustrative (Fig. 56.18).

CASE HISTORY. The patient, a 17-year-old right-handed woman at the time of operation, commenced having seizures 3 years prior to operation. These seizures were first petit mal in nature and culminated in a grand mal seizure, during which she collapsed and suffered a skull fracture. Following that seizure, which occurred 3 years prior to operation, she had imaging studies that showed a lesion present on noncontrast CT scan, slightly enhancing on contrast CT scan, and typical of a cavernous malformation on the MRI scan (Fig. 56.8). An arteriogram through all phases was normal. She was maintained on a therapeutic anticonvulsant regimen. She suffered no further seizures but maintained an abnormal electroencephalogram (EEG). Her neurologic examination was normal.

On July 19, 1990, operation was carried out with the total removal of a cavernous malformation (Fig. 56.18). At operation a large middle cerebral artery branch, identified as normal on the arteriogram, coursed intimately around the convexity surface of the malformation, giving small branches to it. These branches were not visualized as abnormal on the arteriogram. Postoperatively, the patient was maintained on anticonvulsants and was normal. One year postoperatively, the patient continues normal, and consideration is being given to stopping anticonvulsant medication.

VENOUS MALFORMATIONS

Venous malformations, also clinical curiosities, are turning up with a frequency that parallels the increasing use of CT and MRI scanning.[95,99,102,122,125-127] Again, the symptomatology, similar to that in cavernous malformations, is primarily reflected by seizure disorders, headaches, and, rarely, hemorrhage. In some cases, an associated cavernous malformation may be present in the vicinity of the venous malformation, explaining why, in some series of venous malformations, there was a 40% to 50% incidence of hemorrhage.[99,102,122,123,125] When hemorrhage has occurred, it has not been fatal, and often the patient has recovered completely. These lesions may be located in any region of the brain, but have not been reported in the spinal cord. The CT scan and angiographic appearance are pathognomonic.[125] On the CT scan, there is generally a contrast-enhancing linear density representing the draining vein; a comparable image is seen by MRI scan. This appears in the white matter, but may extend to the cortical region. The angiogram, which is pathognomonic, shows a "caput medusae" arrangement of veins deep in the white matter, coalescing to a dilated venous channel, which passes through the white matter, usually toward the cortical surface. These are low-flow systems readily identified on the venous phase of the angiogram. There is no evidence of an arterial contribution to the lesion. At surgery, blood sampled from the draining vein is purely venous, with no evidence of arteriovenous shunting or elevated oxygen content. In most cases, especially those that do not present with hemorrhage, the approach should be conservative and surgery is not indicated. The dilemma arises when the lesion has hemorrhaged. The few cases that have been operated on, especially those located

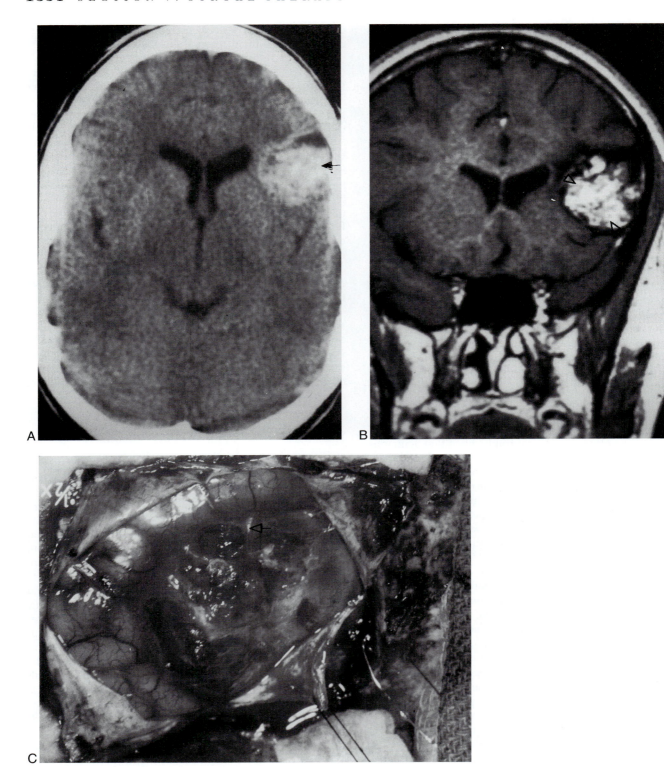

Figure 56.18 (**A**) A CT scan demonstrating a large area of density (arrow) on the noncontrast scan representing the cavernous malformation. (**B**) MRI scan showing the typical pattern of a large cavernous malformation (arrow). (**C**) Operative photograph showing the surface of the cavernous malformation and the middle cerebral branch coursing intimate to the malformation (arrow).

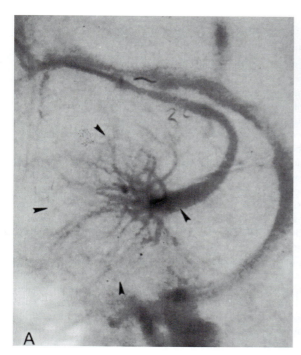
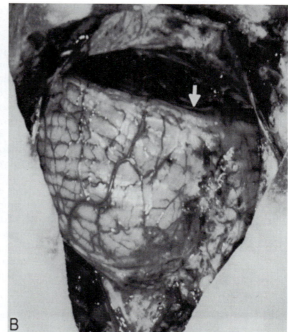

Figure 56.19 Features of a venous malformation. (**A**) Posterior fossa angiogram showing the typical configuration of a venous malformation (arrows). (**B**) Operative photograph demonstrating the paucity of normal veins over the convexity of the right cerebellar hemisphere and the single large draining vein (arrow) representing the venous malformation.

in the cerebellum, would indicate that the venous malformation represents an abnormal, probably congenital, but essential venous drainage for the deep white matter, subserving areas where surface veins are deficient.[127] In such cases, it may be impossible to remove the venous malformation, even if it has hemorrhaged, because of ensuing massive brain swelling due to the obliteration of the only venous drainage for that portion of the brain. Therefore even those venous malformations associated with hemorrhage should be treated with utmost caution and conservatism. It is comforting to note that the few data available on the natural history of these lesions suggest that recurrent hemorrhages are the exception rather than the rule. The following case is instructive (Fig. 56.19).

CASE STUDY. The patient was a 24-year-old right-handed woman who was in excellent health until October 1983, when she developed a right cerebellar hemorrhage. This was operated on and the hemorrhage removed. Following the operation, a CT scan demonstrated the classic appearance of a venous malformation of the right cerebellar hemisphere. In a second operation, part of the malformation was removed, but a postoperative arteriogram still showed the characteristic findings of a venous malformation (Fig. 56.19A). Having fully recovered from the hemorrhage, she was referred to us, and in April 1984 a third operation was carried out on the right cerebellar hemisphere. There was evidence of old hemorrhage surrounding a tangle of veins that coalesced into a large single draining vein gaining the surface of the cerebellum and

draining into the tentorium. Samples of blood from this vein indicated venous blood comparable with a peripheral venous sample. There was no evidence of arterial oxygenation of the blood in this vein. Temporary occlusion of this vein led to swelling of the cerebellar hemisphere, and it was obvious that this was the only visible venous drainage for the posterior and superior surface of the right cerebellar hemisphere (Fig. 56.19B). The vein in the area of old hemorrhage was then coated with a scarifying material and the wound was closed.

It was presumed that the venous drainage of the right cerebellar hemisphere was anomalous, depending primarily on this enlarged vein for drainage of both the white matter and the cortex. The hemorrhage had occurred at a deep portion of the vein. We did not feel that part or all of this abnormal venous system could be obliterated without destroying important venous drainage. Five years after the surgery the patient was well, without recurrent hemorrhage, and an MRI showed no cavernous malformations.

TELANGIECTASIAS

Telangiectasias are clinical curiosities that rarely lead to hemorrhage, but that can result in neurologic deficits.[35] These are not generally removed surgically, since their borders are ill defined and their significance uncertain. These lesions are frequently seen by the neuropathologist and may be associated

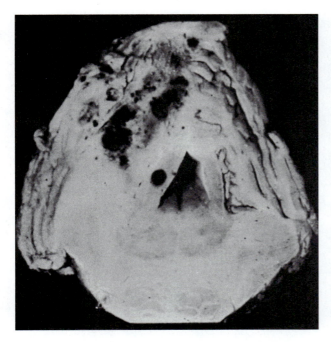

Figure 56.20 A telangiectasia of the brain stem and cerebellum.

with other lesions that make up the Rendu-Osler-Weber syndrome (Fig. 56.20).

VEIN OF GALEN MALFORMATIONS

Some malformations consist of arteriovenous connections in the region of the vein of Galen.[2,15,45,55,92] They are generally represented by large aneurysmal dilatations of the deep venous system in this region; in other instances, an AVM is the major component of the abnormality. In general, they act as a mass, with obstruction to the aqueduct, producing hydrocephalus. Uncommonly, they are associated with intracranial hemorrhage. These congenital lesions, unlike many of the other vascular malformations, become apparent in childhood, commonly in the form of a rapidly progressive hydrocephalus and also cardiac failure in the infant whose juvenile heart is unaccustomed to the high-flow arteriovenous shunts.

Patients with vein of Galen malformations may be divided into three groups: (1) those with direct arterial shunts to the vein of Galen, forming a large venous aneurysm; (2) those with a true AVM located in the posterior third ventricle and midbrain region, with veins draining into the vein of Galen and straight sinus; and (3) those with a combination of these two situations. The practical aspect of this categorization is that the first type of malformation is essentially a large artery to single-vein shunt, whereas the second and third categories represent a true AVM, which forms the major portion of the malformation. This categorization has validity in terms of surgical approach and embolization.

Clinical Presentation

The clinical presentation of these lesions is primarily related to the size of the shunt and the age of the patient; as reported by Amacher and Shillito,[2] it can be divided into four clinical patterns: (1) severe cardiac failure presenting within hours or days of birth, usually before the first week of life; (2) mild to moderate cardiac failure with increasing head size due to hydrocephalus, occurring around 6 months; (3) seizures and hydrocephalus occurring after the first year of life; and (4) subarachnoid hemorrhage in patients who have attained several years of age. It is significant that 64 of the patients become symptomatic before 2 years of age. In those infants who present with severe cardiac failure due to a large shunt and the major size of the aneurysmal dilatation, there is little that can be done. The natural course is invariably fatal and therapeutic measures have generally been futile. These children are so young and their cardiac status so precarious that it has been impossible to use the appropriately sized catheter or amount of fluid required for embolization. Similarly, surgical procedures in this age group are generally fatal. If there is any way possible, and there rarely is, these children should be tided over by medical means directed at compensation for cardiac failure until they are older and better able to withstand the rigors of the various forms of treatment. In the older age group, with mild cardiac failure and signs of hydrocephalus, it is the hydrocephalus that often needs immediate attention. Hydrocephalus is generally due to the obstruction of the posterior third ventricle or aqueductal region and can be alleviated by the usual extracranial shunts. In patients with progressive cardiac failure, therapeutic endeavors designed to reduce or eliminate the arteriovenous shunts may be necessary. As a preliminary, CT scan evaluation and selective intracranial angiography are necessary. Arteriography will demonstrate the major arterial supply, which is generally from the posterior cerebral artery or its branches. In addition, there may be arterial supply of lesser importance from the anterior cerebral, middle cerebral, or superior cerebellar arteries.

Embolization

Some of these malformations, depending on the size of the shunt and the arteriographic anatomy, have been treated successfully by embolization.[54,92] Embolization, although not completely eliminating the shunt, has been effective in reducing it, ameliorating the abnormal cardiac failure. Hilal et al[54] have been successful in utilizing the technique of Silastic pellet embolization.

Surgical Approach

A technique reported by Mickle and Quisling[92] involves the placement of thrombogenic coils via the torcula into the malformation. Conversely, the open surgical approach is fraught with difficulties and a high morbidity and mortality.[15,169] As previously mentioned, the mortality rate for infants who present with severe cardiac decompensation within the first week or two of life has been prohibitive, and, for the most part, operation has been abandoned in this group. Operation becomes useful in those patients whose cardiac situation has been stabilized and who are better able to withstand an operative approach. The aim of the operation is to eliminate the arteriovenous shunts as much as possible, often totally, without injuring the blood supply to the normal structures, such as the midbrain, or interrupting the deep venous system. It is not necessary to excise the enlarged vein of Galen, as this will attenuate over time once the arterial contribution to it is eliminated.

The operation, because of hydrocephalus, is usually carried out with the patient in the prone position and may involve bilateral parietal craniotomies. Initially, the attack should be from the right side with a parietal craniotomy and retraction of the parietal lobe, with the greatest possible exposure of the dilated vein of Galen or AVM in this region. A supratentorial approach is preferred, since the majority of the malformation is located in this region, and it is difficult to work from the posterior fossa on the vascular supply that comes from the anterior cerebral or middle cerebral arteries. As the surgeon approaches the malformation from the right side, various arterial components are gradually eliminated by cautery and division. Subsequently, the remaining margins of the malformation are secured, either with the addition of a left parietal craniotomy or, in the modest- to smaller-sized malformations, entirely from the right side. Once the arterial contributions have been divided, the vein generally collapses, and it may be necessary to plicate it further in order to reduce its volume and thereby eliminate the mass effect created by this large distended vessel. Rarely, it is necessary to resect the entire malformation or veins. In fact, this may lead to venous congestion of the diencephalic region and high morbidity, if not mortality.

With this approach, the mortality of surgery in the older children with hydrocephalus and mild to moderate but stabilized cardiac failure has been in the range of 30%. This may seem somewhat high; however, the natural history of such lesions is universally dismal. The lowest mortality and morbidity have been experienced in older children who present with subarachnoid hemorrhage due to the malformation.

Prognosis

Therefore, malformations in the region of the vein of Galen in children represent a heterogeneous group of lesions ranging from single arteriovenous shunts with huge aneurysmal dilatations to true complex AVMs. The natural history and results of treatment have been uniformly dismal in those cases presenting with severe cardiac failure in the first few weeks of life. The best results are obtained in older children who present with none of the major complications of these malformations, such as cardiac failure or progressive hydrocephalus, but, rather, with a milder syndrome of subarachnoid hemorrhage. In this instance, the lesion can be excised as prophylaxis against future hemorrhage. In the intermediate group presenting with cardiac failure and hydrocephalus, but in the older child, the results of shunting procedures and interruption of feeding arteries have been reasonably encouraging.

DURAL ARTERIOVENOUS MALFORMATIONS

The malformations that involve the dura are similar to those involving the brain in that they have major arterial supply with large venous drainage.[3,5,79,148] These venous channels may be extensive and usually empty into the major sinus. The malformations are generally modest in size, although small ones have been recorded as symptomatic, and in some instances the size of the dural malformations can only be described as horrendous, being comprehensive and involving many of the major sinuses and much of one or both hemispheres. As cerebral AVMs, they appear to have a congenital origin. They are uncommon, constituting less than 10% of cerebral malformations. Their blood supply is most commonly from the external carotid or muscular branches of the vertebral artery, although on occasion they may be associated with cerebral AVMs and in these instances may be fed by the cerebral arteries (Fig. 56.21).

Dural AVMs may hemorrhage, often presenting with an acute subdural hemorrhage that may be severe and even fatal on occasion. Unlike their cerebral counterparts, they may also present with evidence of raised intracranial pressure, including papilledema, headaches, vomiting, and all of the manifestations of intracranial hypertension. These malformations, since they are often large and close to the skull, are more often producers of bruit than the cerebral malformations. Frequently, the patient's initial symptomatology is related to a noise in the ear. In children the massive shunting through the larger dural AVMs may lead to high-output cardiac failure, much as the situation seen with the vein of Galen malformations.

To summarize the clinical symptomatology, the AVMs of the dura, although associated with symptomatology similar to that of their cerebral counterparts, present with a different clinical spectrum; bruits, headaches, and signs of increased intracranial pressure are more common with dural malformations than with cerebral AVMs, whereas seizures and hemorrhage common with cerebral malformations tend to be uncommon with those located in the dura.

Dural malformations of the cranial cavity can be anatomically divided into those occurring supratentorially or in the anterior portion of the cranium, as opposed to those that are generally infratentorial or present in the posterior portion of the cranium. The former tend to drain into the sagittal sinus or the circular or cavernous sinuses, while the latter tend to drain into the posterior sagittal sinus or the straight or lateral sinuses, as well as the torcular region. The malformations can show diffuse small artery to major venous sinus shunting or may be associated with one or two major arteries shunting directly into large venous channels.

The diagnosis is often made from the clinical history; certainly the low incidence of hemorrhage would not lead one to suspect dural malformations as a major cause of intracranial hemorrhage. Definitive diagnosis is made by CT scan and either conventional or digital subtraction angiography. Because of the high flow of these systems and often comprehensive involvement of the dura, it may be difficult to define the location of shunts and detailed anatomy by conventional angiograms. In such cases, it may be necessary to use extra quantities of contrast agent and prolong the filming of the arterial and venous phases of the angiogram.

Surgical Approach

The treatment of these lesions can be more difficult than the treatment of their cerebral counterparts[5,79,148] because these malformations tend to be diffuse and parasitize feeding arter-

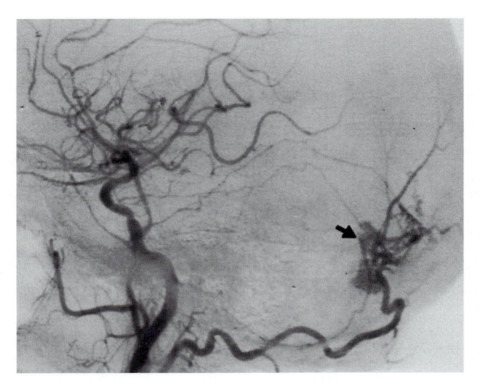

Figure 56.21 Cerebral angiogram demonstrating a large dural malformation (arrow) and also a cerebral malformation somewhat masked by the features of the dural malformation.

ies from many and varied dural surfaces. This makes complete obliteration of the lesion more difficult than the obliteration of a cerebral AVM. It is often necessary to remove all the dura surrounding the shunt into the major sinuses and even on occasion remove the major sinuses, which may lead to catastrophic problems, these channels being critical for normal venous drainage of the brain. However, unlike the case of cerebral AVMs, there have been many reports of spontaneous occlusion of dural AVMs during their natural course. This happens more frequently with those located in the anterior portion of the cranium than with those located posteriorly. Perhaps anteriorly the arterial supply is smaller in caliber and the sinuses into which the arteries flow are not as developed or as cavernous as those located in the posterior cranium. Obviously, it may be virtually impossible to locate and excise a dural malformation in the basal dura around such important structures as the sella turcica, the clivus, cranial nerves, and the blood vessels related to these structures. That in some cases there are both dural and cerebral malformations, interconnected and interdependent, complicates the surgery even further. Both must be removed at the time of surgery. The surgical procedures for the treatment of dural AVMs are primarily directed at those of smaller caliber and consist of cutting and resecting portions of the dura, especially the falx and tentorium.[148] This may be achieved with greater surgical efficiency in those lesions located in the posterior cranium; however, the dilemma occurs when the excision reaches the region of the major sinuses, such as the straight, sagittal, or lateral sinuses. In most instances, these cannot be sacrificed and must be left intact. It is often through the small remaining

dural pedicle adjacent to these sinuses that the malformation acquires new collateral circulation and continues to be a problem. On other occasions, however, removal of the major feeders is related to spontaneous thrombosis of the residual feeding vessels and the fistula closes. This appears to be the case more frequently in those lesions located in the anterior cranium.

Embolization

Embolization procedures have been particularly useful in the treatment of dural AVMs.[7,79] Selective catheterization of the proximal feeding arteries to these malformations can now be accomplished with great efficiency, especially with balloon catheters, which may then be inflated so as to block the distal flow of blood while a solidifying agent or particulate matter is injected distally into the malformation. However, in some cases, such as those malformations located in and around the sella turcica, it may be impossible to direct the blocking agent into the small arteries directly supplying the malformation, and some of the material may be lost to other vessels making up various branches of the extracranial circulation. In most instances, this will cause no problem. However, there have been cases of slough of the cutaneous or subcutaneous tissues. Of greater risk is the proximal migration of particulate matter or solidifying agents into the intracranial circulation. Such a complication can lead to catastrophic neurologic deficits due to cerebral embolization in a multitude of areas. Similarly, collaterals between distal branches of the external carotid circulation and the muscular branches of the vertebral artery may lead to embolization by solidifying substances into the posterior circulation. This has disastrous consequences in the distribution of the vertebral circulation, such as in the brain stem and occipital lobes. Therefore, the embolization procedures cannot be taken lightly, and appropriate material must be used while the procedure is carried out by specialists who have had broad experience in techniques of embolization. When these criteria are met, it has been possible to successfully obliterate some of these dural malformations. There are many dural malformations fed by branches of critical arteries destined for the cerebral circulation, such as those malformations involving the tentorium, where the blood supply is through the meningohypophyseal trunk, a direct branch of the internal carotid artery. It is generally impossible to embolize into these lesions and those fed by muscular branches of the vertebral artery. On some occasions, it may be propitious to follow embolization by surgery in order to secure certain feeding vessels that cannot be successfully embolized.[147]

Risks of Therapy

As previously noted, in many cases therapeutic endeavors short of complete obliteration of the malformation may lead to relief of symptomatology such as bruits, headaches, and raised intracranial pressure. Since the incidence of hemorrhage, especially fatal or disabling hemorrhage, is low in these lesions, therapy short of complete success may be acceptable. The surgeon and the interventional neuroradiologist must realize this and be willing to stop short of total anatomic success, understanding that attempts at total obliteration often lead to a much higher complication rate from the therapeutic endeavors.

CAROTID-CAVERNOUS FISTULAS

Carotid-cavernous fistulas are in the true sense dural arteriovenous shunts.[28,48,57,80,96,107] However, as opposed to most vascular malformations involving the dura, these are anatomically direct single shunts between the internal carotid artery within the cavernous sinus and the various venous channels that make up the cavernous sinus. These fistulas are often associated with trauma, especially fractures through the base of the skull, that distort and lacerate the internal carotid artery, especially at the junction of small branches such as the artery to the cavernous sinus that lies directly within the cavernous sinus. In addition, these fistulas may develop spontaneously without any antecedent history of trauma. The symptom complex is generally classic and leads to the diagnosis in most cases. The symptomatology consists of injection of the sclera of the eye, the presence of dilated vessels around the eye and orbit, a pulsating exophthalmos, chemosis, ophthalmoplegia, and loss of vision in severe cases (Fig. 56.22), all this with a background of an annoying, persistent intracranial bruit. Extradural or intraorbital hemorrhage from these fistulas is extremely rare. The main threat is to the eye and to the patient's psyche because of the consistency of the bruit and the pain and discomfort associated with the ocular pathology.

The history of the therapy of these lesions is the history of neurosurgery, with ingenious attempts being made to stamp out these fistulas, and the degree of success with an intact patient is disturbingly low. Although the fistula is often a single channel between the internal carotid artery and the surrounding veins, attempts to occlude it with the major pressure difference between the artery and the sinus have led to the rapid development of collateral channels to feed the fistula. Therefore, obliteration has often been extremely difficult without sacrifice of the internal carotid artery. Since the primary aim is to save the eye or reduce orbital symptomatology, one must also keep in mind the necessity of preserving the patient's vision. Similarly, measures short of total obliteration will only result in the return of the ocular symptomatology after a brief period of respite.

Parkinson,[107] in elegant anatomic studies, has detailed the anatomy of the carotid-cavernous sinus region, the basis of his study being surgical attempts to cure the fistula by direct intervention under extreme hypotension. His anatomic contributions have formed a foundation for current-day treatment. The treatment modalities fall into three major categories: (1) surgical intervention directed at the obliteration of the fistula and often the involved carotid artery, except for the direct technique developed by Parkinson; (2) techniques aimed at thrombosis of the venous side of the fistula; and (3) intravascular techniques developed by neuroradiologists whereby the carotid artery is occluded at the site of the fistula or the fistula itself is occluded with preservation of the carotid artery. A fourth endeavor might be mentioned, and this is the technique of intermittent manual occlusion of the internal carotid artery in the hopes of spontaneous remission of the fistula, which may occur in rare cases.

Surgical Intervention

The surgical approach, especially that of Parkinson, directly addresses the problem and has been successful in the hands of experienced neurosurgeons, such as Parkinson, but it is not for the faint of heart. It requires meticulous dissection of a high-pressure, high-flow system directly, albeit extreme hypotension and hypothermia have been utilized. It is a major operation and often requires cardiac arrest. In addition, during the stresses of the operation (time being a major factor) the delicate cranial nerves in this area must be preserved if the operation is to reach a successful conclusion with a resultant normal eye. The less direct approaches are the classic neurosurgical approaches and generally result in trapping the internal carotid artery, especially in the area of the fistula. These operations are often multistaged, the first stage being to place a clip across the internal carotid artery, preferably between the ophthalmic artery and the cavernous sinus (not an easy task to preserve the ophthalmic artery), and then occluding the internal carotid artery in the neck, often preceded by embolization with particulate matter stuffing the internal carotid artery in the cavernous and petrous portions to ensure that all potential collaterals have been eliminated. This series of surgeries is laborious for both the surgeon and the patient. Although generally successful this treatment may be associated with the risks attendant to the occlusion of a major artery of the cerebral circulation. On some occasions these fistulas are bilateral, and in these situations both internal carotid arteries cannot be occluded.

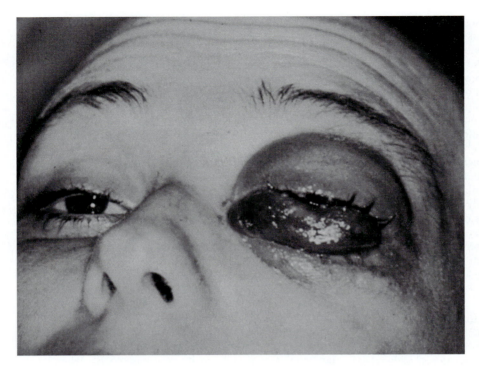

Figure 56.22 Intense proptosis and chemosis secondary to a carotid-cavernous fistula.

Thrombosis Techniques

The technique of thrombosis of the venous portion of the fistula has been developed by Hosobuchi[57] and Mullan.[96] This requires the insertion of fine wires of different metallic content directly into the cavernous sinus. A study of the anatomy of the fistula and of the sinus allows the surgeon to place the wires free of the intracavernous structures of importance, such as the cranial nerves and the internal carotid artery. The coiling of these wires within the sinus, especially wires of a different composition, will provide a nidus for progressive thrombosis of the venous side of the fistula (Fig. 56.23). Unlike arteriovenous fistulas elsewhere, the buttressing effect of the dura prevents explosion of the fistula and thrombosis progresses within the venous side, generally with a smooth occlusion up to the lumen of the internal carotid artery. This procedure results in obliteration of the fistula in a high percentage of cases and preservation of the internal cartoid artery. In Hosobuchi's series of 70 patients with a total of 81 fistulas, 11 of which were bilateral, the fistulas were obliterated in all except 3 cases.[57] In 5 patients the thrombosis extended to the internal carotid artery, with occlusion of that artery; 3 of these patients died and 2 developed a hemiparesis. Among the 67 survivors, none suffered significant morbidity, and many of them showed improvement of extraocular palsies and of impaired vision.

Intravascular Techniques

Intravascular techniques have now been developed by the interventional neuroradiologist.[28,48,66,80,128] Foremost among these procedures is the use of balloon catheters, either to be placed permanently at the site of the fistula, with occlusion and sacrifice of the internal carotid artery, or, more important, to be detached at the level of the fistula, with occlusion of the venous side but preservation of the internal carotid artery. Debrun et al[28] have reported the use of detachable balloons filled with a solidifying material. There has been a high degree of success with this procedure and the benefit is the preservation of the carotid artery while the fistula is obliterated. However, the techniques are successful only in the hands of experienced interventional neuroradiologists, and there may be the hazard of deflation of the balloon and its migration up the internal carotid artery, with disastrous occlusion of the internal carotid or middle cerebral artery. Debrun et al[28] used the detachable balloon in 17 cases with no mortality and only 1 significant morbidity. In all patients, the fistula was successfully occluded. Carotid artery flow was preserved in 12 of the 17 patients, and in the other 5 there were various degrees of occlusion of the internal carotid artery by the balloon. Viñuela et al[157] have reviewed the treatment of these lesions by endovascular methods and emphasize that this method is now the treatment of choice. The approach may be either arterial (carotid artery) or venous (inferior petrosal sinus or superior ophthalmic vein).

Intermittent Manual Occlusion of the Internal Carotid Artery

Finally, the conservative approach to carotid-cavernous fistulas has some merit, considering that a spontaneous disappearance rate of 5% exists in relation to these fistulas. Intermittent compression of the internal carotid artery in the neck by the patient or physician has been recommended to aid in the spon-

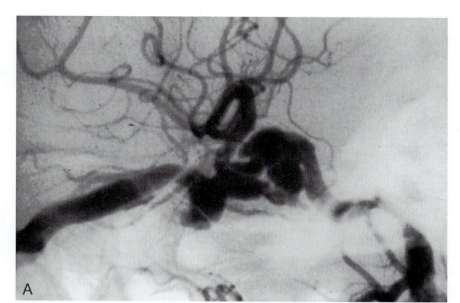

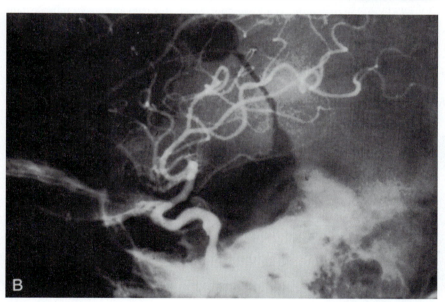

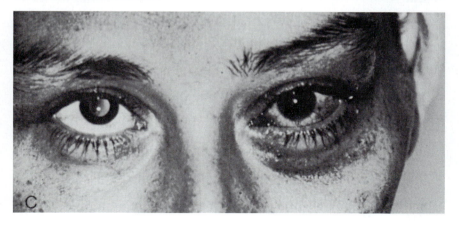

Figure 56.23 Features of the electro-thrombotic technique for carotid-cavernous fistula. (**A**) Cerebral angiogram showing the fistula. (**B**) Cerebral arteriogram demonstrating the obliteration of the fistula by the wire technique of Hosobuchi. (**C**) Regression of ocular abnormalities following obliteration of the fistula (same patient as in Fig. 56.22).

taneous regression of these fistulas. In the milder cases, it may be necessary to take no action, since the ocular symptomatology is minimal and not life threatening. In such cases, one can hope for either spontaneous regression or maintenance of a state of minimal symptomatology that is of no great distress to the patient. Valuable time is not lost while watching and evaluating such fistulas, as they will rarely pick up additional collateral circulation.

Risks of Therapeutic Maneuvers

Whichever method is selected, it is important to place a premium on the preservation of the internal carotid artery and consider the degree of symptomatology in gauging the risks of the various therapeutic maneuvers. For example, it is difficult to justify a trapping procedure that entails obliteration of the internal carotid artery as well as external carotid artery with the result of glaucoma in the involved eye, even though the fistula has been eliminated. The glaucoma may progress to an ophthalmitis that results in the enucleation of that eye. The main purpose, of course, is to preserve vision and improve

the eye, whereas in such an instance the eye is lost and there is a possible threat to the opposite eye from sympathetic ophthalmitis. In such a case the therapeutic endeavors carry a much higher risk than the natural history of the disease process.

CRYPTIC MALFORMATIONS

"Cryptic malformations" comprise a heterogeneous group, traditionally including any vascular anomaly that is visible either on CT scan or histologic evaluation but cannot be identified on angiograms[19,81,90] (Fig. 56.24). It is presumed that the nutrient vasculature is too small to be observed on an angiogram. The lesions are generally discovered when an "apparently spontaneous" hematoma is evacuated from the brain. In the walls of the hematoma cavity, the surgeon may note a discrete nodule, which, when later examined by the neuropathologist, will be found to contain a mixture of thrombosed and patent vascular channels. In fact, the term *cryptic malformation* is a misnomer, since this category may embrace rare small AVMs or more likely cavernous malformations, which are not angiographically visible.

Figure 56.24 A scan demonstrating a cryptic arteriovenous malformation (arrow) (the cause of encephalomalacia following hemorrhage). This was not demonstrable on arteriography. This malformation was successfully removed. Only a minute arterial supply to the malformation was observed at surgery.

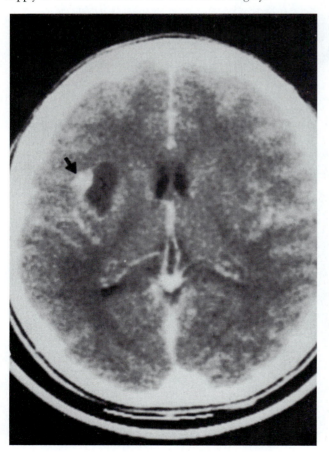

References

1. Amacher AL, Allock JM, Drake CG: Cerebral angiomas: the sequelae of surgical treatment. Neurosurg 37:571, 1972

2. Amacher AL, Shillito J Jr: The syndromes and surgical treatment of aneurysms of the great vein of Galen. J Neurosurg 39:89, 1973

3. Aminoff MJ: Vascular anomalies in the intracranial dura mater. Brain 96:601, 1973

4. Awad IA, Leblanc R, Little JR: Blood flow measurements in intracranial arteriovenous malformations. p. 91. In Barrow DL (ed): Intracranial Vascular Malformations: Neurosurgical Topics. AANS Publications Committee, IL, 1990

5. Awad IA, Little JR: Dural arteriovenous malformations. p. 219. In Barrow DL (ed): Intracranial Vascular Malformations: Neurosurgical Topics. AANS Publications Committee, IL, 1990

6. Barnett GH, Little JR, Ebralium ZY et al: Cerebral circulation during arteriovenous malformation operation. Neurosurgery 20:836, 1987

7. Barnwell SL, Halback VV, Higashida RT et al: Complex dural arteriovenous fistulas: results of combined endovascular and neurosurgical treatment in 16 patients. J Neurosurg 71:352–358, 1989

8. Barrow DL: Intracranial Vascular Malformations: Neurosurgical Topics. AANS Publications Committee, IL, 1990

9. Batjer HH, Devous MD Sr, Seibert GB et al: Intracranial arteriovenous malformation: relationship between clinical factors and surgical complications. Neurosurgery 24:75, 1989

10. Batjer HH, Purdy PD, Giller CA, Samson DS: Evidence of redistribution of cerebral blood flow during treatment for an intracranial arteriovenous malformation. Neurosurgery 25:599, 1989

11. Berenstein A, Kricheff II: Catheter and material selection for transarterial embolization. I. Technical considerations. II. Materials. Radiology 132:631, 1979

12. Betti OO, Munari C, Rosler R: Stereotactic radiosurgery with the linear accelerator: treatment of arteriovenous malformations. Neurosurgery 24:311, 1989

13. Brown RD Jr, Wiebers DO, Forbes C et al: The natural history of unruptured intracranial arteriovenous malformations. J Neurosurg 68:352, 1988

14. Brown RD Jr, Wiebers DO, Forbes GS: Unruptured intracranial aneurysms and arteriovenous malformations: frequency of intracranial hemorrhage and relationship of lesions. J Neurosurg 73:859, 1990

15. Bruce DA: Surgery of the vein of Galen arteriovenous malformation. Contemp Neurosurg 3:1, 1981

16. Burge HJC, Chirela AB, Guevora JA et al: Infratentorial arteriovenous malformations: radiosurgical treatment. p. 169. In Lunsford L: Stereotactic Radiosurgery Update. Elsevier, New York, 1992

17. Chou SN, Erickson DL, Ortiz-Suarez HJ: Surgical treatment of vascular lesions in the brain stem. J Neurosurg 42:23, 1975

18. Coffey RJ, Nichols DA, Shaw EG: Stereotactic radiosurgical treatment of cerebral arteriovenous malformations. Mayo Clin Proc 70:214, 1995

19. Cohen HCM, Tucker WS, Humphreys RP, Perrin RJ: Angiographically cryptic histologically verified cerebrovascular malformations. Neurosurgery 10:704, 1982

20. Colombo F, Benedetti A, Pozza F et al: External stereotactic irradiation by linear accelerator. Neurosurgery 16:154, 1985

21. Colombo F, Benedetti A, Pozza F et al: Linear accelerator radiosurgery of cerebral arteriovenous malformations. Neurosurgery 24:833, 1989

22. Crawford PM, West CR, Chadwick DW, Shaw MD: Arteriovenous malformations of the brain: natural history in unoperated patients. J Neurol Neurosurg Psychiatry 49:1, 1986

23. Cromwell LD, Harris BA: Treatment of cerebral arteriovenous malformations: a combined neurosurgical and neuroradiological approach. J Neurosurg 52:705, 1982

24. Cunha e Sa MJ, Stein BM, Solomon RA, McCormick PC: The treatment of associated intracranial aneurysms and arteriovenous malformations. J Neurosurg 77:853–859, 1992

25. DaPian R, Pasqualin A, Scienza R: Microsurgical treatment of juxtapeduncular angiomas. Surg Neurol 17:16, 1982

26. DaPian R, Pasqualin A, Scienza R, Vivenza C: Microsurgical treatment of ten arteriovenous malformations in critical areas of the cerebrum. J Microsurg 1:305, 1980

27. Debrun GM, Viñuela F, Fox A, Drake CG: Embolization of cerebral arteriovenous malformations with bucrylate: experience in 46 cases. J Neurosurg 56:615, 1982

28. Debrun GM, Viñuela F, Fox AJ et al: Indications for treatment and classification of 132 carotid-cavernous fistulas. Neurosurgery 22:285, 1988

29. Dias MS, Sekhar LN: Intracranial hemorrhage from aneurysms and arteriovenous malformations during pregnancy and the puerperium. Neurosurgery 27:855, 1990

30. Drake CG: Surgical removal of arteriovenous malformations from the brain stem and cerebellopontine angle. J Neurosurg 43:661, 1975

31. Drake CG: Cerebral arteriovenous malformations: considerations for and experience with surgical treatment in 166 cases. Clin Neurosurg 26:145, 1979

32. Drake CG: Arteriovenous malformations of the brain: the options for management. N Engl J Med 309:308, 1983

33. Drake CG, Friedman AH, Peerless SJ: Posterior fossa arteriovenous malformations. J Neurosurg 64:1, 1986

34. Epstein N, Epstein F: Arteriovenous malformation presenting as a first seizure in a 13-year-old child: surgical indications. Neurosurgery 7:391, 1980

35. Farrell DF, Forno LS: Symptomatic capillary telangiectasis of the brainstem without hemorrhage: report of an unusual case. Neurology (NY) 20:341, 1970

36. Forster DMC, Steiner L, Hakanson S: Arteriovenous malformations of the brain: a long-term clinical study. J Neurosurg 37:562, 1972

37. Fournier D, TerBrugge KG, Willinsky R et al: Endovascular treatment of intracerebral arteriovenous malformations: experience in 49 cases. J Neurosurg 75:228, 1991

38. Fox JL, Al Mefty O: Embolization of an arteriovenous malformation of the brain stem. Surg Neurol 8:7, 1977

39. Friedman WA, Bova FJ: Linear accelerator radiosurgery for arteriovenous malformations. J Neurosurg 77:832, 1992

40. Friedman WA, Bova FJ, Mendenhall WM: Linear accelerator radiosurgery for arteriovenous malformations: the relationship of size to outcome. J Neurosurg 82:180, 1995

41. Fults D, Kelly DL: The natural history of arteriovenous malformations of the brain: a clinical study. Neurosurgery 15:658, 1984

42. Garretson HD: Postoperative pressure and flow changes in the feeding arteries of cerebral arteriovenous malformations. Neurosurgery 4:544, 1979

43. Garretson HD: Intracranial arteriovenous malformations. p. 1448. In Wilkins RH, Rengachary SS (eds): Neurosurgery. McGraw-Hill, New York, 1985

44. Garrido E, Stein BM: Removal of an arteriovenous malformation from the basal ganglion. J Neurol Neurosurg Psychiatry 41:992, 1978

45. Gold AP, Ransohoff J, Carter S: Vein of Galen malformation. Acta Neurol Scand suppl. 40:1, 1964

46. Graf CJ, Perret G, Torner JC: Bleeding from cerebral arteriovenous malformations as part of their natural history. J Neurosurg 58:331, 1983

47. Guidetti B, DeLitala A: Intracranial arteriovenous malformations: conservative and surgical treatment. J Neurosurg 53:149, 1980

48. Halbach VV, Higashida RT, Hieshima GB, Hardin CW: Transvenous embolization of direct carotid-cavernous fistulas. AJNR 9:741, 1988

49. Halbach VV, Higashida RT, Yang P et al: Preoperative

balloon occlusion of arteriovenous malformations. Neurosurgery 22:301, 1988

50. Hassler W, Steinmetz H: Cerebral hemodynamics in angioma patients: an intraoperative study. J Neurosurg 67: 822, 1987

51. Hayashi S, Arimoto T, Itakura T et al: The association of intracranial aneurysms and arteriovenous malformation of the brain. J Neurosurg 55:971, 1981

52. Heros RC, Korosue K: Radiation treatment of cerebral arteriovenous malformations. N Engl J Med 323:127, 1990

53. Heros RC, Korosue K, Riebold P: Surgical excision of cerebral arteriovenous malformations: late results. Neurosurgery 26:570, 1990

54. Hilal SK, Sane P, Mawad ME et al: Therapeutic interventional radiologic procedures in neuroradiology. p. 1094. In Abrams HL (ed): Abrams Angiography: Vascular and Interventional Radiology, 3rd Ed. Little, Brown, Boston, 1983

55. Hoffman HJ, Chuang S, Hendrick EB et al: Aneurysms of the vein of Galen. J Neurosurg 57:316, 1982

56. Horton JC, Chambers WA, Lyons SL et al: Pregnancy and the risk of hemorrhage from cerebral arteriovenous malformations. Neurosurgery 27:867, 1990

57. Hosobuchi Y: Electrothrombosis of carotid-cavernous fistula. J Neurosurg 42:76, 1975

58. Hunt B, Suss RA, Samson D: Intracranial arteriovenous malformations associated with aneurysms. Neurosurgery 18:29, 1986

59. Itoyama Y, Uemura S, Ushio Y et al: Natural course of unoperated intracranial arteriovenous malformations: study of 50 cases. J Neurosurg 71:805, 1989

60. Jafar JJ, Davis AJ, Berenstein A et al: The effect of embolization with N-butyl cyanoacrylate prior to surgical resection of cerebral arteriovenous malformations. J Neurosurg 78:60–69, 1993

61. Jane J, Kassell N, Torner J, Winn HR: The natural history of aneurysms and arteriovenous malformations. J Neurosurg 62:321, 1985

62. Kader A, Goodrich JT, Sonstein WJ et al: Recurrent cerebral arteriovenous malformations after negative postoperative angiograms. J Neurosurg 85:14–18, 1996

63. Kader A, Young WL, Pile-Spellman J et al: The influence of hemodynamic and anatomic factors on hemorrhage from cerebral arteriovenous malformations. Neurosurgery 34:801–807, 1994

64. Kemeny AA, Dias PS, Forster DM: Results of stereotactic radiosurgery of arteriovenous malformations: an analysis of 52 cases. J Neurol Neurosurg Psychiatry 52:554, 1989

65. Kerber CW: Use of balloon catheters in the treatment of cranial arterial abnormalities. Stroke 11:210, 1980

66. Kerber CW, Bank WO, Cromwell LD: Cyanoacrylate occlusion of carotid-cavernous fistula with preservation of carotid artery flow. Neurosurgery 4:210, 1979

67. Kjellberg R, Abe M: Stereotactic Bragg Peak proton beam therapy. p. 463. In Lunsford LD (ed): Modern Stereotactic Neurosurgery. Martinus Nijhoff Publishing, Boston, 1988

68. Kjellberg RN, Hanamura T, Davis KR et al: Bragg-Peak proton beam therapy for arteriovenous malformations of the brain. N Engl J Med 309:269, 1983

69. Kondziolka D, Lunsford LD, Coffey RJ et al: Stereotactic radiosurgery of angiographically occult vascular malformations: indications and preliminary experience. Neurosurgery 27:892, 1990

70. Kondziolka D, Lunsford LD, Flickenger JC: Gamma Knife stereotactic radiosurgery for cerebral vascular malformations. p. 136. In Alexander E III, Loeffler JS, Lunsford LD (eds): Stereotactic Radiosurgery. McGraw-Hill, New York, 1993

71. Künc Z: Surgery of arteriovenous malformations in the speech and motor sensory regions. J Neurosurg 40:291, 1974

72. Kvam DA, Michelsen WJ, Quest DO: Intracerebral hemorrhage as a complication of artificial embolization. Neurosurg 7:491, 1980

73. Lindegaard K, Grolimund P, Aaslid R, Nornes H: Evaluation of cerebral AVMs using transcranial Doppler ultrasound. J Neurosurg 65:335, 1986

74. Lindquist C, Steiner L: Stereotactic radiosurgical treatment of malformations of the brain. p. 491. In Lunsford LD (ed): Modern Stereotactic Neurosurgery. Martinus Nijhoff Publishing, Boston, 1988

75. Luessenhop AJ, Presper JH: Surgical embolization of cerebral arteriovenous malformations through internal carotid and vertebral arteries: long-term results. J Neurosurg 42:443, 1975

76. Luessenhop AJ, Rosa L: Cerebral arteriovenous malformations. Indications for and results of surgery, and the role of intravascular techniques. J Neurosurg 60:14, 1984

77. Luessenhop AJ, Spence WT: Artificial embolization of cerebral arteries: report of use in a case of arteriovenous malformation. JAMA 172:1153, 1960

78. Lunsford JD, Siddon RL, Wen PY et al: Stereotactic radiosurgery for arteriovenous malformations of the brain. J Neurosurg 75:512, 1991

79. Manaka S, Izawa M, Nawata H: Dural arteriovenous malformation treated by artificial embolization with liquid silicone. Surg Neurol 7:63, 1977

80. Manelfe C, Berenstein A: Treatment of carotid-cavernous fistulas by venous approach. J Neuroradiol 7:13, 1980

81. Margolis G, Odom GL, Woodhall B, Blon B: Role of small AVM in production of intracerebral hematomas. J Neurosurg 8:564, 1951

82. Marks LB, Spencer DP: The influence of volume on the tolerance of the brain to radiosurgery. J Neurosurg 75: 177, 1991

83. Marks MP, Lane B, Steinberg GK et al: Endovascular treatment of cerebral arteriovenous malformations. AJNR 14:297, 1993

84. Martin NA, Wilson CB: Medial occipital arteriovenous malformations. J Neurosurg 56:798, 1982

85. Mathis JA, Barr JD, Horton JA et al: The efficacy of particulate embolization combined with stereotactic radiosurgery for treatment of large arteriovenous malformations of the brain. AJNR 16:299, 1995

86. Mawad M, Hilal S, Michelsen WJ et al: Occlusive vascular disease associated with cerebral arteriovenous malformations. Radiology 153:401, 1984

87. McCormick PC, Michelsen WJ: Management of intracranial cavernous and venous malformations. p. 197. In Barrow DL (ed): Intracranial Vascular Malformations: Neurosurgical Topics. AANS Publications Committee, IL, 1990

88. McCormick WF: The pathology of vascular ("arteriovenous") malformations. J Neurosurg 24:807, 1966

89. McCormick WF, Hardman JM, Boulter TR: Vascular malformations ("angiomas") of the brain with special reference to those occurring in the posterior fossa. J Neurosurg 28:241, 1968

90. McCormick WF, Nofzinger JD: "Cryptic" vascular malformations of the central nervous system. J Neurosurg 24:865, 1966

91. McCormick WF, Rosenfield DB: Massive brain hemorrhage: a review of 144 cases and an examination of their causes. Stroke 4:946, 1973

92. Mickle JP, Quisling RG: The transtorcular embolization of vein of Galen aneurysms. J Neurosurg 64:731, 1986

93. Morello G, Broghi GP: Cerebral angiomas: a report of the 154 personal cases and a comparison between the results of surgical excision and conservative management. Acta Neurochir (Wien) 28:135, 1973

94. Morgan MK, Johnson I, Besser M et al: Cerebral arteriovenous malformations, steal and the hypertensive breakthrough threshold. J Neurosurg 66:563, 1987

95. Moritake K, Handa H, Mori K et al: Venous angiomas of the brain. Surg Neurol 14:95, 1980

96. Mullan S: Treatment of carotid-cavernous fistulas by cavernous sinus occlusion. J Neurosurg 50:131, 1979

97. Mullan S, Brown FD, Patronas NJ: Hyperemic and ischemic problems of surgical treatment of arteriovenous malformations. J Neurosurg 51:757, 1979

98. Muraszko K, Wang HH, Pelton G, Stein BM: A study of the reactivity of feeding vessels to arteriovenous malformations: correlation with clinical outcome. Neurosurgery 26:190, 1990

99. Nishizaki T, Tamaki N, Matsumoto S et al: Consideration of the operative indications for posterior fossa venous angiomas. Surg Neurol 25:441, 1986

100. Nornes H, Grip A: Hemodynamic aspects of cerebral arteriovenous malformations. J Neurosurg 53:456, 1980

101. Nornes H, Grip A, Wikeby P: Intraoperative evaluation of cerebral hemodynamics using directional Doppler technique. I. Arteriovenous malformations. J Neurosurg 50:145, 1979

102. Numaguchi Y, Kitamura K, Fukui M et al: Intracranial venous angiomas. Surg Neurol 18:193, 1982

103. Nussbaum ES, Heros RC, Camarata PJ: Surgical treatment of intracranial arteriovenous malformations with an analysis of cost-effectiveness. Clin Neurosurg 42:348, 1994

104. Ogilvy CS, Heros RC, Ojemann RG et al: Angiographically occult arteriovenous malformations. J Neurosurg 69:350, 1988

105. Okabe T, Meyer JS, Okayasu H et al: Xenon-enhanced CT CBF measurements in cerebral AVMs before and after excision: contribution to pathogenesis and treatment. J Neurosurg 59:21, 1983

106. Ondra SL, Troupp H, George E, Schwav K: The natural history of symptomatic arteriovenous malformations of the brain: a 24-year follow-up assessment. J Neurosurg 73:387, 1990

107. Parkinson D: Carotid cavernous fistula: direct repair with preservation of the carotid artery: technical note. J Neurosurg 38:99, 1973

108. Parkinson D, Bachers G: Arteriovenous malformations: summary of 100 consecutive supratentorial cases. J Neurosurg 53:285, 1980

109. Pasqualin A, Scienza R, Cioffi F et al: Treatment of cerebral arteriovenous malformation with a combination of preoperative embolization and surgery. Neurosurgery 29:358, 1991

110. Paterson JH, McKissock W: A clinical survey of intracranial angiomas with special reference to their mode of progression and surgical treatment: a report of 110 cases. Brain 79:233, 1956

111. Patronas NJ, Marx WJ, Duda EE, Mullan JJ: Microvascular embolization of arteriovenous malformations: predicting success by cerebral angiography. AJNR 1:459, 1980

112. Pellettieri L: Surgical versus conservative treatment of intracranial arteriovenous malformations: a study in surgical decision-making. Acta Neurochirn (Wien) suppl. 29:1, 1979

113. Perret G: The epidemiology and clinical course of arteriovenous malformations. p. 21. In Pia HW, Gleave JRW, Grote E, Zierski J (eds): Cerebral Angiomas: Advances in Diagnosis and Therapy. Springer-Verlag, New York, 1975

114. Perret G, Nishioka H: Report on the cooperative study of intracranial aneurysms and subarachnoid hemorrhage. VI. Arteriovenous malformations. J Neurosurg 25:467, 1966

115. Pertuiset B, Ancri D, Clergue F: Preoperative evaluation of hemodynamic factors in cerebral arteriovenous malformations for selection of a radical surgical tactic with special reference to vascular autoregulation disorders. Neurol Res 4:209, 1982

116. Pevsner PH, Doppman JL: Therapeutic embolization with a microballoon catheter. AJNR 1:171, 1980

117. Pia HW, Gleave JRW, Grote E, Zierski J (eds): Cerebral Angiomas: Advances in Diagnosis and Therapy. p. 285. Springer-Verlag, New York, 1975

118. Pollock B, Flickinger J, Lunsford L, Zierski J (eds): Hemorrhage risk after stereotactic radiosurgery of cerebral arteriovenous malformations. Neurosurgery 38:652, 1996

119. Pool JL: Excision of cerebral arteriovenous malformations. J Neurosurg 29:312, 1968

120. Post KD, Stein BM: Technique for spinal drainage. Neurosurgery 4:255, 1979

121. Rauch RA, Viñuela F, Dion J et al: Preembolization functional evaluation in brain arteriovenous malformations: the ability of superselective Amytal test to predict neurologic dysfunction before embolization. AJNR 13:309–314, 1992

122. Rigamonti D, Spetzler RF, Drayer BP et al: Appearance of venous malformations on magnetic resonance imaging. J Neurosurg 69:535, 1988

123. Rigamonti D, Spetzler RF, Johnson PC et al: Cerebral vascular malformations. BNI Q 3:18, 1987

124. Rosenblum BR, Bonner RF, Oldfield EH: Intraoperative measurement of cortical blood flow adjacent to cerebral AVMs using laser Doppler velocimetry. J Neurosurg 66:396, 1987

125. Rothfus WE, Albright AL, Casey KF et al: Cerebellar venous angiomas: "benign" entity? AJNR 5:61, 1984

126. Saito Y, Kobayashi N: Cerebral venous angiomas. Radiology 139:87, 1981

127. Senegor M, Dohrmann GJ, Wollman RL: Venous angiomas of the posterior fossa should be considered anomalous venous drainage. Surg Neurol 19:26, 1983

128. Serbinenko FA: Balloon catheterization and occlusion of major cerebral vessels. J Neurosurg 41:125, 1974

129. Simard JM, Garcia-Benjochea F, Ballinger WE et al: Cavernous angioma: a review of 126 collected and 12 new clinical cases. Neurosurgery 18:162, 1986

130. Sisti MB, Kader A, Stein BM: Microsurgery of 67 intracranial arteriovenous malformations less than 3 cm. in diameter. J Neurosurg 79:653, 1993

131. Sisti MB, Solomon RA, Stein BM: Stereotactic craniotomy in the resection of small arteriovenous malformations. J Neurosurg 75:40, 1991

132. Solomon RA, Stein BM: Management of arteriovenous malformations of the brain stem. J Neurosurg 64:857, 1986

133. Solomon RA, Stein BM: Surgical treatment of arteriovenous malformations that follow the tentorial ring. Neurosurgery 18:708, 1986

134. Solomon RA, Stein BM: Interhemispheric approach for the surgical removal of thalamocaudate arteriovenous malformations. J Neurosurg 66:345, 1987

135. Spetzler RF, Martin NA: A proposed grading system for arteriovenous malformations. J Neurosurg 65:476, 1986

136. Spetzler RF, Martin NA, Carter P et al: Surgical management of large AVMs by staged embolization and operative excision. J Neurosurg 67:17, 1987

137. Spetzler RF, Wilson CB, Weinstein P et al: Normal perfusion pressure breakthrough theory. Clin Neurosurg 25:651, 1978

138. Stein BM: Arteriovenous malformations of the medial cerebral hemisphere and the limbic system. J Neurosurg 60:23, 1984

139. Stein BM: General techniques for surgical removal of arteriovenous malformations. p. 143. In Wilson CB, Stein BM (eds): Current Neurosurgical Practice. Intracranial Arteriovenous Malformations. Williams & Wilkins, Baltimore, 1984

140. Stein BM, Solomon RA: Surgical approaches to posterior fossa arteriovenous malformations. Clin Neurosurg 37:353, 1991

141. Stein BM, Wolpert SM: Surgical and embolic treatment of cerebral arteriovenous malformations. Surg Neurol 7:359, 1977

142. Stein BM, Wolpert SM: Arteriovenous malformations of the brain. I. Current concepts and treatment. Arch Neurol 37:1, 1980

143. Stein BM, Wolpert SM: Arteriovenous malformations of the brain. II. Current concepts and treatment. Arch Neurol 37:69, 1980

144. Steinberg GK, Fabrikant JI, Marks MP et al: Stereotactic heavy-charged-particle Bragg-peak radiation for intracranial arteriovenous malformations. N Engl J Med 323:96, 1990

145. Steiner L: Treatment of arteriovenous malformations by radiosurgery. p. 295. In Wilson CB, Stein BM (eds): Current Neurosurgical Practice. Intracranial Arteriovenous Malformations. Williams & Wilkins, Baltimore, 1984

146. Steiner, L: Radiosurgery in cerebral arteriovenous malformations. pp. 1161–1215. In Fein JM, Flamm ES: Cerebrovascular Surgery. Springer-Verlag, New York, 1985

147. Sundt TM Jr, Nichols DA, Piepgras DG, Fode NC: Strategies, techniques and approaches for dural arteriovenous malformations of the posterior dural sinuses. Clin Neurosurg 37:155–170, 1991

148. Sundt TM, Jr, Piepgras DG: The surgical approach to arteriovenous malformations of the lateral and sigmoid dural sinuses. J Neurosurg 59:32, 1983

149. Troupp H: Arteriovenous malformations of the brain: what are the indications for operation? p. 210. In Morley TP (ed): Current Controversies in Neurosurgery. WB Saunders, Philadelphia, 1976

150. Troupp H, Marttila I, Halonen V: Arteriovenous malformations of the brain: prognosis without operation. Acta Neurochir 22:125, 1970

151. Vaquero J, Salazar R, Martinez P et al: Cavernomas of the central nervous system: clinical syndromes, CT scan diagnosis, and prognosis after surgical treatment in 25 cases. Acta Neurochir 85:29, 1987

152. Viale GL, Turtas S, Pau A: Surgical removal of striate arteriovenous malformations. Surg Neurol 14:321, 1980

153. Viñuela F, Dion JE, Duckweiler G et al: Combined endovascular embolization and surgery in the management of cerebral arteriovenous malformations: experience with 101 cases. J Neurosurg 75:856–864, 1991

154. Viñuela F, Dion JE, Fox AJ et al: Interventional neuroradiology for intracranial arteriovenous malformations. p. 169. In Barrow DL (ed): Intracranial Vascular Malformations: Neurosurgical Topics. AANS Publications Committee, IL, 1990

155. Viñuela F, Fox AJ, Debrun G, Pelz D: Preembolization superselective angiography: role in the treatment of brain arteriovenous malformations with isobutyl-2 cyanoacrylate. AJNR 5:765–769, 1984

156. Viñuela FV, Dion J, Lylyk P, Duckweiler G: Update on interventional neuroradiology. AJR 153:23, 1989

157. Viñuela FV, Fox AJ, Pelz D et al: Angiographic follow-up of large cerebral AVMs incompletely embolized with isobutyl 2-cyanoacrylate. AJNR 7:919, 1986

158. Voigt K, Yasargil MG: Cerebral cavernous haemangiomas or cavernomas. Incidence, pathology, localization, diagnosis, clinical features and treatment: review of the literature and report of an unusual case. Neurochirurgia 19:59, 1976

159. Waltimo O: The relationship of size, density, and localization of intracranial arteriovenous malformations to the type of initial symptom. J Neurol Sci 19:13, 1973

160. Weil S, Tew JM, Steiner L: Comparison of radiosurgery and microsurgery for treatment of cavernous malformations of the brainstem, abstracted. J Neurosurg 72:713, 1990

161. Wilkins RH: Natural history of intracranial vascular malformations: a review. Neurosurgery 16:421, 1985

162. Wilson CB, Stein BM: Intracranial Arteriovenous Malformations in Current Neurosurgical Practice. p. 1. Williams & Wilkins, Baltimore, 1984

163. Wilson CB, U HS, Dominque J: Microsurgical treatment of intracranial vascular malformations. J Neurosurg 51:446, 1979

164. Winston KR, Lutz W: Linear accelerator as a neurosurgical tool for stereotactic radiosurgery. Neurosurgery 22:454, 1988

165. Wolpert SM, Stein BM: Catheter embolization of intracranial arteriovenous malformations as an aid to surgical excision. Neuroradiology 10:73, 1975

166. Wolpert SM, Stein BM: Factors governing the course of emboli in the therapeutic embolization of cerebral arteriovenous malformations. Radiology 131;1:125, 1979

167. Yamada S, Brauer FS, Knierim DS: Direct approach to arteriovenous malformations in functional areas of the cerebral hemisphere. J Neurosurg 72:418, 1990

168. Yamamoto Y, Coffey RJ, Nichols DA, Shaw EG: Interim report on the radiosurgical treatment of cerebral arteriovenous malformations. J Neurosurg 83:832, 1995

169. Yasargil MG, Antic J, Lacha R et al: Arteriovenous malformations of vein of Galen: microsurgical treatment. Surg Neurol 6:195, 1976

170. Yasargil MG, Jain KK, Antic J et al: Arteriovenous malformations of the anterior and middle portion of the corpus callosum: microsurgical treatment. Surg Neurol 5:67, 1976

171. Yasargil MG, Jain KK, Antic J, Laciga R: Arteriovenous malformations of the splenium of the corpus callosum: microsurgical treatment. Surg Neurol 5:5, 1976

172. Young WL, Pile-Spellman J, Prohovnik I et al: Evidence for adaptive autoregulatory displacement in hypotensive cortical territories adjacent to arteriovenous malformations. Neurosurgery 34:601–610, 1994

173. Young WL, Prohovnik I, Ornstein E et al: The effect of arteriovenous malformation resection on cerebrovascular reactivity to carbon dioxide. Neurosurgery 27:257, 1990

CHAPTER 57

Management of Spinal Vascular Malformations

PAUL C. McCORMICK

BENNETT M. STEIN

TANVIR F. CHOUDHRI

Spinal arteriovenous (AVMs) and cavernous malformations are the most commonly encountered spinal vascular malformations. While autopsy studies have described spinal venous malformations (angiomas) or capillary telangiectasia, these lesions rarely, if ever, require treatment. Spinal AVMs may be further classified into dural and intradural types according to the location of the fistulas. This simplified classification suffices for a general review of spinal AVMs. More complex terminology is available for those involved in the nuances of treatment and outcome of these rare lesions.

Management of spinal vascular malformations continues to evolve since the introduction of selective spinal angiography some 30 years ago. Since then, a better understanding of the anatomy and pathophysiology of these lesions, combined with advances in imaging, endovascular techniques, refined microsurgical techniques, and intraoperative, spinal monitoring, has resulted in an increasing percentage of the successful elimination of these treacherous lesions.

Arteriovenous Malformations

DURAL FISTULA

The dural malformation (type I, long dorsal AVM) is the most common type of spinal AVM. This lesion accounts for about 75% of AVMs in most reported series.[1,2,8,11] Unlike true AVMs, however, the nidus of this malformation is not a conglomeration of abnormally formed vessels but, rather, a direct, probably acquired, arteriovenous fistula (Fig. 57.1). The fistula is typically located on the superior aspect of the dural root sleeve and consists of a direct communication between a radicular artery and a radicular vein. The absence of venous valves allows retrograde filling of the intradural venous system. Thus, the entire intradural component of the malformation is venous carrying arterialized blood under increased pressure. Elevated intradural venous pressure caused by the fistula, probably in conjunction with an acquired or developmental compromise of intradural venous drainage, contributes to the pathologic venous hypertension and progressive ischemia of the spinal cord. Thus, these lesions may share a similar etiology to the intracranial dural malformations that are frequently associated with dural venous sinus thrombosis. The dural fistula almost exclusively occurs in the lower thoracic and lumbar region in patients of middle and later years. Men are affected four times more commonly than women. The absence of associated metameric anomalies further attests to an acquired etiology. A relentless, progressive paraparesis, often punctuated by an exacerbation of symptoms with exercise or episodic worsening from venous thrombosis, is the well-known history of this lesion.

Treatment of the dural malformation is directed at elimination of the fistula. Stripping of tortuous, dilated, and arterialized veins off the surface of the spinal cord is no longer advocated because it is unnecessary and may further compromise the venous drainage of the spinal cord. While endovascular embolization has been successful in blocking the fistula, the effects are usually short-lived because recanalization frequently occurs.[4] Although more complex, surgical elimination of the fistula represents the treatment of choice. This is a straightforward procedure and may consist either of division of the draining vein near the dural root sleeve or excision of the dural root sleeve, which contains the fistula (Fig. 57.1).

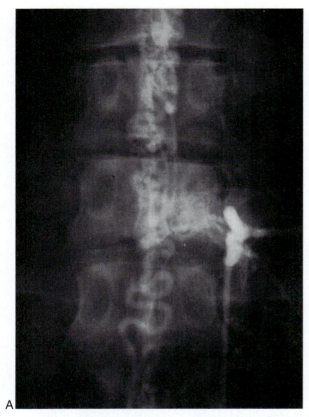

A

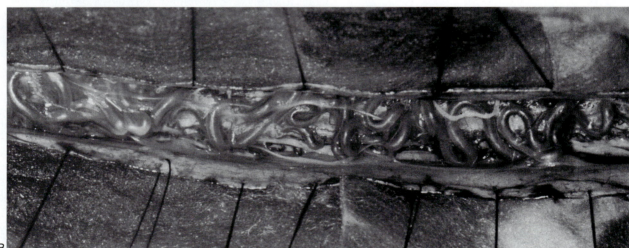

B

Figure 57.1 (**A**) Selective spinal angiogram (right T10 intercostal artery injection) demonstrates an atypical single, long, coiled vessel, which represents the engorged dorsal vein. (**B**) Operative photography shows appearance of the tortuous vein on the dorsal surface of the spinal cord.

Like most other progressive disorders of the spinal cord, outcome is most dependent on the immediate preoperative status. Significant return of neurologic function, which may be dramatic, can be anticipated in patients with mild to moderate deficit or with deficit of short duration. Fixed or long-standing deficits (i.e., several months to years) only rarely are improved by surgery. Thus, a premium is placed on early diagnosis and treatment of these lesions.

INTRADURAL ARTERIOVENOUS MALFORMATIONS

Intradural arteriovenous malformations are further divided into glomus and juvenile types, and the rare direct arteriovenous fistula.[5] These are true arteriovenous malformations, which are similar to their intracranial parenchymal counter-

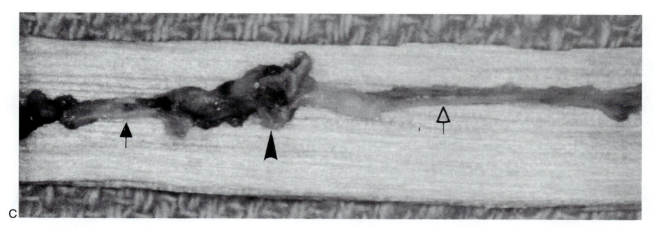

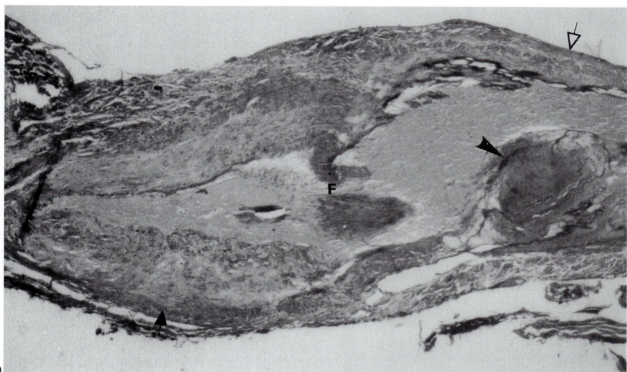

Figure 57.1 (*Continued*) (**C**) Photograph of excised specimen shows feeding artery (closed arrow), draining vein (open arrow), and intervening dural fistula (arrowhead). (**D**) Photomicrograph of longitudinal section of Fig. C. shows fistulous communication between thick-walled artery (closed arrow) and draining vein (open arrow). Note the intimal cushion (arrowhead), which is the morphologic consequence of direct arterial flow into a vein. The fistula site is also demonstrated.

parts. Their occasional association with metameric skin, bone, or other mesenchymal anomalies attests to their congenital origin. While dural fistulas occur more frequently in the thoracic and lumbar regions, intradural malformations occur in proportion to spinal cord vascular supply. Thus, cervical cord and lumbar enlargement/conus are more commonly affected than previously reported, while the thoracic cord is less affected.

The glomus AVM is more common in our experience. We reserve the term *juvenile AVM* to describe those multiple fistula malformations that permeate the spinal cord, occasion-

ally with vertebral and paraspinal involvement. These rare lesions typically present in childhood or adolescence with hemorrhage, pain, or a progressive neurologic deficit, which results from mechanical compression or arterial steal.[3,9] Cardiovascular abnormalities and an audible bruit may be present. Definitive therapy for these "juvenile" lesions is seldom possible.[10] Most commonly, the entire transverse area of the spinal cord is incorporated within the interstices of the malformation. Partial treatment with endovascular techniques, however, may improve pain, cardiac symptoms, and neurologic

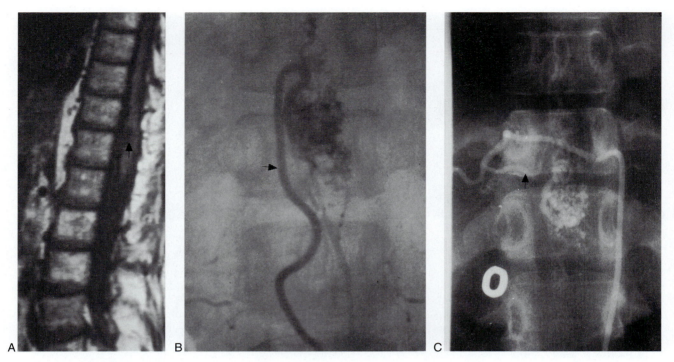

Figure 57.2 (**A**) Sagittal magnetic resonance imaging in 56-year-old woman with acute onset of back pain, urinary dysfunction, and leg weakness, shows intramedullary arteriovenous malformation in ventral conus (arrow). (**B**) Initial selective spinal angiogram showed only one anterior medullary feeder arising from LL2 (arrow). Operative ligation of this feeder at its entry into the malformation was performed with gradual clinical improvement. At 1 year following surgery, urinary symptoms reappeared. (**C**) Repeat selective angiogram shows recurrence of arteriovenous malformation fed through RT1, which did not supply the arteriovenous malformation on angiographic injection 1 year earlier (arrow).

deficit from arterial steal in some cases. These benefits are usually temporary, requiring repeat procedures at variable intervals.

The glomus AVM is a high-flow lesion in comparison with dural fistula, but generally has a slower shunt than seen with most intracranial AVMs. By definition, the glomus should have definable nidus, but this may not always be the case. The nidus may be intramedullary, pial, or both.[3,8,10] The intramedullary nidus most commonly occupies the anterior portion of the spinal cord and invariably fills via branches of anterior spinal artery with supplementary supply via the posterior medullary arteries (Fig. 57.2). Aneurysmal dilatations, which are usually venous, occur in about one-third of intradural AVMs, and in our experience is associated with a higher percentage of hemorrhagic presentation.

Angiography will typically reveal only one or at most two medullary arteries, which fill malformations located below the cervical spinal cord. This is probably a flow-related phenomenon, as other medullary feeders will be recruited if the major feeding vessel is occluded (Fig. 57.2). This is one reason for the failure of embolization to permanently treat the AVM.[4] Cervical glomus AVMs tend to be higher flow, with more feeding vessels demonstrated on angiography. This probably reflects the vascularity of the cervical cord segment. Feeders may arise directly from the vertebral, thyrocervical, costocer-

vical, deep cervical, and supreme intercostal arteries, as well as the descending limb of the anterior spinal artery.

A lateral or dorsolateral location is common for the pial glomus AVM, although a more ventral location is occasionally encountered. Pure dorsal lesions are usually encountered at the cervicomedullary junction. Pial malformations are supplied by circumferential pial branches from both the anterior and posterior spinal arteries, as well as an occasional direct branch from the medullary artery. Deep penetrating branches from the anterior spinal artery are invariably encountered if there are any intramedullary components to the malformation.

Intradural AVMs may present at any age, but the majority (about two-thirds) will become symptomatic during adolescence or early adult years.[9] An ictal event from subarachnoid or intramedullary hemorrhage or venous thrombosis is the most frequent presentation, particularly in the younger patient or in the malformation with an aneurysmal dilatation. Repeat hemorrhage is to be expected.

The neurologic consequence of a hemorrhagic presentation is variable. Purely subarachnoid hemorrhage may produce headache and meningeal irritation indistinguishable from subarachnoid hemorrhage of intracranial origin; even hydrocephalus may result. Sudden complete deficit from subarachnoid hemorrhage does occur, but is typically transitory and probably concussive in nature. Hematomyelia usually produces more devastating and sometimes permanent deficit.

In our experience, the acute or subacute onset of symptoms, as well as the young age and parenchymal location of these well-defined AVMs, makes them equivalent to intracranial AVMs. Accordingly, they are more dangerous to the patient than dural AVMs of the spine, which have a more insidious course.

MANAGEMENT CONSIDERATIONS

The management of intradural spinal AVMs is difficult to standardize for several reasons. First, these are extremely rare lesions whose natural history is not well-defined. Studies on the natural history of spinal AVMs are generally biased to reflect the progressive course of the much more commonly occurring dural fistula.[1,2,8,11] Second, these are potentially treacherous lesions whose initial or subsequent presentation may consist of a catastrophic event. Conversely, however, surgical or endovascular treatment of these lesions also carries significant risk of serious neurologic morbidity. Finally, although

surgery is the cornerstone of treatment, the role of endovascular techniques as an adjunct to surgery or as primary treatment continues to evolve. Advances in catheter technology, rapidly polymerizing low-viscosity liquids, and precisely calibrated particular emboli, allow safer more distal vascular occlusion within the nidus.[4] While these techniques have clearly been indispensable as adjuncts to surgical excision, they have also been utilized as primary treatment. Complete angiographic obliteration has been achieved in many cases. Long-term angiographic and clinical follow-up is needed to determine whether this obliteration is permanent or if recannulation occurs.[4] We have recently seen one patient who suffered repeat subarachnoid hemorrhage from a residual arteriovenous malformation 12 years following complete filling of the entire angioarchitecture of the AVM with liquid Silastic glue.

Determination of the operability of a spinal AVM hinges on the identification and characterization of the nidus. This may be easily identified on angiography with smaller, relatively slow-flow glomus AVMs with one or two medullary feeders, but can be very difficult in high-flow lesions whose early draining veins may obscure and overestimate the size of the nidus. For these lesions, embolization as an initial treatment is advisable. Magnetic resonance imaging (MRI) has become indispensable in defining the precise relationship to the spinal cord.

Figure 57.3 (**A**) Anteroposterior view and (**B**) lateral view of cervical intramedullary arteriovenous malformation supplied through multiple medullary arteries off the vertebral artery.

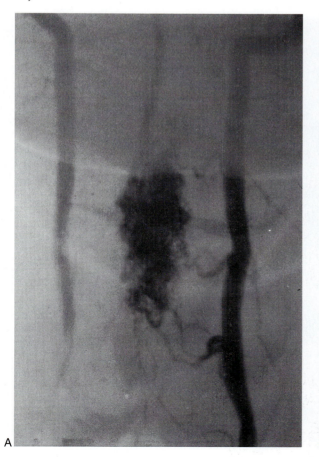
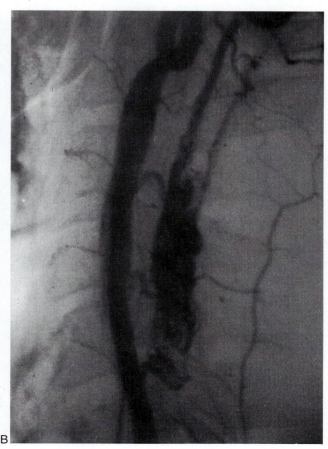

A   B

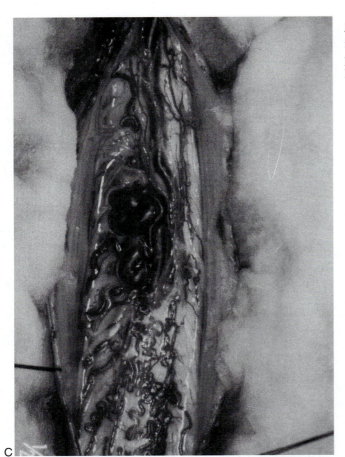

C

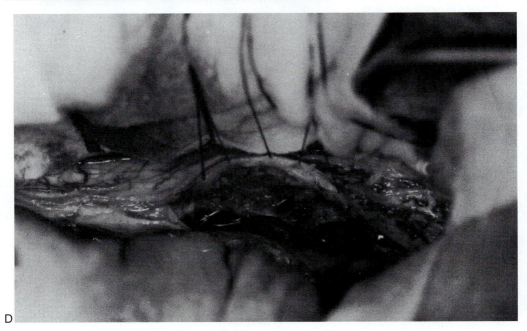

D

Figure 57.3 (*Continued*) (**C**) Intraoperative photograph shows feeding vessels and pial component of the nidus. (**D**) Operative photograph following complete resection of pial and intramedullary nidus.

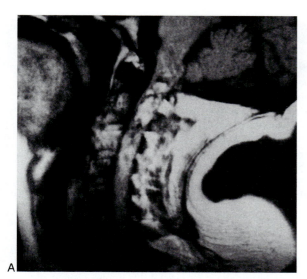

Figure 57.4 (**A**) T$_1$-weighted sagittal magnetic resonance imaging demonstrates intramedullary mass of upper cervical cord. The appearance is characteristic of a cavernous malformation. (**B**) Operative photograph clearly shows the cavernous malformation seen through the dorsal cord surface. (**C**) Operative photograph following complete resection of the cavernous malformation.

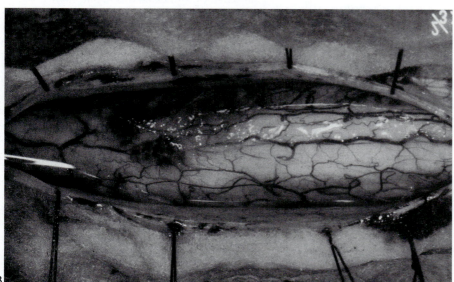

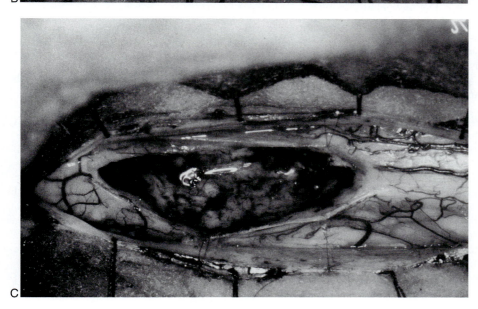

High-quality sagittal and axial MRIs will define the precise relationship ship of the nidus to the spinal cord. This is extremely useful in selecting treatment options, planning operative strategies (i.e., myelotomy), and assessing the risk of intervention. The technique of operative removal of spinal AVMs requires adequate visualization, exposure, and meticulous microsurgical techniques.[2,3,5,6,8,10] Although an intramedullary clot may assist the dissection, subarachnoid hemorrhage does not, so operative intervention should be delayed, if possible following subarachnoid hemorrhage.

The vast majority of these pial or intramedullary glomus AVMs are removed from a dorsal or dorsolateral approach with the patient in the prone position. The anterior vertebrectomy approach should be reserved for single anterior pial fistulas. Somatosensory evoked potentials are routinely employed and may be quite useful in assisting the removal of these vascular lesions. Following laminectomy and dural incision, the arachnoid is carefully dissected free from the underlying vessels and pia. Intermittent fine-needle intravascular pressure determination and/or Doppler sonography can help to distinguish artery from vein and assess the completeness of the resection. Superficial feeding arteries are cauterized and divided as they enter the malformation. The surgeon should resist the temptation to divide a large anterior medullary feeder along its ascending course. The descending limb of these ventrally placed feeders can be identified and divided near their entry into the malformation following dentate ligament section and gentle cord rotation from suture retraction on the proximal ligament stump.

The key to nidus dissection is to maintain the correct plane.[3] Entry into the nidus will cause troublesome bleeding and obscure planes. Conversely, a resection that is too wide increases the risk of neurologic deficit. The dissection should ideally take place right on the surface of the AVM. This will require a longitudinal myelotomy for intramedullary lesions. Gentle tension on the AVM with a suction dissector or bipolar forceps will identify small feeding arteries and draining veins, which are cauterized and divided. Larger draining veins are preserved as long as possible. Gentle cautery on the surface of the AVM will gradually shrink the nidus. The meticulous, often tedious, dissection continues systematically around the malformation. Anteriorly, the branches of the anterior spinal artery are encountered, cauterized, and divided to insure the complete removal of the AVM as it is extracted on the last draining vein (Fig. 57.3). The remaining vein can then be cauterized and divided. Hemostasis must be carefully secured prior to wound closure.

In summary, the dural fistulas are obliterated by either interventional techniques or direct surgery; the intradural glomus AVMs are removed surgically with or without the adjuvant of interventional techniques; anterior pial fistulas are obliterated by anterior spinal approaches, whereas the juvenile AVMs are generally void of therapeutic options. In general, 80% to 90% good or excellent results with total excision (confirmed by angiography) can be anticipated. As with intramedullary tumors, outcome tends to relate to the cord level involved and the clinical grade prior to operation. The most favorable outcome is achieved with cervical lesions and followed by lumbar enlargement/conus malformations. Thoracic cord AVMs, although fortunately rare, present a much greater risk of operative morbidity.

CAVERNOUS MALFORMATIONS

Cavernous malformations are rare congenital lesions that may become symptomatic. They are occasionally multiple or familial in occurrence. About 10% of central nervous system cavernous malformations arise within the spinal cord. The characteristic histologic pattern of cavernous malformations is thin- or thick-walled vessels of capillary structure arranged in a sinusoidal network without intervening parenchyma.

Spinal cavernous malformations may produce an acute, recurrent, or progressive myelopathy. Prior to MRI, many patients were likely erroneously diagnosed as having multiple sclerosis, transverse myelitis, or associated myelopathic disorders. Acute and recurrent presentation probably result from hemorrhage. Unlike hematomyelia neurologic deficit may evolve over several hours or even days. It is rare for a hemorrhage from a cavernous malformation to produce complete paraplegia, although we witnessed this in one 15-year-old patient.[7] A progressive course is probably secondary to enlargement of the malformation, either from repeated internal hemorrhage, vessel dilation, or capillary budding. A neurotoxic effect of hemosiderin or compromise of surrounding microcirculation are alternative proposed mechanisms.

The diagnosis of cavernous malformation is made with MRI. The characteristic appearance consists of a central area of mixed signal intensity surrounded by a hypointense rim of hemosiderin (Fig. 57.4). Myelography followed by a computed tomography (CT) scan is often reported as normal even in the presence of significant deficit.[7] Angiography is unrevealing.

We believe that surgery should be considered for symptomatic lesions. Although cavernous malformations are unencapsulated, there is usually a plane of gliotic/hemosiderin-stained tissue that serves as an adequate dissection plane. Most patients will improve or stabilize following excision.[7] Occasionally, however, the malformation will be quite diffuse and unresectable.

References

1. Aminoff MJ, Logue V: The prognosis of patients with spinal vascular malformations. Brain 97:211, 1974

2. Anson JA, Spetzler RF: Classification of spinal arteriovenous malformations and implications for treatment. BNI Q 8:2, 1992

3. Cogen P, Stein BM: Spinal cord arteriovenous malformations with significant intramedullary components. J Neurosurg 59:471, 1983

4. Hall WA, Oldfield EH, Doppman JL: Recanalization of spinal arteriovenous malformations following embolization. J Neurosurg 70:714, 1989

5. Heros RC, Debrun GM, Ojemann RG et al: Direct spinal arteriovenous fistula: a new type of spinal AVM: Case report. J Neurosurg 64:134, 1986

6. Krayenbühl H, Yasargil MG, McClintock HG: Treatment of spinal cord vascular malformations by surgical excision. J Neurosurg 30:427, 1969

7. McCormick PC, Michelsen WJ, Post KD et al: Cavernous malformations of the spinal cord. Neurosurgery 23:459, 1988

8. Muraszko KM, Oldfield EH: Vascular malformations of the spinal cord and dura. Neurosurg Clin North Am 1:631, 1990

9. Rosenblum B, Oldfield EH, Doppman JL et al: Spinal arteriovenous malformations: a comparison of dural arteriovenous fistulas and intradural AVMs in 81 patients. J Neurosurg 67:795, 1987

10. Spetzler RF, Zabramski JM, Flom RA: Management of juvenile spinal AVMs by embolization and operative excision. J Neurosurg 70:628, 1989

11. Tobin WD, Layton DD: The diagnosis and natural history of spinal cord arteriovenous malformations. Mayo Clin Proc 51:637, 1976

CHAPTER 58

Intracerebral Hemorrhage

Medical Considerations

CHRISTINE A.C. WIJMAN

CARLOS S. KASE

Intracerebral hemorrhage (ICH) accounts for approximately 10% of all strokes.[63] The causes of ICH are multiple. Frequent mechanisms are vascular malformations and illicit drug use in the young, hypertension in the middle-aged, and cerebral amyloid angiopathy in the elderly. Other less common causes include head trauma, tumors, moyamoya disease, vasculitis, anticoagulants, thrombolytics, and bleeding diatheses. On some occasions ICH has been associated with migraine, embolic cerebral infarction, carotid endarterectomy, correction of congenital heart defects in children, spät apoplexy following head trauma, exposure to cold weather, and surgery for trigeminal neuralgia.[12] The location of the hematoma varies with the different causes, and the clinical presentation depends on the location and the size of the hematoma.

The outcome of patients with ICH is generally poor in comparison with those with ischemic infarction. The mortality continues to be high, ranging between 20% and 56%, and many ICH survivors remain severely incapacitated.[46] Of 180 patients from greater Cincinnati who were hospitalized for ICH during 1988, 43% died within 30 days and only 12% were either normal or left with a minor handicap.[10] The prognosis of patients with ICH has been related to age,[31] level of consciousness on presentation,[22,35,75,99] volume of the hematoma,[22,31,35,75,99] and extension of the hemorrhage into the ventricular system.[22,75]

The medical management of patients with ICH commonly includes prevention and treatment of raised intracranial pressure (ICP), ventilatory support, control of elevated mean arterial blood pressure (MAP), and prevention and treatment of the common complications of ICH such as pneumonia and deep vein thrombosis (DVT). Surgical evacuation of the hematoma is employed most commonly in young patients with large hematoma volumes,[10] or in those with a worsening neurologic status. Although some evidence

shows that surgical removal of the hematoma may be of benefit in subgroups of patients with ICH, the absence of data from well-designed, prospective, randomized controlled trials has resulted in a lack of guidelines on the indications and timing for surgical intervention. In a few circumstances surgical treatment is superior to medical treatment alone. This is the case in noncomatose patients with cerebellar hemorrhage and signs of tegmental pontine compression, or with computed tomography (CT) showing a hematoma >3 cm in diameter, with local mass effect and obstructive hydrocephalus.[55,68,91] The current data from clinical trials comparing best medical management with and without surgical treatment in patients with ICH are limited. The availability in recent years of new, less invasive surgical techniques for intracranial clot removal has provided new treatment options,[51] however, their efficacy and safety in comparison with conventional open craniotomy are still untested. These techniques include stereotactic clot removal (with or without clot thrombolysis) and endoscopic clot removal. Because of the limited data on the outcome of patients treated with these various modalities, a well-designed, prospective, randomized multicenter trial is badly needed to determine whether patients with ICH should be treated surgically or nonsurgically. In the meantime, the treatment of ICH needs to be directed toward the individual patient. Variables such as the size and location of the hematoma, the patient's neurologic status, and the presence of accompanying medical complications guide the choice of the treatment approach.

In this chapter we discuss the current nonsurgical management of ICH, with an emphasis on early medical interventions, management and monitoring of raised ICP, as well as treatment of the medical complications encountered in these patients. In addition, the available data comparing the outcome of medical therapy alone versus medical and surgical therapy combined in patients with ICH are summarized.

Initial Evaluation

The initial management of patients with ICH includes medical stabilization of the patient (airway protection and control of vital signs), assessment of the neurologic status, determination of the cause of the hemorrhage, and assessment of the need for specific treatment measures including surgical removal of the hematoma, treatment of the underlying cause, and management of increased ICP.

The level of consciousness should be assessed promptly to determine whether the patient is able to protect the airway and avoid aspiration. In the event of lethargy or coma (i.e., a Glasgow Coma Scale [GCS] score ≤8), early endotracheal intubation is indicated to prevent pooling of oropharyngeal secretions, leading to inadequate oxygenation. Since vomiting frequently occurs early in these patients, aspiration of gastric contents poses an additional threat to airway patency and adequate oxygenation. Hypoxia adversely affects cerebral function and may also increase cerebral blood flow (CBF), resulting in elevation of ICP. Thus, adequate oxygenation should be ensured in patients with ICH, either with oxygen by nasal cannula or, if indicated, by early endotracheal intubation and mechanical ventilation. Unless the patient is unresponsive to tracheal stimulation, endotracheal intubation is best achieved by administration of intravenous thiopental (1 to 5 mg/kg) or lidocaine (1 mg/kg). These short-acting agents effectively block increases in ICP caused by tracheal and oropharyngeal stimulation, without having lasting effects on the level of consciousness or neurologic function.[9,21] Some authors advocate that every patient with ICH who requires endotracheal intubation should be immediately hyperventilated to maintain a PaCO$_2$ between 30 and 35 mmHg and should receive mannitol (0.5 to 1.0 g/kg intravenously) prior to any further diagnostic test.[9,21] In addition, intubated patients require placement of a nasogastric tube to prevent gastric distension.[9]

Another immediate concern in patients with acute ICH is the need for emergency management of abnormal vital signs at presentation. These include hemodynamic instability (which is rarely an issue in the early stages of ICH) and, most importantly, the presence of severe hypertension. Some patients with ICH and severe hypertension present with signs of congestive heart failure that require immediate treatment (oxygen therapy, digitalis, diuretics); however, it is severe hypertension itself that usually needs to be addressed at this stage. Since hypertension is a common cause of ICH[96] and, alternatively, the presence of increased ICP may lead to hypertension (the so-called Cushing effect), many patients will be hypertensive at the time of presentation to the emergency department. Furthermore, circumstances that are associated with acute rises in systemic blood pressure (BP) or CBF, either diffusely or focally, may provoke ICH, such as occurs in instances of illicit drug use, after carotid endarterectomy, after correction of congenital heart lesions, and with severe dental pain and spät apoplexy.[12,13] The BP values that require treatment in the setting of an acute ICH have not been established. There are no useful data derived from either randomized, prospective trials or clinical series linking the quality of BP control in the acute setting to events such as hematoma growth, early mortality, complications, or long-term functional outcome. Some retrospective series suggest that patients with ICH and an elevated MAP on presentation fare worse than those with a normal MAP.[20,95] However, the retrospective character of these data does not allow definite conclusions regarding the impact of BP management in the acute phase of ICH.[54] Even in the area of acute ischemic infarction, published criteria for BP management in the acute setting reflect individual institutional, experience-derived policies rather than guidelines arrived at by consensus based on available evidence.

Hypertension should be treated cautiously in patients with ICH because of the potential risks of excessive lowering of BP, resulting in a reduction of CBF and cerebral ischemia. The ideal antihypertensive agent is short acting and easily titrated and should not increase ICP or cause vasodilatation with the associated risk of excessive hypotension and cerebral ischemia. An appropriate agent is the α- and β-adrenergic blocker labetalol, which is administered intravenously in a 10-mg bolus, followed by doses of 10 to 20 mg after 10 minutes as needed, to a maximum of 160 mg. In a small prospective study of 10 patients with ICH, labetalol at doses between 5 and 25 mg as an adjunct therapy lowered the systolic BP by 6% to 19% and the diastolic BP by 3% to 26%, without having adverse effects on mental status or focal neurologic deficits.[73] Some clinicians recommend the use of labetalol in combination with diuretics.[80] A frequently used agent when BP is severely elevated is intravenous sodium nitroprusside because it is easily titrated and has a rapid and predictable effect on BP. This agent has the potential of causing cerebral vasodilatation, but it has not been reported to raise ICP significantly.[80] Another vasodilator sometimes used as an oral agent is hydralazine, which has the potential of causing excessive hypotension and an increase in ICP.[6] Sublingual nifedipine (10 mg) is a frequently chosen agent to lower high BP in the acute setting, but it may cause an unpredictable and excessive reduction in BP with the risk of inducing brain ischemia. Other agents that may be used include parenteral clonidine, trimethaphan, and angiotensin-converting enzyme inhibitors.[21] Interactions of BP, ICP, and CBF in patients with disturbed cerebral autoregulation are described in detail below.

Coagulation parameters, platelet count, and urine for toxic screen should be obtained as soon as the patient arrives in the emergency room. In addition, a serum fibrinogen level is helpful in patients who recently received thrombolytic therapy. Patients who have an ICH while receiving anticoagulant therapy generally have larger hematomas and a less favorable outcome.[31,49,78] Abnormalities in the coagulation status of these patients should be corrected immediately to prevent further enlargement of the hematoma. Patients who received intravenous heparin therapy and have a prolonged activated partial thromboplastin time should be treated with protamine sulfate at a dose of approximately 1 mg for every 100 units of heparin present in the plasma.[69] The amount of heparin present in the plasma can be estimated from its half-life, which is dose related, and the amount of drug most recently administered.[57] Only the minimal required dose of protamine sulfate should be administered to neutralize the heparin because the drug interacts in vivo with platelets, fibrinogen, and other plasma proteins and may cause an anticoagulant effect of its own.[57] Protamine sulfate should be administered by slow intravenous injection over a 10-minute period in doses not to exceed 50 mg because of the potential risk of severe systemic hypotension.[57] Patients with a prolonged prothrombin time (PT) secondary to warfarin are often treated with subcutaneous or intravenous vitamin K_1 (5 to 25 mg)[57,69]; however, improvement of hemostasis following vitamin K_1 administration does not occur for several hours, regardless of the route of administration, and 24 hours or longer may be needed for maximal effect. Therefore, for an immediate effect, either fresh-frozen plasma (10 to 20 ml/kg) or prothrombin complex concentrate should be administered in large enough quantities to normalize the PT.[57,69] The results of a retrospective study in 17 patients with anticoagulant-related ICH suggest that prothrombin complex concentrate acts more rapidly than fresh-frozen plasma in reversing the anticoagulation effect, but it carries the risk of triggering generalized thromboembolism.[32]

The incidence of ICH following thrombolytic therapy (streptokinase, urokinase, tissue plasminogen activator) is likely to increase with the widespread use of intravenous tissue plasminogen activator for acute myocardial infarction[48] and acute ischemic stroke,[64] including the use in selected patients of intra-arterial thrombolysis for acute intracranial occlusions. Intracerebral hematomas in this setting may occur at multiple sites and frequently have a poor outcome. The risk of ICH in patients who receive thrombolytic therapy varies with the type of agent and dose used, and it increases when anticoagulants are administered simultaneously.[48] Furthermore, patients with low body weight, hypertension, old age, recent ischemic stroke or head injury, previous ICH, recent major surgery, and abnormalities in coagulation status are at increased risk of bleeding complications.[17,77] Hemorrhage secondary to thrombolytic therapy may not only result from lysis of fibrin at a site of vascular injury, but may also be mediated by a systemic lytic state resulting from formation of plasmin, which produces fibrinogenolysis and inactivation of other coagulation factors.[57] Information regarding the treatment of ICH secondary to thrombolytic therapy is scarce.[57] If transfusions are needed, at least 4 units of packed red blood cells, 4 to 6 units of cryoprecipitate or fresh-frozen plasma, and 1 unit of single-donor platelets are recommended.[77] Some authors advocate treatment with aminocaproic acid (5 g over 60 minutes loading dose, followed by 1 g/h until bleeding is controlled), which inhibits the fibrinolytic system by binding to plasminogen and plasmin, thus preventing the binding of plasmin to fibrin.[17,21,26] However, definite benefit from this agent has not been documented and it has the disadvantage of promoting clot formation, with a risk of DVT and pulmonary embolism. This in part results from the fact that blood clots that form during treatment with aminocaproic acid are not lysed by the fibrinolytic system.[57] Patients with ICH in association with dysfunctional platelets or thrombocytopenia should be treated with platelet transfusions; 6 units usually suffice to maintain hemostasis.

A urine toxic screen may be helpful in revealing the mechanism of ICH, in particular in young patients.[98] The occurrence of ICH has been associated with many recreational and over-the-counter drugs including ethanol,[1,53] cocaine hydrochloride,[1,53] "crack" cocaine,[34] amphetamines,[88] Talwin-pyribenzamine ("Ts and blues"),[15] methylphenidate, phencyclidine, and phenylpropanolamine.[29,47,88]

The sequence of neurologic symptoms in conjunction with the findings on the neurologic examination often allows identification of the location and approximate size of the hematoma; these features are discussed in detail in Chapter 25. When evaluating a patient with ICH, it is important to keep in mind that early neurologic deterioration is common[59] and is often the result of progressive hematoma enlargement within a few hours from onset.[11] Serial neurologic assessments are necessary to follow the patient's course, and observation in an intensive care unit is indicated in those with a depressed sensorium and medium-sized or large hematomas.

Imaging of the brain with a noncontrast CT scan is indicated in every patient with suspected ICH. Follow-up CT scans should be obtained if the neurologic status of the patient deteriorates to assess for an increase in hematoma volume and the development of edema and hydrocephalus. CT reliably identifies most hematomas as a hyperdense lesion[24]; however, in patients with severe anemia (hematocrit <20) the hematoma may appear isodense or even hypodense.[44] The mechanism causing the ICH can often be suspected based on the medical history of the patient and the appearance of the hematoma on CT scan.[45] In patients with atypical hemorrhage features (e.g., subdural extension of the hematoma), location suggestive of aneurysmal hemorrhage, or without an identified cause, further imaging with magnetic resonance imaging (MRI) and magnetic resonance angiography is indicated. If these are not diagnostic, cerebral angiography is indicated to determine the presence of an underlying vascular abnormality. Angiography is also appropriate in patients with cocaine-related ICH because vascular abnormalities (arteriovenous malformation, aneurysm, vasculitis) are frequently present. Cerebral angiography is also indicated when a ruptured aneurysm is considered in patients with an intracerebral hematoma in the proximity of the sylvian fissure or with extension into the interhemisperic fissure, suggestive of a middle cerebral artery or anterior communicating artery aneurysm, respectively. In patients with a suspected small vascular malformation, follow-up imaging studies may be required several weeks after initial presentation to allow for visualization of the lesion after resorption of the hematoma. Repeated enhanced MRI studies are sometimes necessary to reveal an underlying primary or metastatic brain tumor presenting with ICH.

The need for emergency neurosurgical evaluation is dictated by the location of the hematoma, its size, and the condition of the patient. In general, neurosurgical consultation is recommended in most patients with intracranial hemorrhage to assess for the need of ventriculostomy, placement of an ICP monitor, and removal of the hematoma either by open craniotomy or by one of the recently available less invasive surgical techniques.

Medical Management

Patients with small (≤20 ml) intracerebral hematomas that do not increase ICP generally do well without specific treatment measures. Conversely, patients with large hematomas (>60 ml) who present in a comatose state generally have a poor outcome regardless of therapy. Patients with hematomas of intermediate size are most likely to benefit from medical and surgical therapy, in particular those patients who have a deterioration in their neurologic status after hospital admission. The following discussion focuses on the management of patients with intracerebral hematomas that are large enough to raise the ICP.

Brain injury in ICH is caused by tissue destruction and by compression and displacement of brain tissue by the rapidly expanding mass lesion. Secondary brain injury may result from ischemia in the area immediately surrounding the hemorrhage, brain herniation, and elevated ICP resulting in a decrease of CBF to ischemic values. The medical management of patients with ICH is primarily directed toward preventing or limiting these mechanisms of secondary injury to healthy cerebral tissue.

PHYSIOLOGY OF INCREASED INTRACRANIAL PRESSURE

A basic knowledge of the relationships among cerebral volume, CBF, BP, cerebral perfusion pressure (CPP), and ICP and the factors that influence these variables is helpful in understanding the rationale of therapies aimed at decreasing raised ICP in patients with ICH.

The pressure inside the rigid skull is determined by the size of its nearly incompressible contents, the brain parenchyma, cerebrospinal fluid (CSF), and blood. The intracranial volume is composed of 80% brain and interstitial fluids, 10% CSF, and 10% blood, which is predominantly contained in the low-pressure, high-capacitance venous system.[85] Under normal circumstances, the blood-brain barrier regulates brain volume by controlling the transport of free water from the blood. Disturbance of this regulatory function after brain injury results in leakage of water into the extracellular space, leading to edema formation and an increase in brain volume.[21] The volume of the CSF is tightly regulated, with production (at a rate of approximately 20 ml/h) matching absorption.[85] Obstruction of CSF flow at the level of the ventricles or at the level of the arachnoidal granulations results in increased CSF volume (hydrocephalus). The production of CSF usually does not change in patients with increased ICP and hydrocephalus, but absorption does increase to some extent under these circumstances.[85]

Cerebral blood volume (CBV) is determined by the CBF and the size of the capacitance vessels within the brain.[21] Therefore, factors that alter CBF or the tone of the capacitance vessels change CBV as well. Normal CBF is approximately 75 ml/100 g/min of gray matter and 45 ml/100 g/min of white matter and is regulated by a number of factors including CPP, $PaCO_2$, PaO_2, and cerebral metabolic rate.[21,85] If CBF is reduced below the 12 to 18 ml/100 g/min range, permanent neuronal damage is likely to occur.[85] Since CBF measurements are difficult to perform in vivo, the CPP is used in clinical practice to guide the adequacy of the cerebral circulation. CPP is defined as the difference between MAP and the greater of either the ICP or the cerebral venous pressure. Under normal circumstances, CPP is in the range 70 to 100 mmHg. In the absence of brain injury, in normotensive adults, cerebral autoregulation maintains CBF constant over a wide range of perfusion pressures, approximately from 50 to 150 mmHg.[21] In long-standing hypertensive patients, both the upper and lower limits of autoregulation are elevated (i.e., a relatively higher CPP is needed to maintain a normal CBF).[21,85] Cerebral autoregulation is frequently disrupted globally or focally in an unpredictable manner in patients with damaged brain areas.[85] Under these circumstances, as well as outside the limits of autoregulation, CBF becomes passively dependent on CPP. Small decreases in BP may then result in ischemia, whereas elevations in BP increase CBF (and CBV), promoting the formation of edema and raising ICP.

CBF increases with increasing $PaCO_2$ within the range of 20 to 80 mmHg. This latter response occurs rapidly, within minutes of changing the $PaCO_2$. The increase of CBF induced by hypercarbia generally lasts <12 hours, in spite of continued elevation of $PaCO_2$, presumably because of a gradual normalization of CSF pH. Raising $PaCO_2$ to 80 mmHg doubles the CBF, and lowering the $PaCO_2$ to 20 mmHg reduces CBF by 40%.[85] This latter response is mediated by decreasing CSF $PaCO_2$ and increasing CSF pH. This mechanism is the basis of therapeutic hyperventilation, one of the most effective measures to reduce ICP.[21] CBF remains constant with changes in PaO_2, until it falls below about 50 mmHg, at which time CBF starts to increase rapidly. CBF is tightly correlated with the metabolic demands of the brain. In circumstances that increase the metabolic demands such as seizures and fever, CBF (and thus CBV) increases. Alternatively, CBF decreases when the metabolic rate decreases, such as during hypothermia and with the use of high-dose intravenous barbiturates.

ICP remains relatively constant under normal conditions (between 10 and 15 mmHg) in spite of changes in intracranial volume. To maintain a constant ICP with increases in volume of any of the contents of the skull, several compensatory mechanisms can take place, including migration of CSF into the spinal subarachnoid space and movement of venous blood into the systemic circulation. This is called the compliance of intracranial tissues. When the compensatory mechanisms are exhausted, ICP starts to increase. How much compensatory ability remains at a given point in time cannot be estimated from the ICP itself as long as it is in the normal range. When the ICP is increased, compensation has obviously failed.[85] In treating patients with ICH, knowledge of the residual compliance may help in anticipating dangerous elevations in ICP. Severe elevations in ICP can decrease the CPP to levels below 50 mmHg, resulting in brain ischemia. In addition, raised ICP may contribute to pressure gradients within the cranial cavity, resulting in tissue shifts and brain herniation. Diffusely raised ICP, which develops slowly over a long period of time, is surprisingly well tolerated in most patients. Management of elevated ICP consists of specific treatment measures aimed at lowering the raised ICP itself as well as treatment measures that prevent or treat the factors that may contribute to an elevated ICP.

INTRACRANIAL PRESSURE MONITORING

The neurologic status of a patient with an acutely developing intracerebral mass lesion must be interpreted in the context of the location and size of the mass, its mechanical effects on other brain areas, and the presence of associated factors such as hydrocephalus and raised ICP. An impaired level of consciousness in patients with ICH is generally a poor prognostic sign associated with increased mortality.[99] Proposed mechanisms for stupor and coma in these patients include direct destruction or distortion of diencephalic structures by extension of the hematoma, acute obstructive hydrocephalus, acutely raised ICP with global ischemia, and brain herniation with downward displacement of brain tissue through the tentorial opening with progressive brain stem compression. Ropper and Gress[81] demonstrated a correlation between level of consciousness and the amount of horizontal displacement of the pineal gland in eight patients with ICH of ≥ 55 cm^3. Coma was associated with ≥ 8 mm displacement of the pineal gland.

Because of the multiple mechanisms that may contribute to a decreased level of consciousness in a patient with ICH, it is impossible to assess the presence of raised ICP reliably on clinical grounds alone, in the absence of ICP measurements. Papo et al[71] did not find a good correlation between ICP and level of consciousness in 66 patients with supratentorial ICH, except at the two extremes of ICP. Patients who were alert had normal or slightly elevated ICP (< 20 mmHg), and patients who were in deep coma had severely increased ICP (> 30 mmHg) with no response to treatment measures. In patients with intermediate levels of ICP, the correlation between ICP and level of consciousness was poor. Ropper and King[83] reported on the ICP of 10 comatose patients with supratentorial ICH. Even though all 10 patients were comatose, ICP varied widely: it was < 20 mmHg in four patients, between 20 and 30 mmHg in four patients, and > 30 mmHg in two. On the other hand, Janny et al[37] found some correlation between level of consciousness and ICP in 60 patients with ICH. Average ICP in 19 patients who were alert was 22.2 mmHg, in 23 patients described as stuporous it was 25.3 mmHg, and in 18 comatose patients it was 37 mmHg. These data indicate that ICP is generally not elevated in patients with ICH who are alert, and it may or may not be elevated in patients with ICH who have depressed level of consciousness. Since the presence or absence of elevated ICP cannot be predicted in the latter group of patients on clinical grounds alone, many clinicians recommend measuring ICP if the GCS score is ≤ 8.[21]

The goal in detecting raised ICP is to prevent the development of critically low CPP, resulting in brain ischemia, and to anticipate and prevent dangerous tissue shifts leading to brain stem compression. Unquestionably, the use of continuous ICP monitoring is helpful in evaluating the treatment measures that are intended to decrease ICP. In addition, knowledge of a normal ICP will prevent the institution of potentially harmful and unnecessary therapies. However, no controlled study has demonstrated a benefit of continuous ICP monitoring on the outcome of patients with ICH.[37] Duff et al[25] reported on the medical management of 12 consecutive patients with ICH with continuous ICP monitoring. Treatment was aimed at maintaining CPP > 50 mmHg and ICP < 40 mmHg. All patients survived except for one who died of a myocardial infarction 2 months after discharge. The authors concluded that treatment based on continuous ICP monitoring and CPP may improve outcome in patients with ICH. Some authors have advocated the use of ICP monitoring to decide which patients should be subjected to surgical drainage

of the hematoma based on limited evidence that patients who fail to respond to maximum medical treatment need to be considered for surgical treatment as the only therapeutic measure likely to provide benefit.[36,83]

The principal techniques used to monitor ICP include intraventricular catheters, epidural/subarachnoid screws, and fiberoptic systems.[4] Intraventricular catheters are especially useful in patients with extension of the hemorrhage into the ventricular system, as they allow for periodic drainage of the CSF.[9] An additional advantage is that information regarding intracranial compliance can be readily obtained. The main problem with ventricular catheters is the occurrence of infection. Early detection of CSF infections can be accomplished by routine CSF collection for glucose, cell count, Gram stain, and culture; however, multiple CSF collections may in turn increase the risk of infection.[4] Prophylactic antibiotics and catheter replacement every 5 to 7 days help reduce the risk of infections.[21] Epidural and subdural hematomas, as well as intraventricular and intracerebral hematomas, may occasionally develop after placement of a ventricular catheter. Obstruction of the catheter may result from intraventricular clot or brain edema with compression of the ventricle.[4] A mostly theoretical concern when using an intraventricular catheter is the occurrence of tissue shifts resulting from the unilateral placement of a ventriculostomy that leads to a differential in pressure between the two ventricles.

The subarachnoid screw (bolt) has the advantage of low infection and hemorrhage rates. Its most common problem is obstruction of the bolt by debris or herniation of brain tissue into the lumen of the bolt. Malfunctioning of the bolt may not be recognized, leading to spurious ICP values and potentially inappropriate treatment measures.[4]

Fiberoptic systems are preferred by most clinicians because they are easy to use, have a low infection rate, and can be easily transported.[4] One problem is that fiberoptic systems cannot be calibrated after insertion.[4,21] Since these systems are subject to 'drift', resulting in inaccurately high or low ICP measurements, replacement of the catheter is recommended every 5 days.[9]

THERAPIES AIMED AT REDUCING ELEVATED INTRACRANIAL PRESSURE

When treating the patient with ICH and raised ICP, it is important to pay close attention to the neurologic status of the patient and to treat elevated ICP in this context. Absolute ICP measurements can be inaccurate at times, and the treatment of the patient should prevail over treatment of the ICP. Treatment of raised ICP is best performed by those who have gained ample experience in this area because the most difficult treatment decisions involve the synergistic effects of the various treatment measures combined. The major medical treatments aimed at reducing raised ICP are hyperventilation, osmotic therapy, removal of CSF, and intravenous barbiturates[80] (Table 58.1).

Hyperventilation

Hyperventilation decreases arterial PaCO$_2$, leading to cerebral vasoconstriction through CSF alkalosis, with reduction in ICP.[52] The vasoconstriction only takes place in the brain areas

Table 58.1 Major Therapies for Acutely Increased Intracranial Pressure

Treatment	Dose	Advantages	Limitations
Hyperventilation	PaCO$_2$ 25–33 mmHg RR 10–16/min	Immediate onset, well tolerated	Hypotension, barotrauma, duration hours or less
Osmotic therapy	Mannitol 0.5–1 g/kg 3% NaCl	Rapid onset, titratable, predictable	Hypotension, hypokalemia, duration hours or days
Intravenous barbiturates	Pentobarbital 1.5 mg/kg	Mutes BP and respiratory fluctuations	Hypotension, small fixed pupils, duration days
Ventriculostomy	—	Allows ICP measurement, rapid ICP reduction	Infection, intracranial hemorrhage resulting from placement

Abbreviations: ICP, intracranial pressure; RR, respiratory rate; BP, blood pressure. (Modified from Ropper.[80])

that are unaffected by the ICH, as the vasculature in affected areas has lost its autoregulation. Hyperventilation can be achieved by using intermittent mandatory ventilation or assist/control ventilation.[21] Hypocarbia is produced by raising the rate of the ventilator with a tidal volume of approximately 12 to 14 ml/kg.[80] The therapeutic goal is to obtain an initial PaCO$_2$ between 28 and 35 mmHg, followed by a PaCO$_2$ between 25 and 30 mmHg if ICP continues to be elevated.[46] Lowering the PaCO$_2$ further may theoretically cause excessive vasoconstriction, leading to ischemia in healthy brain tissue. Hyperventilation decreases ICP in <30 minutes, but this effect is short-lived, probably lasting only for several hours, as the pH of the CSF tends to normalize despite continuing arterial hypocarbia. Therefore, additional measures to decrease ICP should be taken simultaneously. Since prolonged systemic alkalosis may cause complications, the patient should be weaned off hyperventilation after 24 to 72 hours. Because of the risk of rebound increase in ICP after discontinuation of hyperventilation, weaning should be accomplished in small steps over a period of 4 to 24 hours and should be guided by the clinical response.[21] Intubation is usually maintained until the patient is alert, following commands, and capable of protecting the airway.[21]

In some patients hyperventilation may, paradoxically, *increase* ICP, presumably because of transmission of positive pressure from the lungs that results in increased cerebral venous pressure. This effect is minimized by raising the patient's head.[80] Another side effect associated with hyperventilation is hypotension resulting from low filling pressures of the heart, which can be prevented by maintaining adequate intravascular volume, without administering free water.[80]

Osmotic Therapy

Osmotic therapy is used to help reduce ICP by transporting water out of the brain. In patients with hematomas of small volume, fluid restriction and free water reduction may be sufficient to control ICP. However, in patients requiring osmotic agents and/or loop diuretics, iso-osmotic fluids or hypertonic saline should be administered to prevent volume contraction and hypotension. Osmotic therapy aims at increasing serum osmolality, creating an osmotic gradient between the intracellular and extracellular compartments, and drawing water from

the brain into the plasma. Mannitol and loop diuretics are the mainstay of osmotic therapy. Mannitol usually reduces ICP and increases CPP and CBF within 10 to 20 minutes or less. Mannitol acts predominantly on the healthy brain with intact autoregulation.[85] In addition to increasing serum osmolality, mannitol increases CBF and reduces CSF production.[21] The increase in CBF after mannitol administration is probably in part a result of a decrease in blood viscosity.[21,80] The standard dose of mannitol is 0.75 to 1.0 g/kg initially, followed by 0.25 to 0.5 g/kg every 3 to 5 hours depending on ICP, CPP, serum osmolality, and clinical findings.[80] Each bolus should be given slowly, over at least 10 minutes to avoid hemolysis. Lower, more frequent doses may be as effective and are probably easier to use in terms of fluid and electrolyte management. The goal is to obtain an approximate serum osmolality of 320 mosm/L and a euvolemic state. Loop diuretics such as furosemide can be used in combination with mannitol to keep the serum osmolality at the desired level when mannitol alone is inadequate.

The main side effects of mannitol include wide variations in blood volume and electrolytes, leading to hypo- or hypernatremia, hypokalemia, congestive heart failure, volume contraction, or renal failure. Hypokalemia must be corrected with potassium replacement. Volume contraction and hypotension should be avoided, in particular in patients with decreased cardiac filling pressures from mechanical ventilation, by replacing with iso-osmotic or hypertonic fluids. An appropriate choice is normal (0.9%) saline, which has an osmolality of 310 mosm/L. If hypotension cannot be corrected rapidly, treatment with vasopressors is in order to ensure adequate cerebral perfusion. The euvolemic hyperosmolar state should be maintained for several days after stabilization of ICP. Fluid status, serum osmolality, and blood electrolytes should be followed closely to guide therapy. Because of the potential for a rebound increase in ICP after the abrupt discontinuation of mannitol, serum osmolality should be lowered slowly over 1 to 2 weeks. Although other osmotic agents have been used in clinical practice, none has been found to be superior to mannitol. A recent randomized, placebo-controlled trial of intravenous glycerol in patients with ICH, which included 107 patients in the treatment group and 109 controls, showed no difference in mortality or functional outcome between the two groups; however, there was no information on ICP provided in either group to assess the need for and effect of glycerol treatment.[105]

Sedation

Sedation with intravenous agents including benzodiazepines, barbiturates, narcotics, and butyrophenones plays a limited role in the management of patients with raised ICP. These agents reduce brain metabolism and thus decrease CBF and ICP; however, side effects such as hypotension, pulmonary infections, and interference with the neurologic examination greatly limit their clinical usefulness. Intravenous barbiturates probably reduce CBF and metabolism the most, resulting in a decrease in ICP and CBV.[80] In addition, barbiturates act as free radical scavengers and may limit peroxidative damage to lipid membranes.[90] A commonly used agent is thiopental at a dose of 1 to 5 mg/kg, which causes a clinically significant reduction in ICP within seconds and is particularly useful for the prevention of transient increases in ICP in maneuvers such as endotracheal intubation and pulmonary suctioning. Its effects last only for minutes unless repeated large doses are administered.[80] Prolonged sedation can be accomplished with intravenous pentobarbital, which is given in an initial loading dose of 3 to 10 mg/kg followed by 1 to 2 mg/kg/h. Severe hypotension may occur with administration of this agent, requiring the use of inotropic support to maintain BP. No controlled studies have demonstrated an improved clinical outcome in patients with ICH who have been treated with high-dose intravenous barbiturates. Some clinicians believe that a role exists for these agents in the management of patients with raised ICP who are resistant to maximum conventional therapy aimed at reducing raised ICP.[80] A recent study investigated the effect of barbiturate coma with thiopental infusion in 60 patients with increased ICP due to large *ischemic* hemispheric infarctions.[90] Although a significant decrease in ICP was observed in 50 patients, the ICP returned to pretreatment values after 6 hours in most patients. Furthermore, CPP did not improve because of sustained hypotension. Only five (8%) of the patients survived, and the authors concluded that the only indication for barbiturate coma in patients with severe ischemic brain edema is "to buy time for more effective therapies to control ICP."

Ventriculostomy

Ventriculostomy with CSF removal is an effective means of reducing ICP. Ventriculostomy allows for both drainage of CSF and ICP monitoring and is indicated in patients with raised ICP and hydrocephalus, in conjunction with a deteriorating level of alertness. Patients particularly at risk for the development of hydrocephalus are those with thalamic, cerebellar, and caudate hemorrhages, as the proximity of the ICH to the ventricular system allows early ventricular extension of the hemorrhage. In addition, obstructive hydrocephalus can result from a hematoma that causes tissue shifts with subsequent compression of the foramen of Monro, the aqueduct of Sylvius, or the fourth ventricle. The potential complications of ventricular catheters have been discussed above.

Corticosteroids

Corticosteroids (dexamethasone) have not been shown to be of benefit in the management of patients with ICH. Tellez and Bauer[94] in a pre-CT era study compared the outcome of 19 patients with ICH receiving 120 mg of dexamethasone over a 10-day period with 21 patients with ICH receiving placebo. The mortality rate was similar in the two groups: 89.5% in the treatment group and 76.2% in the control group. Poungvarin et al[76] tested the effect of dexamethasone (150 mg over 9 days) on survival in 93 patients with ICH by means of a randomized, double-blind, placebo-controlled trial. Mortality was not different between the two groups after 21 days. However, the trial was terminated prematurely because of a significantly poorer outcome in the dexamethasone-treated patients, mainly as a result of systemic complications from steroid treatment. On the basis of this study, the routine use of corticosteroids in ICH is not recommended.

MEASURES AIMED AT CONTROLLING THE FACTORS THAT CONTRIBUTE TO ELEVATED INTRACRANIAL PRESSURE

Treatable factors that may contribute to elevated ICP are listed in Table 58.2.

Elevated Blood Pressure

Blood pressure management in patients with ICH is of great importance in maintaining a normal CPP. In the absence of autoregulation, modest elevations in MAP may increase CPP, with a potential for exaggerating perihematoma edema and ICP, while moderate reductions in MAP can lead to a decrease in CPP and promotion of cerebral ischemia.[21] Treatment of MAP should be guided by ICP to maintain a CPP of approximately 60 to 70 mmHg.[80]

Many drugs can decrease MAP in the setting of raised ICP. Since ICP itself can raise MAP (Cushing's reflex), treatment of ICP alone sometimes decreases MAP to acceptable values. However, if hypertension persists in association with increased CPP (above approximately 85 to 100 mmHg), then pharmacologic treatment is indicated. The agents that are frequently used in clinical practice to reduce BP in patients with ICH have been discussed above.

Table 58.2 Factors that Contribute to Increased Intracranial Pressure

Hypertension
Hypoxia
Seizures
Fever
Head position
Increased intrathoracic pressure

Hypoxia

Severe hypoxia (PaO$_2$ ≤50 mmHg) induces cerebral vasodilatation with subsequent increase in CBF and CBV in patients with poor intracranial compliance, resulting in an increase in ICP. The value of early endotracheal intubation for the maintenance of adequate oxygenation has already been discussed. Adequate oxygenation (PaO$_2$ of 100 to 150 mmHg), in combination with appropriate hemoglobin levels and cardiac output, is needed to ensure sufficient oxygen delivery to the brain.

Seizures

Seizures often occur in patients with ICH, generally within 24 hours of hemorrhage onset.[14,27,89] They relate to the location of the hemorrhage and are particularly common in patients with lobar hemorrhages.[14,27,50,89,103] Seizures increase the metabolic demands of the brain, resulting in an increase in CBF, CBV, and ICP, even in paralyzed patients.[80] If the increase in metabolic requirements cannot be met by an increase in CBF, ischemia may occur with subsequent brain damage. Therefore, seizures should be treated immediately, initially with intravenous diazepam (5 mg), followed by a loading dose of intravenous fosphenytoin at 15 to 20 mg phenytoin sodium equivalents (PE)/kg under cardiac monitoring. Fosphenytoin is a water-soluble, phosphate ester prodrug of phenytoin. The agent can be infused three times more rapidly than phenytoin at a rate of 100 to 150 mg PE/min. It also causes significantly less irritation at the infusion site compared with intravenous phenytoin. When seizures recur in spite of adequate serum phenytoin levels, loading with intravenous phenobarbital (15 to 18 mg/kg) is indicated, which has the disadvantage of causing somnolence and respiratory depression. If seizures are still not controlled with these two agents, intravenous thiopental should be considered, which has the disadvantage of producing hypotension during its administration.

The need for seizure prophylaxis in patients with ICH is controversial. Some clinicians advocate anticonvulsant therapy in every patient with a lobar or superficial subcortical hemorrhage,[9,21] while others only recommend treatment when seizures occur.[29] We favor the latter approach, as the available evidence suggests that most patients who do not have a seizure within 24 hours of ICH onset do not develop seizures subsequently.[27]

Fever

Fever increases the metabolic rate of the brain (5% to 7% for each centigrade degree), requiring an increase in CBF to meet metabolic demands.[80] Hence, fever should be treated aggressively with acetaminophen and cooling blankets. Infections should be detected and treated as early as possible. Uncontrolled severe hyperthermia of central origin reflects a profound autonomic disturbance and is usually a grave prognostic sign. It commonly occurs in patients with large pontine hemorrhages, generally as a preterminal event.

Head Position

Head position may significantly affect ICP. Raising the head relative to the trunk reduces ICP in most patients; however, occasional patients fail to respond in this manner.[84] In patients with elevated ICP, raising the head may decrease CPP because of a drop in BP with head elevation.[80] Feldman et al[28] studied the effect of elevation of the head to 30 degrees in 22 head-injured patients, observing a significant decrease in ICP without changes in CPP and CBF. In a patient with increased ICP and an ICP monitoring device, direct measurement of ICP and CPP in each body position is recommended to determine optimal positioning of the patient. If these measurements are not available and the patient is well hydrated, 20 to 30 degrees of head elevation is probably beneficial in comparison with the supine position. Elevation of the head can sometimes help reduce the effects of high airway pressures on ICP (see below).[21,80] Care should always be taken to maintain the head in midline position because head rotation produces an increase in ICP by impairing jugular venous drainage.[80]

Increased Intrathoracic Pressure

Increased intrathoracic pressure may raise ICP further in patients with poor intracranial compliance. Positive airway pressure may reduce CPP, either increasing intrathoracic pressure, central venous pressure, and cerebral venous pressure, or decreasing venous return to the heart with lowering of BP.[80] Circumstances that lead to positive airway pressure include coughing, endotracheal suctioning, and ventilation with positive end-expiratory pressure, in particular in patients with poor intracranial compliance. By using hyperventilation with 100% oxygen before and after suctioning, or intravenous thiopental or lidocaine, some of the effects of these maneuvers on ICP may be reduced.[21] In addition, chest physiotherapy should be performed in such a way that coughing, "bucking" against the ventilator, autonomic responses, hypoxia, and hypercarbia are limited.[80]

SYSTEMIC MANAGEMENT

Early institution of nutritional support is important to ensure immunocompetency and to prevent skin breakdown and muscle wasting.[21] Enteral feeding is the preferred mode for nutritional support because it is safer, is easier to manage, prevents stress ulcers, and maintains gut integrity.[16,21] A concentrated formula is preferable in those with increased ICP to avoid the administration of large fluid loads. Careful monitoring of the fluid balance is essential.

Prevention of gastrointestinal hemorrhage is best accomplished by institution of tube feedings[21] and administration of antacids or H$_2$ histamine blockers.[82] One concern with the use of these agents is that they alter gastric acidity, hence promoting nosocomial infection.[82] Increased gastric pH allows for bacterial growth and increases the risk of aspiration pneumonia.[82] Sucralfate has been proposed as an alternative,[23] as it provides gastrointestinal bleeding prophylaxis without changing gastric pH.[82]

Hyperglycemia should be avoided in patients with ICH because of evidence that hyperglycemia may have adverse effects on the injured brain.[102] Therefore, blood glucose should be managed meticulously with appropriate amounts of regular insulin.

The incidence of DVT in neurosurgical patients has been estimated as 29% to 43%; only 17% are symptomatic.[16] The presence of thrombus in the thigh vessels carries a higher risk of pulmonary embolism than DVT in the calf vessels.[16] Measures to prevent DVT are indicated in every immobilized and postoperative patient with ICH either with pneumatic air boots or low-dose subcutaneous heparin. Boer et al[7] reported that early (day 2) low-dose heparin significantly decreased the incidence of pulmonary embolism in patients with spontaneous ICH without increasing the risk of rebleeding. When the patient with ICH develops a DVT in spite of prophylactic therapy, placement of an inferior vena cava filter is indicated to prevent pulmonary embolism, as continuous intravenous heparin therapy is contraindicated in these patients.

Close monitoring and prompt correction of electrolyte imbalances (potassium and sodium) are particularly important in patients who are treated with osmotic therapy as outlined earlier.

Surgical Versus Nonsurgical Management of Intracerebral Hemorrhage

Only a few randomized controlled trials have compared surgical with nonsurgical treatment of patients with ICH. This issue will remain unsettled until the outcomes of specific subgroups of patients with ICH treated with best medical therapy with and without surgery are compared in a randomized controlled trial. The data that are available to date are inconclusive and mostly derived from clinical series with several types of biases. However, some of these studies have provided useful information that serves as a basis for the design of an appropriate prospective controlled randomized clinical trial. The studies discussed below are summarized in Table 58.3.

McKissock et al[60] reported in 1961 the results of a relatively large, well-designed, randomized controlled trial comparing surgical with nonsurgical treatment in patients with supratentorial ICH. Because the study was performed prior to the availability of CT, detailed characteristics on the size and location of the hematoma could not be known. The study included a total of 180 patients, 91 in the nonsurgical group and 89 in the surgical group. Patients were stratified according to level of consciousness, age, BP, and displacement of midline structures as detected by cerebral angiography. Patients with a rapid clinical recovery were not included in the study. Open craniotomy with evacuation of the hematoma was performed within 48 hours in most of the patients. In patients with hematomas confined to the basal ganglia or thalamus, surgery was not performed, but such patients remained in the surgical group for the purpose of analysis. There was no difference in mortality between the medical and the surgical groups, with rates of 51% and 65%, respectively, nor was there a difference in functional outcome. Regardless of treatment, patients with lobar hemorrhages had a better outcome than those with deep (basal ganglionic and thalamic) hemorrhages. Outcome correlated with the level of consciousness, as alert or drowsy patients did better than stuporous or comatose ones.

Table 58.3   Clinical Studies on Outcome of Surgical Management of Intracerebral Hemorrhage (ICH)

Author	Ref. No.	Year	No. of Patients		Mortality (%)	
			Surgical Group	Medical Group	Surgical Group	Medical Group
McKissock et al[a]	60	1961	89	91	65	51
Cook et al[b]	18	1965	57	0	51	
Cuatico et al[b]	19	1965	102	0	8	
Luessenhop et al[b]	56	1967	37	27	32	44
Paillas and Alliez[b]	70	1973	250	0	36	
Kaneko et al[b]	40	1977	38	0	8	
Kanaya et al[b]	39	1980	410	204	26	36
Pásztor et al[b]	72	1980	156	0	17	
Bolander et al[b]	8	1983	39	35	13	20
Kaneko et al[b]	41	1983	100	0	7	
Kanno et al[b]	43	1984	80 with mild putaminal ICH		4[c]	8[c]
			78 with moderate putaminal ICH		17[c]	10[c]
			55 with severe putaminal ICH		15[c]	0[c]
			52 with very severe putaminal ICH		86[c]	96[c]
Volpin et al[b]	100	1984	32	34	19	44
Juvela et al[a]	38	1989	26	26	46	38
Batjer et al[a]	5	1990	8	13	50[c]	85[c]
Piotrowski and Rochowanski[b]	74	1996	300	0	31	

[a] Randomized controlled.

[b] Nonrandomized.

[c] Dead or vegetative.

The results of a number of uncontrolled surgical series for supratentorial ICH were reported subsequently, still prior to the CT era. Cuatico et al[19] documented a surprisingly low mortality rate of 8% in 102 surgically treated patients with ICH; however, the selection criteria for surgical intervention were not well defined, other than a deteriorating neurologic condition. The authors found a more dismal outcome in patients with deeply located hematomas and in patients with a depressed level of consciousness. Cook et al[18] reported a mortality of 51% in 57 surgically treated patients with ICH, of which 19 were comatose and 38 were alert or lethargic. Again, outcome was better in those with a better neurologic status prior to surgery. Luessenhop et al[56] published a series of 64 patients with ICH; 27 patients were treated nonsurgically, and 35 of 37 surgically treated patients underwent craniotomy within 24 hours. Patients were selected for surgery on the surgeon's judgment, based on the clinical status of the patient. Mortality was 32% (12 of 37) in the surgical group and 44% (12 of 27) in the nonsurgical group. Regardless of treatment, mortality was higher in patients with deep basal ganglionic hemorrhages (92%) than in those with lobar hemorrhages (4%). Paillas and Alliez[70] addressed the timing of surgery in a surgical series of 250 patients analyzed retrospectively. Overall mortality rate was 36%; however, the mortality in patients who were operated on between days 5 and 10 (30%) was lower than that of those who had surgery within 5 days (54%). The authors felt that the optimal timing of surgery was between days 5 and 10. However, this conclusion is likely to simply reflect the fact that, by selecting patients for surgery based on survival after 5 to 10 days after onset, one is selecting out those patients with devastating hematomas who die within 5 days from ICH onset. Again, patients with deep-seated hematomas had higher mortality rates (48%) than those with superficial hematomas (21%). Kaneko et al[40] reported a very low mortality rate of 8% in 38 patients with hypertensive ICH treated surgically in the acute stage. Twenty-five patients were operated on within 3 hours, and 13 within 7 hours of symptom onset. The neurologic status was described as stuporous in 23, semicomatose in 12, and lethargic in 3 patients. Of the 35 survivors, 24 returned home and could live an independent life. The authors felt that the outcome of early hematoma evacuation was good because patients were operated on before the development of cerebral edema. Pásztor et al[72] found a relatively low mortality rate of 17% in a series of 156 surgically treated patients with supratentorial ICH. This good result may well be based on the timing of surgery, since 87% of the patients were operated on more than 4 days after onset (and 56% of the patients more than 2 weeks after onset).

Since the introduction of CT in 1973, studies have compared similar groups of patients with ICH in regard to the location and size of the hematoma. Kanaya et al[39] analyzed the outcome of 410 surgical and 204 nonsurgical patients with putaminal hemorrhage. No difference was observed in functional outcome between the two groups in patients who were "alert or confused" or "somnolent." In patients who were in "semicoma with herniation signs" or "deep coma," surgery did not affect functional outcome either, but it did reduce mortality. Most importantly, in patients described as in "stupor" or in "semicoma without herniation signs," both functional outcome and mortality were improved in the surgical group compared with the nonsurgical group (mortality rates of 22% and 54%, respectively). Kaneko et al[41] described the

outcome of "ultra-early" surgery (within 7 hours of symptom onset) in 100 patients with putaminal hemorrhage. Sixty of the 100 patients underwent surgery within 3 hours of presentation. Ten patients were described as somnolent (GCS score of 13), 68 as stuporous (GCS score of 10 to 12), and 22 as semicomatose (GCS score of 6 to 9). Overall mortality was only 7%, and 83 of the 93 (89%) survivors were ambulatory 6 months after surgery. Bolander et al[8] compared the outcome of 39 surgical and 35 nonsurgical patients with supratentorial ICH. Mortality was not different between the two groups (13% and 20%, respectively), nor was functional outcome after a mean follow-up of 15 months. However, analysis of those patients with hematoma volumes of 40 to 80 ml suggested a lower mortality in the surgically treated patients compared with the nonsurgical group (6% versus 25%). Volpin et al[100] reported on the outcome of surgical and medical treatment of 132 patients with supratentorial ICH. All patients with a hematoma volume of ≤26 ml survived with medical treatment alone. Patients with a hematoma volume of ≥85 ml died regardless of treatment. Results of surgical and medical therapy were compared in 66 patients with hematoma volumes between 26 and 85 ml. Mortality was significantly less (19%) in the 32 patients in the surgical group compared with that of 34 patients in the medical group (44%). Kanno et al[43] reported the results of surgical and medical treatment of 459 patients with hypertensive ICH in various locations. In the 265 patients with putaminal hemorrhage, there was no benefit from surgery in those with either small hematomas or very large hematomas. In patients with intermediate-sized hematomas, there was a suggestion of a slightly better outcome in surgically treated patients, in particular when surgery was performed within 6 hours of symptom onset. Fujitsu et al[33] obtained similar results in 111 conservatively and 69 surgically treated patients with putaminal hemorrhage. For patients with a rapid progressive course, surgery offered benefit over nonsurgical treatment. Those with a nonprogressive, slowly progressive, or fulminant course did not benefit from surgery. Piotrowski and Rochowanski[74] analyzed the operative results of 300 patients with hypertensive ICH older than 60 years. Overall mortality was 31.3%, which included patients with lobar, cerebellar, and basal ganglionic hemorrhages. Mortality increased with the size of the hematoma (18.1% in patients with a hematoma diameter <40 mm and 46.7% in those with a hematoma diameter of 60 mm). In addition, mortality was greater in patients with basal ganglionic hemorrhages compared with those with lobar hemorrhages.

In spite of two more recent prospective randomized controlled trials comparing medical versus surgical treatment in patients with supratentorial ICH, the issue continues to be unsettled. In the trial of Batjer et al,[5] randomization was interrupted after enrollment of only 21 patients with putaminal hemorrhage over a period of 5½ years because of poor outcome in all three treatment groups: "best medical management," "best medical management" plus ICP monitoring, and craniotomy with microsurgical hematoma evacuation. Fifteen (71%) patients had died or remained vegetative at 6 months: 78% (7/9) in the "best medical management" group, 100% (4/4) in the "best medical management" plus ICP monitoring group, and 50% (4/8) in the surgical group. Juvela et al[38] randomized 26 patients with supratentorial ICH to surgical and 26 to medical treatment within 48 hours of ICH onset. Patients were enrolled if they were "unconscious and/or had severe hemiparesis or dysphasia." The overall mortality rate at 6 months was similar in both treatment groups (Table 58.3); however, in patients with a GCS score of 7 to 10 mortality was 0% (0/4) in the surgical group versus 80% (4/5) in the medical group. In the patients with a GCS score of 11 to 14, mortality was 27% (3/11) in the surgical group and only 7% (1/15) in the medical group. However, the small numbers of observations in each category preclude any definite conclusions about the value of the two treatments.

In summary, the review of these clinical series suggests that there may be a subgroup of patients with ICH with intermediate-sized hematomas and a moderately depressed level of consciousness who could benefit from surgery. Furthermore, there is the suggestion that early surgery may be beneficial. Surgery appears not to be indicated and may even be harmful in those with small hematomas. Patients with very large hematomas and a severely depressed level of consciousness do poorly regardless of therapy. To test these hypotheses, a prospective controlled randomized trial is needed in which patients should be stratified according to their neurologic status on presentation, the timing of surgery (ideally within a few hours from onset), and the hematoma characteristics (size, location, ventricular extension). Other variables that may prove to be of importance on surgical outcome are the surgical technique (craniotomy, stereotactic aspiration with and without thrombolysis, or stereotactic endoscopic aspiration) and the use of neuroprotective agents in combination with surgery (see below).

Future Directions

New surgical and nonsurgical treatment strategies for patients with ICH have emerged in recent years. The modern surgical techniques are aimed at minimizing surgical trauma associated with craniotomy and evacuation of intracerebral hematomas, and include stereotactic clot aspiration,[3,66,92,93] stereotactic clot aspiration after liquefying the clot with urokinase[58,67] or recombinant tissue plasminogen activator,[86] intraventricular therapy in patients with ventricular extension of the hematoma,[79,97] and ultrasound-guided endoscopic clot removal.[2] The development of these novel, less invasive surgical techniques offers an alternative to conventional craniotomy and may be of benefit in patients with deeply located hematomas. Their value, however, can only be appropriately assessed through a prospective randomized clinical trial, comparing these various surgical techniques with conventional craniotomy.

New approaches to the treatment for ICH have been studied mostly in animal models and are aimed at limiting secondary brain injury caused by the hematoma. Primary injury in ICH is mediated by tissue destruction and compression by the rapidly expanding mass lesion. Experimental studies suggest that an intracerebral hematoma produces secondary injury by inducing edema, ischemia, and cell death in the tissues surrounding the hemorrhage.[101,104] The volume of the peripheral ischemic area may be several times larger than the hematoma itself, in particular in hemorrhages that extend into the subarachnoid or ventricular space.[62] Proposed mechanisms for the induction of ischemia in the area surrounding the hematoma include compression of the microcirculation, vasospasm secondary to the presence of blood, and microcirculatory plugging by white blood cells.[62,65] Neuronal injury may be further promoted by inflammation and free radical production due to the presence of serum proteins and heme in the brain parenchyma.[42,61] The presence of an ischemic region surrounding the hematoma has been demonstrated in humans by single-photon emission computed tomography and positron emission tomography studies.[87] The increasing understanding of the mechanisms that cause cell injury in ICH provides a basis for the development of novel treatment strategies directed at limiting secondary brain injury.[61] A potential role for neuroprotective agents in the treatment of ICH has been suggested based on the results of animal studies showing that pretreatment with nimodipine or an *N*-methyl-D-aspartate receptor antagonist reduces the volume of ischemic brain injury in the region surrounding the hematoma.[62] The benefits of such therapies in comparison with other treatment modalities should be explored in prospective randomized clinical trials.

References

1. Aggerwal SAK, Williams V, Levine SR et al: Cocaine-associated intracranial hemorrhage: absence of vasculitis in 14 cases. Neurology 46:1741, 1996

2. Auer LM, Deinsberger W, Niederkorn K et al: Endoscopic surgery versus medical treatment for spontaneous intracerebral hematoma: a randomized study. J Neurosurg 70:530, 1989

3. Backlund E-O, von Holst H: Controlled subtotal evacuation of intracerebral haematomas by stereotactic technique. Surg Neurol 9:99, 1978

4. Barnett GH: Intracranial pressure monitoring devices: principles, insertion, and care. p. 53. In Ropper AH (ed): Neurological and Neurosurgical Intensive Care. 3rd Ed. Lippincott-Raven, Philadelphia, 1993

5. Batjer HH, Reisch JS, Allen BC et al: Failure of surgery to improve outcome in hypertensive putaminal hemorrhage: a prospective randomized trial. Arch Neurol 47:1103, 1990

6. Bertel O, Marx BE, Conen D: Effects of antihypertensive treatment on cerebral perfusion. Am J Med, suppl. 3B, 82:29, 1987

7. Boeer A, Voth E, Henze T, Prange HW: Early heparin therapy in patients with spontaneous intracerebral haemorrhage. J Neurol Neurosurg Psychiatry 54:466, 1991

8. Bolander HG, Kourtopoulos H, Liliequist B, Wittboldt S: Treatment of spontaneous intracerebral haemorrhage: a retrospective analysis of 74 consecutive cases with special reference to computer tomographic data. Acta Neurochir 67:19, 1983

9. Borges LF: Management of nontraumatic brain hemorrhage. p. 279. In Ropper AH (ed): Neurological and Neurosurgical Intensive Care. 3rd. Ed. Lippincott-Raven, Philadelphia, 1993

10. Broderick J, Brott T, Tomsick T et al: Management of intracerebral hemorrhage in a large metropolitan population. Neurosurgery 34:882, 1994

11. Brott T, Broderick J, Kothari R et al: Early hemorrhage growth in patients with intracerebral hemorrhage. Stroke 28:1, 1997

12. Caplan L: Intracerebral hemorrhage revisited. Neurology 38:624, 1988

13. Caplan LR: Intracerebral hemorrhage. Lancet 339:656, 1992

14. Caplan LR: General symptoms and signs. p. 31. In Kase CS, Caplan LR (eds): Intracerebral Hemorrhage. Butterworth-Heinemann, Boston, 1994

15. Caplan LR, Thomas C, Banks G: Central nervous system complications of addiction to "T's and blues." Neurology 32:623, 1982

16. Chestnut RM, Marshall LF: Management of severe head injury. p. 203. In Ropper AH (ed): Neurological and Neurosurgical Intensive Care. 3rd Ed. Lippincott-Raven, Phildelphia, 1993

17. Conrad AR, Feffer SE, Rajan RT, Freeman I: Intracranial hemorrhage complicating acute myocardial infarction in the era of thrombolytic therapy. South Med J 90: 5, 1997

18. Cook AW, Plaut M, Browder J: Spontaneous intracerebral hemorrhage: factors related to surgical results. Arch Neurol 13:25, 1965

19. Cuatico W, Adib S, Gaston P: Spontaneous intracerebral hematomas: a surgical appraisal. J Neurosurg 22:569, 1965

20. Dandapani BK, Suzuki S, Kelley RE et al: Relation between blood pressure and outcome in intracerebral hemorrhage. Stroke 26:21, 1995

21. Diringer MN: Intracerebral hemorrhage: pathophysiology and management. Crit Care Med 21:1591, 1993

22. Dixon AA, Holness RO, Howes WJ, Garner JB: Spontaneous intracerebral haemorrhage: an analysis of factors affecting prognosis. Can J Neurol Sci 12:267, 1985

23. Driks MR, Craven DE, Celli BR et al: Nosocomial pneumonia in intubated patients given sucralfate as compared with antacids or histamine type 2 blockers. N Engl J Med 317:1376, 1987

24. Drury I, Whisnant JP, Garraway M: Primary intracerebral hemorrhage: impact of CT on incidence. Neurology 34:653, 1984

25. Duff TA, Ayeni S, Levin AB, Javid M: Nonsurgical management of spontaneous intracerebral hematoma. Neurosurgery 9:387, 1981

26. Eleff SM, Borel C, Bell WR et al: Acute management of intracranial hemorrhage in patients receiving thrombolytic therapy: case reports. Neurosurg 26:867, 1990

27. Faught E, Peters D, Bartolucci A et al: Seizures after primary intracerebral hemorrhage. Neurology 39:1089, 1989

28. Feldman Z, Kanter MJ, Robertson CS et al: Effect of head elevation on intracranial pressure, cerebral perfusion pressure, and cerebral blood flow in head-injured patients. J Neurosurg 76:207, 1992

29. Feldmann E: Intracerebral hemorrhage. Stroke 22:31, 1991

30. Franke CL, de Jonge J, van Swieten JC et al: Intracerebral hematomas during anticoagulant treatment. Stroke 21:726, 1990

31. Franke CL, van Swieten JC, Algra A, van Gijn J: Prognostic factors in patients with intracerebral haematoma. J Neurol Neurosurg Psychiatry 55:653, 1992

32. Fredriksson K, Norrving B, Strömblad L: Emergency reversal of anticoagulation after intracerebral hemorrhage. Stroke 23:972, 1992

33. Fujitsu K, Muramoto M, Ikeda Y et al: Indications for surgical treatment of putaminal hemorrhage: comparative study based on serial CT and time-course analysis. J Neurosurg 73:518, 1990

34. Green RM, Kelly KM, Gabrielsen T et al: Multiple intracerebral hemorrhages after smoking "crack" cocaine. Stroke 21:957, 1990

35. Helweg-Larsen S, Sommer W, Strange P et al: Prognosis for patients treated conservatively for spontaneous intracerebral hematomas. Stroke 15:1045, 1984

36. Janny P, Colnet G, Georget A-M, Chazal J: Intracranial pressure with intracerebral hemorrhages. Surg Neurol 10:371, 1978

37. Janny P, Papo I, Chazal J et al: Intracranial hypertension and prognosis in spontaneous intracerebral haematomas: a correlative study of 60 patients. Acta Neurochir 61: 181, 1982

38. Juvela S, Heiskanen O, Poranen A et al: The treatment of spontaneous intracerebral hemorrhage: a prospective randomized trial of surgical and conservative treatment. J Neurosurg 70:755, 1989

39. Kanaya H, Yukawa H, Itoh Z et al: Grading and the indications for treatment in ICH of the basal ganglia (cooperative study in Japan). p. 268. In Pia HW, Langmaid C, Zierski J (eds): Spontaneous Intracerebral Haematomas: Advances in Diagnosis and Therapy. Springer-Verlag, Heidelberg, 1980

40. Kaneko M, Koba T, Yokoyama T: Early surgical treatment for hypertensive intracerebral hemorrhage. J Neurosurg 46:579, 1977

41. Kaneko M, Tanaka K, Shimada T et al: Long-term evaluation of ultra-early operation for hypertensive intracerebral hemorrhage in 100 cases. J Neurosurg 58:838, 1983

42. Kanno T, Nagata J, Nonomura K et al: New approaches in the treatment of hypertensive intracerebral hemorrhage. Stroke, suppl. I, 24:I–96, 1993

43. Kanno T, Sano H, Shinomiya Y et al: Role of surgery in hypertensive intracerebral hematoma: a comparative study of 305 nonsurgical and 154 surgical cases. J Neurosurg 61:1091, 1984

44. Kasdon DL, Scott RM, Adelman LS, Wolpert SM: Cerebellar hemorrhage with decreased absorption values on computed tomography: a case report. Neuroradiology 13:265, 1977

45. Kase CS: Intracerebral hemorrhage: non-hypertensive causes. Stroke 17:590, 1986

46. Kase CS: Lobar hemorrhage. p. 363. In Kase CS, Caplan LR (eds): Intracerebral Hemorrhage, Butterworth-Heinemann, Boston, 1994

47. Kase CS, Foster TE, Reed JE et al: Intracerebral hemorrhage and phenylpropanolamine use. Neurology 37:399, 1987

48. Kase CS, Pessin MS, Zivin JA et al: Intracranial hemor-

rhage after coronary thrombolysis with tissue plasminogen activator. Am J Med 92:384, 1992

49. Kase CS, Robinson RK, Stein RW et al: Anticoagulant-related intracerebral hemorrhage. Neurology 35:943, 1985

50. Kase CS, Williams JP, Wyatt DA, Mohr JP: Lobar intracerebral hematomas: clinical and CT analysis of 22 cases. Neurology 32:1146, 1982

51. Kaufman HH: Treatment of deep spontaneous intracerebral hematomas: a review. Stroke, suppl. I, 24:I–101, 1993

52. Lassen NA: Control of cerebral circulation in health and disease. Circ Res 34:749, 1974

53. Levine SR, Welch KMA: Cocaine and stroke. Stroke 19:779, 1988

54. Leys D, Mounier-Vehier F, Mounier-Vehier C, Carré A: Relationship between blood pressure and outcome in intracerebral hemorrhage. Stroke 26:1126, 1995

55. Little JR, Tubman DE, Ethier R: Cerebellar hemorrhage in adults: diagnosis by computerized tomography. J Neurosurg 48:575, 1978

56. Luessenhop AJ, Shevlin WA, Ferrero AA et al: Surgical management of primary intracerebral hemorrhage. J Neurosurg 27:419, 1967

57. Majerus PW, Broze GJ, Miletich JP, Tollefsen DM: Anticoagulant, thrombolytic, and antiplatelet drugs. p. 1311. In Goodman, Gilman A, Rall TW, Nies AS, Taylor P (eds): Goodman & Gilman's The Pharmacological Basis of Therapeutics. Macmillan, New York, 1990

58. Matsumoto K, Hondo H: CT-guided stereotaxic evacuation of hypertensive intracerebral hematomas. J Neurosurg 61:440, 1984

59. Mayer SA, Sacco RL, Shi T, Mohr JP: Neurologic deterioration in noncomatose patients with supratentorial intracerebral hemorrhage. Neurology 44:1379, 1994

60. McKissock W, Richardson A, Taylor J: Primary intracerebral haemorrhage: a controlled trial of surgical and conservative treatment in 180 unselected cases. Lancet 2:221, 1961

61. Mendelow AD: Spontaneous intracerebral haemorrhage. J Neurol Neurosurg Psychiatry 54:193, 1991

62. Mendelow AD: Mechanisms of ischemic brain damage with intracerebral hemorrhage. Stroke, suppl. I, 24: I–115, 1993

63. Mohr JP, Caplan LR, Melski JW et al: The Harvard Cooperative Stroke Registry: a prospective registry. Neurology 26:754, 1978

64. The National Institute of Neurological Disorders and Stroke rt-PA Stroke Study Group: Tissue plasminogen activator for acute ischemic stroke. N Engl J Med 333:1581, 1995

65. Nehls G, Major M, Mendelow D et al: Experimental intracerebral hemorrhage: progression of hemodynamic changes after production of a spontaneous mass lesion: Neurosurgery 24:1115, 1988

66. Nguyen J-P, Decq P, Brugieres P et al: A technique for stereotactic aspiration of deep intracerebral hematomas under computed tomographic control using a new device. Neurosurgery 31:330, 1992

67. Niizuma H, Otsuki T, Johkura H et al: CT-guided stereotactic aspiration of intracerebral hematoma: result of a hematoma-lysis method using urokinase. Appl Neurophysiol 48:427, 1985

68. Ojemann RG, Heros RC: Spontaneous brain hemorrhage. Stroke 14:468, 1983

69. Olson JD: Mechanisms of hemostasis: effect on intracerebral hemorrhage. Stroke, suppl. I, 24:I–109, 1993

70. Paillas JE, Alliez B: Surgical treatment of spontaneous intracerebral hemorrhage: immediate and long-term results in 250 cases. J Neurosurg 39:145, 1973

71. Papo I, Janny P, Caruselli G et al: Intracranial pressure time course in primary intracerebral hemorrhage. Neurosurgery 4:504, 1979

72. Pásztor E, Áfra D, Orosz É: Experiences with the surgical treatment of 156 ICH (1955–1977). p. 251. In Pia HW, Langmaid C, Zierski J (eds): Spontaneous Intracerebral Haematomas: Advances in Diagnosis and Therapy. Springer-Verlag, Heidelberg, 1980

73. Patel RV, Kertland HR, Jahns BE et al: Labetalol: response and safety in critically ill hemorrhagic stroke patients. Ann Pharmacother 27:180, 1993

74. Piotrowski WP, Rochowanski E: Operative results in hypertensive intracerebral hematomas in patients over 60. Gerontology 42:339, 1996

75. Portenoy RK, Lipton RB, Berger AR et al: Intracerebral haemorrhage: a model for the prediction of outcome. J Neurol Neurosurg Psychiatry 50:976, 1987

76. Poungvarin N, Bhoopat W, Viriyavejakul A et al: Effects of dexamethasone in primary supratentorial intracerebral hemorrhage. N Engl J Med 316:1229, 1987

77. Practice advisory: thrombolytic therapy for acute ischemic stroke—summary statement. Neurology 47:835, 1996

78. Rådberg JA, Olsson JE, Rådberg CT: Prognostic parameters in spontaneous intracerebral hematomas with special reference to anticoagulant treatment. Stroke 22:571, 1991

79. Rohde V, Schaller C, Hassler WE: Intraventricular recombinant tissue plasminogen activator for lysis of intraventricular hemorrhage. J Neurol Neurosurg Psychiatry 58:447, 1995

80. Ropper AH: Treatment of intracranial hypertension. p. 29. In Ropper AH (ed): Neurological and Neurosurgical Intensive Care. 3rd Ed. Lippincott-Raven, Philadelphia, 1993

81. Ropper AH, Gress DR: Computerized tomography and clinical features of large cerebral hemorrhages. Cerebrovasc Dis 1:38, 1991

82. Ropper AH, Kennedy SK: Postoperative neurosurgical care. p. 185. In Ropper AH (ed): Neurological and Neurosurgical Intensive Care. 3rd Ed. Lippincott-Raven, Philadelphia, 1993

83. Ropper AH, King RB: Intracranial pressure monitoring in comatose patients with cerebral hemorrhage. Arch Neurol 41:725, 1984

84. Ropper AH, O'Rourke D, Kennedy SK: Head position, intracranial pressure, and compliance. Neurology 32:1288, 1982

85. Ropper AH, Rockoff MA: Physiology and clinical aspects of raised intracranial pressure. p. 11. In Ropper AH (ed): Neurological and Neurosurgical Intensive Care. 3rd Ed. Lippincott-Raven, Philadelphia, 1993

86. Schaller C, Rohde V, Meyer B, Hassler W: Stereotactic puncture and lysis of spontaneous intracerebral hemorrhage using recombinant tissue-plasminogen activator. Neurosurgery 36:328, 1995

87. Sills C, Villar-Cordova C, Pasteur W et al: Demonstration of hypoperfusion surrounding intracerebral hematoma in humans. J Stroke Cerebrovasc Dis 6:17, 1996

88. Sloan MA, Kittner SJ, Rigamonti D, Price T: Occurrence of stroke associated with use/abuse of drugs. Neurology 41:1358, 1991

89. Sung C, Chu N: Epileptic seizures in intracerebral haemorrhage. J Neurol Neurosurg Psychiatry 52:1273, 1989

90. Swab M, Spranger M, Schwarz S, Hacke W: Barbiturate coma in severe hemispheric stroke: useful or obsolete? Neurology 48:1608, 1997

91. Taneda M, Hayakawa T, Mogami H: Primary cerebellar hemorrhage: quadrigeminal cistern obliteration on CT scans as a predictor of outcome. J Neurosurg 67:545, 1987

92. Tanikawa T, Amano K, Kawamura H et al: CT-guided stereotactic surgery for evacuation of hypertensive intracerebral hematoma. Appl Neurophysiol 48:431, 1985

93. Tanizaki Y, Sugita K, Toriyama T, Hokama M: New CT-guided stereotactic apparatus and clinical experience with intracerebral hematomas. Appl Neurophysiol 48:11, 1985

94. Tellez H, Bauer RB: Dexamethasone as treatment in cerebrovascular disease. 1. A controlled study in intracerebral hemorrhage. Stroke 4:541, 1973

95. Terayama Y, Tanahashi N, Fukuuchi Y, Gotoh F: Prognostic value of admission blood pressure in patients with intracerebral hemorrhage. Stroke 28:1185, 1997

96. Thrift AG, McNeil JJ, Forbes A, Donnan GA: Risk factors for cerebral hemorrhage in the era of well-controlled hypertension. Stroke 27:2020, 1996

97. Todo T, Usui M, Takakura K: Treatment of severe intraventricular hemorrhage by intraventricular infusion of urokinase. J Neurosurg 74:881, 1991

98. Toffel GJ, Biller J, Adams HP: Nontraumatic intracerebral hemorrhage in young adults. Arch Neurol 44:483, 1987

99. Tuhrim S, Dambrosia JM, Price TR et al: Prediction of intracerebral hemorrhage survival. Ann Neurol 24:258, 1988

100. Volpin L, Cervellini P, Colombo F et al: Spontaneous intracerebral hematomas: a new proposal about the usefulness and limits of surgical treatment. Neurosurgery 15:663, 1984

101. Wagner KR, Xi G, Hua Y et al: Lobar intracerebral hemorrhage model in pigs: rapid edema development in perihematomal white matter. Stroke 27:490, 1996

102. Weir CJ, Murray GD, Dyker AG, Lees KR: Is hyperglycaemia an independent predictor of poor outcome after acute stroke? Results of a long term follow up study. BMJ 314:1303, 1997

103. Weisberg LA, Shamsnia M, Elliott D: Seizures caused by non-traumatic parenchymal brain hemorrhages. Neurology 41:1197, 1991

104. Yang G, Betz L, Chenevert T et al: Experimental intracerebral hemorrhage: relationship between brain edema, blood flow, and blood brain barrier permeability in rats. J Neurosurg 81:93, 1994

105. Yu YL, Kumana CR, Lauder IJ et al: Treatment of acute cerebral hemorrhage with intravenous glycerol: a double-blind, placebo-controlled, randomized trial. Stroke 23:967, 1992

Surgical Considerations

CHRISTOPHER S. OGILVY

ROBERT G. OJEMANN

ROBERT M. CROWELL

Spontaneous brain hemorrhage is a rather common form of stroke. About 20 cases/100,000 population occur annually. Brain hemorrhage and subarachnoid hemorrhage (10/100,000) amount to about 15% of all strokes.

Although *evacuation of intracerebral hematoma* is one of the older neurosurgical procedures, the operation is undergoing major re-evaluation in light of technological advances. Computed tomography (CT) now easily detects fresh brain hemorrhage, and magnetic resonance (MR) can sometimes give additional useful information. Classical surgical techniques for removal of clots are being supplemented (or supplanted) by stereotactic aspiration, facilitated by instillation of thrombolytic agents. Properly designed clinical trials have begun to demonstrate the specific situations in which clot removal can (or cannot) be of clinical benefit.

After the effects of acute hemorrhage are dealt with, the *risk of recurrent hemorrhage* requires assessment. CT and MR sometimes demonstrate the cause of hemorrhage, for example, aneurysm, cavernous angioma, or tumor. In questionable cases, angiography is warranted. Surgical correction of bleeding lesions is usually warranted to prevent recurrent hemorrhage. Guidelines for management are evolving, as experience with MR-depicted pathology and its natural history is accumulated.

Historical Perspective

In 1883 MacEwen[84] performed the first successful operation for intracerebral hematoma, thus making it one of the earliest neurosurgical procedures.

The evaluations of McKissock[90] and Richardson[119–122] showed that many patients can also make a good recovery with medical therapy.[34] Subsequently, numerous studies attempted to define the role of surgery in brain hemorrhage. Surgery seems indicated as a lifesaving measure for the patient deteriorating with a large hematoma mass[31] and for some patients with cerebellar hematoma.[55] Beyond these concepts, it has not been proved whether morbidity can be lessened by immediate or by delayed removal of a hematoma. Recent controlled trials have failed to show benefit for evacuation of putaminal hemorrhage.

Etiologies

Spontaneous brain hemorrhage may occur from many causes[25,37,41,42,89] (Fig. 58.1). Hypertension is often associated with hemorrhage into the putamen, cerebellum, thalamus, or pons.[13,19,170] The source of bleeding in these cases seems to be microaneurysm or arteriolar necrosis. Such primary brain hemorrhages are usually distinguished from other causes by clinical and CT findings or MRI. For example, bleeds due to aneurysm (Fig. 58.2) or arteriovenous malformation (AVM) may lead to parenchymal bleeding, but clinical features (age of the patient, history of hypertension or seizures) and CT or MRI changes (subarachnoid blood or draining veins) generally serve to distinguish these from primary brain hemorrhage. Intracranial tumors, especially melanoma and glioma, occasionally present with hemorrhage, but the CT or MRI is usually distinctive.[27,60,79,86,110,115,139] Hemorrhagic infarction is often distinguished by its clinical features and CT/MRI appearance, but this may be underdiagnosed[18,48] Patients on anticoagulants may occasionally have a brain hemorrhage,[77] generally in sites typical for hypertensive hemorrhage. In some instances, embolic infarction in anticoagulated patients may set the stage for more dramatic clinical manifestations due to bleeding into infarcted tissue. Endogenous coagulopathies, especially those caused by leukemia in the pediatric age group, may cause parenchymal hemorrhage.[2] In the elderly patient, amyloid angiopathy may be the cause of brain hemorrhage.[87,108] In some cases, vasculitis can be the cause of bleeding,[17,138] occasionally from exogenous agents such as cocaine or phenylpropanamine.[44] In a number of patients, especially those with a lobar hemorrhage, no source can be demonstrated despite extensive radiographic and pathologic studies.

The initial clinical effects from brain hemorrhage are due to direct destruction and displacement of local tissue.[4,126]

Figure 58.1 Cerebellar hemorrhage. (**A**) Computed tomography shows hematoma. (**B**) Computed tomography after stereotactic drainage. (From Mohadjer et al.,[95] with permission.)

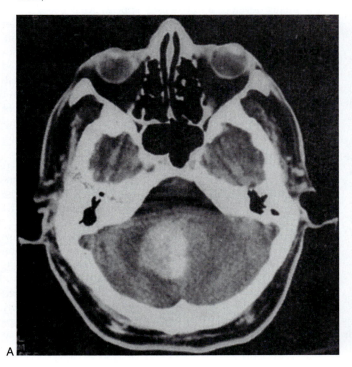
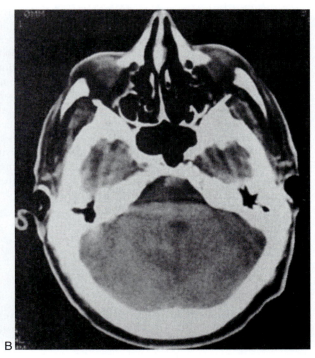

A B

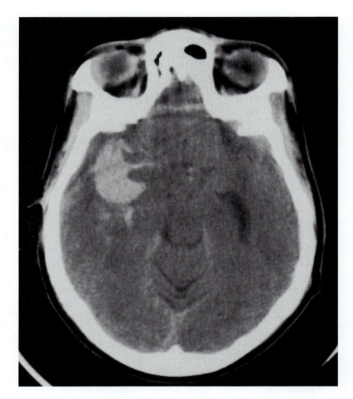

Figure 58.2 Hemorrhage from posterior communicating artery–internal carotid artery aneurysm. Patient in coma with hemiplegia. Surgical clipping of aneurysm without angiography. Complete recovery.

Pathologic studies demonstrate tracking of blood along tissue planes, with displacement of tissue, especially white matter. The mechanism of later deterioration is less certain.[28] Serial imaging studies have shown that rebleeding may be more frequent than previously suspected.[54] Edema and ischemic necrosis around the lesion are probably major factors. Experimental studies show decreased local cerebral blood flow.[99,100,123,124] In addition, hyperemia,[141] dysautoregulation, and blood-brain barrier disruption have been demonstrated.[69,72] Immune mechanisms and blood-derived toxins (such as glutamate and choline) may play a role in causing irreversible tissue damage.[93]

Resorption of the hematoma occurs over a course of months. The process is slow, because macrophage activity must occur along the edge of the mass. After a year, the hematoma site is converted to a slitlike cavity with orange-stained walls representing hemosiderin-laden macrophages.[16]

Evaluation

COAGULATION STUDIES

Routine coagulation studies should be performed in every case. These include prothrombin time, partial thromboplastin time, and platelet count. The bleeding time should be esti-mated in patients receiving aspirin. Although these studies are usually normal, the occasional coagulopathy is detected and can be appropriately treated.

LUMBAR PUNCTURE

There is no indication for a lumbar puncture in a patient suspected of having a brain hemorrhage. CT or MRI establishes the diagnosis noninvasively. In large hematomas, a lumbar puncture can cause brain herniation, whereas in small hemorrhages the cerebrospinal fluid may be clear.[76]

RADIOGRAPHIC STUDIES

CT and MRI have dramatically altered management of brain hemorrhage.[5,49,52,71,85,114,133,158–160] Formerly, diagnosis of the condition was uncertain, and localization and sizing of lesions inferential. Imaging routinely gives precise information about the location, size, and configuration of parenchymal hemorrhage (Figs. 58.1 to 58.5; see Figs. 58.8 and 58.9). The presence and extent of subarachnoid hemorrhage and surrounding edema are depicted. Imaging shows hydrocephalus, intraventricular hematoma, and ventricular compression or displacement. Information regarding volume of hematoma and involvement of posterior limb of internal capsule has been especially valuable in estimation of prognosis. Postoperative residual or recurrent hematoma can be detected.[33]

Because it is rapid with essentially no risk, CT is the initial study of choice for almost all patients suspected of brain hemorrhage. Only rarely does the need for emergency surgery preclude CT evaluation. Over several weeks, the high-density hematoma seen on CT scan gradually becomes isodense and eventually develops a low-density appearance.[33,94]

MRI, formerly more cumbersome but now rapid, can readily image parenchymal hemorrhage, typically showing acute hematoma as bright signal on T_2-weighted sequences.[24,148] The size of a hematoma may be overestimated on T_2 sequences, since edema is also seen as bright signal; thus reference to T_1-weighted images is needed to interpret the findings. As blood products decay over time, images of hematoma on T_1- and T_2-weighted sequences undergo a complex series of changes that have been characterized for acute, subacute, and chronic lesions.

For investigation of the source of hemorrhage, MRI is superior to CT (Fig. 58.3B). AVMs, giant (partially thrombosed) aneurysms, and cavernous angiomas have characteristic appearances.[101] Often tumors can be identified by MRI with contrast enhancement.

In some cases, MR angiography (MRA), done with phase contrast or two-dimensional time-of-flight techniques, may be helpful in evaluation of the etiology of hemorrhage. This is particularly true for sizable aneurysms and AVMs. However, clot and vessels are both bright, thus confusing the issue, and the detail is seldom sufficient to depict parent vessels precisely enough for surgery. Therefore, MRA is so far unable to supplant conventional angiography fully in the evaluation of brain hemorrhage of uncertain etiology.

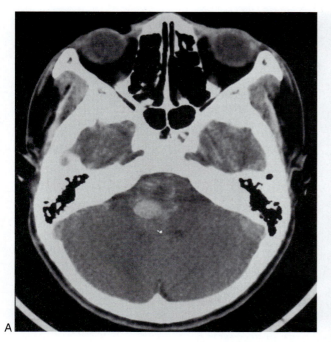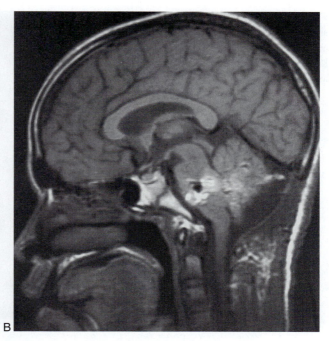

Figure 58.3 Pontine hemorrhage from cavernous angioma. (**A**) Computed tomography shows hematoma. Patient in coma. Hematoma partially removed by emergency transvermian approach followed by clinical improvement. (**B**) Postoperative MRI shows cavernous angioma. Reoperation with total excision of typical cavernous angioma. Recovery to minimal neurologic deficit.

ANGIOGRAPHY

In the typical hypertensive brain hemorrhage, angiography is rarely indicated. When hypertension is not the likely cause, particularly in lobar hemorrhage and in young people, and if CT and MRI are nondiagnostic, angiography is indicated to determine if a vascular abnormality or tumor is present (Fig. 58.4B).[3,112,123] If angiography is negative, then repeat CT, MRI, and angiography a few months later, after resolution of the mass effect, may permit visualization of an AVM or tumor.

Indications for Surgery

Despite numerous series of medically and surgically treated patients with parenchymal hematoma, solid indications for surgery have not been established.[1,29,38,61,66,67,70,83,96,104,105,111,117,118,127] This statement holds for a range of surgical procedures, including open clot evacuation, stereotactic aspiration, and ventriculostomy. Even though some controlled prospective studies have been performed, they are marred by small numbers, lack of adequate controls, and other design flaws. In the absence of adequate controlled studies, only broad guidelines for treatment can be suggested.

When a parenchymal hematoma threatens life, surgical removal of the lesion seems reasonable, especially in a young person with delayed deterioration. On the other hand, an el-derly person with coma from onset and a huge deep dominant hemispheric clot is not a surgical candidate. Most cases lie in between these extremes, making decisions difficult. Although clear-cut indications are not yet available, guidelines for therapy are emerging. Some tentative indications can be offered, beginning with the most firmly established. They are as follows:

1. *Secondary deterioration* suggests reversibility of deficit in that function survived the initial hemorrhage (Fig. 58.4).[4,31] Recurrent hemorrhage appears to be an occasional cause of secondary deterioration. Medical therapy is usually ineffective in this setting. Further downhill progression, probably related to increased intracranial pressure, seems likely in such cases. In 9 to 15 cases headed for almost certain death, surgery was lifesaving to the deteriorating patient.[4,120] Operation seems especially appropriate for lesions extending into accessible lobar sites. Although data from modern controlled studies are unavailable, deterioration appears an eminently logical, fairly well-established, and widely accepted indication for surgery. Surgery is generally not recommended if there is massive hemorrhage with immediate loss of brain stem function and no response to medical therapy.

2. *Cerebellar hemorrhage* is a special management problem for which guidelines are available.[3] With hematoma near the brain stem, rapid and irreversible deterioration may take place without warning (Figs. 58.1 and 58.4). Surgical evacuation of these lesions is associated with low morbidity. To protect against abrupt deterioration, surgery is recommended for all lesions >3 cm in diameter. Most smaller lesions have a benign

Figure 58.4 Hemorrhage from vasculitis. (**A**) CT shows hematoma. (**B**) Vasculitis is demonstrated on angiography. Gradual deterioration with aphasia, hemiparesis, and obtundation. Surgical evacuation and steroid therapy with full recovery.

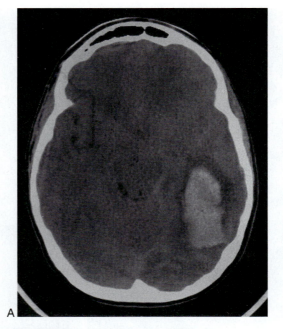

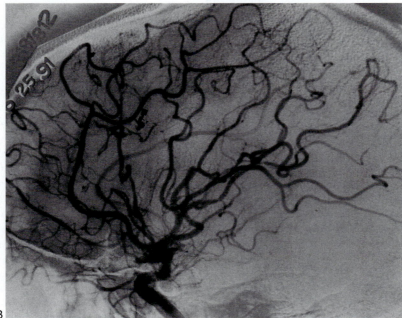

course, and preliminary CT data have indicated that lesions <3 cm may be treated medically with good results. Large lesions may cause sudden coma even after 1 month, and removal should be considered whenever large clots are encountered. One group used a Glasgow Coma Scale score of ≤13 or a hematoma ≥4 cm as criteria for surgical treatment.[73] The role of stereotactic removal has been discussed.

3. *Diagnostic uncertainty* as to etiology sometimes requires exploratory operation.[12,103] CT, MRI, and angiography can generally identify tumors and AVMs, particularly if studies are repeated after mass effect has declined. However, if there is still a question, operation is occasionally warranted to establish the diagnosis of tumor, AVM, or cavernous angioma. This is particularly appropriate in the setting of recurrent hemorrhages with progressive deficit.

4. *Central hemorrhage* (medullary, pontine, and mesencephalic) may occasionally be evacuated with success (Fig. 58.3). This may be appropriate in a young patient with preserved brain stem function. In the case of thalamic and brain stem hemorrhage, a shunt procedure for acute hydrocephalus may be lifesaving.

5. *Stable persistent deficit* may or may not be improved by surgery. For moderate deficits, some authors suggest initial medical therapy.[123,126] If the deficits persist beyond 1 to 4

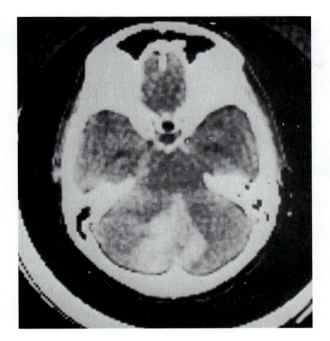

Figure 58.5 Cerebellar hemorrhage. Large paravermian hematoma. Patient in coma. Awakened after surgical evacuation. Mild residual ataxia.

weeks, surgery may be offered on grounds that decompression may restore function to some marginal neurons, and surgery may hasten recovery and improve outcome,[120] as seen experimentally.[100] Reports of single cases and small series suggest that surgery may diminish late morbidity. Prospective clinical studies will be needed to evaluate the role of surgery for such patients. Benefits of early operation and delayed operation have been evaluated, but clear superiority of either approach has not been established. We have usually not recommended surgery in this setting, except when there is reasonable doubt as to the etiology (see above).

6. *Initial coma* has rarely been reversed by emergency operation.[83] Quality of survival has been fair at best, with all 4 survivors in a study of 21 cases requiring full-time care. Emergency operations in this setting rarely seem justified, even in a young person. Patients with clots greater than 85 ml in volume almost always succumb.

Surgical Techniques

OPEN EVACUATION OF HEMATOMA

With increasing use of stereotactic aspiration of intracerebral hematomas, craniotomy for removal of hematoma under direct vision is less frequent. However, in an emergency or when adequate removal cannot be done, one should proceed immediately to open evacuation. In the last few years, localization and determining the best approach to the hematoma have been aided by use of frameless stereotactic procedures. Intraopera-

tive ultrasound has also helped in localization as well as in demonstrating an AVM nidus within a hematoma.[74]

In the deteriorating patient, surgical treatment begins with maximum medical decompression. Mannitol, 100 g, is given intravenously. Intubation and hyperventilation are done. An arterial catheter is inserted, and blood pressure is controlled with sodium nitroprusside.

The craniotomy opening, cortical incision, and hematoma removal are usually done with the aid of loupes and a headlight.[106] The operating microscope is used for deep lesions and inspection of the hematoma cavity wall.[155] A cortical incision is performed in an appropriate noneloquent gyrus (Fig. 58.6). Deep exposure is greatly aided by self-retaining retractors (Fig. 58.7A). Evacuation of the hemorrhage is achieved with gentle suction and irrigation. Most of the hematoma is removed to achieve decompression, but the last adherent bits of clot may be left behind. This is done to avoid injury and bleeding from the walls of the cavity. Tissue suspicious of angioma or tumor warrants careful biopsy or excision. Hemostasis must be meticulous to avoid a recurrence. We raise blood pressure for 5 to 10 minutes to high-normal levels to check hemostasis. Great care must be taken to avoid hypertension, which could cause brain swelling.

STEREOTACTIC ASPIRATION

Backlund and von Holst[8] first suggested stereotactic aspiration of intracerebral hematomas. Over the past decade a host of reports, especially from Japan, have appeared with results of stereotactic aspiration.[51,57–59,65] Postprocedure CT scans have shown impressive reductions in clot size, or even total removal (Fig. 58.1). Clinical results have been encouraging, with infrequent recurrent hemorrhage.

Thrombolytic agents have been added to stereotactic aspiration to permit greater clot removal (Fig. 58.1).[95,131,164]

A related technique is endoscopic clot aspiration, reported by Auer and colleagues.[7] This method utilizes intraoperative ultrasound to localize the hematoma.[125] An excellent controlled study in 100 cases showed a clear advantage for endoscopic evacuation over medical treatment. This method is not widely used, however, and results may be more operator dependent than with stereotactic treatment.

In view of published results, stereotactic aspiration may be considered a reasonable alternative to open surgery when clot evacuation is warranted. In fact, this technique may even supplant craniotomy in the future.[93]

VENTRICULOSTOMY

When hydrocephalus or intraventricular hemorrhage is symptomatic, ventricular drainage is often warranted.[165] (Fig. 58.8). A standard ventricular drain is placed through a frontal bur hole, usually on the right side, but on the left if that ventricle seems more likely to drain satisfactorily. We use continuous drainage through a closed, sterile system, with the spillway set at 10 cm above the foramen of Monro. Within a few days, a decision is made regarding removal of the catheter or conversion to a ventriculoperitoneal shunt. Serial CT scans and a trial clamping of the drain may help make the decision.

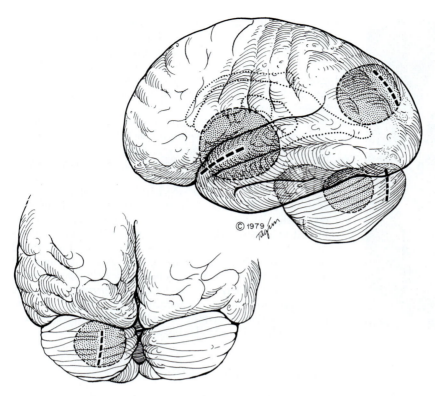

Figure 58.6 Common sites for brain hemorrhage requiring surgery: frontotemporal or basal ganglion areas, parieto-occipital area, and cerebellum. Cortical incisions are indicated.

POSTOPERATIVE CARE

Postoperative care must be meticulous to avoid recurrence. Blood pressure must be controlled, particularly as the anesthesia wears off.[63] Intravenous antihypertensive agents are given as needed to maintain the pressure in the normal range until oral agents can be substituted. Steroids are continued and then tapered approximately 1 week after surgery. If antithrombotic agents are indicated for other conditions (e.g., cardiac valve prosthesis), aspirin can be started after surgery with a low risk of rebleeding. Data are lacking, but warfarin probably can be resumed 1 month after surgery.

To avert seizures, appropriate doses of anticonvulsants are given to patients with supratentorial lesions. The anticonvulsant is tapered after 6 months if an electroencephalogram shows no epileptiform activity. When hydrocephalus is symptomatic, a ventriculoperitoneal shunt may be necessary.

Specific Hemorrhage Locations

PUTAMINAL HEMORRHAGE

The clinical syndrome is well established. Patients are characteristically up and active when they become ill. A hemiparesis develops and may progress to a hemiplegia accompanied in some patients by hemisensory loss, hemianopsia, dysphasia, or unawareness of the deficit, depending on the side involved. The hemorrhage may remain localized or it can track into the white matter of the frontal or temporal lobe, involve the internal capsule, or rupture into the ventricle. The progression of symptoms may cease at any point or continue to coma and death within a few hours. In 27 consecutive patients, a smooth onset characterized 62%, while 30% developed symptoms so rapidly that observers felt the deficit was nearly maximal at onset.[107] None of the patients experienced fluctuation of the deficit. Headache affected only 14% at onset and only 28% at any time, leaving nearly 72% free of headache, even in the presence of substantial focal neurologic deficit.

In evaluation of CT scans in 24 patients with putaminal hemorrhage, three groups were defined.[56] In the first group, patients in coma were found to have massive hemorrhage and poor prognosis. Patients in the second group were alert, with significant neurologic deficit and moderate-sized hematomas. Some made acceptable recoveries, but most were left with a substantial deficit. In the third group, mild deficits were found in relation to small hemorrhages. These patients generally made a good recovery. Whether surgery would have improved the outcome in groups 1 and 2 is not known.

Patients with small or moderate-sized hematomas in the putamen often make a good recovery either spontaneously or with medical management. When hematomas are >3 cm in diameter, the initial treatment is usually medical, but if the patient develops progressive neurologic deficit or drowsiness despite medical treatment, then early surgical removal of the hematoma may be considered.[140,153]

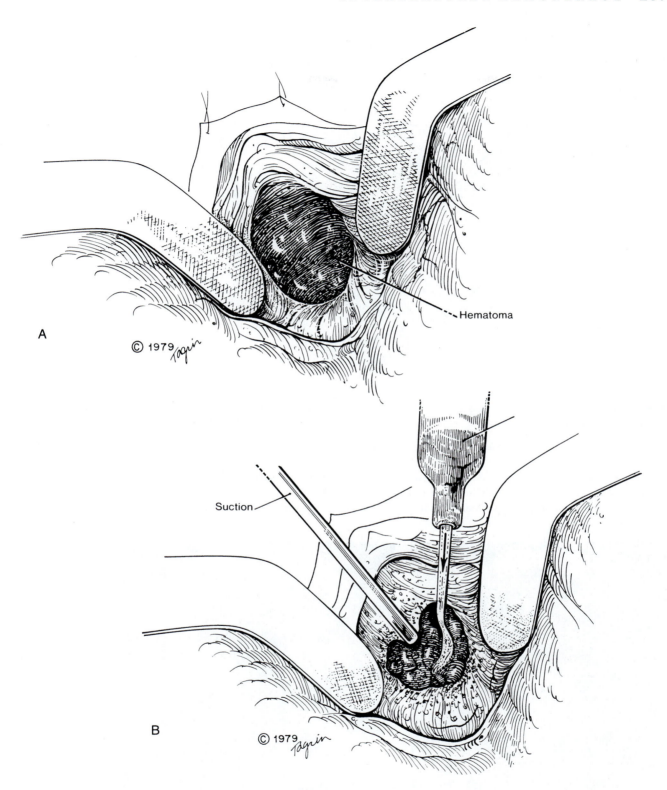

Hematoma

© 1979 Tagrin

A

Suction

© 1979 Tagrin

B

Figure 58.7 Surgical technique for removal of brain hemorrhage. (**A**) Exposure of hematoma with self-retaining retractors. (**B**) Suction removal of hematoma.

Illustration continued on following page

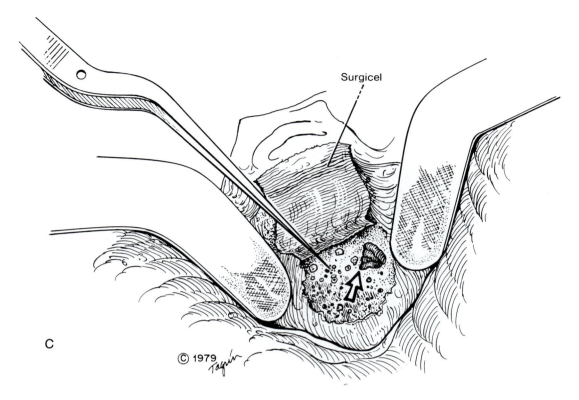

Figure 58.7 *Continued*. (**C**) Hemostasis with bipolar cautery and Surgicel. Suspicious tissue (*arrow*) warrants biopsy.

Figure 58.8 Thalamic hemorrhage. (**A**) CT shows large hematoma extending into ventricular system with hydrocephalus. Patient in coma with fixed pupils. (**B**) CT after initial ventriculostomy and later ventriculoperitoneal shunt. Gradual improvement with residual left hemiparesis.

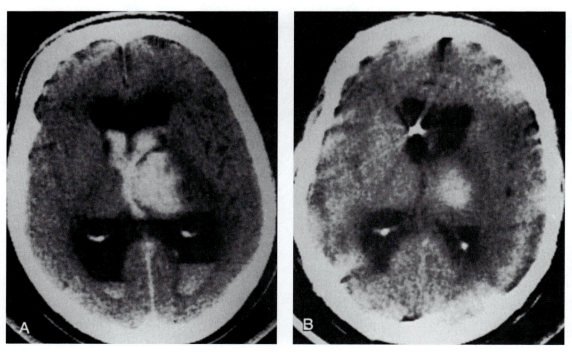

In two major controlled studies of surgical evacuation of putaminal hemorrhages, no clear benefit was demonstrated.[10,64] However, stratification was not done regarding the initial mild deficit that progressed. We continue to consider this group for surgery.

THALAMIC HEMORRHAGE

The classic features of thalamic hemorrhage are well described.[9,40,50] The initial deficit is hemisensory, and if the internal capsule becomes involved, motor weakness supervenes. Extension into the upper brain stem commonly leads to vertical gaze palsy, retraction nystagmus, skew deviation, loss of convergence, ptosis and miosis, anisocoria, or unreactive pupils. Dysphasia has been reported. Headache is rare. Compression of the third ventricle may cause hydrocephalus. In two reports of patients with thalamic hemorrhage, all died when the hematoma was >3.3 cm on the CT scan, while patients harboring smaller hematomas recovered, but frequently with disability. There is no evidence to indicate whether direct surgery would be of benefit to patients with larger hematomas. In general, we have not operated on patients with thalamic hemorrhage except to treat hydrocephalus by emergency ventricular drainage or permanent ventricular peritoneal shunting (Fig. 58.8). The role of stereotactic operation is uncertain, but the less invasive nature of the procedure lends itself to such deep lesions.

LOBAR HEMORRHAGE

Ropper and Davis[123] have characterized the syndromes associated with lobar hemorrhage. Occipital hemorrhage (11 patients) caused severe pain around the ipsilateral eye and dense hemianopsia. Left temporal hemorrhage (7 patients) began with mild pain in or just anterior to the ear, fluent dysphasia with poor comprehension and relatively preserved repetition, and a partial hemianopic deficit. Patients with frontal hemorrhages (4 cases) had severe contralateral arm weakness, minimal leg and face weakness, and frontal headaches. Parietal hematomas (3 patients) began with anterior temporal headache and hemisensory disturbance. In these 26 patients, 8 (31%) were known to have had hypertension prior to hemorrhage, 14 (54%) had documentation of normal blood pressure, 2 (8%) were on anticoagulants, 2 (8%) had an AVM, and 1 (4%) had a metastatic tumor. In another report of 22 patients with lobar hemorrhage, 45% were hypertensive, 14% had a metastatic tumor, 9% had an AVM, and 5% had a blood dyscrasia; in 27% the cause was unknown.[68] Amyloid angiopathy may be the source of bleeding in such patients.

In view of the varied etiologies, angiography is indicated in the evaluation of these lesions if the patient is stable.[68,167] If no etiology is discovered, the CT scan, MRI, and angiography should be repeated some months after hemorrhage, when the effects of compression have subsided, because tumor or AVM may not have been seen on the initial study.

With a deteriorating patient and suspicion of aneurysm, emergency operation without angiography may be warranted (Fig. 58.2).

Most patients with spontaneous or hypertensive lobar hemorrhages will make a good recovery with medical treatment.[144,161] However, if the patient shows signs of progressive neurologic deficit despite medical treatment, surgical removal of the hematoma is clearly indicated.[162,167]

INTRAVENTRICULAR HEMORRHAGE

CT scan demonstrates the degree of intraventricular hemorrhage. Most such hematomas result from the rupture of a parenchymal hematoma into the ventricular system[72]; occasionally, primary intraventricular hemorrhage can occur. Although the traditional teaching has indicated a poor prognosis, intraventricular hemorrhage may be associated with a rather benign clinical course.[78,113,151] A review of 54 patients with intraventricular hemorrhage on the CT scan revealed an association with a number of disorders, such as hypertension, intracranial aneurysm, AVM, tumor, and coagulopathy.[78] In a report of 32 cases of hypertensive intracerebral hemorrhage, 63% had intraventricular rupture.[160] The guidelines for surgical treatment are the same as those suggested for parenchymal hematoma. Ventricular drainage is generally of limited value, because the catheter frequently becomes obstructed. Thrombolytic agents might be of value, but data are lacking. Occasionally, ventriculostomy can be lifesaving and is indicated for neurologic deterioration secondary to acute hydrocephalus. Patients surviving the acute phase often require a ventriculoperitoneal shunt.

CEREBELLAR HEMORRHAGE

Frequently, hemorrhages into the cerebellum lead to a life-threatening downhill course, which may be dramatically reversed by surgical intervention.[20,32,33,43,55,82,109,129] Since there is effective therapy, a patient suspected of having a cerebellar hemorrhage should have an immediate CT scan[115] (Figs. 58.1 and 58.5). The onset of the hemorrhage is usually sudden, with nausea, vomiting, and inability to stand or walk. In a series of 56 patients, headache was present in 75%, dizziness in 55%, and loss of consciousness at onset in 14%. Examination showed appendicular ataxia in 78%, facial palsy in 60%, and ipsilateral gaze palsy in 54%.[138] Cerebellar hemorrhage may occur in childhood.[45]

Cerebellar hematoma represents a special situation regarding treatment.[30] Deterioration due to brain stem compression is unpredictable, and it is important to treat the patient before compression causes alteration in the state of consciousness and an unstable clinical situation. In one report,[109] 10 of 12 patients who were alert or drowsy preoperatively survived operation, while only 4 of 16 who were stuporous or comatose before surgery lived. The relationship of the level of consciousness to prognosis and the importance of not delaying surgery in patients with acute cerebellar hematomas have been stressed in other reviews.[163,166] However, even for a patient in a deep coma, removal of the hematoma can result in good recovery, especially if the time interval between the development of the comatose state and surgery is short. In a report of 10 patients with cerebellar hematomas 6 had a progressive course and all had hematomas ≳3 cm on CT scan.[80] We generally recommend removal of hematomas that are >3 cm in diameter if the patient is seen within the first week of hemorrhage. Patients seen later who have a stable neurologic course may be treated medically with close observation. One group treated patients with surgery if their Glasgow Coma Scale was ≤13 or the hematoma measured ≥4 cm.[73]

Patients with smaller lesions and no signs of brain stem compression are monitored carefully in the intensive care unit. Most patients with small hematomas have a benign course and may be treated medically with a good result.[53,80,91] On the other hand, once the patient shows signs of brain stem compression, deterioration can proceed abruptly. In this clinical setting, operation is indicated even if the hematoma is <3 cm. The hematoma is removed under direct vision via a suboccipital craniectomy. In addition, late deterioration has been reported as late as 1 month.[22] A few patients can be treated by ventricular drainage,[137] but this therapy alone does not relieve brain stem compression and may be followed by later deterioration. Ventricular drainage may be necessary after evacuation of the hematoma to treat persisting hydrocephalus.

MESENCEPHALIC HEMORRHAGE

In patients with mesencephalic hematoma, clinical features, including paralysis of vertical eye movements and a marked tendency to fall backward when standing, allow accurate localization of the lesion.[39,92,128] The etiology may be cavernous malformation or hypertension. Deterioration can result from extension of the hematoma mass. A subtemporal approach allows excellent exposure of the mesencephalon for evacuation of the hematoma, and a few successful cases have been reported.[35] Hydrocephalus can develop due to the obstruction of the aqueduct and can be successfully treated by ventriculoperitoneal shunting. The importance of initial close observation is emphasized along with supportive care in the stable patient. Surgery is recommended for patients demonstrating evidence of deterioration from rebleeding or hydrocephalus.

PONTINE HEMORRHAGE

Hemorrhage into the pons is the most dramatic and least treatable of all brain hemorrhages.[16,46,150] A small hematoma often leads to immediate coma, rapid quadriplegia, with small, barely reactive pupils and extraocular movement disturbances. A "locked-in" syndrome occasionally results. Most patients do not survive the acute phase.

A few cases of successful removal of pontine hematomas have been reported[11,97] (Fig. 58.3). A review of 24 patients with pontine hemorrhage included 4 who had suboccipital craniotomy and several who had ventricular drainage.[128]

MEDULLARY HEMORRHAGE

Bulbar hemorrhage is almost always fatal.[26] In a quadriparetic young woman, we microsurgically removed a small hematoma from the medulla with good recovery. MRI made the diagnosis, but no etiology was ever established.

Special Pathologic Entities

ANEURYSM AND AVM HEMORRHAGE

When either an aneurysm or an AVM is suspected to have caused an intracerebral hematoma, angiography is indicated. The indications for surgical removal of the hematoma are essentially the same as those for other types of intracerebral hemorrhage.

In patients with an aneurysm who urgently require an operation to remove the hematoma, every effort should be made to repair the aneurysm at the same operation. In patients with a ruptured AVM, the incidence of rebleeding is low. If the hematoma has to be removed urgently and the AVM is not readily accessible or would require extensive surgery, excision can be delayed for several weeks until brain swelling has subsided.

TUMOR HEMORRHAGE

Brain tumor is responsible for about 10 percent of all spontaneous intracerebral hemorrhages. Metastatic tumors, particularly melanomas and gliomas, are the cause in most cases.[79,88,102,135,154,171]

Pituitary adenomas bleed frequently, but the bleeding is usually within the tumor and rarely results in intracerebral hemorrhage.[154] Whenever tumor is suspected as the cause of intracerebral hemorrhage because of clinical, MRI, or angiographic findings, the hematoma should be removed, with thorough exploration and biopsy of the wall of the hematoma cavity. If a diagnosis is not established and the suspicion is high, follow-up MRI and possible angiography are indicated.

CAVERNOUS MALFORMATIONS

Usually, these lesions manifest with seizures or mass effect due to small hemorrhages.[98,106,171] On rare occasions, a large hematoma can occur. The general diagnosis may be suspected on the basis of MRI findings.[98,171] If the lesion is accessible, excision generally is warranted.[98,171] For deep lesions (basal ganglia, thalamus, brain stem), initial careful follow-up is a logical approach, with surgical excision reserved for severe deficit, recurrent bleeding, or progressive neurologic deterioration (see Fig. 58.3).[98,145,171]

ANGIITIS

Inflammatory angiitis of the brain may present as spontaneous hemorrhage.[17,138] The diagnosis is established by angiography, which shows a beaded appearance of arteries. Precise etiology is unclear. Steroids may be helpful. Surgery may be dramatically beneficial for the hemorrhage (Fig. 58.4).

DRUG-RELATED HEMORRHAGE

Intravenous methamphetamine administration has been associated with cerebral angiitis and intracerebral hemorrhage.[169] Phencyclidine abuse may also lead to intraparenchymal hemorrhage.[15] There are reports of vasculitis and hemorrhage after phenylpropanolamine ingestion (diet pills).[44]

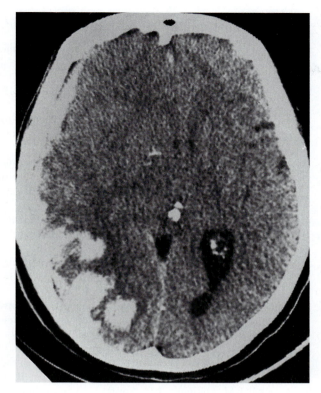

Figure 58.9 Amyloid angiopathy with hemorrhage. CT scan shows multilobular lobar hemorrhage. Surgical removal led to fair recovery. Pathologic confirmation of amyloid angiopathy.

AMYLOID ANGIOPATHY

Amyloid angiopathy may be the cause of spontaneous lobar hemorrhage.[87,108,146,147,152,156] The frequency is probably higher than previously accepted. The problem usually occurs in patients older than 60 years and may be associated with multiple hemorrhages. The diagnosis should be considered in lobar hemorrhage found in a normotensive elderly patient. If such a patient has had multiple hemorrhages, this diagnosis becomes the leading consideration. When amyloid angiopathy is suspected, efforts should be made to treat the patient medically, since surgery may be attended by severe hemorrhage. However, in some patients careful operation can be carried out without further neurologic deterioration (Fig. 58.9). Care should be taken to avoid disturbing the cavity walls, which may harbor fragile, amyloid-laden vessels, although biopsy is essential in establishing the diagnosis.

ANTICOAGULANT THERAPY

With widespread use of anticoagulants for treatment of cardiac and neurologic diseases, the number of patients with brain hemorrhage secondary to this cause has increased.[77] Most such cases are found to have either an excessively prolonged prothrombin time or a focal lesion such as an infarction to account for the bleeding. Such patients should be treated immediately with transfusion of fresh-frozen plasma. In addi-

tion, vitamin K_1 is administered to restore normal coagulation. With these measures, operation can be safely performed. In one patient on warfarin and aspirin, we achieved solid hemostasis only with exchange transfusion of fresh blood atop fresh-frozen plasma, vitamin K_1, and platelet administration.

THROMBOCYTOPENIA

This condition is diagnosed when the platelet count is >80,000/mm^3. Intracerebral hemorrhage due to thrombocytopenia has been reported in idiopathic thrombocytopenic purpura and in a variety of secondary thrombocytopenias.[2,21,23] Usually the hemorrhage is intracerebral, but subdural hematoma has been reported. Surgery is hazardous if the platelet count is <50,000 and is of concern with platelet counts in the 50,000 to 100,000 range. Platelet transfusions and corticosteroid therapy can usually achieve a hemostatic level. Guidelines for surgery are the same as in other conditions, once a hemostatic level of platelets can be achieved. Other hemorrhagic conditions, such as von Willebrand's disease, juvenile diabetic ketoacidosis,[6] and hepatic failure[102] have also been associated with brain hemorrhage.[3]

HEMOPHILIA

The great majority of hemophilia patients are deficient in factor VIII, a small number in factor IX, and an occasional patient in factor XI.[165] Brain hemorrhage is usually associated with mild head trauma. Any patient with hemophilia and a persistent headache should have a CT scan.[134] If hemorrhage is confirmed, then appropriate replacement therapy should be started immediately. To avoid spontaneous, intraoperative, or postoperative hemorrhage, it is necessary to maintain a level of at least 20% of the deficient factor with transfusions of the appropriate concentrate. If an operation is performed, replacement needs to be given until the incision is healed.

Future Directions

The most important question is patient selection for surgery. A properly designed, randomized, controlled study is needed. Because of the variability of the illness, careful stratification must be done in search of subgroups that might benefit from surgery.[116,132,136] Some important factors are age, Glasgow Coma Scale score, location of hematoma, volume of hematoma,[163] and involvement of crucial structures such as the posterior limb of internal capsule.[47,130,143] The number of factors and existing experience suggest the study needs to be large, probably requiring multiple institutions. Stereotactic aspiration and thrombolysis would seem to be attractive surgical techniques for such a study, to minimize operative trauma and maximize technical reproducibility.

References

1. Acampora S, Guarniere L, Troisi F: Spontaneous intracerebellar hematoma: report of ten cases. Acta Neurochir (Wien) 66:83, 1982

2. Almani WS, Awid AS: Spontaneous intracranial bleeding in hemorrhagic diathesis. Surg Neurol 17:137, 1982

3. Almani WS, Awid AS: Spontaneous intracranial hemorrhage secondary to von Willebrand's disease. Surg Neurol 26:457, 1986

4. Arana-Iniquez R, Wilson E, Bastarrica E et al: Cerebral hematomas. Surg Neurol 6:45, 1976

5. Astarloa R, Jimenex-Scrig A, Gimeno A et al: Valor pronostico de la TAC en la hemorragia cerebral supratentorial cerebral hemorrhage: multivariate study in 114 patients. Arch Neurobiol (Madr) 52:234, 1989

6. Atluru VL: Spontaneous intracerebral hematomas in juvenile diabetic ketoacidosis. Pediatr Neurol 2:167, 1986

7. Auer LM, Deinsberger W, Niederkorn K et al: Endoscopic surgery versus medical treatment for spontaneous intracerebral hematoma: a randomized study. J Neurosurg 70:530, 1989

8. Backlund EQ, von Holst H: Controlled subtotal evacuation of intracerebral hematomas by stereotactic technique. Surg Neurol 9:99, 1978

9. Barraquer-Bordes L, Illa A, Escartin J et al: Thalamic hemorrhage: a study of 23 patients with diagnosis by computed tomography. Stroke 12:524, 1981

10. Batjer HH, Reisch JS, Allen BC et al: Failure of surgery to improve outcome in hypertensive putaminal hemorrhage: a prospective randomized trial. Arch Neurol 47:1103, 1990

11. Becker DH, Silverberg GD: Successful evacuation of an acute pontine hematoma. Surg Neurol 10:263, 1978

12. Becker DH, Townsend JJ, Kramer RA et al: Occult cerebrovascular malformations: a series of 18 histologically verified cases with negative angiography. Brain 102:249, 1979

13. Benes V, Koukoik F, Obrovska D: Two types of spontaneous intracerebral hemorrhage due to hypertension. J Neurosurg 37:509, 1972

14. Bertalanffy H, Gilsbach JM, Eggert HR et al: Microsurgery of deep-seated cavernous angiomas: report of 26 cases. Acta Neurochir (Wien) 108:91, 1991

15. Bessen HA: Intracranial hemorrhage associated with phencyclidine abuse. JAMA 248:585, 1982

16. Bewermeyer H, Hojer C, Szelies B et al: Die spontane Ponsblutung: eine Analyse von 38 Fallen. Nervenarzt 59:640, 1988

17. Biller J, Loftus CM, Moore SA: Isolated central nervous system angiitis first presenting as spontaneous intracranial hemorrhage. Neurosurgery 20:310, 1987

18. Bogousslavsky J, Regli F, Uske A et al: Early spontaneous hematoma in cerebral infarct: is primary cerebral hemorrhage overdiagnosed? Neurology (NY) 41:837, 1991

19. Brambilla GL, Sangiovanni G, Rainoldi F et al: Gli ematomi intracerebrali spontanei: trattamento e risultati a distanza. Minerva Med 77:1209, 1986

20. Brennan R, Bergland RM: Acute cerebellar hemorrhage: analysis of clinical findings and outcome in 12 cases. Neurology (NY) 27:527, 1977

21. Brenner B, Guilburd JN, Tatarsky I et al: Spontaneous intracranial hemorrhage in immune thrombocytopenic purpura. Neurosurgery 22:761, 1988

22. Brillman H: Acute hydrocephalus and death one month after nonsurgical treatment for acute cerebellar hemorrhage: case report. J Neurosurg 50:374, 1979

23. Burrows RF, Caco CC, Kelton JG: Neonatal alloimmune thrombocytopenia: spontaneous in utero intracranial hemorrhage. Am J Hematol 28:98; 1988

24. Bydder GM, Steiner RE, Young IR et al: Clinical NMR imaging of the brain: 140 cases. AJNR 3:459, 1982

25. Calandre L, Arnal C, Ortega JF et al: Risk factors for spontaneous cerebral hematomas: case-control study. Stroke 17:1126, 1986

26. Calandre L, Felgueroso B, Bermejo F et al: Hematoma bulbar: presentacion de un caso con parada respiratoris y recuperacion espontanea. Arch Neurobiol (Madr) 49:95, 1986

27. Chee CP, Bailey IC, Refsum SE: Spontaneous massive haemorrhage into acoustic neuroma during anticoagulation therapy. Br J Neurosurg 1:489, 1987

28. Chen ST, Chen SD, Hsu CY et al: Progression of hypertensive intracerebral hemorrhage. Neurology (NY) 39:1509, 1989

29. Coraddu M, Nurchi GC, Floris F et al: Considerations about the surgical indication of the spontaneous cerebral haematomas. J Neurosurg Sci 34:35, 1990

30. Crowell RM, Ojemann RG: Cerebellar hemorrhage. p. 135. In Buchheit WA, Truex, Jr, RC (eds): Surgery of the Posterior Fossa. Lippincott-Raven, Philadelphia, 1979

31. Crowell RM, Ojemann RG: Surgery for brain hemorrhage. p. 233. In Moossy J, Reinmuth OM (eds): Cerebrovascular Diseases. Lippincott-Raven, Philadelphia, 1981

32. Dinsdale HB: Spontaneous hemorrhage in the posterior fossa. Arch Neurol 10:200, 1964

33. Dolinskas CA, Bilaniuk LT, Zimmerman RA et al: Computed tomography of intracerebral hematomas. I. Transmission CT observations on hematoma resolution. AJR Radium Ther Nucl Med 129:681, 1977

34. Duffy TA, Ayeni S, Levin AB, Javid M: Nonsurgical management of spontaneous intracerebral hematoma. Neurosurgery 9:387, 1981

35. Durward QJ, Barnett HJM, Barr HWK: Presentation and management of mesencephalic hematoma: report of 2 cases. J Neurosurg 56:123, 1982

36. el-Gohary EG, Tomita T, Gutierrez FA et al: Angiographically occult vascular malformations in childhood. Neurosurgery 20:759, 1987

37. Espinosa Urrutia J: Hematomas intracerebrales espontaneous. Rev Med Panama 15:81, 1990

38. Fazio C: A neurologist's study of the problem concerning surgical treatment of spontaneous cerebral hemorrhage. Sci Med Ital 1:101, 1950

39. Fingerote RJ, Shuaib A, Brownell AK: Spontaneous midbrain hemorrhage. South Med J 83:280, 1990

40. Fisher CM: The pathologic and clinical aspects of thalamic hemorrhage. Trans Am Neurol Assoc 84:56, 1959

41. Fisher CM: The pathology and pathogenesis of intracerebral hemorrhage. p. 295. In Field WS (ed): Pathogenesis and Treatment of Cerebro-vascular Disease. Charles C Thomas, Springfield, IL, 1961

42. Fisher CM: Clinical syndromes in cerebral hemorrhage. p. 295. In Fields WS (ed): Pathogenesis and Treatment

of Cerebrovascular Disease. Charles C Thomas, Springfield, IL, 1961

43. Fisher CM, Picard EH, Polak A et al: Cerebellar hemorrhage: diagnosis and surgical treatment. J Nerv Ment Dis 140:38, 1965

44. Forman HP, Levin S, Stewart B et al: Cerebral vasculitis and hemorrhage in an adolescent taking diet pills containing phenylpropanolamine: case report and review of literature. Pediatrics 83:737, 1989

45. Freitas PE, Aquini MG: Spontaneous intracerebellar hematoma during childhood. Neurosurgery 21:103, 1987

46. Froment JC, Bascoulergue Y, Crouzet G et al: Apparently isolated, spontaneous haematomas of the brain stem: seven cases explored by CT and MRI. J Neuroradiol 16:38, 1989

47. Fukiishi Y, Arita S, Suzuki T: Predicting recovery of ambulatory function after hypertensive putaminal hemorrhage by multivariate analysis of acute-phase clinical data. Neurol Med Chir (Tokyo) 29:503, 1989

48. Garcia CA, Weisberg LA, McGarry PA et al: Spontaneous hemorrhage in previously ischemic (pale) cerebral infarcts. Comput Radiol 10:55, 1986

49. Godersky JC, Biller J: Diagnosis and treatment of spontaneous intracerebral hemorrhage. Compr Ther 13:22, 1987

50. Goto N, Kaneko M, Muraki M et al: Thalamic hemorrhage—a clinicoanatomic study. Neurol Med Chir (Tokyo) 22:24, 1982

51. Hayashi M, Hawegawa T, Kobayashi H et al: Aspiration of hypertensive intracerebral hematoma by stereotactic technique. Neurol Surg (Tokyo) 9:1365, 1981

52. Hayward RD, O'Reilly GVA: Computerized tomography and intracerebral hemorrhage. Am Heart J 93:126, 1977

53. Heiman TD, Satya-Murti S: Benign cerebellar hemorrhages. Ann Neurol 3:366, 1978

54. Herbstein DS, Schaumberg HH: Hypertensive intracerebral hematoma: an investigation of the initial hemorrhage and rebleeding using chormium CR^5-labeled erythrocytes. Arch Neurol 30:412, 1974

55. Heros RC: Cerebellar hemorrhage and infarction. Stroke 16:17, 1981

56. Hier DB, Davis KR, Richardson EP, Jr et al: Hypertensive putaminal hemorrhage. Ann Neurol 1:152, 1977

57. Higgins AC, Nashold BS: Stereotactic evacuation of large intracerebral hematoma. Appl Neurophysiol 43:3, 1980

58. Hondo H, Matsumoto K, Tomida K, Shichijo F: CT-controlled stereotactic aspiration in hypertensive brain hemorrhage: six-month postoperative outcome. Appl Neurophysiol 50:233, 1987

59. Hondo H, Uno M, Sasaki K et al: Computed tomography controlled aspiration surgery for hypertensive intracranial hemorrhage: experience of more than 400 cases. Stereotact Funct Neurosurg 54–55:432, 1990

60. Husain MM, Metzer WS, Binet EF: Multiple intraparenchymal brain plasmacytomas with spontaneous intratumoral hemorrhage. Neurosurgery 20:619, 1987

61. Jensen G, Mosdal C, Sommer W: Sontane intracerebrale haematomer: en opgorelse over 54 opererede patiener. Ugeskr Laeger 148:2086, 1986

62. Jinkins JR: Current neuroradiological investigation of spontaneous hemorrhage into the craniospinal axis. Neurosurgery 18:664, 1986

63. Johnston JH, Beevers DG, Dunn FG et al: The importance of good blood pressure control in the prevention of stroke recurrence in hypertensive patients. Postgrad Med J 57:690, 1981

64. Juvela S, Heiskanen O, Poranen A et al: The treatment of spontaneous intracerebral hemorrhage: a prospective randomized trial of surgical and conservative treatment. J Neurosurg 70:755, 1989

65. Kandel EI, Peresedov VV: Stereotactic evacuation of spontaneous intracerebral hematomas. Stereotact Funct Neurosurg 54–55:427, 1990

66. Kaneko M, Tanaka K, Shimada T et al: Long-term evaluation of ultra-early operation for hypertensive intracerebral hemorrhage in 100 cases. J Neurosurg 58:838, 1983

67. Kanno T, Nagata J, Hoshino M et al: Evaluation of the hypertensive intracerebral hematoma based on the study of long-term outcome. II. A role of surgery in putaminal hemorrhage. No Shinkei Geka 14:1307, 1986

68. Kase CS, Williams JP, Wyatt DA, Mohr JP: Lobar intracerebral hematomas: clinical and CT analysis of 22 cases. Neurology (NY) 32:1146, 1982

69. Kawakami H, Kutsuzawa T, Uemura K et al: Regional cerebral blood flow in patients with hypertensive intracerebral hemorrhage. Stroke 5:207, 1974

70. Kawamura S, Ohta H, Suzuki A et al: Surgical indication and limitation in hypertensive intracerebral hemorrhage of the basal ganglia. No Shinkei Geka 14:1071, 1986

71. Kendall BE: Computed tomography in spontaneous intracerebral hematomas. Br J Radiol 51:563, 1978

72. Konig HJ: Zur Therapie und Prognose spontaner intrazerebraler Bluntungen mit Ventrikeleinbruch. Neurochirurgia (Stuttg) 29:75, 1986

73. Kobayashi S et al: Treatment of hypertensive cerebellar hemorrhage—surgical or conservative management? Neurosurgery 34:246, 1994

74. Kitazawa K et al: Color Doppler ultrasound imaging in the emergency management of an intracerebral hematoma caused by cerebral arteriovenous malformations: a technical report. Neurosurgery 42:405, 1998

75. LeDoux MS, Aronin PA, Odrezin GT: Surgically treated cavernous angiomas of the brain stem: report of two cases and review of the literature. Surg Neurol 35:395, 1991

76. Lee MX, Heaney LM, Jacobson RL, Klassen AC: Cerebrospinal fluid in cerebral hemorrhage and infarction. Stroke 6:638, 1975

77. Lieberman A, Hass WK, Rinto R et al: Intracranial hemorrhage and infarction in anticoagulated patients with prosthetic heart valves. Stroke 9:18, 1978

78. Little JR, Blomquist GA, Ethier R: Intraventricular hemorrhage in adults. Surg Neurol 8:143, 1977

79. Little JR, Dial B, Belanger G et al: Brain hemorrhage from intracranial tumor. Stroke 10:283, 1979

80. Little JR, Tubman DE, Ethier R: Cerebellar hemorrhage in adults: diagnosis by computerized tomography. J Neurosurg 48:575, 1978

81. Lobato RD, Perez C, Rivas JJ et al: Clinical, radiological, and pathological spectrum of angiographically occult in-

tracranial vascular malformations: analysis of 21 cases and review of the literature. J Neurosurg 68:518, 1988

82. Locatelli D, Messina AL, Bonfanti N et al: Spontaneous cerebellar hemorrhage. Ital J Surg Sci 18:159, 1988

83. Luessenhop AJ, Shevlin WA, Ferrero AA et al: Surgical management of primary intracerebral hemorrhage. J Neurosurg 27:419, 1967

84. MacEwen W: An Address on the surgery of the brain and spinal cord. 2:302, 1988

85. Maiuri F, Corriero G, Passarelli F et al: CT indications for surgery and evaluation of prognosis in patients with spontaneous intracerebral haematomas. Br J Neurosurg 4:155, 1990

86. Mandybur TI: Intracranial hemorrhage caused by metastatic tumors. Neurology (NY) 27:650, 1977

87. Mandybur TI, Bates SRD: Fatal massive intracranial hemorrhage complicating cerebral amyloid angiopathy. Arch Neurol 35:246, 1978

88. Mason I, Aase JM, Orrison WW et al: Familial cavernous angiomas of the brain in a Hispanic family. Neurology (NY) 75:169, 1991

89. McCormick WF, Rosenfield DB: Massive brain hemorrhage: a review of 144 cases and an examination of their causes. Stroke 4:946, 1973

90. McKissock W, Richardson A, Taylor J: Primary intracerebral hemorrhage: a controlled trial of surgical and conservative treatment in 180 unselected cases. Lancet 2:221, 1961

91. McKissock W, Richardson A, Walsh L: Spontaneous cerebellar hemorrhage, a study of 34 consecutive cases treated surgically. Brain 83:1, 1960

92. Mehler MF, Ragone PS: Primary spontaneous mesencephalic hemorrhage. Can J Neurol Sci 15:435, 1988

93. Mendelow AD: Spontaneous intracerebral haemorrhage [editorial]. J Neurol Neurosurg Psychiatry 54:193, 1991

94. Messina AV, Chernik NL: Computed tomograph: the "resolving" intracerebral hemorrhage. Radiology 118:609, 1976

95. Mohadjer M, Eggert R, May J, Mayfrank L: CT-guided stereotactic fibrinolysis of spontaneous and hypertensive cerebellar hemorrhage: long-term results. J Neurosurg 73:217, 1990

96. Mosdal C, Jensen G, Sommer W et al: Spontaneous intracerebral haematomas: clinical and computer tomographic findings and long-term outcome after surgical treatment. Acta Neurochir 83:92, 1986

97. Murphy MG: Successful evacuation of acute pontine hematoma. J Neurosurg 37:224, 1972

98. Ojemann RG, Crowell RM, Ogilvy CS: Management of cranial and spinal cavernous angiomas. Clin Neurosurg 40:98, 1993

99. Nehls DG, Mendelow DA, Graham DI et al: Experimental intracerebral hemorrhage: progression of hemodynamic changes after production of a spontaneous mass lesion. Neurosurgery 23:439, 1988

100. Nehls DG, Mendelow DA, Graham DI et al: Experimental intracerebral hemorrhage: early removal of a spontaneous mass lesion improves late outcome. Neurosurgery 27:674, 1990

101. New PF, Ojemann RG, Davis KR et al: MR and CT of occult vascular malformations of the brain. AJR 147:985, 1986

102. Niizuma H, Suzuki J, Yonemitsu T et al: Spontaneous intracerebral hemorrhage and liver dysfunction. Stroke 19:852, 1988

103. Ogilvy CS, Heros RC, Ojemann RG et al: Angiographically occult arteriovenous malformations. J Neurosurg 69:350, 1988

104. Ojemann RG: Spontaneous brain hemorrhage: what treatment should we recommend? Stroke 14:467, 1983

105. Ojemann RG, Heros RC: Spontaneous brain hemorrhage. Stroke 14:458, 1983

106. Ojemann RG, Crowell RM, Heros RC: Surgical Management of Neurovascular Disease. 3rd Ed. Williams & Wilkins, Baltimore, 1995

107. Ojemann RG, Mohr JP: Hypertensive brain hemorrhage. Clin Neurosurg 23:220, 1975

108. Okazak H, Reagan R, Campbell RJ: Clinicopathologic studies of primary cerebral amyloid angiopathy. Mayo Clin Proc 54:22, 1979

109. Ott KH, Kase CS, Ojemann RG et al: Cerebellar hemorrhage: diagnosis and treatment: a review of 56 cases. Arch Neurol 31:160, 1974

110. Padt JP, Dereuk J, vander Eecken H: Intracerebral hemorrhage as initial symptom of a brain tumor. Acta Neurol Belg 73:241, 1973

111. Paillas JE, Alliez B: Surgical treatment of spontaneous intracerebral hemorrhage: immediate and long-term results in 250 cases. J Neurosurg 39:145, 1973

112. Pecker J, Ioualalen N, Brassier G et al: Place de l'artériographie dans le diagnostic étiologique des hématomes intra-cérébraux spontanés. Neurochirurgie 32:281, 1986

113. Pia HW: The surgical treatment of intracerebral and intraventricular hematomas. Acta Neurochir (Wein) 27:149, 1972

114. Pineda A: Computed tomography in intracerebral hemorrhage. Surg Neurol 8:55, 1977

115. Pressman BD, Kirkwood JR, David DO: Posterior fossa hemorrhage: localization by computerized tomography. JAMA 232:932, 1975

116. Radberg JA, Olsson JE, Radberg CT: Prognostic parameters in spontaneous intracerebral hematomas with special reference to anticoagulant treatment. Stroke 22:571, 1991

117. Ransohoff J, Derby B, Kricheff I: Spontaneous intracerebral hemorrhage. Clin Neurosurg 18:247, 1971

118. Prasad K et al: Surgery in primary supratentorial intracerebral hematoma: a meta-analysis of randomized trials. Acta Neurol Scand 95:103, 1997

119. Richardson A: The management of primary intracranial hemorrhage. Mod Trends Neurol 3:89, 1962

120. Richardson A: Surgical therapy of spontaneous intracerebral hemorrhage. p. 397. In Krayenbuhl H, Maspes PE, Sweet WH (eds): Progress in Neurological Surgery. Vol. 3. Year Book Medical Publications, Chicago, 1969

121. Richardson A: Surgical therapy of spontaneous intracerebral hemorrhage. Clin Neurosurg 18:247, 1971

122. Richardson A: Spontaneous intracerebral and cerebellar hemorrhage. p. 210. In Russell RW (ed): Cerebral Arterial Disease. Churchill Livingstone, New York, 1976

123. Ropper A, Davis K: Lobar cerebral hemorrhage: acute syndromes in 26 cases. Ann Neurol 8:141, 1980

124. Ropper A, Zervas NT: Cerebral blood flow after experimental basal ganglia hemorrhage. Ann Neurol 11:266, 1980

125. Rubin JM, Dohrmann GJ: Use of ultrasonically guided probes and catheters in neurosurgery. Surg Neurol 18:143, 1982

126. Russell DS: The pathology of spontaneous intracranial hemorrhage. Proc R Soc Med 47:689, 1954

127. Sahuquillo J, Vilalta J, Sumalla J et al: Surgical vs. conservative treatment for spontaneous ICH. [letter; comment]. J Neurosurg 72:152, 1990

128. Sano K, Ochiai C: Brain stem hematomas: clinical aspects with reference to indications for treatment. p. 366. In Pia HW, Langmaid C, Zierski J (eds): Spontaneous Intracerebral Hematomas. Springer-Verlag, New York, 1980

129. Sano K, Yoshida S: Cerebellar hematomas. p. 348. In Pia HW, Langmaid C, Zierski J (eds): Spontaneous Intracerebral Hematomas. Springer-Verlag, New York, 1980

130. Sasaki K, Matsumoto K: Relationship between motor disturbance and involvement of internal capsule in hypertensive thalamic hemorrhage. No Shinkei Geka 19:221, 1991

131. Schaller C, Rohde V, Hassler W: Local thrombolytic treatment of spontaneous intracerebral hemorrhage with plasminogen activator (rt-PA). Indications and limits. Nervenarzt 66:275, 1995

132. Schutz H, Bodeker RH, Damian M et al: Age-related spontaneous intracerebral hematoma in a German community. Stroke 21:1412, 1990

133. Scott WR, New PFJ, Davis KR, Schnur JA: Computerized axial tomography of intracerebral and intraventricular hemorrhage. Radiology 112:73, 1974

134. Seeler RA, Imana RB: Intracranial hemorrhage in patients with hemophilia. J Neurosurg 39:181, 1973

135. Scott M: Spontaneous intracerebral hematoma caused by cerebral neoplasms. Report of eight cases. J Neurosurg 12:338, 1975

136. Senant J, Samson M, Proust B: Approache multi-factorielle du pronostic vital des hématomes intracérébraux spontanés. Rev Neurol 144:279, 1988

137. Shenkin HA, Zavala M: Cerebellar strokes: mortality, surgical indications and results of ventricular drainage. Lancet 2:429, 1982

138. Shuangshoti S, Phunthumchinda K: Cerebral acute angiitides and extensive hemorrhages associated with clinically silent acute bacterial endocarditis. J Med Assoc Thai 70:523, 1987

139. Specht CS, Pinto-Lord C, Smith TW et al: Spontaneous hemorrhage in a mixed glioma of the cerebellum: case report. Neurosurgery 19:278, 1986

140. Suzuki J, Sato T: Grading and timing of operation in putaminal ICH. p. 274. In Pia HW, Langmaid C, Zierski J (eds): Spontaneous Intracerebral Hematomas. Springer-Verlag, New York, 1980

141. Suzuki R, Ohno K, Matsushima Y, Inaba Y: Serial changes in focal hyperemia associated with hypertensive putaminal hemorrhage. Stroke 19:322, 1988

142. Tedeschi G, Bernini FP, Cerillo A: Indication for surgical treatment of intracerebral hemorrhage. J Neurosurg 43:590, 1975

143. Thie A, Spitzer K, Lappe H et al: Prognostische Bedeutung initialer klinischer und apparativer Parameter bei spontanen intrazerebralen Blutungen. Fortschr Neurol Psychiatr 56:163, 1988

144. Troncale JA, Close D, Pham XD: Spontaneous hypertensive-arteriosclerotic intracerebral hemorrhage. J Fam Pract 29:243, 1989

145. Tung H, Giannotta SL, Chandrasoma PT et al: Recurrent intraparenchymal hemorrhages from angiographically occult vascular malformations. J Neurosurg 73:174, 1990

146. Tucker WJ, Bilbao J, Klodawsky H: Cerebral amyloid angiopathy and multiple intracranial hematomas. Neurosurgery 7:611, 1982

147. Tyler KL, Poletti CE, Heros RC: Cerebral amyloid angiopathy with multiple intracerebral hemorrhages. Neurosurgery 57:286, 1982

148. Uchino A, Ohnari N, Ohno M: Acute hypertensive intracranial hemorrhage: MR imaging at 1.5T. Nippon Igaku Hoshasen Gakkai Zasshi 49:1243, 1989

149. Uede T, Nonaka T, Takigami M et al: Cavernous malformation of the brain stem: clinical symptom and its surgical indication. No Shinkei Geka 19:27, 1991

150. Veerapen R: Spontaneous lateral pontine hemorrhage with associated trigeminal nerve root hematoma. Neurosurgery 25:451, 453, 1989

151. Verma A, Maheshwari MC, Bhargava S: Spontaneous intraventricular haemorrhage. J Neurol 234:233, 1987

152. Vinters HV, Gilbert JJ: Amyloid angiopathy: its incidence and complications in the aging brain. Stroke 12:118, 1981

153. Waga S, Miyazaki M, Okada M et al: Hypertensive putaminal hemorrhage: analysis of 182 patients. Surg Neurol 26:159, 1986

154. Wakai S et al: Spontaneous intracerebral hemorrhage caused by brain tumor. Its incidence and clinical significance. Neurosurgery 10:437, 1982

155. Wakai S, Ueda Y, Inoh S et al: Angiographically occult angiomas: a report of thirteen cases with an analysis of the cases documented in the literature. Neurosurgery 17:549, 1985

156. Wattendorff AR, Bots GT, Went LN et al: Familial cerebral amyloid angiopathy presenting as recurrent cerebral hemorrhage. J Neurol Sci 55:121, 1982

157. Weil SM, Tew JM, Jr: Surgical management of brain stem vascular malformations. Acta Neurochir (Wien) 105:14, 1990

158. Weisberg L: Multiple spontaneous intracerebral hematomas: clinical and computed tomographic correlations. Neurology (NY) 37:897, 1981

159. Weisberg LA: Computerized tomograph in intracranial hemorrhage. Arch Neurol 36:422, 1979

160. Wiggins WS, Moody DM, Toole JF: Clinical and computerized tomographic study of hypertensive intracerebral hemorrhage. Arch Neurol 35:832, 1978

161. Yarnell P, Earnest MP: Primary non-traumatic intracranial hemorrhage: municipal emergency hospital viewpoint. Stroke 7:608, 1976

162. Yashon D, Kosnik EG: Chronic intracerebral hematoma. Neurosurgery 2:103, 1978

163. Yoshida H, Fujita H, Ohta K et al: Clinical study of hypertensive cerebellar hemorrhage: surgical indication and measurement of volume of hematoma. No Shinkei Geka 17:1105, 1989

164. Yoshida H, Komai N, Nakai E et al: Stereotactic evacuation of hypertensive cerebellar hemorrhage using plasminogen activator. No Shinkei Geka 17:421, 1989

165. Yoshida M, Hayashi T, Kuramoto S et al: Traumatic intracranial hematomas in hemophiliac children. Surg Neurol 12:115, 1979

166. Yoshida N, Kagawa M, Takeshita M et al: Grading and operative indication for hypertensive cerebellar hemorrhage. No Shinkei Geka 14:725, 1986

167. Yoshimoto H, Fujita H, Ohta K et al: Clinical study of hypertensive subcortical hemorrhage: surgical indication and long-term, functional prognosis. No Shinkei Geka 16:1465, 1988

168. Yoshimoto T, Suzuki J: Radical surgery on cavernous angioma of the brainstem. Surg Neurol 26:72, 1986

169. Yu Y, Cooper DR, Wellenstein DE et al: Cerebral angitis and intracerebral hemorrhage associated with methamphetamine abuse: case report. J Neurosurg 58:109, 1983

170. Zulch KJ: Pathologic aspects of cerebral accidents in arterial hypertension. Acta Neurol Belg 71:196, 1971

171. Sepideh A-H, Ogilvy CS, Ojemann RG, Crowell RM: Risk of surgical management for cavernous malformations of the nervous system. Neurosurgery 42:1220, 1998

CHAPTER 59

Rehabilitation of the Stroke Survivor

GLEN E. GRESHAM

WILLIAM B. STASON

The essential goal of rehabilitation is to restore the best possible performance and independence. For the survivor of stroke, relevant functional parameters usually include swallowing, communication, walking, other activities of daily living (ADL), instrumental activities of daily living (IADL), cognitive function, affect, socialization, the living setting in the community, family function, and, when appropriate, return to work.

The processes of medical rehabilitation are well-established in many countries throughout the world. In the United States, a team approach is regularly used, involving physicians (frequently physiatrists), rehabilitation nurses, physical and occupational therapists, speech-language-hearing pathologists, psychologists (including neuropsychologists), social workers, rehabilitation counselors, and recreation therapists. In addition, it is now widely recognized that the patient and family (significant others) are themselves integral members of the "rehabilitation team."[32]

Each rehabilitation professional is licensed to practice his or her specialty, and institutional team programs are accredited by the appropriate agencies. For instance, rehabilitation hospital programs are accredited by the Joint Commission for the Accreditation of Health Care Organizations (JCAHO) and the Commission for the Accreditation of Rehabilitation Facilities (CARF).[11,40] Rehabilitation services for the stroke survivor may be provided by individual professionals (if only one service is required) or by a "team" in a variety of settings, including hospitals (units of general hospitals or free-standing rehabilitation hospitals), nursing homes, home care programs, and outpatient settings.[32] The appropriate matching of stroke survivor to rehabilitation setting has recently been identified as a major priority by the Agency for Health Care Policy and Research (AHCPR) in its 1995 Clinical Practice Guideline on Post-Stroke Rehabilitation.[32]

Role of Rehabilitation Professionals in Acute Care for Stroke

Rehabilitation professionals have specific contributions to make in the acute care of stroke patients, long before a decision can be made concerning formal rehabilitation programs. These include proper positioning of the patient, implementing a regular schedule of turning, good skin care to prevent pressure ulcers, assessment of swallowing function and establishment of a safe and effective program of nutrition, early attention to possible removal of an indwelling urinary catheter, establishment of a regular voiding and bowel evacuation pattern, and passive joint range of motion exercises. Failure to provide these basic elements of good stroke care greatly increases the risk of preventable complications that might impede future functional progress. Joint contractures, pressure ulcers, unmanaged incontinence, and aspiration due to ignored dysphagia should not occur in the well-managed stroke patient. The rehabilitation professionals with special expertise in these areas are rehabilitation nurses, physical therapists, speech-language pathologists (for dysphagia), and registered dieticians.[32]

Once a program of knowledgeable bedside care is established, as a complement to ongoing diagnostic and therapeutic maneuvers by the neurologist or other acute care physician, the basis is in place for formulating a functional prognosis and designing a rehabilitation strategy to achieve the best possible functional outcomes. As soon as the patient's condition stabilizes sufficiently, steps should be taken to facilitate mobilization and to encourage socialization and resumption of responsibility for self-care.

Table 59.1 Neurologic Deficits Manifested by 148 Survivors of Documented Completed Stroke: The Framingham Study (April 1972 through March 1975)

Peripheral Motor Deficit	Hemisensory Defect		Hemianopia		Dysarthria		Dysphasia		All Patients					
									Men		Women		Total	
	Men	Women	Men	Women	Men	Women	Men	Women	#	%	#	%	#	%
None	4	1	3	2	1	2	7	6	31	47.0	46	56.1	77	82.0
Left hemiparesis	8	9	3	4	2	1	2	1	17	25.8	17	20.7	34	23.0
Right hemiparesis	5	5	2	2	8	7	5	5	16	24.2	17	20.7	33	22.3
Bilateral	2	2	1	2	1	1	1	0	2	3.0	2	2.4	4	2.7
Total	19	17	9	10	12	11	15	12	66	100	82	100	148	100

(From Gresham et al,[34] with permission.)

Prognosis for Functional Outcomes in Stroke Survivors

Evidence from community-based studies provides valuable information on the expected clinical courses of stroke survivors as a group. This phenomenon has, perhaps, been best documented by The Framingham Heart Study.[34] This research was carried out on stroke survivors from a community-based cohort (rather than an institution-specific study group with the inherent biases this involves). It was, in addition, conducted with great methodologic rigor, including comparisons with age-sex matched control subjects from the same cohort who were free of stroke. The epidemiologic profile, of 148 persons surviving stroke for at least 6 months, is shown in Tables 59.1 to 59.3.

Table 59.1 displays the neurologic deficits manifested. Over half (52%) had no residual hemiparesis. Of those who did, equal numbers had left and right hemiparesis.[34] Dysarthria and dysphagia were more commonly associated with right hemiparesis. Otherwise, no striking constellations of residual neurologic deficits were observed, and there was no significant difference between men and women.

Stroke survivors had significantly greater cardiovascular comorbidity than the age-sex matched controls with resultant implications for both survival and function (Table 59.2). They also had significantly higher frequency of obesity, diabetes mellitus, and arthritis.

Table 59.3 displays the frequencies of nine different types of disability. Each disability was significantly more common in stroke survivors than in controls. Psychosocial disabilities (such as socialization and vocational function) were much more common than physical disabilities (such as problems with mobility or activities of daily living). The disability profile was not substantially affected after analyses designed to control for comorbidities.[34]

Other recent community-based studies have added to this profile of functional outcomes in stroke survivors. In the Frenchay Health District Stroke Registry, 85% of enrollees were able to walk independently after 6 months and 12% remained aphasic.[64,65] Studies reviewed in the AHCPR guidelines found that two-thirds of survivors were independent in

ADL, results similar to those shown in Table 59.3.[32] A 1984 Finnish study found depression in about 30% of stroke survivors at 12 months[48] and several studies have documented decreased quality of life after stroke.[32] Rates of institutionalization range from 10% to 29%.[34] Gender seems to be a factor

Table 59.2 Frequency of 14 Documented Comorbid Disease Processes in 148 Stroke Survivors and 148 Stroke-Free Matched Controls: The Framingham Study (April 1972 through March 1975)

Type of Comorbid Disease[a]	Stroke Survivors		Matched Controls		P
	N	%	N	%	
Hypertension	99	67	66	45	<0.001
Hypertensive cardiovascular disease[b]	78	53	46	31	<0.001
Coronary heart disease	47	32	30	20	<0.05
Other heart disease	45	30	30	20	<0.05
Obesity	33	22	18	12	<0.05
Diabetes mellitus	32	22	15	10	<0.02
Arthritis	32	22	18	12	<0.05
Left ventricular hypertrophy by ECG	31	21	9	6	<0.001
Congestive heart failure	26	18	7	5	<0.001
Chronic lung disease	26	18	38	26	NS
Peripheral vascular disease	26	18	19	13	NS
Cancer	16	11	14	9	NS
Intermittent claudication	15	10	9	6	NS
Extremity amputation	3	2	0	0	NS
Total number of subjects	148	100	148	100	

Abbreviation: ECG, electrocardiogram.

[a] Not mutually exclusive categories.

[b] Includes cardiac enlargement by radiography or ECG in the hypertensive individual.

(From Gresham et al,[34] with permission.)

Table 59.3 Frequency of Nine Types of Functional Deficit in 148 Stroke Survivors and 148 Stroke-Free Matched Controls: The Framingham Study (April 1972 through March 1975)

Type of Functional Deficit[a]	Stroke Survivors		Matched Controls		P
	N	%	N	%	
Decreased vocational function	93	63	54	36	<0.001
Decreased socialization outside the home	87	59	42	28	<0.001
Limited in household tasks	83	56	30	20	<0.001
Decrease in interests and hobbies	70	47	30	20	<0.001
Decreased ability to use outside transportation	65	44	19	13	<0.001
Decreased socialization at home	64	43	41	28	<0.01
Dependent in ADL[b]	48	32	13	9	<0.001
Dependent in mobility	32	22	9	6	<0.001
Not living at home (nursing home or other institutional setting)	22	15	3	2	<0.001
Total number of subjects	148	100	148	100	

Abbreviation: ADL, activities of daily living.

[a] In descending order of frequency; not mutually exclusive categories.

[b] Dependent in ADL = Katz index score of C, D, E, F, G, or other.

(From Gresham et al,[34] with permission.)

as well, with women more likely to be in institutions than men.[46]

Role of Spontaneous Recovery in Stroke Survivors

Spontaneous recovery occurs most rapidly during the first 3 months after stroke.[47] The community-based Copenhagen Stroke Study, for example, showed that 95% of patients reached maximum neurological recovery within 13 weeks after acute strokes (95% confidence interval [CI] 11.6 to 14.4) and that maximum ADL function was reached within 20 weeks (95% CI 16 to 24).[41] Most stroke rehabilitation services are rendered during this period; hence, it is difficult to differentiate their respective contributions to recovery. Improvements in specific neurologic impairments can be tracked using the National Institutes of Health (NIH)[6] or Canadian Stroke Scales.[12] Improvements in function, however, may be due either to reductions in impairments or as a direct result of rehabilitation interventions. Imaginative future research will be needed to define benefits that are attributable specifically to rehabilitation.

Functional Assessment in Stroke Survivors

Formalized functional assessment, using standardized instruments, is the means by which the levels of different types of disability are documented. This process of functional assessment is used to screen candidates for stroke rehabilitation, establish a baseline, document improvement and establish final outcomes. The AHCPR guideline contains a complete guide to standardized functional assessment instruments used in stroke rehabilitation. The more commonly used global instruments are reviewed below, and those limited to specific functional domains are included in the respective following subsections.

The Rankin scale[55] was the first comprehensive functional assessment instrument published for use on stroke survivors. It is an ordinal scale that provides an overall estimate of the level of functional dependence in a given stroke survivor. It is still widely used today, although it was devised in the late 1950s when Rankin[55] and Adams and Merrett[1] were publishing pioneering studies that indicated that the long-term outcomes of stroke are not nearly as dismal as had previously been generally believed.

Other global or comprehensive functional assessment instruments that are frequently used with stroke survivors and span a spectrum of functional domains include the Functional Independence Measure (FIM),[30] the Patient Evaluation Conference System (PECS),[37] and the PULSES profile.[53]

The two most frequently used functional assessment instruments, in studies of stroke outcome worldwide, are the Barthel index[51] and FIM.[30] Their properties are shown in Table 59.4. The Barthel index is limited to ADL, but its great usefulness has made it a first choice for multiple investigators for 30 years. FIM is newer but has grown rapidly in popularity. In addition to ADL, it contains items for communication and social cognition. It has been the vehicle for generating the large database on medical rehabilitation maintained by the Uniform Data System for Medical Rehabilitation/Data Management Service at the State University of New York at Buffalo.

Patient progress should be monitored throughout rehabilitation using one of these standardized instruments administered at the time of entry into a rehabilitation program, at frequent intervals during rehabilitation, and during the first year after a patient returns to community living. The value of the information will be greatest if the instrument is administered in a consistent fashion by health professionals who are trained in its use. Results self-recorded by patients or their families are likely to differ considerably from those obtained by direct observation of the patient by professionals and need to be cross-validated. Goals of evaluation are to document clinically meaningful progress and to identify areas in which the patient fails to progress. Lack of progress may indicate a need for changes in the treatment regimen or may suggest that further treatment is not warranted. Both FIM and the Barthel index have ceiling effects and, therefore, may not be sensitive enough to measure progress in patients with mild levels of disability.

Table 59.4 Measures of Disability in Basic Activities of Daily Living (ADL)

Instrument	Description	Validity, Reliability, and Sensitivity	Uses and Time to Administer	Strengths and Weaknesses
Barthel index[51,63]	Ordinal scale with total scores from 0 (totally dependent) to 20 (totally independent) (or, 0 to 100 by multiplying each item score by 5). 10 items: bowel, bladder, feeding, grooming, dressing, transfer, toilet use, mobility, stairs, bathing.	Validity[16,33,38,64b] Reliability[60,63b] Sensitivity[16,24,25,33,59b]	Uses Screening, formal assessment, monitoring, maintenance Time 5–10 minutes	Strengths Widely used in stroke disability Excellent reliability and validity Weaknesses "Ceiling" effect in detecting change at higher level functioning Only fair sensitivity to change
Functional independence measure (FIM)[30,31,45,61]	18 items scored on a 7-point ordinal scale (1 = complete independence; 7 = total assistance). Total score ranges from 18 to 126. Subscores for motor function and cognition. Domains for self-care, sphincter control, mobility, locomotion, communication, and social cognition.	Validity[28,31b] Reliability[31,35b] Sensitivity[29,31b]	Uses Screening, formal assessment, monitoring, maintenance Time <40 minutes	Strengths Measures social cognition and functional communication as well as mobility and ADL Use of a 7-point scale increases sensitivity versus other disability scales Widely used in the United States and other countries Weaknesses "Ceiling" and "floor" effects at the upper and lower ends of function

Abbreviation: ADL, activities of daily living.

[a] *Adequately evaluated.*

[b] *Comprehensively evaluated. Additional useful instruments include the Katz index of ADL,[43] the Kenny self-care evaluation,[58] LORS/LAD,[8] and PECS.[37]*

(From Gresham et al,[32] with permission.)

Identifying Candidates for Stroke Rehabilitation

The results of standardized functional assessment must be combined with certain other information to produce a complete evaluation of rehabilitation potential. Intrinsic items include age, sex, race, marital status, a detailed evaluation of neurologic deficits, etiology of stroke, comorbid processes, educational level, vocational status, and financial/insurance/entitlement status. Extrinsic factors are also important. These include the constellation of family or significant others; the physical environment of the home; and the physical environment, resources, attitudes, and services available in the patient's community.

As soon as the patient becomes medically stable after a stroke and the assessment is complete, a knowledgeable and experienced physician should review the profile of patient characteristics and decide whether, and in what type of setting, rehabilitation services or programs are indicated.

Referrals to Rehabilitation Programs

One of the major contributions made by the AHCPR Clinical Practice Guideline on Stroke Rehabilitation was the formulation of a consensus-based decision tree for selecting the most appropriate rehabilitation setting for a stroke survivor[32] (Fig. 59.1). Alternatives range from no rehabilitation to single rehabilitation services to formal rehabilitation programs of varying intensity. Settings can be free-standing rehabilitation hospitals or rehabilitation units in general hospitals, nursing homes, outpatient facilities, or programs delivered in patient's home. The goal is to match the stroke survivor's medical and functional status with the capabilities of available rehabilitation programs. It is imperative that the stroke survivor and his or her family or significant others participate in the decision about if and where stroke rehabilitation services are to be delivered.

Threshold criteria at the top indicate patient characteristics that are essential preconditions for referral to any rehabili-

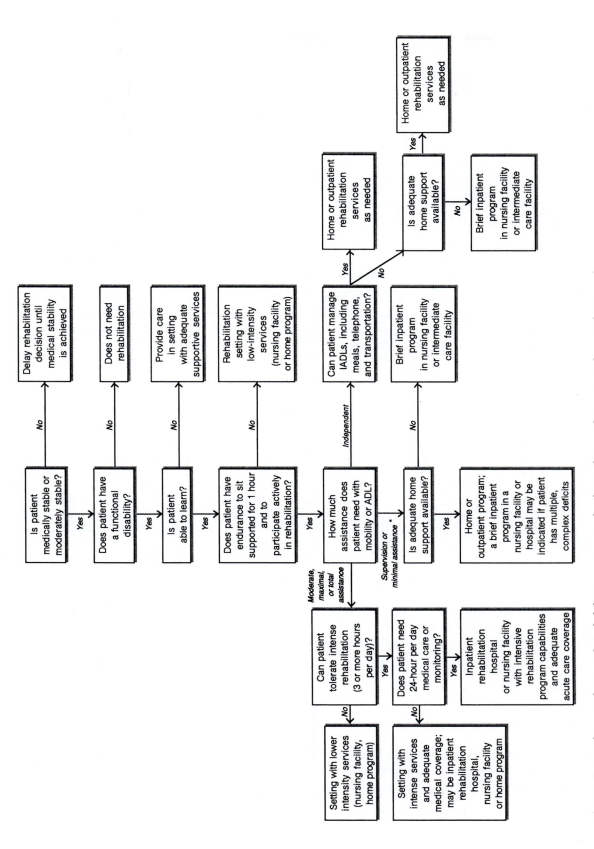

Figure 59.1 Selection of setting for rehabilitation program after hospitalization for acute stroke. [a]Under special circumstances, some patients with multiple, complex, functional deficits may be appropriate for inpatient programs. ADL, activities of daily living; IADL, instrumental activities of daily living. (From Gresham et al,[32] with permission.)

tation program. Reasonable medical stability, some significant functional disability, and the ability to learn and retain new ways of performing daily activities are primary among these. Medical conditions such as severe angina pectoris or inadequately diagnosed or treated infections militate against referral to rehabilitation until they are under control. Neurologic impairments that do not significantly affect the patient's ability to perform daily functions do not usually require rehabilitation therapies. Patients who are unable to participate in rehabilitation treatments because of cognitive deficits that result in the inability to concentrate or to learn adaptive strategies for performing tasks are unlikely to benefit from rehabilitation. At least, some minimal level of physical endurance is also essential.

The choice of rehabilitation setting in a patient who meets threshold criteria depends most importantly on the level of assistance required to perform daily activities, the closeness of medical supervision required, the ability to tolerate intense and frequent therapies, and the availability of caregiver support. A patient who requires moderate or maximal assistance (50% or more of the effort supplied by others) and can tolerate activities requiring intense physical and mental effort several hours a day has the potential to recover function more rapidly if referred to an intense ("acute") rehabilitation program in a hospital or nursing facility. Hospital settings are usually better able to provide round-the-clock medical and nursing care, if this is needed. Patients who are not able to tolerate intense treatments, even if they need moderate or maximal assistance, will be better served in a lower level program in a nursing facility or at home.

Greater flexibility of setting is possible for patients with disabilities requiring lesser levels of assistance. In these situations, the availability of adequate support at home often determines whether an outpatient, home, or nursing home program is best.

Process of Stroke Rehabilitation

Rehabilitation is an integrated learning process aimed at assisting the patient to achieve the greatest possible return of functional independence after a stroke. A treatment plan individualized to each patient's needs aims to

Prevent recurrent strokes and complications of the stroke

Reduce the effects of specific neurologic deficits

Help the patient compensate for disabilities by learning new ways to perform tasks

Help the patient adapt to life in a community setting after discharge from a rehabilitation program and to maintain functional abilities over the long term

The reader is referred to an extensive literature that discusses the process of rehabilitation.[4,13] Current recommendations are largely consensus-based, although some conclusions can be drawn from research studies. In all cases, appropriate

treatment plan documentation is required, periodic evaluation by the team or provider is mandatory, and a smooth transition to a permanent living setting (usually the home) must be effected when an inpatient rehabilitation program has been completed. Each of the following clinical or functional areas will be addressed during rehabilitation and, if indicated, specific treatment will be instituted:

1. Prevention of recurrent stroke
2. Prevention of deep vein thrombosis
3. Management of comorbid diseases
4. Swallowing, nutrition, and hydration
5. Bladder function
6. Bowel function
7. Sleep patterns
8. Cognitive function and perceptual deficits
9. Affective disorders and especially depression
10. Motor function, sensorimotor deficits, and impaired mobility
11. Spasticity treatment and contracture prevention
12. Communication disorders including aphasia and dysarthria
13. Activities of daily living
14. Need for adaptive equipment

Patient and family involvement is vital at all stages of the process. A detailed review of the current consensus approach to each of these areas of concern during the rehabilitation process is given in the AHCPR guideline.[32]

During stroke rehabilitation, the patient is monitored regularly by the use of standardized functional assessment techniques selected from those described earlier. When no evidence of functional improvement is seen in two successive evaluations (every 2 weeks in intensive programs and every 4 weeks in less intensive ones), the patient is usually discharged from a formal rehabilitation program. Individual services, however, may be continued after the return to community living to help the patient maintain the progress made during rehabilitation and achieve greater functional independence. Efficient management of the transition to the community, working with both patient and family, is an important priority in poststroke rehabilitation.[32]

Long-Term Outcomes in Stroke

It is not yet possible to "plug in" the clinical characteristics of an individual stroke survivor and derive, through a predictive formula, the profile of functional outcomes to be expected. There is, however, enough evidence available to enable the clinician to approximate this by combining careful observation and classification of the intrinsic and extrinsic characteristics of the patient with a knowledge of the expected distribution of particular outcomes for stroke survivors generally. Future stroke outcome research is needed on subgroups of patients with different neurologic syndromes and etiologies.

The outcome variables that have been studied in stroke survivors include

1. Survival

2. Location or living setting (e.g., within an institution or independent in the community)

3. Walking (ambulation)—considered independently or as a part of ADL, motor function, and balance

4. ADL—basic self-care including feeding, toileting, dressing, transfers, mobility, bathing, and grooming

5. IADL—more complex tasks needed for independent living, such as use of the telephone or public transportation

6. Communication/speech and language function

7. Psychosocial function, including cognitive performance and affect or mood

8. Sexual function

9. Community transition and social integration

10. Return to work

SURVIVAL

Survival is basic. Early advocates of programs for stroke survivors, such as Rankin[55] and Adams[1] acknowledged the appreciable levels of mortality but emphasized the importance of the ongoing needs of survivors for many kinds of help and understanding. Thus, over the past 30 years, emphasis has shifted from a fatalistic preoccupation with high immediate and excess long-term mortality to positive interest in improving the quality of life of survivors. This interest has also led to an increasing sense of responsibility for identifying and meeting their needs.

Mortality from an acute stroke is about 20% at 30 days after stroke; survivors are significantly more likely to die in each subsequent year than their stroke-free counterparts of the same age.[32] In the Framingham cohort, overall 10-year survival after stroke was 35%, with much better rates of survival for brain infarction in the absence of cardiovascular comorbidity.[56] There is, in addition, good evidence that survival after stroke is steadily increasing.[32] This reminds us that correspondingly greater numbers of individuals with strokes, many of them elderly, will be alive with needs that must be addressed. As acute neurologic care becomes more sophisticated and the various non-neurologic causes of death in stroke survivors (cardiac, thromboembolic, infectious) are more successfully treated, the obvious effect will be an increasing number of persons who will become candidates for stroke rehabilitation. Ongoing sensitivity to their needs and provision of appropriate services to meet them is a fundamental responsibility of rehabilitation and all long-term care providers.

LOCATION OR LIVING SETTING

Location or living setting (i.e., institution or community) of the stroke survivor is an important outcome of stroke. In general, institutional living is regarded as more restrictive, less pleas-

ant, and more expensive than community living (at least in the United States). It was, therefore, of interest that only 15% of long-term stroke survivors in the Framingham cohort were living in an institutional setting.[34] This frequency was even lower in other locales, at that time, probably due to the greater availability and desirability of institutional settings.[34] Finally, Kelly-Hayes and colleagues suggest that specific host characteristics, such as female gender, increase the risk of institutionalization after stroke.[46]

WALKING (AMBULATION)

Stroke does not usually destroy the ability to walk. Independent ambulation, with or without an assistive device but not requiring help from another person, was observed in 78% of long-term stroke survivors in the Framingham study[34] (see Table 59.3). Other studies with highly selected institutional populations (e.g., patients referred for rehabilitation services) have found frequencies for eventual independent ambulation ranging from 52% to 87%.[34] Since the Framingham study data were derived from a large, carefully followed community cohort, its findings should be representative of other populations.

Awareness that up to four out of five long-term stroke survivors will eventually be able to walk independently should encourage both the patient and the clinician. When a patient is not progressing toward independent ambulation, the reasons should be ascertained and appropriate changes made to the rehabilitation program. Only after all reasonable efforts have proved fruitless and the reasons for the inability to walk are clear should the clinician settle for a wheelchair or a lesser level of mobility.

Stroke survivors who are treated in a medical rehabilitation setting (whether it be a hospital, a free-standing clinic, a skilled nursing facility, or a home program) will have had the benefits of thorough assessment and physical therapy. Issues of preserving range of motion, muscle strengthening, improving coordination, gait training, and prescription and provision of the most appropriate ankle-foot orthosis or walking aid, as well as the knowledgeable management of spasticity, will be systematically addressed. It is important to recognize, however, that some patients who have walked well in a sheltered institutional setting may decompensate if discharged abruptly and without preparation into a less ideal environment, especially if continued services are not provided.

An overview of the rehabilitation treatment of motor function is given in the AHCPR clinical guidelines. Recommended functional assessment instruments for use in this area are the Fugl-Meyer Assessment,[23] the Motor Assessment Scale,[9] the Motricity Index,[14] the Berg balance scale,[3] and the Rivermead mobility index.[10]

ACTIVITIES OF DAILY LIVING (ADL)

Activities of daily living (ADL) have received the most attention and are the best-standardized outcomes in stroke. Formally designated as an *Index Medicus* category in 1968,[26] ADL comprises the daily functions that an individual must be able to perform in order to get along without the help of another person in carrying out daily personal care services (with all the expense and loss of personal autonomy that this implies).

Rehabilitation medicine emphasizes maximization of independence in personal care activities as the first step in returning the impaired individual to a meaningful life in the community. Indeed, independence in ADL is the dividing line between those persons who might manage on their own and those who will continue to require either an institutional setting or extended personal care services in the home. For a stroke survivor, the achievement of independence in ADL makes a life of autonomy and manageable costs in a community setting a possibility, unless he or she requires constant supervision because of dementia or emotional disorders. Thus, ADL independence is a major goal toward which the stroke survivor labors, aided by knowledgeable health care, rehabilitation, and human service professionals.

The functional variables that comprise ADL are well-delineated. The most important ADL outcome parameters are dressing (upper and lower body, indoor and outdoor garments, and putting on and taking off clothing), ambulation (already covered above in terms of walking, and including wheelchair mobility where walking is not possible), bathing (autonomy is highly dependent on the type of setting available), feeding, transfers, toileting (both bladder and bowel), and grooming (e.g., combing hair, shaving, and applying makeup). Other variables, such as activities in bed, are useful for assessing progress from postictal helplessness to maximal independence, but the seven variables listed above comprise the basic requirements for being able to leave the institutional setting and manage without direct and daily personal care services.[26]

There has been a major investigative effort since the 1960s to achieve a composite, overall expression of the level of independence in ADL, and a number of functional assessment instruments for this purpose have been devised. The advantages of such an approach include not only the greater ease of managing a single overall expression of ADL independence in documenting a patient's progress (as opposed to a number of separate component ratings), but also the opportunity such instruments provide to use aggregate data for both investigative and administrative purposes.[26,27]

One of the first major studies to use a standardized functional assessment instrument to assess the ADL independence of a group of stroke survivors was published by Katz et al in 1963.[43] This study of 138 elderly patients who had survived a first stroke for 30 days and had been referred to a geriatric rehabilitation hospital found that 43% were independent in ADL, as measured by the Katz Index,[43] at the end of 2 years. In the 1970s, Gresham and co-workers, using the same instrument in long-term survivors of stroke in the Framingham study, found that 68% of stroke survivors and 91% of matched controls were independent in ADL.[34] These two studies not only helped to establish the level of ADL independence to be expected in stroke survivors, but also documented the extent that these levels were truly related to stroke rather than to advanced age. Since the Katz index of ADL was used as the classification instrument in both studies, it could be inferred that the differences in frequencies were due to basic differences in the groups studied (i.e., an elderly institutional

as opposed to a middle-aged community population), rather than to disparate methodologies.

Other investigators, using other instruments, have documented frequencies of ADL independence in stroke survivors within the one-half to two-thirds range. For example, Feigenson found that 54% percent of stroke patients were independent in ADL at the time of discharge from a stroke rehabilitation unit, as measured by the Burke Stroke Time-Oriented Profile (BUSTOP); and Wade et al found that 45% and 62%, respectively, of medical service and stroke unit patients were independent in ADL 16 weeks after admission.[18]

These investigations, using rigorous methodologic approaches, have been able to establish a norm for ADL independence as an outcome variable in stroke. The fact that two of three patients recover considerable function is a powerful argument against a fatalistic, "do-nothing" approach and provides encouragement to those who feel that rewards of independent function warrant an ongoing positive emphasis in the clinical management of stroke survivors.

Another source of normative data on ADL outcomes in stroke is the work of Granger and associates.[26] Building on the earlier work of Moskowitz and McCann,[53] Mahoney and Barthel,[51] and others, they have carried out an elaborate series of studies of outcomes in stroke using adapted versions of the PULSES profile,[53] the Barthel index[51] and FIM.[30]

In 1979, Granger, Albrecht, and Hamilton published a widely recognized study in which their formalized functional assessment approach was used to evaluate a random sample of 658 patients in the 10-center Comprehensive Service Needs Study.[24] Patients were evaluated at admission to medical rehabilitation, at discharge, and 2 years after discharge. For the 134 patients in this group who had focal cerebral disorders, the mean Barthel index scores were 34, 71, and 72 for the three points in time, respectively. Thus, the study documented that ADL scores increased during rehabilitation and, very important, were maintained after discharge. Subsequently, the Uniform Data System for Medical Rehabilitation (UDSMR) has published annually the national database FIM scores, which include ADL as a major component, in the *American Journal of Physical Medicine and Rehabilitation*.[19]

Worldwide popularity of the Barthel index as a measure of ADL independence has been due to the comprehensiveness of component variables, categorical scoring, the ability to retain subscores for each variable, and the fact that a maximum score of 100 signifies the ability of an individual to get along without attendant care (even though fully independent living may be precluded by other factors). This is conceptually consonant with the current process of medical rehabilitation, in which the "maximum benefit" of inpatient physical restoration is usually synonymous with reaching the highest achievable level of independence in ADL.

Since so many different ADL scales had been generated, a 1980 study by Gresham, Phillips, and Labi compared the relative merits of the Katz index of ADL, the Barthel index, and the Kenny self-care evaluation in scoring ADL independence in stroke.[33] By administering the Donaldson ADL evaluation form,[15] which contains the data needed for all three instruments, to the 148 stroke survivors in the Framingham study, they found that there was no statistically significant difference among the overall ratios of perfect ADL independ-

Table 59.5 Frequency of Independence in ADL[a,b] in Stroke Survivors in the Framingham Study

Instrument	Frequency of Full Independence in ADL (%)
Barthel index[51]	35.1
Katz index of ADL[43]	39.2
Kenny self-care evaluation[57]	41.9

Abbreviation: ADL, activities of daily living.

[a] As determined simultaneously by three different instruments in 148 long-term stroke survivors in the Framingham Study Cohort. Independence = a perfect score.

[b] N = 148. Frequencies are not significantly different as determined by the Z test.

(From Gresham et al,[34] with permission.)

ence (Table 59.5). Differences in sensitivity (the Kenny self-care evaluation being the most sensitive and the Katz index of ADL the least) were again demonstrated.

In recent years, FIM[30] has become even more widely used in the United States than the Barthel index.[51] Currently, both are used as methods of documenting stroke patients before, during, and after rehabilitation. The descriptions of the attributes of these instruments is shown in Table 59.4.

New research ideas and innovative clinical interventions that will promote greater independence in ADL and, in so doing, lower the costs of ongoing care continue to be needed. For example, improved technology may be able to increase ADL independence in stroke survivors above the two-thirds level currently documented. It is hoped that such improvements will soon occur.

INSTRUMENTAL ACTIVITIES OF DAILY LIVING

Instrumental activities of daily living (IADL) have been less intensively studied but are of great importance in formulating care plans for survivors of stroke. These activities, such as use of the telephone, homemaking, and shopping, represent an extension of ADL skills into more complex areas of independent living. Such skills obviously depend on cognitive, emotional, and environmental factors, as well as physical competence in motor skills. They comprise the next steps toward truly autonomous living. As with personal ADLs, IADLs are the particular professional purview of occupational therapists in the medical rehabilitation team. Two recommended functional assessment scales for IADL are the PGC Instrumental Activities of Daily Living Scale[50] and the Frenchay activities index.[39]

COMMUNICATION/SPEECH AND LANGUAGE FUNCTION

Communication is of great importance to stroke survivors whose neurologic deficits include dysphasia or dysarthria. In the Framingham cohort, 18% and 16%, of long-term stroke

survivors were found to have dysphasia and dysarthria, respectively. Residual frequencies of these magnitudes emphasize the importance of carrying out adequate assessments and establishing plans for enhancing communication skills for stroke survivors with these problems.

Assessments are best performed by experienced speech pathologists. By combining structured functional assessment of overall communication skills with audiometric screening and good clinical judgment, the speech pathologist can both describe the deficit and suggest the most feasible method for improving overall communication. An excellent summary of functional communication instruments has been published by Frattali and colleagues.[21]

As with physical therapy services for mobility and occupational therapy for ADL, the presence of the speech pathologist on the rehabilitation team facilitates early and coordinated attention to the communication needs of the patient. An increasing body of evidence documents that individual or group treatment for aphasic patients is of value.[32] Since the speech pathologist is the best source of evaluation and recommendations for treatment, stroke survivors with speech problems should be referred for both. The speech pathologist can direct the patient and family to treatment and support groups, as well as provide the best specific therapy.

PSYCHOSOCIAL FUNCTION

Psychosocial function includes the complex and important dimensions of memory, ability to problem solve, and a variety of affective and behavioral disorders. Overall psychosocial disabilities manifested by long-term stroke survivors exceeds anything that could be explained by physical limitations alone[34] (see Table 59.3) and the work of Labi et al showed that even physically restored stroke survivors have excess psychosocial dysfunction.[49]

Cognitive Performance

The assessment of cognitive function is vitally important but often elusive.[32] A sensible beginning is the consistent use of a simple screening instrument for dementia. The most widely used, in stroke, is the mini-mental status examination.[20] Physicians not wishing to rely on such an instrument can always draw their conclusions from in-depth interviews.

Identification of specific cognitive dysfunctions raises the possibility that conventional rehabilitation services, which rely heavily on learning by the patient for their success, may face unusual difficulties and a decreased likelihood for achievement. It is better to face these possibilities directly rather than continue with unsuccessful rehabilitation programs that end up being frustrating to both patient and provider.

In practical terms, it is often difficult for the primary physician to find appropriate cognitive assessment consultants and therapists. While hospital-based rehabilitation programs offer expertise in neuropsychology, many primary physicians may legitimately elect to settle for less sophisticated services that are readily available in the community.

Cognitive remediation is currently a very active field of investigation, greatly stimulated by the present "epidemic" of traumatic closed head injuries.[62] While much is being learned about cerebral dysfunction, it is important for physicians to remember that findings from brain-injured groups with multiple deficits may not be uniformly applicable to stroke survivors, whose cerebral lesions are usually more discrete. Moreover, documented benefits from treatment for cognitive dysfunction are sparse.

Depression and Other Affective Disorders

Depression occurs in 11% to 68% of patients after strokes including major depression in 10% to 27%.[32] A high index of suspicion is needed if the condition is to be diagnosed and treated appropriately. A variety of screening tests may help to raise awareness, but the diagnosis ultimately requires a thorough clinical interview by a knowledgeable health professional. Establishing the diagnosis is important, because effective pharmacologic and psychological treatment is available and because undiagnosed depression will adversely affect the success of rehabilitation.

Once the diagnosis of depression is made, treatment should be sought from the most expert mental health professional available and preferably one who has had experience in working with stroke patients. Depression is a treatable entity that should not be missed or ignored in stroke patients. For screening purposes, four depression scales are recommended in the AHCPR guideline.[32] These are the Beck depression inventory,[2] the Center for Epidemiologic Studies depression scale (CES-D),[54] the geriatric depression scale (GDS),[69] and the Hamilton depression scale.[36]

SEXUAL FUNCTION

Physicians should know that stroke survivors continue to have sexual identities, needs, and capabilities. Since the specific organs involved in sexual activity are bilaterally innervated, there is no neurologic reason why unilateral stroke should permanently impair sexual capabilities. Recently, a number of formal studies have begun to examine sexual function in stroke survivors.[5] Their findings suggest that stroke survivors would benefit from more information and understanding on sexual matters from health care professionals.

COMMUNITY TRANSITION AND SOCIAL INTEGRATION

The period after discharge from the hospital for an acute stroke or from an inpatient rehabilitation program is a difficult one both for the disabled stroke survivor and for caregivers. Adapting to a home environment that does not provide the same level of support as the hospital or nursing facility and the need to resume daily activities and family relationships can be formidable challenges. Prior preparation of the patient and caregivers and evaluation of the home setting lay the groundwork. Follow-up is essential, however, and creative problem solving is frequently required. Continuity of medical and rehabilitative care; coordination of care between patient, family, and providers; and home visits to monitor postdischarge progress are the key elements. Generally, care should be coordinated by a single individual who under different circumstances could be the patient, caregiver, primary care physician, or a rehabilitation specialist. The burdens of caregiving may interfere with family functioning and adversely affect the caregiver's health. Close attention should be paid to these possibilities. The family assessment device (FAD)[17] (Table 59.6), is a useful and recommended functional assessment instrument for this important area.

RETURN TO WORK

Although they may be a minority, many stroke survivors can and do return to work. Weisbroth et al[67] have shown that vocational rehabilitation services can help stroke survivors re-enter the work force. Formal medical rehabilitation programs will routinely consider this possibility. Other providers should remember that if the possibility of return to work exists, the patient should be referred to the state vocational agency (in most states, the Division of Vocational Rehabilitation or the Office of Vocational Rehabilitation), where programs of assessment, training, and placement are available for appropriate candidates.

Classical medical rehabilitation began with the concept that to return handicapped people to work would generate more additional taxes than were expended for rehabilitation services. Only recently has the emphasis in stroke rehabilitation been extended to include consideration of "quality of life" as a valued outcome. The simple facts are that a large number of older people who survive strokes are already retired because of age; some are eager to exercise the option to retire that is presented by a major, disabling illness such as stroke; and still others will face the familiar financial disincentives (loss of disability income and related health insurance benefits) that encourage many handicapped Americans to shy away from employment possibilities. A life of good quality for many stroke survivors, therefore, will have to be achieved outside the workplace. Health professionals treating stroke survivors need to support and facilitate creative, meaningful avocational pursuits. For many stroke patients and their families, the stroke clubs (sponsored by the American Heart Association and other agencies) provide a helpful means of re-entry into community activities.

Summary

Significant numbers of individuals will survive their strokes but face the obstacles of living with varying levels and types of functional limitations. Health and human services providers have a responsibility to meet their needs. A thorough assessment of each individual's problems and strengths is basic to planning the appropriate program of care. Four out of five long-term stroke survivors will walk, more than half will be independent in ADL, and fewer than 2 of 10 will require an

Table 59.6 Family Assessment

Instrument	Description	Validity, Reliability, and Sensitivity	Uses and Time to Administer	Strengths and Weaknesses
Family Assessment Device (FAD)[17]	7 domain scales assessing problem solving, communication, roles, affective responsiveness, affective involvement, behavior control, and general functioning	Validity[7,22,42,52,68a] Reliability[7,17,44,52a] Sensitivity: Not tested.	Uses Formal assessment, monitoring, and maintenance Time <30 minutes	Strengths Widely used in stroke Computer scoring available Excellent validity and reliability Cut-off scores for family functioning Available in multiple languages Weaknesses Assessment subjective Sensitivity not tested

[a] *Adequately evaluated.*

institutional living setting. Psychosocial problems are likely to persist after maximum physical restoration has occurred. Although a minority of stroke survivors will return to work, good social reintegration is a legitimate goal for each. Comprehensive medical rehabilitation programs, in a variety of settings, will systematically address these problems and will work toward the coordinated remediation of deficits.

References

1. Adams GF, Merrett JD: Prognosis and survival in the aftermath of hemiplegia. Br Med J 17:309, 1961
2. Beck AT, Ward CH, Mendelson M et al: An inventory for measuring depression. Arch Gen Psychiatry 4:561, 1961
3. Berg K, Wood-Dauphinee S, Williams JJ et al: Measuring balance in the elderly: validation of an instrument. Can J Public Health, suppl. 2:S7, 1992
4. Braddom RL ed: Physical Medicine and Rehabilitation. WB Saunders, Philadelphia, 1996
5. Bray GP, DeFrank RS, Wolf TL: Sexual functioning in stroke survivors. Arch Phys Med Rehabil 62:286, 1981
6. Brott T, Adams HP, Olinger CP et al: Measurements of acute cerebral infarction: a clinical examination scale. Stroke 20:864, 1989
7. Byles J, Bryne C, Boyle M et al: Ontario child health study: reliability and validity of the general functioning subscale of the McMaster family assessment device. Fam Process 27:97, 1988
8. Carey RG, Posavac EJ: Program evaluation of a physical medicine and rehabilitation unit: a new approach. Arch Phys Med Rehabil 59:330, 1978
9. Carr JH, Shepherd RB, Nordholm L et al: Investigation of a new motor assessment scale for stroke patients. Phys Ther 65:175, 1985
10. Collen FM, Wade DT, Robb GF et al: The Rivermead mobility index: a further development of the Rivermead motor assessment. Int Disabil Stud 13:50, 1991
11. Commission on Accreditation of Rehabilitation Facilities

(CARF): Standards Manual for Organizations Serving People with Disabilities. CARF, Tucson, AZ, 1994
12. Cote R, Hachinski VC, Shurvill BL et al: The Canadian neurological scale: a preliminary study in acute stroke. Stroke 17:731, 1986
13. DeLisa JA, Gans BM: Rehabilitation Medicine: Principles and Practice. 2nd Ed. JB Lippincott, Philadelphia, 1993
14. Demeurisse G, Demol O, Robaye E: Motor evaluation in vascular hemiplegia. Eur Neurol 19:382, 1980
15. Donaldson SW, Wagner C, Gresham GE: A unified ADL evaluation form. Arch Phys Med Rehabil 54:175, 1973
16. Duncan PW: Contemporary management of motor control problems: proceedings of the II Step Conference—stroke: physical therapy assessment and treatment. Ch 21. Foundation for Physical Therapy, Alexandria, VA, 1992
17. Epstein NB, Baldwin LM, Bishop DS: The McMaster family assessment device. J Marital Fam Ther 9:171, 1983
18. Feigenson JS, McCarthy ML, Greenberg SD et al: Factors influencing outcome and length of stay in a stroke rehabilitation unit. 2. Comparison of 318 screened and 248 unscreened patients. Stroke 8:657, 1977
19. Fiedler RC, Granger CV, Ottenbacher KJ: The uniform data system for medical rehabilitation. Report of first admissions for 1994. Am J Phys Med Rehabil 75:125, 1996
20. Folstein MF, Folstein SE, McHugh PR: Mini-mental state exam: a practical method for grading the cognitive state of patients for clinicians. J Psychiatr Res 12:189, 1975
21. Frattali C, Thompson C, Holland A et al: American Speech-Language-Hearing Association Functional Assessment of Communication Skills for Adults (ASHA FACS). ASHA, Rockville, MD, 1995.
22. Fristad MA: A comparison of the McMaster and Circumplex family assessment instruments. J Marital Fam Ther 15:259, 1989
23. Fugl-Meyer AR, Jaasko L, Leyman I et al: The post-stroke hemiplegic patient. I. A method for evaluation of physical performance. Scand J Rehabil Med 7:13, 1975
24. Granger CV, Albrecht GL, Hamilton BB: Outcome of comprehensive medical rehabilitation: measurement by

PULSES profile and the Barthel index. Arch Phys Med Rehabil 60:145, 1979

25. Granger CV, Dewis LS, Peters NC et al: Stroke rehabilitation: analysis of repeated Barthel index measures. Arch Phys Med Rehabil 60:14, 1979

26. Granger CV, Gresham GE: Functional Assessment in Rehabilitation Medicine. Williams & Wilkins, Baltimore, 1984

27. Granger CV, Gresham GE: New Developments in Functional Assessment. Phys Med Rehabil Clin North Am. Vol. 4. WB Saunders, Philadelphia, 1993

28. Granger CV, Hamilton BB: Measurement of stroke rehabilitation outcome in the 1980's. Stroke, 21(suppl. II):S46, 1990

29. Granger CV, Hamilton BB: UDS report: the uniform data system for medical rehabilitation report on the first admissions for 1990. Am J Phys Med Rehabil 71:108, 1992

30. Granger CV, Hamilton BB, Keith RA et al: Advances in functional assessment for medical rehabilitation. Top Geriat Rehabil 1:59, 1986

31. Granger CV, Hamilton BB, Sherwin FS: Guide for the use of the uniform data set for medical rehabilitation. Buffalo General Hospital, Uniform Data System for Medical Rehabilitation Project Office, Buffalo, NY, 1986

32. Gresham GE, Duncan PW, Stason WB et al: Post-Stroke Rehabilitation. Clinical Practice Guideline No. 16. U.S. Department of Health and Human Services, Public Health Service, Agency for Health Care Policy and Research (AHCPR Publication No. 95–0662), Rockville, MD, 1995

33. Gresham GE, Phillips TF, Labi ML: ADL status in stroke: relative merits of three standard indexes. Arch Phys Med Rehabil 61:355, 1980

34. Gresham GE, Phillips TF, Wolf PA et al: Epidemiologic profile of long-term stroke disability: the Framingham study. Arch Phys Med Rehabil 60:487, 1979

35. Hamilton BB, Laughlin JA, Granger CV et al: Interrater agreement of the seven level functional independence measure (FIM). Arch Phys Med Rehabil 72:790, 1991

36. Hamilton M: A rating scale for depression. J Neurol Neurosurg Psychiatry 23:56, 1960

37. Harvey RF, Jellinek HM: Functional performance assessment: a program approach. Arch Phys Med Rehabil 62:456, 1981

38. Hertanu JS, Demopoulos JT, Yang WC et al: Stroke rehabilitation: correlation and prognostic value of computerized tomography and sequential functional assessements. Arch Phys Med Rehabil 65:505, 1984

39. Holbrook M, Skilbeck CE: An activities index for use with stroke patients. Age Aging 12:166, 1983

40. Joint Commission on Accreditation for Healthcare Organizations (JCAHO): 1993 Accreditation Manual for Hospitals. JCAHO, Oakbrook Terrace, IL, 1992

41. Jorgensen H, Nakayama H, Raaschou HO et al: Outcome and time course of recovery in stroke. Part II: time course of recovery. The Copenhagen study. Arch Phys Med Rehabil 76:406, 1995

42. Kabacoff RI, Miller IW, Bishop DS et al: A psychometric study of the McMaster family assessment device in psychiatric, medical, and nonclinical samples. J Fam Psychol 3:431, 1990

43. Katz S, Ford AB, Moskowitz RW et al: Studies of illness in the aged: the index of ADL: a standardized measure of biological and psychosocial function. JAMA 185:914, 1963

44. Kaufman KL, Tarnowksi KJ, Simonian SJ et al: Assessing the readability of family assessment self-report measures. Psychol Assess: A J Consult Clin Psychol 3:697, 1991

45. Keith RA, Granger CV, Hamilton BB et al: The functional independence measure: a new tool for rehabilitation. p. 6. In Eisenberg MG, Grzesiak RC (eds): Advances in Clinical Rehabilitation. Vol. 1. Springer-Verlag, New York, 1987

46. Kelly-Hayes M, Wolf PA, Kannel WB et al: Factors influencing survival and need for institutionalization following stroke: the Framingham study. Arch Phys Med Rehabil 69:415, 1988

47. Kelly-Hayes M, Wolf PA, Kase CS et al: Time course of functional recovery after stroke: the Framimgham study. J Neurol Rehabil 3:65, 1989

48. Kotila M, Waltino O, Niemi ML et al: The profile of recovery from stroke and factors influencing outcome. Stroke 15:1039, 1984

49. Labi MLC, Phillips TB, Gresham GE: Psychosocial disability in physically restored long-term stroke survivors. Arch Phys Med Rehabil 61:561, 1980

50. Lawton MP: Instrumental activities of daily living (IADL) scale: original observer-rated version. Psychopharmacol Bull 24:785, 1988a

51. Mahoney FI, Barthel DW: Functional evaluation: the Barthel index. MD State Med J 14:61, 1965

52. Miller IW, Bishop DS, Epstein NB et al: The McMaster family assessment device: reliability and validity. J Marital Fam Ther 11:345, 1985

53. Moskowitz E, McCann CB: Classification of disability in the chronically ill and aging. J Chronic Dis 5:342, 1957

54. Radloff LS: The CES-D scale: a self-report depression scale for research in the general population. J Appl Psychol Meas 1:385, 1977

55. Rankin J: Cerebral vascular accidents in patients over the age of 60: II. prognosis. Scot Med J 2:200, 1957

56. Sacco RL, Wolf PA, Kannel WB et al: Survival and recurrence following stroke. The Framingham study. Stroke 13:290, 1982

57. Schoening HA, Anderegg L, Bergstrom D et al: Numerical scoring of self-care status of patients. Arch Phys Med Rehabil 46:689, 1965

58. Schoening HA, Iversen IA: Numerical scoring of self-care status: a study of the Kenny self-care evaluation. Arch Phys Med Rehabil 49:221, 1968

59. Shah S, Vanclay F, Cooper B: Improving the sensitivity of the Barthel index for stroke rehabilitation. J Clin Epidemiol 42:703, 1989

60. Shinar D, Gross CR, Bronstein KS et al: Reliability of the activities of daily living scale and its use in telephone interviews. Arch Phys Med Rehabil 68:723, 1987

61. Uniform Data System for Medical Rehabilitation/Data Management Service: Guide for the Uniform Data Set for Medical Rehabilitation (Adult FIM). Version 4.0. State University of New York at Buffalo, Buffalo, NY, 1993

62. Wade DT: Measurement in Neurological Rehabilitation. Oxford University Press, Oxford, 1992

63. Wade DT, Collin C: The Barthel ADL index: a standard measure of physical disability? Int Disabil Stud 10:64, 1988

64. Wade DT, Hewer RL: Functional abilities after stroke: measurement, natural history and prognosis. J Neurol Neurosurg Psychiatry 50:177, 1987a

65. Wade DT, Hewer RL, David RM, Enderby PM: Aphasia after stroke: natural history and associated deficits. J Neurol Neurosurg Psychiatry 49:11, 1986

66. Wade DT, Skilbeck CE, Langton-Hewer R: Predicting Barthel ADL score at 6 months after an acute stroke. Arch Phys Med Rehabil 64:24, 1983

67. Weisbroth S, Esibill N, Zuger RR: Factors in the vocational success of hemiplegic patients. Arch Phys Med Rehabil 52:441, 1971

68. Wenniger WFMdB, Hagemand WJPM, Arrindell WA: Cross-national validity of dimensions of family functioning: first experience with the Dutch version of the McMaster family assessment device (FAD). Pers Indiv Dif 14:769, 1993

69. Yesavage JA, Brink TL, Rose TL et al: Development and validation of a geriatric depression screening scale: a preliminary report. J Psychiatr Res 17:37, 1982

Index

Note: Page numbers followed by f refer to figures; page numbers followed by t refer to tables.